Includes only evidence-based off-label uses

Lists adverse reactions by body system

Indicates level of drug that can be reduced by dialysis

➤ **Acute ischemic stroke presenting 3 to 4.5 hours after symptom onset (Activase)** ◆
Adults: 0.9 mg/kg by IV infusion over 1 hour with 10% of total dose given as an initial IV bolus over 1 minute. Maximum total dose is 90 mg.

Route	Onset	Peak	Duration
PO	15 min	1 hr	6–12 hr
PO (extended-release)	15 min	6–12 hr	24 hr
IV	5 min	20 min	5–8 hr

Half-life: 3 to 10 hours.

ADVERSE REACTIONS

CNS: fatigue, dizziness, depression, headache, insomnia, mental confusion, nightmares, short-term memory loss, hallucinations, vertigo, *stroke.* **CV:** hypotension, *bradycardia*, *HF*, edema, palpitations, Raynaud syndrome, cold extremity, first-degree AV block. **EENT:** blurred vision, tinnitus, rhinitis, dry mouth. **GI:** nausea, diarrhea, constipation, heartburn, flatulence, gastric pain, vomiting. **GU:** decreased libido, erectile dysfunction. **Respiratory:** dyspnea, wheezing, *bronchospasm*. **Skin:** rash, pruritus, gangrene (IV). **Other:** accidental injury.

INTERACTIONS

Drug-drug. *Amiodarone:* May increase bradycardic effects. Monitor therapy.
Barbiturates: May reduce metoprolol effect. Monitor therapy.
Calcium channel blockers: May increase hypotensive effects. Monitor therapy.
Cardiac glycosides: May cause excessive bradycardia and increased depressant effect on myocardium. Use together cautiously.
Catecholamine-depleting drugs (MAO inhibitors): May have additive effect. Monitor patient for hypotension and bradycardia.
Clonidine: May increase risk of bradycardia. If clonidine and a beta blocker are coadministered, withdraw the beta blocker several days before the gradual withdrawal of clonidine.
CYP2D6 inhibitors (fluoxetine, paroxetine, propafenone, quinidine): May increase metoprolol level. Monitor vital signs carefully. Metoprolol dosage reduction may be needed.
Epinephrine: May blunt epinephrine effect during treatment of allergic reaction. Monitor therapy.
Hydralazine: May increase levels and effects of both drugs. Monitor patient closely.

EFFECTS ON LAB TEST RESULTS
• May increase transaminase, ALP, and LDH levels.

CONTRAINDICATIONS & CAUTIONS
• Contraindicated in patients hypersensitive to drug or other beta blockers.
Dialyzable drug: Yes.
⚠ *Overdose S&S:* Bradycardia, nausea, hypotension, bronchospasm, HF, cardiac arrest, coma, AV block, vomiting.

PREGNANCY-LACTATION-REPRODUCTION
• There are no adequate studies during pregnancy. Drug crosses the placental barrier. Use during pregnancy only if clearly needed. Monitor fetal growth.
• Drug appears in human milk in very small quantities. Consider possible infant exposure with use during breastfeeding.

NURSING CONSIDERATIONS
🛈 *Alert:* Always check patient's apical pulse rate before giving drug. If it's slower than 60 beats/minute, withhold drug and contact prescriber immediately to verify dose.
• In patients with diabetes, monitor glucose level closely because drug masks common signs and symptoms of hypoglycemia.
• Monitor BP frequently; drug masks common signs and symptoms of shock.
• Beta blockers may mask tachycardia caused by hyperthyroidism. In patients with suspected thyrotoxicosis, taper off beta blocker to avoid thyroid storm.

Boxed Warning When stopping long-term therapy, taper dosage over 1 to 2 weeks. Abrupt discontinuation may cause exacerbations of angina or MI. Don't discontinue therapy abruptly even in patients treated only for HTN. Restart metoprolol, at least temporarily, if angina markedly worsens or acute coronary insufficiency occurs. ∎
• Beta selectivity is lost at higher doses. Watch for peripheral side effects.
• *Look alike–sound alike:* Don't confuse metoprolol succinate with metoprolol tartrate. Don't confuse metoprolol with metaproterenol, misoprostol, or metolazone. Don't confuse Toprol-XL with Topamax, Tegretol, or Tegretol-XR.

PATIENT TEACHING
• Instruct patient to take drug exactly as prescribed and with meals.
• Caution patient to avoid driving and other tasks requiring mental alertness until

Identifies known signs and symptoms of overdose

Highlights pregnancy, lactation, and reproduction concerns

Points out critical information that can't be overlooked

Lists potential interactions with other drugs, herbs, and lifestyle factors

Easy-to-spot FDA boxed warnings

Identifies drugs with similar appearance or name

Lists most important information patients should know

Lists how results may be affected by taking drug

✦Canada   ◇OTC   ◆Off-label use   ⊜Do not crush   *Liquid contains alcohol   ✻Genetic

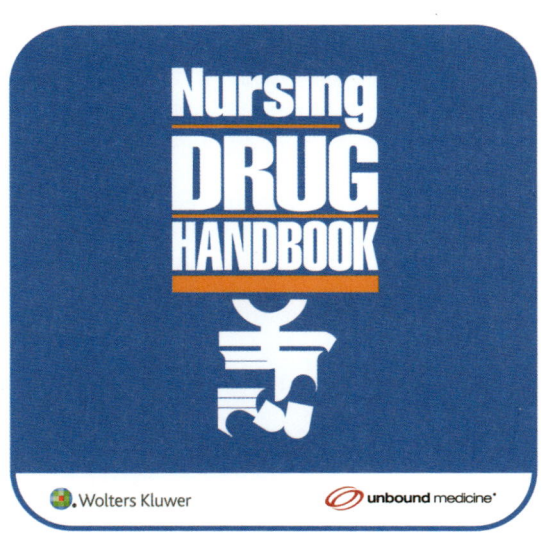

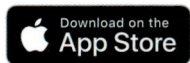
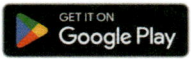
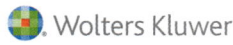

45TH EDITION

Nursing
2025-2026
DRUG
HANDBOOK®

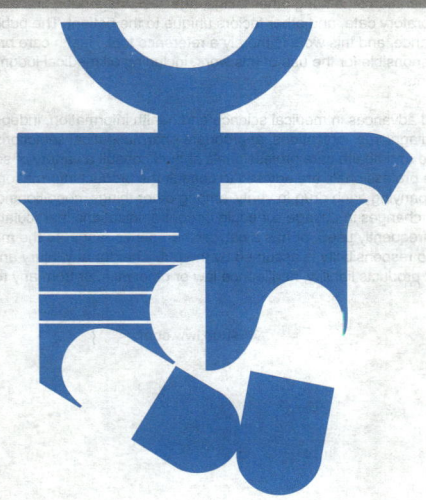

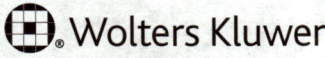

. Wolters Kluwer

Philadelphia • Baltimore • New York • London
Buenos Aires • Hong Kong • Sydney • Tokyo

Chief Nurse: Anne Dabrow Woods, DNP, RN, CRNP, ANP-BC, AGACNP-BC, FAAN
Acquisitions Editor: Susan M. Hartman
Editor-in-Chief: Collette Bishop, RN, MS, MA, CIC
Clinical Project Manager: Janet Rader, RN, BSN
Clinical Editors: John Bodnar, BSN, BS, RN; Emily Hudson, BSN, RN; Meghan Lynch, BSN, RN;
Lisa Merenda, MSN, RN; Linda Lee Phelps, DNP, RN
Managing Editors: Carla A. Rudoy Vitale, PhD; Diane Labus; Ellen Sellers
Editors: Jaime L. Buss, Mary T. Durkin
Editorial Assistant: Linda K. Ruhf
Graphic Arts & Design Manager: Stephen Druding
Senior Production Associate: Bridgett Dougherty
Manufacturing Coordinator: Bernard Tomboc
Production Services: Aptara, Inc.

9 8 7 6 5 4 3 2 1
Printed in China

NDH45-010524
ISSN: 0273-320X
ISBN-13: 978-1-9752-1711-2
ISBN-10: 1-9752-1711-X

shop.lww.com

Contents

Contributors and consultants

Janine Barnaby, RPh, BCOP
Manager, Outpatient Hospital Pharmacy
Lehigh Valley Hospital
Allentown, PA

David Bruch, BS, PharmD
Associate Lecturer
University of Wyoming—School
of Pharmacy
Laramie, WY

Lawrence Carey, PharmD
Assistant Dean for Assessment,
Accreditation, and Quality
Temple University School of Pharmacy
Philadelphia, PA

Jeffrey J. Cies, PharmD, MPH, BCPS, AG-ID,
BCPPS, FCCP, FCCM, FPPA
Pediatric Critical Care and Infectious
Diseases Clinical Pharmacist
St. Christopher's Hospital for Children
Philadelphia, PA

Jason C. Cooper, PharmD
Clinical Specialist, MUSC Drug
Information Center
Medical University of South Carolina
Health
Charleston, SC

Kelsey D. Frederick, PharmD
Assistant Professor, Clinical Pharmacy
& Translational Science
The University of Tennessee Health
Science Center, College of Pharmacy
Nashville, TN

Toshal Hallowell, PharmD
Pharmacist
Edward M. Kennedy Community
Health Center
Worcester, MA

AnhThu Hoang, PharmD
Pharmacist
North York Cardiovascular Centre
North York, Ontario

Jill Krabak, PharmD, MAc, BSPharm
Clinical Pharmacist
Justice Grown
Dickson City, PA

Chung-Shien Lee, PharmD, BCPS, BCOP
Associate Professor
St. John's University
Queens, NY

Hannah McCaffery, PharmD
Manager, Pharmacy Regulations
and Implementations
Health Partners Plans
Philadelphia, PA

Jamie L. McConaha, PharmD, NCTTP,
BCACP, CDCES
Associate Professor of Pharmacy Practice
Duquesne University School of Pharmacy
Pittsburgh, PA

Kimberly E. Ng, PharmD, BCPS
Associate Professor
St. John's University
Queens, NY

Christine K. O'Neil, BS, PharmD, BCPS, BCGP,
FASCP, FCCP, TTS
Professor, Division of Pharmacy Practice
Duquesne University
Pittsburgh, PA

Christine Price, PharmD
Clinical Coordinator, PGY1 Pharmacy
Residency Director
Morton Plant Hospital
Clearwater, FL

Melissa Rinaldi, PharmD
Clinical Pharmacist
Independence Blue Cross
Philadelphia, PA

Kerry Rinato, PharmD, BCPS
Clinical Pharmacist
Sunrise Hospital
Las Vegas, NV

Maha Saad, PharmD, BCGP, BCPS
Associate Clinical Professor/Co-Director
Drug Information Center
St. John's University College of Pharmacy
and Health Sciences
Long Island Jewish Medical
Center-Northwell Health
Queens, NY

Michele F. Shepherd, PharmD, MS, BCPS, FASHP
Clinical Consultant
Jordan, MN

James S. Wheeler, PharmD, BCPS
Associate Professor/Associate Dean
University of Tennessee Health Science
Center, College of Pharmacy
Knoxville, TN

Maggie White-Jones, PharmD
Pharmacist
Walgreens Pharmacy
Berlin, MD

How to use *Nursing2025–2026 Drug Handbook*®

The best-selling nursing drug guide for 45 years, *Nursing Drug Handbook* is meticulously reviewed and updated by pharmacists and nurses to include the most current, relevant information that practicing nurses and students need to know to administer medications safely in any health care setting. As in previous editions, *Nursing2025–2026 Drug Handbook* emphasizes nursing and safety aspects of drug administration without attempting to replace detailed pharmacology texts. Only the most essential information is included, and helpful graphic symbols, logos, and highlighting draw special attention to critical details that nurses shouldn't overlook.

Outstanding features

The 45th edition provides a wealth of the latest drug information right at your fingertips:
• Tabbed "New drugs" section that ensures quick access to 24 completely new drug monographs introduced in this edition
• The latest information on thousands of generic, brand, and combination drugs included in 670 comprehensive drug monographs and 10 appendices
• Drug safety always at the forefront, including prominently displayed safety alerts, drug warnings, and Institute for Safe Medication Practices (ISMP) "tall man" lettering to help differentiate similarly spelled drug names—plus a special chapter on safe drug administration with updated guidelines on administration of opioid analgesics, prevention and treatment of IV extravasation injury, safe handling of hazardous drugs, and best practices to ensure patient safety and reduce drug errors
• Special logos and symbols throughout to emphasize FDA boxed warnings, clinical alerts, new indications, necessary dosage adjustments, overdose signs and symptoms, off-label uses, drugs that shouldn't be crushed or chewed, over-the-counter drugs, biosimilar drugs, Canadian drugs, look alike–sound alike drugs, and the dialyzability status of each drug
• Genetic symbols pinpointing monographs and specific genetic-related information to help select and guide drug therapy
• "Pregnancy-lactation-reproduction" section in each monograph that captures all relevant information in one convenient place
• Thoroughly updated appendices containing indications and dosages of various classes and groupings of drugs—antacids, antidiarrheals, laxatives, vitamins and minerals, additional OTC drugs, common combination drugs, antidotes, ophthalmic drugs, biologicals and blood derivatives, and less commonly used drugs.

Introductory chapters

Chapter 1, "Drug actions, interactions, and reactions," explains how drugs work in the body. It provides a general overview of drug properties (absorption, distribution, metabolism, and excretion) and other significant factors that affect drug action (including protein binding, patient age, underlying disease, dosage form, and route and timing of administration). Also discussed are drug interactions, adverse reactions, and toxic reactions. Chapter 2, "Drug therapy across the lifespan," covers the unique challenges of giving drugs to children and older adults and offers practical suggestions on how to minimize problems with these special populations. This chapter also discusses the danger associated with indiscriminate use of drugs during pregnancy and breastfeeding and the special precautions women should take when medications are necessary. Chapter 3, "Safe drug administration," explores the ongoing involvement of governmental and nongovernmental organizations in drug safety issues and the necessary measures nurses must take to prevent medication errors from occurring.

Drug monographs

Each generic drug monograph in the *Nursing2025–2026 Drug Handbook* includes the most pertinent clinical information nurses must know to administer medications safely, monitor for potential interactions and adverse effects, implement necessary care measures, and provide appropriate patient teaching. Entries are arranged alphabetically, with the generic drug name prominently displayed—along with its ISMP "tall man" lettering (if applicable), pronunciation, corresponding brand (or trade) names, therapeutic class, and pharmacologic class—on a shaded background for quick and easy identification. This highlighted area also includes banners or symbols to identify drugs that warrant a special safety alert or to designate biosimilar drugs.

Specific information for each drug is then systematically organized under the headings below. Special icons and logos are used throughout, as warranted, to point out the drug's safety concerns. For example, a clinical alert logo (🔔) provides important advice about life-threatening effects associated with the drug or its administration; a boxed warning (**Boxed Warning**) represents a specific warning issued by the FDA; and a special icon (ⓄⓃⒸ) indicates oral drug forms that shouldn't be crushed or chewed. (See "Anatomy of a monograph" on the inside book cover for a visual guide to the various symbols that may appear within a drug entry.)

Available forms
This section lists the preparations available for each drug (for example, tablets, capsules, and solutions for injection) and specifies available dosage forms and strengths. Dosage strengths specifically available in Canada are designated with a maple leaf (🍁). Preparations that may be obtained over the counter, without a prescription, are marked with an open diamond (◊). Liquid formulations that contain alcohol are indicated with an asterisk (*). Capsules or tablets that shouldn't be crushed are marked with a "Do Not Crush" symbol (ⓄⓃⒸ).

Indications & dosages
The "Indications & dosages" section contains general dosage information for adults and children. The dosage instructions reflect current trends in therapeutics and can't be considered absolute or universal. For each individual patient, dosage instructions must be considered in light of the patient's condition. Indications and dosages that aren't approved by the FDA are followed by a closed diamond (♦). Only highly evidence-based off-label uses are included in this edition. *Adjust-a-dose* content within this section indicates the need for a special dosage adjustment for certain patient populations, such as older adults or those with kidney or liver impairment. In some cases, a dosage adjustment may apply to all patient populations for all the indications listed; such cases are marked accordingly.

Administration
Here, readers will find guidelines for safely administering drugs by all applicable routes, including PO, IV, IM, subcut, ophthalmic, inhalational, topical, rectal, vaginal, transdermal, and buccal. A special screened background highlights IV administration guidelines (including specific instructions on how to reconstitute,

mix, and store IV medications) and the major potential IV incompatibilities.

Action
This section succinctly describes each drug's mechanism of action—that is, how the drug provides its therapeutic effect. For example, although all antihypertensives lower BP, they don't all do so by the same process. Also included, in table form, are the onset, peak (described in terms of effect or peak blood level), and duration of drug action for each route of administration, if data are available or applicable. Values listed are for patients with normal kidney function, unless otherwise specified. The drug's half-life is also provided when known.

Adverse reactions
In this section, adverse reactions that are known to occur at a frequency of 1% or greater are listed according to body system. Life-threatening reactions appear in ***bold italic*** type.

Interactions
Within this section, readers can find each drug's confirmed, clinically significant interactions (additive effects, potentiated effects, and antagonistic effects) with other drugs, herbs, foods, beverages, and lifestyle behaviors (such as alcohol use, sun exposure, and smoking). Drug interactions are listed under the drug that's adversely affected. For example, because celecoxib, a nonsteroidal anti-inflammatory drug, interacts with candesartan to decrease the antihypertensive effect of candesartan, this interaction is listed under candesartan. To check on the possible effects of using two or more drugs simultaneously, refer to the interaction section for each drug.

Effects on lab test results
This section lists increased and decreased levels, counts, and other values in lab test results that may be caused by the drug's systemic effects. It also indicates false-positive, false-negative, and otherwise altered lab test results a drug may cause.

Contraindications & cautions
The "Contraindications & cautions" section outlines any conditions or special circumstances, such as diseases or conditions, in which use of the drug is undesirable or for which the drug

should be given with caution. This section also contains information about whether the drug is dialyzable. When applicable, specific signs and symptoms of drug overdose are listed as the last bulleted item under this heading and highlighted by a special logo (⚠ *Overdose S&S:*) for easy identification.

Pregnancy-lactation-reproduction
This section provides nurses with targeted, easy-to-understand safety information about each drug's use during pregnancy and breastfeeding. It also provides information about fertility effects, contraception recommendations, and enrollment information for registries that monitor drug safety during pregnancy.

Nursing considerations
Within this section, readers can find practical information on patient-monitoring techniques and suggestions for the prevention and treatment of adverse reactions as well as helpful tips on promoting patient comfort.

Patient teaching
Concise guidelines for explaining the drug's purpose, encouraging compliance, ensuring proper use and storage, and preventing or minimizing adverse reactions are included in this section.

Appendices and other helpful aids
Nursing2025–2026 Drug Handbook includes 10 handy appendices featuring the latest indications and dosages for some of the most commonly prescribed antacids, antidiarrheals, laxatives, vitamins and minerals, combination drugs, antidotes, ophthalmic drugs, and biologicals and blood derivatives and as well as commonly used OTC generic and brand-name drugs and less commonly used drugs.

The book also includes a concise visual "Quick guide to special symbols, logos, and highlighted terms" and "Guide to abbreviations" immediately following this "How to use" piece.

Lippincott NursingCenter®
Readers also have online access to monthly drug updates, including postings of newly FDA-approved drugs, new indications & dosages, new formulations, drug warnings, and drug news abstracts by visiting **NursingCenter.com**. Also included are drug quizzes, best-practice medication safety guidelines, administration tips, real-life medication stories, CE tests, and so much more.

Quick guide to special symbols, logos, and highlighted terms

The following symbols or highlighted features appear throughout drug monographs and select appendices in this edition.

Special symbols, logos, and highlighting	Usage or meaning
SAFETY ALERT!	Drug that presents a heightened risk of avoidable danger
BIOSIMILAR DRUG	FDA-approved biosimilar drug
buPROPion	"Tall man" lettering for FDA-designated generic drug names prone to mix-ups
➤	Indication for drug
✱ *NEW INDICATION:*	New indication for drug
Adjust-a-dose:	Dosage adjustment needed for certain populations
Adjust-a-dose (for all indications):	Dosage adjustment needed for all indications
✖	Genetic considerations used to select and guide drug therapy
☯ *Alert:*	Clinical alert
♣	Available in Canada
◇	Over-the-counter (OTC)
♦	Off-label use
*	Liquid contains alcohol
ONC	Drugs that shouldn't be crushed or chewed
Look alike–sound alike:	Drugs with easily confused names
Boxed Warning	FDA boxed warning
⚠ *Overdose S&S:*	Overdose signs & symptoms
life-threatening	Life-threatening reaction

Guide to abbreviations

ACE	angiotensin-converting enzyme	COPD	chronic obstructive pulmonary disease
ACS	acute coronary syndrome	COVID-19	coronavirus disease 2019
ADH	antidiuretic hormone	COX	cyclooxygenase
ADHD	attention deficit hyperactivity disorder	CrCl	creatinine clearance
		CSF	cerebrospinal fluid
ADLs	activities of daily living	CT	computed tomography
ADP	adenosine 5′ diphosphate	CTCAE	Common Terminology Criteria for Adverse Events
AEDs	antiepileptic drugs		
AIDS	acquired immunodeficiency syndrome	CV	cardiovascular
		CVAD	central venous access device
AKD	acute kidney disease	D_5W	dextrose 5% in water
AKI	acute kidney injury	DEHP	di(2-ethylhexyl) phthalate
ALP	alkaline phosphatase	DIC	disseminated intravascular coagulation
ALS	amyotrophic lateral sclerosis		
ALT	alanine transaminase	dL	deciliter
ANA	antinuclear antibody	DMARD	disease-modifying antirheumatic drug
ANC	absolute neutrophil count		
ARB	angiotensin receptor blocker	DNA	deoxyribonucleic acid
ARDS	acute respiratory distress syndrome	DPP-4	dipeptidyl peptidase-4
		DRESS	drug reaction with eosinophilia and systemic symptoms
AST	aspartate transaminase		
AUC	area under the curve		
AV	atrioventricular	DVT	deep vein thrombosis
BCRP	breast cancer resistance protein	ECG	electrocardiogram
		EEG	electroencephalogram
b.i.d.	twice daily	EENT	eyes, ears, nose, and throat
BMI	body mass index	eGFR	estimated glomerular filtration rate
BP	blood pressure		
BPH	benign prostatic hypertrophy	ET	endotracheal
BRCA	breast cancer gene	FDA	U.S. Food and Drug Administration
BSA	body surface area		
BUN	blood urea nitrogen	FSH	follicle-stimulating hormone
CABG	coronary artery bypass graft	5-FU	fluorouracil
		g	gram
CAD	coronary artery disease	G	gauge
cAMP	cyclic 3′, 5′ adenosine monophosphate	G-CSF	granulocyte colony-stimulating factor
		G6PD	glucose-6-phosphate dehydrogenase
CBC	complete blood count		
CDAD	*Clostridioides difficile*–associated diarrhea	GABA	gamma-aminobutyric acid
		GERD	gastroesophageal reflux disease
CDC	Centers for Disease Control and Prevention		
		GFR	glomerular filtration rate
CK	creatine kinase	GGT	gamma-glutamyltransferase
CKD	chronic kidney disease	GI	gastrointestinal
CKRT	continuous kidney replacement therapy	GnRH	gonadotropin-releasing hormone
CMV	cytomegalovirus	GU	genitourinary
CNS	central nervous system		

GVHD	graft-versus-host disease		M	molar
H$_1$	histamine$_1$		m^2	square meter
H$_2$	histamine$_2$		MAC	*Mycobacterium avium* complex
Hb	hemoglobin		MAO	monoamine oxidase
HbA$_{1c}$	glycosylated hemoglobin		mcg	microgram
HBsAg	hepatitis B virus surface antigen		MD	muscular dystrophy
			MDD	major depressive disorder
HBV	hepatitis B virus		mEq	milliequivalent
HCV	hepatitis C virus		mg	milligram
HDL-C	high-density lipoprotein cholesterol		MI	myocardial infarction
			min	minute
HER2	human epidermal growth factor receptor 2		mL	milliliter
			mm^3	cubic millimeter
HF	heart failure		mo	month
HIV	human immunodeficiency virus		MRI	magnetic resonance imaging
			MRSA	methicillin-resistant *Staphylococcus aureus*
HLA	human leucocyte antigen			
HMG-CoA	3-hydroxy-3-methyl-glutaryl coenzyme A		MS	multiple sclerosis
			msec	millisecond
HPA	hypothalamic-pituitary-adrenal		mTOR	mechanistic target of rapamycin
HPV	human papilloma virus		MUGA	multigated acquisition
hr	hour		NG	nasogastric
HR	heart rate		NMS	neuroleptic malignant syndrome
HTN	hypertension			
IBS	irritable bowel syndrome		NNRTI	non-nucleoside reverse transcriptase inhibitor
ICP	intracranial pressure			
ICU	intensive care unit		NRTI	nucleoside reverse transcriptase inhibitor
ID	intradermal			
Ig	immunoglobulin		NSAID	nonsteroidal anti-inflammatory drug
ILD	interstitial lung disease			
IM	intramuscular		NSCLC	non-small-cell lung cancer
INR	International Normalized Ratio		NSR	normal sinus rhythm
			NSS	normal (0.9%) saline solution
IOP	intraocular pressure		NYHA	New York Heart Association
IPPB	intermittent positive-pressure breathing		OCD	obsessive-compulsive disorder
			ODT	orally disintegrating tablet
ITP	immune thrombocytopenia		OTC	over-the-counter
IV	intravenous		oz	ounce
KF	kidney failure		P-gp	P-glycoprotein
KFRT	kidney failure with replacement therapy		PABA	para-aminobenzoic acid
			PAC	premature atrial contraction
kg	kilogram		PAH	pulmonary arterial hypertension
L	liter			
LABA	long-acting beta-agonist		PCA	patient-controlled analgesia
lb	pound		PCI	percutaneous coronary intervention
LDH	lactate dehydrogenase			
LDL-C	low-density lipoprotein cholesterol		PDE5	phosphodiesterase type 5
			PE	pulmonary embolus
LFTs	liver function tests		PID	pelvic inflammatory disease
LH	luteinizing hormone		PML	progressive multifocal leukoencephalopathy
LVEF	left ventricular ejection fraction			

PO	by mouth	SL	sublingual
PPI	proton pump inhibitor	SLE	systemic lupus erythematosus
PR	by rectum	SNRI	serotonin-norepinephrine
PRES	posterior reversible		reuptake inhibitor
	encephalopathy	SSRI	selective serotonin reuptake
PRN	as needed		inhibitor
PSA	prostate-specific antigen	SSS	sick sinus syndrome
PT	prothrombin time	STI	sexually transmitted infection
PTCA	percutaneous transluminal	subcut	subcutaneous
	coronary angioplasty	T_3	triiodothyronine
PTSD	posttraumatic stress disorder	T_4	thyroxine
PTT	partial thromboplastin time	TB	tuberculosis
PVC	premature ventricular	TCA	tricyclic antidepressant
	contraction	TEN	toxic epidermal necrolysis
PVD	peripheral vascular disease	TIA	transient ischemic attack
q.i.d.	four times daily	t.i.d.	three times daily
RA	rheumatoid arthritis	TLS	tumor lysis syndrome
RAAS	renin-angiotensin-aldosterone	TNF	tumor necrosis factor
	system	TPN	total parenteral nutrition
RBC	red blood cell	TSH	thyroid-stimulating hormone
RDA	recommended daily allowance	tsp	teaspoon
REM	rapid eye movement	ULN	upper limit of normal
REMS	risk evaluation and mitigation	URI	upper respiratory infection
	strategy	USP	United States Pharmacopeia
RNA	ribonucleic acid	UTI	urinary tract infection
RSV	respiratory syncytial virus	UV	ultraviolet
SA	sinoatrial	VLDL-C	very-low-density lipoprotein
SARS-	severe acute respiratory		cholesterol
CoV-2	syndrome coronavirus 2	VTE	venous thromboembolism
SCAR	severe cutaneous adverse	WBC	white blood cell
	reaction	WHO	World Health Organization
SCLC	small cell lung cancer	wk	week
sec	second		
SIADH	syndrome of inappropriate		
	antidiuretic hormone		
SJS	Stevens-Johnson syndrome		

1

Drug actions, interactions, and reactions

Any drug a patient takes causes a series of physical and chemical events in the body. The first event, when a drug combines with cellular drug receptors, is the *drug's mechanism of action*. What happens next is the *drug effect*. Depending on the type of cellular drug receptors affected by a given drug, an effect can be local, systemic, or both. A systemic drug effect can follow a local effect. For example, application of a drug to the skin causes a local effect. But transdermal absorption of that drug can also produce a systemic effect. A local effect can also follow systemic absorption. For example, the peptic ulcer drug cimetidine produces a local effect after it's swallowed by blocking histamine receptors in the stomach's parietal cells. Diphenhydramine, on the other hand, causes a systemic effect by blocking histamine receptors throughout the body.

Drug properties

Drug absorption, distribution, metabolism, and excretion make up a drug's pharmacokinetics. These processes determine a drug's onset of action, peak concentration, duration of action, and bioavailability.

Absorption

After administration, a drug must be absorbed into the bloodstream before it can act in the body. Oral administration is the most common route. Before an oral drug can be absorbed, it must disintegrate into particles small enough to dissolve in GI secretions. Only after dissolving can the drug be absorbed. Most absorption of orally given drugs occurs in the small intestine because the mucosal villi provide extensive surface area. Once absorbed and circulated in the bloodstream, the drug is *bioavailable*, or ready to exert its action and produce a drug effect. The speed and degree of absorption (complete or partial) depend on the drug's effects; dosage form; administration route; interactions with other substances in the GI tract, such as other drugs and food; and various patient characteristics. Oral solutions and syrups bypass the need for disintegration and dissolution and are usually absorbed faster than solid dosage forms. Some tablets have enteric coatings to prevent disintegration in the acidic environment of the stomach; others have coatings of varying thicknesses that simply delay release of the drug.

Drugs given IM must first be absorbed through the muscle into the bloodstream. Rectal suppositories must dissolve to be absorbed through the rectal mucosa. Drugs given IV are injected directly into the bloodstream and are bioavailable completely and immediately.

Distribution

After absorption, a drug moves from the bloodstream into the fluids and tissues in the body, a movement known as *distribution*. The volume into which a drug is distributed throughout the body is known as the *volume of distribution*. Individual patient variations can change the amount of drug distributed throughout the body. For example, in a patient with edema, a given dose is distributed into a larger volume than in a patient without edema. Occasionally, a dose is increased to account for this difference. In such cases, the dose should be decreased after the edema is corrected. Conversely, a dose given to a patient with dehydration may need to be decreased to allow for its distribution into a much smaller volume. Obesity is another important factor when considering drug distribution. Some drugs—such as digoxin, gentamicin, and tobramycin—aren't well-distributed into fatty tissue. For such drugs, doses based on actual body weight may lead to overdose and serious toxicity. In these cases, doses must be based on ideal body weight or adjusted body weight, which can be estimated from mathematical formulas or actuarial tables that give an average weight range for height.

Metabolism

Most drugs are metabolized in the liver. The rate at which a drug is metabolized varies from person to person. Some patients metabolize drugs so quickly that the drug levels in their blood and tissues prove therapeutically inadequate. In other patients, the rate of metabolism is so slow that ordinary doses can produce toxicity or prolonged duration of action. Genetic tests can help to determine whether a patient metabolizes drugs slowly or quickly.

Liver diseases may affect the liver's metabolic functions and may increase or decrease a drug's usual metabolism. Close

1

monitoring for drug effect and toxicity is necessary for all patients with liver disease.

Excretion

Drug excretion is the movement of a drug or its metabolites from the tissues back into circulation and from the circulation into the organs of excretion, where they're removed from the body. Most drugs are excreted by the kidneys, but some can be eliminated through the lungs, exocrine (sweat, salivary, or mammary) glands, liver, skin, or intestinal tract. Drugs also may be removed artificially by direct mechanical intervention, such as peritoneal dialysis or hemodialysis.

Other modifying factors

One important factor that influences a drug's action and effect is its tendency to bind to plasma proteins, especially albumin, and other tissue components. Because only a free, unbound drug molecule can act in the body, protein binding greatly influences the degree and duration of a drug's effect. Malnutrition, kidney failure, and the presence of other protein-bound drugs can influence protein binding. When protein-binding behavior changes, the drug dosage may need to be adjusted accordingly.

The patient's age is another important factor. Older adults usually have decreased liver function, reduced muscle mass, diminished kidney function, and low albumin levels. These patients sometimes need lower doses and longer dosage intervals to avoid toxicity. Neonates have underdeveloped metabolic enzyme systems and inadequate kidney function, so they need highly individualized dosages and careful monitoring.

Underlying disease also may affect drug action and effect. For example, acidosis can cause insulin resistance. Genetic diseases, such as G6PD deficiency and hepatic porphyria, can turn drugs into toxins, with serious consequences. Patients with G6PD deficiency may develop hemolytic anemia when given certain drugs, such as sulfonamides. A patient with genetic susceptibility can develop acute porphyria if given a barbiturate. A patient with a highly active liver enzyme system can develop hepatitis when treated with isoniazid because of the quick buildup of a toxic metabolite in the liver.

Drug administration issues

The dosage form of a drug is important because it can influence the drug's action in the body. Some tablets and capsules are too large

to be easily swallowed by patients with certain conditions. An oral solution may be substituted, but it may produce higher drug levels than other forms because the liquid is more easily and completely absorbed. When a potentially toxic drug (such as digoxin) is given in liquid form, its increased absorption can cause toxicity. Sometimes a change in dosage form also requires a change in dosage.

Routes of administration aren't always interchangeable. For example, diazepam is readily absorbed PO but is slowly and erratically absorbed IM. On the other hand, gentamicin must be given parenterally because oral administration results in drug levels too low to effectively treat systemic infections.

Improper storage can alter a drug's potency. Most drugs must be stored in tight containers protected from direct sunlight and extremes in temperature and humidity that can cause them to deteriorate. Some drugs require special storage conditions, such as refrigeration. Patients should be cautioned not to store drugs in a bathroom because of the constantly changing environment.

The timing of drug administration can be important. Sometimes, giving an oral drug during, shortly before, or after a meal changes the amount of drug absorbed. The presence of food in the GI tract may be desirable to increase absorption (such as with rivaroxaban) or to increase tolerability (such as with aspirin and other irritating drugs). But other drugs (such as penicillins and tetracyclines) shouldn't be taken at mealtimes because certain foods can inactivate them. If unsure about the effect of food on a certain drug, the nurse should check with a pharmacist.

The nurse should always document the patient's age, actual height, and actual weight (in kg). Patient "stated" or "reported" weight isn't appropriate for medication dosing. Prescribers and pharmacists need this information to be as accurate as possible when calculating the dosages for many drugs. Recording of daily weight is especially important for patients who require intensive care, neonates, and infants because their weights frequently change and most medications given to these patients are weight-based.

The patient's medical record should also include all current lab data, especially results of kidney and liver function studies, so the prescriber and pharmacist can adjust drug dosages as needed. The nurse should also watch for metabolic and physiologic changes (such as depressed respiratory function, acidosis, or alkalosis) that might alter drug effects.

The nurse should obtain a comprehensive family history from the patient or family, asking about past reactions to drugs, possible genetic traits that might affect drug response, and current use of other prescription and OTC drugs, illicit drugs, herbal supplements, and vitamin supplements. Multiple drug therapies can cause serious and fatal drug interactions and can dramatically change many drugs' effects.

Drug interactions

A *drug interaction* occurs when giving two drugs concomitantly alters the effects of either or both drugs. Usually, the effect of one drug is increased or decreased. For instance, one drug may inhibit or stimulate the metabolism or excretion of the other or free it for further action by displacing the drug from protein-binding sites.

Combination therapy is based on drug interactions. One drug may be given to complement, enhance, or protect the effects of another. For example, imipenem and cilastatin are given together because cilastatin inhibits a kidney enzyme that would degrade imipenem. In many cases, two drugs with similar actions are given together precisely because of the additive effect. For instance, acetaminophen and codeine are commonly given in combination because together they provide greater pain relief than if either is given alone.

Drug interactions are sometimes used to prevent or antagonize certain adverse reactions. The diuretics hydrochlorothiazide and spironolactone are often given together because the former is potassium-depleting and the latter is potassium-sparing.

Not all drug interactions are beneficial. Many drugs interact to decrease efficacy or increase toxicity. For example, decreased efficacy occurs when tetracycline is given with drugs or foods that contain calcium or magnesium (such as antacids or milk); these electrolytes bind with tetracycline in the GI tract and cause inadequate drug absorption. Increased toxicity can occur when a patient takes an NSAID with an anticoagulant such as warfarin; this combination of drugs increases the risk of GI bleeding. Nurses should avoid drug combinations that produce these effects, if possible.

Sometimes drug interactions occur after a drug that inhibits or increases the metabolism of another drug has been discontinued. After discontinuation of the first drug, the other drug's levels may increase or decrease, so the dosage may need adjustment.

Adverse reactions

Drugs cause adverse *effects;* patients have adverse *reactions.* An adverse reaction may be tolerated to obtain a therapeutic effect, or it may be hazardous and unacceptable. Some adverse reactions subside with continued use. For example, the drowsiness caused by paroxetine and the orthostatic hypotension caused by prazosin usually subside after several days, when the patient develops tolerance. But many adverse reactions are dose related and lessen or disappear only if the dosage is reduced. Most adverse reactions aren't therapeutically desirable, but a few can be put to clinical use. An example is the drowsiness caused by diphenhydramine, which makes it useful as a mild sedative.

Common Terminology Criteria for Adverse Events are standardized definitions that describe adverse events that may occur in the course of cancer therapy. An *adverse event* is any event that's unfavorable or that has an unfavorable outcome to a patient and is caused by a medication and not to the patient's underlying condition. (See *Common Terminology Criteria for Adverse Events,* page 4.)

Drug hypersensitivity, or drug allergy, is the result of an antigen-antibody immune reaction that occurs in the body when a drug is given to a susceptible patient. Signs and symptoms of a drug allergy may include rash, itching, angioedema, and shortness of breath. One of the most dangerous of all drug hypersensitivities is anaphylaxis. In its most severe form, anaphylaxis can rapidly become fatal.

Rarely, idiosyncratic reactions occur. These reactions are highly unpredictable and unusual. One of the best known idiosyncratic adverse reactions is aspirin-induced asthma, which may be life-threatening. A more common idiosyncratic reaction is extreme sensitivity to very low doses of a drug or insensitivity to higher-than-normal doses.

To manage adverse reactions correctly, you need to be aware of changes in the patient's clinical condition, even subtle ones. Such changes may be an early warning of impending toxicity. Listen to the patient's complaints about reactions to a drug, and consider each objectively. You may be able to reduce adverse reactions in several ways. Dosage reduction can help. But, in many cases, so does a simple rescheduling of the dose. For example, the CNS stimulation that pseudoephedrine may produce can be managed by giving the drug early in the day rather than at bedtime. Similarly, drowsiness from antihistamines or tranquilizers can be less disruptive if these drugs are given at bedtime. Most importantly, you need to alert the patient which adverse reactions to expect so that the patient won't become worried or decide to stop taking the drug. Always advise the patient to report all adverse reactions to the prescriber, and teach the patient which adverse reactions to report immediately.

Your ability to recognize signs and symptoms of drug allergies or serious idiosyncratic reactions may save a patient's life. Ask each patient about the drugs currently being taken and those taken in the past and ask whether any unusual reactions occurred while the patient was taking them. If a patient claims to be allergic to a drug, ask for specific examples of what the patient experienced after taking the drug. The patient may be calling a harmless adverse reaction, such as upset stomach, an allergic reaction or may have a true history of anaphylaxis. In either case, you and the prescriber need to be aware of the reaction. Record and report clinical changes throughout the patient's course of treatment. If you suspect a severe adverse reaction, withhold the drug until you can check with a pharmacist and the prescriber.

Toxic reactions

Chronic drug toxicities are usually caused by the cumulative effect and resulting buildup of the drug in the body. These effects may be undesired extensions of the desired therapeutic effect. For example, standard doses of glyburide normalize the blood glucose level, but higher doses can produce hypoglycemia.

Drug toxicities may also occur when a drug level rises as a result of impaired metabolism or excretion. For example, liver dysfunction impairs the metabolism of amiodarone, raising its concentration in the blood. Similarly, kidney dysfunction may cause digoxin toxicity because this drug is eliminated by the kidneys. Excessive dosage can also cause toxic levels. For instance, tinnitus is usually a sign that the safe dose of aspirin has been exceeded.

Many drug toxicities are predictable, dosage-related, and reversible upon dosage adjustment or discontinuation. Monitor patients carefully for physiologic changes that might alter drug effects. Watch especially for liver and kidney impairment. Warn the patient about signs of impending toxicity and tell the patient what to do if a toxic reaction occurs. Also, make sure to emphasize the importance of taking a drug exactly as prescribed. Warn the patient that serious problems could arise if the patient changes the dose or schedule or stops taking the drug without the prescriber's knowledge.

Pharmacogenetics

Prescribers typically follow a standardized approach to prescribing drugs. Although decisions are made based on evidence-based approaches and with the best of intentions, some result in the development of adverse drug reactions. Being able to accurately predict which patients will (and which will not) respond and to what degree they will respond when they take a certain drug would be helpful. Pharmacogenetics—the study of how varied responses to a drug can be caused by genetic differences between individuals—attempts to do just this.

The first pharmacogenetic detection occurred when Pythagoras recognized the dangers of ingesting fava beans in 510 B.C., which eventually led to the discovery of G6PD in 1956. Shortly after, the term *pharmacogenetics* was coined and later defined as the study of variability in drug response due to heredity. The goals of pharmacogenetics include identification of innovative drug targets, consideration of DNA sequence variation on drug effects, development of new agents, and optimization of drug efficacy while minimizing drug toxicity.

Pharmacogenetics considers the existence of *polymorphisms,* which are genetic variations that occur in 1% or more of the population. If clinicians are able to predict which patients express polymorphisms, they can provide targeted therapy. Researchers have learned that many polymorphisms involve cytochrome P450 (CYP450) isoenzymes.

Polymorphisms play a significant role in determining whether a drug will be predictably metabolized. Patients fall into one of four classes of metabolizers: extensive, ultrarapid, intermediate, and poor. Patients considered extensive metabolizers possess an overwhelming capacity to metabolize certain drugs and may exhibit therapeutic failure, whereas patients who are poor metabolizers, such as those with G6PD deficiency, exhibit toxicities due to their inability to metabolize certain drugs. Ethnicity may also play a role in determining how patients are classified in regard to metabolism.

Recognizing the importance of the CYP450 system is vital. Approximately 60 CYP enzymes are found in humans, and many genes that encode for these enzymes are polymorphic. Polymorphism associated with CYP enzymes may be expressed via amino acid substitution (thereby reducing enzymatic activity) or by amplification or duplication of activity (thereby increasing enzymatic activity). Approximately one-third of all medications prescribed today are metabolized by CYP450, including TCAs, antiarrhythmics, beta-receptor antagonists, codeine, warfarin, phenytoin, and nicotine.

In addition, enzymes that metabolize cancer chemotherapy drugs, such as thiopurine S-methyltransferase, dihydropyrimidine dehydrogenase, and UDP-glucuronosyl transferase, can have therapeutic implications; for example, polymorphisms affecting these enzymes can result in serious adverse reactions, such as anemia and neurotoxicity. Finally, miscellaneous polymorphisms affecting drug transport proteins such as P-gp may affect drug response. P-gp acts as a safety mechanism to remove toxins from cells and has a role in the distribution of chemotherapy drugs, digoxin, cyclosporine, and protease inhibitors.

As a nurse, you need to be aware of the clinical ramifications of pharmacogenetics—having an effective knowledge of which drugs, diseases, and ethnic groups are affected by these variations can help you anticipate issues that may arise with patients under your care. For example, some patients of Asian descent have a significant reduction in enzyme activity secondary to amino acid substitution and therefore exhibit slower metabolism of certain drugs than patients from other ethnic groups. This effect influences clinical practice, such as in the dosing of rosuvastatin; patients of Asian descent are typically started at 5 mg/day PO, whereas other patients are started at 10 mg/day. Giving a lower dose helps limit the development of serious adverse reactions in patients of Asian descent.

Another example of how genetic polymorphism affects drug metabolism involves the drug warfarin. Studies show that CYP2C9, which is the primary enzyme responsible for warfarin metabolism, has two genetic variants. These variants are associated with up to an 80% decrease in enzymatic activity that can affect approximately 7% to 11% of patients. Consequently, patients with these variant genotypes retain warfarin longer, have a 2.4 times greater risk of serious or life-threatening bleeding after usual doses of warfarin, and need significantly lower maintenance dosages.

Fortunately, genetic testing for polymorphisms is available when issues such as these arise. Although not every patient undergoes testing, it can be helpful for those who seem to be refractory or overly sensitive to the effects of certain drugs or who meet other criteria.

2

Drug therapy across the lifespan

Drug therapy is a fact of life for millions of people of all ages, and certain aspects of a patient's life, such as age, growth, and development, can affect drug therapy.

Drugs and pregnancy

Drug administration safety during pregnancy has been a source of serious medical concern and controversy since the thalidomide tragedy of the late 1950s, when thousands of malformed infants were born after their mothers received this mild sedative-hypnotic while pregnant. To identify drugs that may cause such teratogenic effects, preclinical drug studies include tests on pregnant lab animals. These studies may reveal gross teratogenicity but don't establish absolute safety because different animal species react to drugs in different ways. Consequently, animal studies can't reveal all possible teratogenic effects in humans. For example, the preliminary animal studies on thalidomide gave no warning of its teratogenic effects, and it was subsequently released for general use in Europe.

Once thought to protect a fetus from drug effects, the placenta isn't much of a barrier. Almost every drug a patient takes during pregnancy crosses the placental barrier and enters fetal circulation, except for drugs with exceptionally large molecular structures, such as heparin, an injectable anticoagulant. By this standard, heparin could be used during pregnancy without fear of harming the fetus, but even heparin carries a warning for cautious use during pregnancy. Conversely, just because a drug crosses the placental barrier doesn't necessarily mean it's harmful to a fetus.

One factor—stage of fetal development—seems clearly related to greater risk during pregnancy. During the first and third trimesters of pregnancy, the fetus is especially vulnerable to damage from maternal use of drugs. During these times, *all* drugs should be given with extreme caution.

Organogenesis—when fetal organs differentiate—occurs in the first trimester, making this the most sensitive period for drug-induced fetal malformation. During this time, patients should not take medications, including OTC drugs and supplements, without first discussing them with a health care provider.

Fetal sensitivity to drugs is also of special concern during the third trimester because, after birth, the neonate's own metabolism must eliminate any remaining drug. Because a neonate's detoxifying systems aren't fully developed, any residual drug may take a long time to be metabolized and thus may induce prolonged toxic reactions. For this reason, patients shouldn't take drugs during the last 3 months of pregnancy, except when absolutely necessary and advised by their prescribers.

In many circumstances, patients must continue to take certain drugs during pregnancy. For example, a patient with a well-controlled seizure disorder may need to keep taking an anticonvulsant during pregnancy. Similarly, a patient with a bacterial infection must receive antibiotics during pregnancy. In such cases, the patient's medical needs outweigh the risk to the fetus, but drugs with lower teratogenic potential should be used whenever possible.

Complying with the following general guidelines can prevent indiscriminate and harmful use of drugs during pregnancy:

● Before a drug is prescribed for a patient of childbearing potential, ask the date of the patient's last menstrual period and ask about the possibility of pregnancy. If a drug is a known teratogen (for example, isotretinoin), some manufacturers recommend special precautions to ensure that the drug isn't given to a patient of childbearing potential until pregnancy is ruled out and may require use of contraceptives throughout the course of therapy.

● Caution a patient to avoid all drugs (including OTC drugs, herbs, and supplements) except those essential to maintain the pregnancy and the patient's health—especially during the first and third trimesters.

● Be aware that topical drugs may be subject to the same warning against use during pregnancy because many topically applied drugs can be absorbed in amounts large enough to be harmful to a fetus.

● When a patient needs to be prescribed a medication during pregnancy, use the safest drug in the lowest dose possible to minimize harm to the fetus.

● Instruct a patient to check with the prescriber before taking any drug during pregnancy.

• Encourage a patient to enroll in the pregnancy exposure registry for drugs that have one. Registries compile data on pregnancy outcomes to further define the risks of drug exposure in human pregnancies.

• During pregnancy, advise a patient to give the prescriber a list of all drugs, herbs, and supplements the patient is currently taking.

• Some drugs are part of a REMS drug safety program to ensure that the benefits of the medication outweigh its risks through restricted access, education, and strict monitoring. Be sure to advise a patient on the necessity to comply with program requirements while taking such medications.

Drugs and breastfeeding

Many drugs a mother takes appear in human milk. Drug levels in human milk tend to be high when drug levels in maternal blood are high, especially after each dose. Many manufacturers' instructions advise the mother to breastfeed *before* taking each drug dose, not *after*. Also, in general, drugs with short half-lives are preferred because they peak quickly and are then eliminated, making their excretion in human milk less likely.

A mother who wants to breastfeed usually may continue to do so with the prescriber's advice. However, breastfeeding should be temporarily interrupted and replaced with bottle-feeding when a mother must take certain drugs, such as a tetracycline, a sulfonamide (during the first 2 weeks postpartum), some oral anticoagulants, a drug that contains iodine, or an antineoplastic.

Caution a patient who is breastfeeding to protect the infant by not taking drugs indiscriminately. Instruct the mother to first check with the prescriber to be sure the patient is taking the safest drug at the lowest dose. Also instruct the patient to give the prescriber a list of all drugs, herbs, and supplements the patient is currently taking.

Drug therapy in children

Providing drug therapy to infants, children, and adolescents is challenging. Physiologic differences between children and adults, including those involving vital organ maturity and body composition, significantly influence drug effectiveness.

Physiologic changes affecting drug action

As a child develops, the processes of absorption, distribution (including drug binding to plasma proteins), metabolism, and excretion undergo profound changes that affect drug dosage. To ensure optimal drug effect and minimal toxicity, consider these factors when giving drugs to a child.

Absorption

Drug absorption in children depends on the form of the drug, its physical properties, simultaneous ingestion of other drugs or food, physiologic changes, and concurrent disease.

The pH of neonatal gastric fluid is neutral or slightly acidic; it becomes more acidic as the infant matures, which affects drug absorption. For example, ampicillin is better absorbed in an infant than in an adult because of the infant's low gastric acidity.

Various infant formulas and milk products may increase gastric pH and impede absorption of acidic drugs. If possible and so advised, give a child oral drugs on an empty stomach.

Gastric emptying time and transit time through the small intestine—which take longer in children than in adults—can affect absorption. Intestinal hypermotility (as occurs in patients with diarrhea) can also diminish a drug's absorption.

A child's comparatively thin epidermis allows increased absorption of topical drugs, increasing the risk of adverse systemic reactions.

Distribution

As with absorption, differences in body weight and physiology during childhood can significantly influence a drug's distribution and effects. In an infant born prematurely, body fluid makes up about 85% of total body weight; in an infant born at term, it makes up 55% to 70%; in an adult, 50% to 55%. Extracellular fluid (mostly blood) constitutes 40% of a neonate's body weight, compared with 20% in an adult. Intracellular fluid remains fairly constant throughout life and has little effect on drug dosage.

Extracellular fluid volume influences a water-soluble drug's concentration and effect because most drugs travel through extracellular fluid to reach their receptors. Compared with adults, distribution volume in children is proportionately greater because their fluid-to-solid body weight proportion is larger.

Because the proportion of fat to lean body mass increases with age, the distribution of fat-soluble drugs is more limited in children than in adults. As a result, a drug's fat or water solubility affects the dosage for a child.

Plasma protein binding
Decreased albumin level or intermolecular attraction between drug and plasma proteins causes many drugs to be less bound to plasma proteins in infants than in adults.

Highly protein-bound drugs may displace endogenous compounds, such as bilirubin and free fatty acids. Displacement of bound bilirubin can increase unbound (free) bilirubin, increasing the risk of kernicterus at normal bilirubin levels. Conversely, an endogenous compound may displace a low protein-bound drug.

Because only an unbound drug molecule has a pharmacologic effect, a change in the ratio of protein-bound to unbound active drug can greatly influence the drug's effect.

Several diseases and disorders, such as nephrotic syndrome and malnutrition, can decrease plasma protein levels and increase the level of an unbound drug, which can either intensify the drug's effect or produce toxicity.

Metabolism
A neonate's ability to metabolize a drug depends on the integrity of the liver's enzyme system, intrauterine exposure to the drug, and the properties of the drug itself.

Certain metabolic mechanisms are underdeveloped in neonates. Glucuronidation is a metabolic process occurring in the liver that renders most drugs more water soluble, facilitating kidney excretion. This process isn't developed enough to permit larger doses of most drugs until an infant is 1 month old. The use of chloramphenicol sodium succinate in a neonate may cause gray baby syndrome because the neonate's immature liver can't metabolize the drug; as a result, toxic levels accumulate in the blood. Reducing the dosage in a neonate and periodically monitoring drug levels are good ways to avoid toxicity. Conversely, intrauterine exposure to drugs may induce early development of the liver's enzyme mechanisms, thereby increasing the infant's capacity to metabolize potentially harmful substances.

Concomitant administration of drugs to a child may change liver metabolism and initiate the production of liver enzymes. Also, older children can metabolize some drugs (theophylline, for example) more rapidly than adults. This ability may arise from their increased metabolic activity in the liver. Doses larger than those recommended for adults may be required.

Excretion
Kidney excretion of a drug is the net result of glomerular filtration, active tubular secretion, and passive tubular reabsorption. Many drugs are excreted in the urine. The degree of kidney development or presence of kidney disease can greatly affect a child's dosage requirements because inability to excrete a drug through the kidneys may allow the drug to accumulate to toxic levels.

Physiologically, an infant's kidneys differ from an adult's in that infants have a high resistance to blood flow and their kidneys receive a smaller proportion of cardiac output. Infants have incomplete glomerular and tubular development and short, incomplete loops of Henle. (A child's GFR reaches an adult value between ages 2½ and 5 months; tubular secretion rate may reach an adult value between ages 7 and 12 months.) Infants also are less able to concentrate urine or reabsorb certain filtered compounds. The proximal tubules in infants also are less able to secrete organic acids.

Children and adults have diurnal variations in urine pH that correlate with sleep patterns. Changes in urine pH can affect the amount of drug excreted into the urine.

Special administration considerations
Biochemically, a drug displays the same mechanisms of action in all people. But the response to a drug can be affected by a child's age and size as well as by the maturity of the target organ. To ensure optimal drug effect and minimal toxicity, consider the following factors when giving drugs to children.

Adjusting dosages for children
When calculating children's dosages, don't use formulas that modify adult dosages. Children aren't scaled-down versions of adults. Base pediatric dosages on either body weight (mg/kg) or BSA (mg/m^2).

Reevaluate dosages at regular intervals to incorporate needed adjustments as a child develops. Although BSA provides a useful standard for adults and older children, use the body weight method in premature and full-term infants. Don't exceed the maximum adult dosage when calculating amounts per kilogram of body weight (except with certain drugs, such as theophylline, if indicated).

Obtain an accurate maternal drug history, including prescription and OTC drugs, vitamins, herbs, and supplements taken during pregnancy.

Drugs passed into human milk can have adverse effects on a breastfeeding infant. Before giving a drug to a breastfeeding mother, investigate its potential effects on the infant. For example, a sulfonamide given to a mother for a UTI appears in human milk and may cause kernicterus in an infant with low levels of unconjugated bilirubin.

Giving oral drugs

Remember the following guidelines when giving oral drugs to a child:

For an infant, give drugs in liquid form, if possible. For accurate administration, measure and give the preparation by oral syringe, never parenteral syringe. Remember to remove the syringe cap to keep the infant from swallowing or aspirating it. Instruct parents to do the same. Never use a vial or cup. Lift the infant's head to prevent aspiration of the drug, and press down on the chin to prevent choking. Or, place the drug in a nipple and allow the infant to suck the contents.

For a toddler, explain how you're going to give the drug. If possible, have the parents enlist the child's cooperation. Never call the drug "candy," even if it has a pleasant taste. Let the child take a liquid drug from a calibrated medication cup rather than a spoon; it's easier and more accurate. If a preparation is available only in tablet form, crush and mix it with an appropriate vehicle, such as applesauce. (First, verify with a pharmacist that the tablet can be crushed and mixed without compromising its effectiveness. For example, most long-acting or extended-release products shouldn't be crushed.)

For an older child who can swallow a tablet or capsule, have the child place the drug on the back of the tongue and swallow it with water or nonacidic fruit juice (such as apple juice), because milk and milk products may interfere with drug absorption.

Giving IV infusions

For IV infusions in infants, use a peripheral vein or a scalp vein in the temporal region. A scalp vein should be used as a last resort, when no other site is available. Foot veins can be used if the patient isn't walking.

The arms are the most accessible insertion sites, but because children tend to move about, take these precautions:

• Protect the insertion site with a site protection device, such as a clear plastic dome, if needed to prevent catheter dislodgement. Use a joint stabilization device, such as an armboard or splint, to facilitate infusion delivery, maintain device patency, and minimize infusion therapy complications. Periodically remove the stabilization device to assess circulation, skin integrity, and range of motion.

• Place the IV tubing clamp out of the child's reach. If extension tubing is used to allow the child greater mobility, securely tape the connection.

• Explain in simple terms to the child why a physical immobilization device is needed, to alleviate anxiety and maintain trust.

During an infusion, monitor flow rate, the child's condition, vascular access device patency, and the condition of the insertion site and surrounding area (hourly or more frequently if the child is receiving a vesicant drug). Flow rate may vary if an electronic infusion device isn't used. Flow should be adequate because some drugs (calcium, for example) can be irritating at low flow rates. Infants, small children, and children with compromised cardiopulmonary status are especially vulnerable to fluid overload with IV administration. To prevent this problem and help ensure that a limited volume of fluid is infused in a controlled manner, use an electronic infusion device.

Giving IM injections

IM injections are preferred when a drug can't be given by other parenteral routes and rapid absorption is needed. The Z-track method is the preferred method for IM injections because it leaves a zig-zag path, which prevents drug leakage into the subcutaneous tissue, helps seal the drug in the muscle, and minimizes irritation.

The vastus lateralis muscle of the anterolateral aspect of the thigh is the preferred injection site in children up to age 3. The deltoid muscle can be used in toddlers, if muscle mass is adequate. For children ages 3 to 18, the deltoid muscle is the preferred site. Though rarely used in children, the ventrogluteal site can be used if the child's condition prevents administration in other sites. To select the correct needle size, consider the child's age, muscle mass, thickness of adipose tissue at the injection site, and drug type, volume, and viscosity.

Record and rotate injection sites. Explain that the injection will hurt but that the drug will help the child feel better. For infants, use a combination of pain management strategies (such as nonnutritive sucking, containment, and breastfeeding, if possible) during injection.

Giving topical drugs and inhalants

When giving a child a topical drug or inhalant, follow these guidelines.

Warm eardrops to room temperature before use because cold drops can cause pain and vertigo. To give eardrops, turn the child on the side, with the affected ear up. If the child is younger than age 3, pull the pinna down and back; if age 3 or older, pull the pinna up and back.

Avoid using inhalants in young children because they commonly don't cooperate. Before giving a drug to an older child through a metered-dose inhaler, explain how to use the inhaler. Then have the child hold the inhaler and close the lips around the mouthpiece. Have the child exhale and pinch the nostrils shut. When the child starts to inhale, release one dose of the drug into the child's mouth. Tell the child to continue inhaling until the lungs feel full; then tell the child to breathe normally and unpinch the nostrils. Most inhaled drugs aren't useful if the drug remains in the mouth or throat—if you doubt the child's ability to use the inhaler correctly, don't use it. Devices such as spacers and assist devices may help. Check with a pharmacist, the prescriber, or a respiratory therapist for suggestions.

Use topical corticosteroids cautiously because prolonged use in children may delay growth. When applying topical corticosteroids to an infant's diaper area, don't cover the area with plastic or rubber pants, which act as an occlusive dressing and may enhance systemic absorption.

Giving parenteral nutrition

Give IV nutrition to pediatric patients who can't take in adequate nutrition orally and to those with hypermetabolic conditions who need supplementation. The latter group includes infants born prematurely, children, and adolescents with burns or other major trauma, intractable diarrhea, malabsorption syndromes, GI abnormalities, mental disorders (such as anorexia nervosa), and congenital abnormalities.

Before giving lipid injectable emulsions to infants and children, weigh the potential benefits against any possible risks. Fats—supplied as 10% or 20% lipid injectable emulsions—are given both peripherally and centrally. Their use is limited by the child's ability to metabolize them. For example, an infant or a child with severe liver insufficiency can't efficiently metabolize fats.

Some fats, however, must be supplied both to prevent essential fatty acid deficiency and

to permit normal growth and development. A minimum of calories (2% to 4%) must be supplied as linoleic acid—an essential fatty acid found in lipids. Nevertheless, fat solutions may decrease oxygen perfusion and may adversely affect a child with pulmonary disease. This risk can be minimized by supplying only the minimum fat needed for essential fatty acid requirements and not the usual intake of 40% to 50% of the child's total calories.

Fatty acids can also displace bilirubin bound to albumin, causing a rise in free, unconjugated bilirubin and an increased risk of kernicterus. Fat solutions may interfere with some bilirubin assays and cause a falsely elevated bilirubin level. To avoid this complication, draw a blood sample 4 hours after infusion of the lipid emulsion or, if the emulsion is infused over 24 hours, be sure the lab is aware so that the blood samples can be centrifuged before the assay is performed.

Giving IV solutions and medications through the same IV catheter as parenteral nutrition isn't usually recommended because of the potential for precipitate formation. Refer to your facility's guidelines or contact a pharmacist for further information.

Drug therapy in older adults

If you're giving drugs to older adults, you need to understand the physiologic and pharmacokinetic changes in this population that may affect drug dosages, cause common adverse reactions, and create adherence problems.

Physiologic changes affecting drug action

As a person ages, gradual physiologic changes occur. Some of these age-related changes can alter the therapeutic and toxic effects of drugs.

Body composition

Proportions of fat, lean tissue, and water in the body change with age. Total body mass and lean body mass tend to decrease, but the proportion of body fat tends to increase.

Body composition varies from person to person, and changes in body composition affect the relationship between a drug's concentration and distribution in the body. For example, a water-soluble drug such as gentamicin isn't distributed to fat. Because older adults have relatively more fat tissue and less lean tissue, more drug remains in the blood. Fat-soluble drugs tend to accumulate in older adults, resulting in prolonged half-lives and more pronounced effects.

Gastrointestinal function
In older adults, decreases in gastric acid secretion and GI motility slow the emptying of stomach contents and movement through the entire intestinal tract. Research suggests that older adults may not absorb drugs as easily as younger people. This problem is especially significant with drugs that have a narrow therapeutic index, such as digoxin, in which any change in absorption can be crucial.

Liver function
The liver's ability to metabolize certain drugs decreases with age. This decrease is caused by diminished blood flow to the liver, which results from an age-related decrease in cardiac output, and from the lessened activity of certain liver enzymes. When an older adult takes a sleep medication such as flurazepam, for example, the liver's reduced ability to metabolize the drug as well as the lipophilic property of the drug can produce residual effects the next morning.

Decreased liver function can result in more intense drug effects caused by higher levels, longer-lasting drug effects because of prolonged levels, and a greater risk of drug toxicity.

Kidney function
Older adults' kidney function is usually sufficient to eliminate excess body fluid and waste, but the ability to eliminate some drugs may be reduced by 50% or more. Many drugs commonly used by older adults, such as digoxin, are primarily excreted through the kidneys. If the kidneys' ability to excrete the drug is decreased, high blood levels and digoxin toxicity may result.

Drug dosages can be modified to compensate for age-related decreases in kidney function. Aided by results of lab tests, such as BUN and creatinine levels and creatinine clearance, adjusted drug dosages help patients receive therapeutic benefits without the risk of toxicity.

Nurses must remember that serum creatinine is a function of muscle mass and that most older adults lose muscle mass as they age. An older adult can have significant kidney impairment even with a serum creatinine level in the normal range. Watching for signs and symptoms of toxicity is important.

Special administration considerations
Aging is usually accompanied by a decline in organ function that can affect drug distribution and clearance. This physiologic decline is likely to be worsened by a disease or chronic disorder. Together, these factors can significantly increase the risk of adverse reactions and drug toxicity as well as nonadherence.

Adverse reactions
Compared with younger people, older adults experience twice as many adverse drug reactions, mostly from increased use of concomitant medications, poor adherence, and physiologic changes.

Signs and symptoms of adverse drug reactions—including confusion, weakness, agitation, and lethargy—are often mistakenly attributed to senility or disease. If an adverse reaction isn't identified, the patient may continue to receive the causal drug and receive other, unnecessary drugs to treat the resulting complications. This prescribing cascade can sometimes result in a pattern of inappropriate and excessive drug prescribing, causing polypharmacy.

Any drug can cause adverse reactions, but most of the serious reactions in older adults are caused by relatively few drugs. Be particularly alert for toxicities resulting from diuretics, antihypertensives, digoxin, corticosteroids, anticoagulants, sleeping aids, and OTC drugs.

Diuretic toxicity
Because total body water content decreases with age, a normal dosage of a potassium-wasting diuretic, such as furosemide or hydrochlorothiazide, may result in fluid loss and even dehydration in an older adult. These diuretics may deplete a patient's potassium level, making the patient feel weak, and they may raise blood uric acid and glucose levels, complicating gout and diabetes.

Antihypertensive toxicity
Many older adults experience light-headedness or fainting when they take antihypertensives, partly in response to atherosclerosis and decreased elasticity of blood vessels. Antihypertensives can lower BP too rapidly, resulting in insufficient blood flow to the brain, which can cause dizziness, fainting, and even a stroke.

Consequently, dosages of antihypertensives must be carefully individualized. In older adults, aggressive treatment of high BP may be harmful. Treatment goals should be reasonable. Elevated BP needs to be reduced slowly in older adults. Patients should change positions slowly and maintain adequate fluid intake to avoid orthostatic hypotension.

Digoxin toxicity

As kidney function and rate of excretion decline, digoxin level in the blood of an older adult may increase to the point of causing nausea, vomiting, diarrhea and, most seriously, cardiac arrhythmias. Monitoring of digoxin level and watching for early signs and symptoms of toxicity, such as appetite loss, confusion, and depression, are important interventions.

Corticosteroid toxicity

Older adults taking a corticosteroid may experience short-term effects, including fluid retention and psychological effects ranging from mild euphoria to acute psychotic reactions. Long-term toxic effects, such as osteoporosis, can be especially severe in older adults who have been taking prednisone or related steroidal compounds for months or even years. Careful monitoring of patients on long-term regimens is necessary to prevent serious toxicity. Observe for subtle changes in appearance, mood, and mobility and for impaired healing and fluid and electrolyte disturbances.

Anticoagulant effects

Older adults taking an anticoagulant are at increased risk for bleeding, especially when they take NSAIDs or aspirin at the same time. Because older adults are more likely to fall, they're also at increased risk for bleeding as a result of a fall. Careful monitoring of INR is necessary for a patient taking warfarin as well as monitoring for bruising and other signs and symptoms of bleeding.

Sleeping aid toxicity

Sedatives and sleeping aids, such as zolpidem and diphenhydramine, can cause excessive sedation and drowsiness. Alcohol consumption may increase these CNS depressant effects, even if the drug was taken the previous evening. These drugs should be used sparingly in older adults.

Over-the-counter drug toxicity

Prolonged ingestion of aspirin, aspirin-containing analgesics, and other OTC NSAIDs (such as ibuprofen and naproxen) may cause GI irritation—even ulcers—and gradual blood loss, resulting in severe anemia. Prescription NSAIDs can cause similar problems. Both OTC and prescription NSAIDs can cause kidney toxicity in older adults. Anemia from prolonged aspirin consumption can affect all age-groups, but older adults may be less able to compensate because of already-reduced iron stores. These drugs should be used very carefully and at the lowest effective doses.

Acetaminophen is found in a variety of prescription and OTC products. Liver injury may occur from inadvertently taking excess acetaminophen from multiple sources.

Laxatives can cause diarrhea in older adults, who are extremely sensitive to drugs such as bisacodyl. Long-term oral use of mineral oil as a lubricating laxative may result in lipoid pneumonia from aspiration of small residual oil droplets in the patient's mouth.

Antihistamines such as diphenhydramine have anticholinergic effects and can cause confusion and mental status changes; they are also more likely to cause dizziness, sedation, and hypotension in older adults. OTC decongestants, including phenylephrine, can have systemic effects, such as hypertension, anxiety, insomnia, and agitation.

Nonadherence

Poor adherence can be a problem with patients of any age. Many hospitalizations result from failure to adhere to a medical regimen. In older adults, factors linked to aging, such as diminished visual acuity, hearing loss, forgetfulness, the need for multiple drug therapy, and socioeconomic factors, can combine to make nonadherence a special problem. About one-third of older adults fail to adhere to their prescribed drug therapy, including failure to take prescribed doses or to follow the correct schedule. They may take drugs prescribed for previous disorders, stop drugs prematurely, or indiscriminately use drugs that should be taken as needed. Older adults may also have multiple prescriptions for the same drug and inadvertently take an overdose.

To prevent adherence-related problems, take these steps:

• Review the patient's prescribed drug regimen. Make sure the patient understands the dose amount, the time and frequency of doses, and the reason the drug has been prescribed. Also, explain in detail if a drug should be taken with food, with water, or separate from other drugs. To verify understanding, ask the patient to repeat the instructions back to you.

• Help prevent drug therapy problems by suggesting the use of drug calendars, pill sorters, and other aids to help with adherence. Refer the patient to the prescriber, a pharmacist, or social services if further information or assistance with drug therapy is needed.

3

Safe drug administration

Medication therapy is a primary intervention for many illnesses. It greatly benefits many patients and yet is involved in many instances of unintended harm to patients and health care workers from either unintended consequences of therapy (adverse drug reactions or exposure to hazardous drugs) or medication-related errors (preventable adverse drug events). (See *Preventing and treating IV vesicant extravasation injury,* page 14.) Medication errors are a significant cause of patient morbidity and mortality in the United States. Each year, 7,000 to 9,000 people die as a result of medication errors. Of all sentinel events reviewed in 2021 (1,197) by The Joint Commission (a nonprofit organization that seeks to improve public health care through the voluntary accreditation of health care institutions), approximately 35 events were attributed to medication management. A *sentinel event* is a patient safety event that results in patient death or permanent harm or requires intervention to sustain life.

Many governmental and nongovernmental organizations are dedicated to improving the safety of drug administration. One mission of the FDA, for example, is to protect the public health by assuring the safety, effectiveness, and security of human drugs, vaccines, and medical devices. In 2007, the Food and Drug Administration Amendments Act expanded the FDA's authority regarding assessing and communicating risks associated with drugs. One of the new provisions of the law granted the FDA authority to require drug manufacturers to submit Risk Evaluation and Mitigation Strategies. (See *Risk Evaluation and Mitigation Strategies*, page 15.) The U.S. Pharmacopeia (USP), a nonprofit, nongovernmental public health organization, sets official public standards for quality, purity, strength, and identity of drugs, food ingredients, and dietary supplements manufactured or sold in the United States.

The Patient Safety and Quality Improvement Act of 2005 authorized the creation of patient safety organizations (PSOs) to improve the quality and safety of U.S. health care delivery. One of these PSOs, the Institute for Safe Medication Practices (ISMP), is a nonprofit organization entirely dedicated to preventing medication errors and using medications safely. In addition, The Joint Commission has established National Patient Safety Goals and standards to improve the safe use of medications in its accredited facilities.

The CDC has a number of campaigns and initiatives to promote medication safety by developing evidence-based guidelines.

Opioid safety

One important initiative of the CDC, FDA, and other organizations is to address the use and misuse of opioids in treating chronic pain (pain not related to cancer or palliative care that lasts longer than 3 months or past the time of normal tissue healing). According to the Substance Abuse and Mental Health Services Administration's National Drug Survey on Drug Use and Health, an estimated 10.1 million people ages 12 and older reported misusing opioids in 2019. In 2018, overdoses involving opioids alone killed nearly 47,000 people; 32% of those deaths involved prescription opioids. (See *Safe opioid administration*, page 16.)

The CDC has developed an evidence-based guideline called "CDC Clinical Practice Guideline for Prescribing Opioids for Pain—United States, 2022" (available at http://dx.doi.org/10.15585/mmwr.rr7103a1), which addresses the following four areas:
- determining whether to initiate opioids for pain
- selecting opioids and determining opioid dosages
- deciding duration of initial opioid prescription and conducting follow-up
- assessing risk and addressing harms of opioid use.

The CDC has also developed the "Checklist for Prescribing Opioids for Chronic Pain" (available at https://www.cdc.gov/drugoverdose/pdf/pdo_checklist-a.pdf), which provides guidance for primary care providers treating adults with chronic pain.

The FDA has developed a comprehensive action plan that focuses on reducing the impact of the opioid abuse epidemic on families and communities while providing patients access to safe and effective pain relief. The FDA opioids action plan includes these steps:
- consulting expert advisory committees before new approvals for opioids without abuse-deterrent properties and for new labeling of appropriate opioid use in children

Preventing and treating IV vesicant extravasation injury

Extravasation injuries occur when vesicant IV solutions or drugs—those with the potential to cause significant tissue injury (such as certain chemotherapy drugs, antibiotics, electrolyte solutions, vasopressors, and antiemetics)—escape from blood vessels into surrounding tissue (extravasate) during administration. Drugs and solutions that produce inflammation rather than serious or lasting tissue injury from extravasation are considered *irritants*. Extravasation injuries may occur when vesicants are given centrally or peripherally. Such injuries can cause significant harm, including necrotic ulcers that may require surgical intervention, infection, loss of a limb or limb function, and complex regional pain syndrome.

Recognizing extravasation

Signs and symptoms of peripheral extravasation include:
- changes in IV site appearance (blanching, bruising) or temperature (coolness, erythema)
- pain, tightness, or itching at or surrounding the insertion site
- IV site fluid leakage
- numbness or tingling, diminished capillary refill, or decreased motor function in the extremity.
  Signs and symptoms of CVAD extravasation include:
- discomfort at the insertion site or along the CVAD path
- fluid leakage from the insertion site
- increased resistance to solution injection
- shoulder, neck, or chest edema.

Preventing extravasation

Use the following measures to prevent extravasation injuries:
- Follow best practices for administering vesicant drugs and solutions. Make sure you've received proper training in prevention measures and extravasation recognition and management.
- When administering vesicants, know the specific antidote for the drug you're giving and make sure that the antidote and equipment needed to manage extravasation are on hand. Some antidotes for vesicants and solutions include sodium thiosulfate for mechlorethamine, calcium, and cisplatin; phentolamine for vasopressors (such as dopamine and

norepinephrine); and terbutaline for vasopressor extravasation when phentolamine is unavailable.
- Ensure that the IV access site or CVAD is patent before giving the drug. Make sure the insertion site is visible, and use an appropriate catheter stabilization device.
- Make sure the drug is given by the proper route. Most vesicants administered by continuous infusion should be given utilizing a CVAD. Know when an electronic infusion device should and shouldn't be used.
- Frequently monitor the patient for extravasation signs and symptoms, and teach the patient to immediately report them.

Treating extravasation

Follow best practices for treatment of extravasation injury:
- Stop the drug, and aspirate any residual drug and blood from the IV catheter or CVAD.
- Note the time the infusion started to provide an estimate of the amount of solution extravasated.
- Notify the practitioner.
- Remove the peripheral IV catheter; don't apply pressure to the site.
- For extravasation from a CVAD, prepare the patient for radiographic tests to identify CVAD tip location.
- For peripheral extravasation, prepare for subcut injections of a drug-specific antidote, if appropriate.
- Elevate the affected extremity.
- Assess the insertion site and surrounding tissue.
- Apply hot (for vasoconstrictors) or cold (for alkylating drugs) compresses, if ordered.
- Use a skin marker or photo for serial documentation of extravasation.
- Monitor the site for pain, erythema progression, induration, tissue necrosis, and possible compartment syndrome. Note that symptom development may be delayed for 48 hours.
- Document the date and time of the infusion, extravasation signs and symptoms, time when signs and symptoms were first noted, type and size of venous access device, estimated extravasation solution volume, treatment instituted, practitioner notification, and the patient's response to treatment.
- Note that patients with significant tissue damage may need surgery.

- developing additional changes and warnings to immediate-release opioid labeling information to provide risk and safe prescribing guidance for prescribers
- strengthening the requirements for drug companies to generate postmarket data on long-term impacts of opioid use to improve treatment of both addiction and pain

- updating REMS requirements for opioids to increase pain management and safe prescribing training of prescribers and to decrease inappropriate opioid prescription
- supporting the development of and expanding the use of abuse-deterrent opioids
- improving access to naloxone and other drug treatment options for opioid use disorders

Risk Evaluation and Mitigation Strategies

REMS is a risk management program that goes beyond the drug's package insert and is used when necessary to make certain that a drug's benefits outweigh its risks. REMS are designed to help reduce the occurrence or severity of certain serious risks by informing or supporting the execution of the safe use conditions described in the medication's FDA-approved prescribing information. The FDA can require a REMS at any stage of a drug's life cycle (as part of a drug's New Drug Application or after approval as new safety information becomes available), and manufacturers who fail to comply with REMS requirements can face substantial monetary penalties. For a list of currently approved REMS, go to https://www.accessdata.fda.gov/scripts/cder/rems/index.cfm.

When evaluating the necessity of REMS, the FDA takes into consideration such factors as:
- the number of patients most likely to use the drug
- the seriousness of the patient's disease
- the drug's benefit
- the projected duration of treatment
- the severity of known or potential adverse events
- whether the drug is a new molecular entity.

The FDA has issued an outline of specific components that manufacturers should use to develop a REMS proposal. These include the development of specific REMS goals and elements to ensure a drug's safe and appropriate use. The REMS must also describe how the manufacturer plans to evaluate whether the REMS goal is being met and the timetable for periodic assessments and reassessments. The results of the evaluations must be reported to the FDA, and the FDA determines whether the REMS must be modified and whether additional actions must be taken.

REMS may contain one or all of the following components:
- **Medication guide:** Written safety information for patients that must be distributed by the pharmacist to each patient receiving the drug
- **Communication plan:** Plan that includes the tools to teach health care professionals how to use the drug safely and appropriately
- **Elements to Assure Safe Use (EASU):** Specific requirements and elements to ensure safe use of the drug, including requirements that each patient be enrolled in a registry, that essential lab monitoring be performed, that the drug may only be prescribed by a prescriber with a specific certification, and that the drug may only be distributed by a specialty pharmacy
- **Implementation plan:** Plan that describes how the EASUs will be put into action.

- reexamining the risks and benefits of opioids and their effects on public health.

Causes of medication errors

The National Coordinating Council for Medication Error Reporting and Prevention (www.nccmerp.org) defines a *medication error* as "any preventable event that may cause or lead to inappropriate medication use or patient harm while the medication is in the control of the health care professional, patient, or consumer. Such events may be related to professional practice, health care products, procedures, and systems, including prescribing; order communication; product labeling, packaging, and nomenclature; compounding; dispensing; distribution; administration; education; monitoring; and use."

Medication errors were once thought to be caused by lapses in an individual's practice. Traditionally, teaching nurses to administer drugs safely focused on the individual nurse's practice and the application of the "rights" of safe medication administration. (See *The eight "rights" of medication administration,* page 17.)

Although individual nursing practice is still an extremely important part of safe drug administration, the focus of prevention efforts has widened. After medication errors were systematically studied by numerous organizations who shared data, it became apparent that these errors are complex events with multiple factors and are most often caused by failures within systems. As a result of these findings, research has shifted to preventing medication errors by identifying their root causes and then developing and validating evidence-based prevention strategies. Organizational processes, management decisions, inadequate medication administration protocols, staffing shortages, environmental conditions, poor communication, inadequate drug knowledge and resources, and individual mistakes or protocol violations may all contribute to medication errors.

The medication administration process

Medication errors can occur within any one or more of the five stages of the medication administration process. Because up to 40% of a nurse's time may be spent on medication administration and nursing practice intersects multiple stages, nurses may often be involved in medication errors. Here are some of the types of errors that have been reported in each stage.

Safe opioid administration

Opioid analgesics are associated with adverse effects, most notably respiratory depression followed by sedation. Additional adverse effects include aspiration pneumonia, constipation, delirium, dizziness, falls, hallucinations, hypotension, nausea, and vomiting. Opioid analgesics are also linked with adverse drug events due to:
- lack of knowledge regarding differing potencies among opioids
- incorrect administration of multiple opioids, including their respective routes of administration
- inadequate monitoring of patients who take opioids.

Nurses can help avoid opioid misuse by:
- identifying conditions that put patients at higher risk for oversedation and respiratory depression, such as sleep disorders, morbid obesity, older age, habitual opioid use, major organ dysfunction or failure, respiratory disorders, smoking, and polypharmacy
- screening patients for respiratory depression risk factors using screening tools, such as the Pasero Opioid-induced Sedation Scale (POSS), Richmond Agitation-Sedation Scale (RASS), Screener and Opioid Assessment for Patients with Pain (SOAPP and SOAPP-R), Opioid Risk Tool (ORT), and Screening Instrument for Substance Abuse Potential (SISAP)
- assessing the patient's opioid history, including possible abuse, adverse effects, and intolerance
- assessing the patient's skin for an existing opioid patch, implanted drug delivery system, or infusion pump
- starting patients who are opioid-naive with a nonopioid pain regimen before moving on to opioids
- starting patients who are opioid-naive with the lowest dosage of opioid possible and titrating upward
- consulting a pharmacist when changing opioid medications or their administration routes
- dosing opioids based on the individual patient's condition and needs
- being mindful of the timing of opioid administration; for instance, not administering opioids before a patient transfer to avoid possible injury to the patient if drug levels peak during the time of transfer
- using PCA devices
- educating patients and caregivers about opioid misuse and steps to take to prevent this occurrence.

Tips for safe opioid administration include the following measures:
- Double-check the medication order, appropriateness of the medication, dose, line placement for infusions, and pump settings.
- Ensure standing orders are available for reversal agents.
- Label all IV and epidural lines to avoid confusion.
- Closely monitor a patient identified as being at high risk for adverse outcomes related to opioid treatment. Frequently assess respiration quality and rate, and observe for signs and symptoms of oversedation.
- Use capnography and pulse oximetry readings to help detect opioid toxicity.
- Keep oxygen and naloxone in areas where opioids are administered.
- Utilize established pain guidelines and standardized formats that are consistent with the patient's age, condition, and ability to understand to monitor and document the patient's pain.
- In collaboration with the multidisciplinary team, involve the patient in the pain management planning process. Develop realistic expectations and measurable goals that the patient understands for the degree, duration, and reduction of pain. Discuss objectives used to evaluate treatment progress (for example, relief of pain and improved physical and psychosocial function).
- Educate patients and caregivers about PCA use before surgical procedures and warn against dosing by proxy.
- Regularly observe and monitor patients who are using PCA.
- Provide patient and caregiver education on pain management, treatment options, and safe use of the prescribed opioid.
- Teach the patient and caregiver about pain management strategies during discharge planning. Include information about the patient's pain management plan and adverse effects of pain management treatment.
- Teach the patient and caregiver about safe use, storage, and disposal of opioids. Instruct patients who use fentanyl patches to store them in a secure manner to prevent access by children, pets, and drug-seekers. Provide education on how to properly apply patches and to protect them from heat.

Stage 1: Ordering and prescribing
- Prescriber orders are incomplete or illegible.
- Contraindicated drugs (such as drugs to which the patient is allergic) are prescribed.

- The prescriber specifies the wrong drug, dose, route, frequency, or duration or fails to specify the indication.
- Drugs are prescribed using inappropriate or inadequate verbal orders.

The eight "rights" of medication administration

Traditionally, nurses have been taught the "five rights" of medication administration. These are broadly stated goals and practices to help individual nurses administer drugs safely and correctly.

1. The *right drug:* Check the drug label and verify that the drug and form to be given match the drug that was prescribed.
2. The *right patient:* Confirm the patient's identity by checking at least two patient identifiers.
3. The *right dose:* Verify that the dose and dosage form to be given are appropriate for the patient, and compare the drug label with the prescriber's order.
4. The *right time:* Ensure that the drug is administered at the correct time and frequency.
5. The *right route:* Verify that the route by which the drug is to be given is specified by the prescriber and is appropriate for the patient.
   In addition to the traditional "five rights" of individual practice, best-practice researchers have added three additional "rights":
6. The *right reason:* Verify that the drug prescribed is appropriate to treat the patient's condition.
7. The *right response:* Monitor the patient's response to the drug administered for the desired effect.
8. The *right documentation:* Completely and accurately document in the patient's medical record the drug administered; monitoring of the patient, including the patient's response; and other nursing interventions.

Stage 2: Transcribing and verifying
• An incorrect drug, dose, route, time, or frequency is transcribed into the medication administration record (MAR) by the pharmacist or nurse.
• Drug verification and documentation in the MAR by the pharmacist or nurse are inadequate.

Stage 3: Dispensing and delivery
• The prescribed drug is filled incorrectly.
• Failure to deliver the right drug to the right place for the right patient occurs.

Stage 4: Administering
• The wrong drug is given to the wrong patient by the nurse or other licensed professional.
• The wrong dose is calculated and given or infused by the nurse or other licensed professional.
• The right drug is incorrectly prepared (such as crushing a drug that shouldn't be crushed)

and is given by the nurse or other licensed professional.
• The correct drug is administered by the wrong route (such as an oral drug that is injected IV) by the nurse or other licensed professional.
• The correct drug is given at the wrong time or frequency by the nurse or other licensed professional.

Stage 5: Monitoring and reporting
• Monitoring of the patient by the nurse before and after medication administration is inadequate.
• Documentation and reporting of the patient's condition by the nurse before and after medication administration are inadequate.
• Hand-off communication between licensed professionals is inadequate.
• Reporting of medication errors is inadequate.

Elements contributing to safer drug administration

Ensuring the safe delivery of medication involves a system-wide, interdisciplinary approach. Research shows that improvements in communication, education, and prevention of hazardous drug exposure can facilitate safe medication delivery.

Communication improvements
Communication issues are implicated in approximately 60% of reported medication errors. Communication can be improved in many ways throughout the medication administration process. The traditional nursing process "rights" of safe drug administration are still important components of safe drug administration, but even when protocols are followed exactly, some medication errors still occur. For example, a nurse who's exactly following the eight "rights" might administer a drug to which a patient is allergic if the allergy information is incomplete or undocumented or hasn't been effectively communicated. Appropriate communication among all members of the health care team, including nurses, is vitally important.

Many health care facilities have instituted measures to help standardize and organize appropriate communication. One tool commonly used is SBAR (Situation, Background, Assessment, and Recommendation); its purpose is to logically organize information to optimize proper communication among health care providers.

Each institution must have processes and tools to document medication administration. Each prescribed medication order must be clearly written or entered into an electronic medical record system, and verbal orders must be used only when absolutely necessary. Each verbal order should be read back and verified with the prescriber before the drug is administered. The patient's condition must be monitored after each medication is given, and the patient's response and any nursing interventions must be appropriately documented. Clear communication through documentation is essential to safe practice.

The Joint Commission has developed goals and standards regarding medication reconciliation—the process of comparing a patient's medication regimen when medications are discontinued, dosages are changed, or new medications are added and at every transition in care (for example, on admission, upon discharge, and between care settings and levels). Medication reconciliation helps ensure that essential information about the patient's medication regimen is communicated to the health care team. Medication reconciliation helps prevent the inadvertent omission of needed medications, prevents medication duplication, and helps identify medications with potentially harmful interactions.

Education improvements

Lack of knowledge has also been implicated in many medication errors; therefore, education about medications is essential to their safe administration. All health care team members involved in the process of medication administration, including the prescriber, pharmacist, and nurse, must have access to accurate information about each drug's indications, appropriate dosing regimen, appropriate route, appropriate frequency, possible drug interactions, appropriate monitoring, any cautions, and possible adverse effects. Each facility should have processes in place to educate staff and communicate important drug information.

Governmental and nongovernmental agencies are doing their part toward educating facilities, prescribers, and nurses. The FDA established the boxed warning system to alert prescribers to drugs with increased risks to patients. These boxed warnings are the strongest labeling requirements for drugs that can have serious reactions. The Joint Commission requires accredited health care facilities to develop a list of abbreviations to avoid in all medication communications. The ISMP maintains a list of high-alert medications that may cause significant patient harm when given incorrectly. (Each facility should have protocols in place for administering high-alert medications, with safeguards built into the process.) The FDA and ISMP have developed a list of drugs with similar names—look-alike, sound-alike (LASA) medications—that can be easily confused with each other. Dissimilarities in each drug's name are highlighted with uppercase letters (so each name has mixed-case letters, called *tall-man lettering*), making such mix-ups less likely to occur for each drug.

Patient education

Patients and their families should be active participants in the patient's care and should understand the patient's plan of care, including the purpose of newly prescribed medications. The patient and family need to learn what to watch for, how the patient's condition will be monitored, what signs and symptoms to report, and what to report, including anything that doesn't seem right, such as unfamiliar medications. Before administering a medication, the nurse must verify with the patient medication allergies and unusual past reactions to medications.

The following general teaching guidelines will help ensure that the patient receives the maximum therapeutic benefit from the medication regimen and will help the patient avoid adverse reactions, accidental overdose, and harmful changes in effectiveness:

• Instruct the patient to learn the brand names, generic names, and dosages of all drugs and supplements (such as herbs and vitamins) being taken.
• Tell the patient to notify the pharmacist and prescriber about all medications the patient is taking, including prescription drugs, OTC drugs, and herbal or other supplements, and about any drug allergies or reactions.
• Advise the patient to always read the label and medication guide before taking a drug, to take it exactly as prescribed, and to never share prescription drugs with others.
• Warn the patient not to change manufacturers of a drug without consulting the prescriber, to avoid harmful changes in effectiveness.
• Tell the patient to check the expiration date before taking a drug.
• Teach the patient how to safely discard drugs that are outdated or no longer needed.
• Caution the patient to keep all drugs safely out of the reach of children and pets.

• Advise the patient to store drugs in their original containers, at the proper temperature, and in areas where they won't be exposed to sunlight or excessive heat or humidity. Sunlight, heat, and humidity can cause drug deterioration and reduce a drug's effectiveness.

• Encourage the patient to report all suspected adverse or unusual reactions to the prescriber, and teach proper techniques for self-monitoring the condition (for example, how to obtain a resting HR before taking digoxin).

• Suggest that the patient have all prescriptions filled at the same pharmacy or pharmacy system so that pharmacists can warn against potentially harmful drug interactions.

• Tell the patient to report the complete medication history to all health care providers involved in the patient's care, including the dentist.

• Instruct the patient to immediately contact the prescriber, pharmacist, or poison control center (1-800-222-1222 or https://www.poison.org/) and seek immediate medical attention if the patient or someone else takes an overdose. Tell the patient to keep emergency numbers handy at all times.

• If the patient is taking an opioid, educate the patient and caregiver on the signs and symptoms of an overdose and the administration of naloxone, as state law permits.

• Advise the patient to take a sufficient supply of drugs when traveling. The patient should personally carry the drugs in their original containers and not pack them in luggage. Also, recommend that the patient carry a letter from the prescriber authorizing use of the drugs, especially if a drug is a controlled substance.

• Encourage the patient to keep a wallet card or cell phone app that lists all medications the patient is taking, including dose, route, frequency, and indication.

Improvements in preventing hazardous drug exposure

Hazardous drugs, as defined by the American Society of Health-System Pharmacists and the National Institute for Occupational Safety and Health (NIOSH), have one or more of the following characteristics:

• carcinogenicity (cause cancer)
• teratogenicity (cause defects in a developing fetus or other developmental toxicities)
• reproductive toxicity
• organ toxicity at low doses
• genotoxicity (cause damage to DNA)

• a structure and toxicity profile that mimics that of existing hazardous drugs.

The NIOSH list of antineoplastics and other hazardous drugs can be found at https://www.cdc.gov/niosh/docs/2016-161/pdfs/2016-161.pdf. Health care workers can be exposed to hazardous drugs through inhalation, ingestion, skin contact and absorption, or injection; exposure is most likely from skin contact and absorption or inhalation. Potential exposure can occur in many ways, such as:

• preparing drugs for administration (reconstituting powdered drugs, crushing tablets for oral liquids, compounding powders, or counting out oral doses from multidose bottles)
• administering hazardous drugs IM, IV, intrathecally, or subcut
• directly contacting drugs on the contaminated exteriors of drug vials, on drug-contaminated work surfaces, and on IV tubing and syringes
• handling body fluids that contain drugs or drug-contaminated dressings, linens, or waste
• transporting hazardous drugs
• removing and disposing of personal protective equipment (PPE)
• cleaning contaminated workspaces and spills.

Protecting workers and minimizing exposure

Engineering and administrative controls and use of appropriate PPE can help protect health care workers by minimizing their exposure to hazardous drugs.

Engineering controls include:
• class II or III biological safety cabinets (also known as *vertical flow hoods* or *ventilated cabinets*) for hazardous drug preparation
• closed-system drug transfer devices
• needleless systems.

Administrative controls include:
• implementing training, retraining, and testing programs to educate and monitor staff about best practices to prevent hazardous drug exposure
• developing and implementing management protocols to reduce staff risk
• using monitoring programs to identify hazardous drugs and staff exposure or development of early disease.

Appropriate use of PPE includes:
• making sure PPE fits and undergoes proper use and disposal
• selecting PPE based on assessment of the potential for hazardous drug exposure:
– Gloves: Gloves should be appropriate for the potential exposure. Double gloving may be

necessary. Polyvinyl chloride exam gloves offer little hazardous drug protection. Test information from the glove manufacturer details the resistance to specific hazardous drugs. Gloves made with latex should not be used with a patient who has a latex allergy.
- Gowns: Gowns should be long-sleeved, with tight-fitting cuffs. Disposable gowns coated with laminate materials provide better protection than noncoated gowns. Refer to the manufacturer for permeation information. Don't reuse gowns; change gowns immediately after a spill or splash.
- Respirators: A properly fit-tested certified N-95 respirator or surgical N-95 respirator provides protection from most airborne particles. Other types of respirators may be necessary to protect from airborne gases. Surgical masks don't provide adequate respiratory protection from drug exposure.
- Face shields: Using face shields with goggles protects against splashes to the face and eyes. Full-face respirators also provide protection. Face shields or eye glasses with side shields don't provide full eye and face protection.
- Sleeve, hair, and shoe covers: These items provide additional protection and may be required in certain environments, such as drug-compounding areas.

Strategies for reducing error rates

In addition to improvements in communication and education, other strategies that can help reduce medication administration error rates include:
• providing adequate nurse-to-patient staffing ratios
• designing drug preparation areas as safety zones that promote making correct choices during the medication administration process based on drug importance, frequency of use, and sequence of use
• improving the medication administration environment (reduce noise to 50 dB, improve lighting to at least 100 foot-candles, obtain nonglare computer screens)
• developing and using protocols that reduce distractions for nursing staff directly involved in medication administration
• dispensing medications in unit-dose or unit-of-use packaging
• restricting high-alert drugs and administration routes (limiting their number, variety, and concentration in patient care areas). For example:
- Remove all neuromuscular blockers from units where patients aren't normally intubated.

- Remove highly concentrated electrolytes from unit stock in patient care units.
- Remove concentrated oral opioids from unit stock and dispensing cabinets.
- Apply additional strong warnings to drug labels.
- Make sure emergency equipment is always available.
• switching from IV to oral or subcut forms as soon as possible
• dispensing IV and epidural infusions only from the pharmacy
• labeling all medications both on and off the sterile field
• posting drug information in patient care units
• having drug information (such as infusion rate and dosing charts) available for all health care providers at the point of care
• avoiding use of unapproved abbreviations
• using leading zeros; for example, use "0.5 mg" rather than ".5 mg"
• avoiding trailing zeros; for example, use "5 mg" rather than "5.0 mg"
• requiring that medication orders be prescribed by metric weight, not by volume (for example, in mg/kg not mL) and never relying on a patient's stated or historical weight (instead, obtain weight as soon as possible, and measure and document actual weight only in metric units in all electronic and written formats)
• establishing protocols and checklists to double-check and document high-alert drugs or unusual drugs, dosages, or regimens
• always recalculating doses before giving drugs to children and neonates. (Make sure the formula is included for calculating the dose; have a second clinician [preferably a pharmacist] double-check the calculations.)
• making sure each patient is appropriately monitored (with appropriate monitoring equipment [cardiac monitors, capnography, pulse oximeters] before and after drug administration).

Using technology to promote safety

Technology is becoming an increasingly important part of providing safer drug administration. The goal of medication administration technology is to enhance individual practice and help build safeguards into the medication administration process. Information about the ISMP and safe medication practices can be found at http://ismp.org/.

Computerized provider order entry

In computerized provider order entry (CPOE), a prescriber enters a medication order into a computerized record, thus eliminating errors due to illegible handwriting. Systems can include such safeguards as immediate order checking for errors (such as incorrect dosing or routes of administration) and drug interactions, allergy checks, and administration protocols. They can immediately transmit orders to appropriate departments and can also be linked to drug information databases. CPOE can help monitor how drugs are utilized and can provide data for quality improvement.

Bar codes

Bar-code technology is widely used and was initially developed to help control and track inventory. The use of this technology for safer drug administration, dispensing, inventory control, and drug storage and preparation has been endorsed by The Joint Commission, ISMP, Institute of Medicine, and Agency for Healthcare Research and Quality. With this technology, the patient wears a bar-code identifier on a wristband; the medication also has a bar code that uses the medication's own unique National Drug Code to identify the name, dose, manufacturer, and type of packaging. The nurse scans the bar code using an optical scanner, verifying the patient's identity and medication. The system supports but does not replace the traditional "rights" of safe medication.

Bar-code systems can reduce medication errors, but they aren't without disadvantages. For example, they don't expedite the medication administration process. Problems with the technology (such as malfunctioning scanners and unreadable wristbands) can actually cause delays in treatment. These problems may tempt nurses to develop dangerous shortcuts, such as attaching patient wristbands to clipboards and giving patients medications before scanning their wristbands.

Automated dispensing cabinets

Automated dispensing cabinets (ADCs) are computer-controlled medication distribution systems in the patient care unit or ancillary department that are used to store, track, and dispense medications. ADCs can provide nurses with near-total access to medications needed in their patient care area and promote the control and security of medications. They electronically track the use of drugs such as controlled substances. They may have bar-code capabilities for restocking and correct medication selection, and can be programmed to provide safeguards such as drug safety alerts. ADCs can also be linked with external databases and billing systems to increase the efficiency of drug dispensing and billing.

"Smart" pumps

"Smart" IV pumps can have such features as programmable drug libraries and dosage limits, can perform automatic calculations, have dose-error reduction software, and can be programmed to signal dosage alerts. The ISMP recommends administering high-alert IV medications using programmable infusion pumps with dose error-reduction software. They can be integrated with bar-code and CPOE technologies and can be wireless. Smart pumps help alert nurses to the selection of incorrect dosages or to dosages that exceed recommended levels.

Smart pumps can't detect or prevent all problems with IV drug infusions, however. For example, with some pumps, a nurse can select an incorrect drug from the library database and then override the safety alerts. Other infusion pump problems include software defects and failure of built-in safety alarms. Some pumps have ambiguous on-screen directions that can lead to dosing errors. The FDA recommends reporting all infusion-related adverse events, planning ahead in case a pump fails, labeling the channels and tubing to prevent errors, checking all settings, and monitoring patients for signs and symptoms of infusion problems. Nurses should perform independent calculation of all doses and infusion rates and not rely solely on the pump. Double-checking each dosage calculation is essential. Nurses shouldn't bypass pump alarms and must verify that a pump is functioning properly before beginning an infusion.

Other technologies

Using oral syringes without luer-locks to administer oral or enteral medications helps prevent administration of oral and enteral medications via the wrong route. (The ISMP has reported cases in which oral medications were drawn into parenteral syringes and inadvertently injected into IV lines, resulting in patient deaths.) Utilizing special tubing that doesn't have side ports for epidural medication administration prevents inadvertent injection of an incorrect drug into an epidural catheter.

Certain drugs such as vincristine should always be dispensed in a minibag (25 to 50 mL) of solution, never in a syringe, to avoid accidental intrathecal (instead of IV) administration. Oral liquid dosing devices, such as syringes, cups, and droppers, should display the metric scale only.

Reporting medication errors

Clearly, medication errors are a major threat to patient safety. Only by sharing and analyzing data and performing more research can evidence-based quality improvements be developed and validated. Several agencies and organizations provide voluntary reporting systems to study the causes and prevalence of medication errors. The FDA has the Adverse Event Reporting System (FAERS), which is part of the MedWatch program. The National Coordinating Council for Medication Error Reporting and Prevention (NCC MERP) has 27 national organization members, including the ISMP and United States Pharmacopeial Convention, cooperating to address interdisciplinary issues. The ISMP has reporting programs for practitioner-based medication errors, vaccine errors, and consumer medication errors. Nurses should report medication errors and "near misses" to help identify problems within systems.

abacavir sulfate ⚕
ah-BAK-ah-veer

Ziagen

Therapeutic class: Antiretrovirals
Pharmacologic class: Nucleoside reverse transcriptase inhibitors

AVAILABLE FORMS
Oral solution: 20 mg/mL
Tablets: 300 mg

INDICATIONS & DOSAGES
➤ **HIV-1 infection, with other antiretrovirals.**
Adults: 300 mg PO b.i.d. or 600 mg PO daily.
Children ages 3 months and older (oral solution): 8 mg/kg PO b.i.d. or 16 mg/kg PO once daily, up to maximum of 600 mg PO daily.
Children weighing 25 kg or more (scored tablets): 300 mg PO b.i.d.
Children weighing 20 to less than 25 kg (scored tablets): 150 mg PO in the morning and 300 mg PO in the evening.
Children weighing 14 to less than 20 kg (scored tablets): 150 mg PO b.i.d.
Adjust-a-dose: In patients with Child-Pugh class A liver impairment, give 200 mg (oral solution) PO b.i.d.

ADMINISTRATION
PO
⚕ **Boxed Warning** Screen for the HLA-B*5701 allele before start of therapy and before reinitiating therapy in patients with unknown status who previously tolerated drug. ∎
⊘ *Alert:* Hazardous drug; use safe handling and disposal precautions.
• Always give drug with other antiretrovirals.
• May give with or without food.
• Give missed dose as soon as possible; don't double dose.

ACTION
Converted intracellularly to the active metabolite carbovir triphosphate, which inhibits activity of HIV-1 reverse transcriptase, terminating viral DNA growth.

Route	Onset	Peak	Duration
PO	Unknown	0.7–1.7 hr	Unknown

Half-life: 1 to 2 hours.

ADVERSE REACTIONS
CNS: bad dreams, fever, headache, insomnia and sleep disorders, anxiety, depressive disorders, malaise, fatigue, dizziness.
EENT: ear, nose, and throat infections. **GI:** diarrhea, nausea, vomiting, abdominal pain.
Hematologic: *neutropenia, thrombocytopenia.* **Hepatic:** elevated transaminase levels.
Metabolic: increased CK, amylase, triglyceride levels; hyperglycemia. **Musculoskeletal:** pain. **Respiratory:** bronchitis, pneumonia, viral infection. **Skin:** rash. **Other:** chills, *hypersensitivity reaction.*

INTERACTIONS
Drug-drug. *Methadone:* May slightly increase methadone elimination. Monitor effectiveness; increase methadone dosage if needed.
Riociguat: May increase riociguat serum concentration. Decrease riociguat dosage if needed.
Drug-lifestyle. *Alcohol use:* May decrease elimination of drug, increasing overall exposure. Monitor alcohol consumption. Discourage use together.

EFFECTS ON LAB TEST RESULTS
• May increase ALT, AST, amylase, CK, glucose, and triglyceride levels.
• May decrease Hb level and platelet and neutrophil counts.

CONTRAINDICATIONS & CAUTIONS
⚕ **Boxed Warning** Contraindicated in patients who carry the HLA-B*5701 allele because of high risk of hypersensitivity reactions. ∎
Boxed Warning Drug can cause serious and sometimes fatal hypersensitivity reactions with multiple organ involvement. Contraindicated in patients with a prior hypersensitivity reaction to abacavir. ∎
• Contraindicated in patients with Child-Pugh class B or C liver impairment.
⊘ *Alert:* Due to increased risk of liver toxicity, use cautiously when giving drug to patients at risk for liver disease. Lactic acidosis and severe liver enlargement with steatosis, including fatal cases, have been reported with the use of nucleoside analogues alone or in combination, including abacavir and other antiretrovirals. Stop treatment with drug and don't restart if events occur.

• Women are more likely than men to experience lactic acidosis and severe liver enlargement with steatosis. Obesity and prolonged nucleoside exposure may be risk factors.
• Use cautiously in older adults and patients with underlying risk of CAD.
Dialyzable drug: Unknown.

PREGNANCY-LACTATION-REPRODUCTION

• Use cautiously during pregnancy; drug crosses placental barrier. Use during pregnancy only if potential benefits outweigh risk.
• Register patients who are pregnant with the Antiretroviral Pregnancy Registry (1-800-258-4263).
• Drug appears in human milk. To avoid postnatal HIV-1 infection transmission, viral resistance in infants who test positive for HIV, and possible adverse reactions, instruct patients not to breastfeed.

NURSING CONSIDERATIONS

Boxed Warning Monitor patient for signs and symptoms of hypersensitivity (fever, rash, fatigue, achiness, generalized malaise, nausea, vomiting, diarrhea, abdominal pain, cough, dyspnea, pharyngitis); if present, immediately stop drug and notify prescriber. ■

Boxed Warning Don't restart drug or any abacavir-containing product after a hypersensitivity reaction, regardless of HLA-B*5701 status, because more severe signs and symptoms can recur within hours, including life-threatening hypotension and death. ■

• Because of a high rate of early virologic resistance, triple antiretroviral therapy with abacavir, lamivudine, and tenofovir shouldn't be used as a new treatment regimen for treatment-naive or pretreated patients. Monitor patients currently controlled with this combination and those who use this combination in addition to other antiretrovirals; consider modification of therapy.
• Monitor patient for immune reconstitution syndrome. Inflammatory response to indolent or residual opportunistic infection (MAC infection, CMV, *Pneumocystis jiroveci* pneumonia, or TB) may occur during initial treatment; autoimmune disorders (Graves disease, polymyositis, or Guillain-Barré syndrome) may occur at any time after start of therapy.
• Assess for CAD risk factors with antiretroviral use; address modifiable risk factors

(such as HTN, hyperlipidemia, diabetes, and smoking).
• Drug may mildly elevate glucose level, especially in children.

PATIENT TEACHING

✪ Alert: Inform patient that drug can cause a life-threatening hypersensitivity reaction. Warn patient who develops signs or symptoms of hypersensitivity (such as fever, rash, severe tiredness, achiness, generally ill feeling, nausea, vomiting, diarrhea, stomach pain, cough, shortness of breath, or sore throat) to stop taking drug and notify prescriber immediately.
• Encourage patient to review drug information leaflet with each new prescription and refill and to carry a warning card with the signs and symptoms of hypersensitivity.
• Inform patient that drug doesn't cure HIV infection or reduce the risk of HIV transmission to others through sexual contact or blood contamination. Explain that long-term drug effects are unknown.
• Caution patient not to stop anti-HIV medicines, even for a short time, because the virus may become harder to treat.
• Warn patient not to restart abacavir or other abacavir-containing drugs without being under medical care because of the risk of serious hypersensitivity reaction.
• Instruct patient in safe medication handling and administration.
• Advise patient of childbearing potential to consult prescriber if pregnant or planning to become pregnant.

abatacept ☒

ab-a-TA-sept

Orencia, Orencia ClickJect

Therapeutic class: Antirheumatics
Pharmacologic class: Selective costimulation modulators

AVAILABLE FORMS

Lyophilized powder for injection: 250 mg single-use vial (25 mg/mL when reconstituted)
Solution for subcut administration: 50 mg/ 0.4 mL, 87.5 mg/0.7 mL, 125 mg/mL single-dose prefilled syringe; 125 mg/mL prefilled autoinjector

INDICATIONS & DOSAGES

➤ **Moderate to severe RA, used alone or with other DMARDs (except biologic DMARDs, Janus kinase [JAK] inhibitors)**
Adults weighing more than 100 kg: 1 g IV over 30 minutes. Repeat 2 and 4 weeks after initial infusion; then every 4 weeks thereafter.
Adults weighing 60 to 100 kg: 750 mg IV over 30 minutes. Repeat 2 and 4 weeks after initial infusion; then every 4 weeks thereafter.
Adults weighing less than 60 kg: 500 mg IV over 30 minutes. Repeat 2 and 4 weeks after initial infusion; then every 4 weeks thereafter.
Adults (subcut): 125 mg subcut once weekly with or without IV loading dose. For patients receiving loading dose, give single IV dose based on weight. Then give 125 mg subcut within a day, followed by 125 mg subcut once weekly. Patients transferring from IV to subcut form should receive the first subcut dose instead of the next scheduled IV dose.

➤ **Moderately to severely active polyarticular juvenile idiopathic arthritis, used alone or with methotrexate**
Children ages 6 and older weighing 75 kg or more: Use adult dosing regimen, not to exceed a maximum dose of 1,000 mg.
Children ages 6 and older weighing less than 75 kg: 10 mg/kg IV over 30 minutes. Repeat 2 and 4 weeks after initial infusion; then every 4 weeks thereafter. Calculate dosing based on body weight before each dose.
Children ages 2 and older weighing 50 kg or more: 125 mg subcut once weekly without an IV loading dose.
Children ages 2 and older weighing 25 to less than 50 kg: 87.5 mg subcut once weekly without an IV loading dose.
Children ages 2 and older weighing 10 to less than 25 kg: 50 mg subcut once weekly without an IV loading dose.

➤ **Psoriatic arthritis, used alone or in combination with nonbiologic DMARDs**
Adults weighing more than 100 kg: 1 g IV over 30 minutes. Repeat 2 and 4 weeks after initial infusion; then every 4 weeks thereafter.
Adults weighing 60 to 100 kg: 750 mg IV over 30 minutes. Repeat 2 and 4 weeks after initial infusion; then every 4 weeks thereafter.
Adults weighing less than 60 kg: 500 mg IV over 30 minutes. Repeat 2 and 4 weeks after initial infusion; then every 4 weeks thereafter.
Adults (subcut): 125 mg subcut once weekly without IV loading dose. Patients transferring from IV to subcut form should receive first subcut dose instead of the next scheduled IV dose.

➤ **Acute GVHD prophylaxis, in combination with a calcineurin inhibitor and methotrexate in patients undergoing hematopoietic stem cell transplantation (HSCT) from a matched or 1 allele-mismatched unrelated donor** ☒
Adults and children ages 6 and older: 10 mg/kg (maximum, 1,000 mg) IV over 60 minutes on day before transplantation; then a dose on days 5, 14, and 28 after transplantation.
Children ages 2 to younger than 6: 15 mg/kg IV over 60 minutes on day before transplantation; then 12 mg/kg on days 5, 14, and 28 after transplantation.

ADMINISTRATION

IV

⚠ *Alert:* Don't use prefilled syringes and autoinjectors for IV administration.

▼ Reconstitute vial with 10 mL of sterile water for injection, using only the silicone-free disposable syringe provided, to yield 25 mg/mL. Use an 18G to 21G needle for preparation.

▼ Gently swirl contents until completely dissolved. Avoid vigorous shaking.

▼ Vent the vial with a needle to clear away foam.

▼ Ensure solution is clear and colorless to pale yellow. Don't use if opaque particles, discoloration, or other foreign particles are present.

▼ Further dilute solution to 100 mL total volume with NSS using silicone-free disposable syringe provided with each vial. Gently mix; don't shake the bag or bottle.

▼ Infuse using an infusion set and a sterile, nonpyrogenic, low–protein-binding 0.2- to 1.2-micron filter.

▼ Store diluted solution at room temperature or refrigerate at 36° to 46° F (2° to 8° C). Complete infusion within 24 hours of reconstituting.

▼ **Incompatibilities:** Don't infuse in the same line with other IV drugs.

Subcutaneous

● Remove prefilled syringe or autoinjector from refrigerator 30 to 60 minutes before administration so that it reaches room temperature.

● Ensure drug is clear and colorless to pale yellow; don't use if particulate matter or discoloration is present.

- Rotate injection sites. Give in abdomen, thighs, or outer area of upper arms.
- Never inject into tender, bruised, red, or hard areas.
- The ability of children to self-inject with the autoinjector hasn't been tested.
- Store at 36° to 46° F (2° to 8° C); don't freeze.

ACTION

Inhibits T-cell activation, decreases T-cell proliferation, and inhibits production of TNF-alpha, interferon-gamma, and interleukin-2.

Route	Onset	Peak	Duration
IV, subcut	Unknown	Unknown	Unknown

Half-life: IV, 13 days; subcut, 14.3 days.

ADVERSE REACTIONS

CNS: headache, dizziness, fever. **CV:** HTN. **EENT:** epistaxis, nasopharyngitis, rhinitis, sinusitis. **GI:** nausea, dyspepsia, diarrhea, abdominal pain. **GU:** acute pyelonephritis, UTI, *AKI.* **Hematologic:** anemia, decreased CD4 lymphocyte count. **Metabolic:** *hypermagnesemia.* **Musculoskeletal:** back pain, limb pain. **Respiratory:** URI, bronchitis, cough, pneumonia, rhonchi, dyspnea, hypoxia. **Skin:** rash, injection-site reaction. **Other:** infections, *malignancies,* herpes simplex, influenza, infusion reactions.

INTERACTIONS

Drug-drug. *Anakinra, TNF antagonists:* May increase risk of infection. Don't use together. *Biologic DMARDs, JAK inhibitors:* Safety and effectiveness when used together haven't been determined. Concurrent use isn't recommended.
Live-virus vaccines: May decrease effectiveness of vaccine. Avoid giving vaccines during and for 3 months after abatacept therapy.
Non-live vaccines: May diminish therapeutic effect of vaccine. If given during treatment, consider revaccination at least 2 to 3 months after therapy.
Drug-herb. *Echinacea:* May diminish the therapeutic effect of immunosuppressants. Avoid concurrent use.

EFFECTS ON LAB TEST RESULTS

- May increase magnesium level.
- May decrease CD4 lymphocyte count and Hb level.

- Glucose dehydrogenase pyrroloquinoline quinone–based glucose monitoring systems may react with maltose present in abatacept, causing falsely elevated blood glucose readings on the day of infusion (IV form only).

CONTRAINDICATIONS & CAUTIONS

- Contraindicated in patients hypersensitive to drug or its components.
- Rare cases of severe hypersensitivity reactions have been reported. Reactions may occur with the first dose or within 24 hours of infusion. Discontinue drug and treat emergently if hypersensitivity occurs.
- Use cautiously in patients with active infection, history of chronic infection, or underlying conditions that may predispose patient to infection; scheduled elective surgery; or COPD.
- Malignancies, including skin cancer, have been reported with abatacept use; periodic skin exams are recommended.
- Ensure patient's vaccination status is current with vaccination guidelines before starting abatacept.
- Safety and effectiveness in polyarticular juvenile idiopathic arthritis or acute GVHD in patients younger than age 2 haven't been established.
Dialyzable drug: Unknown.

PREGNANCY-LACTATION-REPRODUCTION

- Use cautiously during pregnancy and only if benefit to patient justifies fetal risk.
- Register patients who are pregnant with the pregnancy registry (1-877-311-8972).
- Drug appears in human milk. Patient should discontinue breastfeeding or discontinue drug, considering importance of drug to patient.

NURSING CONSIDERATIONS

- Make sure patient has been screened for TB and HBV before giving drug. Treat patient who tests positive for TB before starting drug.
- Ensure patient receives antiviral prophylaxis for Epstein-Barr virus reactivation and continues for 6 months after HSCT. Consider prophylactic antivirals for CMV infection or reactivation during treatment and for 6 months after HSCT.
- Carefully monitor patient, especially an older adult, for infections and malignancies.
- If patient develops a severe infection, notify prescriber; therapy may need to be stopped.

Reactions in bold italics are *life-threatening*.

❸ *Alert:* If patient has COPD, watch for worsening respiratory status.
• Monitor patient for hypersensitivity reactions; ensure supportive measures are available to treat hypersensitivity reactions.
• Ensure that patient's immunizations are up-to-date before therapy.
• *Look alike–sound alike:* Don't confuse Orencia with Oracea.

PATIENT TEACHING
• Instruct patient that TB and HBV screening is necessary before therapy.
• Caution patient to avoid exposure to infections.
• Advise patient to immediately report signs and symptoms of infection, swollen face or tongue, and difficulty breathing.
• Instruct patient with COPD to report worsening signs and symptoms.
• Advise patient to avoid live-virus vaccines during and for 3 months after therapy.
• Caution patient to consult prescriber if pregnant or planning to breastfeed.
• Advise patient to contact prescriber before taking any other drugs or herbal supplements.
• Remind patient to contact prescriber before scheduling surgery.
• Instruct patient or caregiver in subcut administration, drug storage, and syringe disposal.

SAFETY ALERT!

abemaciclib ⚒
a-bem-a-SYE-klib

Verzenio

Therapeutic class: Antineoplastics
Pharmacologic class: Kinase inhibitors

AVAILABLE FORMS
Tablets ⓓ: 50 mg, 100 mg, 150 mg, 200 mg

INDICATIONS & DOSAGES
Adjust-a-dose (for all indications): For Child-Pugh class C liver impairment, reduce abemaciclib dosing frequency to once daily. Refer to manufacturer's instructions for toxicity-related dosage adjustments.

For concomitant use of strong CYP3A inhibitors (except ketoconazole), if recommended starting dose of abemaciclib is 150 or 200 mg b.i.d., reduce abemaciclib dose to 100 mg b.i.d. If a strong CYP3A inhibitor

is begun and abemaciclib dose has been decreased to 100 mg b.i.d. due to adverse reactions, further reduce abemaciclib dose to 50 mg b.i.d. When a strong CYP3A inhibitor has been discontinued, increase abemaciclib dose (after three to five half-lives of the inhibitor) to the dose that was used before the strong CYP3A inhibitor was begun. With concomitant use of moderate CYP3A inhibitors, monitor patient for adverse reactions; consider reducing abemaciclib dose in 50-mg decrements.
➤ **Initial endocrine-based treatment of hormone receptor (HR)–positive, HER2-negative advanced or metastatic breast cancer, in combination with an aromatase inhibitor**
Adults males and adult females after menopause: 150 mg PO b.i.d. Continue treatment until disease progression or unacceptable toxicity occurs. Treat adult males and adult females before and during menopause with a GnRH agonist per clinical practice guidelines.
➤ **HR-positive, HER2-negative advanced or metastatic breast cancer with disease progression after endocrine therapy, in combination with fulvestrant**
Adults: 150 mg PO b.i.d. Continue treatment until disease progression or unacceptable toxicity occurs. Treat adult females before and during menopause with a GnRH agonist per clinical practice standards.
➤ **Monotherapy for the treatment of HR-positive, HER2-negative advanced or metastatic breast cancer with disease progression after endocrine therapy and prior chemotherapy in the metastatic setting**
Adults: 200 mg PO b.i.d. Continue treatment until disease progression or unacceptable toxicity occurs.
➤ **Adjuvant treatment for HR-positive, HER2-negative, node-positive early breast cancer, in combination with endocrine therapy (tamoxifen or aromatase inhibitor), in patients at high risk for recurrence**
Adults: 150 mg PO b.i.d. until completion of 2 years of treatment or disease recurrence or unacceptable toxicity occurs.

ADMINISTRATION
PO
❸ *Alert:* Hazardous drug; use safe handling and disposal precautions.

- Give drug at approximately the same time every day without regard for food.
- Have patient swallow tablets whole; don't crush or cut tablets.
- If patient vomits or misses a dose, give the next dose at its scheduled time.
- Store at 68° to 77° F (20° to 25° C).

ACTION
An inhibitor of cyclin-dependent kinases 4 and 6 (CDK4 and CDK6). In estrogen receptor–positive breast cancer cells, cyclin D1 and CDK4 and CDK6 promote cell-cycle progression and cell proliferation. Drug blocks progression from G1 into S phase of the cell cycle, resulting in cell aging and death.

Route	Onset	Peak	Duration
PO	Unknown	8 hr	Unknown

Half-life: 18.3 hours.

ADVERSE REACTIONS
CNS: fatigue, fever, headache, dysgeusia, dizziness. **CV:** peripheral edema, *VTE.* **EENT:** dry mouth, increased tearing. **GI:** diarrhea, nausea, abdominal pain, vomiting, stomatitis, constipation, decreased appetite. **GU:** UTI, vaginal infection, increased creatinine level. **Hematologic:** *neutropenia,* anemia, *leukopenia, thrombocytopenia, lymphopenia.* **Hepatic:** increased transaminase levels, *liver toxicity.* **Metabolic:** weight loss, dehydration, *hypokalemia.* **Musculoskeletal:** arthralgia. **Respiratory:** cough, dyspnea, ILD, pneumonitis. **Skin:** alopecia, pruritus, rash, nail disorder. **Other:** infections, flulike symptoms, *sepsis.*

INTERACTIONS
Drug-drug. *Ketoconazole:* May significantly increase abemaciclib level. Avoid use together.
Moderate and strong CYP3A inducers (rifampin): May decrease abemaciclib plasma level and lead to reduced activity. Avoid use together; consider alternative agents.
Moderate CYP3A inhibitors (diltiazem, verapamil): May increase abemaciclib level. Monitor patient for adverse reactions; consider reducing abemaciclib dose.
Strong CYP3A inhibitors (clarithromycin, itraconazole): May increase abemaciclib level and increase risk of toxicity. Decrease abemaciclib dosage.

Drug-food. *Grapefruit products:* May increase abemaciclib level. Avoid use together.

EFFECTS ON LAB TEST RESULTS
- May increase ALT, AST, and creatinine levels.
- May decrease potassium level.
- May decrease Hb level and hematocrit and WBC, RBC, neutrophil, lymphocyte, and platelet counts.

CONTRAINDICATIONS & CAUTIONS
🔹 *Alert:* CDK4 or CDK6 inhibitors may cause rare but severe or fatal ILD and pneumonitis.
- Drug may cause GI toxicity (including diarrhea associated with dehydration and infection), bone marrow suppression, and liver toxicity.
- VTE has been reported in patients treated with abemaciclib. Safety and effectiveness haven't been studied in patients with early breast cancer with a history of VTE.
- Use in patients with severe kidney impairment and chronic kidney failure hasn't been studied.
- Use cautiously in patients with Child-Pugh class C liver impairment.
- Safety and effectiveness in children haven't been established.
Dialyzable drug: Unknown.

PREGNANCY-LACTATION-REPRODUCTION
- Drug may cause fetal harm. Advise patient of fetal risk.
- Patients of childbearing potential should use effective contraception during treatment and for at least 3 weeks after final dose.
- Serious adverse reactions may occur in infants who are breastfed. Patient shouldn't breastfeed during treatment and for at least 3 weeks after final dose.
- Based on animal studies, drug may impair fertility in adult males of reproductive potential.

NURSING CONSIDERATIONS
🔹 *Alert:* Monitor patients for new or worsening pulmonary signs or symptoms (hypoxia, cough, dyspnea, interstitial infiltrates on radiologic images); if they occur, interrupt therapy immediately and evaluate patient. If infection, neoplasm, and other causes are excluded, permanently discontinue treatment in patients with severe ILD or pneumonitis.

Reactions in bold italics are *life-threatening*.

- Monitor patients for loose stools and associated dehydration and infection. Initiate antidiarrheal therapy and increase oral fluids at first sign of diarrhea.
- Monitor CBC before therapy begins, every 2 weeks during therapy for the first 2 months, monthly for the next 2 months, then as clinically indicated.
- Monitor patients for signs and symptoms of liver toxicity (fatigue, right upper quadrant abdominal pain, loss of appetite) and bone marrow suppression (fatigue, unusual bleeding or bruising, fever, infection).
- Obtain LFTs before therapy begins, every 2 weeks during therapy for the first 2 months, monthly for the next 2 months, then as clinically indicated.
- Monitor patients for signs and symptoms of thrombosis (pain and swelling of the extremities) and PE (chest pain, dyspnea, tachycardia), and treat appropriately.
- Verify pregnancy status prior to treatment.

PATIENT TEACHING

⬧ *Alert:* Warn patient to immediately report breathing difficulty or discomfort, and shortness of breath while at rest or with low activity, which may indicate ILD or pneumonitis.
- Teach about proper drug administration and handling.
- Tell patient to report all adverse reactions and to immediately report signs and symptoms of liver toxicity or VTE.
- Advise patient to immediately report fever, particularly in association with other signs and symptoms of infection (malaise, pain, cough, shortness of breath, drainage, changes in urine).
- Instruct patient to begin antidiarrheal therapy (such as loperamide) at first sign of loose stools, to increase fluid intake, and to notify prescriber for further instructions and follow-up.
- Warn patient of childbearing potential of fetal risk, to use effective contraception during therapy and for at least 3 weeks after final dose, and to report known or suspected pregnancy.
- Remind patient not to breastfeed during treatment and for at least 3 weeks after final dose.
- Advise adult male patient of reproductive potential that drug may impair fertility.

abiraterone acetate
a-bir-A-ter-one

Yonsa, Zytiga

Therapeutic class: Antineoplastics
Pharmacologic class: Antiandrogen biosynthesis inhibitors

AVAILABLE FORMS

Tablets ⬤*:* 250 mg
Tablets (film-coated) ⬤*:* 500 mg
Tablets (micronized) ⬤*:* 125 mg

INDICATIONS & DOSAGES

Adjust-a-dose (for all indications): For patients with baseline Child-Pugh class B liver impairment, reduce starting dosage of Zytiga to 250 mg PO once daily or Yonsa starting dosage to 125 mg once daily. If liver toxicity develops during treatment, refer to manufacturer's instructions for dosage adjustments.

For patients who must take a strong CYP3A4 inducer, increase dosing frequency to b.i.d. only during coadministration.

➤ **Metastatic, castration-resistant prostate cancer**

Adult men: 1,000 mg Zytiga PO once daily, in combination with 5 mg prednisone PO b.i.d. Or, 500 mg Yonsa PO once daily in combination with 4 mg methylprednisolone PO b.i.d.

➤ **Metastatic, high-risk castration-sensitive prostate cancer (Zytiga only)**

Adult men: 1,000 mg PO once daily in combination with 5 mg prednisone PO daily.

ADMINISTRATION
PO

⬧ *Alert:* Hazardous drug; use safe handling and disposal precautions. Anyone who is pregnant or may become pregnant should wear gloves when handling tablets.
- Patient receiving abiraterone should also receive a GnRH analogue concurrently (or have had a bilateral orchiectomy).
- Zytiga and Yonsa aren't interchangeable; don't substitute formulations.
- Give Zytiga on an empty stomach; patient shouldn't eat for 2 hours before or 1 hour after receiving drug. Give Yonsa without regard to food.

• Have patient swallow tablets whole with water; don't crush or cut tablets.
• Store tablets at room temperature.

ACTION
Inhibits biosynthesis of androgen production and increases mineralocorticoid production by adrenal glands.

Route	Onset	Peak	Duration
PO	Rapid	2 hr	Unknown

Half-life: 7 to 17 hours.

ADVERSE REACTIONS
CNS: fatigue, fever, insomnia, headache. **CV:** edema, hot flushes, HTN, *arrhythmias,* chest pain, *cardiac failure.* **EENT:** nasopharyngitis. **GI:** diarrhea, dyspepsia, constipation, vomiting. **GU:** UTI, hematuria, urinary frequency, nocturia. **Hematologic:** anemia, bruising, *lymphopenia.* **Hepatic:** increased transaminase levels, bilirubinemia, *liver toxicity.* **Metabolic:** *hypokalemia, hypophosphatemia,* hyperglycemia, hyperlipidemia, hypernatremia. **Musculoskeletal:** joint swelling, joint discomfort, muscle discomfort, fractures, groin pain. **Respiratory:** URI, cough, dyspnea. **Skin:** rash. **Other:** falls.

INTERACTIONS
Drug-drug. *CYP2C8 substrates (pioglitazone):* May increase substrate level. Monitor patient closely.
Dextromethorphan, thioridazine, other CYP2D6 substrates: May inhibit metabolism of these drugs, causing higher levels. Avoid use together. If drugs must be used together, consider reducing dosage of substrate drug.
Strong CYP3A4 inducers (carbamazepine, phenobarbital, phenytoin, rifabutin, rifampin, rifapentine): May decrease abiraterone level. If drugs must be used together, increase abiraterone dosage during use together; decrease back to the previous dose and frequency if the CYP3A4 inducer is discontinued.
Drug-food. *Any food:* May significantly increase drug absorption of Zytiga. Patient must take Zytiga on an empty stomach.

EFFECTS ON LAB TEST RESULTS
• May increase ALP, ALT, AST, bilirubin, glucose, sodium, cholesterol, and triglyceride levels.
• May decrease potassium, phosphate, and Hb levels.
• May decrease lymphocyte count.

CONTRAINDICATIONS & CAUTIONS
• Contraindicated in patients hypersensitive to drug or its components and in those with Child-Pugh class C liver impairment.
• Use cautiously in patients with a history of CV disease (HF, recent MI, ventricular arrhythmias), diabetes, or liver disease.
• Avoid use with radium Ra 223 dichloride; combined use increases mortality and fracture risk.
• Safety in patients with LVEF of less than 50% or NYHA Class II to IV HF hasn't been established.
Dialyzable drug: Unknown.

PREGNANCY-LACTATION-REPRODUCTION
• Drug isn't indicated for use in adult females and is contraindicated during pregnancy and breastfeeding.
• Based on animal studies, adult male patients with partners of childbearing potential should use effective contraception during treatment and for at least 3 weeks after final dose.

NURSING CONSIDERATIONS
• Monitor ALT, AST, and bilirubin levels in all patients at baseline, every 2 weeks for first 3 months, then monthly thereafter. For patients with Child-Pugh class B liver impairment, measure at baseline, every week during first month of treatment, every 2 weeks for next 2 months, and monthly thereafter. If AST or ALT level rises above $5 \times$ ULN or bilirubin level rises above $3 \times$ ULN, interrupt treatment and closely monitor liver function.
• Monitor patient for signs and symptoms of liver toxicity (malaise, jaundice, abdominal pain, nausea, vomiting).
• Monitor patient with a history of CV disease at least monthly for HTN, hypokalemia, and fluid retention. Monitor serum potassium level before treatment and at least monthly. Control HTN and correct hypokalemia before and during treatment.
• Monitor blood glucose level in patient with diabetes during and after treatment with abiraterone. Adjust antidiabetic dosage, if needed, to minimize risk of hypoglycemia. Severe hypoglycemia has been reported in patients receiving thiazolidinediones (including pioglitazone) or repaglinide.
• Monitor patient for signs and symptoms of adrenocortical insufficiency (chronic fatigue, loss of appetite, muscle weakness, weight

loss, nausea, vomiting). Patient may need an increased corticosteroid dosage before, during, and after stressful situations.

PATIENT TEACHING
• Teach about proper drug administration and handling.
• Advise that if patient misses a single dose of abiraterone, methylprednisolone, or prednisone, patient should take regular dose the next day; if patient misses more than one dose, patient should inform prescriber.
• Explain that patient must use abiraterone with either prednisone or methylprednisolone.
• Warn patient not to stop abiraterone, prednisone, methylprednisolone, or other chemotherapy drugs without consulting prescriber.
• Teach patient that periodic blood tests will be needed to monitor tolerance to therapy.
• Warn patient, adult female caregivers, and adult female sexual partners about risk of fetal harm from abiraterone therapy.
• Teach adult male patient the importance of using effective birth control method during treatment and for at least 3 weeks after final dose.

---

abrocitinib ⬚
a-broe-SYE-ti-nib

Cibinqo

Therapeutic class: Immunomodulators
Pharmacologic class: Janus kinase inhibitors

AVAILABLE FORMS
Tablets ⬤**⬤**: 50 mg, 100 mg, 200 mg

INDICATIONS & DOSAGES
➤ **Refractory, moderate to severe atopic dermatitis not adequately controlled with other systemic drug products, including biologics, or when use of those therapies is inadvisable**
Adults and children ages 12 and over: 100 mg PO once daily. May increase to 200 mg once daily if inadequate response after 12 weeks. Discontinue drug if inadequate response after 200-mg dose increase. Can use with or without topical corticosteroids.

⬚ *Adjust-a-dose:* For patients with eGFR of 30 to 59 mL/minute or patients who are known or suspected CYP2C19 poor metabolizers, reduce dosage to 50 mg once daily; if inadequate response after 12 weeks, may double the dose. Refer to manufacturer's instructions for toxicity-related dosage adjustments.

ADMINISTRATION
PO
• Give at same time each day without regard to food.
• Have patient swallow tablets whole; don't crush or cut tablets.
• If a dose is missed, give as soon as possible. If missed dose is within 12 hours of the time before next dose, skip the missed dose and resume dosing at regular scheduled time.
• Store tablets at 68° to 77° F (20° to 25° C) in original container.

ACTION
Reversibly inhibits Janus kinase (JAK) by blocking the adenosine triphosphate binding site, possibly reducing inflammation.

Route	Onset	Peak	Duration
PO	Unknown	1 hr	Unknown

Half-life: 3 to 5 hours.

ADVERSE REACTIONS
CNS: dizziness, fatigue, headache. **CV:** HTN. **EENT:** nasopharyngitis, oropharyngeal pain. **GI:** abdominal discomfort, gastroenteritis, nausea, vomiting, upper abdominal pain. **GU:** UTI. **Hematologic:** *thrombocytopenia.* **Metabolic:** increased CK level. **Skin:** acne, contact dermatitis, impetigo. **Other:** flulike symptoms, infections, herpes simplex, herpes zoster.

INTERACTIONS
Drug-drug. *Antiplatelet drugs (clopidogrel, prasugrel, ticagrelor [excluding low-dose aspirin]):* May increase risk of bleeding with thrombocytopenia. Avoid use together during first 3 months of therapy.
Moderate to strong CYP2C19 and CYP2C9 inhibitors (fluconazole): May increase abrocitinib level. Avoid use with drugs that are moderate to strong inhibitors of both CYP2C19 and CYP2C9.
Other JAK inhibitors, biologic immunomodulators, immunosuppressants: May enhance

immunosuppressant effect. Avoid use together.

P-gp substrates (dabigatran, digoxin): May increase P-gp substrate level and risk of adverse reactions of substrate. Small increases may lead to serious or life-threatening toxicities. Monitor patient closely or titrate P-gp substrate dosage.

Strong CYP2C19 and CYP2C9 inducers (rifampin): May decrease abrocitinib level. Avoid use together.

Strong CYP2C19 inhibitors (fluvoxamine): May increase abrocitinib level. Reduce abrocitinib dosage.

Vaccines: May decrease therapeutic effect of inactivated vaccines and increase risk of infection from live vaccines. Give all immunizations, including herpes zoster, according to immunization guidelines before starting drug. Avoid live vaccines immediately before, during, and immediately after therapy.

Drug-lifestyle. *Smoking:* May increase risk of malignancies and CV events. Discourage smoking.

Sun exposure: May increase risk of skin cancer. Encourage limited exposure to sunlight and UV light.

EFFECTS ON LAB TEST RESULTS

• May increase LDL, total cholesterol, HDL, and CK levels.
• May decrease Hb level, ANC, and platelet and lymphocyte counts.

CONTRAINDICATIONS & CAUTIONS

Boxed Warning Drug may increase risk of serious bacterial, fungal, viral, and opportunistic infections, leading to hospitalization or death. The most frequently reported serious infections were herpes simplex, herpes zoster, and pneumonia. Avoid use in patients with active, serious infection, including localized infections. Consider risks and benefits of use in patients with chronic or recurrent infection. ■

• Don't give to patients with active TB. Consider anti-TB treatment in patients with previously untreated latent TB, patients with a history of active TB if an adequate course of treatment can't be confirmed, and patients with a negative latent TB test who have risk factors for TB infection.

Boxed Warning Patients ages 50 and older with RA and at least one CV risk factor treated with a JAK inhibitor are at increased risk for major adverse CV events, including all-cause mortality. A higher rate of major adverse CV events (CV death, MI, stroke) and thrombosis (PE, venous, arterial) have occurred with JAK inhibitors compared with TNF blockers in patients with RA. Patients who are current or past smokers are at additional risk. Discontinue drug in patients with MI, stroke, or signs or symptoms of thrombosis. Abrocitinib isn't approved for use in patients with RA. ■

Boxed Warning Lymphoma and other malignancies have been observed in patients treated with JAK inhibitors. Those receiving JAK inhibitors for RA have a higher rate of malignancies (excluding non-melanoma skin cancer) compared with TNF blockers. Patients who are current or past smokers are at increased risk. ■

Boxed Warning Serious and sometimes fatal thrombosis, including DVT, PE, and arterial thrombosis, have occurred in patients treated with JAK inhibitors. Consider risks and benefits. Use cautiously in patients at risk for thrombosis. ■

• Contraindicated in patients with active HBV or HCV infection.
• Avoid use in patients with Child-Pugh class C liver impairment.
• Use cautiously in patients with moderate kidney impairment.
• Contraindicated in patients with eGFR of 15 to 29 mL/minute or chronic kidney disease with dialysis, platelet count less than 150,000/mm^3, absolute lymphocyte count less than 500/mm^3, ANC less than 1,000/mm^3, or Hb level less than 8 g/dL.
▧ Use cautiously in older adults and patients who are CPY2C19 poor metabolizers.
• Safety and effectiveness in children younger than 12 haven't been established.
Dialyzable drug: Unknown.

PREGNANCY-LACTATION-REPRODUCTION

• Studies during pregnancy are inadequate. It isn't known whether drug increases risk of major birth defects, miscarriage, or adverse maternal or fetal outcomes.
• Enroll patient exposed to drug during pregnancy in the pregnancy exposure registry (1-877-311-3770).
• It isn't known if drug appears in human milk or how drug affects milk production or infants who are breastfed. Patient shouldn't

breastfeed during therapy and for 1 day after final dose.

• Drug may impair fertility in patients of childbearing potential.

NURSING CONSIDERATIONS

Boxed Warning Monitor patient for infection during and after therapy. Stop drug if serious or opportunistic infection occurs. Initiate diagnostic testing and appropriate antimicrobial therapy. Weigh risks and benefits of restarting therapy. ■

Boxed Warning Test patient for latent TB before and during therapy. Treat TB before therapy. Monitor for active TB during therapy, even if patient initially tested negative for latent TB. ■

• Monitor patient for herpes zoster. If reactivation occurs, consider interrupting therapy until episode resolves.

• Screen and monitor patient for HBV infection reactivation before and during therapy. Monitor patient with inactive HBV infection for expression of HBV DNA during therapy. If HBV DNA is detected, consult liver specialist.

• Perform periodic skin exams in patient who is at increased risk for skin cancer.

• Monitor patient for serious CV events. Discontinue drug if MI or stroke occurs.

• Monitor patient for signs and symptoms of PE, DVT, and arterial thrombosis (edema; pain in one leg; sudden, unexplained chest pain; dyspnea). If signs or symptoms occur, stop drug, promptly evaluate, and treat as clinically indicated.

• Monitor patient for signs and symptoms of GI perforation (fever, abdominal pain, changes in bowel habits).

• Monitor CBC at baseline, 4 weeks after starting drug, 4 weeks after dosage increase, and as indicated for patients on long-term abrocitinib therapy who develop hematologic abnormalities.

• Monitor lipid levels 4 weeks after starting drug. Manage hyperlipidemia according to clinical guidelines.

• Ensure that patient is up-to-date with all immunizations, including herpes zoster, before starting drug.

• **Look alike–sound alike:** Don't confuse abrocitinib with axitinib, afatinib, alectinib, abciximab, abemaciclib, or acalabrutinib.

PATIENT TEACHING

• Instruct patient about safe drug administration and storage.

Boxed Warning Inform patient to immediately report signs or symptoms of infection (fever, diaphoresis, chills, shortness of breath, muscle aches, fatigue, weight loss, cough, hemoptysis, burning on urination, stomach pain, diarrhea, skin sores, or red, warm, painful skin). ■

Boxed Warning Tell patient about increased risk of certain cancers, such as skin cancer, and to obtain periodic skin exams during therapy. Advise patient to limit exposure to sunlight and UV light. ■

Boxed Warning Teach about increased risk of MI, stroke, DVT, and PE. Advise patient to seek immediate medical attention if chest or limb pain, extremity edema, dyspnea, numbness, difficulty walking or speaking, sudden headache, or confusion occurs. ■

• Inform patient about immunizations required before therapy.

• Tell patient to immediately report sudden vision changes.

• Counsel patient to avoid receiving livevirus vaccines.

• Instruct patient of childbearing potential to report pregnancy or plans to become pregnant during therapy.

• Advise patient not to breastfeed during therapy and for 1 day after final dose.

• Inform patient of childbearing potential that drug may impair fertility.

acamprosate calcium
a-kam-PROE-sate

Therapeutic class: Alcohol deterrents
Pharmacologic class: Synthetic amino acid neurotransmitter analogues

AVAILABLE FORMS
Tablets (delayed-release) ⓓⓝⓒ: 333 mg

INDICATIONS & DOSAGES
➤ **Adjunct to management of alcohol abstinence**
Adults: 666 mg PO t.i.d.
Adjust-a-dose: A lower dose may be effect in some patients. In patients with CrCl of 30 to 50 mL/minute, give 333 mg t.i.d.

ADMINISTRATION
PO
• Have patient swallow tablets whole; don't crush or break tablets.
• Give drug with food, if possible.

ACTION
Restores the balance of neuronal excitation and inhibition, probably by interacting with glutamate and GABA neurotransmitter systems, thus reducing alcohol dependence.

Route	Onset	Peak	Duration
PO	Unknown	3–8 hr	Unknown

Half-life: 20 to 33 hours.

ADVERSE REACTIONS
CNS: abnormal thinking, abnormal vision, amnesia, anxiety, asthenia, depression, dizziness, headache, insomnia, migraine, pain, paresthesia, somnolence, *suicidality,* syncope, taste disturbance, tremor. **CV:** chest pain, HTN, palpitations, peripheral edema, vasodilation. **EENT:** abnormal vision, dry mouth, pharyngitis, rhinitis. **GI:** abdominal pain, anorexia, constipation, diarrhea, dyspepsia, flatulence, increased appetite, nausea, vomiting. **GU:** erectile dysfunction. **Metabolic:** weight gain. **Musculoskeletal:** arthralgia, back pain, myalgia. **Respiratory:** bronchitis, dyspnea, increased cough. **Skin:** increased sweating, pruritus, rash. **Other:** accidental injury, chills, decreased libido, flulike symptoms, infection.

INTERACTIONS
None significant.

EFFECTS ON LAB TEST RESULTS
• May increase ALT, AST, ALP, bilirubin, blood glucose, creatinine, LDH, and uric acid levels.
• May decrease sodium level.
• May decrease leukocyte count.

CONTRAINDICATIONS & CAUTIONS
• Contraindicated in patients hypersensitive to drug or its components and in those with CrCl of 30 mL/minute or less.
• Don't use in patients with a history of sulfite sensitivity.
• Use cautiously in older adults, patients with moderate kidney impairment, and patients with a history of depression and suicidal thoughts or attempts.

• Safety and effectiveness in children haven't been established.
Dialyzable drug: Unknown.
⚠ *Overdose S&S:* Diarrhea, hypercalcemia (in chronic overdose).

PREGNANCY-LACTATION-REPRODUCTION
• Use cautiously during pregnancy and only if potential benefit justifies fetal risk.
• It isn't known if drug appears in human milk. Use cautiously during breastfeeding.

NURSING CONSIDERATIONS
• Use only after patient successfully becomes abstinent from drinking.
• Note that drug doesn't eliminate or reduce withdrawal symptoms.
🔵 *Alert:* Monitor patient for development of depression or suicidality.
• Drug doesn't cause alcohol aversion or a disulfiram-like reaction if used with alcohol.

PATIENT TEACHING
• Tell patient to continue alcohol abstinence program, including counseling and support.
🔵 *Alert:* Advise patient to notify prescriber if depression, anxiety, thoughts of suicide, or severe diarrhea develops.
• Caution patient's family or caregiver to watch for signs of depression or suicidality.
• Teach about proper drug administration and handling.
• Advise patient to use effective contraception during therapy. Tell patient to report pregnancy or plans to become pregnant.
• Explain that drug may impair judgment, thinking, and motor skills. Urge patient to use caution when driving or performing hazardous activities until drug's effects are known.
• Tell patient to continue taking acamprosate and to contact prescriber if patient resumes drinking alcohol.

Reactions in bold italics are *life-threatening*.

acetaminophen (APAP, paracetamol) ✖

a-seet-a-MIN-a-fen

ACET ✤ ◇, Arthritis Pain Relief ◇, Children's Silapap ◇, FeverAll ◇, Pediatrix ✤ ◇, Rapid Action ✤ ◇, Taminol ✤, Triaminic Fever Reducer ◇, Tylenol ◇

Therapeutic class: Analgesics
Pharmacologic class: Para-aminophenol derivatives

AVAILABLE FORMS

Caplets: 500 mg ◇
Caplets (extended-release) ⓐ: 650 mg ◇
Capsules: 325 mg ◇, 500 mg ◇
Drops: 80 mg/mL ✤ ◇
Elixir: 160 mg/5 mL ✤ ◇
Gelcaps: 350 mg, 500 mg ◇
Injection: 10 mg/mL in vials, premixed containers
Oral liquid: 160 mg/5 mL ✤ ◇, 500 mg/15 mL ◇
Oral solution: 80 mg/mL ✤ ◇, 160 mg/5 mL ◇
Oral suspension: 80 mg/0.8 mL ✤ ◇, 160 mg/5 mL ✤ ◇
Oral syrup: 160 mg/5 mL ◇
Powder: 160 mg ◇, 500 mg ◇
Suppositories: 80 mg ◇, 120 mg ◇, 160 mg ✤ ◇, 325 mg ◇, 650 mg ◇
Tablets: 325 mg ◇, 500 mg ◇, 650 mg ◇
Tablets (chewable): 80 mg ◇, 160 mg ◇
Tablets (dispersible): 80 mg ◇, 160 mg ◇
Tablets (extended-release) ⓐ: 650 mg ◇

INDICATIONS & DOSAGES

Boxed Warning Maximum daily dose includes all routes of administration and all acetaminophen-containing products, including combination products. ▮

➤ **Mild pain or fever (PO)**
Adults: 325 to 650 mg PO every 4 to 6 hours PRN. Or, two extended-release caplets PO every 8 hours PRN. Maximum, 3,250 mg daily unless under health care provider supervision, when 4 g daily (immediate-release) may be used. For long-term therapy, don't exceed 2.6 g daily unless prescribed and monitored closely by health care provider.
Children older than age 12: 325 to 650 mg PO every 4 to 6 hours or 1,300 mg PO every 8 hours (extended-release) PRN. Maximum dose for immediate-release is 3,250 mg/24 hours unless under health care provider supervision, when up to 4 g/24 hours may be used. Maximum dose for extended-release is 3,900 mg/24 hours.
Children ages 6 to 11 (immediate-release): 325 mg PO every 4 to 6 hours PRN. Maximum daily dose, 1,625 mg/day PO. Don't use for more than 5 days unless directed by health care provider.
Children age 11 weighing 32.7 to 43.2 kg: 480 to 500 mg PO (oral suspension or chewable tablets) every 4 hours PRN. Maximum, five doses/day.
Children ages 9 to 10 weighing 27.3 to 32.6 kg: 325 to 400 mg PO (oral suspension or chewable tablets) every 4 hours PRN. Maximum, five doses/day.
Children ages 6 to 8 weighing 21.8 to 27.2 kg: 320 to 325 mg PO (oral suspension or chewable tablets) every 4 hours PRN. Maximum, five doses/day.
Children ages 4 to 5 weighing 16.4 to 21.7 kg: 240 mg PO (oral suspension or chewable tablets) every 4 hours PRN. Maximum, five doses/day.
Children ages 2 to 3 weighing 10.9 to 16.3 kg: 160 mg PO (oral suspension or chewable tablets) every 4 hours PRN. Maximum, five doses/day.
Children ages 1 to 2 weighing 8.2 to 10.8 kg: 120 mg PO (oral suspension or chewable tablets) every 4 hours PRN. Maximum, five doses/day.
Children ages 4 to 11 months weighing 5.4 to 8.1 kg: 80 mg PO (oral suspension, drops, or liquid) every 4 hours PRN. Maximum, five doses/day.
Children ages 0 to 3 months weighing 2.7 to 5.3 kg: 40 mg PO (oral drops) every 4 hours PRN. Maximum, five doses/day.
Adjust-a-dose: For adults with GFR of 10 to 50 mL/minute/1.73 m^2, give every 6 hours; if GFR is less than 10 mL/minute/1.73 m^2, give every 8 hours. For patients receiving CKRT, give every 6 hours. For infants, children, and adolescents with GFR less than 10 mL/minute/1.73 m^2, give every 8 hours. For infants, children, and adolescents receiving hemodialysis or peritoneal dialysis, give every 8 hours.

➤ **Mild pain or fever (Rectal)**
Adults and children ages 12 and older: 325 to 650 mg PR every 4 to 6 hours PRN. Maximum, 3.9 g daily. For long-term therapy, don't exceed 2.6 g daily unless prescribed and monitored closely by health care provider.
Children ages 6 to 11: 325 mg PR every 4 to 6 hours PRN. Maximum, 1,625 mg in 24 hours.
Children ages 3 to 6: 120 mg PR every 4 to 6 hours PRN. Maximum, 600 mg in 24 hours.
Children ages 1 to 3: 80 mg PR every 4 to 6 hours PRN. Maximum, 400 mg in 24 hours.
Children ages 6 to 11 months: 80 mg PR every 6 hours PRN. Maximum, 320 mg in 24 hours.

➤ **Mild to moderate pain; mild to moderate pain with adjunctive opioid analgesics; fever**
Adults and children ages 13 and older weighing 50 kg or more: 1,000 mg IV every 6 hours or 650 mg IV every 4 hours PRN. Maximum, 1,000 mg as a single dose and 4,000 mg/day.
Adults and children ages 13 and older weighing less than 50 kg: 15 mg/kg IV every 6 hours or 12.5 mg/kg IV every 4 hours PRN. Maximum dose, 15 mg/kg (up to 750 mg) as a single dose and 75 mg/kg (up to 3,750 mg)/day.
Children ages 2 to 12: 15 mg/kg IV every 6 hours or 12.5 mg/kg IV every 4 hours PRN. Maximum dose, 15 mg/kg (up to 750 mg) as a single dose and 75 mg/kg (up to 3,750 mg)/day.
Infants ages 29 days to 2 years for fever: 15 mg/kg IV every 6 hours PRN. Maximum dose, 60 mg/kg/day, with minimum dosing interval of 6 hours.
Neonates (32 weeks' gestational age and greater) to age 28 days for fever: 12.5 mg/kg IV every 6 hours PRN. Maximum dose, 50 mg/kg/day, with minimum dosing interval of 6 hours.
Adjust-a-dose: Longer dosing intervals and a reduced total daily dose may be warranted in patients with CrCl of 30 mL/minute or less.

ADMINISTRATION
PO
• Use liquid form for children and patients who have difficulty swallowing.
• Give drug without regard for food.
• Patient should allow dispersible tablet or powder to dissolve in the mouth.
• Shake liquid formulations well before using.

• Give extended-release forms whole; don't crush, dissolve, or allow patient to chew extended-release forms.
IV
▼ Examine solution for injection; don't use if particulate matter or discoloration is observed.
▼ For 1,000-mg dose, give by inserting a vented IV set through the septum of a 100-mL vial.
▼ For doses less than 1,000 mg, withdraw appropriate dose and place into a separate container before administration.
▼ Place small-volume pediatric doses of up to 60 mL in a syringe and use a syringe-pump.
▼ May administer without further dilution.
▼ Don't add other medications to IV solution.
▼ Give over 15 minutes.
▼ Don't use entire 100-mL vial in patients weighing less than 50 kg.
▼ Monitor end of infusion to prevent possibility of air embolism.
▼ Use within 6 hours of penetrating vial seal.
▼ Vials and IV containers are for single use only. Discard unused portion.
▼ **Incompatibilities:** Diazepam, chlorpromazine hydrochloride. Don't admix with other drugs.
Rectal
• If suppository is too soft, refrigerate for 15 minutes or run under cold water in wrapper.

ACTION
Thought to produce analgesia by inhibiting prostaglandin and other substances that sensitize pain receptors. Drug may relieve fever through central action in the hypothalamic heat-regulating center.

Route	Onset	Peak	Duration
PO	<1 hr	30–60 min	4–6 hr
IV	5–30 min	15 min	4–6 hr
PR	Unknown	1.5–5 hr	Unknown

Half-life: PO, 2 to 3 hours; IV, 2.4 hours (adults), 3 hours (children and adolescents), 4.2 hours (infants), 7 hours (neonates); PR, 2 to 3 hours.

ADVERSE REACTIONS
CNS: agitation (IV), anxiety, fatigue, headache, insomnia, fever. **CV:** HTN, hypotension, peripheral edema, periorbital edema, tachycardia (IV). **GI:** nausea,

Reactions in bold italics are ***life-threatening***.

vomiting, abdominal pain, diarrhea, constipation (IV). **GU:** oliguria (IV). **Hematologic:** anemia, hemolytic anemia, *leukopenia, neutropenia, pancytopenia, anemia.* **Hepatic:** jaundice. **Metabolic:** hypoalbuminemia (IV), *hypoglycemia, hypokalemia,* hypervolemia, *hypomagnesemia,* hypophosphatemia (IV). **Musculoskeletal:** muscle spasms, extremity pain (IV). **Respiratory:** abnormal breath sounds, dyspnea, *hypoxia,* atelectasis, pleural effusion, *pulmonary edema, stridor,* wheezing (IV). **Skin:** rash, urticaria; infusion-site pain (IV), pruritus.

INTERACTIONS
Drug-drug. *Barbiturates, carbamazepine, hydantoins, rifampin:* High doses or long-term use of these drugs may reduce therapeutic effects and enhance liver toxic effects of acetaminophen. Avoid use together.
Busulfan: May increase busulfan level. Monitor patient closely.
Cholestyramine resin: May decrease acetaminophen absorption. Give at least 1 hour after acetaminophen or consider therapy change.
Dasatinib: May enhance liver toxic effects of dasatinib and increase acetaminophen level. Avoid use together.
Imatinib: May increase liver toxic effects of these drugs. Monitor patient closely.
Isoniazid: May increase risk of acetaminophen adverse effects. Monitor patient closely.
Lamotrigine: Prolonged acetaminophen use may decrease lamotrigine level. Monitor patient for therapeutic effects; adjust lamotrigine dosage as needed.
Lomitapide: May increase risk of liver toxicity. Limit maximum adult dose of acetaminophen to 4 g or less daily for 3 or fewer days per week or consider therapy change.
Metyrapone, probenecid: May increase acetaminophen level and risk of liver toxicity. Avoid use together.
Warfarin: May increase anticoagulant effects with long-term use with high doses of acetaminophen. Monitor INR closely.
Drug-lifestyle. *Alcohol use:* May increase risk of liver damage. Discourage use together.

EFFECTS ON LAB TEST RESULTS
• May increase AST level. May decrease glucose, potassium, phosphorus, magnesium, albumin, and Hb levels and hematocrit.

• May decrease neutrophil, WBC, RBC, and platelet counts.
• May cause false-positive test result for urinary 5-hydroxyindoleacetic acid. May falsely decrease glucose level in home monitoring systems.

CONTRAINDICATIONS & CAUTIONS
Boxed Warning Drug can cause acute liver failure, which may require a liver transplant or cause death. Most cases of liver injury are associated with drug doses exceeding 4,000 mg/day and often involve more than one acetaminophen-containing product. ■
🕖 *Alert:* May cause serious, potentially fatal skin reactions (SJS, TEN, acute generalized exanthematous pustulosis.) Reaction may occur with first or subsequent use when acetaminophen is used as monotherapy or when it's one component of combination drug therapy. Monitor for reddening of skin, rash, blisters, and detachment of the upper surface of skin. Stop drug immediately if skin reaction is suspected.
• Contraindicated in patients hypersensitive to drug. IV form is contraindicated in patients with Child-Pugh class C liver impairment.
• Use cautiously in patients with any type of liver disease, chronic malnutrition, severe hypovolemia, or CrCl of 30 mL/minute or less.
⚛ Use cautiously in patients with G6PD deficiency.
• Use cautiously in patients with long-term alcohol use because therapeutic doses cause liver toxicity in these patients. Patients with chronic alcoholism shouldn't take more than 2 g of acetaminophen every 24 hours.
Dialyzable drug: Unknown.
⚠ *Overdose S&S:* Stage 1 (up to 24 hours): abdominal pain, diaphoresis, nausea, vomiting, malaise, pallor; stage 2 (24 to 36 hours): right upper quadrant pain, elevated LFT results, prolonged PT; stage 3 (72 to 96 hours): liver failure, encephalopathy, coma.

PREGNANCY-LACTATION-REPRODUCTION
• Use cautiously during pregnancy as directed by health care provider.
• There are no studies of IV acetaminophen use during pregnancy; use only if clearly needed.
• Drug appears in human milk. Use cautiously during breastfeeding.

• Drug may decrease fertility based on animal studies. Reversibility of the effects are unknown.

NURSING CONSIDERATIONS

Boxed Warning Many OTC and prescription products contain acetaminophen; be aware of this fact when calculating total daily dose. ■

Boxed Warning Use caution when prescribing, preparing, and administering IV acetaminophen to avoid dosing errors leading to accidental overdose and death. Don't confuse dose in milliGRAMS and dose in milliLITERS. Be sure to base dose on weight for patients weighing less than 50 kg, to properly program infusion pump, and to ensure that total daily dose of acetaminophen from all sources doesn't exceed maximum daily limit. ■

• Consider reducing total daily dose and increasing dosing intervals in patients with liver or kidney impairment.

PATIENT TEACHING

• Tell parents and caregivers to consult prescriber before giving drug to children younger than age 2.

• Advise parents and caregivers that drug is only for short-term use; urge them to consult prescriber if giving to infants for longer than 3 days, children for longer than 5 days, or adults for longer than 10 days.

Boxed Warning Caution patient or caregiver that many OTC products contain acetaminophen and should be counted when calculating total daily dose. ■

• Tell patient to consult prescriber for fever lasting longer than 3 days or recurrent fever.

❸ *Alert:* Warn patient that high doses or unsupervised long-term use can cause liver damage. Excessive alcohol use may increase the risk of liver damage. Caution patient with long-term alcoholism to limit drug to 2 g/day or less.

• Caution patient to contact health care provider if signs and symptoms of liver damage (illogical thinking, severe dyspepsia, jaundice, inability to eat, weakness) occur.

❸ *Alert:* Warn patient to stop drug and seek medical attention immediately if rash or other reactions occurs while using acetaminophen.

• Advise patient who is pregnant to discuss taking acetaminophen with health care provider before use.

• Tell patient who is breastfeeding that drug appears in human milk in low levels. Drug may be used safely for short-term therapy if recommended doses aren't exceeded.

acetaZOLAMIDE
a-set-a-ZOLE-a-mide

acetaZOLAMIDE sodium

Therapeutic class: Diuretics
Pharmacologic class: Carbonic anhydrase inhibitors

AVAILABLE FORMS

acetazolamide
Capsules (extended-release) ⒹⒷ: 500 mg
Tablets: 125 mg, 250 mg
acetazolamide sodium
Powder for injection: 500-mg vial

INDICATIONS & DOSAGES

➤ **Secondary glaucoma; preoperative treatment of acute angle-closure glaucoma**
Adults: 250 mg PO every 4 hours or 250 mg PO b.i.d. for short-term therapy. In acute cases, 500 mg PO; then 125 to 250 mg PO every 4 hours. Or, for extended-release capsules, 500 mg PO b.i.d. To rapidly lower IOP, initially, 500 mg IV; may repeat in 2 to 4 hours, if needed, followed by 125 to 250 mg PO or IV every 4 hours.

➤ **Chronic open-angle glaucoma**
Adults: 250 mg to 1 g PO daily in divided doses q.i.d., or 250 mg IV every 4 hours, or 500 mg extended-release PO b.i.d.

➤ **To prevent or treat acute mountain sickness (high-altitude sickness)**
Adults and children ages 12 and older: 500 mg to 1 g PO daily in divided doses every 12 hours. Start 24 to 48 hours before ascent and continue for 48 hours while at high altitude. When rapid ascent is required, start with 1,000 mg PO daily.

➤ **Adjunct for epilepsy and myoclonic, refractory, generalized tonic-clonic, absence, or mixed seizures**
Adults: 8 to 30 mg/kg PO (immediate-release only) or IV daily in divided doses; optimum range is 375 mg to 1 g daily. If given with other anticonvulsants, start at 250 mg PO or IV once daily and increase to 375 mg to 1 g daily.

➤ **Edema caused by HF; drug-induced edema**
Adults: 250 to 375 mg (5 mg/kg; immediate-release only) PO daily in the morning. For best results, use every other day or 2 days on followed by 1 to 2 days off. Or, 250 to 375 mg IV once daily for 1 or 2 days, alternating with a day of rest.

ADMINISTRATION
PO
• Give oral drug with food to minimize GI upset.
• Don't crush or open extended-release capsules.
• If patient can't swallow oral form, pharmacist may make a suspension using crushed tablets.
• Refrigeration of suspension improves palatability but doesn't improve stability.
IV
▼ Reconstitute drug in 500-mg vial with at least 5 mL of sterile water for injection. Store reconstituted solution for 3 days under refrigeration or 12 hours at room temperature.
▼ Direct IV injection is the preferred route. Administer in divided doses for amounts more than 250 mg.
▼ IM administration isn't recommended.
▼ Store vials at room temperature.
▼ **Incompatibilities:** Multivitamins.

ACTION
Promotes kidney excretion of sodium, potassium, bicarbonate, and water. As anticonvulsant, drug normalizes neuronal discharge. In mountain sickness, drug stimulates ventilation and increases cerebral blood flow. In glaucoma, drug reduces IOP.

Route	Onset	Peak	Duration
PO	60–90 min	1–4 hr	8–12 hr
PO (extended-release)	2 hr	3–6 hr	18–24 hr
IV	2–10 min	15 min	4–5 hr

Half-life: 2.4 to 5.8 hours.

ADVERSE REACTIONS
CNS: *seizures,* drowsiness, paresthesia, confusion, depression, ataxia, headache, malaise, fever, fatigue, excitement, dizziness, flaccid paralysis, taste alteration. **CV:** flushing. **EENT:** transient myopia, hearing dysfunction, tinnitus. **GI:** nausea, vomiting, anorexia,

diarrhea, melena. **GU:** polyuria, hematuria, crystalluria, glycosuria, kidney stones. **Hematologic:** *aplastic anemia, leukopenia, thrombocytopenia purpura,* hemolytic anemia, *agranulocytosis, pancytopenia.* **Hepatic:** abnormal liver function, cholestatic jaundice, liver insufficiency, *fulminant liver necrosis.* **Metabolic:** *hypokalemia,* hyponatremia, *hypoglycemia,* hyperglycemia, asymptomatic hyperuricemia, hyperchloremic acidosis. **Skin:** pain at injection site, photosensitivity, rash, urticaria. **Other:** growth retardation in children, *anaphylaxis.*

INTERACTIONS
Drug-drug. *Alpha blockers, beta blockers, antihypertensives:* May increase hypotensive effect. Monitor patient carefully.
Amphetamines, quinidine: May decrease kidney clearance of these drugs, increasing toxicity. Monitor patient for toxicity.
Carbamazepine: May increase carbamazepine level. Monitor patient for toxicity.
Carbonic anhydrase inhibitors (brinzolamide, dorzolamide, methazolamide): May have additive toxic effects. Avoid use together.
Cyclosporine: May increase cyclosporine level, causing kidney toxicity and neurotoxicity. Monitor patient for toxicity.
Flecainide: May increase flecainide concentration. Monitor patient for toxicity and cardiac rhythm disturbances.
Folic acid antagonists: May increase adverse effects of folic acid antagonists. Use together cautiously.
Lithium: May increase lithium excretion, decreasing its effect. Monitor lithium level.
Methenamine: May reduce methenamine effect. Avoid use together.
Phenytoin: May increase phenytoin level and risk of osteomalacia. Use together cautiously.
Primidone: May decrease serum and urine primidone levels and decrease anticonvulsant effect. Monitor patient closely.
🜊 *Alert:* *Salicylates (aspirin):* May cause accumulation and toxicity of acetazolamide, resulting in CNS depression, metabolic acidosis, anorexia, and death. Administer with caution; monitor patient for toxicity.
Sodium bicarbonate: May increase risk of kidney stones. Monitor patient closely.
Drug-lifestyle. *Sun exposure:* May increase risk of photosensitivity reactions. Advise patient to avoid excessive sunlight exposure.

🍁 Canada   ◇ OTC   ◆ Off-label use   ⊕ Do not crush   *Liquid contains alcohol   🧬 Genetic

EFFECTS ON LAB TEST RESULTS
• May increase uric acid level. May decrease potassium, sodium, and Hb levels and hematocrit.
• May increase or decrease glucose level.
• May decrease WBC and platelet counts.
• May interfere with the HPLC method of assay for theophylline.
• May give false negative or decrease urinary phenolsulfonphthalein and phenol red elimination values for urinary protein, serum nonprotein, and serum uric acid.

CONTRAINDICATIONS & CAUTIONS
• **Alert:** Cross-sensitivity between sulfonamides and sulfonamide-derivative diuretics such as acetazolamide has been reported.
• **Alert:** Fatalities have occurred due to severe reactions to sulfonamides, including SJS, TEN, fulminant liver necrosis, aplastic anemia, agranulocytosis, and other blood dyscrasias. Sensitizations may recur when a sulfonamide is readministered, irrespective of the route of administration. If signs and symptoms of hypersensitivity or other serious reactions occur, discontinue drug.
• Contraindicated in patients hypersensitive to drug or any of its components and in those with hyponatremia or hypokalemia, marked kidney or liver disease or dysfunction, suprakidney gland failure, hyperchloremic acidosis, or cirrhosis.
• Contraindicated in patients receiving long-term treatment for chronic noncongestive angle-closure glaucoma.
• Use cautiously in patients receiving other diuretics and in those with diabetes, kidney impairment, respiratory acidosis, emphysema, or COPD.
Dialyzable drug: Unknown.
⚠ Overdose S&S: Electrolyte imbalances, acidotic state, CNS effects.

PREGNANCY-LACTATION-REPRODUCTION
• There are no well-controlled studies during pregnancy; use only if potential benefit justifies fetal risk.
• Enroll patients who are pregnant and taking acetazolamide for seizure disorders in the AED Pregnancy Registry (1-888-233-2334).
• Drug appears in human milk. Patient should discontinue breastfeeding or discontinue drug, considering importance of drug to patient. Use during breastfeeding only when benefit to patient justifies risk to infant.

NURSING CONSIDERATIONS
• Monitor fluid intake and output and glucose and electrolyte levels, especially potassium, bicarbonate, and chloride. When drug is used as diuretic therapy, consult prescriber and dietitian about providing a high-potassium diet.
• Monitor an older adult closely due to susceptibility to excessive diuresis.
• Weigh patient daily. Rapid or excessive fluid loss may cause weight loss and hypotension.
• Be aware that diuretic effect decreases when acidosis occurs but can be reestablished by using intermittent administration schedules.
• Monitor patient for signs of hemolytic anemia (pallor, weakness, palpitations).
• Monitor blood glucose level in patients with diabetes or impaired glucose tolerance.
• Monitor patient for hypersensitivity reactions, including SCARs.
• Monitor growth in children.
• **Look alike–sound alike:** Don't confuse acetazolamide with acetaminophen or acyclovir.

PATIENT TEACHING
• Teach about proper drug administration and handling.
• Caution patient not to perform hazardous activities if adverse CNS reactions occur.
• Instruct patient to avoid prolonged exposure to sunlight because drug may cause phototoxicity.
• Instruct patient to notify prescriber of unusual bleeding, bruising, tingling, tremors, rash, fever, kidney stones, or loss of appetite.

acetylcysteine
a-se-teel-SIS-tay-een

Acetadote

Therapeutic class: Mucolytics
Pharmacologic class: L-cysteine derivatives

AVAILABLE FORMS
Inhalation solution: 10%, 20%
IV injection: 200 mg/mL

INDICATIONS & DOSAGES
➤ **Adjunctive therapy for abnormal viscid or thickened mucous secretions in patients with pneumonia, bronchitis, bronchiectasis, primary amyloidosis of the lung, TB, cystic fibrosis, emphysema, atelectasis,**

pulmonary complications of thoracic surgery, or CV surgery
Adults and children: 1 to 2 mL 10% or 20% solution by direct instillation into trachea as often as every hour. Or, 1 to 10 mL of 20% solution or 2 to 20 mL of 10% solution by nebulization every 2 to 6 hours PRN.

➤ **Diagnostic bronchial studies**
Adults and children: Two or three administrations of 1 to 2 mL of 20% solution or 2 to 4 mL of 10% solution by nebulization or intratracheal instillation before procedure.

➤ **Routine tracheostomy care**
Adults and children: 1 to 2 mL of 10% or 20% solution by direct instillation into tracheostomy every 1 to 4 hours.

➤ **Acetaminophen toxicity**
Adults and children: Initially, 140 mg/kg inhalation solution given PO as soon as possible within 24 hours of ingestion; then 70 mg/kg PO 4 hours after initial dose; then every 4 hours for 17 doses (total).
Adults and children weighing 41 to 100 kg or more: 150 mg/kg in 200 mL of diluent IV over 1 hour; then 50 mg/kg in 500 mL of diluent IV over 4 hours; then 100 mg/kg in 1,000 mL of diluent IV over 16 hours.
Adults and children weighing 21 to 40 kg: 150 mg/kg in 100 mL of diluent IV over 1 hour; then 50 mg/kg in 250 mL of diluent IV over 4 hours; then 100 mg/kg in 500 mL diluent IV over 16 hours.
Adults and children weighing 5 to 20 kg: 150 mg/kg in 3 mL/kg diluent IV over 1 hour; then 50 mg/kg in 7 mL/kg diluent IV over 4 hours; then 100 mg/kg in 14 mL/kg diluent IV over 16 hours.
Adjust-a-dose: Refer to manufacturer's instruction for dosing in patients weighing less than 40 kg and requiring fluid restriction.

ADMINISTRATION
PO (inhalation formulation)
• Administer via oral route. Dilute oral dose (used for acetaminophen overdose) with diet cola or other diet soft drink or water. Dilute 20% solution to 5% (add 3 mL of diluent to each milliliter of drug). If patient vomits within 1 hour of receiving loading or maintenance dose, repeat dose. Use diluted solution within 1 hour.
• Drug smells strongly of sulfur. Mixing oral form with juice or cola improves taste.
• Drug delivered through NG tube may be diluted with water.

• Store opened, undiluted oral solution in refrigerator for up to 96 hours.

IV
▼ Drug may turn from colorless liquid to slight pink or purple color once stopper is punctured. Color change doesn't affect drug.
▼ Drug is hyperosmolar and is compatible with D₅W, half-NSS, and sterile water for injection.
▼ Refer to manufacturer's instructions for additional dosage and dilution information.
▼ Reconstituted solution is stable for 24 hours at room temperature.
▼ Vials contain no preservatives; discard after opening.
▼ **Incompatibilities:** None listed by manufacturer. Consult drug compatibility reference for more information.

Inhalational
• Use plastic, glass, stainless steel, or another nonreactive metal when giving by nebulization. Hand-bulb nebulizers aren't recommended because output is too small and particle size too large.
• 20% solution may be diluted with NSS, NSS for inhalation, or sterile water for injection or inhalation. 10% solution may be used undiluted.
• If only a portion of the solution in a vial is used for inhalation, store remainder in refrigerator and use within 96 hours.
• **Incompatibilities:** Physically or chemically incompatible with inhaled tetracyclines, erythromycin lactobionate, amphotericin B, and ampicillin sodium. If given by aerosol inhalation, nebulize these drugs separately. Iodized oil, trypsin, and hydrogen peroxide are physically incompatible with acetylcysteine; don't add to nebulizer.

ACTION
Reduces the viscosity of pulmonary secretions by splitting disulfide linkages between mucoprotein molecular complexes. Also restores liver stores of glutathione to treat acetaminophen toxicity.

Route	Onset	Peak	Duration
Inhalation	5–10 min	1–2 hr	1 hr
IV	Unknown	0.5–1 hr	Unknown

Half-life: Inhalation, 5.6 hours; IV, 5.6 hours.

ADVERSE REACTIONS

CNS: fever, drowsiness. **CV:** chest tightness, flushing, tachycardia, edema. **EENT:** rhinorrhea, pharyngitis, throat tightness. **GI:** nausea, stomatitis, vomiting. **Respiratory:** *bronchospasm,* cough, dyspnea, rhonchi. **Skin:** clamminess, pruritus, rash, urticaria. **Other:** *anaphylactoid reaction,* chills, hypersensitivity reaction.

INTERACTIONS

Drug-drug. *Activated charcoal:* May limit acetylcysteine's effectiveness. Avoid using activated charcoal before or with oral acetylcysteine.

EFFECTS ON LAB TEST RESULTS

None reported.

CONTRAINDICATIONS & CAUTIONS

• Contraindicated in patients hypersensitive to drug.
• *Alert:* Serious anaphylactoid reactions (rash, hypotension, dyspnea, wheezing) have been reported. Reactions usually occur 30 to 60 minutes after start of infusion and may require treatment and drug discontinuation.
• Use cautiously in older adults and patients with debilitation and severe respiratory insufficiency.
• Use IV form cautiously in patients with asthma, history of bronchospasm, weight less than 40 kg, or need for fluid restriction.
Dialyzable drug: Yes.

PREGNANCY-LACTATION-REPRODUCTION

• There are no adequate and well-controlled studies during pregnancy; use cautiously during pregnancy and only if clearly indicated.
• It isn't known if drug appears in human milk. Use cautiously during breastfeeding.

NURSING CONSIDERATIONS

• Monitor cough type and frequency.
• *Alert:* Monitor patient for bronchospasm, especially if patient has asthma.
• Ingestion of more than 150 mg/kg of acetaminophen may cause liver toxicity. Measure acetaminophen level 4 hours after ingestion to determine risk of liver toxicity. See manufacturer's information for nomogram for estimating potential for liver toxicity from acute acetaminophen ingestion and need for acetylcysteine therapy.

• *Alert:* Use drug for acetaminophen overdose within 24 hours of ingestion. Start drug immediately; don't wait for results of acetaminophen level. Give within 8 hours of acetaminophen ingestion for maximal protection against liver injury.
• For suspected acetaminophen overdose, obtain baseline INR and AST, ALT, bilirubin, BUN, creatinine, glucose, and electrolyte levels.
• In acetaminophen overdose, check acetaminophen, ALT, and AST levels and INR after the last maintenance dose. If acetaminophen level is still detectable, or if ALT/AST level is still increasing or INR remains elevated, continue maintenance doses and the prescriber should contact a regional poison control center (1-800-222-1222) or a special health professional assistance line (1-800-525-6115) for assistance with dosing recommendations.
• Half-life elimination increases by 80% in patients with severe liver damage.
• *Alert:* Monitor patient receiving IV form for anaphylactoid reactions. Reactions involving more than simple skin flushing or erythema should be treated as anaphylactoid reactions. If an anaphylactoid reaction occurs, stop infusion and treat reaction with antihistamines and epinephrine, if needed. Once anaphylaxis treatment starts, carefully restart infusion. If anaphylactoid symptoms return, stop drug.
• Flushing and skin erythema may occur within 30 to 60 minutes of starting IV infusion and usually resolve without stopping infusion.
• When acetaminophen level is below toxic level according to nomogram, stop therapy.
• Note that the vial stopper doesn't contain natural rubber latex, dry natural rubber, or blends of natural rubber.
• *Look alike–sound alike:* Don't confuse acetylcysteine with acetylcholine or acetazolamide.

PATIENT TEACHING

• Warn patient that drug may have a foul taste or smell that may be distressing.
• For maximum effect, instruct patient to cough to clear the airway before aerosol administration.

acyclovir
ay-SYE-kloe-ver

Sitavig, Zovirax

acyclovir sodium

Therapeutic class: Antivirals
Pharmacologic class: Nucleosides and
nucleotides

AVAILABLE FORMS
Capsules: 200 mg
Cream: 5%
Ointment: 5%
Solution (IV): 50 mg/mL
Suspension: 200 mg/5 mL
Tablets: 400 mg, 800 mg
Tablets (buccal) ⚫: 50 mg

INDICATIONS & DOSAGES
Adjust-a-dose (for all indications): For patients receiving IV form: If CrCl is 25 to 50 mL/minute/1.73 m^2, give 100% of dose every 12 hours. If CrCl is 10 to 25 mL/minute/1.73 m^2, give 100% of dose every 24 hours. If CrCl is less than 10 mL/minute/1.73 m^2, give 50% of dose every 24 hours.

Adjust-a-dose (for all PO indications): For patients receiving PO form: If normal dose is 200 mg every 4 hours five times daily and CrCl is 10 mL/minute/1.73 m^2 or less, give 200 mg PO every 12 hours. If normal dose is 400 mg every 12 hours and CrCl is 10 mL/minute/1.73 m^2 or less, give 200 mg every 12 hours. If normal dose is 800 mg every 4 hours five times daily and CrCl is 10 to 25 mL/minute/1.73 m^2, give 800 mg every 8 hours; if CrCl is less than 10 mL/minute/1.73 m^2 or less, give 800 mg every 12 hours.

For patients who require hemodialysis, give additional dose after each dialysis.

➤ **First and recurrent episodes of mucocutaneous HSV (HSV-1 and HSV-2) infections in patients who are immunocompromised**
Adults and children ages 12 and older: 5 mg/kg IV over 1 hour every 8 hours for 7 days.
Children ages 3 months to younger than 12 years: 10 mg/kg IV over 1 hour every 8 hours for 7 days.

➤ **Severe first episodes of genital herpes in patients who aren't immunocompromised**
Adults and children ages 12 and older: 5 mg/kg IV over 1 hour every 8 hours for 5 days.

➤ **First genital herpes episode**
Adults: 200 mg PO every 4 hours while awake, five times daily. Continue for 7 to 10 days.

➤ **Initial genital herpes; limited, non-life-threatening mucocutaneous HSV infections in patients who are immunocompromised**
Adults and children ages 12 and older: Adequately cover all lesions every 3 hours six times daily for 7 days with ointment. Although dosage varies depending on total lesion area, use about ½-inch (1.3-cm) ribbon of ointment on each 4-inch (10-cm) square of surface area.

➤ **Intermittent therapy for recurrent genital herpes**
Adults: 200 mg PO every 4 hours while awake, five times daily. Continue for 5 days. Begin therapy at first sign of recurrence.

➤ **Long-term suppressive therapy for recurrent genital herpes**
Adults: 400 mg PO b.i.d. for up to 12 months. Or, 200 mg PO t.i.d. to five times daily for up to 12 months.

➤ **Varicella zoster infections in patients who are immunocompromised**
Adults and children ages 12 and older: 10 mg/kg IV over 1 hour every 8 hours for 7 days. Use ideal body weight for patients with obesity. Don't exceed maximum dosage equivalent of 20 mg/kg every 8 hours.
Children younger than age 12: 20 mg/kg IV over 1 hour every 8 hours for 7 days.

➤ **Varicella (chickenpox) infection in patients who are immunocompetent**
Adults and children weighing more than 40 kg: 800 mg PO q.i.d. for 5 days.
Children ages 2 and older weighing 40 kg or less: 20 mg/kg (maximum, 80 mg/kg/day) PO q.i.d. for 5 days. Start therapy as soon as symptoms appear.

➤ **Acute herpes zoster infection in patients who are immunocompetent**
Adults and children ages 12 and older: 800 mg PO every 4 hours five times daily for 7 to 10 days.

➤ **Herpes simplex encephalitis**
Adults and children ages 12 and older: 10 mg/kg IV over 1 hour every 8 hours for 10 days.

Children ages 3 months to younger than 12 years: 20 mg/kg IV over 1 hour every 8 hours for 10 days.

➤ **Neonatal HSV infections**

Neonates with postmenstrual age of at least 34 weeks: 20 mg/kg IV over 1 hour every 8 hours for 21 days.

Neonates with postmenstrual age of less than 34 weeks: 20 mg/kg IV over 1 hour every 12 hours for 21 days.

➤ **Recurrent herpes labialis in patients who are immunocompetent**

Adults and children ages 12 and older: Apply cream five times daily for 4 days. Start therapy as early as possible after signs and symptoms occur.

Adults: Apply 50-mg buccal tablet as a single dose to upper gum region, on the same side as symptoms, within 1 hour after onset of prodromal symptoms and before appearance of signs of cold sore.

ADMINISTRATION
PO
• Give drug without regard for meals, but give with food if stomach irritation occurs.
Buccal
• Patients shouldn't chew, suck, crush, or swallow tablets.
• Apply with dry finger immediately after taking tablet out of blister pack.
• Place tablet just above incisor tooth on upper gum on same side of mouth as prodromal symptoms appeared.
• Hold tablet in place with slight pressure over upper lip for 30 seconds to ensure adhesion. Place rounded side to gum for comfort, but either side can be applied.
• Tablet stays in place and dissolves gradually.
• Food and drink can be taken normally with tablet in place.
• Patients should avoid chewing gum, touching or pressing tablet, wearing upper denture, brushing teeth, and other activity that may interfere with adhesion.
• Patients should drink plenty of liquids in case of dry mouth.
• If buccal tablet doesn't adhere or falls off within first 6 hours, immediately reposition the same tablet. If tablet doesn't adhere, place a new tablet.
• If patient swallows buccal tablet within first 6 hours, have patient drink a glass of water; then apply a new tablet.

• If buccal tablet falls out or patient swallows it after first 6 hours, don't reapply.
IV
▼ Inspect solution for particulate matter and discoloration before administration.
▼ Once diluted, use each dose within 24 hours.
▼ Solutions concentrated at 7 mg/mL or more may cause a higher risk of phlebitis.
▼ Encourage fluid intake because patient must be adequately hydrated during infusion.
▼ Bolus injection, dehydration (decreased urine output), kidney disease, and use with other kidney-toxic drugs increase the risk of kidney toxicity. Don't give by bolus injection.
▼ Give IV infusion over at least 1 hour to prevent kidney tubular damage.
▼ Monitor intake and output, especially during the first 2 hours after administration.
🔆 *Alert:* Don't give IM or subcut.
▼ Store at room temperature. Precipitate may form if solution is refrigerated.
▼ **Incompatibilities:** None listed by manufacturer. Consult drug compatibility reference for more information.
Topical
• Apply with finger cot or rubber glove to prevent autoinoculation of other body sites and transmission of infection to others.
• Apply as early as possible after onset of prodromal symptoms or lesion appearance.
• Topical form is for cutaneous use only; don't apply to eyes.

ACTION
Interferes with DNA synthesis and inhibits viral multiplication.

Route	Onset	Peak	Duration
PO	Unknown	2.5 hr	Unknown
Buccal	Unknown	7 hr (in saliva)	Unknown
IV	Immediate	Immediate	Unknown
Topical	Unknown	Unknown	Unknown

Half-life: 2 to 3.5 hours with normal kidney function; up to 19 hours with kidney impairment.

ADVERSE REACTIONS
CNS: headache, malaise, *encephalopathic changes (including lethargy, obtundation, tremor, confusion, hallucinations, agitation, seizures, coma).* **EENT:** gum pain, canker sores (buccal tablets). **GI:** nausea, vomiting,

diarrhea. **GU:** *acute kidney injury,* hematuria. **Hematologic:** *leukopenia, neutropenia, thrombocytopenia,* thrombocytosis, anemia. **Hepatic:** bilirubinemia, increased transaminases. **Skin:** inflammation or phlebitis at injection site, rash, urticaria, eczema, dryness, pruritus, contact dermatitis, application-site reaction; mild pain, burning, or stinging (topical or buccal form). **Other:** hypersensitivity reaction.

INTERACTIONS
Drug-drug. *Foscarnet:* May enhance kidney toxicity. Don't use together.
Probenecid: May increase acyclovir level. Monitor patient for possible toxicity.
Varicella vaccine: May diminish therapeutic effect of vaccine. Avoid use of acyclovir within 24 hours before vaccine administration and for 14 days after.
Zidovudine: May increase risk of CNS depression. Use together cautiously.

EFFECTS ON LAB TEST RESULTS
• May increase bilirubin, BUN, and creatinine levels.
• May increase Hb level.
• May decrease ANC and WBC count.
• May increase or decrease platelet count.

CONTRAINDICATIONS & CAUTIONS
• Contraindicated in patients hypersensitive to drug or valacyclovir.
• Use cautiously in patients with neurologic problems, kidney disease, liver disease, electrolyte abnormalities, significant hypoxia, or dehydration and in those receiving other kidney-toxic drugs.
• Drug increases risk of thrombotic thrombocytopenic purpura and hemolytic-uremic syndrome in patients who are immunocompromised, which can be fatal.
Dialyzable drug: Yes.
⚠ **Overdose S&S:** Agitation, coma, seizures, lethargy, elevated BUN and creatinine levels, kidney failure.

PREGNANCY-LACTATION-REPRODUCTION
• Use cautiously during pregnancy and only if potential benefit outweighs fetal risk.
• Drug appears in human milk. Use cautiously during breastfeeding and only when clearly indicated. Patients with active herpetic lesions on or near breasts should avoid breastfeeding.

NURSING CONSIDERATIONS
• Start therapy as early as possible after signs or symptoms occur.
• Note that drug isn't a cure for herpes, but it helps improve signs and symptoms.
❸ *Alert:* Long-term acyclovir use may result in kidney toxicity. In patients with kidney disease or dehydration and in those taking other kidney-toxic drugs, monitor kidney function.
❸ *Alert:* If signs and symptoms of extravasation occur, immediately stop IV infusion and notify prescriber. Hyaluronidase may need to be injected subcut at extravasation site as an antidote.
• Encephalopathic changes are more likely to occur in patients with neurologic disorders and in those who have had neurologic reactions to cytotoxic drugs.
• Monitor patient for hypersensitivity reactions, including SJS, TEN, anaphylaxis, and angioedema.
• Topical formulations aren't expected to cause drug interactions.
• *Look alike–sound alike:* Don't confuse acyclovir sodium with acetazolamide sodium vials. Don't confuse Zovirax with Zyvox.

PATIENT TEACHING
• Tell patient to take drug as prescribed, even after feeling better.
• Inform patient drug is effective in managing herpes infection but doesn't eliminate or cure it. Warn patient that drug won't prevent spread of infection to others.
• Advise patient to avoid sexual contact while visible lesions are present. Virus transmission can occur during treatment.
• Teach patient about early signs and symptoms of herpes infection (tingling, itching, pain). Instruct patient to notify prescriber and get a prescription for drug before infection fully develops. Early treatment is most effective.

BIOSIMILAR DRUG

adalimumab
ay-da-LIM-yoo-mab

Humira

adalimumab-aacf
Idacio

adalimumab-adaz
Hyrimoz

adalimumab-adbm
Cyltezo

adalimumab-afzb
Abrilada

adalimumab-aqvh
Yusimry

adalimumab-atto
Amjevita

adalimumab-bwwd
Hadlima

adalimumab-fkjp

Therapeutic class: Antiarthritics
Pharmacologic class: TNF blockers

AVAILABLE FORMS
Injection: 10 mg/0.1 mL, 10 mg/0.2 mL,
20 mg/0.2 mL, 20 mg/0.4 mL, 40 mg/0.4 mL,
40 mg/0.8 mL, 80 mg/0.8 mL prefilled syringes or pens; 40 mg/0.8 mL single-use vial
(institutional use only)

INDICATIONS & DOSAGES
➤ **RA, psoriatic arthritis, ankylosing
spondylitis**
Adults: 40 mg subcut every other week.
Patient may continue to take methotrexate,
steroids, NSAIDs, salicylates, analgesics, or
other DMARDs during therapy. Patient with
RA who isn't also taking methotrexate may
have dose increased to 40 mg weekly or 80 mg
every other week, if needed.
➤ **Moderate to severe adult Crohn disease
when response to conventional therapy
is inadequate or when response to infliximab is lost or patient can't tolerate drug;
moderate to severe active ulcerative colitis when response to immunosuppressants**
(such as corticosteroids, azathioprine, or
6-mercaptopurine) is inadequate
Adults: Initially, 160 mg subcut on day 1
given in 1 day or split over 2 consecutive
days; then 80 mg 2 weeks later (day 15), followed by a maintenance dose of 40 mg every
other week starting at week 4 (day 29). Patients not taking concomitant methotrexate
may derive additional benefit from increasing
dosage to 40 mg every week or 80 mg every
other week. For ulcerative colitis, only continue in patients who show evidence of clinical remission by 8 weeks (day 57) of therapy.
➤ **Pediatric Crohn disease**
*Children ages 6 and older weighing 40 kg or
more):* Initially, 160 mg subcut on day 1 given
in 1 day or split over 2 consecutive days; then
80 mg 2 weeks later (day 15); then maintenance dose of 40 mg every other week starting at week 4 (day 29).
*Children ages 6 and older weighing between
17 and 40 kg (Humira, Abrilada, Amjevta,
Cyltezo, Hadlima, Hulio only):* 80 mg subcut
on day 1; then 40 mg 2 weeks later (day 15);
then maintenance dose of 20 mg every other
week starting at week 4 (day 29).
➤ **Pediatric moderate to severe active
ulcerative colitis (Humira only)**
*Children ages 5 and older weighing 40 kg or
more:* Initially, 160 mg subcut on day 1 given
in 1 day or split over 2 consecutive days; then
80 mg on day 8 and 80 mg on day 15; then
maintenance dose of 40 mg every week or
80 mg every other week starting at week 4
(day 29).
*Children ages 5 and older weighing from 20
to less than 40 kg:* 80 mg subcut on day 1;
then 40 mg on day 8 and 40 mg on day 15;
then maintenance dose of 20 mg every week
or 40 mg every other week starting at week 4
(day 29).
➤ **To reduce signs and symptoms of moderately to severely active polyarticular
juvenile idiopathic arthritis**
*Children ages 2 and older weighing 30 kg or
more:* 40 mg subcut every other week.
*Children ages 2 and older weighing 15 to less
than 30 kg:* 20 mg subcut every other week.
*Children ages 2 and older weighing 10 to
less than 15 kg:* 10 mg subcut every other
week.
➤ **Moderate to severe chronic plaque
psoriasis**
Adults: 80 mg subcut, followed by 40 mg subcut every other week starting 1 week after

initial dose. Treatment beyond 1 year hasn't been studied.

➤ **Noninfectious intermediate uveitis, posterior uveitis, and panuveitis (Humira only)**

Adults: 80 mg subcut, followed by 40 mg subcut every other week starting 1 week after initial dose.

Children ages 2 and older weighing 30 kg or more: 40 mg subcut every other week.

Children ages 2 and older weighing 15 to less than 30 kg: 20 mg subcut every other week.

Children ages 2 and older weighing 10 kg to less than 15 kg: 10 mg subcut every other week.

➤ **Moderate to severe hidradenitis suppurativa (Humira only)**

Adults and adolescents ages 12 and older weighing 60 kg or more: 160 mg subcut given in 1 day or split over 2 consecutive days; then 80 mg subcut on day 15; then 40 mg subcut weekly or 80 mg every other week (starting on day 29).

Adolescents ages 12 and older weighing 30 to less than 60 kg: 80 mg subcut on day 1; then 40 mg subcut on day 8; then 40 mg subcut every other week.

ADMINISTRATION

Subcutaneous

• Inject subcut into lower abdomen or thigh at separate sites.

• Rotate injection sites.

• Don't give in an area that is bruised, tender, red, or hard.

• May leave drug (don't remove cap or cover) at room temperature for about 15 to 30 minutes before injecting.

• Don't use if particulates or discoloration is noted in autoinjector, pen, prefilled syringe, or single-use institutional-use vial.

• Refrigerate at 36° to 46° F (2° to 8° C); don't freeze. May store at room temperature (maximum, 77° F [25° C]) for up to 14 days, if needed. Discard after 14 days. Protect from light.

🔵 *Alert:* The needle cap or cover of pen and prefilled syringe may contain latex. Check product packaging to confirm.

ACTION

A recombinant human IgG₁ monoclonal antibody that blocks human TNF-alpha. TNF-alpha participates in normal inflammatory and immune responses and in inflammation and joint destruction of RA.

Route	Onset	Peak	Duration
Subcut	Variable	75–187 hr	Unknown

Half-life: 10 to 20 days.

ADVERSE REACTIONS

CNS: headache, syncope, *hypertensive encephalopathy,* confusion, pain, paresthesia, *subdural hematoma,* tremor, myasthenia. **CV:** HTN, arrhythmia, atrial fibrillation, chest pain, CAD, *DVT, cardiac arrest, HF, MI,* palpitations, pericardial effusion, pericarditis, edema. **EENT:** cataract, pharyngitis, caries, sinusitis. **GI:** abdominal pain, nausea, cholecystitis, cholelithiasis, esophagitis, gastroenteritis, *GI hemorrhage,* vomiting, diverticulitis. **GU:** hematuria, UTI, cystitis, pelvic pain, kidney stones, pyelonephritis, menstrual disorder. **Hematologic:** polycythemia, *agranulocytosis,* positive ANA titer, paraproteinemia. **Hepatic:** increased ALP level, *liver necrosis.* **Metabolic:** hypercholesterolemia, hyperlipidemia, dehydration, ketosis, increased CK level. **Musculoskeletal:** back pain, bone disorder, osteonecrosis, joint disorder, muscle cramps, synovitis, tendon disorder, septic arthritis, limb pain, bone fracture. **Respiratory:** URI, dyspnea, decreased lung function, pleural effusion, asthma, *bronchospasm,* pneumonia. **Skin:** rash, injection-site reactions (erythema, itching, pain, swelling), cellulitis, erysipelas. **Other:** accidental injury, *malignancy,* adenoma, abnormal healing, hypersensitivity reactions, flulike syndrome, parathyroid disorder, infection, herpes simplex or zoster infection, *sepsis,* antibody development.

INTERACTIONS

Drug-drug. *Abatacept, anakinra, tocilizumab, other biologic DMARDs:* May increase risk of serious infections and neutropenia in patients with RA. Don't use together.

CYP450 substrates with narrow therapeutic index (cyclosporine, theophylline, warfarin): May affect CYP450 substrate level. Monitor levels closely when initiating or discontinuing adalimumab; adjust substrate dosage as needed.

Live-virus vaccines: No data are available on secondary transmission of infection from live-virus vaccines. Avoid use together.

EFFECTS ON LAB TEST RESULTS
• May increase CK, ALP, and cholesterol levels.
• May decrease platelet and WBC counts.
• May cause positive ANA titer and development of antibodies.

CONTRAINDICATIONS & CAUTIONS
۞ Alert: Anaphylaxis and angioneurotic edema have been reported. If serious reaction occurs, immediately discontinue drug and treat appropriately.

Boxed Warning Patients taking TNF-alpha blockers are at increased risk for developing serious infections that can lead to hospitalization or death (especially if taking concomitant immunosuppressants, such as methotrexate or corticosteroids). Reported infections include *Legionella* and *Listeria* infections, active TB, and invasive fungal infections. Consider empirical antifungal therapy for patients at risk for invasive fungal infections who develop systemic illness. Carefully consider risk and benefits of therapy before starting drug in patients with chronic or recurrent infections. ∎

• Drug may cause reactivation of HBV in chronic carriers.

Boxed Warning Lymphoma and other malignancies, some fatal, have been reported in children and adolescents treated with TNF blockers, including adalimumab. ∎

Boxed Warning Hepatosplenic T-cell lymphoma, a rare type of T-cell lymphoma, has occurred in adolescents and young adults with inflammatory bowel disease treated with TNF blockers, including adalimumab. ∎

• Use cautiously in patients with demyelinating disorders, a history of chronic or recurrent infection, those with underlying conditions that predispose them to infections, those who have been exposed to TB, those who have lived in areas where TB and histoplasmosis are endemic, patients with HF, and older adults.

• Drug may increase risk of new onset or exacerbation of CNS demyelinating disease (MS, optic neuritis, Guillain-Barré syndrome).

Dialyzable drug: Unknown.

PREGNANCY-LACTATION-REPRODUCTION
• Use during pregnancy only if clearly needed. Drug is increasingly transported across the placenta as pregnancy progresses.

• Consider risks and benefits of giving live or live-attenuated vaccines to infants exposed to adalimumab during pregnancy.

• Drug appears in human milk. Use cautiously during breastfeeding.

NURSING CONSIDERATIONS
• Give first dose under supervision of prescriber.

Boxed Warning Patient should be evaluated and treated, if necessary, for latent TB before start of adalimumab therapy. Closely monitor patient for possible development of TB even if patient tested negative before start of therapy. ∎

Boxed Warning Serious infections and sepsis, including TB and invasive fungal infections, may occur. If patient develops new infection during treatment, monitor closely; if infection becomes serious, stop drug. ∎

۞ Alert: Drug may increase the risk of malignancy. Monitor the patient for skin cancer before and during treatment.

۞ Alert: If patient develops anaphylaxis, a severe infection, other serious allergic reaction, or evidence of a lupuslike syndrome, stop drug.

• Monitor blood counts for blood dyscrasias.

۞ Alert: The needle covers or caps may contain latex. Avoid handling by those with latex sensitivity.

• Instruct patient with arthritis to continue to take methotrexate as prescribed.

۞ Look alike–sound alike: Don't confuse Humira with Humulin or Humalog.

PATIENT TEACHING
• Tell patient to report all adverse reactions and any evidence of TB or other infection.

• Teach about proper drug administration and handling.

• Instruct patient not to place used needles and syringes in household trash or recyclables but to dispose of them properly.

۞ Alert: Warn patient to seek immediate medical attention for symptoms of blood dyscrasias or infection (fever, bruising, bleeding, pallor).

• Inform patient of risk of malignancies.

Reactions in bold italics are *life-threatening*.

adenosine
a-DEN-oh-seen

Therapeutic class: Antiarrhythmics
Pharmacologic class: Nucleosides

AVAILABLE FORMS
Injection: 3 mg/mL

INDICATIONS & DOSAGES
➤ **To convert paroxysmal supraventricular tachycardia (PSVT) to sinus rhythm**
Adults and children weighing 50 kg or more: 6 mg IV by rapid bolus injection over 1 to 2 seconds, followed by saline flush. If PSVT isn't eliminated in 1 to 2 minutes, 12 mg by rapid IV push and repeat, if needed.
Children weighing less than 50 kg: Initially, 0.05 to 0.1 mg/kg IV by rapid bolus injection followed by a saline flush. If PSVT isn't eliminated in 1 to 2 minutes, additional bolus injections, increasing the amount given in 0.05- to 0.1-mg/kg increments, followed by a saline flush. Continue, as needed, until conversion of the PSVT or a maximum single dose of 0.3 mg/kg (up to 12 mg) is given.
Adjust-a-dose: Reduce initial adenosine dose to 3 mg IV bolus if patient is currently receiving carbamazepine or dipyridamole or has a transplanted heart, or if adenosine is given via central venous catheter (CVC).
➤ **Stress-testing diagnostic aid** ♦
Adults: 140 mcg/kg/minute IV infusion over 6 minutes (total dose of 0.84 mg/kg).

ADMINISTRATION
IV
▼ Don't give single doses exceeding 12 mg.
▼ Crystals may form if solution is cold; gently warm solution to room temperature. Don't use solutions that aren't clear.
▼ In adults, avoid giving drug through a CVC because central administration hasn't been studied.
▼ For PSVT, give by rapid IV injection to ensure drug action.
▼ Give directly into vein as proximal as possible to trunk. When giving through IV line, use port closest to patient.
▼ Flush immediately and rapidly with NSS to ensure that drug quickly reaches systemic circulation.

▼ Drug lacks preservatives. Discard unused portion. Don't refrigerate.
▼ When used as a diagnostic aid, infuse using syringe pump or volumetric infusion pump. Thallium-201 and adenosine are compatible. Thallium will be administered midway through the adenosine infusion.
▼ **Incompatibilities:** Consult drug compatibility reference for information.

ACTION
Naturally occurring nucleoside that acts on the AV node to slow conduction and inhibit reentry pathways.

Route	Onset	Peak	Duration
IV	Immediate	Immediate	Unknown

Half-life: Less than 10 seconds.

ADVERSE REACTIONS
CNS: dizziness, light-headedness, numbness, headache, nervousness. **CV:** chest discomfort, flushing, hypotension, *arrhythmias,* ST-segment depression, first- or second-degree AV block. **EENT:** throat, neck, or jaw discomfort. **GI:** nausea. **Musculoskeletal:** upper extremity discomfort. **Respiratory:** dyspnea.

INTERACTIONS
Drug-drug. *Aminophylline:* May increase risk of seizures. Avoid use together.
Carbamazepine: May cause high-level heart block. Use together cautiously and consider using a lower initial adenosine dose.
Digoxin, verapamil: May cause ventricular fibrillation. Monitor ECG closely.
Dipyridamole: May increase adenosine's effects. Adenosine dose may need to be reduced. Use together cautiously.
Methylxanthines (caffeine, theophylline): May decrease adenosine's effects. Adenosine dose may need to be increased, or patients may not respond to adenosine therapy.

EFFECTS ON LAB TEST RESULTS
None reported.

CONTRAINDICATIONS & CAUTIONS
• Contraindicated in patients hypersensitive to drug.
• Contraindicated in those with second- or third-degree heart block or sinus node disease (sick sinus syndrome and symptomatic bradycardia), except those with a pacemaker.

• Contraindicated for use as diagnostic aid in patients with known or suspected bronchoconstrictive or bronchospastic lung disease (asthma).
• Use cautiously in patients with obstructive lung disease not associated with bronchoconstriction (emphysema or bronchitis); avoid use for PSVT in those with bronchoconstriction or bronchospasm (asthma).
• Drug may increase risk of seizures.
• Avoid use in patients with signs and symptoms of acute MI (unstable angina, CV instability). Drug may increase risk of serious CV reaction (fatal or nonfatal cardiac arrest, supraventricular tachycardia, MI). Make sure appropriate emergency equipment is readily available.
• Use cautiously in patients with autonomic dysfunction, stenotic valvular heart disease, pericarditis or pericardial effusions, stenotic carotid artery disease with cerebrovascular insufficiency, or uncorrected hypovolemia.
• Drug may increase risk of hypotension and related complications.
Dialyzable drug: Unknown.

PREGNANCY-LACTATION-REPRODUCTION

• No studies have been performed during pregnancy. Use during pregnancy only if clearly indicated.
• There are no well-controlled studies during breastfeeding. Patient should interrupt or discontinue breastfeeding or not receive drug, considering importance of drug to patient.

NURSING CONSIDERATIONS

⚠️ *Alert:* By decreasing conduction through the AV node, drug may produce first-, second-, or third-degree heart block. Patients who develop high-level heart block after a single dose shouldn't receive additional doses.
⚠️ *Alert:* New arrhythmias, including atrial fibrillation, heart block, and transient asystole, may develop; monitor cardiac rhythm and treat as indicated.
• Monitor BP closely. Discontinue drug in patients who develop persistent or symptomatic hypotension. Significant HTN may develop within several minutes or last several hours.
• Monitor patient for seizures during therapy.
• Monitor for hypersensitivity reactions, including anaphylaxis.

⚠️ *Alert:* Don't confuse adenosine with adenosine phosphate.

PATIENT TEACHING

• Instruct patient to report adverse reactions promptly.
• Teach patient to avoid products containing methylxanthines (caffeinated coffee or tea, other caffeinated beverages, caffeine-containing drug products, aminophylline, and theophylline) before an imaging study.
• Tell patient to report discomfort at IV site.
• Inform patient that flushing and chest pain lasting 1 to 2 minutes may occur.

SAFETY ALERT!

ado-trastuzumab emtansine ⚠️
ADD-oh tras-TOOZ-oo-mab em-TAN-seen

Kadcyla

Therapeutic class: Antineoplastics
Pharmacologic class: Antibody drug conjugates

AVAILABLE FORMS

Injection (lyophilized powder for solution): 100 mg, 160 mg in single-use vials

INDICATIONS & DOSAGES

Adjust-a-dose (for all indications): Refer to manufacturer's instructions for toxicity-related dosage adjustments.
➤ **HER2-positive, metastatic breast cancer in patients who previously received trastuzumab and a taxane, separately or in combination. Patients should have either received previous treatment for metastatic disease or developed recurrence during or within 6 months of completing adjuvant treatment**
Adults: 3.6 mg/kg IV every 21 days until disease progression or unacceptable toxicity occurs. Maximum dose, 3.6 mg/kg.
➤ **Adjuvant treatment of HER2-positive early breast cancer with residual invasive disease after neoadjuvant taxane and trastuzumab-based treatment**
Adults: 3.6 mg/kg IV every 21 days for 14 cycles, unless disease recurrence or unacceptable toxicity occurs.

ADMINISTRATION

IV

⚠️ *Alert:* Hazardous drug; use safe handling and disposal precautions.

⚠️ *Alert:* Don't confuse or substitute this drug with trastuzumab (Herceptin). These drugs aren't interchangeable.

⚠️ *Alert:* The manufacturer recommends that the trade name be used and clearly recorded (with batch number) in the patient record to avoid confusion.

▼ To reconstitute, slowly inject 5 mL sterile water for injection into 100-mg vial or 8 mL sterile water for injection into 160-mg vial to yield concentration of 20 mg/mL.

▼ Swirl gently until dissolved. Don't shake. Solution should be colorless to pale brown.

▼ Add reconstituted dose to 250 mL of NSS in infusion bag and administer immediately through IV line containing 0.2- or 0.22-micron in-line nonprotein adsorptive polyethersulfone filter.

▼ Administer initial infusion over 90 minutes. Don't administer as IV push or bolus.

▼ May administer subsequent infusions over 30 minutes if initial infusion was uneventful.

▼ Give at dosage and rate patient tolerated at most recent infusion.

▼ If dose is delayed or missed, give as soon as possible; don't wait for next planned cycle. Adjust schedule to maintain a 3-week interval between doses.

▼ Reconstituted vials can be stored in refrigerator for up to 24 hours at 36° to 46° F (2° to 8° C). Diluted solution can be stored in refrigerator for an additional 24 hours. Don't freeze.

▼ **Incompatibilities:** Dextrose solution, other drugs.

ACTION

Drug contains both trastuzumab and DM1 (a microtubule inhibitor), linked by a covalent bond, and targets the HER2 receptor by combined mechanisms of trastuzumab and DM1. The recombinant monoclonal antibody, trastuzumab, binds to the HER2 receptor and intracellular lysosomal degradation releases the cytotoxic component, DM1, resulting in microtubule disruption and cell death.

Route	Onset	Peak	Duration
IV	Unknown	End of infusion	Unknown

Half-life: 4 days.

ADVERSE REACTIONS

CNS: fatigue, headache, fever, asthenia, dizziness, peripheral neuropathy, taste perversion, insomnia. **CV:** *left ventricular dysfunction,* edema, HTN. **EENT:** dry eye syndrome, blurred vision, conjunctivitis, increased lacrimation, epistaxis, dry mouth. **GI:** nausea, constipation, stomatitis, abdominal pain, vomiting, diarrhea, dyspepsia. **GU:** UTI. **Hematologic:** *thrombocytopenia, neutropenia,* anemia, *hemorrhage.* **Hepatic:** elevated transaminase levels, increased ALP level, bilirubinemia. **Metabolic:** *hypokalemia.* **Musculoskeletal:** pain, arthralgia, myalgia, weakness. **Respiratory:** pneumonitis, dyspnea, cough. **Skin:** pruritus, rash. **Other:** chills, hypersensitivity reactions, infusion reaction.

INTERACTIONS

Drug-drug. *Anthracyclines:* May enhance cardiotoxic effects of anthracyclines. When possible, avoid anthracycline-based therapy for up to 7 months after stopping ado-trastuzumab emtansine. Monitor patient who must receive this combination closely for cardiac dysfunction.

Anticoagulants (clopidogrel, heparin, warfarin), antiplatelet agents: May increase risk of hemorrhagic events. Monitor patient closely.

Strong CYP3A4 inhibitors (atazanavir, clarithromycin, ketoconazole, nefazodone, nelfinavir, ritonavir, telithromycin): May increase ado-trastuzumab level and potential toxicity. Avoid use together. If use together is necessary, stop CYP3A4 inhibitor and delay treatment until inhibitor clears from patient's circulation, or monitor patient carefully for adverse effects.

EFFECTS ON LAB TEST RESULTS

• May increase bilirubin, AST, and ALT levels.
• May decrease potassium level.
• May decrease Hb level and platelet and neutrophil counts.

CONTRAINDICATIONS & CAUTIONS

Boxed Warning Severe liver injury (including fatal liver damage, liver failure, and death) has been reported. Monitor serum transaminase and bilirubin levels before starting drug and before each dose. Dosage modifications or discontinuation of therapy may be necessary. ∎

Boxed Warning Drug may significantly reduce LVEF. Assess LVEF before starting drug and every 3 months during treatment. Withhold or discontinue drug as clinically indicated. ∎

• Contraindicated in patients hypersensitive to drug or its components.

• Avoid use in patients with history of trastuzumab hypersensitivity or infusion-related events.

• Use cautiously in patients with liver failure, risk of liver toxicity, symptomatic HF, serious cardiac arrhythmia, history of MI, or unstable angina.

• Patients with shortness of breath at rest due to advanced malignancy and comorbidities may be at increased risk for pulmonary toxicity.

• Use cautiously in patients with preexisting thrombocytopenia due to increased risk of hemorrhage.

⚕ Patients of Asian ancestry may be at higher risk for thrombocytopenia.

Dialyzable drug: Unknown.

⚠ *Overdose S&S:* Thrombocytopenia, death.

PREGNANCY-LACTATION-REPRODUCTION
Boxed Warning Exposure to drug can result in embryo-fetal death or birth defects. ∎

🟦 *Alert:* Patients of childbearing potential should use effective contraception during treatment and for 7 months after last dose. Adult male patients with partners of childbearing potential should use effective contraception during treatment and for 4 months after last dose.

• May impair fertility in females and males of reproductive potential. It isn't known if the effects are reversible.

🟦 *Alert:* Advise patient to immediately report suspected or confirmed pregnancy during therapy or within 7 months after last dose. Report drug exposure to manufacturer (1-888-835-2555).

• It isn't known if drug appears in human milk. Advise patients not to breastfeed during treatment and for 7 months after final dose.

NURSING CONSIDERATIONS
⚕ Confirm HER2 testing with FDA-approved test by established lab. Only patients with HER2 protein overexpression should receive drug because they're the only patients studied for whom benefit has been shown.

• Verify pregnancy status before start of therapy.

• Infusion-related reactions, including hypersensitivity reactions, may occur. Closely monitor patient during and for 90 minutes after initial infusion and for 30 minutes after subsequent infusions (if tolerated) for fever, chills, flushing, dyspnea, hypotension, wheezing, bronchospasm, and tachycardia. Slow or interrupt infusion as necessary. In most patients, these reactions resolve over course of several hours to a day after infusion termination. Discontinue drug if life-threatening, infusion-related reactions occur.

• Monitor patient for extravasation, which may cause redness, tenderness, skin irritation, pain, or swelling at infusion site.

🟦 *Alert:* Permanently discontinue drug in patients diagnosed with ILD or pneumonitis.

• Monitor platelet count and liver function before treatment and before each dose.

• Discontinue drug in patients diagnosed with nodular regenerative hyperplasia of the liver.

• Monitor patients for peripheral neuropathy.

• *Look alike–sound alike:* Don't confuse ado-trastuzumab emtansine with fam-trastuzumab deruxtecan, pertuzumab, trastuzumab, or trastuzumab–hyaluronidase.

PATIENT TEACHING
• Inform patient that drug may cause severe liver damage that may be life-threatening.

• Tell patient to report unexplained nausea, vomiting, abdominal pain, jaundice, dark urine, generalized itchiness, or anorexia.

• Caution patient that drug may cause heart problems, with or without symptoms. Instruct patient to report new-onset or worsening of shortness of breath, cough, swelling of ankles or legs, palpitations, weight gain of more than 5 lb in 24 hours, fatigue, dizziness, or loss of consciousness.

• Advise patient that drug may cause lung problems. Tell patient to report trouble breathing, cough, or tiredness.

• Alert patient that drug may cause low platelet count. Instruct patient to contact prescriber if excessive bleeding occurs.

• Warn patient that drug may cause nerve damage. Instruct patient to report numbness or tingling, burning or sharp pain, sensitivity to touch, lack of coordination, muscle weakness, or loss of muscle function.

Reactions in bold italics are *life-threatening*.

Boxed Warning Inform patient that drug may cause birth defects and fetal death. Advise patient of the need for effective contraception during and after treatment. ∎

🌜 *Alert:* Advise patient to immediately report suspected or confirmed pregnancy during therapy.

• Advise patient not to breastfeed during treatment and for 7 months after final dose.

albuterol sulfate (salbutamol sulfate)
al-BYOO-ter-ole

Airomir🍁, ProAir Digihaler, ProAir RespiClick, Proventil HFA, Ventolin HFA

Therapeutic class: Bronchodilators
Pharmacologic class: Adrenergics

AVAILABLE FORMS
Inhalation aerosol: 90 mcg/actuation, 100 mcg/actuation🍁
Inhalation powder (base): 90 mcg/actuation, 100 mcg/actuation🍁
Solution for inhalation: 0.021% (0.63 mg/ 3 mL), 0.042% (1.25 mg/3 mL), 0.083% (2.5 mg/3 mL), 0.5% (0.5 mg/mL)
Syrup: 2 mg/5 mL
Tablets: 2 mg, 4 mg

INDICATIONS & DOSAGES
➤ **To prevent or treat bronchospasm in patients with reversible obstructive airway disease**
Adjust-a-dose (for oral forms): For older adults and patients sensitive to sympathomimetic amines, 2 mg PO t.i.d. or q.i.d. as oral tablets or syrup. Maximum, 32 mg daily.
Adults and children older than age 12: For tablets, 2 to 4 mg PO t.i.d. or q.i.d. Maximum, 32 mg daily.
Children ages 6 to 12: For tablets, 2 mg PO t.i.d. or q.i.d. Maximum, 24 mg daily.
Adults and children older than age 14: For syrup, 2 to 4 mg PO t.i.d. or q.i.d. Maximum, 32 mg daily.
Children ages 6 to 14: For syrup, 2 mg PO t.i.d. or q.i.d. Maximum, 24 mg daily.
Children ages 2 to 5: For syrup, initially, 0.1 mg/kg PO t.i.d. Starting dose shouldn't exceed 2 mg t.i.d. Maximum, 12 mg daily.

Adults and children ages 12 and older: For solution for inhalation, 2.5 mg by nebulizer, given over 5 to 15 minutes, t.i.d. or q.i.d. To prepare solution, use 0.5 mL of 0.5% solution diluted with 2.5 mL of NSS. Or, use 3 mL of 0.083% solution.
Children ages 2 to 12 weighing more than 15 kg: For solution for inhalation, 2.5 mg by nebulizer given over 5 to 15 minutes t.i.d. or q.i.d., with subsequent doses adjusted to response. Don't exceed 2.5 mg t.i.d. or q.i.d.
Children ages 2 to 12 weighing 15 kg or less: For solution for inhalation, 0.63 mg or 1.25 mg by nebulizer given over 5 to 15 minutes t.i.d. or q.i.d., with subsequent doses adjusted to response. Don't exceed 2.5 mg t.i.d. or q.i.d.
Adults and children ages 4 and older: For inhalation aerosol, 2 inhalations every 4 to 6 hours as needed. In some patients, 1 inhalation every 4 hours may be sufficient. Regular use for maintenance therapy to control asthma symptoms isn't recommended.
Adults and children ages 4 and older: For inhalation powder, 2 inhalations every 4 to 6 hours. In some patients, 1 inhalation every 4 hours may be sufficient.
➤ **To prevent exercise-induced bronchospasm**
Adults and children ages 4 and older: 2 inhalations 15 to 30 minutes before exercise.
➤ **Adjuvant therapy for acute treatment of moderate to severe hyperkalemia** ♦
Adults: 10 to 20 mg via nebulization over 10 minutes, given in combination with other recommended therapy.

ADMINISTRATION
PO
• Give drug without regard for food.
• Store at room temperature.
Inhalational
• If more than 1 inhalation is ordered, wait 1 minute; then shake the inhaler again if necessary, and repeat procedure.
• Inhalation powder inhaler device doesn't require priming. Use spacer device to improve drug delivery, if appropriate. Don't use ProAir RespiClick with a spacer or volume holding chamber.
• Shake aerosol inhaler well before use and prime inhaler according to manufacturer's instructions before first use, when it has been dropped, or when it hasn't been used for more than 2 weeks.

• Keep cap on inhaler closed during storage.
• For nebulization, empty entire contents of one sterile unit-dose vial into nebulizer reservoir. Connect mouthpiece or face mask; then connect nebulizer to compressor and turn on compressor. Flow rate is regulated for the nebulizer to deliver albuterol inhalation solution over 5 to 15 minutes.
• Patient should breathe calmly, deeply, and evenly through the mouth until mist no longer appears in nebulizer chamber.
• Clean nebulizer or inhaler according to manufacturer's instructions.

ACTION

Relaxes bronchial, uterine, and vascular smooth muscle by stimulating beta$_2$ receptors.

Route	Onset	Peak	Duration
PO	15–30 min	2–3 hr	4–8 hr
Inhalation (aerosol)	5–15 min	30–120 min	3–4 hr
Inhalation (powder)	Rapid	30 min	3–4 hr

Half-life: Oral, 5 to 6 hours; inhalation aerosol, 6 hours; inhalation powder, 5 hours.

ADVERSE REACTIONS

CNS: tremor, excitement, nervousness, anxiety, ataxia, depression, drowsiness, emotional lability, fatigue, headache, tremor, shakiness, hyperactivity, insomnia, dizziness, CNS stimulation, malaise, altered taste, fever. **CV:** tachycardia, palpitations, HTN, chest pain, lymphadenopathy, edema, extrasystoles. **EENT:** conjunctivitis, otitis media, tinnitus, ear disorder, dry and irritated nose and throat (inhaled forms), nasal congestion, epistaxis, hoarseness, pharyngitis, rhinitis, glossitis. **GI:** nausea, vomiting, diarrhea, eructation, flatulence, gastroenteritis, heartburn, anorexia, increased appetite. **GU:** UTI. **Hematologic:** anemia, decreased WBC count, lymphadenopathy. **Hepatic:** increased transaminase levels. **Metabolic:** hyperglycemia, *hypokalemia.* **Musculoskeletal:** pain, hyperkinesia, muscle cramps, back pain. **Respiratory:** *bronchospasm,* exacerbation of asthma, URI, cough, wheezing, dyspnea, bronchitis, increased sputum, viral respiratory tract infection. **Skin:** diaphoresis, pallor, urticaria, rash. **Other:** hypersensitivity reactions, flulike syndrome, cold symptoms, infection.

INTERACTIONS

Drug-drug. *Antiarrhythmics (amiodarone, disopyramide, dofetilide, procainamide, quinidine, sotalol), arsenic trioxide, chlorpromazine, dolasetron, droperidol, mefloquine, mesoridazine, moxifloxacin, pentamidine, pimozide, tacrolimus, thioridazine, ziprasidone:* May prolong QT interval and increase risk of life-threatening arrhythmias, including torsades de pointes. Monitor QT interval and patient.
Beta blockers (labetalol, propranolol): May block pulmonary effect and increase risk of severe bronchospasm in patients with asthma. Avoid use together. If unavoidable, cautiously use cardioselective beta blockers (atenolol, metoprolol).
CNS stimulants: May increase CNS stimulation. Avoid use together.
Digoxin: May decrease digoxin level. Monitor digoxin level closely.
Diuretics (loop diuretics, thiazides): May cause ECG changes and hypokalemia. Monitor potassium level. Use caution when administered with non-potassium-sparing diuretics.
Epinephrine, short-acting sympathomimetic bronchodilators (levalbuterol, pirbuterol): May increase risk of toxicity. Don't use together.
Linezolid, MAO inhibitors, TCAs: May increase adverse CV effects. Consider alternative therapy. Monitor patient closely if used together.

EFFECTS ON LAB TEST RESULTS

• May increase glucose level.
• May decrease potassium level.
• May decrease Hb level, hematocrit, and WBC count.

CONTRAINDICATIONS & CAUTIONS

• Contraindicated in patients hypersensitive to drug or its ingredients and in those with severe hypersensitivity to milk proteins (dry powder inhalers).
• Use cautiously in patients with CV disorders (including coronary insufficiency and HTN), seizure disorders, hyperthyroidism, or diabetes and in those who are unusually responsive to adrenergics.
⊕ *Alert:* Deaths have been reported with excessive use of inhaled sympathomimetic drugs in patients with asthma. Don't exceed recommended dose.
Dialyzable drug: Unknown.

Reactions in bold italics are *life-threatening*.

⚠ Overdose S&S: Exaggeration of adverse reactions, seizures, angina, hypotension, HTN, tachycardia, arrhythmias, nervousness, headache, tremor, dry mouth, palpitations, nausea, dizziness, fatigue, malaise, sleeplessness, hypokalemia, cardiac arrest.

PREGNANCY-LACTATION-REPRODUCTION
• There are no adequate and well-controlled studies during pregnancy. Use during pregnancy only if potential benefit justifies fetal risk.
• Data collection to monitor outcomes during pregnancy in patients with asthma and in infants and medications used to treat asthma in pregnancy is available at MotherToBaby Pregnancy Studies at 866-626-6847 or https://mothertobaby.org.
• It isn't known if drug appears in human milk. Use cautiously during breastfeeding.
• Drug may interfere with uterine contractility; use during labor only when benefits clearly outweigh the risk.

NURSING CONSIDERATIONS
• Drug may decrease sensitivity of spirometry used for diagnosis of asthma.
• Syrup contains no alcohol or sugar and may be taken by children as young as age 2.
• Monitor patient for hypersensitivity reactions, including SJS.
• Monitor patient for effectiveness. Using drug alone may not be adequate to control asthma in some patients. Long-term control medications (corticosteroids) may be needed.
• In patients with COVID-19 who require a bronchodilator for asthma or COPD symptoms, use a pressurized metered-dose inhaler. Nebulized delivery may increase transmission of particles (SARS-CoV2) into the environment and potentially decrease the life of expiratory circuit filter.
• **Alert:** Drug may cause paradoxical bronchospasm. Monitor patient closely; immediately discontinue drug and use alternative therapy if paradoxical bronchospasm occurs. Bronchospasm with inhaled formulations frequently occurs with first use of new canister or vial.
• **Alert:** Patient may use tablets and aerosol together. Monitor closely for signs and symptoms of toxicity.
• **Look alike–sound alike:** Don't confuse albuterol with atenolol.

PATIENT TEACHING
• Warn patient about risk of paradoxical bronchospasm and advise patient to stop drug immediately if it occurs.
• Teach about proper drug administration and handling. Encourage patient to read manufacturer's instructions for use of inhaler.
• Advise patient not to use more than prescribed and not to increase dose or frequency without consulting prescriber.
• Instruct patient to report worsening symptoms.
• Tell patients who are pregnant or breastfeeding to contact their prescriber.

SAFETY ALERT!

alectinib hydrochloride ⬚
al-EK-ti-nib

Alecensa

Therapeutic class: Antineoplastics
Pharmacologic class: Tyrosine kinase inhibitors

AVAILABLE FORMS
Capsules 🚫*:* 150 mg

INDICATIONS & DOSAGES
➤ **Anaplastic lymphoma kinase (ALK)-positive, metastatic NSCLC** ⬚
Adults: 600 mg PO b.i.d. until disease progression or unacceptable toxicity occurs.
Adjust-a-dose: Recommended dosage in patients with Child-Pugh class C liver impairment is 450 mg PO b.i.d. Refer to manufacturer's instructions for toxicity-related dosage adjustments.

ADMINISTRATION
PO
• **Alert:** Hazardous drug; use safe handling and disposal precautions.
• Give drug with food.
• Have patient swallow capsules whole; don't break or open capsules.
• If a dose is missed or vomiting occurs after taking a dose, give next dose at the scheduled time.
• Don't store above 86° F (30° C). Store in the original container to protect from light and moisture.

ACTION

A tyrosine kinase inhibitor that targets *ALK* and *RET* gene abnormalities that alter signaling and expression and result in increased cellular proliferation and survival in tumors that express these fusion proteins. Inhibiting ALK signaling decreases tumor cell viability.

Route	Onset	Peak	Duration
PO	Unknown	4 hr	Unknown

Half-life: 33 hours (parent drug).

ADVERSE REACTIONS

CNS: fatigue, headache, dysgeusia. **CV:** *bradycardia,* edema. **EENT:** vision disorder. **GI:** vomiting, constipation, nausea, diarrhea. **GU:** kidney impairment. **Hematologic:** anemia, *lymphopenia, neutropenia.* **Hepatic:** hyperbilirubinemia, elevated ALP, AST, and ALT levels. **Metabolic:** increased weight, hypoalbuminemia, *hypocalcemia,* hyperglycemia, *hypokalemia, hyperkalemia,* hyponatremia, hypophosphatemia, increased CK and GGT levels. **Musculoskeletal:** myalgia, back pain. **Respiratory:** dyspnea, cough. **Skin:** rash, photosensitivity.

INTERACTIONS

Drug-drug. *Bradycardia-causing drugs:* May increase risk of bradycardia. Monitor patient closely.
Drug-lifestyle. *Sun exposure:* May increase risk of photosensitivity. Discourage sun exposure.

EFFECTS ON LAB TEST RESULTS

- May increase AST, ALT, ALP, CK, bilirubin, glucose, GGT, and creatinine levels.
- May decrease calcium, phosphorus, albumin, and sodium levels.
- May increase or decrease potassium level.
- May decrease WBC and RBC counts.

CONTRAINDICATIONS & CAUTIONS

⚠ Drug is only approved for use in patients with metastatic NSCLC who test positive for the abnormal *ALK* gene.
- Drug may increase risk of liver toxicity, pulmonary toxicity (ILD or pneumonitis), kidney impairment, intestinal perforation, endocarditis, hemolytic anemia, and hemorrhage.
- Safety and effectiveness in children haven't been determined.
Dialyzable drug: Unlikely.

PREGNANCY-LACTATION-REPRODUCTION

- Drug may cause fetal harm. Patients of childbearing potential should use effective contraception during treatment and for 1 week after final dose.
- Adult males with partners of childbearing potential should use effective contraception during treatment and for 3 months after final dose.
- It's unknown if drug appears in human milk. Due to the potential for serious adverse reactions in infants, breastfeeding isn't recommended during treatment and for 1 week after final dose.

NURSING CONSIDERATIONS

- Monitor LFTs (ALT, AST, and total bilirubin levels) every 2 weeks during first 3 months of treatment, then once a month and as clinically indicated during treatment. Monitor patient for signs and symptoms of liver toxicity and intestinal perforation.
- Monitor patient for signs and symptoms of ILD or pneumonitis (worsening of respiratory symptoms, cough, dyspnea, fever). Withhold drug if patient is diagnosed with ILD or pneumonitis and permanently discontinue drug if it's the cause.
- Monitor patient for myalgia or musculoskeletal pain and assess CK level every 2 weeks for first month of treatment and as clinically indicated. Drug may need to be withheld or dosage reduced.
- Monitor patient for chest pain, and assess HR and BP regularly. Dosage modification isn't required in cases of asymptomatic bradycardia. Adjust dosage for non-life-threatening, symptomatic bradycardia and assess for concomitant bradycardia-contributing drugs. Treat life-threatening bradycardia appropriately.
- Monitor kidney function. Drug may need to be withheld or permanently discontinued, or dosage may need to be reduced.
- Monitor patient for abnormal bleeding.
- Monitor patient for signs and symptoms of photosensitivity.

PATIENT TEACHING

- Teach patient to report signs and symptoms of liver injury or intestinal perforation (tiredness, anorexia, jaundice, dark urine, pruritus, nausea, vomiting, right-sided stomach pain, sharp abdominal pain, fever, easy bleeding or bruising); explain the need for blood tests throughout treatment.

• Inform patient of the risks of severe ILD and pneumonitis. Advise patient to contact prescriber immediately for new or worsening respiratory symptoms.

• Educate patient about the possibility of muscle pain, tenderness, and weakness. Instruct patient to immediately report new, worsening, or persistent signs and symptoms of muscle pain or weakness.

• Counsel patient that drug may cause dizziness, light-headedness, syncope and, rarely, chest pain. Instruct patient to immediately these symptoms to prescriber.

• Tell patient to report abnormal bleeding.

• Advise patient to avoid prolonged sun exposure while taking drug and for at least 7 days after last dose. Advise patient to use broad-spectrum sunscreen and lip balm (SPF 50 or higher) to protect from potential sunburn.

• Teach about proper drug administration and handling.

• Caution patient of possible harm if fetus is exposed to drug during pregnancy.

• Advise patient of childbearing potential to use effective contraception during treatment and for 1 week after final dose and to inform prescriber immediately of possible pregnancy.

• Explain to male patient with partner of childbearing potential the need to use effective contraception during treatment and for 3 months after last dose.

• Warn patient not to breastfeed during treatment and for 1 week after last dose.

alendronate sodium
ah-LEN-dro-nate

Binosto, Fosamax

Therapeutic class: Antiosteoporotics
Pharmacologic class: Bisphosphonates

AVAILABLE FORMS
Oral solution: 70 mg/75 mL
Tablets: 5 mg, 10 mg, 35 mg, 70 mg
Tablets (effervescent): 70 mg

INDICATIONS & DOSAGES
➤ **Osteoporosis**
Adult males and adult females after menopause: 10 mg PO daily or 70-mg tablet or solution PO once weekly.

➤ **To prevent osteoporosis (excluding Binosto and oral solution)**
Adult women after menopause: 5 mg PO daily or 35-mg PO once weekly.

➤ **Glucocorticoid-induced osteoporosis in patients receiving glucocorticoids in a daily dose equivalent to 7.5 mg or more of prednisone and who have low bone mineral density (excluding Binosto and oral solution)**
Adult women: 5 mg PO daily.
Adult women after menopausal who aren't receiving estrogen: 10 mg PO daily.

➤ **Paget disease of bone (osteitis deformans) (excluding Binosto and oral solution)**
Adults: 40 mg PO daily for 6 months. May consider retreatment in 6 months.

➤ **Prevention of androgen deprivation therapy–associated osteoporosis in non-metastatic prostate cancer ◆**
Adult males: 70 mg PO once weekly.

ADMINISTRATION
PO
• Give tablets with 180 to 240 mL of plain water.

• Dissolve effervescent tablet in 120 mL of plain room-temperature water. Once effervescence stops, wait 5 minutes or more and stir solution for about 10 seconds before administration.

• Give at least 60 mL of water after oral solution.

• Give all formulations at least 30 minutes before patient's first food or drink of the day to facilitate delivery to stomach and reduce esophageal irritation risk.

• Don't allow patient to lie down for 30 minutes after taking drug and until after first food of the day.

• Don't give at bedtime or before patient arises for the day. Failure to follow these instructions may increase the risk of esophageal adverse effects.

• Give a missed once-weekly dose on the morning after aware of omission and then return to weekly dosing on the chosen day as originally scheduled.

ACTION
Suppresses osteoclast activity on newly formed resorption surfaces, which reduces bone turnover. Bone formation exceeds resorption at remodeling sites, leading to progressive gains in bone mass.

Route	Onset	Peak	Duration
PO	Unknown	Unknown	Unknown

Half-life: More than 10 years.

ADVERSE REACTIONS

CNS: headache. **GI:** abdominal pain, nausea, dyspepsia, constipation, diarrhea, flatulence, acid regurgitation, esophageal reflux, vomiting, dysphagia, abdominal distention, gastritis, gastric ulcer, melena. **Musculoskeletal:** pain, muscle cramp.

INTERACTIONS

Drug-drug. *Antacids, calcium supplements, multivitamins and minerals, many oral drugs:* May interfere with absorption of alendronate. Instruct patient to wait at least 30 minutes after taking alendronate before taking any other drug orally.
Aspirin, NSAIDs: May increase risk of upper GI adverse reactions. Monitor patient closely.
Levothyroxine: May decrease bioavailability of alendronate. Monitor patient.
PPIs: May diminish therapeutic effects of alendronate. Monitor therapy.
Drug-food. *Any food:* May decrease absorption of drug. Advise patient to take with full glass of plain water at least 30 minutes before food, beverages, or ingestion of other drugs.

EFFECTS ON LAB TEST RESULTS

• May decrease calcium and phosphate levels.

CONTRAINDICATIONS & CAUTIONS

• Contraindicated in patients hypersensitive to drug and in those with hypocalcemia or abnormalities of the esophagus that delay esophageal emptying.
• Contraindicated in patients unable to stand or sit upright for at least 30 minutes.
• Oral solution contraindicated in patients at increased risk for aspiration.
• Drug isn't recommended for patients with CrCl of less than 35 mL/minute.
◊ **Alert:** Risk of atypical fractures of the thigh may be increased in patients treated with bisphosphonates.
• Use cautiously in patients with active upper GI problems (dysphagia, symptomatic esophageal diseases, gastritis, duodenitis, ulcers) or mild to moderate kidney insufficiency.
• Use cautiously in patients with known risk factors for osteonecrosis of the jaw (diagnosis of cancer; concomitant treatment with

chemotherapy, radiotherapy, or corticosteroids), invasive dental procedures, poor oral hygiene, and comorbid disorders, such as pre-existing dental disease, anemia, coagulopathy, or infection.
• Use effervescent tablet cautiously in patients who must restrict sodium intake, including some patients with a history of HF, HTN, or other CV diseases. Each effervescent tablet contains 603 mg of sodium, equivalent to approximately 1,532 mg of salt (NaCl).
• Drug isn't indicated for use in children.
Dialyzable drug: No.
⚠ *Overdose S&S:* Hypocalcemia, hypophosphatemia, upset stomach, heartburn, esophagitis, gastritis, ulcer.

PREGNANCY-LACTATION-REPRODUCTION

• No data exist on fetal risk in humans, but there is a theoretical risk of fetal harm. Discontinue use during pregnancy.
• It isn't known if drug appears in human milk. Use cautiously during breastfeeding.

NURSING CONSIDERATIONS

• Correct hypocalcemia and other disturbances of mineral metabolism (such as vitamin D deficiency) before therapy begins.
• Patients at risk for vitamin D deficiency (those who are chronically ill, are nursing home bound, have a GI malabsorption syndrome, or are older than age 70) may require vitamin D supplementation.
• In Paget disease, drug is indicated for patients with ALP level at least $2 \times$ ULN, for those who are symptomatic, and for those at risk for future complications from the disease.
• Monitor patient's calcium and phosphate levels throughout therapy.
• Severe musculoskeletal pain has been associated with bisphosphonate use and may occur within days, months, or years of start of therapy. When drug is stopped, symptoms may resolve partially or completely.
• Patients who develop osteonecrosis of the jaw should receive care by an oral surgeon.
• Optimal length of treatment hasn't been determined. Periodically reevaluate need for continued therapy. Patients at low risk for fracture should be considered for discontinuation after 3 to 5 years of treatment.
• *Look alike–sound alike:* Don't confuse Fosamax with Flomax.

Reactions in bold italics are *life-threatening*.

PATIENT TEACHING

• Teach about proper drug administration and handling. Stress importance of taking drug as directed to avoid adverse effects.

• Warn patient not to lie down for at least 30 minutes after taking drug to facilitate delivery to stomach and to reduce risk of esophageal irritation.

• Advise patient to report adverse reactions immediately, especially chest pain or difficulty swallowing.

• Instruct patient to take supplemental calcium and vitamin D as prescribed.

• Advise patient to discuss usage and timing of OTC medications with prescriber.

• Tell patient about benefits of weight-bearing exercises in increasing bone mass.

• If applicable, explain importance of reducing or eliminating cigarette smoking and alcohol use.

• Warn patient of fetal risk and need for drug discontinuation during pregnancy.

aliskiren hemifumarate
a-lis-KYE-ren

Rasilez ✦, Tekturna

Therapeutic class: Antihypertensives
Pharmacologic class: Renin inhibitors

AVAILABLE FORMS
Tablets: 150 mg, 300 mg

INDICATIONS & DOSAGES
➤ **HTN, alone or with other antihypertensives**
Adults and children ages 6 and older weighing 50 kg or more: 150 mg PO daily; may increase to 300 mg PO daily.

ADMINISTRATION
PO
• Don't give drug with high-fat meal; may decrease drug's effectiveness.
• Give consistently at same time each day with or without meals. However, consistent administration regarding meals is recommended.

ACTION
Decreases renin activity and inhibits conversion of angiotensin to angiotensin I, decreasing vasoconstriction and lowering BP.

Route	Onset	Peak	Duration
PO	Unknown	1–3 hr	Unknown

Half-life: 24 hours.

ADVERSE REACTIONS
CNS: headache, dizziness. **CV:** hypotension. **GI:** abdominal pain, diarrhea, dyspepsia, gastroesophageal reflux. **GU:** increased creatinine and BUN levels. **Metabolic:** *hyperkalemia,* increased CK level. **Respiratory:** cough, URI. **Skin:** rash. **Other:** hypersensitivity reaction.

INTERACTIONS
Drug-drug. ❶ *Alert: ACE inhibitors (benazepril, captopril, lisinopril, moexipril, quinapril), ARBs (azilsartan, candesartan, irbesartan, losartan, telmisartan, valsartan), other drugs that antagonize RAAS:* May increase risk of kidney impairment, hypotension, and hyperkalemia. Use together is contraindicated in patients with diabetes. Avoid use together in patients with GFR less than 60 mL/minute.
Atorvastatin: May increase aliskiren levels. Use together cautiously.
Cyclosporine, itraconazole: May increase aliskiren concentration and risk of adverse reactions. Avoid concurrent use.
Furosemide: May reduce furosemide level. Monitor patient for effectiveness.
NSAIDs: May increase risk of kidney toxicity and decrease effect of aliskiren. Periodically monitor kidney function.
Potassium-sparing diuretics, potassium supplements: May increase risk of hyperkalemia. Use together cautiously.
Drug-food. *Grapefruit juice:* May decrease aliskiren plasma level. Advise patient to avoid products containing fruit juice.
High-fat meals: May substantially decrease aliskiren plasma level. Monitor patient for effectiveness.

EFFECTS ON LAB TEST RESULTS
• May increase potassium, CK, BUN, uric acid, and serum creatinine levels.
• May decrease Hb level and hematocrit.

CONTRAINDICATIONS & CAUTIONS
• Contraindicated in patients hypersensitive to drug or its components and in those with diabetes who are receiving ARBs or ACE inhibitors.

• Contraindicated in children younger than age 2.
• Use cautiously in patients with history of angioedema, GFR of less than 30 mL/minute, HF, MI, volume depletion, history of dialysis, nephrotic syndrome, or renovascular HTN.
Dialyzable drug: No.
⚠ *Overdose S&S:* Hypotension.

PREGNANCY-LACTATION-REPRODUCTION

Boxed Warning Drugs that act on the RAAS can cause injury and death to a developing fetus. Discontinue drug as soon as possible once pregnancy is detected. ∎
• Patients of childbearing potential should avoid becoming pregnant while taking drug.
• It isn't known if drug appears in human milk. Patient should discontinue breastfeeding or discontinue drug, considering importance of drug to patient.

NURSING CONSIDERATIONS

• Monitor BP for hypotension, especially if used in combination with other antihypertensives.
• Monitor potassium level, especially in patients also taking ACE inhibitors.
• *Alert:* Rarely, angioedema may occur at any time during treatment. Discontinue drug for angioedema or anaphylaxis and don't readminister. Early emergency treatment is critical and may include intubation, antihistamines, steroids, and epinephrine.
• Monitor patient for serious skin reactions (SJS, TEN).
• Monitor kidney function. The response of patients with significant kidney disorders to use of this drug is unknown.
• Correct volume or salt depletion before giving drug or start therapy under close monitoring.
• Expect to see effect of any dose within 2 weeks.

PATIENT TEACHING

• Instruct patient not to take drug with a high-fat meal to avoid decreased drug effectiveness.
• Instruct patient to monitor BP daily, if possible, and to report low readings, dizziness, and headaches to prescriber.
• Tell patient to immediately report swelling of face or neck or difficulty breathing.
• Advise patient of need for regular lab tests to monitor for adverse effects.
• Instruct patient to discontinue drug and notify prescriber if pregnancy is detected.

allopurinol ⌧
al-oh-PURE-i-nole

Zyloprim

allopurinol sodium ⌧
Aloprim

Therapeutic class: Antigout drugs
Pharmacologic class: Xanthine oxidase inhibitors

AVAILABLE FORMS
allopurinol
Tablets (scored): 100 mg, 200 mg, 300 mg
allopurinol sodium
Injection: 500-mg vial

INDICATIONS & DOSAGES
Adjust-a-dose (for all indications): For CrCl 10 to 20 mL/minute, 200 mg PO or IV daily; for CrCl 3 to 10 mL/minute, 100 mg PO or IV daily; for CrCl less than 3 mL/minute, maximum of 100 mg PO or IV at extended intervals.
➤ **Gout or hyperuricemia**
Adults: Initially, 100 mg PO daily; then titrate in 100-mg increments weekly until serum urate concentration falls to 6 mg/dL or less. Maximum, 800 mg daily. Dosage varies with severity of disease; can be given as a single dose or divided, but doses greater than 300 mg should be divided.
➤ **Hyperuricemia caused by malignancies**
Adults: 200 to 400 mg/m^2 daily IV as a single infusion or in equally divided doses every 6, 8, or 12 hours beginning 24 to 48 hours before initiation of chemotherapy. Maximum, 600 mg daily.
Children and adolescents: Initially, 200 mg/m^2 daily IV as single infusion or in equally divided doses every 6, 8, or 12 hours beginning 24 to 48 hours before initiation of chemotherapy. Maximum, 400 mg/day. Then titrate according to uric acid level. For children ages 6 to 10, give 300 mg PO daily or in three divided doses; for children younger than age 6, give 150 mg PO daily.
➤ **To prevent uric acid nephropathy (TLS) during cancer chemotherapy**
Adults: 600 to 800 mg PO daily for 2 to 3 days, with high fluid intake.
➤ **Recurrent calcium oxalate calculi**
Adults: 200 to 300 mg PO daily in single or divided doses.

ADMINISTRATION
PO
- Give drug with or immediately after meals to minimize GI upset.
- Store drug at room temperature.
- Protect drug from light.

IV

▼ When possible, initiate therapy 24 to 48 hours before the start of chemotherapy known to cause tumor lysis.

▼ Dissolve contents of each 30-mL vial with 25 mL of sterile water for injection.

▼ Dilute solution to desired concentration of less than 6 mg/mL with NSS for injection or D_5W. Can give as a single daily infusion or in equally divided infusions at 6-, 8-, or 12-hour intervals. Rate of infusion depends on volume of infusate.

▼ Store solution at 68° to 77° F (20° to 25° C) and use within 10 hours.

▼ Don't use solution if it contains particulates or is discolored.

▼ **Incompatibilities:** Amikacin, amphotericin B, carmustine, cefotaxime, chlorpromazine, cimetidine, clindamycin, cytarabine, dacarbazine, daunorubicin, diphenhydramine, doxorubicin, doxycycline, droperidol, floxuridine, gentamicin, haloperidol, hydroxyzine, idarubicin, imipenem–cilastatin, mechlorethamine, meperidine, methylprednisolone, metoclopramide, minocycline, nalbuphine, netilmicin, ondansetron, prochlorperazine, promethazine, sodium bicarbonate (or solutions containing sodium bicarbonate), streptozocin, tobramycin, vinorelbine.

ACTION
Reduces uric acid production by inhibiting xanthine oxidase.

Route	Onset	Peak	Duration
PO	Unknown	1.5 hr (allopurinol); 4.5 hr (oxypurinol)	1–2 wk
IV	Unknown	30 min	Unknown

Half-life: Allopurinol, 1 to 2 hours; oxypurinol, 15 hours.

ADVERSE REACTIONS
GI: nausea, vomiting, diarrhea. **GU:** *kidney failure.* **Hepatic:** increased ALP and transaminase levels. **Musculoskeletal:** acute gout attack. **Skin:** rash, maculopapular rash.

INTERACTIONS
Drug-drug. *Amoxicillin, ampicillin, bendamustine, thiazide diuretics:* May increase possibility of rash. Avoid use together.

Antineoplastics: May increase potential for bone marrow suppression. Monitor patient carefully.

Azathioprine, mercaptopurine: May increase levels of these drugs. Concomitant administration of 300 to 600 mg of oral allopurinol per day requires dosage reduction according to prescribing information for azathioprine or mercaptopurine. Make subsequent dosage adjustments based on therapeutic response and appearance of toxic effects.

Capecitabine, fluorouracil: May decrease effectiveness of these drugs. Avoid use together.

Chlorpropamide: May increase hypoglycemic effect. Avoid use together.

Cyclosporine: May increase cyclosporine level. Monitor cyclosporine level and adjust dosage as necessary.

Ethacrynic acid, thiazide diuretics: May increase risk of allopurinol toxicity. Reduce allopurinol dosage, and closely monitor kidney function.

Pegloticase: May increase risk of pegloticase-related anaphylaxis. Avoid use together.

Theophylline: May increase theophylline level. Adjust theophylline dosage as needed.

Uricosurics (colchicine, probenecid): May have additive effect. May be used to therapeutic advantage.

Warfarin: May increase anticoagulant effect. Monitor INR and adjust warfarin dosage, if needed.

EFFECTS ON LAB TEST RESULTS
- May increase creatinine, uric acid, glucose, phosphorus, ALP, ALT, and AST levels.
- May decrease magnesium level.
- May increase or decrease calcium, potassium, and sodium levels.
- May increase eosinophil count.
- May decrease Hb level, hematocrit, and granulocyte and platelet counts.
- May increase or decrease WBC count.

CONTRAINDICATIONS & CAUTIONS
- Contraindicated in patients hypersensitive to drug.
- 🜲 ❶ *Alert:* To avoid risk of SCARs, avoid use of allopurinol in patients who are HLA-B*5801-positive. Patients of African, Asian (Han Chinese, Korean, Thai), and Native

Hawaiian or Pacific Islander ancestry may be at increased risk. Consider testing for HLA-B*58:1 allele in at-risk populations.

• Drug may increase risk of kidney impairment. Use cautiously in patients with kidney impairment or history of kidney stones.

• Drug may cause reversible liver toxicity and myelosuppression.

Dialyzable drug: Yes.

PREGNANCY-LACTATION-REPRODUCTION

• Drug may cause fetal harm. Use in pregnancy only if clearly needed.

• Drug appears in human milk. Use cautiously during breastfeeding.

NURSING CONSIDERATIONS

⚠ *Alert:* Rash can be followed by more severe hypersensitivity reactions (SJS, vasculitis, irreversible liver toxicity), which can be fatal. Discontinue drug at first sign of rash.

• Monitor uric acid level to evaluate drug's effectiveness.

• Monitor fluid intake and output; daily urine output of at least 2 L and maintenance of neutral or slightly alkaline urine are desirable.

• Periodically monitor CBC and hepatic and kidney function, especially at start of therapy.

• Optimal benefits when used for gout may need 2 to 6 weeks of therapy. Because acute gout attacks may occur during this time, concurrent use of colchicine may be prescribed prophylactically.

• Don't restart drug in patients who have a severe reaction.

• *Look alike–sound alike:* Don't confuse Zyloprim with ZORprin or zolpidem.

PATIENT TEACHING

• To minimize GI adverse reactions, tell patient to take drug with or immediately after meals.

⚠ *Alert:* Advise patient who is known to be HLA-B*5801-positive to avoid allopurinol.

• Encourage patient to drink plenty of fluids while taking drug unless otherwise contraindicated.

• Drug may cause drowsiness; tell patient not to drive or perform hazardous tasks requiring mental alertness until CNS effects of drug are known.

• If patient is taking drug for recurrent calcium oxalate stones, advise patient also to reduce dietary intake of animal protein, sodium,

refined sugars, oxalate-rich foods, and calcium.

• Tell patient to stop drug at first sign of rash, which may precede severe hypersensitivity or other adverse reactions. Rash is more common in patients taking diuretics and in those with kidney disorders. Tell patient to report all adverse reactions.

• Teach patient importance of continuing drug even if asymptomatic.

---

almotriptan malate
al-moh-TRIP-tan

Therapeutic class: Antimigraine drugs
Pharmacologic class: Serotonin 5-HT$_1$ receptor agonists

AVAILABLE FORMS
Tablets: 6.25 mg, 12.5 mg

INDICATIONS & DOSAGES

➤ **Acute migraine with or without aura**
Adults and adolescents ages 12 and older:
6.25 mg or 12.5 mg PO, with one additional dose after 2 hours if headache is unresolved or recurs. The 12.5-mg dose tends to be more effective in adults. Maximum, two doses (total of 25 mg) within 24 hours.

Adjust-a-dose: For patients with liver or kidney impairment, initially 6.25 mg, with maximum daily dose of 12.5 mg.

ADMINISTRATION
PO

• Give drug without regard for food.

• Give only one repeat dose within 24 hours, no sooner than 2 hours after first dose.

ACTION

May act as an agonist at serotonin receptors, which constricts extracerebral intracranial blood vessels, inhibits neuropeptide release, and reduces pain transmission in trigeminal pathways.

Route	Onset	Peak	Duration
PO	1–3 hr	1–3 hr	Unknown

Half-life: 3 to 4 hours.

ADVERSE REACTIONS

CNS: paresthesia, headache, dizziness, somnolence. **EENT:** dry mouth. **GI:** nausea, vomiting.

Reactions in bold italics are *life-threatening*.

INTERACTIONS

Drug-drug. *Antiemetics (5-HT₃ antagonists), antipsychotics, metolazone, methylene blue, metoclopramide, opioid analgesics, tramadol:* May increase serotonergic effects and serotonin syndrome. Monitor therapy.

CYP3A4 inhibitors (such as ketoconazole): May increase almotriptan level. Monitor patient for potential adverse reaction. May need to reduce dosage. Avoid use together in patients with kidney or liver impairment.

Ergot-containing drugs, serotonin 5-HT₁ᵦ/₁ᴅ agonists: May cause additive effects. Contraindicated for use within 24 hours of almotriptan.

MAO inhibitors: May increase risk of serotonin syndrome. Avoid use together.

SSNRIs, SSRIs: May cause additive serotonin effects, resulting in weakness, hyperreflexia, or incoordination. Monitor patient closely if given together.

EFFECTS ON LAB TEST RESULTS

None reported.

CONTRAINDICATIONS & CAUTIONS

• Contraindicated in patients hypersensitive to drug.

• Contraindicated in patients with angina pectoris, history of MI, silent ischemia, coronary artery vasospasm, Prinzmetal variant angina, or other CV disease; uncontrolled HTN; PVD, including ischemic bowel disease; cerebrovascular disease (history of stroke or TIA); and hemiplegic or basilar migraine.

• Use cautiously in patients with kidney or liver impairment and known hypersensitivity to sulfonamide.

• Use cautiously in patients with risk factors for CAD (obesity, diabetes, smoking, hypercholesterolemia, HTN, females after menopause or males older than age 40, family history of CAD). CV evaluation to exclude CV disease is recommended.

• Drug isn't intended for migraine prophylaxis or treatment of cluster headaches.

• Safety of treating more than 4 migraines in a 30-day period hasn't been established.

Dialyzable drug: Unknown.

⚠ **Overdose S&S:** HTN, more serious CV symptoms.

PREGNANCY-LACTATION-REPRODUCTION

• There are no adequate studies of use during pregnancy. Use during pregnancy only if potential benefit justifies fetal risk.

• It isn't known if drug appears in human milk. Use cautiously during breastfeeding.

NURSING CONSIDERATIONS

• Overuse of acute migraine drugs for 10 or more days per month may lead to migraine-like daily headaches or a marked increase in frequency of migraine attacks (medication overuse headache). Withdrawal of the overused drugs may be necessary.

• Consider obtaining ECG with first dose of drug in patients with positive CAD risk factors.

• Assess patients with signs and symptoms of angina after almotriptan dose for CAD and Prinzmetal or variant angina, including ECG monitoring.

• Monitor patient for vasospastic events, such as peripheral ischemia (Raynaud syndrome), blindness, partial vision loss, or GI ischemia (abdominal pain, bloody diarrhea). Consider further evaluation for signs or symptoms suggesting decreased arterial flow after triptan use.

❸ **Alert:** Combining triptans with SSRIs or SSNRIs may cause serotonin syndrome. Monitor patient for signs and symptoms (restlessness, hallucinations, loss of coordination, rapid heartbeat, rapid changes in BP, increased body temperature, overactive reflexes, nausea, vomiting, diarrhea). Serotonin syndrome is more common when starting or increasing the dose of a triptan, SSRI, or SSNRI.

PATIENT TEACHING

• Teach about proper drug administration and handling.

• Advise patient to take drug only when having a migraine; explain that drug isn't taken on a regular schedule.

• Inform patient that other commonly prescribed migraine drugs can interact with almotriptan.

• Caution patient to report chest or throat tightness, pain, or heaviness; weakness; slurred speech; or shortness of breath.

• Instruct patient to notify the prescriber if pregnant or planning to become pregnant or breastfeed.

• Warn patient that drug may cause dizziness, somnolence, visual changes, and other CNS symptoms that can interfere with driving or operating machinery. Advise patient to avoid hazardous activities until drug's effects are known.

alogliptin benzoate
AL-oh-GLIP-tin

Nesina

Therapeutic class: Antidiabetics
Pharmacologic class: DPP-4 inhibitors

AVAILABLE FORMS
Tablets: 6.25 mg, 12.5 mg, 25 mg

INDICATIONS & DOSAGES
➤ **Adjunct to diet and exercise to improve glycemic control in adults with type 2 diabetes**
Adults: 25 mg PO daily.
Adjust-a-dose: For patients with CrCl of 30 to less than 60 mL/minute, 12.5 mg PO daily. For patients with CrCl of 15 to less than 30 mL/minute and for those with CrCl of less than 15 mL/minute or requiring hemodialysis, 6.25 mg PO daily.

ADMINISTRATION
PO
- Give drug without regard for food.
- Don't split tablets.
- Store at room temperature.

ACTION
Slows inactivation of incretin, which increases blood concentrations of incretin and reduces fasting or postprandial glucose in patients with type 2 diabetes.

Route	Onset	Peak	Duration
PO	Unknown	1–2 hr	Unknown

Half-life: 21 hours.

ADVERSE REACTIONS
CNS: headache. **EENT:** nasopharyngitis.
GU: decreased CrCl. **Metabolic:** *hypoglycemia.*
Respiratory: URI.

INTERACTIONS
Drug-drug. *ACE inhibitors:* May enhance adverse effects of ACE inhibitor, especially angioedema. Monitor therapy.
Insulin, sulfonylureas: May enhance hypoglycemic activity. Adjust dosage of insulin or sulfonylurea.
MAO inhibitors, salicylates, SSRIs: May increase hypoglycemic effect. Monitor therapy.

Thiazide diuretics: May diminish hypoglycemic effect. Monitor therapy.

EFFECTS ON LAB TEST RESULTS
- May increase ALT level.
- May decrease CrCl.

CONTRAINDICATIONS & CAUTIONS
- Contraindicated in patients hypersensitive to drug or its components and in those with type 1 diabetes or ketoacidosis.
- Use cautiously in patients with liver disease or injury, history of pancreatitis, gallstones, history of alcoholism, kidney disease, or history of angioedema with another DPP-4 inhibitor.
- **Alert:** Use cautiously in patients with a history of HF or kidney disease. Drug may increase risk of HF in these patients.
- Safety and effectiveness in children haven't been established.
Dialyzable drug: No.

PREGNANCY-LACTATION-REPRODUCTION
- Use cautiously during pregnancy and only if clearly needed.
- It isn't known if drug appears in human milk. Use cautiously during breastfeeding.

NURSING CONSIDERATIONS
- **Alert:** Monitor patient for signs and symptoms of HF (shortness of breath, orthopnea, tiredness, weakness, fatigue, weight gain, peripheral or abdominal edema). Drug discontinuation and treatment with other antidiabetics may be needed.
- Assess kidney function at baseline and periodically during treatment.
- Monitor patient for hypersensitivity reactions, including SJS. Stop drug immediately if hypersensitivity is suspected.
- Monitor for development of blisters or skin erosions; if present, consider referral to dermatologist for diagnosis and treatment.
- Monitor for signs and symptoms (rare) of acute pancreatitis (severe abdominal pain that may radiate to back, with or without vomiting).
- Assess LFTs before treatment. If liver injury is suspected during treatment (fatigue, anorexia, abdominal discomfort, dark urine, jaundice), obtain LFTs. If elevated LFT values are present, persist, or worsen, withhold drug and determine probable cause. Restart drug only if cause isn't alogliptin-related.

- Monitor blood glucose level if patient is receiving concurrent antidiabetics; adjust dosages of these medications if needed.

⟲ *Alert:* Drug may cause joint pain that can be severe and disabling. Report severe and persistent joint pain to prescriber; drug may need to be discontinued.

PATIENT TEACHING

⟲ *Alert:* Instruct patient to immediately report signs and symptoms of HF. Patient shouldn't stop drug without first discussing with prescriber.

- Instruct patient to monitor blood glucose level carefully.
- Advise patient to seek medical attention for hypersensitivity symptoms.
- Caution patient to seek medical attention for signs and symptoms of pancreatitis (severe abdominal pain that may radiate to back, with or without vomiting) or liver injury (fatigue, anorexia, abdominal discomfort, dark urine, jaundice).

SAFETY ALERT!

alpelisib ⚕
al-pe-LIS-ib

Piqray, Vijoice

Therapeutic class: Antineoplastics
Pharmacologic class: Kinase inhibitors

AVAILABLE FORMS

Tablets: 50 mg, 125 mg, 200 mg
Tablets ⓒ: 50 mg, 150 mg, 200 mg

INDICATIONS & DOSAGES

➤ **In combination with fulvestrant for hormone receptor (HR)–positive, HER2-negative, *PIK3CA*-mutated, advanced, or metastatic breast cancer following progression on or after an endocrine-based regimen** ⚕
Adult women after menopause and adult men: 300 mg PO once daily. Continue treatment until disease progression or unacceptable toxicity occurs. When given with alpelisib, recommended fulvestrant dosage is 500 mg IM on days 1, 15, and 29, and once monthly thereafter.
Adjust-a-dose: Refer to manufacturer's instructions for toxicity-related dosage adjustments of alpelisib and fulvestrant.

➤ **Severe manifestations of PIK3CA-related overgrowth spectrum requiring systemic therapy (Vijoice)** ⚕
Adults: 250 mg PO once daily until disease progression or unacceptable toxicity occurs.
Children ages 6 to younger than 18: Initially, 50 mg PO once daily. May increase after 24 weeks to 125 mg for response optimization. Continue until disease progression or unacceptable toxicity occurs.
Children ages 2 to younger than 6: 50 mg PO once daily until disease progression or unacceptable toxicity occurs.
Adjust-a-dose: Refer to manufacturer's instructions for toxicity-related dosage adjustments.

ADMINISTRATION
PO

⟲ *Alert:* Hazardous drug; use safe handling and disposal precautions.

- Give at approximately the same time each day with food.
- Have patient swallow tablets whole; don't crush or cut tablets. Don't give tablets that are broken, cracked, or otherwise not intact.
- For patients unable to swallow Vijoice tablets, place tablets in glass with 60 to 120 mL of water and let stand for 5 minutes then crush tablets with a spoon and stir until an oral suspension is obtained. Give immediately or discard if not given within 60 minutes. After giving, place 30 to 45 mL in same glass, stir with the same spoon to re-suspend any remaining particles and give to patient. Repeat rinse step if particles remain to ensure full dose.
- If a dose is missed, give within 9 hours after the usual time. If dose is more than 9 hours late, skip dose for that day. The next day, give drug at the usual time.
- If patient vomits after taking dose, don't give an additional dose on that day; resume dosing schedule the next day at usual time.
- Store at 68° to 77° F (20° to 25° C).

ACTION

A phosphatidylinositol-3-kinase (PI3K) inhibitor that increases estrogen receptor transcription in breast cancer cells. The combination of alpelisib and fulvestrant provides greater antitumor activity compared with either treatment alone. For PROS, inhibition of the PI3K pathway results in prevention or

---

improvement of organ abnormalities associated with PROS.

Route	Onset	Peak	Duration
PO	Unknown	2–4 hr	Unknown

Half-life: 8 to 9 hours.

ADVERSE REACTIONS

CNS: fatigue, fever, dysgeusia, headache. **CV:** peripheral edema. **GI:** diarrhea, stomatitis, vomiting, nausea, abdominal pain, dyspepsia, decreased appetite. **GU:** UTI, *AKI.* **Hematologic:** *lymphocytopenia,* anemia, prolonged PTT, *thrombocytopenia.* **Hepatic:** increased lipase and transaminase levels, hypoalbuminemia, increased bilirubin. **Metabolic:** weight loss, hyperglycemia, increased HbA$_{1c}$, hypophosphatemia, hyponatremia, increased GGT level, *hypocalcemia, hypoglycemia, hypokalemia, hyperkalemia, hypomagnesemia,* hyperlipidemia. **Musculoskeletal:** osteonecrosis of jaw. **Respiratory:** pneumonitis. **Skin:** rash, alopecia, pruritus, eczema, dry skin, cellulitis, *SCARs (SJS, TEN, erythema multiforme [EM]).* **Other:** mucosal dryness, mucosal inflammation, hypersensitivity reaction.

INTERACTIONS

Drug-drug. *BCRP inhibitors (estrone, omeprazole, saquinavir, verapamil):* May increase alpelisib level and risk of toxicity. Avoid use together. If use together can't be avoided, closely monitor patient for adverse reactions.
CYP2C9 substrates (bosentan, candesartan, celecoxib, diclofenac, glipizide, indomethacin, losartan, phenobarbital, phenytoin, rosuvastatin, warfarin): May decrease substrate plasma concentration and therapeutic effects. Monitor patient closely.
CYP3A4 inducers (carbamazepine, efavirenz, phenytoin, rifampin): May decrease alpelisib level and therapeutic effect. Avoid use together.

EFFECTS ON LAB TEST RESULTS

• May increase bilirubin, creatinine, GGT, ALT, AST, cholesterol, triglyceride, HbA$_{1c}$, and lipase levels.
• May decrease calcium, sodium, albumin, phosphate, and magnesium levels.
• May increase or decrease glucose and potassium levels.
• May prolong PTT.

• May increase eosinophil counts.
• May decrease Hb level and lymphocyte, neutrophil, leukocyte, and platelet counts.

CONTRAINDICATIONS & CAUTIONS

• Contraindicated in patients with severe hypersensitivity to drug or its components; severe reactions (anaphylaxis, anaphylactic shock, angioedema) have been reported.
• SCARs have been reported, including SJS, EM, TEN, and DRESS syndrome.
• Severe hyperglycemia, including ketoacidosis, has been reported.
• Use cautiously in patients with diabetes. The safety of drug in patients with type 1 and uncontrolled type 2 diabetes hasn't been established. Patients with a history of diabetes may require intensified diabetic treatment.
• Drug may increase risk of severe pneumonitis, including acute interstitial pneumonitis and ILD. Consider a diagnosis of noninfectious pneumonitis in patients with nonspecific respiratory signs and symptoms (hypoxia, cough, dyspnea, interstitial infiltrates on radiologic exams) and in whom infectious, neoplastic, and other causes have been excluded by appropriate means.
• Severe diarrhea and colitis have occurred with use of drug in oncology settings.
• Safety and effectiveness of Piqray in children haven't been established.
Dialyzable drug: Unknown.
⚠ *Overdose S&S:* Hyperglycemia, nausea, asthenia, rash.

PREGNANCY-LACTATION-REPRODUCTION

• Drug can cause fetal harm. Advise patient of potential fetal risk if used during pregnancy.
• Advise patients of childbearing potential to use effective contraception during therapy and for 1 week after final dose.
• Advise adult males with partners of childbearing potential to use condoms and effective contraception during treatment and for 1 week after final dose.
• Drug may impair fertility in males and females of reproductive potential.
• It isn't known if drug appears in human milk. Because of the potential for serious adverse reactions in an infant, patients shouldn't breastfeed during treatment and for 1 week after final dose.

NURSING CONSIDERATIONS
• Verify pregnancy status before starting therapy.
• Monitor patient for hypersensitivity reactions (dyspnea, flushing, rash, fever, tachycardia). Permanently discontinue drug for severe hypersensitivity reactions.
• Monitor patient for SCARs, including SJS, EM, TEN, and DRESS syndrome. If signs or symptoms of SCARs occur (severe rash; worsening rash; reddened or peeling skin; blistering of lips, eyes, mouth, or skin; flulike symptoms; fever), interrupt therapy and consult a dermatologist. If SCAR is confirmed, permanently discontinue drug. If SCAR isn't confirmed, dosage modifications and management of rash may be required, per manufacturer's instructions.
• Monitor patient for hyperglycemia, including ketoacidosis. If hyperglycemia occurs, therapy interruption, dosage reduction, or drug discontinuation may be required, per manufacturer's instructions.
• Before starting drug, obtain fasting plasma glucose (FPG) and HbA$_{1c}$ levels and optimize blood glucose level. After initiating drug, monitor blood glucose level, FPG, or both at least once every week for first 2 weeks, then at least once every 4 weeks and as clinically indicated. Monitor HbA$_{1c}$ every 3 months and as clinically indicated.
• If hyperglycemia occurs during therapy, monitor blood glucose or FPG level as clinically indicated and at least twice weekly until blood glucose or FPG level decreases to normal. During treatment with an antidiabetic, continue monitoring blood glucose or FPG level at least once a week for 8 weeks, then once every 2 weeks and as clinically indicated.
• Monitor patient for new or worsening respiratory signs and symptoms or for development of pneumonitis. If signs or symptoms occur, immediately interrupt therapy and evaluate for pneumonitis. Permanently discontinue drug in patients with confirmed pneumonitis.
• Monitor for severe diarrhea, including dehydration and AKI, and colitis, including abdominal pain and mucus or blood in stool. If diarrhea occurs, therapy interruption, dosage reduction, or drug discontinuation may be required. Treat diarrhea as clinically indicated. A patient with colitis may require additional treatment, such as enteric-acting or systemic steroids.

PATIENT TEACHING
• Instruct patient in safe drug administration.
• Teach patient to report all adverse reactions.
• Inform patient to immediately report signs and symptoms of hypersensitivity.
• Warn that severe skin reactions can occur. Teach about and tell patient to immediately report signs and symptoms of SCARs.
• Warn patient that hyperglycemia may develop. Advise patient to closely monitor blood glucose level during therapy and to report signs and symptoms of hyperglycemia (increased thirst, dry mouth, frequent urination, increased appetite with weight loss).
• Inform patient to immediately report respiratory problems, as drug can increase risk of pneumonitis.
• Advise that drug may cause diarrhea, which may be severe. Inform patient to start antidiarrheal treatment, increase fluid intake, and notify prescriber if diarrhea occurs.
• Warn patient of childbearing potential that drug can cause fetal harm and that pregnancy testing will be performed before therapy begins. Advise patient to report known or suspected pregnancy immediately.
• Advise patient of childbearing potential and adult male patient with partner of childbearing potential to use effective contraception during therapy and for 1 week after final dose.
• Caution patient not to breastfeed during treatment and for 1 week after final dose.
• Inform male or female patient of reproductive potential that drug may impair fertility.

SAFETY ALERT!

ALPRAZolam
al-PRAH-zoe-lam

Apo-Alpraz✤, Xanax, Xanax TS✤, Xanax XR

Therapeutic class: Anxiolytics
Pharmacologic class: Benzodiazepines
Controlled substance schedule: IV

AVAILABLE FORMS
Oral solution: 1 mg/mL (concentrate)
Tablets: 0.25 mg, 0.5 mg, 1 mg, 2 mg
Tablets (extended-release) ⓓ: 0.5 mg, 1 mg, 2 mg, 3 mg
Tablets (ODTs): 0.25 mg, 0.5 mg, 1 mg, 2 mg

INDICATIONS & DOSAGES

Adjust-a-dose (for all indications): For older adults and patients with debilitation or advanced liver disease, usual first dose is 0.25 mg PO b.i.d. or t.i.d. For extended-release tablets, 0.5 mg PO once daily.

To discontinue drug or reduce dosage, decrease by no more than 0.5 mg every 3 days. Some patients may benefit from more gradual discontinuation.

Boxed Warning To reduce risk of withdrawal reactions, use a gradual taper to discontinue or reduce dosage. If withdrawal reactions develop, consider pausing the taper or increasing the dosage to the previous tapered dosage level. Subsequently decrease the dosage more slowly. ■

➤ **Anxiety**
Adults: Usual first dose, 0.25 to 0.5 mg (immediate-release) PO t.i.d. Maximum, 4 mg daily in divided doses.

➤ **Panic disorders with or without agoraphobia**
Adults: 0.5 mg PO t.i.d., increased at intervals of 3 to 4 days in increments of no more than 1 mg/day. Maximum, 10 mg daily in divided doses. For extended-release tablets, initially 0.5 to 1 mg PO once daily. Increase by no more than 1 mg/day every 3 to 4 days. Maximum daily dose, 10 mg.

ADMINISTRATION

PO
• Don't break or crush extended-release tablets.
• Mix oral solution with liquids or semisolid food (water, juices, carbonated beverages, applesauce, pudding). Use only calibrated dropper provided with this product. Give drug immediately after mixing.
• Use dry hands to remove ODTs from bottle. Place tablet on top of the tongue and allow to disintegrate; water isn't necessary. Discard cotton from inside bottle.
• Patients treated with divided doses of immediate-release tablets can be switched to extended-release tablets at same total daily dose. Patients should take extended-release tablets in the morning.

ACTION

Unknown. Probably potentiates the effects of GABA, depresses the CNS, and suppresses the spread of seizure activity.

Route	Onset	Peak	Duration
PO	Unknown	1–2 hr	Unknown
PO (extended-release)	Unknown	10 hr	Unknown

Half-life: Immediate-release, 6.3 to 26.9 hours; extended-release, 10.7 to 15.8 hours.

ADVERSE REACTIONS

CNS: insomnia, irritability, dizziness, lightheadedness, headache, anxiety, confusion, drowsiness, sedation, somnolence, difficulty speaking, impaired coordination, memory impairment, fatigue, depression, mental impairment, ataxia, dyskinesia, hypoesthesia, lethargy, vertigo, malaise, tremor, nervousness, restlessness, agitation, nightmare, akathisia, disorientation, derealization, depersonalization, talkativeness, disinhibition, disturbance in attention, equilibrium disturbance, weakness, abnormal involuntary movement. **CV:** palpitations, chest pain, hypotension. **EENT:** blurred vision, dry mouth, increased or decreased salivation, allergic rhinitis, nasal congestion. **GI:** diarrhea, constipation, nausea, increased appetite, anorexia, vomiting, dyspepsia, abdominal pain. **GU:** dysmenorrhea, sexual dysfunction, difficulty urinating, incontinence. **Metabolic:** increased or decreased weight. **Musculoskeletal:** arthralgia, myalgia, limb pain, back pain, muscle cramps, muscle twitch, muscle tone disorders. **Respiratory:** dyspnea, hyperventilation. **Skin:** rash, pruritus, increased sweating, dermatitis, allergic reaction. **Other:** injury, dependence, warm feeling, increased or decreased libido.

INTERACTIONS

Drug-drug. *Anticonvulsants, antidepressants, antihistamines, barbiturates, benzodiazepines, general anesthetics, narcotics, phenothiazines, protease inhibitors:* May increase CNS depressant effects. Avoid use together.
CYP3A inducers (carbamazepine, phenytoin, rifampin): May induce alprazolam metabolism and may reduce therapeutic effects. Increase dosage as needed.
Strong CYP3A inhibitors (atazanavir, clarithromycin, itraconazole, ketoconazole, miconazole, saquinavir, telithromycin): May increase alprazolam level, CNS depression, and psychomotor impairment. Use together is contraindicated.

Reactions in bold italics are ***life-threatening***.

Digoxin: May increase digoxin level, especially in older adults. Monitor level and adjust digoxin dosage, if necessary.

Methadone: May significantly increase risk of CNS depression. Avoid use together, if possible, or monitor patient closely.

Moderate or weak CYP3A inhibitors (cimetidine, fluoxetine, fluvoxamine, hormonal contraceptives): May increase alprazolam level. Use together cautiously; consider alprazolam dosage reduction.

Boxed Warning *Opioids:* May cause slow or difficult breathing, sedation, and death. Avoid use together. If use together can't be avoided, limit dose and duration of each drug to the minimum needed for desired effect. ■

Ritonavir: May increase alprazolam level with short-term use; after 10 days, alprazolam exposure isn't affected. Reduce alprazolam dosage when initiating ritonavir. May increase dosage after 10 to 14 days of concomitant ritonavir dosing.

TCAs (amitriptyline, doxepin, imipramine, nortriptyline): May increase adverse effects. Monitor patient closely.

Drug-herb. *Kava, valerian root:* May increase sedation. Discourage use together.

St. John's wort: May decrease drug level. Discourage use together.

Drug-food. *Grapefruit juice:* May increase drug level. Discourage use together.

Drug-lifestyle. *Alcohol and cannabis use:* May cause additive CNS effects. Discourage use together.

Smoking: May decrease effectiveness of drug. Monitor patient closely.

EFFECTS ON LAB TEST RESULTS

• May increase liver enzyme levels.

CONTRAINDICATIONS & CAUTIONS

Boxed Warning Benzodiazepine use exposes patient to risks of abuse, misuse, and addiction, which can lead to overdose or death. Assess each patient's risk of abuse, misuse, and addiction before prescribing and periodically during therapy. ■

Boxed Warning Abrupt discontinuation or rapid dosage reduction of benzodiazepines after continued use may precipitate acute withdrawal reactions, which can be life-threatening. To reduce risk of withdrawal reactions, gradually taper drug to discontinue or reduce dosage. ■

• Contraindicated in patients hypersensitive to drug or other benzodiazepines and in those with acute angle-closure glaucoma.

Boxed Warning *Opioid class warning:* Opioids should only be prescribed with benzodiazepines or other CNS depressants when alternative treatment options are inadequate, not expected to provide adequate analgesia, haven't been tolerated, or aren't expected to be tolerated. ■

• Use cautiously in patients with liver, kidney, or lung disease or history of substance abuse.

• Use cautiously in older adults.

• Safety and effectiveness in children haven't been established.

Dialyzable drug: No.

⚠ *Overdose S&S:* Somnolence, confusion, impaired coordination, diminished reflexes, coma.

PREGNANCY-LACTATION-REPRODUCTION

• Drug may cause fetal harm. Neonates exposed during late pregnancy may experience sedation, respiratory depression, and neonatal withdrawal. Use during pregnancy isn't recommended.

• Encourage patients who are pregnant to enroll in the National Pregnancy Registry for Psychiatric Medications (866-961-2388 or https://womensmentalhealth.org/research/pregnancyregistry/).

• Drug appears in human milk. Use during breastfeeding isn't recommended.

NURSING CONSIDERATIONS

Boxed Warning Monitor patient also taking an opioid for signs and symptoms of respiratory depression and sedation. ■

• Closely monitor a patient with impaired respiratory function.

• The optimum duration of therapy is unknown.

• Give smallest effective dose to prevent ataxia or oversedation, especially in an older adult or a patient who is debilitated.

• Periodically monitor liver and kidney function in a patient receiving repeated or prolonged therapy.

🔆 *Alert:* Panic disorder is associated with major depressive disorders and increased reports of suicide among patients who are untreated. Monitor a patient with depression for suicidality.

• Consider giving same total daily dose of immediate-release formulation in divided doses more frequently in a patient being treated for panic disorder who experiences early-morning anxiety or anxiety symptoms between doses.

• *Look alike–sound alike:* Don't confuse alprazolam with alprostadil or lorazepam. Don't confuse Xanax with Fanapt.

PATIENT TEACHING

Boxed Warning Caution patient or caregiver of patient taking an opioid with a benzodiazepine, CNS depressant, or alcohol to seek immediate medical attention if patient experiences dizziness, light-headedness, extreme sleepiness, slowed or difficult breathing, or unresponsiveness. ■

Boxed Warning Caution patient that benzodiazepines, even at recommended doses, increase risk of abuse, misuse, and addiction, which can lead to overdose and death, especially when used in combination with other drugs (opioid analgesics), alcohol, or illicit substances. ■

Boxed Warning Instruct patient to seek emergency medical help for signs and symptoms of benzodiazepine abuse, misuse, and addiction (abdominal pain, amnesia, anorexia, anxiety, aggression, ataxia, blurred vision, confusion, depression, disinhibition, disorientation, dizziness, euphoria, impaired concentration and memory, indigestion, irritability, muscle pain, slurred speech, tremors, vertigo, delirium, paranoia, suicidal thoughts or actions, seizures, difficulty breathing, coma). Teach patient proper disposal of unused drug. Advise patient not to take drug at a higher dose, more frequently, or for longer than prescribed. ■

Boxed Warning Tell patient that continued use of drug for several days to weeks may lead to physical dependence and that abrupt discontinuation or rapid dosage reduction may precipitate acute withdrawal reactions (unusual movements, responses, or expressions; seizures; sudden and severe mental or nervous system changes; depression; seeing or hearing things that others don't; homicidal thoughts; extreme increase in activity or talking; losing touch with reality; suicidal thoughts or actions), which can be life-threatening. Instruct patient that discontinuation or dosage reduction may require a slow taper. ■

Boxed Warning Stress the possibility of developing protracted withdrawal syndrome

(anxiety; trouble remembering, learning, or concentrating; depression; problems sleeping; feeling like insects are crawling under the skin; weakness; shaking; muscle twitching; burning or prickling feeling in the hands, arms, legs, or feet; ringing in the ears), with symptoms lasting weeks to more than 12 months. ■

• Warn patient to avoid hazardous activities that require alertness and good coordination (driving, operating machinery) until effects of drug are known.

• Tell patient to avoid use of alcohol while taking drug.

• Advise patient that smoking may decrease drug's effectiveness.

• Teach about proper drug administration and handling.

• Warn patient not to use drug during pregnancy or breastfeeding and to report pregnancy to prescriber.

SAFETY ALERT!

alteplase
al-ti-PLAZE

Activase, Cathflo Activase

Therapeutic class: Thrombolytics
Pharmacologic class: Enzymes

AVAILABLE FORMS
Cathflo Activase injection: 2-mg vials
Injection: 50-mg, 100-mg vials

INDICATIONS & DOSAGES
➤ **Lysis of thrombi obstructing coronary arteries in acute MI (Activase)**
Adults weighing 65 kg or more (3-hour infusion): 6 to 10 mg IV bolus over first 1 to 2 minutes, then 50 to 54 mg IV infusion over remainder of first hour (for a total of 60 mg the first hour); then 20 mg/hour infused for 2 hours. Maximum total dose, 100 mg.
Adults weighing less than 65 kg (3-hour infusion): 0.075 mg/kg IV bolus over 1 to 2 minutes, followed by 0.675 mg/kg for rest of first hour; then 0.25 mg/kg/hour infused for 2 hours. Maximum total dose, 100 mg.
Adults weighing more than 67 kg (accelerated infusion): 15 mg IV bolus over 1 to 2 minutes, followed by 50 mg infused over the next 30 minutes; then 35 mg infused over the next hour. Maximum total dose, 100 mg.

Adults weighing 67 kg or less (accelerated infusion: 15 mg IV bolus over 1 to 2 minutes, followed by 0.75 mg/kg (not to exceed 50 mg) infused over the next 30 minutes; then 0.5 mg/kg (not to exceed 35 mg) infused over the next hour. Maximum total dose, 100 mg.

➤ **To manage acute massive PE (Activase)**
Adults: 100 mg by IV infusion over 2 hours. Begin parenteral anticoagulation at end of infusion when PTT or thrombin time returns to twice normal or less. Don't exceed 100-mg dose. Higher doses may increase risk of intracranial bleeding.

➤ **Acute ischemic stroke within 3 hours of symptom onset (Activase)**
Adults: 0.9 mg/kg by IV infusion over 1 hour with 10% of total dose given as an initial IV bolus over 1 minute. Maximum total dose, 90 mg.

➤ **To restore function to CVADs (Cathflo Activase)**
Adults and children older than age 2: For patients weighing 30 kg or more, instill 2 mg in 2 mL sterile water into catheter. For patients weighing less than 30 kg, instill 110% of the internal lumen volume of catheter, not to exceed 2 mg in 2 mL sterile water. After 30 minutes dwell time, assess catheter function by aspirating blood. If function is restored, aspirate 4 to 5 mL of blood in patients weighing 10 kg or more or 3 mL in patients weighing less than 10 kg to remove drug and residual clot, and gently irrigate catheter with NSS. If catheter function isn't restored after 120 minutes, instill a second dose.

➤ **Acute ischemic stroke presenting 3 to 4.5 hours after symptom onset (Activase)** ◆
Adults: 0.9 mg/kg by IV infusion over 1 hour, with 10% of total dose given as an initial IV bolus over 1 minute. Maximum total dose, 90 mg.

ADMINISTRATION

IV

▼ Immediately before use, reconstitute solution with unpreserved sterile water for injection. Check manufacturer's labeling for specific reconstitution information.
▼ Don't use 50-mg vial if vacuum isn't present; 100-mg vials don't have a vacuum.
▼ Slight foaming is common. Let it settle before giving drug. Solution should be colorless or pale yellow.
▼ Drug may be given reconstituted (at 1 mg/mL) or diluted with an equal volume

of NSS or D_5W to yield 0.5 mg/mL, using polyvinyl chloride bags or glass vials.
▼ Directly infuse the 100-mg dose from the vial after reconstitution using transfer device, per manufacturer's instructions.
▼ Give drug using a controlled infusion device.
▼ Discard any unused drug after 8 hours.
Cathflo Activase
▼ Assess the cause of catheter dysfunction before using drug. Possible causes of occlusion include catheter malposition, mechanical failure, constriction by a suture, and lipid deposits or drug precipitates in the catheter lumen. Don't try to suction catheter to prevent damaging the vessel wall or collapsing a soft-walled catheter.
▼ Reconstitute Cathflo Activase with 2.2 mL sterile water to yield 1 mg/mL. Dissolve completely to produce a colorless to pale yellow solution. Don't shake.
▼ Don't use excessive pressure while instilling drug into catheter; doing so could rupture the catheter or expel a clot into circulation.
▼ Solution remains stable for up to 8 hours at room temperature.
▼ **Incompatibilities:** Bivalirudin, dobutamine, dopamine, heparin, morphine, nitroglycerin. Consult detailed reference for other specific incompatibilities.

ACTION

Converts plasminogen to plasmin by directly cleaving peptide bonds at two sites, causing fibrinolysis.

Route	Onset	Peak	Duration
IV	Unknown	Unknown	Unknown

Half-life: Less than 5 minutes.

ADVERSE REACTIONS

CNS: *cerebral hemorrhage.* **CV:** *VTE.* **GI:** *bleeding.* **GU:** *bleeding.* **Hematologic:** *spontaneous bleeding.* **Skin:** ecchymosis. **Other:** *sepsis (Cathflo Activase),* bleeding at puncture sites, hypersensitivity reactions.

INTERACTIONS

Drug-drug. *ACE inhibitors:* May increase risk of angioedema. Monitor patient closely. *Aspirin, clopidogrel, dipyridamole, drugs affecting platelet activity, heparin, warfarin, anticoagulants:* May increase risk of bleeding. Monitor patient carefully.

Nitroglycerin: May decrease alteplase serum concentration. Monitor therapy.

EFFECTS ON LAB TEST RESULTS
• May alter coagulation and fibrinolytic test results.

CONTRAINDICATIONS & CAUTIONS
• Contraindicated in patients hypersensitive to drug or its components.
• Activase therapy for acute MI or PE is contraindicated in patients with active internal bleeding; history of stroke; recent intracranial or intraspinal surgery or trauma; intracranial neoplasm, AV malformation, or aneurysm; known bleeding diathesis; or severe uncontrolled HTN.
• Activase therapy for acute ischemic stroke is contraindicated in patients with evidence of intracranial hemorrhage; suspected subarachnoid hemorrhage; recent (within 3 months) intracranial or intraspinal surgery; serious head trauma or previous stroke; history of intracranial hemorrhage; uncontrolled HTN at time of treatment; seizure at onset of stroke; active internal bleeding; intracranial neoplasm, AV malformation, or aneurysm; bleeding diathesis (which may include current use of oral anticoagulants, INR greater than 1.7, PT longer than 15 seconds, platelet count less than 100,000/mm³, current use of direct thrombin inhibitors or direct factor Xa inhibitors with elevated sensitive lab tests, or heparin administration within the previous 48 hours with prolonged PTT at presentation).
• In patients with acute ischemic stroke without recent use of oral anticoagulants or heparin, may initiate Activase before available coagulation study results. Discontinue infusion if either pretreatment INR is greater than 1.7 or PTT is prolonged.
• Patients with severe neurologic deficits (National Institutes of Health Stroke Scale greater than 22) or who have major early infarct signs on a CT scan may have increased risk of bleeding.
• Use cautiously in patients who have had a recent major surgery or procedure or who have other conditions in which bleeding constitutes a significant hazard or would be difficult to control because of its location.
• Use cautiously in patients with previous puncture of a noncompressible vessel; concomitant oral anticoagulant therapy; organ biopsy; trauma (including cardiopulmonary

resuscitation); GI or GU bleeding; cerebrovascular disease; systolic pressure of 175 mm Hg or higher or diastolic pressure of 110 mm Hg or higher; mitral stenosis, atrial fibrillation, or other conditions that may lead to left heart thrombus; acute pericarditis or subacute bacterial endocarditis; hemostatic defects caused by liver or kidney impairment; septic thrombophlebitis; or diabetic hemorrhagic retinopathy.
• Use cautiously in patients receiving anticoagulants.
• Use cautiously in patients ages 75 and older.
• Use of thrombolytics can increase risk of thromboembolic events in patients at risk for left heart thrombus, such as patients with mitral stenosis or atrial fibrillation. Drug hasn't been shown to adequately treat underlying DVT in patients with PE. Consider possible risk of reembolization due to lysis of underlying deep venous thrombi in these patients.
• Safety and effectiveness in children haven't been established.
Dialyzable drug: Unknown.

PREGNANCY-LACTATION-REPRODUCTION
• Information related to use during pregnancy is limited; most guidelines consider pregnancy a relative contraindication. Drug shouldn't be withheld during pregnancy in life-threatening situations but should be avoided if safer alternatives are available.
• It isn't known if drug appears in human milk. Use cautiously during breastfeeding.

NURSING CONSIDERATIONS
⊙ *Alert:* When used for acute ischemic stroke, give drug within 3 hours after symptoms occur and only when intracranial bleeding has been ruled out.
• Drug may be given to menstruating patients.
• To recannulize occluded coronary arteries and improve heart function, begin treatment as soon as possible after symptoms start.
• Anticoagulant and antiplatelet therapy is commonly started during or after treatment, to decrease risk of another thrombosis.
• Monitor vital signs and neurologic status carefully. Keep patient on strict bed rest.
• Coronary thrombolysis is linked with arrhythmias caused by reperfusion of ischemic myocardium. Such arrhythmias don't differ from those commonly linked with MI. Have antiarrhythmics readily available, and carefully monitor ECG.

Reactions in bold italics are *life-threatening*.

• Avoid invasive procedures, IM injections, and nonessential handling of patient during thrombolytic therapy. Perform essential venipunctures carefully. Closely monitor for signs of internal bleeding, and frequently check all puncture sites. Bleeding is the most common adverse effect and may occur internally and at external puncture sites.

• If an arterial puncture is necessary during Activase infusion, use an arm vessel that can be manually compressed. Apply pressure for at least 30 minutes followed by a pressure dressing. Regularly check site for bleeding.

• If uncontrollable bleeding occurs, stop infusion (and parenteral anticoagulant) and notify prescriber.

• Don't use the "tPA" abbreviation when ordering this drug. "tPA" has been mistaken for TNKase (tenecteplase), TPN, and TXA (error-prone).

• *Look alike–sound alike:* Don't confuse alteplase with Altace. Don't confuse Activase with Cathflo Activase or TNKase.

PATIENT TEACHING
• Explain use and administration of drug to patient and family.

• Tell patient to promptly report adverse reactions and to immediately report signs and symptoms of bleeding, urinary problems, abdominal pain, nausea, vomiting, confusion, severe headache, one-sided weakness, trouble speaking or thinking, visual disturbances, dizziness, passing out, chest pain, or catheter-site pain.

---

amantadine hydrochloride
a-MAN-ta-deen

Gocovri, Osmolex ER

Therapeutic class: Antivirals
Pharmacologic class: Synthetic cyclic primary amines

AVAILABLE FORMS
Capsules: 100 mg
Capsules (extended-release) ⓓ: 68.5 mg, 137 mg
Oral syrup: 50 mg/5 mL
Tablets: 100 mg
Tablets (extended-release) ⓓ: 129 mg, 193 mg

INDICATIONS & DOSAGES
Adjust-a-dose (for all indications): Lower dosages are recommended for patients with kidney impairment. Refer to the manufacturer's product information.

➤ **Parkinson disease**
Adults: Initially, if used as monotherapy, 100 mg PO b.i.d. In patients with serious illness or in those already receiving high doses of other antiparkinsonian drugs, begin dose at 100 mg PO once daily. Increase to 100 mg b.i.d. if needed after at least 1 week. Some patients may benefit from 400 mg daily in divided doses. For extended-release tablet (Osmolex ER), 129 mg PO once daily; increase weekly to maximum daily dose of 322 mg. For extended-release capsule Y (Gocovri), 137 mg PO once daily; increase in 1 week to maximum daily dose of 274 mg.

➤ **Adjunct to levodopa–carbidopa in patients with Parkinson disease experiencing "off" episodes (Gocovri)**
Adults: 137 mg PO once daily. Increase in 1 week to maximum daily dose of 274 mg.

➤ **Drug-induced extrapyramidal reactions**
Adults: 100 mg PO b.i.d. May increase to 300 mg daily in divided doses. For extended-release tablet (Osmolex ER), 129 mg PO once daily; increase weekly to maximum daily dose of 322 mg.

➤ **Influenza A prophylaxis or treatment**
Adults and children: Refer to manufacturer's instructions of immediate use formulation for recommended dosages. Use for this indication isn't recommended by the Centers for Disease Control and Prevention and Infections Diseases Society of America due to high resistance rates.

ADMINISTRATION
PO
• Give drug without regard for food.
• Give extended-release tablets in the morning; give extended-release capsules at bedtime.
• Don't crush, break, or allow patient to chew extended-release forms. May sprinkle entire contents of capsule on a small amount (tsp) of soft food, such as applesauce, and administer immediately.

ACTION
May exert its antiparkinsonian effect by causing the release of dopamine in the substantia nigra.

Route	Onset	Peak	Duration
PO	Unknown	2–4 hr	Unknown
PO (extended-release)	Unknown	5–12 hr	Unknown

Half-life: About 10 to 25 hours; with kidney dysfunction, up to 10 days.

ADVERSE REACTIONS

CNS: dizziness, delusions, illusion, paranoia, insomnia, irritability, light-headedness, depression, fatigue, confusion, hallucinations, anxiety, ataxia, headache, nervousness, dream abnormalities, agitation, somnolence, dystonia, syncope, apathy, *suicidality.* **CV:** peripheral edema, orthostatic hypotension. **EENT:** blurred vision, cataract, dry eye, dry nose, dry mouth. **GI:** nausea, anorexia, constipation, vomiting, diarrhea. **GU:** UTI, BPH. **Musculoskeletal:** joint swelling, muscle spasms. **Respiratory:** cough. **Skin:** livedo reticularis, contusion, dyschromia. **Other:** falls.

INTERACTIONS

Drug-drug. *Alkalinizing agents, quinidine, sulfamethoxazole–trimethoprim, thiazide diuretics, triamterene:* May increase amantadine level, increasing the risk of toxicity. Use together cautiously.
Anticholinergics: May increase anticholinergic effects. Use together cautiously; reduce dosage of anticholinergic before starting amantadine.
Antipsychotics (clozapine, quetiapine): May decrease therapeutic effect of both drugs. Avoid use together. If use together is unavoidable, decrease antipsychotic dose or consider a non-dopamine antagonist (pimavanserin).
Live attenuated influenza vaccines: May interfere with efficacy of live attenuated influenza vaccines. Use together cautiously.
Urine acidifying drugs (ascorbic acid, potassium acid phosphate): May increase excretion of amantadine. Monitor efficacy.
Drug-lifestyle. *Alcohol use:* May increase CNS effects, including dizziness, confusion, and orthostatic hypotension. Discourage use together.

EFFECTS ON LAB TEST RESULTS

• May increase CK, BUN, creatinine, ALP, LDH, bilirubin, GGT, AST, and ALT levels.

CONTRAINDICATIONS & CAUTIONS

• Contraindicated in patients hypersensitive to drug and in those with chronic kidney failure with dialysis.

• Use cautiously in older adults and in patients with seizure disorders, psychosis, impulse control disorders, HF, peripheral edema, liver disease, psychiatric disorders, substance abuse, eczematoid rash, kidney impairment, orthostatic hypotension, or CV disease.
• Avoid use in patients with untreated angle-closure glaucoma.
• Drug may increase risk of compulsive behaviors and loss of impulse control.
Dialyzable drug: No.
⚠ *Overdose S&S:* Arrhythmias, HTN, tachycardia, pulmonary edema, respiratory distress, increased BUN level, decreased CrCl, kidney insufficiency, insomnia, anxiety, aggressive behavior, hypertonia, hyperkinesia, tremor, confusion, disorientation, depersonalization, fear, delirium, hallucinations, psychotic reactions, lethargy, somnolence, coma, seizures, hyperthermia.

PREGNANCY-LACTATION-REPRODUCTION

• Drug may cause fetal harm. Use during pregnancy isn't recommended.
• Drug appears in human milk. Use during breastfeeding isn't recommended.

NURSING CONSIDERATIONS

• Note that a patient with Parkinson disease who doesn't respond to anticholinergics may respond to this drug.
• Monitor an older adult for mental status changes because older adults are more susceptible to adverse neurologic effects.
⟳ *Alert:* Monitor all patients for suicidality. Suicidal ideation and attempts may occur in any patient, regardless of psychiatric history.
⟳ *Alert:* Sporadic cases of NMS-like symptoms have been reported with dosage reduction or drug withdrawal. Symptoms include fever, muscular rigidity, altered consciousness, and autonomic instability. Observe patient carefully with abrupt dosage reduction or drug discontinuation.
• Discontinue drug gradually. Abrupt discontinuation can cause an increase in signs and symptoms of Parkinson disease as well as delirium, agitation, delusions, hallucinations, paranoid reaction, stupor, anxiety, depression, and slurred speech.
• Monitor liver and kidney function test results.
• *Look alike–sound alike:* Don't confuse amantadine with amiodarone or rimantadine.

PATIENT TEACHING

🕲 *Alert:* Tell patient to take drug exactly as prescribed because not doing so may result in serious adverse reactions or death.

• Advise patient that drug must be stopped gradually. Instruct patient to not stop taking drug or change dose before consulting prescriber.

• Caution patient to report increases in Parkinson disease signs or symptoms or adverse effects.

• Stress importance of taking extended-release capsules at bedtime or extended release tablets in the morning.

• If insomnia occurs, tell patient to take drug several hours before bedtime.

• Warn patient not to stand or change positions too quickly if dizziness occurs when standing up.

• Instruct patient to notify prescriber of adverse reactions, especially dizziness, depression, anxiety, nausea, and urine retention.

• Caution patient to avoid activities that require mental alertness until effects of drug are known.

• Inform patient and caregiver of risk of intense urges (gambling, sexual urges, spending money, binge eating) while taking drug; instruct them to report these urges if they occur.

• Encourage patient with Parkinson disease to gradually increase physical activity as symptoms improve.

• Advise patient to avoid alcohol while taking drug.

SAFETY ALERT!

ambrisentan
am-bree-SEN-tan

Letairis, Volibris✤

Therapeutic class: Vasodilators
Pharmacologic class: Endothelin-receptor antagonists

AVAILABLE FORMS
Tablets 🚫: 5 mg, 10 mg

INDICATIONS & DOSAGES

➤ **PAH (WHO Group 1) to improve exercise ability and delay clinical worsening; in combination with tadalafil to reduce risks of disease progression and hospitalization for worsening PAH, and to improve exercise ability**

Adults: 5 mg PO once daily with or without tadalafil 20 mg once daily; at 4-week intervals, may increase ambrisentan to 10 mg PO once daily or tadalafil to 40 mg once daily, if tolerated.

ADMINISTRATION
PO

🕲 *Alert:* Hazardous drug; use safe handling and disposal precautions.

• Give drug without regard for food.

• Have patient swallow tablets whole; don't crush or cut tablets.

ACTION

Blocks endothelin-1 receptors on vascular endothelin and smooth muscle. Stimulation of these receptors in smooth muscle cells is associated with vasoconstriction and PAH.

Route	Onset	Peak	Duration
PO	Rapid	2 hr	Unknown

Half-life: 9 hours.

ADVERSE REACTIONS

CNS: headache. **CV:** peripheral edema, flushing. **EENT:** nasal congestion, sinusitis. **GI:** dyspepsia. **Hematologic:** anemia. **Hepatic:** liver impairment. **Respiratory:** cough, bronchitis.

INTERACTIONS

Drug-drug. *Cyclosporine:* May increase ambrisentan level. Use together cautiously. Limit ambrisentan dosage to 5 mg daily.

EFFECTS ON LAB TEST RESULTS

• May increase AST, ALT, and bilirubin levels.

• May decrease Hb level and hematocrit.

CONTRAINDICATIONS & CAUTIONS

• Contraindicated in patients hypersensitive to drug or its components and in those with idiopathic pulmonary fibrosis (IPF), including IPF patients with pulmonary HTN.

• Use cautiously in patients with Child-Pugh class A liver impairment. Not recommended in patients with Child-Pugh class B or C liver impairment.

• Use cautiously in those with kidney impairment; drug hasn't been studied in those with severe kidney impairment.

🕲 *Alert:* Patients who develop acute pulmonary edema during initial treatment may have pulmonary veno-occlusive disease. Discontinue drug if pulmonary veno-occlusive disease is confirmed.

Dialyzable drug: Unknown.

⚠ *Overdose S&S:* Headache, flushing, dizziness, nausea, nasal congestion, hypotension.

PREGNANCY-LACTATION-REPRODUCTION

Boxed Warning Contraindicated during pregnancy. May cause birth defects. ■

Boxed Warning Must exclude pregnancy before starting therapy. Obtain monthly pregnancy tests during treatment and for 1 month after final dose. ■

Boxed Warning Patients of childbearing potential must use one highly effective form of contraception (intrauterine device, contraceptive implant, or tubal sterilization) or a combination of methods (hormonal method with a barrier method or two barrier methods) during treatment and for 1 month after treatment ends. If vasectomy is the chosen method of contraception, a hormonal or barrier method must also be used. ■

Boxed Warning Because of risk of embryofetal toxicity, ambrisentan is available to females only through the Ambrisentan REMS Program. Only registered prescribers and pharmacies may prescribe and dispense ambrisentan and only to patients enrolled in and meeting all the conditions of REMS at www.ambrisentanrems.us.com or 1-888-417-3172. ■

• It isn't known if drug appears in human milk. Patient should discontinue breastfeeding or discontinue drug, considering importance of drug to patient.

• Drug may adversely affect spermatogenesis.

NURSING CONSIDERATIONS

• Treat a patient of childbearing potential only after negative pregnancy test.

• Assess Hb level at initiation, at 1 month, and periodically thereafter. Use isn't recommended in a patient with significant anemia.

• Monitor patient for fluid retention; diuretic or fluid management may be needed.

PATIENT TEACHING

Boxed Warning Explain that monthly pregnancy testing is required during therapy. Instruct patient to immediately report suspected pregnancy to prescriber. ■

⊘ *Alert:* Counsel patient of childbearing potential on contraceptive use.

• Tell patient that monthly blood tests are necessary to monitor for adverse effects.

• Teach about proper drug administration and handling.

⊘ *Alert:* Teach patient immediately to notify prescriber of signs or symptoms of liver injury (anorexia, nausea, vomiting, fever, malaise, fatigue, right upper quadrant abdominal discomfort, itching, jaundice).

• Tell patient to report edema and weight gain.

• Inform male patient of potential for decreased sperm count.

amikacin sulfate
am-i-KAY-sin

Therapeutic class: Antibiotics
Pharmacologic class: Aminoglycosides

AVAILABLE FORMS
Injection: 250 mg/mL vial

INDICATIONS & DOSAGES

Adjust-a-dose (for all indications): Adjust dosage to avoid peak drug level above 35 mcg/mL and trough drug level above 10 mcg/mL. For adults with impaired kidney function, initially, 7.5 mg/kg IM or IV. Subsequent doses and frequency determined by amikacin levels and kidney function studies, according to manufacturer's instructions. For adults receiving hemodialysis, monitor drug levels and adjust dosage accordingly.

➤ **Serious infections caused by sensitive strains of** *Pseudomonas aeruginosa, Escherichia coli, Proteus, Klebsiella, Staphylococcus, Providencia, Enterobacter, Serratia,* **or** *Acinetobacter*

Adults, children, and older infants: Maximum dosage, 15 mg/kg/day IM or IV infusion, in divided doses every 8 to 12 hours, for 7 to 10 days. Don't exceed 1.5 g/day.
Neonates: Initially, loading dose of 10 mg/kg IV; then 7.5 mg/kg every 12 hours for 7 to 10 days.

➤ **Uncomplicated UTI caused by organisms not susceptible to less-toxic drugs**
Adults: 250 mg IM or IV b.i.d.

ADMINISTRATION

IV

▼ Obtain specimen for culture and sensitivity tests before giving first dose. Begin therapy while awaiting results.

▼ For adults, dilute IV drug in 100 to 200 mL of D₅W or NSS. For children, amount of fluid depends on the ordered dose.

▼ Other compatible fluids include D₅ with 0.2% or 0.45% sodium chloride, lactated Ringer, Normosol M or R in D₅W, and Plasma-Lyte 56 or 148 injection in D₅W.

▼ In adults and children, infuse over 30 to 60 minutes. In infants, infuse over 1 to 2 hours.

▼ Don't premix with other drugs.

▼ Inspect solution for particulate matter and discoloration before administration.

▼ After infusion, flush line with NSS or D₅W.

▼ Refer to manufacturer's instructions for stability and storage after dilution in D₅W, NSS, and other solutions.

▼ May store vials at room temperature.

▼ **Incompatibilities:** None listed by manufacturer. Consult drug compatibility reference for more information.

IM

● Obtain specimen for culture and sensitivity tests before giving first dose. Begin therapy while awaiting results.

ACTION

Inhibits protein synthesis by binding directly to the 30S ribosomal subunit; bactericidal.

Route	Onset	Peak	Duration
IV	Immediate	30 min	8–12 hr
IM	Unknown	1 hr	8–12 hr

Half-life: Adults, 2 hours; patients with severe kidney damage, 17 to 150 hours.

ADVERSE REACTIONS

CNS: *neuromuscular blockade.* **EENT:** ototoxicity. **GU:** azotemia, *kidney toxicity,* increase in urinary excretion of casts. **Respiratory:** *apnea, respiratory paralysis.*

INTERACTIONS

Drug-drug. Boxed Warning *Acyclovir, amphotericin B, bacitracin, cisplatin, colistin, paromomycin, polymyxin B, vancomycin, other aminoglycosides:* May increase kidney toxicity. Avoid use together. Monitor kidney function test results. ■

Cephalosporins, penicillins: May inactivate each other in vitro. Don't mix.

Boxed Warning *General anesthetics:* May increase neuromuscular blockade. Monitor patient for increased effects. ■

Boxed Warning *IV loop diuretics (ethacrynic acid, furosemide):* May increase ototoxicity. Avoid use together. Monitor patient's hearing. ■

Boxed Warning *Neuromuscular blockers:* May increase effects of nondepolarizing muscle relaxants, including prolonged respiratory depression. Use together only when necessary and expect to reduce dosage of nondepolarizing muscle relaxant. ■

NSAIDs (indomethacin): May increase amikacin level in premature infants. Avoid administering together or monitor amikacin level if unavoidable.

EFFECTS ON LAB TEST RESULTS

● May increase BUN and creatinine levels.

CONTRAINDICATIONS & CAUTIONS

● Contraindicated in patients hypersensitive to drug or other aminoglycosides.

● Use cautiously in patients with sulfite sensitivity.

● Use cautiously in patients with impaired kidney function, hypocalcemia, neuromuscular disorders (myasthenia gravis, parkinsonism), or hearing impairment; neonates and infants; and older adults.

● Drug can cause superinfection, such as CDAD, which can be severe and can occur more than 2 months after therapy ends.

Dialyzable drug: Yes.

⚠ *Overdose S&S:* Kidney toxicity, ototoxicity, neurotoxicity.

PREGNANCY-LACTATION-REPRODUCTION

● There are no well-controlled studies during pregnancy. Other aminoglycosides can cause fetal harm, so not recommended for use during pregnancy. If used during pregnancy or if patient becomes pregnant while taking drug, apprise patient of potential fetal hazard.

● It isn't known if drug appears in human milk. Patient should discontinue breastfeeding or discontinue drug, considering importance of drug to patient.

NURSING CONSIDERATIONS

Boxed Warning Periodically monitor serum amikacin peak and trough levels during therapy. Peak drug levels greater than 35 mcg/mL and trough levels greater than 10 mcg/mL may be linked to a higher risk of toxicity. ■

• Obtain blood for peak level 1 hour after IM injection and 30 minutes to 1 hour after IV infusion ends; for trough level, draw blood just before next dose. Don't collect blood in a heparinized tube; heparin is incompatible with aminoglycosides.

Boxed Warning Due to increased risk of ototoxicity, evaluate patient's hearing before and during therapy if patient will be receiving the drug for longer than 2 weeks. Notify prescriber if patient has tinnitus, vertigo, or hearing loss. ■

Boxed Warning Weigh patient and review kidney function studies before and periodically during therapy. ■

• Correct dehydration before therapy because of increased risk of toxicity.

Boxed Warning Due to increased risk of kidney toxicity, monitor kidney function: urine output, specific gravity, urinalysis, BUN and creatinine levels, and CrCl. Report evidence of declining kidney function to prescriber. Safe use for longer than 14 days hasn't been established. ■

• Watch for signs and symptoms of superinfection (especially of upper respiratory tract), such as continued fever, chills, and increased pulse rate.

• Monitor for CDAD.

Boxed Warning Neuromuscular blockade and respiratory paralysis have been reported after aminoglycoside administration, especially in patients receiving anesthetics, neuromuscular blockers, or massive transfusions of citrate-anticoagulated blood. If blockade occurs, calcium salts may reverse these phenomena, but mechanical ventilation may be necessary. Monitor patient closely. ■

• Therapy usually continues for 7 to 10 days. If no response occurs after 3 to 5 days, stop therapy and obtain new specimens for culture and sensitivity testing.

• *Look alike–sound alike:* Don't confuse amikacin with anakinra.

PATIENT TEACHING

• Instruct patient to promptly report all adverse reactions, especially changes in urine, weight gain, edema, hearing impairment, fever, diarrhea, and abdominal pain.

• Explain that CDAD may occur up to a few months after taking antibiotics. Instruct patient to immediately report abdominal pain,

cramps, or very loose, watery, or bloody stools.

• Warn patient about risks to fetus if drug is taken during pregnancy and instruct patient to immediately report possible pregnancy to prescriber.

• Encourage patient to maintain adequate fluid intake.

---

aMILoride hydrochloride
a-MILL-oh-ride

Midamor ✤

Therapeutic class: Diuretics
Pharmacologic class: Potassium-sparing diuretics

AVAILABLE FORMS
Tablets: 5 mg

INDICATIONS & DOSAGES
➤ **To counteract hypokalemia induced by thiazide or other potassium-wasting diuretics in patients with HTN or HF**
Adults: 5 mg PO daily in addition to patient's antihypertensive or diuretic. May increase to 10 mg daily if needed. If hypokalemia persists with 10 mg, may increase to 15 mg, then 20 mg with careful monitoring of electrolyte levels.

ADMINISTRATION
PO
• Give drug with food to minimize GI upset.
• Store at room temperature.

ACTION
Inhibits sodium reabsorption and potassium excretion in the distal tubules.

Route	Onset	Peak	Duration
PO	2 hr	3–4 hr	24 hr

Half-life: 6 to 9 hours.

ADVERSE REACTIONS
CNS: dizziness, fatigue, headache, weakness, *encephalopathy.* **GI:** abdominal pain, anorexia, appetite changes, constipation, diarrhea, nausea, vomiting, gas pain. **GU:** erectile dysfunction. **Metabolic:** *hyperkalemia.* **Musculoskeletal:** muscle cramps. **Respiratory:** cough, dyspnea.

Reactions in bold italics are *life-threatening*.

INTERACTIONS

Drug-drug. *ACE inhibitors, ARBs, canagliflozin, cyclosporine, eplerenone, indomethacin, potassium supplements, tacrolimus, tolvaptan:* May cause hyperkalemia. Use together cautiously. Monitor potassium level closely.

Digoxin: May affect digoxin clearance and decrease inotropic effects. Monitor digoxin level.

Lithium: May decrease lithium clearance, increasing risk of lithium toxicity. Avoid use together.

NSAIDs: May decrease diuretic effectiveness and cause severe hyperkalemia. Avoid use together.

Spironolactone, triamterene, other potassium-sparing drugs: May cause hyperkalemia. Use together is contraindicated.

Drug-food. *Foods high in potassium (bananas, oranges), salt substitutes containing potassium:* May cause hyperkalemia. Advise patient to choose diet carefully and to use low-potassium salt substitutes.

EFFECTS ON LAB TEST RESULTS

• May increase BUN and potassium levels.
• May decrease pH, chloride, and sodium levels.
• May decrease Hb level and neutrophil count.

CONTRAINDICATIONS & CAUTIONS

• Contraindicated in patients hypersensitive to drug, in those with potassium level greater than 5.5 mEq/L, and in those with anuria, acute or chronic kidney insufficiency, or diabetic nephropathy.
• Use cautiously in patients with diabetes, cardiopulmonary disease, or severe liver insufficiency.
• Use cautiously in older adults or patients who are debilitated.
• Safety and effectiveness in children haven't been established.
Dializable drug: Unknown.
⚠ *Overdose S&S:* Dehydration, electrolyte imbalances.

PREGNANCY-LACTATION-REPRODUCTION

• Use during pregnancy only if clearly needed.
• It isn't known if drug appears in human milk. Patient should discontinue breastfeeding or discontinue drug, considering importance of drug to patient.

NURSING CONSIDERATIONS

Boxed Warning Carefully monitor potassium level because of the risk of hyperkalemia, especially in a patient with kidney impairment or diabetes and in an older adult. Monitor potassium level when drug is initiated, when diuretic dosages are adjusted, and during an illness that could affect kidney function. Immediately alert prescriber if potassium level exceeds 5.5 mEq/L; expect to stop drug. ■
• Drug may cause severe hyperkalemia after glucose tolerance testing in a patient with diabetes; stop drug at least 3 days before testing.
• Monitor serum electrolyte levels and kidney function.
• Monitor acid-base balance in a patient who is severely ill and at risk for respiratory or metabolic acidosis.
• *Look alike–sound alike:* Don't confuse amiloride with amiodarone, amlodipine, or inamrinone.

PATIENT TEACHING

• Instruct patient to take drug with food to minimize GI upset.
• Advise patient to avoid sudden posture changes and to rise slowly to avoid dizziness.
• Caution patient not to perform hazardous activities if adverse CNS reactions occur.
• To prevent serious hyperkalemia, warn patient to avoid eating potassium-rich foods, potassium-containing salt substitutes, and potassium supplements.
• Advise patient to report signs of hyperkalemia (tingling, muscle weakness, muscle cramps, fatigue, limb paralysis).
• Instruct patient to check with prescriber before taking new prescription or OTC drugs.

SAFETY ALERT!

amiodarone hydrochloride
am-ee-OH-dah-rohn

Nexterone, Pacerone

Therapeutic class: Antiarrhythmics
Pharmacologic class: Benzofuran derivatives

AVAILABLE FORMS

Injection: 50 mg/mL vial; 150 mg/100 mL, 360 mg/200 mL, 450 mg/250 mL, 900 mg/500 mL premixed bag
Tablets: 100 mg, 200 mg, 300 mg, 400 mg

INDICATIONS & DOSAGES

Boxed Warning Due to toxicity, amiodarone is intended for use only in patients with life-threatening arrythmias unresponsive to adequate doses of other antiarrhythmics or when alternative drugs can't be tolerated. ■

➤ **Prevention of recurrent life-threatening ventricular arrhythmias, such as ventricular fibrillation or hemodynamically unstable ventricular tachycardia**

Adults: Give loading dose of 800 to 1,600 mg PO daily or divided into two equal doses daily for 1 to 3 weeks until first therapeutic response occurs; then 600 to 800 mg PO daily for 1 month, followed by maintenance dose of 400 mg PO daily or, for patients with severe GI intolerance, 200 mg PO b.i.d. Determine long-term maintenance dose according to antiarrhythmic effect.

Or, give loading dose of 150 mg IV over 10 minutes (15 mg/minute); then 360 mg IV over next 6 hours (1 mg/minute), followed by 540 mg IV over next 18 hours (0.5 mg/minute). After first 24 hours, continue with maintenance IV infusion of 720 mg/24 hours (0.5 mg/minute).

Maintenance infusion can continue cautiously for 2 to 3 weeks. To convert to oral form from IV (based on a 720-mg/day infusion): If IV infusion has been for less than 1 week, initial dose is 800 to 1,600 mg PO daily; if IV infusion has been from 1 to 3 weeks, initial dose is 600 to 800 mg PO daily; if IV infusion has been more than 3 weeks, initial dose is 400 mg PO daily.

If breakthrough episodes of ventricular fibrillation or hemodynamically unstable ventricular tachycardia occur, may give supplemental infusions of 150 mg IV over 10 minutes.

ADMINISTRATION

Boxed Warning Drug can exacerbate arrythmias and should be initiated in a clinical setting where continuous ECG monitoring and cardiac resuscitation are available. ■

PO

• Divide oral loading dose into two or three equal doses and give with meals to decrease GI intolerance. Give maintenance dose once daily or divide into two doses with meals to decrease GI intolerance.

IV

▼ Give drug IV only if continuous ECG and electrophysiologic monitoring are available.

▼ Mix first dose of 150 mg in 100 mL of D_5W solution followed by 360 mg in 200 mL of D_5W solution for maintenance infusion.

▼ If infusion will last 2 hours or longer, mix solution in glass or polyolefin bottles.

▼ If concentration is 2 mg/mL or more, give drug through a CVC. If possible, use a dedicated line.

▼ Drug may be a vesicant; ensure proper needle or catheter placement before and during IV infusion and avoid extravasation.

▼ Use an in-line filter.

▼ Continuously monitor patient's cardiac status. If hypotension occurs, reduce infusion rate.

▼ IV amiodarone leaches out plasticizers from IV tubing and adsorbs to polyvinyl chloride (PVC) tubing, which can adversely affect male reproductive tract development in fetuses, infants, and toddlers when used at concentrations or flow rates outside of recommendations.

▼ **Incompatibilities:** Aminophylline, ampicillin sodium–sulbactam sodium, bivalirudin, cefazolin sodium, ceftazidime, digoxin, furosemide, heparin sodium, imipenem–cilastatin sodium, magnesium sulfate, micafungin, nitroprusside sodium, NSS, piperacillin sodium, piperacillin–tazobactam sodium, quinidine gluconate, sodium bicarbonate, sodium phosphates, potassium phosphates. Consult drug compatibility reference for other drugs.

ACTION

Inhibits adrenergic stimulation and blocks sodium and potassium channels, leading to prolongation of action potential duration.

Route	Onset	Peak	Duration
PO	Variable	3–7 hr	Variable
IV	Unknown	Unknown	Variable

Half-life: Oral, 15 to 142 days; IV single dose mean range, 9 to 36 days.

ADVERSE REACTIONS

CNS: fatigue, malaise, tremor, peripheral neuropathy, ataxia, paresthesia, insomnia, sleep disturbances, headache, dizziness, lack of coordination, abnormal taste, abnormal smell. **CV:** hypotension, *asystole*, atrial fibrillation, *bradycardia*, *ventricular tachycardia*,

---

Reactions in bold italics are *life-threatening*.

cardiogenic shock, arrhythmias, HF, heart block, sinus arrest, edema, flushing. **EENT:** asymptomatic corneal microdeposits, visual disturbances, optic neuropathy or neuritis resulting in visual impairment, abnormal salivation. **GI:** nausea, vomiting, anorexia, constipation, abdominal pain. **Hematologic:** *coagulation abnormalities.* **Hepatic:** *liver failure,* liver dysfunction. **Metabolic:** hypothyroidism, hyperthyroidism. **Respiratory:** *severe pulmonary toxicity.* **Skin:** photosensitivity, blue-gray skin. **Other:** decreased libido.

INTERACTIONS

Drug-drug. *Antiarrhythmics:* May reduce liver or kidney clearance of certain antiarrhythmics, especially flecainide and procainamide. Use of amiodarone with other antiarrhythmics, especially mexiletine, propafenone, disopyramide, and procainamide, may induce torsades de pointes. Avoid use together.

Azole antifungals, disopyramide, pimozide: May increase risk of arrhythmias, including torsades de pointes. Avoid use together.

Beta blockers, calcium channel blockers: May potentiate bradycardia, sinus arrest, and AV block; may increase hypotensive effect. Use together cautiously.

Cimetidine: May increase amiodarone level. Use together cautiously.

Cyclosporine: May increase cyclosporine level, resulting in increased serum creatinine level and kidney toxicity. Monitor cyclosporine level and kidney function tests.

Dabigatran: May increase bleeding risk. Monitor patient closely.

Digoxin: May increase digoxin level 70% to 100%. Monitor digoxin level closely, and reduce digoxin dosage by half or stop drug completely when starting amiodarone therapy.

Fentanyl: May cause hypotension, bradycardia, and decreased cardiac output. Monitor patient closely.

Fluoroquinolones: May increase risk of arrhythmias, including torsades de pointes. Avoid use together.

HMG-CoA reductase inhibitors (lovastatin, simvastatin): May cause myopathy or rhabdomyolysis. Lovastatin dosage shouldn't exceed 40 mg daily. Simvastatin dosage shouldn't exceed 20 mg daily. Lower the dosages of other drugs in this class. Monitor patient carefully.

Loratadine, trazodone: May cause prolonged QT interval and torsades de pointes. Monitor closely.

Macrolide antibiotics (azithromycin, clarithromycin, erythromycin): May cause additive prolongation of the QT interval. Use with caution.

Phenytoin: May decrease phenytoin metabolism and increase phenytoin level. May decrease amiodarone level. Monitor phenytoin level and adjust dosages of drugs if needed.

Protease inhibitors (amprenavir, atazanavir, lopinavir–ritonavir, nelfinavir, ritonavir, saquinavir): May increase risk of amiodarone toxicity. Use of ritonavir or nelfinavir with amiodarone is contraindicated. Use other protease inhibitors cautiously.

Quinidine: May increase quinidine level, causing life-threatening cardiac arrhythmias. Avoid use together, or monitor patient closely if use together can't be avoided. Adjust quinidine dosage as needed.

Rifamycins: May decrease amiodarone level. Monitor patient closely.

Theophylline: May increase theophylline level and cause toxicity. Monitor theophylline level.

Warfarin: May increase anticoagulant response, with the potential for serious or fatal bleeding. Decrease warfarin dosage 33% to 50% when starting amiodarone. Monitor patient closely.

Drug-herb. *St. John's wort:* May decrease amiodarone level. Discourage use together.

Drug-food. *Grapefruit juice:* May inhibit CYP3A4 metabolism of drug in the intestinal mucosa, causing increased level and risk of toxicity. Discourage use together.

Drug-lifestyle. *Sun exposure:* May cause photosensitivity reaction. Advise patient to take precautions.

EFFECTS ON LAB TEST RESULTS

- May increase ALP, ALT, AST, GGT, inactive reverse T_3, and T_4 levels.
- May decrease T_3 level.
- May prolong PT and increase INR.

CONTRAINDICATIONS & CAUTIONS

- Contraindicated in patients hypersensitive to drug or to iodine.
- Contraindicated in those with cardiogenic shock, second- or third-degree AV block, or severe SA node disease resulting in

---

bradycardia (unless an artificial pacemaker is present) and in those for whom bradycardia has caused syncope.

• Use cautiously in patients receiving other antiarrhythmics. Upon starting amiodarone, attempt to gradually discontinue prior antiarrhythmics.

• Use cautiously in patients with pulmonary, liver, or thyroid disease.

Boxed Warning Drug may cause lung and liver toxicity, which can be fatal. ∎

⊘ *Alert:* Avoid use in patients with Wolff-Parkinson-White syndrome and preexcited atrial fibrillation or flutter.

• Safety and effectiveness in children haven't been established. Life-threatening gasping syndrome may occur in neonates given IV solutions containing benzyl alcohol.

Dialyzable drug: No.

⚠ *Overdose S&S:* AV block, bradycardia, hypotension, cardiogenic shock, liver toxicity.

PREGNANCY-LACTATION-REPRODUCTION

• Drug may cause fetal harm. Use during pregnancy only to treat life-threatening or refractory arrhythmias.

• Drug appears in human milk. Breastfeeding isn't recommended during amiodarone therapy.

NURSING CONSIDERATIONS

• Be aware of the high risk of adverse reactions.

• Obtain baseline thyroid function tests.

⊘ *Alert:* Drug may cause hyperthyroidism or hypothyroidism. Hyperthyroidism can result in fatal thyrotoxicosis or arrhythmia. If hyperthyroidism or hypothyroidism occurs, reduce dosage or discontinue drug. Thyroid nodules and thyroid cancer have been reported. Use cautiously in patients with thyroid disease. Monitor thyroid function during treatment, particularly in older adults and patients with underlying thyroid dysfunction.

Boxed Warning Drug is highly toxic. Watch carefully for lung toxicity. Obtain baseline chest X-ray and pulmonary function tests. Reassess history, physical exam, and chest X-ray every 3 to 6 months and as clinically indicated. ∎

• Watch for evidence of pneumonitis, exertional dyspnea, nonproductive cough, and pleuritic chest pain.

Boxed Warning Monitor for hepatotoxicity. Obtain baseline and periodic LFTs. Discontinue or reduce dosage if LFT values exceed

3 × ULN or double in a patient with elevated baseline LFT values. Discontinue if signs or symptoms of liver injury occur. Liver injury is common and is usually mild but has been fatal in a few cases. ∎

• Correct electrolyte imbalances before start of therapy and throughout treatment.

• Monitor electrolyte levels, particularly potassium and magnesium.

• Monitor PT and INR if patient takes warfarin and digoxin level if patient takes digoxin.

• Regular ophthalmic exams are advised to monitor patient for optic neuropathy, optic neuritis, and corneal microdeposits.

• Frequently monitor BP and HR and rhythm. Perform continuous ECG monitoring when starting or changing dosage. Notify prescriber of significant change in assessment results.

⊘ *Alert:* Patient may continue to be at risk for drug-related adverse reactions or drug interactions for several weeks after discontinuation of amiodarone.

⊘ *Alert:* May cause life-threatening or fatal reactions, including SJS and TEN. Immediately discontinue drug if signs or symptoms, such as progressive rash with blisters or mucosal lesions, occur.

• During or after treatment with IV form, patient may be transferred to oral therapy.

• *Look alike–sound alike:* Don't confuse amiodarone with amiloride.

PATIENT TEACHING

• Advise patient to wear sunscreen or protective clothing to prevent sensitivity reaction to the sun. Monitor patient for skin burning or tingling, followed by redness and blistering. Exposed skin may turn blue-gray.

• Advise patient to keep follow-up appointments, including eye exams and blood tests.

• Tell patient to report vision changes, weakness, "pins and needles" or numbness, poor coordination, weight change, heat or cold intolerance, neck swelling, progressive rash, or mucosal lesions.

• Tell patient to take oral drug with food if GI reactions occur.

• Inform patient that adverse effects of drug are more common at high doses and become more frequent with treatment longer than 6 months but are generally reversible when drug is stopped. Resolution of adverse reactions may take up to 4 months.

Reactions in bold italics are *life-threatening*.

- Tell patient not to stop taking drug without consulting prescriber.
- Inform patient of potential hazard to a fetus if drug is used during pregnancy.

amitriptyline hydrochloride
a-mih-TRIP-ti-leen

Elavil✤

Therapeutic class: Antidepressants
Pharmacologic class: TCAs

AVAILABLE FORMS
Tablets: 10 mg, 25 mg, 50 mg, 75 mg, 100 mg, 150 mg

INDICATIONS & DOSAGES
➤ **Depression (outpatients)**
Adults: 75 mg PO daily in divided doses. Or, 50 to 100 mg PO daily as a single dose at bedtime or in divided doses. May increase by 25 to 50 mg, as needed, to a total of 150 mg/day. Make increases preferably in late afternoon or at bedtime. Titrate maintenance dosage to lowest dose that maintains relief of symptoms, usually 40 to 100 mg daily. Continue maintenance therapy for at least 3 months.
Older adults and adolescents: 10 mg PO t.i.d. plus 20 mg at bedtime daily.
➤ **Depression (patients who are hospitalized)**
Adults: Initially, 100 mg PO daily. If necessary, gradually increase to 200 to 300 mg daily.

ADMINISTRATION
PO
- Give drug without regard for food.
- Give higher doses in late afternoon or at bedtime to minimize daytime sedation.
- May give maintenance dose as a single dose at bedtime.

ACTION
Unknown. May increase amount of norepinephrine, serotonin, or both in the CNS by blocking their reuptake by presynaptic neurons.

Route	Onset	Peak	Duration
PO	Unknown	2–5 hr	Unknown

Half-life: 13 to 36 hours.

ADVERSE REACTIONS
CNS: *stroke, seizures, coma,* ataxia, tremor, peripheral neuropathy, anxiety, insomnia, nightmares, restlessness, drowsiness, dizziness, syncope, weakness, fatigue, headache, extrapyramidal reactions, hallucinations, delusions, confusion, incoordination, numbness, tingling, paresthesia, dysarthria, disturbed concentration, excitement, disorientation, fever, peculiar taste. **CV:** orthostatic hypotension, tachycardia, *heart block, arrhythmias, MI,* ECG changes, HTN, edema, palpitations. **EENT:** blurred vision, mydriasis, increased IOP, tinnitus, dry mouth, black tongue, parotid swelling. **GI:** nausea, vomiting, anorexia, epigastric pain, diarrhea, constipation, paralytic ileus, stomatitis. **GU:** urinary retention, urinary frequency, erectile dysfunction, testicular swelling. **Hematologic:** *agranulocytosis, thrombocytopenia, leukopenia,* purpura, eosinophilia. **Metabolic:** *hypoglycemia,* hyperglycemia, SIADH, weight gain or loss. **Skin:** rash, urticaria, alopecia, photosensitivity reactions, diaphoresis. **Other:** hypersensitivity reactions, gynecomastia, female galactorrhea, altered libido.

INTERACTIONS
Drug-drug. *Antiemetics (5HT₃), antipsychotics, linezolid, methylene blue:* May cause serotonin syndrome. Avoid combination.
Barbiturates: May increase amitriptyline metabolism. Consider therapy modification.
Cimetidine: May decrease TCA metabolism. Monitor therapy.
CNS depressants: May enhance CNS depression. Avoid use together.
Disulfiram: May increase amitriptyline level and risk of CNS toxicity. Monitor patient closely.
Drugs that prolong QT interval (antiarrhythmics, chlorpromazine, clarithromycin, haloperidol, levofloxacin, quinolones, thioridazine): May increase risk of life-threatening arrhythmias, including torsades de pointes. Use together cautiously.
Epinephrine, norepinephrine: May increase hypertensive effect. Use together cautiously.
Fluoxetine, fluvoxamine, hormonal contraceptives, paroxetine, sertraline: May increase TCA level. Consider therapy modification.
MAO inhibitors: May cause severe excitation, hyperpyrexia, or seizures, usually with high

doses. Avoid using within 14 days of MAO inhibitor therapy.

Topiramate: May increase amitriptyline level. Adjust amitriptyline dosage if clinically indicated.

Drug-herb. *SAM-e, St. John's wort, yohimbe:* May cause serotonin syndrome and decrease amitriptyline level. Discourage use together.

Drug-lifestyle. *Alcohol use:* May enhance CNS depression. Discourage use together. *Smoking:* May lower drug level. Watch for lack of effect.

Sun exposure: May increase risk of photosensitivity reactions. Advise patient to take precautions.

EFFECTS ON LAB TEST RESULTS
• May increase LFT values.
• May increase or decrease glucose level.
• May increase eosinophil count.
• May decrease granulocyte, platelet, and WBC counts.

CONTRAINDICATIONS & CAUTIONS
• Contraindicated in patients hypersensitive to drug, in those who have received an MAO inhibitor within the past 14 days, and in acute MI recovery phase.

◑ Alert: Concomitant use with linezolid or methylene blue can cause serotonin syndrome (fever, mental status changes, muscle twitching, excessive sweating, shivering or shaking, diarrhea, loss of coordination). Use drug with linezolid or methylene blue only for life-threatening or urgent conditions when the potential benefits outweigh the risks of toxicity.
• Drug isn't approved for use in children younger than age 12.
• Use cautiously in patients with history of seizures, urine retention, angle-closure glaucoma, or increased IOP; in those with hyperthyroidism, CV disease, diabetes, or impaired liver function; and in those receiving thyroid drugs.
• Use cautiously in older adults and in patients with suicidality.
• Use cautiously in those receiving electroconvulsive therapy.
• Avoid use in patients with bipolar disorder; drug may precipitate a shift to mania or hypomania.

Dialyzable drug: No.

⚠ Overdose S&S: Arrhythmias, severe hypotension, seizures, CNS depression, coma, impaired myocardial contractility, confusion,

disturbed concentration, transient visual hallucinations, dilated pupils, disorders of ocular motility, agitation, hyperactive reflexes, stupor, drowsiness, polyradiculoneuropathy, muscle rigidity, vomiting, hypothermia, hyperpyrexia.

PREGNANCY-LACTATION-REPRODUCTION
• There are no adequate and well-controlled studies during pregnancy. Drug crosses the placenta. Use during pregnancy only if potential benefit outweighs fetal risk.
• Drug appears in human milk. Patient should discontinue breastfeeding or discontinue drug, considering importance of drug to patient.

NURSING CONSIDERATIONS
Boxed Warning Drug may increase the risk of suicidal thinking and behavior in children, adolescents, and young adults with major depressive disorder or other psychiatric disorders. Monitor all patients closely for clinical worsening, suicidality, or unusual changes in behavior, especially at start of therapy. ∎

◑ Alert: If linezolid or methylene blue must be given, amitriptyline must be stopped and patient should be monitored for serotonin toxicity for 2 weeks or until 24 hours after the last dose of methylene blue or linezolid, whichever comes first. Treatment with amitriptyline may resume 24 hours after last dose of methylene blue or linezolid.
• Amitriptyline has strong anticholinergic effects and is one of the most sedating TCAs. Anticholinergic effects have rapid onset, even though therapeutic effect is delayed for weeks.
• Older adults may have an increased sensitivity to anticholinergic effects of drug; sedating effects of drug increase risk of falls in this population.
• If signs or symptoms of psychosis occur or increase, expect prescriber to reduce dosage. Record mood changes. Monitor patient for suicidal tendencies and allow only minimum supply of drug.
• Because patients using TCAs may suffer hypertensive episodes and arrhythmias during surgery, stop drug gradually several days before surgery.
• Monitor glucose level.
• Watch for nausea, headache, and malaise after abrupt withdrawal of long-term therapy; these symptoms don't indicate addiction.
• Don't withdraw drug abruptly.

• *Look alike–sound alike:* Don't confuse amitriptyline with nortriptyline or aminophylline. Don't confuse Elavil with enalapril.

PATIENT TEACHING

Boxed Warning Advise family and caregivers to closely observe patient for increased suicidal thinking and behavior. ■

◑ Alert: Teach patient to recognize and immediately report symptoms of serotonin toxicity (fever, mental status changes, muscle twitching, excessive sweating, shivering or shaking, diarrhea, loss of coordination).

• Advise patient to take full dose at bedtime when possible; however, caution patient that morning orthostatic hypotension may occur.

• Tell patient to avoid alcohol during drug therapy.

• Advise patient to consult prescriber before taking other drugs.

• Warn patient to avoid activities that require alertness and psychomotor coordination until CNS effects of drug are known. Explain that drowsiness and dizziness usually subside after a few weeks.

• Inform patient that dry mouth may be relieved with sugarless hard candy or gum. Saliva substitutes may be useful.

• Caution patient to use a sunblock, wear protective clothing, and avoid prolonged exposure to strong sunlight.

• Warn patient not to stop drug abruptly.

• Advise patient that drug may take as long as 30 days to achieve full therapeutic effect.

amLODIPine besylate
am-LOE-di-peen

Katerzia, Norliqva, Norvasc

Therapeutic class: Antihypertensives
Pharmacologic class: Calcium channel blockers

AVAILABLE FORMS
Oral solution: 1 mg/mL*
Oral suspension: 1 mg/mL
Tablets: 2.5 mg, 5 mg, 10 mg

INDICATIONS & DOSAGES
Adjust-a-dose (for all indications): For older adults, patients who are small or frail or have liver insufficiency, and those taking other antihypertensives, initially 2.5 mg PO daily.

➤ **Chronic stable angina; vasospastic angina (Prinzmetal or variant angina); to reduce risk of hospitalization because of angina or to reduce risk of coronary revascularization procedure in patients with recently documented CAD by angiography and without HF or with LVEF less than 40%**
Adults: Initially, 5 to 10 mg PO daily. Titrate over 7 to 14 days according to response and tolerance. Most patients need 10 mg daily.

➤ **HTN**
Adults: Initially, 5 mg PO daily. Titrate over 7 to 14 days according to response and tolerance. Maximum daily dose, 10 mg.
Children ages 6 to 17: 2.5 to 5 mg PO once daily. Maximum daily dose, 5 mg.

ADMINISTRATION
PO
• Give drug without regard for food.

• Give missed dose as soon as possible. If more than 12 hours since missed dose, wait and give next dose at the regular time.

• Shake oral suspension before using.

• Refrigerate oral suspension; don't freeze. Protect from light.

• Store oral solution at room temperature.

ACTION
Inhibits calcium ion influx across cardiac and smooth-muscle cells, dilates coronary arteries and arterioles, and decreases BP and myocardial oxygen demand.

Route	Onset	Peak	Duration
PO	Unknown	6–12 hr	24 hr

Half-life: 30 to 50 hours

ADVERSE REACTIONS
CNS: somnolence, fatigue, dizziness, asthenia. **CV:** edema, flushing, palpitations. **GI:** nausea, abdominal pain. **GU:** sexual dysfunction. **Musculoskeletal:** cramps. **Respiratory:** dyspnea. **Skin:** pruritus, rash.

INTERACTIONS
Drug-drug. *Conivaptan, moderate and strong CYP3A4 inhibitors (clarithromycin, itraconazole, ketoconazole, ritonavir):* May increase amlodipine level. Monitor patient for hypotension and edema. Decrease amlodipine dose as clinically indicated.
Cyclosporine (systemic), tacrolimus: May increase cyclosporine or tacrolimus level. Monitor levels and patient.

Sildenafil: May increase risk of hypotension. Monitor BP closely.

Simvastatin: May increase risk of myopathy, including rhabdomyolysis. Simvastatin dosage shouldn't exceed 20 mg daily.

EFFECTS ON LAB TEST RESULTS
None reported.

CONTRAINDICATIONS & CAUTIONS
• Contraindicated in patients hypersensitive to drug.

• Use cautiously in patients receiving other peripheral vasodilators, especially those with severe aortic stenosis or hypertrophic cardiomyopathy with outflow tract obstruction and in patients with HF with reduced LVEF. Because drug is metabolized by the liver, use cautiously and with reduced dosage in patients with severe liver disease.

• Safety and effectiveness in children younger than age 6 haven't been established.

Dialyzable drug: No.

⚠ **Overdose S&S:** Marked peripheral vasodilation with hypotension and possibly reflex tachycardia.

PREGNANCY-LACTATION-REPRODUCTION
• Use in pregnancy only if potential benefit justifies fetal risk. Other antihypertensives are preferred during pregnancy.

• Drug appears in human milk. Use cautiously during breastfeeding.

NURSING CONSIDERATIONS
🕙 *Alert:* Monitor patient carefully. Some patients, especially those with severe obstructive CAD, have developed increased frequency, duration, or severity of angina or acute MI after initiation of calcium channel blocker therapy or at time of dosage increase.

• Monitor BP frequently during initiation of therapy. Because drug-induced vasodilation has gradual onset, acute hypotension is rare.

• Notify prescriber if signs of HF occur, such as swelling of hands and feet or shortness of breath.

🕙 *Alert:* Abrupt withdrawal of drug may increase frequency and duration of chest pain. Taper dose gradually under medical supervision.

• *Look alike–sound alike:* Don't confuse amlodipine with amiloride.

PATIENT TEACHING
• Caution patient to report all adverse reactions and to continue taking drug, even after feeling better.

• Tell patient SL nitroglycerin may be taken as needed when angina symptoms are acute. If patient continues nitrate therapy during adjustment of amlodipine dosage, urge continued adherence.

• Teach about proper drug administration and handling.

amoxicillin
a-moks-i-SIL-in

Amoxil, Apo-Amoxi❖, Novamoxin❖

Therapeutic class: Antibiotics
Pharmacologic class: Aminopenicillins

AVAILABLE FORMS
Capsules: 250 mg, 500 mg
Oral suspension: 125 mg/5 mL, 200 mg/5 mL, 250 mg/5 mL, 400 mg/5 mL (after reconstitution)
Tablets: 500 mg, 875 mg
Tablets (chewable): 125 mg, 250 mg

INDICATIONS & DOSAGES
Adjust-a-dose (for all indications): Adults with GFR less than 30 mL/minute shouldn't receive 875-mg tablet. Adults with GFR of 10 to 30 mL/minute should receive 250 or 500 mg every 12 hours depending on the infection. Adults with GFR less than 10 mL/minute should receive 250 or 500 mg every 24 hours depending on infection severity. Adults on hemodialysis should receive 250 or 500 mg every 24 hours with extra dose both during and at end of dialysis.

Continue treatment for 48 to 72 hours after patient becomes asymptomatic or evidence of bacterial eradication is obtained. Continue treatment for any *Streptococcus pyogenes* infections for at least 10 days to prevent acute rheumatic fever.

➤ **Mild to moderate infections of the ear, nose, and throat; skin and skin structure; or GU tract**
Adults and children weighing 40 kg or more: 500 mg PO every 12 hours or 250 mg PO every 8 hours.
Children older than age 3 months weighing less than 40 kg: 25 mg/kg/day PO divided

every 12 hours or 20 mg/kg/day PO divided every 8 hours.

Neonates and infants up to age 3 months: Up to 30 mg/kg/day PO divided every 12 hours.

➤ **Mild to severe infections of the lower respiratory tract; severe infections of the ear, nose, and throat or skin and skin structure or GU tract**

Adults and children weighing 40 kg or more: 875 mg PO every 12 hours or 500 mg PO every 8 hours.

Children older than age 3 months weighing less than 40 kg: 45 mg/kg/day PO divided every 12 hours or 40 mg/kg/day PO divided every 8 hours.

Neonates and infants up to age 3 months: Up to 30 mg/kg/day PO divided every 12 hours.

➤ *Helicobacter pylori* **eradication to reduce risk of duodenal ulcer recurrence**

Adults: Amoxicillin 1 g with lansoprazole 30 mg PO every 8 hours for 14 days (dual therapy). Or, amoxicillin 1 g, clarithromycin 500 mg, and lansoprazole 30 mg, all given PO every 12 hours for 14 days (triple therapy). Consult latest guidelines for recommendations due to increasing macrolide resistance.

ADMINISTRATION

PO

• Drug is for treatment of ENT or respiratory infections due to beta-lactamase-negative *Streptococcus* species (alpha- and beta-hemolytic isolates only), *S. pneumoniae*, *Staphylococcus* species, or *Haemophilus influenzae*; GU infection due to *Escherichia coli*, *Porteus mirabilis*, or *Enterococcus faecalis*; or skin infections due to beta-lactamase-negative *Streptococcus* species (alpha- and beta hemolytic isolates only), *S. pneumoniae*, *Staphylococcus* species, or *Escherichia coli*.

• Obtain specimen for culture and sensitivity tests before giving first dose. Begin therapy while awaiting results.

• Before giving, ask patient about allergic reactions to penicillin. A negative history of penicillin allergy is no guarantee against allergic reaction.

• Give drug with or without food.

• Shake oral suspension vigorously after reconstitution and before administration.

• For a child, place drops directly on tongue for swallowing or add to formula, milk, fruit juice, water, ginger ale, or other cold drink for immediate and complete consumption.

• Store reconstituted oral suspension in refrigerator, if possible. Check individual product labels for storage information.

ACTION

Inhibits cell-wall synthesis during bacterial multiplication.

Route	Onset	Peak	Duration
PO	Unknown	1–2 hr	6–8 hr

Half-life: 1 to 1.5 hours (7.5 hours in severe kidney impairment).

ADVERSE REACTIONS

GI: diarrhea, nausea, vomiting, *CDAD.* **Skin:** rash. **Other:** hypersensitivity reactions.

INTERACTIONS

Drug-drug. *Allopurinol:* Increases incidence of rashes from both drugs compared to incidence with use of amoxicillin alone. Monitor patient closely for rashes.

Chloramphenicol, macrolides, sulfonamides, tetracycline: May reduce therapeutic action of penicillins. Monitor therapy.

Live-virus vaccines: May decrease effectiveness of live-virus vaccines. Concurrent use isn't recommended.

Methotrexate: May increase methotrexate serum concentration. Monitor patient closely for toxicity.

Oral anticoagulants (warfarin): May enhance anticoagulant effect. Monitor closely and adjust anticoagulant dose as indicated.

Probenecid: May increase levels of amoxicillin and other penicillins. Probenecid may be used for this purpose.

EFFECTS ON LAB TEST RESULTS

• May increase AST and ALT levels.

• May increase eosinophil count.

• May decrease Hb level and granulocyte, platelet, and WBC counts.

• May alter results of urine glucose tests that use cupric sulfate, such as Benedict reagent and Clinitest.

• May cause transient decrease in total conjugated estriol, estriol glucuronide, conjugated estrone, and estradiol during pregnancy.

CONTRAINDICATIONS & CAUTIONS

• Contraindicated in patients hypersensitive to drug or other penicillins.

- Use cautiously in patients with other drug allergies (especially to cephalosporins) because of possible cross-sensitivity.
- Use isn't recommended in those with mononucleosis because of high risk of maculopapular rash.
- Use cautiously in older adults.

Dialyzable drug: Yes.

⚠ *Overdose S&S:* Oliguric kidney failure.

PREGNANCY-LACTATION-REPRODUCTION
- Use during pregnancy only if clearly needed.
- Drug appears in human milk. Use cautiously during breastfeeding.

NURSING CONSIDERATIONS
- Watch for signs and symptoms of bacterial or fungal superinfection, especially in an older adult or a patient with immunosuppression or debilitation, if doses are large or therapy is prolonged.
- Evaluate patient if diarrhea occurs. CDAD, ranging from mild diarrhea to fatal colitis, has been reported with nearly all antibacterial agents, including amoxicillin. Note amoxicillin usually causes fewer cases of diarrhea than ampicillin.
- Monitor patient for hypersensitivity reactions, including anaphylaxis and SJS.
- Some infections require several weeks of treatment as well as clinical follow-up for several months after the end of therapy.
- *Look alike–sound alike:* Don't confuse amoxicillin with ampicillin, amoxapine.

PATIENT TEACHING
- Tell patient to take entire quantity of drug exactly as prescribed, even after feeling better.
- Teach about proper drug administration and handling.
- Tell patient to report rash, fever, or chills.

amoxicillin–clavulanate potassium
a-mox-i-SILL-in/KLAV-yu-lah-nate

Augmentin, Augmentin ES-600, Clavulin ✦

Therapeutic class: Antibiotics
Pharmacologic class: Aminopenicillins–beta-lactamase inhibitors

AVAILABLE FORMS
Oral suspension (after reconstitution): 125 mg amoxicillin trihydrate, 31.25 mg clavulanic acid/5 mL; 200 mg amoxicillin trihydrate, 28.5 mg clavulanic acid/5 mL; 250 mg amoxicillin trihydrate, 62.5 mg clavulanic acid/5 mL; 400 mg amoxicillin trihydrate, 57 mg clavulanic acid/5 mL; 600 mg amoxicillin trihydrate, 42.9 mg clavulanic acid/5 mL
Tablets (chewable): 200 mg amoxicillin trihydrate, 28.5 mg clavulanic acid; 400 mg amoxicillin trihydrate, 57 mg clavulanic acid
Tablets (extended-release): 1 g amoxicillin trihydrate, 62.5 mg clavulanic acid
Tablets: 250 mg amoxicillin trihydrate, 125 mg clavulanic acid; 500 mg amoxicillin trihydrate, 125 mg clavulanic acid; 875 mg amoxicillin trihydrate, 125 mg clavulanic acid

INDICATIONS & DOSAGES
➤ **Lower respiratory tract infections, otitis media, sinusitis, skin and skin-structure infections, and UTIs caused by susceptible strains of gram-positive and gram-negative organisms**
Adults and children weighing 40 kg or more: 250 mg PO, based on amoxicillin component, every 8 hours; or 500 mg every 12 hours. For more severe infections, 500 mg every 8 hours or 875 mg every 12 hours.
Children ages 3 months and older weighing less than 40 kg: 20 to 45 mg/kg/day PO, based on amoxicillin component and severity of infection, daily in divided doses every 8 to 12 hours.
Children younger than age 3 months: 30 mg/kg/day PO, based on amoxicillin component of the 125 mg/5 mL oral suspension, in divided doses every 12 hours.
Adjust-a-dose: Don't give 875-mg tablet to patients with CrCl less than 30 mL/minute. If CrCl is 10 to 30 mL/minute, give 250 to 500 mg PO every 12 hours. If CrCl is less than 10 mL/minute, give 250 to 500 mg PO every 24 hours. Give patients on hemodialysis 250 to 500 mg PO every 24 hours with an additional dose both during and after dialysis.
➤ **Acute bacterial sinusitis or community-acquired pneumonia caused by** *Haemophilus influenzae, M. catarrhalis, H. parainfluenzae, Klebsiella pneumoniae,* **methicillin-susceptible** *Staphylococcus aureus,* **or** *S. pneumoniae*
Adults and children weighing more than 40 kg: 2 g amoxicillin/125 mg clavulanic acid (two

extended-release tablets) PO every 12 hours for 10 days (sinusitis) or 7 to 10 days (pneumonia).

ADMINISTRATION
PO
• Before giving drug, ask patient about allergic reactions to penicillin. A negative history of penicillin allergy is no guarantee against an allergic reaction.
• Obtain specimen for culture and sensitivity tests before giving first dose. Begin therapy while awaiting results.
• Give drug at the start of a meal to enhance absorption and decrease GI intolerance. Avoid giving extended-release tablet with a high-fat meal, because it reduces clavulanate absorption.
• Give drug at least 1 hour before a bacteriostatic antibiotic.
• Avoid use of 250-mg tablet in children weighing less than 40 kg. Use chewable form or oral suspension instead.
• After reconstitution, refrigerate the oral suspension; discard after 10 days.

ACTION
Amoxicillin prevents bacterial cell-wall synthesis during replication. Clavulanic acid increases amoxicillin's effectiveness by inactivating beta-lactamases, which destroy amoxicillin.

Route	Onset	Peak	Duration
PO	Unknown	1–2.5 hr	Unknown

Half-life: 1 to 1.5 hours. For patients with severe kidney impairment, 7.5 hours for amoxicillin and 4.5 hours for clavulanate.

ADVERSE REACTIONS
GI: nausea, vomiting, diarrhea. **GU:** vaginal candidiasis, vaginitis. **Skin:** rash, candidal diaper rash, diaper rash, urticaria. **Other:** hypersensitivity reactions.

INTERACTIONS
Drug-drug. *Allopurinol:* May increase risk of rash. Monitor patient for rash.
Live-virus vaccines: May decrease effectiveness of live-virus vaccines. Concurrent use isn't recommended.
Methotrexate: May increase risk of methotrexate toxicity. Monitor methotrexate level.

Oral anticoagulants (warfarin): May prolong PT. Monitor PT closely during coadministration.
Probenecid: May increase levels of amoxicillin and other penicillins. Use together isn't recommended.
Tetracyclines: May reduce therapeutic action of penicillins. Avoid administering together.

EFFECTS ON LAB TEST RESULTS
• May decrease platelet, leukocyte, and granulocyte counts.
• May increase or decrease eosinophil count.
• May alter results of urine glucose tests that use cupric sulfate, such as Benedict reagent and Clinitest.

CONTRAINDICATIONS & CAUTIONS
• Contraindicated in patients with serious hypersensitivity to drug's components or other penicillins and in those with a history of amoxicillin-related cholestatic jaundice or liver dysfunction.
• Use cautiously in patients with other drug allergies (especially to cephalosporins) because of possible cross-sensitivity.
• Use cautiously in older adults and patients with liver dysfunction.
• Drug may increase risk of liver dysfunction (hepatitis, cholestatic jaundice), especially in older adults, males, and patients on prolonged treatment.
• Don't give ampicillin-class antibiotics to patients with mononucleosis due to high incidence of erythematous rash.
Dialyzable drug: Yes.
⚠ *Overdose S&S:* Crystalluria, oliguric kidney failure, GI symptoms, rash, hyperactivity or drowsiness.

PREGNANCY-LACTATION-REPRODUCTION
• Use during pregnancy only if clearly needed.
• Drug appears in human milk. Use cautiously during breastfeeding.

NURSING CONSIDERATIONS
🗘 *Alert:* Ratios of amoxicillin and clavulanic acid aren't consistent from product to product. Therefore, formulations aren't equivalent. For example, don't substitute two 250-mg tablets for one 500-mg tablet or substitute one 250-mg tablet for one 250-mg chewable tablet. Don't substitute extended-release tablets mg-to-mg with other formulations.

• Watch for signs and symptoms of bacterial or fungal superinfection, especially in an older adult or a patient with immunosuppression or debilitation, if doses are large or therapy is prolonged.

• Evaluate patient if diarrhea occurs. CDAD, ranging from mild diarrhea to fatal colitis, has been reported with nearly all antibacterial agents, including amoxicillin–clavulanate.

• Note that chewable tablets and powder for oral solution contain phenylalanine.

• Periodically monitor LFTs in patients with liver impairment. Discontinue drug if signs of hepatitis occur.

• Monitor patient closely for SCARs (SJS, TEN, DRESS syndrome, acute generalized exanthematous pustulosis). Discontinue treatment if rash worsens.

• This drug combination is useful in settings with a high prevalence of amoxicillin-resistant organisms.

• *Look alike–sound alike:* Don't confuse amoxicillin with ampicillin, amoxapine, or Azulfidine.

PATIENT TEACHING

• Advise patient to take entire quantity of drug exactly as prescribed, even after feeling better.

• Instruct patient to take drug with food to prevent GI upset.

• Teach patient or caregiver to keep oral suspension refrigerated, to shake it well before taking it, and to discard remaining drug after 10 days.

• Tell patient to report all adverse reactions and to call prescriber if a rash occurs because rash may indicate an allergic reaction.

SAFETY ALERT!

amphotericin B lipid complex
am-foe-TER-i-sin

Abelcet

Therapeutic class: Antifungals
Pharmacologic class: Polyene antibiotics

AVAILABLE FORMS
Suspension for injection: 100 mg/20 mL vial

INDICATIONS & DOSAGES
➤ **Invasive fungal infections, including** *Aspergillus* **and** *Candida* **species, in patients**

refractory to or intolerant of conventional amphotericin B therapy
Adults and children: 5 mg/kg daily IV as a single infusion given at rate of 2.5 mg/kg/hour.
Adjust-a-dose: Determine dosage based on overall clinical condition of individual patient.

ADMINISTRATION
IV
▼ To prepare, shake vial gently until there's no yellow sediment. Withdraw calculated dose into one or more 20-mL syringes using an 18G needle. More than one vial will be needed.

▼ Attach a 5-micron filter needle to syringe and inject dose into IV bag of D_5W. Volume of D_5W should be sufficient to yield 1 mg/mL (May be diluted to 2 mg/mL for children and those with CV disorders). One filter needle can be used for up to four vials of amphotericin B lipid complex.

▼ Don't use an in-line filter.

▼ If infusing through an existing IV line, flush first with D_5W.

▼ If infusion time exceeds 2 hours, mix contents by shaking infusion bag every 2 hours.

▼ Reconstituted drug is stable for up to 48 hours if refrigerated (36° to 46° F [2° to 8° C]) and up to 6 hours at room temperature.

▼ Discard any unused drug because it contains no preservative.

▼ **Incompatibilities:** Electrolytes, other IV drugs, saline solutions.

ACTION
Binds to sterols of fungal cell membranes, altering cell permeability and causing cell death.

Route	Onset	Peak	Duration
IV	Unknown	Unknown	Unknown

Half-life: About 1 week.

ADVERSE REACTIONS
CNS: fever, headache, pain. **CV:** *cardiac arrest,* chest pain, HTN, hypotension. **GI:** *GI hemorrhage,* abdominal pain, diarrhea, nausea, vomiting. **GU:** increased creatinine level, *kidney failure.* **Hematologic:** *leukopenia, thrombocytopenia,* anemia. **Hepatic:** hyperbilirubinemia. **Metabolic:** *hypokalemia.* **Respiratory:** *respiratory failure,* dyspnea, respiratory disorder. **Skin:** rash. **Other:** *multiple organ failure,* chills, *sepsis,* infection.

INTERACTIONS
Drug-drug. *Antineoplastics:* May increase risk of kidney toxicity, bronchospasm, and hypotension. Use together cautiously.
Cardiac glycosides: May increase risk of digitalis toxicity from amphotericin B–induced hypokalemia. Monitor potassium level closely.
Clotrimazole, fluconazole, itraconazole, ketoconazole, miconazole: May counteract effects of amphotericin B by inducing fungal resistance. Monitor patient closely.
Corticosteroids, corticotropin: May enhance hypokalemia, which could lead to cardiac toxicity. Monitor electrolyte levels and cardiac function.
Cyclosporine: May increase kidney toxicity. Closely monitor kidney function test results.
Flucytosine: May increase risk of flucytosine toxicity from increased cellular uptake or impaired kidney excretion. Use together cautiously.
Leukocyte transfusions: May increase risk of pulmonary reactions, such as acute dyspnea, tachypnea, hypoxemia, hemoptysis, and interstitial infiltrates. Don't use together.
Kidney-toxic drugs (such as aminoglycosides, pentamidine): May increase risk of kidney toxicity. Use together cautiously and monitor kidney function closely.
Skeletal muscle relaxants (tubocurarine): May enhance skeletal muscle relaxant effects of amphotericin B–induced hypokalemia. Closely monitor potassium level.
Zidovudine: May increase myelotoxicity and kidney toxicity. Monitor kidney and hematologic function.

EFFECTS ON LAB TEST RESULTS
• May increase ALP, ALT, AST, bilirubin, amylase, uric acid, BUN, creatinine, GGT, and LDH levels.
• May decrease pH, phosphate, magnesium, and potassium levels.
• May increase or decrease glucose level.
• May decrease Hb level and platelet and WBC counts.

CONTRAINDICATIONS & CAUTIONS
• Contraindicated in patients hypersensitive to amphotericin B or its components.
• Anaphylaxis can occur. If patient develops severe respiratory distress, discontinue infusion, treat appropriately, and don't restart drug.

• Use cautiously in patients with kidney impairment. Adjust dosage based on patient's overall condition. Kidney toxicity is more common at higher dosages.
Dialyzable drug: No.
⚠ *Overdose S&S:* Cardiorespiratory arrest.

PREGNANCY-LACTATION-REPRODUCTION
• Use cautiously during pregnancy, considering importance of drug to patient.
• It isn't known if drug appears in human milk. Patient should discontinue breastfeeding or discontinue drug, considering importance of drug to patient.

NURSING CONSIDERATIONS
⚕ *Alert:* Different amphotericin B preparations aren't interchangeable, so dosages vary. Confusing the preparations may cause permanent damage or death.
• Hydrate before infusion to reduce risk of kidney toxicity.
• During therapy, frequently monitor creatinine and electrolyte levels (especially magnesium and potassium), LFT values, and CBC.
• Acute infusion reactions, including fever and chills, may occur 1 to 2 hours after start of infusion and are more common with first few doses. Infusion has rarely been associated with arrhythmias, hypotension, and shock.
• Monitor vital signs closely. Slowing infusion rate may decrease risk of infusion-related reactions.
⚕ *Alert:* Immediately stop infusion if severe respiratory distress occurs. Patient shouldn't receive further infusions.
• *Look alike–sound alike:* Don't confuse Abelcet with AmBisome or amphotericin B lipid complex with conventional amphotericin B.

PATIENT TEACHING
• Inform patient that fever, chills, nausea, and vomiting may develop during infusion, but that these symptoms usually subside with subsequent doses.
• Instruct patient to report redness or pain at infusion site.
• Teach patient to recognize and report to prescriber signs and symptoms of acute hypersensitivity, such as respiratory distress.
• Warn patient that therapy may take several months.
• Tell patient to expect frequent lab testing to monitor kidney and liver function.

amphotericin B liposomal
am-foe-TER-i-sin

AmBisome

Therapeutic class: Antifungals
Pharmacologic class: Polyene antibiotics

AVAILABLE FORMS
Powder for injection: 50-mg vial

INDICATIONS & DOSAGES
➤ **Empirical therapy for presumed fungal infection in patients who are febrile and neutropenic**
Adults and children: 3 mg/kg IV infusion over 2 hours daily.
➤ **Systemic fungal infections caused by *Aspergillus* species, *Candida* species, or *Cryptococcus* species refractory to conventional amphotericin B therapy; patients for whom kidney impairment or unacceptable toxicity precludes use of conventional amphotericin B therapy**
Adults and children: 3 to 5 mg/kg IV infusion over 2 hours daily.
➤ **Visceral leishmaniasis in patients who are immunocompetent**
Adults and children: 3 mg/kg IV infusion over 2 hours daily on days 1 to 5, day 14, and day 21. A repeat course of therapy may be beneficial if initial treatment fails to clear parasites.
➤ **Visceral leishmaniasis in patients who are immunocompromised**
Adults and children: 4 mg/kg IV infusion over 2 hours daily on days 1 to 5, day 10, day 17, day 24, day 31, and day 38.
➤ **Cryptococcal meningitis in patients with HIV infection**
Adults and children: 6 mg/kg/day IV infusion over 2 hours.

ADMINISTRATION
IV
▼ Don't reconstitute with bacteriostatic water for injection, and don't allow bacteriostatic product in solution.
▼ Don't reconstitute with saline solutions, add saline solutions to reconstituted concentration, or mix with other drugs.
▼ Reconstitute each 50-mg vial with 12 mL of sterile water for injection to yield

4 mg/mL. A yellow, translucent suspension will form.
▼ After reconstitution, shake vial vigorously for 30 seconds or until particulate matter disperses.
▼ Dilute to 1 to 2 mg/mL by withdrawing calculated amount of reconstituted solution into a sterile syringe and injecting it through a 5-micron filter into an appropriate amount of D_5W. Use only one filter needle per vial. Concentrations of 0.2 to 0.5 mg/mL may provide sufficient volume of infusion for children.
▼ Flush existing IV line with D_5W before infusing drug. If this isn't possible, give drug through a separate line.
▼ Use a controlled infusion device and an in-line filter with a mean pore diameter of 1 micron or larger.
▼ Initially, infuse drug over at least 2 hours. If drug is tolerated well, reduce infusion time to 1 hour. If discomfort occurs, increase infusion time.
▼ Store unopened vials at temperatures up to 77° F (25° C). Store reconstituted drug for up to 24 hours at 36° to 46° F (2° to 8° C). Use within 6 hours of dilution with D_5W. Don't freeze.
▼ **Incompatibilities:** Other IV drugs, bacteriostatic agents, saline solutions.

ACTION
Binds to sterols of fungal cell membranes, altering cell permeability and causing cell death.

Route	Onset	Peak	Duration
IV	Unknown	Unknown	Unknown

Half-life: About 4 to 6 days.

ADVERSE REACTIONS
CNS: fever, anxiety, confusion, headache, insomnia, asthenia, pain. **CV:** chest pain, hypotension, tachycardia, HTN, edema, phlebitis, flushing. **EENT:** epistaxis, rhinitis. **GI:** anorexia, constipation, nausea, vomiting, abdominal pain, diarrhea, *GI hemorrhage.* **GU:** hematuria, increased BUN and creatinine levels. **Hematologic:** anemia, *thrombocytopenia, leukopenia.* **Hepatic:** increased ALP and transaminase levels, bilirubinemia, *liver toxicity.* **Metabolic:** hyperglycemia, hypernatremia, hyponatremia, *hypocalcemia, hypokalemia,* hypovolemia, *hypomagnesemia.* **Musculoskeletal:** back pain.

Respiratory: increased cough, dyspnea, hypoxia, pleural effusion, lung disorder. **Skin:** pruritus, rash, diaphoresis. **Other:** chills, infection, hypersensitivity reaction, *sepsis,* blood product transfusion reaction, procedural complication.

INTERACTIONS
Drug-drug. *Antineoplastics:* May enhance potential for kidney toxicity, bronchospasm, and hypotension. Use together cautiously.
Cardiac glycosides: May increase risk of digitalis toxicity caused by amphotericin B–induced hypokalemia. Monitor potassium level closely.
Clotrimazole, fluconazole, ketoconazole, miconazole: May induce fungal resistance to amphotericin B. Use together cautiously.
Corticosteroids, corticotropin: May increase potassium depletion, which could cause cardiac dysfunction. Monitor electrolyte levels and cardiac function.
Flucytosine: May increase flucytosine toxicity by increasing cellular reuptake or impairing kidney excretion of flucytosine. Use together cautiously.
Leukocyte transfusions: Increases risk of pulmonary toxicity. Don't use together.
Other kidney-toxic drugs (aminoglycosides, cyclosporine): May cause additive kidney toxicity. Use together cautiously; closely monitor kidney function.
Skeletal muscle relaxants (tubocurarine): May enhance effects of skeletal muscle relaxants resulting from amphotericin B–induced hypokalemia. Monitor potassium level.

EFFECTS ON LAB TEST RESULTS
• May increase ALP, ALT, AST, bilirubin, BUN, creatinine, GGT, glucose, and LDH levels.
• May decrease calcium, magnesium, and potassium levels.
• May increase or decrease sodium level.
• May decrease Hb level and leukocyte and platelet counts.

CONTRAINDICATIONS & CAUTIONS
• Contraindicated in patients hypersensitive to drug or its components, unless benefits of therapy outweigh the risks.
• Use cautiously in older adults and patients with impaired kidney function.
Dialyzable drug: No.
⚠ *Overdose S&S:* Cardiorespiratory arrest.

PREGNANCY-LACTATION-REPRODUCTION
• Use during pregnancy only if potential benefits outweigh fetal risk.
• It isn't known if drug appears in human milk. Patient should discontinue breastfeeding or discontinue drug, considering importance of drug to patient.

NURSING CONSIDERATIONS
• Patients also receiving chemotherapy or bone marrow transplantation and those with HIV disease are at greater risk for additional adverse reactions (cardiac arrest, hallucinations, seizures, arrhythmias, thrombocytopenia). Refer to manufacturer's instructions for a complete list of reactions.
◑ *Alert:* Different amphotericin B preparations aren't interchangeable, and dosages vary. Confusing the preparations may cause permanent damage or death.
• Hydrate before infusion to reduce risk of kidney toxicity.
• Monitor BUN, creatinine, and electrolyte levels (particularly magnesium and potassium), LFT, and CBC.
• Watch for signs and symptoms of hypokalemia (ECG changes, muscle weakness, cramping, drowsiness).
• Patients treated with this drug have a lower risk of chills, elevated BUN level, hypokalemia, HTN, and vomiting than patients treated with conventional amphotericin B.
• Therapy may take several weeks or months.
• Observe patient closely for adverse reactions during infusion. If anaphylaxis occurs, immediately stop infusion, provide supportive therapy, and notify prescriber.
• Consider premedication to prevent infusion-related reactions.
• *Look alike–sound alike:* Don't confuse amphotericin B liposomal with AmBisome or amphotericin B liposomal lipid complex with conventional amphotericin B.

PATIENT TEACHING
• Teach patient signs and symptoms of hypersensitivity, and stress importance of reporting them immediately.
• Warn patient that therapy may take several months.
• Teach personal hygiene and other measures to prevent spread and recurrence of lesions.
• Instruct patient to report any adverse reactions that occur while receiving drug.

• Tell patient to watch for and report signs and symptoms of low blood potassium level (muscle weakness, cramping, drowsiness).
• Advise patient that frequent lab testing will be needed.

ampicillin
am-pi-SIL-in

ampicillin sodium

Therapeutic class: Antibiotics
Pharmacologic class: Aminopenicillins

AVAILABLE FORMS
Capsules: 250 mg✦, 500 mg
Injection: 125 mg, 250 mg, 500 mg, 1 g, 2 g, 10 g

INDICATIONS & DOSAGES
➤ **Respiratory tract infections**
Adults and children weighing more than 20 kg: 250 mg PO every 6 hours.
Children weighing 20 kg or less: 50 mg/kg/day PO in equally divided doses every 6 to 8 hours. Maximum dose, 250 mg q.i.d.
➤ **Respiratory tract and soft-tissue infections**
Adults and children weighing 40 kg or more: 250 to 500 mg IV or IM every 6 hours.
Adults and children weighing less than 40 kg: 25 to 50 mg/kg/day IV or IM in equally divided doses every 6 to 8 hours.
➤ **GI or GU infections (excluding gonorrhea)**
Adults and children weighing 20 kg or more: 500 mg PO every 6 hours. For severe infections, larger doses may be needed.
Children weighing less than 20 kg: 100 mg/kg/day PO in equally divided doses every 6 hours. Maximum dose, 500 mg q.i.d.
➤ **GI and GU tract infections (including gonorrhea in females)**
Adults and children weighing 40 kg or more: 500 mg IV or IM every 6 hours.
Adults and children weighing less than 40 kg: 50 mg/kg/day IV or IM in equally divided doses every 6 to 8 hours.
➤ **Uncomplicated gonorrhea**
Adults and children weighing more than 20 kg: 3.5 g PO with 1 g probenecid given as a single dose.
➤ **Urethritis in males due to gonorrhea**
Adult men: Two doses of 500 mg each IV or IM at 8- to 12-hour intervals. May repeat or extend treatment if necessary.

➤ **Bacterial meningitis or septicemia**
Adults and children: 150 to 200 mg/kg/day IM or IV in divided doses every 3 to 4 hours. May start with IV therapy, then continue with IM injections. For sepsis, give IV at least 3 days before switching to IM.
Neonates gestational age greater than 34 weeks and postnatal 28 days or less: 150 mg/kg/day in divided doses every 8 hours.
Neonates gestational age 34 weeks or less and postnatal 8 to less than 28 days: 150 mg/kg/day in divided doses every 12 hours.
Neonates gestational age 34 weeks or less and postnatal 7 days or less: 100 mg/kg/day in divided doses every 12 hours.

ADMINISTRATION
• Before giving drug, ask patient about allergic reactions to penicillin. A negative history of penicillin allergy is no guarantee against a future allergic reaction.
• Obtain specimen for culture and sensitivity tests before giving. Begin therapy while awaiting results.
PO
• When given orally, drug may cause GI disturbances. Food may interfere with absorption. Give drug with 8 oz of water ½ hour before or 2 hours after meals.
• Give drug IM or IV if infection is severe or if patient can't take oral dose.
IV
▼ Give drug IV only if infection is severe or if patient can't take oral dose.
▼ Give drug intermittently to prevent vein irritation. Change site every 48 hours.
▼ For direct injection, reconstitute with bacteriostatic or sterile water for injection. Use 5 mL for 125-mg, 250-mg or 500-mg vials, 7.4 mL for 1-g vials, and 14.8 mL for 2-g vials. Give 125-mg to 500-mg doses slowly over 3 to 5 minutes. Give 1-g or 2-g doses slowly over at least 10 minutes to avoid seizures. Don't exceed 100 mg/minute.
▼ For intermittent infusion, dilute in 50 to 100 mL of NSS for injection. Give drug over 15 to 30 minutes.
▼ Use first dilution within 1 hour. Follow manufacturer's directions for stability data when drug is further diluted for IV infusion.
▼ **Incompatibilities:** None listed by manufacturer. Consult drug compatibility reference for more information.

IM

- Give drug IM only if infection is severe or patient can't take oral dose.
- Dissolve contents of vial with sterile water or bacteriostatic water for injection. Final concentration is 125 mg or 250 mg/mL.
- Use solution for IM injection within 1 hour of preparation.

ACTION

Inhibits cell-wall synthesis during bacterial multiplication.

Route	Onset	Peak	Duration
PO	Unknown	2 hr	6–8 hr
IV	Immediate	Immediate	Unknown
IM	Unknown	1 hr	Unknown

Half-life: 1 to 1.8 hours (10 to 24 hours in severe kidney impairment).

ADVERSE REACTIONS

CNS: *seizures.* **EENT:** glossitis. **GI:** diarrhea, nausea, *pseudomembranous colitis,* abdominal pain, black hairy tongue, enterocolitis, gastritis, stomatitis, vomiting. **Hematologic:** *leukopenia, thrombocytopenia, thrombocytopenic purpura,* anemia, eosinophilia, hemolytic anemia, *agranulocytosis.* **Skin:** rash, urticaria. **Other:** hypersensitivity reactions, overgrowth of nonsusceptible organisms.

INTERACTIONS

Drug-drug. *Allopurinol:* May increase risk of rash. Monitor patient for rash.
H₂ antagonists, PPIs: May decrease ampicillin absorption and level. Separate administration times. Monitor patient for continued antibiotic effectiveness.
Live-virus vaccines: May decrease effectiveness of live-virus vaccines. Concurrent use isn't recommended.
Methotrexate: May increase methotrexate level, increasing risk of toxicity. Monitor methotrexate level.
Probenecid: May increase levels of ampicillin and other penicillins. Probenecid may be used for this purpose.
Warfarin: May increase bleeding risk. Monitor PT and INR.

EFFECTS ON LAB TEST RESULTS

- May decrease Hb and aminoglycoside level.
- May increase eosinophil count.
- May decrease granulocyte, platelet, and WBC counts.

- May alter results of urine glucose tests that use copper sulfate, such as Benedict reagent and Clinitest.

CONTRAINDICATIONS & CAUTIONS

- Contraindicated in patients hypersensitive to drug or other penicillins and in those with infections caused by penicillinase-producing organisms.
- Use cautiously in patients with other drug allergies (especially to cephalosporins) because of possible cross-sensitivity and in those with mononucleosis because of high risk of maculopapular rash.
- Use cautiously in patients with kidney impairment.
Dialyzable drug: Yes.

PREGNANCY-LACTATION-REPRODUCTION

- Ampicillin crosses the placental barrier. Use during pregnancy only if clearly needed.
- Drug appears in human milk. Use cautiously during breastfeeding.

NURSING CONSIDERATIONS

- Frequently monitor sodium level because each gram of ampicillin sodium injection contains 2.9 mEq of sodium.
- Watch for signs and symptoms of bacterial or fungal superinfection, especially in an older adult or a patient with immunosuppression or debilitation, if doses are large or therapy is prolonged.
- Watch for signs and symptoms of hypersensitivity, such as erythematous maculopapular rash, urticaria, and anaphylaxis.
- Use lowest dosage compatible with effective treatment in neonates and infants because of incompletely developed kidney function in these patients.
- Monitor patient for CDAD, which can be fatal and can occur even more than 2 months after therapy ends. Antibiotic may need to be stopped and other treatment begun.
- Duration of therapy depends on the organism and severity of infection. Follow-up culture from the original site of infection may be obtained 7 to 14 days after therapy.

PATIENT TEACHING

- Tell patient to take entire quantity of drug exactly as prescribed, even after feeling better.
- Instruct patient in safe drug administration.
- Inform patient to report all adverse reactions and to notify prescriber if rash, fever,

or chills develop. A rash is the most common allergic reaction, especially if allopurinol is taken together.

• Instruct patient to report diarrhea.

ampicillin sodium–sulbactam sodium

am-pi-SIL-in/sul-BAK-tam

Unasyn

Therapeutic class: Antibiotics
Pharmacologic class: Aminopenicillins– beta-lactamase inhibitors

AVAILABLE FORMS

Injection: Vials and piggyback vials containing 1.5 g (1 g ampicillin sodium and 0.5 g sulbactam sodium), 3 g (2 g ampicillin sodium and 1 g sulbactam sodium); vial containing 15 g (10 g ampicillin sodium and 5 g sulbactam sodium)

INDICATIONS & DOSAGES

Adjust-a-dose (for all indications): If CrCl in adults is 15 to 29 mL/minute/1.73 m^2, give 1.5 to 3 g every 12 hours; if CrCl is 5 to 14 mL/minute/1.73 m^2, give 1.5 to 3 g every 24 hours. Give dose after hemodialysis.

➤ **Intra-abdominal, gynecologic, and skin-structure infections caused by susceptible strains**

Adults: 1.5 to 3 g IM or IV every 6 hours. Don't exceed 4 g/day of sulbactam.
Children ages 1 and older weighing 40 kg or more (skin and skin-structure infections only): 1.5 to 3 g IV or IM every 6 hours for no longer than 14 days. Don't exceed 4 g/day sulbactam. Continue therapy with an appropriate oral anti-infective agent if necessary.
Children ages 1 and older weighing less than 40 kg (skin and skin-structure infections only): 300 mg/kg/day (200 mg ampicillin/ 100 mg sulbactam) IV in divided doses every 6 hours for no longer than 14 days. Continue therapy with an appropriate oral anti-infective agent if necessary.

ADMINISTRATION

• Before giving, ask patient about allergic reactions to penicillin. A negative history of penicillin allergy is no guarantee against future allergic reaction.

• Obtain specimen for culture and sensitivity tests. Begin therapy while awaiting results.
IV
▼ Reconstitute powder with NSS, sterile water for injection, D$_5$W, lactated Ringer injection, M/6 sodium lactate, dextrose 5% in half-NSS for injection, or 10% invert sugar. Prepare piggyback vial according to manufacturer's instructions.
▼ After reconstitution, let vials stand for a few minutes so foam can dissipate. Inspect solution for particles.
▼ Give drug at least 1 hour before giving a bacteriostatic antibiotic.
▼ For infusion, can give dose by slow IV injection over at least 10 to 15 minutes or can dilute in 50 to 100 mL of compatible diluent and infuse over 15 to 30 minutes.
▼ Stability varies with diluent, temperature, and concentration of solution.
▼ **Incompatibilities:** Acyclovir, aminoglycosides, amiodarone, amphotericin B cholesteryl, amphotericin B lipid complex, amphotericin B liposomal, caspofungin, chlorpromazine, ciprofloxacin, daunorubicin, dobutamine, ganciclovir, ondansetron, phenytoin, prochlorperazine, verapamil. Consult drug compatibility reference for full listing.
IM
• For IM injection, reconstitute with sterile water for injection or 0.5% or 2% lidocaine hydrochloride injection. Add 3.2 mL to a 1.5-g vial (or 6.4 mL to a 3-g vial) to yield 375 mg/mL. Give deep into muscle within 1 hour after preparation.
• IM injection may cause pain at injection site.
• In children, don't use IM route.

ACTION

Inhibits cell-wall synthesis during bacterial multiplication.

Route	Onset	Peak	Duration
IV	Immediate	15 min	Unknown
IM	Unknown	30–52 min	Unknown

Half-life: 1 to 1.5 hours (10 to 24 hours in severe kidney impairment).

ADVERSE REACTIONS

CV: thrombophlebitis, phlebitis. **GI:** diarrhea. **Skin:** pain at injection site, rash, urticaria. **Other:** hypersensitivity reactions.

Reactions in bold italics are *life-threatening*.

INTERACTIONS
Drug-drug. *Allopurinol:* May increase risk of rash. Monitor patient for rash.
Live-virus vaccines: May decrease effectiveness of live-virus vaccines. Use together isn't recommended.
Methotrexate: May increase methotrexate level, increasing risk of toxicity. Monitor methotrexate level.
Oral anticoagulants: May increase risk of bleeding. Monitor PT and INR.
Probenecid: May increase ampicillin level. Probenecid may be used for this purpose.
Tetracycline: May decrease effectiveness of ampicillin–sulbactam. Avoid coadministration if possible.
Drug-herb. *Khat:* May decrease antimicrobial effect of certain penicillins. Discourage khat chewing, or tell patient to take drug 2 hours after khat chewing.

EFFECTS ON LAB TEST RESULTS
• May increase ALP, ALT, AST, bilirubin, BUN, creatinine, and LDH levels.
• May decrease albumin and protein levels.
• May increase eosinophil, lymphocyte, monocyte, and basophil counts.
• May decrease Hb level, hematocrit, and granulocyte, RBC, and WBC counts.
• May increase or decrease platelet count.
• May increase urine RBC and hyaline casts.
• May transiently decrease conjugated estriol, conjugated estrone, estradiol, and estriol glucuronide levels during pregnancy.
• May alter results of urine glucose tests that use cupric sulfate, such as Benedict reagent and Clinitest.

CONTRAINDICATIONS & CAUTIONS
• Contraindicated in patients hypersensitive to drug or other penicillins, in those with other drug allergies (especially to cephalosporins) because of possible cross-sensitivity, and in those with mononucleosis because of high risk of maculopapular rash.
• Contraindicated in patients with a history of cholestatic jaundice or hepatitis.
• Use cautiously in patients with kidney impairment.
Dialyzable drug: Yes.
⚠ *Overdose S&S:* Neuromuscular hyperexcitability, seizures.

PREGNANCY-LACTATION-REPRODUCTION
• There are no adequate and well-controlled studies during pregnancy. Use cautiously during pregnancy and only if clearly needed.
• Drug appears in human milk. Use cautiously during breastfeeding.

NURSING CONSIDERATIONS
• Dosage is expressed as total drug. Each vial contains a 2:1 ratio of ampicillin sodium to sulbactam sodium.
• Monitor LFT results during therapy, especially in patients with impaired liver function.
• Watch for signs and symptoms of bacterial or fungal superinfection, especially in an older adult or a patient with immunosuppression or debilitation, if doses are large or therapy is prolonged.
• Watch for signs and symptoms of hypersensitivity, such as erythematous maculopapular rash, urticaria, and anaphylaxis.
• Monitor patient for CDAD, which can be fatal. Antibiotic may need to be stopped and other treatment begun.

PATIENT TEACHING
• Tell patient to report all adverse reactions, including rash, fever, and chills. A rash is the most common allergic reaction.
• Warn patient that IM injection may cause pain at injection site.

SAFETY ALERT!

anastrozole
an-AS-troe-zole

Arimidex

Therapeutic class: Antineoplastics
Pharmacologic class: Aromatase inhibitors

AVAILABLE FORMS
Tablets: 1 mg

INDICATIONS & DOSAGES
➤ **First-line treatment of adult females after menopause with hormone receptor (HR)–positive or HR–unknown locally advanced or metastatic breast cancer; advanced breast cancer in adult females after menopause with disease progression after tamoxifen therapy; adjunctive treatment of**

adult females after menopause with HR–positive early breast cancer
Adults: 1 mg PO daily.
➤ **Risk reduction for breast cancer in women who are postmenopausal** ♦
Adults: 1 mg PO daily for 5 years.

ADMINISTRATION
PO
🜲 *Alert:* Hazardous drug; use safe handling and disposal precautions.
• Give drug without regard for meals.

ACTION
A selective nonsteroidal aromatase inhibitor that significantly lowers estradiol levels, which inhibits breast cancer cell growth in women who are postmenopausal.

Route	Onset	Peak	Duration
PO	<24 hr	2–5 hr	<7 days

Half-life: 50 hours.

ADVERSE REACTIONS
CNS: headache, fatigue, asthenia, pain, dizziness, fatigue, depression, mood disturbance, paresthesia, anxiety, insomnia, *stroke.* **CV:** hot flashes, *thromboembolic disease,* chest pain, peripheral edema, HTN, vasodilation, *cardiac ischemia, DVT.* **EENT:** cataracts, dry mouth, pharyngitis, sinusitis. **GI:** nausea, vomiting, diarrhea, constipation, abdominal pain, anorexia, dyspepsia, GI disorder. **GU:** vaginal dryness, leukorrhea, vaginitis, vulvovaginitis, *vaginal hemorrhage,* pelvic pain, UTI. **Hematologic:** anemia. **Metabolic:** weight gain, increased cholesterol level. **Musculoskeletal:** bone pain, back pain, arthritis, arthralgia, osteoporosis, fractures, arthrosis, joint disorder, myalgia, carpal tunnel syndrome. **Respiratory:** dyspnea, bronchitis, cough. **Skin:** alopecia, rash, diaphoresis. **Other:** infection, accidental injury, *neoplasm,* tumor flare, lymphedema, flulike symptoms, breast pain, cyst formation.

INTERACTIONS
Drug-drug. *Estrogen:* May decrease pharmacologic action of anastrozole. Use together isn't recommended.
Tamoxifen: May reduce anastrozole plasma level. Don't use together.

EFFECTS ON LAB TEST RESULTS
• May increase calcium, liver enzyme, and cholesterol levels.

CONTRAINDICATIONS & CAUTIONS
• Contraindicated in patients hypersensitive to drug or its components.
• Use cautiously in patients with preexisting ischemic heart disease.
Dialyzable drug: Unknown.

PREGNANCY-LACTATION-REPRODUCTION
• Drug can cause fetal harm. Advise patients of childbearing potential of fetal risk.
• Patients of childbearing potential should use effective contraception during therapy and for at least 3 weeks after final dose.
• It isn't known if drug appears in human milk. Patient shouldn't breastfeed during therapy and for 2 weeks after final dose.
• May impair fertility in patients of childbearing potential.

NURSING CONSIDERATIONS
• Give drug under supervision of a prescriber experienced in use of antineoplastics.
• Patients with HR–negative disease and patients who didn't respond to previous tamoxifen therapy rarely respond to anastrozole.
• For patients with advanced breast cancer, continue anastrozole until tumor progresses.
• Monitor bone mineral density because drug can decrease bone mineral density.
• Use drug only in women who are postmenopausal.
• Rule out pregnancy before starting drug.

PATIENT TEACHING
• Instruct patient to report adverse reactions, especially difficulty breathing, chest pain, and skin lesions or blisters.
• Tell patient to take medication at the same time each day.
• Stress the need for follow-up care.
• Counsel patient about risks of pregnancy during therapy. Advise use of effective contraception during therapy and for at least 3 weeks after final dose.
• Advise patient not to breastfeed during treatment and for 2 weeks after final dose.
• Inform patient that cholesterol level may increase.
• Tell patient that drug lowers estrogen level, which may lead to decreased bone strength and increased risk of fractures.

Reactions in bold italics are *life-threatening*.

apalutamide
a-pa-LOO-ta-mide

Erleada

Therapeutic class: Antineoplastics
Pharmacologic class: Androgen receptor inhibitors

AVAILABLE FORMS
Tablets ⓓⓝⓒ: 60 mg, 240 mg

INDICATIONS & DOSAGES
Adjust-a-dose (for all indications): If grade 3 or greater toxicity occurs, withhold drug until symptoms improve to grade 1 or less or to original grade; then resume at same dosage or a reduced dosage (180 or 120 mg), if warranted.

➤ **Nonmetastatic castration-resistant prostate cancer, metastatic castration-sensitive prostate cancer**
Adult males: 240 mg (four 60-mg tablets) PO once daily.

ADMINISTRATION
PO
🔸 *Alert:* Hazardous drug; use safe handling and disposal precautions.
• Give with or without food.
• Have patient swallow tablets whole; don't crush or cut tablets.
• If patient can't swallow 60 mg tablet, mix whole tablets in 4 oz (120 mL) of applesauce by stirring. Don't crush tablets. Wait 15 minutes; then stir mixture. Wait another 15 minutes; then stir mixture until tablets are well mixed, with no chunks remaining. Using a spoon, have patient swallow mixture right away. Rinse container with 2 oz (60 mL) of water and have patient immediately drink contents. Repeat rinse with 2 oz of water to ensure patient takes entire dose. Give mixture within 1 hour of preparation.
• If patient can't swallow 240-mg tablet, disperse in 10 mL water without crushing or splitting the tablet. Wait 2 minutes then stir and administer with 30 mL of either orange juice, applesauce, or additional water. Give immediately; then rinse cup with enough water to ensure the whole dose is taken and have patient drink immediately. Don't store.

• To give 240-mg tablet through feeding tube, place tablet in 20 mL or larger syringe and draw up 10 mL of water. Wait 10 minutes; then shake vigorously. Administer through feeding tube. Refill syringe with water and repeat administration until no tablet residue is left in syringe or feeding tube.
• Give a missed dose as soon as possible on the same day; then return to the normal schedule on the following day. Don't give extra tablets to make up for a missed dose.
• Store in original container and protect from light and moisture; don't discard desiccant.

ACTION
Binds to androgen receptors to decrease tumor cell proliferation and increase apoptosis, leading to decreased tumor volume.

Route	Onset	Peak	Duration
PO	Unknown	2 hr	Unknown

Half-life: 3 days.

ADVERSE REACTIONS
CNS: fatigue, asthenia, dysgeusia. **CV:** peripheral edema, HTN, hot flashes, *ischemic heart disease, HF.* **GI:** decreased appetite, diarrhea, nausea, vomiting, stomatitis. **GU:** hematuria. **Hematologic:** anemia, *leukopenia, lymphopenia.* **Metabolic:** weight loss, hypothyroidism, hypercholesterolemia, hyperglycemia, hypertriglyceridemia, *hyperkalemia.* **Musculoskeletal:** arthralgia, fracture, muscle spasm. **Skin:** rash, pruritus. **Other:** fall.

INTERACTIONS
Drug-drug. *Strong CYP3A4/CYP2C8 inducers (rifampin):* May decrease apalutamide level. Monitor patient for loss of apalutamide activity.
Strong CYP3A4 (itraconazole, ketoconazole) or CYP2C8 (gemfibrozil) inhibitors: May increase apalutamide level. Monitor patient and reduce apalutamide dosage if necessary.
Substrates of CYP2C9 (warfarin), CYP2C19 (omeprazole), CYP3A4 (midazolam), and uridine diphosphate glycosyltransferase: May reduce levels of these drugs. Use other drugs as substitutes for these drugs, if possible. If use with apalutamide is necessary, monitor patient for loss of activity of these drugs.
Substrates of P-gp (fexofenadine), BCRP, and organic anion transporting polypeptide 1B1 (rosuvastatin): May reduce levels of these

drugs. Use together cautiously if necessary. If use with apalutamide is necessary, monitor patient for loss of activity of these drugs.

EFFECTS ON LAB TEST RESULTS
• May increase TSH, potassium, cholesterol, glucose, and triglyceride levels.
• May decrease RBC, WBC, and lymphocyte counts.

CONTRAINDICATIONS & CAUTIONS
• Drug isn't indicated for use in females.
• Use cautiously in patients with a risk of falls and fractures.
• Drug may increase risk of seizures. Avoid use in patients with a history of seizures or with predisposing factors for seizures and in those receiving drugs known to decrease seizure threshold or to induce seizures.
• Drug may increase risk of hypothyroidism and CV disease.
• Drug may increase risk of cerebrovascular and ischemic CV events, including events leading to death.
• Safety and effectiveness in females and children haven't been established.
Dialyzable drug: Unknown.

PREGNANCY-LACTATION-REPRODUCTION
⚠ *Alert:* Drug isn't indicated for use in females. May cause fetal harm and loss of pregnancy.
• Patients with partners of childbearing potential should use effective contraception (condom) during treatment and for 3 months after final dose.
• Drug may impair fertility in males of reproductive potential.

NURSING CONSIDERATIONS
• Administer a GnRH analogue concurrently unless patient has had a bilateral orchiectomy.
• Use appropriate precautions (such as wearing single gloves) when receiving, handling, administering, and disposing of drug.
• Evaluate patient for risk of falls and fractures. Consider use of bone-targeted agents, if appropriate.
• Monitor patient for seizures. If seizure occurs, permanently discontinue drug.
• Monitor patient for signs and symptoms of cerebrovascular disorders and ischemic heart disease. Optimize management of CV risk factors.
• Monitor patient for SCARs, including SJS, TEN, and DRESS syndrome. Signs and

symptoms may include fever, flulike symptoms, mucosal lesions, progressive skin rash, and lymphadenopathy. Permanently discontinue apalutamide for a confirmed SCAR or other grade 4 skin reaction.
• *Look alike–sound alike:* Don't confuse apalutamide with bicalutamide, flutamide, or nilutamide.

PATIENT TEACHING
• Teach about proper drug administration and handling.
• Inform patient receiving a GnRH analogue to continue this drug while taking apalutamide.
• Warn patient that drug isn't indicated for use in females.
• Tell patient that drug may increase risk of falls and fractures.
• Warn that drug may increase risk of heart disease, stroke, and ministroke. Instruct patient to seek help immediately if chest pain or discomfort; numbness or weakness of the face, arm, or leg; trouble speaking; or loss of balance occurs.
• Caution patient that drug may increase risk of seizures. Instruct patient to use care when involved in activities in which loss of consciousness could cause harm to self or others.
• Tell patient to report all adverse reactions and to immediately report seizure, falls, or rash.
⚠ *Alert:* Advise patient of reproductive potential to use effective contraception during treatment and for 3 months after final dose.
• Caution patient to use condoms while having sex. Drug may cause fetal harm.
• Educate patient of reproductive potential about the risk of impaired fertility. Advise patient not to donate sperm during treatment and for 3 months after final dose.

SAFETY ALERT!

apixaban
a-PIX-a-ban

Eliquis

Therapeutic class: Anticoagulants
Pharmacologic class: Factor Xa inhibitors

AVAILABLE FORMS
Tablets: 2.5 mg, 5 mg

INDICATIONS & DOSAGES

Adjust-a-dose (for all indications): If given with P-gp and strong CYP3A4 inhibitors decrease 5-mg or 10-mg doses by half.

➤ **Reduction of risk of stroke and systemic embolism in patients with nonvalvular atrial fibrillation**

Adults: 5 mg PO b.i.d.

Adjust-a-dose: Reduce dosage to 2.5 mg b.i.d. in patients with any two of the following characteristics: age 80 or older, body weight 60 kg or less, or serum creatinine 1.5 mg/dL or greater.

➤ **DVT prophylaxis after hip or knee replacement surgery**

Adults: 2.5 mg PO b.i.d. beginning 12 to 24 hours after surgery. Continue for 35 days after hip replacement surgery or for 12 days after knee replacement surgery.

➤ **DVT and PE**

Adults: 10 mg PO b.i.d. for 7 days followed by 5 mg PO b.i.d.; then, to reduce risk of recurrence after at least 6 months of treatment, 2.5 mg PO b.i.d.

ADMINISTRATION

PO

• Give drug without regard for food.

• Give a missed dose as soon as possible on the same day; then resume twice-daily administration. Don't double the dose to make up for a missed dose.

• If patient can't swallow tablets, crush and suspend in water, D_5W, or apple juice or mix with applesauce and give promptly PO, or crush and suspend in 60 mL of water or D_5W and give promptly through NG tube. Crushed tablets are stable in water, D_5W, apple juice, or applesauce for up to 4 hours.

• Store at room temperature.

ACTION

Selectively inhibits factor Xa, decreasing thrombin generation and thrombus development.

Route	Onset	Peak	Duration
PO	Unknown	3–4 hr	Unknown

Half-life: 12 hours.

ADVERSE REACTIONS

EENT: epistaxis, bleeding gums. **GI:** nausea, rectal hemorrhage. **GU:** hematuria, menorrhagia. **Hematologic:** *major bleeding,* anemia, hematoma, bruising. **Hepatic:** increased LFTs. **Respiratory:** hemoptysis.

INTERACTIONS

Drug-drug. *Aspirin and other antiplatelet agents/anticoagulants, heparin, NSAIDs, SSNRIs, SSRIs, thrombolytics:* May increase bleeding risk. Avoid use together.

Combined strong dual inducers of CYP3A4 and P-gp (carbamazepine, phenytoin, rifampin): May decrease apixaban concentration. Avoid use together.

Combined strong dual inhibitors of CYP3A4 and P-gp (clarithromycin, itraconazole, ketoconazole, ritonavir): May increase apixaban concentration. Decrease dosage by 50% in patients taking 5 or 10 mg b.i.d.; avoid use together in patients already taking 2.5 mg b.i.d.

Drug-herb. *Alfalfa, anise, bilberry:* May increase bleeding risk. Consider therapy modification.

St. John's wort: May decrease apixaban concentration. Avoid use together.

Drug-food. *Grapefruit juice:* May increase drug level and risk of bleeding. Use cautiously and monitor patient for bleeding.

EFFECTS ON LAB TEST RESULTS

• May increase LFT values.
• May prolong PT, INR, and PTT.

CONTRAINDICATIONS & CAUTIONS

• Contraindicated in patients with severe hypersensitivity to drug or its components and in those with active pathological bleeding.

• Use cautiously in patients at risk for severe bleeding (especially those concomitantly taking drugs that affect hemostasis).

• Use of apixaban isn't recommended in patients with acute PE who are hemodynamically unstable, patients who require thrombolysis or pulmonary embolectomy, or patients with antiphospholipid syndrome.

Boxed Warning Discontinuing drug prematurely increases risk of thrombotic events. If anticoagulation with apixaban must be discontinued for a reason other than pathological bleeding, strongly consider coverage with another anticoagulant. ∎

Boxed Warning Consider potential risk of epidural or spinal hematoma versus benefit in patients scheduled for spinal procedures (spinal or epidural anesthesia, spinal puncture). Hematomas may result in long-term or permanent paralysis. Risk increases with use of indwelling epidural catheters, concomitant use of drugs that affect hemostasis (NSAIDs, platelet inhibitors, anticoagulants), history of traumatic or repeated epidural or spinal punctures, or history of spinal deformity or surgery. ∎

🜂 *Alert:* Discontinue apixaban at least 48 hours before elective surgery or invasive procedures with a moderate or high risk of unacceptable or clinically significant bleeding.

🜂 *Alert:* Discontinue apixaban at least 24 hours before elective surgery or invasive procedures with a low risk of bleeding or when bleeding would be noncritical in location and easily controlled.

• Bridging anticoagulation before the intervention isn't generally required. Restart apixaban as soon as adequate hemostasis has returned.

• Drug isn't recommended for patients with severe liver impairment or prosthetic heart valves.

• Increased risk for bleeding in patients with severe kidney impairment.

• Safety and effectiveness in children haven't been established.

Dialyzable drug: 14%.

⚠ *Overdose S&S:* Increased risk of bleeding.

PREGNANCY-LACTATION-REPRODUCTION

• Drug may cross the placental barrier. Drug may increase risk of bleeding in fetus and neonate and during labor or delivery. Not recommended during pregnancy.

• It isn't known if drug appears in human milk. Patient should discontinue breastfeeding or discontinue drug, considering importance of drug to patient.

NURSING CONSIDERATIONS

• Monitor patient for bleeding. Discontinue drug if acute pathologic bleeding occurs.

🜂 *Alert:* Promptly evaluate signs and symptom of blood loss. Drug can cause serious, potentially fatal bleeding.

Boxed Warning Monitor patient receiving neuraxial anesthesia or undergoing spinal puncture for neurologic impairment (midline back pain; sensory or motor deficits, such as numbness or weakness in lower limbs; bowel or bladder dysfunction). Treat impairment urgently. ∎

🜂 *Alert:* Removal of indwelling epidural or intrathecal catheter should be delayed for at least 24 hours after last dose of apixaban. Next dose of apixaban should be given no earlier than 5 hours after catheter removal. Don't

give drug for at least 48 hours after traumatic or repeated epidural or spinal punctures.

• Administration of activated charcoal may be useful in the management of apixaban overdose or accidental ingestion. Andexanet alfa is available for reversal of the anti-factor Xa activity of apixaban.

• When switching from warfarin to apixaban, discontinue warfarin and start apixaban when INR is below 2.

• If switching from apixaban to warfarin, discontinue apixaban and begin both a parenteral anticoagulant and warfarin at the time the next dose of apixaban would have been taken. Discontinue the parenteral anticoagulant when INR reaches an acceptable range. Initial INR measurements during the transition to warfarin may not be useful because apixaban affects INR.

• If switching between apixaban and anticoagulants other than warfarin, discontinue drug being taken and begin other drug at next scheduled dose.

PATIENT TEACHING

• Warn patient not to discontinue drug without first talking to prescriber because of risk of clot formation and stroke.

• Tell patient to report all adverse reactions and unusual bleeding; caution patient that bruising or bleeding may occur more easily.

• Instruct patient to inform all health care providers (including dentist) about taking this drug as well as other products known to affect bleeding (including nonprescription products, such as aspirin or NSAIDs) before scheduling surgery or medical or dental procedure and before taking any new drug.

• Tell patient to report pregnancy or plans to become pregnant or breastfeed during treatment.

---

apremilast
a-PRE-mil-ast

Otezla

Therapeutic class: Antiarthritics
Pharmacologic class: Phosphodiesterase-4 inhibitors

AVAILABLE FORMS

Tablets ⓞⓝⓒ: 10 mg, 20 mg, 30 mg

INDICATIONS & DOSAGES
➤ **Active psoriatic arthritis; plaque psoriasis in patients who are candidates for phototherapy or systemic therapy; oral ulcers associated with Behçet disease**
Adults: Initially, 10 mg PO in a.m. on day 1; 10 mg PO b.i.d. (a.m. and p.m.) on day 2; 10 mg PO in a.m. and 20 mg PO in p.m. on day 3; 20 mg PO b.i.d. (a.m. and p.m.) on day 4; 20 mg PO in a.m. and 30 mg PO in p.m. on day 5; then 30 mg PO b.i.d. (a.m. and p.m.) on day 6 and thereafter.
Adjust-a-dose: In patients with CrCl less than 30 mL/minute, give doses according to a.m. schedule only (omit p.m. doses) from days 1 through 5. For day 6 and onward, give 30 mg once daily.

ADMINISTRATION
PO
• Give drug without regard to meals.
• Have patient swallow tablets whole; don't crush or cut tablets.
• Store tablets below 86° F (30° C).

ACTION
Increases intracellular cAMP level. Its action in the treatment of psoriatic arthritis and psoriasis isn't well defined.

Route	Onset	Peak	Duration
PO	Unknown	2.5 hr	Unknown

Half-life: 6 to 9 hours.

ADVERSE REACTIONS
CNS: headache, depression, fatigue, insomnia, migraine. **EENT:** nasopharyngitis, tooth abscess. **GI:** diarrhea, frequent bowel movements, nausea, vomiting, upper abdominal pain, decreased appetite, dyspepsia, GERD. **Metabolic:** weight loss. **Musculoskeletal:** back pain, arthralgia. **Respiratory:** URI, bronchitis. **Skin:** folliculitis.

INTERACTIONS
Drug-drug. *Strong CYP450 inducers (carbamazepine, phenobarbital, phenytoin, rifampin):* May decrease apremilast level, causing loss of effectiveness. Use together isn't recommended.
Drug-herb. *St. John's wort:* May decrease apremilast level. Discourage use together.

EFFECTS ON LAB TEST RESULTS
None reported.

CONTRAINDICATIONS & CAUTIONS
• Contraindicated in patients hypersensitive to drug or its components.
⚠ *Alert:* Use cautiously in patients with history of depression or suicidality. Weigh risks and benefits of using drug in these patients.
• Use cautiously in patients with severe kidney impairment.
• Use cautiously in older adults and patients taking medications that can lead to volume depletion or hypotension; they're at increased risk of complications from severe diarrhea, nausea, or vomiting.
• Safety and effectiveness in children haven't been established.
Dialyzable drug: Unknown.

PREGNANCY-LACTATION-REPRODUCTION
• Use cautiously during pregnancy and only if benefits outweigh fetal risk.
• It isn't known if drug appears in human milk. Use cautiously during breastfeeding.

NURSING CONSIDERATIONS
• Titration to maintenance dose is intended to reduce GI symptoms with initial therapy.
• Monitor for complications of diarrhea or vomiting. Severe symptoms may require dosage reductions or drug suspension.
• Monitor for depression and suicidality.
• Regularly monitor patient for unexplained or significant weight loss. Evaluate cause and consider discontinuing drug.

PATIENT TEACHING
• Explain to patient that drug may cause weight loss.
⚠ *Alert:* Warn patient and caregivers to immediately report signs and symptoms of depression or suicidality.
• Teach about proper drug administration and handling, including titration schedule to reduce GI symptoms.

aprepitant
ah-PRE-pit-ant

Aponvie, Cinvanti, Emend

fosaprepitant dimeglumine
Emend

Therapeutic class: Antiemetics
Pharmacologic class: Substance P and neurokinin-1 receptor antagonists

AVAILABLE FORMS
aprepitant
Capsules: 40 mg, 80 mg, 125 mg
Injection (emulsion)*: 32 mg/4.4 mL, 130 mg/18 mL single-dose vial
Powder for oral suspension (kit): 125 mg
fosaprepitant dimeglumine
Injection: 150-mg single-dose vial

INDICATIONS & DOSAGES
➤ **To prevent nausea and vomiting after highly emetogenic chemotherapy (HEC) (including cisplatin) and moderately emetogenic chemotherapy (MEC), with a 5-HT₃ antagonist and a corticosteroid (except Aponvie)**
Adults and children ages 12 and older (capsules): On day 1 of chemotherapy, 125 mg PO 1 hour before treatment; on days 2 and 3, 80 mg PO 1 hour before chemotherapy or, if no chemotherapy is scheduled, in the morning.
Adults unable to swallow capsules and children ages 6 months to younger than 12 years weighing 6 kg or more (oral suspension): On day 1 of chemotherapy, 3 mg/kg PO 1 hour before treatment; maximum dose, 125 mg. On days 2 and 3, 2 mg/kg PO 1 hour before chemotherapy or, if no chemotherapy is scheduled, in the morning; maximum dose, 80 mg.
Adults (fosaprepitant): On day 1, 150 mg IV over 20 to 30 minutes 30 minutes before chemotherapy.
Children ages 12 and older (fosaprepitant): Single-day regimen: On day 1, 150 mg IV over 30 minutes 30 minutes before chemotherapy. For 3-day dosage regimen in children ages 12 to 17: On day 1, 115 mg IV over 30 minutes 30 minutes before chemotherapy; on days 2 and 3, 80 mg IV over 30 minutes or capsules or suspension PO 1 hour before treatment or, if no chemotherapy is scheduled, in the morning.

Children ages 2 to younger than 12 weighing at least 6 kg (fosaprepitant): Single-day regimen: On day 1, 4 mg/kg (maximum dose, 150 mg) IV over 60 minutes 30 minutes before chemotherapy.
Children ages 6 months to younger than 2 years weighing at least 6 kg (fosaprepitat): Single-day regimen: On day 1, 5 mg/kg (maximum dose, 150 mg) IV over 60 minutes 30 minutes before chemotherapy.
Children ages 6 months to younger than 12 years weighing at least 6 kg (fosaprepitant): For 3-day dosing regimen: On day 1, 3 mg/kg (maximum dose, 115 mg) IV over 60 minutes 30 minutes before chemotherapy; on days 2 and 3, 2 mg/kg (maximum dose, 80 mg) IV over 60 minutes or suspension PO 1 hour before chemotherapy or, if no chemotherapy is scheduled, in the morning.
Adults (aprepitant [Cinvanti]): Single-dose regimen for HEC or MEC: On day 1, 130 mg IV over 30 minutes before chemotherapy. For 3-day dosing regimen, on day 1, 100 mg IV emulsion complete 30 minutes before chemotherapy; on days 2 and 3, 80 mg PO aprepitant once daily.
➤ **To prevent postoperative nausea and vomiting**
Adults: 40 mg PO within 3 hours before induction of anesthesia. Or, Aponvie 32 mg IV over 30 seconds prior to induction of anesthesia.

ADMINISTRATION
PO
- Give drug without regard for food.
- Drug may be given with other antiemetics.
- Oral suspension should be prepared by a health care provider according to manufacturer's instructions, but once prepared may be administered by a health care provider, patient, or caregiver.
- Refer to manufacturer's instructions and instructions for concomitant administration with dexamethasone and 5-HT₃ antagonist.
- Refrigerate prepared oral suspension until administered. May store at room temperature for up to 3 hours before use. Discard any dose remaining after 72 hours.
IV
▼ Reconstitute fosaprepitant with 5 mL of NSS. Add NSS along the vial wall to prevent foaming. Swirl gently; avoid shaking.
▼ Add entire reconstituted fosaprepitant volume to infusion bag containing 145 mL of NSS.

Reactions in bold italics are *life-threatening*.

▼ Gently invert the bag two to three times. Total volume will be 150 mL and concentration will be 1 mg/mL.

▼ Final fosaprepitant (Emend) solution is stable for 24 hours at room temperature.

▼ Aprepitant emulsions can be given IV as an injection over 2 minutes or an infusion over 30 minutes

▼ For infusion, add aprepitant emulsion (Civanti only) dose to 100 mL infusion bag of NSS or D₅W and then gently invert four to five times. Avoid shaking.

▼ Before administering, inspect bag for particulate matter and discoloration. Discard if particulates or discoloration is observed.

▼ Flush the infusion line with NSS before and after administration.

▼ Cinvanti is stable for 6 hours in NSS, 12 hours in D₅W at room temperature, or up to 72 hours under refrigeration.

▼ **Incompatibilities:** Solutions containing divalent cations (Ca^{2+}, Mg^{2+}), including lactated Ringer solution and Hartmann solution.

ACTION
Inhibits emesis by selectively antagonizing substance P and neurokinin-1 receptors in the brain; appears to be synergistic with 5-HT₃ antagonists and corticosteroids.

Route	Onset	Peak	Duration
PO	Unknown	3–4 hr	Unknown
IV	Unknown	<30 min	Unknown

Half-life: 9 to 13 hours.

ADVERSE REACTIONS
CNS: asthenia, fatigue, dizziness, headache, peripheral neuropathy, anxiety. **CV:** *bradycardia,* HTN, hypotension. **EENT:** dry mouth. **GI:** anorexia, constipation, diarrhea, nausea, abdominal pain, eructation, flatulence, gastritis, heartburn, vomiting, dyspepsia. **GU:** UTI. **Hematologic:** *neutropenia, leukopenia, thrombocytopenia,* anemia. **Hepatic:** increased ALT level. **Metabolic:** dehydration. **Musculoskeletal:** extremity pain. **Respiratory:** cough, hiccups. **Skin:** pruritus, alopecia, infusion-site reaction. **Other:** candidiasis.

INTERACTIONS
Drug-drug. *Alprazolam, midazolam, triazolam:* May increase levels of these drugs. Watch for CNS effects, such as increased sedation. Decrease benzodiazepine dose.

Atazanavir, clarithromycin, diltiazem, erythromycin, itraconazole, ketoconazole, nefazodone, nelfinavir, ritonavir, troleandomycin, other CYP3A4 inhibitors: May increase aprepitant level and risk of toxicity. Use together cautiously.

Carbamazepine, phenytoin, rifampin, other CYP3A4 inducers: May decrease aprepitant level. Watch for decreased antiemetic effect.

Dexamethasone, methylprednisolone: May increase levels of these drugs and risk of toxicity. Decrease PO corticosteroid dose by 50%; decrease IV methylprednisolone dose by 25%.

Diltiazem: May increase diltiazem level. Monitor HR and BP. Avoid use together.

Docetaxel, etoposide, ifosfamide, imatinib, irinotecan, paclitaxel, vinorelbine, vinblastine, vincristine: May increase levels and risk of toxicity of these drugs. Use together cautiously.

Hormonal contraceptives: May decrease contraceptive effectiveness. Female patients should use additional birth control method during therapy and for 1 month after last dose.

Paroxetine: May decrease paroxetine and aprepitant effects. Monitor for effectiveness.

Pimozide: May increase pimozide level and QT prolongation. Use together is contraindicated.

Warfarin: May decrease warfarin effectiveness. Monitor INR carefully for 2 weeks after each aprepitant treatment.

Drug-herb. *St. John's wort:* May decrease antiemetic effects by inducing CYP3A4. Discourage use together.

Drug-food. *Grapefruit juice:* May increase drug level and risk of toxicity. Discourage use together.

EFFECTS ON LAB TEST RESULTS
• May increase ALP, AST, ALT, BUN, creatinine, glucose, and urine protein levels.
• May decrease sodium level.
• May decrease Hb level and WBC, platelet, and neutrophil counts.

CONTRAINDICATIONS & CAUTIONS
• Contraindicated in patients hypersensitive to fosaprepitant, aprepitant, or their components. Hypersensitivity reactions have been reported.
• Use cautiously in patients receiving chemotherapy drugs metabolized mainly via CYP3A4 and in those with severe liver disease.

• Cinvanti and Aponvie aren't approved for use in children.

Dialyzable drug: No.

⚠ *Overdose S&S:* Drowsiness, headache.

PREGNANCY-LACTATION-REPRODUCTION

• Use during pregnancy only if clearly needed.

• Cinvanti and Aponvie contain alcohol and shouldn't be used during pregnancy.

• Patients taking hormonal contraceptives should use an additional form of contraception during therapy and for 1 month after final dose.

• It isn't known if drug appears in human milk. Use cautiously during breastfeeding.

NURSING CONSIDERATIONS

• Avoid giving drug for more than 3 days per chemotherapy cycle.

🔵 *Alert:* Only give IV form on day 1 of a 3-day antiemetic regimen.

🔵 *Alert:* Before giving drug, carefully screen patient for possible drug and herb interactions.

• Monitor for hypersensitivity reactions (dyspnea, flushing, eye swelling, pruritus and wheezing) directly after administration.

• Don't give drug for established nausea or vomiting.

• Expect to give drug with other antiemetics to treat breakthrough emesis.

• Periodically monitor CBC, LFT results, and creatinine level during therapy.

• *Look alike–sound alike:* Don't confuse aprepitant (oral and IV form) with fosaprepitant (IV form).

PATIENT TEACHING

• Advise patient to report all adverse reactions to prescriber.

• Tell patient that severe hypersensitivity reactions have occurred and that patient will be monitored after therapy.

• If nausea or vomiting occurs, instruct patient to take breakthrough antiemetics rather than more aprepitant.

• Urge patient to report use of any other drugs or herbs.

• Instruct patient in safe oral drug administration.

• Advise patient who takes a hormonal contraceptive to use an additional form of birth control during therapy and for 1 month after last dose.

• Tell patient who takes warfarin that PT and INR will be closely monitored for 2 weeks after therapy starts.

SAFETY ALERT!

argatroban
ahr-GAH-troh-ban

Therapeutic class: Anticoagulants
Pharmacologic class: Direct thrombin inhibitors

AVAILABLE FORMS

Injection: 1 mg/mL in 50-mL; 100 mg/mL in 2.5-mL vial

INDICATIONS & DOSAGES

➤ **To prevent or treat thrombosis in patients with heparin-induced thrombocytopenia**

Adults: 2 mcg/kg/minute, given as a continuous IV infusion; adjust dose until the steady-state PTT is 1½ to 3 times the initial baseline value, not to exceed 100 seconds; maximum dose, 10 mcg/kg/minute. See current manufacturer's label for recommended doses and infusion rates.

Adjust-a-dose: For adults with moderate or severe liver impairment, reduce first dose to 0.5 mcg/kg/minute, given as a continuous infusion. Monitor PTT closely and adjust dosage as needed.

➤ **Anticoagulation in patients with or at risk for heparin-induced thrombocytopenia during PCI**

Adults: Start a continuous IV infusion at 25 mcg/kg/minute and give a 350 mcg/kg IV bolus over 3 to 5 minutes. Check activated clotting time (ACT) 5 to 10 minutes after completion of bolus dose. Proceed with procedure if ACT is more than 300 seconds.

Adjust-a-dose: Use the following table to adjust dosage.

Activated clotting time (ACT)	Additional IV bolus	Continuous IV infusion
<300 sec	150 mcg/kg	30 mcg/kg/min*
>450 sec	None needed	15 mcg/kg/min*

*Check ACT again after 5 to 10 minutes.

Once therapeutic ACT (300 to 450 sec) has been achieved, continue this dose for duration of procedure. In case of dissection, impending abrupt closure, thrombus formation

---

during procedure, or inability to achieve or maintain ACT exceeding 300 seconds, give additional bolus of 150 mcg/kg and increase infusion rate to 40 mcg/kg/minute. Recheck ACT after 5 to 10 minutes.

ADMINISTRATION

IV

▼ Before starting therapy, obtain a complete list of patient's prescription and OTC drugs and supplements, including herbs.

▼ Stop all parenteral anticoagulants before giving drug. Giving with antiplatelets, thrombolytics, and other anticoagulants may increase risk of bleeding.

▼ Before starting drug, get results of baseline coagulation tests, platelet count, Hb level, and hematocrit, and report any abnormalities to prescriber.

▼ Dilute each 2.5-mL vial with 250 mL of NSS, D₅W, or lactated Ringer injection to a final concentration of 1 mg/mL. Dilution isn't required for 50-mL vial.

▼ Mix the solution by repeated inversion of the diluent bag for 1 minute.

▼ Don't expose solution to direct sunlight.

▼ See manufacturer's instructions for storage.

▼ **Incompatibilities:** Other IV drugs.

ACTION

Reversibly binds to the thrombin-active site and inhibits thrombin-catalyzed or thrombin-induced reactions: fibrin formation; coagulation factor V, VIII, and XIII activation; protein C activation; and platelet aggregation. Inhibits the action of free and clot-associated thrombin.

Route	Onset	Peak	Duration
IV	Rapid	1–3 hr	Duration of infusion

Half-life: 39 to 51 minutes.

ADVERSE REACTIONS

CNS: *cerebrovascular disorder, intracranial bleeding,* fever, pain, headache. **CV:** *hemorrhage,* atrial fibrillation, *cardiac arrest,* hypotension, *ventricular tachycardia,* chest pain, angina, *bradycardia, MI,* groin or brachial bleeding. **GI:** abdominal pain, diarrhea, *GI bleeding,* nausea, vomiting. **GU:** abnormal kidney function, hematuria, UTI. **Hematologic:** anemia. **Respiratory:** cough, dyspnea, pneumonia, hemoptysis. **Skin:** *injection-site hemorrhage.* **Other:** allergic reactions, infection, *sepsis.*

INTERACTIONS

Drug-drug. *Glycoprotein IIb/IIIa inhibitors (eptifibatide, tirofiban), thrombolytics:* May increase risk of bleeding, including intracranial bleeding. Avoid use together; safety and effectiveness haven't been established.
Heparin: May increase risk of bleeding. Allow sufficient time for heparin's effect on PTT to decrease before starting argatroban.
Warfarin: May prolong PT and INR and increase risk of bleeding. Monitor patient closely.

Drug-herb. *Herbs with anticoagulant or antiplatelet properties (alfalfa, anise, bilberry, others):* May increase risk of bleeding. Discourage use together.

EFFECTS ON LAB TEST RESULTS

- May decrease Hb level and hematocrit.
- May prolong PTT and ACT.

CONTRAINDICATIONS & CAUTIONS

- Contraindicated in patients who have overt major bleeding or are hypersensitive to drug or any of its components.
- Use cautiously in patients with liver disease or conditions that increase the risk of hemorrhage, such as severe HTN.
- Use cautiously in patients who have just had lumbar puncture, spinal anesthesia, or major surgery, especially of the brain, spinal cord, or eye; patients with hematologic conditions causing increased bleeding tendencies, such as congenital or acquired bleeding disorders; and patients with GI ulcers or other lesions.
- Use cautiously in patients who are critically ill; reduced dosages may be needed.
- Safety and effectiveness in children haven't been established.

Dialyzable drug: 20% during 4-hour hemodialysis session.

⚠ **Overdose S&S:** Excessive anticoagulation, with or without bleeding.

PREGNANCY-LACTATION-REPRODUCTION

- There are no adequate well-controlled studies during pregnancy. Use during pregnancy only if clearly needed.
- It isn't known if drug appears in human milk. Patient should discontinue breastfeeding or discontinue drug, considering importance of drug to patient.

NURSING CONSIDERATIONS

• Check PTT 2 hours after giving drug; dose adjustments may be required to get targeted PTT of 1½ to 3 times baseline, no longer than 100 seconds. Steady state is achieved 1 to 3 hours after starting drug.

• Draw blood for ACT every 20 to 30 minutes during prolonged PCI.

⚠ Alert: Patients can hemorrhage from any site in body. Unexplained decreases in hematocrit or BP and other unexplained symptoms may signify a hemorrhagic event.

• To convert to warfarin therapy, give expected daily dose of warfarin PO with argatroban at up to 2 mcg/kg/minute until INR exceeds 4 on combined therapy. If argatroban infusion rate is greater than 2 mcg/kg/minute, decrease rate to 2 mcg/kg/minute before administering warfarin. After argatroban is stopped, repeat INR in 4 to 6 hours. If repeat INR remains less than desired therapeutic range, resume IV argatroban infusion. Repeat procedure daily until desired therapeutic range on warfarin alone is reached.

• Look alike–sound alike: Don't confuse argatroban with Aggrastat.

PATIENT TEACHING

• Instruct patient who is pregnant, has recently delivered, or is breastfeeding to notify prescriber.

• Advise patient to immediately report bleeding, tarry stools, bruising, rash, or difficulty breathing.

ARIPiprazole ⬤
ar-i-PIP-ra-zole

Abilify, Abilify Maintena, Abilify MyCite

ARIPiprazole lauroxil ⬤
Aristada, Aristada Initio

Therapeutic class: Antipsychotics
Pharmacologic class: Quinolinone derivatives

AVAILABLE FORMS

Oral solution: 1 mg/mL
Suspension for IM use (extended-release): 300-mg or 400-mg vial or prefilled syringe (Abilify Maintena); 441 mg/1.6 mL, 662 mg/2.4 mL, 882 mg/3.2 mL, 1,064 mg/3.9 mL in prefilled syringe (Aristada); 675 mg/2.4 mL in prefilled syringe (Aristada Initio)
Tablets: 2 mg, 5 mg, 10 mg, 15 mg, 20 mg, 30 mg
Tablets (ODTs): 10 mg, 15 mg, 20 mg, 30 mg
Tablets (with sensor [Abilify MyCite]) ⓄⓃⓄ: 2 mg, 5 mg, 10 mg, 15 mg, 20 mg, 30 mg

INDICATIONS & DOSAGES

Adjust-a-dose (for all indications except adjunctive treatment of major depressive disorder): Refer to manufacturer's instructions for drug interactions, CYP2D6 poor metabolizers, and missed-dose dosage adjustments.

➤ Schizophrenia (oral, IM [Abilify Maintena])

Adults: Initially, 10 to 15 mg PO daily; increase to maximum daily dose of 30 mg, if needed, after at least 2 weeks. Continue patients who respond on the lowest dosage needed to maintain remission. Periodically reassess patients to determine the need for maintenance treatment.

Or, 400 mg IM monthly. For patients who have never taken aripiprazole, establish tolerability with aripiprazole PO before initiating treatment with Abilify Maintena. Tolerability may take up to 2 weeks to fully assess. After the first IM injection, administer 10 to 20 mg aripiprazole PO for 14 days. For patients already stable on another oral antipsychotic and known to tolerate aripiprazole, after the first IM injection, continue treatment with the other antipsychotic for 14 days.

Maintenance dosage is 400 mg IM monthly, no sooner than 26 days after previous injection.

Adjust-a-dose: If adverse reactions occur with 400-mg dose or if patient is a poor metabolizer of CYP2D6, consider reducing dosage to 300 mg IM monthly. ⬤

Adolescents ages 13 to 17: Initially, 2 mg PO daily; increase to 5 mg after 2 days, then to recommended dose of 10 mg in 2 more days. May titrate to maximum daily dose of 30 mg in 5-mg increments. Continue patients who respond on the lowest dosage needed to maintain remission. Periodically reassess patients to determine need for maintenance treatment.

➤ Schizophrenia (Aristada, Aristada Initio)

Adults: Establish tolerability with oral aripiprazole before initiating treatment with aripiprazole lauroxil, which may take up to 2 weeks. Base initial monthly dose of Aristada on current oral daily aripiprazole dose. If

---

Reactions in bold italics are *life-threatening*.

current oral aripiprazole dose is 10 mg/day, give 441 mg IM in deltoid or gluteal muscle once per month. If current oral aripiprazole dose is 15 mg/day, give 662 mg once per month, 882 mg once every 6 weeks, or 1,064 mg once every 2 months IM in the gluteal muscle. If current oral aripiprazole dose is 20 mg/day or more, give 882 mg IM in the gluteal muscle once every month. Continue oral aripiprazole for 21 consecutive days after initiation of first monthly dose or give a single injection of 675 mg Aristada Initio in deltoid or gluteal muscle and one dose of oral aripiprazole 30 mg. Avoid injecting both preparations into the same deltoid or gluteal muscle.

The first Aristada injection may be administered on the same day as Aristada Initio or up to 10 days after.

Adolescents ages 13 to 17 years: Initially, 2 mg/day PO for 2 days, then increase to 5 mg/day for 2 days, then increase to target dose of 10 mg/day. Increase subsequent doses, as indicated in 5-mg increments. Maximum dosage, 30 mg/day.

Adjust-a-dose: Adjust dosage as needed; if a dose is required earlier than the recommended interval, don't administer earlier than 14 days after previous injection.

➤ **Bipolar mania, including manic and mixed episodes, with or without psychotic features; adjunctive therapy with either lithium or valproate for treatment of manic and mixed episodes associated with bipolar I disorder with or without psychotic features**

Adults: Initially, 15 mg PO once daily as monotherapy or 10 to 15 mg PO once daily as adjunctive therapy with lithium or valproate. Target dose is 15 mg/day as monotherapy or adjunctive therapy. May increase dose to maximum of 30 mg/day based on clinical response.

Children ages 10 to 17: Initially, 2 mg PO daily; increase to 5 mg PO daily after 2 days, then to recommended dose of 10 mg after 2 additional days. May titrate to maximum daily dose of 30 mg in 5-mg increments every 5 days.

Adjust-a-dose: For maintenance, continue patients who respond on monotherapy on the lowest dosage needed to maintain remission. Periodically reassess patients to determine the long-term usefulness of maintenance treatment.

➤ **Bipolar I disorder maintenance monotherapy (extended-release injection)**

Adults: For patients who have never taken aripiprazole, establish tolerability with oral aripiprazole before initiating treatment with extended-release IM suspension. Once tolerability is established, give 400 mg (extended-release suspension) IM monthly. After first injection, continue oral aripiprazole (10 to 20 mg) for 14 consecutive days to achieve therapeutic aripiprazole concentrations during initiation of therapy. Maintenance dosage is 400 mg IM monthly, given no sooner than 26 days after previous injection.

Adjust-a-dose: If adverse reactions occur with 400-mg dose or if patient is a poor metabolizer of CYP2D6, consider reducing dosage to 300 mg IM monthly. ⌧

➤ **Adjunctive treatment of major depressive disorder**

Adults: Initially, 2 to 5 mg PO daily. Dose range is 2 to 15 mg/day. Dosage adjustments of up to 5 mg/day should occur gradually, at intervals of no less than 1 week.

➤ **Irritability associated with autistic disorder**

Children ages 6 to 17: Initially, 2 mg PO daily for 7 days. Increase dosage to 5 mg/day at intervals of no less than 1 week, with subsequent increases to 10 or 15 mg/day if needed.

➤ **Tourette disorder**

Children ages 6 to 18 weighing 50 kg or more: Initially, 2 mg/day PO for 2 days; then increase to 5 mg/day for 5 days with target dose of 10 mg/day on day 8. If optimal control of tics isn't achieved, increase by 5 mg/day at intervals of no less than 1 week to maximum of 20 mg/day.

Children ages 6 to 18 weighing less than 50 kg: Initially, 2 mg/day PO, increasing to target dose of 5 mg/day after 2 days. If optimal control of tics isn't achieved, increase to 10 mg/day. Adjust dosage at intervals of no less than 1 week.

ADMINISTRATION
PO
• Give drug without regard for food.
• Substitute oral solution on a mg-per-mg basis up to 25 mg. Give patients taking 30-mg tablets 25 mg of solution.
• Keep ODTs in blister package until ready to use. Don't split tablet. Place tablet on tongue and allow to dissolve; no liquid is needed.

• Abilify MyCite drug-device combination system consists of tablets with an embedded ingestible event marker (IEM) to track drug ingestion, a wearable patch containing a sensor that detects the signal from the IEM after ingestion and transmits data to a smartphone, a smartphone application (app) to display patient information, and a Web-based portal for health care professionals and caregivers. Refer to manufacturer's detailed instructions for use.

• Apply MyCite patch when instructed by app to left side of body just above lower edge of rib cage. Don't place patch over skin that is irritated, inflamed, or not intact or overlaps area where last patch was located.

• Have patient swallow tablets with sensor whole; don't divide or crush these tablets.

• Don't repeat dose if tablet with sensor isn't detected after ingestion.

• Store oral solution at room temperature; it can be used up to 6 months after opening.

IM

• Inject slowly into deltoid or gluteal muscle according to manufacturer's instructions; rotate injection sites.

🕃 *Alert:* Don't confuse IM dosage forms (Abilify Maintena, Aristada, Aristada Initio).

ACTION

Thought to exert partial agonist activity at dopamine 2 and 5-HT_{1A} receptors and antagonist activity at 5-HT_{2A} receptors.

Route	Onset	Peak	Duration
PO	Unknown	3–5 hr	Unknown
IM	Unknown	1–3 hr	Unknown
		4–7 days (Abilify Maintena)	
		16 to 35 days (Aristada Initio)	

Half-life: About 75 hours in patients with normal metabolism. Abilify Maintena, 30 to 45 days; Aristada, 54 to 57 days; Aristada Initio, 15 to 18 days.

ADVERSE REACTIONS

CNS: headache, anxiety, insomnia, somnolence, sedation, akathisia, extrapyramidal disorder, tremor, asthenia, fatigue, lethargy, pain, dizziness, irritability, fever, restlessness, agitation, impaired concentration. **CV:** tachycardia, orthostatic hypotension, angina, palpitations. **EENT:** blurred vision, epistaxis, toothache, increased salivation, drooling, nasopharyngitis, dry mouth,

pharyngolaryngeal pain. **GI:** nausea, vomiting, constipation, anorexia, dyspepsia, diarrhea, abdominal pain, increased appetite. **GU:** urinary incontinence. **Hematologic:** *neutropenia.* **Metabolic:** weight gain, weight loss, hyperglycemia, hyperlipidemia, increased CK level. **Musculoskeletal:** stiffness, muscle spasms, muscle rigidity, muscle weakness, dystonia, myalgia, arthralgia, extremity pain. **Respiratory:** cough, URI. **Skin:** rash, application-site rash (patch), injection-site reaction.

INTERACTIONS

Drug-drug. *Antihypertensives:* May enhance antihypertensive effects. Monitor BP.

Benzodiazepines (lorazepam): May cause excessive sedation and orthostatic hypotension. Monitor patient closely.

Carbamazepine and other CYP3A4 inducers: May decrease aripiprazole level and effectiveness. See manufacturer's instructions for dosage adjustments. Monitor patient closely.

CNS depressants: May lead to enhanced CNS depression. Use together with caution.

Ketoconazole and other CYP3A4 inhibitors: May increase risk of serious toxic effects. Start treatment with reduced dose of aripiprazole, and monitor patient closely.

Metoclopramide: May increase risk of extrapyramidal reactions. Use together is contraindicated.

Opioid class warning: May cause slow or difficult breathing, sedation, and death. Avoid use together. If use together is necessary, limit dosage and duration of each drug to the minimum necessary for desired effect.

Strong CYP2D6 inhibitors (fluoxetine, paroxetine, quinidine): May increase aripiprazole level and toxicity. See manufacturer's instructions for dosage adjustments.

Drug-food. *Grapefruit juice:* May increase drug level. Tell patient not to take drug with grapefruit juice.

Drug-lifestyle. *Alcohol use:* May increase CNS effects. Discourage use together.

EFFECTS ON LAB TEST RESULTS

• May increase CK, LDL-C, triglyceride, and glucose levels.

• May decrease HDL-C level.

• May decrease WBC count and ANC.

---

*Reactions in bold italics are **life-threatening**.*

CONTRAINDICATIONS & CAUTIONS

• Contraindicated in patients hypersensitive to drug.

• Safety and effectiveness in children with major depressive disorder haven't been established.

Boxed Warning Older adults with dementia-related psychosis treated with atypical antipsychotics are at an increased risk for death. Drug isn't approved for treatment of patients with dementia-related psychosis. ∎

• Use cautiously in patients with CV disease, cerebrovascular disease, or conditions that could predispose patient to hypotension, such as dehydration or hypovolemia.

⊕ *Alert:* Life-threatening arrhythmias have occurred with therapeutic doses of antipsychotics.

• Use cautiously in patients with history of seizures or with conditions that lower the seizure threshold.

• Use cautiously in patients who engage in strenuous exercise, are exposed to extreme heat, take anticholinergics, or are susceptible to dehydration.

• Use cautiously in patients with Lewy body dementia or Parkinson disease; drug may aggravate motor disturbances.

• Use cautiously in patients at risk for aspiration pneumonia, such as those with Alzheimer disease.

• Use cautiously in patients at risk for falls, including those who have diseases or conditions or are taking medications that may cause somnolence, orthostatic hypotension, or motor or sensory instability.

• Discontinue drug at first sign of blood dyscrasia or if ANC is less than 1,000/mm³.

• Abilify MyCite drug-device product is only approved for use in adults.

Dialyzable drug: Unlikely.

⚠ *Overdose S&S:* Somnolence, tremor, vomiting, acidosis, aggression, atrial fibrillation, bradycardia, coma, confusion, seizures, depressed level of consciousness, HTN, hypokalemia, hypotension, increased AST and blood CK levels, lethargy, loss of consciousness, aspiration pneumonia, prolonged QRS complex, prolonged QT interval, respiratory arrest, status epilepticus, tachycardia.

PREGNANCY-LACTATION-REPRODUCTION

• Drug crosses the placenta. Routine use of aripiprazole isn't recommended. Use during pregnancy only if potential benefit justifies fetal risk.

⊕ *Alert:* Neonates exposed to antipsychotics during third trimester are at risk for developing extrapyramidal signs and symptoms (repetitive muscle movements of face and body) and withdrawal signs and symptoms (agitation, abnormally increased or decreased muscle tone, tremors, sleepiness, severe difficulty breathing, difficulty feeding) after delivery.

• Enroll patients exposed to aripiprazole during pregnancy in the National Pregnancy Registry for Atypical Antipsychotics (1-866-961-2388 or https://womensmentalhealth.org/research/pregnancyregistry/atypicalantipsychotic/).

• Drug appears in human milk. Use during breastfeeding isn't recommended.

NURSING CONSIDERATIONS

⊕ *Alert:* NMS may occur. Monitor patient for hyperpyrexia, muscle rigidity, altered mental status, irregular pulse or BP, tachycardia, diaphoresis, and cardiac arrhythmias.

• If signs and symptoms of NMS occur, immediately stop drug and notify prescriber.

• Monitor patient for signs and symptoms of tardive dyskinesia. Older adults, especially women, are at highest risk for developing this adverse effect.

⊕ *Alert:* Fatal cerebrovascular adverse events (stroke, TIA) may occur in older adults with dementia. Drug isn't safe or effective in these patients.

Boxed Warning Drug may increase risk of suicidal thinking and behavior in children, adolescents, and young adults ages 18 to 24 during the first 2 months of treatment, especially in those with major depressive or other psychiatric disorder. Monitor all patients for worsening or emergence of suicidal thoughts and behaviors. ∎

⊕ *Alert:* Hyperglycemia may occur. Regularly monitor patient with diabetes. Patient with risk factors for diabetes should undergo fasting blood glucose testing at baseline and periodically. Monitor all patients for symptoms of hyperglycemia (increased hunger, thirst, frequent urination, weakness). Hyperglycemia may resolve when patient stops taking drug.

• Monitor patient for symptoms of metabolic syndrome (significant weight gain and increased BMI, HTN, hyperglycemia, hypercholesterolemia, and hypertriglyceridemia).

• Monitor patient for new or increasing compulsive or uncontrollable urges to gamble, binge eat, shop, and have sex. Dosage may need to be reduced or drug discontinued if urges occur.

• Monitor patient with clinically significant neutropenia for fever or other signs and symptoms of infection; treat promptly if they occur. If ANC is less than 1,000/mm³, discontinue drug and monitor WBC count until recovery.

• Assess fall risk at start of treatment and then periodically for patient who has a disease or condition or is taking drug that may cause somnolence, orthostatic hypotension, or motor or sensory instability.

• Monitor patient for abnormal body temperature regulation, especially if patient exercises, is exposed to extreme heat, takes anticholinergics, or is dehydrated.

▨ Dosage adjustments may be indicated in patients who are known CYP2D6 poor metabolizers.

• Treat patient with smallest dose for shortest time; periodically reevaluate for need to continue.

• Give prescriptions only for small quantities of drug to reduce risk of overdose.

• Change Abilify MyCite patch weekly or sooner, as needed. Patient should keep patch on while showering, swimming, or exercising.

• Remove Abilify MyCite patch before MRI or if patch causes skin irritation.

• Detection of tablet by MyCite sensor takes 30 minutes to 2 hours and may not occur in some cases.

• Tracking drug ingestion in "real time" or during an emergency isn't recommended because detection of MyCite sensor may be delayed or not occur, causing false-negative reading.

• *Look alike–sound alike:* Don't confuse aripiprazole with rabeprazole, omeprazole, or pantoprazole. Don't confuse IM dosage forms (Abilify Maintena, Aristada, Aristada Initio).

PATIENT TEACHING

Boxed Warning Advise families and caregivers to closely observe patient for clinical worsening, suicidality, or unusual changes in behavior. ▨

• Caution patient or caregiver of patient taking an opioid with a benzodiazepine, CNS depressant, or alcohol to seek immediate medical attention if patient experiences dizziness, light-headedness, extreme sleepiness, slowed or difficult breathing, or unresponsiveness.

• Advise patient and caregiver to notify prescriber if compulsive or uncontrollable urges occur.

❸ *Alert:* Caution patient not to stop drug without first discussing with prescriber.

• Tell patient to use caution while driving or operating hazardous machinery because psychoactive drugs may impair judgment, thinking, and motor skills.

• Advise patient that gradual improvement in symptoms should occur over several weeks rather than immediately.

❸ *Alert:* Warn patient with phenylketonuria that ODTs contain phenylalanine.

• Advise patient that each milliliter of oral solution contains 400 mg of sucrose and 200 mg of fructose.

• Tell patient to avoid alcohol use while taking drug.

• Advise patient to limit strenuous activity while taking drug to avoid dehydration.

• Instruct patient in safe drug administration and storage.

• Teach patient that Abilify MyCite drug-device combination product is used to track drug ingestion. Ensure that patient is capable and willing to use a smartphone and app and that the app is compatible with the specific phone. Assist patient to download app and encourage patient to follow instructions for use.

• Instruct patient to verify that Abilify MyCite app is paired with sensor patch before use.

• Teach patient that Abilify MyCite app will direct patient how to apply and remove patch correctly. Tell patient to change patch weekly and to keep it on while showering, swimming, or exercising.

• Tell patient that Abilify MyCite patch must be removed before MRI and replaced with new patch as soon as possible afterward.

• Instruct patient to remove patch if skin irritation occurs and to report to prescriber.

• Teach patient that Abilify MyCite tablets are usually detected within 30 minutes but there may be a delay of more than 2 hours for the smartphone app/Web portal to detect it. Inform patient that sometimes the tablet may not be detected at all. If tablet isn't detected, instruct patient not to repeat dose.

• Advise patient not to become pregnant or breastfeed without first discussing with prescriber.

Reactions in bold italics are *life-threatening*.

SAFETY ALERT!

asciminib ☒
as-KIM-i-nib

Scemblix

Therapeutic class: Antineoplastics
Pharmacologic class: Kinase inhibitors

AVAILABLE FORMS
Tablets ⓄⓃⒸ: 20 mg, 40 mg

INDICATIONS & DOSAGES
Adjust-a-dose (for all indications): Refer to manufacturer's instructions for toxicity-related dosage adjustments.
➤ **Philadelphia chromosome–positive chronic myeloid leukemia (CML) in chronic phase previously treated with two or more tyrosine kinase inhibitors** ☒
Adults: 80 mg PO once daily or 40 mg PO every 12 hours if clinical benefit is observed or until unacceptable toxicity occurs.
➤ **Philadelphia chromosome–positive CML in chronic phase with *T315I* mutation** ☒
Adults: 200 mg PO every 12 hours.

ADMINISTRATION
PO
• Give at approximately same time each day or at 12-hour intervals.
• Avoid giving food for at least 2 hours before and 1 hour after each dose.
• Have patient swallow tablets whole; don't crush or cut tablets.
• If a dose is missed by more than 12 hours on a once-daily regimen or by more than 6 hours on a twice-daily regimen, skip dose and take next dose as scheduled.
• Store tablets at 68° to 77° F (20° to 25° C).

ACTION
Inhibits the ABL1 kinase activity of BCR-ABL1 fusion protein.

Route	Onset	Peak	Duration
PO	Unknown	2–3 hr	Unknown

Half-life: 5.5 to 9 hours.

ADVERSE REACTIONS
CNS: dizziness, fatigue, fever, headache, peripheral neuropathy. **CV:** arrhythmias, edema, HF, *hemorrhage,* HTN, palpitations, *prolonged QT interval.* **EENT:** blurred vision, dry eye. **GI:** abdominal pain, constipation, diarrhea, nausea, increased amylase and lipase levels, *pancreatitis,* vomiting. **GU:** increased creatinine level, UTI. **Hematologic:** anemia, *febrile neutropenia, lymphopenia, neutropenia, thrombocytopenia.* **Hepatic:** hyperbilirubinemia, increased ALT and AST levels. **Metabolic:** dyslipidemia, hypercholesterolemia, hypertriglyceridemia, hyperuricemia, *hypocalcemia, hypokalemia,* hypophosphatemia, hypothyroidism, increased CK level. **Musculoskeletal:** arthralgia, musculoskeletal pain. **Respiratory:** cough, dyspnea, pleural effusion, pneumonia, URI. **Skin:** hypersensitivity reaction, pruritus, rash.

INTERACTIONS
Drug-drug. *Certain P-gp substrates:* May increase substrate level. If concomitant use can't be avoided, closely monitor patient for substrate-related adverse reactions.
CYP2C9 substrates (warfarin): May increase risk of substrate-related adverse reactions. Avoid concomitant use with asciminib 80 mg (total) daily; if concomitant use can't be avoided, reduce the substrate dose. Avoid concomitant use with asciminib 200 mg b.i.d.; if concomitant use can't be avoided, consider alternative therapy with a non-CYP2C9 substrate.
CYP3A4 substrates (midazolam): May increase substrate level and risk of adverse reactions. Closely monitor patient treated concomitantly with asciminib 80 mg daily. Avoid concomitant use with asciminib 200-mg b.i.d.
Itraconazole oral solution containing hydroxypropyl-β-cyclodextrin: May reduce asciminib level and effectiveness. Avoid concomitant use.
Strong CYP3A4 inhibitors (clarithromycin): May increase asciminib level and risk of adverse reactions. Closely monitor patient treated with asciminib 200 mg b.i.d.

EFFECTS ON LAB TEST RESULTS
• May increase amylase, AST, ALT, bilirubin, cholesterol, CK, creatinine, lipase, triglyceride, and uric acid levels.
• May decrease phosphate, corrected calcium, and potassium levels.
• May decrease Hb level.
• May decrease lymphocyte, neutrophil, and platelet counts.

CONTRAINDICATIONS & CAUTIONS

• Drug may increase risk of hypersensitivity reactions, HTN, pancreatic toxicity, severe thrombocytopenia, and neutropenia events.

• CV toxicity (arrhythmias; prolonged QT interval; ischemic cardiac and CNS conditions; HF; arterial, thrombotic, and embolic events) may occur. Patients with prior exposure to multiple tyrosine kinase inhibitors, preexisting cardiac conditions, or CV risk factors are at increased risk.

• Safety and effectiveness in children haven't been established.

Dialyzable drug: No.

PREGNANCY-LACTATION-REPRODUCTION

• Drug can cause fetal harm. Advise patients who are pregnant of the risk.

• Patients of childbearing potential should use effective contraception during therapy and for 1 week after final dose.

• It isn't known if drug appears in human milk or how drug affects milk production or infants who are breastfed. Patient shouldn't breastfeed during therapy and for 1 week after final dose.

• Drug may impair fertility in patients of childbearing potential. Reversibility of the effect is unknown.

NURSING CONSIDERATIONS

• Verify pregnancy status in patients of childbearing potential before drug initiation.

• Monitor CBC every 2 weeks for the first 3 months and monthly thereafter, or as clinically indicated.

• Monitor patient for signs and symptoms of myelosuppression (fever, infection, easy bruising, bleeding).

• Monitor serum lipase and amylase levels monthly during therapy and as clinically indicated. Assess patient for pancreatitis when lipase elevation is accompanied by abdominal symptoms (nausea, vomiting, severe abdominal pain or discomfort).

• Monitor BP and manage HTN as clinically indicated.

• Monitor patient for signs and symptoms of hypersensitivity reaction (rash, edema, bronchospasm); initiate appropriate treatment as clinically indicated.

• Monitor patient with CV risk factors for CV toxicity signs and symptoms. Initiate appropriate treatment as clinically indicated.

PATIENT TEACHING

• Teach about proper drug administration and handling.

• Inform patient of the need for routine blood testing during therapy.

• Warn about the potential for low blood cell counts. Instruct patient to immediately report fever, signs or symptoms of infection, bleeding, or easy bruising.

• Inform patient about risk of pancreatitis. Instruct patient to contact prescriber if signs or symptoms occur.

• Inform patient about the risk of HTN. Advise patient to routinely monitor BP and report BP elevations or signs and symptoms of HTN (confusion, headache, dizziness, chest pain, shortness of breath).

• Tell patient to immediately stop drug and report signs or symptoms of hypersensitivity reaction (rash, edema, bronchospasm).

• Inform patient about risk of CV toxicity, especially if patient has CV risk factors. Tell patient to immediately contact prescriber or seek medical help if palpitations, edema, shortness of breath, chest pain, dizziness, weight gain, visual changes, numbness or weakness, trouble talking, severe stomach pain, or headache occurs.

• Advise patient to report pregnancy or plans to become pregnant or to breastfeed.

• Advise patient of childbearing potential to use effective contraception during therapy and for 1 week after final dose.

• Warn patient not to breastfeed during therapy and for 1 week after final dose.

• Caution patient of childbearing potential that drug may impair fertility.

asenapine
a-SEN-a-peen

Saphris, Secuado

Therapeutic class: Antipsychotics
Pharmacologic class: Dopamine–serotonin antagonists

AVAILABLE FORMS

Tablets (SL) ⓄⓃⒸ: 2.5 mg, 5 mg, 10 mg
Transdermal system: 3.8 mg/24 hours, 5.7 mg/24 hours, 7.6 mg/24 hours

---

Reactions in bold italics are *life-threatening*.

INDICATIONS & DOSAGES

➤ **Schizophrenia (acute and maintenance therapy)**

Adults: 5 mg SL b.i.d., increased up to 10 mg b.i.d. after 1 week based on tolerability; for maintenance therapy, 5 to 10 mg SL b.i.d. Or, 3.8 mg/24 hours (transdermal system); may increase to 5.7 mg/24 hours or 7.6 mg/24 hours after 1 week.

➤ **Acute manic or mixed episodes associated with bipolar I disorder as adjunctive therapy with either lithium or valproate**

Adults: 5 mg SL b.i.d. Dosage may be increased to maximum of 10 mg SL b.i.d. as tolerated.

➤ **Acute manic or mixed episodes associated with bipolar I disorder as monotherapy**

Adults: 5 to 10 mg SL b.i.d.

Children ages 10 to 17: Initially, 2.5 mg SL b.i.d. May increase after 3 days to 5 mg SL b.i.d., then to 10 mg SL b.i.d. after 3 additional days based on tolerability.

➤ **Maintenance treatment of bipolar I disorder as monotherapy**

Adults: Continue dosage that patient received during stabilization (5 or 10 mg SL b.i.d.). Based on clinical response and tolerability, can decrease dose of 10 mg SL b.i.d. to 5 mg SL b.i.d.

ADMINISTRATION

Sublingual

• Make sure patient doesn't split, crush, chew, or swallow tablet.

• Peel back colored tab on tablet pack, gently remove tablet, place under patient's tongue, and allow to dissolve completely.

• Make sure patient doesn't eat or drink for 10 minutes after taking drug.

Transdermal

• Don't open pouch until ready to apply patch.

• Apply 1 patch daily to clean, dry, intact skin of upper arm, upper back, abdomen, or hip, and leave on for only 24 hours.

• Patient should wear only 1 patch at a time and not use same application site two times in a row.

• Don't cut patches.

• If patch comes completely off, apply a new one.

• Patient may shower while wearing patch; swimming and bathing haven't been evaluated.

• Don't apply heat over patch; prolonged heat application increases drug's plasma concentration.

ACTION

Unknown. May block dopamine and 5-HT receptors.

Route	Onset	Peak	Duration
SL	Immediate	0.5–1.5 hr	Unknown
Transdermal	Rapid	12–24 hr	Unknown

Half-life: SL, 24 hours; transdermal, 30 hours.

ADVERSE REACTIONS

CNS: akathisia, agitation, anxiety, depression, dizziness, dystonia, extrapyramidal symptoms, fatigue, headache, insomnia, irritability, somnolence, manic symptoms, anger, taste perversion. **CV:** HTN, peripheral edema, tachycardia. **EENT:** dry mouth, oral hypoesthesia, salivary hypersecretion, toothache, glossitis, nasopharyngitis, oropharyngeal pain, nasal congestion. **GI:** constipation, diarrhea, dyspepsia, increased appetite, stomach discomfort, abdominal pain, nausea, vomiting. **GU:** dysmenorrhea. **Hematologic:** anemia. **Hepatic:** increased LFTs. **Metabolic:** weight gain, hyperglycemia, hyperinsulinemia, increased prolactin level, dehydration. **Musculoskeletal:** arthralgia, muscle strain, extremity pain. **Respiratory:** dyspnea, URI. **Skin:** rash, application-site reaction. **Other:** *suicidality.*

INTERACTIONS

Drug-drug. *Antiarrhythmics, class IA (procainamide, quinidine) and class III (amiodarone, sotalol); antibiotics (gatifloxacin, moxifloxacin); antipsychotics (chlorpromazine, thioridazine, ziprasidone); citalopram:* May prolong QTc interval, leading to lethal arrhythmias, such as torsades de pointes. Avoid use together.

Antihypertensives (alpha blockers, diuretics, ACE inhibitors, ARBs, beta blockers): May increase risk of hypotension. Use together cautiously. Adjust dosage of antihypertensive as clinically indicated.

CNS agents: May enhance CNS depression. Use with caution.

CYP2D6 substrates and inhibitors (paroxetine): May increase substrate and inhibitor level. Reduce substrate dosage as needed.

Metoclopramide: May increase risk of extrapyramidal reactions. Avoid administering together.

Opioid class warning: May cause slow or difficult breathing, sedation, and death. Avoid use together. If use together is necessary, limit dosage and duration of each drug to minimum necessary for desired effect.

Strong CYP1A2 inhibitors (fluvoxamine, ciprofloxacin): May increase asenapine level. Monitor therapy; adjust asenapine dose as needed.

Drug-lifestyle. *Alcohol use:* May increase CNS effects. Discourage use together.

EFFECTS ON LAB TEST RESULTS

• May increase glucose, total cholesterol, LDL, ALT, AST, GGT, serum triglyceride, CK, and prolactin levels.
• May decrease sodium and HDL-C level.
• May decrease Hb level and platelet, WBC, and neutrophil counts.

CONTRAINDICATIONS & CAUTIONS

Boxed Warning Older adults with dementia-related psychosis treated with atypical or conventional antipsychotics are at increased risk for death. Antipsychotics aren't approved for treatment of dementia-related psychosis. ■

• *Opioid class warning:* Opioids should only be prescribed with benzodiazepines or other CNS depressants to patients for whom alternative treatment options are inadequate.
• Contraindicated in patients with known hypersensitivity or Child-Pugh class C liver failure. Hypersensitivity reactions may occur as early as the first dose.
• **Alert:** Avoid use in patients with conditions that increase risk of torsades de pointes and in those taking other drugs that prolong QTc interval.
• Use cautiously in patients with or at risk for diabetes; in those with known CV or cerebrovascular disease, preexisting low WBC count, difficulty swallowing, history of leukopenia or neutropenia, Parkinson disease, or history of seizures or conditions that lower seizure threshold; and in patients who are antipsychotic-naive.
• Don't use in patients at risk for aspiration.
• Use cautiously in patients at risk for falls, including those who have diseases or conditions or are taking medications that may cause somnolence, orthostatic hypotension, or motor or sensory instability.
• Safe and effective use for bipolar I disorder in children younger than age 10 or for schizophrenia in children younger than age 12 hasn't been established.
Dialyzable drug: Unknown.

⚠ Overdose S&S: Agitation, confusion, hypotension, circulatory collapse.

PREGNANCY-LACTATION-REPRODUCTION

• Drug may cause fetal harm. Safety of atypical antipsychotic use during pregnancy hasn't been well studied; routine use isn't recommended. Use during pregnancy only if potential benefit justifies fetal risk.
• **Alert:** Neonates exposed to antipsychotics during third trimester are at risk for developing extrapyramidal signs and symptoms (repetitive muscle movements of the face and body) and withdrawal signs and symptoms (agitation, abnormally increased or decreased muscle tone, tremors, sleepiness, severe difficulty breathing, difficulty feeding) after delivery.
• Enroll patients exposed to asenapine during pregnancy in the National Pregnancy Registry for Atypical Antipsychotics (1-866-961-2388 or https://womensmentalhealth.org/research/pregnancyregistry/atypicalantipsychotic/).
• It isn't known if drug appears in human milk. Use cautiously during breastfeeding, weighing benefit to patient against risk to infant.

NURSING CONSIDERATIONS

• Obtain BP before starting drug, and monitor BP regularly. Watch for orthostatic hypotension.
• Monitor waist circumference and BMI.
• Monitor patient for tardive dyskinesia, which may occur after prolonged use. It may disappear spontaneously or persist for life, despite stopping drug.
• **Alert:** Monitor patient for suicidality, especially at start of therapy.
• **Alert:** Watch for signs and symptoms of NMS (extrapyramidal effects, hyperthermia, autonomic disturbance), which are rare but can be fatal. Immediately discontinue drug if they occur, and monitor patient closely.
• Monitor patient for serious allergic reactions (anaphylaxis, angioedema, hypotension, difficulty breathing, wheezing, swollen tongue, rash).
• Monitor glucose level closely in patient with diabetes because drug may alter glucose control.
• Monitor CBC frequently during first few months of therapy in patient with history of

leukopenia or neutropenia. If WBC count decreases, monitor for signs and symptoms of infection; if infection occurs, discontinue drug in the absence of another cause.

• Monitor patient for dysphagia, which can lead to aspiration and aspiration pneumonia.

• Dispense lowest appropriate quantity of drug to reduce risk of overdose.

• Monitor patient for abnormal body temperature regulation, especially if patient exercises, is exposed to extreme heat, takes anticholinergics, or is dehydrated.

• Assess risk of falls at start of treatment and periodically thereafter for patient on long-term therapy who has a disease or condition or is taking medication that may cause somnolence, orthostatic hypotension, or motor or sensory instability.

• When discontinuing antipsychotic therapy, reduce dosage gradually to avoid withdrawal symptoms.

PATIENT TEACHING

• *Opioid class warning:* Caution patient or caregiver of patient taking an opioid with a benzodiazepine, CNS depressant, or alcohol to seek immediate medical attention if patient experiences dizziness, light-headedness, extreme sleepiness, slowed or difficult breathing, or unresponsiveness.

• Teach about proper drug administration and handling.

• Warn patient to avoid activities that require mental alertness, such as operating hazardous machinery and operating a motor vehicle, until drug's effects are known.

• Caution patient to contact prescriber if palpitations or rapid heartbeat occurs.

• Advise patient not to stand up quickly but to get up slowly from a sitting position to avoid dizziness.

• Inform patient that weight gain may occur.

• Warn patient against exposure to extreme heat because drug may impair body's ability to reduce temperature.

• Advise patient to avoid alcohol.

aspirin (acetylsalicylic acid, ASA) 🗶
AS-pir-in

Asaphen✤ ◊, Asatab✤ ◊, Bayer Aspirin ◊, Durlaza, Ecotrin ◊, Entrophen✤ ◊, Rivasa✤ ◊, St. Joseph ◊, Vazalore ◊

Therapeutic class: Anti-inflammatory drugs
Pharmacologic class: Salicylates

AVAILABLE FORMS
Capsules (immediate-release) 🚫: 81 mg ◊, 325 mg ◊
Capsules (extended-release) 🚫: 162.5 mg
Suppositories: 60 mg ◊, 300 mg ◊
Tablets: 80 mg ◊, 325 mg ◊, 500 mg ◊
Tablets (chewable): 80 mg✤ ◊, 81 mg ◊
Tablets (delayed-release): 81 mg ◊, 325 mg ◊, 500 mg ◊
Tablets (enteric-coated): 80 mg✤ ◊, 81 mg ◊, 325 mg ◊, 500 mg ◊

INDICATIONS & DOSAGES
➤ **RA, osteoarthritis, and other polyarthritic or inflammatory conditions**
Adults: Initially, 3 g PO daily in divided doses. Increase as needed, with target plasma salicylate levels of 150 to 300 mcg/mL.
➤ **Juvenile RA**
Children: 90 to 130 mg/kg/day PO in divided doses. Increase as needed, with target plasma salicylate levels of 150 to 300 mcg/mL.
➤ **Mild pain or fever; spondyloarthropathies**
Adults and children ages 12 and older weighing 50 kg or more: 325 to 650 mg PO or PR every 4 hours PRN. Or, for delayed-release products, 1,300 mg PO, followed by 650 to 1,300 mg PO every 8 hours. Maximum dose, 4,000 mg in 24 hours.
Children ages 2 to 11 weighing less than 50 kg: 10 to 15 mg/kg/dose PO or PR every 4 hours up to 90 mg/kg daily.
➤ **Suspected acute MI**
Adults: Initially, 160 to 325 mg PO (non-enteric-coated) chewed or crushed; or 160 to 162.5 mg immediate-release capsule (Vazalore) as soon as MI is suspected. Continue maintenance dose of 162.5 to 325 mg PO daily for 30 days after infarction. After 30 days, consider further therapy for prevention of MI.

➤ **To reduce risk of MI in patients with previous MI, unstable angina, and chronic stable angina pectoris**
Adults: 75 to 325 mg PO daily. Or, 162.5 mg extended-release capsule PO daily.

➤ **To reduce risk of recurrent TIAs and stroke or death in patients at risk**
Adults: 50 to 325 mg PO daily. Or, 162.5 mg extended-release capsule PO daily.

➤ **Acute ischemic stroke**
Adults: 50 to 325 mg PO daily, started within 48 hours of stroke onset. Continue indefinitely.

➤ **CABG**
Adults: 75 to 81 mg PO daily starting 6 hours postprocedure. Continue for up to 1 year.

➤ **VTE extended therapy to prevent recurrence (in patients who have completed anticoagulation treatment and have decided to stop oral anticoagulation)** ◆
Adults: 100 mg immediate-release PO once daily.

➤ **VTE prophylaxis for total hip arthroplasty (THA) or total knee arthroplasty (TKA) (immediate-release)** ◆
Adults: After 5-day course of postoperative rivaroxaban prophylaxis, initiate aspirin 81 mg once daily starting on postoperative day 6 and continue for 9 days for TKA (total duration: 14 days) or 30 days for THA (total duration: 35 days).

ADMINISTRATION
PO
• For patient with swallowing difficulties, crush non-enteric-coated aspirin and dissolve in soft food or liquid. Give liquid immediately after mixing because drug break downs rapidly.
• Give capsules with full glass of water.
• Give tablets with food, milk, antacid, or large glass of water to reduce GI effects.
• Give enteric-coated, immediate-release capsules, or extended-release forms whole; don't break or open capsules.
• For acute MI, have patient chew non-enteric-coated tablet.
Rectal
• Refrigerate suppositories.

ACTION
Thought to produce analgesia and exert its anti-inflammatory effect by inhibiting prostaglandin and other substances that sensitize pain receptors. May relieve fever through central action in hypothalamic heat-regulating center. In low doses, also may interfere with clotting by keeping a platelet-aggregating substance from forming.

Route	Onset	Peak	Duration
PO (buffered)	5–30 min	1–2 hr	1–4 hr
PO (enteric-coated)	5–30 min	Variable	1–4 hr
PO (tablet)	5–30 min	25–40 min	1–4 hr
PO (extended-release)	Unknown	2 hr	4–8 hr
PR	Unknown	3–4 hr	Unknown

Half-life: 15 minutes to 6 hours (dose dependent).

ADVERSE REACTIONS
CNS: agitation, *cerebral edema, coma,* confusion, dizziness, headache, lethargy, hyperthermia, nervousness, *seizures,* subdural or intracranial hemorrhage. **CV:** *arrhythmias,* edema, hypotension, tachycardia, *hemorrhage.* **EENT:** tinnitus, hearing loss. **GI:** nausea, *GI bleeding,* dyspepsia, GI distress, gastritis, GI erosion, heartburn, occult bleeding, *pancreatitis,* vomiting, ulcer. **GU:** *antepartum and postpartum bleeding,* interstitial kidney inflammation, papillary necrosis, prolonged pregnancy and labor, proteinuria, kidney insufficiency, kidney failure. **Hematologic:** anemia, prolonged bleeding time, *leukopenia, thrombocytopenia,* coagulopathy, *DIC.* **Hepatic:** *hepatitis, liver toxicity,* increased transaminase levels. **Metabolic:** dehydration, *hyperkalemia,* hyponatremia, hyperglycemia; *hypoglycemia* (children), *metabolic acidosis,* respiratory alkalosis. **Musculoskeletal:** acetabular bone destruction, rhabdomyolysis, weakness. **Respiratory:** *asthma, bronchospasm,* dyspnea, hyperventilation, *laryngeal edema, noncardiogenic pulmonary edema,* tachypnea. **Skin:** rash, bruising, urticaria, hives. **Other:** *angioedema, Reye syndrome,* hypersensitivity reactions, low birth weight, *stillbirth.*

INTERACTIONS
Drug-drug. *ACE inhibitors:* May decrease antihypertensive effects and increase kidney toxicity. Monitor therapy closely.
Ammonium chloride and other urine acidifiers: May increase levels of aspirin products. Watch for aspirin toxicity.
Antacids in high doses and other urine alkalinizers: May decrease levels of aspirin products. Watch for decreased aspirin effect.

Reactions in bold italics are *life-threatening*.

Anticoagulants, antiplatelet agents: May increase risk of bleeding. Use with extreme caution if these drugs must be used together.

Beta blockers: May decrease antihypertensive effect. Avoid long-term aspirin use if patient is taking antihypertensives.

Corticosteroids: May enhance salicylate elimination and decrease drug level. Watch for decreased aspirin effect. May increase risk of GI ulceration and bleeding. Monitor therapy.

Diuretics: May decrease effectiveness of diuretics in patients with underlying kidney or CV disease. Monitor therapy.

Heparin: May increase risk of bleeding. Monitor coagulation studies and patient closely if used together.

Ibuprofen, other NSAIDs: May negate antiplatelet effect of low-dose aspirin therapy and decrease kidney function. Patients using immediate-release aspirin (not enteric-coated) should take ibuprofen at least 30 minutes after or more than 8 hours before aspirin. Patients using extended-release aspirin should take ibuprofen at least 2 to 4 hours after or more than 8 hours before aspirin. Occasional use of ibuprofen is unlikely to have a negative effect.

Influenza virus vaccine, live; varicella virus vaccine, live: Increased risk of Reye syndrome. Use together is contraindicated in children and adolescents.

Methotrexate: May increase risk of methotrexate toxicity. Avoid use together.

Oral antidiabetics: May increase hypoglycemic effect. Monitor patient closely.

Phenytoin: May decrease phenytoin level. Avoid use together.

Probenecid: May decrease uricosuric effect. Avoid use together.

Valproic acid: May increase valproic acid level. Avoid use together.

Vitamin E: May enhance antiplatelet effect of agents with antiplatelet properties. Monitor patient closely.

Drug-herb. *White willow:* Contains salicylates and may increase risk of adverse effects. Discourage use together.

Drug-food. *Caffeine:* May increase drug absorption. Watch for increased effects.

Drug-lifestyle. *Alcohol use:* May increase risk of GI bleeding. Discourage use together.

EFFECTS ON LAB TEST RESULTS
• May increase LFT values and BUN, creatinine, sodium, and potassium levels.

• May decrease platelet and WBC counts.
• May interfere with urine glucose analysis with Diastix, Chemstrip uG, Clinitest, and Benedict solution; with urinary 5-hydroxyindoleacetic acid and vanillylmandelic acid tests; and with Gerhardt test for urine acetoacetic acid.

CONTRAINDICATIONS & CAUTIONS
• Contraindicated in patients hypersensitive to drug and in those with NSAID-induced sensitivity reactions or bleeding disorders, such as hemophilia, von Willebrand disease, telangiectasia, bleeding ulcers, and hemorrhagic states.
• Use cautiously in patients with GI lesions, impaired kidney function, hypoprothrombinemia, vitamin K deficiency, thrombocytopenia, or thrombotic thrombocytopenic purpura.
⚕ Avoid use in patients with severe liver or kidney impairment, G6PD deficiency, or history of active peptic ulcer disease.
🔆 *Alert:* Oral and rectal OTC products containing aspirin and nonaspirin salicylates shouldn't be given to children or teenagers who have or are recovering from chickenpox or flulike symptoms (with or without fever) because of risk of Reye syndrome.
• Safe use of extended-release capsules in children hasn't been established.
Dialyzable drug: Yes.
⚠ *Overdose S&S:* Severe acid-base and electrolyte disturbances, hyperthermia, dehydration, tinnitus, vertigo, headache, confusion, drowsiness, diaphoresis, hyperventilation, vomiting, diarrhea.

PREGNANCY-LACTATION-REPRODUCTION
• Use in pregnancy only if clearly needed and specifically directed to do so by a practitioner. Avoid use during third trimester.
• Drug appears in human milk. Patients who are breastfeeding should avoid aspirin if possible.
• Use of NSAIDs (including aspirin) at 20 weeks or later in pregnancy may cause fetal kidney dysfunction, leading to oligohydramnios and potential neonatal kidney impairment; use at 30 weeks or later in pregnancy may increase risk of premature closure of the ductus arteriosus.
• Avoid NSAID use during pregnancy starting at 20 weeks' gestation. If potential benefit justifies fetal risk, use lowest effective dose

for shortest duration. Consider ultrasound monitoring of amniotic fluid if NSAID use is longer than 48 hours.

• Use of 81 mg of low-dose aspirin for certain pregnancy-related conditions under prescriber direction is acceptable.

NURSING CONSIDERATIONS

• For inflammatory conditions, rheumatic fever, and thrombosis, give aspirin on a schedule rather than as needed.

• Because enteric-coated tablets are slowly absorbed, they aren't suitable for rapid relief of acute pain, fever, or inflammation. They cause less GI bleeding and may be better suited for long-term therapy, such as for arthritis.

• For patients who can't tolerate oral drugs, ask prescriber about using aspirin rectal suppositories. Watch for rectal mucosal irritation or bleeding.

• Febrile, dehydrated children can rapidly develop toxicity.

• Monitor older adults closely because they are more susceptible to drug's toxic effects.

• Monitor salicylate level. Therapeutic salicylate level for arthritis is 150 to 300 mcg/mL. Tinnitus may occur at levels above 200 mcg/mL but isn't a reliable indicator of toxicity, especially in very young patients and those older than age 60. With long-term therapy, severe toxic effects may occur with levels exceeding 400 mcg/mL.

• During prolonged therapy, periodically assess hematocrit, Hb level, PT, INR, and kidney function.

• Drug irreversibly inhibits platelet aggregation. Stop drug 5 to 7 days before elective surgery to allow time for production and release of new platelets.

• Monitor patient for hypersensitivity reactions, such as anaphylaxis and asthma.

• *Look alike–sound alike:* Don't confuse aspirin with Afrin.

PATIENT TEACHING

• Tell patient who's allergic to tartrazine to avoid aspirin.

• Advise patient on low-salt diet that 1 tablet of buffered aspirin contains 553 mg of sodium.

• Teach about proper drug administration and handling.

• Warn patient not to drink alcohol 2 hours before or 1 hour after taking extended-release

capsule and not to take extra capsule to make up for a missed dose.

• Remind patient taking drug for a chronic condition not to stop drug without first discussing with prescriber.

• Instruct patient to discard aspirin tablets that have a strong vinegar-like odor.

• Tell patient to consult prescriber if giving drug to children for longer than 5 days or adults for longer than 10 days.

• Advise patient receiving prolonged treatment with large doses of aspirin to watch for small, round, red pinprick spots; bleeding gums; and signs of GI bleeding. Advise patient to drink plenty of fluids. Encourage use of soft-bristled toothbrush.

• Because of the many drug interactions with aspirin, warn patient taking prescription drugs to check with prescriber or pharmacist before taking aspirin or OTC products containing aspirin.

• Warn patient who is pregnant not to take NSAIDs at 20 weeks' gestation or later unless instructed to do so by prescriber due to potential fetal risk. Advise patient to consult pharmacist or health care provider about taking OTC medications during pregnancy.

• Note that aspirin is a leading cause of poisoning in children. Caution parents to keep drug out of reach of children. Encourage use of child-resistant containers.

atazanavir sulfate

at-a-za-NA-veer

Reyataz

Therapeutic class: Antiretrovirals
Pharmacologic class: Protease inhibitors

AVAILABLE FORMS

Capsules ⊙: 100 mg, 150 mg, 200 mg, 300 mg
Oral powder: 50 mg

INDICATIONS & DOSAGES

Adjust-a-dose (for all indications): Patients with kidney failure who are treatment-naive and on hemodialysis should receive atazanavir 300 mg with ritonavir 100 mg. Don't give to patients who are treatment-experienced and on hemodialysis.

Significant drug interactions exist requiring dosage adjustment or drug avoidance.

Refer to manufacturer's instructions or interactions reference for dosage adjustments.

➤ **HIV-1 infection, with other antiretrovirals in patients who are treatment-experienced**

Adults: 300 mg once daily, plus 100 mg ritonavir once daily with food. In patients also taking an H_2-receptor antagonist (H2RA) and tenofovir, 400 mg PO once daily, plus 100 mg ritonavir.

Children and adolescents ages 6 to younger than 18 who are treatment-experienced and receiving ritonavir: For patients weighing 35 kg or more, 300 mg with ritonavir 100 mg PO once daily. For patients weighing 15 to 34 kg, 200 mg with ritonavir 100 mg PO once daily. For patients weighing 5 to 15 kg, capsules aren't recommended; use oral powder.

Children at least age 3 months and weighing at least 5 kg and less than 25 kg: For patients weighing 15 to less than 25 kg, 250 mg oral powder PO, immediately followed by 80 mg ritonavir daily. For patients weighing 5 to less than 15 kg, 200 mg oral powder PO, immediately followed by 80 mg ritonavir daily.

➤ **HIV-1 infection, with other antiretrovirals, in patients who are treatment-naive**

Adults: Recommended regimen is 300 mg PO once daily with ritonavir 100 mg. When given with efavirenz, give atazanavir 400 mg and ritonavir 100 mg as a single daily dose with food and efavirenz on an empty stomach, preferably at bedtime. For adults unable to tolerate ritonavir, give 400 mg PO once daily.

Adolescents at least age 13 and weighing at least 40 kg who can't tolerate ritonavir: 400 mg PO once daily with food.

Children and adolescents ages 6 to younger than 18: For patients weighing 35 kg or more, 300 mg with ritonavir 100 mg PO once daily. For patients weighing 15 to 34 kg, 200 mg with ritonavir 100 mg PO once daily. For patients weighing less than 15 kg, capsules aren't recommended; use oral powder.

Children at least age 3 months and weighing at least 5 kg and less than 25 kg: For patients weighing 15 to less than 25 kg, 250 mg oral powder PO, immediately followed by 80 mg ritonavir daily. For patients weighing 5 to less than 15 kg, 200 mg oral powder PO, immediately followed by 80 mg ritonavir daily.

Adjust-a-dose: Administration with ritonavir in patients with any degree of liver impairment isn't recommended. In adults with Child-Pugh class A liver impairment, give 400 mg atazanavir PO daily; for patients with Child-Pugh class B liver impairment, give 300 mg daily; for patients with Child-Pugh class C liver impairment, atazanavir isn't recommended.

➤ **HIV-1 infection, with other antiretrovirals, in patients who are treatment-experienced and pregnant**

Women: 300 mg PO daily with 100 mg ritonavir. For patients who are treatment-experienced during second or third trimester when given with either H2RA or tenofovir, 400 mg PO daily with 100 mg ritonavir.

ADMINISTRATION

PO

• Give drug with food to increase drug bioavailability.

• Have patient swallow capsules whole; don't break or open capsules.

• Mix oral powder with food (such as applesauce or yogurt) or beverage (such as milk, infant formula, or water).

• When mixing with food, mix powder with a minimum of 1 tablespoon of food in small container and feed to child. Add additional tablespoon of food to container, mix, and feed residual mixture to child.

• When mixing with beverage, mix powder with minimum of 30 mL of beverage and give to child to drink. Add additional 15 mL of beverage to the drinking cup, mix, and give to child to drink residual mixture. If water is used, also give food at same time.

• For young infants who can't eat solid food or drink from a cup, mix powder with 10 mL of infant formula in a medicine cup and draw up into oral syringe. Give to infant into either inner cheek. Pour additional 10 mL of formula into medicine cup and mix. Give residual mixture to infant in the same manner. Don't give in an infant bottle.

• Give entire dose of powder after mixing within 1 hour of preparation. Additional food may be given after dose is given.

ACTION

Inhibits viral maturation in HIV-1–infected cells, resulting in the formation of immature noninfectious viral particles.

Route	Onset	Peak	Duration
PO	Unknown	2–3 hr	Unknown

Half-life: Unboosted, 7 to 8 hours; boosted with ritonavir, 9 to 18 hours.

ADVERSE REACTIONS

CNS: headache, depression, dizziness, fever, insomnia, peripheral neuropathy. **CV:** prolonged PR interval, first- and second-degree heart block, peripheral edema. **EENT:** nasal congestion, rhinorrhea, oropharyngeal pain. **GI:** abdominal pain, diarrhea, nausea, vomiting. **Hematologic:** anemia, *neutropenia.* **Hepatic:** hyperbilirubinemia, increased LFT values, jaundice. **Metabolic:** increased CK level, hyperlipidemia, *hypoglycemia.* **Musculoskeletal:** arthralgia, myalgia, limb pain. **Respiratory:** increased cough, wheezing. **Skin:** rash.

INTERACTIONS

Refer to drug interactions resource for both atazanavir and ritonavir for complete information.

Drug-drug. *Alfuzosin:* May increase alfuzosin plasma concentration, increasing risk of hypotension. Use together is contraindicated.

Antacids, buffered medications (didanosine buffered preparation): May reduce atazanavir plasma concentration. Administer atazanavir 2 hours before or 1 hour after these medications.

Antiarrhythmics (amiodarone, bepridil, systemic lidocaine, quinidine): May produce serious or life-threatening adverse reactions. Use cautiously. Monitor antiarrhythmic therapeutic concentration.

Anticoagulants (apixaban, rivaroxaban, warfarin): May cause serious or life-threatening bleeding. Monitor INR.

Antifungals (itraconazole, ketoconazole, posaconazole, voriconazole): May increase risk of toxicity of both antifungal and atazanavir. Use cautiously when high doses of ketoconazole or itraconazole are administered with atazanavir and ritonavir. Administration of voriconazole with atazanavir and ritonavir isn't recommended.

Benzodiazepines (midazolam, triazolam): May increase plasma concentrations of these drugs. Oral midazolam and triazolam are contraindicated because of the potential for serious or life-threatening events, such as prolonged or increased sedation or respiratory depression. Use IV midazolam with caution and close monitoring. Consider reducing the IV midazolam dosage.

Bosentan: May decrease atazanavir plasma concentration when administered without ritonavir; coadministration of atazanavir and bosentan without ritonavir isn't recommended. May increase bosentan plasma concentration. Adjust bosentan dose when used with atazanavir–ritonavir. Consider therapy modification.

Calcium channel blockers (amlodipine, diltiazem, felodipine, nicardipine, nifedipine, verapamil): May prolong PR interval in some patients; use caution. Consider reducing diltiazem dosage by 50% and titrating dosages of other calcium channel blockers. Monitor ECG.

Carbamazepine: May increase carbamazepine level. May decrease atazanavir level, resulting in antiretroviral treatment failure. If coadministration can't be avoided, monitor patient closely. Consider alternative therapy for carbamazepine.

Clarithromycin: May prolong QTc interval; reduce clarithromycin dosage by 50%. Significantly reduces concentration of active metabolite (14-OH clarithromycin); consider alternative therapy for indications other than MAC.

Colchicine: May increase plasma concentrations of colchicine. Don't give colchicine and atazanavir together to patients with liver or kidney impairment. In those with normal kidney and liver function, reduce colchicine dose. Consider therapy modification.

Corticosteroids (fluticasone, prednisone): May increase corticosteroid plasma concentration. Monitor patient for signs and symptoms of adrenal insufficiency. Consider alternatives to fluticasone for long-term use.

Digoxin: May prolong PR interval. Use with caution.

Eplerenone: May increase eplerenone plasma concentration. Avoid combination.

Ergot derivatives (dihydroergotamine, ergonovine, ergotamine, methylergonovine): May cause serious or life-threatening events such as acute ergot toxicity (peripheral vasospasm, ischemia of the extremities). Use together is contraindicated.

Fluoxetine: May increase plasma concentrations of both drugs. Closely monitor patient for adverse reactions, including serotonin syndrome. Fluoxetine or atazanavir dosage reduction may be needed.

Hepatitis C antivirals (elbasvir/grazoprevir, glecaprevir/pibrentasvir): May increase serum concentrations of these drugs, which can lead to increased liver toxicity. Coadministration is contraindicated.

Reactions in bold italics are *life-threatening*.

Hepatitis C antivirals (voxilaprevir/sofosbuvir/velpatasvir): May increase serum concentrations of voxilaprevir. Coadministration isn't recommended.

HMG-CoA reductase inhibitors (atorvastatin, lovastatin, rosuvastatin, simvastatin): May increase serum concentrations of these drugs, possibly increasing their toxicity, including rhabdomyolysis. Administration with simvastatin or lovastatin is contraindicated. If using atorvastatin or rosuvastatin, start with lowest possible dosage with careful monitoring. Consider pravastatin or fluvastatin in combination with atazanavir.

Hormonal contraceptives (ethinyl estradiol, norethindrone, norgestimate): See manufacturer's instructions. Alternative methods of nonhormonal contraception are recommended.

H2RAs (famotidine): May decrease atazanavir plasma concentration, possibly causing development of resistance. See manufacturer's instructions for H2RA administration recommendations.

Immunosuppressants (cyclosporine, sirolimus, tacrolimus): May increase levels of these drugs. Monitor immunosuppressant concentrations.

Irinotecan: May interfere with irinotecan metabolism, resulting in increased toxicity. Use together is contraindicated.

Lurasidone: May increase lurasidone plasma concentration. Use together is contraindicated if administered with ritonavir.

mTOR inhibitors (everolimus, temsirolimus): May increase plasma concentrations of these drugs. If coadmination can't be avoided, monitor clinical response and adjust mTOR inhibitor dosage as needed.

NNRTIs (efavirenz, nevirapine): May decrease atazanavir plasma level. In patients who are treatment-naive, give atazanavir 400 mg with food and ritonavir 100 mg with efavirenz 600 mg on an empty stomach. Don't administer atazanavir with efavirenz in patients who are treatment-experienced. Nevirapine may decrease atazanavir exposure; administering them together may increase nevirapine exposure. Use together is contraindicated.

Opioid analgesics (buprenorphine, fentanyl, oxycodone, sufentanil): May increase plasma concentration and half-life of opioid; reduced opioid dosage may be needed. Closely monitor respiratory function during opioid administration and for a longer period than usual after stopping opioid. Atazanavir without ritonavir shouldn't be administered with buprenorphine.

PDE5 inhibitors (sildenafil, tadalafil, vardenafil): Coadministration of atazanavir and sildenafil for PAH is contraindicated. When used for erectile dysfunction, see manufacturer's instructions for dosage adjustments. Monitor patient closely.

Pimozide: May cause serious or life-threatening reactions (cardiac arrhythmias). Use is contraindicated.

Protease inhibitors (amprenavir, darunavir, indinavir, ritonavir, saquinavir): Drug may increase concentration of other protease inhibitors. Atazanavir–ritonavir isn't recommended with other protease inhibitors. Atazinavir is contraindicated with indinavir. Other combinations may require dosage changes. Consider therapy modification.

PPIs (omeprazole): Substantially decrease atazanavir plasma concentration, possibly causing development of resistance. In patients who are treatment-naive, give PPI 12 hours before atazanavir dose. PPI shouldn't exceed dose equivalent to omeprazole 20 mg. Don't use PPIs in patients who are treatment-experienced and receiving atazanavir.

Quetiapine: May increase quetiapine plasma concentration. Administer cautiously; closely monitor clinical response. Adjust quetiapine dosage to one-sixth of current dose.

Ranolazine: Increases risk of dose-related QTc-interval prolongation, torsades de pointes–type arrhythmias, and sudden death. Avoid use together. Contraindicated with cobicistat-boosted atazanavir.

Rifabutin: May increase rifabutin blood level. Rifabutin dosage reduction of up to 75% (150 mg every other day or three times/week) is recommended.

Rifampin: May decrease atazanavir plasma concentration, possibly causing development of resistance. Use together is contraindicated.

Salmeterol: May increase salmeterol concentration, increasing risk of CV events, including QT-interval prolongation, palpitations, and sinus tachycardia. Use together isn't recommended.

Saxagliptin: May increase saxagliptin plasma concentration. Limit saxagliptin dosage to 2.5 mg daily.

Strong CYP3A4 inhibitors (brentuximab, cabazitaxel, cilostazol, eletriptan, eplerenone, maraviroc, risperidone, romidepsin, trazodone): May increase inhibitor level. Refer to interactions resource for complete information.

TCAs (amitriptyline): May cause serious or life-threatening adverse reactions. Monitor TCA concentration.

Tenofovir: May decrease atazanavir level. Don't administer atazanavir with tenofovir unless also administering ritonavir; administer as atazanavir 300 mg, ritonavir 100 mg, and tenofovir 300 mg. Atazanavir increases tenofovir concentration; watch for tenofovir-associated adverse reactions.

Tyrosine kinase inhibitors (dasatinib, lapatinib, nilotinib, pazopanib, sorafenib, sunitinib): May increase tyrosine kinase inhibitor plasma concentrations. If use together can't be avoided, closely monitor clinical response and adjust tyrosine kinase inhibitor dosage as needed.

Vasopressin receptor antagonists (conivaptan, tolvaptan): May increase plasma concentration of these drugs. Avoid coadministration.

Vemurafenib: May increase vemurafenib plasma concentration. Avoid combination.

Vilazodone: May increase vilazodone plasma concentration. Reduce vilazodone dosage to 20 mg in patients receiving atazanavir.

Vinca alkaloids (vinblastine, vincristine): May increase pharmacologic effects of these drugs and risk of toxicity (characterized by profound neutropenia or severe neuropathy). Consider temporarily withholding or decreased dosage of vinca alkaloid.

Drug-herb. *St. John's wort:* May decrease drug level, reducing therapeutic effect and causing drug resistance. Use together is contraindicated.

EFFECTS ON LAB TEST RESULTS
● May increase ALT, AST, amylase, bilirubin, lipase, CK, triglyceride, and total cholesterol levels.
● May increase or decrease glucose level.
● May decrease Hb level and neutrophil and platelet counts.

CONTRAINDICATIONS & CAUTIONS
● Contraindicated in patients hypersensitive to drug or its ingredients.
● Contraindicated in patients taking drugs cleared mainly by CYP3A4 or drugs that

can cause serious or life-threatening reactions at high levels (alfuzosin, amiodarone [with ritonavir], dihydroergotamine, elbasvir–grazoprevir, ergonovine, ergotamine, glecaprevir–pibrentasvir, irinotecan, lovastatin, lurasidone [with ritonavir], methylergonovine, midazolam [PO], nevirapine, pimozide, quinidine [with ritonavir], rifampin, sildenafil [Revatio], St. John's wort, simvastatin, triazolam).

● Don't use in patients with Child-Pugh class C liver impairment or kidney failure managed with hemodialysis.
● Use cautiously in patients with cardiac conduction system disease, diabetes, liver impairment, or hemophilia type A or B.
● Use cautiously in older adults because of increased likelihood of other disease, additional drug therapy, and decreased liver, kidney, or cardiac function.
● Use isn't recommended in children younger than age 3 months due to risk of kernicterus.
Dialyzable drug: No.
⚠ **Overdose S&S:** Asymptomatic bifascicular block, PR-interval prolongation, jaundice.

PREGNANCY-LACTATION-REPRODUCTION
● Use during pregnancy only if potential benefit justifies fetal risk. U.S. Department of Health and Human Services Perinatal HIV Guidelines recommend atazanavir as a preferred protease inhibitor for patients who are pregnant and antiretroviral-naive when combined with low-dose ritonavir boosting. Enroll patients who are pregnant in the Antiretroviral Pregnancy Registry (1-800-258-4263).
● Drug appears in human milk. Breastfeeding is contraindicated in patients infected with HIV because of risk of postnatal transmission of HIV.

NURSING CONSIDERATIONS
🔔 **Alert:** Drug may prolong PR interval. Monitor ECG, especially in a patient with preexisting conduction system disease.
● Monitor patient for hyperglycemia and new-onset diabetes or worsened diabetes. Insulin and oral antidiabetic dosages may need adjustment.
● Monitor patient with HBV or HCV infection for elevated liver enzyme levels or liver decompensation.
● Monitor patient for immune reconstitution syndrome. Evaluate and treat indolent

or residual opportunistic infections (MAC, CMV, *Pneumocystis jiroveci* pneumonia, TB). Some autoimmune disorders (Graves disease, polymyositis, Guillain-Barré syndrome) have also occurred, even after many months of treatment.
• Watch for life-threatening lactic acidosis syndrome and symptomatic hyperlactatemia, especially in women and patients with obesity.
• If patient has hemophilia, watch for bleeding.
• Drug may cause kidney lithiasis or cholelithiasis. Evaluate patient for signs or symptoms of kidney lithiasis (flank pain) or cholelithiasis (abdominal pain, nausea, vomiting, jaundice); interrupt or discontinue drug as clinically indicated if signs or symptoms occur.
• Monitor patient for rash. Discontinue drug if rash occurs.
• Expect asymptomatic increase in indirect bilirubin, possibly resulting in yellowed skin or sclerae. This hyperbilirubinemia resolves when therapy stops.
• Monitor liver enzyme levels and kidney function before and periodically during treatment.
• Although cross-resistance occurs among protease inhibitors, resistance to drug doesn't preclude use of other protease inhibitors.
🕑 *Alert:* For patients with phenylketonuria, be aware that oral powder contains 35 mg of phenylalanine; capsules don't.

PATIENT TEACHING
• Urge patient to take drug with food every day and to take other antiretrovirals as prescribed.
• Advise patient to maintain adequate hydration to decrease risk of chronic kidney disease.
• Explain that drug doesn't cure HIV infection and that patient may develop opportunistic infections and other complications of HIV disease.
• Caution patient that drug doesn't reduce risk of transmitting HIV to others.
• Tell patient that drug may cause altered or increased body fat, central obesity, buffalo hump, peripheral wasting, facial wasting, breast enlargement, and cushingoid appearance.
• Advise patient to report all adverse drug reactions.
• Caution patient not to take other prescriptions or OTC or herbal medicines without first consulting prescriber due to significant drug interactions.

• Advise patient to discuss pregnancy with prescriber.

SAFETY ALERT!

atenolol
a-TEN-o-loll

Tenormin

Therapeutic class: Antihypertensives
Pharmacologic class: Beta blockers

AVAILABLE FORMS
Tablets: 25 mg, 50 mg, 100 mg

INDICATIONS & DOSAGES
Adjust-a-dose (for all indications): If CrCl is 15 to 35 mL/minute/1.73 m^2, maximum dose is 50 mg daily; if CrCl is below 15 mL/minute/1.73 m^2, maximum dose is 25 mg daily. Patients on hemodialysis need 25 to 50 mg after each dialysis session. For older adults, consider starting initial dose at 25 mg PO daily.
➤ **HTN**
Adults: Initially, 50 mg PO daily alone or in combination with a diuretic as a single dose, increased to 100 mg once daily after 7 to 14 days. Dosages of more than 100 mg daily are unlikely to produce further benefit.
➤ **Angina pectoris**
Adults: 50 mg PO once daily, increased as needed to 100 mg daily after 7 days for optimal effect. Maximum, 200 mg daily.
➤ **Acute MI**
Adults: 100 mg PO daily or 50 mg b.i.d. for at least 7 days; may continue for 1 to 3 years if no contraindications.

ADMINISTRATION
PO
• Give drug without regard for meals.
• Give drug exactly as prescribed, at the same time each day.

ACTION
Selectively blocks beta$_1$-adrenergic receptors, decreases cardiac output and cardiac oxygen consumption, and depresses renin secretion.

Route	Onset	Peak	Duration
PO	1 hr	2–4 hr	24 hr

Half-life: 6 to 7 hours.

ADVERSE REACTIONS

CNS: depression, dizziness, fatigue, lethargy, vertigo, drowsiness, fever, light-headedness, dreaming. **CV:** orthostatic hypotension, *bradycardia, HF, heart block,* bundle-branch block, cold extremities, intermittent claudication, atrial fibrillation, atrial flutter, *supraventricular tachycardia, cardiac arrest, cardiogenic shock, ventricular tachycardia, MI.* **GI:** nausea, diarrhea. **Musculoskeletal:** leg pain. **Respiratory:** *bronchospasm,* dyspnea, *PE,* wheezing. **Skin:** rash. **Other:** *death.*

INTERACTIONS

Drug-drug. *Amiodarone:* May increase risk of bradycardia, AV block, and myocardial depression. Monitor ECG and vital signs.
Antihypertensives: May increase hypotensive effect. Use together cautiously.
Calcium carbonate, calcium citrate: May decrease atenolol level. Separate doses by at least 2 hours. Monitor patient and adjust atenolol dosage as needed.
Calcium channel blockers, hydralazine, methyldopa: May cause additive hypotension and bradycardia. Adjust dosage as needed.
Cardiac glycosides, diltiazem, verapamil: May cause excessive bradycardia and increased depressant effect on myocardium. Use together cautiously.
Catecholamine-depleting drugs (reserpine): May increase risk of hypotension and bradycardia. Use together cautiously.
Clonidine: May exacerbate rebound HTN if clonidine is withdrawn. Withdraw atenolol several days before clonidine or add atenolol several days after clonidine is stopped.
Disopyramide: May increase risk of severe bradycardia, asystole, and HF. Use together cautiously.
Insulin, oral antidiabetics: May alter dosage requirements in patient with diabetes who has been previously stabilized. Observe patient carefully.
IV lidocaine: May reduce liver metabolism of lidocaine, increasing risk of toxicity. Give bolus doses of lidocaine at a slower rate and monitor therapy.
NSAIDs: May decrease antihypertensive effects. Monitor BP.
Prazosin: May increase risk of orthostatic hypotension in early phases of use together.
Rivastigmine: May enhance bradycardic effect of atenolol. Avoid use together.

EFFECTS ON LAB TEST RESULTS

• May increase bilirubin and liver enzyme levels.
• May decrease glucose level.
• May increase platelet count.

CONTRAINDICATIONS & CAUTIONS

• Contraindicated in patients hypersensitive to drug or its components.
• Contraindicated in patients with sinus bradycardia, heart block greater than first degree, overt cardiac failure, untreated pheochromocytoma, and cardiogenic shock.
• Use cautiously in older adults, patients at risk for HF, and those with diabetes, hyperthyroidism, myasthenia gravis, or impaired kidney or liver function.
• Don't routinely use beta blockers in patients with bronchospastic disease. Atenolol may be used cautiously in patients who don't respond to or can't tolerate other antihypertensive treatment. Use lowest possible dosage and have bronchodilator available. Consider divided doses if atenolol dosage must be increased.
• Drug may precipitate or aggravate signs and symptoms of PVD and Raynaud disease and worsen anginal symptoms in a patient with vasospastic angina.
• Don't routinely stop long-term beta blocker therapy before major surgery; however, risks associated with general anesthesia and surgery may be increased due to the heart's impaired ability to respond to reflex adrenergic stimuli.
• Safe use in children hasn't been established.
Dialyzable drug: Yes.
⚠ **Overdose S&S:** Lethargy, decreased respiratory drive, wheezing, sinus pause, bradycardia.

PREGNANCY-LACTATION-REPRODUCTION

• Drug can cause fetal harm. Use cautiously during pregnancy; inform patient of potential fetal hazard.
• Drug appears in human milk. Use cautiously during breastfeeding.
• Neonates born to patients receiving atenolol at parturition and infants being breastfed by patients receiving atenolol may be at risk for hypoglycemia and significant bradycardia.

NURSING CONSIDERATIONS

• Monitor HR and BP, preferably just before next dose, to evaluate effectiveness.

Reactions in bold italics are *life-threatening*.

• Closely monitor patients on hemodialysis for hypotension.
• Beta blockers may mask tachycardia caused by hyperthyroidism. In patients with suspected thyrotoxicosis, withdraw beta blocker gradually to avoid thyroid storm.
• Drug may mask signs and symptoms of hypoglycemia in a patient with diabetes.
• Drug may cause changes in exercise tolerance and ECG.
• Monitor for cardiac failure. Discontinue drug in a patient who develops cardiac failure that doesn't respond to standard treatment.
Boxed Warning Avoid abrupt discontinuation of therapy. Withdraw drug gradually to avoid serious adverse reactions, such as severe exacerbations of angina, MI, and ventricular arrhythmias. Because CAD is common and may be unrecognized, avoid abrupt discontinuation even in patients treated only for HTN. ■
• *Look alike–sound alike:* Don't confuse atenolol with timolol or albuterol.

PATIENT TEACHING

• Instruct patient to take drug exactly as prescribed, at the same time every day.
Boxed Warning Caution patient not to stop drug suddenly. ■
• Advise patient to report all adverse reactions to prescriber.
• Teach patient how to take pulse, when to withhold drug, and when to report HR according to prescriber's instructions.
• Tell patient of childbearing potential to notify prescriber about planned, suspected, or known pregnancy.
• Advise patient who is breastfeeding to contact prescriber; drug may cause hypoglycemia or significant bradycardia in the infant.

atogepant
a-TOE-je-pant

Qulipta

Therapeutic class: Antimigraine drugs
Pharmacologic class: Calcitonin gene-related peptide receptor antagonists

AVAILABLE FORMS
Tablets: 10 mg, 30 mg, 60 mg

INDICATIONS & DOSAGES
➤ **Prevention of episodic migraine headaches**
Adults: 1 tablet PO once daily.
Adjust-a-dose: If used concomitantly with strong CYP3A4 inhibitor, 10 mg PO once daily. If used concomitantly with strong or moderate CYP3A4 inducer, give 30 or 60 mg PO once daily. If used concomitantly with OATP inhibitor, give 10 or 30 mg PO once daily. In patients with CrCl less than 30 mL/minute, give 10 mg PO once daily.
✷ *NEW INDICATION:* **Prevention of chronic migraine headaches**
Adults: 60 mg PO once daily.
Adjust-a-dose: Avoid use with CYP3A4 inducers and strong CYP3A4 inhibitors. If used concomitantly with an OATP inhibitor, give 30 mg PO once daily. Avoid use in patients with CrCl less than 30 mL/minute.

ADMINISTRATION
PO
• Give drug without regard to food.
• If patient is receiving dialysis, give after treatment.
• Store tablets at 68° to 77° F (20° to 25° C).

ACTION
Antagonizes calcitonin gene-related peptide receptors.

Route	Onset	Peak	Duration
PO	Unknown	1–2 hr	Unknown

Half-life: 11 hours.

ADVERSE REACTIONS
CNS: fatigue, somnolence. **GI:** constipation, decreased appetite, nausea. **Hepatic:** elevated transaminase levels. **Metabolic:** weight loss.

INTERACTIONS
Drug-drug. *OATP inhibitors (cyclosporine, rifampin):* May increase atogepant level. Adjust atogepant dosage.
Strong or moderate CYP3A4 inducers (carbamazepine, efavirenz, etravirine, phenytoin, rifampin): May decrease atogepant level. Adjust atogepant dosage.
Strong CYP3A4 inhibitors (clarithromycin, itraconazole, ketoconazole): May increase atogepant level. Adjust atogepant dosage.
Drug-herb. *St. John's wort:* May decrease atogepant level. Adjust atogepant dosage.

EFFECTS ON LAB TEST RESULTS
• May increase liver transaminase levels.

CONTRAINDICATIONS & CAUTIONS
• Avoid use in patients with Child-Pugh class C liver impairment.
• Use cautiously in older adults. Initiate therapy at lowest dose.
• Safety and effectiveness in children haven't been established.
Dialyzable drug: Unknown.

PREGNANCY-LACTATION-REPRODUCTION
• Based on animal studies, drug may cause fetal harm. Advise patients who are pregnant of fetal risk.
• Use during pregnancy only if clearly indicated and benefit outweighs fetal risk.
• It isn't known if drug appears in human milk or how drug affects milk production or infants who are breastfed. Before decision about breastfeeding, consider patient's clinical need and risk to infant.

NURSING CONSIDERATIONS
• Monitor LFT values when appropriate.

PATIENT TEACHING
• Teach about proper drug administration and handling.
• Advise patient to report use of other prescription drugs, OTC drugs, or herbal products to prescriber.
• Inform patient that drug may interact with other drugs and that dosage modifications may be necessary.

atomoxetine hydrochloride ☒
AT-oh-mox-e-teen

Strattera

Therapeutic class: ADHD drugs
Pharmacologic class: Selective norepinephrine reuptake inhibitors

AVAILABLE FORMS
Capsules ⓄⓃⒸ: 10 mg, 18 mg, 25 mg, 40 mg, 60 mg, 80 mg, 100 mg

INDICATIONS & DOSAGES
➤ **ADHD**
Adults and children older than age 6 and adolescents weighing more than 70 kg: Initially, 40 mg PO daily; increase after at least 3 days to a total of 80 mg/day PO, as a single dose in the morning or two evenly divided doses in the morning and late afternoon or early evening. After 2 to 4 weeks, increase total dose to a maximum of 100 mg, if needed.
Children ages 6 and older and adolescents weighing 70 kg or less: Initially, 0.5 mg/kg PO daily; increase after a minimum of 3 days to a target total daily dose of 1.2 mg/kg PO as a single dose in the morning or two evenly divided doses in the morning and late afternoon or early evening. Don't exceed 1.4 mg/kg or 100 mg daily, whichever is less.
Adjust-a-dose: In patients with Child-Pugh class B liver impairment, reduce to 50% of normal dose; in those with Child-Pugh class C liver impairment, reduce to 25% of normal dose.

☒ In children and adults weighing more than 70 kg who are also receiving strong CYP2D6 inhibitors or are known CYP2D6 poor metabolizers, start at 40 mg daily and increase to 80 mg daily only if symptoms don't improve after 4 weeks and if first dose is tolerated.

☒ In children weighing less than 70 kg who are also receiving strong CYP2D6 inhibitors or are known CYP2D6 poor metabolizers, adjust dosage to 0.5 mg/kg daily and increase to 1.2 mg/kg daily only if symptoms don't improve after 4 weeks and if first dose is tolerated.

ADMINISTRATION
PO
• Give drug without regard for meals.
• Have patient swallow capsules whole; don't break or open capsules.
• Give missed dose as soon as possible but give no more than prescribed total daily amount in a 23-hour period.
• May discontinue drug without tapering.
• Store tablets at controlled room temperature of 59° to 86° F (15° to 30° C).

ACTION
May be related to selective inhibition of the presynaptic norepinephrine transporter.

Route	Onset	Peak	Duration
PO	Rapid	1–2 hr	Unknown

Half-life: 5 hours; 24 hours in poor metabolizers.

ADVERSE REACTIONS

CNS: headache, insomnia, dizziness, somnolence, irritability, jittery feeling, mood swings, fatigue, sedation, depression, tremor, early-morning awakening, paresthesia, abnormal dreams, sleep disorder, syncope, anxiety, unexpected therapeutic response. **CV:** orthostatic hypotension, tachycardia, HTN, palpitations, hot flush. **EENT:** mydriasis, conjunctivitis, dry mouth, oropharyngeal pain, pharyngolaryngeal pain, sinus headache. **GI:** abdominal pain, constipation, dyspepsia, nausea, anorexia, vomiting, decreased appetite. **GU:** urine retention, urinary hesitation, ejaculatory problems, difficulty in micturition, dysmenorrhea, erectile dysfunction, menstrual disorder, prostatitis. **Metabolic:** weight loss, thirst. **Skin:** pruritus, excoriation, increased sweating, rash. **Other:** decreased libido, chills.

INTERACTIONS

Drug-drug. *Albuterol:* May increase CV effects. Use together cautiously.
Antihypertensive drugs: May increase hypotensive effect. Use together cautiously.
MAO inhibitors: May cause hyperthermia, rigidity, myoclonus, autonomic instability with possible rapid fluctuations of vital signs, and mental status changes. Avoid use within 2 weeks of MAO inhibitor.
Pressor agents (dopamine, dobutamine): May increase BP. Use together cautiously.
Strong CYP2D6 inhibitors (fluoxetine, paroxetine, quinidine): May increase atomoxetine level. Adjust atomoxetine dosage based on effect and tolerance.

EFFECTS ON LAB TEST RESULTS
None reported.

CONTRAINDICATIONS & CAUTIONS
• Contraindicated in patients hypersensitive to drug or its components; in those with current or history of pheochromocytoma or narrow-angle glaucoma; in those with serious CV disorders who are intolerant of increased BP or HR; and in those who have taken an MAO inhibitor within the past 2 weeks.
• Drug may increase risk of sudden death, stroke, and MI in patients with preexisting structural cardiac disorders or other serious heart problems, including cardiomyopathy, CAD, and arrhythmias.

☒ Use cautiously in patients with HTN, tachycardia, hypotension, urine retention, cerebrovascular disease, or poor CYP2D6 metabolization.
Boxed Warning Drug may increase risk of suicidality in children and adolescents. ∎
• Safety and effectiveness in children younger than age 6 haven't been established.
Dialyzable drug: No.
⚠ *Overdose S&S:* Somnolence, agitation, hyperactivity, abnormal behavior, GI symptoms, mydriasis, tachycardia, dry mouth, prolonged QT interval, disorientation, hallucinations, seizures.

PREGNANCY-LACTATION-REPRODUCTION
• Don't use during pregnancy unless potential benefit justifies fetal risk. Advise patients of childbearing potential to use effective contraception.
• It isn't known if drug appears in human milk. Use cautiously during breastfeeding.
• Register patients in the National Pregnancy Registry for ADHD Medications, which monitors pregnancy outcomes in patients exposed to ADHD medications during pregnancy (1-866-961-2388 or https://womensmentalhealth.org/adhd-medications/).

NURSING CONSIDERATIONS
• Use drug as part of a total treatment program for ADHD, including psychological, educational, and social intervention. Drug may be discontinued without tapering.
Boxed Warning Closely monitor children and adolescents for worsening of condition, agitation, irritability, suicidal thinking or behaviors, and unusual changes in behavior, especially within first few months of therapy and when dosage increases or decreases. ∎
• Periodically monitor patient for changes in HR or BP.
• Carefully assess patient for cardiac disease, including family history of sudden death or ventricular arrhythmia. Promptly evaluate patient with new cardiac symptoms.
• Screen patient for bipolar disorder or risk factors for bipolar disorder before treatment, including family history of mania or depression. Drug may increase risk of emergence or worsening of disorder.
• Periodically reevaluate patient taking drug for extended period to determine drug's usefulness.

• Monitor growth during treatment. If growth or weight gain is unsatisfactory, consider interrupting therapy.

🌓 *Alert:* Severe liver injury may occur and progress to liver failure. Notify prescriber of any sign of liver injury (yellowing of skin or sclerae of eyes, pruritus, dark urine, upper right-sided tenderness, unexplained flulike syndrome).

• Monitor BP and pulse rate at baseline, after each dosage increase, and periodically during treatment.

• Monitor for urinary hesitancy, urine retention, or priapism.

• Monitor patient for appearance or worsening of psychotic or manic symptoms, aggressive behavior, and hostility.

• Monitor for hypersensitivity reactions, including anaphylaxis.

PATIENT TEACHING

Boxed Warning Advise patient or caregivers to immediately report unusual behavior or suicidality. ∎

• Instruct patient to immediately report chest pain, shortness of breath, or fainting.

• Tell patient to use caution when operating a vehicle or machinery until the effects of drug are known.

• Warn male patient to seek prompt medical attention for an erection that lasts more than 4 hours.

• Inform patient that therapy may be periodically interrupted to check ADHD symptoms.

• Tell patient who is pregnant, planning to become pregnant, or breastfeeding to consult prescriber before taking atomoxetine.

atorvastatin calcium 🖂
a-TORE-va-sta-tin

Lipitor

Therapeutic class: Antilipemics
Pharmacologic class: HMG-CoA reductase inhibitors

AVAILABLE FORMS
Tablets ᴼᴺᴳ: 10 mg, 20 mg, 40 mg, 80 mg

INDICATIONS & DOSAGES

Adjust-a-dose (for all indications): Significant drug interactions exist, requiring dosage or frequency adjustment or drug avoidance.

Refer to manufacturer's instructions for dosage adjustments.

➤ **In patients with clinically evident CAD, to reduce risk of nonfatal MI, fatal and nonfatal strokes, angina, HF, and revascularization procedures**
Adults: Initially, 10 to 20 mg PO daily. May increase based on patient response and tolerance; usual dosage, 10 to 80 mg PO daily.

➤ **To reduce risk of MI, stroke, angina, or revascularization procedures in patients with multiple risk factors for CAD who don't yet have the disease; to reduce risk of MI or stroke in patients with type 2 diabetes and multiple risk factors for CAD who don't yet have the disease**
Adults: Initially, 10 to 20 mg PO daily. May increase based on patient response and tolerance; usual dosage, 10 to 80 mg PO daily.

➤ **Adjunct to diet to reduce LDL in patients with primary hyperlipidemia; adjunct to diet in patients with primary dysbetalipoproteineia or hypertriglyceridemia**
Adults: Initially, 10 or 20 mg PO once daily. Patients who require a reduction of more than 45% in LDL level may be started at 40 mg once daily. Increase dose, as needed, to maximum of 80 mg daily as a single dose. Dosage based on lipid levels drawn within 2 to 4 weeks of starting therapy and after dosage adjustment.

➤ **Alone or as an adjunct to lipid-lowering treatments, such as LDL apheresis, to reduce total and LDL cholesterol in patients with homozygous familial hypercholesterolemia** 🖂
Adults and children ages 10 to 17: Initially, 10 to 20 mg PO once daily. Adults who requires a reduction of more than 45% in LDL level may be started at 40 mg once daily. Adjustment intervals should be at least 4 weeks. Maximum daily dose, 80 mg.

➤ **Heterozygous familial hypercholesterolemia** 🖂
Adults: Initially, 10 to 20 mg PO once daily. Patient who requires a reduction of more than 45% in LDL level may be started at 40 mg once daily. Adjustment intervals should be at least 4 weeks. Maximum daily dose, 80 mg.
Children ages 10 to 17: Initially, 10 mg PO once daily. Adjustment intervals should be at least 4 weeks. Maximum daily dose, 20 mg.

Reactions in bold italics are *life-threatening*.

ADMINISTRATION
PO
• Give drug without regard for meals at any time of the day.

ACTION
Inhibits HMG-CoA reductase, an early (and rate-limiting) step in cholesterol biosynthesis.

Route	Onset	Peak	Duration
PO	Unknown	1–2 hr	Unknown

Half-life: 14 hours.

ADVERSE REACTIONS
CNS: insomnia. **EENT:** nasopharyngitis, pharyngolaryngeal pain. **GI:** abdominal pain, diarrhea, dyspepsia, flatulence, nausea. **GU:** UTI. **Hepatic:** increased LFT values. **Metabolic:** *diabetes.* **Musculoskeletal:** *rhabdomyolysis,* arthralgia, myalgia, extremity pain, muscle spasms, musculoskeletal pain. **Skin:** rash.

INTERACTIONS
Drug-drug. *Amiodarone:* May increase risk of severe myopathy or rhabdomyolysis. Avoid use together or decrease atorvastatin dose.
Antacids, cholestyramine, colestipol: May decrease atorvastatin level. Separate administration times.
Colchicine, diltiazem, fibric acid derivatives, nefazodone, niacin, protease inhibitors, verapamil: May decrease metabolism of HMG-CoA reductase inhibitors, increasing toxicity. Monitor patient for adverse effects and report unexplained muscle pain.
Cyclosporine, tacrolimus, telaprevir, tipranavir plus ritonavir: May increase statin level and risk of myopathy and rhabdomyolysis. Avoid use together.
Darunavir and ritonavir, fosamprenavir, fosamprenavir and ritonavir, saquinavir and ritonavir: May increase atorvastatin level and risk of myopathy and rhabdomyolysis. Atorvastatin dosage shouldn't exceed 20 mg daily.
Digoxin: May increase digoxin level. Monitor digoxin level and patient for evidence of toxicity.
Fluconazole, itraconazole, ketoconazole, voriconazole: May increase atorvastatin level and adverse effects. Avoid use together or, if unavoidable, ensure atorvastatin dosage doesn't exceed 20 mg daily.
Gemfibrozil: May increase risk of myopathy and rhabdomyolysis. Avoid use together.

Hormonal contraceptives: May increase norethindrone and ethinyl estradiol levels. Consider increased drug effect when selecting an oral contraceptive.
Lopinavir and ritonavir: May increase statin level and risk of myopathy and rhabdomyolysis. Use together cautiously and at lowest atorvastatin dosage necessary.
Macrolides (azithromycin, clarithromycin, erythromycin, telithromycin): May increase atorvastatin level and risk of myopathy and rhabdomyolysis. Atorvastatin dosage shouldn't exceed 20 mg daily or withhold atorvastatin during macrolide therapy.
Nelfinavir: May increase statin level and risk of myopathy and rhabdomyolysis. Atorvastatin dosage shouldn't exceed 40 mg daily.
Drug-herb. *Jin bu huan, kava:* May increase risk of liver toxicity. Discourage use together.
Drug-food. *Grapefruit juice:* May increase drug levels when consumed in large quantities, increasing risk of adverse reactions. Discourage use together.
Drug-lifestyle. *Alcohol use:* May increase liver toxic effects. Monitor patient closely.

EFFECTS ON LAB TEST RESULTS
• May increase LFT values and CK levels.

CONTRAINDICATIONS & CAUTIONS
• Contraindicated in patients hypersensitive to drug and in those with active liver disease or unexplained persistent elevations of transaminase levels.
• Drug increases risk of myopathy and rhabdomyolysis, especially in patients ages 65 and older, in those with uncontrolled hypothyroidism or kidney impairment, and in those taking certain other drugs.
• Some dosage forms contain polysorbate 80, which can cause delayed hypersensitivity reactions.
• Use cautiously in patients with liver impairment or heavy alcohol use.
• Withhold or stop drug in patients at risk for kidney failure caused by rhabdomyolysis resulting from trauma; in serious, acute conditions that suggest myopathy; and in major surgery, severe acute infection, hypotension, uncontrolled seizures, or severe metabolic, endocrine, or electrolyte disorders.
⚕ Limit use in children to those older than age 10 with familial hypercholesterolemia.
Dialyzable drug: No.

PREGNANCY-LACTATION-REPRODUCTION
• Drug may cause fetal harm.
• Use during pregnancy is contraindicated unless benefits to patient outweigh fetal risk. Consider use in patients at high risk for CV events during pregnancy (homozygous familial hypercholesterolemia, established CV disease) on an individual basis.
• Patients of childbearing potential should use effective contraception during treatment and be apprised of potential hazards to fetus. Discontinue drug when pregnancy is recognized.
• It isn't known if drug appears in human milk. Use is contraindicated during breast-feeding. Patient should discontinue breast-feeding or temporarily discontinue drug.

NURSING CONSIDERATIONS
• Patient should follow a standard cholesterol-lowering diet before and during therapy.
• Before treatment, assess patient for underlying causes for hypercholesterolemia and obtain a baseline lipid profile. Obtain periodic LFT results and lipid levels before starting treatment, at 4 and 12 weeks after initiation, after an increase in dosage, and periodically thereafter.
• Watch for signs of myositis and myopathy (unexplained muscle pain, tenderness, weakness, malaise, dark urine, fever). Drug may need to be discontinued.
• Monitor HbA_{1c} and fasting serum glucose levels.
• *Look alike–sound alike:* Don't confuse atorvastatin with atomoxetine or other statins.

PATIENT TEACHING
• Teach about proper dietary management, weight control, and exercise. Explain their importance in controlling high fat levels.
• Counsel patient to avoid alcohol.
• Tell patient to inform prescriber of all adverse reactions. Stress the risk of myopathy (unexplained muscle pain, tenderness, or weakness, particularly if accompanied by malaise and fever).
• Advise patient that drug can be taken at any time of day, without regard for meals.
• *Alert:* Tell patient to stop drug and notify prescriber immediately if pregnant or breast-feeding.

atovaquone
a-TOE-va-kwone

Mepron

Therapeutic class: Antiprotozoals
Pharmacologic class: Ubiquinone analogues

AVAILABLE FORMS
Oral suspension: 750 mg/5 mL

INDICATIONS & DOSAGES
➤ **Acute, mild to moderate *Pneumocystis jiroveci* pneumonia in patients who can't tolerate sulfamethoxazole–trimethoprim**
Adults and adolescents ages 13 and older: 750 mg (5 mL) PO b.i.d. for 21 days.
➤ **To prevent *P. jiroveci* pneumonia in patients who are unable to tolerate sulfamethoxazole–trimethoprim**
Adults and adolescents ages 13 and older: 1,500 mg (10 mL) PO daily.

ADMINISTRATION
PO
• Give drug with food to enhance absorption.
• Shake bottle gently before using.
• Give entire contents of foil pouch, which can be poured into a dosing spoon or cup or be taken directly into the mouth.

ACTION
May interfere with electron transport in protozoal mitochondria, inhibiting enzymes needed to synthesize nucleic acids and adenosine triphosphate.

Route	Onset	Peak	Duration
PO	Unknown	Unknown	Unknown

Half-life: 2 to 4 days.

ADVERSE REACTIONS
CNS: headache, insomnia, fever, pain, asthenia, anxiety, dizziness, taste perversion, depression, weakness. **CV:** hypotension. **EENT:** sinusitis, rhinitis, oral candidiasis. **GI:** abdominal pain, nausea, diarrhea, vomiting, constipation, anorexia, dyspepsia. **Hematologic:** *neutropenia,* anemia. **Hepatic:** elevated transaminase levels, increased ALP level. **Metabolic:** *hypoglycemia,* hyponatremia, increased amylase level. **Musculoskeletal:** myalgia. **Respiratory:** cough,

dyspnea. **Skin:** rash, diaphoresis, pruritus. **Other:** flulike syndrome.

INTERACTIONS
Drug-drug. *Metoclopramide:* May decrease atovaquone bioavailability. Use another antiemetic.

Rifabutin, rifampin: May decrease atovaquone's steady-state level. Avoid use together.

Tetracycline: May decrease atovaquone level. Monitor patient for continued or reactivated infection.

EFFECTS ON LAB TEST RESULTS
• May increase glucose, BUN, creatinine amylase, ALP, ALT, and AST levels.
• May decrease Hb and sodium levels.
• May decrease neutrophil count.

CONTRAINDICATIONS & CAUTIONS
• Contraindicated in patients hypersensitive to drug. Serious hypersensitivity reactions have been reported.
• Use cautiously in patients with severe liver impairment.
• Use cautiously with other highly protein-bound drugs; if used together, assess patient for toxicity.
◑ **Alert:** Patients with GI disorders may not absorb drug well and may not achieve adequate plasma levels. Consider parenteral therapy with alternative drugs.
• Safety and effectiveness in children ages 12 and younger haven't been established.
Dialyzable drug: Unknown.
⚠ *Overdose S&S:* Methemoglobinemia, rash.

PREGNANCY-LACTATION-REPRODUCTION
• Use cautiously during pregnancy and only if potential benefit justifies fetal risk.
• It isn't known if drug appears in human milk. Breastfeeding by patients with HIV-1 infection isn't recommended due to potential for transmission.

NURSING CONSIDERATIONS
◑ **Alert:** Closely monitor patient during therapy due to risk of pulmonary infection.
• Closely monitor patient with liver impairment.
• Monitor patient for GI disorders (nausea, vomiting, diarrhea) that might affect ability to absorb drug.

PATIENT TEACHING
• Instruct patient to take drug with meals; food significantly enhances absorption.
• Stress importance of taking atovaquone as prescribed.
• Advise patient to report all adverse reactions and to immediately report nausea, vomiting, diarrhea, white mouth patches, flulike symptoms, dark urine, tiredness, lack of appetite, yellow skin, and light stools.

atovaquone–proguanil hydrochloride
a-TOE-va-kwon/pro-GWA-nil

Malarone

Therapeutic class: Antimalarials
Pharmacologic class: Hydroxynaphthoquinone and biguanide derivatives

AVAILABLE FORMS
Tablets (adult-strength): 250 mg atovaquone and 100 mg proguanil hydrochloride
Tablets (pediatric-strength): 62.5 mg atovaquone and 25 mg proguanil hydrochloride

INDICATIONS & DOSAGES
➤ **To prevent *Plasmodium falciparum* malaria, including in areas where chloroquine resistance has been reported, beginning 1 or 2 days before entering a malaria-endemic area and continuing during stay and for 7 days after return**
Adults and children weighing more than 40 kg: 1 adult-strength tablet PO once daily.
Children weighing 31 to 40 kg: 3 pediatric-strength tablets PO once daily.
Children weighing 21 to 30 kg: 2 pediatric-strength tablets PO once daily.
Children weighing 11 to 20 kg: 1 pediatric-strength tablet PO daily.
Adjust-a-dose: Don't use for malaria prophylaxis in patients with severe kidney impairment (CrCl less than 30 mL/minute).
➤ **Acute, uncomplicated *P. falciparum* malaria**
Adults and children weighing more than 40 kg: 4 adult-strength tablets PO once daily for 3 consecutive days.
Children weighing 31 to 40 kg: 3 adult-strength tablets PO once daily for 3 consecutive days.

Children weighing 21 to 30 kg: 2 adult-strength tablets PO once daily for 3 consecutive days.
Children weighing 11 to 20 kg: 1 adult-strength tablet PO once daily for 3 consecutive days.
Children weighing 9 to 10 kg: 3 pediatric-strength tablets PO once daily for 3 consecutive days.
Children weighing 5 to 8 kg: 2 pediatric-strength tablets PO once daily for 3 consecutive days.

ADMINISTRATION
PO
- Give dose at same time each day, with food or milk.
- If patient has difficulty swallowing tablets, crush tablets and mix in condensed milk.
- If vomiting occurs within 1 hour of drug administration, repeat dose.
- Store tablets at room temperature.

ACTION
Thought to interfere with nucleic acid replication in the malarial parasite. Atovaquone selectively inhibits mitochondrial electron transport in the parasite. Cycloguanil, an active metabolite of proguanil hydrochloride, inhibits dihydrofolate reductase. Atovaquone and cycloguanil are active against the erythrocytic and exoerythrocytic stages of *Plasmodium* species.

Route	Onset	Peak	Duration
PO	Unknown	Unknown	Unknown

Half-life: Atovaquone: 2 to 3 days in adults, 1 to 2 days in children; proguanil: 12 to 21 hours in adults and children.

ADVERSE REACTIONS
CNS: headache, asthenia, dizziness, dreams, insomnia. **EENT:** vision changes, oral ulcers. **GI:** abdominal pain, nausea, vomiting, diarrhea, anorexia, dyspepsia, gastritis. **Respiratory:** cough. **Skin:** pruritus.

INTERACTIONS
Drug-drug. *Metoclopramide:* May decrease atovaquone bioavailability. Use another antiemetic.
Rifabutin, rifampin: May significantly decrease atovaquone level. Avoid use together.
Tetracycline: May decrease atovaquone level. Monitor closely for continued or reactivated infection.

Warfarin: May increase anticoagulation effect. Monitor INR.

EFFECTS ON LAB TEST RESULTS
- May increase LFT values.
- May decrease Hb level, hematocrit, and neutrophil count.

CONTRAINDICATIONS & CAUTIONS
- Contraindicated in patients hypersensitive to atovaquone, proguanil hydrochloride, or components of drug and in those with severe kidney impairment or severe or complicated malaria.
- Use cautiously in patients with vomiting or diarrhea; drug absorption may be decreased.
- Use cautiously in older adults because they have a greater frequency of decreased kidney, liver, and heart function.
- Safety and effectiveness haven't been established for prevention in children who weigh less than 11 kg or for treatment in children who weigh less than 5 kg.
Dialyzable drug: Unknown.
⚠ *Overdose S&S:* Rash, methemoglobinemia (atovaquone); epigastric discomfort, vomiting, reversible hair loss, scaling of skin on palms or soles, reversible aphthous ulceration, hematologic adverse effects (proguanil).

PREGNANCY-LACTATION-REPRODUCTION
- Use during pregnancy only if potential benefit justifies fetal risk.
- It isn't known if atovaquone appears in human milk, but proguanil does appear in small amounts. Use cautiously during breastfeeding.

NURSING CONSIDERATIONS
- Monitor patient for persistent diarrhea or vomiting. Patients with these symptoms may need a different antimalarial.
- Monitor patients on prophylactic therapy for elevated liver enzyme levels, hepatitis, and liver failure.
- Monitor for relapse or failure of prophylaxis.

PATIENT TEACHING
- Teach about proper drug administration and handling.
- Advise patient to notify prescriber if patient can't complete the course of therapy as prescribed.
- Instruct patient to supplement preventive antimalarial with use of protective clothing, bed nets, and insect repellents.

Reactions in bold italics are *life-threatening*.

• Caution patient that prophylaxis isn't assured. Instruct patient to seek medical attention for any febrile illness during or after return from malaria-endemic area.

atropine sulfate ⚕
AT-troe-peen

AtroPen

Therapeutic class: Antiarrhythmics
Pharmacologic class: Anticholinergics–belladonna alkaloids

AVAILABLE FORMS
Injection: 0.4 mg/mL, 1 mg/mL vials
Prefilled autoinjectors: 0.25 mg, 0.5 mg, 1 mg, 2 mg
Prefilled syringe: 0.25 mg/5 mL, 0.5 mg/5 mL, 0.8 mg/2 mL, 1 mg/2.5 mL, 1 mg/10 mL

INDICATIONS & DOSAGES
➤ **Bradyasystolic cardiac arrest**
Adults: 1 mg IV (preferred) every 3 to 5 minutes; maximum total dose, 3 mg.
➤ **Symptomatic bradycardia**
Adults: 0.5 mg IV push or IM, repeated every 3 to 5 minutes, not to exceed a total of 3 mg or 0.04 mg/kg.
Children and adolescents: 0.02 mg/kg IV. May repeat once in 3 to 5 minutes; maximum dose, 1 mg.
➤ **Organophosphorus or muscarinic mushroom poisoning**
Adults: 2 to 3 mg IV (preferred), IM, or subcut; may repeat every 20 to 30 minutes.
➤ **Initial treatment of muscarinic symptoms of insecticide (organophosphorus or carbamate) poisoning or organophosphorus nerve agent poisoning**
Adults and children weighing more than 41 kg: For severe symptoms, immediately give three AtroPen 2 mg IM injections in rapid succession. For mild symptoms, give one AtroPen 2 mg IM injection. If patient then develops severe symptoms, give two additional 2 mg IM injections in rapid succession 10 minutes after first injection.
Children weighing 18 to 41 kg: For severe symptoms, immediately give three AtroPen 1 mg IM injections in rapid succession. For mild symptoms, give one AtroPen 1 mg IM injection. If patient then develops severe

symptoms, give two additional 1 mg IM injections in rapid succession 10 minutes after first injection.
Children weighing 7 to 18 kg: For severe symptoms, immediately give three AtroPen 0.5 mg IM injections in rapid succession. For mild symptoms, give one AtroPen 0.5 mg IM injection. If patient then develops severe symptoms, give two additional 0.5 mg IM injections in rapid succession 10 minutes after first injection.
Infants weighing less than 7 kg: For severe symptoms, immediately give three AtroPen 0.25 mg IM injections in rapid succession. For mild symptoms, give one AtroPen 0.25 mg IM injection. If patient then develops severe symptoms, give two additional 0.25 mg IM injections in rapid succession 10 minutes after first injection.
➤ **Preoperatively to diminish secretions and block cardiac vagal reflexes**
Adults: 0.5 to 1 mg IV (preferred), IM, or subcut 30 to 60 minutes before anesthesia. May repeat in 1 to 2 hours PRN. Maximum total dose, 3 mg.
➤ **Stress echocardiography (adjunct chronotropic agent)** ◆
Adults: 0.25 to 0.5 mg IV up to a total dose of 1 to 2 mg until 85% of target HR is achieved.

ADMINISTRATION
IV
▼ Give into a large vein or into IV tubing by rapid injection.
▼ Slow delivery may cause paradoxical bradycardia.
▼ **Incompatibilities:** None listed by manufacturer. Consult drug compatibility reference for more information.
Subcutaneous
• Document administration site.
IM
• Firmly jab autoinjector needle tip into mid-lateral thigh at 90-degree angle, through clothing as needed.
• Hold autoinjector in place for at least 10 seconds to allow time for complete administration.
• Make sure needle is visible after removing autoinjector. If needle didn't engage, repeat injection, jabbing more firmly.
• Massage injection site for several seconds after removing autoinjector.

• In patients who are young or very thin, pinch the skin on the thigh together before injection.

ACTION
Inhibits muscarinic actions of acetylcholine at parasympathetic neuroeffector junction, blocking vagal effects on SA and AV nodes, enhancing conduction through AV node and increasing HR.

Route	Onset	Peak	Duration
IV	Immediate	Unknown	Unknown
IM	Rapid	3–60 min	4 hr
Subcut	Unknown	Unknown	Unknown

Half-life: Adults, 2 to 4 hours; children older than age 2, 1.5 to 3.5 hours; children younger than age 2, 4 to 10 hours; older adults 3 to 17 hours.

ADVERSE REACTIONS
• Severity and frequency of adverse reactions are dose-related.
CNS: headache, restlessness, insomnia, dizziness, ataxia, disorientation, hallucinations, delirium, excitement, agitation, anxiety, amnesia, decreased deep tendon reflex, drowsiness, dysarthria, hyperreflexia, *seizure,* vertigo, confusion, fever, weakness. **CV:** *bradycardia,* palpitations, tachycardia, chest pain, hypotension, *prolonged QT interval, atrial and ventricular arrhythmias.* **EENT:** blurred vision, mydriasis, photophobia, cycloplegia, increased IOP, dry mouth. **GI:** constipation, nausea, vomiting, abdominal distention, abdominal pain, delayed gastric emptying, diminished bowel sounds. **GU:** urinary retention, urinary hesitancy or urgency, erectile dysfunction. **Hematologic:** leukocytosis, anemia, petechiae, increased Hb level. **Metabolic:** hyperglycemia, *hypoglycemia,* hyponatremia, *hypokalemia,* thirst, dehydration. **Musculoskeletal:** muscle twitching. **Respiratory:** *bradypnea,* dyspnea, *pulmonary edema.* **Skin:** rash, anhidrosis, hyperhidrosis, dermatitis, injection-site reaction, cyanosis. **Other:** hypersensitivity reaction, *anaphylaxis.*

INTERACTIONS
Drug-drug. *Anticholinergics, drugs with anticholinergic effects (amantadine, antiarrhythmics, antiparkinsonian drugs, meperidine, phenothiazines, TCAs):* May increase anticholinergic effects. Use together cautiously.

Potassium chloride, potassium citrate: May increase risk of mucosal lesions. Avoid use together.

EFFECTS ON LAB TEST RESULTS
• May increase BUN level.
• May decrease sodium and potassium levels.
• May increase or decrease glucose level.
• May increase or decrease Hb level.
• May increase RBC and WBC counts.

CONTRAINDICATIONS & CAUTIONS
• Contraindicated in patients hypersensitive to drug and in patients with hyperthermia.
• Drug may increase risk of acute angle-closure glaucoma, obstructive uropathy, obstructive disease of GI tract, and paralytic ileus, toxic megacolon, and intestinal atony.
• Use cautiously in patients with hyperthyroidism, CAD, HTN, HF, tachycardia, chronic lung disease, hiatal hernia with reflux esophagitis, prostatic hypertrophy, myasthenia gravis, or kidney or liver impairment and in older adults.
• Drug is ineffective for treatment of bradycardia in patients with heart transplants due to lack of vagal nerve innervation.
Dialyzable drug: No.
⚠ *Overdose S&S:* Delirium, seizures, coma, tachycardia, fever, mydriasis, decreased salivation and sweating, urine retention, HTN, vasodilation, hyperthermia.

PREGNANCY-LACTATION-REPRODUCTION
• Use during pregnancy only if clearly needed.
• Safe use during breastfeeding hasn't been established. Atropine has been reported in human milk. Use cautiously during breastfeeding.

NURSING CONSIDERATIONS
• Doses less than 0.5 mg in adults and less than 0.1 mg in children may increase risk of paradoxical bradycardia.
• Monitor pulse rate, BP, and mental status.
• IV administration requires cardiac monitoring.
🔔 *Alert:* Watch for tachycardia in patients with cardiac conditions because it may lead to ventricular fibrillation.
• Monitor fluid intake and urine output. Drug causes urinary retention and urinary hesitancy.
• Drug may increase respiratory tract mucous plug formation in a patient with chronic lung disease. Monitor closely.

Reactions in bold italics are *life-threatening*.

PATIENT TEACHING
• Instruct patient to report all adverse reactions and to immediately report urinary retention, abnormal heartbeat, dizziness, passing out, difficulty breathing, weakness, tremors, and abdominal edema.
• Teach patient signs and symptoms of insecticide poisoning (nausea, diarrhea, muscle spasms).
• Explain to patient how to use, store, and dispose of AtroPen.

axitinib
ax-i-TI-nib

Inlyta

Therapeutic class: Antineoplastics
Pharmacologic class: Kinase inhibitors

AVAILABLE FORMS
Tablets ⬤: 1 mg, 5 mg

INDICATIONS & DOSAGES
Adjust-a-dose (for all indications): Base adjustments on individual safety and tolerability. If patient tolerates drug for at least 2 consecutive weeks (6 weeks if given with pembrolizumab) with adverse reactions no greater than grade 2 CTCAE guidelines, is normotensive, and isn't receiving antihypertensives, may increase dosage to 7 mg b.i.d., then 10 mg b.i.d. See manufacturer's labeling for dosage adjustment for adverse reactions. For patients with Child-Pugh class B liver impairment, reduce axitinib starting dose by approximately half.
➤ **Advanced renal cell carcinoma (RCC) after failure of one prior systemic therapy**
Adults: 5 mg PO b.i.d.
➤ **First-line treatment of advanced RCC in combination with avelumab**
Adults: 5 mg PO b.i.d. in combination with avelumab 800-mg IV infusion every 2 weeks. Continue until disease progression or unacceptable toxicity occurs. Refer to manufacturer's instructions for avelumab prescribing information.
➤ **First-line treatment of advanced RCC in combination with pembrolizumab**
Adults: 5 mg PO b.i.d. in combination with pembrolizumab 200-mg IV infusion every 3 weeks or 400-mg IV infusion every 6 weeks.

Continue until disease progression or unacceptable toxicity occurs. Refer to manufacturer's instructions for pembrolizumab prescribing information.

ADMINISTRATION
PO
⚠ *Alert:* Hazardous drug; use safe handling and disposal precautions.
• Give drug without regard for food.
• Give tablets approximately 12 hours apart.
• Have patient swallow tablets whole with a glass of water; don't allow patient to crush or cut tablets.
• If a dose is missed or patient vomits, don't give an additional dose; give next prescribed dose at usual time.
• Store at 68° to 77° F (20° to 25° C).

ACTION
Inhibits receptor tyrosine kinase, which decreases cell proliferation, tumor growth, angiogenesis, and cancer progression.

Route	Onset	Peak	Duration
PO	Unknown	2.5–4.1 hr	Unknown

Half-life: 2.5 to 6.1 hours.

ADVERSE REACTIONS
CNS: asthenia, fatigue, headache, dizziness, dysgeusia, TIA. **CV:** *HF, thromboembolism, hemorrhage,* HTN, *DVT.* **EENT:** dysphonia, mucosal inflammation, stomatitis, epistaxis, tinnitus, retinal vein occlusion or thrombosis, glossodynia. **GI:** diarrhea, nausea, vomiting, constipation, mucositis, stomatitis, abdominal pain, dyspepsia, hemorrhoids, *GI perforation,* fistula formation, *rectal hemorrhage.* **GU:** hematuria, increased creatinine level, proteinuria. **Hematologic:** anemia, *lymphocytopenia, thrombocytopenia, polycythemia.* **Hepatic:** increased transaminase levels, bilirubinemia, increased ALP, *liver toxicity.* **Metabolic:** decreased appetite, decreased weight, hypothyroidism, hypernatremia, hyponatremia, *hyperkalemia,* dehydration, hypertriglyceridemia, hypercholesterolemia, decreased bicarbonate level, *hypocalcemia,* hyperglycemia, *hypoglycemia,* increased lipase and amylase levels, hypoalbuminemia, hypophosphatemia. **Musculoskeletal:** arthralgia, musculoskeletal pain, extremity pain, myalgia. **Respiratory:** cough, *hemoptysis,* dyspnea, *PE.* **Skin:** alopecia, hand-foot syndrome, rash, dry skin, pruritus, erythema.

INTERACTIONS

Drug-drug. *Moderate CYP3A4/5 inducers (bosentan, efavirenz, etravirine, modafinil, nafcillin), strong CYP3A4/5 inducers (carbamazepine, dexamethasone, phenobarbital, phenytoin, rifabutin, rifampin, rifapentine):* May reduce axitinib level. Avoid concurrent use.

Strong CYP3A4/5 inhibitors (atazanavir, clarithromycin, itraconazole, ketoconazole, nefazodone, nelfinavir, ritonavir, saquinavir, telithromycin, voriconazole): May increase axitinib level. Avoid concurrent use; if strong CYP3A4/5 inhibitor is necessary, reduce axitinib dosage.

Drug-herb. *St. John's wort:* May decrease axitinib plasma concentration. Discourage concurrent use.

Drug-food. *Grapefruit, grapefruit juice:* May increase axitinib plasma concentration. Discourage concurrent use.

EFFECTS ON LAB TEST RESULTS

• May increase potassium, amylase, lipase, ALP, ALT, AST, bilirubin, cholesterol, triglyceride, and creatinine levels.
• May decrease bicarbonate, calcium, albumin, and phosphate levels.
• May increase or decrease glucose, sodium, and TSH levels.
• May decrease Hb level and lymphocyte, WBC, and platelet counts.

CONTRAINDICATIONS & CAUTIONS

• Use isn't recommended in patients with recent GI bleeding or untreated brain metastases.
• Combination use with avelumab can cause severe and fatal CV events. Optimize management of CV risk factors (HTN, diabetes, dyslipidemia) before use.
• Drug may be associated with impaired wound healing.
• Use cautiously in patients with HTN; in those at risk for GI perforation or fistula formation, HF, thyroid dysfunction, or arterial or venous thromboembolic events; and in patients with Child-Pugh class B liver impairment or CrCl less than 15 mL/minute. Drug hasn't been studied in patients with Child-Pugh class C liver impairment.
• Cases of reversible posterior leukoencephalopathy syndrome (RPLS) have been reported.
• Safety and effectiveness in children haven't been established.

Dialyzable drug: Unknown.
⚠ **Overdose S&S:** Dizziness, HTN, seizures, possible fatal hemoptysis.

PREGNANCY-LACTATION-REPRODUCTION

• Drug can cause fetal harm. Advise patients of childbearing potential of fetal risk and warn to avoid becoming pregnant during therapy.
• Patients of childbearing potential and males with partners of childbearing potential should use effective contraception during therapy and for 1 week after final dose.
• It isn't known if drug appears in human milk. Patient should discontinue breastfeeding or discontinue drug during treatment and for 2 weeks after final dose.
• Drug may impair both female and male fertility.

NURSING CONSIDERATIONS

• Verify pregnancy status in patients of childbearing potential before starting drug.
• HTN should be well controlled before start of therapy. Monitor patient for increased BP; treat as indicated. If HTN persists despite antihypertensive use, decrease axitinib dosage, as ordered.
• Watch for hypotension if drug is withheld for any reason and patient continues antihypertensive use.
• Monitor patient for signs and symptoms of hematologic or neurologic disease, thromboembolic events, and GI disorders.
• Monitor patient for bleeding or hemorrhagic event. Temporarily interrupt treatment if bleeding occurs.
• Monitor for CV events and HF; obtain baseline and periodic evaluations of LVEF.
• Monitor use of all prescription drugs, OTC medications, grapefruit or grapefruit juice, and supplements.
• Obtain LFTs and kidney and thyroid function tests before and periodically during therapy. Consider more frequent monitoring of liver enzymes when therapy is combined with avelumab and pembrolizumab.
• Stop drug at least 2 days before elective surgery; resume at least 2 weeks after major surgery and adequate wound healing. Monitor wound healing carefully.
• Monitor patient for signs and symptoms of RPLS (headache, seizures, lethargy, confusion, blindness, and other visual disturbances)

---

*Reactions in bold italics are **life-threatening**.*

and other neurologic signs and symptoms. Discontinue drug if these occur.
• Monitor patient for proteinuria before and during therapy. For moderate or severe proteinuria, reduce dosage or withhold drug.

PATIENT TEACHING
• Advise patient of childbearing potential and male patient with partner of childbearing potential to use effective birth control during treatment and for 1 week after final dose.
• Instruct patient in safe drug administration.
• Advise patient to report all adverse reactions.
• Caution patient to tell prescriber of planned surgeries.
• Teach patient to consult prescriber before starting new drugs or supplements.
• Instruct patient to keep lab test appointments as requested by prescriber to monitor drug's safety and effectiveness.

azelastine hydrochloride
a-ZEL-as-teen

Astepro Allergy ◊

Therapeutic class: Antihistamines
Pharmacologic class: H_1-receptor antagonists

AVAILABLE FORMS
Intranasal: 0.1% (137 mcg/spray), 0.15% (205.5 mcg/spray) ◊
Ophthalmic solution: 0.05%

INDICATIONS & DOSAGES
➤ **Pruritus from allergic conjunctivitis**
Adults and children ages 3 and older: Instill 1 drop into affected eye b.i.d.
➤ **Perennial allergic rhinitis**
Adults and children ages 12 and older: Instill 2 sprays (0.15%) per nostril b.i.d.
Children ages 6 to 11: Instill 1 spray (0.1% or 0.15%) per nostril b.i.d.
Children ages 6 months to 5 years: Instill 1 spray (0.1%) per nostril b.i.d.
➤ **Seasonal allergic rhinitis**
Adults and children ages 12 and older: Instill 1 to 2 sprays (0.1% or 0.15%) per nostril b.i.d. or 2 sprays (0.15%) per nostril once daily.
Children ages 6 to 11: Instill 1 spray (0.15%) per nostril b.i.d.
Children ages 5 to 11: Instill 1 spray (0.1%) per nostril b.i.d.

➤ **Vasomotor rhinitis**
Adults and adolescents ages 12 and older: Instill 2 sprays (0.1%) per nostril b.i.d.

ADMINISTRATION
Ophthalmic
• Keep bottle tightly closed when not in use.
• Don't touch tip of dropper to any surface.
Intranasal
• Before initial use of nasal spray, prime the delivery system with 4 sprays (0.1%) or 6 sprays (0.15%), or until a fine mist appears.
• Have patient tilt head downward while spraying to help avoid bitter taste.
• If 3 or more days have elapsed since last use, reprime the delivery system with 2 sprays or until a fine mist appears.
• After each use, wipe spray tip with a clean tissue or cloth.
⚠ *Alert:* Be aware of different concentrations of nasal spray because some aren't indicated for use for all indications or in certain age-groups.

ACTION
Inhibits the release of histamine and other mediators from cells involved in the allergic response.

Route	Onset	Peak	Duration
Ophthalmic	3 min	Unknown	8 hr
Intranasal	Unknown	2–4 hr	Unknown

Half-life: 22 to 25 hours.

ADVERSE REACTIONS
CNS: anxiety, depression, dizziness, drowsiness, headache, fatigue, malaise, nervousness, sleep disorder, vertigo, dysesthesia, fever.
CV: flushing, HTN, tachycardia. **EENT:** transient eye burning or stinging, conjunctivitis, eye pain, temporary blurring, otitis media, epistaxis, nasal discomfort, nasal congestion, nasal mucosa ulcer, postnasal drip, rhinitis, pharyngitis, pharyngolaryngeal pain, sinusitis, dry mouth, sneezing, bitter taste.
GI: abdominal pain, constipation, diarrhea, nausea, vomiting, gastroenteritis, increased appetite. **GU:** hematuria, increased urinary frequency. **Metabolic:** weight gain. **Musculoskeletal:** myalgia. **Respiratory:** *asthma, bronchospasm,* dyspnea, cough, URI. **Skin:** pruritus, contact dermatitis. **Other:** flulike syndrome, cold symptoms.

♣Canada   ◊OTC   ◆Off-label use   ⊛Do not crush   *Liquid contains alcohol   ⬚Genetic

INTERACTIONS
Drug-drug. *CNS depressants:* May enhance CNS depressant effect of azelastine. Avoid combination.
Drug-lifestyle. *Alcohol use:* May increase CNS depressant effect of azelastine. Avoid use together.

EFFECTS ON LAB TEST RESULTS
None reported.

CONTRAINDICATIONS & CAUTIONS
• Contraindicated in patients hypersensitive to drug or its components.
Dialyzable drug: Unknown.

PREGNANCY-LACTATION-REPRODUCTION
• Use cautiously during pregnancy and only if potential benefit justifies fetal risk.
• It isn't known if drug appears in human milk. Use cautiously during breastfeeding.

NURSING CONSIDERATIONS
• Drug is for ophthalmic or intranasal use only. Don't inject or give orally.
• Don't use ophthalmic form for irritation caused by contact lenses.

PATIENT TEACHING
• Teach patient to take drug only as prescribed or directed by manufacturer's instructions.
• Instruct patient using ophthalmic form not to touch any surface, eyelid, or surrounding areas with tip of eye dropper.
• Advise patient not to wear contact lens if eye is red.
• Warn patient that soft contact lenses may absorb the preservative benzalkonium.
• Instruct patient using ophthalmic form who wears soft contact lenses and whose eyes aren't red to wait at least 10 minutes after instilling drug before inserting contact lenses.
• Tell patient using intranasal form to report all adverse reactions and to immediately report shortness of breath or severe nose irritation.
• Because drug may cause CNS depression, advise patient using intranasal form to avoid hazardous activities requiring complete mental alertness, such as driving and operating machinery.
• Advise patient and caregivers that different concentrations of nasal spray exist and may not be indicated for use in certain conditions or age-groups.

azelastine hydrochloride–fluticasone propionate
a-ZEL-as-teen/floo-TIK-a-sone

Dymista

Therapeutic class: Antihistamines–corticosteroids
Pharmacologic class: H_1-receptor antagonists–corticosteroids

AVAILABLE FORMS
Nasal spray: 137 mcg azelastine hydrochloride and 50 mcg fluticasone propionate/spray

INDICATIONS & DOSAGES
➤ **Symptoms of seasonal allergic rhinitis**
Adults and children ages 6 and older: 1 spray per nostril b.i.d.

ADMINISTRATION
Intranasal
• Shake gently before each use.
• Prime the spray before initial use; spray six times or until a fine mist appears. If the spray hasn't been used within the past 14 days, prime the spray again with 1 spray or until a fine mist appears.
• Store upright at room temperature with dust cap in place. Don't freeze or refrigerate.
• Protect from light.

ACTION
Azelastine inhibits release of histamine and other mediators from cells involved in the allergic response. Fluticasone may decrease inflammation by inhibiting mast cells, macrophages, and mediators such as leukotrienes.

Route	Onset	Peak	Duration
Intranasal	Rapid	0.5 hr (azelastine), 1 hr (fluticasone)	Unknown

Half-life: Azelastine, 25 hours; fluticasone, 7.8 hours.

ADVERSE REACTIONS
CNS: headache, fever, dysgeusia, pain.
EENT: epistaxis, nasal congestion, rhinitis, pharyngitis, oropharyngeal pain, otitis media, otitis externa. **GI:** diarrhea, nausea, vomiting, upper abdominal pain. **Respiratory:** cough, URI. **Skin:** urticaria. **Other:** viral infection.

INTERACTIONS

Drug-drug. *CNS depressants:* May increase risk of drowsiness. Use together cautiously.
CYP3A4 inhibitors (fluconazole, ketoconazole): May increase fluticasone plasma level. Use together cautiously.
Ritonavir: May increase fluticasone plasma level and risk of systemic corticosteroid effects, including Cushing syndrome and adrenal suppression. Avoid use together.
Drug-lifestyle. *Alcohol use:* May increase risk of somnolence and CNS impairment. Discourage use together.

EFFECTS ON LAB TEST RESULTS

None reported.

CONTRAINDICATIONS & CAUTIONS

• Contraindicated in patients hypersensitive to either drug or its components.
• Avoid use in patients with current nasal ulcers, nasal trauma, or nasal surgery until healing occurs.
• Use cautiously in patients with glaucoma, cataracts, ongoing infection, immunosuppression, or history of adrenal suppression.
• Safety and effectiveness in children younger than age 6 haven't been established.
Dialyzable drug: Unknown.

PREGNANCY-LACTATION-REPRODUCTION

• Use cautiously during pregnancy or breastfeeding and only if benefits outweigh risks to the fetus or infant.

NURSING CONSIDERATIONS

• Monitor patient for fungal, bacterial, or viral infections.
• Monitor for localized nasopharyngeal *Candida albicans* infection with prolonged use.
• Ensure that patient receives regular eye exams to screen for cataracts and glaucoma with long-term use.
• Monitor growth in children using the spray long-term because corticosteroids may slow growth rate.
• Monitor patient for signs and symptoms of adrenal insufficiency (tiredness, weakness, nausea, vomiting, hypotension).

PATIENT TEACHING

• Instruct patient to follow full package directions for use.

• Caution patient to avoid spraying into eyes and, if exposure occurs, to flush eyes with water for 10 minutes.
• Warn patient to watch for changes in vision, which can indicate serious eye problems, such as glaucoma or cataracts. Advise patient to have regular eye exams while taking drug.
• Tell patient to watch for nasal problems (nosebleeds, nasal septal perforation).
• Advise patient that drug can decrease the body's ability to heal or fight infection. Tell patient to report fever, aches or pains, chills, fatigue, or exposure to chickenpox or measles. Caution patient to avoid exposure to communicable diseases.
• Warn that drug can cause drowsiness. Instruct patient to avoid alcohol and other drugs that cause drowsiness while taking this drug.
• Advise patient to avoid driving and tasks that require alertness until drug's effects are known.
• Instruct patient to report pregnancy, plans to become pregnant, or breastfeeding.

azithromycin
ay-zi-thro-MY-sin

AzaSite, Zithromax

Therapeutic class: Antibiotics
Pharmacologic class: Macrolides

AVAILABLE FORMS

Injection: 500 mg
Ophthalmic solution: 1%
Powder for oral suspension: 100 mg/5 mL; 200 mg/5 mL; 1,000 mg/single-dose packet
Tablets: 250 mg, 500 mg, 600 mg

INDICATIONS & DOSAGES

➤ **Acute bacterial worsening of COPD caused by *Haemophilus influenzae*, *Moraxella catarrhalis*, or *Streptococcus pneumoniae*; uncomplicated skin and skin-structure infections caused by *Staphylococcus aureus*, *Streptococcus pyogenes*, or *Streptococcus agalactiae*; second-line therapy for pharyngitis or tonsillitis caused by *S. pyogenes***
Adults: Initially, 500 mg PO as a single dose on day 1, followed by 250 mg daily on days 2 through 5. Total cumulative dose, 1.5 g. Or, for worsening COPD, 500 mg PO daily for 3 days.

➤ **Community-acquired pneumonia caused by *Chlamydophila pneumoniae*, *H. influenzae*, *Mycoplasma pneumoniae*, *S. pneumoniae*, *Legionella pneumophila*, *M. catarrhalis*, or *S. aureus***

Adults: For mild infections, 500 mg PO as a single dose on day 1; then 250 mg PO daily on days 2 through 5. Total dose, 1.5 g. For more severe infections or those caused by *S. aureus*, 500 mg IV as a single daily dose for at least 2 days; then 500 mg PO as a single daily dose to complete a 7- to 10-day course of therapy. Switch from IV to oral therapy based on patient response.

➤ **Community-acquired pneumonia caused by *C. pneumoniae*, *H. influenzae*, *M. pneumoniae*, or *S. pneumoniae***

Children ages 6 months and older: 10 mg/kg oral suspension PO (maximum of 500 mg) as a single dose on day 1, followed by 5 mg/kg (maximum, 250 mg) daily on days 2 through 5.

➤ **Acute bacterial sinusitis caused by *H. influenzae*, *M. catarrhalis*, or *S. pneumoniae***

Adults: 500 mg PO daily for 3 days.
Children ages 6 months and older: 10 mg/kg oral suspension PO once daily for 3 days. Maximum daily dose, 500 mg.

➤ **Chancroid; nongonococcal urethritis or cervicitis caused by *Chlamydia trachomatis***

Adults: 1 g PO as a single dose.

➤ **To prevent disseminated MAC in patients with advanced HIV infection**

Adults: 1.2 g PO once weekly.

➤ **MAC in patients with advanced HIV infection**

Adults: 600 mg PO daily with ethambutol 15 mg/kg daily.

➤ **Urethritis and cervicitis caused by *Neisseria gonorrhoeae***

Adults: 2 g PO as a single dose.

➤ **Pelvic inflammatory disease caused by *C. trachomatis*, *N. gonorrhoeae*, or *Mycoplasma hominis* in patients who need initial IV therapy**

Adults and adolescents age 16 and older: 500 mg IV as a single daily dose for at least 2 days; then 250 mg PO daily to complete a 7-day course of therapy. Switch from IV to oral therapy based on patient response.

➤ **Otitis media**

Children older than age 6 months: 30 mg/kg oral suspension PO as a single dose (maximum dose, 1,500 mg); or 10 mg/kg PO once daily for 3 days (maximum daily dose, 500 mg);

or 10 mg/kg PO on day 1 (maximum dose, 500 mg), then 5 mg/kg once daily on days 2 to 5 (maximum daily dose, 250 mg).

➤ **Pharyngitis, tonsillitis**

Children ages 2 and older: 12 mg/kg oral suspension (maximum, 500 mg) PO daily for 5 days.

➤ **Bacterial conjunctivitis caused by coryneform group G, *H. influenzae*, *Staphylococcus aureus*, *Streptococcus mitis* group, and *S. pneumoniae***

Adults and children ages 1 and older: Instill 1 drop in affected eye(s) b.i.d., 8 to 12 hours apart for first 2 days; then instill 1 drop in affected eye(s) once daily for next 5 days.

➤ **Cat scratch disease (*Bartonella henselae* infection)** ◆

Adults and children weighing 45.5 kg or more: 500 mg PO on day 1, then 250 mg PO daily on days 2 to 5.
Children weighing less than 45.5 kg: 10 mg/kg on day 1, then 5 mg/kg PO daily on days 2 to 5.

➤ **Severe cholera** ◆

Adults: 1 g PO as a single dose.
Children: 20 mg/kg (maximum, 1 g) PO as a single dose.

➤ **COPD, prevention of exacerbations** ◆

Adults: 250 to 500 mg PO three times/week or 250 mg PO once daily.

➤ **Cystic fibrosis to improve lung function and reduce exacerbations** ◆

Adults and children ages 6 and older: 500 mg PO for patients weighing 40 kg or more or 250 mg PO for patients weighing less than 40 kg three times/week or 250 mg PO once daily. Screen patients before treatment; don't give to those who test positive for nontuberculous mycobacterial infection.

➤ **Uncomplicated typhoid and parathyphoid fever** ◆

Adults: 1g PO daily or 1g PO on day 1, followed by 500 mg PO once daily for 5 to 7 days.

ADMINISTRATION
PO

• Obtain specimen for culture and sensitivity tests before giving first dose. Begin therapy while awaiting results.

• Reconstitute suspension packet with 2 oz (60 mL) of water. After patient has taken dose, rinse glass with additional 2 oz of water and have patient drink it to ensure entire dose has been taken. Packets aren't for children.

• Reconstitute oral suspension by adding 9 mL of water to the 300-mg and 600-mg bottles,

---

*Reactions in bold italics are **life-threatening**.*

12 mL of water to the 900-mg bottle, and 15 mL to the 1,200-mg bottle. Shake well after each use. Store at 41° to 86° F (5° to 30° C) for up to 10 days.

IV
▼ Reconstitute drug in 500-mg vial with 4.8 mL of sterile water for injection to yield 100 mg/mL.

▼ Shake well until all drug is dissolved.

▼ Further dilute in 250- or 500-mL NSS solution, half-NSS, D₅W, or lactated Ringer solution to yield a final concentration of 1 or 2 mg/mL, respectively.

▼ Infuse a 250-mL infusion (2-mg/mL dose) over 1 hour or 500-mL infusion (1-mg/mL dose) over 3 hours. Never give it as a bolus or IM injection.

▼ Reconstituted and diluted solutions are stable for 24 hours when stored below 86° F (30° C). Diluted solution is stable for 7 days when refrigerated at 41° F (5° C).

▼ **Incompatibilities:** Amikacin sulfate, aztreonam, cefotaxime, ceftazidime, ceftriaxone sodium, cefuroxime, ciprofloxacin, clindamycin phosphate, famotidine, fentanyl citrate, furosemide, gentamicin sulfate, imipenem–cilastatin sodium, ketorolac tromethamine, levofloxacin, morphine sulfate, piperacillin–tazobactam sodium, potassium chloride, tobramycin sulfate. Consult drug compatibility reference for additional information.

Ophthalmic
• Avoid contaminating applicator tip. Don't allow it to touch eye, fingers, or other surfaces.
• Invert closed bottle and shake once before each use. Remove cap with bottle still in the inverted position. Tilt head back, and with bottle inverted, gently squeeze bottle to instill 1 drop into affected eye(s).
• Store unopened bottle under refrigeration at 36° to 46° F (2° to 8° C). Once bottle has been opened, store at 36° to 77° F (2° to 25° C) for up to 14 days. Discard after 14 days.

ACTION

Binds to the 50S subunit of bacterial ribosomes, blocking protein synthesis; bacteriostatic or bactericidal, depending on concentration.

Route	Onset	Peak	Duration
PO	Unknown	2–5 hr	Unknown
IV, oph- thalmic	Unknown	Unknown	Unknown

Half-life: About 3 days.

ADVERSE REACTIONS

CNS: fatigue, headache, somnolence, dizziness, dysgeusia, fever. **CV:** chest pain, palpitations, edema. **EENT:** eye irritation (ophthalmic), oral candidiasis. **GI:** abdominal pain, anorexia, diarrhea, constipation, nausea, vomiting, stomatitis, dyspepsia, enteritis, gastritis, flatulence, melena. **GU:** candidiasis, kidney inflammation, vaginitis. **Hepatic:** cholestatic jaundice. **Metabolic:** increased LDH level. **Respiratory:** *bronchospasm,* cough, pleural effusion. **Skin:** photosensitivity reactions, rash, injection-site reaction, diaphoresis, eczema, dermatitis, pruritus. **Other:** *angioedema,* fungal infection.

INTERACTIONS

Drug-drug. *Antacids containing aluminum and magnesium:* May lower peak azithromycin level (immediate-release form). Separate doses by at least 2 hours.
Antiarrhythmics (amiodarone, quinidine): May increase risk of life-threatening arrhythmias, including torsades de pointes. Monitor ECG rhythm carefully.
Carbamazepine, phenytoin: May increase levels of these drugs. Use together cautiously.
Cyclosporine: May elevate cyclosporine concentrations, with increased risk of kidney toxicity and neurotoxicity. Monitor cyclosporine levels and kidney function.
Digoxin: May increase digoxin level. Monitor closely.
Drugs that prolong QT interval (fluoroquinolones, lithium, methadone, paliperidone, perflutren, pimozide): May prolong QT interval. Use together with caution and monitor patient. Avoid use with pimozide.
HMG-CoA reductase inhibitors (atorvastatin, lovastatin): May increase HMG-CoA reductase inhibitor levels, resulting in severe myopathy or rhabdomyolysis. Consider alternative therapy.
Nelfinavir: May increase azithromycin level. Monitor for liver enzyme abnormalities and hearing impairment.
Warfarin: May increase INR. Carefully monitor PT and INR.
Drug-lifestyle. *Sun exposure:* May cause photosensitivity reactions. Advise patient to avoid excessive sunlight exposure.

EFFECTS ON LAB TEST RESULTS
• May increase ALT, AST, GGT, glucose, potassium, BUN, creatinine, LDH, CK, and bilirubin levels.
• May decrease platelet and WBC counts.
• May decrease Hb level and hematocrit.

CONTRAINDICATIONS & CAUTIONS
• Contraindicated in patients hypersensitive to azithromycin, erythromycin, or other macrolide or ketolide antibiotics and in those with history of cholestatic jaundice or liver dysfunction from prior use of azithromycin.
• Serious cases of allergic reactions, including angioedema, anaphylaxis, SJS, TEN, and DRESS syndrome, have been reported, some with fatalities. Prolonged observation and symptomatic treatment may be necessary.
• Infantile hypertrophic pyloric stenosis has been reported after use of azithromycin in neonates (treatment up to 42 days of life).
• Use cautiously in patients with impaired liver function or myasthenia gravis.
◔ Alert: Use cautiously in patients at increased risk for torsades de pointes and fatal arrhythmias, including those with known prolonged QT interval, history of torsades de pointes, congenital long QT syndrome, bradyarrhythmias, decompensated HF, uncorrected hypokalemia or hypomagnesemia, clinically significant bradycardia, or concomitant use of drugs known to prolong the QT interval or class IA (procainamide, quinidine) or class III (amiodarone, dofetilide, sotalol) antiarrhythmics.
◔ Alert: Older adults may be at increased risk for drug-associated QT-interval effects.
• Drug may cause CDAD, ranging in severity from mild diarrhea to fatal colitis, which may occur more than 2 months after administration. If CDAD is suspected or confirmed, drug may need to be discontinued and appropriate treatment begun.
• Prolonged use of ophthalmic solution may result in overgrowth of nonsusceptible organisms, including fungi. If superinfection occurs, discontinue drug and institute alternative therapy.
Dialyzable drug: Unknown.

PREGNANCY-LACTATION-REPRODUCTION
• There are no adequate and well-controlled studies during pregnancy. Use during pregnancy only if clearly needed.
• Drug appears in human milk. Use cautiously during breastfeeding.

NURSING CONSIDERATIONS
• Monitor patient for superinfection. Drug may cause overgrowth of nonsusceptible bacteria or fungi.
• Monitor patient for CDAD, which may range in severity from mild diarrhea to fatal colitis.
◔ Alert: Consider full risk profile when choosing appropriate antibiotic therapy. Alternative macrolide or fluoroquinolone class drugs also have the potential to cause QT-interval prolongation and other significant adverse effects.
• Monitor patient for allergic and skin reactions. Discontinue drug if reactions occur. Be aware that allergic symptoms may recur when symptomatic therapy is discontinued; patient may require prolonged monitoring and treatment.
• Monitor patient for jaundice, liver toxicity, and hepatitis. Immediately discontinue drug if signs and symptoms (yellowing of skin or sclera, abdominal pain, nausea, vomiting, dark urine) occur.
• Exacerbation and new onset of myasthenia gravis have occurred with azithromycin use. Monitor patient for neurologic changes.

PATIENT TEACHING
• Tell patient to take drug as prescribed, even after feeling better.
• Advise patient to avoid excessive sunlight and to wear protective clothing and use sunscreen when outside.
• Instruct patient to promptly report adverse reactions.
• Instruct parents and caregivers to contact prescriber if vomiting or irritability with feeding occurs during or after azithromycin use in neonates (treatment up to 42 days of life).
◔ Alert: Warn patient to seek immediate medical care for irregular heartbeat, shortness of breath, dizziness, or fainting.
• Instruct patient to thoroughly wash hands before instilling ophthalmic solution.
• Teach about proper drug administration and handling.
• Inform patient that tablets and suspension can be taken with or without food. Food may reduce GI upset.
• Advise patient to avoid contact lens use when diagnosed with bacterial conjunctivitis.

Reactions in bold italics are *life-threatening*.

aztreonam
AZ-tree-oh-nam

Azactam, Cayston

Therapeutic class: Antibiotics
Pharmacologic class: Monobactams

AVAILABLE FORMS
Inhalation (Cayston): 75-mg ampule
Injection: 1-g, 2-g vials

INDICATIONS & DOSAGES
➤ **UTI; septicemia; infections of lower respiratory tract, skin, and skin structures; intra-abdominal infections, surgical infections, and gynecologic infections caused by susceptible *Escherichia coli*, *Klebsiella pneumoniae*, *Proteus mirabilis*, *Pseudomonas aeruginosa*, *Enterobacter* species, *Klebsiella oxytoca*, *Citrobacter* species, and *Serratia marcescens;* respiratory infections caused by *Haemophilus influenzae***
Adults: 500 mg, 1 g, or 2 g IV or IM every 8 to 12 hours. For severe systemic or life-threatening infections, 2 g every 6 to 8 hours. Maximum dose, 8 g daily.
Children ages 9 months and older: 30 mg/kg IV every 6 to 8 hours. Maximum dose, 120 mg/kg/day.
Adjust-a-dose: For adults with CrCl of 10 to 30 mL/minute/1.73 m², 1 to 2 g; then 50% of usual dose at usual interval. If CrCl is less than 10 mL/minute/1.73 m², 500 mg to 2 g; then 25% of usual dose at usual interval. For serious infections, add ⅛ of initial dose to maintenance doses after each hemodialysis session.
➤ **To improve respiratory symptoms in patients with *P. aeruginosa* infection who have cystic fibrosis (Cayston)**
Adults and children ages 7 and older: 75 mg inhalation t.i.d. at least 4 hours apart for 28 days, followed by 28 days off.

ADMINISTRATION
Inhalational
• Patient should use bronchodilator before Cayston administration.
• Give short-acting bronchodilators 15 minutes to 4 hours before each dose of aztreonam or long-acting bronchodilators 30 minutes to 12 hours before each dose.

• Treatment order for patients on multiple therapies is bronchodilator, mucolytics, then aztreonam.
• Don't reconstitute until ready to give dose.
• Add one ampule of diluent to one amber glass vial of aztreonam. Replace rubber stopper on vial and gently swirl until contents have completely dissolved. Administer immediately.
• Don't use diluent or reconstituted drug if it's cloudy or if particles are in the solution.
• Use only Altera Nebulizer System to administer drug.
• Never mix with other drugs in nebulizer.
• Administration usually takes 2 to 3 minutes.

IV
▼ Obtain specimen for culture and sensitivity tests before giving first dose. Begin therapy while awaiting results.
▼ For direct injection, reconstitute with 6 to 10 mL of sterile water for injection and immediately shake vial vigorously. Constituted solutions aren't for multiple-dose use. Discard unused solution.
▼ To give a bolus, inject drug over 3 to 5 minutes directly into IV tubing.
▼ For infusion, reconstitute with a compatible IV solution to yield 20 mg/mL or less.
▼ Give infusions over 20 minutes to 1 hour.
▼ **Incompatibilities:** Acyclovir, amphotericin B, ampicillin sodium, azithromycin, chlorpromazine, daunorubicin hydrochloride, ganciclovir, lorazepam, metronidazole, mitomycin, mitoxantrone, nafcillin, prochlorperazine, streptozocin, vancomycin. Consult drug compatibility reference for additional information.

IM
• To prepare IM injection, add at least 3 mL of one of the following solutions per gram of aztreonam: sterile water for injection, bacteriostatic water for injection, NSS, or bacteriostatic NSS.
• Give IM injections deep into a large muscle, such as upper outer quadrant of gluteus maximus or side of thigh.
• Give doses larger than 1 g by IV route.
⊙ *Alert:* Don't give IM injection to children.
• Pain and swelling may occur at injection site.

ACTION
Inhibits bacterial cell-wall synthesis, ultimately causing cell-wall destruction; bactericidal.

Route	Onset	Peak	Duration
IV	Unknown	Immediate	Unknown
IM	Unknown	<1 hr	Unknown
Inhalation	Unknown	1 hr	Unknown

Half-life: 1.5 to 2.1 hours.

ADVERSE REACTIONS

CNS: fever. **CV:** phlebitis, thrombophlebitis, chest discomfort (inhalation). **EENT:** (inhalation) nasal congestion, sore throat. **GI:** diarrhea, abdominal pain, nausea, vomiting. **GU:** increased creatinine level. **Respiratory:** (inhalation) bronchospasm, wheezing, cough. **Skin:** discomfort and swelling at IM injection site, rash. **Other:** hypersensitivity reactions.

INTERACTIONS

Drug-drug. *Aminoglycosides:* May have synergistic kidney-toxic effects. Monitor kidney function.
Cefoxitin, imipenem: May have antagonistic effect. Avoid use together.

EFFECTS ON LAB TEST RESULTS

- May increase ALT, AST, BUN, creatinine, and LDH levels.
- May decrease Hb level and neutrophil and RBC counts.
- May increase or decrease platelet and WBC counts.
- May prolong PT and PTT and increase INR.
- May cause false-positive Coombs test result.
- May alter urine glucose determinations using cupric sulfate (Clinitest or Benedict reagent).

CONTRAINDICATIONS & CAUTIONS

- Contraindicated in patients hypersensitive to drug or its components.
- **Alert:** Use cautiously in patients with hypersensitivity to other beta-lactam antibiotics (penicillins, cephalosporins, carbapenems).
- Use cautiously in older adults and in patients with impaired kidney or liver function. Dosage adjustment may be needed. Monitor kidney function test results.
- Drug may cause CDAD, ranging in severity from mild diarrhea to fatal colitis and possibly

occurring up to 2 months after administration. For suspected or confirmed CDAD, drug may need to be discontinued and appropriate treatment begun.

- Rare cases of TEN have been reported in patients undergoing bone marrow transplant with multiple risk factors, including sepsis, radiation therapy, and concomitantly administered drugs associated with TEN.

Dialyzable drug: Yes.

PREGNANCY-LACTATION-REPRODUCTION

- Drug crosses the placental barrier. There are no adequate and well-controlled studies during pregnancy. Use during pregnancy only if clearly needed.
- Drug appears in human milk. Patient should temporarily discontinue breastfeeding.

NURSING CONSIDERATIONS

- Observe patient for signs and symptoms of superinfection.
- **Alert:** Because drug is ineffective against gram-positive and anaerobic organisms, combine it with other antibiotics for immediate treatment of life-threatening illnesses.
- Monitor for hypersensitivity reactions
- Antibiotics may promote overgrowth of nonsusceptible organisms. Monitor patient for signs of superinfection.
- In patients using inhalation, consider monitoring FEV_1 at baseline to determine if posttreatment FEV_1 decreases are due to a pulmonary exacerbation.

PATIENT TEACHING

- Warn patient receiving IM drug that pain and swelling may occur at injection site.
- Tell patient to report discomfort at IV insertion site.
- Instruct patient to report adverse reactions and signs and symptoms of superinfection promptly.
- Teach patient or caregiver in proper administration of drug by nebulizer.
- Advise patient or caregiver to use bronchodilator before using Cayston.

Reactions in bold italics are *life-threatening*.

baclofen
BAK-loe-fen

Fleqsuvy, Gablofen, Lioresal
Intrathecal, Lyvispah, Ozobax

Therapeutic class: Skeletal muscle relaxants
Pharmacologic class: Gamma-aminobutyric
acid derivatives

AVAILABLE FORMS
Intrathecal injection: 50 mcg/mL,
500 mcg/mL, 1,000 mcg/mL, 2,000 mcg/mL
Oral granules: 5-mg, 10-mg, 20-mg packets
Oral solution: 5 mg/5 mL
Oral suspension: 25 mg/5 mL
Tablets: 5 mg, 10 mg, 20 mg

INDICATIONS & DOSAGES
Adjust-a-dose (for all indications): For patients
with impaired kidney function, decrease oral
and intrathecal doses.
➤ **Spasticity in MS; spinal cord injury**
Adults and children ages 12 and older: Initially, 5 mg PO t.i.d. for 3 days; then 10 mg
t.i.d. for 3 days, 15 mg t.i.d. for 3 days, 20 mg
t.i.d. for 3 days. Increase daily dosage, based
on response, to maximum of 80 mg (given as
20 mg q.i.d.).
Adjust-a-dose: For older adults and patients
with psychiatric or brain disorders, increase
dose gradually.
➤ **To manage severe spasticity in patients
who don't respond to or can't tolerate oral
baclofen therapy**
Adults: For screening phase, after test dose
to check responsiveness, give drug via implantable infusion pump. Give test dose of
1 mL of 50 mcg/mL dilution into intrathecal space by barbotage over 1 minute or
longer. Significantly decreased severity or frequency of muscle spasm or reduced muscle
tone should appear within 4 to 8 hours. If response is inadequate, give second test dose of
75 mcg/1.5 mL 24 hours after first. If response is still inadequate, give final test dose
of 100 mcg/2 mL after 24 hours. Patients unresponsive to the 100-mcg dose shouldn't be
considered candidates for implantable pump.
Children ages 4 and older: Initial test dose is
the same as that for adults (50 mcg); for very
small children, initial dose is 25 mcg.
For maintenance therapy: Adjust first dose
based on screening dose that elicited an

adequate response. Double this effective dose
and give over 24 hours. However, if screening
dose effectiveness was maintained for 8 hours
or longer, don't double dose. After first
24 hours, increase dose slowly as needed
and tolerated by 10% to 30% increments at
24-hour intervals in spasticity of spinal cord
origin. In children with spasticity of spinal
cord origin and adults and children with spasticity of cerebral origin, increase by 5% to
15% increments at 24-hour intervals. During prolonged maintenance therapy, increase
daily dose by 10% to 40% in spasticity of
spinal cord origin or increase daily dose by
5% to 20% in spasticity of cerebral origin,
if needed. If patient experiences adverse effects, decrease dose by 10% to 20%. Maintenance dosages range from 12 to 2,003 mcg
daily based on diagnosis, but experience with
dosages of more than 1,000 mcg daily is limited. Most patients need 300 to 800 mcg daily
for spasticity of spinal cord origin and 90
to 703 mcg daily for spasticity of cerebral
origin.

ADMINISTRATION
PO
• Give drug with meals or milk to prevent GI
distress.
• May give granules without water by emptying packet into the mouth and allowing to
dissolve. Or, mix with 15 mL of liquid or soft
food (applesauce, yogurt, pudding) and give
within 2 hours. If giving multiple packets,
mix each packet with a separate volume of
liquid or soft food.
• May give granules through an 8F or larger
feeding tube after mixing well with 15 mL
of liquid; flush tube before and after giving.
Give within 2 hours of mixing suspension and
remix if suspension is left standing for more
than 15 minutes.
• Shake oral suspensions well.
• Discard unused oral solution or suspension
2 months after first opening bottle.
• Use calibrated measuring device to deliver
prescribed dose of solution or suspension.
Intrathecal
Boxed Warning Don't discontinue abruptly.
This can result in high fever, altered mental
status, exaggerated rebound spasticity, and
muscle rigidity, which in rare cases, has led to
rhabdomyolysis, multiple organ-system failure, and death. Carefully program and monitor the infusion system. ∎

• Don't give intrathecal injection by IV, IM, subcut, or epidural route.
• Maintenance infusions that require dilution must be diluted with sterile preservative-free sodium chloride for injection.
• If patient suddenly requires a large intrathecal dose increase, check for catheter complications (kinking, dislodgment).
• With long-term intrathecal use, about 5% of patients may develop tolerance to drug. In some cases, this may be treated by hospitalizing patient and slowly withdrawing drug over 2- to 4-week period. After "drug holiday," drug may be restarted at initial continuous infusion dose.

ACTION
Hyperpolarizes fibers to reduce impulse transmission. Appears to reduce transmission of impulses from spinal cord to skeletal muscle, thus decreasing the frequency and amplitude of muscle spasms in patients with spinal cord lesions.

Route	Onset	Peak	Duration
PO	Unknown	30 min–4 hr	Unknown
Intrathecal	30 min–1 hr	4 hr	4–8 hr

Half-life: Oral, children with cerebral palsy, 4.5 hours; adults, 2.75 to 5.7 hours. Intrathecal, 1.5 hours over first 4 hours.

ADVERSE REACTIONS
CNS: agitation, drowsiness, somnolence, dizziness, headache, weakness, fatigue, hypotonia, tremor, confusion, insomnia, *seizures (with intrathecal use)*, paresthesia, asthenia, pain, speech disorder, depression, *coma.* **CV:** hypotension, peripheral edema. **EENT:** amblyopia, nasal congestion, dry mouth, excessive salivation. **GI:** nausea, constipation, diarrhea, vomiting. **GU:** urinary frequency, urine retention, erectile dysfunction, incontinence. **Metabolic:** hyperglycemia, weight gain. **Musculoskeletal:** muscle rigidity or spasticity, muscle weakness, back pain. **Respiratory:** dyspnea, hypoventilation, pneumonia. **Skin:** rash, pruritus, urticaria, diaphoresis. **Other:** chills, accidental injury, *death (with intrathecal use).*

INTERACTIONS
Drug-drug. *CNS depressants:* May increase CNS depression. Avoid use together.
Opioid class warning: May cause slow or difficult breathing, sedation, and death. Avoid use together. If use together is necessary, limit dosage and duration of each drug to minimum necessary for desired effect.
Drug-lifestyle. *Alcohol use:* May increase CNS depression. Discourage use together.

EFFECTS ON LAB TEST RESULTS
• May increase ALP, AST, and glucose levels.
• May increase urine and serum albumin level.

CONTRAINDICATIONS & CAUTIONS
• Contraindicated in patients hypersensitive to drug.
• Use cautiously in patients with impaired kidney function, respiratory disease, or seizure disorder or when spasticity is used to maintain motor function.
• Use cautiously in patients with psychotic disorders, schizophrenia, confusional states, or autonomic dysreflexia. Drug may exacerbate these conditions.
• Use cautiously in patients who have had a stroke; drug is poorly tolerated and not significantly beneficial.
⚡ *Alert:* Oral drug isn't indicated for treatment of muscle spasm caused by rheumatic disorders, cerebral palsy, Parkinson disease, or stroke because drug's effectiveness for these indications hasn't been established.
• Safety and effectiveness in children younger than age 4 (intrathecal use) and age 12 (oral use) haven't been established.
Dialyzable drug: Yes.
⚠ *Overdose S&S:* Coma, dizziness, lightheadedness, diminished reflexes, vomiting, hypotonia, increased salivation, drowsiness, vision changes, respiratory depression, seizures.

PREGNANCY-LACTATION-REPRODUCTION
• Use during pregnancy only when potential benefits justify fetal risk.
• Drug may increase risk of late-onset neonatal withdrawal symptoms.
• Oral drug appears in human milk. It isn't known if drug appears in human milk after intrathecal administration. Patient should avoid breastfeeding during therapy unless potential benefit justifies risk to infant. Withdrawal symptoms can occur in infant when breastfeeding ceases.

NURSING CONSIDERATIONS
• Life-threatening CNS depression, CV collapse, and respiratory failure may occur with

intrathecal use. Have trained staff and resuscitation equipment available during screening, dosage titration, and pump refill.

• Avoid contamination of sterile surfaces through contact with nonsterile exterior of Gablofen prefilled syringe while refilling implantable intrathecal pumps. Use of prefilled syringe in aseptic setting (such as an operating room) to fill sterile intrathecal pumps before implantation in patients isn't recommended unless external surface of syringe is treated to ensure sterility.

• Reservoir refilling must be performed by fully trained and qualified personnel following directions provided by the pump manufacturer.

♦ **Alert:** Use extreme caution when filling an FDA-approved implantable pump equipped with an injection port that allows direct access to the intrathecal catheter. Direct injection into the catheter through the catheter access port may cause a life-threatening overdose.
Boxed Warning Consult the infusion system's technical manual for postimplant information. ∎

• Watch for sensitivity reactions (fever, skin eruptions, respiratory distress).

• Expect an increased risk of seizures in a patient with seizure disorder.

• Monitor patient's level of relief, which determines ability to reduce dosage (and drowsiness).

• Some degree of muscle tone and spasticity may be necessary to sustain upright posture and balance with movement or to obtain optimal function, help support circulatory function, and prevent formation of DVT.

• When switching to intrathecal baclofen, attempt to discontinue concomitant oral antispasmodics to avoid overdose or increased adverse effects. Reduce oral antispasmodic dosage slowly while monitoring patient closely.
Boxed Warning Don't withdraw intrathecal drug abruptly after long-term use unless severe adverse reactions demand it; doing so may precipitate seizures, high fever, hallucinations, and rebound spasticity. ∎

PATIENT TEACHING
Boxed Warning Advise patient and caregivers, especially patients with spinal cord injuries at T6 or above, communication difficulties, or history of withdrawal symptoms from oral or intrathecal baclofen, of risks

associated with abrupt discontinuation of intrathecal form. Tell them to keep scheduled refill visits and teach them the signs and symptoms of baclofen withdrawal. ∎

• Teach about proper oral drug administration and handling.

• *Opioid class warning:* Caution patient or caregiver of patient taking an opioid with a benzodiazepine, CNS depressant, or alcohol to seek immediate medical attention for dizziness, light-headedness, extreme sleepiness, slowed or difficult breathing, or unresponsiveness.

• Tell patient to avoid activities that require alertness until CNS effects of drug are known. Drowsiness usually is transient.

• Caution patient to avoid alcohol and OTC antihistamines while taking drug.

• Advise patient to follow prescriber's orders regarding rest and physical therapy.

• Instruct patient and caregivers about the signs and symptoms of overdose and what to do if an overdose occurs.

• Teach patient and caregivers proper home care of pump and insertion site.

baloxavir marboxil
bal-OX-a-vir mar-BOX-il

Xofluza

Therapeutic class: Antivirals
Pharmacologic class: Endonuclease inhibitors

AVAILABLE FORMS
Oral suspension (granules): 40 mg/20 mL
Tablets: 40 mg, 80 mg

INDICATIONS & DOSAGES
➤ **Acute, uncomplicated influenza in patients who have been symptomatic for no more than 48 hours who are otherwise healthy or at high risk for developing influenza-related complications; postexposure influenza prophylaxis**
Adults and children ages 5 and older weighing 80 kg or more: 80 mg PO as a single dose.
Adults and children ages 5 and older weighing 20 to 80 kg: 40 mg PO as a single dose.
Children ages 5 and older weighing less than 20 kg: 2 mg/kg oral suspension PO as a single dose.

ADMINISTRATION
PO
• Give drug with or without food. Avoid giving with dairy products and calcium-fortified beverages.
• Give drug as soon as possible within 48 hours of symptom onset or after contact with an individual with influenza.
• Oral suspension may be used for oral or enteral administration.
• Oral suspension contains no preservative and must be given within 10 hours after constitution.
• Prepare oral suspension by gently tapping bottom of the bottle to loosen granules. Add 20 mL of drinking water or sterile water to achieve a final concentration of 2 mg/mL. Gently swirl to ensure that granules are evenly suspended. Don't shake.
• Write the expiration time and date on the bottle label in the space provided.
• Use measuring device (oral syringe, measuring cup) to deliver suspension dose.
• For enteral administration (such as feeding tube), draw up suspension with enteral syringe. Flush with 1 mL of water before and after enteral administration.
• Store drug in original blister card or bottle at 68° to 77° F (20° to 25° C).

ACTION
Inhibits the activity of polymerase acidic protein to halt viral gene transcription.

Route	Onset	Peak	Duration
PO	Unknown	4 hr	Unknown

Half-life: 79.1 hours.

ADVERSE REACTIONS
CNS: headache. **EENT:** sinusitis. **GI:** diarrhea, nausea, vomiting. **Respiratory:** bronchitis.

INTERACTIONS
Drug-drug. *Live attenuated influenza vaccine:* May decrease effectiveness of the vaccine. Avoid use together.
Polyvalent cation–containing antacids, laxatives, or oral supplements (calcium, iron, magnesium, selenium, zinc): May decrease baloxavir level and effectiveness. Avoid use together.
Drug-food. *Calcium-fortified beverages, dairy products, milk:* May decrease baloxavir concentration and effectiveness. Avoid use together.

EFFECTS ON LAB TEST RESULTS
None reported.

CONTRAINDICATIONS & CAUTIONS
• Contraindicated in patients hypersensitive to drug or its components.
• Serious bacterial infections may begin with influenza-like symptoms or may coexist with or occur as a complication of influenza.
• Drug isn't indicated for children younger than age 5 due to increased incidence of treatment-emergent resistance.
Dialyzable drug: Unlikely.

PREGNANCY-LACTATION-REPRODUCTION
• No data exist on use of drug during pregnancy or on developmental risk to a fetus. Due to lack of data, the CDC doesn't recommend use of drug during pregnancy.
• Pregnancy may increase risk of severe complications from influenza, including maternal death, stillbirth, birth defects, preterm delivery, and low-birth-weight and small-for-gestational-age infants.
• It isn't known if drug appears in human milk. Consider the benefits of breastfeeding and the potential adverse effects on the infant before using drug.

NURSING CONSIDERATIONS
• Monitor for secondary bacterial infection, which may begin with influenza-like symptoms or coexist with or occur as a complication of influenza. Treat appropriately.
• Monitor for hypersensitivity reactions (anaphylaxis, erythema multiforme).

PATIENT TEACHING
• Instruct patient that drug should be taken as soon as possible within 48 hours of onset of symptoms or after contact with an individual with influenza.
• Counsel patient on safe drug administration.
• Inform patient that a pharmacist will mix oral suspension before it's dispensed. Instruct patient to take drug before expiration time and date written on bottle label. Caution patient not to take suspension if the expiration time and date have passed.
• Alert patient that the total prescribed dose of oral suspension may require two bottles.
• Tell patient to report all adverse reactions.
• Advise patient to consider postponing receiving live attenuated influenza vaccine while taking drug.

Reactions in bold italics are *life-threatening*.

beclomethasone dipropionate (inhalation)

be-kloe-METH-a-sone

QVAR RediHaler

Therapeutic class: Antiasthmatics
Pharmacologic class: Corticosteroids

AVAILABLE FORMS

Oral inhalation aerosol: 40 mcg/metered spray, 80 mcg/metered spray

INDICATIONS & DOSAGES

➤ Chronic asthma

Adults and children ages 12 and older: Starting dose, 40 to 80 mcg b.i.d. when patient previously used bronchodilators alone, or 40 to 320 mcg b.i.d. when patient previously used inhaled corticosteroids. If patient doesn't respond adequately to initial dosage after 2 weeks, increasing dosage may provide additional asthma control. Maximum, 320 mcg b.i.d.

Children ages 4 to 11: 40 mcg b.i.d. May increase to 80 mcg b.i.d. after 2 weeks if needed. Maximum, 80 mcg b.i.d.

ADMINISTRATION

Inhalational

• No need to prime or shake RediHaler.
• Close the white cap to prepare the inhaler with medicine before each inhalation.
• Instruct patient to hold breath for 5 to 10 seconds to enhance drug action.
• Have patient rinse mouth with water without swallowing after use.
• Space doses 12 hours apart.
• Don't shake inhaler with cap open to avoid possible actuation.
• Don't wash or put any part of the inhaler in water; gently wipe mouthpiece with a clean dry cloth or tissue as needed.
• Don't use with a spacer or volume holding chamber.
• Discard the inhaler when the dose counter displays "0."
• Store drug at room temperature.

ACTION

May decrease inflammation by decreasing the number and activity of inflammatory cells, inhibiting bronchoconstrictor mechanisms, producing direct smooth-muscle relaxation, and decreasing airway hyperresponsiveness.

Route	Onset	Peak	Duration
Inhalation	1–4 wk	0.5 hr	Unknown

Half-life: 4 hours.

ADVERSE REACTIONS

CNS: headache, pain, fever. **EENT:** ear infection, nasopharyngitis, pharyngitis, allergic rhinitis, sinusitis, oral candidiasis, oropharyngeal pain, dry mouth. **GI:** nausea, vomiting, diarrhea, viral gastroenteritis. **Musculoskeletal:** back pain, myalgia. **Respiratory:** cough, URI, viral URI, exacerbation of asthma, wheezing. **Other:** flulike symptoms, hypersensitivity reactions.

INTERACTIONS

None reported by manufacturer.

EFFECTS ON LAB TEST RESULTS

None reported.

CONTRAINDICATIONS & CAUTIONS

• Contraindicated in patients hypersensitive to drug or its ingredients and in those with status asthmaticus or other acute episodes of asthma that require intensive measures.
• Use cautiously, if at all in patients with TB, ocular HSV, or untreated systemic fungal, bacterial, parasitic, or viral infections.
• Use cautiously in patients receiving systemic corticosteroid therapy.
• Safety and effectiveness in children younger than age 4 haven't been established.
Dialyzable drug: No.

PREGNANCY-LACTATION-REPRODUCTION

• Use during pregnancy only when potential benefits justify fetal risk.
• After delivery, evaluate neonates for adrenal suppression if mother received substantial doses during pregnancy.
• Serious adverse reactions may occur in breastfeeding infants. Discontinue breastfeeding or discontinue drug, considering importance of drug to patient.

NURSING CONSIDERATIONS

• Frequently check oral mucous membranes for signs and symptoms of fungal infection.
• During times of stress (trauma, surgery, infection), systemic corticosteroids may be needed to prevent adrenal insufficiency

in patients who have been corticosteroid-dependent.

• Periodic measurement of growth and development may be needed during high-dose or prolonged therapy in children.

• Cataracts and decreases in bone mineral density can occur with long-term use. Closely monitor patients for vision changes and for decreased bone mineral content, especially patients with major risk factors.

🟦 *Alert:* Taper oral corticosteroid therapy slowly. Acute adrenal insufficiency and death may occur in patients with asthma who change abruptly from oral corticosteroids to beclomethasone.

🟦 *Alert:* Bronchospasm may occur after dosing; discontinue drug and immediately treat with a short-acting inhaled bronchodilator.

• Monitor patient for hypersensitivity reactions (urticaria, angioedema, rash, bronchospasm) and infections.

PATIENT TEACHING

• Teach about proper drug administration and handling, including care of inhaler.

• Inform patient that drug doesn't relieve acute asthma attacks.

• Tell patient who needs a bronchodilator to use it several minutes before beclomethasone.

• Instruct patient who hasn't had chickenpox or measles or been properly immunized to use particular care to avoid exposure due to immunosuppression. Advise patient to contact prescriber if exposure occurs.

• Instruct patient to carry or wear medical identification indicating patient's need for supplemental systemic corticosteroids during stress.

• Tell patient drug may take up to 4 weeks to have full effect.

• Advise patient to prevent oral fungal infections by gargling or rinsing mouth with water after each use. Caution patient not to swallow the water.

• Tell patient to report evidence of corticosteroid withdrawal, including fatigue, weakness, arthralgia, orthostatic hypotension, and dyspnea.

beclomethasone dipropionate (intranasal)
be-kloe-METH-a-sone

Beconase AQ, Qnasl

Therapeutic class: Corticosteroids
Pharmacologic class: Corticosteroids

AVAILABLE FORMS
Nasal aerosol solution (Qnasl): 40 mcg/actuation, 80 mcg/actuation
Nasal spray (Beconase AQ): 42 mcg/metered spray

INDICATIONS & DOSAGES
➤ **To relieve symptoms of seasonal or perennial allergic and nonallergic (vasomotor) rhinitis; to prevent nasal polyp recurrence after surgical removal (Beconase AQ)**
Adults and children ages 12 and older: 1 or 2 sprays (42 to 84 mcg Beconase AQ) in each nostril b.i.d.
Children ages 6 to 12: Initially, 1 spray (42 mcg) in each nostril b.i.d. May increase to 2 sprays in each nostril b.i.d. Once adequate control is achieved, decrease to 1 spray in each nostril b.i.d. Maximum, 336 mcg daily.
➤ **To relieve symptoms of seasonal or perennial allergic rhinitis (Qnasl)**
Adults and children ages 12 and older: 2 sprays (160 mcg total) in each nostril once daily. Maximum, 320 mcg/day.
Children ages 4 to 11: 1 spray (40 mcg) in each nostril once daily. Maximum, 80 mcg/day.

ADMINISTRATION
Intranasal
• Pump nasal spray six times or until a fine mist is produced before first use; repeat priming if nasal spray hasn't been used for 7 days (Beconase AQ). Qnasl doesn't need to be primed.

• Shake Beconase AQ well before use.

• Instruct patient to blow nose to clear nasal passages before use.

• Insert nozzle into nostril, pointing away from septum; patient's head should tilt forward slightly for Beconase AQ. Hold other nostril closed while spraying; patient should hold breath for a few seconds, then exhale through the mouth. Repeat in other nostril.

Reactions in bold italics are ***life-threatening***.

• After administering, remove Beconase AQ nasal applicator, wash with cold water, dry, and replace protective cap. Wipe Qnasl nasal tip with clean, dry cloth or tissue and replace protective cap; always keep dry.
• Store at room temperature.

ACTION
May reduce nasal inflammation by inhibiting mediators of inflammation.

Route	Onset	Peak	Duration
Intranasal	5–7 days	3 wk	Unknown

Half-life: About 2.8 hours (major active metabolite).

ADVERSE REACTIONS
CNS: headache, light-headedness, fever.
EENT: mild, transient nasal burning and stinging; dryness, epistaxis, nasal congestion, nasopharyngeal fungal infections, rhinorrhea, sneezing, watery eyes. **GI:** nausea.
Metabolic: growth velocity reduction in children and adolescents. **Respiratory:** URI.

INTERACTIONS
None reported by manufacturer.

EFFECTS ON LAB TEST RESULTS
None reported.

CONTRAINDICATIONS & CAUTIONS
• Contraindicated in patients hypersensitive to drug or its components.
• Use cautiously, if at all, in patients with active or quiescent respiratory tract tuberculous infections, untreated local or systemic fungal or bacterial infections, systemic viral or parasitic infections, or ocular HSV infections.
• Avoid use in patients who have recently had nasal septal ulcers, nasal surgery, or trauma until wound healing occurs.
• Use cautiously in patients receiving systemic corticosteroid therapy.
• Safety and effectiveness in children younger than age 6 (Beconase AQ) or age 4 (Qnasl) haven't been established.
Dialyzable drug: No.
⚠ *Overdose S&S:* Hypercorticism, adrenal suppression.

PREGNANCY-LACTATION-REPRODUCTION
• Use during pregnancy only when potential benefits justify fetal risk.

• After delivery, evaluate neonates for adrenal suppression if patient received substantial doses during pregnancy.
• It isn't known if drug appears in human milk. Use cautiously during breastfeeding.

NURSING CONSIDERATIONS
• Observe patient for signs and symptoms of infection.
• Drug isn't effective for acute exacerbations of rhinitis. Use decongestants or antihistamines as needed.
• Stop drug if no significant symptom improvement occurs after 3 weeks.
• Routinely monitor growth in children; reduced growth rate may occur.
• Glaucoma and cataracts can occur. Closely monitor patients for vision changes and increased IOP.
• Watch for hypercorticism and adrenal suppression with very high doses or with standard doses in patients who are susceptible. If signs and symptoms occur, taper and discontinue drug.
• Monitor patient for hypersensitivity reactions (anaphylaxis, angioedema, urticaria, rash).

PATIENT TEACHING
• Advise patient or caregiver to read package insert for instructions on drug use and canister and applicator care.
• Tell patient not to blow nose for 15 minutes after using Qnasl.
• Advise patient to use drug as prescribed. Explain that drug's effects won't be immediate and depend on regular use.
• Explain that, unlike decongestants, drug doesn't work right away. Most patients notice improvement within a few days, but some require 2 to 3 weeks.
• Warn patient not to exceed recommended dosage because of risk of HPA axis suppression.
• Instruct patient who hasn't had chickenpox or measles or been properly immunized to use particular care to avoid exposure due to immunosuppression. Advise patient to contact prescriber if exposure occurs.
• Tell patient to notify prescriber if signs and symptoms don't improve within 3 weeks or if nasal irritation persists.
• Teach patient good nasal and oral hygiene.

✦ Canada   ◇ OTC   ◆ Off-label use   ⊕ Do not crush   *Liquid contains alcohol   ※ Genetic

belimumab ☒
beh-LIM-oo-mab

Benlysta

Therapeutic class: Immunosuppressants
Pharmacologic class: Human monoclonal
antibodies

AVAILABLE FORMS
IV injection: 120 mg, 400 mg in single-use
vials
Subcut injection: 200 mg/mL single-dose prefilled autoinjector or prefilled syringe

INDICATIONS & DOSAGES
➤ **Active SLE**
Adults and children ages 5 and older: 10 mg/
kg IV infusion every 2 weeks for first three
doses; then every 4 weeks thereafter.
Adults ages 18 and older: 200 mg subcut once
weekly.
➤ **Active lupus nephritis in patients who
are receiving standard therapy**
Adults and children ages 5 and older: 10 mg/
kg IV infusion every 2 weeks for first three
doses; then every 4 weeks thereafter.
Adults ages 18 and older: 400 mg subcut
(two 200-mg injections) once weekly for four
doses; then 200 mg once weekly thereafter.

ADMINISTRATION
IV
▼ Consider premedicating with an antihistamine and antipyretic for prophylaxis
against infusion and hypersensitivity reactions.
▼ Store unopened vials in refrigerator.
▼ Once vial has been at room temperature
for 10 to 15 minutes, reconstitute with sterile
water: 1.5 mL for 120-mg vial and 4.8 mL
for 400-mg vial.
▼ Direct stream of sterile water toward side
of vial to minimize foaming. Gently swirl
for 60 seconds every 5 minutes until dissolved. Don't shake. Protect solution from
sunlight while dissolving. Usual reconstitution time is 10 to 15 minutes but may take up
to 30 minutes.
▼ Solution should be opalescent and colorless to pale yellow. Small air bubbles are
expected and acceptable.
▼ Dilute only in NSS, half-NSS, or lactated
Ringer solution to a volume of 250 mL.

▼ To dilute, withdraw a volume of fluid
equal to amount of drug to be added from
a 250-mL infusion bag, so total volume will
remain at 250 mL when drug is added. Add
drug to the 250-mL infusion bag and gently
invert to mix the solution. Discard any unused drug solution. If patients weigh 40 kg
or less, use 100 mL infusion bag so that final
concentration doesn't exceed 4 mg/mL.
▼ Protect unused reconstituted solution from
light and store in refrigerator. Store NSS,
half-NSS, and lactated Ringer solution in
refrigerator or at room temperature.
▼ Administer as an IV infusion over 1 hour.
Don't give as an IV push or bolus.
▼ Complete infusion within 8 hours of reconstitution.
▼ **Incompatibilities:** Dextrose solution,
other IV drugs.
Subcutaneous
● If changing from IV therapy to subcut administration for SLE, give first subcut dose
1 to 4 weeks after last IV dose. If changing
from IV therapy for lupus nephritis, give first
subcut dose any time after first two IV doses
and 1 to 2 weeks after last IV dose.
● Remove from refrigerator and allow to sit
at room temperature for 30 minutes before
use.
● Visually inspect for particulate matter and
discoloration before administration; use only
if solution appears clear to opalescent and
colorless to pale yellow.
● Administer once a week, preferably on the
same day each week.
● Administer by subcut injection in abdomen
or thigh.
● Allow at least 5 cm between injections
when giving more than one injection at same
site.
● Rotate injection sites weekly; never inject
into areas where skin is tender, bruised, red, or
hard.
● If a dose is missed, administer injection as
soon as possible; then resume schedule or
start a new weekly schedule from the day that
the missed dose was administered. Don't administer two doses on the same day.

ACTION
B-lymphocyte stimulator-specific inhibitor
that inhibits survival of B cells, including au-
toreactive B cells, and reduces their differentiation into Ig-producing plasma cells.

Reactions in bold italics are *life-threatening*.

Route	Onset	Peak	Duration
IV	Unknown	Unknown	Unknown
Subcut	Unknown	2.6 days	Unknown

Half-life: IV, 19.4 days; subcut, 18.3 days.

ADVERSE REACTIONS

CNS: anxiety, headache, insomnia, migraine, depression, fever. **EENT:** nasopharyngitis, pharyngitis. **GI:** nausea, diarrhea, viral gastroenteritis. **GU:** cystitis, UTI. **Hematologic:** *leukopenia.* **Musculoskeletal:** extremity pain. **Respiratory:** bronchitis, URI. **Skin:** injection-site reactions. **Other:** infection, antibody detection, hypersensitivity reactions, infusion reactions.

INTERACTIONS

Drug-drug. *Biologic agents (including B-cell targeted therapies):* Use together hasn't been studied. Don't use together.
Live-virus vaccines: May impair response to vaccines. Don't give live-virus vaccines for 30 days before or at same time as belimumab.

EFFECTS ON LAB TEST RESULTS

• May decrease leukocyte count.

CONTRAINDICATIONS & CAUTIONS

• Contraindicated in patients with a history of anaphylaxis to belimumab.
• Use cautiously in patients with a history of chronic infection, hypersensitivity reactions, infusion reactions, depression, or malignancies.
▧ Use cautiously in patients who are Black because response rate may be lower.
• More deaths occurred with belimumab than with placebo during the controlled period of the main clinical trials. No single cause of death predominated, but possible causes included infection, CV disease, and suicide.
• Use isn't recommended for patients with severe active lupus nephritis or severe active CNS lupus.
• IV administration in children younger than age 5 with SLE isn't indicated.
• Safety and effectiveness of IV administration in patients younger than age 18 with active lupus nephritis haven't been established.
• Safety and effectiveness of subcut administration in patients younger than age 18 haven't been established.
Dialyzable drug: Unknown.

PREGNANCY-LACTATION-REPRODUCTION

• There are insufficient data to determine drug-associated risks during pregnancy. Use cautiously during pregnancy and only if potential benefit outweighs fetal risk.
• Monoclonal antibodies are increasingly transported across the placenta during pregnancy, with the largest amount during the third trimester.
• Patients who are pregnant should enroll in a pregnancy registry that monitors maternal-fetal outcomes of exposure to belimumab (1-866-626-6847 or https://mothertobaby.org/ongoing-study/benlysta-belimumab/).
• Patients of childbearing potential should use adequate contraception during treatment and for at least 4 months after final dose.
• Monitor the infant of a treated patient for B-cell reduction and other immune dysfunction; consider risks and benefits before giving live or live-attenuated vaccines to the infant.
• It isn't known if drug appears in human milk. Patient should discontinue breastfeeding or discontinue drug, considering importance of drug to patient.

NURSING CONSIDERATIONS

• IV drug should be administered only by a health care professional prepared to manage anaphylaxis.
• Patient or caregiver may administer subcut after prescriber approval and proper training.
• Watch for hypersensitivity reactions, even in patients who previously tolerated infusions.
• Monitor patient for signs and symptoms of infection. Serious and sometimes fatal infections have occurred in patients receiving immunosuppressants.
• Monitor patient for depression, suicidality, malignancies, allergic reactions, and infusion reactions.
• Assess patients with new-onset or deteriorating neurologic signs and symptoms for JC virus-associated progressive multifocal leukoencephalopathy (PML). If PML is confirmed, discontinuation of therapy may be necessary.

PATIENT TEACHING

• Warn patient not to skip appointments to ensure that drug is given on schedule to improve effectiveness of treatment.
• Tell patient to immediately report signs and symptoms of an allergic reaction

(itching, hives, shortness of breath, swelling of the face, and throat closure) and new or worsening depression, suicidality, or other mood changes.

• Teach patient infection-prevention measures.
• Instruct patient to immediately report signs and symptoms of infection (fever, body aches, cough, and sore throat).
• Tell patient to report history of cancer to health care provider.
• Instruct patient not to receive live-virus vaccines while taking drug.
• If patient or caregiver will be administering subcut at home, provide training and instruct patient or caregiver to follow directions for administration provided in the "Instructions for Use."
• Counsel patient of childbearing potential to use adequate contraception during treatment and for at least 4 months after final dose.
• Advise patient to tell prescriber if pregnant or breastfeeding.

---

benazepril hydrochloride ℞
ben-A-za-pril

Lotensin

Therapeutic class: Antihypertensives
Pharmacologic class: ACE inhibitors

AVAILABLE FORMS
Tablets: 5 mg, 10 mg, 20 mg, 40 mg

INDICATIONS & DOSAGES
➤ **HTN**
Adults: For patients not receiving a diuretic, 10 mg PO daily initially. Adjust dosage as needed and tolerated; usually 20 to 40 mg daily in one or two divided doses. For patients receiving a diuretic, 5 mg PO daily initially.
Children ages 6 and older: 0.2 mg/kg (between 0.1 and 0.6 mg/kg) PO daily. Adjust as needed up to 0.6 mg/kg (maximum, 40 mg) PO daily.
Adjust-a-dose: In adults, if CrCl is below 30 mL/minute/1.73 m² or serum creatinine level is greater than 3 mg/dL, give 5 mg PO daily. May adjust daily dose up to 40 mg.

ADMINISTRATION
PO
• Protect tablets from moisture.
• Suspension may be prepared by a pharmacist.

• Shake suspension before each use.
• Refrigerate suspension at 36° to 46° F (2° to 8° C). Discard unused portion after 30 days.

ACTION
Inhibits ACE, preventing conversion of angiotensin I to angiotensin II, a potent vasoconstrictor. Less angiotensin II decreases peripheral arterial resistance, decreasing aldosterone secretion, which reduces sodium and water retention and lowers BP. Drug also acts as antihypertensive in patients with low-renin HTN.

Route	Onset	Peak	Duration
PO	1 hr	1–2 hr	24 hr

Half-life: 10 to 11 hours.

ADVERSE REACTIONS
CNS: headache, fatigue, dizziness, postural dizziness, somnolence. **CV:** symptomatic hypotension. **Respiratory:** cough.

INTERACTIONS
Drug-drug. *Aliskiren:* May increase risk of kidney impairment, hypotension, and hyperkalemia in patients with diabetes and those with GFR less than 60 mL/minute. Use together is contraindicated in patients with diabetes. Avoid use together in those with moderate to severe kidney impairment.
Antidiabetics, insulin: May increase risk of hypoglycemia. Monitor patient carefully.
ARBs (telmisartan): May increase risk of kidney dysfunction. Avoid use together.
Azathioprine: May increase risk of anemia or leukopenia. Monitor hematologic study results if used together.
Diuretics, other antihypertensives: May cause excessive hypotension. Stop diuretic or lower dosage of benazepril, as needed.
Everolimus, neprilysin inhibitors (sacubitril), sirolimus, temsirolimus: May increase risk of angioedema. Discontinue one or both agents if an interaction is suspected.
Gold salts: May increase risk of nitritoid reaction. Carefully monitor patient.
Iron salts (parenteral): May increase risk of adverse reactions to iron salts. Monitor patient closely.
Lithium: May increase lithium level and risk of toxicity. Use together cautiously; monitor lithium level.
Nesiritide: May increase risk of hypotension. Monitor BP.

Reactions in bold italics are ***life-threatening***.

NSAIDs (including selective cyclooxygenase-2 inhibitors): May decrease antihypertensive effects. Monitor BP. May also increase risk of kidney dysfunction. Monitor kidney function periodically.

Potassium-sparing diuretics, potassium supplements: May cause hyperkalemia. Monitor potassium level and kidney function.

Salicylates: May decrease hypotensive effects of benazepril and increase risk of nephrotoxicity. Use together cautiously. Consider increasing benazepril dosage or decreasing or stopping salicylate.

Thiazide diuretics: May attenuate potassium loss. Also may increase risk of kidney failure. Monitor serum potassium level and kidney function.

Trimethoprim: May increase risk of hyperkalemia. Monitor serum potassium level and clinical response.

Drug-herb. *Ma huang, yohimbe:* May decrease antihypertensive effects. Discourage use together.

Drug-food. *Salt substitutes containing potassium:* May cause hyperkalemia. Monitor potassium level and kidney function.

EFFECTS ON LAB TEST RESULTS
• May increase BUN, creatinine, potassium, uric acid, glucose, bilirubin, urine protein, and liver enzyme levels.
• May decrease sodium level.
• May increase eosinophil count.
• May lead to false-negative aldosterone/renin ratio.

CONTRAINDICATIONS & CAUTIONS
• Contraindicated in patients hypersensitive to ACE inhibitors and in those with a history of angioedema regardless of prior ACE inhibitor use.
• Use cautiously in patients with impaired liver or kidney function. If jaundice develops or liver enzyme levels are markedly elevated, discontinue drug.
• Use cautiously in patients with history of airway surgery or other risk factors for airway obstruction.
• Use cautiously in older adults.
• Use cautiously in patients at risk for hypovolemia including HF, ischemic heart disease, cerebrovascular disease, hyponatremia, dialysis, severe intravascular volume depletion, or salt depletion.

• Use cautiously in patients at risk for hyperkalemia (patients with kidney insufficiency or diabetes and those using potassium supplements or salt-substitutes).
• Safety and effectiveness in children younger than age 6 or in children with GFR less than 30 mL/minute/1.73 m^2 haven't been established.

Dialyzable drug: Slightly.

PREGNANCY-LACTATION-REPRODUCTION
Boxed Warning Drugs that act on the RAAS can cause injury and death to a developing fetus. Discontinue drug if pregnancy is detected. ▋
• Small amounts of drug appear in human milk. Use cautiously during breastfeeding.

NURSING CONSIDERATIONS
• Monitor patient for hypotension. Excessive hypotension can occur when drug is given with diuretics. If possible, diuretic therapy should be stopped 2 to 3 days before starting benazepril to decrease potential for excessive hypotensive response. If drug doesn't adequately control BP, diuretic may be cautiously reinstituted.
⚥ Although ACE inhibitors reduce BP in patients of all races, they reduce it less in patients who are Black and are taking ACE inhibitors alone. These patients should take drug with a thiazide diuretic for a more favorable response.
• Monitor patient for angioedema and anaphylactoid reactions, including intestinal angioedema (abdominal pain with or without nausea or vomiting).
⚥ Drug may increase risk of angioedema in patients who are Black.
• Measure BP when drug level is at peak (2 to 6 hours after administration) and at trough (just before a dose) to verify adequate BP control.
• Assess kidney and liver function before and periodically during therapy. Monitor potassium level.
• Monitor patient for excessive cough. Therapy may need to be changed if cough is intolerable.
• *Look alike–sound alike:* Don't confuse benazepril with Benadryl. Don't confuse Lotensin with lovastatin.

PATIENT TEACHING
• Instruct patient to avoid salt substitutes because they may contain potassium, which can

cause high potassium level in patients taking drug.

• Inform patient that light-headedness can occur, especially during first few days of therapy. Tell patient to rise slowly to minimize this effect, to report dizziness to prescriber and, if fainting occurs, to immediately stop drug and call prescriber.

• Warn patient to use caution in hot weather and during exercise. Inadequate fluid intake, vomiting, diarrhea, and excessive perspiration can lead to light-headedness and fainting.

• Advise patient to report signs and symptoms of infection (fever, sore throat); easy bruising or bleeding; swelling of tongue, lips, face, eyes, mucous membranes, or extremities; difficulty swallowing or breathing; or hoarseness.

• Caution patient with diabetes to closely monitor blood glucose level.

• **Alert:** Tell patient of childbearing potential to notify prescriber if pregnancy occurs. Drug will need to be stopped.

• Tell patient to contact prescriber if intolerable cough develops.

benztropine mesylate
BENZ-troe-peen

Therapeutic class: Antiparkinsonian drugs
Pharmacologic class: Anticholinergics

AVAILABLE FORMS
Injection: 1 mg/mL
Tablets: 0.5 mg, 1 mg, 2 mg

INDICATIONS & DOSAGES
➤ **Drug-induced extrapyramidal disorders (except tardive dyskinesia)**
Adults: 1 to 4 mg PO, IV, or IM once daily or b.i.d.
➤ **Transient extrapyramidal disorders**
Adults: 1 to 2 mg PO, IV, or IM b.i.d. or t.i.d. After 1 or 2 weeks, withdraw drug to determine continued need.
➤ **Acute dystonic reaction**
Adults: 1 to 2 mg PO, IV, or IM; then 1 to 2 mg PO once daily or b.i.d. to prevent recurrence. IV or IM route is preferred for severe acute reactions.
➤ **Parkinsonism**
Adults: 0.5 to 6 mg PO, IV, or IM daily in a single dose at bedtime or divided in two to four doses. First dose is 0.5 to 1 mg, increased

by 0.5 mg every 5 to 6 days. Adjust dosage to meet individual requirements. Maximum, 6 mg daily.
➤ **Postencephalitic parkinsonism**
Adults: 2 mg PO, IV, or IM daily in one or more doses. For patients who are highly sensitive, may initiate at 0.5 mg PO or IM at bedtime and increase as needed. Maximum, 6 mg daily.

ADMINISTRATION
PO
• May give before or after meals, depending on patient reaction. If patient is prone to excessive salivation, give drug after meals. If patient's mouth dries excessively, give drug before meals, unless it causes nausea.
• Store at room temperature.
IV
▼ Reserve IV delivery for emergencies, such as acute dystonic reactions.
▼ The IV form is seldom used because no significant difference in onset exists between it and the IM form.
▼ Use filtered needle to draw up solution from ampule.
▼ Visually inspect solution for particulate matter and discoloration before administration.
▼ Discard unused portion.
▼ Store drug at room temperature.
▼ **Incompatibilities:** Haloperidol lactate.
IM
• Use filtered needle to draw up solution from ampule.
• Visually inspect solution for particulate matter and discoloration before giving.
• Discard unused portion.
• Store at room temperature.

ACTION
Unknown. May block central cholinergic receptors, helping to balance cholinergic activity in the basal ganglia.

Route	Onset	Peak	Duration
PO	1 hr	7 hr	24 hr
IV, IM	15 min	Unknown	24 hr

Half-life: Unknown.

ADVERSE REACTIONS
CNS: nervousness, depression, listlessness, *toxic psychosis (confusion, disorientation, memory impairment, visual hallucinations)*, fever, finger numbness. **CV:** tachycardia.

EENT: dilated pupils, blurred vision, dry mouth. **GI:** constipation, nausea, vomiting, paralytic ileus. **GU:** urine retention, dysuria. **Musculoskeletal:** muscle weakness. **Skin:** decreased sweating. **Other:** hypersensitivity reaction, hyperthermia, *heat stroke.*

INTERACTIONS
Drug-drug. *Amantadine, haloperidol, phenothiazines, TCAs:* May cause additive anticholinergic adverse reactions, such as confusion, hallucinations, GI effects, fever, or heat intolerance. Reduce dosage before giving.
Cholinergics (donepezil, galantamine, rivastigmine, tacrine): May antagonize the therapeutic effects of these drugs. If used together, monitor patient for therapeutic effect.

EFFECTS ON LAB TEST RESULTS
None reported.

CONTRAINDICATIONS & CAUTIONS
• Contraindicated in patients hypersensitive to drug or its components and in children younger than age 3.
• Drug isn't recommended for use in patients with tardive dyskinesia and in those with angle-closure glaucoma.
• Drug may produce anhidrosis. Use cautiously in hot weather, in patients with mental disorders, in older adults, and in children ages 3 and older.
• Use cautiously in patients with prostatic hyperplasia, arrhythmias, or seizure disorders.
Dialyzable drug: Unknown.
⚠ *Overdose S&S:* CNS depression preceded or followed by stimulation; confusion, nervousness, listlessness, intensification of mental symptoms or toxic psychosis (in patients with mental illness being treated with neuroleptic drugs), hallucinations, dizziness, muscle weakness, ataxia, dry mouth, mydriasis, blurred vision, palpitations, tachycardia, HTN, nausea, vomiting, dysuria, numbness of fingers, dysphagia, allergic reactions, headache, delirium, coma, shock, seizures, respiratory arrest, anhidrosis, hyperthermia, glaucoma, constipation; hot, dry, flushed skin.

PREGNANCY-LACTATION-REPRODUCTION
• Safe use during pregnancy hasn't been established.
• It isn't known if drug appears in human milk. Anticholinergic agents may suppress lactation.

NURSING CONSIDERATIONS
• Monitor vital signs carefully.
• Watch closely for adverse reactions, especially in older adults and patients who are debilitated. Report adverse reactions promptly.
• At certain doses, drug produces atropine-like toxicity, which may aggravate tardive dyskinesia.
• Watch for intermittent constipation and abdominal distention and pain, which may indicate onset of paralytic ileus.
🔶 *Alert:* Never stop drug abruptly. Reduce dosage gradually.
• *Look alike–sound alike:* Don't confuse benztropine with bromocriptine.

PATIENT TEACHING
• Warn patient to avoid activities that require alertness until CNS effects of drug are known.
• Advise patient who takes a single daily dose to do so at bedtime.
• Caution patient to report signs and symptoms of urinary hesitancy or urine retention.
• Tell patient to relieve dry mouth with cool drinks, ice chips, sugarless gum, or hard candy.
• Advise patient to limit hot weather activities because drug-induced lack of sweating may cause overheating.

betamethasone dipropionate
bay-ta-METH-a-sone

Diprolene, Sernivo

betamethasone valerate
Luxiq

Therapeutic class: Corticosteroids
Pharmacologic class: Corticosteroids

AVAILABLE FORMS
betamethasone dipropionate
Cream: 0.05%
Gel: 0.05%
Lotion: 0.05%
Ointment: 0.05%
Spray: 0.05%
betamethasone valerate
Cream: 0.1%
Foam: 0.12%
Lotion: 0.1%
Ointment: 0.1%

INDICATIONS & DOSAGES

➤ **Inflammation and pruritus from corticosteroid-responsive dermatoses**

Adults and children older than age 12: Clean area; apply cream, ointment, lotion, or gel sparingly. Give dipropionate products once daily to b.i.d.; give valerate 0.1% lotion b.i.d. or valerate 0.1% cream or ointment once daily to t.i.d. Maximum dosage of augmented betamethasone dipropionate 0.05% ointment, cream, gel, or lotion is 45 g, 45 g, 50 g, or 50 mL per week, respectively. Therapy with augmented formulations shouldn't exceed 2 weeks.

➤ **Inflammation and pruritus from corticosteroid-responsive dermatoses of scalp (valerate foam only)**

Adults: Gently massage small amounts of foam into affected scalp areas b.i.d., morning and evening, until control is achieved. If no improvement is seen in 2 weeks, reassess diagnosis.

➤ **Mild to moderate plaque psoriasis**

Adults: Apply spray to affected skin areas b.i.d. for up to 4 weeks; rub in gently. Discontinue when control is achieved.

ADMINISTRATION

Topical

• Apply sparingly to affected areas. To prevent skin damage, rub in gently, leaving a thin coat.
• May decrease dosing frequency of cream or ointment to once daily as directed by prescriber, if clinical improvement occurs.
• Avoid applying near eyes or mucous membranes or in ear canal, groin area, or armpit.
• Don't dispense foam directly into warm hands because foam will begin to melt on contact; dispense onto a plate or other cool surface and pick up small amounts of foam with fingers to apply immediately.
❸ **Alert:** Foam product is flammable. Avoid fire, flame, or smoking during use. Don't expose to heat.
• For patients with eczematous dermatitis whose skin may be irritated by adhesive material, hold dressing in place with gauze, elastic bandages, stockings, or stockinette.
❸ **Alert:** Don't use occlusive dressings unless directed by prescriber.
• Shake spray well before use.
• Avoid use on face, scalp, axilla, groin, or other skinfold areas or if skin atrophy is present at treatment site.
• Store at room temperature.

ACTION

Unclear. Diffuses across cell membranes to form complexes with receptors. Has antiinflammatory, antipruritic, vasoconstrictive, and antiproliferative activity. Considered a medium-potency to very-high-potency drug (depending on product), according to vasoconstrictive properties.

Route	Onset	Peak	Duration
Topical	Unknown	Unknown	Unknown

Half-life: Unknown.

ADVERSE REACTIONS

GU: glucosuria (with dipropionate).
Metabolic: hyperglycemia. **Skin:** burning, pruritus, irritation, dryness, erythema, folliculitis, striae, acneiform eruptions, scaling, perioral dermatitis, hypopigmentation, hypertrichosis, allergic contact dermatitis, maceration, atrophy, alopecia, miliaria with occlusive dressings, application-site pain. **Other:** *HPA axis suppression,* Cushing syndrome, secondary infection.

INTERACTIONS

None significant.

EFFECTS ON LAB TEST RESULTS

• May increase glucose level.
• May suppress wheal and flare reactions to skin test antigens.

CONTRAINDICATIONS & CAUTIONS

• Contraindicated in patients hypersensitive to corticosteroids.
• Don't use as monotherapy in primary bacterial infections (impetigo, paronychia, erysipelas, cellulitis, angular cheilitis); rosacea; perioral dermatitis; or acne.
• Don't use augmented betamethasone dipropionate 0.05% ointment; betamethasone dipropionate 0.05% gel, cream, and ointment; betamethasone 0.05% spray; or betamethasone valerate 0.1% ointment on the face, groin, or axilla.
Dialyzable drug: No.
⚠ **Overdose S&S:** Systemic effects.

PREGNANCY-LACTATION-REPRODUCTION

• There are no adequate and well-controlled studies during pregnancy. Use during pregnancy only if potential benefit justifies fetal risk.
• Use cautiously during breastfeeding.

NURSING CONSIDERATIONS
• Drug isn't for ophthalmic use.
• Because of alcohol content of vehicle, gel products may cause mild, transient stinging, especially when used on or near excoriated skin.
• If antifungal or antibiotic combined with corticosteroid fails to provide prompt improvement, stop corticosteroid until infection is controlled.
• Monitor patient for allergic contact dermatitis, often identified as failure to heal.
• Systemic absorption is likely with prolonged or extensive body surface treatment. Watch for symptoms of HPA axis suppression, manifestations of Cushing syndrome, hyperglycemia, and glucosuria. If HPA axis suppression occurs, attempt to withdraw drug or substitute a less potent steroid. Withdraw gradually.
• Evaluate patient for HPA axis suppression by using the urinary free cortisol and corticotropin stimulation tests.
• Drug may increase risk of posterior subcapsular cataracts and glaucoma. Consider referral to an ophthalmologist for evaluation if symptoms develop.
• **Alert:** Children may demonstrate greater susceptibility to HPA axis suppression and Cushing syndrome.
• Avoid using plastic pants or tight-fitting diapers on treated areas in young children. Children may absorb larger amounts of drug and be more susceptible to systemic toxicity.
• **Alert:** Don't replace Diprolene with generics because other products have different potencies.

PATIENT TEACHING
• Teach patient how to apply drug.
• Emphasize that drug is for external use only.
• Tell patient to wash hands after application.
• Advise patient to stop drug and report signs of systemic absorption, skin irritation or ulceration, hypersensitivity, visual changes, or infection.
• Instruct patient not to use occlusive dressings unless directed by prescriber.
• Discuss personal hygiene measures to reduce chance of infection.

bethanechol chloride
be-THAN-e-kole

Therapeutic class: Urinary stimulants
Pharmacologic class: Cholinergic agonists

AVAILABLE FORMS
Tablets: 5 mg, 10 mg, 25 mg, 50 mg

INDICATIONS & DOSAGES
➤ **Acute postoperative and postpartum nonobstructive (functional) urine retention, neurogenic atony of urinary bladder with urine retention**
Adults: 10 to 50 mg PO t.i.d. to q.i.d. Determine minimum effective dose by giving 5 or 10 mg and repeating same amount at hourly intervals until satisfactory response or maximum of 50 mg.

ADMINISTRATION
PO
• Give drug 1 hour before or 2 hours after meals because drug may cause nausea and vomiting if taken soon after eating.
• Store at room temperature.

ACTION
Directly stimulates muscarinic cholinergic receptors, mimicking acetylcholine action, increasing GI tract tone and peristalsis and contraction of the detrusor muscle of the urinary bladder.

Route	Onset	Peak	Duration
PO	30 min	60–90 min	1 hr

Half-life: Unknown.

ADVERSE REACTIONS
CNS: headache, malaise, *seizures.* **CV:** *bradycardia,* profound hypotension with reflexive tachycardia, flushing. **EENT:** excessive salivation, lacrimation, miosis. **GI:** abdominal cramps, diarrhea, nausea, belching, borborygmus. **GU:** urinary urgency. **Respiratory:** *bronchoconstriction, asthma attack.* **Skin:** diaphoresis.

INTERACTIONS
Drug-drug. *Anticholinergics, atropine, belladonna alkaloids, procainamide, quinidine:* May reverse cholinergic effects. Observe patient for lack of drug effect.

Cholinesterase inhibitors (donepezil), cholinergic agonists: May cause additive effects or increase toxicity. Avoid use together.
Ganglionic blockers (pentolinium): May cause critical drop in BP, usually preceded by severe abdominal pain. Avoid use together.

EFFECTS ON LAB TEST RESULTS
None reported.

CONTRAINDICATIONS & CAUTIONS
• Contraindicated in patients hypersensitive to drug or its components and in those with uncertain strength or integrity of bladder wall, mechanical obstruction of GI or urinary tract, hyperthyroidism, peptic ulceration, latent or active bronchial asthma, obstructive pulmonary disease, pronounced bradycardia or hypotension, vasomotor instability, cardiac disease or CAD, seizure disorder, Parkinson disease, spastic GI disturbances, acute inflammatory lesions of the GI tract, peritonitis, or marked vagotonia.
• Safe use in children hasn't been established.
Dialyzable drug: Unknown.
⚠ *Overdose S&S:* Abdominal discomfort, excessive salivation, flushing, hot feeling, diaphoresis, nausea, vomiting.

PREGNANCY-LACTATION-REPRODUCTION
• It isn't known if drug affects reproduction. Use during pregnancy only if clearly needed.
• It isn't known if drug appears in human milk. Patient should discontinue breastfeeding or discontinue drug, considering importance of drug to patient.

NURSING CONSIDERATIONS
• Monitor patient for orthostatic hypotension.
• Monitor for UTI related to reflux of urine into the kidney pelvis.
• Watch closely for adverse reactions that may indicate drug toxicity.

PATIENT TEACHING
• Tell patient to take drug on an empty stomach and at regular intervals.
• Inform patient that drug is usually effective 30 to 90 minutes after use.

SAFETY ALERT!
BIOSIMILAR DRUG

bevacizumab
be-vuh-SIZ-uh-mab

Avastin

bevacizumab-adcd
Vegzelma

bevacizumab-awwb
Mvasi

bevacizumab-bvzr
Zirabev

bevacizumab-maly
Alymsys

Therapeutic class: Antineoplastics
Pharmacologic class: Monoclonal antibodies

AVAILABLE FORMS
Intravitrial: 2.5 mg/mL in 0.1-mL, 0.13-mL, 0.15-mL prefilled syringes
Solution: 25 mg/mL in 4-mL, 16-mL vials

INDICATIONS & DOSAGES
Adjust-a-dose (for all indications): Although there are no recommended dosage reductions, temporarily suspend or stop drug in patients with severe infusion reactions (GI perforations and fistulae, wound healing complications, hemorrhage, thromboembolic events, PRES, kidney injury and proteinuria, HF), severe HTN that isn't controlled with medical management, or moderate to severe proteinuria.
➤ **Platinum-resistant recurrent epithelial ovarian, fallopian tube, or primary peritoneal cancer**
Adults: 10 mg/kg IV every 2 weeks in combination with paclitaxel, pegylated liposomal doxorubicin, or weekly topotecan; or 15 mg/kg IV every 3 weeks in combination with topotecan.
➤ **Platinum-sensitive recurrent epithelial ovarian, fallopian tube, or primary peritoneal cancer**
Adults: Initially, 15 mg/kg IV every 3 weeks in combination with carboplatin and paclitaxel for 6 to 8 cycles, followed by continued use of bevacizumab 15 mg/kg IV every 3 weeks as a single agent until disease progression. Or, 15 mg/kg IV every 3 weeks

---

*Reactions in bold italics are **life-threatening**.*

in combination with carboplatin and gemcitabine for 6 cycles up to 10 cycles, followed by continued use of bevacizumab 15 mg/kg IV every 3 weeks as a single agent until disease progression.

➤ **Stage III or IV epithelial ovarian, fallopian tube, or primary peritoneal cancer after initial surgical resection**
Adults: 15 mg/kg every 3 weeks with carboplatin and paclitaxel for up to 6 cycles, followed by 15 mg/kg every 3 weeks as a single agent, for a total of up to 22 cycles.

➤ **Persistent, recurrent, or metastatic cervical cancer**
Adults: 15 mg/kg IV infusion once every 3 weeks with paclitaxel and cisplatin or paclitaxel and topotecan.

➤ **First- or second-line treatment, with 5-FU–based chemotherapy, for metastatic colon or rectal cancer**
Adults: If used with bolus irinotecan, 5-FU, and leucovorin (IFL) regimen, give 5 mg/kg IV every 14 days. If used with oxaliplatin, 5-FU, and leucovorin (FOLFOX 4) regimen, 10 mg/kg IV every 14 days. Infusion rate varies by patient tolerance and number of infusions.

➤ **Metastatic colorectal cancer with fluoropyrimidine-irinotecan-based or fluoropyrimidine-oxaliplatin-based chemotherapy for second-line treatment after progression on a first-line bevacizumab-containing regimen**
Adults: 5 mg/kg IV every 2 weeks or 7.5 mg/kg IV every 3 weeks.

➤ **With carboplatin and paclitaxel as first-line treatment of unresectable, locally advanced, recurrent, or metastatic nonsquamous NSCLC**
Adults: 15 mg/kg IV infusion once every 3 weeks.

➤ **With interferon alfa for metastatic renal cell carcinoma; as single agent for progressive glioblastoma following prior therapy**
Adults: 10 mg/kg IV every 14 days.

➤ **Unresectable or metastatic hepatocellular carcinoma in combination with atezolizumab in patients who haven't received prior systemic therapy (Avastin only)**
Adults: 15 mg/kg IV infusion after 1,200-mg IV infusion of atezolizumab on the same day, every 3 weeks until disease progression or unacceptable toxicity occurs. Refer to manufacturer's instructions for atezolizumab prescribing information.

➤ **Unresectable malignant pleural mesothelioma** ◆
Adults: 15 mg/kg IV every 3 weeks in combination with pemetrexed and cisplatin for up to 6 cycles, followed by bevacizumab maintenance therapy at 15 mg/kg once every 3 weeks until disease progression or unacceptable toxicity occurs.

➤ **Age-related macular degeneration** ◆
Adults: Intravitreal bevacizumab 1.25 mg (0.05 mL) monthly for 3 months; then may give scheduled (monthly) or as needed based on monthly ophthalmologic assessment.

➤ **Diabetic macular edema** ◆
Adults: Initially, intravitreal bevacizumab 1.25 mg (0.05 mL); repeat every 4 weeks depending on ophthalmologic response.

ADMINISTRATION
IV
▼ Don't freeze or shake vials.
▼ Dilute drug using aseptic technique. Withdraw proper dose and mix in a total volume of 100 mL NSS in an IV bag.
▼ Don't give by IV push or bolus.
▼ Give first infusion over 90 minutes and, if tolerated, second infusion over 60 minutes. Give later infusions over 30 minutes if previous infusions were tolerated.
▼ Discard unused portion; drug is preservative-free.
▼ Diluted drug is stable 8 hours if refrigerated at 36° to 46° F (2° to 8° C).
▼ Protect from light.
▼ **Incompatibilities:** Dextrose solutions.
Intravitreal
● Give adequate local anesthesia and topical antimicrobial prior to procedure.

ACTION
A recombinant humanized vascular endothelial growth factor inhibitor.

Route	Onset	Peak	Duration
IV	Unknown	Unknown	Unknown
Intravitreal	Unknown	Unknown	Unknown

Half-life: About 20 days (IV), about 5 to 10 days (intravitreal).

ADVERSE REACTIONS
Includes adverse reactions as part of chemotherapy regimens.
CNS: asthenia, dysarthria, dizziness, headache, taste disorder, anxiety, pain, syncope, fatigue, insomnia, myasthenia,

fever. **CV:** *intra-abdominal thrombosis,* HTN, *arterial thrombosis, thromboembolism, DVT, hemorrhage,* edema, chest pain, left ventricular dysfunction, *PE.* **EENT:** excess lacrimation, blurred vision, tinnitus, deafness, epistaxis, rhinitis, rhinorrhea, nasal congestion, sinusitis, gum bleeding, voice alteration, oropharyngeal pain, oral ulceration, tooth abscess. **GI:** anorexia, constipation, diarrhea, stomatitis, vomiting, *GI hemorrhage,* abdominal pain, gastritis, nausea, bile duct fistula, rectal fistula, rectal pain, tracheoesophageal fistula. **GU:** *vaginal hemorrhage,* increased creatinine level, proteinuria, UTI, ovarian failure, pelvic pain, bladder fistula, vaginal fistula, kidney fistula. **Hematologic:** *leukopenia, neutropenia, thrombocytopenia.* **Hepatic:** bilirubinemia, increased liver enzyme levels. **Metabolic:** *hypokalemia, hyperkalemia,* weight loss, hyperglycemia, *hypomagnesemia,* hyponatremia, hypoalbuminemia, *hypocalcemia,* dehydration. **Musculoskeletal:** back pain, limb pain, myalgia, arthralgia, muscle weakness. **Respiratory:** *hemoptysis, pulmonary hemorrhage,* dyspnea, cough, bronchopleural fistula. **Skin:** dry skin, bruise, acne, cellulitis, exfoliative dermatitis, nail disorder, palmar-plantar erythrodysesthesia. **Other:** postoperative wound complication, infection, infusion-related reaction.

INTERACTIONS
Drug-drug. *Bisphosphonate derivatives:* May increase risk of osteonecrosis of the jaw. Monitor therapy.
Sunitinib: May increase bevacizumab toxicities, including microangiopathic hemolytic anemia and HTN. Avoid combination.

EFFECTS ON LAB TEST RESULTS
• May increase AST, ALT, ALP, bilirubin, glucose, and urine protein levels.
• May decrease albumin, magnesium, calcium, and sodium levels.
• May increase or decrease potassium level.
• May decrease neutrophil, platelet, and WBC counts.

CONTRAINDICATIONS & CAUTIONS
• Use cautiously in patients hypersensitive to drug or its components and in those who need surgery, have a bowel obstruction or fistulae, have received pelvic radiation, are at increased risk for kidney failure, are taking

anticoagulants, or have significant CV disease (HTN, HF, thromboembolism).
• Use cautiously in patients with prior anthracycline-based chemotherapy because the incidence of HF and decreased LVEF may increase with use of bevacizumab. Discontinue drug in patients who develop HF.
• Use cautiously in older adults; adverse reactions occur more often in these patients.
• Drug increases risk of severe or fatal hemorrhage, hemoptysis, GI bleeding, CNS hemorrhage, and vaginal bleeding. Don't give to patients with serious hemorrhage or recent hemoptysis.
• Safety and effectiveness in children haven't been established.
Dialyzable drug: Unknown.
⚠ *Overdose S&S:* Headache.

PREGNANCY-LACTATION-REPRODUCTION
• Drug has shown teratogenic effects in animal studies. Avoid use during pregnancy.
• Because of bevacizumab's long half-life, patients of childbearing potential should use adequate contraception during therapy and for 6 months after final dose.
🔹 *Alert:* May increase risk of ovarian failure and may impair fertility. Long-term effects on fertility are unknown.
• It isn't known if drug appears in human milk. Patients should avoid breastfeeding during therapy and for 6 months after final dose.

NURSING CONSIDERATIONS
🔹 *Alert:* PRES-associated symptoms (HTN, headache, visual disturbances, altered mental function, seizures) may occur 16 hours to 1 year after starting drug. PRES can be confirmed only by MRI. Monitor patient closely. If syndrome occurs, stop drug and provide supportive care.
🔹 *Alert:* Monitor patient for arterial thromboembolic events and VTE. Permanently discontinue drug for grade 4 VTE, including PE.
🔹 *Alert:* Drug may increase risk of developing fistula, including non-GI fistulae (tracheoesophageal, bronchopleural, biliary, vaginal, kidney, or bladder), which can be fatal.
• Permanently stop drug if patient develops any fistula of an internal organ.
• Hypersensitivity reactions can occur during infusion. Monitor patient closely for signs

and symptoms of hypertensive crisis (neurologic changes), wheezing, oxygen desaturation, chest pain, headache, rigors, and diaphoresis.

• Drug may cause fatal GI perforation. Monitor patient closely.

• Monitor patient's BP every 2 to 3 weeks.

• If patient develops severe HTN, hypertensive crisis, serious hemorrhage, or GI perforation that needs intervention, stop drug.

🕒 **Alert:** Drug may increase risk of serious arterial thromboembolic events, including MI, TIAs, stroke, HF, diabetes, and angina. At highest risk are patients ages 65 and older, those with a history of arterial thromboembolism, and those who have taken drug before. If patient has an arterial thromboembolic event, permanently stop drug.

• Bevacizumab can result in life-threatening wound dehiscence. Permanently discontinue bevacizumab therapy in patients who experience wound dehiscence that requires medical intervention. Discontinue drug at least 28 days before elective surgery and don't restart drug for at least 28 days after surgery and until the surgical wound is fully healed.

• Monitor urinalysis for worsening proteinuria. Patients with 2+ or greater urine dipstick test should undergo 24-hour urine collection. Discontinue use in patients with nephrotic syndrome.

PATIENT TEACHING

• Inform patient about potential adverse reactions. Tell patient to immediately report adverse reactions, especially abdominal pain, constipation, and vomiting.

• Advise patient that BP and urinalysis will be monitored during treatment.

• Caution patient of childbearing potential to avoid pregnancy during treatment and for 6 months after final dose.

• Tell patient not to breastfeed during therapy and for 6 months after final dose.

🕒 **Alert:** Inform patient of the potential for ovarian failure and impaired fertility before starting treatment.

• Urge patient to alert other health care providers about bevacizumab therapy and to avoid elective surgery during treatment.

bisoprolol fumarate
bis-OH-proe-lol

Therapeutic class: Antihypertensives
Pharmacologic class: Selective beta blockers

AVAILABLE FORMS
Tablets: 5 mg, 10 mg

INDICATIONS & DOSAGES
Adjust-a-dose (for all indications): In patients with bronchospastic disease or liver insufficiency or CrCl less than 40 mL/minute, initially give 2.5 mg; then titrate with caution.

➤ **HTN**
Adults: Initially, 2.5 to 5 mg PO daily alone or with other antihypertensives. May increase to 10 mg daily, then to 20 mg once daily if needed.

➤ **HF with reduced ejection fraction** ◆
Adults: 1.25 mg PO once daily. Titrate gradually up to 10 mg/day.

➤ **Angina** ◆
Adults: 10 mg PO once daily; may increase to maximum dose of 20 mg once daily after at least 1 week if needed.

ADMINISTRATION
PO
• Give drug without regard to meals.
• Store at room temperature.
• Protect from moisture.

ACTION
Selectively blocks cardiac adrenoceptors, reducing resting and exercise HR, decreasing cardiac output, depressing renin secretion, and decreasing tonic sympathetic outflow from vasomotor centers in the brain.

Route	Onset	Peak	Duration
PO	1–2 hr	2–4 hr	Unknown

Half-life: 9 to 12 hours.

ADVERSE REACTIONS
CNS: headache, dizziness, hypoesthesia, insomnia, asthenia, fatigue. **CV:** chest pain, peripheral edema, *bradycardia*. **EENT:** dry mouth, pharyngitis, rhinitis, sinusitis. **GI:** diarrhea, nausea, vomiting. **Hepatic:** increased transaminase levels. **Musculoskeletal:** arthralgia. **Respiratory:** cough, dyspnea, URI. **Skin:** diaphoresis.

INTERACTIONS

Drug-drug. *Antiarrhythmics (disopyramide), calcium channel blockers (diltiazem, verapamil):* May increase myocardial depression or conduction delay. Use together cautiously.
Beta blockers: May increase beta blocker effects to unsafe level. Use together cautiously.
Catecholamine-depleting drugs (guanethidine, reserpine): May cause hypotension or bradycardia. Monitor patient closely.
Clonidine: May cause rebound HTN if clonidine is discontinued. Stop bisoprolol for several days before discontinuing clonidine.
Digoxin: May increase risk of slow AV conduction and bradycardia. Use together cautiously.
Insulin, oral antidiabetics: May mask signs and symptoms of hypoglycemia, particularly tachycardia. Use together cautiously.
Rifampin: May increase bisoprolol metabolism. Monitor patient for decreased bisoprolol effects.

EFFECTS ON LAB TEST RESULTS

• May increase serum triglyceride, AST, ALT, uric acid, creatinine, BUN, potassium, glucose, and phosphorus levels.
• May decrease WBC and platelet counts.
• May cause ANA conversion.

CONTRAINDICATIONS & CAUTIONS

• Contraindicated in patients hypersensitive to drug and in those with cardiogenic shock, overt cardiac failure, second- or third-degree AV block, or marked sinus bradycardia.
• Use cautiously in patients with liver or kidney insufficiency, hyperthyroidism, HF, arterial insufficiency, PVD, or diabetes.
• Use cautiously in patients with a history of severe anaphylactic reaction to a variety of allergens. Patients may be more sensitive if allergen is reintroduced; usual epinephrine doses may not be effective.
• Use cautiously in patients with bronchospastic disease who don't tolerate or respond to other antihypertensive treatment. Patients should have a bronchodilator on hand in the event of an episode.
• Safety and effectiveness in children haven't been established.
Dialyzable drug: No.
⚠ *Overdose S&S:* Bradycardia, hypotension.

PREGNANCY-LACTATION-REPRODUCTION

• There are no adequate and well-controlled studies during pregnancy. Use during pregnancy only if potential benefit justifies fetal risk.
• It isn't known if drug appears in human milk. Use cautiously during breastfeeding.

NURSING CONSIDERATIONS

• Monitor BP closely.
• Avoid use in patients with acute HF because of worsening of disease. If bisoprolol administration is necessary, monitor patient closely.
• Use cautiously in patients with known compensated HF. In patients without a history of HF, drug may precipitate signs and symptoms of new HF. Consider stopping drug at first indication of new HF. Drug may be continued while HF is being treated with other drugs.
• Drug interruption or abrupt discontinuation may exacerbate angina pectoris, MI, or ventricular arrhythmia and may exacerbate the signs and symptoms of hyperthyroidism, possibly leading to thyroid storm. If drug is to be discontinued, taper over approximately 1 week while monitoring patient. If withdrawal signs and symptoms occur, restart drug at least temporarily.
• Drug may mask tachycardia caused by hyperthyroidism. In patients with suspected thyrotoxicosis, withdraw drug gradually to avoid thyroid storm.
• A long-term bisoprolol regimen shouldn't be discontinued before major surgery. However, the impaired ability of the heart to respond to reflex adrenergic stimuli may increase risks of general anesthesia and surgical procedures.
• Drug may mask signs and symptoms of hypoglycemia in patients with diabetes.
• Drug may cause or aggravate signs and symptoms of arterial insufficiency in patients with PVD.

PATIENT TEACHING

• Tell patient to report slowed heartbeat, difficulty breathing, and other signs of HF.
• Caution patient not to discontinue bisoprolol without first consulting health care provider.
• Warn patient with diabetes that bisoprolol may mask signs and symptoms of hypoglycemia (tachycardia, dizziness, weakness).
• Urge patient to use caution when operating automobiles or machinery and performing activities that require alertness.

Reactions in bold italics are *life-threatening*.

SAFETY ALERT!

bivalirudin
bye-VAL-ih-roo-din

Angiomax

Therapeutic class: Anticoagulants
Pharmacologic class: Direct thrombin inhibitors

AVAILABLE FORMS
Injection: 250-mg lyophilized powder/vial;
5 mg/mL solution in 50-mL single-dose vial

INDICATIONS & DOSAGES
➤ **Anticoagulation in patients undergoing PCI, including patients with heparin-induced thrombocytopenia and heparin-induced thrombocytopenia and thrombosis syndrome**
Adults: 0.75 mg/kg IV bolus followed by a continuous infusion of 1.75 mg/kg/hour during the procedure. Check activated clotting time 5 minutes after giving bolus dose. May give additional 0.3 mg/kg bolus dose if needed. Infusion may continue for up to 4 hours after procedure in patients with ST-segment elevation MI.
Adjust-a-dose: For patients with CrCl of 30 mL/minute or less, decrease maintenance infusion rate to 1 mg/kg/hour; for patients on hemodialysis, reduce infusion rate to 0.25 mg/kg/hour. No reduction of bolus dose is needed.

ADMINISTRATION
IV
▼ Lyophilized powder must be reconstituted and diluted. Reconstitute each 250-mg vial with 5 mL of sterile water for injection. Gently swirl until all material is dissolved.
▼ Reconstituted material should be a clear to slightly opalescent, colorless to slightly yellow solution.
▼ Withdraw and discard 5 mL from a 50-mL infusion bag containing D₅W or NSS. Then add contents of reconstituted vial to infusion bag to yield a final concentration of 5 mg/mL.
▼ Store unopened vials at room temperature. Keep reconstituted vials at room temperature or refrigerate for up to 24 hours; don't freeze.
▼ Store premixed solution at 36° to 46° F (2° to 8° C). Use immediately once removed from refrigerator.
▼ Discard remaining unused solution.

▼ **Incompatibilities:** Alteplase, amiodarone, amphotericin B, chlorpromazine, diazepam, dobutamine, prochlorperazine, reteplase, streptokinase, vancomycin.

ACTION
Binds specifically and rapidly to thrombin, inhibiting its effects, thereby producing an anticoagulant effect.

Route	Onset	Peak	Duration
IV	Rapid	Immediate	1–2 hr

Half-life: 25 minutes in patients with normal kidney function.

ADVERSE REACTIONS
CV: *thrombosis.* **Hematologic:** *severe, spontaneous bleeding (cerebral, retroperitoneal, GU, GI).*

INTERACTIONS
Drug-drug. *GPIIa/IIIb inhibitors (abciximab, eptifibatide, tirofiban), heparin, thrombolytics, warfarin:* May increase risk of hemorrhage. Use together cautiously.
Drug-herb. *Herbs with anticoagulant or antiplatelet properties (alfalfa, anise, bilberry, ginseng):* May increase risk of bleeding. Discourage use together.

EFFECTS ON LAB TEST RESULTS
• May decrease Hb level, hematocrit, and platelet count.
• May increase INR.

CONTRAINDICATIONS & CAUTIONS
• Contraindicated in patients hypersensitive to drug or its components and in patients with significant active bleeding.
• Use cautiously in patients undergoing brachytherapy due to an increased risk of thrombus formation and in those with diseases linked to increased bleeding risk.
• Use cautiously in older adults; bleeding events are more common in these patients.
• Safety and effectiveness in children haven't been established.
Dialyzable drug: 25%.
⚠ *Overdose S&S:* Bleeding, death due to hemorrhage.

PREGNANCY-LACTATION-REPRODUCTION
• Use cautiously during pregnancy and only if clearly indicated.

- It's unknown if drug appears in human milk. Use cautiously during breastfeeding.

NURSING CONSIDERATIONS
- Drug has no antidote.
- Monitor coagulation test results, Hb level, and hematocrit before starting therapy and periodically thereafter.
- ⚠ **Alert:** Hemorrhage can occur at any site in the body. If patient has unexplained decrease in hematocrit, decrease in BP, or other unexplained symptoms, suspect hemorrhage.
- Monitor venipuncture sites for bleeding, hematoma, or inflammation.
- Don't give drug IM.

PATIENT TEACHING
- Inform patient that drug can cause bleeding. Instruct patient to immediately report unusual bruising or bleeding (nosebleeds, bleeding gums) or melena.
- Explain that drug is given with aspirin. Caution patient to avoid other aspirin-containing drugs and NSAIDs while receiving this drug.
- Advise patient to consult with prescriber before initiating any herbal therapy; many herbs have anticoagulant, antiplatelet, and fibrinolytic properties.
- Caution patient to avoid activities that carry a risk of injury. Instruct patient to use soft toothbrush and electric razor while taking drug.

SAFETY ALERT!

bleomycin sulfate
blee-oh-MYE-sin

Therapeutic class: Antineoplastics
Pharmacologic class: Cytotoxic glycopeptide antibiotics

AVAILABLE FORMS
Injection: 15-unit vials, 30-unit vials

INDICATIONS & DOSAGES
Adjust-a-dose (for all indications): For patients with CrCl of 40 to 50 mL/minute, give 70% of dose; for CrCl of 30 to 39 mL/minute, give 60% of dose; for CrCl of 20 to 29 mL/minute, give 55% of dose; for CrCl of 10 to 19 mL/minute, give 45% of dose; and for CrCl of 5 to 9 mL/minute, give 40% of dose.

➤ **Squamous cell carcinoma (head, neck, skin, penis, cervix, and vulva), non-Hodgkin lymphoma, testicular carcinoma**
Adults: Because an anaphylactoid reaction is possible, treat patients with lymphoma with 2 units or less for first two doses. If no acute reaction occurs, then follow regular dosage schedule: 0.25 to 0.5 units/kg (10 to 20 units/m^2) IV, IM, or subcut once or twice weekly to maximum total of 400 units.

➤ **Hodgkin lymphoma**
Adults: Because an anaphylactoid reaction is possible, treat patients with lymphoma with 2 units or less for first two doses. If no acute reaction occurs, then follow regular dosage schedule: 0.25 to 0.5 units/kg (10 to 20 units/m^2) IV, IM, or subcut one or two times weekly. After 50% response, maintenance dose is 1 unit IV or IM daily or 5 units IV or IM weekly. Total cumulative dose is 400 units.

➤ **Malignant pleural effusion**
Adults: 60 units given as single-dose bolus intrapleural injection.

ADMINISTRATION
IV
- ⚠ **Alert:** Preparing and giving parenteral form of drug may be mutagenic, teratogenic, and carcinogenic. Use safe handling and disposal.
- ▼ Reconstitute 15-unit or 30-unit vial with 5 or 10 mL, respectively, of NSS yielding 3 units/mL solution.
- ▼ Administer slowly over 10 minutes.
- ▼ Use reconstituted solution within 24 hours.
- ▼ Refrigerate unopened vials containing dry powder.
- ▼ Drug is an irritant and may cause phlebitis. It isn't known to cause tissue damage with extravasation. If signs or symptoms of extravasation occur, immediately stop infusion and institute appropriate care.
- ▼ **Incompatibilities:** Amino acids; aminophylline; amphotericin B conventional/lipid complex/liposome; ascorbic acid injection; cefazolin; dantrolene; diazepam; drugs containing sulfhydryl groups; fluids containing dextrose; furosemide; hydrocortisone; methotrexate; mitomycin; nafcillin; penicillin G; phenytoin; riboflavin; solutions containing divalent and trivalent cations, especially calcium salts and copper; terbutaline sulfate.

Reactions in bold italics are *life-threatening*.

IM
- Dilute 15-unit vial in 1 to 5 mL or 30-unit vial in 2 to 10 mL of sterile water for injection, bacteriostatic water for injection, or NSS for injection.
- Monitor injection site for irritation.

Subcutaneous
- Dilute 15-unit vial in 1 to 5 mL or 30-unit vial in 2 to 10 mL of sterile water for injection, bacteriostatic water for injection, or NSS for injection.
- Monitor injection site for irritation.

Intrapleural
- Dilute 60 units of drug in 50 to 100 mL NSS for injection.
- Give drug through thoracotomy tube.
- If patient's condition requires sclerosis, instill drug when chest tube drainage is 100 to 300 mL/24 hours; ideally, drainage should be less than 100 mL/24 hours. After instillation, clamp thoracotomy tube and move patient from the back to the left then right side several times for the next 4 hours. Remove clamp and reestablish suction. Length of time chest tube is left in place after sclerosis depends on patient's condition.

ACTION
May inhibit DNA synthesis and cause scission of single- and double-stranded DNA; also inhibits RNA and protein synthesis.

Route	Onset	Peak	Duration
IV, IM, subcut	Unknown	30–60 min	Unknown

Half-life: 2 hours.

ADVERSE REACTIONS
CNS: fever. **CV:** chest pain, phlebitis. **GI:** stomatitis, anorexia, nausea, vomiting, diarrhea. **Metabolic:** weight loss, hyperuricemia. **Respiratory:** *pneumonitis, pulmonary fibrosis.* **Skin:** erythema, hyperpigmentation, acne, rash, striae, skin tenderness, pruritus, reversible alopecia, hyperkeratosis, nail changes. **Other:** chills, tumor pain, *anaphylactoid reactions.*

INTERACTIONS
Drug-drug. *Anesthesia:* May increase oxygen requirements. Monitor patient closely.
Brentuximab: May increase risk of pulmonary toxicity. Avoid use together.

Cisplatin: May decrease bleomycin elimination. Monitor kidney function and adjust bleomycin dosage as needed.
Fosphenytoin, phenytoin: May decrease phenytoin and fosphenytoin levels. Monitor drug levels closely.
Nephrotoxic drugs: May decrease bleomycin elimination and increase risk of pulmonary toxicity. Monitor patient closely.
Other antineoplastics: May increase risk of pulmonary toxicities at lower doses. Monitor patient closely.
Oxygen: May increase risk of pulmonary toxicity during surgery due to increased sensitization of lung tissue from bleomycin. Use together cautiously.

EFFECTS ON LAB TEST RESULTS
None reported.

CONTRAINDICATIONS & CAUTIONS
- Contraindicated in patients hypersensitive to drug.
- Use cautiously in patients with kidney or pulmonary impairment.
- **Alert:** Adverse pulmonary reactions are more common in patients older than age 70. Pulmonary toxic adverse effects may be increased in patients receiving radiation therapy, patients with lung disease, and patients who need oxygen therapy.
Dialyzable drug: Unknown.

PREGNANCY-LACTATION-REPRODUCTION
- Drug can cause fetal harm when administered during pregnancy. Inform patient of the fetal risk.
- Patient of childbearing potential should avoid becoming pregnant during therapy.
- It isn't known if drug appears in human milk. Patient should discontinue breastfeeding during therapy, considering importance of drug to patient.

NURSING CONSIDERATIONS
Boxed Warning Drug should be administered under the supervision of a physician experienced in the use of cancer chemotherapeutic agents. ▉
- Pulmonary toxicities are common. Obtain pulmonary function tests before start of treatment and at regular intervals during treatment. If tests show a marked decline, stop drug.

Boxed Warning Fatal pulmonary fibrosis may occur, especially when cumulative dose exceeds 400 units. ■

• Monitor chest X-rays every 1 to 2 weeks and listen to lungs regularly.

Boxed Warning Monitor patient with lymphoma for idiosyncratic reactions (hypotension, confusion, fever, chills, wheezing) after receiving drug. ■

• Severe idiosyncratic reactions can occur, usually after first or second dose. Monitor patient carefully.

• Monitor liver and kidney function.

• Watch for fever, which may be treated with antipyretics. Fever usually occurs within 3 to 6 hours of administration.

• Hodgkin disease and testicular tumor commonly respond within 2 weeks. Response is unlikely after 2 weeks. Squamous cell cancers sometimes require up to 3 weeks for notable improvement.

🔷 *Alert:* Watch for hypersensitivity reactions, which may be delayed for several hours, especially in patients with lymphoma. (Give test dose of 1 to 2 units before first two doses in patients with lymphoma. If no reaction occurs, follow regular dosage schedule.)

PATIENT TEACHING

• Warn patient that hair loss may occur but is usually reversible.

• Tell patient to report adverse reactions promptly and to take infection-control and bleeding precautions.

• Advise patient who is to receive anesthesia to inform anesthesiologist about taking this drug. High oxygen levels inhaled during surgery may enhance pulmonary toxicity of drug.

SAFETY ALERT!

bortezomib
bore-TEZ-oh-mib

Velcade

Therapeutic class: Antineoplastics
Pharmacologic class: Proteasome inhibitors

AVAILABLE FORMS
Powder for injection: 1 mg, 2.5 mg, 3.5 mg
Solution: 3.5 mg/1.4 mL vial

INDICATIONS & DOSAGES

Adjust-a-dose (for all indications): Refer to manufacturer's instructions for toxicity-related dosage adjustments and adjustments for patients on combination therapies.

➤ **Previously untreated multiple myeloma**
Adults: 1.3 mg/m^2 IV bolus over 3 to 5 seconds or subcut in combination with oral melphalan and oral prednisone for nine 6-week treatment cycles. In cycles 1 to 4, give bortezomib twice weekly (days 1, 4, 8, 11, 22, 25, 29, and 32). In cycles 5 to 9, give bortezomib once weekly (days 1, 8, 22, and 29). Separate consecutive doses of drug by at least 72 hours. Prior to initiating any cycle, platelet count should be 70×10^9/L or greater, ANC should be 1×10^9/L or greater, and non-hematologic toxicities should have resolved to grade 1 or baseline.

➤ **Previously untreated mantle cell lymphoma**
Adults: 1.3 mg/m^2 IV bolus over 3 to 5 seconds in combination with IV rituximab, cyclophosphamide, doxorubicin, and oral prednisone for six 3-week treatment cycles. Administer bortezomib first, followed by rituximab. Give bortezomib twice weekly for 2 weeks (days 1, 4, 8, and 11), followed by 10-day rest period on days 12 to 21. Patients who respond at cycle 6 should receive two additional cycles for a total of 8 cycles. Separate consecutive doses of drug by at least 72 hours. Before initiating any cycle other than cycle 1, platelet count should be 100×10^9/L or greater, ANC should be 1.5×10^9/L or greater, Hb level should be at least 8 g/dL or greater, and non-hematologic toxicities should have resolved to grade 1 or baseline.

➤ **Multiple myeloma or mantle cell lymphoma that still progresses after at least one therapy**
Adults: 1.3 mg/m^2 by IV bolus over 3 to 5 seconds or subcut twice weekly for 2 weeks (days 1, 4, 8, and 11), followed by a 10-day rest period (days 12 through 21). This 3-week period is a treatment cycle. For therapy longer than eight cycles, may adjust dosage schedule to once weekly for 4 weeks (days 1, 8, 15, and 22), followed by a 13-day rest period (days 23 through 35). Separate consecutive doses of drug by at least 72 hours.

ADMINISTRATION
🔷 *Alert:* Hazardous drug; use safe handling and disposal precautions.

Reactions in bold italics are *life-threatening*.

• Use caution and aseptic technique when preparing and handling drug. Wear gloves and protective clothing to prevent skin contact.
• Inspect solution before administration. Don't give if solution is discolored or contains particles.
◑ **Alert:** Be aware that the IV and subcut concentrations are different. Confirm that patient is receiving appropriate concentration of drug before administration.

IV

▼ Reconstitute with 3.5 mL of NSS to a final concentration of 1 mg/mL.
▼ Give by IV bolus over 3 to 5 seconds within 8 hours of preparation.
▼ Store reconstituted drug in original vial or a syringe at 77° F (25° C); total storage time must not exceed 8 hours.
▼ Store unopened vial at a controlled room temperature, in original packaging, protected from light.
▼ **Incompatibilities:** None listed by manufacturer. Consult drug compatibility reference for more information.

Subcutaneous

• Reconstitute with 1.4 mL of NSS to a final concentration of 2.5 mg/mL.
• Give within 8 hours of preparation.
• Store reconstituted drug in original vial or a syringe at 77° F (25° C); total storage time must not exceed 8 hours.
• Rotate injection sites. Give new injections at least 1 inch (2.5 cm) from old sites and never in areas that are tender, bruised, reddened, or hard.
• If an injection-site reaction occurs, use a less-concentrated solution (1 mg/mL).

ACTION

Disrupts intracellular homeostatic mechanisms by inhibiting the 26S proteasome, which regulates intracellular levels of certain proteins, causing cells to die.

Route	Onset	Peak	Duration
IV, subcut	Unknown	Unknown	Unknown

Half-life: 40 to 193 hours (1-mg/m^2 dose); 76 to 108 hours (1.3-mg/m^2 dose).

ADVERSE REACTIONS

CNS: anxiety, asthenia, dizziness, dysesthesia, fatigue, fever, headache, insomnia, paresthesia, peripheral neuropathy, neuralgia, rigors, weakness. **CV:** edema, HTN, hypotension, cardiac disease, *hemorrhage.*

EENT: blurred vision. **GI:** abdominal pain, constipation, decreased appetite, diarrhea, dysgeusia, dyspepsia, nausea, vomiting. **Hematologic:** *neutropenia, thrombocytopenia,* anemia, *leukopenia,* lymphopenia. **Hepatic:** *acute liver failure, hepatitis,* hyperbilirubinemia, increased liver enzyme levels. **Metabolic:** dehydration, anorexia, hyperglycemia. **Musculoskeletal:** arthralgia, back pain, bone pain, limb pain, muscle cramps, myalgia. **Respiratory:** cough, dyspnea, pneumonia, URI. **Skin:** alopecia, pruritus, rash, injection-site reaction. **Other:** infection, herpes zoster, herpes simplex.

INTERACTIONS

Drug-drug. *Antihypertensives:* May increase risk of hypotension. Monitor patient's BP closely.
Drugs linked to peripheral neuropathy (amiodarone, antivirals, isoniazid, nitrofurantoin, statins): May worsen neuropathy. Use together cautiously.
Drugs that prolong QT interval (antiarrhythmics [disopyramide, dofetilide, procainamide, quinidine, sotalol], chlorpromazine, dolasetron, droperidol, mefloquine, mesoridazine, moxifloxacin, pentamidine, pimozide, tacrolimus, thioridazine, ziprasidone): May prolong QT interval and increase risk of life-threatening ventricular arrhythmias. Use together with caution.
Oral antidiabetics: May cause hypoglycemia or hyperglycemia. Monitor glucose level closely.
Strong CYP3A4 inducers (rifampin): May reduce drug's effects. Avoid use together.
Strong CYP3A4 inhibitors (ketoconazole): May increase risk of toxicity. Monitor patient closely; consider bortezomib dosage reduction.
Drug-herb. *St. John's wort:* May decrease bortezomib exposure. Avoid use together.
Drug-food. *Grapefruit:* May increase risk of toxicity. Discourage use together.
Green tea: May decrease therapeutic effect of drug. Avoid use together.

EFFECTS ON LAB TEST RESULTS

• May increase liver enzyme, bilirubin, and uric acid levels.
• May decrease calcium level.
• May increase or decrease potassium, sodium, and glucose levels.
• May decrease Hb level and neutrophil and platelet counts.

CONTRAINDICATIONS & CAUTIONS
• Contraindicated in patients hypersensitive to bortezomib, boron, or mannitol.
• Intrathecal administration is contraindicated.
• Use cautiously in patients with liver or kidney impairment or a history of syncope and in those who are dehydrated or receiving other drugs known to cause hypotension.
• Use cautiously in patients with risk factors for, or existing, heart disease. Closely monitor patients for acute HF development or exacerbation and new-onset decreased LVEF.
• Use cautiously in older adults, who may be at greater risk for adverse effects.
Dialyzable drug: Yes.
⚠ *Overdose S&S:* Symptomatic hypotension, thrombocytopenia.

PREGNANCY-LACTATION-REPRODUCTION
• There are no adequate and well-controlled studies during pregnancy. Drug may cause fetal harm. Use during pregnancy isn't recommended.
• Patients of childbearing potential should avoid becoming pregnant and should use effective contraception during treatment and for 7 months after final dose.
• Males with partners of childbearing potential should use effective contraception during treatment and for at least 4 months after final dose.
• It isn't known if drug appears in human milk. Patients shouldn't breastfeed during treatment and for 2 months after final dose.
• Drug may effect fertility.

NURSING CONSIDERATIONS
• Verify pregnancy status before treatment.
• Monitor patient for evidence of neuropathy (burning sensation, hyperesthesia, hypoesthesia, paresthesia, discomfort, neuropathic pain).
• Consider subcut administration for a patient at high risk for or with preexisting peripheral neuropathy.
• Monitor patient closely for PRES-associated symptoms (HTN, headache, visual disturbances, altered mental function, seizures), which may occur after starting drug. PRES can be confirmed only by MRI. If syndrome occurs, stop drug and provide supportive care.

• Monitor for signs and symptoms of TLS (hyperuricemia, hyperkalemia, hyperphosphatemia, hypocalcemia, AKI).
• Monitor for pulmonary and cardiac toxicity (HF, pneumonitis, lung infiltrates).
• Monitor for thrombotic microangiopathy (anemia, thrombocytopenia, confusion, HTN, decreased urine output, edema, fever).
• Monitor glucose level in a patient with diabetes who is taking oral antidiabetics.
• Watch carefully for adverse effects, especially in an older adult.
• Be sure patient has an order for an antiemetic, antidiarrheal, or both to treat drug-induced nausea, vomiting, or diarrhea.
• Provide fluid and electrolyte replacement to prevent dehydration.
• To manage orthostatic hypotension, adjust antihypertensive dosage, maintain hydration status, and give mineralocorticoids or sympathomimetics.
• Dialysis may reduce drug level; give after dialysis.
🔵 *Alert:* Because thrombocytopenia is common, monitor patient's CBC and platelet count carefully during treatment, before each dose, and especially on day 11.

PATIENT TEACHING
• Instruct patient to report all adverse effects.
• Tell patient to notify prescriber about new or worsening peripheral neuropathy.
• Urge patient to use effective contraception during treatment and for 7 months after final dose and not to breastfeed during treatment and for 2 months after final dose.
• Teach patient how to avoid dehydration. Stress need to tell prescriber about dizziness, light-headedness, or fainting spells.
• Tell patient to use caution when driving and performing other hazardous activities because drug may cause fatigue, dizziness, faintness, light-headedness, and doubled or blurred vision.
• Advise patient with diabetes to check blood glucose level frequently if using an oral antidiabetic and to report changes in blood glucose level.
• Caution patient to immediately report bleeding or signs or symptoms of infection.

Reactions in bold italics are *life-threatening*.

B

bosentan ⚚
bow-SEN-tan

Tracleer

Therapeutic class: Vasodilators
Pharmacologic class: Endothelin-receptor antagonists

AVAILABLE FORMS
Tablets: 62.5 mg, 125 mg
Tablets (for suspension): 32 mg

INDICATIONS & DOSAGES
Adjust-a-dose (for all indications): Refer to manufacturer's instructions for toxicity-related dosage adjustments. Discontinue bosentan at least 36 hours before start of ritonavir; at least 10 days after ritonavir start, resume bosentan at recommended initial dose once daily or every other day based on tolerability.

➤ **PAH (WHO Group 1) in patients with WHO/NYHA Class II to IV symptoms to improve exercise ability and decrease rate of clinical worsening** ⚚
Adults: 62.5 mg PO b.i.d. for 4 weeks. If patient weighs 40 kg or more, may increase to maintenance dosage of 125 mg PO b.i.d. If patient weighs less than 40 kg, maintenance dosage is 62.5 mg PO b.i.d.

➤ **To improve pulmonary vascular resistance in PAH (idiopathic or congenital) in children** ⚚
Children older than age 12 weighing more than 40 kg: Initially, 62.5 mg PO b.i.d. After 4 weeks, increase to 125 mg PO b.i.d.
Children older than age 12 weighing less than 40 kg: Initial and maintenance dosage is 62.5 mg PO b.i.d.
Children ages 3 to 12 weighing more than 24 to 40 kg: Initial and maintenance dosage is 64 mg PO b.i.d.
Children ages 3 to 12 weighing more than 16 to 24 kg: Initial and maintenance dosage is 48 mg PO b.i.d.
Children ages 3 to 12 weighing more than 8 to 16 kg: Initial and maintenance dosage is 32 mg PO b.i.d.
Children ages 3 to 12 weighing 4 to 8 kg: Initial and maintenance dosage is 16 mg PO b.i.d.

ADMINISTRATION
PO
❶ *Alert:* Hazardous drug; use safe handling and disposal precautions.
• Give drug in the morning and evening without regard for meals.
• Disperse tablets for oral suspension or dispersible tablet half in a minimal amount of water immediately before administration.
• Store divided dispersible tablet pieces at 68° to 77° F (20° to 25° C) in opened blister for up to 7 days.

ACTION
Specific and competitive antagonist for endothelin-1 (ET-1). ET-1 levels are elevated in patients with PAH, suggesting a pathogenic role for ET-1 in this disease.

Route	Onset	Peak	Duration
PO	Unknown	3–5 hr	Unknown

Half-life: About 5 hours.

ADVERSE REACTIONS
CNS: headache, fatigue, syncope. **CV:** edema, flushing, hypotension, palpitations, chest pain. **EENT:** sinusitis. **GU:** decreased sperm count. **Hematologic:** anemia. **Hepatic:** abnormal transaminase levels, *liver toxicity.* **Musculoskeletal:** arthralgia. **Respiratory:** respiratory tract infection.

INTERACTIONS
Drug-drug. *Clarithromycin:* May increase risk of bosentan liver toxicity and increase active metabolite of clarithromycin. Consider alternate antimicrobial. Monitor patient closely if used together. Stop one or both drugs if an interaction is suspected.
Cyclosporine: May increase bosentan level and decrease cyclosporine level. Use together is contraindicated.
CYP2C9 inhibitor (amiodarone, fluconazole) plus moderate CYP3A inhibitor (amprenavir, diltiazem, erythromycin, fluconazole) or strong CYP3A inhibitor (ketoconazole, itraconazole): May cause large increase in bosentan plasma concentration. Administration of bosentan with a CYP2C9 inhibitor plus a strong or moderate CYP3A inhibitor isn't recommended.
Glyburide: May increase risk of elevated LFT values and decrease levels of both drugs. Use together is contraindicated.

Hormonal contraceptives: May cause contraceptive failure. Patient should use two reliable methods of birth control during treatment and for 1 month after stopping drug.

Ketoconazole: May increase bosentan effect. Watch for adverse effects.

PDE5 inhibitors (sildenafil): May increase bosentan level and decrease sildenafil level. Use together with caution.

Rifampin: May alter bosentan level. Monitor liver function weekly for 4 weeks followed by routine monitoring.

Ritonavir: May increase risk of bosentan toxicity. Dosage adjustment may be needed.

Simvastatin, other statins: May decrease levels of these drugs. Monitor cholesterol levels to assess need to adjust statin dose.

Tacrolimus: May decrease tacrolimus level. Use together cautiously.

Warfarin: May decrease warfarin level. Monitor coagulation tests and adjust warfarin dosage as needed.

EFFECTS ON LAB TEST RESULTS

Boxed Warning May increase AST, ALT, and bilirubin levels. ∎
• May decrease Hb level and hematocrit.

CONTRAINDICATIONS & CAUTIONS

Boxed Warning Only prescribers and pharmacies registered with the Bosentan REMS Program may prescribe and distribute bosentan. ∎
• Contraindicated in patients hypersensitive to drug; reactions may include DRESS syndrome, anaphylaxis, rash, and angioedema.

Boxed Warning Generally avoid using in patients with moderate to severe liver impairment or in those with elevated aminotransferase levels greater than $3 \times$ ULN. ∎
• Use cautiously in patients with Child-Pugh class A liver impairment.

Dialyzable drug: Unlikely.

⚠ *Overdose S&S:* Headache, nausea, vomiting, hypotension, dizziness, blurred vision.

PREGNANCY-LACTATION-REPRODUCTION

Boxed Warning Drug is likely to cause major birth defects. Contraindicated in pregnancy. Verify pregnancy status of patients of childbearing potential before starting drug, monthly during treatment, and 1 month after final dose. ∎

Boxed Warning Patients of childbearing potential must use one highly effective form of contraception (intrauterine device [IUD] or tubal sterilization) or a combination of methods (hormone method with a barrier method or two barrier methods). If a partner's vasectomy is the chosen method of contraception, patient should also use a hormone or barrier method. Ensure patient continues contraception until 1 month after completion of bosentan therapy. ∎

Boxed Warning Contraception failure may result when bosentan is administered with hormonal contraceptives; patient shouldn't use hormonal contraceptives alone when taking bosentan. ∎
• Decreased sperm counts have been observed in patients receiving drug.
• It isn't known if drug appears in human milk. Use during breastfeeding isn't recommended.

NURSING CONSIDERATIONS

Boxed Warning Use of this drug can cause serious liver injury. AST and ALT level elevations may be dose dependent and reversible, so measure these levels before treatment and monthly thereafter, adjusting dosage accordingly. If elevations are accompanied by symptoms of liver injury (nausea, vomiting, fever, abdominal pain, jaundice, unusual lethargy or fatigue) or if bilirubin level increases by $2 \times$ ULN or greater, immediately discontinue drug and notify prescriber. ∎
• Fluid retention and HF may occur. Patient may require diuretics, fluid management, or hospitalization for decompensating HF.
• Monitor patient for pulmonary edema.
• Monitor Hb level after 1 and 3 months of therapy; then every 3 months.
• Gradually reduce dosage before stopping drug.

PATIENT TEACHING

• Teach about proper drug administration and handling.

Boxed Warning Warn patient to avoid becoming pregnant while taking this drug and for 1 month after final dose. Hormonal contraceptives (oral, implantable, and injectable methods) may not be effective when used with this drug. Advise patient to use two acceptable methods of contraception during and for 1 month after treatment with bosentan. A monthly pregnancy test must be performed. ∎
• Inform patient of risk of low sperm count.
• Advise patient of need for regular LFTs and blood counts.

brentuximab vedotin ⌧
bren-TUK-see-mab ve-DOE-tin

Adcetris

Therapeutic class: Antineoplastics
Pharmacologic class: CD30-directed
antibodies

AVAILABLE FORMS
Powder for injection: 50 mg single-use vial

INDICATIONS & DOSAGES
Adjust-a-dose (for all indications): Refer to
manufacturer's instructions for toxicity-
related dosage adjustments and dosage adjustments for patients with liver and kidney
impairment.
➤ **Classic Hodgkin lymphoma (cHL) in
patients at high risk for relapse or progression after autologous hematopoietic stem
cell transplantation (auto-HSCT) consolidation**
Adult: Within 4 to 6 weeks after auto-HSCT
or recovery from auto-HSCT, 1.8 mg/kg IV
every 3 weeks for a maximum of 16 cycles or
until disease progression or toxicity occurs.
Maximum dose, 180 mg.
➤ **Previously untreated stage III or IV
cHL, in combination with chemotherapy**
Adults: 1.2 mg/kg IV infusion every 2 weeks
for a maximum of 12 doses or until disease
progression or unacceptable toxicity occurs.
Maximum dose, 120 mg.
✳ *NEW INDICATION:* **Previously untreated
high-risk cHL, in combination with
doxorubicin, vincristine, etoposide,
prednisone, and cyclophosphamide**
Children ages 2 and older: 1.8 mg/kg IV every 3 weeks for a maximum of 5 doses or until disease progression or unacceptable toxicity occurs. Maximum dose, 180 mg. Give
G-CSF beginning with cycle 1.
Adjust-a-dose: Refer to prescribing information for chemotherapy agents for additional
information.
➤ **Hodgkin lymphoma after failure of
auto-HSCT or after failure of at least two
multiagent chemotherapy regimens in patients who aren't auto-HSCT candidates;
systemic anaplastic large cell lymphoma
(ALCL) after failure of at least one multiagent chemotherapy regimen**
Adults: 1.8 mg/kg IV infusion every 3 weeks
or until disease progression or toxicity occurs.
Maximum dose, 180 mg.
➤ **Relapsed primary cutaneous ALCL or
CD30-expressing mycosis fungoides**
Adults: 1.8 mg/kg IV infusion every 3 weeks
for a maximum of 16 cycles or until disease
progression or toxicity occurs. Maximum
dose, 180 mg.
➤ **Previously untreated systemic ALCL or
other CD30-expressing peripheral T-cell
lymphomas (PTCL), including angioim-
munoblastic T-cell lymphoma and PTCL
not otherwise specified, in combination
with cyclophosphamide, doxorubicin, and
prednisone ⌧**
Adults: 1.8 mg/kg IV infusion every 3 weeks,
with each cycle of chemotherapy for six to
eight doses. Maximum dose, 180 mg.

ADMINISTRATION
IV
🛑 *Alert:* Hazardous drug; use safe handling
and disposal precautions.
▼ Reconstitute each 50-mg vial with 10.5 mL
sterile water for injection to yield a single-
use solution containing 5 mg/mL.
▼ Gently swirl contents; don't shake vial.
Inspect for particulates and discoloration.
▼ Dilute further to yield 0.4 to 1.8 mg/mL
in infusion bag of NSS injection, 5% dextrose injection, or lactated Ringer injection.
Gently mix by inverting bag.
▼ After reconstitution, infuse immediately
or store at 36° to 46° F (2° to 8° C) and use
within 24 hours of reconstitution. Don't
freeze. Discard unused portion left in vial.
▼ Administer drug only by IV infusion over
30 minutes; don't give by IV push or bolus.
▼ **Incompatibilities:** Don't mix or administer drug with other medications or fluids.

ACTION
Disrupts microtubule network of cancer cells,
which induces cell-cycle arrest and apoptotic
death of the cells.

Route	Onset	Peak	Duration
IV	Rapid	1–3 days	Unknown

Half-life: 4 to 6 days.

ADVERSE REACTIONS
CNS: peripheral neuropathy (sensory,
motor), headache, dizziness, fatigue, chills,
insomnia, anxiety, pain, fever. **CV:** peripheral

edema, *PE, supraventricular arrhythmia,* lymphadenopathy. **EENT:** oropharyngeal pain. **GI:** nausea, diarrhea, abdominal pain, vomiting, constipation, decreased appetite. **GU:** pyelonephritis, UTI. **Hematologic: *neutropenia,*** anemia, ***thrombocytopenia.*** **Metabolic:** decreased weight, hyperglycemia. **Musculoskeletal:** arthralgia, myalgia, back pain, extremity pain, muscle spasms. **Respiratory:** URI, cough, dyspnea, pneumonitis, pneumothorax. **Skin:** rash, pruritus, alopecia, night sweats, dry skin, cellulitis. **Other: *septic shock, anaphylaxis,*** immunogenicity, infusion-related reactions.

INTERACTIONS
Drug-drug. *Bleomycin:* Increases risk of pulmonary toxicity. Use together is contraindicated.
Strong CYP3A4 inducers (rifampin): May decrease brentuximab level. Monitor patient for brentuximab effectiveness.
Strong CYP3A4 inhibitors (ketoconazole): May increase brentuximab level. Monitor patient for increased adverse effects.

EFFECTS ON LAB TEST RESULTS
• May increase glucose, transaminase, and bilirubin levels.
• May decrease RBC, WBC, platelet, and neutrophil counts.

CONTRAINDICATIONS & CAUTIONS
• Contraindicated in patients hypersensitive to drug.
Boxed Warning John Cunningham virus infection resulting in progressive multifocal leukoencephalopathy (PML) and death can occur in patients receiving brentuximab. ■
❸ *Alert:* Infusion-related reactions, including anaphylaxis, have occurred. If anaphylaxis occurs, immediately and permanently discontinue drug and initiate appropriate therapy. Interrupt infusion for other infusion-related reactions and treat appropriately. Premedicate (acetaminophen, antihistamine, corticosteroid) patients with prior infusion-related reactions for subsequent infusions.
• Avoid use in patients with severe kidney impairment or moderate or severe liver impairment.
• Serious infections (pneumonia, bacteremia, sepsis, fatal septic shock) have been reported.
Dialyzable drug: Unknown.

PREGNANCY-LACTATION-REPRODUCTION
• Drug may cause fetal harm. Patients of childbearing potential should avoid pregnancy during therapy and for 6 months after therapy ends.
• Drug may damage spermatozoa and testicular tissue, resulting in possible genetic abnormalities. Males with partners of childbearing potential should use effective contraception during therapy and for 6 months after therapy ends.
• Drug may compromise male fertility.
• It isn't known if drug appears in human milk. Use during breastfeeding isn't recommended.

NURSING CONSIDERATIONS
• Drug may cause severe peripheral neuropathy. Monitor patient for new or worsening signs and symptoms.
• Drug may cause liver toxicity, which can be fatal, especially in patients with preexisting liver disease or elevated baseline liver enzymes and in those taking concomitant medications. Monitor patient's liver enzyme and bilirubin levels. Delay or reduce dose, or discontinue drug as clinically indicated.
• Monitor patient closely for infusion-related adverse effects; interrupt therapy and treat as necessary.
• Monitor patient for signs and symptoms of neutropenia and anemia. Monitor CBC before each dose and more frequently if patient exhibits grade 3 or 4 neutropenia. Delay or reduce dose, or discontinue drug as required. May give G-CSF prophylaxis.
• Monitor patient for TLS, characterized by electrolytes changes and kidney damage.
• Monitor patient for skin reactions, especially SJS. Discontinue drug if reactions occur.
Boxed Warning Monitor patient for vision loss, impaired speech, muscle weakness or paralysis, and cognitive deterioration, which may indicate PML. Hold drug for suspected PML; discontinue if diagnosis is confirmed. ■
• Monitor patient for noninfectious pulmonary toxicity (pneumonitis, ILD, ARDS). Hold drug during evaluation of new or worsening pulmonary symptoms and until symptoms improve.
• Monitor patient for infection (bacterial, fungal, or viral) during treatment.
• Monitor for new or worsening GI signs and symptoms of perforation, hemorrhage, erosion, ulcer, intestinal obstruction, enterocolitis, neutropenic colitis, and ileus.

Reactions in bold italics are *life-threatening*.

- Monitor patient for hyperglycemia, exacerbation of preexisting diabetes, and ketoacidosis. Give antidiabetic agent as clinically indicated.
- Verify pregnancy status before therapy.

PATIENT TEACHING
- Tell patient to report muscle weakness or numbness or tingling of the hands or feet.
- Advise patient to report signs or symptoms of possible infection, including temperature of 100.5° F (38° C) or greater, chills, cough, and pain on urination.
- Warn patient to report signs or symptoms of possible infusion-related reactions, including fever; chills; rash; breathing problems (wheezing, cough, chest tightness); blue skin color; and swelling of face, lips, tongue, or throat.
- Instruct patient to immediately report signs or symptoms of PML (changes in mood or unusual behavior, confusion, thinking problems, memory loss, vision changes, altered speech, gait abnormalities, decreased strength on one side of the body).
- Tell patient to report all adverse effects.
- Explain that drug may cause fetal harm. Caution patient to avoid becoming pregnant during and for 6 months after therapy ends and to immediately report possible pregnancy.
- Advise patient that breastfeeding during therapy isn't recommended.
- Caution patient with partner of childbearing potential to use effective contraception during and for 6 months after therapy ends.

brexpiprazole ⚕
brex-PIP-ra-zole

Rexulti

Therapeutic class: Antipsychotics
Pharmacologic class: Atypical antipsychotics

AVAILABLE FORMS
Tablets: 0.25 mg, 0.5 mg, 1 mg, 2 mg, 3 mg, 4 mg

INDICATIONS & DOSAGES
Adjust-a-dose (for all indications): Refer to manufacturer's instructions for drug-interaction dosage adjustments. Reduce

dosage by half in patients who are CYP2D6 poor metabolizers.
➤ **Adjunctive treatment of major depressive disorder (MDD)**
Adults: Initially, 0.5 or 1 mg PO once daily. If starting at 0.5 mg, increase to 1 mg PO once daily after 1 week based on patient's response and tolerability. Then increase to target dose of 2 mg PO once daily after 1 week. Maximum daily dose, 3 mg.
Adjust-a-dose: If Child-Pugh score is 7 or more or CrCl is less than 60 mL/minute, maximum daily dose is 2 mg.
➤ **Schizophrenia**
Adults: Initially, 1 mg PO once daily on days 1 through 4; then titrate to 2 mg PO once daily on days 5 through 7; then increase to 4 mg PO once daily on day 8 based on patient's response and tolerability. Recommended target dose is 2 to 4 mg daily. Maximum daily dose, 4 mg.
Children ages 13 and older: Initially, 0.5 mg PO once daily on days 1 through 4; then titrate to 1 mg PO once daily on days 5 through 7; then increase to 2 mg PO once daily on day 8 based on response and tolerability. Increase by 1 mg weekly, if indicated. Recommended target dose, 2 to 4 mg daily. Maximum dose, 4 mg.
Adjust-a-dose: If Child-Pugh score is 7 or more or CrCl is less than 60 mL/minute, maximum daily dose is 3 mg.

ADMINISTRATION
PO
- Give without regard for food.
- If a dose is missed, give it as soon as possible. If it's close to the time for next dose, skip missed dose and give next dose at the regular time. Don't double-dose.
- Store at 68° to 77° F (20° to 25° C).

ACTION
Exact mechanism unknown. Effect may occur through partial agonist activity at serotonin 5-HT$_{1A}$ and dopamine D$_2$ receptors as well as antagonist activity at serotonin 5-HT$_{2A}$ receptors.

Route	Onset	Peak	Duration
PO	Unknown	4 hr	Unknown

Half-life: 91 hours.

ADVERSE REACTIONS
CNS: fatigue, drowsiness, akathisia, headache, tremor, dizziness, anxiety, restlessness, somnolence, sedation, abnormal dreams, insomnia, extrapyramidal reactions. **EENT:** blurred vision, nasopharyngitis, dry mouth, sialorrhea. **GI:** constipation, dyspepsia, increased appetite, diarrhea, nausea, abdominal pain, flatulence. **GU:** UTI. **Metabolic:** weight gain, increased CK level, increased prolactin level, decreased cortisol level. **Musculoskeletal:** myalgia. **Skin:** hyperhidrosis.

INTERACTIONS
Drug-drug. *Anticholinergics (diphenhydramine, meclizine, scopolamine):* May increase risk of body temperature dysregulation. Use together cautiously.
CNS depressants: May increase CNS depressant effects. Monitor therapy.
Strong CYP2D6 inhibitors (bupropion, fluoxetine, paroxetine, quinidine), strong CYP3A4 inhibitors (clarithromycin, itraconazole, ketoconazole, ritonavir): May increase brexpiprazole concentration. Reduce brexpiprazole dosage.
Strong CYP3A4 inducers (carbamazepine, phenytoin, rifampin): May decrease brexpiprazole concentration. Increase brexpiprazole dosage.
Drug-herb. *St. John's wort:* May decrease brexpiprazole concentration. Increase brexpiprazole dosage.

EFFECTS ON LAB TEST RESULTS
• May increase CK, glucose, triglyceride, and prolactin levels.
• May decrease cortisol level.
• May decrease WBC count.

CONTRAINDICATIONS & CAUTIONS
• Contraindicated in patients hypersensitive to drug or its components.
Boxed Warning Older adults with dementia-related psychosis treated with antipsychotics are at increased risk for death. Drug isn't approved for treatment of patients with dementia-related psychosis. ∎
Boxed Warning Antidepressants increase risk of suicidality in patients younger than age 24. Safety and effectiveness in children with MDD haven't been established. ∎
• Antipsychotics can cause NMS, which can be fatal.

• Antipsychotics can cause possibly irreversible tardive dyskinesia, especially in older adults.
• Atypical antipsychotics are associated with metabolic changes (weight gain, dyslipidemia, hyperglycemia, diabetes).
• Antipsychotics may increase the risk of seizures. Use cautiously in patients with a history of seizures or conditions that could lower the seizure threshold.
• Drug may alter the body's ability to lower the core temperature.
▧ Use cautiously in patients who are poor metabolizers of CYP2D6, in patients with Child-Pugh score of 7 or more liver impairment, and in those with CrCl less than 60 mL/minute; adjust dosage appropriately.
• Use cautiously in patients with preexisting hypotension, CV, or cerebrovascular disease and those who are taking other antihypertensives; drug can cause orthostatic hypotension and syncope.
• Use cautiously in patients at risk for aspiration pneumonia. Esophageal dysmotility and aspiration have been associated with antipsychotic use.
• Antipsychotics can impair thinking, judgment, and motor skills.
• Drug may cause intense impulsive or compulsive behavior urges, particularly for gambling, and the inability to control these urges. Other less frequently reported compulsive urges include sexual urges, shopping, and eating or binge eating.
• Drug may cause somnolence, orthostatic hypotension, and motor and sensory instability, which may lead to falls and, consequently, fractures and other injuries.
• Tablets may contain lactose; avoid use in patients with lactose-intolerant conditions.
• Use cautiously in older adults because of the increased risk of adverse events.
Dialyzable drug: Unlikely.

PREGNANCY-LACTATION-REPRODUCTION
• There are no adequate studies in pregnancy. Neonates exposed to antipsychotics during the third trimester are at risk for extrapyramidal or withdrawal signs and symptoms, which can vary in severity but may require prolonged hospitalization. Routine use during pregnancy isn't recommended; risks and benefits should be considered.
• Enroll patients exposed to drug during pregnancy in the National Pregnancy

Registry for Atypical Antipsychotics by calling 1-866-961-2388 or visiting https://womensmentalhealth.org/research/pregnancyregistry/atypicalantipsychotic/).
• It's unknown if drug appears in human milk. Consider risks and benefits before using during breastfeeding.

NURSING CONSIDERATIONS

Boxed Warning Monitor patient for suicidality, especially during the first few months of treatment and after dosage changes. Consider discontinuing drug in a patient who experiences worsening depression or suicidality. ■

• Monitor for signs and symptoms of NMS (hyperpyrexia, muscle rigidity, mental status changes, tachycardia, BP or pulse changes, diaphoresis, arrhythmias, elevated CK level, rhabdomyolysis, AKI). Discontinue drug if reactions appear, and treat appropriately.
• Monitor blood glucose, triglyceride, and lipid levels; observe for weight changes.
• Regularly monitor patient with diabetes for worsening of glucose control.
• Monitor patient at risk for diabetes (obesity, family history) before and periodically during treatment.
• Monitor patient for seizures, difficulty swallowing, and aspiration.
• Avoid exposing patient to extreme heat; ensure adequate hydration.
• Monitor patient for tardive dyskinesia (involuntary, dyskinetic movements). Periodically reassess need for continued treatment. If tardive dyskinesia develops, consider discontinuing drug.
• Monitor patient with a history of significantly low WBC count or ANC or drug-induced neutropenia frequently during first few months of therapy. Consider discontinuing drug at first sign of significant decline in WBC count; monitor patient for fever and other signs or symptoms of infection. Discontinue drug in patient with severe neutropenia (ANC less than $1,000/mm^3$).
• Monitor for orthostatic hypotension and syncope, especially if patient has dehydration, hypovolemia, history of CV or cerebrovascular disease; is taking antihypertensives; or is antipsychotic-naive. Use lower starting dose and slower titration as needed.
• Complete fall risk assessment when initiating antipsychotic treatment and periodically for patient on long-term therapy, especially if patient has diseases or conditions or is taking other medications that could exacerbate fall risk.
• Monitor patient for impulsive or compulsive behavior urges; consider reducing dosage or stopping drug if any develop.
• Check with pharmacist regarding potential interactions with other drugs that are metabolized via the CYP450 enzyme system in the liver.
• *Look alike–sound alike:* Don't confuse Rexulti with Maxalt.

PATIENT TEACHING

❸ *Alert:* Counsel family members or caregivers to monitor for changes in behavior and to immediately report suicidality to prescriber.
• Explain the potential for dystonic or extrapyramidal symptoms (involuntary, abnormal movements). Instruct patient to immediately report symptoms to prescriber.
• Teach patient with diabetes to closely monitor and report changes in blood glucose level.
• Advise patient to report lactose intolerance before starting therapy.
• Educate patient about risk of metabolic changes, ways to recognize hyperglycemia, and the need for blood tests for glucose and lipid levels.
• Encourage patient to report weight gain.
• Caution patient about risk of orthostatic hypotension and syncope, especially at start of therapy and with dosage changes.
• Advise patient to immediately contact prescriber if patient is or plans to become pregnant or is breastfeeding.
• Remind patient to avoid strenuous exercise, dehydration, and exposure to extreme heat. Encourage patient to drink plenty of water while taking drug.
• Instruct patient to report muscle rigidity, diaphoresis, changes in BP, or irregular heartbeats.
• Warn patient about potential for drug interactions. Advise patient to report to prescriber all OTC drugs, prescription medications, and supplements being taken before start of therapy.
• Advise patient or caregivers to watch for and report new or intense gambling urges, compulsive sexual urges, compulsive shopping, binge or compulsive eating, or other urges.

• Caution patient about risk of impaired judgment, thinking, and motor skills. Advise patient not to perform activities that require mental alertness (operating hazardous machinery and motor vehicles) until drug's effects are known.

brimonidine tartrate
bri-MOE-ni-deen

Alphagan P, Lumify ◊, Mirvaso, Onreltea✦

Therapeutic class: Antiglaucoma drugs–dermatologic agents
Pharmacologic class: Selective alpha₂ agonists

AVAILABLE FORMS
Ophthalmic solution: 0.025% ◊, 0.1%, 0.15%, 0.2%
Topical gel: 0.33%

INDICATIONS & DOSAGES
➤ **To reduce IOP in open-angle glaucoma or ocular HTN**
Adults and children ages 2 and older: 1 drop in affected eye t.i.d., about 8 hours apart.
➤ **Relief of redness of the eye due to minor irritations (OTC only)**
Adults and children ages 5 and older: Instill 1 drop in affected eye every 6 to 8 hours. Don't use more often than q.i.d.
➤ **Persistent facial erythema of rosacea (Mirvaso)**
Adults: Apply a pea-size amount to five areas of the face (central forehead, chin, nose, and each cheek) once daily.

ADMINISTRATION
Ophthalmic
• Don't touch tip of dropper to eye or surrounding tissue.
• If more than one ophthalmic product is being used, give them at least 5 minutes apart.
• Patient should remove contact lenses before administration and wait 10 minutes before reinserting or, if using products that contain benzalkonium chloride, wait 15 minutes.
Topical
• Apply a thin layer across entire face, avoiding the lips and eyes.
• Don't apply to open wounds or irritated skin.

• Wash hands immediately after applying.
• Store at room temperature.

ACTION
Ophthalmic form reduces aqueous humor production and increases uveoscleral outflow. Topical form may reduce erythema through direct vasoconstriction.

Route	Onset	Peak	Duration
Ophthalmic	Unknown	1–4 hr	Unknown
Topical	Unknown	15 days	Unknown

Half-life: Ophthalmic, 3 hours; topical, unknown.

ADVERSE REACTIONS
CNS: asthenia, dizziness, headache, fatigue, somnolence, paresthesia, abnormal taste. **CV:** HTN, hypotension, flushing, chest pain, palpitations. **EENT:** allergic conjunctivitis; ocular hyperemia; pruritus; abnormal vision; allergic reaction; blepharitis; burning; conjunctival edema; conjunctival blanching, corneal staining, corneal erosion; ocular pain, hemorrhage, or inflammation; ocular dryness; eyelid crusting; eyelid edema or erythema; foreign body sensation; increased tearing; pain; photophobia; stinging (ophthalmic only); nasal congestion; nasopharyngitis; rhinitis; sinusitis; dry mouth. **GI:** dyspepsia. **Musculoskeletal:** pain. **Respiratory:** bronchitis, cough, dyspnea. **Skin:** rash; acne rosacea, acne vulgaris, allergic contact dermatitis, dermatitis, erythema, burning sensation, pain (topical only). **Other:** infection, flulike symptoms.

INTERACTIONS
Drug-drug. *Antihypertensives, beta blockers, cardiac glycosides:* May further decrease BP or pulse rate. Monitor vital signs.
Apraclonidine, dorzolamide, pilocarpine, timolol: May have additive IOP-lowering effects. Use together cautiously.
CNS depressants: May increase effects of depressant. Use together cautiously.
Linezolid, MAO inhibitors: May increase effects of brimonidine. Use together cautiously.
TCAs: May interfere with brimonidine's effect. Use together cautiously.
Drug-lifestyle. *Alcohol use:* May increase CNS depressant effect. Discourage use together.

EFFECTS ON LAB TEST RESULTS
None reported.

CONTRAINDICATIONS & CAUTIONS
• Ophthalmic form is contraindicated in patients hypersensitive to drug or its components and in neonates, infants, and children younger than age 2.
• Topical gel is contraindicated in patients hypersensitive to drug or its components; reactions include angioedema, urticaria, and contact dermatitis.
• Use cautiously in patients with CV disease, cerebral or coronary insufficiency, liver or kidney impairment, depression, Raynaud phenomenon, Sjögren syndrome, orthostatic hypotension, or thromboangiitis obliterans.
Dialyzable drug: Unknown.
⚠ *Overdose S&S:* Hypotension.

PREGNANCY-LACTATION-REPRODUCTION
• Use during pregnancy only if potential benefit justifies fetal risk.
• It isn't known if drug appears in human milk. Discontinue drug or discontinue breastfeeding, considering importance of drug to patient.

NURSING CONSIDERATIONS
• Monitor IOP because drug effect may diminish over time.
• Erythema, intermittent flushing, or pallor or excessive whitening may occur after topical application and may resolve when therapy is discontinued.

PATIENT TEACHING
• Teach about proper drug administration and handling.
• Caution patient to avoid hazardous activities because of risk of decreased mental alertness, fatigue, and drowsiness.
• Advise patient to avoid alcohol.

brodalumab
broe-DAL-ue-mab

Siliq

Therapeutic class: Immunomodulators
Pharmacologic class: Interleukin receptor antagonists

AVAILABLE FORMS
Injection: 210 mg/1.5 mL in single-dose, prefilled syringe

INDICATIONS & DOSAGES
➤ **Moderate to severe plaque psoriasis in patients who are candidates for systemic therapy or phototherapy and have failed to respond or have lost response to other systemic therapies**
Adults: 210 mg subcut at weeks 0, 1, and 2; then every 2 weeks. If adequate response doesn't occur after 12 to 16 weeks of treatment, consider discontinuing therapy as success is less likely.

ADMINISTRATION
Subcutaneous
• Allow syringe to reach room temperature (approximately 30 minutes) before injecting. Don't warm in any other way. Don't remove gray needle cap until ready to inject.
• Once syringe has reached room temperature, don't rerefrigerate.
• Don't use drug if cloudy or discolored or if foreign matter is present. A few translucent to white particles may be present.
• Inject the 1.5 mL contained in the single-dose, prefilled syringe to administer a 210-mg dose.
• Inject subcut into thigh, abdomen, or upper outer arm.
• Don't inject into area where skin is tender, bruised, red, hard, thick, scaly, or affected by psoriasis.
• Store drug refrigerated at 36° to 46° F (2° to 8° C) in original carton to protect from light and damage during storage. When necessary, store drug at room temperature up to a maximum of 77° F (25° C) for a maximum single period of 14 days. Discard after 14 days at room temperature.
• Don't freeze or shake syringe or carton filled with syringes.

ACTION
A monoclonal antibody that binds to interleukin-17RA and inhibits proinflammatory cytokines and other inflammatory mediators, leading to decreased inflammation.

Route	Onset	Peak	Duration
Subcut	Unknown	3 days	Unknown

Half-life: Unknown.

ADVERSE REACTIONS
CNS: headache, fatigue. **EENT:** oropharyngeal pain. **GI:** diarrhea, nausea. **Hematologic:** *neutropenia.* **Musculoskeletal:**

arthralgia, myalgia. **Skin:** injection-site reactions, tinea infections. **Other:** flulike symptoms, infections.

INTERACTIONS

Drug-drug. *Cyclosporine:* May decrease effect of cytokines on cyclosporine, a CYP450 substrate. Monitor cyclosporine level; adjust cyclosporine dosage as clinically indicated.
CYP450 substrates: May decrease effect of cytokines on CYP450 substrates. Adjust CYP450 substrate dosage as clinically indicated by drug concentration or therapeutic effect.
Live-virus vaccines: May affect ability to elicit immune response. Avoid use together.
Warfarin: May decrease effect of cytokines on warfarin, a CYP450 substrate. Monitor INR; adjust warfarin dosage as clinically indicated.

EFFECTS ON LAB TEST RESULTS
• May decrease ANC.

CONTRAINDICATIONS & CAUTIONS
• Contraindicated in patients with Crohn disease; drug may worsen disease.
Boxed Warning Suicidality, including completed suicides, have occurred in patients treated with this drug. Before therapy, consider risks and benefits in patients with history of depression or suicidality. ∎
Boxed Warning Because of suicide risk, drug is available only through the restricted SILIQ REMS Program. ∎
• Drug increases risk of infections, including serious infections.
• Drug increases risk of latent TB reactivation.
• Use cautiously in patients with chronic infection or history of recurrent infection.
• Safety and effectiveness in children haven't been evaluated.
Dialyzable drug: Unknown.

PREGNANCY-LACTATION-REPRODUCTION
• There are no human data concerning use during pregnancy. Because human IgG antibodies cross the placental barrier, drug may be transmitted from patient to developing fetus.
• It isn't known if drug appears in human milk. Drug's effects on infants who are breastfed and on milk production are also unknown.

Use only if benefit clearly outweighs risk to infant.

NURSING CONSIDERATIONS
• Discontinue drug if patient develops Crohn disease during therapy.
Boxed Warning Assess for new or worsening suicidality, new-onset or worsening depression, anxiety, and other mood changes. Refer patient to mental health professional, as appropriate. Reevaluate continued use of drug if changes occur. ∎
• Evaluate patient for TB before therapy begins. Consider anti-TB therapy before starting drug in patient with history of latent TB or active TB when an adequate course of TB treatment can't be confirmed.
• Closely monitor for signs and symptoms of active TB during and after treatment.
• Monitor for signs and symptoms of infection (fever, malaise, cough, pain, skin changes, wound or rash with drainage). If a serious infection develops or patient isn't responding to standard treatment for the infection, discontinue drug until infection resolves.
• *Look alike–sound alike:* Don't confuse Siliq with Actiq.

PATIENT TEACHING
Boxed Warning Instruct patient and caregivers to watch for suicidality, new or worsening depression, anxiety, and other mood changes. Tell patient to carry provided Siliq patient wallet card and to call National Suicide Prevention Lifeline (988) if suicidality occurs. ∎
• Explain that drug may lower the ability to fight infection. Tell patient to report signs and symptoms of infection.
• Teach patient to report signs and symptoms of Crohn disease (diarrhea, bloody stools, stomach pain or cramping, sudden or uncontrollable bowel movements, constipation, loss of appetite, weight loss, fever, fatigue).
• Show patient or caregiver drug injection technique, if appropriate. Explain need to follow manufacturer's instructions for use.
• Tell patient not to use a syringe that has been dropped on a hard surface because syringe may have a break (which may or may not be obvious). Instruct patient to use a new syringe and to call 1-800-321-4576.

Reactions in bold italics are *life-threatening*.

budesonide (inhalation, intranasal)
byoo-DES-oh-nide

Pulmicort Flexhaler, Pulmicort Nebuamp✦, Pulmicort Respules, Pulmicort Turbuhaler✦, Rhinocort Allergy ◇

Therapeutic class: Corticosteroids
Pharmacologic class: Corticosteroids

AVAILABLE FORMS
Dry powder inhaler: 90 mcg/dose, 100 mcg/dose✦, 180 mcg/dose, 200 mcg/dose✦, 400 mcg/dose✦
Inhalation suspension (Respules): 0.25 mg/2 mL, 0.5 mg/2 mL, 1 mg/2 mL
Nasal spray: 32 mcg/metered spray ◇, 64 mcg/metered spray✦

INDICATIONS & DOSAGES
➤ **As a preventative in maintenance of asthma**
Adjust-a-dose: For all inhaled formulations, use lowest effective dose after stabilizing asthma.
Adults (Flexhaler): Initially, inhaled dose of 360 mcg b.i.d. to maximum of 720 mcg b.i.d. Starting dose of 180 mcg b.i.d. may be adequate in some adults.
Adults and children ages 12 and older when treatment with inhaled glucocorticoids is started, during periods of severe asthma, and while oral glucocorticoids are being reduced or discontinued (Turbuhaler): Initially, inhaled dose of 400 to 2,400 mcg daily divided into two to four administrations. Maintenance dose is usually 200 to 400 mcg b.i.d. Use lowest dose needed to control symptoms.
Children ages 6 to 17 (Flexhaler): Initially, inhaled dose of 180 mcg b.i.d. to maximum of 360 mcg b.i.d. Starting dose of 360 mcg b.i.d. may be appropriate in some children.
Children ages 6 to 12 when beginning budesonide, during periods of severe asthma, and while oral corticosteroids are being reduced or discontinued (Turbuhaler): Initially, inhaled dose of 100 to 200 mcg b.i.d. For maintenance, use lowest dose necessary to control symptoms.
Children ages 1 to 8 previously taking bronchodilator alone: 0.5 mg daily or 0.25 mg b.i.d. suspension via jet nebulizer. Maximum dose, 0.5 mg/day.
Children ages 1 to 8 previously taking inhaled corticosteroid: 0.5 mg daily or 0.25 mg b.i.d. suspension via jet nebulizer to maximum dose of 1 mg/day.
Children ages 1 to 8 previously taking oral corticosteroid: 1 mg daily or 0.5 mg b.i.d. suspension via jet nebulizer. Maximum dose, 1 mg/day.
Adjust-a-dose: Symptomatic children not responding to nonsteroidal therapy may require starting dose of 0.25 mg suspension daily.
➤ **Symptoms of seasonal or perennial allergic rhinitis**
Adults and children ages 12 and older: 1 to 2 sprays in each nostril once daily. Once allergy symptoms improve, reduce to 1 spray in each nostril daily. Maximum dose, 4 sprays (256 mcg) per nostril once daily.
Children age 6 to younger than age 12: 1 spray per nostril daily. If allergy symptoms don't improve, may increase to 2 sprays per nostril daily. Once allergy symptoms improve, reduce to 1 spray in each nostril daily. Maximum dose for 32 mcg/actuation, 2 sprays per nostril daily (128 mcg). Maximum dose for 64 mcg/actuation, 2 sprays per nostril daily (256 mcg).

ADMINISTRATION
Inhalational
• Give inhalation suspension at regular intervals daily or b.i.d., as directed.
• Give suspension with a jet nebulizer connected to a compressor with adequate airflow. Make sure that it's equipped with a mouthpiece or suitable face mask.
• Total daily dose may be increased or given as a divided dose to improve control if needed. Titrate dosage downward again after asthma is stabilized.
• When aluminum foil envelope has been opened, the shelf-life of unused ampules is 2 weeks when protected from light.
• Refer to manufacturer's instructions before use. Prime inhaler before first use. Have patient inhale deeply and forcefully each time unit is used.
• Remind patient to rinse mouth with water without swallowing after inhalation.
• Discard inhaler after 60 (90-mcg dose) or 120 (180-mcg dose) actuations.

Intranasal

• Prime pump by actuating eight times before first use. Reprime pump with one spray or until a fine spray appears if not used for 2 or more days. Discard bottle after 120 sprays.

• If applicator hasn't been used for 14 days or more, rinse it and reprime with two sprays or until a fine mist appears.

• Shake before each actuation.

• To instill intranasal drug, have patient blow nose to clear nasal passages and tilt head slightly forward. Insert nozzle into nostril, pointing away from septum. Have patient hold other nostril closed and inhale gently during spraying. Next, shake container and repeat in other nostril. Instruct patient to avoid blowing nose for 15 minutes after administration.

• Wipe spray tip clean with a clean tissue.

• Store nasal canister with valve upward and away from extreme heat or cold.

ACTION

Exhibits potent glucocorticoid activity and weak mineralocorticoid activity. Inhibits mast cells, macrophages, and mediators (such as leukotrienes) involved in inflammation.

Route	Onset	Peak	Duration
Inhalation, powder	24 hr	1–2 wk	Unknown
Inhalation, Respules	2–8 days	4–6 wk	Unknown
Intranasal	10 hr	2 wk	Unknown

Half-life: Inhalation and intranasal, 2 to 3 hours.

ADVERSE REACTIONS

CNS: headache, asthenia, fever, hypertonia, insomnia, pain, syncope, taste perversion, fatigue, emotional lability. **CV:** chest pain. **EENT:** conjunctivitis, nasopharyngitis, nasal congestion, oral candidiasis, otitis media, otitis externa, sinusitis, rhinitis, voice alteration, dry mouth (inhalation), epistaxis and nasal irritation (intranasal). **GI:** abdominal pain, dyspepsia, diarrhea, gastroenteritis, nausea, vomiting, anorexia. **Metabolic:** weight gain. **Musculoskeletal:** back pain, fractures, myalgia. **Respiratory:** respiratory tract infection, *bronchospasm,* increased cough, stridor. **Skin:** ecchymoses, rash, dermatitis, pruritus, eczema. **Other:** flulike symptoms, hypersensitivity reactions, viral infection, cervical lymphadenopathy.

INTERACTIONS

Drug-drug. *Strong CYP3A4 inhibitors (atazanavir, clarithromycin, itraconazole, ketoconazole, nefazodone, nelfinavir, ritonavir, saquinavir, telithromycin):* May inhibit metabolism and increase level of budesonide. Monitor patient for adverse reactions and adjust dosage as needed.

EFFECTS ON LAB TEST RESULTS

None reported.

CONTRAINDICATIONS & CAUTIONS

• Contraindicated in patients hypersensitive to drug, in those with severe hypersensitivity to milk proteins (powder for inhalation), and in those with status asthmaticus or other acute asthma episodes.

• Use nasal formulation cautiously in patients with septal ulcers, nasal surgery, nasal trauma, or untreated localized nasal mucosa infections.

• Use cautiously, if at all, in patients with active or inactive TB, ocular HSV infections, or untreated systemic fungal, bacterial, viral, or parasitic infections.

Dialyzable drug: Unlikely.

⚠ *Overdose S&S:* Hyperadrenocorticism.

PREGNANCY-LACTATION-REPRODUCTION

• Hypoadrenalism may occur in infants of patients who received corticosteroids during pregnancy. Monitor these infants carefully.

• Studies during pregnancy of patients using inhaled or intranasal form haven't shown increased risk of abnormalities. Inhaled corticosteroids are recommended for treatment of asthma during pregnancy.

• Drug appears in human milk. Patient should use lowest possible dose immediately after breastfeeding to maximize time between dose and breastfeeding.

NURSING CONSIDERATIONS

🔹 *Alert:* When transferring from systemic corticosteroid to inhalation drug, use caution and gradually decrease corticosteroid dose to prevent adrenal insufficiency.

• Inhalation drug doesn't remove the need for systemic corticosteroid therapy in some situations.

• Systemic effects of corticosteroid therapy may occur if recommended daily dosage is exceeded.

Reactions in bold italics are *life-threatening*.

- If bronchospasm occurs after inhalation use, stop therapy and treat with a bronchodilator.
- Lung function may improve within 24 hours of starting therapy, but maximum benefit may not occur for 1 to 2 weeks or longer.
- For Pulmicort Respules, lung function improves in 2 to 8 days, but maximum benefit may not occur for 4 to 6 weeks.
- Watch for *Candida* infections of the mouth or pharynx.
- ⚠️ *Alert:* Corticosteroids may increase risk of developing serious or fatal infections in patients exposed to viral illnesses, such as chickenpox and measles.
- In rare cases, inhaled corticosteroids have been linked to increased IOP and cataract development. Stop drug if local irritation occurs.
- Monitor bone mineral density in patient at risk for decreased bone mineral content (prolonged immobilization, family history of osteoporosis, postmenopausal status).
- Monitor a child for reduction in growth velocity. Use lowest effective dose.
- Monitor patient for hypercorticism and adrenal suppression and, if they occur, slowly reduce dosage.
- Rare cases of vasculitis (eosinophilic granulomatosis with polyangiitis) and other eosinophilic conditions have occurred when systemic corticosteroids have been reduced or withdrawn. Monitor patient for eosinophilia, vasculitic rash, worsening pulmonary symptoms, cardiac symptoms, and neuropathy.

PATIENT TEACHING
- Tell patient that budesonide inhaler isn't a bronchodilator and isn't intended to treat acute episodes of asthma.
- Instruct patient to use inhaler according to manufacturer's instructions at regular intervals because effectiveness depends on twice-daily use on a regular basis.
- Tell patient that improvement in asthma control may occur within 24 hours but maximum benefit may not occur for 1 to 2 weeks. Instruct patient to contact prescriber if signs or symptoms worsen during this time.
- Advise that drug may increase risk of infection. Instruct patient to avoid exposure to TB, chickenpox, and measles and to contact prescriber if exposure occurs.
- Instruct patient using inhaler to carry or wear medical identification indicating need

for supplementary corticosteroids during periods of stress or an asthma attack.
- Tell patient to read and follow patient information leaflet contained in package.
- Advise patient using nasal formula to notify prescriber if signs or symptoms don't improve or if they worsen in 2 weeks.
- Teach patient good nasal and oral hygiene. Instruct patient not to share drug to prevent spread of infection.

budesonide (oral, rectal)
byoo-DES-oh-nide

Ortikos, Tarpeyo, Uceris

Therapeutic class: Corticosteroids
Pharmacologic class: Glucocorticoids

AVAILABLE FORMS
Capsules (delayed-release 🚫*:* 3 mg, 4 mg, 6 mg, 9 mg
Foam: 2 mg/actuation
Tablets (extended-release 🚫*:* 9 mg

INDICATIONS & DOSAGES
Adjust-a-dose (for all indications): In patients with moderate to severe liver disease who have increased signs or symptoms of hypercorticism, reduce dosage or avoid use.
➤ **Mild to moderate active Crohn disease involving the ileum, ascending colon, or both (capsules)**
Adults: 9 mg PO once daily in the morning for up to 8 weeks. For recurrent episodes of active Crohn disease, may repeat 8-week course.
Children ages 8 to 17 weighing more than 25 kg: 9 mg PO once daily in the morning for up to 8 weeks, followed by 6 mg once daily in the morning for 2 weeks.
➤ **To maintain remission in mild to moderate Crohn disease that involves the ileum or ascending colon (capsules)**
Adults: 6 mg PO daily in the morning for up to 3 months. Taper dosage to complete cessation after 3 months. Therapy for longer than 3 months doesn't have added benefit.
➤ **Induction of remission in active mild to moderate ulcerative colitis (tablets)**
Adults: 9 mg PO once daily in the morning for up to 8 weeks.
➤ **Induction of remission in mild to moderate distal ulcerative colitis (rectal foam)**

Adults: 2 mg (1 metered dose) PR b.i.d. for 2 weeks then 2 mg PR once daily for 4 weeks.

➤ **Proteinuria in patients with primary IgA neuropathy at risk for rapid disease progression (Tarpeyo)**
Adults: 16 mg PO daily in the morning at least 1 hour before a meal for 9 months.
Adjust-a-dose: Reduce dosage to 8 mg daily for 2 weeks before discontinuing drug.

ADMINISTRATION
PO
• Have patient swallow drug whole; don't break, crush or cut capsules or tablets.
• For patients unable to swallow an intact capsule: Open capsule containing pellets, mix contents with 1 tablespoon of applesauce, and have patient consume within 30 minutes of mixing. Follow with a full glass of water. Verify formulation with pharmacist before opening capsule. For other formulations (Ortikos, Uceris, Tarpeyo): Instruct patient to swallow whole and not chew, crush, or open.
Rectal
• Have patient empty bowels before use. When giving in the evening, patient should try not to empty bowels again before morning.
• Attach applicator to canister nozzle. Warm canister in the hands while shaking it for 10 to 15 seconds.
• Unlock canister top; then turn it upside down and insert applicator tip into rectum.
• Push down on pump dome for 2 seconds and hold applicator in place for 10 to 15 seconds.
• Withdraw and discard used applicator.

ACTION
Significant glucocorticoid effects caused by drug's high affinity for glucocorticoid receptors.

Route	Onset	Peak	Duration
PO	Unknown	0.5–10 hr	Unknown
PO (extended-release)	Unknown	7.4–19.2 hr	Unknown
Rectal	Unknown	Unknown	Unknown

Half-life: 2 to 8 hours.

ADVERSE REACTIONS
CNS: headache, dizziness, asthenia, hyperkinesia, paresthesia, tremor, weakness, vertigo, fatigue, malaise, agitation, confusion, drowsiness, insomnia, nervousness, somnolence, pain, sleep disorder, fever. **CV:** chest pain, HTN, edema, palpitations, tachycardia,

flushing. **EENT:** facial edema, eye abnormality, abnormal vision, ear infection, sinusitis, rhinitis, pharyngeal disorder, glossitis, tooth disorder. **GI:** nausea, diarrhea, dyspepsia, abdominal pain, flatulence, vomiting, anal disorder, aggravated Crohn disease, enteritis, epigastric pain, fistula, glossitis, hemorrhoids, intestinal obstruction, increased appetite, abdominal distention, constipation. **GU:** dysuria, micturition frequency, nocturia, intermenstrual bleeding, menstrual disorder, hematuria, pyuria, UTI. **Hematologic:** leukocytosis, anemia. **Metabolic:** hypercorticism, adrenocortical insufficiency, *hypokalemia,* increased weight. **Musculoskeletal:** back pain, aggravated arthritis, cramps, arthralgia, myalgia. **Respiratory:** respiratory tract infection, bronchitis, dyspnea. **Skin:** acne, alopecia, dermatitis, eczema, skin disorder, diaphoresis, purpura, hirsutism, bruising. **Other:** flulike disorder, candidiasis, viral infection.

INTERACTIONS
Drug-drug. *CYP3A4 inhibitors (cyclosporine, erythromycin, itraconazole, ketoconazole, ritonavir, saquinavir):* May increase effects of budesonide. If use together is unavoidable, reduce budesonide dosage.
Gastric acid secretion inhibitors (antacids, H_2 blockers, PPIs): May affect dissolution of extended-release budesonide. Avoid use together or separate administration times by as much as possible and monitor clinical response to budesonide.
Drug-food. *Grapefruit juice:* May increase drug effects. Discourage use together.

EFFECTS ON LAB TEST RESULTS
• May increase ALP and C-reactive protein levels. May decrease potassium, cortisol, and Hb levels.
• May increase erythrocyte sedimentation rate and WBC count.

CONTRAINDICATIONS & CAUTIONS
• Contraindicated in patients hypersensitive to drug.
• Use cautiously in patients with HTN, diabetes, osteoporosis, liver impairment, peptic ulcer disease, glaucoma, or cataracts; those with a family history of diabetes or glaucoma; and those with any other condition in which glucocorticoids may have unwanted effects.

Reactions in bold italics are *life-threatening*.

• Use cautiously, if at all, in patients with active or inactive TB, ocular HSV infection, or untreated systemic fungal, bacterial, viral, or parasitic infection.
Dialyzable drug: Unlikely.
⚠ *Overdose S&S:* Hypercorticism, adrenal suppression.

PREGNANCY-LACTATION-REPRODUCTION
• Drug may be used cautiously during pregnancy for induction of remission in patients with inflammatory bowel disease. Use only if potential benefit justifies fetal risk.
• Monitor infants born to patients receiving corticosteroids during pregnancy for signs and symptoms of hypoadrenalism (poor feeding, irritability, weakness, vomiting).
• Glucocorticoids appear in human milk, and infants may have adverse reactions. Use cautiously during breastfeeding and only if benefits outweigh risks.

NURSING CONSIDERATIONS
• Reduced liver function affects elimination of this drug; systemic availability of drug may increase in patient with liver cirrhosis. Consider dosage reduction or discontinue drug in patient with severe liver dysfunction.
• Patient undergoing surgery or other stressful situation may need systemic glucocorticoid supplementation in addition to budesonide therapy.
• Carefully monitor for signs and symptoms of corticosteroid withdrawal in patient transferred from systemic glucocorticoid therapy to budesonide.
• Watch for immunosuppression, especially in patient who hasn't had chickenpox or measles; these diseases can be fatal in patients who are immunosuppressed or receiving glucocorticoids.
• Replacement of systemic glucocorticoids with this drug may unmask allergies, such as eczema and rhinitis, which were previously controlled by systemic drug.
• Long-term use of drug may cause hypercorticism and adrenal suppression.

PATIENT TEACHING
• Teach about proper drug administration and handling, including the need to keep foam away from flame.
• Advise patient to avoid grapefruit juice while taking drug.

• Tell patient to immediately notify prescriber of exposure to TB, chickenpox, or measles or development of signs and symptoms of infection during treatment.

bumetanide
byoo-MET-a-nide

Burinex ✤

Therapeutic class: Diuretics
Pharmacologic class: Loop diuretics

AVAILABLE FORMS
Injection: 0.25 mg/mL
Tablets: 0.5 mg, 1 mg, 2 mg, 5 mg ✤

INDICATIONS & DOSAGES
➤ **Edema caused by HF or liver or kidney disease**
Adults: 0.5 to 2 mg PO once daily. If diuretic response isn't adequate, give second and third doses at 4- to 5-hour intervals. Or (recommended as safest and most effective method for continued control of edema) give on an intermittent-dose schedule on alternate days or for 3 to 4 days with rest periods of 1 to 2 days in between. Maximum, 10 mg daily.
  May give parenterally if oral route isn't possible or if risk of impaired GI absorption exists. Usual first dose is 0.5 to 1 mg IV or IM. If response isn't adequate, give second and third doses at 2- to 3-hour intervals. Maximum, 10 mg daily. Institute oral treatment as soon as possible.

ADMINISTRATION
PO
• To prevent nocturia, give drug in the morning. If second dose is needed, give in the early afternoon.
IV
▼ For direct injection, give drug over 1 to 2 minutes.
▼ For intermittent infusion, give diluted drug through an intermittent infusion device or piggyback into an IV line containing a free-flowing, compatible solution.
▼ Solutions should be freshly prepared and used within 24 hours. Protect from light.
▼ **Incompatibilities:** None listed by manufacturer. Consult drug compatibility reference for more information.

IM
• Document injection site.

ACTION
Inhibits sodium and chloride reabsorption in the ascending loop of Henle.

Route	Onset	Peak	Duration
PO	30–60 min	1–2 hr	4–6 hr
IV	Within min	15–30 min	2–3 hr
IM	40 min	Unknown	5–6 hr

Half-life: 1 to 1.5 hours.

ADVERSE REACTIONS
CNS: dizziness, headache. **CV:** hypotension. **EENT:** impaired hearing. **GU:** increased creatinine level, azotemia. **Hepatic:** increased LDH level. **Metabolic:** volume depletion, dehydration, *hypokalemia,* hypochloremia, *hypomagnesemia,* hyperuricemia, hyponatremia, hyperglycemia. **Musculoskeletal:** muscle cramps.

INTERACTIONS
Drug-drug. *Aminoglycoside antibiotics:* May increase ototoxicity risk. Avoid use together if possible.
Antidiabetics: May decrease hypoglycemic effects. Monitor glucose level.
Antihypertensives: May increase hypotensive effects. Consider dosage adjustment.
Cardiac glycosides: May increase risk of digoxin toxicity from bumetanide-induced hypokalemia. Monitor potassium and digoxin levels.
Cisplatin: May increase risk of ototoxicity and nephrotoxicity. Monitor patient closely.
Lithium: May decrease lithium clearance, increasing risk of lithium toxicity. Monitor lithium level.
Neuromuscular blockers: May prolong neuromuscular blockade. Monitor patient closely.
NSAIDs, probenecid: May inhibit diuretic response. Avoid use together.
Other potassium-wasting drugs (amphotericin B, corticosteroids): May increase risk of hypokalemia. Use together cautiously.
Drug-herb. *Licorice:* May cause unexpected, rapid potassium loss. Discourage use together.

EFFECTS ON LAB TEST RESULTS
• May increase ALP, ALT, AST, bilirubin, protein, cholesterol, creatinine, glucose, LDH, BUN, and urine urea levels.

• May decrease calcium, magnesium, potassium, sodium, and chloride levels.
• May decrease platelet count.

CONTRAINDICATIONS & CAUTIONS
• Contraindicated in patients hypersensitive to drug and in patients with anuria, hepatic coma, or severe electrolyte depletion.
• Patients allergic to sulfonamides may show hypersensitivity to bumetanide.
• Use cautiously in patients with cirrhosis and ascites or decreased kidney function and in older adults.
Dialyzable drug: Unknown.
⚠ *Overdose S&S:* Electrolyte depletion, weakness, dizziness, confusion, anorexia, lethargy, vomiting, cramps, dehydration, circulatory collapse, vascular thrombosis, and embolism.

PREGNANCY-LACTATION-REPRODUCTION
• There are no adequate well-controlled studies during pregnancy. Use during pregnancy only if potential benefits justify fetal risk.
• Use during breastfeeding isn't recommended.

NURSING CONSIDERATIONS
Boxed Warning Profound diuresis with electrolyte depletion can occur. Adjust dosage and dosing schedule to individual patient's needs; careful medical supervision is required. ▪
• Frequently monitor fluid intake and output, weight, and electrolyte, BUN, creatinine, and carbon dioxide levels, especially in older adults.
• Watch for evidence of hypokalemia, such as muscle weakness and cramps.
• Consult prescriber and dietitian about a high-potassium diet.
• Monitor glucose level in patient with diabetes.
• Monitor uric acid level, especially in patient with history of gout.
• If oliguria or azotemia develops or increases, prescriber may stop drug.
• Drug can be safely used in patient allergic to furosemide; 1 mg of bumetanide equals about 40 mg of furosemide.
• Monitor patient for ototoxicity, especially when drug is given IV, at high doses, and in combination with other ototoxins.

PATIENT TEACHING
• Instruct patient to weigh self daily to monitor fluid status.

Reactions in bold italics are *life-threatening*.

- Advise patient to take drug in the morning to avoid need to urinate at night. Tell patient who needs second dose to take it in the early afternoon.
- Caution patient to avoid sudden posture changes and to rise slowly to avoid dizziness upon standing quickly.
- Teach patient to eat foods rich in potassium, such as citrus fruits, tomatoes, bananas, dates, and apricots.
- Instruct patient to notify prescriber about extreme thirst, muscle weakness, cramps, nausea, or dizziness.

SAFETY ALERT!

buprenorphine
byoo-pre-NOR-feen

Brixadi, Butrans, Sublocade

buprenorphine hydrochloride
Belbuca, Buprenex

Therapeutic class: Opioid analgesics
Pharmacologic class: Opioid agonist-antagonists–opioid partial agonists
Controlled substance schedule: III

AVAILABLE FORMS
Buccal film: 75 mcg, 150 mcg, 300 mcg, 450 mcg, 600 mcg, 750 mcg, 900 mcg
Injection: 0.324 mg (equivalent to 0.3 mg base/mL)
Injection (extended-release): 100 mg/0.5 mL, 300 mg/1.5 mL prefilled syringes
Injection (extended-release weekly): 8 mg/0.16 mL, 16 mg/0.32 mL, 24 mg/0.48 mL, 32 mg/0.64 mL prefilled syringes
Injection (extended-release monthly): 64 mg/0.18 mL, 96 mg/0.27 mL, 128 mg/0.36 mL prefilled syringes
Sublingual tablets ⓪ 2 mg, 8 mg
Transdermal patch: 5 mcg/hour, 7.5 mcg/hour, 10 mcg/hour, 15 mcg/hour, 20 mcg/hour

INDICATIONS & DOSAGES
➤ **Moderate to severe pain**
Adults and children ages 13 and older: 0.3 mg IM or slow IV (over at least 2 minutes) every 6 hours PRN or around the clock; repeat dose once (up to 0.3 mg), as needed, 30 to 60 minutes after first dose.

Children ages 2 to 12: 2 to 6 mcg/kg IM or slow IV (over at least 2 minutes) every 4 to 6 hours.
Adjust-a-dose: In patients at high risk, such as older adults and patients who are debilitated, use minimum dose required. May increase a single IM dose to 0.6 mg for severe pain in adults who aren't high risk.
➤ **Moderate to severe chronic pain in patients requiring continuous opioid analgesia for an extended period of time for whom alternative treatment options are inadequate**
Adults (opioid-naive): 5 mcg/hour transdermal patch once every 7 days. May titrate dosage to maximum of 20 mcg/hour. Allow a minimum of 72 hours between dosage increases. Or, 75 mcg buccal film once daily or, if tolerated, every 12 hours for at least 4 days; then increase to 150 mcg every 12 hours. May titrate dosage as needed in increments of 150 mcg every 12 hours, no more frequently than every 4 days. Maximum, 450 mcg every 12 hours.
Adults (non-opioid-naive): Buprenorphine may precipitate withdrawal in patients already on opioids. For conversion from other opioids to transdermal buprenorphine, taper patient's current around-the-clock opioids for up to 7 days to no more than morphine 30 mg or equivalent per day before beginning treatment with buprenorphine. Patients may use short-acting analgesics as needed until analgesic efficacy with buprenorphine is attained. For patients whose daily dose was less than morphine 30 mg PO or equivalent, initiate treatment with buprenorphine transdermal patch 5 mcg/hour. For patients whose daily dose was between 30 and 80 mg of morphine equivalents, initiate treatment with buprenorphine transdermal patch 10 mcg/hour.

For patients whose daily dose was greater than 80 mg of morphine equivalents, buprenorphine transdermal system 20 mcg/hour may not provide adequate analgesia. Consider use of an alternative analgesic.

May titrate dosage to maximum of 20 mcg/hour transdermal patch once every 7 days. Allow minimum of 72 hours between dosage increases. If patch must be discontinued, gradually taper dosage every 7 days to prevent withdrawal in patient who is physically dependent; consider initiating immediate-release opioids, if needed.

Or, for conversion from other opioids to buccal buprenorphine, taper dosage to no more than 30 mg PO morphine sulfate equivalents (MSE) per day. For patients taking less than 30 mg PO MSE per day, start treatment with 75 mcg buccal film once daily or every 12 hours. For patients taking between 30 and 89 mg PO MSE, start treatment with 150 mcg every 12 hours. For patients taking between 90 and 160 mg PO MSE, start treatment with 300 mg every 12 hours. Buccal buprenorphine may not provide adequate analgesia for patients requiring greater than 160 mg PO MSE per day. Consider using an alternative analgesic. Titrate dosage in increments of 150 mcg every 12 hours, no more frequently than every 4 days to a maximum dose of 900 mcg every 12 hours.

To discontinue buccal therapy, gradually taper dosage while carefully monitoring patient for signs and symptoms of withdrawal. If patient develops withdrawal signs or symptoms, increase dosage to previous level and taper more slowly by increasing the interval between decreases, decreasing the amount of change in dose, or both.

Adjust-a-dose: Transdermal buprenorphine hasn't been evaluated in patients with Child-Pugh class C liver impairment. Consider use of an alternative analgesic that may permit more dosing flexibility in these patients.

Adjust-a-dose: In patients with Child-Pugh class C liver impairment, reduce buccal starting dose and reduce buccal titration dose by half that of patients with normal liver function, from 150 to 75 mcg. In patients with known or suspected mucositis, reduce starting dosage and titration incremental dosage by half compared to patients without mucositis.

➤ **Opioid use disorder**

Adults: 8 mg SL on day 1 and 16 mg SL on day 2. Titrate buprenorphine dosage in increments or decrements of 2 or 4 mg to a level that holds patient in treatment and suppresses opioid withdrawal signs and symptoms. Maintenance dose is generally in the range of 4 to 24 mg SL per day. Recommended target dosage is 16 mg as a single daily dose. Continue treatment for as long as patient is benefiting and drug contributes to intended treatment goals.

✱ *NEW INDICATION:* **Moderate to severe opioid use disorder in patients who have initiated treatment with a single dose of a transmucosal buprenorphine-containing product, or who are already being treated with buprenorphine (Brixadi)**

Adults: Individualize dose based on tolerability or efficacy. After a test dose of 4 mg transmucosally to establish tolerance without withdrawal, begin weekly dosing subcut every 7 days. Or, in patients currently treated with other buprenorphine-containing products, switch to either weekly subcut dosing every 7 days or monthly dosing subcut every 28 days.

Adjust-a-dose: May give weekly dose up to 2 days before or after the weekly time point. May give monthly dose up to 1 week before or after the monthly time point.

➤ **Moderate to severe opioid use disorder in patients who have initiated treatment with a transmucosal buprenorphine-containing product, followed by dosage adjustment for a minimum of 7 days (Sublocade)**

Adults: 300 mg (extended-release) subcut monthly for first 2 months, followed by 100 mg (extended-release) subcut maintenance dose monthly. May increase maintenance dose to 300 mg monthly for patients who tolerate 100-mg dose but don't demonstrate a satisfactory clinical response. Administer drug with a minimum of 26 days between doses.

Adjust-a-dose: For patients on long-term treatment of 100 mg monthly, may give a single 300-mg dose to cover a 2-month period when patient may not be available for injection (such as extended travel). Thereafter, resume 100-mg monthly regimen.

ADMINISTRATION

IV

▼ For direct injection, give slowly over at least 2 minutes into a vein or through tubing of a free-flowing, compatible IV solution.

▼ **Incompatibilities:** None listed by manufacturer. Consult drug compatibility reference for more information.

IM

● Inspect drug for particulate matter and discoloration.

● Give drug as deep IM injection.

Subcutaneous

Boxed Warning Sublocade may cause serious harm or death if given IV. Don't administer Sublocade IV or IM. ∎

Boxed Warning Brixadi may cause serious harm or death if given IV. Drug is only available through a REMS program to prevent risk of IV self-administration. ∎

• Only health care providers should prepare and administer Sublocade or Brixadi.

🔷 *Alert:* Weekly and monthly formulations aren't interchangeable. Weekly formulation can't be combined to yield a monthly dose.

• Use only the syringe and safety needle supplied.

• Remove drug from refrigerator at least 15 minutes before use. Don't open foil pack until ready for use. Discard drug if left at room temperature for longer than 7 days.

• Don't use if particles or discoloration is present.

• Remove excess air from syringe and inject drug subcut in abdomen only. Select a site between the transpyloric and transtubercular planes, avoiding areas where skin is irritated, red, bruised, infected, or scarred.

• Don't rub skin after injection. A lump may be palpable for several weeks but will shrink over time.

• Rotate injection sites.

• Give a missed dose as soon as possible, with the next dose no sooner than 26 days later. Occasional dosing delays up to 2 weeks aren't expected to significantly impact treatment.

Sublingual

• Place all tablets of the dose under the tongue until dissolved. Only give tablets whole.

• Patient shouldn't eat or drink anything until the tablets are completely dissolved.

• After transmucosal medicine has completely dissolved, assist patient with gently rinsing teeth and gums with water and then swallowing the water. Have patient wait at least 1 hour before brushing teeth.

Transdermal

🔷 *Alert:* Avoid exposing patch or surrounding area to direct external heat source or direct sunlight. Such exposure may increase amount of drug released, which can result in overdose and death.

• Each patch is intended to be worn for 7 days. If patch falls off during 7-day dosing interval, apply new patch to different site.

• Don't use if pouch seal is broken or patch is cut, damaged, or altered. Apply patch to intact skin immediately after opening.

• Appropriate application sites are upper outer arm, upper chest, upper back, or side of the chest (eight total available sites).

• Application site should be hairless or nearly hairless; clip hair if needed but don't shave site. If needed, clean selected site with water only and allow to dry completely before applying patch.

• Edges of patch may be taped to the skin if needed. Or, cover with waterproof or semipermeable adhesive dressing suitable for 7 days of wear.

• After removing patch, fold it in half, seal it in patch-disposal unit, and place it in trash.

• Wait a minimum of 3 weeks before applying new patch to same application site.

• Exposure of patch to water, such as while bathing or showering, is acceptable.

Buccal

• Don't use film if package seal is broken or film is cut, damaged, or altered.

• To administer, first have patient moisten inside of cheek with tongue or water.

• Apply film immediately after removal from sealed package. Place yellow side of film against inside of cheek and hold in place with dry fingers for 5 seconds; then leave in place until film fully dissolves (about 30 minutes).

• Make sure patient doesn't chew or swallow film and doesn't eat or drink until film has dissolved.

🔷 *Alert:* After medication completely dissolves, assist patient with gently rinsing teeth and gums with water and then swallowing the water. Have patient wait at least 1 hour before brushing teeth.

ACTION

Unknown. Binds with opioid receptors in the CNS, altering perception of and emotional response to pain.

Route	Onset	Peak	Duration
IV	Immediate	2 min	6 hr
IM	15 min	1 hr	6 hr
Subcut	Unknown	24 hr	Unknown
SL	Unknown	30–60 min	Unknown
Transdermal	17 hr	3–6 days	7 days
Buccal	Unknown	0.5–4 hr	Unknown

Half-life: 1 to 7 hours; subcut, 43 to 60 days; transdermal, 26 hours; buccal, 16 to 39 hours.

ADVERSE REACTIONS

CNS: dizziness, sedation, vertigo, depression, dreaming, fatigue, headache, insomnia, anxiety, pain, paresthesia, weakness, somnolence, fever. **CV:** HTN, hypotension, peripheral edema. **EENT:** conjunctivitis, diplopia, miosis, nasopharyngitis, sinus congestion, sinusitis, dry mouth, oropharyngeal pain. **GI:** nausea, abdominal pain, constipation, diarrhea, vomiting, anorexia, dyspepsia, gastroenteritis, decreased appetite. **GU:** urine retention, UTI. **Hematologic:** anemia. **Hepatic:** increased AST and ALT levels. **Metabolic:** increased GGT and CK levels. **Musculoskeletal:** arthralgia, back pain, muscle spasm, joint swelling, extremity pain. **Respiratory:** *respiratory depression,* dyspnea, hypoventilation, URI, bronchitis. **Skin:** application-site rash or erythema (patch), diaphoresis, injection-site reactions, pruritus, rash, bruising. **Other:** chills, hot flashes, infection, withdrawal syndrome, flulike symptoms, falls.

INTERACTIONS
Drug-drug. *Anticholinergics:* May increase risk of constipation and urine retention. Monitor therapy.

Atazanavir: May increase buprenorphine level. Monitor patient and reduce buprenorphine dose as clinically indicated.

Boxed Warning *Benzodiazepines, CNS depressants:* May cause slow or difficult breathing, sedation, and death. Avoid use together. If use together is necessary, limit dosage and duration of each drug to the minimum needed for desired effect. ■

Class IA or III antiarrhythmics: May increase risk of prolonged QT syndrome. Monitor patient closely.

CYP3A4 inducers (carbamazepine, phenobarbital, phenytoin, rifampin): May increase clearance of buprenorphine. Monitor patient for clinical effects of drug. If patient is taking Sublocade, patient may need to be transitioned back to a formulation that permits dosage adjustments.

CYP3A4 inhibitors (erythromycin, ketoconazole, ritonavir, saquinavir): May decrease clearance of buprenorphine. Monitor for increased adverse effects.

Diuretics: May decrease therapeutic effects of diuretics. Monitor therapy.

MAO inhibitors: May cause additive effects and increase risk of serotonin syndrome. Avoid use within 14 days of each other.

Mixed agonist/antagonist, partial agonist opioid analgesics (butorphanol, nalbuphine, pentazocine): May reduce analgesic effect or precipitate withdrawal symptoms. Avoid use together.

NNRTIs (delavirdine, efavirenz, etravirine, nevirapine): May increase or decrease therapeutic effects of Sublocade. Monitor therapy closely.

🚱 *Alert: Serotonergic drugs (amoxapine, antiemetics [dolasetron, granisetron, ondansetron, palonosetron], antimigraine drugs, buspirone, cyclobenzaprine, dextromethorphan, linezolid, lithium, maprotiline, methylene blue, mirtazapine, nefazodone, SSNRIs, SSRIs, TCAs, trazodone, tryptophan, vilazodone):* Can increase risk of serotonin syndrome. Use together cautiously; monitor patient for serotonin syndrome.

Skeletal muscle relaxants: May enhance neuromuscular blocking action and increase respiratory depression. Use together cautiously.

Drug-lifestyle. **Boxed Warning** *Alcohol use, illicit drug use:* May cause slow or difficult breathing, sedation, and death. Discourage use together. ■

EFFECTS ON LAB TEST RESULTS
• May increase amylase, ALT, AST, GGT, and CK levels.

CONTRAINDICATIONS & CAUTIONS
• Contraindicated in patients hypersensitive to drug.
• Buprenorphine for injection and transdermal system are contraindicated in patients with paralytic ileus, GI obstruction, or significant respiratory depression as well as in patients with acute or severe bronchial asthma in an unmonitored setting or setting without resuscitative equipment.

Boxed Warning Use exposes patient and others to risk of opioid addiction, abuse, and misuse, which can lead to overdose and death. These effects can occur at any dose or duration. Assess patient risk before prescribing and regularly reassess patient for these behaviors and conditions. ■

Boxed Warning Serious, life-threatening, or fatal respiratory depression may occur, especially during drug initiation or after a dosage increase. Misuse or abuse of drug by chewing, swallowing, snorting, or injecting buprenorphine extracted from the transdermal system results in uncontrolled delivery of buprenorphine and poses a significant risk of overdose and death. ■

Boxed Warning *Opioid class warning:* Opioids should only be prescribed with benzodiazepines or other CNS depressants to patients for whom alternative treatment options are inadequate. ■

Boxed Warning Prescribers are strongly encouraged to complete a REMS-compliant education program. Drug should be prescribed only by prescribers with knowledge of opioid use and ways to reduce associated risks. ■

Boxed Warning Never inject Sublocade IV. Serious harm or death can occur because drug forms a solid mass upon contact with body fluids. If given IV, local tissue damage and thromboembolic events can occur. ■

• To achieve adequate analgesia and minimize adverse effects, consider patient's tolerance, condition, and other medications.

Alert: Use lowest effective dose for shortest period consistent with patient's treatment goals.

Alert: Because risk of overdose increases as opioid dose increases, reserve titration to higher doses for patients in whom lower doses are ineffective and in whom expected benefits of higher opioid dose outweigh risks.

Alert: Drug shouldn't be used for an extended period unless pain remains severe enough to require an opioid analgesic and alternative treatment options are inadequate to treat pain.

Alert: Long-acting or extended-release formulations are indicated for severe, persistent pain for which extended treatment with a daily opioid analgesic is required and for which alternative treatment options are inadequate. Use isn't indicated for as-needed analgesia.

Alert: Don't exceed dose of one 20-mcg/hour transdermal patch every 7 days or 900 mcg every 12 hours for buccal film due to risk of prolonging QTc interval.

Alert: Patients are at increased risk for oversedation and respiratory depression if they snore or have a history of sleep apnea, haven't used opioids recently or are first-time opioid users, have increased opioid dosage requirements or opioid habituation, received general anesthesia for longer lengths of time, received other sedating drugs, have thoracic or other surgical incisions that may impair breathing, or have preexisting pulmonary or cardiac disease. Monitor these patients carefully.

Boxed Warning Accidental ingestion of even one dose of an opioid, especially by children, can result in a fatal overdose. ■

Alert: Drug may lead to rare but serious decrease in adrenal gland cortisol production.

Alert: Combined use of medication-assisted treatment (MAT) drugs methadone or buprenorphine with benzodiazepines or other CNS depressants increases risk of serious adverse effects; however, the harm caused by untreated opioid addiction may outweigh these risks. Patients may require MAT for opioid addiction indefinitely, and use of these drugs should continue for as long as patients are benefiting and their use contributes to the intended treatment goals.

• Use cautiously in older adults; patients who are debilitated; patients with morbid obesity; patients with opioid dependence; patients undergoing biliary tract surgery; patients with biliary tract disease or pancreatitis; patients with head injury, intracranial lesions, or increased ICP; patients with severe respiratory, liver, or kidney impairment; patients with CNS depression or coma; patients at risk for hypotension and circulatory shock; and patients with thyroid irregularities, adrenal insufficiency, prostatic hypertrophy, urethral stricture, acute alcoholism, delirium tremens, or kyphoscoliosis.

• Don't use Sublocade in patients with preexisting Child-Pugh class B or C liver impairment because buprenorphine levels can't be rapidly adjusted. If patient develops Child-Pugh class B or C liver impairment during treatment and buprenorphine toxicity or overdose occurs within 2 weeks of drug administration, surgical removal of the depot may be needed.

Dialyzable drug: Unknown.

⚠ Overdose S&S: Respiratory depression; pinpoint pupils; sedation; hypotension; death; snoring; bradycardia; cool, clammy skin; partial or complete airway obstruction; skeletal muscle flaccidity; somnolence.

PREGNANCY-LACTATION-REPRODUCTION

• There are no adequate and controlled studies during pregnancy. Use during pregnancy only if potential benefits justify fetal risk.

Boxed Warning Prolonged use during pregnancy can result in neonatal opioid withdrawal syndrome, which may be life-threatening. It requires management with expert neonatology protocols. If prolonged use is needed, advise patient of risks and ensure availability of proper treatment. ■

• Drug appears in human milk. Use during breastfeeding isn't recommended.

• Monitor infants exposed to large doses of opioids during breastfeeding for apnea and sedation. Withdrawal symptoms can occur in infants when drug or breastfeeding is stopped.

• Chronic opioid use may reduce fertility.

NURSING CONSIDERATIONS
Boxed Warning May cause life-threatening or fatal respiratory depression at any time during therapy. Monitor patient closely, especially when starting or increasing doses. Proper dosing and titration are essential to reduce risk. ■

Boxed Warning Regularly monitor all patients for opioid addiction, abuse, and misuse, which can lead to overdose and death. ■

• Don't stop drug abruptly; withdraw slowly and individualize the gradual taper plan to prevent signs and symptoms of withdrawal, worsening pain, and psychological distress in patients who are physically dependent. Refer to manufacturer's label for specific tapering instructions.

• When tapering opioids, watch closely for signs and symptoms of opioid withdrawal. Such symptoms may indicate a need to taper more slowly. Also monitor for suicidality, use of other substances, and mood changes.

⊗ *Alert:* Carefully monitor vital signs, pain level, respiratory status, and sedation level in patients receiving opioids, especially those receiving IV opioids postoperatively.

⊗ *Alert:* Drug may cause opioid-induced hyperalgesia (OIH). Symptoms include increased pain level with opioid dose increase, decreased pain level with opioid dose reduction, pain from ordinarily nonpainful stimuli without underlying disease progression, opioid tolerance or withdrawal, and addictive behavior. For suspected OIH, decrease opioid dose or switch patient to alternative opioid.

⊗ *Alert:* If patient is taking opioids with serotonergic drugs, watch for signs and symptoms of serotonin syndrome (agitation, hallucinations, rapid HR, fever, diaphoresis, shivering or shaking, muscle twitching or stiffness, trouble with coordination, nausea, vomiting, diarrhea), especially when starting treatment or increasing dosages. Signs and symptoms may occur within several hours of coadministration but may also occur later, especially after dosage increase. Discontinue the opioid,

serotonergic drug, or both if serotonin syndrome is suspected.

• Monitor patient for signs and symptoms of adrenal insufficiency (nausea, vomiting, loss of appetite, fatigue, weakness, dizziness, low BP). Perform diagnostic testing if adrenal insufficiency is suspected. If adrenal insufficiency is confirmed, treat with corticosteroids and wean patient off opioids if appropriate. Discontinue corticosteroids when clinically appropriate.

• Monitor patient for signs and symptoms of decreased sex hormone levels (low libido, erectile dysfunction, amenorrhea, infertility); drug may cause decreased sex hormone levels with long-term use. If signs or symptoms occur, evaluate patient and obtain lab testing.

• Work with patient to develop strategies to manage the use of prescribed or illicit benzodiazepines or other CNS depressants when starting MAT. Taper benzodiazepine or CNS depressant to discontinuation, if possible.

⊗ *Alert:* If patient is receiving prescribed benzodiazepines or other CNS depressants for anxiety or insomnia, verify diagnosis and consider other treatment options for these conditions, if possible.

• Drug should be used as part of a complete treatment program that includes counseling and psychosocial support.

⊗ *Alert:* Coordinate care to ensure other prescribers are aware of patient's MAT.

• Monitor patient for illicit drug use, including urine and blood screening.

• Assess patient's oral health history before transmucosal use. Tooth decay, cavities, oral infections, and loss of teeth have been reported in patients taking transmucosal buprenorphine. These problems can be serious and can occur in patients with no history of dental issues.

• Drug may prolong QT interval and increase risk of ventricular arrhythmias. Avoid use in patient with a personal or family history of long QT syndrome. Use caution and periodically monitor ECGs in patient with hypomagnesemia; hypokalemia; or unstable cardiac disease, including atrial fibrillation, unstable HF, or active myocardial ischemia.

• For patient at risk for liver toxicity, monitor LFTs before and during treatment.

• Drug may worsen increased ICP and mask its signs and symptoms. Carefully monitor patient's pupillary reflexes and level of consciousness.

Reactions in bold italics are *life-threatening*.

• Monitor patient with history of seizure disorders for worsening of condition.

• Monitor for signs and symptoms of hypotension after initiating therapy or increasing dosage.

• Monitor patient with fever or increased core body temperature after exertion; adjust dosage if signs or symptoms of respiratory or CNS depression occur.

• Watch for worsening of symptoms in patient with biliary tract disease, including acute pancreatitis; drug may cause spasm of sphincter of Oddi.

• Reassess patient's pain level 15 and 30 minutes after parenteral administration.

⚠️ *Alert:* Naloxone won't completely reverse the respiratory depression caused by buprenorphine overdose; an overdose may require mechanical ventilation. Larger-than-usual doses of naloxone (more than 0.4 mg) and doxapram also may be indicated.

• Drug may cause constipation. Assess bowel function and need for stool softeners and stimulant laxatives.

⚠️ *Alert:* Drug's opioid antagonist properties may cause withdrawal syndrome in patient who is opioid dependent.

• If dependence occurs, withdrawal symptoms may appear up to 14 days after drug is stopped.

• If Sublocade depot must be surgically removed or treatment discontinued, monitor patient for signs and symptoms of withdrawal and treat appropriately.

• Regularly monitor Sublocade subcut injection site for evidence of tampering or attempted removal of the drug depot.

• In patient with oral mucositis using the buccal film, consider reducing dose; oral mucositis may lead to faster absorption and higher blood concentration of drug.

• *Look alike–sound alike:* Don't confuse buprenorphine with bupropion.

PATIENT TEACHING

Boxed Warning Counsel patient and caregiver on serious risks, safe use, and importance of reading the medication guide with each prescription. ∎

• Advise patient to take drug exactly as prescribed and to use lowest dose possible for shortest time needed.

• Inform patient that, for acute pain, drug may only be needed for a few days. Teach patient about safe disposal of unused drug.

• Warn patient that extended-release and long-acting formulations aren't to be taken on an "as needed" basis.

• Instruct patient to contact health care provider if prescribed dosage isn't controlling pain.

⚠️ *Alert:* Warn patient to withhold drug and inform prescriber if pain level worsens, pain sensitivity increases, or new pain occurs after taking drug.

⚠️ *Alert:* Counsel patient who has been regularly taking drug not to discontinue without first discussing the need for gradual tapering with prescriber.

⚠️ *Alert:* Encourage patient to report all medications being taken, including prescription and OTC drugs and supplements.

⚠️ *Alert:* Caution patient to immediately report signs and symptoms of hypersensitivity reaction (rash, hives, itching, facial swelling, wheezing, dizziness), serotonin syndrome, adrenal insufficiency, decreased sex hormone levels, or liver impairment (yellowing of skin or eyes, dark urine, light-colored stools, abdominal pain, nausea).

• Tell patient and family to immediately report adverse reactions to prescriber.

⚠️ *Alert:* Teach patient to avoid nonprescribed benzodiazepines, sedatives, or alcohol when taking MAT due to increased risk of overdose and death.

• Stress to patient taking transmucosal formulations the importance of oral care and potential for dental problems. Instruct patient in proper oral care after transmucosal dose.

• Tell patient to obtain a dental evaluation before starting transmucosal drug and to establish a dental caries prevention plan with regular dental checkups.

• Advise patient to notify all prescribers of MAT and not to stop MAT or other prescribed drugs without first consulting prescriber to determine need for gradual tapering regimen.

• Caution patient who is ambulatory about quickly getting out of bed or chair and walking because hypotension can occur.

• Teach patient not to drive, operate heavy machinery, or perform dangerous activities until drug's effects are known.

• When drug is used after surgery, encourage patient to turn, cough, and breathe deeply to prevent breathing problems.

• Explain assessment and monitoring process to patient and family. Instruct them to immediately report difficulty breathing or other signs or symptoms of potential adverse opioid-related reaction.

• Teach about proper drug administration, storage, handling, and disposal.

• Advise patient to treat accidental skin exposure of household members (including children) or other close contacts with transdermal drug by removing exposed clothing and rinsing skin with water only. Use of naloxone may be necessary.

• Caution patient not to apply heat to patch application site or to cut patch.

• Warn patient not to take other long-acting opioids while using transdermal system or buccal film.

• Teach patient that naloxone may be prescribed with the opioid when beginning and renewing therapy to reduce risk of opioid overdose and death.

• Caution patient to report to prescriber pregnancy or plan to become pregnant.

buPROPion hydrobromide
byoo-PROE-pee-on

Aplenzin

buPROPion hydrochloride
Forfivo XL, Wellbutrin SR, Wellbutrin XL

Therapeutic class: Antidepressants
Pharmacologic class: Aminoketones

AVAILABLE FORMS
bupropion hydrobromide
Tablets (extended-release) 🔵: 174 mg, 348 mg, 522 mg
bupropion hydrochloride
Tablets (extended-release 12-hour) 🔵: 100 mg, 150 mg, 200 mg
Tablets (extended-release 24-hour) 🔵: 150 mg, 300 mg, 450 mg
Tablets (immediate-release) 🔵: 75 mg, 100 mg

INDICATIONS & DOSAGES
Adjust-a-dose (for all indications): In patients with GFR less than 90 mL/minute or Child-Pugh score 5 to 6 liver impairment, consider reduced frequency or dosage. In patients with Child-Pugh score 7 to 15 liver impairment, don't exceed 174 mg every other day (bupropion hydrobromide [HBr]); 100 mg

per day or 150 mg every other day (bupropion hydrochloride [HCl] sustained-release tablets); 150 mg every other day (bupropion hydrochloride extended-release tablets); or 75 mg per day (bupropion HCl immediate-release tablets). Forfivo XL isn't recommended in patients with kidney or liver impairment.

➤ **Major depressive disorder (Aplenzin only)**
Adults: Initially, 174 mg PO (equivalent to 150 mg/day bupropion HCl) given as a single daily dose in the morning. After 4 days of dosing, may increase to target dose of 348 mg once daily. Full antidepressant effect may not be evident for several months of treatment or longer. When switching patients from Wellbutrin SR or Wellbutrin XL to Aplenzin, give the equivalent total daily dose when possible (522 mg bupropion HBr is equivalent to 450 mg bupropion HCl; 348 mg bupropion HBr is equivalent to 300 mg bupropion HCl; 174 mg bupropion HBr is equivalent to 150 mg bupropion HCl).

➤ **Major depressive disorder (except Aplenzin)**
Adults: For immediate-release, initially, 100 mg PO b.i.d.; increase to 100 mg PO t.i.d. after 3 days, if needed. If patient doesn't improve after several weeks of therapy, increase dosage to 150 mg t.i.d. No single dose should exceed 150 mg. Allow at least 6 hours between successive doses. Maximum dose, 450 mg daily. For sustained-release, initially, 150 mg PO every morning; increase to target dose of 150 mg PO b.i.d., as tolerated, as early as day 4 of dosing. Allow at least 8 hours between successive doses. Maximum dose, 400 mg daily. For extended-release, initially, 150 mg PO every morning; increase to target dosage of 300 mg PO daily, as tolerated, as early as day 4 of dosing. Allow at least 24 hours between successive doses. Maximum dose, 450 mg daily. Don't initiate treatment with Forfivo XL.

➤ **Seasonal affective disorder**
Adults: Start treatment in autumn before depressive symptoms appear. Wellbutrin XL: Initially, 150 mg extended-release PO once daily in the morning. After 1 week, may increase to 300 mg once daily, if tolerated. Continue 300 mg daily during autumn and winter and taper to 150 mg daily before stopping drug in early spring. Aplenzin: 174 mg PO daily in the morning. May increase to 348 mg

PO once daily after 7 days. Taper and discontinue drug in early spring.

➤ **Aid to smoking-cessation treatment (extended-release tablets 12-hour)**

Adults: 150 mg PO daily for 3 days; increased to maximum of 300 mg daily in two divided doses at least 8 hours apart. Begin therapy at least 1 week before target cessation date; continue therapy for at least 12 weeks. Some patients may need continued treatment.

ADMINISTRATION

PO
• Have patient swallow tablets whole; don't crush or cut chew tablets.
• Give drug without regard to meals.
• When switching patients from immediate-release or sustained-release tablets to extended-release tablets, give the same total daily dose (when possible) as the once-daily dosage provided.

ACTION

Unknown. Drug doesn't inhibit MAO, but it weakly inhibits norepinephrine, dopamine, and serotonin reuptake. Noradrenergic or dopaminergic mechanisms, or both, may cause drug's effect.

Route	Onset	Peak	Duration
PO (extended-release)	Unknown	5 hr	Unknown
PO (immediate-release)	Unknown	2 hr	Unknown
PO (sustained-release)	Unknown	3 hr	Unknown

Half-life: 12 to 30 hours.

ADVERSE REACTIONS

CNS: abnormal dreams, insomnia, headache, migraine, sedation, tremor, agitation, dizziness, *suicidality,* anxiety, confusion, delusions, euphoria, fever, hostility, impaired concentration, decreased memory, impaired sleep quality, akinesia, akathisia, asthenia, paresthesia, abnormal thinking, depression, fatigue, syncope, taste disturbance, somnolence. **CV:** tachycardia, *arrhythmias,* HTN, hypotension, palpitations, chest pain, flushing. **EENT:** blurred vision, tinnitus, auditory disturbances, epistaxis, rhinitis, pharyngitis, nasopharyngitis, sinusitis, dry mouth, dysphagia. **GI:** constipation, nausea, vomiting, anorexia, dyspepsia, diarrhea, abdominal pain, flatulence. **GU:** erectile dysfunction, decreased libido, menstrual complaints,

urinary frequency, urinary urgency, urine retention. **Metabolic:** increased appetite, weight loss, weight gain. **Musculoskeletal:** arthritis, myalgia, arthralgia, muscle spasm or twitch. **Respiratory:** URI, bronchitis, cough. **Skin:** diaphoresis, pruritus, rash, dry skin, cutaneous temperature disturbance, urticaria. **Other:** chills, accidental injury, hot flashes, infection.

INTERACTIONS

Drug-drug. *Amantadine, levodopa:* May increase risk of adverse reactions. If used together, give small first doses of bupropion and increase dosage gradually.

Antidepressants (desipramine, fluoxetine, imipramine, nortriptyline, sertraline), antipsychotics (haloperidol, risperidone, thioridazine), systemic corticosteroids, theophylline: May lower seizure threshold. Use together cautiously.

Beta blockers, class IC antiarrhythmics: May increase levels of these drugs and risk of adverse reactions. Use a reduced dose if used with bupropion.

Bupropion-containing drugs: May increase risk of seizures when used with other bupropion products. Use together is contraindicated.

Carbamazepine, phenobarbital, phenytoin: May enhance metabolism of bupropion and decrease its effect. Monitor patient closely.

Clopidogrel, ticlopidine: May decrease bupropion metabolite exposure. Avoid use together.

CYP2B6 substrates or inhibitors (cyclophosphamide, orphenadrine, thiotepa), efavirenz, fluvoxamine, nelfinavir, norfluoxetine, paroxetine, sertraline: May increase bupropion activity. Monitor patient for expected therapeutic effects and adverse effects.

Linezolid, methylene blue: May increase hypertensive effect of bupropion. Use together is contraindicated.

MAO inhibitors: May increase hypertensive effect of bupropion. Use of these drugs within 14 days of each other is contraindicated.

Nicotine replacement agents: May increase risk of HTN. Monitor BP.

SSRIs: May increase risk of suicidality in children, adolescents, and young adults with major depressive disorder. Use together cautiously.

Drug-lifestyle. *Alcohol use:* May alter seizure threshold. Discourage use together.

Sun exposure: May increase risk of photosensitivity reactions. Advise patient to avoid excessive sunlight exposure.

EFFECTS ON LAB TEST RESULTS
• May increase LFT values.
• May cause false-positive results for urine detection of amphetamines.

CONTRAINDICATIONS & CAUTIONS
• Contraindicated in patients hypersensitive to drug and in those with seizure disorders or history of bulimia or anorexia nervosa because of a higher risk of seizures.
• Hypersensitivity reactions (anaphylaxis, pruritus, urticaria, angioedema, dyspnea, erythema multiforme, SJS) have occurred.
◊ *Alert:* Concomitant use with SSRIs, linezolid, or methylene blue can cause serotonin syndrome (fever, mental status changes, muscle twitching, diaphoresis, shivering or shaking, diarrhea, loss of coordination). Use drug with SSRIs, linezolid, or methylene blue only for life-threatening or urgent conditions when potential benefits outweigh risks of toxicity.
• Contraindicated in patients abruptly stopping use of alcohol, sedatives (including benzodiazepines), or antiepileptics.
• Don't initiate therapy with Forfivo XL or taper Forfivo XL dosage; use another bupropion formulation for initial dosage titration and for tapering dosage before discontinuation.
◊ *Alert:* Bupropion isn't approved for use in children.
• Use cautiously in patients with recent history of MI; unstable heart disease; kidney or liver impairment; or history of seizures, head trauma, or other predisposition to seizures and in those being treated with drugs that lower seizure threshold.
Dialyzable drug: Unknown.
⚠ *Overdose S&S:* Seizures, ECG changes, hallucinations, loss of consciousness, sinus tachycardia, coma, fever, hypotension, muscle rigidity, rhabdomyolysis, respiratory failure, stupor.

PREGNANCY-LACTATION-REPRODUCTION
• Use during pregnancy only when potential benefits justify fetal risk.
• Health care providers are encouraged to register patients who are pregnant in the National Pregnancy Registry for Antidepressants (1-866-961-2388 or https://womensmentalhealth.org/clinical-and-research-programs/pregnancyregistry/antidepressants/).
• Drug and its metabolites appear in human milk. Recommendations for breastfeeding vary by individual product; refer to manufacturer's labeling for recommendations.

NURSING CONSIDERATIONS
• Note that many patients experience a period of increased restlessness, including agitation, insomnia, and anxiety, especially at start of therapy.
◊ *Alert:* To minimize the risk of seizures, don't exceed maximum recommended dose.
◊ *Alert:* Patient with major depressive disorder may experience a worsening of depression and suicidality. Carefully monitor patient for worsening depression or suicidality, especially at the beginning of therapy and during dosage changes.
Boxed Warning Drug may increase risk of suicidality in children, adolescents, and young adults with major depressive disorder or other psychiatric disorders. ∎
◊ *Alert:* If SSRIs, linezolid, or methylene blue must be given, bupropion must be stopped and patient monitored for serotonin toxicity for 2 weeks or until 24 hours after the last dose of SSRIs, methylene blue, or linezolid, whichever comes first. Treatment with bupropion may resume 24 hours after last dose of SSRIs, methylene blue, or linezolid.
• Closely monitor patient with history of bipolar disorder. Antidepressants can cause manic episodes during depressed phase of bipolar disorder (may be less likely to occur with bupropion than with other antidepressants).
• Begin smoking-cessation treatment while patient is still smoking; about 1 week is needed to achieve steady-state drug levels.
• Stop smoking-cessation treatment if patient hasn't progressed toward abstinence by week 7. Treatment usually lasts up to 12 weeks. Patient can stop taking drug without tapering off.
• Monitor patients without iridectomy for narrow-angle glaucoma.
• Monitor BP for HTN before and periodically during treatment.
• Monitor for hypersensitivity reactions.
• *Look alike–sound alike:* Don't confuse bupropion with buspirone. Don't confuse Wellbutrin SR with Wellbutrin XL.

Reactions in bold italics are *life-threatening*.

PATIENT TEACHING

Boxed Warning Advise family or caregivers to closely observe patient for increased suicidality as well as hostility, agitation, and depressed mood. Instruct them to immediately contact health care provider should these effects occur. ∎

🕓 *Alert:* Explain that excessive use of alcohol, abrupt withdrawal from alcohol or other sedatives, and addiction to cocaine, opiates, or stimulants during therapy may increase risk of seizures. Seizure risk is also greater in patients using OTC stimulants or anorectic drugs and in patients with diabetes using oral antidiabetics or insulin.

🕓 *Alert:* Teach patient to recognize and immediately report symptoms of serotonin toxicity (fever, mental status changes, muscle twitching, diaphoresis, shivering or shaking, diarrhea, loss of coordination).

• Teach about proper drug administration and handling.

• Inform patient that tablets may have an odor.

• Tell patient taking extended-release form that the empty shell may appear in stool.

• Advise patient to avoid hazardous activities that require alertness and good psychomotor coordination until effects of drug are known.

• Tell patient that drug may take 4 weeks or longer to reach full antidepressant effect.

busPIRone hydrochloride
byoo-SPYE-rone

Therapeutic class: Anxiolytics
Pharmacologic class: Azaspirodecanedione derivatives

AVAILABLE FORMS
Tablets: 5 mg, 7.5 mg, 10 mg, 15 mg, 30 mg

INDICATIONS & DOSAGES
➤ **Generalized anxiety disorder**
Adults: Initially, 7.5 mg PO b.i.d. Increase dosage by 5 mg daily at 2- to 3-day intervals. Usual maintenance dosage is 20 to 30 mg daily in divided doses. Don't exceed 60 mg daily.

ADMINISTRATION
PO
• Give drug at the same times each day, and always with or always without food.

ACTION
May inhibit neuronal firing and reduce serotonin and dopamine turnover in cortical, amygdaloid, and septohippocampal tissue.

Route	Onset	Peak	Duration
PO	Unknown	40–90 min	Unknown

Half-life: 2 to 3 hours.

ADVERSE REACTIONS
CNS: dizziness, drowsiness, headache, nervousness, insomnia, light-headedness, fatigue, numbness, excitement, confusion, depression, anger, decreased concentration, paresthesia, incoordination, tremor, hostility, weakness, dream disturbance. **CV:** tachycardia, nonspecific chest pain. **EENT:** blurred vision, dry mouth, tinnitus sore throat, nasal congestion. **GI:** nausea, diarrhea, abdominal distress, constipation, vomiting. **Musculoskeletal:** aches and pains. **Skin:** rash, diaphoresis, clamminess.

INTERACTIONS
Drug-drug. *Azole antifungals:* May inhibit first-pass metabolism of buspirone. Monitor patient closely for adverse effects; adjust dosage as needed.
CNS depressants: May increase CNS depression. Use together cautiously.
CYP3A4 inducers (carbamazepine, dexamethasone, phenobarbital, phenytoin, rifabutin, rifampin): May decrease buspirone level. Adjust dosage as needed.
Drugs metabolized by CYP3A4 (clarithromycin, diltiazem, erythromycin, fluvoxamine, itraconazole, ketoconazole, nefazodone, ritonavir, verapamil): May increase buspirone level. Monitor patient; decrease buspirone dosage and adjust carefully.
Linezolid, methylene blue: May cause serotonin syndrome. Use extreme caution and monitor closely.
MAO inhibitors: May elevate BP and increase risk of serotonin syndrome. Use of MAO inhibitors within 14 days of stopping or starting buspirone is contraindicated.
Nefazodone: May increase levels of both drugs. If used together, lower buspirone dosage.
Drug-food. *Grapefruit juice:* May increase drug level, increasing adverse effects. Discourage use together.
Drug-lifestyle. *Alcohol use:* May increase CNS depression. Discourage use together.

EFFECTS ON LAB TEST RESULTS
• May interfere with urinary metanephrine/catecholamine assay testing for pheochromocytoma, resulting in false-positive result.

CONTRAINDICATIONS & CAUTIONS
• Contraindicated in patients hypersensitive to drug.
❸ *Alert:* Concomitant use with linezolid or methylene blue can cause serotonin syndrome (fever, mental status changes, muscle twitching, diaphoresis, shivering or shaking, diarrhea, loss of coordination). Use drug with linezolid or methylene blue only for life-threatening or urgent conditions when the potential benefits outweigh the risks of toxicity.
• Drug isn't recommended for patients with severe liver or kidney impairment.
Dialyzable drug: No.
⚠ *Overdose S&S:* Nausea, vomiting, dizziness, drowsiness, miosis, gastric distress.

PREGNANCY-LACTATION-REPRODUCTION
• Use during pregnancy and breastfeeding isn't recommended. Use during pregnancy only if clearly needed.

NURSING CONSIDERATIONS
• Monitor patient closely for adverse CNS reactions. Drug is less sedating than other anxiolytics, but CNS effects may be unpredictable.
❸ *Alert:* Before starting therapy, don't stop a previous benzodiazepine regimen abruptly because a withdrawal reaction may occur.
❸ *Alert:* If linezolid or methylene blue must be given, buspirone must be stopped and patient should be monitored for serotonin toxicity for 2 weeks or until 24 hours after the last dose of methylene blue or linezolid, whichever comes first. Treatment with buspirone may resume 24 hours after last dose of methylene blue or linezolid.
• Drug shows no potential for abuse and isn't classified as a controlled substance.
• *Look alike–sound alike:* Don't confuse buspirone with bupropion or risperidone.

PATIENT TEACHING
❸ *Alert:* Teach patient to recognize and immediately report symptoms of serotonin toxicity (fever, mental status changes, muscle twitching, diaphoresis, shivering or shaking, diarrhea, loss of coordination).

• Warn patient to avoid hazardous activities that require alertness and good coordination until effects of drug are known.
• Remind patient that drug effects may not be noticeable for several weeks.
• Warn patient not to abruptly stop a benzodiazepine because of risk of withdrawal symptoms.
• Tell patient to avoid use of alcohol and grapefruit juice during therapy.
• Advise patient to take consistently, always with or always without food.

SAFETY ALERT!

butorphanol tartrate
byoo-TOR-fa-nole

Therapeutic class: Opioid analgesics
Pharmacologic class: Opioid agonist-antagonists–opioid partial agonists

AVAILABLE FORMS
Injection: 1 mg/mL, 2 mg/mL
Nasal spray: 10 mg/mL (1 mg/spray)

INDICATIONS & DOSAGES
➤ **Moderate to severe pain**
Adults: Initially, 2 mg IM every 3 to 4 hours PRN or around the clock; then individualize dose to 1 to 4 mg, not to exceed 4 mg per dose. Or initially, 1 mg IV every 3 to 4 hours PRN; then individualize dose to 0.5 to 2 mg. Or, 1 mg by nasal spray every 3 to 4 hours (1 spray in one nostril); repeat in 60 to 90 minutes if pain relief is inadequate. For severe pain, 2 mg (1 spray in each nostril) every 3 to 4 hours.
Adjust-a-dose: For patients with kidney or liver impairment, increase dosage interval to 6 to 8 hours and give 50% of the normal dose. For older adults, give 1 mg IM or 0.5 mg IV; wait 6 hours before repeating dose. For nasal use, 1 mg (1 spray in one nostril). May give another 1 mg in 1.5 to 2 hours. Wait 6 hours before repeating sequence.
➤ **Labor for patients at full term; early labor (without signs of fetal distress)**
Adults: 1 or 2 mg IV or IM; repeat after 4 hours as needed. Don't give dose less than 4 hours before anticipated delivery.
➤ **Preoperative anesthesia or preanesthesia**
Adults: 2 mg IM 60 to 90 minutes before surgery.

➤ **Adjunct to balanced anesthesia**
Adults: 2 mg IV shortly before induction, or
0.5 to 1 mg IV in increments during anesthesia.
Older adults: One-half usual dose, with repeat doses determined by patient's response.

ADMINISTRATION
IV
▼ Compatible solutions include D₅W and NSS.

▼ Give by direct injection into a vein or into
the tubing of a free-flowing IV solution.
▼ **Incompatibilities:** None listed by manufacturer. Consult drug compatibility reference for more information.
IM
• Give drug IM; don't give subcut.
Intranasal
• Prime pump before initial use; if not used
for 2 days or more, reprime with one or two
strokes.
• Have patient blow nose gently to clear both
nostrils.
• Insert spray tip into one nostril, pointing toward back of the nose; have patient
close other nostril with fingertip and tilt head
slightly forward.
• Have patient sniff gently with mouth closed
during spray, then tilt head backward and sniff
gently a few more seconds. Repeat with other
nostril, if prescribed.
• Store at room temperature.

ACTION
May bind with opioid receptors in the CNS,
altering perception of and emotional response
to pain.

Route	Onset	Peak	Duration
IV	1 min	30–60 min	3–4 hr
IM	15 min	30–60 min	3–4 hr
Nasal	15 min	1–2 hr	4–5 hr

Half-life: About 2 to 9 hours.

ADVERSE REACTIONS
CNS: dizziness, insomnia, somnolence, anxiety, asthenia, confusion, euphoria, floating
feeling, headache, lethargy, nervousness,
pain, paresthesia, tremor, weakness, sensation of heat, unpleasant taste. **CV:** flushing,
hypotension, HTN, palpitations, vasodilation.
EENT: blurred vision, tinnitus, earache, nasal
congestion, nasal irritation, epistaxis, pharyngitis, sinus congestion, sinusitis, rhinitis,
dry mouth. **GI:** nausea, vomiting, anorexia,
constipation, diarrhea, stomach pain.

Respiratory: bronchitis, cough, dyspnea,
URI. **Skin:** clamminess, diaphoresis, pruritus.

INTERACTIONS
Drug-drug. ▐Boxed Warning▐ *Benzodiazepines, CNS depressants:* May cause slow
or difficult breathing, sedation, and death.
Avoid use together. If use together is necessary, limit dosage and duration of each drug
to the minimum necessary for desired effect. ▐
▐Boxed Warning▐ *CYP3A4 inducers (carbamazepine, phenytoin, rifampin):* May decrease level of intranasally administered drug,
causing decreased effectiveness or drug withdrawal syndrome. Discontinuation of inducer
may increase butorphanol level. Monitor patient closely. ▐
▐Boxed Warning▐ *CYP3A4 inhibitors (azole
antifungals, macrolide antibiotics, protease
inhibitors):* May increase level of intranasally
administered drug, resulting in increased or
prolonged adverse reactions; may also cause
potentially fatal respiratory depression. Avoid
use together. ▐
⊕ *Alert: Serotonergic drugs:* May increase
risk of serotonin syndrome. Use together
cautiously; monitor patient for serotonin
syndrome.
Drug-herb. ⊕ *Alert: St. John's wort:* May increase risk of serotonin syndrome. Use together cautiously; monitor patient for serotonin syndrome.
Drug-lifestyle. *Alcohol use:* May cause slow
or difficult breathing, sedation, and death.
Discourage use together.

EFFECTS ON LAB TEST RESULTS
None reported.

CONTRAINDICATIONS & CAUTIONS
• Contraindicated in patients hypersensitive to drug or to preservative, benzotho-
nium chloride; in those with severe bronchial
asthma in an unmonitored setting or in the absence of resuscitative equipment, and in those
with known or suspected GI obstruction, including paralytic ileus.
▐Boxed Warning▐ Prescribers are strongly encouraged to complete a REMS-compliant education program. Drug should be prescribed
only by prescribers with knowledge of opioid
use and ways to reduce associated risks. ▐
▐Boxed Warning▐ Drug exposes patients and
other users to risks of opioid addiction, abuse,
and misuse, which can lead to overdose and

death. These effects can occur at any dose or duration. Assess patient risk before prescribing and regularly reassess patient for these behaviors and conditions. ■

❸ *Alert:* Use lowest effective dose for shortest period consistent with patient's treatment goals.

❸ *Alert:* Because risk of overdose increases as opioid dose increases, reserve titration to higher doses for patients in whom lower doses are ineffective and in whom expected benefits of higher opioid dose outweigh risks.

Boxed Warning *Opioid class warning:* Opioids should only be prescribed with benzodiazepines or other CNS depressants to patients for whom alternative treatment options are inadequate, not expected to provide adequate analgesia, haven't been tolerated, or aren't expected to be tolerated. ■

❸ *Alert:* Drug shouldn't be used for an extended period unless pain remains severe enough to require an opioid analgesic and alternative treatment options are inadequate to treat pain.

❸ *Alert:* Drug may lead to rare but serious decrease in adrenal gland cortisol production.

• Drug may cause decreased sex hormone levels with long-term use.

• Use cautiously in patients with head injury, increased ICP, acute MI, ventricular dysfunction, coronary insufficiency, respiratory disease or depression, thyroid dysfunction, seizure disorder, mental health disorder, prostatic hyperplasia, urinary stricture, and kidney or liver dysfunction.

• Use cautiously in patients who have recently received repeated doses of opioid analgesic.

• Safety and efficacy in patients younger than age 18 haven't been established.

• Older adults may have increased sensitivity to drug. Use caution when selecting a dosage for such patients, and usually start at low end of dosing range.

Dialyzable drug: Unknown.

⚠ *Overdose S&S:* Respiratory depression, CNS depression, CV insufficiency, coma, death.

PREGNANCY-LACTATION-REPRODUCTION

• There are no adequate and well-controlled studies in pregnancy before 37 weeks' gestation. Use during pregnancy only if potential benefit justifies fetal risk.

• There have been rare reports of infant respiratory distress and apnea after butorphanol administration during labor. These reports have been associated with administration of a dose within 2 hours of delivery, use of multiple doses, use with additional analgesics or sedatives, or use during preterm delivery.

• If fetal HR pattern is abnormal, use butorphanol cautiously.

• The decision to continue therapy or discontinue breastfeeding should take into account risks versus benefits to mother and infant.

❸ *Alert:* Monitor patients who are breastfeeding and infants for psychomimetic reactions. Monitor infants exposed to drug during breastfeeding for apnea and sedation. Withdrawal symptoms can occur in infants when drug or breastfeeding is stopped.

Boxed Warning Prolonged use during pregnancy can result in neonatal opioid withdrawal syndrome, which may be life-threatening. It requires management with expert neonatology protocols. If prolonged use is needed, advise patient of risks and ensure availability of proper treatment ■

NURSING CONSIDERATIONS

Boxed Warning May cause life-threatening or fatal respiratory depression at any time during therapy. Monitor patient closely, especially when starting or increasing doses. Proper dosing and titration are essential to reduce risk. ■

Boxed Warning Regularly monitor all patients for opioid addiction, abuse, and misuse, which can lead to overdose and death. ■

❸ *Alert:* If patient is taking opioids with serotonergic drugs, monitor for signs and symptoms of serotonin syndrome, especially when starting treatment or increasing dosages. Signs and symptoms may occur within several hours of coadministration but may also occur later, especially after dosage increase. Discontinue the opioid, serotonergic drug, or both if serotonin syndrome is suspected.

Boxed Warning Use of any coadministered CYP3A4 inhibitors or inducers can cause an increase or decrease in drug levels, leading to fatal adverse effects. ■

• Don't stop drug abruptly; withdraw slowly and individualize the gradual taper plan to prevent signs and symptoms of withdrawal, worsening pain, and psychological distress in patients who are physically dependent. Refer to manufacturer's label for specific tapering instructions.

Reactions in bold italics are *life-threatening*.

• When tapering opioids, watch closely for signs and symptoms of opioid withdrawal. Such symptoms may indicate a need to taper more slowly. Monitor patient for suicidality, use of other substances, and mood changes.

⚠️ *Alert:* Monitor patient for signs and symptoms of adrenal insufficiency. Perform diagnostic testing if adrenal insufficiency is suspected. If adrenal insufficiency is confirmed, treat with corticosteroids and wean patient off opioids, if appropriate. Discontinue corticosteroids when clinically appropriate.

⚠️ *Alert:* Monitor patient for signs and symptoms of decreased sex hormone levels. If signs and symptoms occur, evaluate patient and obtain specimens for lab testing.

• Drug may cause constipation. Assess bowel function and need for stool softener and stimulant laxatives.

• Periodically monitor postoperative vital signs and bladder function. Because drug decreases both rate and depth of respirations, monitor arterial oxygen saturation to help assess respiratory depression.

⚠️ *Alert:* Drug may cause opioid-induced hyperalgesia (OIH). Symptoms include increased pain level with opioid dose increase, decreased pain level with opioid dose reduction, pain from ordinarily nonpainful stimuli without underlying disease progression, opioid tolerance or withdrawal, and addictive behavior. For suspected OIH, decrease opioid dose or switch patient to alternative opioid.

PATIENT TEACHING

Boxed Warning Counsel patient and caregiver on serious risks, safe use, and importance of reading the medication guide with each prescription. ∎

• Advise patient to take drug exactly as prescribed and to use lowest dose possible for shortest time needed.

• Inform patient that, for acute pain, drug may only be needed for a few days. Teach patient about safe disposal of unused drug.

• Instruct patient to contact health care provider if prescribed dosage isn't controlling pain.

⚠️ *Alert:* Encourage patient to report all medications being taken, including prescription and OTC drugs and supplements.

• Advise patient to avoid alcohol during therapy.

⚠️ *Alert:* Counsel patient who has been regularly taking drug not to discontinue without first discussing the need for gradual tapering with prescriber.

⚠️ *Alert:* Caution patient to immediately report signs and symptoms of serotonin syndrome, adrenal insufficiency, and decreased sex hormone levels.

⚠️ *Alert:* Warn patient to withhold drug and inform prescriber if pain level worsens, pain sensitivity increases, or new pain occurs after taking drug.

• Teach patient who is ambulatory to use care when getting out of bed or walking due to possible dizziness or light-headedness.

• Warn outpatient to avoid driving and other hazardous activities that require mental alertness until drug's effects on the CNS are clear.

Boxed Warning Accidental ingestion of even one dose of an opioid, especially by children, can result in a fatal overdose. ∎

• Tell patient how to take nasal spray and how to store it in child-resistant container.

• Teach patient that naloxone may be prescribed with the opioid when beginning and renewing therapy to reduce risk of opioid overdose and death.

• Caution patient to report to prescriber pregnancy or plan to become pregnant.

cabotegravir

ka-boe-TEG-ra-vir

Apretude, Vocabria

Therapeutic class: Antiretrovirals
Pharmacologic class: HIV-1 integrase strand transfer inhibitors

AVAILABLE FORMS

Injection (extended-release): 600 mg/3 mL single-dose vial
Tablets: 30 mg

INDICATIONS & DOSAGES

➤ **Short-term treatment of HIV-1 infection in combination with rilpivirine in patients who are virologically suppressed (HIV-1 RNA less than 50 copies/mL) while on a stable antiretroviral regimen with no history of treatment failure and with no known or suspected resistance to either cabotegravir or rilpivirine**
Adults and adolescents ages 12 and older weighing at least 35 kg (lead-in therapy): 30 mg PO daily in combination with oral rilpivirine for at least 28 days as lead-in

therapy to assess cabotegravir tolerability before starting cabotegravir and rilpivirine extended-release injections. Give final oral dose the same day as starting cabotegravir and rilpivirine injections.

Adults (bridging therapy): 30 mg PO daily in combination with oral rilpivirine for up to 2 months as bridging therapy for patients who plan to miss a scheduled injection by more than 7 days. Start first dose of bridging therapy 1 month after final cabotegravir and rilpivirine injection for patients on a monthly schedule and about 2 months after last injection for patients on an every-2-month schedule. Continue oral dosing until injections are restarted.

➤ **Short-term preexposure prophylaxis (PrEP) to reduce risk of sexually acquired HIV-1 infection in patients at risk**

Adults and adolescents weighing at least 35 kg (lead-in therapy): 1 tablet PO daily for at least 28 days as lead-in therapy before starting cabotegravir extended-release injections. Give final oral dose on same day of or within 3 days after initiating cabotegravir injections.

Adults and adolescents ages 12 and older weighing at least 35 kg (bridging therapy): 1 tablet PO daily to replace one every-2-month injection as bridging therapy for patients who plan to miss cabotegravir injection by more than 7 days. Start first dose of bridging therapy 2 months after final cabotegravir injection dose and continue until or within 3 days after injections are restarted. An alternative oral PrEP regimen is recommended when duration exceeds 2 months.

➤ **PrEP to reduce risk of sexually acquired HIV-1 infection in patients at risk, with or without an oral lead-in with oral cabotegravir**

Adults and adolescents weighing at least 35 kg: Initially, 600 mg IM on the last day of or within 3 days after oral lead-in therapy (if used), followed by a second injection 1 month later. Continue with injections every 2 months thereafter.

ADMINISTRATION

• **Boxed Warning** Don't initiate drug for PrEP unless negative infection status is confirmed. ∎

PO
• Give at same time each day with food.
• Give missed dose as soon as possible.
• Store tablets below 86° F (30° C).

IM
• Drug is provided in a kit with vial adapter, needle, and syringe.
• Allow vial to reach room temperature if stored in refrigerator.
• Inspect for particulate matter and discoloration. Discard if present.
• Shake vial vigorously until suspension appears uniform. Small air bubbles are expected and acceptable.
• Give as soon as possible. Suspension may remain in syringe for up to 2 hours. After 2 hours, discard drug and syringe. Don't refrigerate filled syringe.
• Inject into ventrogluteal area (preferred) or dorsogluteal area (upper outer quadrant).
• May need longer needle lengths sufficient to reach gluteus muscle for patients with BMI greater than 30 kg/m².
• May give injection up to 7 days before or after the date patient is to receive the injection.
• If patient plans to miss a scheduled every-2-month injection by more than 7 days, give oral cabotegravir bridge doses.
• If injection is missed or delayed more than 7 days and oral therapy hasn't been given, reassess patient to determine if resumption of injection dosing remains appropriate. Refer to manufacturer's instructions for recommendations on repeated missed injections and time since prior injection.
• Store suspension at 36° to 77° F (2° to 25° C). Don't freeze.

ACTION

Inhibits HIV integrase by binding to the integrase active site and blocking the strand transfer step of retroviral DNA integration.

Route	Onset	Peak	Duration
PO	Unknown	3 hr	Unknown
IM	Unknown	7 days	Unknown

Half-life: PO, 41 hours; IM, 5.6 to 11.5 weeks.

ADVERSE REACTIONS

CNS: abnormal dreams, asthenia, depressive disorders, dizziness, fatigue, fever, headache, mood swings, sleep disorder, somnolence. **GI:** abdominal pain, decreased appetite, diarrhea, flatulence, nausea, vomiting. **GU:** increased creatinine level. **Hepatic:** increased AST and ALT. **Metabolic:** increased CK level, increased lipase level. **Musculoskeletal:** back pain, myalgia. **Respiratory:** URI. **Skin:** rash. **Other:** injection-site reactions.

Reactions in bold italics are *life-threatening*.

INTERACTIONS

Drug-drug. *Antacids containing aluminum, calcium carbonate, or magnesium:* May decrease oral cabotegravir level. Administer antacids at least 2 hours before or 4 hours after cabotegravir.

Methadone: May decrease methadone level. Monitor patient and adjust methadone dosage as needed.

Other antiretrovirals: Avoid use of other antiretrovirals with cabotegravir when used as monotherapy for PrEP or in combination with rilpivirine for treatment of HIV-1.

Rifabutin: May decrease cabotegravir level when given with extended-release injection. If used together, give second injection of extended-release cabotegravir 2 weeks after initial dose, and give maintenance doses monthly while patient is receiving rifabutin.

Strong inducers of UGT1A1 or UGT1A9 (carbamazepine, oxcarbazepine, phenobarbital, phenytoin, rifampin, rifapentine): May significantly decrease cabotegravir level and cause loss of virologic response. Avoid use together.

EFFECTS ON LAB TEST RESULTS

• May increase AST, ALT, lipase, creatinine, fasting lipid, and CK levels.
• May decrease HDL level.

CONTRAINDICATIONS & CAUTIONS

• Contraindicated in patients hypersensitive to drug or its components.
• Contraindicated for PrEP in patients with unknown or positive HIV-1 status. Monotherapy with drug isn't a complete regimen for HIV-1 treatment.
• Time from initiation of HIV-1 PrEP to maximal protection is unknown.

Boxed Warning Risk of drug resistance may occur with use for HIV PrEP in patients with undiagnosed HIV-1 infection. Drug-resistant variants have been identified in patients with undiagnosed HIV-1 infections with use of cabotegravir injections. ■

• Serious or severe hypersensitivity reactions may occur with cabotegravir. Discontinue drug if hypersensitivity reactions occur.
• Drug may cause liver toxicity in patients with or without known preexisting liver disease or other risk factors. Use cautiously in patients with underlying liver disease or marked transaminase elevations before drug initiation.

• Residual extended-release formulation of drug may remain in circulation for 12 months or longer.
• Use cautiously in older adults and patients with severe or end-stage kidney disease. Use in patients with Child-Pugh class C liver impairment hasn't been studied.
• Safety and efficacy in children younger than age 12 or weighing less than 35 kg haven't been established.

Dialyzable drug: Unlikely.

PREGNANCY-LACTATION-REPRODUCTION

• There are no studies during pregnancy. Cabotegravir injections aren't recommended for use in patients planning to become pregnant. Consider risks and benefits of therapy in patients of childbearing potential or who are pregnant.
• Enroll patients exposed to drug during pregnancy in the Antiretroviral Pregnancy Registry (1-800-258-4263).
• It isn't known if drug appears in human milk or how drug affects milk production or infants who are breastfed.
• Breastfeeding isn't recommended in patients who are HIV positive. For uninfected patients taking drug for PrEP, assess risks and benefits of therapy during breastfeeding. Extended-release formulation may appear in human milk 12 months or more after discontinuing drug.

NURSING CONSIDERATIONS

Boxed Warning Before starting drug (oral or IM) for PrEP and before each subsequent injection, test for HIV-1 infection using an FDA-approved or FDA-cleared test for diagnosis of acute primary HIV-1 infection. Patients who become infected with HIV-1 while receiving injections for PrEP must transition to a complete HIV-1 therapy regimen. ■

• Evaluate patient for potential exposure events and signs and symptoms of acute HIV-1 infection. Test patient for HIV-1 infection if diagnosed with other STIs.
• Monitor for signs and symptoms of hypersensitivity reactions (severe rash; rash with fever; general malaise; fatigue; muscle or joint aches; blisters, including oral blisters or lesions; conjunctivitis; facial edema; hepatitis; eosinophilia; angioedema; difficulty breathing); immediately discontinue drug if any occur and treat patient as appropriate.

• Monitor LFT values during therapy and as clinically indicated. Discontinue cabotegravir if liver toxicity is suspected.

• Monitor patient for depressive symptoms, and promptly evaluate for relation to cabotegravir.

• Refer to rilpivirine's prescribing information if rilpivirine is used with cabotegravir.

PATIENT TEACHING

• Inform patient taking cabotegravir for PrEP that it's part of an overall HIV-1 infection prevention strategy that includes adherence to dosing schedule and safer sex practices, including condoms, to reduce risk of STIs.

• Tell patient taking cabotegravir for PrEP that testing for HIV-1 is needed before therapy, before each injection, and if patient is diagnosed with other STIs.

• Inform patient that drug isn't always effective in preventing HIV-1 infection.

• Advise patient to immediately contact prescriber if signs and symptoms of hypersensitivity reaction (severe rash, rash with fever, tiredness, muscle or joint aches, blisters, facial swelling, difficulty breathing, liver problems [jaundice, dark urine, pale-colored stools, nausea, vomiting, right upper abdominal pain]) occur.

• Inform patient that LFT values and HIV-1 infection testing will be monitored during therapy.

• Tell patient to promptly report depressive symptoms to prescriber.

• Advise patient to follow testing schedule, take drug as prescribed, and avoid missed doses as doing so increases the risk of acquiring HIV-1 infection and developing drug resistance.

• Counsel patient of childbearing potential to report pregnancy or plans to become pregnant or breastfeed.

cabotegravir–rilpivirine
ka-boe-TEG-ra-vir/ril-pi-VIR-een

Cabenuva

Therapeutic class: Antiretrovirals
Pharmacologic class: HIV-1 integrase strand transfer inhibitors/HIV-1 NNRTIs

AVAILABLE FORMS

Injection (extended-release suspension):
400 mg cabotegravir and 600 mg rilpivirine single-dose vials (kit); 600 mg cabotegravir and 900 mg rilpivirine single-dose vials (kit)

INDICATIONS & DOSAGES

➤ **HIV-1 infection to replace current antiretroviral regimen in patients who are virologically suppressed on a stable antiretroviral regimen with no history of treatment failure and no known or suspected resistance to cabotegravir or rilpivirine**

Adults and adolescents ages 12 and older weighing at least 35 kg: Initially, cabotegravir 30 mg PO daily and rilpivirine 25 mg PO daily for at least 28 days to assess tolerability. On the last day of oral dosing, initiate injections with cabotegravir 600 mg IM and rilpivirine 900 mg IM as separate gluteal injections. Starting 1 month after initial injections, give cabotegravir 400 mg IM and rilpivirine 600 mg IM as separate gluteal injections once monthly.

Alternatively, on last day of current antiretroviral therapy, initiate injections with cabotegravir 600 mg IM and rilpivirine 900 mg IM as separate gluteal injections and repeat monthly.

Adjust-a-dose: If switching from monthly to every-2-month regimen, give cabotegravir 600 mg IM and rilpivirine 900 mg IM 1 month after last monthly injection, then every 2 months thereafter. If switching from every-2-month to monthly regimen, give cabotegravir 400 mg IM and rilpivirine 600 mg IM 2 months after last every-2-month injection, then every month thereafter.

ADMINISTRATION
IM

• Complete dose requires an injection of cabotegravir and an injection of rilpivirine during the same visit. Order of injections isn't important.

• Don't further dilute or reconstitute vials. Don't mix with other products or diluents.

• Before use, remove vials from refrigerator; allow products to reach room temperature (not to exceed 77° F [25° C]) for 15 minutes.

• Inspect vials for particulate matter and discoloration. Don't use if present. Note cabotegravir vial has a brown tint, which may limit inspection.

• Shake vials vigorously until suspension looks uniform before withdrawing into syringes. Small air bubbles are expected and acceptable.

C

• Give as soon as possible; suspension may remain in syringe for up to 2 hours. After 2 hours, discard drug and syringe.
• Give each injection at separate gluteal sites on opposite sides or at least 2 cm apart using the Z-track technique. Ventrogluteal site is preferred. Don't give by other routes or in other anatomic sites. May need longer needle lengths to reach the gluteus muscle in patients with high BMI.
• May give dose up to 7 days before or after the date patient is scheduled to receive maintenance injections.
• If patient plans to miss a scheduled injection by more than 7 days, give oral therapy to replace up to two consecutive months of injections. Recommended dose is cabotegravir 30 mg PO daily and rilpivirine 25 mg PO daily, with the first dose starting when the next injection is due and continued until the day injection dosing is restarted. If oral therapy lasts for more than 2 months, an alternative regimen is recommended.
• Refer to manufacturer's instructions for unplanned missed injections.
• Store vials at 36° to 46° F (2° to 8° C) in original carton. Don't freeze. Vials may remain in original carton at room temperature for up to 6 hours; discard vials after 6 hours.

ACTION

Cabotegravir inhibits the integrase strand transfer step of retroviral DNA integration essential for HIV-1 replication. Rilpivirine inhibits HIV-1 replication by noncompetitive inhibition of HIV-1 reverse transcriptase.

Route	Onset	Peak	Duration
IM (cabotegravir)	Unknown	7 days	Unknown
IM (rilpivirine)	Unknown	3–4 days	Unknown

Half-life: Cabotegravir, 5.6 to 11.5 weeks; rilpivirine, 13 to 28 weeks.

ADVERSE REACTIONS

CNS: abnormal dreams, anxiety, depressive disorders, dizziness, fatigue, fever, headache, sleep disorder. **GI:** abdominal pain, diarrhea, dyspepsia, flatulence, gastritis, nausea, vomiting. **Hepatic:** increased transaminases, *hepatotoxicity.* **Metabolic:** weight gain, increased CK and lipase levels. **Musculoskeletal:** bone and muscle pain. **Skin:** rash,

injection-site reaction. **Other:** hypersensitivity reaction.

INTERACTIONS

Drug-drug. *Anticonvulsants (carbamazepine, oxcarbazepine, phenobarbital, phenytoin):* May decrease cabotegravir and rilpivirine levels and decrease antiviral effect. Use together is contraindicated.
Antimycobacterials (rifabutin, rifampin, rifapentine): May decrease cabotegravir and rilpivirine levels and decrease antiviral effect. Use together is contraindicated.
Drugs that prolong the QT interval and increase risk of torsades de pointes (amiodarone, ciprofloxacin, haloperidol, SSRIs): May increase risk of prolonged QTc interval. Use together cautiously.
Macrolide or ketolide antibiotics (azithromycin, clarithromycin, erythromycin): May increase rilpivirine level and risk of torsades de pointes. Consider alternatives or use other macrolides with less effect on rilpivirine level (azithromycin).
Methadone: May decrease methadone level. Monitor patient closely and adjust methadone maintenance dosage as needed.
Other antiretrovirals: May increase risk of adverse effects. Avoid use together.
Systemic glucocorticoids (dexamethasone): May decrease rilpivirine level and decrease antiviral effect if more than one dose is given. Use together is contraindicated.
Drug-herb. *St. John's wort:* May decrease rilpivirine level and decrease antiviral effect. Use together is contraindicated.

EFFECTS ON LAB TEST RESULTS

• May increase ALT, AST, CK, and lipase levels.

CONTRAINDICATIONS & CAUTIONS

• Contraindicated in patients with previous hypersensitivity reaction to cabotegravir or rilpivirine.
• Hypersensitivity reactions to rilpivirine, including DRESS syndrome, have been reported. Skin reactions may be accompanied by constitutional symptoms (fever, organ dysfunction).
• Drug may increase risk of liver toxicity in patients with preexisting liver disease or identifiable risk factors.
• Use in patients with CrCl of less than 30 mL/minute or Child-Pugh class C liver

impairment hasn't been studied. Use cautiously and monitor for adverse effects.
• Residual levels of cabotegravir and rilpivirine may remain in systemic circulation for 12 months or longer.
• Use only in patients who agree to required injections because nonadherence to injections or missed doses could lead to viral resistance. To minimize risk of viral resistance, initiate an alternative, suppressive antiretroviral regimen no later than when injection is due. If virologic failure is suspected, switch patient to an alternative regimen as soon as possible.
• Safety and effectiveness in children younger than age 12 or weighing less than 35 kg haven't been established.
• Use cautiously in older adults.
Dialyzable drug: No.

PREGNANCY-LACTATION-REPRODUCTION
• It isn't known if drug increases risk of birth defects or miscarriage. Consider benefits and risks when using in patients of childbearing potential or during pregnancy.
• Enroll patients exposed to drug during pregnancy in the Antiretroviral Pregnancy Registry (1-800-258-4263).
• It isn't known if drug appears in human milk or how drug affects milk production or infants who are breastfed. Patients with HIV-1 infection shouldn't breastfeed to avoid transmission to infant.

NURSING CONSIDERATIONS
• Follow injection instructions carefully to avoid accidental IV administration.
• Monitor patient for about 10 minutes after injection. If postinjection reaction occurs (dyspnea, agitation, abdominal cramping, flushing, sweating, oral numbness, and changes in BP), treat as indicated.
• Monitor for signs and symptoms of hypersensitivity (severe rash, rash accompanied by fever, general malaise, fatigue, muscle or joint aches, blisters, mucosal involvement [oral blisters or lesions], conjunctivitis, facial edema, hepatitis, eosinophilia, angioedema, difficulty breathing, dark urine); if any occur, immediately discontinue drug and treat patient as appropriate.
• Routinely monitor LFT values and discontinue drug for suspected liver toxicity.
• Monitor patient with depressive symptoms to assess whether symptoms are related to drug and to determine risk of continued therapy.

PATIENT TEACHING
🛈 *Alert:* Stress importance of maintaining viral suppression by adhering to medication regimen and scheduled visits. Tell patient to contact prescriber if patient plans to or misses a scheduled injection, and explain that oral therapy may be used to replace up to two consecutive monthly injections.
• Inform patient that injection-site reactions (pain, erythema, tenderness, pruritus, local swelling) and systemic reactions (fever, pain [musculoskeletal pain, sciatica]) may occur.
• Teach patient to immediately report signs and symptoms of hypersensitivity reaction.
• Advise patient of the need for lab tests to monitor liver function.
• Tell patient to immediately report depressive symptoms (depressed mood, depression, major depression, altered mood, mood swings, feeling tense, negative thoughts, suicidality).
• Advise patient that if drug is stopped, other medicine will be given to treat HIV-1 infection.
• Warn patient of reproductive potential about the long duration of drug exposure; explain that drug's effect in pregnancy is still under study.

calcitonin salmon
kal-si-TOE-nin

Miacalcin

Therapeutic class: Antiosteoporotics
Pharmacologic class: Polypeptide hormones

AVAILABLE FORMS
Injection: 200 units/mL in 2-mL vials
Nasal spray: 200 units/activation

INDICATIONS & DOSAGES
➤ **Paget disease of bone (osteitis deformans)**
Adults: 100 units daily IM or subcut.
➤ **Hypercalcemia**
Adults: 4 units/kg every 12 hours IM or subcut. If response is inadequate after 1 or 2 days, increase dosage to 8 units/kg every 12 hours. If response remains unsatisfactory after 2 additional days, increase dosage to maximum of 8 units/kg every 6 hours.

C

➤ **Postmenopausal osteoporosis in patients more than 5 years after menopause**
Adults: 200 units (one activation) daily intranasally, alternating nostrils daily. Or, 100 units IM or subcut daily. Patient should receive adequate vitamin D and calcium supplements (at least 1,000 mg elemental calcium and 400 units of vitamin D) daily.

ADMINISTRATION
IM
• IM route is preferred if volume of dose exceeds 2 mL; use multiple injection sites.
• Visually inspect solution for particles, cloudiness, or discoloration. If present, discard.
• Store in refrigerator between 36° and 46° F (2° and 8° C).
Intranasal
• Alternate nostrils daily.
• Allow bottle to reach room temperature and prime pump before first use by releasing until a full spray is produced. Don't prime pump every day. Don't shake bottle.
• Carefully insert nozzle into nostril with patient's head upright and firmly depress pump toward bottle.
• Wipe nozzle with a clean, damp cloth and dry.
• Discard spray container after 14 doses (2 mL bottle) or 30 doses (3.7 mL bottle).
• Keep bottle refrigerated between 36° and 46° F (2° and 8° C) while unopened; store in an upright position at room temperature after opening.
Subcutaneous
• Visually inspect solution for particles, cloudiness, or discoloration. If present, discard.
• Alternate injection sites.
• Store in refrigerator between 36° and 46° F (2° and 8° C).

ACTION
Decreases osteoclastic activity by inhibiting osteocytic osteolysis; decreases mineral release and matrix or collagen breakdown in bone.

Route	Onset	Peak	Duration
IM, subcut	2 hr	23 min	6–8 hr
Intranasal	Rapid	10–13 min	Unknown

Half-life: IM and subcut, 58 to 64 minutes. intranasal, 18 minutes.

ADVERSE REACTIONS
CNS: depression, headache, dizziness, paresthesia, fatigue. **CV:** flushing, pedal edema. **EENT:** eye pain, abnormal tearing,

conjunctivitis, epistaxis, nasal congestion, rhinitis, sinusitis, facial edema. **GI:** transient nausea, salty taste, anorexia, nausea, abdominal pain. **GU:** increased urinary frequency, nocturia. **Hematologic:** infection, lymphadenopathy. **Musculoskeletal:** arthrosis, myalgia, back pain, osteoarthritis. **Respiratory:** *bronchospasm,* URI, shortness of breath, sinusitis. **Skin:** rash, pruritus of ear lobes, injection-site reaction. **Other:** hypersensitivity reactions, flulike symptoms, *malignancy.*

INTERACTIONS
Drug-drug. *Lithium:* May reduce plasma lithium level due to increased urinary clearance of lithium. Monitor level and adjust lithium dosage as needed.
Zoledronic acid: May enhance hypocalcemic effect of zoledronic acid. Monitor therapy.

EFFECTS ON LAB TEST RESULTS
• May reduce calcium level.
• May increase urine sediment.

CONTRAINDICATIONS & CAUTIONS
• Contraindicated in patients hypersensitive to drug or any of its components.
• For Paget disease or osteoporosis, reserve use for patients with contraindications or intolerance to alternative agents.
• Safety and effectiveness in children haven't been established.
Dialyzable drug: Unknown.
⚠ *Overdose S&S:* Hypocalcemic tetany (increased neuromuscular irritability, repetitive neuromuscular movements after a single stimulus).

PREGNANCY-LACTATION-REPRODUCTION
• Use during pregnancy only if potential benefit justifies fetal risk.
• Nasal spray isn't indicated for use in patients of childbearing potential.
• It isn't known if drug appears in human milk, but it has been shown to decrease milk production in animals. Before use during breastfeeding, consider risk of infant exposure, benefits of breastfeeding to infant, and benefits of treatment to patient.

NURSING CONSIDERATIONS
• Skin testing is usually done before therapy in patient with suspected drug sensitivity.

• Calcium and vitamin D supplements are recommended in patients with osteoporosis or Paget disease who have inadequate dietary intake.

🕓 *Alert:* Systemic allergic reactions are possible because the hormone is a protein. Monitor patient for hypersensitivity reactions, including anaphylaxis, and prepare for emergency treatment if needed.

🕓 *Alert:* Observe patient for signs of hypocalcemic tetany during therapy (muscle twitching, tetanic spasms, and seizures when hypocalcemia is severe).

🕓 *Alert:* Periodically reevaluate need for continued therapy because of the possible association between malignancy and long-term calcitonin salmon use.

• Monitor calcium level closely. Watch for symptoms of hypercalcemia relapse (bone pain, kidney stones, polyuria, anorexia, nausea, vomiting, thirst, constipation, lethargy, bradycardia, muscle hypotonicity, pathologic fracture, psychosis, coma).

• Be aware that periodic exams of urine sediment are recommended.

• Be aware that periodic nasal exams with visualization of nasal mucosa, turbinates, septum, and mucosal blood vessel status are recommended to assess for ulceration in patient using intranasal form.

• Be aware that nasal reactions occur more commonly in older adults.

• Monitor periodic ALP and 24-hour urine hydroxyproline levels to evaluate drug effect. Be aware that, in patient with Paget disease, maximum reductions of ALP and urinary hydroxyproline excretion may take 6 to 24 months of continuous treatment.

• In patient with good first response to drug who has a relapse, expect to evaluate antibody response to the hormone protein.

• If symptoms have been relieved after 6 months, treatment may be stopped until symptoms or radiologic signs recur.

• *Look alike–sound alike:* Don't confuse calcitonin with calcifediol or calcitriol.

PATIENT TEACHING

• When drug is given for Paget disease or postmenopausal osteoporosis, remind patient to take adequate calcium and vitamin D supplements.

• Inform patient that local inflammatory reactions at subcut or IM injection sites and facial flushing and warmth may occur within minutes of injection and usually last about 1 hour.

• Tell patient that nausea may occur at the onset of therapy.

• Instruct patient to promptly report signs and symptoms of hypercalcemia.

• Advise patient who is breastfeeding that drug may inhibit lactation.

• Teach about proper drug administration and handling, including storage and disposal of injection supplies.

calcitriol (1,25-dihydroxycholecalciferol)
kal-SIH-trye-ol

Rocaltrol, Vectical

Therapeutic class: Antihypocalcemics
Pharmacologic class: Vitamin D analogues

AVAILABLE FORMS
Capsules: 0.25 mcg, 0.5 mcg
Injection: 1 mcg/mL
Oral solution: 1 mcg/mL
Topical ointment: 3 mcg/g

INDICATIONS & DOSAGES
➤ **Hypocalcemia in patients undergoing long-term dialysis (PO)**
Adults: Initially, 0.25 mcg PO daily. Increase by 0.25 mcg daily at 4- to 8-week intervals. Maintenance oral dosage is 0.25 mcg every other day up to 1 mcg daily (most patients undergoing hemodialysis respond to doses between 0.5 and 1 mcg/day).
➤ **Hypocalcemia in patients undergoing long-term dialysis (IV)**
Adults and children ages 13 and older: Usual IV dosage is 1 to 2 mcg IV three times weekly (approximately every other day). Increase dose by 0.5 to 1 mcg at 2- to 4-week intervals.
➤ **Management of secondary hyperparathyroidism and resulting metabolic bone disease in patients with CrCl of 15 to 55 mL/minute**
Adults and children ages 3 and older: Initially, 0.25 mcg PO daily. Increase to 0.5 mcg PO daily, if needed.
Children younger than age 3: Initially, 0.01 to 0.015 mcg/kg PO daily.

Reactions in bold italics are *life-threatening*.

➤ **Hypoparathyroidism, pseudohy-poparathyroidism**
Adults and children ages 6 and older: Initially, 0.25 mcg PO daily in the morning. Dosage may be increased at 2- to 4-week intervals. Maintenance dosage, 0.5 to 2 mcg PO daily.
➤ **Hypoparathyroidism**
Children ages 1 to 5: 0.25 to 0.75 mcg PO daily.
➤ **Mild to moderate plaque psoriasis**
Adults and children ages 7 and older: Apply ointment topically to affected area b.i.d., morning and evening. Maximum weekly dose, 200 g.
Children ages 2 to 6: Apply ointment topically to affected area b.i.d., morning and evening. Maximum weekly dose, 100 g.

ADMINISTRATION
PO
• Give drug without regard for food.
IV
▼ Give by rapid injection through catheter at end of hemodialysis session.
▼ Discard unused portion.
▼ Store at room temperature.
▼ **Incompatibilities:** None listed by manufacturer. Consult drug compatibility reference for more information.
Topical
• Topical form isn't for oral, ophthalmic, or intravaginal use. Don't use on facial skin.
• Gently rub into skin until no longer visible.
• Don't apply an occlusive dressing.

ACTION
Stimulates calcium absorption from GI tract and promotes movement of calcium from bone to blood.

Route	Onset	Peak	Duration
PO	2–6 hr	3–6 hr	3–5 days
IV	Immediate	Unknown	3–5 days
Topical	Unknown	Unknown	Unknown

Half-life: 5 to 8 hours.

ADVERSE REACTIONS
CNS: headache, somnolence, weakness, irritability, apathy. **CV:** HTN, *arrhythmias.* **EENT:** conjunctivitis, photophobia, dry mouth, metallic taste, rhinorrhea. **GI:** nausea, vomiting, constipation, polydipsia, *pancreatitis,* anorexia, abdominal pain, epigastric discomfort. **GU:** polyuria, nocturia,

nephrocalcinosis, hypercalciuria, decreased libido, UTI. **Hepatic:** increased transaminases. **Metabolic:** weight loss, dehydration, hypercholesterolemia. **Musculoskeletal:** bone and muscle pain, arrested growth. **Skin:** pruritus, skin discomfort at application area or injection site. **Other:** hyperthermia.

INTERACTIONS
Drug-drug. *Aluminum hydroxide:* May increase aluminum level. Don't use together.
Calcium supplements: May increase risk of hypercalcemia. Avoid unmonitored calcium use.
Cardiac glycosides: May increase risk of arrhythmias. Monitor therapy.
Cholestyramine, colestipol, excessive use of mineral oil: May decrease absorption of oral vitamin D analogues. Avoid use together.
Corticosteroids: May diminish vitamin D analogue effects. Monitor therapy.
Magnesium-containing antacids: May cause hypermagnesemia, especially in patients with KF. Avoid use together.
Phenobarbital, phenytoin: May accelerate metabolism of calcitriol. Dose may need to be increased.
Phosphate binders (lanthanum carbonate, sevelamer): May alter phosphate level. Monitor phosphate level and adjust binder dosage, as needed.
Sucralfate: May increase serum sucralfate and aluminum levels. Avoid use together.
Thiazide, thiazide-like diuretics: May cause hypercalcemia. Use together cautiously.
Vitamin D: May cause additive effects and hypercalcemia. Avoid use together.

EFFECTS ON LAB TEST RESULTS
• May increase AST, ALT, BUN, creatinine, cholesterol, urine albumin, and calcium levels.

CONTRAINDICATIONS & CAUTIONS
• Contraindicated in patients with hypercalcemia or vitamin D toxicity. Withhold all preparations containing vitamin D.
• Contraindicated in patients hypersensitive to drug or its components or to drugs in the same class.
• Use cautiously in patients with sarcoidosis or hyperparathyroidism.
Dialyzable drug: Unknown.
⚠ **Overdose S&S:** Hypercalcemia, hyperphosphatemia, hypercalciuria.

PREGNANCY-LACTATION-REPRODUCTION

• Use during pregnancy only if potential benefit justifies fetal risk.

• Ingested calcitriol may appear in human milk. Patients shouldn't breastfeed during therapy.

• Use topical calcitriol cautiously in patients who are breastfeeding. If patient use of a topical vitamin D analogue is needed, patient should ensure infant doesn't come in contact with treated area.

NURSING CONSIDERATIONS

• Effective therapy requires adequate calcium intake.

• Monitor calcium level (multiplied by phosphate level, shouldn't exceed 70). After dosage adjustment, determine calcium level daily until level returns to normal. Once level falls within normal limits, monitor calcium level at least twice weekly. If hypercalcemia occurs, stop drug and notify prescriber but resume after calcium level returns to normal. Patient should receive adequate daily intake of calcium. Observe for hypocalcemia, bone pain, and weakness before and during therapy.

• Monitor phosphate level, especially in patient with hypoparathyroidism or on dialysis.

• Reduce dose as parathyroid hormone level decreases in response to therapy.

• Ensure patient taking calcitriol maintains adequate fluid status.

• Watch for symptoms of vitamin D intoxication (headache, somnolence, weakness, irritability, HTN, arrhythmias, conjunctivitis, photophobia, rhinorrhea, nausea, vomiting, constipation, polydipsia, pancreatitis, metallic taste, dry mouth, anorexia, nephrocalcinosis, polyuria, nocturia, weight loss, bone and muscle pain, pruritus, hyperthermia, decreased libido).

• *Look alike–sound alike:* Don't confuse calcitriol with calcifediol or calcitonin.

PATIENT TEACHING

• Tell patient to report all adverse reactions and to immediately report early signs and symptoms of vitamin D intoxication.

• Instruct patient to adhere to diet and calcium supplementation and to avoid OTC drugs and antacids that contain magnesium.

• *Alert:* Warn patient that drug is the most potent form of vitamin D available and shouldn't be taken by anyone except patient.

calcium acetate
Calphron ◊, Phoslyra

calcium chloride

calcium citrate ◊
Cal-Citrate ◊, Cal-C-Cap ◊, Citracal ◊

calcium gluconate

calcium lactate

Therapeutic class: Calcium supplements
Pharmacologic class: Calcium salts

AVAILABLE FORMS
1 mEq of elemental calcium equals 20 mg
calcium acetate
Contains 169 mg or 8.45 mEq of elemental calcium/g
Capsules: 667 mg
Gelcaps: 667 mg
Solution: 667 mg/5 mL
Tablets OTC: 667 mg, 668 mg ◊
calcium chloride
Contains 273 mg or 13.6 mEq of elemental calcium/g
Injection: 10% solution in 10-mL ampules, vials, and syringes
calcium citrate
Contains 211 mg or 10.6 mEq of elemental calcium/g
Capsules: 180 mg ◊, 225 mg ◊
Powder for oral solution: 760 mg/3.5 g
Tablets: 200 mg ◊, 250 mg ◊, 950 mg ◊
calcium gluconate
Contains 93 mg or 4.5 mEq of elemental calcium/g
Capsules: 500 mg ◊
Injection: 10 mg/mL, 20 mg/mL, 100 mg/mL
Tablets: 50 mg ◊, 500 mg ◊
calcium lactate
Contains 130 mg or 6.5 mEq of elemental calcium/g
Capsules: 100 mg ◊, 500 mg ◊
Tablets: 100 mg ◊, 325 mg ◊, 648 mg ◊

INDICATIONS & DOSAGES
➤ **Hypocalcemia**
Adults: 7 to 14 mEq elemental calcium IV. May give as a 10% calcium chloride solution. Or, initially, 1 to 2 g calcium gluconate IV.
Children: 0.136 to 0.252 mEq elemental calcium/kg IV. Or, initially, 29 to 200 mg/kg

calcium gluconate IV based on age and serum calcium level.

➤ **Adjunctive treatment of magnesium intoxication**
Adults: Initially, 7 mEq IV. Base subsequent doses on patient's response.

➤ **During exchange transfusions**
Adults: 1.35 mEq IV with each 100 mL citrated blood.
Neonates: 0.45 mEq IV after each 100 mL citrated blood.

➤ **Hyperphosphatemia**
Adults: Initially, 2 capsules or tablets or 10 mL oral solution PO t.i.d. with meals. Titrate dose every 2 to 3 weeks until an acceptable serum phosphorus level is reached; watch for hypercalcemia. Most patients on dialysis need 3 to 4 capsules or tablets or 15 to 20 mL oral solution with each meal.

➤ **Dietary supplement**
Adults: 500 mg to 2 g PO daily.

ADMINISTRATION
PO
• Give drug with a full glass of water.
• Give 1 to 1.5 hours after meals if GI upset occurs.
IV
▼ Give calcium chloride and gluconate only by IV route.
▼ Dilute calcium gluconate before use in 5% dextrose or NSS per manufacturer's instructions and assess for potential drug or IV fluid incompatibilities, especially with concurrent phosphate administration.
▼ Monitor ECG when giving calcium IV. Stop drug and notify prescriber if patient complains of discomfort.
⊕ *Alert:* Extravasation may cause severe necrosis and tissue sloughing. Calcium gluconate is less irritating to veins and tissues than calcium chloride.
Direct injection
▼ Don't use scalp veins in children.
▼ Warm solution to body temperature before giving it.
▼ For calcium chloride, give at 0.5 to 1 mL/minute (1.36 mEq/minute). For calcium gluconate bolus injection, don't exceed an infusion rate of 200 mg/minute in adults and 100 mg/minute in children, including neonates.
▼ Give slowly through a small needle into a large vein or through an IV line containing a free-flowing, compatible solution.

▼ After injection, keep patient recumbent for 15 minutes.
Intermittent infusion
▼ Infuse diluted solution through an IV line containing a compatible solution.
▼ **Incompatibilities:** *Calcium chloride:* None listed by manufacturer. Consult drug compatibility reference for more information. *Calcium gluconate.* Ceftriaxone, fluids containing bicarbonate or phosphate, lipid products, methylprednisolone, minocycline.

ACTION
Replaces calcium and maintains calcium level.

Route	Onset	Peak	Duration
PO	Unknown	Unknown	Unknown
IV	Immediate	Immediate	30 min–2 hr

Half-life: Unknown.

ADVERSE REACTIONS
CNS: anxiety; tingling sensations, sense of oppression or heat waves (IV use), syncope (rapid IV use). **CV:** *bradycardia, arrhythmias, cardiac arrest (rapid IV use),* decreased BP, vasodilation. **GI:** constipation, irritation, chalky taste, *hemorrhage,* nausea, vomiting, thirst, abdominal pain. **GU:** polyuria, kidney stones. **Metabolic:** hypercalcemia. **Skin:** infusion-site reactions.

INTERACTIONS
Drug-drug. *Bisphosphonates:* May reduce absorption of bisphosphonate from GI tract. Give calcium salts at least 30 minutes after alendronate or risedronate, at least 60 minutes after ibandronate, and not within 2 hours of tiludronate or etidronate.
Calcium channel blockers: May diminish therapeutic effects of calcium channel blocker. Monitor therapy.
Cardiac glycosides: May increase digoxin toxicity. Give calcium cautiously, if at all, to patients taking cardiac glycosides.
Deferiprone: May decrease deferiprone serum level. Separate administration of deferiprone and oral calcium medications or supplements by at least 4 hours.
Fluoroquinolones: Oral calcium may decrease absorption of oral quinolones. Consider therapy modification. Give at least 2 hours before or 6 hours after Phoslyra.
Iron supplements: May reduce iron absorption. Separate drug administration by 2 hours.

Levothyroxine: May decrease effects of thyroid products. Separate by at least 4 hours.
Raltegravir: May decrease raltegravir serum level. Give raltegravir 2 hours before or 6 hours after calcium or avoid use together.
Sodium polystyrene sulfonate: May cause metabolic acidosis in patients with kidney disease and a reduction of the resin's binding of potassium. Separate drugs by several hours.
Tetracyclines: May decrease serum level of tetracyclines. Avoid use together or, if use together can't be avoided, consider separating administration of each agent by several hours.
Thiazide diuretics: May cause hypercalcemia. Avoid use together.
Drug-food. *Foods containing oxalic acid (rhubarb, spinach), phytic acid (bran, whole-grain cereals), or phosphorus (dairy products, milk):* May interfere with calcium absorption. Discourage use together.

EFFECTS ON LAB TEST RESULTS
• May increase calcium level.
• May decrease phosphorus level.

CONTRAINDICATIONS & CAUTIONS
• Contraindicated in those with ventricular fibrillation, existing digoxin toxicity, or hypercalcemia.
• Use calcium products with extreme caution in patients taking cardiac glycosides and in those with cancer who have bone metastases, sarcoidosis, kidney or cardiac disease, kidney stones, or electrolyte disturbances, including hyperphosphatemia hypokalemia and hypomagnesemia.
• Use calcium chloride cautiously in patients with cor pulmonale, respiratory acidosis, or respiratory failure.
Dialyzable drug: Yes.
⚠ **Overdose S&S:** Hypercalcemia, confusion, delirium, stupor, coma.

PREGNANCY-LACTATION-REPRODUCTION
• It isn't known if drug causes fetal harm when used during pregnancy or if it affects reproductive capacity. Use during pregnancy only if clearly needed; monitor serum calcium level.
• Calcium appears in human milk but is thought to be compatible with breastfeeding. Monitor patient serum calcium level.

NURSING CONSIDERATIONS
⚠ *Alert:* Double-check that you're giving the correct form of calcium; resuscitation cart may contain both calcium gluconate and calcium chloride.
• Monitor calcium level frequently. Hypercalcemia may result after large doses in KF. Report abnormalities.
• Signs and symptoms of severe hypercalcemia include stupor, confusion, delirium, and coma. Signs and symptoms of mild hypercalcemia include anorexia, nausea, and vomiting.
• *Look alike–sound alike:* Don't confuse calcium with calcitriol. Don't confuse calcium chloride with calcium gluconate.

PATIENT TEACHING
• Tell patient to take oral calcium 1 to 1½ hours after meals if GI upset occurs.
• Instruct patient to take oral calcium with a full glass of water.
• Teach patient to report anorexia, nausea, vomiting, constipation, abdominal pain, dry mouth, thirst, or polyuria.
• Advise patient to notify prescriber if taking OTC products such as iron.
• Warn patient not to eat rhubarb, spinach, bran or whole-grain cereals, and dairy products in the meal before taking calcium; these foods may interfere with calcium absorption.
• Inform patient that some products may contain phenylalanine or tartrazine.

SAFETY ALERT!

canagliflozin
kan-a-gli-FLOE-zin

Invokana

Therapeutic class: Antidiabetics
Pharmacologic class: Sodium-glucose cotransporter 2 inhibitors

AVAILABLE FORMS
Tablets: 100 mg, 300 mg

INDICATIONS & DOSAGES
Adjust-a-dose (for all indications): Refer to manufacturer's instructions for use in patients with kidney impairment and drug interaction dosage adjustments.
➤ **Adjunct to diet and exercise to improve glycemic control in patients with type 2**

Reactions in bold italics are *life-threatening*.

diabetes; to reduce risk of major adverse CV events in patients with type 2 diabetes and established CV disease

Adults: 100 mg PO once daily before first meal of the day. May increase to 300 mg/day.

➤ **To reduce risk of CKD, doubling of serum creatinine level, CV death, and hospitalization for HF in patients with type 2 diabetes and diabetic nephropathy with albuminuria greater than 300 mg/day**

Adults: 100 mg PO once daily. May increase to 300 mg/day only in patients with eGFR 60 mL/minute/1.73 m^2 or greater.

ADMINISTRATION
PO
- Give before first meal of the day.
- Give missed dose as soon as possible unless it's close to time of next regularly scheduled dose. Don't give two doses at the same time.
- Store tablets at room temperature.

ACTION
Inhibits SGLT2, which reabsorbs glucose filtered by the kidneys, increasing urinary glucose excretion.

Route	Onset	Peak	Duration
PO	Unknown	1–2 hr	Unknown

Half-life: 10.6 hours for 100-mg dose; 13.1 hours for 300-mg dose.

ADVERSE REACTIONS
CNS: fatigue, asthenia, syncope, postural dizziness. **CV:** hypotension, orthostatic hypotension. **GI:** thirst, constipation, nausea, abdominal pain, dehydration, *pancreatitis.* **GU:** genital fungal infection, UTI, increased urination, vulvovaginal pruritus, kidney impairment. **Hematologic:** increased Hb level. **Metabolic:** *hypoglycemia, hyperkalemia,* hypercholesterolemia, hyperphosphatemia. **Musculoskeletal:** bone fracture, increased risk of lower limb amputation. **Other:** hypersensitivity reactions, falls.

INTERACTIONS
Drug-drug. *Digoxin:* May increase digoxin level. Monitor digoxin level periodically.
Fosphenytoin, phenytoin: May decrease canagliflozin level. Consider increasing canagliflozin to 200 mg/day in patients tolerating 100 mg/day and to 300 mg/day in patients with eGFR of 60 mL/minute/1.73 m^2 or greater.

Insulin and insulin secretagogues (glipizide, repaglinide): May increase risk of hypoglycemia. Consider lower dosage of insulin or insulin secretagogue.
Lithium: May decrease lithium level. Monitor level more frequently during canagliflozin initiation and dosage change.
Salicylates: May increase hypoglycemic effects. Monitor patient closely.
SSRIs (citalopram, fluoxetine, sertraline): May increase canagliflozin level. Monitor patient closely. Canagliflozin dosage may need adjustment if SSRI is discontinued.
UGT inducers (phenobarbital, rifampin, ritonavir): May decrease canagliflozin level. Adjust canagliflozin dosage based on estimated GFR.
Drug-herb. *St. John's wort:* May decrease canagliflozin level. Consider increasing canagliflozin dosage based on GFR.

EFFECTS ON LAB TEST RESULTS
- May increase serum creatinine, potassium, phosphate, Hb, LDL-C, non-HDL-C, and urine glucose levels.
- May decrease GFR and serum glucose level.
- May cause positive test for glycosuria and interfere with 1,5-anhydroglucitol assay. Use other methods to monitor glycemic control.

CONTRAINDICATIONS & CAUTIONS
- Contraindicated in patients with serious hypersensitivity to drug or its components.
- Contraindicated in patients with eGFR of less than 30 mL/minute/1.73 m^2.
- Drug isn't recommended for patients with Child-Pugh class C liver impairment, type 1 diabetes, or diabetic ketoacidosis.
- For patients who will undergo scheduled surgery, consider temporarily stopping drug for at least 3 days before surgery.
- **Alert:** Drug may cause acidosis, which may require emergency department care or hospitalization. Temporarily stop drug and resolve ketoacidosis before restarting drug.
- Drug may increase risk of bone fracture as early as 12 weeks after start of treatment and has been linked to decreased bone mineral density. Consider factors that may contribute to bone fracture risk prior to prescribing.
- **Alert:** Drug may increase risk of severe UTI, including urosepsis and pyelonephritis. Monitor patient and treat promptly if indicated.
- **Alert:** SGLT2 inhibitors such as canagliflozin increase the risk of a rare but

---

✚Canada   ◇OTC   ◆Off-label use   ⬤Do not crush   *Liquid contains alcohol   � Genetic

serious necrotizing fasciitis of the perineum (Fournier gangrene). If necrotizing fasciitis is suspected, immediately discontinue SGL2 drug and begin broad-spectrum antibiotics. Surgical debridement may be necessary. Monitor blood glucose level and start alternative therapy for glycemic control. Serious outcomes have included hospitalization, multiple surgeries, and death.

• Drug increases serum creatinine level and decreases eGFR; patients with hypovolemia may be more susceptible to these changes. Kidney function abnormalities can occur after drug initiation. More frequent kidney function monitoring is recommended in patients with an eGFR of less than 60 mL/minute/1.73 m².

• Use cautiously in older adults; in patients with volume depletion, impaired kidney function, chronic low systolic BP, or hypotension; and in those on concurrent diuretics.

• Safety and effectiveness in children haven't been established.

Dialyzable drug: No.

PREGNANCY-LACTATION-REPRODUCTION

• Studies during pregnancy are inadequate. Use during pregnancy only if potential benefit justifies fetal risk.

• Due to adverse effects on kidney development seen in animal studies, use of canagliflozin during second and third trimesters isn't recommended.

• It isn't known if drug appears in human milk. Due to potential for serious adverse reactions in the infant, use of drug during breastfeeding isn't recommended.

NURSING CONSIDERATIONS

• Monitor patient for infections, new pain or tenderness, and sores or ulcers of the lower limbs. Discontinue drug if these complications occur.

⚠ *Alert:* Drug can increase risk of AKI. Before start of therapy, assess for factors that may predispose patient to AKI (decreased blood volume, CKD, HF, or concurrent use of other medications [diuretics, ACE inhibitors, metformin, ARBs, NSAIDs]). Assess kidney function before starting drug and monitor patient periodically. If AKI occurs, discontinue drug and treat kidney impairment.

• Correct volume depletion before initiating drug. Observe for hypotension during therapy.

⚠ *Alert:* Monitor patient for ketoacidosis, especially with major illness, reduced food or fluid intake, or reduced insulin dose. Elevated urine or serum ketone levels without associated very high glucose levels have occurred with SGLT2 inhibitor use.

⚠ *Alert:* Immediately report signs and symptoms of necrotizing fasciitis of the perineum (temperature above 100.4° F [38° C]); general feeling of unwellness; tenderness, redness, or swelling of area from genitals to rectum). Signs and symptoms can worsen quickly. Immediately stop drug and prepare to administer broad-spectrum antibiotics; surgical debridement may be necessary. Monitor blood glucose level and start alternative therapy for glycemic control.

• Monitor blood glucose level. Assess for signs and symptoms of hypoglycemia.

• Be aware that because of drug's mechanism of action, urine test will be positive for glucose.

• Drug may increase lipid levels. Assess levels periodically and treat as clinically indicated.

• Assess for genital mycotic (fungal) infections, especially in patient with a history of infection and in uncircumcised male. Treat appropriately.

• Monitor patient for hypersensitivity reaction (urticaria); reaction may occur hours to days after start of therapy. Discontinue drug and treat appropriately if hypersensitivity reaction occurs.

PATIENT TEACHING

• Counsel patient about increased risk of lower limb amputations. Explain importance of routine preventive foot care, and instruct patient to immediately report infections, new pain or tenderness, and sores or ulcers involving the lower limbs.

• Advise patient to discontinue drug and immediately report hypersensitivity reaction (generalized urticarial rash).

⚠ *Alert:* Teach about signs and symptoms of necrotizing fasciitis (temperature above 100.4° F [38° C]; general feeling of unwellness; and tenderness, redness, or swelling of area from genitals to rectum). Instruct patient to seek immediate medical attention if any occur.

⚠ *Alert:* Advise patient to seek immediate medical attention for signs and symptoms of ketoacidosis (difficulty breathing, hyperventilation, anorexia, nausea, vomiting, abdominal pain, confusion, unusual fatigue or sleepiness).

⚠ *Alert:* Instruct patient to seek medical attention for signs and symptoms of UTI (dysuria, frequency, urgency, pelvic or back pain, hematuria, fever, nausea, vomiting).

🜊 *Alert:* Advise patient to seek immediate medical attention for signs and symptoms of AKI (decreased urine output, swelling in legs or feet). Warn patient not to stop drug without first discussing with prescriber.

• Warn patient of possible risks to fetus and infant during pregnancy and breastfeeding. Instruct patient who is breastfeeding to discontinue drug or discontinue breastfeeding.

• Caution patient to avoid dehydration, which can cause hypotension. Promote adequate fluid intake, and instruct patient to report signs and symptoms of hypotension (postural dizziness, weakness, syncope).

• Advise patient to use care during first few weeks of therapy because of increased risk of falls.

• Instruct patient on general diabetes care, including importance of diet and exercise and monitoring of blood glucose and HbA$_{1c}$ levels; signs and symptoms and management of hypoglycemia and hyperglycemia; and assessment for diabetes complications.

• Advise patient to seek medical advice promptly during periods of stress (such as fever, trauma, infection, or surgery) because medication requirements may change.

• Teach about proper drug administration and handling.

candesartan cilexetil
kan-de-SAR-tan

Atacand

Therapeutic class: Antihypertensives
Pharmacologic class: ARBs

AVAILABLE FORMS
Tablets: 4 mg, 8 mg, 16 mg, 32 mg

INDICATIONS & DOSAGES
Adjust-a-dose (for all indications): If patient, especially patient with impaired kidney function, is taking a diuretic, administer under close medical supervision and consider a lower starting dose.

➤ **HTN (used alone or with other antihypertensives)**
Adults: Initially, 16 mg PO once daily when used alone in patients who aren't volume-depleted; usual dosage range, 8 to 32 mg PO

daily as a single dose or in two divided doses. Adjust dosage about every 2 weeks, as tolerated, to target effect.

Adjust-a-dose: In patients with Child-Pugh class B liver impairment, initially give 8 mg PO once daily.

➤ **Pediatric HTN (used alone or with other antihypertensives)**
🜊 *Alert:* Don't use in children with GFR less than 30 mL/minute/1.73 m^2.

Children ages 6 to younger than 17: Initially for patients weighing more than 50 kg, 8 to 16 mg PO once daily. May adjust dosage to between 4 and 32 mg PO as single dose or divided doses as indicated.

Initially for patients weighing less than 50 kg, 4 to 8 mg PO once daily. May adjust dosage to between 2 and 16 mg PO as single dose or divided doses as needed.

Children ages 1 to younger than 6: Initially, 0.2 mg/kg PO once daily. Dosage range, 0.05 to 0.4 mg/kg/day PO as single dose or divided doses.

➤ **HF with reduced ejection fraction (NYHA Class II to IV)**
Adults: Initially, 4 mg PO once daily. Double dose about every 2 weeks as tolerated to target dose of 32 mg once daily.

ADMINISTRATION
PO

• Give drug without regard for food.

• Pharmacist may make tablets into suspension for patients unable to swallow pills.

• Shake suspension well before each use.

• Suspension may be stored unopened at room temperature for 100 days.

• Use suspension within 30 days of opening bottle.

ACTION
Inhibits vasoconstrictive action of angiotensin II by blocking angiotensin II receptor on the surface of vascular smooth muscle and other tissue cells.

Route	Onset	Peak	Duration
PO	Unknown	3–4 hr	24 hr

Half-life: 9 hours.

ADVERSE REACTIONS
CNS: dizziness, headache. **CV:** hypotension. **EENT:** pharyngitis, rhinitis. **GU:** kidney function abnormality. **Metabolic:** *hyperkalemia.*

Musculoskeletal: back pain. **Respiratory:** URI.

INTERACTIONS

Drug-drug. *ACE inhibitors, other ARBs:* May increase risk of hypotension, hyperkalemia, and changes in kidney function (including AKI) when used with other drugs that cause blockade of the RAAS. Consider therapy modification.

Aliskiren: May increase risk of kidney impairment, hypotension, and hyperkalemia in patients with diabetes and those with GFR less than 60 mL/minute. Use together is contraindicated in patients with diabetes. Avoid use together in those with GFR less than 60 mL/minute.

Lithium: May increase lithium level. Monitor lithium level closely.

NSAIDs (celecoxib, ibuprofen): May decrease antihypertensive effect of candesartan. Coadministration in patients who are volume-depleted (including those taking diuretics) or with decreased kidney function and in older adults may result in deteriorating kidney function. Monitor BP and kidney function.

Potassium-sparing diuretics, potassium supplements: May cause hyperkalemia. Monitor patient closely.

Drug-food. *Salt substitutes containing potassium:* May cause hyperkalemia. Monitor patient closely.

EFFECTS ON LAB TEST RESULTS
• May increase potassium, BUN, and serum creatinine levels.
• May cause false-negative aldosterone-to-renin ratio.

CONTRAINDICATIONS & CAUTIONS
• Contraindicated in patients hypersensitive to drug or its components, in children with GFR of less than 30 mL/min/1.73 m^2, and in children younger than age 1.
• Use cautiously in patients whose kidney function depends on the RAAS (such as patients with HF) because of risk of oliguria and progressive azotemia with AKI or death.
• Use cautiously in patients who are volume or salt depleted; may cause symptoms of hypotension. Start therapy with a lower dosage range, and monitor BP carefully.
• Don't use for HTN in children younger than age 1 because of potential effects on the developing immature kidneys.

Dialyzable drug: No.
⚠ **Overdose S&S:** Hypotension, dizziness, tachycardia; possible bradycardia from parasympathetic stimulation.

PREGNANCY-LACTATION-REPRODUCTION
Boxed Warning Drugs such as candesartan that act directly on the RAAS can cause injury and death to a developing fetus. Discontinue candesartan as soon as possible if pregnancy occurs. ∎
• It isn't known if drug appears in human milk. Use of drug during breastfeeding isn't recommended.

NURSING CONSIDERATIONS
• Most of drug's antihypertensive effect occurs within 2 weeks. Maximal effect may take 4 to 6 weeks. Diuretic may be added if BP isn't controlled by drug alone.
• Monitor BP during dosage escalation and periodically thereafter.
• If hypotension occurs after a candesartan dose, position patient supine and treat appropriately.
• Periodically monitor kidney function and serum potassium level.

PATIENT TEACHING
Boxed Warning Inform patient of childbearing potential of consequences of drug exposure during pregnancy. Instruct patient to immediately report suspected pregnancy. ∎
• Advise patient who is breastfeeding to discuss risks with prescriber.
• Teach about proper drug administration and handling.
• Inform patient to report all adverse reactions without delay.

SAFETY ALERT!

cangrelor
KAN-grel-or

Kengreal

Therapeutic class: Antiplatelet drugs
Pharmacologic class: Platelet aggregation inhibitors

AVAILABLE FORMS
Lyophilized powder for injection: 50 mg

---

*Reactions in bold italics are **life-threatening**.*

INDICATIONS & DOSAGES
➤ **Adjunct to PCI for reducing risk of periprocedural MI, repeat coronary revascularization, and stent thrombosis in patients who haven't been treated with a P2Y$_{12}$ platelet inhibitor and aren't receiving a glycoprotein IIb/IIIa inhibitor**

Adults: 30 mcg/kg IV bolus before PCI followed immediately by a 4 mcg/kg/minute IV infusion continued for at least 2 hours or for duration of PCI, whichever is longer. Transition patient to oral P2Y$_{12}$ platelet inhibitor to maintain platelet inhibition. Recommended inhibitors include ticagrelor 180 mg PO at any time during infusion or immediately after discontinuation; or, prasugrel 60 mg or clopidogrel 600 mg immediately after infusion discontinuation.

ADMINISTRATION
IV

▼ For each 50-mg vial, reconstitute by adding 5 mL sterile water for injection. Swirl gently until dissolved; avoid vigorous mixing. Ensure contents are fully dissolved, clear, colorless to pale yellow, and free from particulate matter.

▼ Immediately dilute reconstituted drug. Don't use without dilution.

▼ Further dilute each reconstituted vial by withdrawing contents from one reconstituted vial and adding to one 250-mL NSS or dextrose 5% bag. Mix bag thoroughly. This dilution results in a concentration of 200 mcg/mL and should be sufficient for at least 2 hours of dosing. Patients weighing 100 kg or more require a minimum of two bags.

▼ Discard any unused portion of reconstituted solution remaining in vial.

▼ Administer via a dedicated IV line.

▼ Administer bolus volume rapidly (over less than 1 minute) from the diluted bag via manual IV push or pump. Ensure bolus is completely administered before start of PCI. Start infusion immediately after bolus administration.

▼ Diluted drug remains stable for up to 12 hours in 5% dextrose injection and 24 hours in NSS at room temperature.

▼ **Incompatibilities:** None listed by manufacturer. Consult drug compatibility reference for more information.

ACTION
Direct P2Y$_{12}$ platelet receptor inhibitor that blocks ADP-induced platelet activation and aggregation. Binds selectively and reversibly to P2Y$_{12}$ platelet receptor to prevent further signaling and platelet activation.

Route	Onset	Peak	Duration
IV	2 min	2 min	1 hr after discontinuation of infusion

Half-life: 3 to 6 minutes.

ADVERSE REACTIONS
CNS: *intracranial hemorrhage.* **CV:** *hemorrhage.* **GU:** worsening kidney function in patients with CrCl less than 30 mL/minute. **Respiratory:** dyspnea.

INTERACTIONS
Drug-drug. *Agents with antiplatelet properties (NSAIDs, SSRIs):* May enhance antiplatelet effects. Monitor therapy.
Anticoagulants: May increase anticoagulant effects. Monitor therapy.
Thienopyridines (P2Y$_{12}$ platelet inhibitors clopidogrel, prasugrel, and ticagrelor): Negate antiplatelet effect. Don't give thienopyridines until cangrelor infusion has been discontinued.

EFFECTS ON LAB TEST RESULTS
• May inhibit platelet aggregation.

CONTRAINDICATIONS & CAUTIONS
• Contraindicated in patients hypersensitive to drug or its components and in those with significant active bleeding.
• Drug can cause serious hypersensitivity reactions (anaphylaxis, bronchospasm, angioedema, stridor).
• Safety and effectiveness in children haven't been established.
Dialyzable drug: Unlikely.

PREGNANCY-LACTATION-REPRODUCTION
• Studies during pregnancy are inadequate. Untreated MI can be fatal.
• When possible, discontinue cangrelor 1 hour before labor, delivery, or neuraxial blockade.
• It isn't known if drug appears in human milk. Use cautiously during breastfeeding.

NURSING CONSIDERATIONS

• Monitor patient for hypersensitivity reactions (anaphylactic reactions, anaphylactic shock, bronchospasm, angioedema, stridor). Discontinue drug immediately and treat emergently.
• Monitor patient for signs of overt bleeding and symptoms of active bleeding.
• Note that platelet function will normalize 1 hour after discontinuation of infusion.

PATIENT TEACHING

• Explain that drug is used to inhibit platelet function during PCI and that platelet function and clot formation normalize 1 hour after infusion.
• Warn patient of risk of bleeding; advise patient to immediately report signs and symptoms of bleeding (mental status changes, light-headedness, low BP, blood in stool or urine, bleeding from gums, joint pain and swelling, abnormal bruising, abdominal or chest pain).
• Caution that hypersensitivity reactions may occur. Instruct patient to immediately report difficulty breathing, swelling of throat and lips, faintness, hives, or rash.

SAFETY ALERT!

capecitabine ⚠
kap-ah-SEAT-ah-been

Xeloda

Therapeutic class: Antineoplastics
Pharmacologic class: Pyrimidine analogues

AVAILABLE FORMS

Tablets ⬛: 150 mg; 500 mg

INDICATIONS & DOSAGES

Adjust-a-dose (for all indications): Round to nearest dose that gives a whole tablet; don't cut tablets in half.
For patients with CrCl of 30 to 50 mL/minute: Reduce starting dose to 75% of usual starting dose PO b.i.d. Dosage for severe kidney impairment (CrCl less than 30 mL/minute) hasn't been established.
  Refer to prescribing information for dosing of agents used in combination.
  Refer to manufacturer's instructions for toxicity-related dosage adjustments.

➤ **Advanced or metastatic breast cancer as a single agent if anthracycline- or taxane-containing chemotherapy isn't indicated or in combination with docetaxel after disease progression on prior anthracycline-containing chemotherapy**
Adults: 1,000 mg/m² or 1,250 mg/m² PO b.i.d. on days 1 to 14 of each 21-day cycle until disease progression or unacceptable toxicity occurs. When used in combination with docetaxel, give docetaxel 75 mg/m² IV on day 1 of each cycle.
Adjust-a-dose: Individualize dose based on patient risk factors and adverse reactions.
➤ **Adjuvant treatment of stage III colon cancer as a single agent or as part of combination chemotherapy with oxaliplatin-containing regimen**
Adults: 1,250 mg/m² PO b.i.d. as a single agent or 1,000 mg/m² PO b.i.d. as part of combination chemotherapy on days 1 to 14 of each 21-day cycle for a maximum of 8 cycles. When used in combination therapy, give oxaliplatin 130 mg/m² IV on day 1 of each cycle.
✴ *NEW INDICATION:* **Perioperative treatment of locally advanced rectal cancer as part of chemoradiotherapy**
Adults: 825 mg/m² PO b.i.d. with concomitant radiation therapy or 1,250 mg/m² PO b.i.d. without concomitant radiation therapy.
✴ *NEW INDICATION:* **Unresectable or metastatic colorectal cancer as a single agent or as part of combination chemotherapy**
Adults: 1,250 mg/m² PO b.i.d. on days 1 to 14 as a single agent or 1,000 mg/m² in combination with oxaliplatin on days 1 to 14 of each 21-day cycle until disease progression or unacceptable toxicity occurs. When used in combination with oxaliplatin, give oxaliplatin 130 mg/m² IV on day 1 of each cycle.
✴ *NEW INDICATION:* **Unresectable or metastatic gastric, esophageal, or gastroesophageal junction cancer as part of combination chemotherapy**
Adults: 625 mg/m² PO b.i.d. on days 1 to 21 of each 21-day cycle for a maximum of 8 cycles, in combination with platinum-containing chemotherapy. Or, 850 mg/m² or 1,000 mg/m² PO b.i.d. on days 1 to 14 of each 21-day cycle until disease progression or unacceptable toxicity occurs, in combination with oxaliplatin 130 mg/m² IV on day 1 of each cycle.

Adjust-a-dose: Individualize capecitabine dose for combination chemotherapy based on patient risk factors and adverse reactions.

✳ *NEW INDICATION:* **Previously untreated HER2-overexpressing metastatic gastric or gastroesophageal junction adenocarcinoma as part of combination chemotherapy**
Adults: 1,000 mg/m^2 PO b.i.d. on days 1 to 14 of each 21-day cycle until disease progression or unacceptable toxicity occurs, in combination with cisplatin and trastuzumab.

✳ *NEW INDICATION:* **Pancreatic adenocarcinoma as part of combination adjuvant therapy**
Adults: 830 mg/m^2 PO b.i.d. on days 1 to 21 of each 28-day cycle until disease progression or unacceptable toxicity occurs or for a maximum of 6 cycles in combination with gemcitabine 1,000 mg/m^2 IV on days 1, 8, and 15 of each cycle.

➤ **Breast cancer (adjuvant therapy) in patients with HER2-negative primary breast cancer who had residual invasive disease after neoadjuvant therapy (containing an anthracycline, taxane, or both) and surgery** ◆
Adults: 1,250 mg/m^2 PO b.i.d. on days 1 to 14 of a 21-day treatment cycle for six to eight cycles.

➤ **Pancreatic cancer (locally advanced or metastatic)** ◆
Adults: 1,250 mg/m^2 PO b.i.d. on days 1 to 14 of a 3-week cycle until disease progression occurs or for up to 1 year; or, 830 mg/m^2 PO b.i.d. (in combination with gemcitabine) on days 1 to 21 of a 4-week cycle until disease progression or unacceptable toxicity occurs.

ADMINISTRATION
PO
⚠ *Alert:* Hazardous drug; use safe handling and disposal precautions.
• Give drug at same time each day.
• Give drug while with water within 30 minutes after a meal.
• Have patient swallow tablets whole; don't crush or cut tablets.
• Don't give a missed dose. Don't give additional dose if vomiting occurs. Continue with next scheduled dose.
• Store at room temperature.

ACTION
Converts to active 5-FU, which causes cellular injury by interfering with DNA synthesis to inhibit cell division and with RNA processing and protein synthesis.

Route	Onset	Peak	Duration
PO	Unknown	90–120 min	Unknown

Half-life: About 45 minutes.

ADVERSE REACTIONS
CNS: asthenia, confusion, depression, dizziness, dysarthria, dysphasia, *encephalopathy,* fatigue, fever, headache, impaired balance, insomnia, lethargy, mood alteration, pain, paresthesia, peripheral neuropathy, taste perversion, tremor, vertigo, weakness. **CV:** *arrhythmias,* chest pain, edema, myocarditis, *venous thrombosis.* **EENT:** abnormal vision, conjunctivitis, epistaxis, eye irritation, increased lacrimation, oral discomfort, pharyngeal disorder, rhinorrhea. **GI:** abdominal pain, anorexia, constipation, diarrhea, dyspepsia, gastric ulcer, *GI hemorrhage,* GI motility disorder, gastroenteritis, ileus, nausea, stomatitis, vomiting. **GU:** kidney impairment. **Hematologic:** anemia, *coagulation disorder, lymphopenia, neutropenia, thrombocytopenia.* **Hepatic:** altered LFT values, fibrosis, *hepatitis,* hyperbilirubinemia. **Metabolic:** dehydration, *hypocalcemia, hypokalemia, hypomagnesemia,* hypercalcemia, hypertriglyceridemia. **Musculoskeletal:** arthralgia, back pain, limb pain, myalgia. **Respiratory:** bronchitis, cough, dyspnea, hemoptysis, pneumonia, *respiratory distress.* **Skin:** alopecia, dermatitis, erythema, increased diaphoresis, nail disorder, palmar-plantar erythrodysesthesia (hand-foot syndrome), photosensitivity reaction, pruritus, radiation recall syndrome, rash, skin discoloration. **Other:** cachexia, fungal infection, hypersensitivity reaction, *sepsis,* viral infection.

INTERACTIONS
Drug-drug. *Allopurinol:* May decrease capecitabine metabolite concentration. Avoid use together.
Antacids containing aluminum hydroxide or magnesium hydroxide: May increase exposure to capecitabine and its metabolites. Monitor patient.
Clozapine: May enhance neutropenia. Monitor use together.
CYP2C9 substrates (celecoxib, glimepiride, torsemide): May increase substrate exposure and risk of adverse reactions. Monitor patient

closely when minimal substrate level changes may lead to serious adverse reactions.

Fosphenytoin, phenytoin: May increase fosphenytoin or phenytoin level and risk of toxicity. Monitor phenytoin level closely.

Leucovorin: May increase risk of fluoropyrimidine (capecitabine) toxicity. Monitor patient closely.

Kidney-toxic drugs (irinotecan, IV bisphosphonates, methotrexate, platinum salts): May increase risk of kidney failure. Use together cautiously.

Boxed Warning *Vitamin K antagonists (warfarin) :* May decrease clearance of warfarin and increase risk of bleeding. Frequently monitor PT and INR. ∎

EFFECTS ON LAB TEST RESULTS

• May increase triglyceride, ALT, and bilirubin levels.
• May decrease potassium and magnesium levels.
• May increase or decrease calcium level.
• May decrease Hb level.
• May decrease neutrophil, platelet, and WBC counts.

CONTRAINDICATIONS & CAUTIONS

• Contraindicated in patients hypersensitive to 5-FU.
• Severe bone marrow suppression can occur and is more common when drug is used in combination therapy. Dosage adjustment may be needed.
• Use cautiously in older adults and patients with history of CAD, mild to moderate liver dysfunction, hyperbilirubinemia, or abnormal kidney function.
• Patients with certain homozygous or heterozygous mutations of *DPYD* gene have increased risk of acute early-onset toxicity and severe, life-threatening, or fatal adverse reactions. Use isn't recommended in patients with known complete DPD deficiency. Consider testing for variants of *DPYD* gene before initiating drug.
• Safety and effectiveness in children haven't been established.

Dialyzable drug: Unknown.

PREGNANCY-LACTATION-REPRODUCTION

• Drug may cause fetal harm. Females of childbearing potential should use effective contraception during therapy and for 6 months after final dose.

• Males with female partners of childbearing potential should use effective contraception during therapy and for 3 months after final dose.
• It isn't known whether drug appears in human milk. Patient shouldn't breastfeed during therapy and for 1 week after final dose.
• Drug may impair fertility.

NURSING CONSIDERATIONS

• Monitor patient for hypersensitivity reactions.
• Assess for severe diarrhea; notify prescriber if it occurs. Give fluid and electrolyte replacement if dehydration occurs. Drug may need to be immediately interrupted until diarrhea resolves or becomes less intense.
• Note that older adults may be at increased risk for adverse GI effects.
• Monitor patient for neutropenia at baseline and before each cycle using CBC. Drug isn't recommended if baseline neutrophil count is less than 1.5×10^9/L or platelet count is less than 100×10^9/L.
• Monitor for cardiotoxicity (MI, angina, arrhythmias, cardiac arrest ECG changes, cardiomyopathy).
• Monitor for new or worsening skin reactions. Discontinue drug for SCARs, such as SJS and TEN, which can be fatal.
• Monitor patient for hand-foot syndrome (numbness, paresthesia, painless or painful swelling, erythema, desquamation, blistering, and severe pain of hands or feet), hyperbilirubinemia, and severe nausea. Drug therapy requires immediate adjustment.
• Optimize hydration before initiating drug. Assess patient's hydration status and kidney function at baseline and as clinically indicated.

Boxed Warning Frequently monitor INR and PT in patient taking capecitabine and oral vitamin K antagonist therapy; adjust anticoagulant dosage accordingly. Altered coagulation parameters, bleeding, and death have occurred with concomitant use. ∎

❸ *Alert:* Monitor carefully for toxicity, which may be managed by symptomatic treatment, dose interruptions, and dosage adjustments.
• *Look alike–sound alike:* Don't confuse capecitabine with cabozantinib or capmatinib. Don't confuse Xeloda with Xenical or Xpovio.

PATIENT TEACHING

• Teach about proper drug administration and handling.

Reactions in bold italics are *life-threatening*.

C

◆ Alert: Tell patient who also takes warfarin to report significant bleeding or bruising.
• If patient is prescribed a combination of tablets, teach about importance of correctly identifying tablets to avoid dosing errors.
• Inform patient and caregiver about expected adverse effects of drug (especially nausea, vomiting, diarrhea, and hand-foot syndrome) and self-management steps (such as antidiarrheal treatment). Explain that patient-specific dosage adaptations during therapy are expected and needed.
◆ Alert: Instruct patient to immediately stop taking drug and contact prescriber if diarrhea (more than four bowel movements daily or diarrhea at night), bloody diarrhea, vomiting (two to five episodes in 24 hours), nausea, appetite loss or decrease in amount of food intake each day, decreased urinary output, stomatitis (pain, redness, swelling, or sores in mouth), jaundice, hand-foot syndrome, cardiac symptoms (chest pain, shortness of breath, dizziness), temperature of 100.5° F (38° C) or higher, or other evidence of infection develops.
• Caution patient to seek immediate medication attention for hypersensitivity reactions.
• Explain that most adverse effects improve within 3 days after stopping drug. Advise patient who doesn't improve to contact prescriber.
• Inform patient of fetal risk and contraception recommendations.
• Tell patient that drug may impair fertility.
• Advise patient not to breastfeed during therapy and for 1 week after final dose.

captopril ⚹
KAP-toe-pril

Therapeutic class: Antihypertensives
Pharmacologic class: ACE inhibitors

AVAILABLE FORMS
Tablets: 12.5 mg, 25 mg, 50 mg, 100 mg

INDICATIONS & DOSAGES
Adjust-a-dose (for all indications): Patients with impaired kidney function may respond to smaller or less-frequent doses. In patients with significant kidney impairment, reduce initial daily dosage, and use smaller increments for a slow titration (1- to 2-week intervals). Slowly back-titrate dosage after desired

therapeutic effect has been achieved to determine the minimal effective dose. A loop diuretic such as furosemide, rather than a thiazide diuretic, is preferred in patients with severe kidney impairment when concomitant diuretic therapy is required.
➤ **HTN (alone or in combination with other antihypertensives)**
Adults: Initially, 25 mg PO b.i.d. or t.i.d. If dosage doesn't satisfactorily control BP in 1 or 2 weeks, increase to 50 mg b.i.d. or t.i.d. If that dosage doesn't satisfactorily control BP after another 1 or 2 weeks, expect to add a diuretic. If patient needs further BP reduction, may increase dosage to 100 mg b.i.d. or t.i.d.; then if necessary to 150 mg b.i.d. or t.i.d. while continuing diuretic. Usual dosage range, 25 to 150 mg b.i.d. or t.i.d. Maximum daily dosage, 450 mg.
➤ **Diabetic nephropathy**
Adults: 25 mg PO t.i.d.
➤ **HF**
Adults: Initially, 25 mg PO t.i.d. Patients with normal or low BP who have been vigorously treated with diuretics and who may be hyponatremic or hypovolemic may start with 6.25 or 12.5 mg PO t.i.d.; starting dosage may be adjusted over several days. Gradually increase dosage to 50 mg PO t.i.d.; once patient reaches this dosage, delay further dosage increases for at least 2 weeks to assess satisfactory response. Usual dosage is 50 to 100 mg PO t.i.d.; maximum dosage, 450 mg daily. Generally used in conjunction with a diuretic and, in select patients, possibly a cardiac glycoside.
➤ **Left ventricular dysfunction after acute MI**
Adults: Start therapy as early as 3 days after MI with 6.25 mg PO for one dose, followed by 12.5 mg PO t.i.d. Increase over several days to 25 mg PO t.i.d.; then increase to 50 mg PO t.i.d. over several weeks.

ADMINISTRATION
PO
• Give 1 hour before meals to enhance drug absorption.
• Pharmacist may compound drug into a suspension if patient can't swallow tablets.
• Refrigerate suspension. Suspension is stable for 56 days if refrigerated.
• Shake suspension well before use.

ACTION
Inhibits ACE, preventing conversion of angiotensin I to angiotensin II, a potent vasoconstrictor. Less angiotensin II decreases peripheral arterial resistance, decreasing aldosterone secretion, which reduces sodium and water retention and lowers BP.

Route	Onset	Peak	Duration
PO	Within 15 min	60–90 min	Unknown

Half-life: Less than 2 hours.

ADVERSE REACTIONS
CNS: dizziness, headache, malaise, fatigue, fever, insomnia, dysgeusia, paresthesia. **CV:** tachycardia, hypotension, chest pain, palpitations. **EENT:** oral ulceration, dry mouth. **GI:** gastritis, abdominal pain, anorexia, constipation, diarrhea, nausea, vomiting, peptic ulcer. **GU:** proteinuria. **Hematologic:** *leukopenia, agranulocytosis, thrombocytopenia, pancytopenia,* anemia. **Metabolic:** hyperkalemia. **Respiratory:** dry, persistent, nonproductive cough; dyspnea. **Skin:** rash, pruritus, alopecia.

INTERACTIONS
Drug-drug. *Aliskiren:* May increase risk of kidney impairment, hypotension, and hyperkalemia in patients with diabetes and those with GFR less than 60 mL/minute. Use together is contraindicated in patients with diabetes. Avoid use together in those with GFR less than 60 mL/minute.
Antacids: May decrease captopril effect. Separate dosage times.
ARBs (candesartan, valsartan), other ACE inhibitors: May increase toxic effects of captopril. Consider alternative therapy.
Diuretics, other antihypertensives: May cause excessive hypotension. May need to stop diuretic or reduce captopril dosage.
Gold: May cause nitritoid reactions (facial flushing, nausea, vomiting, hypotension). Monitor therapy.
Lithium: May increase lithium level; symptoms of toxicity possible. Monitor lithium level and patient closely.
Neprilysin inhibitors (sacubitril): May increase risk of angioedema. Use together is contraindicated. Don't give within 36 hours of switching to or from sacubitril.
NSAIDs: May reduce antihypertensive effect. Monitor BP.
Potassium-sparing diuretics, potassium supplements: May cause hyperkalemia. Avoid use together unless hypokalemia is confirmed.
Vasodilators (nitrates): May have additive effect. Discontinue nitrates before starting captopril. If resumed during captopril therapy, use together cautiously at lower dosage.
Drug-food. *Salt substitutes containing potassium:* May cause hyperkalemia. Monitor patient closely.

EFFECTS ON LAB TEST RESULTS
• May increase ALP, bilirubin, liver transaminase, BUN, serum creatinine, and potassium levels.
• May decrease serum sodium level.
• May decrease Hb level, hematocrit, and granulocyte, platelet, RBC, and WBC counts.
• May cause positive ANA titer.
• May cause false-positive urine acetone test results.

CONTRAINDICATIONS & CAUTIONS
• Contraindicated in patients hypersensitive to drug or other ACE inhibitors and in patients who had angioedema related to previous treatment with an ACE inhibitor.
• Use cautiously in patients with aortic stenosis, impaired kidney function, or collagen vascular disease (SLE, scleroderma) and in those who have been exposed to other drugs that affect WBC counts or immune response.
Dialyzable drug: Yes (hemodialysis in adults only).
⚠ **Overdose S&S:** Hypotension.

PREGNANCY-LACTATION-REPRODUCTION
Boxed Warning Use during pregnancy can cause injury and death to a developing fetus. When pregnancy is detected, stop drug as soon as possible. ∎
• Drug appears in human milk. Patient should discontinue breastfeeding or discontinue drug, considering importance of drug to patient.

NURSING CONSIDERATIONS
⚕ Patients who are Black and taking ACE inhibitors as monotherapy for HTN have a smaller reduction in BP than patients of other ethnicities.
⚕ Patients who are Black and taking ACE inhibitors have a higher incidence of angioedema than patients of other ethnicities.
• Frequently monitor BP and pulse rate.
🜛 **Alert:** Older adults may be more sensitive to drug's hypotensive effects.

Reactions in bold italics are ***life-threatening***.

- Assess for signs of angioedema.
- Drug causes cough, most frequently of all ACE inhibitors.
- In patients with impaired kidney function or collagen vascular disease, monitor WBC and differential counts before starting treatment, every 2 weeks for the first 3 months of therapy, and periodically thereafter.
- *Look alike–sound alike:* Don't confuse captopril with carvedilol.

PATIENT TEACHING

- Teach about proper drug administration and handling.
- Inform patient that light-headedness is possible, especially during first few days of therapy; instruct patient to rise slowly to minimize this effect and to report occurrence to prescriber. If fainting occurs, tell patient to stop drug and call prescriber immediately.
- Tell patient to use caution in hot weather and during exercise. Lack of fluids, vomiting, diarrhea, and excessive perspiration can lead to light-headedness and syncope.
- Advise patient to report signs and symptoms of infection (fever, sore throat).
- **Boxed Warning** Tell patient to notify prescriber if pregnancy occurs. Discontinuation of drug is necessary. ■
- Urge patient to promptly report difficulty breathing or swelling of face, lips, or mouth.
- Advise patient not to use potassium-sparing diuretics, ARBs, potassium supplements, or potassium-containing salt substitutes without first consulting prescriber.

carBAMazepine ⚥
kar-ba-MAZ-e-peen

Carbatrol, Epitol, Equetro, TEGretol, TEGretol-XR

Therapeutic class: Anticonvulsants
Pharmacologic class: Iminostilbene derivatives

AVAILABLE FORMS

Capsules (extended-release) ⊝: 100 mg, 200 mg, 300 mg
Oral suspension: 100 mg/5 mL
Tablets ⊝: 100 mg, 200 mg, 300 mg, 400 mg
Tablets (chewable): 100 mg, 200 mg
Tablets (extended-release) ⊝: 100 mg, 200 mg, 400 mg

INDICATIONS & DOSAGES

➤ **Generalized tonic-clonic and complex partial seizures, mixed seizure patterns**
Adults and children older than age 12: Initially, 200 mg PO b.i.d. (conventional or extended-release tablets or capsules), or 100 mg suspension PO q.i.d. with meals. May be increased at weekly intervals by 200 mg daily in divided doses at 12-hour intervals for extended-release tablets or capsules or 6- to 8-hour intervals for conventional tablets or suspension, adjusted to minimum effective level.

After 2 to 3 months of treatment, serum level may decrease due to liver enzyme autoinduction and dosage may need to further increase to 15 to 20 mg/kg/day; doses up to approximately 2 g/day may be needed in some patients for optimal effect.

Maximum, 1,000 mg daily in children ages 12 to 15 and 1,200 mg daily in patients older than age 15. Doses up to 1,600 mg daily have been used in adults in rare instances. Usual maintenance dosage is 800 to 1,200 mg daily.
Children younger than age 12 (extended-release capsules): Children taking total daily dosages of immediate-release carbamazepine of 400 mg or greater may be converted to the same total daily dosage of extended-release capsules, using a twice-daily regimen. Usually, optimal clinical response is achieved at daily doses below 35 mg/kg.
Children ages 6 to 12: Initially, 100 mg PO b.i.d. (conventional or extended-release tablets) or 50 mg suspension PO q.i.d. with meals, increased at weekly intervals by up to 100 mg PO in three to four divided doses daily (in two divided doses for extended-release form). Maximum, 1,000 mg daily. Usual maintenance dosage is 400 to 800 mg daily.
Children younger than age 6: 10 to 20 mg/kg/day in two to three divided doses (conventional tablets) or four divided doses (suspension). Increase at weekly intervals to achieve therapeutic response. Maximum dosage, 35 mg/kg in 24 hours.
➤ **Acute manic and mixed episodes associated with bipolar I disorder**
Adults: Initially, 100 to 400 mg PO daily in divided doses. Increase by 200 mg every 1 to 4 days to achieve therapeutic response. Doses up to 1,800 mg daily may be needed in some patients.

♣ Canada   ◇ OTC   ◆ Off-label use   ⊝ Do not crush   *Liquid contains alcohol   ⚥ Genetic

Adults (Equetro): Initially, 200 mg Equetro PO b.i.d. Increase by 200 mg daily to achieve therapeutic response. Doses higher than 1,600 mg daily haven't been studied.

➤ **Trigeminal neuralgia**

Adults: Initially, 100 mg PO b.i.d. (conventional or extended-release tablets) or 50 mg suspension PO q.i.d. with meals, increased by 100 mg every 12 hours for tablets or 50 mg q.i.d. for suspension until pain is relieved. Maximum, 1,200 mg daily. Maintenance dosage is usually 200 to 400 mg PO b.i.d.

ADMINISTRATION
PO

⚠ *Alert:* Hazardous drug; use safe handling and disposal precautions.

• Shake oral suspension well before measuring dose.

• When converting from tablets to suspension, administer the same number of milligrams per day in smaller, more frequent doses.

• When converting from immediate-release to extended-release tablets, administer same total daily dosage.

• Give chewable, immediate-release, and extended-release tablets and suspension with meals.

• Contents of extended-release capsules may be sprinkled over applesauce if patient has difficulty swallowing capsules. Extended-release capsules may be administered with or without food. Capsules and tablets shouldn't be crushed or chewed, unless labeled as chewable form.

• When giving by NG tube, mix dose with an equal volume of water, NSS, or D₅W. Flush tube with 100 mL of diluent after giving dose.

• Don't crush or split extended-release form or give broken or chipped tablets.

ACTION
Thought to stabilize neuronal membranes and limit seizure activity by either increasing efflux or decreasing influx of sodium ions across cell membranes in motor cortex during generation of nerve impulses.

Route	Onset	Peak	Duration
PO	Unknown	1.5–12 hr	Unknown
PO (extended-release)	Unknown	4–8 hr	Unknown

Half-life: 25 to 65 hours with single dose; 8 to 29 hours with long-term use.

ADVERSE REACTIONS
CNS: ataxia; dizziness; drowsiness; somnolence; vertigo; *worsening of seizures;* confusion; fatigue; fever; headache; pain; syncope; depression, including *suicidality;* speech disorder; asthenia; abnormal thinking; paresthesia; twitching; tremor; weakness; disturbances of coordination; hallucinations. **CV:** *arrhythmias, AV block, HF,* edema, aggravation of CAD, HTN, hypotension, thrombophlebitis, embolism, lymphadenopathy. **EENT:** blurred vision, cortical lens opacities, increased IOP, conjunctivitis, diplopia, nystagmus, tinnitus, hyperacusis, dry pharynx, dry mouth. **GI:** nausea, vomiting, constipation, abdominal pain, anorexia, diarrhea, dyspepsia, glossitis, stomatitis, *pancreatitis.* **GU:** albuminuria, glycosuria, erectile dysfunction, urinary frequency, urine retention. **Hematologic:** *agranulocytosis, aplastic anemia, thrombo-cytopenia, pancytopenia, leukopenia,* eosinophilia, leukocytosis, porphyria. **Hepatic:** abnormal LFT values, jaundice, *hepatitis.* **Metabolic:** hyponatremia, *hypocalcemia.* **Musculoskeletal:** leg cramps, arthralgia, myalgia. **Respiratory:** pulmonary hypersensitivity. **Skin:** *erythema multiforme, SJS, TEN,* diaphoresis, rash, urticaria, pruritus, photosensitivity reactions, skin disorder, alopecia, nail disorder. **Other:** SIADH, chills.

INTERACTIONS
Drug-drug. *Aripiprazole:* May decrease aripiprazole serum level. Double aripiprazole dose over 1 or 2 weeks when carbamazepine is added; then base additional dosage increases on clinical evaluation. If carbamazepine is later withdrawn, reduce aripiprazole dose.

Atracurium, cisatracurium, pancuronium, rocuronium, vecuronium: May decrease the effects of nondepolarizing muscle relaxant, causing it to be less effective. May need to increase the dose of the nondepolarizing muscle relaxant.

CYP1A2 and CYP3A4 substrates (acetaminophen, alprazolam, doxycycline, felbamate, haloperidol, hormonal contraceptives, phenytoin, sirolimus, theophylline, tiagabine, topiramate, valproate): May decrease levels of these drugs. Watch for decreased effect.

CYP3A4 inducers (phenytoin, rifampin, theophylline): May decrease carbamazepine level.

Reactions in bold italics are *life-threatening*.

C

Increase carbamazepine dosage as clinically indicated.

CYP3A4 inhibitors (erythromycin, cimetidine, gluvoxamine, loratadine): Increases plasma carbamazepine level. Monitor carbamazepine level; adjust carbamazepine dosage as necessary.

Lapatinib: May decrease lapatinib serum level; increase lapatinib dosage as clinically indicated. Avoid use together when possible.

Lithium: May increase CNS toxicity of lithium. Avoid use together.

MAO inhibitors: May increase depressant and anticholinergic effects. Avoid use together. Discontinue MAO inhibitors at least 14 days before starting carbamazepine.

Nefazodone: May increase carbamazepine level and toxicity while reducing nefazodone level and therapeutic benefits. Use together is contraindicated.

Oral and other hormonal contraceptives: May cause breakthrough bleeding and reduce contraceptive effectiveness. Consider back-up method of birth control.

SSRIs, TCAs: May increase carbamazepine level and decrease level of antidepressant. Closely monitor patient and adjust dosage as needed.

Warfarin: May reduce anticoagulant effect. Monitor PT when starting or stopping carbamazepine.

Drug-herb. *Plantains (psyllium seed):* May inhibit GI absorption of drug. Discourage use together.

Drug-food. *Grapefruit juice:* May increase carbamazepine level. Don't use together.

EFFECTS ON LAB TEST RESULTS
• May increase BUN and urine albumin levels and LFT values.
• May decrease sodium level and thyroid function test values.
• May increase eosinophil and WBC counts.
• May decrease granulocyte and platelet counts.
• May interact with some pregnancy tests.

CONTRAINDICATIONS & CAUTIONS
• Contraindicated in patients hypersensitive to this drug or TCAs and in those with a history of bone marrow suppression.
• Use cautiously in patients with mixed seizure disorders because they may experience an increased risk of generalized seizures. Also use cautiously in patients with myasthenia gravis or kidney or liver dysfunction.

• Avoid use in patients with porphyria.
▧ **Boxed Warning** Serious, sometimes fatal, dermatologic reactions (TEN, SJS) have been reported. Patients of Asian ancestry with HLA-B*1502 allele are at increased risk. Screen patients with ancestry in genetically at-risk populations for HLA-B*1502 before carbamazepine treatment. Don't use drug in patients testing positive unless benefit clearly outweighs risk. ■
• Drug may cause AV heart block conduction abnormalities. Use cautiously in patients at risk for conduction abnormalities, in those with abnormal ECGs, and in patients with preexisting heart damage.
• Drug can cause hyponatremia. Risk appears dose-related and may be increased in older adults and patients taking diuretics. For symptomatic hyponatremia, drug may need to be discontinued.
▧ Oral suspension may contain sorbitol; avoid use in patients with hereditary fructose intolerance.
• Safety and effectiveness of Equetro in children and adolescents haven't been established for indications other than epilepsy.

Dialyzable drug: Yes.

⚠ *Overdose S&S:* Conduction disorders; HTN or hypotension; impairment of consciousness; irregular breathing; respiratory depression; tachycardia; shock; seizures; adiadochokinesia; ataxia; athetoid movements; ballism; dizziness; drowsiness; dysmetria; motor restlessness; muscular twitching; mydriasis; nystagmus; opisthotonos; psychomotor disturbances; tremor; hyperreflexia followed by anuria or oliguria, hyporeflexia, nausea, vomiting, and urine retention.

PREGNANCY-LACTATION-REPRODUCTION
• Drug can cause fetal harm, including major congenital malformations. Weigh benefits against risks. If used during pregnancy, monotherapy (rather than use in combination with other anticonvulsants) is recommended to possibly reduce risk of teratogenic effects.
• Consider tests to detect fetal defects as part of routine prenatal care in patients receiving drug during pregnancy.
• Patients taking carbamazepine during pregnancy should enroll in the North American Antiepileptic Drug Pregnancy Registry (1-888-233-2334 or www.aedpregnancyregistry.org).

• Drug and its metabolite appear in human milk. Patient should discontinue breastfeeding or discontinue drug, considering importance of drug to patient.
• Drug may impair male fertility.

NURSING CONSIDERATIONS
• Watch for worsening of seizures, especially in patients with mixed seizure disorders, including atypical absence seizures.
• *Alert:* Closely monitor all patients taking or starting AEDs for changes in behavior indicating worsening of depression or suicidality. Symptoms such as anxiety, agitation, hostility, mania, and hypomania may be precursors to emerging suicidality.
• Obtain baseline determinations of urinalysis, kidney function, iron level, electrolyte levels, liver function, CBC, and platelet and reticulocyte counts. Monitor these values periodically thereafter.
Boxed Warning Aplastic anemia and agranulocytosis have been reported in association with carbamazepine therapy. Obtain complete pretreatment hematologic testing as a baseline. If patient exhibits low or decreased WBC or platelet counts during treatment, monitor patient closely. Consider discontinuing drug if significant bone marrow depression develops. ∎
• Never stop drug suddenly when treating seizures. Notify prescriber immediately if adverse reactions occur.
• Adverse reactions may be minimized by increasing dosages gradually.
• Therapeutic level is 4 to 12 mcg/mL. Monitor level and effects closely. Ask patient when last dose was taken to better evaluate drug level.
• When managing seizures, take appropriate precautions.
• *Alert:* Watch for signs of anorexia or subtle appetite changes, which may indicate excessive drug level.
• *Look alike–sound alike:* Don't confuse carbamazepine with oxcarbazepine. Don't confuse Tegretol or Tegretol-XR with Topamax or Toprol-XL. Don't confuse Carbatrol with carvedilol.

PATIENT TEACHING
• Tell patient that genetic testing may be needed before start of therapy.
• Teach about proper drug administration, handling, and storage.

• Tell patient that TEGretol-XR tablet coating may appear in stool because it isn't absorbed.
• Inform patient using drug for trigeminal neuralgia that an attempt should be made to decrease dosage or withdraw drug every 3 months.
• Advise patient to report adverse reactions and to immediately report fever, sore throat, mouth ulcers, and easy bruising or bleeding.
• Warn that drug may cause mild to moderate dizziness and drowsiness when first taken. Instruct patient to avoid hazardous activities until effects disappear, usually within 3 to 4 days.
• Advise patient that periodic eye exams are recommended.
• Warn of risks to fetus if pregnancy occurs while taking carbamazepine; advise patient to enroll in the North American Antiepileptic Drug Pregnancy Registry.
• Advise patient that breastfeeding isn't recommended during therapy.

SAFETY ALERT!

CARBOplatin
KAR-boe-pla-tin

Therapeutic class: Antineoplastics
Pharmacologic class: Platinum-containing compounds

AVAILABLE FORMS
Aqueous solution for injection: 10 mg/mL in 5-mL, 15-mL, 45-mL, 60-mL, 100-mL vials

INDICATIONS & DOSAGES
➤ **Advanced ovarian cancer**
Adults: 360 mg/m^2 IV on day 1 every 4 weeks as a single agent. Or, 300 mg/m^2 on day 1 every 4 weeks for six cycles when used with other chemotherapy drugs, such as cyclophosphamide. Or, use Calvert formula to calculate initial dosage:

$$\text{Total dose (mg)} = (\text{target AUC in mg/mL/minute}) \times (\text{GFR in mL/minute} + 25)$$

where *target AUC* is usually 4 to 6 mg/mL/minute.

Don't repeat doses until platelet count exceeds 100,000/mm^3 and neutrophil count exceeds 2,000/mm^3. Subsequent doses are based on blood counts: If platelet count is greater than 100,000/mm^3 and neutrophil

C

count is greater than 2,000/mm³, give 125% of prior dose. If platelet count is 50,000/mm³ to 100,000/mm³ and neutrophil count is 500/mm³ to 2,000/mm³, keep same dose. If platelet count is less than 50,000/mm³ and neutrophil count is less than 500/mm³, give 75% of dose.

Adjust-a-dose: If CrCl is 41 to 59 mL/minute, first dose is 250 mg/m². If CrCl is 16 to 40 mL/minute, first dose is 200 mg/m². Drug isn't recommended for patients with CrCl of 15 mL/minute or less.

➤ **Neuroblastoma, localized and unresectable ◆**

Children weighing 10 kg or more: 200 mg/m²/day IV on days 1, 2, and 3 every 21 days for two cycles (in combination with etoposide for two cycles, followed by cyclophosphamide, doxorubicin, and vincristine).

Children younger than age 1: 6.6 mg/kg/day IV on days 1, 2, and 3 (in combination with etoposide for two cycles, followed by cyclophosphamide, doxorubicin, and vincristine).

➤ **Glioma ◆**

Children and adolescents ages 3 months and older: For induction, 175 mg/m² IV weekly for 4 weeks every 6 weeks for two cycles, with a 2-week recovery period between courses (in combination with vincristine).

For maintenance, 175 mg/m² IV weekly for 4 weeks (in combination with vincristine) for up to 12 cycles, with a 3-week recovery period between cycles.

➤ **Breast cancer, cervical cancer, endometrial cancer, esophageal cancer, gastric cancer, head and neck cancer, NSCLC, small-cell lung cancer, and testicular cancer ◆**

Adults: Refer to individual treatment protocol.

ADMINISTRATION

IV

Boxed Warning Anaphylaxis may occur within minutes of administration. Keep epinephrine, corticosteroids, and antihistamines available when giving carboplatin. ∎

ⓤ *Alert:* Hazardous drug; use safe handling and disposal precautions.

▼ Don't use aluminum needles or IV administration sets because drug may precipitate or lose potency.

▼ For ready-to-use aqueous solution of 10 mg/mL, may further dilute with NSS or D₅W to a concentration as low as 0.5 mg/mL.

▼ Give drug by continuous or intermittent infusion over at least 15 minutes.

▼ Store unopened vials at room temperature. Protect from light.

▼ Once diluted, drug remains stable at room temperature for 8 hours.

▼ Because drug contains no preservatives, discard after 8 hours.

▼ **Incompatibilities:** None listed by manufacturer. Consult drug compatibility reference for more information.

ACTION

May cross-link strands of cellular DNA and interfere with RNA transcription, causing an imbalance of growth that leads to cell death. Not specific to cell cycle.

Route	Onset	Peak	Duration
IV	Unknown	Unknown	Unknown

Half-life: Carboplatin, about 2.5 to 6 hours; platinum, 5 or more days.

ADVERSE REACTIONS

CNS: dizziness, confusion, *stroke,* peripheral neuropathy, *central neurotoxicity,* pain, asthenia, taste perversion, fever. **CV:** *HF, embolism, bleeding.* **EENT:** ototoxicity. **GI:** abdominal pain, constipation, diarrhea, nausea, vomiting, mucositis, stomatitis. **GU:** kidney toxicity, increased BUN and creatinine levels. **Hematologic:** *thrombocytopenia, leukopenia, neutropenia,* anemia, *bone marrow suppression, bleeding.* **Hepatic:** hyperbilirubinemia, elevated LFT values. **Metabolic:** hyponatremia, *hypokalemia, hypocalcemia, hypomagnesemia.* **Skin:** alopecia, injection-site reactions. **Other:** hypersensitivity reactions, infection.

INTERACTIONS

Drug-drug. *Bone marrow suppressants, including radiation therapy:* May increase hematologic toxicity. Closely monitor CBC with differential.

Live-virus vaccines: May diminish vaccine's effect. Don't give live-virus vaccines for 3 months after last dose of carboplatin.

Kidney-toxic drugs, especially aminoglycosides and amphotericin B: May enhance kidney toxicity of carboplatin. Use together cautiously.

Phenytoin: May decrease phenytoin level. Monitor serum level, and watch patient for decreased effectiveness.

Drug-herb. *Echinacea:* May diminish therapeutic effects of carboplatin. Avoid use together.

EFFECTS ON LAB TEST RESULTS
• May increase ALP, AST, BUN, and creatinine levels.
• May decrease calcium, sodium, magnesium, and potassium levels.
• May decrease Hb level, hematocrit, and neutrophil, platelet, RBC, and WBC counts.

CONTRAINDICATIONS & CAUTIONS
• Contraindicated in patients with severe bone marrow suppression or bleeding and in patients with history of hypersensitivity to cisplatin or platinum-containing compounds
• Patients older than age 65 and those previously treated with cisplatin are at greater risk for neurotoxicity.
• Safety and effectiveness in children haven't been established.
Dialyzable drug: Yes.
⚠ *Overdose S&S:* Bone marrow suppression, liver toxicity.

PREGNANCY-LACTATION-REPRODUCTION
• Drug may cause fetal harm when administered during pregnancy. Patients shouldn't become pregnant during therapy.
• It's unknown if drug appears in human milk. Patient should discontinue breastfeeding during therapy due to risk of toxicity to infant.
• Drug may increase risk of infertility.

NURSING CONSIDERATIONS
Boxed Warning Carboplatin should be administered under the supervision of a physician experienced in the use of chemotherapeutic agents. Appropriate management of therapy and complications is possible only when adequate treatment facilities are readily available. ■
• Determine electrolyte, creatinine, and BUN levels; CBC with differential; platelet count; and CrCl before first infusion and before each course of treatment.
🔵 *Alert:* Note that, when using the Calvert formula, the total dose is calculated in mg, not mg/m^2.
• Monitor CBC with differential and platelet count frequently during therapy and, when indicated, until recovery. Lowest WBC and

platelet counts usually occur by day 21. Levels usually return to baseline by day 28. Don't repeat unless platelet count exceeds 100,000/mm^3.
Boxed Warning Anaphylactic-like reactions to carboplatin injection have been reported and may occur within minutes of administration. Epinephrine, corticosteroids, and antihistamines have been employed to alleviate symptoms. ■
Boxed Warning Bone marrow suppression is dose related and may be severe, resulting in infection or bleeding. Anemia may be cumulative and require transfusion support. ■
Boxed Warning Vomiting is a frequent, sometimes severe drug-related adverse effect. ■
• Antiemetics are recommended to prevent nausea and vomiting.
• Bone marrow suppression may be more severe in patients with CrCl below 60 mL/minute; adjust dosage.
🔵 *Alert:* Carefully check ordered dose against lab test results. Only one increase in dosage is recommended. Subsequent doses shouldn't exceed 125% of starting dose.
• Therapeutic effects are commonly accompanied by toxicity.
• To prevent bleeding, avoid all IM injections when platelet count is below 50,000/mm^3.
• Monitor vital signs during infusion.
• Monitor patient for hearing and vision changes.
• *Look alike–sound alike:* Don't confuse carboplatin with cisplatin.

PATIENT TEACHING
• Advise patient of most common adverse reactions (nausea, vomiting, bone marrow suppression, anemia, reduced platelets).
• Instruct patient to watch for signs of infection (fever, sore throat, fatigue) and bleeding (easy bruising, nosebleeds, bleeding gums, melena). Tell patient to take temperature daily.
• Counsel patient about risk of infertility before starting therapy.
• Recommend that patient consult prescriber before becoming pregnant.
• Advise patient to stop breastfeeding during therapy because of risk of toxicity to infant.

Reactions in bold italics are *life-threatening*.

C

cariprazine hydrochloride
kar-IP-ra-zeen

Vraylar

Therapeutic class: Antipsychotics
Pharmacologic class: Atypical antipsychotics

AVAILABLE FORMS
Capsules: 1.5 mg, 3 mg, 4.5 mg, 6 mg

INDICATIONS & DOSAGES
Adjust-a-dose (for all indications): If a strong CYP3A4 inhibitor is initiated while patient is on a stable dose of cariprazine, reduce cariprazine dosage by half; if patient is taking 4.5 mg daily, reduce to 1.5 or 3 mg daily; if patient is taking 1.5 mg daily, give every other day. Adjust cariprazine dosage when CYP3A4 inhibitor is discontinued. If initiating cariprazine while patient is on a strong CYP3A4 inhibitor, give 1.5 mg on days 1 and 3 (with no dose on day 2); from day 4 onward, give 1.5 mg daily and increase to maximum dose of 3 mg daily. Adjust cariprazine dosage when CYP3A4 inhibitor is discontinued. Concomitant use of cariprazine and CYP3A4 inducers hasn't been studied and isn't recommended.

➤ **Schizophrenia; manic or mixed episodes associated with bipolar I disorder**
Adults: Initially, 1.5 mg PO once daily on day 1. May increase to 3 mg PO once daily on day 2. Based on patient's response and tolerability, may make further dosage adjustments in 1.5- or 3-mg increments. Recommended dosage range for schizophrenia is 1.5 to 6 mg once daily. Recommended dosage for bipolar I disorder is 3 to 6 mg once daily. Maximum, 6 mg daily.

➤ **Depressive episodes associated with bipolar I disorder (bipolar depression)**
Adults: Initially, 1.5 mg PO once daily. May increase to 3 mg PO once daily on day 15 based on response and tolerability. Maximum, 3 mg daily.

✳ *NEW INDICATION:* **Adjunctive therapy to antidepressant treatment of major depressive disorder (MDD)**
Adults: Initially, 1.5 mg PO once daily. May increase to 3 mg PO once daily on day 15. Maximum, 3 mg daily.

ADMINISTRATION
PO
- May give with or without food.
- Store at room temperature.
- Protect 3- and 4.5-mg capsules from light to prevent potential color fading.

ACTION
Exact mechanism unknown. Action thought to occur through partial agonist activity at central dopamine D_2 and serotonin 5-HT_{1A} receptors as well as antagonist activity at serotonin 5-HT_{2A} receptors.

Route	Onset	Peak	Duration
PO	Unknown	3–6 hr	Unknown

Half-life: 48 to 96 hours (parent compound); 1 day to 3 weeks (major metabolites).

ADVERSE REACTIONS
CNS: fatigue, fever, extrapyramidal symptoms, akathisia, headache, somnolence, dizziness, agitation, insomnia, restlessness, anxiety. **CV:** tachycardia, HTN, edema. **EENT:** blurred vision, nasopharyngitis, toothache, oropharyngeal pain, dry mouth. **GI:** abdominal pain, constipation, diarrhea, dyspepsia, nausea, vomiting, decreased appetite. **GU:** UTI. **Hepatic:** increased liver enzyme levels. **Metabolic:** weight gain, increased CK level. **Musculoskeletal:** arthralgia, back pain, extremity pain. **Respiratory:** cough. **Skin:** rash, hyperhidrosis

INTERACTIONS
Drug-drug. *Antiparkinsonian drugs (dopamine agonists):* May diminish therapeutic effect of dopamine agonists; when possible in patients with Parkinson disease, consider use of alternative anti-psychotic, such as clozapine or quetiapine, which may convey lowest interaction risk.
CNS depressants: May increase CNS depression. Monitor therapy.
CYP3A4 inducers (carbamazepine, rifampin): May increase or decrease cariprazine level. Use together isn't recommended.
Opioid class warning: May cause slow or difficult breathing, sedation, and death. Avoid use together. If use together can't be avoided, limit dosage and duration of each drug to the minimum needed for desired effect.
Strong CYP3A4 inhibitors (itraconazole, ketoconazole): May increase cariprazine level. Reduce cariprazine dosage.

✤ Canada   ◇OTC   ◆Off-label use   ⊜Do not crush   *Liquid contains alcohol   ✂ Genetic

Drug-herb. *Kava kava:* May enhance adverse or toxic effects of cariprazine. Monitor use together.

St. John's wort: May decrease cariprazine concentration. Discourage use together.

Drug-food. *Grapefruit juice (CYP3A4 inhibitor):* May increase cariprazine concentration. Discourage use together.

EFFECTS ON LAB TEST RESULTS
• May increase CK and liver enzyme levels.
• May decrease WBC count.

CONTRAINDICATIONS & CAUTIONS
• Contraindicated in patients hypersensitive to drug or its components.

Boxed Warning Antipsychotics increase the risk of death in older adults with dementia-related psychosis. Drug isn't approved to treat patients with dementia-related psychosis. ∎

Boxed Warning *Opioid class warning:* Opioids should only be prescribed with benzodiazepines or other CNS depressants when alternative treatment options are inadequate, aren't expected to provide adequate analgesia, haven't been tolerated, or aren't expected to be tolerated. ∎

Boxed Warning Antidepressants increase the risk of suicidality in children and young adults. Closely monitor all patients treated with antidepressants for clinical worsening and emergence of suicidality. ∎

✪ **Alert:** Antipsychotics can cause leukopenia, neutropenia, and agranulocytosis, which can be fatal. Use cautiously in patients with preexisting low WBC count or ANC or history of drug-induced leukopenia or neutropenia.

• Antipsychotics can cause orthostatic hypotension and syncope. Drug hasn't been evaluated in patients with a recent history of MI or unstable CV disease.

• Use cautiously in patients at risk for aspiration; antipsychotics can cause esophageal dysmotility and aspiration.

• Antipsychotics can cause NMS, which can be fatal.

• Drug may cause irreversible tardive dyskinesia, especially in older adults, most notably older women.

• Antipsychotics can disrupt the body's ability to reduce core body temperature; impair judgment, thinking, or motor skills; and increase risk of metabolic changes (hyperglycemia, diabetes, dyslipidemia, weight gain), esophageal dysmotility, aspiration, aspiration pneumonia, and falls.

• Antipsychotics increase risk of seizures, especially in patients with a history of seizures or with conditions that lower seizure threshold.

• Drug is associated with dystonia, especially in males and younger age-groups, most commonly during first few days of treatment.

• Use isn't recommended in patients with Child-Pugh class C liver impairment or CrCl less than 30 mL/minute.

Boxed Warning Safety and effectiveness in children haven't been established. ∎

Dialyzable drug: Unlikely.

⚠ ***Overdose S&S:*** Orthostasis, sedation.

PREGNANCY-LACTATION-REPRODUCTION
• Drug may cause fetal harm. Neonates exposed to antipsychotics during the third trimester are at risk for extrapyramidal and withdrawal signs and symptoms, which can vary in severity and require prolonged hospitalization.

• Encourage patients exposed to drug during pregnancy to enroll in the National Pregnancy Registry for Atypical Antipsychotics (1-866-961-2388 or https://womensmentalhealth.org/research/pregnancyregistry/atypicalantipsychotic/).

• It isn't known if drug appears in human milk. Consider risks and benefits before using during breastfeeding.

NURSING CONSIDERATIONS
• Because of drug's long half-life, dosage changes aren't fully reflected in plasma drug level for several weeks. Monitor for adverse reactions and treatment response for several weeks after initiation and any dosage change.

• Monitor for hypersensitivity reactions (rash, pruritus, urticaria, swollen tongue or lips, facial edema, pharyngeal edema).

• Monitor for signs and symptoms of NMS (hyperpyrexia, muscle rigidity, delirium, autonomic instability, elevated CK level, rhabdomyolysis, acute kidney injury); discontinue drug immediately if reactions appear. Provide intensive symptomatic treatment and monitoring.

• Monitor for signs and symptoms of tardive dyskinesia (potentially irreversible, involuntary, dyskinetic movements). Drug may need to be discontinued.

Reactions in bold italics are ***life-threatening***.

- Monitor for signs and symptoms of dystonia (throat tightness, difficulty swallowing or breathing, tongue protrusion).
- Monitor blood glucose, triglyceride, and lipid levels, and watch for changes in weight, waist circumference, and BMI.
- Monitor patient for clinically significant leukopenia, neutropenia, agranulocytosis, fever, or other signs and symptoms of infection; treat promptly. Discontinue drug for ANC less than 1,000/mm^3 and monitor WBC count until abnormalities resolve.
- Monitor for orthostatic hypotension, especially in an older adult or patient with dehydration, hypovolemia, concomitant treatment with antihypertensives, or known CV or cerebrovascular disease. Assess fall risk at baseline and periodically during treatment.
- Ask about a history of seizures and review patient's medications for those that might lower the seizure threshold because drug may increase risk of seizures.
- Monitor a patient who is exposed to strenuous exercise or extreme heat, is dehydrated, or is taking anticholinergics for elevated core body temperature.
- Monitor patient for clinical worsening and emergence of suicidality.

PATIENT TEACHING

- *Opioid class warning:* Caution patient or caregiver of patient taking an opioid with a benzodiazepine, CNS depressant, or alcohol to seek immediate medical attention for dizziness, light-headedness, extreme sleepiness, slowed or difficult breathing, or unresponsiveness.
- Counsel patient on importance of following dosage escalation instructions.
- Explain potential for dystonic or extrapyramidal signs and symptoms (involuntary, abnormal movements). Advise patient to immediately report signs and symptoms to prescriber because drug may need to be discontinued.
- Instruct patient to report signs and symptoms of NMS.
- Educate patient about risk of metabolic changes and signs and symptoms of hyperglycemia and diabetes. Explain that lab monitoring of blood glucose and lipid levels and weight monitoring may be necessary.
- Advise patient to report fever or other signs or symptoms of infection, which may indicate blood dyscrasias.

- Remind patient to avoid strenuous exercise or exposure to extreme heat and to drink plenty of water because drug may impair body temperature–regulating ability.
- Counsel patient on risk of orthostatic hypotension and syncope, especially during treatment initiation and dosage increases.
- Warn about potential for drug interactions and advise patient to report to prescriber all OTC and prescription drugs and natural supplements being taken.
- Caution patient about operating hazardous machinery, including motor vehicles, until drug's effects on cognitive and motor skills are known.
- Advise patient who is pregnant, considering pregnancy, or is breastfeeding to discuss risks and benefits with prescriber.

SAFETY ALERT!

carmustine (BCNU)
kar-MUS-teen

BiCNU, Gliadel Wafer

Therapeutic class: Antineoplastics
Pharmacologic class: Nitrosoureas

AVAILABLE FORMS
Injection: 100-mg vial (lyophilized), with a 3-mL vial of dehydrated alcohol diluent
Wafer: 7.7 mg, for intracavitary use

INDICATIONS & DOSAGES
➤ **Brain tumor, Hodgkin lymphoma, non-Hodgkin lymphoma, multiple myeloma**
Adults: 150 to 200 mg/m^2 IV by slow infusion every 6 weeks; may be divided into daily injections of 75 to 100 mg/m^2 on 2 successive days. Repeat dose every 6 weeks if platelet count is greater than 75,000/mm^3 and WBC count is greater than 3,000/mm^3.
Adjust-a-dose: Reduce dose by 30% when WBC nadir is 2,000 to 2,999/mm^3 and platelet nadir is 25,000 to 74,999/mm^3. Reduce dose by 50% when WBC nadir is less than 2,000/mm^3 and platelet nadir is less than 25,000/mm^3.
➤ **Adjunct to surgery in patients with recurrent glioblastoma for whom surgical resection is indicated; adjunct to surgery and radiation in patients with newly diagnosed high-grade malignant glioma**

Adults: Place 8 wafers in resection cavity if size and shape of cavity allow. If 8 wafers don't fit, use maximum number allowed.

ADMINISTRATION

IV

🜲 *Alert:* Hazardous drug; use safe handling and disposal precautions. Wear gloves when handling any form of drug.

▼ Prepare drug only in polypropylene or glass containers. Ensure containers used are polyvinyl chloride (PVC) free and DEHP free. Solution is unstable in PVC IV bags.

▼ If powder liquefies or appears oily, discard because decomposition has occurred.

▼ To reconstitute, dissolve 100 mg of drug in 3 mL of dehydrated alcohol provided by manufacturer.

▼ Dilute solution with 27 mL of sterile water for injection. Resulting solution should be clear and colorless to yellowish and contains 3.3 mg of carmustine/mL in 10% alcohol.

▼ For infusion, further dilute in 500 mL D_5W or NSS in polypropylene or glass container to a concentration of 0.2 mg/mL.

▼ Don't use PVC IV tubing. May use polyethylene IV tubing.

▼ Don't mix with other drugs during administration.

▼ Give over at least 2 hours; don't exceed rate of 1.66 mg/m²/minute.

▼ To reduce pain on infusion, dilute further, slow infusion rate, or administer via central catheter.

▼ Reconstituted solution may be stored in refrigerator for 24 hours. Once further diluted in D_5W or NSS, store at room temperature and give within 8 hours. Solution is also stable for 24 hours refrigerated, followed by 6 additional hours at room temperature. Protect from light.

▼ **Incompatibilities:** Sodium bicarbonate. Consult drug compatibility reference for more information.

Intracavitary

🜲 *Alert:* Hazardous drug; use safe handling and disposal precautions.

• Use double gloves when handling wafers. Discard outer gloves into a biohazard waste container after use.

• May keep unopened foil pouches of wafers at room temperature for a maximum of 6 hours. Open only in operating room immediately before implantation.

• Wafers broken in half may be used; however, discard wafers as hazardous waste if broken into more than two pieces.

ACTION

Inhibits enzymatic reactions involved with DNA synthesis, cross-links strands of cellular DNA, and interferes with RNA transcription, causing an imbalance of growth that leads to cell death. Not specific to cell cycle.

Route	Onset	Peak	Duration
IV, intracavitary	Unknown	Unknown	Unknown

Half-life: IV, 15 to 75 minutes.

ADVERSE REACTIONS

IV only

CNS: headache, encephalopathy, *seizures.*
CV: tachycardia, chest pain, veno-occlusive disease. **EENT:** conjunctival edema, conjunctival hemorrhage, visual disturbances. **GI:** nausea, vomiting, anorexia, diarrhea. **GU:** *kidney toxicity,* kidney impairment, decreased kidney size, azotemia. **Hematologic:** *leukopenia, thrombocytopenia, acute leukemia or bone marrow dysplasia,* anemia. **Hepatic:** increased transaminase levels, increased ALP level, hyperbilirubinemia, *liver toxicity.* **Metabolic:** hyperglycemia, *hypokalemia,* hyponatremia. **Respiratory:** pneumonitis, ILD. **Skin:** alopecia, hyperpigmentation, erythema, burning sensation; injection-site pain, burning, erythema, swelling, tissue necrosis. **Other:** hypersensitivity reaction, opportunistic infection, gynecomastia.

Intracavitary wafer only

CNS: fever, depression, *intracranial HTN,* pain, asthenia, *seizures, cerebral edema, cerebral hemorrhage,* brain abscess, brain cyst, hydrocephalus, meningitis. **CV:** chest pain, *PE.* **GI:** nausea, vomiting, constipation, abdominal pain. **GU:** UTI. **Musculoskeletal:** back pain. **Other:** abnormal healing.

INTERACTIONS

Drug-drug. *Cimetidine:* May increase carmustine's bone marrow toxicity. Avoid use together.

Clozapine: May increase risk of neutropenia. Monitor use together.

Live-virus vaccines: May increase risk of infection in patients who are immunocompromised. Don't use together;

don't give for at least 3 months after carmustine.

Myelosuppressants: May increase myelosuppression. Monitor patient.

Phenobarbital: Induces carmustine metabolism, reducing exposure and possibly leading to reduced carmustine efficacy. Consider alternative to phenobarbital.

Phenytoin: May decrease phenytoin level. Monitor patient. Consider alternative to phenytoin.

Drug-herb. *Echinacea:* May diminish therapeutic effect of immunosuppressants. Consider therapy modification.

EFFECTS ON LAB TEST RESULTS
• May increase ALP, AST, bilirubin, Hb, and urine uric acid levels.
• May decrease platelet and WBC counts.

CONTRAINDICATIONS & CAUTIONS
• Contraindicated in patients hypersensitive to drug.

Boxed Warning Bone marrow suppression (thrombocytopenia, and leukopenia), the most common and severe toxic effect, may cause bleeding and overwhelming infections in patients who are already immunocompromised. ∎

Boxed Warning Lung toxicity appears to be dose related. Patients receiving greater than 1,400 mg/m² cumulative dose are at higher risk. Lung toxicity can occur years after treatment and can result in death, particularly in patients treated in childhood. ∎

• Drug may increase risk of secondary malignancies.
• Injection-site reactions may occur, especially during rapid IV infusion. Intense skin flushing and suffusion of conjunctivae may occur within 2 hours, lasting about 4 hours.
• Use cautiously in older adults.
• Safety and effectiveness in children haven't been established.

Dialyzable drug: No.

PREGNANCY-LACTATION-REPRODUCTION
• Drug may cause fetal harm. Patients of childbearing potential should use effective contraception during treatment and for at least 6 months after final dose.
• Males of reproductive potential should use effective contraception during treatment and for 3 months after final dose.
• Drug may impair male fertility.

• It isn't known if drug appears in human milk. Patient should discontinue breastfeeding during IV treatment or not breastfeed for at least 7 days after wafer implantation.

NURSING CONSIDERATIONS
⚠ *Alert:* Carmustine injection should be administered under the supervision of a physician experienced in the use of cancer chemotherapeutic agents.
• Obtain pulmonary function tests before and during therapy.

Boxed Warning Bone marrow suppression is delayed with carmustine. Blood counts should be monitored weekly for at least 6 weeks after a dose and drug shouldn't be given more often than every 6 weeks. ∎

• Bone marrow toxicity of carmustine for injection is cumulative; dosage adjustment must be considered based on nadir blood cell counts from prior dose. Don't administer a repeat course of drug until blood counts recover.
• Drug is associated with moderate to high emetic potential (dose-related); give antiemetic before drug to reduce nausea.
• Avoid contact with skin. If drug touches skin, wash off thoroughly. Drug stains skin brown and skin contact may increase extravasation risk.
• Monitor infusion site for possible infiltration during drug administration.
• Periodically obtain LFT values and kidney function test results.
• Monitor CBC with differential. May use ANC to assess patient's immunosuppressive state.
• Monitor uric acid level. To prevent hyperuricemia with resulting uric acid nephropathy, allopurinol may be used with adequate hydration.
• Therapeutic levels are commonly toxic.
• Note that acute leukemia or bone marrow dysplasia may occur after long-term use.
• Anticipate blood transfusions during treatment because of cumulative anemia.
• Monitor for secondary malignancies.

PATIENT TEACHING
• Advise patient about common adverse reactions to drug.
• Tell patient to watch for signs and symptoms of infection (fever, sore throat, fatigue), stiff neck, and bleeding (easy bruising, nosebleeds, bleeding gums, melena) and to take temperature daily.

- Instruct patient to avoid OTC products containing aspirin and NSAIDs unless prescribed by health care provider.
- Advise patient to stop breastfeeding during IV therapy because of possible risk of toxicity to infant.
- Caution patient of childbearing potential to avoid becoming pregnant during therapy and for 6 months after final dose and to consult prescriber before becoming pregnant.
- Instruct male patient of reproductive potential to use effective contraception during treatment and for 3 months after final dose.

carvedilol
kar-VAH-da-lol

Coreg

carvedilol phosphate
Coreg CR

Therapeutic class: Antihypertensives
Pharmacologic class: Alpha-nonselective beta blockers

AVAILABLE FORMS
Capsules (extended-release) ⓄⓃⒸ: 10 mg, 20 mg, 40 mg, 80 mg
Tablets: 3.125 mg, 6.25 mg, 12.5 mg, 25 mg

INDICATIONS & DOSAGES
Adjust-a-dose (for all indications): In patients with pulse rate below 55 beats/minute, reduce dosage.

➤ **HTN**
Adults: Dosage highly individualized. For immediate-release tablets, initially, 6.25 mg PO b.i.d. Measure standing BP 1 hour after first dose. If tolerated, continue dosage for 7 to 14 days. May increase to 12.5 mg PO b.i.d. for 7 to 14 days, following same BP monitoring protocol as before. Maximum dose, 25 mg PO b.i.d. as tolerated. May switch to extended-release capsule after controlled on immediate-release tablets.

For extended-release capsule, initially 20 mg PO once daily. Measure standing BP 1 hour after dose. May increase by 20 mg every 7 to 14 days to maximum of 80 mg PO once daily if needed and tolerated, using standing systolic pressure 1 hour after dosing as a guide for tolerance.

➤ **Left ventricular dysfunction after MI**
Adults: Dosage individualized. Start therapy after patient is hemodynamically stable and fluid retention has been minimized. For immediate-release tablets, initially, 3.125 to 6.25 mg PO b.i.d. Increase after 3 to 10 days to 12.5 mg b.i.d. as tolerated, then again after 3 to 10 days to a target dose of 25 mg b.i.d. May switch to extended-release capsule after controlled on immediate-release tablets.

For extended-release capsule, 10 to 20 mg PO once daily. May increase after 3 to 10 days to 20 to 40 mg PO once daily; continue increasing dose every 3 to 10 days, as tolerated, until target dose of 80 mg PO once daily is reached.

➤ **Mild to severe HF**
Adults: Dosage highly individualized. For immediate-release tablets, initially, 3.125 mg PO b.i.d. for 2 weeks; if tolerated, may increase to 6.25 mg PO b.i.d. Dosage may be doubled every 2 weeks, as tolerated. Maximum dose for patients in severe HF or who weigh less than 85 kg is 25 mg PO b.i.d.; for those weighing more than 85 kg, dose is 50 mg PO b.i.d. May switch to extended-release capsule after controlled on immediate-release tablets.

For extended-release capsule, 10-mg PO once daily for 2 weeks. May increase to 20, 40, and 80 mg over successive intervals of at least 2 weeks to maximum tolerated dose.

ADMINISTRATION
PO
- Give drug with food.
- Make sure patient doesn't crush, chew, or take capsules in divided doses.
- If needed, open capsules, sprinkle contents on cool applesauce, and give immediately; don't store.
- Give capsules in the morning.
- Be aware extended-release equivalent of 3.125 mg immediate-release b.i.d. is 10 mg once daily, 6.25 mg immediate-release b.i.d. is 20 mg once daily, 12.5 mg immediate-release b.i.d. is 40 mg once daily, and 25 mg immediate-release b.i.d. is 80 mg once daily.
- Administer extended-release form and drugs that contain alcohol 2 hours apart.

ACTION
Nonselective beta blocker with alpha-blocking activity.

Route	Onset	Peak	Duration
PO	Rapid	1–2 hr	7–10 hr
PO (extended-release)	30 min	5 hr	Unknown

Half-life: Immediate-release, 7 to 10 hours; extended-release, unknown.

ADVERSE REACTIONS

CNS: asthenia, dizziness, fatigue, headache, malaise, fever, hypoesthesia, hypotonia, vertigo, somnolence, depression, insomnia, syncope, paresthesia, abnormal thinking, nervousness, sleep disorder. **CV:** hypotension, orthostatic hypotension, *AV block, bradycardia,* edema, angina pectoris, HTN, palpitations, PVD, peripheral ischemia, tachycardia. **EENT:** abnormal vision, blurred vision, tinnitus, periodontitis, dry mouth, nasopharyngitis, nasal congestion, sinus congestion. **GI:** diarrhea, vomiting, nausea, melena, GI pain. **GU:** erectile dysfunction, kidney insufficiency, increased BUN level, increased creatinine level, albuminuria, glycosuria, hematuria, UTI, decreased libido. **Hematologic:** *thrombocytopenia,* purpura, hypoprothrombinemia. **Hepatic:** increased transaminase levels, increase ALP level, hyperbilirubinemia, increased liver enzyme levels. **Metabolic:** hyperglycemia, weight gain or loss, *hyperkalemia, hypoglycemia,* hypercholesterolemia, hyperuricemia, hypovolemia, fluid overload, hyponatremia, diabetes, gout. **Musculoskeletal:** arthralgia, muscle cramps. **Respiratory:** cough, dyspnea, rales. **Skin:** diaphoresis, rash, pruritus, photosensitivity. **Other:** hypersensitivity reactions, flulike symptoms.

INTERACTIONS

Drug-drug. *Amiodarone:* May increase risk of bradycardia, AV block, and myocardial depression. Monitor patient's ECG and vital signs.
Calcium channel blockers (diltiazem, verapamil): May cause isolated conduction disturbances. Monitor patient's heart rhythm and BP.
Catecholamine-depleting drugs (MAO inhibitors, reserpine), clonidine: May cause bradycardia or severe hypotension. Monitor patient closely.
Cimetidine: May increase bioavailability of carvedilol. Monitor vital signs closely.
Cyclosporine: May increase cyclosporine level. Monitor cyclosporine level.

CYP2D6 inhibitors (fluoxetine, paroxetine, propafenone, quinidine): May increase carvedilol level. Monitor patient for hypotension and dizziness.
Digoxin: May increase digoxin level by about 15% when given together. Monitor digoxin level.
Insulin, oral antidiabetics: May enhance hypoglycemic properties. Monitor glucose level.
NSAIDs, salicylates: May decrease antihypertensive effects. Monitor BP.
Rifamycins (except rifabutin): May significantly reduce carvedilol level. Monitor vital signs closely.

EFFECTS ON LAB TEST RESULTS

• May increase ALP, ALT, AST, BUN, bilirubin, cholesterol, creatinine GGT, nonprotein nitrogen, potassium, triglyceride, sodium, and uric acid levels.
• May increase or decrease glucose level.
• May shorten PT and decrease platelet and leukocyte counts.

CONTRAINDICATIONS & CAUTIONS

• Contraindicated in patients hypersensitive to drug and in those with NYHA Class IV decompensated cardiac failure or cardiogenic shock requiring IV inotropic therapy.
• Contraindicated in patients with bronchial asthma or related bronchospastic conditions, second- or third-degree AV block, sick sinus syndrome or severe bradycardia (unless a pacemaker is in place), or Child-Pugh class C liver impairment.
• Use cautiously in patients with left-sided HF who have HTN, perioperative patients who receive anesthetics that depress myocardial function, patients with diabetes receiving insulin or oral antidiabetics, and those subject to spontaneous hypoglycemia.
• Use cautiously in patients with thyroid disease (may mask hyperthyroidism; withdrawal may precipitate thyroid storm or exacerbation of hyperthyroidism), myasthenia gravis, untreated pheochromocytoma, Prinzmetal or variant angina, bronchospastic disease (in those who can't tolerate other antihypertensives), or PVD (may precipitate or aggravate symptoms of arterial insufficiency).
• Safety and effectiveness in children younger than age 18 haven't been established.
Dialyzable drug: No.
⚠ *Overdose S&S:* Hypotension, bradycardia, cardiac insufficiency, cardiogenic shock,

cardiac arrest, respiratory problems, bronchospasm, vomiting, lapses of consciousness, generalized seizures.

PREGNANCY-LACTATION-REPRODUCTION
• Studies during pregnancy are inadequate. Use during pregnancy only if potential benefit justifies fetal risk.
• Beta blocker use in the third trimester may increase risk of hypotension, bradycardia, hypoglycemia, and respiratory depression in the neonate.
• It's unknown if drug appears in human milk. Patient should discontinue breastfeeding or discontinue drug, considering importance of drug to patient.

NURSING CONSIDERATIONS
🛈 *Alert:* Patients who have a history of severe anaphylactic reaction to several allergens may be more reactive to repeated challenge (accidental, diagnostic, or therapeutic). They may also be unresponsive to dosages of epinephrine typically used to treat allergic reactions.
• If drug must be stopped, do so gradually over 1 to 2 weeks, if possible.
• Monitor patient with HF for worsened condition, kidney dysfunction, and fluid retention; diuretics may need to be increased.
• Monitor patient with diabetes closely; drug may mask signs of hypoglycemia or hyperglycemia may worsen.
• Hypotension can occur. Observe patient for dizziness and light-headedness for 1 hour after giving each new dose. Reduce dose in patient with HR less than 55 beats/minute.
• Monitor an older adult carefully; drug levels are about 50% higher in older adults.
• *Look alike–sound alike:* Don't confuse carvedilol with captopril.

PATIENT TEACHING
• Tell patient not to interrupt or stop drug without medical approval.
• Inform patient that improvement of HF symptoms might take several weeks of drug therapy.
• Advise patient with HF to call prescriber if weight gain or shortness of breath occurs.
• Inform patient that low BP when standing may occur. If patient feels dizzy or faint (rare), advise sitting or lying down. Instruct patient to notify prescriber if symptoms persist.

• Caution patient against performing hazardous tasks during start of therapy.
• Advise patient with diabetes to promptly report changes in glucose level.
• Inform patient who wears contact lenses that eyes may feel dry.
• Teach about proper drug administration and handling.
• Instruct patient considering cataract surgery to inform ophthalmologist of carvedilol use due to risk of intraoperative floppy iris syndrome.

caspofungin acetate
KAS-po-fun-gin

Cancidas

Therapeutic class: Antifungals
Pharmacologic class: Echinocandins

AVAILABLE FORMS
Lyophilized powder for injection: 50 mg, 70 mg in single-dose vials

INDICATIONS & DOSAGES
Adjust-a-dose (for all indications): For adults receiving rifampin, give 70 mg IV once daily. Adults receiving other CYP inducers may also require 70 mg IV once daily. Also consider giving 70 mg/m^2 IV once daily (not to exceed 70 mg) for children receiving other CYP inducers. For adults with Child-Pugh class B liver impairment, after initial 70-mg loading dose (when indicated), give 35 mg/day. There's no clinical experience in adults with Child-Pugh score of more than 9 or in children with any degree of liver impairment.

➤ **Invasive aspergillosis in patients who are refractory to or intolerant of other therapies; candidemia and *Candida*-caused intra-abdominal abscesses, peritonitis, and pleural space infections**
Adults: 70-mg IV loading dose on day 1, then 50 mg IV once daily. Base treatment duration on severity of patient's underlying disease, recovery from immunosuppression, and clinical response.
Children ages 3 months to 17 years: 70-mg/m^2 IV loading dose on day 1, then 50 mg/m^2 daily thereafter. May increase daily maintenance dose to 70 mg/m^2. Maximum loading dose and daily maintenance dose shouldn't exceed 70 mg.

Reactions in bold italics are *life-threatening*.

➤ **Empirical treatment of presumed fungal infections in patients who are febrile and neutropenic**

Adults: 70-mg IV loading dose on day 1, then 50 mg IV once daily thereafter. Continue therapy until neutropenia resolves. If fungal infection is confirmed, treat for at least 14 days after the last positive culture and continue therapy for at least 7 days after neutropenia and symptoms resolve. May increase daily dose to 70 mg if the 50-mg dose is well tolerated but clinical response is suboptimal.

Children ages 3 months to 17 years: 70-mg/m^2 IV loading dose on day 1, then 50 mg/m^2 daily thereafter. May increase daily maintenance dose to 70 mg/m^2. Maximum loading dose and daily maintenance dose shouldn't exceed 70 mg.

➤ **Esophageal candidiasis**

Adults: 50 mg IV daily for 7 to 14 days after symptoms resolve. May transition to oral fluconazole once oral intake is tolerable.

Children ages 3 months to 17 years: 70-mg/m^2 IV loading dose on day 1, then 50 mg/m^2 daily thereafter. May increase daily maintenance dose to 70 mg/m^2. Maximum loading dose and daily maintenance dose shouldn't exceed 70 mg.

Adjust-a-dose: Consider suppressive oral therapy in adults with HIV infection due to risk of oropharyngeal candidiasis relapse.

ADMINISTRATION

IV

▼ Let refrigerated vial warm to room temperature.

▼ Reconstitute drug by adding 10.8 mL of NSS, sterile water for injection, bacteriostatic water for injection with methylparaben and propylparaben, or bacteriostatic water for injection with benzyl alcohol 0.9% to vial. Resulting solution will be clear.

▼ Reconstitution leads to a concentration of 5 mg/mL for 50-mg vial and 7 mg/mL for 70-mg vial.

▼ Use reconstituted vials within 1 hour of reconstitution, or discard them. Vials are for single dose only. Discard unused portion.

▼ Transfer appropriate volume (mL) of reconstituted drug to an IV bag containing 250 mL of NSS, 0.45% or 0.225% sodium chloride, or lactated Ringer solution. Or, for patients on fluid restrictions, may add reconstituted volume of drug to a reduced volume of solution, not to exceed final concentration of 0.5 mg/mL.

▼ Give drug by slow infusion over about 1 hour. Don't administer as IV bolus.

▼ Monitor site carefully for phlebitis.

▼ The final product for infusion (solution in IV bag) can be stored at room temperature for 24 hours or at 36° to 46° F (2° to 8° C) for 48 hours.

▼ **Incompatibilities:** Don't mix or infuse with other drugs or dextrose solutions.

ACTION

Inhibits synthesis of 1,3-β-D-glucan, an essential component of the cell wall, in susceptible *Aspergillus* and *Candida* species. Drug is extensively distributed and has a prolonged half-life.

Route	Onset	Peak	Duration
IV	Unknown	Unknown	Unknown

Half-life: 9 to 11 hours; terminal, 40 to 50 hours.

ADVERSE REACTIONS

CNS: fever, headache, asthenia, fatigue, *seizure,* dizziness, somnolence, tremor, anxiety, confusion, depression, insomnia. **CV:** edema, tachycardia, phlebitis, infused vein complications, hypotension, HTN, flushing, arrythmia, *bradycardia.* **EENT:** epistaxis. **GI:** anorexia, nausea, vomiting, diarrhea, abdominal pain, abdominal distention, constipation, dyspepsia, mucosal inflammation. **GU:** proteinuria, increased creatinine level, increased BUN level, hematuria, UTI, *AKI.* **Hematologic:** anemia, eosinophilia, coagulopathy, *neutropenia, thrombocytopenia.* **Hepatic:** increased transaminase levels, increased ALP level, hyperbilirubinemia, *hepatotoxicity.* **Metabolic:** *hypokalemia, hypomagnesemia,* hyperglycemia, hypercalcemia, fluid overload. **Musculoskeletal:** arthralgia, back pain, extremity pain. **Respiratory:** dyspnea, *hypoxia,* cough, pneumonia, tachypnea. **Skin:** rash, pruritus, erythema. **Other:** chills, hypersensitivity reaction, infusion reaction, *sepsis.*

INTERACTIONS

Drug-drug. *Cyclosporine:* May increase caspofungin level. May increase risk of elevated ALT level. Avoid use together unless benefit outweighs risk.

CYP inducers (carbamazepine, dexamethasone, efavirenz, nevirapine, phenytoin,

rifampin): May reduce caspofungin level. May need to adjust dosage upward to 70 mg in patients who are clinically unresponsive.
Tacrolimus: May reduce tacrolimus level. Monitor tacrolimus level; expect to adjust dosage.

EFFECTS ON LAB TEST RESULTS
• May increase glucose, calcium, BUN, creatinine, bilirubin, ALP, and liver enzyme levels.
• May decrease albumin, potassium, magnesium, and protein levels.
• May decrease Hb level, hematocrit, and neutrophil and platelet counts.

CONTRAINDICATIONS & CAUTIONS
• Contraindicated in patients hypersensitive to drug or its components.
• Anaphylaxis, other hypersensitivity reactions, and possible histamine-mediated adverse reactions (rash, facial swelling, angioedema, pruritus, sensation of warmth, bronchospasm) have been reported during administration.
• Cases of SJS and TEN, some with a fatal outcome, have been reported.
• Safety and effectiveness in neonates and infants younger than age 3 months aren't known.
Dialyzable drug: No.

PREGNANCY-LACTATION-REPRODUCTION
• Based on animal data, drug may cause fetal harm. Use during pregnancy only if potential benefit justifies fetal risk. Other antifungals are recommended for *Aspergillus* or *Candida* infections during pregnancy.
• It's unknown if drug appears in human milk. Drug was found in study of animal milk. Use cautiously during breastfeeding; use of other antifungals is recommended. Monitor infants for signs and symptoms of histamine release (facial swelling, rash, GI symptoms).

NURSING CONSIDERATIONS
• Observe patient for histamine-mediated reactions (rash, facial swelling, pruritus, sensation of warmth).
• Discontinue drug at first sign or symptom of hypersensitivity reaction, and administer appropriate treatment.
• Monitor patient who develops abnormal LFT values during therapy for evidence of worsening liver function, and evaluate risks and benefits of continuing therapy.

PATIENT TEACHING
• Instruct patient to report signs and symptoms of phlebitis.
• Caution patient to immediately report signs or symptoms of a hypersensitivity reaction, rash, or other skin reactions.
• Advise patient to report to prescriber pregnancy, breastfeeding, or plan to become pregnant.

cefadroxil
sef-a-DROX-ill

Therapeutic class: Antibiotics
Pharmacologic class: First-generation cephalosporins

AVAILABLE FORMS
Capsules: 500 mg
Oral suspension: 250 mg/5 mL, 500 mg/5 mL
Tablets: 1 g

INDICATIONS & DOSAGES
➤ **UTIs caused by *Escherichia coli, Proteus mirabilis*, and *Klebsiella* species; skin and soft-tissue infections caused by staphylococci and streptococci; pharyngitis or tonsillitis caused by group A beta-hemolytic streptococci *(Streptococcus pyogenes)***
Adults: 1 to 2 g PO daily, depending on infection being treated. Usually given once daily or in two divided doses. For pharyngitis and tonsillitis, treat for 10 days.
Children: 30 mg/kg PO daily in a single dose or in two divided doses every 12 hours for tonsillitis, pharyngitis, and impetigo, and in two divided doses every 12 hours for other skin infections and UTIs. For beta-hemolytic strep infection, treat for at least 10 days.
Adjust-a-dose: In adults with kidney impairment, give first dose of 1 g. Reduce additional doses based on CrCl. If CrCl is 25 to 50 mL/minute, give 500 mg PO every 12 hours. If CrCl is 10 to 25 mL/minute, give 500 mg PO every 24 hours; if CrCl is less than 10 mL/minute, give 500 mg PO every 36 hours.

ADMINISTRATION
PO
• Before administration, ensure patient isn't allergic to penicillins or cephalosporins.
• Obtain specimen for culture and sensitivity tests before giving first dose. Begin therapy while awaiting results.

Reactions in bold italics are *life-threatening*.

- Administer without regard to meals but can give drug with food or milk to lessen GI discomfort.
- Keep oral suspension refrigerated; discard unused portion after 14 days. Shake well before using.

ACTION
Inhibits cell-wall synthesis, promoting osmotic instability; usually bactericidal.

Route	Onset	Peak	Duration
PO	Unknown	70–90 min	Unknown

Half-life: About 1 to 2 hours.

ADVERSE REACTIONS
GI: diarrhea. **Other:** hypersensitivity reactions.

INTERACTIONS
Drug-drug. *Aminoglycosides (gentamicin, amikacin):* May increase risk of kidney toxicity. Avoid use together.
Live-virus vaccines: May decrease vaccine effectiveness. Don't give together.
Probenecid: May inhibit excretion and increase cefadroxil level. Use together cautiously.
Warfarin: May enhance anticoagulant effects. Monitor therapy.

EFFECTS ON LAB TEST RESULTS
- May increase ALP, ALT, AST, bilirubin, and LDH levels.
- May increase eosinophil count.
- May decrease Hb level and granulocyte, neutrophil, platelet, and WBC counts.
- May prolong PT.
- May falsely increase serum or urine creatinine level in tests using Jaffé reaction.
- May cause false-positive results of Coombs test and urine glucose tests that use cupric sulfate (Benedict reagent, Clinitest).

CONTRAINDICATIONS & CAUTIONS
- Contraindicated in patients hypersensitive to drug or other cephalosporins.
- To reduce development of drug-resistant bacteria and maintain effectiveness of antibacterial drugs, use drug only to treat or prevent infections proven or strongly suspected to be caused by bacteria.
- Use cautiously in patients with a history of sensitivity to penicillins or GI diseases (colitis).
- Use cautiously in patients with impaired kidney function; adjust dosage as needed.

⚠ Alert: Seizures have occurred, particularly in patients with kidney impairment when dosage wasn't reduced. If seizures occur, discontinue drug and treat as clinically indicated.
⚠ Alert: Drug can cause CDAD and pseudomembranous colitis, ranging from mild to life-threatening, which can occur more than 2 months after treatment.
Dialyzable drug: Yes.

PREGNANCY-LACTATION-REPRODUCTION
- Studies during pregnancy are inadequate. Use during pregnancy only if potential benefit justifies fetal risk.
- It isn't known if drug appears in human milk. Use cautiously during breastfeeding.

NURSING CONSIDERATIONS
- If CrCl is less than 50 mL/minute, lengthen dosage interval so drug doesn't accumulate. Monitor kidney function in patient with kidney dysfunction.
- If patient receives large doses, therapy is prolonged, or patient is at high risk, monitor for signs and symptoms of superinfection.
- Monitor patient for diarrhea and treat appropriately.
- *Look alike–sound alike:* Don't confuse drug with other cephalosporins that sound alike.

PATIENT TEACHING
- Teach about proper drug administration and handling.
- Tell patient to take entire amount of drug exactly as prescribed, even if feeling better.
- Advise patient to notify prescriber if rash or diarrhea develops or if signs and symptoms of superinfection (recurring fever, chills, malaise) appear.

ceFAZolin sodium
sef-AH-zoe-lin

Therapeutic class: Antibiotics
Pharmacologic class: First-generation cephalosporins

AVAILABLE FORMS
Infusion: 1 g, 2 g/50 in 50-mL bag; 2 g, 3 g in 100-mL bag
Injection (parenteral): 500 mg, 1 g, 2 g, 3g

INDICATIONS & DOSAGES

Adjust-a-dose (for all indications): If CrCl is 35 to 54 mL/minute, give full dose every 8 hours or longer; if CrCl is 11 to 34 mL/minute, give 50% of usual dose every 12 hours; if CrCl is below 10 mL/minute, give 50% of usual dose every 18 to 24 hours.

For children with CrCl of 40 to 70 mL/minute, give 60% of normal daily dose divided every 12 hours; if CrCl is 20 to 40 mL/minute, give 25% of usual daily dose divided every 12 hours; if CrCl is 5 to 20 mL/minute, give 10% of usual dose every 24 hours.

➤ **Perioperative prevention in contaminated surgery**
Adults: 1 to 2 g IM or IV 30 to 60 minutes before surgery; then 0.5 to 1 g IM or IV every 6 to 8 hours for 24 hours. In operations lasting longer than 2 hours, give another 0.5- to 1-g dose IM or IV intraoperatively. Continue treatment for 3 to 5 days if life-threatening infection is likely.

➤ **Infections of respiratory, biliary, and GU tracts; skin, soft-tissue, bone, and joint infections; septicemia; endocarditis caused by** *Escherichia coli,* **Enterobacteriaceae, gonococci,** *Haemophilus influenzae,* **Klebsiella species,** *Proteus mirabilis, Staphylococcus aureus, Streptococcus pneumoniae,* **and group A beta-hemolytic streptococci** *(Streptococcus pyogenes)*
Adults: 250 to 500 mg IM or IV every 8 hours for mild infections or 500 mg to 1.5 g IM or IV every 6 to 8 hours for moderate to severe or life-threatening infections. 1 g IM or IV every 12 hours for uncomplicated UTI. 500 mg IM or IV every 12 hours for pneumococcal pneumonia. Maximum, 12 g/day in life-threatening situations.
Children older than age 1 month: 25 to 50 mg/kg/day IM or IV in three or four divided doses. In severe infections, dose may be increased to 100 mg/kg/day.

ADMINISTRATION

● Before giving first dose, obtain specimen for culture and sensitivity tests. Begin therapy while awaiting results.

IV
▼ Before giving drug, ensure patient isn't allergic to penicillins or cephalosporins.
▼ Give commercially available frozen solutions in D₅W only by intermittent or continuous IV infusion.

▼ Reconstitute drug with sterile water, bacteriostatic water, or NSS according to manufacturer's instructions.
▼ Shake well until dissolved.
▼ For direct injection, further dilute with 5 mL of sterile water for injection.
▼ Inject into large vein or into tubing of free-flowing IV solution over 3 to 5 minutes or as intermittent infusion over 30 to 60 minutes.
▼ For intermittent infusion, add reconstituted drug to 50 to 100 mL of compatible solution or use premixed solution.
▼ If IV therapy lasts longer than 3 days, alternate injection sites. Use of small IV needles in larger available veins may be preferable.
▼ Reconstituted drug remains stable for 24 hours at room temperature or 7 to 10 days refrigerated. Refer to manufacturer's instructions.
▼ **Incompatibilities:** None listed by manufacturer. Consult drug compatibility reference for more information.

IM
● After reconstitution, inject drug IM without further dilution. This drug isn't as painful as other cephalosporins. Give injection deep into a large muscle.
● Not all products can be given by IM injection. Refer to manufacturer's instructions.

ACTION

Inhibits cell-wall synthesis, promoting osmotic instability; usually bactericidal.

Route	Onset	Peak	Duration
IV	Immediate	Immediate	Unknown
IM	Unknown	0.5–2 hr	Unknown

Half-life: About 2 hours.

ADVERSE REACTIONS

CNS: dizziness, syncope, confusion, weakness, fatigue, headache, somnolence. **CV:** hypotension, phlebitis, thrombophlebitis (IV injection). **EENT:** oral candidiasis, oral ulcers. **GI:** diarrhea, *CDAD,* anorexia, glossitis, dyspepsia, abdominal cramps, anal pruritus, vomiting, nausea, epigastric pain, flatus. **GU:** genital pruritus, candidiasis, vaginitis. **Hematologic:** *neutropenia, leukopenia, thrombocytopenia,* eosinophilia. **Skin:** maculopapular and erythematous rashes, urticaria, pruritus, pain, induration, sterile abscesses, tissue sloughing at injection site, *SJS.*

Reactions in bold italics are *life-threatening*.

Other: *anaphylaxis,* hypersensitivity reactions, drug fever.

INTERACTIONS
Drug-drug. *Aminoglycosides:* May increase risk of kidney toxicity. Avoid use together.
Live-virus vaccines: May decrease effectiveness of live-virus vaccines. Use together isn't recommended.
Phenytoin: May decrease protein binding of phenytoin. Monitor phenytoin level.
Probenecid: May inhibit excretion and increase cefazolin level. Use together isn't recommended.
Warfarin: May enhance anticoagulant effects. Monitor therapy.

EFFECTS ON LAB TEST RESULTS
• May increase ALP, ALT, and AST levels.
• May increase eosinophil count.
• May decrease neutrophil, platelet, and WBC counts.
• May prolong INR.
• May falsely increase serum or urine creatinine level in tests using Jaffé reaction.
• May cause false-positive results of Coombs test and urine glucose tests that use cupric sulfate (Benedict reagent, Clinitest).

CONTRAINDICATIONS & CAUTIONS
• Contraindicated in patients hypersensitive to drug or other cephalosporins and in those with immediate hypersensitivity reactions (anaphylaxis, serious skin reactions) to penicillins or other beta-lactams.
• Use cautiously in patients hypersensitive to penicillins because of the risk of cross-sensitivity with other beta-lactam antibiotics.
• Solutions containing dextrose may be contraindicated in patients with hypersensitivity to corn products.
• Use cautiously in patients with a history of colitis, seizure disorders, or kidney insufficiency.
• To reduce development of drug-resistant bacteria and maintain effectiveness of antibacterial drugs, use drug only to treat or prevent infections proven or strongly suspected to be caused by bacteria.
• Prolonged use may result in fungal or bacterial superinfection, including CDAD and pseudomembranous colitis, which can occur more than 2 months after treatment ends.
Dialyzable drug: Yes.
⚠ *Overdose S&S:* Pain, inflammation, and phlebitis at injection site; dizziness;

paresthesia; headache; seizures; elevated creatinine, BUN, liver enzyme, and bilirubin levels; positive Coombs test; thrombocytosis; thrombocytopenia; eosinophilia; leukopenia; prolonged PT.

PREGNANCY-LACTATION-REPRODUCTION
• Studies during pregnancy are inadequate. Use during pregnancy only if clearly needed and potential benefit justifies fetal risk.
• Drug appears in very low concentrations in human milk. Use cautiously during breast-feeding.

NURSING CONSIDERATIONS
• If CrCl falls below 55 mL/minute in adults or 70 mL/minute in children, adjust dosage.
• If patient receives large doses, therapy is prolonged, or patient is at high risk, monitor for signs and symptoms of superinfection.
• Monitor patient for diarrhea and treat appropriately.
• Monitor for hypersensitivity reactions.
• *Look alike–sound alike:* Don't confuse drug with other cephalosporins that sound alike.

PATIENT TEACHING
• Instruct patient to promptly report adverse reactions.
• Tell patient to report discomfort at the IV injection site.
• Advise patient to notify prescriber if diarrhea or a rash develops or if signs and symptoms of superinfection (recurring fever, chills, malaise) appear.

---

cefdinir
sef-DIN-er

Therapeutic class: Antibiotics
Pharmacologic class: Third-generation cephalosporins

AVAILABLE FORMS
Capsules: 300 mg
Oral suspension: 125 mg/5 mL, 250 mg/5 mL

INDICATIONS & DOSAGES
Adjust-a-dose (for all indications): If CrCl is less than 30 mL/minute, reduce dosage to 300 mg PO once daily for adults and 7 mg/kg (up to 300 mg) PO once daily for children ages 6 months to 12 years. In patients receiving long-term hemodialysis, give 300 mg or

7 mg/kg PO at end of each dialysis session and then every other day.

➤ **Mild to moderate infections caused by susceptible strains of microorganisms in community-acquired pneumonia, acute worsening of chronic bronchitis, acute maxillary sinusitis, acute bacterial otitis media, and uncomplicated skin and skin-structure infections caused by susceptible strains of _Haemophilus influenzae, Haemophilus parainfluenzae, Streptococcus pneumoniae, Moraxella catarrhalis, Staphylococcus aureus, Streptococcus pyogenes_**

Adults and children ages 13 and older: 300 mg PO every 12 hours or 600 mg PO every 24 hours. Give every 12 hours for pneumonia and skin infections. Treat for 5 to 10 days based on type of infection.

Children ages 6 months to 12 years: For otitis media and skin and skin-structure infections only, 7 mg/kg PO every 12 hours or 14 mg/kg PO every 24 hours for 10 days, up to maximum dose of 600 mg daily. Give every 12 hours for skin infections. Treat for 5 to 10 days based on type of infection.

➤ **Pharyngitis, tonsillitis caused by _Streptococcus pyogenes_**

Adults and children ages 13 and older: 300 mg PO every 12 hours for 5 to 10 days or 600 mg PO every 24 hours for 10 days.

Children ages 6 months to 12 years: 7 mg/kg PO every 12 hours for 5 to 10 days; or 14 mg/kg PO every 24 hours for 10 days.

ADMINISTRATION

PO

• Before administration, ensure patient isn't allergic to penicillins or cephalosporins.
• Give drug without regard for meals.
• Give twice-daily doses every 12 hours.
• Shake suspension well before use.
• Suspension can be stored at room temperature for 10 days.

ACTION

Inhibits cell-wall synthesis, promoting osmotic instability; usually bactericidal.

Route	Onset	Peak	Duration
PO	Unknown	2–4 hr	Unknown

Half-life: 1.75 hours.

ADVERSE REACTIONS

CNS: headache. **GI:** diarrhea, abdominal pain, nausea, vomiting. **GU:** vaginal moniliasis, vaginitis, increased urine proteins. **Hematologic:** increased platelet, WBC, and RBC counts. **Hepatic:** increased LDH level, increased ALP level. **Skin:** rash. **Other:** hypersensitivity reactions, _**anaphylaxis.**_

INTERACTIONS

Drug-drug. _Aminoglycosides:_ May increase risk of kidney toxicity. Avoid use together.
Antacids containing aluminum and magnesium, iron supplements, multivitamins containing iron: May decrease rate of absorption and bioavailability of cefdinir. Give such preparations 2 hours before or after cefdinir.
Live-virus vaccines: May decrease effectiveness of live-virus vaccines. Use together isn't recommended.
Probenecid: May inhibit kidney excretion of cefdinir. Monitor for adverse reactions.
Warfarin: May enhance anticoagulant effects. Monitor therapy.

EFFECTS ON LAB TEST RESULTS

• May increase ALP, GGT, bilirubin, potassium, and LDH levels.
• May decrease bicarbonate level.
• May increase WBC, RBC, eosinophil, lymphocyte, and platelet counts.
• May decrease Hb level.
• May falsely increase serum or urine creatinine level in tests using Jaffé reaction.
• May cause false-positive results of Coombs test and urine glucose tests that use cupric sulfate (Benedict reagent, Clinitest).

CONTRAINDICATIONS & CAUTIONS

• Contraindicated in patients hypersensitive to drug or other cephalosporins.
• To reduce development of drug-resistant bacteria and maintain effectiveness of antibacterial drugs, use drug only to treat or prevent infections proven or strongly suspected to be caused by bacteria.
• Use cautiously in patients hypersensitive to penicillins because of the possibility of cross-sensitivity with other beta-lactam antibiotics.
• Use cautiously in patients with history of colitis or kidney insufficiency.
Dialyzable drug: 63%.

PREGNANCY-LACTATION-REPRODUCTION

• Studies during pregnancy are inadequate. Use during pregnancy only if clearly needed.

Reactions in bold italics are _**life-threatening.**_

• Drug didn't appear in human milk after a single 600-mg dose. Use cautiously during breastfeeding.

NURSING CONSIDERATIONS
• Prolonged drug treatment may result in emergence and overgrowth of resistant organisms. Monitor patient for signs and symptoms of superinfection.
• Monitor for pseudomembranous colitis and CDAD, which can occur more than 2 months after therapy ends. Monitor for diarrhea in patients after antibiotic therapy and in those with history of colitis.
• Monitor patient for hypersensitivity reactions.
• *Look alike–sound alike:* Don't confuse drug with other cephalosporins that sound alike.

PATIENT TEACHING
• Teach about proper drug administration and handling.
• Inform patient with diabetes that suspension contains sucrose.
• Instruct patient to take drug as prescribed, even if feeling better.
• Advise patient to report severe diarrhea or diarrhea with abdominal pain.
• Tell patient to promptly report all adverse reactions and signs and symptoms of superinfection.

cefepime hydrochloride
SEF-e-pim

Therapeutic class: Antibiotics
Pharmacologic class: Fourth-generation cephalosporins

AVAILABLE FORMS
Injection: 500-mg, 1-g, 2-g vials; 1-g, 2-g ready-to-use dual chamber IV bag; 1 g/50 mL, 2 g/100 mL premixed IV bag

INDICATIONS & DOSAGES
Adjust-a-dose (for all indications): Refer to manufacturer's instructions for adjustments to adult dosage based on CrCl of 60 mL/minute or less. Because pediatric and adult cefepime pharmacokinetics are similar, change pediatric dosing regimen proportional to adult regimen.
➤ **Mild to moderate UTI caused by** *Escherichia coli, Klebsiella pneumoniae,* **or** *Proteus mirabilis,* **including concurrent bacteremia with these microorganisms**

Adults and children ages 16 and older: 0.5 to 1 g IM or IV over 30 minutes every 12 hours for 7 to 10 days. Use IM only for *E. coli* infection when IM route is considered more appropriate route of administration.
➤ **Severe UTI, including pyelonephritis, caused by** *E. coli, P. mirabilis,* **or** *K. pneumoniae*
Adults and children ages 16 and older: 2 g IV over 30 minutes every 12 hours for 10 days.
➤ **Moderate to severe pneumonia caused by** *Streptococcus pneumoniae, Pseudomonas aeruginosa, K. pneumoniae,* **or** *Enterobacter* **species**
Adults and children ages 16 and older: 1 to 2 g IV over 30 minutes every 8 to 12 hours for 10 days. For *P. aeruginosa,* 2 g IV every 8 hours for 10 days.
➤ **Moderate to severe skin infection, uncomplicated skin infection, and skin-structure infection caused by** *Streptococcus pyogenes* **or methicillin-susceptible strains of** *Staphylococcus aureus*
Adults and children ages 16 and older: 2 g IV over 30 minutes every 12 hours for 10 days.
➤ **Complicated intra-abdominal infection caused by** *E. coli,* **viridans streptococci,** *P. aeruginosa, K. pneumoniae, Enterobacter* **species, or** *Bacteroides fragilis*
Adults and children ages 16 and older: 2 g IV over 30 minutes every 8 to 12 hours for 7 to 10 days. Give with metronidazole. For *P. aeruginosa,* 2 g IV every 8 hours.
➤ **Empirical therapy for febrile neutropenia**
Adults and children ages 16 and older: 2 g IV every 8 hours for 7 days or until neutropenia resolves. If fever resolves but patient remains neutropenic for more than 7 days, frequently reevaluate the need for continued antimicrobial therapy.
➤ **Uncomplicated and complicated UTI (including pyelonephritis), uncomplicated skin and skin-structure infection, pneumonia, empirical therapy for febrile neutropenic children**
Children ages 2 months to 16 years weighing up to 40 kg: 50 mg/kg/dose IV over 30 minutes every 12 hours for 7 to 10 days. For febrile neutropenia or moderate to severe pseudomonal pneumonia, 50 mg/kg IV every 8 hours for 7 days or until neutropenia resolves (10 days for pseudomonal pneumonia). For UTI, treat for 7 to 10 days. Don't exceed 2 g/dose. May consider IM route only for

mild to moderate, uncomplicated or complicated UTIs due to *E. coli*.

ADMINISTRATION

• Before giving, ensure patient isn't allergic to penicillins or cephalosporins.
• Obtain specimen for culture and sensitivity tests before giving first dose. Start therapy while awaiting results.

IV

▼ When reconstituting drug, closely follow manufacturer's guidelines, which vary with concentration of drug ordered and how drug is packaged.

▼ Type of diluent varies with product used. Use only solutions recommended by manufacturer.

▼ Give intermittent IV infusion with a Y-type administration set and compatible solutions over 30 minutes.

▼ Interrupt flow of primary IV solution while drug is infusing.

▼ May also give by direct IV injection over 5 minutes after vial reconstitution.

▼ Give cefepime after hemodialysis and at the same time each day.

▼ **Incompatibilities:** Aminophylline, ciprofloxacin, netilmicin sulfate, gentamicin, metronidazole, tobramycin, vancomycin.

IM

• Reconstitute drug using sterile water for injection, NSS for injection, D_5W injection, 0.5% or 1% lidocaine hydrochloride, or bacteriostatic water for injection with parabens or benzyl alcohol. Follow manufacturer's guidelines for quantity of diluent to use.

• Inspect solution for particulate matter before use. The powder and its solutions tend to darken, depending on storage conditions. If stored as recommended, potency isn't adversely affected.

• Pain may occur at injection site. Give deep IM into a large muscle.

ACTION

Inhibits bacterial cell-wall synthesis, promotes osmotic instability, and destroys bacteria.

Route	Onset	Peak	Duration
IV	Unknown	30 min	Unknown
IM	Unknown	1–2 hr	Unknown

Half-life: Adults, 2 to 2.5 hours.

ADVERSE REACTIONS

CNS: fever, headache. **CV:** injection-site phlebitis. **GI:** diarrhea, nausea, vomiting. **Hematologic:** increase eosinophil count, abnormal PTT and PT. **Hepatic:** increased transaminase levels. **Metabolic:** hypophosphatemia. **Skin:** rash, pruritus. **Other:** injection-site reactions (pain, inflammation), hypersensitivity reactions.

INTERACTIONS

Drug-drug. *Aminoglycosides, potent diuretics:* May increase risk of kidney toxicity. Monitor kidney function closely.
Live-virus vaccines: May decrease effectiveness of live-virus vaccines. Use together isn't recommended.
Probenecid: May inhibit kidney excretion of cefepime. Monitor for adverse reactions.
Warfarin: May enhance anticoagulant effects. Monitor therapy.

EFFECTS ON LAB TEST RESULTS

• May increase BUN, creatinine, potassium, bilirubin, ALK, ALT, and AST levels.
• May increase or decrease phosphorus and calcium levels.
• May increase eosinophil count.
• May decrease hematocrit and neutrophil, platelet, and WBC counts.
• May alter PT and PTT.
• May falsely increase serum or urine creatinine level in tests using Jaffé reaction.
• May cause false-positive results of Coombs test and urine glucose tests that use cupric sulfate (Benedict reagent, Clinitest).

CONTRAINDICATIONS & CAUTIONS

• Contraindicated in patients hypersensitive to drug or other cephalosporins and in patients with immediate hypersensitivity reactions to beta-lactam antibiotics or penicillins.
• Use cautiously in patients sensitive to penicillins because they may also be sensitive to other beta-lactam antibiotics.
• Dextrose solutions may be contraindicated in patients with hypersensitivity to corn products.
• To reduce development of drug-resistant bacteria and maintain effectiveness of antibacterial drugs, use drug only to treat or prevent infections proven or strongly suspected to be caused by bacteria.

Reactions in bold italics are *life-threatening*.

C

◐ *Alert:* Drug may increase risk of neurotoxicity (altered mental status, confusion, decreased responsiveness, hallucinations, aphasia, monoclonus, seizures, and nonconvulsive status epilepticus), especially in patients with kidney impairment. To decrease risk, follow dosage adjustment guidelines for patients with CrCl of 60 mL/minute or less. Discontinue drug in patients with neurotoxicity associated with drug.

• Use cautiously in patients with history of colitis or kidney insufficiency.

Dialyzable drug: 68%.

⚠ *Overdose S&S:* Encephalopathy, myoclonus, seizures, neuromuscular excitability, nonconvulsive status epilepticus.

PREGNANCY-LACTATION-REPRODUCTION

• Studies during pregnancy are inadequate. Use during pregnancy only if clearly needed and potential benefit justifies fetal risk.

• Drug appears in human milk in very low concentrations. Use cautiously during breastfeeding.

NURSING CONSIDERATIONS

• Monitor patient for superinfection, including CDAD and pseudomembranous colitis, which can occur more than 2 months after final dose. Drug may cause overgrowth of nonsusceptible bacteria or fungi.

• Drug may alter PT and increase bleeding risk. Patients at risk include those with kidney or liver impairment or poor nutrition and those receiving prolonged therapy. Monitor PT and INR in these patients. Give vitamin K, as indicated.

• Monitor patient for neurologic changes.

• Monitor for hypersensitivity reactions.

• *Look alike–sound alike:* Don't confuse drug with other cephalosporins that sound alike.

PATIENT TEACHING

• Warn patient receiving drug IM that pain may occur at injection site.

• Advise patient to promptly report all adverse reactions, including rash, and signs and symptoms of superinfection (recurring fever, chills, malaise, diarrhea).

cefotaxime sodium
sef-oh-TAKS-eem

Therapeutic class: Antibiotics
Pharmacologic class: Third-generation cephalosporins

AVAILABLE FORMS
Injection: 500 mg, 1 g, 2 g

INDICATIONS & DOSAGES

Adjust-a-dose (for all indications): For patients with CrCl less than 20 mL/minute/1.73 m^2, give half of usual dose at regular time interval.

➤ **Perioperative prophylaxis in contaminated surgery**

Adults: 1 g IM or IV 30 to 90 minutes before surgery. In patients undergoing bowel surgery, provide preoperative mechanical bowel cleansing and give a nonabsorbable anti-infective, such as neomycin. In patients undergoing cesarean delivery, give 1 g IM or IV as soon as the umbilical cord is clamped; then 1 g IM or IV 6 and 12 hours later.

➤ **Uncomplicated gonorrhea caused by penicillinase-producing strains or nonpenicillinase-producing strains of *Neisseria gonorrhoeae***

Adults and adolescents: 500 mg IM as a single dose.

➤ **Rectal gonorrhea**

Adult and adolescent males: 1 g IM as a single dose.

Adult and adolescent females: 500 mg IM as a single dose.

➤ **Serious infection of lower respiratory and urinary tract, CNS, skin, bone, and joints; gynecologic and intra-abdominal infection; bacteremia; septicemia caused by susceptible microorganisms, such as streptococci (including *Streptococcus pneumoniae* and *Streptococcus pyogenes*, *Staphylococcus aureus* [penicillinase- and nonpenicillinase-producing] and *Staphylococcus epidermidis*), *Escherichia coli*, *Klebsiella*, *Haemophilus influenzae*, *Serratia marcescens*, and species of *Pseudomonas* (including *P. aeruginosa*), *Enterobacter*, *Proteus*, and *Peptostreptococcus***

Adults and children weighing 50 kg or more: 1 to 2 g IV or IM every 6 to 8 hours. Up to 2 g every 4 hours (12 g) IV daily can be given for life-threatening infections.

Children ages 1 month to 12 years weighing less than 50 kg: 50 to 180 mg/kg/day IM or IV in four to six divided doses.

Neonates ages 1 to 4 weeks: 50 mg/kg IV every 8 hours.

Neonates to age 1 week: 50 mg/kg IV every 12 hours.

Adjust-a-dose: Duration of therapy depends on clinical response.

ADMINISTRATION
● Before giving, ensure patient isn't allergic to penicillins or cephalosporins.
● Obtain specimen for culture and sensitivity tests before giving first dose. Begin therapy while awaiting results.

IV
▼ For direct injection, reconstitute drug in 500-mg, 1-g, or 2-g vials with at least 10 mL of sterile water for injection. Solutions containing 1 g/14 mL are isotonic.
▼ Inject drug over 3 to 5 minutes into large vein or into tubing of free-flowing IV solution. Potentially life-threatening arrhythmias have been reported with more-rapid administration.
▼ For infusion, reconstitute drug in infusion vials with 50 to 100 mL of D_5W or NSS.
▼ Interrupt flow of primary IV solution, and infuse this drug over 15 to 30 minutes.
▼ **Incompatibilities:** Allopurinol, azithromycin, doxapram, filgrastim, fluconazole, pentamidine, sodium bicarbonate injection, vancomycin.

IM
● Reconstitute 500-mg vial with 2 mL, 1-g vial with 3 mL, and 2-g vial with 5 mL sterile water for injection.
● For doses of 2 g, divide the dose and give at different sites.
● Inject deep into a large muscle, such as gluteus maximus or side of thigh.

ACTION
Inhibits cell-wall synthesis, promoting osmotic instability; usually bactericidal.

Route	Onset	Peak	Duration
IV	Immediate	Immediate	Unknown
IM	Unknown	30 min	Unknown

Half-life: 1 to 2 hours.

ADVERSE REACTIONS
CNS: fever, headache. **GI:** colitis, diarrhea, nausea, vomiting. **Hematologic:**

eosinophilia. **Skin:** rash, pruritus, IM site pain and induration, IV site inflammation. **Other:** hypersensitivity reactions.

INTERACTIONS
Drug-drug. *Aminoglycosides, NSAIDS, diuretics:* May increase risk of kidney toxicity. Monitor kidney function tests.
Live-virus vaccines: May decrease effectiveness of live-virus vaccines. Use together isn't recommended.
Probenecid: May inhibit excretion and increase cefotaxime level. Use together cautiously.
Warfarin: May enhance anticoagulant effects. Monitor therapy.

EFFECTS ON LAB TEST RESULTS
● May increase BUN, ALP, ALT, AST, bilirubin, and LDH levels.
● May decrease Hb level.
● May increase eosinophil count.
● May decrease granulocyte, neutrophil, and platelet counts.
● May falsely increase serum or urine creatinine level in tests using Jaffé reaction.
● May cause false-positive results of Coombs test and urine glucose tests that use cupric sulfate (Benedict reagent, Clinitest).

CONTRAINDICATIONS & CAUTIONS
● Contraindicated in patients hypersensitive to drug or other cephalosporins.
● Use cautiously in patients hypersensitive to penicillins because of possibility of cross-sensitivity with other beta-lactam antibiotics.
● CDC guidelines for STIs don't recommend cefotaxime as treatment option for uncomplicated or rectal gonorrhea; ceftriaxone is preferred.
● Prolonged use may result in fungal or bacterial superinfection, including CDAD and pseudomembranous colitis, which can occur more than 2 months after treatment ends.
● To reduce development of drug-resistant bacteria and maintain effectiveness of antibacterial drugs, use drug only to treat or prevent infections proven or strongly suspected to be caused by bacteria.
● Use cautiously in patients with history of colitis or kidney insufficiency.
Dialyzable drug: Yes.
⚠ *Overdose S&S:* Elevated BUN and creatinine levels.

Reactions in bold italics are *life-threatening*.

C

PREGNANCY-LACTATION-REPRODUCTION
• Studies during pregnancy are inadequate. Use during pregnancy only if clearly needed.
• Low concentrations of drug appear in human milk. Use cautiously during breastfeeding.

NURSING CONSIDERATIONS
• If patient receives large doses, therapy is prolonged, or patient is at high risk, monitor for signs and symptoms of superinfection.
• Monitor for diarrhea and treat appropriately.
• Monitor for signs and symptoms of allergic reaction.
• For treatment lasting longer than 10 days, monitor blood counts. Granulocytopenia and, more rarely, agranulocytosis may develop during prolonged treatment.
• *Look alike–sound alike:* Don't confuse drug with other cephalosporins that sound alike.

PATIENT TEACHING
• Tell patient to promptly report adverse reactions and signs and symptoms of superinfection, including diarrhea.
• Instruct patient to report discomfort at IV insertion site.

cefpodoxime proxetil
sef-pode-OKS-eem

Therapeutic class: Antibiotics
Pharmacologic class: Third-generation cephalosporins

AVAILABLE FORMS
Granules for oral suspension: 50 mg/5 mL or 100 mg/5 mL when reconstituted
Tablets (film-coated): 100 mg, 200 mg

INDICATIONS & DOSAGES
Adjust-a-dose (for all indications): For patients with CrCl less than 30 mL/minute, increase dosage interval to every 24 hours. Give to patients receiving hemodialysis three times weekly after hemodialysis.
➤ **Acute community-acquired pneumonia caused by strains of *Haemophilus influenzae* or *Streptococcus pneumoniae***
Adults and children ages 12 and older: 200 mg PO every 12 hours for 14 days.
➤ **Acute bacterial worsening of chronic bronchitis caused by *S. pneumoniae* or *H. influenzae* (strains that don't produce beta-lactamase only), or *Moraxella catarrhalis* (tablets only)**
Adults and children ages 12 and older: 200 mg PO every 12 hours for 10 days.
➤ **Uncomplicated gonorrhea; rectal gonococcal infections in females**
Adults and children ages 12 and older: 200 mg PO as a single dose.
➤ **Uncomplicated skin and skin-structure infections caused by *Staphylococcus aureus* or *Streptococcus pyogenes***
Adults and children ages 12 and older: 400 mg PO every 12 hours for 7 to 14 days.
➤ **Acute otitis media caused by *S. pneumoniae* (penicillin-susceptible strains only), *S. pyogenes*, *H. influenzae*, or *M. catarrhalis***
Children ages 2 months to 12 years: 5 mg/kg oral suspension PO every 12 hours for 5 days. Don't exceed 200 mg per dose.
➤ **Pharyngitis or tonsillitis caused by *S. pyogenes***
Adults: 100 mg PO every 12 hours for 5 to 10 days.
Children ages 2 months to 12 years: 5 mg/kg PO every 12 hours for 5 to 10 days. Don't exceed 100 mg per dose.
➤ **Uncomplicated UTIs caused by *Escherichia coli*, *Klebsiella pneumoniae*, *Proteus mirabilis*, or *Staphylococcus saprophyticus***
Adults and adolescents ages 12 and older: 100 mg PO every 12 hours for 7 days.
➤ **Mild to moderate acute maxillary sinusitis caused by *H. influenzae*, *S. pneumoniae*, or *M. catarrhalis***
Adults and adolescents ages 12 and older: 200 mg PO every 12 hours for 10 days.
Children ages 2 months to 12 years: 5 mg/kg PO every 12 hours for 10 days; maximum, 200 mg/dose.

ADMINISTRATION
PO
• Before administration, ensure patient isn't allergic to penicillins or cephalosporins.
• Obtain specimen for culture and sensitivity tests before giving first dose. Begin therapy while awaiting results.
• Give tablets with food to enhance absorption. May give oral suspension without regard to food.
• Shake suspension well before using.
• Store suspension in refrigerator (36° to 46° F [2° to 8° C]). Discard unused portion after 14 days.

ACTION
Inhibits cell-wall synthesis, promoting osmotic instability; usually bactericidal.

Route	Onset	Peak	Duration
PO	Unknown	2–3 hr	Unknown

Half-life: 2 to 3 hours.

ADVERSE REACTIONS
CNS: headache. **GI:** diarrhea, *CDAD*, nausea, abdominal pain. **GU:** vaginal fungal infections, vulvovaginal infections. **Skin:** rash, diaper rash. **Other:** hypersensitivity reactions.

INTERACTIONS
Drug-drug. *Aminoglycosides, NSAIDs, diuretics:* May increase risk of kidney toxicity. Monitor kidney function tests.
Antacids, H_2-receptor antagonists: May decrease absorption of cefpodoxime. Separate H_2-receptor antagonist and cefpodoxime doses by at least 2 hours. Monitor therapy.
Live-virus vaccines: May decrease effectiveness of live-virus vaccines. Use together isn't recommended.
Probenecid: May decrease excretion of cefpodoxime. Monitor patient for signs and symptoms of toxicity.
Warfarin: May prolong PT and increase INR. Monitor levels closely, and adjust warfarin dosage.

EFFECTS ON LAB TEST RESULTS
• May increase AST, ALT, GGT, ALP, bilirubin, potassium, and LDH levels.
• May decrease albumin, protein, and sodium levels.
• May increase or decrease glucose level.
• May decrease Hb level, hematocrit, ANC, and WBC, platelet, and lymphocyte counts.
• May prolong PT and PTT.
• May falsely increase serum or urine creatinine level in tests using Jaffé reaction.
• May cause false-positive results of Coombs test and urine glucose tests that use cupric sulfate (Benedict reagent, Clinitest).

CONTRAINDICATIONS & CAUTIONS
• Contraindicated in patients hypersensitive to drug or other cephalosporins.
⚠ *Alert:* Drug can cause CDAD and pseudomembranous colitis, ranging from mild to life-threatening, due to overgrowth of nonsusceptible bacteria or fungi.

• To reduce development of drug-resistant bacteria and maintain effectiveness of antibacterial drugs, use drug only to treat or prevent infections proven or strongly suspected to be caused by bacteria.
• Use cautiously in patients with a history of penicillin hypersensitivity because of risk of cross-sensitivity.
• For children with otitis media, American Academy of Pediatrics guidelines recommend basing duration on patient age. For patients younger than age 2 or with severe symptoms (any age), 10-day course; for patients ages 2 to 5 with mild to moderate symptoms, 7-day course; for patients ages 6 and older with mild to moderate symptoms, 5-day course.
⚠ *Alert:* Some dosage forms may contain benzoate, a metabolite of benzyl alcohol. Benzyl alcohol in large amounts has been linked to potentially fatal gasping syndrome in neonates. Avoid dosage forms with benzyl alcohol derivatives in neonates. Refer to manufacturer's labeling.
• Safety and effectiveness in children younger than age 2 months haven't been established.
Dialyzable drug: 23%.

PREGNANCY-LACTATION-REPRODUCTION
• Studies during pregnancy are inadequate. Use during pregnancy only if clearly needed.
• Drug appears in human milk. Patient should discontinue breastfeeding or discontinue drug, considering importance of drug to patient.

NURSING CONSIDERATIONS
• Monitor kidney function closely.
• Monitor patient for signs and symptoms of superinfection and diarrhea, and treat appropriately. Use extreme caution when using drug in patients at increased risk for antibiotic-induced pseudomembranous colitis due to exposure to health care settings with endemic *Clostridioides difficile* infection.
• Monitor for hypersensitivity reactions.
• *Look alike–sound alike:* Don't confuse drug with other cephalosporins that sound alike.

PATIENT TEACHING
• Tell patient to take drug as prescribed, even if feeling better.
• Teach about proper drug administration and handling.

Reactions in bold italics are ***life-threatening***.

C

- Tell patient to report all adverse reactions, especially rash and signs or symptoms of superinfection.
- Advise patient to promptly report loose stools or diarrhea.

cefprozil
sef-PRO-zil

Therapeutic class: Antibiotics
Pharmacologic class: Second-generation cephalosporins

AVAILABLE FORMS
Powder for oral suspension: 125 mg/5 mL, 250 mg/5 mL when reconstituted
Tablets: 250 mg, 500 mg

INDICATIONS & DOSAGES
Adjust-a-dose (for all indications): If CrCl is less than 30 mL/minute, give 50% of standard dose at standard intervals. If patient is receiving dialysis, give dose after hemodialysis.

➤ **Pharyngitis or tonsillitis caused by *Streptococcus pyogenes***
Adults and children ages 13 and older: 500 mg PO daily for at least 10 days.
Children ages 2 to 12: 7.5 mg/kg PO every 12 hours for 10 days. Don't exceed 500 mg/day.

➤ **Otitis media caused by *Streptococcus pneumoniae, Haemophilus influenzae,* or *Moraxella catarrhalis***
Infants and children ages 6 months to 12 years: 15 mg/kg PO every 12 hours for 10 days. Don't exceed 500 mg/dose. American Academy of Pediatrics guidelines don't routinely recommend cefprozil use.

➤ **Secondary bacterial infections of acute bronchitis and acute bacterial worsening of chronic bronchitis caused by *S. pneumoniae, H. influenzae,* or *M. catarrhalis***
Adults and children ages 13 and older: 500 mg PO every 12 hours for 10 days.

➤ **Acute sinusitis caused by *Streptococcus pneumoniae, Haemophilus influenzae,* and *Moraxella catarrhalis.***
Adults and children ages 13 and older: 250 mg PO every 12 hours for 10 days. For moderate to severe infections, increase dose to 500 mg PO every 12 hours for 10 days.
Infants and children ages 6 months to 12 years: 7.5 mg/kg PO every 12 hours for 10 days. For moderate to severe

infections, increase dose to 15 mg/kg PO every 12 hours for 10 days.

➤ **Uncomplicated skin and skin-structure infections caused by *Staphylococcus aureus* or *S. pyogenes***
Adults and children ages 13 and older: 250 or 500 mg PO every 12 hours or 500 mg PO daily for 10 days.
Children ages 2 to 12: 20 mg/kg PO every 24 hours for 10 days. Don't exceed adult dose.

ADMINISTRATION
PO
- Obtain specimen for culture and sensitivity tests before giving first dose. Start therapy while awaiting results.
- Before giving, ensure patient isn't allergic to penicillins or cephalosporins.
- Give without regard to meals.
- Give around the clock to limit variation in peak and trough serum levels.
- Shake suspension well before using.
- Refrigerate suspension and discard after 14 days.

ACTION
Inhibits cell-wall synthesis, promoting osmotic instability; usually bactericidal.

Route	Onset	Peak	Duration
PO	Unknown	1.5 hr	Unknown

Half-life: 1.25 hours in adults with normal kidney function; 1.5 hours in children; 2 hours in patients with impaired liver function; 6 to 6 hours in patients with kidney impairment or CKD.

ADVERSE REACTIONS
CNS: dizziness. **GI:** diarrhea, nausea, vomiting, abdominal pain. **GU:** genital pruritus, vaginitis. **Hematologic:** eosinophilia. **Hepatic:** increased transaminase levels. **Skin:** rash, diaper rash. **Other:** superinfection, hypersensitivity reaction, including *anaphylaxis.*

INTERACTIONS
Drug-drug. *Aminoglycosides, cephalosporins:* May increase risk of kidney toxicity. Monitor kidney function tests closely.
Live-virus vaccines: May decrease effectiveness of live-virus vaccines. Use together isn't recommended.

Probenecid: May inhibit excretion and increase cefprozil level. Use together cautiously.

Warfarin: May enhance anticoagulant effects. Monitor therapy.

EFFECTS ON LAB TEST RESULTS
• May increase ALP, ALT, AST, bilirubin, BUN, creatinine, and LDH levels.
• May increase eosinophil count.
• May decrease platelet and WBC counts.
• May prolong PT and PTT.
• May provide false-negative reaction in ferricyanide test for blood glucose.
• May falsely increase serum or urine creatinine level in tests using Jaffé reaction.
• May cause false-positive results of Coombs test and urine glucose tests that use cupric sulfate (Benedict reagent, Clinitest).

CONTRAINDICATIONS & CAUTIONS
• Contraindicated in patients hypersensitive to drug or other cephalosporins.
• To reduce development of drug-resistant bacteria and maintain effectiveness of antibacterial drugs, use drug only to treat or prevent infections proven or strongly suspected to be caused by bacteria.
• Use cautiously in patients hypersensitive to penicillins because of possibility of cross-sensitivity with other beta-lactam antibiotics.
۞ Alert: May cause mild to life-threatening CDAD and pseudomembranous colitis, which can occur even more than 2 months after therapy; drug may need to be discontinued and other treatment initiated. Use cautiously in patients with a history of GI disease, especially colitis.
• Use cautiously in patients with history of kidney insufficiency.
Dialyzable drug: Yes.

PREGNANCY-LACTATION-REPRODUCTION
• Studies during pregnancy are inadequate. Use during pregnancy only if clearly needed.
• Small amounts of drug appear in human milk. Use cautiously during breastfeeding.

NURSING CONSIDERATIONS
• Monitor kidney function test results.
• Drug may cause overgrowth of nonsusceptible bacteria or fungi. Monitor for signs and symptoms of superinfection.
• Monitor patient for diarrhea and treat accordingly.

• Monitor for hypersensitivity reactions.
• *Look alike–sound alike:* Don't confuse drug with other cephalosporins that sound alike.

PATIENT TEACHING
• Advise patient to take drug as prescribed, even if feeling better.
• Inform patient with phenylketonuria that product may contain phenylalanine.
• Teach about proper drug administration and handling.
• Instruct patient to report all adverse reactions and to immediately report rash and signs or symptoms of superinfection, including diarrhea.

cefTAZidime
sef-TAZ-i-deem

Tazicef

Therapeutic class: Antibiotics
Pharmacologic class: Third-generation cephalosporins

AVAILABLE FORMS
Infusion: 1 g, 2 g in 50-mL ready-to-use dual chamber IV bag
Injection (with sodium carbonate): 500 mg, 1 g, 2 g

INDICATIONS & DOSAGES
Adjust-a-dose (for all indications): If CrCl is 31 to 50 mL/minute, give 1 g every 12 hours; if CrCl is 16 to 30 mL/minute, give 1 g every 24 hours; if CrCl is 6 to 15 mL/minute, give 500 mg every 24 hours; if CrCl is less than 5 mL/minute, give 500 mg every 48 hours. Give a loading dose of 1 g, followed by 1 g after each hemodialysis period. If patient is receiving continuous ambulatory peritoneal dialysis, give a loading dose of 1 g, followed by 500 mg every 24 hours. Or, add 250 mg per 2 L of dialysis fluid. Duration of therapy depends on clinical response. Generally, therapy is continued for 2 days after signs and symptoms of infection have disappeared.
➤ **Serious lower respiratory tract infection; skin and skin structure, gynecologic, intra-abdominal, bone and joint, and CNS infection; bacterial septicemia caused by susceptible microorganisms, such as streptococci (including *Streptococcus pneumoniae* and *Streptococcus***

pyogenes), penicillinase- and non-penicillinase-producing *Staphylococcus aureus, Escherichia coli, Klebsiella, Proteus, Enterobacter, Haemophilus influenzae, Pseudomonas,* and some strains of *Bacteroides*

Adults and children ages 12 and older: 1 to 2 g IV or IM every 8 to 12 hours. Route and dosage are determined by susceptibility of the organism, severity of infection, and condition of patient. Give up to 6 g daily in life-threatening infections.

Children ages 1 month to 12 years: 30 to 50 mg/kg IV every 8 hours. Maximum dose, 6 g/day.

Neonates up to age 4 weeks: 30 mg/kg IV every 12 hours.

➤ **Uncomplicated UTI**
Adults: 250 mg IV or IM every 12 hours.

➤ **Complicated UTI**
Adults and children ages 12 and older: 500 mg to 1 g IV or IM every 8 to 12 hours.

➤ **Uncomplicated pneumonia; mild skin and skin-structure infections**
Adults and children ages 12 and older: 500 mg to 1 g IV or IM every 8 hours.

➤ **Lung infections caused by *Pseudomonas* in patients with cystic fibrosis with normal kidney function**
Adults and children ages 12 and older: 30 to 50 mg/kg IV every 8 hours. Maximum dose, 6 g/day.

➤ **Very severe life-threatening infections, especially in patients who are immunocompromised**
Adults and children older than age 12: 2 g IV every 8 hours.

ADMINISTRATION

IV

▼ Before administration, ensure patient isn't allergic to penicillins or cephalosporins.

▼ Obtain specimen for culture and sensitivity tests before giving first dose. Begin therapy while awaiting results.

▼ Each brand of drug includes specific instructions for reconstitution. Read and follow them carefully.

▼ Inspect solution for particulate matter and discoloration before giving. Use only if solution is clear.

▼ Infuse drug over 15 to 30 minutes.

▼ **Incompatibilities:** Aminophylline, amiodarone, azithromycin, clarithromycin, fluconazole, idarubicin, midazolam, pentamidine, ranitidine, sargramostim, vancomycin.

IM

• Before administration, ensure patient isn't allergic to penicillins or cephalosporins.

• Obtain specimen for culture and sensitivity tests before giving first dose. Begin therapy while awaiting results.

• Inject deep into a large muscle, such as gluteus maximus or side of thigh.

ACTION

Inhibits cell-wall synthesis, promoting osmotic instability; usually bactericidal.

Route	Onset	Peak	Duration
IV	Immediate	Immediate	Unknown
IM	Unknown	1 hr	Unknown

Half-life: 2 hours.

ADVERSE REACTIONS

CNS: headache, dizziness, paresthesia, fever. **CV:** injection-site phlebitis and thrombophlebitis. **GI:** *CDAD,* nausea, vomiting, diarrhea, abdominal cramps. **Hematologic:** *agranulocytosis, leukopenia, thrombocytopenia,* eosinophilia, thrombocytosis. **Skin:** rash, pruritus, pain, injection-site inflammation. **Other:** hypersensitivity reactions, candidiasis.

INTERACTIONS

Drug-drug. *Aminoglycosides, cephalosporins, diuretics:* May cause additive or synergistic effect against some strains of *Pseudomonas aeruginosa* and *Enterobacteriaceae;* may increase risk of kidney toxicity. Monitor patient for effects, and monitor kidney function.
Chloramphenicol: May cause antagonistic effect. Avoid use together.
Live-virus vaccines: May decrease effectiveness of live-virus vaccines. Use together isn't recommended.
Probenecid: May increase serum concentrations of cephalosporins. Monitor therapy.
Warfarin: May increase anticoagulation effect. Monitor PT and INR closely.

EFFECTS ON LAB TEST RESULTS

• May increase BUN, creatinine, ALP, ALT, AST, bilirubin, GGT, and LDH levels.
• May decrease Hb level.
• May increase eosinophil count.
• May decrease granulocyte and WBC counts.
• May increase or decrease platelet count.

- May prolong PTT and PT and increase INR.
- May falsely increase serum or urine creatinine level in tests using Jaffé reaction.
- May cause false-positive results of Coombs test and urine glucose tests that use cupric sulfate (Benedict reagent, Clinitest).

CONTRAINDICATIONS & CAUTIONS
- Contraindicated in patients hypersensitive to drug or other cephalosporins.
- To reduce development of drug-resistant bacteria and maintain effectiveness of antibacterial drugs, use drug only to treat or prevent infections proven or strongly suspected to be caused by bacteria.
- Use cautiously in patients hypersensitive to penicillins; may cause cross-sensitivity with other beta-lactam antibiotics.
- Prolonged use can result in superinfection, including CDAD and pseudomembranous colitis, which can occur even more than 2 months after treatment ends.
- Use cautiously in patients with history of colitis, kidney impairment, or seizures.
Dialyzable drug: Yes.
⚠ *Overdose S&S:* Seizures, encephalopathy, asterixis, neuromuscular excitability, coma (in patients with KF).

PREGNANCY-LACTATION-REPRODUCTION
- Studies during pregnancy are inadequate. Use during pregnancy only if clearly needed.
- Drug appears in human milk in low concentrations. Use cautiously during breastfeeding.

NURSING CONSIDERATIONS
- If patient receives large doses, therapy is prolonged, or patient is at high risk, monitor for signs and symptoms of superinfection.
- Monitor for diarrhea and treat appropriately.
- Monitor for hypersensitivity reactions.
- Monitor kidney function with prolonged use.
- *Look alike–sound alike:* Don't confuse drug with other cephalosporins that sound alike.

PATIENT TEACHING
- Tell patient to promptly report adverse reactions and signs or symptoms of superinfection.
- Instruct patient to report discomfort at IV insertion site.
- Advise patient to notify prescriber about loose stools or diarrhea.

- Instruct patient to report to prescriber pregnancy, plans to become pregnant, or breastfeeding.

cefTAZidime–avibactam sodium
sef-TAZ-i-deem/A-vi-BAK-tam sodium

Avycaz

Therapeutic class: Antibiotics
Pharmacologic class: Cephalosporins–beta-lactamase inhibitors

AVAILABLE FORMS
Injection (single-use vials): 2 g ceftazidime and 0.5 g avibactam per vial

INDICATIONS & DOSAGES
❸ *Alert:* Dosage recommendations are expressed as total grams of the ceftazidime–avibactam combination.

Adjust-a-dose (for all indications): For adults: If CrCl is 31 to 50 mL/minute, give 1.25 g every 8 hours; if CrCl is 16 to 30 mL/minute, give 0.94 g every 12 hours; if CrCl is 6 to 15 mL/minute, give 0.94 g every 24 hours; if CrCl is 5 mL/minute or less, give 0.94 g every 48 hours.

For children ages 2 and older: If eGFR is 31 to 50 mL/minute/1.73 m^2, give 31.25 mg/kg to maximum of 1.2 g every 8 hours; if eGFR is 16 to 30 mL/minute/1.73 m^2, give 23.75 mg/kg to maximum of 0.94 g every 12 hours; if eGFR is 6 to 15 mL/minute/1.73 m^2, give 23.75 mg/kg to maximum of 0.94 g every 24 hours; if eGFR is 5 mL/minute/1.73 m^2 or less, give 23.75 mg/kg to maximum of 0.94 g every 48 hours. Dosing for children younger than age 2 years with kidney impairment hasn't been established.

➤ **Complicated intra-abdominal infections caused by susceptible microorganisms (*Escherichia coli, Klebsiella pneumoniae, Proteus mirabilis, Providencia stuartii, Enterobacter cloacae, Klebsiella oxytoca,* or *Pseudomonas aeruginosa*) in combination with metronidazole**
Adults: 2.5 g IV every 8 hours for 5 to 14 days.
Children ages 2 to 18: 62.5 mg/kg IV every 8 hours for 5 to 14 days. Maximum dose, 2.5 g.
Children ages 6 months to 2 years: 62.5 mg/kg IV every 8 hours for 5 to 14 days.

C

Children ages 3 to 6 months: 50 mg/kg IV every 8 hours for 5 to 14 days.

➤ **Complicated UTI, including pyelonephritis, caused by susceptible microorganisms (*E. coli, K. pneumoniae, Citrobacter koseri, Enterobacter aerogenes, E. cloacae, Citrobacter freundii, Proteus* spp., or *P. aeruginosa*)**

Adults: 2.5 g IV every 8 hours for 7 to 14 days.
Children ages 2 to 18: 62.5 mg/kg IV every 8 hours for 7 to 14 days. Maximum dose, 2.5 g.
Children ages 6 months to 2 years: 62.5 mg/kg IV every 8 hours for 7 to 14 days.
Children ages 3 to 6 months: 50 mg/kg IV every 8 hours for 7 to 14 days.

➤ **Hospital-acquired bacterial pneumonia and ventilator-associated bacterial pneumonia caused by susceptible microorganisms (*K. pneumoniae, E. cloacae, E. coli, Serratia marcescens, P. mirabilis, P. aeruginosa,* or *Haemophilus influenzae*)**

Adults: 2.5 g IV every 8 hours for 7 to 14 days.
Children ages 2 years to less than 18 years: 62.5 mg/kg IV every 8 hours for 7 to 14 days. Maximum dose, 2.5 g.
Children ages 6 months to less than 2 years: 62.5 mg/kg IV every 8 hours for 7 to 14 days.
Children ages 3 months to less than 6 months: 50 mg/kg IV every 8 hours for 7 to 14 days.

ADMINISTRATION

IV

▼ Store unconstituted vials at room temperature. Protect from light.

▼ Reconstitute vial with 10 mL of sterile water for injection, NSS, 5% dextrose, lactated Ringer solution, or all combinations of dextrose injection and sodium chloride injection containing up to 2.5% dextrose and 0.45% sodium chloride. Mix gently.

▼ After reconstitution, transfer appropriate volume from the vial within 30 minutes to an infusion bag for further dilution.

▼ Further dilute constituted solution with the same diluent used for constitution to achieve a total volume between 50 and 250 mL. Mix gently.

▼ Inspect for particulate matter and discoloration (the color of solution ranges from clear to light yellow).

▼ Final admixed solution is stable for 12 hours at room temperature and for 24 hours if refrigerated at 36° to 46° F (2° to 8° C).

▼ Infuse final solution over 2 hours.

▼ If patient is receiving dialysis, give dose after hemodialysis.

▼ **Incompatibilities:** Solutions other than those listed above. Refer to manufacturer's instructions for list of compatible drugs or consult drug compatibility reference for more information.

ACTION

Ceftazidime is a bactericidal agent that inhibits cell-wall synthesis, promoting osmotic instability. Avibactam increases ceftazidime's effectiveness by inactivating certain beta-lactamases, which destroy ceftazidime.

Route	Onset	Peak	Duration
IV	Rapid	Unknown	Unknown

Half-life: Ceftazidime, about 3 hours; avibactam, about 2.5 hours.

ADVERSE REACTIONS

CV: injection-site phlebitis. **GI:** nausea, diarrhea, vomiting, constipation, abdominal pain. **Skin:** rash, pruritus. **Other:** hypersensitivity reaction.

INTERACTIONS

Drug-drug. *Aminoglycosides:* May increase risk of kidney toxicity. Monitor closely.
Live-virus vaccines: May decrease effectiveness of live-virus vaccines. Use together isn't recommended.
Probenecid: May decrease ceftazidime–avibactam excretion. Avoid use together.
Vitamin K antagonists (warfarin): May enhance anticoagulation effects. Monitor therapy.

EFFECTS ON LAB TEST RESULTS

• May increase ALP, GGT, and ALT levels.
• May decrease potassium level.
• May decrease leukocyte count.
• May increase or decrease platelet count.
• May prolong PT.
• May cause false-positive reaction for glucose in urine with certain methods.
• May result in seroconversion from a negative to a positive direct Coombs test.

CONTRAINDICATIONS & CAUTIONS

• Contraindicated in patients hypersensitive to cephalosporins or avibactam.
• To reduce development of drug-resistant bacteria and maintain effectiveness of antibacterial drugs, use drug only to treat or

prevent infections proven or strongly suspected to be caused by susceptible bacteria.

• Use cautiously in patients with penicillins or other beta-lactam allergy because of cross-sensitivity.

⚠️ **Alert:** Drug may cause severe neurologic reactions (encephalopathy, myoclonus, seizures, nonconvulsive status epilepticus). Risk may increase in patients with kidney impairment; ensure dosage adjustment for kidney function. Discontinue drug if neurotoxicity occurs.

⚠️ **Alert:** Serious and fatal hypersensitivity reactions and anaphylaxis can occur.

• Use cautiously in patients with kidney impairment.

⚠️ **Alert:** CDAD has been reported with use of nearly all systemic antibacterial drugs and may range in severity from mild diarrhea to fatal colitis. CDAD may occur more than 2 months after use of antibacterial drugs.

• Safety and effectiveness in children younger than age 3 months haven't been established.

• Use cautiously in older adults, who are more likely to have kidney dysfunction.

Dialyzable drug: Yes.

PREGNANCY-LACTATION-REPRODUCTION

• Studies during pregnancy are inadequate. Use during pregnancy only if clearly needed.

• Ceftazidime appears in human milk in low concentrations; it isn't known if avibactam appears in human milk. Use cautiously during breastfeeding.

NURSING CONSIDERATIONS

⚠️ **Alert:** Monitor kidney function at baseline and at least daily in patients with kidney impairment.

⚠️ **Alert:** Monitor for CNS reactions (seizures, nonconvulsive status epilepticus, encephalopathy, coma, asterixis, myoclonia, and neuromuscular excitability), particularly in those with kidney impairment. Adjust dosage based on CrCl level or discontinue therapy as clinically indicated.

• Watch for CDAD in patients who develop diarrhea. If CDAD is suspected or confirmed, antibacterial drugs not directed against CDAD may need to be discontinued.

• Assess carefully for previous hypersensitivity reactions to cephalosporins, penicillins, or carbapenems.

• Monitor closely for hypersensitivity reaction. Discontinue drug if allergic reactions occur.

• Urine glucose tests based on enzymatic glucose oxidase reactions are recommended. False-positive reactions may occur with other methods.

• *Look alike–sound alike:* Don't confuse ceftazidime with other cephalosporins that sound alike. Don't confuse avibactam with aztreonam.

PATIENT TEACHING

• Instruct patient to immediately report changes in CNS status (disturbance of consciousness [confusion, hallucinations, stupor, coma]; myoclonus, seizures).

• Advise patient that diarrhea, including frequent watery or bloody diarrhea, may occur even months after antibacterial treatment ends and to consult health care provider for evaluation.

• Teach patient to report signs and symptoms of hypersensitivity reactions.

• Inform patient that blood tests to assess kidney function will be needed during treatment.

• Counsel patient, family, and caregivers that antibacterial drugs should be used to treat bacterial infections only and aren't effective in treating viral infections (such as the common cold).

• Advise patient that it's common to feel better early in the course of therapy but to take the full course of the drug as prescribed.

• Instruct patient to report pregnancy, plans to become pregnant, or breastfeeding.

---

ceftolozane sulfate–tazobactam sodium
sef-TOL-oh-zane/taz-oh-BAK-tam

Zerbaxa

Therapeutic class: Antibiotics
Pharmacologic class: Cephalosporins–beta-lactamase inhibitors

AVAILABLE FORMS

Powder for injection: 1 g ceftolozane and 0.5 g tazobactam in single-dose vial

INDICATIONS & DOSAGES

⚠️ **Alert:** Dosage recommendations are expressed as total grams of the ceftolozane–tazobactam combination.

Adjust-a-dose (for all indications): For patients with changing kidney function, monitor CrCl at least daily and adjust dosage accordingly.

➤ **Complicated intra-abdominal infections caused by *Enterobacter cloacae, Escherichia coli, Klebsiella oxytoca, Klebsiella pneumoniae, Proteus mirabilis, Pseudomonas aeruginosa, Bacteroides fragilis, Streptococcus anginosus, Streptococcus constellatus,* or *Streptococcus salivarius* in combination with metronidazole***

Adults: 1.5 g IV every 8 hours for 4 to 14 days based on infection severity and clinical response.

Children from birth to younger than age 18: 30 mg/kg (to maximum 1.5 g) IV every 8 hours for 5 to 14 days.

Adjust-a-dose: In adults, if CrCl is 30 to 50 mL/minute, give 750 mg IV every 8 hours; if CrCl is 15 to 29 mL/minute, give 375 mg IV every 8 hours; if on hemodialysis or with CKD, give single loading dose of 750 mg IV followed by maintenance dose of 150 mg IV every 8 hours for remainder of treatment period. Use isn't recommended in children with eGFR of 50 mL/minute/1.73 m^2 or less.

Refer to metronidazole manufacturer's instructions for additional information.

➤ **Complicated UTIs, including pyelonephritis, caused by *E. coli, K. pneumoniae, P. mirabilis,* or *P. aeruginosa***

Adults: 1.5 g IV every 8 hours for 7 days.

Children from birth to younger than age 18: 30 mg/kg (to maximum 1.5 g) IV every 8 hours for 7 to 14 days.

Adjust-a-dose: In adults, if CrCl is 30 to 50 mL/minute, give 750 mg IV every 8 hours; if CrCl is 15 to 29 mL/minute, give 375 mg IV every 8 hours; if on hemodialysis or with CKD, give single loading dose of 750 mg IV, then maintenance dose of 150 mg IV every 8 hours for remainder of treatment period. Use isn't recommended in children with eGFR of 50 mL/minute/1.73 m^2 or less.

➤ **Hospital-acquired bacterial pneumonia and ventilator-associated bacterial pneumonia caused by susceptible gram-negative bacteria (*E. cloacae, E. coli, Haemophilus influenzae, K. oxytoca, K. pneumoniae, P. mirabilis, P. aeruginosa, Serratia marcescens*)**

Adults: 3 g IV infusion every 8 hours for 8 to 14 days (may need longer duration) based on infection severity and clinical response.

Adjust-a-dose: If CrCl is 30 to 50 mL/minute, give 1.5 g IV every 8 hours; if CrCl is 15 to 29 mL/minute, give 750 mg IV every 8 hours; for patients with CKD on hemodialysis, give single loading dose of 2.25 g, then 450 mg maintenance dose IV every 8 hours for remainder of treatment.

ADMINISTRATION

IV

▼ Reconstitute vial with 10 mL of sterile water for injection or NSS; gently shake to dissolve. The final volume is approximately 11.4 mL and must be added to a larger volume for infusion.

▼ To prepare required dose, withdraw appropriate volume from vial and add withdrawn volume to infusion bag containing 100 mL NSS or D$_5$W.

▼ Administer by infusion over 60 minutes.

▼ On hemodialysis days, give maintenance dose immediately after completion of dialysis.

▼ Once reconstituted, vials are stable for 1 hour; once placed in infusion bag, drug is stable for 24 hours at room temperature or 7 days under refrigeration. Don't freeze vials or infusion bags that contain drug.

▼ Infusions range from clear, colorless solutions to solutions that are clear and slightly yellow. Variations in color within this range don't affect product's potency.

▼ Vial doesn't contain a bacteriostatic preservative. Discard unused portion.

▼ **Incompatibilities:** Don't mix with other drugs or solutions except D$_5$W or NSS.

ACTION

Ceftolozane inhibits cell-wall synthesis by binding to penicillin-binding proteins. Tazobactam is an irreversible inhibitor of some beta-lactamases.

Route	Onset	Peak	Duration
IV	Unknown	1 hr	Unknown

Half-life: Ceftolozane, 3 to 4 hours; tazobactam, 2 to 3 hours.

ADVERSE REACTIONS

CNS: headache, insomnia, anxiety, dizziness, fever, *intracranial hemorrhage.* **CV:** hypotension, atrial fibrillation, phlebitis, HTN. **GI:** nausea, diarrhea, *CDAD,* constipation, vomiting, gastritis, abdominal pain. **GU:** kidney impairment. **Hematologic:** anemia, *thrombocytosis, leukopenia.* **Hepatic:** increased AST and ALT levels. **Metabolic:** *hypokalemia.* **Respiratory:** bradypnea. **Skin:** rash.

INTERACTIONS

Drug-drug. *Aminoglycosides:* May increase risk of kidney toxicity. Monitor patient closely.
Live-virus vaccines: May decrease effectiveness of live-virus vaccines. Use together isn't recommended.
Probenecid: May increase tazobactam serum concentration. Monitor therapy.
Vitamin K antagonists (warfarin): May enhance anticoagulant effects. Monitor PT and INR.

EFFECTS ON LAB TEST RESULTS

• May increase ALT, AST, GGT, ALP, glucose levels.
• May decrease potassium, magnesium, and phosphate levels.
• May increase or decrease platelet count.
• May decrease Hb level, hematocrit, leukocytes, and RBC count.
• May cause positive Coombs test.

CONTRAINDICATIONS & CAUTIONS

• Contraindicated in patients with serious hypersensitivity to ceftolozane–tazobactam, piperacillin–tazobactam, or other members of the beta-lactam class.
• Use cautiously in patients hypersensitive to cephalosporins, penicillins, or tazobactam because of the risk of cross-sensitivity.
• To reduce development of drug-resistant bacteria and maintain effectiveness of antibacterial drugs, use drug only to treat or prevent infections proven or strongly suspected to be caused by bacteria.
• May cause fungal or bacterial superinfection, including CDAD and pseudomembranous colitis. Stop drug and take appropriate measures if diarrhea develops. CDAD has occurred more than 2 months after antibacterial treatment.
• Use cautiously in older adults.
• Safety and effectiveness in children with pneumonia haven't been established.
• Use isn't recommended in children with eGFR of 50 mL/minute/1.73 m^2 or less. Infants may not have sufficient eGFR in the first few months of life.
Dialyzable drug: Ceftolozane, 66%; tazobactam, 56%.

PREGNANCY-LACTATION-REPRODUCTION

• Use during pregnancy hasn't been studied. Use cautiously and only if potential benefit justifies fetal risk.

• It isn't known if drug appears in human milk. Use cautiously during breastfeeding.

NURSING CONSIDERATIONS

• Obtain kidney function tests at least daily in patients with changing kidney function. Adjust dosage as necessary based on CrCl.
• Monitor patient for signs and symptoms of hypersensitivity; institute appropriate therapy if needed. Discontinue drug if anaphylactic reaction occurs.
• Monitor patient for signs and symptoms of superinfection, including diarrhea.
• *Look alike–sound alike:* Don't confuse Zerbaxa with Pradaxa.

PATIENT TEACHING

• Teach patient that drug is given IV.
• Instruct patient to immediately report signs and symptoms of allergic reactions (wheezing; chest tightness; itching; swelling of face, lips, tongue, or throat).
• Advise patient not to skip doses even if feeling better to avoid decreasing treatment effectiveness.
• Counsel patient to report GI adverse effects, such as severe watery or bloody diarrhea, even months after therapy ends.
• Instruct patient to report to prescriber pregnancy, plans to become pregnant, or breastfeeding.

cefTRIAXone sodium
sef-try-AX-ohn

Therapeutic class: Antibiotics
Pharmacologic class: Third-generation cephalosporins

AVAILABLE FORMS

Infusion: 1 g/50 mL, 2 g/50 mL premixed and dual-chamber, single-dose container
Injection: 250 mg, 500 mg, 1 g, 2 g

INDICATIONS & DOSAGES

Adjust-a-dose (for all indications): In patients with significant kidney disease and liver dysfunction, maximum dose is 2 g/day. In patients receiving intermittent hemodialysis, no dosage adjustment is necessary as drug is poorly dialyzed.

➤ **Uncomplicated gonorrhea**
Adults: 250 mg IM as a single dose, plus azithromycin 1 g PO as a single dose or doxycycline 100 mg PO b.i.d. for 7 days.

➤ **UTI; lower respiratory tract, gynecologic, bone or joint, intra-abdominal, skin, or skin-structure infection; septicemia caused by susceptible microorganisms, including** *Streptococcus pneumoniae, Staphylococcus aureus, Haemophilus influenzae, Haemophilus parainfluenzae, Klebsiella pneumoniae, Klebsiella oxytoca, Escherichia coli, Enterobacter aerogenes, Proteus mirabilis, Serratia marcescens, Morganella morganii, Bacteroides fragilis, Acinetobacter calcoaceticus,* **and** *Neisseria gonorrhoeae*
Adults and children older than age 12: 1 to 2 g IM or IV daily or in equally divided doses every 12 hours. Total daily dose shouldn't exceed 4 g. Treat for 4 to 14 days. Complicated infections may require longer treatment.
Children ages 12 and younger: 50 to 75 mg/kg IM or IV daily or in divided doses every 12 hours. Total daily dose not to exceed 2 g.

➤ **Meningitis caused by** *H influenzae, Neisseria meningitidis,* **or** *S. pneumoniae*
Adults: 2 g IV b.i.d. Usual duration of therapy is 7 to 21 days depending on clinical response.
Children: Initially, 100 mg/kg IM or IV; then 100 mg/kg/day as a single dose or in divided doses every 12 hours for 7 to 14 days. Maximum dose, 4 g/day.

➤ **Perioperative prophylaxis**
Adults: 1 g IV as a single dose 30 minutes to 2 hours before surgery.

➤ **Acute bacterial otitis media caused by** *S. pneumoniae, H. influenzae,* **or** *Moraxella catarrhalis*
Adults: 1 to 2 g IM or IV once daily or in two equally divided doses daily for 3 days.
Children: 50 mg/kg IM as a single dose. Don't exceed 1 g.

ADMINISTRATION
• Before giving drug, ensure patient isn't allergic to penicillins or cephalosporins.
• Obtain specimen for culture and sensitivity testing before giving first dose. Begin therapy while awaiting results.

IV
▼ Reconstitute drug with sterile water for injection, NSS for injection, D_5W, or a combination of NSS and dextrose injection and other compatible solutions.

▼ Add 2.4 mL of diluent to the 250-mg vial, 4.8 mL to the 500-mg vial, 9.6 mL to the 1-g vial, and 19.2 mL to the 2-g vial. All reconstituted solutions average 100 mg/mL. For intermittent infusion, dilute further to achieve desired concentration, and give over 30 minutes.
▼ Allow refrigerated solutions to come to room temperature before infusing.
▼ Diluted IV preparation is stable for 48 hours at room temperature or 10 days if refrigerated.
⚠ **Alert:** Don't mix or administer ceftriaxone with calcium-containing IV solutions, including parenteral nutrition.
▼ **Incompatibilities:** Aminoglycosides, aminophylline, azithromycin, calcium-containing solutions, clindamycin phosphate, filgrastim, fluconazole, gentamicin, labetalol, linezolid, pentamidine, theophylline, vancomycin, vinorelbine tartrate. Consult drug compatibility reference for more information.

IM
• Reconstitute powder with sterile water for injection, NSS, or bacteriostatic water to final concentration of 250 or 350 mg/mL.
• Can also dilute with 1% lidocaine to decrease discomfort.
• Inject deep into a large muscle, such as gluteus maximus or lateral aspect of thigh.
• Reconstituted solution remains stable for 2 days at room temperature or 10 days refrigerated. If reconstituted with lidocaine or bacteriostatic water, solution remains stable for 24 hours at room temperature.

ACTION
Inhibits cell-wall synthesis, promoting osmotic instability; usually bactericidal.

Route	Onset	Peak	Duration
IV	Immediate	Immediate	Unknown
IM	Unknown	2–3 hr	Unknown

Half-life: Adults 5 to 9 hours.

ADVERSE REACTIONS
GI: diarrhea. **GU:** increased BUN level.
Hematologic: eosinophilia, *thrombocytosis, leukopenia.* **Hepatic:** increased transaminase levels. **Skin:** pain, induration, tenderness at injection site; rash. **Other:** hypersensitivity reactions.

INTERACTIONS

Drug-drug. *Aminoglycosides:* May increase kidney toxicity and cause synergistic effect against some strains of *Enterobacteriaceae* species. Monitor patient.

Live-virus vaccines: May decrease effectiveness of live-virus vaccines. Use together isn't recommended.

Probenecid: May increase ceftriaxone concentration. Monitor therapy.

Warfarin: May increase anticoagulation effect. Closely monitor PT and INR.

EFFECTS ON LAB TEST RESULTS

• May increase ALP, ALT, AST, bilirubin, BUN, creatinine, and LDH levels.
• May increase eosinophil and platelet counts.
• May decrease Hb level and WBC count.
• May prolong PTT and PT.
• May increase INR.
• May falsely increase serum or urine creatinine level in tests using Jaffé reaction. May cause false-positive results of Coombs test and urine glucose tests that use cupric sulfate (Benedict reagent, Clinitest).

CONTRAINDICATIONS & CAUTIONS

• Contraindicated in patients hypersensitive to drug or other cephalosporins.
• Contraindicated in premature neonates up to postmenstrual age of 41 weeks (gestational age + chronological age), neonates with hyperbilirubinemia, and neonates requiring calcium-containing IV solutions.
• May cause ceftriaxone-calcium precipitates, causing stones to form in the urinary tract and gallbladder, especially in children.
• Use cautiously in patients hypersensitive to penicillins because of possibility of cross-sensitivity with other beta-lactam antibiotics.
• Hypersensitivity reactions can occur in patients receiving dextrose from corn-derived solution.
• To reduce development of drug-resistant bacteria and maintain effectiveness of antibacterial drugs, use drug only to treat or prevent infections proven or strongly suspected to be caused by bacteria.
• **Alert:** May cause fungal or bacterial superinfection, including CDAD and pseudomembranous colitis. Stop drug and take appropriate measures if diarrhea develops. CDAD has occurred more than 2 months after antibacterial treatment.

• **Alert:** May cause hemolytic anemia, which can be fatal. If anemia develops during therapy, stop drug until cause is determined.
• **Alert:** Drug may cause severe neurologic reactions (encephalopathy, myoclonus, seizures, nonconvulsive status epilepticus). Risk may increase in patients with kidney impairment; ensure dosage adjustment for kidney function. Discontinue drug if neurotoxicity occurs.
• Drug may increase risk of pancreatitis.
• Use cautiously in patients with history of colitis, kidney insufficiency, or GI or gallbladder disease.
Dialyzable drug: No.

PREGNANCY-LACTATION-REPRODUCTION

• Studies during pregnancy are inadequate. Drug crosses the placenta. Use during pregnancy only if clearly needed.
• Drug appears in human milk in low concentrations. Use cautiously during breastfeeding.

NURSING CONSIDERATIONS

• If patient receives large doses, therapy is prolonged, or patient is at high risk, monitor for signs and symptoms of superinfection.
• Monitor PT and INR in patient with impaired vitamin K synthesis or low vitamin K stores. Vitamin K therapy may be needed.
• Monitor patient for diarrhea and anemia, and treat appropriately.
• Monitor for hypersensitivity reactions.
• Monitor for signs and symptoms of gallbladder disease, urolithiasis, oliguria, and AKI. Ensure patient is adequately hydrated.
• *Look alike–sound alike:* Don't confuse drug with other cephalosporins that sound alike.

PATIENT TEACHING

• Tell patient to promptly report adverse reactions.
• Warn that neurotoxicity can occur. Instruct patient to immediately report signs and symptoms (somnolence, lethargy, confusion, seizures).
• Instruct patient to report discomfort at IV insertion site.
• If patient with diabetes is receiving home care and is testing urine for glucose, explain that drug may affect results of cupric sulfate tests and patient should use enzymatic test instead.
• Tell patient to notify prescriber about watery and bloody stools with or without

stomach cramps and fever even if months after treatment.

cefuroxime axetil
se-fyoor-OX-eem

cefuroxime sodium

Therapeutic class: Antibiotics
Pharmacologic class: Second-generation cephalosporins

AVAILABLE FORMS
cefuroxime axetil
Tablets: 125 mg, 250 mg, 500 mg
cefuroxime sodium
Infusion: 750 mg, 1.5 g vials and ready-to-use dual chamber IV bag
Injection: 750 mg, 1.5 g vials

INDICATIONS & DOSAGES

Adjust-a-dose (for all indications): For injectable form in adults with CrCl of 10 to 20 mL/minute, give 750 mg IV or IM every 12 hours; if CrCl is less than 10 mL/minute, give 750 mg IV or IM every 24 hours. For injectable form in children with CrCl of 10 to 20 mL/minute, give standard weight-based dose every 12 hours; if CrCl is less than 10 mL/minute, give every 24 hours. For oral form in adults with CrCl of 10 to less than 30 mL/minute, give standard dose every 24 hours; if CrCl is less than 10 mL/minute without hemodialysis, give standard dose every 48 hours. Give patients on hemodialysis an additional dose IV, IM, or PO after hemodialysis.

➤ **Serious lower respiratory tract infection, UTI, skin or skin-structure infection, bone or joint infection, septicemia, meningitis, and gonorrhea**
Adults: 750 mg to 1.5 g cefuroxime sodium IV or IM every 8 hours for 5 to 10 days. For life-threatening infections and infections caused by less susceptible organisms, 1.5 g IV or IM every 6 hours; for bacterial meningitis, up to 3 g IV every 8 hours.
Children ages 3 months and older: 50 to 100 mg/kg/day cefuroxime sodium IV or IM in equally divided doses every 6 to 8 hours. Use higher dosage of 100 mg/kg/day, not to exceed maximum adult dosage, for more severe or serious infections. For bacterial meningitis, 200 to 240 mg/kg/day cefuroxime sodium IV in divided doses every 6 to 8 hours.

➤ **Perioperative prophylaxis**
Adults: 1.5 g IV 30 to 60 minutes before initial incision; in lengthy operations, 750 mg IV or IM every 8 hours. For open-heart surgery, 1.5 g IV at induction of anesthesia and then every 12 hours for a total dose of 6 g.
➤ **Mild to moderate acute bacterial exacerbations of chronic bronchitis**
Adults and children ages 13 and older: 250 or 500 mg PO every 12 hours for 10 days.
➤ **Acute bacterial maxillary sinusitis**
Adults and children ages 13 and older: 250 mg PO every 12 hours for 10 days.
Children ages 12 and younger able to swallow pills: 250 mg every 12 hours for 10 days.
➤ **Pharyngitis and tonsillitis**
Adults and children ages 13 and older: 250 mg PO every 12 hours for 10 days.
➤ **Otitis media**
Children ages 12 and younger able to swallow pills: 250 mg PO every 12 hours for 10 days.
➤ **Uncomplicated skin and skin-structure infection**
Adults and children ages 13 and older: 250 or 500 mg PO every 12 hours for 10 days.
➤ **Uncomplicated UTI**
Adults and children age 13 and older: 250 mg PO every 12 hours for 7 to 10 days.
➤ **Uncomplicated gonorrhea**
Adults: 1,000 mg PO as a single dose. Or, 1.5 g IM with 1 g probenecid PO for one dose.
➤ **Early Lyme disease**
Adults and children ages 13 and older: 500 mg PO every 12 hours for 20 days.

ADMINISTRATION
• Obtain specimen for culture and sensitivity tests before giving first dose. Begin therapy while awaiting results.
• Before giving drug, ensure patient isn't allergic to penicillins or cephalosporins.
PO
• Give tablets without regard for meals.
• Don't crush tablets due to bitter taste.
IV
▼ Reconstitute each 750-mg vial with 8.3 mL and each 1.5-g vial with 16 mL of sterile water for injection.
▼ Withdraw entire contents of vial for a 750-mg or 1.5-g dose.
▼ For direct injection, inject over 3 to 5 minutes into large vein or into tubing of free-flowing IV solution.
▼ For intermittent infusion, add reconstituted drug in D_5W, NSS for injection, or

other compatible IV solution to final concentration of 30 mg/mL or less.

▼ Infuse over 15 to 30 minutes.

▼ May story diluted solution for 24 hours at room temperature or 7 days under refrigeration.

▼ **Incompatibilities:** Azithromycin, ciprofloxacin, cisatracurium, clarithromycin, doxapram, filgrastim, fluconazole, gentamicin, midazolam, ranitidine, sodium bicarbonate injection, vancomycin, vinorelbine tartrate.

IM

• Reconstitute 750-mg vial with 3 mL of sterile water for injection.

• Inject deep into a large muscle, such as gluteus maximus or side of thigh.

ACTION

Inhibits cell-wall synthesis, promoting osmotic instability; usually bactericidal.

Route	Onset	Peak	Duration
PO	Unknown	2–4 hr	Unknown
IV	Immediate	2–3 min	Unknown
IM	Unknown	15–60 min	Unknown

Half-life: 1 to 2 hours.

ADVERSE REACTIONS

CV: local thrombophlebitis. **GI:** diarrhea, nausea, vomiting. **GU:** vaginitis. **Hematologic:** anemia, *thrombocytopenia, transient neutropenia,* eosinophilia. **Hepatic:** transient elevated LFT values. **Metabolic:** increased LDH level. **Skin:** rash. **Other:** hypersensitivity reactions.

INTERACTIONS

Drug-drug. *Aminoglycosides:* May increase kidney toxicity. Monitor patient's kidney function closely.

Antacids: May decrease cefuroxime serum level. Give oral drug at least 1 hour before or 2 hours after short-acting antacids.

Live-virus vaccines: May decrease effectiveness of live-virus vaccines. Use together isn't recommended.

Loop diuretics: May increase risk of adverse kidney reactions. Monitor kidney function.

Probenecid: May inhibit excretion and increase cefuroxime level. Probenecid may be used for this effect.

Warfarin: May increase anticoagulation effects. Monitor PT and INR closely.

EFFECTS ON LAB TEST RESULTS

• May increase ALP, ALT, AST, bilirubin, and LDH levels.

• May decrease Hb level and hematocrit.

• May increase INR and eosinophil count.

• May decrease neutrophil, leukocyte, and platelet counts.

• May prolong PT.

• May falsely increase serum or urine creatinine level in tests using Jaffé reaction.

• May cause false-positive results of Coombs test and urine glucose tests that use cupric sulfate (Benedict reagent, Clinitest).

CONTRAINDICATIONS & CAUTIONS

• Contraindicated in patients hypersensitive to drug or other cephalosporins.

• Use cautiously in patients hypersensitive to penicillins because of possibility of cross-sensitivity with other beta-lactam antibiotics.

• Solutions containing dextrose may be contraindicated in patients with hypersensitivity to corn.

• Use cautiously in patients with history of colitis and in those with kidney insufficiency.

• Be aware that some products contain phenylalanine or sodium.

⚠ *Alert:* Drug may cause mild to life-threatening CDAD and pseudomembranous colitis, which can occur even 2 months after therapy.

• Some cephalosporins have been associated with seizures in patients with kidney impairment when the dosage wasn't reduced. If drug-associated seizures occur, discontinue drug and treat with anticonvulsant therapy if indicated.

Dialyzable drug: Yes.

PREGNANCY-LACTATION-REPRODUCTION

• Studies during pregnancy are inadequate. Use during pregnancy only if clearly needed.

• Drug appears in human milk. Patient should consider temporarily discontinuing breast-feeding during treatment.

NURSING CONSIDERATIONS

• Monitor patient for signs and symptoms of superinfection and diarrhea; treat appropriately.

• Drug may increase INR and risk of bleeding. Monitor patient.

• Monitor for hypersensitivity reactions.

• *Look alike–sound alike:* Don't confuse drug with other cephalosporins that sound alike.

Reactions in bold italics are *life-threatening*.

PATIENT TEACHING
- Tell patient to take drug as prescribed, even if feeling better.
- Instruct patient to notify prescriber about rash, loose stools, diarrhea (even months after treatment), or evidence of superinfection.
- Tell patient to report hypersensitivity reactions.
- Advise patient receiving drug IV to report discomfort at IV insertion site.

---

celecoxib ☒
sell-ah-COCKS-ib

CeleBREX, Elyxyb

Therapeutic class: NSAIDs
Pharmacologic class: Cyclooxygenase-2 inhibitors

AVAILABLE FORMS
Capsules: 50 mg, 100 mg, 200 mg, 400 mg
Solution: 120 mg/4.8 mL (25 mg/mL)

INDICATIONS & DOSAGES
☒ *Adjust-a-dose (for all indications):* For older adults and patients weighing less than 50 kg, start at lowest dosage. For patients with Child-Pugh class B liver impairment, reduce dosage by about 50%. For patients who are poor metabolizers of CYP2C9, start treatment at half the lowest recommended dose.
➤ **To relieve signs and symptoms of osteoarthritis**
Adults: 200 mg PO daily as a single dose or in two equally divided doses.
➤ **To relieve signs and symptoms of RA**
Adults: 100 to 200 mg PO b.i.d.
➤ **To relieve signs and symptoms of ankylosing spondylitis**
Adults: 200 mg PO once daily or in two divided doses. If no response after 6 weeks, may increase dose to 400 mg daily. If no response after 6 more weeks, consider other treatment.
➤ **To relieve signs and symptoms of juvenile RA**
Children ages 2 and older weighing 10 to 25 kg: 50 mg PO b.i.d.
Children ages 2 and older weighing more than 25 kg: 100 mg PO b.i.d.
➤ **Acute pain and primary dysmenorrhea**
Adults: Initially, 400 mg PO, then another 200-mg dose if needed on the first day. On subsequent days, 200 mg PO b.i.d. as needed.

➤ **Acute migraine (Elyxyb only)**
Adults: 120 mg PO, as needed. Maximum dosage, 120 mg/day. Use for fewest number of days per month.
Adjust-a-dose: For patients with Child-Pugh class B liver impairment or patients who are poor CYP2C9 metabolizers, give 60-mg dose.

ADMINISTRATION
PO
- May give without regard to meals.
- For patient with difficulty swallowing capsules, may add capsule contents to applesauce. Carefully empty entire contents of capsule onto a level teaspoon of cool or room-temperature applesauce and give immediately with water. The capsule contents sprinkled on applesauce are stable for up to 6 hours under refrigeration.
- Use calibrated medication measuring device to measure and deliver solution.
- Store at room temperature.

ACTION
Thought to inhibit prostaglandin synthesis, impeding cyclooxygenase-2, to produce anti-inflammatory, analgesic, and antipyretic effects.

Route	Onset	Peak	Duration
PO	Unknown	3 hr	Unknown
PO (solution)	Unknown	1 hr	Unknown

Half-life: capsules, 11 hours; solution, 6 hours.

ADVERSE REACTIONS
CNS: headache, dizziness, insomnia, dysgeusia, fever. **CV:** HTN, peripheral edema. **EENT:** eye disorder, pharyngitis, rhinitis, sinusitis. **GI:** abdominal pain, diarrhea, dyspepsia, flatulence, GERD, nausea. **GU:** nephrolithiasis. **Metabolic:** hyperchloremia. **Musculoskeletal:** back pain, arthralgia. **Respiratory:** dyspnea, URI, cough. **Skin:** rash. **Other:** accidental injury, hypersensitivity reaction.

INTERACTIONS
Drug-drug. *ACE inhibitors, ARBs, beta blockers (propranolol):* May decrease antihypertensive effects. Monitor BP.
Antacids containing aluminum or magnesium: May decrease celecoxib level. Separate doses.
Anticoagulants, antiplatelets (clopidogrel, prasugrel), SSNRIs, SSRIs: May increase bleeding risk. Use cautiously.

Aspirin: May increase risk of bleeding; low aspirin dosages can be used safely to reduce the risk of CV events. Monitor patient for signs and symptoms of GI bleeding.

Corticosteroids: May increase risk of GI bleeding. Use together cautiously.

Cyclosporine: May increase risk of kidney toxicity. Monitor kidney function.

CYP2C9 inducers (rifampin): May decrease effect of celecoxib. Monitor therapy.

CYP2C9 inhibitors (amiodarone, fluconazole, metronidazole, ritonavir, zafirlukast): May increase celecoxib level and risk of toxicity. Use together cautiously.

CYP2D6 substrates (atomoxetine): May increase exposure and toxicity of substrates. Monitor therapy.

Digoxin: May increase digoxin serum level. Monitor use together.

Lithium: May increase lithium level. Monitor patient for lithium toxicity.

Loop and thiazide diuretics: May increase kidney toxicity; may decrease antihypertensive effects. Monitor therapeutic effects and kidney function.

Methotrexate: May increase risk of methotrexate toxicity (neutropenia, thrombocytopenia, kidney dysfunction). Monitor patient.

Boxed Warning *NSAIDs:* Can increase risk of serious CV thrombotic events, including MI or stroke, which can be fatal. Risk may occur early in treatment and may increase with duration of use in patients with or without heart disease or risk factors for heart disease. Risk appears greater at higher doses. Use lowest effective dose for shortest duration possible. ■

Pemetrexed: May increase risk of myelosuppression and kidney and GI toxicity. Monitor patient closely, especially patients with kidney impairment.

Warfarin: May prolong PT and risk of bleeding complications. Monitor PT and INR, and check for signs and symptoms of bleeding.

Drug-herb. *Alfalfa, anise, bilberry:* May increase risk of bleeding. Discourage use together.

White willow: Herb and drug contain similar components. Discourage use together.

Drug-lifestyle. *Long-term alcohol use, smoking:* May cause GI irritation or bleeding. Check for signs and symptoms of bleeding.

EFFECTS ON LAB TEST RESULTS
• May increase ALT, AST, BUN, creatinine, CK, glucose, uric acid, and potassium levels.
• May decrease Hb level and hematocrit.
• May prolong PTT.

CONTRAINDICATIONS & CAUTIONS
Boxed Warning Contraindicated for treatment of perioperative pain after CABG. ■
• Contraindicated in patients hypersensitive to drug; in patients who experienced asthma, urticaria, or allergic-type reactions after taking aspirin or other NSAIDs; and in those who have demonstrated allergic-type reactions to sulfonamides.
• Avoid use in patients with recent MI.
• Use in patients with severe kidney or Child-Pugh C liver impairment isn't recommended.
• Use may lead to new-onset HTN or worsening of preexisting HTN.
• Drug may increase risk of DIC in children with juvenile RA.
⊙ *Alert:* NSAIDs increase risk of HF.
⊠ Use cautiously in patients with history of ulcers or GI bleeding, advanced kidney disease, dehydration, anemia, symptomatic liver disease, HTN, edema, HF, or asthma and in poor CYP2C9 metabolizers.
⊠ Consider alternative therapies for treatment of juvenile RA in patients identified to be poor CYP2C9 metabolizers.
• Use cautiously in older adults and patients who are debilitated.
Boxed Warning Older adults and patients with a history of peptic ulcer disease or GI bleeding are at greater risk for serious GI events, which can be fatal. ■
Dialyzable drug: Unlikely.
⚠ *Overdose S&S:* Lethargy, drowsiness, nausea, vomiting, epigastric pain, GI bleeding, HTN, AKI, respiratory depression, coma, anaphylaxis.

PREGNANCY-LACTATION-REPRODUCTION
⊙ *Alert:* Use of NSAIDs at 20 weeks or later in pregnancy may cause fetal kidney dysfunction, leading to oligohydramnios and potential neonatal kidney impairment. NSAID use at 30 weeks or later in pregnancy may increase risk of premature closure of the ductus arteriosus. Avoid use during pregnancy starting at 20 weeks' gestation. If potential benefit justifies fetal risk, use lowest effective dose for shortest duration. Consider ultrasound monitoring of amniotic fluid if NSAID use

is longer than 48 hours. Use of low-dose aspirin (81 mg) for certain pregnancy-related conditions under the direction of a prescriber is acceptable.

• Drug appears in human milk. Use cautiously during breastfeeding. Patient should consider temporarily discontinuing breastfeeding during treatment.

• Long-term use of NSAIDs in patients of childbearing potential may be associated with infertility that's reversible on discontinuation of NSAID.

NURSING CONSIDERATIONS

Boxed Warning NSAIDs increase risk of serious GI adverse events, including bleeding, ulceration, and perforation of stomach or intestines, which can be fatal. ■

• Additional risk factors for GI bleeding include treatment with corticosteroids or anticoagulants, longer duration of NSAID treatment, smoking, alcohol use disorder, advanced age, and poor overall health.

• Although drug may be used with low-aspirin dosages, the combination may increase risk of GI bleeding.

• Watch for signs and symptoms of overt and occult bleeding and abnormal clotting.

⊕ **Alert:** Watch for and immediately evaluate signs and symptoms of heart attack (chest pain, shortness of breath, trouble breathing) or stroke (weakness in one part or side of the body, slurred speech).

• Drug can cause fluid retention; monitor patient with HTN, edema, or HF.

• Drug may impair response of antihypertensives. Monitor BP.

• Drug may mask signs and symptoms of infection and fever due to anti-inflammatory effect.

• Assess patient for CV risk factors before therapy.

• Drug may be toxic to liver; watch for signs and symptoms of liver toxicity.

• Before starting drug therapy, rehydrate patient who is dehydrated.

• Monitor patient's kidney function. Long-term administration may cause kidney papillary necrosis and other kidney injury.

• Monitor patient for hypersensitivity reactions, including serious skin reactions (SJS, exfoliative dermatitis, DRESS syndrome). Discontinue at first appearance of rash.

• *Look alike–sound alike:* Don't confuse Celebrex with Cerebyx or Celexa.

PATIENT TEACHING

• Instruct patient to promptly report signs of GI bleeding (melena; blood in vomit, urine, or stool).

• Tell patient to report pregnancy or plans to become pregnant during therapy.

⊕ *Alert:* Warn patient who is pregnant not to take NSAIDs at 20 weeks' gestation or later unless instructed to do so by prescriber, due to potential fetal risk. Advise patient to discuss taking OTC medications with a pharmacist or health care provider during pregnancy.

⊕ *Alert:* Advise patient to immediately report rash, unexplained weight gain, or swelling.

⊕ *Alert:* Advise patient to immediately seek medical attention if chest pain, shortness of breath or trouble breathing, weakness in one part or side of the body, or slurred speech occurs.

• Teach about proper drug administration and handling.

• Advise patient that using OTC NSAIDs with celecoxib may increase the risk of GI toxicity.

• Tell patient that drug may harm the liver. Advise patient to stop therapy and immediately notify prescriber if signs or symptoms of liver toxicity (nausea, fatigue, lethargy, itching, yellowing of skin or eyes, right upper quadrant tenderness, flulike syndrome) occur.

• Inform patient that it may take several days before consistent pain relief occurs.

SAFETY ALERT!

cemiplimab-rwlc
se-MIP-li-mab

Libtayo

Therapeutic class: Antineoplastics
Pharmacologic class: Programmed death receptor-1 blocking antibodies

AVAILABLE FORMS

Injection: 350 mg/7 mL (50 mg/mL) single-dose vial

INDICATIONS & DOSAGES

Adjust-a-dose (for all indications): Refer to manufacturer's instructions for toxicity-related dosage adjustments.

➤ **Metastatic cutaneous squamous cell carcinoma (CSCC) or locally advanced CSCC**

---

in patients who aren't candidates for curative surgery or curative radiation
Adults: 350 mg IV infusion over 30 minutes every 3 weeks until disease progression or unacceptable toxicity occurs.

➤ **Locally advanced or metastatic basal cell carcinoma previously treated with a hedgehog pathway inhibitor or when a hedgehog pathway inhibitor isn't appropriate**
Adults: 350 mg IV infusion over 30 minutes every 3 weeks until disease progression or unacceptable toxicity occurs.

➤ **First-line treatment of patients with advanced NSCLC (locally advanced, in which patients aren't candidates for surgical resection or definitive chemoradiation or who have metastatic disease) whose tumors have high PD-L1 expression, with no *EGFR, ALK,* or *ROS1* alterations**
Adults: 350 mg IV infusion over 30 minutes every 3 weeks until disease progression or unacceptable toxicity occurs.

✳ *NEW INDICATION:* **Locally advanced or metastatic NSCLC with no *EGFR, ALK,* or *ROS1* aberrations as first-line treatment in combination with platinum-based chemotherapy**
Adults: 350 mg IV infusion over 30 minutes every 3 weeks until disease progression or unacceptable toxicity occurs.

ADMINISTRATION

IV

▼ Inspect vial for particulate matter and discoloration. Drug should appear clear to slightly opalescent, colorless to pale yellow and may contain trace amounts of translucent to white particles. Discard vial if solution is cloudy, is discolored, or contains other particulate matter.

▼ Withdraw 7 mL from vial and dilute with NSS or D_5W to a final concentration between 1 and 20 mg/mL; mix diluted solution by gentle inversion but don't shake. Discard any unused drug.

▼ Infuse over 30 minutes through an IV line containing an in-line filter or add-on 0.2- to 5-micron filter.

▼ Store at room temperature up to 77° F (25° C) for no more than 8 hours or refrigerate at 36° to 46° F (2° to 8° C) for no more than 24 hours from time of preparation to end of infusion. Allow diluted solution to come to room temperature before administration; don't freeze.

▼ Store unopened vials at 36° to 46° F (2° to 8° C) in original carton and protected from light; don't freeze or shake.

▼ **Incompatibilities:** Don't give with solutions other than NSS or D_5W.

ACTION
IgG4 monoclonal antibody that binds to programmed death-receptor (PD) antibodies, thereby blocking PD-1 activity and decreasing tumor growth.

Route	Onset	Peak	Duration
IV	Unknown	Unknown	Unknown

Half-life: 20.3 days.

ADVERSE REACTIONS
CNS: fatigue, headache. **CV:** HTN. **GI:** diarrhea, nausea, constipation, vomiting, decreased appetite, immune-mediated colitis. **GU:** UTI, increased creatinine level. **Hematologic:** anemia, *lymphocytopenia, prolonged bleeding time.* **Hepatic:** hyperbilirubinemia, increased transaminase levels, *hepatitis.* **Metabolic:** decreased appetite, *endocrinopathies,* hyponatremia, *hypokalemia, hyperkalemia,* hypercalcemia, *hypocalcemia,* hypophosphatemia, hypoalbuminemia, hypermagnesemia, hypothyroidism. **Musculoskeletal:** pain, arthralgia, muscular weakness. **Respiratory:** URI, dyspnea, pneumonia, *pneumonitis,* cough. **Skin:** rash, pruritus, cellulitis, skin infection, immune-mediated dermatologic reactions (rash, dermatitis). **Other:** *sepsis,* antibody development.

INTERACTIONS
None reported.

EFFECTS ON LAB TEST RESULTS
• May increase ALT, AST, ALP, bilirubin, creatinine, and magnesium levels.
• May decrease albumin, phosphate, and sodium levels.
• May increase or decrease calcium and potassium levels.
• May increase INR.
• May decrease Hb level, hematocrit, and lymphocyte and RBC counts.

CONTRAINDICATIONS & CAUTIONS
🔸 *Alert:* Immune-mediated adverse reactions, which may be severe or fatal, can

occur in any organ system or tissue and include pneumonitis, GI toxicities (colitis, hepatitis, pancreatitis), endocrinopathies (adrenal insufficiency, hypophysitis, hypothyroidism, hyperthyroidism, type 1 diabetes), nephritis with kidney dysfunction, dermatologic toxicities (erythema multiforme, SJS, pemphigoid, TEN), myocarditis, neurologic toxicities (meningitis, encephalitis, myelitis and demyelination, myasthenic syndrome, myasthenia gravis, Guillain-Barré syndrome, nerve paresis, autoimmune neuropathy), ocular inflammatory toxicities (uveitis, iritis, retinal detachment, vision loss), musculoskeletal toxicities (myositis, rhabdomyolysis, arthritis, polymyalgia rheumatica), and hematologic and immunologic toxicities (hemolytic anemia, aplastic anemia, hemophagocytic lymphohistiocytosis, systemic inflammatory response syndrome, histiocytic necrotizing lymphadenitis, Kikuchi lymphadenitis, sarcoidosis, and immune thrombocytopenic purpura). Monitor patient closely.

🕭 *Alert:* Fatal and other serious complications can occur in patients who receive allogeneic hematopoietic stem cell transplantation (HSCT) despite intervening therapy between drug administration and allogeneic HSCT. Consider risk versus benefit.

• Drug may cause rejection of a transplanted organ. Monitor patient closely.

• Safety and effectiveness in children haven't been established.

Dialyzable drug: Unknown.

PREGNANCY-LACTATION-REPRODUCTION

• Drug can cause fetal harm based on mechanism of action. Advise patients of childbearing potential about fetal risk and the need to use effective contraception during treatment and for at least 4 months after final dose.

• It isn't known if drug appears in human milk. Patient shouldn't breastfeed during treatment and for at least 4 months after final dose.

NURSING CONSIDERATIONS

• Monitor patient for infusion-related reactions (chills, rash, pruritus, flushing, shortness of breath, dizziness, fever, syncope, back or neck pain, facial swelling). Interrupt or slow rate of infusion or permanently discontinue infusion based on severity of the reaction.

• Monitor patient for development of immune-mediated adverse reactions.

• If immune-mediated adverse reactions occur, withhold or discontinue drug as needed and administer corticosteroids until resolved, followed by a corticosteroid taper over 1 month.

• Consider use of other systemic immunosuppressants when immune-mediated adverse reactions aren't controlled with corticosteroids, and begin hormone replacement therapy for endocrinopathies as warranted.

• Evaluate LFTs, creatinine level, and thyroid function tests at baseline and periodically during treatment.

• Assess pregnancy status before start of treatment.

PATIENT TEACHING

• Teach patient to report all adverse reactions.

• Counsel patient to immediately report immune-mediated adverse reactions or infusion-related reactions.

• Advise patient of childbearing potential that drug can harm fetus. Instruct patient to inform prescriber of known or suspected pregnancy.

• Warn patient of childbearing potential to use effective contraception during treatment and for at least 4 months after final dose.

• Instruct patient not to breastfeed while taking drug and for at least 4 months after final dose.

cephalexin
sef-a-LEX-in

Apo-Cephalex ✤

Therapeutic class: Antibiotics
Pharmacologic class: First-generation cephalosporins

AVAILABLE FORMS
Capsules: 250 mg, 333 mg, 500 mg, 750 mg
Oral suspension: 125 mg/5 mL, 250 mg/5 mL
Tablets: 250 mg, 500 mg

INDICATIONS & DOSAGES
➤ **Respiratory tract infections caused by susceptible isolates of *Streptococcus pneumoniae* and *Streptococcus pyogenes;* GU tract infections caused by susceptible isolates of *Escherichia coli, Proteus mirabilis,* and *Klebsiella pneumoniae;* skin and skinstructure infections caused by susceptible**

isolates of *Staphylococcus aureus* or *S. pyogenes;* bone infections caused by susceptible isolates of *S. aureus* and *P. mirabilis;* and otitis media caused by susceptible isolates of *S. pneumoniae, Haemophilus influenzae, S. aureus, S. pyogenes,* and *Moraxella catarrhalis*
Adults and children ages 15 and older: 250 mg to 1 g PO every 6 hours or 500 mg every 12 hours for 7 to 14 days. Maximum, 4 g daily.
Children older than age 1: 25 to 50 mg/kg/ day PO in two to four equally divided doses for 7 to 14 days. For otitis media, 75 to 100 mg/kg PO in equally divided doses every 6 hours. For severe infections, 50 to 100 mg/kg PO in equally divided doses. Don't exceed recommended adult dosage.
Adjust-a-dose: For adults and children ages 15 and older with CrCl of 30 to 59 mL/minute, no dosage adjustment is needed but maximum daily dose shouldn't exceed 1 g; for CrCl of 15 to 29 mL/minute, reduce dosage to 250 mg every 8 or 12 hours; for CrCl of 5 to 14 mL/minute in patients not yet on dialysis, reduce dosage to 250 mg every 24 hours; for CrCl of 1 to 4 mL/minute in patients not yet on dialysis, reduce dosage to 250 mg every 48 or 60 hours.

ADMINISTRATION
PO
• Before giving, ensure patient isn't allergic to penicillins or cephalosporins.
• Obtain specimen for culture and sensitivity tests before giving first dose. Begin therapy while awaiting results.
• To prepare oral suspension, add required amount of water to powder in two portions. Shake well after each addition. After mixing, store in refrigerator. Mixture will remain stable for 14 days. Keep tightly closed and shake well before using.
• May give without regard to meals but give with food or milk to lessen GI discomfort.

ACTION
Inhibits cell-wall synthesis, promoting osmotic instability; usually bactericidal.

Route	Onset	Peak	Duration
PO	Unknown	1 hr	Unknown

Half-life: Adults, 30 minutes to 1.25 hours; children ages 3 to 12 months, 2.5 hours; neonates, 5 hours.

ADVERSE REACTIONS
CNS: dizziness, headache, fatigue, agitation, confusion, hallucinations. **GI:** anorexia, nausea, vomiting, diarrhea, *CDAD,* gastritis, glossitis, dyspepsia, abdominal pain, anal pruritus. **GU:** genital pruritus, candidiasis, vaginitis, vaginal discharge, interstitial nephritis. **Hematologic:** *neutropenia, thrombocytopenia,* eosinophilia, anemia. **Musculoskeletal:** arthritis, arthralgia, joint pain. **Skin:** rash, urticaria. **Other:** hypersensitivity reactions.

INTERACTIONS
Drug-drug. *Aminoglycosides:* May increase risk of kidney toxicity. Avoid use together.
Live-virus vaccines: May decrease effectiveness of live-virus vaccines. Use together isn't recommended.
Metformin: May increase metformin level. Monitor blood glucose level closely.
Multivitamins containing zinc: May decrease cephalexin absorption. Consider administering at least 3 hours after cephalexin. Consider therapy modification.
Probenecid: May increase cephalosporin level. Use together isn't recommended.
Warfarin: May enhance anticoagulant effects. Monitor therapy.

EFFECTS ON LAB TEST RESULTS
• May increase ALP, ALT, AST, bilirubin, and LDH levels.
• May increase eosinophil count.
• May decrease Hb level and neutrophil and platelet counts.
• May prolong PT.
• May falsely increase serum or urine creatinine level in tests using Jaffé reaction. May cause false-positive results of Coombs test and urine glucose tests that use cupric sulfate (Benedict reagent, Clinitest).

CONTRAINDICATIONS & CAUTIONS
• Contraindicated in patients hypersensitive to cephalosporins.
• Use cautiously in patients hypersensitive to penicillins because of possibility of cross-sensitivity with other beta-lactam antibiotics.
• Severe hypersensitivity reactions, including anaphylaxis and SCARs (SJS, erythema multiforme), can occur. If an allergic reaction occurs, discontinue drug immediately and treat appropriately.

Reactions in bold italics are *life-threatening*.

• Drug may increase risk of seizures. Use cautiously in patients with history of seizures.

• Use cautiously in older adults, patients with history of colitis, and those with kidney or liver impairment.

⚕ Alert: Drug can cause mild to life-threatening superinfection, CDAD, and pseudomembranous colitis, which can occur even 2 months after therapy.

Dialyzable drug: Unknown.

⚠ Overdose S&S: Nausea, vomiting, epigastric distress, diarrhea, hematuria.

PREGNANCY-LACTATION-REPRODUCTION

• Studies during pregnancy are inadequate. Use during pregnancy only if clearly needed and potential benefit justifies fetal risk.

• Drug appears in human milk. Use cautiously during breastfeeding.

NURSING CONSIDERATIONS

• If patient receives large doses, therapy is prolonged, or patient is at high risk, monitor for signs and symptoms of superinfection, including diarrhea.

• Treat group A beta-hemolytic streptococcal infections for a minimum of 10 days.

• If anemia develops during or after cephalexin therapy, obtain a diagnostic work-up for drug-induced hemolytic anemia, discontinue drug, and institute appropriate therapy.

• Monitor PT in patient with kidney impairment, liver impairment, or poor nutritional state; in patient on prolonged therapy; and in patient taking anticoagulants.

• Monitor for hypersensitivity reactions.

• *Look alike–sound alike:* Don't confuse drug with other cephalosporins that sound alike.

PATIENT TEACHING

• Tell patient to take drug exactly as prescribed, even if feeling better.

• Teach about proper drug administration and handling.

• Tell patient to report all adverse reactions and to immediately report rash and signs and symptoms of superinfection or diarrhea.

---

certolizumab pegol
cer-to-LIZ-u-mab PEG-ol

Cimzia

Therapeutic class: Immunomodulators
Pharmacologic class: TNF blockers

AVAILABLE FORMS
Lyophilized powder for injection: 200 mg
Prefilled syringe: 200 mg/mL

INDICATIONS & DOSAGES
➤ **Crohn disease when response to conventional therapy is inadequate**
Adults: Initially and at weeks 2 and 4, 400 mg subcut (given as two injections of 200 mg); then maintenance dose of 400 mg every 4 weeks, if response is adequate.

➤ **RA; psoriatic arthritis; active ankylosing spondylitis; nonradiographic axial spondyloarthritis, with objective signs of inflammation**
Adults: Initially and at weeks 2 and 4, 400 mg subcut (given as two injections of 200 mg); then maintenance dose of 200 mg every other week or may consider 400 mg every 4 weeks.

➤ **Plaque psoriasis in patients who are candidates for systemic therapy or phototherapy**
Adults: 400 mg (given as 2 subcut injections of 200 mg) every other week.
Adults weighing 90 kg or less: Consider initial doses of 400 mg (given as 2 subcut injections of 200 mg) at weeks 0, 2, and 4; then 200 mg every other week.

ADMINISTRATION
Subcutaneous
• Bring drug to room temperature for 30 minutes before reconstituting. Bring drug in prefilled syringe to room temperature before administration.

• Each 400-mg dose requires two vials. Reconstitute each vial with 1 mL of sterile water for injection, using provided 20G needle. Gently swirl vial without shaking. May take up to 30 minutes to fully reconstitute. Inspect vial for particulate matter and discoloration; discard if present.

• Draw up each vial in its own syringe, switching each 20G needle to a 23G needle.

• Inject prepared or prefilled syringes into separate sites in abdomen or thigh. Don't

---

inject in areas where skin is tender, bruised, red, or hard. Discard unused portion of vial or syringe.

• Reconstituted drug is stable for 2 hours at room temperature or for up to 24 hours if refrigerated. Don't freeze.

• May store prefilled syringes at room temperature for up to 7 days; write date removed from refrigerator and discard if not used within 7 days. Store in original carton (to protect from light) and don't return to refrigerator.

• The needle shield inside the removable cap of prefilled syringe contains natural rubber latex, which may cause an allergic reaction in latex-sensitive individuals.

ACTION

Selectively neutralizes TNFα, a proinflammatory cytokine responsible for stimulating the production of inflammatory mediators.

Route	Onset	Peak	Duration
Subcut	Unknown	54–171 hr	Unknown

Half-life: 14 days.

ADVERSE REACTIONS

CNS: anxiety, bipolar disorder, *suicidality,* fever, headache, *stroke,* TIA. **CV:** angina pectoris, *arrhythmias, HF,* HTN, *MI,* pericardial effusion, pericarditis, vasculitis, thrombophlebitis, *hemorrhage.* **EENT:** optic neuritis, retinal hemorrhage, uveitis, nasopharyngitis. **GI:** abdominal pain. **GU:** UTI, nephrotic syndrome, impaired kidney function, menstrual disorder. **Hematologic:** anemia, *leukopenia,* lymphadenopathy, *pancytopenia, thrombophilia, hepatic:* elevated liver enzyme levels, *hepatitis.* **Musculoskeletal:** arthralgia, extremity pain. **Respiratory:** URI, cough, bronchitis. **Skin:** rash, alopecia, dermatitis, peripheral edema, erythema nodosum, urticaria, injection-site reactions. **Other:** viral infection (herpes), bacterial infection (TB).

INTERACTIONS

Drug-drug. *Abatacept, anakinra, natalizumab, rilonacept, rituximab:* May increase risk of serious infection and neutropenia. Avoid use together.
Live-virus vaccines: May cause infection. Avoid use together.
Immunosuppressants (pimecrolimus, tacrolimus [topical], tocilizumab, tofacitinib, vedolizumab): May enhance adverse or toxic effects of immunosuppressants. Avoid use together.
Drug-herb. *Echinacea:* May diminish therapeutic effects. Consider therapy modification.

EFFECTS ON LAB TEST RESULTS

• May falsely prolong PTT.

CONTRAINDICATIONS & CAUTIONS

• Contraindicated in patients with a history of hypersensitivity reaction (angioedema, anaphylactoid reaction, serum sickness, and urticaria) to drug or its components.

• Use cautiously in patients with known hypersensitivity to other TNF blockers and those with underlying conditions that may increase risk of infection.

• Use cautiously in patients with underlying hematologic disorders because significant hematologic abnormalities have occurred.

• Use in combination with biological DMARDs or other TNF-blocker therapy isn't recommended.

Boxed Warning Patients treated with certolizumab are at increased risk for serious infections that may lead to hospitalization or death. Most patients who developed these infections were taking concomitant immunosuppressants, such as methotrexate or corticosteroids. ∎

Boxed Warning Consider empirical antifungal therapy for patients at risk for invasive fungal infections who develop severe systemic illness. ∎

• Use cautiously in patients with a history of recurrent infections or concomitant immunosuppressive therapy and in those who have resided in regions where TB and histoplasmosis are endemic. Don't begin drug in patients with active infection.

• Use cautiously in patients with a history of CNS demyelinating disorder, hematologic disorders, or HF.

• Drug may increase risk of malignancies. Perform periodic skin exams in patients with risk factors for skin cancer.

• Rare reactivation of HBV infection can occur, usually in chronic carriers who are also receiving immunosuppressants. Evaluate patient for HBV infection before initiating treatment. Monitor HBV carriers for clinical signs and symptoms of active infection and altered lab values during and for several months after therapy ends.

Reactions in bold italics are *life-threatening*.

Boxed Warning Certolizumab isn't indicated for use in children or adolescents because of the risk of lymphoma and other malignancies reported with the use of TNF blockers. ■

• Use cautiously in older adults because of increased risk of infection.

Dialyzable drug: Unknown.

PREGNANCY-LACTATION-REPRODUCTION

• Use during pregnancy only when clearly needed and if benefit outweighs fetal risk.

• Enroll patients exposed to certolizumab pegol during pregnancy in Autoimmune Diseases in Pregnancy Study (1-877-311-8972 or https://mothertobaby.org/pregnancy-studies/).

• Drug may affect immune response in an in utero–exposed newborn or infant.

• It isn't known if drug appears in human milk. Before use during breastfeeding, prescriber should consider importance of drug to patient and potential adverse effects on infant.

NURSING CONSIDERATIONS

Boxed Warning Carefully consider risks and benefits of treatment before initiating therapy in patient with chronic or recurrent infection. ■

Boxed Warning Monitor patient for signs and symptoms of invasive fungal infection (such as histoplasmosis) and other opportunistic infections during and after treatment. Discontinue treatment if serious infection or sepsis develops. Fatal infections have occurred. ■

Boxed Warning Be aware that bacterial, viral, and other infections due to opportunistic pathogens, including *Legionella* and *Listeria*, have occurred. ■

Boxed Warning Test patient for latent TB before and during therapy; active TB, including reactivation of latent TB, has occurred. Initiate treatment for latent infection before starting therapy. ■

Boxed Warning Closely monitor patient for signs and symptoms of infection during and after treatment, including possible development of TB in patients who tested negative for latent TB before starting therapy. ■

• Before therapy, evaluate patient at risk for HBV infection and test for previous HBV infection.

• Monitor for hypersensitivity reactions, including severe skin reactions.

• Monitor for new or worsening neurologic disorders, including seizures, optic neuritis, and peripheral neuropathy.

• Monitor for signs and symptoms of blood dyscrasias (bruising, bleeding, pallor).

PATIENT TEACHING

Boxed Warning Teach patient to seek prompt medical attention for signs and symptoms of infection, such as persistent fever, cough, shortness of breath, or fatigue. ■

• Advise patient to seek immediate medical attention for unusual bruising or bleeding.

• Instruct patient to seek immediate medical attention if symptoms of allergic reaction develop.

• Tell patient to report signs and symptoms of HF or neurologic changes.

• Advise patient of the risk of lymphoma and other malignancies.

• Teach about safe drug administration technique, storage, and syringe disposal.

SAFETY ALERT!

cetuximab ✄

seh-TUX-eh-mab

Erbitux

Therapeutic class: Antineoplastics
Pharmacologic class: Monoclonal antibodies

AVAILABLE FORMS

Injection: 2 mg/mL

INDICATIONS & DOSAGES

Adjust-a-dose (for all indications): If patient develops grade 1 or 2 CTCAE infusion reaction, permanently reduce infusion rate by 50%. If patient develops grade 3 or 4 CTCAE infusion reaction, immediately and permanently stop drug. Refer to manufacturer's instructions for dosage modifications for other toxicities.

➤ **Squamous cell carcinoma of head and neck, in combination with radiation therapy**

Adults: Loading dose of 400 mg/m² IV infusion over 120 minutes, then weekly maintenance dose of 250 mg/m² IV infusion over 60 minutes. Begin drug 1 week before radiation course. Complete administration 1 hour before radiation. Continue for duration (6 or

---

7 weeks) of radiation therapy or until disease progression or unacceptable toxicity occurs.

➤ **Squamous cell carcinoma of head and neck, as single-agent or in combination with platinum-based therapy and 5-FU**
Adults: 500 mg/m² IV infusion over 2 hours every 2 weeks. Or, initially, 400 mg/m² IV infusion over 120 minutes, then weekly maintenance dose of 250 mg/m² IV infusion over 60 minutes. Complete infusion 1 hour before platinum-based therapy with 5-FU. Continue therapy until disease progression or unacceptable toxicity occurs.

➤ *KRAS* **mutation-negative (wild type), epidermal growth factor receptor (EGFR)–expressing, metastatic colorectal cancer in combination with FOLFIRI (irinotecan, 5-FU, leucovorin) chemotherapy regimen for first-line treatment, or in combination with irinotecan in patients refractory to irinotecan-based chemotherapy, or as a single agent in patients who have failed oxaliplatin- and irinotecan-based chemotherapy or who are intolerant to irinotecan** 🔍
Adults: 500 mg/m² IV infusion over 2 hours every 2 weeks. Or, initially, 400 mg/m² IV infusion over 120 minutes, then weekly maintenance dose of 250 mg/m² IV infusion over 60 minutes. Complete infusion 1 hour before irinotecan or FOLFIRI regimen. Continue therapy until disease progression or unacceptable toxicity occurs.

➤ **Metastatic colorectal cancer with** *BRAF* **V600E mutation after prior therapy, in combination with encorafenib** 🔍
Adults: Initially, 400 mg/m² IV infusion over 120 minutes, then 250 mg/m² infusion over 60 minutes weekly with encorafenib 300 mg PO daily until disease progression or unacceptable toxicity occurs. Refer to encorafenib prescribing information.

ADMINISTRATION
IV

⚠ *Alert:* Hazardous drug; use safe handling and disposal precautions. Drug is a potential teratogen.

▼ Premedicate with an H₁-antagonist such as diphenhydramine 50 mg IV 30 to 60 minutes before first dose. Premedication before subsequent doses should be based on clinical judgment and severity of prior infusion reactions.

▼ Solution should be clear and colorless and may contain a small number of particulates.

▼ Don't shake or dilute.

▼ Drug may be given by infusion pump or syringe pump, piggybacked into infusion line. Don't give by IV push or bolus.

▼ Give initial loading dose over 120 minutes and subsequent infusions over 60 minutes. Don't exceed infusion rate of 10 mg/minute.

▼ Give drug through a low-protein-binding 0.22-micron in-line filter.

▼ Flush line with NSS at end of infusion.

▼ Store vials at 36° to 46° F (2° to 8° C). Don't freeze.

▼ Solution in infusion container is stable up to 12 hours at 36° to 46° F (2° to 8° C) and up to 8 hours at 68° to 77° F (20° to 25° C).

▼ **Incompatibilities:** Don't dilute with other solutions.

ACTION
An EGFR antagonist that binds to the EGFR on normal and tumor cells.

Route	Onset	Peak	Duration
IV	Unknown	Unknown	Unknown

Half-life: 3 to 10 days.

ADVERSE REACTIONS
CNS: asthenia, depression, fever, headache, fatigue, insomnia, anxiety, confusion, pain, peripheral neuropathy, taste disturbance. **CV:** *cardiopulmonary arrest, PE.* **EENT:** conjunctivitis, pharyngitis. **GI:** abdominal pain, anorexia, constipation, diarrhea, dyspepsia, dysphagia, mucositis, nausea, stomatitis, vomiting, dry mouth. **Hematologic:** anemia, *neutropenia, leukopenia.* **Hepatic:** increased transaminase levels, increased ALP level. **Metabolic:** dehydration, *hypomagnesemia, hypocalcemia, hypokalemia,* weight loss. **Musculoskeletal:** back pain, bone pain, arthralgia. **Respiratory:** cough, dyspnea. **Skin:** alopecia, rash, pruritus, nail changes, hand-foot syndrome, skin fissures, dry skin. **Other:** antibody development, chills, infection, infusion reaction, *sepsis.*

INTERACTIONS
Drug-lifestyle. *Sun exposure:* May worsen skin reactions. Advise patient to avoid excessive sun exposure.

EFFECTS ON LAB TEST RESULTS
• May increase LFT values and PTT.

Reactions in bold italics are *life-threatening*.

• May decrease magnesium, calcium, and potassium levels.
• May decrease Hb level and lymphocyte and neutrophil counts.

CONTRAINDICATIONS & CAUTIONS

• Use cautiously in patients hypersensitive to drug, its components, or murine proteins.
• If used with radiation, use cautiously in patients with history of CAD, arrhythmias, or HF.
• Risk of anaphylactic reactions may be increased in patients with history of tick bites or red meat allergy or in the presence of IgE antibodies directed against galactose-α-1, 3-galactose (alpha-gal).
▧ Determine *RAS* mutation and EGFR-negative expression status before initiating treatment for colorectal cancer. Drug isn't indicated for treatment of *RAS*-mutant colorectal cancer or when results of *RAS* mutation tests are unknown; increased tumor progression, increased mortality, or lack of benefit may occur in patients with *RAS*-mutant metastatic colorectal cancer.
• ILD has been reported in patients using drug.
• Dermatologic toxicity has been reported in most patients. Acneiform rash usually develops in first 2 weeks of therapy and may require dosage modification and treatment with topical or oral antibiotics.
• Life-threatening and fatal SCARs have been observed in patients treated with cetuximab.
• Adverse reactions may occur more frequently when drug is given with cisplatin and radiation.
• Electrolyte abnormalities are common, especially hypomagnesemia.
Dialyzable drug: No.

PREGNANCY-LACTATION-REPRODUCTION

• Drug may cause fetal harm and isn't recommended for use during pregnancy. Inform patient of fetal risk.
• Patients of childbearing potential should use effective contraception during treatment and for 2 months after final dose.
• Patients shouldn't breastfeed during therapy and for at least 2 months after final dose.
• Drug may impair female fertility.

NURSING CONSIDERATIONS

• Verify pregnancy status in patients of child-bearing potential before starting drug.
Boxed Warning Severe and fatal infusion reactions, including acute airway obstruction, urticaria, and hypotension, may occur, usually with the first infusion. If a severe infusion reaction occurs, stop drug immediately and permanently and provide symptomatic treatment. ▪
• Keep epinephrine, corticosteroids, IV antihistamines, bronchodilators, and oxygen available for severe infusion reactions.
• Manage mild to moderate infusion reactions by decreasing infusion rate and premedicating with an antihistamine before subsequent infusions.
• Monitor patient for infusion reactions for 1 hour after infusion ends.
• Assess for acute onset or worsening of pulmonary symptoms. If ILD is confirmed, interrupt therapy or stop drug.
• Monitor for skin toxicity, which starts most often during first 2 weeks of therapy. Treat with topical and oral antibiotics.
• Monitor magnesium, calcium, and potassium levels weekly during treatment and for at least 8 weeks after therapy ends.
Boxed Warning In patients also receiving radiation therapy or platinum-based therapy with 5-FU, closely monitor electrolytes, especially magnesium, potassium, and calcium, during and after therapy. Cardiopulmonary arrest and sudden death have occurred. ▪

PATIENT TEACHING

• Tell patient to promptly report adverse reactions (dyspnea, chest pain, new or worsening cough, chills, fever).
• Inform patient that skin reactions may occur, typically during the first 2 weeks of treatment, and may last more than 28 days after final cetuximab dose.
• Advise patient to avoid prolonged or unprotected sun exposure during and for 2 months after final dose.
• Instruct patient not to breastfeed during therapy and for at least 2 months after final dose.
• Advise patient of childbearing potential to use adequate contraception during therapy and for 2 months after final dose.

---

chloroquine phosphate ⊠
KLO-ro-kwin

Therapeutic class: Antimalarials
Pharmacologic class: Aminoquinolines

AVAILABLE FORMS
Tablets: 250 mg (equivalent to 150 mg base),
500 mg (equivalent to 300 mg base)

INDICATIONS & DOSAGES
❸ *Alert:* Prescribers should be completely
familiar with this drug before prescribing.
➤ **Acute malarial attacks caused by susceptible strains of *Plasmodium vivax, Plasmodium malariae, Plasmodium ovale,* and
*Plasmodium falciparum***
Adults: Initially, 1 g (600 mg base) PO; then
500 mg (300 mg base) at 6, 24, and 48 hours.
Adults of low body weight and children:
Initially, 16.7 mg/kg (10 mg/kg base) PO;
then 8.3 mg/kg (5 mg/kg base) at 6, 24, and
36 hours. Don't exceed adult dose of 1,000 mg
(600 mg base) for initial dosage and 500 mg
(300 mg base) for subsequent doses.
Adjust-a-dose: For adults and children,
for treatment of chloroquine-sensitive
P. vivax and *P. malariae,* use with an
8-aminoquinoline (primaquine) is necessary.
➤ **To prevent malaria**
Adults: 500 mg (300 mg base) PO once
weekly on the same day each week, for 1 to
2 weeks before entering a malaria-endemic
area and continued for 4 weeks after leaving
the area. If beginning after entering a malaria-
endemic area, initially 1 g (600 mg base) PO
in two divided doses 6 hours apart and continued for 8 weeks after leaving the area.
Children: Initially, 8.3 mg/kg (5 mg/kg base)
PO once weekly on the same day each week,
for 1 to 2 weeks before entering a malaria-
endemic area and continued for 4 weeks after leaving the area. Don't exceed 500 mg
(300 mg base). If beginning after entering a
malaria-endemic area, initially 16.7 mg/kg
(10 mg/kg base) PO in two divided doses
6 hours apart, followed by usual dosing regimen. Continue for 8 weeks after leaving the
endemic area.
➤ **Extraintestinal amebiasis**
Adults: 1 g (600 mg base) PO once daily for
2 days; then 500 mg (300 mg base) daily for
2 to 3 weeks. Treatment is usually combined
with an intestinal amebicide.

ADMINISTRATION
PO
❸ *Alert:* Drug dosage may be discussed in
"mg" or "mg base"; be aware of the difference.
• To improve adherence when drug is used
for prevention, advise patient to take drug immediately before or after a meal on the same
day each week.
• Give drug with food to decrease GI adverse
effects.
• Pharmacist can prepare an oral suspension
if patient can't swallow pills.
• Shake suspension before use.

ACTION
May bind to and alter the properties of DNA
in susceptible parasites.

Route	Onset	Peak	Duration
PO	Unknown	1–2 hr	Unknown

Half-life: 3 to 5 days.

ADVERSE REACTIONS
CNS: *seizures,* agitation, anxiety, confusion,
mild and transient headache, psychic stimulation, neuropathy, acute extrapyramidal reactions, hallucinations. **CV:** hypotension, ECG
changes, *cardiomyopathy.* **EENT:** blurred vision; difficulty focusing; reversible corneal
changes; typically irreversible, sometimes
progressive or delayed retinal changes (narrowing of arterioles, macular lesions, pallor
of optic disk, optic atrophy, and patchy retinal
pigmentation, typically leading to blindness);
ototoxicity; nerve deafness; vertigo; tinnitus.
GI: anorexia, abdominal cramps, diarrhea,
nausea, vomiting. **Hematologic:** *agranulocytosis, aplastic anemia, thrombocytopenia.*
Hepatic: *hepatitis.* **Musculoskeletal:** myopathy or neuromyopathy, leading to progressive weakness and atrophy of proximal muscle groups. **Skin:** pruritus, lichen planus eruptions, skin and mucosal pigmentary changes,
pleomorphic skin eruptions, *erythema multiforme, SJS, TEN,* exfoliative dermatitis,
urticaria, DRESS syndrome, hair loss and
bleaching of hair pigment. **Other:** *anaphylaxis, angioedema.*

INTERACTIONS
Drug-drug. *Aluminum salts (kaolin),
antacids, magnesium:* May decrease GI absorption. Separate dose times by 4 hours.

Reactions in bold italics are ***life-threatening.***

Ampicillin: May significantly reduce bioavailability of ampicillin. Separate dose times by 2 hours.

Cimetidine: May decrease metabolism of chloroquine. Avoid use together.

Cyclosporine: May increase serum cyclosporine level. Monitor patient closely. If necessary, discontinue chloroquine.

Drugs that prolong QT interval (amiodarone, moxifloxacin): May have additive effects on QT interval and increase risk of life-threatening arrhythmias. Avoid use together if possible.

Insulin, other antidiabetics: May increase hypoglycemic effect. Adjust antidiabetic dosage.

Lumefantrine: May enhance adverse and toxic effects of lumefantrine. Don't use artemether–lumefantrine combination concurrently with chloroquine unless no option exists.

Mefloquine: May increase seizure risk. Avoid use together and, when possible, delay administration of mefloquine until at least 12 hours after last dose of chloroquine.

Praziquantel: May reduce praziquantel bioavailability. Monitor patient.

Tamoxifen: May increase risk of retinal toxicity. Monitor patient.

Drug-lifestyle. *Sun exposure:* May cause drug-induced dermatoses. Advise patient to avoid sun exposure.

EFFECTS ON LAB TEST RESULTS

• May increase liver enzyme levels.
• May decrease glucose level.
• May decrease Hb level and granulocyte, neutrophil, and platelet counts.

CONTRAINDICATIONS & CAUTIONS

• Contraindicated in patients hypersensitive to drug or 4-aminoquinoline compounds and in those with retinal or visual field changes or porphyria.

▨ Use cautiously in patients with severe GI, neurologic, or blood disorders; cardiac disease; history of ventricular arrhythmia; uncorrected hypokalemia or hypomagnesemia; bradycardia; liver disease; alcohol use disorder; or G6PD deficiency.

• Don't use to treat *Plasmodium* species acquired in an area of known chloroquine resistance or when chloroquine prophylaxis has failed. Use other antimalarials if patient has a resistant strain of plasmodia.

• Drug may worsen psoriasis or porphyria; use only if benefit outweighs risk.

• Risk of toxic reactions may be greater in older adults and in patients with impaired kidney function because drug is largely excreted by the kidneys. Closely monitor kidney function.

Dialyzable drug: Unknown.

⚠ *Overdose S&S:* Headache, drowsiness, visual disturbances, nausea, vomiting, CV collapse, seizures, sudden and early respiratory and cardiac arrest, atrial standstill, nodal rhythm, prolonged intraventricular conduction time, progressive bradycardia leading to ventricular fibrillation or arrest.

PREGNANCY-LACTATION-REPRODUCTION

• Safety and effectiveness of chloroquine during pregnancy aren't known. Avoid use during pregnancy except in suppression or treatment of malaria when benefit outweighs fetal risk.

• Serious adverse reactions may occur in breastfed infants. Patient should discontinue breastfeeding or discontinue drug, considering importance of drug to patient.

NURSING CONSIDERATIONS

• Ensure patient undergoes baseline and periodic ophthalmic exams. Periodically check for ocular muscle weakness after long-term use. Risk factors for development of retinopathy during treatment include advanced age, subnormal glomerular filtration, concomitant use of tamoxifen citrate or concurrent macular disease, duration of treatment, and high daily or accumulated dosage.

• Make sure patient undergoes audiometer testing before, during, and after therapy, especially if therapy is long-term.

• Periodically monitor CBC and LFT values during long-term therapy. If a severe blood disorder—not caused by the disease—develops, drug may need to be stopped.

• Monitor patient for hypoglycemia and muscle weakness.

◑ *Alert:* Monitor patient for overdose, which can quickly lead to toxic symptoms. Children are extremely susceptible to toxicity; avoid long-term treatment.

PATIENT TEACHING

• Teach about proper drug administration and handling as well as duration of therapy.

- Advise patient to avoid excessive sun exposure to prevent worsening of drug-induced dermatoses.
- Tell patient to promptly report adverse reactions, especially blurred vision, increased sensitivity to light, tinnitus, hearing loss, and muscle weakness.
- Instruct patient to keep drug out of reach of children. Overdose may be fatal.
- Caution that hypoglycemia may occur with or without antidiabetic medication use. Instruct patient to immediately report hypoglycemia signs and symptoms (dizziness, headache, weakness, shaking, fast heartbeat, confusion, hunger, sweating).
- Advise patient of childbearing potential to discuss pregnancy and breastfeeding with provider.

ciclesonide (inhalation, intranasal)
sik-le-SON-ide

Alvesco, Omnaris, Zetonna

Therapeutic class: Corticosteroids
Pharmacologic class: Corticosteroids

AVAILABLE FORMS
Nasal aerosol solution: 37 mcg/metered spray
Nasal suspension: 50 mcg/metered spray
Oral inhalation aerosol: 80 mcg, 160 mcg

INDICATIONS & DOSAGES
➤ **Preventative during asthma maintenance (Alvesco)**
Adults and children ages 12 and older who were previously taking bronchodilators alone: Initially, inhaled dose of 80 mcg b.i.d.; increase to maximum of 160 mcg b.i.d. after 4 weeks if not controlled.
Adults and children ages 12 and older who were previously taking inhaled corticosteroids: Initially, 80 mcg b.i.d.; may increase in 4-week intervals to maximum of 320 mcg b.i.d.
Adults and children ages 12 and older who were previously taking oral corticosteroids: 320 mcg b.i.d.
Adjust-a-dose: After asthma stability has been achieved, titrate to lowest effective dosage to reduce risk of adverse effects.

➤ **Signs and symptoms of perennial allergic rhinitis**
Adults and children ages 12 and older: 2 sprays of Omnaris in each nostril once daily (200 mcg/day). Or, 1 actuation of Zetonna per nostril once daily.
➤ **Signs and symptoms of seasonal allergic rhinitis**
Adults and children ages 12 and older: 1 actuation of Zetonna per nostril once daily.
Adults and children ages 6 and older: 2 sprays of Omnaris in each nostril once daily (200 mcg/day).

ADMINISTRATION
Inhalational
- Before first use or when inhaler hasn't been used for more than 10 days, prime by actuating three times.
- Have patient rinse mouth without swallowing after inhalation.
Intranasal
- Before first use of Omnaris, gently shake container, then prime by spraying eight times. If not used for 4 consecutive days, gently shake and reprime with 1 spray or until a fine mist appears.
- Before first use of Zetonna, prime by actuating three times. If not used for 10 consecutive days, prime by actuating three times. If product is dropped, canister and actuator may become separated; if this happens, instruct patient to reassemble product and test spray once into the air before using.

ACTION
May decrease inflammation by inhibiting macrophages, eosinophils, and mediators such as leukotrienes involved in the asthmatic response.

Route	Onset	Peak	Duration
Inhalation	>4 wk	1 hr	Unknown
Intranasal	1–2 days	1–5 wk	Unknown

Half-life: Inhalation drug, less than 1 hour; inhalation drug's active metabolite, 6 to 7 hours; intranasal drug, unknown.

ADVERSE REACTIONS
CNS: headache. **EENT:** ear pain, nasopharyngitis, pharyngolaryngeal pain, sinusitis, nasal congestion or discomfort, epistaxis, nasal mucosal or septum disorders. **GI:** nausea. **GU:** UTI. **Metabolic:** growth retardation. **Musculoskeletal:** arthralgia, extremity or back

pain. **Respiratory:** URI, cough, bronchitis. **Other:** flulike symptoms.

INTERACTIONS

Drug-drug. *Desmopressin:* May enhance hyponatremic effect of desmopressin. Avoid use together.

Esketamine: Nasal corticosteroids may diminish therapeutic effect of intranasal esketamine. Give ciclesonide at least 1 hour before esketamine.

Ketoconazole, other inhibitors of CYP450: May increase ciclesonide metabolite level and adverse effects. Use together cautiously; adjust ciclesonide dosage as needed.

EFFECTS ON LAB TEST RESULTS
None reported.

CONTRAINDICATIONS & CAUTIONS
• Contraindicated as primary treatment of status asthmaticus or other acute asthmatic episodes.
• Contraindicated in patients hypersensitive to drug or its components.
• Intranasal form is contraindicated in patients who have had recent nasal septal ulcers, nasal surgery, or nasal trauma until healing has occurred.
• Use cautiously in patients who have changed from systemic to inhaled corticosteroids because AKI, steroid withdrawal (pain, lassitude, depression), and acute worsening of symptoms may occur.
• Use cautiously in patients who are immunosuppressed and in those with wounds; corticosteroids suppress the immune system.
• Use cautiously in children; may cause a decline in growth rate.
• Use cautiously, if at all, in patients with active or quiescent respiratory TB infection; untreated systemic fungal, bacterial, viral, or parasitic infections; or ocular HSV infection.
Dialyzable drug: Unknown.
⚠ *Overdose S&S:* Hyperadrenocorticism.

PREGNANCY-LACTATION-REPRODUCTION
• Studies during pregnancy are inadequate. Use during pregnancy only if potential benefit justifies fetal risk.
• If patient takes a corticosteroid during pregnancy, monitor neonate for hypoadrenalism.
• It isn't known if drug appears in human milk. Use cautiously during breastfeeding.

NURSING CONSIDERATIONS
⚠ *Alert:* Don't use inhaler for acute bronchospasm or acute asthma.
• Assess patient for bone loss during long-term use.
• Watch for evidence of localized mouth infections, glaucoma, cataracts, and immunosuppression.
• Monitor patient who switches from systemic to inhaled corticosteroids for worsening of signs and symptoms and other adverse effects of withdrawal. Wean patient off oral corticosteroids slowly.
• Monitor child for decline in growth rate; the potential to regain growth after drug cessation hasn't been studied.
• Monitor for nasal adverse effects.

PATIENT TEACHING
• Teach about proper drug administration and handling.
• Inform patient that drug isn't indicated for relief of acute bronchospasm.
• Instruct patient to rinse mouth with water and spit out after oral inhalation to decrease risk of oral candidiasis.
• Advise patient to use drug at regular intervals or about the same time every day, as directed.
• Instruct patient using intranasal form to contact prescriber if no relief from symptoms occurs after 1 week.
• Explain that asthma-related therapeutic results may take several weeks. Instruct patient to contact prescriber if symptoms don't improve after 4 weeks of treatment or if condition worsens.
• Warn patient to avoid exposure to chickenpox, measles, and other infections and, if exposed, to immediately consult prescriber.
• Advise parents of child receiving long-term therapy that child should have periodic growth measurements.

cilostazol
sil-OH-sta-zol

Therapeutic class: Antiplatelet drugs
Pharmacologic class: cAMP phosphodiesterase inhibitors

AVAILABLE FORMS
Tablets: 50 mg, 100 mg

INDICATIONS & DOSAGES

➤ **To reduce symptoms of intermittent claudication**

Adults: 100 mg PO b.i.d.

Adjust-a-dose: Decrease dosage to 50 mg PO b.i.d. when giving with CYP3A4 or CYP2C19 inhibitors.

ADMINISTRATION

PO

• Give drug at least 30 minutes before or 2 hours after breakfast and dinner.

ACTION

Thought to inhibit the enzyme phosphodiesterase III, thus inhibiting platelet aggregation and causing vasodilation.

Route	Onset	Peak	Duration
PO	2–4 wk	Unknown	Unknown

Half-life: 11 to 13 hours.

ADVERSE REACTIONS

CNS: dizziness, headache, vertigo. **CV:** palpitations, peripheral edema, tachycardia. **EENT:** pharyngitis, rhinitis. **GI:** abnormal stools, diarrhea, abdominal pain, dyspepsia, flatulence, nausea. **Musculoskeletal:** back pain, myalgia. **Respiratory:** cough. **Other:** infection.

INTERACTIONS

Drug-drug. *Anticoagulants, antiplatelet agents:* May increase bleeding risk. Use together cautiously.

CYP2C19 inhibitors (fluconazole, omeprazole, ticlopidine), strong or moderate CYP3A4 inhibitors (diltiazem, erythromycin, itraconazole, ketoconazole): May increase level of cilostazol and its metabolites. Reduce cilostazol dosage to 50 mg b.i.d.

Drug-herb. *Herbs with anticoagulant properties (alfalfa, anise, bilberry):* May prolong bleeding time. Discourage use together.

Drug-food. *Grapefruit juice:* May increase drug level. Discourage use together.

Drug-lifestyle. *Smoking:* May decrease drug exposure. Discourage smoking.

EFFECTS ON LAB TEST RESULTS

• May reduce triglyceride levels.
• May increase HDL-C level.

CONTRAINDICATIONS & CAUTIONS

• Contraindicated in patients hypersensitive to drug or its components.

Boxed Warning Contraindicated in patients with HF of any severity. Cilostazol and similar drugs that inhibit the enzyme phosphodiesterase decrease likelihood of survival compared with placebo in patients with class III and IV HF. ∎

• Drug hasn't been studied in patients with hemostatic disorders or active bleeding. Avoid use in these patients.
• Use cautiously in patients with ischemic heart disease. Drug may increase risk of angina exacerbation or MI.
• Use cautiously in patients with CrCl less than 25 mL/minute and in those with Child-Pugh class B or C liver impairment.

Dialyzable drug: No.

⚠ *Overdose S&S:* Severe headache, diarrhea, hypotension, tachycardia, cardiac arrhythmias.

PREGNANCY-LACTATION-REPRODUCTION

• Studies during pregnancy are inadequate. Fetal risk is unknown.
• Drug may appear in human milk. Patient should discontinue breastfeeding or discontinue drug considering importance of drug to patient.

NURSING CONSIDERATIONS

• Beneficial effects may not be seen for up to 12 weeks after therapy starts. If symptoms haven't improved after 3 months, discontinue drug.
• Monitor patient for new cardiac signs or symptoms.
• Be aware that dosage can be reduced or stopped without such rebound effects as platelet hyperaggregation.
• Periodically monitor platelet and WBC counts.

PATIENT TEACHING

• Teach about proper drug administration and handling.
• Tell patient that beneficial effect of drug on cramping pain isn't likely to be noticed for 2 to 4 weeks and may take as long as 12 weeks.
• Inform patient that CV risk is unknown in patients who use drug on a long-term basis.
• Tell patient that drug may cause dizziness. Caution patient not to drive or perform other activities that require alertness until response to drug is known.

Reactions in bold italics are *life-threatening*.

cimetidine
sye-MET-i-deen

Tagamet HB ◇

cimetidine hydrochloride

Therapeutic class: Antiulcer drugs
Pharmacologic class: H$_2$-receptor antagonists

AVAILABLE FORMS
Oral liquid: 300 mg/5 mL*
Tablets: 200 mg ◇; 300 mg; 400 mg; 800 mg

INDICATIONS & DOSAGES
Adjust-a-dose (for all indications): In patients with abnormal kidney function, decrease dosage to 300 mg PO every 12 hours, increasing frequency to every 8 hours with caution. Further reduce dosage in patient with abnormal kidney function who also has liver dysfunction as needed.

➤ **Short-term treatment of duodenal ulcer; maintenance therapy**
Adults and children ages 16 and older: 800 mg PO at bedtime or as prescribed. Treatment lasts 4 to 8 weeks. Alternatively, higher doses of 1,600 mg at bedtime for 4 weeks may be beneficial for patients with larger duodenal ulcers (larger than 1 cm defined endoscopically) who are also heavy smokers (1 pack/ day or more) when it's important to ensure healing within 4 weeks for this subpopulation. For maintenance therapy, 400 mg at bedtime.

➤ **Active benign gastric ulceration**
Adults: 800 mg PO at bedtime or 300 mg PO q.i.d. (with meals and at bedtime) for up to 8 weeks.

➤ **Pathologic hypersecretory conditions, such as Zollinger-Ellison syndrome, systemic mastocytosis, and multiple endocrine adenomas**
Adults and children ages 16 and older: 300 mg PO q.i.d. with meals and at bedtime, adjusted to patient's needs. Maximum oral amount, 2,400 mg daily.

➤ **GERD with erosive esophagitis**
Adults: 800 mg PO b.i.d. or 400 mg PO q.i.d. before meals and at bedtime for up to 12 weeks.

➤ **Heartburn ◆**
Adults and children ages 12 and older: 200 mg PO with water as symptoms occur, or as directed, up to b.i.d. For prevention, 200 mg PO right before or up to 30 minutes before eating food or drinking beverages that cause heartburn. Maximum, 400 mg daily. Drug shouldn't be taken daily for longer than 2 weeks.

ADMINISTRATION
PO
- Give dose after hemodialysis.
- Store at room temperature.
- Protect from light.

ACTION
Competitively inhibits action of histamine on the H$_2$ receptor sites of parietal cells, decreasing gastric acid secretion.

Route	Onset	Peak	Duration
PO	1 hr	45–90 min	4–5 hr

Half-life: 2 hours.

ADVERSE REACTIONS
CNS: dizziness, headache, somnolence.
GI: mild and transient diarrhea. **Other:** mild gynecomastia if used longer than 1 month, hypersensitivity reactions.

INTERACTIONS
Drug-drug. *Amiodarone:* May increase amiodarone level. Avoid use together if possible. Monitor for increased amiodarone concentrations and effects. Consider therapy modification.
Antacids: May interfere with cimetidine absorption. Separate doses by at least 1 hour, if possible.
Cefpodoxime, cefuroxime, digoxin, fluconazole, indomethacin, iron salts, ketoconazole, tetracycline: May decrease drug absorption. Separate doses by at least 2 hours.
Fosphenytoin, phenytoin, some benzodiazepines, theophylline: May inhibit hepatic microsomal enzyme metabolism of these drugs. Monitor drug level.
IV lidocaine: May decrease clearance of lidocaine, increasing the risk of toxicity. Consider using a different H$_2$ antagonist, if possible. Monitor lidocaine level closely.
Metformin: May increase metformin concentration and related toxicities. Consider alternative H$_2$ antagonist.
Metoprolol, propranolol, timolol: May increase the effects of beta blocker. Consider another H$_2$ antagonist or decrease the beta blocker dosage.

Procainamide: May increase procainamide level. Avoid this combination, if possible. Monitor procainamide level closely and adjust the dosage as necessary.

Warfarin-type anticoagulants: May increase blood levels of these drugs. Closely monitor PT and INR, and adjust anticoagulant dosage if necessary.

Drug-lifestyle. *Alcohol use:* May increase blood alcohol level. Discourage use together. *Smoking:* May decrease drug's ability to inhibit nocturnal gastric secretion. Urge patient to quit smoking.

EFFECTS ON LAB TEST RESULTS

• May increase ALT, AST, and creatinine levels.
• May antagonize pentagastrin's effect during gastric acid secretion tests.
• May cause false-negative results in skin tests using allergen extracts.
• May impair interpretation of Hemoccult and Gastroccult test results on gastric content aspirate because of FD&C blue dye #2 used in tablets.

CONTRAINDICATIONS & CAUTIONS

• Contraindicated in patients hypersensitive to drug.
• Use cautiously in older adults and patients who are debilitated because they may be more susceptible to drug-induced confusion.
• Use cautiously in patients with abnormal kidney or liver function and patients who are immunocompromised.
• Prolonged treatment (2 years or more) increases risk of vitamin B_{12} malabsorption and deficiency, especially in adult females and patients younger than age 30.
• Drug may increase risk of acute gastroenteritis and community-acquired pneumonia in children.
Dializable drug: Yes.
⚠ *Overdose S&S:* Mental deterioration, unresponsiveness, death.

PREGNANCY-LACTATION-REPRODUCTION

• Studies during pregnancy are inadequate. Use during pregnancy only if clearly needed and potential benefit justifies fetal risk.
• Drug appears in human milk. As a general rule, patient shouldn't breastfeed while taking drug.

NURSING CONSIDERATIONS

• Assess patient for abdominal pain. Note blood in emesis, stool, or gastric aspirate. Relief of symptoms doesn't eliminate the presence of a gastric malignancy.
• Wait at least 15 minutes after giving tablet before drawing sample for Hemoccult or Gastroccult test, and follow test manufacturer's instructions closely.
• Treatment of gastric ulcer isn't as effective as treatment of duodenal ulcer.
• *Look alike–sound alike:* Don't confuse cimetidine with simethicone.

PATIENT TEACHING

• Teach about proper drug administration and handling.
• Instruct patient taking OTC formulation not to exceed recommended dosage and not to take daily for longer than 14 days.
• Urge patient to avoid cigarette smoking because it may increase gastric acid secretion and worsen disease.
• Advise patient to report all adverse reactions, including abdominal pain, blood in stools or emesis, black tarry stools, and coffee-ground emesis.
• Tell patient to check with prescriber or pharmacist before taking other drugs.

cinacalcet hydrochloride
sin-ah-KAL-set

Sensipar

Therapeutic class: Hyperparathyroidism drugs
Pharmacologic class: Calcimimetics

AVAILABLE FORMS
Tablets ⊙: 30 mg, 60 mg, 90 mg

INDICATIONS & DOSAGES
Adjust-a-dose (for all indications): Patients with Child-Pugh class B or C liver impairment may experience increased exposure to cinacalcet and increased half-life. Dosage adjustments may be necessary based on serum calcium, serum phosphorus, or intact parathyroid hormone (iPTH) level.
➤ **Primary hyperparathyroidism; hypercalcemia in patients with parathyroid carcinoma**

C

Adults: Initially, 30 mg PO b.i.d. Titrate every 2 to 4 weeks through sequential doses of 30 mg, 60 mg, and 90 mg PO b.i.d. and 90 mg PO t.i.d. or q.i.d. to normalize calcium level.

➤ **Secondary hyperparathyroidism in patients with chronic kidney disease undergoing dialysis**

Adults: Initially, 30 mg PO once daily; adjust no more than every 2 to 4 weeks through sequential doses of 30 mg, 60 mg, 90 mg, 120 mg, and 180 mg PO once daily to reach target range of 150 to 300 picograms (pg)/mL for iPTH level.

ADMINISTRATION

PO

• Have patient swallow tablets whole; don't crush or cut tablets.

• Give drug with food or shortly after meal.

• Stop etelcalcetide at least 4 weeks before starting cinacalcet. Ensure corrected serum calcium level is at or above lower limit of normal (LLN) before cinacalcet use.

ACTION

Increases sensitivity of calcium-sensing receptor on the parathyroid gland to extracellular calcium, which lowers PTH level and subsequently lowers serum calcium level.

Route	Onset	Peak	Duration
PO	Unknown	2–6 hr	Unknown

Half-life: Terminal half-life, 30 to 40 hours.

ADVERSE REACTIONS

CNS: dizziness, asthenia, *seizures,* depression, fatigue, headache, paresthesia. **CV:** hypotension, HTN. **GI:** diarrhea, nausea, vomiting, anorexia, constipation, abdominal pain, dyspepsia. **Hematologic:** anemia. **Metabolic:** *hypocalcemia,* hypercalcemia, dehydration, *hyperkalemia,* hypoparathyroidism. **Musculoskeletal:** myalgia, arthralgia, fracture, limb pain, noncardiac chest pain, muscle spasms. **Respiratory:** URI, cough, dyspnea. **Skin:** rash. **Other:** hypersensitivity reaction, dialysis access infection.

INTERACTIONS

Drug-drug. *CYP2D6 substrates (carvedilol, desipramine, metoprolol), especially with a narrow therapeutic index (flecainide, thioridazine, most TCAs, vinblastine):* May increase levels of these drugs. Adjust dosage of substrate, as needed.

Etelcalcetide: May enhance hypocalcemic effect of etelcalcetide. Avoid use together.

Strong CYP3A4 inhibitors (erythromycin, itraconazole, ketoconazole): May increase cinacalcet level. Use together cautiously, monitoring PTH and calcium level closely and adjusting cinacalcet dosage, as needed.

EFFECTS ON LAB TEST RESULTS

• May decrease phosphorus level.

• May increase potassium level.

• May increase or decrease calcium level.

CONTRAINDICATIONS & CAUTIONS

• Contraindicated in patients hypersensitive to drug or its components and in patients with calcium level less than LLN range.

• Use cautiously in patients with history of seizures and in those with Child-Pugh class B or C liver impairment.

• Use cautiously in patients with known gastritis, esophagitis, ulcers, or severe vomiting who are at increased risk for upper GI bleeding.

• Isolated, idiosyncratic cases of hypotension, worsening HF, or arrhythmia have been reported in patients with impaired cardiac function.

• Safety and effectiveness in children haven't been established.

Dialyzable drug: No.

⚠ *Overdose S&S:* Hypocalcemia.

PREGNANCY-LACTATION-REPRODUCTION

• Studies during pregnancy are inadequate. Use during pregnancy only if potential benefit justifies fetal risk.

• It isn't known if drug appears in human milk. Patient should discontinue breastfeeding or discontinue drug, considering importance of drug to patient.

NURSING CONSIDERATIONS

🔵 *Alert:* Monitor calcium level closely. Hypocalcemia can prolong QT interval, potentially resulting in ventricular arrhythmia, and lower seizure threshold.

• Measure calcium level within 1 week after starting therapy or adjusting dosage. After maintenance dose is established, measure calcium level monthly for patient with CKD who is receiving dialysis and every 2 months for patient with primary hyperparathyroidism or parathyroid carcinoma.

• Monitor patient for worsening of common GI adverse reactions (nausea, vomiting) and for signs and symptoms of GI bleeding and ulcerations. Promptly evaluate and treat suspected GI bleeding.

• Patient with Child-Pugh class C liver impairment may need dosage adjustment based on PTH and calcium level. Monitor patient closely.

• Give drug alone or with vitamin D sterols, phosphate binders, or both.

• Watch carefully for evidence of hypocalcemia (paresthesia, myalgia, cramping, tetany, seizures).

• For patient with secondary hyperparathyroidism: If calcium level is 7.5 to 8.4 mg/dL or patient develops symptoms of hypocalcemia, give calcium-containing phosphate binders, vitamin D sterols, or both, to raise calcium level. If calcium level is below 7.5 mg/dL or hypocalcemia symptoms persist and the vitamin D dose can't be increased, withhold drug until calcium level reaches 8.0 mg/dL, hypocalcemia symptoms resolve, or both. Resume therapy with the next lowest dose.

• Measure iPTH level 1 to 4 weeks after therapy starts or with dosage changes (wait at least 12 hours after dose before measuring iPTH level). After the maintenance dose is established, monitor PTH level every 1 to 3 months. Level in patient with CKD who is receiving dialysis should be 150 to 300 pg/mL.

• If iPTH level is less than 150 pg/mL, reduce cinacalcet or vitamin D sterols dosage or discontinue therapy.

• Adynamic bone disease may develop if iPTH levels are suppressed below 100 pg/mL. If this occurs, notify prescriber.

🕉 *Alert:* Don't use drug in patients with CKD who aren't receiving dialysis because they have an increased risk of hypocalcemia.

PATIENT TEACHING

• Teach about proper drug administration and handling.

• Advise patient to report to prescriber adverse reactions and signs of hypocalcemia (paresthesia, muscle weakness, muscle cramping, muscle spasm).

• Caution patient to immediately report signs or symptoms of GI bleeding (black or tarry stool, bright-red blood in vomit, dark or bright-red blood in stool, abdominal cramps).

• Emphasize importance of regular blood tests to monitor safety and efficacy.

• Inform patient with HF that drug may worsen condition and monitoring may be required.

ciprofloxacin
si-proe-FLOX-a-sin

Cipro

Therapeutic class: Antibiotics
Pharmacologic class: Fluoroquinolones

AVAILABLE FORMS
Infusion (premixed): 200 mg in 100 mL, 400 mg in 200 mL
Injection: 200 mg/20 mL, 400 mg/40 mL
Suspension (oral): 250 mg/5 mL, 500 mg/5 mL
Tablets: 100 mg, 250 mg, 500 mg, 750 mg

INDICATIONS & DOSAGES
Boxed Warning Use in patients with acute sinusitis, acute exacerbations of chronic bronchitis, and acute uncomplicated cystitis isn't recommended because of risk of serious adverse effects. Use in these patients only when no other treatment options are available. ■

Adjust-a-dose (for all indications): Dosage and duration of treatment vary by severity of infection, susceptibility of microorganism, and patient's health status. For adults with CrCl of 30 to 50 mL/minute, give 250 to 500 mg PO every 12 hours or the usual IV dose; if CrCl is 5 to 29 mL/minute, give 250 to 500 mg PO every 18 hours or 200 to 400 mg IV every 18 to 24 hours. If patient is receiving hemodialysis or peritoneal dialysis, give 250 to 500 mg PO every 24 hours.

➤ **Complicated intra-abdominal infection**
Adults: 500 mg PO or 400 mg IV every 12 hours for 7 to 14 days. Give with metronidazole.

➤ **Bone or joint infection, skin or skin-structure infection**
Adults: 500 to 750 mg PO every 12 hours or 400 mg IV every 8 to 12 hours. Continue treatment for bone or joint infection for 4 to 8 weeks and for skin or skin-structure infections for 7 to 14 days.

➤ **Infectious diarrhea; typhoid fever**
Adults: 500 mg PO every 12 hours. Continue treatment for infectious diarrhea for 5 to 7 days; for typhoid fever, 10 days.

➤ **Health care–associated pneumonia**
Adults: 400 mg IV every 8 hours for 10 to 14 days.
➤ **UTI**
Adults: 250 to 500 mg PO or 200 to 400 mg IV every 12 hours for 7 to 14 days.
➤ **Complicated UTI or pyelonephritis**
Children ages 1 to 17: 6 to 10 mg/kg IV every 8 hours for 10 to 21 days. Maximum IV dose, 400 mg. Or, 10 to 20 mg/kg PO every 12 hours. Maximum PO dose, 750 mg. Treat for 10 to 21 days. Don't exceed maximum dose, even in patients who weigh more than 51 kg.
➤ **Acute uncomplicated cystitis**
Adults: 250 mg PO every 12 hours for 3 days.
➤ **Uncomplicated urethral and cervical gonococcal infection**
Adults: 250 mg PO as a single dose.
➤ **Chronic bacterial prostatitis**
Adults: 500 mg PO every 12 hours or 400 mg IV every 12 hours for 28 days.
➤ **Lower respiratory tract infections; acute exacerbation of chronic bronchitis**
Adults: 500 to 750 mg PO every 12 hours or 400 mg IV every 8 to 12 hours for 7 to 14 days.
➤ **Acute sinusitis**
Adults: 500 mg PO or 400 mg IV every 12 hours for 10 days.
➤ **Empirical therapy in patients who are febrile and neutropenic**
Adults: 400 mg IV every 8 hours used with piperacillin 50 mg/kg IV every 4 hours (not to exceed 24 g/day of piperacillin) for 7 to 14 days.
➤ **Inhalation anthrax (postexposure)**
Adults: 400 mg IV every 12 hours initially until susceptibility test results are known; then 500 mg PO every 12 hours. Give drug with one or two additional antimicrobials. Switch to oral therapy when appropriate. Treat for 60 days (IV and PO combined).
Children: 10 mg/kg IV every 12 hours; then 15 mg/kg PO every 12 hours. Don't exceed 800 mg/day IV or 1,000 mg/day PO. Give drug with one or two additional antimicrobials. Switch to oral therapy when appropriate. Treat for 60 days (IV and PO combined).
➤ **Plague due to *Yersinia pestis*; plague prophylaxis as soon as possible after suspected or confirmed exposure**
Adults: 400 mg IV every 8 to 12 hours or 500 to 750 mg PO every 12 hours for 14 days.
Children ages 1 to 17: 10 mg/kg IV or 15 mg/kg PO every 8 to 12 hours for 10 to 21 days.

Maximum dosage, 500 mg/dose PO and 400 mg/dose IV.

ADMINISTRATION
• Obtain specimen for culture and sensitivity tests before giving first dose. Begin therapy while awaiting results.
PO
• To avoid decreasing effects of ciprofloxacin, give at least 2 hours before or 6 hours after certain drugs and vitamins. Food doesn't affect absorption but may delay peak levels.
• Give drug with plenty of fluids to reduce risk of urine crystals.
• Shake oral suspension vigorously each time before use for approximately 15 seconds; don't give through feeding tube.
• Give dose after dialysis.
• Give missed PO dose up to 6 hours prior to the next scheduled dose. Omit missed dose if less than 6 hours remain.
IV
▼ Dilute drug to 1 to 2 mg/mL using D_5W or NSS for injection.
▼ If giving drug through a Y-type set, stop the other IV solution while infusing.
▼ Infuse over 1 hour into a large vein to minimize discomfort and vein irritation.
▼ **Incompatibilities:** Aminophylline, ampicillin–sulbactam, azithromycin, cefepime, clindamycin phosphate, dexamethasone sodium phosphate, furosemide, heparin sodium, methylprednisolone sodium succinate, phenytoin sodium. Consult drug compatibility reference for complete listing.

ACTION
Inhibits bacterial DNA synthesis, mainly by blocking DNA gyrase; bactericidal.

Route	Onset	Peak	Duration
PO	Unknown	30–120 min	Unknown
IV	Unknown	Immediate	Unknown

Half-life: 4 hours

ADVERSE REACTIONS
CNS: dizziness, drowsiness, insomnia, nervousness, neurologic changes, confusion, headache, restlessness, fever. **GI:** abdominal pain, dyspepsia, diarrhea, nausea, vomiting. **GU:** vulvovaginal candidiasis. **Hematologic:** *leukopenia, neutropenia, thrombocytopenia, thrombocytosis,* eosinophilia. **Hepatic:** abnormal LFT values. **Musculoskeletal:** musculoskeletal symptoms. **Respiratory:**

asthma. **Skin:** rash, injection-site reaction.
Other: hypersensitivity reactions.

INTERACTIONS

Drug-drug. *Aluminum hydroxide, aluminum-magnesium hydroxide, calcium carbonate, didanosine (chewable tablets, buffered tablets, or pediatric powder for oral solution), iron salts, magnesium hydroxide, products containing zinc:* May decrease ciprofloxacin absorption and effects. Give ciprofloxacin 2 hours before or 6 hours after these drugs.
Cyclosporine: May increase risk of cyclosporine toxicity. Monitor kidney function and cyclosporine level.
Drugs primarily metabolized by CYP1A2 (clozapine, olanzapine, ropinirole, zolpidem): May increase level of coadministered drug and risk of adverse reactions. Monitor patient for adverse reactions. Avoid use with zolpidem.
Drugs that prolong QT interval (amiodarone, procainamide, TCAs): May additionally increase QT interval and risk of life-threatening cardiac arrhythmias. Avoid use together.
Duloxetine: May significantly increase duloxetine level. Avoid use together.
Methotrexate: May increase methotrexate-associated toxicity. Monitor patient closely.
NSAIDs: May increase risk of CNS stimulation. Monitor patient closely.
Oral antidiabetics (glimepiride, glyburide): May increase risk of hypoglycemia. Monitor glucose level closely if used together.
Phenytoin: May increase or decrease phenytoin level. Monitor phenytoin level during and after use together.
Probenecid: May elevate ciprofloxacin level. Monitor patient for signs and symptoms of toxicity.
Boxed Warning *Steroids:* May increase risk of tendinitis and tendon rupture. ∎
Sildenafil: May increase sildenafil level. Use together cautiously and monitor for signs and symptoms of sildenafil toxicity.
Sucralfate: May decrease ciprofloxacin absorption, reducing anti-infective response. If use together can't be avoided, give at least 6 hours apart.
Theophylline: May increase theophylline level and prolong theophylline half-life. If use together can't be avoided, monitor theophylline level and watch for adverse effects.
Tizanidine: Increases tizanidine level, hypotension, and sedative effects. Use together is contraindicated.

Warfarin: May increase anticoagulant effects. Closely monitor PT and INR.
Drug-food. *Caffeine:* May increase effect of caffeine. Discourage use together.
Dairy products, other foods: May delay peak drug levels. Advise patient to take drug on an empty stomach.
Orange juice fortified with calcium: May decrease GI absorption of drug, reducing its effects. Discourage use together.
Drug-lifestyle. *Sun, UV light exposure:* May cause photosensitivity reactions. Advise patient to avoid excessive sunlight and UV light exposure.

EFFECTS ON LAB TEST RESULTS

• May increase calcium, ALP, ALT, AST, bilirubin, BUN, creatinine, LDH, and GGT levels.
• May decrease Hb, hematocrit, serum protein, and albumin levels.
• May increase or decrease glucose and potassium levels.
• May increase eosinophil count.
• May decrease WBC, leukocyte, neutrophil, and platelet counts.
• May increase crystals in urine.

CONTRAINDICATIONS & CAUTIONS

• Contraindicated in patients sensitive to quinolones.
⊕ *Alert:* Serious and occasionally fatal hypersensitivity reactions, some after first dose, have been reported. Emergency treatment for anaphylaxis may be necessary. Immediately discontinue drug at first appearance of rash, pharyngeal or facial edema, dyspnea, or other signs and symptoms of hypersensitivity.
⊕ *Alert:* Cases of severe liver toxicity, including fatal events, have been reported. Acute liver injury can be rapid and is frequently associated with hypersensitivity. If signs and symptoms of hepatitis occur, immediately discontinue drug.
⊕ *Alert:* Patients receiving systemic drug have an increased risk of hyperglycemia and hypoglycemia, which can result in coma. Hypoglycemia has been reported more often in older adult and patients with diabetes.
⊕ *Alert:* Drug may increase risk of aortic dissection or rupture when used systemically. Avoid use in patients with known aortic aneurysm; patients at risk for aortic aneurysm, including those with peripheral atherosclerotic vascular diseases, HTN, or

certain genetic conditions (Marfan syndrome, Ehlers-Danlos syndrome); and older adults. Use drug in these patients only if no other treatment options are available.

• Use cautiously in patients with CNS disorders, such as severe cerebral arteriosclerosis or seizure disorders, and in those at risk for seizures. Drug may cause CNS stimulation.

Boxed Warning Drug may exacerbate muscle weakness in patients with myasthenia gravis. Avoid use of fluoroquinolones in patients with known history of myasthenia gravis. ∎

• Oral or parenteral fluoroquinolones may increase the risk of peripheral neuropathy. Symptoms can occur anytime during treatment and can last for months to years or be permanent. If patient develops symptoms, immediately stop drug and switch to a nonfluoroquinolone antibacterial drug unless benefits of continued treatment outweigh risks.

Boxed Warning Fluoroquinolones have been associated with disabling and potentially irreversible serious adverse reactions that have occurred together, including tendinitis and tendon rupture, peripheral neuropathy, and CNS effects. Drug is associated with increased risk of serious adverse CNS reactions (seizures, toxic psychoses, increased ICP, tremors, pseudotumor cerebri, restlessness, anxiety, light-headedness, confusion, hallucinations, paranoia, depression, nightmares, insomnia, disturbances in attention, disorientation, agitation, memory impairment, delirium and, rarely, suicidality). If any of these serious adverse reactions occur, immediately discontinue drug. ∎

Boxed Warning The risk of tendinitis and tendon rupture is increased in patients older than age 60 and in those who have had heart, kidney, or lung transplants. ∎

Boxed Warning Reserve drug for use in patients who have no alternative treatment options for acute exacerbation of chronic bronchitis, acute sinusitis, and acute uncomplicated cystitis. ∎

• Drug may cause CDAD, ranging in severity from mild diarrhea to fatal colitis and possibly occurring more than 2 months after therapy ends. Drug may need to be discontinued if CDAD develops during therapy.

• Drug isn't the first choice for use in children due to increased risk of adverse reactions, including joint and surrounding tissue reactions.

Dialyzable drug: Less than 10%.

PREGNANCY-LACTATION-REPRODUCTION

• Studies during pregnancy are inadequate. Use during pregnancy only if potential benefit justifies fetal risk.

• During pregnancy, patients should receive the usual doses and regimens for anthrax postexposure prophylaxis.

• Drug appears in human milk; the amount absorbed by infant is unknown. Because of risk of serious adverse reactions (including articular damage), a decision should be made to discontinue breastfeeding or discontinue drug, considering importance of drug to patient.

• Patients who are breastfeeding may pump and discard human milk during and for 2 days after treatment.

NURSING CONSIDERATIONS

• Patients who are immunocompromised should receive the usual doses and regimens for anthrax postexposure prophylaxis.

• Monitor patient's intake and output, and observe patient for signs of crystalluria.

Boxed Warning Monitor patients receiving systemic drug for CNS (seizures, increased ICP, pseudotumor cerebri, dizziness, tremors) and psychiatric (disturbances in attention, disorientation, agitation, nervousness, memory impairment, delirium) adverse reactions. Discontinue drug for CNS adverse effects, including psychiatric adverse reactions. ∎

Boxed Warning Monitor for tendon rupture in patients receiving quinolones. If pain or inflammation or tendon rupture occurs, stop drug. ∎

⚠ *Alert:* Monitor patients for signs and symptoms of aortic aneurysm, dissection, and rupture (sudden, severe, and constant pain in stomach, chest, or back; throbbing in stomach area, deep pain in back or side of stomach; steady, gnawing pain in stomach that lasts for hours or days; pain in jaw, neck, back, or chest; coughing or hoarseness; shortness of breath, trouble swallowing). Discontinue drug immediately if any of these aortic disorders are suspected.

• Monitor for symptoms of peripheral neuropathy (pain; burning; tingling; numbness; weakness; change in sensation to light touch, pain, temperature, or sense of body position); immediately report them to practitioner if any occur.

⚠ *Alert:* Immediately report signs and symptoms of hepatitis (anorexia, jaundice, dark urine, pruritus, abdominal tenderness) and discontinue drug.

• Long-term therapy may result in overgrowth of drug-resistant organisms.

• Patients with cutaneous anthrax and signs and symptoms of systemic involvement, extensive edema, or lesions on head or neck need IV therapy and a multidrug approach.

☺ *Alert:* Monitor patients receiving systemic drug for symptoms of hypoglycemia (confusion, pounding or rapid heartbeat, dizziness, pale skin, shakiness, diaphoresis, unusual hunger, trembling, headache, weakness, irritability, unusual anxiety). Immediately discontinue drug for blood glucose disturbances, and switch to a nonfluoroquinolone antibiotic if possible.

PATIENT TEACHING

• Tell patient to take drug as prescribed, even after feeling better.

• Advise patient to drink plenty of fluids to reduce risk of urine crystals.

• Instruct patient in safe drug administration.

☺ *Alert:* Warn patient to seek immediate medical attention for signs or symptoms of aortic aneurysm.

☺ *Alert:* Warn patient to immediately notify prescriber of signs and symptoms of serious adverse reactions (unusual joint or tendon pain, muscle weakness, "pins and needles" tingling or pricking sensation, numbness in arms or legs, confusion, hallucinations).

☺ *Alert:* Caution patients that significantly low blood sugar levels can occur. Instruct patients how to manage symptoms and to immediately report any occurrence to the prescriber.

☺ *Alert:* Advise patients with diabetes that they may need to monitor blood glucose level more frequently during therapy.

☺ *Alert:* Inform patients to immediately report psychiatric adverse reactions and that these effects can occur after just one dose.

• Warn patient to avoid hazardous tasks that require alertness, such as driving, until effects of drug are known.

• Advise patient that hypersensitivity reactions may occur even after first dose. Tell patient to stop drug immediately and notify prescriber if rash or other allergic reaction occurs.

• Explain that tendon rupture can occur with drug. Instruct patient to notify prescriber if pain or inflammation occurs.

• Caution patient to avoid excessive sunlight and artificial UV light during therapy.

SAFETY ALERT!

CISplatin
SIS-pla-tin

Therapeutic class: Antineoplastics
Pharmacologic class: Platinum-containing compounds

AVAILABLE FORMS
Injection: 1 mg/mL
Lyophilized powder for injection: 50 mg

INDICATIONS & DOSAGES

☺ *Alert:* Dosages greater than 100 mg/m^2/cycle are rarely used and should be confirmed with prescriber.

Adjust-a-dose (for all indications): Other dosage regimens may be used. Consider alternative treatment or dosage reductions for impaired CrCl, myelosuppression, or neuropathy. Consider permanent discontinuation for grade 3 or 4 neuropathy.

Don't give repeat course of cisplatin until serum creatinine level is below 1.5 mg/dL or BUN level is below 25 mg/dL, platelets are 100,000/mm^3 or higher, WBCs are 4,000/mm^3 or higher, and audiometric analysis indicates that auditory acuity is within normal limits.

➤ **Adjunctive therapy in advanced testicular cancer**
Adults: 20 mg/m^2 IV daily for 5 days in combination with other approved chemotherapeutic agents.

➤ **Adjunctive therapy in advanced ovarian cancer**
Adults: 75 to 100 mg/m^2 IV once every 3 to 4 weeks on day 1.

➤ **Advanced bladder cancer**
Adults: 50 to 70 mg/m^2 IV every 3 to 4 weeks. Give 50 mg/m^2 every 4 weeks in patients who have received other antineoplastics or radiation therapy.

ADMINISTRATION
IV

☺ *Alert:* Hazardous drug; use safe handling and disposal precautions. Drug may be mutagenic, teratogenic, or carcinogenic.

▼ Hydrate with 1 to 2 L of fluid for 8 to 12 hours before giving drug, with continued hydration for 24 hours after administration.

🕒 *Alert:* Don't use needles or IV sets containing aluminum parts for preparation or administration.

▼ Infusions are most stable in solutions containing chloride (such as NSS or half-NSS and 0.22% sodium chloride). Don't use D₅W alone.

▼ Reconstitute 50-mg powder vial with 50 mL sterile water for injection to produce a 1-mg/1 mL clear or colorless to slightly yellow solution. Don't refrigerate reconstituted solution.

▼ Visually inspect solution for particulate matter and discoloration before administration, whenever solution and container permit.

▼ Further dilute reconstituted solution in 1 to 2 L of a compatible infusion solution with or without 37.5 g of mannitol. Refer to detailed references for specific infusion solution stability and compatibility information.

▼ Reconstituted solution is stable for 20 hours at controlled room temperature; don't refrigerate. Protect solution removed from amber vial from light if not used within 6 hours.

▼ Administer over 6 to 8 hours.

Boxed Warning Premedicate with highly effective antiemetic. Drug can cause severe nausea and vomiting. Posttreatment antiemetics may be necessary. ∎

▼ Solutions in vials that have been entered are stable for 7 days at room temperature under fluorescent light; if protected from light, stability is 28 days. Don't refrigerate.

▼ **Incompatibilities:** None listed by manufacturer. Consult drug compatibility reference for more information.

ACTION

May cross-link strands of cellular DNA and interfere with RNA transcription, causing an imbalance of growth that leads to cell death. Not specific to cell cycle.

Route	Onset	Peak	Duration
IV	Rapid	Unknown	Several days

Half-life: Initial phase, 14 to 49 minutes; beta, 0.7 to 4.6 hours; gamma, 24 to 127 hours.

ADVERSE REACTIONS

CNS: peripheral neuropathy, loss of taste.
EENT: ototoxicity (tinnitus, hearing loss).
GI: anorexia, diarrhea, nausea, vomiting. **GU:** *kidney toxicity.* **Hematologic:** *myelosuppression, leukopenia, thrombocytopenia,*

anemia. **Hepatic:** increased liver enzyme levels. **Metabolic:** *hypomagnesemia, hypokalemia, hypocalcemia.* **Skin:** local irritation. **Other:** hypersensitivity reactions.

INTERACTIONS

Drug-drug. *Aminoglycosides (gentamicin, tobramycin):* May increase kidney toxicity. Avoid use together.

Aminoglycosides, bumetanide, ethacrynic acid, furosemide, torsemide: May increase ototoxicity. Avoid use together, if possible.

Aspirin, NSAIDs: May increase risk of kidney toxicity. Avoid use together.

Clozapine: May increase neutropenic risk. Monitor use together.

Fosphenytoin, phenytoin: May decrease phenytoin and fosphenytoin levels. Monitor levels.

Live-virus vaccines: May increase vaccine-associated infection and decrease chemotherapy effectiveness. Use together isn't recommended.

Myelosuppressants (chemotherapy, radiation therapy): May increase myelosuppression. Monitor patient.

Drug-herb. *Echinacea:* May diminish drug's therapeutic effect. Monitor patient.

EFFECTS ON LAB TEST RESULTS

• May increase uric acid, transaminases, LDH, and bilirubin levels. May decrease calcium, Hb, magnesium, phosphate, potassium, and sodium levels.

• May decrease platelet and WBC counts.

CONTRAINDICATIONS & CAUTIONS

• Hypersensitivity reactions, including anaphylaxis have been reported. Facial edema, bronchoconstriction, tachycardia, and hypotension may occur within minutes of administration. Epinephrine, corticosteroids, and antihistamines have been effective in alleviating symptoms.

• Contraindicated in patients hypersensitive to drug or other platinum-containing compounds and in those with preexisting kidney impairment, hearing impairment, or myelosuppression.

• Use cautiously in patients previously treated with radiation or cytotoxic drugs and in those with peripheral neuropathies; also use cautiously with other ototoxic and kidney toxic drugs.

Boxed Warning Drug can cause severe kidney toxicity, including AKI, which is dose-related and cumulative. Ensure adequate hydration and monitor kidney function and electrolyte levels. Consider dosage reductions or alternative treatment in patients with kidney impairment. ■

Boxed Warning Drug can cause dose-related peripheral neuropathy that becomes more severe with repeated courses of drug. ■

• Secondary malignancies have been reported.
• Drug can cause hyperuricemia and TLS, requiring antihyperuricemia therapy to reduce uric acid levels, especially with dosages higher than 50 mg/m^2.
• Use cautiously in older adults.
• Safe use in children hasn't been established.

Dialyzable drug: No.

△ Overdose S&S: Kidney failure, liver failure, deafness, ocular toxicity, significant myelosuppression, intractable nausea and vomiting, neuritis, death.

PREGNANCY-LACTATION-REPRODUCTION

• Drug can cause fetal harm when used during pregnancy. Patients of childbearing potential should use effective contraception during and for 14 months after treatment.
• Males with partners of childbearing potential should use effective contraception during and for 11 months after treatment.
• Drug may cause ovarian failure, premature menopause, impaired spermatogenesis, and decreased fertility.
• Drug appears in human milk. Patients shouldn't breastfeed during therapy.

NURSING CONSIDERATIONS

• Drug should be administered under the supervision of a physician experienced in the use of cancer chemotherapeutic agents.

Boxed Warning Severe myelosuppression with fatalities due to infection can occur. Monitor blood counts accordingly. Therapy interruption may be required. ■

◑ Alert: Cisplatin is considered a vesicant if more than 20 mL is administered or if it's given at a concentration of 0.5 mg/mL or more. Monitor infusion site; immediately stop infusion and notify prescriber if extravasation occurs. Don't flush the line.
• Monitor CBC, electrolyte levels (especially potassium and magnesium), platelet count, and kidney function studies before initial and subsequent doses.

• Ototoxicity, which may be more pronounced in children, is manifested by tinnitus or loss of high-frequency hearing and, occasionally, deafness.
• To detect hearing loss, obtain audiometry tests before initial and subsequent doses.
• Prehydration and mannitol diuresis may significantly reduce kidney toxicity and ototoxicity. Maintain adequate hydration and urine output for 24 hours after drug administration.
• Therapeutic effects are frequently accompanied by toxicity.
• Drug is highly emetogenic. Nausea and vomiting may occur immediately or may be delayed. Give antiemetics. Monitor intake and output. Continue IV hydration until patient can tolerate adequate oral intake.

Boxed Warning Kidney toxicity is cumulative; don't give next dose until kidney function returns to normal. ■

• To prevent bleeding, avoid all IM injections when platelet count is less than 50,000/mm^3.
• Anticipate need for blood transfusions during treatment because of cumulative anemia.
• Monitor patient for hypersensitivity reactions; treat as clinically indicated.
• Verify pregnancy status before treatment.
• *Look alike–sound alike:* Don't confuse cisplatin with carboplatin; they aren't interchangeable.

PATIENT TEACHING

• Teach patient to report all adverse reactions, including nausea, vomiting, and infusion-site discomfort.
• Instruct patient in management of nausea and vomiting, and need to maintain hydration.
• Advise patient to watch for signs and symptoms of infection (fever, sore throat, fatigue) and bleeding (easy bruising, nosebleeds, bleeding gums, tarry stools). Tell patient to take temperature daily.
• Tell patient to immediately report ringing in the ears, hearing loss, vertigo, or numbness in hands or feet.
• Instruct patient to avoid OTC products containing aspirin or other NSAIDs.
• Advise patient to stop breastfeeding during therapy because of risk of toxicity to infant.
• Warn patient of childbearing potential about need for contraception due to risk of fetal harm and patients of reproductive age of the risk for infertility.
• Inform patient that drug can cause hair loss.

Reactions in bold italics are *life-threatening*.

citalopram hydrobromide ⬓
si-TAL-oh-pram

CeleXA

Therapeutic class: Antidepressants
Pharmacologic class: SSRIs

AVAILABLE FORMS
Capsules: 30 mg
Solution: 10 mg/5 mL
Tablets: 10 mg, 20 mg, 40 mg

INDICATIONS & DOSAGES
⬓ *Adjust-a-dose (for all indications):* For patients with liver impairment, those who are CYP2C19 poor metabolizers, those who are taking a CYP2C19 inhibitor, and older adults, maximum dosage is 20 mg/day.

➤ **MDD**
Adults: Initially, 20 mg PO once daily, increasing to maximum of 40 mg daily after no less than 1 week.
Adults older than age 60: 20 mg PO daily.

ADMINISTRATION
PO
• Give without regard for food.
• Capsules are only available in 30-mg strength. Use of tablets or solution is necessary for initial dosage and titration.

ACTION
Probably linked to potentiation of serotonergic activity in CNS resulting from inhibition of neuronal reuptake of serotonin.

Route	Onset	Peak	Duration
PO	1–4 wk	4 hr	1–2 days

Half-life: 35 hours.

ADVERSE REACTIONS
CNS: somnolence, insomnia, *suicidality,* anxiety, agitation, dizziness, paresthesia, migraine, impaired concentration, amnesia, depression, apathy, tremor, confusion, fatigue, fever, asthenia, taste perversion, yawning. **CV:** tachycardia, orthostatic hypotension, hypotension, *prolonged QT interval.* **EENT:** rhinitis, sinusitis, dry mouth, increased saliva, abnormal vision. **GI:** nausea, diarrhea, anorexia, dyspepsia, vomiting, abdominal pain, flatulence, increased appetite. **GU:** dysmenorrhea, amenorrhea, ejaculation disorder, erectile dysfunction, anorgasmia, polyuria, decreased libido. **Metabolic:** decreased or increased weight. **Musculoskeletal:** arthralgia, myalgia. **Respiratory:** URI, coughing. **Skin:** rash, pruritus, diaphoresis.

INTERACTIONS
Drug-drug. *Amphetamines, antiemetics, antipsychotics, buspirone, dextromethorphan, dihydroergotamine, opioids, other SSRIs or SSNRIs (duloxetine, venlafaxine), TCAs, tramadol, trazodone, triptans:* May increase risk of serotonin syndrome. Avoid other drugs that increase availability of serotonin in CNS; monitor patient closely if used together.
Antiarrhythmics (Class IA [procainamide, quinidine], Class III [amiodarone, sotalol]), antibiotics (clarithromycin, erythromycin, levofloxacin, moxifloxacin), antipsychotics (chlorpromazine, thioridazine), drugs that prolong QTc interval (dolasetron, methadone, ondansetron, pentamidine): May cause QTc prolongation and increase risk of torsades de pointes. Use together isn't recommended.
Anticoagulants, antiplatelet agents, NSAIDs: May increase bleeding risk. Monitor therapy.
CYP2C19 inhibitors: May increase risk of QT-interval prolongation or ventricular arrhythmias. Limit citalopram dosage to 20 mg daily.
MAO inhibitors (phenelzine, selegiline, tranylcypromine, linezolid, methylene blue): May cause serotonin syndrome or signs and symptoms resembling NMS. Use together is contraindicated. Avoid using within 14 days of MAO inhibitor therapy.
Pimozide: May increase pimozide level and risk of QT-interval prolongation or ventricular arrhythmias. Use together is contraindicated.
Drug-lifestyle. *Alcohol use:* May increase CNS effects. Discourage use together.

EFFECTS ON LAB TEST RESULTS
None reported.

CONTRAINDICATIONS & CAUTIONS
• Contraindicated in patients hypersensitive to drug or its inactive components.
⬓ ❸ *Alert:* Drug isn't recommended for patients with congenital long QT syndrome, bradycardia, hypokalemia, hypomagnesemia, recent acute MI, or uncompensated HF.
⬓ ❸ *Alert:* High doses can prolong the QT interval and cause torsades de pointes. Don't exceed recommended maximum dosage.

🜂 *Alert:* Discontinue drug in patients with persistent QTc interval measurement longer than 500 msec.

🜂 *Alert:* Using together with linezolid or methylene blue can cause serotonin syndrome (fever, mental status changes, muscle twitching, diaphoresis, shivering or shaking, diarrhea, loss of coordination). Use together is contraindicated.

• Use cautiously in patients with history of mania, seizures, suicidality, or significant liver or kidney impairment.

• Avoid use in patients with untreated narrow-angle glaucoma.

Dialyzable drug: No.

⚠ *Overdose S&S:* Dizziness, diaphoresis, nausea, vomiting, tremor, somnolence, sinus tachycardia, amnesia, confusion, coma, seizures, hyperventilation, cyanosis, rhabdomyolysis, ECG changes.

PREGNANCY-LACTATION-REPRODUCTION

• Studies during pregnancy are inadequate. Use during pregnancy only if potential benefit justifies fetal risk.

• Encourage patients who are pregnant to register in National Pregnancy Registry for Antidepressants (1-866-961-2388 or https://womensmentalhealth.org/research/pregnancyregistry/antidepressants).

• Use in third trimester may be linked to neonatal complications at birth requiring respiratory support and tube feeding. Consider risk versus benefit of treatment during this time.

• Drug appears in human milk. Infants exposed in utero may have irritability, restlessness, excessive somnolence, decreased feeding, and weight loss. Monitor infant closely. Consider patient's clinical need and risk to infant before use.

NURSING CONSIDERATIONS

• Correct electrolyte disturbances before starting drug; periodically monitor patient at high risk for electrolyte disturbances during therapy.

• Although drug hasn't been shown to impair psychomotor performance, any psychoactive drug has the potential to impair judgment, thinking, and motor skills.

Boxed Warning The possibility of a suicide attempt is inherent in depression and may persist until significant remission occurs. Closely supervise patient for clinical worsening,

suicidality, or unusual changes in behavior at start of drug therapy. ■

Boxed Warning Drug may increase risk of suicidality in children, adolescents, and young adults with major depressive disorder or other psychiatric disorders. Drug isn't approved for use in children. ■

• Reduce risk of overdose by limiting amount of drug available per refill.

🜂 *Alert:* Monitor for signs and symptoms of serotonin syndrome (restlessness, hallucinations, loss of coordination, fast heartbeat, rapid changes in BP, increased body temperature, overactive reflexes, nausea, vomiting, diarrhea). Serotonin syndrome may be more likely to occur when starting or increasing the dose of the triptan, SSRI, or SSNRI.

🜂 *Alert:* If linezolid or methylene blue must be given, stop citalopram and monitor for signs and symptoms of serotonin toxicity for 2 weeks, or until 24 hours after the last dose of methylene blue or linezolid, whichever comes first. Treatment may resume 24 hours after last dose of methylene blue or linezolid.

• Don't abruptly discontinue citalopram because a discontinuation syndrome can develop, with varying symptoms.

• *Look alike–sound alike:* Don't confuse CeleXA with Zyprexa, CeleBREX, or Cerebyx.

PATIENT TEACHING

Boxed Warning Advise families and caregivers to closely observe patient for increased suicidality. ■

🜂 *Alert:* Teach patient to recognize and immediately report symptoms of serotonin toxicity (fever, mental status changes, muscle twitching, excessive sweating, shivering or shaking, diarrhea, loss of coordination).

• Caution patient against use of MAO inhibitors while taking citalopram.

• Although improvement may take 1 to 4 weeks, inform patient to continue therapy as prescribed.

• Advise patient not to stop drug abruptly.

• Tell patient that drug may be taken in the morning or evening without regard to meals. If drowsiness occurs, patient should take drug in evening.

• Instruct patient to exercise caution when driving or operating hazardous machinery; drug may impair judgment, thinking, and motor skills.

Reactions in bold italics are *life-threatening*.

- Advise patient to consult prescriber before taking other prescription or OTC drugs.
- Warn patient to avoid alcohol during therapy.
- Advise patient of childbearing potential to consult prescriber before breastfeeding.
- Instruct patient of childbearing potential to immediately notify prescriber if pregnancy is planned or suspected.

clarithromycin
kla-RITH-roe-mye-sin

Therapeutic class: Antibiotics
Pharmacologic class: Macrolides

AVAILABLE FORMS
Suspension: 125 mg/5 mL, 250 mg/5 mL
Tablets (extended-release) ⓘ: 500 mg
Tablets (film-coated): 250 mg, 500 mg

INDICATIONS & DOSAGES
Adjust-a-dose (for all indications): In patients with CrCl of less than 30 mL/minute, reduce dosage by 50%. For use together with atazanavir or ritonavir in patients with CrCl of 30 to 60 mL/minute, reduce dosage by 50%; if CrCl is less than 30 mL/minute, reduce dosage by 75%. In patients with normal kidney function, decrease clarithromycin dose by 50% when administered with atazanavir.
➤ **Pharyngitis or tonsillitis caused by** *Streptococcus pyogenes*
Adults: 250 mg PO every 12 hours for 10 days.
Children ages 6 months and older: 7.5 mg/kg PO every 12 hours for 10 days.
➤ **Acute maxillary sinusitis caused by** *Streptococcus pneumoniae, Haemophilus influenzae,* **or** *Moraxella catarrhalis*
Adults: 500 mg PO every 12 hours for 14 days. Or, if using extended-release form, two 500-mg tablets PO daily for 14 days.
Children ages 6 months and older: 7.5 mg/kg PO every 12 hours for 10 days.
➤ **Acute worsening of chronic bronchitis caused by** *M. catarrhalis* **or** *S. pneumoniae*
Adults: 250 mg PO every 12 hours for 7 to 14 days. Or, two 500-mg extended-release tablets PO daily for 7 days.
➤ **Acute worsening of chronic bronchitis caused by** *H. influenzae* **or** *Haemophilus parainfluenzae*
Adults: 500 mg PO every 12 hours for 7 days (*H. parainfluenzae*) or 7 to 14 days

(*H. influenzae*). Or, two 500-mg extended-release tablets PO daily for 7 days.
➤ **Mild to moderate community-acquired pneumonia caused by** *H. influenzae, S. pneumoniae, Chlamydophila pneumoniae,* **or** *Mycoplasma pneumoniae*
Adults: 250 mg PO every 12 hours for 7 days (*H. influenzae*) or 7 to 14 days (other bacteria).
➤ **Mild to moderate community-acquired pneumonia caused by** *H. influenzae, H. parainfluenzae, M. catarrhalis, S. pneumoniae, C. pneumoniae,* **or** *M. pneumoniae*
Adults: Two 500-mg extended-release tablets PO once daily for 7 days.
➤ **Mild to moderate community-acquired pneumonia caused by** *S. pneumoniae, C. pneumoniae,* **or** *M. pneumoniae*
Children ages 6 months and older: 7.5 mg/kg PO every 12 hours for 10 days.
➤ **Uncomplicated skin and skin-structure infections caused by** *Staphylococcus aureus* **or** *S. pyogenes*
Adults: 250 mg PO every 12 hours for 7 to 14 days.
Children ages 6 months and older: 7.5 mg/kg PO every 12 hours for 10 days.
➤ **Acute otitis media**
Children ages 6 months and older: 7.5 mg/kg PO every 12 hours for 10 days.
➤ **To prevent and treat disseminated infection caused by MAC in patients with advanced HIV infection**
Adults: 500 mg PO every 12 hours.
Children ages 20 months and older: 7.5 mg/kg PO every 12 hours, up to 500 mg every 12 hours.
Adjust-a-dose: Therapy should continue if clinical response is observed; can be discontinued when patient is considered at low risk for disseminated infection.
➤ **To reduce risk of duodenal ulcer recurrence in** *Helicobacter pylori* **infection**
Adults: 500 mg clarithromycin with 30 mg lansoprazole and 1 g amoxicillin, all given PO every 12 hours for 10 to 14 days. Or, 500 mg clarithromycin with 20 mg omeprazole and 1 g amoxicillin, all given PO every 12 hours for 10 days. Or, two-drug regimen with 500 mg clarithromycin PO every 8 hours and 40 mg omeprazole PO once daily for 14 days. Continue omeprazole for 14 additional days for symptom relief and ulcer healing. *Note:* Avoid use of clarithromycin triple therapy in patients with risk factors for macrolide resistance (prior macrolide exposure, local

clarithromycin resistance rates of 15% or more).

ADMINISTRATION
PO
- Certain bacterial infections caused by *S. pneumoniae* and *S. aureus* show resistance to macrolides. Obtain specimen for culture and sensitivity tests before giving. Begin therapy while awaiting results.
- Give immediate-release form with or without food; give extended-release tablets with food.
- Don't crush extended-release tablets.
- Don't refrigerate suspension form; discard unused portion after 14 days.

ACTION
Binds to the 50S subunit of bacterial ribosomes, blocking protein synthesis; bacteriostatic or bactericidal, depending on concentration.

Route	Onset	Peak	Duration
PO	Unknown	2–3 hr	Unknown
PO (extended-release)	Unknown	5–8 hr	Unknown

Half-life: 3 to 7 hours; 5 to 9 hours (extended-release).

ADVERSE REACTIONS
CNS: headache, insomnia, taste perversion. **GI:** abdominal pain or discomfort, diarrhea, nausea, dyspepsia, flatulence, vomiting. **GU:** increased BUN level. **Hematologic:** coagulation abnormalities. **Hepatic:** abnormal LFT values. **Skin:** rash. **Other:** hypersensitivity reaction, candidiasis.

INTERACTIONS
Drug-drug. *Alfuzosin, alprazolam, midazolam, triazolam:* May decrease clearance of these drugs, causing adverse reactions. Use together cautiously.
Almotriptan: May increase almotriptan serum level. Limit initial almotriptan adult dose to 6.25 mg and maximum adult dose to 12.5 mg/24 hours. Avoid use together in patients with impaired liver or kidney function. Consider therapy modification.
Apixaban, dabigatran, edoxaban, rivaroxaban: May increase levels of these drugs. Apixaban, dabigatran, rivaroxaban, or edoxaban dosage reductions or avoidance of combination may be necessary. Consider therapy modification.

Atazanavir, ritonavir: May increase clarithromycin level. Reduce clarithromycin dosage in patients with kidney impairment and in all patients taking atazanavir.
Carbamazepine, phenytoin: May inhibit metabolism of these drugs, increasing serum levels and risk of toxicity. Use together cautiously.
Colchicine: May increase colchicine level. Use together is contraindicated in patients with kidney or liver impairment. In those with normal kidney or liver function, reduce colchicine dose.
Cyclosporine: May increase cyclosporine level. Monitor cyclosporine level.
CYP3A4 inducers (efavirenz, nevirapine, rifabutin, rifampin): May decrease clarithromycin level. Consider alternative antibacterial treatment.
CYP3A inhibitors (itraconazole): May increase inhibitor level. Use together cautiously.
CYP3A4 substrates (amlodipine, diltiazem, nifedipine, verapamil): May increase substrate concentration. Avoid use together or reduce substrate dosage.
Digoxin, other P-gp substrates: May increase digoxin and substrate levels. Monitor for signs and symptoms of toxicity.
Dihydroergotamine, ergotamine: May cause acute ergot toxicity. Use together is contraindicated.
Fluconazole: May increase clarithromycin level. Monitor patient closely.
HMG-CoA reductase inhibitors: Lovastatin and simvastatin are contraindicated. Use with other statins may increase levels of these drugs and may rarely cause rhabdomyolysis. Use together cautiously. For adults, limit atorvastatin to a maximum dose of 20 mg/day and pravastatin to 40 mg/day.
Oral antidiabetic agents (nateglinide, pioglitazone, repaglinide, rosiglitazone), insulin: May result in significant hypoglycemia. Monitor patient.
Other drugs that prolong QTc interval (amiodarone, antipsychotics, disopyramide, dofetilide, fluoroquinolones, fluoxetine, procainamide, quinidine, sotalol, TCAs): May have additive effects. Monitor ECG for QTc interval prolongation. Avoid use together if possible.
PDE5 inhibitors (sildenafil, tadalafil, vardenafil): May increase level of PDE5 inhibitor. Coadministration not recommended. Consider reduced PDE5 inhibitor dosage.

Reactions in bold italics are ***life-threatening***.

Pimozide: May cause torsades de pointes. Use together is contraindicated.
Theophylline: May increase theophylline level. Monitor drug level.
Warfarin: May prolong PT and increase INR. Carefully monitor PT and INR.
Zidovudine: May alter zidovudine level. Separate doses by at least 2 hours.
Drug-herb. *St. John's wort:* May decrease clarithromycin level. Avoid use.

EFFECTS ON LAB TEST RESULTS
• May increase BUN level and LFT values.
• May decrease WBC count.
• May prolong PT and increase INR.

CONTRAINDICATIONS & CAUTIONS
⚠️ *Alert:* Use in patients with CAD has shown an increased risk of all-cause mortality 1 year or more after the end of treatment. Consider risk versus benefits before using in patients with suspected or confirmed heart disease. Use of an alternative antibiotic is recommended.
• Severe acute hypersensitivity reactions (anaphylaxis, SJS, TEN, DRESS, Henoch-Schönlein purpura) have been reported. Discontinue drug and begin immediate treatment if these reactions occur.
• Contraindicated in patients hypersensitive to clarithromycin, erythromycin, or other macrolides and in those receiving pimozide or other drugs that prolong QT interval or cause cardiac arrhythmias.
• Contraindicated in patients with history of cholestatic jaundice or liver impairment associated with prior use of clarithromycin.
• Avoid use in patients with ongoing proarrhythmic conditions (uncorrected hypokalemia or hypomagnesemia, clinically significant bradycardia) and in patients receiving Class IA or Class III antiarrhythmics. Older adults may be more susceptible to drug-associated effects on the QT interval.
• Use cautiously in patients with liver or kidney impairment.
• May exacerbate or cause new signs and symptoms in patients with myasthenia gravis. Use cautiously in these patients.
• Drug may cause CDAD and pseudomembranous colitis, which can occur more than 2 months after therapy ends.
• Safety in patients with MAC infection younger than age 20 months hasn't been studied.

• Safety and effectiveness for pharyngitis, tonsillitis, community-acquired pneumonia, sinusitis, otitis media, and skin and skin-structure infections in children younger than age 6 months haven't been established.
• Safety and effectiveness of extended-release tablets in children haven't been established.
Dialyzable drug: No.

PREGNANCY-LACTATION-REPRODUCTION
• Studies during pregnancy are inadequate; animal studies show adverse pregnancy outcome and embryo-fetal risk. Use during pregnancy only in clinical circumstances in which no alternative therapy is appropriate. Inform patient of fetal risk.
• Drug appears in human milk. Use cautiously during breastfeeding and weigh benefits against risks. Rash, diarrhea, loss of appetite, and somnolence may occur in infant.

NURSING CONSIDERATIONS
⚠️ *Alert:* Be sure to use extended-release form to only treat infections for which it is approved.
• Monitor for signs and symptoms of superinfection. Drug may cause overgrowth of non-susceptible bacteria or fungi.
• Monitor for hypersensitivity reactions and diarrhea.
• For MAC treatment, use drug in combination with other antimycobacterial drugs.

PATIENT TEACHING
• Tell patient to take drug as exactly prescribed, even after feeling better.
• Caution patient to report all adverse reactions.
• Instruct patient to notify prescriber of signs and symptoms of CDAD (watery, bloody stools with or without cramps and fever), which can occur as late as 2 months after treatment.
• Advise patient of the importance of taking immediate-release product every 12 hours.
• Teach about proper drug administration and handling.
• Warn patient to inform prescriber of concurrent drugs patient is taking because of risk of significant drug interactions.
• Caution patient that drug may cause dizziness, vertigo, and confusion, which should be considered before driving or using machinery.

clascoterone
klas-KOE-ter-one

Winlevi

Therapeutic class: Antiacne drugs
Pharmacologic class: Androgen receptor inhibitors

AVAILABLE FORMS
Cream: 1%

INDICATIONS & DOSAGES
➤ **Acne vulgaris**
Adults and children ages 12 and older: Apply thin uniform layer to affected area b.i.d., in morning and evening.

ADMINISTRATION
Topical
• Gently wash and dry affected area before applying drug.
• For topical use only; not for ophthalmic, oral, or vaginal use.
• Avoid getting drug in eyes, mouth, and mucous membranes; if contact occurs, rinse thoroughly with water.
• Avoid applying to cuts, abrasions, or eczematous or sunburned skin.
• Wash hands after applying drug.
• Store at room temperature. Discard drug 180 days after date prescription was filled or 1 month after first opening, whichever is sooner.

ACTION
Inhibits androgen receptors and decreases sebum production and inflammation.

Route	Onset	Peak	Duration
Topical	Unknown	Unknown	Unknown

Half-life: Unknown.

ADVERSE REACTIONS
CV: edema. **GU:** amenorrhea, polycystic ovaries. **Metabolic:** *hyperkalemia,* HPA axis suppression. **Skin:** dryness, erythema, pruritus, scaling, skin atrophy, stinging or burning, striae rubrae, telangiectasia.

INTERACTIONS
Drug-drug. *Astringents, medicated soaps and cleansers:* May increase skin irritation. Avoid use together.

EFFECTS ON LAB TEST RESULTS
• May increase potassium level.
• May decrease cortisol level.

CONTRAINDICATIONS & CAUTIONS
• HPA axis suppression may occur with prolonged use on large surface areas or use of occlusive dressings over drug.
• Avoid use with other potentially irritating topical products (medicated or abrasive soaps and cleansers, soaps and cosmetics with strong drying effect, products with high alcohol content, astringents, spices, or lime).
• Safety and effectiveness in children younger than age 12 haven't been established. Use cautiously in children as they are more prone to systemic toxicity.
• Use cautiously in older adults.
Dialyzable drug: Unknown.

PREGNANCY-LACTATION-REPRODUCTION
• Studies during pregnancy are lacking. It's unknown if drug increases risk of major birth defects, miscarriage, or adverse patient or fetal outcomes.
• It isn't known if drug appears in human milk or how drug affects milk production or infants who are breastfed. Consider benefit to the mother against risk to the infant.

NURSING CONSIDERATIONS
• Monitor patient for local skin reactions. Avoid using with other potentially irritating topical products.
• Monitor patient for signs of HPA axis suppression (decreased cortisol level, fatigue, muscle and joint pain, hypotension, irregular menstruation); if HPA suppression occurs, attempt to withdraw drug.

PATIENT TEACHING
• Instruct patient to gently wash and dry affected area before applying drug and to wash hands well after application.
• Advise patient to keep drug away from eyes, mouth, and mucous membranes. If contact occurs, tell patient to rinse areas thoroughly with water.
• Warn patient to avoid applying drug to cuts and abrasions, eczematous areas, and sunburned skin.
• Tell patient to avoid using with other potentially irritating topical products.

Reactions in bold italics are *life-threatening*.

clevidipine
clev-ID-i-peen

Cleviprex

Therapeutic class: Antihypertensives
Pharmacologic class: Dihydropyridine
calcium channel blockers

AVAILABLE FORMS
Injection: 0.5 mg/mL in 50- and 100-mL
single-use vials

INDICATIONS & DOSAGES
➤ **To lower BP when oral therapy isn't feasible or desirable**
Adults: Begin infusion at 1 to 2 mg/hour and
titrate by doubling dose every 90 seconds.
When BP approaches goal, titrate every 5
to 10 minutes at less than double the dose.
Maintenance dose is usually 4 to 6 mg/hour.
Maximum dose, 1,000 mL (average of
21 mg/hour) per 24-hour period. Drug isn't
recommended for use beyond 72 hours.

ADMINISTRATION
IV
▼ Store vials in cartons in refrigerator because drug is photosensitive. May store unopened vials at controlled room temperature
(77° F [25° C]) for up to 2 months.
▼ Upon transfer to room temperature, mark
vials in cartons with date. Don't return to
refrigerated storage after beginning room
temperature storage.
▼ Invert vial several times to mix emulsion
before use.
▼ Inspect solution and discard if particulate
matter or discoloration is present before use.
Don't dilute.
▼ Use a continuous infusion pump to regulate flow.
▼ Maintain aseptic technique when handling
solution. Drug can support growth of microorganisms.
▼ Discard unused portion within 12 hours
after stopper puncture.
▼ **Incompatibilities:** Don't administer drug
in same IV line with other medications.

ACTION
Inhibits calcium ion influx across cardiac and
smooth-muscle cells, decreasing contractility
and oxygen demand. Dilates coronary arteries

and arterioles, decreasing systemic vascular
resistance.

Route	Onset	Peak	Duration
IV	2–4 min	Unknown	5–15 min

Half-life: 15 minutes; metabolite, 9 hours.

ADVERSE REACTIONS
CNS: headache. **CV:** atrial fibrillation, hypotension, reflex tachycardia. **GI:** nausea,
vomiting. **GU:** *AKI.*

INTERACTIONS
None reported.

EFFECTS ON LAB TEST RESULTS
None reported.

CONTRAINDICATIONS & CAUTIONS
• Contraindicated in patients hypersensitive to soybeans, soy products, eggs, or egg
products and in those with defective lipid
metabolism (pathologic hyperlipidemia,
lipoid nephrosis, acute pancreatitis) or severe
aortic stenosis.
• Use cautiously in patients with HF and
older adults.
• Safety and effectiveness in children
younger than age 18 haven't been established.
Dialyzable drug: Unknown.
⚠ *Overdose S&S:* Hypotension, reflex tachycardia.

PREGNANCY-LACTATION-REPRODUCTION
• Studies during pregnancy are inadequate.
Use during pregnancy only if potential benefit
justifies fetal risk.
• It isn't known if drug appears in human
milk. Consider the possibility of infant exposure during breastfeeding; monitor infant
for adverse effects.

NURSING CONSIDERATIONS
• Monitor BP and HR continuously, especially when starting drug and during dosage
adjustments.
• Drug may exacerbate HF; monitor patient
closely.
• Titrate dose slowly; rapid titration may
cause hypotension and reflex tachycardia. If
either occurs, decrease clevidipine dosage.
• Monitor patient who received prolonged infusion for rebound HTN for at least 8 hours
after infusion is stopped if no other antihypertensive is prescribed.

• To convert to oral therapy, discontinue or titrate drug downward while appropriate oral therapy is established. When an oral antihypertensive is started, consider the lag time of onset of the oral agent's effect and continue BP monitoring until desired effect is achieved.

• Drug isn't a beta blocker; if given with beta blocker, gradually reduce beta blocker dosage to avoid withdrawal symptoms.

• Drug contains 0.2g of lipid/mL. Lipid intake may need to be limited in patients with significant lipid metabolism disorders.

PATIENT TEACHING
• Tell patient to promptly report adverse reactions.

• Advise patient to immediately seek medical attention if signs and symptoms of hypertensive emergency occur (visual changes, neurologic symptoms, HF).

clindamycin hydrochloride
klin-da-MYE-sin

Cleocin Hydrochloride, Dalacin C✜

clindamycin palmitate hydrochloride
Cleocin Pediatric, Dalacin C Flavored Granules✜

clindamycin phosphate (injection)
Cleocin Phosphate, Dalacin C Phosphate✜

Therapeutic class: Antibiotics
Pharmacologic class: Lincomycin derivatives

AVAILABLE FORMS
clindamycin hydrochloride
Capsules: 75 mg, 150 mg, 300 mg
clindamycin palmitate hydrochloride
Granules for oral solution: 75 mg/5 mL
clindamycin phosphate (injection)
Infusion (premixed): 300 mg (50 mL), 600 mg (50 mL), 900 mg (50 mL)
Injection: 150 mg/mL

INDICATIONS & DOSAGES
➤ **Infections caused by sensitive staphylococci, streptococci, pneumococci,** *Prevotella*
elaninogenica, Fusobacterium, Clostridium perfringens, **or other sensitive aerobic and anaerobic organisms**
Adults: 150 to 300 mg PO every 6 hours; or 600 to 1,200 mg IM or IV in two, three, or four equal doses. In more severe infections, dosage may be increased to 450 mg PO every 6 hours; or 1,200 to 2,700 mg/day IM or IV in two, three, or four equal doses. In life-threatening infections, dosages as high as 4,800 mg IV daily can be given.
Children able to swallow capsules: 8 to 20 mg/kg/day PO divided in three or four equal doses.
Children weighing more than 10 kg: 8 to 25 mg/kg/day suspension PO divided in three or four equal doses.
Children weighing 10 kg or less: Minimum recommended dosage, 37.5 mg suspension PO every 8 hours.
Children ages 1 month to 16 years: 20 to 40 mg/kg/day or 350 to 450 mg/m^2/day IM or IV in three or four equal doses. In beta-hemolytic streptococcal infections, continue treatment for at least 10 days.
Neonates younger than age 1 month: 15 to 20 mg/kg/day IM or IV in three or four equal doses. Consider 15 mg/kg/day for small premature infants.

ADMINISTRATION
PO
• Obtain specimen for culture and sensitivity tests before giving first dose. Begin therapy while awaiting results.

• Give capsule form with a full glass of water to prevent esophageal irritation.

• Don't refrigerate reconstituted oral solution because it will thicken. Drug is stable for 2 weeks at room temperature.

IV
▼ Obtain specimen for culture and sensitivity tests before giving first dose. Begin therapy while awaiting results.

▼ Never give undiluted as a bolus.

▼ For infusion, dilute each 300 mg in 50-mL solution and give over 10 to 60 minutes at no more than 30 mg/minute.

▼ Check site daily for phlebitis and irritation.

▼ Drug may contain benzyl alcohol. Benzyl alcohol has been associated with fatal gasping syndrome in premature infants.

Reactions in bold italics are *life-threatening*.

▼ Incompatibilities: Aminophylline, ampicillin, barbiturates, calcium gluconate, magnesium sulfate, phenytoin.

IM

• Obtain specimen for culture and sensitivity tests before giving first dose. Begin therapy while awaiting results.

• IM administration uses undiluted solution.

• Inject deep into muscle. Rotate sites. Don't exceed 600 mg per injection.

ACTION

Inhibits bacterial protein synthesis by binding to 50S subunit of ribosome.

Route	Onset	Peak	Duration
PO	Unknown	45–60 min	Unknown
IV	Immediate	Immediate	Unknown
IM	Unknown	1–3 hr	Unknown

Half-life: 2.5 to 3 hours.

ADVERSE REACTIONS

CNS: metallic taste. **CV:** thrombophlebitis. **GI:** nausea, *CDAD,* abdominal pain, diarrhea, vomiting, esophageal ulcer, esophagitis. **GU:** AKI, vaginitis. **Hematologic:** *thrombocytopenia, transient leukopenia,* eosinophilia. **Hepatic:** jaundice, elevated LFT values. **Skin:** rash, urticaria, pruritus, dermatitis, injection site reactions. **Other:** hypersensitivity reactions.

INTERACTIONS

Drug-drug. *CYP3A4 inducers (phenytoin, rifampin):* May decrease clindamycin level. Monitor patient for loss of efficacy.
CYP3A4 and CYP3A5 inhibitors (diltiazem, erythromycin, itraconazole, ritonavir, saquinavir, verapamil): May increase clindamycin level. Monitor patient for adverse effects.
Live-virus vaccines: May decrease vaccine effectiveness. Don't give together.
Neuromuscular blockers: May increase neuromuscular blockade. Monitor patient closely.

EFFECTS ON LAB TEST RESULTS

• May increase BUN, creatinine, ALP, AST, and bilirubin levels.

• May increase eosinophil count.

• May decrease platelet and WBC counts.

CONTRAINDICATIONS & CAUTIONS

• Contraindicated in patients hypersensitive to drug or lincomycin. Severe hypersensitivity

reactions requiring emergency treatment have been reported. Discontinue drug if these occur.

• Use only to treat or prevent infections proven or strongly suspected to be caused by bacteria to reduce development of drug-resistant bacteria.

• Clindamycin use may result in overgrowth of nonsusceptible organisms, particularly yeasts. Monitor for signs and symptoms of superinfection.

• Use cautiously in neonates and patients with kidney or liver disease, asthma, history of GI disease, or significant allergies.

• Severe or fatal reactions, such as TEN, DRESS syndrome, and SJS, have been reported. Discontinue drug if severe skin reaction occurs.

Boxed Warning Clindamycin has been associated with development of CDAD, which may evolve into severe, possibly fatal, colitis; its use should be reserved for serious infections. Don't use drug in nonbacterial infections. ▮

Dialyzable drug: No.

PREGNANCY-LACTATION-REPRODUCTION

• Use during the first trimester of pregnancy only if clearly needed. Use in second and third trimesters hasn't been associated with increased congenital abnormalities.

• Clindamycin phosphate formulations may contain benzyl alcohol which crosses the placenta.

• Drug appears in human milk. Use during breastfeeding isn't recommended. Monitor infant who is breastfed for diarrhea and candidiasis.

NURSING CONSIDERATIONS

• IM injection may raise CK level in response to muscle irritation.

• Monitor kidney, liver, and hematopoietic functions during prolonged therapy.

• Observe patient for signs and symptoms of superinfection.

❸ Alert: Don't give opioid antidiarrheals to treat drug-induced diarrhea; they may prolong and worsen this condition.

Boxed Warning Diarrhea, colitis, and pseudomembranous colitis have developed up to 2 months after cessation of drug therapy. If CDAD is suspected or confirmed, the antibiotic not directed against *C. difficile* may need to be discontinued. Initiate fluid and electrolyte management, protein supplementation, antibiotic treatment of *C. difficile*, and surgical evaluation as clinically indicated. ■

• Drug doesn't penetrate blood-brain barrier.

PATIENT TEACHING

• Advise patient to take capsule form with a full glass of water to prevent esophageal irritation.

• Warn patient that IM injection may be painful.

• Tell patient to report discomfort at IV insertion site.

• Instruct patient to report all adverse reactions (especially diarrhea and hypersensitivity reactions). Warn patient not to self-treat diarrhea because drug may cause life-threatening colitis.

clindamycin phosphate (intravaginal, topical)
klin-da-MYE-sin

Cleocin, Cleocin T, Clinda-Derm, Clindagel, Clindesse, Clindets, Dalacin ✦, Evoclin, Xaciato

Therapeutic class: Antibiotics
Pharmacologic class: Lincomycin derivatives

AVAILABLE FORMS
Foam: 1%
Gel: 1%
Lotion: 1%
Pledget (swab): 1%*
Topical cream: 2%
Topical solution: 1%*
Vaginal cream: 2%
Vaginal gel: 2%
Vaginal suppositories: 100 mg

INDICATIONS & DOSAGES
➤ **Inflammatory acne vulgaris**
Adults and children ages 12 and older: Apply to skin b.i.d., morning and evening, or once daily, as prescribed.
➤ **Bacterial vaginosis**
Adults: 1 applicatorful vaginally at bedtime for 3 to 7 days in patients who aren't pregnant or 7 days in patients who are pregnant, or 1 suppository vaginally at bedtime for 3 days, or 1 applicatorful of Clindesse vaginally as a single dose.
Adults and children ages 12 and older: 1 applicatorful of 2% gel vaginally as a single dose.

ADMINISTRATION
Topical
• Wash area with warm water and soap, rinse, pat dry, and wait 30 minutes after washing or shaving to apply.
• Avoid excessive washing of affected area.
• Apply to entire area, but avoid contact with eyes, nose, mouth, and other mucous membranes.
• Remove pledgets from foil just before use.
• Use pledgets only once and then discard; more than 1 pledget may be used per application.
• If using foam or Clindagel, discontinue use if no improvement occurs after 6 to 8 weeks or if condition worsens.
Vaginal
• Make sure patient knows how to use applicators that come with drug following manufacturer's instructions.

ACTION
Bacteriostatic or bactericidal based on drug level and susceptibility of organism; suppresses growth of susceptible organisms in sebaceous glands by blocking protein synthesis.

Route	Onset	Peak	Duration
Topical, vaginal	Unknown	Unknown	Unknown
Vaginal (2% gel)	Unknown	6 hr	Unknown

Half-life: Topical and vaginal cream, 1.5 to 2.5 hours; vaginal suppositories, 11 hours.

ADVERSE REACTIONS
CNS: headache. **EENT:** pharyngitis. **GI:** constipation. **GU:** vulvovaginal disease, vulvovaginitis, vulvar irritation, vaginal discomfort, vaginal candidiasis, UTI. **Musculoskeletal:** back pain. **Skin:** dryness, redness, burning, irritation, pruritus, swelling, oily skin, exfoliation. **Other:** moniliasis (body).

INTERACTIONS
Drug-drug. *Erythromycin (topical or systemic):* May diminish clindamycin's effect. Avoid use together.
Isotretinoin: May cause cumulative dryness, resulting in excessive skin irritation. Use together cautiously.
Neuromuscular blockers: May increase action of neuromuscular blocker. Use together cautiously.

Reactions in bold italics are *life-threatening*.

Drug-lifestyle. *Abrasive or medicated soaps or cleansers, acne products, or other preparations containing peeling drugs (benzoyl peroxide, resorcinol, salicylic acid, sulfur, tretinoin); alcohol-containing products (aftershave, cosmetics, perfumed toiletries, shaving creams or lotions); astringent soaps or cosmetics; medicated cosmetics or cover-ups:* May cause cumulative dryness, resulting in excessive skin irritation. Urge caution.

EFFECTS ON LAB TEST RESULTS
• May increase liver enzyme levels.

CONTRAINDICATIONS & CAUTIONS
• Contraindicated in patients hypersensitive to clindamycin or lincomycin and in those with history of ulcerative colitis, regional enteritis, or antibiotic-related colitis.
• Intravaginal form can be absorbed systemically and cause CDAD even 2 months after therapy ends.
Dialyzable drug: No.
⚠ *Overdose S&S:* Systemic effects.

PREGNANCY-LACTATION-REPRODUCTION
• Refer to manufacturer's instructions. Recommendations vary by product. Systemic formulations are recommended for use during the first trimester of pregnancy only if clearly needed. Systemic use in second and third trimesters hasn't been associated with increased congenital abnormalities.
• Drug appears in human milk. Use cautiously during breastfeeding. If topical drug is applied to chest, patient should avoid accidental ingestion by the infant.

NURSING CONSIDERATIONS
• For treating acne, drug may be used with tretinoin or benzoyl peroxide as well as systemic antibiotics.
• Drug can cause excessive dryness.
• Topical solution and pledgets contain alcohol base, which may irritate eyes.
• Monitor an older adult for systemic effects.
• Monitor patient for diarrhea.
• Monitor patient for vulvovaginal candidiasis, which may require antifungal treatment in patient receiving vaginal form.

PATIENT TEACHING
• Teach about proper drug administration and handling.

• Tell patient to wash area with warm water and soap, rinse, pat dry, and wait 30 minutes after washing or shaving before applying topically.
• Warn patient to avoid excessive washing of area. Tell patient to cover entire affected area but to avoid contact with eyes, nose, mouth, and other mucous membranes.
• Instruct patient to use other prescribed acne medicines at a different time.
• Teach patient to dab, not roll, applicator-tipped bottle. If tip becomes dry, patient should invert bottle and depress tip several times to moisten.
• Warn patient not to smoke while applying topical solution or foam.
• Advise patient that some vaginal forms contain mineral oil, which can weaken latex or rubber products (condoms, diaphragms), and that patient should use another form of birth control during and within 3 days (Cleocin) or 5 days (Clindesse) of therapy. Polyurethane condoms aren't recommended during or for 7 days after treatment with Xaciato; patient may use latex or polyisoprene condoms.
• Advise patient to avoid sexual intercourse and use of tampons and douches during vaginal treatment.
• Instruct patient to immediately notify prescriber if abdominal pain or diarrhea occurs. Inform patient that an antidiarrheal may worsen condition and should only be used as directed by prescriber.
• Advise patient to complete entire course of therapy.

clobetasol propionate
kloe-BAY-ta-sol

Clobex, Clodan, Dermovate✦, Impeklo, Olux-E, Tovet

Therapeutic class: Corticosteroids
Pharmacologic class: Corticosteroids

AVAILABLE FORMS
Cream: 0.025%, 0.05%
Cream (emollient): 0.05%
Foam: 0.05%*
Gel: 0.05%
Lotion: 0.05%
Ointment: 0.05%
Scalp application: 0.05%*

Shampoo: 0.05%*
Solution: 0.05%*
Spray: 0.05%*

INDICATIONS & DOSAGES

➤ **Short-term topical treatment for moderate to severe plaque-type psoriasis of non-scalp regions, excluding face and intertriginous areas**

Adults: Apply thin layer of lotion or cream to affected areas b.i.d., morning and evening, for up to 14 days. Or, apply spray directly onto affected areas b.i.d. and rub in gently and completely. For localized lesions (less than 10% of BSA) that haven't sufficiently improved, continue treatment for up to 2 more weeks. Total dose shouldn't exceed 50 g (50 mL) weekly.

Adolescents ages 16 and older: Apply thin layer of emollient cream to affected areas b.i.d. and rub in gently and completely. If applied to 5% to 10% of BSA, can be used for up to 4 consecutive weeks. Total dosage shouldn't exceed 50 g (50 mL) weekly.

➤ **Inflammation and pruritus from corticosteroid-responsive dermatoses**

Adults: Apply thin layer of cream, emollient cream, foam, gel, lotion, solution, or ointment to affected areas b.i.d., morning and evening, for maximum of 14 days. Total dose shouldn't exceed 50 g (50 mL) weekly.

Children ages 12 and older: Apply thin layer of cream, emollient cream, foam, gel, solution, or ointment to affected areas b.i.d., morning and evening, for maximum of 14 days. Total dose shouldn't exceed 50 g (50 mL) weekly.

➤ **Short-term topical treatment of mild to moderate plaque-type psoriasis of non-scalp regions, excluding face and intertriginous areas**

Adults and children ages 12 and older: Apply thin layer of foam to affected areas b.i.d., morning and evening, for maximum of 14 days. Total dose shouldn't exceed 50 g (21 capfuls) weekly.

➤ **Inflammation and pruritus of moderate to severe corticosteroid-responsive dermatoses of scalp**

Adults and children ages 12 and older: Apply thin layer of solution to the affected scalp area b.i.d., morning and evening. Massage into affected scalp area gently and completely. Limit treatment to 14 days, with no more than 50 g (50 mL) weekly.

➤ **Moderate to severe scalp psoriasis**

Adults: Apply thin film of shampoo to affected areas of dry scalp once daily. Leave in place for 15 minutes before lathering and rinsing. Limit treatment to 4 consecutive weeks. If complete disease control isn't achieved after 4 weeks, substitute treatment with a less potent topical steroid. Maximum dose, 50 g (50 mL) weekly. Or, apply thin layer of foam to scalp b.i.d. for up to 2 weeks. Maximum dose, 50 g (21 capfuls) weekly.

Children ages 12 and older: Apply thin layer of foam to scalp b.i.d. for up to 2 weeks. Maximum dose, 50 g (21 capfuls) weekly.

ADMINISTRATION
Topical

● Apply the smallest amount that will cover affected area.

● Apply shampoo to dry scalp.

● Gently wash skin before applying. To prevent skin damage, rub medication in gently and completely. When treating hairy sites, part hair and apply directly to lesions.

● To dispense foam, hold can upside down and depress actuator.

● Avoid applying near eyes or mucous membranes or in ear canal.

🕤 *Alert:* Don't use occlusive dressings or bandages. Don't cover or wrap treated areas unless directed by prescriber.

ACTION

Unclear. Diffuses across cell membranes to form complexes with receptors, showing anti-inflammatory, antipruritic, vasoconstrictive, and antiproliferative activity. Considered a very-high-potency to high-potency drug, according to vasoconstrictive properties.

Route	Onset	Peak	Duration
Topical	Unknown	Unknown	Unknown

Half-life: Unknown.

ADVERSE REACTIONS
CNS: headache, finger numbness. **EENT:** nasopharyngitis, streptococcal pharyngitis (spray). **GU:** glycosuria. **Metabolic:** hyperglycemia. **Skin:** burning, pruritus, irritation, dryness, erythema, folliculitis, skin fissure, stinging, perioral dermatitis, allergic contact dermatitis, hypertrichosis, hypopigmentation, acneiform eruptions, eczema, skin atrophy, telangiectasia. **Respiratory:** URI (spray).

Reactions in bold italics are *life-threatening*.

Other: *HPA axis suppression,* Cushing syndrome.

INTERACTIONS
None significant.

EFFECTS ON LAB TEST RESULTS
• May increase serum and urine glucose level.

CONTRAINDICATIONS & CAUTIONS
• Contraindicated in patients hypersensitive to corticosteroids and in those with primary scalp infections (scalp solution only).
• Topical corticosteroids may be absorbed and cause hyperadrenocorticism (Cushing syndrome), hyperglycemia, glycosuria, or suppression of the HPA axis, particularly in younger children and in patients receiving high doses for prolonged periods.
• Rarely, prolonged treatment with corticosteroids is associated with development of Kaposi sarcoma.
• Don't use as monotherapy for primary bacterial infections (impetigo, paronychia, erysipelas, cellulitis, angular cheilitis, erythrasma), rosacea, perioral dermatitis, or acne.
• Don't use very-high-potency or high-potency agents on the face, groin, or axilla areas.
• Drug isn't for ophthalmic use. Avoid contact with eyes as drug may increase risk of posterior subcapsular cataracts and glaucoma.
• Use cautiously in children. Use in children younger than age 12 isn't recommended. Lotion, shampoo, and spray formulations aren't recommended for use in children ages 17 and younger.
Dialyzable drug: Unknown.
⚠ *Overdose S&S:* Systemic effects.

PREGNANCY-LACTATION-REPRODUCTION
• Studies during pregnancy are inadequate. Use during pregnancy only if potential benefit justifies fetal risk. Extensive use during pregnancy isn't recommended.
• It isn't known if drug appears in human milk. Use cautiously during breastfeeding. Avoid direct infant exposure to treated skin.

NURSING CONSIDERATIONS
• If antifungal or antibiotic combined with corticosteroid fails to provide prompt improvement, stop corticosteroid until infection is controlled.

• Stop drug and notify prescriber if skin infection, striae, or atrophy occurs.
• Monitor children closely for HPA axis suppression. Suppression can occur at prescribed doses.

PATIENT TEACHING
• Teach patient how to apply drug, including avoiding contact with eyes and washing hands after application.
• Caution patient to stop drug and report signs of systemic absorption, skin irritation or ulceration, hypersensitivity, or infection.
• Warn patient not to use drug for longer than prescribed.
• Instruct patient to carefully follow manufacturer's instructions for use.
• Advise patient to report any vision changes.
• Instruct patient to inform health care provider if contemplating surgery.
• Tell patient using foam that contents are flammable and under pressure. Instruct patient to avoid smoking during and immediately after application and to keep can away from flames. Also tell patient not to puncture or incinerate container.
• Advise patient to inform prescriber if pregnant or breastfeeding.

SAFETY ALERT!

clonazePAM
kloe-NAZ-e-pam

KlonoPIN

Therapeutic class: Anticonvulsants
Pharmacologic class: Benzodiazepines
Controlled substance schedule: IV

AVAILABLE FORMS
Tablets: 0.5 mg, 1 mg, 2 mg
Tablets (ODTs): 0.125 mg, 0.25 mg, 0.5 mg, 1 mg, 2 mg

INDICATIONS & DOSAGES
➤ **Lennox-Gastaut syndrome, atypical absence seizures, akinetic and myoclonic seizures**
Adults and children older than age 10 or weighing more than 30 kg: Initially, no more than 1.5 mg/day PO in three divided doses. May be increased by 0.5 to 1 mg every 3 days until seizures are controlled or adverse effects

prevent further increases. Maximum recommended daily dose, 20 mg.

Children ages 10 and younger or weighing 30 kg or less: Initially, 0.01 to 0.03 mg/kg PO daily (not to exceed 0.05 mg/kg daily) in two or three divided doses. Increase by 0.25 to 0.5 mg every third day to maximum maintenance dosage of 0.1 to 0.2 mg/kg PO daily divided into three equal doses, as needed.

➤ **Panic disorder**

Adults: Initially, 0.25 mg PO b.i.d. Increase in increments of 0.125 to 0.25 mg b.i.d. every 3 days until panic disorder is controlled, or adverse reactions occur, to target dose of 1 mg daily. Some patients may benefit from dosages up to maximum of 4 mg daily. To achieve 4 mg daily, increase dosage in increments of 0.125 to 0.25 mg b.i.d. every 3 days, as tolerated, until panic disorder is controlled or adverse effects make further increases undesired. Taper drug with decrease of 0.125 mg b.i.d. every 3 days until drug is stopped.

ADMINISTRATION

PO

• Have patient swallow tablets whole with water. Give ODT to patient with or without water.

• Peel back foil of ODT pouch carefully. Don't push ODT through foil.

• Pharmacist can prepare oral suspension from tablets if necessary for younger patients.

• Give one dose at bedtime to reduce the inconvenience of somnolence.

ACTION

Unknown. Probably acts by facilitating the effects of the inhibitory neurotransmitter GABA.

Route	Onset	Peak	Duration
PO	20–40 min	1–4 hr	6–12 hr

Half-life: Adults, 17 to 60 hours; children, 22 to 33 hours; neonates, 22 to 81 hours.

ADVERSE REACTIONS

CNS: amnesia, aphonia, choreiform movements, confusion, depression, emotional lability, drowsiness, fatigue, memory impairment, dysarthria, dysdiadochokinesis, "glassy-eyed" appearance, headache, hemiparesis, hypotonia, hysteria, insomnia, psychosis, slurred speech, tremor, vertigo, paradoxical reactions (aggressive behavior, agitation, anxiety, excitability, hostility, irritability, nervousness, nightmares and vivid dreams, sleep disturbances), fever, ataxia, abnormal coordination, somnolence, dizziness, reduced intellectual ability. **CV:** edema, palpitations. **EENT:** abnormal eye movements, diplopia, nystagmus, blurred vision, pharyngitis, rhinitis, rhinorrhea, sinusitis, coated tongue, dry mouth, sore gums. **GI:** constipation, diarrhea, fecal incontinence, gastritis, nausea, increased or decreased appetite, abdominal pain. **GU:** dysuria, enuresis, nocturia, urine retention, dysmenorrhea, vaginitis, delayed ejaculation, erectile dysfunction, increased or decreased libido, urinary frequency, UTI. **Hematologic:** anemia, eosinophilia, *leukopenia, thrombocytopenia.* **Hepatic:** liver enlargement, transient elevations of serum transaminases and ALP. **Metabolic:** dehydration, weight loss or gain. **Musculoskeletal:** muscle weakness, myalgia. **Respiratory:** chest congestion, hypersecretion in upper respiratory tract passages, respiratory depression, shortness of breath, bronchitis, URI, cough. **Skin:** hair loss, hirsutism, rash. **Other:** hypersensitivity reaction, general deterioration, lymphadenopathy, flulike symptoms.

INTERACTIONS

Drug-drug. *Carbamazepine, phenobarbital:* May lower clonazepam levels. Monitor patient closely.

Clozapine: May increase clozapine-related toxicities. Consider therapy modification.

CNS depressants: May increase CNS depression. Avoid use together.

Digoxin: May increase digoxin level and toxicity. Monitor digoxin level.

Fluconazole, itraconazole, ketoconazole, miconazole: May increase and prolong clonazepam level, CNS depression, and psychomotor impairment. Use together cautiously.

Methadone: May increase CNS depression. Use together cautiously.

Olanzapine: May enhance olanzapine-related toxicity. Avoid use of drug with IM olanzapine due to risks of additive adverse events.

Boxed Warning *Opioids:* May cause slow or difficult breathing, sedation, coma, and death. Avoid use together. If use together can't be avoided, limit dosage and duration of each drug to the minimum needed for desired effect. ■

Reactions in bold italics are *life-threatening*.

Phenytoin: May lower clonazepam level or increase phenytoin level. Monitor serum concentrations of both drugs.

Theophylline: May decrease clonazepam effects. Monitor patient closely.

Valproic acid: May increase clonazepam toxicity and absence status and increase seizure risk and teratogenic effects of both drugs in first trimester. Use cautiously.

Drug-herb. *Kava kava:* May enhance adverse or toxic effects of drug. Use cautiously.

St. John's wort: May decrease clonazepam serum concentration, resulting in decreased drug effects. Consider therapy modification.

Drug-lifestyle. *Alcohol use:* May cause additive CNS effects. Discourage use together.

EFFECTS ON LAB TEST RESULTS
- May increase ALP and transaminase levels.
- May increase eosinophil count.
- May decrease Hb level.
- May decrease platelet and WBC counts.

CONTRAINDICATIONS & CAUTIONS
Boxed Warning *Opioid class warning:* Opioids should only be prescribed with benzodiazepines or other CNS depressants when alternative treatment options are inadequate, aren't expected to provide adequate analgesia, haven't been tolerated, or aren't expected to be tolerated. ∎

Boxed Warning Benzodiazepine use exposes patients to risks of abuse, misuse, and addiction, which can lead to overdose or death. Assess each patient's risk of abuse, misuse, and addiction before prescribing and periodically during therapy. ∎

Boxed Warning Continued use of benzodiazepines, including clonazepam, may lead to clinically significant physical dependence. Risk increases with longer treatment duration and higher daily dose. ∎

Boxed Warning Abrupt discontinuation or rapid dosage reduction of benzodiazepines after continued use may precipitate acute withdrawal reactions, which can be life-threatening. To reduce risk of withdrawal reactions, gradually taper drug to discontinue or reduce dosage. ∎

- Contraindicated in patients hypersensitive to benzodiazepines and in those with significant liver disease or acute angle-closure glaucoma.
- Use cautiously in patients with mixed-type seizures because drug may cause generalized tonic-clonic seizures.

- Use cautiously in children; in patients with chronic respiratory disease, open-angle glaucoma, porphyria, or a history of drug or alcohol addiction; in patients who are debilitated; and in those at risk for falls.
- Use cautiously in older adults. Drug may accumulate due to potential decrease in liver and kidney function.

Dialyzable drug: No.

⚠ *Overdose S&S:* Somnolence, confusion, coma, diminished reflexes.

PREGNANCY-LACTATION-REPRODUCTION
- Drug may cause fetal harm. Use during pregnancy only if clearly needed and potential benefit justifies fetal risk.
- Drug may cause neonatal flaccidity, respiratory and feeding difficulties, and hypothermia in infants born to patients who received benzodiazepines late in pregnancy. In addition, neonates born to patients who received benzodiazepines late in pregnancy may be at some risk for experiencing withdrawal symptoms during the postnatal period.
- Encourage patients who are taking drug during pregnancy to register in the North American Antiepileptic Drug Pregnancy Registry (1-888-233-2334 or www.aedpregnancyregistry.org); patients must register themselves.
- Drug appears in human milk. Patient should discontinue breastfeeding or discontinue drug, considering importance of drug to patient.

NURSING CONSIDERATIONS
⚡ *Alert:* Closely monitor all patients for changes in behavior that may indicate worsening of suicidality or depression.
- Don't stop drug abruptly because doing so may worsen seizures. Notify prescriber at once if adverse reactions develop.
- Closely assess response of older adults, who are more sensitive to drug's CNS effects.
- Monitor patient for oversedation.
- Monitor CBC and LFT values.
- Withdrawal symptoms are similar to those of barbiturates.

Boxed Warning Monitor patient taking an opioid with clonazepam for signs and symptoms of respiratory depression and sedation. ∎
- *Look alike–sound alike:* Don't confuse clonazepam with clonidine, clozapine, or lorazepam. Don't confuse Klonopin with clonidine.

PATIENT TEACHING

Boxed Warning Caution patient that benzodiazepines, even at recommended doses, increase risk of abuse, misuse, and addiction, which can lead to overdose and death, especially when used with other drugs (opioid analgesics), alcohol, or illicit substances. Warn patient or caregiver of patient taking an opioid with a benzodiazepine, CNS depressant, or alcohol to seek immediate medical attention for dizziness, light-headedness, extreme sleepiness, slowed or difficult breathing, or unresponsiveness. ■

Boxed Warning Teach patient signs and symptoms of benzodiazepine abuse, misuse, and addiction (abdominal pain, amnesia, anorexia, anxiety, aggression, ataxia, blurred vision, confusion, depression, disinhibition, disorientation, dizziness, euphoria, impaired concentration and memory, indigestion, irritability, muscle pain, slurred speech, tremors, vertigo, delirium, paranoia, suicidality, seizures, difficulty breathing, coma) and instruct patient to seek emergency medical help if they occur. Demonstrate proper disposal of unused drug. Advise patient not to take drug at a higher dose, more frequently, or for longer than prescribed. ■

Boxed Warning Tell patient that continued use of drug for several days to weeks may lead to physical dependence and that abrupt discontinuation or rapid dosage reduction may precipitate acute withdrawal reactions (unusual movements, responses, or expressions; seizures; sudden and severe mental or nervous system changes; depression; seeing or hearing things that others don't; homicidal thoughts; extreme increase in activity or talking; losing touch with reality; suicidality), which can be life-threatening. Instruct patient that drug discontinuation or dosage reduction may require a slow taper. ■

Boxed Warning Stress the possibility of development of protracted withdrawal syndrome (anxiety; trouble remembering, learning, or concentrating; depression; problems sleeping; feeling like insects are crawling under the skin; weakness; shaking; muscle twitching; burning or prickling feeling in hands, arms, legs, or feet; ringing in ears), with symptoms lasting weeks to more than 12 months. ■

• Advise patient to avoid driving and other hazardous activities that require mental alertness until drug's CNS effects are known.

• Instruct parent to monitor child's school performance because drug may interfere with attentiveness.

• Warn patient and parents not to stop drug abruptly because seizures may occur.

• Caution patient to immediately report pregnancy, plans to become pregnant, breastfeeding, or intent to breastfeed during treatment.

• Teach about proper drug administration and handling.

cloNIDine
KLOE-ni-deen

Catapres-TTS

cloNIDine hydrochloride
Duraclon, Kapvay, Nexiclon XR

Therapeutic class: Antihypertensives
Pharmacologic class: Centrally acting alpha agonists

AVAILABLE FORMS
Injection for epidural use: 100 mcg/mL
Injection for epidural use, concentrate: 500 mcg/mL
Tablets: 0.1 mg, 0.2 mg, 0.3 mg
Tablets (extended-release) **DNC**: 0.1 mg, 0.2 mg
Tablets (scored extended-release): 0.17 mg, 0.26 mg
Transdermal: 0.1 mg/24 hours, 0.2 mg/24 hours, 0.3 mg/24 hours

INDICATIONS & DOSAGES
➤ **HTN**
Adults: Initially, 0.1 mg PO b.i.d.; then increase by 0.1 mg daily on a weekly basis. Usual range is 0.2 to 0.6 mg daily in divided doses; rarely, dosages as high as 2.4 mg daily are used. Or, 0.17 mg Nexiclon XR PO daily; then increase by 0.09 mg daily on a weekly basis. Doses higher than 0.52 mg daily not recommend.

Or, apply transdermal patch once every 7 days, starting with 0.1-mg system and adjusting with another 0.1-mg or larger system after 1 or 2 weeks if desired BP reduction isn't achieved. Don't exceed concurrent use of two clonidine 0.3-mg systems.

Adjust-a-dose: Consider a lower initial dose and slower titration in older adults and patients with kidney impairment. In patients with CKD on KRT, initially 0.09 mg Nexiclon XR PO daily; then titrate as tolerated.

➤ **Severe cancer pain that is unresponsive to opiate analgesia alone**
Adults: Initially, 30 mcg/hour by continuous epidural infusion. Cautiously adjust dosage according to response and tolerance. Experience with rates greater than 40 mcg/hour is limited.
Children old enough to tolerate placement and management of an epidural catheter: Initially, 0.5 mcg/kg/hour by epidural infusion. Dosage should be cautiously adjusted, based on response and tolerance.
Adjust-a-dose: Decrease dosage in patients with kidney impairment.

➤ **ADHD as monotherapy or as adjunctive therapy to stimulant medications**
Children ages 6 to 17: Initially, 0.1 mg extended-release tablet (Kapvay) PO at bedtime. Adjust by 0.1 mg/day at weekly intervals to desired response. With first dosage increase, give tablets b.i.d., with equal or higher dose given at bedtime. Maximum dose, 0.4 mg/day.

ADMINISTRATION
PO
• Don't crush, break, or allow patient to chew extended-release tablets except Nexiclon XR tablets, which are scored to be broken.
• Immediate- and extended-release forms can't be substituted on a milligram-per-milligram basis.
• Give initial extended-release dose at bedtime.
• Give last dose immediately before bedtime.
• Skip a missed extended-release dose and give the next dose as scheduled.
• Reduce dosage gradually over 2 to 4 days before discontinuing. Decrease dosage of extended-release form by no more than 0.1 mg every 3 to 7 days.
Transdermal
• Apply patch to nonhairy area of intact skin on upper arm or torso. Apply each new patch to different site than previous site.
• If patch loosens during the 7-day period, apply an adhesive cover and ensure good adhesion.
• When converting from oral to patch form, place patch on patient and gradually decrease oral dose over several days. Antihypertensive effect of patch takes 2 to 3 days to appear.
Epidural
Boxed Warning The injection form concentrate, containing 500 mcg/mL, must be diluted in NSS injection before use to yield 100 mcg/mL. ∎

◑ Alert: The injection form must not be used with a preservative.

ACTION
Unknown. Thought to stimulate alpha$_2$ receptors and inhibit the central vasomotor centers, decreasing sympathetic outflow to the heart, kidneys, and peripheral vasculature and lowering peripheral vascular resistance, BP, and HR.

Route	Onset	Peak	Duration
PO (immediate-release)	30–60 min	1–3 hr	6–10 hr
PO (extended-release)	1–2 wk	7–8 hr	Unknown
Transdermal	2–3 days	3 days	7 days
Epidural	Unknown	30–60 min	Unknown

Half-life: Immediate- and extended-release, 12 to 16 hours; transdermal, 20 hours; epidural, 1 to 2 hours (in CSF).

ADVERSE REACTIONS
CNS: drowsiness, dizziness, confusion, lethargy, sedation, fatigue, irritability, malaise, hallucinations, agitation, depression, nightmares, night terrors, restless sleep, emotional disorder, aggression, tearfulness, headache, insomnia, tremor, somnolence, nervousness, taste alteration. **CV:** *bradycardia,* chest pain, edema, hypotension, orthostatic hypotension, tachycardia. **EENT:** otitis media, tinnitus, nasal congestion, sore throat, dry mouth. **GI:** constipation, nausea, vomiting, anorexia, abdominal pain, viral GI infection. **GU:** enuresis, nocturia, urine retention, erectile dysfunction, loss of libido. **Metabolic:** weight gain. **Musculoskeletal:** myalgia, arthralgia, weakness. **Respiratory:** hypoventilation. **Skin:** pruritus; dermatitis; burning sensation, contact allergy, or localized blanching with transdermal patch; hyperpigmentation; diaphoresis; rash. **Other:** withdrawal syndrome, gynecomastia.

INTERACTIONS
Drug-drug. *Amitriptyline, amoxapine, other TCAs:* May decrease antihypertensive effect of clonidine. Avoid use together.
Beta blockers: May increase risk of sinus node dysfunction. May increase rebound HTN if clonidine is withdrawn abruptly. Use together cautiously and closely monitor BP.

Calcium channel blockers (verapamil), digoxin: May cause AV block and severe hypotension. Monitor BP and ECG.

CNS depressants (barbiturates, cannabinoid-containing products, opioids): May increase CNS depression. Use together cautiously.

Diuretics, other antihypertensives: May increase hypotensive effect. Monitor patient closely.

Levodopa: May increase hypotensive effects. Monitor patient.

Drug-herb. *Capsicum:* May reduce antihypertensive effectiveness. Discourage use together.

Ma huang: May decrease antihypertensive effects. Discourage use together.

Drug-lifestyle. *Alcohol use:* May increase CNS depression and clonidine level. Discourage use together.

EFFECTS ON LAB TEST RESULTS
• None.

CONTRAINDICATIONS & CAUTIONS
• Contraindicated in patients hypersensitive to drug.

Boxed Warning Epidural clonidine isn't recommended for obstetric, postpartum, or perioperative pain management due to the risk of hemodynamic instability, especially hypotension and bradycardia, except in rare cases in which the potential benefits outweigh the risks. ■

• Transdermal form is contraindicated in patients hypersensitive to any component of the adhesive layer of transdermal system.

• Epidural form is contraindicated in patients receiving anticoagulant therapy, in those with bleeding diathesis, in those with an injection-site infection, and for use above the C4 dermatome. Use isn't recommended in those who are hemodynamically unstable or have severe CV disease.

• Use cautiously in patients with severe coronary insufficiency, conduction disturbances, recent MI, cerebrovascular disease, CKD, or impaired liver function.

• Safety and effectiveness in children for HTN haven't been established in adequate and well-controlled trials.

Dialyzable drug: Minimal.

⚠ *Overdose S&S:* Early HTN, then hypotension; bradycardia; respiratory and CNS depression; hypothermia; drowsiness; decreased or absent reflexes; weakness; irritability;

miosis. *With large overdoses:* Reversible cardiac conduction defects or arrhythmias, apnea, coma, seizures.

PREGNANCY-LACTATION-REPRODUCTION
• Studies during pregnancy are inadequate. Drug crosses the placental barrier. Use during pregnancy only if clearly needed.

• Register patient exposed to ADHD medications during pregnancy in the National Pregnancy Registry for ADHD Medications (1-866-961-2388 or https://womensmentalhealth.org/adhd-medications/).

• Drug appears in human milk. Use cautiously during breastfeeding; monitor infant for sedation, lethargy, tachypnea, and poor feeding.

NURSING CONSIDERATIONS
• Drug may be given to rapidly lower BP in some hypertensive emergencies.

• Frequently monitor BP and pulse rate. Dosage is usually adjusted to patient's BP and tolerance.

• Observe patient for tolerance to drug's therapeutic effects, which may require increased dosage.

🔵 *Alert:* Remove transdermal patch before defibrillation or cardioversion to prevent arcing.

• Stop drug gradually to avoid rapid rebound in BP, agitation, headache, and tremor. When stopping therapy in patient receiving both clonidine and a beta blocker, gradually withdraw beta blocker several days before gradually stopping clonidine to minimize adverse reactions.

• Don't stop drug before surgery because of risk of rebound HTN from abrupt withdrawal. Withhold immediate-release forms within 4 hours of surgery and restart as soon as possible afterward. May give Nexiclon XR up to 28 hours before surgery and resume the following day. Consider transitioning to transdermal patch at least 3 days before surgery if patients aren't expected to resume PO medications within 12 hours of surgery.

• When drug is given epidurally, carefully monitor infusion pump and inspect catheter tubing for obstruction or dislodgment.

• *Look alike–sound alike:* Don't confuse clonidine with clonazepam, clozapine, Klonopin, quinidine, or clomiphene.

Reactions in bold italics are *life-threatening*.

C

PATIENT TEACHING
• Instruct patient to take drug exactly as prescribed and to report adverse reactions.
• Advise patient that abruptly stopping drug may cause severe rebound HTN; dosage must be reduced gradually as instructed by prescriber.
• Tell patient to take the last dose of the day immediately before bedtime.
• Reassure patient that the transdermal patch usually remains attached despite showering and other routine daily activities. Instruct patient on use of the adhesive overlay to provide additional skin adherence, if needed. Also tell patient to place patch at a different site each week.
• Caution patient that drug may cause drowsiness but that this adverse effect usually diminishes over 4 to 6 weeks.
• Inform patient that dizziness upon standing can be minimized by rising slowly from a sitting or lying position and avoiding sudden position changes.
• If an MRI is scheduled, advise patient to alert the facility about wearing a transdermal patch.
• Instruct patient to immediately report pregnancy, plans to become pregnant, breastfeeding, or intent to breastfeed during treatment.

clopidogrel bisulfate ▓
cloe-PID-oh-grel

Plavix

Therapeutic class: Antiplatelet drugs
Pharmacologic class: Platelet aggregation inhibitors

AVAILABLE FORMS
Tablets: 75 mg, 300 mg

INDICATIONS & DOSAGES
➤ **To reduce rate of MI and stroke in patients with established peripheral arterial disease or history of recent MI or stroke**
Adults: 75 mg PO daily.
➤ **Acute coronary syndrome to reduce rate of MI and stroke**
Adults: Initially, a single 300-mg PO loading dose; then 75 mg PO once daily. Clopidogrel should be given with aspirin. Initiating clopidogrel without a loading dose delays (by several days) antiplatelet effects.

ADMINISTRATION
PO
• Give drug without regard to meals.

ACTION
Inhibits the binding of the P2Y$_{12}$ component of ADP to its platelet receptor, impeding ADP-mediated activation and subsequent platelet aggregation, and irreversibly modifies the platelet ADP receptor.

Route	Onset	Peak	Duration
PO	2 hr	45 min	5 days

Half-life: 6 hours.

ADVERSE REACTIONS
CV: hematoma, *hemorrhage.* **EENT:** epistaxis. **Other:** hypersensitivity reactions.

INTERACTIONS
Drug-drug. *Apixaban, dabigatran, edoxaban, rivaroxaban:* May increase risk of bleeding. Use together cautiously.
Aspirin, NSAIDs: May increase risk of GI bleeding. Monitor patient.
CYP2C19 inducers (rifamycins): May increase antiplatelet effect and risk of bleeding. Avoid use together. If use is necessary, carefully monitor platelet function when starting, stopping, or changing rifamycin dosage. Adjust clopidogrel dosage as needed.
CYP2C8 substrates (repaglinide): May increase substrate level. Avoid use together or adjust substrate dosage and monitor patient closely.
Opioids: May delay and reduce clopidogrel absorption. Consider parenteral antiplatelet agents in patients with ACS requiring opioids.
SNRIs, SSRIs: May increase bleeding risk. Use together cautiously.
Strong or moderate CYP2C19 inhibitors (cimetidine, esomeprazole, etravirine, felbamate, fluconazole, ketoconazole, omeprazole, ticlopidine, voriconazole), PPIs: May decrease effects of clopidogrel. Avoid use together.
Warfarin: May increase risk of bleeding. Use together cautiously.
Drug-herb. *Herbs with antiplatelet activity (capsicum, fenugreek, garlic, ginkgo biloba, turmeric, many others):* May increase risk of bleeding. Discourage use together.
Drug-food. *Grapefruit, grapefruit juice:* May reduce drug's antiplatelet effects. Avoid use together.

EFFECTS ON LAB TEST RESULTS
• May increase LFT values and creatinine level.
• May decrease Hb level and platelet and granulocyte counts.

CONTRAINDICATIONS & CAUTIONS
• Contraindicated in patients hypersensitive to drug or its components, in those with a history of hypersensitivity or hematologic reaction to other thienopyridines, and in those with pathologic bleeding (such as peptic ulcer or intracranial hemorrhage).
• Hypersensitivity reactions (rash, angioedema, hematologic reactions) have been reported, including in patients hypersensitive to other thienopyridines.
• Drug has shown to be effective in patients with unstable angina and non-ST-elevation MI (NSTEMI), including those managed medically and those managed with coronary revascularization, and in patients with acute ST-elevation MI (STEMI) who are to be managed medically.
• Consider discontinuing drug 5 days before elective surgery, including elective CABG, except in patients with cardiac stents who haven't completed the full course of dual antiplatelet therapy; discuss patient-specific situations with cardiologist. Platelet aggregation won't return to normal for at least 5 days after drug has been stopped.
• Premature interruption of therapy may result in stent thrombosis with subsequent fatal or nonfatal MI. Duration of therapy, in general, is determined by type of stent placed (bare metal or drug eluting) and whether an ACS event was ongoing at time of placement.
• Use cautiously in patients at risk for increased bleeding from trauma, surgery, or other pathologic conditions and in those with kidney or liver impairment.
Dialyzable drug: Unknown.
⚠ *Overdose S&S:* Prolonged bleeding time, bleeding complications.

PREGNANCY-LACTATION-REPRODUCTION
• Information related to use during pregnancy is limited. Use cautiously during pregnancy and only if clearly needed.
• It isn't known if drug appears in human milk. Drug is present in animal milk. Patient should discontinue breastfeeding or discontinue drug, considering importance of drug to patient.

NURSING CONSIDERATIONS
🗶 **Boxed Warning** Drug effectiveness depends on the drug's activation to an active metabolite by the cytochrome P450 system, principally CYP2C19. Patients who are poor metabolizers form less of the active metabolite and the effects of the drug on platelet activity are reduced. Tests are available to assess a patient's CYP2C19 genotype. Consider alternative treatment for patients identified as poor metabolizers. ∎
🗶 Approximately 2% of White patients and 4% of Black patients are poor metabolizers of CYP2C19; prevalence is higher in patients of Asian descent (14% of patients of Chinese descent).
🔆 *Alert:* Drug may cause life-threatening thrombotic thrombocytopenic purpura (thrombocytopenia, hemolytic anemia, neurologic findings, kidney dysfunction, fever) that requires urgent treatment, including plasmapheresis.
• *Look alike–sound alike:* Don't confuse Plavix with Paxil.

PATIENT TEACHING
• Advise patient that it may take longer than usual to stop bleeding and to refrain from activities in which trauma and bleeding may occur. Encourage patient to wear a seat belt when in a car.
• Instruct patient to notify prescriber if unusual bleeding or bruising occurs.
• Tell patient to inform all health care providers, including dentists, before undergoing procedures or starting new drug therapy about taking drug.
• Caution patient not to stop drug without first discussing with prescriber.
• Caution patient to immediately report pregnancy, plans to become pregnant, breastfeeding, or intent to breastfeed during treatment.

clotrimazole
kloe-TRIM-a-zole

Alvazol ◇, Canesten✳,
Clotrimaderm✳, Gyne-Lotrimin ◇,
Lotrimin ◇

Therapeutic class: Antifungals
Pharmacologic class: Imidazole derivatives

AVAILABLE FORMS
Topical cream: 1% ◇
Topical foam: 1% ◇
Topical ointment: 1% ◇
Topical solution: 1% ◇
Troches (lozenges) ⓓⓝⓒ: 10 mg
Vaginal cream: 1% ◇, 2% ◇
Vaginal tablets: 200 mg❧ ◇, 500 mg❧ ◇

INDICATIONS & DOSAGES
➤ **Superficial fungal infections (tinea corporis, tinea cruris, tinea pedis, tinea versicolor, candidiasis)**
Adults and children ages 2 and older: Apply thin film and massage into affected and surrounding area b.i.d., morning and evening, for 2 to 4 weeks, or as directed by prescriber. Continue treatment of tinea pedis until 1 week after clinical resolution. If improvement doesn't occur after 2 to 4 weeks, reevaluate patient.
➤ **Vulvovaginal candidiasis**
Adults and children ages 12 and older: 1 applicatorful of vaginal cream daily at bedtime for 3 days (2%) or 7 days (1%). A small amount of cream may be applied to opening of vagina for additional relief of external symptoms. Or, one 500-mg vaginal tablet at bedtime for 1 dose or one 200-mg vaginal tablet at bedtime for 3 days.
➤ **Oropharyngeal candidiasis**
Adults and children ages 3 and older: 1 lozenge dissolved in mouth over 15 to 30 minutes five times daily for 14 consecutive days.
➤ **To prevent oropharyngeal candidiasis in patients immunocompromised by chemotherapy, radiotherapy, or corticosteroid therapy in the treatment of leukemia, solid tumors, or kidney transplantation**
Adults: 1 lozenge dissolved in mouth over 15 to 30 minutes t.i.d. for duration of chemotherapy or until corticosteroid is reduced to maintenance levels.

ADMINISTRATION
PO
• Lozenges should dissolve in mouth, and not be chewed, for full benefit.
Topical
• Clean and dry area before applying drug.
• Don't use occlusive wrappings or dressings.
Vaginal
• If applicator for cream isn't disposable, wash applicator with soap and warm water immediately after use. Rinse thoroughly and dry.

• Use applicator supplied with vaginal tablet to ensure placement high in the vagina.

ACTION
Fungistatic or fungicidal, depending on drug level. Alters fungal cell-wall permeability and produces osmotic instability.

Route	Onset	Peak	Duration
PO	Unknown	Unknown	3 hr
Topical, vaginal	Unknown	Unknown	Unknown

Half-life: Unknown.

ADVERSE REACTIONS
GI: lower abdominal cramps, nausea and vomiting (lozenges). **GU:** mild vaginal burning or irritation, urinary frequency. **Hepatic:** elevated AST level (lozenges). **Skin:** erythema, blistering, burning, edema, general irritation, peeling, pruritus, skin fissures, stinging, urticaria.

INTERACTIONS
Drug-drug. *Sirolimus, tacrolimus:* May increase level of these drugs when used with vaginal clotrimazole. Monitor patient.

EFFECTS ON LAB TEST RESULTS
• May increase liver enzyme levels.

CONTRAINDICATIONS & CAUTIONS
• Contraindicated in patients hypersensitive to drug.
• Contraindicated for ophthalmic use.
Dialyzable drug: Unknown.

PREGNANCY-LACTATION-REPRODUCTION
• Studies during pregnancy are inadequate. Use lozenges during pregnancy only if potential benefit justifies fetal risk.
• Use topical clotrimazole during first trimester only if clearly indicated.
• Manual insertion may be preferred over use of vaginal applicator during pregnancy. Use only on advice of physician.
• It's unknown if drug appears in human milk. Patient should consider discontinuing breastfeeding.

NURSING CONSIDERATIONS
• Consult prescriber before using topical preparations in children younger than age 2. Don't use troches in children younger than age 3. Don't use vaginal preparations in children younger than age 12.

• Watch for irritation and sensitivity; stop drug and notify prescriber if irritation occurs.
• Improvement of topical conditions usually occurs within 1 week; if no improvement occurs within 2 to 4 weeks, review diagnosis.

PATIENT TEACHING
• Reassure patient that hypopigmentation from tinea versicolor will resolve gradually.
• Warn patient not to use occlusive wrappings or dressings.
• Warn patient to avoid contact with eyes.
• Caution patient that frequent or persistent yeast infections may suggest a more serious medical problem.
• Tell patient to refrain from sexual intercourse during vaginal treatment.
• Warn patient that topical preparation may stain clothing.
• Tell patient that using a sanitary napkin protects clothing when using vaginal preparation.
• Stress need to continue use of vaginal preparations, as prescribed, even if menstruation begins.
• Tell patient with athlete's foot to change shoes and cotton socks daily and to dry between the toes after bathing.
• Instruct patient to allow lozenges to dissolve in mouth and not to chew them, for full benefit.
• Stress the need to continue treatment for full course and to notify prescriber if no improvement occurs after 2 to 4 weeks.

SAFETY ALERT!

cloZAPine §
KLOE-za-peen

Clozaril, Versacloz

Therapeutic class: Antipsychotics
Pharmacologic class: Dibenzapine derivatives

AVAILABLE FORMS
Oral suspension: 50 mg/mL
Tablets: 25 mg, 50 mg, 100 mg, 200 mg
Tablets (ODTs): 12.5 mg, 25 mg, 100 mg, 150 mg, 200 mg

INDICATIONS & DOSAGES
➤ **Treatment-resistant schizophrenia; to reduce risk of recurrent suicidality in schizophrenia or schizoaffective disorders**

Adults: Initially, 12.5 mg PO once daily or b.i.d. Adjust dose upward by 25 to 50 mg daily (if tolerated) to 300 to 450 mg daily in one to three doses by end of 2 weeks. Individual dosage is based on clinical response, patient tolerance, and adverse reactions. Subsequent dosage shouldn't be increased more than once or twice weekly and shouldn't exceed 100-mg increments. Don't exceed 900 mg daily.

§ For the general population, if ANC is 1,500/mm³ or greater (normal baseline range), treatment may be initiated. Confirm all initial reports of ANC less than 1,500/mm³ with a repeat ANC within 24 hours. For patients with benign ethnic neutropenia (BEN), obtain two baseline ANC levels before initiating treatment (normal ANC range for those with BEN is 1,000/mm³ or greater). For patients with BEN, if ANC is 1,000/mm³ or greater, treatment may be initiated

§ *Adjust-a-dose:* Refer to manufacturer's instructions for ANC monitoring and dosage interruption for neutropenia and for concurrent use with CYP1A2, CYP2D6, or CYP3A4 inhibitors or CYP1A2 or CYP3A4 inducers. Reduce dosages in those with significant kidney or liver impairment and in those who are poor metabolizers of CYP2D6.

In older adults, start with 12.5 mg once daily for 3 days; then increase to 25 mg once daily for 3 days as tolerated. May further increase, as tolerated, in increments of 12.5 to 25 mg daily every 3 days to desired response, up to 700 mg/day (mean dose is 300 mg/day).

Discontinue drug in patients with QT interval greater than 500 msec, those with symptoms of ventricular arrhythmias, and those with cardiomyopathy, myocarditis, or NMS.

When restarting drug in patients who have discontinued clozapine for 2 days or more, reinitiate at 12.5 mg once daily or b.i.d. to minimize risk of hypotension, bradycardia, and syncope. If that dose is well tolerated, may increase dose to the previously therapeutic dose more quickly than recommended for initial treatment.

ADMINISTRATION
PO
• Give drug with or without food.
• May divide total daily dose into uneven doses, with larger dose given at bedtime.

• Peel foil from ODT blister and gently remove tablet immediately before giving. Don't push tablet through foil.
• Give ODT with or without water.
• Shake bottle for 10 seconds before withdrawing suspension using provided oral syringe and syringe adaptor.
• If patient has missed more than 2 days of treatment, restart drug at 12.5 mg once daily or b.i.d. and retitrate. May titrate more quickly than initial treatment, if tolerated.

ACTION
Unknown. Binds selectively to dopaminergic receptors in the CNS and may interfere with adrenergic, cholinergic, histaminergic, and serotonergic receptors.

Route	Onset	Peak	Duration
PO	Unknown	1–6 hr	4–12 hr

Half-life: Proportional to dose; may range from 4 to 66 hours.

ADVERSE REACTIONS
CNS: drowsiness, sedation, dizziness, vertigo, headache, *seizures,* syncope, tremor, disturbed sleep or nightmares, restlessness, hypokinesia or akinesia, agitation, rigidity, akathisia, confusion, fatigue, insomnia, lethargy, ataxia, slurred speech, depression, myoclonus, anxiety, fever. **CV:** tachycardia, hypotension, HTN, chest pain, ECG changes, orthostatic hypotension. **EENT:** visual disturbances, hypersalivation, dry mouth. **GI:** constipation, nausea, vomiting, heartburn, diarrhea. **GU:** urinary frequency or urgency, urine retention, incontinence, abnormal ejaculation. **Hematologic:** *leukopenia, neutropenia,* eosinophilia. **Metabolic:** hyperglycemia, weight gain, hypercholesterolemia, hypertriglyceridemia. **Musculoskeletal:** hypokinesia, muscle rigidity, muscle weakness. **Skin:** rash, diaphoresis.

INTERACTIONS
Drug-drug. *Anticholinergics (benztropine, diphenhydramine):* May potentiate anticholinergic effects of clozapine. Use together cautiously.
Antihypertensives: May potentiate hypotensive effects. Monitor BP.
☣ *Alert: Benzodiazepines other psychotropic drugs:* May increase risk of sedation and CV and respiratory arrest. Use together cautiously.

Bone marrow suppressants: May increase bone marrow toxicity. Avoid use together.
CYP2D6 or CYP3A4 inhibitors (bupropion, cimetidine, duloxetine, erythromycin, escitalopram, fluoxetine, paroxetine, quinidine, sertraline, terbinafine); moderate or weak CYP1A2 inhibitors (caffeine, oral contraceptives): Monitor patient for adverse reactions. Reduce clozapine oral dosage if necessary.
CYP2D6 substrates (carbamazepine, flecainide, phenothiazines, propafenone): May increase substrate level. Use together cautiously.
Digoxin, other highly protein-bound drugs, warfarin: May increase levels of these drugs. Monitor patient closely for adverse reactions.
Drugs that prolong the QT interval (antiarrhythmics, citalopram, ziprasidone): May increase risk of prolonged QT interval and ventricular arrhythmias. Avoid use together.
Opioid class warning: May cause slow or difficult breathing, sedation, and death. Avoid use together. If use together can't be avoided, limit dosage and duration of each drug to the minimum needed for desired effect.
Psychoactive drugs: May cause additive effects. Use together cautiously.
Strong CYP3A4 inducers (carbamazepine, phenytoin, rifampin): May decrease clozapine effectiveness. Use together isn't recommended. If coadministration is necessary, consider increasing clozapine dosage.
Strong CYP1A2 inhibitors (ciprofloxacin, fluvoxamine): May increase clozapine level. Reduce clozapine dosage to one-third during coadministration.
Drug-herb. *St. John's wort:* May decrease clozapine level. Discourage use together.
Drug-lifestyle. *Alcohol use:* May increase CNS depression. Discourage use together.
Smoking: May decrease drug level. Urge patient to quit smoking. Monitor patient for effectiveness and adjust dosage.

EFFECTS ON LAB TEST RESULTS
• May increase glucose, cholesterol, and triglyceride levels.
• May increase eosinophil count.
• May decrease granulocyte and WBC counts and ANC.

CONTRAINDICATIONS & CAUTIONS
Boxed Warning Because of risk of severe neutropenia, which can lead to fatal

infections, drug is available only through the Clozapine REMS Program. ∎

• *Opioid class warning:* Opioids should only be prescribed with benzodiazepines or other CNS depressants when alternative treatment options are inadequate, aren't expected to provide adequate analgesia, haven't been tolerated, or aren't expected to be tolerated.

• Contraindicated in patients with history of serious hypersensitivity to drug or its components, in patients who experienced clozapine-induced agranulocytosis or severe granulocytopenia, and in patients with uncontrolled epilepsy.

• Closely monitor patients taking other drugs that suppress bone marrow function.

• Use cautiously in patients with prostatic hyperplasia or angle-closure glaucoma because drug has potent anticholinergic effects. Severe GI reactions (constipation, intestinal obstruction, fecal impaction, paralytic ileus) can also occur.

Boxed Warning Fatal myocarditis and cardiomyopathy may occur at any time during treatment. If signs or symptoms (chest pain, tachycardia, palpitations, dyspnea, fever, flulike symptoms, hypotension, ECG changes) occur, obtain a cardiac evaluation and discontinue drug. Generally, patients with clozapine-related myocarditis or cardiomyopathy shouldn't be re-challenged with the drug. ∎

• Eosinophilia associated with organ involvement (myocarditis, pancreatitis, hepatitis, colitis, nephritis) frequently develops during first month of treatment. If eosinophilia develops, evaluate for systemic reactions and, if clozapine-related disease is suspected, immediately discontinue drug. If clozapine isn't the cause, treat underlying cause before continuing clozapine.

• Drug may cause QT-interval prolongation and life-threatening ventricular arrhythmias. Use caution in those with risk factors for QT-interval prolongation or serious CV reactions and in those taking drugs known to prolong QT interval. Consider obtaining baseline ECG and serum chemistry panel, and correct electrolyte abnormalities before starting treatment. Discontinue clozapine if QTc interval is greater than 500 msec. Obtain cardiac evaluation and discontinue drug if patient has symptoms of torsades de pointes or other arrhythmias (syncope, presyncope, dizziness, palpitations).

• Drug can cause NMS, which can be fatal. If signs and symptoms of NMS (hyperpyrexia, muscle rigidity, altered mental status, irregular pulse, fluctuating BP, tachycardia, diaphoresis, cardiac arrhythmias, elevated CK level, myoglobinuria, rhabdomyolysis, AKI) occur, discontinue drug and begin appropriate treatment and monitoring.

• Tardive dyskinesia (TD), a syndrome of potentially irreversible, involuntary dyskinetic movements, has occurred in patients taking antipsychotics. Use the lowest effective dosage for the shortest duration possible. Consider discontinuing drug if TD occurs. (*Note:* Some patients require treatment despite TD.)

• Somnolence, orthostatic hypotension, and motor and sensory instability have been reported, which may lead to falls and, consequently, fractures and other fall-related injuries.

• Older adults may have an increased sensitivity to anticholinergic effects of drug; sedating effects of drug may increase the risk of falls in this population.

Boxed Warning Drug isn't indicated for use in older adults with dementia-related psychoses because of an increased risk of death from CV disease or infection. ∎

• Safe and effective use in children hasn't been established.

Dialyzable drug: No.

⚠ *Overdose S&S:* Altered state of consciousness, drowsiness, delirium, coma, tachycardia, hypotension, respiratory depression or failure, hypersalivation, aspiration pneumonia, cardiac arrhythmias, seizures.

PREGNANCY-LACTATION-REPRODUCTION
• Studies during pregnancy are inadequate. Use during pregnancy only if clearly needed and potential benefit justifies fetal risk.

⚠ *Alert:* Neonates exposed to antipsychotics during the third trimester are at risk for developing extrapyramidal signs and symptoms (repetitive muscle movements of face and body) and withdrawal symptoms (agitation, abnormally increased or decreased muscle tone, tremors, sleepiness, severe difficulty breathing, and difficulty feeding) after delivery.

• Drug appears in human milk. Patient shouldn't breastfeed during therapy.

Reactions in bold italics are *life-threatening*.

C

NURSING CONSIDERATIONS

☼ Alert: Drug may cause hyperglycemia. Regularly monitor patient with diabetes. In patient with risk factors for diabetes, obtain fasting blood glucose test results at baseline and periodically.

☼ Alert: Monitor patient for signs and symptoms of metabolic syndrome (significant weight gain, increased BMI, HTN, hyperglycemia, hypercholesterolemia, and hypertriglyceridemia).

• Monitor for signs and symptoms of liver toxicity (fatigue, anorexia, nausea, jaundice, bilirubinemia, coagulopathy). Regularly evaluate LFT values during therapy.

• Monitor for signs and symptoms of myocarditis and cardiomyopathy.

• Monitor for anticholinergic effects, including constipation and urine retention.

Boxed Warning Monitor patient for neutropenia. Obtain ANC before and regularly during treatment to continue treatment. ■

Boxed Warning Orthostatic hypotension, syncope, bradycardia, and cardiac arrest can occur. Orthostatic hypotension is more likely to occur during initial titration with rapid dose escalation and can occur with the first dose and with doses as low as 12.5 mg. Start treatment with 12.5 mg once daily or b.i.d. and titrate slowly using divided dosages. Use cautiously in patient with CV or cerebrovascular disease or a condition that may cause hypotension. ■

Boxed Warning Seizures may occur, especially in patient receiving high doses. Begin treatment at 12.5 mg, titrate gradually, and use divided dosing. Use caution with patient with a history of seizures or risk factors for seizures (CNS pathology, drugs that lower seizure threshold, alcohol abuse). ■

• Some patients experience transient fever with temperature higher than 100.4° F (38° C), especially in the first 3 weeks of therapy. Monitor such a patient closely.

☼ Alert: Fever may be the first sign of neutropenic infection. Interrupt therapy and obtain ANC level in patient who develops fever (temperature of 101.3° F [38.5° C]). If fever occurs in patient with ANC less than 1,000/mm³, initiate appropriate workup and treatment and appropriately monitor and manage patient.

☒ If drug is to be discontinued and patient doesn't have moderate to severe neutropenia, gradually reduce dose over 1 to 2 weeks.

To abruptly discontinue drug for a reason unrelated to neutropenia, continue to monitor ANC until it is 1,500/mm³ or greater (for the general population) or until ANC is 1,000/mm³ or greater or above patient's baseline (for those with BEN).

• If patient reports onset of fever (temperature 101.3° F or greater) while discontinuing drug, continue to monitor ANC for an additional 2 weeks after discontinuation of drug.

• When discontinuing drug, carefully monitor patient for recurrence of psychotic symptoms and symptoms related to cholinergic rebound (diaphoresis, headache, nausea, vomiting, diarrhea).

• PE and DVT have occurred in patients taking clozapine. It isn't known whether these effects can be attributed to the drug or to some other patient characteristic. Monitor for PE if patient develops DVT, acute dyspnea, chest pain, or other respiratory signs and symptoms.

• Drug can cause sedation and impair cognitive and motor performance. Carefully monitor patient for CNS changes.

• Assess fall risk when initiating therapy and recurrently for patient on long-term therapy, especially an older adult or patient who has a disease or condition that could exacerbate fall risk.

☼ Look alike–sound alike: Don't confuse clozapine with clonidine, clonazepam, or Klonopin. Don't confuse Clozaril with Colazal.

PATIENT TEACHING

Boxed Warning Tell patient about need for regular blood tests to check for low ANC. Advise patient to report flulike symptoms, fever, sore throat, lethargy, weakness, malaise, or other signs of neutropenia or infection. ■

Boxed Warning Warn patient taking drug to avoid hazardous activities that require alertness and good coordination and during which sudden loss of consciousness and falls could cause serious risk to patient or others. ■

• Tell patient to check with prescriber before taking alcohol or OTC drugs.

• Advise patient that smoking may decrease drug effectiveness.

• Caution patient to rise slowly to avoid dizziness and to immediately report feeling faintness, loss of consciousness, or irregular or slow heartbeat.

• Inform patient that drug may cause somnolence, orthostatic hypotension, and motor and sensory instability, which may lead to falls and, consequently, fractures or other injuries.
• Teach about proper drug administration and handling.
• Inform patient about risk of metabolic changes, seizures, and TD.

SAFETY ALERT!

codeine phosphate–acetaminophen ▨
koe-DEEN/a-seet-a-MIN-a-fen

Therapeutic class: Opioid analgesics
Pharmacologic class: Opioids–para-aminophenol derivatives
Controlled substance schedule: III (tablets); V (liquid)

AVAILABLE FORMS
Oral solution: 12 mg codeine and 120 mg acetaminophen/5 mL*
Tablets: 15 mg codeine and 300 mg acetaminophen, 30 mg codeine and 300 mg acetaminophen, 60 mg codeine and 300 mg acetaminophen

INDICATIONS & DOSAGES
➤ **Mild to moderately severe pain**
Adults: Codeine 15 to 60 mg and acetaminophen 300 to 1,000 mg PO every 4 hours as needed for pain; adjust dosage based on pain severity and patient response. Maximum total daily dosage: codeine 360 mg and acetaminophen 4,000 mg.
Adjust-a-dose: Initiate dosing regimen for each patient individually, taking into consideration pain severity, patient response, prior analgesic treatment experience, and risk factors for addiction, abuse, and misuse. Consider decreased dosage in patients with kidney impairment, older adults, and patients overly sensitive to effects of opioids. For patients with liver impairment, consider dosage adjustment to total daily of acetaminophen.

ADMINISTRATION
PO
• Store tablets at room temperature.
• Give with milk or meals to avoid GI upset.
• For oral solution or suspension, be sure to use a calibrated measuring device.

ACTION
Codeine may bind with opioid receptors in the CNS, altering perception and emotional response to pain. Acetaminophen is thought to produce analgesia by inhibiting prostaglandin and other substances that sensitize pain receptors.

Route	Onset	Peak	Duration
PO (codeine)	30–45 min	1–2 hr	4–6 hr
PO (acetaminophen)	Rapid	0.5–2 hr	3–4 hr

Half-life: Codeine, 2.9 hours; acetaminophen, 1.25 to 3 hours.

ADVERSE REACTIONS
CNS: drowsiness, light-headedness, dizziness, sedation, euphoria, dysphoria. **GI:** nausea, vomiting, constipation, abdominal pain. **Hematologic:** *thrombocytopenia, agranulocytosis.* **Metabolic:** adrenal insufficiency. **Respiratory:** shortness of breath, *respiratory depression.* **Skin:** pruritus, rash, diaphoresis. **Other:** hypersensitivity reactions.

INTERACTIONS
Drug-drug. *Anticholinergics (scopolamine, diphenhydramine):* May increase risk of urinary retention or severe constipation. Monitor patient closely.
Antipsychotics, general anesthetics, opioid analgesics, sedative-hypnotics, tranquilizers, other CNS depressants: May increase CNS depression. Use together cautiously.
Boxed Warning *Benzodiazepines, CNS depressants:* May cause slow or difficult breathing, sedation, and death. Avoid use together. If use together can't be avoided, limit dosage and duration of each drug to the minimum needed for desired effect. ∎
CYP2D6 inducers: May decrease analgesic effects or result in opioid withdrawal. Use cautiously.
Boxed Warning *CYP3A4 inducers and inhibitors (erythromycin, ketoconazole, ritonavir), CYP2D6 inhibitors (amiodarone, quinidine):* Effects of concomitant use or discontinuation of these drugs with codeine are complex. Their use with codeine requires careful consideration of the effects on the parent drug, codeine, and the active metabolite, morphine. Refer to prescribing information of drugs used along with the drug. ∎

Reactions in bold italics are *life-threatening*.

Diuretics: May decrease effect of diuretic. Monitor patient for diminished diuresis or effects on BP.

MAO inhibitors: May cause serotonin syndrome or opioid toxicity (respiratory depression, coma). Use together or within 14 days is contraindicated. If urgent use of an opioid is necessary, use test doses and frequent titration of small doses of other opioids (such as oxycodone, hydrocodone, oxymorphone, or buprenorphine) to treat pain while closely monitoring BP and signs and symptoms of CNS and respiratory depression.

Muscle relaxants (baclofen, methocarbamol): May increase neuromuscular blocking effect and risk of respiratory depression. Monitor patient closely.

Serotonergic drugs (amoxapine, antiemetics [dolasetron, granisetron], antimigraine drugs, buspirone, cyclobenzaprine, dextromethorphan, lithium, maprotiline, methylene blue, mirtazapine, nefazodone, SSNRIs, SSRIs, TCAs, trazodone, tryptophan, vilazodone): May increase risk of serotonin syndrome. Use together cautiously, and monitor for signs and symptoms of serotonin syndrome.

Drug-herb. *St. John's wort:* May increase risk of serotonin syndrome. Use together cautiously.

Drug-lifestyle. **Boxed Warning** *Alcohol use:* May cause slow or difficult breathing, sedation, and death. Discourage use together. ∎

EFFECTS ON LAB TEST RESULTS
• May increase serum amylase level.
• May cause false-positive results for urinary 5-hydroxyindoleacetic acid.
• May cause urine drug screen to be positive for morphine.

CONTRAINDICATIONS & CAUTIONS
• Contraindicated in patients hypersensitive to codeine or acetaminophen; in patients with significant respiratory depression or acute or severe bronchial asthma in an unmonitored setting or in the absence of resuscitative equipment; and in those with known or suspected GI obstruction, including paralytic ileus.

Boxed Warning Use exposes patient and others to the risk of opioid addiction, abuse, and misuse. These effects can occur at any dose or duration. Assess each patient risk before prescribing and regularly reassess patient for these behaviors and conditions. ∎

Boxed Warning Prescribers are strongly encouraged to complete a REMS-compliant education program. Drug should be prescribed only by prescribers with knowledge of opioid use and ways to reduce associated risks. ∎

Boxed Warning *Opioid class warning:* Opioids should only be prescribed with benzodiazepines or other CNS depressants when alternative treatment options are inadequate, aren't expected to provide adequate analgesia, haven't been tolerated, or aren't expected to be tolerated. ∎

§ **Boxed Warning** *Opioid class warning:* Life-threatening respiratory depression and death have occurred in children who received codeine. Most reported cases occurred after tonsillectomy or adenoidectomy, and many of the children had evidence of being an ultrarapid metabolizer of codeine due to CYP2D6 polymorphism. Codeine phosphate–acetaminophen is contraindicated in children younger than age 12 and in children younger than age 18 after tonsillectomy or adenoidectomy. Avoid use in adolescents ages 12 to 18 who have other risk factors that may increase their sensitivity to the respiratory depressant effects of codeine, unless benefits outweigh risks. Risk factors include conditions associated with hypoventilation (postoperative status, obstructive sleep apnea, obesity, severe pulmonary disease, neuromuscular disease, and use with other drugs that cause respiratory depression). ∎

Boxed Warning Accidental ingestion of even one dose of codeine–acetaminophen, especially by children, can result in a fatal overdose. ∎

🚱 *Alert:* Patients are at increased risk for oversedation and respiratory depression if they snore or have a history of sleep apnea, have no recent history of opioid use or are first-time opioid users, have increased opioid dose requirements or opioid habituation, received general anesthesia for longer lengths of time, received other sedating drugs, have preexisting pulmonary or cardiac disease, or have thoracic or other surgical incisions that may impair breathing. Monitor these patients carefully.

🚱 *Alert:* Use lowest effective dose for shortest period consistent with patient's treatment goals.

🚱 *Alert:* Because risk of overdose increases as opioid dose increases, reserve titration to higher doses for patients in whom lower doses are ineffective and in whom expected benefits of higher opioid dose outweigh risks.

🌢 *Alert:* Drug shouldn't be used for an extended period unless pain remains severe enough to require an opioid analgesic and alternative treatment options are inadequate to treat pain.

🌢 *Alert:* Drug may cause opioid-induced hyperalgesia (OIH). Symptoms include increased pain level with opioid dose increase, decreased pain level with opioid dose reduction, pain from ordinarily nonpainful stimuli without underlying disease progression, opioid tolerance or withdrawal, and addictive behavior. For suspected OIH, decrease opioid dose or switch patient to alternative opioid.

• Drug may increase risk of severe hypotension, including orthostatic hypotension and syncope. Reduced blood volume and concurrent use of CNS depressant drugs increase risk.

🌢 *Alert:* For managing pain (not associated with tonsillectomy or adenoidectomy), codeine should be used in children only if benefits outweigh risks.

• Safety and effectiveness in children younger than age 18 haven't been established. Use in children younger than age 12 is contraindicated.

• Drug may lead to a rare but serious decrease in adrenal gland cortisol production.

• Drug may decrease sex hormone levels with long-term use.

• Use cautiously in patients with head injury, intracranial lesions, increased ICP, or acute abdominal conditions.

Boxed Warning Acetaminophen has been associated with acute liver failure, usually at doses greater than 4,000 mg/day and often when more than one acetaminophen-containing product is used. Liver failure may result in liver transplant or death. ∎

🌢 *Alert:* May cause SCAR, including SJS, TEN, and acute generalized exanthematous pustulosis. Reaction may occur with first or subsequent use. Monitor for reddening of skin, rash, blisters, and detachment of upper surface of skin. Stop drug immediately if skin reaction is suspected.

• Use cautiously in patients with asthma or sulfite sensitivity because allergy-type reactions, anaphylaxis, and asthmatic episodes may occur.

⚕ Use cautiously in older adults and patients who are debilitated; in those with severe kidney or liver impairment, seizure disorders, hypothyroidism, urethral stricture, Addison disease, or prostatic hypertrophy; in patients identified as ultra-rapid codeine metabolizers; and in those with identified polymorphism of CYP2D6 genotype.

Dialyzable drug: Unknown.

⚠ *Overdose S&S:* Extreme sleepiness, confusion, shallow breathing. *Codeine:* Pinpoint pupils, respiratory depression, loss of consciousness, seizures. *Acetaminophen:* Liver necrosis, nausea, vomiting, diaphoresis, malaise, renal tubular necrosis, hypoglycemia, coma, coagulation defects.

PREGNANCY-LACTATION-REPRODUCTION

Boxed Warning Prolonged use during pregnancy can result in neonatal opioid withdrawal syndrome, which may be life-threatening. It requires management with expert neonatology protocols. If prolonged use is needed, advise patient of risks and ensure availability of proper treatment. ∎

🌢 *Alert:* Studies during pregnancy are inadequate. Use during pregnancy only if potential benefit justifies fetal risk.

• Don't administer drug during labor when delivery of a premature infant is anticipated.

🌢 *Alert:* Codeine and its metabolites and acetaminophen appear in human milk. Breastfeeding isn't recommended for patients taking codeine due to risk of serious adverse reactions in infants, such as excess sleepiness, difficulty breastfeeding, or serious breathing problems that could result in death.

NURSING CONSIDERATIONS

Boxed Warning May cause life-threatening or fatal respiratory depression at any time during therapy. Monitor patient closely, especially when starting or increasing doses. Proper dosing and titration are essential to reduce risk. ∎

Boxed Warning Regularly monitor all patients for opioid addiction, abuse, and misuse, which can lead to overdose and death. ∎

• Inform patient of risks and signs and symptoms of acetaminophen and codeine toxicity.

• Ensure accuracy when prescribing, dispensing, and administering codeine 12 mg–acetaminophen 120 mg/5 mL. Dosing errors due to confusion between mg and mL and other codeine–acetaminophen oral liquids of different concentrations can result in accidental overdose and death.

⟐ Alert: If patient is taking opioids with serotonergic drugs, watch for signs and symptoms of serotonin syndrome (agitation, hallucinations, rapid HR, fever, diaphoresis, shivering or shaking, muscle twitching or stiffness, trouble with coordination, nausea, vomiting, diarrhea), especially at start of treatment and after dosage increases. Signs and symptoms may occur within several hours of coadministration or later, especially after dosage increase. Discontinue opioid, serotonergic drug, or both for suspected serotonin syndrome.

⟐ Alert: Monitor for signs and symptoms of adrenal insufficiency (nausea, vomiting, loss of appetite, fatigue, weakness, dizziness, low BP). Perform diagnostic testing for suspected adrenal insufficiency. For confirmed adrenal insufficiency, treat with corticosteroids and wean patient off opioids, if appropriate. Discontinue corticosteroids when clinically appropriate.

• Monitor patient for signs and symptoms of decreased sex hormone levels (low libido, erectile dysfunction, amenorrhea, infertility). If signs and symptoms occur, evaluate patient and obtain specimens for lab testing.

⟐ Alert: Carefully monitor vital signs, pain level, respiratory status, and sedation level in all patients receiving opioids (especially IV), even those given postoperatively.

⚶ Carefully monitor patients identified as ultrarapid metabolizers of codeine and those with identified polymorphism of CYP2D6 genotype. Overdose signs and symptoms and exaggerated adverse effects may occur at normal doses in these patients.

• Monitor serial kidney function test results or LFT values in patients with severe liver or kidney impairment.

⟐ Alert: Don't stop drug abruptly; withdraw slowly and individualize gradual taper plan to prevent signs and symptoms of withdrawal, worsening pain, and psychological distress in patients who are physically dependent. Refer to manufacturer's label for specific tapering instructions.

⟐ Alert: When tapering opioids, monitor patient closely for signs and symptoms of opioid withdrawal (restlessness, lacrimation, rhinorrhea, yawning, perspiration, chills, myalgia, mydriasis, irritability, anxiety, insomnia, backache, joint pain, weakness, abdominal cramps, anorexia, nausea, vomiting, diarrhea, increased BP or HR, increased respiratory rate). Such symptoms may indicate a need to taper more slowly. Also monitor patient for suicidality, use of other substances, and mood changes.

PATIENT TEACHING
Boxed Warning Counsel patient and caregiver on serious risks, safe use, and importance of reading the medication guide with each prescription. ∎

Boxed Warning Caution patient or caregiver of patient taking an opioid with a benzodiazepine, CNS depressant, or alcohol to seek immediate medical attention for dizziness, light-headedness, extreme sleepiness, slowed or difficult breathing, or unresponsiveness. ∎

⟐ Alert: Warn patient and caregiver of patient taking codeine to watch for slow or shallow breathing, difficult or noisy breathing, confusion, excessive sleepiness, or trouble breastfeeding or limpness (in infant). If any of these signs occur, tell patient or caregiver to stop drug and immediately seek emergency medical attention.

• Instruct patient to contact prescriber if prescribed dosage isn't controlling pain.

⟐ Alert: Warn patient to withhold drug and inform the prescriber if pain level worsens, pain sensitivity increases, or new pain occurs after taking drug.

• Warn patient to immediately stop drug and seek medical attention if skin rash or reaction occurs while using acetaminophen.

• Encourage patient to report all medications being taken, including prescriptions and OTC medications and supplements.

• Caution patient to immediately report signs and symptoms of serotonin syndrome, adrenal insufficiency, and decreased sex hormone levels.

⟐ Alert: Counsel patient who has been taking the drug regularly not to discontinue without first discussing the need for gradual tapering of the regimen with prescriber.

• Teach patient that naloxone may be prescribed in conjunction with the opioid when beginning and renewing treatment as a preventive measure to reduce opioid overdose and death.

• Inform patient with severe liver or kidney disease that serial kidney function tests or LFTs will be needed.

• Caution patient not to drive a car or operate heavy machinery while taking drug.

- Inform patient that, for acute pain, drug may only be needed for a few days. Teach about safe disposal of unused drug.
- Advise patient to take drug exactly as prescribed and to use lowest dose possible for shortest time needed.
- Instruct patient who is pregnant or planning to become pregnant to inform health care provider.
- Advise patient who is breastfeeding and is an ultrarapid metabolizer to obtain emergency treatment if the infant shows signs and symptoms of codeine toxicity (sleepiness, difficulty breastfeeding or breathing, limpness).

SAFETY ALERT!

codeine sulfate ⚛

Therapeutic class: Opioid analgesics
Pharmacologic class: Opioids
Controlled substance schedule: II

AVAILABLE FORMS
Tablets: 15 mg, 30 mg, 60 mg

INDICATIONS & DOSAGES
➤ **Mild to moderately severe pain**
Adults: 15 to 60 mg PO up to every 4 hours PRN for pain. Adjust dosage to obtain appropriate balance between pain management and opioid-related adverse reactions. Maximum, 360 mg/24 hours.
Adjust-a-dose: For older adults and patients with kidney or liver impairment, begin with lower-than-normal dosages or with longer dosing intervals and titrate slowly while monitoring for respiratory depression, sedation, and hypotension. Initiate individual dosing regimen for each patient, considering pain severity, patient response, prior analgesic treatment experience, and risk factors for addiction, abuse, and misuse.

ADMINISTRATION
PO
- Give drug with milk or meals to avoid GI upset.
- Pharmacist may compound drug into an oral suspension if patient can't swallow tablets.
- Store at room temperature.

ACTION
May bind with opioid receptors in the CNS, altering perception of and emotional response to pain. Also suppresses the cough reflex by direct action on the cough center in the medulla.

Route	Onset	Peak	Duration
PO	30–60 min	1–2 hr	4–6 hr

Half-life: 2.5 to 3.5 hours.

ADVERSE REACTIONS
CNS: drowsiness, sedation, dizziness, euphoria, dysphoria, light-headedness, syncope. **CV:** *bradycardia,* flushing, hypotension. **EENT:** dry mouth. **GI:** constipation, nausea, vomiting, abdominal pain, anorexia. **GU:** urine retention. **Respiratory:** shortness of breath, *respiratory depression.* **Skin:** diaphoresis, pruritus. **Other:** hypersensitivity reaction.

INTERACTIONS
Drug-drug. *Anticholinergic drugs (diphenhydramine, scopolamine):* May increase risk of urinary retention or severe constipation. Monitor patient closely.
Boxed Warning *Benzodiazepines, CNS depressants:* May cause respiratory depression, sedation, coma, and death. Avoid use together. If use together can't be avoided, limit dosage and duration of each drug to the minimum needed for desired effect. ▌
CNS depressants, general anesthetics, hypnotics, other opioid analgesics, sedatives, TCAs, tranquilizers: May cause additive effects. Use together cautiously; monitor patient response.
Boxed Warning *CYP3A4 inducers (carbamazepine, phenytoin, rifampin) and inhibitors (azole antifungals, macrolide antibiotics, protease inhibitors), CYP2D6 inhibitors (bupropion, paroxetine):* Effects of concomitant use or discontinuation of these drugs with codeine use are complex. Their use with codeine sulfate requires careful consideration of effects on the parent drug, codeine, and the active metabolite, morphine. Refer to prescribing information of drugs used together with the drug. ▌
Diuretics: May decrease effect of diuretic. Monitor patient for diminished diuresis or effects on BP.
MAO inhibitors (linezolid, phenelzine): May cause serotonin syndrome or opioid toxicity (respiratory depression, coma). Use together or within 14 days is contraindicated. If urgent use of an opioid is necessary, use test doses

and frequent titration of small doses of other opioids (oxycodone, hydrocodone, oxymorphone, or buprenorphine) to treat pain while closely monitoring BP and signs and symptoms of CNS and respiratory depression.

Muscle relaxants (baclofen, methocarbamol): May increase neuromuscular blocking effect and risk of respiratory depression. Monitor patient closely.

Opioid antagonists (nalbuphine, pentazocine): May reduce analgesic effect or precipitate withdrawal symptoms. Avoid use together.

☺ *Alert:* *Serotonergic drugs (amoxapine, antiemetics [dolasetron, granisetron, ondansetron, palonosetron], antimigraine drugs, buspirone, cyclobenzaprine, dextromethorphan, lithium, maprotiline, methylene blue, mirtazapine, nefazodone, SSNRIs, SSRIs, TCAs, trazodone, tryptophan, vilazodone):* May increase risk of serotonin syndrome. Use together cautiously, and monitor for signs and symptoms of serotonin syndrome.

Drug-herb. *St. John's wort:* May increase risk of serotonin syndrome. Use together cautiously.

Drug-lifestyle. **Boxed Warning** *Alcohol use:* May cause slow or difficult breathing, sedation, and death. Avoid use together. ∎

EFFECTS ON LAB TEST RESULTS
• May increase amylase level.
• May cause urine drug screen to be positive for morphine.

CONTRAINDICATIONS & CAUTIONS
• Contraindicated in patients hypersensitive to drug; in patients with significant respiratory depression or acute or severe bronchial asthma in an unmonitored setting or in the absence of resuscitative equipment; and in those with known or suspected GI obstruction, including paralytic ileus.

Boxed Warning *Opioid class warning:* Opioids should only be prescribed with benzodiazepines or other CNS depressants when alternative treatment options are inadequate, aren't expected to provide adequate analgesia, haven't been tolerated, or aren't expected to be tolerated. ∎

Boxed Warning Use exposes patient and others to risk of opioid addiction, abuse, and misuse, which can lead to overdose and death. These effects can occur at any dose or duration. Assess patient risk before prescribing

and regularly reassess patient for these behaviors and conditions.

Boxed Warning Prescribers are strongly encouraged to complete a REMS-compliant education program. Drug should be prescribed only by prescribers with knowledge of opioid use and ways to reduce associated risks. ∎

☺ *Alert:* Use lowest effective dose for shortest period consistent with patient's treatment goals.

☺ *Alert:* Because risk of overdose increases as opioid dose increases, reserve titration to higher doses for patients in whom lower doses are ineffective and in whom expected benefits of higher opioid dose outweigh risks.

☺ *Alert:* Drug shouldn't be used for an extended period unless pain remains severe enough to require an opioid analgesic and alternative treatment options are inadequate to treat pain.

☺ *Alert:* Safety and effectiveness and pharmacokinetics of codeine in children younger than age 18 haven't been established. Use is contraindicated in children younger than age 12.

✄ **Boxed Warning** Children who receive codeine for pain relief after a tonsillectomy or adenoidectomy and are ultrarapid metabolizers due to a CYP2D6 polymorphism are at increased risk for death. Codeine is contraindicated for pain management after these surgeries in children younger than age 18. ∎

• Drug may lead to a rare but serious decrease in adrenal gland cortisol production.
• Drug may decrease sex hormone levels with long-term use.

☺ *Alert:* Patients are at increased risk for oversedation and respiratory depression if they snore or have a history of sleep apnea, have no recent opioid use or are first-time opioid users, have increased opioid dose requirements or opioid habituation, received general anesthesia for longer lengths of time, received other sedating drugs, have preexisting pulmonary or cardiac disease, or have thoracic or other surgical incisions that may impair breathing. Monitor these patients carefully.

• Drug may increase risk of severe hypotension, including orthostatic hypotension and syncope. Reduced blood volume or concurrent use of CNS depressant drug increases risk.

Boxed Warning Accidental ingestion of even one dose of codeine sulfate tablets, especially by children, can result in a fatal overdose. ∎

3 *Alert:* Drug may cause opioid-induced hyperalgesia (OIH). Symptoms include increased pain level with opioid dose increase, decreased pain level with opioid dose reduction, pain from ordinarily nonpainful stimuli without underlying disease progression, opioid tolerance or withdrawal and addictive behavior. For suspected OIH, decrease opioid dose or switch patient to alternative opioid.

• Use cautiously in older adults, patients who are debilitated, and in those with head injury, increased ICP, increased CSF pressure, liver or kidney disease, hypothyroidism, Addison disease, acute alcoholism, seizures, severe CNS depression, bronchial asthma, COPD, respiratory depression, or shock.

Dialyzable drug: Unknown.

⚠ Overdose S&S: CNS depression, respiratory depression, apnea, flaccid skeletal muscles, bradycardia, hypotension, circulatory collapse, death.

PREGNANCY-LACTATION-REPRODUCTION

3 *Alert:* Studies during pregnancy are inadequate. Use during pregnancy only if potential benefit justifies fetal risk.

Boxed Warning Prolonged use during pregnancy can cause neonatal withdrawal syndrome, which can be life-threatening and requires management by neonatology experts. If used during pregnancy, advise patient of risks and ensure appropriate treatment is available. ■

• Don't administer drug during labor when delivery of a premature infant is anticipated.

3 *Alert:* Breastfeeding isn't recommended for patients taking codeine because of the risk of serious adverse reactions in breastfed infants, such as excess sleepiness, difficulty breastfeeding, and serious breathing problems that could result in death.

NURSING CONSIDERATIONS

Boxed Warning May cause life-threatening or fatal respiratory depression at any time during therapy. Monitor patient closely, especially when starting or increasing doses. Proper dosing and titration are essential to reduce risk. ■

Boxed Warning Regularly monitor all patients for opioid addiction, abuse, and misuse, which can lead to overdose and death. ■

• If patient is taking opioids with serotonergic drugs, watch for signs and symptoms of serotonin syndrome (agitation, hallucinations, rapid HR, fever, diaphoresis, shivering or shaking, muscle twitching or stiffness, trouble with coordination, nausea, vomiting, diarrhea), especially at start of treatment and after dosage increases. Signs and symptoms may occur within several hours of coadministration or later, especially after dosage increase. Discontinue opioid, serotonergic drug, or both if serotonin syndrome is suspected.

• Monitor for signs and symptoms of adrenal insufficiency (nausea, vomiting, loss of appetite, fatigue, weakness, dizziness, low BP). Perform diagnostic testing if adrenal insufficiency is suspected. If adrenal insufficiency is confirmed, treat with corticosteroids and wean patient off opioids, if appropriate. Discontinue corticosteroids when clinically appropriate.

• Monitor for signs and symptoms of decreased sex hormone levels (low libido, erectile dysfunction, amenorrhea, infertility). If signs and symptoms occur, evaluate patient and obtain specimens for lab testing.

3 *Alert:* Don't stop drug abruptly; withdraw slowly and individualize gradual taper plan to prevent signs and symptoms of withdrawal, worsening pain, and psychological distress in patients who are physically dependent. Refer to manufacturer's label for specific tapering instructions.

3 *Alert:* When tapering opioids, monitor patient closely for signs and symptoms of opioid withdrawal (restlessness, lacrimation, rhinorrhea, yawning, perspiration, chills, myalgia, mydriasis, irritability, anxiety, insomnia, backache, joint pain, weakness, abdominal cramps, anorexia, nausea, vomiting, diarrhea, increased BP or HR, increased respiratory rate). Such symptoms may indicate a need to taper more slowly. Also monitor patient for suicidality, use of other substances, and mood changes.

• Reassess patient's level of pain at least 15 and 30 minutes after use.

• For full analgesic effect, give drug before patient has intense pain.

• Drug is an antitussive; don't use when cough is a valuable diagnostic sign or is beneficial (as after thoracic surgery). Monitor cough type and frequency.

• Monitor respiratory and circulatory status.

• Opioids may cause constipation. Assess bowel function and need for stool softeners and stimulant laxatives.

Reactions in bold italics are *life-threatening*.

• Codeine may delay gastric emptying, increase biliary tract pressure from contraction of the sphincter of Oddi, and interfere with hepatobiliary imaging studies.

• *Look alike–sound alike:* Don't confuse codeine with Cardene or Cordran.

PATIENT TEACHING

Boxed Warning Counsel patient and caregiver on serious risks, safe use, and the importance of reading the medication guide with each prescription. ■

Boxed Warning Caution patient or caregiver of patient taking an opioid with a benzodiazepine, CNS depressant, or alcohol to seek immediate medical attention for dizziness, light-headedness, extreme sleepiness, slowed or difficult breathing, or unresponsiveness. ■

◑ *Alert:* Warn patient and caregiver of patient taking codeine to watch for slow or shallow breathing, difficult or noisy breathing, confusion, or excessive sleepiness. If any of these signs occur, tell patient or caregiver to stop drug and immediately seek emergency medical attention.

• Inform patient that, for acute pain, drug may only be needed for a few days. Teach about safe disposal of unused drug.

• Instruct patient to contact prescriber if prescribed dosage isn't controlling pain.

◑ *Alert:* Warn patient to withhold drug and inform prescriber if pain level worsens, pain sensitivity increases, or new pain occurs after taking drug.

• Advise patient to take drug exactly as prescribed and to use the lowest dose possible for the shortest time needed.

◑ *Alert:* Counsel patient who has been regularly taking drug not to discontinue without first discussing the need for gradual tapering with prescriber.

◑ *Alert:* Encourage patient to report all medications being taken, including prescriptions and OTC medications and supplements.

• Caution patient to immediately report signs and symptoms of serotonin syndrome, adrenal insufficiency, or decreased sex hormone levels.

• Teach patient that naloxone may be prescribed with the opioid when beginning and renewing therapy to reduce risk of opioid overdose and death.

• Advise patient that GI distress caused by taking drug orally can be eased by taking drug with milk or meals.

• Instruct patient to ask for or to take drug before pain becomes intense.

• Caution patient who is ambulatory about getting out of bed or walking. Warn outpatient to avoid driving and other hazardous activities that require mental alertness until drug's effects on CNS are known.

• Advise patient to avoid alcohol during therapy.

Boxed Warning Warn patient that accidental ingestion of even one dose of codeine sulfate, especially by children, can result in a fatal overdose of codeine. ■

• Caution patient to report to prescriber pregnancy or plan to become pregnant.

• Warn patient who is breastfeeding to watch for increased sleepiness, difficulty breastfeeding or breathing, or limpness (in infant). Tell patient to immediately seek medical attention if these signs occur.

---

colchicine ⚹
KOL-chi-seen

Colcrys, Gloperba, Mitigare

Therapeutic class: Antigout drugs
Pharmacologic class: Colchicum autumnale alkaloids

AVAILABLE FORMS
Capsules: 0.6 mg
Oral solution: 0.6 mg/5 mL
Tablets: 0.6 mg

INDICATIONS & DOSAGES
Adjust-a-dose (for all indications): Administration of CYP3A4 or P-gp inhibitors or inhibitors of both CYP3A4 and P-gp with colchicine in patients who are on or have recently completed treatment (within past 14 days) may cause colchicine toxicity and fatal drug interactions, particularly in patients with liver or kidney impairment. If coadministration of either a CYP3A4 or a P-gp inhibitor is required, colchicine dose may need to be reduced or therapy interrupted; carefully monitor patient for colchicine toxicity. Refer to Colcrys manufacturer's instructions for dosage adjustments by drug and indication for CYP3A4, P-gp, and protease inhibitors.

➤ **Prevention of gout flares**
Adults: 0.6 mg PO once daily or b.i.d. Maximum daily dose, 1.2 mg.

Children older than age 16 (Colcrys): 0.6 mg PO once daily or b.i.d. Maximum daily dose, 1.2 mg.

Adjust-a-dose: For patients taking Colcrys with CrCl of less than 30 mL/minute, give 0.3 mg/day. Closely monitor patient after dosage increases. For patients on dialysis, starting doses should be 0.3 mg twice a week with close monitoring. Closely monitor patients with Child-Pugh class A or B liver impairment; no dosage adjustment is required. Consider dosage reduction in patients with Child-Pugh class C liver impairment.

For patients taking Mitigare or Gloperba, consider dosage reduction or alternative drug in patients with CrCl of less than 30 mL/minute; closely monitor patients undergoing hemodialysis for signs and symptoms of toxicity. Consider dosage reduction or alternative drug in patients with Child-Pugh class C liver impairment.

➤ **Gout flares (Colcrys)**
Adults and adolescents older than age 16: 1.2 mg PO at first sign of a flare, followed by 0.6 mg 1 hour later. Maximum dosage, 1.8 mg over a 1-hour period. Wait 12 hours before resuming gout prophylaxis.
Adjust-a-dose: For patients with CrCl of less than 30 mL/minute or Child-Pugh class C liver impairment, no dosage adjustment is needed but treatment course should be repeated no more than once every 2 weeks. For patients with CrCl of less than 30 mL/minute or Child-Pugh class C liver impairment requiring repeated courses for treatment of gout flares, consider alternative therapy. For patients on dialysis, reduce total recommended dose for treatment of gout flares to a single dose of 0.6 mg (one tablet) no more than once every 2 weeks.

➤ **Familial Mediterranean fever (Colcrys)**
Adults: 1.2 to 2.4 mg PO daily; may increase by 0.3 mg/day to maximum daily dosage given once daily or in two divided doses.
Adolescents ages 13 and older: 1.2 to 2.4 mg PO once daily or in two divided doses.
Children ages 6 to 12: 0.9 to 1.8 mg PO once daily or in two divided doses.
Children ages 4 to 6: 0.3 to 1.8 mg PO once daily or in two divided doses.
Adjust-a-dose: For patients with CrCl of less than 30 mL/minute or CKD requiring dialysis, initially 0.3 mg/day, carefully increasing dosage as needed. For patients with Child-Pugh class C liver impairment consider

dosage reduction with careful monitoring. Decrease dosage by 0.3 mg/day, if adverse effects are intolerable.

➤ **Behçet syndrome with arthritis, cutaneous lesions, or mucocutaneous ulcers ◆**
Adults: 1.2 to 1.8 mg/day in two or three divided doses.

➤ **Pericarditis, acute and recurrent, in combination with aspirin or NSAIDs ◆**
Adults: For maintenance, with or without loading dose: In patients weighing 70 kg or more, 0.6 mg b.i.d.; for those weighing less than 70 kg or unable to tolerate higher dosing regimen, 0.6 mg once daily.

ADMINISTRATION
PO
⬥ *Alert:* Hazardous drug; use safe handling and disposal precautions.
• Give drug with or without food.
• Give missed dose as soon as possible; then return to normal dosing schedule. Don't double dose.

ACTION
Exact mechanism of action is not fully known; thought to involve a reduction in lactic acid produced by leukocytes, reducing uric acid deposits and phagocytosis, thereby decreasing the inflammatory process.

Route	Onset	Peak	Duration
PO	Unknown	30–180 min	Unknown

Half-life: 27 to 31 hours.

ADVERSE REACTIONS
CNS: fatigue, headache. **EENT:** pharyngolaryngeal pain. **GI:** diarrhea, nausea, vomiting, abdominal discomfort. **Hematologic:** *aplastic anemia, granulocytopenia, leukopenia, pancytopenia, thrombocytopenia.* **Metabolic:** gout.

INTERACTIONS
Drug-drug. *Digoxin, HMG-CoA reductase inhibitors (atorvastatin, simvastatin), fibrates, gemfibrozil:* May increase risk of myopathy or rhabdomyolysis. Avoid use together. If coadministration can't be avoided, monitor patient carefully. Discontinue colchicine if signs or symptoms occur.
Moderate CYP3A4 inhibitors (aprepitant, diltiazem, erythromycin, fluconazole, fosamprenavir, verapamil), P-gp inhibitors (cyclosporine, ranolazine), strong CYP3A4

C

inhibitors (atazanavir, clarithromycin, keto-conazole, nefazodone, nelfinavir, ritonavir, saquinavir; fixed combination of elvitegravir–cobicistat–emtricitabine–tenofovir): May increase colchicine level, increasing risk of toxic effects. Reduce colchicine dosage if alternative treatment isn't available. Use together in patients with kidney or liver impairment is contraindicated.

Drug-food. *Grapefruit, grapefruit juice:* May increase drug level. Discourage use together.

EFFECTS ON LAB TEST RESULTS
• May increase AST, ALT, and CK levels.
• May decrease Hb level, hematocrit, and leukocyte, granulocyte, and platelet counts.
• May cause false-positive results when testing urine for RBCs or Hb.

CONTRAINDICATIONS & CAUTIONS
• Contraindicated in patients with both kidney and liver impairment and in those with kidney or liver impairment taking drugs that inhibit both P-gp and CYP3A4.
• Myelosuppression has been reported. Use cautiously in patients with hematologic disorders.
• **Alert:** Fatal overdoses, both accidental and intentional, have been reported in adults and children who have ingested colchicine.
Dialyzable drug: No.
⚠ **Overdose S&S:** Abdominal pain, nausea, vomiting, diarrhea, hypovolemia, multiorgan failure, death.

PREGNANCY-LACTATION-REPRODUCTION
• Colchicine crosses the human placenta. Use during pregnancy only if potential benefit justifies fetal risk.
• Drug appears in human milk. Use cautiously during breastfeeding and observe infant for adverse effects.

NURSING CONSIDERATIONS
• Safety and effectiveness of repeat treatment for gout flares haven't been established.
• Drug isn't an analgesic and shouldn't be used to treat pain from other causes.
• Obtain baseline lab studies, including CBC, before starting therapy and periodically thereafter.
• Monitor patient who has used drug for a prolonged period for neuromuscular toxicity and rhabdomyolysis.

• **Look alike–sound alike:** Don't confuse colchicine with Cortrosyn.

PATIENT TEACHING
• Teach about proper drug administration and handling.
• Advise patient to take drug as prescribed even if feeling better and not to alter dosage or discontinue drug without first discussing with prescriber.
• Caution patient that many drugs and other substances may interact with colchicine. Instruct patient to tell prescriber and pharmacist all prescription and OTC medications and supplements used and to check with prescriber before starting new medications, especially antibiotics.
• Tell patient to keep drug out of the reach of children due to risk of fatal overdose.
• Advise patient to report all adverse reactions, including muscle pain or weakness, tingling or numbness in fingers or toes, unusual bleeding or bruising, increased infections, weakness, tiredness, cyanosis, nausea, vomiting, or diarrhea; advise patient to discontinue drug.

crisaborole
kris-a-BOR-ole

Eucrisa

Therapeutic class: Dermatologic agents
Pharmacologic class: Phosphodiesterase 4 inhibitors

AVAILABLE FORMS
Topical ointment: 2%

INDICATIONS & DOSAGES
➤ **Mild to moderate atopic dermatitis**
Adults and children ages 3 months and older: Apply thin film to affected areas b.i.d.

ADMINISTRATION
Topical
• Drug is for external use only; not for ophthalmic, oral, or intravaginal use.
• Store at room temperature.
• Keep tube tightly closed.

ACTION
Exact mechanism unknown. Drug is a phosphodiesterase 4 inhibitor that increases intracellular cAMP levels.

Route	Onset	Peak	Duration
Topical	Unknown	Unknown	Unknown

Half-life: Unknown.

ADVERSE REACTIONS
Skin: application-site pain, burning, stinging.

INTERACTIONS
None reported.

EFFECTS ON LAB TEST RESULTS
None reported.

CONTRAINDICATIONS & CAUTIONS
• Contraindicated in patients hypersensitive to drug or its components.
• Hypersensitivity reactions have been reported, including contact urticaria.
• Safety and effectiveness in children younger than age 3 months haven't been established.
Dialyzable drug: Unlikely.

PREGNANCY-LACTATION-REPRODUCTION
• Drug hasn't been studied during pregnancy. Animal studies revealed no adverse developmental effects.
• Drug is systemically absorbed; risk of harm in infants who are breastfed is unknown. Consider benefits to patient and risks to infant before use.

NURSING CONSIDERATIONS
• Monitor for hypersensitivity reactions (severe pruritus, swelling, erythema). If any occur, discontinue drug.

PATIENT TEACHING
• Advise patient to discontinue drug and immediately report signs or symptoms of hypersensitivity reaction (hives, itching, swelling, redness).
• Warn patient that effects of drug during pregnancy and breastfeeding are unknown.
• Remind patient and caregivers to wash hands after applying drug, unless patient's hands are being treated.

cyclobenzaprine hydrochloride
sye-kloe-BEN-za-preen

Amrix, Fexmid

Therapeutic class: Skeletal muscle relaxants
Pharmacologic class: TCA derivatives

AVAILABLE FORMS
Capsules (extended-release) **ⓒ**: 15 mg, 30 mg
Tablets: 5 mg, 7.5 mg, 10 mg

INDICATIONS & DOSAGES
➤ **Adjunct to rest and physical therapy to relieve muscle spasm from acute, painful musculoskeletal conditions**
Adults and children ages 15 and older: 5 mg PO t.i.d. Based on response, may increase to 7.5 or 10 mg t.i.d. Don't exceed 30 mg/day. Or, initially, 15 mg extended-release capsule PO once daily; may increase to 30 mg daily (adults only). Use for longer than 2 or 3 weeks isn't recommended.
Adjust-a-dose: In older adults and patients with Child-Pugh class A liver impairment, start with 5-mg conventional tablets and adjust slowly upward; consider less-frequent dosing. Don't use extended-release capsules in children, older adults, or patients with impaired liver function.

ADMINISTRATION
PO
• Have patient swallow extended-release capsules whole; don't crush or break capsules.
• In patients able to reliably swallow applesauce without chewing, sprinkle capsule contents onto a tablespoon of applesauce; have patient consume immediately without chewing and then rinse mouth to ensure all of the contents have been swallowed.

ACTION
Unknown. Relieves skeletal muscle spasm of local origin without disrupting muscle function.

Route	Onset	Peak	Duration
PO	1 hr	4 hr	12–24 hr
PO (extended-release)	1.5 hr	7–8 hr	Unknown

Half-life: Tablets, 18 hours; extended-release capsules, 32 hours.

---

*Reactions in bold italics are **life-threatening**.*

ADVERSE REACTIONS

CNS: dizziness, irritability, somnolence, drowsiness, *seizures,* headache, tremor, insomnia, fatigue, asthenia, nervousness, decreased mental acuity, attention disturbances, dysgeusia. **CV:** palpitations. **EENT:** visual disturbances, blurred vision, pharyngitis, dry mouth. **GI:** dyspepsia, constipation, nausea, diarrhea, abdominal pain. **Respiratory:** URI.

INTERACTIONS

Drug-drug. *CNS depressants:* May increase CNS depression. Avoid use together.
MAO inhibitors: May cause serotonin syndrome. Use within 2 weeks of MAO inhibitor therapy is contraindicated.
Boxed Warning *Opioid class warning:* Use with opioids may cause slow or difficult breathing, sedation, and death. Avoid use together. If use together can't be avoided, limit dosage and duration of each drug to the minimum needed for desired effect. ∎
Naproxen: May increase drowsiness. Make patient aware of this interaction.
Tramadol: May increase risk of seizures. Use together cautiously.
Drug-lifestyle. *Alcohol use:* May increase CNS depression. Discourage use together.

EFFECTS ON LAB TEST RESULTS

• May cause false-positive serum TCA screen.

CONTRAINDICATIONS & CAUTIONS

• Contraindicated in patients hypersensitive to drug; in those with hyperthyroidism, heart block, arrhythmias, conduction disturbances, or HF; and in those in the acute recovery phase of an MI.
• Drug isn't recommended in patients with Child-Pugh class B and C liver impairment.
• The risk of potentially life-threatening serotonin syndrome is increased when drug is used in combination with SSRIs, SSNRIs, other TCAs, tramadol, bupropion, meperidine, or verapamil.
• Use cautiously in older adults, patients who are debilitated, and patients with a history of urine retention, acute angle-closure glaucoma, or increased IOP.
• Safety and effectiveness of immediate-release form in children younger than age 15 and extended-release in all children haven't been established.

Dialyzable drug: Unknown.
⚠ *Overdose S&S:* Drowsiness, coma, tachycardia, tremor, agitation, ataxia, HTN, slurred speech, confusion, dizziness, nausea, vomiting, hallucinations, cardiac arrest, chest pain, cardiac arrhythmias, ECG changes (changes in QRS axis or width).

PREGNANCY-LACTATION-REPRODUCTION

• Studies during pregnancy are inadequate. Use during pregnancy only if clearly needed.
• It isn't known if drug appears in human milk. Use cautiously during breastfeeding.

NURSING CONSIDERATIONS

• Drug may cause toxic reactions similar to those caused by TCAs, including arrhythmias and prolonged conduction time, leading to MI and stroke. Observe same precautions as when giving TCAs.
• Monitor patient for nausea, headache, and malaise, which may occur if drug is stopped abruptly after long-term use.
• Monitor for signs and symptoms of serotonin syndrome (mental status changes, diaphoresis, tachycardia, labile BP, hyperthermia, neuromuscular abnormalities, GI symptoms).
⚠ *Alert:* Immediately notify prescriber of signs and symptoms of overdose, including cardiac toxicity.

PATIENT TEACHING

Boxed Warning Caution patient or caregiver of patient taking an opioid with a benzodiazepine, CNS depressant, or alcohol to seek immediate medical attention for dizziness, light-headedness, extreme sleepiness, slowed or difficult breathing, or unresponsiveness. ∎
• Advise patient to report urinary hesitancy or urine retention. If constipation is a problem, suggest that patient increase fluid intake and use a stool softener.
• Warn patient to avoid activities that require alertness until CNS effects of drug are known.
• Caution patient not to combine with alcohol or other CNS depressants, including OTC cold or allergy remedies.
• Teach about proper drug administration and handling.
• Advise patient that using drug for longer than 2 to 3 weeks isn't recommended.

SAFETY ALERT!

cyclophosphamide
sye-kloe-FOSS-fa-mide

Procytox✚

Therapeutic class: Antineoplastics
Pharmacologic class: Nitrogen mustards

AVAILABLE FORMS
Capsules ⓞⓝⓒ*:* 25 mg, 50 mg
Injection (powder): 200-mg✚, 500-mg, 1-g,
2-g vials
Injection (solution): 500-mg, 1-g, 2-g vials

INDICATIONS & DOSAGES
Adjust-a-dose (for all indications): Consider
dosage reduction in patients with kidney or
liver impairment. Withhold drug in patients
with ANC of 1,500/mm³ or less or platelets
less than 50,000/mm³.
➤ **Leukemias, breast cancer, Hodgkin
lymphoma, mycosis fungoides, multiple myeloma, neuroblastoma, malignant
lymphomas, Hodgkin lymphoma, non-
Hodgkin lymphomas (including Burkitt
lymphoma), ovarian adenocarcinoma, and
retinoblastoma, multiple myeloma**
Adults and children: Initially for induction,
40 to 50 mg/kg IV in divided doses over 2
to 5 days. Or, 10 to 15 mg/kg IV every 7 to
10 days, 3 to 5 mg/kg IV twice weekly, or 1
to 5 mg/kg PO daily, based on patient tolerance. Adjust subsequent doses according to
evidence of antitumor activity or leukopenia.
Adjust-a-dose: Cyclophosphamide is included
in cytotoxic regimens. Follow prescribed
treatment protocol.
➤ **Minimal-change nephrotic syndrome in
patients who failed to adequately respond
to or are unable to tolerate adrenocorticos-
teroid therapy**
Children: 2 mg/kg PO daily for 8 to 12 weeks.
Maximum cumulative dose, 168 mg/kg.

ADMINISTRATION
🔾 *Alert:* Hazardous drug; use safe handling
and disposal precautions.
PO
• Give oral form in the morning; infrequent
urination during the night may increase possibility of cystitis.

• Drug is associated with moderate to high
emetic potential. Consider use of antiemetics
to prevent nausea and vomiting.
• Make sure patient receives adequate fluids
to force diuresis to reduce risk of urinary tract
toxicity.
• Have patient swallow capsules whole; don't
crush or cut capsules.
• Pharmacist can prepare solution for oral
administration. Refrigerate solution for up to
14 days. Shake before use.
IV
▼ Follow manufacturer's instructions for initial dilution of solution or reconstitution of
powder.
▼ Check reconstituted solution for small
particles. Filter solution, if needed.
▼ For infusion, further dilute with D₅W, dextrose 5% in NSS for injection, or half-NSS
for injection to minimum concentration of
2 mg/mL.
▼ Give by direct IV injection slowly or by
IV infusion, as prescribed. Infusion rate
varies by infusion volume.
▼ Storage time varies by product. Refer to
manufacturer's instructions for storage time.
▼ **Incompatibilities:** None listed by manufacturer. Consult drug compatibility reference for more information.

ACTION
Cross-links strands of cellular DNA and interferes with RNA transcription, causing an
imbalance of growth that leads to cell death.
Not specific to cell cycle.

Route	Onset	Peak	Duration
PO	Unknown	Unknown	Unknown
IV	Unknown	2–3 hr	Unknown

Half-life: 3 to 12 hours.

ADVERSE REACTIONS
GI: nausea, vomiting, anorexia, abdominal discomfort, stomatitis. **Hematologic:**
leukopenia, neutropenia, thrombocytopenia,
anemia. **Hepatic:** *liver toxicity.* **Metabolic:**
hyperuricemia, hyponatremia. **Skin:** alopecia,
rash. **Other:** hypersensitivity reactions.

INTERACTIONS
Drug-drug. *ACE inhibitors, allopurinol,
clozapine, natalizumab, paclitaxel, thiazide
diuretics, zidovudine:* May increase hema-
totoxicity and immunosuppression. Monitor
therapy.

Reactions in bold italics are *life-threatening*.

Amiodarone, G-CSF drugs: May increase risk of lung toxicity. Monitor therapy.

Amphotericin B, indomethacin: May increase risk of kidney toxicity. Monitor patient closely.

Azathioprine: May increase risk of liver necrosis. Monitor patient closely.

Busulfan: May increase risk of veno-occlusive liver disease. Monitor patient closely.

Cardiotoxic drugs (anthracycline), cytarabine, pentostatin, trastuzumab): May increase adverse cardiac effects. Monitor patient for signs and symptoms of toxicity.

Cyclosporine: May decrease cyclosporine level and increase risk of GVHD. Monitor patient closely.

Etanercept: May increase risk of malignant solid tumors in patients with Wegener granulomatosis. Use cautiously.

Leflunomide: May increase risk of hematologic toxicity (pancytopenia, agranulocytosis, thrombocytopenia). Don't use leflunomide loading dose and monitor patient for bone marrow suppression at least monthly.

Live-virus vaccines: May increase vaccine-induced adverse reactions. Don't give together.

Metronidazole: May increase risk of acute encephalopathy. Monitor patient response.

Protease inhibitors: May increase cyclophosphamide-related toxicities and mucositis. Monitor therapy.

Succinylcholine: May prolong neuromuscular blockade and cause apnea. Avoid use together and alert anesthesiologist if drug has been given within 10 days of general anesthesia.

Tamoxifen: May increase risk of thromboembolism. Monitor patient closely.

Warfarin: May increase or decrease warfarin effects. Monitor PT closely.

Drug-herb. *Echinacea:* May decrease effect of cyclophosphamide. Consider alternative agents.

EFFECTS ON LAB TEST RESULTS

• May increase uric acid, bilirubin, LFT values, LDH, C-reactive protein, and urine blood levels.

• May decrease Hb, sodium, and pseudo-cholinesterase levels.

• May decrease platelet, RBC, and WBC counts.

• May increase or decrease glucose level.

• May suppress positive reaction to *Candida*, mumps, *Trichophyton*, and tuberculin skin test results.

• May cause a false-positive Papanicolaou test result.

CONTRAINDICATIONS & CAUTIONS

• Contraindicated in patients hypersensitive to drug and in those with urinary outflow obstruction.

• Use cautiously in patients with hypersensitivity to other alkylating agents; cross-sensitivity can occur.

• Use cautiously in patients with leukopenia, thrombocytopenia, malignant cell infiltration of bone marrow, or liver, cardiac, or kidney disease and in those who have recently undergone radiation therapy or chemotherapy.

• Drug may increase risk of cardiotoxicity. Myocarditis, pericardial effusion, cardiac tamponade, HF, and arrhythmias have occurred. Radiation therapy of cardiac region may increase risk of cardiotoxicity.

• Combined effect of cyclophosphamide and past or concomitant radiation treatment may increase risk of hemorrhagic cystitis.

• Drug may increase risk of secondary malignancies and veno-occlusive liver disease.

Dialyzable drug: Yes.

⚠ *Overdose S&S:* Infection, myelosuppression, cardiotoxicity.

PREGNANCY-LACTATION-REPRODUCTION

• Drug may cause fetal harm if used during pregnancy. Patients of childbearing potential should avoid pregnancy while receiving cyclophosphamide and for up to 1 year after completion of treatment. Male patients who are sexually active with partners of childbearing potential should use a condom during and for at least 4 months after treatment.

• Transient or permanent amenorrhea develops in some patients treated with drug. The risk of premature menopause increases with age.

• Males treated with drug may develop oligospermia or azoospermia. Development of sterility appears to depend on dose, duration of therapy, and state of gonadal function at time of treatment. Sterility may be irreversible in some patients. Treatment for nephrotic syndrome beyond 90 days in boys increases the probability of sterility.

• Drug appears in human milk. Patient should discontinue breastfeeding or discontinue drug, considering importance of drug to patient.

NURSING CONSIDERATIONS
• If cystitis occurs, stop drug and notify prescriber. Cystitis can occur months after therapy ends. Mesna may be given to reduce frequency and severity of bladder toxicity. Test urine for blood.
• Adequately hydrate patient before and after dose to decrease risk of cystitis.
• Use caution to ensure correct dose to decrease risk of cardiac toxicity.
• Monitor CBC, electrolytes, and kidney function test and LFT results.
• Monitor closely for leukopenia (nadir between days 8 and 15, recovery in 17 to 28 days). Withhold drug in patient whose ANC is less than 1,500/mm³.
• Monitor for infection. Drug may need to be interrupted or dose reduced in patient with serious infection. G-CSF may be given.
• Monitor uric acid level. To prevent hyperuricemia with resulting uric acid nephropathy, allopurinol may be used with adequate hydration.
• To prevent bleeding, avoid all IM injections when platelet count is less than 50,000/mm³.
• Monitor patient for kidney, pulmonary, and cardiac toxicities; veno-occlusive liver disease; secondary malignancies; impaired wound healing; and hyponatremia.
• Anticipate blood transfusions because of cumulative anemia.
• Therapeutic effects are often accompanied by toxicity.
• Drug is associated with a moderate to high emetic potential (depending on dose, regimen, and administration route); antiemetics are recommended to prevent nausea and vomiting.

PATIENT TEACHING
• Warn patient that hair loss is likely to occur but is reversible.
• Advise patient to report all adverse reactions, especially signs and symptoms of infection (fever, sore throat, fatigue) and bleeding (easy bruising, nosebleeds, bleeding gums, tarry stools, bloody urine), dyspnea, cough, edema, and dizziness. Tell patient to take temperature daily.
• Instruct patient to avoid OTC products that contain aspirin.

• To minimize risk of hemorrhagic cystitis, encourage patient to urinate every 1 to 2 hours while awake and to drink at least 3 L of fluid daily.
• Tell patient taking capsules to take them in the morning because infrequent urination during night increases risk of cystitis.
• Advise patient that drug is associated with a moderate to high emetic potential and that antiemetics are recommended.
• Caution patients to practice contraception during therapy and for 4 months afterward for males and 12 months for females; drug may cause birth defects.
• Advise patient to stop breastfeeding during therapy because of risk of toxicity to infant.
• Drug can cause irreversible sterility. Before therapy, counsel patient who is considering parenthood. Also recommend that patient consult prescriber before becoming pregnant.

cycloSPORINE
sye-kloe-SPOR-een

Sandimmune

cycloSPORINE (modified)
Gengraf, Neoral

Therapeutic class: Immunosuppressants
Pharmacologic class: Immunosuppressants

AVAILABLE FORMS
Capsules for microemulsion (modified): 25 mg, 100 mg*
Capsules (nonmodified): 25 mg, 50 mg, 100 mg
Injection: 50 mg/mL
Oral solution (modified and nonmodified): 100 mg/mL*

INDICATIONS & DOSAGES
➤ **To prevent organ rejection in kidney, liver, or cardiac transplantation**
Adults and children: 15 mg/kg PO 4 to 12 hours before transplantation, continued daily for 1 to 2 weeks postoperatively. Then reduce dosage by 5% each week to maintenance level of 5 to 10 mg/kg daily. Or, 5 to 6 mg/kg IV concentrate 4 to 12 hours before transplantation as slow IV infusion over 2 to 6 hours. Postoperatively, repeat dose daily until patient can tolerate oral forms.

Reactions in bold italics are *life-threatening*.

For conversion from Sandimmune to Gengraf or Neoral, use same daily dose as previously used for Sandimmune. Monitor blood levels every 4 to 7 days after conversion; monitor BP and creatinine level every 2 weeks during the first 2 months.

➤ **Severe, active RA that hasn't adequately responded to methotrexate (Gengraf or Neoral)**
Adults: 1.25 mg/kg PO b.i.d. Onset of action generally occurs between 4 and 8 weeks. Dosage may be increased by 0.5 to 0.75 mg/kg daily after 8 weeks and again after 12 weeks to a maximum of 4 mg/kg daily. If no response occurs after 16 weeks, stop therapy.
Adjust-a-dose: Decrease dosage by 25% to 50% to control adverse reactions (such as HTN, serum creatinine elevations [30% above patient's pretreatment level], or clinically significant lab abnormalities). If dosage reduction doesn't control abnormalities or if adverse reaction or abnormality is severe, discontinue drug.

➤ **Psoriasis (Gengraf or Neoral)**
Adults: 1.25 mg/kg daily PO b.i.d. for at least 4 weeks. Increase dosage by 0.5 mg/kg daily once every 2 weeks as needed to a maximum of 4 mg/kg daily.
Adjust-a-dose: Decrease dosage by 25% to 50% to control adverse reactions (such as HTN, serum creatinine elevations [25% above patient's pretreatment level], or clinically significant lab abnormalities). If dosage reduction doesn't control abnormalities or if adverse reaction or abnormality is severe, discontinue drug.

ADMINISTRATION
⏺ *Alert:* Hazardous drug; use safe handling and disposal precautions.
PO
• Give Neoral or Gengraf on an empty stomach in two divided doses. Give on a consistent schedule.
• Measure oral solution doses carefully in an oral syringe. Don't rinse dosing syringe with water. If syringe is cleaned, ensure it is completely dry before reuse.
• To improve the taste of Sandimmune oral solution, mix it with milk, chocolate milk, or orange juice. Gengraf or Neoral oral solution may be mixed with orange or apple juice (not grapefruit juice); it's less palatable when mixed with milk.

• Use a glass container to mix, and have patient drink at once.
IV
▼ IV form is usually reserved for patients who can't tolerate oral drugs.
▼ Immediately before use, dilute each milliliter of concentrate in 20 to 100 mL of D₅W or NSS for injection. Give at one-third the oral dose.
▼ Infuse over 2 to 6 hours.
▼ Protect diluted drug from light.
▼ **Incompatibilities:** Amphotericin B cholesteryl sulfate complex, magnesium sulfate.

ACTION
May inhibit proliferation and function of T lymphocytes and inhibit production and release of lymphokines.

Route	Onset	Peak	Duration
PO	Unknown	90 min–3 hr	Unknown
IV	Unknown	Unknown	Unknown

Half-life: Initial phase, about 1 hour; terminal phase, 8.5 to 27 hours.

ADVERSE REACTIONS
CNS: tremor, headache, confusion, dizziness, fatigue, fever, rigors, pain, insomnia, depression, migraine, paresthesia, *seizures.*
CV: HTN, flushing, edema, chest pain, arrhythmias, purpura. **EENT:** rhinitis, sinusitis, gum hyperplasia, gingivitis, ear disorder.
GI: anorexia, nausea, vomiting, diarrhea, abdominal discomfort, dyspepsia, flatulence, *rectal hemorrhage,* stomatitis. **GU:** increased creatinine level, UTI, urinary frequency, menstrual disorder, *kidney dysfunction.* **Hematologic:** anemia, *leukopenia, thrombocytopenia, lymphoma.* **Hepatic:** *liver toxicity.*
Metabolic: *hypomagnesemia,* hyperglycemia, hypertriglyceridemia. **Musculoskeletal:** leg cramps, arthralgia. **Respiratory:** URI, pneumonia, cough, dyspnea, *bronchospasm.* **Skin:** hirsutism, acne, rash.
Other: infections, hypersensitivity, gynecomastia, flulike symptoms, accidental trauma.

INTERACTIONS
Drug-drug. *Acyclovir, aminoglycosides, amphotericin B, cimetidine, diclofenac, gentamicin, ketoconazole, melphalan, NSAIDs, sulfamethoxazole–trimethoprim, tacrolimus, tobramycin, vancomycin:* May increase risk of kidney toxicity. Avoid use together.

---

*Allopurinol, azathioprine, **azole antifungals**, bromocriptine, calcium channel blockers, **caspofungin**, cimetidine, clarithromycin, corticosteroids, cyclophosphamide, danazol, erythromycin, imipenem–cilastatin, metoclopramide, **micafungin**:* May increase cyclosporine level and immunosuppression. Monitor patient closely.

*Carbamazepine, isoniazid, nafcillin, octreotide, **orlistat**, phenobarbital, **phenytoin**, **rifabutin**, **rifampin**, ticlopidine:* May decrease immunosuppressant effect from low cyclosporine level. Cyclosporine dosage may need to be increased.

Digoxin, HMG-CoA reductase inhibitors (lovastatin, other statins), prednisolone: May decrease clearance of these drugs. Use together cautiously.

Mycophenolate mofetil: May decrease mycophenolate level. Monitor patient closely when cyclosporine is added to or removed from therapy.

Potassium-sparing diuretics: May induce hyperkalemia. Avoid use together.

Pravastatin: May increase levels of both drugs. Limit pravastatin to 20 mg/day.

Protease inhibitors (indinavir, ritonavir): May increase cyclosporine level. Use together cautiously.

Rosuvastatin: May decrease clearance of statin. Limit rosuvastatin dose to 5 mg/day.

Sirolimus: May increase sirolimus level. Take sirolimus at least 4 hours after cyclosporine dose. If separating doses isn't possible, monitor patient for increased adverse effects.

Vaccines: May decrease immune response. Delay routine immunization.

Drug-herb. *Astragalus, echinacea, licorice:* May interfere with drug's effect. Discourage use together.

St. John's wort: May reduce drug level, resulting in transplant failure. Discourage use together.

Drug-food. *Grapefruit and grapefruit juice:* May increase drug level and cause toxicity. Advise patient to avoid use together.

Drug-lifestyle. *Sun exposure:* May increase risk of sensitivity to sunlight. Advise patient to avoid excessive sun exposure.

EFFECTS ON LAB TEST RESULTS
• May increase ALT, AST, bilirubin, BUN, creatinine, potassium, triglyceride, cholesterol, and LDL-C levels.
• May decrease Hb and magnesium levels.

• May increase or decrease glucose level.
• May decrease platelet and WBC counts.

CONTRAINDICATIONS & CAUTIONS
• Contraindicated in patients hypersensitive to drug or polyoxyethylated castor oil.
• Contraindicated in patients with RA or psoriasis with abnormal kidney function, uncontrolled HTN, or malignancies (Neoral or Gengraf).
• Contraindicated with psoralen and UVA light (PUVA), methotrexate or other immunosuppressive agents, UVB light, coal tar, or radiation therapy in patients with psoriasis (Neoral or Gengraf).
• Obtain biopsy of skin lesions not typical for psoriasis before starting drug. Use in patients with malignant or premalignant skin changes only after appropriate treatment of such lesions and if no other treatment option exists.
• PRES has occurred. Use cautiously in patients with hypomagnesemia, hypocholesterolemia, or GVHD; in patients on corticosteroids; and in patients with high cyclosporine levels.

Boxed Warning Only experienced prescribers should prescribe this drug. Manage patients receiving drug in facilities equipped and staffed with adequate lab and supportive medical resources. ■

Dialyzable drug: No.

PREGNANCY-LACTATION-REPRODUCTION
• Studies during pregnancy are inadequate. Use during pregnancy isn't recommended. If drug is needed during pregnancy, use only if potential benefit justifies fetal risk.
• Alcohol is present in cyclosporine preparations; consider this fact when using drug during pregnancy.
• Drug and ethanol present in cyclosporine preparations appear in human milk. Patient should discontinue breastfeeding or discontinue drug, considering importance of drug to patient.

NURSING CONSIDERATIONS
Boxed Warning Patient with psoriasis previously treated with PUVA, methotrexate or other immunosuppressive agents, UVB, coal tar, or radiation therapy is at an increased risk

---

Reactions in bold italics are *life-threatening*.

C

for skin malignancies when taking Neoral or Gengraf. ■

• Drug can cause liver toxicity.

Boxed Warning Cyclosporine may increase the patient's susceptibility to infection and the development of neoplasia. ■

☻ *Alert:* Drugs that cause immunosuppression increase risk of opportunistic infections, including activation of latent viral infections such as BK virus-associated neuropathy, which may lead to serious outcomes, including kidney graft loss.

Boxed Warning Monitor patient's kidney function. ■

Boxed Warning Monitor cyclosporine level at regular intervals with prolonged use. Absorption of capsules and oral solution can be erratic during long-term use. ■

Boxed Warning Neoral and Gengraf have greater bioavailability than Sandimmune. A lower dose of Neoral or Gengraf may be needed to provide blood level similar to that achieved with Sandimmune. Monitor blood level when switching patients between these brands. ■

• Gengraf is bioequivalent to and interchangeable with Neoral capsules.

Boxed Warning Always give Sandimmune with corticosteroids; however, don't give Sandimmune with other immunosuppressants. ■

Boxed Warning Drug can cause systemic HTN and kidney toxicity; risk increases with increasing dosage and duration of therapy. ■

• Monitor for signs and symptoms of PRES (seizures, vision changes, change in consciousness, loss of motor functions, movement disorders, psychiatric disturbances.)

RA

• Before starting treatment, measure BP at least twice and obtain two creatinine levels to estimate baseline.

• Evaluate BP and creatinine level ever 2 weeks during first 3 months and then monthly if patient is stable.

• Monitor BP and creatinine level after an increase in NSAID dosage or introduction of a new NSAID. Monitor CBC and LFT values monthly if patient also receives methotrexate.

Psoriasis

• Measure BP at least twice to determine a baseline. Monitor BP after dosage changes.

• Evaluate patient for occult infection and tumors initially and throughout treatment.

• Obtain baseline creatinine level (on two occasions), CBC, and BUN, magnesium, uric acid, potassium, and lipid levels.

• Evaluate BP, CBC, and uric acid, potassium, lipid, magnesium, creatinine, and BUN levels every 2 weeks during first 3 months and then monthly thereafter if patient is stable.

• Monitor creatinine level after increasing NSAID dose or starting a new NSAID.

• Improvement in psoriasis takes 12 to 16 weeks of therapy.

• *Look alike–sound alike:* Don't confuse cyclosporine with cyclophosphamide or cycloserine. Don't confuse Sandimmune with Sandostatin.

PATIENT TEACHING

• Encourage patient to take drug at same time each day and to be consistent with relation to meals.

• Teach patient safe medication administration and handling.

• Tell patient being treated for psoriasis that improvement may not occur until after 12 to 16 weeks of therapy.

• Stress that drug shouldn't be stopped without prescriber's approval.

• Inform patient of increased risk of tumors, high BP, and kidney problems.

• Explain to patient the importance of frequent lab monitoring while receiving therapy.

• Tell patient to avoid people with infections because drug lowers resistance to infection.

• Advise patient to perform careful oral care and to see a dentist regularly because drug can cause gum disease.

• Inform patient of childbearing potential to use barrier contraception, not hormonal contraceptives, during therapy. Advise patient of potential risk during pregnancy.

• Warn patient to wear protection in the sun and to avoid excessive sun exposure.

dabigatran etexilate mesylate
da-BIG-a-tran e-TEX-i-late

Pradaxa

Therapeutic class: Anticoagulants
Pharmacologic class: Direct thrombin inhibitors

AVAILABLE FORMS
Capsules ⓄⓉⒸ: 75 mg, 110 mg, 150 mg
Oral pellets: 20 mg, 30 mg, 40 mg, 50 mg, 110 mg, 150 mg packets

INDICATIONS & DOSAGES
➤ **To reduce risk of stroke and systemic embolism in patients with nonvalvular atrial fibrillation**
Adults with CrCl greater than 30 mL/minute: 150 mg PO b.i.d.
Adjust-a-dose: For patients with CrCl of 15 to 30 mL/minute or for those with CrCl of 30 to 50 mL/minute who are taking dronedarone or oral ketoconazole concurrently, give 75 mg PO b.i.d. Avoid use in patients with CrCl of less than 30 mL/minute also taking P-gp inhibitors. Don't use in patients on dialysis or in those with CrCl of less than 15 mL/minute.
➤ **To treat DVT and PE in patients who have been treated with a parenteral anticoagulant for 5 to 10 days; to reduce risk of recurrence of DVT and PE in patients who have been previously treated**
Adults with CrCl greater than 30 mL/minute: 150 mg PO b.i.d.
Adjust-a-dose: There are no dosing recommendations for patients with CrCl of 30 mL/minute or less or for those on dialysis. Avoid use in patients with CrCl of less than 50 mL/minute also taking P-gp inhibitors.
➤ **Prophylaxis of DVT and PE after hip replacement surgery**
Adults with CrCl greater than 30 mL/minute: 110 mg PO 1 to 4 hours after surgery and after hemostasis has been achieved; then 220 mg once daily for 28 to 35 days. If drug isn't started on day of surgery, after hemostasis has been achieved, start treatment with 220 mg once daily.
Adjust-a-dose: There are no dosing recommendations for patients with CrCl of less

than 30 mL/minute or for those on dialysis. Avoid use in patients with CrCl less than 50 mL/minute also taking P-gp inhibitors.
➤ **VTE in children previously treated with parenteral anticoagulant for at least 5 days; to reduce risk of VTE recurrence in previously treated children**
Children ages 8 to younger than 18 (capsules): If 81 kg or more, 260 mg PO b.i.d.; if 61 to less than 81 kg, 220 mg PO b.i.d.; if 41 to less than 61 kg, 185 mg PO b.i.d.; if 26 to less than 41 kg, 150 mg PO b.i.d.; if 16 to less than 26 kg, 110 mg PO b.i.d.; if 11 to less than 16 kg, 75 mg PO b.i.d.
Children ages 3 months to younger than 12 years (pellets): Weight-based dose PO b.i.d. according to manufacturer's instructions.
Adjust-a-dose: Avoid use in children with eGFR less than 50 mL/minute/1.73 m².

ADMINISTRATION
PO
• Refer to manufacturer's instructions when converting to and from warfarin or parenteral anticoagulants.
• Give without regard to food as close to 12 hours apart as possible. Give with food if GI distress occurs with capsules.
• Dosages for capsules and oral pellets are not equivalent.
• Have patient swallow capsules whole with full glass of water; don't crush or cut capsules.
• Give pellets before a meal to ensure patient takes full dose.
• Mix pellets in 2 tsp (10 mL) of applesauce or mashed carrots or bananas. Or, spoon pellets directly into patient's mouth and have patient swallow with apple juice, or add to approximately 1 to 2 oz (30 to 60 mL) of apple juice for drinking.
• Don't mix pellets with milk, milk products, or soft foods containing milk products.
• Don't give pellets via syringe or feeding tube.
• Give pellets within 30 minutes of mixing; discard dose after 30 minutes if not given.
• Give missed dose as soon as possible on same day; if less than 6 hours before next scheduled dose, skip missed dose.
• If patient ingests a partial dose of pellets, don't give additional dose; give next dose as scheduled.

Reactions in bold italics are *life-threatening*.

ACTION

Reversible, direct thrombin inhibitor that prevents thrombus development.

Route	Onset	Peak	Duration
PO	Unknown	1–2 hr	Unknown

Half-life: Adults, 12 to 17 hours; children, 12 to 14 hours; children (pellets), 9 to 11 hours.

ADVERSE REACTIONS

EENT: epistaxis. **GI:** abdominal pain or discomfort, gastritis-like symptoms (GERD, esophagitis, erosive gastritis, *gastric hemorrhage, hemorrhagic erosive gastritis*, GI ulcer), diarrhea, nausea, vomiting, *GI bleeding.* **GU:** menorrhagia. **Hematologic:** *major bleeding event,* minor bleeding.

INTERACTIONS

Drug-drug. *Antiplatelet drugs, aspirin, fibrinolytic therapy, heparin, NSAIDs:* May increase risk of bleeding. Carefully consider risks and benefits of use together, monitor closely, and consider therapy modification.
P-gp inducers (rifampin): May reduce dabigatran level. Generally, avoid use together. Refer to individual inducer's manufacturer's instructions or interactions reference for further recommendations.
P-gp inhibitors (dronedarone, systemic ketoconazole): May increase effectiveness of dabigatran; dosage reductions may be needed. Refer to indication-specific dosage adjustments above and manufacturer's instructions for additional information.
Drug-herb. *Herbs with anticoagulant/antiplatelet properties (alfalfa, anise, bilberry):* May increase risk of bleeding. Consider therapy modification.

EFFECTS ON LAB TEST RESULTS

• May increase PTT, ecarin clotting time (ECT), and thrombin time.

CONTRAINDICATIONS & CAUTIONS

Boxed Warning Consider risk of epidural or spinal hematoma in patients scheduled for spinal procedures (spinal or epidural anesthesia, spinal puncture). Hematomas may result in long-term or permanent paralysis. Risk may increase with use of indwelling epidural catheters; use with drugs that affect hemostasis (NSAIDs, platelet inhibitors, anticoagulants); history of traumatic or repeated epidural or spinal punctures; or history of spinal

deformity or surgery. Optimal timing between administration of drug and spinal or epidural procedure isn't known. ■
• Contraindicated in patients hypersensitive to drug and in those with active pathologic bleeding.
• Contraindicated in patients with mechanical prosthetic valves. Use in patients with atrial fibrillation in the setting of other forms of valvular heart disease, including the presence of a bioprosthetic heart valve, isn't recommended.
• Use isn't recommended in patients with triple-positive antiphospholipid syndrome; drug may increase risk of recurrent thrombotic events.
• Use cautiously in older adults, in patients with history of bleeding, and when used with other drugs that increase risk of bleeding.
• Because of risk of clot formation and stroke, avoid lapses in therapy when possible. Restart therapy as soon as possible.
Boxed Warning Discontinuing drug prematurely increases risk of thrombotic events. If drug must be discontinued for a reason other than pathologic bleeding or completion of a course of therapy, consider coverage with another anticoagulant. ■
• Use in children with an eGFR less than 50 mL/minute/1.73 m² hasn't been studied; avoid use in these patients.
Dialyzable drug: Approximately 49% to 57%.
⚠ Overdose S&S: Hemorrhagic complications.

PREGNANCY-LACTATION-REPRODUCTION

• Studies during pregnancy are inadequate. Consider risks of bleeding and stroke if drug is used during pregnancy.
• Patients of childbearing potential may be at risk for severe uterine bleeding.
• Drug may increase bleeding risk in the fetus and neonate. Monitor neonates for bleeding.
• It isn't known if drug appears in human milk. Breastfeeding isn't recommended during treatment.

NURSING CONSIDERATIONS

• Monitor patient for signs of bleeding. If bleeding occurs, stop drug, investigate cause, and provide supportive measures.
• A specific reversal agent (idarucizumab) is available. Refer to idarucizumab prescribing information for more information.

• Monitor ECT or PTT to assess treatment effectiveness.

Boxed Warning After spinal procedure, monitor patient for neurologic impairment (midline back pain; sensory or motor deficits, such as numbness or weakness in lower limbs; bowel or bladder dysfunction). Treat impairment urgently. ∎

• Discontinue dabigatran 1 to 2 days before invasive or surgical procedures in patients with CrCl of 50 mL/minute or more and 3 to 5 days in patients with CrCl of less than 50 mL/minute. Consider longer times for patients undergoing major surgery, spinal puncture, or placement of a spinal or epidural catheter or port, in whom complete hemostasis may be required. Restart drug as soon as medically appropriate.

• For children, discontinue drug 24 hours before elective surgery if GFR is greater than 80 mL/minute/1.73 m² or 2 days before elective surgery if eGFR is 50 to 80 mL/minute/1.73 m².

PATIENT TEACHING

◑ *Alert:* Advise patient to keep drug in original bottle to protect from moisture, to remove only one capsule from opened bottle at the time of use, to tightly close bottle immediately after removing drug, and to not put drug in pillboxes or pill organizers.

• Teach about proper drug administration and handling.

• Caution patient to take drug as prescribed and to not stop or change dosage without first consulting prescriber.

• Advise patient to tell all health care providers about taking drug.

• Tell patient to inform prescriber about use of other drugs, including OTC medications, vitamins, and herbs.

• Warn patient that bruising may occur more easily and bleeding may last longer during therapy.

• Instruct patient to report bleeding when brushing teeth or shaving; blood in vomit, urine, or stool; heavier-than-normal menstrual bleeding; or nosebleeds.

• Explain that patient will need to undergo regular blood tests to monitor drug's effects.

• Instruct patient to inform health care provider of scheduled invasive procedures, including dental work. Drug may need to be temporarily stopped.

SAFETY ALERT!

dalteparin sodium
DAHL-tep-ah-rin

Fragmin

Therapeutic class: Anticoagulants
Pharmacologic class: Low-molecular-weight heparins

AVAILABLE FORMS

◑ *Alert:* Strengths expressed as antifactor Xa international unit/mL.
Injection (multidose vial): 95,000/3.8 mL vial*
Injection (prefilled syringe): 2,500/0.2 mL; 5,000/0.2 mL; 7,500/0.3 mL; 10,000/1 mL; 12,500/0.5 mL; 15,000/0.6 mL; 18,000/0.72 mL
Injection (single-dose graduated syringe): 10,000/1 mL
Injection (single-dose vial): 10,000/4 mL

INDICATIONS & DOSAGES

➤ **To prevent DVT in patients undergoing abdominal surgery who are at moderate to high risk for thromboembolic complications**
Adults: 2,500 international units subcut daily, starting 1 to 2 hours before surgery and repeated once daily for 5 to 10 days postoperatively. Or, for patients at high risk, 5,000 international units subcut the evening before surgery and then once-daily postoperatively for 5 to 10 days. Or, in patients with malignancy, 2,500 international units subcut 1 to 2 hours before surgery, followed by 2,500 international units subcut 12 hours later, then 5,000 international units subcut once daily for 5 to 10 days postoperatively.

➤ **To prevent DVT in patients undergoing hip replacement surgery**
Adults: 2,500 international units subcut within 2 hours before surgery and second dose of 2,500 international units subcut the evening after surgery (4 to 8 hours after surgery or later if hemostasis hasn't been achieved). Starting on first postoperative day, allowing a minimum of 6 hours after postoperative dose, 5,000 international units subcut once daily for 5 to 10 days. Or, 5,000 international units subcut 10 to 14 hours before surgery; then 5,000 international units subcut once daily starting 4 to 8 hours after surgery

and continuing for 5 to 10 days postoperatively. Allow approximately 24 hours between preoperative and first postoperative doses.

If starting postoperatively, 2,500 international units subcut the evening after surgery (4 to 8 hours after surgery, or later if hemostasis hasn't been achieved). Starting on first postoperative day, allowing a minimum of 6 hours after postoperative dose, 5,000 international units subcut once daily for 5 to 10 days.

➤ **Prophylaxis of ischemic complications in patients with unstable angina; non-Q-wave MI**

Adults: 120 international units/kg subcut every 12 hours PO. Give with aspirin (75 to 165 mg daily), unless contraindicated. Maximum dose, 10,000 international units. Treatment usually lasts 5 to 8 days.

➤ **To prevent DVT in patients at risk for thromboembolic complications because of severely restricted mobility during acute illness**

Adults: 5,000 international units subcut once daily for 12 to 14 days.

➤ **Symptomatic VTE in patients with cancer**

Adults: Initially, 200 international units/kg (maximum, 18,000 international units) subcut daily for 30 days; then 150 international units/kg (maximum, 18,000 international units) subcut daily months 2 through 6.

Adjust-a-dose: In patients with platelet count of 50,000 to 100,000/mm^3, reduce dose by 2,500 international units until platelet count exceeds 100,000/mm^3. In patients with platelet count less than 50,000/mm^3, stop drug until platelet count exceeds 50,000/mm^3. In patients with CrCl of 30 mL/minute or less, monitor anti-Xa levels to determine appropriate dose. Target anti-Xa range is 0.5 to 1.5 international units/mL. Draw anti-Xa 4 to 6 hours after dose and only after patient has received three to four doses.

➤ **Symptomatic VTE in children**

Children ages 8 to younger than 17: 100 international units/kg b.i.d. for three doses; then assess anti-Xa level.

Children ages 2 to younger than 8: 125 international units/kg b.i.d. for three doses; then assess anti-Xa level.

Children ages 4 weeks to younger than 2 years: 150 international units/kg b.i.d. for three doses; then assess anti-Xa level.

Adjust-a-dose: Adjust dosage in increments of 25 international units/kg to achieve target anti-Xa level between 0.5 and 1 international

unit/mL. If platelet count is 50,000 to 100,000/mm^3, reduce dosage by 50% until platelet count exceeds 100,000/mm^3. If platelet count is less than 50,000/mm^3, stop drug until platelet count exceeds 50,000/mm^3.

➤ **Acute symptomatic superficial vein thrombosis** ◆

Adults: 5,000 units subcut every 12 hours for 45 days.

ADMINISTRATION
Subcutaneous

• Injection sites include U-shaped area around navel, upper outer side of thigh, and upper outer quadrangle of buttock. Rotate sites daily.

• Give subcut injection deeply, inserting entire length of needle at 45- to 90-degree angle.

• After first penetration of rubber stopper, store multidose vial at room temperature for up to 2 weeks. Discard any unused solution after 2 weeks.

• Whenever possible, use benzyl alcohol–free formulations (prefilled syringes) in children.

• The needle shield of the prefilled syringe may contain natural rubber latex. Use cautiously in patients with latex allergies.

• Prepare graduated syringe by expelling air bubble and discarding extra solution to achieve desired dose. Be sure to give entire dose of graduated syringe or needle guard will not activate.

• Don't mix with other injections or infusions unless specific compatibility data support such mixing.

• Store at room temperature.

ACTION

Inhibition of factor Xa and thrombin by antithrombin.

Route	Onset	Peak	Duration
Subcut	1–2 hr	4 hr	>12 hr

Half-life: 2 to 5 hours.

ADVERSE REACTIONS

EENT: epistaxis. **GU:** hematuria. **Hematologic:** *thrombocytopenia, hemorrhage,* ecchymoses, bleeding complications. **Hepatic:** elevated transaminase levels. **Skin:** hematoma at injection site, wound hematoma, injection-site pain. **Other:** hypersensitivity reaction (pruritus, rash, fever).

INTERACTIONS

Drug-drug. *Antiplatelet drugs (aspirin, NSAIDs, clopidogrel, dipyridamole, ticlopidine), oral anticoagulants, SSRIs (fluoxetine), thrombolytics:* May increase risk of bleeding. Use together cautiously.

Drug-herb. *Herbs with anticoagulant/antiplatelet properties (alfalfa, anise, bilberry, willow):* May increase risk of bleeding. Discourage use together.

EFFECTS ON LAB TEST RESULTS

- May increase ALT and AST levels.
- May decrease Hb level and platelet count.

CONTRAINDICATIONS & CAUTIONS

- Contraindicated in patients hypersensitive to drug, heparin, or pork products; in those with active major bleeding; and in those with a history of heparin-induced thrombocytopenia or heparin-induced thrombocytopenia with thrombosis.
- Contraindicated in patients with unstable angina or non-Q-wave MI or prolonged VTE prophylaxis who are undergoing epidural/neuraxial anesthesia.
- Use cautiously in patients at increased risk for hemorrhage, such as those with severe uncontrolled HTN, bacterial endocarditis, congenital or acquired bleeding disorders, active ulceration, angiodysplastic GI disease, or hemorrhagic stroke; also use with caution shortly after brain, spinal, or ophthalmic surgery. Monitor vital signs.
- Use cautiously in patients with bleeding diathesis, thrombocytopenia, platelet defects, liver or kidney insufficiency, hypertensive or diabetic retinopathy, or recent GI bleeding.
- Use cautiously in patients at risk for DVT following abdominal surgery and candidates for therapy, including those older than age 40, those who are obese, those undergoing surgery under general anesthesia lasting longer than 30 minutes, and those who have additional risk factors (such as malignancy or history of DVT or PE).
- Use preservative-free dalteparin in neonates and infants because serious and fatal adverse reactions, including gasping syndrome, can occur in neonates and low-birth-weight infants treated with medications containing benzyl alcohol.

Dialyzable drug: Unknown.

⚠ **Overdose S&S:** Hemorrhagic complications.

PREGNANCY-LACTATION-REPRODUCTION

- Studies during pregnancy are inadequate. Use during pregnancy only if clearly needed.
- Use preservative-free formulations without benzyl alcohol (not multidose vial) when possible during pregnancy and only if clearly needed. Benzyl alcohol may cross the placental barrier.
- Small amounts of anti-Xa activity have been detected in human milk; clinical implications, if any, for a breastfeeding infant are unknown. Use cautiously during breastfeeding.

NURSING CONSIDERATIONS

Boxed Warning Patients who have received epidural or spinal anesthesia or spinal puncture are at increased risk for developing an epidural or spinal hematoma, which may result in long-term or permanent paralysis. Increased risk may occur with use of indwelling epidural catheters, use with drugs that affect hemostasis (NSAIDs, platelet inhibitors, anticoagulants), history of traumatic or repeated epidural or spinal punctures, or history of spinal deformity or surgery. Monitor these patients closely for neurologic impairment and treat urgently. ∎

Boxed Warning Monitor patients for neurologic impairment (midline back pain; sensory or motor deficits, such as numbness or weakness in lower limbs; bowel or bladder dysfunction). Treat impairment urgently. ∎

Boxed Warning Optimal timing between administration of drug and neuraxial procedures isn't known. Consider benefits and risks before neuraxial intervention in patients anticoagulated or to be anticoagulated for thromboprophylaxis. ∎

- Never give drug IM.

⚠ *Alert:* Drug isn't interchangeable (unit for unit) with unfractionated heparin or other low-molecular-weight heparin.

- Periodic, routine CBC and fecal occult blood tests are recommended during therapy. Patients don't need regular monitoring of PT or PTT.
- Closely monitor patient for thrombocytopenia.
- Stop drug if a thromboembolic event occurs despite dalteparin prophylaxis.

PATIENT TEACHING

- Instruct patient and family to watch for and report signs and symptoms of bleeding (bruising, blood in stools) and to promptly report all adverse reactions.

Reactions in bold italics are *life-threatening*.

- Inform patient it may take longer than usual to stop bleeding.
- Tell patient to avoid OTC drugs containing aspirin or other salicylates unless ordered by prescriber.
- Advise patient to consult with prescriber before initiating any herbal therapy; many herbs have anticoagulant, antiplatelet, and fibrinolytic properties.
- Tell patient to inform physicians and dentists of all medications being taken.
- Instruct patient to use a soft toothbrush and electric razor during treatment.
- Teach about proper drug administration and handling, including syringe disposal if appropriate.
- Urge patient to inform prescriber if patient or caregiver giving the injection has an allergy to natural rubber latex.

SAFETY ALERT!

dapagliflozin
dap-a-gli-FLOE-zin

Farxiga

Therapeutic class: Antidiabetics
Pharmacologic class: Sodium-glucose cotransporter 2 inhibitors

AVAILABLE FORMS
Tablets: 5 mg, 10 mg

INDICATIONS & DOSAGES
➤ **Adjunct to diet and exercise to improve glycemic control in patients with type 2 diabetes**
*Adults with eGFR of 45 mL/minute/1.73 m²
or greater:* Initially, 5 mg PO once daily; may increase to 10 mg daily for patients who require additional glycemic control.
➤ **To reduce risk of CV death and hospitalization for HF in patients with NYHA Class II, III, or IV HF with reduced ejection fraction**
*Adults with eGFR of 25 mL/minute/1.73 m²
or greater:* 10 mg PO once daily.
➤ **To reduce risk of hospitalization for HF in patients with type 2 diabetes and established CV disease or multiple CV risk factors**
*Adults with eGFR of 45 mL/minute/1.73 m²
or greater:* 10 mg PO once daily.
➤ **To reduce risk of sustained eGFR decline, CKD, CV death, and hospitalization for**

HF in patients with CKD at risk for progression
*Adults with eGFR of 25 mL/minute/1.73 m²
or greater:* 10 mg PO once daily.
Adjust-a-dose: Drug isn't recommended for initiation when eGFR is less than 25 mL/
minute/1.73 m²; however, patient may continue 10 mg PO once daily to reduce risk of eGFR decline, CKD, CV death, and hospitalization for HF.

ADMINISTRATION
PO
- Give dose in the morning.
- May give without regard for food.
- Give missed dose as soon as possible unless it's almost time for next dose; don't double dose.
- Store at room temperature.

ACTION
Inhibitor of sodium-glucose cotransporter 2 (SGLT2), which reduces reabsorption of filtered glucose from the proximal kidney tubule and lowers the kidney threshold for glucose, resulting in increased urine glucose excretion.

Route	Onset	Peak	Duration
PO	Unknown	2 hr	Unknown

Half-life: About 12.9 hours.

ADVERSE REACTIONS
CV: volume depletion (dehydration, hypovolemia, orthostatic hypotension, hypotension). **EENT:** nasopharyngitis. **GI:** nausea, constipation. **GU:** genital mycotic infection, UTI, increased urination, dysuria. **Metabolic:** dyslipidemia. **Musculoskeletal:** back pain, extremity pain. **Other:** flu-like symptoms.

INTERACTIONS
Drug-drug. *Insulin, insulin secretagogues (glimepiride, glipizide, glyburide, nateglinide, repaglinide):* May increase risk of hypoglycemia. Monitor patient closely and adjust insulin and secretagogue dosages as necessary.
Loop diuretics: May increase risk of volume depletion or hypotension. Monitor patient closely.

EFFECTS ON LAB TEST RESULTS
- May increase creatinine level, LDL-C level, and hematocrit.

- May decrease eGFR level.
- May cause positive urine glucose test.
- May interfere with 1,5-AG assay. Use alternative methods to monitor glycemic control.

CONTRAINDICATIONS & CAUTIONS
- Contraindicated in patients who are on dialysis and in patients with history of serious hypersensitivity reactions (anaphylaxis, angioedema, SCAR) to dapagliflozin-containing products.
- Use isn't recommended in patients with an eGFR less than 45 mL/minute/1.73 m^2 in patients without CV disease or risk factors.
- Not recommended for use in patients with type 1 diabetes or for treatment of diabetic ketoacidosis.
- Not recommended for treatment of CKD in patients with polycystic kidney disease or those with current or recent immunosuppressive therapy for kidney disease.
- Use cautiously in older adults because of increased risk of adverse events.
- Drug increases serum creatinine level and decreases eGFR; older adults and patients with hypovolemia may be more susceptible to these changes.
- **Alert:** SGLT2 inhibitors such as dapagliflozin increase the risk of necrotizing fasciitis of the perineum (Fournier gangrene), a rare but serious and life-threatening infection requiring urgent surgical intervention.
- **Alert:** Drug may cause ketoacidosis, which may require emergency department care or hospitalization. Elevated urine or serum ketone level without associated very high glucose level has occurred with SGLT2 inhibitor use.

Dialyzable drug: Unknown.

PREGNANCY-LACTATION-REPRODUCTION
- Studies during pregnancy are inadequate. Use during pregnancy, especially second and third trimesters, isn't recommended. If needed during pregnancy, use only if potential benefit justifies fetal risk.
- It isn't known if drug appears in human milk. Use while breastfeeding isn't recommended.

NURSING CONSIDERATIONS
- **Alert:** Drug increases risk of AKI. Before starting therapy, assess patient for factors that may predispose to AKI (decreased blood volume; CKD; HF; concurrent use of other medications, such as diuretics, ACE inhibitors, ARBs, and NSAIDs). Assess kidney function before start of therapy and monitor periodically. Correct volume depletion before starting drug. If AKI occurs, discontinue drug and treat kidney impairment.
- Drug may increase risk of severe UTI, including urosepsis and pyelonephritis. Monitor patient and treat promptly, if indicated.
- **Alert:** Monitor for and immediately report signs and symptoms of necrotizing fasciitis of the perineum (temperature above 100.4° F [38° C], general feeling of unwellness; tenderness, redness, or swelling of the area from genitals to rectum). Signs and symptoms can worsen quickly. Immediately discontinue drug and prepare to administer broad-spectrum antibiotics. Surgical debridement may be necessary. Monitor blood glucose level and start alternative therapy for glycemic control.
- Monitor glucose level closely, especially if patient is taking antidiabetics concurrently. Adjust hypoglycemic dosages if needed.
- Monitor patient for signs and symptoms of diabetic ketoacidosis (dehydration, nausea, vomiting abdominal pain, malaise, anorexia, confusion, shortness of breath).
- Monitor for genital mycotic infections.
- Stop drug immediately if hypersensitivity or reduced kidney function is suspected.
- Monitor volume status and watch for signs and symptoms of hypotension, particularly in patients with eGFR less than 60 mL/minute/1.73 m^2, older adults, and patients taking loop diuretics. Increased urine glucose excretion also results in increased urine volume.
- Consider temporarily discontinuing drug for at least 3 days before scheduled surgery or other clinical situations known to predispose patient to ketoacidosis (prolonged fasting due to acute illness, postsurgery). Ensure risk factors are resolved before resuming therapy.

PATIENT TEACHING
- Warn patient to use drug only as directed.
- **Alert:** Advise patient to seek immediate medical attention for signs and symptoms of AKI (decreased urine output, swelling in legs or feet). Warn patient not to stop taking drug without first discussing with prescriber.
- **Alert:** Review signs and symptoms of necrotizing fasciitis. Instruct patient to seek immediate medical attention if any occur.

- Instruct patient to promptly report signs and symptoms of yeast infections (itching, burning, discharge).
- Counsel patient on importance of diet and exercise in addition to medication for diabetes control.
- Teach patient to obtain periodic blood testing as requested by prescriber.

❸ *Alert:* Instruct patient to immediately seek medical attention for signs and symptoms of ketoacidosis.

- Inform patient of increased UTI risk. Instruct patient to seek medical attention for signs and symptoms of UTI (painful urination, urinary frequency, blood in urine, urgency, pelvic pain, fever, back pain, nausea, vomiting).
- Advise patient to watch for signs and symptoms of hypoglycemia (fatigue, weakness, confusion, headache, pallor, or profuse sweating) when taking drug with insulin or insulin secretagogues.
- Caution patient to maintain adequate fluid intake to decrease risk of hypotension.
- Warn patient to contact prescriber for signs and symptoms of hypotension, such as lightheadedness (especially with position change) and weakness.
- Advise patient to promptly seek medical attention for fever, trauma, or infection and when surgery is needed; dosage adjustment may be needed due to stress.
- Caution patient to immediately report pregnancy, plans to become pregnant, breastfeeding, or intent to breastfeed during treatment.

DAPTOmycin
dap-toe-MYE-sin

Cubicin

Therapeutic class: Antibiotics
Pharmacologic class: Cyclic lipopeptides

AVAILABLE FORMS
Powder for injection: 350-mg, 500-mg vial

INDICATIONS & DOSAGES
➤ **Bacteremia caused by** *Staphylococcus aureus* **(including right-sided endocarditis caused by methicillin-susceptible and methicillin-resistant strains)**
Adults: 6 mg/kg IV infusion over 30 minutes or IV injection over 2 minutes every 24 hours

for at least 2 to 6 weeks based on patient response.
Adjust-a-dose: For patients with bacteremia and CrCl of less than 30 mL/minute, including those on CKRT, give 6 mg/kg IV every 48 hours. When possible, give drug after hemodialysis on hemodialysis days.
➤ **Bacteremia caused by** *S. aureus* **in children with normal kidney function**
Children ages 12 to 17: 7 mg/kg IV infusion over 30 minutes once every 24 hours for up to 42 days.
Children ages 7 to 11: 9 mg/kg IV infusion over 30 minutes once every 24 hours for up to 42 days.
Children ages 1 to 6: 12 mg/kg IV infusion over 60 minutes once every 24 hours for up to 42 days.
➤ **Complicated skin or skin-structure infection (cSSSI) caused by susceptible strains of** *S. aureus* **(including MRSA),** *Streptococcus pyogenes, Streptococcus agalactiae, Streptococcus dysgalactiae,* **and** *Enterococcus faecalis* **(vancomycin-susceptible strains only)**
Adults: 4 mg/kg IV infusion over 30 minutes or IV injection over 2 minutes every 24 hours for 7 to 14 days.
Children ages 12 to 17: 5 mg/kg IV infusion over 30 minutes once every 24 hours for up to 14 days.
Children ages 7 to 11: 7 mg/kg IV infusion over 30 minutes once every 24 hours for up to 14 days.
Children ages 2 to 6: 9 mg/kg IV infusion over 60 minutes once every 24 hours for up to 14 days.
Children ages 1 to younger than 2: 10 mg/kg IV infusion over 60 minutes once every 24 hours for up to 14 days.
Adjust-a-dose: In adults with cSSSI and CrCl of less than 30 mL/minute, including those on CKRT, give 4 mg/kg IV every 48 hours. When possible, give drug after hemodialysis on hemodialysis days. Dosage adjustment for children with kidney impairment hasn't been established.

ADMINISTRATION
IV
▼ Obtain specimen for culture and sensitivity tests before giving first dose. Begin therapy while awaiting results.

🔵 *Alert:* Refer to and carefully follow manufacturer's instructions for reconstitution and storage because formulations vary.

▼ Remove reconstituted liquid from the vial with a 21-gauge or smaller needle.

▼ Withdraw the appropriate volume.

▼ For IV injection over 2 minutes, give at a concentration of 50 mg/mL (adults only).

▼ Further dilute the appropriate volume in 50 mL NSS for IV infusion. Infuse over 30 minutes in adults and children ages 7 and older. For children ages 1 to 6, infuse over 60 minutes.

▼ Vials are for single use; discard excess.

▼ Don't use drug with ReadyMED elastomeric infusion pumps (Cardinal Health); an impurity may leach from the pump into the solution.

▼ **Incompatibilities:** Dextrose-containing solutions and other IV drugs. If an IV line is used for several drugs, flush the line with NSS or lactated Ringer solution injection between drugs.

ACTION

Bactericidal; binds to and depolarizes susceptible bacterial membranes to inhibit protein, DNA, and RNA synthesis.

Route	Onset	Peak	Duration
IV	Rapid	<1 hr	Unknown

Half-life: About 3.7 to 9 hours.

ADVERSE REACTIONS

CNS: dizziness, fever, headache, insomnia. **CV:** chest pain, edema, HTN, hypotension. **EENT:** sore throat. **GI:** abdominal pain, diarrhea, nausea, vomiting. **GU:** UTI. **Hepatic:** abnormal LFT values. **Metabolic:** increase CK level. **Respiratory:** cough, dyspnea. **Skin:** injection-site reactions, pruritus, rash, diaphoresis. **Other:** infection, bacteremia, *sepsis.*

INTERACTIONS

Drug-drug. *HMG-CoA reductase inhibitors (simvastatin):* May increase risk of myopathy. Consider stopping these drugs while giving daptomycin.

Warfarin: May falsely prolong PT and elevate INR with certain recombinant thromboplastin assay reagents. Draw specimen for INR and PT just before next dose of daptomycin. If PT and INR remain substantially elevated,

consider evaluation of INR and PT using an alternative method.

EFFECTS ON LAB TEST RESULTS

• May increase ALP and CK levels and LFT values.

• May decrease Hb level, platelet count, and hematocrit.

• May cause false elevation of INR and false prolongation of PT.

CONTRAINDICATIONS & CAUTIONS

• Contraindicated in patients hypersensitive to drug.

• Use cautiously in patients with kidney insufficiency and in older adults.

• Safety and effectiveness haven't been established in children younger than age 1 year. Avoid use in children with kidney impairment and those younger than age 1 year because of risk of potential effects on muscular, neuromuscular, or nervous systems (peripheral or central).

Dialyzable drug: Yes.

PREGNANCY-LACTATION-REPRODUCTION

• Studies during pregnancy are inadequate. Use during pregnancy only if potential benefit justifies fetal risk.

• Drug appears in human milk in low amounts. Use cautiously during breastfeeding.

NURSING CONSIDERATIONS

• Periodically monitor CBC, kidney function test results, and LFT values.

• Monitor patient for muscle pain and weakness, particularly of distal extremities.

🔵 *Alert:* Because drug may increase risk of myopathy, monitor CK level weekly or more frequently if patient has kidney impairment. If CK level rises, monitor it more often. In patient with unexplained signs and symptoms of myopathy with CK level greater than 1,000 units/L (approximately 5 × ULN) and in patients without reported signs and symptoms with CK level greater than 2,000 units/L (10 × ULN or greater), stop drug. Consider stopping all other drugs linked with myopathy (such as HMG-CoA reductase inhibitors) during therapy.

• Monitor for signs and symptoms of superinfection as drug may cause overgrowth of nonsusceptible organisms.

🔵 *Alert:* Drug may cause eosinophilic pneumonia, a rare type of pneumonia in which

---

Reactions in bold italics are ***life-threatening***.

eosinophil-type WBCs fill the lungs, causing fever, cough, shortness of breath, and difficulty breathing. Monitor patient closely.

• DRESS syndrome has been reported. Monitor patient for rash, fever, peripheral eosinophilia, and systemic organ impairment. If DRESS syndrome is suspected, discontinue drug and start appropriate treatment.

• Tubulointerstitial nephritis (TIN) has been reported. Monitor patient for new or worsening kidney impairment. If TIN is suspected, discontinue drug and start appropriate treatment.

• Monitor patient for signs and symptoms of neuropathy; consider stopping drug if neuropathy occurs.

• Watch for evidence of CDAD, which can occur more than 2 months after therapy.

• *Look alike–sound alike:* Don't confuse daptomycin with dactinomycin. Don't confuse Cubicin with Cleocin.

PATIENT TEACHING

• Inform patient about possible adverse reactions.

• Advise patient to immediately report muscle weakness, tingling or numbness of extremities, and infusion-site irritation.

• Tell patient to report all adverse reactions, especially severe diarrhea, rash, fever, cough, shortness of breath, and infection.

• Teach patient importance of completing full course of treatment.

• Advise patient to report watery and bloody stools, with or without stomach cramps and fever, as late as 2 or more months after antibiotic treatment.

SAFETY ALERT!

darbepoetin alfa
dar-bah-poe-E-tin

Aranesp

Therapeutic class: Colony-stimulating factors
Pharmacologic class: Recombinant human erythropoietins

AVAILABLE FORMS

Injection: 25 mcg/mL, 40 mcg/mL, 60 mcg/mL, 100 mcg/mL, 200 mcg/mL, 300 mcg/mL in single-dose vials

Injection (prefilled syringe): 10 mcg/0.4 mL, 25 mcg/0.42 mL, 40 mcg/0.4 mL, 60 mcg/ 0.3 mL, 100 mcg/0.5 mL, 150 mcg/0.3 mL, 200 mcg/0.4 mL, 300 mcg/0.6 mL, 500 mcg/mL

INDICATIONS & DOSAGES

➤ **Anemia due to CKD**
Adults: Initiate drug only if Hb level is less than 10 g/dL. For patients on dialysis, 0.45 mcg/kg IV (preferred) or subcut once weekly, or 0.75 mcg/kg IV (preferred) or subcut once every 2 weeks. For patients not on dialysis, 0.45 mcg/kg IV or subcut at 4-week intervals. Give the lowest effective dose to gradually increase Hb to a level at which blood transfusion isn't necessary. Refer to manufacturer's instructions for specific dosing. Don't increase dose more often than once every 4 weeks.

Children younger than age 18: Initiate drug only if Hb level is less than 10 g/dL. For children on dialysis, 0.45 mcg/kg IV or subcut once weekly. For children not on dialysis, 0.75 mcg/kg IV or subcut once every 2 weeks.

Adults and children older than age 1 who are on dialysis and converting from epoetin alfa: Refer to manufacturer's instructions.

Adjust-a-dose: For patients with CKD who aren't on dialysis, if Hb level exceeds 10 g/dL, reduce dosage or interrupt therapy; use the lowest dosage sufficient to reduce the need for RBC transfusions. For adults with CKD who are on dialysis, if Hb level approaches or exceeds 11 g/dL, reduce dosage or interrupt therapy. For children with CKD, if Hb level approaches or exceeds 12 g/dL, reduce or interrupt dose.

➤ **Anemia due to chemotherapy in patients with nonmyeloid malignancies**
Adults: Initiate drug only if Hb level is less than 10 g/dL and if chemotherapy is planned for at least 2 additional months; 2.25 mcg/kg subcut once weekly or 500 mcg subcut once every 3 weeks until completion of chemotherapy course.

Adjust-a-dose: For either dosing schedule, adjust dose to maintain a target Hb level necessary to avoid RBC transfusions. Give the lowest effective dose to gradually increase Hb to a level at which blood transfusion isn't necessary. Refer to manufacturer's instructions for dosing adjustment.

If after 8 weeks of therapy patient has no response (as measured by Hb level) or if transfusions are still required, discontinue drug. Discontinue drug after completion of chemotherapy course.

ADMINISTRATION

IV

🜲 *Alert:* The needle cover of the prefilled syringe contains dry natural rubber (a derivative of latex). Assess patient for history of latex allergy.

▼ Don't shake. Shaking can denature drug.
▼ If drug contains particles or is discolored, don't use.
▼ Give drug undiluted by IV injection.
▼ Single-dose vials contain no preservatives; don't pool unused portions.
▼ Store drug in refrigerator; don't freeze. Don't use if drug has been frozen.
▼ Protect drug from light.
▼ **Incompatibilities:** Other IV drugs and solutions.

Subcutaneous

🜲 *Alert:* The needle cover of the prefilled syringe contains dry natural rubber (a derivative of latex). Assess patient for history of latex allergy.

• Don't shake. Shaking can denature drug.
• Store drug in refrigerator; don't freeze.
• Protect drug from light.

ACTION

Stimulates erythropoiesis by same mechanism as endogenous erythropoietin.

Route	Onset	Peak	Duration
IV	Unknown	Unknown	Unknown
Subcut	Slow	48 hr (CKD); 71 hr (cancer)	Unknown

Half-life: IV: 21 hours. Subcut: patients with CKD on dialysis, 46 hours; patients with CKD not on dialysis, 70 hours; patients with cancer, 74 hours.

ADVERSE REACTIONS

CNS: *stroke.* **CV:** edema, HTN, hypotension, *PE, acute MI, HF, thrombosis,* angina, vascular access complications. **GI:** abdominal pain. **Metabolic:** fluid overload. **Respiratory:** cough, dyspnea. **Skin:** pruritus, rash, erythema. **Other:** injection-site pain, hypersensitivity reactions.

INTERACTIONS

Drug-drug. *Lenalidomide, pomalidomide, thalidomide:* May increase thrombogenic effects. Monitor therapy.

EFFECTS ON LAB TEST RESULTS

• May increase Hb level.

CONTRAINDICATIONS & CAUTIONS

• Contraindicated in patients hypersensitive to drug or its components, in those with uncontrolled HTN, and in patients with pure red cell aplasia that begins after treatment with Aranesp or other erythropoietin protein drugs.
• Use cautiously in patients with CV disease and stroke.
• Some forms contain polysorbate 80, which may cause hypersensitivity reactions.
• Not indicated for use in patients with cancer receiving hormonal agents, biologic products, or radiotherapy unless patients are also receiving myelosuppressive chemotherapy; in those receiving myelosuppressive chemotherapy when the anemia can be managed by transfusion; or as a substitute for RBC transfusions in patients who require immediate correction of anemia.

Boxed Warning Drug isn't indicated for patients receiving myelosuppressive therapy when the anticipated outcome is cure. ∎

Boxed Warning Erythropoiesis-stimulating agents increase risk of death, MI, stroke, VTE, vascular access thrombosis, and tumor progression or recurrence. No trial has identified an Hb target level, drug dose, or dosing strategy that doesn't increase these risks. ∎

• Blistering and skin exfoliation reactions (erythema multiforme, SJS, TEN) have been reported. Immediately discontinue therapy if SCAR is suspected.
• Safety and effectiveness in children with cancer haven't been established.

Dializable drug: No.

⚠ *Overdose S&S:* CV and thrombotic reactions, polycythemia.

PREGNANCY-LACTATION-REPRODUCTION

• Studies during pregnancy are inadequate. Animal studies show that drug may cause fetal harm. Use during pregnancy only if potential benefit justifies fetal risk.
• It isn't known if drug appears in human milk. Use cautiously during breastfeeding.

NURSING CONSIDERATIONS

Boxed Warning Patients with CKD have an increased risk of death and serious CV events, including stroke, when erythropoiesis-stimulating agents are used to increase Hb level to greater than 11 g/dL. Therapy should be individualized for each patient; use the lowest possible dose sufficient to reduce the need for RBC transfusions. ∎

Boxed Warning Patient with NSCLC and breast, head and neck, lymphoid, or cervical cancers have a risk of tumor growth and shortened survival when Hb levels exceed the lowest dose needed to avoid RBC transfusion. Target for the lowest dosage needed to avoid RBC transfusions. Use only for treatment of anemia due to concomitant myelosuppressive chemotherapy, and discontinue drug after chemotherapy course. ∎

• Evaluate iron status in all patients before and during treatment. Administer supplemental iron when serum ferritin level is less than 100 mcg/L or when serum transferrin saturation is less than 20%. The majority of patients with CKD require supplemental iron during the course of erythropoietin-stimulating agent therapy.

• When initiating therapy or adjusting dosage, monitor Hb level at least weekly until stable; then, at least monthly.

• Hb level may not increase until 2 to 6 weeks after starting therapy.

• If patient has a minimal response or lack of response at recommended dose, check for deficiency in folic acid, iron, or vitamin B_{12}. Other contributing factors include infection, malignancy, and occult blood loss.

⊘ **Alert:** If patient develops a sudden loss of response with severe anemia and low reticulocyte count, withhold drug and test patient for antierythropoietin antibodies. If antibodies are present, stop treatment. Don't switch to another erythropoietic protein because a cross-reaction is possible.

• Control BP and monitor it carefully.

• Monitor kidney function and electrolyte levels in patients in predialysis.

• Monitor patency of vascular and dialysis access; immediately report problems.

• Patients who are marginally dialyzed may need adjustments in dialysis prescriptions.

• Serious allergic reactions, including skin rash and urticaria, may occur. If an anaphylactic reaction occurs, stop drug and give appropriate therapy.

• Drug increases risk of seizures in a patient with CKD. Monitor closely for premonitory neurologic signs and symptoms during first few months of therapy.

PATIENT TEACHING

• Teach about proper drug administration and handling, including proper storage and disposal of supplies.

• Advise patient of possible side effects and allergic reactions.

• Inform patient of the need for frequent monitoring of BP and Hb level; stress adherence with treatment for high BP.

• Advise patient to report new-onset seizures or symptoms or change in seizure frequency.

daridorexant
dar-i-doe-REX-ant

Quviviq

Therapeutic class: Hypnotics
Pharmacologic class: Orexin receptor antagonists
Controlled substance schedule: IV

AVAILABLE FORMS
Tablets: 25 mg, 50 mg

INDICATIONS & DOSAGES
➤ **Insomnia characterized by difficulties with sleep onset or sleep maintenance**
Adults: 25 to 50 mg PO nightly.
Adjust-a-dose: In patients with Child Pugh class B liver impairment or when drug is used with moderate CYP3A4 inhibitor, maximum dosage is 25 mg once nightly.

ADMINISTRATION
PO
• Give within 30 minutes of bedtime; ensure at least 7 hours remain before planned time of awakening.
• May delay sleep onset if drug is given with or soon after a meal.
• Store tablets at 68° to 77° F (20° to 25° C).

ACTION
Blocks orexin receptors, suppressing the system responsible for promoting wakefulness.

Route	Onset	Peak	Duration
PO	Unknown	1–2 hr	Unknown

Half-life: 8 hours.

ADVERSE REACTIONS
CNS: dizziness, fatigue, headache, somnolence. **GI:** nausea.

INTERACTIONS

Drug-drug. *CNS depressants (alprazolam, oxycodone):* May increase risk of CNS depression. Adjust daridorexant or CNS depressant dosage to limit additive effects.

Strong and moderate CYP3A4 inducers (efavirenz, phenytoin, rifampin): May decrease daridorexant level. Avoid use together.

Strong or moderate CYP3A4 inhibitors (clarithromycin, diltiazem, itraconazole): May increase daridorexant level and risk of adverse reactions. Avoid use with strong CYP3A4 inhibitors. Decrease daridorexant dosage to 25 mg once nightly with use of moderate CYP3A4 inhibitors.

Drug-food. *High-caloric, high-fat meals:* May delay sleep onset. Patient should avoid ingesting drug with or soon after a meal.

Drug-lifestyle. *Alcohol use:* May increase CNS depression. Discourage use together.

EFFECTS ON LAB TEST RESULTS

None reported.

CONTRAINDICATIONS & CAUTIONS

• Contraindicated in patients with narcolepsy.
• Use in patients with Child-Pugh class C liver impairment isn't recommended.
• Use cautiously in patients with psychiatric disorders; drug may worsen depression or suicidality.
• Use cautiously in patients with a history of abuse of or addiction to alcohol or other substances.
• Use cautiously in patients with compromised respiratory function (obstructive sleep apnea, COPD).
• Use cautiously in older adults.
• Safety and effectiveness in children haven't been established.

Dialyzable drug: Unlikely.

⚠ *Overdose S&S:* Somnolence, muscle weakness, cataplexy-like symptoms, sleep paralysis, disturbance in attention, fatigue, headache, constipation.

PREGNANCY-LACTATION-REPRODUCTION

• There are no studies during pregnancy.
• Enroll patients exposed to drug during pregnancy in the pregnancy exposure registry (1-833-400-9611).
• It isn't known if drug appears in human milk or how drug affects milk production or infants who are breastfed. Drug was detected in animal milk studies.

• Before initiating breastfeeding, consider patient's clinical need and risk to infant. Monitor infant who is breastfed for excessive sedation.

NURSING CONSIDERATIONS

• Evaluate comorbid diseases as cause of insomnia before starting drug or if insomnia persists after 7 to 10 days of treatment.
• Monitor patient for sleep paralysis, hallucinations, and cataplexy-like symptoms (periods of leg weakness lasting from seconds to a few minutes that may not be associated with an identified triggering event [laughter or surprise]).
• Monitor patient for complex sleep behaviors (sleepwalking; sleep-driving; engaging in activities while not fully awake, including preparing and eating food, making phone calls, having sex). Discontinue drug if complex sleep behaviors occur.
• Monitor patient for worsening insomnia or emergence of new cognitive or behavioral abnormalities; report these changes to prescriber. Abnormalities may be related to unrecognized underlying psychiatric or medical disorder and may become evident during therapy.
• Monitor respiratory status as clinically indicated.

PATIENT TEACHING

• Teach about proper drug administration and handling.
• Tell patient and family to alert prescriber if adverse effects occur.

⚠ *Alert:* Caution patient to immediately report suicidality or new behavioral signs or symptoms.

• Warn patient not to increase dose unless directed by prescriber.
• Tell patient about risk of decreased awareness and alertness. Warn patient to avoid performing activities that require mental alertness or physical coordination (driving, operating heavy machinery) until fully awake.
• Inform patient and family about the risk of sleep paralysis, hallucinations, and complex sleep behaviors.
• Tell patient to contact prescriber if insomnia worsens or hasn't improved within 7 to 10 days after starting drug.
• Warn patient to avoid alcohol while taking drug.

Reactions in bold italics are *life-threatening*.

• Instruct patient of childbearing potential to report pregnancy or plans to become pregnant or to breastfeed.

darifenacin hydrobromide
dar-i-FEN-a-sin

Therapeutic class: Antispasmodics
Pharmacologic class: Anticholinergics

AVAILABLE FORMS
Tablets (extended-release) ⓄⒹⒸ: 7.5 mg, 15 mg

INDICATIONS & DOSAGES
➤ **Urge incontinence, urgency, and frequency from overactive bladder**
Adults: Initially, 7.5 mg PO once daily. After 2 weeks, may increase to 15 mg PO once daily if needed.
Adjust-a-dose: If patient has Child-Pugh class B liver impairment or when drug is administered with strong CYP3A4 inhibitor, don't exceed 7.5 mg PO once daily. Drug isn't recommended for use in patients with Child-Pugh class C liver impairment.

ADMINISTRATION
PO
• Have patient swallow tablets whole with water; don't crush or cut tablets.
• Give drug without regard for food.

ACTION
Relaxes smooth muscle of bladder by selectively antagonizing M3 muscarinic receptors.

Route	Onset	Peak	Duration
PO	Unknown	7 hr	Unknown

Half-life: 13 to 19 hours.

ADVERSE REACTIONS
CNS: asthenia, dizziness, pain, headache. **CV:** HTN, peripheral edema. **EENT:** abnormal vision, dry eyes, rhinitis, sinusitis, pharyngitis, dry mouth. **GI:** constipation, abdominal pain, diarrhea, dyspepsia, nausea, vomiting. **GU:** urinary tract disorder, UTI, vaginitis, urine retention. **Metabolic:** weight gain. **Musculoskeletal:** arthralgia, back pain. **Respiratory:** bronchitis. **Skin:** dry skin, pruritus, rash. **Other:** accidental injury, flulike syndrome.

INTERACTIONS
Drug-drug. *Anticholinergics:* May increase anticholinergic effects (dry mouth, blurred vision, constipation). Monitor patient closely.
Drugs metabolized by CYP2D6 (flecainide, TCAs, thioridazine): May increase levels of these drugs. Use together cautiously.
Strong CYP3A4 inhibitors (clarithromycin, ketoconazole, nefazodone, ritonavir): May increase darifenacin level. Maintain dosage no higher than 7.5 mg PO daily.
Drug-lifestyle. *Hot weather:* May cause heat exhaustion or heat stroke from decreased sweating. Urge caution.

EFFECTS ON LAB TEST RESULTS
None reported.

CONTRAINDICATIONS & CAUTIONS
• Contraindicated in patients hypersensitive to drug or its components. Angioedema can be life-threatening and has been reported after the first dose. If angioedema occurs, discontinue drug, start appropriate therapy, and ensure patent airway.
• Contraindicated in patients with or at risk for urine retention, gastric retention, or uncontrolled angle-closure glaucoma.
• Use cautiously in patients with bladder outflow or GI obstruction, ulcerative colitis, myasthenia gravis, severe constipation, controlled angle-closure glaucoma, decreased GI motility, or Child-Pugh class B liver impairment.
Dialyzable drug: Unknown.
⚠ **Overdose S&S:** Severe antimuscarinic effects (mydriasis, decreased secretions, ileus, urine retention, tachycardia, altered mental status).

PREGNANCY-LACTATION-REPRODUCTION
• There are no studies during pregnancy. Use only if potential benefit justifies fetal risk.
• It isn't known if drug appears in human milk; drug appears in animal milk. Use cautiously during breastfeeding.

NURSING CONSIDERATIONS
• Assess bladder function, and monitor drug effects.
• If patient has bladder outlet obstruction, watch for urine retention.
• Assess patient for decreased gastric motility and constipation.

• Monitor for CNS anticholinergic effects (headache, confusion, hallucinations, somnolence), particularly after starting treatment or increasing dosage.

• Monitor for hypersensitivity reactions, including angioedema.

PATIENT TEACHING

• Teach about proper drug administration and handling.

• Tell patient to use caution, especially when performing hazardous tasks, until drug effects are known.

• Advise patient to report blurred vision, constipation, and urine retention and to immediately report swelling of face, lips, or tongue or difficulty speaking.

• Discourage use of other drugs that may cause dry mouth, constipation, urine retention, or blurred vision.

• Tell patient that drug increases risk of heat exhaustion or heat stroke (decreased sweating, dizziness, fatigue, nausea, fever). Advise cautious use in hot environments and during strenuous activity.

dasiglucagon
das-i-GLOO-ka-gon

Zegalogue

Therapeutic class: Antihypoglycemics
Pharmacologic class: Glucagon receptor agonists

AVAILABLE FORMS

Injection: 0.6 mg/0.6 mL single-dose autoinjector; 0.6 mg/0.6 mL single-dose prefilled syringe

INDICATIONS & DOSAGES

➤ **Severe hypoglycemia in patients with diabetes**

Adults and children ages 6 and older: 0.6 mg subcut. If no response after 15 minutes, may repeat with additional 0.6 mg subcut.

ADMINISTRATION
Subcutaneous

🔵 *Alert:* The needle shield of the autoinjector and needle cap of the syringe contain dry natural rubber (a derivative of latex) and may cause allergic reactions in patients sensitive to latex.

• Inspect drug for particulate matter or discoloration before administration.

• Inject into lower abdomen, buttock, thigh, or outer upper arm.

• Store in protected case refrigerated at 36° to 46° F (2° to 8° C) until expiration date. Don't freeze.

• May store at room temperature for up to 12 months. Discard after 12 months.

• Protect from light.

• Don't refrigerate drug after storing at room temperature.

ACTION

Increases blood glucose concentration by activating liver glucagon receptors and stimulating glycogen breakdown and liver glucose release.

Route	Onset	Peak	Duration
Subcut	Unknown	35 min	Unknown

Half-life: 30 minutes.

ADVERSE REACTIONS

CNS: headache. **CV:** *bradycardia,* HTN, hypotension, palpitations, presyncope, orthostatic intolerance. **GI:** diarrhea, nausea, vomiting. **Skin:** injection-site pain. **Other:** hypersensitivity reactions.

INTERACTIONS

Drug-drug. *Beta blockers:* May transiently increase pulse rate and BP. Monitor vital signs.

Indomethacin: May decrease antihypoglycemic effect of dasiglucagon or may produce hypoglycemia. Use together cautiously.

Warfarin: May increase anticoagulant effect of warfarin. Monitor patient closely.

EFFECTS ON LAB TEST RESULTS

• May increase or decrease blood glucose level.

CONTRAINDICATIONS & CAUTIONS

• Contraindicated in patients with pheochromocytoma. In patients with suspected undiagnosed pheochromocytoma who have substantial increase in BP, consider giving 5 to 10 mg of IV phentolamine mesylate.

• Contraindicated in patients with insulinoma. Drug may stimulate exaggerated insulin release from an insulinoma and cause hypoglycemia. If patients develop signs or

symptoms of hypoglycemia after a dose, give PO or IV glucose.
• Allergic reactions have been reported with glucagon products.
• Drug is effective in treating hypoglycemia only if sufficient liver glycogen stores are present. Patients in a starvation state or with adrenal insufficiency or chronic hypoglycemia may not have adequate levels of liver glycogen for drug to be effective. Treat these patients with glucose.
• Safety and effectiveness in children younger than age 6 haven't been established.
Dialyzable drug: Unknown.
⚠ *Overdose S&S:* Nausea, vomiting, inhibition of GI tract motility, increased BP and HR, decreased serum potassium level.

PREGNANCY-LACTATION-REPRODUCTION
• There are no studies during pregnancy. Untreated hypoglycemia during pregnancy can cause complications and may be fatal.
• It isn't known if drug appears in human milk or how drug affects milk production or infants who are breastfed. Dasiglucagon is expected to be broken down in infant's GI tract and unlikely to cause harm.

NURSING CONSIDERATIONS
• Call for emergency assistance immediately after administering the dose.
• Once patient responds to treatment, give carbohydrates PO to prevent recurrence of hypoglycemia and restore liver glycogen level.
• Monitor patient for allergic reactions (generalized rash, anaphylactic shock with breathing difficulties, hypotension).
• *Look alike–sound alike:* Don't confuse dasiglucagon with glucagon.

PATIENT TEACHING
🔵 *Alert:* Educate patient and caregivers about signs and symptoms of severe hypoglycemia (confusion, sleepiness, slurred speech, blurred vision, seizures) and risks of prolonged hypoglycemia.
• Tell patient about allergic reactions, and instruct patient to seek immediate medical attention if signs or symptoms of serious hypersensitivity reactions occur.
• Advise patient and caregiver to read the information and instructions for use before drug is needed.
• Teach patient and caregiver how to store and dispose of injectors and syringes.

• Instruct patient and caregiver to immediately seek emergency medical help or call health care provider after injection, even if patient awakens.
• Educate patient and caregiver that if no response occurs within 15 minutes, patient may receive another dose of drug.
• Instruct patient and caregiver that, when safely able, patient should ingest a fast-acting source of sugar (fruit juice) and a long-acting source of sugar (crackers with cheese or peanut butter).

SAFETY ALERT!

degarelix acetate
deg-a-REL-ix

Firmagon

Therapeutic class: Antineoplastics
Pharmacologic class: GnRH receptor antagonists

AVAILABLE FORMS
Injection: 80-mg, 120-mg vial

INDICATIONS & DOSAGES
➤ **Advanced prostate cancer**
Adult men: Initially, 240 mg subcut, administered as two 120-mg injections at a concentration of 40 mg/mL. Maintenance dose, 80 mg subcut given as one injection at a concentration of 20 mg/mL every 28 days, starting 28 days after first dose.

ADMINISTRATION
Subcutaneous
🔵 *Alert:* Hazardous drug; use safe handling and disposal precautions.
• Attach vial adaptor and reconstitute with provided prefilled syringe containing preservative-free sterile water for injection (reconstitute each 120-mg vial with 3 mL; reconstitute 80-mg vial with 4.2 mL). Leave syringe in place.
• Do not use if the vial has no powder or the sterile water for injection is discolored.
• Keeping vial in an upright position, swirl it very gently until liquid looks clear and has no undissolved powder or particles. If powder adheres to vial over the liquid surface, slightly tilt vial to dissolve powder. Avoid shaking to prevent foam formation. A ring of small air bubbles on surface of liquid is acceptable.

The reconstitution procedure may take up to 15 minutes.

• To withdraw for administration, turn vial completely upside down and pull down on plunger to withdraw all of reconstituted solution from vial to syringe; expel all air bubbles. Detach syringe by unscrewing it from vial adaptor.

• While holding syringe with tip pointing up, screw injection needle onto syringe.

• Inject drug only in areas of abdomen that won't be exposed to pressure, not close to waistband or belt or close to ribs.

• Give drug within 1 hour of reconstitution.

• Pinch skin of abdomen, and elevate subcutaneous tissue. Insert needle deeply (all the way to the hub) at angle of not less than 45 degrees. Gently pull back plunger to check for blood aspiration. If blood appears in syringe, reconstituted product can no longer be used. Discontinue procedure and discard syringe and needle. Reconstitute new dose. Slowly inject over 30 seconds.

• Remove needle; then release skin.

• Lock needle into shield.

• Repeat reconstitution procedure for second 120-mg initial dose.

• Choose different injection site and inject.

ACTION

Binds to and antagonizes GnRH receptors, which reduces the release of gonadotropins and, consequently, testosterone.

Route	Onset	Peak	Duration
Subcut	Unknown	2 days	Unknown

Half-life: Loading dose, about 53 days; maintenance dose, about 31 days.

ADVERSE REACTIONS

CNS: asthenia, dizziness, fatigue, fever, headache, insomnia. **CV:** HTN, hot flashes. **GI:** constipation, diarrhea, nausea. **GU:** erectile dysfunction, UTI, testicular atrophy. **Hepatic:** increased transaminase and GGT levels. **Metabolic:** weight gain, weight loss, increased GGT. **Musculoskeletal:** arthralgia, back pain. **Skin:** injection-site reactions (including pain, erythema, swelling, induration, and nodule formation), night sweats, hyperhidrosis. **Other:** chills, gynecomastia.

INTERACTIONS

Drug-drug. *Class IA, Class III antiarrhythmics (amiodarone, procainamide, quinidine, sotalol), other drugs known to prolong QT interval:* May prolong QT interval. Avoid use together.

EFFECTS ON LAB TEST RESULTS

• May increase PSA, AST, ALT, and GGT levels.

CONTRAINDICATIONS & CAUTIONS

• Contraindicated in patients hypersensitive to drug or its components. Discontinue drug for serious hypersensitivity reactions and don't rechallenge.

• Androgen deprivation therapy may increase risk of CV disease, anemia, decreased bone density, and diabetes.

• Androgen deprivation therapy may prolong QT interval. Prescribers should consider whether benefits of therapy outweigh potential risks. Use cautiously in patients with congenital long QT syndrome, electrolyte abnormalities, or HF and in those taking drugs known to prolong QT interval.

• Use cautiously in patients with CrCl of less than 50 mL/minute or Child-Pugh class C liver impairment.

Dialyzable drug: Unknown.

PREGNANCY-LACTATION-REPRODUCTION

• Drug may cause fetal harm and loss of pregnancy. Drug isn't indicated for use in patients of childbearing potential.

• Drug may impair fertility in patients of reproductive potential.

NURSING CONSIDERATIONS

• Drug is only to be administered by a health care professional.

• Monitor QT interval and electrolyte levels in patients with congenital long QT syndrome, electrolyte abnormalities, or HF and in those taking drugs known to prolong QT interval.

• Monitor PSA level; if level is elevated, monitor testosterone level.

• Periodically monitor bone density tests.

• Monitor LFT values in patients with liver impairment.

• Monitor patient for mental status changes.

PATIENT TEACHING

• Advise patient about possible adverse effects (hot flashes, skin flushing, weight gain, decreased sex drive, difficulties with erectile function). Explain that injection-site reactions

are usually mild, self-limiting, and decrease within 3 days.
• Inform patient that drug may cause infertility.
• Stress importance of reporting heart problems, such as HF, irregular heart rhythm, or salt imbalance, before taking drug.
• Advise patient to inform all health care providers about taking drug.

delafloxacin meglumin
del-a-FLOKS-a-sin

Baxdela

Therapeutic class: Antibiotics
Pharmacologic class: Fluoroquinolones

AVAILABLE FORMS
Injection: 300 mg in single-dose vial
Tablets: 450 mg

INDICATIONS & DOSAGES
Adjust-a-dose (for all indications): If eGFR is between 15 and 29 mL/minute/1.73 m^2, no dosage adjustment is needed for tablets but decrease IV dosage to 200 mg every 12 hours, or give 200 mg IV every 12 hours, then switch to 450 mg PO every 12 hours at prescriber's discretion.

➤ **Acute bacterial skin and skin-structure infections caused by susceptible bacteria, including gram-positive organisms (*Staphylococcus aureus* [including MRSA and methicillin-susceptible isolates], *Staphylococcus haemolyticus, Staphylococcus lugdunensis, Streptococcus agalactiae, Streptococcus anginosus* group [including *S. anginosus, Streptococcus intermedius,* and *Streptococcus constellatus*], *Streptococcus pyogenes,* and *Enterococcus faecalis*) and gram-negative organisms (*Escherichia coli, Enterobacter cloacae, Klebsiella pneumoniae,* and *Pseudomonas aeruginosa*)**
Adults: 300 mg IV infusion or 450 mg PO every 12 hours for 5 to 14 days. May switch from IV to PO dosing at prescriber's discretion.

➤ **Community-acquired bacterial pneumonia caused by susceptible microorganisms (*Streptococcus pneumoniae, S. aureus* [methicillin-susceptible [MSSA] isolates only]), *K. pneumoniae, E. coli, P. aeruginosa, Haemophilus influenzae, H. parainfluenzae, Chlamydia pneumoniae,***

Legionella pneumophila, **and** *Mycoplasma pneumoniae*)
Adults: 300 mg IV infusion or 450 mg PO every 12 hours for 5 to 10 days. May switch from IV to PO dosing at prescriber's discretion.

ADMINISTRATION
PO
• Give drug without regard to food.
• May give missed dose any time up to 8 hours before next scheduled dose. If less than 8 hours remain before next dose, wait until next scheduled dose.
IV
▼ Reconstitute vial using 10.5 mL of D$_5$W or NSS for each 300-mg vial.
▼ Shake vial vigorously until contents are completely dissolved. Final concentration is 300 mg/12 mL (25 mg/mL) as a clear yellow to amber solution.
▼ Withdraw 12 mL from reconstituted vial for 300-mg dose and 8 mL for 200-mg dose. Add volume withdrawn to total volume of 250 mL using either NSS or D$_5$W to achieve a final concentration of 1.2 mg/mL before administration.
▼ Infuse over 60 minutes. If a common IV line is used to administer other drugs, flush line before and after infusion with NSS or D$_5$W.
▼ Inspect for particulate matter and discoloration before administration.
▼ Store unopened vials at room temperature.
▼ Store reconstituted vials or diluted IV bag either refrigerated at 36° to 46° F (2° to 8° C) or at room temperature for up to 24 hours; don't freeze.
▼ **Incompatibilities:** Magnesium, other multivalent cations given through same IV line, and other drugs.

ACTION
Inhibits bacterial topoisomerase IV and DNA gyrase enzymes.

Route	Onset	Peak	Duration
PO	Unknown	0.75–1 hr	Unknown
IV	Unknown	1 hr	Unknown

Half-life: Oral, 4.2 to 8.5 hours; IV, 3.7 hours.

ADVERSE REACTIONS
CNS: headache, dizziness, hypoesthesia, paresthesia, presyncope, syncope, anxiety, dysgeusia, insomnia, abnormal dreams. **CV:** sinus tachycardia, palpitations, bradycardia,

hypotension, HTN, flushing. **EENT:** blurred vision, tinnitus, vertigo, oral candidiasis. **GI:** nausea, diarrhea, vomiting, abdominal pain, dyspepsia, *CDAD.* **GU:** vulvovaginal candidiasis, kidney impairment, *AKI.* **Hepatic:** elevated transaminase levels. **Metabolic:** *hypoglycemia,* hyperglycemia. **Musculoskeletal:** myalgia. **Skin:** infusion-site extravasation, infusion-site reactions (bruising, discomfort, edema, erythema, irritation, pain, phlebitis, swelling, thrombosis), pruritus, urticaria, dermatitis, rash. **Other:** hypersensitivity reaction, fungal infection.

INTERACTIONS
Drug-drug. *Antacids containing aluminum or magnesium, didanosine, iron, multivitamins containing iron or zinc, sucralfate:* May lower delafloxacin level when taken with PO formulation. Separate delafloxacin dose by at least 2 hours before or 6 hours after these drugs.
Corticosteroids: May increase risk of tendon injury. Avoid concurrent use.
Insulin, oral antidiabetics (glyburide): May increase risk of hypoglycemia. Closely monitor glucose level.

EFFECTS ON LAB TEST RESULTS
• May increase liver transaminase, ALP, creatinine, and CK levels.
• May decrease Hb level.
• May increase or decrease blood glucose level.
• May decrease granulocyte, leukocyte, and neutrophil counts.

CONTRAINDICATIONS & CAUTIONS
• Contraindicated in patients hypersensitive to drug, its components, or other fluoroquinolones.
🌙 *Alert:* Patients receiving systemic delafloxacin have an increased risk of hyperglycemia and hypoglycemia, which can result in coma. Hypoglycemia has been reported more frequently in older adults and in patients with diabetes.
🌙 *Alert:* Drug may increase risk of aortic dissection or rupture when used systemically. Avoid use in patients with known aortic aneurysm; in patients at risk for aortic aneurysm, including those with peripheral atherosclerotic vascular diseases, HTN, or certain genetic conditions (Marfan syndrome, Ehlers-Danlos syndrome); and in older adults.

Drug should only be used in these patients if no other treatment options are available.
• Use should be limited to infections that are proven or strongly suspected to be caused by susceptible bacteria to reduce risk of drug-resistant bacteria and to maintain drug's effectiveness.

Boxed Warning Fluoroquinolones have been associated with disabling and potentially irreversible serious adverse reactions that have occurred together, including tendinitis and tendon rupture, peripheral neuropathy, and CNS effects. Immediately discontinue drug if signs and symptoms occur; avoid using fluoroquinolones in patients who experience any of these serious adverse reactions. ∎

Boxed Warning Fluoroquinolones may exacerbate muscle weakness in patients with myasthenia gravis. Avoid using fluoroquinolones in patients with known history of myasthenia gravis. ∎

Boxed Warning Oral or parenteral fluoroquinolones may increase risk of peripheral neuropathy of arms or legs. Signs and symptoms can occur anytime during treatment and can last for months to years or be permanent. Immediately discontinue drug if patient develops signs or symptoms. Avoid use in patients who have previously experienced peripheral neuropathy. ∎

Boxed Warning Use cautiously in patients with history of known or suspected CNS disorders (severe cerebral arteriosclerosis, epilepsy) or other risk factors that increase risk of seizures or lower seizure threshold. Drug may increase risk of CNS reactions, including seizures, increased ICP (including pseudotumor cerebri), dizziness, and tremors. If these reactions occur, immediately discontinue drug and institute appropriate measures. ∎

Boxed Warning Fluoroquinolones have been associated with an increased risk of psychiatric adverse reactions (toxic psychosis; hallucinations; paranoia; depression; suicidality; delirium, disorientation, confusion, or disturbances in attention; anxiety, agitation, or nervousness; insomnia or nightmares; and memory impairment). These adverse reactions may occur after first dose. Immediately stop drug and institute appropriate measures if patient develops any of these reactions. ∎
• Drug isn't indicated for patients with eGFR of less than 15 mL/minute/1.73 m^2, including patients receiving CKRT.

• Drug may cause CDAD, ranging in severity from mild diarrhea to fatal colitis and possibly occurring more than 2 months after therapy ends. Drug may need to be discontinued if signs or symptoms of CDAD develop during therapy.

• Use cautiously in older adults; patients taking corticosteroids; patients with history of kidney, heart, or lung transplant; patients with kidney impairment; patients with previous tendon disorders, including RA; and those participating in strenuous physical activity due to increased risk of tendinitis or tendon rupture.

• Drug isn't approved for children younger than age 18.

Dialyzable drug: Yes, 19%.

PREGNANCY-LACTATION-REPRODUCTION

• Data are limited on the safety of delafloxacin during pregnancy. Use cautiously and only if potential benefit justifies fetal risk.

• It isn't known if drug appears in human milk; drug appears in animal milk. Weigh benefits of therapy and risks of breastfeeding.

NURSING CONSIDERATIONS

• Whenever possible, obtain specimen for culture and sensitivity tests before first dose. Begin therapy while awaiting results.

⚠️ *Alert:* Monitor patients for signs and symptoms of aortic aneurysm, dissection, or rupture (sudden, severe, and constant pain in the stomach, chest, or back; throbbing in stomach area; deep pain in back or side of stomach; steady, gnawing pain in stomach that lasts for hours or days; pain in jaw, neck, back, or chest; coughing or hoarseness; shortness of breath or trouble swallowing). Immediately discontinue drug if any of these aortic disorders are suspected.

• Monitor for tendinitis (pain, swelling, inflammation), tendon rupture, arthralgia, and myalgia. Symptoms may occur from hours after starting drug to several months after therapy ends. Immediately discontinue drug if symptoms occur.

• Monitor for peripheral neuropathy (pain; burning; tingling; numbness; weakness; alterations in light touch, pain, temperature, position sense, vibratory sensation, and motor strength) and CNS effects (seizures, increased ICP, pseudotumor cerebri, severe headaches, dizziness, tremors). Signs and symptoms may

occur hours or weeks after initial dose. Discontinue drug if these reactions occur.

• Monitor patients with myasthenia gravis for exacerbation of muscle weakness; immediately discontinue drug if symptoms occur.

• Monitor patients for rash and other signs and symptoms of hypersensitivity. Stop drug at first appearance of reaction.

• Monitor patients for CDAD, which has been reported in users of nearly all systemic antibacterial drugs. Stop drug and provide appropriate therapy if CDAD occurs.

⚠️ *Alert:* Monitor patients receiving systemic drug for symptoms of hypoglycemia (confusion, pounding or rapid heartbeat, dizziness, pale skin, shakiness, diaphoresis, unusual hunger, trembling, headache, weakness, irritability, unusual anxiety). Immediately discontinue drug for blood glucose disturbances, and switch to a nonfluoroquinolone antibiotic if possible.

⚠️ *Alert:* Monitor patients receiving systemic drug for psychiatric adverse reactions (toxic psychosis, hallucinations, paranoia, depression, suicidality, confusion, insomnia, nightmares, disturbances in attention, disorientation, agitation, nervousness, memory impairment, delirium). Discontinue drug if these reactions occur.

PATIENT TEACHING

• Discuss importance of completing a full treatment course to prevent antibacterial resistance and to avoid decreasing drug's effectiveness. If drug is stopped because of adverse effects, patient should discuss with prescriber completing treatment with another antibacterial drug.

⚠️ *Alert:* Warn patient to seek immediate medical attention for signs or symptoms of aortic aneurysm, dissection, or rupture.

Boxed Warning Tell patient that tendon rupture can occur during therapy. Instruct patient to notify prescriber if pain, swelling, or inflammation of tendon or weakness or inability to use a joint occurs. Advise patient to stop drug and to rest and refrain from exercise. ∎

Boxed Warning Inform patient with myasthenia gravis that drug may exacerbate signs and symptoms of muscle weakness, including respiratory difficulties. Instruct patient to immediately report worsening. ∎

Boxed Warning Caution patient to immediately report signs and symptoms of peripheral neuropathy to prescriber and to stop drug. ∎

🍁Canada   ◇OTC   ◆Off-label use   ⓓⓞ Do not crush   *Liquid contains alcohol   ⬚ Genetic

Boxed Warning Explain risk of CNS adverse effects (seizures, dizziness, lightheadedness, increased ICP, headache with or without blurred vision) with use of drug. Advise patient to immediately notify prescriber if these occur. ∎

• Warn patient to avoid hazardous tasks that require alertness, such as driving, until drug's effects are known.

• Advise patient to report all adverse reactions and to immediately report hypersensitivity reactions (rash, hives, and other skin reactions; tachycardia; difficulty swallowing or breathing; tightness of throat, hoarseness; swelling of lips, tongue, or face), which can occur even after a single dose.

☉ Alert: Caution patient that significantly low blood sugar level can occur. Teach patient how to manage symptoms, and instruct patient to immediately report any occurrence to the prescriber.

☉ Alert: Advise patient with diabetes of need to monitor blood glucose level more frequently during therapy.

Boxed Warning Instruct patient to immediately report psychiatric adverse reactions. Explain that these reactions can occur after just one dose. ∎

• Caution patient to immediately report watery or bloody stools with or without abdominal cramping and fever. Diarrhea may occur during therapy or 2 months or more after last dose.

denosumab
den-OH-sue-mab

Prolia, Xgeva

Therapeutic class: Antiosteoporotics–antiresorptives
Pharmacologic class: Monoclonal antibodies

AVAILABLE FORMS
Injection: 60 mg/mL in prefilled syringe (Prolia); 120 mg/1.7 mL (70 mg/mL) in single-use vial (Xgeva)

INDICATIONS & DOSAGES
➤ **Osteoporosis in patients at risk for fracture (Prolia only)**
Adult males and adult females after menopause: 60 mg subcut every 6 months.

All patients should receive 1,000 mg of calcium daily and at least 400 international units of vitamin D daily.
➤ **To increase bone mass in males at high risk for fracture who are receiving androgen deprivation therapy for nonmetastatic prostate cancer and in females who are receiving adjuvant aromatase inhibitor therapy for breast cancer (Prolia only)**
Adults: 60 mg subcut once every 6 months. All patients should receive calcium 1,000 mg daily and at least 400 international units of vitamin D daily.
➤ **Glucocorticoid-induced osteoporosis in patients at high risk for fracture who are either initiating or continuing systemic glucocorticoids in a daily dosage equivalent to 7.5 mg or greater of prednisone and expected to remain on glucocorticoids for at least 6 months (Prolia only)**
Adults: 60 mg subcut once every 6 months. All patients should receive calcium 1,000 mg daily and at least 400 international units of vitamin D daily.
➤ **Giant cell tumor of bone (Xgeva only)**
Adults and skeletally mature adolescents ages 13 and older: 120 mg subcut every 4 weeks with additional 120-mg doses on days 8 and 15 of first month of therapy. Administer calcium and vitamin D as necessary to prevent or treat hypocalcemia.
➤ **Hypercalcemia of malignancy refractory to bisphosphonate therapy (Xgeva only)**
Adults: 120 mg subcut every 4 weeks with additional 120-mg doses on days 8 and 15 of first month of therapy.
➤ **Bone metastases from solid tumors; prevention of skeletal-related events in patients with multiple myeloma (Xgeva only)**
Adults: 120 mg subcut every 4 weeks, with calcium and vitamin D as necessary to prevent or treat hypocalcemia.

ADMINISTRATION
Subcutaneous

• Drug should only be administered by a health care professional.

• Don't use if solution is discolored or cloudy or contains many particles or foreign particulate matter.

• Before administration, drug may be removed from refrigerator and brought to room temperature by letting stand in original container. This generally takes 15 to 30 minutes.

Reactions in bold italics are *life-threatening*.

Don't warm drug in any other way. Avoid vigorous shaking of drug. Once removed from refrigerator, use within 14 days. Discard after 14 days if not used.

• Protect from direct light and heat.

• Use 27G needle to withdraw drug from single-use vial, and inject entire contents of vial. Don't reenter vial.

• Administer via subcut injection in upper arm, upper thigh, or abdomen.

• Don't give IV, IM, or intradermally.

�ா]**Alert:** Needle cap on single-use syringe contains latex; keep away from patients with latex allergy.

• If a Prolia dose is missed, give as soon as convenient. Schedule injections every 6 months from date of last injection.

ACTION

Inhibits osteoclast activity, thereby decreasing bone resorption and increasing bone mass and strength.

Route	Onset	Peak	Duration
Subcut	Unknown	10 days	4–5 mo

Half-life: About 25 to 28 days.

ADVERSE REACTIONS

CNS: asthenia, insomnia, sciatica, headache, fatigue. **CV:** angina, atrial fibrillation, peripheral edema. **EENT:** vertigo, pharyngitis, nasopharyngitis, toothache. **GI:** flatulence, GERD, upper abdominal pain, nausea, decreased appetite, vomiting, constipation, diarrhea. **GU:** cystitis. **Hematologic:** anemia, *thrombocytopenia.* **Metabolic:** hypercholesterolemia, *hypocalcemia,* hypophosphatemia. **Musculoskeletal:** osteonecrosis of jaw, back pain, bone pain, extremity pain, musculoskeletal pain, myalgia, spinal osteoarthritis. **Respiratory:** pneumonia, URI, dyspnea, cough, bronchitis. **Skin:** pruritus, rash, dermatitis. **Other:** infection, herpes zoster.

INTERACTIONS

Drug-drug. *Calcimimetic drugs, calcium-lowering drugs:* May worsen hypocalcemia risk. Closely monitor serum calcium level.
Immunosuppressants: May enhance adverse effects of immunosuppressants and increase risk of serious infections. Monitor patient closely.

EFFECTS ON LAB TEST RESULTS

• May increase cholesterol level.

• May decrease calcium, magnesium, and phosphate levels.

• May decrease Hb level and platelet count.

CONTRAINDICATIONS & CAUTIONS

🔰]**Alert:** Drug may increase risk of hypocalcemia in patients on dialysis. The risks of hypocalcemia should be considered before use. Adequate calcium and vitamin D supplementation and frequent blood calcium monitoring may help decrease the likelihood or severity of these risks.

• Contraindicated in patients with history of systemic hypersensitivity to components of the product. Reactions include anaphylaxis, facial swelling, and urticaria.

• Contraindicated in patients with hypocalcemia.

• Discontinue use if severe bone, joint, or muscle pain occurs.

• Use cautiously in patients with history of hypoparathyroidism, thyroid surgery, parathyroid surgery, malabsorption syndromes, excision of small intestine, or CrCl less than 30 mL/minute.

• Clinically significant hypercalcemia requiring hospitalization and complicated by AKI has been reported within the first year after treatment discontinuation in patients with giant cell tumor of bone being treated with Xgeva and in patients with growing skeletons.

• Use cautiously in older adults and patients with an impaired immune system.

• Safety and effectiveness in children haven't been established, except for Xgeva in skeletally mature adolescents (ages 12 to 16) with giant cell tumor of bone.
Dialyzable drug: Unknown.

PREGNANCY-LACTATION-REPRODUCTION

• Drug may cause fetal harm; use is contraindicated during pregnancy. Inform patient of fetal risk.

• Caution patients of childbearing potential to use highly effective contraception during therapy and for at least 5 months after last dose.

• It isn't known if drug appears in human milk. Use cautiously during breastfeeding, considering benefit to patient and risk to infant.

NURSING CONSIDERATIONS

• Verify pregnancy status of patient of childbearing potential before starting drug.

🍁Canada   ◇OTC   ◆Off-label use   💊Do not crush   *Liquid contains alcohol   🧬Genetic

• Make sure patient has adequate intake of calcium and vitamin D.
• Monitor calcium (especially in first weeks of therapy), vitamin D, magnesium, and phosphorus levels before and during therapy. Administer calcium, magnesium, and vitamin D as needed.
• Drug can cause severe symptomatic hypocalcemia; fatal cases have been reported. Correct hypocalcemia before starting drug.
• Multiple vertebral fractures have been reported after treatment ends. Evaluate patient's individual risk of vertebral fractures and consider transitioning to an alternative antiresorptive therapy.
• Drug may cause osteonecrosis of jaw, which can occur spontaneously and is commonly associated with tooth extraction, local infection with delayed healing, or both. Monitor for signs and symptoms. Perform an oral exam and ensure appropriate preventive dentistry before starting drug and periodically during therapy.
• Consider stopping drug if severe skin reactions occur.
• When treatment is discontinued, monitor patient for signs and symptoms of hypercalcemia (nausea, vomiting, headache, decreased alertness), assess serum calcium level periodically, reevaluate patient's calcium and vitamin D supplementation requirements, and treat appropriately.
🜂 **Alert:** Prolia and Xgeva contain the same active ingredient, denosumab. Patients receiving Prolia should not receive Xgeva.

PATIENT TEACHING
🜂 **Alert:** Warn patient to immediately seek help if symptoms of hypocalcemia (unusual tingling or numbness in hands, arms, legs, or feet; painful muscle spasms or cramps; laryngeal or lung spasms causing difficulty breathing; vomiting; seizures; or irregular heart rhythm) occur. Emphasize the importance of maintaining normal calcium level.
• Advise patient to have a dental exam before treatment and to follow good oral hygiene practices during therapy.
• Instruct patient to tell dentist before dental procedures about taking drug and to inform dentist or prescriber if persistent pain or slow healing of mouth or jaw occurs after dental surgery.
• Tell patient to report jaw pain, swelling, or numbness; loose teeth; or dramatic gum loss.

• Advise patient to seek prompt medical care if signs and symptoms of severe infection occur, including cellulitis or skin reactions (dermatitis, rash, eczema).
• Caution patient to contact health care provider if severe bone, joint, or muscle pain occurs.
• Tell patient to take calcium and vitamin D supplement as directed by prescriber.
• Advise patient of childbearing potential to use highly effective contraception during therapy and for at least 5 months after final dose.

desmopressin acetate
des-moe-PRESS-in

DDAVP, Nocdurna

Therapeutic class: Hemostatics, antidiuretic hormones
Pharmacologic class: Posterior pituitary hormones

AVAILABLE FORMS
Injection: 4 mcg/mL
Metered nasal spray: 10 mcg/spray
Tablets: 0.1 mg, 0.2 mg
Tablets (SL): 27.7 mcg, 55.3 mcg

INDICATIONS & DOSAGES
➤ **Nonnephrogenic diabetes insipidus, temporary polyuria, and polydipsia related to pituitary trauma**
Adults and children older than age 12: 2 to 4 mcg (0.5 to 1 mL) IV or subcut daily, usually in two divided doses.
Adults and children older than age 4: Initially, 0.05 mg (half of the 1-mg tablet) PO b.i.d.; adjust dosage to patient response. If patient previously received drug intranasally, begin oral therapy 12 hours after last intranasal dose. Maximum dose, 1.2 mg/day (divided into two or three doses) for patients with diabetes insipidus.
Adults and children older than age 12: 10 to 40 mcg (0.1 to 0.4 mL) intranasally daily in one to three doses. Most adults need 20 mcg (0.2 mL) daily in two divided doses.
Children ages 4 to 12: 10 to 30 mcg (0.1 to 0.3 mL) intranasally daily in one or two doses.
➤ **Hemophilia A and von Willebrand disease**
Adults and children ages 3 months and older: 0.3 mcg/kg (maximum dose, 20 mcg) diluted

in NSS and infused IV over 15 to 30 minutes. If used preoperatively, give 30 minutes before scheduled procedure. Repeat dose after 8 to 12 hours and once daily thereafter, if needed, as indicated by lab response and patient's condition.

➤ **Primary nocturnal enuresis**
Adults and children ages 6 and older: Initially, 0.2 mg PO at bedtime; adjust dose up to 0.6 mg to achieve desired response.

➤ **Nocturnal polyuria in adults who awaken at least two times per night to void (Nocdurna)**
Adult females: 27.7 mcg SL daily without water, 1 hour before bedtime.
Adult males: 55.3 mcg SL daily without water, 1 hour before bedtime.

ADMINISTRATION
PO
• Discontinue in patient with acute illness that may result in fluid or electrolyte imbalance.
• Store at controlled room temperature.
IV
▼ When given IV push for diabetes insipidus, dilution isn't required.
▼ Don't give injection to patients with hemophilia A with factor VIII activity of up to 5% or with severe von Willebrand disease.
▼ For adults and children weighing more than 10 kg, dilute with 50 mL NSS. For children weighing 10 kg or less, 10 mL of diluent is recommended. Infuse over 15 to 30 minutes.
▼ Inspect drug for particulates and discoloration before infusing.
▼ Monitor BP and pulse rate during infusion.
▼ Comparable antidiuretic dose of injection is about one-tenth of intranasal dose.
▼ Solution and injection must be refrigerated.
▼ **Incompatibilities:** None listed by manufacturer. Consult drug compatibility reference for more information.
Intranasal
• Ensure nasal passages are intact, clean, and free of obstruction before giving intranasally.
• Nasal spray pump delivers only doses of 10 mcg DDAVP (per 0.1-mL dose). If doses other than these are required, use injection.
• Prime spray pump before first use. To prime pump, press down four times. If pump isn't used for 1 week, reprime by pressing down on pump once. Discard bottle after 50 doses (10 mcg/spray) because the amount delivered

thereafter per spray may be substantially less than the required dose.
• Nasal spray may be stored at room temperature.
Subcutaneous
• Dilution isn't required before injection.
• Teach patient to rotate injection sites to prevent tissue damage.
Sublingual
• Patient should empty bladder immediately before bedtime and limit fluid intake to a minimum from 1 hour before until 8 hours after administration.
• Patient should keep tablet under tongue until it has fully dissolved.

ACTION
Synthetic analogue of ADH that increases the permeability of the kidney tubular epithelium to adenosine monophosphate and water, enabling the epithelium to promote reabsorption of water and produce a concentrated urine. Also increases factor VIII activity by releasing endogenous factor VIII from plasma storage sites.

Route	Onset	Peak	Duration
PO	1 hr	0.9–1.5 hr	12 hr
IV	30 min	1.5–2 hr	6–14 hr
Intranasal	15–30 min	0.25–1.5 hr	6–14 hr
Subcut	Unknown	Unknown	Unknown
SL	30 min	Unknown	6 hr

Half-life: PO, 1.5 to 2.5 hours; IV, 3 hours; intranasal (DDAVP), 7.8 minutes (initial phase) and 75.5 minutes (terminal phase); intranasal, 3.3 to 3.5 hours; SL (Nocdurna), 2.8 hours.

ADVERSE REACTIONS
CNS: headache, dizziness, asthenia. **CV:** flushing, HTN, fluid retention. **EENT:** conjunctivitis, edema around eyes, abnormal lacrimation, nasal discomfort or congestion, epistaxis, rhinitis, nasopharyngitis, sore throat, dry mouth. **GI:** nausea, abdominal cramps. **GU:** vulvar pain. **Metabolic:** *hyponatremia.* **Musculoskeletal:** back pain. **Respiratory:** cough, bronchitis. **Skin:** local erythema, swelling, or burning after injection. **Other:** chills.

INTERACTIONS
Drug-drug. *Chlorpromazine, lamotrigine, NSAIDs, opioid analgesics, oxybutynin, SSRIs, TCAs:* May increase risk of water

intoxication with hyponatremia. Monitor patient closely.

Demeclocycline, lithium, tolvaptan: May decrease effect of desmopressin. Use together cautiously. Avoid use with tolvaptan.

Boxed Warning *Loop diuretics, systemic or inhaled glucocorticoids:* May increase risk of hyponatremia. Use with Nocdurna or IV formulation is contraindicated. Drug can be started or resumed 3 days or 5 half-lives after discontinuation of glucocorticoid, whichever is longer. ■

Pressor agents: May enhance pressor effects with large doses of desmopressin. Monitor patient closely.

Drug-lifestyle. *Alcohol use:* May increase risk of adverse effects. Discourage use together.

EFFECTS ON LAB TEST RESULTS
• May decrease sodium level.

CONTRAINDICATIONS & CAUTIONS
⚕ Contraindicated in patients hypersensitive to drug and in those with type IIB von Willebrand disease, CrCl less than 50 mL/minute, hyponatremia, or a history of hyponatremia.

Boxed Warning Nocdurna and IV formulation are contraindicated in patients at increased risk for severe hyponatremia, such as patients with excessive fluid intake or illnesses that can cause fluid or electrolyte imbalances (gastroenteritis, salt-wasting nephropathies, systemic infection). ■

• Nocdurna and IV formulation are contraindicated in patients with HF (NYHA Class II to IV), uncontrolled HTN, hyponatremia or a history of hyponatremia, polydipsia, primary nocturnal enuresis, eGFR less than 50 mL/minute/1.73 m², and known or suspected SIADH secretion due to increased risk of severe hyponatremia.

Boxed Warning Nocdurna and IV formulation can cause hyponatremia. Severe hyponatremia can be life-threatening, leading to seizures, coma, respiratory arrest, or death. ■

• Use cautiously in patients with coronary artery insufficiency, hypertensive CV disease, and conditions linked to fluid and electrolyte imbalances, such as cystic fibrosis, because these patients are susceptible to hyponatremia.

• Use cautiously in patients at risk for water intoxication with hyponatremia.

Dialyzable drug: Unknown.

⚠ *Overdose S&S:* Confusion, drowsiness, continuing headache, problems passing urine, rapid weight gain due to fluid retention.

PREGNANCY-LACTATION-REPRODUCTION
• Studies during pregnancy are inadequate. Use during pregnancy only if clearly needed.

• Drug appears in small amounts in human milk and is poorly absorbed orally by infants. Use cautiously during breastfeeding.

• Drug isn't recommended for nocturia caused by normal physiologic changes that occur during pregnancy.

NURSING CONSIDERATIONS
• Before starting Nocdurna, evaluate patient for possible causes of nocturia, including excessive fluid intake before bedtime, and optimize treatment of underlying conditions that may be contributing to nocturia. Confirm diagnosis of nocturnal polyuria with 24-hour urine collection, if not previously obtained.

Boxed Warning Ensure serum sodium level is normal before starting or resuming Nocdurna or IV formulation or increasing the dosage. Measure serum sodium level within 7 days and approximately 1 month after initiating therapy or increasing the dosage as well as periodically during treatment. Monitor serum sodium level more frequently in patients ages 65 and older and in patients at increased risk for hyponatremia. ■

Boxed Warning If hyponatremia occurs, Nocdurna or IV formulation may need to be temporarily or permanently discontinued. ■

• Adjust morning and evening doses separately to achieve adequate diurnal rhythm of water turnover as well as adequate sleep duration.

• Intranasal use can cause changes in the nasal mucosa, resulting in erratic, unreliable absorption. Report worsening condition to prescriber, who may recommend alternate route.

• Restrict fluid intake to reduce risk of water intoxication and sodium depletion, especially in children or older adults.

⚠ *Alert:* Overdose may cause oxytocic or vasopressor activity. Withhold drug and notify prescriber. If fluid retention is excessive, give furosemide.

• *Look alike–sound alike:* Don't confuse desmopressin with vasopressin.

D

PATIENT TEACHING

• Advise patient with nocturia or nocturnal enuresis to moderate fluid intake in the evening and nighttime hours to decrease risk of hyponatremia and to avoid caffeine and alcohol before bedtime.

• Teach patient to immediately report signs or symptoms associated with hyponatremia (headache; nausea; vomiting; weight gain; restlessness; fatigue; lethargy; depressed reflexes; disorientation; loss of appetite; irritability; muscle weakness, spasms, or cramps; abnormal mental status [hallucinations]; decreased consciousness; confusion). Severe symptoms may include seizure, coma, and respiratory arrest.

• Some patients may have trouble measuring and inhaling drug into nostrils. Teach patient and caregivers correct administration method.

• Instruct patient to clear nasal passages before using nasal spray.

• Advise patient to report nasal congestion, allergic rhinitis, or URI to prescriber; dosage adjustment of nasal spray may be needed.

• Warn patient to drink only enough water to satisfy thirst.

▧ Inform patient with hemophilia A or von Willebrand disease that taking desmopressin may prevent hazards associated with using blood products.

• Advise patient to carry medical identification indicating use of drug.

---

desoximetasone
de-soks-i-MET-a-sone

Topicort

Therapeutic class: Corticosteroids
Pharmacologic class: Corticosteroids

AVAILABLE FORMS
Cream: 0.05%, 0.25%
Gel: 0.05%*
Ointment: 0.05%, 0.25%
Spray: 0.25%

INDICATIONS & DOSAGES
➤ **Inflammation and pruritus from corticosteroid-responsive dermatoses (except spray)**
Adults and children: Clean area; apply a thin film and rub in gently b.i.d. Don't use 0.25% ointment on children younger than age 10. If

no improvement occurs within 4 weeks, contact prescriber.
➤ **Plaque psoriasis (spray only)**
Adults: Apply a thin film to affected areas and rub in gently b.i.d. Treatment beyond 4 weeks isn't recommended.

ADMINISTRATION
Topical
• Gently wash skin before applying. To prevent skin damage, rub in gently, leaving thin coat. When treating hairy sites, part hair and apply directly to lesions.

• Avoid applying near eyes, near mucous membranes, or in ear canal.

• Avoid using spray on face, axilla, or groin or if atrophy is present.

• Don't bandage, cover, or wrap treated skin area unless ordered; adverse reactions may occur more frequently.

• Stop drug and notify prescriber if skin infection, striae, or atrophy occurs.

• Discontinue therapy when control is achieved.

• Discard unused portion of spray after 30 days.

ACTION
Diffuses across cell membranes to form complexes with receptors, showing antiinflammatory, antipruritic, vasoconstrictive, and antiproliferative activity.

Route	Onset	Peak	Duration
Topical	Unknown	Unknown	Unknown

Half-life: 13 to 17 hours (urine).

ADVERSE REACTIONS
Skin: burning, pruritus, irritation, dryness, erythema, folliculitis, hypertrichosis, acneiform eruptions, perioral dermatitis, hypopigmentation, allergic contact dermatitis, maceration, secondary infection, atrophy, striae, miliaria. **Other:** *HPA axis suppression.*

INTERACTIONS
None significant.

EFFECTS ON LAB TEST RESULTS
• May increase serum or urine glucose level.

CONTRAINDICATIONS & CAUTIONS
• Contraindicated in patients hypersensitive to drug or its components.

• Don't use as monotherapy for primary bacterial infections (impetigo, paronychia,

erysipelas, cellulitis, angular cheilitis), rosacea, perioral dermatitis, or acne.
• Don't use very-high-potency or high-potency agents on face, groin, or axillae.
• Don't use spray if atrophy is present at treatment site.
• Drug isn't for ophthalmic use.
• Use cautiously in children. Don't use ointment in children under age 10. Spray isn't recommended for use in children.
Dialyzable drug: Unknown.
⚠ *Overdose S&S:* Systemic effects.

PREGNANCY-LACTATION-REPRODUCTION
• Studies during pregnancy are inadequate. Use during pregnancy only if potential benefit justifies fetal risk.
• During pregnancy or breastfeeding, use on the smallest area of skin for the shortest duration possible.
• It isn't known if topical corticosteroids are sufficiently absorbed systemically to produce detectable quantities in human milk. If used during breastfeeding, don't apply on chest to avoid accidental ingestion by infant.

NURSING CONSIDERATIONS
• If antifungal or antibiotic combined with corticosteroid fails to provide prompt improvement, stop corticosteroid until infection is controlled.
• Systemic absorption is likely with use of occlusive dressings, prolonged treatment, or extensive body surface treatment. Watch for symptoms of HPA axis suppression, Cushing syndrome, hyperglycemia, and glycosuria.
• Avoid using plastic pants and tight-fitting diapers on treated areas in young children. Children may absorb larger amounts of drug and be more susceptible to systemic toxicity.
• Gel contains alcohol and may cause burning or irritation in open lesions.
• *Look alike–sound alike:* Don't confuse desoximetasone with dexamethasone.

PATIENT TEACHING
• Teach about proper drug administration and handling.
• Instruct patient to report all adverse reactions.
• Tell patient to use drug for external use only and to avoid contact with the eyes.
• If an occlusive dressing is ordered, advise patient to leave it in place for no longer than 12 hours each day and not to use the dressing on infected or weeping lesions.

• Tell patient to stop drug and report signs of systemic absorption, skin irritation or ulceration, hypersensitivity, or infection.
• Inform patient that spray is flammable, and instruct patient to keep away from heat, flame, or smoke while applying.

desvenlafaxine succinate
des-ven-la-FAX-een

Pristiq

Therapeutic class: Antidepressants
Pharmacologic class: SSNRIs

AVAILABLE FORMS
Tablets (extended-release) ⓄⓃⒸ: 25 mg, 50 mg, 100 mg

INDICATIONS & DOSAGES
Adjust-a-dose (for all indications): For patients with CrCl of 30 to 50 mL/minute, maximum of 50 mg PO once daily. For patients with CrCl of less than 30 mL/minute, 25 mg PO daily or 50 mg PO every other day. Don't give supplemental doses after dialysis. For patients with Child-Pugh class B or C liver impairment, 50 mg PO daily; dosage escalation above 100 mg/day isn't recommended. Use 25-mg/day dose for gradual reduction when discontinuing treatment to minimize discontinuation symptoms.
➤ **Major depressive disorder**
Adults: 50 mg PO once daily.
➤ **Vasomotor symptoms associated with menopause ◆**
Adults: Initially, 50 mg once daily. Titrate by 25 to 50 mg a day to target dose of 100 mg once daily; 150 mg once daily has also been studied and has been shown to be effective.

ADMINISTRATION
PO
• Administer at approximately the same time each day with or without food.
• Have patient swallow tablets whole with fluid; don't crush or cut tablets.

ACTION
Thought to potentiate serotonin and norepinephrine in the CNS through inhibition of their reuptake.

Route	Onset	Peak	Duration
PO	Unknown	Unknown	Unknown

Half-life: About 10 to 11 hours.

ADVERSE REACTIONS

CNS: abnormal dreams, anxiety, asthenia, dizziness, dysgeusia, fatigue, jittery feeling, headache, insomnia, paresthesia, somnolence, tremor, disturbance in attention, nervousness. **CV:** increased BP, hot flashes, HTN, palpitations, tachycardia. **EENT:** blurred vision, mydriasis, tinnitus, vertigo, dry mouth. **GI:** decreased appetite, constipation, diarrhea, nausea, vomiting. **GU:** proteinuria, sexual dysfunction. **Metabolic:** weight loss, hyperlipidemia. **Skin:** hyperhidrosis, rash. **Other:** chills, yawning.

INTERACTIONS

Drug-drug. *Amphetamines, buspirone, fentanyl, lithium, SSNRIs, SSRIs, TCAs, tramadol, triptans, tryptophan:* May increase risk of serotonin syndrome. Monitor patient closely if used together.
Aspirin, NSAIDs, warfarin, other drugs that affect coagulation: May increase risk of bleeding. Use together cautiously.
CNS drugs: Drug may cause additive CNS effects. Avoid use together.
Linezolid, methylene blue: Increases risk of serotonin syndrome. Use together is contraindicated. If urgent treatment with either of these drugs is needed, immediately stop desvenlafaxine; then administer linezolid or methylene blue. Watch for signs and symptoms of serotonin syndrome for 7 days or until 24 hours after last dose of linezolid or methylene blue. Restart desvenlafaxine 24 hours after last dose of linezolid or methylene blue.
MAO inhibitors: May cause serotonin syndrome or signs and symptoms resembling NMS. Contraindicated for use together. Allow at least 14 days between discontinuation of an MAO inhibitor and starting desvenlafaxine, and 7 days after stopping desvenlafaxine before starting an MAO inhibitor.
Venlafaxine: Drug is a major active metabolite of venlafaxine. Avoid use together.
Drug-lifestyle. *Alcohol:* May enhance CNS depression. Discourage use together.

EFFECTS ON LAB TEST RESULTS

- May increase total cholesterol, LDL-C, triglyceride, and urine protein levels.
- May decrease sodium level.
- May cause false-positive test for phencyclidine and amphetamines.

CONTRAINDICATIONS & CAUTIONS

- Contraindicated in patients hypersensitive to drug.
- **⚠ Alert:** Use with linezolid or methylene blue is contraindicated due to risk of serotonin syndrome (fever, mental status changes, muscle twitching, diaphoresis, shivering or shaking, diarrhea, loss of coordination).
- Potentially life-threatening serotonin syndrome has been reported with desvenlafaxine alone, but particularly with concomitant use of other serotonergic drugs and with drugs that impair serotonin metabolism.
- Use cautiously in older adults and in patients with kidney impairment, diseases or conditions that could affect hemodynamic responses or metabolism, and in those with a history of mania or seizures.
- Drug may increase risk of bleeding events, ranging from bruising, hematoma, epistaxis, and petechiae to life-threatening hemorrhage.
- Angle-closure glaucoma has occurred in patients with untreated anatomically narrow angles who have taken antidepressants.

Boxed Warning Desvenlafaxine isn't approved for use in children. ∎
Dialyzable drug: No.
⚠ Overdose S&S: Headache, vomiting, agitation, dizziness, nausea, constipation, diarrhea, dry mouth, paresthesia, tachycardia, change in level of consciousness, mydriasis, seizures, ECG changes.

PREGNANCY-LACTATION-REPRODUCTION

- Studies during pregnancy are inadequate. Use during pregnancy only if clearly needed and potential benefit justifies fetal risk.
- Health care providers are encouraged to register patients in the National Pregnancy Registry for Antidepressants (1-866-961-2388 or https://womensmentalhealth.org/research/pregnancyregistry/antidepressants/).
- Drug appears in human milk. Use cautiously during breastfeeding and monitor infant for excessive sedation and abnormal feeding pattern.

NURSING CONSIDERATIONS

Boxed Warning Closely monitor all patients being treated for depression for signs and symptoms of clinical worsening and suicidality, especially at beginning of therapy and with dosage adjustments. Signs and symptoms include agitation, insomnia, anxiety, aggressiveness, or panic attacks. ■

• Carefully monitor BP. Drug may cause dose-related increases in BP.

• Monitor IOP in patient at risk for angle-closure glaucoma.

• Record mood changes. Monitor patient for suicidality and allow patient only a minimal supply of drug.

• Monitor for signs and symptoms of bleeding.

• Monitor lipid and sodium levels before and during therapy.

• Hyponatremia can occur with desvenlafaxine use. Consider stopping drug in patients with symptomatic hyponatremia; institute appropriate medical intervention.

⚠ *Alert:* Don't stop drug abruptly. Withdrawal or discontinuation syndrome may occur. Signs and symptoms of withdrawal syndrome include dizziness, nausea, headache, irritability, insomnia, diarrhea, anxiety, fatigue, abnormal dreams, and hyperhidrosis. Taper drug slowly.

• Monitor respiratory status. Drug may cause ILD or eosinophilic pneumonia. If patient develops dyspnea, cough, or chest discomfort, discontinue drug.

• Monitor for signs and symptoms of serotonin syndrome (mental status changes, autonomic instability, neuromuscular symptoms, seizures, and GI symptoms).

PATIENT TEACHING

Boxed Warning Warn family members to closely monitor patient for signs and symptoms of worsening condition or suicidality. ■

⚠ *Alert:* Teach patient to recognize and immediately report symptoms of serotonin toxicity (fever, mental status changes, muscle twitching, diaphoresis, shivering or shaking, diarrhea, loss of coordination).

• Teach about proper drug administration and handling.

• Tell patient to avoid alcohol and to consult prescriber before taking other prescription or OTC drugs.

• To discontinue drug, tell patient to stop gradually by tapering dosage as instructed by prescriber and not to abruptly stop taking drug.

• Teach patient to report all adverse reactions, including abnormal bleeding.

• Warn patient to avoid hazardous activities that require alertness and good coordination until effects of drug are known.

• Advise patient of childbearing potential to inform prescriber if pregnant or breastfeeding or if planning to become pregnant.

• Explain that drug may cause symptoms of sexual dysfunction. Advise patient to discuss management strategies with prescriber.

• Inform patient that inert matrix tablet may pass through stool, but active medication has already been absorbed.

dexamethasone (oral)
dex-a-METH-a-sone

Dexamethasone Intensol*, Hemady

dexamethasone sodium phosphate injection

Therapeutic class: Corticosteroids
Pharmacologic class: Glucocorticoids

AVAILABLE FORMS
dexamethasone
Elixir: 0.5 mg/5 mL*
Oral concentrate: 1 mg/mL*
Oral solution: 0.5 mg/5 mL
Tablets: 0.5 mg, 0.75 mg, 1 mg, 1.5 mg, 2 mg, 4 mg, 6 mg, 20 mg
dexamethasone sodium phosphate
Injection: 4-mg/mL, 10-mg/mL vials and prefilled syringes

INDICATIONS & DOSAGES
Adjust-a-dose (for all indications): Dosage requirements are variable. Usual adult IV or IM dosage is 4 to 20 mg/day. Usual initial adult PO dosage is 0.75 to 9 mg/day. Usual initial children's IV, IM, or PO dosage is 0.02 to 0.3 mg/kg/day in divided doses.
➤ **Cerebral edema**
Adults: Initially, 10 mg IV; then 4 mg IM every 6 hours until symptoms subside (usually 2 to 4 days). Replace IM dosing with oral therapy (1 to 3 mg t.i.d.) as soon as possible; then taper over 5 to 7 days.
➤ **Palliative management of recurrent or inoperable brain tumors**
Adults: 2 mg PO, IM, or IV b.i.d. or t.i.d. for maintenance therapy.

➤ **Inflammatory conditions, neoplasias**
Adults: 0.75 to 9 mg/day PO or 0.5 to 9 mg/day IM or IV, depending on size and location of affected area.

➤ **Acute, self-limited allergic disorders; acute exacerbations of chronic allergic disorders**
Adults: On day 1, 4 or 8 mg IM (using 4 mg/mL preparation). On days 2 and 3, four 0.75-mg tablets PO in two divided doses. On day 4, two 0.75-mg tablets PO in two divided doses. On days 5 and 6, one 0.75-mg tablet PO. Follow-up visit on day 8.

➤ **Shock**
Adults: 1 to 6 mg/kg IV as single dose. Or, 40 mg IV every 2 to 6 hours, as needed, while shock persists.

➤ **Dexamethasone suppression test for Cushing syndrome**
Adults: Determine baseline 24-hour urine level of 17-hydroxycorticosteroids; then give 0.5 mg PO every 6 hours for 48 hours. Repeat 24-hour urine collection to determine 17-hydroxycorticosteroid excretion during second 24 hours of dexamethasone administration. Or, 1 mg PO as single dose at 11:00 p.m. with determination of plasma cortisol at 8 a.m. the next morning.

➤ **Adrenocortical insufficiency**
Children: 0.02 to 0.3 mg/kg/day or 0.6 to 9 mg/m²/day PO in three or four divided doses.

➤ **Acute exacerbation of MS**
Adults: 30 mg PO daily for 1 week, followed by 4 to 12 mg every other day for 1 month.

➤ **Adjunctive therapy for short-term administration in synovitis of osteoarthritis, RA, bursitis, acute gouty arthritis, epicondylitis, acute nonspecific tenosynovitis, posttraumatic osteoarthritis; lesions (keloids; localized, hypertrophic, infiltrated, inflammatory lesions of lichen planus; psoriatic plaques; granuloma annulare; or lichen simplex chronicus; discoid lupus erythematosus; necrobiosis lipoidica diabeticorum; alopecia areata; cystic tumors of an aponeurosis or tendon [ganglia])**
Adults: 0.2 to 4 mg intra-articular, soft tissue, or intralesional injection ranging from one single injection to injection every 3 to 5 days to once every 2 to 3 weeks. Dosage and frequency of injection vary depending on condition and site of injection.

➤ **Multiple myeloma, in combination with other antimyeloma products (Hemady only)**
Adults: 20 or 40 mg PO once daily on specific days, depending on treatment regimen. Refer to prescribing information of other antimyeloma products used in combination for specific dosing.

Adjust-a-dose: Reduce dosage in older adults because of increased risk of toxicity.

ADMINISTRATION
PO
• Give oral dose with food when possible. As needed, institute measures to prevent GI irritation.
• Only give concentrated oral solution using calibrated dropper supplied with product. Discard opened bottle after 90 days.
• Mix concentrated oral solution with liquid or semisolid food (water, juice, soda or soda-like beverages, applesauce, pudding). Have patient consume immediately.
IV
▼ For direct injection, inject undiluted over at least 1 minute (doses 10 mg or less).
▼ For intermittent or continuous infusion, dilute solution according to manufacturer's instructions and give over prescribed duration.
▼ During continuous infusion, change solution every 24 hours.
▼ **Incompatibilities:** Ciprofloxacin, diphenhydramine, doxapram, glycopyrrolate, idarubicin, midazolam, vancomycin.
IM
• Give IM injection deep into gluteal muscle. Rotate injection sites to prevent muscle atrophy. Avoid subcut injection because atrophy and sterile abscesses may occur.
Intra-articular, soft tissue, intralesional
• Use only dexamethasone sodium phosphate formulation.
• Frequent intra-articular injection may damage joint tissues.
• Use when affected joints or areas are limited to one or two sites.

ACTION
Decreases inflammation, mainly by stabilizing leukocyte lysosomal membranes; suppresses immune response; stimulates bone marrow; and influences protein, fat, and carbohydrate metabolism.

Route	Onset	Peak	Duration
PO	1–2 hr	1–2 hr	2.5 days
IV	1 hr	1 hr	Variable
IM	1 hr	1 hr	6 days
Intra-articular, intralesional, soft tissue	Unknown	Unknown	Unknown

Half-life: PO, 3 to 5 hours; IV, 1 to 5 hours (adults), 2 to 9.5 hours (children).

ADVERSE REACTIONS

CNS: euphoria, insomnia, psychotic behavior, *pseudotumor cerebri,* vertigo, syncope, headache, paresthesia, *seizures,* depression. **CV:** *HF,* HTN, edema, *arrhythmias,* cardiomegaly, vasculitis, thrombophlebitis, *thromboembolism.* **EENT:** cataracts, glaucoma, increase IOP. **GI:** peptic ulceration, abdominal distention, GI irritation, increased appetite, *pancreatitis,* nausea, vomiting. **GU:** menstrual irregularities, increased urine glucose and calcium levels. **Metabolic:** *hypokalemia,* alkalosis, carbohydrate intolerance, hypercholesterolemia, hyperglycemia, *hypocalcemia,* sodium retention, fluid retention, weight gain. **Musculoskeletal:** growth suppression in children, muscle weakness, loss of muscle mass, osteoporosis, vertebral compression fracture, aseptic necrosis of femoral and humeral heads, pathologic long bone fracture, tendon rupture, myopathy, hiccups. **Skin:** hirsutism, delayed wound healing, acne, various skin eruptions, atrophy at IM injection site, thin fragile skin, increased or decreased pigmentation, facial erythema, diaphoresis, petechiae, ecchymosis, sterile abscess. **Other:** susceptibility to infections, cushingoid state, acute adrenal insufficiency after increased stress or abrupt withdrawal after long-term therapy, *angioedema, anaphylaxis.* **After abrupt withdrawal:** rebound inflammation, fatigue, weakness, arthralgia, fever, dizziness, lethargy, fainting, orthostatic hypotension, dyspnea, anorexia, *hypoglycemia.*

INTERACTIONS

Drug-drug. *Antidiabetics, including insulin:* May decrease response. May need dosage adjustment.
Aspirin, indomethacin, other NSAIDs: May increase risk of GI distress and bleeding. Use together cautiously.

Cardiac glycosides: May increase risk of arrhythmia resulting from hypokalemia. May need dosage adjustment.
Cyclosporine: May increase toxicity. Monitor patient closely.
CYP3A4 inducers (barbiturates, carbamazepine, phenytoin, rifampin): May decrease corticosteroid effect. Increase corticosteroid dosage.
CYP3A4 inhibitors (clarithromycin, ketoconazole, itraconazole), estrogens: May decrease metabolism of dexamethasone and increase risk of corticosteroid-related adverse effects. Consider therapy modification.
Oral anticoagulants: May alter dosage requirements. Closely monitor PT and INR.
Potassium-depleting drugs such as thiazide diuretics: May enhance potassium-wasting effects of dexamethasone. Monitor potassium level.
Salicylates: May decrease salicylate level. Monitor for lack of salicylate effectiveness.
Skin-test antigens: May decrease response. Postpone skin testing until therapy is completed.
Toxoids, vaccines: May decrease antibody response and increase risk of neurologic complications. Avoid use together.
Drug-herb. *Echinacea:* May reduce drug's therapeutic effects. Avoid use together.
Drug-lifestyle. *Alcohol use:* May increase risk of gastric irritation and GI ulceration. Discourage use together.

EFFECTS ON LAB TEST RESULTS

• May increase cholesterol and glucose levels.
• May decrease calcium, potassium, T_3, and T_4 levels.
• May decrease ^{131}I uptake and protein-bound iodine levels in thyroid function tests.
• May cause false-negative result in nitro blue tetrazolium test for systemic bacterial infection.
• May alter reactions to skin tests.

CONTRAINDICATIONS & CAUTIONS

• Contraindicated in patients hypersensitive to drug or its ingredients, in those with systemic fungal infections, and in those receiving immunosuppressive doses together with live-virus vaccines. IM administration is contraindicated in patients with ITP.
• Use cautiously in patients with recent MI.
• Use cautiously in patients with GI ulcer, kidney disease, liver impairment, HTN, osteoporosis, diabetes, hypothyroidism,

---

Reactions in bold italics are *life-threatening*.

diverticulitis, nonspecific ulcerative colitis, thromboembolic disorders, recent intestinal anastomoses, pheochromocytoma, seizures, myasthenia gravis, HF, TB, active hepatitis, hepatitis B (reactivation can occur), ocular HSV infection, emotional instability, or psychotic tendencies.

• Some forms contain sulfite preservatives; use cautiously in patients sensitive to sulfites.

• Some forms contain benzyl alcohol, which has been associated with life-threatening neonatal gasping syndrome. Avoid use in neonates.

Dialyzable drug: No.

PREGNANCY-LACTATION-REPRODUCTION

• Dexamethasone crosses the placental barrier. Use during pregnancy only if potential benefit justifies fetal risk. When systemic corticosteroids are needed during pregnancy, use lowest effective dose for shortest duration of time, avoiding high doses during first trimester.

• Use together with antineoplastics for multiple myeloma during pregnancy is contraindicated. Obtain pregnancy test before start of therapy. Patients of reproductive potential should use effective contraception during treatment and for 1 month after final dose.

• Drug appears in human milk. Patients shouldn't breastfeed during treatment and for 2 weeks after final dose or should discontinue drug, considering importance of drug to patient.

• Steroids can increase or decrease motility and number of spermatozoa.

NURSING CONSIDERATIONS

❸ *Alert:* Epidural corticosteroid injections for neck pain, back pain, or radiating pain in arms and legs may result in rare but serious adverse events (vision loss, stroke, paralysis, death). Use of epidural corticosteroid injections isn't approved by the FDA.

• Most adverse reactions to corticosteroids are dose- or duration-dependent.

• For better results and less toxicity, give once-daily dose in morning.

• Always adjust to lowest effective dose.

• Monitor patient's weight, BP, and electrolyte levels.

• Monitor for cushingoid effects (moon face, buffalo hump, central obesity, thinning hair, HTN, increased susceptibility to infection).

• Watch for depression or psychotic episodes, especially with high-dose therapy.

• Patient with diabetes may need increased insulin; monitor glucose level.

• Be aware that drug may mask or worsen infections, including latent amebiasis.

• Older adults may be more susceptible to osteoporosis with long-term use.

• Inspect patient's skin for petechiae.

• Gradually reduce dosage after long-term therapy.

• *Look alike–sound alike:* Don't confuse dexamethasone with desoximetasone.

PATIENT TEACHING

• Instruct patient to take drug with food or milk.

❸ *Alert:* Counsel patient to discuss benefits, risks, and other possible treatments with provider before undergoing epidural corticosteroid injection and to seek immediate medical attention for loss of vision or vision changes; tingling in arms or legs; sudden weakness or numbness of face, arm, or leg on one or both sides of body; dizziness; severe headache; or seizures.

• Tell patient not to stop drug abruptly or without prescriber's consent.

• Teach patient signs and symptoms of early adrenal insufficiency (fatigue, muscle weakness, joint pain, fever, anorexia, nausea, shortness of breath, dizziness, and fainting).

• Instruct patient to carry medical identification indicating the need for supplemental systemic glucocorticoids during stress, especially when dosage is decreased. Card should contain prescriber's name, drug name, and drug dosage.

• Warn patient on long-term therapy about cushingoid effects (moon face, buffalo hump) and the need to notify prescriber about sudden weight gain or swelling.

• Warn patient about easy bruising.

• Advise patient receiving long-term therapy to consider exercise or physical therapy.

• Tell patient to ask prescriber about vitamin D or calcium supplement.

• Instruct patient receiving long-term therapy to have periodic eye exams.

• Advise patient to avoid exposure to infections (such as measles and chickenpox) and to notify prescriber if exposure occurs.

• Caution patient to avoid alcohol.

• Counsel patient to immediately report pregnancy, plans to become pregnant, breastfeeding, or intent to breastfeed during treatment.

• Advise patient of reproductive potential who is taking Hemady to use effective contraception during treatment and for at least 1 month after final dose.

dexmethylphenidate hydrochloride
dex-meth-il-FEN-i-date

Focalin, Focalin XR

Therapeutic class: CNS stimulants
Pharmacologic class: Methylphenidate derivatives
Controlled substance schedule: II

AVAILABLE FORMS
Capsules (extended-release) ⓄⓃⒸ: 5 mg, 10 mg, 15 mg, 20 mg, 25 mg, 30 mg, 35 mg, 40 mg
Tablets: 2.5 mg, 5 mg, 10 mg

INDICATIONS & DOSAGES
➤ **ADHD**
Adults and children ages 6 and older (immediate-release tablets): For patients who aren't currently taking methylphenidate, initially, 2.5 mg PO b.i.d., given at least 4 hours apart. Increase weekly by 2.5 to 5 mg daily, up to a maximum of 20 mg daily in divided doses.

For patients who are currently taking methylphenidate, initially give half the current methylphenidate dosage, up to a maximum of 20 mg PO daily in divided doses at least 4 hours apart.

Adults (extended-release capsules):
For patients who aren't currently taking dexmethylphenidate or methylphenidate, or who are on stimulants other than methylphenidate, 10 mg PO once daily in the morning. May adjust in weekly increments of 10 mg to maximum dose of 40 mg daily.

For patients who are currently taking methylphenidate, initially give half the total daily dose of methylphenidate. Patients who are currently taking the immediate-release form of dexmethylphenidate may be switched to the same daily dose of extended-release form. Maximum daily dose, 40 mg.
Children ages 6 and older (extended-release capsules): For patients who aren't currently taking dexmethylphenidate or methylphenidate or who are on stimulants

other than methylphenidate, 5 mg PO daily in the morning. May adjust in weekly increments of 5 mg to a maximum daily dose of 30 mg.

For patients who are currently taking methylphenidate, initially give half the total daily dose of methylphenidate. Patients currently taking immediate-release form of dexmethylphenidate may be switched to same daily dose of extended-release form. Maximum daily dose, 30 mg.

ADMINISTRATION
PO
• Patient may swallow capsules whole with or without food or may sprinkle contents on a small amount of applesauce and eat immediately without chewing.
• Don't crush or divide the capsule or its contents.
• Separate tablet twice-daily dosing by at least 4 hours.

ACTION
Blocks presynaptic reuptake of norepinephrine and dopamine and increases their release, increasing concentration in the synapse.

Route	Onset	Peak	Duration
PO (immediate-release)	Unknown	1–1.5 hr	Unknown
PO (extended-release)	Unknown	1–4 hr; 4.5–7 hr	Unknown

Half-life: Extended-release, about 3 hours (adults), 2 to 3 hours (children); immediate-release, 2.2 hours.

ADVERSE REACTIONS
CNS: headache, anxiety, jitteriness, insomnia, fever, dizziness, mood swings, depression, irritability. **CV:** tachycardia. **EENT:** nasal congestion, pharyngolaryngeal pain, dry mouth. **GI:** anorexia, abdominal pain, nausea, dyspepsia, vomiting. **Musculoskeletal:** twitching (motor or vocal tics). **Skin:** pruritus. **Other:** hypersensitivity reactions.

INTERACTIONS
Drug-drug. *Antacids, acid suppressants:* May alter the release of extended-release form. Avoid use together.
Antihypertensives (ACE inhibitors, ARBs, beta blockers, calcium channel blockers, centrally acting alpha-2 receptor agonists, potassium-sparing and thiazide diuretics): May decrease effectiveness of these drugs.

Reactions in bold italics are *life-threatening*.

Monitor BP and adjust dose of antihypertensive as needed.

Halogenated anesthetics (halothane, isoflurane): May increase risk of sudden BP and HR increase during surgery. Avoid dexmethylphenidate in patients being treated with anesthetics on day of surgery.

MAO inhibitors (isocarboxazid, linezolid, methylene blue, selegiline): May increase risk of hypertensive crisis. Use together within 14 days of MAO inhibitor therapy is contraindicated.

Risperidone: May increase risk of extrapyramidal symptoms with dosage change of either agent. Monitor patient closely.

EFFECTS ON LAB TEST RESULTS
• May decrease Hb level and leukocyte and platelet counts.
• May increase LFT values.

CONTRAINDICATIONS & CAUTIONS
• Contraindicated in patients hypersensitive to methylphenidate or other components.
🕭 *Alert:* Avoid use in patients with known serious structural cardiac abnormalities, cardiomyopathy, serious heart rhythm abnormalities, CAD, and other serious heart problems. Sudden death, stroke, and MI have been reported.
Boxed Warning Stimulants carry a high risk of abuse and misuse, which can lead to substance use disorder, including addiction, which can lead to overdose and death. The risk increases with high doses or unapproved administration methods, such as snorting or injection. ■
• Drug may cause tolerance, requiring a higher dose to produce the same effect a lower dose once provided.
• Use cautiously in patients with psychiatric illness, bipolar disorder, depression, or family history of suicide and in patients with seizures, HTN, hyperthyroidism, HF, stroke, or recent MI.
• Rare cases of priapism have been reported.
• Safety and effectiveness in children less than 6 years old haven't been established.
Dialyzable drug: Unknown.
⚠ *Overdose S&S:* Delirium, dryness of mucous membranes, euphoria, flushing, headache, hyperreflexia, muscle twitching, mydriasis, palpitations, diaphoresis, tremors, vomiting, tachyarrhythmias, HTN or hypotension, vasospasm, MI, aortic dissection,

cardiomyopathy, psychomotor agitation, confusion, hallucinations, serotonin syndrome, seizures, stroke, coma, life-threatening hyperthermia, rhabdomyolysis, death.

PREGNANCY-LACTATION-REPRODUCTION
• Studies during pregnancy are inadequate. Use during pregnancy only if clearly needed and potential benefit justifies fetal risk.
• Drug appears in human milk. Use cautiously during breastfeeding. Long-term neurodevelopmental effects on infants are unknown.
• Enroll patients in National Pregnancy Registry for ADHD Medications (1-866-961-2388 or https://womensmentalhealth.org/adhd-medications/).

NURSING CONSIDERATIONS
• Diagnosis of ADHD must be based on complete history and evaluation of patient by psychological and educational experts.
• Obtain detailed patient history, including family history of mental disorders, family suicide, ventricular arrhythmias, and sudden death.
• Refer patient for psychological, educational, and social support.
Boxed Warning Assess patient's risk of abuse, misuse, and addiction before therapy. Reassess risk during therapy. Monitor for signs and symptoms of drug abuse, misuse, and addiction (increased HR, respiratory rate, or BP; sweating; dilated pupils; hyperactivity; restlessness; insomnia; decreased appetite; loss of coordination; tremors; flushing; vomiting; abdominal pain). Anxiety, psychosis, hostility, aggression, suicidality, and homicidal ideation may also occur. ■
• Abrupt drug stoppage or dose reduction may cause withdrawal symptoms (dysphoria, depression, fatigue, vivid and unpleasant dreams, insomnia or hypersomnia, increased appetite, psychomotor retardation or agitation) in patient with physical dependence.
• Periodically reevaluate long-term usefulness of drug.
• Monitor CBC and differential and platelet counts during prolonged therapy.
• Don't use for severe depression or normal fatigue states.
• Stop treatment or reduce dosage if symptoms worsen or adverse reactions occur.
• Long-term stimulant use may temporarily suppress growth. Monitor children for growth

and weight gain. If growth slows or weight gain is lower than expected, stop drug.

🔵 *Alert:* Periodically monitor patient for changes in HR or BP. Promptly evaluate chest pain, unexplained syncope, or other signs or symptoms of cardiac disease.

• If seizures occur, stop drug.

• Monitor for digital vascular changes during therapy. Drug is associated with peripheral vasculopathy, including Raynaud phenomenon.

• *Look alike–sound alike:* Don't confuse dexmethylphenidate with methadone, methylphenidate, or dextroamphetamine.

PATIENT TEACHING

• Advise patient and caregiver to read the medication guide.

Boxed Warning Teach patient and caregiver about risk of abuse, misuse, and addiction, which can lead to overdose and death. Advise patient to store drug in a safe (preferably locked) place. Teach about proper disposal of unused drug. Instruct patient not to give drug to anyone else. ∎

• Stress the importance of taking the correct dose of drug at the same time every day. Immediately report accidental overdose.

🔵 *Alert:* Instruct patient to immediately report chest pain, shortness of breath, or fainting.

• Advise parents to monitor child for medication abuse or sharing. Also inform parents to watch for increased aggression or hostility and to report worsening behavior.

• Warn patient to seek immediate medical attention for prolonged or painful erections.

• Instruct parents to monitor child's height and weight and to tell prescriber if they suspect growth is slowing.

• Advise patient or caregivers to report new numbness, pain, skin color change, or sensitivity to temperature in fingers or toes, because of risk of peripheral vasculopathy, including Raynaud phenomenon.

• Warn that blurred vision or difficulty with accommodation may occur. Advise patient to exercise caution while performing activities that require a clear visual field and to report blurred vision to prescriber.

dextroamphetamine
dex-troe-am-FET-a-meen

Xelstrym

dextroamphetamine sulfate
Dexedrine, ProCentra, Zenzedi

Therapeutic class: CNS stimulants
Pharmacologic class: Amphetamines
Controlled substance schedule: II

AVAILABLE FORMS

Capsules (extended-release) 🅞🅝🅒: 5 mg, 10 mg, 15 mg
Oral solution: 5 mg/5 mL
Tablets: 2.5 mg, 5 mg, 7.5 mg, 10 mg, 15 mg, 20 mg, 30 mg
Transdermal system: 4.5 mg/9 hours, 9 mg/9 hours, 13.5 mg/9 hours, 18 mg/9 hours

INDICATIONS & DOSAGES

➤ **Narcolepsy**
Adults: 5 to 60 mg/day PO in divided doses or once-daily extended-release capsule.
Children ages 12 and older: 10 mg PO daily. Increase by 10 mg at weekly intervals until optimal response is obtained. Give first dose on awakening; give additional doses (one or two) at intervals of 4 to 6 hours.
Children ages 6 to 12: 5 mg PO daily. Increase by 5 mg at weekly intervals as needed until optimal response is obtained. Give first dose on awakening; give additional doses (one or two) at intervals of 4 to 6 hours.

➤ **ADHD**
Adults: Initially, 9 mg/9 hours transdermal system daily. May titrate to maximum dose of 18 mg/9 hours.
Children ages 6 and older: 5 mg PO once daily or b.i.d. Increase by 5 mg at weekly intervals until optimal response is obtained (rarely necessary to exceed 40 mg/day). Or, initially, 4.5 mg/9 hours transdermal system daily. Titrate weekly by 4.5 mg up to maximum recommended dose of 18 mg/9 hours.
Children ages 3 to 5: Initially, 2.5 mg immediate-release tablets or solution PO daily. May increase daily dosage in increments of 2.5 mg at weekly intervals until optimal response is obtained.

Adjust-a-dose: If GFR is 15 to less than 30 mL/minute/1.73 m^2, maximum transdermal dose is 13.5 mg/9 hours. If eGFR less than 15 mL/minute/1.73 m^2, maximum transdermal dose is 9 mg/9 hours.

ADMINISTRATION
PO
• Avoid late-evening doses, particularly with extended-release capsules, due to resulting insomnia. Give initial dose upon awakening.
• Some formulations contain tartrazine (immediate-release tablets) or benzoic acid, which is a derivative of benzyl alcohol (oral solution). Derivatives of benzyl alcohol are associated with potentially fatal gasping syndrome in neonates.
• Make sure patient doesn't chew or crush extended-release capsules.
Transdermal
• Apply to clean, dry, intact skin of hip, upper arm, chest, upper back, or flank.
• Select a different site with application of each new system.
• Apply system 2 hours before an effect is needed; remove within 9 hours after application.
• Don't touch adhesive side of system to avoid absorption of drug.
• If adhesive is touched, immediately wash hands with soap and water. If system lifts at edges, reattach by firmly and smoothly pressing down on edges. If system comes off, apply new system; don't reapply with dressing, tape, or other common adhesive.
• Avoid exposing application site to direct external heat source (hair dryer, heating pad, electric blanket, heated water bed); heat increases both rate and extent of absorption.
• After removing system, fold so that adhesive adheres to itself and place in a lidded container. Don't flush down toilet.
• Don't substitute for other amphetamine products on a mg-per-mg basis because of differing pharmacokinetics.

ACTION
Promotes release of dopamine and norepinephrine from nerve terminals in the brain and, to a lesser extent, promotes the reuptake of catecholamines.

Route	Onset	Peak	Duration
PO	Unknown	3 hr	4–6 hr
PO (extended-release)	Unknown	8 hr	8 hr
Transdermal	Unknown	9 hr	9 hr

Half-life: PO, 10 to 12 hours; transdermal, 6.4 to 11.5 hours.

ADVERSE REACTIONS
CNS: insomnia, nervousness, anxiety, restlessness, tremor, dizziness, headache, chills, overstimulation, dysphoria, euphoria, dyskinesia, aggressive behavior, taste perversion, fatigue, irritability, labile affect. **CV:** tachycardia, palpitations, *arrhythmias,* elevated BP. **EENT:** blurred vision, dry mouth. **GI:** diarrhea, constipation, anorexia, other GI disturbances, abdominal pain, nausea, vomiting. **GU:** changes in libido, erectile dysfunction. **Hematologic:** *neutropenia, leukopenia.* **Metabolic:** weight loss. **Musculoskeletal:** exacerbation of motor and phonic tics, *rhabdomyolysis.* **Skin:** urticaria, alopecia, application-site reaction (pain, pruritus, burning, erythema, edema). **Other:** slowed growth rate.

INTERACTIONS
Drug-drug. *Acetazolamide, alkalizing drugs, antacids, sodium bicarbonate:* May increase kidney reabsorption. Monitor patient for enhanced amphetamine effects.
Acidifying drugs, ammonium chloride, ascorbic acid: May decrease level and increase kidney clearance of dextroamphetamine. Monitor patient for decreased amphetamine effects.
Adrenergic blockers: May inhibit adrenergic blocking effects. Avoid use together.
Antihypertensives: May diminish antihypertensive effects. Monitor BP.
Lithium: May inhibit central stimulant effects of amphetamines. Monitor therapy.
MAO inhibitors: May cause severe HTN or hypertensive crisis. Avoid using within 14 days of MAO inhibitor therapy.
Opioid agonists (meperidine): May potentiate analgesic effect. Use together cautiously.
Methenamine: May increase urinary excretion of amphetamines and reduce effectiveness. Monitor drug effects.
Serotonergic drugs (SSNRIs, SSRIs, TCAs, triptans, CYP2D6 inhibitors): Increases risk of serotonin syndrome. Start dextroamphetamine at lower doses and monitor patient for signs and symptoms of serotonin syndrome, especially during initiation or dosage increases.
TCAs: May increase adverse amphetamine effects and potentiate CV effects. Monitor patient closely; adjust dosage or use alternative therapy.

Drug-food. *Acidic foods, fruit juice:* Decreases amphetamine absorption. May decrease effectiveness. Avoid use together.

EFFECTS ON LAB TEST RESULTS
• May increase corticosteroid levels.
• May interfere with urinary steroid determinations.

CONTRAINDICATIONS & CAUTIONS
• Contraindicated in patients hypersensitive to or with idiosyncratic reactions to sympathomimetic amines; in those hypersensitive to amphetamine; in those with hyperthyroidism, moderate to severe HTN, symptomatic CV disease, glaucoma, advanced arteriosclerosis, or history of drug abuse; and in those in an agitated state.

Boxed Warning Stimulants carry a high risk of abuse and misuse, which can lead to substance use disorder, including addiction, which can lead to overdose and death. The risk increases with high doses or unapproved administration methods, such as snorting or injection. ■

• Drug may cause tolerance, requiring a higher dose to produce the same effect a lower dose once provided.
🔵 *Alert:* Use cautiously in patients with motor tics, phonic tics, or Tourette syndrome. Also use cautiously in patients whose underlying condition may be worsened by an increase in BP or HR (preexisting HTN, HF, recent MI); patients with a psychiatric illness, bipolar disorder, depression, or family history of suicide; and those with a seizure disorder.
• Don't use in children or adolescents with structural cardiac abnormalities or other serious heart problems.
• Drug isn't indicated for use in children under age 3.
Dialyzable drug: Unknown.
⚠ *Overdose S&S:* Assaultiveness, hyperreflexia, rapid respiration, restlessness, tremor, panic states, fatigue, depression, circulatory collapse, nausea, vomiting, diarrhea, abdominal cramps, tachyarrhythmias, HTN or hypotension, vasospasm, MI, aortic dissection, cardiomyopathy, psychomotor agitation, confusion, hallucinations, serotonin syndrome, seizures, stroke, coma, life-threatening hyperthermia, rhabdomyolysis, death.

PREGNANCY-LACTATION-REPRODUCTION
• Studies during pregnancy are inadequate. Use during pregnancy only if potential benefit justifies fetal risk.
• Enroll patients in the National Pregnancy Registry for Psychiatric Medications (866-961-2388 or https://womensmentalhealth.org/research/pregnancyregistry/).
• Infants born to patients dependent on amphetamines are at increased risk for premature delivery and low birth weight and may experience signs and symptoms of withdrawal, as demonstrated by dysphoria (agitation, significant drowsiness).
• Drug appears in human milk. Use during breastfeeding isn't recommended.

NURSING CONSIDERATIONS
• Obtain a detailed patient history, including family history of mental disorders, family suicide, ventricular arrhythmias, or sudden death.
• Monitor patient beginning treatment for ADHD for aggressive behavior and hostility.
• Don't use drug to prevent fatigue.
Boxed Warning Assess patient's risk of abuse, misuse, and addiction before therapy. Reassess risk during therapy. Monitor for signs and symptoms of drug abuse, misuse, and addiction (increased HR, respiratory rate, or BP; sweating; dilated pupils; hyperactivity; restlessness; insomnia; decreased appetite; loss of coordination; tremors; flushing; vomiting; abdominal pain). Anxiety, psychosis, hostility, aggression, suicidality, and homicidal ideation may also occur. ■

• Abrupt drug stoppage or dose reduction may cause withdrawal symptoms (dysphoria, depression, fatigue, vivid and unpleasant dreams, insomnia or hypersomnia, increased appetite, psychomotor retardation or agitation) in patient with physical dependence.
• Periodically monitor patient for changes in HR or BP.
• Monitor for growth retardation in children.
• *Look alike–sound alike:* Don't confuse Dexedrine with dextran or Excedrin. Don't confuse ProCentra with Kcentra.

PATIENT TEACHING
• Advise patient and caregiver to read the medication guide.
Boxed Warning Teach patient and caregiver about risk of abuse, misuse, and addiction, which can lead to overdose and death.

Reactions in bold italics are *life-threatening*.

Advise patient to store drug in a safe (preferably locked) place. Teach about proper disposal of unused drug. Instruct patient not to give drug to anyone else. ∎

🜂 **Alert:** Instruct patient to immediately report chest pain, shortness of breath, or fainting.

• Warn patient to avoid activities that require alertness, a clear visual field, or good coordination until CNS effects of drug are known.

• Tell patient fatigue may occur as drug effects wear off.

• Ask patient to report signs and symptoms of excessive stimulation.

• Inform caregiver that child may show increased aggression or hostility. Instruct them to report worsening behavior.

• Warn patient with a seizure disorder that drug may decrease seizure threshold. Instruct patient to notify prescriber if seizures occur.

• Caution patient to immediately report pregnancy, plans to become pregnant, breastfeeding, or intent to breastfeed during treatment.

dextroamphetamine sulfate–dextroamphetamine saccharate–amphetamine aspartate–amphetamine sulfate

dex-tro-am-PHET-ta-meen/
am-PHET-ta-meen

Adderall, Adderall XR, Mydayis

Therapeutic class: CNS stimulants
Pharmacologic class: Amphetamines
Controlled substance schedule: II

AVAILABLE FORMS

Capsules (extended-release) 🄳🄽🄶: 5 mg, 10 mg, 12.5 mg, 15 mg, 20 mg 25 mg, 30 mg, 37.5 mg, 50 mg
Tablets: 5 mg, 7.5 mg, 10 mg, 12.5 mg, 15 mg, 20 mg, 30 mg

INDICATIONS & DOSAGES

➤ **Narcolepsy**

Adults and children ages 12 and older: Initially, 10 mg (immediate-release) tablet PO daily. May increase daily dose by 10 mg at weekly intervals to maximum of 60 mg/day. Give in one to three divided doses per day.
Children ages 6 to younger than 12: Initially, 5 mg (immediate-release) tablet PO daily. May increase daily dose by 5 mg at weekly

intervals until optimal response is achieved. Give in one to three divided doses per day.
Adjust-a-dose: For adverse reactions (insomnia or anorexia), reduce dosage.

➤ **ADHD**

Adults: Initially, 5 mg (immediate-release) tablet PO once daily or b.i.d. May increase daily dose by 5 mg at weekly intervals until optimal response achieved; maximum dose, 40 mg/day. Or, 20-mg extended-release capsule PO once daily in morning. Maximum dose, 30 mg/day. Or, in adults ages 18 to 55, 12.5 to 25 mg Mydayis PO once daily in the morning. May increase daily dose by 12.5 mg at weekly intervals until optimal response achieved; maximum dose, 50 mg/day.
Adolescents ages 13 to 17 (extended-release): Initially, 10 mg PO daily in morning. May increase to 20 mg/day after 1 week if symptoms aren't controlled. Or, 12.5 mg Mydayis PO daily in the morning. May increase to maximum of 25 mg/day after 1 week if symptoms aren't controlled.
Children ages 6 and older (immediate-release): Initially, 5 mg PO once daily or b.i.d. May increase daily dose by 5 mg at weekly intervals until optimal response is achieved. Give in one to three divided doses per day. Rarely necessary to exceed total of 40 mg/day.
Children ages 6 to 12 (extended-release): Initially, 5 to 10 mg PO once daily in morning. May increase daily dose by 5 or 10 mg at weekly intervals. Maximum dose, 30 mg/day.
Children ages 3 to 5 (immediate-release): Initially, 2.5 mg PO daily. May increase daily dose by 2.5 mg at weekly intervals until optimal response is achieved. Give in one to three divided doses per day.
Adjust-a-dose: In patients with GFR of 15 to less than 30 mL/minute/1.73 m³, dosage reduction may be needed. Refer to manufacturer's instructions.

ADMINISTRATION
PO

• May give with or without food. Give Mydayis consistently either with or without food.

• Give extended-release dose upon awakening; don't give immediate-release dose in late evening to avoid insomnia.

• Make sure patient takes extended-release capsules whole, or open capsules and sprinkle entire contents on applesauce and have patient consume immediately without chewing.

• Don't give missed Mydayis dose later in the day because effects may last up to 16 hours.

ACTION
Promotes release of dopamine and norepinephrine from nerve terminals in the brain and, to a lesser extent, promotes the reuptake of catecholamines.

Route	Onset	Peak	Duration
PO (immediate-release)	Unknown	3 hr	4–6 hr
PO (extended-release)	Unknown	7–8 hr	Unknown

Half-life: Immediate-release, 9 to 14 hours; extended-release, 10 to 14 hours.

ADVERSE REACTIONS
CNS: headache, insomnia, agitation, anxiety, dizziness, drowsiness, emotional lability, nervousness, irritability, jitteriness, fatigue, speech disturbance, twitching, fever, depression. **CV:** systolic HTN, palpitations, tachycardia, Raynaud phenomenon. **EENT:** dry mouth, teeth clenching, tooth infection. **GI:** abdominal pain, anorexia, constipation, diarrhea, dyspepsia, nausea, vomiting. **GU:** decreased libido, erectile dysfunction, UTI, dysmenorrhea. **Metabolic:** weight loss. **Respiratory:** dyspnea. **Skin:** diaphoresis, photosensitivity. **Other:** infection, accidental injury, hypersensitivity reaction.

INTERACTIONS
Drug-drug. *Acidifying agents (ammonium chloride, ascorbic acid, glutamic acid, methenamine, reserpine, sodium acid phosphate):* May lower amphetamine absorption and blood level. Don't use together.
Adrenergic blockers, antihistamines, antihypertensives, ethosuximide, phenobarbital, phenytoin: Amphetamines may reduce therapeutic effects of these drugs. Monitor patient response.
Alkalizing agents (acetazolamide, sodium bicarbonate, thiazides): May increase amphetamine level through decreased urine excretion. Monitor patient response.
CYP2D6 inhibitors (fluoxetine, paroxetine, ritonavir): May increase amphetamine level and risk of serotonin syndrome. Monitor patient, especially during amphetamine initiation and dosage increase.
MAO inhibitors (isocarboxazid, linezolid, methylene blue, selegiline): May increase risk of hypertensive crisis. Concurrent use or use within 14 days of MAO inhibitors is contraindicated.
PPIs (omeprazole): May increase amphetamine absorption rate. Monitor therapy.
Serotonergic agents (buspirone, fentanyl, lithium, SSNRIs, SSRIs, TCAs, tramadol, triptans): May increase risk of serotonin syndrome. Monitor patient. If syndrome occurs, discontinue both drugs and provide supportive care.
TCAs (desipramine, protriptyline): May increase amphetamine level and risk of CV effects. Monitor patient closely.
Drug-herb. *Ephedra:* May cause HTN or arrhythmias. Don't use together.
St. John's wort: May increase risk of serotonin syndrome. Use together cautiously.
Drug-lifestyle. *Alcohol use:* May increase risk of drug dependency. Concurrent use is contraindicated in patients with history of ethanol or drug dependency.

EFFECTS ON LAB TEST RESULTS
• May increase plasma corticosteroid level.
• May interfere with urinary steroid testing.

CONTRAINDICATIONS & CAUTIONS
Boxed Warning Stimulants carry a high risk of abuse and misuse, which can lead to substance use disorder, including addiction, which can lead to overdose and death. The risk increases with high doses or unapproved administration methods, such as snorting or injection. ∎
• Drug may cause tolerance, requiring a higher dose to produce the same effect a lower dose once provided.
• Contraindicated in patients with advanced arteriosclerosis, symptomatic CV disease, moderate to severe HTN, hyperthyroidism, known hypersensitivity or idiosyncrasy to amphetamines, glaucoma, agitated states, or history of drug addiction.
🛇 *Alert:* Sudden death has been reported at usual doses in patients with structural cardiac abnormalities and other serious heart problems. Stimulants generally should not be used in patients with structural cardiac abnormalities, cardiomyopathy, serious heart rhythm abnormalities, or other serious cardiac problems.
• Drug can increase BP. Use cautiously in patients with underlying medical conditions (preexisting HTN, HF, recent MI, ventricular

---

arrhythmia) that might be compromised by increases in BP or HR.

• Use cautiously in patients with a history of seizures, tics or Tourette syndrome, or mental problems, including psychosis, bipolar illness, mania, or depression.

• Drug may cause peripheral vasculopathy, including Raynaud phenomenon, which may improve after dosage reduction or drug discontinuation.

• Drug hasn't been studied in older adults.

• Immediate-release tablets aren't recommended for children with ADHD younger than age 3 or for children with narcolepsy younger than age 6. Use of extended-release capsules in children younger than age 6 hasn't been studied.

• Safety and effectiveness of Mydayis in children ages 12 and younger haven't been established.

Dialyzable drug: Unknown.

⚠ *Overdose S&S:* Restlessness, tremor, hyperreflexia, rapid respiration, assaultiveness, panic states, fatigue, depression, circulatory collapse; nausea, vomiting, diarrhea, abdominal cramps, tachyarrhythmias, HTN or hypotension, vasospasm, MI, aortic dissection, cardiomyopathy, psychomotor agitation, confusion, hallucinations, serotonin syndrome, seizures, stroke, coma, life-threatening hyperthermia, rhabdomyolysis, death.

PREGNANCY-LACTATION-REPRODUCTION

• Current data have not shown drug-associated risk of major birth defects and miscarriage. Use during pregnancy only if potential benefit justifies fetal risk.

• Infants born to patients on amphetamines have an increased risk of premature delivery and low birth weight. These infants may also experience signs and symptoms of withdrawal, such as dysphoria (agitation, excessive drowsiness).

• Register patients in the National Pregnancy Registry for ADHD Medications (1-866-961-2388 or https://womensmentalhealth.org/research/pregnancyregistry/adhd-medications/).

• Drug appears in human milk. Don't use during breastfeeding.

NURSING CONSIDERATIONS

Boxed Warning Assess patient's risk of abuse, misuse, and addiction before therapy. Reassess risk during therapy. Monitor for

signs and symptoms of drug abuse, misuse, and addiction (increased HR, respiratory rate, or BP; sweating; dilated pupils; hyperactivity; restlessness; insomnia; decreased appetite; loss of coordination; tremors; flushing; vomiting; abdominal pain). Anxiety, psychosis, hostility, aggression, suicidality, and homicidal ideation may also occur. ■

• Abrupt drug stoppage or dose reduction may cause withdrawal symptoms (dysphoria, depression, fatigue, vivid and unpleasant dreams, insomnia or hypersomnia, increased appetite, psychomotor retardation or agitation) in patient with physical dependence.

• Interrupt therapy occasionally to assess if ADHD behavioral symptoms warrant continued therapy, if possible.

• Perform a careful history and physical exam in all patients to assess for presence of cardiac disease. Further cardiac evaluation may be needed. All patients who develop cardiac signs and symptoms (chest pain, syncope) during therapy should undergo prompt cardiac evaluation.

• Monitor HR and BP during therapy.

• Screen patient for family history of suicide, bipolar disorder, and depression before use. Monitor patient for increased aggression, worsening of existing psychiatric signs and symptoms, or psychosis.

• When used long term, drug may slow growth rate in children. Monitor growth rate; interrupt treatment for child who is not growing or gaining weight as expected.

• Monitor patient for risk of vasculopathies, including Raynaud phenomenon. Evaluate unexplained wounds on fingers and toes.

• When switching from other dextroamphetamine–amphetamine preparations to Mydayis, discontinue previous formulation and titrate per package labeling. Don't substitute on a milligram-per-milligram basis.

• *Look alike–sound alike:* Don't confuse Adderall with Inderal.

PATIENT TEACHING

• Advise patient and caregiver to read the medication guide.

Boxed Warning Teach patient and caregiver about risk of abuse, misuse, and addiction, which can lead to overdose and death. Advise patient to store drug in a safe (preferably locked) place. Teach about proper disposal of unused drug. Instruct patient not to give drug to anyone else. ■

• Tell patient to report all drugs and supplements being taken before start of therapy.

• Explain that serious cardiac effects are possible during therapy. Advise patient to immediately report chest pain, shortness of breath, or fainting.

• Advise patient to report development of such conditions as glaucoma, high BP, or hyperthyroidism.

• Instruct patient to keep regular follow-up appointments for monitoring of HR, BP, and growth (in children). Patient who isn't growing or gaining weight as expected may need treatment interruption.

• Advise patient to report worsening of psychiatric signs and symptoms or behavioral changes during therapy.

• Explain that drug may cause circulatory problems. Advise patient to immediately report unexplained wounds on fingers or toes.

• Caution patient that abruptly stopping drug may cause withdrawal signs and symptoms (extreme fatigue, depression, increased appetite, agitation, abnormal dreams).

SAFETY ALERT!

diazePAM ⊗
dye-AZ-e-pam

Diastat*, Diastat AcuDial*, Diazepam Intensol*, Valium, Valtoco

Therapeutic class: Anxiolytics
Pharmacologic class: Benzodiazepines
Controlled substance schedule: IV

AVAILABLE FORMS
Injection: 5 mg/mL vials and prefilled syringes
Nasal spray: 5 mg/spray, 7.5 mg/spray, 10 mg/spray
Oral solution: 5 mg/5 mL, 5 mg/mL*
Rectal gel twin packs: 2.5 mg (pediatric); 10 mg, 20 mg (adult)
Tablets: 2 mg, 5 mg, 10 mg

INDICATIONS & DOSAGES
Adjust-a-dose (for all indications): For older adults and patients who are debilitated, give 2 to 2.5 mg PO daily or b.i.d. initially; increase gradually as needed and tolerated. When using injection, use lower doses (2 to 5 mg) and increase dosage more gradually. When using nasal spray or rectal gel, consider reducing dosage due to increased half-life in older adults.

➤ **Anxiety**
Adults: Depending on severity, 2 to 10 mg PO b.i.d. to q.i.d. or 2 to 10 mg IM or IV. May repeat in 3 to 4 hours if needed.
Children ages 6 months and older: 1 to 2.5 mg PO t.i.d. or q.i.d., increased gradually, as needed and tolerated.

➤ **Acute alcohol withdrawal**
Adults: 10 mg PO t.i.d. or q.i.d. during first 24 hours; reduce to 5 mg PO t.i.d. or q.i.d. PRN. Or, 10 mg IV or IM initially; then 5 to 10 mg IV or IM again in 3 to 4 hours PRN.

➤ **Before endoscopic procedures**
Adults: Adjust IV dose to desired sedative response (up to 20 mg). If IV can't be used, 5 to 10 mg IM 30 minutes before procedure.

➤ **Muscle spasm**
Adults: 2 to 10 mg PO b.i.d. to q.i.d. as an adjunct. Or, 5 to 10 mg IV or IM initially; then 5 to 10 mg IV or IM again in 3 to 4 hours if needed.

➤ **Muscle spasm associated with tetanus**
Adults: Initially, 5 to 10 mg IV or IM then 5 to 10 mg in 3 to 4 hours if needed. Larger doses may be required.
Children ages 5 and older: 5 to 10 mg IM or IV repeated every 3 to 4 hours PRN.
Children ages 30 days to younger than 5 years: 1 to 2 mg IM or IV slowly repeated every 3 to 4 hours PRN.

➤ **Preoperative sedation**
Adults: 10 mg IM or IV before surgery.

➤ **Adjunctive treatment for seizure disorders**
Adults: 2 to 10 mg PO b.i.d. to q.i.d.
Children ages 6 months and older: 1 to 2.5 mg PO t.i.d. or q.i.d. initially; increase as needed and as tolerated.

➤ **Status epilepticus, severe recurrent seizures**
Adults: 5 to 10 mg IV or IM initially. Use IM route only if IV access is unavailable. Repeat every 10 to 15 minutes PRN, up to maximum dose of 30 mg. Repeat every 2 to 4 hours PRN.
Children ages 3 months and older: 0.2 mg/kg IV slowly to a maximum of 8 mg. May give a second dose of 0.1 mg/kg (maximum 4 mg) 5 minutes after first dose.

➤ **Patients on stable regimens of antiepileptic drugs who need diazepam**

intermittently to control bouts of increased seizure activity (rectal)

Adults and children ages 12 and older:
0.2 mg/kg PR, rounding up to nearest available dose form. A second dose may be given 4 to 12 hours later.

Children ages 6 to 11: 0.3 mg/kg PR, rounding up to nearest available dose form. A second dose may be given 4 to 12 hours later.

Children ages 2 to 5: 0.5 mg/kg PR, rounding up to nearest available dose form. A second dose may be given 4 to 12 hours later.

➤ **Acute treatment of intermittent, stereotypic episodes of frequent seizure activity that are distinct from usual seizure pattern in patients with epilepsy (intranasal)**

Adults and children ages 12 and older weighing 76 kg or more: 10 mg intranasally in both nostrils (20 mg total).

Adults and children ages 12 and older weighing 51 to 75 kg: 7.5 mg intranasally in both nostrils (15 mg total).

Adults and children ages 12 and older weighing 28 to 50 kg: 10 mg intranasally in one nostril (10 mg total).

Adults and children ages 12 and older weighing 14 to 27 kg: 5 mg intranasally in one nostril (5 mg total).

Children ages 6 to 11 weighing 56 to 74 kg: 10 mg intranasally in both nostrils (20 mg total).

Children ages 6 to 11 weighing 38 to 55 kg: 7.5 mg intranasally in both nostrils (15 mg total).

Children ages 6 to 11 weighing 19 to 37 kg: 10 mg intranasally in one nostril (10 mg total).

Children ages 6 to 11 weighing 10 to 18 kg: 5 mg intranasally in one nostril (5 mg total).

Adjust-a-dose: If a second dose is needed, give at least 4 hours after initial dose. Don't use more than two doses to treat a single episode.

ADMINISTRATION
PO
• When using concentrated oral solution, dilute dose just before giving with liquid or semisolid food (water, juice, soda or sodalike beverages, applesauce, pudding). Use provided calibrated dropper to draw up the prescribed dose.
• Store at room temperature.
• Discard opened bottle of solution after 90 days.

IV
▼ Keep emergency resuscitation equipment and oxygen at bedside.
▼ For adults, give at no more than 5 mg/minute.
▼ For children with status epilepticus, administer slowly over 1 minute. For other indications, give at no more than 5 mg/minute.
▼ Avoid infusion sets and containers made from polyvinyl chloride.
▼ If possible, inject directly into a large vein. If not, inject slowly through infusion tubing as near to insertion site as possible. Watch closely for phlebitis at injection site.
▼ Monitor respirations every 5 to 15 minutes and before each dose.
▼ Don't store parenteral solution in plastic syringes.
▼ **Incompatibilities:** All other IV drugs, most IV solutions.

IM
• Use the IM route if IV administration is impossible.

Rectal
• Use Diastat rectal gel to treat no more than five episodes per month and no more than one episode every 5 days.
• Lubricate tip of rectal syringe before use with provided lubricant packet.
• Give gel over 3 seconds, wait 3 seconds before removing syringe from rectum, then wait 3 seconds while holding buttocks together to prevent leakage.
⚠ *Alert:* Only caregivers who can distinguish the distinct cluster of seizures or events from patient's ordinary seizure activity, who have been instructed and can give the treatment competently, who understand which seizures may be treated with Diastat, and who can monitor the clinical response and recognize when immediate professional medical evaluation is needed should give Diastat rectal gel.

Intranasal
• Use nasal spray to treat no more than five episodes per month and no more than one episode every 5 days.
• Each single-use nasal spray device delivers 1 spray and cannot be reused. Do not prime or attempt to use for more than one administration per device.
• Don't open blister packs or test devices before use.
• Store at 20° C to 25° C (68° F to 77° F). Don't freeze.
• Protect from light.

ACTION
Potentiates the effects of GABA, depresses the CNS, and suppresses the spread of seizure activity.

Route	Onset	Peak	Duration
PO	30 min	0.25–2.5 hr	20–80 hr
IV	1–5 min	1–5 min	15–60 min
IM	Unknown	1 hr	Unknown
Intranasal	Unknown	90 min	Unknown
PR	2–10 min	90 min	Unknown

Half-life: About 1 to 12 days. Varies with route and patient age.

ADVERSE REACTIONS
CNS: drowsiness, abnormal thinking, agitation, emotional lability, euphoria, nervousness, asthenia, dysarthria, slurred speech, tremor, transient amnesia, fatigue, ataxia, headache, insomnia, nightmares, paradoxical anxiety, disinhibition, hallucinations, minor changes in EEG patterns, pain, vertigo, confusion, depression, dysgeusia (nasal form). **CV:** hypotension, vasodilation. **EENT:** diplopia, blurred vision, nystagmus; with nasal form: nasal discomfort, nasal congestion, epistaxis, dry mouth. **GI:** nausea, abdominal pain, constipation, diarrhea with rectal form. **GU:** altered libido, incontinence, urine retention. **Hematologic:** *neutropenia.* **Hepatic:** jaundice. **Respiratory:** hiccups. **Skin:** rash, phlebitis at injection site. **Other:** physical or psychological dependence.

INTERACTIONS
Drug-drug. *CNS depressants:* May increase CNS and respiratory depression. Use together cautiously.
CYP2C19 inducers (rifampin), CYP3A4 inducers (carbamazepine, phenytoin, dexamethasone, phenobarbital): May decrease diazepam level. Monitor therapy.
CYP2C19 inhibitors (cimetidine, quinidine), CYP3A4 inhibitors (troleandomycin, ketoconazole): May increase diazepam level and increase risk of adverse effects. Monitor patient for excessive sedation and impaired psychomotor function.
Boxed Warning *Opioids:* May cause slow or difficult breathing, sedation, and death. Avoid use together. If use together can't be avoided, limit dosage and duration of each drug to the minimum necessary for desired effect. ∎

Drug-herb. *Kava kava:* May increase sedation. Discourage use together.
Drug-lifestyle. **Boxed Warning** *Alcohol use:* May cause additive CNS effects. Don't use together. ∎

EFFECTS ON LAB TEST RESULTS
- May increase LFT values.
- May decrease neutrophil count.

CONTRAINDICATIONS & CAUTIONS
Boxed Warning Opioids should only be prescribed with benzodiazepines or other CNS depressants to patients for whom alternative treatment options are inadequate. Limit doses and durations to the minimum required. ∎
Boxed Warning Benzodiazepine use exposes patients to risks of abuse, misuse, and addiction, which can lead to overdose or death. Assess each patient's risk of abuse, misuse, and addiction before prescribing and periodically during therapy. ∎
Boxed Warning Abrupt discontinuation or rapid dosage reduction of benzodiazepines after continued use may precipitate acute withdrawal reactions, which can be life-threatening. To reduce risk of withdrawal reactions, gradually taper drug to discontinue or reduce dosage. ∎
- Contraindicated in patients hypersensitive to drug, patients with acute angle-closure glaucoma, and children younger than age 6 months (oral form).
- Diazepam (oral form) is contraindicated in patients with myasthenia gravis, severe respiratory insufficiency, Child-Pugh class C liver insufficiency, or sleep apnea syndrome.
- Use cautiously in patients experiencing shock, coma, or acute alcohol intoxication (parenteral form).
- Use cautiously in older adults; patients who are debilitated; patients at risk for falls; and patients with liver or kidney impairment, depression, history of substance abuse, impaired gag reflex, or chronic open-angle glaucoma (who are receiving appropriate therapy).
- Some injectable forms may contain propylene glycol; large amounts are potentially toxic and have been associated with hyperosmolality, lactic acidosis, seizures, and respiratory depression.
- Safety and effectiveness and approval for use in children vary by formulation. Use only for ages indicated.
Dialyzable drug: No.

Reactions in bold italics are *life-threatening*.

⚠ Overdose S&S: Somnolence, confusion, coma, diminished reflexes.

PREGNANCY-LACTATION-REPRODUCTION

• Drug crosses the placenta. Use during pregnancy isn't recommended, especially during first and third trimesters. If drug is needed during pregnancy, use only if potential benefit justifies fetal risk.

• Neonatal flaccidity, respiratory and feeding difficulties, hypothermia, and withdrawal symptoms have been reported in infants born to patients who received benzodiazepines late in pregnancy.

• Drug appears in human milk. Don't use during breastfeeding. Monitor infant exposed to drug for sedation, poor feeding, and poor weight gain.

• Enroll patient in North American Antiepileptic Drug Pregnancy Registry (1-888-233-2334 or https://www.aedpregnancyregistry.org/).

NURSING CONSIDERATIONS

• Periodically monitor LFT values, CBC, and kidney function in patient receiving repeated or prolonged therapy.

• Monitor HR, BP, and mental status changes. Patient is at increased risk for falls.

• **Look alike–sound alike:** Don't confuse diazepam with diazoxide or Ditropan. Don't confuse Valium with Valcyte.

PATIENT TEACHING

Boxed Warning Caution patient or caregiver of a patient taking an opioid with a benzodiazepine, CNS depressant, or alcohol to seek immediate medical attention for dizziness, light-headedness, extreme sleepiness, slowed or difficult breathing, or unresponsiveness. ■

Boxed Warning Caution patient that benzodiazepines, even at recommended doses, increase risk of abuse, misuse, and addiction, which can lead to overdose and death, especially when used with other drugs (opioid analgesics), alcohol, or illicit substances. ■

⊕ Alert: Teach about signs and symptoms of benzodiazepine abuse, misuse, and addiction (abdominal pain, amnesia, anorexia, anxiety, aggression, ataxia, blurred vision, confusion, depression, disinhibition, disorientation, dizziness, euphoria, impaired concentration and memory, indigestion, irritability, muscle pain, slurred speech, tremors, vertigo, delirium, paranoia, suicidality, seizures, difficulty

breathing, coma); instruct patient to seek emergency help if any occur.

• Teach about proper drug administration, handling, and disposal.

• Caution patient not to take drug at a higher dose, more frequently, or for longer than prescribed.

Boxed Warning Tell patient that continued use of drug may lead to physical dependence and that abrupt discontinuation or rapid dosage reduction may precipitate acute withdrawal reactions (unusual movements, responses, or expressions; seizures; sudden and severe mental or nervous system changes; depression; seeing or hearing things that others don't; homicidal thoughts; extreme increase in activity or talking; losing touch with reality; suicidality), which can be life-threatening. Instruct patient that discontinuation or dosage reduction may require a slow taper. ■

• Inform patient of possibility of development of protracted withdrawal syndrome (anxiety; trouble remembering, learning or concentrating; depression; problems sleeping; feeling of insects crawling under skin; weakness, shaking, muscle twitching; burning or prickling feeling in hands, arms, legs, or feet; ringing in ears), with symptoms lasting weeks to more than 12 months.

• Warn patient to report all adverse reactions.

• Caution patient to avoid activities that require alertness and good coordination until effects of drug are known.

• Tell patient to avoid alcohol while taking drug.

• Instruct caregivers not to administer a second dose if concerned about patient's breathing.

• Advise patient to avoid use during pregnancy due to fetal risk; instruct patient to notify prescriber of pregnancy or intention to become pregnant.

---

diclofenac potassium
dye-KLOE-fen-ak

Cambia, Voltaren Rapide✚, Zipsor

diclofenac sodium (oral)
Voltaren

Therapeutic class: NSAIDs
Pharmacologic class: NSAIDs

AVAILABLE FORMS
diclofenac potassium
Capsules: 25 mg*
Powder for solution: 50 mg/packet
Tablets: 25 mg, 50 mg
diclofenac sodium (oral)
Tablets (delayed-release) [ONC]: 25 mg, 50 mg, 75 mg
Tablets (extended-release) [ONC]: 100 mg

INDICATIONS & DOSAGES
Adjust-a-dose (for all indications): Patients with liver impairment may require lower initial dosages. Initiate treatment with diclofenac potassium capsules at the lowest dosage; if efficacy isn't achieved with the lowest dosage, discontinue drug.

➤ **Ankylosing spondylitis**
Adults: 25 mg delayed-release diclofenac sodium PO q.i.d.; may add another 25-mg dose at bedtime if needed.

➤ **Osteoarthritis**
Adults: 50 mg diclofenac potassium tablet or delayed-release diclofenac sodium PO b.i.d. or t.i.d., or 75 mg delayed-release diclofenac sodium PO b.i.d.; or 100 mg extended-release diclofenac sodium PO daily.

➤ **RA**
Adults: 50 mg diclofenac potassium tablet or delayed-release diclofenac sodium PO t.i.d. or q.i.d.; or 75 mg delayed-release diclofenac sodium PO b.i.d.; or 100 mg extended-release diclofenac sodium PO daily or b.i.d.

➤ **Analgesia**
Adults: 50 mg diclofenac potassium tablet PO t.i.d. For some patients, first dose on first day may be 100 mg, followed by 50 mg for second and third doses; maximum dose for first day is 200 mg. Don't exceed 150 mg daily after the first day. Or, 25 mg Zipsor capsule PO q.i.d.
Children ages 12 and older (Zipsor): 25 mg PO q.i.d.

➤ **Primary dysmenorrhea**
Adults: 50 mg diclofenac potassium tablet PO t.i.d. For some patients, first dose on first day may be 100 mg, followed by 50 mg for second and third doses; maximum dose for first day is 200 mg. Don't exceed 150 mg daily after first day.

➤ **Migraine**
Adults: 50 mg solution (1 packet) PO as a single dose.

ADMINISTRATION
PO
- Give drug (except powder) with milk, meals, or antacids.
- Don't crush or break delayed- or extended-release tablets.
- Mix powder in 30 to 60 mL water only. Use no other liquid.
- Mix solution well and have patient drink immediately.
- Powder may be less effective if taken with food.

⊕ **Alert:** Different formulations of oral diclofenac are not bioequivalent even if the milligram strength is the same.

ACTION
Reversibly inhibits cyclooxygenase 1 and 2 enzymes, which decreases proinflammatory processes. Has analgesic, anti-inflammatory, and antipyretic properties.

Route	Onset	Peak	Duration
PO (delayed-release)	30 min	2–3 hr	8 hr
PO (extended-release)	Unknown	5–6 hr	Unknown
PO	10 min	1 hr	8 hr

Half-life: 1 to 2.3 hours.

ADVERSE REACTIONS
CNS: dizziness, drowsiness, headache. **CV:** edema, fluid retention, HF, HTN, syncope, tachycardia. **EENT:** tinnitus, sinusitis, nasopharyngitis. **GI:** abdominal pain, *bleeding or perforation,* constipation, diarrhea, flatulence, heartburn, nausea, peptic ulceration, vomiting, dyspepsia. **GU:** UTI, increased creatinine level, kidney function abnormality. **Hepatic:** increased transaminase levels. **Hematologic:** anemia, increased bleeding time. **Musculoskeletal:** osteoarthritis, arthralgia, back or limb pain. **Respiratory:** URI, cough, bronchitis. **Skin:** bruising, pruritus, rash, diaphoresis. **Other:** falls, flulike symptoms, hypersensitivity reactions.

INTERACTIONS
Drug-drug. *ACE inhibitors, ARBs:* May enhance adverse or toxic effect of NSAIDs and result in a significant decrease in kidney function. May diminish antihypertensive effect of ACE inhibitors and ARBs. Monitor therapy.

Reactions in bold italics are *life-threatening*.

Anticoagulants, antiplatelet agents, SSNRIs, SSRIs, warfarin: May cause bleeding. Monitor patient closely.

Aspirin: May decrease effectiveness of diclofenac and increase GI toxicity. Avoid use together.

Beta blockers: May decrease antihypertensive effects. Monitor patient closely.

Cyclosporine, digoxin, lithium, methotrexate: May reduce kidney clearance of these drugs and increase risk of toxicity. Monitor patient closely.

CYP2C9 inducers (rifampin): May decrease diclofenac effect. Monitor therapy; adjust dosage as needed.

CYP2C9 inhibitors (voriconazole): May increase diclofenac level and risk of toxicity. Monitor therapy; adjust dosage as needed.

Diuretics: May decrease effectiveness of diuretics and risk of kidney toxicity. Avoid use together.

NSAIDs, salicylates: May increase risk of GI toxicity. Avoid use together.

Pemetrexed: May increase risk of pemetrexed-associated myelosuppression and kidney and GI toxicity. Monitor patient closely.

Potassium-sparing diuretics: May enhance retention and increase level of potassium. Monitor potassium level.

Drug-herb. *Alfalfa, anise, bilberry, willow:* May cause bleeding. Don't use together.

Drug-lifestyle. *Sun exposure:* May cause photosensitivity reactions. Advise patient to avoid excessive sunlight exposure.

EFFECTS ON LAB TEST RESULTS

• May increase ALT, AST, bilirubin, BUN, potassium, glucose, and creatinine levels.
• May decrease Hb level and platelet, leukocyte, and eosinophil counts.

CONTRAINDICATIONS & CAUTIONS

Boxed Warning Contraindicated for the treatment of pain after CABG surgery. ∎
• Contraindicated in patients hypersensitive to drug and in those with hepatic porphyria or history of asthma, urticaria, or other allergic reactions after taking aspirin or other NSAIDs. Zipsor capsules are contraindicated in patients hypersensitive to bovine protein.
Boxed Warning NSAID use increases risk of serious CV thrombotic events, including MI and stroke, which can be fatal. This risk may occur early in treatment and increase

with duration of use. Risk appears greater at higher doses and in patients with CV disease or risk factors for CV disease. Use lowest effective dose for shortest duration possible. ∎
⚠ *Alert:* NSAIDs increase the risk of HF. Don't use in patients with severe HF unless the benefits are expected to outweigh risks.
• Use cautiously in patients with history of peptic ulcer disease, liver dysfunction, cardiac disease, HTN, fluid retention, or impaired kidney function.
Dialyzable drug: Unknown.
⚠ *Overdose S&S:* Drowsiness, confusion, GI bleeding, hypotonia, loss of consciousness, vomiting, aspiration, pneumonitis, increased ICP.

PREGNANCY-LACTATION-REPRODUCTION

⚠ *Alert:* Drug can cause fetal harm when administered at 30 weeks' gestation or later. Use during pregnancy before 30 weeks' gestation only if potential benefit justifies fetal risk.
⚠ *Alert:* Use of NSAIDs at 20 weeks or later in pregnancy may cause fetal kidney dysfunction, leading to oligohydramnios and potential neonatal kidney impairment. Use at 30 weeks or later in pregnancy may increase risk of premature closure of the ductus arteriosus. Avoid use starting at 20 weeks' gestation. If potential benefit justifies fetal risk, use lowest effective dose for shortest duration. Consider ultrasound monitoring of amniotic fluid if NSAID use is longer than 48 hours. Use of low-dose aspirin (81 mg) for certain pregnancy-related conditions under direction of prescriber is acceptable.
• Drug may appear in human milk. Use cautiously during breastfeeding.
• May increase risk of reversible infertility in females.

NURSING CONSIDERATIONS

⚠ *Alert:* Monitor patient and immediately evaluate signs and symptoms of heart attack (chest pain, shortness of breath, trouble breathing) or stroke (weakness in one part or side of the body, slurred speech).
• Because NSAIDs impair synthesis of kidney prostaglandins, they can decrease kidney blood flow and lead to reversible kidney impairment, especially in patients with CKD, HF, or liver dysfunction; in older adults; and in patients taking diuretics. Monitor these patients closely.

• LFT values may increase during therapy. Periodically monitor transaminase levels in patient undergoing long-term therapy. Make first transaminase measurement no later than 8 weeks after therapy begins.

• Discontinue drug immediately if liver impairment occurs, including persistent or worsening abnormal LFT values, clinical signs or symptoms consistent with liver disease, or systemic manifestations of liver disease.

Boxed Warning NSAIDs increase risk of serious GI adverse events, including bleeding, ulceration, and perforation of stomach or intestines, which can occur at any time during use without warning and be fatal. Older adults are at greater risk. ■

• Because of their antipyretic and anti-inflammatory actions, NSAIDs may mask the signs and symptoms of infection.

• Consider periodic CBC and chemistry profile monitoring with long-term NSAID treatment because serious GI bleeding, liver toxicity, and kidney injury can occur without warning.

• Monitor BP and fluid balance.

• Monitor for photosensitivity as well as SCAR (exfoliative dermatitis, SJS, TEN), which can be fatal. Discontinue at first sign of rash or hypersensitivity.

• Closely monitor older adult patient due to increased risk of adverse reactions.

• *Look alike–sound alike:* Don't confuse diclofenac with Diflucan.

PATIENT TEACHING

• Teach about proper drug administration and handling.

☉ Alert: Advise patient to immediately seek medical attention if chest pain, shortness of breath or trouble breathing, weakness in one part or side of the body, or slurred speech occurs.

☉ Alert: Warn patient who is pregnant not to take NSAIDs at 20 weeks' gestation or later unless instructed to do so by prescriber due to potential fetal risk. Advise patient to discuss taking OTC medications with pharmacist or health care provider during pregnancy.

• Advise patient not to take drug with other diclofenac-containing products, other NSAIDs, or salicylates (salsalate, diflunisal).

• Teach patient signs and symptoms of GI bleeding (blood in vomit, urine, or stool; coffee-ground vomit; black, tarry stools).

Instruct patient to notify prescriber immediately if any occur.

• Teach patient signs and symptoms of damage to the liver (nausea, fatigue, lethargy, itching, yellowed skin or eyes, right upper quadrant tenderness, flulike symptoms). Tell patient to immediately contact prescriber if any occur.

• Advise patient to avoid drinking alcohol and taking aspirin during drug therapy.

• Tell patient to wear sunscreen or protective clothing because drug may cause sensitivity to sunlight.

• Warn patient to avoid hazardous activities that require alertness until CNS effects of drug are known.

• Advise patient that use of OTC NSAIDs (which may be present in OTC medications for treatment of colds, fever, or insomnia) and diclofenac may increase risk of GI toxicity.

diclofenac epolamine
dye-KLOE-fen-ak

Flector, Licart

diclofenac sodium (topical)
Pennsaid, Voltaren ◇

Therapeutic class: NSAIDs
Pharmacologic class: NSAIDs

AVAILABLE FORMS
Topical gel: 1% ◇, 3%
Topical solution: 1.5%, 2%
Transdermal patch: 1.3%

INDICATIONS & DOSAGES
➤ **Actinic keratosis (3% gel only)**
Adults: Apply gel to lesion b.i.d. for 60 to 90 days.

➤ **Osteoarthritis**
Adults: Apply 4 g of 1% gel to affected foot, knee, or ankle q.i.d.; maximum dose of 16 g to any single joint of lower extremities. Or apply 2 g of 1% gel to affected hand, elbow, or wrist q.i.d.; maximum dose of 8 g to any single joint of upper extremities. Total dose shouldn't exceed 32 g daily for all affected joints.

➤ **Acute pain due to minor strains, sprains, and contusions**
Adults and children ages 6 and older (Flector): Apply 1 patch to most-painful area b.i.d.

Reactions in bold italics are *life-threatening*.

Adults (Licart): Apply 1 topical system to most-painful area once daily.

➤ **Osteoarthritis of the knee**

Adults: Count 10 drops at a time of 1.5% topical solution onto hand or directly onto knee. Apply to each side, front and back, spreading evenly, using a total of 40 drops q.i.d. Or, 2 pump actuations (40 mg) of 2% topical solution on each painful knee b.i.d. Dispense solution directly onto knee or first into hand and then onto knee. Spread evenly around front, back, and sides of knee.

ADMINISTRATION
Topical
- Apply to clean, dry skin.
- Don't apply to open wounds or broken skin.
- Avoid contact with eyes.
- Use enough gel to cover the lesion; for example, use 0.5 g of gel on a 5-cm × 5-cm lesion.
- Don't apply Flector or Licart patch to nonintact or damaged skin (exudative dermatitis, eczema, infected lesions, burns, wounds).
- Patient shouldn't wear patch while bathing or showering.
- If patch begins to peel off, the edges may be taped down.
- Measure gel using supplied dosing cards in package.
- Wash hands after applying. If treatment area is the hands, patient should wait at least 1 hour before washing hands.
- Don't cover area with clothing for at least 10 minutes after applying gel.
- Wait at least 1 hour before showering or bathing after applying gel and 30 minutes after applying solution.
- Don't cover treated area with an occlusive dressing or apply heat.
- Pump for 2% topical solution must be primed before first use. Depress pump four times while holding bottle upright; discard solution obtained during priming.

ACTION
Reversibly inhibits cyclooxygenase 1 and 2 enzymes, which decreases proinflammatory processes. Has analgesic, anti-inflammatory, and antipyretic properties.

Route	Onset	Peak	Duration
Topical	Unknown	4–14 hr	Unknown
Transdermal	Unknown	4–20 hr	Unknown

Half-life: 1 to 3 hours; 12 hours for patch.

ADVERSE REACTIONS
CNS: paresthesia, headache, hyperesthesia, pain, asthenia, migraine, hypokinesia, dysgeusia, somnolence. **CV:** chest pain, HTN. **EENT:** conjunctivitis, eye pain, sinusitis, pharyngitis, rhinitis. **GI:** diarrhea, dyspepsia, abdominal pain, flatulence, nausea. **GU:** hematuria, kidney impairment. **Hepatic:** increased transaminase levels. **Metabolic:** hypercholesterolemia, hyperglycemia, increased CK level. **Musculoskeletal:** arthralgia, osteoarthritis, back pain, myalgia, neck pain. **Respiratory:** *asthma,* dyspnea, pneumonia. **Skin:** application-site reaction, contact dermatitis, dry skin, localized pain, pruritus, rash, vesicles, erythema, localized edema, acne, alopecia, photosensitivity reactions, skin ulcer, skin carcinoma. **Other:** *anaphylaxis,* flulike syndrome, infection, hypersensitivity reaction.

INTERACTIONS
Drug-drug. *ACE inhibitors, ARBs:* May enhance adverse or toxic effect of NSAIDs and result in a significant decrease in kidney function. May diminish antihypertensive effect of ACE inhibitors and ARBs. Monitor therapy.

Anticoagulants, antiplatelet agents, SSNRIs, SSRIs, warfarin: May cause bleeding. Monitor patient closely.

Aspirin: May decrease effectiveness of diclofenac and increase GI toxicity. Avoid use together.

Beta blockers: May decrease antihypertensive effects. Monitor patient closely.

Cyclosporine, digoxin, lithium, methotrexate: May reduce kidney clearance of these drugs and increase risk of toxicity. Monitor patient closely.

Diuretics: May decrease effectiveness of diuretics. Avoid use together.

Insulin, oral antidiabetics: May alter requirements for antidiabetics. Monitor patient closely.

Oral NSAIDs: May increase diclofenac effects. Minimize use together.

Pemetrexed: May increase risk of pemetrexed-associated myelosuppression and kidney and GI toxicity. Avoid topical NSAID use 2 days before, day of, and 2 days after pemetrexed.

Potassium-sparing diuretics: May enhance retention and increase potassium level. Monitor potassium level.

Herb-drug. *Alfalfa, anise, bilberry, willow:* May cause bleeding. Don't use together.
Drug-lifestyle. *Sun exposure:* May increase risk of photosensitivity reactions. Advise patient to avoid excessive sun exposure.

EFFECTS ON LAB TEST RESULTS
• May increase ALT, AST, cholesterol, creatinine, glucose, and transaminase levels.

CONTRAINDICATIONS & CAUTIONS
• Contraindicated in patients hypersensitive to diclofenac. Diclofenac 3% sodium gel is also contraindicated in patients with a known hypersensitivity to benzyl alcohol, polyethylene glycol monomethyl ether 350, or hyaluronate sodium.
• Contraindicated in patients with a history of asthma, urticaria, or other allergic reactions after taking aspirin or other NSAIDs.
Boxed Warning Contraindicated for perioperative pain for CABG surgery. ■
Boxed Warning NSAIDs can increase risk of MI or stroke in patients with or without heart disease or risk factors for heart disease. Risk of MI or stroke can occur as early as the first weeks of NSAID use and can be fatal. ■
• Risk of MI or stroke appears greater at higher doses. Use lowest effective dose for shortest duration possible.
☉ Alert: NSAIDs increase risk of HF. Don't use in patients with severe HF unless benefits are expected to outweigh risks.
• Use cautiously in patients with aspirin triad; these patients are usually asthmatics who develop rhinitis, with or without nasal polyps, after taking aspirin or other NSAIDs.
• Use cautiously in patients with active GI bleeding or ulceration and in those with CKD or Child-Pugh class C liver impairment.
Dialyzable drug: Unknown.

PREGNANCY-LACTATION-REPRODUCTION
☉ Alert: Drug can cause fetal harm when administered at 30 weeks' gestation or later. Use during pregnancy before 30 weeks' gestation only if potential benefit justifies fetal risk.
☉ Alert: Use of NSAIDs at 20 weeks or later in pregnancy may cause fetal kidney dysfunction, leading to oligohydramnios and potential neonatal kidney impairment. Use at 30 weeks or later in pregnancy may increase risk of premature closure of the ductus arteriosus. Avoid use starting at 20 weeks' gestation. If potential benefit justifies fetal risk, use lowest effective dose for shortest duration. Consider ultrasound monitoring of amniotic fluid if NSAID use is longer than 48 hours. Use of low-dose aspirin (81 mg) for certain pregnancy-related conditions under direction of prescriber is acceptable.
• Drug may appear in human milk. Use cautiously during breastfeeding.
• Drug may increase risk of reversible infertility in females.

NURSING CONSIDERATIONS
Boxed Warning NSAIDs may increase the risk of serious CV thrombotic events. Risk may increase with duration of use. Patients with CV disease or risk factors for CV disease may be at greater risk. ■
Boxed Warning NSAIDs increase the risk of serious GI adverse reactions, including bleeding, ulceration, and perforation of the stomach or intestines, which can be fatal. These reactions can occur at any time and without warning. Older adults and patients with a history of peptic ulcer disease or GI bleeding are at greater risk. ■
☉ Alert: Monitor patient and immediately evaluate signs and symptoms of MI (chest pain, shortness of breath, trouble breathing) or stroke (weakness in one part or side of the body, slurred speech).
• Avoid use in patient with recent MI unless benefits are expected to outweigh risk of recurrent CV thrombotic events. If used in patient with recent MI, watch for signs and symptoms of cardiac ischemia.
• Avoid use in patient with severe HF unless benefits are expected to outweigh risk of worsening HF. If used in patient with severe HF, watch for signs and symptoms of worsening HF.
• Evaluate patient with signs or symptoms of liver dysfunction or with abnormal LFT results for development of more severe liver reaction while taking drug.
• If clinical signs or symptoms of liver disease develop, discontinue drug.
• Safety and effectiveness of sunscreens, cosmetics, or other topical medications used with drug are unknown.
• Complete healing or optimal therapeutic effect may not be seen until 30 days after therapy is complete.
• Reevaluate treatment if signs or symptoms worsen or don't respond to therapy.

Reactions in bold italics are ***life-threatening***.

• Monitor for SCAR (exfoliative dermatitis, SJS, TEN), which can be fatal. Discontinue use at first sign of rash or hypersensitivity.

PATIENT TEACHING
• Inform patient about risk of skin reactions (rash, itchiness, pain, irritation) at the application site. Urge patient to seek medical attention if adverse reactions occur.

🕒 *Alert:* Advise patient to immediately seek medical attention if chest pain, shortness of breath or trouble breathing, weakness in one part or side of the body, or slurred speech occurs.

• Teach about proper drug administration and handling.

• Encourage patient to minimize sun exposure during therapy. Explain that sunscreen may be helpful but that the safety of using sunscreen with drug is unknown.

• Advise patient needing an MRI to inform the facility about wearing a transdermal patch.

• Tell patient using diclofenac 3% gel that complete healing or optimal therapeutic effect may not occur for up to 30 days after stopping therapy.

• Instruct patient not to apply other topical drugs or cosmetics to affected area while using drug, unless directed.

• Instruct patients to avoid contact with the eyes and mucosa. If eye contact occurs, immediately wash out the eye with water or saline and consult a practitioner if irritation persists for more than an hour.

• Tell patient to notify prescriber if pregnant or breastfeeding.

dicyclomine hydrochloride
dye-SYE-kloe-meen

Bentyl

Therapeutic class: Antispasmodics
Pharmacologic class: Anticholinergics–antimuscarinics

AVAILABLE FORMS
Capsules: 10 mg
Injection: 10 mg/mL
Solution: 10 mg/5 mL
Tablets: 10 mg ✤, 20 mg

INDICATIONS & DOSAGES
➤ **IBS, other functional GI disorders**
Adults: Initially, 20 mg PO q.i.d.; may increase to 40 mg PO q.i.d. after 1 week unless adverse effects limit dosage escalation. If efficacy isn't achieved within 2 weeks or adverse effects require doses below 80 mg per day, discontinue drug.

Or, 10 to 20 mg IM q.i.d. Don't use IM form for longer than 1 to 2 days.

ADMINISTRATION
PO
• Give drug without regard to food.
• Protect from excessive heat. Store in light-resistant container.
IM
• Don't give subcut or IV. Thrombosis and injection-site reaction may occur if drug is inadvertently injected IV.
• Visually inspect for particulate matter and discoloration before giving.

ACTION
Inhibits action of acetylcholine on postganglionic, parasympathetic muscarinic receptors, decreasing GI motility. Drug possesses local anesthetic properties that may be partly responsible for spasmolysis.

Route	Onset	Peak	Duration
PO, IM	Unknown	1–1.5 hr	Unknown

Half-life: Initially, about 1.8 hours.

ADVERSE REACTIONS
CNS: asthenia, dizziness, somnolence, nervousness. **EENT:** blurred vision, dry mouth. **GI:** nausea.

INTERACTIONS
Drug-drug. *Amantadine, antihistamines, antiparkinsonian drugs, disopyramide, glutethimide, meperidine, phenothiazines, procainamide, quinidine, TCAs:* May have additive adverse anticholinergic effects. Avoid use together.
Antacids: May interfere with dicyclomine absorption. Give dicyclomine at least 1 hour before antacid.
Antiglaucoma drugs: May decrease therapeutic effect of these drugs. Use together is contraindicated.
GI motility agents (metoclopramide): May decrease effectiveness of motility agents. Monitor therapy.

EFFECTS ON LAB TEST RESULTS
None reported.

CONTRAINDICATIONS & CAUTIONS
• Contraindicated in patients hypersensitive to anticholinergics, in children younger than age 6 months, and in those with obstructive uropathy, obstructive disease of the GI tract, reflux esophagitis, severe ulcerative colitis, salmonella dysentery, myasthenia gravis, unstable CV status in acute hemorrhage, or glaucoma.
• Use cautiously in patients with tachycardia secondary to cardiac insufficiency or thyrotoxicosis.
• Don't use in patients with myasthenia gravis except to reduce adverse muscarinic effects of an anticholinesterase.
• Use cautiously in patients with autonomic neuropathy, hyperthyroidism, CAD, arrhythmias, HF, HTN, hiatal hernia, liver or kidney disease, prostatic hyperplasia, known or suspected GI infection, and ulcerative colitis.
• Use cautiously in patients in hot or humid environments; drug can cause heatstroke.
• May affect GI absorption of various drugs (such as slowly dissolving dosage forms of digoxin) by affecting GI motility, which may increase serum level.
• Drug may increase risk of intestinal dilation and perforation when given to patients with *Salmonella* dysentery.
• **Alert:** Use cautiously in patient sensitive to anticholinergic drugs, especially older adult or patient with mental illness, because of the risk of psychosis and delirium. When present, these signs and symptoms usually resolve within 12 to 24 hours after discontinuation of drug.
• Safety and effectiveness in children haven't been established.
Dialyzable drug: Unknown.
Overdose S&S: Headache; nausea; vomiting; blurred vision; dilated pupils; hot, dry skin; dry mouth; dysphagia; CNS stimulation; muscle weakness; paralysis.

PREGNANCY-LACTATION-REPRODUCTION
• Use during pregnancy only if clearly needed.
• Drug appears in human milk. Contraindicated during breastfeeding.

NURSING CONSIDERATIONS
• Adjust dosage based on patient's needs and response. Safety and effectiveness for longer than 2 weeks haven't been established.

• IM injection is about twice as bioavailable as oral form.
• Dicyclomine may have atropine-like adverse reactions.
• **Alert:** Overdose may cause curare-like effects, such as respiratory paralysis. Keep emergency equipment available.
• Carefully monitor patient's vital signs and urine output.
• **Look alike–sound alike:** Don't confuse dicyclomine with dyclonine or doxycycline. Don't confuse Bentyl with Benadryl.

PATIENT TEACHING
• Tell patient when to take drug, and stress importance of doing so on time and at evenly spaced intervals.
• Advise patient to report all adverse reactions.
• Instruct patient to contact a practitioner, poison control center (1-800-222-1222), or emergency room in case of overdose.
• Advise patient to avoid driving and other hazardous activities if drowsiness, dizziness, or blurred vision occurs; to drink plenty of fluids to help prevent constipation; and to report hypersensitivity reactions, including rash or other skin eruption.
• Warn patient that heat prostration may occur during therapy when environmental temperatures are high. If signs and symptoms (fever, decreased sweating) occur, instruct patient to stop drug and contact prescriber.
• Caution patient not to breastfeed during therapy.

SAFETY ALERT!

digoxin
di-JOX-in

Lanoxin*

Therapeutic class: Inotropes
Pharmacologic class: Cardiac glycosides

AVAILABLE FORMS
Injection: 0.1 mg/mL (pediatric), 0.25 mg/mL
Oral elixir: 0.05 mg/mL
Tablets: 0.0625 mg, 0.125 mg, 0.25 mg

INDICATIONS & DOSAGES
• **Alert:** Factors to consider when selecting a digoxin dosing regimen include body weight, age, kidney function, concomitant

D

drugs, and disease. Toxic levels of digoxin are only slightly higher than therapeutic levels. In newborns, kidney clearance of digoxin is diminished and suitable dosage adjustments must be observed, especially in preterm infants. Beyond the immediate newborn period, children generally require proportionally larger doses than adults on the basis of body weight or surface area.

Adjust-a-dose (for all indications): Refer to manufacturer's information for recommended dosage adjustments based on kidney function and weight. May adjust dose every 2 weeks based on clinical response, serum drug levels, and toxicity.

➤ **HF, rapid digitalization**

🕭 *Alert:* Initially, give half the total loading dose followed by one-quarter of the loading dose every 6 to 8 hours twice. Carefully assess clinical response and toxicity before each dose. Follow loading dose with daily or b.i.d. maintenance dosing.

Adults and children older than age 10: Total loading dose is 10 to 15 mcg/kg tablets PO or 8 to 12 mcg/kg IV in divided doses.

Children older than age 10: Total loading dose is 10 to 15 mcg/kg solution PO in divided doses.

Children ages 5 to 10: Total loading dose is 20 to 45 mcg/kg tablets PO or 20 to 35 mcg/kg solution PO or 15 to 30 mcg/kg IV in divided doses.

Children ages 2 to 5: Total loading dose is 30 to 45 mcg/kg solution PO or 25 to 35 mcg/kg IV given in divided doses.

Infants ages 1 to 24 months: Total loading dose is 35 to 60 mcg/kg solution PO or 30 to 50 mcg/kg IV given in divided doses.

Full-term infants: Total loading dose is 25 to 35 mcg/kg solution PO or 20 to 30 mcg/kg IV in divided doses.

Preterm infants: Loading dose is 20 to 30 mcg/kg solution PO or 15 to 25 mcg/kg IV in divided doses.

Adjust-a-dose: If patient's clinical response necessitates a change from the calculated loading dose of digoxin, base the calculation of the maintenance dose on the amount actually given as the loading dose.

➤ **HF maintenance or gradual digitalization**

Adults and children older than age 10: Give starting maintenance dose of 3.4 to 5.1 mcg/kg tablets PO or 3 to 4.5 mcg/kg solution PO or 2.4 to 3.6 mcg/kg IV once daily.

Children ages 5 to 10: Give starting maintenance dose of 3.2 to 6.4 mcg/kg/dose tablets PO or 2.8 to 5.6 mcg/kg/dose solution PO or 2.3 to 4.5 mcg/kg/dose IV b.i.d.

Children ages 2 to 5: 4.7 to 6.6 mcg/kg/dose solution PO or 3.8 to 5.3 mcg/kg/dose IV b.i.d.

Infants ages 1 to 24 months: 5.6 to 9.4 mcg/kg/dose solution PO or 4.5 to 7.5 mcg/kg/dose IV b.i.d.

Full-term infants: 3.8 to 5.6 mcg/kg/dose solution PO or 3 to 4.5 mcg/kg/dose IV b.i.d.

Preterm infants: 2.3 to 3.9 mcg/kg/dose solution PO or 1.9 to 3.1 mcg/kg/dose IV b.i.d.

➤ **Atrial fibrillation (chronic)**

Adults: PO or IV: If a loading dose is used, give half the total loading dose followed by one-quarter of the loading dose every 6 to 8 hours twice. Carefully assess clinical response and toxicity before each dose. Total loading dose is 10 to 15 mcg/kg PO (tablets, solution) or 8 to 12 mcg/kg IV in divided doses. Recommended starting maintenance dosage for patients with normal kidney function is 3.4 to 5.1 mcg/kg (tablets) PO once daily or 3 to 4.5 mcg/kg (elixir) PO once daily or 2.4 to 3.6 mcg/kg IV once daily.

Or, for more gradual digitalization in patients with normal kidney function, begin with the starting maintenance dosage of 3.4 to 5.1 mcg/kg (tablets) PO once daily or 3 to 4.5 mcg/kg (oral elixir) PO once daily or 2.4 to 3.6 mcg/kg IV. May increase every 2 weeks based on clinical response, serum drug level, and toxicity.

ADMINISTRATION

● Before giving loading dose, obtain baseline data (HR and rhythm, BP, and electrolyte levels) and ask patient about use of cardiac glycosides within the previous 2 to 3 weeks.

● Before giving drug, take apical-radial pulse for 1 minute. Record and notify prescriber of significant changes (sudden increase or decrease in pulse rate, pulse deficit, irregular beats and, particularly, regularization of a previously irregular rhythm). If these occur, check BP and obtain a 12-lead ECG.

PO

● Use calibrated measuring device to give oral solution.

● Bioavailability of PO formulation is 60% to 80% of IV formulation, which should be

taken into consideration when switching between forms.
- Store tablets and solution at room temperature.

IM
- Use of IM route isn't recommended because injection can cause severe pain.
- If no other route is available, inject IV dosage deep into muscle, followed by massage.
- Don't inject more than 500 mcg for adults or 200 mcg for children into a single site.

IV
▼ May administer undiluted or diluted with a fourfold or greater volume of D₅W, NSS, or sterile water for injection; use immediately. Using less than a fourfold volume of diluent could lead to precipitation of digoxin.
▼ Infuse drug slowly over at least 5 minutes or longer.
▼ Protect solution from light.
▼ **Incompatibilities:** Other IV drugs.

ACTION
Inhibits sodium-potassium-activated adenosine triphosphatase, promoting movement of calcium from extracellular to intracellular cytoplasm and strengthening myocardial contraction. Also acts on CNS to enhance vagal tone, slowing conduction through the SA and AV nodes.

Route	Onset	Peak	Duration
PO	30–120 min	2–6 hr	3–4 days
IV	5–30 min	1–4 hr	3–4 days

Half-life: With normal kidney function: adults, 36 to 48 hours; children, 18 to 36 hours.

ADVERSE REACTIONS
CNS: apathy, confusion, weakness, mental disturbances (anxiety, hallucinations, depression, delirium), dizziness, headache. **CV:** *arrhythmias, heart block.* **EENT:** blurred vision, diplopia, light flashes, photophobia, yellow-green color disturbance, halos around visual images. **GI:** anorexia, nausea, diarrhea, vomiting. **Other:** gynecomastia (prolonged use).

INTERACTIONS
Drug-drug. *ACE inhibitors, ARBs, COX-2 inhibitors, NSAIDs, other drugs that affect kidney function:* May increase digoxin level. Monitor therapy.

Amiloride: May decrease digoxin effect and increase kidney clearance of digoxin. Monitor patient for altered digoxin effect.
Amiodarone, diltiazem, indomethacin, nifedipine, protease inhibitors, quinidine, verapamil: May increase digoxin level. Monitor patient for toxicity.
Amphotericin B, carbenicillin, corticosteroids, diuretics (chlorthalidone, loop diuretics, metolazone), ticarcillin: May cause hypokalemia and hypomagnesemia, predisposing patient to cardiac glycoside toxicity. Monitor electrolyte levels.
Antacids: May decrease absorption of oral digoxin. Separate doses as much as possible.
Antibiotics (azole antifungals, macrolides, telithromycin, tetracyclines), propafenone, ritonavir: May increase risk of cardiac glycoside toxicity. Monitor patient for toxicity.
Beta blockers, calcium channel blockers: May have additive effects on AV node conduction, causing advanced or complete heart block. Use cautiously.
Cholestyramine, colestipol, metoclopramide: May decrease absorption of oral digoxin. Monitor patient for decreased digoxin level and effect. Give digoxin 1.5 hours before or 2 hours after other drugs.
Dronedarone: May significantly increase digoxin level and risk of sudden death. Monitor patient closely or consider therapy modification.
Parenteral calcium, thiazides: May cause hypercalcemia and hypomagnesemia, predisposing patient to digoxin toxicity. Monitor calcium and magnesium levels.
P-gp inducers or inhibitors: May alter digoxin level and effect. Consult interactions resource for specific drug.
Sotalol: May increase proarrhythmic effect. Use together cautiously.
Sympathomimetics (dopamine, epinephrine, norepinephrine): May increase risk of arrhythmias. Use together cautiously.
Drug-herb. *Foxglove, fumitory, goldenseal, hawthorn:* May increase cardiac effects. Discourage use together.
Licorice, Siberian ginseng: May increase toxicity. Monitor patient closely.
St. John's wort: May decrease digoxin serum level. Monitor therapy.

EFFECTS ON LAB TEST RESULTS
- May prolong PR interval or depress ST segment on ECG.

Reactions in bold italics are *life-threatening*.

D

CONTRAINDICATIONS & CAUTIONS
• Contraindicated in patients hypersensitive to drug and those with ventricular fibrillation.
• Don't use in patients with Wolff-Parkinson-White syndrome unless the conduction accessory pathway has been pharmacologically or surgically disabled.
• Avoid use in patients with sinus node dysfunction or sinoatrial block unless patients has a functioning artificial pacemaker.
• Use with extreme caution in older adults and patients with sinus bradycardia, PVCs, kidney impairment, severe pulmonary disease, or hypothyroidism.
• Avoid use in patients with myocarditis or acute MI and those with HF with preserved left ventricular ejection fraction (restrictive cardiomyopathy, constrictive pericarditis, amyloid heart disease, acute cor pulmonal, and idiopathic hypertrophic subaortic stenosis).
• Loading doses to initiate digoxin therapy in patients with HF aren't recommended by the American College of Cardiology Foundation/American Heart Association for management of HF. For patients who are older than age 70, have impaired kidney function, or have a low lean body mass, initially use low doses (0.125 mg daily or every other day).
• Safety and effectiveness in control of ventricular rate in children with atrial fibrillation haven't been established.
Dialyzable drug: No.
⚠ *Overdose S&S:* Ventricular tachycardia, ventricular fibrillation, bradycardia, heart block, cardiac arrest, hyperkalemia.

PREGNANCY-LACTATION-REPRODUCTION
• Drug isn't known to cause fetal harm. Use during pregnancy only if clearly needed.
• Drug crosses the placenta. If given during pregnancy, monitor neonate for signs and symptoms of digoxin toxicity (vomiting, cardiac arrhythmias).
• Drug appears in human milk; however, an infant who is breastfed is exposed to an amount estimated to be far below the usual infant maintenance dose. Use cautiously during breastfeeding.

NURSING CONSIDERATIONS
• Drug-induced arrhythmias may increase the severity of HF and hypotension.
• In children, cardiac arrhythmias, including sinus bradycardia, are usually early signs of toxicity.

• Patients with hypothyroidism are extremely sensitive to cardiac glycosides and may need lower doses.
• Monitor patient for signs and symptoms of toxicity (anorexia, nausea, vomiting, visual changes, cardiac arrhythmias). Toxic effects on the heart may be life-threatening and require immediate attention. Patient with low body weight, advanced age, kidney impairment, or electrolyte disturbances is at increased risk.
• Monitor digoxin level. Therapeutic level ranges from 0.5 to 2 nanograms/mL. Obtain blood for digoxin level at least 6 to 8 hours after last oral dose, preferably just before next scheduled dose.
❸ *Alert:* Excessively slow pulse rate (60 beats/minute or less) may be a sign of digitalis toxicity. Withhold drug and notify prescriber.
• Carefully monitor potassium level. Take corrective action before hypokalemia occurs. Hyperkalemia may result from digoxin toxicity.
• Reduce dose or discontinue drug for 1 or 2 days before elective cardioversion. Adjust dosage after cardioversion.
• *Look alike–sound alike:* Don't confuse digoxin with doxepin. Don't confuse Lanoxin with levothyroxine, Levoxyl or Lasix.

PATIENT TEACHING
• Teach patient and a responsible family member about drug action, dosage regimen, pulse monitoring, reportable signs, and follow-up care.
• Tell patient to report pulse rate less than 60 beats/minute or more than 110 beats/minute as well as skipped beats or other rhythm changes.
• Instruct patient to promptly report all adverse reactions. Explain that nausea, vomiting, diarrhea, appetite loss, and visual disturbances may indicate toxicity.
• Caution caregivers that signs and symptoms of toxicity in infants and children include weight loss, failure to thrive, abdominal pain and behavior disturbances.
• Encourage patient to eat a consistent amount of potassium-rich foods.
• Tell patient not to substitute one brand for another without discussing with prescriber.
• Advise patient to avoid using herbal supplements and to consult prescriber before taking one.
• Inform patient that blood tests are necessary to ensure appropriateness of digoxin dose.

dilTIAZem hydrochloride

dil-TYE-a-zem

Cardizem, Cardizem CD, Cardizem LA, Cartia XT, Matzim LA, Taztia XT, Tiazac, Tiazac XC✦

Therapeutic class: Antihypertensives
Pharmacologic class: Calcium channel blockers

AVAILABLE FORMS

Capsules (extended-release) ⓄⓃⒸ: 60 mg, 90 mg, 120 mg, 180 mg, 240 mg, 300 mg, 360 mg, 420 mg
Injection: 5 mg/mL
Powder for injection: 100 mg
Tablets: 30 mg, 60 mg, 90 mg, 120 mg
Tablets (extended-release) ⓄⓃⒸ: 120 mg, 180 mg, 240 mg, 300 mg, 360 mg, 420 mg

INDICATIONS & DOSAGES

➤ **To manage Prinzmetal or variant angina or chronic stable angina pectoris**
Adults: 30 mg PO q.i.d. (immediate-release tablets) before meals and at bedtime. Increase dose gradually to maximum of 360 mg/day divided into three or four doses, as indicated. Or, 120- or 180-mg extended-release capsule or 180-mg extended-release tablet PO once daily. Adjust over a 7- to 14-day period as needed and tolerated up to a maximum dose of 360 mg/day extended-released tablets (Cardizem LA, Matzim LA), 480 mg/day extended-release capsules (Cardizem CD, Cartia XT), or 540 mg/day (Tiazac, Taztia XT).
➤ **HTN, alone or as combination therapy**
Adults: Initially 180 to 240 mg extended-release capsules PO once daily. Adjust dosage based on patient response to a maximum dose of 480 mg/day. Or, 120 to 240 mg extended-release capsules PO once daily. Adjust dosage based on patient response to a maximum dose of 540 mg/day (Tiazac, Taztia XT, Matzim LA). Or, 180 to 240 mg extended-release tablet PO once daily. Dosage can be adjusted approximately every 14 days to a maximum of 540 mg daily.
➤ **To control rapid ventricular rate in atrial fibrillation or atrial flutter; to rapidly convert paroxysmal supraventricular tachycardia (PSVT) to sinus rhythm**
Adults: 0.25 mg/kg IV bolus. If after 15 minutes rate control is insufficient, repeat with dose of 0.35 mg/kg IV bolus. If patient with atrial fibrillation or flutter responds after one to two bolus doses, begin continuous infusion of 5 mg/hour. May increase infusion rate in 5-mg/hour increments according to ventricular response up to maximum of 15 mg/hour. If patient with PSVT fails to respond, consider alternative therapy.

ADMINISTRATION

PO

• Have patient swallow extended-release tablets or capsules whole; don't crush.
• Tiazac and Taztia extended-release capsules can be opened and contents sprinkled onto a spoonful of applesauce. Applesauce must be eaten immediately and without chewing, followed by a glass of cool water.

IV

▼ For direct injection, no need to dilute 5-mg/mL injection. Give over 2 minutes.
▼ For continuous infusion, refer to manufacturer's instructions for dilution and administration. Compatible solutions include NSS, D_5W, or 5% dextrose and half-NSS.
▼ Continuous infusion rate ranges from 5 to 15 mg/hour.
▼ For direct injection or continuous infusion, give slowly while continuously monitoring ECG and BP.
▼ Don't infuse for longer than 24 hours.
▼ **Incompatibilities:** Acetazolamide, acyclovir, aminophylline, ampicillin, ampicillin sodium–sulbactam sodium, diazepam, furosemide, heparin, hydrocortisone, insulin, methylprednisolone, nafcillin, phenytoin, rifampin, sodium bicarbonate, thiopental.

ACTION

Inhibits calcium ion influx across cardiac and smooth-muscle cells, decreasing myocardial contractility and oxygen demand. Drug also dilates coronary arteries and arterioles.

Route	Onset	Peak	Duration
PO	30–60 min	2–4 hr	6–8 hr
PO (extended-release capsule)	2–3 hr	10–14 hr	12–24 hr
PO (LA)	3–4 hr	11–18 hr	6–9 hr
IV	<3 min	2–7 min	1–10 hr

Half-life: 3 to 9 hours.

ADVERSE REACTIONS

CNS: headache, dizziness, asthenia, nervousness. **CV:** edema, *arrhythmias, AV block,* *bradycardia, HF,* flushing, hypotension, conduction abnormalities, abnormal ECG, palpitations, vasodilation. **EENT:** conjunctivitis, sinus congestion, pharyngitis, rhinitis. **GI:** nausea, vomiting, constipation, diarrhea, dyspepsia, abdominal discomfort. **GU:** erectile dysfunction. **Metabolic:** gout. **Respiratory:** bronchitis, cough, dyspnea. **Skin:** rash, injection-site reaction. **Other:** infection, flu-like symptoms.

INTERACTIONS

Drug-drug. *Anesthetics:* May increase effects of anesthetics. Monitor patient.
Atazanavir, cimetidine: May inhibit diltiazem metabolism, increasing additive AV node conduction slowing. Monitor patient for toxicity.
Beta blockers (propranolol): May increase risk of bradycardia, AV block, and depressed contractility. Use together cautiously.
Buspirone, quinidine, sirolimus, tacrolimus: May increase level of these drugs. Monitor drug levels and patient for toxicity.
Carbamazepine: May increase level of carbamazepine. Monitor carbamazepine level, and watch for signs and symptoms of toxicity.
Cyclosporine: May increase cyclosporine level. Monitor cyclosporine level with each dosage change.
CYP3A inducers (rifampin): May lower diltiazem level significantly. Avoid use together.
Diazepam, midazolam, triazolam: May increase CNS depression and prolong effects of these drugs. Use lower dose of these benzodiazepines.
Digoxin: May have additive effect that slows AV node conduction and increases digoxin level. Monitor patient for digoxin toxicity.
HMG-CoA reductase inhibitors (lovastatin, simvastatin): May increase risk of myopathy, rhabdomyolysis, and kidney failure. Use lower starting and maintenance doses of diltiazem and statins.
Ivabradine: May increase ivabradine level, which may exacerbate bradycardia and conduction disturbances. Avoid use together.

EFFECTS ON LAB TEST RESULTS

• May increase CK, glucose, ALT, AST, LDH, bilirubin, and ALP levels.
• May decrease Hb level and leukocyte and platelet counts.
• May increase urine crystals and uric acid level.

CONTRAINDICATIONS & CAUTIONS

• Contraindicated in patients hypersensitive to drug and in those with sick sinus syndrome or second- or third-degree AV block in absence of artificial pacemaker, hypotension (systolic BP less than 90 mm Hg), acute MI, and pulmonary congestion.
• Additional contraindications for IV form include atrial fibrillation or flutter with an accessory bypass tract, as in Wolff-Parkinson-White syndrome or short PR interval syndrome; cardiogenic shock; and ventricular tachycardia. IV form also contraindicated within a few hours of IV beta blocker therapy.
• Use cautiously in older adults and patients with HF, hypertrophic obstructive cardiomyopathy, or impaired liver or kidney function.
• Safety and effectiveness in children haven't been established.
Dialyzable drug: No.
⚠ *Overdose S&S:* Bradycardia, hypotension, heart block, cardiac failure.

PREGNANCY-LACTATION-REPRODUCTION

• Studies during pregnancy are inadequate. Use during pregnancy only if clearly needed.
• Drug appears in human milk. Patient should discontinue breastfeeding or discontinue drug considering importance of drug to patient.

NURSING CONSIDERATIONS

• Monitor BP and HR when starting therapy and during dosage adjustments.
• Be aware that maximal antihypertensive effect may not occur for 14 days.
• If systolic BP is below 90 mm Hg or HR is below 60 beats/minute, withhold dose and notify prescriber.
• Monitor ECG and liver and kidney function.
• *Look alike–sound alike:* Don't confuse Tiazac with Ziac.

PATIENT TEACHING

• Teach about proper drug administration and handling.
• Instruct patient to take drug as prescribed, even when feeling better.
• Tell patient to report all adverse reactions.
• Advise patient to avoid hazardous activities during start of therapy.
• If nitrate therapy is prescribed during dosage adjustment, stress patient adherence. Tell patient that SL nitroglycerin may be taken with drug, as needed, when angina symptoms are acute.

• Advise patient to consult prescriber if pregnant or planning to become pregnant or breastfeed.

diphenhydrAMINE hydrochloride
dye-fen-HYE-drah-meen

Banophen ◇, Benadryl ◇, Children's Benadryl Allergy ◇, Sominex ◇, Unisom SleepMelts ◇, ZzzQuil ◇

Therapeutic class: Antihistamines
Pharmacologic class: Ethanolamines

AVAILABLE FORMS
Capsules: 25 mg ◇, 50 mg ◇
Elixir: 12.5 mg/5 mL * ◇
Injection: 50 mg/mL
Liquid: 12.5 mg/5 mL * ◇, 50 mg/30 mL * ◇
Tablets: 25 mg ◇, 50 mg ◇
Tablets (chewable): 12.5 mg ◇
Tablets (ODTs): 25 mg ◇

INDICATIONS & DOSAGES
➤ **Rhinitis, allergy symptoms, motion sickness, Parkinson disease**
Adults and children ages 12 and older: 25 to 50 mg PO every 4 to 6 hours. Maximum, 300 mg PO daily. Or, 10 to 50 mg IV or deep IM. May give 100 mg if needed. Maximum IV or IM dosage, 400 mg daily. Don't exceed 25 mg/minute when giving IV.
Children ages 6 to 11: 12.5 to 25 mg PO every 4 to 6 hours. Maximum dose, 150 mg daily.
Children other than premature infants and neonates: 5 mg/kg/24 hours deep IM or IV divided into four doses. Don't exceed 25 mg/minute when giving IV. Maximum dose, 300 mg daily.
➤ **Nighttime sleep aid**
Adults and children ages 12 and older: 25 to 50 mg PO at bedtime.
➤ **Nonproductive cough**
Adults and children ages 12 and older: 25 to 50 mg (liquid) PO every 4 hours. Don't exceed 300 mg daily.
Children ages 6 to 11: 12.5 to 25 mg (liquid) PO every 4 to 6 hours or as directed. Don't exceed six doses in 24 hours.

ADMINISTRATION
PO
• Give drug with food or milk to reduce GI distress.
• Give 30 minutes before bedtime when given for insomnia or 30 minutes before exposure when given for motion sickness.
IV
▼ For injection, don't exceed 25 mg/minute.
▼ May further dilute and give as an intermittent infusion over 10 to 15 minutes for children.
▼ **Incompatibilities:** Allopurinol, amobarbital, amphotericin B, cefepime, dexamethasone, foscarnet, haloperidol, pentobarbital, phenobarbital, phenytoin, thiopental.
IM
• Give IM injection deep into large muscle; alternate injection sites to prevent irritation.

ACTION
Competes with histamine for H_1-receptor sites. Prevents, but doesn't reverse, histamine-mediated responses, particularly those of the bronchial tubes, GI tract, uterus, and blood vessels.

Route	Onset	Peak	Duration
PO	15 min	1–4 hr	3–6 hr
IV	Immediate	1–4 hr	3–6 hr
IM	Unknown	1–4 hr	3–6 hr

Half-life: About 4 to 18 hours.

ADVERSE REACTIONS
CNS: ataxia, drowsiness, euphoria, sedation, sleepiness, dizziness, incoordination, *seizures,* confusion, insomnia, headache, vertigo, fatigue, restlessness, tremor, nervousness, irritability, paradoxical excitation, paresthesia, vertigo, neuritis. **CV:** palpitations, hypotension, tachycardia, chest tightness. **EENT:** diplopia, blurred vision, tinnitus, dry mouth, nasal congestion, pharyngeal edema, labyrinthitis. **GI:** nausea, epigastric distress, vomiting, diarrhea, constipation, anorexia. **GU:** dysuria, urine retention, urinary frequency, early menses. **Hematologic:** *thrombocytopenia, agranulocytosis,* hemolytic anemia. **Respiratory:** thickening of bronchial secretions, wheezing. **Skin:** urticaria, photosensitivity, diaphoresis, rash. **Other:** chills, dry mucous membranes, *anaphylactic shock.*

Reactions in bold italics are *life-threatening.*

INTERACTIONS

Drug-drug. *CNS depressants:* May increase sedation. Use together cautiously.

MAO inhibitors: May increase anticholinergic effects. Avoid use together.

Other products that contain diphenhydramine (including topical therapy): May increase risk of adverse reactions. Avoid use together.

Drug-lifestyle. *Alcohol use:* May increase CNS depression. Discourage use together.

Sun exposure: May cause photosensitivity reactions. Advise patient to avoid extensive sunlight exposure.

EFFECTS ON LAB TEST RESULTS

• May decrease Hb level and hematocrit.
• May decrease granulocyte and platelet counts.
• May prevent, reduce, or mask positive result in diagnostic skin test.
• May produce false-positives in urine detection of methadone and phencyclidine and in serum TCA screens.

CONTRAINDICATIONS & CAUTIONS

• Contraindicated in patients hypersensitive to drug and other similar antihistamines, in newborns, and in premature neonates.
• Don't use parenteral form as a local anesthetic due to risk of local necrosis.
• Use cautiously in older adults and patients with stenosing peptic ulcer, bladder neck obstruction, pyloroduodenal obstruction, prostatic hyperplasia, asthma, increased IOP, angle-closure glaucoma, thyroid dysfunction, CV disease, and HTN.
• Children younger than age 6 should use drug only as directed by prescriber.
Dialyzable drug: Unlikely.
⚠ *Overdose S&S:* Dry mouth, fixed or dilated pupils, flushing, GI symptoms.

PREGNANCY-LACTATION-REPRODUCTION

• Studies during pregnancy are inadequate. Use during pregnancy only if clearly needed.
• Drug appears in human milk. Contraindicated during breastfeeding.

NURSING CONSIDERATIONS

• Stop drug 4 days before diagnostic skin testing, or as directed.
• Be aware that dizziness, excessive sedation, syncope, toxicity, paradoxical stimulation, and hypotension are more likely to occur in an older adult.

• *Look alike–sound alike:* Don't confuse diphenhydramine with dimenhydrinate. Don't confuse Benadryl with Bentyl or benazepril.

PATIENT TEACHING

• Advise patient to consult prescriber before using OTC sleep and cold products (drug is in many of these products).
• Warn patient not to take drug with any other products that contain diphenhydramine (including topical therapy) because of increased risk of adverse reactions.
• Teach about proper drug administration and handling.
• Warn patient to avoid alcohol and hazardous activities that require alertness until CNS effects of drug are known.
• Tell patient to notify prescriber if tolerance develops because a different antihistamine may need to be prescribed.
• Warn patient of possible photosensitivity reactions. Advise use of sunblock.

dipyridamole
dye-peer-IH-duh-mohl

Therapeutic class: Antiplatelet drugs
Pharmacologic class: Pyrimidine analogues

AVAILABLE FORMS

Injection: 5 mg/mL
Tablets: 25 mg, 50 mg, 75 mg

INDICATIONS & DOSAGES

➤ **To inhibit platelet adhesion in prosthetic heart valves (given together with warfarin)**
Adults and children ages 12 and older: 75 to 100 mg PO q.i.d.
➤ **Alternative to exercise in evaluation of CAD during thallium myocardial perfusion scintigraphy**
Adults: 0.57 mg/kg (total dose) by IV infusion at a constant rate over 4 minutes (0.142 mg/kg/minute). Maximum dose, 60 mg.

ADMINISTRATION

PO
• Pharmacist can prepare oral suspension for patients unable to swallow tablets. Shake well before use.
IV
▼ For use as a diagnostic drug, dilute in half-NSS, NSS, or D_5W in at least a 1:2 ratio for a total volume of 20 to 50 mL.

▼ Inject thallium-201 within 5 minutes after completing the 4-minute dipyridamole infusion.
▼ Don't mix in same syringe or infusion container with other drugs.
▼ **Incompatibilities:** Other drugs.

ACTION

Inhibits adenosine deaminase and phosphodiesterase, which increases adenosine, a coronary vasodilator and platelet aggregation inhibitor.

Route	Onset	Peak	Duration
PO	Unknown	75 min	Unknown
IV	Unknown	2 min	Unknown

Half-life: 1 to 12 hours; alpha half-life of oral form, 40 minutes; beta half-life of oral form, 10 hours.

ADVERSE REACTIONS

CNS: dizziness, headache, fatigue, pain, paresthesia. **CV:** angina pectoris (IV), chest pain, *ECG abnormalities (IV)*, flushing, hypotension, HTN, labile BP. **GI:** nausea, abdominal distress, diarrhea, vomiting. **Respiratory:** dyspnea (IV). **Skin:** rash, pruritus.

INTERACTIONS

Drug-drug. *Adenosine:* May increase level and cardiac effects of adenosine. Adjust adenosine dose as needed.
Anticoagulants, apixaban, dabigatran, drugs with antiplatelet properties (NSAIDs, P2Y₁₂ inhibitors, SSRIs), edoxaban, heparin, rivaroxaban, salicylates, thrombolytics: May increase bleeding risk. Monitor therapy.
Cholinesterase inhibitors: May counteract anticholinesterase effects and aggravate myasthenia gravis. Monitor patient.
Theophylline, caffeine, other xanthine derivatives: May prevent coronary vasodilation by IV dipyridamole, causing a false-negative thallium-imaging result. Avoid use together.

EFFECTS ON LAB TEST RESULTS

• May increase liver enzyme levels.

CONTRAINDICATIONS & CAUTIONS

• Contraindicated in patients hypersensitive to drug.
• Use cautiously in patients with hypotension, liver impairment, or severe CAD.
⊙ **Alert:** IV drug is associated with cardiac death, fatal and nonfatal MI, ventricular fibrillation, symptomatic ventricular

tachycardia, stroke, transient cerebral ischemia, seizures, anaphylactoid reaction, and bronchospasm.
• Safety and effectiveness of oral dipyridamole in children younger than age 12 or IV dipyridamole in children haven't been established.
Dialyzable drug: Unlikely.
⚠ *Overdose S&S:* Hypotension, warm feeling, flushes, diaphoresis, restlessness, weakness, dizziness, tachycardia.

PREGNANCY-LACTATION-REPRODUCTION

• Studies during pregnancy are inadequate. Use during pregnancy only if clearly needed.
• Drug appears in human milk. Use cautiously during breastfeeding.

NURSING CONSIDERATIONS

• Observe for adverse reactions, especially with large doses. Monitor BP.
• Observe for signs and symptoms of bleeding.
• Be aware that dipyridamole injection may contain tartrazine, which can cause allergic reactions in some patients.
• *Look alike–sound alike:* Don't confuse dipyridamole with disopyramide.

PATIENT TEACHING

• Instruct patient to take drug exactly as prescribed.
• Advise patient to promptly report adverse reactions.
• Tell patient receiving drug IV to report discomfort at IV insertion site.

SAFETY ALERT!

DOBUTamine hydrochloride
doe-BYOO-ta-meen

Therapeutic class: Inotropes
Pharmacologic class: Adrenergics–beta₁ agonists

AVAILABLE FORMS

Dobutamine in 5% dextrose: 250 mg (1 mg/mL), 500 mg (2 mg/mL), 1,000 mg (4 mg/mL) in 250 mL
Injection: 12.5 mg/mL

INDICATIONS & DOSAGES

➤ **To increase cardiac output during short-term treatment of cardiac decompensation caused by depressed contractility from**

Reactions in bold italics are *life-threatening*.

heart disease; adjunctive therapy in cardiac surgery

Adults: Initially, 0.5 to 1 mcg/kg/minute IV infusion, titrating to optimum dosage of 2 to 20 mcg/kg/minute. Usual effective range to increase cardiac output is 2 to 20 mcg/kg/minute. Rarely, rates up to 40 mcg/kg/minute may be needed.

ADMINISTRATION

IV

▼ Before starting therapy, give a plasma volume expander to correct hypovolemia and, in patients who have atrial fibrillation with rapid ventricular response, a cardiac glycoside.

▼ Dilute concentrate before injecting in D_5W, D_5W and NSS injection, D_5W and half-NSS injection, NSS, or other compatible solution

▼ Oxidation may slightly discolor admixture. This doesn't indicate a significant loss of potency, provided drug is used within 24 hours of reconstitution.

▼ Don't administer unless solution is clear and container is undamaged.

▼ Give through a CVAD or large peripheral vein using an infusion pump.

▼ Titrate rate according to patient's condition.

▼ Infusions lasting up to 72 hours produce no more adverse effects than shorter infusions.

▼ Watch for irritation and infiltration; extravasation can cause tissue damage and necrosis. Change IV sites regularly to avoid phlebitis.

▼ Solution remains stable for 24 hours. Don't freeze.

▼ **Incompatibilities:** Diluents containing both sodium bisulfite and ethanol and other drugs; 5% sodium bicarbonate injection and other strongly alkaline solutions. Consult drug compatibility reference for more information.

ACTION

Stimulates heart's $beta_1$ receptors to increase myocardial contractility and stroke volume. At therapeutic dosages, drug increases cardiac output by decreasing peripheral vascular resistance, reducing ventricular filling pressure, and facilitating AV node conduction.

Route	Onset	Peak	Duration
IV	1–2 min	10 min	<5 min after infusion

Half-life: 2 minutes.

ADVERSE REACTIONS

CNS: headache. **CV:** increased BP, increased HR, angina, PVCs, phlebitis, nonspecific chest pain, palpitations, ventricular ectopy, hypotension. **GI:** nausea, vomiting. **Respiratory:** shortness of breath. **Other:** hypersensitivity reactions.

INTERACTIONS

Drug-drug. *Beta blockers:* May antagonize dobutamine effects. Avoid use together.
Oxytocic drugs: May increase pressor response, causing severe HTN. Closely monitor BP.
Linezolid: May increase hypertensive effect of sympathomimetics. May need to decrease initial doses of dobutamine and titrate to effect.

EFFECTS ON LAB TEST RESULTS

• May decrease potassium level.
• May decrease platelet count.

CONTRAINDICATIONS & CAUTIONS

• Contraindicated in patients hypersensitive to drug or its components and in those with idiopathic hypertrophic subaortic stenosis.
• Solutions containing dextrose may be contraindicated in patients with known allergy to corn or corn products.
• Use cautiously in patients with history of HTN because drug may increase pressor response.
• Use cautiously after acute MI.
• Use cautiously in patients with history of sulfite sensitivity. Anaphylaxis or asthmatic episodes can occur.
• May precipitate or exacerbate ventricular ectopic activity, but rarely has caused ventricular tachycardia.
Dialyzable drug: Unknown.
⚠ *Overdose S&S:* Anorexia, nausea, vomiting, tremor, anxiety, palpitations, headache, shortness of breath, anginal and nonspecific chest pain, HTN, myocardial ischemia, tachyarrhythmias, ventricular fibrillation, hypotension.

PREGNANCY-LACTATION-REPRODUCTION

• Studies during pregnancy are inadequate. Use during pregnancy only if clearly needed.
• It isn't known if drug appears in human milk. Discontinue breastfeeding for duration of therapy.

NURSING CONSIDERATIONS

🌢 *Alert:* Because drug increases AV node conduction, patients with atrial fibrillation may develop a rapid ventricular rate.

• Continuously monitor ECG, BP, pulmonary artery wedge pressure, cardiac output, and urine output during therapy.

• Correct hypovolemia before therapy.

• Monitor electrolyte levels. Drug may lower potassium level.

• *Look alike–sound alike:* Don't confuse dobutamine with dopamine.

PATIENT TEACHING

• Tell patient to promptly report all adverse reactions, especially labored breathing, angina, palpitations, dizziness, and drug-induced headache.

• Instruct patient to report discomfort at IV insertion site.

SAFETY ALERT!

DOCEtaxel
dohs-eh-TAX-ell

Therapeutic class: Antineoplastics
Pharmacologic class: Taxoids

AVAILABLE FORMS

Injection concentrate: 20 mg/mL* vials
Injection solution: 20 mg/2 mL*, 80 mg/8 mL*, 160 mg/16 mL* vials

INDICATIONS & DOSAGES

Adjust-a-dose (for all indications): Refer to manufacturer's instructions for toxicity-related dosage adjustments and treatment.

➤ **Locally advanced or metastatic breast cancer after failure of previous chemotherapy**
Adults: 60 to 100 mg/m² IV over 1 hour every 3 weeks.

➤ **Adjuvant postsurgery treatment of operable, node-positive breast cancer**
Adults: 75 mg/m² IV as a 1-hour infusion given 1 hour after doxorubicin 50 mg/m² and cyclophosphamide 500 mg/m² every 3 weeks for six cycles. May use prophylactic G-CSF therapy to decrease risk of hematologic toxicities.

➤ **Locally advanced or metastatic NSCLC after failure of previous cisplatin-based chemotherapy**
Adults: 75 mg/m² IV over 1 hour every 3 weeks.

➤ **With cisplatin, unresectable, locally advanced, or metastatic NSCLC not previously treated with chemotherapy**
Adults: 75 mg/m² docetaxel IV over 1 hour, immediately followed by cisplatin 75 mg/m² IV over 30 to 60 minutes every 3 weeks.

➤ **Metastatic castration-resistant prostate cancer, with prednisone**
Adults: 75 mg/m² IV, as a 1-hour infusion every 3 weeks, given with 5 mg prednisone PO b.i.d. continuously. Premedicate with dexamethasone 8 mg PO at 12 hours, 3 hours, and 1 hour before docetaxel infusion.

➤ **Advanced gastric adenocarcinoma, in combination with cisplatin and 5-FU**
Adults: Premedicate with antiemetics and hydration per cisplatin recommendations. Give 75 mg/m² docetaxel IV over 1 hour, followed by cisplatin 75 mg/m² IV over 1 to 3 hours both on day 1 only, then 5-FU 750 mg/m² IV daily as a 24-hour continuous infusion for 5 days beginning at the end of cisplatin infusion. Repeat cycle every 3 weeks.

➤ **Induction treatment of inoperable locally advanced squamous cell cancer of the head and neck (SCCHN), with cisplatin and 5-FU**
Adults: Premedicate with antiemetics and hydration per cisplatin recommendations. Use prophylaxis for neutropenic infections. Give 75 mg/m² IV infusion over 1 hour, followed by cisplatin 75 mg/m² IV infusion over 1 hour, on day 1, followed by 5-FU 750 mg/m² daily as a continuous IV infusion for 5 days. Repeat this regimen every 3 weeks for four cycles. After chemotherapy, patients should receive radiotherapy.

➤ **Induction treatment for locally advanced (unresectable, low surgical cure, or organ preservation) SCCHN with cisplatin and 5-FU before chemoradiotherapy**
Adults: Premedicate with antiemetics and hydration per cisplatin recommendations. Give 75 mg/m² IV infusion over 1 hour, followed by cisplatin 100 mg/m² IV infusion over 30 minutes to 3 hours on day 1, followed by 5-FU 1,000 mg/m² daily as a continuous IV infusion from day 1 to day 4. Repeat this regimen every 3 weeks for three cycles. After chemotherapy, patients should receive chemoradiotherapy.

Reactions in bold italics are *life-threatening*.

ADMINISTRATION

IV

⚠ *Alert:* Hazardous agent; use safe handling and disposal precautions.

▼ Give oral corticosteroid such as dexamethasone 16 mg PO (8 mg b.i.d.) daily for 3 days, starting 1 day before docetaxel administration, to reduce risk or severity of fluid retention and hypersensitivity reactions.

⚠ *Alert:* Carefully read package instructions and confirm concentration being used; admixture errors have occurred due to the availability of various concentrations.

▼ If using the 2-vial formulation, dilute using supplied diluent. Let drug and diluent stand at room temperature for 5 minutes before mixing. After adding all the diluent to drug vial, gently rotate vial for about 45 seconds. Let solution stand for a few minutes so foam dissipates. All foam need not dissipate before preparing infusion solution.

▼ If using the 1-vial formulation, no dilution is needed. The product comes ready to add to the infusion solution.

▼ Prepare infusion solution by withdrawing needed amount of premixed solution from vial and injecting it into 250 mL NSS or D₅W using a 21-gauge needle to yield 0.3 to 0.74 mg/mL. Doses of more than 200 mg need a larger volume to stay below 0.74 mg/mL of drug. Mix infusion thoroughly by manual rotation.

▼ Prepare and store infusion solution in bottles (glass, polypropylene) or plastic bags (polypropylene, polyolefin), and give through polyethylene-lined administration sets.

▼ Contact between undiluted concentrate and polyvinyl chloride equipment or devices isn't recommended.

▼ If solution isn't clear or contains precipitate, discard it.

▼ Infuse over 1 hour.

⚠ *Alert:* When indicated, cisplatin dose should follow docetaxel dose.

▼ Store unopened vials between 36° and 77° F (2° and 25° C).

⚠ *Alert:* Mark all waste materials with CHEMOTHERAPY HAZARD labels.

▼ **Incompatibilities:** None listed by manufacturer. Consult drug compatibility reference for more information.

ACTION

Promotes formation and stabilization of nonfunctional microtubules, preventing mitosis and leading to cell death.

Route	Onset	Peak	Duration
IV	Rapid	Unknown	Unknown

Half-life: Terminal phase, 11.1 hours.

ADVERSE REACTIONS

CNS: asthenia, paresthesia, dysesthesia, fatigue, dizziness, peripheral neuropathy, weakness, dysgeusia, drug fever, syncope. **CV:** peripheral edema, HF, *arrhythmias,* chest tightness, flushing, vasodilation, hypotension, lymphedema, phlebitis, left ventricular dysfunction. **EENT:** tearing, conjunctivitis, altered hearing. **GI:** anorexia, diarrhea, dysphagia, esophagitis, nausea, stomatitis, abdominal pain, vomiting. **GU:** amenorrhea. **Hematologic:** *febrile neutropenia, leukopenia, myelosuppression, neutropenia, thrombocytopenia,* anemia. **Hepatic:** *liver toxicity.* **Metabolic:** fluid retention, weight gain. **Musculoskeletal:** myalgia, arthralgia. **Respiratory:** dyspnea, cough, *pulmonary edema.* **Skin:** alopecia, skin toxicity, nail disorder, rash, reaction at injection site. **Other:** infection, chills, hypersensitivity reactions, *death.*

INTERACTIONS

Drug-drug. *Compounds that induce or are metabolized by CYP3A4 (phenytoin, rifampicin, tacrolimus, midazolam):* May modify metabolism of docetaxel. Use together cautiously.

CYP3A4 inhibitors (ketoconazole, ritonavir): May increase docetaxel level and toxicity, including neutropenia. Monitor patient closely. Consider docetaxel dosage reduction if administration with strong CYP3A4 inhibitors can't be avoided.

EFFECTS ON LAB TEST RESULTS

• May increase ALP, ALT, AST, and bilirubin levels.
• May decrease Hb level and platelet and WBC counts.

CONTRAINDICATIONS & CAUTIONS

Boxed Warning Contraindicated in patients with neutrophil counts less than 1,500/mm³. Frequently monitor blood cell counts during therapy. ■

D

Boxed Warning Treatment-related mortality increases in patients with abnormal liver function, those receiving higher doses, and patients with NSCLC and a history of prior treatment with platinum-based chemotherapy who receive docetaxel as a single agent at a dose of 100 mg/m^2. ■

Boxed Warning Avoid use in patients with bilirubin levels exceeding the ULN or those with ALT or AST levels above $1.5 \times$ ULN and ALP levels above $2.5 \times$ ULN. LFT elevations increase the risk of severe or life-threatening complications. Obtain LFT values before each treatment cycle. ■

Boxed Warning Contraindicated in patients severely hypersensitive to drug or with a history of hypersensitivity to polysorbate 80. Some dosage forms may contain polysorbate 80. ■

• SCAR (SJS, TEN, acute generalized exanthematous pustulosis) has occurred.

• Safety and effectiveness in children haven't been established.

• Discontinue treatment if cystoid macular edema develops.

⚠ *Alert:* Some drug formulations may contain alcohol. Use cautiously in patients with liver impairment and in those in whom ethanol intake should be avoided or minimized. Some medications, such as pain relievers and sleep aids, may interact with the alcohol in the docetaxel infusion and worsen intoxicating effects. A generic, nonalcoholic form of docetaxel is available.

Dialyzable drug: No.

⚠ *Overdose S&S:* Severe neutropenia, mild asthenia, cutaneous reactions, mild paresthesia, bone marrow suppression, peripheral neurotoxicity, mucositis.

PREGNANCY-LACTATION-REPRODUCTION

• Drug can cause fetal harm. Advise patients of childbearing potential to avoid becoming pregnant during therapy.

• Patients of childbearing potential should use effective contraception during treatment and for 6 months after final dose. Males with partners of childbearing potential should use effective contraception during treatment and for 3 months after final dose.

• It isn't known if drug appears in human milk. Advise patient not to breastfeed during treatment with docetaxel injection and for 1 week after the last dose.

• Drug may impair male fertility.

NURSING CONSIDERATIONS

⚠ *Alert:* Drug should be administered only under the supervision of a physician experienced with antineoplastics and in a facility equipped to handle anaphylaxis.

• Verify pregnancy status before starting therapy.

• Bone marrow toxicity is the most frequent and dose-limiting toxicity. Frequent blood count monitoring is needed during therapy.

Boxed Warning Monitor patient closely for hypersensitivity reactions, especially during first and second infusions. Severe and even fatal reactions have occurred in patients who have received recommended steroid premedication. For severe reactions, immediately discontinue docetaxel and administer appropriate therapy. ■

• Cross sensitivity with paclitaxel may occur, including severe or fatal reactions such as anaphylaxis. Closely monitor patient with a history of hypersensitivity to paclitaxel during initiation of therapy. Reactions may occur within a few minutes after infusion is started. If minor reactions (flushing, localized skin reactions) occur, therapy interruption isn't required.

Boxed Warning Fluid retention is dose related and may be severe. Monitor patient closely. ■

• Enterocolitis and neutropenic colitis have occurred in patients treated with docetaxel alone and in combination with other chemotherapeutic agents, despite the coadministration of G-CSF. Use cautiously in patient with neutropenia, particularly one at risk for developing GI complications. Enterocolitis and neutropenic colitis may develop at any time and lead to death as early as the first day of symptom onset. Closely monitor patient from onset of signs and symptoms of GI toxicity.

⚠ *Alert:* Evaluate patient for history of problems with alcohol or drinking, liver disease, or other conditions that may be affected by alcohol intake.

⚠ *Alert:* Monitor for signs and symptoms of alcohol intoxication during and after treatment (appearance of being drunk, confusion, stumbling, somnolence). Consider using formulation with lowest alcohol content for patients who experience adverse reactions. Slowing infusion rate during administration may help resolve signs and symptoms of alcohol intoxication.

Reactions in bold italics are *life-threatening*.

• Closely monitor for TLS. Correct dehydration and treat high uric acid level before start of therapy.

• Monitor for vision changes. If they occur, arrange for patient to undergo prompt, comprehensive eye exam.

• Monitor patient who received docetaxel, doxorubicin, and cyclophosphamide for delayed myelodysplasia or myeloid leukemia.

• Monitor patient closely for signs and symptoms of SJS and TEN (fever, blistering and peeling of skin, eye irritation and redness) and acute generalized exanthematous pustulosis (sudden high fever and rash). Consider permanently discontinuing drug in patient who experiences these types of reactions.

• **Look alike–sound alike:** Don't confuse docetaxel with paclitaxel.

PATIENT TEACHING

Alert: Caution patient to avoid driving, operating machinery, and performing other hazardous activities for 1 to 2 hours after treatment.

Alert: Instruct patient to immediately report signs and symptoms of alcohol intoxication that may occur during or 1 to 2 hours after treatment.

• Caution patient of childbearing potential to avoid pregnancy or breastfeeding during therapy.

• Inform patient of potential hazard to fetus if drug is used during pregnancy.

• Advise patient to report pain or burning at injection site during or after administration.

• Warn patient that hair loss occurs in almost 80% of patients and, although it usually reverses when treatment stops, cases of permanent hair loss have been reported.

• Tell patient to report all adverse reactions and to promptly report neurologic reactions, vision changes, sore throat, fever, skin reactions, and unusual bruising or bleeding as well as signs and symptoms of fluid retention (swelling, shortness of breath).

• Tell patient to report new or worsening signs or symptoms of GI toxicity.

• Advise patients that periodic blood work is necessary.

• Explain the need for premedication and the importance of compliance.

---

dofetilide
doe-FE-ti-lyed

Tikosyn

Therapeutic class: Antiarrhythmics
Pharmacologic class: Antiarrhythmics

AVAILABLE FORMS
Capsules: 125 mcg, 250 mcg, 500 mcg

INDICATIONS & DOSAGES

➤ **To maintain normal sinus rhythm in patients with symptomatic atrial fibrillation or atrial flutter lasting longer than 1 week who have been converted to normal sinus rhythm; to convert atrial fibrillation and atrial flutter to normal sinus rhythm**

Adults: Individualized dosage based on CrCl and baseline QTc interval (or QT interval if HR is below 60 beats/minute), determined before first dose; usually 500 mcg PO b.i.d.

Adjust-a-dose: If CrCl is 40 to 60 mL/minute, starting dose is 250 mcg PO b.i.d.; if CrCl is 20 to 39 mL/minute, starting dose is 125 mcg PO b.i.d. Don't use drug if CrCl is less than 20 mL/minute.

Determine QTc or QT (if heart rate less than 60 beats/minute) interval 2 to 3 hours after first dose. If QTc or QT interval has increased by more than 15% above baseline or if it's more than 500 msec (550 msec in patients with ventricular conduction abnormalities), adjust dosage as follows: If starting dose based on CrCl was 500 mcg PO b.i.d., give 250 mcg PO b.i.d. If starting dose based on CrCl was 250 mcg b.i.d., give 125 mcg b.i.d. If starting dose based on CrCl was 125 mcg b.i.d., give 125 mcg once a day.

Determine QTc interval 2 to 3 hours after each subsequent dose while patient is in hospital. If at any time after second dose the QTc interval exceeds 500 msec (550 msec in patients with ventricular conduction abnormalities), stop drug.

ADMINISTRATION
PO
• Give drug without regard to food or antacid administration.

• Protect drug from moisture and humidity.

• If a dose is missed, don't double the dose. Give next dose at the usual time.

ACTION

Prolongs repolarization without affecting conduction velocity (Vaughan-Williams Class III antiarrhythmic). Doesn't affect sodium channels, alpha-adrenergic receptors, or beta-adrenergic receptors.

Route	Onset	Peak	Duration
PO	Unknown	2–3 hr	Unknown

Half-life: 10 hours.

ADVERSE REACTIONS

CNS: headache, *stroke,* dizziness, insomnia, anxiety, migraine, *cerebral ischemia,* asthenia, paresthesia, syncope, pain. **CV:** chest pain, *ventricular fibrillation, ventricular tachycardia, torsades de pointes, AV block, heart block, bradycardia, cardiac arrest, MI,* bundle-branch block, angina, atrial fibrillation, supraventricular tachycardia, HTN, palpitations, peripheral edema. **GI:** nausea, diarrhea, abdominal pain. **GU:** UTI. **Hepatic:** liver damage. **Musculoskeletal:** back pain, arthralgia, facial paralysis. **Respiratory:** respiratory tract infection, dyspnea, increased cough. **Skin:** rash, diaphoresis. **Other:** *angioedema,* flulike syndrome, accidental injury.

INTERACTIONS

Drug-drug. *Amiodarone:* May increase risk of adverse effects. Don't give drug after amiodarone therapy until amiodarone level falls below 0.3 mcg/mL or until amiodarone has been stopped for at least 3 months.

Antiarrhythmics (Class I and III): May increase dofetilide adverse effects. Withhold other antiarrhythmics for at least three plasma half-lives before giving dofetilide.

CYP3A4 inhibitors (amiodarone, azole antifungals, cannabinoids, diltiazem, macrolides, nefazodone, norfloxacin, protease inhibitors, quinine, SSRIs, zafirlukast): May decrease metabolism and increase dofetilide level. Use together cautiously.

Drugs secreted by kidney tubular cationic transport (amiloride, metformin, triamterene): May increase dofetilide level. Use together cautiously; monitor patient for adverse effects.

Drugs that prolong QT interval: May increase risk of QT interval prolongation. Avoid use together.

Hydrochlorothiazide: May significantly increase dofetilide level and prolong QT interval. Use together is contraindicated.

Inhibitors of kidney cationic secretion (cimetidine, ketoconazole, megestrol, prochlorperazine, sulfamethoxazole–trimethoprim), trimethoprim, verapamil: May increase dofetilide level. Use together is contraindicated.

Potassium-depleting diuretics: May increase risk of hypokalemia or hypomagnesemia. Monitor potassium and magnesium levels.

Thiazide diuretics: May cause hypokalemia and arrhythmias. Use together is contraindicated.

Drug-food. *Grapefruit juice:* May decrease liver metabolism and increase drug level. Discourage use together.

EFFECTS ON LAB TEST RESULTS

None reported.

CONTRAINDICATIONS & CAUTIONS

• Contraindicated in patients hypersensitive to drug, in those with congenital or acquired long QT interval syndromes or with baseline QTc interval greater than 440 msec (500 msec in patients with ventricular conduction abnormalities), and in those with CrCl less than 20 mL/minute.

• Use cautiously in patients with Child-Pugh Class C liver impairment.

• Safety and effectiveness in children haven't been studied.

Dialyzable drug: Unknown.

⚠ **Overdose S&S:** Prolonged QT interval, ventricular fibrillation, torsades de pointes, cardiac arrest.

PREGNANCY-LACTATION-REPRODUCTION

• Studies during pregnancy are inadequate. Use during pregnancy only if clearly needed and if potential benefit justifies fetal risk.

• It isn't known if drug appears in human milk. Patients shouldn't breastfeed during therapy.

NURSING CONSIDERATIONS

Boxed Warning When dofetilide is initiated or reinitiated, patients should be hospitalized for a minimum of 3 days in a facility that can provide calculations of CrCl, continuous ECG monitoring, and cardiac resuscitation. ■

• Don't discharge patient within 12 hours of conversion to normal sinus rhythm.

• Before discharge, ensure patient has an adequate supply of medication to allow

---

Reactions in bold italics are *life-threatening*.

uninterrupted dosing until patient can fill a prescription as an outpatient.
• Monitor patient for prolonged diarrhea, diaphoresis, and vomiting. Report these signs to prescriber because electrolyte imbalance may increase the potential for arrhythmia development.
• Monitor kidney function and QTc interval every 3 months. Drug can cause torsades de pointes ventricular arrhythmia.
• Use of potassium-depleting diuretics may cause hypokalemia and hypomagnesemia, increasing the risk of torsades de pointes. Give dofetilide after potassium level reaches and stays in normal range.
• If dofetilide must be stopped to allow dosing with interacting drugs, allow at least 2 days before starting other drug therapy.

PATIENT TEACHING
• Tell patient to report any change in OTC drug, prescription drug, supplement, or herb use.
• Teach about proper drug administration and handling.
• Tell patient to immediately report chest pain, dyspnea, palpitations, excessive or prolonged diarrhea, diaphoresis, vomiting, or loss of appetite or thirst.
• Instruct patient to notify prescriber of pregnancy.
• Advise patient not to breastfeed while taking dofetilide.

dolutegravir–rilpivirine
doe-loo-TEG-ra-vir/ril-pi-VIR-een

Juluca

Therapeutic class: Antiretrovirals
Pharmacologic class: Integrase strand transfer inhibitors–NNRTIs

AVAILABLE FORMS
Tablets: 50 mg dolutegravir base/25 mg rilpivirine base

INDICATIONS & DOSAGES
➤ **HIV-1 infection in patients who are virologically suppressed (HIV-1 RNA less than 50 copies/mL) on a stable antiretroviral regimen for at least 6 months with no history of treatment failure and no known**

substitutions associated with resistance to the individual components of the drug
Adults: 1 tablet PO once daily.
Adjust-a-dose: If administered with rifabutin, give an additional 25-mg rilpivirine tablet once daily for the duration of rifabutin coadministration.

ADMINISTRATION
PO
• Give with a meal.
• If a dose is missed, give it as soon as possible. Don't double the next dose.
• Store in original bottle; don't remove desiccant. Protect from moisture.
• Store at 68° to 77° F (20° to 25° C).

ACTION
Dolutegravir inhibits HIV integrase by binding to the integrase active site and blocking retroviral DNA integration essential for HIV replication. Rilpivirine inhibits HIV-1 replication by noncompetitive inhibition of HIV-1 reverse transcriptase.

Route	Onset	Peak	Duration
PO (dolutegravir)	Unknown	3 hr	Unknown
PO (rilpivirine)	Unknown	4 hr	Unknown

Half-life: Dolutegravir, 14 hours; rilpivirine, 50 hours.

ADVERSE REACTIONS
CNS: headache, depressive disorders (including *suicidality*), fatigue, dizziness, somnolence, anxiety, insomnia, sleep disorders, abnormal dreams. **GI:** diarrhea, abdominal pain or discomfort, flatulence, nausea, vomiting, decreased appetite. **GU:** membranous glomerulonephritis, mesangioproliferative glomerulonephritis, nephrolithiasis, kidney impairment. **Hepatic:** *liver toxicity,* cholecystitis, cholelithiasis, *hepatitis.* **Metabolic:** hyperglycemia. **Musculoskeletal:** myositis, decreased bone mineral density. **Skin:** rash, pruritus. **Other:** immune reconstitution syndrome.

INTERACTIONS
Drug-drug. *Antacids (aluminum hydroxide, magnesium hydroxide); drugs containing polyvalent cations (aluminum, magnesium) such as buffered drugs, cation-containing products or laxatives, sucralfate:* May decrease rilpivirine level. Administer drug 4 hours before or 6 hours after antacids or cation-containing drug.

Anticonvulsants (carbamazepine, oxcarbazepine, phenobarbital, phenytoin): May decrease dolutegravir and rilpivirine levels, resulting in loss of virologic response. Use together is contraindicated.

Calcium and iron supplements (oral), multivitamins containing calcium or iron: May decrease dolutegravir level. Administer supplements and dolutegravir–rilpivirine together with a meal or give supplements 4 hours before or 6 hours after dolutegravir–rilpivirine.

Clarithromycin, erythromycin: May increase rilpivirine level. Consider alternative antibiotics, such as azithromycin.

Dalfampridine: May increase dalfampridine level and risk of seizures. Weigh benefits of concomitant therapy against seizure risk. Consider alternative treatments.

Dexamethasone (systemic): May decrease rilpivirine level when dexamethasone is given as more than a single-dose treatment, resulting in loss of virologic response. Use together is contraindicated except for a single dose of dexamethasone.

Dofetilide: May increase dofetilide level, causing serious or life-threatening events. Use together is contraindicated.

Drugs known to prolong QTc interval and increase risk of torsades de pointes (amiodarone, erythromycin, haloperidol, oxycodone): May increase risk of QT-interval prolongation and torsades de pointes. Avoid use together.

H₂-receptor antagonists (cimetidine, famotidine): May decrease rilpivirine level. Give dolutegravir–rilpivirine at least 4 hours before or 12 hours after H₂-receptor antagonist.

Metformin: May increase metformin level. When used together, limit metformin to 1,000 mg daily when starting metformin or dolutegravir–rilpivirine. When starting or stopping dolutegravir–rilpivirine, monitor glucose level and adjust metformin dosage. Monitor glucose level when initiating concomitant use and after withdrawal of dolutegravir–rilpivirine.

Methadone: May decrease methadone level. No dosage adjustments are required when starting administration of methadone. Monitor patients on methadone maintenance therapy because dosage adjustments may be needed.

Other antiretrovirals to treat HIV-1: Dolutegravir–rilpivirine is a complete regimen. Use with other antiretrovirals isn't recommended.

PPIs (lansoprazole, omeprazole): May decrease rilpivirine level due to gastric pH increase, which may result in loss of virologic response. Use together is contraindicated.

Rifabutin: May decrease rilpivirine level. Give an additional 25-mg tablet of rilpivirine once daily for duration of rifabutin coadministration.

Rifampin, rifapentine: May decrease dolutegravir and rilpivirine levels, resulting in loss of virologic response. Use together is contraindicated.

Drug-herb. *St. John's wort:* May decrease dolutegravir and rilpivirine levels, resulting in loss of virologic response. Use together is contraindicated.

EFFECTS ON LAB TEST RESULTS
• May increase creatinine, ALT, AST, total bilirubin, CK, lipase, and glucose levels.
• May decrease cortisol level.

CONTRAINDICATIONS & CAUTIONS
• Contraindicated in patients hypersensitive to dolutegravir, rilpivirine, or other components of the tablet.
• Use cautiously in patients with underlying HBV or HCV infection or marked elevations in transaminase levels before treatment. Drug may increase risk of worsening or development of transaminase elevations, immune reconstitution syndrome, or HBV reactivation.
• Use cautiously in older adults and in patients with CKD or Child-Pugh class C liver impairment.
• Safety and effectiveness in children haven't been established.
Dialyzable drug: Unlikely.

PREGNANCY-LACTATION-REPRODUCTION
🔹 *Alert:* Dolutegravir may increase risk of neural tube birth defects, especially when taken at the time of conception and during the first trimester. Prescribers should weigh risks and benefits of drug and consider use of alternative antiretrovirals before prescribing dolutegravir–rilpivirine to patients of childbearing potential.
🔹 *Alert:* Patients of childbearing potential using drug should use consistent, effective contraception.

Reactions in bold italics are *life-threatening*.

❸ *Alert:* Enroll patients exposed to drug during pregnancy in the Antiretroviral Pregnancy Registry (1-800-258-4263).
• The CDC recommends that patients infected with HIV-1 shouldn't breastfeed due to the potential risk of HIV-1 transmission to the infant. Dolutegravir is present in human milk.

NURSING CONSIDERATIONS

❸ *Alert:* Verify pregnancy status before start of therapy. Don't start drug in patient actively trying to become pregnant unless no suitable alternative is available.
❸ *Alert:* Drug may cause hypersensitivity reactions such as DRESS syndrome with organ dysfunction, including liver injury. Monitor LFT values and initiate appropriate therapy.
❸ *Alert:* Monitor patient for severe rash (or rash accompanied by fever, general malaise, skin blisters or skin peeling, oral blisters or lesions, conjunctivitis, facial edema, hepatitis, eosinophilia, angioedema, or difficulty breathing). Immediately discontinue drug if these signs or symptoms occur; delay in stopping drug may result in a life-threatening reaction.
• Monitor patient for severe depressive symptoms (depressed mood, depression, dysphoria, major depression, altered mood, negative thoughts, suicidality). Promptly evaluate symptoms to assess whether they are related to drug and to determine whether risks of continued therapy outweigh benefits.
• Monitor patient for signs and symptoms of liver toxicity (elevated LFT values, yellowing of skin or whites of eyes, dark urine, pale-colored stools, nausea, vomiting, loss of appetite, right-sided abdominal pain or tenderness), especially in patients with HBV or HCV infection, who may be at increased risk. Liver toxicity has also occurred in patients without preexisting liver disease or identifiable risk factors.
• *Look alike–sound alike:* Don't confuse rilpivirine with ritonavir. Don't confuse Juluca with Januvia.

PATIENT TEACHING

• Teach patient to report all adverse reactions and to immediately stop drug and report a rash with signs or symptoms of hypersensitivity, DRESS syndrome, or liver toxicity.
• Tell patient to report all drugs and supplements being taken before start of therapy because drug interactions can lead to loss of therapeutic effect, development of resistance, and an increase in adverse reactions.
• Advise patient that drug isn't a cure for HIV or AIDS. Stress the importance of taking drug as directed and staying on continuous antiretroviral therapy to control HIV infection and prevent resistance to therapy.
• Teach about proper drug administration and handling.
• Caution patient and caregiver to immediately report depressive symptoms (depressed mood, depression, dysphoria, major depression, altered mood, negative thoughts, suicidality).
• Advise patient to immediately report pregnancy, plans to become pregnant, breastfeeding, or intent to breastfeed during treatment.
• Caution patient not to breastfeed during therapy.

donepezil hydrochloride
doe-NEP-eh-zill

Adlarity, Aricept, Aricept ODT

Therapeutic class: Anti-Alzheimer drugs
Pharmacologic class: Acetylcholinesterase inhibitors

AVAILABLE FORMS
Tablets: 5 mg, 10 mg, 23 mg
Tablets (ODTs): 5 mg, 10 mg
Transdermal patch: 5 mg/day, 10 mg/day

INDICATIONS & DOSAGES
➤ **Mild to moderate Alzheimer dementia**
Adults: 5 mg PO once daily for 4 to 6 weeks; may then increase dosage to 10 mg PO once daily.
➤ **Moderate to severe Alzheimer dementia**
Adults: Initially, 5 mg PO once daily for 4 to 6 weeks; may then increase dose to 10 mg PO once daily. After 3 months, may increase dose to 23 mg PO once daily.
➤ **Mild, moderate, or severe Alzheimer dementia**
Adults: 5 mg/day transdermal patch applied once weekly. After 4 to 6 weeks, may increase to maximum dose of 10 mg/day. May switch patients taking 5 or 10 mg of PO donepezil to once-weekly transdermal patch at the same dose. May switch patients taking 5 mg PO donepezil for at least 4 weeks immediately to once weekly 10 mg/day transdermal system.

ADMINISTRATION
PO
• Allow ODT to dissolve on tongue; then follow with water.
• Give drug at bedtime, without regard for food.
• Don't split or crush tablets.
Transdermal
• When switching from PO, apply first patch with the last oral dose.
• Remove from refrigerator and allow pouch to reach room temperature before opening. Don't apply a cold patch. Don't use heat source to warm patch.
• Use within 24 hours of warming.
• At the end of 7 days, remove patch and apply a new one; apply only one patch at a time.
• Apply to back (avoid spine) or, if needed, may apply to upper buttocks or upper outer thigh on skin that won't be rubbed by tight clothing.
• Don't apply to same location for at least 2 weeks.
• Apply patch immediately after removing from pouch to clean, dry, intact skin with minimal hair.
• Press down firmly for 30 seconds to ensure good contact at edges of patch.
• Don't apply where medication, cream, lotion, or powder has recently been applied and don't apply to reddened, irritated, or cut skin. Don't shave the site.
• Patch may remain on for bathing.
• Avoid prolonged exposure of patch to external heat sources (sunlight, saunas, heating pads).
• If patch falls off or a dose is missed, immediately apply new patch; then replace 7 days later.
• Store in refrigerator at 36° to 46° F (2° to 8° C).

ACTION
Inhibits acetylcholinesterase, the enzyme that causes acetylcholine hydrolysis, resulting in increased acetylcholine available for synaptic transmission in the CNS.

Route	Onset	Peak	Duration
PO	Unknown	3–8 hr	Unknown
Transdermal	Unknown	7 days	Unknown

Half-life: 70 hours (oral); 91 hours (patch).

ADVERSE REACTIONS
CNS: headache, insomnia, *seizures,* dizziness, fatigue, depression, somnolence, syncope, pain, hallucinations, abnormal dreams, hostility, nervousness, fever, confusion, emotional lability, personality disorder. **CV:** chest pain, HTN, hypotension, *hemorrhage.* **GI:** nausea, diarrhea, vomiting, anorexia, abdominal pain, *GI bleeding.* **GU:** urinary incontinence, urinary frequency, UTI. **Metabolic:** weight loss, dehydration, increased CK level, hyperlipidemia. **Musculoskeletal:** muscle cramps, arthritis, back pain. **Respiratory:** dyspnea, bronchitis. **Skin:** eczema, diaphoresis, ecchymosis, laceration; application-site pruritus, dermatitis, or pain. **Other:** accidental injury, infection.

INTERACTIONS
Drug-drug. *Anesthesia:* May exaggerate succinylcholine-type muscle relaxation during anesthesia. Use together cautiously.
Anticholinergics (diphenhydramine, scopolamine): May decrease donepezil effects. Avoid use together.
Drugs that prolong QT interval: May increase risk of QT-interval prolongation. Monitor patient; consider therapy modification.
Neuromuscular blocking agents (succinylcholine): May have synergistic effect. Monitor patient closely.
NSAIDs: May increase gastric acid secretions. Monitor for active or occult GI bleeding.

EFFECTS ON LAB TEST RESULTS
• May increase CK and lipid levels.

CONTRAINDICATIONS & CAUTIONS
• Contraindicated in patients hypersensitive to drug or piperidine derivatives.
• Patches are contraindicated in patients with a history of allergic contact dermatitis with transdermal donepezil.
• Use cautiously in patients who have CV disease, are at risk for rhabdomyolysis and kidney failure, or have asthma, obstructive pulmonary disease, seizure disorders, or urinary outflow impairment.
• Drug may increase gastric acid secretion. Use cautiously in patients with a history of GI bleeding or ulcer disease.
• Drug may prolong QT interval and increase risk of torsades de pointes and may cause vagotonic bradycardia, heart block, or syncope. Use cautiously in patients with sick

---

Reactions in bold italics are *life-threatening*.

sinus syndrome, bradycardia, or conduction abnormalities.
• Some products contain aspartame; avoid use or use cautiously in patients with phenylketonuria.
Dialyzable drug: Unknown.
⚠ *Overdose S&S:* Severe nausea, vomiting, salivation, diaphoresis, bradycardia, hypotension, respiratory depression, collapse, seizures, increasing muscle weakness.

PREGNANCY-LACTATION-REPRODUCTION
• Studies during pregnancy are inadequate. Use during pregnancy only if clearly needed and potential benefit justifies fetal risk.
• It isn't known if drug appears in human milk. Use cautiously during breastfeeding.

NURSING CONSIDERATIONS
• Monitor patient for evidence of active or occult GI bleeding.
• Monitor patient for bradycardia because of potential for vagotonic effects.
• Monitor patient for signs and symptoms of GI intolerance (nausea, vomiting, diarrhea) at start of therapy and after dosage increases.
• Monitor patient who weighs less than 55 kg for increased nausea, vomiting, and weight loss.
• Monitor for application site reaction. Suspect contact dermatitis if reaction spreads beyond size of patch, if reaction is intense (increasing erythema, edema, papules, vesicles), or if symptoms don't improve within 48 hours of patch removal.
• *Look alike–sound alike:* Don't confuse Aricept with Ascriptin, Aciphex, or Azilect.

PATIENT TEACHING
• Stress that drug doesn't alter underlying degenerative disease but can temporarily stabilize or relieve symptoms. Effectiveness depends on taking drug at regular intervals.
• Teach about proper drug administration and handling.
• Advise patient and caregiver to immediately report significant adverse effects or changes in overall health status and to inform health care team that patient is taking drug before patient receives anesthesia.
• Tell patient to avoid OTC cold or sleep remedies because of risk of increased anticholinergic effects.

DOPamine hydrochloride
DOE-pa-meen

Therapeutic class: Vasopressors
Pharmacologic class: Adrenergics

AVAILABLE FORMS
Injection: 40 mg/mL; 80 mg/mL for IV infusion
Injection (premixed in D_5W): 0.8 mg/mL, 1.6 mg/mL, 3.2 mg/mL

INDICATIONS & DOSAGES
➤ **To treat shock and correct hemodynamic imbalances, to improve perfusion to vital organs, to increase cardiac output, to correct hypotension**
Adults: Initially, 2 to 5 mcg/kg/minute by IV infusion. Titrate dosage to desired hemodynamic or kidney response. In patients who are seriously ill, start with 5 mcg/kg/minute and increase gradually in increments of 5 to 10 mcg/kg/minute to a rate of 20 to 50 mcg/kg/minute, as needed.
Adjust-a-dose: In patients with occlusive vascular disease, consider decreasing dosage for changes in extremity skin color or temperature. Initial dopamine dosages shouldn't exceed one-tenth of the usual dosage in patients who have received MAO inhibitors within the prior 2 to 3 weeks.

ADMINISTRATION
IV
▼ Dilute vials (concentrated solution) before administration. Dilute with D_5W, NSS, D_5W in NSS or half-NSS, lactated Ringer solution, D_5W in lactated Ringer solution, or sodium lactate injection. Mix just before use.
▼ Use a central line or large vein (such as the antecubital fossa) to minimize risk of extravasation.
▼ Use a continuous infusion pump to regulate flow rate. Avoid inadvertent administration of a bolus of the drug.
Boxed Warning Watch infusion site carefully for extravasation; if it occurs, immediately stop infusion and call prescriber. To prevent sloughing and necrosis in ischemic areas, infiltrate the area with 5 to 10 mg phentolamine in 10 to 15 mL NSS as soon as possible. ∎

▼ Because solution rapidly deteriorates, discard after 24 hours or earlier if it's discolored.

▼ Don't use product if it's darker than slightly yellow or discolored in another way.

▼ **Incompatibilities:** Alkalies (including sodium bicarbonate), oxidizing agents, iron salts.

ACTION

Stimulates dopaminergic, alpha, and beta receptors of the sympathetic nervous system, resulting in a positive inotropic effect and increased cardiac output. Action is dose-related; large doses cause mainly alpha stimulation.

Route	Onset	Peak	Duration
IV	5 min	Unknown	<10 min after infusion

Half-life: 2 minutes.

ADVERSE REACTIONS

CNS: headache, anxiety. **CV:** hypotension, HTN, *arrhythmias,* ectopic beats, tachycardia, angina, palpitations, conduction abnormalities, *bradycardia,* vasoconstriction. **GI:** nausea, vomiting. **Metabolic:** azotemia. **Respiratory:** dyspnea. **Skin:** necrosis and tissue sloughing with extravasation, piloerection.

INTERACTIONS

Drug-drug. *Alpha and beta blockers:* May diminish vasocontricting effects. Monitor patient closely.

Ergot alkaloids: May cause extremely high BP. Avoid use together.

Haloperidol: May suppress kidney and mesenteric vasodilation. Monitor therapy.

Inhaled anesthetics (enflurane, isofluane): May increase risk of arrhythmias or HTN. Monitor patient closely.

⟲ *Alert:* MAO inhibitors (phenelzine, selegiline): May cause fever, hypertensive crisis, or severe headache. Avoid use together. If patient received MAO inhibitor in past 2 to 3 weeks, initial dopamine dose should be less than or equal to 10% of usual dose.

Oxytocics, vasopressors: May cause severe, persistent HTN. Use together cautiously.

Phenytoin: May cause severe hypotension, bradycardia, and cardiac arrest. Monitor patient carefully.

TCAs (amitriptyline, doxepin): May increase pressor response. Monitor patient closely.

EFFECTS ON LAB TEST RESULTS
• May increase catecholamine level.

CONTRAINDICATIONS & CAUTIONS
• Contraindicated in patients with uncorrected tachyarrhythmias, pheochromocytoma, or ventricular fibrillation.
• Use cautiously in patients with sulfite sensitivity. Hypersensitivity reactions, including anaphylaxis and asthmatic episodes, may occur.
• Use cautiously in patients with occlusive vascular disease, cold injuries, diabetic endarteritis, or arterial embolism and in those taking MAO inhibitors.
Dialyzable drug: Unlikely.
⚠ *Overdose S&S:* Excessive BP elevation.

PREGNANCY-LACTATION-REPRODUCTION
• Studies during pregnancy are inadequate. Use during pregnancy only if potential benefit justifies fetal risk.
• If vasopressors are used to correct hypotension or are added to a local anesthetic solution during labor or delivery, the interaction with some oxytocics may cause severe persistent HTN. Monitor patient closely.
• It isn't known if drug appears in human milk. Use cautiously during breastfeeding.

NURSING CONSIDERATIONS
• Most patients receive less than 20 mcg/kg/minute. Doses of 0.5 to 2 mcg/kg/minute mainly stimulate dopamine receptors and dilate the kidney vasculature. Doses of 2 to 10 mcg/kg/minute stimulate beta receptors for a positive inotropic effect. Higher doses also stimulate alpha receptors, constricting blood vessels and increasing BP.
• Correct hypovolemia, acidosis, and hypoxia before giving dopamine. Acidosis decreases effectiveness of drug.
• During infusion, frequently monitor ECG, BP, cardiac output, central venous pressure, pulmonary artery occlusion pressure, pulse rate, urine output, and color and temperature of limbs.
• If diastolic pressure rises disproportionately with a significant decrease in pulse pressure, decrease infusion rate and watch carefully for further evidence of predominant vasoconstrictor activity, unless such an effect is desired.
• Closely observe patient for adverse reactions; dosage may need to be adjusted or drug stopped.

Reactions in bold italics are *life-threatening*.

• Check urine output often. If urine flow decreases without hypotension, notify prescriber because dosage may need to be reduced.
⚡ *Alert:* After stopping drug, watch closely for sudden drop in BP. Taper dosage slowly to evaluate stability of BP, and provide IV fluids as clinically indicated to expand blood volume.
• *Look alike–sound alike:* Don't confuse dopamine with dobutamine.

PATIENT TEACHING
• Tell patient to promptly report adverse reactions.
• Instruct patient to immediately report discomfort at IV insertion site.

doxazosin mesylate
dox-AY-zo-sin

Cardura, Cardura XL

Therapeutic class: Antihypertensives
Pharmacologic class: Alpha blockers

AVAILABLE FORMS
Tablets (immediate-release): 1 mg, 2 mg, 4 mg, 8 mg
Tablets (extended-release) ⬛: 4 mg, 8 mg

INDICATIONS & DOSAGES
➤ **Essential HTN**
Adults: Initially, 1 mg immediate-release tablet PO daily. After initial dose and with each dosage increase, monitor BP for at least 6 hours. May increase to 2 mg and thereafter 4 mg and 8 mg once daily, if needed. Maximum daily dose is 16 mg, but doses over 4 mg daily increase the risk of adverse reactions. Don't use extended-release formulation to treat HTN.
➤ **BPH**
Adults: Initially, 1 mg immediate-release tablet PO once daily in the morning or evening; may increase at 1- or 2-week intervals to 2 mg and, thereafter, 4 mg and 8 mg once daily, if needed. Or, one 4-mg extended-release tablet once daily with breakfast. May increase to 8 mg in 3 to 4 weeks.

ADMINISTRATION
PO
• Have patient swallow extended-release tablets whole; don't crush or cut tablets.
• Give extended-release tablet with breakfast.

• Don't give evening dose the night before switching to extended-release tablets from immediate-release formula. Start extended-release tablets at lowest dose (4 mg once daily) the next morning.
• If therapy is interrupted for several days, restart drug at initial dosing regimen.

ACTION
Alpha$_1$ blocker that acts on the peripheral vasculature to reduce peripheral vascular resistance and produce vasodilation. Also decreases smooth muscle tone in the prostate and bladder neck.

Route	Onset	Peak	Duration
PO	Unknown	2–3 hr	24 hr
PO (XL)	Unknown	8–9 hr	24 hr

Half-life: Extended-release, 15 to 19 hours; immediate-release, 22 hours.

ADVERSE REACTIONS
CNS: dizziness, asthenia, headache, vertigo, somnolence, malaise, drowsiness, pain, fatigue. **CV:** orthostatic hypotension, *arrhythmias,* hypotension, edema. **EENT:** rhinitis, dry mouth. **GI:** abdominal pain, nausea, dyspepsia. **GU:** polyuria, UTI. **Hematologic:** *leukopenia, neutropenia.* **Musculoskeletal:** myalgia. **Respiratory:** dyspnea, respiratory tract infection.

INTERACTIONS
Drug-drug. *Antihypertensives, diuretics:* May increase hypotensive effects. Adjust dosages as necessary.
PDE5 inhibitors (sildenafil, tadalafil, vardenafil): May cause additive hypotensive effects and symptomatic hypotension. Initiate PDE5 therapy at lowest possible dosage.
Strong CYP3A4 inhibitors (atazanavir, clarithromycin, ketoconazole, ritonavir): May increase doxazosin level. Use together with caution; monitor BP and watch for hypotension signs and symptoms.
Drug-herb. *Ma huang:* May decrease antihypertensive effects. Discourage use together.

EFFECTS ON LAB TEST RESULTS
• May decrease WBC and neutrophil counts.

CONTRAINDICATIONS & CAUTIONS
• Contraindicated in patients hypersensitive to drug and quinazoline derivatives (including prazosin and terazosin).

• Use cautiously in patients with impaired liver function. Drug isn't recommended for use in patients with Child-Pugh class C liver impairment.
• Intraoperative floppy iris syndrome has been observed during cataract surgery in some patients on or previously treated with alpha₁ blockers.
• Rarely, drug has been associated with priapism (painful penile erection, sustained for hours and unrelieved by sexual intercourse or masturbation), which can lead to permanent erectile dysfunction if not promptly treated.
• Safety and effectiveness in children haven't been established.
Dialyzable drug: No.
⚠ *Overdose S&S:* Hypotension.

PREGNANCY-LACTATION-REPRODUCTION
• Studies during pregnancy are inadequate. Use immediate-release form during pregnancy only if clearly needed; extended-release form isn't indicated for use in females.
• Drug may appear in human milk. Use immediate-release form cautiously.

NURSING CONSIDERATIONS
• Monitor BP closely. Observe for signs and symptoms of hypotension.
• If syncope occurs, place patient in a recumbent position and treat supportively. A transient hypotensive response isn't considered a contraindication to continued therapy.
• Rule out prostate cancer before starting treatment for BPH.
• Watch for new or worsening angina, especially in patient with acute MI within the last 6 months, or HF.
• *Look alike–sound alike:* Don't confuse doxazosin with doxapram, doxorubicin, or doxepin. Don't confuse Cardura with Cardene.

PATIENT TEACHING
• Instruct patient to take drug exactly as prescribed.
🔔 *Alert:* Advise patient that a first-dose effect (marked low BP on standing up, with dizziness or fainting) may occur. This effect is most common after first dose but can also occur during dosage adjustment or interruption of therapy.
• Instruct patient to consult prescriber if dizziness or palpitations are bothersome.
• Caution patient to rise slowly from sitting or lying position.

• Advise patient to avoid driving and other hazardous activities until drug's effects are known.
• Instruct patient to inform surgeon of alpha₁-blocker therapy before having cataract surgery.
• Inform patient that drug has been associated with rare, but serious, priapism. Instruct patient to seek immediate medical treatment for a painful penile erection lasting longer than 4 hours.
• Advise patient not to be concerned if an extended-release tablet occasionally appears in stool. Explain that drug is contained within nonabsorbable shell designed to release drug at controlled rate. Empty tablet is eliminated from body through the stool.

doxepin hydrochloride
DOKS-eh-pin

Silenor

Therapeutic class: Antidepressants
Pharmacologic class: TCAs

AVAILABLE FORMS
Capsules: 10 mg, 25 mg, 50 mg, 75 mg, 100 mg, 150 mg
Oral concentrate: 10 mg/mL
Tablets: 3 mg, 6 mg

INDICATIONS & DOSAGES
➤ **Depression; anxiety**
Adults: Initially, 75 mg PO daily. Usual dosage range is 75 to 150 mg daily to maximum of 300 mg daily in divided doses. Mild symptoms may require only 25 to 50 mg/day. Or, may give entire maintenance dose once daily to a maximum dose of 150 mg/day at bedtime.
➤ **Insomnia (Silenor only)**
Adults: 6 mg PO once daily within 30 minutes of bedtime.
Adjust-a-dose: For older adults, give 3 mg PO once daily within 30 minutes of bedtime. May increase daily dose to 6 mg if indicated. For patients with liver impairment, initial dose is 3 mg PO once daily. For administration with cimetidine, give maximum dose of 3 mg once daily.

ADMINISTRATION
PO
• Dilute oral concentrate with 4 oz (120 mL) of water, milk, or juice (orange, grapefruit, tomato, prune, or pineapple, but not grape);

don't mix preparation with carbonated beverages.
• Give at bedtime, if possible, because it may cause drowsiness and dizziness.
• Don't give Silenor within 3 hours of a meal to minimize potential for next-day effect.

ACTION
Increases amount of norepinephrine, serotonin, or both in the CNS by blocking their reuptake by presynaptic neurons.

Route	Onset	Peak	Duration
PO	Unknown	3.5 hr	Unknown

Half-life: About 15 hours.

ADVERSE REACTIONS
CNS: drowsiness, dizziness, *seizures,* confusion, numbness, hallucinations, paresthesia, ataxia, weakness, headache, extrapyramidal reactions, tardive dyskinesia, tremor, taste disturbance, fatigue. **CV:** hypotension, HTN, tachycardia, flushing. **EENT:** blurred vision, closed-angle glaucoma, mydriasis, tinnitus, dry mouth, aphthous stomatitis. **GI:** constipation, nausea, vomiting, indigestion, diarrhea, anorexia, gastroenteritis. **GU:** urine retention, change in libido, testicular swelling. **Hepatic:** jaundice. **Metabolic:** *hypoglycemia,* hyperglycemia, weight gain. **Respiratory:** asthma exacerbation, URI. **Skin:** diaphoresis, rash, urticaria, photosensitivity reactions, alopecia. **Other:** hypersensitivity reactions, breast enlargement, galactorrhea, chills.

INTERACTIONS
Drug-drug. *Barbiturates, CNS depressants:* May enhance CNS depression. Avoid use together.
Cimetidine: May increase doxepin level. If Silenor is used with cimetidine, maximum Silenor dose of 3 mg is recommended in adults and patients who are older.
Drugs metabolized by CYP2D6 (flecainide, phenothiazines, propafenone, quinidine, SSRIs [fluoxetine, fluvoxamine, paroxetine, sertraline]): May increase doxepin level. Monitor drug levels and watch for signs and symptoms of toxicity.
Linezolid, methylene blue: May cause serotonin syndrome. Use with extreme caution and monitor patient closely.
MAO inhibitors: May increase risk of serotonin syndrome. Contraindicated within 14 days of MAO inhibitor therapy.

Quinolones: May increase risk of life-threatening arrhythmias. Avoid use together.
Tolazamide: May increase risk of severe hypoglycemia. Monitor patient closely.
Drug-herb. *Evening primrose oil:* May cause additive or synergistic effect, resulting in lower seizure threshold and increasing the risk of seizure. Discourage use together.
St. John's wort, SAM-e, yohimbe: May cause serotonin syndrome. Discourage use together.
Drug-lifestyle. *Alcohol use:* May enhance CNS depression. Discourage use together.
Sun exposure: May increase risk of photosensitivity reactions. Advise patient to avoid excessive sunlight exposure.

EFFECTS ON LAB TEST RESULTS
• May increase or decrease glucose level.
• May increase LFT values.

CONTRAINDICATIONS & CAUTIONS
• Contraindicated in patients hypersensitive to drug and in those with glaucoma or tendency toward urine retention.
Boxed Warning Doxepin isn't approved for use in children. Clinicians considering use of doxepin in a child, adolescent, or young adult must weigh risk against clinical need. ∎
Boxed Warning Drug may increase risk of suicidality in children, adolescents, and young adults ages 18 to 24, especially during the first few months of treatment, especially in those with major depressive disorder or other psychiatric disorder. ∎
🔹 *Alert:* Use with linezolid or methylene blue can cause serotonin syndrome. Use together only for life-threatening or urgent conditions when the potential benefits outweigh the risks of toxicity.
• Avoid use in patients with bipolar disorder. Drug isn't approved to treat bipolar depression.
• Drug may increase risk of SIADH and hyponatremia, especially in females, older adults, and patients who are volume depleted; in those with concurrent diuretic use; and in patients with low body weight or debilitation.
Dialyzable drug: No.
⚠ *Overdose S&S:* Cardiac arrhythmias, severe hypotension, seizures, CNS depression, coma, confusion, disturbed concentration, transient visual hallucinations, dilated pupils, agitation, hyperactive reflexes, stupor, drowsiness, muscle rigidity, vomiting, hypothermia, hyperpyrexia.

PREGNANCY-LACTATION-REPRODUCTION

• Studies during pregnancy are inadequate. Use during pregnancy only if clearly needed and potential benefit justifies fetal risk.

• Drug appears in human milk. Patients shouldn't breastfeed due to risk of excess sedation and respiratory depression.

NURSING CONSIDERATIONS

• Don't withdraw drug abruptly; gradually taper dosage to minimize withdrawal symptoms.

• Monitor patient for nausea, headache, and malaise after abrupt withdrawal of long-term therapy; these symptoms don't indicate addiction.

⚠ Alert: If linezolid or methylene blue must be given, stop drug and monitor patient for serotonin toxicity for 2 weeks, or until 24 hours after the last dose of methylene blue or linezolid, whichever comes first. Signs and symptoms include fever, mental status changes, muscle twitching, diaphoresis, shivering or shaking, diarrhea, and loss of coordination. Treatment may resume 24 hours after last dose of methylene blue or linezolid.

• If signs or symptoms of psychosis occur or increase, expect prescriber to reduce dosage. Record mood changes. Monitor patient for suicidality, and allow only a minimum supply of drug.

• If using drug for insomnia and symptoms don't resolve after 10 days, evaluate for primary psychiatric or medical illness.

Boxed Warning Monitor all patients for clinical worsening, suicidality, or unusual changes in behavior. ∎

• Drug has strong anticholinergic effects and is one of the most sedating TCAs. Adverse anticholinergic effects can occur rapidly.

• **Look alike–sound alike:** Don't confuse doxepin with doxazosin, digoxin, or doxapram.

PATIENT TEACHING

⚠ Alert: Teach patient to recognize and immediately report symptoms of serotonin toxicity.

• Teach about proper drug administration and handling.

• Warn patient not to stop drug suddenly.

Boxed Warning Advise families and caregivers to closely observe patient for increased suicidality. ∎

• Tell patient to take full dose at bedtime whenever possible but to watch for possible morning dizziness on standing up quickly.

• Advise patient to consult prescriber before taking other prescription or OTC drugs.

• Warn patient to avoid hazardous activities that require alertness and good psychomotor coordination until effects of drug are known. Drowsiness and dizziness usually subside after a few weeks.

• Advise patient to report episodes of complex sleep behaviors (driving, preparing and eating food, making phone calls, or having sex while not fully awake, with amnesia of the event).

• Caution patient to avoid alcohol during drug therapy.

• Tell patient that antianxiety effect is apparent before antidepressant effect; maximal effect may not be evident for 2 to 3 weeks.

• To prevent sensitivity to the sun, advise patient to use sunblock, wear protective clothing, and avoid prolonged exposure to strong sunlight.

• Recommend use of sugarless hard candy or gum to relieve dry mouth.

SAFETY ALERT!

DOXOrubicin hydrochloride
dox-oh-ROO-bi-sin

Adriamycin

Therapeutic class: Antineoplastics
Pharmacologic class: Anthracycline glycoside antibiotics

AVAILABLE FORMS

Injection (preservative-free): 2 mg/mL
Powder for injection: 10 mg, 20 mg, 50 mg

INDICATIONS & DOSAGES

Adjust-a-dose (for all indications): Refer to manufacturer's instructions for toxicity-related dosage adjustments.

➤ **Metastatic bladder, breast, lung, ovarian, stomach, and thyroid cancers; non-Hodgkin lymphoma; Hodgkin lymphoma; acute lymphoblastic or myeloblastic leukemia; Wilms tumor; neuroblastoma; lymphoma; soft-tissue and bone sarcomas**
Adults and children: 60 to 75 mg/m^2 IV as single dose every 21 days, or 40 to 75 mg/m^2 IV every 21 to 28 days when used in combination with other chemotherapy drugs.

➤ **Adjuvant treatment as a component of multiagent chemotherapy in females with evidence of axillary lymph node**

D

involvement after resection of primary breast cancer

Adult females: 60 mg/m² IV bolus on day 1 of each 21-day treatment cycle in combination with cyclophosphamide for a total of four cycles.

➤ **Endometrial carcinoma ◆**

Adults: 60 mg/m² IV on day 1 of each 21-day treatment cycle for eight cycles in combination with cisplatin, or as a single agent until disease progression or unacceptable toxicity occurs.

➤ **Multiple myeloma ◆**

Adults: In combination with other chemotherapy drugs, 9 mg/m²/day IV on days 1 to 4 for three cycles or 10 mg/m²/day IV as a continuous infusion on days 1 to 4 of each cycle.

➤ **Uterine sarcoma ◆**

Adults: 60 mg/m² IV on day 1 of each 21-day treatment cycle; maximum cumulative dose, 480 mg/m². Or, 50 mg/m² IV (over 15 minutes) on day 1 of each 21-day treatment cycle in combination with ifosfamide/mesna; maximum cumulative dose, 450 mg/m².

➤ **Waldenström macroglobulinemia ◆**

Adults: 50 mg/m² IV on day 1 of each 21-day treatment cycle for four to eight cycles in combination with other chemotherapy drugs.

ADMINISTRATION

IV

⚠ *Alert:* Hazardous drug; use safe handling and disposal precautions.

▼ Never give drug IM or subcut.

Boxed Warning If extravasation occurs, immediately stop infusion, apply ice to affected area, and notify prescriber. Extravasation can result in severe local tissue injury and necrosis requiring wide excision and skin grafting. ∎

▼ Reconstitute with preservative-free NSS for injection to yield 2 mg/mL; add 5 mL to 10-mg vial, 10 mL to 20-mg vial, or 25 mL to 50-mg vial. Shake vial to dissolve drug.

▼ Don't place IV catheter over joints or in limbs with poor venous or lymphatic drainage.

▼ Give by direct injection over 3 to 10 minutes through CVAD or into tubing of free-flowing IV solution containing D₅W or NSS for injection.

▼ Give continuous IV infusion only through CVAD.

▼ If vein streaking proximal to the site of infusion or facial flushing occurs, slow

administration rate. If welts appear, stop drug and notify prescriber.

▼ Refrigerated, reconstituted solution is stable for 15 days; at room temperature, it's stable for 7 days.

▼ Protect reconstituted solution from light following preparation and until completion of infusion.

▼ **Incompatibilities:** Other drugs and alkaline solutions.

ACTION

Interferes with DNA-dependent RNA synthesis by intercalation.

Route	Onset	Peak	Duration
IV	Unknown	Unknown	Unknown

Half-life: Initial, 5 minutes; terminal, 20 to 48 hours.

ADVERSE REACTIONS

CNS: malaise. **CV:** cardiac depression, *arrhythmias, HF, acute left ventricular failure, irreversible cardiomyopathy, shock, myocarditis, pericarditis.* **GI:** nausea, vomiting, diarrhea, abdominal pain, stomatitis, esophagitis, anorexia, ulcer, mucositis. **GU:** transient red urine. **Hematologic:** anemia, *myelosuppression.* **Metabolic:** hyperuricemia, weight loss, weight gain. **Skin:** alopecia, severe cellulitis and tissue sloughing (extravasation), discolored sweat, pruritus, urticaria, rash, photosensitivity, facial flushing, radiation recall effect. **Other:** chills, systemic infection, *sepsis, anaphylaxis, secondary malignancy (acute myelogenous leukemia [AML], myelodysplastic syndrome).*

INTERACTIONS

Drug-drug. *CYP2D6, CYP3A4, or P-gp inhibitors (cyclosporine, erythromycin, ketoconazole, ritonavir, verapamil):* May increase doxorubicin level. Avoid use together. *CYP3A4 or P-gp inducers (carbamazepine, phenobarbital, phenytoin, rifampin):* May decrease doxorubicin level. Avoid use together. *Dexrazoxane:* May decrease tumor response and time to progression. Don't give dexrazoxane as a cardioprotectant at start of doxorubicin therapy. May consider use as a cardioprotectant in patients who have received a cumulative doxorubicin dose of 300 mg/m² and who will continue to receive doxorubicin.

Mercaptopurine: May increase risk of liver toxicity. Use together cautiously.

Paclitaxel: May decrease doxorubicin clearance. Give doxorubicin before paclitaxel if used together.

Trastuzumab: May increase risk of cardiac dysfunction. Avoid use together.

Vaccines (inactivated): May diminish therapeutic effect of vaccines. If patient is vaccinated during therapy, revaccinate 3 months after stopping immunosuppressant.

Vaccines (live-virus): May increase vaccine-related toxicities and decrease vaccine's therapeutic effects. Avoid use of live-virus vaccines with immunosuppressants.

Drug-herb. *St. John's wort:* May decrease doxorubicin level. Avoid use together.

EFFECTS ON LAB TEST RESULTS
• May increase transaminase, bilirubin, and uric acid levels.
• May decrease platelet and WBC counts.

CONTRAINDICATIONS & CAUTIONS
• Contraindicated in patients with history of sensitivity reactions to drug or its components.
• Contraindicated in patients with severe myocardial insufficiency, recent (past 4 to 6 weeks) MI, severe persistent drug-induced myelosuppression, Child-Pugh class C liver impairment, or serum bilirubin level above 5 mg/dL.
• Don't use in patients who had previous treatment with complete cumulative doses of doxorubicin, daunorubicin, idarubicin, or other anthracyclines or anthracenediones.
Boxed Warning Risk of secondary AML or myelodysplastic syndrome increases with anthracyclines, including doxorubicin. ■
Dialyzable drug: No.

PREGNANCY-LACTATION-REPRODUCTION
• May cause fetal harm. Advise patients of risk. Patients of childbearing potential and male patients with partners of childbearing potential should avoid pregnancy.
• Advise patients of childbearing potential to use effective nonhormonal contraception during and for 6 months after therapy ends. Advise male patients with partners of childbearing potential to use effective contraception during and for 6 months after therapy ends.
• Drug appears in human milk. Patient shouldn't breastfeed during therapy.

• Drug may cause oligospermia, azoospermia, and permanent loss of fertility in males. Sperm counts have returned to normal levels in some patients, which may occur several years after stopping treatment.
• Drug may cause amenorrhea, infertility, and premature menopause in females. Recovery of menses and ovulation is related to age at time of treatment.

NURSING CONSIDERATIONS
❸ **Alert:** Drug should be administered under the supervision of a physician experienced with cancer chemotherapeutic agents.
• Verify pregnancy status before starting treatment.
Boxed Warning Cardiomyopathy risk is proportional to the cumulative exposure, with incidence rates of 1% to 20% for cumulative doses ranging from 300 to 500 mg/m^2 when drug is given every 3 weeks. Cardiomyopathy risk is further increased with concomitant cardiotoxic therapy. Assess LVEF before, regularly during, and after doxorubicin treatment. ■
• Perform cardiac function studies, including a MUGA or echocardiogram, ECG, and LVEF, before treatment, periodically throughout therapy, and after therapy is completed.
• Monitor ECG for changes, such as sinus tachycardia, T-wave flattening, ST-segment depression, and voltage reduction.
• Take preventive measures, including adequate hydration of patient, before starting treatment. Rapid lysis of leukemic cells may cause hyperuricemia and TLS. Allopurinol may be ordered.
• Premedicate with antiemetic to reduce nausea.
• If skin or mucosal contact occurs, immediately wash with soap and water.
• Monitor LFT values at baseline and during therapy. Reduce dosage or discontinue drug in patients with elevated bilirubin level.
Boxed Warning Severe myelosuppression may occur, possibly resulting in hospitalization or death. ■
• Monitor CBC with differential, electrolyte levels, and kidney function values; monitor ECG during therapy.
• Leukopenia may occur during days 10 to 14, with recovery by day 21.
• If tachycardia develops, stop drug or slow rate of infusion, and notify prescriber.
Boxed Warning Myocardial toxicity, including acute left ventricular failure, may occur

---

Reactions in bold italics are *life-threatening*.

during therapy or months to years after termination of therapy. Assess LVEF regularly, during, and after treatment with doxorubicin. Children are at increased risk for developing delayed cardiotoxicity. ■

⟳ Alert: If signs of HF develop, stop drug and notify prescriber. HF can often be prevented by increasing frequency of ECG assessments or multigated radionuclide angiography as the cumulative dose exceeds 300 mg/m² when patient is also receiving or has received cyclophosphamide, trastuzumab, or radiation therapy to cardiac area.

• Esophagitis is common in patients who also have received radiation therapy.

⟳ Alert: Patient who has previously received radiation therapy is susceptible to radiation recall effect.

⟳ Alert: Reddish color of drug is similar to that of daunorubicin; don't confuse the two drugs.

• **Look alike–sound alike:** Don't confuse doxorubicin with doxorubicin liposomal, daunorubicin, or idarubicin.

PATIENT TEACHING

⟳ Alert: Advise patient to immediately report pain or burning at injection site during or after administration.

• Tell patient to report all adverse effects.

• Inform patient of increased risk of treatment-related leukemia.

• Instruct patient to watch for signs and symptoms of infection (fever, sore throat, fatigue) and bleeding (easy bruising, nosebleeds, bleeding gums, tarry stools) and to take temperature daily.

• Advise patient that orange to red urine for 1 to 2 days is normal and doesn't indicate presence of blood.

• Inform patient that hair loss may occur but that it's usually reversible. Hair may regrow 2 to 5 months after drug is stopped.

• Counsel patient to take antiemetics on a regular basis to avoid nausea and vomiting.

• Warn of fetal risk. Advise patient to use effective contraception during and after treatment.

• Caution patient not to breastfeed during therapy.

• Inform patient of changes to fertility.

• Warn patient that drug can cause irreversible heart muscle damage that may lead to HF and serious heart rhythm problems that may lead to death.

DOXOrubicin hydrochloride liposomal
dox-oh-ROO-bi-sin

Doxil

Therapeutic class: Antineoplastics
Pharmacologic class: Anthracycline glycoside antibiotics

AVAILABLE FORMS
Injection: 2 mg/mL

INDICATIONS & DOSAGES

Adjust-a-dose (for all indications): Refer to manufacturer's instructions for toxicity-related dosage adjustments.

➤ **Ovarian cancer that has progressed or recurred after platinum-based chemotherapy**
Adults: 50 mg/m² IV. Repeat treatment once every 28 days until disease progression or unacceptable toxicity occurs.

➤ **AIDS-related Kaposi sarcoma after failure of prior systemic chemotherapy or intolerance to such therapy**
Adults: 20 mg/m² IV every 21 days until disease progression or unacceptable toxicity occurs.

➤ **Multiple myeloma in patients who haven't previously received bortezomib and have received at least one prior therapy**
Adults: 30 mg/m² IV on day 4 of every 21-day cycle (administer after bortezomib) for eight cycles or until disease progression or unacceptable toxicity occurs.

➤ **Refractory metastatic breast cancer ◆**
Adults: 50 mg/m² IV every 4 weeks.

ADMINISTRATION
IV

⟳ Alert: Hazardous drug; use safe handling and disposal precautions. Immediately wash thoroughly with soap and water if drug contacts skin or mucosa.

▼ Don't give as undiluted suspension or IV bolus. Don't give IM or subcut.

▼ Dilute doses up to 90 mg in 250 mL D₅W using aseptic technique. Dilute doses exceeding 90 mg in 500 mL D₅W.

⟳ Alert: Carefully check label on IV bag before giving drug. Accidentally substituting doxorubicin hydrochloride liposomal for conventional doxorubicin hydrochloride may cause severe adverse reactions. The two products can't be substituted on a milligram-per-milligram basis.

▼ Don't use an in-line filter.

▼ Inspect product for particulate matter and discoloration before administration; don't use if precipitate or foreign matter is present.

▼ Initiate infusion at 1 mg/minute and, if no infusion-related reactions occur, increase rate to complete administration over 60 minutes. Monitor patient carefully during infusion. Never give as bolus injection.

Boxed Warning Serious, sometimes fatal, allergic infusion reactions can occur. Make sure emergency equipment and medications are available. Acute infusion-related reactions include flushing, shortness of breath, facial swelling, headache, chills, back pain, tightness in chest or throat, and hypotension. ■

▼ If extravasation occurs, immediately stop infusion and attempt to aspirate extravasated fluid before removing needle. Don't flush line or apply pressure to site. Apply ice to site intermittently for 15 minutes four times a day for 3 days. If extravasation is in an extremity, elevate the extremity. Restart infusion in another vein.

▼ Refrigerate diluted solution at 36° to 46° F (2° to 8° C) and give within 24 hours.

▼ **Incompatibilities:** Other IV drugs.

ACTION

Consists of doxorubicin hydrochloride encapsulated in liposomes. Inhibits DNA and RNA synthesis through intercalation.

Route	Onset	Peak	Duration
IV	Unknown	Unknown	Unknown

Half-life: 3.6 to 6.6 hours in first phase; 46.7 to 59.8 hours in second phase with doses of 10 to 20 mg/m^2.

ADVERSE REACTIONS

CNS: asthenia, paresthesia, headache, somnolence, dizziness, depression, insomnia, anxiety, malaise, emotional lability, fatigue, neuralgia, peripheral neuropathy, taste perversion, fever. **CV:** vasodilation, *DVT,* chest pain, hypotension, tachycardia, flushing, peripheral edema, *cardiomyopathy, HF, arrhythmias, cardiac arrest.* **EENT:** conjunctivitis, dry eyes, optic neuritis, retinitis, epistaxis, rhinitis, pharyngitis, sinusitis,

oral moniliasis, oral ulcers, glossitis. **GI:** nausea, vomiting, constipation, anorexia, diarrhea, abdominal pain, dyspepsia, enlarged abdomen, esophagitis, dysphagia, stomatitis, rectal bleeding, ileus. **GU:** UTI, hematuria, vaginal candidiasis. **Hematologic:** *leukopenia, neutropenia, thrombocytopenia,* anemia. **Hepatic:** hyperbilirubinemia, increased ALP level, increased transaminase levels. **Metabolic:** dehydration, weight loss, hypercalcemia, *hypokalemia,* hyponatremia. **Musculoskeletal:** myalgia, back pain. **Respiratory:** dyspnea, increased cough, pneumonia. **Skin:** rash, alopecia, dry skin, pruritus, ecchymosis, skin discoloration, skin disorder, exfoliative dermatitis, fungal dermatitis, acne, diaphoresis, palmar-plantar erythrodysesthesia. **Other:** allergic reaction, chills, herpes zoster, herpes simplex, infection, *infusion-related reactions.*

INTERACTIONS

No formal drug interaction studies have been conducted. However, doxorubicin hydrochloride liposomal may interact with drugs that interact with the conventional form of doxorubicin hydrochloride.

Drug-drug. *Other antineoplastics:* May increase toxicity of other antineoplastics. Use together cautiously.

EFFECTS ON LAB TEST RESULTS

• May increase bilirubin, calcium, ALT, and ALP levels.

• May decrease potassium and sodium levels.

• May decrease Hb level and neutrophil, platelet, and WBC counts.

• May prolong PT and increase INR.

CONTRAINDICATIONS & CAUTIONS

• Contraindicated in patients hypersensitive to conventional formulation of doxorubicin hydrochloride or any component of the liposomal form.

Boxed Warning May cause myocardial damage, including acute left ventricular failure. Risk is 11% when total cumulative doxorubicin dose is between 450 mg/m^2 and 550 mg/m^2. Risk of cardiomyopathy may be increased at lower cumulative doses in patients with prior mediastinal irradiation. Prior use of other anthracyclines or anthracenediones should be included in calculations of total cumulative dosage. ■

Reactions in bold italics are *life-threatening.*

• Give drug to patient with history of CV disease only when benefit outweighs risk.
• Safety and effectiveness in children haven't been established.
Dialyzable drug: Unknown.
⚠ *Overdose S&S:* Leukopenia, mucositis, thrombocytopenia.

PREGNANCY-LACTATION-REPRODUCTION
• Drug may cause fetal harm. Advise patients of fetal risk.
• Patients of childbearing potential and male patients with partners of childbearing potential should use effective contraception during therapy and for 6 months after final dose.
• It isn't known if drug appears in human milk. Patient should discontinue breastfeeding during treatment.
• Drug may cause oligospermia, azoospermia, and permanent loss of fertility.
• Drug may cause amenorrhea, infertility, and premature menopause in females. Recovery of menses and ovulation is related to age at time of treatment.

NURSING CONSIDERATIONS
• Verify pregnancy status before starting treatment.
• Consider previous or current therapy with related compounds such as daunorubicin when calculating total dose of drug to be given. HF and cardiomyopathy may occur after therapy ends.
Boxed Warning Assess left ventricular cardiac function (via multigated radionuclide angiogram scan or echocardiogram) before drug initiation, during treatment to detect acute changes, and after treatment to detect delayed cardiotoxicity. ■
• Monitor for infusion reactions (flushing, dyspnea, facial swelling, headache, chills, chest pain, back pain, chest and throat tightness, fever, tachycardia, pruritus, rash, cyanosis, syncope, bronchospasm, asthma, apnea, hypotension). Most reactions occur with first infusion. Ensure emergency equipment is readily available.
• Monitor for signs and symptoms of hand-foot syndrome, hematologic toxicity, and stomatitis. Manage these adverse reactions with dosage delays and adjustments.
Boxed Warning If an infusion-related reaction occurs, temporarily stop drug until resolution, then resume at a reduced infusion

rate. Discontinue infusion for serious or life-threatening reactions. ■
• Evaluate liver function before therapy, and reduce dosage for serum bilirubin level of 1.2 mg/dL or higher.
• Monitor CBC, including platelets, before each dose and frequently throughout therapy. Leukopenia is usually transient. Persistent severe myelosuppression may result in superinfection or hemorrhage. Patient may need G-CSF to support blood counts.
• Secondary oral cancers, primarily squamous cell carcinoma, have been reported during treatment and for up to 6 years after last dose in patients with long-term exposure to drug. Assess patients at regular intervals for the presence of oral ulceration or any oral discomfort that may indicate secondary oral cancer.
• *Look alike–sound alike:* Don't confuse doxorubicin with daunorubicin. Don't confuse Doxil with Paxil. Don't confuse regular formulation of doxorubicin with liposomal formulation.

PATIENT TEACHING
• Tell patient to notify prescriber of all adverse reactions, including signs and symptoms of hand-foot syndrome (tingling, burning, redness, flaking, bothersome swelling, small blisters, or small sores on palms of hands or soles of feet).
• Advise patient to report signs and symptoms of stomatitis (painful redness, swelling, sores in mouth).
• Inform patient of risk of secondary oral cancers.
• Warn patient to avoid exposure to people with infections. Tell patient to report temperature of 100.5° F (38° C) or higher.
• Tell patient to report nausea, vomiting, tiredness, weakness, rash, or hair loss.
• Advise patient of childbearing potential to avoid pregnancy and to use effective contraception during treatment and for 6 months after final dose. Instruct patient to discontinue breastfeeding during therapy.
• Caution male patient with partner of childbearing potential to use effective contraception during treatment and for 6 months after final dose.

---

doxycycline calcium
dox-i-SYE-kleen

Vibramycin

doxycycline hyclate
Doryx, Doryx MPC, Doxy 100, Vibramycin

doxycycline monohydrate
Apprilon✣, Oracea, Vibramycin

Therapeutic class: Antibiotics
Pharmacologic class: Tetracyclines

AVAILABLE FORMS
doxycycline calcium
Syrup: 50 mg/5 mL
doxycycline hyclate
Capsules: 50 mg, 100 mg
Injection: 100 mg, 200 mg
Tablets: 20 mg, 50 mg, 75 mg, 100 mg, 150 mg
Tablets (delayed-release) 🆕: 50 mg, 60 mg, 75 mg, 80 mg, 100 mg, 120 mg, 150 mg, 200 mg
doxycycline monohydrate
Capsules: 50 mg, 75 mg, 100 mg, 150 mg
Capsules (Oracea): 40 mg (30 mg immediate-release and 10 mg delayed release)
Oral suspension: 25 mg/5 mL
Tablets: 50 mg, 75 mg, 100 mg, 150 mg

INDICATIONS & DOSAGES
➤ **Infections caused by susceptible gram-positive and gram-negative organisms (including *Haemophilus ducreyi, Yersinia pestis, Francisella tularensis,* and *Campylobacter fetus*), *Rickettsiae* species, *Mycoplasma pneumoniae, Chlamydia trachomatis,* or *Borrelia burgdorferi* (Lyme disease); *Chlamydophila psittacosis;* granuloma inguinale; adjunctive therapy in acute intestinal amebiasis or severe acne (PO)**
Adults and children older than age 8 weighing 45 kg or more: 100 mg PO or 120 mg (Doryx MPC) PO every 12 hours on first day; then 100 mg PO or 120 mg Doryx MPC daily as a single dose or in two divided doses. Or, 200 mg IV on first day in one or two infusions; then 100 to 200 mg IV daily. Daily doses of 200 mg IV can be given as a single dose or in two divided doses.

Children older than age 8 weighing less than 45 kg for severe or life-threatening infections: 2.2 mg/kg PO or IV or 2.6 mg/kg Doryx MPC PO every 12 hours.
Children older than age 8 weighing less than 45 kg for less severe infections: 4.4 mg/kg PO or IV divided into two doses on first day of treatment, followed by maintenance dose of 2.2 mg/kg PO given as a single daily dose or divided into twice-daily doses or 2.2 to 4.4 mg/kg/day IV given as one or two infusions, depending on infection severity. Or, 5.3 mg/kg Doryx MPC PO divided into two doses on first day of treatment, followed by maintenance dose of 2.6 mg/kg given as a single daily dose or divided into twice-daily doses.

Give IV infusion slowly (minimum 1 hour). Refer to manufacturer's instructions for duration of therapy.
➤ **Uncomplicated gonococcal infections (except anorectal infections in men)**
Adults: 100 mg PO b.i.d. for 7 days. Or, 300 mg PO once, followed in 1 hour with a second 300-mg PO dose. Alternately, 120 mg Doryx MPC PO b.i.d. for 7 days. Or, 360 mg Doryx MPC PO followed by 360 mg PO in 1 hour.
➤ **Acute epididymo-orchitis caused by *Neisseria gonorrhoeae* or *C. trachomatis* (Doryx MPC)**
Adults: 120 mg PO b.i.d. for at least 10 days.
➤ **Syphilis in patients allergic to penicillins**
Adults: 100 mg PO or 120 mg Doryx MPC PO b.i.d. for 14 days (early). If more than 1-year duration, 100 mg PO or 120 mg Doryx MPC PO b.i.d. for 4 weeks.
➤ **Primary or secondary syphilis in patients allergic to penicillins**
Adults: 300 mg IV daily in divided doses for 14 days. Switch to oral therapy when possible.
➤ **Uncomplicated urethral, endocervical, or rectal infections caused by *C. trachomatis* or *Ureaplasma urealyticum***
Adults: 100 mg PO or 120 mg Doryx MPC b.i.d. for at least 7 days.
➤ **To prevent malaria**
Adults: 100 mg PO or 120 mg Doryx MPC PO daily beginning 1 to 2 days before travel to endemic area and continuing for 4 weeks after travel.
Children older than age 8: 2 mg/kg (2.4 mg/kg for Doryx MPC) PO once daily beginning 1 to 2 days before travel to endemic area and continuing for 4 weeks after travel. Don't

Reactions in bold italics are *life-threatening*.

exceed daily dose of 100 mg (excluding Doryx MPC).

➤ **Adjunct to other antibiotics for inhalation, GI, and oropharyngeal anthrax**
Adults: 100 mg every 12 hours IV initially until susceptibility test results are known. Switch to 100 mg PO or 120 mg Doryx MPC PO b.i.d. when appropriate. Treat for 60 days total.
Children older than age 8 weighing more than 45 kg: 100 mg every 12 hours IV; then switch to 100 mg PO b.i.d. when appropriate. Treat for 60 days total.
Children older than age 8 weighing 45 kg or less: 2.2 mg/kg every 12 hours IV; then switch to 2.2 mg/kg (up to 100 mg) PO b.i.d. when appropriate. Treat for 60 days total.
Children ages 8 and younger: 2.2 mg/kg IV every 12 hours; then switch to 2.2 mg/kg (up to 100 mg) PO b.i.d. when appropriate. Treat for 60 days total.

➤ **Inhalational anthrax (postexposure) (Doryx MPC)**
Adults and children weighing 45 kg or more: 120 mg PO b.i.d. for 60 days.
Children weighing less than 45 kg: 2.6 mg/kg PO b.i.d. for 60 days.

➤ **Cutaneous anthrax** ◆
Adults: 100 mg PO every 12 hours for 60 days.
Children older than age 8 weighing more than 45 kg: 100 mg PO every 12 hours for 60 days.
Children older than age 8 weighing 45 kg or less: 2.2 mg/kg (up to 100 mg) PO every 12 hours for 60 days.
Children ages 8 and younger: 2.2 mg/kg (up to 100 mg) PO every 12 hours for 60 days.

➤ **Inflammatory lesions of rosacea (Oracea)**
Adults: 40 mg PO once daily in the morning, 1 hour before or 2 hours after a meal. Reevaluate treatment after 16 weeks.

ADMINISTRATION
PO
• Obtain specimen for culture and sensitivity tests before giving first dose. Begin therapy while awaiting results.
• Doryx MPC and Oracea can't be substituted on a milligram-per-milligram basis with other oral doxyclines.
🛈 *Alert:* Check expiration date. Outdated or deteriorated tetracyclines may cause reversible kidney toxicity (Fanconi syndrome).
• Give drug with food or milk if stomach upset occurs.

• Increase fluid intake and don't administer tablets or capsules within 1 hour of bedtime because of possible esophageal irritation or ulceration.
• Give Oracea with a full glass of water.
• Don't crush delayed-release tablets or capsules. Delayed-released tablets can be cut into small pieces and capsules can be carefully broken apart and their contents sprinkled onto a spoonful of applesauce and swallowed without chewing.

IV
▼ Obtain specimen for culture and sensitivity tests before giving first dose. Begin therapy while awaiting results.
▼ Reconstitute powder for injection with sterile water for injection. Use 10 mL in 100-mg vial and 20 mL in 200-mg vial. Further dilute solution to a concentration of 0.1 mg/mL to 1 mg/mL; don't infuse solution that contains more than 1 mg/mL. Refer to manufacturer's instructions for compatible solutions.
▼ Don't expose drug to light or heat. Protect it from sunlight during infusion.
▼ Infusion time varies with dose but usually ranges from 1 to 4 hours.
▼ Monitor infusion site for evidence of thrombophlebitis.
▼ Reconstituted injectable solution is stable 72 hours if refrigerated and protected from light. After dilution, infusion must be completed within 12 hours or within 6 hours in lactated Ringer solution or dextrose 5% in lactated Ringer solution.
▼ **Incompatibilities:** Allopurinol, drugs that are unstable in acidic solutions (such as barbiturates), erythromycin lactobionate, heparin, meropenem, nafcillin, penicillin G potassium, piperacillin–tazobactam, riboflavin, sulfonamides. Refer to IV drug compatibilities reference for full listing.

ACTION
Exerts bacteriostatic effect by binding to the 30S and possibly 50S ribosomal subunits of microorganisms and inhibiting protein synthesis.

Route	Onset	Peak	Duration
PO	Unknown	1.5–4 hr	Unknown
PO (delayed-release)	Unknown	2–4 hr	Unknown
IV	Immediate	Unknown	Unknown

Half-life: About 1 day after multiple dosing.

ADVERSE REACTIONS

CNS: *intracranial HTN,* headache, anxiety, pain. **CV:** HTN, pericarditis, thrombophlebitis. **EENT:** nasopharyngitis, sinusitis, nasal congestion, dry mouth, glossitis, permanent tooth discoloration, enamel defects. **GI:** diarrhea, epigastric distress, nausea, anorexia, dysphagia, vomiting, oral candidiasis, enterocolitis, anogenital inflammatory lesions, esophagitis, abdominal distention, abdominal pain, *pancreatitis.* **GU:** vaginitis, vulvovaginal mycotic infection. **Hematologic:** *neutropenia, thrombocytopenia,* eosinophilia, hemolytic anemia. **Hepatic:** increased transaminase levels. **Metabolic:** hyperglycemia, increased LDH level. **Musculoskeletal:** back pain, bone growth retardation (in children younger than age 8). **Skin:** rash, photosensitivity reactions, increased pigmentation, urticaria. **Other:** superinfection, flulike symptoms, hypersensitivity reactions, *including anaphylaxis.*

INTERACTIONS

Drug-drug. *Antacids and laxatives containing aluminum, magnesium, or calcium; antidiarrheals:* May decrease antibiotic absorption. Give antibiotic 1 hour before or 2 hours after these drugs.

Barbiturates, carbamazepine, phenobarbital, phenytoin, rifamycins: May decrease antibiotic effect. Consider therapy modification.

Ferrous sulfate and other iron products, zinc: May decrease antibiotic absorption. Give drug 2 hours before or 3 hours after iron.

Isotretinoin: May increase risk of pseudotumor cerebri. Avoid use together.

Methoxyflurane: May cause kidney toxicity with tetracyclines. Avoid use together.

Penicillins: May interfere with bactericidal action of penicillins. Avoid use together.

Warfarin: May increase anticoagulant effect. Monitor PT and INR; adjust dosage.

Drug-lifestyle. *Alcohol use:* May decrease drug's effect. Discourage use together.

Sun exposure: May cause photosensitivity reactions. Advise patient to avoid excessive sunlight exposure.

EFFECTS ON LAB TEST RESULTS

• May increase BUN and liver enzyme levels and eosinophil count.

• May decrease Hb level and platelet, neutrophil, and WBC counts.

• May falsely elevate fluorometric tests for urine catecholamines. May cause false-negative results in urine glucose tests using glucose oxidase reagent (Diastix or Chem-strip uG). Parenteral form may cause false-positive Clinitest results.

CONTRAINDICATIONS & CAUTIONS

• Contraindicated in patients hypersensitive to drug or other tetracyclines.

• Use cautiously in patients with impaired kidney or liver function.

• CDAD ranging in severity from mild diarrhea to fatal colitis has been reported.

• In fetus in last half of gestation or in child younger than age 8, drug may cause permanently discolored teeth, enamel defects, and bone growth retardation. Don't use drug in this age-group unless other drugs aren't likely to be effective or are contraindicated.

• Use in patients ages 8 and younger only when potential benefits are expected to outweigh risks in severe or life-threatening conditions, such as anthrax or Rocky Mountain spotted fever, particularly when no alternative therapies are available.

• Drug doesn't completely suppress malaria of *Plasmodium* strains. Patients may still transmit infection to mosquitoes outside endemic areas.

• Don't use Oracea for treatment or prevention of infections. Oracea should only be used as indicated for rosacea.

Dialyzable drug: No.

⚠ *Overdose S&S:* Dizziness, nausea, vomiting.

PREGNANCY-LACTATION-REPRODUCTION

• Tetracyclines cross the placental barrier. Drug is generally considered a second-line antibiotic during pregnancy and use should be avoided. Use during pregnancy only when other drugs are contraindicated or ineffective.

• During pregnancy, use the usual dosage schedule for anthrax.

• Drug appears in human milk. Patient should take into account benefits of breastfeeding versus risk of exposure to infant.

NURSING CONSIDERATIONS

• If patient receives large doses or prolonged therapy or if patient is at high risk, watch for signs and symptoms of superinfection. If superinfection occurs, discontinue drug and institute appropriate therapy.

- Use usual dosage schedule for anthrax in patient who is immunocompromised.
- Use IV therapy and multidrug approach for cutaneous anthrax with signs of systemic involvement, extensive edema, or lesions on the head or neck.
- Ciprofloxacin and doxycycline are first-line therapies for anthrax. If patient with anthrax also has meningitis, ciprofloxacin is preferred because of better distribution to the CNS.
- Drug may increase risk of intracranial HTN (IH) and pseudotumor cerebri, especially in adult females who are overweight or have a history of IH. Monitor patient for headache, blurred vision, diplopia, and vision loss. If visual changes occur, prompt ophthalmic evaluation is needed.
- Monitor for signs and symptoms of autoimmune syndrome (fever, rash, arthralgia, malaise). If symptoms are present, evaluate LFT values, ANA, CBC, and other test results as appropriate.
- Check patient's tongue for signs of fungal infection. Emphasize good oral hygiene.
- Photosensitivity reactions may occur within a few minutes to several hours after exposure and may last after therapy ends. Discontinue drug at first evidence of skin erythema.
- Monitor for diarrhea. If CDAD is suspected or confirmed, ongoing antibiotic use not directed against *Clostridioides difficile* may need to be discontinued. Institute appropriate treatment.
- ***Look alike–sound alike:*** Don't confuse doxycycline with doxylamine or dicyclomine. Don't confuse Oracea with Orencia.

PATIENT TEACHING
- Tell patient to take entire amount of drug exactly as prescribed, even if feeling better.
- Instruct patient to promptly report adverse reactions, especially signs or symptoms of hypersensitivity or IH. If drug is being given IV, tell patient to report discomfort at IV site.
- Teach about proper drug administration and handling.
- Warn patient to avoid direct sunlight and UV light, wear protective clothing, and use sunscreen.
- Tell patient to report signs and symptoms of superinfection or CDAD to prescriber. CDAD has occurred over 2 months after antibiotic treatment.

doxylamine succinate–pyridoxine hydrochloride
docks-ILL-ah-meen/peer-reh-DOCK-seen

Bonjesta, Diclectin ✦, Diclegis

Therapeutic class: Antiemetics
Pharmacologic class: Antihistamines–vitamin B$_6$ analogues

AVAILABLE FORMS
Tablets (delayed-release) ⓄⓃⒸ*:* doxylamine succinate 10 mg/pyridoxine hydrochloride 10 mg
Tablets (extended-release) ⓄⓃⒸ*:* doxylamine succinate 20 mg/pyridoxine hydrochloride 20 mg

INDICATIONS & DOSAGES
➤ **Nausea and vomiting of pregnancy in patients who don't respond to conservative management**
Adult (delayed-release): 2 tablets at bedtime on day 1, then daily if that dosage adequately controls symptoms the next day. If symptoms persist into the afternoon of day 2, patients should take 2 tablets at bedtime that night, then take 1 tablet in the morning and 2 tablets at bedtime on day 3. If that dosage adequately controls symptoms on day 4, patients should continue taking 1 tablet in the morning and 2 tablets at bedtime. Otherwise, they should take 1 tablet in the morning, 1 tablet in the midafternoon, 2 tablets at bedtime on day 4. Maximum dose, 4 tablets/day.
Adult (extended-release): Initially, 1 tablet at bedtime on day 1. If symptoms aren't adequately controlled on day 2, increase dose to 1 tablet in the morning and 1 tablet at bedtime. Maximum dose is 1 tablet b.i.d.

ADMINISTRATION
PO
- Have patient swallow tablets whole with a glass of water on an empty stomach; don't crush or cut tablets.
- Patient should take tablets daily and not PRN.
- Store bottle at room temperature. Keep bottle tightly closed and protect from moisture. Don't remove desiccant canister from bottle.

ACTION
Unknown. The combination of antihistamine and vitamin B_6 may cause anticholinergic effects, decreasing nausea.

Route	Onset	Peak	Duration
PO (doxylamine)	Unknown	1.7–8.5 hr	Unknown
PO (pyridoxine)	Unknown	0.5–4.7 hr	Unknown

Half-life: Doxylamine, 11.9 hours (Bonjest), 12.5 hours (Diclegis); pyridoxine, 0.4 hour.

ADVERSE REACTIONS
CNS: somnolence.

INTERACTIONS
Drug-drug. *CNS depressants (sedative-hypnotics and tranquilizers):* May have additive effects. Don't use together.
MAO inhibitors (selegiline, tranylcypromine): May prolong and intensify CNS anticholinergic effects. Use together is contraindicated.
Other ethanolamine derivative antihistamines (diphenhydramine): May have additive effects. Avoid use together.
Drug-food. *Any food:* May delay onset and reduce absorption. Patient should take drug on an empty stomach.
Drug-lifestyle. *Alcohol use:* May cause additive CNS depression. Alcohol isn't recommended during pregnancy.

EFFECTS ON LAB TEST RESULTS
• May cause false-positive urine screening tests for methadone, opiates, and phencyclidine.

CONTRAINDICATIONS & CAUTIONS
• Contraindicated in patients hypersensitive to drug, its components, and other ethanolamine-derivative antihistamines.
• Use cautiously in patients with asthma, increased IOP, angle-closure glaucoma, stenosing peptic ulcer, or pyloroduodenal or urinary bladder neck obstruction because of anticholinergic effects.
• Safety and effectiveness in children haven't been established.
Dialyzable drug: Unknown.

PREGNANCY-LACTATION-REPRODUCTION
• Drug is intended for use during pregnancy. Drug hasn't been studied in patients with hyperemesis gravidarum.

• Drug appears in human milk and shouldn't be used during breastfeeding.

NURSING CONSIDERATIONS
• Reassess for continued need for drug as pregnancy progresses.
• Monitor patient for anticholinergic effects (dry mouth, tachycardia, urine retention, constipation, ataxia).
• Monitor patient for somnolence, increased falls, and other CNS depressant effects.

PATIENT TEACHING
• Warn patient about adverse reactions (somnolence, increased falls, other CNS depressant effects, dry mouth, dilated pupils, dizziness, confusion, fast heartbeat, fluid retention).
• Explain that patient should take drug as prescribed and not on an as-needed basis.
• Advise patient to avoid alcohol and sedating medications, including antihistamine cough and cold products, opioids, and sleep aids, while taking this drug because of increased risk of additive effects.
• Caution patient to avoid driving and operating heavy equipment or other activities that require complete mental alertness.

dronabinol (delta-9-tetrahydrocannabinol)
droe-NAB-i-nol

Marinol, Syndros

Therapeutic class: Antiemetics
Pharmacologic class: Cannabinoids
Controlled substance schedule: III (Marinol); II (Syndros)

AVAILABLE FORMS
Capsules: 2.5 mg, 5 mg, 10 mg
Oral solution: 5 mg/mL*

INDICATIONS & DOSAGES
➤ **Nausea and vomiting from cancer chemotherapy after failure of conventional antiemetics**
Adults and children: 5 mg/m^2 (capsules) PO 1 to 3 hours before chemotherapy session, then 5 mg/m^2 (capsules) PO every 2 to 4 hours after chemotherapy, for a total of four to six doses per day. If needed, increase dosage in 2.5-mg/m^2 increments to maximum of 15 mg/m^2 (capsules) per dose.

Reactions in bold italics are ***life-threatening***.

Adults: 4.2 mg/m^2 (oral solution) 1 to 3 hours before chemotherapy, then every 2 to 4 hours after chemotherapy for a total of four to six doses per day. If needed, increase oral solution dosage as tolerated in increments of 2.1 mg/m^2. Maximum dosage, 12.6 mg/m^2 (oral solution)/dose.

Adjust-a-dose: For older adults, initiate capsules at low end of dosing range; may initiate oral solution at 2.1 mg/m^2 once daily before chemotherapy to reduce risk of CNS symptoms.

➤ **Anorexia and weight loss in patients with AIDS**

Adults: 2.5 mg (capsules) PO b.i.d. 1 hour before lunch and dinner. If patient can't tolerate twice-daily dosing, decrease to 2.5 mg (capsules) PO given as a single dose daily before dinner or at bedtime. May gradually increase to maximum of 20 mg (capsules) daily given in divided doses. Or, 2.1 mg (oral solution) PO b.i.d. 1 hour before lunch and dinner. If needed, may gradually increase dosage to 2.1 mg (oral solution) PO 1 hour before lunch and 4.2 mg 1 hour before dinner. If needed, may further increase dosage to 4.2 mg (oral solution) PO 1 hour before lunch and 4.2 mg 1 hour before dinner. Maximum dosage, 8.4 mg b.i.d.

Adjust-a-dose: For older adults, initiate capsules at low end of dosing range; may initiate at 2.1 mg (oral solution) PO once daily 1 hour before dinner or at bedtime to reduce risk of CNS symptoms. For patients with severe or persistent CNS symptoms, may reduce dosage to 2.5 mg (capsules) PO or 2.1 mg (oral solution) PO once daily 1 hour before dinner or at bedtime.

ADMINISTRATION
PO
• Give 1 to 3 hours before chemotherapy.
• For nausea and vomiting, give first dose on an empty stomach at least 30 minutes before patient eats; can give subsequent doses without regard to meals.
• When giving for nausea and vomiting, keep timing of dosing in relation to meal times consistent for each chemotherapy cycle, once dosage has been determined from the titration process.
• Dosing later in the day may reduce frequency of CNS adverse reactions.
• Always use the calibrated oral dosing syringe when administering oral solution.

Patient should take each dose with 180 to 240 mL of water.
• Can give Syndros via a silicone enteral feeding tube, #14 French or greater. Don't use tubes made of polyurethane. If prescribed dose is greater than 5 mg, divide total dose and draw up in two or more portions using oral syringe. Flush feeding tube with 30 mL of water after administration.
• Store capsules in cool environment at 46° to 59° F (8° to 15°C) or refrigerator, but protect from freezing. May store opened bottle of oral solution at 77° F (25° C); discard unused oral solution 42 days after opening.

ACTION
Cannabinoid that potentiates the activity of CB-1 and CB-2 receptors.

Route	Onset	Peak	Duration
PO	30–60 min	0.5–4 hr	4–6 hr (psychoactive effect); >24 hr (appetite stimulation)

Half-life: 25 to 36 hours.

ADVERSE REACTIONS
CNS: ataxia, dizziness, euphoria, paranoia, amnesia, asthenia, confusion, depersonalization, hallucinations, abnormal thinking, somnolence, anxiety, nervousness. **CV:** orthostatic hypotension, palpitations, tachycardia, vasodilation, facial flushing. **GI:** abdominal pain, nausea, vomiting.

INTERACTIONS
Drug-drug. *CNS depressants, psychomimetic substances, sedatives, TCAs:* May cause additive CNS depression. Avoid use together. *CYP2C9 inhibitors (amiodarone, fluconazole), CYP3A4 inhibitors (clarithromycin, erythromycin, itraconazole, ketoconazole, ritonavir):* May increase dronabinol-related adverse reactions. Monitor carefully. *Disulfiram, metronidazole (Syndros only):* May cause disulfiram-like reaction. Discontinue products containing disulfiram or metronidazole at least 14 days before starting treatment and don't give them within 7 days of completing treatment. *Drugs with cardiac effects (anticholinergics, TCAs):* May have additive effects. Use together cautiously.
Drug-food. *Grapefruit juice:* May increase dronabinol-related adverse reactions. Discourage use together.

Drug-lifestyle. *Alcohol use:* May cause additive CNS depression. Discourage use together.

EFFECTS ON LAB TEST RESULTS
• May increase LFT values.

CONTRAINDICATIONS & CAUTIONS
• Contraindicated in patients hypersensitive to drug.
• Capsules are contraindicated in patients hypersensitive to sesame oil.
• Oral solution is contraindicated in patients hypersensitive to alcohol and within 14 days of products containing disulfiram or metronidazole.
• Oral solution contains propylene glycol; large amounts are toxic and are associated with hyperosmolarity, lactic acidosis, kidney toxicity, CNS depression, seizures, cardiac arrhythmias, ECG changes, and hemolysis. Use caution.
• Use cautiously in older adults and patients with heart disease, seizure disorders, or history of substance abuse disorder.
• Safety and effectiveness in children haven't been established.
Dialyzable drug: Unknown.
⚠ *Overdose S&S:* Drowsiness, euphoria, heightened sensory awareness, altered time perception, reddened conjunctivae, dry mouth, tachycardia, memory impairment, depersonalization, mood alteration, panic reactions, urine retention, decreased bowel motility, decreased motor coordination, lethargy, slurred speech, orthostatic hypotension; lactic acidosis, hypoglycemia, CNS depression, coma, seizures.

PREGNANCY-LACTATION-REPRODUCTION
• Drug may cause fetal harm. Avoid use during pregnancy.
• Data are limited on presence of dronabinol in human milk, its effects on infant who is breastfed, and its effects on milk production. Patients with HIV shouldn't breastfeed due to risk of postnatal HIV transmission. Use cautiously in patients with nausea and vomiting; closely monitor weight of breastfed infant.

NURSING CONSIDERATIONS
• Expect drug to be prescribed only for patient who hasn't responded satisfactorily to other antiemetics.

⚱ *Alert:* Drug is the principal active substance in *Cannabis sativa* (marijuana), which can produce both physiologic and psychological dependence and has a high risk of abuse. Use cautiously in patient receiving sedative, hypnotic, or other psychoactive drug.
• Assess patient's risk of abuse or misuse before drug is prescribed. Monitor patient for abuse or misuse behaviors during treatment.
▓ Patient who is known to carry genetic variants associated with CYP2C9 function (CYP2C9 polymorphism) has increased risk of adverse drug-related effects.
• Monitor patient for hypotension, HTN, syncope, and tachycardia.
• Monitor patient with history of seizure disorder for worsening of seizure control.
• Drug can exacerbate mania, depression, and schizophrenia. Screen patient for these illnesses before giving drug. If drug must be used, monitor patient for worsening signs and symptoms of psychiatric illness. Older adult may be more sensitive to drug's effects.
• CNS effects are intensified at higher dosages.
• Drug effects may persist for days after treatment ends.
• New or worsening nausea, vomiting, or abdominal pain can occur during treatment. Ask patient about these symptoms because patient may not recognize they're abnormal.
• *Look alike–sound alike:* Don't confuse dronabinol with droperidol.

PATIENT TEACHING
• Tell patient to report all adverse reactions; tell patient that drug may induce unusual changes in mood or other adverse behavioral effects.
• Advise patient to report new or worsening nausea, vomiting, or abdominal pain.
• Caution patient that oral solution can't be taken within 14 days of disulfiram or metronidazole.
• Advise patient against performing activities that require alertness until CNS effects of drug are known.
• Warn caregivers to supervise patient during and immediately after treatment.
• Caution patient to store drug securely.
• Instruct patient to immediately report pregnancy, plans to become pregnant, breastfeeding, or intent to breastfeed during treatment.

Reactions in bold italics are *life-threatening*.

dronedarone
dro-neh-DAR-rone

Multaq

Therapeutic class: Antiarrhythmics
Pharmacologic class: Benzofuran
derivatives

D

AVAILABLE FORMS
Tablets: 400 mg

INDICATIONS & DOSAGES
➤ **To reduce risk of hospitalization for atrial fibrillation in patients in sinus rhythm with a history of paroxysmal or persistent atrial fibrillation**
Adults: 400 mg PO b.i.d.

ADMINISTRATION
PO
• Give drug with morning and evening meals.
• Omit a missed dose and give next regularly scheduled dose.
• Store at room temperature.

ACTION
Blocks sodium and potassium channels and decreases atrial ventricular node and sinus node conduction by blocking calcium and beta$_1$ channels.

Route	Onset	Peak	Duration
PO	Unknown	3–6 hr	Unknown

Half-life: 13 to 19 hours.

ADVERSE REACTIONS
CNS: asthenia. **CV:** *bradycardia, HF, QT-interval prolongation.* **GI:** abdominal pain, diarrhea, dyspepsia, nausea, vomiting. **GU:** prerenal azotemia, *AKI,* elevated creatinine level. **Metabolic:** hypovolemia. **Skin:** allergic dermatitis, dermatitis, eczema, pruritus, rash.

INTERACTIONS
Drug-drug. *Beta blockers:* May increase risk of bradycardia. Initially, give low dose of beta blocker and increase dosage only after monitoring ECG for tolerance.
Calcium channel blockers: May cause additive AV-blocking effects. Reduce initial dosage of calcium channel blocker; increase dosage only after monitoring ECG for tolerance.

CYP3A inducers (carbamazepine, phenobarbital, phenytoin, rifampin): May decrease dronedarone level. Avoid use together.
CYP3A substrates with narrow therapeutic range (sirolimus, tacrolimus): May increase levels of these drugs. Monitor drug levels.
Dabigatran: May increase dabigatran level. Reduce dabigatran dose. Avoid use together in patients with severe kidney impairment.
Digoxin: May increase electrophysiologic effects of dronedarone. Avoid use together; if use is unavoidable, decrease digoxin dosage, monitor level, and observe for toxicity.
Drugs that prolong QT interval (Class I and III antiarrhythmics, macrolide antibiotics, phenothiazines, TCAs): May further increase QT interval, leading to torsades de pointes. Use together is contraindicated.
Potassium-depleting diuretics (furosemide): May cause hypokalemia and hypomagnesemia. Use together cautiously.
Statins: May increase statin level. Use together cautiously. Limit simvastatin dosage to 10 mg once daily. For other statins, follow statin label recommendations for use with CYP3A and P-gp inhibitors.
Strong CYP3A inhibitors (clarithromycin, erythromycin, itraconazole, ketoconazole, ritonavir, voriconazole): May increase dronedarone level. Use together is contraindicated.
Warfarin: May increase warfarin level. Monitor INR.
Drug-herb. *St John's wort:* May decrease drug level. Discourage use together.
Drug-lifestyle. *Grapefruit juice:* May increase drug level. Avoid use together.

EFFECTS ON LAB TEST RESULTS
• May increase serum creatinine level and LFT values.

CONTRAINDICATIONS & CAUTIONS
Boxed Warning Contraindicated in patients with NYHA Class IV HF or Class II to III HF with recent decompensation requiring hospitalization or referral to HF clinic. Drug doubles risk of death in these patients. ∎
Boxed Warning Contraindicated in patients with atrial fibrillation who won't or can't be restored to normal sinus rhythm. Drug doubles risk of death, stroke, and hospitalization for HF in patients with permanent atrial fibrillation. ∎

✚Canada   ◇OTC   ◆ Off-label use   ⓓⓝⓒDo not crush   *Liquid contains alcohol   ▨ Genetic

• Contraindicated in patients hypersensitive to drug or its components.
• Contraindicated in patients with second- or third-degree AV block or sick sinus syndrome (unless a functioning pacemaker is in place), bradycardia (less than 50 beats/minute), Child-Pugh class C liver impairment, QTc interval of 500 msec or greater, or PR interval greater than 280 msec.
• Contraindicated in patients with previous liver or pulmonary toxicity with amiodarone use.
• **Alert:** Drug may increase risk of severe liver injury or failure.
• Use cautiously in patients with new or worsening HF.
• ILD has been reported. Discontinue drug if pulmonary toxicity is confirmed.
• Marked increase in serum creatinine level, prerenal azotemia, and AKI, frequently in the setting of HF or hypovolemia, have been reported. Effects appear to be reversible upon drug discontinuation and with appropriate medical treatment.
• Safety and effectiveness in children haven't been established.
Dialyzable drug: Unknown.
Overdose S&S: QTc-interval prolongation.

PREGNANCY-LACTATION-REPRODUCTION
• Drug may cause fetal harm. Use during pregnancy is contraindicated.
• Patients of childbearing potential should use effective contraception during therapy.
• It isn't known if drug appears in human milk. Drug is contraindicated during breast-feeding.

NURSING CONSIDERATIONS
• Potassium-depleting diuretics may cause hypokalemia and hypomagnesemia, increasing the risk of torsades de pointes. Initiate dronedarone therapy after potassium and magnesium levels reach and stay within normal range.
• Ensure that patients discontinue Class I or III antiarrhythmics or drugs that are strong inhibitors of CYP3A before starting drug.
• Routinely monitor CV status, ECG, electrolyte levels, and QTc interval.
• Regularly monitor kidney function. Kidney impairment can occur.
• Monitor liver serum enzyme levels, especially during first 6 months of therapy. Discontinue drug if liver injury is suspected.

PATIENT TEACHING
• Teach about proper drug administration and handling.
• Advise patient to report weight gain, dyspnea, fatigue, and peripheral edema, which may indicate worsening HF.
• Tell patient to report changes in OTC drug, prescription drug, supplement, or herb use.
• Instruct patient to report slowed heartbeat, diarrhea, nausea, vomiting, abdominal pain, indigestion, fatigue, or rash.
• Advise patient of childbearing potential to use an effective method of birth control while taking drug and to notify prescriber if becoming pregnant or thinking of becoming pregnant.
• Warn patient not to breastfeed while taking dronedarone because drug may appear in human milk.

drospirenone–estetrol
droh-SPYE-re-none/ES-te-trol

Nextstellis

Therapeutic class: Contraceptives
Pharmacologic class: Estrogen-progestin combinations

AVAILABLE FORMS
Tablets: 3 mg drospirenone/14.2 mg estetrol as 24 active tablets and 4 inert tablets per pack

INDICATIONS & DOSAGES
➤ **Prevention of pregnancy**
Adults with no current use of hormonal contraceptives: 1 active tablet PO daily for 24 days beginning on day 1 of menstrual cycle. Then 1 inert tablet PO daily on days 25 through 28. Begin each subsequent 28-day pack on same day of week on which first regimen began, following same schedule. Restart active tablets on next day after last inert tablet.
Adjust-a-dose: Refer to manufacturer's instructions for patients switching from another contraceptive method or starting after delivery, abortion, or miscarriage.

ADMINISTRATION
PO
• Give 1 tablet at same time each day without regard to food. Give tablets in the order directed on the blister pack.

Reactions in bold italics are *life-threatening*.

• If 1 active tablet is missed, give missed tablet as soon as possible and next tablet at scheduled time, even if 2 active tablets are taken on same day; then continue 1 tablet a day until pack is finished.

• If 2 or more active tablets are missed in weeks 1 or 2, give 1 missed tablet as soon as possible with tablet for current day and discard other missed tablet(s). Continue 1 tablet a day until pack is finished. Give additional nonhormonal contraceptive until active tablets are taken for 7 consecutive days.

• If 2 active tablets are missed in week 3, give 1 missed tablet as soon as possible and the tablet for current day; discard other missed tablets. Finish active tablets and discard inert tablets in pack. Start new pack of tablets on next day. Give additional nonhormonal contraceptive until active tablets are taken for 7 consecutive days.

• If 1 or more inert tablets are missed, skip missed tablet days and continue taking 1 tablet a day until pack is finished.

• If patient vomits or acute diarrhea occurs within 3 to 4 hours after giving an active tablet, give active tablet scheduled for next day as soon as possible and within 12 hours of usual time of tablet-taking if possible. If more than 2 tablets are missed, follow above information on missed tablets, including use of additional nonhormonal contraceptives.

• Store tablets at 68° to 77° F (20° to 25° C).

ACTION
Prevents pregnancy primarily by suppressing ovulation.

Route	Onset	Peak	Duration
PO (drospirenone)	Unknown	1–3 hr	Unknown
PO (estetrol)	Unknown	30 min–2 hr	Unknown

Half-life: 34 hours (drospirenone); 27 hours (estetrol).

ADVERSE REACTIONS
CNS: headache, mood disturbance. **CV:** *thromboembolism.* **GU:** dysmenorrhea, decreased libido. **Hematologic:** bleeding irregularities. **Metabolic:** weight gain. **Skin:** acne. **Other:** breast symptoms.

INTERACTIONS
Drug-drug. *Antidiabetics:* May decrease blood glucose-lowering effect of antidiabetic. Increase frequency of glucose monitoring and increase antidiabetic dose, as needed, based on glucose level.

Bile acid sequestrants (cholestyramine, colesevelam, colestipol): May cause contraceptive failure or increase breakthrough bleeding. Separate administration times. Refer to sequestrant prescribing information for additional information.

Drugs that may increase serum potassium level (ACE inhibitors, ARBs, NSAIDs, potassium supplements, spironolactone): May increase serum potassium level. Monitor serum potassium level.

Hepatitis C drug combinations containing ombitasvir/paritaprevir/ritonavir with or without dasabuvir: May increase liver enzyme levels. Use together is contraindicated. May initiate drospirenone–estetrol 2 weeks after completion of hepatitis C combination drug regimen.

Lamotrigine: May decrease effect of lamotrigine. Adjust lamotrigine dosage according to prescribing information based on hormonal contraceptive initiation or discontinuation.

Moderate and weak CYP3A4 inducers (dabrafenib, dexamethasone, modafinil, nafcillin): May cause contraceptive failure. Advise use of additional contraceptive method during use together and for 28 days after discontinuing CYP3A inducer, unless prescribing information of inducer indicates no clinically significant interaction.

Strong CYP3A inducers (dexamethasone, phenobarbital, phenytoin, rifampin, rifamycin): May lead to contraceptive failure. Avoid use together. If use together is unavoidable, advise use of alternative contraceptive method or additional nonhormonal contraceptive during use together and for 28 days after discontinuing inducer.

Strong CYP3A inhibitors (diltiazem, ketoconazole, loperamide, saquinavir): May increase risk of adverse drug reactions. Monitor serum potassium level in patients taking concomitantly long term.

Systemic corticosteroids: May increase risk of corticosteroid-related adverse reactions. Monitor patient closely. Follow recommendation for corticosteroid according to its prescribing information.

Thyroid hormone replacement therapy: May increase thyroid-binding globulin level. Monitor TSH level and follow recommendation for thyroid hormone replacement according to its prescribing information.

Drug-herb. *St. John's wort:* May decrease contraceptive effect or increase breakthrough bleeding. Discourage use together or recommend alternative contraceptive method.

Drug-lifestyle. **Boxed Warning** *Smoking:* May increase risk of CV events. Use is contraindicated in females older than age 35 who smoke. ■

Sunlight, UV light: May increase risk of chloasma. Encourage patient to limit exposure and wear sunscreen while taking drug.

EFFECTS ON LAB TEST RESULTS
• May increase fibrinogen, potassium, liver enzyme, blood glucose, triglyceride, corticosteroid-binding globulin, aldosterone, and total T_3 and total T_4 levels.
• May decrease LDL-C level.
• May increase platelet count.
• May decrease PT, PTT, and platelet aggregation time.

CONTRAINDICATIONS & CAUTIONS
• Contraindicated in patients at risk for arterial or venous thrombotic events. Evaluate patient for personal or family history of thrombotic or thromboembolic disorders and consider whether history suggests inherited or acquired hypercoagulopathy before starting drug.
• Contraindicated in patients with current or history of hormonally sensitive malignancy (breast cancer), liver adenoma, hepatocellular carcinoma, acute hepatitis, or decompensated cirrhosis.
• Contraindicated in patients with uterine bleeding of undiagnosed etiology.
• Contraindicated in patients at risk for hyperkalemia, such as those with kidney impairment, liver impairment, or adrenal insufficiency.
• Contraindicated in patients with uncontrolled HTN or HTN with vascular disease.
• Contraindicated in patients with migraine headaches with aura. Discontinue drug in patients who develop new migraines that are recurrent, persistent, or severe, or who experience increased frequency or severity of migraines while taking drug.
▧ Avoid use in patients with hereditary angioedema; drug may induce or exacerbate symptoms.
• Avoid use in patients with history of chloasma gravidarum or increased sensitivity to sun or UV exposure.

• Drug may be ineffective in patients with BMI of 30 kg/m^2 or greater. Safety and effectiveness in patients with BMI of 35 kg/m^2 or greater haven't been established.
• Drug may increase risk of CV events, especially in patients older than age 40; those with HTN, dyslipidemia, diabetes, or obesity; and those who use nicotine-containing products.
• Drug may decrease glucose tolerance. Use cautiously in patients who are prediabetic or diabetic.
• Drug may increase triglyceride levels and risk of pancreatitis. Consider alternative contraceptive method in patients with history of hypertriglyceridemia.
• Drug may increase risk of development or worsening of gallbladder disease. Consider discontinuing drug in patients with symptomatic gallbladder or cholestatic disease.
Dialyzable drug: Unknown.
⚠ *Overdose S&S:* Nausea, vomiting, severe headache, thromboembolic complications, vaginal bleeding.

PREGNANCY-LACTATION-REPRODUCTION
• Use during pregnancy isn't indicated. Discontinue if pregnancy is confirmed.
• Drug appears in human milk and may decrease milk production. Patient should use other forms of contraception while breastfeeding. Evaluate benefits of breastfeeding, keeping in mind patient's clinical need and potential adverse effects on infant.

NURSING CONSIDERATIONS
• Monitor patient for thrombotic and thromboembolic events; discontinue drug if an event occurs.
• Monitor patient for unexplained vision changes. Stop drug and immediately evaluate patient for retinal vein thrombosis.
• Stop drug during prolonged periods of immobilization.
• Monitor patient with history of depression; stop drug if depression recurs to a serious degree.
• In patient at high risk for hyperkalemia and patient in whom taking drug may increase potassium level, check serum potassium level during first treatment cycle.
• Periodically monitor BP. Stop drug if BP rises significantly.
• Monitor liver enzyme levels. Withhold or permanently discontinue drug for significant liver enzyme elevations.

Reactions in bold italics are *life-threatening*.

• Monitor glucose level in patients who are prediabetic or diabetic.
• Irregular bleeding and spotting may occur especially during the first 4 months of use. Amenorrhea may occur even if not pregnant. Evaluate patient for other causes if irregular bleeding or amenorrhea persists.

PATIENT TEACHING

Boxed Warning Inform patient that smoking increases risk of a serious CV event when combined with drug and that hormonal contraceptives are contraindicated in females older than age 35 who smoke. ■
• Instruct patient in proper drug administration (including managing missed doses) and storage.
• Warn patient about increased risk of arterial or venous thrombotic or thromboembolic events while taking drug, especially if patient has HTN, dyslipidemia, diabetes, or obesity.
• Instruct patient to immediately report limb pain or swelling, sudden shortness of breath, sudden change in vision, chest pain, sudden severe headache, weakness or numbness in arm or leg, or trouble speaking.
• Tell patient to contact prescriber if prolonged immobilization occurs.
• Teach patient to report signs or symptoms of hyperkalemia (weakness, palpitations or irregular heartbeat, nausea, vomiting, severe chest pain, dyspnea).
• Inform patient about need for regular BP checks. Instruct patient to report BP increases to prescriber.
• Alert patient that drug may cause elevated liver enzyme levels and can increase risk of liver tumors. Instruct patient to report signs or symptoms of liver disease (jaundice).
• Instruct patient who is prediabetic or diabetic to contact prescriber for signs or symptoms of hyperglycemia (increased thirst, dry mouth, frequent urination, increased appetite with weight loss).
• Warn patient about risk of development or worsening of gallbladder disease. Advise patient to report signs or symptoms of gallbladder disease (rapidly intensifying pain in upper portion of abdomen or in center of abdomen just below breastbone, back pain between shoulder blades, pain in right shoulder, nausea, vomiting).
• Inform patient that drug may cause unscheduled bleeding and spotting.

• Tell patient to contact prescriber if amenorrhea occurs in two or more consecutive cycles or signs and symptoms of pregnancy occur (morning sickness, unusual breast tenderness). Inform patient to stop drug if pregnancy is confirmed.
• Inform patient that drug may cause chloasma (dark patches of facial skin), especially in patient with history of chloasma gravidarum.
• Instruct patient to avoid exposure to UV light or prolonged exposure to sunlight and to wear sunscreen while taking drug.

drospirenone–ethinyl estradiol
droh-SPYE-re-none/ETH-i-nill es-tra-DYE-ole

Loryna, Lo-Zumandimine, Mya✦, Nikki, Ocella, Syeda, Yasmin, Yaz, Zamine 21✦, Zamine 28✦, Zumandimine

Therapeutic class: Contraceptives
Pharmacologic class: Estrogen–progestin combinations

AVAILABLE FORMS
Tablets: 3 mg drospirenone and 0.02 mg ethinyl estradiol as 24 active tablets and 4 inert tablets (Loryna, Lo-Zumandimine, Mya, Nikki, Yaz). Or, 3 mg drospirenone and 0.03 mg ethinyl estradiol as 21 active tablets (Zamine 21) and 7 inert tablets (Ocella, Syeda, Yasmin, Zamine 28, Zumandimine).

INDICATIONS & DOSAGES
➤ **Contraception**
Adult females: 1 active tablet PO daily for 21 days beginning on day 1 of menstrual cycle or first Sunday after onset of menstruation; then 1 inert tablet PO daily on days 22 through 28. Or 1 active tablet PO daily for 24 days beginning on day 1 of menstrual cycle or first Sunday after onset of menstruation; then 1 inert tablet PO daily on days 25 through 28. Begin next and all subsequent 28-day regimens on same day of week that first regimen began, following same schedule. Restart active tablets on next day after last inert tablet.

➤ **Premenstrual dysphoric disorder (Loryna, Lo-Zumandimine, Nikki, Yaz)**
Adult females: 1 active tablet PO daily for 24 days beginning on day 1 of menstrual cycle or first Sunday after menstruation begins; then 1 inert tablet PO daily on days 25 through 28. Begin next and all subsequent 28-day regimens on same day of week that first regimen began, following same schedule. Restart active tablets on next day after last inert tablet.

➤ **Acne in females at least age 14 and only if patient desires an oral contraceptive for birth control (Loryna, Lo-Zumandimine, Mya, Nikki, Yaz, Zamine)**
Females: Follow guidelines of use for contraception. The 28-day dosing regimen consists of 1 active tablet PO for 24 consecutive days followed by 1 inert tablet PO daily for 4 days. After 28 tablets are taken, new course is started next day.

ADMINISTRATION
PO
• Give drug at same time each day.
• Give tablets in order directed on blister pack.

ACTION
Reduces chance of conception by inhibiting ovulation, inhibiting sperm progression, and reducing chance of implantation.

Route	Onset	Peak	Duration
PO	Unknown	1–2 hr	Unknown

Half-life: Drospirenone, 30 hours; ethinyl estradiol, 24 hours.

ADVERSE REACTIONS
CNS: depression, dizziness, emotional lability, headache, migraine, irritability, nervousness, mood changes. **CV:** *arterial thromboembolism or VTE,* HTN, fluid retention. **EENT:** cataracts, steepening of corneal curvature, intolerance to contact lenses, retinal thrombosis. **GI:** abdominal pain, abdominal cramping, bloating, changes in appetite, colitis, diarrhea, nausea, vomiting, gallbladder disease. **GU:** amenorrhea, breakthrough bleeding, change in cervical erosion and secretion, change in menstrual flow, cystitis, cystitis-like syndrome, dysmenorrhea, impaired kidney function, leukorrhea, menstrual disorder, premenstrual syndrome, spotting, temporary infertility after discontinuing treatment, vaginal candidiasis, vaginitis. **Hepatic:** *Budd-Chiari syndrome, liver adenomas,*

cholestatic jaundice, benign liver tumors. **Metabolic:** reduced glucose tolerance, porphyria, weight change, *hyperkalemia.* **Musculoskeletal:** back pain. **Skin:** *erythema multiforme,* acne, erythema nodosum, hemorrhagic eruption, hirsutism, loss of scalp hair, melasma, pruritus, rash. **Other:** hypersensitivity reaction, changes in libido, breast tenderness.

INTERACTIONS
Drug-drug. *ACE inhibitors, aldosterone antagonists, ARBs, NSAIDs, potassium-sparing diuretics:* May increase risk of hyperkalemia. Monitor potassium level.
Acetaminophen: May increase level of contraceptive and decrease effectiveness of acetaminophen. Monitor patient for adverse effects. Adjust acetaminophen dose as needed.
Ascorbic acid, atorvastatin: May increase level of contraceptive. Monitor patient for adverse effects.
CYP3A4 inducers (barbiturates, carbamazepine, phenytoin): May increase metabolism of ethinyl estradiol and decrease contraceptive effectiveness. Advise patient to use another method of birth control.
CYP3A4 inhibitors (azole antifungals, verapamil, erythromycin): May increase level of contraceptive. Monitor patient for adverse effects.
Cyclosporine, omeprazole, prednisolone, theophylline: May increase levels of these drugs. Monitor patient for adverse effects and toxicity.
Hepatitis C drug combinations containing ombitasvir, paritaprevir, ritonavir, dasabuvir: May increase ALT level. Use together is contraindicated. Discontinue drospirenone–ethinyl estradiol before starting therapy due to risk of significant liver enzyme level increases. May restart approximately 2 weeks after completion of the combination drug regimen.
Lamotrigine: May decrease lamotrigine level and reduce seizure control. Dosage adjustment may be necessary.
Rifampin: May decrease contraceptive effectiveness and increase menstrual irregularities. Advise patient to use another method of birth control.
Warfarin, other anticoagulants: May increase or decrease anticoagulation effect. Monitor INR or consider therapy modification.
Drug-herb. *St. John's wort:* May decrease contraceptive effectiveness and increase

Reactions in bold italics are *life-threatening*.

breakthrough bleeding. Discourage use together, or advise use of additional method of birth control.

Drug-lifestyle. Boxed Warning *Smoking:* May increase the risk of adverse CV effects. Advise patient to avoid smoking. ■

Sunlight, UV light: May increase risk of chloasma. Encourage patient to limit exposure and wear sunscreen while taking drug.

EFFECTS ON LAB TEST RESULTS

• May increase potassium, corticoid, prothrombin, thyroid-binding globulin, total circulating sex steroid, total thyroid hormone, triglyceride, amylase, GGT, transferrin, prolactin, renin activity, vitamin A, and factor VII, VIII, IX, and X levels, as well as iron-binding capacity.

• May decrease antithrombin III, folate, albumin, zinc, and vitamin B_{12} levels.

• May increase norepinephrine-induced platelet aggregation.

• May decrease glucose tolerance and free T_3 resin uptake.

CONTRAINDICATIONS & CAUTIONS

Boxed Warning Smoking increases the risk of serious CV adverse effects. Risk increases with age, especially in females older than age 35, and with the number of cigarettes smoked. Use is contraindicated in females over age 35 who smoke. ■

• Contraindicated in females with liver dysfunction, tumor, or disease; kidney or adrenal insufficiency; thrombophlebitis, thromboembolic disorders, or history of DVT or thromboembolic disorders; inherited hypercoagulopathies; cerebrovascular disease or CAD; uncontrolled HTN; diabetes with vascular disease; thrombogenic valvular or thrombogenic rhythm diseases of the heart; headaches with focal neurologic symptoms or migraine headaches with or without aura (if older than age 35); known, suspected, or history of breast cancer, endometrial cancer, or other estrogen-dependent neoplasia; undiagnosed abnormal uterine bleeding; or cholestatic jaundice of pregnancy or jaundice with other hormonal contraceptive use.

• Contraindicated in patients hypersensitive to components of formulation and in females ages 65 and older.

• Contraindicated after major surgery with prolonged immobilization.

• Use cautiously in patients with CV risk factors (HTN, hyperlipidemia, obesity, and diabetes).

• Don't use in patients predisposed to hyperkalemia; drug may increase potassium level.

• Use cautiously in patients with depression and in those with conditions aggravated by fluid retention.

⚕ Drug may induce or exacerbate symptoms of angioedema in patients with hereditary angioedema.

Dialyzable drug: Unknown.

⚠ *Overdose S&S:* Nausea, withdrawal uterine bleeding.

PREGNANCY-LACTATION-REPRODUCTION

• Contraindicated in patients who are pregnant. There is little or no increased risk of birth defects with inadvertent use of combined oral contraceptives during early pregnancy.

• Small amounts of hormonal contraceptives appear in human milk. Use of drug during breastfeeding isn't recommended; may reduce milk production.

NURSING CONSIDERATIONS

🕒 *Alert:* Use of contraceptives increases risk of MI, thromboembolism, stroke, liver neoplasia, gallbladder disease, and HTN. Risk further increases in patient with HTN, diabetes, hyperlipidemia, or obesity.

• Relationship between use of hormonal contraceptives and breast and cervical cancers is unclear. Encourage patient to schedule a complete gynecologic exam at least yearly and to perform breast self-exams monthly.

• In patient scheduled to have elective surgery that may increase the risk of thromboembolism, stop contraceptive use from at least 4 weeks before until 2 weeks after surgery. Also stop use during and after prolonged immobilization.

• Because of increased risk of thromboembolism in the postpartum period, don't start contraceptive earlier than 4 to 6 weeks after delivery.

• Stop use and evaluate patient if loss of vision, proptosis, diplopia, papilledema, or retinal vascular lesions occur. Recommend that contact lens wearers be evaluated by an ophthalmologist if visual changes or lens intolerance occurs.

• If patient misses two consecutive periods, obtain a negative pregnancy test result before continuing use of contraceptive.

• Immediately stop use if pregnancy is confirmed.

• Closely monitor patient with diabetes. Glucose intolerance may occur.

• Closely monitor patient with HTN or history of depression. Stop drug if these events occur.

• In patient at high risk for hyperkalemia and patient taking medications that may increase potassium, check potassium level during the first treatment cycle.

• Stop drug and evaluate patient if persistent, severe headaches occur or if migraines occur or worsen.

• Evaluate for malignancy or pregnancy if patient experiences breakthrough bleeding or spotting.

• Closely monitor patient with hyperlipidemia.

• Stop use if jaundice occurs.

• Monitor patient on thyroid replacement therapy because estrogens may lead to decreased total thyroid hormone levels. Thyroid medication dosage may need to be increased while patient is taking estrogens.

• *Look alike–sound alike:* Don't confuse Yaz with Yasmin.

PATIENT TEACHING

• Advise patient to use additional method of birth control during first 7 days of first cycle of hormonal contraceptive.

• Inform patient that pills don't protect against STIs such as HIV.

Boxed Warning Advise patient of the dangers of smoking while taking hormonal contraceptives. Suggest a smoker choose a different form of birth control. ■

• Tell patient to schedule gynecologic exams yearly and to perform breast self-exam monthly.

• Inform patient that spotting, light bleeding, and stomach upset may occur while taking first one to three packs of pills. Tell patient to continue taking pills and to notify health care provider if these symptoms persist.

• Teach about proper drug administration and handling.

• Explain that risk of pregnancy increases with each missed active tablet. Inform patient what to do in case of missed pills.

• Advise patient to use an additional method of birth control and to notify health care provider if uncertain what to do about missed pills.

• Tell patient to immediately report sharp chest pain, coughing of blood or sudden

shortness of breath, calf pain, crushing chest pain or chest heaviness, sudden severe headache or vomiting, dizziness or fainting, visual or speech disturbances, weakness or numbness in arm or leg, vision loss, breast lumps, severe stomach pain or tenderness, difficulty sleeping, lack of energy, fatigue, change in mood, or jaundice with fever, fatigue, loss of appetite, dark urine, or light-colored bowel movements.

• If patient wears contact lenses, instruct patient to notify health care provider if change in vision or trouble wearing lenses occurs.

• Advise patient that amenorrhea may occur. Rule out pregnancy if amenorrhea occurs in two or more consecutive cycles.

• Caution patient who is breastfeeding to use an alternative method of birth control until infant is completely weaned. In patient taking drug, quality and quantity of human milk may decrease and breastfed neonate may experience yellowing of skin and eyes (jaundice) and breast enlargement.

• Inform patient that drug may cause chloasma (dark patches of facial skin), especially with history of chloasma gravidarum.

• Instruct patient to avoid exposure to UV light or prolonged exposure to sunlight and to wear sunscreen while taking drug.

SAFETY ALERT!

dulaglutide
doo-la-GLOO-tide

Trulicity

Therapeutic class: Antidiabetics
Pharmacologic class: Glucagon-like peptide-1 receptor agonists

AVAILABLE FORMS
Injection: 0.75 mg/0.5 mL, 1.5 mg/0.5 mL, 3 mg/0.5 mL, 4.5 mg/0.5 mL in single-dose pens

INDICATIONS & DOSAGES
➤ **Type 2 diabetes as adjunct to diet and exercise to improve glycemic control; to reduce risk of major adverse CV events in patients with type 2 diabetes who have established CV disease or multiple CV risk factors**
Adults: 0.75 mg subcut once weekly. Increase dosage to 1.5 mg once weekly for additional

glycemic control. If additional glycemic control is needed, increase to 3 mg once weekly after at least 4 weeks on 1.5-mg dose. If further glycemic control is needed, increase dosage to maximum dose of 4.5 mg once weekly after at least 4 weeks on 3-mg dose.

✳ *NEW INDICATION:* **Type 2 diabetes as adjunct to diet and exercise to improve glycemic control**
Children ages 10 and older: 0.75 mg subcut one weekly. If after at least 4 weeks additional glycemic control is needed, may increase dosage to maximum of 1.5 mg weekly.

ADMINISTRATION
Subcutaneous
• Inject into abdomen, thigh, or upper arm once weekly any time of day. Use a different injection site each week.
• Give drug without regard to meals.
• **Alert:** Don't mix dulaglutide with insulin. Give as separate injections in nonadjacent areas.
• Don't give IM or IV.
• Inspect for particulate matter and discoloration before administration. Don't give if present.
• If a dose is missed, give within 3 days of missed dose; then resume prior schedule. If less than 3 days remain until next scheduled dose, skip the missed dose and give the next dose on schedule.
• The day of weekly administration may be changed if necessary as long as the last dose was 3 or more days before the new day.
• Refrigerate at 36° to 46° F (2° to 8° C). May store at room temperature for a total of 14 days if temperature doesn't exceed 86° F (30° C).
• Don't freeze. Don't use drug if it has been frozen.
• Protect from light by storing in original carton until time of administration.
• Discard injection device after each use in puncture-resistant container.

ACTION
Human glucagon-like peptide-1 (GLP-1) receptor agonist that, like endogenous GLP-1, binds to and activates the GLP-1 receptor in the pancreatic beta cells, leading to glucose-dependent insulin release. Also decreases glucagon secretion and slows gastric emptying.

Route	Onset	Peak	Duration
Subcut	Unknown	24–72 hr	Unknown

Half-life: About 5 days.

ADVERSE REACTIONS
CNS: fatigue. **CV:** tachycardia, increased PR interval, first-degree AV block. **GI:** nausea; diarrhea; vomiting; decreased appetite; dyspepsia; constipation; flatulence; GERD; eructation; abdominal pain, tenderness, or distention. **GU:** kidney impairment. **Hepatic:** elevated lipase and amylase levels. **Metabolic:** *hypoglycemia.* **Other:** antidrug antibody formation.

INTERACTIONS
Drug-drug. *Insulin, insulin secretagogues (meglitinides, sulfonylureas):* May increase risk of hypoglycemia. Consider reducing insulin or insulin secretagogue dosage; closely monitor blood glucose level.
Oral medications: May affect absorption of oral medications because dulaglutide delays gastric emptying. Monitor effects, especially when given with other drugs with a narrow therapeutic index, such as warfarin.

EFFECTS ON LAB TEST RESULTS
• May increase lipase and amylase levels.
• May decrease glucose level.

CONTRAINDICATIONS & CAUTIONS
Boxed Warning Contraindicated in patients with personal or family history of medullary thyroid carcinoma (MTC) and in patients with multiple endocrine neoplasia syndrome type 2. ∎
Boxed Warning Thyroid C-cell adenomas and carcinomas occurred in animal studies. It isn't known if dulaglutide causes thyroid C-cell tumors, including MTC, in humans. ∎
• Contraindicated in patients with a serious hypersensitivity reaction to drug or its components.
• Hypersensitivity reactions (including anaphylaxis and angioedema) have been reported with other GLP-1 receptor agonists. Use cautiously in patients with a history of angioedema or anaphylaxis with another GLP-1 receptor agonist.
• Drug hasn't been studied in patients with a history of pancreatitis. Consider alternative antidiabetic therapy.

• Drug shouldn't be used in patients with type 1 diabetes or for treatment of diabetic ketoacidosis. Drug isn't a substitute for insulin.

• To reduce risk of hypoglycemia, consider dosage reduction of concomitantly administered secretagogues or insulin when initiating dulaglutide.

• Avoid use in patients with severe GI disease, including severe gastroparesis; drug slows gastric emptying and hasn't been studied in this population.

• Use cautiously in patients with liver or kidney insufficiency.

• Drug may cause diabetic retinopathy complications, especially in patients with a history of diabetic retinopathy.

• Safety and effectiveness in children younger than age 10 haven't been established.

Dialyzable drug: Unknown.

⚠ *Overdose S&S:* Mild or moderate GI symptoms, nonsevere hypoglycemia.

PREGNANCY-LACTATION-REPRODUCTION

• Studies during pregnancy are inadequate. Use cautiously during pregnancy and only if potential benefit justifies fetal risk.

• It isn't known if drug appears in human milk. Use cautiously during breastfeeding after considering risks.

NURSING CONSIDERATIONS

• Use caution when initiating dulaglutide therapy or escalating dosage in patient with kidney insufficiency. Monitor kidney function, especially in patient who reports severe GI adverse reactions (nausea, vomiting, diarrhea, dehydration).

• Monitor for hypoglycemia; patient also using an insulin secretagogue or insulin is at increased risk.

• Monitor for signs and symptoms of pancreatitis (persistent severe abdominal pain, sometimes radiating to back, which may or may not be accompanied by vomiting). Discontinue drug if pancreatitis is suspected. Don't restart drug if pancreatitis is confirmed.

• Monitor patient for tachycardia; monitor ECG for PR-interval prolongation.

• Refer patient with elevated serum calcitonin level or thyroid nodules on exam or neck imaging to an endocrinologist.

• Monitor patient with history of diabetic retinopathy for disease progression.

• *Look alike–sound alike:* Don't confuse dulaglutide with duloxetine or dutasteride.

PATIENT TEACHING

• Explain to patient that dulaglutide isn't a substitute for insulin. Educate patient on general diabetes care, including the need to monitor glucose and HbA_{1c} levels, signs and symptoms of hypoglycemia and hyperglycemia, importance of diet and exercise, and impact stress and trauma may have on glucose level.

• Warn patient to immediately discontinue drug and inform prescriber if hypersensitivity reactions occur.

• Advise patient to report heart palpitations or feelings of a racing heartbeat while at rest.

• Inform patient of risk of dehydration due to GI adverse reactions, including the associated risk of worsening kidney function. Counsel patient to take precautions to avoid fluid depletion.

• Review signs and symptoms of acute pancreatitis (persistent severe abdominal pain, sometimes radiating to the back, which may or may not be accompanied by vomiting). Instruct patient to promptly discontinue drug and contact prescriber if any of these signs and symptoms occur.

Boxed Warning Inform patient of risk of MTC. Review signs and symptoms of thyroid tumors (mass in neck, dysphagia, dyspnea, persistent hoarseness). ■

• Teach about proper drug administration and handling (rotating sites, inspecting solution for particles, discarding needles, storing pens and syringes, handling a missed dose).

• Caution patient never to mix insulin and dulaglutide but to give as separate injections. Although dulaglutide and insulin may be injected in the same body area, they shouldn't be injected adjacent to each other.

• Instruct patient to report pregnancy or plans to become pregnant or breastfeed.

DULoxetine hydrochloride
doo-LOX-ah-teen

Cymbalta

Therapeutic class: Antidepressants
Pharmacologic class: SSNRIs

AVAILABLE FORMS

Capsules (delayed-release) ⒹⓇ: 20 mg, 30 mg, 40 mg, 60 mg

INDICATIONS & DOSAGES

Adjust-a-dose (for all indications): If possible, gradually taper dosage when discontinuing drug to avoid adverse reactions.

➤ **Major depressive disorder**

Adults: Initially, 20 mg PO b.i.d. to 60 mg PO once daily or divided in two equal doses. May also start at 30 mg/day for 1 week to allow patients to adjust to medication. Maximum, 120 mg daily.

➤ **Generalized anxiety disorder**

Adults: 60 mg PO daily. Or, 30 mg PO daily for 1 week; then increase to 60 mg PO daily. May increase in increments of 30 mg daily to 120 mg PO once daily.

Children ages 7 to 17: 30 mg PO once daily for 2 weeks; may increase to 60 mg once daily. For doses greater than 60 mg/day, increase dosage in increments of 30 mg/day. Maximum, 120 mg daily.

Adjust-a-dose: In older adults, initially give 30 mg PO once daily for 2 weeks before considering an increase to target dose of 60 mg once daily. If needed, further increase dosage in increments of 30 mg once daily. Maximum, 120 mg daily.

➤ **Fibromyalgia**

Adults: Initially, 30 mg PO once daily for 1 week; increase to 60 mg PO once daily after a week. Some patients may respond to the starting dose. Maximum, 60 mg daily. Base continued treatment on individual patient response.

Children ages 13 to 17: 30 mg PO once daily. May increase to 60 mg PO once daily based on response and tolerability.

➤ **Neuropathic pain related to diabetic peripheral neuropathy**

Adults: 60 mg PO once daily.

Adjust-a-dose: Consider a lower starting dose and a gradual increase in dose for patients with kidney impairment.

➤ **Chronic musculoskeletal pain**

Adults: Initially, 30 mg PO once daily for 1 week; then increase to 60 mg PO once daily.

ADMINISTRATION

PO

• Give drug without regard to meals.
• Have patient swallow capsules whole; don't crush or cut capsules.

ACTION

Inhibits serotonin and norepinephrine reuptake and is a weak inhibitor of dopamine reuptake in the CNS.

Route	Onset	Peak	Duration
PO	Unknown	6 hr (fasting)	Unknown

Half-life: 8–17 hours.

ADVERSE REACTIONS

CNS: dizziness, fatigue, headache, insomnia, somnolence, *suicidality,* fever, hypoesthesia, paresthesia, irritability, lethargy, nervousness, abnormal dreams, insomnia, restlessness, sleep disorder, anxiety, asthenia, tremor, agitation, dysgeusia, vertigo. **CV:** flushing, increased BP, palpitations. **EENT:** blurred vision, nasopharyngitis, pharyngolaryngeal pain, dry mouth. **GI:** constipation, diarrhea, nausea, dyspepsia, gastritis, vomiting, flatulence, abdominal pain, increased or decreased appetite, viral gastroenteritis. **GU:** decreased libido, abnormal orgasm, urinary frequency, ejaculatory disorder, dysuria, erectile dysfunction, urinary hesitation. **Hepatic:** increased ALT level. **Metabolic:** weight gain or loss, hyponatremia. **Musculoskeletal:** myalgia, muscle spasms. **Respiratory:** cough, URI. **Skin:** diaphoresis, night sweats, pruritus, rash. **Other:** hot flash, chills, rigors, yawning, flu-like symptoms.

INTERACTIONS

Drug-drug. *Anticoagulants (aspirin, NSAIDs, warfarin):* May increase bleeding risk. Monitor patient closely.

Class IC antiarrhythmics (flecainide, propafenone), phenothiazines: May increase levels of these drugs. Use together cautiously.

CNS drugs: May increase adverse effects. Use together cautiously.

CYP1A2 inhibitors (cimetidine, fluvoxamine, certain quinolones): May increase duloxetine level. Avoid use together.

CYP1A2 substrates (caffeine, theophylline): May increase substrate level. Use together cautiously.

CYP2D6 inhibitors (fluoxetine, paroxetine, quinidine): May increase duloxetine level. Use together cautiously.

Drugs that reduce gastric acidity: May cause premature breakdown of duloxetine's protective coating and early release of drug. Monitor patient for effects.

Linezolid, methylene blue: May increase risk of serotonin syndrome. Don't use together.
Lithium, SSNRIs, SSRIs, tramadol: May increase risk of serotonin syndrome. Avoid use together.

⊙ *Alert: MAO inhibitors (phenelzine, rasagiline, selegiline):* May cause hyperthermia, rigidity, myoclonus, autonomic instability, rapid fluctuations of vital signs, agitation, delirium, and coma. Avoid use within 2 weeks after MAO inhibitor therapy; wait at least 5 days after stopping duloxetine before starting MAO inhibitor.

TCAs (amitriptyline, imipramine, nortriptyline): May increase levels of these drugs. Reduce TCA dose, and monitor drug levels closely.

Thioridazine: May prolong QT interval and increase risk of serious ventricular arrhythmias and sudden death. Avoid use together.

Triptans: May cause serotonin syndrome (restlessness, hallucinations, loss of coordination, fast heartbeat, rapid changes in BP, increased body temperature, hyperreflexia, nausea, vomiting, and diarrhea) or NMS. Use cautiously and with increased monitoring, especially when starting or increasing dosages.

Drug-herb. *St. John's wort:* May increase risk of serotonin syndrome. Discourage use together.

Drug-lifestyle. *Alcohol use:* May increase risk of liver damage. Discourage use together.

EFFECTS ON LAB TEST RESULTS
• May increase ALP, ALT, AST, bilirubin, glucose, bicarbonate, cholesterol, and CK levels.
• May decrease sodium level.
• May increase or decrease potassium level.

CONTRAINDICATIONS & CAUTIONS
• Contraindicated in patients hypersensitive to drug or its ingredients.
• Drug isn't recommended for patients with chronic liver disease, cirrhosis, or GFR less than 30 mL/minute.

⊙ *Alert:* Before using duloxetine in a child or adolescent, balance potential risks with clinical need.
• Safety and effectiveness in children younger than age 7 for generalized anxiety disorder or younger than age 13 for fibromyalgia haven't been established. Use for other indications hasn't been studied.

• Use cautiously in patients with a history of mania or seizures, patients who drink substantial amounts of alcohol, patients with HTN, patients with controlled angle-closure glaucoma, and those with conditions that slow gastric emptying.
• Pupil dilation that occurs after duloxetine use may trigger an angle-closure attack in a patient with anatomically narrow angles who doesn't have a patent iridectomy.
• Drug may increase risk of bleeding events and sexual dysfunction.
• Orthostatic hypotension, falls, and syncope have been reported with therapeutic doses and tend to occur within first week of therapy but can occur at any time during treatment, particularly after dosage increases. Fall risk appears to increase steadily with age and be related to degree of orthostatic decrease in BP as well as other factors that may increase the underlying risk of falls. Consider dosage reduction or discontinuing drug if falls occur.
Dialyzable drug: Unlikely.
⚠ *Overdose S&S:* Coma, hypotension, HTN, seizures, serotonin syndrome, somnolence, syncope, tachycardia, vomiting.

PREGNANCY-LACTATION-REPRODUCTION
• Drug may increase risk of postpartum hemorrhage if used in the month before delivery.
• Enroll patients exposed to drug during pregnancy in the National Pregnancy Registry for Antidepressants (866-961-2388 or https://womensmentalhealth.org/research/pregnancyregistry/antidepressants/).
• Use during the third trimester may cause neonatal complications (respiratory distress, cyanosis, apnea, seizures, vomiting, hypoglycemia, hypotonia, hyperreflexia), which may require prolonged hospitalization, respiratory support, and tube feeding. Use during pregnancy only if potential benefit justifies fetal risk.
• Drug appears in human milk. Use cautiously during breastfeeding and only when benefits outweigh risks to infant, which include sedation, poor feeding, and poor weight gain.

NURSING CONSIDERATIONS
Boxed Warning Drug may increase risk of suicidality in children, adolescents, and young adults, especially during the first few months of treatment, and in those with major depressive disorder or other psychiatric disorder. ■

D

Boxed Warning Monitor all patients for worsening of depression or emergence of suicidality, especially when therapy starts or dosage changes. ▪

⚠️ *Alert:* Use with linezolid or methylene blue can cause serotonin syndrome (fever, mental status changes, muscle twitching, diaphoresis, shivering or shaking, diarrhea, loss of coordination). If linezolid or methylene blue must be given, stop drug and monitor patient for serotonin toxicity for 5 days or until 24 hours after last dose of methylene blue or linezolid, whichever comes first. May resume treatment 24 hours after last dose of methylene blue or linezolid.

• If taken with TCAs, duloxetine metabolism is prolonged and patient requires extended monitoring.

• Severe skin reactions, including erythema multiforme and SJS, can occur. Discontinue at first sign of blisters, peeling rash, mucosal erosions, or other signs or symptoms of hypersensitivity if no other etiology can be identified.

• Periodically reassess patient to determine the need for continued therapy.

• Don't stop drug abruptly. Decrease dosage gradually, and watch for symptoms that may arise when drug is stopped (dizziness, nausea, headache, paresthesia, vomiting, irritability, nightmares).

• If intolerable symptoms arise when decreasing or stopping drug, restart at previous dose and decrease more gradually.

• Periodically monitor BP during treatment.

• Monitor patient for orthostatic hypotension, falls, and syncope, especially during initial use and dose escalations.

• Older adult may be more sensitive to drug effects than a younger adult.

• Monitor for urinary hesitancy and retention.

• Monitor for signs and symptoms of hyponatremia (headache, difficulty concentrating, memory impairment, confusion, weakness unsteadiness). Severe cases include hallucination, syncope, seizure, coma, respiratory arrest, and death.

• Monitor for signs and symptoms of liver impairment (itching, abdominal pain, dark urine, jaundice).

⚠️ *Alert:* Combining triptans with an SSRI or an SSNRI may cause serotonin syndrome or NMS-like reactions. Signs and symptoms of serotonin syndrome include restlessness, hallucinations, loss of coordination, fast heartbeat,

rapid changes in BP, increased body temperature, overactive reflexes, nausea, vomiting, and diarrhea. Serotonin syndrome may be more likely to occur when starting or increasing the dose of triptan, SSRI, or SSNRI.

• May worsen glycemic control in patient with diabetes. Monitor blood glucose level.

• Ask patient about changes to sexual function. Sexual dysfunction can occur, and patient may not spontaneously report the signs and symptoms.

• *Look alike–sound alike:* Don't confuse duloxetine with fluoxetine or paroxetine. Don't confuse Cymbalta with Symbyax.

PATIENT TEACHING
Boxed Warning Warn families or caregivers to immediately report signs of worsening depression (such as agitation, irritability, insomnia, hostility, impulsivity) and signs of suicidality to prescriber. ▪

⚠️ *Alert:* Teach patient to recognize and immediately report signs and symptoms of serotonin toxicity.

• Tell patient to immediately contact prescriber and to discontinue drug at first sign of hypersensitivity (blisters, peeling rash, mucosal erosions).

• Instruct patient to report urinary retention or hesitancy, and signs and symptoms of low sodium level or liver impairment.

• Advise patient that blood pressure should be measured prior to initiating and periodically throughout treatment because drug may increase blood pressure.

• Caution patient to not stop drug abruptly; dosage must be gradually reduced to avoid adverse effects.

• Tell patient to consult prescriber or pharmacist before taking other prescription drugs, OTC drugs, or herbal or other dietary supplements.

• Urge patient to avoid activities that are hazardous or require mental alertness until drug's effects are known.

• Warn against drinking alcohol during therapy.

• If patient takes drug for depression, explain that it may take 1 to 4 weeks to notice an effect.

• Advise patient with diabetes to closely monitor blood glucose level.

• Counsel patient to report signs and symptoms of sexual dysfunction, including decreased libido.

• Instruct patient to report pregnancy or plans to become pregnant or breastfeed.

dutasteride
doo-TAS-teh-ride

Avodart

Therapeutic class: BPH drugs
Pharmacologic class: 5-alpha-reductase enzyme inhibitors

AVAILABLE FORMS
Capsules ⬤ℕℂ: 0.5 mg

INDICATIONS & DOSAGES
➤ **To treat and improve symptoms of BPH, reduce risk of acute urine retention, and reduce need for BPH-related surgery**
Adult males: 0.5 mg PO once daily as monotherapy. May be given with tamsulosin 0.4 mg PO once daily as combination therapy.

ADMINISTRATION
PO
⚠ *Alert:* Drug is considered a teratogen. Follow safe handling and disposal procedures.
⚠ *Alert:* Because drug may be absorbed through the skin, anyone who is or may become pregnant shouldn't handle drug, especially avoiding contact with crushed or broken tablets. If contact occurs, immediately wash contact area with soap and water.
• Have patient swallow capsules whole; don't crush or cut capsules. Contact with contents may cause oropharyngeal irritation.
• Give drug without regard for food.

ACTION
Inhibits conversion of testosterone to dihydrotestosterone, the androgen primarily responsible for initial development and subsequent enlargement of prostate gland.

Route	Onset	Peak	Duration
PO	Unknown	2–3 hr	Unknown

Half-life: About 5 weeks.

ADVERSE REACTIONS
GU: impotence, erectile dysfunction, decreased libido, ejaculation disorder.
Other: gynecomastia, breast tenderness.

INTERACTIONS
Drug-drug. *CYP3A4 inhibitors (cimetidine, ciprofloxacin, diltiazem, ketoconazole, ritonavir, verapamil):* May increase dutasteride

level. Use together cautiously and monitor therapy.

EFFECTS ON LAB TEST RESULTS
• May increase total testosterone and TSH levels.
• May lower PSA level.

CONTRAINDICATIONS & CAUTIONS
• Contraindicated in patients hypersensitive to dutasteride or its ingredients or to other 5-alpha-reductase inhibitors.
⚠ *Alert:* 5-alpha-reductase inhibitors may increase the risk of high-grade prostate cancer.
• Drug isn't indicated for use in females or children.
• Use cautiously in patients with liver disease.
Dialyzable drug: Unknown.

PREGNANCY-LACTATION-REPRODUCTION
• Drug isn't indicated for use in females. Contraindicated during pregnancy.
• It isn't known if drug appears in human milk. Contraindicated for use during breastfeeding.
• Drug appears in semen. Effects on male fertility are unknown.

NURSING CONSIDERATIONS
• Carefully monitor patient with a large residual urine volume, severely diminished urine flow, or both for obstructive uropathy.
• Patient should wait at least 6 months after last dose before donating blood.
• Establish a new baseline PSA level at least 3 months after start of treatment, and use it to assess potentially cancer-related changes in PSA level.
• To interpret PSA values in patient treated for 3 months or more, double the PSA value for comparison with normal values in untreated patients. Any increase in PSA level in patient receiving dutasteride should be considered significant; evaluate patient for prostate cancer.
• Evaluate patient for prostate cancer and other urologic conditions that may cause similar signs and symptoms before initiating therapy and periodically thereafter.

PATIENT TEACHING
• Teach about proper drug administration and handling.

- Inform patient that ejaculate volume may decrease but that sexual function should remain normal. Effect on fertility is unknown.
- Inform patient that an increase in high-grade prostate cancer occurred in patients treated with 5 alpha-reductase inhibitors (which are indicated for BPH treatment), including Avodart.
- Caution caregiver who is pregnant or may become pregnant not to handle drug. A male fetus exposed to drug may be born with abnormal sex organs.
- **Alert:** Tell patient not to donate blood for at least 6 months after final dose to prevent drug administration to a transfusion recipient who is pregnant.
- Advise patient that drug is present in semen.
- Tell patient periodic blood tests will be needed to monitor therapeutic effects.

SAFETY ALERT!

edoxaban tosylate
e-DOX-a-ban

Savaysa

Therapeutic class: Factor Xa inhibitors
Pharmacologic class: Anticoagulants

AVAILABLE FORMS
Tablets: 15 mg, 30 mg, 60 mg

INDICATIONS & DOSAGES
Adjust-a-dose (for all indications): If CrCl is 15 to 50 mL/minute, decrease dosage to 30 mg PO once daily.
➤ **To reduce risk of stroke and systemic embolism in patients with nonvalvular atrial fibrillation (NVAF)**
Adults: 60 mg PO once daily. Refer to manufacturer's instructions for transitioning to or from other anticoagulants.
Boxed Warning Don't use for treatment of NVAF in patients with CrCl greater than 95 mL/minute because of increased risk of ischemic stroke. ∎
➤ **VTE**
Adults weighing more than 60 kg: 60 mg PO once daily after 5 to 10 days of therapy with a parenteral anticoagulant. Refer to manufacturer's instructions for transitioning to or from other anticoagulants.

Adjust-a-dose: If patient weighs 60 kg or less or is also taking certain P-gp inhibitors, decrease dosage to 30 mg PO once daily.

ADMINISTRATION
PO
- Give drug without regard to meals.
- For patients who can't swallow whole tablets, crush tablets and mix with applesauce or 60 to 90 mL water; give immediately.
- For patients with a gastric tube, crush tablets and mix with 60 to 90 mL water; give immediately.
- If a dose is missed, give as soon as possible on the same day. Resume normal schedule the following day. Don't double the dose to make up for missed dose.

ACTION
Inhibits free factor Xa, prothrombinase activity, and thrombin-induced platelet aggregation. Inhibition of factor Xa in the coagulation cascade reduces thrombin generation and thrombus formation.

Route	Onset	Peak	Duration
PO	Unknown	1–2 hr	Unknown

Half-life: 10 to 14 hours.

ADVERSE REACTIONS
CNS: *intracranial hemorrhage, hemorrhagic stroke, epidural or spinal hematoma.* **CV:** *hemorrhage.* **EENT:** epistaxis, *oral hemorrhage.* **GI:** *GI hemorrhage.* **GU:** *vaginal hemorrhage,* hematuria. **Hematologic:** anemia, bruising. **Hepatic:** abnormal LFT values. **Skin:** rash, puncture-site bleeding.

INTERACTIONS
Drug-drug. *Anticoagulants, antiplatelet drugs, NSAIDs, omega-3-fatty acids, SSNRIs, SSRIs, thrombolytics, vitamin E, vorapaxar:* May increase risk of bleeding. Monitor patient for bleeding during therapy.
Aspirin: May increase risk of bleeding. Monitor patient on long-term low-dose aspirin therapy for bleeding.
Digoxin: May increase digoxin level. Closely monitor digoxin level.
P-gp inducers (rifampin): May increase P-gp inducer exposure and decrease edoxaban serum level. Avoid use together.
P-gp inhibitors (itraconazole, ketoconazole [systemic], macrolide antibiotics, quinidine, verapamil): May increase edoxaban level

when edoxaban is used for VTE; reduce edoxaban dose to 30 mg if patient is receiving P-gp inhibitor. Edoxaban dosage adjustment isn't recommended when edoxaban is used to treat NVAF.

Drug-herb. *Alfalfa, anise, bilberry:* May increase bleeding risk. Avoid use together.

EFFECTS ON LAB TEST RESULTS
• May increase LFT values.
• May increase PT, PTT, and INR.
• May decrease thrombocyte and RBC counts.

CONTRAINDICATIONS & CAUTIONS
• Contraindicated in patients hypersensitive to drug or its components and in those with active pathological bleeding.
• Drug isn't recommended in patients with triple positive antiphospholipid syndrome due to increased risk of thrombotic events.
• Drug hasn't been studied in patients with mechanical heart valves or moderate to severe mitral stenosis or when CrCl is less than 15 mL/minute. Use isn't recommended in these patients.
• Use isn't recommended in patients with Child-Pugh class B or C liver impairment because of possible intrinsic coagulation abnormalities.

Boxed Warning Epidural or spinal hematomas may occur in patients taking edoxaban who are receiving neuraxial anesthesia or undergoing spinal puncture. Risk increases with indwelling epidural catheter use, use together with drugs that affect hemostasis (NSAIDs, platelet inhibitors, anticoagulants), spinal surgery or deformity, or history of traumatic or repeated epidural or spinal punctures. The optimal timing between edoxaban administration and neuraxial procedures isn't known. Weigh risks and benefits before neuraxial intervention in patients who are or will be anticoagulated. ∎

• Safety and effectiveness in children haven't been established.

Dialyzable drug: Less than 7%.

⚠ *Overdose S&S:* Bleeding.

PREGNANCY-LACTATION-REPRODUCTION
• Studies during pregnancy are inadequate. Use during pregnancy only if potential benefits outweigh fetal risk.
• It isn't known if drug appears in human milk. Discontinue breastfeeding or discontinue drug, considering importance of drug to patient.

NURSING CONSIDERATIONS
Boxed Warning Premature discontinuation of drug increases risk of ischemic events. If drug is stopped for a reason other than pathological bleeding or completion of treatment, consider transitioning to an alternative anticoagulant. ∎
• Monitor patient for bleeding. Immediately evaluate signs and symptoms of blood loss; discontinue drug if acute pathological bleeding occurs. Drug can cause serious and potentially fatal bleeding.
• A reversal agent for edoxaban isn't available. Vitamin K, protamine, tranexamic acid, and dialysis aren't expected to reverse the effects of edoxaban.
• Discontinue edoxaban at least 24 hours before invasive or surgical procedures. If surgery can't be delayed, weigh risk of bleeding against urgency of intervention.
• After surgery or another procedure, may restart edoxaban as soon as hemostasis has been achieved and patient can take oral medication.
⚕ *Alert:* Don't remove an indwelling epidural or intrathecal catheter earlier than 12 hours after last dose of edoxaban. Don't give next dose earlier than 2 hours after catheter removal.
Boxed Warning After spinal or epidural anesthesia or puncture, frequently monitor patient for signs and symptoms of neurologic impairment (numbness or weakness of legs, bowel or bladder dysfunction). Evaluate impairment urgently. Epidural or spinal hematoma can result in long-term or permanent paralysis. ∎

PATIENT TEACHING
• Warn patient that bruising and bleeding may occur more easily and that bleeding may last longer during therapy.
• Instruct patient to immediately report unusual bleeding to prescriber.
• Warn patient to immediately report signs and symptoms of hemorrhage or adverse reactions, such as one-sided weakness, problems thinking or speaking, dizziness, balance changes, blurred vision, severe headache, and pale skin.
• Teach patient to take drug exactly as prescribed.

Reactions in bold italics are *life-threatening*.

- Advise patient not to discontinue drug without first consulting prescriber.
- Caution patient to inform health care providers about taking edoxaban before scheduling surgery or other procedures.
- Instruct patient to inform health care providers and dentists about prescription medications, OTC drugs, or herbal products currently being taken or that may be taken.
- Advise patient to immediately report pregnancy, plans to become pregnant, or intent to breastfeed during treatment.
- Warn patient having neuraxial anesthesia or spinal puncture to watch for signs and symptoms of spinal or epidural hematoma (back pain, tingling, numbness [especially in the lower limbs], muscle weakness, stool or urine incontinence) and to immediately contact health care provider if any occur.

efavirenz
eff-ah-VYE-renz

Sustiva

Therapeutic class: Antiretrovirals
Pharmacologic class: NNRTIs

AVAILABLE FORMS
Capsules ⚫: 50 mg, 200 mg
Tablets ⚫: 600 mg

INDICATIONS & DOSAGES
➤ **HIV-1 infection, with other antiretrovirals**
Adults and children ages 3 months and older weighing 40 kg or more: 600 mg (three 200-mg capsules or one 600-mg tablet) PO once daily.
Children ages 3 months and older weighing 32.5 to less than 40 kg: 400 mg PO once daily.
Children ages 3 months and older weighing 25 to less than 32.5 kg: 350 mg PO once daily.
Children ages 3 months and older weighing 20 to less than 25 kg: 300 mg PO once daily.
Children ages 3 months and older weighing 15 to less than 20 kg: 250 mg PO once daily.
Children ages 3 months and older weighing 7.5 to less than 15 kg: 200 mg PO once daily.
Children ages 3 months and older weighing 5 to less than 7.5 kg: 150 mg PO once daily.
Children ages 3 months and older weighing 3.5 to less than 5 kg: 100 mg PO once daily.

Adjust-a-dose: For adults also taking voriconazole, increase voriconazole maintenance dose to 400 mg every 12 hours and decrease efavirenz dose to 300 mg once daily using capsule formulation. For adults and children weighing 50 kg or more who are also taking rifampin, recommended efavirenz dosage is 800 mg once daily.

ADMINISTRATION
PO
- Drug must be given in combination with other antiretrovirals.
- Give drug at bedtime to decrease CNS adverse effects.
- In a child, consider prophylaxis with antihistamine before initiating therapy to prevent rash.
- Have patient swallow tablets whole; don't crush or cut tablets. Don't crush capsules.
- Give once daily on an empty stomach.
- For patient who can't swallow capsules or tablets, sprinkle capsule contents over a small amount (1 or 2 tsp) of food and mix gently. For patient who can tolerate solid foods, mix with soft food (applesauce, grape jelly, yogurt).
- For young infant, gently mix dose from capsules into 10 mL of reconstituted room-temperature infant formula in 30-mL medicine cup. If more than 1 capsule is needed for a dose, add contents of all capsules needed to 10 mL of formula; don't add more formula. Draw up mixture into 10-mL dosing syringe to administer; then add an additional 10 mL to mixing cup and stir to disperse any remaining residue. Administer to infant.
- Give efavirenz mixture within 30 minutes of mixing. Patient shouldn't consume any additional food or additional formula for 2 hours after administration.

ACTION
Inhibits nonnucleoside reverse transcriptase, which inhibits the transcription of HIV-1 RNA to DNA, a critical step in viral replication, suppressing viral replication.

Route	Onset	Peak	Duration
PO	Unknown	3–5 hr	Unknown

Half-life: Single dose, 52 to 76 hours; multiple doses, 40 to 55 hours.

ADVERSE REACTIONS
CNS: dizziness, abnormal dreams or thinking, anxiety, agitation, amnesia, confusion, depersonalization, depression, euphoria,

fever, fatigue, pain, hallucinations, headache, hypoesthesia, impaired concentration, insomnia, nervousness, somnolence. **GI:** diarrhea, nausea, abdominal pain, anorexia, dyspepsia, vomiting. **Hematologic:** *neutropenia.* **Hepatic:** increased transaminase levels, increased GGT level. **Metabolic:** increased amylase level, hyperglycemia, hypertriglyceridemia. **Skin:** rash, *erythema multiforme,* pruritus.

INTERACTIONS

❂ *Alert:* Efavirenz can interact with many drugs. Consult a drug compatibility resource or pharmacist for more information.

Drug-drug. *Amprenavir, itraconazole, lopinavir:* May decrease levels of these drugs. Consider alternative therapy or dosage adjustment. Refer to prescribing information for these drugs.

Atorvastatin, calcium channel blockers, pravastatin, simvastatin: May decrease levels of these drugs. Monitor therapy. Dosage adjustments may be necessary.

Bupropion, sertraline: May decrease plasma levels and clinical effects of these drugs. Guide dosage by clinical response.

Carbamazepine, phenytoin, phenobarbital: May decrease levels of these drugs. Monitor therapy.

CYP2B6 (propofol, nortriptyline) or CYP3A substrates (corticosteroids): May decrease substate level. Some combinations may be contraindicated. Consult manufacturer labeling. Consider therapy modification.

CYP3A4 inducers (phenobarbital, phenytoin, rifampin): May decrease efavirenz level. Avoid use together. Refer to manufacturer's instructions for contraindications.

Drugs that prolong QT interval (amiodarone, haloperidol, lithium, procainamide, thioridazine): May increase risk of torsades de pointes. Consider alternative to efavirenz.

Elbasvir, grazoprevir: May lead to loss of virologic response of these drugs. Use together is contraindicated.

Hormonal contraceptives (ethinyl estradiol–norgestimate, etonogestrel): May decrease norgestimate and etonogestrel levels. Advise use of a reliable method of barrier contraception in addition to use of hormonal contraceptives.

Immunosuppressants (cyclosporine, tacrolimus): May decrease level of immunosuppressant. Monitor closely and adjust immunosuppressant dosage, as indicated.

Macrolide antibiotics (clarithromycin): May prolong QT interval. Use alternative antibiotic.

Methadone: May decrease methadone level. Monitor for methadone withdrawal and increase dose to alleviate withdrawal symptoms.

Psychoactive drugs (caffeine, amphetamines): May cause additive CNS effects. Avoid use together.

Ranolazine: May decrease ranolazine level. Avoid use together.

Rifabutin: May decrease rifabutin level. Increase daily rifabutin dosage by 50%. Consider doubling rifabutin dosage when rifabutin is given two to three times per week.

Ritonavir: May increase levels of both drugs. Closely monitor patient and liver function.

Saquinavir: May decrease saquinavir level and efavirenz exposure to the body. Don't use with saquinavir as sole protease inhibitor.

Voriconazole (in standard doses): Significantly decreases voriconazole level, while efavirenz level significantly increases. Avoid use together without dosage adjustments to each drug.

Warfarin: May increase or decrease warfarin level and effects. Monitor INR.

Drug-herb. *St. John's wort:* May decrease response and lead to possible resistance to efavirenz or all same-class drugs. Avoid use together.

Ginkgo biloba: May decrease efavirenz level. Monitor use together.

Kava: May enhance adverse or toxic effect of CNS depressants. Monitor therapy.

Drug-food. *High-fat meals:* May increase drug absorption. Instruct patient to maintain a proper low-fat diet.

Drug-lifestyle. *Alcohol use:* May enhance CNS effects. Discourage use together.

EFFECTS ON LAB TEST RESULTS

• May increase ALT, AST, GGT, triglyceride, glucose, amylase, and cholesterol levels.

• May decrease neutrophil count.

• May cause false-positive urine cannabinoid and benzodiazepine test results.

CONTRAINDICATIONS & CAUTIONS

• Contraindicated in patients hypersensitive to drug or its components.

• Use in patients with Child-Pugh class B or C liver impairment isn't recommended.

• Use cautiously in patients with Child-Pugh class A liver impairment and in those receiving liver-toxic drugs.

Reactions in bold italics are *life-threatening*.

• Administration with Atripla (efavirenz 600 mg/emtricitabine 200 mg/tenofovir disoproxil fumarate 300 mg) isn't recommended unless needed for dosage adjustment (with rifampin) because efavirenz is one of its active ingredients.

• Serious psychiatric adverse reactions have been reported, including aggressive behavior, severe depression, suicidality, nonfatal suicide attempts, paranoia, and mania. Use cautiously in patients with a history of mental illness or substance abuse.

• Drug may prolong QT interval. Avoid use in patients at increased risk for or with other drugs with known risk of torsades de pointes. Consider alternative to efavirenz.

• Use cautiously in patients with history of seizures.

• Immune reconstitution syndrome has been reported in patients treated with combination antiretroviral therapy.

• Late-onset neurotoxicity, including ataxia and encephalopathy (impaired consciousness, confusion, psychomotor slowing, psychosis, delirium), may occur months to years after therapy.

Dialyzable drug: No.

⚠ *Overdose S&S:* Increased nervous system symptoms, involuntary muscle contractions.

PREGNANCY-LACTATION-REPRODUCTION

• Because of risk of neural tube defects, don't use drug in first trimester. Advise patients who are pregnant of fetal risk. Strongly consider other antiretrovirals.

• Register patients who are pregnant in the Antiretroviral Pregnancy Registry at 1-800-258-4263 or www.apregistry.com.

• Patients should avoid breastfeeding because of risk of HIV transmission.

• Patients of childbearing potential should use barrier contraception in combination with other hormonal contraceptives during therapy and for 12 weeks after therapy.

NURSING CONSIDERATIONS

⚠ *Alert:* Drug shouldn't be used as monotherapy or added on as a single drug to a regimen failing because of viral resistance.

• Verify pregnancy status before treatment.

• Note that using drug with ritonavir may increase liver enzyme levels and adverse effects (dizziness, nausea, paresthesia).

• Monitor LFT values before and during treatment in all patients. Consider discontinuing

drug in patient with persistent elevation of serum transaminase levels greater than 5 × ULN. Discontinue drug if elevation is accompanied by clinical signs or symptoms of hepatitis or liver decompensation.

• Monitor for neurologic symptoms, which often begin during the first 2 days of therapy and resolve after 2 to 4 weeks of therapy.

• Monitor for psychiatric symptoms.

• Be aware that a child is more prone to adverse reactions, especially diarrhea, nausea, vomiting, and rash. Consider prophylaxis with antihistamines before initiating therapy to prevent rash in this population.

• Monitor for rash, which usually begins 1 to 2 weeks after start of therapy and resolves within 4 weeks. Discontinue drug if severe rash (SJS) develops (blistering, mucosal involvement, desquamation, or fever).

• Monitor for elevated triglyceride and cholesterol levels before therapy and periodically during treatment.

PATIENT TEACHING

• Tell patient to take drug exactly as prescribed and not to stop drug without medical approval.

• Instruct patient to report adverse reactions.

• Instruct patient to immediately report signs and symptoms of serious psychiatric adverse effects.

• Inform patient about need for blood tests to monitor LFT values and triglyceride levels.

• Advise patient of childbearing potential of fetal risk. Review contraceptive use and need to immediately notify prescriber of suspected pregnancy.

• Inform patient that drug doesn't cure HIV infection, that opportunistic infections and other complications of HIV infection may continue to occur, and that transmission of HIV to others through sexual contact or blood contamination is still possible.

• Explain that rash is a common adverse effect. Tell patient to immediately report rash because it may be serious in rare cases.

• Instruct patient to report use of other drugs, including OTC drugs and herbal supplements.

• Tell patient to avoid alcohol.

• Advise patient that dizziness, difficulty sleeping or concentrating, drowsiness, or unusual dreams may occur. Reassure patient that these symptoms typically resolve after 2 to 4 weeks and may be less problematic if drug is taken at bedtime.

• Tell patient to avoid driving and operating machinery until drug's effects are known.

elagolix
el-a-GOE-lix

Orilissa

Therapeutic class: Endocrine drugs
Pharmacologic class: GnRH receptor antagonists

AVAILABLE FORMS
Tablets: 150 mg, 200 mg

INDICATIONS & DOSAGES
Adjust-a-dose (for all indications): For patients with Child-Pugh class B liver impairment, give 150 mg PO once daily for up to 6 months. Use of 200 mg b.i.d. isn't recommended.
➤ **Management of moderate to severe pain associated with endometriosis**
Females ages 18 and older: 150 mg PO once daily for up to 24 months.
➤ **Management of moderate to severe pain associated with endometriosis with dyspareunia**
Females ages 18 and older: 200 mg PO b.i.d. for up to 6 months.

ADMINISTRATION
PO
• Exclude pregnancy before starting drug or start drug within 7 days from menses onset.
• Limit duration of use based on dose and coexisting condition because of risk of bone loss.
• Give drug at the same time each day, with or without food.
• Give missed dose on the same day as soon as possible; then resume regular dosing schedule.
• Store at 36° to 86° F (2° to 30° C).

ACTION
A GnRH receptor antagonist that suppresses the pituitary gland and decreases ovarian sex hormone, estradiol, and progesterone levels.

Route	Onset	Peak	Duration
PO	Unknown	1 hr	Unknown

Half-life: 4 to 6 hours.

ADVERSE REACTIONS
CNS: headache, insomnia, anxiety, depression, mood changes, exacerbation of mood disorders, dizziness, irritability. **GI:** nausea, diarrhea, abdominal pain, constipation. **GU:** changes in menstrual bleeding pattern, amenorrhea, decreased libido. **Metabolic:** night sweats, weight gain. **Musculoskeletal:** arthralgia, bone loss. **Skin:** rash. **Other:** hot flashes, hypersensitivity reactions.

INTERACTIONS
Drug-drug. *CYP3A inducers (carbamazepine, phenytoin):* May decrease elagolix level. Monitor therapy.
Hormonal contraceptives: May reduce efficacy of elagolix if contraceptive contains estrogen. Use of nonhormonal contraception is recommended during treatment and for at least 28 days after final dose.
Midazolam: May decrease midazolam level. Monitor patient for effectiveness; adjust midazolam dosage as clinically indicated.
Rifampin: May increase elagolix level. Limit elagolix dosage to 150 mg once daily, and limit concomitant use to 6 months.
Rosuvastatin: May decrease rosuvastatin level. Consider increasing rosuvastatin dosage.
Strong CYP3A inhibitors (cobicistat, conivaptan, danoprevir, elvitegravir, itraconazole, ketoconazole, lopinavir, ritonavir, saquinavir, voriconazole): May increase elagolix level. Limit 200-mg b.i.d. regimen to 1 month, and limit concomitant use of 150-mg once-daily regimen to 6 months.
Strong OATP1B1 inhibitors (cyclosporine, gemfibrozil): May increase elagolix level. Use together is contraindicated.
Substrates of CYP3A (alprazolam, atorvastatin, buspirone, colchicine, darunavir, rivaroxaban, saquinavir, simvastatin, tipranavir): May decrease levels of these drugs. Monitor patient for therapeutic effect; adjust substrate dosage as clinically indicated.
Substrates of P-gp (digoxin): May increase digoxin level. Monitor digoxin level; adjust dosage as indicated.

EFFECTS ON LAB TEST RESULTS
• May increase transaminase, total cholesterol, LDL-C, HDL-C, and triglyceride levels.

Reactions in bold italics are *life-threatening*.

CONTRAINDICATIONS & CAUTIONS

• Contraindicated in patients hypersensitive to drug and in those with Child-Pugh class C liver impairment or known osteoporosis.

🔵 *Alert:* Use cautiously in patients with a history of suicidality or depression. Drug may increase risk of suicidality and mood disorders.

• Drug can cause liver impairment and should be used at lowest effective dose.

• Drug may cause bone loss, which may not be completely reversible. Assess bone mineral density (BMD) in patients with other risk factors for osteoporosis. Limit duration of use in all patients.

• Safety and effectiveness in patients younger than age 18 haven't been studied.

Dialyzable drug: No.

PREGNANCY-LACTATION-REPRODUCTION

• Contraindicated during pregnancy. Drug may increase risk of early pregnancy loss. Discontinue drug if pregnancy occurs during treatment.

• Patients who become pregnant during treatment should enroll in the pregnancy registry (1-833-782-7241 or https://www.bloompregnancyregistry.com/).

• Patients should use nonhormonal contraception during treatment and for 28 days after final dose.

• It isn't known whether drug appears in human milk or how drug affects milk production or infants who are breastfed. Weigh benefit to patient against risk to infant before use.

NURSING CONSIDERATIONS

🔵 *Alert:* Monitor patient for suicidality and exacerbation of existing mood disorders.

🔵 *Alert:* Promptly evaluate patient with depressive symptoms to determine whether risks of continued therapy outweigh benefits.

🔵 *Alert:* Refer patient with new or worsening depression, anxiety, or other mood changes to a mental health professional for assessment.

• Exclude pregnancy before start of treatment and obtain pregnancy test for suspected pregnancy during treatment.

• Monitor BMD in patient with history of low-trauma fracture or other risk factors for osteoporosis or bone loss.

• Consider supplementation with calcium and vitamin D. The benefits of taking these supplements during treatment with elagolix

haven't been studied, but supplements may benefit all patients.

• Monitor patient for changes in menstrual bleeding (reduction in amount, intensity, or duration). These changes can make it difficult to recognize pregnancy. Perform pregnancy testing if pregnancy is suspected; discontinue treatment if confirmed.

• Monitor for signs and symptoms of liver injury (jaundice, abdominal pain, dark amber-colored urine, fatigue, nausea, vomiting, generalized swelling, easy bruising). Obtain LFT values if signs and symptoms occur.

PATIENT TEACHING

🔵 *Alert:* Advise patient to seek immediate medical attention for suicidality, new-onset or worsening depression, anxiety, or other mood changes.

🔵 *Alert:* Counsel family caregivers to watch for changes in behavior and to immediately report suicidality to prescriber.

• Advise patient that drug may cause menstrual changes, which can make it difficult to detect an early pregnancy. Counsel patient to obtain a pregnancy test if pregnancy is suspected and to discontinue drug if pregnancy is confirmed.

• Caution patient to avoid pregnancy while using drug and to use nonhormonal contraceptives during and for 28 days after treatment, even if taking oral contraceptives.

• Inform patient that estrogen-containing contraceptives may reduce drug's efficacy.

• Inform patient about risk of bone loss. Advise adequate intake of calcium and vitamin D and supplementation if prescribed.

• Counsel patient to immediately report signs and symptoms of liver injury.

• Teach about proper drug administration and handling.

---

elbasvir–grazoprevir 🔒

ELB-as-vir/graz-OH-pre-vir

Zepatier

Therapeutic class: Antivirals
Pharmacologic class: HCV NS5A inhibitors/HCV NS3/4A protease inhibitors

AVAILABLE FORMS

Tablets: elbasvir 50 mg/grazoprevir 100 mg

INDICATIONS & DOSAGES

➤ **Chronic HCV genotypes 1 or 4 infection, with or without ribavirin** ▓

Adults and children ages 12 and older or weighing at least 30 kg: 1 tablet PO once daily. See manufacturer's instructions for recommended dosing regimens and durations for treatment of HCV genotype 1 or 4 in patients with or without cirrhosis.

Adjust-a-dose: If ALT level is greater than 10 × ULN, consider discontinuing drug. If ALT level is elevated and accompanied by signs or symptoms of liver inflammation, increased conjugated bilirubin or ALP level, or increased INR, discontinue drug. If CrCl is 50 mL/minute or less and ribavirin is used, refer to ribavirin prescribing information for ribavirin dosage adjustment.

ADMINISTRATION
PO
• Give drug without regard to food.
• Store at 68° to 77° F (20° to 25° C).
• Store in original container. Protect from moisture.

ACTION
Elbasvir inhibits HCV NS5A, an enzyme needed for viral RNA replication and assembly of virions. Grazoprevir inhibits HCV NS3/4A protease, an enzyme that is essential for viral replication and is responsible for HCV protein cleavage.

Route	Onset	Peak	Duration
PO (elbasvir)	Unknown	3 hr	Unknown
PO (grazoprevir)	Unknown	2 hr	Unknown

Half-life: Elbasvir, 24 hours; grazoprevir, 31 hours.

ADVERSE REACTIONS
CNS: headache, fatigue, insomnia, irritability, depression. **GI:** nausea, diarrhea, abdominal pain. **Hematologic:** anemia. **Hepatic:** ALT elevation, bilirubin elevation. **Musculoskeletal:** arthralgia (with ribavirin). **Respiratory:** dyspnea (with ribavirin). **Skin:** rash or pruritus (with ribavirin).

INTERACTIONS
❂ *Alert:* Elbasvir–grazoprevir can interact with many drugs. Consult a drug compatibility reference or pharmacist for more information.
Drug-drug. *Antibiotics (nafcillin):* May decrease levels and therapeutic effects of

elbasvir and grazoprevir. Use together isn't recommended.

HIV medications (cobicistat, elvitegravir, emtricitabine, etravirine, tenofovir): May increase elbasvir–grazoprevir levels. Use together isn't recommended. Etravirine may decrease elbasvir–grazoprevir level and lead to decreased effectiveness. Use together isn't recommended.

HMG-CoA reductase inhibitors (atorvastatin, rosuvastatin): May increase atorvastatin and rosuvastatin levels. Maximum recommended dosages are atorvastatin 20 mg/day and rosuvastatin 10 mg/day.

HMG-CoA reductase inhibitors (fluvastatin, lovastatin, simvastatin): May increase levels of HMG-CoA reductase inhibitors. Use lowest necessary statin dosage and monitor patient closely for statin-associated adverse effects such as myopathy.

Immunosuppressants (tacrolimus): May increase tacrolimus level. Frequently monitor kidney function and tacrolimus level, and watch for tacrolimus-associated adverse effects.

Moderate CYP3A inducers (bosentan, modafinil): May decrease elbasvir–grazoprevir plasma levels. Use together isn't recommended.

OATP1B1/3 inhibitors (atazanavir, cyclosporine, darunavir, lopinavir, saquinavir, tipranavir): May increase risk of ALT elevation. Use together is contraindicated.

Strong CYP3A inducers (carbamazepine, efavirenz, phenytoin, rifampin): May cause loss of virologic response. Use together is contraindicated.

Strong CYP3A inhibitors (clarithromycin, ketoconazole, nefazodone, nelfinavir, ritonavir): May increase elbasvir or grazoprevir level. Use together isn't recommended.

Drug-herb. *St. John's wort:* May decrease elbasvir–grazoprevir levels and cause loss of virologic response. Use together is contraindicated.

EFFECTS ON LAB TEST RESULTS
• May increase ALT and bilirubin levels.
• May decrease Hb level.

CONTRAINDICATIONS & CAUTIONS
▓ Patients with HCV genotype 1a infection should undergo testing for NS5A resistance-associated polymorphisms before starting treatment to determine need for ribavirin as well as treatment duration.

E

• If elbasvir–grazoprevir is administered with ribavirin, the contraindications for ribavirin also apply.

Boxed Warning Reactivation of HBV may occur in patients who are coinfected with HCV, resulting in fulminant hepatitis, liver failure, and death. Screen all patients for current or prior HBV infection before treatment and, if positive for HBV infection, assess baseline HBV DNA. ■

• Contraindicated in patients with Child-Pugh class B or C liver impairment.

🔵 *Alert:* Use cautiously in patients with risk factors for liver failure (hepatocellular carcinoma, alcohol abuse).

🔶 Female patients, patients of Asian descent, and patients ages 65 and older are at increased risk for elevated ALT level.

• Safe use in children younger than age 12 or weighing less than 35 kg, recipients of liver transplants, and patients with HBV and HCV coinfection hasn't been established.

Dialyzable drug: No.

PREGNANCY-LACTATION-REPRODUCTION

• Studies during pregnancy are inadequate. If drug is used with ribavirin, the combination regimen is contraindicated in patients who are pregnant and in males whose partners are pregnant.

• It isn't known if elbasvir or grazoprevir appears in human milk. Use cautiously during breastfeeding.

NURSING CONSIDERATIONS

Boxed Warning Monitor patient with current or prior HBV infection for hepatitis flare or HBV reactivation with lab testing and watch for signs and symptoms of liver injury during active and posttreatment follow-up. Begin appropriate HBV treatment as clinically indicated. ■

• If drug is given with ribavirin, a negative pregnancy test is required immediately before initiation, monthly during therapy, and for 6 months after treatment ends.

• Obtain LFT values before start of therapy, at treatment week 8, at week 12 in patient receiving 16 weeks of treatment, and as clinically indicated.

🔵 *Alert:* Monitor patient closely for liver failure; discontinue drug if signs and symptoms of decompensation develop or as clinically indicated.

• Monitor for signs and symptoms of liver inflammation (fatigue, weakness, lack of appetite, abdominal pain, nausea, vomiting, jaundice, and discolored feces).

PATIENT TEACHING

🔵 *Alert:* Warn patient to immediately report signs and symptoms of liver injury.

• Instruct patient to report current or new prescription or OTC medications or supplements before taking them because of possible interactions.

• Explain importance of taking drug around the same time every day, without missing or skipping doses. Advise patient to contact prescriber if a dose is missed and to not double a dose.

• Teach patient importance of adherence and regular follow-up with prescriber during therapy.

• Advise patient of childbearing potential and male patient's partner of childbearing potential to avoid pregnancy during and after therapy when drug is used concomitantly with ribavirin.

eletriptan hydrobromide
ell-ah-TRIP-tan

Relpax

Therapeutic class: Antimigraine drugs
Pharmacologic class: Serotonin 5-HT$_1$ receptor agonists

AVAILABLE FORMS
Tablets: 20 mg, 40 mg

INDICATIONS & DOSAGES
➤ **Acute migraine with or without aura**
Adults: 20 to 40 mg PO at first migraine symptom. If headache recurs, dose may be repeated at least 2 hours later to a maximum of 80 mg in any 24-hour period.

ADMINISTRATION
PO
• Give drug without regard to food.
• Store at room temperature.

ACTION
Binds to 5-HT$_{1B/1D/1F}$ receptors and may constrict intracranial blood vessels and inhibit proinflammatory neuropeptide release.

Route	Onset	Peak	Duration
PO	0.5 hr	1.5–2 hr	Unknown

Half-life: About 4 hours.

ADVERSE REACTIONS

CNS: asthenia, dizziness, drowsiness, headache, paresthesia, somnolence. **CV:** chest tightness, pain, and pressure; flushing. **EENT:** dry mouth, pharyngitis. **GI:** abdominal pain, discomfort, or cramps; dyspepsia; dysphagia; nausea.

INTERACTIONS

Drug-drug. *CYP3A4 inhibitors (clarithromycin, itraconazole, ketoconazole, nefazodone, nelfinavir, ritonavir):* May increase eletriptan metabolism. Use within 72 hours of these drugs is contraindicated.

Ergotamine-containing or ergot-type drugs (dihydroergotamine), other 5-HT$_1$ antagonists: May prolong vasospastic reactions. Use within 24 hours of these drugs is contraindicated.

Linezolid: May enhance serotonergic effect of eletriptan, possibly resulting in serotonin syndrome. If urgent initiation of linezolid is needed, immediately discontinue eletriptan and monitor patient.

MAO inhibitors: May increase risk of serotonin syndrome. Avoid use together.

Methylene blue: May increase risk of serotonin syndrome. Avoid use together.

SSNRIs, SSRIs, TCAs: May increase risk of serotonin syndrome. Monitor patient closely.

EFFECTS ON LAB TEST RESULTS

None reported.

CONTRAINDICATIONS & CAUTIONS

• Contraindicated in patients hypersensitive to drug or its components. Hypersensitivity reactions, including anaphylaxis, have been reported. Anaphylactic reactions are more likely in patients with history of sensitivity to multiple allergens.

• Contraindicated in patients with severe liver impairment; ischemic heart disease; history of MI; silent ischemia; coronary artery vasospasm, including Prinzmetal variant angina; Wolff-Parkinson-White syndrome or arrhythmias associated with other cardiac accessory conduction pathway disorders; and other significant CV conditions.

• Contraindicated in patients with cerebrovascular syndromes, such as stroke or TIA; PVD, including ischemic bowel disease; uncontrolled HTN; or hemiplegic or basilar migraine.

• Use cautiously in older adults.

• Safety of treating more than three migraine headaches in 30 days hasn't been established.

• Safety and effectiveness in children haven't been established.

Dialyzable drug: Unknown.

⚠ *Overdose S&S:* HTN, serious CV reactions.

PREGNANCY-LACTATION-REPRODUCTION

• Data related to eletriptan use during pregnancy are limited. Use of other agents for migraine management is preferred.

• Drug appears in human milk. Use cautiously during breastfeeding.

NURSING CONSIDERATIONS

• Drug isn't intended for migraine prevention.

🔵 *Alert:* Combining a triptan with an SSRI or SSNRI, TCA, linezolid, methylene blue, or MAO inhibitor may cause serotonin syndrome. Signs and symptoms (restlessness, hallucinations, loss of coordination, fast heartbeat, rapid BP changes, increased body temperature, hyperreflexia, nausea, vomiting, diarrhea) occur within minutes to hours of patient receiving a new or increased dosage of the serotonergic drug; signs and symptoms are more likely to occur at start of therapy or when serotonergic drug dosage is increased.

• Use drug only when patient has a clear diagnosis of migraine. If first use produces no response, reconsider migraine diagnosis.

• Significant HTN can occur, even in patient with no history of HTN. Closely monitor BP.

• Prior to use, patient with risk factors for CAD should undergo CV evaluation. If evaluation is negative, closely monitor patient and ECG after first dose.

PATIENT TEACHING

• Teach about proper drug administration and handling.

• Warn patient to avoid driving and operating machinery if dizziness or fatigue occurs.

• Tell patient to immediately report signs or symptoms of MI (pain, tightness, heaviness, or pressure in chest, throat, neck, or jaw); stroke (trouble speaking, change in balance, one-sided weakness); or vasospasm (change in color or sensation of fingers or toes, GI cramps or pain, bloody diarrhea, leg cramps or pain, burning or aching pain in feet while resting, numbness or tingling in legs).

eluxadoline
el-ux-AD-oh-leen

Viberzi

Therapeutic class: Anti–IBS drugs
Pharmacologic class: Mu-opioid receptor agonists, delta-opioid receptor antagonists, kappa-opioid receptor agonists
Controlled substance schedule: IV

AVAILABLE FORMS
Tablets: 75 mg, 100 mg

INDICATIONS & DOSAGES
➤ **IBS with diarrhea (IBS-D)**
Adults: 100 mg PO b.i.d.
Adjust-a-dose: Reduce dosage to 75 mg b.i.d. in patients who can't tolerate 100-mg dose, are receiving concomitant OATP1B1 inhibitors, have Child-Pugh class A or B liver impairment, or have eGFR less than 60 mL/minute/1.73 m² and in patients with eGFR less than 15 mL/minute/1.73 m² who are not yet on dialysis.

ADMINISTRATION
PO
• Give drug with food.
• If a dose is missed, give next dose at the regular time. Don't give two doses at the same time to make up for a missed dose.
• Store at room temperature.

ACTION
Mu-opioid receptor agonist, delta-opioid receptor antagonist, and kappa-opioid receptor agonist that decreases peristaltic action of the intestines. Acts locally to reduce abdominal pain and IBS-D without constipating adverse effects.

Route	Onset	Peak	Duration
PO (with food)	Unknown	1.5 hr (range, 1–8 hr)	Unknown

Half-life: 3.7 to 6 hours.

ADVERSE REACTIONS
CNS: dizziness, fatigue, drowsiness, euphoria, intoxicated feeling, sedation, somnolence.
EENT: nasopharyngitis. **GI:** constipation, nausea, vomiting, abdominal pain, abdominal distention, flatulence, viral gastroenteritis, GERD. **Hepatic:** elevated ALT and AST levels. **Respiratory:** URI, bronchitis, *asthma, bronchospasm, respiratory failure,* wheezing. **Skin:** rash. **Other:** hypersensitivity reactions.

INTERACTIONS
Drug-drug. *Drugs that cause constipation (alosetron, anticholinergics, opioids):* May increase risk of constipation-related adverse reactions. Avoid use together.
OATP1B1 inhibitors (atazanavir, cyclosporine, eltrombopag, gemfibrozil, lopinavir, rifampin, ritonavir, saquinavir, tipranavir): May increase eluxadoline level. Decrease eluxadoline dose; monitor patient for eluxadoline-related adverse reactions.
Rosuvastatin: May increase rosuvastatin level and risk of myopathy and rhabdomyolysis. Use lowest effective rosuvastatin dose.
Drug-lifestyle. *Alcohol use:* May increase risk of acute pancreatitis. Patient should avoid prolonged or acute excessive alcohol use while taking drug. Monitor patient closely.

EFFECTS ON LAB TEST RESULTS
• May increase ALT and AST levels.

CONTRAINDICATIONS & CAUTIONS
• Contraindicated in patients hypersensitive to drug or its components.
• Contraindicated in patients without a gallbladder, with known or suspected biliary duct obstruction, or sphincter of Oddi disease or dysfunction.
• Contraindicated in patients with alcohol abuse, alcohol addiction, alcoholism, or consumption of more than three alcoholic beverages each day; history of pancreatitis or structural diseases of the pancreas or suspected pancreatic duct obstruction; Child-Pugh class C liver impairment; history of chronic or severe constipation or sequelae from constipation; or known or suspected mechanical GI obstruction.
• Drug has potential for abuse and psychological dependence. Consider naloxone in the event of overdose.
• Safety and effectiveness in children haven't been established.

• Use cautiously in older adults, who are at increased risk for adverse reactions.
Dialyzable drug: Unlikely.

PREGNANCY-LACTATION-REPRODUCTION
• Use cautiously during pregnancy. Risk to fetus is unknown.
• It isn't known if drug appears in human milk. Use cautiously during breastfeeding, considering maternal benefits and fetal risk.

NURSING CONSIDERATIONS
• Monitor patient with liver impairment for impaired mental or physical abilities needed to perform potentially hazardous activities, such as driving and operating machinery.
• Monitor patient for sphincter of Oddi spasm (unusual or severe epigastric or upper right quadrant abdominal pain that may radiate to the back or shoulder, with or without nausea and vomiting and with liver or pancreatic enzyme elevations). Discontinue drug if signs or symptoms develop.
• Monitor patient, especially one with excessive alcohol intake, for pancreatitis (new or worsening abdominal or epigastric pain that may radiate to the back, associated with elevated pancreatic enzyme levels). Discontinue drug if signs and symptoms occur.
• Monitor patient for constipation. Immediately discontinue drug if severe constipation develops.
• Watch for signs and symptoms of abuse of drug, including psychological dependence.

PATIENT TEACHING
• Advise patient to read the medication guide.
• Teach about proper drug administration and handling.
• Warn patient to stop drug and seek medical attention for new or worsening upper right quadrant abdominal pain that radiates to the shoulder or back or if nausea or vomiting occurs.
• Advise patient to avoid prolonged and acute excessive alcohol use while taking drug.
• Counsel patient to discontinue drug and immediately contact prescriber for severe constipation.
• Instruct patient to avoid taking drug with other medications that may cause constipation and to ask prescriber for a list of these medications.
• Inform patient that loperamide may occasionally be used with eluxadoline but must be stopped if constipation develops.

• Caution patient with liver impairment not to drive, operate machinery, or perform other dangerous activities until effects of drug are known.

elvitegravir–cobicistat–emtricitabine–tenofovir disoproxil fumarate
el-vye-TEG-ra-veer/koe-BIK-i-stat/em-tra-SYE-tah-ben/te-NOE-fo-veer

Stribild

Therapeutic class: Antiretrovirals
Pharmacologic class: Antivirals

AVAILABLE FORMS
Tablet: 150 mg elvitegravir, 150 mg cobicistat, 200 mg emtricitabine, and 300 mg tenofovir disoproxil fumarate per tablet

INDICATIONS & DOSAGES
➤ **HIV-1 infection in patients who are antiretroviral treatment–naive or to replace current antiretroviral regimen in patients who are virologically suppressed (HIV-1 RNA fewer than 50 copies/mL) on a stable regimen for at least 6 months with no history of treatment failure and no known substitutions associated with resistance to individual components**
Adults and children ages 12 and older weighing at least 35 kg: 1 tablet PO once daily.
Adjust-a-dose: Discontinue drug in adult patients whose estimated CrCl declines to less than 50 mL/minute. No recommendations exist for children with kidney impairment.

ADMINISTRATION
PO
• Give drug with food.
• Drug is used as a complete treatment; don't give with other antiretrovirals.

ACTION
Combination of agents with differing mechanisms of action (integrase strand transfer inhibition, pharmacokinetic enhancement, nucleoside and nucleotide analogue HIV-1 reverse transcriptase inhibition) working together to inhibit HIV replication.

Route	Onset	Peak	Duration
PO (elvitegravir)	Unknown	4 hr	Unknown
PO (cobicistat, emtricitabine)	Unknown	3 hr	Unknown
PO (tenofovir)	Unknown	2 hr	Unknown

Half-life: Elvitegravir, 12.9 hours; cobicistat, 3.5 hours; emtricitabine, 10 hours; tenofovir, 12 to 18 hours.

ADVERSE REACTIONS

CNS: headache, dizziness, insomnia, abnormal dreams, fatigue, somnolence, depression. **GI:** diarrhea, nausea, flatulence. **GU:** increased creatinine level, proteinuria, hematuria. **Hepatic:** increased transaminase levels. **Metabolic:** increased amylase, lipase, CK, lipid levels. **Musculoskeletal:** bone fracture. **Respiratory:** cough, pneumonia. **Skin:** rash.

INTERACTIONS

🌣 *Alert:* Drug can interact with many drugs. Consult a drug compatibility reference or pharmacist for additional information.

Drug-drug. *Acyclovir, cidofovir, ganciclovir, valacyclovir, valganciclovir, aminoglycosides (gentamicin), NSAIDs:* May increase levels of these drugs, emtricitabine, and tenofovir due to competition for kidney excretion. Use together carefully.

Additional antiretrovirals: May increase risk of drug interactions and altered pharmacokinetics of drug components. Use together is contraindicated.

Alfuzosin: May increase alfuzosin level and risk of severe hypotension. Use together is contraindicated.

Antacids, calcium or iron supplements, cation-containing laxatives, buffered medications: May decrease elvitegravir level. Separate administration times by 2 hours.

Antiarrhythmics, digoxin: May increase levels of these drugs. Use together cautiously and monitor drug levels if possible.

Antidepressants (SSRIs, TCAs, trazodone): May increase levels of these drugs. Use together cautiously and titrate antidepressant according to response.

Antifungals (itraconazole, ketoconazole, voriconazole): May increase levels of these drugs, elvitegravir, and cobicistat. Use together cautiously. Don't exceed 200 mg/day of ketoconazole or itraconazole.

Antiplatelet drugs (clopidogrel, ticagrelor): May increase ticagrelor level or decrease clopidogrel level. Use together isn't recommended.

Beta blockers (metoprolol, timolol): May increase beta blocker level. Monitor patient carefully and decrease beta blocker dosage as necessary.

Bosentan: May increase bosentan level. Give bosentan dose based on manufacturer's instructions and adjust according to patient tolerance.

Calcium channel blockers (amlodipine, diltiazem, nicardipine, nifedipine, verapamil): May increase level of calcium channel blocker. Use together cautiously and monitor patient closely.

Carbamazepine, oxcarbazepine, phenobarbital, phenytoin: May significantly decrease elvitegravir and cobicistat levels; may increase carbamazepine level. Use together is contraindicated.

Clarithromycin: May increase clarithromycin and cobicistat levels. Use together cautiously. Decrease clarithromycin dosage by 50% if CrCl falls between 50 and 60 mL/minute.

Clonazepam, ethosuximide: May increase levels of these drugs. Use together cautiously.

Colchicine: May increase colchicine level. Adjust dosage according to manufacturer's instructions. Use together is contraindicated in patients with kidney or liver impairment.

CYP2D6, CYP3A, P-gp substrates: May alter plasma levels of the four drug components (elvitegravir, cobicistat, emtricitabine, and tenofovir). Use together cautiously.

Dexamethasone: May significantly decrease cobicistat and elvitegravir levels. Monitor patient carefully for loss of therapeutic effect (elvitegravir, cobicistat) and development of resistance. Consider alternative corticosteroid.

Direct oral anticoagulants (apixaban, dabigatran, edoxaban, rivaroxaban): May increase bleeding risk. Adjust anticoagulant dosage.

Ergot derivatives (dihydroergotamine, ergotamine, methylergonovine): May increase levels of these drugs. Use together is contraindicated.

Fluticasone: May increase fluticasone level. Choose an alternative corticosteroid.

HMG-CoA reductase inhibitors (atorvastatin, lovastatin, simvastatin): May increase statin drug level and risk of myopathy. Start atorvastatin at lowest dosage and titrate carefully.

E

Use with lovastatin and simvastatin is contraindicated.

Hormonal contraceptives: May alter levels of these drugs. Consider nonhormonal forms of birth control.

Immunosuppressants (cyclosporine, sirolimus, tacrolimus): May increase immunosuppressant level. Use together cautiously.

Lomitapide: May significantly increase transaminase levels. Use together is contraindicated.

Lurasidone, pimozide: May increase risk of cardiac adverse effects. Use together is contraindicated.

Midazolam: May increase midazolam level. Use with oral midazolam is contraindicated. Use parenteral form cautiously and monitor patient closely.

Neuroleptics (perphenazine, quetiapine, risperidone, thioridazine): May increase neuroleptic drug levels. Decrease neuroleptic dosage as needed.

Opioid analgesics (fentanyl, tramadol): May increase sedation and respiratory depression. Use together cautiously.

PDE5 inhibitors (sildenafil, tadalafil, vardenafil): May increase effects of PDE5 inhibitors. Adjust dosage according to manufacturer's instructions. Use with sildenafil for PAH is contraindicated.

Rifabutin, rifapentine: May decrease cobicistat and elvitegravir levels. Avoid use together.

Rifampin: May decrease elvitegravir and cobicistat levels, decreasing therapeutic effect. Use together is contraindicated.

Salmeterol: May increase risk of CV effects of salmeterol, including QT-interval prolongation, palpitations, and tachycardia. Avoid use together.

Sedative-hypnotics (buspirone, clorazepate, diazepam, estazolam, flurazepam, zolpidem): May increase levels of sedative-hypnotics. Use together cautiously and monitor patient carefully.

Triazolam: May increase triazolam level. Use together is contraindicated.

Warfarin: Effect on warfarin level isn't known. Monitor INR carefully.

Drug-herb. *St. John's wort:* May reduce levels of drug components and decrease therapeutic effect. Use together is contraindicated.

EFFECTS ON LAB TEST RESULTS
- May increase AST, ALT, GGT, amylase, creatinine, CK, total cholesterol, HDL-C, LDL-C, and triglyceride levels.
- May decrease potassium and phosphate levels.
- May increase urine RBC count.

CONTRAINDICATIONS & CAUTIONS
- Contraindicated in patients hypersensitive to drugs or their components and in those with CrCl of less than 70 mL/minute or Child-Pugh class C liver impairment.
- Contraindicated for use together with drugs that are highly dependent on CYP3A for clearance or strongly induce CYP3A.
- Use cautiously in patients with new-onset or worsening kidney impairment, including AKI and Fanconi syndrome. Avoid administering with other kidney-toxic agents.
- Use cautiously in patients with history of pathologic fracture or other risk factors for osteoporosis or bone loss. Consider calcium and vitamin D supplementation.

Boxed Warning Drug isn't approved for treatment of chronic HBV infection; safety and effectiveness of drug haven't been established in patients infected with both HBV and HIV-1. Severe acute exacerbations of HBV have been reported in patients who are infected with both HBV and HIV-1 and who have discontinued emtricitabine (Emtriva) or tenofovir (Viread). Monitor liver function closely with both clinical and lab follow-up for at least several months in patients who are infected with both HBV and HIV-1 and who discontinue this drug. If appropriate, initiation of anti-hepatitis B therapy may be warranted. ■

Alert: Lactic acidosis and severe liver enlargement with steatosis, including fatal cases, have been reported with use of nucleoside analogues (tenofovir, emtricitabine) in combination with other antiretrovirals.
- Drug may cause immune reconstitution syndrome.
- Safety and effectiveness in children younger than age 12 or weighing less than 35 kg haven't been established.

Dialyzable drug: Elvitegravir, unlikely; cobicistat, unlikely; emtricitabine, 30% hemodialysis; tenofovir, 10% hemodialysis.

PREGNANCY-LACTATION-REPRODUCTION
• Register patients who are pregnant in the Antiretroviral Pregnancy Registry at 1-800-258-4263 or www.apregistry.com.
• Drug is not recommended for use during pregnancy.
• Drug components (emtricitabine, tenofovir) appear in human milk. Because of risk of HIV transmission, patient shouldn't breastfeed.

NURSING CONSIDERATIONS
• Monitor LFT values.
• Suspend treatment in patient who develops signs and symptoms or lab findings suggestive of lactic acidosis or pronounced liver toxicity (nausea, vomiting, unusual or unexpected stomach discomfort, weakness).
• Test for HBV before starting therapy; severe acute exacerbations of hepatitis B have been reported in patients infected with both HBV and HIV-1.
• Assess CrCl, urine glucose, and urine protein before initiating and periodically during treatment.
• Monitor serum phosphorus and potassium levels in patient at risk for kidney impairment.
• Closely monitor patient with increased serum creatinine level of greater than 0.4 mg/dL from baseline for kidney safety.
• Consider assessing bone mineral density (BMD) in patient with history of pathologic bone fracture or other risk factors for osteoporosis or bone loss because of risk of drug-related decreased BMD.
• Monitor patient for infection and development of immune reconstitution syndrome (inflammatory response to indolent or residual opportunistic infections, such as MAC infection, CMV, *Pneumocystis jiroveci* pneumonia, or TB), which may necessitate further evaluation and treatment.
• Autoimmune disorders (Graves disease, polymyositis, Guillain-Barré syndrome) have also been reported in the setting of immune reconstitution; however, time to onset varies, and the disorder can occur many months after initiation of treatment.

PATIENT TEACHING
• Caution patient to remain under the care of a health care provider and to comply with routine monitoring to decrease risk of adverse events.
• Inform patient that this drug isn't a cure for HIV-1 infection; patient must stay on continuous HIV therapy to control HIV-1 infection and decrease HIV-related illnesses.
• Instruct patient to avoid behaviors that can spread HIV-1 infection to others (sharing needles and other injection equipment; sharing personal items that may have blood or body fluids on them, such as toothbrushes and razor blades; having sex without a latex or polyurethane condom).
• Warn patient not to breastfeed because HIV-1 can pass to infant in human milk.
• Teach patient to take drug on a regular dosing schedule with food and not to miss doses to decrease the risk of resistance.
• Instruct patient not to change dose or stop drug without first consulting health care provider.
• Advise patient to immediately report nausea, vomiting, unusual or unexpected stomach discomfort, and weakness.
• Caution patient to report signs and symptoms of infection.
• Teach patient to report yellowing of skin or sclerae, dark urine, light-colored stools, loss of appetite, or nausea.

SAFETY ALERT!

empagliflozin
em-pa-gli-FLOE-zin

Jardiance

Therapeutic class: Antidiabetics
Pharmacologic class: Sodium-glucose cotransporter 2 inhibitors

AVAILABLE FORMS
Tablets: 10 mg, 25 mg

INDICATIONS & DOSAGES
Adjust-a-dose (for all indications): Discontinue drug if GFR is less than 30 mL/minute/1.73 m^2 for treatment of DM and if GFR is less than 20 mL/minute/1.73 m^2 in those with HF.
➤ **Adjunct to diet and exercise to improve glycemic control in patients with type 2 diabetes**
Adults: 10 mg PO daily in the morning. May increase to 25 mg daily after as needed and tolerated for additional glycemic control.
➤ **To reduce risk of CV death in patients with type 2 diabetes and established CV disease; to reduce risk of CV death and hospitalization in patients with HF**
Adults: 10 mg PO daily in the morning.

ADMINISTRATION
PO
- Give drug without regard to food.
- Store at room temperature.

ACTION
Inhibits kidney reabsorption of glucose and lowers kidney threshold for glucose, resulting in increased urinary excretion of glucose.

Route	Onset	Peak	Duration
PO	Unknown	1.5 hr	Unknown

Half-life: 12.4 hours.

ADVERSE REACTIONS
GI: nausea. **GU:** genital mycotic infections, UTI, kidney impairment, increased urination. **Hematologic:** increased hematocrit. **Metabolic:** dyslipidemia, increased thirst. **Musculoskeletal:** arthralgia. **Respiratory:** URI.

INTERACTIONS
Drug-drug. *Diuretics:* May enhance diuretic effect. Closely monitor patient for volume depletion.
Insulin, insulin secretagogues, sulfonylureas, other antidiabetics: May increase hypoglycemic risk. Monitor patient closely.
Lithium: May decrease serum lithium level; monitor lithium level more frequently during empagliflozin initiation and dosage changes.

EFFECTS ON LAB TEST RESULTS
- May increase serum creatinine level.
- May increase hematocrit.
- May decrease GFR.
- May cause false-positive urine glucose test.
- Interferes with 1,5-anhydroglucitol assay.

CONTRAINDICATIONS & CAUTIONS
- Contraindicated in patients with history of serious hypersensitivity reaction to drug or its components.
- Contraindicated in patients with CKD on CKRT.
- Drug isn't recommended for glycemic control in patients with eGFR of less than 30 mL/minute/1.73 m^2.
- Dosing recommendations haven't been determined for patients with type 2 diabetes and established CV disease with eGFR of less than 30 mL/minute/1.73 m^2 or for patients who have HF with reduced ejection fraction with eGFR of less than 20 mL/minute/1.73 m^2.

- Drug isn't indicated for treatment of type 1 diabetes or diabetic ketoacidosis.
- Serious hypersensitivity reactions, including angioedema, have been reported in patients treated with empagliflozin.
- **Alert:** Sodium-glucose cotransporter 2 (SGLT2) inhibitors increase risk of rare but serious necrotizing fasciitis of perineum (Fournier gangrene).
- **Alert:** Drug may cause ketoacidosis, which may require emergency department care or hospitalization for treatment.
- Consider temporarily discontinuing drug at least 3 days before scheduled surgery to reduce risk of ketoacidosis.
- Use cautiously in patients with low BP or CrCl of 30 to less than 60 mL/minute and in those taking diuretics; drug may increase risk of hypotension.
- Drug may increase risk of adverse events related to volume depletion and reduced kidney function, especially in older adults and patients with kidney impairment.
- Drug may increase incidence of bone fractures. Per American Diabetes Association guidelines, avoid use of SGLT2 inhibitors in patients with fracture risk factors.
- Use cautiously in patients with elevated hematocrit at baseline, as value may increase.
- Safety and effectiveness in children haven't been established.
Dialyzable drug: Unknown.

PREGNANCY-LACTATION-REPRODUCTION
- Drug hasn't been studied in patients who are pregnant. Drug isn't recommended during second and third trimesters. Use during pregnancy only if benefit justifies fetal risk.
- It isn't known if drug appears in human milk. Patient should discontinue breastfeeding or discontinue drug, considering importance of drug to patient.

NURSING CONSIDERATIONS
- Assess kidney function before initiating therapy and periodically during treatment. Don't start therapy if GFR is less than 30 mL/minute. Closely monitor patient with GFR of less than 60 mL/minute.
- Assess fluid status. Correct volume depletion before starting therapy and monitor during therapy.
- Monitor patient for signs and symptoms of hypotension (fatigue, dizziness, blurred vision, clammy skin) during therapy. Drug may

increase risk of hypotension due to intravascular volume contraction.

• Closely monitor glucose level during drug initiation. Concomitant use of insulin and other antidiabetics may increase risk of hypoglycemia.

• Monitor for ketoacidosis, especially in patient with major illness, reduced food or fluid intake, or reduced insulin dose. Elevated urine or serum ketone levels without very high glucose levels have occurred with SGLT2 inhibitor use.

• Monitor for hypersensitivity reactions. Discontinue drug if a reaction occurs, treat promptly, and monitor patient until signs and symptoms resolve.

• Watch for genital mycotic infections and treat appropriately.

🜂 *Alert:* Monitor patient and immediately report signs and symptoms of necrotizing fasciitis of the perineum (temperature above 100.4° F [38° C]; malaise; genital or perianal pain, tenderness, erythema, or swelling). Symptoms can quickly worsen. Immediately discontinue drug and prepare to administer broad-spectrum antibiotics. Surgical debridement may be necessary. Monitor blood glucose level and start alternative therapy for glycemic control.

🜂 *Alert:* Drug may increase risk of severe UTI, including urosepsis and pyelonephritis. Monitor patient and treat promptly if indicated.

• Monitor LDL-C periodically; treat appropriately.

• Drug causes positive urine glucose tests. Avoid urine glucose testing for glycemic control monitoring.

• *Look alike–sound alike:* Don't confuse empagliflozin with canagliflozin or dapagliflozin. Don't confuse Jardiance with Januvia, Jantoven, or Janumet.

PATIENT TEACHING

• Teach about proper drug administration and handling.

• Stress importance of adhering to diet, weight reduction, exercise, personal hygiene, and blood glucose monitoring while on therapy.

• Instruct patient to report all adverse reactions.

• Teach patient how to identify and manage signs and symptoms of hypoglycemia (shaking, dizziness, weakness, fast heartbeat) and hypotension (fatigue, dizziness, blurred vision, clammy skin).

• Encourage patient to maintain adequate fluid intake.

🜂 *Alert:* Teach about signs and symptoms of necrotizing fasciitis. Instruct patient to seek immediate medical attention if any occur.

🜂 *Alert:* Instruct patient to immediately seek medical attention for signs and symptoms of ketoacidosis (difficulty breathing, hyperventilation, anorexia, nausea, vomiting, abdominal pain, confusion, unusual fatigue or sleepiness) or necrotizing fasciitis (fever or malaise along with genital or perianal pain, tenderness, erythema, swelling).

• Instruct patient to seek medical advice during periods of stress or illness because medication requirements may change.

🜂 *Alert:* Instruct patient to seek medical attention for signs and symptoms of UTI (difficulty urinating, frequency, urgency, pelvic or back pain, blood in urine, fever, nausea, vomiting).

• Inform patient that periodic monitoring of blood glucose and HbA_{1c} levels and kidney function is necessary.

• Advise patient that urine glucose tests will be falsely positive because drug increases glucose excretion. Recommend alternative methods to monitor glycemic control.

• Counsel patient to consult prescriber before starting new prescription or OTC medications or supplements.

• Tell patient to report pregnancy or plans to become pregnant or breastfeed during treatment.

emtricitabine

em-tra-SYE-tah-ben

Emtriva

Therapeutic class: Antiretrovirals
Pharmacologic class: NRTIs

AVAILABLE FORMS
Capsules: 200 mg
Oral solution: 10 mg/mL

INDICATIONS & DOSAGES
➤ **HIV-1 infection, with other antiretrovirals**
Adults: One 200-mg capsule or 240 mg (24 mL) oral solution PO once daily.
Children ages 3 months to 17 years: 6 mg/kg up to maximum dose of 240 mg (24 mL) oral solution PO once daily. Or, for children weighing more than 33 kg who can swallow a capsule, 200-mg capsule PO once daily.

Children younger than age 3 months: 3 mg/kg oral solution PO once daily.

Adjust-a-dose: In adults with CrCl of 30 to 49 mL/minute, give one 200-mg capsule every 48 hours or 120 mg oral solution every 24 hours; if CrCl is 15 to 29 mL/minute, give one 200-mg capsule every 72 hours or 80 mg oral solution every 24 hours; if CrCl is less than 15 mL/minute or patient is receiving hemodialysis, give one 200-mg capsule every 96 hours or 60 mg oral solution every 24 hours. Give dose after hemodialysis session. In children with kidney insufficiency, consider a dose reduction or increased dosing interval.

ADMINISTRATION

PO
- Give drug with or without food.
- Refrigerate oral solution; or, patient may store at room temperature for up to 3 months.
- Dispense in original container; keep container tightly closed.

ACTION
Inhibits replication of HIV by blocking viral DNA synthesis and inhibits reverse transcriptase by acting as an alternative for the enzyme's substrate, deoxycytidine triphosphate.

Route	Onset	Peak	Duration
PO	Unknown	1–2 hr	Unknown

Half-life: About 10 hours.

ADVERSE REACTIONS
CNS: abnormal dreams, asthenia, dizziness, headache, insomnia, depression, fatigue, neuritis, paresthesia, peripheral neuropathy, fever. **EENT:** rhinitis, sinusitis, otitis media. **GI:** abdominal pain, diarrhea, nausea, dyspepsia, vomiting, gastroenteritis. **GU:** hematuria. **Hematologic:** anemia. **Hepatic:** increased transaminase and ALP levels, hyperbilirubinemia, *liver toxicity.* **Metabolic:** hyperglycemia, *hypoglycemia,* increased amylase and lipase levels, increased CK level, hypertriglyceridemia. **Musculoskeletal:** arthralgia, myalgia. **Respiratory:** increased cough, pneumonia, URI. **Skin:** allergic skin reaction, hyperpigmentation, rash, pruritus, urticarial and purpuric lesions. **Other:** infection.

INTERACTIONS
Drug-drug. *Orlistat:* May decrease serum level of antiretrovirals. Monitor use together.

EFFECTS ON LAB TEST RESULTS
- May increase ALT, AST, ALP, amylase, bilirubin, CK, lipase, and triglyceride levels.
- May increase or decrease glucose level.
- May decrease Hb level and neutrophil count.
- May increase urine glucose level.

CONTRAINDICATIONS & CAUTIONS
- Contraindicated in patients hypersensitive to drug or its ingredients.
- Use cautiously in older adults because of the potential for other diseases and drug therapies and for decreased liver, kidney, or cardiac function.

Boxed Warning Severe acute exacerbations of HBV infection have been reported in patients infected with both HBV and HIV-1 who have discontinued emtricitabine. Monitor liver function closely with both clinical and lab follow-up for at least several months in patients infected with both HIV-1 and HBV who discontinue this drug. If appropriate, initiation of anti–HBV therapy may be warranted. ■

⚠ Alert: Lactic acidosis and severe liver enlargement with steatosis, including fatal cases, have been reported with use of nucleoside analogues, alone or in combination with other antiretrovirals.

Dialyzable drug: 30% over 3-hour hemodialysis period.

PREGNANCY-LACTATION-REPRODUCTION
- Use drug during pregnancy only if clearly needed.
- Register patients who are pregnant in the Antiretroviral Pregnancy Registry at 1-800-258-4263 or www.apregistry.com.
- Patients should avoid breastfeeding because of potential for HIV-1 transmission and serious adverse reactions in breastfed infants.

NURSING CONSIDERATIONS
- Test patient for HBV before starting drug.
- Suspend treatment in patient who develops signs and symptoms or lab findings suggestive of lactic acidosis or pronounced liver toxicity (nausea, vomiting, unusual or unexpected stomach discomfort, weakness).

Boxed Warning Monitor liver function closely with both clinical and lab follow-up for at least several months in patient infected with both HIV-1 and HBV who discontinues this drug. ■

Reactions in bold italics are *life-threatening.*

- Monitor patient for infection and development of immune reconstitution syndrome (inflammatory response to opportunistic infections, such as MAC infection, CMV, *Pneumocystis jiroveci* pneumonia, or TB), which may necessitate further evaluation and treatment.
- Hyperpigmentation is more common in children.

PATIENT TEACHING

- Teach about proper drug administration and handling.
- Remind patient that anti-HIV medicine must be taken for life.
- Inform patient that drug doesn't cure HIV infection, that opportunistic infections and other complications of HIV infection may continue to occur, and that transmission of HIV to others through sexual contact or blood contamination is still possible.
- Explain possible adverse reactions, including lactic acidosis and liver toxicity; advise patient to report all adverse reactions.
- Tell patient to immediately notify prescriber of known or suspected pregnancy.
- Warn patient against breastfeeding.

emtricitabine–rilpivirine–tenofovir alafenamide fumarate
em-tra-SYE-ta-ben/ril-pi-VIR-een/te-NOE-fo-veer

Odefsey

Therapeutic class: Antiretrovirals
Pharmacologic class: NRTIs–NNRTIs

AVAILABLE FORMS
Tablets: 200 mg emtricitabine, 25 mg rilpivirine, and 25 mg tenofovir alafenamide fumarate

INDICATIONS & DOSAGES
➤ **HIV-1 infection as initial therapy in patients with no antiretroviral treatment history and HIV-1 RNA of 100,000 copies/mL or less; or to replace a stable antiretroviral regimen in patients who are virologically suppressed (HIV-1 RNA less than 50 copies/mL) for at least 6 months with no history of treatment failure and no known substitutions associated with resistance to the individual components**

Adults and children ages 12 and older weighing at least 35 kg: 1 tablet PO once daily with a meal.
Adjust-a-dose: For patients on hemodialysis, give 1 tablet once daily; give after hemodialysis on dialysis days. Drug isn't recommended for patients with CrCl of less than 30 mL/minute or in patients with CKD who aren't receiving long-term dialysis.

ADMINISTRATION
PO
- Give drug once daily with a meal.
- Store below 86° F (30° C).
- Keep only in tightly closed, original container.

ACTION
Nucleoside, nonnucleoside, and nucleotide inhibitor combination of reverse transcriptase that inhibits viral replication.

Route	Onset	Peak	Duration
PO (emtricitabine)	Unknown	1–2 hr	Unknown
PO (rilpivirine)	Unknown	4–5 hr	Unknown
PO (tenofovir)	Unknown	0.48 hr	Unknown

Half-life: Emtricitabine, 10 hours; rilpivirine, 50 hours; tenofovir, 0.51 hour.

ADVERSE REACTIONS
CNS: abnormal dreams, headache, insomnia, sleep disturbances, depression, somnolence, dizziness. **GI:** flatulence, diarrhea, nausea, vomiting, abdominal pain. **Metabolic:** hypophosphatemia, increased lipid levels. **Musculoskeletal:** decreased bone mineral density. **Skin:** rash. **Other:** hypersensitivity reaction.

INTERACTIONS
❸ *Alert:* Drug combination can interact significantly with many drugs. Consult a drug compatibility reference or pharmacist for additional information.
Drug-drug. *Acyclovir, aminoglycosides, cidofovir, ganciclovir, valacyclovir, valganciclovir:* May increase Odefsey (specifically tenofovir) level. Monitor patient for Odefsey-related increased adverse effects. Tenofovir products may increase ganciclovir or valganciclovir serum level. Monitor therapy.
Antacids (aluminum, magnesium hydroxide, calcium carbonate): May decrease rilpivirine level. Give antacids at least 2 hours before or at least 4 hours after Odefsey.

Anticonvulsants (carbamazepine, oxcarbazepine, phenobarbital, phenytoin): May decrease rilpivirine level, resulting in loss of virologic response and possible drug resistance. Use together is contraindicated.

Antimycobacterial drugs (rifabutin, rifampin, rifapentine): May decrease rilpivirine and tenofovir levels, resulting in loss of virologic response and possible drug resistance. Use together is contraindicated.

Azole antifungals (fluconazole, itraconazole, ketoconazole): May decrease azole level. Monitor patient for breakthrough fungal infections.

CYP3A inducers: May decrease rilpivirine level, resulting in loss of virologic response and possible drug resistance. Use together is contraindicated.

CYP3A inhibitors: May increase rilpivirine level and risk of adverse events. Monitor therapy.

Dexamethasone (systemic): May decrease rilpivirine level, resulting in loss of virologic response and possible drug resistance. Use of more than a single dose of dexamethasone is contraindicated.

Didanosine: May decrease didanosine serum level. Give didanosine on an empty stomach at least 2 hours before or 4 hours after Odefsey due to the requirement that rilpivirine be administered with food.

H₂-receptor antagonists (cimetidine, famotidine): May decrease rilpivirine level. Administer H_2-receptor antagonist at least 12 hours before or 4 hours after Odefsey. Consider therapy modification.

Macrolide antibiotics (clarithromycin, erythromycin): May increase rilpivirine level. Consider using alternative antibiotic.

Methadone: May increase methadone metabolism. Adjust methadone dosage as clinically indicated.

NSAIDs: May increase risk of kidney toxicity and adverse effects, especially at high doses. Use alternatives if possible.

P-gp inducers: May decrease tenofovir level, which may lead to loss of therapeutic effect and resistance. Monitor patient closely.

P-gp inhibitors (colchicine, diltiazem): May increase tenofovir level. Monitor patient for increased Odefsey-related adverse effects.

PPIs (dexlansoprazole, esomeprazole, lansoprazole, omeprazole, pantoprazole): May decrease rilpivirine level, resulting in loss of virologic response and possible drug resistance. Use together is contraindicated.

QTc interval-prolonging agents (amiodarone, haloperidol, moxifloxacin, quinidine): May enhance QTc interval-prolonging effect. Consider alternative medications to Odefsey in patients with known risk of torsades de pointes.

Drug-herb. *St. John's wort:* May decrease Odefsey serum level, resulting in loss of virologic response and possible resistance to drug combination. Discourage use together.

EFFECTS ON LAB TEST RESULTS
• May increase phosphorus, triglyceride, lipid, and serum lactate levels.

CONTRAINDICATIONS & CAUTIONS
Boxed Warning Severe acute exacerbations of HBV infection have been reported in patients coinfected with HIV-1 and HBV after discontinuation of antiretroviral therapy with emtricitabine or tenofovir. ▪

• Contraindicated in patients hypersensitive to drug or its components.

• Consider alternative therapy in patients at high risk for torsades de pointes or when administered with medications known to increase risk of torsades de pointes. Supratherapeutic dosages of Odefsey have been shown to prolong QTc interval and may increase risk of ventricular arrhythmias.

• Use isn't recommended in patients with CrCl of less than 15 mL/minute unless they are receiving long-term hemodialysis.

• Use cautiously in patients at risk for kidney dysfunction. Hypophosphatemia has been reported secondary to proximal kidney tubulopathy; in patients at risk for or with CKD, assess serum phosphorus level.

• Use cautiously in patients at risk for liver disease. Liver adverse events have been reported.

• Use in patients with Child-Pugh class C liver impairment hasn't been studied.

🜚 *Alert:* Drug may cause lactic acidosis and liver enlargement with steatosis, including fatal cases. These effects may occur without elevated transaminase levels and in patients with no known risk factors (long-term antiretroviral use, obesity, and female sex). Monitor all patients closely.

• May increase risk of immune reconstitution syndrome, resulting in an inflammatory response to an indolent or opportunistic infection or activation of autoimmune disorders (MAC infection, CMV, *Pneumocystis jiroveci*

---

pneumonia, TB, Graves disease, polymyositis, Guillain-Barré syndrome).

• Safety and effectiveness in children younger than age 12 or weighing less than 35 kg haven't been established.

Dialyzable drug: Emtricitabine, 30%; rilpivirine, unlikely; tenofovir, 54%.

PREGNANCY-LACTATION-REPRODUCTION

• Well-controlled studies during pregnancy are lacking. Use cautiously during pregnancy.

• Patients who become pregnant during therapy and who are virologically suppressed (HIV-1 RNA less than 50 copies per mL) may continue drug. Closely monitor viral load.

• To monitor pregnancy outcomes, health care providers are encouraged to register patients who are pregnant in the Antiretroviral Pregnancy Registry (1-800-258-4263 or www.apregistry.com).

• Some components of drug appear in human milk. It isn't known if Odefsey affects lactation or has effects on infant.

NURSING CONSIDERATIONS

Boxed Warning Monitor liver function during and for several months after discontinuation of treatment. If appropriate, initiate anti-HBV therapy ■

• Discontinue Odefsey if clinical or lab findings suggestive of lactic acidosis or liver toxicity develop.

• Test for HBV before initiation of antiretroviral therapy in all patients.

• Assess CD4 count and HIV-1 RNA plasma, serum creatinine, urine glucose, and urine protein levels before initiation and during therapy in all patients. Assess serum phosphorus level in patients at risk for or with CKD.

• In patient who is virologically suppressed, additional monitoring of HIV-1 RNA and regimen tolerability is recommended after replacing therapy to assess for potential virologic failure or rebound.

• Monitor patient for hypersensitivity, rash, and severe skin reactions, including DRESS syndrome (severe rash or rash accompanied by fever, blisters, mucosal involvement, conjunctivitis, facial edema, angioedema, hepatitis, eosinophilia). Most rashes occur within first 4 to 6 weeks of therapy. Monitor lab parameters and clinical status. Immediately stop drug if hypersensitivity or rash develops.

• Odefsey may increase risk of Fanconi syndrome. Discontinue drug in patient who develops clinically significant decrease in kidney function or evidence of Fanconi syndrome.

• Calcium and vitamin D supplementation may be beneficial for all patients.

• Monitor for depression, dysphoria, mood changes, negative thoughts, suicidality, and suicide attempts. Promptly evaluate patient who develops these symptoms; consider risks versus benefits of continued treatment.

• Monitor patient for infection.

PATIENT TEACHING

⏱ *Alert:* Counsel patient, family members, and caregivers to watch for signs and symptoms of depression and to immediately report depression, negative thoughts, dysphoria, or suicidality to prescriber.

• Advise that Odefsey can cause buildup of lactic acid in the blood. Instruct patient to seek immediate medical attention for weakness, fatigue, muscle pain, trouble breathing, stomachache with nausea and vomiting, dizziness, chills, or fast or irregular heartbeat.

• Caution patient that Odefsey may cause liver problems. Instruct patient to seek immediate medical attention for yellowing of the skin or eyes, dark-colored urine, loss of appetite, light-colored stool, nausea, or pain or tenderness on right side of stomach.

⏱ *Alert:* Warn patient to stop taking drug and immediately seek medical attention for allergic reactions, including severe skin reactions.

• Caution patient not to discontinue drug combination without first discussing with prescriber. Advise patient of importance of not running out of medication and not missing doses.

Boxed Warning Inform patient that severe acute exacerbations of hepatitis B have been reported in patients who are coinfected and who discontinue drug. ■

• Remind patient to notify prescriber about other prescription and OTC drugs, including herbal and vitamin supplements, patient is taking or plans to take.

• Inform patient that blood tests will be needed to check for effectiveness and adverse effects of therapy.

• Advise patient to immediately report signs and symptoms of infection.

• Tell patient of childbearing potential to notify prescriber about planned, suspected, or known pregnancy.

• Advise patient not to breastfeed during therapy.

emtricitabine–tenofovir alafenamide
em-tra-SYE-tah-ben/te-NOE-fo-veer

Descovy

Therapeutic class: Antiretrovirals
Pharmacologic class: NNRTIs

AVAILABLE FORMS
Tablets: 120 mg emtricitabine and 15 mg tenofovir alafenamide, 200 mg emtricitabine and 25 mg tenofovir alafenamide

INDICATIONS & DOSAGES
Adjust-a-dose (for all indications): In adults with CrCl below 15 mL/minute who are receiving long-term hemodialysis, give daily dose on days of hemodialysis after completion of hemodialysis treatment. Use isn't recommended in patients with CrCl of 15 to less than 30 mL/minute or with CrCl below 15 mL/minute who are not receiving hemodialysis.

➤ **HIV-1 infection in combination with other antiretrovirals**
Adults and children weighing 35 kg or more: One 200 mg/25 mg tablet PO once daily.

➤ **HIV-1 infection in combination with other antiretrovirals (other than protease inhibitors that require CYP3A inhibitor)**
Children weighing at least 25 to less than 35 kg: One 200 mg/25 mg tablet PO once daily.
Children weighing at least 14 to less than 25 kg: One 120 mg/15 mg tablet PO once daily.

➤ **Preexposure prophylaxis (PrEP) in patients who are at risk and have negative HIV-1 test immediately before treatment to reduce risk of HIV-1 infection from sexual acquisition, excluding those at risk from receptive vaginal sex**
Adults and adolescents weighing at least 35 kg: One 200 mg/25 mg tablet PO once daily.

ADMINISTRATION
PO
• Give drug with or without food.
• Give missed dose as soon as possible. If it's close to time for next dose, skip missed dose. Don't give two doses at the same time or extra doses.
• Keep only in tightly closed, original container.

ACTION
Interferes with HIV viral RNA-dependent DNA polymerase activities, resulting in inhibition of viral replication.

Route	Onset	Peak	Duration
PO (emtricitabine)	Unknown	1–2 hr	Unknown
PO (tenofovir)	Unknown	0.48 hr	Unknown

Half-life: Emtricitabine, 10 hours; tenofovir, 0.51 hour.

ADVERSE REACTIONS
CNS: headache, fatigue. **GI:** nausea, diarrhea, vomiting, abdominal pain. **Metabolic:** increased triglyceride levels. **Musculoskeletal:** decreased bone mineral density.

INTERACTIONS
❸ *Alert:* Drug combination can interact significantly with many drugs. Consult a drug compatibility reference or pharmacist for additional information.
Drug-drug. *Acyclovir, valacyclovir:* May increase serum level of tenofovir products. Tenofovir products may increase serum level of acyclovir or valacyclovir. Monitor therapy.
Adefovir: May diminish therapeutic effect of tenofovir products. Tenofovir products may increase adefovir serum level. Avoid use together.
Aminoglycosides: May increase serum level of tenofovir products and aminoglycosides. Monitor therapy.
Anticonvulsants (carbamazepine, oxcarbazepine, phenobarbital, phenytoin, primidone): May decrease tenofovir serum level. Consider alternative anticonvulsant.
Antimycobacterial drugs (rifabutin, rifampin, rifapentine): May decrease tenofovir level. Use together isn't recommended.
Cidofovir: May increase serum levels of tenofovir products and cidofovir. Monitor therapy.
Cobicistat: May increase risk of adverse effects of tenofovir. Monitor therapy.
Ganciclovir, valganciclovir: May increase serum level of tenofovir, ganciclovir, or valganciclovir level. Monitor patient closely for increased adverse effects.
Lamivudine: May increase risk of adverse effects of emtricitabine. Avoid use together.
NSAIDs: May enhance kidney toxic effect of tenofovir. Seek alternatives to this combination whenever possible. Avoid use of tenofovir with multiple NSAIDs or with any NSAID given at a high dose.

Reactions in bold italics are *life-threatening*.

P-gp inducers: May decrease tenofovir absorption, causing loss of therapeutic effect and development of resistance. Monitor therapy closely or consider therapy modification.
P-gp inhibitors: May increase tenofovir level. Use together cautiously.
Protease inhibitors (ritonavir, tipranavir): May decrease tenofovir serum level. Use together isn't recommended.
Ribavirin (oral inhalation, systemic): May increase risk of liver toxicity. Use together cautiously.
Drug-herb. *St. John's wort:* May decrease tenofovir serum level. Discourage use together.

EFFECTS ON LAB TEST RESULTS
• May increase total cholesterol, LDL-C, HDL-C, triglyceride, ALT, amylase, AST, bilirubin, CK, lipase, serum creatinine, and glucose levels.
• May decrease phosphate level.
• May decrease neutrophil count.

CONTRAINDICATIONS & CAUTIONS
• Contraindicated for use for PrEP in individuals with unknown or positive HIV-1 status.
Boxed Warning Safety and effectiveness haven't been established for patients coinfected with HIV and HBV. Acute, severe exacerbations of HBV infection (liver decompensation, liver failure) have been reported after discontinuation of antiretroviral therapy. ∎
Boxed Warning When used for HIV-1 PrEP, drug must only be prescribed to individuals confirmed to be HIV-negative immediately before drug initiation and at least every 3 months during use. Drug-resistant HIV-1 variants have been identified with use of emtricitabine–tenofovir for HIV-1 PrEP after undetected acute HIV-1 infection. Don't use for HIV-1 PrEP in patients with signs or symptoms of acute HIV-1 infection unless HIV-1 negative infection status is confirmed. ∎
• Drug may increase risk of AKI and Fanconi syndrome. Those with preexisting kidney impairment or who are taking kidney toxic agents (including NSAIDs) are at increased risk.
• Use in patients with Child-Pugh class C liver impairment hasn't been studied.
• Immune reconstitution syndrome may occur, resulting in inflammatory response to opportunistic infection (MAC infection, CMV, *Pneumocystis jiroveci* pneumonia, TB) or autoimmune disorder (Graves disease,

polymyositis, Guillain-Barré syndrome); evaluate and treat appropriately.
🕓 *Alert:* Lactic acidosis and severe liver enlargement with steatosis, including fatal cases, have been reported with nucleoside analogues (tenofovir) in combination with other antiretrovirals.
• Safety and effectiveness when administered with an HIV-1 protease inhibitor that's given with either ritonavir or cobicistat haven't been established in children weighing less than 35 kg or adults with CrCl below 15 mL/minute, with or without hemodialysis.
• Safety and effectiveness in children with HIV infection weighing less than 14 kg or in children weighing less than 35 kg treated for HIV-1 PrEP haven't been established.
Dialyzable drug: Emtricitabine, 30%; tenofovir alafenamide, 54%.

PREGNANCY-LACTATION-REPRODUCTION
• If indicated, drug shouldn't be withheld because of pregnancy.
• Emtricitabine and tenofovir appear in human milk. Both drugs are contraindicated during breastfeeding.
• To monitor pregnancy outcomes, health care providers are encouraged to register patients in the Antiretroviral Pregnancy Registry (1-800-258-4263 or www.apregistry.com).

NURSING CONSIDERATIONS
• Test for HBV before initiation of antiretroviral therapy. Drug isn't approved for treatment of chronic HBV infection.
• Descovy must be given as part of a regimen with other antiretrovirals, unless used for PrEP.
• Screen all patients for HIV-1 infection immediately before initiating drug for HIV-1 PrEP, at least once every 3 months during treatment, and upon diagnosis of other STIs.
• If recent (less than 1 month) exposure to HIV-1 is suspected or clinical symptoms are consistent with acute HIV-1 infection, use a test approved or cleared by the FDA to help diagnose acute or primary HIV-1 infection.
• Use drug for HIV-1 PrEP to reduce risk of HIV-1 infection as part of a comprehensive prevention strategy, including adherence to daily administration and safer sex practices, including condoms, to reduce risk of STIs.
• Monitor CD4 counts and HIV RNA plasma level to evaluate effectiveness of treatment.

• Assess serum creatinine, estimated CrCl, urine protein, and urine glucose levels before initiation and during therapy.

• Monitor serum phosphorus level in patient with CKD due to increased risk of developing Fanconi syndrome. Discontinue drug in patient who develops clinically significant decrease in kidney function or evidence of Fanconi syndrome.

Boxed Warning Clinically monitor patient and monitor LFT values for at least several months after discontinuation of antiretroviral in patient with HBV. Begin anti-HBV therapy, as appropriate. ■

• Interrupt treatment in patient who develops clinical or lab findings suggestive of lactic acidosis or liver toxicity (liver enlargement and steatosis with or without transaminase elevations). Some cases of liver toxicity have occurred in patients with no liver disease before treatment.

• Evaluate patient with persistent or worsening bone or muscle signs and symptoms for kidney dysfunction (including Fanconi syndrome), hypophosphatemia, and osteomalacia.

• Periodically monitor lipid levels.

Boxed Warning Monitor patients with HIV and HBV coinfection for several months after therapy discontinuation for acute exacerbations of HBV infection. Monitor liver function by clinical assessment and lab testing. Start anti-hepatitis B therapy as clinically indicated, especially in patients with advanced liver disease or cirrhosis. ■

• Due to potential to decrease bone mineral density, calcium and vitamin D supplements may benefit all patients.

PATIENT TEACHING

Boxed Warning Inform patient that severe acute exacerbations of hepatitis B have been reported in patients who are coinfected and who discontinue drug. ■

• Caution patient not to stop drug without first discussing with prescriber.

• Advise patient of importance of taking drug without missing doses to avoid loss of treatment effectiveness.

• Warn patient to report signs and symptoms of kidney problems (inability to pass urine, change in amount of urine passed, blood in urine, weight gain).

Boxed Warning Instruct patient to report signs and symptoms of liver problems (dark urine, loss of appetite, nausea, right upper quadrant abdominal pain, achiness or tenderness, light-colored stools, vomiting, yellowing of skin or eyes). ■

• Advise patient to report signs and symptoms of lactic acidosis (trouble breathing, fast or irregular heartbeat, stomach pain with nausea or vomiting, fatigue, shortness of breath, weakness, dizziness or lightheadedness, feeling cold, muscle pain or cramps).

• Instruct patient to report signs and symptoms of infection (fever, sore throat, weakness, cough, shortness of breath).

• Teach patient to avoid behaviors that can spread HIV-1 infection to others, including sharing or reusing needles, sharing razors or toothbrushes, or having sex without using a latex or polyurethane condom.

• Instruct patient about the use of other prevention measures (consistent and correct condom use, knowledge of partners' HIV-1 status [including viral suppression status], regular testing for STIs that can facilitate HIV-1 transmission). Inform uninfected individuals about potential for HIV-1 infection and support their efforts in reducing sexual risk behavior.

• Caution patient not to breastfeed to avoid transmitting HIV-1 to infant.

enalaprilat ⚥
eh-NAH-leh-prel-at

enalapril maleate ⚥
Epaned, Vasotec

Therapeutic class: Antihypertensives
Pharmacologic class: ACE inhibitors

AVAILABLE FORMS
enalaprilat
Injection: 1.25 mg/mL
enalapril maleate
Oral solution: 1 mg/mL
Tablets: 2.5 mg, 5 mg, 10 mg, 20 mg

INDICATIONS & DOSAGES
➤ **HTN**
Adults: In patients not taking diuretics, initially, 5 mg PO once daily; then adjusted based on response. Usual dosage ranges from 10 to 40 mg daily as a single dose or two divided doses. Or, 1.25 mg IV infusion over 5 minutes every 6 hours.

Children ages 1 month to 16 years: 0.08 mg/kg (up to 5 mg) PO once daily; dosage should be adjusted as needed up to 0.58 mg/kg (maximum 40 mg). Don't use if GFR is less than 30 mL/minute/1.73 m^2.

Adjust-a-dose: If adult patient is taking diuretics or CrCl is 30 mL/minute or less, initially, 2.5 mg PO once daily and titrate to a maximum dose of 40 mg daily. Or, 0.625 mg IV over 5 minutes, and repeat in 1 hour, if needed; then 1.25 mg IV every 6 hours. For adult patients on dialysis, give 2.5 mg PO on dialysis days; adjust dosage on dialysis days based on BP response.

➤ **To manage symptomatic HF**
Adults: Initially, 2.5 mg PO b.i.d., increased gradually as tolerated over a few days or weeks. Maintenance is 5 to 40 mg daily in two divided doses. Maximum daily dose is 40 mg in two divided doses.

Adjust-a-dose: For patients with hyponatremia (serum sodium level less than 130 mEq/L) or serum creatinine level greater than 1.6 mg/dL, recommended initial dose is 2.5 mg once daily.

➤ **Asymptomatic left ventricular dysfunction**
Adults: Initially, 2.5 mg PO b.i.d. Increase as tolerated to target daily dose of 20 mg PO in divided doses.

ADMINISTRATION
PO
• Give drug without regard to food.
• Request oral suspension for patients who have difficulty swallowing.

IV
▼ Inspect solution for particulate matter and discoloration before administration.
▼ Compatible solutions include D$_5$W, NSS for injection, dextrose 5% in lactated Ringer injection, and dextrose 5% in NSS for injection.
▼ Inject drug slowly over at least 5 minutes, or dilute in 50 mL of a compatible solution and infuse over 15 minutes.
▼ **Incompatibilities:** Amphotericin B, cefepime, phenytoin.

ACTION
Inhibits ACE, preventing conversion of angiotensin I to angiotensin II, a potent vasoconstrictor. Less angiotensin II decreases peripheral arterial resistance, decreasing aldosterone secretion, reducing sodium and water retention, and lowering BP.

Route	Onset	Peak	Duration
PO	1 hr	3–4 hr	12–24 hr
IV	15 min	1–4 hr	6 hr

Half-life: 11 hours, but varies by age and comorbidities.

ADVERSE REACTIONS
CNS: asthenia, headache, dizziness, fatigue, vertigo, syncope, weakness. **CV:** hypotension, orthostatic hypotension, chest pain, angina, *MI.* **GI:** anorexia, diarrhea, nausea, abdominal pain, vomiting. **GU:** UTI. **Respiratory:** bronchitis; dry, persistent, tickling, nonproductive cough; dyspnea; pneumonia. **Skin:** rash. **Other:** hypersensitivity reactions.

INTERACTIONS
Drug-drug. *ACE inhibitors, ARBs (candesartan, telmisartan):* May increase risk of hypotension, hyperkalemia, and kidney failure. Avoid use together; if use together is unavoidable, closely monitor BP, kidney function, and electrolyte levels.
Aldosterone blockers (eplerenone): May increase risk of hyperkalemia. Monitor therapy.
Aliskiren: May increase risk of hypotension, hyperkalemia, and kidney failure. Use together is contraindicated in patients with diabetes.
Azathioprine: May increase risk of anemia or leukopenia. Monitor hematologic study results if used together.
Diuretics: May excessively reduce BP. Use together cautiously.
Gold sodium thiomalate: May increase risk of nitritoid reactions. Use together cautiously.
Insulin, oral antidiabetics: May cause hypoglycemia, especially at start of enalapril therapy. Monitor patient closely.
Lithium: May cause lithium toxicity. Monitor lithium level.
mTOR inhibitors (sirolimus, temsirolimus): May increase risk of angioedema. Monitor patient closely.
Neprilysin inhibitors (sacubitril): May increase risk of angioedema. Use together is contraindicated. Don't give within 36 hours of switching to or from sacubitril–valsartan, a neprilysin inhibitor.
NSAIDs: May increase risk of kidney failure in older adults or patients with volume depletion or impaired kidney function. Monitor kidney function.
Potassium-sparing diuretics, potassium supplements: May cause hyperkalemia. Avoid use together unless hypokalemia is confirmed.

Drug-herb. *Capsaicin:* May cause cough. Discourage use together.

Ma huang: May decrease antihypertensive effects. Discourage use together.

Drug-food. *Salt substitutes containing potassium:* May cause hyperkalemia. Monitor patient closely.

EFFECTS ON LAB TEST RESULTS

• May increase bilirubin, BUN, creatinine, and potassium levels and LFT values.
• May decrease sodium and Hb levels and hematocrit.

CONTRAINDICATIONS & CAUTIONS

⬛ Contraindicated in patients hypersensitive to drug, in those with history of angioedema related to previous treatment with an ACE inhibitor, and in patients with hereditary or idiopathic angioedema.
• Safety and effectiveness of IV use in children haven't been established.
• Oral drug isn't recommended in neonates (younger than age 1 month), preterm infants who haven't reached a corrected postconceptual age of 44 weeks, and in children with GFR of less than 30 mL/minute/1.73 m^2.
• Use cautiously in patients with kidney impairment and those with aortic stenosis or hypertrophic cardiomyopathy.
Dialyzable drug: Yes.
⚠ *Overdose S&S:* Hypotension.

PREGNANCY-LACTATION-REPRODUCTION

Boxed Warning Use during pregnancy can cause injury and death to the developing fetus. If pregnancy is detected, stop drug as soon as possible. ∎
• Drug appears in human milk. Breastfeeding isn't recommended.

NURSING CONSIDERATIONS

• Closely monitor BP response to drug.
• Monitor CBC with differential counts before and during therapy.
• Monitor potassium intake and potassium level in patient with diabetes, impaired kidney function, or HF or if patient is receiving drugs that can increase potassium level due to risk of hyperkalemia.
• Monitor kidney function, especially in patient who had an MI or has bilateral kidney artery stenosis, CKD, volume depletion, or HF.
• Monitor patient for angioedema and anaphylactoid reactions (airway obstruction;

edema of face, extremities, lips, and tongue; abdominal pain with or without nausea or vomiting).
• Monitor for signs and symptoms of liver toxicity (jaundice, increased LFT values).
⬛ Be aware that a patient who is Black and is taking ACE inhibitor as monotherapy for HTN may have a smaller-than-usual reduction in BP. Also patient who is Black and taking ACE inhibitor is at higher risk for angioedema.
• *Look alike–sound alike:* Don't confuse enalapril with Anafranil.

PATIENT TEACHING

• Instruct patient to report breathing difficulty or swelling of face, eyes, lips, or tongue. Swelling of face and throat (including swelling of larynx) may occur, especially after first dose.
• Advise patient to report signs and symptoms of infection (fever, sore throat).
• Instruct patient to report persistent nonproductive cough.
• Inform patient that light-headedness can occur, especially during first few days of therapy. Tell patient to rise slowly to minimize this effect and to notify prescriber if symptoms develop. If fainting occurs, advise patient to immediately stop drug and call prescriber.
• Tell patient to use caution in hot weather and during exercise. Inadequate fluid intake, vomiting, diarrhea, and excessive perspiration can lead to light-headedness and fainting.
• Advise patient to avoid salt substitutes; these products may contain potassium, which can cause high potassium level in patient taking this drug.
Boxed Warning Tell patient of childbearing potential to notify prescriber if pregnancy occurs. Drug will need to be stopped. ∎

SAFETY ALERT!

enfuvirtide
en-foo-VEER-tide

Fuzeon

Therapeutic class: Antiretrovirals
Pharmacologic class: Fusion inhibitors

AVAILABLE FORMS

Powder for injection: 108-mg single-use vials (90 mg/mL after reconstitution)

Reactions in bold italics are *life-threatening*.

INDICATIONS & DOSAGES
➤ **HIV-1 infection, with other antiretrovirals, in patients who have continued HIV-1 replication despite antiretroviral therapy**
Adults: 90 mg subcut b.i.d.
Children weighing at least 11 kg: 2 mg/kg subcut b.i.d. Maximum, 90 mg/dose.

ADMINISTRATION
Subcutaneous
• Reconstitute vial with 1 mL sterile water for injection. Tap vial with fingertip for 10 seconds, then gently roll, making sure powder doesn't adhere to vial wall. Let drug stand for up to 45 minutes to ensure reconstitution. When completely mixed, solution should be clear, colorless, and without bubbles or particulate matter. If solution appears foamy or jelled, allow more time for it to dissolve. Then draw up correct dose and inject drug.
• If drug isn't used immediately after reconstitution, refrigerate in original vial and use within 24 hours. Don't inject drug until it's at room temperature.
• Vial is for single use; discard unused portion.
• Inject into upper arm, anterior thigh, or abdomen. Rotate injection sites. Don't inject into same site for two consecutive doses, and don't inject into moles, scar tissue, bruises, tattoos, or the navel, where large nerves course close to the skin.
• Store unreconstituted vials at room temperature.

ACTION
Interferes with entry of HIV-1 into cells by inhibiting fusion of HIV-1 to CD4 cell membranes.

Route	Onset	Peak	Duration
Subcut	Unknown	4–8 hr	Unknown

Half-life: 3.8 hours.

ADVERSE REACTIONS
CNS: fatigue, insomnia, anxiety, asthenia.
EENT: conjunctivitis, sinusitis, dry mouth.
GI: diarrhea, nausea, *pancreatitis,* abdominal pain, anorexia, constipation. **Hematologic:** eosinophilia. **Hepatic:** increased transaminase levels. **Metabolic:** weight loss, increased CK level. **Musculoskeletal:** myalgia, limb pain. **Respiratory:** pneumonia, cough. **Skin:** injection-site reactions, folliculitis. **Other:** herpes simplex, flulike illness.

INTERACTIONS
Drug-drug. *Orlistat:* May decrease enfuvirtide serum level. Monitor therapeutic response.

EFFECTS ON LAB TEST RESULTS
• May increase CK, ALT, AST, GGT, lipase, amylase, and triglyceride levels.
• May increase eosinophil count.
• May decrease Hb level.

CONTRAINDICATIONS & CAUTIONS
• Contraindicated in patients hypersensitive to drug and in those not infected with HIV.
• Safety and effectiveness in children weighing less than 11 kg haven't been determined.
Dialyzable drug: Unlikely.

PREGNANCY-LACTATION-REPRODUCTION
• Well-controlled studies during pregnancy are lacking. Use during pregnancy only if clearly needed.
• Register patients who are pregnant in the Antiretroviral Pregnancy Registry at 1-800-258-4263 or www.apregistry.com.

NURSING CONSIDERATIONS
• Injection-site reactions (pain, discomfort, induration, erythema, pruritus, nodules, cysts, ecchymosis), which are common, may require analgesics or rest.
• Monitor patient for infection and development of immune reconstitution syndrome (inflammatory response to opportunistic infections, such as MAC infection, CMV, *Pneumocystis jiroveci* pneumonia, and TB), which may necessitate further evaluation and treatment. Autoimmune disorders (such as Graves disease, polymyositis, and Guillain-Barré syndrome) have also been reported in the setting of immune reconstitution; however, onset varies and can occur months after initiation of treatment.
• Nerve pain (neuralgia or paresthesia) lasting up to 6 months and associated with administration at sites where large nerves course close to the skin, bruising, and hematomas have occurred. Be aware that risk of postinjection bleeding may be higher if patient is receiving anticoagulant or has hemophilia or another coagulation disorder.
• *Alert:* Monitor patient closely for evidence of bacterial pneumonia. Patients at high risk include those with a low initial CD4 count or high initial viral load, those who use IV drugs or smoke, and those with history of lung disease.

- Hypersensitivity may occur with first dose or later doses. If systemic symptoms occur, stop drug and don't rechallenge.

PATIENT TEACHING
- Teach patient how to prepare and give drug and how to safely dispose of used needles and syringes.
- Tell patient to rotate injection sites and to watch for cellulitis or local infection.
- Urge patient to immediately report evidence of pneumonia, such as cough with fever, rapid breathing, or shortness of breath.
- Tell patient to stop taking drug and seek medical attention if evidence of hypersensitivity develops (rash, fever, nausea, vomiting, chills, rigor, hypotension).
- Teach patient that drug doesn't cure HIV infection and that it must be taken with other antiretrovirals.
- Tell patient to inform prescriber of pregnancy or plans to become pregnant or to breastfeed while taking drug.
- Inform patient that drug may affect the ability to drive or operate machinery.
- Tell patient that information on self-administration is available at 1-877-4FUZEON (1-877-438-9366).

SAFETY ALERT!

enoxaparin sodium
en-OCKS-a-par-in

Lovenox

Therapeutic class: Anticoagulants
Pharmacologic class: Low-molecular-weight heparins

AVAILABLE FORMS
Multidose vial: 300 mg/3 mL*
Syringes (graduated prefilled): 60 mg/0.6 mL, 80 mg/0.8 mL, 100 mg/mL, 120 mg/0.8 mL, 150 mg/mL
Syringes (prefilled): 30 mg/0.3 mL, 40 mg/0.4 mL

INDICATIONS & DOSAGES
➤ **To prevent PE and DVT after hip or knee replacement surgery**
Adults: 30 mg subcut every 12 hours for 7 to 10 days. Treatment for up to 14 days has been well tolerated. Give initial dose between 12 and 24 hours postoperatively, as long as

hemostasis has been established. Continue treatment during postoperative period until risk of DVT has diminished. Before hip replacement surgery, patients may receive 40 mg subcut 12 hours (range, 9 to 15 hours) preoperatively then 40 mg subcut daily for 3 weeks.
Adjust-a-dose: In patients with CrCl of less than 30 mL/minute, give 30 mg subcut once daily.
➤ **To prevent PE and DVT after abdominal surgery**
Adults: 40 mg subcut daily with initial dose 2 hours before surgery. Give subsequent dose, as long as hemostasis has been established, 24 hours after initial preoperative dose, and continue once daily for 7 to 10 days. Treatment for up to 12 days has been well tolerated. Continue treatment during postoperative period until risk of DVT has diminished.
Adjust-a-dose: In patients with CrCl of less than 30 mL/minute, give 30 mg subcut once daily.
➤ **To prevent PE and DVT in patients with acute illness who are at increased risk because of decreased mobility**
Adults: 40 mg subcut once daily for 6 to 11 days. Treatment for up to 14 days has been well tolerated.
Adjust-a-dose: In patients with CrCl of less than 30 mL/minute, give 30 mg subcut once daily.
➤ **To prevent ischemic complications of unstable angina and non-Q-wave MI with oral aspirin therapy**
Adults: 1 mg/kg subcut every 12 hours until clinical stabilization (minimum 2 days) with aspirin 100 to 325 mg PO once daily. Usual duration of treatment is 2 to 8 days.
Adjust-a-dose: In patients with CrCl of less than 30 mL/minute, give 1 mg/kg subcut once daily.
➤ **Acute ST-segment elevation MI**
Adults younger than age 75: 30 mg single IV bolus plus 1 mg/kg subcut, followed by 1 mg/kg subcut every 12 hours (maximum of 100 mg for first two doses only) with aspirin 75 to 325 mg PO once daily. When given with thrombolytic, give enoxaparin from 15 minutes before to 30 minutes after start of fibrinolytic therapy. For patients undergoing PCI, if last subcut dose was given less than 8 hours before balloon inflation, no additional dose is needed. If last dose was given more than 8 hours before balloon inflation, 0.3 mg/kg IV bolus.

Adults ages 75 and older: No initial IV bolus; 0.75 mg/kg subcut every 12 hours (maximum 75 mg for first two doses only).

Adjust-a-dose: In adults younger than age 75 with CrCl of less than 30 mL/minute, give 30 mg single IV bolus plus 1 mg/kg subcut, followed by 1 mg/kg subcut once daily. In adults ages 75 and older with CrCl of less than 30 mL/minute, give 1 mg/kg subcut once daily with no initial bolus. Give with aspirin.

➤ **Inpatient treatment of acute DVT with or without PE when given with warfarin sodium**

Adults: 1 mg/kg subcut every 12 hours or 1.5 mg/kg subcut once daily (at same time daily) for 5 to 7 days until therapeutic oral anticoagulant effect (INR 2 to 3) is achieved. Warfarin sodium therapy is usually started within 72 hours of enoxaparin injection.

Adjust-a-dose: In patients with CrCl of less than 30 mL/minute, give 1 mg/kg subcut once daily.

➤ **Outpatient treatment of acute DVT without PE when given with warfarin sodium**

Adults: 1 mg/kg subcut every 12 hours for 5 to 7 days until therapeutic oral anticoagulant effect (INR 2 to 3) is achieved. Warfarin sodium therapy usually is started within 72 hours of enoxaparin injection.

Adjust-a-dose: In patients with CrCl of less than 30 mL/minute, give 1 mg/kg subcut once daily.

ADMINISTRATION

● Solution should appear clear and colorless to pale yellow; discard it if it is discolored or contains particulate matter.

IV

▼ Use multidose vial for IV injections.

▼ Flush IV access with sufficient amount of saline or dextrose solution before and after IV bolus administration.

▼ **Incompatibilities:** Don't mix or administer with other IV drugs.

Subcutaneous

● With patient lying down, give by deep subcut injection, alternating doses between left and right anterolateral and posterolateral abdominal walls. Don't expel air bubble from prefilled syringe before injecting to prevent drug loss and an incorrect dose. Hold skinfold between thumb and forefinger and insert entire length of needle. Push plunger to bottom of syringe.

● Don't massage after subcut injection.
● Watch for signs of bleeding at site.
● Rotate sites and keep record.

ACTION

Accelerates formation of antithrombin III–thrombin complex and deactivates thrombin, preventing conversion of fibrinogen to fibrin. Drug has a higher antifactor-Xa-to-antifactor-IIa activity ratio than heparin.

Route	Onset	Peak	Duration
IV	Unknown	Unknown	Unknown
Subcut	Unknown	4 hr	Unknown

Half-life: 4.5 hours after a single dose; 7 hours after repeated dosing.

ADVERSE REACTIONS

CNS: confusion, fever, pain. **CV:** edema, peripheral edema. **GI:** nausea, diarrhea. **GU:** hematuria. **Hematologic:** *thrombocytopenia, hemorrhage,* bleeding complications, anemia. **Hepatic:** increased transaminase levels. **Respiratory:** dyspnea. **Skin:** irritation, pain, hematoma, ecchymosis, and erythema at injection site.

INTERACTIONS

Drug-drug. *Anticoagulants, antiplatelet drugs, NSAIDs:* May increase risk of bleeding. Discontinue use before starting enoxaparin, if possible. If necessary, use together cautiously and monitor patient for bleeding. *SSRIs:* May increase risk of severe bleeding. Monitor patient for bleeding. Adjust therapy as needed.

Drug-herb. *Alfalfa, anise, bilberry:* May increase risk of bleeding. Discourage use together.

EFFECTS ON LAB TEST RESULTS

● May increase potassium, ALT, and AST levels.
● May decrease Hb level and platelet count.

CONTRAINDICATIONS & CAUTIONS

● Contraindicated in patients hypersensitive to drug, heparin, pork products, or benzyl alcohol (multidose vial only); in those with active major bleeding; and in those with history of immune-mediated heparin-induced thrombocytopenia (HIT) within the past 100 days or in the presence of circulating antibodies.
● Use drug in patients with a history of HIT only if more than 100 days have elapsed since

the prior HIT episode and no circulating antibodies are present. Because HIT may still occur in these circumstances, the decision to use enoxaparin in such a case must be made only after a careful benefit-risk assessment and after nonheparin alternative treatments have been considered.

• Use cautiously in patients with history of aneurysms, cerebrovascular hemorrhage, spinal or epidural punctures, uncontrolled HTN, or threatened abortion.

• Use cautiously in older adults and in patients with conditions that place them at increased risk for hemorrhage (bacterial endocarditis; congenital or acquired bleeding disorders; ulcer disease; angiodysplastic GI disease; hemorrhagic stroke; recent spinal, eye, or brain surgery).

Boxed Warning Consider risks and benefits before neuraxial intervention (neuraxial anesthesia or spinal puncture) in patients who are or will be anticoagulated for thrombus prevention. ■

• Use cautiously in patients with prosthetic heart valves, blood dyscrasias, pericarditis, pericardial effusion, kidney insufficiency, or severe CNS trauma as well as those who are receiving regional or lumbar block anesthesia or recently underwent childbirth.

• Safety and effectiveness in children haven't been established.

Dialyzable drug: No.

⚠ *Overdose S&S:* Hemorrhagic complications.

PREGNANCY-LACTATION-REPRODUCTION

• Well-controlled studies during pregnancy are lacking. Closely monitor patients who are pregnant for evidence of bleeding or excessive coagulation. Warn patients about risk of therapy during pregnancy.

• Consider using a shorter-acting anticoagulant as delivery approaches.

• Avoid use of multidose vial in patients who are pregnant due to benzyl alcohol content and risk of gasping syndrome in premature infants.

• It isn't known if drug appears in human milk. Use cautiously during breastfeeding.

NURSING CONSIDERATIONS

• It's important to achieve hemostasis at the puncture site after PCI. The vascular access sheath for instrumentation should remain in place for 6 hours after enoxaparin dose if manual compression method is used; give next dose no sooner than 6 to 8 hours after sheath removal. Monitor vital signs and site for hematoma and bleeding.

• Obtain baseline coagulation studies before therapy.

• Monitor anti-Xa levels if abnormal coagulation parameters or bleeding occurs. PT and PTT aren't adequate for monitoring drug's anticoagulant effects.

• Monitor anti-Xa levels during pregnancy in patients with mechanical heart valves and in patients with CrCl less than 30 mL/minute.

Boxed Warning Patients who receive epidural or spinal anesthesia or spinal puncture during therapy are at increased risk for developing an epidural or spinal hematoma, which may result in long-term or permanent paralysis. Factors that can increase risk include use of indwelling epidural catheters, concurrent use of other drugs that affect hemostasis, history of traumatic or repeated epidural or spinal puncture, and history of spinal deformity or spinal surgery. Monitor these patients closely for neurologic impairment, as urgent treatment is necessary. ■

Boxed Warning The optimal timing between administration of enoxaparin and spinal procedures isn't known. ■

⊙ *Alert:* For spinal procedures, consider both dose and elimination half-life of drug. Delay placement or removal of a spinal catheter for at least 12 hours after prophylactic doses or for 24 hours for higher therapeutic doses of 0.75 mg/kg b.i.d., 1 mg/kg b.i.d., or 1.5 mg/kg daily. Give postprocedure doses no sooner than 4 hours after catheter removal.

• Never give drug IM.

• Avoid IM injections of other drugs to prevent or minimize hematoma.

• Regularly monitor platelet counts. Patients with normal coagulation won't need close monitoring of PT or PTT.

• Regularly inspect patient for bleeding gums, bruises on arms or legs, petechiae, nosebleeds, melena, hematuria, and hematemesis.

• To treat severe overdose, give protamine sulfate (a heparin antagonist) by slow IV injection. Refer to manufacturer's instructions for protamine use.

⊙ *Alert:* Drug isn't interchangeable with heparin or other low-molecular-weight heparins.

PATIENT TEACHING

• Instruct patient and family to watch for and immediately notify prescriber of signs and symptoms of bleeding or abnormal bruising.

Boxed Warning Tell patient to immediately report signs and symptoms of spinal or epidural hematoma, such as numbness (especially of lower limbs) and muscle weakness. ∎

• Advise patient to consult prescriber before initiating herbal therapy because many herbs have anticoagulant, antiplatelet, or fibrinolytic properties.

• Show patient how to properly administer subcut injection and dispose of syringe.

• Inform patient that longer-than-usual time may be needed to stop bleeding and that bruising or bleeding may occur more easily.

• Instruct patient to inform health care providers and dentists of all medications being taken, including OTC products.

• Tell patient to avoid OTC drugs containing aspirin or other salicylates unless ordered by prescriber.

• Advise patient to inform prescriber of pregnancy or plans to become pregnant or to breastfeed during therapy.

---

entecavir
en-TEK-ah-veer

Baraclude

Therapeutic class: Antivirals
Pharmacologic class: Nucleosides–
nucleotides

AVAILABLE FORMS
Oral solution: 0.05 mg/mL
Tablets: 0.5 mg, 1 mg

INDICATIONS & DOSAGES
➤ **Chronic HBV infection in patients with active viral replication and either persistently increased aminotransferase levels or histologically active disease**
Adults and adolescents ages 16 and older with no previous nucleoside treatment: 0.5 mg PO once daily for patients with compensated liver disease and 1 mg PO once daily for patients with decompensated liver disease.
Adjust-a-dose: If CrCl is 30 to less than 50 mL/minute, give 0.25 mg PO once daily or 0.5 mg PO every 48 hours. If CrCl is 10 to less than 30 mL/minute, give 0.15 mg PO once daily or 0.5 mg PO every 72 hours. If CrCl is less than 10 mL/minute or patient is undergoing hemodialysis or continuous ambulatory peritoneal dialysis (CAPD), give

0.05 mg PO once daily or 0.5 mg PO every 7 days.
Children age 2 to younger than age 16 and weighing at least 10 kg who have had no previous nucleoside treatment: For children weighing more than 30 kg, 0.5 mg PO once daily. For children weighing more than 26 to 30 kg, 9 mL (0.45 mg) oral solution PO once daily. For children weighing more than 23 to 26 kg, 8 mL (0.4 mg) oral solution PO once daily. For children weighing more than 20 to 23 kg, 7 mL (0.35 mg) oral solution PO once daily. For children weighing more than 17 to 20 kg, 6 mL (0.3 mg) oral solution PO once daily. For children weighing more than 14 to 17 kg, 5 mL (0.25 mg) oral solution PO once daily. For children weighing more than 11 to 14 kg, 4 mL (0.2 mg) oral solution PO once daily. For children weighing more than 10 to 11 kg, 3 mL (0.15 mg) oral solution PO once daily.
Adjust-a-dose: Insufficient data are available for specific dosage adjustments in children with kidney impairment. Consider reducing dosage or increasing dosing interval similar to adjustments for adults.
☉ Alert: While an FDA-approved indication, treatment of lamivudine-refractory or lamivudine- or telbivudine-resistant HBV infection isn't recommended by American Association for the Study of Liver Disease. If needed, refer to manufacturer's instructions for dosing.

ADMINISTRATION
PO
☉ Alert: Hazardous drug; use safe handling and disposal precautions.
• Give on an empty stomach at least 2 hours after a meal and 2 hours before next meal to increase absorption.
• Store tablets at room temperature in tightly closed container.
• Use oral solution for patients weighing up to 30 kg and for doses less than 0.5 mg.
• Only give oral solution with provided dosing spoon.
• Don't mix oral solution with other liquids.
• Protect oral solution from light by storing in the outer carton.
• After oral solution has been opened, it can be used up to expiration date on the bottle.
• Give missed dose as soon as possible unless it's almost time for the next dose.

✦Canada   ◇OTC   ◆Off-label use   ⓓ Do not crush   *Liquid contains alcohol   ✄ Genetic

ACTION
Reduces viral DNA level by inhibiting HBV viral polymerase, which blocks reverse transcriptase activity.

Route	Onset	Peak	Duration
PO	Unknown	0.5–1.5 hr	Unknown

Half-life: About 5 to 6 days.

ADVERSE REACTIONS
CNS: dizziness, fatigue, headache, fever, hepatic encephalopathy. **CV:** edema. **GI:** abdominal pain, diarrhea, dyspepsia, nausea, vomiting. **GU:** glycosuria, hematuria, increased creatinine level. **Hepatic:** increased transaminase levels, ascites, hyperbilirubinemia, liver enlargement. **Metabolic:** increased lipase level, hyperglycemia. **Respiratory:** URI. **Skin:** rash.

INTERACTIONS
Drug-drug. *Drugs that reduce kidney function or compete for active tubular secretion:* May increase level of either drug. Monitor kidney function, and watch for adverse effects. *Orlistat:* May decrease entecavir serum level. Monitor therapy.
Drug-food. *All foods:* Delay absorption and decrease drug level. Give drug on an empty stomach.

EFFECTS ON LAB TEST RESULTS
• May increase ALT, amylase, AST, blood glucose, creatinine, lipase, and total bilirubin levels.
• May decrease platelet count.

CONTRAINDICATIONS & CAUTIONS
• Contraindicated in patients hypersensitive to drug or its components.
Boxed Warning Don't use in patients infected with both HIV and HBV who aren't also receiving highly active antiretroviral therapy due to risk of resistance.∎
• Use cautiously in patients with kidney impairment and in patients who have had a liver transplant.
• Safety and effectiveness in children younger than age 2 haven't been established.
Dialyzable drug: 13% after 4-hour hemodialysis.

PREGNANCY-LACTATION-REPRODUCTION
• Use cautiously during pregnancy and only if benefit outweighs fetal risk.

• Register patients who are pregnant in the Antiretroviral Pregnancy Registry at 1-800-258-4263 or www.apregistry.com.
• It isn't known if drug appears in human milk. Use cautiously during breastfeeding.

NURSING CONSIDERATIONS
Boxed Warning Drug may cause life-threatening lactic acidosis and severe liver enlargement with steatosis when used alone or in combination with antiretrovirals.∎
• Monitor for liver toxicity with physical assessment and LFTs.
Boxed Warning HBV infection may worsen severely after therapy stops. Monitor liver function for several months in patients who stop therapy. If appropriate, start therapy for HBV infection.∎
• In older adults, adjust dosage for age-related decrease in kidney function.

PATIENT TEACHING
• Teach about proper drug administration and handling.
• Tell patient to report all adverse effects of this drug and to report all other drugs being taken.
• Explain that drug doesn't reduce the risk of HBV transmission to others.
• Review signs and symptoms of lactic acidosis (muscle pain, weakness, dyspnea, GI distress, cold hands and feet, dizziness, fast or irregular heartbeat).
• Teach patient signs and symptoms of liver toxicity (jaundice, dark urine, light-colored stool, loss of appetite, nausea, stomach pain).
• Warn patient that missed doses increase risk of resistance. Instruct patient to be sure to refill drug before it runs out.

SAFETY ALERT!

EPINEPHrine (adrenaline)
ep-i-NEF-rin

EPINEPHrine hydrochloride
Adrenaclick, Adrenalin, Auvi-Q, EpiPen, EpiPen Jr, Symjepi

Therapeutic class: Vasopressors
Pharmacologic class: Adrenergics

AVAILABLE FORMS
Injection: 0.1 mg/mL, 1 mg/mL

Reactions in bold italics are *life-threatening*.

Injection (premixed for infusion): 2 mg, 4 mg, 5 mg, or 8 mg in 250 mL NSS
Injection device: 0.15 mg/delivery, 0.3 mg/delivery

INDICATIONS & DOSAGES

➤ **Anaphylaxis**

Adults and children weighing 30 kg or more: 0.3 to 0.5 mg IM or subcut, repeated every 5 to 10 minutes as needed; maximum single dose, 0.5 mg. Or, 0.3 mg IM or subcut with autoinjector to maximum of 0.5 mg per injection, repeated every 5 to 10 minutes as needed.
Children weighing 15 to less than 30 kg: 0.01 to 0.15 mg/kg IM or subcut to maximum of 0.3 mg per injection, repeated every 5 to 10 minutes as needed. May use 0.15 mg autoinjector.
Children weighing 7.5 to less than 15 kg: 0.01 mg/kg IM or subcut to maximum of 0.3 mg per injection, repeated every 5 to 10 minutes as needed.

➤ **Hypotension associated with septic shock**

Adults: 0.05 to 2 mcg/kg/minute IV infusion titrated to achieve desired mean arterial pressure. May adjust dosage every 10 to 15 minutes in increments of 0.05 to 0.2 mcg/kg/minute to achieve desired BP goal. Titrate to patient response. After hemodynamic stabilization, wean incrementally over time, such as by decreasing epinephrine dosages every 10 minutes, to determine patient tolerance.

➤ **Cardiac resuscitation**

Adults: 1 mg IV or intraosseously every 3 to 5 minutes until return of spontaneous circulation.
Children: 0.01 mg/kg IV or intraosseously, up to 1 mg, repeated every 3 to 5 minutes until return of spontaneous circulation.

ADMINISTRATION

• Discard solution if it's discolored or contains precipitate.

IV

▼ Keep solution in light-resistant container, and don't remove before use.
▼ For IV infusion, just before use, mix with D_5W, combinations of dextrose in saline solution, or NSS as ordered or use premixed bags. Concentration may vary by indication.
▼ Monitor BP, HR, and ECG when therapy starts and frequently thereafter.

▼ Discard solution after 4 hours at room temperature or after 24 hours if refrigerated.
▼ When giving as a continuous infusion, use a central line with an infusion pump. Extravasation can cause tissue necrosis.
▼ Don't give autoinjectors IV.
▼ **Incompatibilities:** Don't mix with alkaline solutions (such as sodium bicarbonate). Consult a drug compatibility reference for more information.

IM

• Give in anterolateral aspect of thigh, through clothing if necessary. Repeat injection every 5 to 15 minutes, if necessary.
• Massage site after IM injection to counteract vasoconstriction. Repeated local injection can cause necrosis at injection site.

Subcutaneous

• Follow manufacturer's instructions for administration.
• Store drug at room temperature. Don't freeze.
• Protect drug from light.

ACTION

Potentiates alpha and beta receptors. Relaxes bronchial smooth muscle by stimulating $beta_2$ receptors. Stimulates alpha and beta receptors in the sympathetic nervous system.

Route	Onset	Peak	Duration
IV	Immediate	5 min	Short
IM	Rapid	Unknown	1–4 hr
Subcut	5–15 min	30 min	1–4 hr

Half-life: IV injection, less than 5 minutes. IM and subcut, unknown.

ADVERSE REACTIONS

CNS: drowsiness, headache, nervousness, tremor, *cerebral hemorrhage, stroke,* vertigo, pain, disorientation, agitation, asthenia, tremor, anxiety, apprehensiveness, fear, restlessness, dizziness, weakness, somnolence, paresthesia, *subarachnoid hemorrhage.* **CV:** palpitations, *ventricular fibrillation, shock,* widened pulse pressure, HTN, *MI,* tachycardia, anginal pain, *arrhythmias,* altered ECG (including decreased T-wave amplitude), limb ischemia. **GI:** nausea, vomiting. **GU:** kidney insufficiency. **Metabolic:** hyperglycemia, *hypoglycemia, hypokalemia, lactic acidosis,* insulin resistance. **Respiratory:** dyspnea, *pulmonary edema,* respiratory difficulties. **Skin:** urticaria, hemorrhage or necrosis at injection site, pallor, diaphoresis.

✤Canada   ◇OTC   ◆Off-label use   ⓜDo not crush   *Liquid contains alcohol   ⚖ Genetic

INTERACTIONS

Drug-drug. *Alpha blockers (phentolamine):* May cause hypotension from unopposed beta-adrenergic effects. Avoid use together.

Antihistamines, thyroid hormones: When given with sympathomimetics, may cause severe adverse cardiac effects. Avoid use together.

Beta-adrenergic blockers (propranolol): May increase BP and decrease HR. Use together cautiously.

Beta blockers (carteolol, nadolol, penbutolol, pindolol, pindol, timolol): May cause HTN, followed by bradycardia. Stop beta blocker 3 days before starting epinephrine.

Cardiac glycosides, diuretics, general anesthetics (halogenated hydrocarbons): May increase risk of ventricular arrhythmias. Monitor ECG closely.

Doxapram, methylphenidate: May enhance CNS stimulation or pressor effects. Monitor patient closely.

Ergot alkaloids: May decrease vasoconstrictor activity. Monitor patient closely.

Levodopa: May enhance risk of arrhythmias. Monitor ECG closely.

MAO inhibitors: May increase risk of hypertensive crisis. Monitor BP closely.

Potassium-depleting diuretics, corticosteroids, theophylline: May increase hypokalemic effects of epinephrine. Monitor potassium level.

TCAs: May potentiate pressor response and cause arrhythmias. Use together cautiously.

EFFECTS ON LAB TEST RESULTS

- May increase BUN, glucose, and lactic acid levels.
- May decrease potassium level.
- May increase or decrease glucose level.
- Interferes with tests for urinary catecholamines.

CONTRAINDICATIONS & CAUTIONS

- There are no absolute contraindications in lifesaving situations.
- Contraindicated in patients with shock (other than anaphylactic shock), organic brain damage, HF, cardiac dilation, arrhythmias, coronary insufficiency, or cerebral arteriosclerosis.
- Contraindicated in patients receiving general anesthesia with halogenated hydrocarbons or cyclopropane and in patients in labor (may delay second stage).

- Some products contain sulfites. Use is contraindicated in patients with sulfite allergies, except when epinephrine is used to treat serious allergic reactions or other emergency situations.
- Don't use epinephrine with local anesthetic in fingers, toes, ears, nose, or genitalia.
- Use cautiously in patients with longstanding bronchial asthma or emphysema who have developed degenerative heart disease.
- Use cautiously in older adults and in patients with hyperthyroidism, CV disease, HTN, psychoneurosis, pheochromocytoma, and diabetes.

Dialyzable drug: Unknown.

⚠ *Overdose S&S:* Precordial distress, vomiting, headache, dyspnea, HTN, peripheral vascular constriction, pulmonary edema, cerebral hemorrhage, arrhythmias, extreme pallor and coldness of the skin, metabolic acidosis, kidney failure.

PREGNANCY-LACTATION-REPRODUCTION

- Use during pregnancy only if potential benefit justifies fetal risk.
- Parenteral administration of epinephrine, if used to support BP during spinal anesthesia for delivery, can cause accelerated fetal HR and shouldn't be used in obstetric patients when BP exceeds 130/80 mm Hg.
- It isn't known if drug appears in human milk. Use cautiously during breastfeeding.

NURSING CONSIDERATIONS

- Use phentolamine to prevent tissue sloughing and necrosis if epinephrine extravasation occurs.
- In patients with Parkinson disease, drug temporarily increases rigidity and tremors.
- Epinephrine is drug of choice in emergency treatment of acute anaphylactic reactions.
- Closely observe patient for and notify prescriber of adverse reactions; adjusting dosage or stopping drug may be necessary.
- If BP increases sharply, give rapid-acting vasodilators, such as nitrates and alpha blockers, to counteract the marked pressor effect of large doses.
- Oxidizing products, such as iodine, chromates, nitrites, oxygen, and salts of easily reducible metals (such as iron), rapidly destroy drug.
- When treating patient with reactions caused by other drugs given IM or subcut, inject this drug into the site where the other drug was given to minimize further absorption.

Reactions in bold italics are *life-threatening*.

• *Look alike–sound alike:* Don't confuse epinephrine with ephedrine or norepinephrine.

PATIENT TEACHING

• If patient has acute hypersensitivity reactions (such as to bee stings), it may be necessary to teach patient how to self-inject.
• Instruct patient in autoinjector use and disposal. Tell patient to give autoinjector in outer thigh and not into buttock.
• Caution patient or caregiver to only give two sequential doses unless under direct medical supervision. Patient should seek immediate medical care for acute hypersensitivity reactions.
• Tell patient to promptly report all adverse reactions.

SAFETY ALERT!

epiRUBicin hydrochloride
ep-i-ROO-bi-sin

Ellence

Therapeutic class: Antineoplastics
Pharmacologic class: Anthracycline glycoside antibiotics

AVAILABLE FORMS
Injection: 50 mg/25 mL, 200 mg/100 mL single-dose vials

INDICATIONS & DOSAGES
➤ **Adjuvant therapy in patients with evidence of axillary node tumor involvement after resection of primary breast cancer**
Adults: 100 to 120 mg/m^2 IV infusion on day 1 of each cycle, or divided equally in two doses on days 1 and 8 of each cycle; cycle repeated every 3 to 4 weeks for six cycles; used with regimens containing cyclophosphamide and 5-FU.
Adjust-a-dose: For patients with bone marrow dysfunction (patients heavily pretreated and those with bone marrow depression or neoplastic bone marrow infiltration), start at lower dose of 75 to 90 mg/m^2.

For patients with liver dysfunction, if bilirubin is 1.2 to 3 mg/dL or AST is 2 to 4 × ULN, give half recommended starting dose. If bilirubin level is above 3 mg/dL or AST is more than 4 × ULN, give one-quarter the recommended starting dose.

For patients with creatinine level over 5 mg/dL, consider lower doses.

Refer to manufacturer's instructions for toxicity-related dosage adjustment.

ADMINISTRATION
IV
✪ *Alert:* Hazardous drug; use safe handling and disposal precautions.
▼ Wear protective clothing (goggles, gown, disposable gloves) when handling a vesicant drug.
Boxed Warning Extravasation can result in severe local tissue injury and necrosis, requiring wide excision and skin grafting. Immediately terminate drug and apply ice to affected area. ∎
Boxed Warning If burning or stinging occurs, indicating infiltration, stop infusion immediately and restart in another vein. ∎
▼ Never give drug IM or subcut; severe tissue necrosis may result.
▼ Always give IV in free-flowing NSS or D$_5$W over 3 to 20 minutes, depending on dosage and volume of infusion solution. Don't give by direct injection. Infuse doses of 100 to 120 mg/m^2 over 15 to 20 minutes.
▼ Avoid veins over joints or in limbs with compromised venous or lymphatic drainage.
▼ Avoid repeated injection into same vein.
▼ Facial flushing and erythematous streaking along vein may indicate overly rapid delivery.
▼ After vial has been penetrated, discard unused solution after 24 hours.
▼ Store refrigerated solution between 36° and 46° F (2° and 8° C). Don't freeze.
▼ Protect from light.
▼ **Incompatibilities:** 5-FU, heparin, any alkaline pH solutions, other IV drugs.

ACTION
Known to form a complex with DNA by getting between nucleotide base pairs, inhibiting DNA, RNA, and protein synthesis; DNA cleavage occurs, resulting in cytocidal activity. Drug may also interfere with replication and transcription of DNA and may generate cytotoxic free radicals.

Route	Onset	Peak	Duration
IV	Unknown	Unknown	Unknown

Half-life: 33 hours.

ADVERSE REACTIONS

CNS: lethargy, fever. **CV:** *cardiomyopathy, HF.* **EENT:** conjunctivitis, keratitis. **GI:** nausea, vomiting, diarrhea, anorexia, mucositis. **GU:** amenorrhea, red urine. **Hematologic:** *leukopenia, neutropenia, febrile neutropenia, thrombocytopenia,* anemia. **Skin:** alopecia, rash, pruritus, skin changes, local toxicity. **Other:** hot flashes, infection.

INTERACTIONS

Drug-drug. *Calcium channel blockers, other cardioactive compounds:* May increase risk of HF. Monitor cardiac function closely.
Cimetidine: May significantly increase epirubicin level. Don't use together.
Cytotoxic drugs (anthracyclines, trastuzumab): May cause additive toxicities.
Live-virus vaccines: May increase risk of vaccine-induced adverse reactions. Avoid use together; don't give for at least 3 months after drug.
Pimecrolimus, tacrolimus (topical): May enhance adverse and toxic effects of epirubicin. Don't use together.
Taxanes (doxorubicin, paclitaxel): May increase level of epirubicin metabolites and risk of toxicity. Monitor patient closely for CV toxicity and separate administration times as much as possible.

EFFECTS ON LAB TEST RESULTS

• May decrease Hb level and neutrophil, platelet, and WBC counts.

CONTRAINDICATIONS & CAUTIONS

• Contraindicated in patients hypersensitive to drug, other anthracyclines, or anthracenediones and in those with persistent drug-induced myelosuppression, severe myocardial insufficiency, recent MI, cardiomyopathy or HF, serious arrhythmias, previous treatment with anthracyclines up to the maximum cumulative dose, Child-Pugh class C liver impairment, or bilirubin level greater than 5 mg/dL.
• Use cautiously in patients with active or dormant cardiac disease, previous or current radiotherapy to mediastinal and pericardial areas, or previous therapy with other anthracyclines or anthracenediones.
Boxed Warning Secondary acute myeloid leukemia and myelodysplastic syndromes have been reported in patients with breast cancer treated with anthracyclines, including epirubicin. ∎

⊌ Alert: Drug may increase risk of thrombophlebitis and thromboembolic events, including fatal PE. Venous sclerosis may result from injection into a small vessel or repeated injections into the same vein.
• Safety and effectiveness in children haven't been established.
Dialyzable drug: Unknown.
⚠ Overdose S&S: Bone marrow aplasia, grade 4 mucositis, GI bleeding, hyperthermia, multiple organ failure, lactic acidosis, increased LDH level, anuria, death.

PREGNANCY-LACTATION-REPRODUCTION

• Drug can cause fetal harm. If drug is used during pregnancy or if patient becomes pregnant during therapy, inform patient of fetal risk.
• Patients of childbearing potential should use effective contraception during treatment and for 6 months after final dose.
• Males with partners of childbearing potential should use effective contraception during treatment and for 3 months after final dose. Males with partners who are pregnant should use condoms during treatment and for at least 7 days after final dose.
• It isn't known if drug appears in human milk. Patient shouldn't breastfeed during treatment and for at least 7 days after final dose.
• Drug may impair fertility and induce premature menopause. Drug may permanently impair fertility in males.

NURSING CONSIDERATIONS

• Verify pregnancy status before starting drug.
• Don't handle drug if pregnant.
• For patient taking 120 mg/m^2 regimen, give prophylactic antibiotic therapy.
• Drug is moderately to highly emetogenic; give antiemetic before drug to reduce nausea and vomiting.
Boxed Warning Myocardial damage, including acute left ventricular failure, can occur. Cardiomyopathy risk is proportional to cumulative exposure, with incidence rates from 0.9% at a cumulative dose of 550 mg/m^2, 1.6% at 700 mg/m^2, and 3.3% at 900 mg/m^2. Risk of cardiomyopathy increases with concomitant cardiotoxic therapy. Assess LVEF before and regularly during and after treatment. ∎
• Stop drug at first sign of impaired cardiac function. Early signs of cardiac toxicity

---

include sinus tachycardia, ECG abnormalities, tachyarrhythmias, bradycardia, AV block, and bundle-branch block.

Boxed Warning Severe myelosuppression resulting in serious infection, septic shock, requirement for transfusions, hospitalization, and death may occur. ∎

• Obtain total and differential WBC, CBC, and platelet counts and LFT values before and during each cycle of therapy.

• WBC nadir is usually reached 10 to 14 days after drug administration, and WBC count returns to normal by day 21.

• Monitor uric acid, potassium, calcium, phosphate, and creatinine levels immediately after initial chemotherapy administration in patients susceptible to TLS. Hydration, urine alkalinization, and prophylaxis with allopurinol may prevent hyperuricemia and minimize potential complications of TLS.

• Drug may enhance the effects of radiation therapy or cause an inflammatory cell reaction at irradiation site. Monitor patient closely.

PATIENT TEACHING

• Advise patient to report any pain or burning at injection site during or after administration.

• Instruct patient to report nausea, vomiting, mouth inflammation, dehydration, fever, evidence of infection, or symptoms of HF (rapid heartbeat, labored breathing, swelling).

• Tell patient that urine will be reddish pink for 1 to 2 days after treatment.

• Inform patient of risk of heart damage and treatment-related leukemia with use of drug.

• Advise patient of fetal and fertility risk. Provide contraception and breastfeeding recommendations.

• Tell patient that hair usually regrows within 2 to 3 months after final dose.

---

eplerenone
ep-LER-eh-nown

Inspra

Therapeutic class: Antihypertensives
Pharmacologic class: Selective aldosterone receptor antagonists

AVAILABLE FORMS
Tablets: 25 mg, 50 mg

INDICATIONS & DOSAGES
➤ **HTN**
Adults: 50 mg PO once daily. If response is inadequate after 4 weeks, increase dosage to 50 mg PO b.i.d. Maximum daily dose, 100 mg/day. May use in combination with other antihypertensives.

Adjust-a-dose: In patients taking moderate CYP3A4 inhibitors, reduce eplerenone starting dose to 25 mg PO once daily. If BP response is inadequate, may increase dosage to a maximum of 25 mg b.i.d.

➤ **HF with reduced ejection fraction after MI**
Adults: Initially, 25 mg PO once daily. Increase within 4 weeks, as tolerated and according to potassium level, to 50 mg PO once daily.

Adjust-a-dose: Once treatment begins, if potassium level is less than 5 mEq/L, increase dosage from 25 mg every other day to 25 mg daily; or increase dosage from 25 mg daily to 50 mg daily. If potassium level is 5 to 5.4 mEq/L, don't adjust dosage. If potassium level is 5.5 to 5.9 mEq/L, decrease dosage from 50 mg daily to 25 mg daily; or decrease dosage from 25 mg daily to 25 mg every other day; or if dosage was 25 mg every other day, withhold drug. If potassium level is 6 mEq/L or greater, withhold drug. May restart drug at 25 mg every other day when potassium level is less than 5.5 mEq/L. In patients receiving a moderate CYP3A inhibitor, don't exceed 25 mg once daily.

➤ **HF (NYHA Class II to IV) with reduced LVEF of 40% or less in patients already taking optimal doses of other HF medications** ◆
Adults: Initially, 25 mg once daily. May double the dose after 4 weeks, if serum potassium level remains less than 5 mEq/L and kidney function is stable, to a maximum target dose of 50 mg once daily.

ADMINISTRATION
PO
• Give drug without regard to meals.

ACTION
Binds to mineralocorticoid receptors and blocks aldosterone, which increases BP through induction of sodium reabsorption and possibly other mechanisms.

Route	Onset	Peak	Duration
PO	Unknown	1.5–2 hr	Unknown

Half-life: 3 to 6 hours.

ADVERSE REACTIONS

CNS: headache, dizziness. **CV:** angina, *MI.*
GU: increased creatinine level, abnormal
vaginal bleeding. **Metabolic:** *hyperkalemia.*
Other: gynecomastia.

INTERACTIONS

Drug-drug. *ACE inhibitors, ARBs:* May increase risk of hyperkalemia. Use together
cautiously.
Canagliflozin: May increase risk of hyperkalemia. Monitor therapy.
Lithium: May increase risk of lithium toxicity.
Monitor lithium level.
*Moderate CYP3A4 inhibitors (erythromycin,
fluconazole, saquinavir, verapamil):* May increase eplerenone level. Reduce eplerenone
starting dose to 25 mg PO once daily.
NSAIDs: May reduce the antihypertensive effect and cause severe hyperkalemia in patients
with impaired kidney function. Monitor BP
and potassium level.
*Potassium supplements, potassium-sparing
diuretics (amiloride, spironolactone, triamterene):* May increase risk of hyperkalemia
and sometimes-fatal arrhythmias. Use together is contraindicated.
*Strong CYP3A inhibitors (azole antifungals
[fluconazole, ketoconazole], macrolides
[clarithromycin], nefazodone, protease inhibitors [nelfinavir, ritonavir]):* Increase
eplerenone level. Use together is contraindicated.
Drug-herb. *St. John's wort:* May decrease
eplerenone level over time. Discourage use
together.
Drug-food. *Grapefruit juice:* May increase
eplerenone level. Discourage use together.

EFFECTS ON LAB TEST RESULTS

● May increase BUN, creatinine, GGT, and
potassium levels.
● May decrease sodium level.

CONTRAINDICATIONS & CAUTIONS

● When used for HTN, contraindicated in patients with type 2 diabetes with microalbu-
minuria, creatinine level greater than 2 mg/dL
in males or greater than 1.8 mg/dL in females,
or CrCl of less than 50 mL/minute.
● Contraindicated in all patients with potassium level greater than 5.5 mEq/mL at initiation or CrCl of 30 mL/minute.
● Use cautiously in patients with Child-Pugh
class B or C liver impairment.

Dialyzable drug: No.
⚠ *Overdose S&S:* Hypotension, hyperkalemia.

PREGNANCY-LACTATION-REPRODUCTION

● Use during pregnancy only if potential benefits justify fetal risk.
● It isn't known if drug appears in human milk.
Patient should discontinue breastfeeding or
discontinue drug, considering importance of
drug to patient.
● Drug may impair male fertility.

NURSING CONSIDERATIONS

● Full therapeutic effect of the drug occurs in
4 weeks.
● Measure potassium level at baseline, within
first week or after dosage adjustment, at
1 month after starting therapy, and periodically thereafter.
● Monitor patient for signs and symptoms of
hyperkalemia (dizziness, diarrhea, vomiting,
rapid or irregular heartbeat, lower extremity
edema, or difficulty breathing).
● *Look alike–sound alike:* Don't confuse
Inspra with Spiriva.

PATIENT TEACHING

● Teach about proper drug administration and
handling.
● Advise patient to avoid potassium supplements and salt substitutes during treatment.
● Inform male patient that drug may compromise fertility.
● Tell patient to report adverse reactions.

SAFETY ALERT!

epoetin alfa (erythropoietin)
i-POE-i-tin

Epogen, Eprex❋, Procrit

epoetin alfa-epbx
Retacrit

Therapeutic class: Colony-stimulating factors
Pharmacologic class: Recombinant human
erythropoietins

AVAILABLE FORMS

Injection (prefilled syringe): 1,000 units/
0.5 mL❋, 2,000 units/0.5 mL❋, 3,000 units/
0.3 mL❋, 4,000 units/0.4 mL❋, 5,000 units/
0.5 mL❋, 6,000 units/0.5 mL❋, 8,000 units/

Reactions in bold italics are *life-threatening*.

0.8 mL✤, 20,000 units/0.5 mL✤,
30,000 units/0.75 mL✤, 40,000 units/mL✤
Injection (single-use vial): 2,000 units/mL,
3,000 units/mL, 4,000 units/mL,
10,000 units/mL, 40,000 units/mL
Injection (multidose vial)* (Epogen, Procrit):
20,000 units/mL, 20,000 units/2 mL

INDICATIONS & DOSAGES
➤ **Anemia caused by CKD**
Adults: Dosage is individualized. For patients
on hemodialysis, start treatment only if Hb
level is less than 10 g/dL. For patients not
on hemodialysis, start treatment only if Hb
level is less than 10 g/dL, the rate of decline
of Hb level indicates that patient will require
an RBC transfusion, and reducing the risk of
alloimmunization and other RBC transfusion-
related risks is a treatment goal. Starting dose
is 50 to 100 units/kg subcut or IV three times
weekly. IV route is preferred for patients receiving hemodialysis.
 Maintenance dosage is highly individualized. Give lowest effective dose to gradually
increase Hb to a level at which blood transfusion isn't necessary.
Children ages 1 month and older: Initially,
50 units/kg IV or subcut three times weekly.
Start treatment only if Hb level is less than
10 g/dL. IV route is preferred for patients receiving hemodialysis.
 Maintenance dosage is highly individualized to keep Hb level within target range.
Give lowest effective dose to gradually increase Hb to a level at which blood transfusion isn't necessary.
Adjust-a-dose: For all patients, don't increase
dosage more frequently than every 4 weeks.
Reduce dosage by 25% or more as needed
to reduce rapid responses if Hb level rises
more than 1 g/dL in any 2-week period. Increase dosage by 25% if Hb hasn't increased
by more than 1 g/dL after 4 weeks or falls
below 10 g/dL. For adults on dialysis, if Hb
level approaches or exceeds 11 g/dL, reduce
dosage or interrupt therapy. For adults not on
dialysis, if Hb level exceeds 10 g/dL, reduce
dosage or interrupt therapy. For children, if
Hb level approaches or exceeds 12 g/dL, reduce dosage or interrupt therapy.
➤ **Anemia from zidovudine therapy
(4,200 mg/week or less) in patients infected
with HIV**
Adults: Initially, 100 units/kg IV or subcut three
times weekly until Hb level reaches target

level. Evaluate response every 4 to 8 weeks;
increase dosage in increments of 50 to
100 units/kg three times weekly, up to maximum
of 300 units/kg IV or subcut. Give lowest
effective dose to gradually increase Hb to a
level where blood transfusion isn't necessary.
Adjust-a-dose: Withhold drug if Hb level exceeds 12 g/dL. Restart drug at 25% below the
previous dosage if Hb level declines to less
than 11 g/dL. Discontinue if an increase in Hb
isn't achieved at 300 units/kg for 8 weeks.
➤ **Anemia from chemotherapy**
Adults: Start therapy if Hb level is less than
10 g/dL and a minimum of 2 additional
months of chemotherapy is planned. Initially,
150 units/kg subcut three times weekly or
40,000 units subcut weekly until completion of a chemotherapy course. If Hb level
hasn't increased by at least 1 g/dL (in the absence of RBC transfusion) and remains below
10 g/dL after initial 4 weeks of therapy, increase dosage up to 300 units/kg subcut three
times weekly or 60,000 units weekly. Give
lowest effective dose to gradually increase Hb
to a level at which blood transfusion isn't necessary. Discontinue drug after 8 weeks if no
response, as measured by Hb level, or if transfusions are still required.
Children ages 5 to 18: 600 units/kg IV once
weekly until completion of a chemotherapy course. If Hb level hasn't increased by
at least 1 g/dL (in the absence of RBC transfusion) and remains below 10 g/dL after initial 4 weeks of therapy, increase dosage to
900 units/kg IV (maximum, 60,000 units).
Discontinue drug after 8 weeks if no response, as measured by Hb level, or if transfusions are still required.
Adjust-a-dose: Withhold drug if Hb level exceeds level needed to avoid an RBC transfusion. Restart drug at dosage 25% below
previous dosage when Hb level approaches
a level at which an RBC transfusion may be
required. Reduce dosage by 25% if Hb level
increases more than 1 g/dL in a 2-week period
or reaches a level needed to avoid an RBC
transfusion.
➤ **To reduce need for allogenic blood
transfusion in patients with anemia scheduled to have elective, noncardiac, nonvas-
cular surgery**
Adults: 300 units/kg subcut daily for 10 days
before surgery, on day of surgery, and for
4 days after surgery. Or, 600 units/kg subcut in once-weekly doses (21, 14, and 7 days

before surgery), plus a fourth dose on day of surgery. DVT prophylaxis is recommended for patients undergoing surgery during epoetin therapy.

➤ **Symptomatic anemia in myelodysplastic syndromes ◆**
Adults: 150 to 300 units/kg subcut once daily; 450 to 1,000 units/kg/week in divided doses, three to seven times a week; or 60,000 units once weekly.

ADMINISTRATION

IV
▼ Store solution in refrigerator. Don't freeze.
▼ Protect from light.
▼ Don't shake.
▼ Give by direct injection without dilution.
▼ If patient is having dialysis, drug may be given into venous return line after dialysis session.
▼ Single-dose vials contain no preservatives. Discard unused portion. Don't re-enter preservative-free vials.
▼ Don't use prefilled syringes for IV use.
▼ Store unused portions of multidose vials at 36° to 46° F (2° to 8° C). Discard 21 days after initial entry.
🜚 *Alert:* Multidose vials contain benzyl alcohol, which has been associated with sometimes fatal neurologic and other complications in premature infants.
▼ **Incompatibilities:** Other IV drugs.
Subcutaneous
• Store solution in refrigerator. Don't freeze.
• Protect from light.
• Don't shake.
• Don't use if solution is discolored or has particulate matter.
• Give in upper arm, abdomen, midthigh, or outer buttocks.
• Single-use vial without preservative may be admixed in a syringe with bacteriostatic NSS for injection with benzyl alcohol 0.9% (bacteriostatic saline) at a 1:1 ratio to provide local anesthetic.
• Single-use prefilled syringes contain no preservatives. Discard any unused portion.
• Rotate injection sites and document.

ACTION

Functions as a growth factor and as a differentiating factor, enhancing RBC production.

Route	Onset	Peak	Duration
IV	Immediate	Immediate	Unknown
Subcut	Unknown	5–24 hr	Unknown

Half-life. 4 to 13 hours.

ADVERSE REACTIONS

CNS: asthenia, dizziness, depression, fatigue, headache, insomnia, paresthesia, fever, chills, *seizures.* **CV:** edema, HTN, vascular occlusion by clot of arteriovenous graft, *PE, DVT, thrombosis.* **EENT:** pharyngitis. **GI:** diarrhea, nausea, vomiting, stomatitis, dysphagia. **Hematologic:** *leukopenia.* **Metabolic:** hyperglycemia, *hypokalemia,* hyperuricemia, weight loss. **Musculoskeletal:** arthralgia, myalgia, bone pain, muscle spasm. **Respiratory:** cough, congestion, shortness of breath, URI. **Skin:** injection-site reactions, rash, urticaria, pruritus. **Other:** medical device malfunction (clotting), chills.

INTERACTIONS

Drug-drug. *Lenalidomide, pomalidomide, thalidomide:* May enhance thrombogenic effects of these drugs. Monitor therapeutic response.

EFFECTS ON LAB TEST RESULTS

• May increase BUN, creatinine, potassium, Hb, and uric acid levels.
• May decrease leukocyte count.

CONTRAINDICATIONS & CAUTIONS

• Contraindicated in patients hypersensitive to products derived from mammal cells or albumin (human) and in those with uncontrolled HTN or pure RBC aplasia that begins after treatment with epoetin.
Boxed Warning In patients with NSCLC or breast, head and neck, lymphoid, or cervical cancers, there is a risk of tumor growth or recurrence and shortened survival. Use lowest dosage needed to avoid RBC transfusions. Use only for treatment of anemia due to concomitant myelosuppressive chemotherapy and discontinue drug after chemotherapy course. Erythropoiesis-stimulating agents aren't indicated for patients receiving myelosuppressive therapy when the anticipated outcome is cure. ■
Boxed Warning Patients with CKD have an increased risk of death, serious adverse CV events, and stroke when erythropoiesis-stimulating agents are used to increase Hb level to more than 11 g/dL. Individualize

---

*Reactions in bold italics are **life-threatening**.*

therapy and use lowest dosage needed to reduce the need for RBC transfusion. ■

• Drug isn't indicated for patients scheduled for surgery who are willing to donate autologous blood, for patients undergoing cardiac or vascular surgery, or as a substitute for RBC transfusion in patients who need immediate correction of anemia.

• SCAR (erythema multiforme, SJS, and TEN) may occur with use of erythropoiesis-stimulating agents; discontinue drug if SCAR is suspected.

Dialyzable drug: Unknown.

⚠ *Overdose S&S:* Severe HTN.

PREGNANCY-LACTATION-REPRODUCTION

• Use single-dose formulations during pregnancy only if potential benefit justifies fetal risk.

• Multidose vials contain benzyl alcohol and are contraindicated during pregnancy and breastfeeding and in neonates and infants. Patients shouldn't breastfeed for at least 2 weeks after final dose containing benzyl alcohol.

• It isn't known if drug appears in human milk. Use single-dose vials cautiously during breastfeeding.

NURSING CONSIDERATIONS

• Before starting therapy, evaluate patient's iron status. Patient should receive adequate iron supplementation beginning no later than when epoetin alfa treatment starts and continuing throughout therapy. Patient also may need vitamin B_{12} and folic acid.

• Monitor BP before therapy. Most patients with CKD have HTN. BP may increase, especially when hematocrit increases in the early part of therapy.

• Institute diet restrictions or drug therapy to control BP.

• Monitor Hb level twice weekly until it stabilizes in the target range and maintenance dose is established; then continue to monitor at least monthly. Resume twice-weekly testing after any dosage adjustments.

• When used in HIV-infected adult, follow dosage recommendations for those with endogenous erythropoietin levels of 500 milliunits/mL or less and cumulative zidovudine doses of 4.2 g/week or less.

• Monitor blood counts; elevated hematocrit may cause excessive clotting. For patient with CKD, monitor Hb level weekly until stable and then at least monthly.

• Monitor patient for hypersensitivity reactions, including SCAR.

• For patient who doesn't respond adequately over a 12-week escalation period, further increasing dosage may increase risks and not improve response. Evaluate other causes of anemia and discontinue drug if responsiveness doesn't improve.

• Patient may need additional heparin to prevent clotting during dialysis treatments.

• Drug increases risk of seizures in patients with CKD. Monitor patient closely for neurologic signs and symptoms.

Boxed Warning Due to increased risk of DVT, prophylaxis is recommended perisurgery. ■

🛈 *Alert:* Evaluate patient who experiences a lack or loss of effect for pure red cell aplasia.

• *Look alike–sound alike:* Don't confuse Epogen with Neupogen.

PATIENT TEACHING

• Teach about safe drug administration, storage, and disposal.

• Inform patient that pain or discomfort in limbs (long bones) and pelvis, feelings of cold, and diaphoresis may occur after injection (usually within 2 hours). Symptoms may last for 12 hours and then disappear.

• Counsel patient on the increased risks of mortality, CV reactions, thromboembolic events, stroke, and tumor progression.

• Teach patient that routine blood tests will be needed to monitor drug effect.

• Advise patient to avoid driving and operating heavy machinery at start of therapy. A too-rapid increase in hematocrit may cause seizures.

• Tell patient to monitor BP at home and to adhere to dietary restrictions.

SAFETY ALERT!

eptifibatide
ep-tiff-IB-ah-tide

Therapeutic class: Antiplatelet drugs
Pharmacologic class: Glycoprotein IIb/IIIa inhibitors

AVAILABLE FORMS

Injection (bolus): 20 mg/10 mL (2 mg/mL) vial
Injection (premixed for infusion): 75 mg/ 100 mL (0.75 mg/mL)

INDICATIONS & DOSAGES

➤ **ACS (unstable angina or non–ST-segment-elevation MI) in patients receiving drug therapy and in those undergoing PCI**

Adults: 180 mcg/kg IV bolus as soon as possible after diagnosis, followed by continuous IV infusion at a rate of 2 mcg/kg/minute until hospital discharge or start of CABG surgery, for up to 72 hours. Give aspirin (160 to 325 mg) daily and heparin (target PTT, 50 to 70 sec) unless PCI is scheduled.

Adjust-a-dose: If CrCl is less than 50 mL/minute, give 180 mcg/kg IV bolus as soon as possible after diagnosis, followed by continuous IV infusion at 1 mcg/kg/minute.

➤ **PCI**

Adults: 180 mcg/kg IV bolus given just before the procedure, immediately followed by infusion of 2 mcg/kg/minute and second IV bolus of 180 mcg/kg given 10 minutes after first bolus. Continue infusion until hospital discharge or for 18 to 24 hours, whichever comes first. Minimum duration of infusion is 12 hours; maximum duration is 96 hours. Give aspirin 160 to 325 mg PO 1 to 24 hours before PCI and daily thereafter; give heparin to maintain ACT target of 200 to 300 seconds before PCI (but not after).

Adjust-a-dose: If CrCl is less than 50 mL/minute, give 180 mcg/kg IV bolus just before the procedure, immediately followed by continuous IV infusion at 1 mcg/kg/minute and second bolus of 180 mcg/kg given 10 minutes after first bolus.

ADMINISTRATION

IV

▼ Inspect solution for particles before use; if they appear, drug may not be sterile. Discard it.

▼ Protect drug from light before giving.

▼ May give drug in same line with NSS, D₅NSS, alteplase, atropine, dobutamine, heparin, lidocaine, meperidine, metoprolol, midazolam, morphine, nitroglycerin, or verapamil. Main infusion may also contain up to 60 mEq/L of potassium chloride.

▼ For IV push, withdraw bolus dose from 10-mL vial into a syringe and give over 1 or 2 minutes. Discard unused drug left in vial.

▼ For infusion, give undiluted drug directly from 100-mL vial or container using an infusion pump. Vials require a vented infusion set.

▼ Administer drug with heparin titrated to dosing parameters.

▼ If patient needs thrombolytics, stop infusion.

▼ Refrigerate vials at 36° to 46° F (2° to 8° C). Store vials at room temperature for no longer than 2 months; afterward, discard.

▼ **Incompatibilities:** Furosemide.

ACTION

Reversibly binds to the glycoprotein IIb/IIIa (GPIIb/IIIa) receptor on human platelets and inhibits platelet aggregation.

Route	Onset	Peak	Duration
IV	Immediate	Immediate	4–8 hr

Half-life: 2.5 hours.

ADVERSE REACTIONS

CV: hypotension. **GU:** hematuria. **Hematologic:** ***thrombocytopenia, major bleeding,*** minor bleeding. **Other:** bleeding at femoral artery access site.

INTERACTIONS

Drug-drug. *Apixaban, clopidogrel, dabigatran, dipyridamole, edoxaban, NSAIDs, oral anticoagulants (warfarin), rivaroxaban, SSRIs, thrombolytics, ticlopidine:* May increase risk of bleeding. Monitor closely for signs of bleeding.

Other inhibitors of GPIIb/IIIa: May cause serious bleeding. Avoid use together.

EFFECTS ON LAB TEST RESULTS

● May decrease platelet count.

CONTRAINDICATIONS & CAUTIONS

● Contraindicated in patients hypersensitive to drug or its components and in those with history of bleeding diathesis or evidence of active abnormal bleeding within previous 30 days; severe HTN (systolic BP higher than 200 mm Hg or diastolic BP higher than 110 mm Hg) not adequately controlled with antihypertensives; history of major surgery within previous 6 weeks; history of stroke within 30 days or any history of hemorrhagic stroke; current or planned use of another parenteral GPIIb/IIIa inhibitor; or dependency on dialysis.

● There is no clinical experience with drug use in patients with a baseline platelet count less than 100,000/mm³.

● Safety and effectiveness in children haven't been established.

Dialyzable drug: Yes.

Reactions in bold italics are ***life-threatening***.

PREGNANCY-LACTATION-REPRODUCTION
• Use during pregnancy only if clearly needed.
• It isn't known if drug appears in human milk. Use cautiously during breastfeeding.

NURSING CONSIDERATIONS
• Drug is intended for use with heparin and aspirin.
• At least 4 hours before hospital discharge, stop eptifibatide and heparin and achieve sheath hemostasis using standard compressive techniques.
• Remove sheath during infusion only after heparin has been stopped and its effects largely reversed.
• Stop infusion at least 4 hours before CABG surgery.
• Minimize use of arterial and venous punctures, IM injections, urinary catheters, and nasotracheal and NG tubes.
• When obtaining IV access, avoid use of noncompressible sites (such as subclavian or jugular vein).
• Monitor patient for bleeding.
• **Alert:** If platelet count falls below 100,000/mm^3, stop eptifibatide and heparin. Monitor patient closely.
• Obtain baseline lab tests (including Hb level, hematocrit, PT, INR, PTT, platelet count, and creatinine level) before start of drug therapy.
• Obtain platelet count 2 to 4 hours after initiation and at 24 hours or before discharge, whichever comes first.

PATIENT TEACHING
• Advise patient to inform health care provider of all drugs and supplements being taken.
• Counsel patient that benefits of drug outweigh risk of serious bleeding.
• Tell patient to immediately report chest discomfort or other adverse effects to prescriber.
• Instruct patient to report unusual bleeding, bruising, or blood in stools.

---

erenumab-aooe
e-REN-ue-mab

Aimovig

Therapeutic class: Antimigraine drugs
Pharmacologic class: Monoclonal antibodies

AVAILABLE FORMS
Injection: 70 mg/mL, 140 mg/mL prefilled autoinjectors or syringes

INDICATIONS & DOSAGES
➤ **Migraine prevention**
Adults: 70 mg subcut once monthly. If ineffective, 140 mg subcut once monthly.

ADMINISTRATION
Subcutaneous
• **Alert:** The needle shield of the autoinjector and the needle cap of the syringe may contain dry natural rubber (a derivative of latex), which can cause allergic reactions in patients sensitive to latex. Manufacturer is transitioning to nonlatex product. Check package label.
• Before administration, allow product to sit at room temperature for at least 30 minutes protected from direct sunlight. Don't warm by using a heat source, such as hot water or microwave.
• Don't shake product.
• Visually inspect solution for discoloration or particulate matter. Don't use if solution is cloudy, discolored, or contains flakes or particles.
• Products are for single use; give entire contents.
• Administer subcut in abdomen, thigh, or upper arm. Don't inject into areas where skin is tender, bruised, red, or hard.
• Give missed dose as soon as possible; then schedule monthly from date of the last dose.
• Store product refrigerated at 36° to 46° F (2° to 8° C) in original carton to protect it from light until time of use. Don't freeze.
• If removed from the refrigerator, store at room temperature (up to 77° F [25° C]) in original carton and use within 7 days. Don't return product to refrigerator after it has been warmed. Discard product if left at room temperature for more than 7 days.

ACTION
Human monoclonal antibody that binds to the calcitonin gene-related peptide (CGRP) receptor and antagonizes CGRP receptor function.

Route	Onset	Peak	Duration
Subcut	Unknown	6 days	Unknown

Half-life: 28 days.

ADVERSE REACTIONS

CV: HTN. **GI:** constipation. **Musculoskeletal:** muscle spasms, cramps. **Skin:** injection-site reaction (pain, erythema, pruritus). **Other:** antibody development.

INTERACTIONS

None reported.

EFFECTS ON LAB TEST RESULTS

None reported.

CONTRAINDICATIONS & CAUTIONS

• Hypersensitivity reactions (rash, angioedema, anaphylaxis) have been reported; discontinue use if serious reaction occurs.
• Safety and effectiveness in children haven't been established.
• Use cautiously in patients ages 65 and older.
Dialyzable drug: Unknown.

PREGNANCY-LACTATION-REPRODUCTION

• Studies during pregnancy are lacking. Data suggest that patients with migraines may be at increased risk for preeclampsia and gestational hypertension during pregnancy.
• It isn't known if drug appears in human milk or how drug affects an infant who is breastfed. Before use during breastfeeding, consider patient's need for the drug and potential adverse effects on the infant.

NURSING CONSIDERATIONS

• Monitor patient for injection-site and other adverse reactions.
• Monitor BP.

PATIENT TEACHING

🜚 *Alert:* Warn patient who is latex-sensitive about risk of allergic reaction. Instruct patient to check packaging to determine if latex is present.
• Teach about proper drug administration, storage, and handling as well as safe syringe disposal.
• Advise patient to report injection-site reactions, allergic reactions, or other adverse effects.
• Caution patient that development of HTN and worsening of preexisting HTN can occur. Instruct patient to contact prescriber if BP is elevated.
• Warn patient not to use an autoinjector or syringe that has been dropped on a hard surface as it may have broken, even if no damage is visible. Tell patient to use a new autoinjector

or syringe and to call 1-800-77-AMGEN (1-800-772-6436).

SAFETY ALERT!

erlotinib ☒
er-LOE-tye-nib

Tarceva

Therapeutic class: Antineoplastics
Pharmacologic class: Epidermal growth factor receptor inhibitors

AVAILABLE FORMS

Tablets ⓄⓃⒸ: 25 mg, 100 mg, 150 mg

INDICATIONS & DOSAGES

Adjust-a-dose (for all indications): Refer to manufacturer's instructions for toxicity-related dosage adjustments.
➤ **With gemcitabine, first-line treatment of locally advanced, unresectable, or metastatic pancreatic cancer**
Adults: 100 mg PO once daily on an empty stomach. Continue until disease progresses or intolerable toxicity occurs.
➤ **Metastatic NSCLC in patients with tumors with epidermal growth factor receptor (*EGFR*) exon 19 deletions or exon 21 (L858R) substitution mutations receiving first-line, maintenance, or second-line or greater treatment after progression following at least one prior chemotherapy regimen** ☒
Adults: 150 mg PO once daily on an empty stomach. Continue until disease progresses or intolerable toxicity occurs.

ADMINISTRATION
PO

🜚 *Alert:* Hazardous drug; use safe handling and disposal precautions.
• Give drug on an empty stomach 1 hour before or 2 hours after a meal.
• For patients unable to swallow tablets whole, tablets may be dissolved in 100 mL of water and given orally or via feeding tube (silicone-based). To ensure patients receive full dose, rinse container with 40 mL water, administer residue, and repeat rinse.
• Store tablets and suspension at room temperature. Suspension remains stable for at least 28 days.

Reactions in bold italics are ***life-threatening***.

ACTION
Inhibits tyrosine kinase activity in EGFRs, which are expressed on the surface of normal and cancer cells.

Route	Onset	Peak	Duration
PO	Unknown	4 hr	Unknown

Half-life: 36.2 hours.

ADVERSE REACTIONS
CNS: fatigue, syncope, *stroke*, anxiety, depression, dizziness, headache, insomnia, fever. **CV:** chest pain, *arrhythmias,* edema, *MI, DVT.* **EENT:** conjunctivitis, keratoconjunctivitis sicca, decreased tear production, abnormal eyelash growth. **GI:** anorexia, diarrhea, nausea, stomatitis, vomiting, constipation, *pancreatitis.* **GU:** kidney insufficiency. **Hematologic:** anemia, *thrombocytopenia, leukopenia, lymphocytopenia.* **Hepatic:** increased ALT level, hyperbilirubinemia. **Metabolic:** weight loss. **Musculoskeletal:** pain, weakness, back pain, arthralgia, myalgia. **Respiratory:** cough, dyspnea. **Skin:** dry skin, pruritus, rash, paronychia. **Other:** infection, mucosal inflammation.

INTERACTIONS
Drug-drug. *Antacids:* May reduce bioavailability of drug. Separate doses by several hours if an antacid is necessary.
Ciprofloxacin: May increase erlotinib level. Consider reducing erlotinib dosage if severe adverse reactions occur; avoid use together if possible.
CYP3A4 inducers (carbamazepine, phenobarbital, phenytoin, rifabutin, rifampin): May increase erlotinib metabolism. Avoid use if possible or increase erlotinib dosage by 50-mg increments at 2-week intervals to a maximum of 450 mg, as tolerated.
H₂-receptor antagonists (cimetidine, famotidine): May reduce bioavailability of drug. Give erlotinib 10 hours after and at least 2 hours before H₂-antagonist dosing.
PPIs (esomeprazole, omeprazole): May reduce bioavailability of drug. Dose separation may not eliminate interaction; avoid use together if possible.
Strong CYP3A4 inhibitors (atazanavir, clarithromycin, ketoconazole, nefazodone, nelfinavir, ritonavir, saquinavir): May decrease erlotinib metabolism. Avoid use together if possible or reduce erlotinib dosage by 50-mg decrements.

Warfarin: May increase risk of bleeding. Monitor PT and INR.
Drug-herb. *St. John's wort:* May increase drug metabolism. Drug dosage may need to be increased. Discourage use together.
Drug-food. *Any food:* May increase bioavailability of drug. Give drug 1 hour before or 2 hours after meals.
Grapefruit or grapefruit juice: May increase drug level. Avoid use together.
Drug-lifestyle. *Cigarette smoking:* May decrease drug level. Increase drug dosage by 50-mg increments at 2-week intervals to a maximum of 300 mg. Immediately reduce dosage to recommended dose (100 or 150 mg daily) upon smoking cessation.
Sun exposure: May cause photosensitivity reactions. Patient should use alcohol-free emollient cream and sunscreen and avoid sun exposure.

EFFECTS ON LAB TEST RESULTS
- May increase ALT, AST, bilirubin, BUN, and creatinine levels.
- May decrease Hb level and platelet and WBC counts.
- May increase INR and prolong PT.

CONTRAINDICATIONS & CAUTIONS
- Use cautiously in patients with pulmonary disease or liver impairment.
- Use cautiously in patients who have received or are receiving chemotherapy; drug may worsen adverse pulmonary effects.
- Use cautiously in patients receiving other antiangiogenic agents, corticosteroids, NSAIDs, or taxane-based chemotherapy and in those with history of peptic ulcer disease because of increased risk of GI perforation.
- Interrupt therapy or discontinue drug in patients with liver impairment or dehydration, which increases risk of kidney failure.
- SCARs (SJS, TEN, exfoliative dermatitis) can occur.
- Safety and effectiveness in children haven't been established.
Dialyzable drug: Unknown.
⚠ *Overdose S&S:* Severe adverse reactions (diarrhea, ALT or AST elevation, rash).

PREGNANCY-LACTATION-REPRODUCTION
- Drug may cause fetal harm. If used during pregnancy or if patient becomes pregnant during therapy, inform patient of fetal risk.

• Patients of childbearing potential should use effective contraception during therapy and for 1 month after final dose.
• It isn't known if drug appears in human milk. Patients shouldn't breastfeed during treatment and for 2 weeks after final dose.

NURSING CONSIDERATIONS
• Periodically monitor kidney function test and LFT values during therapy.
⚠️ *Alert:* GI perforation with fatalities has been reported. Permanently discontinue drug if GI perforation occurs.
⚠️ *Alert:* Rarely, serious ILD may occur. If patient develops dyspnea, cough, and fever, notify prescriber. Therapy may need to be interrupted or stopped.
• Monitor patient for severe diarrhea; give loperamide, if needed.
• Monitor patient for eye ulcers, bullous blistering, and exfoliative skin conditions.

PATIENT TEACHING
⚠️ *Alert:* Tell patient to immediately report new or worsened cough, shortness of breath, eye irritation or pain, or severe or persistent diarrhea, nausea, anorexia, or vomiting.
• Teach about proper drug administration and handling.
• Explain the likelihood of serious interactions with other drugs and herbal supplements and the need to tell prescriber about any change in drugs and supplements.
• Counsel patient about smoking cessation; smoking may decrease drug level and effectiveness.
• Advise patient to notify prescriber of suspected or current pregnancy or plans to breastfeed.

---

ertapenem sodium
er-tah-PEN-em

INVanz

Therapeutic class: Antibiotics
Pharmacologic class: Carbapenems

AVAILABLE FORMS
Injection: 1 g

INDICATIONS & DOSAGES
Adjust-a-dose (for all indications): In adults with CrCl of 30 mL/minute/1.73 m^2 or less,

give 500 mg/day. In patients on hemodialysis receiving daily 500-mg dose less than 6 hours before hemodialysis, give supplementary 150-mg dose afterward. In patients on hemodialysis receiving dose 6 hours or more before hemodialysis, no supplementary dose is needed.
➤ **Complicated intra-abdominal infection caused by** *Escherichia coli, Clostridium clostridioforme, Eubacterium lentum, Peptostreptococcus* **species,** *Bacteroides fragilis, Bacteroides distasonis, Bacteroides ovatus, Bacteroides thetaiotaomicron,* **or** *Bacteroides uniformis*
Adults and children ages 13 and older: 1 g IV or IM once daily for 5 to 14 days.
Infants and children ages 3 months to 12 years: 15 mg/kg IV or IM every 12 hours for 5 to 14 days. Maximum, 1 g daily.
➤ **Complicated skin or skin-structure infection, including diabetic foot infections without osteomyelitis, caused by** *Staphylococcus aureus* **(methicillin-susceptible strains),** *Streptococcus agalactiae, Streptococcus pyogenes, E. coli, Klebsiella pneumoniae, Proteus mirabilis, B. fragilis, Peptostreptococcus* **species,** *Porphyromonas asaccharolytica,* **or** *Prevotella bivia*
Adults and children ages 13 and older: 1 g IV or IM once daily for 7 to 14 days. Diabetic foot infections may need up to 28 days of treatment, which may include switching to oral therapy.
Infants and children ages 3 months to 12 years: 15 mg/kg IV or IM every 12 hours for 7 to 14 days. Maximum, 1 g daily.
➤ **Community-acquired pneumonia from** *S. pneumoniae* **(penicillin-susceptible strains),** *Haemophilus influenzae* **(beta-lactamase-negative strains), or** *Moraxella catarrhalis;* **complicated UTI, including pyelonephritis caused by** *E. coli* **or** *K. pneumoniae*
Adults and children ages 13 and older: 1 g IV or IM once daily for 10 to 14 days. If patient improves after at least 3 days of treatment, use appropriate oral therapy to complete the full course of therapy.
Infants and children ages 3 months to 12 years: 15 mg/kg IV or IM every 12 hours for 10 to 14 days. Maximum, 1 g daily. If patient improves after at least 3 days of treatment, use appropriate oral therapy to complete the full course of therapy.

Reactions in bold italics are *life-threatening*.

➤ **Acute pelvic infection, including post-partum endomyometritis, septic abortion, and postsurgical gynecologic infection caused by** *S. agalactiae, E. coli, B. fragilis, P. asaccharolytica, Peptostreptococcus* **species, or** *P. bivia*
Adults and children ages 13 and older: 1 g IV or IM once daily for 3 to 10 days.
Infants and children ages 3 months to 12 years: 15 mg/kg IV or IM every 12 hours for 3 to 10 days. Maximum, 1 g daily.
➤ **Prevention of surgical site infection after elective colorectal surgery**
Adults: 1 g IV 1 hour before surgical incision.

ADMINISTRATION

• Obtain specimens for culture and sensitivity testing before giving. Begin therapy while awaiting results.
• Before giving first dose, check for previous hypersensitivity to penicillin, cephalosporin, beta-lactam, or local amide-type anesthetics.
IV
▼ May give IV infusions for up to 14 days.
▼ Reconstitute 1-g vial with 10 mL of sterile water for injection, NSS for injection, or bacteriostatic water for injection.
▼ Shake well to dissolve; then immediately transfer contents to 50 mL of NSS.
▼ For children ages 3 months to 12 years, immediately withdraw a volume equal to 15 mg/kg (not to exceed 1 g/day); dilute in NSS to a final concentration of 20 mg/mL or less.
▼ Infuse over 30 minutes.
▼ Complete the infusion within 6 hours of reconstitution or refrigerate for up to 24 hours. Infuse within 4 hours once removed from refrigeration. Don't freeze.
▼ **Incompatibilities:** Diluents containing dextrose, other IV drugs.
IM
• May give IM injections for up to 7 days.
• Reconstitute 1-g vial with 3.2 mL of 1% lidocaine hydrochloride injection (without epinephrine). Shake vial thoroughly to form solution. Immediately withdraw volume equal to 15 mg/kg of body weight (not to exceed 1 g/day) and give by deep IM injection into a large muscle, such as the gluteal muscles or lateral part of the thigh. Use the reconstituted IM solution within 1 hour after preparation. Don't give reconstituted solution IV.

ACTION

Inhibits cell-wall synthesis through binding to penicillin-binding proteins.

Route	Onset	Peak	Duration
IV	Immediate	30 min	24 hr
IM	Unknown	2.3 hr	24 hr

Half-life: 4 hours.

ADVERSE REACTIONS

CNS: altered mental status, anxiety, dizziness, fatigue, fever, headache, insomnia. **CV:** edema, HTN, hypotension, phlebitis, tachycardia, thrombophlebitis. **EENT:** pharyngitis, oral candidiasis. **GI:** diarrhea, abdominal pain, constipation, nausea, vomiting. **GU:** kidney dysfunction, vaginitis. **Hematologic:** *leukopenia, neutropenia, thrombocytopenia,* anemia, coagulation abnormalities, eosinophilia, *thrombocytosis.* **Hepatic:** jaundice, increased transaminase levels, increased ALP level. **Metabolic:** *hyperkalemia, hypokalemia,* hyperglycemia. **Musculoskeletal:** leg pain. **Respiratory:** cough, dyspnea, URI, crackles, *respiratory distress,* rhonchi. **Skin:** erythema, extravasation, infusion-site pain and redness, pruritus, rash, diaper dermatitis. **Other:** hypersensitivity reactions, infused vein complications, *death.*

INTERACTIONS

Drug-drug. *Probenecid:* May reduce kidney clearance; may increase half-life. Use together isn't recommended.
Valproic acid: May decrease valproic acid level, leading to loss of seizure control. Monitor valproic acid level, and observe patient for signs of seizure activity. Use together isn't recommended.

EFFECTS ON LAB TEST RESULTS

• May increase albumin, ALT, ALP, AST, bilirubin, creatinine, glucose, and potassium levels.
• May increase eosinophil count, urine RBC count, or urine WBC count.
• May decrease Hb level and hematocrit.
• May decrease segmented neutrophil and serum WBC counts.
• May increase or decrease platelet count.
• May prolong PT.

CONTRAINDICATIONS & CAUTIONS

• Contraindicated in patients hypersensitive to components of the drug or to other drugs in

the same class and in patients who have had anaphylactic reactions to beta-lactams.
• IM use is contraindicated in patients hypersensitive to local anesthetics of amide type because of use of lidocaine as diluent.
• Drug may cause CDAD, ranging in severity from mild to fatal colitis, which can occur during treatment or 2 months or more after treatment. Drug may need to be discontinued for suspected CDAD.
• Use cautiously in patients with CNS disorders and compromised kidney function, as CNS reactions (including seizures) may occur in these patients.
• Use cautiously in older adults.
Dialyzable drug: Yes.
⚠ *Overdose S&S:* Nausea, diarrhea, dizziness.

PREGNANCY-LACTATION-REPRODUCTION
• Studies during pregnancy are inadequate. Use during pregnancy only if clearly needed.
• Drug appears in human milk. Use cautiously during breastfeeding.

NURSING CONSIDERATIONS
• If patient has diarrhea during therapy, notify prescriber and collect stool specimen for culture to rule out CDAD.
• Vomiting occurs more frequently in children than adults. Monitor child closely for signs and symptoms of dehydration and electrolyte imbalances.
• If allergic reaction occurs, stop drug immediately.
• Anaphylactic reactions require immediate emergency treatment with epinephrine, oxygen, IV steroids, and airway management.
• Anticonvulsants may continue in patient with seizure disorder. If focal tremors, myoclonus, or seizures occur, notify prescriber. Dosage may need to be decreased or drug stopped.
• Monitor kidney, liver, and hematopoietic function during prolonged therapy.
• MRSA and *Enterococcus* species are resistant to drug.

PATIENT TEACHING
• Tell patient to report all adverse reactions.
• Instruct patient to report discomfort at injection site.
• Advise patient to report diarrhea as soon as possible.

• Inform patient that CDAD can occur 2 months or more after last dose of an antibiotic. Instruct patient to immediately report watery or bloody stools.

SAFETY ALERT!

ertugliflozin
er-too-gli-FLOE-zin

Steglatro

Therapeutic class: Antidiabetics
Pharmacologic class: Sodium-glucose cotransporter 2 inhibitors

AVAILABLE FORMS
Tablets: 5 mg, 15 mg

INDICATIONS & DOSAGES
➤ **Adjunct to diet and exercise to improve glycemic control in patients with type 2 diabetes**
Adults: 5 mg PO once daily in the morning. May increase to 15 mg once daily.

ADMINISTRATION
PO
• Give drug with or without food.
• Give a missed dose as soon as possible. If it's almost time for the next dose, skip the missed dose and give at the next regularly scheduled time. Don't give two doses at the same time.
• Store in a dry place at room temperature.

ACTION
Increases excretion of urinary glucose by inhibiting sodium-glucose cotransporter 2 (SGLT2), which reabsorbs glucose through the kidneys.

Route	Onset	Peak	Duration
PO	Unknown	1–2 hr	Unknown

Half-life: 16.6 hours.

ADVERSE REACTIONS
CNS: headache. **EENT:** nasopharyngitis. **GI:** thirst. **GU:** genital fungal infections, UTI, vaginal pruritus, increased urination, kidney impairment. **Metabolic:** volume depletion, weight loss, hyperphosphatemia, increased LDL-C level, *hypoglycemia.* **Musculoskeletal:** back pain.

INTERACTIONS
Drug-drug. *ACE inhibitors (enalapril, lisinopril), ARBs (candesartan, losartan, valsartan), diuretics, NSAIDs:* May increase risk of AKI. Monitor patient closely and use together cautiously.
Insulin, insulin secretagogues (glipizide, repaglinide): May increase risk of hypoglycemia. Consider lower dosage of insulin or insulin secretagogue.
Lithium: May decrease lithium level. Monitor lithium level more frequently during ertugliflozin initiation and dose changes.

EFFECTS ON LAB TEST RESULTS
● May increase serum creatinine, LDL-C, phosphate, and Hb levels.
● Causes false-positive urine glucose tests. Use alternative methods to monitor glycemic control.
● May cause unreliable 1,5-AG assay results. Use alternative methods to monitor glycemic control.

CONTRAINDICATIONS & CAUTIONS
● Contraindicated in patients hypersensitive to drug or its components and in patients on dialysis.
● Drug isn't indicated in patients with type 1 diabetes or for the treatment of ketoacidosis.
● Use in patients with Child-Pugh class C liver impairment isn't recommended.
● Use cautiously in patients with an eGFR less than 60 mL/minute/1.73 m^2, in patients with low systolic BP, and in patients on diuretics because these patients are at increased risk for hypotension due to drug's intravascular volume contraction effect.
● Drug isn't recommended in patients with eGFR less than 45 mL/minute/1.73 m^2. Drug hasn't shown improved glycemic control in patients whose eGFR is persistently 30 to 60 mL/minute/1.73 m^2.
● Use cautiously in patients with pancreatic insulin deficiency, individuals on calorie restrictions, and patients with history of alcohol abuse, as ketoacidosis is more likely to occur in these individuals.
● Consider temporarily discontinuing drug for at least 4 days before scheduled surgery to reduce risk of ketoacidosis.
● Use cautiously in patients with hypovolemia, CKD, or HF, as kidney impairment and AKI can occur.

● Drug may increase risk of serious UTIs, including urosepsis and pyelonephritis.
● Use cautiously in patients with history of amputation, peripheral vascular disease, neuropathy, or diabetic foot ulcers. Studies show an increased risk of lower limb amputation with another SGLT2 inhibitor.
● Safety and effectiveness in children haven't been established.
● Use cautiously in older adults, who may be at greater risk for hypovolemia and hypotension.
⚠ Alert: SGLT2 inhibitors increase risk of rare but serious necrotizing fasciitis of perineum (Fournier gangrene). If Fournier gangrene is suspected, immediately discontinue SGLT2 inhibitor and begin broad-spectrum antibiotics. Surgical debridement may be necessary. Monitor blood glucose level and start alternative therapy for glycemic control.
Dialyzable drug: Unknown.

PREGNANCY-LACTATION-REPRODUCTION
● Drug may cause adverse kidney effects. Use isn't recommended during second and third trimesters.
● There are no data regarding the presence of drug in human milk, effects on breastfed infant, or effects on milk production. Because of the potential for serious adverse reactions in breastfed infants, patients shouldn't breastfeed during therapy.

NURSING CONSIDERATIONS
● Correct fluid volume depletion before starting drug, if clinically indicated.
● Monitor for signs and symptoms of hypovolemia (dehydration, dizziness, orthostatic hypotension, presyncope, syncope, hypotension, AKI).
● Monitor for signs and symptoms of AKI. Assess kidney function at baseline and periodically throughout therapy.
● Monitor for signs and symptoms of UTI. Treat promptly, if indicated.
● Monitor for signs and symptoms of genital mycotic infection, especially if patient is uncircumcised male or has history of genital mycotic infection. Treat promptly.
⚠ Alert: Watch for and immediately report signs and symptoms of necrotizing fasciitis of perineum (temperature above 100.4° F [38° C], general feeling of unwellness, and tenderness, redness, or swelling of area from genitals to rectum). Signs and symptoms can worsen quickly. Immediately discontinue

drug and prepare to administer broad-spectrum antibiotics.

• Monitor blood glucose level. Assess for signs and symptoms of hypoglycemia.

• Monitor for signs and symptoms of ketoacidosis (dehydration, severe metabolic acidosis, nausea, vomiting, abdominal pain, generalized malaise, shortness of breath), even if glucose level is less than 250 mg/dL. Discontinue drug for suspected ketoacidosis and treat appropriately.

• Consider temporarily discontinuing therapy in patient with reduced oral intake (such as in acute illness or prolonged fasting for surgery) or fluid losses (such as from GI illness or excessive heat exposure) because kidney impairment and AKI can occur.

• Drug may increase LDL-C level. Assess periodically and treat if clinically indicated.

• Monitor for signs and symptoms of infection, new pain or tenderness, and sores or ulcers of lower limbs. Treat as indicated; discontinue drug if these complications occur.

• *Look alike–sound alike:* Don't confuse ertugliflozin with canagliflozin, dapagliflozin, or empagliflozin. Don't confuse Steglatro with Segluromet or Steglujan.

PATIENT TEACHING

• Teach about proper drug administration and handling.

• Stress importance of adherence to dietary instructions, regular physical activity, periodic blood glucose monitoring, and HbA$_{1c}$ testing.

• Advise patient to report all adverse reactions.

• Teach patient how to recognize and manage hypoglycemia, hyperglycemia, and other diabetic complications.

• Advise patient to promptly seek medical advice during periods of stress, such as fever, trauma, infection, or surgery, because drug requirements may change.

• Caution patient to avoid dehydration, which can cause hypotension. Tell patient to maintain adequate fluid intake and to report signs and symptoms of hypotension.

• Instruct patient to immediately stop drug and seek medical attention if signs and symptoms of ketoacidosis occur.

• Explain that AKI has been reported, and instruct patient to immediately report reduced oral intake (due to acute illness or fasting) or increased fluid losses (due to vomiting, diarrhea, or excessive heat exposure) because

ertugliflozin may need to be temporarily discontinued.

• Advise patient that lab monitoring of kidney function is necessary.

• Teach about signs and symptoms of UTIs (changes in urination, frequent urination, burning with urination). Instruct patient to seek medical attention if they occur.

• Inform patient of increased risk of amputation. Review the importance of routine preventive foot care.

• Instruct patient to watch for and immediately report new pain or tenderness, sores or ulcers, or infections involving the leg or foot.

• Teach patient to recognize and report signs and symptoms of genital yeast infections (redness or rash of glans or foreskin of penis or vulva, burning with urination, discharge).

⚠ *Alert:* Teach patient signs and symptoms of necrotizing fasciitis, and instruct patient to seek immediate medical attention if any of these signs and symptoms occur.

• Advise patient of fetal risk. Instruct patient to immediately report pregnancy or plans to become pregnant.

• Caution patient not to breastfeed during therapy.

• Inform patient that urine will test positive for glucose during therapy.

SAFETY ALERT!

ertugliflozin–metformin hydrochloride
er-too-gli-FLOE-zin/met-FORE-min

Segluromet

Therapeutic class: Antidiabetics
Pharmacologic class: Sodium-glucose cotransporter 2 inhibitors–biguanides

AVAILABLE FORMS
Tablets: 2.5 mg ertugliflozin/500 mg metformin hydrochloride; 2.5 mg ertugliflozin/1,000 mg metformin hydrochloride; 7.5 mg ertugliflozin/500 mg metformin hydrochloride; 7.5 mg ertugliflozin/1,000 mg metformin hydrochloride

INDICATIONS & DOSAGES
➤ **Adjunct to diet and exercise to improve glycemic control in patients with type 2 diabetes**

Adults: In patients taking metformin, switch to tablets containing 2.5 mg ertugliflozin with a similar total daily dose of current metformin regimen and give PO in divided doses b.i.d. In patients taking ertugliflozin, switch to tablets containing 500 mg metformin with a similar total daily dose of current ertugliflozin regimen and give PO in divided doses b.i.d. In patients taking ertugliflozin and metformin, switch to tablets containing the same total daily dose of current ertugliflozin regimen and a similar daily dose of current metformin regimen and give PO in divided doses b.i.d. Gradually escalate dose based on effectiveness and tolerability to a maximum daily dose of 15 mg ertugliflozin and 2,000 mg metformin.

ADMINISTRATION
PO
- Give drug with meals.
- Give missed dose as soon as possible. If it's almost time for the next dose, skip the missed dose and give drug at the next regularly scheduled time. Don't give two doses at the same time.
- Store at controlled room temperature (68° to 77° F [20° to 25° C]).
- Protect from moisture; store in a dry place.

ACTION
Ertugliflozin increases excretion of urinary glucose by inhibiting sodium-glucose cotransporter 2 (SGLT2), which reabsorbs glucose through the kidneys. Metformin decreases liver glucose production and intestinal absorption of glucose and improves insulin sensitivity by increasing peripheral glucose uptake and utilization.

Route	Onset	Peak	Duration
PO (ertugliflozin)	Unknown	1–2 hr	Unknown
PO (metformin hydrochloride)	Unknown	2–3 hr	Unknown

Half-life: Ertugliflozin, 16.6 hours; metformin hydrochloride, 6.2 hours.

ADVERSE REACTIONS
CNS: headache, asthenia. **CV:** hypotension. **EENT:** nasopharyngitis. **GI:** diarrhea, nausea, vomiting, flatulence, abdominal discomfort, indigestion. **GU:** genital fungal infections, UTI, vaginal pruritus, increased urination, kidney impairment. **Metabolic:** volume depletion, weight loss, increased LDL-C level, decreased vitamin B_{12} level,

hyperphosphatemia, *hypoglycemia, lactic acidosis.* **Musculoskeletal:** back pain.

INTERACTIONS
Drug-drug. *Calcium channel blockers, corticosteroids, estrogens, isoniazid, nicotinic acid, oral contraceptives, phenothiazines, phenytoin, sympathomimetics, thiazides and other diuretics, thyroid products:* May increase risk of hyperglycemia and lead to loss of glycemic control. Closely monitor glycemic control.
Carbonic anhydrase inhibitors (acetazolamide, dichlorphenamide, topiramate, zonisamide): May increase risk of lactic acidosis. Consider more-frequent monitoring of patient.
Drugs that reduce metformin clearance (cimetidine, dolutegravir, ranolazine, vandetanib): May increase systemic exposure to metformin and risk of lactic acidosis. Consider benefits and risks of concomitant use.
Insulin, insulin secretagogues (sulfonylureas): May increase risk of hypoglycemia. Lower insulin or insulin secretagogue dosages may be needed.
Lithium: Ertugliflozin may decrease lithium level. Monitor lithium level closely during ertugliflozin initiation and dosage changes.
Radiologic contrast dye: May cause acute decrease in kidney function and increase risk of lactic acidosis. Stop drug at time of, or before, iodinated contrast imaging procedure in patients with eGFR of less than 60 mL/minute/1.73 m^2. Reevaluate eGFR 48 hours after imaging procedure. May restart drug if kidney function stabilizes.
Drug-lifestyle. *Alcohol use (excessive):* May increase risk of lactic acidosis. Discourage use together.

EFFECTS ON LAB TEST RESULTS
- May increase serum creatinine, LDL-C, phosphate, and Hb levels.
- May decrease vitamin B_{12} level and eGFR.
- May cause unreliable 1,5-AG assay results and false-positive urine glucose test results.

CONTRAINDICATIONS & CAUTIONS
Boxed Warning Metformin-containing drugs increase the risk of lactic acidosis and can result in hypothermia, hypotension, resistant bradyarrhythmias, and death. For suspected metformin-associated lactic acidosis, immediately discontinue drug. Prompt hemodialysis is recommended. ■

Boxed Warning Risk factors for metformin-associated lactic acidosis include kidney impairment, use of certain drugs, age 65 or older, radiologic study with contrast, surgery or other procedures, and hypoxic states (HF, MI, sepsis, shock). ■

Boxed Warning Patients with liver impairment are at increased risk for developing metformin-associated lactic acidosis. Avoid use in these patients. ■

• Contraindicated in patients hypersensitive to ertugliflozin, metformin, product components.

• Contraindicated in patients with eGFR less than 30 mL/minute/1.73 m^2 and those on dialysis. Use isn't recommended in patients with eGFR less than 45 mL/minute/1.73 m^2.

• Contraindicated in patients with acute or chronic metabolic acidosis, including diabetic ketoacidosis, with or without coma.

• Consider temporarily discontinuing drug for at least 4 days before scheduled surgery to reduce risk of ketoacidosis.

• Drug isn't indicated for treatment of type 1 diabetes or diabetic ketoacidosis.

• Use cautiously in patients with eGFR of less than 60 mL/minute/1.73 m^2, in patients ages 65 and older, in patients with low systolic BP, and in patients on diuretics, as intravascular volume contraction and hypotension can occur.

• Use cautiously in patients with pancreatic insulin deficiency, patients with calorie restrictions, and patients with a history of excessive alcohol intake, as ketoacidosis is more likely to occur.

• Use cautiously in patients with HF or hypovolemia and in those receiving concomitant diuretic, ACE inhibitor, ARB, or NSAID therapy, as kidney impairment and AKI can occur.

• Use cautiously in patients with history of amputation, peripheral vascular disease, neuropathy, or diabetic foot ulcers, as increased risk of lower limb amputation (primarily of toe) was observed in clinical studies with another SGLT2 inhibitor.

• Use cautiously in patients with history of genital mycotic infection and in patients who aren't circumcised, as they are more likely to develop genital mycotic infections.

❸ *Alert:* SGLT2 inhibitors increase risk of rare but serious necrotizing fasciitis of perineum (Fournier gangrene).

• Use cautiously in patients with inadequate vitamin B$_{12}$ or calcium intake or absorption. Drug may decrease vitamin B$_{12}$ level.

• Safety and effectiveness in children haven't been established.

Dialyzable drug: Ertugliflozin, unknown; metformin hydrochloride, yes.

⚠ *Overdose S&S:* Hypoglycemia, lactic acidosis.

PREGNANCY-LACTATION-REPRODUCTION

• Drug isn't recommended during the second and third trimesters; animal studies suggest increased risk of adverse kidney effects from ertugliflozin.

• It isn't known if ertugliflozin appears in human milk or how drug affects milk production or infant who is breastfed. Metformin is present in human milk. Because of the potential for serious adverse reactions in infants, patients shouldn't breastfeed.

• Metformin may cause ovulation in some patients who are premenopausal and anovulatory. Advise patients of the potential for unintended pregnancy.

NURSING CONSIDERATIONS

• Correct volume depletion before start of treatment. Monitor for signs and symptoms of hypovolemia (hypotension, dizziness, syncope, thirst) after initiating therapy.

• Monitor patient for signs and symptoms of AKI, and assess kidney function, including eGFR, at baseline and periodically throughout therapy. If AKI occurs, discontinue drug and begin treatment.

• Monitor patient for signs and symptoms of genital mycotic infections; treat promptly if indicated.

❸ *Alert:* Watch for and immediately report signs and symptoms of necrotizing fasciitis of perineum (temperature above 100.4° F [38° C], general feeling of unwellness, and tenderness, redness, or swelling of area from genitals to rectum). Signs and symptoms can worsen quickly. Immediately discontinue drug and prepare to administer broad-spectrum antibiotics. Surgical debridement may be necessary. Monitor blood glucose level and start alternative therapy for glycemic control.

• Monitor blood glucose level. Assess for signs and symptoms of hypoglycemia.

• Drug may increase LDL-C level. Assess periodically and treat if clinically indicated.

Reactions in bold italics are *life-threatening*.

• Monitor vitamin B_{12} level every 2 to 3 years in patient at high risk; monitor hematologic parameters annually in all patients to assess for anemia.

• Monitor for signs and symptoms of infection, osteomyelitis, new pain, and lower limb ulcers. Discontinue drug if these occur.

• Monitor patient for peripheral vascular disease, neuropathy, and diabetic foot ulcers. Treat as indicated.

• Monitor for signs and symptoms of UTI. Treat promptly.

Boxed Warning Monitor for signs and symptoms of metformin-associated lactic acidosis (hypothermia, hypotension, resistant bradyarrhythmias), including subtle, non-specific signs and symptoms and lab abnormalities (elevated blood lactate levels, anion gap acidosis, increased lactate/pyruvate ratios, metformin level greater than 5 mcg/mL). Treat suspected lactic acidosis as clinically indicated and immediately discontinue drug. Hemodialysis may reverse symptoms and lead to recovery. ∎

• Drug may need to be temporarily discontinued during times of reduced oral intake (such as in acute illness or prolonged fasting for surgery) or fluid losses (such as from GI illness or excessive heat exposure). Kidney impairment and AKI can occur.

• Don't use urine tests to monitor glycemic control.

• *Look alike–sound alike:* Don't confuse ertugliflozin with canagliflozin, dapagliflozin, or empagliflozin. Don't confuse Segluromet with Steglatro or Steglujan.

PATIENT TEACHING

Boxed Warning Inform patient of risks of lactic acidosis due to metformin component. Teach patient signs and symptoms of lactic acidosis and conditions that predispose to lactic acidosis. Advise patient to discontinue drug immediately and report unexplained hyperventilation, malaise, myalgia, unusual somnolence, slow or irregular heartbeat, sensation of feeling cold (especially in the extremities), or other nonspecific symptoms. Stress importance of adhering to dietary instructions, regular physical activity, periodic blood glucose and HbA_{1c} monitoring, and kidney function testing. ∎

• Teach patient to report all adverse reactions.

• Teach patient how to recognize and manage hypoglycemia, hyperglycemia, and other diabetic complications.

• Advise patient to promptly seek medical advice during periods of stress (such as fever, trauma, infection, or surgery) because drug requirements may change.

• Caution patient to avoid dehydration, which can cause hypotension. Instruct patient to maintain adequate fluid intake and to immediately report signs and symptoms of hypotension (postural dizziness, weakness, temporary loss of consciousness).

• Instruct patient to seek immediate medical advice if signs and symptoms of ketoacidosis (nausea, vomiting, abdominal pain, tiredness, labored breathing) occur.

• Inform patient that AKI has been reported. Instruct patient to immediately seek medical advice if reduced oral intake (due to acute illness or fasting) or increased fluid losses (due to vomiting, diarrhea, or excessive heat exposure) occur because drug may need to be temporarily discontinued.

• Instruct patient to recognize and immediately report signs and symptoms of UTIs (abdominal, pelvic, or back pain; frequent urination; burning with urination; fever; nausea; vomiting).

• Inform patient that drug may increase risk of amputation. Stress importance of routine preventive foot care. Instruct patient to watch for and immediately report new pain or tenderness, sores or ulcers, or infections involving the leg or foot.

• Tell patient to report signs and symptoms of genital yeast infections (itching, redness, rash, discharge, genital pain).

🜂 *Alert:* Teach patient signs and symptoms of necrotizing fasciitis and to seek immediate medical attention if any of these signs and symptoms occur.

• Inform patient that urine glucose tests shouldn't be used for monitoring glycemic control during therapy because patient's urine will test positive for glucose.

• Advise patient of fetal risk. Instruct patient to immediately report pregnancy or plans to become pregnant.

• Caution patient not to breastfeed during therapy.

• Inform patient who is premenopausal and anovulatory that metformin therapy may result in ovulation.

ertugliflozin–sitagliptin
er-too-gli-FLOE-zin/sit-a-GLIP-tin

Steglujan

Therapeutic class: Antidiabetics
Pharmacologic class: Sodium-glucose cotransporter 2 inhibitors–DPP-4 enzyme inhibitors

AVAILABLE FORMS
Tablets: 5 mg ertugliflozin/100 mg sitagliptin; 15 mg ertugliflozin/100 mg sitagliptin

INDICATIONS & DOSAGES
➤ **Adjunct to diet and exercise to improve glycemic control in adults with type 2 diabetes**
Adults: Initially, 5 mg ertugliflozin/100 mg sitagliptin PO once daily in the morning. May increase to a maximum dose of 15 mg/100 mg PO once daily if tolerated and additional glycemic control is needed. For patients already treated with ertugliflozin, maintain current ertugliflozin dose when switching to combination product.

ADMINISTRATION
PO
• Give drug with or without food.
• If a dose is missed, give it as soon as possible. If it's almost time for the next dose, skip the missed dose and give drug at the next regularly scheduled time. Don't give two doses at the same time.
• Store at room temperature.

ACTION
Ertugliflozin increases excretion of urinary glucose by inhibiting sodium-glucose cotransporter 2 (SGLT2), which reabsorbs glucose through the kidneys. Sitagliptin inhibits DPP-4. By increasing and prolonging active incretin levels, sitagliptin helps increase insulin release and decrease circulating glucose.

Route	Onset	Peak	Duration
PO (ertugliflozin)	Unknown	1–2 hr	Unknown
PO (sitagliptin)	Rapid	1–4 hr	Unknown

Half-life: Ertugliflozin, 16.6 hours; sitagliptin, 12.4 hours.

ADVERSE REACTIONS
CNS: headache. **CV:** peripheral edema. **EENT:** nasopharyngitis. **GI:** thirst, abdominal pain, nausea, diarrhea. **GU:** genital fungal infections, UTI, vaginal pruritus, increased urination, kidney impairment. **Hematologic:** increased Hb level. **Metabolic:** volume depletion, weight loss, increased LDL-C level, *hypoglycemia,* hyperphosphatemia. **Musculoskeletal:** back pain. **Respiratory:** URI.

INTERACTIONS
Drug-drug. *ACE inhibitors, ARBs, diuretics, NSAIDs:* May increase risk of kidney impairment and AKI. Use together cautiously.
Digoxin: May increase digoxin level. Monitor digoxin level.
Insulin, insulin secretagogues: May increase risk of hypoglycemia. Consider lower insulin or insulin secretagogue dosage.
Lithium: Ertugliflozin may decrease lithium level. Monitor lithium level more closely during ertugliflozin initiation and dosage changes.

EFFECTS ON LAB TEST RESULTS
• May increase serum creatinine, LDL-C, phosphate, and digoxin levels.
• May increase Hb level.
• May decrease eGFR.
• May cause false-positive urine glucose tests and unreliable 1,5-AG assay results.

CONTRAINDICATIONS & CAUTIONS
• Contraindicated in patients hypersensitive to sitagliptin, ertugliflozin, or components of product; in patients with eGFR less than 30 mL/minute/1.73 m^2; and in patients on dialysis.
• Rare but serious allergic and hypersensitivity reactions (anaphylaxis, angioedema, and exfoliative skin conditions, including SJS), have been reported with use of sitagliptin and other DPP-4 inhibitors. If reactions occur, discontinue drug and begin appropriate monitoring and treatment.
• Drug isn't indicated for treatment of type 1 diabetes or diabetic ketoacidosis.
• Drug hasn't been studied in patients with a history of pancreatitis. Acute pancreatitis, including fatal and nonfatal hemorrhagic or necrotizing pancreatitis, has been reported in patients taking sitagliptin. It's unknown if a history of pancreatitis increases risk of sitagliptin-related pancreatitis.

• Drug may increase risk of symptomatic hypotension from intravascular volume depletion. Use cautiously in patients with eGFR less than 60 mL/minute/1.73 m² or preexisting hypotension and in patients ages 65 and older.

• Drug isn't recommended in patients with eGFR less than 45 mL/minute/1.73 m². Drug increases serum creatinine level and decreases eGFR. Monitor these patients more frequently.

• Consider temporarily discontinuing drug for at least 4 days before scheduled surgery to reduce risk of ketoacidosis.

• HF has occurred with other DPP-4 inhibitors. Before starting drug, consider risks and benefits of therapy in patient with known risk factors for HF.

• Serious and life-threatening ketoacidosis has been reported in patients taking SGLT2 inhibitors and in patients taking ertugliflozin. In some cases, risk factors for ketoacidosis (insulin dosage reduction, acute febrile illness, reduced calorie intake due to illness or surgery, pancreatic insulin deficiency, or alcohol abuse) were identified.

• Use cautiously in patients with hypovolemia or HF because drug may increase risk of kidney impairment and AKI.

• Use cautiously in patients with history of amputation, peripheral vascular disease, neuropathy, or diabetic foot ulcers, as an increased risk of lower limb amputation (primarily of the toe) was observed in clinical studies with another SGLT2 inhibitor.

• Use cautiously in patients with history of genital mycotic infection and in patients who aren't circumcised, as they are more likely to develop genital mycotic infections.

🔄 *Alert:* SGLT2 inhibitors increase risk of rare but serious necrotizing fasciitis of perineum (Fournier gangrene).

• Drug may increase risk of severe and disabling arthralgia, which may occur soon after therapy begins or years later. If disabling joint pain occurs, discontinue drug, if appropriate.

• Cases of bullous pemphigoid requiring hospitalization have been reported.

• Safety and effectiveness in children haven't been determined.

Dialyzable drug: Ertugliflozin, unknown; sitagliptin, 13.5%.

PREGNANCY-LACTATION-REPRODUCTION

• Drug isn't recommended during the second and third trimesters, as animal studies suggest increased risk of adverse kidney effects from ertugliflozin.

• It isn't known if drug appears in human milk or how drug affects milk production or an infant who is breastfed. Because of the potential for serious adverse reactions in infants who are breastfed, patient shouldn't breastfeed during therapy.

NURSING CONSIDERATIONS

• Assess for volume depletion at baseline and correct fluid balance before initiating therapy. Monitor patient for hypovolemia during therapy.

• Monitor for signs and symptoms of AKI. Assess kidney function at baseline and periodically during therapy.

🔄 *Alert:* Drug may need to be temporarily discontinued during times of reduced oral intake (such as in acute illness or prolonged fasting for surgery) or fluid losses (such as from GI illness or excessive heat exposure). Kidney impairment and AKI can occur.

• Monitor patients for signs and symptoms of UTIs, urosepsis, and pyelonephritis; treat promptly, if indicated.

• Monitor for signs and symptoms of genital mycotic infections; treat promptly, if indicated.

🔄 *Alert:* Watch for and immediately report signs and symptoms of necrotizing fasciitis of perineum (temperature above 100.4° F [38° C], general feeling of being unwell, and tenderness, redness, or swelling of the genitals back to the rectum). Signs and symptoms can worsen quickly. Immediately discontinue drug and prepare to administer broad-spectrum antibiotics. Surgical debridement may be necessary. Monitor blood glucose levels and start alternative therapy for glycemic control.

• Monitor blood glucose level. Assess for signs and symptoms of hypoglycemia.

• For suspected ketoacidosis, discontinue drug, assess patient, and treat promptly.

• Drug may increase LDL-C level. Assess periodically and treat if clinically indicated.

• Monitor patients for signs and symptoms of infection, osteomyelitis, new pain, and ulcers of the lower limbs. Discontinue drug if these occur.

• Monitor patients for PVD, neuropathy, and diabetic foot ulcers. Treat as indicated.

• Monitor patients for acute pancreatitis; if suspected, promptly discontinue drug and treat appropriately.

• Monitor patients for signs and symptoms of HF. If HF develops, treat as clinically indicated; drug may need to be discontinued.

• Monitor patients for serious allergic and hypersensitivity reactions. If reactions occur, discontinue drug and institute appropriate monitoring and treatment.

• Monitor patients for arthralgia. If severe joint pain occurs, drug may need to be discontinued.

• Monitor patients for blisters or erosions, as this may indicate bullous pemphigoid. For suspected bullous pemphigoid, discontinue drug and refer patient to a dermatologist for diagnosis and treatment.

• Urine tests shouldn't be used to monitor glycemic control.

• *Look alike–sound alike:* Don't confuse ertugliflozin with canagliflozin, dapagliflozin, or empagliflozin. Don't confuse sitagliptin with saxagliptin, linagliptin, or alogliptin. Don't confuse Steglujan with Steglatro or Segluromet.

PATIENT TEACHING

• Advise patient to report all adverse reactions.

• Stress importance of adhering to dietary instructions, regular physical activity, periodic blood glucose and HbA$_{1c}$ monitoring, and kidney function testing.

• Teach patient how to recognize and manage hypoglycemia, hyperglycemia, and other diabetic complications. Caution patient that use with insulin and insulin secretagogues may increase risk of hypoglycemia.

• Advise patient to discontinue drug and seek immediate medical attention for allergic reactions (rash; hives; swelling of the face, lips, tongue, and throat; difficulty swallowing or breathing).

• Caution patient to promptly seek medical advice during periods of stress (such as fever, trauma, infection, or surgery), as drug requirements may change.

• Teach patient to avoid dehydration, which can cause hypotension. Instruct patient regarding adequate fluid intake and to report signs and symptoms of hypotension (postural dizziness, weakness, temporary loss of consciousness).

• Instruct patient to immediately seek medical advice if signs and symptoms of ketoacidosis (nausea, vomiting, abdominal pain, tiredness, and labored breathing) occur.

• Inform patient that AKI has been reported and to immediately seek medical advice if reduced oral intake (due to acute illness or fasting) or increased fluid losses (due to vomiting, diarrhea, or excessive heat exposure) occur, as drug may need to be temporarily discontinued.

• Caution patient to immediately report symptoms of HF (increasing shortness of breath, rapid increase in weight, or swelling of the feet).

• Advise patient that acute pancreatitis can occur. Tell patient to discontinue drug and immediately report severe, persistent abdominal pain that may radiate to the back, with or without vomiting.

• Instruct patient to recognize and immediately report signs and symptoms of UTIs (abdominal, pelvic, or back pain; frequent urination; burning with urination; fever; nausea; vomiting).

• Inform patient of the increased risk of amputations. Counsel patient about the importance of routine preventive foot care.

• Instruct patient to watch for and immediately report new pain or tenderness, sores or ulcers, or infections involving the leg or foot.

• Advise patient that arthralgia can occur at any time during treatment and to report severe joint pain to prescriber.

• Advise patient that bullous pemphigoid requiring hospitalization can occur and to immediately report blisters or skin erosions.

• Tell patient to report signs and symptoms of genital yeast infections (itching, redness, rash, discharge, genital pain).

• *Alert:* Teach patient signs and symptoms of necrotizing fasciitis, and instruct patient to seek immediate medical attention if any of these signs and symptoms occur.

• Inform patient that urine glucose tests shouldn't be used for monitoring glycemic control during therapy because patient's urine will test positive for glucose.

• Advise patient of fetal risk. Instruct patient to immediately report pregnancy or plans to become pregnant.

• Caution patient not to breastfeed during therapy.

Reactions in bold italics are *life-threatening*.

erythromycin (ophthalmic, topical)
er-ith-roe-MYE-sin

Erygel, Ery 2% Pads

Therapeutic class: Antibiotics
Pharmacologic class: Macrolides

AVAILABLE FORMS
Ophthalmic ointment: 0.5%
Topical gel: 2%
Topical pad: 2%
Topical solution: 2%*

INDICATIONS & DOSAGES
➤ **Superficial ocular infections involving the conjunctiva or cornea caused by organisms susceptible to erythromycin (ophthalmic ointment)**
Adults and children: Apply a ribbon of ointment about 1 cm long directly to infected eye up to six times daily, depending on severity of infection.
➤ **Prevention of ophthalmia neonatorum caused by *Neisseria gonorrhoeae* or *Chlamydia trachomatis* (ophthalmic ointment)**
Neonates: Apply a ribbon of ointment about 1 cm long in lower conjunctival sac of each eye shortly after birth.
➤ **Inflammatory acne vulgaris (topical gel, topical pads, topical solution)**
Adults and children: Apply pads and solution to affected areas b.i.d., morning and evening. Apply gel once daily or b.i.d. If no improvement in 6 to 8 weeks, discontinue drug; prescriber should reevaluate treatment.

ADMINISTRATION
Ophthalmic
• Don't use to treat infection unless causative organism has been identified.
• Clean eye area of excessive discharge before application.
• To prevent ophthalmia neonatorum, apply ointment no later than 1 hour after birth. Use drug in neonates born either vaginally or by cesarean birth. Gently massage eyelids for 1 minute to spread ointment.
• Use new tube for each neonate.
• Store ophthalmic ointment at room temperature in tightly closed, light-resistant container.

Topical
• Wash, rinse, and pat affected areas dry before application.
• Apply solution using supplied applicator top.
• Spread gel lightly; don't rub.
• Wash hands after each application.
• Avoid contact with eyes, nose, mouth, other mucous membranes, and broken skin.

ACTION
Inhibits RNA-dependent protein synthesis by binding to bacterial 50s ribosomal subunits.

Route	Onset	Peak	Duration
Ophthalmic, topical	Unknown	Unknown	Unknown

Half-life: Unknown.

ADVERSE REACTIONS
EENT: minor ocular irritations, redness.
Skin: burning, dryness, itching, erythema, irritation, oily skin, peeling, sensitivity reactions, leather appearance, tenderness.
Other: hypersensitivity reactions.

INTERACTIONS
Drug-drug. *Clindamycin (topical):* Topical form may antagonize clindamycin's effect. Avoid use together.
Isotretinoin (topical): May increase adverse effects of erythromycin. Use together cautiously.
Drug-lifestyle. *Abrasive or medicated soaps or cleansers, acne products or other preparations containing peeling drugs (benzoyl peroxide, resorcinol, salicylic acid, sulfur, tretinoin), alcohol-containing products (aftershave, cosmetics, perfumed toiletries, shaving creams or lotions), astringent soaps or cosmetics, medicated cosmetics or cover-ups:* May cause cumulative dryness, resulting in excessive skin irritation. Urge caution.

EFFECTS ON LAB TEST RESULTS
None reported.

CONTRAINDICATIONS & CAUTIONS
• Contraindicated in patients hypersensitive to drug.
• Safety and effectiveness of topical drug in children haven't been established.
Dialyzable drug: Unknown.

PREGNANCY-LACTATION-REPRODUCTION
• Use during pregnancy only if clearly needed.
• It isn't known if drug appears in human milk after topical application. Use cautiously during breastfeeding.

NURSING CONSIDERATIONS
• Topical formulations are intended only for treatment of inflammatory acne and not for treatment of superficial skin infections.
⚠️ *Alert:* Prolonged topical use may result in fungal or bacterial superinfection, including pseudomembranous colitis and CDAD, during and up to 2 months after treatment. Consider these diagnoses in patients who present with diarrhea; stop drug for significant diarrhea, abdominal cramps, or passage of blood or mucus.

PATIENT TEACHING
• Teach about proper drug administration and handling. Warn patient not to touch tip of applicator to eye or surrounding tissue.
• Instruct patient to wash hands before and after applying ointment.
• Tell patient that vision may be blurred for a few minutes after applying ophthalmic ointment. Instruct patient to keep eyes closed for 1 to 2 minutes after applying drug.
• Advise patient to watch for and report signs and symptoms of sensitivity (itching lids, redness, swelling, or constant burning of eyes or skin).
• Tell patient not to share drug, washcloths, or towels with family members and to notify prescriber if anyone develops same signs or symptoms.
• Stress importance of adherence with recommended therapy.
• Teach patient to wash, rinse, and dry face thoroughly before each topical use.
• Advise patient to avoid topical use near eyes, nose, mouth, or other mucous membranes.
• Tell patient to stop using drug and notify prescriber if condition worsens or if no improvement occurs.
• Caution patient to keep topical drug away from heat and open flame.
• Advise patient to immediately report diarrhea.

erythromycin base
er-ith-roe-MYE-sin

Eryc, Ery-Tab

erythromycin ethylsuccinate
E.E.S. Granules, EryPed

erythromycin lactobionate
Erythrocin

erythromycin stearate
Erythrocin Stearate

Therapeutic class: Antibiotics
Pharmacologic class: Macrolides

AVAILABLE FORMS
erythromycin base
Capsules (delayed-release): 250 mg
Tablets: 250 mg, 500 mg
Tablets (delayed-release): 250 mg, 333 mg, 500 mg
erythromycin ethylsuccinate
Oral suspension (after reconstitution): 200 mg/5 mL, 400 mg/5 mL
Tablets: 400 mg
erythromycin lactobionate
Injection: 500 mg*
erythromycin stearate
Tablets (film-coated): 250 mg

INDICATIONS & DOSAGES
➤ **Acute PID caused by** *Neisseria gonorrhoeae* **in females with history of penicillin sensitivity**
Adults: 500 mg IV every 6 hours for 3 days; then 500 mg (base) PO every 12 hours or 333 mg (base) PO every 8 hours for 7 days.
➤ **Intestinal amebiasis caused by** *Entamoeba histolytica*
Adults: 500 mg (base or stearate) PO every 12 hours, or 333 mg (base) PO every 8 hours, or 250 mg (base or stearate) PO every 6 hours, or 400 mg (ethylsuccinate) q.i.d. for 10 to 14 days.
Children: 30 to 50 mg/kg PO daily in divided doses for 10 to 14 days. Maximum, 4 g/day.
➤ **To prevent rheumatic fever recurrence in patients allergic to penicillin and sulfonamides**
Adults: 250 mg (base or stearate) PO b.i.d., or 400 mg (ethylsuccinate) PO b.i.d.

Reactions in bold italics are *life-threatening*.

► **Mild to moderately severe respiratory tract, skin, or soft-tissue infection from sensitive group A beta-hemolytic streptococci, *Streptococcus pneumoniae, Streptococcus pyogenes, Mycoplasma pneumoniae, Corynebacterium diphtheriae,* or *Bordetella pertussis; Listeria monocytogenes* infection**

Adults: 250 mg PO every 6 hours, 333 mg PO every 8 hours, or 500 mg PO every 12 hours. Maximum, 4 g/day. Or 15 to 20 mg/kg IV daily, as continuous infusion or in divided doses every 6 hours for 10 days (3 weeks for *Mycoplasma* species infection). Maximum, 4 g/day.

Children: 30 to 50 mg/kg PO daily in divided doses every 6 hours or 15 to 20 mg/kg IV daily in divided doses every 4 to 6 hours for 10 days (3 weeks for *Mycoplasma* species infection).

► **Legionnaires disease**

Adults: 1 to 4 g (base or stearate) or 1.6 to 4 g (ethylsuccinate) PO daily in divided doses for 10 to 14 days alone or with rifampin. IV route may be used initially in severe cases.

► **Nongonococcal urethritis caused by *Ureaplasma urealyticum* when tetracycline is contraindicated or not tolerated**

Adults: 500 mg (base or stearate) PO every 6 hours, 666 mg (base) PO every 8 hours, or 800 mg (ethylsuccinate) PO every 8 hours for at least 7 days.

► **Uncomplicated urethral, endocervical, or rectal infection caused by *Chlamydia trachomatis* when tetracyclines are contraindicated**

Adults: 500 mg base PO q.i.d. for at least 7 days, 666 mg PO every 8 hours for at least 7 days, or 250 mg PO q.i.d. for 14 days if patient can't tolerate higher doses.

► **Urogenital *C. trachomatis* infection during pregnancy**

Women: 500 mg (base or stearate) PO q.i.d. or 666 mg (base) PO every 8 hours for at least 7 days. Patients who can't tolerate this regimen may receive 500 mg (base or stearate) PO every 12 hours, 333 mg (base) PO every 8 hours, or 250 mg (base or stearate) PO q.i.d. for at least 14 days.

► **Conjunctivitis of newborn caused by *C. trachomatis***

Neonates: 50 mg/kg/day PO in 4 divided doses for at least 2 weeks.

► **Pneumonia in infants caused by *C. trachomatis***

Infants: 50 mg/kg/day (base or stearate) PO in four divided doses for 21 days.

► **Pertussis**

Adults: 40 to 50 mg/kg/day PO in divided doses for 5 to 14 days.

► **Preoperative prophylaxis for elective colorectal surgery**

Adults: Two 500-mg tablets, three 333-mg tablets, or four 250-mg tablets PO at 1 p.m., 2 p.m., and 11 p.m. on preoperative day 1 before 8 a.m. surgery. Protocols may vary.

► **Primary syphilis**

Adults: 30 to 40 g (base or stearate) PO or 48 to 64 g (ethylsuccinate) PO in divided doses for 10 to 15 days. (CDC guidelines don't recommend erythromycin for this indication.)

ADMINISTRATION

• Obtain specimen for culture and sensitivity tests before administration. Begin therapy while awaiting results.

PO

• When giving suspension, note the concentration.

• Give base or stearate with full glass of water at least ½ hour and preferably 2 hours before meals for best absorption; may give ethylsuccinate, solution, or delayed release without regard to meals.

• Give drug with food if GI upset occurs. Don't give drug with milk, soda, or fruit juice.

• Consider coated tablets or encapsulated pellets for patients who have trouble tolerating drug because these forms cause less GI upset.

• Protect capsules from moisture and excessive heat.

IV

▼ Reconstitute drug according to manufacturer's directions.

▼ Dilute each to 1 g per liter (1 mg/mL) for continuous infusion or 1 to 5 mg/mL for intermittent infusions. Don't give IV push.

▼ Infuse intermittent dose over 20 to 60 minutes.

▼ **Incompatibilities:** None listed by manufacturer. Consult drug compatibility reference for more information.

ACTION

Inhibits bacterial protein synthesis by binding to the 50S subunit of the ribosome. Bacteriostatic or bactericidal, depending on concentration.

Route	Onset	Peak	Duration
PO	Unknown	0.5–4 hr	Unknown
IV	Immediate	2.5 hr	Unknown

Half-life: 1.5 to 2 hours.

ADVERSE REACTIONS

CNS: fever. **CV:** vein irritation or thrombophlebitis after IV injection, *ventricular arrhythmias, prolonged QT interval.* **GI:** *CDAD,* abdominal pain and cramping, diarrhea, nausea, vomiting, anorexia. **Hepatic:** liver dysfunction. **Skin:** eczema, rash, urticaria. **Other:** hypersensitivity reactions, including *anaphylaxis;* overgrowth of nonsusceptible bacteria or fungi.

INTERACTIONS

Drug-drug. *Azole antifungals (ketoconazole):* May increase erythromycin and antifungal levels, leading to increased risk of adverse reactions, including sudden death from cardiac causes. Avoid use together.

Astemizole, terfenadine: May increase risk of CV events, including QT prolongation, ventricular arrhythmias, and cardiac arrest. Use together is contraindicated.

Benzodiazepines (midazolam, triazolam): May increase effects of these drugs. Monitor patient closely.

Carbamazepine: May inhibit metabolism of carbamazepine, increasing blood level and risk of toxicity. Avoid use together.

Clarithromycin: May increase QTc interval and risk of arrhythmias. Avoid use together.

Clindamycin, lincomycin: May be antagonistic. Avoid use together.

Clopidogrel: May inhibit antiplatelet effect of clopidogrel. Monitor platelet function when starting or stopping erythromycin. Adjust clopidogrel dosage as needed.

Colchicine: May increase colchicine level and risk of colchicine-related adverse reactions. Use cautiously and monitor patient for colchicine-related toxicity.

Cyclosporine: May increase cyclosporine level. Monitor drug level.

Digoxin: May increase digoxin level. Monitor patient for digoxin toxicity.

Dihydroergotamine, ergotamine: May increase ergot toxicity. Use together is contraindicated.

Disopyramide: May increase disopyramide level, which may cause arrhythmias and prolonged QT intervals. Monitor ECG.

Fluoroquinolones, other drugs that prolong QTc interval (amiodarone, antipsychotics, procainamide, quinidine, sotalol, TCAs): May have additive effects. Monitor ECG for QTc interval prolongation. Avoid use together, if possible.

HMG-CoA reductase inhibitors (atorvastatin, lovastatin, simvastatin): May increase statin level; rhabdomyolysis has occurred. Monitor CK and serum transaminase levels. Don't use with lovastatin or simvastatin.

Oral anticoagulants (warfarin): May increase anticoagulant effect. Closely monitor PT and INR.

Pimozide, cisapride: May increase QTc interval and risk of ventricular arrhythmias. Use together is contraindicated.

Rifamycins (rifabutin, rifampin, rifapentine): May decrease therapeutic effects of erythromycin while increasing adverse effects of rifamycin. Monitor patient.

Sildenafil: May increase sildenafil level. Consider reducing sildenafil dosage.

Strong CYP3A inhibitors (diltiazem, verapamil): May increase risk of sudden death from cardiac causes. Don't use together.

Theophylline: May decrease erythromycin level and increase theophylline toxicity. Use together cautiously.

Drug-food. *Grapefruit juice:* May inhibit drug's metabolism. Caution patient to avoid grapefruit juice during therapy.

EFFECTS ON LAB TEST RESULTS

• May increase ALP, ALT, AST, and bilirubin levels.

• May interfere with fluorometric determination of urine catecholamines and with colorimetric assays.

CONTRAINDICATIONS & CAUTIONS

• Contraindicated in patients hypersensitive to drug or other macrolides.

• *Alert:* Drug has been associated with prolonged QT interval and infrequent cases of arrhythmias, including torsades de pointes. Avoid drug in patients with known prolonged QT interval, proarrhythmic conditions, or clinically significant bradycardia and in those receiving class IA (quinidine, procainamide) or class III (dofetilide, amiodarone, sotalol) antiarrhythmics.

• Use erythromycin salts cautiously in patients with impaired liver function.

• May cause infantile hypertrophic pyloric stenosis (IHPS) requiring surgery. Weigh benefit of therapy against risk of IHPS.

• Prolonged or repeated use may result in superinfection. If superinfection occurs, discontinue drug.

Reactions in bold italics are *life-threatening*.

• Drug may cause CDAD, ranging in severity from mild to life-threatening colitis, during treatment and for up to 2 months after treatment. Drug may need to be discontinued for suspected or confirmed CDAD.

• Use cautiously in older adults, who are at increased risk for developing drug-induced hearing loss, fluid retention, and QT prolongation.

• Don't use drug to treat neurosyphilis.
Dialyzable drug: No.

PREGNANCY-LACTATION-REPRODUCTION

• Use drug during pregnancy only if clearly needed.

• Drug may not reach the fetus adequately to prevent congenital syphilis; a penicillin regimen is recommended.

☉ Alert: Some IV formulations contain benzyl alcohol, which is associated with sometimes fatal neonatal gasping syndrome.

• Drug appears in human milk. Use cautiously during breastfeeding.

NURSING CONSIDERATIONS

• Monitor for diarrhea and signs and symptoms of superinfection. Drug may cause overgrowth of nonsusceptible bacteria and fungi.

• Monitor liver function. Drug may cause liver toxicity.

• Monitor patient for new hearing loss.

• Monitor patient for fluid retention.

PATIENT TEACHING

• Teach about proper drug administration and handling.

• Tell patient to take drug as prescribed, even after feeling better.

• Caution patient to report all adverse reactions, especially diarrhea, nausea, abdominal pain, vomiting, and fever.

• Inform patient that CDAD can occur 2 months or more after last dose of an antibiotic. Instruct patient to immediately report watery or bloody stools.

• Instruct parents or caregivers of infants to immediately report signs and symptoms of IHPS (vomiting or irritability with feeding).

• Advise patient to use cautiously if breastfeeding.

Lexapro

Therapeutic class: Antidepressants
Pharmacologic class: SSRIs

AVAILABLE FORMS

Oral solution: 5 mg/5 mL
Tablets: 5 mg, 10 mg, 20 mg

INDICATIONS & DOSAGES

Adjust-a-dose (for all indications): For older adults and patients with liver impairment, 10 mg PO daily, initially and as maintenance dosages.

➤ **Acute and maintenance therapy for patients with MDD**
Adults and adolescents ages 12 and older: Initially, 10 mg PO once daily, increasing to 20 mg if needed after at least 1 week in adults and 3 weeks in adolescents.

➤ **Generalized anxiety disorder**
Adults and children ages 7 and older: Initially, 10 mg PO once daily, increasing to 20 mg if needed after at least 1 week.

➤ **Obsessive-compulsive disorder ◆**
Adults and adolescents ages 12 and older: Initially, 10 mg PO once daily. May increase dose in 10-mg increments at 1-week or greater intervals up to 30 mg once daily.

➤ **Premenstrual dysphoric disorder ◆**
Adult women: Continuous daily dosing regimen: Initially, 5 to 10 mg PO once daily. Over the first month, may increase dose, based on response and tolerability, up to 20 mg once daily.
Luteal phase dosing regimen: 5 to 10 mg PO once daily, starting 14 days before anticipated onset of menstruation and continuing to onset of menses. Over the first month, may increase dose to 20 mg once daily during luteal phase.
Symptom-onset dosing regimen: 5 to 10 mg PO once daily from day of symptom onset until a few days after start of menses. Over the first month, may increase dose, based on response and tolerability, up to 20 mg once daily.

ADMINISTRATION

PO

• Give drug without regard to food.

• Give in the morning or evening.

ACTION
Selectively inhibits reuptake of serotonin.

Route	Onset	Peak	Duration
PO	Unknown	5 hr	Unknown

Half-life: 27 to 32 hours.

ADVERSE REACTIONS
CNS: fever, insomnia, dizziness, somnolence, paresthesia, headache, light-headedness, migraine, tremor, vertigo, abnormal dreams, irritability, impaired concentration, fatigue, lethargy. **CV:** palpitations, HTN, flushing, chest pain. **EENT:** blurred vision, tinnitus, earache, rhinitis, sinusitis, dry mouth, toothache. **GI:** nausea, diarrhea, constipation, indigestion, abdominal pain, vomiting, increased or decreased appetite, flatulence, heartburn, cramps, gastroesophageal reflux. **GU:** ejaculation disorder, erectile dysfunction, anorgasmia, decreased libido, menstrual cramps, UTI, urinary frequency. **Metabolic:** weight gain or loss, hyponatremia. **Musculoskeletal:** arthralgia; myalgia; muscle cramps; pain in neck, shoulder, arms, or legs. **Respiratory:** bronchitis, cough. **Skin:** rash, diaphoresis. **Other:** yawning, flulike symptoms.

INTERACTIONS
Drug-drug. *Aspirin, NSAIDs, other drugs known to affect coagulation:* May increase risk of bleeding. Use together cautiously.
Beta blockers (metoprolol): May cause bradycardia and increase risk of CNS toxicity. Monitor patient closely.
Carbamazepine: May decrease escitalopram level. Monitor patient for expected antidepressant effect. Adjust dose as needed.
Cimetidine: May increase escitalopram level. Monitor for increased adverse reactions to escitalopram.
Citalopram: May cause additive effects. Use together is contraindicated.
CNS drugs: May cause additive effects. Use together cautiously.
Desipramine, other drugs metabolized by CYP2D6 substrates: May increase levels of these drugs. Use together cautiously.
Linezolid, methylene blue: May cause serotonin syndrome. Avoid use together.
MAO inhibitors: May cause fatal serotonin syndrome or signs and symptoms resembling NMS. Avoid use within 14 days of MAO inhibitor therapy.

Pimozide: May increase risk of QTc-interval prolongation. Use together is contraindicated.
Serotonergic drugs (amphetamines, buspirone, fentanyl, lithium, rasagiline, selegiline, SSRIs, TCAs, tramadol, triptans): May increase risk of serotonin syndrome. Use together cautiously, especially at the start of therapy and at dosage increases.
Drug-herb. *St. John's wort:* May cause serotonin syndrome. Use with caution.
Drug-lifestyle. *Alcohol use:* May increase CNS effects. Discourage use together.

EFFECTS ON LAB TEST RESULTS
• May increase bilirubin and cholesterol levels and LFT values.
• May decrease serum potassium and sodium levels.
• May increase or decrease glucose level.
• May decrease prothrombin level.
• May increase INR.

CONTRAINDICATIONS & CAUTIONS
• Contraindicated in patients hypersensitive to escitalopram, citalopram, or any of its inactive ingredients.
• Use cautiously in patients with history of mania, seizure disorders, suicidality, or kidney or liver impairment.
• Use cautiously in patients with diseases that produce altered metabolism or hemodynamic responses.
• Drug may increase risk of angle-closure glaucoma in patients with anatomically narrow angles without iridectomy.
• Use cautiously in older adults because they may have greater sensitivity to drug.
Boxed Warning Escitalopram isn't approved for use in children younger than age 7. ■
• Safety and effectiveness in children younger than age 7 with generalized anxiety disorder haven't been established.
Dializable drug: Unknown.
⚠ *Overdose S&S:* Seizures, coma, dizziness, ECG changes, hypotension, insomnia, nausea, sinus tachycardia, somnolence, vomiting, AKI.

PREGNANCY-LACTATION-REPRODUCTION
• Use during pregnancy only if potential benefit justifies fetal risk.
• Prescriber should consider tapering dosage in the third trimester by carefully weighing established benefit of treating depression with an antidepressant against risks; decision can only be made on a case-by-case basis.

Reactions in bold italics are *life-threatening*.

- Health care providers are encouraged to register patients in the National Pregnancy Registry for Antidepressants (1-866-961-2388 or https://womensmentalhealth.org/research/pregnancyregistry/antidepressants).
- Drug appears in human milk. Use cautiously during breastfeeding; monitor infants for adverse reactions.

NURSING CONSIDERATIONS

Boxed Warning Drug may increase risk of suicidality in children, adolescents, and young adults ages 18 to 24, especially during the first few months of treatment, especially in patients with major depressive disorder or other psychiatric disorder. ■

Boxed Warning Closely monitor all patients for clinical worsening and for emergence of suicidality. ■

- Evaluate patient for history of drug abuse, and observe for signs of misuse or abuse.
- When discontinuing drug, taper gradually and monitor patient for reemerging signs and symptoms.
- Periodically reassess patient to determine need for maintenance treatment and appropriate dosing.
- Monitor for signs and symptoms of hyponatremia (headache, difficulty concentrating, memory impairment, confusion, weakness, unsteadiness, falls). If severe, symptoms may include hallucinations, syncope, seizure, coma, respiratory arrest, and death.
- Monitor for abnormal bleeding.

☀ Alert: Concomitant use with methylene blue or linezolid can cause serotonin syndrome (fever, mental status changes, muscle twitching, diaphoresis, shivering, shaking, diarrhea, loss of coordination). If linezolid or methylene blue must be given, stop escitalopram and monitor patient for serotonin toxicity for 2 weeks or until 24 hours after last dose of methylene blue or linezolid, whichever comes first. May resume escitalopram 24 hours after last dose of methylene blue or linezolid.

☀ Alert: Combining triptans with an SSRI or an SSNRI may cause serotonin syndrome or NMS-like reactions. Serotonin syndrome may be more likely to occur when starting or increasing dose of triptan, SSRI, or SSNRI.

☀ Look alike–sound alike: Don't confuse escitalopram with estazolam or citalopram

PATIENT TEACHING

- Teach about proper drug administration and handling.
- Inform patient that symptoms should improve gradually over several weeks, rather than immediately.
- Instruct patient to continue drug as prescribed, even though improvement may occur within 1 to 4 weeks.

Boxed Warning Caution patient and family to immediately report signs of worsening depression (agitation, irritability, insomnia, hostility, impulsivity) and suicidality to prescriber. ■

☀ Alert: Teach patient to recognize and immediately report symptoms of serotonin toxicity.

- Inform patient that drug may cause symptoms of sexual dysfunction. Advise patient to discuss management strategies with health care provider.
- Tell patient to use caution while driving or operating hazardous machinery because of drug's potential to impair judgment, thinking, and motor skills.
- Advise patient to consult health care provider before taking other prescription or OTC drugs.
- Encourage patient to avoid alcohol while taking drug.
- Advise patient to report pregnancy or breastfeeding before starting therapy.

esketamine
es-KET-a-meen

Spravato

Therapeutic class: Antidepressants
Pharmacologic class: Noncompetitive
N-methyl-D-aspartate receptor antagonists
Controlled substance schedule: III

AVAILABLE FORMS
Nasal spray: 28 mg (2 sprays)/device

INDICATIONS & DOSAGES
➤ Treatment-resistant depression in conjunction with an oral antidepressant
Adults: Induction phase (weeks 1 to 4): On day 1, starting dose is 56 mg intranasal with a subsequent dose that week of 56 or 84 mg based on efficacy and tolerability. For weeks 2 to 4, 56 or 84 mg intranasal twice per week. For maintenance phase weeks 5 to 8, 56 or

84 mg intranasal once weekly. For maintenance phase week 9 and after, 56 or 84 mg intranasal once weekly or once every 2 weeks. Individualize to the least frequent dosing to maintain response.

Adjust-a-dose: If patient misses treatment sessions and depression symptoms worsen, consider returning patient to previous dosing schedule.

➤ **Depressive symptoms in patients with MDD with acute suicidality**
Adults: 84 mg intranasal twice per week for 4 weeks. May reduce dosage to 56 mg twice per week, based on tolerability. After 4 weeks, assess for therapeutic benefit to determine need for continued treatment. Use together with an oral antidepressant beyond 4 weeks hasn't been systematically evaluated.

ADMINISTRATION
Intranasal
• Drug must be administered under direct supervision of a health care provider.
• A treatment session consists of nasal administration and postadministration observation under supervision.
• Patients should avoid food for at least 2 hours and liquids for at least 30 minutes before administration due to the risk of nausea and vomiting.
• Patients should blow nose before first dose to clear nasal passages. Patients shouldn't blow nose between doses.
• Patients taking a nasal corticosteroid or nasal decongestant on dosing day should use these medications at least 1 hour before administration of esketamine.
• Don't prime device before use.
• Use two devices for a 56-mg dose or three devices for an 84-mg dose, with a 5-minute rest period between use of each device.
• Ensure indicator shows two green dots. If it doesn't, dispose of device and obtain a new one.
• Recline patient's head to about 45 degrees during administration.
• Insert tip straight into nostril until nose rest touches the skin between the nostrils; close opposite nostril. Have patient inhale while pushing in plunger until it stops. Repeat to deliver dose to other nostril. Instruct patient to sniff gently to keep drug inside nose.
• Ensure administration by confirming that the indicator shows no green dots when the device is empty. When one dose is delivered,

one green dot will indicate that a dose remains in the device.
• Dab patient's nose with a tissue if liquid drops out. Caution patient not to blow nose.
• If patient misses treatment sessions and there is no worsening of depressive symptoms, continue current dosing schedule. If patient misses maintenance-phase treatment sessions and depression symptoms worsen, consider returning to previous dosing schedule.
• Store at room temperature.

ACTION
Mechanism for antidepressant effect is unknown.

Route	Onset	Peak	Duration
Intranasal	Unknown	20–40 min	Unknown

Half-life: 7 to 12 hours.

ADVERSE REACTIONS
CNS: dissociation, dizziness, sedation, vertigo, hypoesthesia, anxiety, depression, lethargy, feeling drunk, feeling abnormal, dysarthria, headache, tremor, euphoric mood, insomnia, mental impairment, intentional self-injury, dysphoria, taste disorder. **CV:** increased BP, tachycardia. **EENT:** nasal discomfort, oropharyngeal pain, throat irritation, dry mouth, toothache. **GI:** nausea, vomiting, constipation, diarrhea. **GU:** urinary frequency. **Musculoskeletal:** myalgia. **Skin:** hyperhidrosis.

INTERACTIONS
Drug-drug. *CNS depressants (benzodiazepines, opioids):* May increase sedation. Use together cautiously and monitor closely for additive sedative effects.
MAO inhibitors (rasagiline, selegiline), psychostimulants (amphetamines, armodafinil, methylphenidate, modafinil): May increase BP. Use together cautiously and monitor BP closely.
Drug-lifestyle. *Alcohol use:* May increase sedation. Avoid use together.

EFFECTS ON LAB TEST RESULTS
None reported.

CONTRAINDICATIONS & CAUTIONS
• Contraindicated in patients hypersensitive to esketamine, ketamine, or components and in those with aneurysmal vascular disease (including thoracic and abdominal aorta and

intracranial and peripheral arterial vessels), AV malformation, or history of intracerebral hemorrhage.

• Use cautiously in patients with history of hypertensive encephalopathy.

Boxed Warning Drug can cause delayed or prolonged sedation. ∎

Boxed Warning Dissociative or perceptual changes (including distortion of time and space and illusions), derealization, and depersonalization may occur. Because of drug's potential to induce dissociative effects, carefully assess patients with psychosis before giving drug. Initiate treatment only if benefit outweighs risk. ∎

Boxed Warning Drug is a controlled substance with potential for abuse, misuse, and diversion. Assess patient's risk of abuse or misuse before prescribing and monitor all patients for development of these behaviors or conditions, including drug-seeking behavior, during therapy. Individuals with history of drug abuse or dependence are at greater risk. ∎

Boxed Warning Drug is only available through a REMS program because of the risks of serious adverse effects. ∎

Boxed Warning Risk of suicidality is increased in children and young adults who take antidepressants. Drug isn't approved for use in children. ∎

• Drug may increase risk of short- or long-term cognitive or memory impairment.

• Use cautiously in patients with moderate liver impairment because of increased risk of adverse reactions.

• Drug hasn't been studied in patients on dialysis or in those with Child-Pugh class C liver impairment.

• Drug's effectiveness in preventing suicide or reducing suicidality hasn't been proven. Patient may still require in-patient treatment.

• Drug hasn't been studied or approved for use as an anesthetic.

Dialyzable drug: Unknown.

PREGNANCY-LACTATION-REPRODUCTION

• Drug may cause fetal harm and isn't recommended for use during pregnancy.

• If pregnancy occurs during treatment, discontinue drug and counsel patient about fetal risk.

• Patients of childbearing potential should consider pregnancy planning and prevention during treatment.

• Prescribers should register patients who are pregnant in the National Pregnancy Registry for Antidepressants (1-866-961-2388 or https://womensmentalhealth.org/research/pregnancyregistry/antidepressants).

• Drug appears in human milk. Breastfeeding isn't recommended during treatment.

NURSING CONSIDERATIONS

• Assess BP before administration. If baseline BP is greater than 140 mm Hg systolic or 90 mm Hg diastolic, consider risks of short-term increases in BP and benefit of treatment.

• Don't give if an increase in BP or ICP poses a serious risk.

• After administration, reassess BP for at least 2 hours, beginning at approximately 40 minutes. If BP drops and patient appears clinically stable for at least 2 hours, may discharge patient at end of postdose monitoring period; if not, continue to monitor.

• Assess for signs and symptoms of hypertensive crisis (chest pain, shortness of breath) or hypertensive encephalopathy (sudden severe headache, visual disturbances, seizures, diminished consciousness, or focal neurologic deficits). Provide emergency care as indicated.

Boxed Warning Because of risks of sedation and dissociation, health care provider must monitor patient for at least 2 hours at each treatment session and assess to determine whether patient is stable and ready to leave the health care setting. ∎

Boxed Warning Closely monitor patient who is also using CNS depressants for sedation. ∎

Boxed Warning Monitor all patients for signs and symptoms of abuse, misuse, dependence, and tolerance. ∎

Boxed Warning Closely monitor patient for clinical worsening and emergence of suicidality. Consider changing the therapeutic regimen, including possibly discontinuing drug or the concomitant oral antidepressant, in patient whose depression is persistently worse or who experiences emergent suicidality. ∎

• Drug may increase risk of ulcerative or interstitial cystitis. Monitor patient for urinary tract and bladder signs and symptoms (urinary frequency, dysuria, urinary urgency, nocturia, cystitis). Refer for appropriate follow-up as clinically indicated.

• *Look alike–sound alike:* Don't confuse esketamine with ketamine or escitalopram.

PATIENT TEACHING

• Advise patient to report all adverse reactions.

Boxed Warning Inform patient that sedation, dissociative symptoms, perception disturbances, dizziness, vertigo, anxiety, and increased BP may occur and that monitoring by a health care provider is necessary until these effects resolve. ■

Boxed Warning Advise patient that drug is a federally controlled substance because it can be abused and misused or lead to dependence. ■

Boxed Warning Tell patient that drug is available only through a REMS program. ■

Boxed Warning Advise patient and caregivers to look for emergence of suicidality, especially early during treatment and when dosage is adjusted. Instruct patient to immediately contact prescriber if changes occur. ■

• Because drug may impair the ability to drive or operate machinery, caution patient to avoid potentially hazardous activities requiring complete mental alertness and motor coordination (driving, operating machinery) until the next day after a restful sleep.

• Warn patient that someone must be available to drive patient home after each treatment session.

• Caution patient of childbearing potential about risk to a fetus. Advise patient to report pregnancy or plan to become pregnant during treatment.

• Advise patient not to breastfeed during treatment.

SAFETY ALERT!

esmolol hydrochloride
ES-moe-lol

Brevibloc

Therapeutic class: Antiarrhythmics
Pharmacologic class: Selective beta blockers

AVAILABLE FORMS

Injection: 10 mg/mL vial
Premixed IV bags in sodium chloride:
10 mg/mL in 250-mL bags; 20 mg/mL in 100-mL bags

INDICATIONS & DOSAGES

➤ **Supraventricular tachycardia; noncompensatory sinus tachycardia**

Adults: 500 mcg/kg as loading dose by IV infusion over 1 minute; then 4-minute maintenance infusion of 50 mcg/kg/minute. If adequate response doesn't occur within 5 minutes, may repeat loading dose and follow with maintenance infusion of 100 mcg/kg/minute for 4 minutes. May repeat loading dose and increase maintenance infusion by increments of 50 mcg/kg/minute. Maintenance dose general range, 50 to 200 mcg/kg/minute. Maximum maintenance infusion for tachycardia is 200 mcg/kg/minute. May continue maintenance infusions for up to 48 hours.

➤ **Intraoperative and postoperative tachycardia or HTN**

Adults: For immediate control: 1,000 mcg/kg as bolus dose over 30 seconds, followed by 150 mcg/kg/minute IV infusion, if needed.
For gradual control (stepwise dosing): Loading dose of 500 mcg/kg over 1 minute, then 50 mcg/kg/minute for 4 minutes. Optional loading dose, if needed; then 100 mcg/kg/minute for 4 minutes. Optional loading dose, if needed; then 150 mcg/kg/minute for 4 minutes. If necessary, increase to 200 mcg/kg/minute. Maximum dose, 200 mcg/kg/minute for tachycardia and 300 mcg/kg/minute for HTN.

ADMINISTRATION

IV

▼ Don't dilute single-dose vials or premixed containers.

▼ Give with an infusion-control device rather than by IV push. Administer by continuous IV infusion with or without a loading dose and titrate based on ventricular rate or BP at 4-minute or more intervals. Avoid infusing into small veins or through a butterfly catheter.

▼ If concentration exceeds 10 mg/mL, give drug through a central line.

▼ Don't use for longer than 48 hours. Watch infusion site carefully for signs of extravasation; if they occur, immediately stop infusion and call prescriber.

▼ **Incompatibilities:** Amphotericin B cholesteryl sulfate complex, diazepam, furosemide, procainamide, sodium bicarbonate 5%.

Reactions in bold italics are *life-threatening*.

ACTION
A class II antiarrhythmic and ultra-short-acting selective beta-1 blocker that decreases HR, contractility, and BP.

Route	Onset	Peak	Duration
IV	Immediate	5 min (with loading dose); 30 min (without loading dose)	30 min after discontinuation of infusion

Half-life: About 9 minutes.

ADVERSE REACTIONS
CNS: dizziness, somnolence, headache, agitation, confusion. **CV:** hypotension, peripheral ischemia. **GI:** nausea, vomiting. **Skin:** inflammation or induration at infusion site, hyperhidrosis.

INTERACTIONS
Drug-drug. *Antidiabetic agents:* May increase blood glucose-lowering effect of antidiabetic. Closely monitor blood glucose level.
Calcium channel blockers (diltiazem, nicardipine, nifedipine, verapamil), flecainide: May potentiate pharmacologic effects of both drugs. IV administration in close proximity is contraindicated. Monitor cardiac function closely and adjust therapy as needed.
Clonidine: May cause life-threatening BP increases. Closely monitor BP. Discontinue either agent gradually, preferably esmolol first.
Digoxin: May increase digoxin level and bradycardia. Monitor digoxin level.
Lidocaine: May increase lidocaine level. Monitor patient closely and adjust dosage as needed.
MAO inhibitors: May worsen bradycardia or HTN. Discontinue esmolol or reduce esmolol dosage, if needed.
Morphine: May increase esmolol level. Adjust esmolol dosage carefully.
NSAIDs: May impair antihypertensive effect of esmolol. Monitor BP and adjust esmolol dosage as needed.
Prazosin: May increase risk of orthostatic HTN. Help patient to stand slowly until effects are known.
Salicylates (aspirin): May impair antihypertensive effect of esmolol. Monitor patient and consider alternative therapy as needed.
Succinylcholine: May prolong neuromuscular blockade. Monitor patient closely.

Vasoconstrictive and positive inotropic agents (dopamine, epinephrine, norepinephrine): May increase risk of reduced cardiac contractility in presence of high systemic vascular resistance. Don't use together.

EFFECTS ON LAB TEST RESULTS
• May increase serum potassium level.

CONTRAINDICATIONS & CAUTIONS
• Contraindicated in patients hypersensitive to drug or its components, in those with severe sinus bradycardia, second- or third-degree heart block, sick sinus syndrome, cardiogenic shock, decompensated HF, and pulmonary HTN.
• Use cautiously in patients with kidney impairment, hypovolemia, peripheral circulatory disorders, hypoglycemia, diabetes, or bronchospasm.
• May cause myocardial ischemia when abruptly discontinued in patients with CAD. Avoid use in patients with Prinzmetal angina.
🔹 **Alert:** Don't withdraw drug abruptly, as angina, MI, and ventricular arrhythmias can occur.
• Use in combination with an alpha blocker (after starting alpha blocker) in patients with pheochromocytoma to avoid paradoxical BP increases.
• Safety and effectiveness in children haven't been established.
Dialyzable drug: Unknown.
⚠ **Overdose S&S:** Bradycardia, hypotension, loss of consciousness, cardiac arrest, pulseless electrical activity.

PREGNANCY-LACTATION-REPRODUCTION
• Use during third trimester can cause fetal bradycardia. Use during pregnancy only if potential benefit justifies fetal risk.
• It isn't known if drug appears in human milk. Patient should discontinue breastfeeding or discontinue drug, considering importance of drug to patient.

NURSING CONSIDERATIONS
🔹 **Alert:** Continuously monitor ECG and BP during infusion. Nearly half of patients develop hypotension. Diaphoresis and dizziness may accompany hypotension. Monitor patient closely, especially if patient had low BP before treatment.
• Hypotension can usually be reversed within 30 minutes by decreasing the dose or, if

needed, by stopping the infusion. Notify prescriber if this action becomes necessary.

• If local reaction develops at infusion site, change to another site. If extravasation occurs, immediately stop infusion and disconnect tubing from cannula. Gently aspirate extravasated solution without flushing catheter; then remove the IV catheter and elevate the extremity.

• When HR stabilizes, replace IV drug with an alternative antiarrhythmic. Reduce esmolol infusion rate by 50% 30 minutes after first dose of the new drug. Monitor patient response and, if HR is controlled for 1 hour after administration of second dose of the replacement drug, stop esmolol infusion.

• Monitor serum electrolyte levels, as hyperkalemia can occur, especially in patients with kidney impairment.

• Drug can mask signs and symptoms of hyperthyroidism. Monitor patient for thyrotoxicosis when withdrawing drug.

• Drug can mask hypoglycemia-related tachycardia. Monitor patient.

• Monitor patient for and correct hypovolemia.

PATIENT TEACHING

• Instruct patient to promptly report all adverse reactions.

• Tell patient to report discomfort at IV site.

esomeprazole magnesium
ess-oh-ME-pray-zol

Nexium, Nexium 24 HR ◊

esomeprazole sodium
Nexium IV

Therapeutic class: Antiulcer drugs
Pharmacologic class: PPIs

AVAILABLE FORMS
esomeprazole magnesium
Capsules (delayed-release) **ONC**: 20 mg ◊, 40 mg
Powder for suspension (delayed-release): 2.5 mg, 5 mg, 10 mg, 20 mg, 40 mg
Tablets (delayed-release): 20 mg ◊
esomeprazole sodium
Powder for injection: 40-mg single-use vials

INDICATIONS & DOSAGES

Adjust-a-dose (for all indications): For patients with Child-Pugh class C liver impairment, maximum daily dose is 20 mg.

➤ **GERD; to heal erosive esophagitis**
Adults and adolescents ages 12 to 17: 20 or 40 mg PO daily for 4 to 8 weeks. May continue for an additional 4 to 8 weeks in adults, as needed. Adult maintenance dose for healing erosive esophagitis is 20 mg PO daily for up to 6 months.
Children ages 1 to 11 weighing 20 kg or more: 10 or 20 mg PO once daily for up to 8 weeks.
Children ages 1 to 11 weighing less than 20 kg: 10 mg PO once daily for up to 8 weeks.

➤ **Symptomatic GERD**
Adults: 20 mg PO daily for 4 weeks. If symptoms are unresolved, may continue treatment for 4 more weeks.
Adolescents ages 12 to 17: 20 mg PO once daily for up to 4 weeks.
Children ages 1 to 11: 10 mg PO once daily for up to 8 weeks.

➤ **Heartburn occurring 2 or more days per week**
Adults: 20 mg (OTC only) PO daily for 14 days. May repeat 14-day course every 4 months.

➤ **Erosive esophagitis due to acid-mediated GERD only**
Infants ages 1 to 11 months weighing more than 7.5 to 12 kg: 10 mg PO once daily for up to 6 weeks.
Infants ages 1 to 11 months weighing more than 5 to 7.5 kg: 5 mg PO once daily for up to 6 weeks.
Infants ages 1 to 11 months weighing 3 to 5 kg: 2.5 mg PO once daily for up to 6 weeks.

➤ **Short-term treatment (up to 10 days) of GERD in patients with history of erosive esophagitis who can't take drug orally**
Adults: 20 or 40 mg IV bolus once daily over at least 3 minutes. Or, dilute to a total volume of 50 mL and give by IV infusion over 10 to 30 minutes once daily.
Children ages 1 to 17 weighing 55 kg or more: 20 mg IV infusion once daily over 10 to 30 minutes.
Children ages 1 to 17 weighing less than 55 kg: 10 mg IV infusion once daily over 10 to 30 minutes.
Children ages 1 month to younger than 1 year: 0.5 mg/kg IV infusion once daily over 10 to 30 minutes.

Adjust-a-dose: Switch patient to oral therapy as soon as tolerated.

➤ **To reduce risk of gastric ulcers in patients receiving continuous NSAID therapy**
Adults: 20 or 40 mg PO once daily for up to 6 months.

➤ **Long-term treatment of pathologic hypersecretory conditions, including Zollinger-Ellison syndrome**
Adults: 40 mg PO b.i.d. Adjust dosage based on patient response.

➤ **To eliminate *Helicobacter pylori***
Adults: 40 mg (magnesium) PO daily, 1,000 mg amoxicillin PO b.i.d., and 500 mg clarithromycin PO b.i.d., given together for 10 days to reduce duodenal ulcer recurrence.

➤ **To reduce risk of rebleeding of gastric or duodenal ulcers after therapeutic endoscopy**
Adults: 80 mg IV infusion over 30 minutes, followed by continuous infusion of 8 mg/hour for a total IV treatment duration of 72 hours, followed by oral acid-suppressive therapy.
Adjust-a-dose: In patients with Child-Pugh classes A and B liver impairment, maximum continuous infusion rate is 6 mg/hour. In patients with Child-Pugh class C liver impairment, maximum continuous infusion rate is 4 mg/hour.

ADMINISTRATION
PO
• Give drug at least 1 hour before meals. If patient has difficulty swallowing capsule, empty contents of capsule, mix with 1 tablespoon of applesauce, and have patient swallow (without chewing enteric-coated pellets).
• If giving capsule via NG tube, open capsule and empty the granules into a 60-mL syringe. Mix with 50 mL of water. Replace the plunger and shake vigorously for 15 seconds. Flush NG tube with additional water after use. Don't give if pellets have dissolved or disintegrated.
• For oral suspension, mix contents of 2.5- or 5-mg packet with 5 mL of water; mix contents of 10-, 20-, or 40-mg packet with 15 mL of water. Then let it sit for 2 to 3 minutes to thicken. Stir the suspension and drink within 30 minutes.
• To give oral suspension via NG tube, add 5 mL of water to a syringe, then add contents of 2.5- or 5-mg packet; or add 15 mL of water to a syringe, then add contents of 10-, 20-, or 40-mg packet. Shake syringe and leave for 2 to 3 minutes to thicken. Shake syringe again and inject through NG or gastric tube

(6 French or larger) within 30 minutes. Flush any remaining contents into stomach with additional 5 to 15 mL of water.
• Give a missed dose as soon as possible; if it's almost time for the next dose, skip missed dose and take the next dose at the regular scheduled time.
IV
▼ For IV bolus in adults only, reconstitute powder with 5 mL of NSS and inject over at least 3 minutes.
▼ For IV infusion, reconstitute powder with 5 mL of NSS, lactated Ringer injection, or D₅W. Further dilute with 45 mL of NSS, lactated Ringer injection, or D₅W. Infuse over 10 to 30 minutes.
▼ For continuous IV infusion, add two 40-mg vials reconstituted with NSS to 100 mL NSS. Infuse at 8 mg/hour for 71.5 hours.
▼ Flush IV line with D₅W, NSS, or lactated Ringer injection before and after administration.
▼ Use reconstituted powder within 12 hours.
▼ Use admixture diluted with D₅W within 6 hours.
▼ If diluted with NSS or lactated Ringer injection, use within 12 hours.
▼ Store reconstituted solution and admixture at room temperature.
▼ **Incompatibilities:** Other IV drugs.

ACTION
Reduces gastric acid secretion and decreases gastric acidity.

Route	Onset	Peak	Duration
PO	Unknown	1.5 hr	13–17 hr
IV	Unknown	Unknown	Unknown

Half-life: 1 to 1.5 hours.

ADVERSE REACTIONS
CNS: headache, dizziness, fever. **EENT:** dry mouth. **GI:** abdominal pain, constipation, diarrhea, flatulence, nausea, vomiting. **Respiratory:** cough. **Skin:** pruritus, injection-site reaction.

INTERACTIONS
Drug-drug. *Calcium salts (calcium carbonate):* May interfere with GI absorption of calcium salts. Closely monitor clinical response to calcium; larger dosages of calcium may be needed.
Cilostazol: May increase level of cilostazol and its active metabolite. Consider a cilostazol

dose reduction when giving concurrently with esomeprazole.

Clopidogrel: May decrease antiplatelet activity. Use esomeprazole magnesium or esomeprazole sodium cautiously with clopidogrel.

Dabigatran: May decrease level of active metabolite of dabigatran. Monitor patient closely.

Diazepam: May decrease clearance of diazepam. Monitor patient for diazepam toxicity.

Digoxin: May increase serum digoxin level. Monitor digoxin level and clinical response. For suspected interaction, adjust digoxin dosage as needed.

Drugs metabolized by CYP2C19: May alter clearance of esomeprazole, especially in older adults or patients with liver insufficiency. Monitor patient for toxicity.

Fluvoxamine: May increase risk of adverse reactions. Use cautiously.

Iron salts (ferrous sulfate): May interfere with absorption of iron salts. May need to temporarily stop esomeprazole to achieve response to oral iron. If stopping esomeprazole isn't an option, parenteral iron may be needed.

Ketoconazole, voriconazole: May increase esomeprazole level. Monitor therapy.

Methotrexate: May increase methotrexate level and risk of toxicity. Monitor patient closely.

Mycophenolate: May decrease mycophenolate level and effects. Monitor clinical response and adjust mycophenolate dosage as needed.

Protease inhibitors (atazanavir, nelfinavir, saquinavir): May reduce atazanavir or nelfinavir plasma level. Use together isn't recommended. May increase saquinavir level. Monitor patient carefully. Refer to protease inhibitor prescribing information.

Rilpivirine: May cause loss of virologic response or resistance. Use together is contraindicated.

Strong CYP2C19 or CYP3A4 inducers (ritonavir, rifampin): May decrease esomeprazole level. See prescribing information for specific drugs.

Tacrolimus: May increase pharmacologic effects of tacrolimus and risk of adverse reactions. Closely monitor tacrolimus trough level when starting or stopping esomeprazole. Adjust tacrolimus dosage as needed.

Warfarin: May prolong PT and increase INR, causing abnormal bleeding. Monitor patient, PT, and INR.

Drug-herb. *St. John's wort:* May decrease esomeprazole level. Avoid use together.

Drug-food. *Any food:* May reduce drug level. Advise patient to take drug 1 hour before food.

EFFECTS ON LAB TEST RESULTS

• May decrease magnesium and vitamin B_{12} levels.

• May cause false-positive results in diagnostic investigations for neuroendocrine tumors (CgA level).

• May cause false-positive results for urine screening for tetrahydrocannabinol (THC).

• May cause a hyperresponse in gastrin secretion in response to secretin stimulation test, falsely suggesting gastrinoma.

CONTRAINDICATIONS & CAUTIONS

• Contraindicated in patients hypersensitive to drug or components of esomeprazole or omeprazole.

🔵 *Alert:* PPIs may be associated with an increased risk of osteoporosis-related hip, wrist, and spine fractures. Risk is increased in patients who received high-dose and long-term (longer than 1 year) therapy. Use the lowest dosage for shortest duration. Consider vitamin D and calcium supplementation.

• Use cautiously in patients receiving continuous NSAID therapy who are at increased risk for gastric ulcers (those ages 60 and older and those with history of gastric ulcers).

• Symptomatic response to drug doesn't preclude the presence of gastric malignancy. Consider reevaluating patients with suboptimal response or early relapse.

• SCARs (SJS, TEN, DRESS, and acute generalized exanthematous pustulosis) have been reported with PPI use. Discontinue drug at first signs or symptoms.

• Cutaneous and systemic lupus erythematosus have been reported in patients taking PPIs. Exacerbations of existing autoimmune disease and new onset have both occurred. Avoid use of PPIs for longer than medically indicated.

Dialyzable drug: Unlikely.

⚠ *Overdose S&S:* Blurred vision, confusion, tremor, ataxia, intermittent clonic seizures, diaphoresis, drowsiness, flushing, headache, nausea, tachycardia.

PREGNANCY-LACTATION-REPRODUCTION
• Use during pregnancy only if potential benefit justifies fetal risk.
• It isn't known if drug appears in human milk, but omeprazole does. Use cautiously during breastfeeding.

NURSING CONSIDERATIONS
• Antacids can be used while taking drug, unless otherwise directed by prescriber.
• Monitor patient for rash and signs of symptoms of hypersensitivity. Monitor GI symptoms for improvement or worsening. Monitor LFT values, especially in patients with preexisting liver disease.
❸ *Alert:* Prolonged use may cause low magnesium level. Monitor magnesium level before treatment and periodically during treatment; supplement magnesium or discontinue drug as indicated. Monitor for signs and symptoms of low magnesium level (abnormal HR or heart rhythm, palpitations, muscle spasms, tremor, seizures). In children, abnormal HR may present as fatigue, upset stomach, dizziness, and light-headedness.
❸ *Alert:* Drug may increase risk of CDAD. Evaluate for CDAD in patients who develop diarrhea that doesn't improve.
❸ *Alert:* Prolonged treatment (at least 3 years or more) may lead to vitamin B_{12} malabsorption and subsequent vitamin B_{12} deficiency, which is dose-related and more severe in females and those younger than age 30; prevalence decreases after discontinuation of therapy.
• Monitor patient for signs and symptoms of acute tubulointerstitial nephritis (rash, fever, arthralgia, decreased kidney function, malaise, nausea, anorexia).
• Drug-induced decreases in gastric acidity may increase serum chromogranin A (CgA) level, possibly causing false-positive results in diagnostic testing for neuroendocrine tumors. Temporarily stop esomeprazole at least 14 days before assessing CgA level; consider repeating test if initial CgA level is high.
• *Look alike–sound alike:* Don't confuse esomeprazole with ARIPiprazole or omeprazole. Don't confuse Nexium with NexAVAR.

PATIENT TEACHING
• Teach about proper drug administration and handling.
• Instruct patient to take drug exactly as prescribed.

• Tell patient to inform prescriber of worsening signs and symptoms, pain, or diarrhea that doesn't improve.
• Instruct patient to alert prescriber if rash or other signs and symptoms of allergy occur.
• Warn patient to immediately report symptoms of low magnesium level (involuntary muscle movements, seizures).

E

esterified estrogens
es-TER-i-fied ES-troe-jenz

Menest

Therapeutic class: Estrogens
Pharmacologic class: Estrogens

AVAILABLE FORMS
Tablets (film-coated): 0.3 mg, 0.625 mg, 1.25 mg, 2.5 mg

INDICATIONS & DOSAGES
➤ **Inoperable progressing prostate cancer**
Adult males: 1.25 to 2.5 mg PO t.i.d.
➤ **Palliative treatment for metastatic breast cancer**
Adult males and postmenopausal adult females: 10 mg PO t.i.d. for 3 or more months.
➤ **Hypoestrogenism due to hypogonadism**
Adult females: 2.5 to 7.5 mg PO daily in divided doses in cycles of 20 days on, 10 days off.
➤ **Hyperestrogenism due to female castration, primary ovarian failure**
Adult females: 1.25 mg PO daily in cycles of 3 weeks on, 1 week off. Adjust for symptoms. Can be given continuously.
➤ **Vasomotor menopausal symptoms**
Adult females: 1.25 mg PO daily in cycles of 3 weeks on, 1 week off. If patient is menstruating, cyclic administration is started on day 5 of bleeding.
➤ **Moderate to severe menopausal vulvar and vaginal atrophy**
Adult females: 0.3 to 1.25 mg or more PO daily, depending on tissue response of individual patient, in cycles of 3 weeks on, 1 week off.

ADMINISTRATION
PO
❸ *Alert:* Hazardous drug; use safe handling and disposal precautions.
• Use lowest effective dose needed for specific indication.
• Give drug without regard to food.

ACTION

Mimics the actions of endogenous estrogens; increases synthesis of DNA, RNA, and protein in responsive tissues; reduces release of FSH and LH from pituitary gland.

Route	Onset	Peak	Duration
PO	Unknown	Unknown	Unknown

Half-life: Unknown.

ADVERSE REACTIONS

CNS: headache, migraine, dizziness, chorea, depression, nervousness, mood disturbance, irritability, exacerbation of epilepsy, dementia exacerbation, *stroke, seizure exacerbation.* **CV:** thrombophlebitis, *VTE,* HTN, edema, *MI.* **EENT:** worsening myopia or astigmatism, intolerance of contact lenses, retinal thrombosis. **GI:** nausea, vomiting, abdominal cramps, bloating, anorexia, increased appetite, *pancreatitis,* gallbladder disease. **GU:** breakthrough bleeding, altered menstrual flow, dysmenorrhea, amenorrhea, premenstrual-like syndrome, *endometrial cancer, ovarian cancer,* endometrial hyperplasia, cervical erosion, altered cervical secretions, enlargement of uterine fibromas, vaginal candidiasis, testicular atrophy, impotence, change in libido, cystitis-like syndrome. **Hepatic:** cholestatic jaundice, benign liver adenoma. **Metabolic:** hypercalcemia, weight gain or loss, hypertriglyceridemia, carbohydrate intolerance. **Respiratory:** asthma exacerbation. **Skin:** melasma, chloasma, rash, pruritus, urticaria, hirsutism or hair loss, erythema nodosum, *erythema multiforme,* dermatitis. **Other:** breast tenderness, enlargement, or secretion; gynecomastia; *breast cancer;* hypersensitivity reaction, including *anaphylaxis.*

INTERACTIONS

Drug-drug. *Anastrozole:* May interfere with anastrozole effectiveness. Avoid use together.
Clarithromycin, erythromycin, itraconazole, ketoconazole, ritonavir: May increase estrogen plasma levels and side effects. Monitor patient.
Corticosteroids: May increase corticosteroid effects. Monitor patient closely.
CYP3A4 inducers (carbamazepine, fosphenytoin, phenobarbital, phenytoin, rifampin): May decrease effects of estrogen therapy. Monitor patient closely.

Dantrolene, liver toxic drugs: May increase risk of liver toxicity. Closely monitor liver function.
Exemestane: May interfere with exemestane effectiveness. Avoid use together.
Oral anticoagulants: May decrease anticoagulant effects. Adjust dosage if needed. Monitor PT and INR.
Ospemifene: May enhance adverse or toxic effect of and interfere with effectiveness of ospemifene. Avoid use together.
Thyroid replacement therapy: May decrease thyroid hormone levels. Higher doses of thyroid hormone may be required.
Tranexamic acid: May enhance thrombogenic effect. Avoid if possible.
Drug-herb. *Red clover:* May increase estrogen effects. Discourage use together.
St. John's wort: May decrease effects of drug. Discourage use together.
Drug-food. *Folic acid:* May decrease absorption of folic acid. Monitor levels.
Grapefruit, grapefruit juice: May increase risk of adverse effects. Discourage use together.
Drug-lifestyle. *Alcohol use:* May increase estrogen level and risk of breast cancer and osteoporosis. Avoid concurrent use.
Smoking: May increase risk of CV effects. Recommend smoking cessation. If smoking continues, consider alternative therapy.

EFFECTS ON LAB TEST RESULTS

• May increase calcium, thyroid-binding globulin, circulating thyroid hormone, serum triglyceride, HDL-C, and serum phospholipid levels.
• May decrease LDL-C level.
• May increase platelet count.
• May alter clotting factors.
• May accelerate PT, PTT, and platelet aggregation time.
• May reduce response to metyrapone test.
• May cause impaired glucose tolerance.

CONTRAINDICATIONS & CAUTIONS

• Contraindicated in patients hypersensitive to drug and in patients with breast cancer (except metastatic disease), estrogen-dependent neoplasia, active thrombophlebitis, thromboembolic disorders, undiagnosed abnormal genital bleeding, liver dysfunction or disease, or history of thromboembolic disease.
• Use cautiously in patients with history of HTN, mental depression, cardiac or kidney

dysfunction, gallbladder disease, bone disease, migraine, seizures, SLE, porphyria, asthma, or diabetes.

• Patients who use estrogen replacement for longer than 5 years after menopause may be at increased risk for endometrial cancer. Taking the lowest possible estrogen dose and using cyclic rather than continuous therapy reduces the risk. Adding progestins to regimen decreases risk of endometrial hyperplasia. Progestins' effect on endometrial cancer risk is unknown.

Boxed Warning Don't use drug for prevention of CV disease. Drug is associated with dementia in patients ages 65 and older who are postmenopausal. Estrogen, with or without progestin, should be prescribed at lowest effective dose for shortest duration consistent with treatment goals. ■

Dialyzable drug: Unknown.

⚠ *Overdose S&S:* Nausea, withdrawal bleeding in females.

PREGNANCY-LACTATION-REPRODUCTION

• Use is contraindicated during pregnancy.

• There is no indication for use during pregnancy. Use of estrogen and progestin (as in combination hormonal contraceptives) hasn't been associated with teratogenic effects when inadvertently taken early in pregnancy.

• Estrogen appears in and decreases the quantity and quality of human milk. Use only if clearly needed; closely monitor infant's growth.

NURSING CONSIDERATIONS

🜂 *Alert:* Drug is a high-risk medication for older adults.

Boxed Warning Close clinical surveillance of all patients taking estrogens is important because estrogens have been reported to increase risk of endometrial cancer. Adequate diagnostic measures, including endometrial sampling when indicated, should be undertaken to rule out malignancy in all cases of undiagnosed persistent or recurring abnormal vaginal bleeding. ■

• Reevaluate therapy as clinically appropriate to determine treatment necessity.

• When given for short-term use, administration should be cyclic and attempts to discontinue or taper the medication should be made at 3- to 6-month intervals.

• Make sure patient undergoes thorough physical exam before starting estrogen

therapy. Patient receiving long-term therapy should undergo annual exams. Periodically monitor body weight, BP, lipid levels, and liver function.

• Notify pathologist about patient's estrogen therapy when sending specimens to the lab for evaluation.

🜂 *Alert:* Because of risk of VTE, stop therapy at least 4 to 6 weeks before procedures that cause prolonged immobilization or increased risk of VTE.

• May impair glucose tolerance. Closely monitor glucose level in patient with diabetes.

• Monitor calcium level in patient with breast cancer or bone metastases. If hypercalcemia occurs, stop drug and treat appropriately to reduce calcium level.

• Monitor for vision changes. Stop drug pending examination if sudden partial or complete vision loss, migraine, double vision, or other changes occur.

PATIENT TEACHING

• Advise patient to promptly report all adverse reactions.

• Emphasize the importance of regular physical exams.

🜂 *Alert:* Warn patient to immediately report abdominal pain; pain, numbness, or stiffness in legs or buttocks; pressure or pain in chest or shortness of breath; severe headaches; visual disturbances, such as blind spots, flashing lights, or blurriness; vaginal bleeding or discharge; breast lumps; swelling of hands or feet; yellow skin or sclera; dark urine; or light-colored stools.

• Tell patient with diabetes to report elevated glucose level so that antidiabetic dosage can be adjusted.

• Explain to patient receiving cyclic therapy for postmenopausal symptoms that withdrawal bleeding may occur during week off drug. Tell patient to report unusual vaginal bleeding.

• Teach patient to perform routine breast self-exam.

• Advise patient of childbearing potential to consult prescriber before taking drug and to immediately inform prescriber of pregnancy.

• Teach patient methods to decrease risk of blood clots.

• Encourage smoking cessation to reduce risk of CV complications, as applicable.

estradiol ⚕
es-tra-DYE-ole

Alora, Climara, Dotti, Estrace, Estring Vaginal Ring, Evamist, Imvexxy, Menostar, Minivelle, Vagifem, Vivelle, Vivelle-Dot, Yuvafem

estradiol acetate
Femring

estradiol cypionate
Depo-Estradiol

estradiol gel
Divigel, Elestrin, EstroGel

estradiol valerate
Delestrogen

Therapeutic class: Estrogens
Pharmacologic class: Estrogens

AVAILABLE FORMS
estradiol
Spray, topical solution: 1.53 mg/spray
Tablets: 0.5 mg, 1 mg, 2 mg
Transdermal: 0.014 mg/24 hours, 0.025 mg/24 hours, 0.0375 mg/24 hours, 0.05 mg/24 hours, 0.06 mg/24 hours, 0.075 mg/24 hours, 0.1 mg/24 hours
Vaginal cream: 0.1 mg/g (0.01%)
Vaginal ring (extended-release): 2 mg (0.0075 mg/24 hours)
Vaginal tablets: 4 mcg, 10 mcg
estradiol acetate
Vaginal ring: 0.05 mg/24 hours; 0.1 mg/24 hours
estradiol cypionate
Injection (in oil): 5 mg/mL
estradiol gel
Transdermal gel: 0.06% (0.87 g/activation), 0.06% (1.25 g/activation), 0.1% (in 0.25 mg, 0.5 mg, 0.75 mg, 1 mg, and 1.25 mg single-dose packets)
estradiol valerate
Injection (in oil): 10 mg/mL, 20 mg/mL, 40 mg/mL

INDICATIONS & DOSAGES
➤ **Vasomotor menopausal symptoms, female hypogonadism, female castration, primary ovarian failure**
Adult females: 1 to 2 mg PO estradiol daily. Or, for vasomotor symptoms, 1 to 5 mg

cypionate IM once every 3 to 4 weeks or 10 to 20 mg valerate IM once every 4 weeks. For female hypogonadism, 1.5 to 2 mg cypionate IM or 10 to 20 mg valerate IM once every month.
Adult females (transdermal patch): Apply patch according to manufacturer's instructions. Adjust dosage, if necessary, after the first 2 or 3 weeks of therapy. Attempt to taper or discontinue at 3- to 6-month intervals.
➤ **Moderate to severe vasomotor symptoms from menopause**
Adult females: Start with Divigel 0.25 g transdermally daily and adjust dosage based on patient response (range, up to 1.25 g/day). Or, 1 pump per day of Elestrin transdermally applied to the upper arm. Or, Evamist 1 spray transdermally per day initially; may adjust dose based on clinical response (1 to 3 sprays/day). Or, 1.25 g EstroGel applied transdermally once daily to arm. Or, 0.05 to 0.1 mg daily by vaginal ring; replace vaginal ring every 3 months.
➤ **Vulvar and vaginal atrophy**
Adult females: 0.025 to 0.05 mg/24 hours transdermal patch applied once or twice weekly continuously or as directed following in a cyclic regimen (3 weeks on, 1 week off). Adjust dosage based on clinical response. Or, 1.25 g EstroGel applied once daily to skin. Or, 2 to 4 g vaginal applications of cream daily for 1 to 2 weeks; then gradually reduce to one-half initial dosage for 1 to 2 weeks. When vaginal mucosa is restored, maintenance dosage is 1 g one to three times weekly in a cyclic regimen. Or, 10 to 20 mg valerate IM every 4 weeks as needed. Or, vaginal ring retained for 90 days; replace vaginal ring every 3 months.
Adjust-a-dose: Attempt to taper dose or discontinue drug at 3- to 6-month intervals.
➤ **Atrophic vaginitis due to menopause**
Adult females: 10-mcg tablet vaginally once daily for 2 weeks. Maintenance dose is 1 tablet inserted vaginally twice weekly. Periodically reevaluate need for treatment.
➤ **Dyspareunia due to menopause-related vulvar and vaginal atrophy**
Adult females: Initially, 4 mcg Imvexxy tablet vaginally once daily for 2 weeks; then 1 tablet twice weekly. May increase to 10-mcg tablets based on clinical response.
➤ **Palliative treatment of advanced, inoperable breast cancer**
Adult males and postmenopausal adult females: 10 mg PO estradiol t.i.d. for 3 months.

Reactions in bold italics are ***life-threatening***.

➤ **Palliative treatment of advanced, inoperable prostate cancer**
Adult males: 30 mg valerate IM every 1 to 2 weeks or 1 to 2 mg estradiol PO t.i.d.
➤ **To prevent postmenopausal osteoporosis**
Adult females: Place 6.5-cm^2 (0.025 mg/24 hours) Climara patch once weekly on clean, dry skin of lower abdomen or upper quadrant of buttock. Or, place 3.25-cm^2 (0.014 mg/24 hours) Menostar patch once weekly to clean, dry area of lower abdomen. Or, place 0.025 mg/24 hours patch twice weekly in cyclic regimen in patients with intact uterus. In patients who have had hysterectomy, apply one patch twice weekly in a continuous regimen. Or, 0.025-mg/24 hours Vivelle, Vivelle-Dot, or Alora system applied to a clean, dry area of the trunk twice weekly. Or, 0.5 mg PO daily for 23 days, followed by 5 days without drug.

ADMINISTRATION
PO
• Give drug without regard to food. If stomach upset occurs, give with food.
• Store at controlled room temperature.
IM
• To give IM injection, roll vial between palms to disperse drug.
• Visually inspect solution to ensure that it's clear and colorless to pale yellow. If solution is stored at low temperature, some crystals may form that redissolve with warming.
• Inject deep into upper outer quadrant of gluteal muscle. Rotate injection sites to prevent muscle atrophy. Never give IV.
• Topical applications are preferred over IM for treatment of vulval and vaginal atrophy.
Transdermal
• Apply Elestrin once daily to upper arm.
• Apply EstroGel over entire area of one arm on the inside and outside from wrist to shoulder. Don't massage or rub EstroGel. Allow gel to dry for 5 minutes before patient dresses.
• Apply Evamist each morning to adjacent, nonoverlapping areas on inner surface of forearm, starting near elbow. Allow to dry for 2 minutes; do not wash site for 30 minutes.
• Apply Divigel once daily on skin of either right or left upper thigh. Application surface area should be about 5 × 7 inches (12.5 × 18 cm), or the size of two palm prints. Apply entire contents of unit-dose packet each day. To avoid potential skin irritation, apply Divigel to right or left upper thigh on alternating days.

Don't apply Divigel on face, breasts, or irritated skin or in or around vagina. After application, allow gel to dry before dressing. Don't wash application site within 1 hour after applying Divigel. Avoid contact of gel with eyes. Wash hands after application.
• Apply transdermal patch to clean, dry, hairless, intact skin on abdomen or buttock. Don't apply to breasts, waistline, or other areas where clothing can loosen patch. When applying, ensure thorough contact between patch and skin, especially around edges, and hold in place for about 10 seconds. Apply patch immediately after opening and removing protective cover. Rotate application sites.
• Dispose of patches by folding adhesive ends together and discarding properly in trash away from children and pets.
Vaginal
• Using the applicator, insert vaginal tablet as far into vagina as it can comfortably go, without using force. Insert Imvexxy with smaller end up to a depth of about 2 inches into vaginal canal.
• Remove vaginal ring from its pouch. Squeeze sides together and insert ring into vagina where comfortable.
• Rinse vaginal ring in lukewarm water and reinsert if ring falls out or is removed before end of treatment.
• Attach applicator to vaginal cream tube and squeeze tube from the bottom to expel prescribed amount of cream into applicator. Remove applicator from tube and insert deeply into vagina. Press plunger downward to its original position.
• Cleanse vaginal cream applicator by washing in mild soap and water; allow it to dry thoroughly.

ACTION
Increases synthesis of DNA, RNA, and protein in responsive tissues; reduces release of FSH and LH from pituitary gland.

Route	Onset	Peak	Duration
PO, IM, vaginal	Unknown	Unknown	Unknown
Transdermal gel (EstroGel)	Immediate	1 hr	24–36 hr

Half-life: Alora transdermal patch, 1.75 ± 2.87 hours; Vivelle transdermal patch, 4.4 ± 2.3 hours; Vivelle-Dot transdermal patch, 5.9 to 7.7 hours; other forms, unknown. Estradiol apparent elimination half-life, 21 to 26 hours. Estradiol apparent terminal half-life, about 10 hours after Divigel administration.

ADVERSE REACTIONS

CNS: *stroke,* headache, migraine, pain, asthenia, dizziness, fatigue, anxiety, nervousness, mood disturbance, irritability, dementia, chorea, depression, *seizure exacerbation.* **CV:** thrombophlebitis, *VTE,* HTN, edema, *MI.* **EENT:** worsening myopia or astigmatism, intolerance of contact lenses, retinal thrombosis, sinusitis, nasopharyngitis. **GI:** nausea, vomiting, abdominal pain or cramps, bloating, constipation, flatulence, gastroenteritis, *pancreatitis,* gallbladder disease, dyspepsia. **GU:** UTI, breakthrough bleeding, altered menstrual flow, dysmenorrhea, *endometrial cancer,* cervical erosion (ring), altered cervical secretions, uterine pain, enlargement of uterine fibromas, vaginal candidiasis, genital pruritus, vaginal discomfort, vaginal discharge, vaginitis. **Hepatic:** cholestatic jaundice. **Metabolic:** weight gain, hypothyroidism, hypercalcemia (in patients with breast cancer and bone metastases). **Musculoskeletal:** arthralgia, back pain, myalgia, neck pain, limb pain, fractures. **Respiratory:** URI, asthma exacerbation, bronchitis. **Skin:** application-site reaction, acne, rash, melasma, erythema nodosum, dermatitis, hair loss, hirsutism, pruritus. **Other:** gynecomastia, *breast cancer,* hot flashes, breast tenderness or enlargement, nipple pain or discharge, flulike syndrome, accidental injury.

INTERACTIONS

Drug-drug. *Anastrozole:* May interfere with anastrozole effectiveness. Avoid use together.
Carbamazepine, fosphenytoin, phenobarbital, phenytoin, rifampin: May decrease effectiveness of estrogen therapy. Monitor patient closely.
Clarithromycin, erythromycin, itraconazole, ketoconazole, ritonavir: May increase estrogen plasma level and side effects. Monitor patient.
Corticosteroids: May enhance effects of corticosteroids. Monitor patient closely.
Cyclosporine: May increase risk of toxicity. Use together with caution, and frequently monitor cyclosporine level.
Dantrolene, other liver-toxic drugs: May increase risk of liver toxicity. Closely monitor liver function.
Exemestane: May interfere with exemestane effectiveness. Avoid use together.
Lamotrigine: May decrease lamotrigine level. Monitor therapy.

Oral anticoagulants: May decrease anticoagulant effect. Dosage adjustments may be needed. Monitor PT and INR.
Ospemifene: May enhance adverse or toxic effects of ospemifene and interfere with its effectiveness. Avoid use together.
Thyroid hormones: May decrease therapeutic effect. Monitor therapy.
Drug-herb. *Red clover:* May increase estrogen effects. Discourage use together.
Saw palmetto: May negate drug's effects. Discourage use together.
St. John's wort: May decrease effects of drug. Discourage use together.
Drug-food. *Caffeine:* May increase caffeine level. Advise patient to avoid or minimize use of caffeine.
Folic acid: May decrease absorption of folic acid. Monitor levels.
Grapefruit juice: May elevate drug level. Tell patient to take drug with liquid other than grapefruit juice.
Drug-lifestyle. *Alcohol use:* May increase estrogen level and risk of breast cancer and osteoporosis. Avoid concurrent use.
Smoking: May increase risk of adverse CV effects. Recommend smoking cessation. If smoking continues, consider alternative therapy.

EFFECTS ON LAB TEST RESULTS

- May increase LFT values and total T_4, thyroid-binding globulin, HDL-C, and triglyceride levels.
- May decrease LDL-C level.
- May increase platelet count.
- May alter clotting factors.
- May accelerate PT, PTT, and platelet aggregation times.
- May decrease metyrapone test results.
- May impair glucose tolerance.

CONTRAINDICATIONS & CAUTIONS

- Contraindicated in patients with active or history of thrombophlebitis or thromboembolic disorders, estrogen-dependent neoplasia, breast or reproductive organ cancer, or undiagnosed abnormal genital bleeding.
- ⌧ Contraindicated in patients with protein C, protein S, or antithrombin deficiency or other known thrombophilic disorders.
- Contraindicated in patients with liver dysfunction or disease.
- ⌧ Contraindicated in patients with known anaphylactic reaction or angioedema caused by drug. Exogenous estrogens may exacerbate

signs and symptoms of angioedema in adult females with hereditary angioedema.
• Use cautiously in patients with cerebrovascular disease or CAD, asthma, bone disease, diabetes, gallbladder disease, hypothyroidism, porphyria, SLE, migraines, seizures, or cardiac or kidney dysfunction.
🧬 Use cautiously in patients with strong family history (grandmother, mother, sister) of breast cancer, breast nodules, fibrocystic breasts, or abnormal mammogram findings.
Boxed Warning Patients ages 50 to 79 who are postmenopausal and are taking estrogen and progestin have an increased risk of MI, stroke, invasive breast cancer, PE, and thrombosis. Patients ages 65 and older who are postmenopausal also have an increased risk of dementia. ■
Dialyzable drug: Unknown.
⚠ *Overdose S&S:* Nausea, vomiting, withdrawal uterine bleeding.

PREGNANCY-LACTATION-REPRODUCTION
• Use is contraindicated during pregnancy.
• Use of estrogen and progestin (as in combination hormonal contraceptives) hasn't been associated with teratogenic effects when inadvertently taken early in pregnancy.
• Estrogen appears in and decreases the quantity and quality of human milk. Use only if clearly needed; closely monitor infant's growth.

NURSING CONSIDERATIONS
• Ensure that patient undergoes physical exam before starting therapy. Patients receiving long-term therapy should have yearly exams. Monitor lipid levels, BP, body weight, and liver function.
Boxed Warning Estrogen increases the risk of endometrial cancer. Use diagnostic tests, including endometrial sampling when indicated, to rule out malignancy in cases of undiagnosed persistent or recurring abnormal vaginal bleeding. ■
Boxed Warning Don't use estrogen, with or without progestin, to prevent CV disease or dementia. Use lowest effective dose for shortest duration consistent with treatment goals. ■
• When estrogen is prescribed for patient with uterus who is postmenopausal, also initiate progestin to reduce risk of endometrial cancer.
🔆 *Alert:* EstroGel contains alcohol. Avoid fire, flame, or smoking until area dries (in 2 to 5 minutes).

• In patient also taking oral estrogen, treatment with transdermal patch can begin 1 week after withdrawal of oral therapy, or sooner if menopausal symptoms appear before the end of the week.
• Transdermal system may be used continually rather than cyclically in patient without an intact uterus. Other alternative regimens include 10 to 20 mg valerate IM every 4 weeks, as needed.
• Prescriber should assess patient's need to continue estradiol therapy. Make attempts to stop or taper at 3- to 6-month intervals.
• Because of risk of VTE, stop therapy at least 1 month before high-risk procedures or those that cause prolonged immobilization.
• Glucose tolerance may be impaired. Closely monitor glucose level in patient with diabetes.
• Notify pathologist about estrogen therapy when sending specimens for lab evaluation.

PATIENT TEACHING
• Tell patient to read package insert describing estrogen's adverse effects, and explain those effects.
• Emphasize importance of regular physical exams. Using estrogen replacement for longer than 5 years after menopause may increase risk of endometrial cancer. Using cyclic rather than continuous therapy and lowest possible dosages of estrogen reduces risk. Adding progestins to regimen decreases risk of endometrial hyperplasia; however, it isn't known whether progestins affect risk of endometrial cancer. No increased risk of breast cancer has been reported.
Boxed Warning Advise patient not to allow contact between children and Evamist application site. Accidental exposure may cause breast budding and breast masses in prepubertal females and gynecomastia and breast masses in prepubertal males. ■
• Teach about proper drug administration and handling. Instruct patient to follow package insert for prescribed product.
• Instruct patient or caregiver how to inject estradiol valerate, if able to administer.
• Caution patient using vaginal tablet who has severely atrophic vaginal mucosa to be careful to avoid abrasions when inserting applicator.
• After gynecologic surgery, tell patient to use any vaginal applicator cautiously and only if clearly indicated.

❶ Alert: Warn patient to immediately report abdominal pain, chest pressure or pain, shortness of breath, severe headaches, visual disturbances, vaginal bleeding or discharge, breast lumps, swelling of hands or feet, yellow skin or sclerae, dark urine, light-colored stools, and pain, numbness, or stiffness in legs or buttocks.

• Explain to patient receiving cyclic therapy for postmenopausal symptoms that withdrawal bleeding may occur during week off drug. Instruct patient to report unusual vaginal bleeding.

• Tell patient with diabetes to report elevated glucose level so that antidiabetic drug dosage can be adjusted.

• Teach patient how to perform routine breast self-exam.

• Advise patient not to become pregnant during estrogen therapy.

• Encourage smoking cessation to reduce risk of CV complications, as applicable.

• Advise patient not to allow pets to lick or touch Evamist application site. If signs of illness occur, instruct patient to contact veterinarian.

estradiol–norethindrone acetate transdermal system ℞

ess-tra-DYE-ole/nor-ETH-in-drone

CombiPatch

Therapeutic class: Estrogens
Pharmacologic class: Estrogen–progestin combinations

AVAILABLE FORMS

Transdermal: 9-cm² system releasing 0.05 mg estradiol and 0.14 mg norethindrone acetate/day; 16-cm² system releasing 0.05 mg estradiol and 0.25 mg norethindrone acetate/day

INDICATIONS & DOSAGES

➤ **Moderate to severe vasomotor symptoms from menopause; vulval and vaginal atrophy; hypoestrogenemia from hypogonadism, castration, or primary ovarian failure in patient with intact uterus**
Adult females (continuous combined regimen): Continuously wear 9-cm² patch system on lower abdomen. Replace system twice weekly

during 28-day cycle. May increase to 16-cm² patch.
Adult females (continuous sequential regimen): In sequential regimen with estradiol transdermal system, wear 0.05-mg estradiol transdermal patch for first 14 days of 28-day cycle; replace system twice weekly. Wear 9-cm² estradiol/norethindrone patch on lower abdomen for rest of 28-day cycle; replace system according to product directions. May increase to 16-cm² patch.

ADMINISTRATION
Transdermal

❶ Alert: Hazardous drug; use safe handling and disposal precautions.

• Keep patch sealed until ready to apply.

• Apply patch system to smooth (fold-free), clean, dry, nonirritated area of skin on lower abdomen, avoiding waistline. Rotate application sites, with interval of at least 1 week between applications to same site.

• Don't apply patch on or near breasts.

• Avoid applying to areas that may get prolonged sun exposure.

• If patch falls off, reapply to another area of lower abdomen. If patch fails to adhere, replace with new patch in a different area.

• Remove patch slowly to avoid skin irritation.

• Fold patch so that it sticks to itself, and discard in trash out of reach of children and pets. Don't flush patch down toilet.

ACTION

Estrogen replacement therapy can reduce menopausal symptoms and release of FSH and LH by binding to nuclear receptors in estrogen-responsive tissues in patients who are postmenopausal. Norethindrone blocks gonadotropin, which inhibits ovulation.

Route	Onset	Peak	Duration
Transdermal	12–24 hr	Unknown	Unknown

Half-life: Estradiol, 2 to 3 hours; norethindrone, 6 to 8 hours.

ADVERSE REACTIONS

CNS: asthenia, depression, insomnia, nervousness, dizziness, headache, weakness, pain. **CV:** HTN, edema. **EENT:** pharyngitis, rhinitis, sinusitis, tooth disorder. **GI:** abdominal pain, diarrhea, dyspepsia, flatulence, nausea, constipation, gallbladder disease. **GU:** dysmenorrhea, leukorrhea, menstrual disorder, changes in libido, suspicious

Reactions in bold italics are *life-threatening*.

Papanicolaou smears, vaginitis, menorrhagia, *vaginal hemorrhage.* **Metabolic:** hypercalcemia (in patients with breast cancer and bone metastases). **Musculoskeletal:** arthralgia, back pain. **Respiratory:** respiratory disorder, bronchitis. **Skin:** application-site reactions, acne, rash. **Other:** accidental injury, flulike syndrome, breast pain, breast enlargement, infection.

INTERACTIONS

Drug-drug. *Anastrozole:* May interfere with anastrozole effectiveness. Avoid use together.

Carbamazepine, fosphenytoin, phenobarbital, phenytoin, rifampin: May decrease estrogen therapy effectiveness. Monitor patient closely.

Clarithromycin, erythromycin, itraconazole, ketoconazole, ritonavir: May increase estrogen plasma level and adverse effects. Monitor patient.

Corticosteroids: May enhance effects of corticosteroids. Monitor patient closely.

Cyclosporine: May increase risk of toxicity. Use together with caution; frequently monitor cyclosporine level.

Dantrolene, liver toxic drugs: May increase risk of liver toxicity. Monitor liver function closely.

Exemestane: May interfere with exemestane effectiveness. Avoid use together.

Oral anticoagulants: May decrease effect of anticoagulant, requiring dosage adjustment. Monitor PT and INR.

Ospemifene: May enhance adverse effects of ospemifene and interfere with its effectiveness. Avoid use together.

Drug-herb. *Red clover:* May increase estrogen effects. Discourage use together.

Saw palmetto: May cause antiestrogenic effects. Discourage use together.

St. John's wort: May decrease effects of drug. Discourage use together.

Drug-food. *Caffeine:* May increase caffeine level. Advise patient to avoid or minimize use of caffeine.

Folic acid: May decrease absorption of folic acid. Monitor folic acid level.

Grapefruit juice: May elevate estrogen level. Advise patient to avoid taking drug with grapefruit juice.

Drug-lifestyle. *Alcohol use:* May increase estrogen level and risk of breast cancer and osteoporosis. Instruct patient to avoid use together.

Smoking: May increase risk of adverse CV effects. Recommend smoking cessation. If smoking continues, consider alternative therapy.

Sun exposure: May cause photosensitivity reactions. Don't expose patch to sun for long periods of time.

EFFECTS ON LAB TEST RESULTS

- May increase T_3, T_4, HDL-C, triglyceride, and transaminase levels.
- May decrease LDL-C level.
- May increase fibrinogen activity and platelet count.
- May decrease T_3 resin uptake.
- May accelerate PT, PTT, and platelet aggregation time.
- May reduce response to metyrapone test. May alter glucose tolerance test results.

CONTRAINDICATIONS & CAUTIONS

- Contraindicated in patients with known anaphylactic reaction or angioedema to estrogen, progestin, or any component of the patch and in patients with known, suspected, or history of breast cancer; known or suspected estrogen-dependent neoplasia; known liver impairment or disease; undiagnosed abnormal genital bleeding; active thrombophlebitis; or thromboembolic disorders, including MI, VTE, or stroke.

- Contraindicated in patients with known protein C, protein S, or antithrombin deficiency or other thrombophilic disorders.

Boxed Warning Don't use estrogen, with or without progestin, to prevent CV disease or dementia. Use drug with or without progestin at lowest effective doses and for shortest duration consistent with treatment goals. ∎

Boxed Warning Patients ages 50 to 79 who are postmenopausal and taking estrogen and progestin have an increased risk of MI, stroke, invasive breast cancer, and VTE. Patients ages 65 and older who are postmenopausal also have an increased risk of dementia. ∎

- Exogenous estrogens may exacerbate angioedema in patients with hereditary angioedema.

- Use cautiously in patients with asthma, epilepsy, migraines, SLE, porphyria, diabetes, liver hemangiomas, or cardiac or kidney dysfunction.

- Drug may increase risk of gallbladder disease after menopause.

Dialyzable drug: Unknown.

⚠ *Overdose S&S:* Nausea, withdrawal bleeding.

PREGNANCY-LACTATION-REPRODUCTION
• Contraindicated with known or suspected pregnancy.
• Estrogen appears in and decreases the quantity and quality of human milk. Use cautiously in patients who are breastfeeding.

NURSING CONSIDERATIONS
• Treatment of postmenopausal symptoms often starts when vasomotor symptoms begin.
• Combined estrogen-progestin regimen is indicated for patient with intact uterus. Progestin taken with estrogen reduces risk of endometrial cancer linked to use of estrogen alone.

Boxed Warning Estrogen increases risk of endometrial cancer. Adding a progestin to estrogen therapy reduces risk of endometrial hyperplasia. For patient who is postmenopausal, use diagnostic tests, including endometrial sampling when indicated, to rule out malignancy if undiagnosed persistent or recurring abnormal vaginal bleeding occurs. ■

• Patient not receiving continuous estrogen or combined estrogen-progestin therapy may start therapy at any time.
• Patient receiving continuous hormone replacement therapy should complete the current cycle before starting therapy. Withdrawal bleeding commonly occurs with cycle completion; first day of withdrawal bleeding is an appropriate time to start therapy.
• Reevaluate therapy at 3- to 6-month intervals.
• Stop therapy at least 4 to 6 weeks before surgery associated with an increased risk of VTE and during periods of prolonged immobilization.
• BP increases have been linked to estrogen use. Regularly monitor patient's BP.
• Closely monitor glucose level in patient with diabetes.
• **Alert:** Don't interchange CombiPatch with other estrogen patches. Verify therapy before application.

PATIENT TEACHING
• Teach patient how to properly apply, remove, and dispose of patch.
• Tell patient that oil-based cream or lotion may help remove adhesive from the skin after patch has been removed and area allowed to dry for 15 minutes.
• Advise patient not to use patch if pregnant or planning to become pregnant.

• Inform patient that continuous combined regimen may lead to irregular bleeding, particularly in first 6 months, but bleeding often decreases with time and stops completely.
• Explain that monthly withdrawal bleeding commonly occurs with continuous sequential regimen.
• Advise patient to alert prescriber and remove patch at first sign of clotting disorder (cerebrovascular disorder, VTE).
• Instruct patient to stop using patch and call prescriber about any loss of vision, sudden onset of eyeball protrusion (proptosis), double vision, or migraine.
• Encourage smoking cessation to reduce risk of CV complications, as applicable.
• Advise patient to perform monthly breast self-exams and to have annual gynecologic and breast exams by a health care provider.
• Tell patient undergoing MRI to alert facility of transdermal patch.

estradiol–progesterone ✕
ES-tra-dye-ole/proe-JES-te-rone

Bijuva

Therapeutic class: Menopause drugs
Pharmacologic class: Estrogen–progestin combinations

AVAILABLE FORMS
Capsules: 1 mg estradiol/100 mg progesterone

INDICATIONS & DOSAGES
➤ **Moderate to severe vasomotor symptoms due to menopause**
Patients with intact uterus: 1 capsule PO once daily.

ADMINISTRATION
PO
• Give drug with food in the evening.
• Give a missed dose as soon as possible, unless it's within 2 hours of the next dose.
• Store drug at room temperature.

ACTION
Circulating estrogens modulate the pituitary secretion of the gonadotropins LH and FSH through a negative feedback mechanism. Estrogens reduce elevated levels of these hormones seen in patients who are postmenopausal. Progesterone opposes the action

of estrogen by decreasing estrogen receptor level, increasing metabolism of estrogen to less-active metabolites, or blunting the response to estrogen at the cellular level.

Route	Onset	Peak	Duration
PO	Unknown	Estradiol, 5 hr; progesterone, 3 hr	Unknown

Half-life: Estradiol, 26 hours; progesterone, 10 hours.

ADVERSE REACTIONS
CNS: headache. **GI:** nausea. **GU:** vaginal bleeding, vaginal discharge, pelvic pain. **Other:** breast tenderness.

INTERACTIONS
Drug-drug. *CYP3A4 inducers (carbamazepine, phenobarbital, rifampin):* May decrease estrogen and progestin levels, decreasing therapeutic effect and causing changes in uterine bleeding. Monitor patient closely.
CYP3A4 inhibitors (clarithromycin, erythromycin, itraconazole, ketoconazole, ritonavir): May increase estrogen and progestin levels and increase adverse effects. Monitor patient closely.
Drug-herb. *St. John's wort:* May decrease estrogen and progestin levels, decreasing therapeutic effect and causing changes in uterine bleeding. Monitor patient closely.
Drug-food. *Grapefruit juice:* May increase plasma levels of estrogen and progestin. Discourage use together.
Drug-lifestyle. *Smoking:* May increase risk of adverse CV effects. Recommend smoking cessation. If smoking continues, consider alternative therapy.

EFFECTS ON LAB TEST RESULTS
• May increase HDL-C and triglyceride levels.
• May decrease LDL-C level.
• May increase or decrease calcium level.
• May accelerate PT, PTT, and platelet aggregation time.
• May increase platelet count and clotting factors.
• May decrease antifactor Xa and antithrombin III levels.
• May increase fibrinogen and plasminogen levels and activity.
• May increase circulating total thyroid hormone, corticosteroid binding globulin, sex hormone-binding globulin, free testosterone,

and free estradiol levels as well as other plasma protein test results.
• May impair glucose tolerance.

CONTRAINDICATIONS & CAUTIONS
• Contraindicated in patients with undiagnosed abnormal genital bleeding; known, suspected, or history of breast cancer; known or suspected estrogen-dependent neoplasia; active DVT, PE, arterial thromboembolic disease or history of these conditions; known anaphylactic reaction, angioedema, or hypersensitivity to estrogen or progesterone or capsule ingredients; or known liver impairment or disease.
▧ Contraindicated in patients with known protein C, protein S, or antithrombin deficiency or other known thrombophilic disorders.
Boxed Warning Patients ages 50 to 79 who are postmenopausal and are taking estrogen and progestin have an increased risk of VTE, stroke, MI, and invasive breast cancer. Patients ages 65 and older who are postmenopausal also have an increased risk of dementia. ■
Boxed Warning Estrogen plus progestin therapy shouldn't be used to prevent CV disease or dementia. ■
Boxed Warning Unopposed estrogen therapy increases risk of endometrial cancer in patients with a uterus. Adding a progestin to estrogen therapy reduces risk of endometrial hyperplasia, which may lead to endometrial cancer. ■
Boxed Warning Use lowest effective dose for shortest duration consistent with treatment goals and individual risks. Reevaluate patients as clinically appropriate to determine continuing need for treatment. ■
• Estrogen therapy may cause retinal vascular thrombosis.
• Drug may increase risk of gallbladder disease after menopause.
• Drug may increase risk of pancreatitis in patients with preexisting hypertriglyceridemia. If pancreatitis occurs, consider discontinuing drug.
• Drug may be poorly metabolized by patients with impaired liver function. Use cautiously in patients with history of cholestatic jaundice associated with estrogen use or with pregnancy. If cholestatic jaundice recurs, discontinue drug.
▧ Use cautiously in patients with history of asthma, diabetes, cardiac or kidney

dysfunction, epilepsy, migraines, porphyria, SLE, liver hemangiomas, or hereditary angioedema. Estrogen therapy may exacerbate these conditions.

• Drug isn't indicated for use in children.

Dialyzable drug: Unknown.

⚠ *Overdose S&S:* Nausea, vomiting, breast tenderness, abdominal pain, drowsiness, fatigue, withdrawal bleeding.

PREGNANCY-LACTATION-REPRODUCTION

• Drug isn't indicated for use during pregnancy or in patients of childbearing potential.

• Estrogen appears in and decreases the quantity and quality of human milk. Use cautiously in patients who are breastfeeding.

NURSING CONSIDERATIONS

Boxed Warning Assess patient who is postmenopausal with undiagnosed persistent or recurring abnormal genital bleeding to rule out malignancy. ∎

• Assess baseline risk of breast cancer and CV disease before starting drug.

• Monitor BP, fluid status, lipid levels, LFT values, and thyroid function during therapy as clinically indicated. Patient on thyroid replacement therapy may require a higher dose of thyroid hormone.

• Monitor calcium level in patient with breast cancer and bone metastases. Discontinue drug for hypercalcemia and treat calcium level as appropriate.

• Ensure that patient receives age-appropriate breast and pelvic exams.

• Monitor patient for vision abnormalities. If sudden partial or complete loss of vision or sudden onset of proptosis, diplopia, or migraine occurs, discontinue drug and obtain eye exam. If eye exam reveals papilledema or retinal vascular lesions, permanently discontinue drug.

• Discontinue estrogen therapy at least 4 to 6 weeks before surgery associated with an increased risk of VTE and during periods of prolonged immobilization.

• *Look alike–sound alike:* Don't confuse this product with other estrogen or progesterone products.

PATIENT TEACHING

• Teach about proper drug administration and handling.

• Instruct patient to report all adverse reactions.

Boxed Warning Warn patient of possible serious adverse reactions related to drug, including CV disorders, malignant neoplasms, and age-related probable dementia. ∎

• Instruct patient to immediately report abnormal vaginal bleeding; new breast lumps; changes in vision or speech; sudden, new headaches; severe chest or leg pain with or without shortness of breath; weakness and fatigue; or vomiting.

• Inform patient that drug may need to be stopped before surgery or bed rest.

• Tell patient that prescriber will evaluate continued need for treatment every 3 to 6 months.

• Instruct patient to have yearly pelvic and breast exams and mammograms, unless otherwise directed by prescriber.

estradiol valerate–estradiol valerate with dienogest ℞

ess-tra-DYE-ole VAL-er-ate/dye-EN-oh-jest

Natazia

Therapeutic class: Estrogens
Pharmacologic class: Estrogen–progestin combinations

AVAILABLE FORMS

Tablets: 28-day blister pack containing two 3-mg estradiol valerate, five 2-mg estradiol valerate with 2-mg dienogest, seventeen 2-mg estradiol valerate with 3-mg dienogest, two 1-mg estradiol valerate, and two inert tablets

INDICATIONS & DOSAGES

➤ **Prevention of pregnancy; treatment of heavy menstrual bleeding in patients without organic pathology who choose to use an oral contraceptive**

Females after menarche: 1 tablet PO daily beginning on first day of menstrual cycle bleeding in order directed on blister pack. When changing from another combination hormonal contraceptive, begin on first day of withdrawal bleeding. When changing from combination hormonal vaginal ring or transdermal patch, begin on day of vaginal ring or transdermal patch removal. When changing from progestin-only contraceptive, begin on day patient would have taken the next progestin-only pill. When changing from implant contraceptive or intrauterine system, begin on day of implant or intrauterine system removal. When changing from injection contraceptive, begin day next injection is due.

ADMINISTRATION
PO
❸ *Alert:* Hazardous drug; use safe handling and disposal precautions.
• Give at same the time each day; don't skip or delay intake by more than 12 hours.
• Follow manufacturer's detailed instructions if 1 or 2 tablets are missed; patient should use additional backup nonhormonal forms of contraception, if necessary.
• If patient experiences severe vomiting or diarrhea within 3 to 4 hours after taking a colored tablet, treat as a missed tablet.
• Must give tablets in order indicated on blister pack.

ACTION
Prevents pregnancy by suppressing ovulation. May also cause changes in endometrium and cervical mucus, inhibiting sperm penetration and reducing likelihood of implantation.

Route	Onset	Peak	Duration
PO	Unknown	3 hr (estradiol); 1.5 hr (dienogest)	Unknown

Half-life: Estradiol, 14 hours; dienogest, 11 hours.

ADVERSE REACTIONS
CNS: mood changes (depression, mood swings, dysthymic disorder, crying), headache or migraine. **GI:** nausea, vomiting. **GU:** menstrual disorder (amenorrhea, irregular uterine bleeding, metrorrhagia, *uterine hemorrhage*). **Metabolic:** weight gain. **Skin:** acne. **Other:** breast pain, tenderness, or discomfort; hypersensitivity reaction.

INTERACTIONS
Drug-drug. *HIV protease inhibitors, NNRTIs:* May either increase or decrease estrogen and progesterone levels. Use together cautiously and monitor patient for effectiveness of hormone treatment.
Lamotrigine: May decrease lamotrigine serum level, reducing seizure control. Adjust lamotrigine dosage as necessary.
Strong CYP3A4 inducers (barbiturates, carbamazepine, felbamate, griseofulvin, oxcarbazepine, phenytoin, rifampin, topiramate): May reduce contraceptive effectiveness or

increase breakthrough bleeding. Instruct patient to use alternative birth control method.
Strong and moderate inhibitors of CYP3A4 (cimetidine, clarithromycin, diltiazem, erythromycin, fluconazole, itraconazole, ketoconazole, SSRIs, verapamil, voriconazole): May increase levels of hormones. Avoid use together. If drugs must be used together, monitor patient for adverse effects.
Thyroid hormone: May increase serum level of thyroid-binding globulin, leading to decreased effectiveness of thyroid replacement therapy. Monitor patient; thyroid hormone dosage may need adjustment.
Drug-herb. *Red clover:* May increase estrogen effects. Discourage use together.
St. John's wort: May reduce contraceptive effectiveness or increase breakthrough bleeding. Recommend alternative birth control method.
Drug-food. *Grapefruit juice:* May increase hormone levels. Avoid use together.
Drug-lifestyle. **Boxed Warning** *Smoking:* Increases risk of serious CV events, such as stroke, emboli, and heart disease. Recommend smoking cessation. ■

EFFECTS ON LAB TEST RESULTS
• May increase thyroid-binding globulin, glucose, cholesterol, and triglyceride levels.
• May alter clotting factors.
• May affect glucose tolerance test results.

CONTRAINDICATIONS & CAUTIONS
• Contraindicated in patients with benign or malignant liver tumors; liver disease; current or history of breast cancer or other estrogen- or progestin-sensitive cancer; undiagnosed abnormal uterine bleeding; headaches with focal neurologic symptoms or migraines with or without aura if older than age 35; diabetes with vascular disease; uncontrolled HTN; HTN with vascular disease; thrombogenic valvular or thrombogenic rhythm disease of heart, such as endocarditis or atrial fibrillation; CAD; cerebrovascular disease; and current or past VTE.
⚵ Contraindicated in patients with inherited or acquired hypercoagulopathies.
Boxed Warning Contraindicated in patients who smoke and who are older than age 35. ■
• Use cautiously in females with CV disease risk factors, history of cholestasis, history of well-controlled HTN, prediabetes or well-controlled diabetes, history of

hyperlipidemia, new-onset headaches, history of bleeding irregularities, or history of emotional disorders, angioedema, or chloasma.

⚕ Exogenous estrogens may exacerbate signs and symptoms of angioedema in patients with hereditary angioedema.

• Drug may increase risk of gallbladder disease.
• Use isn't recommended in patients with complicated solid organ transplant or SLE.
• Safety and effectiveness in females with BMI greater than 30 kg/m² haven't been evaluated.
• Drug isn't indicated in patients who are postmenopausal.

Dialyzable drug: Unknown.

⚠ *Overdose S&S:* Nausea, withdrawal bleeding.

PREGNANCY-LACTATION-REPRODUCTION

• Use is contraindicated during pregnancy.
• Use of estrogen and progestin (as in combination hormonal contraceptives) hasn't been associated with teratogenic effects when inadvertently taken early in pregnancy.
• Estrogen appears in and decreases the quantity and quality of human milk. Use cautiously during breastfeeding.
• Use before menarche isn't indicated.

NURSING CONSIDERATIONS

• Start drug no earlier than 4 weeks after delivery in patient who isn't breastfeeding. Risk of postpartum VTE decreases and ovulation risk increases after third postpartum week.
• Monitor BP; elevations are possible in females who are nonhypertensive.
• Monitor coagulation factors as appropriate.
• Regularly monitor glucose and cholesterol levels, especially in patient who is prediabetic or has history of elevated lipid levels.
• Monitor patient for headache. New-onset headaches may require discontinuing oral contraceptives.
• Carefully monitor patient with history of depression for recurrence or exacerbation.
• Stop drug if arterial or deep VTE occurs. Highest risk of VTE occurs during first year of contraceptive use. If feasible, stop tablets at least 4 weeks before and for 2 weeks after major surgery.
• Oral contraceptives are associated with increased risk of thrombotic and hemorrhagic strokes, especially in females older than age 35, in those with HTN, and in smokers. Stop drug if unexplained vision loss, proptosis, diplopia, papilledema, or retinal vascular

changes occur. Immediately evaluate retinal vein thrombosis.
• Risk of drug causing breast, cervical, or endometrial cancer remains uncertain. As a precaution, patient should have regular Papanicolaou tests, breast exams, and mammograms.
• Discontinue drug if jaundice develops. Patients who take oral contraceptives are at higher risk for liver tumors and gallstones. Monitor patient for skin color changes and pain in right upper quadrant.
• Ensure that patient uses a nonhormonal contraceptive method, such as a condom or spermicide, for the first 9 days.

PATIENT TEACHING

• Teach about proper drug administration and handling. Ensure patient reads patient guide for information on missed tablets and reasons to contact pharmacist or prescriber; tell patient that backup contraception must be used.
• Tell patient starting drug for first time to begin taking tablets on day 1 of menses and to use backup contraception for first 9 days.
• Inform patient that spotting or light bleeding may occur at first.
• Advise patient that nausea is possible, especially during first few months, but that this symptom usually disappears. Instruct patient not to stop taking tablets. Tell patient to report to prescriber if nausea doesn't resolve.
• Warn patient to start drug no earlier than 4 weeks after giving birth.
• Advise patient to notify prescriber if pregnant before taking drug.
• Tell patient that breastfeeding while taking tablets isn't recommended because milk production may be reduced and small amounts of drug appear in human milk.
• Inform patient taking tablets that blood tests may be needed to assess blood clotting and blood glucose and cholesterol levels and that BP monitoring may also be needed.
• Tell patient to inform prescriber if taking prescription or OTC medications or herbal supplements.
• Advise patient to quit smoking before taking drug, as appropriate.

Boxed Warning Inform patient who smokes of increased risk of serious CV events from combination oral contraceptive use. Risk increases with age, especially after age 35, and with number of cigarettes smoked. ∎

• Warn patient that contraceptive use doesn't protect against HIV infection or other STIs.
• Tell patient that a missed period may occur but that pregnancy should be ruled out for two or more consecutive missed menstrual cycles.
• Advise patient to immediately report persistent leg pain; sudden shortness of breath; sudden blindness (partial or complete); severe chest pain; sudden, severe headache; weakness or numbness in arm or leg; trouble speaking; or yellowing of skin or eyes.
• Inform patient with tendency to chloasma to avoid sun exposure and UV radiation.

estrogens (conjugated) (estrogenic substances, conjugated; oestrogens, conjugated) ☒
Premarin

Therapeutic class: Estrogens
Pharmacologic class: Estrogens

AVAILABLE FORMS
Injection: 25-mg vial
Tablets: 0.3 mg, 0.45 mg, 0.625 mg, 0.9 mg, 1.25 mg
Vaginal cream: 0.625 mg/g

INDICATIONS & DOSAGES
➤ **Abnormal uterine bleeding (hormonal imbalance)**
Adult females: 25 mg slow IV (preferred) or IM. Repeat dose in 6 to 12 hours, if needed.
➤ **Vulvar or vaginal atrophy; kraurosis vulvae**
Adult females: 0.5 to 2 g cream intravaginally once daily in cycles of 21 days on, 7 days off.
➤ **Moderate to severe dyspareunia due to menopause-related vulvar and vaginal atrophy**
Adult females: 0.5 g cream intravaginally twice weekly as a continuous regimen. Or, 0.5 g intravaginally once daily for 21 days, followed by 7 days off.
➤ **Moderate to severe vasomotor symptoms with or without moderate to severe symptoms of vulvar and vaginal atrophy associated with menopause**
Adult females: Initially, 0.3 mg PO daily. May give continuously or cyclically 25 days on, 5 days off. Adjust dosage based on patient response.

➤ **Hypoestrogenism due to castration or primary ovarian failure**
Adult females: Initially, 1.25 mg PO daily in cycles of 3 weeks on, 1 week off. Adjust dose as needed.
➤ **Hypoestrogenism due to female hypogonadism**
Adult females: 0.3 to 0.625 mg PO daily, given cyclically 3 weeks on, 1 week off. Adjust dose depending on symptom severity and responsiveness of the endometrium.
➤ **Prevention of osteoporosis**
Females who are postmenopausal: 0.3 mg PO daily or cyclically 25 days on, 5 days off. Adjust dose based on response of bone mineral density testing.
➤ **Palliative treatment of inoperable prostatic cancer**
Adult males: 1.25 to 2.5 mg PO t.i.d. Judge effectiveness based on phosphatase determinations and symptomatic improvement.
➤ **Palliative treatment of breast cancer**
Adult males and females: 10 mg PO t.i.d. for at least 3 months.

ADMINISTRATION
⚠️ *Alert:* Hazardous drug; use safe handling and disposal precautions.
PO
• Give drug at same time each day.
• May give with or without food.
• Store tablets at controlled room temperature.
IV
▼ IV use is preferred over IM use due to more-rapid response.
▼ Refrigerate drug before reconstituting it.
▼ Store injection in refrigerator (36° to 46° F [2° to 8° C]).
▼ Reconstitute slowly with 5 mL sterile water for injection. Gently agitate; don't shake.
▼ Drug is compatible with NSS and dextrose and invert sugar solutions.
▼ Use solution immediately after reconstitution.
▼ Give direct injection slowly to avoid flushing reaction.
▼ **Incompatibilities:** Acidic solutions, ascorbic acid, protein hydrolysate.
IM
• Reconstitute with sterile water for injection. Agitate gently after adding diluent.
• Inject deep into large muscle.
• Rotate injection sites to prevent muscle atrophy.

Vaginal

- Wash vaginal area with soap and water
- Attach applicator to tube.
- Gently squeeze tube from bottom to fill tube with prescribed dose.
- Insert about two-thirds of applicator length into vagina, and release drug.
- Separate applicator's barrel and plunger. Wash them with mild soap and warm water.
- Give drug at bedtime or when patient will lie flat for 30 minutes after use to minimize drug loss.
- Store cream at room temperature.

ACTION

Increases synthesis of DNA, RNA, and protein in responsive tissues. Also reduces release of FSH and LH from pituitary gland.

Route	Onset	Peak	Duration
PO, IV, IM, vaginal	Unknown	7 hr	Unknown

Half-life: 27 hours.

ADVERSE REACTIONS

CNS: asthenia, headache, pain, dizziness, migraine, anxiety, depression, emotional lability, insomnia, nervousness, *exacerbation of seizures.* **CV:** flushing with rapid IV administration; palpitations, vasodilation, HTN, edema, *VTE.* **EENT:** worsening myopia or astigmatism, intolerance of contact lenses. **GI:** nausea, vomiting, abdominal pain or cramps, bloating, flatulence, constipation, diarrhea, dyspepsia, increased appetite. **GU:** *vaginal hemorrhage,* breakthrough bleeding, altered menstrual flow, dysmenorrhea, amenorrhea, leukorrhea, cervical disorder, endometrial disorder, enlargement of uterine fibromas, uterine spasm, vaginal candidiasis, vaginal dryness, vaginitis, vulvovaginal disorder, pelvic pain, dysuria, urinary frequency, UTI, impotence, changes in libido. **Hepatic:** cholestatic jaundice. **Metabolic:** weight gain, hypercalcemia, hyperlipidemia, hypertriglyceridemia. **Musculoskeletal:** arthralgia, back or chest pain, muscle cramps, myalgia. **Skin:** skin discoloration, diaphoresis, acne, erythema, pruritus, rash, urticaria, hirsutism or hair loss, erythema nodosum. **Other:** breast tenderness or secretion, gynecomastia, *breast cancer.*

INTERACTIONS

Drug-drug. *Anastrozole:* May interfere with anastrozole effectiveness. Avoid use together.
Corticosteroids: May enhance corticosteroid effects. Monitor patient closely.
Cyclosporine: May increase risk of toxicity. Use together with caution, and frequently monitor cyclosporine level.
CYP3A4 inducers (carbamazepine, fosphenytoin, phenobarbital, phenytoin, rifampin): May decrease effectiveness of estrogen therapy. Monitor patient closely.
CYP3A4 inhibitors (itraconazole, ketoconazole, macrolide antibiotics, ritonavir): May increase estrogen plasma level and risk of adverse effects. Monitor patient.
Dantrolene, other liver toxic drugs: May increase risk of liver toxicity. Monitor liver function closely.
Exemestane: May interfere with exemestane effectiveness. Avoid use together.
Oral anticoagulants: May decrease anticoagulant effects, requiring dosage adjustment. Monitor PT and INR.
Ospemifene: May enhance adverse or toxic effects of ospemifene and interfere with its effectiveness. Avoid use together.
Thyroid hormones: May increase serum thyroxine-binding globulin level, which may increase thyroid hormone requirements.
Drug-herb. *Red clover:* May increase estrogen effects. Discourage use together.
Saw palmetto: May have antiestrogenic effects. Discourage use together.
St. John's wort: May decrease effects of drug. Discourage use together.
Drug-food. *Caffeine:* May increase caffeine level. Advise caution.
Grapefruit juice: May increase estrogen level. Instruct patient to avoid use together.
Drug-lifestyle. *Smoking:* May increase risk of adverse CV effects. Recommend smoking cessation. If smoking continues, recommend nonhormonal contraception.

EFFECTS ON LAB TEST RESULTS

- May increase T_3, total T_4, phospholipid, thyroid-binding globulin, HDL-C, and triglyceride levels.
- May decrease LDL-C level.
- May increase platelet count.
- May alter clotting factors.
- May accelerate PT, PTT, and platelet aggregation time.

Reactions in bold italics are *life-threatening*.

• May cause false-positive metyrapone test result.

• May interfere with glucose tolerance test.

CONTRAINDICATIONS & CAUTIONS

• Contraindicated in patients with liver dysfunction, thrombophlebitis, thromboembolic disorders, active or history of DVT or PE, known or suspected estrogen-dependent neoplasia, breast or reproductive cancer (except for palliative treatment), undiagnosed abnormal genital bleeding, and known anaphylactic reaction or angioedema to conjugated estrogens.

🔬 Contraindicated in patients with known protein C, protein S, or antithrombin deficiency or other thrombophilic disorders.

Boxed Warning Don't use to prevent CV disease. In patients who are postmenopausal receiving therapy for more than 5 years, drug may increase risks of MI, stroke, invasive breast cancer, and VTE. Use lowest effective dose for shortest duration, considering benefits and risks. ∎

Boxed Warning In patients who are postmenopausal receiving therapy for more than 5 years, drug may increase risk of endometrial cancer. Use cyclic therapy and lowest possible dose to reduce risk. Adding progestin decreases risk of endometrial hyperplasia but effect on endometrial cancer risk is unknown. ∎

Boxed Warning Drug shouldn't be used to prevent dementia. Drug may increase risk of dementia in patients after menopause who are ages 65 and older and receiving conjugated estrogens plus medroxyprogesterone acetate for 4 years. ∎

• Use cautiously in patients with cerebrovascular disease or CAD, asthma, bone disease, migraines, seizures, SLE, porphyria, liver hemangioma, gallbladder disease, diabetes, hypoparathyroidism, or kidney dysfunction.

🔬 Use cautiously in patients with strong family history (mother, grandmother, sister) of breast or reproductive tract cancer, breast nodules, fibrocystic breasts, or abnormal mammogram findings.

🔬 Exogenous estrogens may exacerbate signs and symptoms of angioedema in females with hereditary angioedema.

• Drug may increase risk of gallbladder disease.

Dialyzable drug: Unknown.

⚠ *Overdose S&S:* Nausea, vomiting, breast tenderness, abdominal pain, drowsiness or fatigue, withdrawal uterine bleeding.

PREGNANCY-LACTATION-REPRODUCTION

• Contraindicated with known or suspected pregnancy.

• Estrogen appears in and decreases the quantity and quality of human milk. Drug shouldn't be used during breastfeeding.

NURSING CONSIDERATIONS

• Make sure patient has thorough physical exam before starting therapy; patient receiving long-term therapy should have yearly exams. Periodically monitor lipid levels, BP, body weight, and liver function.

• Rapid treatment of dysfunctional uterine bleeding or reduction of surgical bleeding usually requires delivery by IV or IM route.

• Periodically reevaluate need for therapy.

• When used solely to treat vulval and vaginal atrophy, consider topical products.

• Ensure adequate calcium and vitamin D intake to prevent osteoporosis.

• Monitor calcium level in patient with breast cancer and bone metastases. Discontinue drug for hypercalcemia, and treat calcium level as appropriate.

• Because of VTE risk, stop therapy at least 4 to 6 weeks before procedures that prolong immobilization or raise risk of VTE.

• Notify pathologist about estrogen therapy when sending specimens for lab evaluation.

• Glucose tolerance may be impaired. Closely monitor glucose level in patient with diabetes.

• *Look alike–sound alike:* Don't confuse Premarin with Primaxin, Provera, or Remeron.

PATIENT TEACHING

• Teach about proper drug administration and handling.

• Instruct patient to promptly report adverse effects.

• Emphasize importance of regular physical exams.

• Explain that cyclic therapy for postmenopausal symptoms may cause withdrawal bleeding during week off drug. Tell patient to report unusual vaginal bleeding.

🔔 *Alert:* Warn patient to immediately report abdominal pain; pain, numbness, or stiffness in legs or buttocks; chest pressure or pain;

shortness of breath; severe headaches; visual disturbances, such as blind spots, flashing lights, or blurriness; vaginal bleeding or discharge; breast lumps; swelling of hands or feet; yellow skin or sclerae; dark urine; and light-colored stools.
- Tell patient with diabetes to report elevated glucose level so that antidiabetic drug dosage can be adjusted.
- Teach patient how to perform routine breast self-exam.
- Advise patient not to become pregnant during estrogen therapy.
- Encourage smoking cessation to reduce risk of CV complications, as applicable.
- Tell patient using drug for osteoporosis prevention to ensure adequate intake of calcium and vitamin D.
- Inform patient that vaginal cream may weaken latex condoms. Instruct patient to use alternative method of contraception.

SAFETY ALERT!

eszopiclone
es-zoe-PIK-lone

Lunesta

Therapeutic class: Hypnotics
Pharmacologic class: Pyrrolopyrazine derivatives
Controlled substance schedule: IV

AVAILABLE FORMS
Tablets: 1 mg, 2 mg, 3 mg

INDICATIONS & DOSAGES
➤ **Insomnia**
Adults: 1 mg PO immediately before bedtime. Increase to 2 or 3 mg as needed.
Adjust-a-dose: In older adults, patients who are debilitated, patients with Child-Pugh Class C liver impairment, and those also taking a potent CYP3A4 inhibitor, don't exceed 2-mg dose.

ADMINISTRATION
PO
- Don't give drug with or immediately after a meal.
- Give drug immediately before bedtime because drug may cause dizziness or lightheadedness.

ACTION
Probably interacts with GABA receptors at allosteric binding sites close to or connected to benzodiazepine receptors.

Route	Onset	Peak	Duration
PO	Rapid	1 hr	Unknown

Half-life: 6 hours.

ADVERSE REACTIONS
CNS: abnormal dreams, anxiety, confusion, depression, dizziness, hallucinations, headache, migraine, nervousness, pain, somnolence, neuralgia, unpleasant taste.
CV: chest pain, edema. **EENT:** dry mouth.
GI: diarrhea, dyspepsia, nausea, vomiting.
GU: dysmenorrhea, UTI, decreased libido.
Respiratory: URI. **Skin:** pruritus, rash.
Other: accidental injury, viral infection, infection, gynecomastia.

INTERACTIONS
Drug-drug. *CNS depressants:* May have additive CNS effects. Adjust dosage of either drug as needed.
CYP3A4 inducers (rifampin): May decrease eszopiclone level and effects. Monitor therapy.
Boxed Warning *Opioid class warning:* May cause slow or difficult breathing, sedation, and death. Avoid use together. If use together can't be avoided, limit dose and duration of each drug to the minimum needed for desired effect. ■
Strong CYP3A4 inhibitors (clarithromycin, itraconazole, ketoconazole, nefazodone, nelfinavir, ritonavir): May decrease eszopiclone elimination, increasing toxicity risk. Use together cautiously. Limit eszopiclone dose.
Drug-herb. *St. John's wort:* May decrease eszopiclone level. Discourage use together.
Drug-food. *High-fat meals:* May delay drug's effects. Discourage high-fat meals with or just before taking drug.
Drug-lifestyle. *Alcohol use:* May decrease psychomotor ability. Discourage taking drug if patient drank alcohol that evening or before bed.

EFFECTS ON LAB TEST RESULTS
None reported.

CONTRAINDICATIONS & CAUTIONS
- Contraindicated in patients with known hypersensitivity to eszopiclone.

Boxed Warning Drug may cause rare but serious injury, including death, due to complex sleep behaviors, such as sleepwalking, sleep driving, and engaging in other activities while not fully awake. These behaviors can occur at the lowest recommended dosages and after just one dose. Drug is contraindicated in patients with a history of complex sleep behavior after taking eszopiclone. ■

• Rarely, drug may cause angioedema and anaphylaxis that require emergency treatment and can be fatal. Don't rechallenge patients who develop angioedema after drug therapy.

Boxed Warning *Opioid class warning:* Opioids should only be prescribed with benzodiazepines or other CNS depressants when alternative treatment options are inadequate, aren't expected to provide adequate analgesia, haven't been tolerated, or aren't expected to be tolerated. ■

• Use cautiously in older adults and patients who are debilitated, in patients with diseases or conditions that could affect metabolism or hemodynamic responses, and in patients with compromised respiratory function or severe liver impairment. Also use cautiously in patients with signs and symptoms of depression because of increased suicide risk.

• Safety and effectiveness in children haven't been established.

⚠ *Overdose S&S:* CNS depression.

PREGNANCY-LACTATION-REPRODUCTION
• Use during pregnancy only if potential benefit justifies fetal risk.
• It isn't known if drug appears in human milk. Breastfeeding isn't recommended.

NURSING CONSIDERATIONS
🔹 *Alert:* Anaphylaxis and angioedema may occur as early as the first dose; monitor patient closely.

🔹 *Alert:* Drug may increase risk of next-day impairment of driving and other activities that require full alertness. Risk increases with dosage and if drug is taken with less than 7 or 8 hours of sleep. Patient taking 3-mg dose shouldn't drive or perform activities requiring mental alertness during the morning after use.
• Evaluate patient for physical and psychiatric disorders before treatment.
• Use lowest effective dose.
• Give drug immediately before patient goes to bed or after patient has gone to bed and has trouble falling asleep.

• Use only for short periods (for example, 7 to 10 days). If patient still has trouble sleeping, check for other psychological disorders.
• Risk of abuse and dependence increases with dose and duration of treatment and concurrent use of other psychoactive drugs. Abrupt discontinuation may cause withdrawal symptoms.
• Monitor patient for changes in behavior (decreased inhibition, aggression, agitation), including those that suggest depression or suicidality. Amnesia and other neuropsychiatric symptoms may occur unpredictably.

PATIENT TEACHING
Boxed Warning *Opioid class warning:* Caution patient or caregiver of patient taking an opioid with a benzodiazepine, CNS depressant, or alcohol to seek immediate medical attention for dizziness, light-headedness, extreme sleepiness, slowed or difficult breathing, or unresponsiveness. ■

Boxed Warning Warn patient of risk of injury or death related to complex sleep behaviors. Direct patient to stop drug and immediately inform prescriber if an episode of complex sleep behavior occurs or if patient doesn't remember activities performed while taking drug. ■

• Warn patient that drug may cause allergic reactions (rash, shortness of breath, facial swelling).

🔹 *Alert:* Caution patient taking 3 mg of eszopiclone not to drive or engage in activities that are hazardous or require complete mental alertness the day after use.
• Caution patient not to take drug unless a full night's sleep is possible.
• Advise patient to avoid taking drug after a high-fat meal and to avoid alcohol.
• Tell patient to avoid activities that require mental alertness until drug's effects are known.
• Urge patient to immediately report changes in behavior and thinking.
• Warn patient not to stop drug abruptly or change dose without consulting prescriber.
• Inform patient that tolerance or dependence may develop if drug is taken for a prolonged period.
• Teach about proper drug administration, handling, storage, and disposal.

BIOSIMILAR DRUG

etanercept
ee-TAN-er-sept

Enbrel

etanercept-szzs
Erelzi

etanercept-ykro
Eticovo

Therapeutic class: Antiarthritics
Pharmacologic class: TNF blockers

AVAILABLE FORMS
Injection (powder): 25 mg multidose vial
Injection (solution): 25 mg/0.5 mL single-dose vial
Prefilled autoinjector: 50 mg/mL
Prefilled single-dose syringe: 25 mg/0.5 mL, 50 mg/mL

INDICATIONS & DOSAGES
➤ **Polyarticular juvenile idiopathic arthritis**
Children ages 2 to 17: For children weighing 63 kg or more, 50 mg subcut once weekly. For children weighing less than 63 kg (Enbrel only), 0.8 mg/kg subcut once weekly. Maximum dosage, 50 mg/week. Glucocorticoids, NSAIDs, or analgesics may be continued during treatment. Use with methotrexate hasn't been studied in children.
➤ **RA, ankylosing spondylitis, psoriatic arthritis**
Adults: 50 mg subcut once weekly. Methotrexate, glucocorticoids, salicylates, NSAIDs, and analgesics may be continued during treatment.
➤ **Chronic moderate to severe plaque psoriasis in patients who are candidates for systemic therapy or phototherapy**
Adults: 50 mg subcut twice weekly for 3 months; then reduce dosage to 50 mg subcut once weekly.
Children ages 4 and older: For patients weighing 63 kg or more, 50 mg subcut once weekly. For patients weighing less than 63 kg, 0.8 mg/kg (Enbrel or Erelzi) subcut once weekly. Maximum dosage, 50 mg/week.

ADMINISTRATION
Subcutaneous
• Give 50-mg dose as one subcut injection using 50-mg/mL single-use prefilled syringe or prefilled autoinjector or as two 25-mg subcut injections using prefilled syringe or multidose vial. May give the two 25-mg injections on the same day or 3 to 4 days apart.
• No dosage form for Erelzi or Eticovo allows weight-based dosing for children weighing less than 63 kg.
• To achieve pediatric doses other than 25 or 50 mg, use reconstituted Enbrel.
• Store single-dose vial, prefilled syringe, or prefilled autoinjector under refrigeration at 36° to 46° F (2° to 8° C), but warm to room temperature (15 to 30 minutes) before use. Don't remove needle cover or vial cap while allowing drug to reach room temperature.
• Don't return prefilled syringe, prefilled autoinjector, or single-dose vial to refrigerator after it has reached room temperature. Protect from light and heat and, if not used, discard after 30 days (Enbrel), 28 days (Erelzi), or 14 days (Eticovo).
• Reconstitute multidose vial aseptically with 1 mL of supplied sterile bacteriostatic water for injection (0.9% benzyl alcohol). Use a 25G needle rather than the supplied vial adapter if the vial will be used for multiple doses, but use a 27G needle for injection. Don't filter reconstituted solution when preparing or giving drug. Inject diluent slowly into vial. Refrigerate reconstituted vial for up to 14 days at 36° to 46° F (2° to 8° C); discard after 14 days.
• Minimize foaming by gently swirling, rather than shaking, during dissolution. Dissolution takes less than 10 minutes.
• Don't use solution if it's discolored or cloudy or contains particulate matter.
• Separate injection sites by at least 1 inch (2.5 cm), rotate regularly, and never use areas where skin is tender, bruised, red, or hard. Use sites on thigh, abdomen, and upper arm.
⚠ *Alert:* Needle covers of diluent syringe, prefilled syringe, and needle within cap of the pen contain latex and shouldn't be handled by persons sensitive to latex.

ACTION
Binds specifically to TNF and blocks its action with cell-surface TNF receptors, reducing inflammatory and immune responses found in RA.

Reactions in bold italics are *life-threatening*.

Route	Onset	Peak	Duration
Subcut	Unknown	72 hr	Unknown

Half-life: About 5 days.

ADVERSE REACTIONS
CNS: dizziness, fever. **Respiratory:** URI, lower respiratory infection. **Skin:** injection-site reaction, rash, urticaria, pruritus. **Other:** infection, antibody development, hypersensitivity.

INTERACTIONS
Drug-drug. *Antidiabetics:* Increase risk of hypoglycemia. Antidiabetic drug dosage reduction may be needed.
Cyclophosphamide: May increase risk of solid malignancies. Use together not recommended.
Immunomodulators (abatacept, anakinra, belimumab, canakinumab, certolizumab pegol, infliximab, natalizumab, vedolizumab): Increases risk of serious infection. Use together isn't recommended.
Sulfasalazine: May cause decreased neutrophil count. Monitor patient carefully.
Vaccines (inactivated): May reduce vaccine effectiveness. Complete all age-appropriate vaccinations at least 2 weeks before start of immunosuppressive therapy.
Vaccines (live-virus): May affect normal immune response. Postpone live-virus vaccination until 3 months after etanercept discontinuation.
Drug-herb. *Echinacea:* May diminish drug's therapeutic effect. Discourage use together. If used together, monitor patient for decreased effect of etanercept.

EFFECTS ON LAB TEST RESULTS
• May decrease RBC, ANC, thrombocyte, and WBC counts.

CONTRAINDICATIONS & CAUTIONS
• Contraindicated in patients hypersensitive to drug or its components and in those with sepsis.
• Use cautiously in patients ages 65 and older and in patients with underlying diseases that predispose them to infection, such as diabetes, HF, or history of active or chronic infections.
• Rare cases of new-onset or exacerbations of CNS and peripheral nervous system demyelinating disorders (transverse myelitis, optic neuritis, MS, Guillain-Barré syndrome) and seizure disorders have occurred.
• Use cautiously in patients with history of HF or moderate to severe alcoholic hepatitis.
• Don't start drug in patients with an active infection, patients who have been exposed to TB, or patients with history of opportunistic infection, including clinically important localized infections, because of increased risk of serious infections that may lead to hospitalizations or death.
• Use cautiously in patients who reside in or have traveled to areas of endemic TB or endemic mycoses (histoplasmosis, coccidioidomycosis, blastomycosis).
• Use cautiously in patients previously infected with HBV.
• Avoid use in patients with Wegener granulomatosis who are receiving immunosuppressants; drug may increase risk of malignancy.
• Ensure children are up-to-date with all immunizations before start of therapy.
Dialyzable drug: Unknown.

PREGNANCY-LACTATION-REPRODUCTION
• Use during pregnancy only if clearly needed.
• Drug is present in low levels in human milk and is minimally absorbed by an infant who is breastfed. Use cautiously during breastfeeding.

NURSING CONSIDERATIONS
• Based on their conditions of use, no clinical differences exist between biosimilar product and reference product. However, they aren't interchangeable.
Boxed Warning Patients treated with anti-TNF therapies are at increased risk for serious, sometimes fatal, infections (TB; invasive fungal infections; bacterial, viral, and other infections). Most patients who developed serious infections are also receiving immunosuppressants, such as methotrexate or corticosteroids. Monitor patient carefully; if serious infection or sepsis occurs, stop therapy, and notify prescriber. ∎
Boxed Warning Infections, including bacterial sepsis and TB, have been reported. Evaluate patient's risk factors and test for latent TB. Begin treatment for latent TB before therapy with etanercept and monitor patient for active TB during treatment, even if initial latent TB test is negative. ∎

⚠ *Alert:* Don't give live-virus vaccines during therapy.

• Temporarily interrupt treatment in patients with varicella virus exposure; consider preventive treatment with varicella zoster immune globulin.

Boxed Warning Histoplasmosis, coccidioidomycosis, blastomycosis, and other opportunistic infections may develop with use of drug. Consider empirical antifungal therapy in patient at risk for invasive fungal infection with severe systemic illness. ∎

Boxed Warning Lymphoma and other, sometimes fatal, malignancies have been reported in children and adolescents. ∎

• Evaluate patient at increased risk for HBV infection before treatment, and monitor patient for reactivation during and for several months after therapy ends. If reactivation occurs, drug may need to be stopped and antiviral therapy begun.

• Monitor for hypersensitivity reactions and signs and symptoms of new or worsening HF.

• *Look alike–sound alike:* Don't confuse etanercept-szzs (Erelzi) or etanercept-ykro (Eticovo) with the reference drug etanercept (Enbrel).

PATIENT TEACHING

• Teach patient who is self-administering drug about mixing and injection techniques, including the need to rotate injection sites.

• Explain that injection-site reactions usually disappear in 3 to 5 days. Tell patient to contact prescriber if they persist.

• Instruct patient to avoid live-virus vaccine administration during therapy.

• Advise patient to report signs or symptoms of pancytopenia (bruising, bleeding, persistent fever, pallor).

• Instruct patient to report signs or symptoms of new or worsening medical conditions, such as CNS demyelinating disorders (numbness, tingling, vision changes, weakness of arms and legs, dizziness), seizures, or HF.

• Stress importance of alerting other health care providers about this therapy.

• Instruct patient to promptly report signs of infection (persistent fever, cough, shortness of breath, fatigue).

• Advise patient to discuss pregnancy, plans to become pregnant, and breastfeeding with prescriber.

ethacrynate sodium
eth-a-KRIH-nayt

Edecrin

ethacrynic acid
Edecrin

Therapeutic class: Diuretics
Pharmacologic class: Loop diuretics

AVAILABLE FORMS
ethacrynate sodium
Injection: 50 mg/vial
ethacrynic acid
Tablets: 25 mg

INDICATIONS & DOSAGES
➤ **Edema (rapid diuresis)**
Adults: 50 mg or 0.5 to 1 mg/kg IV. Usually only one dose is needed; give a second dose PRN.
➤ **Edema**
Adults: 50 to 200 mg PO daily. May increase to 200 mg b.i.d. if needed for desired effect in 25- to 50-mg increments. May give continuously or intermittently.
Children ages 13 months and older: First dose is 25 mg PO, increased cautiously by 25 mg daily until desired effect is achieved.
Adjust-a-dose: If added to existing diuretic regimen, first dose is 25 mg and dosage adjustments are made in 25-mg increments.

ADMINISTRATION
PO
• Give drug in morning to prevent nocturia.
• Give after meals.
IV
▼ Add 50 mL of D_5W or NSS to vial.
▼ Don't use cloudy or opalescent solution.
▼ Give over several minutes through tubing of running infusion.
▼ If more than one IV dose is needed, use a new injection site to avoid thrombophlebitis.
▼ Discard unused solution after 24 hours.
▼ **Incompatibilities:** Hydralazine, Normosol-M, procainamide, ranitidine, solutions or drugs with pH below 5, whole blood and its derivatives.

ACTION
Potent loop diuretic; inhibits sodium and chloride reabsorption at proximal and distal tubules and ascending loop of Henle.

Route	Onset	Peak	Duration
PO	30 min	2 hr	6–8 hr
IV	5 min	15–30 min	2 hr

Half-life: 2 to 4 hours.

ADVERSE REACTIONS

CNS: malaise, confusion, fatigue, apprehension, vertigo, headache, fever. **CV:** orthostatic hypotension, thrombophlebitis (IV). **EENT:** transient or permanent deafness (over-rapid IV injection), blurred vision, tinnitus. **GI:** cramping, diarrhea, anorexia, nausea, vomiting, abdominal discomfort, dysphagia, *GI bleeding*. **GU:** hematuria, azotemia. **Hematologic:** *agranulocytosis, neutropenia, thrombocytopenia*. **Metabolic:** hyperuricemia, gout, *hypokalemia*, hypochloremic alkalosis, *hyponatremia, hypomagnesemia*, hyperglycemia and impaired glucose tolerance, dehydration. **Skin:** rash. **Other:** chills.

INTERACTIONS

Drug-drug. *Aminoglycoside and some cephalosporin antibiotics, cisplatin:* May increase ototoxicity and kidney toxicity. Use together cautiously.
Antidiabetics: May decrease hypoglycemic effects. Monitor glucose level.
Antihypertensives: May increase risk of hypotension. Use together cautiously.
Cardiac glycosides (digoxin): May increase risk of digoxin toxicity from ethacrynate-induced hypokalemia. Monitor potassium and digoxin levels.
Chlorothiazide, chlorthalidone, hydrochlorothiazide, indapamide, metolazone: May cause excessive diuretic response, causing serious electrolyte abnormalities or dehydration. Adjust doses carefully, and monitor patient closely for signs and symptoms of excessive diuretic response.
Furosemide: May increase risk of ototoxicity. Avoid use together.
Lithium: May decrease lithium clearance, increasing risk of lithium toxicity. Monitor lithium level.
Neuromuscular blockers: May alter neuromuscular blockade. Monitor patient closely.
NSAIDs: May decrease diuretic effect. Use together cautiously.
Other potassium-wasting drugs (amphotericin B, corticosteroids): May increase risk of hypokalemia and hypocalcemia. Use cautiously.

Probenecid: May decrease diuretic effect. Avoid use together.
Risperidone: May enhance adverse or toxic effect of risperidone. Consider therapy modification and maintain adequate hydration.
Warfarin: May increase anticoagulant effect. Use together cautiously.
Drug-herb. *Dandelion:* May increase diuresis. Discourage use together.
Licorice: May cause unexpected rapid potassium loss. Discourage use together.

EFFECTS ON LAB TEST RESULTS
• May increase glucose and uric acid levels.
• May decrease calcium, magnesium, potassium, and sodium levels.
• May decrease granulocyte, neutrophil, and platelet counts.

CONTRAINDICATIONS & CAUTIONS
• Contraindicated in infants, patients hypersensitive to drug, and patients with anuria.
• Use cautiously in patients with electrolyte abnormalities or liver impairment.
• Ototoxicity has been reported, most often with IV use and with excessive doses.
• Rarely, pancreatitis has been reported.
Dialyzable drug: Unknown.
⚠ *Overdose S&S:* Dehydration, electrolyte depletion.

PREGNANCY-LACTATION-REPRODUCTION
• Use during pregnancy only if clearly needed.
• It isn't known if drug appears in human milk. Patient should discontinue breastfeeding or discontinue drug, considering importance of drug to patient.

NURSING CONSIDERATIONS
🛈 *Alert:* Drug is a potent diuretic and can cause severe diuresis with water and electrolyte depletion. Monitor patient closely.
• Monitor fluid intake and output, weight, BP, and electrolyte levels.
• Watch for signs and symptoms of orthostatic hypotension (dizziness, vertigo, syncope) and hypokalemia (muscle weakness and cramps).
• Monitor glucose level in patient with diabetes.
• Consult prescriber and dietitian about providing a high-potassium diet. Potassium chloride and sodium supplements may be needed.
• Dosage may be on an alternate-day schedule, or more-prolonged periods of diuretic

therapy may be interspersed with rest periods. Intermittent dosage schedule allows time to correct electrolyte imbalances and may provide a more-efficient diuretic response.

• Drug may increase risk of gastric hemorrhage caused by steroid treatment.

• Monitor an older adult, who is more susceptible to hypotension and other effects of excessive diuresis.

• Monitor uric acid level, especially in patient with history of gout.

⚠️ *Alert:* If patient develops severe diarrhea, stop drug. Patient shouldn't receive drug again after diarrhea has resolved.

PATIENT TEACHING

• Instruct patient to take drug with food to minimize GI upset.

• Advise patient to take drug in morning to avoid need to urinate at night. If second dose is needed, tell patient to take it in early afternoon.

• Warn patient to avoid sudden position changes and to rise slowly to avoid dizziness upon standing quickly.

• Tell patient to notify prescriber about muscle weakness, cramps, nausea, diarrhea, or dizziness.

• Caution patient not to perform hazardous activities if drug causes drowsiness.

• Advise patient with diabetes to closely monitor glucose level.

---

ethambutol hydrochloride
e-THAM-byoo-tole

Etibi✲, Myambutol

Therapeutic class: Antituberculotics
Pharmacologic class: Synthetic antituberculotics

AVAILABLE FORMS
Tablets: 100 mg, 400 mg

INDICATIONS & DOSAGES

➤ **Adjunctive treatment for pulmonary TB**
Adults and children ages 13 and older: In patients who haven't received prior antituberculotics, 15 mg/kg PO daily as single dose once every 24 hours, combined with other antituberculotic therapy. For retreatment, 25 mg/kg PO every 24 hours as single dose for 60 days (or until bacteriologic smears and cultures become negative) with at least one other antituberculotic; after 60 days, decrease to 15 mg/kg/day as single dose every 24 hours.

ADMINISTRATION
PO

• Always give drug with other antituberculotics to prevent development of resistant organisms.

• Give without regard to food; if GI upset occurs, give with food.

ACTION

May inhibit synthesis of one or more metabolites of susceptible bacteria, changing cell metabolism during cell division; bacteriostatic.

Route	Onset	Peak	Duration
PO	Unknown	2–4 hr	Unknown

Half-life: About 2.5 to 3.6 hours.

ADVERSE REACTIONS

CNS: dizziness, fever, disorientation, hallucinations, headache, malaise, confusion, peripheral neuritis. **EENT:** optic neuritis, irreversible blindness, decreased visual acuity. **GI:** abdominal pain, anorexia, GI upset, nausea, vomiting. **Hematologic:** *thrombocytopenia, leukopenia, neutropenia,* lymphadenopathy. **Hepatic:** abnormal LFT values. **Metabolic:** hyperuricemia, precipitation of acute gout. **Musculoskeletal:** joint pain. **Respiratory:** pulmonary infiltrates. **Skin:** *erythema multiforme,* dermatitis, pruritus. **Other:** *anaphylactoid reactions,* hypersensitivity reactions.

INTERACTIONS

Drug-drug. *Aluminum salts:* May delay and reduce ethambutol absorption. Separate doses by at least 4 hours.

EFFECTS ON LAB TEST RESULTS

• May increase ALT, AST, bilirubin, and uric acid levels.

• May decrease WBC and platelet counts.

CONTRAINDICATIONS & CAUTIONS

• Contraindicated in children younger than age 13, patients hypersensitive to drug, patients with known optic neuritis, and those who can't report vision changes, including unconscious patients.

• Use cautiously in patients with impaired kidney function, cataracts, recurrent eye inflammation, gout, or diabetic retinopathy. Irreversible blindness has occurred.
• Liver toxicities, including fatalities, have been reported.
Dialyzable drug: Unknown.

PREGNANCY-LACTATION-REPRODUCTION
• Drug crosses the placental barrier. Ophthalmic abnormalities have occurred in infants exposed to antituberculotics in utero. Use during pregnancy only if benefit justifies fetal risk.
• Patients of childbearing potential should use effective contraception during treatment for multidrug-resistant TB.
• Drug appears in human milk. Use only if expected benefit to patient outweighs risk to the infant. Monitor infant for jaundice.
• Patients with multidrug-resistant TB and positive sputum smear shouldn't breastfeed.

NURSING CONSIDERATIONS
• Perform visual acuity and color discrimination tests before and during therapy. Urge patient taking more than 15 mg/kg/day to have monthly eye exams.
• Ensure that any changes in vision don't result from an underlying condition.
• Obtain AST and ALT levels before therapy; monitor them every 3 to 4 weeks.
• In patient with impaired kidney function, base dosage on drug level.
• Monitor uric acid level; observe patient for signs and symptoms of gout.

PATIENT TEACHING
• Tell patient to immediately report all vision changes; explain that eye exams will be necessary. Advise patient that visual disturbances usually disappear several weeks to months after drug is stopped. Inflammation of the optic nerve is related to dosage and duration of treatment.
• Inform patient that drug is given with other antituberculotics.
• Stress importance of adherence with drug therapy.
• Instruct patient to report adverse reactions to prescriber.
• Advise patient of childbearing potential to use effective contraception during treatment of multidrug-resistant TB.

ethinyl estradiol–desogestrel
ETH-in-il/DAY-so-jest-rul

Monophasic
Isibloom, Kalliga

Biphasic
Kariva, Pimtrea, Simliya, Viorele, Volnea

Triphasic
Cyclessa, Velivet

ethinyl estradiol–ethynodiol diacetate
Monophasic
Kelnor 1/35, Kelnor 1/50, Zovia 1/35

ethinyl estradiol–levonorgestrel
Monophasic
Afirmelle, Altavera, Ashlyna, Aviane, Ayuna, Balcoltra, Falmina, Iclevia, Introvale, Kurvelo, Lessina, Levora, Marlissa, Portia, Setlakin, Tyblume, Vienva

Biphasic
Daysee, Jaimiess, LoSeasonique, Lo Simpesse, Seasonique, Simpesse

Triphasic
Enpresse, Levonest, Trivora

Four-phasic
Quartette, Rivelsa

ethinyl estradiol–norethindrone
Monophasic
Alyacen 1/35, Balziva, Briellyn, Cyonanz, Dasetta 1/35, Kaitlib Fe, Nexesta Fe, Nortrel 0.5/35, Nortrel 1/35, Nylia 1/35, Philith, Vyfemla, Wera

Triphasic
Alyacen 7/7/7, Aranelle, Dasetta 7/7/7, Nortrel 7/7/7, Nylia 7/7/7

E

ethinyl estradiol–norethindrone acetate
Monophasic
Activella, Fyavolv, Junel 1/20, Junel 1.5/30, Larin 1/20, Larin 1.5/30, Taytulla

ethinyl estradiol–norgestimate
Monophasic
Estarylla, Mili, Mono-Linyah, Previfem, Sprintec

Triphasic
Tri-Estarylla, Tri-Linyah, Tri-Lo-Estarylla, Tri-Lo-Mili, Tri-Lo-Sprintec, Tri-Mili, Tri-Sprintec

ethinyl estradiol–norgestrel
Monophasic
Cryselle, Elinest, Low-Ogestrel

ethinyl estradiol–norethindrone acetate–ferrous fumarate
Monophasic
Blisovi 24 Fe, Blisovi Fe 1.5/30, Blisovi Fe 1/20, Gemmily, Junel Fe 1/20, Junel Fe 1.5/30, Larin 24 Fe, Larin Fe 1/20, Larin Fe 1.5/30, Lo Loestrin Fe, Merzee, Minastrin 24 Fe

Triphasic
Tri-Legest Fe

Therapeutic class: Contraceptives
Pharmacologic class: Estrogen–progestin combinations

AVAILABLE FORMS
Monophasic hormonal contraceptives
ethinyl estradiol–desogestrel
Tablets: ethinyl estradiol 30 mcg and desogestrel 0.15 mg
ethinyl estradiol–ethynodiol diacetate
Tablets: ethinyl estradiol 35 mcg and ethynodiol diacetate 1 mg; ethinyl estradiol 50 mcg and ethynodiol diacetate 1 mg
ethinyl estradiol–levonorgestrel
Tablets: ethinyl estradiol 20 mcg and levonorgestrel 0.1 mg; ethinyl estradiol 30 mcg and levonorgestrel 0.15 mg; ethinyl estradiol 30 mcg and levonorgestrel 0.15 mg (84 tablets)

ethinyl estradiol–norethindrone
Tablets: ethinyl estradiol 20 mcg and norethindrone 1 mg, ethinyl estradiol 35 mcg and norethindrone 0.4 mg; ethinyl estradiol 25 mcg and norethindrone 0.8 mg; ethinyl estradiol 35 mcg and norethindrone 0.5 mg; ethinyl estradiol 35 mcg and norethindrone 0.75 mg; ethinyl estradiol 35 mcg and norethindrone 1 mg
ethinyl estradiol–norethindrone acetate
Tablets: ethinyl estradiol 20 mcg and norethindrone acetate 1 mg; ethinyl estradiol 30 mcg and norethindrone acetate 1.5 mg
Tablets for menopausal symptoms or osteoporosis: ethinyl estradiol 0.0025 mg and norethindrone acetate 0.5 mg; ethinyl estradiol 0.005 mg and norethindrone acetate 1 mg; ethinyl estradiol 0.5 mg and norethindrone acetate 0.1 mg; ethinyl estradiol 1 mg and norethindrone acetate 0.5 mg
ethinyl estradiol–norgestimate
Tablets: ethinyl estradiol 35 mcg and norgestimate 0.25 mg
ethinyl estradiol–norgestrel
Tablets: ethinyl estradiol 30 mcg and norgestrel 0.3 mg
ethinyl estradiol–norethindrone acetate–ferrous fumarate
Chewable tablets: norethindrone 0.4 mg and ethinyl estradiol 35 mcg; inactive tablets contain ferrous fumarate 75 mg
Tablets: ethinyl estradiol 10 mcg, norethindrone acetate 1 mg, and ferrous fumarate 75 mg; ethinyl estradiol 20 mcg, norethindrone acetate 1 mg, and ferrous fumarate 75 mg; ethinyl estradiol 30 mcg, norethindrone acetate 1.5 mg, and ferrous fumarate 75 mg.
Biphasic hormonal contraceptives
ethinyl estradiol–desogestrel
Tablets: ethinyl estradiol 20 mcg and desogestrel 0.15 mg (21 days), then inert tablets (2 days), then ethinyl estradiol 10 mcg (5 days)
ethinyl estradiol–levonorgestrel
Tablets: ethinyl estradiol 0.02 mg and levonorgestrel 0.1 mg (84 days), then ethinyl estradiol 0.01 mg (7 days); ethinyl estradiol 30 mcg and levonorgestrel 0.15 mg (84 days), then ethinyl estradiol 10 mcg (7 days)
ethinyl estradiol–norethindrone
Tablets: ethinyl estradiol 35 mcg and norethindrone 0.5 mg (12 tablets), then ethinyl estradiol 35 mcg and norethindrone 1 mg (9 tablets)

Reactions in bold italics are *life-threatening*.

Triphasic hormonal contraceptives
ethinyl estradiol–desogestrel
Tablets: 0.1 mg desogestrel and 25 mcg
ethinyl estradiol (7 tablets), 0.125 mg
desogestrel and 25 mcg ethinyl estradiol
(7 tablets), 0.15 mg desogestrel and 25 mcg
ethinyl estradiol (7 tablets)
ethinyl estradiol–levonorgestrel
Tablets: ethinyl estradiol 30 mcg and levonorgestrel 0.05 mg (6 days), ethinyl estradiol
40 mcg and levonorgestrel 0.075 mg (5 days),
ethinyl estradiol 30 mcg and levonorgestrel
0.125 mg (10 days); ethinyl estradiol 20 mcg
and 0.15 mg levonorgestrel (42 days), ethinyl
estradiol 25 mcg and 0.15 mg levonorgestrel
(21 days), ethinyl estradiol 30 mcg and
0.15 mg levonorgestrel (21 days), ethinyl
estradiol 10 mcg (7 days)
ethinyl estradiol–norethindrone
Tablets: ethinyl estradiol 30 mcg and
norethindrone 0.5 mg (7 days), ethinyl estradiol 35 mcg and norethindrone 1 mg (9 days),
ethinyl estradiol 35 mcg and norethindrone
0.5 mg (5 days); ethinyl estradiol 35 mcg
and norethindrone 0.5 mg (7 days), ethinyl
estradiol 35 mcg and norethindrone 0.75 mg
(7 days), ethinyl estradiol 35 mcg and
norethindrone 1 mg (7 days)
ethinyl estradiol–norgestimate
Tablets: ethinyl estradiol 25 mcg and norgestimate 0.18 mg (7 days), ethinyl estradiol
25 mcg and norgestimate 0.215 mg (7 days),
ethinyl estradiol 25 mcg and norgestimate
0.25 mg (7 days); ethinyl estradiol 35 mcg
and norgestimate 0.18 mg (7 days), ethinyl
estradiol 35 mcg and norgestimate 0.215 mg
(7 days), ethinyl estradiol 35 mcg and norgestimate 0.25 mg (7 days)
**ethinyl estradiol–norethindrone
acetate–ferrous fumarate**
Tablets: ethinyl estradiol 20 mcg and
norethindrone acetate 1 mg (5 days), ethinyl
estradiol 30 mcg and norethindrone acetate
1 mg (7 days), ethinyl estradiol 35 mcg and
norethindrone acetate 1 mg (9 days), 75-mg
ferrous fumarate tablets (7 days)
Four-phasic hormonal contraceptives
ethinyl estradiol–levonorgestrel
Tablets: ethinyl estradiol 20 mcg and levonorgestrel 0.15 mg (42 days), ethinyl estradiol
25 mcg and levonorgestrel 0.15 mg (21 days),
ethinyl estradiol 30 mcg and levonorgestrel
0.15 mg (21 days), ethinyl estradiol 10 mcg
(7 days).

INDICATIONS & DOSAGES

➤ **Pregnancy prevention (monophasic hormonal contraceptives)**
Females after menarche: 1 tablet PO daily beginning on first day of menstrual cycle or first
Sunday after menstrual cycle begins. With
20- and 21-tablet package, new cycle begins
7 days after last tablet taken. With 28-tablet
package, dosage is 1 tablet daily without interruption; extra tablets taken on days 22 to
28 are placebos or contain iron. Or, for Sea-
sonale, 1 pink tablet PO daily beginning on
first Sunday after menstrual cycle begins, for
84 consecutive days, followed by 7 days of
white (inert) tablets. Or, for Taytulla, once-
daily active pink capsules for 24 days, followed by 4 reminder maroon inert capsules
(without hormones) one daily for the next
4 days.

When changing from 21-day or 28-day
combination oral contraceptive, begin on
first day of withdrawal bleeding, at the latest
7 days after last active tablet. When changing from progestin-only pill, begin the next
day. When changing from implant contraceptive, begin the day of implant removal. When
changing from injection contraceptive, begin
the day when next injection is due.

✱ *NEW INDICATION:* **Pregnancy prevention
(biphasic hormonal contraceptives)**
Females after menarche: 1 color tablet PO
daily for 10 days; then next color tablet for
11 days. With 21-tablet packages, new cycle begins 7 days after last tablet taken. With
28-tablet packages, 1 tablet daily without interruption. Or, for Seasonique, 1 light blue-
green tablet PO once daily for 84 consecutive
days, followed by 1 yellow tablet for 7 consecutive days; then repeat cycle.
➤ **Pregnancy prevention (triphasic hormonal contraceptives)**
Females after menarche: 1 tablet PO daily
in sequence specified on package. With
21-tablet packages, new dosing cycle begins
7 days after last tablet taken. With 28-tablet
packages, 1 tablet daily without interruption.
➤ **Pregnancy prevention (four-phasic hormonal contraceptives)**
Females after menarche: 1 tablet PO daily in
91-day sequence specified on package. Begin
next 91-day sequence without interruption.
➤ **Moderate acne vulgaris in females ages
14 and older who have no known contraindications to hormonal contraceptive therapy, who want oral contraception**

E

for at least 6 months, who have reached menarche, and who are unresponsive to topical antiacne drugs (ethinyl estradiol–norgestimate, ethinyl estradiol–norethindrone acetate–ferrous fumarate)

Females ages 15 and older: 1 tablet PO daily.

➤ **Menopausal signs and symptoms; to prevent osteoporosis (Activella, Fyavolv)**

Adult females with intact uterus: 1 tablet PO daily.

ADMINISTRATION
PO
- Give drug at the same time each day; give at night to reduce nausea and headaches.
- Patient may swallow chewable tablet whole and follow with a full glass of liquid.
- Refer to manufacturer's instructions for missed doses. Recommendations vary based on number of doses missed and timing during the cycle.

ACTION
Inhibits ovulation and may prevent transport of ovum (if ovulation should occur) through fallopian tubes.

Estrogen suppresses FSH, blocking follicular development and ovulation.

Progestin suppresses LH so that ovulation can't occur even if follicle develops; it also thickens cervical mucus, interfering with sperm migration, and prevents implantation of fertilized ovum.

Route	Onset	Peak	Duration
PO	Unknown	2 hr (ethinyl estradiol), 0.5–4 hr (varies by progestin)	Unknown

Half-life: 6 to 20 hours (ethinyl estradiol); 5 to 45 hours (varies by progestin).

ADVERSE REACTIONS
CNS: headache, dizziness, depression, fatigue, insomnia, lethargy, migraine, mood changes, anxiety, ***stroke, cerebral hemorrhage, suicidality.*** **CV:** *VTE,* HTN, chest pain, edema, *MI.* **EENT:** worsening myopia or astigmatism, intolerance of contact lenses, exophthalmos, diplopia. **GI:** nausea, vomiting, abdominal cramps, bloating, anorexia, changes in appetite, gallbladder disease, *pancreatitis.* **GU:** breakthrough bleeding, spotting, granulomatous colitis, dysmenorrhea, amenorrhea, cervical erosion or abnormal secretions, enlargement of uterine fibromas, vaginal candidiasis, *ectopic pregnancy.* **Hepatic:** cholestatic jaundice, *liver tumors,* gallbladder disease. **Metabolic:** weight change, additive insulin resistance in those with diabetes. **Skin:** rash, acne, *erythema multiforme,* melasma, hirsutism, alopecia. **Other:** hypersensitivity reaction, breast tenderness, enlargement, secretion.

INTERACTIONS
Drug-drug. *Anastrozole:* May inhibit anastrozole effect. Avoid use together.
Atorvastatin: May increase norethindrone and ethinyl estradiol levels. Monitor patient for adverse effects.
Benzodiazepines: May decrease or increase benzodiazepine level. Adjust dosage, if necessary.
Beta blockers: May increase beta blocker level. Adjust dosage, if necessary.
Carbamazepine, fosphenytoin, phenobarbital, phenytoin, rifampin: May decrease estrogen effect. Use together cautiously.
Corticosteroids: May enhance corticosteroid effect. Monitor patient closely.
Exemestane: May interfere with exemestane effectiveness. Avoid use together.
Insulin, sulfonylureas: Glucose intolerance may decrease antidiabetic effects. Monitor these effects.
Iron supplements: Increase risk of iron-related toxicity if blister card contains iron. Don't use together.
Lamotrigine: May decrease lamotrigine level. Adjust dosage of lamotrigine, if needed.
NNRTIs, protease inhibitors: May decrease hormonal contraceptive effect. Avoid use together, if possible.
Oral anticoagulants: May decrease anticoagulant effect. Dosage adjustments may be needed. Monitor PT and INR.
Ospemifene: May enhance adverse or toxic effects of ospemifene and interfere with its effectiveness. Avoid use together.
Drug-herb. *Red clover:* May interfere with drug. Discourage use together.
St. John's wort: May decrease drug effect because of increased liver metabolism. Discourage use together, or advise patient to use additional method of contraception.
Drug-food. *Caffeine:* May increase caffeine level. Urge caution.
Grapefruit juice: May increase estrogen level. Advise patient to take with liquid other than grapefruit juice.

Drug-lifestyle. **Boxed Warning** *Smoking:* May increase risk of adverse CV effects. Use of hormonal contraceptives is contraindicated in females over age 35 who smoke. ■

EFFECTS ON LAB TEST RESULTS
• May increase thyroid-binding globulin, total T$_4$, lipid, and triglyceride levels.
• May alter clotting factors.
• May increase norepinephrine-induced platelet aggregation and prolong PT.
• May reduce response to metyrapone test.
• May cause false-positive result in nitroblue tetrazolium test.

CONTRAINDICATIONS & CAUTIONS
• Contraindicated in patients with thromboembolic disorders, cerebrovascular disease, CAD, diplopia or ocular lesions arising from ophthalmic vascular disease, classic migraine, MI, known or suspected breast cancer, known or suspected estrogen-dependent neoplasia, benign or malignant liver tumors, active liver disease or history of cholestatic jaundice with pregnancy or previous use of hormonal contraceptives, or undiagnosed abnormal vaginal bleeding. Also contraindicated in patients receiving hepatitis C drug combinations containing ombitasvir–paritaprevir–ritonavir, with or without dasabuvir.
• Use cautiously in patients with asthma, hyperlipidemia, HTN, migraines, seizure disorders, bleeding irregularities, gallbladder disease, ocular disease, diabetes, emotional disorders, and cardiac, kidney, or liver insufficiency.
Dialyzable drug: Unknown.
⚠ *Overdose S&S:* Nausea, withdrawal uterine bleeding.

PREGNANCY-LACTATION-REPRODUCTION
• Use is contraindicated during pregnancy.
• Use of estrogen and progestin (as in combination hormonal contraceptives) hasn't been associated with teratogenic effects when inadvertently taken early in pregnancy.
• Estrogen appears in and decreases the quantity and quality of human milk. Patient should use other forms of contraception during breastfeeding.

NURSING CONSIDERATIONS
Boxed Warning Cigarette smoking increases risk of serious CV adverse effects

from oral contraceptives. Females over age 35 who use oral contraceptives shouldn't smoke. ■
• Triphasic hormonal contraceptives may cause fewer adverse reactions, such as breakthrough bleeding and spotting.
• The CDC reports that use of hormonal contraceptives may decrease risk of ovarian and endometrial cancers and doesn't seem to increase risk of breast cancer. However, the FDA reports that some studies suggest that hormonal contraceptives may be linked to increased risk of cervical cancer.
• Monitor lipid levels, BP, body weight, and liver function.
⚠ *Alert:* Many hormonal contraceptives share similar names. Make sure to verify hormone strength.
• Estrogens and progestins may alter glucose tolerance, thus changing dosage requirements for antidiabetics. Monitor glucose level.
• Stop hormonal contraceptive for a few weeks before adrenal function testing.
• Stop hormonal contraceptive and notify prescriber if patient develops granulomatous colitis.
• Stop drug at least 1 week before surgery to decrease risk of VTE. Tell patient to use alternative birth control method.
• Patients who are nonlactating or have had a second-trimester abortion must wait 28 days before starting oral contraception.

PATIENT TEACHING
• Tell patient to take tablets or capsules at same time each day; nighttime doses may reduce nausea and headaches.
• Advise patient to use additional method of birth control, such as condom or diaphragm with spermicide, for first week of first cycle.
• Inform patient that missing doses in midcycle greatly increases likelihood of pregnancy.
• Teach patient that missing a dose may cause spotting or light bleeding.
• Instruct patient to follow manufacturer's instructions for missed doses or to contact prescriber for instructions. An additional method of contraception may be necessary.
• Counsel patient that hormonal contraceptives don't protect against HIV or other STIs.
• Tell patient using 91-day method that four planned menses occur per year, but

spotting or bleeding between menses may occur.

• Warn patient of common adverse effects (headache, nausea, dizziness, breast tenderness, spotting, breakthrough bleeding), which usually diminish after 3 to 6 months.

• Instruct patient to obtain weight at least twice per week and to report any sudden weight gain or swelling to prescriber.

• Caution patient to avoid exposure to UV light or prolonged exposure to sunlight.

◑ *Alert:* Warn patient to immediately report abdominal pain; numbness, stiffness, or pain in legs or buttocks; pressure or pain in chest; shortness of breath; severe headache; visual disturbances (blind spots, blurriness, flashing lights); undiagnosed vaginal bleeding or discharge; two consecutive missed menstrual periods; breast lumps; swelling of hands or feet; or severe pain in abdomen (tumor rupture in liver).

• Advise patient of increased risks created by simultaneous use of cigarettes and hormonal contraceptives.

• If one menstrual period is missed and tablets or capsules have been taken on schedule, tell patient to continue taking them. If two consecutive menstrual periods are missed, tell patient to stop drug and have pregnancy test. Progestins may cause birth defects if taken early in pregnancy.

• Tell patient to chew chewable tablet and follow with full glass of liquid or swallow whole.

• Caution patient not to take same drug for longer than 12 months without consulting prescriber. Stress importance of Papanicolaou tests and annual gynecologic exams.

• Advise patient to check with prescriber about how soon pregnancy may be attempted after hormonal therapy is stopped. Many prescribers recommend that patients not become pregnant within 2 months after stopping drug.

• Warn patient of possible delay in achieving pregnancy when drug is stopped.

• Teach patient methods to decrease risk of VTE.

• Advise patient taking hormonal contraceptives to use additional form of birth control during concurrent treatment with certain antibiotics.

• Inform patient that hormonal contraceptives may change the fit of contact lenses.

etonogestrel–ethinyl estradiol vaginal ring
et-oh-noe-JES-trel/ETH-in-il

EluRyng, Haloette, NuvaRing

Therapeutic class: Contraceptives
Pharmacologic class: Progestin–estrogen combinations

AVAILABLE FORMS
Vaginal ring: Delivers 0.12 mg/day etonogestrel and 0.015 mg/day ethinyl estradiol

INDICATIONS & DOSAGES
➤ **Pregnancy prevention**
Females: Insert 1 ring into vagina and leave in place for 3 weeks. Insert new ring 1 week after removal of previous ring.

ADMINISTRATION
Vaginal
• In patients who didn't use hormonal contraception during the previous month, initiate therapy on first day of menstrual cycle; may also insert on days 2 to 5, even if bleeding isn't complete, but use of barrier method, such as male condoms or spermicide, is necessary for the following 7 days. Patients using a combination oral contraceptive may switch to a vaginal ring on any day, but at the latest on the day after the usual hormone-free interval. See manufacturer's instructions for use after progestin-only methods, abortion, miscarriage, or childbirth.

• Leave ring in place continuously for a full 3 weeks to maintain effect; then remove for 1 week. During this time, withdrawal bleeding occurs (usually starting 2 or 3 days after removal). Insert a new ring 1 week after removal of previous ring, at approximately the same time of day, regardless of whether patient is still menstruating.

• Before dispensing to user, store refrigerated (36° to 46° F [2° to 8° C]). After dispensing, can store for up to 4 months at room temperature.

ACTION
Suppresses gonadotropins, which inhibits ovulation; increases the viscosity of cervical mucus (decreasing the ability of sperm to enter the uterus); and alters the endometrial lining (reducing potential for implantation).

Reactions in bold italics are *life-threatening*.

Route	Onset	Peak	Duration
Vaginal	Rapid	200 hr (etono-gestrel); 59 hr (ethinyl estradiol)	Unknown

Half-life: Etonogestrel, 29 hours; ethinyl estradiol, 45 hours.

ADVERSE REACTIONS

CNS: headache, emotional lability, mood changes, depression, migraine. **GI:** nausea, vomiting, abdominal pain. **GU:** vaginitis, leukorrhea, device-related events (for example, foreign body sensation, coital difficulties, device expulsion), vaginal discomfort, breakthrough bleeding, vaginal discharge, dysmenorrhea, decreased libido. **Metabolic:** weight gain. **Skin:** acne. **Other:** breast pain or tenderness.

INTERACTIONS

Drug-drug. *Acetaminophen:* May decrease acetaminophen level and increase ethinyl estradiol level. Monitor patient for effects.
Ampicillin, barbiturates, carbamazepine, felbamate, griseofulvin, oxcarbazepine, phenytoin, rifampin, tetracyclines, topiramate: May decrease contraceptive effect and increase risk of pregnancy, breakthrough bleeding, or both. Tell patient to use an additional form of contraception while taking these drugs.
Anastrozole: May diminish therapeutic effect of anastrozole. Avoid use together.
Ascorbic acid, atorvastatin, itraconazole: May increase ethinyl estradiol level. Monitor patient for adverse effects.
Morphine, salicylic acid, temazepam: May increase clearance of these drugs. Monitor patient for effectiveness.
Cyclosporine, prednisolone, theophylline: May increase levels of these drugs. Monitor levels if appropriate and adjust dosage.
Exemestane: May interfere with exemestane effectiveness. Avoid use together.
HCV combination products (ombitasvir–paritaprevir–ritonavir with or without dasabuvir): May elevate liver enzyme levels. Use together is contraindicated.
HIV protease inhibitors (lopinavir, ritonavir), NNRTIs (efavirenz, nevirapine): May affect contraceptive effect. Refer to drug literature for specific protease inhibitor. May need to use a backup method of contraception.
Lamotrigine: May decrease lamotrigine level and reduce seizure control. Increase lamotrigine dose, as necessary.

Miconazole (oil-based vaginal capsule): May increase level of etonogestrel and ethinyl estradiol. Monitor patient for adverse effects.
Ospemifene: May enhance adverse or toxic effects of ospemifene and interfere with its effectiveness. Avoid use together.
Drug-herb. *St. John's wort:* May reduce drug effectiveness and increase risk of breakthrough bleeding and pregnancy. Discourage use together.
Drug-lifestyle. Boxed Warning *Smoking:* May increase risk of serious CV adverse effects. Urge patient to avoid smoking. ∎

EFFECTS ON LAB TEST RESULTS

• May increase coagulation factors, thyroid-binding globulin (leading to increased circulating total thyroid hormone levels), sex hormone-binding globulin (and other binding proteins), and lipid levels.
• May decrease T_3 resin uptake and glucose tolerance.

CONTRAINDICATIONS & CAUTIONS

• Contraindicated in patients hypersensitive to components of drug and in patients older than age 35 who smoke 15 or more cigarettes daily.
• Contraindicated in patients with thrombophlebitis, thromboembolic disorder, inherited or acquired hypercoagulopathy, history of DVT, cerebrovascular disease, CAD, valvular heart disease with complications, severe HTN, diabetes with vascular complications, headache with focal neurologic symptoms or migraine headaches with aura, known or suspected cancer of endometrium or breast, estrogen-dependent neoplasia, abnormal undiagnosed genital bleeding, jaundice related to pregnancy or previous use of hormonal contraceptives, active liver disease, or benign or malignant liver tumors.
• Avoid use in those undergoing major surgery with prolonged immobilization.
• Use cautiously in patients with HTN, hyperlipidemias, obesity, or diabetes.
• Use cautiously in patients with conditions that could be aggravated by fluid retention and in patients with history of depression.
• **Alert:** Drug may increase risk of MI, VTE, stroke, liver neoplasia, and gallbladder disease.
• Ring may not be suitable for patients with conditions that make the vagina more susceptible to vaginal irritation or ulceration.

Vaginal and cervical erosion and ulceration have been reported.
- Ring may interfere with correct placement and position of barrier contraceptive methods (diaphragm, cervical cap, female condom). These methods aren't recommended as backup methods with ring use.
- Ring breakage has occurred when used together with intravaginal antimycotic, antibiotic, or lubricant products.

Dialyzable drug: Unknown.

PREGNANCY-LACTATION-REPRODUCTION
- Use is contraindicated during pregnancy.
- Use of estrogen and progestin (as in combination hormonal contraceptives) hasn't been associated with teratogenic effects when inadvertently taken early in pregnancy.
- Drug appears in and decreases the quantity and quality of human milk. Patients who are breastfeeding should use other forms of contraception.
- Drug isn't indicated before menarche.

NURSING CONSIDERATIONS
Boxed Warning Cigarette smoking increases the risk of serious adverse cardiac effects, especially in patients older than age 35. Risk increases with age and in patients who smoke 15 or more cigarettes daily. ∎
- Stop drug at least 4 weeks before and for 2 weeks after procedures that may increase risk of VTE and during and after prolonged immobilization.
- Stop drug and notify prescriber if patient develops unexplained partial or complete loss of vision, proptosis, diplopia, papilledema, retinal vascular lesions, migraines, depression, or jaundice.
- Closely monitor BP if patient has HTN or kidney disease.
- Rule out pregnancy if patient hasn't adhered to prescribed regimen and misses a period, if patient has adhered to prescribed regimen and misses two periods, or if patient retains ring for longer than 4 weeks.

PATIENT TEACHING
- Stress importance of having regular annual physical exams to check for adverse effects or developing contraindications.
- Tell patient that drug doesn't protect against HIV and other STIs.
- Advise patient not to smoke while using contraceptive.

- Caution patient to use backup method of contraception until ring has been used continuously for 7 days. Tell patient not to use diaphragm, cervical cap, or female condom as backup method.
- Inform patient who wears contact lenses to contact an ophthalmologist if vision or lens tolerance changes.
- Advise patient to follow manufacturer's instructions for use if switching from different form of hormonal contraceptive.
- Teach patient to insert ring into vagina (using fingers) and keep it in place continuously for 3 weeks to maintain effect, saving foil package for later disposal. Explain that, after ring removal, withdrawal bleeding occurs (usually starting 2 or 3 days after removal). Tell patient to insert new ring 1 week after removing previous one at approximately the same time of day, regardless of menstrual bleeding.
- Advise patient to regularly check for presence of ring in vagina and not to deviate from recommended regimen.
- Inform patient that, if ring is removed or expelled (such as while removing a tampon, straining, or moving bowels), it should be washed with cool to lukewarm (not hot) water and immediately reinserted. Stress that contraceptive effect may be compromised if ring stays out for longer than 3 hours. Instruct patient to use a backup method of contraception until newly reinserted ring has been used continuously for 7 days.
- Tell patient that there's no danger of vaginal ring being pushed too far up in vagina or getting lost.

SAFETY ALERT!

etoposide
e-toe-POE-side

etoposide phosphate
Etopophos

Therapeutic class: Antineoplastics
Pharmacologic class: Podophyllotoxin derivatives

AVAILABLE FORMS
etoposide
Capsules: 50 mg
Injection: 20 mg/mL in 5-mL, 25-mL, 50-mL multidose vials

etoposide phosphate

Injection: 114-mg vials equivalent to 100 mg etoposide

INDICATIONS & DOSAGES

Adjust-a-dose (for all indications): For patients with CrCl of 15 to 50 mL/minute, reduce dose by 25%. For patients with CrCl of less than 15 mL/minute, consider further dosage reduction. Adjust dosage to account for myelosuppressive effects of coadministered drugs or effects of prior radiation therapy or chemotherapy.

➤ **Refractory testicular cancer, in combination with other chemotherapeutic agents**
Adults: 50 to 100 mg/m^2 daily IV on 5 consecutive days every 21- to 28-day cycle. Or, 100 mg/m^2 daily IV on days 1, 3, and 5 every 21- to 28-day cycle.

➤ **Small-cell carcinoma of lung, in combination with other chemotherapeutic agents**
Adults: 35 mg/m^2 daily IV for 4 days or 50 mg/m^2 daily IV for 5 days. Repeat cycles every 3 to 4 weeks. Oral dose is two times IV dose (70 mg/m^2 for 4 days to 100 mg/m^2 for 5 days), rounded to nearest 50 mg.

ADMINISTRATION

PO

⚠ *Alert:* Hazardous drug; use safe handling and disposal precautions.
• Consider antiemetics because oral etoposide is associated with mild to moderate emetic potential.
• Give drug without regard to food.
• Refrigerate capsules at 36° to 46° F (2° to 8° C). Don't freeze. Capsules are stable for 36 months under refrigeration.

IV

⚠ *Alert:* Preparing and giving parenteral drug may be mutagenic, teratogenic, or carcinogenic. Use gloves.
▼ Plastic devices made of acrylic or acrylonitrile butadiene styrene (ABS) have been reported to crack and leak when used with undiluted etoposide injection.
▼ Drug is an irritant; monitor IV site to avoid extravasation.
▼ For etoposide infusion, dilute to 0.2 or 0.4 mg/mL in either D$_5$W or NSS. Higher concentrations may crystallize.
▼ Give etoposide by slow infusion over at least 30 to 60 minutes to prevent severe hypotension. Never give by rapid injection.

▼ For etoposide phosphate, reconstitute each vial with sterile water for injection, D$_5$W, NSS, bacteriostatic water for injection with benzyl alcohol, or bacteriostatic sodium chloride for injection with benzyl alcohol to concentration of 10 mg/mL or 20 mg/mL. After reconstitution, give without further dilution or dilute to as low as 0.1 mg/mL in either D$_5$W or NSS.
▼ Give etoposide phosphate over 5 minutes to 3.5 hours.
▼ Check BP every 15 minutes during infusion. Hypotension may occur if infusion is too rapid. If systolic pressure falls below 90 mm Hg, stop infusion and notify prescriber.
▼ Etoposide diluted to 0.2 mg/mL is stable for 96 hours at room temperature in plastic or glass, unprotected from light; at 0.4 mg/mL, it's stable for 24 hours under same conditions. Diluted etoposide phosphate solution stored in glass or plastic containers is stable under refrigeration for 7 days or for 24 to 48 hours at room temperature, depending on diluent. Further diluted solutions are stable under refrigeration or at room temperature for 24 hours.
▼ **Incompatibilities:** Cefepime, diazepam, filgrastim, gallium nitrate, idarubicin.

ACTION

Inhibits topoisomerase II enzyme, causing inability to repair DNA strand breaks, which leads to cell death. Cell-cycle specific to G$_2$ portion of cell cycle.

Route	Onset	Peak	Duration
PO, IV	Unknown	Unknown	Unknown

Half-life: Terminal phase, 4 to 11 hours.

ADVERSE REACTIONS

CNS: peripheral neuropathy, fatigue, aftertaste, fever, *seizures.* **CV:** hypotension. **EENT:** transient cortical blindness, optic neuritis. **GI:** anorexia, diarrhea, nausea, vomiting, abdominal pain, stomatitis, mucositis, constipation, dysphagia, esophagitis. **Hematologic:** *leukopenia, neutropenia, thrombocytopenia, secondary leukemia,* anemia, *myelosuppression.* **Hepatic:** *liver toxicity.* **Respiratory:** interstitial pneumonitis, pulmonary fibrosis. **Skin:** reversible alopecia, rash, radiation recall dermatitis, pigmentation, *SJS, TEN.* **Other:** hypersensitivity reactions, including *anaphylaxis-like reaction.*

INTERACTIONS

Drug-drug. *Cyclosporine:* May increase etoposide level and toxicity. Monitor CBC and adjust etoposide dose.

CYP3A4 inducers (carbamazepine, fosphenytoin, rifampin): May decrease etoposide phosphate level. Use alternative when possible.

Live-virus vaccines: May increase risk of adverse reactions to live-virus vaccine. Concurrent use isn't recommended.

Warfarin: May further prolong PT. Closely monitor PT and INR.

Drug-food. *Grapefruit juice:* May reduce etoposide level. Avoid use together.

EFFECTS ON LAB TEST RESULTS

- May decrease Hb level and neutrophil, platelet, RBC, and WBC counts.
- May increase LFT values.

CONTRAINDICATIONS & CAUTIONS

- Contraindicated in patients hypersensitive to drug.
- Use cautiously in patients with liver or kidney impairment.
- Secondary leukemias have occurred with long-term use.
- Safety and effectiveness in children haven't been established.

Dialyzable drug: No.

PREGNANCY-LACTATION-REPRODUCTION

- Drug can cause fetal harm if used during pregnancy. Advise patient of childbearing potential to use effective contraception during treatment and for at least 6 months after final dose. If drug is used during pregnancy or if patient becomes pregnant during therapy, apprise patient of fetal hazard.
- Males with partners of childbearing potential should use effective contraception during treatment and for 4 months after final dose.
- Drug appears in human milk. Patient should discontinue breastfeeding or discontinue drug, considering importance of drug to patient.
- In females, drug may cause infertility and result in amenorrhea. Recovery of menses and ovulation is related to age at treatment.
- In males, drug may result in oligospermia, azoospermia, and permanent loss of fertility. Sperm counts have been reported to return to normal levels in some males; in some cases, normal levels have occurred several years after therapy ends.

NURSING CONSIDERATIONS

Boxed Warning Give drug under the supervision of a physician experienced in the use of cancer chemotherapy. Severe myelosuppression with infection or bleeding may occur. ∎

- Obtain baseline BP before starting and monitor during therapy.
- Anticipate the need for antiemetics.
- Have diphenhydramine, hydrocortisone, epinephrine, and emergency equipment available to establish an airway in case anaphylaxis occurs.
- Monitor CBC. Watch for evidence of bone marrow suppression, which could lead to infection or bleeding.
- Patients with low serum albumin level may be at increased risk for etoposide toxicities.
- Inspect patient's mouth for ulcers.
- To prevent bleeding, avoid all IM injections when platelet count falls below 50,000/mm^3.

PATIENT TEACHING

- Tell patient to report all adverse reactions and to watch for signs and symptoms of infection (fever, sore throat, fatigue) and bleeding (easy bruising, nosebleeds, bleeding gums, melena). Tell patient to take temperature daily.
- Inform patient of need for frequent BP readings during IV administration.
- Advise patient of risk of secondary cancers with long-term etoposide use.
- Caution patient of childbearing potential to avoid pregnancy and breastfeeding during therapy and to use effective contraception during treatment and for 6 months after final dose.
- Advise male patient to use effective contraception for 4 months after final dose.

etravirine
eh-trah-VIGH-reen

Intelence

Therapeutic class: Antiretrovirals
Pharmacologic class: NNRTIs

AVAILABLE FORMS

Tablets ⓞⓝⓒ: 25 mg, 100 mg, 200 mg

INDICATIONS & DOSAGES

➤ **HIV-1 in patients who are treatment-experienced, in combination with other antiretrovirals**

Adults, including patients who are pregnant: 200 mg PO b.i.d.

Children ages 2 and older weighing 30 kg or more: 200 mg PO b.i.d.

Children ages 2 and older weighing 25 to less than 30 kg: 150 mg PO b.i.d.

Children ages 2 and older weighing 20 to less than 25 kg: 125 mg PO b.i.d.

Children ages 2 and older weighing 10 to less than 20 kg: 100 mg PO b.i.d.

ADMINISTRATION

PO

• Give drug after meals.
• Have patient swallow tablets whole with a liquid such as water.
• If patient can't swallow whole tablets, place tablets in a glass with 5 mL of water. Stir water well until it looks milky. May add 15 mL more water, orange juice, or milk to glass (avoid grapefruit juice, fluids warmer than 104° F [40° C], and carbonated beverages). Have patient drink immediately. Rinse glass with water several times and have patient swallow each rinse completely.

ACTION

Binds to reverse transcriptase, an enzyme that replicates HIV.

Route	Onset	Peak	Duration
PO	Unknown	2.5–4 hr	Unknown

Half-life: About 41 ± 20 hours.

ADVERSE REACTIONS

CNS: abnormal dreams, amnesia, anxiety, confusion, disorientation, fatigue, headache, hypoesthesia, insomnia, paresthesia, peripheral neuropathy, *seizures,* sluggishness, syncope, tremors. **CV:** angina, *atrial fibrillation,* HTN, *MI.* **EENT:** blurred vision, vertigo, dry mouth. **GI:** abdominal distention, abdominal pain, anorexia, constipation, diarrhea, flatulence, gastritis, GERD, *hematemesis,* nausea, *pancreatitis,* retching, stomatitis, vomiting. **GU:** *kidney failure.* **Hematologic:** anemia, hemolytic anemia. **Hepatic:** *hepatitis,* enlarged liver, increased LFTs. **Metabolic:** hyperglycemia, hypercholesterolemia, diabetes, dyslipidemia. **Respiratory:** *bronchospasm,* dyspnea. **Skin:** rash, night sweats, hyperhidrosis, dry skin, lipohypertrophy, itchy lesions. **Other:** hypersensitivity reactions, immune reconstitution syndrome, gynecomastia.

INTERACTIONS

Etravirine can interact with many drugs. Consult a drug compatibility reference or pharmacist for more information.

Drug-drug. *Antiarrhythmics (amiodarone, bepridil, disopyramide, flecainide, lidocaine, mexiletine, propafenone, quinidine):* May decrease levels of these drugs. Use caution, and monitor patient closely.

Atazanavir: May decrease atazanavir level and increase etravirine level. Avoid use unless atazanavir is boosted with ritonavir.

Atorvastatin, lovastatin, simvastatin: May decrease levels of these drugs. Adjust dosage, if needed.

Clarithromycin: May decrease clarithromycin level and increase etravirine level. Consider using azithromycin for treating MAC.

CYP3A4 inhibitors (itraconazole, ketoconazole): May decrease levels of these drugs and increase etravirine level. Adjust inhibitor dosage, if needed.

CYP450 inducers (carbamazepine, phenobarbital, phenytoin): May decrease etravirine level. Avoid use together.

Delavirdine: May increase etravirine level. Avoid use together.

Dexamethasone: May decrease etravirine level. Avoid use together.

Diazepam: May increase diazepam level. Reduce diazepam dose, as needed.

Dolutegravir: May decrease dolutegravir level. Use only when administered with atazanavir–ritonavir, darunavir–ritonavir, or lopinavir–ritonavir.

Efavirenz, nevirapine: May decrease etravirine level. Avoid use together.

Fluconazole, posaconazole: May increase etravirine level. Use together cautiously.

Fluvastatin: May increase fluvastatin level. Adjust dosage, if needed.

Immunosuppressants (cyclosporine, sirolimus, tacrolimus): May decrease levels of these drugs. Use together cautiously, and monitor patient closely.

Lopinavir–ritonavir: May decrease etravirine level. Use together cautiously.

Methadone: May cause withdrawal symptoms. Monitor patient, and consider increasing methadone dosage.

NNRTIs (delavirdine, efavirenz, nevirapine, rilpivirine): May alter etravirine level and hasn't been shown to be beneficial. Administration with other NNRTIs isn't recommended.

PDE5 inhibitors (sildenafil, tadalafil, vardenafil): May decrease effectiveness of these drugs. Adjust inhibitor dosage, as needed.

Protease inhibitors (atazanavir, fosamprenavir, nelfinavir): May alter protease inhibitor level if given without ritonavir. Avoid use together unless given with low-dose ritonavir.

Rifabutin: May decrease etravirine and rifabutin levels. If etravirine isn't given with a protease inhibitor and ritonavir, give rifabutin 300 mg daily. If etravirine is given with darunavir and ritonavir or with saquinavir and ritonavir, avoid rifabutin.

Rifampin, rifapentine: May decrease etravirine level. Avoid use together.

Ritonavir: May decrease etravirine level. Avoid use together.

Ritonavir and tipranavir: May decrease etravirine level. Avoid use together.

Warfarin: May increase warfarin level. Monitor INR closely, and adjust warfarin dosage if needed.

Drug-herb. *St. John's wort:* May decrease etravirine level. Discourage use together.

EFFECTS ON LAB TEST RESULTS

• May increase amylase, lipase, creatinine, total cholesterol, LDL-C, triglyceride, AST, ALT, and glucose levels.
• May decrease Hb level and WBC, neutrophil, and platelet counts.

CONTRAINDICATIONS & CAUTIONS

• Contraindicated in patients hypersensitive to etravirine or its components.
• Hypersensitivity reactions, including DRESS syndrome (ranging from rash to organ dysfunction), and SCARs (SJS, TEN, erythema multiforme) have been reported. Immediately discontinue drug if signs or symptoms of hypersensitivity reactions or severe skin reactions develop.
• Immune reconstitution syndrome has been reported with combination antiretroviral therapy. Autoimmune disorders (such as Graves disease, polymyositis, Guillain-Barré syndrome, and autoimmune hepatitis) have also been reported with immune reconstitution. Onset time varies and can occur many months after start of therapy.

• Use cautiously in older adults and patients with liver impairment or HBV or HCV infection.
• For children, don't exceed adult dosage or give to children younger than age 2.
Dialyzable drug: Unlikely.

PREGNANCY-LACTATION-REPRODUCTION

• Drug is approved for use during pregnancy; use only if potential benefit outweighs fetal risk. Drug may cross placenta.
• Register patients who are pregnant in the Antiretroviral Pregnancy Registry (1-800-258-4263 or www.apregistry.com).
• It isn't known if drug appears in human milk. Patients with HIV infection shouldn't breastfeed.

NURSING CONSIDERATIONS

⚠ **Alert:** Etravirine may interact with many drugs. Review patient's complete drug regimen.
⚠ **Alert:** Monitor patient closely for skin reactions. Fatalities have occurred due to TEN, SJS, erythema multiforme, and hypersensitivity reactions that may be accompanied by liver failure. Discontinue drug if severe skin or hypersensitivity reactions develop.
• Monitor patient for signs of fat redistribution (central obesity, buffalo hump, peripheral wasting, breast enlargement, cushingoid appearance).
• Immune reconstitution syndrome can occur. Monitor patient for inflammatory response to indolent or residual infections or autoimmune disorders.
• Notify prescriber if signs, symptoms, or lab abnormalities suggest pancreatitis. Monitor amylase and lipase levels.
• Monitor patient's CBC, platelet count, LFT values, and kidney function test results. Report abnormalities.

PATIENT TEACHING

• Teach about proper drug administration and handling.
• Warn patient to tell prescriber about any other prescription drugs, OTC drugs, and herbal supplements being taken.
• Advise patient to report adverse effects to prescriber.
• Inform patient that drug doesn't cure HIV infection, that opportunistic infections and other complications of HIV infection may still occur, and that HIV may still be transmitted to others through sexual contact or blood contamination.

Reactions in bold italics are *life-threatening*.

- Advise patient to take drug as prescribed and not to alter dose or stop drug without medical approval.
- Stress importance of taking every dose; missed doses can result in resistance.
- Tell patient that routine blood tests are needed to assess tolerance of drug therapy.

SAFETY ALERT!

everolimus ⚕
eh-ver-OH-lih-mus

Afinitor, Afinitor Disperz, Zortress

Therapeutic class: Antineoplastics
Pharmacologic class: Kinase inhibitors

AVAILABLE FORMS
Tablets (Afinitor) ⓄⓃⒸ: 2.5 mg, 5 mg, 7.5 mg, 10 mg
Tablets (Zortress) ⓄⓃⒸ: 0.25 mg, 0.5 mg, 0.75 mg, 1 mg
Tablets for oral suspension (Afinitor Disperz) ⓄⓃⒸ: 2 mg, 3 mg, 5 mg

INDICATIONS & DOSAGES
➤ **Advanced renal cell carcinoma after treatment with sunitinib or sorafenib fails; tuberous sclerosis complex (TSC)–associated renal angiomyolipoma; advanced hormone-receptor positive, HER2-negative breast cancer in patients who are postmenopausal in combination with exemestane for recurrence or progression after treatment with letrozole or anastrozole; progressive neuroendocrine tumors of pancreatic origin (unresectable, locally advanced, or metastatic); progressive, well-differentiated, nonfunctional neuroendocrine tumors of GI or lung origin (locally advanced or metastatic) (Afinitor)**
Adults: 10 mg PO once daily. Continue until disease progression or unacceptable toxicity occurs.
Adjust-a-dose: Refer to manufacturer's instructions for dosage modifications for adverse effects, for patients with liver impairment, and for those taking drugs that inhibit or induce P-gp and CYP3A4.
➤ **TSC-associated subependymal giant cell astrocytoma in patients who aren't surgical candidates (Afinitor or Afinitor Disperz)**
Adults and children ages 1 and older: Initially, 4.5 mg/m² PO once daily until

disease progression or unacceptable toxicity occurs; round dose to nearest strength. Adjust dosage per manufacturer's instructions in 1- to 2-week intervals to trough level of 5 to 15 ng/mL. Maximum dose increment at any titration must not exceed 5 mg. Don't combine the two dosage forms (Afinitor tablets and Afinitor Disperz tablets) to achieve the desired dose. Use one dosage form or the other. Once a stable dose is attained, monitor trough levels every 3 to 6 months in patients with changing BSA or every 6 to 12 months in patients with stable BSA for duration of treatment.
Adjust-a-dose: Refer to manufacturer's instructions for dosage modifications for adverse effects, for patients with liver impairment, and for those taking drugs that inhibit or induce P-gp and CYP3A4.
➤ **Adjunctive treatment of patients with TSC-associated partial-onset seizures (Afinitor Disperz)** ⚕
Adults and children ages 2 and older: Initially, 5 mg/m² PO once daily. Titrate dosage to attain trough level 5 to 15 ng/mL. Maximum dose increase is 5 mg every 1 to 2 weeks. Once a stable dose is attained, monitor trough levels every 3 to 6 months in patients with changing BSA or every 6 to 12 months in patients with stable BSA for duration of treatment.
Adjust-a-dose: For patients with Child-Pugh class C liver impairment, initially, 2.5 mg/m² once daily; adjust dosage based on trough levels, as recommended. Refer to manufacturer's instructions for toxicity-related dosage adjustments and for dosage adjustments when drug is used concurrently with P-gp and CYP3A4 inhibitors and P-gp and CYP3A4 inducers.
➤ **Prevention of organ rejection in liver transplantation (Zortress only)**
Adults: 1 mg PO b.i.d. starting at least 30 days after transplant in combination with reduced-dose tacrolimus and corticosteroids. Adjust dosage based on trough levels obtained 4 to 5 days after previous dosing.
Adjust-a-dose: In patients with Child-Pugh class A liver impairment, reduce initial dose by one-third. In patients with Child-Pugh class B or C liver impairment, reduce initial dose by half and monitor blood levels.

➤ **Prevention of kidney transplant rejection in patients at low to moderate immunologic risk (Zortress only)**

Adults: Initially, 0.75 mg PO b.i.d. in combination with basiliximab induction and a reduced dose of cyclosporine and corticosteroids as soon as possible after transplantation. Dosage adjustments may be made at 4- to 5-day intervals based on patient response and clinical situation.

Adjust-a-dose: In patients with Child-Pugh class A liver impairment, reduce initial dose by one-third. In patients with Child-Pugh class B or C liver impairment, reduce initial dose by half and monitor blood levels.

ADMINISTRATION
PO

🜂 *Alert:* Hazardous drug; use safe handling and disposal precautions.

Afinitor, Zortress

• Give drug at same time(s) each day, consistently with or without food. Give Zortress about 12 hours apart at the same time as cyclosporine or tacrolimus.

• Have patient swallow tablets whole; don't crush or cut tablets.

Afinitor Disperz

• Wear gloves to avoid possible contact with everolimus when preparing suspension.

• Give as a suspension only.

• Don't break or crush dispersible tablets.

• Give drug once daily at the same time, either consistently with or without food.

• Prepare suspension in water only and give immediately after preparation. Discard suspension if not administered within 60 minutes after preparation.

• To give drug using an oral syringe, place prescribed dose in 10-mL syringe. Don't exceed total of 10 mg per syringe. If higher doses are required, prepare an additional syringe. Draw approximately 5 mL of water and 4 mL of air into syringe. Place filled syringe into a container (tip up) for 3 minutes, until tablets are in suspension. Gently invert syringe five times immediately before giving. After giving suspension, draw approximately 5 mL of water and 4 mL of air into same syringe, and swirl contents to suspend remaining particles. Give entire contents of syringe.

• To give using a small drinking glass, place prescribed dose into small drinking glass containing approximately 25 mL of water. Don't exceed total of 10 mg per glass. If higher doses are required, prepare an additional glass. Allow 3 minutes for suspension to occur. Stir contents gently with spoon, immediately prior to drinking. Give prepared suspension; then add 25 mL of water to glass and stir with same spoon to resuspend remaining particles. Give entire contents of glass.

• May give a missed Afinitor dose up to 6 hours after the normally scheduled dose. If more than 6 hours have elapsed, omit that day's dose, and give it at the usual time the next day.

ACTION

Binds to an intracellular protein, thereby inhibiting mammalian target rapamycin (mTOR), a kinase. Inhibiting mTOR reduces cancer cell proliferation, angiogenesis, and glucose uptake.

Route	Onset	Peak	Duration
PO	Unknown	1–2 hr	Unknown

Half-life: 30 hours.

ADVERSE REACTIONS

CNS: asthenia, dizziness, headache, insomnia, paresthesia, fever, fatigue, dysgeusia, *seizures,* tremor. **CV:** chest pain, edema, *HF,* HTN, hypotension, atrial fibrillation, tachycardia, palpitations, hot flush, *hemorrhage, DVT.* **EENT:** conjunctivitis, eyelid edema, epistaxis, nasopharyngitis, oropharyngeal pain, rhinitis, dry mouth, blurred vision, cataract. **GI:** abdominal pain, anorexia, diarrhea, dyspepsia, dysphagia, GERD, hemorrhoids, nausea, stomatitis, vomiting, constipation. **GU:** increased creatinine level, kidney failure, UTI, hematuria, dysuria, menstrual irregularities, erectile dysfunction. **Hematologic:** anemia, *leukopenia, neutropenia, thrombocytopenia.* **Hepatic:** elevated ALP, AST, ALT levels. **Metabolic:** diabetes (new onset or exacerbation), weight loss, *hypokalemia, hyperkalemia,* hyperglycemia, hypercholesterolemia, dyslipidemia, *hypomagnesemia,* hypertriglyceridemia, hypophosphatemia. **Musculoskeletal:** extremity pain, jaw pain, arthralgia, back pain. **Respiratory:** cough, dyspnea, pleural effusion, URI, *pneumonitis.* **Skin:** acneiform

Reactions in bold italics are *life-threatening*.

dermatitis, dry skin, erythema, hand-foot syndrome, nail disorder, pruritus, onychoclasis, rash, alopecia, skin lesion. **Other:** chills, infection, hypersensitivity reactions.

INTERACTIONS

☉ Alert: Everolimus may interact with many drugs. Consult a drug compatibility reference or pharmacist for more information.

Drug-drug. *Ace inhibitors (captopril, lisinopril):* May increase risk of angioedema. Avoid use together.

Clozapine: May enhance risk of neutropenia. Monitor patient response.

Boxed Warning *Cyclosporine:* Increased kidney toxicity can occur with standard cyclosporine dosing in combination with Zortress. Decrease cyclosporine dosage, and monitor serum cyclosporine and everolimus levels. ∎

Strong CYP3A4 inducers (carbamazepine, dexamethasone, phenobarbital, phenytoin, rifabutin, rifampin): May decrease everolimus level. Avoid use together; if use together is necessary, increase everolimus dosage per manufacturer's instructions.

Strong or moderate CYP3A4 inhibitors (amprenavir, aprepitant, atazanavir, clarithromycin, delavirdine, diltiazem, erythromycin, fosamprenavir, itraconazole, ketoconazole, nefazodone, ritonavir, saquinavir, verapamil, voriconazole) and P-gp inhibitors (amiodarone, spironolactone): May increase everolimus level. Avoid use together; if use together is necessary, reduce everolimus dosage per manufacturer's instructions.

Vaccines (live-virus): Toxic effects of vaccines may increase and drug's therapeutic effects diminish. Avoid use together.

Drug-herb. *St. John's wort:* May alter drug level. Discourage use together.

Drug-food. *Grapefruit, grapefruit juice:* May increase drug level. Discourage use together.

EFFECTS ON LAB TEST RESULTS

• May increase AST, ALT, urinary protein and creatinine, cholesterol, triglyceride, LDL-C, and glucose levels.

• May decrease phosphate and magnesium levels.

• May increase or decrease potassium level.

• May decrease Hb level and lymphocyte, neutrophil, and platelet counts.

• May increase PT.

CONTRAINDICATIONS & CAUTIONS

Boxed Warning Zortress should only be prescribed by providers experienced in immunosuppressive therapy and management of patients who have undergone organ transplantation. ∎

Boxed Warning Use of Zortress has been shown to increase mortality in a heart transplant clinical trial. Use in patients after heart transplantation isn't recommended. ∎

Boxed Warning Zortress increases risk of infection and malignancies, such as lymphoma and skin cancer. ∎

Boxed Warning Zortress increases risk of arterial and venous kidney thrombosis, mainly during the 30 days after transplantation. ∎

• Contraindicated in patients hypersensitive to drug, its components, or other rapamycin derivatives.

• Afinitor isn't indicated to treat functional carcinoid tumors.

• Use cautiously in patients with liver impairment.

• Avoid use in patients with severe infection.

• New-onset diabetes has occurred with use of Zortress after transplantation.

• Patients younger than age 6 have a higher incidence of serious infections.

• Safety and effectiveness in children with organ transplantation haven't been established.

Dialyzable drug: No.

PREGNANCY-LACTATION-REPRODUCTION

• Avoid use during pregnancy because of fetal risk.

• Patients of childbearing potential should avoid pregnancy and use highly effective contraception during treatment and for 8 weeks after last dose.

• Males with partners of childbearing potential should use effective contraception during treatment and for 4 weeks after final dose.

• The Transplant Pregnancy Registry International encourages reporting of all immunosuppressant exposures during pregnancy in patients who have undergone solid organ transplantation (1-877-955-6877 or www.transplantpregnancyregistry.org).

• Drug may cause male and female infertility.

• It isn't known if drug appears in human milk.

NURSING CONSIDERATIONS

• Avoid direct contact with skin and mucous membranes. If contact occurs, wash area thoroughly.

• Monitor for hypersensitivity reactions, including angioedema.
• Monitor for stomatitis. Ensure patient uses alcohol-free dexamethasone mouthwash when starting treatment.
• Drug can adversely affect wound healing. Withhold drug for at least 1 week before elective surgery. Don't give for at least 2 weeks after major surgery and until adequate wound healing occurs.
• Monitor patient for signs and symptoms of infection (fever, chills, sore throat, fatigue).
⊕ **Alert:** Drug may cause immunosuppression, predisposing patient to bacterial, fungal, viral, and protozoal infections, including reactivation of HBV. Complete treatment of preexisting invasive fungal infections before starting therapy. Consider holding or stopping everolimus if infection occurs. Discontinue drug if invasive systemic fungal infection is diagnosed, and treat infection appropriately.
• Monitor kidney function studies, glucose and lipid levels, and CBC before and during therapy.
• Monitor respiratory status for signs and symptoms of noninfectious pneumonitis (hypoxia, pleural effusion, cough, dyspnea), including radiologic changes. For severe cases, discontinue therapy and administer corticosteroids.
• Monitor for radiation sensitization and recall involving skin and organs (including esophagitis and pneumonitis).

PATIENT TEACHING

• Advise patient of need for contraception.
• Inform patient that use may impair fertility.
• Teach about proper drug administration and handling.
• Inform patient of increased risk of lymphomas and other cancers, especially of the skin. Advise patient to limit sun and UV light exposure, use sunscreen, and wear protective clothing.
• Instruct patient to report mouth ulcers, fever, shortness of breath, cough, rash, headache, loss of appetite, nausea, vomiting, diarrhea, swelling of extremities or face, weakness, tiredness, and nosebleeds.
• Tell patient not to receive live-virus vaccines and to avoid close contact with anyone who has received live-virus vaccine.

SAFETY ALERT!

exenatide ☒
eks-EHN-uh-tyde

Bydureon BCise, Byetta

Therapeutic class: Antidiabetics
Pharmacologic class: Incretin mimetics

AVAILABLE FORMS
Injection: 5 mcg/dose in 1.2-mL; 10 mcg/dose in 2.4-mL prefilled multidose pen
Injection (extended-release): 2 mg/dose in single-dose pen

INDICATIONS & DOSAGES
➤ **Adjunct to diet and exercise to improve glycemic control in patients with type 2 diabetes**
Adults: 5 mcg (immediate-release) subcut b.i.d. within 60 minutes before morning and evening meals. Give doses at least 6 hours apart. If needed, increase to 10 mcg b.i.d. after 1 month. Or, 2 mg (extended-release) subcut once every 7 days any time of day, with or without a meal.
Adjust-a-dose: Use caution when escalating doses of Byetta (injection) from 5 to 10 mcg in patients with CrCl of 30 to 50 mL/minute.

When converting from Byetta immediate-release to Bydureon BCise extended-release formulation, initiate weekly administration of extended-release exenatide the day after discontinuing exenatide immediate-release. Patient may experience increased blood glucose levels for approximately 2 to 4 weeks after conversion. Pretreatment with exenatide immediate-release isn't required before initiating extended-release exenatide.

ADMINISTRATION
Subcutaneous
⊕ **Alert:** Multidose pens are for single patient use only. Never share pens, even if needle is changed. Clearly label with patient-identifying information where it will not obstruct the dosing window, warning, or other product information.
Bydureon BCise
• Give Bydureon BCise at any time during the day and without regard to meals.
• Remove autoinjector from refrigerator 15 minutes before mixing the injection to allow drug to reach room temperature.

• Mix by shaking vigorously for at least 15 seconds. After mixing, Bydureon BCise should appear as an opaque, white to off-white suspension, evenly mixed with no residual medicine along the side, bottom, or top of the inspection window. Don't use if foreign particulate matter or discoloration is visible.

• Give immediately as subcut injection in thigh, abdomen, or back of upper arm. Rotate injection sites each week.

• Hold autoinjector straight up with orange cap toward ceiling. Turn knob on bottom from lock to unlock position until you hear a click; then unscrew and discard orange cap.

• Push autoinjector against skin. Listen for a Beta click when the injection begins.

• Keep holding autoinjector against skin for 15 seconds, until orange rod appears in the window, to ensure delivery of the full dose.

• Give missed dose of extended-release form as soon as noticed, provided next regularly scheduled dose is due 3 or more days later. Then resume usual dosing schedule of once every 7 days. If a dose is missed and the next regularly scheduled dose is due 1 or 2 days later, don't give the missed dose; instead, resume treatment with the next regularly scheduled dose.

• Store autoinjector flat in the refrigerator between 36° and 46° F (2° and 8° C). Can keep at room temperature below 86° F (30° C) for no more than a total of 4 weeks, if needed.

Byetta

• Drug comes in two strengths; check cartridge carefully before use.

• Don't give after a meal.

• Give as subcut injection in thigh, abdomen, or upper arm.

• Inject subcut within 60 minutes before morning and evening meals or before two main meals of the day, approximately 6 hours or more apart.

• If a dose is missed, resume treatment with the next scheduled dose.

• Before first use, store drug in refrigerator at 36° to 46° F (2° to 8° C). After first use, keep drug at room temperature up to 77° F (25° C). Don't freeze, and don't use drug if it has been frozen.

• Protect drug from light.

• Discard pen 30 days after first use, even if some drug remains.

• Don't mix with insulin.

ACTION

Reduces fasting and postprandial glucose levels in type 2 diabetes, as an incretin analogue (glucagon-like peptide 1), by stimulating insulin production in response to elevated glucose level, inhibiting glucagon release after meals, and slowing gastric emptying.

Route	Onset	Peak	Duration
Subcut	Unknown	2.1 hr	Unknown
Subcut (extended-release)	Unknown	2 wk, 6–7 wk	10 wk

Half-life: 2.4 hours; extended-release, about 2 weeks.

ADVERSE REACTIONS

CNS: dizziness, headache, fatigue, jittery feeling, nervousness, asthenia. **GI:** anorexia, constipation, decreased appetite, diarrhea, dyspepsia, nausea, vomiting, GERD, abdominal distention, flatulence. **Hepatic:** gallbladder disease. **Metabolic:** *hypoglycemia.* **Skin:** diaphoresis, injection-site nodule, injection-site pruritus or erythema. **Other:** anti-exenatide antibodies.

INTERACTIONS

Drug-drug. *Oral drugs that need to maintain threshold level to maintain effectiveness (antibiotics, hormonal contraceptives):* May reduce rate and extent of absorption of these drugs. Give these drugs at least 1 hour before giving exenatide.
Other antidiabetics (insulin, meglitinides [repaglinide], sulfonylureas): May increase risk of hypoglycemia. Closely monitor blood glucose level when exenatide is started or stopped, and reinforce patient instructions for hypoglycemia management, especially in patients receiving insulin. Reduce insulin or sulfonylurea dose as needed, and monitor patient closely.
Warfarin: May increase INR and increase bleeding risk when administered together. Frequently monitor INR, especially when starting drug or changing dosage.

EFFECTS ON LAB TEST RESULTS

• Decreases glucose level.
• May increase INR.

CONTRAINDICATIONS & CAUTIONS

▨ **Boxed Warning** Extended-release form is contraindicated in patients with personal or family history of medullary thyroid carcinoma and in patients with multiple endocrine neoplasia syndrome type 2. ■

Boxed Warning Exenatide extended-release causes an increased incidence of thyroid C-cell tumors in rats. It isn't known whether drug increases risk of thyroid C-cell tumors in humans. ■

• Contraindicated in patients hypersensitive to drug or its components. Serious reactions (anaphylaxis, angioedema) have been reported.

• Contraindicated in patients with history of drug-induced immune-mediated thrombocytopenia from exenatide products.

• Possibly fatal bleeding from drug-induced immune-mediated thrombocytopenia has been reported with exenatide use.

• Exenatide extended-release isn't recommended as first-line therapy for patients with inadequate glycemic control on diet and exercise.

• Drug isn't recommended for patients with CrCl of less than 30 mL/minute. Use cautiously in patients with kidney transplantation or CrCl of 30 to 60 mL/minute.

• Drug has been associated with acute pancreatitis, including fatal and nonfatal hemorrhagic or necrotizing pancreatitis. Immediately discontinue drug if pancreatitis is suspected. Don't restart if pancreatitis is confirmed.

• Don't use in patients with type 1 diabetes or diabetic ketoacidosis.

• Don't use in patients with severe GI disease (including gastroparesis).

• Safety and effectiveness in children younger than age 10 haven't been established.

Dialyzable drug: Unknown.

⚠ *Overdose S&S:* Severe nausea, severe vomiting, hypoglycemia.

PREGNANCY-LACTATION-REPRODUCTION

• Use only if potential benefit justifies fetal risk.

• It isn't known if drug appears in human milk. Patient should discontinue breastfeeding or discontinue drug, considering importance of drug to patient.

NURSING CONSIDERATIONS

• Assess GI and kidney function before and during treatment.

◑ *Alert:* Drug-related nausea, vomiting, and diarrhea, resulting in dehydration, have led to increased serum creatinine level and AKI.

• Monitor patient receiving extended-release form for serious injection-site reactions (abscess, cellulitis, necrosis with or without subcutaneous nodules).

• Monitor for hypersensitivity reaction; discontinue drug if it occurs.

• Monitor glucose level regularly and HbA$_{1c}$ level periodically.

◑ *Alert:* Stop drug if pancreatitis is suspected. Initiate appropriate treatment, and monitor patient carefully. Drug shouldn't be readministered.

• *Look alike–sound alike:* Don't confuse exenatide with ezetimibe.

PATIENT TEACHING

Boxed Warning Explain to patient taking extended-release exenatide the risk and signs and symptoms of thyroid tumors (neck mass, dysphagia, dyspnea, persistent hoarseness). ■

• Advise the patient to report any adverse effects.

• Review proper use of medication, particularly one-time setup for each new pen or reconstitution procedure for powder.

• Stress importance of proper storage (refrigeration), infection prevention, and timing of exenatide dose in relation to other oral drugs.

◑ *Alert:* Warn patient not to share multidose pen device with other people, even if needle is changed, due to risk of transmission of bloodborne pathogens, including HIV and hepatitis viruses.

• Advise patient that drug may decrease appetite, food intake, and body weight. Explain that these changes don't warrant a change in dosage.

• Caution patient to seek immediate medical care if unexplained, persistent, severe abdominal pain, with or without vomiting, occurs.

• Inform patient receiving extended-release form about risk of serious injection-site reactions. Instruct patient to immediately report signs and symptoms (erythema, pain, drainage, skin color changes).

Reactions in bold italics are *life-threatening*.

• Review steps for managing hypoglycemia, especially if patient takes a sulfonylurea or insulin.
• Inform patient of risk of worsening kidney function and signs and symptoms of kidney dysfunction.
• Tell patient changing from immediate-release to extended-release form that transient blood glucose elevations are possible during first 2 to 4 weeks of therapy.

ezetimibe ⬥
ee-ZET-ah-mibe

Zetia

Therapeutic class: Antilipemics
Pharmacologic class: Selective cholesterol absorption inhibitors

AVAILABLE FORMS
Tablets: 10 mg

INDICATIONS & DOSAGES
➤ **Adjunct to diet to reduce total cholesterol, LDL-C, and apolipoprotein B (apo B) levels in patients with primary hypercholesterolemia, alone or combined with HMG-CoA reductase inhibitors (statins); adjunct to other lipid-lowering drugs (combined with atorvastatin or simvastatin) to reduce total cholesterol and LDL-C levels in patients with homozygous familial hypercholesterolemia; adjunct to diet in patients with homozygous sitosterolemia to reduce sitosterol and campesterol levels; adjunct to fenofibrate and diet to reduce total cholesterol, LDL-C, apo B, and non-HDL-C levels in patients with mixed hyperlipidemia ⬥**
Adults and children ages 10 and older: 10 mg PO daily.

ADMINISTRATION
PO
• Give drug without regard to meals.
• May give dose at same time as an HMG-CoA reductase inhibitor or fenofibrate.
• Give at least 2 hours before or at least 4 hours after administration of a bile acid sequestrant.

ACTION
Inhibits absorption of cholesterol by small intestine, unlike other drugs used for cholesterol reduction; causes reduced liver cholesterol stores and increased cholesterol clearance from blood.

Route	Onset	Peak	Duration
PO	Within 1 wk; max effect in 2–4 wk	4–12 hr	Unknown

Half-life: 22 hours.

ADVERSE REACTIONS
CNS: fatigue. **EENT:** nasopharyngitis, sinusitis. **GI:** diarrhea. **Musculoskeletal:** arthralgia, back pain, extremity pain, myalgia. **Respiratory:** URI. **Other:** viral infection, flulike symptoms.

INTERACTIONS
Drug-drug. *Bile acid sequestrant (cholestyramine):* May decrease ezetimibe level. Give ezetimibe at least 2 hours before or 4 hours after cholestyramine.
Coumarin anticoagulants (warfarin): May alter anticoagulant effects. Monitor INR.
Cyclosporine: May increase levels of both drugs. Monitor cyclosporine level and patient for adverse reactions.
Fenofibrate: May increase risk of cholelithiasis. Monitor patient; consider alternative therapy if cholelithiasis occurs.
Fibrates: May increase excretion of cholesterol into gallbladder bile. Avoid use together.
Gemfibrozil: May increase ezetimibe level and risk of myopathy and cholelithiasis. Avoid use together.

EFFECTS ON LAB TEST RESULTS
• May increase LFT values and CK level.

CONTRAINDICATIONS & CAUTIONS
• Contraindicated in patients hypersensitive to components of drug.
• Contraindicated in combination with HMG-CoA reductase inhibitors in patients with active liver disease or unexplained increased transaminase levels.
• Rarely, myopathy (including rhabdomyolysis) has been reported. Risk may increase with concurrent use of fibrate drugs or high-dose statins, age greater than 65, hypothyroidism, or kidney impairment.
Dialyzable drug: Unknown.

PREGNANCY-LACTATION-REPRODUCTION
• Use only if potential benefit justifies fetal risk.
• When drug is used with a statin in patient of childbearing potential, refer to pregnancy information and product labeling for the statin.
• It isn't known if drug appears in human milk. Use drug in patient who is breastfeeding only if potential benefit justifies risk to infant.

NURSING CONSIDERATIONS
• Before starting treatment, assess patient for underlying causes of dyslipidemia.
• Obtain baseline triglyceride and total cholesterol, LDL-C, and HDL-C levels.
• Using drug with an HMG-CoA reductase inhibitor significantly decreases total cholesterol, LDL-C, apo B, and triglyceride levels and (except with pravastatin) increases HDL-C level more than use of an HMG-CoA reductase inhibitor alone. Check LFT values when therapy starts and thereafter according to the HMG-CoA reductase inhibitor manufacturer's recommendations.
• Patient should maintain a cholesterol-lowering diet during treatment.
• Monitor patient for muscle pain, weakness, or tenderness. Discontinue drug if signs or symptoms of myopathy occur with CK more than $10 \times$ ULN.

PATIENT TEACHING
• Emphasize importance of following a cholesterol-lowering diet during drug therapy.
• Teach about safe drug administration.
• Advise patient to report unexplained muscle pain, weakness, or tenderness.
• Urge patient to tell prescriber about any herbal or dietary supplements being taken.
• Advise patient to visit prescriber for routine follow-ups and to obtain monitoring blood tests.
• Tell patient to report pregnancy or plans to become pregnant.

famciclovir ⚕
fam-SYE-kloe-vir

Therapeutic class: Antivirals
Pharmacologic class: Nucleosides–nucleotides

AVAILABLE FORMS
Tablets: 125 mg, 250 mg, 500 mg

INDICATIONS & DOSAGES
➤ **Acute herpes zoster infection (shingles)**
Adults: 500 mg PO every 8 hours for 7 days.
Adjust-a-dose: For patients with CrCl of 40 to 59 mL/minute, give 500 mg PO every 12 hours; if CrCl is 20 to 39 mL/minute, give 500 mg PO every 24 hours; if CrCl is less than 20 mL/minute, give 250 mg PO every 24 hours. For patients on hemodialysis, give 250 mg PO after each hemodialysis session.
➤ **Recurrent genital herpes**
Adults: 1,000 mg PO b.i.d. for a single day. Begin therapy at first sign or symptom.
Adjust-a-dose: For patients with CrCl of 40 to 59 mL/minute, give 500 mg every 12 hours for 1 day; for CrCl of 20 to 39 mL/minute, give 500 mg PO as single dose; if CrCl is less than 20 mL/minute, give 250 mg as single dose. For patient on hemodialysis, give 250 mg single dose after hemodialysis session.
➤ **Suppression of recurrent genital herpes**
Adults: 250 mg PO b.i.d. for up to 1 year.
Adjust-a-dose: For patients with CrCl of 20 to 39 mL/minute, give 125 mg PO every 12 hours; if CrCl is less than 20 mL/minute, give 125 mg PO every 24 hours. For patients on hemodialysis, give 125 mg PO after each hemodialysis session.
➤ **Recurrent mucocutaneous (orolabial/genital) herpes simplex infections in patients infected with HIV**
Adults: 500 mg PO b.i.d. for 7 days.
Adjust-a-dose: For patients with CrCl of 20 to 39 mL/minute, give 500 mg PO every 24 hours; if CrCl is less than 20 mL/minute, give 250 mg PO every 24 hours. For patients on hemodialysis, give 250 mg PO after each hemodialysis session.
➤ **Recurrent herpes labialis (cold sores)**
Adults: 1,500 mg PO for one dose. Give at first sign or symptom of cold sore.
Adjust-a-dose: For patients with CrCl of 40 to 59 mL/minute, give 750 mg as single dose; for CrCl of 20 to 39 mL/minute, give 500 mg PO as single dose; if CrCl is less than 20 mL/minute, give 250 mg as single dose. For patient on hemodialysis, give 250 mg single dose after hemodialysis session.

ADMINISTRATION
PO
• Give drug without regard to meals.
• Store at 68° to 77° F (20° to 25° C).

ACTION
A guanosine nucleoside that is converted to penciclovir, which enters viral cells and inhibits DNA polymerase and viral DNA synthesis.

Route	Onset	Peak	Duration
PO	Unknown	1 hr	Unknown

Half-life: Penciclovir, 2 to 4 hours.

ADVERSE REACTIONS
CNS: headache, migraine, fatigue, dizziness, paresthesia, somnolence. **GI:** nausea, abdominal pain, diarrhea, vomiting, flatulence. **GU:** dysmenorrhea. **Hematologic:** *leukopenia, neutropenia.* **Hepatic:** elevated AST and ALT levels, bilirubinemia. **Metabolic:** increased amylase and lipase levels. **Skin:** pruritus, rash.

INTERACTIONS
Drug-drug. *Varicella virus vaccine, zoster vaccine (live, attenuated):* May diminish effect of vaccines. When possible, discontinue famciclovir for at least 24 hours before and 14 days after vaccinations.

EFFECTS ON LAB TEST RESULTS
• May increase AST, ALT, amylase, lipase, and bilirubin levels.
• May decrease Hb level and leukocyte and neutrophil counts.

CONTRAINDICATIONS & CAUTIONS
• Contraindicated in patients hypersensitive to drug, its components, or penciclovir cream.
• Use cautiously in patients with kidney or liver impairment and in older adults.
⚕ Efficacy and safety haven't been established for patients with first episode of genital herpes or ophthalmic zoster; patients who are immunocompromised, other than for treatment of recurrent episodes of orolabial or genital herpes in patients infected with HIV; and patients who are Black or African American with recurrent genital herpes.
• Efficacy in children hasn't been established.
Dialyzable drug: Yes.

PREGNANCY-LACTATION-REPRODUCTION
• Use drug during pregnancy only if benefit clearly outweighs fetal risk.
• It isn't known if drug appears in human milk. Use only if benefits outweigh risk to infant.

NURSING CONSIDERATIONS
• Monitor LFT and kidney function test results.
• Periodically monitor CBC during long-term therapy.

PATIENT TEACHING
• Inform patient that drug doesn't cure herpes but can decrease the duration and severity of symptoms.
• Teach patient how to avoid spreading infection to others.
• Urge patient to recognize and report early signs and symptoms of herpes infection (tingling, itching, burning, pain, or lesion). Therapy is more effective if started within 48 hours of rash onset.
• Drug may contain lactose. If patient is lactose-intolerant, advise patient to notify prescriber before taking drug.
• Advise patient with dizziness, somnolence, confusion, or other CNS disturbance to refrain from driving or operating machinery.

famotidine
fa-MOE-ti-deen

Pepcid, Pepcid AC ◊, Zantac 360° ◊

Therapeutic class: Antiulcer drugs
Pharmacologic class: H₂-receptor antagonists

AVAILABLE FORMS
Injection: 0.4 mg/mL in NSS (premixed), 10 mg/mL
Powder for oral suspension: 40 mg/5 mL after reconstitution
Tablets: 10 mg ◊, 20 mg ◊, 40 mg

INDICATIONS & DOSAGES
Adjust-a-dose (for all indications): For patients with CrCl below 60 mL/minute, refer to manufacturer's product information because dosage varies based on form being administered, indication, and CrCl value.
➤ **Short-term treatment for duodenal ulcer**
Adults, adolescents, and children weighing at least 40 kg: For acute therapy, 40 mg PO once daily at bedtime or 20 mg PO b.i.d. for up to 8 weeks. Healing usually occurs within 4 weeks.

For maintenance therapy (adults), 20 mg PO once daily at bedtime for 1 year or as clinically indicated.

➤ **Short-term treatment for benign gastric ulcer**

Adults, adolescents, and children weighing more than 40 kg: 40 mg PO daily at bedtime for up to 8 weeks.

Children ages 1 to 16: 0.5 mg/kg/day oral suspension PO at bedtime or in two divided doses (maximum dose, 40 mg/day). Dosages up to 1 mg/kg/day have been used.

➤ **Pathologic hypersecretory conditions (such as Zollinger-Ellison syndrome)**

Adults: 20 mg PO every 6 hours, up to 160 mg every 6 hours as clinically indicated. Maximum, 640 mg/day.

➤ **Patients who are hospitalized who can't take oral drug or who have intractable ulcers or hypersecretory conditions**

Adults: 20 mg IV every 12 hours.

Children ages 1 to 16: 0.25 mg/kg IV every 12 hours (maximum dose, 40 mg/day). Dosages up to 0.5 mg/kg every 12 hours have been used.

➤ **GERD**

Adults, adolescents, and children weighing at least 40 kg: Short-term therapy: 20 mg PO b.i.d. for up to 6 weeks. For esophagitis caused by GERD, 20 to 40 mg b.i.d. for up to 12 weeks.

Children ages 1 to 16: Short-term therapy: 0.5 mg/kg/dose PO b.i.d. (maximum dose, 40 mg b.i.d.). Dosages up to 1 mg/kg/dose b.i.d. have been used.

Children ages 3 months to younger than 1 year: Short-term therapy: 0.5 mg/kg/dose oral suspension PO b.i.d.

Children younger than age 3 months: Short-term therapy: 0.5 mg/kg/dose oral suspension once daily for up to 8 weeks.

➤ **To prevent or treat heartburn (only indication for OTC)**

Adults and children ages 12 and older: 10 to 20 mg PO up to b.i.d. Maximum, 40 mg/day.

ADMINISTRATION

PO

• Give drug without regard to meals.
• May give OTC tablets 10 to 60 minutes before patient eats food or drinks beverages that cause heartburn.
• Patient shouldn't chew regular tablets.
• May give with antacids.
• Shake oral suspension before use.
• Store reconstituted oral suspension below 77° F (25° C). Don't freeze. Discard after 30 days.
• Store tablets at 68° to 77° F (20° to 25° C). Protect from light.

IV

▼ Compatible solutions include sterile water for injection, NSS for injection, D_5W or dextrose 10% in water for injection, 5% sodium bicarbonate injection, and lactated Ringer injection. Drug also can be added to TPN solutions.

▼ Before use, store at 36° to 46° F (2° to 8° C). If solution freezes, allow to solubilize at room temperature.

▼ Protect from light.

▼ For direct injection, dilute 2 mL (20 mg) with compatible solution to total volume of either 5 or 10 mL. Inject over at least 2 minutes.

▼ For intermittent infusion, dilute 20 mg (2 mL) in 100-mL compatible solution. The premixed 50-mL solution doesn't need further dilution. Infuse over 15 to 30 minutes.

▼ After dilution, solution is stable for 7 days at room temperature.

▼ **Incompatibilities:** Amphotericin B cholesteryl sulfate complex, azathioprine, cefepime, chloramphenicol, dantrolene, diazepam, ganciclovir, gemtuzumab, lansoprazole, mitomycin, pantoprazole, piperacillin–tazobactam, trimethoprim–sulfamethoxazole.

ACTION

Competitively inhibits action of histamine on H_2-receptor sites of parietal cells, decreasing gastric acid secretion.

Route	Onset	Peak	Duration
PO	1 hr	1–3 hr	10–12 hr
IV	30 minutes	1–4 hr	10–12 hr

Half-life: 2.5 to 3.5 hours (adults), 5 to 15 hours (infants 0 to 3 months).

ADVERSE REACTIONS

CNS: headache, dizziness; irritability, agitation (younger than age 1). **GI:** constipation, diarrhea; vomiting (younger than age 1).

INTERACTIONS

Drug-drug. *Cefditoren, dasatinib, delavirdine, fosamprenavir:* May decrease absorption of these drugs due to reduced gastric acidity. Avoid use together.

Drugs dependent on gastric pH for absorption (atazanavir, cefuroxime, erlotinib, ketoconazole, rilpivirine): May decrease absorption of these drugs. Refer to prescribing information of individual drug.

Reactions in bold italics are *life-threatening*.

Drugs that prolong QT interval (antiarrhythmics, chlorpromazine, citalopram, clarithromycin, fluoxetine, levofloxacin): May increase risk of cardiac arrhythmias, including torsades de pointes. Use together cautiously unless specifically contraindicated. Refer to prescribing information of individual drug.
Risedronate (delayed-release): May increase risedronate level. Avoid combination.
Tizanidine: May increase tizanidine level. Avoid use together. Monitor for hypotension, bradycardia, and excessive drowsiness if use together is unavoidable.

EFFECTS ON LAB TEST RESULTS
• May increase liver enzyme levels.
• May cause false-negative results in skin tests using allergen extracts. May antagonize pentagastrin in gastric acid secretion tests.

CONTRAINDICATIONS & CAUTIONS
• Contraindicated in patients with history of serious hypersensitivity to drug and other H_2-receptor antagonists.
• Use for OTC self-medication is contraindicated in patients with trouble or pain when swallowing, vomiting with blood, bloody or black stools, allergic reactions to other acid reducers, or kidney impairment and in those using other acid reducers, unless directed by health care provider.
• Drug may cause reversible confusional states that clear 3 to 4 days after discontinuation. Patients older than age 50 and those with kidney or liver impairment may be at greater risk.
🟢 **Alert:** Symptomatic response doesn't preclude the presence of gastric malignancy. Consider further evaluation in patients with suboptimal response or an early symptomatic relapse after drug treatment.
🟢 **Alert:** QT-interval prolongation and torsades de pointes have been reported (rarely) in patients with kidney dysfunction.
• Treatment lasting 2 years can cause vitamin B_{12} deficiency, which is dose-related and more likely to occur in females and those younger than age 30.
🟢 **Alert:** Some forms contain benzyl alcohol, which is linked to gasping syndrome (metabolic acidosis, respiratory distress, CNS dysfunction, hypotension, CV collapse) in neonates.
Dialyzable drug: No.
⚠ **Overdose S&S:** Similar to adverse reactions with use at recommended dosages.

PREGNANCY-LACTATION-REPRODUCTION
• Drug crosses placental barrier and appears in human milk. Use cautiously during pregnancy and breastfeeding.

NURSING CONSIDERATIONS
• Assess patient for abdominal pain.
• Look for blood in emesis, stool, or gastric aspirate.
• Monitor patient with kidney dysfunction for QT-interval prolongation.

PATIENT TEACHING
• Instruct patient in proper use of OTC product, if appropriate.
• Advise patient to limit use of prescription drug to no longer than 8 weeks, unless ordered by prescriber, and OTC drug to no longer than 2 weeks.
• With prescriber's knowledge, patient may take with an antacid, especially at beginning of therapy when pain is severe.
• Urge patient to avoid cigarette smoking because it may increase gastric acid secretion and worsen disease.
• Advise patient to report abdominal pain, blood in stools or vomit, melena, or coffee-ground emesis.

---

febuxostat
feb-UX-oh-stat

Uloric

Therapeutic class: Antigout drugs
Pharmacologic class: Xanthine oxidase inhibitors

AVAILABLE FORMS
Tablets: 40 mg, 80 mg

INDICATIONS & DOSAGES
Boxed Warning Only use drug in patients who have an inadequate response to a maximally titrated dose of allopurinol, who are intolerant to allopurinol, or for whom treatment with allopurinol isn't advisable.
➤ **Chronic management of hyperuricemia associated with gout**
Adults: 40 mg PO daily. May increase dosage to 80 mg after 2 weeks if uric acid level remains above 6 mg/dL.
Adjust-a-dose: In patients with CrCl of less than 30 mL/minute, maximum dose is 40 mg/day.

🍁Canada   ◇OTC   ◆Off-label use   🚫Do not crush   *Liquid contains alcohol   ⚡Genetic

ADMINISTRATION
PO
• Give drug without regard to food or antacid use.
• Store at 77° F (25° C).
• Protect from light.

ACTION
Reduces uric acid production by inhibiting xanthine oxidase.

Route	Onset	Peak	Duration
PO	Rapid	1–1.5 hr	Unknown

Half-life: 5 to 8 hours.

ADVERSE REACTIONS
CNS: dizziness. **GI:** nausea. **Hepatic:** liver function abnormalities. **Musculoskeletal:** arthralgia. **Skin:** rash.

INTERACTIONS
Drug-drug. *Azathioprine, didanosine, mercaptopurine:* May increase levels of these drugs, leading to toxicity. Use together is contraindicated.
Pegloticase: May increase toxic effects of pegloticase. Avoid use together.
Rosuvastatin: May increase rosuvastatin level. Limit rosuvastatin dose to 20 mg daily when combined and monitor for adverse effects.
Theophylline: May increase theophylline level. Use together cautiously.

EFFECTS ON LAB TEST RESULTS
• May increase ALP, AST, and ALT levels.

CONTRAINDICATIONS & CAUTIONS
• Contraindicated in patients hypersensitive to drug or its components.
Boxed Warning Drug may increase risk of CV death in patients with CV disease compared to those treated with allopurinol. Consider risks and benefits of drug when deciding to prescribe or continue patients on febuxostat. ■
• Use in patients with secondary hyperuricemia (including organ transplant recipients and patients with malignancy) hasn't been studied. Use isn't recommended.
• Use cautiously in patients with Child-Pugh class C liver impairment or CrCl of less than 30 mL/minute.
• Use cautiously in patients who report serious skin reactions to allopurinol.

• Not recommended for treatment of asymptomatic hyperuricemia.
• Safety and effectiveness in children haven't been established.
• Drug may contain lactose. Consider alternative agent in patients who are lactose-intolerant, if necessary.
Dialyzable drug: Unlikely.

PREGNANCY-LACTATION-REPRODUCTION
• It isn't known if drug crosses the placental barrier. Use during pregnancy only if potential benefit justifies fetal risk.
• It isn't known if drug appears in human milk. Use cautiously during breastfeeding.

NURSING CONSIDERATIONS
Boxed Warning Monitor all patients for signs and symptoms of CV events. ■
• Watch for acute gout flares during first 6 weeks of therapy; colchicine or another anti-inflammatory may be added prophylactically, and drug should be continued.
• Monitor liver function at baseline, 2 months and 4 months after starting therapy, and periodically thereafter.
• Monitor for signs and symptoms of hypersensitivity or severe skin reactions (SJS, DRESS syndrome, TEN). If suspected, discontinue drug.
⚠ *Alert:* Patients with unexplained serum ALT level greater than $3 \times$ ULN with total bilirubin level greater than $2 \times$ ULN are at risk for severe drug-induced liver injury. Stop drug in these patients and don't restart.
• Monitor uric acid level.

PATIENT TEACHING
Boxed Warning Advise patient of risk of CV events. Teach patient to seek immediate emergency medical care for chest pain, shortness of breath, dizziness, fainting, lightheadedness, fast or irregular heartbeat, numbness or weakness on one side of the body, slurred speech, blurred vision, or sudden severe headache. ■
• Warn patient about risk of gout flares and importance of taking an NSAID or colchicine during first 6 weeks of treatment.
• Advise patient to report all adverse reactions, including abnormal bleeding, nausea, malaise, light-colored stools, yellowing of eyes or skin, and rash.
• Instruct patient to immediately report signs or symptoms of severe skin reactions.

Reactions in bold italics are *life-threatening*.

felodipine
fe-LOE-di-peen

Plendil✤

Therapeutic class: Antihypertensives
Pharmacologic class: Calcium channel
blockers

AVAILABLE FORMS
Tablets (extended-release) ⓓⓝⓒ: 2.5 mg, 5 mg,
10 mg

INDICATIONS & DOSAGES
➤ **HTN**
Adults: Initially, 5 mg PO daily. Adjust
dosage based on patient response, usually
at intervals of not less than 2 weeks. Dosage
range, 2.5 to 10 mg daily.
Older adults: 2.5 mg PO daily; adjust dosage
as for adults. Maximum dosage, 10 mg daily.
Adjust-a-dose: Patients with impaired liver
function may respond to lower doses.
➤ **Chronic stable angina (alternative
agent)** ◆
Adults: Initially, 5 to 10 mg PO once daily; if
initiated at 5 mg, increase to 10 mg once daily
as tolerated after 2 to 4 weeks.

ADMINISTRATION
PO
• Have patient swallow tablets whole; don't
crush or break tablets.
• Give drug without food or with a light meal
low in fat and carbohydrates.
• Store at room temperature.
• Protect from light.

ACTION
Dihydropyridine-derivative calcium channel blocker that prevents entry of calcium
ions into vascular smooth muscle and cardiac
cells; shows some selectivity for smooth muscle compared with cardiac muscle.

Route	Onset	Peak	Duration
PO	2–5 hr	2.5–5 hr	24 hr

Half-life: 11 to 16 hours.

ADVERSE REACTIONS
CNS: headache, dizziness, paresthesia, asthenia, warm sensation. **CV:** peripheral edema,
tachycardia, palpitations, flushing. **EENT:**
rhinorrhea. **GI:** abdominal pain, nausea,
constipation, diarrhea, dyspepsia. **Musculoskeletal:** arthralgia, muscle cramps, back
or limb pain. **Respiratory:** URI, cough,
sneezing. **Skin:** rash.

INTERACTIONS
Drug-drug. *Anticonvulsants (long-term
phenytoin, carbamazepine):* May decrease
felodipine level. Avoid use together.
*Atypical second-generation antipsychotics
(risperidone):* May enhance hypotensive effects. Monitor therapy.
*CYP3A4 inhibitors (azole antifungals, cimeti-
dine, erythromycin):* May decrease clearance
of felodipine. Reduce felodipine dose; monitor patient for toxicity.
Metoprolol: May alter pharmacokinetics of
metoprolol. Monitor for adverse reactions.
Tacrolimus: May increase tacrolimus level.
Monitor patient closely.
Drug-herb. *Herbs with hypertensive or hypotensive properties (ginseng, licorice):* May
increase or decrease antihypertensive effects.
Discourage use together.
Drug-food. *Grapefruit:* May increase drug
level and adverse effects. Discourage use together.
Drug-lifestyle. *Alcohol use:* May increase
felodipine absorption. Monitor patient for increased hypotensive effect.

EFFECTS ON LAB TEST RESULTS
• May lead to false-negative aldosterone-
renin ratio.

CONTRAINDICATIONS & CAUTIONS
• Contraindicated in patients hypersensitive
to drug.
• Drug may cause significant hypotension
and, rarely, syncope.
• Safe use in patients with HF hasn't been established. Use cautiously in patients with HF
or decreased ventricular function.
• Use cautiously and in lower doses in older
adults and in patients with liver impairment.
• Drug may contain lactose. If necessary,
consider alternative agent in patients who are
lactose-intolerant.
• Safety and effectiveness in children haven't
been established.
Dialyzable drug: Unlikely.
⚠ **Overdose S&S:** Peripheral vasodilation,
hypotension, bradycardia.

PREGNANCY-LACTATION-REPRODUCTION

• Well-controlled studies during pregnancy are lacking, but animal studies show potential fetal hazards. If treatment for HTN during pregnancy is needed, other agents are preferred.

• It isn't known if drug appears in human milk. Patient should discontinue breastfeeding or discontinue drug, considering importance of drug to patient.

NURSING CONSIDERATIONS

• Monitor BP and HR for response.

• Monitor for peripheral edema, which appears to be both dose- and age-related. It's more common in patients taking higher doses, especially those older than age 60.

PATIENT TEACHING

• Teach about proper drug administration and handling.

• Advise patient to continue taking drug even when feeling better, to watch diet, and to check with prescriber or pharmacist before taking other drugs, including OTC drugs, nutritional supplements, and herbal remedies.

• Teach patient to report all adverse reactions.

• Advise patient to observe good oral hygiene and to regularly see a dentist; use of drug may cause mild gum problems.

• Instruct patient to report pregnancy or plans to become pregnant or to breastfeed.

fenofibrate
fee-no-FYE-brate

Antara, Fenoglide, Lipofen, TriCor

fenofibrate acid (choline fenofibrate)
Trilipix

Therapeutic class: Antilipemics
Pharmacologic class: Fibric acid derivatives

AVAILABLE FORMS
fenofibrate
Capsules ⬤: 50 mg, 150 mg
Capsules (micronized) ⬤: 43 mg, 67 mg, 90 mg, 130 mg, 134 mg, 200 mg
Tablets ⬤: 40 mg, 48 mg, 54 mg, 120 mg, 145 mg, 160 mg
Fenofibrate acid (choline fenofibrate)
Capsules (delayed-release) ⬤: 45 mg, 135 mg
Tablets: 35 mg, 105 mg

INDICATIONS & DOSAGES
Adjust-a-dose (for all indications): Refer to specific product information for guidelines regarding dosing for patients with kidney impairment.

➤ **Hypertriglyceridemia (Fredrickson types IV and V hyperlipidemia) in patients who don't respond adequately to diet alone**
Adults: For Antara and generics, initial dose is 43 to 130 mg PO daily, with maximum dose of 130 mg daily. For fenofibrate acid tablets, initial dose is 35 to 105 mg daily, with maximum dose of 105 mg daily. For fenofibrate (micronized), initial dose is 43 to 130 mg once daily, with maximum dose of 130 mg daily. For Fenoglide and generics, initial dose is 40 to 120 mg/day, with maximum dose of 120 mg daily. For Lipofen and generics, initial dose is 50 to 150 mg daily, with maximum dose of 150 mg daily. For TriCor and generics, initial dose is 48 to 145 mg daily, with maximum dose of 145 mg daily. For Trilipix and generics, initial dose is 45 to 135 mg once daily, with maximum dose of 135 mg once daily. For all forms, adjust dose based on patient response and repeat lipid determinations every 4 to 12 weeks.

➤ **Primary hypercholesterolemia or mixed dyslipidemia (Fredrickson types IIa and IIb) in patients who don't respond adequately to diet alone**
Adults: For Antara and generics, initial dose is 130 mg PO daily. For Fenoglide, initial dose is 120 mg/day. For fenofibrate (micronized), initial dose is 130 mg once daily. For fenofibrate acid tablets, dose is 105 mg PO daily. For Lipofen and generics, initial dose is 150 mg daily. For TriCor and generics, initial dose is 145 mg daily. For Trilipix and generics, initial dose is 45 to 135 mg once daily, with maximum dose of 135 mg once daily. May reduce dose if lipid levels fall significantly below target range.

ADMINISTRATION
PO
• Administer Fenoglide and Lipofen with meals.

• Administer Antara, fenofibrate acid tablets, TriCor, and Trilipix with or without food.

• Have patient swallow tablets whole; don't dissolve, crush, or break tablets, or open capsules.

• Store at room temperature.

Reactions in bold italics are *life-threatening*.

ACTION
May lower triglyceride levels by inhibiting triglyceride synthesis with less VLDL-C released into circulation. May also stimulate breakdown of triglyceride-rich protein.

Route	Onset	Peak	Duration
PO	Unknown	2–8 hr	Unknown

Half-life: 20 hours.

ADVERSE REACTIONS
CNS: dizziness, headache, localized pain. **CV:** *PE,* thrombophlebitis. **EENT:** rhinitis, sinusitis, nasopharyngitis. **GI:** abdominal pain, constipation, diarrhea, dyspepsia, nausea. **Hepatic:** elevated AST and ALT levels. **Metabolic:** increased CK level. **Musculoskeletal:** arthralgia, back pain, limb pain, myalgia. **Respiratory:** URI. **Skin:** urticaria, rash.

INTERACTIONS
Drug-drug. *Bile acid sequestrants:* May bind and inhibit absorption of fenofibrate. Give drug 1 hour before or 4 to 6 hours after bile acid sequestrants.
Colchicine: May increase risk of myopathy. Use together cautiously.
Coumarin-type anticoagulants (warfarin): May increase anticoagulant effect, prolonging PT and INR. Closely monitor PT and INR.
Cyclosporine, immunosuppressants, kidney-toxic drugs: May induce kidney dysfunction. Use together cautiously.
HMG-CoA reductase inhibitors (statins): May increase risk of statin adverse effects. Monitor therapy.
Drug-food. *Any food:* May increase capsule absorption. Advise patient to take capsules with meals. Refer to specific product for more information.
Drug-lifestyle. *Alcohol use:* May increase triglyceride levels. Discourage use together.

EFFECTS ON LAB TEST RESULTS
• May increase ALT, AST, BUN, CK, and creatinine levels.
• May decrease uric acid and Hb levels, hematocrit, and platelet and WBC counts.

CONTRAINDICATIONS & CAUTIONS
• Contraindicated in patients hypersensitive to drug and in those with gallbladder disease, liver dysfunction, primary biliary cirrhosis, CKD (including those receiving dialysis), or unexplained persistent liver function abnormalities.
• Some formulations contain peanut oil or soya lecithin and are contraindicated in patients with allergies. Refer to individual products.
• Use cautiously in older adults and patients with history of pancreatitis or kidney impairment.
• Anaphylaxis and angioedema have been reported with fenofibrate use. In some cases, reactions were life-threatening and required emergency treatment.
• Safety and effectiveness in children haven't been established.
Dialyzable drug: No.

PREGNANCY-LACTATION-REPRODUCTION
• Triglyceride and lipid concentrations increase during pregnancy for normal fetal development. Consider using fenofibrate beginning in second trimester to treat severe hypertriglyceridemia. Use other agents for hypercholesterolemia, if necessary. Refer to individual manufacturer's instructions for use during pregnancy.
• Contraindicated during breastfeeding.

NURSING CONSIDERATIONS
• Obtain baseline lipid levels and LFT results before therapy. Periodically monitor liver function during therapy. Stop drug if enzyme levels persist above $3 \times$ ULN.
• Monitor kidney function in patient with current or risk of kidney impairment.
• **Alert:** Watch for signs and symptoms of pancreatitis, myositis, rhabdomyolysis, liver impairment, cholelithiasis, and kidney failure. Monitor for muscle pain, tenderness, or weakness, especially with malaise or fever.
• Watch for SCARs (SJS, TEN, DRESS syndrome), which can occur days to weeks after drug initiation. Discontinue drug and treat appropriately.
• If adequate response isn't obtained after 2 to 3 months of treatment with maximum daily dose, stop therapy.
• Drug lowers uric acid level by increasing uric acid excretion in patient with or without hyperuricemia.
• Beta blockers, estrogens, and thiazide diuretics may increase triglyceride levels. Evaluate need for continued use of these drugs.
• Hb level, hematocrit, and WBC count may decrease when therapy starts but stabilize with long-term administration.

• Discontinue if gallbladder studies reveal gallstones.

• Discontinue if patient develops markedly elevated CK concentration or if myopathy or myositis is suspected or diagnosed.

• Monitor HDL-C level, and permanently discontinue drug if HDL-C level becomes severely depressed.

PATIENT TEACHING

• Teach about proper drug administration and handling.

• Inform patient that drug therapy doesn't reduce need to follow a triglyceride-lowering diet.

• Advise patient to promptly report all adverse reactions, especially unexplained muscle weakness, pain, or tenderness; abdominal pain; and yellowing of skin or eyes, particularly with malaise or fever.

• Warn patient to immediately report development of skin reactions, such as a rash or exfoliative dermatitis.

• Advise patient to continue weight control measures, including diet and exercise, and to limit alcohol before therapy.

SAFETY ALERT!

fentaNYL citrate
FEN-ta-nil

fentaNYL transdermal system

fentaNYL transmucosal
Actiq, Fentora

Therapeutic class: Opioid analgesics
Pharmacologic class: Opioid agonists
Controlled substance schedule: II

AVAILABLE FORMS

Injection: 50 mcg/mL
Transdermal system: Patches that release 12.5 mcg, 25 mcg, 37.5 mcg, 50 mcg, 62.5 mcg, 75 mcg, 87.5 mcg, or 100 mcg of drug per hour
Transmucosal (buccal tablet) ⬛: 100 mcg, 200 mcg, 400 mcg, 600 mcg, 800 mcg
Transmucosal (lozenge) ⬛: 200 mcg, 400 mcg, 600 mcg, 800 mcg, 1,200 mcg, 1,600 mcg

INDICATIONS & DOSAGES

➤ **Adjunct to general anesthetic**
Adults: For low-dose therapy, 2 mcg/kg IV. For moderate-dose therapy, 2 to 20 mcg/kg IV; then 25 to 100 mcg IV or IM PRN. For high-dose therapy, 20 to 50 mcg/kg IV; then 25 mcg to one-half initial loading dose IV PRN.

➤ **Adjunct to regional anesthesia**
Adults: 50 to 100 mcg IM or slowly IV over 1 to 2 minutes PRN.

➤ **To induce and maintain anesthesia**
Children ages 2 to 12 years: 2 to 3 mcg/kg IV every 1 to 2 hours as needed.

➤ **Postoperative pain, restlessness, tachypnea, and emergence delirium**
Adults: 50 to 100 mcg IM every 1 to 2 hours PRN.

➤ **Preoperative medication**
Adults: 50 to 100 mcg IM 30 to 60 minutes before surgery.

➤ **Management of persistent, moderate to severe chronic pain in patients who are opioid-tolerant and require around-the-clock opioid analgesics for extended time**
Adults and children ages 2 and older: When converting to transdermal system, base first dose on daily dose, potency, and characteristics of current opioid therapy; reliability of the relative potency estimates used to calculate the needed dose; degree of opioid tolerance; and patient's condition. Patient may wear each patch for 72 hours, although some adult patients may need a patch to be applied every 48 hours during the first dosage period. May increase dose 3 days after first dose, then every 6 days thereafter.
Adjust-a-dose: For older adults and patients who are cachectic or debilitated, start transdermal system doses at no higher than 25 mcg/hour, unless these patients are already tolerating an around-the-clock opioid at a dose and potency comparable to fentanyl 25 mcg/hour transdermal system. For patients with Child-Pugh class A or B liver impairment or CrCl of 30 to 90 mL/minute, initiate therapy at one-half the usual transdermal dosage. Avoid use in patients with Child-Pugh class C liver impairment or CrCl less than 30 mL/minute.

➤ **Management of breakthrough cancer pain in patients already receiving and tolerating an opioid**
Adults and adolescents ages 16 and older: 200 mcg Actiq lozenge initially; possible

second dose 15 minutes after completing first dose (30 minutes after first lozenge is placed in mouth). Maximum dose, 2 lozenges per breakthrough episode. At least 4 hours must pass before treating another episode. If several episodes of breakthrough pain requiring 2 lozenges occur, dose may be increased to the next available strength. After an effective dosage has been reached (one lozenge per episode), patient should limit use to no more than 4 lozenges daily.

Adults: Initially 100 mcg buccal tablet between the upper cheek and gum. May repeat same dose once per breakthrough episode after at least 30 minutes. At least 4 hours must pass before treating another episode. Adjust in 100-mcg increments. Doses above 400 mcg can be increased by 200 mcg. Generally, dosage should be increased when patient requires more than one dose per breakthrough episode. Once an effective maintenance dose has been established, reevaluate if patient experiences more than four breakthrough episodes per day.

Adjust-a-dose: For patients with kidney or liver impairment, use lowest possible dose.

➤ **Transition from Actiq to Fentora to manage breakthrough cancer pain in patients who are opioid-tolerant**

Adults: If current Actiq dose is 200 to 400 mcg, start with 100 mcg Fentora; if current Actiq dose is 600 to 800 mcg, use 200 mcg Fentora; if current Actiq dose is 1,200 to 1,600 mcg, use 400 mcg Fentora. Refer to manufacturer's information for titration instructions, if needed. Actiq and Fentora aren't bioequivalent.

ADMINISTRATION

Boxed Warning Substantial differences exist between the pharmacokinetic profiles of fentanyl buccal and SL and other fentanyl products that result in clinically important differences in the extent of fentanyl absorption, which could result in fatal overdose. When prescribing, don't convert patients on a mcg-per-mcg basis from other fentanyl products to fentanyl buccal. When dispensing, don't substitute a fentanyl buccal prescription for other fentanyl products. ∎

IV

▼ Only those trained to give IV anesthetics and manage adverse effects should give this form.

▼ Keep opioid antagonist (naloxone) and resuscitation equipment available.

▼ IV form often used with droperidol to produce neuroleptanalgesia.

▼ Inject slowly over 1 to 2 minutes.

▼ **Incompatibilities:** Azithromycin, dantrolene, gemtuzumab ozogamicin, pantoprazole, phenytoin, sulfamethoxazole–trimethoprim. Compatibility of many other drugs is undetermined.

IM

• Document administration site.

Transdermal

• Dosage equivalent charts are available to calculate fentanyl transdermal dose based on daily morphine intake; for example, for every 60 mg of oral morphine or 15 mg of IM morphine per 24 hours, 25 mcg/hour of transdermal fentanyl is needed.

• Clip hair at application site but don't use a razor, which may irritate skin. Wash area with clear water, if needed, but not with soaps, oils, lotions, alcohol, or other substances that may irritate skin or prevent adhesion. Dry area completely before application.

• Always wear gloves when handling transdermal system.

• Remove transdermal system from package just before applying, hold in place for 30 seconds, and be sure edges of patch stick to skin.

• Don't cut or otherwise alter transdermal patch before applying.

• Place transdermal patch on the upper back for a child or patient who's cognitively impaired to reduce the chance the patch will be removed and placed in the mouth.

• If another patch is needed after 48 to 72 hours, apply it to a different skin site.

Boxed Warning Heat from fever, heating pads, electric blankets, heat lamps, hot tubs, or water beds may increase transdermal delivery and cause toxicity. ∎

• Dispose of removed transdermal patch by folding it so the adhesive side adheres to itself and then flushing it down the toilet.

Transmucosal

• Remove foil just before giving.

• For Actiq: Place lozenge between patient's cheek and gum and allow to dissolve over about 15 to 20 minutes; it must not be bitten, sucked, or chewed. Lozenge should be moved from one side to the other using stick. Discard stick in trash after use; if any drug matrix remains on stick, place under hot running tap water until dissolved and then place in trash.

F

Or, place in child-resistant container provided and discard as for Schedule II drugs.
• For buccal tablet: Place tablet between patient's cheek and gum or under tongue and leave there until disintegrated, usually 14 to 25 minutes. Patient shouldn't suck, chew, or swallow tablet; doing so results in lower plasma levels. After 30 minutes, if remnants from tablet remain, they may be swallowed with a glass of water. Alternate side of mouth with subsequent doses.

ACTION

Binds with opioid receptors in the CNS, altering perception of and emotional response to pain.

Route	Onset	Peak	Duration
IV	1–2 min	3–5 min	30–60 min
IM	7–15 min	20–30 min	1–2 hr
Transdermal	12–24 hr	1–3 days	Variable
Transmucosal	5–15 min	20–90 min	Unknown

Half-life: Parenteral, 3.5 hours; transmucosal, 5 to 15 hours; transdermal, 18 hours.

ADVERSE REACTIONS

CNS: abnormal thinking, asthenia, clouded sensorium, confusion, euphoria, lethargy, sedation, somnolence, *seizures,* anxiety, depression, dizziness, fatigue, pain, hallucinations, headache, migraine, hypertonia, hypoesthesia, insomnia, agitation, nervousness, dysgeusia, fever, tremor. **CV:** edema, *bradycardia,* tachycardia, vasodilation, chest pain, HTN, hypotension, *DVT.* **EENT:** dry eyes, dry mouth, abnormal vision, ptosis, pharyngitis, oral ulcer, vertigo. **GI:** constipation, abdominal pain, anorexia, diarrhea, dyspepsia, flatulence, ileus, nausea, vomiting, stomatitis. **GU:** urine retention. **Hematologic:** anemia, *neutropenia.* **Hepatic:** jaundice, increased ALP, increased AST. **Metabolic:** *hypokalemia,* dehydration, weight loss, hypercalcemia, hyperglycemia, hypoalbuminemia, *hypocalcemia, hypomagnesemia,* hyponatremia, *lactic acidosis.* **Musculoskeletal:** back pain, abnormal gait, rigidity. **Respiratory:** *apnea, hypoventilation, respiratory depression,* dyspnea, cough, URI, bronchitis. **Skin:** diaphoresis, pruritus, rash, pressure injury, erythema at application site (transdermal). **Other:** accidental injury, hypersensitivity reactions, chills, infection, physical dependence.

INTERACTIONS

Drug-drug. *Amiodarone:* May cause hypotension, bradycardia, and decreased cardiac output. Monitor patient closely.
Anticholinergics (benztropine, cyclopentolate, dicyclomine, fesoterodine): May increase risk of urine retention, severe constipation, and paralytic ileus. Monitor patient closely.
Boxed Warning *Benzodiazepines, CNS depressants:* May cause slow or difficult breathing, sedation, and death. Avoid use together. If use together can't be avoided, limit dose and duration of each drug to the minimum needed for desired effect. ∎
Buprenorphine, butorphanol, nalbuphine, pentazocine: May reduce analgesic effect of fentanyl or precipitate withdrawal signs and symptoms. Avoid use together.
Boxed Warning *CYP3A4 inducers (carbamazepine, phenytoin, rifampin):* May decrease fentanyl level and result in decreased efficacy or precipitate withdrawal syndrome in patients with physical dependence on fentanyl. If CYP3A4 inducer is discontinued, fentanyl level may increase and cause fentanyl-related adverse reactions. Taper CYP3A4 inducers cautiously and adjust fentanyl dosage as needed. ∎
Boxed Warning *CYP3A4 inhibitors (erythromycin, ketoconazole, ritonavir):* May increase fentanyl level and result in fatal overdose. Use together cautiously and monitor patient closely. ∎
Diuretics: Opioids may decrease diuresis or BP effects. Monitor therapy.
Droperidol: May cause hypotension and decrease pulmonary arterial pressure. Use together cautiously.
General anesthetics, hypnotics, other opioid analgesics, sedatives, TCAs: May cause additive effects. Use together cautiously. Consider dosage reduction of one or both drugs if adverse effects occur.
Muscle relaxants (cyclobenzaprine, metaxalone): May enhance neuromuscular blocking effect of relaxant and risk of respiratory depression. Use together cautiously.
Protease inhibitors: May increase fentanyl levels and adverse effects. Monitor patient closely for respiratory depression.
Serotonergic drugs (antiemetics [dolasetron, granisetron, ondansetron, palonosetron], amoxapine, antimigraine drugs, buspirone, cyclobenzaprine, dextromethorphan, linezolid, lithium, MAO inhibitors, maprotiline,

---

Reactions in bold italics are *life-threatening.*

methylene blue, mirtazapine, nefazodone, SSNRIs, SSRIs, TCAs, trazodone, tryptophan, vilazodone): May increase risk of serotonin syndrome. Use together cautiously; monitor for signs and symptoms of serotonin syndrome. Don't use fentanyl while patient is taking an MAO inhibitor or within 14 days of stopping one.

Drug-herb. 🔂 *Alert: St. John's wort:* May increase risk of serotonin syndrome. Use together cautiously; monitor for serotonin syndrome.

Drug-lifestyle. **Boxed Warning** *Alcohol use:* May cause slow or difficult breathing, sedation, and death. Discourage use together. ∎

EFFECTS ON LAB TEST RESULTS
• May increase ALP, AST, and amylase levels.
• May decrease albumin, magnesium sodium, and potassium levels.
• May increase or decrease calcium and glucose levels.

CONTRAINDICATIONS & CAUTIONS
• Contraindicated in patients hypersensitive to drug or its components and in those with acute or severe bronchial asthma in an unmonitored setting or in the absence of resuscitative equipment, respiratory depression, or known or suspected GI obstruction, including paralytic ileus.

Boxed Warning *Opioid class warning:* Opioids should only be prescribed with benzodiazepines or other CNS depressants when alternative treatment options are inadequate, aren't expected to provide adequate analgesia, haven't been tolerated, or aren't expected to be tolerated. ∎

🔂 *Alert:* Immediate-release formulations shouldn't be used for an extended period unless pain remains severe enough to require an opioid analgesic and alternative treatment options are inadequate to treat pain.

🔂 *Alert:* Long-acting or extended-release formulations are indicated for severe, persistent pain for which extended treatment with a daily opioid analgesic is required and for which alternative treatment options are inadequate. Use isn't indicated for as-needed analgesia.

Boxed Warning Transdermal and transmucosal forms are contraindicated in those who need acute or postoperative pain management or who aren't opioid tolerant. ∎

Boxed Warning Use exposes patient and others to risk of opioid addiction, abuse, and misuse, which can lead to overdose and death. These effects can occur at any dose or duration. Assess patient risk before prescribing and regularly reassess patient for these behaviors and conditions. ∎

Boxed Warning Prescribers are strongly encouraged to complete a REMS-compliant education program. Drug should be prescribed only by prescribers with knowledge of opioid use and ways to reduce associated risks. ∎

🔂 *Alert:* Use lowest effective dose for shortest period consistent with patient's treatment goals.

🔂 *Alert:* Because risk of overdose increases as opioid dose increases, reserve titration to higher doses for patients in whom lower doses are ineffective and in whom expected benefits of higher opioid dose outweigh risks.

🔂 *Alert:* Drug may lead to rare but serious decrease in adrenal gland cortisol production.
• Drug may cause decreased sex hormone levels with long-term use.
• Fentora is contraindicated in patients with mucositis more severe than grade 1.
• Avoid use in patients with impaired consciousness or coma.
• Use with caution in patients with brain tumors, increased ICP, known seizure disorder, COPD, decreased respiratory reserve, potentially compromised respirations, liver or kidney disease, or cardiac bradyarrhythmias.
• Use with caution in older adults and patients who are debilitated.
• Opioids can cause sleep-related breathing disorders, including central sleep apnea (CSA) and sleep-related hypoxemia. In patients who present with CSA, consider decreasing opioid dosage using best practices for opioid taper.

Boxed Warning Accidental ingestion or transdermal exposure of even one dose of an opioid, especially by children, can result in a fatal overdose. ∎

Dialyzable drug: Unknown.

⚠ *Overdose S&S:* CNS depression, respiratory depression, apnea, flaccid skeletal muscles, bradycardia, hypotension, circulatory collapse.

PREGNANCY-LACTATION-REPRODUCTION
• Studies during pregnancy are inadequate. Use during pregnancy only if potential benefit justifies fetal risk.

Boxed Warning Prolonged maternal use of opioids during pregnancy can cause neonatal withdrawal syndrome, which may be life-threatening. It requires management with expert neonatology protocols. If prolonged use is needed, advise patient of risks, and ensure availability of proper treatment. ∎

• Drug appears in human milk. Refer to individual manufacturer's instructions for use during breastfeeding.

NURSING CONSIDERATIONS

Boxed Warning May cause life-threatening or fatal respiratory depression at any time during therapy. Monitor patient closely, especially when starting or increasing doses. Proper dosing and titration are essential to reduce risk. ∎

Boxed Warning Regularly monitor all patients for opioid addiction, abuse, and misuse, which can lead to overdose and death. ∎

• Monitor patient closely, and provide immediate care for evidence of overdose, such as slow or shallow breathing, slow heartbeat, severe sleepiness, cold and clammy skin, trouble walking and talking, and feeling faint, dizzy, or confused.

🌙 **Alert:** If patient is taking opioids with serotonergic drugs, monitor for signs and symptoms of serotonin syndrome (agitation, hallucinations, rapid HR, fever, diaphoresis, shivering, shaking, muscle twitching or stiffness, trouble with coordination, nausea, vomiting, diarrhea), especially when starting treatment or increasing dosage. Symptoms may occur within several hours of coadministration but may also occur later, especially after dosage increase. Discontinue opioid, serotonergic drug, or both if serotonin syndrome is suspected.

🌙 **Alert:** Monitor patient for signs and symptoms of adrenal insufficiency (nausea, vomiting, loss of appetite, fatigue, weakness, dizziness, low BP). Perform diagnostic testing if adrenal insufficiency is suspected. If adrenal insufficiency is confirmed, treat with corticosteroids and wean patient off opioids, if appropriate. Discontinue corticosteroids when clinically appropriate.

🌙 **Alert:** Don't stop drug abruptly; individualize gradual taper plan to prevent signs and symptoms of withdrawal, worsening pain, and psychological distress in patient who is physically dependent. Refer to manufacturer's label for tapering instructions.

🌙 **Alert:** When tapering opioids, monitor patient closely for signs and symptoms of opioid withdrawal (restlessness, lacrimation, rhinorrhea, yawning, perspiration, chills, myalgia, mydriasis, irritability, anxiety, insomnia, backache, joint pain, weakness, abdominal cramps, anorexia, nausea, vomiting, diarrhea, increased BP or HR, increased respiratory rate). Such signs and symptoms may indicate a need to taper more slowly. Also watch for suicidality, use of other substances, and mood changes.

• Monitor patient for signs and symptoms of decreased sex hormone levels (low libido, erectile dysfunction, amenorrhea, infertility). If signs and symptoms occur, evaluate patient and obtain lab testing.

• For better analgesic effect, give drug before patient has intense pain.

🌙 **Alert:** High doses can produce muscle rigidity, which can be reversed with neuromuscular blockers; however, patient must be artificially ventilated.

🌙 **Alert:** Watch for sedation and respiratory depression in patients with increased ICP, brain tumors, head injury, or impaired consciousness.

• Carefully monitor circulatory and respiratory status and urinary function. Drug may cause respiratory depression, hypotension, urine retention, nausea, vomiting, ileus, and altered level of consciousness.

• Identify all drugs taken by patient, particularly CYP3A4 inhibitors, which may increase fentanyl levels.

• Drug may cause constipation. Assess bowel function and need for stool softeners and stimulant laxatives.

🌙 **Alert:** Drug may cause opioid-induced hyperalgesia (OIH). Symptoms include increased pain level with opioid dose increase, decreased pain level with opioid dose reduction, pain from ordinarily nonpainful stimuli without underlying disease progression, opioid tolerance or withdrawal, and addictive behavior. For suspected OIH, decrease opioid dose or switch patient to alternative opioid.

Transdermal

• Transdermal drug level peaks between 24 and 72 hours after initial application and dose increases. Monitor patient for life-threatening hypoventilation, especially during these times.

• Because drug level rises for first 24 hours after application, analgesic effect can't be evaluated on the first day. Make sure patient has adequate supplemental analgesic to prevent breakthrough pain.

• When converting patient from another opioid, determine the initial fentanyl dosage with great care; overestimating the dosage could be dangerous or fatal.

• Make dosage adjustments gradually in patient using transdermal system. Reaching steady-state level of a new dosage may take up to 6 days; delay dosage adjustment until after at least two applications.

• Monitor patient who develops adverse reactions to transdermal system for at least 12 hours after removal. Drug level drops gradually; it may take as long as 17 hours to decline by 50%.

• Most patients experience good control of pain for 3 days while wearing transdermal system, but a few may need a new application after 48 hours.

• When reducing opioid therapy or switching to a different analgesic, withdraw transdermal system gradually. Because drug level drops gradually after removal, give half the equianalgesic dose of the new analgesic 12 to 18 hours after removal.

Transmucosal

Boxed Warning Transmucosal forms aren't bioequivalent and can't be substituted on a microgram-per-microgram basis. ∎

• *Look alike–sound alike:* Don't confuse fentanyl with alfentanil.

PATIENT TEACHING

Boxed Warning Counsel patient and caregiver on serious risks, safe use, and importance of reading the medication guide with each prescription. ∎

• Advise patient to take drug exactly as prescribed and to use lowest dose possible for shortest time needed.

• Inform patient that, for acute pain, drug may only be needed for a few days. Teach patient about safe disposal of unused drug.

• Warn patient that extended-release and long-acting formulations shouldn't be taken on an "as needed" basis.

• Instruct patient to contact health care provider if prescribed dosage isn't controlling pain.

⚕ *Alert:* Warn patient to withhold drug and inform prescriber if pain level worsens, pain sensitivity increases, or new pain occurs after taking drug.

Boxed Warning Caution patient or caregiver of patient taking an opioid with a

benzodiazepine, CNS depressant, or alcohol to seek immediate medical attention for dizziness, light-headedness, extreme sleepiness, slowed or difficult breathing, or unresponsiveness. ∎

Boxed Warning Advise patient that drug increases risk of opioid addiction, abuse, and misuse, which can lead to overdose and death. Teach patient proper use of drug. ∎

• When drug is used for pain control, instruct patient to request drug before pain becomes intense.

• Encourage patient to report all medications being taken, including prescription and OTC medications and supplements.

• Instruct patient to immediately report signs and symptoms of serotonin syndrome, adrenal insufficiency, and decreased sex hormone levels to health care provider.

⚕ *Alert:* Counsel patient not to discontinue opioids without first discussing need for a gradual tapering regimen with prescriber.

• Tell patient to avoid drinking alcohol and taking other CNS-type drugs, unless specifically prescribed by practitioner, because additive effects can occur.

⚕ *Alert:* Teach patient about proper application and disposal of transdermal patch. Proper use, storage, and disposal of transdermal patches is necessary to prevent poisoning and other harm, especially to children and pets.

⚕ *Alert:* Teach patient not to alter the transdermal patch (such as by cutting it) before application.

• Tell patient that pain relief with the patch may not occur for several hours after application. Oral, immediate-release opioids may be needed for initial pain relief.

Boxed Warning Inform patient that heat from fever or environment, such as from heating pads, electric blankets, heat lamps, hot tubs, and water beds, may increase transdermal delivery and cause toxicity, requiring dosage adjustment. Instruct patient to notify prescriber if fever occurs or if patient will be spending time in hot climate. ∎

⚕ *Alert:* Warn that, if an MRI is required, patient must inform facility of transdermal patch.

• Teach patient proper administration of transmucosal forms.

• Advise patient that transmucosal lozenge contains 2 g sugar per unit.

• Inform patient that naloxone may be prescribed with the opioid when beginning and renewing therapy to reduce risk of opioid overdose and death.

● Caution patient to report to prescriber pregnancy or plans to become pregnant.

ferric carboxymaltose
FER-ik car-box-ee-MAL-tose

Injectafer

Therapeutic class: Iron supplements
Pharmacologic class: Hematinics

AVAILABLE FORMS
Injection: 100 mg/2 mL, 500 mg/10 mL, 750 mg/15 mL, 1,000 mg/20 mL. Each mL contains 50 mg of elemental iron.

INDICATIONS & DOSAGES
➤ **Iron deficiency anemia in patients with non-dialysis-dependent CKD**
Adults: For patients weighing at least 50 kg, 750 mg IV on day 1; repeat dose after at least 7 days. For patients weighing less than 50 kg, give 15 mg/kg body weight on day 1; repeat dose after at least 7 days. May repeat course of therapy if anemia recurs. Maximum cumulative dose, 1,500 mg per treatment course.
➤ **Iron deficiency anemia in patients who are intolerant to or have had an unsatisfactory response to oral iron**
Adults: For patients weighing at least 50 kg, 750 mg IV on day 1; repeat dose after at least 7 days. For patients weighing less than 50 kg, 15 mg/kg body weight on day 1; repeat dose after at least 7 days. May repeat course of therapy if anemia recurs. Maximum cumulative dose, 1,500 mg per treatment course.
Children ages 1 and older weighing 50 kg or more: 750 mg IV on day 1; repeat dose after at least 7 days. May repeat course of therapy if anemia recurs. Maximum cumulative dose, 1,500 mg per course.
Children ages 1 and older weighing less than 50 kg: 15 mg/kg IV on day; repeat dose after at least 7 days. May repeat course of therapy if anemia recurs.
✳ *NEW INDICATION:* **Iron deficiency in patients with NYHA class II/III HF to improve exercise capacity**
Adults weighing at least 70 kg: If Hb is 14 g/dL or less, 1,000 mg IV on day 1. If Hb is more than 14 g/dL to less than 15 g/dL,

500 mg IV on day 1. At week 6, if Hb is less than 10 g/dL, 1,000 mg; or 500 mg if Hb is 10 to 14 g/dL. No additional dose needed if Hb is greater than 14 g/dL at week 6.
Adults weighing less than 70 kg: If Hb is 14 g/dL or less, 1,000 mg IV on day 1. If Hb is more than 14 g/dL to less than 15 g/dL, 500 mg IV on day 1. At week 6, if Hb is less than 10 g/dL, 500 mg. No additional dose needed if Hb is greater than 14 g/dL at week 6.
Adjust-a-dose: Give additional maintenance dose of 500 mg IV at weeks 12, 24, and 36 if ferritin level is less than 100 ng/mL or ferritin is 100 to 300 ng/ML with transferrin saturation of less than 20%. May repeat treatment if iron deficiency recurs.

ADMINISTRATION
IV
▼ Inspect vial for particulate matter and discoloration before administration.
▼ Give either as an undiluted slow IV push (at 100 mg [2 mL]/minute) or as an infusion. To administer by infusion, dilute up to 1,000 mg iron in maximum of 250 mL sterile NSS. Infusion concentration must be not less than 2 mg iron/mL.
▼ Give infusion over at least 15 minutes.
▼ Infusion is stable for 72 hours at room temperature at 2- to 4-mg/mL concentrations.
▼ Store vials at 68° to 77° F (20° to 25° C). Don't freeze vials.
▼ Vials are single-use and have no preservative. Discard any excess drug remaining in vial.
▼ **Incompatibilities:** None listed by manufacturer. Consult drug compatibility reference for more information.

ACTION
Colloidal iron (III) hydroxide acts in complex with carboxymaltose, a carbohydrate polymer that releases iron, an essential component in Hb formulation.

Route	Onset	Peak	Duration
IV	Unknown	15 min–1.21 hr	Unknown

Half-life: 7 to 12 hours.

ADVERSE REACTIONS
CNS: dizziness, headache, fever, chills, dysgeusia, syncope. **CV:** HTN, hypotension, flushing, tachycardia, chest discomfort.

Reactions in bold italics are *life-threatening*.

EENT: nasopharyngitis. **GI:** nausea, vomiting, constipation, GI infection. **Hepatic:** increased liver enzyme levels. **Hematologic:** decreased platelet and WBC counts. **Metabolic:** hypophosphatemia. **Skin:** rash, injection-site reactions (discomfort, erythema, discoloration, pruritus, extravasation).

INTERACTIONS

Drug-drug. *Dimercaprol:* May enhance kidney-toxic effect of iron salts. Avoid combination.

EFFECTS ON LAB TEST RESULTS

- May increase ALT and GGT levels.
- May decrease phosphorus level.
- May decrease platelet and WBC counts.
- May falsely elevate serum iron and transferrin-bound iron levels in the 24 hours after administration.

CONTRAINDICATIONS & CAUTIONS

- Contraindicated in patients hypersensitive to drug or its components, in patients with evidence of iron overload, and in those with anemia not caused by iron deficiency.
- Symptomatic hypophosphatemia has been reported in patients at risk for low serum phosphate levels, mostly after repeated exposure to ferric carboxymaltose in patients with no reported history of kidney impairment.
- Transient HTN has been reported immediately after administration.
- Serious hypersensitivity reactions, including anaphylaxis, have been reported.
- Safety and effectiveness in children with abnormal kidney function and children younger than age 1 haven't been established.
Dialyzable drug: No.
⚠ **Overdose S&S:** Hemosiderosis, hypophosphatemic osteomalacia.

PREGNANCY-LACTATION-REPRODUCTION

- Hypersensitivity reaction to infusion may have serious consequences, such as fetal bradycardia. Use during pregnancy only if potential benefit justifies fetal risk.
- Drug appears in human milk. Use cautiously during breastfeeding.

NURSING CONSIDERATIONS

- Before administering, assess patient for prior history of reactions to parenteral iron products.
- Monitor patient for hypersensitivity reactions during infusion and for at least 30 minutes after infusion or until patient's condition

stabilizes. Only administer drug when personnel and therapies are immediately available to treat serious hypersensitivity reactions.
- Monitor serum phosphate level in patient at risk for low serum phosphate who requires a repeat course of treatment.
- Monitor patient for extravasation during administration. Extravasation may cause persistent discoloration. If extravasation occurs, discontinue infusion at that site.
- Monitor vital signs before and after each dose. Monitor for HTN after each dose.
- Frequently monitor iron status (Hb level, hematocrit, serum ferritin level, iron saturation) during therapy.

PATIENT TEACHING

- Advise patient to report signs and symptoms of hypersensitivity reactions (rash, itching, dizziness, light-headedness, swelling, breathing problems).
- Caution patient not to take oral iron supplements while receiving iron by infusion.
- Advise patient to report pregnancy or plans to become pregnant.

---

fidaxomicin
fye-DAX-oh-MYE-sin

Dificid

Therapeutic class: Antibiotics
Pharmacologic class: Macrolides

AVAILABLE FORMS

Granules for oral suspension: 40 mg/mL
Tablets: 200 mg

INDICATIONS & DOSAGES

➤ **CDAD**

Adults and children weighing 12.5 kg or more and able to swallow tablets: 200 mg PO b.i.d. for 10 days.
Children ages 6 months to younger than 18 years: For those weighing 9 to less than 12.5 kg, 160 mg (4 mL) oral solution PO b.i.d. for 10 days; for 7 to less than 9 kg, 120 mg (3 mL) oral solution PO b.i.d. for 10 days; for 4 to less than 7 kg, 80 mg (2 mL) oral solution PO b.i.d. for 10 days.

ADMINISTRATION

PO

- Give drug without regard to food.

• Remove reconstituted oral solution from refrigerator 15 minutes before administration. Shake vigorously; then give using oral dosing syringe.
• Store tablets at room temperature.
• Store reconstituted oral suspension in refrigerator; discard after 12 days.

ACTION

Acts on *Clostridioides difficile* locally in the GI tract by inhibiting RNA synthesis through RNA polymerases.

Route	Onset	Peak	Duration
PO	<1 hr	1–5 hr	Unknown

Half-life: About 12 hours.

ADVERSE REACTIONS

CNS: fever. **GI:** nausea, vomiting, abdominal pain or discomfort, abdominal distention, *GI bleeding,* dyspepsia, dysphagia, flatulence, intestinal obstruction, megacolon. **Hematologic:** anemia, *neutropenia.* **Hepatic:** increased ALP and liver enzyme levels. **Metabolic:** hyperglycemia, *metabolic acidosis.* **Skin:** drug eruption, rash, pruritus.

INTERACTIONS

None significant.

EFFECTS ON LAB TEST RESULTS

• May increase ALP, liver enzyme, and blood glucose levels.
• May decrease serum bicarbonate level.
• May decrease WBC, RBC, and platelet counts.

CONTRAINDICATIONS & CAUTIONS

• Contraindicated in patients hypersensitive to drug.
• Acute hypersensitivity reactions have been reported. Discontinue drug and treat appropriately. Patients with known macrolide allergies may have increased risk.
• Drug isn't an effective treatment for systemic infections. Don't prescribe fidaxomicin unless *C. difficile* infection has been proven or is strongly suspected to prevent bacterial drug resistance.
• Safety and effectiveness in children younger than age 6 months haven't been determined.
Dialyzable drug: Unknown.

PREGNANCY-LACTATION-REPRODUCTION

• Use drug in pregnancy only if clearly needed.

• It isn't known if drug appears in human milk. Use cautiously during breastfeeding.

NURSING CONSIDERATIONS

• Obtain specimen for culture before start of treatment.
• Monitor response to treatment.
• Monitor glucose level, especially in patient with diabetes.
• Monitor for abdominal pain and bleeding.
• Monitor patient for acute hypersensitivity.

PATIENT TEACHING

• Teach about proper drug administration and handling.
• Advise patient that drug is used to treat CDAD only and shouldn't be used to treat other infections.
• Counsel patient to take drug exactly as directed. Missing doses, skipping doses, or not completing the full course of therapy may lead to reinfection, continued infection, or bacterial resistance.

BIOSIMILAR DRUG

filgrastim (G-CSF)
fill-GRASS-tim

Grastofil✦, Neupogen

filgrastim-aafi
Nivestym

filgrastim-ayow
Releuko

filgrastim-sndz
Zarxio

tbo-filgrastim
Granix

Therapeutic class: Colony-stimulating factors
Pharmacologic class: Hematopoietics

AVAILABLE FORMS

Injection: 300 mcg/mL, 480 mcg/1.6 mL vials; 300 mcg/0.5 mL, 480 mcg/0.8 mL prefilled syringes

INDICATIONS & DOSAGES

➤ **Acute exposure to myelosuppressive doses of radiation (hematopoietic syndrome of acute radiation syndrome) (Neupogen)**

Reactions in bold italics are *life-threatening*.

Adults and children: 10 mcg/kg subcut as soon as possible after suspected or confirmed exposure to radiation doses greater than 2 gray (Gy). Continue daily administration until ANC remains greater than 1,000/mm³ for three consecutive CBCs or exceeds 10,000/mm³ after a radiation-induced nadir.

➤ **To decrease incidence of infection in patients with nonmyeloid malignancies receiving myelosuppressive chemotherapy associated with risk of severe febrile neutropenia; to reduce time to neutrophil recovery and duration of fever after induction or consolidation chemotherapy for acute myeloid leukemia (Neupogen, Nivestym, Releuko, Zarxio)**
Adults and children: 5 mcg/kg by single subcut injection or short IV infusion (15 to 30 minutes) or continuous IV infusion once daily at least 24 hours after chemotherapy. Give daily for up to 2 weeks, until ANC reaches 10,000/mm³.
Adjust-a-dose: May increase dosage by increments of 5 mcg/kg for each chemotherapy cycle, depending on duration and severity of ANC nadir.

➤ **To decrease duration of severe neutropenia in patients with nonmyeloid malignancies receiving myelosuppressive chemotherapy associated with risk of severe febrile neutropenia (Granix)**
Adults and children ages 1 month and older: 5 mcg/kg/day subcut. Continue until anticipated nadir has passed and neutrophil count has recovered to normal range.

➤ **To decrease risk of infection in patients with nonmyeloid malignant disease receiving myelosuppressive antineoplastics followed by bone marrow transplantation (Neupogen, Nivestym, Releuko, Zarxio)**
Adults and children: 10 mcg/kg daily IV infusion for no longer than 24 hours or as continuous 24-hour subcut infusion at least 24 hours after cytotoxic chemotherapy and bone marrow infusion. Adjust subsequent dosages based on neutrophil response.
Adjust-a-dose: For patients with ANC above 1,000/mm³ for 3 consecutive days, reduce dosage to 5 mcg/kg/day. If ANC decreases to less than 1,000/mm³ with 5-mcg/kg/day dose, increase dosage to 10 mcg/kg/day. If ANC remains above 1,000/mm³ for 3 more consecutive days, stop drug. If ANC decreases to below 1,000/mm³, resume therapy at 5 mcg/kg daily.

➤ **Chronic severe neutropenia (Neupogen, Nivestym, Releuko, Zarxio)**
Adults and children: For patients with congenital neutropenia, starting dose is 6 mcg/kg subcut b.i.d. For patients with idiopathic or cyclic neutropenia, starting dose is 5 mcg/kg as single daily subcut injection. Adjust dosage based on patient response.

➤ **Peripheral blood progenitor cell collection and therapy in patients with cancer (Neupogen, Nivestym, Zarxio)**
Adults and children: 10 mcg/kg/day subcut (bolus or continuous infusion). Begin treatment at least 4 days before leukapheresis and continue until last leukapheresis.
Adjust-a-dose: Monitor daily neutrophil count after 4 days of treatment; discontinue drug for WBC count above 100,000/mm³.

➤ **Hematopoietic stem cell mobilization in autologous transplantation in patients with non-Hodgkin lymphoma or multiple myeloma (in combination with plerixafor) (Neupogen)** ◆
Adults: 10 mcg/kg subcut daily; begin 4 days before plerixafor initiation and continue on each day before apheresis for up to 8 days.

ADMINISTRATION
● Give drug at least 24 hours after cytotoxic chemotherapy. Don't give within 24 hours prior to chemotherapy.
🕔 *Alert:* Direct administration of less than 0.3 mL isn't recommended because of potential for dosing errors.
🕔 *Alert:* Removable needle cap in prefilled syringes contains natural rubber latex. Don't use in patients with latex allergies.
● Store in refrigerator at 36° to 46° F (2° to 8° C) in original pack to protect from light.
● Avoid freezing; if frozen, thaw in refrigerator before administering. Discard drug if frozen more than once.
● Don't shake.
● Before use, allow drug to reach room temperature for at least 30 minutes to a maximum of 24 hours. (If beyond 24 hours, discard drug.)
● Solution should be clear and colorless to slightly yellow. Discard solution if it is discolored or contains particulate matter.
● Discard unused portion of prefilled syringes.
● Refer to manufacturer's instructions for further administration details.

IV

▼ Dilute in 50 to 100 mL of D_5W. Dilution to less than 5 mcg/mL isn't recommended.

▼ Don't dilute with NSS; product may precipitate.

▼ If drug yield is 5 to 15 mcg/mL, add albumin at 2 mg/mL (0.2%) to minimize binding of drug to plastic containers or tubing.

▼ Give by intermittent infusion over 15 to 30 minutes or by continuous infusion over 24 hours.

▼ Once a dose is withdrawn, don't reuse vial. Discard unused portion. Vials are for single-dose use only.

▼ **Incompatibilities:** Sodium solutions. No other incompatibilities are listed by manufacturer. Consult drug compatibility reference for more information.

Subcutaneous

• Rotate and record administration sites.

• Administer in outer upper arms, abdomen, thighs, or upper outer areas of buttocks.

• Don't inject into areas that are tender, red, bruised, hardened, or scarred or into sites with stretch marks.

ACTION

Binds cell receptors to stimulate proliferation, differentiation, commitment, and end-cell function of neutrophils.

Route	Onset	Peak	Duration
IV	1–2 days	Unknown	4 days
Subcut	1–2 days	2–8 hr	4 days
Subcut (tbo-filgrastim)	3–5 days to max ANC	4–6 hr	21 days to baseline ANC return after chemotherapy completion

Half-life: 3 to 3.5 hours.

ADVERSE REACTIONS

CNS: fever, headache, weakness, fatigue, malaise, dizziness, insomnia, pain, hypoesthesia. **CV:** chest pain, HTN, peripheral edema. **EENT:** epistaxis, sore throat, oral pain. **GI:** nausea, vomiting, diarrhea, decreased appetite, constipation. **GU:** UTI. **Hematologic:** *thrombocytopenia,* anemia, leukocytosis, splenomegaly, *neutropenic fever.* **Hepatic:** increased ALP level. **Metabolic:** increased LDH level. **Musculoskeletal:** bone pain, back pain, extremity pain, arthralgia, myalgia, muscle spasms. **Respiratory:** dyspnea, cough, bronchitis, URI. **Skin:** alopecia, rash, erythema,

cutaneous vasculitis. **Other:** hypersensitivity reactions, transfusion reaction, *sepsis,* antibody development.

INTERACTIONS

Drug-drug. *Bleomycin, cyclophosphamide:* May increase pulmonary toxicity. Monitor therapy.

Chemotherapeutic drugs: Rapidly dividing myeloid cells may be sensitive to cytotoxic drugs. Don't use within 24 hours before or after a dose of one of these drugs.

EFFECTS ON LAB TEST RESULTS

• May increase ALP, creatinine, LDH, and uric acid levels.

• May increase WBC count.

• May decrease Hb level and platelet count.

CONTRAINDICATIONS & CAUTIONS

• Contraindicated in patients hypersensitive to drug or its components or to proteins derived from *Escherichia coli.*

• Severe allergic reactions, including anaphylaxis, are possible. Permanently discontinue drug if any occur.

• Splenic rupture (including fatal cases), sickle cell crisis (including fatal cases), ARDS, cutaneous vasculitis, glomerulonephritis, and capillary leak syndrome (possibly life-threatening) have been reported.

• Use cautiously in severe chronic neutropenia; confirm diagnosis before initiating drug. Drug may increase risk of myelodysplastic syndrome and acute myelogenous leukemia.

• G-CSF drugs may act as a growth factor on any type of tumor. Transmission of tumor cells by peripheral blood progenitor cell therapy infusion may occur and hasn't been well studied.

• Avoid concurrent radiation therapy with filgrastim products; safety and efficacy haven't been established.

• Studies regarding safety and effectiveness in children are limited. Use cautiously in children.

Dialyzable drug: Unknown.

⚠ **Overdose S&S:** Excessive leukocytosis.

PREGNANCY-LACTATION-REPRODUCTION

• Adverse effects have been seen in animal studies. Use during pregnancy only if potential benefit justifies fetal risk.

• It isn't known if drug appears in human milk. Use with extreme caution during breastfeeding.

Reactions in bold italics are *life-threatening.*

NURSING CONSIDERATIONS

❸ **Alert:** Obtain baseline CBC after exposure to myelosuppressive doses of radiation; don't delay administration if CBC isn't readily available. Monitor CBC every third day until ANC remains greater than 1,000/mm^3 for three consecutive CBCs.

• Obtain baseline CBC and platelet count before therapy.

• Obtain CBC and platelet count two to three times weekly during therapy. Patients who receive drug may also receive high doses of chemotherapy, which increase risk of toxicities.

• A transiently increased neutrophil count is common 1 or 2 days after therapy starts. Continue to give daily for up to 2 weeks or until ANC returns to 10,000/mm^3 after expected chemotherapy-induced neutrophil nadir.

• For severe chronic neutropenia, monitor CBC with differential and platelet count during initial 4 weeks of treatment and during the 2 weeks after dosage adjustments. Once patient is clinically stable, monitor monthly during first year of treatment, then as clinically indicated. Consider risks and benefits of continued treatment if abnormal cytogenetics or myelodysplasia occurs.

• Glomerulonephritis can occur; dosage reduction or drug discontinuation may be necessary.

• Monitor patient with left upper abdominal or shoulder pain for enlarged spleen or splenic rupture.

• Monitor for signs and symptoms of capillary leak syndrome (hypotension, hypoalbuminemia, edema, hemoconcentration), which can be life-threatening. Monitor patient closely; intensive care may be needed.

• Assess patient with fever, lung infiltrates, or respiratory distress for ARDS. Discontinue drug if ARDS is confirmed.

• Watch for sickle cell crisis in patient with sickle cell trait or sickle cell disease.

• Monitor for signs and symptoms of cutaneous vasculitis (purpura, erythema), especially if patient is on long-term therapy. Withhold drug if cutaneous vasculitis develops. Consider restarting drug at a reduced dosage when signs and symptoms have resolved and ANC has decreased.

• **Look alike–sound alike:** Don't confuse Neupogen with Epogen or Neumega. Don't confuse filgrastim biosimilars with filgrastim.

PATIENT TEACHING

• Teach about proper timing, administration, and disposal of subcut self-administered drug.

• Warn that patient with latex allergy shouldn't administer or receive drug in pre-filled syringes that contain latex. Check manufacturer's instructions for latex content.

• Instruct patient to promptly report all adverse reactions.

• Review signs and symptoms of allergic reaction (rash, facial edema, wheezing, dyspnea, hypotension, rapid HR); advise patient to seek immediate medical attention if any occur.

• Advise patient to immediately report purpura or erythema.

• Warn patient to seek immediate medical attention if swelling, decreased urination, shortness of breath, abdominal swelling or feeling of fullness, dizziness, or fatigue occurs.

❸ **Alert:** Rarely, splenic rupture may occur. Advise patient to immediately report left upper abdominal or shoulder tip pain.

• Tell patient that routine blood tests are needed before and during treatment to monitor for effectiveness and safe use.

• Warn patient who is pregnant or breastfeeding about drug's risks.

finasteride
fin-AS-teh-ride

Propecia, Proscar

Therapeutic class: BPH drugs
Pharmacologic class: 5-alpha reductase inhibitors

AVAILABLE FORMS
Tablets: 1 mg, 5 mg

INDICATIONS & DOSAGES

➤ **To improve symptoms of BPH and reduce risk of acute urine retention and need for surgery, including transurethral resection of prostate and prostatectomy; to reduce risk of BPH, with or without doxazosin (Proscar)**
Adult males: 5 mg PO daily.

➤ **Male pattern hair loss (androgenetic alopecia) in men only (Propecia)**
Adult males: 1 mg PO daily.

ADMINISTRATION
PO
🔵 *Alert:* Hazardous drug; use safe handling and disposal precautions.
- Give drug without regard to food.
- Store at room temperature.
- Protect from moisture and light.

ACTION
Inhibits 5-alpha reductase, resulting in inhibition of the conversion of testosterone to dihydrotestosterone (DHT), the androgen primarily responsible for initial development and subsequent enlargement of the prostate gland. In male pattern baldness, decreases scalp DHT levels in hair follicles.

Route	Onset	Peak	Duration
PO	Unknown	1–2 hr	24 hr

Half-life: 6 hours; 8 hours in older adults.

ADVERSE REACTIONS
CNS: dizziness, drowsiness, asthenia, headache. **CV:** hypotension, orthostatic hypotension, peripheral edema. **EENT:** rhinitis. **GU:** ejaculation dysfunction, erectile dysfunction, decreased volume of ejaculate, decreased libido. **Respiratory:** dyspnea. **Skin:** rash. **Other:** gynecomastia, breast tenderness.

INTERACTIONS
None reported.

EFFECTS ON LAB TEST RESULTS
- May decrease PSA level.

CONTRAINDICATIONS & CAUTIONS
- Contraindicated in patients hypersensitive to drug or to other 5-alpha reductase inhibitors, such as dutasteride.
🔵 *Alert:* Drug may increase risk of high-grade prostate cancer.
- Use cautiously in patients with liver dysfunction.
- Drug isn't indicated for use in children or females.
Dialyzable drug: Unknown.

PREGNANCY-LACTATION-REPRODUCTION
- Contraindicated in pregnancy and in patients of childbearing potential.
- Patients who are pregnant should avoid contact with drug and with semen from a male partner taking drug.
- It isn't known if drug appears in human milk.

Reactions in bold italics are *life-threatening*.

NURSING CONSIDERATIONS
- Before therapy, evaluate patient for conditions that mimic BPH (hypotonic bladder, prostate cancer, infection, stricture).
- Evaluate patient for prostate cancer if PSA level increases during therapy.
- Carefully monitor patient who has a large residual urine volume or severely diminished urine flow.
- Sustained increase in PSA level could indicate nonadherence with therapy.
- At least 6 months of therapy may be needed for treatment of BPH.
- At least 3 months of therapy may be needed to see the benefits of treatment for hair loss. Periodically reevaluate benefit. Effects reverse within 12 months after treatment ends.

PATIENT TEACHING
- Teach about proper drug administration and handling.
- Warn patient who is or may become pregnant not to handle crushed or broken tablets because of risk of adverse effects on male fetus and to avoid contact with semen from a male partner exposed to finasteride.
- Inform patient that signs of improvement may require at least 3 months of daily use when drug is used to treat hair loss or at least 6 months when drug is used for BPH.
- Reassure patient that drug may decrease volume of ejaculate without impairing normal sexual function.
- Instruct patient to report breast changes (lumps, pain, nipple discharge).

finerenone
fin-ER-e-none

Kerendia

Therapeutic class: Miscellaneous GU drugs
Pharmacologic class: Mineralocorticoid receptor antagonists

AVAILABLE FORMS
Tablets: 10 mg, 20 mg

INDICATIONS & DOSAGES
➤ **To reduce risk of sustained eGFR decline, kidney failure, CV death, nonfatal MI, and hospitalization for HF in patients with CKD associated with type 2 diabetes**

Adults: Initially, 10 or 20 mg PO once daily based on eGFR and serum potassium thresholds. Don't initiate drug if serum potassium level is more than 5.0 mEq/L. If eGFR is 60 mL/minute/1.73 m^2 or more, start at 20 mg once daily; if eGFR is 25 to less than 60 mL/minute/1.73 m^2, start at 10 mg once daily. If starting with 10 mg, increase dosage after 4 weeks to target dosage of 20 mg once daily, based on eGFR and serum potassium thresholds.

Adjust-a-dose: Adjust dosage as needed based on every-4-week eGFR and potassium level. If current serum potassium level is 4.8 mEq/L or less and patient is taking 10 mg, increase to 20 mg daily, unless eGFR has decreased by more than 30% compared to previous measurement; if so, maintain 10-mg dose. If patient is already taking 20-mg dose, maintain 20 mg daily.

If current serum potassium level is more than 4.8 to 5.5 mEq/L and patient is taking 10 mg daily, stay at 10 mg daily. If patient is already taking 20-mg dose, stay at 20 mg daily.

If current serum potassium level is more than 5.5 mEq/L and patient is taking 10 mg, withhold drug and consider restarting at 10 mg once daily when serum potassium level is 5.0 mEq/L or less. If patient is already taking 20-mg dose, withhold drug and restart at 10 mg once daily when serum potassium level is 5.0 mEq/L or less.

ADMINISTRATION
PO
• Give drug without regard to food.
• If patient can't swallow, crush tablet and mix with applesauce or water; give immediately.
• Give a missed dose as soon as possible but only on same day; if not on same day, skip dose and continue with regular dosing schedule next day.
• Store tablets at 68° to 77° F (20° to 25° C).

ACTION
Blocks mineralocorticoid-mediated sodium reabsorption and mineralocorticoid activation in kidney, cardiac, and vascular tissue, reducing fibrosis and inflammation.

Route	Onset	Peak	Duration
PO	Unknown	0.5–1.25 hr	Unknown

Half-life: 2 to 3 hours.

ADVERSE REACTIONS
CV: hypotension. **Metabolic:** *hyperkalemia,* hyponatremia.

INTERACTIONS
Drug-drug. *Drugs that may increase potassium level (ACE inhibitors, ARBs, potassium-sparing diuretics):* May increase potassium retention. Frequently monitor potassium level.
Moderate (erythromycin) and weak (amiodarone) CYP3A inhibitors: May increase finerenone level and risk of adverse reactions. Use together cautiously and monitor potassium level.
Strong (rifampin) or moderate (efavirenz) CYP3A inducers: May decrease finerenone level. Avoid use together.
Strong CYP3A inhibitors (itraconazole): May significantly increase finerenone level. Use together is contraindicated.
Drug-herb. *St. John's wort:* May decrease finerenone level. Discourage use together.
Drug-food. *Grapefruit, grapefruit juice:* May increase finerenone level. Discourage use together.

EFFECTS ON LAB TEST RESULTS
• May increase potassium level.
• May decrease sodium level and eGFR.

CONTRAINDICATIONS & CAUTIONS
• Contraindicated in patients with adrenal insufficiency.
• Drug isn't recommended if eGFR is less than 25 mL/minute/1.73 m^2.
• Drug increases risk of hyperkalemia in patients who have higher baseline potassium levels, risk factors for hyperkalemia (use of concomitant drugs that increase serum potassium level or impair its excretion), or decreased kidney function.
• Avoid use in patients with Child-Pugh class C liver impairment. Consider additional potassium monitoring in patients with Child-Pugh class B liver impairment.
• Use cautiously in older adults.
• Safety and effectiveness in children haven't been established.
Dialyzable drug: Unlikely.

PREGNANCY-LACTATION-REPRODUCTION
• Studies during pregnancy are lacking.
• It isn't known if drug appears in human milk or how drug affects milk production or infants who are breastfed. Patient shouldn't

breastfeed during therapy and for 1 day after final dose.

NURSING CONSIDERATIONS

• Monitor serum potassium level and eGFR at baseline, at 4 weeks, after dosage adjustment, and periodically during therapy.

• Consider monitoring serum potassium levels more often during the first 4 weeks of therapy in patient with serum potassium level higher than 4.8 to 5.0 mEq/L. Base frequency on clinical judgement and serum potassium level.

PATIENT TEACHING

• Advise patient of the need for periodic monitoring of serum potassium level.

• Caution patient to consult prescriber before using potassium supplements or salt substitutes that contain potassium.

• Instruct patient to inform prescriber if taking other prescription and OTC medications, herbs, and supplements.

• Tell patient to avoid grapefruit and grapefruit juice while taking drug.

• Warn patient not to breastfeed during therapy and for 1 day after final dose.

fingolimod
fin-GOL-ih-mod

Gilenya, Tascenso ODT

Therapeutic class: Immunomodulators
Pharmacologic class: Sphingosine 1-phosphate receptor modulators

AVAILABLE FORMS

Capsules: 0.25 mg, 0.5 mg
ODTs: 0.25 mg, 0.5 mg

INDICATIONS & DOSAGES

➤ **Relapsing MS**

Adults and children ages 10 and older weighing more than 40 kg: 0.5 mg PO once daily.
Children ages 10 and older weighing 40 kg or less: 0.25 mg PO once daily.

ADMINISTRATION

PO

❂ *Alert:* Hazardous drug; use safe handling and disposal precautions.

• Give drug without regard to food.

• May give ODT with or without water.

• Place ODT directly on tongue and allow it to dissolve before patient swallows it.

• Give ODT as soon as it's removed from blister pack; don't store outside of blister pack.

• Store at room temperature.

• Protect from moisture.

ACTION

Blocks activity of lymphocytes leaving lymph nodes, which reduces number of lymphocytes in the peripheral blood.

Route	Onset	Peak	Duration
PO	Unknown	12–16 hr	Unknown

Half-life: 6 to 9 days.

ADVERSE REACTIONS

CNS: asthenia, depression, dizziness, headache, migraine, *seizures.* **CV:** *bradycardia,* HTN. **EENT:** sinusitis, blurred vision, eye pain. **GI:** abdominal pain, gastroenteritis, diarrhea, nausea. **Hematologic:** *lymphopenia, leukopenia.* **Hepatic:** increased transaminase levels, *liver toxicity.* **Metabolic:** weight loss, hypertriglyceridemia. **Musculoskeletal:** back pain, extremity pain. **Respiratory:** bronchitis, cough, dyspnea. **Skin:** tinea infections, alopecia, actinic keratosis, basal cell carcinoma, skin papilloma. **Other:** flulike symptoms, herpes viral infections.

INTERACTIONS

Drug-drug. *Antineoplastics, immunomodulators, immunosuppressants (corticosteroids):* May increase risk of immunosuppression. Use together cautiously.

❂ *Alert: Beta blockers, HR-lowering calcium channel blockers (diltiazem, verapamil), digoxin:* May increase risk of severe bradycardia or heart block. If possible, switch patient to cardiac drug that doesn't cause bradycardia before starting fingolimod. If change isn't possible, monitor patient with continuous ECG overnight after first dose to determine effects.

Carbamazepine: May decrease fingolimod level. Monitor therapy.

Drugs that prolong QT interval (class IA or III antiarrhythmics [amiodarone, procainamide, quinidine, sotalol], citalopram, chlorpromazine, erythromycin, haloperidol, methadone): May increase risk of QT-interval prolongation and torsades de pointes. Use together is contraindicated.

Reactions in bold italics are *life-threatening.*

Ketoconazole: May increase fingolimod level and risk of adverse effects. Use together cautiously and monitor patient closely.
Live attenuated virus vaccines: May decrease vaccination effects or increase infection risk. Don't use together or give vaccine within 60 days of prior fingolimod use.
Drug-lifestyle. *Sun exposure:* May cause photosensitivity reactions. Advise patient to wear protective clothing and use sunscreen with a high sun protection factor.

EFFECTS ON LAB TEST RESULTS
• May increase ALT, AST, GGT, and triglyceride levels.
• May decrease lymphocyte and neutrophil counts.

CONTRAINDICATIONS & CAUTIONS
• Contraindicated in patients hypersensitive to drug and in those with active acute or chronic infection.
🌙 *Alert:* Contraindicated in patients with MI, unstable angina, stroke, decompensated HF requiring hospitalization, TIA, or class III/IV HF within the past 6 months; in those with history or presence of Mobitz Type II second- or third-degree AV block or sick sinus syndrome, unless patient has a functioning pacemaker; in those with cardiac arrhythmias requiring treatment with class IA or class III antiarrhythmics; and in those with baseline QTc interval of 500 msec or greater.
🌙 *Alert:* Use cautiously after cardiac evaluation in patients with ischemic heart disease, history of MI, HF, history of cardiac arrest, cerebrovascular disease, history of symptomatic bradycardia, recurrent syncope, severe untreated sleep apnea, AV block, or SA heart block.
• Use cautiously in patients with sick sinus syndrome and in patients taking beta blockers or calcium channel blockers.
• Use cautiously in patients with history of infection, macular edema, decreased pulmonary function test results, or liver disease.
• Use cautiously in patients older than age 65 who have concomitant disease or are taking other drugs.
• Safety and effectiveness in children younger than age 10 haven't been established.
Dialyzable drug: No.
⚠ *Overdose S&S:* Chest tightness or discomfort.

PREGNANCY-LACTATION-REPRODUCTION
• Drug may cause fetal harm. Use during pregnancy only if benefit justifies fetal risk.
• Patients who are pregnant should enroll in Gilenya Pregnancy Registry (1-877-598-7237 or www.gilenyapregnancyregistry.com).
• Patients of childbearing potential should use effective contraception during therapy and for 2 months after final dose.
• Patients planning to become pregnant should stop drug 2 months before planned conception.
• It isn't known if drug appears in human milk. Use cautiously during breastfeeding.

NURSING CONSIDERATIONS
• Verify pregnancy status before treatment.
🌙 *Alert:* Monitor HR and BP hourly for at least 6 hours after first dose in all patients. Obtain ECG before first dose and at end of observation period. Monitor BP routinely during treatment.
🌙 *Alert:* Monitor patients at high risk and those who may not tolerate bradycardia with continuous ECG overnight in a setting with resources and personnel that can manage symptomatic bradycardia. Patients at high risk include those who develop severe bradycardia after receiving first dose, those with preexisting conditions who may not tolerate bradycardia, those receiving other drugs that slow HR or AV conduction, those with QT-interval prolongation before taking fingolimod or prolonged QT interval that occurs during monitoring period, those receiving other drugs that prolong QT interval, and those at risk for QT-interval prolongation due to hypokalemia, hypomagnesemia, or congenital long-QT syndrome.
🌙 *Alert:* If CV symptoms occur (HR less than 45 beats/minute in adults, less than 55 beats/minute in children ages 12 and older, or less than 60 beats/minute in children age 10 or 11; HR at its lowest value 6 hours after dose; or new-onset second-degree or higher AV block 6 hours after dose), continue monitoring until symptoms resolve.
🌙 *Alert:* Repeat first-dose monitoring guidelines after second dose in patients who required pharmacologic intervention for symptomatic bradycardia after first dose.
• Obtain baseline ECG if one wasn't done within 6 months before start of therapy, especially in patients receiving antiarrhythmics, beta blockers, or calcium channel blockers

and in those with cardiac risk factors or slow or irregular HR on physical exam.

❸ *Alert:* Drug may cause PML, which can cause severe disability or death. Monitor for progressive and diverse symptoms of PML (progressive weakness on one side of body, clumsiness, vision problems, confusion, and changes in thinking, personality, memory, and orientation). Stop drug and perform diagnostic evaluation, including MRI, if PML is suspected.

• Test for varicella antibodies before treatment initiation, especially if patient has no history of chickenpox or immunization; consider vaccination against varicella zoster 1 month before start of fingolimod therapy.

• Obtain baseline ophthalmic exam and monitor patient for macular edema at 3 to 4 months after treatment initiation and if patient complains of visual disturbances. Although macular edema is a rare adverse reaction, patients with uveitis and diabetes are at increased risk.

• Drug may increase risk of infections. Monitor for signs and symptoms of infection during treatment and for 2 months after therapy ends. Obtain baseline CBC with differential within 6 months of beginning therapy. Stop treatment if patient has active infection.

• HPV infections, including papilloma, dysplasia, warts, and HPV-related cancer, have been reported in patients treated with fingolimod. Consider vaccination against HPV before treatment initiation. Cancer screening, including Papanicolaou testing, is recommended for patients receiving immunosuppressive therapy.

• Monitor for liver impairment (unexplained nausea, vomiting, abdominal pain, fatigue, anorexia, jaundice, dark urine). Obtain LFTs within 6 months before start of treatment, promptly in patients who report symptoms that may indicate liver injury, and periodically until 2 months after therapy ends. Most enzyme elevations occur within 3 to 4 months of treatment initiation. Drug discontinuation may be needed if severe liver injury occurs.

• Monitor patient for respiratory changes. Obtain spirometry and diffusion lung capacity tests if clinically indicated.

• Drug increases risk of basal cell carcinoma and melanoma. Monitor for and promptly evaluate suspicious skin lesions.

• Restart therapy at initial dose if patient discontinues treatment for longer than 2 weeks.

PATIENT TEACHING

❸ *Alert:* Teach patient to immediately contact health care provider if signs and symptoms of slowing HR (dizziness, tiredness, irregular heartbeat, palpitations) occur.

❸ *Alert:* Advise patient to immediately report signs and symptoms of PML. Tell patient not to stop drug without first discussing with prescriber.

• Instruct patient to report visual disturbances, trouble breathing, changes in HR (low HR, dizziness, fatigue, chest pain) or rhythm (palpitations), infection (pain, fever, malaise), or suspicious skin lesions.

• Tell patient to immediately report unexplained nausea, vomiting, abdominal pain, fatigue, anorexia, jaundice, or dark urine.

• Advise patient to notify prescriber of any medication changes.

• Warn patient of childbearing potential about fetal risk; advise patient to use effective contraception during treatment and for 2 months after treatment ends.

• Instruct patient to immediately report pregnancy or plans to become pregnant.

• Advise patient to promptly report suspicious skin lesions and to limit exposure to sun and UV light by wearing protective clothing and using a sunscreen with a high sun protection factor.

---

flecainide acetate
FLEH-kay-nide

Therapeutic class: Antiarrhythmics
Pharmacologic class: Benzamide derivatives

AVAILABLE FORMS
Tablets: 50 mg, 100 mg, 150 mg

INDICATIONS & DOSAGES
➤ **Prevention of paroxysmal supraventricular tachycardia (PSVT) or paroxysmal atrial fibrillation or flutter (PAF) in patients without structural heart disease; prevention of life-threatening ventricular arrhythmias such as sustained ventricular tachycardia**
Adults: For PSVT or PAF, 50 mg PO every 12 hours. Increase in increments of 50 mg b.i.d. every 4 days until desired effect occurs. Maximum dose, 300 mg/day. For life-threatening ventricular arrhythmias, 100 mg

---

PO every 12 hours. Increase in increments of 50 mg b.i.d. every 4 days until desired effect occurs. Maximum dose for most patients, 400 mg/day.

Children older than age 6 months: Initially, 100 mg/m²/day in divided doses every 8 to 12 hours. May titrate dosage at 4-day intervals. Maximum dosage, 200 mg/m²/day.

Children ages 6 months and younger: 50 mg/m²/day in divided doses every 8 to 12 hours. May titrate dosage at 4-day intervals. Maximum dosage is 200 mg/m²/day.

Adjust-a-dose: For adults, if CrCl is 35 mL/minute or less, first dose is 100 mg PO once daily or 50 mg PO b.i.d. Titrate dose cautiously in children, because small dose changes may disproportionately increase drug levels.

ADMINISTRATION
PO
• Give drug without regard to food.
• Oral suspension can be prepared by a pharmacist. Shake well before use. May refrigerate or keep at room temperature, protected from light, for 60 days.
• Store tablets at room temperature in a tight, light-resistant container.

ACTION
A class IC antiarrhythmic that decreases excitability, conduction velocity, and automaticity by slowing atrial, AV node, His-Purkinje system, and intraventricular conduction; prolongs refractory periods in these tissues.

Route	Onset	Peak	Duration
PO	Unknown	1–6 hr	Unknown

Half-life: 12 to 27 hours (adults); 11 to 12 hours (adolescents ages 12 to 15); 8 hours (children); 6 hours (12 months [infants]); 11 to 12 hours (3 months [infants]); 29 hours or less (newborns).

ADVERSE REACTIONS
CNS: dizziness, headache, light-headedness, syncope, fatigue, fever, tremor, anxiety, insomnia, hypoesthesia, depression, malaise, paresis, paresthesia, ataxia, asthenia, somnolence. **CV:** *new or worsened arrhythmias, bradycardia, HF, cardiac pause or arrest,* tachycardia, chest pain, palpitations, edema, flushing. **EENT:** blurred vision and other visual disturbances, tinnitus, vertigo. **GI:** nausea, constipation, abdominal pain, dyspepsia, vomiting, diarrhea, anorexia. **Respiratory:** dyspnea. **Skin:** diaphoresis, rash.

INTERACTIONS
Drug-drug. *Amiodarone, cimetidine, CYP2D6 inhibitors (clozapine, quinidine):* May increase level of flecainide. Watch for toxicity. In the presence of amiodarone, reduce usual flecainide dose by 50% and monitor patient for adverse effects.
Digoxin: May increase digoxin level. Monitor digoxin level.
Disopyramide, verapamil: May increase negative inotropic properties. Avoid use together.
Propranolol, other beta blockers: May increase flecainide and propranolol levels. Watch for negative inotropic effects.
QTc interval–prolonging drugs (fluoroquinolones, ondansetron, posaconazole): May increase risk of cardiotoxicity and arrhythmias. Consider therapy modification.
Ritonavir: May increase flecainide levels and toxicity. Use together is contraindicated.
Drug-food. *Milk, milk-based formulas:* May interfere with drug absorption. Monitor trough drug levels during major changes in dietary milk intake.

EFFECTS ON LAB TEST RESULTS
None reported.

CONTRAINDICATIONS & CAUTIONS
• Contraindicated in patients hypersensitive to drug and in those with second- or third-degree AV block or right bundle-branch block with left hemiblock (in absence of artificial pacemaker), structural heart disease, or cardiogenic shock.

Boxed Warning Patients who receive flecainide for atrial fibrillation or flutter are at increased risk for ventricular tachycardia and ventricular fibrillation. Use of drug in patients with chronic atrial fibrillation isn't recommended. ■

Boxed Warning Drug may increase risk of mortality and nonfatal cardiac arrest in patients with MI within 2 years. When used to prevent ventricular arrhythmias, reserve drug for patients with documented life-threatening arrhythmias. ■

• Due to safety risks, flecainide should be reserved for symptomatic supraventricular tachycardia in patients without structural or ischemic heart disease who aren't candidates for, or prefer not to undergo, catheter ablation and in whom other therapies have failed or are contraindicated.

• Use cautiously in patients with severe kidney disease, prolonged QT interval, sick sinus syndrome, or blood dyscrasia. Avoid use in patients with HF.
• In patients with liver disease, use drug only if potential benefits outweigh risk, and use frequent and early drug-level monitoring to guide dosage.
• When transferring patients from another antiarrhythmic to flecainide, allow two to four plasma half-lives to elapse for the drug being discontinued before starting flecainide at usual dosage. Consider hospitalizing patients in whom withdrawal of a previous antiarrhythmic produced life-threatening arrhythmias.
• Safety and effectiveness in children haven't been determined.
Dialyzable drug: No.

PREGNANCY-LACTATION-REPRODUCTION
• Studies during pregnancy are inadequate. Use during pregnancy only if potential benefit justifies fetal risk.
• Drug appears in human milk. Consider discontinuing breastfeeding or drug.

NURSING CONSIDERATIONS
• For patients with sustained ventricular tachycardia, initiate therapy in the hospital and monitor rhythm.
Boxed Warning Patients treated with flecainide for atrial flutter have 1:1 AV conduction due to slowing of atrial rate. A paradoxical increase in ventricular rate may occur. Concomitant negative chronotropic therapy with digoxin or beta blockers may lower risk of this complication. ∎
• Check that pacing threshold was determined 1 week before and after starting therapy in patient with a pacemaker; flecainide can alter endocardial pacing thresholds.
• Correct hypokalemia or hyperkalemia before giving flecainide; these electrolyte disturbances may alter drug's effect.
• Monitor ECG for proarrhythmic effects.
• Most patients can be maintained on an every-12-hours dosing schedule; some need to receive flecainide every 8 hours.
• Monitor flecainide level, especially if patient has KF or HF. Therapeutic flecainide levels range from 0.2 to 1 mcg/mL. Risk of adverse effects increases when trough blood level exceeds 1 mcg/mL.

PATIENT TEACHING
• Stress importance of taking drug exactly as prescribed.
• Instruct patient to promptly report adverse reactions and to limit fluid and sodium intake to minimize fluid retention.
• Advise patient to immediately report pregnancy, plans to become pregnant, breastfeeding, or plans to breastfeed during treatment.

fluconazole ℞
floo-KON-a-zole

Diflucan

Therapeutic class: Antifungals
Pharmacologic class: Triazoles

AVAILABLE FORMS
Injection: 100 mg/50 mL, 200 mg/100 mL, 400 mg/200 mL ready-to-use container
Powder for oral suspension: 50 mg/5 mL, 200 mg/5 mL
Tablets: 50 mg, 100 mg, 150 mg, 200 mg

INDICATIONS & DOSAGES
Adjust-a-dose (for all indications except vulvovaginal candidiasis): If CrCl is less than 50 mL/minute and patient isn't receiving dialysis, give initial loading dose of 50 to 400 mg for patients about to receive multiple doses; then reduce dosage by 50%. Patients receiving regular hemodialysis treatment should receive usual dose after each dialysis session.
➤ **Oropharyngeal candidiasis**
Adults: 200 mg PO or IV on first day, then 100 mg once daily for at least 2 weeks.
Children: 6 mg/kg PO or IV on first day, then 3 mg/kg daily for 2 weeks.
Adjust-a-dose (for premature neonates [gestational age, 26 to 29 weeks]): For first 2 weeks of life, give same dosage as for older children every 72 hours. After first 2 weeks, give dose once daily. Maximum daily dose, 600 mg.
➤ **Esophageal candidiasis**
Adults: 200 mg PO or IV on first day, then 100 mg once daily. Up to 400 mg daily has been used, depending on patient's condition and tolerance of treatment. Patients should receive drug for at least 3 weeks and for 2 weeks after symptoms resolve.
Children: 6 mg/kg PO or IV on first day, then 3 to 12 mg/kg daily for at least 3 weeks

---

and for at least 2 weeks after symptoms resolve. Maximum daily dose, 12 mg/kg (or 600 mg).

Adjust-a-dose (for premature neonates [gestational age, 26 to 29 weeks]): For first 2 weeks of life, give same dosage as for older children every 72 hours. After first 2 weeks, give dose once daily.

➤ **Vaginal candidiasis**
Adults: 150 mg PO for one dose only.

➤ **Systemic candidiasis**
Adults: Optimal therapeutic dosage and duration of therapy haven't been established; doses of up to 400 mg PO or IV daily have been used.
Children: 6 to 12 mg/kg/day PO or IV. Maximum daily dose, 600 mg.

Adjust-a-dose (for premature neonates [gestational age, 26 to 29 weeks]): For first 2 weeks of life, give same dosage as for older children every 72 hours. After first 2 weeks, give dose once daily.

➤ **Cryptococcal meningitis**
Adults: 400 mg PO or IV on first day, then 200 mg once daily for 10 to 12 weeks after CSF culture result is negative. Doses up to 400 mg/day may be used.
Children: 12 mg/kg/day PO or IV on first day, then 6 to 12 mg/kg/day for 10 to 12 weeks after CSF culture result is negative. Maximum daily dose, 600 mg.

Adjust-a-dose (for premature neonates [gestational age, 26 to 29 weeks]): For first 2 weeks of life, administer the same dosage as for older children every 72 hours. After first 2 weeks, administer dose once daily.

➤ **Suppression of cryptococcal meningitis relapse in patients with AIDS**
Adults: 200 mg PO or IV daily.
Children: 6 mg/kg/day PO or IV once daily.

Adjust-a-dose (for premature neonates [gestational age, 26 to 29 weeks]): For first 2 weeks of life, give same dosage as for older children every 72 hours. After first 2 weeks, give dose once daily.

➤ **Prevention of candidiasis in patients receiving bone marrow transplant and patients with cancer**
Adults: 400 mg PO or IV once daily. Start treatment several days before anticipated agranulocytosis, and continue for 7 days after neutrophil count exceeds 1,000/mm³.

➤ *Candida*-**related peritonitis; UTI**
Adults: 50 to 200 mg PO or IV once daily.

ADMINISTRATION

PO
⚠ *Alert:* Hazardous drug; use safe handling and disposal precautions.
• Give drug without regard to food.
• Add 24 mL of distilled or purified water to bottle and shake oral suspension well before giving.
• Store tablets and powder for oral suspension below 86° F (30° C). Store reconstituted suspension between 41° and 86° F (5° and 30° C). Discard unused portion after 2 weeks.
• Protect from freezing.

IV
⚠ *Alert:* Hazardous drug; use safe handling and disposal precautions.
▼ To ensure product sterility, don't remove protective wrap from IV bag until just before use.
▼ The plastic container may show some opacity from moisture absorbed during sterilization. This doesn't affect drug and diminishes over time.
▼ To prevent air embolism, don't connect in series with other infusions.
▼ Use an infusion pump.
▼ Give by continuous infusion at no more than 200 mg/hour.
▼ Don't use if solution is cloudy or precipitated.
▼ Store ready-to-use containers at room temperature.
▼ **Incompatibilities:** Many other IV drugs are incompatible. Consult drug compatibility reference for more information. Don't add other drugs to IV bag.

ACTION

Interferes with fungal CYP450 activity, decreasing ergosterol synthesis and inhibiting cell membrane formation.

Route	Onset	Peak	Duration
PO	Rapid	1–2 hr	30 hr
IV	Immediate	Immediate	Unknown

Half-life: 20 to 50 hours.

ADVERSE REACTIONS

CNS: headache, dizziness, dysgeusia. **GI:** nausea, vomiting, abdominal pain, diarrhea, dyspepsia. **Skin:** rash.

INTERACTIONS

• Fluconazole can significantly interact with many drugs. Consult a drug compatibility reference or pharmacist for additional information.

Drug-drug. *Alprazolam, chlordiazepoxide, clonazepam, clorazepate, diazepam, estazolam, flurazepam, midazolam, quazepam, triazolam:* Fluconazole may increase levels of these drugs and may cause increased CNS depression and psychomotor impairment. Avoid use together.

Carbamazepine, celecoxib, cyclosporine, phenytoin, theophylline: Fluconazole may increase levels of these drugs. Monitor carbamazepine, cyclosporine, phenytoin, and theophylline levels. Consider reducing celecoxib dosage by half when using with fluconazole.

Cimetidine: May decrease fluconazole level. Monitor patient's response to fluconazole.

CYP3A4 substrates that may lead to QT-interval prolongation (erythromycin, pimozide, quinidine): May cause prolonged QT interval and sudden death. Use together is contraindicated.

HMG-CoA reductase inhibitors (atorvastatin, fluvastatin, lovastatin, pravastatin, simvastatin): May increase levels and adverse effects of these drugs. Avoid use together or reduce dosage of HMG-CoA reductase inhibitor.

Hydrochlorothiazide: May increase fluconazole level. Monitor patient for fluconazole toxicity.

Isoniazid, oral sulfonylureas, phenytoin, rifampin, valproic acid: May increase liver transaminase level. Monitor LFT values closely.

Oral sulfonylureas (glipizide, glyburide): May increase levels of these drugs. Monitor patient for enhanced hypoglycemic effect.

Rifampin: May enhance fluconazole metabolism. Monitor patient for lack of response to fluconazole.

Tacrolimus: May increase tacrolimus level and kidney toxicity. Monitor patient carefully.

Warfarin: May increase risk of bleeding. Monitor PT and INR.

Zidovudine: May increase zidovudine-related toxicities. Monitor patient closely. Zidovudine dosage decrease may be needed.

Zolpidem: May increase therapeutic effects of zolpidem. Monitor patient closely. A decrease in dosage may be needed.

EFFECTS ON LAB TEST RESULTS
• May increase ALP, ALT, AST, GGT, cholesterol, and triglyceride levels.
• May decrease potassium level.
• May decrease platelet and WBC counts.

CONTRAINDICATIONS & CAUTIONS
• Contraindicated in patients hypersensitive to drug. Rarely, anaphylaxis has been reported.
• Some formulations contain benzyl alcohol, which has been associated with fatal "gasping syndrome" in neonates; use cautiously or avoid use.
• Use cautiously in patients hypersensitive to other antifungal azole compounds.
• Use cautiously in patients with kidney dysfunction or proarrhythmic conditions.
• Reversible adrenal insufficiency has been reported in patients receiving fluconazole.
⬚ Oral suspension contains sucrose and shouldn't be used in patients with hereditary fructose, glucose, or galactose malabsorption or sucrase-isomaltase deficiency.
Dialyzable drug: 50%.
⚠ *Overdose S&S:* Hallucinations, paranoid behavior.

PREGNANCY-LACTATION-REPRODUCTION
• Contraindicated for most indications during pregnancy. Long-term treatment with high doses (400 to 800 mg/day) during first trimester may be associated with birth defects.
• Patients of childbearing potential should use effective contraception during treatment and for 1 week after final dose.
• Drug appears in human milk. Use cautiously during breastfeeding.

NURSING CONSIDERATIONS
⬥ **Alert:** Serious liver toxicity has occurred in patients with underlying medical conditions. Monitor LFT values and discontinue drug if liver dysfunction develops.
• Rare cases of exfoliative skin disorders have been reported. Closely monitor patients who develop mild rash. Stop drug if lesions progress.
• Monitor kidney function during treatment; dosage adjustment may be necessary.
• Monitor potassium level.
• Monitor for signs and symptoms of adrenal insufficiency (fatigue, weakness, anorexia, weight loss, abdominal pain).
• Likelihood of adverse reactions may be greater in patients with HIV infection.

PATIENT TEACHING
• Tell patient to take drug as directed, even after feeling better.
• Instruct patient to promptly report all adverse reactions.

Reactions in bold italics are *life-threatening*.

• Instruct patient to report pregnancy or plans to become pregnant or to breastfeed.

flumazenil
FLOO-ma-zeh-nil

Therapeutic class: Antidotes
Pharmacologic class: Benzodiazepine antagonists

AVAILABLE FORMS
Injection: 0.1 mg/mL in 5-mL and 10-mL multiple-dose vials

INDICATIONS & DOSAGES
➤ **Complete or partial reversal of sedative effects of benzodiazepines after anesthesia (adults) or conscious sedation (adults and children)**
Adults: Initially, 0.2 mg IV over 15 seconds. If patient doesn't reach desired level of consciousness after 45 seconds, repeat dose. Repeat at 1-minute intervals, if needed, until cumulative dose of 1 mg has been given (first dose plus four more doses). Most patients respond after 0.6 to 1 mg of drug. In case of resedation, repeat dosage after 20 minutes, but don't give more than 1 mg at any one time or exceed 3 mg in any 1 hour.
Children ages 1 year and older: 0.01 mg/kg (up to 0.2 mg) IV over 15 seconds. If patient doesn't reach desired level of consciousness after 45 seconds, repeat dose. Repeat at 1-minute intervals, if needed, until cumulative dose of 0.05 mg/kg or 1 mg, whichever is lower, has been given (first dose plus four more doses).
➤ **Suspected benzodiazepine overdose**
Adults: Initially, 0.2 mg IV over 30 seconds. If patient doesn't reach desired level of consciousness after 30 seconds, give 0.3 mg over 30 seconds. If patient still doesn't respond adequately, give 0.5 mg over 30 seconds. Repeat 0.5-mg doses, as needed, at 1-minute intervals until cumulative dose of 3 mg has been given. Most patients with benzodiazepine overdose respond to cumulative doses between 1 and 3 mg; rarely, patients who respond partially after 3 mg may need additional doses, up to 5 mg total. If patient doesn't respond in 5 minutes after receiving 5 mg, sedation is unlikely to be caused by benzodiazepines. In case of resedation, may repeat dose after 20 minutes, but never give more than 1 mg

(give as 0.5 mg/minute) at any one time or exceed 3 mg in any 1 hour.

ADMINISTRATION
IV
▼ Make sure airway is secure and patent.
▼ Compatible solutions include D_5W, lactated Ringer injection, and NSS.
▼ To minimize pain at injection site, inject drug over 15 to 30 seconds into large vein through free-flowing solution.
▼ Monitor patient for signs and symptoms of extravasation.
▼ Drug remains stable in a syringe for 24 hours.
▼ Store drug in vial at 68° to 77° F (20° to 25° C) until use.
▼ Protect from light.
▼ **Incompatibilities:** None listed by manufacturer. Consult drug compatibility reference for more information.

ACTION
Competitively inhibits the actions of benzodiazepines on the GABA-benzodiazepine receptor complex.

Route	Onset	Peak	Duration
IV	1–2 min	6–10 min	1 hr (variable range: 19–50 min)

Half-life: Adults: 40 to 80 minutes (terminal); children: 20 to 75 minutes (terminal).

ADVERSE REACTIONS
CNS: dizziness, headache, agitation, anxiety, nervousness, tremor, insomnia, fatigue, paresthesia, emotional lability (depersonalization, depression, dysphoria, euphoria, paranoia). **CV:** cutaneous vasodilation, thrombophlebitis, palpitations, flushing. **EENT:** abnormal or blurred vision, lacrimation, dry mouth. **GI:** nausea, vomiting. **Respiratory:** dyspnea, hyperventilation. **Skin:** diaphoresis, rash. **Other:** pain at injection site, injection-site reaction.

INTERACTIONS
None significant.

EFFECTS ON LAB TEST RESULTS
None reported.

CONTRAINDICATIONS & CAUTIONS
• Contraindicated in patients hypersensitive to flumazenil or benzodiazepines, in those

with evidence of serious TCA overdose, and in those who have received benzodiazepines to treat a potentially life-threatening condition, such as status epilepticus or increased ICP.

🕗 *Alert:* Don't use in patients with mixed-drug overdose who are seriously ill when seizures from any cause are likely.

• Use cautiously in patients with head injury, psychiatric disorders, or alcohol dependence.

• Use cautiously in patients at high risk for developing seizures and in those who have recently received multiple doses of a parenteral benzodiazepine, who display signs of seizure activity, or who may be at risk for benzodiazepine dependence, such as patients in the ICU.

Dialyzable drug: No.

⚠️ *Overdose S&S:* Anxiety, agitation, increased muscle tone, hyperesthesia, seizures.

PREGNANCY-LACTATION-REPRODUCTION
• Studies during pregnancy are inadequate. Use during pregnancy only if benefit outweighs fetal risk.

• It isn't known if drug appears in human milk. Use cautiously during breastfeeding.

NURSING CONSIDERATIONS
• Monitor patient closely for resedation, respiratory depression, or other residual effects that may occur after reversal of benzodiazepine effects; drug's duration of action is the shortest of all benzodiazepines. Length of monitoring depends on specific drug being reversed. Monitor patient closely after doses of long-acting benzodiazepines such as diazepam, or after high doses of short-acting benzodiazepines, such as 10 mg of midazolam. In most cases, severe resedation and respiratory depression are unlikely in patients who fail to show signs of resedation 2 hours after a 1-mg dose.

• Repeat doses of flumazenil in patients with liver disease should be reduced in size or frequency, except when used for initial reversal of benzodiazepine effects.

Boxed Warning Monitor patients for seizures, especially those who have been on benzodiazepines for long-term sedation or in overdose cases in which patients are showing signs of serious TCA overdose. Practitioners should individualize flumazenil dosage and be prepared to manage seizures. ∎

PATIENT TEACHING
• Warn patient not to perform hazardous activities within 24 hours of procedure because of risk of residual sedative effects of benzodiazepine.

• Instruct patient to avoid alcohol, CNS depressants, and OTC drugs for 24 hours.

• Tell patient to report all adverse reactions.

• Give family necessary instructions and provide patient with written instructions. Patient may not be able to recall information given after the procedure; drug doesn't reverse amnesic effects of benzodiazepines.

fluocinolone acetonide
floo-oh-SIN-oh-lone

Capex, Derma-Smoothe/FS, DermOtic, Flac, Synalar

Therapeutic class: Corticosteroids
Pharmacologic class: Corticosteroids

AVAILABLE FORMS
Cream: 0.01%, 0.025%
Oil: 0.01%
Oil/drops (otic): 0.01%
Ointment: 0.025%
Shampoo: 0.01%
Topical solution: 0.01%

INDICATIONS & DOSAGES
➤ **Inflammation from corticosteroid-responsive dermatoses (cream, ointment, solution)**
Adults and children: Clean area; apply product sparingly b.i.d. to q.i.d.

➤ **Atopic dermatitis**
Adults: Apply thin film of body oil t.i.d.
Children ages 3 months and older: Moisten skin; then apply thin film of body oil b.i.d. for maximum of 4 weeks. Avoid face and diaper area.

➤ **Scalp psoriasis**
Adults: Thoroughly wet or dampen hair and scalp. Apply thin film of scalp oil and massage into scalp. Cover with supplied shower cap overnight or for a minimum of 4 hours before thoroughly washing with regular shampoo and then thoroughly rinsing with water.

➤ **Seborrheic dermatitis of the scalp**
Adults: Apply no more than 30 mL of 0.01% shampoo to the scalp once daily,

lather, and thoroughly rinse with water after 5 minutes.

➤ **Eczematous external otitis**
Adults and children ages 2 and older: Apply 5 drops of oil (otic) into affected ear b.i.d. for 7 to 14 days.

ADMINISTRATION
Otic
• Tilt head to one side so the affected ear is facing up. Gently pull earlobe backward and upward and apply 5 drops of oil into ear. Keep head tilted for at least 1 minute.
• Gently pat excess material dripping out of ear using a clean cotton ball.
• Otic formulation isn't for ophthalmic use.

Topical
• Gently wash skin before applying. To prevent skin damage, rub in gently, leaving a thin coat. When treating hairy sites, part hair and apply directly to lesions.
• Avoid application near eyes and mucous membranes; in armpits, groin, and rectal area; and in ear canal if eardrum is perforated.
• Do not use occlusive dressing unless ordered.
• For patients with eczematous dermatitis whose skin may be irritated by adhesive material, hold dressing in place with gauze, elastic bandages, stockings, or stockinette.
• Change dressing as prescribed. Stop drug and notify prescriber if skin infection, striae, or atrophy occurs.
• Shake shampoo well before use. Discard shampoo after 2 months.

ACTION
Unclear. Diffuses across cell membranes to form complexes with receptors, resulting in decreased formation, release, and activity of inflammatory mediators.

Route	Onset	Peak	Duration
Otic, topical	Unknown	Unknown	Unknown

Half-life: Unknown.

ADVERSE REACTIONS
CNS: fever. **CV:** telangiectasias. **EENT:** ear infection, nasopharyngitis, rhinorrhea. **GI:** diarrhea, vomiting. **Respiratory:** URI, cough. **Skin:** burning, pruritus, irritation, dryness, erythema, folliculitis, hypertrichosis, hypopigmentation, hyperpigmentation, acneiform eruptions, perioral dermatitis, keratosis pilaris, papules, pustules, skin atrophy, shiny skin, allergic contact dermatitis,

maceration, secondary infection, atrophy, striae, miliaria with occlusive dressings, abscess. **Other:** herpes simplex, secondary infection.

INTERACTIONS
None significant.

EFFECTS ON LAB TEST RESULTS
• May increase glucose level.

CONTRAINDICATIONS & CAUTIONS
• Contraindicated in patients hypersensitive to drug or its components.
• Don't use as monotherapy in treatment of primary bacterial infections (impetigo, paronychia, erysipelas, cellulitis, angular cheilitis), rosacea, perioral dermatitis, or acne.
• Children are at higher risk for HPA-axis suppression and Cushing syndrome than adults when treated with topical corticosteroids. Linear growth retardation, delayed weight gain, and intracranial HTN have been reported.
• Drug isn't indicated for use in children younger than age 3 months.
Dialyzable drug: Unknown.
⚠ *Overdose S&S:* Systemic effects.

PREGNANCY-LACTATION-REPRODUCTION
• Use lowest effective dose during pregnancy and breastfeeding.

NURSING CONSIDERATIONS
• If an occlusive dressing has been applied and fever develops, notify prescriber and remove dressing.
• If antifungal or antibiotic combined with corticosteroid fails to provide prompt improvement, stop corticosteroid until infection is controlled.
• Systemic absorption is likely with use of occlusive dressings, prolonged treatment, or extensive body surface treatment. Watch for symptoms (hyperglycemia, glycosuria, HPA axis suppression, Cushing syndrome).
• Avoid using plastic pants or tight-fitting diapers on treated areas in young children. Children may absorb larger amounts of drug and be more susceptible to systemic toxicity.
🔹 *Alert:* Body oil and scalp oil formulations contain peanut oil.
• *Look alike–sound alike:* Don't confuse fluocinolone with fluocinonide or fluticasone.

PATIENT TEACHING

• Teach patient or family how to apply drug using gloves or sterile applicator.

• Tell patient to wash hands after application.

• Caution patient to use an occlusive dressing only if directed by prescriber. If an occlusive dressing is used, advise patient to leave it in place for no longer than 12 hours each day and not to use dressing on infected or weeping lesions.

• Tell patient to stop using solution and notify prescriber if signs of systemic absorption, skin irritation or ulceration, hypersensitivity, or infection develop.

• Advise patient using the shampoo not to bandage, cover, or wrap the treated scalp area, unless directed.

• Instruct patient to report pregnancy or plans to become pregnant or to breastfeed.

fluocinonide
floo-oh-SIN-oh-nide

Lidemol❦, Lidex❦, Lyderm❦, Tiamol❦, Vanos

Therapeutic class: Corticosteroids
Pharmacologic class: Corticosteroids

AVAILABLE FORMS
Cream: 0.05%, 0.1%
Gel: 0.05%
Ointment: 0.05%
Topical solution: 0.05%

INDICATIONS & DOSAGES
➤ **Inflammation and pruritis from corticosteroid-responsive dermatoses**
Adults and children ages 12 and older: Clean area; then apply cream, gel, ointment, or topical solution sparingly b.i.d. to q.i.d. In children, use lowest dosage that promotes healing. If using Vanos 0.1% cream in adults and children ages 12 and older, apply a thin layer once daily or b.i.d. for up to 2 weeks. Maximum, 60 g/week.

ADMINISTRATION
Topical
• Gently wash skin before applying. To prevent skin damage, rub in gently, leaving a thin coat. When treating hairy sites, part hair and apply directly to lesion.

• Avoid applying 1% cream to face, groin, or axillae. Use 0.05% formulations cautiously on face or opposing skin surfaces that may rub or touch, such as skinfolds of the groin, axilla, and breast.

• Occlusive dressings may be used in severe or resistant dermatoses.

• For patients with eczematous dermatitis whose skin may be irritated by adhesive material, hold dressing in place with gauze, elastic bandages, stockings, or stockinette.

• Change dressing as prescribed. Stop drug and notify prescriber if skin infection, striae, or atrophy occurs.

• Continue treatment for a few days after lesions clear.

ACTION
Diffuses across cell membranes to form complexes with cytoplasmic receptors.

Route	Onset	Peak	Duration
Topical	Unknown	Unknown	Unknown

Half-life: Unknown.

ADVERSE REACTIONS
CNS: headache. **CV:** telangiectasia. **EENT:** nasopharyngitis, nasal congestion. **Skin:** burning, pruritus, irritation, dryness, erythema, folliculitis, hypertrichosis, hypopigmentation, acneiform eruptions, perioral dermatitis, allergic contact dermatitis, maceration, secondary infection, atrophy, striae, miliaria with occlusive dressings.

INTERACTIONS
None significant.

EFFECTS ON LAB TEST RESULTS
• May increase glucose level.

CONTRAINDICATIONS & CAUTIONS
• Contraindicated in patients hypersensitive to drug or its components.

• Don't use as monotherapy in treatment of primary bacterial infections (impetigo, paronychia, erysipelas, cellulitis, angular cheilitis), rosacea, perioral dermatitis, or acne.

• Don't use very-high-potency or high-potency agents on the face, groin, breasts, or armpits.

• Children are at higher risk for HPA-axis suppression and Cushing syndrome than adults when treated with topical corticosteroids. Linear growth retardation, delayed weight gain, and intracranial HTN have been reported.

• Safety and effectiveness in children younger than age 12 haven't been established.

Dialyzable drug: Unknown.

⚠ *Overdose S&S:* Systemic effects.

PREGNANCY-LACTATION-REPRODUCTION

• Use lowest effective dose in pregnancy and only if potential benefit justifies fetal risk.

• It isn't known if drug appears in human milk. Patient should discontinue breastfeeding or discontinue drug, considering importance of drug to patient.

NURSING CONSIDERATIONS

• If an occlusive dressing has been applied and fever develops, notify prescriber and remove dressing.

• If antifungal or antibiotic combined with corticosteroid fails to provide prompt improvement, stop corticosteroid until infection is controlled.

• Systemic absorption is likely with use of occlusive dressings, prolonged treatment, or extensive body surface treatment. Watch for such symptoms as hyperglycemia, glycosuria, and HPA axis suppression.

• Avoid using plastic pants or tight-fitting diapers on treated areas in young children. Children may absorb larger amounts of drug and be more susceptible to systemic toxicity.

• *Look alike–sound alike:* Don't confuse fluocinonide with fluocinolone or fluticasone.

PATIENT TEACHING

• Teach patient and family how to apply drug using careful hand washing and gloves or sterile applicator.

• If an occlusive dressing is ordered, advise patient to leave it in place for no more than 12 hours each day and not to use the dressing on infected or weeping lesions.

• Tell patient to stop drug and report signs of systemic absorption, skin irritation or ulceration, hypersensitivity, or infection.

• Instruct patient to report pregnancy or plans to become pregnant or to breastfeed.

fluorouracil (5-FU) ▧
flure-oh-YOOR-a-sill

Carac, Efudex, Tolak

Therapeutic class: Antineoplastics
Pharmacologic class: Pyrimidine analogues

AVAILABLE FORMS

Cream: 0.5%, 4%, 5%
Injection: 50 mg/mL
Topical solution: 2%, 5%

INDICATIONS & DOSAGES

Adjust-a-dose (for all IV indications): Individualize 5-FU dosage and dosing schedule based on tumor type, specific regimen administered, disease state, response to treatment, and patient risk factors. Refer to manufacturer's instructions for toxicity-related dosage adjustments.

➤ **Multiple actinic (solar) keratoses**
Adults: 0.5% cream once daily for up to 4 weeks as tolerated. 4% cream once daily for 4 weeks as tolerated. Or, 5% cream or 2% or 5% fluorouracil topical solution b.i.d. for 2 to 6 weeks.

➤ **Superficial basal cell carcinoma**
Adults: 5% cream or 5% fluorouracil topical solution b.i.d., usually for 3 to 6 weeks. Maximum, 12 weeks.

➤ **Colon and rectal adenocarcinoma**
Adults (infusional regimen in combination with leucovorin alone or in combination with leucovorin and oxaliplatin or irinotecan): 400 mg/m² by IV bolus on day 1, followed by 2,400 to 3,000 mg/m² IV as a continuous infusion over 46 hours every 2 weeks.
Adults (bolus dosing regimen in combination with leucovorin): 500 mg/m² by IV bolus on days 1, 8, 15, 22, 29, and 36 in 8-week cycles.
Adjust-a-dose: Various other regimens exist. Refer to guidelines or institutional protocols for further information.

➤ **Breast adenocarcinoma**
Adults: 500 or 600 mg/m² IV on days 1 and 8 every 28 days for six cycles as part of a cyclophosphamide-based multidrug regimen.

➤ **Gastric adenocarcinoma**
Adults: 200 to 1,000 mg/m² IV as continuous infusion over 24 hours as part of a platinum-containing multidrug chemotherapy regimen. Frequency of dosing in each cycle and length

F

of each cycle depend on dose of 5-FU injection and specific regimen administered.

➤ **Pancreatic adenocarcinoma**
Adults: 400 mg/m² IV bolus on day 1, followed by 2,400 mg/m² IV as continuous infusion over 46 hours every 2 weeks in combination with leucovorin or as a component of a multidrug chemotherapy regimen that includes leucovorin. ◆

➤ **Anal carcinoma** ◆
Adults: 1,000 mg/m²/day continuous IV infusion days 1 to 4 and days 29 to 32, in combination with mitomycin and radiation.

➤ **Muscle-invasive bladder cancer** ◆
Adults: 500 mg/m²/day continuous IV infusion during radiation therapy fractions 1 to 5 and 16 to 20, in combination with mitomycin.

➤ **Cervical cancer** ◆
Adults: 1,000 mg/m²/day continuous IV infusion days 1 to 4 every 3 weeks for three cycles, in combination with cisplatin and radiation.

➤ **Esophageal cancer** ◆
Adults: 800 mg/m²/day continuous IV infusion on days 1 to 5 every 4 weeks in combination with cisplatin and nivolumab until disease progression or unacceptable toxicity occurs; nivolumab can be continued for up to 2 years.
Adjust-a-dose: Various other regimens exist. Refer to guidelines or institutional protocols for further information.

➤ **Head and neck cancer** ◆
Adults: 1,000 mg/m²/day continuous IV infusion days 1 to 4 every 3 weeks (in combination with cisplatin) for at least six cycles, or 600 mg/m²/day continuous IV infusion days 1 to 4, 22 to 25, and 43 to 46 (in combination with carboplatin and radiation).

Or, 1,000 mg/m²/day continuous IV infusion days 1 to 4 every 3 weeks (in combination with docetaxel and cisplatin) for three cycles, followed by chemoradiotherapy.

Or, 1,000 mg/m²/day continuous infusion days 1 to 4 every 3 weeks (in combination with either carboplatin or cisplatin and pembrolizumab) for 6 cycles, followed by up to 24 months of pembrolizumab monotherapy.
Adjust-a-dose: Other regimens exist. Refer to guidelines or institutional protocols for further information.

ADMINISTRATION

⚠ Alert: Hazardous drug; use safe handling and disposal precautions.

IV
▼ To reduce nausea, give antiemetic before 5-FU.
▼ Don't use cloudy solution. If crystals form, redissolve by warming and shaking vigorously. Allow solution to cool to body temperature before administration.
▼ May give drug by direct injection without dilution or as a continuous infusion. IV administration rates vary by protocol. Refer to specific reference for protocol.
▼ For infusion, dilute drug with D₅W, sterile water for injection, or NSS for injection.
▼ For continuous infusion, use plastic IV containers. Solution is more stable in plastic than in glass bottles.
▼ For IV infusion regimens, administer through CVAD using an infusion pump.
⚠ Alert: Serious dosing errors involving continuous ambulatory infusion pumps have occurred. Carefully select the device and double-check flow rate. Drug should be prescribed in single daily doses (not course doses) and include instructions to infuse over a specific period. Utilize independent double-checks during administration.
▼ Don't refrigerate vials.
▼ Protect drug from sunlight.
▼ Can store diluted solutions and syringes (nondiluted) at room temperature for up to 4 hours.
▼ **Incompatibilities:** Don't administer in same IV line concomitantly with other medicinal products.

Topical
● Apply topical form cautiously near eyes, nose, and mouth.
● Topical form is not for vaginal use.
● Apply 10 minutes after washing, rinsing, and drying affected area.
● Avoid occlusive dressings with topical form because they increase risk of inflammatory reactions in adjacent normal skin.
● Apply topical form with nonmetal applicator or suitable gloves. Wash hands immediately after handling topical form.
● Store at room temperature.

ACTION
Nucleoside metabolic inhibitor that interferes with DNA and RNA synthesis, which affects rapidly growing cells and may lead to cell death.

Route	Onset	Peak	Duration
IV, topical	Unknown	Unknown	Unknown

Half-life: 8 to 20 minutes (IV).

ADVERSE REACTIONS

CNS: malaise, acute cerebellar syndrome, headache, disorientation, confusion, ataxia. **CV:** *cardiotoxicity.* **EENT:** visual changes, nystagmus, lacrimal duct stenosis, photophobia, sinusitis, eye irritation. **GI:** stomatitis, GI ulcer, nausea, vomiting, diarrhea, anorexia, *GI bleeding.* **Hematologic:** *leukopenia, thrombocytopenia, agranulocytosis,* anemia. **Musculoskeletal:** Muscle soreness. **Skin:** application site reaction (erythema, crusting, scarring, scaling, pruritus, erythematous contact dermatitis, pain, burning, soreness, purulent drainage, swelling, dryness, erosion), dermatitis, rash, desquamative rash of hands and feet, hand-foot syndrome, photosensitivity reactions, reversible alopecia, nail changes, pigmented palmar creases. **Other:** hypersensitivity reactions, cold symptoms.

INTERACTIONS

Drug-drug. *Brivudine:* May enhance adverse effects of fluorouracil. Avoid use with both topical and IV 5-FU formulations.
Leucovorin calcium: May increase cytotoxicity and toxicity of 5-FU. Monitor patient closely.
Live-virus vaccines: May increase risk of vaccine-induced adverse reactions. Use together isn't recommended.
Warfarin: May prolong PT and increase INR. Closely monitor PT and INR; adjust warfarin dosage accordingly.
Drug-lifestyle. *Sun exposure:* May cause photosensitivity reactions. Advise patient to avoid excessive sunlight exposure.

EFFECTS ON LAB TEST RESULTS

• May increase ammonia, ALP, AST, ALT, bilirubin, and LDH levels.
• May decrease Hb level and granulocyte, platelet, RBC, and WBC counts.

CONTRAINDICATIONS & CAUTIONS

• Contraindicated in patients hypersensitive to drug. Some topical dosage forms contain peanut oil.
⚕ Patients with dihydropyrimidine dehydrogenase gene mutations have increased risk of acute early-onset of toxicity and severe,

life-threatening, or fatal adverse reactions. Drug may need to be withheld or permanently discontinued based on clinical assessment of toxicities.
• Use cautiously in patients who have received high-dose pelvic radiation or alkylating drugs and in those with impaired liver or kidney function or widespread neoplastic infiltration of bone marrow.
• Safety and effectiveness in children haven't been established.
Dialyzable drug: Yes.
⚠ **Overdose S&S:** Nausea, vomiting, diarrhea, GI ulceration and bleeding, bone marrow depression (thrombocytopenia, leukopenia, agranulocytosis).

PREGNANCY-LACTATION-REPRODUCTION

• Studies during pregnancy are inadequate. Drug may cause fetal harm. Use during pregnancy only if potential benefit justifies fetal risk. Inform patient about potential fetal hazard.
• Topical formulations are contraindicated in patients who are or may become pregnant during therapy.
• Patients of childbearing potential and males with partners of childbearing potential should use effective contraception during therapy and for 3 months after final dose.
• It isn't known if drug appears in human milk. Patient should discontinue breastfeeding or discontinue drug, considering importance of drug to patient.

NURSING CONSIDERATIONS

🕭 *Alert:* IV drug should be administered under the supervision of a physician experienced in cancer chemotherapy. Patient should be hospitalized, at least during the initial course of IV therapy.
• Ingestion and systemic absorption of topical form may cause leukopenia, thrombocytopenia, stomatitis, diarrhea, or GI ulceration, bleeding, and hemorrhage. Application to large ulcerated areas may cause systemic toxicity.
• Monitor patient. Withhold IV drug and notify prescriber for signs and symptoms of cardiotoxicity (angina, MI, ischemia, arrhythmia, HF), neurologic toxicity (confusion, disorientation, ataxia, visual disturbances), GI toxicities (severe diarrhea, mucositis, stomatitis, esophagopharyngitis with mucosal sloughing or ulceration), hyperammonemic

encephalopathy (altered mental status, confusion, disorientation, coma, ataxia, with elevated serum ammonia level), hand-foot syndrome (tingling pain, edema, erythema with tenderness, skin desquamation), and severe hematologic toxicity (neutropenia, thrombocytopenia, anemia).

• Encourage diligent oral hygiene to prevent superinfection of denuded mucosa.

• Monitor CBC with differential and platelet count before each treatment cycle and as clinically indicated. Myelosuppression can be fatal.

• Watch for ecchymoses, petechiae, easy bruising, and anemia, especially in patients taking warfarin.

• To prevent bleeding, avoid IM injections when platelet count is below 50,000/mm³.

• Anticipate blood transfusions because of cumulative anemia.

• The WBC count nadir occurs 9 to 14 days after first dose; the platelet count nadir occurs in 7 to 14 days.

• Monitor fluid intake and output, LFT values, and kidney function test results.

🚫 *Alert:* Signs and symptoms of toxicity may be delayed for 1 to 3 weeks.

• Long-term use may cause erythematous, desquamative rash of hands and feet (hand-foot syndrome). Syndrome gradually resolves over 5 to 7 days after therapy interruption.

• Dermatologic adverse effects are reversible when drug is stopped.

• For overdose, give uridine triacetate within 96 hours of 5-FU infusion.

⚕ *Alert:* Drug may be ordered as "5-fluorouracil" or "5-FU." The numeral "5" is part of the drug name and shouldn't be confused with dosage units.

• *Look alike–sound alike:* Don't confuse fluorouracil with floxuridine, fludarabine, or flucytosine.

PATIENT TEACHING

• Advise patient to immediately report all adverse reactions, especially infection, bleeding, chest pain, palpitations, swelling, dyspnea, severe nausea, vomiting, diarrhea, dark urine, yellowing of skin or eyes, malaise, confusion, visual or gait disturbances, or redness of hands or feet.

• Instruct patient to take temperature daily and to immediately report signs or symptoms of infection.

• Warn patient that hair loss may occur but usually is reversible after drug is stopped.

• Caution patient to avoid prolonged exposure to sunlight and UV light when topical form is used.

• Tell patient to use highly protective sunblock to avoid inflammatory skin irritation.

• Warn patient that topically treated area may be unsightly during therapy and for several weeks afterward. Complete healing may take 1 to 2 months.

• Advise patient of childbearing potential and male patient with partner of childbearing potential to use effective contraception during therapy and for 3 months after final dose.

• Counsel patient not to breastfeed.

FLUoxetine hydrochloride
floo-OX-e-teen

Prozac

Therapeutic class: Antidepressants
Pharmacologic class: SSRIs

AVAILABLE FORMS
Capsules (delayed-release) **OTC**: 90 mg
Capsules: 10 mg, 20 mg, 40 mg
Oral solution: 20 mg/5 mL
Tablets: 10 mg, 20 mg, 60 mg

INDICATIONS & DOSAGES
Adjust-a-dose (for all indications): For patients with kidney or liver impairment and those taking several drugs at the same time, reduce dose or increase dosing interval.

➤ **MDD, OCD**
Adults: Initially, 20-mg immediate release formulations. May increase dosage after several weeks based on patient response. Doses over 20 mg/day can be given once daily in the morning or divided into b.i.d. dosing (morning and noon). OCD target dose is 20 to 60 mg/day. Maximum daily dose, 80 mg.
Children ages 8 to 18 (MDD): 10 or 20 mg PO once daily for 1 week; then increase to 20 mg daily. Due to higher plasma levels in lower weight children, the starting and target dose in this group may be 10 mg/day. Consider a dosage increase to 20 mg/day after several weeks if clinical improvement is insufficient.
Children ages 7 to 17 (OCD): 10 mg PO daily. After 2 weeks, increase to 20 mg daily. Dosage range is 20 to 60 mg daily. In lower weight children, initially 10 mg/day. Consider additional dosage increases after several more

---

weeks if clinical improvement is insufficient. Dosage range of 20 to 30 mg/day is recommended.

➤ **Maintenance therapy for depression in patients who are stabilized (not for newly diagnosed depression)**

Adults: 90-mg delayed-release capsules PO once weekly. Start once-weekly doses 7 days after last daily dose of fluoxetine 20 mg.

➤ **Bulimia nervosa**

Adults: 60 mg PO daily in the morning. For some patients, it may be advisable to titrate up to this target dose over several days.

➤ **Short-term treatment of panic disorder with or without agoraphobia**

Adults: 10 mg PO once daily for 1 week; then increase dose as needed to 20 mg daily. Maximum daily dose, 60 mg.

➤ **Depressive episodes associated with bipolar I disorder (with olanzapine)**

Adults: 20 mg PO with 5 mg PO olanzapine once daily in the evening. Dosage adjustments can be made based on efficacy and tolerability within ranges of fluoxetine 20 to 50 mg and olanzapine 5 to 12.5 mg.

Children ages 10 to 17: Initially, 20 mg PO with 2.5 mg olanzapine PO once daily in evening. Dosage adjustments can be made based on efficacy and tolerability. Safety of doses above 50 mg fluoxetine with 12 mg olanzapine hasn't been evaluated in children.

➤ **Treatment-resistant depression**

Adults: 20 mg PO with 5 mg PO olanzapine once daily in the evening. Dosage adjustments can be made based on efficacy and tolerability within ranges of fluoxetine 20 to 50 mg and olanzapine 5 to 20 mg.

ADMINISTRATION

PO

• Give drug without regard to food.
• Avoid giving drug in the afternoon, whenever possible, because doing so commonly causes nervousness and insomnia.
• Have patient swallow delayed-release capsules whole; don't crush or open capsules.

ACTION

Thought to be linked to drug's inhibition of CNS neuronal uptake of serotonin.

Route	Onset	Peak	Duration
PO	Unknown	6–8 hr	Unknown

Half-life: Acute administration, 1 to 3 days; long-term administration, 4 to 6 days.

ADVERSE REACTIONS

CNS: nervousness, somnolence, anxiety, insomnia, headache, drowsiness, tremor, dizziness, asthenia, abnormal thinking, abnormal dreams, sleep disorder, amnesia, personality disorder, fatigue, fever, emotional lability, dysgeusia, yawning. **CV:** chest pain, HTN, palpitations, vasodilation, hot flashes, *prolonged QT interval.* **EENT:** epistaxis, dry mouth, pharyngitis, sinusitis, abnormal vision. **GI:** nausea, diarrhea, anorexia, dyspepsia, constipation, abdominal pain, vomiting, flatulence, increased appetite. **GU:** sexual dysfunction, decreased libido, micturition disorder, urinary frequency. **Metabolic:** weight loss, increased thirst, hyponatremia. **Musculoskeletal:** muscle pain, hyperkinetic muscle activity. **Skin:** rash, pruritus, diaphoresis. **Other:** flulike syndrome, chills, hypersensitivity reaction.

INTERACTIONS

Drug-drug. *Antiplatelet agents, aspirin, NSAIDs:* May increase risk of bleeding. Use together cautiously.

Benzodiazepines, lithium, TCAs: May increase levels of these drugs, resulting in additional CNS effects. Monitor patient closely.

Beta blockers, carbamazepine, flecainide, vinblastine: May increase levels of these drugs. Monitor drug levels and monitor patient for adverse reactions.

Cyproheptadine: May reverse or decrease fluoxetine effect. Monitor patient closely.

Dextromethorphan: May cause unusual side effects, such as visual hallucinations. Advise use of cough suppressant that doesn't contain dextromethorphan while taking fluoxetine.

Drugs that prolong QT interval (chlorpromazine, droperidol, erythromycin, moxifloxacin, quinidine procainamide, amiodarone, sotalol, methadone, tacrolimus): May increase risk of ventricular arrhythmias, including torsades de pointes. Avoid use together.

Highly protein-bound drugs: May increase level of fluoxetine and other highly protein-bound drugs. Monitor patient closely.

Insulin, oral antidiabetics: May alter glucose level and antidiabetic requirements. Adjust dosage.

Linezolid, methylene blue: May cause serotonin syndrome. Use extreme caution and monitor closely.

F

MAO inhibitors (phenelzine, selegiline, tranylcypromine): May cause serotonin syndrome and signs and symptoms resembling NMS. Use of an MAO inhibitor intended to treat psychiatric disorders with fluoxetine or within 5 weeks of stopping fluoxetine is contraindicated. Use of fluoxetine within 14 days of stopping an MAO inhibitor intended to treat psychiatric disorders is contraindicated.

Phenytoin: May increase phenytoin level and risk of toxicity. Monitor phenytoin level and adjust dosage.

Pimozide, thioridazine: May increase levels of these drugs, increasing risk of serious ventricular arrhythmias and sudden death. Don't use together and don't use thioridazine for at least 5 weeks after stopping fluoxetine.

Serotonergic drugs (amphetamines, antiemetics, antipsychotics, buspirone, dextromethorphan, dihydroergotamine, lithium salts, meperidine, opioids, other SSRIs or SSNRIs [duloxetine, venlafaxine], TCAs, tramadol, trazodone, triptans): May increase risk of serotonin syndrome. Avoid combinations of drugs that increase availability of serotonin in the CNS. Monitor patient closely if used together.

Tamoxifen: May decrease tamoxifen plasma level, leading to breast cancer recurrence. Monitor patient carefully.

Warfarin: May increase risk of bleeding. Monitor PT and INR.

Drug-herb. *Kava hyperammonemia, St. John's wort, tryptophan, valerian:* May increase sedative and hypnotic effects. May cause serotonin syndrome. Discourage use together.

Drug-lifestyle. *Alcohol use:* May increase CNS depression. Discourage use together.

EFFECTS ON LAB TEST RESULTS
• May decrease sodium level.

CONTRAINDICATIONS & CAUTIONS
• Contraindicated in patients hypersensitive to drug.

Boxed Warning Drug may increase risk of suicidality in children, adolescents, and young adults with MDD or other psychiatric disorders. ■

Boxed Warning Fluoxetine is approved for use in children with MDD and OCD. Fluoxetine isn't approved for use in children younger than age 7. ■

⚕ *Alert:* Concomitant use with linezolid or methylene blue can cause serotonin syndrome (fever, mental status changes, muscle twitching, diaphoresis, shivering, shaking, diarrhea, loss of coordination). Use drug with linezolid or methylene blue only for life-threatening or urgent conditions when the potential benefits outweigh the risks of toxicity.

• Use cautiously in patients at high risk for suicide and in those with history of diabetes, glaucoma, seizures, mania, or liver, kidney, or CV disease.

Dialyzable drug: No.

⚠ *Overdose S&S:* Nausea, seizures, somnolence, tachycardia, HTN, vomiting, coma, delirium, ECG abnormalities, hypotension, mania, NMS-like reactions, fever, stupor, syncope.

PREGNANCY-LACTATION-REPRODUCTION
• Use cautiously during pregnancy and only if benefit justifies fetal risk.

• Enroll patients who are pregnant in the National Pregnancy Registry for Antidepressants (1-866-961-2388 or https://womensmentalhealth.org/research/pregnancyregistry/antidepressants).

• Drug appears in human milk. Use during breastfeeding isn't recommended. Monitor infants exposed to drug for agitation, irritability, poor feeding, and poor weight gain.

NURSING CONSIDERATIONS
Boxed Warning Monitor all patients for worsening or emerging suicidality. ■

• Monitor mental status for depression, suicidality (especially at beginning of therapy and with dosage changes), anxiety, social functioning, mania, and panic attacks.

⚕ *Alert:* If linezolid or methylene blue must be given, fluoxetine must be stopped and patient monitored for serotonin toxicity for 5 weeks or until 24 hours after final dose of linezolid or methylene blue, whichever comes first. Treatment with fluoxetine may resume 24 hours after final dose of linezolid or methylene blue.

• Use antihistamines or topical corticosteroids to treat rashes or pruritus.

• Watch for weight change during therapy, particularly in patients who are underweight or bulimic.

• Drug has a long half-life; monitor patient for adverse effects for up to 2 weeks after drug is stopped.

Reactions in bold italics are *life-threatening*.

• Monitor patient for serotonin syndrome, particularly when drug is used in combination with other serotonergic agents.

◑ Alert: Combining triptans with an SSRI or SSNRI may cause serotonin syndrome or NMS-like reactions. Serotonin syndrome is more likely to occur when starting or increasing dose of triptan, SSRI, or SSNRI.

• Monitor blood glucose level (in patients with diabetes) and liver and kidney function (at baseline and as clinically indicated).

• Obtain ECG and monitor periodically in patients with risk factors for QT-interval prolongation and ventricular arrhythmias.

• Observe patient for signs or symptoms of abnormal bleeding, akathisia, or sleep disturbances.

• When discontinuing drug, taper dosage over 2 weeks to 1 month to avoid withdrawal syndrome.

• Evaluate patient for sexual dysfunction before and periodically during treatment.

• **Look alike–sound alike:** Don't confuse fluoxetine with fluvoxamine or fluvastatin. Don't confuse Prozac with Proscar or Prilosec.

PATIENT TEACHING

Boxed Warning Advise family and caregivers to carefully observe patient for worsening suicidality. ■

◑ Alert: Teach patient to recognize and immediately report symptoms of serotonin toxicity (fever, mental status changes, muscle twitching, diaphoresis, shivering, shaking, diarrhea, loss of coordination).

• Tell patient to avoid taking drug in the afternoon whenever possible because doing so commonly causes nervousness and insomnia.

• Drug may cause dizziness or drowsiness. Warn patient to avoid driving and other hazardous activities that require alertness and good psychomotor coordination until effects of drug are known.

• Instruct patient to report adverse effects and to not stop drug suddenly without first discussing with prescriber due to risk of discontinuation reactions.

• Tell patient to consult prescriber before taking other prescription or OTC drugs.

• Advise patient that full therapeutic effect may not occur for 4 weeks or longer.

• Instruct patient to report pregnancy or plans to become pregnant or to breastfeed.

fluticasone furoate
floo-TIK-a-sone

Arnuity Ellipta, Flonase Sensimist Allergy Relief ◇

fluticasone propionate
ArmonAir Digihaler, Flonase Allergy Relief ◇, Flovent Diskus, Flovent HFA, Xhance

Therapeutic class: Corticosteroids
Pharmacologic class: Corticosteroids

AVAILABLE FORMS

Nasal spray (furoate): 27.5 mcg/spray
Nasal spray (propionate): 50 mcg/metered spray, 93 mcg/metered spray
Oral inhalation aerosol: 44 mcg, 110 mcg, 220 mcg
Oral inhalation powder: 50 mcg, 100 mcg, 200 mcg, 250 mcg
Oral inhalation powder (ArmonAir): 55 mcg, 113 mcg, 232 mcg

INDICATIONS & DOSAGES

➤ **Preventive in maintenance of chronic asthma in patients requiring an oral corticosteroid**

Adults and children ages 12 and older not on an inhaled corticosteroid (ICS): For Flovent Diskus, initially, inhaled dose of 100 mcg b.i.d. approximately 12 hours apart. For patients who don't respond adequately to starting dosage after 2 weeks of therapy, may increase dosage to maximum of 1,000 mcg b.i.d.

For Flovent HFA, initially, inhaled dose of 88 mcg b.i.d. approximately 12 hours apart. For patients who don't respond adequately to starting dosage after 2 weeks of therapy, may increase dosage to maximum of 880 mcg b.i.d.

For Arnuity Ellipta, base starting dosage on patient's asthma severity. Recommended starting dose is 100 mcg given as 1 inhalation at the same time every day. May increase to 200 mcg given as 1 inhalation after 2 weeks to provide additional asthma control.

For ArmonAir Digihaler, 55 mcg by oral inhalation b.i.d. Patients with greater asthma severity may use 113 mcg or 232 mcg by oral inhalation b.i.d. Maximum dose, 232 mcg b.i.d.

Children ages 5 to 11 not on an ICS: Recommended starting dosage is 50 mcg Arnuity Ellipta given as 1 inhalation daily.

Children ages 4 to 11 not on an ICS: Recommended starting dosage is 50 mcg b.i.d. for Flovent Diskus or 88 mcg inhaled b.i.d. for Flovent HFA, approximately 12 hours apart. For patients who don't respond adequately to starting dosage after 2 weeks of therapy, may increase Flovent Diskus dosage to maximum of 100 mcg b.i.d.

Adults and children ages 12 and older previously taking an ICS: Base dosage on strength of previous ICS and disease severity, including consideration of patient's current control of asthma symptoms and risk of future exacerbation, to maximum of 1,000 mcg b.i.d. for Flovent Diskus; maximum of 880 mcg b.i.d. for Flovent HFA; maximum of 200 mcg daily for Arnuity Ellipta; or maximum of 232 mcg b.i.d. for ArmonAir Digihaler.

Children ages 4 to 11 previously taking an ICS: Base dosage on strength of previous ICS and disease severity, including consideration of patient's current control of asthma symptoms and risk of future exacerbation, to maximum of 100 mcg b.i.d. for Flovent Diskus.

Adjust-a-dose: For patients who don't respond adequately to starting dose after 2 weeks of therapy, an increased dose may improve control.

➤ **Nasal symptoms of seasonal and perennial allergic and nonallergic rhinitis**
Adults: Initially, 2 sprays (100 mcg) fluticasone propionate in each nostril daily or 1 spray b.i.d. Once symptoms are controlled, decrease to 1 spray in each nostril daily.

Adolescents and children ages 4 and older: Initially, 1 spray (50 mcg) fluticasone propionate in each nostril daily. If not responding, increase to 2 sprays in each nostril daily. Once symptoms are controlled, decrease to 1 spray in each nostril daily. Maximum dose is 2 sprays in each nostril daily.

Adults and children ages 12 and older: 110 mcg fluticasone furoate (OTC) once daily administered as 2 sprays (27.5 mcg/spray) in each nostril for 1 week. For week 2 through 6 months, 1 or 2 sprays in each nostril once daily, as needed. Reevaluate treatment after 6 months of daily use.

Children ages 2 to 11: 55 mcg fluticasone furoate (OTC) once daily administered as 1 spray (27.5 mcg/spray) in each nostril. Use for shortest amount of time necessary to achieve symptom relief. Reevaluate treatment if child needs to use spray for longer than 2 months a year.

➤ **Nasal polyps (Xhance)**
Adults: 1 spray (93 mcg/spray) in each nostril b.i.d. May increase to 2 sprays in each nostril b.i.d. (maximum dose).

ADMINISTRATION
Inhalational
• For best results, store aerosol canister at room temperature.
• Prime and shake well before each use.
• Instruct patient to rinse mouth after inhalation.
• Refer to specific manufacturer's guideline for discard date and storage.

Intranasal
• Prime and shake well before use.

ACTION
Anti-inflammatory and vasoconstrictor that may decrease inflammation by inhibiting mast cells, macrophages, and mediators such as leukotrienes.

Route	Onset	Peak	Duration
Inhalation (nasal)	12 hr	Several days	1–2 wk
Inhalation (oral)	24 hr	0.5-1 hr	1–2 wk

Half-life: 7.8 to 24 hours, depending on formulation.

ADVERSE REACTIONS
CNS: headache, dizziness, fever, migraine, nervousness, fatigue, malaise, pain, voice disorder. **CV:** HTN. **EENT:** cataracts, conjunctivitis, dry eye, eye irritation, nasal burning or irritation, nasal discharge, blood in nasal mucus, epistaxis, nasal congestion, rhinitis, oral candidiasis, sinusitis, sinus infection, pharyngitis, hoarseness, laryngitis, mouth irritation, toothache. **GI:** abdominal discomfort, abdominal pain, diarrhea, nausea, viral gastroenteritis, vomiting. **GU:** UTI. **Hematologic:** eosinophilia. **Metabolic:** weight gain. **Musculoskeletal:** arthralgia, symptoms of neck sprain or strain, joint pain, muscular soreness or spasm, muscle injury, osteoporosis. **Respiratory:** URI, *bronchospasm,* asthma symptoms, bronchitis, chest congestion, cough, dyspnea. **Skin:** dermatitis, urticaria, rash, pruritus. **Other:** *angioedema,* flulike symptoms, viral infections.

Reactions in bold italics are *life-threatening*.

INTERACTIONS

Drug-drug. *Cobicistat:* May increase serum concentration of oral inhalation drug. Avoid use together.

Ketoconazole, other CYP3A4 inhibitors: May increase mean fluticasone level and systemic corticosteroid adverse effects. Avoid use together.

Ritonavir: May cause systemic corticosteroid effects, such as Cushing syndrome and adrenal suppression. Avoid use together.

EFFECTS ON LAB TEST RESULTS

● May cause abnormal response to the 6-hour cosyntropin stimulation test in patients taking high fluticasone doses.

CONTRAINDICATIONS & CAUTIONS

● Contraindicated in patients hypersensitive to components in these preparations, including milk proteins in oral inhalers. Immediate hypersensitivity reactions, including anaphylaxis, can occur.

● Contraindicated as primary treatment of status asthmaticus or other acute, intense episodes of asthma.

● Use cautiously in patients at risk for decreased bone mineralization.

● Drug can increase risk of infections, vasculitis, Kaposi sarcoma, psychiatric disturbances, HTN, fluid retention, GI perforation, hyperglycemia, and IOP.

● Avoid intranasal use in patients with recent nasal septal ulcers, nasal surgery, or nasal trauma until healing has occurred.

Dialyzable drug: Unknown.

⚠ **Overdose S&S:** Hypercorticism.

PREGNANCY-LACTATION-REPRODUCTION

● Use during pregnancy only if potential benefit justifies fetal risk.

● Use cautiously during breastfeeding.

NURSING CONSIDERATIONS

● Because of risk of systemic absorption of ICSs, observe patient carefully for evidence of systemic corticosteroid effects.

🔵 **Alert:** Monitor patient, especially postoperatively, during periods of stress or severe asthma attack for evidence of inadequate adrenal response.

🔵 **Alert:** During withdrawal from oral corticosteroids, some patients may experience signs and symptoms of systemically active corticosteroid withdrawal (joint or muscle pain, lassitude, depression), despite maintenance or even improvement of respiratory function. Deaths due to adrenal insufficiency have occurred with transfer from active corticosteroids to fluticasone propionate inhaler.

● For patients starting therapy who are currently receiving oral corticosteroid therapy, reduce dose of prednisone to no more than 2.5 mg/day on a weekly basis, beginning after at least 1 week of therapy with fluticasone.

🔵 **Alert:** As with other inhaled asthma drugs, bronchospasm may occur, with an immediate increase in wheezing after a dose. If bronchospasm occurs after a dose of inhalation aerosol, immediately treat with a fast-acting inhaled bronchodilator.

● Drug may increase risk of glaucoma and cataracts. Monitor patient.

● ICSs can reduce growth trajectory in children. Monitor growth.

● If a dosage regimen fails to provide adequate asthma control, reevaluate the therapeutic regimen and consider additional therapeutic options, such as replacing current strength with a higher strength, initiating an ICS and long-acting beta$_2$-agonist combination product, or initiating oral corticosteroids.

● After asthma stability has been achieved, titrate to lowest effective dosage to reduce possibility of adverse effects.

PATIENT TEACHING

● Teach about proper drug administration, handling, and storage.

● Advise patient to report all adverse reactions.

● Tell patient that inhalation drug isn't indicated for relief of acute bronchospasm.

● Instruct patient to use drug at regular intervals, as directed.

● Advise patient that maximum inhalation benefit may not occur for 1 to 2 weeks or longer after starting treatment.

● Instruct patient to contact prescriber if nasal spray doesn't improve condition after 4 days of treatment.

● Caution patient to immediately contact prescriber if asthma episodes unresponsive to bronchodilators occur during treatment with fluticasone. During such episodes, patient may need therapy with oral corticosteroids.

● Warn patient to avoid exposure to chickenpox or measles and, if exposed, to immediately consult prescriber.

● Tell patient to carry or wear medical identification indicating that patient may need supplementary corticosteroids during stress or a severe asthma attack.

🔹 *Alert:* During periods of stress or a severe asthma attack, instruct patient who has been withdrawn from systemic corticosteroids to immediately resume prescribed oral corticosteroids and to contact prescriber for further instruction.

• Advise patient to rinse mouth without swallowing after oral inhalation to reduce risk of oropharyngeal candidiasis.

fluticasone furoate–vilanterol trifenatate
floo-TIK-a-sone/vye-LAN-ter-ol

Breo Ellipta

Therapeutic class: Corticosteroids–bronchodilators
Pharmacologic class: Corticosteroids–beta₂-adrenergic agonists

AVAILABLE FORMS
Powder for inhalation: Inhaler containing two double-foil blister strips of powder formulation: One strip contains fluticasone furoate 50 mcg/blister, 100 mcg/blister, or 200 mcg/blister; the other contains vilanterol 25 mcg/blister

INDICATIONS & DOSAGES
➤ **Asthma**
Adults: 1 inhalation of 100 mcg fluticasone furoate–25 mcg vilanterol trifenatate or 200 mcg fluticasone furoate–25 mcg vilanterol trifenatate once daily.
Adolescents ages 12 to 17: 1 inhalation of 100 mcg fluticasone furoate–25 mcg vilanterol trifenatate once daily.
Children ages 5 to 11: 1 inhalation of 50 mcg fluticasone furoate–25 mcg vilanterol trifenatate once daily.
➤ **Maintenance treatment of COPD**
Adults: 1 inhalation of 100 mcg fluticasone furoate–25 mcg vilanterol trifenatate once daily.

ADMINISTRATION
Inhalational
• Give at the same time every day and not more than one time every 24 hours.
• Have patient exhale fully before taking one long, steady, deep breath through the

mouthpiece (patient shouldn't breathe through the nose), hold breath for 3 to 4 seconds, and exhale slowly and gently.
• After use, have patient rinse mouth with water without swallowing to help reduce the risk of oropharyngeal candidiasis.
• Store at room temperature between 68° and 77° F (20° and 25° C) in a dry place away from heat and sunlight.
• Keep drug stored inside the unopened moisture-protective foil tray; remove from tray immediately before initial use.
• Discard drug 6 weeks after opening foil tray or when the counter reads "0" (after all blisters have been used).
• Note that inhaler isn't reusable.
• Don't attempt to take inhaler apart.

ACTION
Fluticasone is an anti-inflammatory and vasoconstrictor that may decrease inflammation by inhibiting mast cells, macrophages, and mediators such as leukotrienes. Vilanterol trifenatate relaxes bronchial smooth muscle and inhibits inflammatory mediators, especially mast cells.

Route	Onset	Peak	Duration
Inhalation (fluticasone)	Unknown	30–60 min	Unknown
Inhalation (vilanterol)	Unknown	10 min	Unknown

Half-life: Fluticasone, 24 hours; vilanterol, 21 hours.

ADVERSE REACTIONS
CNS: headache, fever. **CV:** HTN, peripheral edema, extrasystoles. **EENT:** nasopharyngitis, oropharyngeal candidiasis, oropharyngeal pain, pharyngitis, rhinitis, sinusitis, dysphonia. **GI:** diarrhea, upper abdominal pain. **Musculoskeletal:** back pain, arthralgia. **Respiratory:** URI, pneumonia, bronchitis, cough. **Other:** flulike symptoms.

INTERACTIONS
Drug-drug. *CYP3A4 inhibitors (clarithromycin, conivaptan, itraconazole, ketoconazole, lopinavir, nefazodone, nelfinavir, ritonavir, saquinavir, voriconazole):* May increase systemic effects of corticosteroids, and increased CV adverse effects may occur. Use together cautiously.
Loop or thiazide diuretics (furosemide, hydrochlorothiazide, torsemide): May increase risk of hypokalemia or ECG changes. Monitor patient closely with concurrent use.

Reactions in bold italics are ***life-threatening***.

MAO inhibitors, TCAs, other drugs known to prolong QTc interval: May increase adrenergic effects or risk of ventricular arrhythmias. Don't use together.

Nonselective beta blockers (carvedilol, propranolol, sotalol): May increase risk of bronchospasm. Use cardioselective agents only if absolutely needed.

Other LABAs (arformoterol tartrate, formoterol fumarate, indacaterol, salmeterol): May increase risk of overdose. Don't use together.

Theophylline: May increase risk of adverse effects of theophylline and hypokalemic effect of vilanterol. Monitor therapy.

EFFECTS ON LAB TEST RESULTS
- May increase glucose level.
- May decrease potassium level.

CONTRAINDICATIONS & CAUTIONS
- Contraindicated in patients with severe hypersensitivity to milk proteins and in those who have demonstrated hypersensitivity to fluticasone furoate, vilanterol, or their components.
- ⚠ *Alert:* Contraindicated as primary treatment of status asthmaticus or other acute episodes of COPD or asthma when other intensive measures are required.
- Use of LABAs as monotherapy (without inhaled corticosteroid [ICS]) for asthma is associated with an increased risk of asthma-related death and asthma-related hospitalization in children and adolescents. Use in fixed-dose combination with ICS eliminates a significant increase in the risk compared with ICS alone.
- ⚠ *Alert:* Don't exceed recommended dosage; serious adverse events, including fatalities, have been associated with excessive use of inhaled sympathomimetics.
- Use cautiously in patients with existing TB; fungal, bacterial, viral, or parasitic infections; or ocular herpes simplex. Drug may suppress the immune system and infection may worsen.
- Use cautiously in patients with thyrotoxicosis, diabetes, ketoacidosis, or CV disorders (coronary insufficiency, arrhythmias, HTN).
- Use cautiously in patients with increased IOP, cataracts, or glaucoma. Increased IOP, glaucoma, and cataracts have occurred with prolonged use.

- Use cautiously in patients with seizure disorders; beta agonists may cause CNS stimulation.
- Safety and effectiveness in children haven't been established.
- *Dialyzable drug:* Unknown.

PREGNANCY-LACTATION-REPRODUCTION
- Use cautiously during pregnancy and breastfeeding.
- Avoid use during labor; drug may interfere with uterine contractility.

NURSING CONSIDERATIONS
- If not already prescribed, initiate an inhaled, short-acting beta$_2$ agonist in patient taking this drug.
- Patient who has been taking an oral or inhaled short-acting beta$_2$ agonist on a regular basis (q.i.d.) should discontinue regular use of this drugs and use it only for relief of acute respiratory symptoms.
- Determine if patient has an allergy or intolerance to lactose; anaphylactic reactions have occurred in patients with severe milk protein allergies.
- Monitor short-acting beta$_2$ agonist rescue use. Increased use signals disease deterioration.
- Slowly wean patient who requires oral corticosteroid from systemic corticosteroid use after switch to an inhaler. Reduce daily prednisone dosage by 2.5 mg on a weekly basis during therapy with inhaled drug.
- Patient may require supplemental corticosteroid during times of stress when weaning from systemic corticosteroid.
- Monitor lung function and watch for signs and symptoms of COPD and adrenal insufficiency (fatigue, lassitude, weakness, nausea, vomiting, hypotension).
- Discontinue drug slowly if hypercortisolism or adrenal suppression is suspected.
- Periodically monitor patient for candidal infections of the mouth.
- Monitor for pneumonia.
- If paradoxical bronchospasm occurs, discontinue drug and institute alternative therapy.
- Monitor patient for increased IOP and for development or worsening of glaucoma or cataracts.
- Monitor patient for hypokalemia and hyperglycemia.

• Serious or even fatal courses of chickenpox or measles can occur in patients who are susceptible.
• Monitor patient for CV effects (tachycardia, HTN, supraventricular tachycardia, extrasystoles).
• Monitor patient for reduced bone mineral density (BMD) initially and periodically with long-term use. Patients who use tobacco and those with prolonged immobilization, family history of osteoporosis, postmenopausal status, advanced age, poor nutrition, or long-term use of other drugs that can reduce BMD (anticonvulsants, oral corticosteroids) are at increased risk.
◑ Alert: Orally ICSs may slow growth rate when given to children and adolescents.

PATIENT TEACHING
• Teach patient to rinse mouth without swallowing after inhalation to help reduce the risk of candidal infections.
• Caution patient not to use drug for acute symptoms or asthma.
• Warn patient not to use drug with other LABAs.
• Instruct patient to immediately notify health care provider if adverse reactions occur, symptoms worsen, more inhalations than usual of rescue medication are needed, or lung function significantly decreases.
• Instruct patient not to discontinue drug without the guidance of health care provider.
• Advise patient to obtain regular eye exams.
• Caution patient to report pregnancy to health care provider as soon as possible.

fluticasone propionate (topical)
floo-TIK-a-sone

Therapeutic class: Corticosteroids
Pharmacologic class: Corticosteroids

AVAILABLE FORMS
Cream: 0.05%
Lotion: 0.05%
Ointment: 0.005%

INDICATIONS & DOSAGES
➤ **Inflammation and pruritus from dermatoses responsive to corticosteroids**
Adults: Apply thin film of cream or ointment to affected area b.i.d.; rub in gently and completely. Don't use for longer than 4 weeks.

Children ages 3 months and older: Apply thin film of cream to affected areas b.i.d. Rub in gently. Don't use for longer than 4 weeks.
➤ **Inflammation and pruritus from atopic dermatitis**
Adults and children ages 3 months and older: Apply thin film of cream to affected areas once daily or b.i.d. Or, apply thin film of lotion to affected areas once daily. Rub in gently. Don't use for longer than 4 weeks.

ADMINISTRATION
Topical
• Don't use drug with an occlusive dressing or in diaper area.
• Topical form is not for ophthalmic, oral, or intravaginal use.

ACTION
Diffuses across cell membranes to form complexes with cytoplasmic receptors. Shows anti-inflammatory, antipruritic, vasoconstrictive, and antiproliferative activity. Considered a medium-potency drug, according to vasoconstrictive properties.

Route	Onset	Peak	Duration
Topical	Rapid	Unknown	10 hr

Half-life: About 7.5 hours.

ADVERSE REACTIONS
CNS: finger numbness, light-headedness, headache, fever. **EENT:** ear infection. **GI:** diarrhea, vomiting. **GU:** glycosuria. **Metabolic:** hyperglycemia. **Respiratory:** cough, URI. **Skin:** urticaria, burning, eczema, hypertrichosis, pruritus, irritation, erythema, hives, dryness, rash, stinging, telangiectasia, application site herpes simplex or bacterial infection. **Other:** *HPA-axis suppression,* cold symptoms, flulike symptoms.

INTERACTIONS
Other corticosteroids: Use of more than one corticosteroid product may increase systemic absorption of topical form. Use together cautiously.

EFFECTS ON LAB TEST RESULTS
• May increase serum and urine glucose levels.

CONTRAINDICATIONS & CAUTIONS
• Contraindicated in patients hypersensitive to drug or its components.

Reactions in bold italics are *life-threatening*.

• Don't use as monotherapy in primary bacterial, viral, fungal, herpetic, or tubercular skin infections or for treatment of rosacea, perioral dermatitis, or acne.

• Cushing syndrome, hyperglycemia, and appearance of latent diabetes may occur with systemic absorption of topical corticosteroids.

• Safety and effectiveness of ointment haven't been established in children. Safety and effectiveness of lotion and cream haven't been established in children younger than age 3 months.

Dialyzable drug: Unknown.

⚠ *Overdose S&S:* Systemic effects (including reversible HPA axis suppression, Cushing syndrome, hyperglycemia, glycosuria).

PREGNANCY-LACTATION-REPRODUCTION
• Use during pregnancy only if potential benefit justifies fetal risk.
• Use cautiously during breastfeeding.

NURSING CONSIDERATIONS
• Drug should be discontinued when control is achieved. If no improvement occurs within 2 weeks, reassessment of diagnosis may be necessary.
• If adverse reactions occur, prescriber may order less-potent drug.
• Stop drug if local irritation or systemic infection, absorption, or hypersensitivity occurs.
• May cause suppression of HPA axis in patients receiving high doses, covering large treatment areas; with prolonged use; or with use of occlusive dressings, particularly in children.
• Absorption of corticosteroid is increased when drug is applied to inflamed or damaged skin, eyelids, or scrotal area; it's lowest when applied to intact normal skin, palms of hands, or soles of feet.
• May increase risk of posterior subcapsular cataracts and glaucoma. Monitor for ocular symptoms. Avoid contact with eyes.
• *Look alike–sound alike:* Don't confuse fluticasone with fluconazole, fluocinolone, or fluocinonide.

PATIENT TEACHING
• Teach patient or family member how to apply drug using gloves and sterile applicator. Review need to perform careful hand washing before and after application.

• Caution patient to avoid prolonged use and contact with eyes. Warn patient not to apply to face, in skin creases, or around eyes, genitals, underarms, or rectum.

• Instruct patient to notify prescriber of all adverse reactions, if condition persists or worsens, or if burning or irritation develops.

fluticasone propionate–salmeterol (inhalation)
floo-TIK-a-sone/sal-MEE-ter-ol

Advair Diskus, Advair HFA, AirDuo Digihaler, AirDuo RespiClick, Wixela Inhub

Therapeutic class: Antiasthmatics
Pharmacologic class: Corticosteroids–LABAs

AVAILABLE FORMS
Inhalation powder: 55 mcg fluticasone propionate and 14 mcg salmeterol, 100 mcg fluticasone propionate and 50 mcg salmeterol, 113 mcg fluticasone propionate and 14 mcg salmeterol, 232 mcg fluticasone propionate and 14 mcg salmeterol, 250 mcg fluticasone propionate and 50 mcg salmeterol, 500 mcg fluticasone propionate and 50 mcg salmeterol
Aerosol spray: 45 mcg fluticasone propionate and 21 mcg salmeterol, 115 mcg fluticasone propionate and 21 mcg salmeterol, 230 mcg fluticasone propionate and 21 mcg salmeterol

INDICATIONS & DOSAGES
➤ **Asthma in patients not adequately controlled on a long-term asthma control medication such as inhaled corticosteroid (ICS) or whose disease warrants initiation of treatment with both ICS and LABA**
Adults and children ages 12 and older: 1 inhalation of Advair Diskus, AirDuo Digihaler, AirDuo RespiClick, or Wixela Inhub b.i.d. about 12 hours apart, or 2 inhalations of Advair HFA b.i.d. about 12 hours apart. Starting doses are based on patient's disease severity, previous asthma therapy (including ICS dosage), current control of asthma symptoms, and risk of future exacerbation. May increase dose after 2 weeks in patients without adequate control. Maximum dose of Advair Diskus or Wixela Inhub is 1 inhalation of fluticasone 500 mcg and salmeterol 50 mcg b.i.d. Maximum dosage of AirDuo Digihaler

or RespiClick is 232 mcg/14 mcg b.i.d. Maximum dose of Advair HFA is 2 inhalations of fluticasone 230 mcg and salmeterol 21 mcg b.i.d.

Or, for patients without adequate control on a long-term asthma control medication (such as ICS) or whose disease warrants initiation of treatment with both ICS and LABA, base starting dose on patient's asthma severity; usual recommended starting dose for patients not on ICS is 55 mcg fluticasone/14 mcg salmeterol b.i.d. approximately 12 hours apart. For other patients, base starting dose on previous asthma drug therapy and disease severity.

For patients switching from another ICS, base initial Airduo dose strength on strength of previous ICS and disease severity.
Children ages 4 to 11 not controlled on ICS: 1 inhalation of Advair Diskus or Wixela Inhub fluticasone 100 mcg and salmeterol 50 mcg b.i.d. about 12 hours apart.
➤ **Maintenance therapy for airflow obstruction in patients with COPD; reduced exacerbations of COPD in patients with history of exacerbations**
Adults: 1 inhalation of Advair Diskus or Wixela Inhub 250/50 only b.i.d. about 12 hours apart.

ADMINISTRATION
Inhalational
• Prime Advair HFA before first use by releasing 4 test sprays into the air, away from the face, shaking well for 5 seconds before each spray. If inhaler hasn't been used for 4 weeks or has been dropped, prime inhaler again by shaking well before each spray and releasing 2 test sprays into the air.
• Discard Advair HFA canister when counter reads "000."
• AirDuo RespiClick and AirDuo Digihaler don't require priming. Never place inhaler in water; clean mouthpiece with dry cloth or tissue as needed.
• Don't use spacer with Advair Diskus, AirDuo Digihaler, AirDuo RespiClick, or Wixela.
• Discard Advair Diskus, AirDuo Digihaler, AirDuo RespiClick, and Wixela Inhub 1 month after removal from foil pouch or when counter reads "0," whichever comes first.
• After administration, have patient rinse mouth without swallowing.

ACTION
Fluticasone is a synthetic corticosteroid with potent anti-inflammatory activity. Salmeterol, an LABA, relaxes bronchial smooth muscle and inhibits release of mediators.

Route	Onset	Peak	Duration
Inhalation (fluticasone)	Unknown	1–2 hr	Unknown
Inhalation (salmeterol)	Unknown	5 min	Unknown

Half-life: Fluticasone, 8 hours; salmeterol, 5.5 to 12.6 hours.

ADVERSE REACTIONS
CNS: headache, dizziness, fatigue, malaise, migraine, sleep disorders, pain. **CV:** *arrhythmia, MI,* tachycardia, palpitations. **EENT:** eye redness, keratitis, congestion, nasal irritation, nasal dryness, rhinorrhea, rhinitis, sinusitis, pharyngitis, dental discomfort and pain, decreased salivation, hoarseness or dysphonia, oral candidiasis, oral discomfort and pain, oral erythema and rashes, oral ulcerations, EENT infections. **GI:** abdominal pain and discomfort, diarrhea, gastroenteritis, nausea, unusual taste, vomiting. **Metabolic:** weight gain. **Musculoskeletal:** arthralgia, bone and cartilage disorders, musculoskeletal pain, muscle stiffness, muscle cramps and spasms, rigidity, tightness. **Respiratory:** URI, bronchitis, cough, lower respiratory tract infection, pneumonia. **Skin:** dermatologic disorders (dermatosis, disorders of sweat and sebum), dermatitis, eczema, contact dermatitis, pruritus, infection, skin flakiness. **Other:** allergic reactions, fluid retention, viral or bacterial infections.

INTERACTIONS
Drug-drug. *Beta blockers:* Blocked pulmonary effect of salmeterol may produce severe bronchospasm in patients with asthma. Avoid use together. If necessary, use cardioselective beta blocker cautiously.
Loop diuretics, thiazide diuretics: Potassium-wasting diuretics may cause or worsen ECG changes or hypokalemia. Use together cautiously.
MAO inhibitors, TCAs: May potentiate action of salmeterol on vascular system. Separate doses by 2 weeks.
Strong inhibitors of CYP3A4 (ketoconazole, ritonavir, clarithromycin): May increase fluticasone level and CV adverse effects. Avoid use together.

Reactions in bold italics are *life-threatening*.

EFFECTS ON LAB TEST RESULTS
• May increase liver enzyme levels.

CONTRAINDICATIONS & CAUTIONS
• Contraindicated in patients hypersensitive to drug or its components, as primary treatment of status asthmaticus or other acute episodes of asthma or COPD that require intensive measures, and in those with severe hypersensitivity to milk proteins.
• Use of LABA as monotherapy (without ICS) for asthma is associated with increased risk of asthma-related death as well as asthma-related hospitalization in children and adolescents. Use as a fixed-dose combination with ICS doesn't significantly increase the risk of serious asthma-related events (hospitalizations, intubations, death) compared with ICS alone.
⚠ Alert: Patient shouldn't be switched from systemic corticosteroids to ICSs because of HPA axis suppression. Deaths from adrenal insufficiency have occurred in patients with asthma during and after transfer from systemic corticosteroids to less systemically available ICSs. Several months are required for recovery of HPA function after withdrawal of systemic corticosteroids.
• Use cautiously, if at all, in patients with active or quiescent respiratory TB infection; untreated systemic fungal, bacterial, viral, or parasitic infection; or ocular herpes simplex.
• Use cautiously in patients with CV disorders, seizure disorders, diabetes, or thyrotoxicosis; in patients unusually responsive to sympathomimetic amines; and in patients with liver impairment.
• Glaucoma, increased IOP, and cataracts have been reported in patients with asthma and COPD after long-term ICS use. Consider referral to an ophthalmologist in patients who develop ocular symptoms or use drug long term.
Dialyzable drug: Unknown.
⚠ Overdose S&S: Hypercorticism, angina, arrhythmias, dizziness, dry mouth, fatigue, headache, HTN, hypotension, insomnia, malaise, muscle cramps, nausea, nervousness, palpitations, seizures, tachycardia, prolonged QTc interval, hypokalemia, hyperglycemia, cardiac arrest, death.

PREGNANCY-LACTATION-REPRODUCTION
• Use during pregnancy only if potential benefit justifies fetal risk.

• Avoid use during labor because drug can interfere with uterine contractility.
• Use cautiously during breastfeeding.

NURSING CONSIDERATIONS
• Don't start therapy during rapidly deteriorating or potentially life-threatening asthma episodes. Serious acute respiratory events, including fatality, can occur.
• Don't use this drug to stop an asthma attack. Patients should carry an inhaled, short-acting beta$_2$ agonist (such as albuterol) for acute symptoms.
• Monitor patient for increased use of inhaled short-acting beta$_2$ agonist. Dose of fluticasone and salmeterol may need to be increased.
• Periodically reevaluate patient with COPD to assess for benefits and risks of therapy.
• Monitor patient for urticaria, angioedema, rash, bronchospasm, and other signs of hypersensitivity.
• If drug causes paradoxical bronchospasm, immediately treat with a short-acting inhaled bronchodilator (such as albuterol), and notify prescriber.
• Closely monitor children for growth suppression.

PATIENT TEACHING
• Instruct patient on proper use of the prescribed inhaler to provide effective treatment. Also teach about proper handling and storage. Remind patient to read and follow instructions for use.
• Tell patient to activate and use the dry-powder multidose inhaler in a level, horizontal position. Warn patient to avoid exhaling into it.
• Instruct patient to rinse mouth after inhalation to prevent oral candidiasis.
• Inform patient that improvement may occur within 30 minutes after dose, but full benefit may not occur for 1 week or more.
• Advise patient not to exceed recommended prescribed dose.
• Warn patient not to relieve acute symptoms with drug. Instruct patient to treat acute symptoms with inhaled short-acting beta$_2$ agonist.
• Instruct patient to report decreasing effects or use of increasing doses of inhaled short-acting beta$_2$ agonist.
• Tell patient to report all adverse reactions, especially palpitations, chest pain, rapid HR, tremor, and nervousness.
• Instruct patient to immediately call prescriber if exposed to chickenpox or measles.

fluvastatin sodium ⊠
flue-va-STA-tin

Lescol XL

Therapeutic class: Antilipemics
Pharmacologic class: HMG-CoA reductase inhibitors

AVAILABLE FORMS
Capsules ⓄⒹⒸ*:* 20 mg, 40 mg
Tablets (extended-release) ⓄⒹⒸ*:* 80 mg

INDICATIONS & DOSAGES
➤ **Adjunct to diet to reduce LDL-C, total cholesterol, triglycerides, and apolipoprotein B (apo B) and increase HDL-C in patients with primary hypercholesterolemia and mixed dyslipidemia (types IIa and IIb)**
Adults: Initially, 20 to 40 mg PO at bedtime, increasing if needed to maximum of 80 mg daily in divided doses; 80 mg extended-release tablet PO at bedtime for patients requiring LDL-C reduction to a goal of at least 25%; or 20 mg daily for patients requiring LDL-C reduction to a goal of less than 25%.
➤ **Adjunct to diet to reduce LDL-C, total cholesterol, and apo B in children with heterozygous familial hypercholesterolemia who haven't had an adequate response to dietary restriction and whose LDL-C remains at 190 mg/dL or more or LDL-C remains at 160 mg/dL or more and a positive family history of premature CV disease or two or more other CV disease risk factors are present** ⊠
Adolescent males and adolescent females (who are at least 1 year postmenarche) ages 10 to 16: 20 mg PO once daily at bedtime. Dosage adjustments may be made at 6-week intervals up to maximum of 40 mg (capsule) PO b.i.d. or 80 mg extended-release tablet PO once daily.
➤ **To reduce risk of undergoing coronary revascularization procedures and slow progression of coronary atherosclerosis**
Adults: In patients who must reduce LDL-C level by at least 25%, initially 40 mg PO once daily or b.i.d.; or one 80-mg extended-release tablet as a single dose at any time of the day. In patients who must reduce LDL-C level by less than 25%, initially 20 mg PO daily. Dosages range from 20 to 80 mg daily.

ADMINISTRATION
PO
● Give drug without regard to meals.
● For once-daily dosage, give immediate-release capsules in the evening.
● Have patient swallow tablets or capsules whole; don't crush or break tablets and don't open or crush capsules.
● Administer extended-release tablet as a single dose at any time of the day.
● Don't give two 40-mg capsules at one time.

ACTION
Inhibits HMG-CoA reductase, an early (and rate-limiting) step in the cholesterol synthesis pathway.

Route	Onset	Peak	Duration
PO	Unknown	1 hr	Unknown

Half-life: About 3 hours.

ADVERSE REACTIONS
CNS: dizziness, fatigue, headache, insomnia, syncope. **CV:** atrial fibrillation, HTN, edema, intermittent claudication. **EENT:** pharyngitis, rhinitis, sinusitis, tooth disorder. **GI:** abdominal pain, constipation, diarrhea, dyspepsia, flatulence, nausea, vomiting, gastric disorder. **GU:** UTI. **Hematologic:** *leukopenia, thrombocytopenia,* hemolytic anemia. **Musculoskeletal:** *rhabdomyolysis,* arthralgia, arthritis, back pain, myalgia, arthropathy, extremity pain. **Respiratory:** URI, bronchitis, cough, exertional dyspnea. **Other:** hypersensitivity reactions, accidental trauma, flulike illness.

INTERACTIONS
Drug-drug. *Cholestyramine, colestipol:* May bind with fluvastatin in the GI tract and decrease absorption. Separate doses by at least 4 hours.
Cimetidine, omeprazole: May decrease fluvastatin metabolism. Monitor patient for enhanced effects.
Cyclosporine and other immunosuppressants, colchicine, erythromycin, niacin: May increase risk of polymyositis and rhabdomyolysis. Avoid use together. Don't exceed 20 mg b.i.d. in patients taking cyclosporine.
Digoxin: May alter digoxin pharmacokinetics. Carefully monitor digoxin level.
Erythromycin, nicotinic acid: May increase risk of myopathy and rhabdomyolysis. Don't use together.

Reactions in bold italics are *life-threatening*.

Fibric acids (fenofibrate, gemfibrozil): May cause severe myopathy or rhabdomyolysis. If coadministration is unavoidable, closely monitor CK.

Fluconazole, itraconazole, ketoconazole: May increase fluvastatin level and adverse effects. Use together cautiously or, if given together, reduce dose of fluvastatin. Don't exceed 20 mg b.i.d. in patients taking fluconazole.

Glyburide: May increase levels of both drugs. Monitor serum glucose, and watch for signs and symptoms of toxicity.

Phenytoin: May increase phenytoin level. Monitor phenytoin level.

Protease inhibitors (atazanavir, darunavir, fosamprenavir, nelfinavir, ritonavir, saquinavir, tipranavir): May increase fluvastatin level and risk of myopathy and rhabdomyolysis. Use together cautiously.

Rifampin: May enhance fluvastatin metabolism and decrease level. Monitor patient for lack of effect.

Warfarin: May increase anticoagulant effect with bleeding. Monitor PT and INR.

Drug-herb. *Eucalyptus, jin bu huan, kava:* May increase risk of liver toxicity. Discourage use together.

Red yeast rice: May increase risk of adverse reactions because herb contains compounds similar to those in drug. Discourage use together.

Drug-lifestyle. *Alcohol use:* May increase risk of liver toxicity. Discourage use together.

EFFECTS ON LAB TEST RESULTS
• May increase ALT, AST, GGT, bilirubin, HbA$_{1c}$, fasting glucose, and CK levels.
• May cause thyroid function abnormalities.
• May decrease Hb level, hematocrit, and platelet and WBC counts.

CONTRAINDICATIONS & CAUTIONS
• Contraindicated in patients hypersensitive to drug and in those with active liver disease or unexplained persistent elevations of transaminase levels.
• Drug may cause rhabdomyolysis with AKI secondary to myoglobinuria or myopathy.
• Use cautiously in patients with CrCl less than 30 mL/minute or history of liver disease or heavy alcohol use, in those with inadequately treated hypothyroidism, and in patients ages 65 and older.

• Drug may increase risk of immune-mediated necrotizing myopathy, which persists despite stopping statin treatment and requires immunosuppressive agents.

Dialyzable drug: Unknown.

⚠ *Overdose S&S:* GI complaints, elevated AST and ALT levels.

PREGNANCY-LACTATION-REPRODUCTION
• Contraindicated during pregnancy for most patients.
• The FDA has determined that statin use in patients at high risk for CV events during pregnancy (such as established CV disease) may be considered on an individual basis.
• Contraindicated during breastfeeding.

NURSING CONSIDERATIONS
• Patient should follow a diet restricted in saturated fat and cholesterol during therapy.
• Exercise caution when giving to patient with history of liver disease or heavy alcohol ingestion. Closely monitor patient.
• Obtain LFT values before initiating therapy and if signs and symptoms of liver injury occur.
• Monitor lipid levels before starting therapy, at 4 weeks, at times of dosage changes, and periodically thereafter.
• Watch for signs and symptoms of myopathy. Monitor patient for muscle pain or weakness with malaise and fever. Discontinue drug for markedly elevated CK level or if myopathy is suspected or confirmed.
• Temporarily withhold drug in patient experiencing an acute or serious condition that predisposes patient to development of KF secondary to rhabdomyolysis (sepsis; hypotension; major surgery; trauma; severe metabolic, endocrine, or electrolyte disorder; uncontrolled epilepsy).
• May rarely worsen or precipitate myasthenia gravis (MG); monitor for worsening MG if treatment is initiated.
• *Look alike–sound alike:* Don't confuse fluvastatin with fluoxetine.

PATIENT TEACHING
• Teach about proper drug administration and handling.
• Advise patient who is also taking a bile acid sequestrant (such as cholestyramine) to take fluvastatin at bedtime, at least 4 hours after taking the sequestrant.

- Teach about proper dietary management, weight control, and exercise. Explain their importance in controlling elevated cholesterol and triglyceride levels.
- Warn patient to avoid alcohol.
- Tell patient to notify prescriber of adverse reactions, especially muscle aches and pains.
- Explain that drug may take up to 4 weeks to be completely effective.
- Instruct patient to report pregnancy or plans to become pregnant or to breastfeed.

fluvoxaMINE maleate ℞

floo-VOX-a-meen

Luvox ✦

Therapeutic class: Antidepressants
Pharmacologic class: SSRIs

AVAILABLE FORMS

Capsules (extended-release) ⓞⓝⓒ*:* 100 mg, 150 mg
Tablets: 25 mg, 50 mg, 100 mg

INDICATIONS & DOSAGES

Adjust-a-dose (for all indications): In older adults and patients with liver impairment, give lower first dose and adjust dose more slowly. When using extended-release capsules, titrate dosage more slowly after initial 100-mg dose.

➤ **OCD**

Adults: Initially, 50 mg (tablet) PO daily at bedtime; increase by 50 mg every 4 to 7 days. Maximum, 300 mg/day. Give total daily amounts above 100 mg in two divided doses. Or, 100-mg extended-release capsule PO once per day as single daily dose at bedtime. Increase in 50-mg increments every week, as tolerated, until maximum therapeutic benefit is achieved. Maximum, 300 mg/day.
Children ages 8 to 17: Initially, 25 mg PO daily at bedtime; increase by 25 mg every 4 to 7 days. Maximum, 200 mg/day for children ages 8 to 11 and 300 mg/day for children ages 12 to 17. Give total daily amounts over 50 mg in two divided doses.

ADMINISTRATION
PO

- Give drug without regard to food.
- If b.i.d. tablet doses aren't equal, give the larger dose at bedtime.

- Have patient swallow capsules whole; don't crush or cut capsules.
- Give extended-release capsules at bedtime.
- Store drug at room temperature.
- Protect from high humidity and light.

ACTION

Unknown. Selectively inhibits presynaptic neuronal uptake of serotonin, which may improve OCD.

Route	Onset	Peak	Duration
PO (capsules)	Unknown	Unknown	Unknown
PO (tablets)	Unknown	3–8 hr	Unknown

Half-life: 14 to 16 hours.

ADVERSE REACTIONS

CNS: agitation, apathy, headache, malaise, asthenia, somnolence, insomnia, nervousness, pain, dizziness, tremor, anxiety, emotional lability, hypertonia, depression, psychoneurosis, twitching, amnesia, CNS stimulation, hyperkinesia, hypokinesia, abnormal dreams, abnormal thinking, paresthesia, yawning, dysgeusia, manic reaction, myoclonus, syncope, weakness. **CV:** palpitations, chest pain, HTN, edema, hypotension, vasodilation. **EENT:** amblyopia, epistaxis, pharyngitis, laryngitis, sinusitis, tooth disorder, dry mouth, gingivitis. **GI:** nausea, diarrhea, constipation, dyspepsia, vomiting, anorexia, flatulence, dysphagia. **GU:** abnormal ejaculation, urinary frequency, polyuria, erectile dysfunction, anorgasmia, UTI, urine retention, dysmenorrhea, decreased libido. **Hepatic:** abnormal LFT values. **Metabolic:** weight gain or loss. **Musculoskeletal:** myalgia. **Respiratory:** URI, dyspnea, cough, bronchitis. **Skin:** diaphoresis, acne, ecchymoses. **Other:** flulike syndrome, viral infection, chills, accidental injury.

INTERACTIONS

❸ *Alert:* Fluvoxamine can significantly interact with many drugs. Consult a drug compatibility reference or pharmacist for additional information.
Drug-drug. *Alosetron (and other 5-HT$_3$ inhibitors), pimozide, thioridazine:* May prolong QTc interval. Use together is contraindicated.
Benzodiazepines (alprazolam, diazepam, midazolam, triazolam): May reduce clearance of these drugs. Use together cautiously (except for diazepam, which shouldn't be used with

Reactions in bold italics are *life-threatening*.

fluvoxamine). Adjust benzodiazepine dosage as needed. Initial alprazolam dosage should be at least halved; titration to the lowest effective dosage is recommended. Lorazepam, oxazepam, and temazepam may be given with fluvoxamine.

Carbamazepine, clozapine, methadone, metoprolol, propranolol, tacrine, TCAs, theophylline: May increase levels of these drugs. Use together cautiously, and monitor patient closely for adverse reactions. Dosage adjustments may be needed.

Diltiazem: May cause bradycardia. Monitor HR.

Linezolid, methylene blue: May cause serotonin syndrome. Don't start drug in patients receiving linezolid or methylene blue.

MAO inhibitors (phenelzine, selegiline, tranylcypromine): May increase risk of serotonin syndrome. Use together is contraindicated. Avoid using within 2 weeks of MAO inhibitor.

Mexiletine: May increase mexiletine level. Monitor level.

Ramelteon: May increase ramelteon level. Avoid use together.

Serotonergic drugs (amphetamines, buspirone, fentanyl, lithium, TCAs, tramadol, triptans, tryptophan): May increase risk of serotonin syndrome. Avoid use together. Monitor patient closely if use can't be avoided.

Tizanidine: May significantly increase drowsiness and impair psychomotor skills. Use together is contraindicated.

Warfarin, other drugs that interfere with hemostasis (aspirin, NSAIDs): May increase levels of these drugs and risk of bleeding and prolong PT. Monitor INR and adjust anticoagulant dosage accordingly.

Drug-herb. *Alfalfa, anise, bilberry:* May increase antiplatelet activity. Avoid use together.

Kava, SAM-e, St. John's wort, tryptophan, valerian: May increase sedative-hypnotic effects and risk of serotonin syndrome. Avoid use together.

Melatonin: May increase melatonin bioavailability. Avoid use together.

Drug-lifestyle. *Alcohol use:* May increase CNS effects. Discourage use together.

Smoking: May decrease drug's effectiveness. Urge patient to stop smoking.

EFFECTS ON LAB TEST RESULTS
• May decrease sodium level.

CONTRAINDICATIONS & CAUTIONS
• Contraindicated in patients hypersensitive to drug or to other phenyl piperazine antidepressants; in those receiving pimozide, alosetron, tizanidine, ramelteon, or thioridazine therapy; and within 2 weeks of MAO inhibitor administration.

🕔 **Alert:** Concomitant use with linezolid or methylene blue can cause serotonin syndrome (fever, mental status changes, muscle twitching, diaphoresis, shivering, shaking, diarrhea, loss of coordination). Use drug with linezolid or methylene blue only for life-threatening or urgent conditions when the potential benefits outweigh the risks of toxicity.

• Use cautiously in patients with liver dysfunction, other conditions that may affect hemodynamic responses or metabolism, or history of mania or seizures.

Boxed Warning Fluvoxamine tablets aren't approved for use in children, except for those with OCD. Fluvoxamine extended-release capsules shouldn't be used in children. ∎

• Use cautiously in patients with CV disease. Fluvoxamine hasn't been systemically evaluated in patients with recent history of MI or unstable heart disease.

⚥ Use cautiously in CYP2D6 poor metabolizers.

• Bone fractures have been associated with antidepressant use. Consider the possibility of fragility fracture if patient treated with an antidepressant presents with unexplained bone pain, point tenderness, swelling, or bruising.

Dialyzable drug: Unlikely.

⚠ **Overdose S&S:** Nausea, vomiting, diarrhea, coma, hypokalemia, hypotension, respiratory difficulties, somnolence, tachycardia, ECG abnormalities, seizures, dizziness, liver function disturbances, tremor, increased reflexes, unsteady gait, hypoxic encephalopathy.

PREGNANCY-LACTATION-REPRODUCTION
• Neonates exposed to drug late in third trimester have developed complications requiring prolonged hospitalization, respiratory support, and tube feeding. Neonates exposed to SSRIs in late pregnancy may be at increased risk for persistent pulmonary HTN of the newborn, which is associated with substantial neonatal morbidity and mortality. Carefully consider risks and benefits of treatment on case-by-case basis.

• Register patients in the National Pregnancy Registry for Antidepressants

(1-866-961-2388 or https://womensmentalhealth.org/research/pregnancyregistry/antidepressants).

• Drug appears in human milk. Patient should discontinue breastfeeding or discontinue drug, considering importance of drug to patient.

NURSING CONSIDERATIONS

Boxed Warning Drug may increase risk of suicidality in young adults ages 18 to 24, especially during first few months of treatment. Monitor all patients closely for clinical worsening. ■

• Record mood changes. Monitor patient for suicidality.

⊙ *Alert:* Combining an SSRI with a triptan may cause serotonin syndrome or NMS-like reactions. Serotonin syndrome is more likely to occur when starting or increasing triptan dose.

⊙ *Alert:* If linezolid or methylene blue must be given, fluvoxamine must be stopped and patient should be monitored for serotonin toxicity for 2 weeks or until 24 hours after final dose of linezolid or methylene blue, whichever comes first. Treatment with fluvoxamine may resume 24 hours after final dose of linezolid or methylene blue.

• Patients shouldn't stop drug without first consulting prescriber; abruptly stopping drug may cause withdrawal syndrome (headache, muscle ache, flulike symptoms).

• Glucose control may be impaired; monitor for signs and symptoms of loss of glucose control, particularly in patient with diabetes.

• Monitor for signs and symptoms of hyponatremia (headache, difficulty concentrating, memory impairment, confusion, weakness, unsteadiness). Severe hyponatremia may also cause hallucinations, syncope, seizure, coma, respiratory arrest, and death.

• Monitor for bleeding events, ranging from ecchymosis, epistaxis, and petechiae to life-threatening hemorrhage.

• Consider age and sex differences when determining dosages in children and adult females; therapeutic effect in females may be achieved with lower doses.

• *Look alike–sound alike:* Don't confuse fluvoxamine with fluoxetine.

PATIENT TEACHING

Boxed Warning Advise families and caregivers to closely observe patient for increased suicidality. ■

• Teach about proper drug administration and handling.

• Caution patient to avoid alcohol.

⊙ *Alert:* Teach patient to recognize and immediately report signs and symptoms of serotonin toxicity (fever, mental status changes, muscle twitching, rigidity, hyperflexes, labile BP, increased HR, diaphoresis, shivering, shaking, nausea, vomiting, diarrhea, loss of coordination).

• Warn patient to avoid hazardous activities until CNS effects of drug are known.

• Advise patient to notify prescriber about planned, suspected, or known pregnancy.

• Tell patient who develops a rash, hives, or related allergic reaction to notify prescriber.

• Advise that drug may cause sexual dysfunction. Instruct patient to discuss changes and management with health care provider.

• Inform patient that drug may take several weeks to obtain full therapeutic effect. Once improvement occurs, advise patient not to stop drug until directed by prescriber.

• Suggest that patient keep a diary of changes in mood or behavior. Tell patient to immediately report suicidality.

• Caution patient to check with prescriber before taking OTC medications, supplements, and other prescription drugs. Drug interactions can occur.

SAFETY ALERT!

fondaparinux sodium
fon-da-PAR-i-nuks

Arixtra

Therapeutic class: Anticoagulants
Pharmacologic class: Activated factor X inhibitors

AVAILABLE FORMS
Injection: 2.5 mg/0.5 mL, 5 mg/0.4 mL, 7.5 mg/0.6 mL, 10 mg/0.8 mL in single-dose, prefilled syringe

INDICATIONS & DOSAGES
➤ **Prevention of DVT, which may lead to PE, in patients undergoing surgery for hip fracture, hip replacement, knee replacement, or abdominal surgery**
Adults weighing 50 kg or more: 2.5 mg subcut once daily for 5 to 9 days. Give first dose after hemostasis is established, 6 to 8 hours after

surgery. Giving dose earlier than 6 hours after surgery increases risk of major bleeding. Patients undergoing hip fracture surgery should receive extended prophylaxis course of up to 24 additional days.

➤ **Acute VTE (with warfarin) when treatment is started in hospital**
Adults weighing more than 100 kg: 10 mg subcut daily.
Adults weighing 50 to 100 kg: 7.5 mg subcut daily.
Adults weighing less than 50 kg: 5 mg subcut daily.
Adjust-a-dose: Continue treatment for 5 to 9 days and until INR reaches 2 to 3. Begin warfarin therapy as soon as possible, usually within 72 hours. Optimal duration of therapy is unknown.

➤ **Acute symptomatic superficial vein thrombosis (at least 5 cm in length) of legs** ◆
Adults: 2.5 mg subcut once daily for 45 days.

➤ **ACS (non-ST-elevation ACS [NSTE-ACS] or ST-elevation MI [STEMI])** ◆
Adults: For NSTE-ACS, 2.5 mg subcut once daily for duration of hospitalization or until PCI occurs. For STEMI, 2.5 mg IV once; then 2.5 mg subcut once daily starting the following day. Treat for duration of hospitalization, up to 8 days, or until PCI occurs.

ADMINISTRATION
Subcutaneous
• Give subcut only, never IM. Inspect the single-dose, prefilled syringe for particulate matter and discoloration before giving.
⚠ *Alert:* To avoid loss of drug, don't expel air bubble from syringe.
• Give drug in fatty tissue of lower abdomen, rotating injection sites. If drug has been properly injected, the needle will pull back into the syringe security sleeve and the white safety indicator will appear above the blue upper body. A soft click may be heard or felt when the syringe plunger is fully released. After injection of syringe contents, plunger automatically rises while needle withdraws from skin and retracts into security sleeve. Don't recap needle.

ACTION
Binds to antithrombin III (AT-III) and potentiates neutralization of factor Xa by AT-III, which interrupts coagulation and inhibits formation of thrombin and blood clots.

Route	Onset	Peak	Duration
Subcut	Unknown	2–3 hr	Unknown

Half-life: 17 to 21 hours.

ADVERSE REACTIONS
CNS: insomnia, dizziness, confusion. **CV:** hypotension. **EENT:** epistaxis. **Hematologic:** *hemorrhage,* anemia, hematoma, *postoperative hemorrhage, thrombocytopenia.* **Hepatic:** increased AST and ALT levels. **Metabolic:** *hypokalemia.* **Skin:** mild local irritation (injection-site bleeding, rash, pruritus), bullous eruption, purpura, rash, increased wound drainage and infection.

INTERACTIONS
Drug-drug. *Drugs that increase risk of bleeding (anticoagulants, NSAIDs, platelet inhibitors):* May increase risk of hemorrhage. Stop these drugs before starting fondaparinux. If use together is unavoidable, monitor patient closely.
Drug-herb. *Herbal products with anticoagulant or antiplatelet effects (alfalfa, anise, bilberry, angelica [dong quai], ginkgo, ginseng, willow):* May increase risk of bleeding. Discourage use together.

EFFECTS ON LAB TEST RESULTS
• May increase AST, ALT, and bilirubin levels.
• May decrease potassium level.
• May decrease Hb level, hematocrit, and platelet count.

CONTRAINDICATIONS & CAUTIONS
• Contraindicated in patients with CrCl of less than 30 mL/minute and for VTE prophylaxis in patients weighing less than 50 kg.
• Contraindicated in patients with history of serious hypersensitivity reaction (angioedema, anaphylactoid, or anaphylactic reactions) to fondaparinux.
• Contraindicated in patients with active major bleeding, bacterial endocarditis, or thrombocytopenia with a positive test result for antiplatelet antibody after taking fondaparinux.
• Use cautiously in patients being treated with platelet inhibitors; in those at increased risk for bleeding (such as those with congenital or acquired bleeding disorders); in those with active ulcerative and angiodysplastic GI disease; in those with hemorrhagic stroke; and in patients shortly after brain, spinal, or ophthalmologic surgery.

• Use cautiously in older adults, in patients with CrCl of 30 to 50 mL/minute, and in those with a history of heparin-induced thrombocytopenia, a bleeding diathesis, uncontrolled arterial HTN, or history of recent GI ulceration, diabetic retinopathy, or hemorrhage.

🜂 *Alert:* Use cautiously in patients who are latex-sensitive; the packaging (needle guard) contains dry natural rubber.

• Safety and effectiveness in children haven't been established.

Dialyzable drug: Yes.

⚠ *Overdose S&S:* Hemorrhagic complications.

PREGNANCY-LACTATION-REPRODUCTION
• Use cautiously during pregnancy and only if benefit justifies fetal risk.
• It isn't known if drug appears in human milk. Use cautiously during breastfeeding.

NURSING CONSIDERATIONS
• Don't use interchangeably with heparin, low-molecular-weight heparins, or heparinoids.

Boxed Warning Patients who receive epidural or spinal anesthesia, epidural catheters, or spinal puncture or have history of spine deformity or surgery are at increased risk for developing epidural or spinal hematoma, which may result in long-term or permanent paralysis. Other factors that increase risk include concurrent use of NSAIDs, platelet inhibitors, and other anticoagulants; use of indwelling epidural catheters; and history of traumatic or repeated epidural or spinal surgery. Monitor these patients closely for neurologic impairment, and treat urgently. Consider the risk before neuraxial intervention in patients anticoagulated or to be anticoagulated for thromboprophylaxis. Optimal timing between fondaparinux dose and neuraxial procedures isn't known. ∎

• Periodically monitor kidney function, and stop drug in patients who develop unstable kidney function or CrCl less than 30 mL/minute while receiving therapy.
• Routinely assess for signs and symptoms of bleeding, and regularly monitor CBC, platelet count, creatinine level, and stool occult blood test results. Stop use if platelet count falls below 100,000/mm³.
• Anticoagulant effects may last for 2 to 4 days after stopping drug in patients with normal kidney function.

• PT and PTT aren't suitable monitoring tests to measure drug activity. If coagulation parameters change unexpectedly or patient develops major bleeding, stop drug.
• Drug has been given safely for up to 26 days in clinical trials of VTE treatment.
• Refer to label and local protocol for additional details for transitioning between anticoagulants.

PATIENT TEACHING
• Tell patient to report all adverse reactions, especially signs and symptoms of bleeding or neurologic impairment.
• Instruct patient to avoid OTC products that contain aspirin or other salicylates.
• Advise patient to consult with prescriber before starting herbal therapy; many herbs have anticoagulant, antiplatelet, or fibrinolytic properties.
• Teach patient the correct technique for subcut use, if needed.

---

formoterol fumarate
for-MOH-te-rol

Perforomist

Therapeutic class: Bronchodilators
Pharmacologic class: Selective beta₂-adrenergic agonists

AVAILABLE FORMS
Inhalation solution: 20 mcg/2 mL vial

INDICATIONS & DOSAGES
➤ **Maintenance treatment of bronchoconstriction in patients with COPD (chronic bronchitis, emphysema)**
Adults: 20 mcg by oral inhalation every 12 hours. Maximum dose, 40 mcg/day.

ADMINISTRATION
Inhalational
• Give inhalational solution through a standard jet nebulizer connected to an air compressor.
• Solution doesn't require dilution before giving; don't mix other medications with formoterol solution.
• Patient should breathe deeply and evenly until all medication has been inhaled, about 9 minutes.

F

• Skip a missed dose and give the next dose at the usual time.
• Store in foil pouch and remove immediately before use. Drug is colorless; discard drug if solution isn't colorless.
• Store in refrigerator at 36° to 46°F (2° to 8°C) until expiration date or at room temperature for up to 3 months.
• Clean nebulizer after use.

ACTION
Long-acting selective beta$_2$ agonist that causes bronchodilation. Ultimately increases cAMP, leading to relaxation of bronchial smooth muscle and inhibition of mediator release from mast cells.

Route	Onset	Peak	Duration
Inhalation solution	12 min	1–3 hr	12 hr

Half-life: 7 hours.

ADVERSE REACTIONS
CNS: tremor, dizziness, insomnia, nervousness, headache, fatigue, malaise, anxiety.
CV: *arrhythmias,* chest pain, angina, HTN, hypotension, tachycardia, palpitations.
EENT: nasopharyngitis, sinusitis, dysphonia, dry mouth, tonsillitis. **GI:** nausea, vomiting, diarrhea. **Metabolic:** *metabolic acidosis, hypokalemia,* hyperglycemia.
Musculoskeletal: muscle cramps. **Respiratory:** bronchitis, respiratory tract infection, dyspnea. **Skin:** rash, pruritus. **Other:** viral infection.

INTERACTIONS
Drug-drug. *Adrenergics:* May potentiate sympathetic effects of formoterol. Use together cautiously.
Beta blockers: May antagonize effects of both drugs, causing bronchospasm in patients with COPD. Avoid use except when benefit outweighs risk. Use cardioselective beta blockers with caution to minimize risk of bronchospasm.
Diuretics, steroids, xanthine derivatives: May increase hypokalemic effect of formoterol. Use together cautiously.
MAO inhibitors, TCAs, other drugs that prolong QT interval: May increase risk of ventricular arrhythmias. Use together cautiously.
Non-potassium-sparing diuretics, such as loop or thiazide diuretics: May worsen ECG changes or hypokalemia. Use together cautiously. Monitor patient for toxicity.

EFFECTS ON LAB TEST RESULTS
• May increase glucose level.
• May decrease potassium level.

CONTRAINDICATIONS & CAUTIONS
• Contraindicated in patients hypersensitive to drug or its components.
• Contraindicated with use of other LABAs.
• Use of a LABA without an inhaled corticosteroid is contraindicated in patients with asthma. Drug isn't indicated for treatment of asthma.
• Use of a LABA as monotherapy for asthma is associated with an increased risk of asthma-related hospitalizations and death.
• Don't begin drug in patients with acutely deteriorating COPD, which may be life-threatening.
• Don't use drug to relieve acute symptoms (such as rescue therapy for acute episodes of bronchospasm). Treat acute symptoms with an inhaled short-acting beta$_2$ agonist.
• Use cautiously in patients with CV disease, especially coronary insufficiency, cardiac arrhythmias, and HTN, and in those who are unusually responsive to sympathomimetic amines.
• Use cautiously in patients with diabetes because hyperglycemia and ketoacidosis have occurred rarely with use of beta agonists.
• Use cautiously in patients with seizure disorders or thyrotoxicosis.
• Safety and effectiveness in children haven't been established.
Dialyzable drug: Unknown.
⚠ *Overdose S&S:* Exaggeration of adverse reactions, hypotension, cardiac arrest.

PREGNANCY-LACTATION-REPRODUCTION
• Use cautiously during pregnancy and only if benefit outweighs fetal risk.
• Drug may interfere with uterine contractility if used during labor; use only if clearly needed.
• Use cautiously during breastfeeding.

NURSING CONSIDERATIONS
⊕ *Alert:* If maintenance regimen fails to provide usual response, contact prescriber immediately, as this indicates COPD destabilization.
⊕ *Alert:* As with all beta$_2$ agonists, drug may produce life-threatening paradoxical bronchospasm. If bronchospasm occurs, treat immediately and notify prescriber promptly.

🜄 *Alert:* If patient develops tachycardia, HTN, or other adverse CV effects, drug may need to be stopped.

• Watch for immediate hypersensitivity reactions (anaphylaxis, urticaria, angioedema, rash, bronchospasm).

PATIENT TEACHING

• Teach about proper drug administration, handling, and storage.

• Tell patient not to increase dosage or frequency of use without medical advice and to only use drug with a nebulizer.

• Show patient how to use nebulizer according to manufacturer's instructions.

• Caution that drug isn't to be used for acute asthmatic episodes. Prescriber should give short-acting beta₂ agonist for this use.

• Advise patient to immediately report worsening symptoms, treatment that becomes less effective, or increased use of short-acting beta₂ agonist.

• Tell patient to report nausea, vomiting, shakiness, headache, fast or irregular heartbeat, or sleeplessness.

• Instruct patient to report pregnancy or plans to become pregnant or to breastfeed.

foscarnet sodium (phosphonoformic acid [PFA])

foss-CAR-net

Foscavir

Therapeutic class: Antivirals
Pharmacologic class: Pyrophosphate analogues

AVAILABLE FORMS

Injection: 24 mg/mL

INDICATIONS & DOSAGES

Adjust-a-dose (for all indications): Adjust dosage when CrCl is less than 1.4 mL/minute/kg. If CrCl falls below 0.4 mL/minute/kg, stop drug. Consult manufacturer's package insert for specific dosage adjustments.

Boxed Warning Drug is only indicated for use in patients who are immunocompromised with CMV retinitis and mucocutaneous acyclovir-resistant HSV infections. ∎

➤ **CMV retinitis in patients with AIDS**
Adults: Initially, for induction, 60 mg/kg IV over a minimum of 1 hour every 8 hours or 90 mg/kg IV over 1 to 2 hours every 12 hours for 2 to 3 weeks, depending on patient response. Follow with maintenance infusion of 90 to 120 mg/kg over 2 hours daily. Maximum dosage, 180 mg/kg/day (initial dosage) and 120 mg/kg/day (maintenance dosage).

➤ **Acyclovir-resistant HSV infections**
Adults: 40 mg/kg IV over at least 1 hour every 8 to 12 hours for 2 to 3 weeks or until healed. Maximum dosage, 120 mg/kg/day.

ADMINISTRATION

IV

Boxed Warning To minimize kidney toxicity, make sure patient is adequately hydrated before and during infusion. ∎

▼ Don't exceed recommended dosage, rate, or frequency of infusion. Doses must be individualized to patient's kidney function.

▼ Drug may be infused via a central or peripheral vein with enough blood flow for rapid distribution and dilution. If infusing into a central vein, don't dilute the commercially available form (24 mg/mL). If infusing into a peripheral vein, dilute to 12 mg/mL with D_5W or NSS to decrease risk of local irritation. Use an infusion pump. Use diluted solutions within 24 hours.

▼ Give induction treatment over 1 to 2 hours, depending on dose, and maintenance CMV infusions over 2 hours and at no more than 1 mg/kg/minute.

▼ **Incompatibilities:** Acyclovir, amphotericin B, dextrose 30%, diazepam, digoxin, ganciclovir, lactated Ringer solution, leucovorin, midazolam, pentamidine, phenytoin, prochlorperazine, promethazine, solutions containing calcium (such as TPN), sulfamethoxazole–trimethoprim, vancomycin. Other drugs may also be incompatible. Consult drug compatibility reference for more information.

ACTION

Inhibits herpes virus replication in vitro by blocking the pyrophosphate-binding site on DNA polymerases and reverse transcriptases.

Route	Onset	Peak	Duration
IV	Unknown	Immediate	Unknown

Half-life: 3 to 4 hours.

ADVERSE REACTIONS

CNS: asthenia, dizziness, fatigue, fever, headache, hypoesthesia, malaise, *seizures,* neuropathy, paresthesia, agitation, abnormal coordination, aggression, amnesia, anxiety, aphasia, ataxia, cerebrovascular disorder, confusion, dementia, depression, EEG abnormalities, generalized spasms, hallucinations, insomnia, meningitis, peripheral neuropathy, nervousness, pain, sensory disturbances, somnolence, stupor, dysgeusia, tremor. **CV:** ECG abnormalities, first-degree AV block, flushing, HTN, hypotension, palpitations, sinus tachycardia, chest pain, edema, *thrombosis.* **EENT:** conjunctivitis, eye pain, visual disturbances, pharyngitis, rhinitis, sinusitis, dry mouth. **GI:** abdominal pain, anorexia, diarrhea, nausea, vomiting, *pancreatitis,* constipation, dysphagia, dyspepsia, flatulence, melena, rectal hemorrhage, ulcerative stomatitis. **GU:** *AKI,* abnormal kidney function, albuminuria, candidiasis, dysuria, polyuria, nocturia, urethral disorder, urine retention, UTI. **Hematologic:** anemia, *bone marrow suppression, granulocytopenia, leukopenia, thrombocytopenia,* thrombocytosis. **Hepatic:** abnormal liver function. **Metabolic:** hyperphosphatemia, *hypocalcemia, hypokalemia, hypomagnesemia,* hypophosphatemia, hyponatremia, *acidosis,* thirst, cachexia, weight loss. **Musculoskeletal:** arthralgia, back pain, leg cramps, myalgia. **Respiratory:** *bronchospasm,* cough, dyspnea, hemoptysis, pneumonia, pneumonitis, *pneumothorax,* pulmonary infiltration, *respiratory insufficiency, stridor.* **Skin:** diaphoresis, rash, pruritus, erythematous rash, facial edema, seborrhea, skin discoloration, skin ulceration. **Other:** *sarcoma, sepsis, death,* abscess, bacterial or fungal infections, flulike symptoms, pain and inflammation at infusion site, lymphadenopathy, lymphoma-like disorder, rigors.

INTERACTIONS

Drug-drug. *Loop diuretics:* May increase foscarnet level. Thiazide diuretics are preferred to loop diuretics. Monitor patients receiving loop diuretics for toxicity.
Kidney-toxic drugs (acyclovir, aminoglycosides, amphotericin B, cyclosporine, methotrexate, tacrolimus): May increase risk of kidney toxicity. Avoid use together.
Pentamidine: May increase risk of kidney toxicity; severe hypocalcemia also has been reported. Monitor kidney function test results and electrolyte levels.
❸ *Alert: QT-interval prolonging drugs (amiodarone, dofetilide, fluoroquinolones, phenothiazines, procainamide, quinidine, some macrolides, sotalol, TCAs):* May increase risk of prolonged QT interval and torsades de pointes. Avoid use together.

EFFECTS ON LAB TEST RESULTS

• May increase ALP, ALT, AST, bilirubin, creatinine, and phosphate levels.
• May decrease calcium, magnesium, phosphate, potassium, and sodium levels.
• May decrease Hb level and granulocyte and WBC counts.
• May increase or decrease platelet count.

CONTRAINDICATIONS & CAUTIONS

• Contraindicated in patients hypersensitive to drug.
Boxed Warning In patients with abnormal kidney function, use cautiously, maintain adequate hydration, and reduce dosage. ∎
• Drug may cause QT-interval prolongation and increase risk of ventricular arrhythmias. Use cautiously in patients with history of or at risk for QT-interval prolongation.
• Drug contains sodium. Use cautiously in patients with HF or cardiomyopathy. Avoid use in patients on sodium-controlled diet.
Dialyzable drug: Yes.
⚠ *Overdose S&S:* Seizures, kidney impairment, paresthesia (limb or perioral), calcium and phosphate electrolyte disturbances.

PREGNANCY-LACTATION-REPRODUCTION

• Use cautiously in pregnancy and only if clearly needed.
• Monitoring of amniotic fluid volumes by ultrasound is recommended weekly after 20 weeks' gestation to detect oligohydramnios.
• Patient should discontinue breastfeeding or discontinue drug, considering importance of drug to patient.

NURSING CONSIDERATIONS

❸ *Alert:* Drug is highly toxic. Use lowest effective maintenance dose.
Boxed Warning Frequently monitor serum creatinine level, with dosage adjustment for changes in kidney function. ∎
• Obtain a baseline 24-hour CrCl. Monitor level two to three times weekly during

induction and at least once every 1 to 2 weeks during maintenance.

Boxed Warning Drug can cause seizures related to altered mineral and electrolyte levels; monitor levels using a schedule similar to that established for monitoring of CrCl. Assess patient for tetany and seizures, and correct imbalances if necessary. ■

• Monitor patient's Hb level and hematocrit. Anemia occurs in about one-third of patients and may require transfusions.

• Drug may cause a dose-related transient decrease in ionized calcium, which may not always show up in patient's lab values. Monitor for neurologic and cardiac changes.

• Closely monitor hydration status before and after infusion.

PATIENT TEACHING
• Explain the importance of adequate hydration throughout therapy.

• Advise patient to report all adverse reactions, including tingling around mouth, numbness in arms or legs, pins-and-needles sensations, chest pain, palpitations, dyspnea, and changes in urine volume or color.

• Tell patient to report discomfort at IV insertion site.

• Instruct patient to report pregnancy or plans to become pregnant or to breastfeed.

fosinopril sodium ☒
foe-SIN-oh-pril

Therapeutic class: Antihypertensives
Pharmacologic class: ACE inhibitors

AVAILABLE FORMS
Tablets: 10 mg, 20 mg, 40 mg

INDICATIONS & DOSAGES
➤ **HTN**
Adults: Initially, 10 mg PO daily; adjust dosage based on BP response at peak and trough levels. Usual dosage is 20 to 40 mg daily; maximum is 80 mg/day. Dosage may be divided.

Children ages 6 and older weighing more than 50 kg: Initially, 5 to 10 mg PO once daily. Maximum dosage is 40 mg/day.

➤ **Adjunct therapy for HF**
Adults: Initially, 10 mg PO once daily. Increase dosage over several weeks to a maximum of 40 mg PO daily, if needed.

Adjust-a-dose: Decrease initial dosage to 5 mg in patients with CrCl less than 60 mL/minute.

ADMINISTRATION
PO
• Give drug without regard to meals.
• 10-mg tablets are scored for 5-mg dose.

ACTION
Inhibits ACE, preventing conversion of angiotensin I to angiotensin II, a potent vasoconstrictor. Less angiotensin II decreases peripheral arterial resistance, thus decreasing aldosterone secretion, which reduces sodium and water retention and lowers BP.

Route	Onset	Peak	Duration
PO	1 hr	3 hr	24 hr

Half-life: 11.5 to 14 hours.

ADVERSE REACTIONS
CNS: asthenia, dizziness, headache, fatigue, somnolence, insomnia, depression, paresthesia, weakness, fever. **CV:** chest pain, hypotension, orthostatic hypotension, edema. **GI:** nausea, vomiting, diarrhea. **GU:** sexual dysfunction. **Metabolic:** hyperkalemia. **Respiratory:** URI; dry, persistent, tickling, nonproductive cough.

INTERACTIONS
Drug-drug. *Aliskiren:* Increases risk of hypotension, hyperkalemia, and kidney dysfunction. Don't use together in patients with GFR less than 60 mL/minute. Contraindicated in patients with diabetes.
Antacids: May impair absorption. Separate dosage times by at least 2 hours.
ARBs: May increase toxic effects of ACE inhibitors. Avoid use together when possible.
Azathioprine: May increase risk of anemia or leukopenia. Monitor hematologic studies if used together.
Diuretics, other antihypertensives: May cause excessive hypotension. Stop diuretic or lower fosinopril dosage.
Everolimus: May increase risk of angioedema. Use extreme caution.
Insulin: May alter insulin requirements in patients with diabetes. Monitor patient closely.
Lithium: May increase lithium level and lithium toxicity. Monitor lithium level.
NSAIDs: May decrease antihypertensive effects and increase potential for kidney dysfunction. Monitor BP.

Reactions in bold italics are *life-threatening*.

Potassium-sparing diuretics, potassium sup-plements: May cause hyperkalemia. Use cautiously and monitor patient closely.
Drug-herb. *Capsaicin:* May cause cough. Discourage use together.
Ma huang: May decrease antihypertensive effects. Discourage use together.
Drug-food. *Salt substitutes containing potassium:* May increase risk of hyperkalemia. Discourage use together.

EFFECTS ON LAB TEST RESULTS
• May increase BUN, creatinine, and potassium levels and LFT values.
• May decrease sodium level.
• May increase Hb level and hematocrit.
• May cause falsely low digoxin level with Digi-Tab radioimmunoassay kit for digoxin.

CONTRAINDICATIONS & CAUTIONS
• Contraindicated in patients hypersensitive to drug or other ACE inhibitors.
• Use cautiously in patients with impaired kidney or liver function and cardiac-related diseases.
• Safety and effectiveness in children with HF or children younger than age 6 with HTN haven't been established.
Dialyzable drug: 2% to 7%.
⚠ **Overdose S&S:** Hypotension.

PREGNANCY-LACTATION-REPRODUCTION
• Use during pregnancy and breastfeeding isn't recommended.
Boxed Warning Use during pregnancy can cause fetal injury and death. When pregnancy is detected, stop drug as soon as possible. ∎

NURSING CONSIDERATIONS
• Monitor BP for drug effect.
• Drug can increase risk of angioedema, including intestinal angioedema. Monitor patient for facial swelling, airway obstruction, and abdominal pain.
▧ Patients who are Black and who take ACE inhibitors as monotherapy for HTN have a smaller reduction in BP and a higher incidence of angioedema than patients who are non-Black.
• Monitor potassium intake and potassium level. Patients with diabetes, those with impaired kidney function, and those receiving drugs that can increase potassium level may develop hyperkalemia.

• ACE inhibitors may cause agranulocytosis and neutropenia. Monitor CBC with differential counts before therapy and periodically thereafter.
• Assess kidney and liver function before and periodically throughout therapy.
• *Look alike–sound alike:* Don't confuse fosinopril with lisinopril.

PATIENT TEACHING
• Tell patient to avoid potassium-containing salt substitutes, which may increase risk of hyperkalemia when taken with fosinopril.
• Instruct patient to contact prescriber if light-headedness or fainting occurs.
• Advise patient to report evidence of infection (fever, sore throat).
• Instruct patient to report easy bruising or bleeding; swelling of tongue, lips, face, eyes, mucous membranes, arms, or legs; difficulty swallowing or breathing; cough; or hoarseness.
• Urge patient to use caution in hot weather and during exercise. Inadequate fluid intake, vomiting, diarrhea, and excessive perspiration can lead to light-headedness and fainting.
• Tell patient with diabetes using oral antidiabetics or insulin who is starting an ACE inhibitor to closely watch for hypoglycemia, especially during first month of combined use.
• Tell patient of childbearing potential to notify prescriber if pregnancy occurs. Drug will need to be stopped.

fosphenytoin sodium ▧
FOS-fen-i-toyn

Cerebyx

Therapeutic class: Anticonvulsants
Pharmacologic class: Hydantoin derivatives

AVAILABLE FORMS
Injection: 50 mg phenytoin sodium equivalent (PE)/mL in 2-mL and 10-mL vials

INDICATIONS & DOSAGES
Adjust-a-dose (for all indications): Phenytoin clearance is decreased slightly in older adults; lower or less frequent dosing may be required.
➤ **Status epilepticus**
Adults: Loading dose, 15 to 20 mg PE/kg IV at infusion rate of 100 to 150 mg PE/minute; then 4 to 6 mg PE/kg/day IV or IM in divided

doses as maintenance dose. Don't exceed maximum rate of 150 mg PE/minute.
Children from birth to younger than age 17: Loading dose, 15 to 20 mg PE/kg IV at 2 mg PE/minute or 150 mg PE/minute, whichever is slower; then initial maintenance dose of 2 to 4 mg PE/kg IV 12 hours after loading dose; then continue 2 to 4 mg PE/kg once every 12 hours at 1 to 2 mg PE/kg/minute or 100 mg PE/minute, whichever is slower.

➤ **Prevention and treatment of seizures during neurosurgery (nonemergent loading or maintenance dosing)**
Adults: Loading dose, 10 to 20 mg PE/kg IM or IV at infusion rate not exceeding 150 mg PE/minute. Maintenance dose is 4 to 6 mg PE/kg/day IV or IM in divided doses.
Children from birth to younger than age 17: Loading dose, 10 to 15 mg PE/kg IV at 1 to 2 mg PE/minute or 150 mg PE/minute, whichever is slower; then initial maintenance dose of 2 to 4 mg PE/kg IV 12 hours after loading dose; then continue 2 to 4 mg PE/kg once every 12 hours at 1 to 2 mg PE/kg/minute or 100 mg PE/minute, whichever is slower.

➤ **Parenteral substitutions for oral phenytoin**
Adults and children: Substitute for oral phenytoin when oral dosing isn't possible at the same total daily PE dose. Give IV at infusion rate not exceeding 150 mg PE/minute for adults and at 2 mg PE/kg/minute or 150 mg PE/minute, whichever is slower, for children. Dosing may be once daily or more frequently as divided doses.

➤ **Traumatic brain injury; prevention of early posttraumatic seizure (alternative agent)** ◆
Adults: Loading dose, 17 to 20 mg PE/kg IV at 100 to 150 mg PE/minute; usual maximum dose, 2 g PE. Begin maintenance dose 8 to 12 hours after loading dose. Maintenance dose, 100 mg PE IV every 8 hours or 5 mg PE/kg/day (rounded to nearest 100 mg PE) IV in divided doses every 8 hours. Duration of prophylaxis varies but is generally short term.

ADMINISTRATION

🔆 *Alert:* Don't confuse the amount of drug to be given in PE with the concentration of drug in the vial. Be sure to withdraw the appropriate volume from the vial when preparing for administration.

IV

▼ If rapid phenytoin loading is a main goal, IV form is preferred.
▼ For status epilepticus, give IV rather than IM because therapeutic phenytoin level occurs more rapidly.
▼ IV administration generates phenytoin levels similar enough to oral phenytoin sodium to allow interchangeable use.
▼ For infusion, dilute in D_5W or NSS for injection to yield 1.5 to 25 mg PE/mL.
Boxed Warning Don't give more than 150 mg PE/minute in adults and 2 mg PE/kg/minute (or 150 mg PE/minute) in children because of risk of severe hypotension and cardiac arrhythmias. Careful cardiac monitoring is needed during and after administering IV drug. Although risk of CV toxicity increases with infusion rates above the recommended infusion rate, these events have also been reported at or below the recommended infusion rate. Reducing rate of administration or discontinuing drug may be needed. ■
▼ Maintenance infusion rates in children shouldn't exceed 1 to 2 mg PE/kg/minute (or 100 mg PE/minute, whichever is slower).
▼ Patients receiving 20 mg PE/kg at 150 mg PE/minute typically feel discomfort, usually in the groin. To reduce discomfort, slow or temporarily stop infusion.
▼ Continuously monitor patient's ECG, BP, and respirations during maximum phenytoin level—about 10 to 20 minutes after end of fosphenytoin infusion. Severe CV complications are most common in older adults and patients who are gravely ill. If needed, decrease rate or stop infusion.
▼ Store drug under refrigeration. Don't store at room temperature longer than 48 hours. Discard vials that develop particulate matter.
▼ **Incompatibilities:** Other IV drugs.

IM

● Use IM route only when IV route isn't available. Avoid use in children and for treatment of status epilepticus whenever possible.
● Depending on dose ordered, may require two separate IM injections.
● IM administration generates systemic phenytoin levels similar enough to oral phenytoin sodium to allow essentially interchangeable use.
● Store drug under refrigeration. Don't store at room temperature longer than 48 hours.
● Discard vials that develop particulate matter.

Reactions in bold italics are *life-threatening*.

ACTION
May stabilize neuronal membranes and limit seizure activity either by increasing efflux or decreasing influx of sodium ions across cell membranes in the motor cortex during generation of nerve impulses.

Route	Onset	Peak	Duration
IV	Unknown	End of infusion	Unknown
IM	Unknown	30 min	Unknown

Half-life: Fosphenytoin, 15 minutes; phenytoin, 12 to 29 hours.

ADVERSE REACTIONS
CNS: ataxia, dizziness, somnolence, ***brain edema, intracranial HTN,*** agitation, asthenia, dysarthria, extrapyramidal syndrome, fever, headache, hypesthesia, incoordination, increased or decreased reflexes, nervousness, paresthesia, speech disorders, stupor, thinking abnormalities, tremor, dysgeusia, vertigo. **CV:** HTN, hypotension, tachycardia, vasodilation. **EENT:** nystagmus, amblyopia, diplopia, deafness, tinnitus, tongue disorder, dry mouth. **GI:** constipation, nausea, vomiting. **Metabolic:** *hypokalemia.* **Musculoskeletal:** back pain, myasthenia. **Respiratory:** pneumonia. **Skin:** pruritus, ecchymoses, injection-site reaction and pain, rash. **Other:** chills, facial edema, infection, pelvic pain.

INTERACTIONS
Drug-drug. *Amiodarone, azoles (fluconazole, ketoconazole) capecitabine, chloramphenicol, chlordiazepoxide, cimetidine, disulfiram, estrogens, ethosuximide, felbamate, 5-FU, fluoxetine, fluvastatin, fluvoxamine, H₂-receptor antagonists, isoniazid, methylphenidate, omeprazole, oxcarbazepine, phenothiazines, salicylates, sertraline, succinimides, sulfonamides, ticlopidine, tolbutamide, topiramate, trazodone, warfarin:* May increase phenytoin level and effect. Use together cautiously.
Bleomycin, carbamazepine, carboplatin, cisplatin, diazepam, diazoxide, doxorubicin, folic acid, fosamprenavir, methotrexate, nelfinavir, reserpine, rifampin, ritonavir, theophylline, vigabatrin: May decrease phenytoin level. Monitor patient.
Cisatracurium, corticosteroids, doxycycline, estrogens, azoles (fluconazole, ketoconazole), furosemide, hormonal contraceptives, irinotecan, paclitaxel, pancuronium, paroxetine, quinidine, rifampin, rocuronium, sertraline,

teniposide, theophylline, vecuronium, vitamin D, warfarin: May decrease effects of these drugs because of increased liver metabolism. Monitor patient closely.
Delavirdine: May cause loss of virologic response and possible resistance to delavirdine and NNRTIs. Use together is contraindicated.
Lithium: May increase lithium toxicity. Closely monitor patient's neurologic status. Marked neurologic symptoms have been reported despite normal lithium level.
Phenobarbital, valproate sodium, valproic acid: May increase or decrease phenytoin level. May increase or decrease levels of these drugs. Monitor patient.
Drug-herb. *St. John's wort:* May decrease phenytoin level. Monitor patient.
Drug-lifestyle. *Alcohol use:* Acute intoxication may increase phenytoin level and effect. Discourage use together.
Long-term alcohol use: May decrease phenytoin level. Monitor patient and strongly discourage use together.

EFFECTS ON LAB TEST RESULTS
- May increase ALP, GGT, and glucose levels.
- May decrease folate, phosphate, and T₄ levels.
- May increase or decrease potassium level.
- May cause falsely low dexamethasone and metyrapone test results.

CONTRAINDICATIONS & CAUTIONS
- Contraindicated in patients hypersensitive to drug or its components, phenytoin, or other hydantoins.
- Contraindicated in patients with history of acute liver toxicity attributable to fosphenytoin or phenytoin.
- Contraindicated in patients with sinus bradycardia, SA block, second- or third-degree AV block, or Adams-Stokes syndrome.
- Use cautiously in patients with porphyria and in those with history of hypersensitivity to similarly structured drugs, such as barbiturates, oxazolidinediones, and succinimide.
- Use cautiously in patients with kidney or liver impairment or low albumin level due to increased risk of adverse effects.
- **⊕ Alert:** Serious and sometimes fatal TEN and SJS have been reported; onset of symptoms usually occurs within 28 days but sometimes later.
- *Dialyzable drug:* Unknown.
- **⚠ Overdose S&S:** Asystole, bradycardia, cardiac arrest, hypocalcemia, hypotension,

lethargy, metabolic acidosis, nausea, syncope, tachycardia, vomiting, death.

PREGNANCY-LACTATION-REPRODUCTION

• Prenatal exposure may increase risk of congenital malformations and other adverse developmental outcomes. Use with extreme caution during pregnancy and only if potential benefits justify fetal risk.

• A potentially life-threatening bleeding disorder related to decreased levels of vitamin K-dependent clotting factors may occur in newborns exposed to phenytoin in utero. This drug-induced condition can be prevented with vitamin K administration to patient before delivery and to neonate after birth.

• Encourage patient taking drug during pregnancy to enroll in the North American Antiepileptic Drug Pregnancy Registry (1-888-233-2334 or www.aedpregnancyregistry.org).

• It isn't known if fosphenytoin appears in human milk but phenytoin does. Weigh benefits of breastfeeding with patient's need for drug and potential adverse effects on infant.

NURSING CONSIDERATIONS

🜲 *Alert:* Because of risk of cardiac and local toxicity with IV fosphenytoin administration, use oral phenytoin whenever possible.

• Angioedema has been reported in patients treated with phenytoin and fosphenytoin. Discontinue immediately if symptoms of angioedema (such as facial, perioral, or upper airway swelling) occur.

🜲 *Alert:* Drug should always be prescribed and dispensed in PE units. Don't adjust recommended doses when substituting fosphenytoin for phenytoin and vice versa.

• In status epilepticus, phenytoin may be used as maintenance instead of fosphenytoin, using the appropriate dose.

• Phosphate load provided by fosphenytoin (0.0037 millimole phosphate/mg PE) must be considered when treating patients who need phosphate restriction, such as those with severe kidney impairment. Monitor lab values.

🜲 Some patients metabolize phenytoin slowly, which appears to be genetically determined. If early dose-related CNS toxicity develops, immediately check serum level.

🜲 Patients with Chinese ancestry who have tested positive for allele HLA-B*1502 have an increased risk of SCAR, including SJS and TEN. Monitor these patients carefully.

• If patient develops exfoliative, purpuric, or bullous rash or signs and symptoms of SLE, DRESS, SJS, or TEN, stop drug and notify prescriber. If rash is mild (measles-like or scarlatiniform), therapy may resume after rash disappears. If rash recurs when therapy is resumed, further fosphenytoin or phenytoin administration is contraindicated. Document that patient is allergic to drug.

• Stop drug in patients with acute liver toxicity.

• Doses are usually selected to attain serum total phenytoin concentrations of 10 to 20 mcg/mL (unbound phenytoin concentrations of 1 to 2 mcg/mL). Trough levels provide effective serum level range and are obtained just before patient's next scheduled dose.

• After administration, phenytoin level shouldn't be monitored until conversion to phenytoin is essentially complete—about 2 hours after the end of an IV infusion or 4 hours after IM administration.

• Interpret total phenytoin levels cautiously in patients with kidney or liver disease or hypoalbuminemia caused by an increased fraction of unbound phenytoin. Monitoring unbound phenytoin level may be more useful in these patients.

• Closely monitor glucose level in patient with diabetes; drug may cause hyperglycemia.

🜲 *Alert:* Abrupt withdrawal of drug may precipitate status epilepticus.

🜲 *Look alike–sound alike:* Don't confuse Cerebyx with Cerezyme, Celexa, or Celebrex.

PATIENT TEACHING

• Warn patient that sensory disturbances may occur with IV administration.

• Instruct patient to immediately report adverse reactions, especially rash, palpitations, dyspnea, chest pain, and dizziness.

• Instruct patient to discuss drug therapy with prescriber if considering pregnancy or breastfeeding.

frovatriptan succinate
frow-vah-TRIP-tan

Frova

Therapeutic class: Antimigraine drugs
Pharmacologic class: Serotonin 5-HT$_1$ receptor agonists

AVAILABLE FORMS
Tablets: 2.5 mg

INDICATIONS & DOSAGES

➤ **Acute treatment of migraine attacks with or without aura**

Adults: 2.5 mg PO taken at first sign of migraine attack. If headache recurs after initial relief, second tablet may be taken at least 2 hours after first dose. Total daily dose shouldn't exceed 7.5 mg.

➤ **Short-term prevention of migraines associated with menstruation** ♦

Adults: 2.5 mg PO daily for 6 days prior to anticipated start of menstruation.

ADMINISTRATION

PO
• Give drug without regard to food.
• Give drug with fluids as soon as signs or symptoms appear.

ACTION

May cause vasoconstriction in response to excessive dilation of extracerebral and intracranial arteries during migraine headaches.

Route	Onset	Peak	Duration
PO	Unknown	2–4 hr	Unknown

Half-life: 26 hours.

ADVERSE REACTIONS

CNS: dizziness, headache, fatigue, paresthesia, insomnia, anxiety, somnolence, dysesthesia, hypoesthesia, hot or cold sensation, pain, drowsiness. **CV:** chest pain, palpitations, flushing. **EENT:** abnormal vision, tinnitus, sinusitis, rhinitis, dry mouth. **GI:** dyspepsia, vomiting, abdominal pain, diarrhea, nausea. **Musculoskeletal:** skeletal pain. **Skin:** diaphoresis.

INTERACTIONS

Drug-drug. *Ergotamine-containing or ergot-type drugs (dihydroergotamine):* May cause prolonged vasospastic reactions. Use within 24 hours is contraindicated.

5-HT₁ agonists (such as triptans): May cause additive effects. Use within 24 hours is contraindicated.

MAO inhibitors, SNRIs, SSRIs (citalopram, fluoxetine, fluvoxamine, paroxetine, sertraline), TCAs: May cause serotonin syndrome. Discontinue drug if suspected.

EFFECTS ON LAB TEST RESULTS

None reported.

CONTRAINDICATIONS & CAUTIONS

• Contraindicated in patients hypersensitive to drug or its components.
• Contraindicated in patients with history or symptoms of ischemic heart disease or coronary artery vasospasm, including Prinzmetal variant angina, Wolff-Parkinson-White syndrome, or other cardiac accessory conduction pathway disorders; in those with history of stroke, TIA, or PVD, including ischemic bowel disease; in those with uncontrolled HTN; and in those with hemiplegic or basilar migraine.
• Before use in patients at risk for CAD (HTN, hypercholesterolemia, smoking, obesity, diabetes, strong family history of CAD), postmenopausal females, or males older than age 40, obtain a CV evaluation and show patient is free from cardiac disease. If drug is used in such a patient, monitor patient closely and consider obtaining an ECG after first dose. Intermittent, long-term users of triptans and those with risk factors should undergo periodic cardiac evaluation while using drug.
• Drug may cause vasospastic reactions, such as peripheral vascular ischemia, GI vascular ischemia and infarction, splenic infarction, and Raynaud syndrome.
• Safety of treating an average of more than four migraine headaches in a 30-day period hasn't been established.
• If patient doesn't respond to first dose, second dose probably will not be effective against the same headache.
• Safety and effectiveness in patients younger than age 18 haven't been established.
Dialyzable drug: Unknown.

PREGNANCY-LACTATION-REPRODUCTION

• Studies during pregnancy are inadequate. Use during pregnancy only if potential benefit justifies fetal risk.
• It isn't known if drug appears in human milk. Patient should discontinue breastfeeding or discontinue drug, considering importance of drug to patient.

NURSING CONSIDERATIONS

❶ **Alert:** Rare but serious cardiac events (acute MI, life-threatening cardiac arrhythmias, death) may occur within a few hours of a triptan dose.
• Use drug only when patient has a clear diagnosis of migraine. If patient has no response to first migraine attack treated with frovatriptan, reconsider migraine diagnosis.

• Headache exacerbation can occur when acute migraine drugs (ergotamine, triptans, opioids) are used for 10 or more days per month. Patients may need detoxification and treatment of withdrawal symptoms.

🜨 *Alert:* Combining triptan with SSRI, SSNRI, TCA, MAO inhibitor, or agent that reduced frovatriptan's metabolism may cause serotonin syndrome. Signs and symptoms include restlessness, loss of coordination, hallucinations, fast heartbeat, rapid changes in BP, increased body temperature, hyperreflexia, nausea, vomiting, and diarrhea. Serotonin syndrome is more likely when starting or increasing dosage of a serotonergic drug and usually occurs within minutes to hours.

• Monitor BP in patient taking 5-HT_1 agonist.
• Monitor for hypersensitivity reactions.

PATIENT TEACHING

• Teach about proper drug administration and handling.
• Instruct patient to take drug with a full glass of fluid.
• Caution patient to take extra care or avoid driving and operating machinery if dizziness or fatigue develops after taking drug.
• Stress importance of reporting all adverse reactions. Advise patient to immediately report pain, tightness, heaviness, or pressure in chest, throat, neck, or jaw; rash; or itching after taking drug.
• Instruct patient not to take drug within 24 hours of taking another serotonin-receptor agonist or ergot-type drug.

SAFETY ALERT!

fulvestrant 🜨
full-VES-trant

Faslodex

Therapeutic class: Antineoplastics
Pharmacologic class: Estrogen antagonists

AVAILABLE FORMS

Injection: 50 mg/mL in 5-mL prefilled syringes*

INDICATIONS & DOSAGES

Adjust-a-dose (for all indications): For patients with Child-Pugh class B liver impairment, give 250 mg IM slowly as one 5-mL injection on days 1, 15, and 29, then monthly thereafter.

➤ **Hormone receptor (HR)-positive advanced breast cancer with disease progression after endocrine therapy; HR-positive, HER2-negative advanced breast cancer in patients not previously treated with endocrine therapy** 🜨
Females who are postmenopausal: 500 mg IM slowly into buttocks (over 1 to 2 minutes per injection) as two 5-mL injections, one in each buttock on days 1, 15, and 29, then once monthly thereafter.

➤ **HR-positive, HER2-negative advanced or metastatic breast cancer in combination with palbociclib or abemaciclib in patients with disease progression after endocrine therapy** 🜨
Adult females: 500 mg IM slowly into buttocks (1 to 2 minutes per injection) as two 5-mL injections, one in each buttock, on days 1, 15, 29, and then once monthly thereafter. Recommended palbociclib dose is 125-mg capsule PO once daily for 21 consecutive days, followed by 7 days off each 28-day cycle. Recommended abemaciclib dosage is one 150-mg tablet PO b.i.d. Patients who are premenopausal and perimenopausal treated with this combination should be treated with luteinizing hormone-releasing hormone agonists according to current clinical practice standards.
Adjust-a-dose: Refer to palbociclib or abemaciclib prescribing information for dosage adjustments and management of toxicity, use with concomitant medications, and other relevant safety information related to palbociclib and abemaciclib.

➤ **HR-positive, HER2-negative advanced or metastatic breast cancer in combination with ribociclib, as initial endocrine-based therapy or after disease progression on endocrine therapy** 🜨
Adult females who are postmenopausal: 500 mg IM slowly into buttocks (over 1 to 2 minutes per injection) as two 5-mL injections, one in each buttock on days 1, 15, and 29, then once monthly thereafter. Recommended ribociclib dose is 600 mg PO once daily for 21 consecutive days, followed by 7 days off treatment for each 28-day cycle until disease progression or unacceptable toxicity occurs.
Adjust-a-dose: Refer to ribociclib prescribing information for dosage adjustments and management of ribociclib-related toxicities.

Reactions in bold italics are *life-threatening*.

ADMINISTRATION

IM

🜂 **Alert:** Hazardous drug; use safe handling and disposal precautions.

• Drug may be warmed before use by storing at room temperature for 1 hour or gently rolling injection in hands.
• Expel gas bubble from syringe before giving.
• Give slowly over 1 to 2 minutes per injection into buttocks.

ACTION

Competitively binds estrogen receptors and downregulates estrogen-receptor protein in human breast cancer cells. Is effective in treating estrogen receptor-positive breast tumors.

Route	Onset	Peak	Duration
IM	Unknown	7 days	1 mo

Half-life: About 40 days.

ADVERSE REACTIONS

CNS: asthenia, headache, pain, dizziness, insomnia, fever, paresthesia, depression, anxiety, fatigue. **CV:** chest pain, peripheral edema, vasodilation. **EENT:** pharyngitis. **GI:** nausea, vomiting, constipation, abdominal pain, diarrhea, anorexia. **GU:** UTI. **Hematologic:** anemia. **Hepatic:** elevated AST and ALT levels. **Musculoskeletal:** bone pain, back pain, extremity pain, arthralgia, musculoskeletal pain, myalgia, pelvic pain, arthritis. **Respiratory:** dyspnea, cough. **Skin:** injection-site pain, rash, diaphoresis. **Other:** accidental injury, hot flashes, flulike syndrome.

INTERACTIONS

None reported.

EFFECTS ON LAB TEST RESULTS

• May increase ALT and AST levels.
• May decrease Hb level and hematocrit.
• May interfere with estradiol measurement by immunoassay, resulting in falsely elevated estradiol levels.

CONTRAINDICATIONS & CAUTIONS

• Contraindicated in patients allergic to drug or its components.
• Use cautiously in patients with Child-Pugh class B or C liver impairment.
• When drug is used with palbociclib or abemaciclib, leukopenia, thrombocytopenia, neutropenia, and febrile neutropenia may occur.
Dialyzable drug: Unknown.

PREGNANCY-LACTATION-REPRODUCTION

• Drug can cause fetal harm. Patients shouldn't become pregnant during therapy. If drug is used during pregnancy or patient becomes pregnant during therapy, apprise patient of potential fetal hazard. Patients should use effective contraception during therapy and for 1 year after final dose.
• It isn't known if drug appears in human milk. Patients shouldn't breastfeed during therapy and for 1 year after final dose.
• Drug may impair male and female fertility.

NURSING CONSIDERATIONS

• Because drug is given IM, use cautiously in patient with bleeding diathesis or thrombocytopenia and in patient taking an anticoagulant.
• Pregnancy testing is recommended within 7 days before initiating drug.

PATIENT TEACHING

• Caution patient to avoid pregnancy and breastfeeding during therapy and for 1 year after final dose. Instruct patient to immediately report suspected pregnancy.
• Inform patient of the most common adverse effects (pain at injection site, headache, GI symptoms, back pain, hot flashes, sore throat). Advise patient to report all adverse reactions.

---

furosemide

fur-OH-se-mide

Furoscix, Lasix, Lasix Special ✦

Therapeutic class: Antihypertensives
Pharmacologic class: Loop diuretics

AVAILABLE FORMS

Injection: 10 mg/mL
Oral solution: 8 mg/mL, 10 mg/mL
Tablets: 20 mg, 40 mg, 80 mg, 500 mg ✦
Subcut kit: 80 mg/10 mL

INDICATIONS & DOSAGES

➤ **Acute pulmonary edema**
Adults: 40 mg IV injected slowly over 1 to 2 minutes; then 80 mg IV over 1 to 2 minutes after 1 hour if needed.
➤ **Edema**
Adults: 20 to 80 mg PO daily in the morning. If response is inadequate, give a second dose, and each succeeding dose, every 6 to 8 hours. Carefully increase dose in 20- to 40-mg

---

increments up to 600 mg daily. Once effective dose is attained, may give once daily or b.i.d. Or, 20 to 40 mg IV or IM. Dose may be repeated or increased by 20 mg 2 hours or more after previous dose until desired effect is achieved. *Infants and children:* 2 mg/kg PO daily, increased by 1 to 2 mg/kg in 6 to 8 hours if needed; carefully adjusted up to maximum of 6 mg/kg if needed. Or, 1 mg/kg slowly IV or IM. May increase dosage by 1 mg/kg 2 hours after previous dose if needed up to 6 mg/kg. Maximum dose for premature infants, 1 mg/kg/day.

✴ *NEW INDICATION:* **Fluid overload in patients with New York Heart Association class II and class III chronic HF (Furoscix)**
Adults: Subcutaneous on-body infusor with prefilled cartridge preprogrammed to deliver 30 mg over first hour, followed by 12.5 mg per hour for subsequent 4 hours. Total dose, 80 mg over 5 hours.

▶ **HTN**
Adults: 20 to 40 mg PO b.i.d. Dosage adjusted based on response. Usual dose, 40 to 80 mg/day in two divided doses. May use as adjunct to other antihypertensives, if needed.

ADMINISTRATION
PO
• To prevent nocturia, give in the morning. Give second dose, if ordered, in early afternoon, 6 to 8 hours after morning dose.
• Store tablets in light-resistant container to prevent discoloration.
• Discard open bottle of solution after 90 days.
IV
▼ If discolored yellow, don't use.
▼ For direct injection, give over 1 to 2 minutes.
⊙ *Alert:* For high-dose (160 mg or more), intermittent infusion in adults, dilute with D_5W, NSS, or lactated Ringer solution. To avoid ototoxicity, infuse at a rate no greater than 4 mg/minute.
▼ Use prepared solution within 24 hours.
▼ **Incompatibilities:** Acidic solutions, amrinone, ciprofloxacin, milrinone, and various others. Consult drug compatibility reference for more information.
IM
• To prevent nocturia, give in the morning. Give second dose if ordered in early afternoon, 6 to 8 hours after morning dose.
• Give solution undiluted.
• Record administration site.
• IV administration is preferred over IM.

Subcut
• Subcut infusor isn't for chronic use. Replace with oral diuretics as soon as practical.
• Load prefilled cartridge into on-body infusor and close cartridge holder.
• Peel away adhesive liner on infusor and apply onto clean dry area of abdomen at least 2.5 inches (6 cm) above top of beltline and below bottom of ribcage.
• Start injection by pressing and releasing blue start button.
• Rotate site of each subcut injection.
• Don't remove infusor until solid green status light signals, a beep sounds, and white plunger rod fills the cartridge window.
• Infusor unit is for single use only.

ACTION
Inhibits sodium and chloride reabsorption at the proximal and distal tubules and ascending loop of Henle.

Route	Onset	Peak	Duration
PO	20–60 min	1–2 hr	6–8 hr
IV	Within 5 min	30 min	2 hr
IM	Unknown	30 min	2 hr
Subcut	Unknown	4 hr	Unknown

Half-life: 2 hours.

ADVERSE REACTIONS
CNS: vertigo, headache, dizziness, paresthesia, weakness, restlessness, fever. **CV:** orthostatic hypotension, thrombophlebitis (IV). **EENT:** blurred or yellowed vision, transient deafness, tinnitus. **GI:** abdominal discomfort and pain, GI irritation, diarrhea, anorexia, nausea, vomiting, constipation, *pancreatitis.* **GU:** azotemia, nocturia, polyuria, frequent urination, bladder spasm, oliguria, interstitial nephritis. **Hematologic:** *agranulocytosis, aplastic anemia, leukopenia, thrombocytopenia,* anemia. **Hepatic:** liver dysfunction, jaundice, increased liver enzyme levels. **Metabolic:** volume depletion and dehydration, asymptomatic hyperuricemia, increased cholesterol and triglyceride levels, impaired glucose tolerance, *hypokalemia,* hypochloremic alkalosis, hyperglycemia, dilutional hyponatremia, *hypocalcemia, hypomagnesemia.* **Musculoskeletal:** muscle spasm. **Skin:** dermatitis, purpura, rash, pruritus, photosensitivity reactions, transient pain at IM injection site, subcut site reactions (erythema, bruising, edema, pain). **Other:** hypersensitivity reactions, gout.

Reactions in bold italics are *life-threatening*.

INTERACTIONS

Drug-drug. *Aminoglycoside antibiotics, cisplatin:* May increase ototoxicity. Use together cautiously.

Amphotericin B, corticosteroids, corticotropin, metolazone: May increase risk of hypokalemia. Closely monitor potassium level.

Antidiabetics: May decrease hypoglycemic effects. Monitor glucose level.

Antihypertensives: May increase risk of hypotension. Use together cautiously. Decrease antihypertensive dose if needed.

Cardiac glycosides, neuromuscular blockers: May increase toxicity of these drugs from furosemide-induced hypokalemia. Monitor potassium level.

Chlorothiazide, chlorthalidone, hydrochlorothiazide, indapamide, metolazone: May cause excessive diuretic response, causing serious electrolyte abnormalities or dehydration. Adjust doses carefully, and monitor patient closely for excessive diuretic response.

Ethacrynic acid: May increase risk of ototoxicity. Avoid use together.

Lithium: May decrease lithium excretion, resulting in lithium toxicity. Monitor lithium level.

NSAIDs: May inhibit diuretic response. Use together cautiously.

Phenytoin: May decrease diuretic effects of furosemide. Use together cautiously.

Propranolol: May increase propranolol level. Monitor patient closely.

Salicylates: May cause salicylate toxicity, including ototoxicity. Use together cautiously.

Sucralfate: May reduce diuretic and antihypertensive effect. Separate doses by 2 hours.

Drug-herb. *Aloe:* May increase drug effect. Discourage use together.

Bayberry, blue cohosh, cayenne, ephedra, ginger, ginseng (American), kola, licorice: May worsen HTN. Discourage use together.

Licorice: May cause unexpected rapid potassium loss. Discourage use together.

Drug-lifestyle. *Sun exposure:* May increase risk of photosensitivity reactions. Advise patient to avoid excessive sunlight exposure.

EFFECTS ON LAB TEST RESULTS

• May increase cholesterol, triglyceride, glucose, BUN, creatinine, liver enzyme, and uric acid levels.

• May decrease calcium, magnesium, potassium, and sodium levels.

• May decrease Hb level and granulocyte, platelet, and WBC counts.

CONTRAINDICATIONS & CAUTIONS

• Contraindicated in patients hypersensitive to drug and in those with anuria.

• Use cautiously in patients with liver cirrhosis, kidney impairment, or allergy to sulfonamides.

🜂 **Alert:** Drug may cause tinnitus and reversible or irreversible hearing loss. Ototoxicity is associated with rapid injection, kidney impairment, use of higher-than-recommended doses, hypoproteinemia, and use with other ototoxic drugs.

• Drug may exacerbate or activate SLE.

• Premature infants may be at increased risk for persistent patent ductus arteriosus with furosemide treatment during first weeks of life.

Dialyzable drug: No.

⚠ **Overdose S&S:** Dehydration, blood volume reduction, hypotension, electrolyte imbalances.

PREGNANCY-LACTATION-REPRODUCTION

• Drug crosses placental barrier. Use during pregnancy only if potential benefit justifies fetal risk.

• Drug may decrease birth weight; monitor fetal growth.

• Drug appears in human milk. Avoid use during breastfeeding.

NURSING CONSIDERATIONS

🜂 **Alert:** Monitor weight, BP, and pulse rate routinely with long-term use.

Boxed Warning Drug is potent diuretic and can cause severe diuresis with water and electrolyte depletion. Monitor patient closely and adjust dose carefully. ∎

• If oliguria or azotemia develops or increases, drug may need to be stopped.

• Frequently monitor fluid intake and output and electrolyte, BUN, and carbon dioxide levels.

• Watch for signs of hypokalemia (muscle weakness, cramps).

• Consult prescriber and dietitian about patient's need for high-potassium diet or potassium supplements.

• Monitor glucose level in patient with diabetes.

• Drug may not be well absorbed orally in patient with severe HF. Drug may need to be given IV even if patient is taking other oral drugs.

• Monitor uric acid level, especially in patient with history of gout.

• Closely monitor an older adult, who is especially susceptible to excessive diuresis, because circulatory collapse and thromboembolic complications are possible.

• Monitor patient with severe symptoms of urine retention due to bladder emptying disorders, prostate enlargement, or urethral narrowing or worsening of symptoms, especially during initial treatment.

• Kidney stones and calcium deposits have occurred in infants born prematurely and in children younger than age 4 on long-term furosemide therapy. Monitor kidney function and kidney ultrasounds.

• *Look alike–sound alike:* Don't confuse furosemide with torsemide.

PATIENT TEACHING

• Advise patient to take drug in morning to prevent need to urinate at night. If second dose is needed, tell patient to take it in early afternoon, 6 to 8 hours after morning dose.

• Inform patient of possible need for potassium or magnesium supplements.

• Instruct patient to stand slowly to prevent dizziness and to limit alcohol intake and strenuous exercise in hot weather to avoid worsening dizziness upon standing quickly.

• Advise patient to report all adverse reactions and to immediately report ringing in ears, severe abdominal pain, or sore throat and fever; these symptoms may indicate toxicity.

❂ *Alert:* Discourage patient from storing different types of drugs in the same container, increasing risk of drug errors. (The most popular strengths of furosemide and digoxin are white tablets that are about equal in size.)

• Tell patient to consult prescriber or pharmacist before taking OTC drugs.

• Teach patient to avoid direct sunlight and to use protective clothing and sunblock because of risk of photosensitivity reactions.

---

gabapentin
gab-ah-PEN-tin

Gralise, Neurontin

gabapentin enacarbil
Horizant

Therapeutic class: Anticonvulsants
Pharmacologic class: GABA structural analogues

AVAILABLE FORMS
Capsules: 100 mg, 300 mg, 400 mg
Oral solution: 250 mg/5 mL

Tablets Ⓞ: 100 mg, 300 mg, 400 mg, 600 mg, 800 mg
Tablets (extended-release) Ⓞ: 300 mg, 450 mg, 600 mg, 700 mg, 900 mg

INDICATIONS & DOSAGES
Adjust-a-dose (for all indications): For immediate-release formulation in patients ages 12 and older with CrCl of 30 to 59 mL/minute, give 400 to 1,400 mg daily divided into two doses. For CrCl of 15 to 29 mL/minute, give 200 to 700 mg daily in a single dose. For CrCl of less than 15 mL/minute, give 100 to 300 mg daily in a single dose. Reduce daily dosage in proportion to CrCl (patients with CrCl of 7.5 mL/minute should receive half the daily dosage of those with CrCl of 15 mL/minute). For patients receiving hemodialysis, base dosage on CrCl estimates. Give supplemental dose of 125 to 350 mg after each 4 hours of hemodialysis. Gradually reduce dose or discontinue drug over at least 1 week.

➤ **Adjunct treatment of partial seizures with or without secondary generalization in patients with epilepsy (excluding Gralise and Horizant)**
Adults and children ages 12 and older: Initially, 300 mg PO t.i.d.; increased as needed and tolerated to 1,800 mg daily in three divided doses. Dosages up to 3,600 mg daily have been well tolerated.
Starting dosage, children ages 3 to 11: 10 to 15 mg/kg daily PO in three divided doses, adjusted over 3 days to reach effective dosage.
Effective dosage, children ages 5 to 11: 25 to 35 mg/kg daily PO in three divided doses.
Effective dosage, children ages 3 to 4: 40 mg/kg daily PO in three divided doses.

➤ **Moderate to severe primary restless legs syndrome (Horizant)**
Adults: 600 mg extended-release tablet PO daily at about 5 p.m. If dose isn't taken at recommended time, next dose should be taken the following day as prescribed.
Adjust-a-dose: If CrCl is 30 to 59 mL/minute, give 300 mg daily (may increase to 600 mg, if needed). If CrCl is 15 to 29 mL/minute, give 300 mg daily. If CrCl is less than 15 mL/minute, give 300 mg every other day. Don't give to patients receiving hemodialysis.

➤ **Postherpetic neuralgia (immediate-release)**
Adults: Day 1 give 300 mg PO; day 2 give 300 mg b.i.d.; and day 3 give 300 mg t.i.d.

Titrate as needed for pain relief up to 1,800 mg daily in three divided doses.

➤ **Postherpetic neuralgia (Gralise)**
Adults: Titrate dosage to 1,800 mg PO once daily. On day 1, give 300 mg; on day 2, 600 mg; on days 3 to 6, 900 mg; on days 7 to 10, 1,200 mg; on days 11 to 14, 1,500 mg; and on day 15 and thereafter, 1,800 mg.
Adjust-a-dose: For patients with reduced kidney function, initiate at daily dose of 300 mg. For patients with CrCl of 30 to 60 mL/minute, titrate dosage to 600 to 1,800 mg daily as tolerated. Don't give Gralise to patients with CrCl of less than 30 mL/minute or to those receiving hemodialysis.

➤ **Postherpetic neuralgia (Horizant)**
Adults: 600 mg extended-release PO in morning for 3 days; increase to 600 mg b.i.d. on day 4. If dose isn't taken at recommended time, skip dose and take next dose at time of next scheduled dose.
Adjust-a-dose: If CrCl is 30 to 59 mL/minute, give 300 mg in the morning for 3 days; then increase to 300 mg b.i.d. (may increase to 600 mg b.i.d. as needed). If CrCl is 15 to 29 mL/minute, give 300 mg in the morning on days 1 and 3, then 300 mg daily in the morning (increase to 300 mg b.i.d. if needed). If CrCl is less than 15 mL/minute, give 300 mg in the morning every other day (increase to 300 mg daily in the morning if needed). If CrCl is less than 15 mL/minute and patient is on hemodialysis, give 300 mg after each dialysis treatment (increase to 600 mg after every dialysis if needed).

➤ **Neuropathic pain ◆**
Adults: Initially 100 to 300 mg immediate-release 1 to 3 times daily. Increase to 300 to 1,200 mg t.i.d. based on response and tolerability. Or, initially, 300 mg extended-release at bedtime. Increase dose to 900 to 3,600 mg once daily based on response and tolerability.

ADMINISTRATION
PO
• Give immediate-release forms without regard to food.
• Give extended-release tablets with food.
• Give Gralise tablets with the evening meal.
• When giving drug t.i.d., ensure maximum interval between doses is no more than 12 hours.
• Refrigerate oral solution.
• Have patient swallow capsules and extended-release tablets whole; don't cut or crush them.

• May divide scored 600- or 800-mg Neurontin tablets and give as half-tablets. Use half-tablets within 28 days of dividing or discard.
• Don't use Gralise, Horizant, and other gabapentin products interchangeably.

ACTION
Unknown. Structurally related to GABA but doesn't interact with GABA receptors, isn't converted into GABA or GABA agonist, doesn't inhibit GABA reuptake, and doesn't prevent degradation.

Route	Onset	Peak	Duration
PO (immediate-release)	Unknown	2–4 hr	Unknown
PO (extended-release)	Unknown	8 hr	Unknown
PO (enacarbil)	Unknown	5–7.3 hr	Unknown

Half-life: Gabapentin, 5 to 7 hours; gabapentin enacarbil, 5.1 to 6 hours.

ADVERSE REACTIONS
CNS: asthenia, ataxia, dizziness, fatigue, somnolence, abnormal thinking, amnesia, depression, fever, dysarthria, incoordination, tremor, headache, drowsiness, irritability, hostility, emotional lability, abnormal or drunken feeling, insomnia, hyperkinesia, vertigo. **CV:** peripheral edema, vasodilation. **EENT:** amblyopia, diplopia, nystagmus, vertigo, otitis media, pharyngitis, nasopharyngitis. dental abnormalities, dry throat, dry mouth. **GI:** constipation, dyspepsia, increased appetite, flatulence, nausea, vomiting, diarrhea. **GU:** decreased libido, erectile dysfunction, UTI (Gralise). **Hematologic:** *leukopenia.* **Metabolic:** weight gain, hyperglycemia. **Musculoskeletal:** back pain, fractures, myalgia, limb pain. **Respiratory:** coughing, bronchitis, URI. **Skin:** abrasion, pruritus. **Other:** viral infections, infection, accidental injury.

INTERACTIONS
Drug-drug. *Antacids:* May decrease absorption of gabapentin. Separate dosage times by at least 2 hours.
CNS depressants: May increase risk of CNS depressant-related adverse effects. Monitor therapy.
Hydrocodone: May decrease hydrocodone level and increase gabapentin level. Monitor therapy.
Opioid analgesics (morphine): May enhance CNS depressant effect of opioid analgesics.

G

♣Canada   ◇OTC   ◆Off-label use   ⏺Do not crush   *Liquid contains alcohol   ⚡Genetic

Consider therapy modification or limit dosages and duration of each drug.

Drug-herb. *Kava Horizon:* May enhance adverse or toxic CNS effects. Monitor therapy.

Drug-lifestyle. ⚫ *Alert: Alcohol use:* May increase risk of CNS depression and respiratory difficulties. Discourage use together.

EFFECTS ON LAB TEST RESULTS

- May decrease WBC count.
- May increase glucose level.
- May cause false-positive results with Ames N-Multistix SG dipstick test for urine protein when used with other anticonvulsants.

CONTRAINDICATIONS & CAUTIONS

- Contraindicated in patients with known hypersensitivity to drug or its ingredients.
- In older adults, adjust dosage based on CrCl values.
- Gabapentin enacarbil isn't recommended for patients who must sleep during the day and remain awake at night.
- Anaphylaxis and angioedema can occur any time during therapy and require emergency treatment and discontinuation of drug.

⚫ *Alert:* May cause life-threatening and fatal respiratory depression in older adults and in patients with respiratory risk factors (CNS depressant or opioid use, COPD). Begin treatment at lowest dose and monitor patient closely.

- Potentially life-threatening DRESS syndrome (fever, rash, lymphadenopathy, and other organ system involvement) can occur. Evaluate patient immediately if symptoms occur and discontinue drug.

Dialyzable drug: Yes.

⚠ *Overdose S&S:* Double vision, slurred speech, drowsiness, lethargy, diarrhea.

PREGNANCY-LACTATION-REPRODUCTION

- Use during pregnancy only if potential benefit justifies fetal risk.
- Drug is excreted in human breast milk. Use during breastfeeding only if benefit to patient outweighs risk to the infant.
- Encourage patients who are pregnant to enroll in the North American Antiepileptic Drug Pregnancy Registry (1-888-233-2334 or www.aedpregnancyregistry.org).

NURSING CONSIDERATIONS

⚫ *Alert:* Closely monitor all patients taking or starting AEDs for changes in behavior indicating worsening of suicidality or depression.

Such symptoms as anxiety, agitation, hostility, mania, and hypomania may be precursors to emerging suicidality.

⚫ *Alert:* Don't suddenly withdraw AEDs because of risk of increased seizure frequency.

- Routine monitoring of drug levels isn't necessary. Drug doesn't appear to alter levels of other anticonvulsants.
- Monitor patient for hypersensitivity reactions (anaphylaxis, angioedema, SCAR).
- Monitor patient for CNS depression.

PATIENT TEACHING

⚫ *Alert:* Caution patients and their caregivers that drug may increase suicidality. Instruct them to watch for new or worsening depression, changes in mood or behavior, new suicidal thoughts behaviors, and thoughts of self-harm. Tell them to immediately notify prescriber of behavioral concerns.

- Teach about proper drug administration, handling, and storage.
- Advise patient to take first dose at bedtime to minimize adverse reactions.
- Warn that extended-release formulas can cause significant dizziness and sleepiness.
- Warn patient to report all adverse reactions and to avoid driving and operating heavy machinery until drug's CNS effects are known.

⚫ *Alert:* Caution patient or caregiver to seek immediate medical attention for confusion or disorientation; unusual dizziness or lightheadedness; lethargy; extreme sleepiness; slow, shallow, or difficult breathing; unresponsiveness; or cyanosis of lips, fingers, or toes.

- Advise patient not to take gabapentin with alcohol or other drugs that may cause sleepiness or dizziness.
- Warn patient not to stop drug abruptly.
- Instruct patient to discuss drug therapy with prescriber if considering pregnancy.

---

ganaxolone ⚥
gan-AXE-oh-lone

Ztalmy

Therapeutic class: Anticonvulsants
Pharmacologic class: Neuroactive steroid GABA-A receptor modulators
Controlled substance schedule: V

AVAILABLE FORMS

Oral suspension: 50 mg/mL

INDICATIONS & DOSAGES

➤ **Seizures associated with cyclin-dependent kinase-like 5 deficiency disorder** ⚥
Patients ages 2 and older weighing more than 28 kg: Initially, 150 mg PO t.i.d. (450 mg daily). Titrate to 300 mg t.i.d., then 450 mg t.i.d. to maximum dose of 600 mg t.i.d. (1,800 mg daily) based on tolerability. Titrate no more frequently than every 7 days.
Patients ages 2 and older weighing 28 kg or less: Initially, 6 mg/kg PO t.i.d. (18 mg/kg/day). Titrate to 11 mg/kg t.i.d., then 16 mg/kg t.i.d. to maximum dose of 21 mg/kg t.i.d. (63 mg/kg/daily) based on tolerability. Titrate no more frequently than every 7 days.
Adjust-a-dose: When discontinuing drug, reduce dosage gradually to minimize risk of increased seizure frequency and status epilepticus. Monitor patients with liver impairment for adverse reactions; reduce dosage as needed.

ADMINISTRATION
PO
• Shake bottle for 1 minute; then wait 1 minute before measuring and giving drug.
• Use oral syringe provided to measure dose. Don't use household spoon.
• Give drug with food.
• Store upright in original bottle at 59° to 86° F (15° to 30° C). Keep bottle tightly closed.
• Discard unused drug 30 days after opening or by "Discard After" date on bottle, whichever is sooner.

ACTION
Unknown. Thought to result from positive allosteric modulation of the GABA type A receptor in the CNS.

Route	Onset	Peak	Duration
PO	Unknown	2–3 hr	Unknown

Half-life: 34 hours.

ADVERSE REACTIONS
CNS: fever, *seizures,* somnolence, sedation.
EENT: nasal congestion. **GI:** salivary hypersecretion. **Musculoskeletal:** gait disturbance. **Respiratory:** bronchitis, URI. **Other:** flulike syndrome, seasonal allergy.

INTERACTIONS
Drug-drug. *CNS depressants (antidepressants, opioids):* May cause somnolence and sedation. Use cautiously together.

Strong or moderate CYP450 inducers (antiepileptic drugs [carbamazepine, phenobarbital, phenytoin, primidone], rifampin): May decrease ganaxolone level. Avoid use together. If use together is unavoidable, consider increasing ganaxolone dosage; don't exceed maximum daily dose. May need to increase ganaxolone dosage in patients on stable ganaxolone dosage who are starting or increasing enzyme-inducing antiepileptic drug doses; don't exceed maximum daily dose.
Drug-lifestyle. *Alcohol use:* May increase somnolence and sedation. Discourage use together.

EFFECTS ON LAB TEST RESULTS
None reported.

CONTRAINDICATIONS & CAUTIONS
• Use cautiously in patients with liver impairment or depression.
⚠ *Alert:* Drug may increase risk of suicidality as soon as first week of treatment.
• Drug has potential for abuse. Don't abruptly discontinue antiepileptic drugs due to risk of seizures.
• Safety and effectiveness in children younger than age 2 haven't been established.
Dialyzable drug: Unknown.

PREGNANCY-LACTATION-REPRODUCTION
• Studies during pregnancy are inadequate.
• Enroll patient exposed to drug during pregnancy in the North American Antiepileptic Drug Pregnancy Registry (1-888-233-2334 or www.aedpregnancyregistry.org).
• Drug appears in human milk. It isn't known how drug affects milk production or infant who is breastfed. Use cautiously during breastfeeding.

NURSING CONSIDERATIONS
• Monitor patient for somnolence and sedation.
⚠ *Alert:* Avoid abruptly discontinuing drug.
⚠ *Alert:* Monitor patient for emergence or worsening of depression, suicidality, or unusual changes in mood or behavior.
• Monitor patient for potential drug abuse or dependence. Taper drug as recommended, unless symptoms warrant immediate discontinuation.
• Monitor patient with liver impairment for adverse reactions.
• *Look alike–sound alike:* Don't confuse ganaxolone with oxandrolone or gabapentin. Don't confuse Ztalmy with Xtandi.

G

PATIENT TEACHING

• Teach about proper drug administration and handling.

• Explain that drug may cause somnolence. Caution patient not to drink alcohol, drive, or operate heavy machinery until drug's effects are known.

🕃 *Alert:* Instruct patient to avoid abrupt discontinuation of drug.

🕃 *Alert:* Warn that drug may increase risk of suicidality. Advise patient and family to report emergence or worsening of depression, suicidality, and unusual changes in mood or behavior.

• Caution patient about risk of abuse and dependence during therapy.

• Advise patient to report pregnancy or plans to become pregnant during therapy.

ganciclovir (DHPG)
gan-SYE-kloe-vir

Zirgan

Therapeutic class: Antivirals
Pharmacologic class: Nucleosides–nucleotides

AVAILABLE FORMS

Injection: 500 mg/vial; 500 mg/250 mL single-dose bag
Ophthalmic gel: 0.15%

INDICATIONS & DOSAGES

🕃 *Alert:* IV ganciclovir is indicated only for treatment of CMV retinitis in patients who are immunocompromised and for prevention of CMV disease in patients who have received a transplant and are at risk for CMV disease.

Adjust-a-dose (for all indications): Adjust IV dosage in patients with kidney impairment according to the table. If patient is receiving hemodialysis, give dose shortly after session is complete.

Initial IV therapy

CrCl (mL/min)	Dose (mg/kg)	Interval
50–69	2.5	12 hr
25–49	2.5	24 hr
10–24	1.25	24 hr
<10	1.25	3 times weekly after hemodialysis

Maintenance IV therapy

CrCl (mL/min)	Dose (mg/kg)	Interval
50–69	2.5	24 hr
25–49	1.25	24 hr
10–24	0.625	24 hr
<10	0.625	3 times weekly after hemodialysis

➤ **CMV retinitis in patients who are immunocompromised, including those with AIDS**
Adults: Induction treatment, 5 mg/kg IV every 12 hours for 14 to 21 days. Maintenance treatment, 5 mg/kg IV daily 7 days per week or 6 mg/kg IV once daily five times weekly.

➤ **Prevention of CMV disease in transplant recipients**
Adults: Initially, 5 mg/kg IV every 12 hours for 7 to 14 days; then 5 mg/kg daily 7 days per week or 6 mg/kg once daily five times weekly. Duration of therapy is 100 to 120 days posttransplantation.

➤ **Acute herpetic keratitis (Zirgan)**
Adults and children ages 2 and older: 1 drop in affected eye five times daily (approximately every 3 hours while awake) until corneal ulcer heals; then 1 drop t.i.d. for 7 days.

ADMINISTRATION

IV

🕃 *Alert:* Hazardous drug; use safe handling and disposal precautions.

▼ Avoid direct contact with skin and mucous membranes. If contact occurs, wash area thoroughly with soap and water; thoroughly rinse eyes with plain water.

▼ Inspect vial; discard if particulate matter or discoloration is visible.

▼ To reconstitute, add 10 mL of sterile water for injection to 500-mg vial. Gently swirl vial until solution appears clear. Don't use bacteriostatic water containing parabens because precipitation can result.

▼ Further dilute in 50 to 250 mL (usually 100 mL) of compatible IV solution.

▼ If fluids are being restricted, dilute to no more than 10 mg/mL.

▼ Don't give as rapid or bolus injection.

▼ Use an infusion pump.

▼ Infuse slowly over at least 1 hour at a constant rate. Infusing drug too rapidly increases toxicity.

▼ Redissolve any crystals that formed in premixed bag by gently shaking. Solution must be clear at time of use.

Reactions in bold italics are *life-threatening*.

G

⟁ Alert: Don't give subcut or IM.
▼ Flush IV line with NSS before and after administration.
▼ Reconstituted solution in vial is stable at room temperature for 12 hours. Don't refrigerate or freeze. Use solution within 24 hours of dilution to reduce risk of bacterial contamination.
▼ Diluted solutions for infusion should be refrigerated and used within 24 hours of preparation; don't freeze.
▼ Store commercially premixed solution at room temperature.
▼ **Incompatibilities:** None listed by manufacturer. Consult drug compatibility reference for more information.

Ophthalmic
• Store at 59° to 77° F (15° to 25° C). Don't freeze.

ACTION
Inhibits binding of deoxyguanosine triphosphate to DNA polymerase, resulting in inhibition of viral DNA synthesis.

Route	Onset	Peak	Duration
IV	Unknown	Immediate	Unknown
Ophthalmic	Unknown	Unknown	Unknown

Half-life: IV, about 2.6 to 4.4 hours; ophthalmic, unknown.

ADVERSE REACTIONS
CNS: fever, asthenia, headache, peripheral neuropathy. **EENT:** retinal detachment in patients with CMV retinitis; blurred vision, eye irritation, punctate keratitis, conjunctival hyperemia (ophthalmic). **GI:** abdominal pain, anorexia, diarrhea, nausea, vomiting. **GU:** increased serum creatinine level. **Hematologic:** anemia, *agranulocytosis, leukopenia, thrombocytopenia, neutropenia.* **Respiratory:** cough, dyspnea. **Skin:** diaphoresis, pruritus, pain and phlebitis at injection site. **Other:** *catheter sepsis,* catheter infection, *sepsis,* chills, infection.

INTERACTIONS
Drug-drug. *Amphotericin B, cyclosporine, other kidney-toxic drugs:* May increase risk of kidney toxicity. Monitor kidney function.
Cytotoxic drugs: May increase toxic effects, especially hematologic effects and stomatitis. Use together only if benefits outweigh risks; monitor patient closely.
Didanosine: May increase ganciclovir level. Monitor for adverse effects and decrease ganciclovir level as needed.

Imipenem–cilastatin: May increase seizure activity. Use together only if potential benefits outweigh risks.
Immunosuppressants (azathioprine, corticosteroids, cyclosporine, mycophenolate mofetil): May enhance immune and bone marrow suppression. Use together cautiously.
Probenecid: May increase ganciclovir level. Monitor patient closely.
Tenofovir products: May increase serum concentration of both drugs. Monitor therapy.
Zidovudine: May increase risk of agranulocytosis. Use together cautiously; monitor hematologic function closely.

EFFECTS ON LAB TEST RESULTS
• May increase ALP, ALT, AST, creatinine, and GGT levels.
• May decrease Hb level and granulocyte, neutrophil, platelet, and WBC counts.

CONTRAINDICATIONS & CAUTIONS
Boxed Warning Clinical toxicity of IV ganciclovir includes granulocytopenia, anemia, thrombocytopenia, and pancytopenia. Animal studies indicate that drug is carcinogenic and mutagenic. ■
• Contraindicated in patients hypersensitive to ganciclovir, valganciclovir, acyclovir, or components of the formulation.
• Drug isn't recommended in patients with ANC below 500/mm³, Hb below 8 g/dL, or platelet count below 25,000/mm³.
• Use cautiously and reduce dosage in patients with kidney dysfunction. Monitor kidney function test results.
Dialyzable drug: About 50%.
⚠ Overdose S&S: Myelosuppression, bone marrow failure, hepatitis, kidney toxicity, seizures (all with IV form).

PREGNANCY-LACTATION-REPRODUCTION
Boxed Warning Based on animal studies, IV ganciclovir may be teratogenic or embryotoxic at recommended doses. ■
• Use during pregnancy only if potential benefits justify fetal risk.
• Patients of childbearing potential should use effective contraception during treatment and for 30 days after final dose. Males should practice barrier contraception during treatment and for at least 90 days after final dose.
• Breastfeeding isn't recommended during treatment or by patient who tests positive for

HIV. Timing of safe resumption of breastfeeding after final dose isn't known.

Boxed Warning Based on animal data, IV drug at recommended doses may cause temporary or permanent aspermatogenesis in males and may cause suppression of fertility in females. ∎

NURSING CONSIDERATIONS

• Verify pregnancy status before start of treatment.
• Frequently monitor CBC and platelet count, especially in patient with prior drug-induced cytopenia or baseline ANC below 1,000/mm^3.
• Carefully monitor kidney function before and during treatment, particularly in older adult or patient taking other kidney-toxic drugs.
• Monitor ophthalmologic disease status during treatment.

PATIENT TEACHING

• Explain importance of drinking plenty of fluids during therapy.
• Instruct patient to promptly report adverse reactions.
• Tell patient to report discomfort at IV insertion site.
Boxed Warning Advise patient that IV use may impair fertility. ∎
• Warn patient of fetal risk. Instruct about contraceptive use.
• With IV use, advise patient to use soft toothbrush and electric razor because of increased bleeding risk.
• Emphasize importance of adhering to blood work as requested by prescriber.
• Instruct patient not to let sterile eye dropper touch any surface.
• Caution patient not to wear contact lenses while undergoing ophthalmic treatment.
• Advise patient undergoing ophthalmic treatment to notify prescriber if eye pain, redness, itching, or inflammation becomes aggravated.

SAFETY ALERT!

gemcitabine hydrochloride
jem-SITE-ah-been

Infugem

Therapeutic class: Antineoplastics
Pharmacologic class: Pyrimidine analogues

AVAILABLE FORMS

Injection: 10 mg/mL premixed infusion bag
Powder for injection: 200-mg, 1-g vials
Solution for injection: 200-mg, 1-g, 1.5-g, 2-g vials

INDICATIONS & DOSAGES

Adjust-a-dose (for all indications): If patient is on hemodialysis, begin hemodialysis 6 to 12 hours after drug infusion. If serum bilirubin level is greater than 1.6 mg/dL, use initial dose of 800 mg/m^2 and escalate if tolerated. Refer to manufacturer's instructions for toxicity-related dosage adjustments. Refer to prescribing information for carboplatin, cisplatin, or paclitaxel for more information about combination therapy.

➤ **Locally advanced (nonresectable stage II or III) or metastatic (stage IV) adenocarcinoma of pancreas in patients previously treated with 5-FU**
Adults: 1,000 mg/m^2 IV over 30 minutes once weekly for 7 weeks, followed by 1 week rest, unless toxicity occurs. Subsequent cycles should consist of infusions once weekly on days 1, 8, and 15 of each 28-day cycle.

➤ **With cisplatin, first-line treatment of inoperable, locally advanced (stage IIIA or IIIB) or metastatic (stage IV) NSCLC**
Adults: For 28-day cycle, 1,000 mg/m^2 IV over 30 minutes on days 1, 8, and 15 of each cycle; cisplatin 100 mg/m^2 IV on day 1 after gemcitabine infusion. For 21-day cycle, 1,250 mg/m^2 IV over 30 minutes on days 1 and 8 of each cycle; cisplatin 100 mg/m^2 IV on day 1 after gemcitabine infusion.

➤ **With carboplatin, treatment of advanced ovarian cancer that relapsed at least 6 months after platinum-based therapy**
Adults: 1,000 mg/m^2 IV over 30 minutes on days 1 and 8 of each 21-day cycle; carboplatin IV on day 1 after gemcitabine infusion.

➤ **With paclitaxel, metastatic breast cancer (first-line treatment after failure of adjuvant anthracycline chemotherapy)**
Adults: 1,250 mg/m^2 IV over 30 minutes on days 1 and 8 of each 21-day cycle; paclitaxel 175 mg/m^2 as 3-hour IV infusion on day 1 before gemcitabine.

➤ **Pancreatic cancer (adjuvant therapy)** ◆
Adults: 1,000 mg/m^2 IV on days 1, 8, and 15 every 28 days (combination with capecitabine) for six cycles beginning within 12 weeks of resection.

Reactions in bold italics are *life-threatening*.

➤ **Bladder cancer (advanced or metastatic)** ◆

Adults: 1,000 mg/m^2 IV over 30 to 60 minutes days 1, 8, and 15; repeat cycle every 28 days (in combination with cisplatin); or, 1,000 mg/m^2 IV over 30 minutes days 1 and 8; repeat cycle every 21 days (in combination with carboplatin) until disease progression or unacceptable toxicity occurs.

➤ **Biliary tract cancer (advanced or metastatic)** ◆

Adults: 1,000 mg/m^2 IV over 30 minutes days 1 and 8; repeat cycle every 21 days (in combination with cisplatin). Or, 1,000 mg/m^2 IV over 30 minutes days 1 and 8; repeat cycle every 21 days (in combination with capecitabine). Or, 1,000 mg/m^2 IV infused at 10 mg/m^2/minute every 2 weeks (in combination with oxaliplatin).

ADMINISTRATION

IV

⟲ *Alert:* Hazardous drug; use safe handling and disposal precautions.

▼ Reconstitute lyophilized powder by adding 5 mL of preservative-free NSS for injection to 200-mg vial, 25 mL to 1-g vial, or 50 mL to 2-g vial, resulting in a concentration of 38 mg/mL. Concentration higher than 40 mg/mL isn't recommended.

▼ Further dilute reconstituted powder or concentrated solution with NSS to concentration of at least 0.1 mg/mL.

▼ Make sure solution is clear to light straw-colored and free of particles.

▼ Drug remains stable for 24 hours at room temperature.

▼ Don't refrigerate reconstituted drug because it may crystallize.

▼ Premixed bags remain stable until package expiration date when stored at 68° to 77° F (20° to 25° C). Don't freeze premixed bags; crystallization can occur.

▼ **Incompatibilities:** None listed by manufacturer. Consult drug compatibility reference for more information.

ACTION

Cytotoxic and specific to the S-phase of the cell cycle; inhibits DNA synthesis.

Route	Onset	Peak	Duration
IV	Unknown	30 min	Unknown

Half-life: About 1.7 to 19.4 hours for active metabolite (influenced by length of the infusion, age, and sex).

ADVERSE REACTIONS

CNS: drowsiness, paresthesia, fever. **CV:** edema, peripheral edema, *hemorrhage.* **GI:** stomatitis, nausea, vomiting, diarrhea. **GU:** proteinuria, hematuria, increased BUN, increased creatinine. **Hematologic:** anemia, *neutropenia, thrombocytopenia.* **Hepatic:** *liver toxicity,* increased AST and ALT levels, increased alkaline phosphatase level, hyperbilirubinemia. **Respiratory:** dyspnea, *bronchospasm.* **Skin:** alopecia, rash. **Other:** flulike syndrome, infection, injection-site reactions.

INTERACTIONS

Drug-drug. *Bleomycin:* May increase risk of pulmonary toxicity. Monitor therapy.

Clozapine: May increase risk of neutropenia. Monitor therapy.

Inactivated vaccines: May decrease effectiveness of vaccines. Give inactivated vaccine at least 2 weeks before gemcitabine therapy or revaccinate at least 3 months after therapy completion.

Live-virus vaccines: May increase risk of vaccine-induced adverse reactions. Defer use of live-virus vaccines.

Warfarin: May increase anticoagulant effect of warfarin. Monitor patient and INR.

EFFECTS ON LAB TEST RESULTS

● May increase ALP, ALT, AST, bilirubin, BUN, creatinine, and urine protein levels.

● May decrease Hb level and neutrophil, platelet, and WBC counts.

CONTRAINDICATIONS & CAUTIONS

● Contraindicated in patients hypersensitive to drug.

● Use cautiously in patients with kidney or liver impairment.

● Use cautiously when given within 7 days of radiation therapy. Life-threatening mucositis can occur with concurrent use. Radiation recall has been reported with prior radiation therapy.

● Prolonging infusion duration beyond 60 minutes or administering more frequently than weekly has resulted in an increased incidence of toxicities, including hypotension, severe flulike symptoms, myelosuppression, and asthenia.

● Drug increases risk of capillary leak syndrome, hemolytic-uremic syndrome (HUS), and PRES.

G

• Myelosuppression (manifested by neutropenia, thrombocytopenia, and anemia) occurs when gemcitabine is used alone; risk increases when combined with other cytotoxic drugs.

• Pulmonary toxicity (interstitial pneumonitis, pulmonary fibrosis, pulmonary edema, ARDS) has been reported; it may lead to sometimes fatal respiratory failure despite discontinuation of therapy.

• Serious liver toxicity, including liver failure and death, has been reported with gemcitabine alone or in combination with other potentially liver-toxic drugs. Use cautiously in patients with concurrent liver metastases or preexisting medical history of hepatitis, alcoholism, or liver cirrhosis.

• Safety and effectiveness in children haven't been determined.

Dialyzable drug: 50% for dFdU metabolite. Unknown for peritoneal dialysis.

⚠ *Overdose S&S:* Myelosuppression, paresthesia, severe rash.

PREGNANCY-LACTATION-REPRODUCTION
• Studies during pregnancy are inadequate. Drug can cause fetal harm. If drug is used during pregnancy or if patient becomes pregnant during therapy, apprise patient of potential fetal hazard.

• Patient should discontinue breastfeeding during treatment and for at least 1 week after final dose.

• Advise patient of childbearing potential to use effective contraception during treatment and for 6 months after final dose.

• Advise males with partners of childbearing potential to use effective contraception during treatment and for 3 months after final dose.

• May impair fertility in males of reproductive potential.

NURSING CONSIDERATIONS
• Verify pregnancy status before start of treatment.

• Monitor patient closely. Modify dosage according to toxicity and degree of myelosuppression. Age, gender, and presence of kidney impairment may predispose patient to toxicity.

• Monitor CBC with differential and platelet count before each dose. Increase monitoring as needed during combination therapy.

• Obtain baseline and periodic LFTs.

• Monitor for HUS. Monitor for anemia with microangiopathic hemolysis (elevated bilirubin

or LDH level, reticulocytosis, severe thrombocytopenia, KF), and monitor kidney function at baseline and periodically during treatment. Permanently discontinue if HUS or severe kidney impairment occurs; KF may not be reversible despite discontinuation.

• Monitor for pulmonary toxicity. Onset of pulmonary symptoms may occur up to 2 weeks after last dose of gemcitabine. Discontinue for unexplained dyspnea, with or without bronchospasm, or other evidence of pulmonary toxicity.

• Monitor for PRES (headache, seizure, lethargy, HTN, confusion, blindness, other visual and neurologic disturbances). Confirm PRES diagnosis with MRI; discontinue gemcitabine if PRES develops during therapy.

• *Look alike–sound alike:* Don't confuse gemcitabine with gemtuzumab.

PATIENT TEACHING
• Advise patient to report all adverse reactions and to immediately report evidence of infection (fever, sore throat, fatigue) and bleeding (easy bruising, nosebleeds, bleeding gums, melena). Tell patient to take temperature daily.

• Caution patient to immediately report changes in color or volume of urine output.

• Instruct patient to promptly report flulike symptoms, breathing problems, abdominal pain, or yellowing of skin.

• Tell patient that adverse effects may continue after treatment ends.

• Instruct patient to report pregnancy or plans to become pregnant or to breastfeed. Counsel patient with reproductive potential about contraceptive use.

---

gemfibrozil
jem-FI-broe-zil

Lopid

Therapeutic class: Antilipemics
Pharmacologic class: Fibric acid derivatives

AVAILABLE FORMS
Tablets: 600 mg

INDICATIONS & DOSAGES
➤ **Adjunct to diet in adults with hypertriglyceridemia (types IV and V hyperlipidemia)**

who are unresponsive to diet and at risk for pancreatitis; to reduce risk of CAD in patients without CAD symptoms and with type IIb hyperlipidemia who are refractory to treatment with diet, exercise, and other drugs and who have low HDL-C levels and elevated LDL-C and triglyceride levels
Adults: 600 mg PO b.i.d.

ADMINISTRATION

PO
- Give drug 30 minutes before breakfast and dinner.
- Store at room temperature.

ACTION

Inhibits peripheral lipolysis and reduces triglyceride synthesis in the liver; lowers triglyceride and VLDL-C levels and increases HDL-C levels.

Route	Onset	Peak	Duration
PO	2–5 days	1–2 hr	Unknown

Half-life: 1.5 hours.

ADVERSE REACTIONS

CNS: fatigue, headache, vertigo. **GI:** abdominal pain, dyspepsia, acute appendicitis, constipation, diarrhea, nausea, vomiting. **Hepatic:** cholelithiasis, cholecystitis. **Skin:** dermatitis, eczema, pruritus, rash.

INTERACTIONS

Drug-drug. *Bile acid sequestrants (colestipol):* May decrease absorption of fibric acid derivatives. Separate doses by at least 2 hours to minimize interaction; fenofibric acid labeling recommends giving drug 1 hour before or 4 to 6 hours after a bile acid sequestrant.
Colchicine: May increase risk of myopathy, especially in patients with kidney dysfunction and in older adults. Use cautiously.
Cyclosporine: May decrease cyclosporine level and increase risk of kidney toxicity. Monitor kidney function and cyclosporine level, and adjust dose as needed.
CYP2C8, CYP2C9, CYP2C19, OATP1B1 substrates (bosentan, dabrafenib, glyburide, loperamide, montelukast, olmesartan, paclitaxel, rosiglitazone, rifampin): May increase levels of substrates metabolized through these enzymes. Consider therapy modification or decrease substrate dose.

Dasabuvir: May prolong QT interval and increase risk of ventricular arrhythmias. Use together is contraindicated.
Enzalutamide: May increase enzalutamide exposure and risk of seizures. If use together is unavoidable, reduce enzalutamide dose.
Ezetimibe: May enhance adverse or toxic effect of ezetimibe; may increase risk of myopathy and cholelithiasis. Avoid combination.
Glyburide, pioglitazone: May increase hypoglycemic effects. Monitor glucose level, and watch for signs of hypoglycemia.
HMG-CoA reductase inhibitors: May cause myopathy with rhabdomyolysis. Avoid use together. Use with simvastatin is contraindicated.
Repaglinide: May increase risk of severe hypoglycemia. Use together is contraindicated.
Selexipag: May increase selexipag exposure. Use together is contraindicated.
Warfarin: May prolong PT and increase bleeding risk. Reduce warfarin dosage and monitor PT and INR.

EFFECTS ON LAB TEST RESULTS

- May increase ALT, AST, ALP, bilirubin, and CK levels.
- May decrease Hb level, hematocrit, and eosinophil, WBC, and platelet counts.

CONTRAINDICATIONS & CAUTIONS

- Contraindicated in patients hypersensitive to drug and in those with liver (including primary biliary cirrhosis) or severe kidney dysfunction or gallbladder disease.
- Evaluate patient for secondary causes of hyperlipidemia before use.
- May increase risk of malignancy, gallstones, and myositis.
- Safety and effectiveness in children haven't been established.

Dialyzable drug: Unknown.

⚠ *Overdose S&S:* Abdominal cramps, abnormal LFT values, diarrhea, increased CK level, joint and muscle pain, nausea, and vomiting.

PREGNANCY-LACTATION-REPRODUCTION

- Drug may cause fetal harm based on animal studies. Use in pregnancy only if potential benefit justifies fetal risk.
- Patient should discontinue breastfeeding or discontinue drug, considering importance of drug to patient.

NURSING CONSIDERATIONS

- Periodically check CBC and LFT values during first 12 months of therapy.
- Monitor serum cholesterol level. If drug shows no benefit after 3 months of therapy, stop drug.
- Assess for signs of myopathy. If suspected or diagnosed, discontinue therapy.

PATIENT TEACHING

- Instruct patient to take drug 30 minutes before breakfast and dinner.
- Teach patient about proper dietary management of cholesterol and triglycerides. When appropriate, recommend weight control, exercise, and smoking cessation programs.
- Because of possible dizziness and blurred vision, advise patient to avoid driving and other hazardous activities until effects of drug are known.
- Tell patient to observe bowel movements and to report evidence of excess fat in feces or other signs of bile duct obstruction.
- Advise patient to report all adverse reactions and muscle pain to prescriber.
- Instruct patient to report pregnancy or plans to become pregnant or to breastfeed.

gentamicin sulfate (injection)
jen-ta-MYE-sin

Therapeutic class: Antibiotics
Pharmacologic class: Aminoglycosides

AVAILABLE FORMS
Injection: 10 mg/mL, 40 mg/mL
IV infusion (premixed): 60 mg, 80 mg, 100 mg in 50 mL NSS; 80 mg, 100 mg, 120 mg in 100 mL NSS

INDICATIONS & DOSAGES
➤ **Serious infections caused by sensitive strains of** *Pseudomonas aeruginosa,* *Escherichia coli, Proteus, Klebsiella,* *Enterobacter, Serratia, Citrobacter,* **or** *Staphylococcus*
Adults: 3 mg/kg IM or IV infusion daily in three divided doses every 8 hours. For life-threatening infection, up to 5 mg/kg daily in divided doses every 6 to 8 hours; reduced to 3 mg/kg daily as soon as patient improves.
Children: 2 to 2.5 mg/kg IM or IV infusion every 8 hours.

Neonates older than 1 week and infants: 2.5 mg/kg IM or IV infusion every 8 hours.
Neonates 1 week of age or younger and preterm infants: 2.5 mg/kg IM or IV infusion every 12 hours.
Adjust-a-dose: For adults with impaired kidney function, dosages and frequency are determined by serum drug level and creatinine level. Refer to manufacturer's instructions for kidney function dosage adjustments. To maintain therapeutic levels, adults should receive 1 to 1.7 mg/kg IM or IV infusion after each dialysis session, and children should receive 2 to 2.5 mg/kg IM or IV infusion after each dialysis session, depending on severity of the infection.

ADMINISTRATION
- Obtain specimen for culture and sensitivity tests before giving. Begin therapy while awaiting results.
IV
▼ For intermittent infusion, dilute vial with 50 to 200 mL of D₅W or NSS for injection. For infants and children, the diluent volume should be less, but allow for accurate measurement and administration. Maximum concentration isn't addressed by the manufacturer; the concentration of the pediatric-specific product is 10 mg/mL.
▼ Infuse over 30 minutes to 2 hours.
▼ After completing infusion, flush the line with NSS or D₅W.
▼ Premixed, single-dose, flexible containers should be administered IV only.
▼ Store at room temperature.
▼ **Incompatibilities:** Don't physically premix gentamicin with other drugs; administer separately according to the recommended route of administration and dosage schedule.
IM
- Give undiluted. Gentamicin in NSS isn't intended for IM administration.

ACTION
Inhibits protein synthesis by binding directly to the 30S ribosomal subunit; bactericidal.

Route	Onset	Peak	Duration
IV	Immediate	30–60 min	Unknown
IM	Unknown	30–90 min	Unknown

Half-life: 2 to 3 hours; longer in patients with kidney impairment and in infants.

Reactions in bold italics are *life-threatening*.

ADVERSE REACTIONS

CNS: fever, headache, lethargy, confusion, dizziness, numbness, depression, peripheral neuropathy, tingling, vertigo, pseudotumor cerebri. **CV:** hypotension, HTN. **EENT:** vision disturbance, tinnitus, ototoxicity, increased salivation. **GI:** vomiting, nausea, decreased appetite, stomatitis. **GU:** increased BUN and creatinine levels; oliguria; *kidney toxicity;* increased urine protein, cells, or casts. **Hematologic:** *granulocytopenia, transient agranulocytosis, leukopenia, thrombocytopenia,* anemia, eosinophilia. **Metabolic:** weight loss. **Musculoskeletal:** muscle twitching, joint pain. **Respiratory:** laryngeal edema, pulmonary fibrosis. **Skin:** rash, urticaria, pruritus, burning sensation, alopecia, purpura, injection-site pain. **Other:** *anaphylactoid reaction.*

INTERACTIONS

Drug-drug. **Boxed Warning** *Amikacin, cephaloridine, cisplatin, colistin, kanamycin, neomycin, polymyxin B, streptomycin, tobramycin, vancomycin, viomycin, other potentially neurotoxic or kidney-toxic drugs:* May increase kidney toxicity and neurotoxicity (manifested by ototoxicity). Monitor hearing, serum drug levels, and kidney function test results. Avoid concurrent or sequential use. ■

Atracurium, pancuronium, rocuronium, vecuronium: May increase effects of nondepolarizing muscle relaxants, including prolonged respiratory depression. Use together only when necessary, and expect to reduce dosage of nondepolarizing muscle relaxant.

Bisphosphonate derivatives: May enhance hypocalcemic effect of bisphosphonate derivatives. Monitor therapy.

General anesthetics: May increase neuromuscular blockade. Monitor patient closely.

Boxed Warning *IV loop diuretics (ethacrynic acid, furosemide):* May increase risk of ototoxicity. Avoid use together. ■

Parenteral penicillins (ampicillin): May inactivate gentamicin in vitro. Don't mix together.

EFFECTS ON LAB TEST RESULTS

• May increase ALT, AST, bilirubin, BUN, creatinine, LDH, and nonprotein nitrogen levels.
• May decrease serum calcium, magnesium, sodium, and potassium levels.
• May increase eosinophil count.
• May decrease Hb level and platelet and WBC counts.

CONTRAINDICATIONS & CAUTIONS

• Contraindicated in patients hypersensitive to drug or other aminoglycosides.
• Use cautiously in neonates, infants, older adults, and patients with impaired kidney function or neuromuscular disorders.
• Use drug for short-term treatment, if possible. Prolonged use may result in toxicity or fungal or bacterial superinfection, including CDAD.

Dializable drug: 50%.

⚠ *Overdose S&S:* Kidney toxicity, neurotoxicity, ototoxicity.

PREGNANCY-LACTATION-REPRODUCTION

Boxed Warning Aminoglycosides can cause fetal harm when used during pregnancy. ■
• If drug is used during pregnancy or if patient becomes pregnant during therapy, apprise patient of risk to fetus (deafness).
• Drug appears in human milk. Use cautiously during breastfeeding.

NURSING CONSIDERATIONS

Boxed Warning Evaluate patient's hearing before and during therapy. Notify prescriber if patient complains of tinnitus, vertigo, or hearing loss. Anticipate dosage adjustment or drug discontinuation. ■
• Weigh patient and review kidney function studies before therapy begins.

🔆 *Alert:* Use preservative-free form for intrathecal or intraventricular route when used adjunctively for serious CNS infections, such as meningitis and ventriculitis.

Boxed Warning Maintain peak levels at 4 to 12 mcg/mL and trough levels at 1 to 2 mcg/mL. Prolonged peak levels above 12 mcg/mL or prolonged trough levels greater than 2 mcg/mL may increase risk of toxicity. Hemodialysis may help remove gentamicin, especially with compromised kidney function. Peritoneal dialysis is considerably less effective than hemodialysis. ■
• Obtain blood for peak level 1 hour after IM injection or 30 minutes after IV infusion finishes; for trough levels, draw blood just before next dose. Don't collect blood in a heparinized tube; heparin is incompatible with aminoglycosides.

G

♣Canada ◇OTC ♦Off-label use 🔵Do not crush *Liquid contains alcohol ✂Genetic

Boxed Warning Kidney toxicity risk is greater in patients with kidney impairment and in those who receive high-dosage or prolonged therapy. Monitor kidney function (urine output, specific gravity, urinalysis, BUN and creatinine levels, CrCl). Report declining kidney function to prescriber. ∎

Boxed Warning Older adults and patients with dehydration are at increased risk for toxicity. ∎

• Watch for signs and symptoms of superinfection (continued fever, chills, increased pulse rate, diarrhea).

• Therapy usually continues for 7 to 10 days. If no response occurs in 3 to 5 days, stop therapy and obtain new specimens for culture and sensitivity testing.

PATIENT TEACHING

• Instruct patient to promptly report adverse reactions (vision changes, dizziness, vertigo, unsteady gait, ringing in ears, hearing loss, numbness, tingling, muscle twitching, seizures, changes in urine amount, edema).

• Encourage patient to drink plenty of fluids to avoid dehydration.

• Warn patient to avoid hazardous activities if adverse CNS reactions occur.

SAFETY ALERT!

glatiramer acetate
gla-TIR-a-mer

Copaxone, Glatopa

Therapeutic class: MS drugs
Pharmacologic class: Biological response modifiers

AVAILABLE FORMS

Injection: 20 mg glatiramer acetate and 40 mg mannitol (20 mg/mL); 40 mg glatiramer acetate and 40 mg mannitol (40 mg/mL) single-use prefilled syringe

INDICATIONS & DOSAGES

➤ **Relapsing forms of MS, including clinically isolated syndrome, relapsing-remitting disease, and active secondary progressive disease**
Adults: 20 mg subcut daily, or 40 mg subcut three times per week given at least 48 hours apart.

ADMINISTRATION
Subcutaneous

⚠ *Alert:* 20 mg/mL and 40 mg/mL formulations of glatiramer aren't interchangeable.

• Give drug only subcut in arms, abdomen, hips, or thighs; rotate injection sites to prevent lipoatrophy. Don't give IV.

• Give 40-mg dose on same 3 days each week (Monday, Wednesday, Friday) at least 48 hours apart.

• Allow drug to warm for 20 minutes at room temperature before use.

• Drug doesn't contain preservatives; discard if solution appears cloudy or contains particulate matter.

• Don't try to expel air bubble from prefilled syringe; doing so can lead to loss of drug and incorrect dose.

• An optional autoinjector is available by separate prescription for use with Copaxone or Glatopa. Ensure autoinjector is compatible before use to avoid administering a partial dose or other medication error.

• Store drug in refrigerator (36° to 46° F [2° to 8° C]). Don't freeze; discard if syringe freezes.

• If refrigeration isn't available, store at room temperature for up to 1 month.

• Avoid exposure to higher temperatures, and protect from intense light.

ACTION

May modify immune processes responsible for the pathogenesis of MS.

Route	Onset	Peak	Duration
Subcut	Unknown	Unknown	Unknown

Half-life: Unknown.

ADVERSE REACTIONS

CNS: anxiety, asthenia, abnormal dreams, emotional lability, fever, migraine, nervousness, pain, speech disorder, stupor, syncope, tremor. **CV:** chest pain, palpitations, vasodilation, HTN, tachycardia, edema. **EENT:** eye disorder, diplopia, visual field deficit, rhinitis, oral candidiasis, salivary gland enlargement, dental caries, *laryngospasm,* nasopharyngitis. **GI:** nausea, dysphagia, bowel urgency, gastroenteritis, ulcerative stomatitis, vomiting. **GU:** urinary urgency, *vaginal hemorrhage,* abnormal Papanicolaou smear, amenorrhea, hematuria, erectile dysfunction, menorrhagia, vaginal candidiasis. **Hematologic:** lymphadenopathy. **Metabolic:** weight gain. **Musculoskeletal:** arthralgia, back pain. **Respiratory:** dyspnea, cough, bronchitis, hyperventilation. **Skin:** diaphoresis, injection-site reaction, pruritus, rash, eczema, erythema, residual mass at injection site, benign neoplasm (cyst, polyp), skin atrophy, urticaria, warts. **Other:** infection, hypersensitivity, flulike syndrome, abscess, chills, hay fever, herpes simplex and zoster.

INTERACTIONS

Drug-drug. *Denosumab, natalizumab, roflumilast:* May increase risk of serious infection. Consider therapy modification.
Leflunomide: May increase risk of hematologic toxicity, such as pancytopenia, agranulocytosis, or thrombocytopenia. Consider therapy modification.
Live-virus vaccines: Immunosuppressants may enhance adverse or toxic effects of live-virus vaccines. Avoid use for at least 3 months after immunosuppressive therapy.
Pimecrolimus, tacrolimus (topical): May enhance adverse or toxic effect of immunosuppressants. Avoid this combination.
Tofacitinib: May enhance immunosuppressive effect of tofacitinib. Avoid combination.
Trastuzumab: May enhance neutropenic effect of immunosuppressants. Monitor therapy.
Drug-herb. *Echinacea:* May diminish therapeutic effect of immunosuppressants. Consider therapy modification.

EFFECTS ON LAB TEST RESULTS

• May increase cholesterol level and LFT values.
• May diminish diagnostic effect of coccidioidin skin test.

CONTRAINDICATIONS & CAUTIONS

• Contraindicated in patients hypersensitive to drug or mannitol.
• Drug may increase risk of infection and liver injury.
• Safety and effectiveness in children haven't been established.
Dialyzable drug: Unknown.

PREGNANCY-LACTATION-REPRODUCTION

• Studies during pregnancy are inadequate. Use in pregnancy only if clearly needed.

• It's unknown if drug is present in human milk. Use cautiously during breastfeeding.

NURSING CONSIDERATIONS

• Immediate postinjection reactions (flushing, chest pain, palpitations, anxiety, dyspnea, throat constriction, urticaria) may occur. They typically are transient and self-limiting and don't need specific treatment. Onset of postinjection reaction may occur several months after treatment starts, and patient may have more than one episode.
• Patient may experience at least one episode of transient chest pain, which usually begins at least 1 month after treatment starts and isn't accompanied by other signs or symptoms.
• Monitor patient for injection-site reactions (lipoatrophy, skin necrosis).
• Monitor patient for signs or symptoms of liver dysfunction (nausea, anorexia, fatigue, jaundice, dark-colored urine, pale stools, increased bleeding or bruising).

PATIENT TEACHING

• Instruct patient or caregiver how to self-inject drug. Supervise first injection.
• Tell patient to rotate injection sites daily.
• Explain need for aseptic self-injection techniques, and warn patient against reuse of needles and syringes.
• Periodically review proper disposal of needles, syringes, drug containers, and unused drug.
• Instruct patient to notify prescriber about planned, suspected, or known pregnancy or plans to breastfeed.
• Advise patient not to change drug or dosage schedule or to stop drug without medical approval.
• Tell patient to notify prescriber of all adverse reactions and to immediately report dizziness, flushing, fast heartbeat, anxiety, breathing problems or tightness in throat, swelling, rash, itching, hives, diaphoresis, chest pain, or severe pain after drug injection.
• Warn patient to seek medical attention for chest pain of unusual duration or intensity.
• Explain that an autoinjector may be prescribed for Copaxone or Glatopa. Instruct patient to ensure syringe compatibility before use.

glecaprevir–pibrentasvir ⓄⓃⒸ
glek-A-pre-vir/pi-BRENT-as-vir

Mavyret

Therapeutic class: Antivirals
Pharmacologic class: HCV NS3/4A
protease inhibitors–HCV NS5A inhibitors

AVAILABLE FORMS
Oral pellets ⓄⓃⒸ: 50 mg glecaprevir/20 mg
pibrentasvir
Tablets: 100 mg glecaprevir/40 mg
pibrentasvir

INDICATIONS & DOSAGES
Adjust-a-dose (for all indications): In patients
ages 3 and older who have received a liver or
kidney transplant, a 12-week treatment duration is recommended. In patients with a genotype 1 infection who are NS5A inhibitor–
experienced without prior treatment with an
NS3/4A protease inhibitor or patients with
genotype 3 infection, a 16-week treatment duration is recommended.

➤ **Chronic HCV genotype 1, 2, 3, 4, 5, or
6 infection in patients who are treatment-
naive without cirrhosis or with compensated cirrhosis (Child-Pugh class A)** ▧
*Adults and children ages 12 and older or
weighing at least 45 kg:* 3 tablets (total daily
dose of 300 mg glecaprevir/120 mg pibrentasvir) PO once daily for 8 weeks.
*Children ages 3 and older or weighing at
least 45 kg:* 300 mg glecaprevir/120 mg pibrentasvir PO once daily for 8 weeks.
*Children ages 3 and older or weighing 30 to
less than 45 kg:* 250 mg glecaprevir/100 mg
pibrentasvir PO once daily for 8 weeks.
*Children ages 3 and older weighing 20 to
less than 30 kg:* 200 mg glecaprevir/80 mg
pibrentasvir PO once daily for 8 weeks.
*Children ages 3 and older weighing less than
20 kg:* 150 mg glecaprevir/60 mg pibrentasvir
PO once daily for 8 weeks.

➤ **HCV genotype 1 infection with or without compensated cirrhosis (Child-Pugh
class A) in patients previously treated with
regimen containing an HCV NS5A inhibitor but without an NS3/4A protease
inhibitor (PI)** ▧
*Adults and children ages 12 and older or
weighing at least 45 kg:* 3 tablets (total daily
dose of 300 mg glecaprevir/120 mg pibrentasvir) PO once daily for 16 weeks.
*Children ages 3 and older or weighing at
least 45 kg:* 300 mg glecaprevir/120 mg pibrentasvir PO once daily for 16 weeks.
*Children ages 3 and older or weighing 30 to
less than 45 kg:* 250 mg glecaprevir/100 mg
pibrentasvir PO once daily for 16 weeks.
*Children ages 3 and older weighing 20 to
less than 30 kg:* 200 mg glecaprevir/80 mg
pibrentasvir PO once daily for 16 weeks.
*Children ages 3 and older weighing less than
20 kg:* 150 mg glecaprevir/60 mg pibrentasvir
PO once daily for 16 weeks.

➤ **HCV genotype 1 infection with or without compensated cirrhosis (Child-Pugh
class A) in patients who previously received
an NS3/4A PI without prior treatment with
an NS5A inhibitor** ▧
*Adults and children ages 12 and older or
weighing at least 45 kg:* 3 tablets (total daily
dose of 300 mg glecaprevir/120 mg pibrentasvir) PO once daily for 12 weeks.
*Children ages 3 and older or weighing at
least 45 kg:* 300 mg glecaprevir/120 mg pibrentasvir PO once daily for 12 weeks.
*Children ages 3 and older or weighing 30 to
less than 45 kg:* 250 mg glecaprevir/100 mg
pibrentasvir PO once daily for 12 weeks.
*Children ages 3 and older weighing 20 to
less than 30 kg:* 200 mg glecaprevir/80 mg
pibrentasvir PO once daily for 12 weeks.
*Children ages 3 and older weighing less than
20 kg:* 150 mg glecaprevir/60 mg pibrentasvir
PO once daily for 12 weeks.

➤ **HCV genotype 1, 2, 4, 5, or 6 infection
without cirrhosis in patients who previously received regimens containing interferon, pegylated interferon, ribavirin, or
sofosbuvir but have no prior treatment experience with an HCV NS3/4A PI or NS5A
inhibitor** ▧
*Adults and children ages 12 and older or
weighing at least 45 kg:* 3 tablets (total daily
dose of 300 mg glecaprevir/120 mg pibrentasvir) PO once daily for 8 weeks.
*Children ages 3 and older or weighing at
least 45 kg:* 300 mg glecaprevir/120 mg pibrentasvir PO once daily for 8 weeks.
*Children ages 3 and older or weighing 30 to
less than 45 kg:* 250 mg glecaprevir/100 mg
pibrentasvir PO once daily for 8 weeks.
*Children ages 3 and older weighing 20 to
less than 30 kg:* 200 mg glecaprevir/80 mg
pibrentasvir PO once daily for 8 weeks.

Children ages 3 and older weighing less than 20 kg: 150 mg glecaprevir/60 mg pibrentasvir PO once daily for 8 weeks.

➤ **HCV genotype 1, 2, 4, 5, or 6 infection and compensated cirrhosis (Child-Pugh class A) in patients who previously received regimen containing interferon, pegylated interferon, ribavirin, or sofosbuvir but have no prior treatment experience with an HCV NS3/4A PI or NS5A inhibitor** ▧

Adults and children ages 12 and older or weighing at least 45 kg: 3 tablets (total daily dose of 300 mg glecaprevir/120 mg pibrentasvir) PO once daily for 12 weeks.

Children ages 3 and older or weighing at least 45 kg: 300 mg glecaprevir/120 mg pibrentasvir PO once daily for 12 weeks.

Children ages 3 and older or weighing 30 to less than 45 kg: 250 mg glecaprevir/100 mg pibrentasvir PO once daily for 12 weeks.

Children ages 3 and older weighing 20 to less than 30 kg: 200 mg glecaprevir/80 mg pibrentasvir PO once daily for 12 weeks.

Children ages 3 and older weighing less than 20 kg: 150 mg glecaprevir/60 mg pibrentasvir PO once daily for 12 weeks.

➤ **HCV genotype 3 infection with or without cirrhosis (Child-Pugh class A) in patients who previously received regimen containing interferon, pegylated interferon, ribavirin, or sofosbuvir but have no prior treatment experience with an HCV NS3/4A PI or NS5A inhibitor** ▧

Adults and children ages 12 and older or weighing at least 45 kg: 3 tablets (total daily dose of 300 mg glecaprevir/120 mg pibrentasvir) PO once daily for 16 weeks.

Children ages 3 and older or weighing at least 45 kg: 300 mg glecaprevir/120 mg pibrentasvir PO once daily for 16 weeks.

Children ages 3 and older or weighing 30 to less than 45 kg: 250 mg glecaprevir/100 mg pibrentasvir PO once daily for 16 weeks.

Children ages 3 and older weighing 20 to less than 30 kg: 200 mg glecaprevir/80 mg pibrentasvir PO once daily for 16 weeks.

Children ages 3 and older weighing less than 20 kg: 150 mg glecaprevir/60 mg pibrentasvir PO once daily for 16 weeks.

ADMINISTRATION
PO
- Give drug with food.

- Sprinkle pellets on a small amount of soft food low in water content that sticks to a spoon (peanut butter, chocolate hazelnut spread, cream cheese, thick jam, Greek yogurt); pellets mixed in liquid or food that would slide off a spoon may dissolve and become less effective.
- Give pellets with food within 15 minutes of preparation and have patient swallow dose without chewing.
- Give a missed dose as soon as possible if less than 18 hours have passed since the scheduled time; then resume normal schedule. If more than 18 hours have passed since the scheduled time, skip missed dose; then resume normal schedule.
- Store at or below 86° F (30° C).

ACTION
Glecaprevir is an HCV NS3/4A protease inhibitor; pibrentasvir is an HCV NS5A inhibitor. Both are direct-acting antivirals that prevent viral replication of HCV.

Route	Onset	Peak	Duration
PO	Unknown	5 hr	Unknown

Half-life: Glecaprevir, 6 hours; pibrentasvir, 13 hours.

ADVERSE REACTIONS
CNS: headache, fatigue, asthenia. **GI:** nausea, diarrhea. **Hepatic:** hyperbilirubinemia. **Skin:** pruritus.

INTERACTIONS
Drug-drug. *Atazanavir:* May increase glecaprevir and pibrentasvir levels and ALT level. Use together is contraindicated.

Atorvastatin, lovastatin, simvastatin: May increase statin level, increasing risk of myopathy and rhabdomyolysis. Use together isn't recommended.

Carbamazepine, efavirenz: May decrease glecaprevir and pibrentasvir levels. Use together isn't recommended.

Cyclosporine: May increase glecaprevir and pibrentasvir levels. Coadministration isn't recommended in patients who require more than 100 mg cyclosporine/day.

Dabigatran: May increase dabigatran level. Refer to dabigatran prescribing information for dosage modifications necessary for patients with kidney impairment who are also taking P-gp inhibitors.

Darunavir, lopinavir, ritonavir: May increase glecaprevir and pibrentasvir levels. Use together isn't recommended.

Digoxin: May increase digoxin level. Measure digoxin level before therapy with glecaprevir and pibrentasvir. Decrease digoxin dosage by 50% or by modifying dosing and frequency; continue monitoring.

Efavirenz: May decrease glecaprevir and pibrentasvir levels. Avoid use together.

Ethinyl estradiol: May increase ALT level. Use together isn't recommended.

Fluvastatin, pitavastatin: May increase fluvastatin and pitavastatin levels, increasing risk of myopathy and rhabdomyolysis. Use lowest approved dosage of fluvastatin and pitavastatin. If higher doses are needed, use lowest dosage necessary based on risk and benefit analysis.

Pravastatin: May increase pravastatin level, increasing risk of myopathy and rhabdomyolysis. Reduce pravastatin dosage by 50%.

Rifampin: May decrease glecaprevir and pibrentasvir levels and their therapeutic effect. Use together is contraindicated.

Rosuvastatin: May increase rosuvastatin level, increasing risk of myopathy and rhabdomyolysis. Don't exceed 10 mg of rosuvastatin.

Warfarin: May alter INR. Monitor INR closely.

Drug-herb. *St. John's wort:* May decrease glecaprevir and pibrentasvir levels and reduce their therapeutic effects. Discourage use together.

EFFECTS ON LAB TEST RESULTS
• May increase total bilirubin level.

CONTRAINDICATIONS & CAUTIONS
• Contraindicated in patients with Child-Pugh class B or C liver impairment and in those with history of liver decompensation.

🔵 *Alert:* Use cautiously in patients with risk factors for liver failure (hepatocellular carcinoma, alcohol abuse, portal hypertension).

Boxed Warning HBV reactivation may occur and can result in fulminant hepatitis, liver failure, and death. ∎

• Safety and effectiveness in children younger than age 3 haven't been studied.

Dialyzable drug: No.

PREGNANCY-LACTATION-REPRODUCTION
• Studies during pregnancy are inadequate. Patients should postpone pregnancy until therapy completion.

• It isn't known if drug appears in human milk. Consider benefit to patient against possible risk to infant.

NURSING CONSIDERATIONS
Boxed Warning Before initiating treatment, test all patients for evidence of current or prior HBV infection by measuring HBsAg and hepatitis B core antigen (anti-HBc). ∎

Boxed Warning Monitor patients coinfected with HCV and HBV for hepatitis flare or HBV reactivation during HCV treatment and posttreatment follow-up. Initiate appropriate management for HBV infection as clinically indicated. ∎

🔵 *Alert:* Closely monitor for liver failure; discontinue drug if patient develops signs and symptoms of decompensation or as clinically indicated.

• Monitor LFT values at baseline and periodically when clinically indicated.

• Monitor patient for changes in glucose tolerance. Modify antidiabetic therapy, if needed.

• *Look alike–sound alike:* Don't confuse Mavyret with Mavik.

PATIENT TEACHING
Boxed Warning Teach patient about risk of HBV reactivation in patients coinfected with HBV during or after treatment of HCV infection. Advise patient to tell prescriber about any history of HBV infection. ∎

• Advise patient to report all medications being taken, including OTC and herbal agents, because of risk of drug interactions.

• Inform patient of risk of hypoglycemia, particularly within first 3 months of therapy. Explain that antidiabetic dosage modification may be necessary.

• Tell patient to report all adverse reactions and to immediately report signs and symptoms of liver impairment (fatigue, abdominal pain, nausea, vomiting, dark urine, light-colored stools, yellowing of skin or eyes).

• Instruct patient not to skip doses and to take drug for entire treatment duration.

• Counsel patient to report pregnancy or plans to become pregnant or to breastfeed.

glimepiride ⚶
glye-MEH-per-ide

Amaryl

Therapeutic class: Antidiabetics
Pharmacologic class: Sulfonylureas

AVAILABLE FORMS
Tablets: 1 mg, 2 mg, 3 mg, 4 mg, 6 mg, 8 mg

INDICATIONS & DOSAGES
➤ **Adjunct to diet and exercise to lower glucose level in patients with type 2 diabetes**
Adults: Initially, 1 or 2 mg PO once daily; usual maintenance dose is 1 to 4 mg PO once daily. After reaching 2 mg, dosage is increased in increments not exceeding 2 mg every 1 to 2 weeks, based on patient's glucose level response. Maximum dose, 8 mg daily.
Adjust-a-dose: For patients with kidney impairment, those at risk for hypoglycemia, and older adults, initially give 1 mg PO once daily; then adjust cautiously to appropriate dosage, if needed. If transferring to glimepiride from longer half-life sulfonylurea (such as chlorpropamide), overlapping drug effect may occur for 1 to 2 weeks; monitor closely for hypoglycemia.

ADMINISTRATION
PO
• Give drug with breakfast or first main meal of the day.
• Patients on nothing-by-mouth status and those requiring decreased caloric intake may need doses withheld to avoid hypoglycemia.

ACTION
Lowers glucose level by stimulating release of insulin from functioning pancreatic beta cells and reduces glucose output from the liver; may lead to increased sensitivity of peripheral tissues to insulin.

Route	Onset	Peak	Duration
PO	1 hr	2–3 hr	24 hr

Half-life: 5 to 9 hours.

ADVERSE REACTIONS
CNS: dizziness, asthenia, headache. **GI:** nausea. **Hepatic:** increased ALT level. **Metabolic:** *hypoglycemia,* weight gain. **Other:** accidental injury, flulike symptoms.

INTERACTIONS
• Many drugs affect glucose metabolism, which may require glimepiride dosage adjustment. Monitor glycemic control closely. Consult manufacturer's product information for additional information.
Drug-drug. *Beta blockers, clonidine:* May mask symptoms of hypoglycemia. Monitor glucose level.
Colesevelam: May decrease glimepiride serum concentration. Give glimepiride at least 4 hours before colesevelam. Consider therapy modification.
CYP2C9 inducers (rifampin) or inhibitors (fluconazole): Inducers may increase glimepiride metabolism, leading to worsening glycemic control; inhibitors may decrease glimepiride metabolism, leading to hypoglycemia. Monitor therapy.
Drugs that tend to produce hyperglycemia (corticosteroids, estrogens, fosphenytoin, hormonal contraceptives, isoniazid, nicotinic acid, phenothiazines, phenytoin, thyroid products): May lead to loss of glucose control. Adjust dosage.
Insulin: May increase risk of hypoglycemia. Use together cautiously.
Miconazole (oral): May increase serum concentration and enhance hypoglycemic effect of glimepiride. Monitor therapy.
NSAIDs, other drugs that are highly protein-bound (beta blockers, chloramphenicol, coumarin, MAO inhibitors, probenecid, sulfonamides): May increase hypoglycemic action of sulfonylureas such as glimepiride. Monitor glucose level carefully.
Rifamycins, thiazide diuretics: May increase risk of hyperglycemia. Monitor glucose level.
Salicylates: May increase hypoglycemic effects of sulfonylurea. Monitor glucose level.
Warfarin: Sulfonylureas may enhance anticoagulant effect of vitamin K antagonists; vitamin K antagonists may enhance hypoglycemic effect of sulfonylureas. Monitor therapy.
Drug-herb. *Herbs with hypoglycemic properties (ginger, turmeric):* May enhance hypoglycemic effect of glimepiride. Monitor therapy.
Drug-lifestyle. *Alcohol use:* May alter glycemic control, most commonly causing hypoglycemia. May also cause disulfiram-like reaction. Discourage use together.

G

EFFECTS ON LAB TEST RESULTS
• May increase ALT, AST, BUN, and creatinine levels.
• May decrease glucose and sodium levels.
• May decrease Hb level and granulocyte, platelet, RBC, and WBC counts.

CONTRAINDICATIONS & CAUTIONS
• Contraindicated in patients hypersensitive to drug or sulfonamides.
• Contraindicated for treatment of type 1 diabetes and diabetic ketoacidosis; drug wouldn't be effective.
• **Alert:** Use of oral antidiabetics may carry higher risk of CV mortality than use of diet alone or of diet and insulin therapy.
• Use cautiously in patients who are debilitated or malnourished and in those with adrenal, pituitary, or kidney insufficiency; these patients are more susceptible to the hypoglycemic action of glucose-lowering drugs.
• Use cautiously with other drugs that can cause hypoglycemia.
• Use cautiously in older adults.
▧ Patients with G6PD deficiency may be at increased risk for sulfonylurea-induced hemolytic anemia. Use cautiously and consider therapy modification.
• Not recommended for use in children due to adverse effects on body weight and hypoglycemia.
Dialyzable drug: Unknown.
⚠ Overdose S&S: Hypoglycemia.

PREGNANCY-LACTATION-REPRODUCTION
• Use in pregnancy only if potential benefit justifies fetal risk.
• **Alert:** Prolonged severe hypoglycemia (4 to 10 days) has been reported in neonates born to patients receiving a sulfonylurea at time of delivery. Discontinue drug at least 2 weeks before expected delivery.
• May cause hypoglycemia in infants who are breastfed. Consider risk of exposure to the infant, benefits of breastfeeding, and benefits of treatment for patient. Monitor infant who is breastfeeding for signs and symptoms of hypoglycemia (jitters, cyanosis, apnea, hypothermia, excessive sleepiness, poor feeding, seizures).

NURSING CONSIDERATIONS
• Glimepiride and insulin may be used together in patient who loses glucose control after first responding to therapy.

• Periodically monitor fasting glucose level to determine therapeutic response. Also monitor HbA_{1c} level, usually every 3 to 6 months, to precisely assess long-term glycemic control.
• When changing patient from other sulfonylurea to glimepiride, a transition period isn't needed. Monitor patient carefully for 1 to 2 weeks when changing from longer half-life sulfonylureas, such as chlorpropamide.
• **Look alike–sound alike:** Don't confuse glimepiride with glyburide or glipizide. Don't confuse Amaryl with Altace.

PATIENT TEACHING
• Teach about proper drug administration and handling.
• Make sure patient understands that therapy relieves symptoms but doesn't cure the disease. Patient should also understand risks and advantages of taking drug and of other treatment methods.
• Stress importance of adhering to diet, weight reduction, exercise, and personal hygiene programs. Explain to patient and family how and when to monitor glucose level, and teach recognition of and intervention for signs and symptoms of high and low glucose levels.
• Advise patient to always wear or carry medical identification.
• Instruct patient to consult prescriber before taking OTC products or supplements.
• Tell patient to carry candy or other simple sugars to treat mild low glucose level. Warn that a severe episode may require hospital treatment.
• Advise patient to avoid alcohol, which lowers glucose level.

SAFETY ALERT!

glipiZIDE ▧
GLIP-i-zide

Glucotrol XL

Therapeutic class: Antidiabetics
Pharmacologic class: Sulfonylureas

AVAILABLE FORMS
Tablets (extended-release) 🅞🅝🅒: 2.5 mg, 5 mg, 10 mg
Tablets (immediate-release): 5 mg, 10 mg

INDICATIONS & DOSAGES

➤ **Adjunct to diet and exercise to lower glucose level in patients with type 2 diabetes**

Adults (immediate-release tablets): Initially, 5 mg PO daily. Titrate by 2.5- to 5-mg increments no less than every few days based on blood glucose level. Maximum once-daily dose, 15 mg. Divide doses of more than 15 mg. Maximum total daily dose, 40 mg.

Adjust-a-dose: For patients with liver or kidney insufficiency, patients older than age 65, and patients who are debilitated or malnourished, initially give 2.5 mg PO daily.

Adults (extended-release tablets): Initially, 2.5 to 5 mg PO daily. Increase by 5 mg every 3 months, depending on level of glycemic control. Maximum daily dose, 20 mg.

Adjust-a-dose: For patients with liver or kidney insufficiency, patients older than age 65, and patients who are debilitated or malnourished, initially give 2.5 mg PO daily.

➤ **To replace insulin therapy (immediate-release)**

Adults: If insulin dosage is 20 units or less daily, insulin may be stopped when glipizide starts. If insulin dosage is more than 20 units daily, start patient at usual dosage in addition to 50% of insulin dose. In some cases, especially if insulin dose exceeds 40 units daily, consider transitioning to glipizide in a hospital setting.

ADMINISTRATION

PO

• Give immediate-release tablet about 30 minutes before meals.

• Give extended-release tablet with breakfast.

• Have patient swallow tablets whole; don't crush or break tablets.

• Patients on nothing-by-mouth status and those requiring decreased caloric intake may need doses withheld to avoid hypoglycemia.

ACTION

Stimulates insulin release from pancreatic beta cells, reduces glucose output by the liver, and increases peripheral sensitivity to insulin.

Route	Onset	Peak	Duration
PO (immediate-release)	15–30 min	1–3 hr	12–24 hr
PO (extended-release)	2–3 hr	6–12 hr	12–24 hr

Half-life: 2 to 5 hours.

ADVERSE REACTIONS

CNS: dizziness, drowsiness, headache, nervousness, tremor. **GI:** nausea, dyspepsia, flatulence, constipation, diarrhea, vomiting. **Hematologic:** *leukopenia,* hemolytic anemia, *agranulocytosis, thrombocytopenia.* **Metabolic:** *hypoglycemia.* **Skin:** rash, pruritus, urticaria, photosensitivity reactions.

INTERACTIONS

• Many drugs affect glucose metabolism, which may require glipizide dosage adjustment. Monitor glycemic control closely. Consult manufacturer's product information for more information.

Drug-drug. *Antifungals, chloramphenicol, MAO inhibitors, NSAIDs, probenecid, quinolones, ranitidine, salicylates, sulfonamides:* May increase hypoglycemic activity. Monitor glucose level.

Beta blockers, clonidine: May prolong hypoglycemic effect and mask symptoms of hypoglycemia. Use together cautiously.

Colesevelam: May decrease glipizide serum level. Give glipizide at least 4 hours before colesevelam. Consider therapy modification.

Corticosteroids, glucagon, phenytoin, rifamycins, thiazide diuretics: May decrease hypoglycemic response. Monitor glucose level.

Fluconazole: May increase glipizide serum level, leading to hypoglycemia. Monitor patient closely.

Miconazole (oral): May increase serum level and enhance hypoglycemic effect of glipizide. Monitor therapy.

Oral anticoagulants: May increase hypoglycemic activity or enhance anticoagulant effect. Monitor glucose level, PT, and INR.

Drug-herb. *Herbs with hypoglycemic properties (ginger, turmeric):* May enhance hypoglycemic effect of glipizide. Monitor therapy.

Drug-lifestyle. *Alcohol use:* May alter glycemic control, most commonly causing hypoglycemia. May cause disulfiram-like reaction. Discourage use together.

EFFECTS ON LAB TEST RESULTS

• May increase ALP, AST, ALT, LDH, BUN, and creatinine levels.

• May decrease glucose level.

• May decrease Hb level and granulocyte, platelet, and WBC counts.

CONTRAINDICATIONS & CAUTIONS
• Contraindicated in patients hypersensitive to drug or sulfonamides and in those with type 1 diabetes or diabetic ketoacidosis with or without coma.

⚠ *Alert:* Use of oral antidiabetics may carry a higher risk of CV mortality than use of diet alone or of diet and insulin therapy.

▧ Patients with G6PD deficiency may be at increased risk for sulfonylurea-induced hemolytic anemia. Use cautiously and consider therapy modification.

• Use cautiously in patients with severe GI disease or kidney or liver disease, in older adults, and in patients who are debilitated or malnourished.

Dialyzable drug: Unknown.

⚠ *Overdose S&S:* Hypoglycemia.

PREGNANCY-LACTATION-REPRODUCTION
• Insulin is drug of choice to control diabetes during pregnancy. If glipizide is used, discontinue at least 1 month before expected delivery date because prolonged severe hypoglycemia (4 to 10 days) has been reported in neonates born to mothers receiving a sulfonylurea at the time of delivery.

• Drug may cause hypoglycemia in infants who are breastfed. Consider risk of exposure to infant, benefits of breastfeeding, and benefits of treatment for patient. Monitor infant who is breastfeeding for signs and symptoms of hypoglycemia (jitters, cyanosis, apnea, hypothermia, excessive sleepiness, poor feeding, seizures).

NURSING CONSIDERATIONS
• Some patients attain effective control on once-daily regimen, whereas others respond better with divided dosing.

• Patient may switch from immediate-release to extended-release tablets at the nearest equivalent total daily dose.

• Drug is a second-generation sulfonylurea. Adverse reactions are less common with second-generation drugs than with first-generation drugs such as chlorpropamide.

• During periods of increased stress, patient may need insulin therapy. Monitor closely for hyperglycemia in these situations.

• Check glucose level at least three times a day before meals for patient switching from insulin therapy to an oral antidiabetic.

• *Look alike–sound alike:* Don't confuse glipizide with glyburide or glimepiride.

PATIENT TEACHING
• Instruct patient about disease and importance of following therapeutic regimen, adhering to diet, losing weight, getting exercise, and avoiding infection.

• Explain the risks, symptoms, and treatment of hypoglycemia.

• Review glucose monitoring.

• Tell patient to carry candy or other simple sugars to treat mild low glucose level. Warn that a severe episode may require hospital treatment.

• Caution patient not to change drug dosage without prescriber's consent and to report abnormal blood or urine glucose test results.

• Tell patient not to take other drugs, including OTC drugs, without first checking with prescriber.

• Advise patient to always wear or carry medical identification.

• Warn patient to avoid alcohol, which lowers glucose level.

• Inform patient that something resembling a tablet may appear in stool; assure patient that it's the nonabsorbable shell of the extended-release tablet.

SAFETY ALERT!

glyBURIDE (glibenclamide) ▧
GLYE-byoor-ide

Glynase

Therapeutic class: Antidiabetics
Pharmacologic class: Sulfonylureas

AVAILABLE FORMS
Tablets: 1.25 mg, 2.5 mg, 5 mg
Tablets (micronized): 1.5 mg, 3 mg, 4.5 mg, 6 mg

INDICATIONS & DOSAGES
➤ **Adjunct to diet and exercise to lower glucose level in patients with type 2 diabetes**
Adults (nonmicronized form): Initially, 2.5 to 5 mg PO once daily with breakfast or first main meal. Adjust to maintenance dose at no more than 2.5-mg increments at weekly intervals. Usual daily maintenance dose is 1.25 to 20 mg, in single dose or divided doses. For dosages exceeding 10 mg daily, b.i.d. dosing

may achieve better response. Maximum daily dose, 20 mg PO.

Adults (micronized form): Initially, 1.5 to 3 mg PO daily with breakfast or first main meal. Adjust to maintenance dose at no more than 1.5-mg increments at weekly intervals. Usual daily maintenance dose is 0.75 to 12 mg as a single dose or in divided doses. Dosages exceeding 6 mg daily may have better response with b.i.d. dosing. Maximum dose, 12 mg PO daily.

Adjust-a-dose: Older adults, debilitated or malnourished patients, and those with kidney, liver, adrenal, or pituitary insufficiency should start with 1.25 mg (nonmicronized) or 0.75 mg (micronized) daily.

➤ **To replace insulin therapy**
Adults: If insulin dose is less than 40 units/day, may switch patient directly to glyburide when insulin is stopped. If insulin dose is less than 20 units/day, initial dose is 2.5 to 5 mg (1.5 to 3 mg micronized) PO daily. If insulin dose is 20 to 40 units/day, initial dose is 5 mg (3 mg micronized) PO daily. If insulin dose is 40 or more units/day, initially, 5 mg (3 mg micronized) PO once daily in addition to 50% of insulin dose. Gradually taper insulin while increasing glyburide dose.

ADMINISTRATION
PO
• Give drug with breakfast or first main meal.
• Patients on nothing-by-mouth status and those requiring decreased caloric intake may need doses withheld to avoid hypoglycemia.

ACTION
Stimulates insulin release from pancreatic beta cells, reduces glucose output by the liver, and increases peripheral sensitivity to insulin.

Route	Onset	Peak	Duration
PO (micronized)	1 hr	2–3 hr	≤24 hr
PO (nonmi-cronized)	1 hr	4 hr	≤24 hr

Half-life: 4 to 10 hours.

ADVERSE REACTIONS
GI: nausea, epigastric fullness, heartburn. **Hematologic:** *leukopenia,* hemolytic anemia, *agranulocytosis, thrombocytopenia, aplastic anemia.* **Metabolic:** *hypoglycemia,* weight gain. **Musculoskeletal:** arthralgia, myalgia. **Skin:** rash, pruritus, other allergic reactions. **Other:** *angioedema.*

INTERACTIONS
• Many drugs affect glucose metabolism, which may require glyburide dosage adjustment. Monitor glycemic control closely. Consult manufacturer's product information for more information.

Drug-drug. *Azole antifungals, chloramphenicol, fluoroquinolones, MAO inhibitors, NSAIDs, probenecid, salicylates, sulfonamides:* May increase hypoglycemic activity. Monitor glucose level.
Beta blockers: May prolong hypoglycemic effect and mask symptoms of hypoglycemia. Use together cautiously.
Bosentan: Increases risk of elevated LFT values. Use together is contraindicated.
*Corticosteroids, glucagon, phenytoin, **thiazide diuretics:*** May decrease hypoglycemic response. Monitor glucose level.
Colesevelam: May decrease glyburide serum concentration. Give glyburide at least 4 hours before colesevelam.
CYP2C9 inducers (rifampin): May increase glyburide metabolism, leading to worsening glycemic control. Monitor therapy.
CYP2C9 inhibitors (fluconazole): May decrease glyburide metabolism, leading to hypoglycemia. Monitor therapy.
Miconazole (oral): May increase serum concentration and enhance hypoglycemic effect of glyburide. Monitor therapy.
Oral anticoagulants: May increase hypoglycemic activity or enhance anticoagulant effect. Monitor glucose level, PT, and INR.
Drug-herb. *Herbs with hypoglycemic properties (ginger, turmeric):* May enhance hypoglycemic effect of glyburide. Monitor therapy.
Drug-lifestyle. *Alcohol use:* May alter glycemic control, most commonly causing hypoglycemia. May cause disulfiram-like reaction. Discourage use together.

EFFECTS ON LAB TEST RESULTS
• May increase ALP, AST, ALT, bilirubin, and BUN levels.
• May decrease glucose level.
• May decrease Hb level and granulocyte, platelet, and WBC counts.

CONTRAINDICATIONS & CAUTIONS
• Contraindicated in patients hypersensitive to drug and in those with type 1 diabetes or diabetic ketoacidosis with or without coma.

G

❸ *Alert:* Oral antidiabetics may have a higher risk of CV mortality than use of diet alone or of diet and insulin therapy.

• Use cautiously in patients with liver or kidney impairment, in older adults, in patients who are debilitated or malnourished, and in patients allergic to sulfonamides.

▧ Patients with G6PD deficiency may be at increased risk for sulfonylurea-induced hemolytic anemia. Use cautiously and consider therapy modification.

• Safety and effectiveness in children haven't been established.

Dialyzable drug: Unknown.

⚠ *Overdose S&S:* Hypoglycemia.

PREGNANCY-LACTATION-REPRODUCTION

• Insulin is drug of choice to control diabetes during pregnancy. If glyburide is used during pregnancy, discontinue at least 2 weeks before expected delivery date.

❸ *Alert:* Prolonged severe hypoglycemia (4 to 10 days) has been reported in neonates born to mothers receiving a sulfonylurea at the time of delivery.

• Drug may cause hypoglycemia in infants who are breastfed. Patient should discontinue breastfeeding or discontinue drug, considering importance of drug to patient.

NURSING CONSIDERATIONS

❸ *Alert:* Micronized glyburide (Glynase) contains drug in a smaller particle size and isn't bioequivalent to regular glyburide tablets. In patients who have been taking nonmicronized form, adjust dosage.

• Drug is a second-generation sulfonylurea. Adverse effects are less common with second-generation drugs than with first-generation drugs such as chlorpropamide.

• During periods of increased stress, such as infection, fever, surgery, and trauma, patient may need insulin therapy. Monitor closely for hyperglycemia in these situations.

• Patient switching from insulin therapy to an oral antidiabetic should check glucose level at least three times a day before meals. Patient may require hospitalization during transition.

• *Look alike–sound alike:* Don't confuse glyburide with glimepiride or glipizide.

PATIENT TEACHING

• Teach patient about diabetes and the importance of following therapeutic regimen, adhering to specific diet, losing weight, getting exercise, following personal hygiene programs, and avoiding infection. Explain how and when to monitor glucose level, and teach recognition of and intervention for low and high glucose levels.

• Tell patient not to change drug dosage without prescriber's consent and to report abnormal blood or urine glucose test results.

• Tell patient to carry candy or other simple sugars to treat mild low glucose level. Warn that a severe episode may require hospital treatment.

• Advise patient not to take supplements or other drugs, including OTC drugs, without first checking with prescriber.

• Caution patient to always wear or carry medical identification.

❸ *Alert:* Instruct patient to immediately report episodes of low glucose to prescriber; a severely low glucose level is sometimes fatal in patients receiving as little as 2.5 mg daily.

• Advise patient to avoid alcohol, which may lower glucose level.

golimumab
go-LIM-ue-mab

Simponi, Simponi Aria

Therapeutic class: Antiarthritics
Pharmacologic class: TNF blockers

AVAILABLE FORMS
Injection (IV): 50 mg/4 mL single-dose vial
Injection (subcut): 50 mg/0.5 mL,
100 mg/mL prefilled syringe or prefilled autoinjector

INDICATIONS & DOSAGES
➤ **Moderate to severe active RA in combination with methotrexate; active psoriatic arthritis or active ankylosing spondylitis alone or in combination with methotrexate or other nonbiologic DMARDs**
Adults: 50 mg subcut monthly. Or, 2 mg/kg IV infusion over 30 minutes at weeks 0 and 4, then every 8 weeks thereafter.
➤ **Moderate to severe ulcerative colitis in patients who have demonstrated an inadequate response or intolerance to prior treatment or who require continuous steroid therapy**

Adults: Initially, 200 mg subcut, followed by 100 mg subcut at week 2, then 100 mg subcut every 4 weeks.

➤ **Active polyarticular juvenile idiopathic arthritis; active psoriatic arthritis**
Children ages 2 and older: 80 mg/m^2 IV infusion over 30 minutes at weeks 0 and 4 and every 8 weeks thereafter.

ADMINISTRATION
• The efficacy and safety of switching between IV and subcut formulations and routes of administration haven't been established.
• Store at 36° F to 46° F (2° C to 8° C) or at room temperature for up to 30 days. Don't return to refrigerator after storing at room temperature.

IV
▼ Dilute with NSS or half-NSS to a final volume of 100 mL.
▼ Confirm vial solution is colorless to light yellow. Don't use if discoloration or opaque particles are present.
▼ Administer over 30 minutes. Use a 0.22-micron low protein-binding filter.
▼ Solutions diluted for infusion may be stored at room temperature for 4 hours.
▼ **Incompatibilities:** Don't infuse together in same IV line with other agents; compatibility studies are lacking.

Subcutaneous
• Remove drug from refrigerator and carton 30 minutes before administration, allowing it to reach room temperature.
• Inspect solution before administration. Don't use solution if it's discolored or cloudy or if foreign particles are present. Drug is normally colorless to slightly opalescent to light yellow.
• Prefilled syringe and prefilled autoinjector needle covers contain latex. Don't handle if sensitive to latex.
• To administer, hold autoinjector firmly against skin and inject subcut into thigh, lower abdomen (below navel), or upper arm. Listen for a loud click when injection begins. Continue to hold autoinjector against skin until second click occurs (may take 3 to 15 seconds). After second click, lift autoinjector from injection site.
• Don't use any leftover product remaining in prefilled syringe or prefilled autoinjector.
• Rotate injection sites. Don't inject drug into areas where skin is tender, bruised, red, or hard.

• If multiple injections are required, administer injections at different body sites.

ACTION
Binds to human TNF-alpha, inhibiting its binding with receptors, thereby neutralizing its activity. Ultimately reduces infiltration of inflammatory cells.

Route	Onset	Peak	Duration
IV	Unknown	12 weeks	Unknown
Subcut	Unknown	2–6 days	Unknown

Half-life: 2 weeks.

ADVERSE REACTIONS
CNS: fever. **CV:** HTN. **Hematologic:** *leukopenia.* **Hepatic:** increased AST and ALT levels. **Respiratory:** bronchitis, URI. **Skin:** injection site reactions, rash. **Other:** infection (viral, bacterial), antibody development.

INTERACTIONS
Drug-drug. *Abatacept, anakinra, other immunosuppressants:* May increase risk of serious infection. Avoid use together.
CYP450 substrates (cyclosporine, theophylline, warfarin): May alter levels of these drugs. Monitor patient closely and adjust dosages as needed.
Live-virus vaccines: May increase risk of infection. Don't give together.

EFFECTS ON LAB TEST RESULTS
• May increase LFT values.
• May decrease platelet, WBC, and neutrophil counts.
• May diminish diagnostic effect of coccidioidin skin test.
• May cause positive ANA titer.

CONTRAINDICATIONS & CAUTIONS
Boxed Warning Consider risks and benefits of treatment before start of therapy in patients with chronic or recurrent infection. ∎
• Treatment shouldn't be initiated in patients with active infection.
• Use cautiously in patients with malignancies, hematologic abnormalities, or HF and in patients who are also receiving immunosuppressants.
Boxed Warning Lymphoma and other malignancies (some fatal) have been reported in children and adolescents treated with TNF blockers, including golimumab. ∎

• Drug may increase risk or worsening of demyelinating disorders, including MS and Guillain-Barré syndrome. Use cautiously in patients with preexisting or recent onset of CNS or peripheral demyelinating disorders. *Dialyzable drug:* Unknown.

PREGNANCY-LACTATION-REPRODUCTION
• Use during pregnancy only if benefit justifies fetal risk and only if clearly needed.
• Administration of live-virus vaccines to infants exposed to golimumab in utero isn't recommended for 6 months after mother's last dose during pregnancy.
• It isn't known if drug appears in human milk. Patient should discontinue breastfeeding or discontinue drug, considering importance of drug to patient.

NURSING CONSIDERATIONS
Boxed Warning Monitor patient closely for signs and symptoms of infection before and after treatment. TB, invasive fungal infection, and other bacterial and viral opportunistic infections, which are sometimes fatal, may occur in patients receiving golimumab. Stop drug if serious infection or sepsis develops. ■
Boxed Warning Evaluate patient for latent TB with tuberculin skin test before initiating treatment. Treat latent TB before therapy with golimumab. Monitor all patients for active TB during treatment even if initial latent TB test is negative. ■
• Drug increases risk of reactivation of HBV infection, which can be fatal, in HBV carriers. Before starting therapy, test for HBV infection.
• Monitor patient for new or worsening HF; stop drug if signs or symptoms occur.
• Monitor patient for lymphomas and other malignancies, especially if patient is also receiving immunosuppressants.
• Pancytopenia and other significant cytopenias, including aplastic anemia, can occur. Regularly monitor CBC during therapy. May discontinue drug if hematologic abnormalities develop.

PATIENT TEACHING
• Teach patient or caregiver how to give subcut injection. First self-injection should occur under supervision of qualified health care practitioner.
• Advise patient that prefilled syringes and prefilled autoinjector needle covers contain latex or a latex derivative.

• Instruct patient to report all adverse reactions, especially signs and symptoms of infection, new or worsening HF, or liver or nervous system problems.
• Tell patient to avoid live-virus vaccines while taking drug.
• Instruct patient to report pregnancy or plans to become pregnant or to breastfeed.

granisetron
gran-IZ-e-tron

Sancuso, Sustol

granisetron hydrochloride

Therapeutic class: Antiemetics
Pharmacologic class: 5-HT$_3$ receptor antagonists

AVAILABLE FORMS
Injection: 0.1 mg/mL, 1 mg/mL single-dose, preservative-free vials; 4-mL multidose vials containing benzyl alcohol
Injection (extended-release): 10 mg/0.4 mL prefilled syringe
Tablets: 1 mg
Transdermal patch: 3.1 mg per 24 hours

INDICATIONS & DOSAGES
➤ **Prevention of nausea and vomiting from emetogenic cancer chemotherapy**
Adults and children ages 2 to 16: 10 mcg/kg IV undiluted given by direct injection over 30 seconds or diluted and infused over 5 minutes. Start giving at least 30 minutes before chemotherapy.
    Or, for adults, 1 mg PO up to 1 hour before chemotherapy and repeated 12 hours later. Or, for adults, 2 mg PO daily given up to 1 hour before chemotherapy.
    Or, for adults, apply a single patch to the upper outer arm 24 to 48 hours before chemotherapy; remove patch a minimum of 24 hours after completion of chemotherapy or a maximum of 7 days.
    Or, for adults, 10 mg extended-release form subcut with dexamethasone at least 30 minutes before chemotherapy on day 1. Don't give extended-release form more frequently than once every 7 days. Refer to manufacturer's instructions for dexamethasone dosages.

Reactions in bold italics are *life-threatening*.

Adjust-a-dose: In patients with CrCl of 30 to 59 mL/minute, don't give extended-release form more frequently than once every 14 days. Don't give extended-release form to patients if CrCl of less than 30 mL/minute.

➤ **Prevention of nausea and vomiting from radiation**

Adults: 2 mg PO once daily within 1 hour of radiation.

➤ **Prevention of postoperative nausea and vomiting**

Adults: 1 mg IV over 30 seconds, before anesthetic induction or immediately before reversal of anesthesia.

➤ **Postoperative nausea and vomiting**

Adults: 1 mg IV over 30 seconds, after surgery.

ADMINISTRATION

PO
- Oral suspension may be compounded by a pharmacist for patients who can't swallow tablets.
- Store tablets at room temperature.
- Protect drug from light.

IV
▼ For direct injection, give drug undiluted over 30 seconds.
▼ For intermittent infusion, dilute with NSS for injection or D_5W to a volume of 20 to 50 mL.
▼ Infuse over 5 minutes, starting within 30 minutes before chemotherapy and only on days chemotherapy is given.
▼ Diluted solutions are stable for 24 hours at room temperature. Don't freeze vials.
▼ Use contents of multiuse vial within 30 days after vial penetration.
▼ **Incompatibilities:** Other IV drugs.

Subcutaneous
- Extended-release form is for subcut injection only.
- Drug should only be administered by a health care provider.
- Remove extended-release form kit from refrigerator 1 hour before administration.
- Refer to manufacturer's syringe preparation instructions for warming syringe to body temperature using syringe warming pouches included in kit.
- Don't give drug if discoloration or particulate matter is visible in syringe; be aware that syringe is amber-colored glass.
- Give drug by subcut injection in skin of the back of upper arm or in skin of abdomen at least 1 inch (2.54 cm) from umbilicus.

- Topical anesthetic may be used at injection site before giving drug.
- Avoid injecting into skin that's burned, hardened, inflamed, swollen, or otherwise compromised.
- Give drug as a slow, sustained subcut injection over 20 to 30 seconds.
- Store in refrigerator at 36° to 46° F (2° to 8° C). Don't freeze.
- Once drug has been removed from refrigerator, it can remain at room temperature for up to 7 days.

Transdermal
- Each patch is packed in a pouch and should be applied directly after opening pouch.
- Apply patch to clean, intact, healthy skin on upper outer arm.
- Don't cut patch into pieces.
- Don't apply heating pad or heat lamp over or in vicinity of transdermal system; avoid extended exposure to heat.
- Cover transdermal system application site with clothing if exposure to direct natural or artificial sunlight is possible while patch is applied and for 10 days after its removal.
- Fold removed patch in half with sticky side together and discard to avoid accidental contact or ingestion by others.

ACTION

Selectively blocks $5\text{-}HT_3$ in the CNS in the chemoreceptor trigger zone and in the peripheral nervous system on nerve terminals of the vagus nerve.

Route	Onset	Peak	Duration
PO	Unknown	Unknown	24 hr
IV	1–3 min	Unknown	24 hr
Subcut (extended-release)	Unknown	11–12 hr	7 days
Transdermal	Unknown	48 hr	Unknown

Half-life: PO, IV, transdermal, 5 to 9 hours; extended-release, 24 hours.

ADVERSE REACTIONS

CNS: asthenia, headache, fatigue, fever, agitation, anxiety, CNS stimulation, dizziness, insomnia, somnolence, pain, weakness, drowsiness, dysgeusia. **CV:** HTN. **GI:** constipation, nausea, vomiting, abdominal pain, decreased appetite, diarrhea, dyspepsia, flatulence, GERD. **Hematologic:** *leukopenia.*

Hepatic: increased ALT and AST levels.
Skin: alopecia, rash, dermatitis, injection-site reactions, application-site reactions.

INTERACTIONS
Drug-drug. *Apomorphine:* May increase risk of profound hypotension and loss of consciousness. Avoid use together.
Drugs that prolong QT interval: May increase risk of life-threatening cardiac arrhythmias, including torsades de pointes. Use together cautiously and monitor patient.
Serotonin modulators (fentanyl, lithium, MAO inhibitors, methylene blue IV, mirtazapine, SNRIs, SSRIs, tramadol): May increase risk of serotonin syndrome. Monitor therapy.

EFFECTS ON LAB TEST RESULTS
• May increase ALT and AST levels.
• May alter fluid and electrolyte levels with prolonged use.
• May decrease Hb level, hematocrit, and platelet and WBC counts.
• May increase leukocyte count.

CONTRAINDICATIONS & CAUTIONS
• Contraindicated in patients hypersensitive to drug or other 5-HT₃ receptor antagonists.
• Hypersensitivity reactions, including anaphylaxis, may occur up to 7 days or longer after administration of extended-release form.
• **Alert:** QT-interval prolongation has been reported, and drug may increase risk of ventricular arrhythmias. Use cautiously in patients with preexisting arrhythmias, cardiac conduction disorders, cardiac disease, or electrolyte abnormalities; in patients receiving cardiotoxic chemotherapy; and in those receiving medications that prolong QT interval.
• May increase risk of serotonin syndrome, which can be fatal, especially if drug is used with other serotonergic drugs.
• Use of extended-release form with successive emetogenic chemotherapy cycles for more than 6 months isn't recommended.
• Injection-site bruising and hematoma, which can be severe, may occur more than 5 days after administration of extended-release form. Patients receiving anticoagulants or antiplatelet drugs may be at greater risk.
• Safety and effectiveness in children haven't been established.

Dialyzable drug: Unknown.
⚠ Overdose S&S: Headache.

PREGNANCY-LACTATION-REPRODUCTION
• Use during pregnancy only if clearly needed.
• Some injection forms contain benzyl alcohol, which may cause neonatal gasping syndrome.
• It's unknown if drug is excreted in human milk. Use cautiously during breastfeeding.

NURSING CONSIDERATIONS
• Drug regimen is given only on days when patient receives chemotherapy. Treatment at other times isn't useful.
• Monitor patient for signs and symptoms of serotonin syndrome (mental status changes, neuromuscular signs and symptoms, autonomic instability, seizures, GI symptoms). If any occur, discontinue drug and initiate treatment.
• Monitor patient receiving extended-release form for injection-site infections, bruising, and hematoma.
• Monitor patient receiving extended-release form for signs and symptoms of hypersensitivity reactions (dyspnea, wheezing, rash, hives, fever, swelling).
• Monitor patient for constipation and decreased bowel activity, especially if patient is at risk for GI obstruction.

PATIENT TEACHING
• Stress the importance of taking second dose of oral drug 12 hours after first dose for maximum effectiveness.
• Teach about proper drug administration and handling, including safe patch disposal, if applicable.
• Tell patient to immediately report adverse reactions.
• Inform patient receiving extended-release form that hypersensitivity reactions can occur up to 7 days or later after subcut administration, and advise patient to immediately report signs and symptoms.
• Teach patient signs and symptoms of serotonin syndrome, and advise patient to immediately report them.
• Tell patient to report injection-site reactions (infection, bruising, hematoma, pain, warmth, bleeding) to prescriber.

haloperidol
ha-loe-PER-i-dole

haloperidol decanoate
Haldol Decanoate

haloperidol lactate

Therapeutic class: Antipsychotics
Pharmacologic class: Butyrophenone
derivatives

AVAILABLE FORMS
haloperidol
Tablets: 0.5 mg, 1 mg, 2 mg, 5 mg, 10 mg,
20 mg
haloperidol decanoate
Injection: 50 mg/mL*, 100 mg/mL*
haloperidol lactate
Injection: 5 mg/mL
Oral solution (concentrate): 2 mg/mL

INDICATIONS & DOSAGES
Adjust-a-dose (for all indications): For oral
dosing in older adults and patients who are
debilitated, initially, 0.5 to 2 mg PO b.i.d. or
t.i.d.; increase gradually, as needed.
➤ **Manifestations of psychotic disorders
such as schizophrenia**
Adults and children older than age 12:
Dosage varies for each patient. Initially, 0.5 to
2 mg PO b.i.d. or t.i.d. For severe symptoms,
initially, 3 to 5 mg PO b.i.d. or t.i.d. Maximum dosage, 100 mg PO daily. Or, 2 to 5 mg
lactate IM every 4 to 8 hours (although hourly
administration may be needed until control is
obtained). Maximum dosage, 20 mg/day.
Children ages 3 to 12 weighing 15 to 40 kg:
Initially, 0.5 mg PO in two or three divided
doses daily. May increase dosage by 0.5 mg
at 5- to 7-day intervals, depending on therapeutic response and patient tolerance. Maintenance dosage, 0.05 to 0.15 mg/kg PO daily in
two or three divided doses. Children who are
severely disturbed may need higher dosages.
Maximum dosage, 6 mg/day.
➤ **Chronic schizophrenia requiring prolonged therapy (haloperidol decanoate)**
*Adults stable on low daily oral dosage, older
adults, and patients who are debilitated:* Initial and maintenance dosages, 10 to 15 times
daily oral dosage, given IM every 4 weeks.
*Adults on high oral dosage, at risk for re-
lapse, or tolerant to oral haloperidol:* Initial

dosage, 10 to 20 times daily oral dosage;
maintenance dosage, 10 to 15 times daily oral
dosage, given IM every 4 weeks.
Adjust-a-dose: Adjust dosing interval and
dose based on individual response.
➤ **Nonpsychotic behavior disorders**
Children ages 3 to 12 weighing 15 to 40 kg:
0.05 to 0.075 mg/kg PO daily in two or three
divided doses. Maximum dosage, 6 mg daily.
Children with severe mental illness who don't
have psychosis or are hyperactive with conduct disorders may only require short-term
use.
➤ **Tourette syndrome**
Adults: Initially, 0.5 to 5 mg PO b.i.d., t.i.d.,
or as needed. Maximum dosage, 100 mg/day.
Children ages 3 to 12 weighing 15 to 40 kg:
0.05 to 0.075 mg/kg PO daily in two or three
divided doses. Maximum dosage, 6 mg daily.

ADMINISTRATION
PO
● Give drug with food or milk to decrease GI
distress.
● Avoid skin contact with oral solution; may
cause contact dermatitis.
IM
🛈 *Alert:* Haloperidol isn't approved for IV or
subcut use. Never administer haloperidol decanoate IV.
● Protect drug from light. Slight yellowing
of solution is common and doesn't affect potency. Discard very discolored solution.
● For haloperidol decanoate, use 21G needle.
Ensure maximum volume per injection site
doesn't exceed 3 mL. Give in gluteal muscle by deep IM injection; Z-track technique is
recommended.
● When switching from tablets to IM decanoate injection, if initial dose conversion
requires more than 100 mg, give in two injections (100 mg maximum) separated by 3 to
7 days.

ACTION
A butyrophenone that probably exerts antipsychotic effects by blocking postsynaptic
dopamine receptors in the brain.

Route	Onset	Peak	Duration
PO	Unknown	2–6 hr	Unknown
IM (decanoate)	Unknown	6 days	Unknown
IM (lactate)	Unknown	10–20 min	Unknown

Half-life: PO, 14 to 37 hours; IM (decanoate), 3 weeks;
IM (lactate), 20 hours.

ADVERSE REACTIONS

CNS: agitation, extrapyramidal reactions, dystonia, drowsiness, headache, restlessness, hallucinations, parkinsonian-like syndrome, tremor, hypertonia, dystonia, bradykinesia, hyperkinesia. **EENT:** oculogyric crisis, dry mouth, salivary hypersecretion. **GI:** constipation, abdominal pain. **Metabolic:** hyperglycemia, hyponatremia.

INTERACTIONS

Drug-drug. *Anticholinergics (benztropine, scopolamine, solifenacin):* May increase anticholinergic effects and glaucoma. Use together cautiously.

Antiparkinsonian drugs (dopamine agonists): May diminish therapeutic effects of both haloperidol and antiparkinsonian drug (dopamine agonist). Avoid use together. If use together can't be avoided, monitor for decreased effects of both agents.

Buspirone, CYP2D6 inhibitors (chlorpromazine, paroxetine, quinidine, sertraline), CYP3A4 inhibitors (alprazolam, itraconazole, nefazodone, ritonavir): May increase haloperidol level and risk of adverse effects. Monitor QTc interval and adverse reactions. Dosage reduction may be needed.

CNS depressants: May increase CNS depression. Use together cautiously.

Corticosteroids, diuretics: May cause electrolyte imbalances and increase risk of QT-interval prolongation. Monitor electrolyte levels.

CYP2D6 substrates (desipramine, other TCAs): May increase substrate level. Monitor patient closely.

CYP3A4 inducers (carbamazepine, phenytoin, rifampin): May decrease haloperidol level and effectiveness. Monitor patient for clinical effect.

Lithium: May enhance neurotoxic effects and cause lethargy and confusion after high doses. Monitor patient.

Opioids: May increase CNS depression. Avoid use together. If use together is necessary, limit dosage and duration of each drug to minimum necessary for desired effect.

QT-interval-prolonging drugs (amiodarone, ondansetron, quinidine, erythromycin, levofloxacin, methadone): May prolong QT interval. Monitor ECG. Consider therapy modification.

Drug-herb. *St. John's wort:* May decrease haloperidol level. Discourage use together.

Drug-lifestyle. *Alcohol use, cannabidiol use:* May increase CNS depression. Discourage use together.

Smoking: May decrease haloperidol level. Monitor therapy.

EFFECTS ON LAB TEST RESULTS

- May increase LFT values and prolactin level.
- May decrease sodium level and platelet count.
- May increase or decrease glucose level and WBC count.

CONTRAINDICATIONS & CAUTIONS

- Contraindicated in patients hypersensitive to drug and in those with dementia with Lewy bodies, Parkinson disease, coma, or CNS depression.

Boxed Warning Older adults with dementia-related psychosis treated with atypical or conventional antipsychotics are at increased risk for death. Antipsychotics aren't approved for the treatment of dementia-related psychosis. ■

- Use cautiously in older adults; patients who are debilitated; and patients with history of seizures, EEG abnormalities, prolonged QT interval or other severe CV disorders, allergies, glaucoma, myasthenia gravis, or urine retention.

- Use cautiously in patients at risk for falls, including those who are taking drugs or have diseases or conditions that may cause somnolence, orthostatic hypotension, or motor or sensory instability.

- Endocrine disorders (including breast engorgement, lactation, and erectile dysfunction) have been reported.

- Esophageal dysmotility and aspiration can occur. Use cautiously in patients at risk.

- Decanoate form contains benzyl alcohol.

- Off-label IV administration of lactate form requires ECG monitoring for arrhythmias and prolonged QT interval.

- Blood dyscrasias have been reported. Discontinue drug for ANC less than 1,000/mm³ or for leukopenia or agranulocytosis.

Dialyzable drug: Unknown.

⚠ *Overdose S&S:* Severe extrapyramidal reactions; hypotension; sedation; EEG abnormalities, including torsades de pointes.

PREGNANCY-LACTATION-REPRODUCTION

🜚 *Alert:* Antipsychotic use during third trimester may result in extrapyramidal and withdrawal symptoms in newborns. May cause limb malformation if used during first trimester. Alternative agents are recommended. Use during pregnancy only if benefits outweigh fetal risk and at minimum effective dosage.

• Drug appears in human milk. Breastfeeding isn't recommended.

NURSING CONSIDERATIONS

• Monitor patient for tardive dyskinesia, which may occur after prolonged use. It may not appear until months or years later and may disappear spontaneously or persist for life, despite ending drug.

◐ *Alert:* Watch for signs and symptoms of NMS (mental status changes, muscle rigidity, hyperthermia, autonomic disturbances [arrhythmias, labile BP, tachycardia, diaphoresis], elevated CK level, rhabdomyolysis, AKI), which are rare but commonly fatal.

◐ *Alert:* Monitor ECG when drug is given in high dosages or when patient is taking other QT interval-prolonging drugs because of increased risk of QT-interval prolongation and torsades de pointes.

• Don't withdraw drug abruptly unless required by severe adverse reactions.

• Complete fall risk assessments at start of antipsychotic treatment and recurrently for patients on long-term therapy, especially those at increased risk for falls.

• *Look alike–sound alike:* Don't confuse Haldol with Halcion.

PATIENT TEACHING

◐ *Alert:* Caution patient or caregiver of patient taking an opioid with benzodiazepine, CNS depressant, or alcohol to seek immediate medical attention for dizziness, lightheadedness, extreme sleepiness, slowed or difficult breathing, or unresponsiveness.

• Advise patient to report all adverse reactions.

• Although drug is the least sedating of the antipsychotics, warn patient to avoid activities that require alertness and good coordination until effects of drug are known. Drowsiness and dizziness usually subside after a few weeks.

• Advise patient that drug may cause somnolence, orthostatic hypotension, and motor and sensory instability, which may lead to falls.

• Tell patient to relieve dry mouth with sugarless gum or hard candy.

• Caution patient to report changes in medications to prescribers and pharmacist.

• Instruct patient to report pregnancy or plans to become pregnant or to breastfeed.

SAFETY ALERT!

heparin sodium
HEP-a-rin

Therapeutic class: Anticoagulants
Pharmacologic class: Anticoagulants

AVAILABLE FORMS
Injection: 1,000 units/mL, 5,000 units/mL, 10,000 units/mL, 20,000 units/mL
Premixed IV solutions: Units of heparin and type of solution vary by manufacturer.
Syringes: 1,000 units/mL, 5,000 units/0.5 mL, 5,000 units/mL

INDICATIONS & DOSAGES
➤ **Full-dose continuous IV infusion therapy for VTE**
Adults: 80 units/kg by IV bolus; then 18 units/kg/hour by IV infusion with pump. Titrate hourly rate based on PTT results (every 4 to 6 hours in early stages of treatment).
Children: Initially, 75 to 100 units/kg IV over 10 minutes; then, for infants, maintenance dosage of 25 to 30 units/kg/hour IV. For children older than age 1 year, maintenance dosage, 18 to 20 units/kg/hour IV. Titrate dosage based on PTT.
➤ **Full-dose subcut therapy for VTE**
Adults: Initially, 5,000 units IV bolus and 10,000 to 20,000 units in a concentrated solution subcut; then 8,000 to 10,000 units subcut every 8 hours or 15,000 to 20,000 units in a concentrated solution subcut every 12 hours.
➤ **Full-dose intermittent anticoagulation IV therapy for VTE**
Adults: Initially, 10,000 units by IV bolus; then 5,000 to 10,000 units (or 50 to 70 units/kg) IV every 4 to 6 hours titrated according to PTT.
➤ **Fixed low-dose therapy to prevent VTE, embolism associated with atrial fibrillation, and postoperative DVT**
Adults: 5,000 units subcut every 12 hours. For patients undergoing surgery, give first dose 2 hours before procedure; then 5,000 units subcut every 8 to 12 hours for 5 to 7 days or until patient can walk.

H

ADMINISTRATION

IV

▼ Confirm selection of the correct formulation and strength before administration.

▼ Establish baseline coagulation parameters before therapy.

▼ For continuous infusion, use an infusion pump to provide maximum safety. Check infusions regularly, even when pumps are in good working order, to ensure correct dosing. Place notice above patient's bed to caution IV team or lab personnel to apply pressure dressings after venipuncture.

▼ When adding heparin to infusion solution, invert IV container at least six times to adequately mix solution.

▼ During intermittent administration, always draw blood 30 minutes before next scheduled dose to avoid falsely prolonged PTT. Blood for PTT may be drawn 4 hours after continuous IV heparin therapy starts. Never draw blood for PTT from tubing of heparin infusion or from infused vein because PTT will be falsely prolonged. Always draw blood from opposite arm.

▼ Don't skip a dose or try to "catch up" with a solution containing heparin. If solution runs out, restart it as soon as possible and immediately reschedule bolus dose. Monitor PTT.

▼ Note that concentrated heparin solutions (more than 100 units/mL) can irritate blood vessels.

▼ Never piggyback other drugs into an infusion line while heparin infusion is running. Never mix another drug and heparin in same syringe when giving bolus.

▼ **Incompatibilities:** Alteplase, amiodarone, ciprofloxacin, diazepam, doxycycline hyclate, droperidol, ergotamine, erythromycin, filgrastim, gentamicin, haloperidol, idarubicin, levofloxacin, nesiritide, phenytoin sodium, reteplase. For additional information, consult drug compatibility reference.

Subcutaneous

● Give low-dose injections sequentially between iliac crests in lower abdomen deep into subcutaneous fat. Inject drug subcut slowly into fat pad.

● Don't massage injection site.

● Watch for signs of bleeding at injection site.

● Alternate sites. Record location.

ACTION

Accelerates formation of antithrombin III-thrombin complex and deactivates thrombin, preventing conversion of fibrinogen to fibrin.

Route	Onset	Peak	Duration
IV	Immediate	Immediate	Variable
Subcut	20–30 min	2–4 hr	Variable

Half-life: 0.5 to 2 hours. Half-life is dose-dependent and nonlinear and may be disproportionately prolonged at higher doses.

ADVERSE REACTIONS

CNS: fever. **CV:** *hemorrhage.* **EENT:** rhinitis. **Hematologic:** *heparin-induced thrombocytopenia, thrombocytopenia.* **Metabolic:** *hyperkalemia,* hypoaldosteronism. **Musculoskeletal:** osteoporosis. **Skin:** irritation, mild pain, hematoma, ulceration, cutaneous or subcutaneous necrosis, pruritus, urticaria, transient alopecia. **Other:** hypersensitivity reactions, heparin resistance.

INTERACTIONS

Drug-drug. *Antihistamines, digoxin, nicotine, nitrates, IV nitroglycerin, tetracyclines:* May decrease heparin effect. Monitor coagulation test results.

Antiplatelet drugs, salicylates: May increase anticoagulant effect. Use together cautiously. Closely monitor coagulation test results and patient.

Oral anticoagulants: May increase additive anticoagulation. Monitor PT, INR, and PTT. Avoid combination use unless bridging for long-term warfarin use.

Oritavancin, telavancin: May diminish therapeutic effect of heparin; may artificially increase results of lab tests commonly used to monitor IV heparin. Avoid combination.

Thrombolytics: May increase risk of hemorrhage. Monitor patient closely.

Drug-lifestyle. *Smoking:* May interfere with anticoagulant effect of heparin. Discourage smoking.

EFFECTS ON LAB TEST RESULTS

● May increase ALT, AST, and potassium levels.

● May increase INR and prolong PT and PTT.

● May decrease platelet count.

● May cause false elevations in some tests for thyroxine level.

CONTRAINDICATIONS & CAUTIONS

• Contraindicated in patients hypersensitive to heparin, except in life-threatening situations when alternative anticoagulation isn't possible.

• Contraindicated in patients with history of heparin-induced thrombocytopenia (HIT) and heparin-induced thrombocytopenia and thrombosis (HITT), in those with uncontrolled bleeding state (except DIC), and when blood coagulation tests can't be performed at appropriate intervals (for full-dose heparin).

• Some products are derived from animal tissues and may be contraindicated in patients with pork allergy; consult manufacturer's instructions.

• Use cautiously in patients at increased risk for hemorrhage, such as those with hemophilia, thrombocytopenia, vascular purpuras, subacute bacterial endocarditis, severe HTN, hereditary antithrombin III deficiency receiving concurrent antithrombin III therapy, ulcerative lesions and continuous tube drainage of stomach or small intestine, liver disease with impaired hemostasis, as well as during and immediately after spinal tap or spinal anesthesia or major surgery (especially involving brain, spinal cord, or eye).

• Drug may reduce bone mineral density with prolonged use (longer than 6 months).

• Drug may increase risk of bleeding in females older than age 60.

Dialyzable drug: Unknown.

⚠ *Overdose S&S:* Bleeding, nosebleeds, hematuria, melena, easy bruising, petechiae.

PREGNANCY-LACTATION-REPRODUCTION

• Drug doesn't cross placental barrier. Use during pregnancy only if potential benefit justifies fetal risk.

• Heparin doesn't appear in human milk.

• Use preservative-free formulations (without benzyl alcohol) in patients who are pregnant or breastfeeding and in neonates. Benzyl alcohol may cause gasping syndrome in neonates.

NURSING CONSIDERATIONS

⚕ *Alert:* Some commercially available heparin injections contain benzyl alcohol.

• Drug requirements are higher in early phases of thrombogenic diseases and febrile states; they are lower when patient's condition stabilizes.

• Older adults usually start at lower dosage.

• Monitor for hyperkalemia during therapy.

⚕ *Alert:* Check order and vial carefully; heparin comes in various concentrations. Label must clearly state the strength of the entire container, followed by how much medication is in 1 mL.

⚕ *Alert:* USP and international units are equivalent for heparin.

⚕ *Alert:* Heparin and low-molecular-weight heparins aren't interchangeable.

⚕ *Alert:* Don't change concentrations of infusions unless necessary. This is a common source of dosage errors.

⚕ *Alert:* Delayed onset of HIT, a serious antibody-mediated reaction resulting from irreversible aggregation of platelets, is possible. HIT may progress to development of venous and arterial thromboses, a condition referred to as HITT. Thrombotic events may be the initial presentation for HITT, which can occur up to several weeks after stopping heparin therapy. Evaluate patients presenting with thrombocytopenia or thrombosis after stopping heparin for HIT and HITT.

• Draw blood for PTT 4 to 6 hours after subcut dose or after starting infusion.

• Avoid IM injections of other drugs to prevent or minimize hematoma.

• Regularly monitor PTT. Anticoagulation is present when PTT values are 1½ to 2 times normal control values.

• Regularly monitor platelet count. When new thrombosis accompanies thrombocytopenia (white clot syndrome), stop heparin.

• Regularly inspect patient for bleeding gums, bruises on arms or legs, petechiae, nosebleeds, melena, hematuria, and hematemesis.

• Monitor vital signs.

⚕ *Alert:* To treat severe overdose, use protamine sulfate, a heparin antagonist. Base dosage on dose of heparin, its route of administration, and time since it was given. Generally, 1 mg of protamine neutralizes 100 USP units of heparin. Don't give more than 50 mg protamine in a 10-minute period. Protamine can cause severe hypotension and anaphylactoid reactions. Ensure emergency treatment is available.

• Abrupt withdrawal may cause increased coagulability; warfarin therapy usually overlaps heparin therapy for continued prophylaxis or treatment.

• *Look alike–sound alike:* Don't confuse heparin with Hespan or low-molecular-weight heparin.

PATIENT TEACHING

• Instruct patient to report all drug and food allergies.

• Caution patient and family to report all adverse reactions.

• Advise patient and family to watch for and immediately report signs and symptoms of bleeding (abnormal bleeding or bruising, red or black vomit or feces, abdominal pain, change in mental status, headache).

• Tell patient to avoid OTC drugs containing aspirin, other salicylates, or drugs that may interact with heparin, unless ordered by prescriber.

• Advise patient to consult prescriber before starting herbal therapy; many herbs have anticoagulant, antiplatelet, or fibrinolytic properties.

• Counsel patient to inform practitioners and dentists about receiving heparin before scheduling surgical procedures.

---

hydrALAZINE hydrochloride
hye-DRAL-a-zeen

Apresoline✤

Therapeutic class: Antihypertensives
Pharmacologic class: Peripheral vasodilators

AVAILABLE FORMS

Injection: 20 mg/mL
Tablets: 10 mg, 25 mg, 50 mg, 100 mg

INDICATIONS & DOSAGES

➤ **HTN**

Adults: Initially, 10 mg PO q.i.d. for first 2 to 4 days, then 25 mg q.i.d. for balance of first week; 50 mg q.i.d. from second week on, based on patient tolerance and response. Maximum dosage, 300 mg/day.

Children ages 1 and older: Initially, 0.75 mg/kg PO in two to four divided doses; gradually increase over 3 to 4 weeks to maximum of 7.5 mg/kg/day in four divided doses or 200 mg/day.

Adjust-a-dose: For maintenance dosage, adjust to lowest effective dosage.

➤ **Hypertensive emergency**

Adults: 10 to 20 mg IM or IV; repeat as needed every 4 to 6 hours. May increase to maximum of 40 mg/dose if necessary. Switch to oral form as soon as possible.

Children: 1.7 to 3.5 mg/kg/day IM or IV divided into four to six doses.

➤ **HF with reduced ejection fraction ♦**

Adults: Initially, 25 mg PO t.i.d. in combination with isosorbide dinitrate. Target dosage is 75 mg t.i.d.

ADMINISTRATION

PO

• May give with or without food but giving with food increases absorption. Give consistently with regard to meals.

IV

▼ Give drug as rapid bolus directly into vein only when it can't be given orally. Don't add drug to infusion solutions.

▼ Repeat PRN, generally every 4 to 6 hours.

▼ For children, give drug over 1 to 2 minutes; maximum rate, 5 mg/minute.

▼ Drug may discolor upon contact with metal; discard discolored solutions. Should use immediately after opening vial.

▼ **Incompatibilities:** None.

IM

• Administer undiluted as IM injection.

ACTION

Not fully understood. A direct-acting peripheral vasodilator that relaxes arteriolar smooth muscle.

Route	Onset	Peak	Duration
PO	20–30 min	1–2 hr	2–4 hr
IV	5–20 min	10–80 min	2–6 hr
IM	10–30 min	Within 1 hr	2–6 hr

Half-life: 3 to 7 hours.

ADVERSE REACTIONS

CNS: anxiety, headache, depression, dizziness, peripheral neuritis, *increased ICP,* psychosis, fever. **CV:** angina pectoris, palpitations, tachycardia, orthostatic hypotension, edema, flushing, paradoxical hypertensive response. **EENT:** conjunctivitis, nasal congestion, lacrimation. **GI:** nausea, vomiting, diarrhea, anorexia, constipation, paralytic ileus. **GU:** difficult urination. **Hematologic:** anemia, *neutropenia, leukopenia, agranulocytosis,* eosinophilia, *thrombocytopenia with or without purpura.* **Musculoskeletal:** muscle cramps, arthralgia. **Respiratory:** dyspnea. **Skin:** diaphoresis, pruritus, urticaria, rash. **Other:** hypersensitivity reactions, chills.

Reactions in bold italics are *life-threatening*.

INTERACTIONS

Drug-drug. *Diazoxide, MAO inhibitors:* May cause severe hypotension. Use together cautiously.

Diuretics, other hypotensive drugs: May cause excessive hypotension. Dosage adjustment may be needed.

NSAIDs: May decrease effects of hydralazine. Monitor BP.

Drug-food. *Any food:* Food may increase drug absorption. Encourage patient to take drug with food.

EFFECTS ON LAB TEST RESULTS

- May decrease Hb level and neutrophil, WBC, granulocyte, platelet, and RBC counts.
- May cause positive ANA titers.

CONTRAINDICATIONS & CAUTIONS

- Contraindicated in patients hypersensitive to drug and in those with CAD or mitral valvular rheumatic heart disease.
- Drug may contain tartrazine and cause allergic reactions, especially in patients hypersensitive to aspirin.
- Drug may produce a clinical picture consistent with SLE.
- Use cautiously in patients with suspected cardiac disease, stroke, or kidney impairment and in those taking other antihypertensives.
- May cause blood dyscrasias. Discontinue drug if they occur.

Dialyzable drug: Unknown.

⚠ **Overdose S&S:** Hypotension, tachycardia, headache, flushing.

PREGNANCY-LACTATION-REPRODUCTION

- Drug crosses placental barrier. Use during pregnancy only if expected benefit justifies fetal risk.
- Drug is excreted in human milk. Use cautiously during breastfeeding.

NURSING CONSIDERATIONS

- Frequently monitor patient's BP standing, sitting, and supine; HR; and body weight.
- Drug may be given with diuretics and beta blockers to decrease sodium retention and tachycardia and to prevent angina attacks.
- Older adults may be more sensitive to drug's hypotensive effects.
- Obtain CBC, lupus erythematosus cell preparation, and ANA titer determination before therapy and periodically during long-term therapy.

⚠ *Alert:* Monitor patient closely for signs and symptoms of lupuslike syndrome (sore throat, fever, muscle and joint aches, rash), and immediately notify prescriber if they develop. Long-term steroid therapy may be necessary.
- *Look alike–sound alike:* Don't confuse hydralazine with hydroxyzine.

PATIENT TEACHING

- Instruct patient to take oral form consistently with meals to increase absorption.
- Inform patient that low BP and dizziness upon standing can be minimized by rising slowly and avoiding sudden position changes.
- Tell patient to report all adverse reactions, including unexplained prolonged general tiredness or fever, muscle or joint aches, and chest pain.
- Instruct patient to report pregnancy or plans to become pregnant or to breastfeed.

---

hydroCHLOROthiazide
hye-droe-klor-oh-THYE-a-zide

Therapeutic class: Diuretics
Pharmacologic class: Thiazide diuretics

AVAILABLE FORMS

Capsules: 12.5 mg
Tablets: 12.5 mg, 25 mg, 50 mg

INDICATIONS & DOSAGES

Adjust-a-dose (for all indications): In patients older than age 65, give 12.5 mg daily initially. Adjust in increments of 12.5 mg, if needed.

▶ **Edema**

Adults: 25 to 100 mg PO daily in one or two divided doses.

Children ages 6 months to 12 years: Initially, 1 to 2 mg/kg/day PO in a single dose or two divided doses. May increase to maximum of 37.5 mg/day for children ages 6 months to 2 years and 100 mg/day for children ages 2 to 12 years.

Children younger than age 6 months: 1 to 2 mg/kg/day PO in single dose or two divided doses. Dosages up to 3 mg/kg/day in two divided doses may be needed. Maximum dosage, 37.5 mg/day.

Adjust-a-dose: May give on intermittent schedule (every other day or 3 to 5 days each week) to decrease risk of excessive response and electrolyte imbalances.

➤ HTN
Adults: 12.5 to 50 mg PO daily in one or two divided doses. Increase or decrease daily dosage based on BP.

Children ages 6 months to 12 years: Initially, 1 to 2 mg/kg/day PO in a single dose or two divided doses. May increase to maximum dosage of 37.5 mg/day for children ages 6 months to 2 years and 100 mg/day for children ages 2 to 12 years.

Children younger than age 6 months: 1 to 2 mg/kg/day PO in single dose or two divided doses. Dosages up to 3 mg/kg/day in two divided doses may be needed. Maximum dosage, 37.5 mg/day.

ADMINISTRATION
PO
• Give drug without regard to food.
• To prevent nocturia, give drug in morning. If second dose is needed, give in early afternoon, preferably no later than 6 p.m.
• Capsules aren't indicated for use in children.

ACTION
Increases sodium and water excretion by inhibiting sodium and chloride reabsorption in distal segment of the nephron.

Route	Onset	Peak	Duration
PO	2–6 hr	1–5 hr	6–12 hr

Half-life: About 6 to 15 hours.

ADVERSE REACTIONS
CNS: dizziness, vertigo, headache, paresthesia, weakness, restlessness, asthenia, fever. **CV:** hypotension, vasculitis. **EENT:** blurred vision, yellowing of vision, salivary gland infection. **GI:** *pancreatitis,* anorexia, nausea, epigastric distress, vomiting, abdominal pain, diarrhea, constipation, abdominal cramps. **GU:** *KF,* polyuria, frequent urination, glycosuria, interstitial nephritis, erectile dysfunction. **Hematologic:** *aplastic anemia, agranulocytosis, leukopenia, thrombocytopenia,* hemolytic anemia. **Hepatic:** jaundice. **Metabolic:** asymptomatic hyperuricemia; hyperglycemia and impaired glucose tolerance; fluid and electrolyte imbalances, including hyponatremia, *hypomagnesemia, hypokalemia,* hypochloremia; metabolic alkalosis; hypercalcemia; dehydration. **Musculoskeletal:** muscle spasms. **Respiratory:** *respiratory distress,* pneumonitis. **Skin:** dermatitis, photosensitivity reactions, rash, purpura, alopecia, *erythema multiforme,* exfoliative dermatitis, urticaria. **Other:** *anaphylactic reactions,* hypersensitivity reactions, gout.

INTERACTIONS
Drug-drug. *Allopurinol:* May increase allopurinol level and enhance potential for allergic or hypersensitivity reactions to allopurinol. Monitor allopurinol level.

Amphotericin B, corticosteroids, topiramate: May increase risk of hypokalemia. Closely monitor potassium level.

Antidiabetics: May decrease hypoglycemic effects. Adjust dosage if needed. Monitor glucose level.

Antihypertensives: May have additive antihypertensive effect. Use together cautiously.

Barbiturates, opioids: May increase orthostatic hypotensive effect. Monitor patient closely.

Cardiac glycosides: May increase risk of digoxin toxicity from diuretic-induced hypokalemia. Monitor potassium and digoxin levels.

Cholestyramine, colestipol: May decrease intestinal absorption of thiazides. Separate doses by 2 hours.

Diazoxide: May increase antihypertensive, hyperglycemic, and hyperuricemic effects. Use together cautiously.

Dofetilide: May enhance QTc-prolonging effect of dofetilide. Use is contraindicated.

Lithium: May decrease lithium excretion, increasing risk of lithium toxicity. Consider therapy modification.

Multivitamins and minerals (vitamin D₃): May increase calcium level and effects of digoxin. Monitor patient closely.

NSAIDs: May increase risk of KF. May decrease diuretic and antihypertensive effects. Monitor kidney function and BP.

Drug-herb. *Licorice:* May cause unexpected rapid potassium loss. Discourage use together.

Drug-lifestyle. *Alcohol use:* May increase orthostatic hypotensive effect. Discourage use together.

EFFECTS ON LAB TEST RESULTS
• May increase glucose, cholesterol, triglyceride, calcium, and uric acid levels.
• May decrease potassium, sodium, chloride, magnesium, and serum protein-bound iodine levels.
• May decrease Hb level and granulocyte, WBC, and platelet counts.

Reactions in bold italics are *life-threatening*.

CONTRAINDICATIONS & CAUTIONS
• Contraindicated in patients with anuria and patients hypersensitive to other thiazides or other sulfonamide derivatives.
• Drug can cause systemic lupus activation or exacerbation.
• Use cautiously in patients with gout. Drug may reduce clearance of uric acid.
• Use cautiously in children, older adults, and patients with CrCl less than 30 mL/minute, gout, hypercholesterolemia, diabetes, impaired liver function, or progressive liver disease.
• Drug isn't effective in patients with CrCl less than 10 mL/minute.
Dialyzable drug: No.
⚠ *Overdose S&S:* Electrolyte imbalances, dehydration.

PREGNANCY-LACTATION-REPRODUCTION
• Studies during pregnancy are inadequate; use during pregnancy only if clearly needed.
• Drug crosses placental barrier; maternal use may adversely affect fetus.
• Thiazides appear in human milk. Discontinue drug or discontinue breastfeeding, considering importance of drug to patient.

NURSING CONSIDERATIONS
• Monitor fluid intake and output, weight, BP, and electrolyte levels; correct electrolyte disturbances before start of therapy.
• Watch for signs and symptoms of hypokalemia (muscle weakness, cramps).
• Drug may be used with potassium-sparing diuretic to prevent potassium loss.
• Consult prescriber and dietitian about a high-potassium diet or potassium supplement.
• Regularly monitor creatinine and BUN levels. Cumulative effects of drug may occur with impaired kidney function.
• Monitor uric acid level, especially in patient with history of gout.
• Monitor glucose level, especially in patient with diabetes.
• Closely monitor older adult, who is especially susceptible to excessive diuresis.
• Stop thiazides and thiazide-like diuretics before parathyroid function tests.
• In patient with HTN, therapeutic response may be delayed several weeks.
• Monitor patient for vision changes and ocular pain. Drug may increase risk of acute myopia and secondary angle-closure glaucoma.

PATIENT TEACHING
• Teach about proper drug administration and handling.
• Advise patient to report all adverse reactions, to avoid sudden posture changes, and to rise slowly to avoid dizziness upon standing quickly.
• Encourage sunblock use to prevent photosensitivity reactions.
• Tell patient to check with prescriber or pharmacist before using OTC drugs.
• Advise patient to report pregnancy, plans to become pregnant, breastfeeding, or plans to breastfeed.

SAFETY ALERT!

HYDROcodone bitartrate
hye-droe-KOE-done

Hysingla ER

Therapeutic class: Opioid analgesics
Pharmacologic class: Opioid analgesics
Controlled substance schedule: II

AVAILABLE FORMS
Capsules (extended-release) ⓓⓝⓒ: 10 mg, 15 mg, 20 mg, 30 mg, 40 mg, 50 mg
Tablets (extended-release) ⓓⓝⓒ: 20 mg, 30 mg, 40 mg, 60 mg, 80 mg, 100 mg, 120 mg

INDICATIONS & DOSAGES
➤ **Management of pain severe enough to require daily, around-the-clock, long-term opioid treatment and for which alternative treatment options are inadequate**
Adults who are opioid naive or who aren't opioid tolerant: Initially, 10 mg extended-release capsule PO every 12 hours. Gradually adjust dosage, preferably in increments of 10 mg every 12 hours every 3 to 7 days, until adequate pain relief and acceptable adverse reactions have been achieved.

Or, 20 mg extended-release tablet PO once daily. Increase dosage in increments of 10 to 20 mg once daily every 3 to 5 days as needed to achieve adequate analgesia.
Adults who are opioid tolerant: Discontinue all other around-the-clock opioids before initiating therapy. Refer to manufacturer's instructions when converting from other oral opioids to hydrocodone; doses aren't equianalgesic.

♣Canada   ◇OTC   ◆Off-label use   ⓓⓝⓒDo not crush   *Liquid contains alcohol   ✂Genetic

Adjust-a-dose: In patients with CrCl less than 60 mL/minute, start with 50% of the extended-release tablet initial dose or initiate treatment with low-dose extended-release capsule, and monitor patient closely.

Adjust-a-dose: For patients with Child-Pugh class C liver impairment, start with 10 mg extended-release capsule PO every 12 hours or use 50% of initial dose of extended-release tablet.

Adjust-a-dose: Decrease initial dose in older adults, who may be more sensitive to adverse effects.

ADMINISTRATION

PO
• Have patient swallow tablets whole; don't crush or break tablets. Don't alter capsules or tablets because of risk of rapid release and absorption of potentially fatal drug dose.
• Give capsules or tablets one at a time with enough water to ensure complete swallowing immediately after placing in mouth.
• Don't presoak, wet, or allow patient to lick tablets before administration, which may increase risk of choking and uncontrolled drug delivery.
• Store at room temperature.

ACTION
Acts as a full agonist primarily at the mu opioid receptor, binding to and activating opioid receptors at various sites in the CNS to produce analgesia.

Route	Onset	Peak	Duration
PO (tablet)	Unknown	6–30 hr	Unknown
PO (capsule)	Unknown	5 hr	Unknown

Half-life: Tablet, 7 to 9 hours; capsule, about 8 hours.

ADVERSE REACTIONS
CNS: somnolence, tremor, lethargy, anxiety, depression, insomnia, fatigue, dizziness, drowsiness, headache, migraine, pain, paresthesia, sedation, fever. **CV:** peripheral edema, hot flush, HTN. **EENT:** tinnitus, nasopharyngitis, nasal congestion, oropharyngeal pain, sinusitis, dry mouth. **GI:** constipation, nausea, vomiting, abdominal pain, GERD, decreased appetite, diarrhea, dyspepsia, gastroenteritis. **GU:** UTI. **Hepatic:** increased GGT level. **Metabolic:** dehydration, hypercholesterole-mia, *hypokalemia.* **Musculoskeletal:** muscle spasms, back pain,

foot fracture, joint injury, joint sprain, muscle strain, arthralgia, musculoskeletal pain, myalgia, neck pain, extremity pain, noncardiac chest pain, osteoarthritis. **Respiratory:** URI, bronchitis, cough, dyspnea. **Skin:** pruritus, skin laceration, hyperhidrosis, night sweats, rash. **Other:** fall, flulike syndrome, chills.

INTERACTIONS
Drug-drug. *Anticholinergics (scopolamine, diphenhydramine):* May increase risk of urine retention, severe constipation, or paralytic ileus. Monitor patient for signs and symptoms of urine retention and constipation in addition to respiratory and CNS depression. Use together cautiously.

Boxed Warning *Benzodiazepines, CNS depressants:* May cause slow or difficult breathing, sedation, and death. Avoid use together. If use together is necessary, limit dosage and duration of each drug to the minimum necessary for desired effect. ■

Boxed Warning *CYP3A4 inhibitors (amiodarone, erythromycin, ketoconazole, nefazodone, protease inhibitors, ritonavir):* May increase hydrocodone level and prolong opioid effects, especially with concomitant CYP3A4 inhibitor use. Monitor patient for respiratory depression and sedation; consider dosage adjustments until drug effects are stable. ■

Boxed Warning *CYP3A4 inducers (carbamazepine, phenytoin, rifampin):* May induce metabolism and decrease hydrocodone level, decreasing efficacy and potentially causing withdrawal symptoms. Monitor patient for effectiveness of drug and for opioid withdrawal symptoms. Consider dosage adjustments until stable. If CYP3A4 inducer is stopped, monitor patient for increased therapeutic and adverse effects, especially respiratory depression. ■

Diuretics (furosemide): May reduce diuretic effect. Monitor patient for clinical effect and increase diuretic dosage as indicated.

Laxatives: May increase GI motility and decrease hydrocodone absorption. Monitor patient for hydrocodone therapeutic effect.

MAO inhibitors: May potentiate effects of opioid analgesics or result in serotonin syndrome. Don't use in patients who have received MAO inhibitors within past 14 days.

Mixed agonist/antagonists (butorphanol, nalbuphine, pentazocine), partial agonists

Reactions in bold italics are *life-threatening*.

(buprenorphine): May reduce analgesic effect of hydrocodone or precipitate withdrawal symptoms. Avoid use together.

Muscle relaxants: May enhance effects of skeletal muscle relaxants and increase respiratory depression. Dosage adjustment may be needed. Monitor patient.

🌣 *Alert: Serotonergic drugs (amoxapine, antimigraine drugs, buspirone, cyclobenzaprine, dextromethorphan, linezolid, lithium, maprotiline, methylene blue, mirtazapine, nefazodone, SSNRIs, SSRIs, TCAs, trazodone, tryptophan, vilazodone):* May increase risk of serotonin syndrome; may enhance toxic effect of hydrocodone. Use together cautiously. Monitor patient for serotonin syndrome.

Drug-herb. 🌣 *Alert: St. John's wort:* May decrease hydrocodone level. Use together cautiously.

Drug-lifestyle. **Boxed Warning** *Alcohol use:* May cause slow or difficult breathing, sedation, and death. Discourage use together. ∎

EFFECTS ON LAB TEST RESULTS
- May increase cholesterol and GGT levels.
- May decrease potassium level.

CONTRAINDICATIONS & CAUTIONS
Boxed Warning Use exposes patient and others to risk of opioid addiction, abuse, and misuse, which can lead to overdose and death. These effects can occur at any dose or duration. Assess patient risk before prescribing and regularly reassess patient for these behaviors and conditions. ∎

Boxed Warning Accidental ingestion of even one dose of this drug, especially by children, can result in a fatal overdose. ∎

Boxed Warning *Opioid class warning:* Opioids should only be prescribed with benzodiazepines or other CNS depressants when alternative treatment options are inadequate, aren't expected to provide adequate analgesia, haven't been tolerated, or aren't expected to be tolerated. ∎

Boxed Warning Prescribers are strongly encouraged to complete a REMS-compliant education program. Drug should be prescribed only by prescribers with knowledge of opioid use and ways to reduce associated risks. ∎

🌣 *Alert:* Use lowest effective dose for shortest period consistent with patient's treatment goals.

🌣 *Alert:* Because risk of overdose increases as opioid dose increases, reserve titration to higher doses for patients in whom lower doses are ineffective and in whom expected benefits of higher opioid dose outweigh risks.

🌣 *Alert:* Long-acting or extended-release formulations are indicated for severe, persistent pain for which extended treatment with a daily opioid analgesic is required and for which alternative treatment options are inadequate. Use isn't indicated for as-needed analgesia.

- Contraindicated in patients with significant respiratory depression, acute or severe bronchial asthma, known or suspected paralytic ileus, or hypersensitivity to drug or its components.
- Use cautiously in patients with hypersensitivity to morphine, oxycodone, and codeine because cross-reactivity may occur.
- Use cautiously in patients who are cachectic or debilitated; critical respiratory depression is a risk even at therapeutic dosages.
- Use cautiously in patients with history of seizures and adrenal insufficiency.

🌣 *Alert:* Drug may lead to rare but serious decrease in adrenal gland cortisol production.

- Use cautiously in older adults and in patients with chronic pulmonary disease, seizure disorder, hypotension or depleted blood volume, or liver or kidney impairment.

🌣 *Alert:* Avoid use in patients with head injuries, increased ICP, brain tumors, impaired consciousness, or coma. Drug reduces respiratory drive, increasing carbon dioxide retention and ICP.

- Drug may reduce sex hormone levels with long-term use.
- QTc interval may be prolonged with dosages greater than 160 mg daily. Use cautiously in patients with HF, bradyarrhythmias, or electrolyte abnormalities and in patients using other drugs known to prolong the QTc interval. Don't use in those with congenital long QT syndrome. If QTc-interval prolongation occurs, consider dosage reduction of 33% to 50% or change to another analgesic.
- Esophageal obstruction, dysphagia, and choking have occurred with use of extended-release tablets. Patients with underlying GI disorders or a small GI lumen are at greater risk. Consider another analgesic in these patients.
- Safety and effectiveness in children younger than age 18 haven't been established.

Dialyzable drug: Unknown.

⚠ *Overdose S&S:* Respiratory depression; somnolence (can lead to stupor or coma); skeletal muscle flaccidity; cold, clammy skin; constricted pupils (although mydriasis rather than miosis may occur due to severe hypoxia in overdose situations); pulmonary edema; bradycardia; hypotension; death.

PREGNANCY-LACTATION-REPRODUCTION

• Use during pregnancy only if benefit outweighs fetal risk.

Boxed Warning Prolonged use during pregnancy can result in neonatal opioid withdrawal syndrome, which may be life-threatening. It requires management with expert neonatology protocols. If prolonged use is needed, advise patient of risks and ensure availability of proper treatment. ■

• Don't use during labor and delivery; neonatal respiratory depression may occur.

• Opioids may appear in human milk. Use cautiously during breastfeeding.

• Monitor infants exposed to drug through human milk for excess sedation and respiratory depression.

• Watch for withdrawal symptoms in infants who are breastfed when patient stops opioid analgesic or stops breastfeeding.

• Prolonged opioid use may reduce fertility in individuals of reproductive potential. It's unknown whether these effects on fertility are reversible.

NURSING CONSIDERATIONS

• Be aware that drug may be targeted for theft, diversion, and misuse.

🕏 *Alert:* When giving first dose, it's preferable to underestimate patient's 24-hour oral hydrocodone requirements and provide rescue medication (immediate-release opioid) than to overestimate the 24-hour oral hydrocodone requirements, which could result in adverse reactions.

Boxed Warning May cause life-threatening or fatal respiratory depression at any time during therapy. Monitor patient closely, especially when starting or increasing doses. Proper dosing and titration are essential to reduce risk. ■

Boxed Warning Regularly monitor all patients for opioid addiction, abuse, and misuse, which can lead to overdose and death. ■

🕏 *Alert:* Drug may cause opioid-induced hyperalgesia (OIH). Symptoms include increased pain level with opioid dose increase, decreased pain level with opioid dose reduction, pain from ordinarily nonpainful stimuli without underlying disease progression, opioid tolerance or withdrawal, and addictive behavior. For suspected OIH, decrease opioid dose or switch patient to alternative opioid.

🕏 *Alert:* If patient is taking opioids with serotonergic drugs, watch for signs and symptoms of serotonin syndrome (agitation, hallucinations, rapid HR, fever, diaphoresis, shivering or shaking, muscle twitching or stiffness, trouble with coordination, nausea, vomiting, diarrhea), especially when starting treatment or increasing dosages. Signs and symptoms may occur within several hours of coadministration but may also occur later, especially after dosage increase. Discontinue opioid, serotonergic drug, or both if serotonin syndrome is suspected.

🕏 *Alert:* Monitor for signs and symptoms of adrenal insufficiency (nausea, vomiting, loss of appetite, fatigue, weakness, dizziness, low BP). Perform diagnostic testing if adrenal insufficiency is suspected. If adrenal insufficiency is confirmed, treat with corticosteroids, and wean patient off opioids, if appropriate. Discontinue corticosteroids when clinically appropriate.

• Monitor patient for signs and symptoms of decreased sex hormone levels (low libido, erectile dysfunction, amenorrhea, infertility). If signs and symptoms occur, evaluate patient and obtain specimens for lab testing.

🕏 *Alert:* Don't stop drug abruptly; withdraw slowly and individualize the gradual tapering plan to prevent signs and symptoms of withdrawal, worsening pain, and psychological distress in patients who are physically dependent. Refer to manufacturer's label for specific tapering instructions.

🕏 *Alert:* When tapering opioids, monitor patients closely for signs and symptoms of opioid withdrawal (restlessness, lacrimation, rhinorrhea, yawning, perspiration, chills, myalgia, mydriasis, irritability, anxiety, insomnia, backache, joint pain, weakness, abdominal cramps, anorexia, nausea, vomiting, diarrhea, increased BP or HR, increased respiratory rate). Such signs and symptoms may indicate a need to taper more slowly. Also monitor patients for suicidality, use of other substances, and mood changes.

• Patients considered opioid tolerant are those receiving for 1 week or longer at least

60 mg morphine per day, 25 mcg/hour transdermal fentanyl, 30 mg oral oxycodone per day, 8 mg oral hydromorphone per day, 25 mg oral oxymorphone per day, 60 mg oral hydrocodone per day, or an equianalgesic dose of another opioid.

• Closely monitor patients converting from methadone because methadone has a long half-life and can accumulate in plasma, causing significant respiratory depression.

• Closely monitor patient converting from fentanyl patches because of risk of additive effects.

• Note that older adult receiving drug, especially one with impaired liver or kidney function, may become confused and oversedated. Start with low doses of hydrocodone and closely watch for adverse events, such as respiratory depression.

• Watch for decreased bowel motility in patient who has undergone surgery and for biliary spasm in patients with biliary tract disease or acute pancreatitis.

• Monitor patient with history of seizure disorder for worsening seizure control.

• Use lowest initial dose in patient with kidney or liver impairment, and monitor closely for adverse events, such as respiratory depression.

• Periodically reevaluate patient's need for therapy.

• *Look alike–sound alike:* Don't confuse hydrocodone extended-release with hydrocodone standard release. Don't confuse hydrocodone with oxycodone, oxymorphone, or hydromorphone.

PATIENT TEACHING
Boxed Warning Counsel patient and caregiver on serious risks, safe use, and importance of reading the medication guide with each prescription. ∎

• Advise patient to take drug exactly as prescribed and to use lowest dose possible for shortest time needed.

• Warn patient that extended-release and long-acting formulations aren't to be taken on an "as needed" basis.

• Instruct patient to contact health care provider if prescribed dosage isn't controlling pain.

• *Alert:* Warn patient to withhold drug and inform prescriber if pain level worsens, pain sensitivity increases, or new pain occurs after taking drug.

• Teach patient that naloxone may be prescribed with the opioid when beginning and renewing therapy to reduce risk of opioid overdose and death.

• *Alert:* Encourage patient to report all medications being taken, including prescription and OTC medications and supplements.

• *Alert:* Caution patient to immediately report signs and symptoms of serotonin syndrome, adrenal insufficiency, and decreased sex hormone levels.

• *Alert:* Counsel patient who has been regularly taking drug not to discontinue without first discussing the need for gradual tapering with prescriber.

• Caution patient not to share drug and to protect it from theft or misuse.

• Inform patient that potentially serious additive effects may occur if drug is used with other CNS depressants. Warn patient to avoid such drugs unless supervised by health care provider.

• Advise patient to report signs and symptoms of respiratory depression (respiratory rate less than 12 breaths/minute, shortness of breath, confusion, excessive drowsiness, nausea, vomiting) and to seek immediate medical attention. Risk of respiratory depression is greatest at drug initiation and with dosage increases.

• Warn patient that use of drug, even when taken as recommended, can result in addiction, abuse, and misuse, which can lead to overdose or death.

• Caution patient not to drive or operate dangerous machinery until drug's effects are known.

• Warn patient about potential for severe constipation; teach management instructions and when to seek medical attention.

• Inform patient that drug may cause orthostatic hypotension and fainting. Teach how to recognize signs and symptoms of low BP and how to reduce risk of serious consequences of hypotension (sit or lie down, carefully rise from sitting or lying position).

• Caution patient to immediately seek medical attention if hypersensitivity reactions, including anaphylaxis, occur.

• Inform patient to dispose of unused drug through a drug take-back program. If such a program isn't available in patient's area, instruct patient to flush drug down a toilet.

• Caution patient to report to prescriber pregnancy or plan to become pregnant.

SAFETY ALERT!

HYDROcodone bitartrate–acetaminophen
hye-droe-KOE-done/a-seet-a-MIN-oh-fen

Therapeutic class: Opioid analgesics
Pharmacologic class: Opioid analgesics–
para-aminophenol derivatives
Controlled substance schedule: II

AVAILABLE FORMS
Oral solution*: 7.5 mg hydrocodone/
325 mg acetaminophen per 15 mL, 10 mg hydrocodone/300 mg acetaminophen per 15 mL
Tablets: 2.5 mg hydrocodone/325 mg acetaminophen, 5 mg hydrocodone/300 mg acetaminophen, 5 mg hydrocodone/325 mg acetaminophen, 7.5 mg hydrocodone/300 mg acetaminophen, 7.5 mg hydrocodone/325 mg acetaminophen, 10 mg hydrocodone/300 mg acetaminophen, 10 mg hydrocodone/325 mg acetaminophen

INDICATIONS & DOSAGES
➤ **Moderate to moderately severe pain**
Adults: 1 to 2 tablets (hydrocodone 2.5 to 5 mg/
acetaminophen 300 to 325 mg) PO every 4
to 6 hours PRN or 1 tablet (hydrocodone 7.5
to 10 mg/acetaminophen 300 to 325 mg) PO
every 4 to 6 hours PRN. Or, for oral solution,
15 mL (hydrocodone 7.5 mg/acetaminophen
325 mg) or 11.25 mL (hydrocodone 10 mg/
acetaminophen 300 mg) PO every 4 to 6 hours
PRN. Refer to manufacturer's instructions for
maximum dosages.
Children ages 2 and older (solution only):
Refer to manufacturer's instructions for specific weight- and age-based dosing.
Adjust-a-dose: Adjust dosage according to
severity of pain and patient response. Use a
low initial dosage in older adults and in patients with liver or kidney impairment; monitor closely for adverse events, such as respiratory depression and sedation.
Boxed Warning Total acetaminophen intake
shouldn't exceed 4,000 mg/day in adults and
in children ages 14 and older. ■

ADMINISTRATION
PO
• Give drug with food or milk.
🕛 *Alert:* Ensure accuracy when prescribing, dispensing, and administering oral solution. Dosing errors due to confusion between

mg and mL, and among other hydrocodone
bitartrate–acetaminophen oral solutions of
different concentrations, can result in accidental overdose and death.
• Administer oral solution by a calibrated device, such as syringe or dropper.
🕛 *Alert:* Only oral solution is approved for
pediatric use.

ACTION
Inhibits synthesis of prostaglandins and binds
to opiate receptors in CNS and peripherally
blocks pain impulse generation; may produce
generalized CNS depression.

Route	Onset	Peak	Duration
PO (hydro-codone)	10–20 min	1–1.6 hr	4–8 hr
PO (aceta-minophen)	Unknown	0.5–1 hr	4–6 hr

Half-life: Hydrocodone, 3.5 to 4.1 hours; acetaminophen, 1.25 to 3 hours.

ADVERSE REACTIONS
CNS: light-headedness, dizziness, sedation,
drowsiness, mental clouding, lethargy, impairment of mental and physical performance,
anxiety, fear, dysphoria, psychological dependence, mood changes, stupor, *coma.*
CV: *bradycardia, cardiac arrest, circulatory shock,* hypotension. **EENT:** hearing impairment, permanent hearing loss. **GI:** nausea, vomiting, constipation, abdominal pain,
heartburn, peptic ulcer. **GU:** urethral spasms,
vesical sphincter spasms, urine retention, *kidney toxicity.* **Hematologic:** iron deficiency
anemia, prolonged bleeding time, hemolytic
anemia, *thrombocytopenia, agranulocytosis.*
Hepatic: increased LFT values. **Metabolic:**
hypoglycemia. **Musculoskeletal:** muscle
flaccidity. **Respiratory:** *respiratory depression, acute airway obstruction, apnea,* dyspnea. **Skin:** rash; pruritus; diaphoresis; cold,
clammy skin. **Other:** hypersensitivity reaction.

INTERACTIONS
Drug-drug. *Anticholinergics (scopolamine,
diphenhydramine):* May increase risk of urine
retention, severe constipation, or paralytic
ileus. Avoid use together.
Boxed Warning *Benzodiazepines, CNS depressants:* May cause slow or difficult breathing, sedation, and death. Avoid use together.
If use together can't be avoided, limit dose

and duration of each drug to the minimum needed for desired effect. ■

Barbiturates, metyrapone, mipomersen: May increase risk of liver toxicity from acetaminophen. Monitor therapy.

Carbamazepine, dasatinib, hydantoins, isoniazid: May increase risk of liver toxicity from acetaminophen. Use together cautiously. Consider alternative therapy.

Boxed Warning *CYP3A4 inhibitors (amiodarone, erythromycin, ketoconazole, nefazodone, protease inhibitors, ritonavir):* May increase hydrocodone level and prolong opioid effects, especially if use of CYP3A4 inhibitors is concomitant. These effects may be more pronounced with concomitant use of both CYP3A4 and CYP2D6 inhibitors, particularly when an inhibitor is added after a stable dosage is achieved. Monitor patient for respiratory depression and sedation; consider dosage adjustments until drug effects are stable. ■

Boxed Warning *CYP3A4 inducers (carbamazepine, phenytoin, rifampin):* May decrease hydrocodone level, decreasing efficacy and potentially causing withdrawal symptoms. Monitor patient for effectiveness of drug and for opioid withdrawal symptoms. Consider dosage adjustments until stable. If CYP3A4 inducer is stopped, monitor patient for increased therapeutic and adverse effects, especially respiratory depression. ■

Diuretics (furosemide): May reduce diuretic effects. Monitor clinical response.

MAO inhibitors: May potentiate effects of opioid analgesic and increase risk of serotonin syndrome. Don't use in patients who have received MAO inhibitor within past 14 days.

Mixed agonist/antagonists (butorphanol, nalbuphine, pentazocine), partial agonists (buprenorphine): May reduce analgesic effect of hydrocodone or precipitate withdrawal symptoms. Avoid use together.

Muscle relaxants: May increase neuromuscular blocking action and respiratory depression. Avoid use together. If use together is necessary, decrease dosage of either drug.

⊕ *Alert:* *Serotonergic drugs (amoxapine, antimigraine drugs, buspirone, cyclobenzaprine, dextromethorphan, linezolid, lithium, maprotiline, methylene blue, mirtazapine, nefazodone, SSNRIs, SSRIs, TCAs, trazodone, tryptophan, vilazodone):* May increase risk of serotonin syndrome. Use together cautiously. Monitor patient for serotonin syndrome.

Drug-herb. *Kava, valerian:* May increase risk of excessive sedation. Avoid use together.

⊕ *Alert:* *St. John's wort:* May decrease hydrocodone serum level. Use together cautiously.

Drug-lifestyle. **Boxed Warning** *Alcohol use:* May cause slow or difficult breathing, sedation, and death. Discourage use together. ■

EFFECTS ON LAB TEST RESULTS

- May increase amylase level.
- May decrease Hb level.
- May decrease platelet and WBC counts.
- Acetaminophen may produce false-positive results on urinary 5-hydroxyindoleacetic acid test.

CONTRAINDICATIONS & CAUTIONS

Boxed Warning Acetaminophen has been associated with acute liver failure, at times resulting in need for liver transplant and death. Most cases of liver injury have been associated with use of acetaminophen at dosages exceeding 4,000 mg/day or more than one acetaminophen-containing product. ■

Boxed Warning *Opioid class warning*: Opioids should only be prescribed with benzodiazepines or other CNS depressants when alternative treatment options are inadequate, aren't expected to provide adequate analgesia, haven't been tolerated, or aren't expected to be tolerated. ■

Boxed Warning Use exposes patient and others to risk of opioid addiction, abuse, and misuse, which can lead to overdose and death. These effects can occur at any dose or duration. Assess patient risk before prescribing and regularly reassess patient for these behaviors and conditions. ■

Boxed Warning Prescribers are strongly encouraged to complete a REMS-compliant education program. Drug should be prescribed only by prescribers with knowledge of opioid use and ways to reduce associated risks. ■

⊕ *Alert:* Use lowest effective dose for shortest period consistent with patient's treatment goals.

⊕ *Alert:* Because risk of overdose increases as opioid dose increases, reserve titration to higher doses for patients in whom lower doses are ineffective and in whom expected benefits of higher opioid dose outweigh risks.

⊕ *Alert:* Immediate-release formulations shouldn't be used for an extended period

H

unless pain remains severe enough to require an opioid analgesic and alternative treatment options are inadequate to treat pain.

Boxed Warning Accidental ingestion of even one dose of this drug, especially by children, can result in a fatal hydrocodone overdose. ■

• Contraindicated in patients hypersensitive to hydrocodone or acetaminophen and in those with significant respiratory depression, acute or severe bronchial asthma in an unmonitored setting or in the absence of resuscitative equipment, or known or suspected GI obstruction, including paralytic ileus.

🔹 *Alert:* May cause serious, potentially fatal skin reactions, including SJS, TEN, and acute generalized exanthematous pustulosis. Reaction may occur with first or subsequent use when acetaminophen is used as monotherapy or when it's one component of combination drug therapy.

🔹 *Alert:* Patients with any of the following conditions are at increased risk for oversedation and respiratory depression and require close monitoring: snoring or sleep apnea, first-time opioid use or previous (nonrecent) opioid use, opioid habituation or need for increased opioid doses, need for prolonged general anesthesia or other sedating drugs, preexisting pulmonary or cardiac disease, or thoracic or other surgical incisions that may impair breathing.

• Use cautiously in patients who are allergic to other opioids because cross-sensitivity may occur.

• Use cautiously in patients with a history of respiratory depression, drug abuse, head injury or increased ICP, seizures, acute abdominal conditions, liver disease, recent anesthesia, pulmonary disease, kidney impairment, hypothyroidism, Addison disease, or BPH and urethral stricture.

• Use cautiously in older adults or patients who are debilitated and those sensitive to CNS depressants.

🔹 *Alert:* Drug may lead to rare but serious decrease in adrenal gland cortisol production.

• Drug may reduce sex hormone levels with long-term use.

Dialyzable drug: Unknown.

⚠ *Overdose S&S: Hydrocodone:* Loss of consciousness; pinpoint pupils; respiratory depression; stupor; coma; skeletal muscle flaccidity; cold, clammy skin; bradycardia; hypotension; apnea; circulatory collapse;

cardiac arrest; death. *Acetaminophen:* Fatal liver necrosis, kidney tubular necrosis, hypoglycemic coma, thrombocytopenia, nausea, vomiting, diaphoresis, general malaise.

PREGNANCY-LACTATION-REPRODUCTION

• Use during pregnancy only if benefit outweighs fetal risk.

Boxed Warning Prolonged use during pregnancy can result in neonatal opioid withdrawal syndrome, which may be life-threatening. It requires management with expert neonatology protocols. If prolonged use is needed, advise patient of risks and ensure availability of proper treatment. ■

• Don't use during labor and delivery; neonatal respiratory depression may occur.

• Opioids may appear in human milk. Use cautiously during breastfeeding.

• Monitor infants exposed to drug through human milk for excess sedation and respiratory depression.

• Watch for withdrawal symptoms in infants who are breastfed when patient stops opioid analgesic or stops breastfeeding.

• Prolonged opioid use may cause reduced fertility in individuals of reproductive potential. It's unknown whether these effects on fertility are reversible.

NURSING CONSIDERATIONS

• Monitor closely for allergic reaction, particularly in patient who is allergic to other opioids.

• Be aware that drug may be targeted for theft, diversion, and misuse.

Boxed Warning May cause life-threatening or fatal respiratory depression at any time during therapy. Monitor patient closely, especially when starting or increasing doses. Proper dosing and titration are essential to reduce risk. ■

Boxed Warning Regularly monitor all patients for opioid addiction, abuse, and misuse, which can lead to overdose and death. ■

🔹 *Alert:* Drug may cause opioid-induced hyperalgesia (OIH). Symptoms include increased pain level with opioid dose increase, decreased pain level with opioid dose reduction, pain from ordinarily nonpainful stimuli without underlying disease progression, opioid tolerance or withdrawal, and addictive behavior. For suspected OIH, decrease opioid dose or switch patient to alternative opioid.

🔹 *Alert:* Carefully monitor vital signs, pain level, respiratory status, and sedation level in all patients receiving opioids, especially those receiving IV drugs, even those given postoperatively.

⊙ *Alert:* If patient is taking opioids with serotonergic drugs, watch for signs and symptoms of serotonin syndrome (agitation, hallucinations, rapid HR, fever, diaphoresis, shivering or shaking, muscle twitching or stiffness, trouble with coordination, nausea, vomiting, diarrhea), especially when starting treatment or increasing dosages. Signs and symptoms may occur within several hours of coadministration but may also occur later, especially after dosage increase. Discontinue opioid, serotonergic drug, or both if serotonin syndrome is suspected.

⊙ *Alert:* Monitor for signs and symptoms of adrenal insufficiency (nausea, vomiting, loss of appetite, fatigue, weakness, dizziness, low BP). Perform diagnostic testing if adrenal insufficiency is suspected. If adrenal insufficiency is confirmed, treat with corticosteroids and wean patient off opioid, if appropriate. Discontinue corticosteroid when clinically appropriate.

• Monitor patient for signs and symptoms of decreased sex hormone levels (low libido, erectile dysfunction, amenorrhea, infertility). If signs and symptoms occur, evaluate patient and obtain specimens for lab testing.

⊙ *Alert:* Don't stop drug abruptly; withdraw slowly and individualize gradual tapering plan to prevent signs and symptoms of withdrawal, worsening pain, and psychological distress in patient who is physically dependent. Refer to manufacturer's label for specific tapering instructions.

⊙ *Alert:* When tapering opioids, monitor patients closely for signs and symptoms of opioid withdrawal (restlessness, lacrimation, rhinorrhea, yawning, perspiration, chills, myalgia, mydriasis, irritability, anxiety, insomnia, backache, joint pain, weakness, abdominal cramps, anorexia, nausea, vomiting, diarrhea, increased BP or HR, increased respiratory rate). Such signs and symptoms may indicate a need to taper more slowly. Also monitor patients for suicidality, use of other substances, and mood changes.

• Note that older adult receiving drug, especially one with impaired liver or kidney function, may become confused and oversedated. Start with low doses of hydrocodone and closely watch for adverse events, such as respiratory depression.

• Monitor patient with head injury, intracranial lesion, or elevated ICP. Drug may exaggerate ICP elevation.

• Use of opioids in patients with acute abdominal disorders may mask symptoms.

• Monitor patient for constipation; treat aggressively, if present.

• Monitor patient with history of seizure disorder for worsening seizure control.

• Use lowest initial dose in patient with kidney or liver impairment, and observe closely for adverse events, such as respiratory depression.

• Monitor liver and kidney function. Acetaminophen elimination may be increased in patients with liver impairment.

• Monitor patient's ability to urinate; report urine retention.

• Regularly monitor BP and pulse.

• Monitor for reddening of skin, rash, blisters, and detachment of upper surface of skin. Stop drug immediately for suspected skin reaction.

• Periodically reevaluate patient's need for therapy.

PATIENT TEACHING

Boxed Warning Counsel patient and caregiver on serious risks, safe use, and importance of reading the medication guide with each prescription. ∎

• Advise patient to take drug exactly as prescribed and to use lowest dose possible for shortest time needed.

• Inform patient that, for acute pain, drug may only be needed for a few days. Teach about safe disposal of unused drug.

• Instruct patient to contact health care provider if prescribed dosage isn't controlling pain.

⊙ *Alert:* Warn patient to withhold drug and inform prescriber if pain level worsens, pain sensitivity increases, or new pain occurs after taking drug.

• Teach patient that naloxone may be prescribed with hydrocodone with acetaminophen when beginning and renewing therapy to reduce risk of opioid overdose and death.

⊙ *Alert:* Counsel patient who has been regularly taking drug not to discontinue without first discussing the need for gradual tapering with prescriber.

• Caution patient not to share drug and to protect it from theft or misuse.

• Warn patient that use of drug, even when taken as recommended, can result in addiction, abuse, and misuse, which can lead to overdose or death.

• Inform patient that drug may cause orthostatic hypotension and fainting. Teach patient how to recognize signs and symptoms of low BP and to reduce risk of serious consequences of hypotension by sitting or lying down when symptomatic or by carefully rising from a sitting or lying position.

• Explain the assessment and monitoring process to patient and family. Instruct them to immediately report difficulty breathing or other signs of a potential adverse opioid-related reaction.

• Explain that drug may impair judgment. Warn patient not to operate heavy machinery or drive until drug's effects are known.

• Instruct patient to avoid alcohol while taking drug.

Boxed Warning Warn patient that drug contains acetaminophen (or Tylenol). Caution patient not to take more than 4,000 mg of acetaminophen daily (including from all medications being taken). Instruct patient to look for "acetaminophen" or "APAP" on package labels, not to use more than one product that contains acetaminophen, and to contact health care provider if patient has taken more than 4,000 mg in a day, even if feeling well. ■

❸ Alert: Encourage patient to report all medications being taken, including prescription and OTC medications and supplements.

❸ Alert: Caution patient to immediately report signs and symptoms of serotonin syndrome, adrenal insufficiency, and decreased sex hormone levels.

• Teach patient to eat high-fiber diet, drink plenty of fluids, and use stool softener or bulk laxative to prevent constipation.

• Tell patient to stop drug and immediately report blurred vision, rash, or yellowing of the skin.

• Inform patient to dispose of unused tablets through a drug take-back program. If such a program isn't available in patient's area, instruct patient to flush unused tablets down a toilet.

❸ Alert: Warn patient to immediately stop drug and seek medical attention if rash or reaction occurs while using acetaminophen.

• Caution patient to report to prescriber pregnancy or plan to become pregnant.

---

hydrocortisone (oral, injection, rectal)
hye-droe-KOR-ti-sone

Alkindi Sprinkle, Cortef, Cortenema

hydrocortisone sodium succinate (injection)
Solu-Cortef

Therapeutic class: Corticosteroids
Pharmacologic class: Glucocorticoids

AVAILABLE FORMS
hydrocortisone
Enema: 100 mg/60 mL
Sprinkle capsules ⒹⒽⒸ: 0.5 mg, 1 mg, 2 mg, 5 mg
Tablets: 5 mg, 10 mg, 20 mg
hydrocortisone sodium succinate
Injection:* 100-mg vial, 250-mg vial, 500-mg vial, 1,000-mg vial

INDICATIONS & DOSAGES
➤ **Rheumatic disorders (adjunctive therapy for short-term administration in psoriatic arthritis; RA, including juvenile RA; ankylosing spondylitis; acute and subacute bursitis; acute nonspecific tenosynovitis; acute gouty arthritis; posttraumatic osteoarthritis; synovitis of osteoarthritis; epicondylitis); collagen diseases (SLE, acute rheumatic carditis, systemic dermatomyositis); dermatologic diseases (pemphigus, bullous dermatitis herpetiformis, severe erythema multiforme, exfoliative dermatitis, mycosis fungoides, severe psoriasis, severe seborrheic dermatitis)**
Adults: 20 to 240 mg PO daily. Or, initially, 100 to 500 mg succinate IM or IV; repeat every 2, 4, or 6 hours.
Children: 0.56 to 8 mg/kg/day IV or IM in three or four divided doses.
➤ **Severe or intractable allergic states (seasonal or perennial allergic rhinitis, bronchial asthma, contact dermatitis, atopic dermatitis, serum sickness, drug hypersensitivity reactions, transfusion reactions)**
Adults: 20 to 240 mg PO daily. Or, initially, 100 to 500 mg succinate IM or IV; repeat every 2, 4, or 6 hours.
Children: 0.56 to 8 mg/kg/day IV or IM in three or four divided doses.

➤ Severe acute and chronic allergic and inflammatory processes involving the eye and its adnexa (allergic conjunctivitis, keratitis, allergic corneal marginal ulcers, herpes zoster ophthalmicus, iritis and iridocyclitis, chorioretinitis, anterior segment inflammation, diffuse posterior uveitis and choroiditis, optic neuritis, sympathetic ophthalmia)

Adults: 20 to 240 mg PO daily. Or, initially, 100 to 500 mg succinate IM or IV; repeat every 2, 4, or 6 hours.

Children: 0.56 to 8 mg/kg/day IV or IM in three or four divided doses.

➤ Respiratory diseases (symptomatic sarcoidosis, Loeffler syndrome not manageable by other means, berylliosis, fulminating or disseminated pulmonary TB when used concurrently with appropriate antituberculous chemotherapy, aspiration pneumonitis)

Adults: 20 to 240 mg PO daily. Or, initially, 100 to 500 mg succinate IM or IV; repeat every 2, 4, or 6 hours.

➤ Hematologic disorders (ITP in adults [IM form is contraindicated], secondary thrombocytopenia in adults, acquired [autoimmune] hemolytic anemia, erythroblastopenia, congenital [erythroid] hypoplastic anemia)

Adults: 20 to 240 mg PO daily. Or, initially, 100 to 500 mg succinate IM or IV; repeat every 2, 4, or 6 hours.

Children: 0.56 to 8 mg/kg/day IV or IM in three or four divided doses.

➤ Neoplastic diseases (palliative management of leukemias and lymphomas in adults and acute leukemia of childhood)

Adults: 20 to 240 mg PO daily. Or, initially, 100 to 500 mg succinate IM or IV; repeat every 2, 4, or 6 hours as needed.

Children older than age 1 month: 0.56 to 8 mg/kg/day IV or IM in three or four divided doses.

➤ Edematous states (to induce diuresis or remission of proteinuria in nephrotic syndrome, without uremia, of the idiopathic type or that is due to SLE)

Adults: 20 to 240 mg PO daily. Or, initially, 100 to 500 mg succinate IM or IV; repeat every 2, 4, or 6 hours.

Children older than age 2: 0.56 to 8 mg/kg/day IV or IM in three or four divided doses.

➤ Nervous system disorders (cerebral edema associated with brain tumors or craniotomy [IV], tuberculous meningitis with subarachnoid block or impending block when used concurrently with appropriate antituberculotics, trichinosis with neurologic or myocardial involvement)

Adults: 20 to 240 mg PO daily. Or, initially, 100 to 500 mg succinate IM or IV; repeat every 2, 4, or 6 hours.

Children: 0.56 to 8 mg/kg/day IV or IM in three or four divided doses.

➤ Endocrine disorders (adrenal insufficiency, congenital adrenal hyperplasia, nonsuppurative thyroiditis, hypercalcemia associated with cancer)

Adults: 20 to 240 mg PO daily. Or, initially, 100 to 500 mg succinate IM or IV; repeat every 2, 4, or 6 hours.

➤ Ulcerative colitis; regional enteritis

Adults: 20 to 240 mg PO daily. Or, initially, 100 to 500 mg succinate IM or IV; repeat every 2, 4, or 6 hours.

➤ Adjunctive treatment for ulcerative colitis and proctitis

Adults: 1 enema (100 mg) PR nightly for 21 days.

➤ Replacement therapy in adrenocortical insufficiency

Children: Initially, 8 to 10 mg/m^2/day (sprinkle capsules) t.i.d. in three divided doses. Higher dosages may be needed based on child's age and disease symptoms. Individualize to lowest possible dosage and round dose to nearest 0.5 or 1 mg. In older children, may divide daily dose into two doses b.i.d.

ADMINISTRATION

PO

• Give drug with milk or food when possible. Patient may need another drug to prevent GI irritation.

• Use same dose when switching from tablets to sprinkle capsules.

• Don't give sprinkle capsule granules through NG or other gastric tube because granules may obstruct tube.

• Don't get sprinkle capsule wet because granules may remain in capsule.

• Have patient swallow granules; don't crush them. Don't allow patient to swallow capsules.

• To administer capsules: Hold sprinkle capsule with printed strength at top; tap capsule to move granules to bottom of capsule. Squeeze bottom of capsule, twist off top portion, then pour granules onto patient's tongue or place granules on spoon or spoonful of soft cold or room temperature food before placing in patient's mouth. Follow with fluid (water, milk, human milk, or formula). Don't add granules to liquid as this can result in reductions in the dose administered and may result in a bitter taste.

IV

▼ Reconstitute hydrocortisone sodium succinate with no more than 2 mL bacteriostatic water or bacteriostatic saline solution before adding to IV solutions. Further dilution isn't necessary, but solution may then be added to 100 to 1,000 mL D5W, NSS, or dextrose 5% NSS.

▼ For doses of 500 mg or more, administer over 10 minutes. For direct injection, inject over 30 seconds to 10 minutes. Give intermittent IV infusion over 20 to 30 minutes.

▼ IV solutions are stable for 4 hours.

▼ Not for intrathecal use.

▼ **Incompatibilities:** Solutions other than D₅W, NSS, or dextrose 5% in NSS, and other drugs.

IM

● Reconstitute hydrocortisone sodium succinate with no more than 2 mL bacteriostatic water or bacteriostatic saline solution per vial.

● Inject deep into gluteal muscle. Rotate injection sites to prevent muscle atrophy. Avoid IM injection into deltoid muscle as subcutaneous atrophy and sterile abscesses may occur.

● Don't use injectable forms for alternate-day therapy.

Rectal

● Have patient lie on the left side during administration and for 30 minutes afterward to allow fluid to distribute throughout left colon. Have patient try to retain enema for at least 1 hour but preferably all night.

ACTION

Not clearly defined. Decreases inflammation, mainly by stabilizing leukocyte lysosomal membranes; suppresses immune response; stimulates bone marrow; and influences protein, fat, and carbohydrate metabolism.

Route	Onset	Peak	Duration
PO	Variable	1 hr	Variable
IV, IM, PR	Variable	Variable	Variable

Half-life: Oral, 78 to 128 minutes; IV, 60 to 180 minutes.

ADVERSE REACTIONS

CNS: euphoria, depression, insomnia, psychotic behavior, *pseudotumor cerebri,* vertigo, mood swings, headache, malaise, myasthenia, neuritis, neuropathy, personality changes, paresthesia, fever, syncope, *seizures.* **CV:** *HF, HTN,* edema, *arrhythmias,* thrombophlebitis, *thromboembolism, bradycardia,* tachycardia, vasculitis, cardiomegaly, *circulatory shock.* **EENT:** cataracts, glaucoma, conjunctivitis, otitis media, tonsillitis, pharyngitis, rhinitis, dental caries. **GI:** abdominal distention, gastroenteritis, peptic ulceration, GI irritation, increased appetite, hiccups, *pancreatitis,* nausea, vomiting, diarrhea, *GI perforation.* **GU:** menstrual irregularities, increased urine calcium levels. **Hematologic:** easy bruising, leukocytosis. **Metabolic:** *hypokalemia,* hyperglycemia, carbohydrate intolerance, hypercholesterolemia, *hypocalcemia.* **Hepatic:** increased LFT values, enlarged liver. **Musculoskeletal:** growth suppression in children, muscle weakness, osteoporosis, tendon rupture, vertebral compression fracture. **Respiratory:** URI, *pulmonary edema.* **Skin:** hirsutism, delayed wound healing, acne, atopic dermatitis, atrophic striae, burning sensation, diaphoresis, ecchymosis, petechiae, erythema, hyperpigmentation or hypopigmentation, rash, thinning hair, urticaria, dry skin, skin eruptions, injection-site atrophy. **Other:** *anaphylaxis, angioedema,* hypersensitivity reactions, cushingoid state, susceptibility to infections, *acute adrenal insufficiency after increased stress or abrupt withdrawal after long-term therapy.*

INTERACTIONS

Drug-drug. *Antacids:* May decrease bioavailability of corticosteroids. Separate doses by 2 hours.

Antidiabetics: May increase glucose level and alter antidiabetic needs. Monitor therapy.

Aspirin, indomethacin, other NSAIDs: May increase risk of GI distress and bleeding. Use together cautiously.

Cyclosporine: May increase toxicity of both drugs. Monitor patient closely.

CYP3A4 inducers (barbiturates, carbamazepine, efavirenz, nevirapine, phenytoin, phenobarbital, rifabutin, rifampin): May decrease hydrocortisone (systemic) level. Increase hydrocortisone dosage.

Reactions in bold italics are *life-threatening*.

CYP3A4 inhibitors (erythromycin, ketoconazole, ritonavir): May increase corticosteroid (systemic) level. Decrease corticosteroid dosage.

Estrogen-containing products (oral contraceptives, oral estrogen): May reduce effect of hydrocortisone. Increase hydrocortisone dosage as needed.

Live attenuated virus vaccines, other toxoids, and vaccines: May decrease antibody response and increase risk of infection and neurologic complications. Avoid use together.

Mifepristone: May cause adrenal insufficiency and require high glucocorticoid doses. Increase glucocorticoid dosage.

Oral anticoagulants: May alter dosage requirements. Closely monitor PT and INR.

Potassium-depleting drugs (thiazide diuretics, amphotericin B): May enhance potassium-wasting effects of hydrocortisone. Monitor potassium level.

Skin-test antigens: May decrease response. Postpone skin testing until after therapy.

Tacrolimus (systemic): May decrease tacrolimus level. Conversely, when corticosteroid therapy is discontinued, tacrolimus level may increase. Monitor therapy.

Tacrolimus (topical): May enhance adverse or toxic effect of immunosuppressants. Avoid combination.

Drug-herb. *Echinacea, ginseng:* May diminish therapeutic effect of immunosuppressants. Discourage use together.

EFFECTS ON LAB TEST RESULTS
• May increase glucose and cholesterol levels.
• May decrease potassium and calcium levels.
• May cause decreased ^{131}I uptake and protein-bound iodine levels in thyroid function tests.
• May cause false-negative results in nitroblue tetrazolium test for systemic bacterial infections.
• May alter reactions to coccidioidin skin tests.

CONTRAINDICATIONS & CAUTIONS
• Contraindicated in patients hypersensitive to drug or its ingredients, in those with systemic fungal infections, and in those receiving immunosuppressive doses together with live-virus vaccines.
• IM corticosteroids are contraindicated for ITP.
• Use with caution in patients with recent MI. High IV doses aren't recommended to treat traumatic brain injury.

• Use cautiously in patients with GI ulcer, kidney disease, HTN, osteoporosis, diabetes, hypothyroidism, cirrhosis, diverticulitis, nonspecific ulcerative colitis, active hepatitis, recent intestinal anastomoses, thromboembolic disorders, seizures, myasthenia gravis, HF, TB, ocular herpes simplex, emotional instability, and psychotic tendencies.
• Drug can cause hypercorticism or suppression of the HPA axis, particularly in younger children or patients receiving high-dose therapy. Withdraw drug slowly.
• Kaposi sarcoma has been reported. Clinical remission may occur after discontinuation of corticosteroids.
⚠ *Alert:* Epidural corticosteroid injections to treat neck and back pain and radiating pain in arms and legs may result in rare but serious adverse events (vision loss, stroke, paralysis, death). Use of epidural corticosteroid injections isn't approved by FDA.
Dialyzable drug: Unknown.

PREGNANCY-LACTATION-REPRODUCTION
• Use cautiously during pregnancy and breastfeeding. When essential during pregnancy, use lowest possible dose for shortest duration. Avoid high doses in first trimester.
• Monitor infants exposed to drug in utero for hypoadrenalism.
• Drug appears in human milk and could cause adverse effects, including growth suppression. Breastfeeding isn't recommended.
• Steroids may alter the motility and number of sperm in some patients.

NURSING CONSIDERATIONS
• Determine whether patient is sensitive to other corticosteroids.
• Most adverse reactions to corticosteroids are dose- or duration-dependent.
• For better results and less toxicity, give a once-daily dose in the morning.
⚠ *Alert:* Salts aren't interchangeable.
⚠ *Alert:* Only hydrocortisone sodium succinate can be given IV.
• Enema may produce same systemic effects as other forms of hydrocortisone. If enema therapy must exceed 21 days, taper off by giving every other night for 2 to 3 weeks.
• High-dose therapy usually isn't continued beyond 48 hours.
• Always adjust to lowest effective dose.
• Monitor patient's weight, BP, and electrolyte levels.

• Monitor patient for cushingoid effects (moon face, buffalo hump, central obesity, thinning hair, HTN, increased susceptibility to infection).

• Unless contraindicated, give a low-sodium diet that's high in potassium and protein. Give potassium supplements.

• Drug may mask or worsen infections, including latent amebiasis.

• Stress (fever, trauma, surgery, and emotional problems) may increase adrenal insufficiency. Increase dosage.

• Watch for depression or psychotic episodes, especially during high-dose therapy.

• Inspect patient's skin for petechiae.

• Patient with diabetes may need increased antidiabetic medication; monitor glucose level.

• Periodic measurement of growth and development may be needed during high-dose or prolonged therapy in children.

• Older adults may be more susceptible to osteoporosis with prolonged use.

• Gradually reduce dosage after long-term therapy.

• Monitor for adrenal insufficiency (fatigue, weakness, arthralgia, fever, dizziness, lethargy, depression, fainting, hypotension, dyspnea, anorexia, nausea, vomiting, electrolyte disturbances, hypoglycemia) after abrupt withdrawal or withdrawal after prolonged treatment. Rebound inflammation can also occur. After prolonged use, sudden withdrawal may be fatal.

• *Look alike–sound alike:* Don't confuse Solu-Cortef with Solu-Medrol. Don't confuse hydrocortisone with hydrocodone, hydroxychloroquine, or hydrochlorothiazide. Don't confuse Cortef with Coreg.

PATIENT TEACHING

• Tell patient not to stop drug abruptly or without prescriber's consent.

• Teach about proper drug administration and handling.

• Warn patient on long-term therapy about cushingoid effects (moon face, buffalo hump) and the need to notify prescriber about sudden weight gain or swelling.

• Review signs and symptoms of early adrenal insufficiency (fatigue, muscle weakness, joint pain, fever, anorexia, nausea, shortness of breath, dizziness, fainting).

• Instruct patient to carry a card with prescriber's name and name and dosage of drug, indicating the need for supplemental systemic glucocorticoids during stress.

• Warn patient about easy bruising.

• Urge patient receiving long-term therapy to consider exercise or physical therapy. Also, tell patient to ask prescriber about vitamin D or calcium supplementation.

• Advise patient receiving long-term therapy to have periodic eye exams.

• Caution patient to avoid exposure to infections (such as chickenpox and measles) and to notify prescriber if such exposure occurs.

⚠ *Alert:* Advise patient to discuss benefits and risks along with other possible treatments with health care provider before undergoing epidural corticosteroid injection.

hydrocortisone (topical)
hye-droe-KOR-ti-sone

Ala-Cort, Ala-Scalp, Anusol HC, Cortizone-10 ◇, Preparation H ◇, Proctocort, Scalpicin ◇, Texacort stie-cort

hydrocortisone acetate (topical, rectal)
Anusol HC ◇, Cortaid ◇, Cortifoam, Micort-HC

hydrocortisone butyrate
Locoid, Locoid Lipocream

hydrocortisone probutate
Pandel

hydrocortisone valerate

Therapeutic class: Corticosteroids
Pharmacologic class: Corticosteroids

AVAILABLE FORMS
hydrocortisone
Cream: 0.5% ◇, 1% ◇, 2.5%
Lotion: 1% ◇, 2%, 2.5%
Ointment: 0.5% ◇, 1% ◇, 2.5%
Rectal cream: 1% ◇, 2.5%
Rectal ointment: 1%
Topical solution: 1% ◇, 2.5%
hydrocortisone acetate
Cream: 1%, 2%, 2.5%, 2.5% ◇
Lotion: 1% ◇, 2%
Rectal foam: 90 mg per application
Rectal suppositories: 25 mg, 30 mg
hydrocortisone butyrate
Cream: 0.1%

Lotion: 0.1%
Ointment: 0.1%
Solution: 0.1%
hydrocortisone probutate
Cream: 0.1%
hydrocortisone valerate
Cream: 0.2%
Ointment: 0.2%

INDICATIONS & DOSAGES

➤ **Inflammation and pruritus from corticosteroid-responsive dermatoses, adjunctive topical management of seborrheic dermatitis of scalp**
Adults and children: Clean area; apply cream, lotion, ointment, or topical solution sparingly daily to q.i.d. as directed until acute phase is controlled; then reduce dosage to one to three times weekly as needed. Give children lowest dose that provides positive results.

➤ **Inflammation from proctitis; inflamed hemorrhoids; adjunctive treatment of chronic ulcerative colitis, cryptitis**
Adults: 1 applicatorful of rectal foam PR daily or b.i.d. for 2 to 3 weeks; then every other day as needed. Or, 1 suppository PR b.i.d. to t.i.d. or 2 suppositories PR b.i.d. for 2 weeks. For post-radiation proctitis, give drug for 6 to 8 weeks.

ADMINISTRATION
Rectal
• Refer to manufacturer's instructions to properly fill applicator barrel.
• Wash hands before and after application.
• After filling applicator, gently insert tip into anus, push plunger to expel foam, and then withdraw applicator.
• Thoroughly clean all applicator parts after each use.
• Avoid excessive handling of suppository, which is designed to melt at body temperature.
• Insert suppository, pointed end first, into rectum using gentle pressure.
Topical
• Gently wash skin before applying. To prevent skin damage, rub in gently, leaving a thin coat. When treating hairy sites, part hair and apply directly to lesions.
• Check individual products or prescription for frequency of administration.
• Avoid applying near eyes or mucous membranes or in ear canal; may be safely used on face, groin, and armpits and under breasts.
• Shake lotion well before use.

• For optimal absorption, apply to moist skin immediately after bathing or wet soak.
• Use occlusive dressing only if prescribed.
• Change dressing as prescribed. Stop drug and tell prescriber if skin infection, striae, or atrophy occurs.
• Continue treatment for a few days after lesions clear.

ACTION
Unclear. Diffuses across cell membranes to form complexes with cytoplasmic receptors, showing anti-inflammatory, antipruritic, vasoconstrictive, and antiproliferative activity.

Route	Onset	Peak	Duration
Topical, PR	Unknown	Unknown	Unknown

Half-life: Unknown.

ADVERSE REACTIONS
Topical
Skin: burning sensation, pruritus, irritation, dryness, erythema, folliculitis, hypertrichosis, hypopigmentation, acneiform eruptions, allergic contact dermatitis, atrophy, maceration, secondary infection, striae, miliaria with occlusive dressings.
Rectal
GI: local burning, itching, irritation. **Skin:** dryness, folliculitis, hypopigmentation, allergic contact dermatitis, impaired wound healing, fragile skin, petechiae, erythema, diaphoresis. **Other:** secondary infection.

INTERACTIONS
None significant.

EFFECTS ON LAB TEST RESULTS
• May increase glucose level.

CONTRAINDICATIONS & CAUTIONS
• Contraindicated in patients hypersensitive to drug or its components. Rectal formulations are contraindicated in patients with some GI conditions and after surgery. Refer to individual product information.
• Drug can cause hypercorticism or suppression of the HPA axis, which can lead to adrenal crisis.
• Don't use as monotherapy in primary bacterial infections (impetigo, paronychia, erysipelas, cellulitis, angular cheilitis), treatment of rosacea, perioral dermatitis, or acne.

- Drug isn't for ophthalmic use.
- Use in children varies by product.

Dialyzable drug: Unknown.

⚠ *Overdose S&S:* Systemic effects.

PREGNANCY-LACTATION-REPRODUCTION

- Well-controlled studies during pregnancy are lacking. Use during pregnancy only if potential benefit justifies fetal risk.
- Use cautiously during breastfeeding. Avoid applying drug to breast area that comes in contact with the infant.

NURSING CONSIDERATIONS

🔵 *Alert:* Adverse reactions and drug interactions similar to those that occur with systemic hydrocortisone have occurred.

- If an occlusive dressing is applied and a fever develops, notify prescriber and remove dressing.
- If antifungal or antibiotic combined with corticosteroid fails to provide prompt improvement, stop corticosteroid until infection is controlled.
- Systemic absorption is likely with use of occlusive dressings, prolonged treatment, or extensive body surface treatment. Watch for symptoms (hyperglycemia, glycosuria, HPA-axis suppression).
- Avoid using plastic pants or tight-fitting diapers on treated areas in a young child. Children may absorb larger amounts of drug and be more susceptible to systemic toxicity.
- Monitor patient for fluid and electrolyte disturbances (sodium and fluid retention, potassium loss, hypokalemic alkalosis, negative nitrogen balance from catabolism of protein).
- Drug may suppress skin reaction testing.
- *Look alike–sound alike:* Don't confuse hydrocortisone with hydrocodone, hydroxychloroquine, or hydrochlorothiazide.

PATIENT TEACHING

- Teach about proper drug administration and handling.
- Tell patient to wash hands after application.
- If an occlusive dressing is ordered, advise patient to leave it in place for no longer than 12 hours each day and not to use the dressing on infected or weeping lesions.
- Teach patient how to use rectal foam applicator or suppository if needed.
- Tell patient to stop drug and report signs of systemic absorption, skin irritation or

ulceration, hypersensitivity, infection, or lack of improvement.

- For perianal application, instruct patient to place small amount of drug on a tissue and gently rub in.
- Instruct patient to disassemble applicator and clean with warm water after each use.
- Tell patient to stop using drug if condition worsens or symptoms persist for more than 7 days.

HYDROmorphone hydrochloride (dihydromorphinone hydrochloride)
hye-droe-MOR-fone

Dilaudid, Hydromorph Contin ✦

Therapeutic class: Opioid analgesics
Pharmacologic class: Opioids
Controlled substance schedule: II

AVAILABLE FORMS

Capsules (extended-release) ✦: 3 mg, 4.5 mg, 6 mg, 9 mg, 10 mg, 12 mg, 18 mg, 20 mg, 24 mg, 30 mg
Injection: 0.2 mg/mL, 0.5 mg/0.5 mL, 1 mg/mL, 2 mg/mL, 4 mg/mL, 10 mg/mL
Injection (prefilled syringes): 0.2 mg/mL, 0.5 mg/0.5 mL, 1 mg/mL, 2 mg/mL, 4 mg/mL
Oral liquid: 5 mg/5 mL
Suppository: 3 mg
Tablets: 2 mg, 4 mg, 8 mg
Tablets (extended-release) ⓄⓃⒸ: 8 mg, 12 mg, 16 mg, 32 mg

INDICATIONS & DOSAGES

➤ **Management of pain severe enough to require opioid treatment and for which alternative treatment options are inadequate**
Adults: For patients who are opioid naive, 1 to 4 mg immediate-release tablets PO every 4 to 6 hours PRN. Or, 2.5 to 10 mg oral liquid every 3 to 6 hours PRN. Or, 1 to 2 mg IM or subcut every 2 to 3 hours PRN. Or, 0.2 to 1 mg IV (slowly over at least 2 to 3 minutes) every 2 to 3 hours PRN. Or, one suppository every 6 to 8 hours PRN. For adults who are opioid tolerant, currently on immediate-release hydromorphone, and require continuous analgesia for an extended period, starting dose of extended-release form is equivalent to total daily dosage of immediate-release form.

May increase by 4 to 8 mg every 3 to 4 days as needed to achieve adequate analgesia.

Adjust-a-dose: For older adults, use cautiously and reduce initial oral starting dose. Initial IV starting dose for older adults or patients who are debilitated should be 0.2 mg. For those with kidney or liver impairment, reduce dose to 25% to 50% of usual starting dose of immediate-acting forms. For extended-release forms, give patients with Child-Pugh class B liver impairment 25% of usual starting dose; give patients with CrCl of 40 to 60 mL/minute 50%, and patients with CrCl less than 30 mL/minute 25% of usual starting dose. Extended-release form isn't recommended for those with Child-Pugh class C liver impairment.

ADMINISTRATION
PO
• Give drug with food if GI upset occurs.
🔄 *Alert:* Have patient swallow extended-release tablets whole; don't break, dissolve, crush, or inject them.
🔄 *Alert:* Ensure accuracy when prescribing, dispensing, and administering oral solution to avoid dosing errors due to confusion between mg and mL, which could result in accidental overdose and death.
• For oral solution, use only a calibrated device that can accurately measure and deliver prescribed dose.
IV
🔄 *Alert:* Don't confuse standard hydromorphone for injection with high potency formulation or other opioids; overdose and death could result.
▼ Give by direct injection over no less than 2 minutes.
▼ Respiratory depression and hypotension can occur. Give slowly, and monitor patient constantly. Keep resuscitation equipment available.
▼ A slightly yellowish discoloration may develop. Discoloration doesn't indicate loss of potency.
▼ **Incompatibilities:** None listed by manufacturer. Consult drug compatibility reference for more information.
IM
• Document administration site.
Subcutaneous
• Rotate injection sites to avoid induration with subcut injection.

PR
• Insert tapered end first.
• Ensure patient retains suppository.

ACTION
Unknown. Binds with opioid receptors in the CNS, altering perception of and emotional response to pain. Also suppresses the cough reflex by direct action on the cough center in the medulla.

Route	Onset	Peak	Duration
PO	15–30 min	30–60 min	3–4 hr
PO (extended-release)	Gradually over 6–8 hr	12–16 hr	13 hr
IV	5 min	10–20 min	3–4 hr
IM	15 min	30–60 min	4–5 hr
PR	Unknown	Unknown	Unknown
Subcut	15 min	30–90 min	4 hr

Half-life: Immediate-release, 2 to 3 hours; PO (extended-release), 11 hours.

ADVERSE REACTIONS
CNS: sedation, somnolence, dizziness, dysphoria, euphoria, light-headedness, insomnia, headache, confusion, syncope, taste alteration, weakness, tremors, paresthesia, increased ICP, agitation, nervousness, anxiety, depression, hallucination, disorientation, abnormal dreams. **CV:** hypotension, HTN, flushing, *bradycardia,* extrasystoles, palpitations, chest discomfort, edema, tachycardia. **EENT:** blurred vision, diplopia, nystagmus, dry eye syndrome, miosis, tinnitus, dry mouth, rhinorrhea. **GI:** nausea, vomiting, constipation, anorexia, increased appetite, weight loss, diarrhea, ileus, intestinal obstruction, abdominal pain, abdominal distention, eructation, flatulence, gastroenteritis, delayed gastric emptying, biliary colic. **GU:** urine retention, urinary frequency, urinary hesitancy, bladder spasm, ureteral spasm, dysuria, erectile dysfunction, sexual disorder, hypogonadism. **Hepatic:** increased liver enzyme levels, biliary colic. **Musculoskeletal:** arthralgia, muscle contractions. **Respiratory:** oxygen desaturation, hyperventilation, *hypoxia, apnea, respiratory depression, bronchospasm.* **Skin:** diaphoresis, pruritus, hyperhidrosis, rash, urticaria, pain at injection site. **Other:** chills, induration with repeated subcut injections, physical dependence, pain. drug withdrawal syndrome (extended-release form).

INTERACTIONS

Drug-drug. *Anticholinergics (scopolamine, diphenhydramine):* May increase risk of urine retention or severe constipation. Use together cautiously.

Boxed Warning *Benzodiazepines, CNS depressants:* May cause slow or difficult breathing, sedation, and death. Avoid use together. If use together can't be avoided, limit dose and duration of each drug to the minimum needed for desired effect. ∎

Diuretics: May reduce efficacy of diuretics by inducing release of ADH. Monitor patient.

Droperidol, general anesthetics, minocycline, nabilone, neuromuscular blockers, other opioid analgesics, TCAs, tranquilizers: May cause additive effects. Monitor therapy carefully.

🖲 *Alert: MAO inhibitors:* May manifest as serotonin syndrome or opioid toxicity (respiratory depression, coma). Use together or within 14 days of MAO inhibitors isn't recommended. If administration with MAO inhibitors is unavoidable, monitor patient carefully for respiratory and CNS depression.

Muscle relaxants: May enhance neuromuscular blocking action of skeletal muscle relaxants and produce increased degree of respiratory depression. Monitor patient.

Opioids (mixed agonist/antagonist and partial agonists [butorphanol, buprenorphine, nalbuphine]): May diminish analgesic effect of opioid analgesics or cause withdrawal signs and symptoms. Avoid use together.

🖲 *Alert: Serotonergic drugs (amoxapine, antimigraine drugs, buspirone, cyclobenzaprine, dextromethorphan, linezolid, lithium, maprotiline, methylene blue, mirtazapine, nefazodone, SSNRIs, SSRIs, TCAs, trazodone, tryptophan, vilazodone):* May increase risk of serotonin syndrome. Use together cautiously and monitor patient for serotonin syndrome.

Drug-herb. *Kava, valerian:* May increase CNS depression. Avoid use together.

🖲 *Alert: St. John's wort:* May increase risk of serotonin syndrome. Use together cautiously and monitor patient for serotonin syndrome.

Drug-lifestyle. Boxed Warning *Alcohol use:* May cause slow or difficult breathing, sedation, and death. Discourage use together. ∎

EFFECTS ON LAB TEST RESULTS
• May increase amylase level.
• May interfere with hepatobiliary imaging studies because delayed gastric emptying and contraction of sphincter of Oddi may increase biliary tract pressure.

CONTRAINDICATIONS & CAUTIONS

Boxed Warning *Opioid class warning:* Opioids should only be prescribed with benzodiazepines or other CNS depressants when alternative treatment options are inadequate, aren't expected to provide adequate analgesia, haven't been tolerated, or aren't expected to be tolerated. ∎

• Contraindicated in patients hypersensitive to drug; in those with intracranial lesions that cause increased ICP; in those with paralytic ileus or narrowed or obstructed GI tract; for obstetric analgesia; and in those with depressed ventilation, such as in status asthmaticus, COPD, cor pulmonale, emphysema, and kyphoscoliosis.

Boxed Warning Use exposes patient and others to risk of opioid addiction, abuse, and misuse, which can lead to overdose and death. These effects can occur at any dose or duration. Assess patient risk before prescribing and regularly reassess patient for these behaviors and conditions. ∎

Boxed Warning Prescribers are strongly encouraged to complete a REMS-compliant education program. Drug should be prescribed only by prescribers with knowledge of opioid use and ways to reduce associated risks. ∎

🖲 *Alert:* Use lowest effective dose for shortest period consistent with patient's treatment goals.

🖲 *Alert:* Because risk of overdose increases as opioid dose increases, reserve titration to higher doses for patients in whom lower doses are ineffective and in whom expected benefits of higher opioid dose outweigh risks.

🖲 *Alert:* Immediate release formulations shouldn't be used for an extended period unless pain remains severe enough to require an opioid analgesic and alternative treatment options are inadequate to treat pain.

🖲 *Alert:* Long-acting or extended-release formulations are indicated for severe, persistent pain for which extended treatment with a daily opioid analgesic is required and for which alternative treatment options are inadequate. Use isn't indicated for as-needed analgesia.

Boxed Warning Accidental ingestion of even one dose of an opioid, especially by children, can result in a fatal overdose. ∎

---

*Reactions in bold italics are **life-threatening**.*

❸ *Alert:* Patients with any of the following conditions are at increased risk for oversedation and respiratory depression and require close monitoring: sleep-disordered breathing; first-time opioid use or nonrecent previous opioid use; opioid habituation or need for increased opioid doses; need for prolonged general anesthesia or other sedating drugs; preexisting pulmonary or cardiac disease; or thoracic or other surgical incisions that may impair breathing.

❸ *Alert:* Drug may lead to rare but serious decrease in adrenal gland cortisol production.

• Use cautiously in patients with a history of seizures and adrenal insufficiency.

• Drug may reduce sex hormone levels with long-term use.

• Drug may contain a sulfite that can cause allergic-type reactions, including anaphylactic symptoms and life-threatening or less severe asthmatic episodes in certain patients who are susceptible.

❸ *Alert:* Drug may cause severe hypotension, including orthostatic hypotension and syncope, in patients who are ambulatory. Patients with reduced blood volume and those receiving CNS depressants (phenothiazines or general anesthetics) are at increased risk.

❸ *Alert:* Drug may reduce respiratory drive and the resultant CO_2 retention may increase ICP. Use cautiously in patients with a head injury.

• Use cautiously in older adults, patients who are debilitated, and those with liver or kidney disease, hypothyroidism, Addison disease, prostatic hyperplasia, or urethral stricture. Consider alternative to extended-release form in patients with CrCl less than 30 mL/minute.

• Safety and effectiveness in children haven't been determined. Drug has been used off label.

Dialyzable drug: Unknown.

⚠ *Overdose S&S:* Constricted pupils; cold, clammy skin; extreme somnolence, progressing to stupor or coma; respiratory depression; skeletal muscle flaccidity; bradycardia; hypotension; apnea; cardiac arrest; circulatory collapse; death.

PREGNANCY-LACTATION-REPRODUCTION

❸ *Alert:* Drug crosses placental barrier. Carefully weigh benefits and risks of using drug during pregnancy.

Boxed Warning Prolonged use during pregnancy can result in neonatal opioid withdrawal syndrome, which may be life-threatening. It requires management with expert neonatology protocols. If prolonged use is needed, advise patient of risks and ensure availability of proper treatment. ∎

• Don't use during labor and delivery; neonatal respiratory depression may occur.

• Drug appears in human milk in low concentrations. Breastfeeding isn't recommended during treatment. Monitor infants who are breastfed and exposed to opioids for excess sedation and respiratory depression. Also watch for withdrawal signs and symptoms in infants when maternal administration of an opioid analgesic is stopped or when breastfeeding is stopped.

• Long-term use can cause hypogonadism and infertility.

NURSING CONSIDERATIONS

❸ *Alert:* Vial stopper may contain latex.

• Reassess patient's level of pain at least 15 and 30 minutes after administration.

• For better analgesic effect for chronic pain, give drug at regularly scheduled intervals, before patient has intense pain.

Boxed Warning Regularly monitor all patients for opioid addiction, abuse, and misuse, which can lead to overdose and death. ∎

Boxed Warning May cause life-threatening or fatal respiratory depression at any time during therapy. Monitor patient closely, especially when starting or increasing doses. Proper dosing and titration are essential to reduce risk. ∎

❸ *Alert:* Drug may cause opioid-induced hyperalgesia (OIH). Symptoms include increased pain level with opioid dose increase, decreased pain level with opioid dose reduction, pain from ordinarily nonpainful stimuli without underlying disease progression, opioid tolerance or withdrawal, and addictive behavior. For suspected OIH, decrease opioid dose or switch patient to alternative opioid.

❸ *Alert:* Carefully monitor vital signs, pain level, respiratory status, and sedation level in all patients receiving opioids, especially those receiving IV drugs, even those given postoperatively.

❸ *Alert:* If patient is taking opioids with serotonergic drugs, watch for signs and symptoms of serotonin syndrome (agitation, hallucinations, rapid HR, fever, diaphoresis, shivering or shaking, muscle twitching or stiffness, trouble with coordination, nausea, vomiting, diarrhea), especially when starting treatment

H

or increasing dosages. Signs and symptoms may occur within several hours of coadministration but may also occur later, especially after dosage increase. Discontinue the opioid, serotonergic drug, or both if serotonin syndrome is suspected.

● *Alert:* Monitor patient for signs and symptoms of adrenal insufficiency (nausea, vomiting, loss of appetite, fatigue, weakness, dizziness, low BP). Perform diagnostic testing if adrenal insufficiency is suspected. If adrenal insufficiency is confirmed, treat with corticosteroids and wean patient off opioids, if appropriate. Discontinue corticosteroids when clinically appropriate.

● Monitor patient for signs and symptoms of decreased sex hormone levels (low libido, erectile dysfunction, amenorrhea, infertility). If signs and symptoms occur, evaluate patient and obtain specimens for lab testing.

● *Alert:* Don't stop drug abruptly; withdraw slowly and individualize the gradual tapering plan to prevent signs and symptoms of withdrawal, worsening pain, and psychological distress in patient who is physically dependent. Refer to manufacturer's label for tapering instructions.

● *Alert:* When tapering opioid, monitor closely for signs and symptoms of opioid withdrawal (restlessness, lacrimation, rhinorrhea, yawning, perspiration, chills, myalgia, mydriasis, irritability, anxiety, insomnia, backache, joint pain, weakness, abdominal cramps, anorexia, nausea, vomiting, diarrhea, increased BP or HR, increased respiratory rate). Such signs and symptoms may indicate a need to taper more slowly. Also monitor patient for suicidality, use of other substances, and mood changes.

● Monitor patient with history of seizure disorder for worsening seizure control.

● Patients considered opioid tolerant are those receiving, for 1 week or longer, at least 60 mg morphine per day, 25 mcg/hour transdermal fentanyl, 30 mg oral oxycodone per day, 8 mg oral hydromorphone per day, 25 mg oral oxymorphone per day, or an equianalgesic dose of another opioid.

● Discontinue all other extended-release opioids before giving extended-release form of hydromorphone.

● Keep opioid antagonist (naloxone) available.

● Discontinue use of extended-release form if stopped for more than 3 days.

● Drug may worsen or mask gallbladder pain.

● Drug may cause constipation. Assess bowel function and need for stool softeners and stimulant laxatives.

● *Look alike–sound alike:* Don't confuse hydromorphone with morphine or oxymorphone. Don't confuse Dilaudid with Dilantin.

PATIENT TEACHING

Boxed Warning Counsel patient and caregiver on serious risks, safe use, and importance of reading the medication guide with each prescription. ∎

● Advise patient to take drug exactly as prescribed and to use lowest dose possible for shortest time needed.

● Teach patient to request or take drug before pain becomes intense.

● Tell patient to report all adverse reactions.

● Instruct patient to contact health care provider if prescribed dosage isn't controlling pain.

● Inform patient that, for acute pain, drug may only be needed for a few days. Teach about safe disposal of unused drug.

● Warn that extended-release and long-acting formulations shouldn't be taken on an "as needed" basis.

● *Alert:* Counsel patient who has been regularly taking drug not to discontinue without first discussing the need for gradual tapering with prescriber.

● *Alert:* Teach patient that naloxone may be prescribed with the opioid when beginning and renewing therapy to reduce risk of opioid overdose and death.

● *Alert:* Warn patient to withhold drug and inform prescriber if pain level worsens, pain sensitivity increases, or new pain occurs after taking drug.

● Encourage patient to report all medications being taken, including prescription and OTC medications and supplements.

● *Alert:* Caution patient to immediately report signs and symptoms of serotonin syndrome, adrenal insufficiency, and decreased sex hormone levels.

● *Alert:* Counsel patient not to discontinue opioids without first discussing the need for a gradual tapering regimen with prescriber.

● Warn patient that use of drug, even when taken as recommended, can result in addiction, abuse, and misuse, which can lead to overdose or death. Instruct patient not to discontinue drug without first discussing the need for a tapering regimen with prescriber.

Reactions in bold italics are *life-threatening*.

• Inform patient of the risk of severe constipation and measures to prevent it. Advise patient when to seek medical attention if prevention measures are ineffective.

• Explain the assessment and monitoring process to patient and family. Instruct them to immediately report if patient has difficulty breathing or other signs of a potential adverse opioid-related reaction.

• Advise patient to take drug with food if GI upset occurs.

• When drug is used after surgery, encourage patient to turn, cough, and breathe deeply to avoid lung problems.

• Teach patient how to recognize signs and symptoms of low BP and how to reduce risk of serious consequences of hypotension (by sitting or lying down or by carefully rising from a sitting or lying position).

• Warn outpatient to avoid hazardous activities that require mental alertness until drug's CNS effects are known.

• Caution patient to report to prescriber pregnancy or plan to become pregnant.

hydroxychloroquine sulfate
hye-droks-ee-KLOR-oh-kwin

Plaquenil

Therapeutic class: Antimalarials
Pharmacologic class: Aminoquinolines

AVAILABLE FORMS
Tablets ⓓⓝⓒ: 100 mg, 200 mg, 300 mg, 400 mg (each 200 mg is equivalent to 155 mg base)

INDICATIONS & DOSAGES
➤ **Suppressive prevention of malaria**
Adults: 400 mg PO weekly on the same day each week, beginning 2 weeks before entering malaria-endemic area and continuing for 4 weeks after leaving area.
Children weighing 31 kg or more: 6.5 mg/kg PO weekly on the same day each week, beginning 2 weeks before entering malaria-endemic area and continuing for 4 weeks after leaving area. Maximum, 400 mg weekly.
➤ **Uncomplicated malaria caused by** *Plasmodium vivax, Plasmodium malariae, Plasmodium ovale,* **and susceptible strains of** *Plasmodium falciparum*
Adults: Initially, 800 mg PO; then 400 mg at 6 hours, 24 hours, and 48 hours after first dose.

Children weighing 31 kg or more: Initially, 13 mg/kg (up to 800 mg) PO; then 6.5 mg/kg (up to 400 mg) at 6 hours, 24 hours, and 48 hours after first dose.
➤ **SLE; chronic discoid lupus erythematosus**
Adults: 200 mg PO daily as a single dose or 400 mg PO daily in two divided doses.
➤ **RA**
Adults: Initially, 400 to 600 mg PO daily as a single dose or in two divided doses. When good response occurs, continue at 200 to 400 mg daily in one or two divided doses. Maximum dosage is 600 mg or 5 mg/kg per day, whichever is lower.

ADMINISTRATION
PO
⚠ *Alert:* Drug dosage may be discussed in "mg" or "mg base"; be aware of the difference. Hydroxychloroquine sulfate salt 200 mg is equivalent to hydroxychloroquine base 155 mg.
• Give drug with food or milk to minimize GI upset.
• Have patient swallow film-coated tablets whole; don't crush or break tablets.
• To improve adherence when drug is used for prevention, advise patient to take drug immediately before or after a meal on the same day each week.

ACTION
Concentrates in parasite's acid vesicles and inhibits polymerization of heme. Can also inhibit certain enzymes by its interaction with DNA. Mechanisms of the anti-inflammatory and immunomodulatory effects in treatment of RA, chronic discoid lupus erythematosus, and SLE aren't fully known.

Route	Onset	Peak	Duration
PO	Unknown	3–4 hr	Unknown

Half-life: 40 to 50 days.

ADVERSE REACTIONS
CNS: *seizures,* irritability, nightmares, ataxia, psychosis, vertigo, dizziness, emotional lability, hypoactive deep tendon reflexes, abnormal nerve conduction, headache, fatigue, extrapyramidal disorders, fever. **CV:** *cardiomyopathy, HF, QT-interval prolongation, ventricular arrhythmias, torsades de pointes,* bundle-branch block, AV block, *sick sinus syndrome,* pulmonary HTN.
EENT: blurred vision, retinopathy, difficulty

H

focusing, reversible corneal changes, typically irreversible nystagmus, tinnitus, sensorineural hearing loss. **GI:** decreased appetite, abdominal cramps, diarrhea, nausea, vomiting. **Hematologic:** *agranulocytosis, leukopenia, thrombocytopenia,* anemia, porphyria, *aplastic anemia, hyperleukocytosis.* **Hepatic:** *acute liver failure,* abnormal LFT values. **Metabolic:** *hypoglycemia,* weight loss. **Musculoskeletal:** proximal myopathy. **Respiratory:** bronchospasm. **Skin:** pruritus, lichen planus eruptions, skin and mucosal pigmentary changes, pleomorphic skin eruptions, worsened psoriasis, alopecia, photosensitivity, bleaching of hair, urticaria. **Other:** hypersensitivity reactions.

INTERACTIONS

Drug-drug. *Antacids, kaolin, magnesium:* May decrease GI absorption. Separate dose times by 4 hours.

Antidiabetics, insulin: May enhance effects of hypoglycemic treatment. Decrease insulin or antidiabetic dosage as required.

Antiepileptic drugs (carbamazepine): May decrease antiepileptic effect. Monitor patient.

Beta blockers: May increase CV effects of certain beta blockers (metoprolol). Carefully monitor patient. Consider using alternative beta blocker.

Cimetidine: May increase chloroquine exposure. Avoid use together.

Cyclosporine: May increase cyclosporine level. Monitor level closely.

Digoxin: May increase digoxin level. Monitor drug levels; monitor patient for toxicity.

Drugs that prolong QTc interval: May enhance QTc-prolonging effect of highest-risk QTc-prolonging drugs. Avoid combination.

Mefloquine: May increase QTc-interval prolongation and seizure risk when used concurrently. Avoid use together.

Phenothiazines: May increase serum level of phenothiazines. Monitor therapy.

Rifampin: May decrease hydroxychloroquine effect. Avoid use together.

EFFECTS ON LAB TEST RESULTS

• May increase LFT values.
• May decrease Hb level and granulocyte, WBC, and platelet counts.

CONTRAINDICATIONS & CAUTIONS

• Contraindicated in patients hypersensitive to drug.

• Use cautiously in patients with retinal or visual field changes, psoriasis, or porphyria.
• Daily dosages exceeding 5 mg/kg (actual weight) of hydroxychloroquine increase incidence of retinopathy.
• Use cautiously in patients with severe GI, neurologic, or blood disorders.
• Use cautiously in patients with diabetes or low blood glucose level. Drug may cause hypoglycemia.
• Use cautiously in patients with liver disease or alcoholism or when used with liver-toxic drugs.
⚕ Use cautiously in patients with G6PD deficiency. Drug may cause hemolysis.
❸ Alert: Use cautiously in patients with cardiac disease or QT-interval prolongation. Drug prolongs QT interval and may cause cardiotoxicity.
❸ Alert: Suicidality has been reported in very rare cases.
• Don't give drug to children who weigh less than 31 kg because film-coated tablets can't be crushed or divided.
• Use cautiously for long-term treatment in children.
• Safety and effectiveness of drug haven't been established in children for treatment of RA, chronic discoid lupus erythematosus, or SLE.
Dialyzable drug: Unknown.
⚠ Overdose S&S: Headache, drowsiness, visual disturbances, CV collapse, seizures, sudden and early respiratory and cardiac arrest, atrial standstill, nodal rhythm, prolonged intraventricular conduction time, progressive bradycardia, leading to ventricular fibrillation or arrest.

PREGNANCY-LACTATION-REPRODUCTION

• Drug doesn't appear to pose a significant risk to the fetus, especially with lower doses.
• Drug appears in human milk. Use cautiously during breastfeeding.

NURSING CONSIDERATIONS

• Guidelines for treating and preventing malaria are available at CDC malaria website (www.cdc.gov/parasites/malaria).
• Ensure that baseline and periodic ophthalmic exams are performed at baseline and annually. Periodically check for ocular muscle weakness after long-term use. Retinal toxicity is largely dose-related.

Reactions in bold italics are *life-threatening*.

- Periodically monitor CBC and LFTs during long-term therapy; if severe blood disorder not caused by disease develops, drug may need to be stopped.

♦ Alert: Monitor patient for possible overdose, which can quickly lead to toxic signs or symptoms. Children are extremely susceptible to toxicity.

PATIENT TEACHING

- Teach about proper drug administration and handling and importance of adherence.
- Advise patient to report adverse reactions, infection, and signs and symptoms of liver failure (dark urine, feeling tired, yellowing of skin or eyes) or bleeding.
- Instruct patient to report changes in medications as many drug interactions exist.
- Warn that dizziness may occur. Advise patient to use caution while driving and performing other tasks that require alertness, coordination, or physical dexterity.

SAFETY ALERT!

hydroxyurea

hye-droks-ee-yoor-EE-a

Droxia, Hydrea, Siklos

Therapeutic class: Antineoplastics
Pharmacologic class: Antimetabolites

AVAILABLE FORMS

Capsules: 200 mg, 300 mg, 400 mg, 500 mg
Tablets: 100 mg, 1,000 mg

INDICATIONS & DOSAGES

Adjust-a-dose (for all indications): Base dosage on patient's actual or ideal weight, whichever is less. If CrCl is less than 60 mL/minute, give 50% of usual dose. If patient is on hemodialysis, give 50% of usual dose after dialysis on dialysis days.

➤ **Carcinoma of the head (excluding lip) and neck, with radiation (Hydrea); resistant chronic myelocytic leukemia (Hydrea)**
Adults: Initially, 1.5 mg/kg PO daily. Individualize treatment regimen based on tumor type, response, and current clinical practice standards.

➤ **To reduce frequency of painful crises and need for blood transfusions in adults with sickle cell anemia with recurrent moderate to severe painful crises (Droxia, Siklos)**

Adults (Droxia): 15 mg/kg PO once daily. Monitor blood counts every 2 weeks. If blood counts are in acceptable range, may increase dosage by 5 mg/kg daily every 12 weeks until maximum tolerated dosage or 35 mg/kg daily has been reached. If blood counts are considered toxic, withhold drug until counts recover. Resume treatment after reducing dosage by 2.5 mg/kg daily. May titrate up or down every 12 weeks in 2.5-mg/kg/day increments. Patient should be at stable dosage with no hematologic toxicity for 24 weeks. Permanently discontinue if hematologic toxicity recurs. See manufacturer's instructions for blood count parameters.

Adults and children ages 2 and older (Siklos): 15 mg/kg (adults) or 20 mg/kg (children) PO once daily. Monitor blood counts every 2 weeks. If blood counts are in acceptable range, may increase dosage by 5 mg/kg daily every 8 weeks or if a painful crisis occurs until mild myelosuppression (ANC 2,000 to 4,000/mm³) is achieved, up to maximum dosage of 35 mg/kg/day. If blood counts are considered toxic, withhold drug until counts recover. Resume treatment after reducing dosage by 5 mg/kg daily. Every 8 weeks thereafter, may adjust dosage up or down in 5-mg/kg daily increments until patient is at a stable, nontoxic dosage for 24 weeks. Permanently discontinue if hematologic toxicity develops twice. See manufacturer's instructions for blood count parameters.

➤ **Thrombocythemia ♦**
Adults: 500 to 1,000 mg PO daily. Adjust dosage to maintain platelet count at less than 400,000/mm³.

ADMINISTRATION
PO

♦ Alert: Hazardous drug; use safe handling and disposal precautions.

- Wear gloves when handling drug or its container, and wash hands before and after contact with bottle or capsule. If powder from capsule spills, immediately wipe up with damp towel. Dispose of towel in closed container (such as plastic bag). Then clean spill areas three times using detergent solution followed by clean water.
- Have patient swallow capsules whole; don't crush or break capsules.
- Give tablets with a glass of water.
- The 1,000-mg tablets have three score lines and can be split into four parts (each 250 mg).

The 100-mg tablets can be split into two parts (each 50 mg). Calculate the rounded doses to the nearest 50- or 100-mg strength based on clinical judgment.

• For patients who can't swallow tablets, disperse them immediately before use in a small quantity of water in a teaspoon.

ACTION
May inhibit DNA synthesis.

Route	Onset	Peak	Duration
PO	Unknown	1–4 hr	24 hr

Half-life: 2 to 4 hours.

ADVERSE REACTIONS
CNS: malaise, fever, drowsiness, headache, dizziness, asthenia, fatigue. **CV:** *hemorrhage,* edema. **GI:** anorexia, nausea, vomiting, diarrhea, stomatitis, constipation. **Hematologic:** *bone marrow suppression including leukopenia, thrombocytopenia,* anemia, macrocytosis, megaloblastosis. **Metabolic:** hyperuricemia, vitamin D deficiency, weight gain. **Musculoskeletal:** arthralgia, back pain, extremity pain. **Respiratory:** cough, lung disorder, dyspnea. **Skin:** rash, itching, alopecia, dry skin, vasculitic toxicities (including vasculitic ulcerations and gangrene), nail discoloration. **Other:** chills, infection.

INTERACTIONS
Drug-drug. **⊘** *Alert: Antiretrovirals (didanosine, stavudine):* May cause liver toxicity and liver failure, resulting in death. When given with didanosine to patients infected with HIV, severe peripheral neuropathy or fatal pancreatitis may occur. Avoid use with didanosine and stavudine.
Cytotoxic drugs, radiation therapy: May enhance toxicity of hydroxyurea. Use together cautiously.
Interferon: May increase risk of cutaneous vasculitic toxicities, including vasculitic ulcerations and gangrene. Stop drug.
Live-virus vaccines: May increase risk of vaccine-related adverse reactions, viral replication, and severe infection. Avoid vaccinations during therapy and for 3 months after therapy ends.

EFFECTS ON LAB TEST RESULTS
• May increase BUN, creatinine, liver enzyme, and uric acid levels.

• May decrease Hb level and WBC, RBC, and platelet counts.
• May interfere with lactic acid, urea, and uric acid assays, resulting in falsely elevated results.

CONTRAINDICATIONS & CAUTIONS
• Contraindicated in patients hypersensitive to drug or its components.
• Don't initiate treatment if bone marrow function is markedly depressed. Bone marrow suppression may occur, and leukopenia is generally its first and most common manifestation. Thrombocytopenia and anemia occur less often.
• Use cautiously in patients with kidney dysfunction and in older adults.
• Safety and effectiveness of Hydrea use in children haven't been established.
Dialyzable drug: Yes.
⚠ Overdose S&S: Acute mucocutaneous toxicity; soreness; violet erythema on palms and soles, followed by scaling of hands and feet; severe generalized hyperpigmentation of skin; stomatitis.

PREGNANCY-LACTATION-REPRODUCTION
• Drug can cause fetal harm. Don't use during pregnancy.
• Patients of childbearing potential should use effective contraception during therapy and for at least 6 months after final dose. Males with partners of childbearing potential should use effective contraception during therapy and for at least 6 months (Siklos) or 1 year (Droxia, Hydrea) after final dose.
• Discontinue breastfeeding or discontinue drug, considering importance of drug to patient.
• Azoospermia or oligospermia, sometimes reversible, has been observed.

NURSING CONSIDERATIONS
Boxed Warning Droxia and Siklos may cause severe myelosuppression. Don't give if bone marrow function is markedly depressed. Monitor blood counts at baseline and throughout therapy. Treatment interruption and dosage reductions may be needed. ∎
Boxed Warning Droxia and Siklos are carcinogenic. Monitor patient for malignancies. ∎
• Verify pregnancy status before treatment.

Reactions in bold italics are *life-threatening*.

• Routinely measure BUN, uric acid, liver enzyme, and creatinine levels; monitor blood counts every 2 weeks.
• Use fetal Hb (HbF) level to evaluate drug's efficacy in sickle cell anemia. Obtain HbF level every 3 to 4 months. Monitor patient for an increase in HbF level of at least twofold over baseline.
• Hydroxyurea may dramatically lower WBC count in 24 to 48 hours.
🜂 Alert: Patients who have received or are currently receiving interferon may be at greater risk for developing cutaneous vasculitic toxicities. Monitor patient closely; discontinue drug if toxicities occur.
• Monitor patient for pancreatitis. If it occurs, permanently discontinue drug.
• Drug may increase risk of hyperuricemia. Monitor fluid intake and output; keep patient hydrated.
• To prevent bleeding, avoid all IM injections when platelet count falls below 50,000/mm³.
• Blood transfusions may be necessary for cumulative anemia.
• Dosage change may be needed after chemotherapy or radiation therapy.

PATIENT TEACHING
• Teach about proper drug administration and special handling precautions.
Boxed Warning Advise patient that blood counts must be checked throughout therapy to monitor for toxicity. ∎
• Advise patient to watch for signs and symptoms of infection (fever, sore throat, fatigue) and bleeding (easy bruising, nosebleeds, bleeding gums, melena) and to take temperature daily.
• Instruct patient in the use of effective contraception during and after therapy, as appropriate.
• Counsel patient to discontinue breastfeeding.
• Inform male patient about possible sperm conservation before therapy. Azoospermia or oligospermia, sometimes reversible, has occurred.
• Advise patient to inform prescriber if patient has HIV or is taking antiretrovirals.
Boxed Warning Advise patient to use sun protection and that monitoring for secondary malignancies will be needed. ∎

hydrOXYzine hydrochloride
hye-DROKS-i-zeen

Atarax ✤

hydrOXYzine pamoate
Vistaril

Therapeutic class: Antihistamines
Pharmacologic class: Piperazine derivatives

AVAILABLE FORMS
hydroxyzine hydrochloride
Injection: 25 mg/mL, 50 mg/mL
Syrup: 10 mg/5 mL
Tablets: 10 mg, 25 mg, 50 mg
hydroxyzine pamoate
Capsules: 25 mg, 50 mg, 100 mg
Oral suspension: 25 mg/5 mL

INDICATIONS & DOSAGES
Adjust-a-dose (for all indications): In older adults, initiate drug at the lower end of dosage range and observe closely.
➤ **Anxiety**
Adults: 50 to 100 mg PO q.i.d. Or, 50 to 100 mg IM t.i.d. or q.i.d.
Children ages 6 and older: 50 to 100 mg PO daily in divided doses.
Children younger than age 6: 50 mg PO daily in divided doses.
➤ **Preoperative and postoperative adjunctive therapy for sedation**
Adults: 50 to 100 mg PO.
Children: 0.6 mg/kg/dose PO.
➤ **Preoperative and postoperative and prepartum and postpartum adjunctive therapy to permit reduction in narcotic dosage, allay anxiety, and control emesis**
Adults: 25 to 100 mg IM.
Children: 1.1 mg/kg/dose IM.
➤ **Pruritus**
Adults: 25 mg PO t.i.d. or q.i.d.
Children ages 6 and older: 50 to 100 mg PO daily in divided doses.
Children younger than age 6: 50 mg PO daily in divided doses.
➤ **Nausea and vomiting**
Adults: 25 to 100 mg/dose IM.
Children: 1.1 mg/kg/dose IM.

H

ADMINISTRATION

PO
- Give drug without regard for meals.
- Shake suspension well before giving.

IM
- Parenteral form (hydroxyzine hydrochloride) is for IM use only, preferably by Z-track injection.
- ⚠ *Alert:* Never give drug IV, subcut, or intraarterially.
- Inject deeply into large muscle (don't inject into lower or mid-third of upper arm).

ACTION

Suppresses activity in certain essential regions of the subcortical area of the CNS.

Route	Onset	Peak	Duration
PO	15–30 min	2 hr	Varies
IM	Rapid	Unknown	Varies

Half-life: Children ages 1 to 14, 4 to 11 hours; adults, 20 hours; older adults, 29 hours.

ADVERSE REACTIONS

CNS: drowsiness. **GI:** dry mouth. **Respiratory:** *respiratory depression (high doses).* **Skin:** pain at IM injection site.

INTERACTIONS

Drug-drug. *Anticholinergics (scopolamine, diphenhydramine):* May cause additive anticholinergic effects. Use together cautiously.
CNS depressants: May increase CNS depression. Use together cautiously; dosage adjustments may be needed.
QT interval-prolonging drugs: May prolong QT interval and induce torsades de pointes. Monitor ECG.
Drug-lifestyle. *Alcohol use, cannabidiol, cannabis use:* May increase CNS depression. Discourage use together.

EFFECTS ON LAB TEST RESULTS

- May cause false-negative skin allergen tests by reducing or inhibiting the cutaneous response to histamine.
- May cause false-positive serum TCA screen.

CONTRAINDICATIONS & CAUTIONS

- Contraindicated in patients hypersensitive to drug, in those with known hypersensitivity to cetirizine hydrochloride or levocetirizine hydrochloride, and in patients with prolonged QTc interval.
- Drug can prolong QTc interval. Use cautiously in patients with risk factors for QTc-interval prolongation and in patients with conditions that predispose to QTc-interval prolongation and ventricular arrhythmias as well as in those with recent MI, uncompensated HF, or bradyarrhythmias. Use cautiously during concomitant use of drugs known to prolong QTc interval.
- Use cautiously in older adults and in patients with glaucoma, BPH, urinary stricture, asthma, or COPD.
Dialyzable drug: Unknown.
⚠ *Overdose S&S:* Hypersedation.

PREGNANCY-LACTATION-REPRODUCTION

- Contraindicated during early pregnancy. Studies during pregnancy are inadequate.
- It's unknown if drug appears in human milk. Use during breastfeeding isn't recommended.

NURSING CONSIDERATIONS

- If patient takes other CNS drugs, watch for oversedation.
- Drug may rarely cause acute generalized exanthematous pustulosis (AGEP), a serious skin reaction involving fever, pustules, and large areas of edematous erythema. Discontinue at first sign of rash, worsening of preexisting skin reactions, or other signs or symptoms of hypersensitivity. If signs or symptoms suggest AGEP, don't resume therapy.
- Older adults may be more sensitive to adverse anticholinergic effects; monitor these patients for dizziness, excessive sedation, confusion, hypotension, syncope, and dysuria.
- *Look alike–sound alike:* Don't confuse hydroxyzine with hydroxyurea, Hydrogesic, or hydralazine.

PATIENT TEACHING

- Warn patient to avoid hazardous activities that require alertness and good coordination until effects of drug are known.
- Advise patient to avoid simultaneous use of other CNS depressants and use of alcohol during therapy to avoid increased risk of CNS depression.
- Tell patient to report all adverse reactions, especially heart palpitations, dizziness, fainting, difficulty breathing, difficulty urinating, and vision changes.
- Instruct patient to report pregnancy or plans to become pregnant or to breastfeed during therapy.

Reactions in bold italics are *life-threatening*.

ibandronate sodium
eye-BAN-droh-nate

Therapeutic class: Antiosteoporotics
Pharmacologic class: Bisphosphonates

AVAILABLE FORMS
Injection: 3 mg/3 mL prefilled syringes
Tablets ⒹⓃⒸ: 150 mg

INDICATIONS & DOSAGES
Adjust-a-dose (for all indications): In patients
with CrCl less than 30 mL/minute, drug isn't
recommended.
➤ **To treat or prevent postmenopausal
osteoporosis**
Adult females: 150 mg PO once monthly on
same day each month. 3 mg IV bolus once
every 3 months.
➤ **Metastatic bone disease due to breast
cancer ◆**
Adults: 6 mg IV over 1 to 2 hours every 3 to
4 weeks for up to 4 years.

ADMINISTRATION
PO
• Give drug 1 hour before first food or drink of
the day and before any other drugs or supplements (including calcium, antacids, and vitamins).
• Make sure patient doesn't lie down for at
least 1 hour after receiving drug.
• Give drug with 6 to 8 oz of plain water
only; avoid mineral water.
• Have patient swallow tablets whole; don't
crush or cut tablets. Chewing or sucking
tablets may cause oropharyngeal ulceration.
• Ensure patient doesn't eat or drink anything
except plain water, including includes other
oral medications, for 1 hour after taking drug.
• If dose is missed and it's more than 7 days
before next scheduled dose, give dose the
next morning; if next scheduled dose is 7 days
or less away, omit missed dose.
IV
▼ Prefilled syringes are for single use only.
▼ Give undiluted using needle provided with
the syringe.
▼ Give by IV bolus over 15 to 30 seconds.
▼ Don't use drug if it is discolored or contains particulate matter.
▼ If IV dose is missed, reschedule missed
dose as soon as possible. Schedule subsequent injections once every 3 months from
that dose.

▼ Store at room temperature.
▼ **Incompatibilities:** Calcium-containing
solutions and other IV drugs.

ACTION
Inhibits bone breakdown and removal to reduce bone loss and increase bone mass.

Route	Onset	Peak	Duration
PO	Unknown	0.5–2 hr	Unknown
IV	Rapid	Unknown	Unknown

Half-life: PO, 37 to 157 hours for the 150-mg dose;
IV, about 4.6 to 25.5 hours for the 2- to 4-mg dose.

ADVERSE REACTIONS
CNS: asthenia, dizziness, depression, fatigue, headache, insomnia, vertigo. **CV:** HTN.
EENT: nasopharyngitis, pharyngitis, tooth
disorder. **GI:** dyspepsia, abdominal pain, constipation, diarrhea, gastritis, nausea, vomiting, gastroenteritis. **GU:** cystitis, UTI. **Musculoskeletal:** back pain, arthralgia, arthritis, joint disorder, limb pain, localized osteoarthritis, muscle cramps, myalgia. **Respiratory:** bronchitis, URI, pneumonia. **Skin:**
rash. **Other:** infusion site reaction (redness,
swelling), allergic reaction, infection, flulike
symptoms.

INTERACTIONS
Drug-drug. *Angiogenesis inhibitors (systemic
monoclonal antibodies):* May enhance adverse effects of bisphosphonate derivatives,
especially risk of osteonecrosis of jaw. Monitor patient for adverse effects.
Aspirin, NSAIDs: May increase GI irritation
and risk of kidney toxicity. Use together cautiously.
Deferasirox: May enhance adverse effects of
deferasirox, especially risk of GI ulceration,
irritation, and bleeding. Monitor patient for
adverse effects.
Drugs that prolong QTc interval: May enhance QTc-prolonging effects. For high-
risk QTc-prolonging agents, consider therapy modification. For moderate-risk QTc-
prolonging drugs, monitor therapy.
Potassium-competitive acid blockers, PPIs:
May decrease ibandronate therapeutic effects.
Monitor therapy.
*Products containing aluminum, calcium,
magnesium, or iron:* May decrease ibandronate absorption. Give oral ibandronate
at least 1 hour before vitamins, minerals, or
antacids.

I

Drug-food. *Food, milk, beverages (except water):* May decrease drug absorption. Give oral drug on an empty stomach with plain water.

EFFECTS ON LAB TEST RESULTS
- May decrease calcium level and CrCl.
- May interfere with bone-imaging agents.

CONTRAINDICATIONS & CAUTIONS
- Contraindicated in patients hypersensitive to drug and in those with uncorrected hypocalcemia.
- Oral form is contraindicated in patients with abnormalities of the esophagus that delay esophageal emptying, such as stricture or achalasia, and in those who can't stand or sit upright for 60 minutes.
- ❸ **Alert:** An increased risk of atypical fractures of the thigh is possible in patients treated with bisphosphonates.
- ❸ **Alert:** Drug may cause osteonecrosis, mainly in the jaw. Avoid invasive dental procedures if possible.
- Drug may cause hypocalcemia, especially if dietary intake of calcium or vitamin D is inadequate.
- Don't give to patients with CrCl less than 30 mL/minute.
- Use cautiously in patients with history of GI disorders.
- Safety and effectiveness in children haven't been established.
- *Dialyzable drug:* Yes.
- ⚠ **Overdose S&S:** Hypocalcemia, hypophosphatemia, hypomagnesemia, upset stomach, dyspepsia, esophagitis, gastritis, ulcer.

PREGNANCY-LACTATION-REPRODUCTION
- Not indicated for use in patients of childbearing potential.
- Studies during pregnancy are inadequate.
- It isn't known if drug appears in human milk.

NURSING CONSIDERATIONS
- Correct hypocalcemia or other disturbances of bone and mineral metabolism before therapy.
- Make sure patient has adequate intake of calcium and vitamin D.
- For patient receiving IV ibandronate, obtain serum creatinine level and perform an oral exam before each dose.
- Watch for signs of esophageal irritation (dysphagia, painful swallowing, retrosternal pain, heartburn).

- Monitor for bone, joint, and muscle pain, which may be severe and incapacitating and may occur within days or months of start of therapy. When drug is stopped, symptoms may resolve.
- Watch for signs of uveitis and scleritis.
- Use care to avoid intra-arterial or paravenous injection, which can lead to tissue damage; only administer IV.

PATIENT TEACHING
- For oral form, teach about proper drug administration and handling.
- Advise patient to take calcium and vitamin D supplements as prescribed.
- Tell patient to report any bone, joint, or muscle pain.
- Caution patient to stop drug and immediately report signs and symptoms of esophageal irritation.
- Advise patient to have periodic dental exams to monitor for osteonecrosis of jaw.
- Instruct patient to seek medical attention if severe allergic reaction occurs.

ibrexafungerp
eye-brex-a-FUNJ-erp

Brexafemme

Therapeutic class: Antifungals
Pharmacologic class: Triterpenoid antifungals

AVAILABLE FORMS
Tablets: 150 mg

INDICATIONS & DOSAGES
Adjust-a-dose (for all indications): If used together with strong CYP3A inhibitor, give one 150-mg tablet about 12 hours apart for 1 day for a total daily dosage of 300 mg.
➤ **Vulvovaginal candidiasis**
Adults and pediatric patients who are postmenarchal: 300 mg (two 150-mg tablets) PO approximately 12 hours apart for 1 day, for a total daily dosage of 600 mg (total of 4 tablets for a course of therapy).
✷ *NEW INDICATION:* **To reduce incidence of recurrent vulvovaginal candidiasis (RVVC)**
Adults and pediatric females who are postmenarchal: 300 mg (two 150-mg tablets) PO about 12 hours apart for 1 day for total daily dosage of 600 mg monthly for 6 months.

Reactions in bold italics are *life-threatening*.

ADMINISTRATION
PO
- Give drug without regard to food.
- Store at room temperature.

ACTION
Inhibits glucan synthase, an enzyme involved in formation of the fungal cell wall.

Route	Onset	Peak	Duration
PO	Unknown	4–6 hr	Unknown

Half-life: 20 hours.

ADVERSE REACTIONS
CNS: dizziness, fatigue, headache. **GI:** abdominal pain, diarrhea, flatulence, nausea, vomiting. **GU:** dysmenorrhea, vaginal bleeding, UTI. **Hepatic:** elevated transaminase levels. **Musculoskeletal:** back pain. **Skin:** rash. **Other:** hypersensitivity reaction.

INTERACTIONS
Drug-drug. *Strong or moderate CYP3A inducers (bosentan, carbamazepine, efavirenz, etravirine, long-acting barbiturates, phenytoin, rifampin):* May significantly reduce ibrexafungerp level. Avoid use together.
Strong CYP3A inhibitors (itraconazole, ketoconazole): May significantly increase ibrexafungerp level. Reduce ibrexafungerp dosage.
Drug-herb. *St. John's wort:* May significantly reduce drug level. Discourage use together.

EFFECTS ON LAB TEST RESULTS
- May increase transaminase levels.

CONTRAINDICATIONS & CAUTIONS
- Contraindicated in patients hypersensitive to drug or its components.
- Safety in patients who are premenarchal hasn't been established.
Dialyzable drug: No.

PREGNANCY-LACTATION-REPRODUCTION
- Drug may cause fetal harm; contraindicated during pregnancy.
- If drug is given during pregnancy or if pregnancy is detected within 4 days after patient takes drug, report drug exposure to Scynexis, Inc. (1-888-982-SCYX [7299]).
- Patients of childbearing potential should use effective contraception during therapy and for 4 days after final dose.
- It isn't known if drug appears in human milk or how drug affects milk production

or infants who are breastfed. Weigh risk to infant.

NURSING CONSIDERATIONS
- Verify pregnancy status in patients of childbearing potential before start of therapy and before each dose during 6-month therapy.
- If specimens for fungal culture are obtained before therapy, may start antifungal therapy before culture results are known. Adjust therapy once culture result is known.

PATIENT TEACHING
- Teach about proper drug administration and handling.
- Instruct patient to report known or suspected pregnancy. Tell patient about pregnancy registry.
- Counsel patient of childbearing potential to use effective contraception during therapy and for 4 days after final dose.
- Advise patient to report taking other medications, which may interfere with drug.

SAFETY ALERT!

ibrutinib ⬚
eye-BROO-ti-nib

Imbruvica

Therapeutic class: Antineoplastics
Pharmacologic class: Kinase inhibitors

AVAILABLE FORMS
Capsules ⬚: 70 mg, 140 mg
Oral suspension: 70 mg/mL
Tablets ⬚: 140 mg, 280 mg, 420 mg

INDICATIONS & DOSAGES
Adjust-a-dose (for all indications): Refer to manufacturer's instructions for toxicity-related and drug interaction dosage adjustments.
➤ **Chronic lymphocytic leukemia (CLL) or small lymphocytic lymphoma (SLL); CLL or SLL with 17p deletion** ⬚
Adults: 420 mg PO once daily as single agent, in combination with rituximab or obinutuzumab, or in combination with bendamustine and rituximab until disease progression or unacceptable toxicity occurs.
Adjust-a-dose: For patient with Child-Pugh class A liver impairment, give 140 mg daily. For patient with Child-Pugh class B liver impairment, give 70 mg daily. Avoid use in

patients with Child-Pugh class C liver impairment.

➤ **Waldenström macroglobulinemia**

Adults: 420 mg PO once daily as single agent or in combination with rituximab until disease progression or unacceptable toxicity occurs.

Adjust-a-dose: For patient with Child-Pugh class A liver impairment, give 140 mg daily. For patient with Child-Pugh class B liver impairment, give 70 mg daily.

➤ **Chronic GVHD**

Adults and children ages 12 and older: 420 mg PO once daily until GVHD progresses, underlying malignancy recurs, unacceptable toxicity occurs, or patient no longer requires treatment.

Children age 1 to younger than age 12: 240 mg/m^2 PO once daily (up to 420 mg) until GVHD progresses, underlying malignancy recurs, unacceptable toxicity occurs, or patient no longer requires treatment.

Adjust-a-dose: For bilirubin level greater than 1.5 to 3 times ULN in patients ages 12 and older, give 140 mg daily. For those age 1 to younger than age 12, give 80 mg/m^2 daily. Don't adjust dosage for bilirubin elevations due to nonliver cause or Gilbert syndrome.

ADMINISTRATION
PO

🔆 *Alert:* Hazardous drug; use safe handling and disposal precautions.

• Give capsules and tablets with a glass of water at approximately same time each day.

• Have patient swallow tablets whole; don't crush or break tablets.

• For oral suspension, use only the two supplied dosing syringes. Shake suspension well before use and give as soon as possible after drawing into syringe. After use, remove plunger, rinse dosing syringe with water, and let air dry.

• Consider giving ibrutinib before rituximab or obinutuzumab, if applicable, when given on the same day.

• If dose is missed, administer as soon as missed dose is remembered on same day; return to normal scheduling the following day. Don't give extra dose to make up for missed dose.

• Store tablets and capsules at room temperature in original package.

• Store suspension at 36° to 77° F (2° to 25° C); don't freeze.

ACTION

Inhibits Bruton tyrosine kinase activity, resulting in decreased malignant B-cell proliferation and survival.

Route	Onset	Peak	Duration
PO	Unknown	1–2 hr	Unknown

Half-life: 4 to 6 hours.

ADVERSE REACTIONS

CNS: dizziness, headache, fatigue, fever, asthenia, insomnia, pain, anxiety, *ischemic cerebrovascular event.* **CV:** atrial fibrillation, atrial flutter, tachycardia, *ventricular tachyarrhythmias,* HTN, peripheral edema, *hemorrhage.* **EENT:** blurred vision, decreased visual acuity, dry eye, increased lacrimation, epistaxis, sinusitis, oropharyngeal pain. **GI:** diarrhea, nausea, constipation, abdominal pain, vomiting, stomatitis, dyspepsia, decreased appetite, GERD. **GU:** UTI, hematuria, increased creatinine level. **Hematologic:** *neutropenia, thrombocytopenia,* anemia. **Hepatic:** increased ALT, increased bilirubin level. **Metabolic:** dehydration, hyperuricemia, *hypokalemia,* hypoalbuminemia. **Musculoskeletal:** arthropathy, musculoskeletal pain, muscle spasms, arthralgia, weakness, osteonecrosis. **Respiratory:** URI, pneumonia, dyspnea, cough. **Skin:** skin infections, bruising, rash, petechiae, pruritus. **Other:** fall, chills, flulike symptoms, *secondary malignancies,* infection, *sepsis,* decreased immunoglobulin or antibody levels.

INTERACTIONS

Drug-drug. *Anticoagulants, antiplatelet agents, omega-3 fatty acids, vitamin E (systemic):* May increase risk of bleeding. Monitor bleeding risk and patient closely.

Digoxin: May increase digoxin level. Monitor drug level.

Moderate CYP3A inhibitors (amprenavir, aprepitant, atazanavir, ciprofloxacin, crizotinib, darunavir, diltiazem, erythromycin, fluconazole, fosamprenavir, imatinib, verapamil): May increase ibrutinib level. Avoid concurrent use. If ibrutinib must be used, refer to manufacturer's product information for dosage adjustments and monitor patient for toxicities.

Moderate CYP3A inducers (efavirenz): May decrease ibrutinib level. Monitor therapy.

Strong CYP3A inducers (carbamazepine, phenytoin, rifampin): May decrease ibrutinib level. Avoid concurrent use and consider agents with less CYP3A induction.

Strong CYP3A inhibitors (clarithromycin, ketoconazole, nefazodone, nelfinavir, ritonavir, saquinavir, voriconazole): May increase ibrutinib level. Avoid concurrent use or withhold ibrutinib for antibiotic or antifungal regimens lasting less than 7 days. Monitor patient closely for toxicities.

Drug-herb. *Flaxseed oil:* May enhance antiplatelet effect. Monitor therapy.

St. John's wort: May decrease ibrutinib level. Avoid use together.

Drug-food. *Grapefruit products, Seville oranges:* May increase ibrutinib level. Avoid use together.

EFFECTS ON LAB TEST RESULTS

• May increase uric acid, ALT, bilirubin, and creatinine levels.
• May increase lymphocyte count.
• May decrease Hb level and platelet and neutrophil counts.

CONTRAINDICATIONS & CAUTIONS

• Contraindicated in patients hypersensitive to drug or its components.
• Drug may increase risk of KF. Fatalities have been reported.
• Avoid use for B-cell malignancies in patients with Child-Pugh class C liver impairment.
• Avoid use for GVHD in patients with total bilirubin level greater than 3 times ULN, unless of nonliver origin or due to Gilbert syndrome.
• Drug may cause cardiac arrythmias and HF, including serious and fatal cases, particularly in patients with cardiac risk factors, HTN, acute infections, or history of arrythmias.
• Use cautiously in older adults because of increased risk of adverse effects.
Dialyzable drug: Unknown.

PREGNANCY-LACTATION-REPRODUCTION

• Drug may cause fetal harm; avoid use during pregnancy. Patient should avoid pregnancy for 1 month after therapy ends.
• Male patient with partner of child-bearing potential should use effective contraception during therapy and for 1 month after final dose.
• It isn't known if drug appears in human milk. Patient shouldn't breastfeed during therapy and for 1 week after final dose.

NURSING CONSIDERATIONS

• Verify pregnancy status before treatment.
• Monitor for signs and symptoms of hypersensitivity reactions and SJS.
• Fatal bleeding events have occurred. Monitor patient for bleeding and evaluate risk-benefit of use in patient receiving anticoagulant or antiplatelet drug.
• Consider interrupting therapy for 3 to 7 days before and after surgery, depending on procedure type and risk of bleeding.
• Monitor patient closely for fever and other signs of infection. Serious, sometimes fatal, infections have occurred.
• Monitor blood counts monthly and as indicated.
• Monitor for hyperuricemia and evaluate kidney function; maintain hydration.
• Evaluate patient for new malignancy during treatment.
• Monitor for HTN and start or adjust antihypertensives as clinically indicated.
• Assess ECG and evaluate patient for arrhythmias and HF at baseline and periodically during therapy. Obtain ECG for arrhythmic signs or symptoms (palpitations, lightheadedness, syncope, chest pain) or newonset dyspnea.
• Assess patient's baseline risk of TLS (high tumor burden) and take appropriate precautions. Monitor patient closely and treat appropriately.

PATIENT TEACHING

• Teach about proper drug administration and handling.
• Caution patient to immediately report signs and symptoms of significant hypersensitivity reaction (wheezing; chest tightness; fever; itching; heavy cough; blue-colored skin; seizures; swelling of face, lips, tongue, or throat).
• Instruct patient to contact prescriber if palpitations, light-headedness, syncope, chest pain, swelling of extremities, new-onset shortness of breath, diarrhea, nausea, vomiting, abdominal pain, fever, infection, bleeding, or easy bruising occurs.
• Caution patient to avoid becoming pregnant during therapy and for 1 month after therapy ends. Counsel patient to use effective birth control during treatment because drug may cause harm to fetus.

ibuprofen
eye-byoo-PROH-fen

Advil ◇, Caldolor, Motrin ◇

ibuprofen lysine
NeoProfen

Therapeutic class: Anti-inflammatory drugs
Pharmacologic class: NSAIDs

AVAILABLE FORMS
ibuprofen
Capsules: 200 mg ◇
Injection: 800 mg/8 mL (100 mg/mL) in single-dose vials; 800 mg/200 mL in single-dose IV bags
Oral drops: 40 mg/mL ◇
Oral suspension: 50 mg/1.25 mL ◇, 100 mg/5 mL ◇
Tablets: 100 mg ◇, 200 mg ◇, 400 mg, 600 mg, 800 mg
Tablets (chewable): 100 mg ◇
ibuprofen lysine
Injection: 10 mg/mL

INDICATIONS & DOSAGES
➤ **RA, osteoarthritis, arthritis**
Adults: 400 to 800 mg PO t.i.d. or q.i.d. Maximum daily dosage, 3.2 g.
➤ **Mild to moderate pain; moderate to severe pain as an adjunct to opioid analgesics; fever reduction in children**
Children ages 12 to 17: 400 mg IV every 4 to 6 hours PRN. Infuse over at least 10 minutes. Maximum daily dosage, 2,400 mg.
Children ages 6 months to younger than 12 years: 10 mg/kg IV up to maximum single dose of 400 mg every 4 to 6 hours PRN. Infuse over at least 10 minutes. Maximum daily dosage, 40 mg/kg or 2,400 mg, whichever is less.
Children ages 3 months to younger than 6 months: 10 mg/kg IV, up to maximum single dose of 100 mg. Infuse over at least 10 minutes.
➤ **Mild to moderate pain, fever**
Adults: 200 to 400 mg PO every 4 to 6 hours PRN. Or, for pain, 400 to 800 mg IV every 6 hours PRN; for fever, 400 mg IV, followed by 400 mg IV every 4 to 6 hours or 100 to 200 mg IV every 4 hours PRN. Infuse over at least 30 minutes. Maximum daily dosage, 3,200 mg. Use smallest effective dosage.

Children ages 12 and older: 200 to 400 mg PO every 4 to 6 hours. Maximum daily dosage, 1.2 g. Use smallest effective dosage.
Children age 11 weighing 32.7 to 43.2 kg: 300 mg chewable tablets or 15 mL (300 mg) oral suspension PO every 6 to 8 hours up to q.i.d.
Children ages 9 to 10 weighing 27.3 to 32.6 kg: 250 mg chewable tablets or 12.5 mL (250 mg) oral suspension PO every 6 to 8 hours up to q.i.d.
Children ages 6 to 8 weighing 21.8 to 27.2 kg: 200 mg chewable tablets or 10 mL (200 mg) oral suspension PO every 6 to 8 hours up to q.i.d.
Children ages 4 to 5 weighing 16.4 to 21.7 kg: 150 mg chewable tablets or 7.5 mL (150 mg) oral suspension PO every 6 to 8 hours up to q.i.d.
Children ages 2 to 3 weighing 10.9 to 16.3 kg: 100 mg chewable tablet or 100 mg (5 mL) oral suspension PO every 6 to 8 hours up to q.i.d.
Children ages 12 to 23 months weighing 8.2 to 10.8 kg: 75 mg (1.875 mL) oral drops PO every 6 to 8 hours up to q.i.d.
Children ages 6 to 11 months weighing 5.4 to 8.1 kg: 50 mg (1.25 mL) oral drops PO every 6 to 8 hours up to q.i.d.
Adjust-a-dose: For children ages 6 months to 11 years, use weight to determine dosage if possible; otherwise, use age. If needed, dose may be repeated every 6 to 8 hours but no more frequently than q.i.d. or maximum of 30 mg/kg in 24 hours. Consult health care provider before giving ibuprofen 100 mg chewable tablets to children younger than age 6 or those weighing less than 22 kg, 50 mg chewable tablets to children younger than age 4 or those weighing less than 16 kg, 50 mg oral suspension to children younger than age 2 or those weighing less than 11 kg, or 50 mg oral drops to infants younger than age 6 months or those weighing less than 5 kg. Ibuprofen oral drops should be dosed at 7.5 mg/kg of body weight.
➤ **Relief of signs and symptoms of juvenile arthritis**
Children: Recommended dosage is 30 to 40 mg/kg/day of oral suspension PO divided into three or four doses; patients with milder disease may be adequately treated with 20 mg/kg/day. Dosages above 50 mg/kg/day aren't recommended because they haven't been studied and may increase risk of serious adverse events. Lower to smallest dosage needed to maintain adequate symptom

control when clinical effect is obtained. Maximum single dose, 800 mg; maximum daily dosage, 2,400 mg/day.

➤ **Migraine**

Adults: 400 mg (2 capsules) PO at onset of symptoms. Maximum dosage, 400 mg in 24 hours, unless otherwise directed by health care provider.

➤ **Clinically significant patent ductus arteriosus (PDA) when usual medical management is ineffective (ibuprofen lysine)**

Premature infants weighing between 500 and 1,500 g who are no more than 32 weeks' gestational age: 10 mg/kg IV, then 5 mg/kg IV 24 hours later, then third dose of 5 mg/kg IV 24 hours after second dose. Base doses on birth weight.

Adjust-a-dose: If anuria or marked oliguria (urine output less than 0.6 mL/kg/hour) is evident at the scheduled time of the second or third dose, don't give additional dose until kidney function returns to normal. If ductus arteriosus closes or its size reduces significantly after first course of ibuprofen lysine, no further doses are necessary.

ADMINISTRATION

PO

• Give drug with milk or meals to decrease GI upset.

• Shake oral suspension and drops well before using. Give with calibrated oral syringe, dropper, or measuring cup.

• Store at room temperature.

IV

▼ Dilute drug with NSS, 5% dextrose, or lactated Ringer solution to 4 mg/mL or less. In adults, give over at least 30 minutes; in children, over at least 10 minutes.

▼ Dilute lysine with dextrose or NSS. Give through the port nearest the insertion site.

▼ For weight-based dosing at 10 mg/kg, ensure that drug concentration is 4 mg/mL or less.

▼ Diluted solutions are stable for 24 hours at room temperature, except lysine injection.

▼ Give ibuprofen lysine within 30 minutes of preparation and infuse over at least 15 minutes. Lysine injections don't contain preservatives.

▼ Correct dehydration before administering drug.

▼ Store at room temperature. Protect lysine injection vials from light.

▼ **Incompatibilities:** TPN solutions.

ACTION

May inhibit prostaglandin synthesis to produce anti-inflammatory, analgesic, and antipyretic effects.

Route	Onset	Peak	Duration
PO	Variable	1–2 hr	4–6 hr
IV	Unknown	10–12 min	Unknown

Half-life: 2 to 4 hours; half-life is more than 10 times longer in infants.

ADVERSE REACTIONS

CNS: dizziness, headache, nervousness. **CV:** edema, fluid retention, HTN, hypotension, *hemorrhage* (lysine). **EENT:** tinnitus. **GI:** abdominal pain, abdominal cramps, bloating, constipation, decreased appetite, diarrhea, dyspepsia, epigastric distress, flatulence, heartburn, nausea, vomiting. **GU:** *AKI,* azotemia, cystitis, hematuria, urine retention. **Hematologic:** *agranulocytosis, aplastic anemia, leukopenia, neutropenia, pancytopenia, thrombocytopenia,* anemia, prolonged bleeding time. **Metabolic:** *hyperkalemia, hypokalemia, hypoglycemia, hypocalcemia,* hypoproteinemia, hypernatremia, hypoalbuminemia. **Respiratory:** cough, pneumonia. **Skin:** pruritus, rash, injection-site irritation, *wound hemorrhage.* **Other:** *sepsis.*

INTERACTIONS

Drug-drug. *Anticoagulants (warfarin):* May increase risk of serious GI bleeding. Use with extreme caution if use together can't be avoided. Monitor patient closely.

Antihypertensives (ACE inhibitors, ARBs, beta blockers), furosemide, thiazide diuretics: May decrease effectiveness of diuretics or antihypertensives. Monitor patient closely.

Aspirin: May negate antiplatelet effect of low-dose aspirin therapy. Advise patient on appropriate spacing of doses.

Aspirin, corticosteroids: May cause adverse GI reactions. Avoid use together.

Bisphosphonates: May increase risk of gastric ulceration. Monitor patient for signs of gastric irritation or bleeding.

Cyclosporine: May increase kidney toxicity of both drugs. Avoid use together.

Digoxin, lithium: May increase levels or effects of these drugs. Monitor patient for toxicity.

Direct thrombin inhibitors (dabigatran, desirudin), factor Xa inhibitors (apixaban,

---

edoxaban, rivaroxaban): May increase risk of bleeding. Use together with caution.

Methotrexate: May decrease methotrexate clearance and increase toxicity. Use together cautiously.

Pemetrexed: May increase risk of pemetrexed myelosuppression and kidney and GI toxicity. Consider therapy modification or monitor patient closely if used together.

SSNRIs (desvenlafaxine, duloxetine, venlafaxine), SSRIs (fluoxetine, sertraline): May increase risk of upper GI bleeding. If use together can't be avoided, closely watch for signs of GI bleeding. Consider acid suppression therapy.

Triamterene: May increase risk of AKI. Avoid use together; if unavoidable, closely monitor kidney function.

Drug-herb. *Dong quai, feverfew, garlic, ginger, ginkgo biloba, horse chestnut, red clover:* May increase risk of bleeding, based on the known effects of components. Discourage use together.

White willow: Herb and drug contain similar components. Discourage use together.

Drug-lifestyle. *Alcohol use:* May cause adverse GI reactions. Discourage use together.

Sun exposure: May cause photosensitivity reactions. Advise patient to avoid excessive sunlight exposure.

EFFECTS ON LAB TEST RESULTS

• May increase BUN, creatinine, ALT, AST, and LDH levels.

• May decrease glucose, calcium, protein, and albumin levels.

• May increase or decrease potassium level.

• May decrease Hb level, hematocrit, and neutrophil, WBC, RBC, platelet, and granulocyte counts.

CONTRAINDICATIONS & CAUTIONS

• Contraindicated in patients hypersensitive to drug and in those with history of asthma, urticaria, or other allergic-type reactions to aspirin or other NSAIDs.

Boxed Warning Contraindicated for the treatment of perioperative pain after CABG surgery. ■

Boxed Warning NSAIDs can increase risk of MI or stroke in patients with or without heart disease or risk factors for heart disease. Risk of MI or stroke can occur as early as the first weeks of using an NSAID. Risk appears greater at higher doses. Use lowest effective dose for shortest duration possible. ■

Boxed Warning NSAIDs may increase risk of serious GI adverse events, including bleeding, ulceration, and perforation of the stomach or intestines, which can be fatal. These events can occur at any time during use, without warning symptoms. Older adults are at greater risk for serious GI events. ■

• Ibuprofen lysine injection is contraindicated in preterm infants with significant kidney impairment, proven or suspected untreated infection or necrotizing enterocolitis, thrombocytopenia, coagulation defects, active bleeding, and congenital heart disease in whom patency of the ductus arteriosus is needed for satisfactory pulmonary or systemic blood flow.

🕒 *Alert:* NSAIDs increase risk of HF.

• Use cautiously in older adults and patients with GI disorders, history of peptic ulcer disease, liver or kidney disease, cardiac decompensation, HTN, asthma, or intrinsic coagulation defects.

• Long-term NSAID use may result in kidney papillary necrosis and other kidney injury.

• May increase risk of aseptic meningitis, with fever and coma, particularly in patients with SLE and related connective tissue disease. If signs or symptoms of meningitis occur, consider whether they're related to ibuprofen therapy.

Dialyzable drug: Unknown.

⚠ *Overdose S&S:* Abdominal pain, nausea, vomiting, lethargy, drowsiness, headache, tinnitus, nystagmus, CNS depression, seizures, hypotension, bradycardia, tachycardia, atrial fibrillation, metabolic acidosis, coma, AKI, hyperkalemia, respiratory depression and failure.

PREGNANCY-LACTATION-REPRODUCTION

• Studies during pregnancy are inadequate. Drug can cause fetal harm.

🕒 *Alert:* Use of NSAIDs at 20 weeks or later in pregnancy may cause fetal kidney dysfunction, leading to oligohydramnios and potential neonatal kidney impairment; use at 30 weeks or later in pregnancy may increase risk of premature closure of ductus arteriosus. Avoid use during pregnancy starting at 20 weeks' gestation. If potential benefit justifies fetal risk, use lowest effective dose for shortest duration. Consider ultrasound monitoring of amniotic fluid if NSAID therapy is longer than 48 hours. It's acceptable to use aspirin 81 mg for certain pregnancy-related conditions under the direction of a prescriber.

• Drug appears in human milk. Use cautiously during breastfeeding as directed by prescriber.

• Drug may cause reversible infertility in females.

NURSING CONSIDERATIONS

• Periodically check kidney and liver function in patient on long-term therapy. Stop drug and notify prescriber if abnormalities occur.

• Monitor BP because drug can lead to new-onset HTN or worsening of preexisting HTN, which may contribute to increased incidence of CV events.

• Because of their antipyretic and anti-inflammatory actions, NSAIDs may mask signs and symptoms of infection.

• Blurred or diminished vision and changes in color vision may occur.

• Full anti-inflammatory effects may take 1 or 2 weeks to develop.

🜂 *Alert:* Watch for and immediately evaluate signs and symptoms of MI (chest pain, shortness of breath or trouble breathing) or stroke (weakness in one part or side of the body, slurred speech).

• Monitor for signs or symptoms of aseptic meningitis (fever, headache, sensitivity to light, vomiting), and immediately report if they occur.

• Monitor for rash, fever, lymphadenopathy, and facial swelling. DRESS syndrome has been reported in patients taking NSAIDs. If signs and symptoms of DRESS syndrome occur, immediately discontinue drug and evaluate patient.

PATIENT TEACHING

• Tell patient to take drug with meals or milk to reduce adverse GI reactions.

🜂 *Alert:* Drug is available OTC. Instruct patient not to exceed 3.2 g daily for adults and children ages 12 and older or 30 mg/kg for children ages 6 months to 11 years, not to give to children younger than age 6 months, and not to take for extended periods (longer than 3 days for fever or longer than 10 days for pain) without consulting prescriber.

🜂 *Alert:* Warn patient who is pregnant not to take NSAIDs at 20 weeks' gestation or later unless instructed to do so by prescriber due to fetal risk. Advise patient to discuss taking any OTC medication with a pharmacist or health care provider during pregnancy.

• Tell patient that full therapeutic effect for arthritis may be delayed for 2 to 4 weeks. Although pain relief occurs at low dosage levels, inflammation doesn't improve at dosages less than 400 mg q.i.d.

• Caution patient that use with aspirin, anticoagulants, alcohol, or corticosteroids may increase risk of GI adverse reactions.

• Teach patient to watch for and immediately report to prescriber signs and symptoms of GI bleeding, including blood in vomit, urine, or stool; coffee-ground vomit; and melena.

🜂 *Alert:* Advise patient to immediately seek medical attention if chest pain, shortness of breath, trouble breathing, weakness in one part or side of the body, or slurred speech occurs.

• Tell patient to contact prescriber before using this drug if fluid intake hasn't been adequate or if fluids have been lost as a result of vomiting or diarrhea.

• Warn patient to avoid hazardous activities that require mental alertness until effects of drug on CNS are known.

• Tell patient taking drug not to take other OTC NSAIDs, such as naproxen, as these drugs are in the same class.

• Advise patient to wear sunscreen to avoid hypersensitivity to sunlight.

• Inform patient that oral liquid products are available in two concentrations. Instruct patient to read package carefully.

SAFETY ALERT!

ibutilide fumarate
i-BYOO-ti-lide

Corvert

Therapeutic class: Antiarrhythmics
Pharmacologic class: Methanesulfonanilide derivatives

AVAILABLE FORMS
Injection: 1 mg/10 mL vials

INDICATIONS & DOSAGES

➤ **Rapid conversion of recent-onset atrial fibrillation or atrial flutter to sinus rhythm**
Adults weighing 60 kg or more: 1 mg IV infusion over 10 minutes. May repeat dose if arrhythmia doesn't respond within 10 minutes after completing first dose.
Adults weighing less than 60 kg: 0.01 mg/kg IV infusion over 10 minutes. May repeat dose

if arrhythmia doesn't respond within 10 minutes after completing first dose.

ADMINISTRATION

IV

▼ Give drug undiluted or diluted in 50 mL of NSS or D_5W injection before infusion. Add contents of 10-mL vial (0.1 mg/mL) to 50-mL infusion bag to form admixture of about 0.017 mg ibutilide/mL. Drug is compatible with polyvinyl chloride plastic bags or polyolefin bags.

▼ Give drug over 10 minutes.

▼ Stop infusion if arrhythmia terminates or patient develops ventricular tachycardia or marked prolongation of QT or QTc interval.

▼ Don't infuse parenteral products that contain particulate matter or are discolored.

▼ **Incompatibilities:** None listed by manufacturer. Consult drug compatibility reference for more information.

ACTION

Prolongs action potential in isolated cardiac myocytes and increases atrial and ventricular refractoriness, namely class III electrophysiologic effects.

Route	Onset	Peak	Duration
IV	≤90 min	Unknown	Unknown

Half-life: Averages about 6 hours.

ADVERSE REACTIONS

CNS: headache. **CV:** *sustained polymorphic ventricular tachycardia, AV block, bradycardia, HF,* ventricular extrasystoles, *nonsustained ventricular tachycardia,* hypotension, bundle-branch block, HTN, *prolonged QT interval,* palpitations, tachycardia. **GI:** nausea.

INTERACTIONS

Drug-drug. *Class IA antiarrhythmics (disopyramide, procainamide, quinidine), other class III antiarrhythmics (amiodarone, sotalol):* May increase potential for prolonged refractoriness. Don't give these drugs for at least five half-lives before and 4 hours after ibutilide dose.

Digoxin: Supraventricular arrhythmias may mask cardiotoxicity from excessive digoxin level. Use with caution in patients who may have an increased digoxin therapeutic range.

H_1-receptor antagonists, phenothiazines, TCAs, tetracyclic antidepressants, other drugs that prolong QT interval: May increase risk of proarrhythmia. Monitor patient closely.

EFFECTS ON LAB TEST RESULTS

None reported.

CONTRAINDICATIONS & CAUTIONS

Boxed Warning Administer drug only when the benefits of maintaining sinus rhythm outweigh the immediate risks of ibutilide administration and the risks of maintenance therapy. ■

• Contraindicated in patients hypersensitive to drug or its components.

• Use isn't recommended in patients with history of polymorphic ventricular tachycardia.

• Use cautiously in patients with HF, decreased left ventricular ejection fraction, or liver or kidney dysfunction.

• Drug's effectiveness hasn't been determined in patients with arrhythmias of more than 90 days' duration.

• Safety and effectiveness of drug haven't been established in children.

Dialyzable drug: Unknown.

⚠ *Overdose S&S:* Ventricular ectopy, ventricular tachycardia, third-degree AV block.

PREGNANCY-LACTATION-REPRODUCTION

• Drug causes fetal harm in animals. Use during pregnancy only if clearly needed and potential benefit justifies fetal risk.

• It isn't known if drug appears in human milk. Use isn't recommended during breastfeeding.

NURSING CONSIDERATIONS

Boxed Warning Drug can cause potentially fatal arrhythmias. Only skilled personnel trained in identification and treatment of acute ventricular arrhythmias, particularly polymorphic ventricular tachycardia, should give drug. ■

• Before therapy, correct hypokalemia and hypomagnesemia to reduce arrhythmia risk.

Boxed Warning Patients with atrial fibrillation lasting longer than 2 to 3 days must be adequately anticoagulated, generally over at least 2 weeks. ■

• Monitor ECG continuously during administration and for at least 4 hours afterward or until QTc interval returns to baseline; drug can induce or worsen ventricular arrhythmias. Longer monitoring is required if ECG shows arrhythmia or patient has liver insufficiency.

Reactions in bold italics are *life-threatening*.

PATIENT TEACHING
• Tell patient to promptly report adverse reactions.
• Instruct patient to alert nurse of discomfort at injection site.

idaruCIZUmab ✂
eye-da-roo-SIZ-uh-mab

Praxbind

Therapeutic class: Antidotes
Pharmacologic class: Humanized monoclonal antibody fragments

AVAILABLE FORMS
Injection: 2.5 g/50 mL in single-use vials

INDICATIONS & DOSAGES
➤ **To reverse anticoagulant effects of dabigatran etexilate mesylate (Pradaxa) for emergency surgery or urgent procedures; for life-threatening or uncontrolled bleeding**
Adults: 5 g (two 2.5-g vials) as two consecutive IV infusions by hanging the vials or as two bolus injections, injecting contents of both vials consecutively, one after the other, using syringes.

ADMINISTRATION
IV
▼ Inspect both vials for discoloration and particulate matter before administration. Solution is colorless to slightly yellow and clear to slightly opalescent.
▼ Don't shake vial.
▼ Give drug promptly once removed from vial.
▼ Administer dose undiluted as either an IV bolus via syringe or an infusion by hanging the vials.
▼ Each infusion should take no longer than 5 to 10 minutes.
▼ Administer second vial or infusion within 15 minutes from end of first vial or infusion.
▼ A preexisting IV line may be used for administration, but line must be flushed with NSS before infusion.
▼ Don't administer other infusions at the same time using the same IV access.
▼ Store vials in refrigerator at 36° to 46° F (2° to 8° C). Don't freeze or shake.
▼ Before use, unopened vial may be kept at room temperature for up to 48 hours if stored in original package to protect from light or up to 6 hours when exposed to light.
▼ **Incompatibilities:** Other IV drugs and infusions.

ACTION
A humanized monoclonal antibody fragment that binds specifically to dabigatran and its acyl glucuronide metabolites with higher affinity than binding affinity of dabigatran to thrombin, neutralizing dabigatran's anticoagulant effects within minutes.

Route	Onset	Peak	Duration
IV	Rapid	Unknown	24 hr

Half-life: 10.3 hours.

ADVERSE REACTIONS
CNS: headache. **GI:** constipation, nausea.

INTERACTIONS
None reported.

EFFECTS ON LAB TEST RESULTS
• May prolong PTT and ecarin clotting time.

CONTRAINDICATIONS & CAUTIONS
• Hypersensitivity and anaphylactoid reactions (fever, bronchospasm, hyperventilation, rash, pruritus) may occur.
• Reversing dabigatran therapy exposes patients to the thrombotic risk of their underlying disease. To reduce this risk, consider resumption of anticoagulant therapy as soon as medically appropriate. Dabigatran therapy can be started 24 hours after idarucizumab administration.
✂ Drug contains sorbitol. Use cautiously in patients with hereditary fructose intolerance, as serious and even fatal reactions, including hypoglycemia, hypophosphatemia, metabolic acidosis, increased uric acid level, and acute liver failure, have been reported. The minimum amount of sorbitol that causes serious adverse reactions isn't known.
• Drug hasn't been studied in patients with liver impairment.
• Safety and effectiveness in children haven't been established.
Dialyzable drug: Unknown.

PREGNANCY-LACTATION-REPRODUCTION
• Studies during pregnancy are inadequate. It isn't known if drug can cause fetal harm

or affect reproductive capacity. Use during pregnancy only if clearly needed.

• It isn't known if drug appears in human milk. Use cautiously during breastfeeding.

NURSING CONSIDERATIONS

• For patient with elevated coagulation parameters and reappearance of clinically relevant bleeding or patient who requires a second emergency surgery or urgent procedure, an additional 5 g of drug may be considered. Safety and effectiveness of repeat treatment haven't been established.

⌧ Assess patient for history of hereditary fructose intolerance before giving drug.

• Monitor for hypersensitivity reactions. Discontinue drug if serious hypersensitivity reaction occurs.

• Monitor for signs and symptoms of thrombotic events, including DVT, stroke, and MI. Resume anticoagulant therapy as soon as possible.

PATIENT TEACHING

• Warn patient to immediately report signs and symptoms of hypersensitivity and anaphylactoid reactions (fever, dyspnea, bronchospasm, rash, itching). Explain that drug will need to be discontinued.

• Instruct patient to seek immediate medical attention for signs or symptoms of bleeding.

• Warn patient that reversing dabigatran therapy exposes patient to the thromboembolic risk of the underlying disease. Advise patient that anticoagulant therapy may resume as soon as possible to reduce this risk.

⌧ Teach patient with hereditary fructose intolerance to report this condition before receiving drug because drug contains sorbitol and may cause serious and even fatal reactions.

iloperidone ⌧
eye-loe-PER-ih-done

Fanapt

Therapeutic class: Antipsychotics
Pharmacologic class: Dopamine–serotonin antagonists

AVAILABLE FORMS

Tablets: 1 mg, 2 mg, 4 mg, 6 mg, 8 mg, 10 mg, 12 mg

INDICATIONS & DOSAGES

➤ Schizophrenia

Adults: Initially, 1 mg PO b.i.d. Increase dosage daily as needed according to the following dosing schedule: 2 mg PO b.i.d. on day 2; 4 mg PO b.i.d. on day 3; 6 mg PO b.i.d. on day 4; 8 mg PO b.i.d. on day 5; 10 mg PO b.i.d. on day 6; 12 mg PO b.i.d. on day 7. Maximum dosage, 12 mg PO b.i.d.

Adjust-a-dose: For patients who are poor metabolizers of CYP2D6 and those taking CYP2D6 inhibitors or CYP3A4 inhibitors, reduce dosage by 50%. Patients with Child-Pugh class C liver impairment may need dosage reduction if clinically indicated. ⌧

ADMINISTRATION
PO

• Give drug without regard to food.

• When restarting drug after dosing interruption of more than 3 days, follow initial titration schedule.

ACTION

Actual mechanism unknown. May antagonize dopamine type 2 (D$_2$) and serotonin type 2 (5-HT$_2$) receptors.

Route	Onset	Peak	Duration
PO	Unknown	2–4 hr	Unknown

Half-life: 18 to 37 hours.

ADVERSE REACTIONS

CNS: aggression, delusions, dizziness, extrapyramidal effects, fatigue, lethargy, restlessness, somnolence, tremor. **CV:** hypotension, orthostatic hypotension, palpitations, tachycardia. **EENT:** blurred vision, conjunctivitis, dry mouth, nasal congestion, nasopharyngitis. **GI:** abdominal discomfort, diarrhea, nausea. **GU:** ejaculation failure, erectile dysfunction, urinary incontinence. **Hematologic:** hyperprolactinemia. **Metabolic:** weight gain. **Musculoskeletal:** arthralgia, muscle spasm, musculoskeletal stiffness, myalgia. **Respiratory:** dyspnea, URI. **Skin:** rash.

INTERACTIONS

Drug-drug. *Antihypertensives:* May enhance antihypertensive effects. Use together cautiously.
CNS depressants (barbiturates, droperidol, opioids): May increase depressant effect. Avoid use together. If use together is necessary,

limit dosage and duration of each drug to minimum necessary for desired effect.
CYP3A4 or CYP2D6 inhibitors (clarithromycin, fluoxetine, ketoconazole, paroxetine, quinidine): May increase iloperidone level. Reduce dosage by half.
Drugs that prolong QT interval (amiodarone, methadone, moxifloxacin, procainamide, quinidine, sotalol, thioridazine): May cause lethal arrhythmias. Avoid together.
Drug-lifestyle. *Alcohol use:* May increase CNS effects. Discourage use together.

EFFECTS ON LAB TEST RESULTS
• May increase lipid and glucose levels.
• May decrease WBC count, Hb level, and hematocrit.
• May increase neutrophil count.

CONTRAINDICATIONS & CAUTIONS
• Contraindicated in patients hypersensitive to drug or its components; anaphylaxis, angioedema, and other hypersensitivity reactions have been reported.
Boxed Warning Fatal CV events may occur in older adults with dementia. Drug isn't approved for use in patients with dementia-related psychosis. ■
• Avoid use in patients with history of cardiac arrhythmias, QT-interval prolongation, recent acute MI, or uncompensated HF. Discontinue drug for persistent QTc measurement greater than 500 milliseconds.
• Use cautiously in patients with history of stroke, TIA, diabetes, seizures, orthostatic hypotension, NMS, tardive dyskinesia, leukopenia, neutropenia, agranulocytosis, suicidality, or priapism.
• Use cautiously in patients at risk for falls, including those who have diseases or conditions or are taking drugs that may cause somnolence, orthostatic hypotension, or motor or sensory instability.
• Use cautiously in patients with Child-Pugh class B liver impairment; these patients may require dosage reduction. Use in patients with Child-Pugh class C liver impairment isn't recommended.
• Atypical antipsychotics have been associated with metabolic changes, including hyperglycemia, dyslipidemia, and weight gain, that may increase CV and cerebrovascular risk.
Dialyzable drug: Unknown.

⚠ Overdose S&S: Prolonged QT interval, drowsiness, extrapyramidal symptoms, sedation, tachycardia, hypotension.

PREGNANCY-LACTATION-REPRODUCTION
• Studies during pregnancy are inadequate. Use during pregnancy only if potential benefit justifies fetal risk.
• Encourage enrollment in National Pregnancy Registry for Atypical Antipsychotics (1-866-961-2388 or https://womensmentalhealth.org/research/pregnancyregistry/atypicalantipsychotic/).
Alert: Neonates exposed to antipsychotics during the third trimester are at risk for developing extrapyramidal symptoms (repetitive muscle movements of face and body) and withdrawal symptoms (agitation, abnormally increased or decreased muscle tone, tremors, sleepiness, severe difficulty breathing, difficulty feeding) after delivery.
• It isn't known if drug appears in human milk. Use during breastfeeding isn't recommended.

NURSING CONSIDERATIONS
• Symptom control may be delayed during the first 1 to 2 weeks of treatment compared to other antipsychotics that don't require similar titration.
Alert: Obtain baseline BP measurements before starting therapy and monitor BP regularly. Watch for orthostatic hypotension, especially during first dosage adjustments.
Alert: Watch for evidence of NMS (hyperthermia, muscle rigidity, altered mental status, autonomic instability), which is rare but can be fatal.
Alert: Life-threatening hyperglycemia may occur in patient taking atypical antipsychotics. Regularly monitor patient with diabetes. Monitor fasting blood glucose level at drug initiation and periodically during therapy in patient with risk factors for diabetes.
• Monitor patient for tardive dyskinesia, which may occur with prolonged use of drug. If tardive dyskinesia occurs, discontinue drug unless patient's condition warrants continued use.
• Monitor patient for suicidality.
• Complete fall risk assessments when initiating drug and recurrently for patient on long-term therapy, especially for patient who has disease or condition that increases fall risk or is taking other drugs that could increase fall risk.

- Dispense lowest appropriate quantity of drug to reduce risk of overdose.
- Monitor patient for weight gain.
- Periodically reassess patient to determine continued need for therapy.
- Frequently monitor CBC during first few months of therapy and discontinue drug if WBC count drops with no other underlying cause.
- Monitor potassium and magnesium levels at baseline and periodically in patient at risk for electrolyte imbalances.
- Drug may lower seizure threshold in patient with history of seizures; monitor patient closely.

PATIENT TEACHING

- Teach about proper drug administration and handling.
- Warn patient to avoid driving and other hazardous activities that require mental alertness until drug effects are known.
- Caution patient to rise slowly, avoid hot showers, and use other precautions to avoid fainting and to reduce risk of falls.
- Advise patient to avoid becoming overheated or dehydrated.
- Tell patient to notify prescriber about planned, suspected, or known pregnancy.
- Advise patient not to breastfeed during therapy.
- Instruct patient to report dizziness, palpitations, or fainting to prescriber.
- Advise patient to avoid alcohol use while taking drug.
- Tell patient to seek emergency medical care if an erection lasts more than 4 hours.
- Warn patient and caregiver about risk of NMS; advise them to seek emergency medical care if symptoms occur.
- Tell patient to notify prescriber about other prescription or OTC drugs that patient is taking or plans to take.

iloprost
EYE-loe-prost

Ventavis

Therapeutic class: Pulmonary vasodilators
Pharmacologic class: Prostacyclin analogues

AVAILABLE FORMS
Inhalation solution: 10 mcg/mL, 20 mcg/mL in single-dose ampules

INDICATIONS & DOSAGES
➤ **PAH in patients with NYHA Class III or IV symptoms**
Adults: Initially, 2.5 mcg inhaled using I-neb Adaptive Aerosol Delivery (AAD) device. As tolerated, increase to 5 mcg inhaled six to nine times daily while patient is awake, as needed, but no more than every 2 hours. Maximum dosage, 5 mcg nine times daily.

ADMINISTRATION
Inhalational
- Use only I-neb AAD delivery device, per manufacturer's instructions.
- Don't mix with other medications.
- The 20-mcg/mL concentration is intended for patients receiving the 5-mcg dose who have extended treatment times.
- Discard unused medication.
- Keep drug away from skin and eyes.

ACTION
Lowers pulmonary arterial pressure by dilating systemic and pulmonary arterial vascular beds. Drug also affects platelet aggregation, although effect in PAH treatment isn't known.

Route	Onset	Peak	Duration
Inhalation	Unknown	Within 5 min	30–60 min

Half-life: 20 to 30 minutes.

ADVERSE REACTIONS
CNS: headache, insomnia, syncope. **CV:** hypotension, vasodilation, chest pain, *HF, supraventricular tachycardia,* palpitations, peripheral edema. **EENT:** inability to open jaw (trismus). **GI:** nausea, tongue pain, vomiting. **GU:** *KF.* **Hepatic:** increased ALP and GGT levels. **Musculoskeletal:** back pain, muscle cramps. **Respiratory:** cough, dyspnea, hemoptysis, pneumonia. **Other:** flulike syndrome.

INTERACTIONS
Drug-drug. *Anticoagulants, antiplatelet drugs:* May increase risk of bleeding. Monitor patient closely.
Antihypertensives, vasodilators: May increase hypotensive effects of these drugs. Monitor BP.

EFFECTS ON LAB TEST RESULTS
- May increase ALP and GGT levels.

CONTRAINDICATIONS & CAUTIONS

• No known contraindications. Avoid use in patients whose systolic BP is less than 85 mm Hg.

• Use cautiously in older adults, patients with liver or kidney impairment, and patients with COPD, severe asthma, acute pulmonary infection, or bleeding disorders.

• Safety and effectiveness in children haven't been established.

• PAH may worsen if drug is withdrawn abruptly or dosages are reduced.

Dialyzable drug: Unknown.

⚠ *Overdose S&S:* Diarrhea, dizziness, flushing, headache, hypotension, nausea, vomiting, jaw pain, back pain.

PREGNANCY-LACTATION-REPRODUCTION

• Studies during pregnancy are inadequate. Use during pregnancy only if potential benefit justifies fetal risk.

• It isn't known if drug appears in human milk. Patient should discontinue breastfeeding or discontinue drug, considering importance of drug to patient.

NURSING CONSIDERATIONS

• Monitor patient's vital signs carefully at start of treatment. Monitor for syncope.

• If patient develops evidence of pulmonary edema, immediately stop treatment.

PATIENT TEACHING

• Warn patient not to drink drug. Explain that drug is for inhalation only.

• Caution patient to take drug exactly as prescribed.

• Advise patient to keep a backup I-neb AAD device in case original malfunctions.

• Tell patient to keep drug away from skin and eyes and to immediately rinse the area if contact occurs.

• Inform patient that drug may cause dizziness and fainting. Urge patient to stand up slowly from sitting or lying position and to report to prescriber worsening of symptoms.

• Tell patient to take drug before physical exertion, no more than every 2 hours.

• Advise patient to adjust administration times to cover planned activities because drug benefits may not last 2 hours.

• Tell patient not to expose others, especially those who are pregnant and infants, to drug.

• Teach patient how to clean equipment and safely dispose of used ampules after each

treatment. Caution patient not to save or use leftover solution.

SAFETY ALERT!

imatinib mesylate ✄
eye-MAT-eh-nib

Gleevec

Therapeutic class: Antineoplastics
Pharmacologic class: Kinase inhibitors

AVAILABLE FORMS

Tablets ⬤ : 100 mg, 400 mg

INDICATIONS & DOSAGES

Adjust-a-dose (for all indications): For patients with CrCl of 40 to 59 mL/minute, don't exceed 600 mg daily; if CrCl is 20 to 39 mL/minute, decrease starting dose by 50% and don't exceed 400 mg daily; if CrCl is less than 20 mL/minute, don't exceed 100 mg daily. For patients with Child-Pugh class C liver impairment, reduce dosage by 25%. If use with a strong CYP3A4 inducer can't be avoided, increase imatinib dosage by at least 50% and closely monitor clinical response. See manufacturer's package insert for full details on dosage adjustments for children; patients with neutropenia, thrombocytopenia, or liver toxicity; and those with adverse reactions. Continue treatment until disease progression or unacceptable toxicity occurs.

➤ **Relapsed or refractory Philadelphia chromosome-positive (Ph+) acute lymphoblastic leukemia (ALL)** ✄
Adults: 600 mg PO daily.

➤ **Newly diagnosed Ph+ ALL in children, in combination with chemotherapy** ✄
Children ages 1 and older: 340 mg/m² PO daily. Maximum dosage, 600 mg daily.

➤ **Aggressive systemic mastocytosis (ASM) without the D816V c-*Kit* mutation or with c-*Kit* mutational status unknown** ✄
Adults: 400 mg PO daily.

Adjust-a-dose: For patients with ASM associated with eosinophilia, a clonal hematologic disease related to the fusion kinase FIP1L1-PDGFRα, initial dose is 100 mg/day. Increase dosage from 100 mg to 400 mg/day if no adverse drug reactions occur and if response to therapy is insufficient.

♣ Canada   ◇ OTC   ◆ Off-label use   ⬤ Do not crush   *Liquid contains alcohol   ✄ Genetic

> ➤ **Hypereosinophilic syndrome (HES), chronic eosinophilic leukemia (CEL), or both** ⚕

Adults: 400 mg PO daily.

Adjust-a-dose: In patients with HES or CEL and demonstrated FIP1L1-PDGFRα fusion kinase, initial dose is 100 mg/day. Increase dosage from 100 mg to 400 mg/day if response is insufficient and no adverse drug reactions occur.

> ➤ **Myelodysplastic syndrome (MDS) or myeloproliferative disease (MPD) with *PDGFR* gene rearrangements** ⚕

Adults: 400 mg PO daily.

> ➤ **Unresectable, recurrent, or metastatic dermatofibrosarcoma protuberans** ⚕

Adults: 400 mg PO b.i.d. (800 mg/day).

> ➤ **Chronic myeloid leukemia (CML) in blast crisis, in accelerated phase, or in chronic phase after failure of alfa interferon therapy; newly diagnosed Ph+ chronic-phase CML** ⚕

Adults: For chronic-phase CML, 400 mg PO daily as single dose. For accelerated-phase CML or blast crisis, 600 mg PO daily as single dose. Continue treatment if patient continues to benefit. May increase daily dosage to 600 mg PO in chronic phase or to 800 mg PO (400 mg PO b.i.d.) in accelerated phase or blast crisis.

Children ages 1 and older: For newly diagnosed Ph+ chronic-phase CML only, give 340 mg/m^2 daily PO. May be given once daily or b.i.d. Don't exceed 600 mg/day.

> ➤ **Kit (CD117)-positive or GI stromal tumors (GISTs) after resection** ⚕

Adults: 400 mg PO daily.

> ➤ **Kit-positive unresectable or metastatic malignant GISTs** ⚕

Adults: 400 mg PO daily. May consider a dosage increase up to 800 mg daily (given as 400 mg b.i.d.), as clinically indicated, in patients with clear signs or symptoms of disease progression at a lower dosage and in absence of severe adverse drug reactions.

ADMINISTRATION
PO
• Give with a meal and large glass of water.
• Administer 400-mg or 600-mg dose once daily. Give 800-mg dose as 400 mg b.i.d.
• For daily dosing of 800 mg and above, use the 400-mg tablet to reduce exposure to iron.
• For patients unable to swallow tablets, disperse tablets in water or apple juice (50 mL

for 100-mg tablet and 200 mL for 400-mg tablet). Stir and have patient drink immediately.

🔵 **Alert:** Hazardous drug; use safe handling and disposal precautions.
• If dose is missed, give next scheduled dose at its regular time.
• Store at room temperature.
• Protect drug from moisture.

ACTION
Inhibits the abnormal tyrosine kinase created by the Philadelphia chromosome abnormality in CML; inhibits tumor growth of murine myeloid cells and leukemia lines from patients with CML in blast crisis; also inhibits other kinases for growth and stem cell factors and may inhibit proliferation and induce apoptosis in GIST cells.

Route	Onset	Peak	Duration
PO	Unknown	2–4 hr	Unknown

Half-life: Adults, 18 hours (parent drug), 40 hours (active metabolite); children, 15 hours (parent drug).

ADVERSE REACTIONS
CNS: *cerebral hemorrhage,* fatigue, headache, fever, asthenia, weakness, depression, dizziness, insomnia, anxiety, paresthesia, rigors, peripheral neuropathy, taste alteration. **CV:** *hemorrhage,* edema, fluid retention, HTN, chest pain, flushing, palpitations, pericardial effusion. **EENT:** periorbital edema, increased lacrimation, blurred vision, nasopharyngitis, sinusitis, rhinitis, conjunctivitis, epistaxis, pharyngolaryngeal pain, oropharyngeal pain, dry mouth. **GI:** *GI hemorrhage,* abdominal pain, anorexia, constipation, diarrhea, dyspepsia, nausea, vomiting, gastroenteritis, flatulence, stomatitis, GERD. **Hematologic:** *neutropenia, thrombocytopenia,* anemia, *lymphopenia, pancytopenia,* eosinophilia. **Hepatic:** increased LFT results, *liver toxicity.* **Metabolic:** *hypokalemia; hyperkalemia;* weight increase or decrease; hypoproteinemia; increased CK, lipase, and amylase levels. **Musculoskeletal:** arthralgia, myalgia, muscle cramps, growth suppression in children, musculoskeletal pain, bone pain, limb pain, back pain. **Respiratory:** cough, dyspnea, pneumonia, URI, pleural effusion. **Skin:** petechiae, rash, pruritus, alopecia, dry skin, diaphoresis, exfoliative rash, dermatitis, photosensitivity reaction. **Other:** night sweats, flulike symptoms, infection.

Reactions in bold italics are *life-threatening*.

INTERACTIONS

Drug-drug. *CYP3A4 substrates (alprazolam, certain HMG-CoA reductase inhibitors [simvastatin], cyclosporine, dihydropyridine–calcium channel blockers, pimozide, triazolam):* May increase levels of these drugs. Monitor patient for toxicity, and obtain drug levels, if appropriate.

CYP2D6 substrates with narrow therapeutic window (clonidine, nortriptyline, sotalol): May increase substrate level. Use together cautiously.

CYP3A4 inducers (carbamazepine, dexamethasone, phenobarbital, phenytoin, rifampin): May decrease imatinib level. Avoid concurrent use when possible. If combination must be used, increase imatinib dosage by at least 50%; monitor patient closely.

CYP3A4 inhibitors (clarithromycin, erythromycin, itraconazole, ketoconazole): May decrease metabolism and increase imatinib level. Monitor patient for toxicity.

Levothyroxine: May increase levothyroxine clearance, causing increased TSH levels and symptoms of hypothyroidism. Monitor thyroid function.

Warfarin: May alter metabolism of warfarin. Avoid use together; use standard heparin or a low-molecular-weight heparin.

Drug-herb. *Ginseng:* May increase risk of liver toxicity. Avoid use together.

St. John's wort: May decrease drug effects. Discourage use together.

Drug-food. *Grapefruit juice:* May increase imatinib level. Discourage use together.

EFFECTS ON LAB TEST RESULTS

• May increase CK, amylase, lipase, glucose, protein, creatinine, bilirubin, ALP, AST, and ALT levels.
• May decrease phosphate, albumin, and sodium levels.
• May increase or decrease potassium level.
• May increase eosinophil count.
• May decrease Hb level and neutrophil and platelet counts.

CONTRAINDICATIONS & CAUTIONS

• Contraindicated in patients hypersensitive to drug or its components.
• Use cautiously in older adults and in patients with liver or kidney impairment.
• Severe HF and left ventricular dysfunction have occurred in patients taking imatinib. Use

cautiously in patients with cardiac disease or risk factors for HF.
• Use cautiously in patients with risk factors for kidney dysfunction, including diabetes, HTN, HF, and preexisting kidney impairment.
• Growth retardation has occurred in children and preadolescents receiving imatinib; long-term effects of prolonged treatment are unknown.
• Safety and effectiveness in children younger than age 1 haven't been established.
Dialyzable drug: Unknown.

⚠ **Overdose S&S:** Muscle cramps; ascites; increased creatinine, AST, ALT, and bilirubin levels; nausea; vomiting; diarrhea; weakness; myalgia.

PREGNANCY-LACTATION-REPRODUCTION

• Drug can harm fetus. Patients of childbearing potential should use highly effective contraception during therapy and for 14 days after final dose.
• Drug appears in human milk. Patient shouldn't breastfeed during treatment and for 1 month after final dose.

NURSING CONSIDERATIONS

☒ In adult with MDS, MPD, or ASM, determine *PDGFRB* gene rearrangements status or D816V c-*Kit* mutational status, respectively, before starting therapy.
• Verify pregnancy status before treatment
• Monitor patient closely for possibly severe fluid retention. Older adults may have increased risk of edema.
• Severe bullous skin reactions have been reported. Monitor patient for skin reactions. Drug may need to be withheld.
• Fatal TLS can occur. Correct dehydration and treat high uric acid levels before starting therapy.
• Monitor weight daily. Report unexpected, rapid weight gain.
• Monitor CBC weekly for first month, every other week for second month, and periodically thereafter.
• Monitor LFTs carefully because liver toxicity (occasionally severe) may occur; decrease dosage as needed.
• Monitor kidney function before and periodically during therapy.
• Monitor growth of child being treated with imatinib.
• May increase dosage if no severe adverse reactions or severe non-leukemia-related

neutropenia or thrombocytopenia occur in the following circumstances: disease progression, failure to achieve a satisfactory hematologic response after at least 3 months of treatment, or loss of a previously achieved hematologic response.

⌘ In patient with HES and cardiac involvement, cases of cardiogenic shock and left ventricular dysfunction have been associated with initiation of imatinib therapy. The condition is reversible with administration of systemic steroids and circulatory support measures and by temporarily withholding imatinib. Monitor echocardiogram and serum troponin in patient with HES or CEL and in patient with MDS, MPD, or ASM associated with high eosinophil level.

⌘ Grade 3 or 4 hemorrhage has been reported in patients with newly diagnosed CML and with GIST. GI tumor sites may be the source of GI bleeds in GIST.

• GI perforations, some fatal, have been reported.

• Monitor TSH level in patient who has had thyroidectomy and receives levothyroxine replacement.

PATIENT TEACHING

• Teach about proper drug administration, handling, and disposal.

• Advise patient to report adverse effects, such as fluid retention and sudden weight gain.

• Tell patient that periodic lab tests will be needed to monitor therapy.

• Inform patient and caregivers that growth retardation has occurred in children and preadolescents receiving imatinib and that long-term effects of prolonged treatment are unknown. Growth must be monitored closely.

• Warn of risk of dizziness, blurred vision, and somnolence during treatment. Advise patient to use caution when driving a car or operating machinery.

• Warn patient of childbearing potential that drug may cause fetal harm. Caution patient to avoid pregnancy during therapy and for 14 days after final dose by using highly effective contraceptives.

• Teach patient to report suspected pregnancy.

• Advise patient not to breastfeed during therapy and for 1 month after final dose.

• Instruct patient to tell provider about current medications and use of or plans to take iron supplements.

imipenem–cilastatin sodium
i-mi-PEN-em/sye-la-STAT-in

Primaxin IV

Therapeutic class: Antibiotics
Pharmacologic class: Carbapenems–beta-lactams

AVAILABLE FORMS
Powder for injection: 250 mg imipenem/250 mg cilastatin; 500 mg imipenem/500 mg cilastatin

INDICATIONS & DOSAGES
Adjust-a-dose (for all indications): If CrCl is less than 90 mL/minute, adjust dosage and monitor kidney function test results. Consult manufacturer's package insert for specific dosage adjustments. For patients on hemodialysis, administer dose after hemodialysis and at intervals timed from the end of that dialysis session. Drug isn't recommended in children with kidney impairment who weigh less than 30 kg.

➤ **Serious lower respiratory tract, bone and joint, intra-abdominal, gynecologic, skin and skin structure infections; UTIs; endocarditis; and bacterial septicemia caused by susceptible bacterial species, including *Acinetobacter*, *Enterococcus*, *Staphylococcus aureus*, *Streptococcus*, *Escherichia coli*, *Haemophilus*, *Klebsiella*, *Morganella*, *Proteus*, *Enterobacter*, *Pseudomonas aeruginosa*, or *Bacteroides*, including *B. fragilis*, *Fusobacterium***
Adults: For susceptible bacterial species, 500 mg IV every 6 hours or 1,000 mg IV every 8 hours. For intermediate susceptibility bacterial species, 1,000 mg IV every 6 hours. Refer to manufacturer's package insert for susceptibility test interpretive criteria. Maximum daily dosage, 4,000 mg.
Children ages 3 months and older: 15 to 25 mg/kg IV every 6 hours. Maximum daily dosage, 4 g.
Infants ages 4 weeks to 3 months weighing 1.5 kg or more: 25 mg/kg IV every 6 hours.
Neonates ages 1 to 4 weeks weighing 1.5 kg or more: 25 mg/kg IV every 8 hours.
Neonates younger than age 1 week weighing 1.5 kg or more: 25 mg/kg IV every 12 hours.

➤ **Neutropenic fever ♦**
Adults: 500 mg IV every 6 hours until patient is afebrile for at least 48 hours and ANC reaches 500 cells/mm³ and continues to increase.

ADMINISTRATION

IV

▼ Obtain specimens for culture and sensitivity testing before giving first dose. Begin therapy while awaiting results.

🜂 *Alert:* Don't use diluents containing benzyl alcohol to reconstitute drug for administration to neonates; benzyl alcohol has been associated with toxicity in neonates. While toxicity hasn't been demonstrated in children older than age 3 months, small children in this age range may also be at risk for benzyl alcohol toxicity.

▼ Reconstitute powder by adding approximately 10 mL of appropriate diluent to vial; shake until solution is clear. Solution may be colorless to yellow; color variations within this range don't affect drug's potency.

▼ After reconstitution, transfer resulting suspension to 100 mL of an appropriate infusion solution. Repeat transfer of resulting suspension with an additional 10 mL of infusion solution to ensure complete transfer of vial contents to infusion solution. Agitate resulting mixture until clear before administering by IV infusion.

▼ Reconstituted solution remains stable for 4 hours at room temperature and for 24 hours when refrigerated. Don't freeze drug solutions.

▼ Refer to manufacturer's instructions for reconstitution, preparation, and storage instructions for ADD-Vantage vials.

▼ Don't give by direct IV bolus injection.

▼ For adults with normal kidney function, give each 500-mg dose by IV infusion over 20 to 30 minutes. Infuse each 1-g dose over 40 to 60 minutes. For adults with kidney impairment, refer to manufacturer's instructions for infusion rates.

▼ For children, infuse doses of 500 mg or less over 20 to 30 minutes. Infuse doses greater than 500 mg over 40 to 60 minutes. If nausea occurs, the infusion may be slowed.

▼ **Incompatibilities:** Allopurinol, antibiotics, amiodarone, azithromycin, fluconazole, gemcitabine, lorazepam, meperidine, midazolam, milrinone, sargramostim, sodium bicarbonate. Numerous incompatibilities exist. Consult drug compatibility reference for more information.

ACTION

Inhibits bacterial cell-wall synthesis. Cilastatin prevents kidney metabolism of imipenem.

Route	Onset	Peak	Duration
IV	Unknown	Unknown	Unknown

Half-life: 1 hour after IV dose (adults), 1.2 hours (infants and children), 1.7 to 2.4 hours imipenem and 3.9 to 6.3 hours cilastatin (neonates).

ADVERSE REACTIONS

CNS: *seizures.* **CV:** thrombophlebitis, phlebitis, tachycardia. **EENT:** oral candidiasis. **GI:** diarrhea, nausea, vomiting, gastroenteritis. **GU:** urine discoloration, proteinuria, oliguria, increased creatinine level, *anuria.* **Hematologic:** anemia, eosinophilia, *thrombocytopenia.* **Hepatic:** increased ALP level, increased or decreased bilirubin level. **Skin:** injection-site irritation, rash.

INTERACTIONS

Drug-drug. *Cyclosporine:* May increase CNS adverse effects. Use together cautiously.
Ganciclovir: May cause seizures. Avoid use together.
Probenecid: May increase imipenem level. Don't give concurrently.
Valproic acid: May decrease valproic acid level and increase risk of seizures. Use together isn't recommended; consider using an alternative antibiotic. If use together is necessary, consider supplemental anticonvulsant therapy, and monitor patient carefully.

EFFECTS ON LAB TEST RESULTS

● May increase BUN, creatinine, ALT, AST, ALP, chloride, potassium, and LDH levels.
● May increase or decrease bilirubin level.
● May increase eosinophil count.
● May decrease sodium, Hb, and hematocrit levels.
● May increase or decrease WBC and platelet counts.
● May interfere with urinary glucose determination by Benedict solution, Fehling solution, or Clinitest.
● May result in a false-positive direct Coombs test.

CONTRAINDICATIONS & CAUTIONS

● Contraindicated in patients hypersensitive to drug or its components and in those with CrCl less than 15 mL/minute, unless hemodialysis is begun within 48 hours.

• Patients with CrCl of 15 to less than 30 mL/minute may have an increased risk of seizures.
• Use cautiously in patients allergic to penicillins or cephalosporins because drug has similar chemical structure. Also use cautiously in patients with a history of sensitivity to multiple allergens. Serious anaphylactic reactions require immediate emergency measures.
• Use cautiously in patients with history of seizure disorders, especially if they also have compromised kidney function.
• Drug may cause CDAD, ranging in severity from mild to fatal colitis and occurring even 2 months after drug administration.
• Prolonged use may result in superinfection. Repeated evaluation of patient's condition is essential.
• Use cautiously in children younger than age 3 months. Drug isn't recommended in children with impaired kidney function who weigh less than 30 kg or have CNS infections.
• Drug isn't indicated in patients with meningitis; safety and effectiveness haven't been established.
Dialyzable drug: Yes.

PREGNANCY-LACTATION-REPRODUCTION
• Studies during pregnancy are inadequate. Use during pregnancy only if potential benefit justifies fetal risk.
• It isn't known if drug appears in human milk. Use cautiously during breastfeeding.

NURSING CONSIDERATIONS
🕐 *Alert:* If seizures develop and persist despite anticonvulsant therapy, stop drug.
• For patient receiving hemodialysis, drug is recommended only when benefits outweigh possible risk of seizures.
• Monitor patient for superinfections, including CDAD, during and after therapy.
• Monitor organ system functions, including kidney, liver, and hematopoietic, during prolonged therapy.
• Monitor for hypersensitivity reactions.

PATIENT TEACHING
• Instruct patient to promptly report adverse reactions.
• Advise patient of importance of taking antibiotics exactly as directed and to complete therapy without skipping doses.
• Tell patient to report discomfort at IV insertion site.

• Urge patient to notify prescriber as soon as possible about loose stools or diarrhea.
• Advise patient taking valproic acid or divalproex sodium that seizure therapy may need adjustment.

imipramine hydrochloride
im-IP-ra-meen

imipramine pamoate

Therapeutic class: Antidepressants
Pharmacologic class: TCAs

AVAILABLE FORMS
imipramine hydrochloride
Tablets: 10 mg, 25 mg, 50 mg
imipramine pamoate
Capsules: 75 mg, 100 mg, 125 mg, 150 mg

INDICATIONS & DOSAGES
➤ **Depression**
Adults: Initially, 75 mg PO daily (outpatients); may increase to 150 mg daily. Don't exceed 200 mg/day. Maintenance outpatient dosage is 50 to 150 mg/day. Or, initially 100 mg PO daily (inpatients) in divided doses; gradually increase to 200 mg/day as required. If no response after 2 weeks, increase to 250 to 300 mg/day. Maximum daily dosage, 300 mg for patients who are hospitalized.
Older adults and adolescents: 30 to 40 mg tablets PO once daily, preferably at bedtime, or in divided doses if necessary. Dosage increases above 100 mg daily are generally unnecessary. May switch to capsules when total daily dosage is 75 mg or higher.
➤ **Childhood enuresis**
Children ages 6 and older: Initially, 25 mg imipramine hydrochloride PO 1 hour before bedtime. If patient doesn't improve within 1 week, increase dose to a maximum of 50 mg if child is younger than age 12; increase dose to a maximum of 75 mg for children ages 12 and older. Maximum dosage, 2.5 mg/kg/day.
Adjust-a-dose: Drug may also be given in divided doses for early-night bed-wetting (25 mg midafternoon, 25 mg at bedtime).

ADMINISTRATION
PO
• Give drug without regard to food.
• Bedtime dosing is preferred for depression.
• For childhood enuresis, give 1 hour before bedtime.

ACTION
Unknown. Increases norepinephrine, serotonin, or both in the CNS by blocking their reuptake by presynaptic neurons. Mechanism for enuresis unknown but thought to be separate from drug's antidepressant effects.

Route	Onset	Peak	Duration
PO	Unknown	2–6 hr	Unknown

Half-life: 8 to 21 hours.

ADVERSE REACTIONS
CNS: drowsiness, dizziness, *seizures, stroke,* excitation, tremor, confusion, hallucinations, delusions, anxiety, ataxia, fatigue, peripheral neuropathy, restlessness, headache, paresthesia, nervousness, extrapyramidal reactions, agitation, sleep disorders, nightmares, tiredness, psychosis, taste disturbance, tingling sensation, EEG pattern change. **CV:** orthostatic hypotension, tachycardia, ECG changes, *MI, heart block, arrhythmias,* HTN, *precipitation of HF,* palpitations. **EENT:** blurred vision, mydriasis, angle-closure glaucoma, tinnitus, parotid swelling, black tongue, dry mouth. **GI:** constipation, nausea, vomiting, anorexia, *paralytic ileus,* abdominal cramps, diarrhea. **GU:** urine retention, urinary frequency, urinary tract dilation, impotence, testicular swelling, increased or decreased libido. **Hematologic:** *bone marrow depression, thrombocytopenia.* **Hepatic:** jaundice, altered LFT values. **Metabolic:** *hypoglycemia,* hyperglycemia, weight loss or gain, SIADH. **Skin:** rash, urticaria, photosensitivity reactions, pruritus, diaphoresis, alopecia. **Other:** falls, hypersensitivity reactions, gynecomastia, galactorrhea, breast enlargement.

INTERACTIONS
Drug-drug. *Aclidinium:* May enhance anticholinergic effects. Avoid use together.
Antihypertensives: May potentiate hypotensive effect. Use together cautiously.
Barbiturates, CNS depressants: May enhance CNS depression. Avoid use together.
Cimetidine, fluoxetine, fluvoxamine, paroxetine, sertraline: May increase imipramine level. Monitor drug levels and patient for signs of toxicity.
Clonidine: May cause life-threatening HTN. Avoid use together.
⬙ *Drugs metabolized by CYP2D6 (propafenone, phenothiazines):* May increase

TCA levels in poor metabolizers when given usual dosages. Monitor therapy.
Epinephrine, norepinephrine: May increase hypertensive effect. Use together cautiously.
Linezolid, methylene blue: May cause serotonin syndrome. Use with extreme caution, and monitor patient closely.
MAO inhibitors: May cause hyperpyretic crisis, severe seizures, and death. Don't use within 14 days of MAO inhibitor therapy.
QTc-prolonging drugs (quinidine, quinolones): May increase the risk of life-threatening arrhythmias. Avoid use together.
Drug-herb. *SAM-e, St. John's wort, yohimbe:* May cause serotonin syndrome. Discourage use together.
Drug-lifestyle. *Alcohol use:* May enhance CNS depression. Discourage use together.
Smoking: May lower level of drug. Monitor patient for lack of effect.
Sun exposure: May increase risk of photosensitivity reactions. Advise patient to avoid excessive sunlight exposure.

EFFECTS ON LAB TEST RESULTS
• May increase or decrease glucose level.
• May increase LFT values.
• May decrease granulocyte, eosinophil, and platelet counts.

CONTRAINDICATIONS & CAUTIONS
Boxed Warning Antidepressants increase risk of suicidality in children, adolescents, and young adults with major depressive disorder and other psychiatric disorders. Imipramine isn't approved for use in children, except for those with nocturnal enuresis. ∎
• Contraindicated in patients hypersensitive to drug and during acute recovery phase of MI.
• Drug isn't approved for treating bipolar depression. Evaluate patients carefully for risk of bipolar disorder, including family history of suicide, bipolar disorder, and depression.
⚡ *Alert:* Use with extreme caution in patients at risk for suicide; in older adults and in patients with history of urine retention, angle-closure glaucoma, or seizure disorders; in patients with increased IOP, CV disease, impaired liver or kidney function, or hyperthyroidism; and in patients receiving thyroid drugs.
⚡ *Alert:* Concomitant use with linezolid or methylene blue can cause serotonin syndrome (fever, mental status changes, muscle twitching, diaphoresis, shivering or shaking, diarrhea, loss of coordination). Use imipramine with

linezolid or methylene blue only for life-threatening or urgent conditions when potential benefits outweigh risks of toxicity.

⊕ Alert: Don't use imipramine pamoate in children of any age because of increased risk of acute overdose.

Dialyzable drug: No.

⚠ Overdose S&S: Cardiac arrhythmias, severe hypotension, seizures, CNS depression, coma, ECG changes, drowsiness, stupor, ataxia, restlessness, agitation, hyperactive reflexes, muscle rigidity, athetoid and choreiform movements, tachycardia, HF, respiratory depression, cyanosis, shock, vomiting, hyperpyrexia, mydriasis, diaphoresis.

PREGNANCY-LACTATION-REPRODUCTION

• Studies during pregnancy are inadequate; however, fetal risk can't be excluded. Use during pregnancy only if potential benefit clearly justifies fetal risk.

• Drug appears in human milk. Use during breastfeeding isn't recommended.

NURSING CONSIDERATIONS

Boxed Warning Monitor all patients for clincial worsening, suicidality, or unusal changes in behavior. ■

⊕ Alert: If linezolid or methylene blue must be given, discontinue imipramine and monitor patient for serotonin toxicity for 2 weeks (5 weeks if fluoxetine was taken) or until 24 hours after the last dose of methylene blue or linezolid, whichever comes first. May resume imipramine 24 hours after last dose of methylene blue or linezolid.

• Don't withdraw drug abruptly due to risk of discontinuation syndrome (GI symptoms, diaphoresis, chills, tremors, sleep disturbances).

• Monitor patient for nausea, headache, and malaise after abrupt withdrawal of long-term therapy; these symptoms don't indicate addiction.

• To prevent relapse in child receiving drug for enuresis, withdraw drug gradually.

• Safety of long-term use as adjunctive therapy for nocturnal enuresis in children ages 6 and older hasn't been established. Consider a drug-free period after an adequate therapeutic trial with a favorable response.

• Monitor WBC count during therapy. Also monitor patient for fever and sore throat. Discontinue drug if neutrophil depression occurs.

• Because of hypertensive episodes during surgery in patients receiving TCAs, stop drug gradually several days before elective surgery.

• Recommend sugarless hard candy or gum to relieve dry mouth. Saliva substitutes may be useful.

⊕ Alert: Tofranil may contain tartrazine.

• **Look alike–sound alike:** Don't confuse imipramine with desipramine.

PATIENT TEACHING

Boxed Warning Advise families and caregivers to closely observe patient for increased suicidality, worsening condition, and unusual behavior changes. Instruct them to report these findings to the prescriber. ■

⊕ Alert: Teach patient to recognize and immediately report symptoms of serotonin toxicity (fever, mental status changes, muscle twitching, diaphoresis, shivering or shaking, diarrhea, loss of coordination).

• Tell patient to take full dose at bedtime whenever possible, but caution patient about possible morning dizziness upon standing up quickly.

• If early-night bed-wetting occurs, recommend caregivers divide dose and give first dose earlier in the day.

• Tell patient to avoid alcohol while taking drug.

• Advise patient to consult prescriber before taking other prescription or OTC drugs.

• Warn patient to avoid hazardous activities that require alertness and good coordination until drug effects are known. Drowsiness and dizziness usually subside after a few weeks.

• Warn patient not to stop drug suddenly.

• To prevent oversensitivity to the sun, advise patient to use sunblock, wear protective clothing, and avoid prolonged exposure to strong sunlight.

• Instruct patient to report pregnancy or plans to become pregnant or to breastfeed.

---

immune globulin intramuscular (gamma globulin, Ig, IGIM)
GamaSTAN

immune globulin intravenous (IGIV) 🖾

Asceniv, Bivigam, Flebogamma DIF, Gammagard Liquid, Gammagard S/D, Gammaked, Gammaplex, Gamunex-C, IGIVnex❧, Octagam, Panzyga, Privigen

---

Reactions in bold italics are *life-threatening*.

immune globulin subcutaneous (IGSC, SCIG) ⌧
Cutaquig, Cuvitru, Gammagard, Gammaked, Gamunex-C, Hizentra, HyQvia, IGIVnex ♥, Xembify

Therapeutic class: Antibodies
Pharmacologic class: Immune serums

AVAILABLE FORMS
immune globulin intramuscular
Injection: 15% to 18% in 2-mL and 10-mL single-dose vials
immune globulin intravenous
Solution for injection (preservative-free): 5% in 20-mL, 50-mL, 100-mL, 200-mL, 400-mL, 500-mL vials; 10% in 10-mL, 25-mL, 50-mL, 100-mL, 200-mL, 300-mL, 400-mL vials
Powder for injection (preservative-free): 5-g, 10-g vials
immune globulin subcutaneous
Solution for injection (kit with hyaluronidase vials): 10% in 25-mL, 50-mL, 100-mL, 200-mL, 300-mL vials
Solution for injection (preservative-free): 10% in 10-mL, 25-mL, 50-mL, 100-mL, 200-mL, 300-mL, 400-mL vials; 16.5% in 6-mL, 10-mL, 12-mL, 20-mL, 24-mL, 48-mL vials; 20% in 5-mL, 10-mL, 20-mL, 40-mL, 50-mL vials and 5-mL, 10-mL, 20-mL, 50-mL prefilled syringes

INDICATIONS & DOSAGES
Boxed Warning Drug increases risk of thrombosis. Don't exceed recommended dosage. ■

➤ **Primary humoral immunodeficiency (PI)** ⌧
Adults and adolescents ages 12 to 17 (Asceniv): 300 to 800 mg/kg IV every 3 to 4 weeks. Begin IV infusion at rate of 0.5 mg/kg/minute for first 15 minutes. Increase every 15 minutes, if tolerated, to maximum of 8 mg/kg/minute.
Adults and children ages 6 and older (Bivigam): 300 to 800 mg/kg IV every 3 to 4 weeks. Begin IV infusion at a rate of 0.5 mg/kg/minute for first 10 minutes. Increase every 20 minutes, if tolerated, by 0.8 mg/kg/minute, to maximum of 6 mg/kg/minute.
Adults and children ages 2 and older (Cutaquig, Cuvitru): Individualize subcut infusion dose based on patient's pharmacokinetic and clinical response as monitored by IgG trough levels. Infuse at regular intervals from daily to up to every other week. Infusion

rate varies by manufacturer based on patient's age, weight volume of solution, and tolerance.
Adults (Flebogamma DIF 10%): 300 to 600 mg/kg 10% solution IV every 3 to 4 weeks. Infuse at 1 mg/kg/minute. After 30 minutes, if tolerated, may gradually increase to maximum rate of 8 mg/kg/minute.
Adults and children ages 2 and older (Flebogamma DIF 5%): 300 to 600 mg/kg 5% solution IV every 3 to 4 weeks. Infuse at 0.5 mg/kg/minute. After 30 minutes, if tolerated, may gradually increase to maximum rate of 5 mg/kg/minute.
Adults and children ages 2 and older (Gammagard Liquid, Gammaked): 300 to 600 mg/kg IV every 3 to 4 weeks. Infuse at 0.8 mg/kg/minute and increase every 30 minutes, if tolerated, to 8 mg/kg/minute. May give maintenance therapy weekly by subcut infusion starting 1 week after last IGIV infusion. Initial subcut dose is 1.37 × current IV dose in mg/kg ÷ number of weeks between IV doses. See package insert for dosage adjustments, recommended number of subcut sites, and infusion rates.
Adults and children ages 2 and older (Gammagard S/D): 300 to 600 mg/kg IV every 3 to 4 weeks. Initially, infuse in a 5% solution at 0.5 mL/kg/hour; may increase gradually, as tolerated, to maximum rate of 4 mL/kg/hour. Can give patients who tolerate 5% solution 10% solution starting at 0.5 mL/kg/hour and gradually increase to maximum of 8 mL/kg/hour as tolerated.
Adults and children ages 2 and older (Gammaplex): 300 to 800 mg/kg IV every 3 to 4 weeks. Initially, infuse at 0.5 mg/kg/minute for first 15 minutes. Increase every 15 minutes, if tolerated, to 4 mg/kg/minute for 5% solution and 8 mg/kg/minute for 10% solution.
Adults and children ages 2 and older (Gamunex-C): 300 to 600 mg/kg IV every 3 to 4 weeks. Initially, infuse at 1 mg/kg/minute for first 30 minutes. Increase gradually, if tolerated, to maximum of 8 mg/kg/minute. May give maintenance therapy subcut starting 1 week after last IGIV infusion. Initial subcut dose is 1.37 × current IV dose in mg/kg ÷ number of weeks between IV doses. See package insert for recommended number of subcut sites and infusion rates.
Adults and children ages 2 and older (Hizentra): Calculate initial weekly dose by dividing previous IGIV dose in grams by the number

of weeks between doses during patient's IGIV treatment; then multiply this by the dose adjustment factor of 1.37. Or give the same weekly dose in grams as the prior IGSC treatment. Multiply dose in grams by 5 to obtain dose in milliliters. Adjust dose based on clinical response. Give by subcut infusion at regular intervals from daily up to every 2 weeks. See prescribing information for full dosage adjustment guidelines, recommended number of subcut sites, and infusion rates.

Adults and children ages 2 to 16 (HyQvia): See manufacturer's labeling for initial 7-week subcut infusion ramp-up schedule to increase dose and frequency from a previous 1-week dose to a 3- or 4-week dose. Begin ramp-up 1 week after last infusion of previous treatment. In patients naive to IgG therapy or switching from another IG subcut therapy, give 300 to 600 mg/kg subcut infusion every 3 to 4 weeks, after initial dose ramp-up. In patients switching from IGIV therapy, give by subcut infusion at same dose and frequency as previous IGIV therapy every 3 to 4 weeks after initial dose ramp-up. For subsequent dosage adjustments, refer to manufacturer's instructions.

Adults and children ages 1 and older (IGIVnex): 100 to 600 mg/kg IV infusion every 3 to 4 weeks individualized to achieve serum IgG level at trough of at least 5 g/L. May give maintenance therapy as weekly subcut infusion. Initial subcut dose is $1.37 \times$ current IV dose in mg/kg $\div$ number of weeks between IV doses.

Adults and children ages 6 and older (Octagam 5%): 300 to 600 mg/kg IV every 3 to 4 weeks. Start infusion at 0.5 mg/kg/minute for 30 minutes. Increase rate, as tolerated, to 1 mg/kg/minute for 30 minutes, then to 2 mg/kg/minute for 30 minutes. May then increase to maximum rate of 3.33 mg/kg/ minute, as tolerated.

Adults and children ages 2 and older (Panzyga): 300 to 600 mg/kg IV every 3 to 4 weeks. Start infusion at 1 mg/kg/minute, for 30 minutes. Then if tolerated, may increase every 15 to 30 minutes to maximum rate of 14 mg/kg/minute.

Adults and children ages 3 and older (Privigen): 200 to 800 mg/kg IV every 3 to 4 weeks. Start infusion at 0.5 mg/kg/minute and increase slowly to 8 mg/kg/minute.

Adults and children ages 2 and older (Xembify): Initial weekly dose is previous IGIV dose in

grams divided by the number of weeks between IGIV doses $\times$ 1.37. Multiply dose in grams by 5 to obtain dose in milliliters. Or give the same weekly dose in grams as the prior IGSC treatment. Adjust dose based on clinical response and IgG trough levels. Give by subcut infusion two to seven times per week. See package insert for full dosage adjustment guidelines, recommended number of subcut sites, and infusion rates.

➤ **Measles exposure in patients with PI (IGIV [Flebogamma, Gammagard Liquid, Gamunex-C, Gammagard S/D, Gammaplex, Octagam, Panzyga, Privigen])**
Adults and children: If patient has been exposed to measles, consider giving 400 mg/kg IV as soon as possible within 6 days of exposure to provide a measles antibody serum level greater than 240 mIU/mL for at least 2 weeks. If patient is at risk for future measles exposure and receives a dose of less than 530 mg/kg every 3 to 4 weeks, increase dose to at least 530 mg/kg IV (or give 400 mg/kg IV for Gamunex-C) to provide a measles antibody serum level of 240 mIU/mL for at least 22 days after infusion.

➤ **Measles exposure in patients with PI (IGSC [Cutaquig, Cuvitru, Hizentra, HyQvia])**
Adults and children: If patient has been exposed to measles, consider giving 400 mg/kg subcut infusion as soon as possible within 6 days of exposure to provide a measles antibody serum level greater than 240 mIU/mL for at least 2 weeks.

Cutaquig: If patient is at risk for future measles exposure and receives a dosage of less than 245 mg/kg every week, increase dosage to at least 245 mg/kg/week.

Cuvitru: If patient is at risk for future measles exposure and receives a dosage of less than 230 mg/kg every week, increase dosage to at least 230 mg/kg/week.

HyQvia: If patient is at risk for future measles exposure and receives a dose of less than 530 mg/kg every 3 to 4 weeks, increase dose to at least 530 mg/kg to provide a measles antibody serum level of 240 mIU/mL for at least 22 days after infusion.

➤ **Measles exposure (IGIM)**
Adults and children: 0.25 mL/kg IM within 6 days after exposure.
Children who are immunocompromised: 0.5 mL/kg IM immediately after exposure. Maximum dose, 15 mL.

Reactions in bold italics are *life-threatening*.

➤ **Rubella exposure during pregnancy in patients not considering therapeutic abortion (IGIM)**
Adults: 0.55 mL/kg IM. Not for routine prophylaxis in unexposed patients during pregnancy.

➤ **Chronic inflammatory demyelinating polyneuropathy (CIDP)**
Adults (Gammaked, Gamunex-C, IGIVnex): 2,000 mg/kg IV in divided doses over 2 to 4 days. May administer as a maintenance infusion of 1,000 mg/kg IV over 1 day every 3 weeks or 500 mg/kg IV on 2 consecutive days every 3 weeks. Recommended initial infusion rate is 2 mg/kg/minute, which may be gradually increased to maximum of 8 mg/kg/minute for Gammaked or Gamunex-C or 14 mg/kg/minute for IGIVnex if well tolerated.
Adults (Hizentra): For maintenance therapy, begin subcut infusion 1 week after the last IGIV infusion. Give 200 mg/kg/week (1 mL/kg) or 400 mg/kg/week (2 mL/kg) subcut using an infusion pump in one or two sessions over 1 or 2 consecutive days to prevent relapse. Base duration of therapy on clinical response. Refer to package insert for recommended number of subcut sites, infusion rates, and dosage adjustments if symptoms worsen during treatment.
Adults (Panzyga): Give loading dose of 2,000 mg/kg (20 mL/kg) IV divided into two daily doses of 1,000 mg/kg (10 mL/kg) IV on 2 consecutive days. Maintenance dosage is 1,000 to 2,000 mg/kg (10 to 20 mL/kg) IV every 3 weeks divided in two doses over 2 consecutive days. Initial infusion rate is 1 mg/kg/minute for 30 minutes; may gradually increase every 15 to 30 minutes to maximum of 12 mg/kg/minute if well tolerated.
Adults (Privigen): 2,000 mg/kg IV in divided doses over 2 to 5 days. May give as maintenance dosage of 1,000 mg/kg IV administered in one or two infusions on consecutive days every 3 weeks. Recommended initial infusion rate is 0.5 mg/kg/minute, which may be gradually increased to maximum of 8 mg/kg/minute if infusion is well tolerated. Maintenance therapy with Privigen hasn't been studied beyond 6 months.

➤ **Chronic ITP**
Adults and children ages 2 and older (Flebogamma DIF 10%, Panzyga): 1 g/kg (10 mL/kg) IV daily for 2 consecutive days. Initial infusion rate is 0.01 mL/kg/minute (1 mg/kg/minute) for first 30 minutes. If

tolerated, rate may be gradually increased to 0.04 mL/kg/minute (4 mg/kg/minute) and, if tolerated, gradually increased to maximum of 0.08 mL/kg/minute (8 mg/kg/minute).
Adults (Gammagard S/D): 1,000 mg/kg IV. May give up to three separate doses on alternate days, if needed, as determined by clinical response and platelet count. Initially, infuse in a 5% solution at 0.5 mL/kg/hour; may increase gradually, as tolerated, to maximum rate of 4 mL/kg/hour. For patients who tolerate 5% solution, can give 10% solution starting at 0.5 mL/kg/hour and gradually increase to maximum of 8 mL/kg/hour, as tolerated.
Adults and children (Gammaked, Gamunex-C, IGIVnex): 2,000 mg/kg IV in two divided doses of 1,000 mg/kg given on 2 consecutive days or 400 mg/kg IV in five doses over 5 consecutive days. Initial infusion rate is 1 mg/kg/minute. If infusion is well tolerated, may gradually increase to maximum of 8 mg/kg/minute for Gammaked or Gamunex-C or 14/mg/kg/minute for IGIVnex. If adequate platelet count increase occurs within 24 hours after first dose, may withhold second dose.
Adults (Gammaplex 5% or 10%): 1,000 mg/kg IV for 2 consecutive days. Initial infusion rate is 0.5 mg/kg/minute for 15 minutes. If tolerated, may gradually increase rate every 15 minutes to maximum of 4 mg/kg/minute for 5% solution or 8 mg/kg/minute for 10% solution.
Adults (Octagam 10%): 2,000 mg/kg IV in two divided doses of 1,000 mg/kg given on 2 consecutive days. Initial infusion rate is 1 mg/kg/minute for first 30 minutes. If tolerated, may gradually increase rate every 30 minutes to 2 mg/kg/minute, then 4 mg/kg/minute, then 8 mg/kg/minute, then to maximum of 12 mg/kg/minute.
Adults and adolescents ages 15 and older (Privigen): 1 g/kg IV daily for 2 consecutive days. Initial infusion rate is 0.5 mg/kg/minute. If tolerated, may gradually increase rate 4 mg/kg/minute.

➤ **Multifocal motor neuropathy (MMN) (Gammagard Liquid)**
Adults: 500 to 2,400 mg/kg/month IV based on response. Initial infusion rate is 0.8 mg/kg/minute. If tolerated, may gradually increase rate every 30 minutes to 9 mg/kg/minute.

➤ **Kawasaki syndrome to prevent associated coronary artery aneurysms (Gammagard S/D)**

Children: 400 mg/kg IV daily for 4 consecutive days, or a single dose of 1,000 mg/kg. Start 5% infusion at 0.5 mL/kg/hour. May gradually increase rate to maximum of 4 mL/kg/hour, as tolerated. For patients who tolerate 5% solution, can give 10% solution starting at 0.5 mL/kg/hour and gradually increase to maximum of 8 mL/kg/hour, as tolerated. Begin treatment within 7 days of onset of fever. Give with aspirin (80 to 100 mg/kg PO daily in four divided doses).

➤ **Hepatitis A exposure (IGIM)**
Adults and children: 0.1 mL/kg IM as soon as possible after household or institutional exposure. Not indicated in patients with clinical manifestations of hepatitis A or in those exposed more than 2 weeks prior. Before travel to areas where hepatitis A is common, 0.1 mL/kg IM if length of stay will be up to 1 month or 0.2 mL/kg if length of stay will be up to 2 months; repeat every 2 months for longer stays.

➤ **Chickenpox (varicella) exposure (IGIM)**
Adults and children: 0.6 to 1.2 mL/kg IM as soon as possible after exposure only if varicella-zoster immune globulin is unavailable.

➤ **Prevention of bacterial infections in patients with acquired hypogammaglobulinemia or recurrent bacterial infections secondary to B-cell chronic lymphocytic leukemia (Gammagard S/D)**
Adults and children: 400 mg/kg IV every 3 to 4 weeks for patients with hypogammaglobulinemia or recurrent bacterial infections. Initially, infuse in 5% solution at rate of 0.5 mL/kg/hour; may increase gradually, as tolerated, to maximum of 4 mL/kg/hour. For patients who tolerate 5% solution, can give 10% solution starting at 0.5 mL/kg/hour and gradually increase to maximum of 8 mL/kg/hour, as tolerated.

➤ **Dermatomyositis (Octagam 10%)**
Adults: 2 g/kg IV divided in equal doses given over 2 to 5 consecutive days every 4 weeks. Initial infusion rate is 1 mg/kg/minute for first 30 minutes. If tolerated, may gradually increase to 2 mg/kg/minute and then to maximum of 4 mg/kg/minute.

🔁 *Alert:* Patients with dermatomyositis are at increased risk for thromboembolic events; don't exceed infusion rate of 4 mg/kg/minute.

➤ **Guillain-Barré syndrome (IGIV)** ◆
Adults: 2,000 mg/kg IV over 2 to 5 days within 2 to 4 weeks of onset.

ADMINISTRATION
● Refer to each product's manufacturer's instructions for reconstitution, dilution, and storage information.

IM
🔁 *Alert:* Carefully verify drug, route, and dose before administration.
● Give in anterolateral aspects of upper thigh and deltoid muscle of upper arm. Divide doses larger than 10 mL and inject into several muscle sites to reduce pain and discomfort.
● Don't administer IV or subcut because of risk of serious reactions.
● Give drug soon after reconstitution.
● Don't routinely use gluteal region. If necessary, use only upper outer quadrant.

IV
▼ Infusion rates vary by manufacturer based on patient's age, weight, volume of solution, and tolerance.
Boxed Warning For patients at risk for kidney dysfunction or thrombotic events, give at minimum infusion rate practicable. ∎
▼ Inspect each vial for particulate matter and discoloration before administration.
▼ Don't mix products from different manufacturers together.
▼ **Incompatibilities:** Other IV drugs and IV solutions. Don't mix with immune globulin from other manufacturers.

Subcutaneous
● Give IGSC by subcut infusion.
● Refer to each product's manufacturer for instructions on switching between formulations.
● Inspect each vial for particulate matter and discoloration before administration.
● Infusion sites include abdomen, thighs, upper arms, lateral hip and, for Gammagard Liquid, IGIVnex, and Xembify, lower back.
● May use multiple infusion sites at same time. Refer to each product's manufacturer's instructions for the number of infusion sites allowed, spacing between sites, amounts to infuse per site, and infusion rate.
● Complete Cuvitru and Xembify infusions within 2 hours to prevent formation of particles in siliconized syringes.
● Don't mix with other products.
● Don't shake vials.

HyQvia only
● Infusion sites include abdomen and thighs.
● If using two sites simultaneously, ensure infusion sites are on opposite sides of body.

• Administer components (immune globulin and hyaluronidase) sequentially, beginning with hyaluronidase; don't use either component alone.

• Administer hyaluronidase at an initial rate per site of approximately 1 to 2 mL/minute, or as tolerated.

• Initiate infusion of full dose of immune globulin through same hyaluronidase subcut needle set within approximately 10 minutes of hyaluronidase infusion.

• Refer to manufacturer's instructions for weight-based initial and subsequent infusion rates.

ACTION

Provides passive immunity by increasing antibody titer. The primary component is IgG. It's unknown how it works for ITP.

Route	Onset	Peak	Duration
IV	Immediate	Immediate	3–4 wk
IM	Unknown	2 days	3–4 wk
Subcut	Unknown	2–5 days	Unknown

Half-life: 26 to 40 days in patients who are immunocompromised.

ADVERSE REACTIONS

CNS: headache, fever, lethargy, malaise, dizziness, fatigue, myasthenia syndrome, asthenia, pain, insomnia, depression, vertigo. **CV:** chest pain, chest tightness, HTN, hypotension, tachycardia, decreased HR, edema, heart murmur. **EENT:** eye irritation, conjunctivitis, eye discharge, ear pain, otitis media, nasal congestion, epistaxis, rhinorrhea, sinusitis, pharyngitis, nasopharyngitis, postnasal drip, sore throat, oropharyngeal pain. **GI:** diarrhea, abdominal pain, nausea, vomiting. **GU:** UTI, vulvovaginal candidiasis, cystitis, dysuria, nephrolithiasis, increased creatinine level. **Hematologic:** anemia, leukopenia, hemolysis. **Hepatic:** increased ALT level, hyperbilirubinemia, increased or decreased ALP level. **Musculoskeletal:** back pain, arthralgia, limb pain, hip pain, muscle cramps, muscle stiffness at injection site. **Respiratory:** dyspnea, wheezing, cough, pneumonia, *asthma.* **Skin:** erythema, pain, urticaria, purpura, petechiae, local infusion-site reactions, rash, flushing, hematoma, bruise, cellulitis, excoriation, diaphoresis, allergic dermatitis, eczema. **Other:** *anaphylaxis, angioedema, hypersensitivity,* antibody development, infection, chills, rigors, accidental injury, flulike symptoms.

INTERACTIONS

Drug-drug. *Live-virus vaccines:* May decrease therapeutic effect of vaccine. Length of time to wait before giving live-virus vaccinations varies with immune globulin dosage.

EFFECTS ON LAB TEST RESULTS

• May falsely elevate serum glucose level (for IGIV preparations containing maltose such as Octagam).

• May increase ALT, bilirubin, and creatinine levels.

• May increase or decrease ALP level.

• May decrease hematocrit and leukocyte and neutrocyte counts.

• May cause positive Coombs test.

• Gammagard may produce false-positive readings in assays that depend on detection of beta-D-glucans for diagnosis of fungal infections; this may persist during the weeks after product infusion.

CONTRAINDICATIONS & CAUTIONS

• Contraindicated in patients hypersensitive to drug or its components and in those with IgA deficiency, especially those who have known antibodies against IgA or history of hypersensitivity.

• Octagam is contraindicated in patients hypersensitive to corn or maltose.

• Hizentra is contraindicated in patients hypersensitive to polysorbate 80 and in patients with hyperprolinemia.

• Privigen is contraindicated in patients with hyperprolinemia.

• HyQvia is contraindicated in patients with known systemic hypersensitivity to hyaluronidase or human albumin.

• GamaSTAN is contraindicated in patients with severe thrombocytopenia or any coagulation disorder that would contraindicate IM injections.

▧ Gammaplex 5% is contraindicated in patients with hereditary intolerance to fructose and in infants and neonates for whom sucrose or fructose tolerance hasn't been established. Gammaplex 10% doesn't contain sucrose or fructose.

▧ Don't use Flebogamma DIF in patients with hereditary fructose intolerance because it contains sorbitol, which increases risk of adverse reactions.

• Aseptic meningitis syndrome (AMS) may occur with immune globulin treatment administered IV or subcut. Risk may be higher in females. Syndrome usually begins within several hours to 2 days after immune globulin treatment.

• Use IGIV cautiously in patients with history of CV disease or thrombotic episodes.

Boxed Warning Drug increases risk of thrombosis, especially in older adults; those with prolonged immobilization, hypercoagulable conditions, history of venous or arterial thrombosis, hyperviscosity, CV risk factors, or indwelling central venous catheters; and patients using estrogens. Thrombosis may also occur without these risk factors. Don't exceed recommended dosage. ■

Boxed Warning Kidney dysfunction, AKI, osmotic nephrosis, and death may occur with IGIV products in patients who are predisposed. Patients at increased risk include those with any degree of preexisting kidney insufficiency, diabetes, age greater than 65, volume depletion, sepsis, or paraproteinemia and patients receiving known kidney toxic drugs. Kidney dysfunction and AKI occur more commonly in patients receiving immune globulin IV products containing sucrose. (*Note:* The following IV products don't contain sucrose: Asceniv, Bivigam, Flebogamma 5% DIF, Flebogamma 10% DIF, Gammagard Liquid, Gammagard S/D, Gammaked, Gammaplex, Gamunex-C, Octagam 5%, Octagam 10%, Panzyga, and Privigen.) For patients at risk, administer IGIV products at the minimum concentration dose and infusion rate practicable and ensure adequate hydration. ■

• Subcut and IV formulations can cause hemolysis and hemolytic anemia.

Dialyzable drug: Unknown.

PREGNANCY-LACTATION-REPRODUCTION

• It isn't known if drug causes fetal harm when used during pregnancy. Use during pregnancy only if clearly needed and potential benefit justifies fetal risk. Refer to individual manufacturer's instructions for use.

• Use of IGIM for rubella exposure during pregnancy in patients not considering a therapeutic abortion is FDA approved but not recommended. Congenital rubella has occurred in infants born to patients who received immune globin after exposure.

• Drug may appear in human milk. Use cautiously during breastfeeding and only if clearly indicated. Refer to individual manufacturer's instructions for use.

NURSING CONSIDERATIONS

Boxed Warning For patient at increased risk for thrombosis, give minimum concentration available at minimum rate of infusion practicable. ■

Boxed Warning Ensure adequate hydration before administration. ■

Boxed Warning Monitor for signs and symptoms of thrombosis (pain or swelling of extremity with warmth over affected area, discoloration, unexplained dyspnea, chest pain or discomfort that worsens on deep inspiration, tachycardia, chest pain, numbness or weakness on one side of the body), and assess blood viscosity in patient at risk for hyperviscosity. ■

• Obtain history of allergies and reactions to immunizations. Keep epinephrine available to treat anaphylaxis.

• Monitor for signs and symptoms of AMS (severe headache, nuchal rigidity, fever, drowsiness, photophobia, painful eye movements, nausea, vomiting). Conduct a thorough neurologic examination on patient exhibiting such signs and symptoms, including CSF studies, to rule out other causes of meningitis.

• Transfusion-related acute lung injury (TRALI) can occur after IGIV treatment and typically appears within 1 to 6 hours after therapy. Monitor patient for severe respiratory distress, hypoxemia, pulmonary edema, and fever with normal LVEF. Provide respiratory support and perform tests for the presence of anti-neutrophil antibodies and anti-human leukocyte antigen antibodies in product and patient's serum.

• Monitor kidney function test results and urine output in patient at risk for developing AKI.

• In patient receiving subcut or IV therapy, monitor CBC, and watch for signs and symptoms of hemolysis and hemolytic anemia (weakness, pallor, dark urine, fever, dyspnea, abdominal pain).

• Products made from human plasma may contain infectious agents, such as viruses and, potentially, Creutzfeldt-Jakob disease agent.

• Hyaluronidase infusion included in the HyQvia kit increases dispersion and absorption of IGSC.

PATIENT TEACHING

❸ *Alert:* Warn patient of thrombosis risk. Instruct patient to immediately report signs or symptoms.

• Teach about drug administration.

• Teach patient to immediately report all adverse reactions, especially signs and symptoms of hypersensitivity reactions, thrombosis, AMS, TRALI, kidney injury, and hemolytic anemia.

• Caution patient that local reactions may occur at injection site. Instruct patient to promptly report adverse reactions that persist or become severe.

• Tell patient that lab blood tests will be needed to monitor therapy.

• Inform patient of possible need for therapy more than once monthly to maintain adequate IgG levels.

• Tell patient to report pregnancy or plans to become pregnant before therapy begins.

• Advise patient who is breastfeeding or planning to breastfeed to discuss breastfeeding before therapy begins.

---

inclisiran ▧
in-kli-SIR-an

Leqvio

Therapeutic class: Antilipemics
Pharmacologic class: Small interfering RNA agent

AVAILABLE FORMS
Injection: 284 mg/1.5 mL (189 mg/mL) prefilled syringe

INDICATIONS & DOSAGES

➤ **Adjunct to diet and maximally tolerated statin therapy for treatment of heterozygous familial hypercholesterolemia or clinical atherosclerotic CV disease in patients who require additional lowering of LDL-C** ▧
Adults: 284 mg subcut for one dose. Repeat dose at 3 months, then every 6 months thereafter.

ADMINISTRATION
Subcutaneous

• Inspect solution before use. Solution is clear and colorless to pale yellow. Don't use if particulate matter or discoloration is present.

• Inject subcut into abdomen, upper arm, or thigh. Avoid areas with active skin disease or injury.

• If dose is missed by less than 3 months, give dose and maintain original dosing schedule. If missed dose is beyond 3 months, give dose, repeat at 3 months, and then give every 6 months thereafter.

• Store at room temperature.

ACTION
Targets PCSK9 mRNA, which increases the breakdown of LDL receptors and results in lower LDL-C level in the blood.

Route	Onset	Peak	Duration
Subcut	Unknown	4 hr	Unknown

Half-life: 9 hours.

ADVERSE REACTIONS
GI: diarrhea. **GU:** UTI. **Musculoskeletal:** arthralgia, extremity pain. **Respiratory:** bronchitis, dyspnea. **Skin:** injection-site reactions (pain, erythema, rash).

INTERACTIONS
None reported by manufacturer.

EFFECTS ON LAB TEST RESULTS
None reported.

CONTRAINDICATIONS & CAUTIONS
• Use in patients with KFRT or Child-Pugh class C liver impairment hasn't been studied.

• Drug's effect on CV morbidity and mortality hasn't been established.

• Safety and effectiveness in children haven't been established.

Dialyzable drug: Unknown.

PREGNANCY-LACTATION-REPRODUCTION
• Studies during pregnancy are inadequate. Drug may cause fetal harm.

• Discontinue drug if pregnancy occurs.

• It isn't known if drug appears in human milk or how drug affects milk production or infants who are breastfed. Before patient initiates breastfeeding, consider patient's clinical need for drug and risk to infant.

NURSING CONSIDERATIONS
• Drug should only be given by a health care professional.

• Periodically monitor LDL-C level, beginning as early as 30 days after initiation.

PATIENT TEACHING
• Instruct patient of childbearing potential to report pregnancy or plans to become pregnant during therapy.
• Warn that injection-site reactions can occur.

indomethacin
in-doe-METH-a-sin

Indocin

indomethacin sodium trihydrate

Therapeutic class: Anti-inflammatory drugs
Pharmacologic class: NSAIDs

AVAILABLE FORMS
indomethacin
Capsules: 25 mg, 50 mg
Capsules (extended-release) ⓄⓃⒼ: 75 mg
Injection: 1 mg base/vial
Oral suspension: 25 mg/5 mL
Suppositories: 50 mg, 100 mg ✿
indomethacin sodium trihydrate
Injection: 1 mg base/vial

INDICATIONS & DOSAGES
➤ **Moderate to severe RA or osteoarthritis, ankylosing spondylitis**
Adults and children ages 15 and older: 25 mg PO b.i.d. or t.i.d. with food or antacids or 25 mg PR b.i.d. or t.i.d.; increase daily dosage by 25 or 50 mg every 7 days until satisfactory response is obtained, up to total daily dosage of 150 to 200 mg. Or, 75 mg extended-release capsules PO to start, in morning or at bedtime; then 75 mg extended-release capsules b.i.d. if needed.
➤ **Acute gouty arthritis**
Adults and children ages 15 and older: 50 mg PO or PR t.i.d. Reduce dosage as soon as possible; then stop therapy. Don't use extended-release form.
➤ **Acute painful shoulders (bursitis or tendinitis)**
Adults and children ages 15 and older: 75 to 150 mg PO or PR daily in divided doses t.i.d. or q.i.d. for 7 to 14 days. Or, 75 mg (extended-release) PO daily or b.i.d. for 7 to 14 days.

➤ **To close a hemodynamically significant patent ductus arteriosus in premature neonates**
Neonates older than age 7 days: 0.2 mg/kg IV; then two doses of 0.25 mg/kg at 12- to 24-hour intervals.
Neonates ages 2 to 7 days: 0.2 mg/kg IV; then two doses of 0.2 mg/kg at 12- to 24-hour intervals.
Neonates younger than 48 hours: 0.2 mg/kg IV; then two doses of 0.1 mg/kg IV at 12- to 24-hour intervals.
Adjust-a-dose: If anuria or marked oliguria (urine output less than 0.6 mL/kg/hour) is evident at scheduled time of second or third dose of indomethacin for injection, don't give additional doses until lab studies indicate kidney function has returned to normal.

ADMINISTRATION
PO
• Give drug with food, milk, or antacid.
• Have patient swallow extended-release capsules whole; don't crush or cut capsules.
• Shake suspension well before use.
• Measure suspension with oral medication syringe or calibrated cup.
IV
▼ Reconstitute powder for injection with sterile water or NSS. For each 1-mg vial, add 1 or 2 mL of diluent for a solution containing 1 mg/mL or 0.5 mg/mL, respectively. Give over 20 to 30 minutes.
▼ Avoid IV bolus administration or infusion via an umbilical catheter into vessels near the superior mesenteric artery as these may cause vasoconstriction and can compromise blood flow to the intestines.
❸ *Alert:* Use only preservative-free sterile saline solution or sterile water to prepare. Never use diluents containing benzyl alcohol because it has been linked to toxicity in newborns.
▼ Because injection contains no preservatives, reconstitute drug immediately before use and discard unused solution.
▼ Watch carefully for bleeding and reduced urine output.
▼ **Incompatibilities:** None listed by manufacturer. Consult drug compatibility reference for more information.
Rectal
• If suppository is too soft, place in refrigerator for 15 minutes or run under cold water in wrapper.

Reactions in bold italics are *life-threatening*.

ACTION
May inhibit prostaglandin synthesis to produce anti-inflammatory, analgesic, and antipyretic effects.

Route	Onset	Peak	Duration
PO	30 min	2 hr	4–6 hr
IV	Immediate	Immediate	4–6 hr
PR	Unknown	Unknown	4–6 hr

Half-life: Adults (mean), 4.5 hours; neonates, 12 to 20 hours

ADVERSE REACTIONS
PO and rectal
CNS: headache, dizziness, depression, fatigue, somnolence, syncope, malaise, vertigo. **CV:** edema, *postprocedural hemorrhage.* **EENT:** tinnitus. **GI:** abdominal pain, constipation, diarrhea, dyspepsia, nausea, vomiting. **Skin:** pruritus, rash, diaphoresis. **Other:** hypersensitivity reactions, hot flush.
IV
CV: *hemorrhage,* pulmonary HTN, fluid retention. **GI:** *GI bleeding,* vomiting, abdominal distention, transient ileus, gastric perforation, necrotizing enterocolitis. **Hematologic:** decreased platelet aggregation, *DIC.* **Metabolic:** hyponatremia, *hyperkalemia, hypoglycemia.*

INTERACTIONS
Drug-drug. *ACE inhibitors (benazepril, enalaprilat), angiotensin II receptor blockers (candesartan, valsartan):* May reduce antihypertensive effects; may worsen kidney function in those with impaired kidney function. Monitor patient closely.
Aminoglycosides (amikacin, gentamicin), cyclosporine, methotrexate, pemetrexed, triamterene: May enhance toxicity of these drugs. Avoid use together.
Anticoagulants: May increase bleeding risk. Monitor patient closely.
Antihypertensives: May decrease antihypertensive effect. Monitor patient closely.
Antihypertensives, furosemide, thiazide diuretics: May impair response to both drugs. Avoid use together, if possible.
Aspirin: May increase adverse reactions, including risk of GI toxicity. Avoid use together.
Bisphosphonates: May increase risk of gastric ulceration. Monitor for symptoms of gastric irritation or GI bleeding.
Corticosteroids: May increase indomethacin adverse effects. Avoid use together.

Diflunisal, probenecid: May decrease indomethacin excretion. Watch for increased indomethacin adverse effects.
Digoxin: May prolong half-life of digoxin. Use together cautiously.
Dipyridamole: May enhance fluid retention. Avoid use together.
Drospirenone: May increase hyperkalemic effect of drospirenone. Use together cautiously.
Lithium: May increase lithium level. Monitor patient for toxicity.
Methotrexate: May increase methotrexate toxicity. Use together cautiously.
Phenytoin: May increase phenytoin level. Monitor patient closely.
Probenecid: May increase indomethacin level. Consider decreasing indomethacin dosage in small increments, if necessary.
SSRIs: May increase antiplatelet effect of indomethacin and antidepressant effect of SSRI. Consider alternative to indomethacin or monitor patient for bleeding and decreased antidepressant effect.
Drug-herb. *Alfalfa, anise, bilberry, dong quai, garlic:* May cause bleeding. Discourage use together.
White willow: Herb and drug contain similar components. Don't use together.
Drug-lifestyle. *Alcohol use:* May cause GI toxicity. Discourage use together.

EFFECTS ON LAB TEST RESULTS
• May increase potassium and BUN levels and LFT values.
• May decrease Hb level and hematocrit.
• May cause false-negative results in dexamethasone suppression test.

CONTRAINDICATIONS & CAUTIONS
• Contraindicated in patients hypersensitive to drug and in those with history of aspirin- or NSAID-induced asthma, rhinitis, or urticaria.
• Contraindicated in neonates with untreated infection, active bleeding, coagulation defects or thrombocytopenia, congenital heart disease needing patency of the ductus arteriosus, necrotizing enterocolitis, or significant kidney impairment.
Boxed Warning NSAIDs may increase risk of serious thrombotic events, including MI or stroke, which can be fatal. Risk may be greater with longer use or in patients with CV disease or risk factors for CV disease. ▪
Boxed Warning Risk of MI or stroke can occur as early as the first weeks of NSAID

use. Risk appears greater at higher doses. Use lowest effective dose for shortest duration possible. ■

Boxed Warning NSAIDs may increase risk of serious GI adverse events, including bleeding, ulceration, and perforation of the stomach or intestines, which can be fatal. These events can occur at any time during use and without warning symptoms. Older adults and patients with a prior history of peptic ulcer disease or GI bleeding are at greater risk for serious GI events. ■

⊙ Alert: Avoid use in patients with severe HF unless benefits are expected to outweigh risk of worsening HF.

• Suppositories are contraindicated in patients with history of proctitis or recent rectal bleeding.

Boxed Warning Drug is contraindicated for treatment of perioperative pain after CABG surgery. ■

• Use cautiously in older adults, patients with a history of GI disease, and those with epilepsy, parkinsonism, liver or kidney disease, CV disease, infection, and mental illness or depression.

• Safety and effectiveness of oral and suppository formulations in children ages 14 and younger haven't been established.

Dialyzable drug: Unknown.

⚠ Overdose S&S: Drowsiness, lethargy, nausea, vomiting, paresthesia, epigastric pain, GI bleeding.

PREGNANCY-LACTATION-REPRODUCTION

⊙ Alert: Use of NSAIDs at 20 weeks or later in pregnancy may cause fetal kidney dysfunction, leading to oligohydramnios and potential neonatal kidney impairment; use at 30 weeks or later in pregnancy may increase risk of premature closure of ductus arteriosus. Avoid use during pregnancy, starting at 20 weeks' gestation. If potential benefit justifies fetal risk, use lowest effective dose for shortest duration. Consider ultrasound monitoring of amniotic fluid if NSAID therapy is longer than 48 hours. Use of 81 mg of low-dose aspirin for certain pregnancy-related conditions under direction of prescriber is acceptable.

• Drug appears in human milk. Use during breastfeeding isn't recommended by most manufacturers.

• Long-term use of NSAIDs in patients of childbearing potential may be associated with

infertility that's reversible upon drug discontinuation.

NURSING CONSIDERATIONS

• Because of the high risk of adverse effects from long-term use, drug shouldn't be used routinely as analgesic or antipyretic.

⊙ Alert: Watch for and immediately evaluate signs and symptoms of MI (chest pain, shortness of breath or trouble breathing) or stroke (weakness in one part or side of the body, slurred speech).

• If ductus arteriosus reopens, a second course of one to three doses may be given. If ineffective, surgery may be needed.

• Watch for bleeding in patients receiving anticoagulants, patients with coagulation defects, and neonates.

• Monitor patient for GI adverse effects.

• Because NSAIDs impair synthesis of kidney prostaglandins, they can decrease kidney blood flow and lead to reversible kidney impairment, especially in patients with KF, HF, or liver dysfunction; in older adults; and in patients taking diuretics. Monitor these patients closely.

• Drug causes sodium retention; watch for weight gain (especially in older adults) and increased BP in patients with HTN.

• Monitor patient for rash and respiratory distress, which may indicate a hypersensitivity reaction.

• Because of their antipyretic and antiinflammatory actions, NSAIDs may mask signs and symptoms of infection.

• Monitor patient on long-term oral therapy for toxicity by conducting regular eye exams, hearing tests, CBCs, and liver and kidney function tests.

PATIENT TEACHING

• Tell patient to take oral dose with food, milk, or antacid to prevent GI upset.

⊙ Alert: Advise patient to immediately seek medical attention if chest pain, shortness of breath, trouble breathing, weakness in one part or side of the body, or slurred speech occurs.

⊙ Alert: Warn patient who is pregnant not to take NSAIDs at 20 weeks' gestation or later, unless instructed to do so by prescriber, due to fetal risk. Advise patient to discuss taking any OTC medication with pharmacist or health care provider during pregnancy.

• Alert patient that using oral form with aspirin, alcohol, other NSAIDs, or

corticosteroids may increase risk of adverse GI reactions.
• Teach patient signs and symptoms of GI bleeding (blood in vomit, urine, or stool; coffee-ground vomit; and melena). Instruct patient to immediately notify prescriber if any occur.
• Review warning signs and symptoms of liver toxicity (nausea, fatigue, lethargy, pruritus, diarrhea, jaundice, right upper quadrant tenderness, and flulike symptoms). Instruct patient to stop drug if any occur.
• Warn patient to avoid hazardous activities that require mental alertness until CNS effects are known.
• Tell patient to immediately notify prescriber if visual or hearing changes occur.
• Tell patient to notify prescriber if unexplained weight gain or edema occurs.

BIOSIMILAR DRUG

infliximab
in-FLICKS-ih-mab

Remicade

inFLIXimab-abda
Renflexis

inFLIXimab-axxq
Avsola

inFLIXimab-dyyb
Inflectra

inFLIXimab-qbtx
Ixifi

Therapeutic class: Anti-inflammatory drugs
Pharmacologic class: TNF blockers

AVAILABLE FORMS
Lyophilized powder for injection: 100-mg vials

INDICATIONS & DOSAGES
➤ **Moderately to severely active Crohn disease; reduction in number of draining enterocutaneous and rectovaginal fistulas and maintenance of fistula closure in adults with fistulizing Crohn disease**
Adults: 5 mg/kg IV infusion. Repeat at 2 and 6 weeks, then every 8 weeks thereafter. For

patients who respond and then lose their response, consider 10 mg/kg every 8 weeks. Patients who don't respond by week 14 are unlikely to respond with continued therapy; in those patients, consider stopping drug.
➤ **Ulcerative colitis**
Adults: Induction dose, 5 mg/kg IV. Repeat at 2 and 6 weeks, then every 8 weeks thereafter.
➤ **Pediatric Crohn disease; pediatric ulcerative colitis**
Children ages 6 and older: Initially, 5 mg/kg IV infusion. Repeat at 2 and 6 weeks, then every 8 weeks thereafter.
➤ **Moderately to severely active RA (in conjunction with methotrexate)**
Adults: Initially, 3 mg/kg IV infusion. Repeat at 2 and 6 weeks, then every 8 weeks thereafter. Dose may be increased to 10 mg/kg every 8 weeks, or doses may be given every 4 weeks, if response is inadequate.
➤ **Ankylosing spondylitis**
Adults: 5 mg/kg IV infusion. Repeat at 2 and 6 weeks, then every 6 weeks thereafter.
➤ **Psoriatic arthritis, with or without methotrexate**
Adults: Initially, 5 mg/kg IV infusion. Repeat at 2 and 6 weeks, then every 8 weeks thereafter.
➤ **Chronic severe plaque psoriasis**
Adults: Initially, 5 mg/kg IV. Repeat at 2 and 6 weeks, then give 5 mg/kg every 8 weeks thereafter.

ADMINISTRATION
IV
▼ Reconstitute with 10 mL sterile water for injection, using syringe with 21G or smaller needle. Don't shake; gently swirl to dissolve powder. Allow reconstituted solution to stand for 5 minutes. Solution should be colorless to light yellow and opalescent. It may also develop a few translucent particles; don't use if other types of particles develop or discoloration occurs.
▼ Dilute total volume of reconstituted drug to 250 mL with NSS for injection. Infusion concentration ranges from 0.4 to 4 mg/mL.
▼ Use an in-line, sterile, nonpyrogenic, low-protein-binding filter with a pore size smaller than 1.2 microns.
▼ Begin infusion within 3 hours of preparation and give over at least 2 hours.
▼ **Incompatibilities:** Other IV drugs. Don't infuse with other drugs.

ACTION

Binds to human TNF-alpha to neutralize its activity and inhibit its binding with receptors, thereby reducing the infiltration of inflammatory cells and TNF-alpha production in inflamed areas of the intestine.

Route	Onset	Peak	Duration
IV	Unknown	Unknown	Unknown

Half-life: 7 to 12 days.

ADVERSE REACTIONS

CNS: fatigue, fever, headache, pain. **CV:** HTN, chest pain, flushing, *bradycardia.* **EENT:** sinusitis, pharyngitis. **GI:** diarrhea, abdominal pain, dyspepsia, nausea. **GU:** UTI. **Hematologic:** anemia, *leukopenia, neutropenia.* **Hepatic:** increased ALT level. **Musculoskeletal:** arthralgia, back pain, arthritis, myalgia, bone fracture. **Respiratory:** URI, bronchitis, dyspnea, pneumonia, cough, respiratory tract allergic reaction. **Skin:** rash, pruritus, candidiasis. **Other:** hypersensitivity reactions, infusion reactions, serum sickness, development of antibodies, infection, *sepsis,* candidiasis, chills, flulike syndrome.

INTERACTIONS

Drug-drug. *CYP450 substrates (cyclosporine, theophylline, warfarin):* May normalize formation of CYP450 enzymes upon initiation or discontinuation of infliximab. Monitor effect or drug concentration; may adjust individual dosage of drug product as needed.

Live-virus vaccines: May affect normal immune response. Postpone live-virus vaccine until therapy stops. Withhold live-virus vaccines for at least 6 months in infants born to patients treated with infliximab.

Methotrexate: May decrease anti-infliximab antibody production and increase infliximab level. Monitor patient.

TNF blockers (abatacept, anakinra, golimumab, rilonacept): May increase risk of serious infections and neutropenia. Use together isn't recommended.

Tocilizumab, tofacitinib: May increase immunosuppressive effects and increase risk of infection. Avoid use together.

Drug-herb. *Echinacea:* May diminish therapeutic effect of immunosuppressants. Consider therapy modification.

EFFECTS ON LAB TEST RESULTS

• May increase liver enzyme levels.
• May decrease Hb level, hematocrit, and RBC, WBC, and platelet counts.
• May produce false-negative TB test result.
• May cause false-positive ANA test result.

CONTRAINDICATIONS & CAUTIONS

• Contraindicated in patients hypersensitive to murine proteins or other components of drug. Doses greater than 5 mg/kg are contraindicated in patients with moderate to severe HF.

Boxed Warning Drug increases risk of serious infections that may lead to hospitalization or death, especially in patients taking a concomitant immunosuppressant, such as methotrexate or a corticosteroid. Discontinue drug if serious infection or sepsis occurs. ■

Boxed Warning Carefully consider risks and benefits of treatment before initiating infliximab therapy in patients with chronic or recurrent infection. ■

Boxed Warning Lymphoma and other malignancies, some fatal, have occurred in children and adolescents treated with TNF blockers, including infliximab. ■

Boxed Warning Hepatosplenic T-cell lymphoma, a rare type of lymphoma that can be fatal, has occurred in adolescents and young adult males with inflammatory bowel disease treated with TNF blockers, including infliximab. ■

Alert: Drug increases risk of serious infections, including TB, histoplasmosis, coccidioidomycosis, blastomycosis, bacterial sepsis, *Listeria, Legionella*, and other opportunistic infections. Patients with histoplasmosis or other invasive fungal infections may present with disseminated rather than localized disease. Antigen and antibody testing for histoplasmosis may be negative in some patients with active infection. Consider antifungal therapy in patients at risk for invasive fungal infections who develop severe systemic illness.

• Depending on the product, each vial contains between 50 and 500 mg of sucrose.
• Use cautiously in older adults; in patients with active infection, a history of hematologic abnormalities, or preexisting or recent-onset CNS demyelinating or seizure disorders; and in those who have lived in regions where histoplasmosis is endemic.

Reactions in bold italics are ***life-threatening.***

• Rare cases of severe liver reactions with or without elevations in aminotransferase levels have been reported.

• Use cautiously in patients with hematologic abnormalities. Serious and sometimes fatal cases of leukopenia, neutropenia, thrombocytopenia, and pancytopenia have been reported. *Dialyzable drug:* Unknown.

PREGNANCY-LACTATION-REPRODUCTION

• Drug crosses placental barrier but it isn't known if drug causes fetal harm or affects reproductive capacity. Use during pregnancy only if clearly needed.

• Drug may be present in serum of infants up to 6 months after birth. Exposed infants may be at increased risk for infection.

• It isn't known if drug appears in human milk. Patient should discontinue breastfeeding or discontinue drug, considering importance of drug to patient.

NURSING CONSIDERATIONS

• No clinically meaningful differences exist between the biosimilar product and reference product (Remicade) based on the conditions of their use. However, these drugs aren't considered interchangeable and can't be automatically substituted.

• Premedication with antihistamines, acetaminophen, and corticosteroids may be considered at prescriber's discretion to prevent infusion-related reactions.

• Monitor for signs and symptoms of hypersensitivity reactions (urticaria, dyspnea, hypotension), which may occur during or within 2 hours of infusion and may be severe. Discontinue drug for severe reactions and treat appropriately.

⚠ Alert: Watch for infusion-related reactions (fever, chills, pruritus, urticaria, dyspnea, hypotension, HTN, chest pain) during administration and for 2 hours afterward. If an infusion-related reaction occurs, stop drug, notify prescriber, and prepare to give acetaminophen, antihistamines, corticosteroids, and epinephrine.

• Don't give live-virus vaccines to infants exposed to drug in utero for at least 6 months after birth because of increased risk of infection, including disseminated infection, which can be fatal.

• Give for Crohn disease and ulcerative colitis only after patient has an inadequate response to conventional therapy.

• Consider stopping treatment in patient who develops significant hematologic abnormalities or CNS adverse reactions.

• Notify prescriber for symptoms of new or worsening HF.

Boxed Warning Discontinue drug if serious infection or sepsis develops. ■

Boxed Warning Watch for development of lymphoma and infection. Patients with chronic Crohn disease and long-term exposure to immunosuppressants are more likely to develop lymphoma and infection. ■

• Drug may affect normal immune responses. Patient may develop autoimmune antibodies and lupuslike syndrome; stop drug if this happens. Symptoms should resolve.

Boxed Warning Drug may cause disseminated or extrapulmonary TB and fatal opportunistic infections. ■

Boxed Warning Evaluate patient for latent TB infection with a tuberculin skin test. Treat latent TB infection before therapy. ■

Boxed Warning Closely monitor for signs and symptoms of infection during and after infliximab treatment, including possible development of TB in patient who tested negative for latent TB infection before start of therapy. ■

• TNF blockers may increase risk of reactivation of HBV in patients who are chronic carriers. Patients taking concomitant immunosuppressants are at increased risk. Test for HBV infection before therapy begins. Monitor HBV carriers during and for several months after therapy. If HBV reactivation occurs, discontinue infliximab.

• Monitor patient for liver toxicity (jaundice, liver enzyme elevations 5 × ULN or more). Stop drug and closely evaluate patient if these signs or symptoms occur.

• **Look alike–sound alike:** Don't confuse Remicade with Renacidin or Rituxan. Don't confuse infliximab with rituximab or idarucizumab. Don't confuse Inflectra with Injectafer.

PATIENT TEACHING

Boxed Warning Inform patient that TB testing will occur before therapy. Instruct patient to immediately report signs and symptoms of infection. ■

Boxed Warning Counsel patient about risk of lymphoma and other malignancies. ■

• Tell patient about infusion-reaction symptoms and adverse effects and the need to report them promptly.

• Advise patient to report all adverse reactions and to seek immediate medical attention for signs and symptoms of infection (persistent fever, cough, shortness of breath, fatigue, unusual bleeding, bruising).

• Instruct patients to seek medical attention for signs and symptoms of liver toxicity.

• Instruct patient to report pregnancy or plans to become pregnant before start of therapy. Tell patient not to breastfeed during therapy.

• Tell patient to alert prescriber to therapy before receiving vaccines.

• Advise patient or caregiver to make sure all vaccines are up-to-date before therapy.

SAFETY ALERT!

insulin degludec–liraglutide
IN-su-lin de-GLOO-dek/lir-ah-GLOO-tide

Xultophy 100/3.6

Therapeutic class: Antidiabetics
Pharmacologic class: Insulins–glucagon-like peptide-1 receptor agonists

AVAILABLE FORMS
Injection (prefilled pen): 100 units insulin degludec/3.6 mg liraglutide per mL in 3-mL pens

INDICATIONS & DOSAGES
➤ **Adjunct to diet and exercise to improve glycemic control in patients with type 2 diabetes**
Adults: In patients naive to basal insulin or a glucagon-like peptide-1 (GLP-1) agonist, initially give 10 units (insulin degludec 10 units/liraglutide 0.36 mg) subcut once daily. In patients currently on basal insulin or a GLP-1 agonist, initially give 16 units (insulin degludec 16 units/liraglutide 0.58 mg) subcut once daily. Titrate dosage upward or downward by 2 units (insulin degludec 2 units/liraglutide 0.072 mg) every 3 to 4 days until desired fasting plasma glucose level is achieved. Maximum dose, 50 units (insulin degludec 50 units/liraglutide 1.8 mg/day).
Adjust-a-dose: Titrate dosage to minimize risk of hypoglycemia or hyperglycemia; with changes in physical activity or meal pattern; in patients with kidney or liver function; during acute illness; and when drug is used with other drugs that affect glucose level.

ADMINISTRATION
Subcutaneous
• Discontinue other liraglutide products and basal insulins before start of therapy.

⚠️ *Alert:* Pens are for single-patient use only; never share pens.

• Dose counter displays numbers for insulin units. Numbers display for even units and lines display for odd units.

• Don't mix this product with other insulin products or solutions.

• Give at the same time each day with or without food.

• Visually inspect drug for particulate matter and discoloration before administration.

• Inject subcut into thigh, upper arm, or abdomen; don't give IV or IM or use in an insulin infusion pump.

• Rotate injection sites within same region from one injection to the next to reduce risk of lipodystrophy.

• Don't split the dose; give once daily.

• Keep needle in patient's skin after pressing dose button and allowing dose counter to return to "0" while slowly counting to 6 to allow delivery of full dose.

• If dose is missed, omit missed dose and resume drug at next scheduled dose. Don't give an extra injection or increase dosage to make up for the missed dose.

• If more than 3 days have elapsed since the last dose, reinitiate drug at starting dose to avoid GI symptoms associated with treatment reinitiation.

• Before first use, store pens between 36° and 46° F (2° and 8° C) until expiration date printed on label. Don't freeze.

• After first use, pens can be stored for 21 days at controlled room temperature (59° to 86° F [15° to 30° C]) or in refrigerator (36° to 46° F [2° to 8° C]); keep all pens away from direct heat and light.

ACTION
Insulin degludec lowers blood glucose level by stimulating peripheral glucose uptake, especially by skeletal muscle and fat, and by inhibiting liver glucose production. Insulin also inhibits lipolysis and proteolysis while enhancing protein synthesis. Liraglutide is a GLP-1 receptor agonist that increases glucose-dependent insulin release, decreases glucagon secretion, and slows gastric emptying.

Reactions in bold italics are *life-threatening*.

Route	Onset	Peak	Duration
Subcut	Unknown	Unknown	Unknown

Half-life: Insulin degludec, 25 hours; liraglutide, 13 hours.

ADVERSE REACTIONS

CNS: headache. **CV:** peripheral edema. **EENT:** nasopharyngitis. **GI:** nausea, diarrhea, gallbladder disease. **Metabolic:** *hypoglycemia, hypokalemia,* weight gain, increased lipase level. **Respiratory:** URI. **Skin:** injection-site reactions, lipodystrophy. **Other:** antibody formation, hypersensitivity reactions.

INTERACTIONS

Drug-drug. *ACE inhibitors, antidiabetics, ARBs, disopyramide, fibrates, fluoxetine, MAO inhibitors, octreotide, pentoxifylline, pramlintide, salicylates, sulfonamide antibiotics:* May increase hypoglycemia risk. Closely monitor glucose level, and adjust Xultophy dosage accordingly.
Atypical antipsychotics (olanzapine, clozapine), corticosteroids, danazol, diuretics, estrogens, glucagon, isoniazid, niacin, oral contraceptives, phenothiazines, progestogens in oral contraceptives, protease inhibitors, somatropin, sympathomimetic agents (albuterol, epinephrine, terbutaline), thyroid hormones: May decrease glucose-lowering effects. Closely monitor glucose level, and adjust Xultophy dosage accordingly.
Beta blockers, clonidine: May blunt or mask signs and symptoms of hypoglycemia. Closely monitor glucose level.
Beta blockers, clonidine, lithium salts, pentamidine: May increase risk of hypoglycemia or hyperglycemia. Closely monitor glucose level and adjust Xultophy dosage as needed.
Oral medications: May affect gastric absorption of other oral medications taken at the same time. Monitor effectiveness of oral medications.
Potassium-lowering drugs (loop and thiazide diuretics, theophylline): May increase risk of hypokalemia. Monitor potassium level.
Thiazolidinediones (TZDs; pioglitazone, rosiglitazone): May cause fluid retention that can lead to HF. Monitor patient closely and adjust or stop TZDs as clinically indicated.
Drug-lifestyle. *Alcohol use:* May alter glucose level and insulin needs. Discourage use together.

Smoking: May decrease insulin absorption and increase insulin resistance. Discourage use together.

EFFECTS ON LAB TEST RESULTS

- May increase bilirubin, calcitonin, lipase, and amylase levels.
- May decrease potassium level.
- May develop antibodies against insulin degludec and liraglutide.

CONTRAINDICATIONS & CAUTIONS

Boxed Warning Liraglutide causes dose-dependent and treatment duration-dependent thyroid C-cell tumors at clinically relevant exposures in rats and mice. It isn't known if drug causes thyroid C-cell tumors, including medullary thyroid carcinoma (MTC), in humans, as the human relevance of liraglutide-induced rodent thyroid C-cell tumors hasn't been determined. ∎

Boxed Warning Contraindicated in patients with a personal or family history of MTC and in patients with multiple endocrine neoplasia syndrome type 2 (MEN 2). ∎

- Contraindicated during episodes of hypoglycemia and in patients with hypersensitivity to insulin degludec or liraglutide.
- Severe, life-threatening allergic reactions, including anaphylaxis, angioedema, bronchospasm, urticaria, rash, and pruritus, have been reported. If hypersensitivity reactions occur, discontinue drug. Use cautiously in patients with a history of angioedema resulting from use of another GLP-1 receptor agonist.
- Drug isn't recommended as first-line therapy for patients who have inadequate glycemic control with diet and exercise because of the uncertain relevance of the rodent C-cell tumor findings in humans.
- Use cautiously in patients at risk for pancreatitis. Pancreatitis has been observed in patients taking liraglutide. Drug hasn't been studied in patients with a history of pancreatitis; consider other antidiabetic therapies in these patients.
- Use cautiously in patients with visual impairment, who may rely on audible clicks to dial their dose.
- Drug isn't indicated for use in patients with type 1 diabetes or diabetic ketoacidosis.
- Drug isn't indicated for use in combination with prandial insulin.

• Drug isn't recommended for use in combination with other products containing liraglutide or other GLP-1 receptor agonists.
• Postmarketing reports indicate incidences of AKI and worsening of CKD, sometimes requiring hemodialysis, in patients treated with liraglutide. In most cases, these events occurred in patients who experienced nausea, vomiting, diarrhea, or dehydration.
• Drug can cause hypokalemia that, if untreated, can cause respiratory paralysis, ventricular arrhythmias, and death.
• Safety and effectiveness in children haven't been established.
• Use cautiously in older adults because they may be more sensitive to drug's effects.
Dialyzable drug: No.
⚠ *Overdose S&S:* Hypoglycemia, hypokalemia, GI adverse reactions (severe nausea and vomiting).

PREGNANCY-LACTATION-REPRODUCTION
• Animal studies suggest drug may increase fetal adverse events. Use during pregnancy only if potential benefit justifies fetal risk.
• It isn't known if drug appears in human milk. Consider both potential adverse effects to infant who is breastfed and developmental and health benefits of breastfeeding.

NURSING CONSIDERATIONS
• Adjust dosages cautiously and only under medical supervision with frequent glucose monitoring.
• Monitor patient for dehydration. Drug can cause dehydration due to GI adverse reactions; take precautions to avoid fluid depletion.
• Monitor patient for signs and symptoms of pancreatitis (persistent severe abdominal pain that may radiate to the back, with or without vomiting). Discontinue drug for confirmed pancreatitis.
• Monitor patient for URI and signs and symptoms of gallbladder disease (stomach pain, fever, nausea, vomiting, jaundice).
• Monitor for hypersensitivity reactions (urticaria, rash, pruritus, anaphylactic reaction, angioedema).
• Evaluate patient with changes to thyroid gland or significantly elevated serum calcitonin level.
• Monitor kidney function and blood glucose, amylase, and lipase levels.
• Monitor serum potassium level in patient at risk for hypokalemia (patients taking potassium-lowering medication or medications sensitive to potassium level).
• Monitor patient for lipodystrophy; hyperglycemia may result from alterations at injection site.
• *Look alike–sound alike:* Don't confuse insulin degludec with other insulin products.

PATIENT TEACHING
• Explain that dose selector on pen shows the number of insulin units to be injected. Instruct patient to consult manufacturer's instructions to determine how much drug is left in pen. Dose selector should read "0" after dose delivery.
• Teach patient how to use dosage pen and how to administer drug, including rotating injection sites.
• Warn patient against sharing pens with other individuals because of risk of contracting bloodborne pathogens.
• Instruct patient not to take more than 50 units of drug per day and not to use with other GLP-1 receptor agonists.
• Advise patient not to split doses into two injections and not to mix other insulin or GLP-1 products in the same syringe.
• Emphasize to patient that regular glucose monitoring will be necessary and that glucose level will need to be checked more carefully with changes in amount of activity, meal pattern, and acute illness.
• Caution patient that dosage changes should only be made under medical supervision.
• Teach patient the signs and symptoms of hypoglycemia (confusion, dizziness, feeling shaky, rapid pulse) and how to manage it.
• Instruct patient to report all adverse effects and to immediately report edema, chest pain, or palpitations.
Boxed Warning Inform patient of risk of thyroid tumors, including cancer. Instruct patient to immediately report neck lump or swelling, hoarseness, trouble swallowing, or shortness of breath. ∎
• Warn patient to immediately report severe pain in abdomen that may or may not radiate to the back (with or without vomiting), as this type of pain may indicate pancreatitis.
• Instruct patient to report signs and symptoms of liver and gallbladder disorders.
• Counsel patient to avoid becoming dehydrated, as AKI may occur.

SAFETY ALERT!

insulin glargine–lixisenatide
IN-su-lin GLAR-jeen/lix-i-SEN-a-tide

Soliqua 100/33

Therapeutic class: Antidiabetics
Pharmacologic class: Long-acting insulins–glucagon-like peptide-1 (GLP-1) receptor agonists

AVAILABLE FORMS
Injection: insulin glargine 100 units/mL and lixisenatide 33 mcg/mL in 3-mL pens

INDICATIONS & DOSAGES
➤ **Adjunct to diet and exercise to improve glycemic control in patients with type 2 diabetes**
Adults naive to basal insulin or to a GLP-1 receptor agonist, currently on a GLP-1 receptor agonist, or currently on less than 30 units of basal insulin daily: Initially, 15 units (insulin glargine 15 units/lixisenatide 5 mcg) subcut once daily within the hour before first meal of the day.
Adults inadequately controlled on 30 to 60 units of basal insulin, with or without a GLP-1 receptor agonist: Initially, 30 units (insulin glargine 30 units/lixisenatide 10 mcg) subcut once daily within the hour before the first meal of the day.
Adjust-a-dose: Titrate dosage up or down by 2 to 4 units every week based on patient's metabolic needs, blood glucose monitoring results, and glycemic goal until desired fasting glucose level is achieved. Dosage titration may also be needed with changes in activity, meal pattern, or kidney or liver function; during acute illness or stress; or when used with other medications that affect glucose level. Use alternative antidiabetic products if patients require a Soliqua 100/33 daily dosage below 15 units or above 60 units. Maximum dosage, 60 units (insulin glargine 60 units/lixisenatide 20 mcg) daily.

ADMINISTRATION
Subcutaneous
• Discontinue therapy with a GLP-1 receptor agonist or basal insulin before starting Soliqua 100/33.
• Prefilled pen delivers doses from 15 to 60 units in a single injection.

• Refer to manufacturer's instructions and perform a safety test before each injection to check that pen and needle are working correctly and to ensure that correct dose will be delivered.
• Inspect pen before use. Solution should be clear and colorless to almost colorless.
• Inject into abdominal area, thigh, or upper arm, rotating injection sites within the same region to reduce risk of lipodystrophy.
• Give dose within the hour before first meal of the day.
• Don't administer IV, IM, or via an insulin pump.
• Don't dilute or mix with other insulins or solution.
• Don't administer drug in split doses.
• Remove needle after each injection and store pen without needle attached. Always use a new needle for each injection to prevent contamination.
• If dose is missed, resume the once-daily regimen as prescribed with the next scheduled dose. Don't administer extra dose or increase dose to make up for missed dose.
🕙 *Alert:* Pen is for single-patient use only because of risk of transmission of bloodborne pathogens (even if needle is changed).
• Store drug in refrigerator at 36° to 46° F (2° to 8° C) before first use. Don't freeze. Discard drug if pen has been frozen. Protect from light.
• After first use, store pen at room temperature below 77° F (25° C). Replace pen cap after each use to protect from light. Discard pen 28 days after first use.

ACTION
Insulin glargine lowers blood glucose level by stimulating peripheral glucose uptake and by inhibiting liver glucose production. Lixisenatide increases glucose-dependent insulin release, decreases glucagon secretion, and slows gastric emptying.

Route	Onset	Peak	Duration
Subcut	Insulin glargine: 3–4 hr	Insulin glargine: no pronounced peak Lixisenatide: 2.5–3 hr	Insulin glargine: about 24 hr

Half-life: 3 hours (lixisenatide).

ADVERSE REACTIONS
CNS: headache. **CV:** peripheral edema. **EENT:** nasopharyngitis. **GI:** diarrhea, nausea,

vomiting. **Metabolic:** *hypoglycemia, hypokalemia,* weight gain. **Respiratory:** URI. **Skin:** injection-site reactions, lipodystrophy. **Other:** antibody development, hypersensitivity reactions.

INTERACTIONS

Drug-drug. *ACE inhibitors, antidiabetics, ARBs, disopyramide, fibrates, fluoxetine, MAO inhibitors, pentoxifylline, pramlintide, salicylates, somatostatin analogues (octreotide), sulfonamide antibiotics:* May increase risk of hypoglycemia. Closely monitor glucose level, and adjust dosage as necessary.
Acetaminophen, antibiotics and other oral medications dependent on threshold concentrations for efficacy: Lixisenatide may reduce rate of absorption of coadministered oral drugs. Give other drugs at least 1 hour before Soliqua 100/33.
Atypical antipsychotics (clozapine, olanzapine), corticosteroids, danazol, diuretics, estrogens, glucagon, isoniazid, niacin, phenothiazines, protease inhibitors, somatropin, sympathomimetic agents (albuterol, epinephrine, terbutaline), thyroid hormones: May decrease blood glucose-lowering effect of Soliqua 100/33. Closely monitor glucose level, and adjust Soliqua 100/33 dosage as needed.
Beta blockers, clonidine: May mask signs and symptoms of hypoglycemia. Closely monitor glucose level, and adjust Soliqua 100/33 dosage as needed.
Beta blockers, clonidine, lithium salts: May increase or decrease blood glucose-lowering effect of Soliqua 100/33. Closely monitor glucose level, and adjust Soliqua 100/33 dosage as necessary.
GLP-1 receptor agonists: May increase risk of overdose and hypoglycemia. Use together isn't recommended.
Oral contraceptives, progesterones: May delay rate of contraceptive absorption. Patient should take contraceptive at least 1 hour before or 11 hours after Soliqua 100/33.
Pentamidine: May cause hypoglycemia, which may be followed by hyperglycemia. Closely monitor glucose level, and adjust Soliqua 100/33 dosage as needed.
Thiazolidinediones (TZDs; pioglitazone, rosiglitazone): May cause fluid retention that can lead to HF. Monitor patient closely and adjust or stop TZDs, if indicated.

Drug-lifestyle. *Alcohol use:* May increase or decrease blood glucose-lowering effect of Soliqua 100/33. Discourage use together. *Smoking:* May decrease insulin absorption and increase insulin resistance. Discourage use together.

EFFECTS ON LAB TEST RESULTS

• May decrease glucose, HbA_{1c}, and potassium levels.
• May cause an immune response and positive antibodies.

CONTRAINDICATIONS & CAUTIONS

• Contraindicated during hypoglycemia episodes.
• Contraindicated in patients hypersensitive to either of the active drug substances or their components.
• Rarely, allergic reactions (urticaria, angioedema, anaphylaxis, bronchospasm, hypotension, shock) have been reported. Use cautiously in patients with a history of anaphylaxis or angioedema with use of another GLP-1 receptor agonist.
• Drug isn't indicated for use in patients with type 1 diabetes or for treatment of diabetic ketoacidosis.
• Acute pancreatitis has been reported with GLP-1 receptor agonists. Consider other antidiabetics in patients with history of pancreatitis.
• Acute cholelithiasis or cholecystitis has been reported with GLP-1 receptor agonists.
• Not recommended in patients with eGFR less than 15 mL/minute/1.73 m^2 or in patients with severe gastroparesis. Consider other antidiabetics.
• Use with prandial insulin hasn't been studied.
• Use cautiously in patients with visual impairment, who may rely on audible clicks to dial their dose.
• Safety and effectiveness in children haven't been established.
• Use cautiously in older adults. Initial dosing, dose increments, and maintenance dosing should be conservative to avoid hypoglycemia.
Dialyzable drug: Unknown.
⚠ *Overdose S&S: Insulin glargine:* hypoglycemia, hypokalemia. *Lixisenatide:* increased incidence of GI disorders.

PREGNANCY-LACTATION-REPRODUCTION
- Exposure to lixisenatide during pregnancy may cause fetal harm. Use during pregnancy only if potential benefits justify fetal risk.
- It isn't known if insulin glargine or lixisenatide appears in human milk. Effects on milk production and infant who is breastfed are unknown. Weigh benefits of breastfeeding and patient's clinical need for drug against potential adverse effects on infant.

NURSING CONSIDERATIONS
- Monitor patient for signs and symptoms of hypoglycemia; the long-acting effect of insulin glargine may delay recovery from hypoglycemia.
- Frequently monitor blood glucose level during dosage changes, which may predispose patient to hypoglycemia or hyperglycemia. Adjust concomitant oral antidiabetics as needed.
- Always check insulin label before giving drug, as accidental mix-ups among insulin products have been reported.
- Increase frequency of glucose monitoring with changes to meal pattern or physical activity and in patients with kidney or liver impairment and hypoglycemia unawareness.
- Monitor patient for signs and symptoms of pancreatitis and cholecystitis (persistent severe abdominal pain, sometimes radiating to the back, with or without vomiting). For suspected pancreatitis, discontinue drug and treat appropriately. For confirmed pancreatitis, don't restart drug.
- AKI and worsening of CKD have been reported. Monitor kidney function and watch for dehydration due to GI adverse effects when starting drug or increasing dosage in patients with kidney impairment and in those reporting severe GI reactions. Closely monitor fluid status.
- Monitor patient for worsening glycemic control or failure to achieve targeted glycemic control, significant injection-site reactions, or allergic reactions, which may indicate antibody formation. Consider alternative antidiabetic therapy.
- Insulin-containing products may cause potassium to shift into the intracellular space, resulting in hypokalemia. Monitor potassium level in patient at risk for hypokalemia (patients using potassium-lowering drugs or drugs sensitive to serum potassium level).

- *Look alike–sound alike:* Don't confuse insulin glargine with other insulin products.

PATIENT TEACHING
- Inform patient that serious hypersensitivity reactions, including anaphylaxis, have been reported. Instruct patient to stop drug and immediately seek medical attention for signs and symptoms of hypersensitivity reactions.
- Advise patient of risk of pancreatitis and acute gallbladder disease. Instruct patient to discontinue drug and report persistent abdominal pain, with or without vomiting.
- Teach patient to never share the pen with another person (even if needle is changed) because of risk of transmission of bloodborne pathogens.
- Inform patient that hypoglycemia is the most common adverse reaction, and review signs and symptoms of hypoglycemia. Explain that regimen changes can predispose patient to hypoglycemia or hyperglycemia.
- Warn that hypoglycemia may impair mental alertness. Instruct patient to use caution while driving or operating machinery.
- Advise patient of risk of dehydration due to GI adverse reactions. Instruct patient to take precautions to avoid fluid depletion.
- Inform patient of risk of worsening kidney function, which may require dialysis.
- Instruct patient to always check label before each injection to avoid medication errors due to confusion with other insulin products.
- Caution patient that administering more than 60 units of Soliqua 100/33 daily or concurrent use with other GLP-1 inhibitors can result in lixisenatide overdose.
- Instruct patient on self-management procedures, including glucose monitoring and management of hypoglycemia and hyperglycemia.
- Teach patient how to handle special situations, such as concurrent illness, stress, or emotional disturbances; inadequate or missed insulin dose; inadvertent administration of an increased insulin dose; inadequate food intake; and missed meals.
- Instruct patient on proper administration and handling. Caution patient not to dilute drug or mix drug with other insulin products or solutions.
- Advise patient to report pregnancy or plans to become pregnant or breastfeed.

SAFETY ALERT!

insulins (fixed combinations)
IN-su-lins

insulin lispro protamine–insulin lispro
HumaLOG Mix 50/50, HumaLOG Mix 75/25

isophane insulin suspension–insulin injection combinations
HumuLIN 70/30 ◊, NovoLIN 70/30 ◊

insulin aspart (rDNA origin) protamine suspension–insulin aspart (rDNA origin) injection
NovoLOG Mix 70/30

Therapeutic class: Antidiabetics
Pharmacologic class: Insulins

AVAILABLE FORMS
Injection: Humalog Mix 50/50 (50% insulin lispro protamine suspension and 50% insulin lispro) and 75/25 (75% insulin lispro protamine suspension and 25% insulin lispro) 100 units/mL (U-100) in 10-mL vials, 3-mL prefilled pens
Injection: Humulin 70/30 (70% isophane insulin suspension and 30% regular insulin) 100 units/mL (U-100) in 3-mL and 10-mL vials, 3-mL prefilled pens
Injection: Novolog Mix 70/30 (70% insulin aspart protamine suspension and 30% insulin aspart) 100 units/mL (U-100) in 10-mL vials, 3-mL prefilled pens
Injection: Novolin 70/30 (70% isophane insulin suspension and 30% regular insulin) 100 units/mL (U-100) in 10-mL vials, 3-mL prefilled pens

INDICATIONS & DOSAGES
Adjust-a-dose (for all indications): Individualize dosage based on metabolic needs, blood glucose monitoring, and glycemic control goal. Insulin requirements may be altered during acute illness, emotional distress, or stress. Adjust as needed in older adults, in patients with kidney or liver dysfunction, in patients with obesity, with changes in physical activity or meal pattern, during puberty, and in patients concurrently taking drugs that lower blood glucose level. Refer to manufacturer's instructions for dosage adjustments when converting from other insulin regimens and formulations.

➤ **To improve glycemic control in patients with diabetes**
Adults: For Novolog Mix 70/30, individualize dosage and give subcut b.i.d. within 15 minutes before a meal or, in type 2 diabetes, give up to 15 minutes after start of a meal.
Adults: For Humalog Mix 50/50 and 75/25, individualize dosage and give subcut b.i.d. within 15 minutes before a meal.
Adults: For Humulin 70/30, individualize dosage and give subcut typically b.i.d. about 30 to 45 minutes before a meal.
Adults and children: For Novolin 70/30, individualize dosage and give subcut b.i.d. about 30 minutes before a meal.

ADMINISTRATION
Subcutaneous
• Inspect vials and syringes. Drug should appear uniformly white and cloudy. Don't use if it looks clear or contains solid particles.
• Administer all insulin mixtures at room temperature.
• Don't freeze vials or pens; discard if frozen.
• Drug is a suspension; administer only subcut, never IV.
• Don't use in insulin infusion pumps.
• Don't mix with other insulins.
• Keep away from direct heat and sunlight.
• Discard insulin exposed to temperatures above 86° F (30° C).
• Follow product-specific pen device directions for preparation and administration.
• Rotate injection sites to reduce risk of lipodystrophy.
• Give subcut into thighs, arms, buttocks, or abdomen.
🕒 *Alert:* Multidose pens are for single-patient use only. Never share pens (even if needle is changed). Clearly label with patient-identifying information where it won't obstruct dosing window, warning, or other product information.
Novolog Mix 70/30
• Keep all unopened Novolog Mix 70/30 refrigerated between 36° and 46° F (2° and 8° C) until expiration date.
• Once multidose vial is opened or has been unopened but stored at room temperature, use within 28 days.
• Once a Novolog Mix 70/30 FlexPen has been punctured, keep it at temperature below 86° F (30° C) for up to 14 days. Don't store

a Novolog Mix 70/30 FlexPen that's in use in refrigerator.

Humulin 70/30
• Discard opened or unopened vials stored at room temperature after 31 days.
• Store unopened pen or KwikPen in refrigerator at 36° to 46° F (2° to 8° C). Discard unopened pens stored at room temperature after 10 days.
• Store opened pen or KwikPen at room temperature; discard after 10 days, even if syringe contains insulin.

Novolin 70/30
• Store unopened vials in refrigerator at 36° to 46° F (2° to 8° C).
• If refrigeration isn't possible, may keep unopened vials at room temperature for up to 6 weeks (42 days), if temperature is at or below 77° F (25° C). Keep unopened vials in carton to protect from light.
• If unopened vials are stored in refrigerator, follow expiration date on label.
• Keep open vials at room temperature.
• Throw away open vial after 6 weeks (42 days) of use, even if insulin remains in vial.
• Store FlexPen at room temperature (up to 86° F [30° C]) for up to 28 days

Humalog Mix 75/25 and Humalog Mix 50/50
• Refrigerate vials and pens at 36° to 46° F (2° to 8° C) until ready to use.
• Unrefrigerated (below 86° F [30° C]) vials must be used within 28 days or discarded.
• Unrefrigerated (below 86° F [30° C]) KwikPen and pen must be used within 10 days or discarded, even if syringe contains insulin.

ACTION
Regulates glucose metabolism by stimulating peripheral glucose uptake and inhibiting liver glucose production.

Route	Onset	Peak	Duration
Subcut (Novolog Mix 70/30)	10–20 min	1.8–3.6 hr	Up to 24 hr
Subcut (Humulin 70/30)	30–90 min	2.2 hr	Up to 24 hr
Subcut (Humalog Mix 75/25 and 50/50)	15 min	60 min	11–22 hr
Subcut (Novolin 70/30)	30 min	0.8–10 hr	18–24 hr

Half-life: Novolog Mix 70/30, 8 to 9 hours; Humulin 70/30 and Novolin 70/30, unknown; Humalog Mix 50/50 and 75/25, unknown.

ADVERSE REACTIONS
CNS: headache, neuropathy. **CV:** peripheral edema. **EENT:** pharyngitis, rhinitis. **GI:** abdominal pain, diarrhea, nausea, dyspepsia. **Metabolic:** *hypoglycemia, hypokalemia,* weight gain. **Musculoskeletal:** myalgia. **Respiratory:** bronchitis, cough, URI. **Skin:** lipodystrophy, injection-site reactions, rash. **Other:** hypersensitivity reactions, insulin antibody production, flulike syndrome, infection.

INTERACTIONS
Drug-drug. *ACE inhibitors, antidiabetics (oral), ARBs, disopyramide, fibrates, fluoxetine, MAO inhibitors, octreotide, pentoxifylline, pramlintide, salicylates, sulfonamide antibiotics:* May increase risk of hypoglycemia. Closely monitor glucose level, and adjust insulin dosage as needed.
Atypical antipsychotics, corticosteroids, danazol, diuretics, estrogens, glucagon, hormonal contraceptives, isoniazid, niacin, phenothiazines, protease inhibitors, sympathomimetics (albuterol, epinephrine, terbutaline), somatropin, thyroid hormones: May decrease blood glucose-lowering effects. Closely monitor glucose level, and adjust insulin dosage as needed.
Beta blockers, clonidine: May mask signs and symptoms of hypoglycemia. Avoid concurrent use, if possible, or monitor patient closely.
Beta blockers, clonidine, lithium salts, pentamidine: May cause hypoglycemia or hyperglycemia. Closely monitor glucose level.
Drugs that lower potassium level (diuretics) or affect potassium level (IV insulin): May increase risk of hypokalemia. Monitor potassium level.
Thiazolidinediones (TZDs; pioglitazone, rosiglitazone): May cause fluid retention that can lead to HF. Monitor patient closely and adjust or stop TZDs as clinically indicated.
Drug-herb. *Ginseng:* May increase drug's effects. Discourage use together.
Drug-lifestyle. *Alcohol use:* May cause hyperglycemia or hypoglycemia. Closely monitor glucose level. Discourage concurrent use.

EFFECTS ON LAB TEST RESULTS
• May decrease blood glucose and potassium levels.
• May develop antibodies that react with human insulin.

CONTRAINDICATIONS & CAUTIONS
• Contraindicated during episodes of hypoglycemia or ketoacidosis.
• Contraindicated in patients with history of hypersensitivity to drug or its components. Severe, life-threatening, generalized allergy, including anaphylaxis, can occur with insulin use.
• Changes in insulin or oral antidiabetic dosages may affect glycemic control and should be made only under medical supervision.
• Use cautiously in patients susceptible to hypokalemia. Untreated hypokalemia can cause respiratory paralysis, ventricular arrhythmias, and death.
• Hypoglycemia is the most common adverse reaction; signs and symptoms may differ. Severe hypoglycemia can cause seizures and may be life-threatening or fatal. Hypoglycemia can occur suddenly. Risk is greater in patients with kidney or liver impairment and increases with intensity of glycemic control; changes in glycemic treatment, meal pattern, or physical activity; and concomitant use of certain medications.
• Use pens cautiously in patients with visual impairment, who may rely on audible clicks to dial their dose.
• Use cautiously in older adults, who may be at increased risk for adverse effects. Signs and symptoms of hypoglycemia may be more difficult to recognize in these patients.
• Safety and effectiveness in children haven't been determined, except with Novolin 70/30.
Dialyzable drug: Unknown.
⚠ *Overdose S&S:* Hypoglycemia, hypokalemia.

PREGNANCY-LACTATION-REPRODUCTION
• Use cautiously during pregnancy and only if clearly needed.
• Closely monitor blood glucose level in patients who are pregnant, in patients who have recently given birth, and in patients who are breastfeeding; insulin requirements may change.
• It isn't known if insulin appears in human milk. Use cautiously during breastfeeding.

NURSING CONSIDERATIONS
• The time course of the action of insulin mixtures may vary among patients and in the same patient depending on time of day, injection site, blood supply, temperature, and physical activity.

• Observe injection sites for reactions, such as redness, swelling, itching, and burning. These reactions should resolve within a few days or weeks.
• Assess patient and notify prescriber of signs and symptoms of hypoglycemia (diaphoresis, shaking, trembling, confusion, headache, irritability, hunger, rapid, pulse, nausea) and hyperglycemia (drowsiness, fruity breath odor, frequent urination, thirst).
• Signs and symptoms of hypoglycemia may occur in patients with diabetes regardless of glucose level.
• Symptom awareness may be decreased in patients with long-standing diabetes, diabetic nerve disease, kidney disease, or liver impairment and in patients who have experienced recurrent hypoglycemia. Treat according to individual facility protocol, if necessary.
• May treat mild episodes of hypoglycemia with oral glucose. May treat more severe episodes of hypoglycemia, such as coma, seizure, or neurologic impairment, with IM or subcut glucagon or concentrated IV glucose.
• Monitor blood glucose level and adjust insulin dosages as needed with medical supervision.
• Closely monitor patient also taking other medications because other drugs can mask signs and symptoms of hypoglycemia or cause an increase or decrease in blood glucose level.
• Increase frequency of glucose monitoring in patient who is acutely ill, is under emotional stress, or has a change in diet, exercise, or medication regimen. These situations may affect the rate of insulin absorption.
• Increase frequency of glucose monitoring when initiating therapy or when changes in insulin strength, dosage, manufacturer, or type or method of administration are made. Such changes may affect glycemic control and increase risk of hypoglycemia.
• Monitor potassium level in patient at risk for hypokalemia (those receiving potassium-depleting drugs or IV insulin).
• Monitor patient for generalized allergic reactions, rash (including pruritus) over entire body, shortness of breath, wheezing, hypotension, rapid pulse, diaphoresis, and anaphylaxis.
• Periodically measure HbA_{1c} level.
• *Look alike–sound alike:* Don't confuse Novolog with Novolin. Don't confuse Humalog with Humulin.

Reactions in bold italics are *life-threatening*.

PATIENT TEACHING

• Caution patient not to mix insulin combination products with other insulins.

🜂 *Alert:* Warn patient not to share multidose pen with other people (even if needle is changed) because of risk of bloodborne pathogen transmission, including HIV and hepatitis.

• Advise patient that hypoglycemic episodes can impair the ability to concentrate and react; advise patient to use caution while driving and operating machinery.

• Instruct patient to keep hard candy or glucose tablets on hand to treat mild cases of hypoglycemia.

• Advise patient to keep a log of glucose levels.

• Instruct patient on long-term sequelae of improperly managed diabetes.

• Recommend patient carry identification or wear jewelry indicating that patient has diabetes.

• Warn that allergic and hypersensitivity reactions can occur, including injection-site reactions (local pain, redness, swelling). Instruct patient to report symptoms to health care provider. Review signs and symptoms of anaphylaxis, and instruct patient to promptly seek emergency medical attention if any occur.

• Instruct patient on self-management procedures, including glucose monitoring, proper preparation and administration techniques, and management of hypoglycemia and hyperglycemia.

• Warn patient about special situations, such as concurrent conditions (illness, stress, or emotional disturbances), inadequate or skipped insulin dose, inadvertent administration of an increased insulin dose, inadequate food intake, and skipped meals.

• Caution patient to inform prescriber of pregnancy or plans to become pregnant.

• Advise patient that insulin requirements may change during pregnancy and after childbirth.

• Teach patient that alcohol and some medications may increase or decrease glucose level. Advise patient to inform prescriber of all medications and supplements being taken.

• Caution patient not to stop insulin abruptly or change amount taken without consulting prescriber.

• Advise patient that any insulin change should be made cautiously and only under medical supervision. Changes in insulin strength, manufacturer, type (regular, NPH,

or insulin analogues), species (animal, human), or method of manufacture (rDNA versus animal-source insulin) may result in the need for a dosage change. Dosage of concomitant oral antidiabetic may need adjustment.

• Teach patient to give insulin at appropriate time around a meal, depending on product.

• Instruct patient to rotate injection sites to prevent lipodystrophy.

• Teach patient to store insulin products properly, depending on individual products.

• Explain importance of checking insulin label before each injection, as accidental mix-ups among insulin types have been reported.

SAFETY ALERT!

insulins (intermediate-acting)

IN-su-lins

isophane insulin suspension (NPH)

HumuLIN N ◇, HumuLIN N KwikPen ◇, NovoLIN N ◇, NovoLIN N FlexPen ◇

Therapeutic class: Antidiabetics
Pharmacologic class: Insulins

AVAILABLE FORMS

Injection: 100 units/mL in 3-mL and 10-mL vials, 3-mL prefilled pens (Humulin N); 100 units/mL in 10-mL vials, 3-mL prefilled pens (Novolin N)

INDICATIONS & DOSAGES

➤ **To improve glycemic control in type 1 or type 2 diabetes**

Adults and children: Individualized dosage given subcut once or twice daily.

Adjust-a-dose: Individualize dosage based on metabolic needs, blood glucose monitoring, and glycemic control goal. Insulin requirements may be altered during acute illness, emotional distress, or stress. Adjust as needed in older adults, in patients who have kidney or liver dysfunction, with changes in physical activity or meal pattern, and in patients concurrently taking drugs that lower blood glucose level. Refer to manufacturer's instructions for dosage adjustments when converting from other insulin regimens and formulations.

ADMINISTRATION
Subcutaneous
• NPH is an intermediate-acting insulin usually used concomitantly with rapid- or short-acting insulin.
• Give by subcut injection only; not for IM, IV, or insulin pump administration.
• Give injection in abdominal region, buttock, thigh, or upper arm. Subcut injection into abdominal wall is generally associated with faster absorption than other injection sites.
• Rotate injection sites within same region to reduce risk of lipodystrophy. A general rule is to not administer within 1 inch (2.5 cm) of same site for 1 month.
• Injection into a lifted skin fold minimizes risk of IM injection.
• Gently roll vial between the hands before each dose to uniformly disperse NPH insulin. Avoid vigorous shaking that may cause air bubbles or foam.
• NPH insulin should be uniformly cloudy or milky after gentle mixing and shouldn't contain particulate matter.
• When mixing NPH insulin with regular insulin, always draw clear regular insulin into syringe first. Give injection immediately after mixing.
• NPH insulin is typically given within 60 minutes of a meal. However, time of administration depends on patient-specific variables; NPH insulin may be given with mealtime regular or Humalog insulin if indicated.
◐ *Alert:* Multidose pens are for single patient use only. Never share pens (even if needle is changed). Clearly label with patient-identifying information where it won't obstruct dosing window, warning, or other product information.
• Store Humulin N at room temperature, below 86° F (30° C), if not exposed to direct sunlight, for 31 days (vial) or 14 days (pen). May store opened vials and unopened vials and pens in refrigerator at 36° to 46° F (2° to 8° C); don't refrigerate opened pens. Discard opened pens after 14 days, even if pen still contains drug. Don't freeze vials or pens.
• Store opened or unopened Novolin N away from direct heat or light at room temperature, below 77° F (25° C) for up to 42 days (vial) or below 86° F (30° C) for up to 28 days (pen). Store unopened Novolin N vials and pens in refrigerator at 36° to 46° F (2° to 8° C) and use until expiration date on label. Don't freeze.

ACTION
Lowers blood glucose level by stimulating peripheral glucose uptake and inhibiting liver glucose production; also inhibits lipolysis and proteolysis and enhances protein synthesis.

Route	Onset	Peak	Duration
Subcut	1–1.5 hr	4–12 hr	Up to 24 hr

Half-life: About 4.4 hours.

ADVERSE REACTIONS
CV: peripheral edema. **EENT:** visual disturbances. **Metabolic:** *hypoglycemia, hypokalemia,* weight gain. **Skin:** injection-site reaction, lipodystrophy, pruritus, rash. **Other:** hypersensitivity reactions, immunogenicity.

INTERACTIONS
Drug-drug. *ACE inhibitors, antidiabetics (oral), ARBs, disopyramide, fibrates, fluoxetine, MAO inhibitors, octreotide, pentoxifylline, pramlintide, salicylates, sulfonamide antibiotics:* May increase risk of hypoglycemia. Closely monitor glucose level, and adjust insulin dosage as needed.
Atypical antipsychotics, corticosteroids, danazol, diuretics, estrogens, glucagon, hormonal contraceptives, isoniazid, niacin, phenothiazines, protease inhibitors, sympathomimetics (albuterol, epinephrine, terbutaline), somatropin, thyroid hormones: May decrease blood glucose-lowering effects. Closely monitor glucose level, and adjust insulin dosage as needed.
Beta blockers, clonidine: May mask signs and symptoms of hypoglycemia. Avoid concurrent use, if possible, and monitor patient closely.
Beta blockers, clonidine, lithium salts, pentamidine: May cause hypoglycemia or hyperglycemia. Closely monitor glucose level.
Drugs that lower potassium level (diuretics) or affect potassium level (IV insulin): May increase risk of hypokalemia. Monitor potassium level.
Thiazolidinediones (TZDs; pioglitazone, rosiglitazone): May cause fluid retention that can lead to HF. Monitor patient closely, and adjust or stop TZDs as clinically indicated.
Drug-lifestyle. *Alcohol use:* May cause hyperglycemia or hypoglycemia. Closely monitor glucose level. Discourage concurrent use.

Reactions in bold italics are *life-threatening*.

EFFECTS ON LAB TEST RESULTS
• May decrease blood glucose and potassium levels.
• May develop antibodies that react with human insulin.

CONTRAINDICATIONS & CAUTIONS
• Contraindicated during episodes of hypoglycemia or ketoacidosis.
• Contraindicated in patients with history of hypersensitivity to drug or its components. Severe, life-threatening, generalized allergy, including anaphylaxis, can occur with insulin use.
• Use cautiously in patients susceptible to hypokalemia. Untreated hypokalemia can cause respiratory paralysis, ventricular arrhythmias, and death.
• Hypoglycemia is the most common adverse reaction. Severe hypoglycemia can cause seizures and may be life-threatening or fatal. Hypoglycemia can occur suddenly, and symptoms may differ. Risk is greater in patients with kidney or liver impairment and increases with intensity of glycemic control; changes in glycemic treatment, meal pattern, or physical activity; and concomitant use of certain medications.
• Use cautiously in older adults, who may be at increased risk for adverse effects; signs and symptoms of hypoglycemia may be more difficult to recognize in these patients.
Dialyzable drug: Unknown.
⚠ *Overdose S&S:* Hypoglycemia, hypokalemia.

PREGNANCY-LACTATION-REPRODUCTION
• Use cautiously in patients who are pregnant, and monitor patients closely.
• Closely monitor glucose level in patients who are pregnant, in patients who have recently given birth, and in patients who are breastfeeding; insulin requirements may change.
• It isn't known if insulin appears in human milk. Use cautiously during breastfeeding.

NURSING CONSIDERATIONS
• Monitor blood glucose level, and adjust insulin dosage as needed.
• Closely monitor patients after changes to insulin dosage.
• Closely monitor patient taking other medications with insulin because other drugs may mask signs and symptoms of hypoglycemia or cause an increase or decrease in blood glucose level.

• Increase frequency of glucose monitoring when patient is acutely ill or under emotional stress and if changes in diet, exercise, or medication regimen occur because these conditions may affect insulin absorption.
• Monitor patients carefully for signs and symptoms of hypoglycemia. Treat according to individual facility protocol, if necessary.
• Treat mild episodes of hypoglycemia with oral glucose. Treat more severe episodes, such as those involving coma, seizure, or neurologic impairment, with IM or subcut glucagon or concentrated IV glucose.
• Monitor potassium level in patients at risk for hypokalemia, especially those taking potassium-depleting drugs.
• Assess for signs and symptoms of hypoglycemia (seizures, diaphoresis, shaking, trembling, confusion) and hyperglycemia (drowsiness, fruity breath odor, frequent urination, thirst). Notify prescriber if any occur.
• Periodically measure HbA$_{1c}$ level.
• Monitor patient for generalized allergic reactions, including anaphylaxis.
• *Look alike–sound alike:* Don't confuse Humulin with Humalog. Don't confuse Novolin with Novolog.

PATIENT TEACHING
• Instruct patient in self-management, including glucose monitoring; injection preparation and technique; proper storage of insulin; and recognition and management of hypoglycemia and hyperglycemia.
• Explain that insulin requirements may vary due to illness, stress, emotional disturbance, inadequate food intake, and skipped meals.
• Advise patient that hypoglycemic episodes can impair ability to concentrate and react; advise patient to use caution while driving and operating machinery.
• Warn that allergic and hypersensitivity reactions can occur, including injection-site reactions (local pain, redness, swelling). Instruct patient to report signs and symptoms to health care provider. Review signs and symptoms of anaphylaxis, and instruct patient to promptly seek emergency medical attention if any occur.
• Caution patient to rotate injection sites to avoid developing lipodystrophy.
• *Alert:* Warn patient not to share multidose pen with other people (even if needle is changed) because of risk of bloodborne

pathogen transmission, including HIV and hepatitis.

• Explain importance of checking insulin label before each injection, as accidental mix-ups among insulin types have been reported.

• Teach patient that alcohol and some other medications may increase or decrease glucose level. Advise patient to inform health care provider of all medications and supplements being taken.

• Instruct patient not to stop insulin abruptly or change amount injected without consulting prescriber.

• Advise patient that any insulin changes should be made cautiously and only under medical supervision. Changes in insulin strength, manufacturer, type (regular, NPH, or insulin analogues), species (animal, human), or method of manufacture (rDNA versus animal-source insulin) may result in the need for a dosage change. Dosage of concomitant oral antidiabetic may need adjustment.

• Tell patient to report pregnancy or plans to become pregnant. Explain importance of maintaining tight glucose control.

• Inform patient of the change in insulin requirements that may occur during pregnancy and after childbirth.

SAFETY ALERT!

insulins (long-acting)

IN-su-lins

insulin degludec
Tresiba

insulin detemir (rDNA origin)
Levemir

insulin glargine (rDNA origin)
Basaglar, Lantus, Toujeo

insulin glargine-aglr (rDNA origin)
Rezvoglar

insulin glargine-yfgn (rDNA origin)
Semglee

Therapeutic class: Antidiabetics
Pharmacologic class: Insulins

AVAILABLE FORMS

Injection (degludec): 100 units/mL in 10-mL vials and 3-mL pens, 200 units/mL in 3-mL pens

Injection (detemir): 100 units/mL in 10-mL vials and 3-mL pens

Injection (glargine, glargine-aglr, glargine-yfgn): 100 units/mL in 10-mL vials and 3-mL pens, 200 units/mL in 3-mL pens, 300 units/mL in 1.5-mL and 3-mL pens

INDICATIONS & DOSAGES

Adjust-a-dose (for all indications): Individualize dosage based on metabolic needs, blood glucose monitoring, and glycemic control goal. Insulin requirements may be altered during acute illness, emotional distress, or stress. Adjust dosage as needed in older adults, in patients who have kidney or liver dysfunction, with changes in physical activity or meal pattern, and in patients who are concurrently taking drugs that lower blood glucose level. Refer to manufacturer's instructions for dosage adjustments when converting from other insulin regimens and formulations.

➤ **To improve glycemic control in patients with type 1 diabetes**

Adults (degludec, detemir, glargine) and children ages 2 and older (detemir), ages 6 and older (glargine), or ages 1 and older requiring 5 units or more daily (degludec): In patients who are insulin naive, initially, approximately one-third (Basaglar, Lantus, Rezvoglar, Semglee) or one-third to one-half (Levemir, Toujeo, Tresiba) of total daily insulin requirements subcut once daily.

Satisfy remainder of the daily insulin requirements with rapid- or short-acting premeal insulin.

➤ **To improve glycemic control in patients with type 2 diabetes**

Adults: Initial insulin degludec dosage is 10 units once daily subcut at any time of day. Initial insulin detemir dosage is 10 units (0.1 to 0.2 unit/kg) subcut once daily in evening or divided into two daily doses in patients inadequately controlled on oral antidiabetics, or once daily in the evening in patients inadequately controlled on a glucagon-like peptide 1 (GLP-1) receptor antagonist. Initial insulin glargine dosage is 0.2 unit/kg (up to 10 units) subcut once daily. Adjust dosage as needed. *Children ages 1 and older (degludec only):* Initially, in children who are insulin naive, 10 units subcut once daily at same time every day. Or, in children already receiving insulin therapy, start at 80% of total daily long- or intermediate-acting insulin unit dose to minimize risk of hypoglycemia.

ADMINISTRATION
Subcutaneous
General

• Don't give long-acting insulin by insulin infusion pumps or by IM or IV injection.

• Administer by subcut injection only in the thigh, abdominal wall, or upper arm. Rotate site within same region (abdomen, thigh, or deltoid) from one injection to the next to reduce risk of lipodystrophy.

• Don't mix or dilute long-acting insulins with other insulins or solutions because the pharmacokinetic and pharmacodynamic profile (onset of action, time to peak effect) of the insulin may be altered unpredictably.

• Visually inspect for particulate matter and discoloration before administration, whenever solution and container permit; use only if solution appears clear and colorless.

• Instructions for priming and using pens vary from one to another, are very detailed, and involve multiple steps. Refer to manufacturer's instructions for use.

🚫 **Alert:** Multidose pens are for single patient use only. Never share pens (even if needle is changed). Clearly label with patient-identifying information where it won't obstruct dosing window, warning, or other product information.

Insulin degludec

• In adults, give insulin degludec once daily at any time of day; in children, give once daily at the same time each day.

• Individualize and titrate dosage every 3 to 4 days based on patient's metabolic needs, blood glucose monitoring results, and glycemic control goal.

• Don't perform dose conversion when using FlexTouch pen. The dose window for both 100-unit and 200-unit pens shows the number of insulin units to be delivered and no conversion is needed.

• In adults with type 1 or type 2 diabetes already on insulin therapy, start insulin degludec at the same unit dose as the total daily long- or intermediate-acting insulin unit dose.

• In children ages 1 and older already on insulin therapy, start at 80% of the total daily long- or intermediate-acting insulin unit dose to minimize risk of hypoglycemia.

• For children requiring less than 5 units of drug each day, use U-100 vials.

• Always use a new needle for each injection to help ensure sterility and prevent blocked needles.

• Store unused pens in refrigerator at 36° to 46° F (2° to 8° C); may use until expiration date on label. Don't freeze or use if pens have been frozen.

• Store open pen away from heat and light at room temperature, below 86° F (30° C). Discard after 56 days, even if pen still contains insulin and expiration date hasn't passed.

Insulin detemir

• Give insulin detemir once daily or b.i.d. For patients treated with insulin detemir once daily, give dose with evening meal or at bedtime. For patients who require b.i.d. dosing, administer evening dose with evening meal, at bedtime, or 12 hours after morning dose.

• When using insulin detemir with a GLP-1 receptor agonist, give as separate injections; never mix. Insulin detemir and a GLP-1 receptor agonist may be injected in same body region, but the injections shouldn't be adjacent to each other.

• If converting from insulin glargine or NPH insulin to insulin detemir, maintain the same unit dose. Closely monitor glucose level during transition.

• Store unused (unopened) insulin detemir vials and pens between 36° and 46° F (2° and 8° C). Don't freeze and don't use if vials or pens have been frozen. Keep in carton so that vials or pens stay clean and protected from light.

• If refrigeration isn't possible, can keep unused (unopened) insulin detemir unrefrigerated at room temperature, below 86° F (30° C), if it's kept as cool as possible and away from direct heat and light. Discard unrefrigerated insulin detemir 42 days after it's first kept out of the refrigerator, even if the pen or vial still contains insulin.

• After initial use, store vials in refrigerator; never freeze. If refrigeration isn't possible, can keep in-use vial unrefrigerated at room temperature, below 86° F (30° C), if it's kept as cool as possible and away from direct heat and light. Discard refrigerated insulin detemir vials 42 days after initial use.

• After initial use, don't store insulin detemir pen in refrigerator and don't store with needle in place; keep opened insulin detemir pen away from direct heat and light at room temperature, below 86° F (30° C). Discard unrefrigerated insulin detemir pens 42 days after they're first kept out of refrigerator.

Insulin glargine
• Give subcut once daily at same time every day, at any time during the day.
• If converting from insulin detemir to insulin glargine, maintain the same unit dose. Closely monitor glucose level during transition.
• Store unopened insulin glargine vials and pens at 36° to 46° F (2° to 8° C). Don't freeze; discard if frozen. If refrigeration isn't possible, the open vial in use can be kept unrefrigerated for up to 28 days away from direct heat and light, if the room temperature isn't above 86° F (30° C).
• Use opened vials, refrigerated or not, within a 28-day period or discard them.
• Don't refrigerate opened pens but keep them at room temperature, below 86° F (30° C), away from direct heat and light; discard opened pens kept at room temperature after 28 days.

ACTION
Lowers blood glucose level by stimulating peripheral glucose uptake by binding to insulin receptors on skeletal muscle and in fat cells and by inhibiting liver glucose production; also inhibits lipolysis and proteolysis and enhances protein synthesis.

Route	Onset	Peak	Duration
Subcut (degludec)	1 hr	9 hr	24+ hr
Subcut (detemir)	3–4 hr	3–9 hr	24 hr
Subcut (glargine)	3–6 hr	Constant	24 hr

Half-life: Degludec, 25 hours; detemir, 5 to 7 hours; glargine, unknown.

ADVERSE REACTIONS
CNS: headache, fever, depression. **CV:** peripheral edema, HTN. **EENT:** cataract, retinopathy, nasopharyngitis, pharyngitis, rhinitis, sinusitis. **GI:** abdominal pain, gastroenteritis, nausea, vomiting, diarrhea. **GU:** UTI. **Metabolic:** *hypoglycemia, hypokalemia,* weight gain. **Musculoskeletal:** back pain, arthralgia, limb pain. **Respiratory:** URI, bronchitis, cough. **Skin:** injection-site reactions, lipodystrophy, pruritus, rash. **Other:** hypersensitivity reactions, flulike symptoms, infection, antibody development, accidental injury.

INTERACTIONS
Drug-drug. *ACE inhibitors, antidiabetics (oral), ARBs, disopyramide, fibrates,* *fluoxetine, MAO inhibitors, octreotide, pentoxifylline, pramlintide, salicylates, sulfonamide antibiotics:* May increase blood glucose-lowering effect of insulin, increasing risk of hypoglycemia. Monitor glucose level and patient closely. Adjust insulin dosage as necessary.
Antiadrenergics (beta blockers, clonidine): May mask signs and symptoms of hypoglycemia. Avoid concurrent use, if possible, and monitor patient closely.
Atypical antipsychotics, corticosteroids, danazol, diuretics, estrogens, glucagon, hormonal contraceptives, isoniazid, niacin, phenothiazines, protease inhibitors, somatropin, sympathomimetics (albuterol, epinephrine, terbutaline), thyroid hormones: May decrease blood glucose-lowering effect of insulin, increasing risk of hyperglycemia. Monitor glucose level and patient closely. Adjust insulin dosage as necessary.
Beta blockers, clonidine, lithium salts, pentamidine: May increase risk of either hypoglycemia or hyperglycemia. Closely monitor glucose level.
Drugs that lower potassium level (diuretics) or affect potassium level (IV insulin): May increase risk of hypokalemia. Monitor potassium level.
GLP-1 receptor agonists (albiglutide, exenatide, liraglutide): May increase risk of hypoglycemia. Closely monitor glucose level, and decrease insulin dosage if necessary.
Thiazolidinediones (TZDs; pioglitazone, rosiglitazone): May cause fluid retention that can lead to HF. Monitor patient closely; adjust or stop TZD as clinically necessary.
Drug-lifestyle. *Alcohol use:* May cause hyperglycemia or hypoglycemia. Monitor glucose level. Discourage concurrent use.

EFFECTS ON LAB TEST RESULTS
• May decrease potassium and blood glucose levels.
• May develop antibodies that react with human insulin.

CONTRAINDICATIONS & CAUTIONS
• Contraindicated during episodes of hypoglycemia or diabetic ketoacidosis.
• Contraindicated in patients hypersensitive to drug or its components. Severe, life-threatening, generalized allergy, including anaphylaxis, can occur with insulin use.

⑤ Alert: Adjust insulin regimen only with appropriate glucose monitoring under medical supervision.

• Use cautiously in patients susceptible to hypokalemia, such as patients who are fasting, are taking potassium-lowering drugs, or are concurrently taking drugs that may affect potassium level. Untreated hypokalemia can cause respiratory paralysis, ventricular arrhythmias, and death.

• Hypoglycemia is the most common adverse reaction. Severe hypoglycemia can cause seizures and may be life-threatening or fatal. Hypoglycemia can occur suddenly, and symptoms may differ. Risk is greater in patients with kidney or liver impairment and increases with intensity of glycemic control; changes in glycemic treatment, meal pattern, or physical activity; and concomitant use of certain medications.

• Use cautiously in older adults, who may be at risk for increased sensitivity to drug's effects. Signs and symptoms of hypoglycemia may be more difficult to recognize in these patients.

• Use prefilled pens cautiously in patients with visual impairment, who may rely on audible clicks to dial their dose.

Dialyzable drug: Unknown.

⚠ Overdose S&S: Hypoglycemia, hypokalemia, coma, seizure, neurologic impairment.

PREGNANCY-LACTATION-REPRODUCTION

• Use cautiously during pregnancy.

• Closely monitor glucose level during pregnancy, after recent birth, and during breastfeeding; insulin requirements may change.

• It isn't known if insulin appears in human milk. Use cautiously during breastfeeding. Insulin dosage may need adjustment.

NURSING CONSIDERATIONS

• Insulin glargine-yfgn (Semglee) and insulin glargine-aglr (Rezvoglar) are biosimilar to the FDA-approved reference product Lantus. There are no clinically meaningful differences between biosimilar product and reference product based on the conditions of their use. Semglee is also interchangeable with Lantus and can be substituted without approval of prescriber. Rezvoglar isn't considered interchangeable and can't be automatically substituted.

• Prolonged effect of long-acting insulin may delay recovery from hypoglycemia. Monitor patient carefully.

• Monitor patient taking other medications with insulin more closely because other drugs can mask signs and symptoms of hypoglycemia or cause an increase or a decrease in blood glucose level.

• Adjust dosages regularly, depending on patient-specific glucose measurements.

• Closely monitor patient after changes to insulin dosage.

• Monitor patient carefully for signs and symptoms of hypoglycemia, especially in long-standing disease. Treat according to individual facility protocol, if necessary.

• Assess for signs and symptoms of hypoglycemia (diaphoresis, shaking, trembling, confusion) and hyperglycemia (drowsiness, fruity breath odor, frequent urination, thirst). Notify prescriber if any occur.

• Mild episodes of hypoglycemia may be treated with oral glucose. More severe episodes of hypoglycemia, such as coma, seizure, or neurologic impairment, may be treated with IM or subcut glucagon or concentrated IV glucose.

• Periodically measure HbA_{1c} level.

• Increase frequency of glucose monitoring when patient is acutely ill or under emotional stress and if changes in diet, exercise, or medication regimen occur; these conditions may affect insulin absorption.

• *Look alike–sound alike:* Don't confuse insulin glargine with insulin glulisine.

PATIENT TEACHING

• Instruct patient in self-management, including glucose monitoring, injection technique, proper storage of insulin, and recognition and management of hypoglycemia and hyperglycemia.

• Explain that insulin requirements may vary due to illness, stress, emotional disturbance, change in activity level, inadequate food intake, and skipped meals.

• Teach patient to watch for signs and symptoms of hypoglycemia (diaphoresis, shaking, trembling, confusion) and hyperglycemia (drowsiness, frequent urination, thirst).

• Advise patient that hypoglycemic episodes may impair the ability to concentrate and

react; advise patient to use caution while driving and operating machinery.
- Instruct patient to keep hard candy or glucose tablets on hand to treat mild cases of hypoglycemia.
- Warn that allergic and hypersensitivity reactions can occur, including injection-site reactions (local pain, redness, swelling) and generalized reactions. Instruct patient to report signs and symptoms to health care provider. Review signs and symptoms of anaphylaxis, and instruct patient to promptly seek emergency medical attention if any occur.
- Instruct patient to rotate injection sites within same region to reduce risk of lipodystrophy.
- **Alert:** Warn patient not to share multidose pen with other people (even if needle is changed) because of risk of bloodborne pathogen transmission, including HIV and hepatitis.
- Review proper storage of insulin products, and instruct patient to use solution only if it appears clear and colorless.
- Explain importance of checking insulin label before each injection; accidental mix-ups among insulin types have been reported.
- Instruct patient that long-acting insulins shouldn't be diluted or mixed with other insulins or drugs.
- Teach patient that alcohol may affect glucose level and should be avoided.
- Inform patient that any insulin change should be made cautiously and only under medical supervision. Changes in insulin strength, manufacturer, type (regular, NPH, or insulin analogues), species (animal, human), or method of manufacture (rDNA versus animal-source insulin) may result in need for a dosage change. Dosage of concomitant oral antidiabetics may need adjustment.
- Instruct patient not to stop insulin abruptly or change amount injected without consulting prescriber.
- Warn patient to report pregnancy or plans to become pregnant.
- Advise patient of the change in insulin requirements that may occur during pregnancy and after childbirth.

SAFETY ALERT!

insulins (rapid-acting)
IN-su-lins

insulin aspart (rDNA origin)
Fiasp, Kirsty✦, NovoLOG, NovoRapid✦, Trurapi✦

insulin glulisine (rDNA origin)
Apidra

insulin (human)
Afrezza

insulin (lispro)
Admelog, HumaLOG, Liprelog✦

insulin (lispro-aabc)
Lyumjev

Therapeutic class: Antidiabetics
Pharmacologic class: Insulins

AVAILABLE FORMS
Inhalation powder (Afrezza): 4-unit, 8-unit, 12-unit single-use cartridges
Injection (aspart): 100 units/mL in 10-mL vials, 3-mL prefilled pens and cartridges
Injection (glulisine): 100 units/mL in 10-mL vials, 3-mL prefilled pens
Injection (lispro, lispro-aabc): 100 units/mL in10-mL vials, 3-mL prefilled pens and cartridges; 200 units/mL in 3-mL prefilled pens

INDICATIONS & DOSAGES
Adjust-a-dose (for all indications): Individualize dosage based on metabolic needs, blood glucose monitoring, and glycemic control goal. Insulin requirements may be altered during acute illness, emotional distress, or stress. Adjust as needed in older adults, in patients who have kidney or liver dysfunction, with changes in physical activity or meal pattern, and in those who are concurrently taking drugs that lower blood glucose level. Refer to manufacturer's instructions for dosage adjustments when converting from other insulin regimens or formulations. Patients with obesity and children during puberty may need increased maintenance doses.
➤ **To improve glycemic control in patients with diabetes (aspart, glulisine, lispro)**
Adults and children ages 1 and older (lispro-aabc), adults and children ages 2 and older

---

Reactions in bold italics are *life-threatening*.

(aspart), ages 3 and older (lispro), ages 4 and older (glulisine): For insulin aspart, inject individualized dose subcut at the start of or within 20 minutes after starting a meal (Fiasp) or within 5 to 10 minutes before a meal (Novolo). When using a continuous subcut infusion pump, follow health care provider recommendations for setting basal and mealtime infusion rates. Usual IV concentration is 0.05 to 1 unit/mL in NSS infused under close medical supervision.

For insulin glulisine, inject individualized dose subcut within 15 minutes before or 20 minutes after starting a meal. When continuous subcut infusion pump is used, base initial dosing on total daily insulin dose of previous regimen. Usual IV concentration is 0.05 to 1 unit/mL in NSS infused under close medical supervision.

For lispro, inject individualized dose subcut within 15 minutes before a meal or immediately after a meal or, for lispro-aabc, at the start of a meal or within 20 minutes after starting a meal. When continuous subcut infusion pump is used, follow health care provider recommendations when setting basal and mealtime infusion rates. Usual IV concentration is 0.1 to 1 unit/mL in NSS infused under close medical supervision.

➤ **To improve glycemic control in patients with diabetes (inhalation)**
Adults: For patients who are insulin naive, initially 4 units inhaled at beginning of each meal. To convert to inhaled insulin from subcut mealtime insulin, refer to manufacturer's instructions. For patients using subcut premixed insulin, estimate mealtime injected dose by dividing half of total daily injected premixed insulin dose equally among the three meals of the day; then convert each estimated injected mealtime dose to an appropriate inhaled dose according to manufacturer's instructions. Administer half of total daily injected premixed dose as an injected basal insulin dose. Inhaled insulin must be used in combination with a long-acting insulin in patients with type 1 diabetes.

ADMINISTRATION
General
• Rapid-acting insulins are usually given in a regimen that includes an intermediate-acting or a long-acting insulin.
• Don't use viscous or cloudy solution; use only if clear and colorless.

• Multidose pens are for single-patient use only. Never share pens (even if needle is changed). Clearly label with patient-identifying information where it won't obstruct dosing window, warning, or other product information.
• Store unopened insulin aspart vials, cartridges, and pens under refrigeration (36° to 46° F [2° to 8° C]) until expiration date or at room temperature of less than 86° F (30° C) for 28 days; don't freeze. Keep away from heat and sunlight. Once opened, store vials under refrigeration or at room temperature of less than 86° F (30° C); use within 28 days. Store cartridges and pens that have been opened at temperatures less than 86° F (30° C) and use within 28 days; don't freeze or refrigerate.
• Store insulin glulisine under refrigeration at 36° to 46° F (2° to 8° C) and protect from light. Don't store in freezer. Don't allow insulin glulisine to freeze; discard if it has been frozen. Use unopened vials and cartridge systems not stored in refrigerator within 28 days. Use opened vials, refrigerated or not, within 28 days. If refrigeration isn't possible, can keep open vials at room temperature of less than 77° F (25° C) for up to 28 days away from direct heat and light. Don't refrigerate opened cartridge system, but keep below 77° F (25° C) and away from direct heat and light. Discard opened cartridge systems after 28 days. Don't store pen, with or without cartridge system, in refrigerator at any time.
• Store lispro in refrigerator (36° to 46° F [2° to 8° C]), but not in freezer. Protect from direct heat and light. Don't use if frozen. Store unopened vials and pens in refrigerator until expiration date; if stored unopened at room temperature, discard after 28 days. May store opened vials for 28 days under refrigeration or at room temperature; may store opened pens and cartridges for 28 days at room temperature. Discard if exposed to temperatures greater than 98.6° F (37° C).
• **Incompatibilities:** Don't mix with any other insulin except NPH.
IV
▼ Rapid-acting insulin may be administered IV with close monitoring of blood glucose and serum potassium levels under appropriate medical supervision.
▼ Flush IV tubing with priming infusion of 20 mL from insulin infusion whenever new

---

IV tubing set is added to insulin infusion container to avoid adsorption to IV tubing.

▼ Use NSS and polyvinyl chloride or polypropylene infusion bags for IV infusions.

▼ Always administer IV infusions using an infusion pump.

Subcutaneous

• Administer by subcut injection in abdominal region, buttock, thigh, or upper arm. Subcut injection into abdominal wall is generally associated with faster absorption than other injection sites.

• Rotate injection sites within same region to reduce risk of lipodystrophy.

• Injection into a lifted skin fold minimizes risk of IM injection.

⚠️ *Alert:* Don't transfer 200 unit/mL insulin from a pen to a standard insulin syringe; overdose and severe hypoglycemia can result.

• NovoLog may be diluted with Insulin Diluting Medium for NovoLog for subcut injection. Diluting one part NovoLog to nine parts diluent will yield a concentration one-tenth that of NovoLog (equivalent to U-10). Diluting one part NovoLog to one part diluent will yield a concentration one-half that of NovoLog (equivalent to U-50).

• When used for continuous subcut insulin infusion, replace insulin in reservoir every 6 days (Fiasp) or 7 days (NovoLog) or according to manufacturer's instructions, whichever is shorter. Change infusion sets and insertion site according to manufacturer's instructions.

• When using for continuous subcut insulin infusion, change insulin glulisine in reservoir and infusion set (reservoirs, tubing, and catheters) every 48 hours or after exposure to temperatures greater than 98.6° F (37° C).

• When using for continuous subcut insulin infusion, change lispro in reservoir at least every 7 days, and change infusion sets and insertion site every 3 days.

• Don't dilute or use mixed insulins in external insulin pumps.

Inhalational

• Administer by single inhalation per cartridge using Afrezza inhaler only. Inhaler can be used for all cartridge strengths.

• Administer at beginning of a meal.

• Keep inhaler level, with white mouthpiece on top and purple base on bottom, after inserting cartridge into inhaler.

• Loss of drug effect can occur if inhaler is turned upside down, held with mouthpiece pointing down, or shaken or dropped after

cartridge insertion but before dose administration. If any of these occur, replace cartridge before use.

• May mix and match between 4-unit (blue), 8-unit (green), and 12-unit (yellow) cartridges to obtain correct dose.

• Store unused foil packages of inhalation powder until expiration date under refrigeration (36° to 46° F [2° to 8° C]); if at room temperature, use within 10 days. If in use, unopened blister cards and strips must be used within 10 days and opened strips must be used within 3 days.

• Inhaler can be refrigerated but should be at room temperature before use. Cartridges should be at room temperature for 10 minutes before use.

• Replace inhaler after 15 days of use.

ACTION

Lowers blood glucose level by stimulating peripheral glucose uptake by binding to insulin receptors on skeletal muscle and in fat cells and by inhibiting liver glucose production; also inhibits lipolysis and proteolysis and enhances protein synthesis.

Route	Onset	Peak	Duration
Aspart (IV)	Immediate	Unknown	3–5 hr
Aspart (subcut)	15 min	1–3 hr	3–5 hr
Glulisine (IV)	Immediate	Unknown	5 hr
Glulisine (subcut)	5–15 min	1 hr	5 hr
Lispro (IV)	Immediate	Unknown	Unknown
Lispro (subcut)	15–30 min	30–90 min	≤5 hr
Inhalation	Unknown	12–15 min	180 min

Half-life: Aspart IV, unknown; aspart subcut, 81 minutes; glulisine IV, 13 minutes; glulisine subcut, 42 minutes; lispro IV, 51 to 55 minutes; lispro subcut, 1 hour; inhalation, 28 to 39 minutes.

ADVERSE REACTIONS

CNS: headache, asthenia, fever, fatigue (inhalation), pain, sensory disturbance. **CV:** HTN, peripheral edema. **EENT:** rhinitis, nasopharyngitis, pharyngitis. **GI:** nausea, diarrhea, abdominal pain. **GU:** UTI, dysmenorrhea. **Metabolic:** *hypoglycemia, hypokalemia,* weight gain. **Musculoskeletal:** arthralgia, myalgia. **Respiratory:** URI, bronchitis, cough; bronchospasm, decreased pulmonary function, productive cough (inhalation). **Skin:** injection- or infusion-site reactions, lipodystrophy, pruritus, rash.

Reactions in bold italics are *life-threatening*.

Other: accidental injury, infection, insulin antibody production, flulike symptoms.

INTERACTIONS
Drug-drug. *ACE inhibitors, antidiabetics (oral), ARBs, disopyramide, fibrates, fluoxetine, MAO inhibitors, octreotide, pentoxifylline, pramlintide, salicylates, sulfonamide antibiotics:* May increase risk of hypoglycemia. Closely monitor glucose level, and adjust insulin dosage as needed.
Atypical antipsychotics, corticosteroids, danazol, diuretics, estrogens, glucagon, hormonal contraceptives, isoniazid, niacin, phenothiazines, protease inhibitors, somatropin, sympathomimetics (albuterol, epinephrine, terbutaline), thyroid hormones: May decrease blood glucose-lowering effects. Closely monitor glucose level, and adjust insulin dosage as needed.
Beta blockers, clonidine: May mask signs and symptoms of hypoglycemia. Avoid concurrent use, if possible, or monitor patient closely.
Beta blockers, clonidine, lithium salts, pentamidine: May cause hypoglycemia or hyperglycemia. Closely monitor glucose level.
Drugs that lower potassium level (diuretics) or affect potassium level (IV insulin): May increase risk of hypokalemia. Monitor potassium level.
Thiazolidinediones (TZDs; pioglitazone, rosiglitazone): May cause fluid retention that can lead to HF. Monitor patient closely; adjust or stop TZDs as clinically indicated.
Drug-lifestyle. *Alcohol use:* May cause hyperglycemia or hypoglycemia. Closely monitor glucose level. Discourage use together.

EFFECTS ON LAB TEST RESULTS
• May decrease glucose and potassium levels.
• May develop antibodies that react with human insulin.

CONTRAINDICATIONS & CAUTIONS
Boxed Warning Inhaled insulin is contraindicated in patients with chronic lung disease (asthma, COPD); acute bronchospasm has been observed in these patients. ∎
• Contraindicated during episodes of hypoglycemia.
• Contraindicated in patients with history of hypersensitivity to drug or its components. Severe, life-threatening, generalized allergic reaction, including anaphylaxis, can occur with insulin use.

• Inhaled insulin may increase risk of diabetic ketoacidosis (DKA). Closely monitor patients at risk for DKA. Change route of insulin delivery, if needed.
• Inhaled insulin isn't recommended in patients who smoke or who have recently stopped smoking.
• Use cautiously in patients susceptible to hypokalemia, such as patients who are fasting, are taking potassium-lowering drugs, or are concurrently taking drugs that may affect potassium level. Untreated hypokalemia can cause respiratory paralysis, ventricular arrhythmias, and death.
• Hypoglycemia is the most common adverse reaction. Severe hypoglycemia can cause seizures and may be life-threatening or fatal. Hypoglycemia can occur suddenly, and symptoms may differ. Risk is greater in patients with kidney or liver impairment and increases with intensity of glycemic control; changes in glycemic treatment, meal pattern, or physical activity; and concomitant use of certain medications.
• Use cautiously in older adults, who may be at increased risk for adverse effects. Signs and symptoms of hypoglycemia may be more difficult to recognize in these patients.
• Use prefilled pens cautiously in patients with visual impairment, who may rely on audible clicks to dial their dose.
Dialyzable drug: Unknown.
⚠ *Overdose S&S:* Hypoglycemia, hypokalemia.

PREGNANCY-LACTATION-REPRODUCTION
• Studies during pregnancy are inadequate. Poorly controlled diabetes increases maternal and fetal risk of adverse outcomes. Use cautiously during pregnancy.
• Closely monitor glucose level during pregnancy, after recent birth, and during breastfeeding; insulin requirements may change.
• It isn't known if insulin appears in human milk. Refer to manufacturer's instructions for use during breastfeeding.

NURSING CONSIDERATIONS
Boxed Warning Before initiating inhaled insulin, perform a detailed medical history, physical exam, and spirometry (forced expiratory volume in 1 second [FEV₁]) to identify potential lung disease in all patients. ∎
• Assess pulmonary function (via spirometry) after 6 months of inhalation therapy and

then annually, even in absence of pulmonary symptoms.

• Increase frequency of pulmonary assessment in patients with such symptoms as wheezing, bronchospasm, breathing difficulties, or persistent or recurring cough. Switch to another form of drug for persistent symptoms or decline of 20% or more in FEV_1 from baseline.

• Monitor blood glucose level, and adjust insulin dosage as needed.

• Increase glucose monitoring frequency when initiating therapy or when changing insulin strength, dosage, manufacturer, or type or method of administration. Changes may affect glycemic control and increase risk of hypoglycemia.

• Closely monitor patient also taking other medications; other drugs can mask signs and symptoms of hypoglycemia or cause an increase or decrease in blood glucose level.

• Increase frequency of glucose monitoring when patient is acutely ill or under emotional stress and if changes in diet, exercise, or medication regimen occur; these conditions may affect insulin absorption.

• Closely monitor patient at risk for DKA from acute illness or infection; consider changing from inhalation to alternative route of insulin delivery.

• Closely monitor for signs and symptoms of hypoglycemia. Symptom awareness may be decreased in patients with long-standing diabetes, diabetic nerve disease, or kidney or liver impairment and in patients who have experienced recurrent hypoglycemia. Treat according to individual facility protocol, if necessary.

• Notify prescriber of signs or symptoms of hypoglycemia (diaphoresis, shaking, trembling, confusion) or hyperglycemia (drowsiness, fruity breath odor, frequent urination, thirst).

• Mild episodes of hypoglycemia may be treated with oral glucose. More severe episodes of hypoglycemia, such as coma, seizure, or neurologic impairment, may be treated with IM or subcut glucagon or concentrated IV glucose.

• Monitor potassium level in patients at risk for hypokalemia (those receiving potassium-depleting drugs or IV insulin).

• Monitor patient for generalized allergic reactions, including anaphylaxis.

• Periodically measure HbA_{1c} level.

• Monitor external pump for malfunction, which can cause rapid decline in blood glucose level.

• *Look alike–sound alike:* Don't confuse NovoLog with Novolog 70/30. Don't confuse Humalog with Humalog 50/50 or 75/25. Don't confuse insulin glulisine with insulin glargine.

PATIENT TEACHING
General

• Advise patient that hypoglycemic episodes can impair ability to concentrate and react; advise patient to use caution while driving and operating machinery.

• Instruct patient to keep hard candy or glucose tablets on hand to treat mild cases of hypoglycemia.

• Advise patient to keep a log of glucose levels.

• Instruct patient on long-term sequelae of diabetes if not managed properly.

• Instruct patient to carry identification or wear jewelry indicating that patient has diabetes.

• Warn that allergic and hypersensitivity reactions can occur, including injection-site reactions (local pain, redness, swelling). Instruct patient to report signs and symptoms to health care provider. Review signs and symptoms of anaphylaxis, and instruct patient to promptly seek emergency medical attention if any occur.

• Instruct patient on self-management procedures, including glucose monitoring, proper administration, and management of hypoglycemia and hyperglycemia.

• Warn patient that insulin requirements may vary due to illness, stress, emotional disturbances, inadequate or skipped insulin dose, inadvertent administration of increased insulin dose, inadequate food intake, or skipped meals.

• Instruct patient to report pregnancy or plans to become pregnant.

• Advise patient of change in insulin requirements that may occur during pregnancy and after childbirth.

• Teach patient that alcohol and some other medications may increase or decrease glucose level. Advise patient to inform health care provider of all medications and supplements being taken.

• Caution patient not to stop insulin abruptly or change amount taken without consulting prescriber.

Reactions in bold italics are *life-threatening*.

- Advise patient that any change of insulin should be made cautiously and only under medical supervision. Changes in insulin strength, manufacturer, type (regular, NPH, or insulin analogues), species (animal, human), or method of manufacture (rDNA versus animal-source insulin) may result in need for a dosage change. Dosage of concomitant oral antidiabetics may need adjustment.

Injection

- Teach patient to give insulin at appropriate time around a meal, depending on product.
- Caution patient to rotate injection sites to prevent lipodystrophy.
- Instruct patient mixing two types of insulin to always draw up shorter-acting insulin first, followed by NPH insulin, and to inject immediately.
- Teach patient to properly use external insulin pump, to use appropriate insulin in pump, not to dilute it or mix it with other insulin formulations, to change infusion set as directed, and to rotate infusion sites.
- Advise patient to have a backup external insulin pump available in case of malfunction.
- Teach patient proper insulin storage.
- Explain importance of checking insulin label before each injection; accidental mix-ups among insulin types have been reported.
- **Alert:** Warn patient not to share multidose pen (even if needle is changed) because of risk of bloodborne pathogen transmission, including HIV and hepatitis.

Inhalational

- Instruct patient to read inhaler's medication guide before starting inhalation therapy and to reread it with each prescription renewal.
- Caution patient not to open cartridges, place cartridges in mouth, or swallow cartridges.
- Inform patient that inhaled insulin can decrease lung function and that lung function will be evaluated by spirometry before initiation of treatment and periodically during treatment.
- Advise patient to promptly report respiratory difficulty or signs or symptoms of lung cancer (hemoptysis, cough).
- Inform patient to store unused inhaled product in refrigerator. If inhaler is being used, tell patient to leave it at room temperature and use unopened strips within 10 days and opened strips within 3 days.
- Instruct patient never to wash inhaler but to wipe it with a clean, dry cloth.

- Advise patient to discard and replace inhaler every 15 days.

SAFETY ALERT!

insulins (short-acting)

IN-su-lins

insulin (regular)

HumuLIN R ◇, HumuLIN R U-500 (concentrated), Myxredlin, NovoLIN R ◇

Therapeutic class: Antidiabetics
Pharmacologic class: Insulins

AVAILABLE FORMS

Infusion: 100 units in 100 mL NSS single-dose container
Injection: 100 units/mL in 3-mL, 10-mL vials, 3-mL pens ◇; 500 units/mL in 3-mL pens and 20-mL vials

INDICATIONS & DOSAGES

➤ **Adjunct to diet and exercise to improve glycemic control in patients with type 1 and type 2 diabetes**

Adults and children: Inject individualized total daily insulin requirements subcut in three or more divided doses. Initial doses may be lower, and maintenance doses in patients with obesity and children during puberty may be higher. Give 30 minutes before start of a meal. May give IV under medical supervision with close monitoring of blood glucose and potassium levels to avoid hypoglycemia and hypokalemia.

- **Alert:** U-500 concentrate is used for treatment of patients with diabetes who are insulin resistant and require daily doses of more than 200 units because large dose may be given subcut in reasonable volume. Don't give U-500 concentrated insulin IV or IM.

Adjust-a-dose: Individualize dosage based on metabolic needs, blood glucose monitoring, and glycemic control. Insulin requirements may be altered during acute illness, emotional distress, or stress. Adjust dosage as needed in older adults, in patients with kidney or liver dysfunction, with changes in physical activity or meal pattern, and in patients who are concurrently taking drugs that lower blood glucose level. Dosage may also need adjustment when switching from another insulin formulation, manufacturer, or strength. IV administration of regular insulin is possible under medical supervision with close monitoring of blood glucose and potassium levels to avoid hypoglycemia and hypokalemia. IV administration of insulin is commonly used in treatment of diabetic ketoacidosis, perioperative management of diabetes, and maintenance of glycemic control during labor in patients with diabetes.

ADMINISTRATION
General
● Store unopened vials and pens in refrigerator at 36° to 46° F (2° to 8° C). Don't freeze and don't use if vial has been frozen.

◑ **Alert:** Multidose pens are for single patient use only. Never share pens (even if needle is changed). Clearly label with patient-identifying information where it won't obstruct dosing window, warning, or other product information.

● Keep Novolin R vials at room temperature (not greater than 77° F [25° C]), away from heat or light, for up to 42 days; don't refrigerate after first use. Discard after 42 days even if vial is unopened or isn't empty.

● Keep opened (in use) Humulin R vials at room temperature (not greater than 86° F [30° C]), away from heat or light, for up to 31 days. Discard after 31 days even if vial is unopened or isn't empty.

● Keep opened and unopened Humulin R U-500 vials at room temperature, below 86° F (30° C); discard after 40 days. Also discard opened refrigerated vials after 40 days.

● Keep opened and unopened pens at room temperature, below 86° F (30° C); discard after 28 days. Don't store opened pens in refrigerator.

IV

▼ Don't use if solution is viscous or cloudy; use only if clear and colorless.

▼ Closely monitor blood glucose and serum potassium levels. Appropriate medical supervision is required.

▼ Onset of action when administered IV is more rapid than onset via subcut administration.

▼ For IV use, administer Humulin R U-100 at a concentration of 0.1 to 1 unit/mL in NSS using polyvinyl chloride infusion bags. Use Novolin R at concentrations of 0.05 to 1 unit/mL in infusion systems using polypropylene infusion bags and one of the following infusion solutions: NSS, 5%

dextrose, or 10% dextrose with potassium chloride 40 mmol/L.

▼ Always administer IV infusions using an infusion pump.

▼ Infusion bags prepared with Humulin R are stable when stored in refrigerator for 48 hours at 36° to 46° F (2° to 8° C) and may be used at room temperature for up to an additional 48 hours.

▼ Infusion bags prepared with Novolin R are stable at room temperature for 24 hours.

▼ Store Myxredlin IV solution at 36° to 46° F (2° to 8° C) in original carton until expiration date. May also store at room temperature up to 77° F (25° C) for up to 30 days; don't return to refrigerator after stored at room temperature. Don't freeze or shake.

▼ **Incompatibilities:** Don't mix regular insulin with any other insulin except NPH; don't mix regular concentrated insulin with any other insulin.

Subcutaneous
● Regular insulin administered by subcut injection should generally be used in regimens that include an intermediate- or long-acting insulin. It may also be used in combination with oral antidiabetics.

● Subcut injection should be followed by a meal within 30 minutes of administration.

● Administer by subcut injection in abdominal region, buttock, thigh, or upper arm. Subcut injection into abdominal wall is generally associated with faster absorption than other injection sites.

● Rotate injection sites within same region to reduce risk of lipodystrophy.

● Injection into a lifted skin fold minimizes risk of IM injection.

● Don't perform dose conversion when using Humulin R U-500 KwikPen. Dose window of pen shows number of units of Humulin R U-500 to be injected; no dose conversion is required.

● Don't transfer Humulin R U-500 from pen into syringe for administration because overdose and severe hypoglycemia can occur.

● Don't use if solution is viscous or cloudy; use only if clear and colorless.

● Don't use regular insulin in external subcut insulin pumps because of precipitation risk.

ACTION
Lowers blood glucose level by stimulating peripheral glucose uptake by binding to insulin receptors on skeletal muscle and in fat cells

and by inhibiting liver glucose production; also inhibits lipolysis and proteolysis, and enhances protein synthesis.

Route	Onset	Peak	Duration
IV	10–15 min	Unknown	4 hr
U-100 (subcut)	30 min	0.5–2.5 hr	8 hr
U-500 (subcut)	15 min	4–8 hr	13–24 hr

Half-life: IV, 30 to 60 minutes; subcut, 1.5 hours.

ADVERSE REACTIONS

CV: peripheral edema. **Metabolic:** *hypoglycemia, hypokalemia,* weight gain. **Skin:** injection-site reactions, lipodystrophy, pruritus. **Other:** hypersensitivity reactions, *anaphylaxis,* insulin antibody production.

INTERACTIONS

Drug-drug. *ACE inhibitors, antidiabetics (oral), ARBs, disopyramide, fibrates, fluoxetine, MAO inhibitors, octreotide, pentoxifylline, pramlintide, salicylates, sulfonamide antibiotics:* May cause hypoglycemia. Monitor glucose level, and adjust insulin dosage as needed.

Atypical antipsychotics, corticosteroids, danazol, diuretics, estrogens, glucagon, hormonal contraceptives, isoniazid, niacin, phenothiazines, protease inhibitors, somatropin, sympathomimetics (albuterol, epinephrine, terbutaline), thyroid hormones: May cause hyperglycemia. Monitor glucose level, and adjust insulin dosage as needed.

Beta blockers, clonidine: May mask signs and symptoms of hypoglycemia. Avoid concurrent use, if possible, or monitor patient closely.

Beta blockers, clonidine, lithium salts, pentamidine: May cause hypoglycemia or hyperglycemia. Monitor glucose level.

Drugs that lower potassium level (diuretics) or affect potassium level (IV insulin): May increase risk of hypokalemia. Monitor potassium level.

Thiazolidinediones (TZDs; pioglitazone, rosiglitazone): May cause fluid retention that can lead to HF. Monitor patient closely; adjust or stop TZD as clinically necessary.

Drug-lifestyle. *Alcohol use:* May cause hyperglycemia or hypoglycemia. Closely monitor glucose level. Discourage concurrent use.

EFFECTS ON LAB TEST RESULTS
• May decrease glucose and potassium levels.
• May develop antibodies that react with human insulin.

CONTRAINDICATIONS & CAUTIONS
• Contraindicated during episodes of hypoglycemia.
• Contraindicated in patients with history of hypersensitivity to drug or its components. Severe, life-threatening, generalized hypersensitivity reactions, including anaphylaxis, can occur with insulin use.
• Use cautiously in patients susceptible to hypokalemia, such as patients who are fasting, are taking potassium-lowering drugs, or are concurrently taking drugs that may affect potassium level. Untreated hypokalemia can cause respiratory paralysis, ventricular arrhythmias, and death.
• Hypoglycemia is the most common adverse reaction. Severe hypoglycemia can cause seizures and may be life-threatening or fatal. Hypoglycemia can occur suddenly, and symptoms may differ. Risk is greater in patients with kidney or liver impairment and increases with intensity of glycemic control; changes in glycemic treatment, meal pattern, or physical activity; and concomitant use of certain medications.
• Human insulin differs from animal-source insulin. Change between insulin types cautiously, and monitor patient closely.
• Use cautiously in older adults, who may be at increased risk for adverse effects. Signs and symptoms of hypoglycemia may be more difficult to recognize in these patients.
• Use insulin pens cautiously in patients with visual impairment, who may rely on audible clicks to dial their dose.
Dialyzable drug: Unknown.
⚠ *Overdose S&S:* Hypoglycemia, hypokalemia.

PREGNANCY-LACTATION-REPRODUCTION
• Use cautiously during pregnancy.
• Closely monitor glucose level during pregnancy, after recent birth, and during breastfeeding; insulin requirements may change.
• It isn't known if insulin appears in human milk. Use cautiously during breastfeeding. Adjust insulin dose as needed.

NURSING CONSIDERATIONS

• Monitor patient carefully when initiating therapy. Time course of insulins varies with each patient.

• Monitor blood glucose level and adjust insulin dosage as needed for patient-specific goals.

• Closely monitor patient after changes to insulin dosage.

• Increase frequency of glucose monitoring when patient is acutely ill or under emotional stress and if changes in diet, exercise, or medication regimen occur; these conditions may affect insulin absorption.

• Closely monitor for signs and symptoms of hypoglycemia, especially in long-standing disease. Treat according to individual facility protocol, if necessary.

• Mild episodes of hypoglycemia may be treated with oral glucose. More severe episodes of hypoglycemia, such as coma, seizure, or neurologic impairment, may be treated with IM or subcut glucagon or concentrated IV glucose.

• Assess patient and notify prescriber of signs and symptoms of hypoglycemia (diaphoresis, shaking, trembling, confusion) or hyperglycemia (drowsiness, fruity breath odor, frequent urination, thirst).

• Periodically measure HbA$_{1c}$ level.

• Monitor potassium level in patients at risk for hypokalemia, including those taking potassium-depleting drugs.

• Monitor patient for generalized allergic reactions, including anaphylaxis.

• Verify product label before giving drug to avoid medication errors.

• **Alert:** Medication errors associated with U-500 vial have resulted in hyperglycemia, hypoglycemia, and death; read labels closely to prevent errors.

• **Alert:** Use only a U-500 insulin syringe with U-500 vials to avoid administration errors. Don't use any other type of syringe to administer U-500 insulin.

• *Look alike–sound alike:* Don't confuse Humulin with Humalog. Don't confuse Novolin with NovoLog.

PATIENT TEACHING

• Instruct patient in self-management, including glucose management, injection technique, proper storage of insulin, and recognition and management of hypoglycemia and hyperglycemia.

• Teach patient to eat within 30 minutes of injecting short-acting insulin.

• Instruct patient to only use syringes calibrated for their concentration of insulin.

• **Alert:** Warn patient not to share multidose pen (even if needle is changed) because of risk of bloodborne pathogen transmission, including HIV and hepatitis.

• Teach patient to rotate injection sites to prevent lipodystrophy.

• Instruct patient mixing two types of insulin to always draw up shorter-acting insulin first, followed by NPH, and inject immediately.

• Explain importance of checking insulin label before each injection; accidental mix-ups among insulin types have been reported.

• Instruct patient to keep hard candy or glucose tablets on hand to treat mild cases of hypoglycemia.

• Caution patient that hypoglycemic episodes can impair ability to concentrate and react; advise patient to use caution while driving and operating machinery.

• Advise patient to track glucose level.

• Instruct patient on long-term risks of improperly managed diabetes.

• Counsel patient to carry identification or wear jewelry indicating diabetes status.

• Warn that allergic reactions, including injection-site reactions (local pain, redness or swelling) and generalized allergic reaction and anaphylaxis (whole-body rash, shortness of breath, wheezing, reduced BP, fast pulse, diaphoresis) can occur. Teach patient to immediately seek emergency medical attention for generalized reactions.

• Explain that insulin requirements may vary due to illness, stress, emotional disturbances, inadequate or skipped insulin dose, inadvertent administration of an increased insulin dose, inadequate food intake, skipped meals, or pregnancy.

• Caution patient not to stop insulin abruptly or to change amount injected without consulting prescriber.

• Warn patient that any change in insulin should be made cautiously and only under medical supervision. Changes in insulin strength, manufacturer, type (regular, NPH, or insulin analogues), species (animal, human), or method of manufacture (rDNA, animal-source insulin) may result in the need for a dosage change.

Reactions in bold italics are ***life-threatening***.

• Caution patient to discuss adjustments to administration schedule if traveling across more than two time zones.
• Instruct patient to report pregnancy or plans to become pregnant or to breastfeed.

interferon alfa-2b (recombinant) (IFN-alpha 2b)
in-ter-FEER-on

Intron A

Therapeutic class: Antivirals
Pharmacologic class: Biological response modifiers

AVAILABLE FORMS
Powder for injection: 10, 18, and 50 million international units/vial with diluent
Solution for injection: 18 and 25 million international units/vial (6 and 10 million international units/mL)

INDICATIONS & DOSAGES
Adjust-a-dose (for all indications): For all indications except condylomata acuminata, if adverse effects occur, stop drug until they abate; then resume drug at 50% of previous dose. If intolerance persists, stop drug. See package insert for specific guidance.
➤ **Hairy cell leukemia**
Adults: 2 million international units/m^2 IM or subcut three times weekly for up to 6 months or more if patient is responding to treatment. Give subcut if platelet count is less than 50,000/mm^3.
➤ **AIDS-related Kaposi sarcoma**
Adults: 30 million international units/m^2 subcut or IM three times weekly. Maintain dose until disease progression or maximal response has been achieved after 16 weeks of treatment. Don't use solution for injection in vials for this indication.
➤ **Chronic HBV infection**
Adults: 30 to 35 million international units IM or subcut weekly, given as 5 million international units daily or 10 million international units three times weekly for 16 weeks.
Children ages 1 to 17: 3 million international units/m^2 subcut three times weekly for first week; then increase to 6 million international units/m^2 subcut three times weekly (maximum, 10 million international

units three times weekly) for total of 16 to 24 weeks.
Adjust-a-dose: If WBC count is less than 1.5×10^9/L, granulocyte count is less than 0.75×10^9/L, or platelet count is less than 50×10^9/L, reduce dose by 50%. Permanently discontinue drug if WBC count is less than 1×10^9/L, granulocyte count is less than 0.5×10^9/L, or platelet count is less than 25×10^9/L.
➤ **Chronic HCV infection**
Adults: 3 million international units IM or subcut three times weekly. In patients tolerating therapy with normalization of ALT at 16 weeks of therapy, continue for 18 to 24 months. In patients without normalized ALT or with persistently high levels of HCV RNA after 16 weeks of therapy, consider stopping therapy.
➤ **Adjunct to surgical treatment in patients with malignant melanoma who are free of disease but at high risk for systemic recurrence for up to 8 weeks after surgery**
Adults: Induction dose, 20 million international units/m^2 by IV infusion over 20 minutes 5 consecutive days weekly for 4 weeks; then maintenance dosage of 10 million international units/m^2 subcut three times weekly for 48 weeks. Solution for injection in vials isn't recommended for IV administration and shouldn't be used for induction phase.
Adjust-a-dose: Refer to manufacturer's instructions for toxicity-related dosage adjustments.
➤ **First treatment of clinically aggressive follicular non-Hodgkin lymphoma with chemotherapy containing anthracycline**
Adults: 5 million international units subcut three times weekly for up to 18 months in conjunction with anthracycline-containing chemotherapy regimen.
Adjust-a-dose: Refer to manufacturer's instructions for toxicity-related dosage adjustments.
➤ **Condylomata acuminata (genital or perianal warts)**
Adults: 1 million international units for each lesion (maximum five lesions in a single course) intralesionally three times weekly for 3 weeks. Additional course may be given at 12 to 16 weeks. Don't use 18-million or 50-million international units powder for injection or 18-million international units multidose solution for injection for this indication.

ADMINISTRATION

- Reconstitute powder with 1 mL of sterile water; swirl gently. Solution should be clear and colorless to light yellow.
- Reconstituted powder doesn't contain preservative and must be used immediately. Don't reenter vial after withdrawing dose. Discard unused portion.
- Solution in multidose vials should be clear and colorless and may be injected IM, subcut, or intralesionally. Don't give IV.

IV

▼ Prepare infusion solution immediately before use.

▼ Bring solution to room temperature before use.

▼ Based on desired dose, reconstitute appropriate vial strength of drug with diluent provided. Withdraw dose and inject into 100-mL bag of NSS. Final yield of drug shouldn't be less than 10 million international units/100 mL.

▼ Infuse over 20 minutes.

▼ Give in the evening, when possible, to enhance tolerability.

▼ Store solution in refrigerator. Store powder before and after reconstitution in refrigerator. Use within 24 hours.

▼ **Incompatibilities:** Dextrose solutions.

IM

- Carefully monitor injection sites in patients with thrombocytopenia. Avoid IM injections, if possible.
- Give IM injection in anterior thigh, deltoid, or superolateral buttock.
- In patients whose platelet count falls below 50,000/mm^3, give subcutaneously.
- Give drug at bedtime to minimize daytime drowsiness.

Subcutaneous

- Give subcut injection in thigh, upper outer arm, or abdomen.

Intralesional

- For condylomata acuminata intralesional injection, use only 10 million-international unit vial because dilution of other strengths for intralesional use results in a hypertonic solution.
- Don't reconstitute drug in 10 million-international unit vial with more than 1 mL of diluent.
- Use tuberculin or similar syringe and 25G to 30G needle.

- Don't inject too deep beneath lesion (subcutaneously) or too superficially. As many as five lesions can be treated at one time.
- To ease discomfort, give in evening with acetaminophen.

ACTION

Unknown. May inhibit tumor or viral cell replication and modulate host immune response by enhancing macrophage activity and improving specific lymphocytes' cytotoxicity for target cells.

Route	Onset	Peak	Duration
IV	Unknown	30 min	4 hr
IM, subcut	Unknown	3–12 hr	16 hr
Intralesional	Unknown	Unknown	Unknown

Half-life: IV, 2 hours; IM, subcut, 2 to 3 hours.

ADVERSE REACTIONS

CNS: apathy, amnesia, agitation, abnormal dreams, asthenia, depression, difficulty thinking or concentrating, confusion, dizziness, vertigo, drowsiness, fatigue, insomnia, paresthesia, somnolence, anxiety, aggression, lethargy, nervousness, fever, weakness, abnormal gait, headache, malaise, hypothermia, irritability, taste alteration, smell alteration, voice disorder, dysphagia, emotional lability, pain, *stroke, suicidality.* **CV:** angina, arteritis, arrhythmia, atrial fibrillation, *bradycardia, HF,* cardiomegaly, *cardiomyopathy,* CAD, chest pain, cyanosis, edema, extrasystoles, heart valve disorder, HTN, flushing, hypotension, palpitations, phlebitis, orthostatic hypotension, *PE,* Raynaud disease, tachycardia, *thrombosis,* varicose veins. **EENT:** conjunctivitis, abnormal vision, earache, epistaxis, nasal congestion, rhinorrhea, rhinitis, sinusitis, pharyngitis, gingivitis, dry mouth. **GI:** anorexia, diarrhea, dyspepsia, nausea, vomiting, abdominal pain, constipation, esophagitis, flatulence, stomatitis. **GU:** increased BUN level, decreased libido, impotence, amenorrhea. **Hematologic:** *leukopenia, thrombocytopenia,* anemia, *neutropenia, granulocytopenia.* **Hepatic:** increased LFT values, jaundice, *hepatitis.* **Metabolic:** weight loss, hypercalcemia, thirst, hyperglycemia. **Musculoskeletal:** myalgia, arthralgia, back pain, musculo-skeletal pain. **Respiratory:** coughing, dyspnea, bronchitis. **Skin:** alopecia, dryness, injection-site reaction, diaphoresis, pruritus, purpura, rash, dermatitis. **Other:** flulike syndrome, chills, rigors, infection.

Reactions in bold italics are *life-threatening*.

INTERACTIONS

Drug-drug. *Aldesleukin, telbivudine:* May enhance adverse or toxic effects of these drugs. Avoid use together.

CNS depressants: May increase CNS effects. Avoid use together.

Myelosuppressants (zidovudine), clozapine: May increase risk of neutropenia. Carefully monitor WBC count.

Ribavirin: May enhance adverse effects, including hemolytic anemia. Monitor therapy.

Theophylline: May reduce theophylline clearance. Monitor theophylline level.

Vitamin K antagonists (warfarin): May increase anticoagulant effect. Closely monitor PT and INR.

EFFECTS ON LAB TEST RESULTS

• May increase calcium, phosphate, AST, ALT, LDH, ALP, triglyceride, creatinine, BUN, and fasting glucose levels.

• May increase or decrease TSH level.

• May increase INR and prolong PT and PTT.

• May decrease Hb level and WBC and platelet counts.

CONTRAINDICATIONS & CAUTIONS

• Contraindicated in patients hypersensitive to drug or its components and in those with autoimmune hepatitis or decompensated liver disease.

• Combination therapy with ribavirin is additionally contraindicated in patients hypersensitive to ribavirin or other components of product and in those with hemoglobinopathies or CrCl less than 50 mL/minute.

• Use cautiously in older adults and in patients with history of CV disease, cerebrovascular disorders, pulmonary disease, diabetes, coagulation disorders, kidney impairment, or severe myelosuppression.

• Depression, psychosis, and suicidality have been linked to drug use; patients with psychotic disorders, especially depression, shouldn't continue drug treatment.

🜂 *Alert:* Neurotoxicity and cardiotoxicity are more common in older adults, especially those with underlying CNS or cardiac impairment.

• Safety and effectiveness in children haven't been established except for HBV and chronic HCV.

Dialyzable drug: No.

⚠ *Overdose S&S:* Abnormal liver enzyme levels, kidney failure, hemorrhage, MI.

PREGNANCY-LACTATION-REPRODUCTION

• Studies during pregnancy are inadequate. Use during pregnancy only if potential benefit justifies fetal risk.

🜂 *Alert:* Combination therapy with ribavirin is contraindicated during pregnancy and in men whose partners are pregnant. Use of two forms of contraception is recommended.

• It isn't known if drug appears in human milk. Patient should discontinue breastfeeding or discontinue drug.

NURSING CONSIDERATIONS

Boxed Warning Alpha interferons cause or aggravate fatal or life-threatening neuropsychiatric, autoimmune, ischemic, and infectious disorders. Monitor patients closely with periodic clinical and lab evaluations. Withdraw patients with persistently severe or worsening signs or symptoms of these conditions from therapy. ∎

🜂 *Alert:* Not all dosage forms are appropriate for all indications. Refer to manufacturer's instructions for approved indications before use.

• Verify pregnancy status before treatment.

• Ensure patient is well hydrated, especially at beginning of treatment.

• At start of treatment, monitor patient for flulike signs and symptoms, which tend to diminish with continued therapy. Premedicate patient with acetaminophen to minimize these symptoms.

• Periodically check for adverse CNS reactions (decreased mental status, dizziness) during therapy.

• Monitor CBC with differential, platelet count, and blood chemistry and electrolyte studies. Monitor ECG before and during treatment if patient has cardiac disorder or advanced stages of cancer.

• Monitor liver function (serum bilirubin, ALT, AST, ALP, and LDH) at 2, 8, and 12 weeks after start of therapy, then every 6 months during therapy. Permanently stop drug for evidence of severe (grade 3) liver injury or Child-Pugh classes B and C liver impairment.

• If patient develops thrombocytopenia, exercise extreme care when performing invasive procedures; frequently inspect injection site and skin for signs and symptoms of bruising; limit frequency of IM injections; and test urine, emesis fluid, stool, and secretions for occult blood.

• Severe adverse reactions may need dosage reduction to half or withholding of drug until reactions subside.

• Use with blood dyscrasia-causing drugs, bone marrow suppressants, or radiation therapy may increase bone marrow suppression. Dosage reduction may be needed.

• For condylomata acuminata, maximum response usually occurs in 4 to 8 weeks.

PATIENT TEACHING

• Advise patient to avoid contact with persons with viral illness; patient is at increased risk for infection during therapy.

• Inform patient that lab tests will be performed before and periodically during therapy.

• Teach patient proper oral hygiene during treatment because bone marrow suppressant effects of interferon may lead to microbial infection, delayed healing, and bleeding gums. Drug also may decrease saliva.

• Advise patient to check with prescriber for instructions after missing a dose.

• Stress need to follow prescriber's instructions about taking and recording temperature and how and when to take acetaminophen.

• Teach patient who will self-administer drug how to prepare injection and how to use and dispose of syringe. Provide information on drug stability.

• Tell patient that drug may cause temporary partial hair loss; hair should return after drug is stopped.

• Advise patient to report all adverse reactions and to immediately report neuropsychiatric symptoms (depression, mania, psychosis, suicidality).

• Warn patient of reproductive potential of fetal risk. Counsel about contraception use.

SAFETY ALERT!

interferon beta-1a
in-ter-FEER-on

Avonex, Rebif

Therapeutic class: Antivirals
Pharmacologic class: Biological response modifiers

AVAILABLE FORMS
Avonex (IM use only)
Injection: 30 mcg (6 million international units)/0.5 mL prefilled syringe or autoinjector

Rebif (subcut use only)
Injection: 8.8 mcg (2.4 million international units)/0.2 mL, 22 mcg (6 million international units)/0.5 mL, 44 mcg (12 million international units)/0.5 mL prefilled syringe or autoinjector

INDICATIONS & DOSAGES
➤ **Relapsing forms of MS**
Adults: Initially, 7.5 mcg IM (week 1); then increase in increments of 7.5 mcg once weekly (weeks 2 to 4) up to recommended dosage (30 mcg once weekly). Or, initially, 4.4 or 8.8 mcg subcut three times weekly for 2 weeks; then increase dosage to 11 or 22 mcg three times weekly for another 2 weeks. Then increase to a maintenance dosage of 22 or 44 mcg subcut three times weekly.
Adjust-a-dose: For Rebif, in patients with decreased blood counts or elevated LFT values (ALT level greater than $5 \times$ ULN), reduce dosage or withhold drug until toxicity resolves. Stop treatment if jaundice or other signs of liver injury occur.

ADMINISTRATION
• Visually inspect for particulate matter and discoloration before administration.

• Rotate sites of injection. Don't inject into areas of redness, bruising, or irritation.
Subcutaneous
• Administer Rebif at same time on same 3 days at least 48 hours apart each week (late afternoon or evening on Monday, Wednesday, and Friday).

• Use only prefilled syringes for titration to 22 mcg prescribed dose of Rebif. Prefilled syringes or autoinjectors may be used to titrate to 44 mcg dose.

• Give missed dose as soon as possible, then resume normal schedule; if next dose is less than 48 hours away, check with prescriber.

• Store Rebif in refrigerator between 36° and 46° F (2° and 8° C). Don't freeze. Rebif may be stored at or below 77° F (25° C) for up to 30 days if away from heat and light, but refrigeration is preferred.
IM
⚠ *Alert:* Syringe tip cap contains natural rubber latex, which may cause allergic reactions.

• Assess injection site after 2 hours for redness, swelling, or tenderness.

• Give missed dose as soon as possible, then resume normal schedule; don't give 2 days in a row.

Reactions in bold italics are *life-threatening*.

• Store Avonex prefilled syringes and autoinjectors in refrigerator at 36° to 46° F (2° and 8° C). If refrigeration is unavailable, may store at room temperature for up to 7 days. Once refrigerated, syringes and autoinjectors must not be stored above 77° F. Once removed from refrigerator, warm to room temperature (about 30 minutes). Don't use external heat sources, such as hot water, to warm syringe, or expose to high temperatures. If product has been exposed to conditions other than those recommended after removal from refrigerator, discard product. Don't freeze. Protect from light.

• After giving each dose, discard any remaining product in syringe or autoinjector.

ACTION
Unknown. Interacts with specific cell receptors found on the surface of cells. Binding of these receptors causes expression of a number of interferon-induced gene products believed to mediate the biological actions of interferon beta-1a.

Route	Onset	Peak	Duration
Subcut	Unknown	16 hr	Unknown
IM	12 hr	15 hr	4 days

Half-life: Subcut, 69 hours; IM, 19 hours.

ADVERSE REACTIONS
CNS: dizziness, fatigue, asthenia, fever, headache, migraine, pain, depression, *seizures, suicidality,* abnormal coordination, ataxia, hypertonia, malaise, somnolence, rigors. **CV:** chest pain, vasodilation. **EENT:** abnormal vision, dry eyes, dry mouth, sinusitis, toothache. **GI:** abdominal pain. **GU:** UTI, urinary frequency, urinary incontinence. **Hematologic:** *leukopenia, pancytopenia, thrombocytopenia,* anemia, lymphadenopathy. **Hepatic:** increased transaminase levels, bilirubinemia, liver injury. **Metabolic:** hyperthyroidism, hypothyroidism. **Musculoskeletal:** back pain, myalgia, skeletal pain, arthralgia, muscle spasm. **Respiratory:** URI, dyspnea, bronchitis. **Skin:** injection-site reaction, injection-site necrosis, alopecia, ecchymosis at injection site, urticaria, rash, diaphoresis. **Other:** chills, flulike syndrome, infection, hypersensitivity reactions, neutralizing antibodies.

INTERACTIONS
Drug-drug. *Liver-toxic drugs (allopurinol, erythromycin, statins):* May increase risk of liver injury. Use together cautiously.

EFFECTS ON LAB TEST RESULTS
• May increase liver enzyme levels.
• May increase eosinophil count.
• May decrease Hb level, hematocrit, and WBC and platelet counts.
• May increase or decrease thyroid function test levels.

CONTRAINDICATIONS & CAUTIONS
• Contraindicated in patients hypersensitive to natural or recombinant interferon beta, human albumin (Rebif), or other components of drug.
• Use cautiously in patients with depression, seizure disorders, HF, cardiac conditions, liver disease, or alcohol use disorder.
• Thrombotic microangiopathy (TMA), including thrombotic thrombocytopenic purpura and hemolytic-uremic syndrome, sometimes fatal, has been reported with interferon beta products and may occur several weeks to years after start of therapy.
• Autoimmune disorders, including ITP, thyroid disorders, and autoimmune hepatitis have been reported.
• Safety and effectiveness of drug in patients with chronic progressive MS and in children haven't been established.
Dialyzable drug: Unknown.

PREGNANCY-LACTATION-REPRODUCTION
• Studies during pregnancy are inadequate. Use during pregnancy only if potential benefit justifies fetal risk.
• Drug appears in human milk at low levels. Use cautiously during breastfeeding.

NURSING CONSIDERATIONS
• Monitor patient closely for depression and suicidality. It isn't known if these symptoms are related to underlying neurologic basis of MS or to drug.
• Monitor thyroid function tests, WBC count, platelet count, and blood chemistry results, including LFTs.
• Monitor patient for TMA and discontinue drug if clinical signs and symptoms (bruises, bleeding, confusion, decreased urine output, edema, HTN) and lab findings (hemolytic

anemia, thrombocytopenia) consistent with TMA occur; manage as clinically indicated.
• Give analgesics or antipyretics to decrease flulike symptoms.
• Monitor patient for hypersensitivity reactions, including anaphylaxis.
• Monitor patient for injection-site reactions, including necrosis. Antibiotics or surgical intervention may be necessary. Don't inject into affected area until completely healed; if multiple lesions occur, may discontinue drug until lesions heal.

PATIENT TEACHING
• Advise patient to read medication guide that comes with drug.
• Teach about safe drug administration, storage, and needle disposal.
• Instruct patient to keep syringes and needles away from children, not to reuse needles or syringes, and to discard them in a syringe-disposal unit.
• Caution patient not to change dosage or schedule of administration unless directed by prescriber.
• Inform patient that flulike signs and symptoms (fever, fatigue, muscle aches, headache, chills, joint pain) aren't uncommon at start of therapy and that analgesics or antipyretics may be prescribed on treatment days to lessen their severity.
• Advise patient to report depression, suicidality, or other adverse reactions.
• If pregnancy occurs, instruct patient to notify prescriber immediately.

SAFETY ALERT!

interferon beta-1b (recombinant)
in-ter-FEER-on

Betaseron, Extavia

Therapeutic class: Immunomodulators
Pharmacologic class: Biological response modifiers

AVAILABLE FORMS
Powder for injection: 0.3 mg

INDICATIONS & DOSAGES
➤ **Relapsing forms of MS, including clinically isolated syndrome, relapsing-remitting**

disease, and active secondary progressive disease
Adults: 0.0625 mg subcut every other day for weeks 1 and 2; then 0.125 mg subcut every other day for weeks 3 and 4; then 0.1875 mg subcut every other day for weeks 5 and 6; then 0.25 mg subcut every other day thereafter.

ADMINISTRATION
Subcutaneous
⚠ *Alert:* The removable rubber cap of Extavia diluent prefilled syringe contains natural rubber latex, which may cause allergic reactions and shouldn't be handled by latex-sensitive individuals.
• To reconstitute, slowly inject 1.2 mL of supplied diluent (half-NSS for injection) into vial and gently swirl to dissolve drug.
• Don't shake. Discard vial that contains particulates or discolored solution.
• Each mL of reconstituted solution contains 0.25 mg of interferon beta-1b.
• Inject immediately after preparation.
• Rotate injection sites to minimize local reactions and observe site for necrosis. Don't inject into red, sore, or infected skin.
• Give missed dose as soon as possible; give next injection 48 hours after that dose. Don't give drug on two consecutive days.
• Store at room temperature. After reconstitution, if not used immediately, may refrigerate drug for up to 3 hours. Don't freeze.

ACTION
Exact mechanism unknown. A naturally occurring antiviral and immunoregulatory drug derived from human fibroblasts. Attaches to membrane receptors and causes cellular changes, including increased protein synthesis.

Route	Onset	Peak	Duration
Subcut	Unknown	1–8 hr	Unknown

Half-life: 8 minutes to 4.3 hours.

ADVERSE REACTIONS
CNS: depression, asthenia, migraine, headache, pain, malaise, fever, insomnia, incoordination. **CV:** chest pain, peripheral edema, HTN. **GI:** abdominal pain. **GU:** menstrual disorder, urinary urgency, impotence. **Hepatic:** increased transaminase levels. **Hematologic:** *leukopenia, lymphocytopenia, neutropenia,* lymphadenopathy.

Reactions in bold italics are *life-threatening*.

Musculoskeletal: myalgia, hypertonia. **Respiratory:** dyspnea. **Skin:** inflammation, pain, necrosis at injection site; rash, skin disorder. **Other:** flulike syndrome, chills.

INTERACTIONS

• *Liver toxic drugs (allopurinol, erythromycin, statins):* May increase risk of liver toxicity. Use together cautiously.

EFFECTS ON LAB TEST RESULTS

• May increase ALT, AST, and bilirubin levels.
• May decrease WBC and neutrophil counts.

CONTRAINDICATIONS & CAUTIONS

• Contraindicated in patients hypersensitive to interferon beta, human albumin, mannitol, or components of drug.
• Use cautiously in patients with HF.
• Drug-induced lupus erythematosus has been reported and has occurred with positive serologic testing (including positive antinuclear or anti-double-stranded DNA antibody testing).
• Thrombotic microangiopathy (TMA), including thrombotic thrombocytopenic purpura and hemolytic-uremic syndrome, sometimes fatal, has been reported with interferon beta products and may occur several weeks to years after start of therapy.
• Seizures have been reported with beta interferon use; however, it's unknown if they're related to a primary seizure disorder, the effects of MS, other causes of seizures (fever), or use of the drug.
• Safety and effectiveness in children haven't been established.
Dialyzable drug: Unknown.

PREGNANCY-LACTATION-REPRODUCTION

• Studies during pregnancy are inadequate; however, spontaneous abortions have been reported in clinical trials. Use during pregnancy only if potential benefit justifies fetal risk.
• It isn't known if drug appears in human milk. Use cautiously during breastfeeding.

NURSING CONSIDERATIONS

⚠ **Alert:** Serious liver damage, including liver failure requiring transplant, can occur. Monitor liver function at 1, 3, and 6 months after therapy starts and periodically thereafter.
• Drug is intended for use under guidance and supervision of a prescriber. Administer first injection under supervision of a health care provider. If patient or caregiver will administer drug, train them in proper self-administration technique.
• Monitor for signs and symptoms of drug-induced lupus erythematosus (rash, serositis, polyarthritis, Raynaud phenomenon, nephritis); discontinue therapy if any occur.
• Monitor patient for TMA and discontinue drug if clinical signs and symptoms (bruising, bleeding, HTN, edema, decreased urine output, confusion) and lab findings (hemolytic anemia, thrombocytopenia) consistent with TMA occur; manage as clinically indicated.
• Monitor patient for symptoms of depression and severe psychiatric effects (mania, suicidality, psychosis).
• Monitor CBC and blood chemistry results at 1, 3, and 6 months after therapy starts and periodically thereafter.
• Monitor thyroid function tests every 6 months in patient being treated for thyroid disorder.
• Use of analgesics and antipyretics on treatment days may help improve flulike symptoms associated with interferon beta-1b use.
• Monitor for injection-site reactions, including necrosis. Antibiotics or surgical intervention may be necessary. Don't inject into affected area until completely healed; if multiple lesions occur, may discontinue drug until lesions heal.

PATIENT TEACHING

• Warn patient about dangers to a fetus. Instruct patient to notify prescriber if pregnancy occurs during therapy.
• Advise patient to read medication guide that comes with drug.
• Teach patient how to perform subcut injections, including solution preparation, aseptic technique, injection-site rotation, and equipment disposal. Periodically reevaluate patient's technique.
• Tell patient to take drug at bedtime to minimize mild flulike symptoms.
• Advise patient to stay well hydrated.
• Tell patient to report sign and symptoms of drug-induced lupus erythematosus.
• Advise patient to report suicidality or depression.
• Urge patient to immediately report signs or symptoms of tissue death at injection site.
• Advise patient of importance of obtaining routine blood tests.

SAFETY ALERT!

ipilimumab ⚸
ip-ih-LIM-yoo-mab

Yervoy

Therapeutic class: Antineoplastics
Pharmacologic class: Monoclonal antibodies

AVAILABLE FORMS
Injection: 5 mg/mL in 10 mL and 40 mL vials

INDICATIONS & DOSAGES
Adjust-a-dose (for all indications): Refer to manufacturer's instructions for toxicity-related dosage adjustments.

➤ **Unresectable or metastatic melanoma**
Adults and children ages 12 and older:
3 mg/kg IV infusion every 3 weeks for a total of four doses. All treatment must be administered within 16 weeks of first dose.

➤ **Combination therapy for unresectable or metastatic melanoma**
Adults and children ages 12 and older:
3 mg/kg IV every 3 weeks immediately after nivolumab 1 mg/kg on same day for four combination doses. Continue nivolumab as a single agent until disease progression or unacceptable toxicity occurs.

➤ **Adjuvant treatment of cutaneous melanoma with pathologic involvement of regional lymph nodes of more than 1 mm after complete resection, including total lymphadenectomy**
Adults: 10 mg/kg IV over 90 minutes every 3 weeks for four doses; then 10 mg/kg every 12 weeks for up to 3 years or until disease recurrence or unacceptable toxicity occurs.

➤ **Intermediate- or poor-risk, previously untreated advanced renal cell carcinoma in combination with nivolumab**
Adults: 1 mg/kg IV infusion every 3 weeks with nivolumab 3 mg/kg IV infusion every 3 weeks for maximum of four doses. Continue nivolumab as a single agent until disease progression or unacceptable toxicity occurs.

➤ **Microsatellite instability-high or mismatch repair-deficient metastatic colorectal cancer that has progressed after treatment with a fluoropyrimidine, oxaliplatin, and irinotecan, in combination with nivolumab**

Adults and children ages 12 and older:
1 mg/kg IV infusion every 3 weeks with nivolumab 3 mg/kg every 3 weeks for up to four doses. Continue nivolumab as single agent until disease progression or unacceptable toxicity occurs.

➤ **Hepatocellular carcinoma in combination with nivolumab after treatment with sorafenib**
Adults: 3 mg/kg IV infusion with nivolumab 1 mg/kg IV infusion every 3 weeks for up to four combination doses. Continue nivolumab as single agent until disease progression or unacceptable toxicity occurs.

➤ **First-line combination therapy for metastatic NSCLC when tumors express PD-L1 according to FDA-approved testing, with no *EGFR* or *ALK* genomic tumor aberrations ⚸**
Adults: 1 mg/kg IV infusion every 6 weeks with nivolumab 360 mg IV infusion every 3 weeks. Continue until disease progression or unacceptable toxicity occurs, or for up to 2 years in patients without disease progression.

➤ **Metastatic or recurrent NSCLC with no *EGFR* or *ALK* genomic tumor aberrations in combination with nivolumab and platinum-doublet chemotherapy ⚸**
Adults: 1 mg/kg IV infusion every 6 weeks with nivolumab 360 mg IV infusion every 3 weeks and two cycles of chemotherapy every 3 weeks. Continue until disease progression or unacceptable toxicity occurs, or up to 2 years in patients without disease progression.

➤ **Unresectable malignant pleural mesothelioma in combination with nivolumab**
Adults: 1 mg/kg IV infusion every 6 weeks with nivolumab 360 mg IV infusion every 3 weeks. Continue until disease progression or unacceptable toxicity occurs, or up to 2 years in patients without disease progression.

➤ **Unresectable advanced or metastatic esophageal squamous cell carcinoma as first-line treatment, in combination with nivolumab**
Adults: 1 mg/kg IV infusion every 6 weeks with nivolumab 3 mg/kg IV infusion every 2 weeks or 360 mg IV infusion every 3 weeks until disease progression or unacceptable toxicity occurs, or up to 2 years in patients without disease progression.

Reactions in bold italics are *life-threatening*.

ADMINISTRATION

IV

▼ Store vials in refrigerator at 36° to 46° F (2° to 8° C). Don't freeze or shake vials. Protect from light.

▼ Visually inspect solution, which may be clear to pale yellow. Discard if cloudy or discolored or if particles (other than translucent-to-white, amorphous particles) are present.

▼ Allow vials to come to room temperature for 5 minutes before preparing infusion.

▼ Withdraw required volume of drug and transfer into IV bag of NSS or D_5W. Final concentration should range from 1 to 2 mg/mL. Gently invert bag to mix.

▼ Store diluted solution for up to 24 hours under refrigeration or at room temperature.

▼ Administer diluted solution over 30 minutes or 90 minutes (for adjuvant melanoma treatment only) through IV line containing a sterile, nonpyrogenic, low-protein-binding in-line filter.

▼ When given in combination with nivolumab, infuse nivolumab first followed by ipilimumab on same day. If ordered, follow with platinum-based doublet chemotherapy (all on the same day). Use separate infusion bags and filters for each infusion.

▼ After each dose, flush IV line with NSS or D_5W.

▼ Discard unused portion of vial.

▼ **Incompatibilities:** Other IV drugs and solutions other than NSS or D_5W.

ACTION

Binds to the cytotoxic T-lymphocyte-associated antigen 4; this blockade has been shown to augment T-cell-mediated antitumor immune responses.

Route	Onset	Peak	Duration
IV	Rapid	Unknown	Unknown

Half-life: 15.4 days.

ADVERSE REACTIONS

Note: Includes reported adverse reactions during nivolumab combination therapy
CNS: fatigue, malaise, neuropathy, fever, headache, insomnia. **CV:** hypotension, HTN, edema. **EENT:** dry mouth. **GI:** diarrhea, colitis, enterocolitis, nausea, vomiting, decreased appetite, constipation, stomatitis, abdominal pain. **GU:** nephritis, increased creatinine level. **Hematologic:** anemia, *lymphopenia.* **Hepatic:** ascites, increased transaminase

levels, increased ALP level, hyperbilirubinemia, *liver toxicity.* **Metabolic:** endocrinopathy (hypothyroidism, hyperthyroidism, adrenal insufficiency, hypopituitarism), *hyperkalemia, hypokalemia, hypomagnesemia,* hyperglycemia, hyponatremia, increased lipase and amylase levels, *hypocalcemia,* weight loss. **Musculoskeletal:** pain, arthralgia. **Respiratory:** cough, URI, dyspnea, pneumonitis. **Skin:** pruritus, rash, vitiligo, dermatitis, urticaria. **Other:** flulike symptoms, chills.

INTERACTIONS

None reported.

EFFECTS ON LAB TEST RESULTS

● May increase ALT, AST, ALP, bilirubin, amylase, lipase, and creatinine levels.

● May decrease magnesium, sodium, calcium, and Hb levels.

● May increase or decrease potassium or thyroid hormone levels.

● May increase eosinophil, neutrophil, lymphocyte, and platelet counts.

CONTRAINDICATIONS & CAUTIONS

● Contraindicated in patients hypersensitive to drug or its components.

● Drug can cause severe and fatal immune-mediated adverse reactions involving any organ system, especially such reactions as enterocolitis, hepatitis, dermatitis (including TEN, SJS, DRESS syndrome), neuropathy, pneumonitis, kidney dysfunction, and endocrinopathy. Reactions usually occur during treatment but may present weeks to months after therapy ends. If severe immune-mediated reactions occur, permanently discontinue ipilimumab and initiate systemic high-dose corticosteroid therapy. Assess patient for these reactions.

● Drug may increase risk of fatal or serious GVHD before or after allogeneic hematopoietic stem cell transplantation. Consider risks and benefits; monitor patient closely.

● Refer to nivolumab prescribing information for additional risk information.

● Safety and effectiveness in children younger than age 12 haven't been determined. *Dialyzable drug:* Unknown.

PREGNANCY-LACTATION-REPRODUCTION

● Based on its mechanism of action and data from animal studies, drug can cause fetal

harm when given during pregnancy. Report pregnancy to Bristol-Myers Squibb at 1-844-593-7869.
• Advise patients of childbearing potential to use effective contraception during treatment and for 3 months after last dose.
• Drug may appear in human milk. Because of the risk of serious adverse reactions in breastfeeding infants, patient shouldn't breastfeed during treatment and for 3 months after final dose.

NURSING CONSIDERATIONS
• Verify pregnancy status before treatment.
• Monitor patient for infusion reactions; interrupt or slow rate of infusion in patient with mild or moderate reactions.
• Assess patient for signs and symptoms of enterocolitis, dermatitis, neuropathy, and endocrinopathy, and evaluate clinical chemistry values, including ACTH level and thyroid function test results, at baseline and before each dose.
• Monitor LFT results and assess for signs and symptoms of liver toxicity (jaundice, dark urine, nausea, vomiting, right upper quadrant pain, abnormal bleeding, or bruising) before each dose.
• Monitor for signs and symptoms of enterocolitis and bowel perforation (abdominal pain, fever, ileus, peritoneal signs and symptoms, increase in stool frequency to seven or more over patient's baseline, fecal incontinence, need for IV hydration for more than 24 hours, GI hemorrhage, perforation). Rule out infection and consider endoscopic evaluation for persistent or severe symptoms.
• Monitor for signs and symptoms of motor or sensory neuropathy. Withhold ipilimu-mab in patient with moderate neuropathy. Permanently discontinue drug in patient with severe neuropathy that interferes with daily activities, such as Guillain-Barré-like syndromes (unilateral or bilateral weakness, sensory changes, paresthesia).
• Monitor for signs and symptoms of dermatitis (rash, pruritus); consider these symptoms immune-mediated unless an alternative cause is identified. Permanently discontinue ipilimumab in patient with SJS, TEN, or rash complicated by full-thickness dermal ulceration or necrotic, bullous, or hemorrhagic manifestations.

• Monitor for signs and symptoms of hypophysitis, adrenal insufficiency (including adrenal crisis), and hyperthyroidism or hypothyroidism (headaches, fatigue, feeling cold, weight gain, changes in mood or behavior, dizziness, fainting). Endocrinopathies should be considered immune-mediated unless an alternative cause is identified.
• Monitor for ocular symptoms (vision changes, eye pain or redness). Administer corticosteroid eyedrops to patient who develops uveitis, iritis, or episcleritis. Permanently discontinue drug in patient with immune-mediated ocular disease unresponsive to local immunosuppressive therapy.

PATIENT TEACHING
• Instruct patient to report history of immune system disorders, such as ulcerative colitis, Crohn disease, lupus, or sarcoidosis; organ transplant; or liver damage.
• Teach patient signs and symptoms of serious immune-mediated adverse reactions, and advise patient to immediately report them to prescriber.
• Advise patient that blood chemistry studies will be needed before start of therapy and before each dose.
• Instruct patient to read the Yervoy medication guide before taking each dose.
• Warn patient that ipilimumab can cause fetal harm. Instruct patient to immediately report pregnancy.
• Advise patient of childbearing potential to use effective contraception during treatment and for 3 months after final dose.
• Tell patient not to breastfeed during therapy and for 3 months after final dose.

ipratropium bromide
i-pra-TROE-pee-um

Atrovent HFA, Ipravent✤

Therapeutic class: Bronchodilators
Pharmacologic class: Anticholinergics

AVAILABLE FORMS
Inhaler: 17 mcg/metered dose
Nasal spray: 0.03% (21 mcg/metered dose), 0.06% (42 mcg/metered dose)
Solution (for inhalation): 0.02% 500 mcg/ 2.5 mL vials

INDICATIONS & DOSAGES

➤ **Bronchospasm in chronic bronchitis and emphysema**
Adults: Usually, 2 inhalations q.i.d.; patient may take additional inhalations as needed but shouldn't exceed 12 inhalations in 24 hours. Or, 500 mcg every 6 to 8 hours via oral nebulizer.
Children ages 12 and older: 500 mcg every 6 to 8 hours via oral nebulizer.

➤ **Rhinorrhea caused by allergic and non-allergic perennial rhinitis**
Adults and children ages 6 and older: Two 0.03% nasal sprays (42 mcg) per nostril b.i.d. or t.i.d. Total dosage, 168 to 252 mcg/day.

➤ **Rhinorrhea caused by common cold**
Adults and children ages 12 and older: Two 0.06% nasal sprays (84 mcg) per nostril t.i.d. or q.i.d. Total dosage, 672 mcg/day.
Children ages 5 to 11: Two 0.06% nasal sprays (84 mcg) per nostril t.i.d. Total dosage, 504 mcg/day.

➤ **Rhinorrhea caused by seasonal allergic rhinitis**
Adults and children ages 5 and older: Two 0.06% nasal sprays (84 mcg) per nostril q.i.d. Total dosage is 672 mcg/day.

➤ **Acute asthma exacerbations, in combination with a short-acting beta agonist ◆**
Adults and adolescents ages 13 and older: 500 mcg via oral nebulizer every 20 minutes for three doses; then as needed. Or 4 to 8 inhalations with spacer of inhalation aerosol every 20 minutes as needed for up to 3 hours.
Children ages 6 to 12: 250 to 500 mcg via oral nebulizer every 20 minutes for three doses; then as needed. Or 4 to 8 inhalations of inhalation aerosol every 20 minutes as needed for up to 3 hours.
Children ages 5 and younger: 250 mcg via oral nebulizer every 20 minutes for 1 hour. Or 2 inhalations of inhalation aerosol every 20 minutes if needed for 1 hour.

ADMINISTRATION
Inhalational
• Prime inhaler before initial use by releasing 2 test sprays into air. If inhaler is not used for more than 3 days, reprime.
• If more than 1 inhalation is ordered, wait at least 15 seconds between inhalations.
• Use spacer device to improve drug delivery, if appropriate.
• Wash mouthpiece once a week for 30 seconds in warm water only and let air dry.

• Don't puncture inhaler, throw into a fire or incinerator, or use or store near heat or open flame.
• Inhalation solution is for use with oral nebulizer. Refer to manufacturer's instructions for use.
• Protect solution from light. Store unused vials in foil pouch.
• Store inhaler and solution between 59° and 86° F (15° and 30° C).
Intranasal
• Prime nasal spray with 7 sprays of pump before first use; prime with 2 sprays after pump hasn't been used for more than 24 hours. If pump hasn't been used for 7 days, reprime with 7 sprays.
• Tilt patient's head backward after dose to allow drug to spread to back of nose.
• Store between 59° and 77° F (15° and 25° C); avoid freezing.

ACTION
Inhibits vagally mediated reflexes by antagonizing acetylcholine at muscarinic receptors on bronchial smooth muscle.

Route	Onset	Peak	Duration
Inhalation	15 min	1–2 hr	2–8 hr
Intranasal	15 min	Unknown	Unknown

Half-life: Inhalation, about 2 hours; intranasal, 1.6 hours.

ADVERSE REACTIONS
CNS: dizziness, headache, taste perversion, pain. **CV:** palpitations, chest pain. **EENT:** blurred vision, epistaxis, rhinitis, sinusitis, pharyngitis, nasal dryness, nasal irritation, nasal congestion, dry mouth and throat. **GI:** nausea, diarrhea, dyspepsia. **GU:** UTI, urine retention. **Musculoskeletal:** back pain. **Respiratory:** URI, COPD exacerbation, bronchitis, *bronchospasm,* cough, dyspnea, increased sputum. **Skin:** rash. **Other:** flulike symptoms, hypersensitivity reactions.

INTERACTIONS
Drug-drug. *Anticholinergics (dicyclomine, scopolamine):* May increase anticholinergic effects. Avoid use together.

EFFECTS ON LAB TEST RESULTS
None reported.

CONTRAINDICATIONS & CAUTIONS
• Contraindicated in patients hypersensitive to drug, atropine, or its derivatives.

• Use cautiously in patients with angle-closure glaucoma, prostatic hyperplasia, bladder neck obstruction, or liver or kidney impairment.

⊕ Alert: Drug isn't indicated for initial treatment of acute episodes of bronchospasm, for which rescue therapy is required for rapid response.

• Safety and effectiveness of intranasal use beyond 4 days in patients with a common cold or 3 weeks in patients with seasonal allergic rhinitis haven't been established.

• Safety and effectiveness of nebulization or inhaler use in children younger than age 12 haven't been established.

• Safety and effectiveness of 0.03% nasal solution in children younger than age 6 and 0.06% nasal solution in children younger than age 5 haven't been established.

Dialyzable drug: Unknown.

PREGNANCY-LACTATION-REPRODUCTION
• Studies during pregnancy are inadequate. Use during pregnancy only if clearly needed and if potential benefit justifies fetal risk.

• It isn't known if drug appears in human milk. Use cautiously during breastfeeding.

NURSING CONSIDERATIONS
• If patient uses a face mask for a nebulizer, take care to prevent leakage around the mask because eye pain or temporary blurring of vision may occur.

• Monitor for hypersensitivity reactions.

• Inhalation form may cause paradoxical bronchospasm. Treat emergently, and discontinue drug.

PATIENT TEACHING
• Warn patient that, when used alone, drug isn't effective for treating acute episodes of bronchospasm when rapid response is needed.

• Teach patient to correctly use metered-dose inhaler (MDI) or oral nebulizer. Refer to manufacturer's instructions for use.

• Instruct patient to prime inhaler and clean mouthpiece according to manufacturer's instructions.

• Inform patient that use of a spacer device with an MDI may improve drug delivery to lungs.

• Warn patient to avoid accidentally spraying drug into eyes. Temporary blurring of vision may result.

• If more than 1 inhalation is prescribed, tell patient to wait at least 15 seconds before repeating procedure.

• Advise patient who is also using a corticosteroid inhaler to use ipratropium first and then to wait about 5 minutes before using the corticosteroid. This lets the bronchodilator open air passages for maximal effectiveness of the corticosteroid.

• Teach about proper drug administration and handling. Instruct patient to prime nasal spray as directed by manufacturer.

---

irbesartan
ir-be-SAR-tan

Avapro

Therapeutic class: Antihypertensives
Pharmacologic class: Angiotensin II receptor antagonists

AVAILABLE FORMS
Tablets: 75 mg, 150 mg, 300 mg

INDICATIONS & DOSAGES
Adjust-a-dose (for all indications): For patients who are volume- and sodium-depleted, initially, 75 mg PO daily.

➤ **HTN**
Adults: Initially, 150 mg PO daily, increased to maximum of 300 mg daily, if needed.

➤ **Nephropathy in patients with type 2 diabetes**
Adults: 300 mg PO once daily.

ADMINISTRATION
PO
• Give drug without regard to meals.
• May give with other antihypertensives.

ACTION
Produces antihypertensive effect by competitive antagonist activity at the angiotensin II receptor.

Route	Onset	Peak	Duration
PO	1–2 hr	1.5–2 hr	>24 hr

Half-life: 11 to 15 hours.

ADVERSE REACTIONS
CNS: fatigue, dizziness. **CV:** orthostatic hypotension. **GI:** diarrhea, dyspepsia. **Metabolic:** *hyperkalemia.*

Reactions in bold italics are *life-threatening*.

INTERACTIONS

Drug-drug. *ACE inhibitors:* May increase risk of hypotension, kidney dysfunction, and hyperkalemia. Use together cautiously; closely monitor BP, kidney function, and potassium level.

🔵 *Alert: Aliskiren:* May increase risk of kidney impairment, hypotension, and hyperkalemia in patients with diabetes and those with GFR less than 60 mL/minute. Use together is contraindicated in patients with diabetes. Avoid use together in those with GFR less than 60 mL/minute.

Lithium: May increase lithium level, possibly causing toxicity. Monitor lithium level, and monitor patient.

NSAIDs, selective cyclooxygenase-2 inhibitors (celecoxib): May result in deterioration of kidney function. May decrease antihypertensive effect of irbesartan. Periodically monitor kidney function during coadministration.

Potassium-sparing diuretics, potassium supplements, trimethoprim: May increase risk of hyperkalemia. Closely monitor potassium level.

EFFECTS ON LAB TEST RESULTS

• May increase potassium level.
• May lead to false-negative aldosterone-to-renin ratio.

CONTRAINDICATIONS & CAUTIONS

• Contraindicated in patients hypersensitive to drug or its components.
• Use cautiously in older adults and patients with volume depletion, impaired kidney function, HF, or kidney artery stenosis.
• Drug isn't approved for use in children.
Dialyzable drug: No.
⚠ *Overdose S&S:* Hypotension, tachycardia, bradycardia.

PREGNANCY-LACTATION-REPRODUCTION

Boxed Warning Use during pregnancy can cause injury and death to the developing fetus. When pregnancy is detected, stop drug as soon as possible. ∎

• It isn't known if drug appears in human milk. Use during breastfeeding isn't recommended because of potential for adverse effects on infant.

NURSING CONSIDERATIONS

• Drug may be given with a diuretic or other antihypertensive, if needed, for control of HTN.

• Symptomatic hypotension may occur in patients who are volume- or sodium-depleted (vigorous diuretic use or dialysis). Correct cause of volume depletion before administration and before lowering dose.
• If hypotension occurs, place patient in supine position and give IV infusion of NSS, if needed. Once BP stabilizes after transient hypotensive episode, continue drug.
• Dizziness and orthostatic hypotension may occur more frequently in patients with type 2 diabetes and kidney disease.

PATIENT TEACHING

• Warn of consequences of drug exposure to fetus. Instruct patient to immediately notify prescriber if pregnancy is suspected.
• Teach about proper drug administration and handling.
• Tell patient to report all adverse reactions.
• Instruct patient to inform prescriber of other prescription and OTC drugs and supplements being taken.
• Caution patient not to use potassium supplements or salt substitutes containing potassium without consulting prescriber.

irinotecan hydrochloride ✂
eye-rye-no-TEE-kan

Camptosar

Therapeutic class: Antineoplastics
Pharmacologic class: DNA topoisomerase inhibitors

AVAILABLE FORMS

Injection: 20 mg/mL in 2-, 5-, 15-, and 25-mL vials

INDICATIONS & DOSAGES

Adjust-a-dose (for all indications): Consider reducing starting dose by at least one level for patients with homozygous (*28/*28, *6/*6) or compound heterozygous for the UGT1A1*28 or *6 alleles (*6/*28) genotypes. Consider reducing starting dose in patients ages 65 and older, in those who have received pelvic or abdominal radiation, and in those who have a performance status of 2 or increased bilirubin level. See manufacturer's instructions for details on dosage adjustments due to toxicities. ✂

➤ **Colorectal cancer, metastatic (single-agent regimen)**
Adults: Initially, 125 mg/m^2 by IV infusion over 90 minutes on days 1, 8, 15, and 22; then 2-week rest period. Thereafter, additional courses of treatment may be repeated every 6 weeks with 4 weeks on and 2 weeks off. Subsequent doses may be adjusted to low of 50 mg/m^2 or maximum of 150 mg/m^2 in 25- to 50-mg/m^2 increments based on patient's tolerance. Or, 350 mg/m^2 by IV infusion over 90 minutes once every 3 weeks. May adjust subsequent doses as low as 200 mg/m^2 in 50-mg/m^2 decrements, depending on individual patient tolerance. Additional courses may continue indefinitely in patients who respond favorably and in those whose disease remains stable, provided intolerable toxicity doesn't occur.

➤ **Colorectal cancer, metastatic (combination regimen and 5-FU and leucovorin)**
Regimen 1
Adults: 125 mg/m^2 IV infusion on days 1, 8, 15, and 22; followed by leucovorin 20 mg/m^2 IV bolus on days 1, 8, 15, and 22 and 5-FU 500 mg/m^2 IV bolus on days 1, 8, 15, and 22. Repeat course every 6 weeks.
Regimen 2
Adults: 180 mg/m^2 IV infusion on days 1, 15, and 29; followed by leucovorin 200 mg/m^2 IV over 2 hours on days 1, 2, 15, 16, 29, and 30 and 5-FU 400 mg/m^2 IV bolus on days 1, 2, 15, 16, 29, and 30 and 5-FU 600 mg/m^2 IV infusion over 22 hours on days 1, 2, 15, 16, 29, and 30.

➤ **Esophageal cancer, metastatic or locally advanced ◆**
Adults: 65 mg/m^2 IV infusion on days 1, 8, 15, and 22 of a 6-week cycle (in combination with cisplatin), or 180 mg/m^2 IV infusion every 2 weeks (in combination with leucovorin and 5-FU), or 250 mg/m^2 IV every 3 weeks (in combination with capecitabine).

➤ **Gastric cancer, metastatic or locally advanced ◆**
Adults: 150 mg/m^2 IV infusion (as a single agent) on days 1 and 15 of a 4-week cycle, or 65 mg/m^2 IV infusion on days 1, 8, 15, and 22 of a 6-week cycle (in combination with cisplatin), or 70 mg/m^2 IV infusion on days 1 and 15 of a 4-week cycle (in combination with cisplatin) for up to six cycles, or 180 mg/m^2 IV infusion over 90 minutes every 2 weeks (in combination with leucovorin and 5-FU), or 250 mg/m^2 IV every 3 weeks (in combination with capecitabine).

➤ **Pancreatic cancer, advanced ◆**
Adults: 180 mg/m^2 IV infusion every 2 weeks (in combination with oxaliplatin, leucovorin, and 5-FU).

➤ **Pancreatic cancer, potentially curable, adjuvant therapy ◆**
Adults: 150 mg/m^2 IV every 2 weeks (in combination with 5-FU, leucovorin, and oxaliplatin; modified FOLFIRINOX [mFOLFIRINOX] regimen) for 24 weeks.

➤ **Small-cell lung cancer, extensive stage ◆**
Adults: 60 mg/m^2 IV infusion on days 1, 8, and 15 every 4 weeks (in combination with cisplatin), or 65 mg/m^2 IV on days 1 and 8 every 3 weeks (in combination with cisplatin), or 175 mg/m^2 IV on day 1 every 3 weeks (in combination with carboplatin), or 50 mg/m^2 IV on days 1, 8, and 15 every 4 weeks (in combination with carboplatin).

➤ **Rhabdomyosarcoma (metastatic or relapsed/progressive) ◆**
Children: 50 mg/m^2 (maximum, 100 mg/dose) IV once daily for 5 days during protocol-specific weeks (in combination with ifosfamide, etoposide, vincristine, doxorubicin, cyclophosphamide, dactinomycin, and radiation [high-risk disease]) or 50 mg/m^2 IV once daily for 5 days at weeks 1 and 4 (in combination with vincristine).

ADMINISTRATION
IV

🜨 *Alert:* Hazardous drug; use safe handling and disposal precautions. Wear gloves while handling and preparing infusion solutions. If drug contacts skin, wash thoroughly with soap and water. If drug contacts mucous membranes, flush thoroughly with water.

▼ Dilute drug in D$_5$W injection (preferred) or NSS for injection before infusion to yield a final concentration of 0.12 to 2.8 mg/mL.

▼ Administer by IV infusion, usually over 90 minutes.

▼ Prepare infusion solution immediately before use and infuse as soon as possible after preparation. Discard infusion solution if particulates are visible. If infusion solution can't be used immediately, store for up to 24 hours at 35.6° to 46.4° F (2° to 8° C) or discard it. Solutions diluted with NSS may precipitate if refrigerated.

▼ Premedicate patient with antiemetic drugs on day of treatment starting at least 30 minutes before giving irinotecan.

Reactions in bold italics are *life-threatening*.

▼ Watch for irritation and infiltration; extravasation can cause tissue damage. If extravasation occurs, flush site with sterile water and apply ice. Notify prescriber.

▼ Store vial at 59° to 86° F (15° to 30° C). Protect from light. Vials are single use only; discard unused portion.

▼ **Incompatibilities:** Numerous incompatibilities exist. Consult drug compatibility reference for more information.

ACTION

Interacts with topoisomerase I, inducing reversible single-strand DNA breaks. Drug binds to the topoisomerase I-DNA complex and prevents religation of these single-strand breaks.

Route	Onset	Peak	Duration
IV	Unknown	1 hr	Unknown

Half-life: About 6 to 12 hours; active metabolite, 10 to 20 hours.

ADVERSE REACTIONS

CNS: asthenia, dizziness, fever, headache, insomnia, pain, akathisia, confusion, somnolence. **CV:** edema, vasodilation, orthostatic hypotension, ***thromboembolic event.*** **EENT:** rhinitis. **GI:** diarrhea, abdominal cramping, abdominal pain and enlargement, anorexia, constipation, dyspepsia, flatulence, nausea, stomatitis, vomiting. **Hematologic:** anemia, *leukopenia, neutropenia, thrombocytopenia.* **Hepatic:** bilirubinemia, increased ALP and AST levels. **Metabolic:** dehydration, weight loss. **Musculoskeletal:** back pain. **Respiratory:** dyspnea, increased cough, pneumonia. **Skin:** alopecia, rash, diaphoresis. **Other:** chills, infection.

INTERACTIONS

Drug-drug. *Diuretics:* May increase risk of dehydration and electrolyte imbalances. Consider stopping diuretic during active periods of nausea and vomiting.

Laxatives: May increase risk of diarrhea. Avoid use together.

Live-virus vaccines: May cause serious or fatal infection. Don't give together.

Neuromuscular blockers: May prolong neuromuscular-blocking effects of succinylcholine and antagonize neuromuscular blockade of nondepolarizing drugs. Monitor patient for prolonged effects of succinylcholine if given together.

Other antineoplastics: May cause additive adverse effects, such as myelosuppression and diarrhea. Monitor patient closely.

Prochlorperazine: May increase risk of akathisia. Monitor patient closely.

Strong CYP3A4 inducers (anticonvulsants [carbamazepine, phenobarbital, phenytoin], rifabutin, rifampin): May significantly decrease irinotecan level. Avoid use together. For patients requiring anticonvulsant treatment, consider substituting non-enzyme-inducing anticonvulsants at least 2 weeks before start of irinotecan therapy.

Strong CYP3A4 inhibitors (clarithromycin, ketoconazole, lopinavir, nefazodone, ritonavir, telaprevir); UGT1A1 inhibitors (atazanavir, gemfibrozil, indinavir): May increase systemic exposure to irinotecan. Discontinue strong CYP3A4 inhibitors at least 1 week before starting irinotecan. Don't give strong CYP3A4 or UGT1A1 inhibitors with irinotecan unless no therapeutic alternatives are available.

Vaccines (killed or inactivated virus): May diminish response to vaccine. Avoid use together.

Drug-herb. *St. John's wort:* May decrease drug levels. Use together is contraindicated.

Drug-food. *Grapefruit juice:* May increase irinotecan level. Avoid combination.

EFFECTS ON LAB TEST RESULTS

• May increase ALP, AST, and bilirubin levels.

• May decrease Hb level and platelet, WBC, and neutrophil counts.

CONTRAINDICATIONS & CAUTIONS

• Contraindicated in patients hypersensitive to drug.

⬥ Patients with UGT1A1*28 allele or UGT1A1 *6 alleles (*28/*28, *6/*6) genotype are at increased risk for neutropenia.

• Use cautiously in patients with liver impairment. See prescribing information for further guidance.

• Radiation to pelvis or abdomen may increase risk of severe myelosuppression. Avoid use of drug in patients undergoing radiation therapy.

• Early and late diarrhea can occur, and late diarrhea can be fatal.

• Fatal interstitial pulmonary disease (IPD) has been reported. Patients with preexisting lung disease, patients taking pulmonary toxic drugs or colony-stimulating factors, and patients receiving radiation therapy are at increased risk. If IPD is diagnosed, all chemotherapy will be discontinued.

• Rare cases of kidney impairment and AKI have been identified, usually in patients who became volume-depleted from severe vomiting or diarrhea.

• Safety and effectiveness in children haven't been established.

• Use cautiously in older adults.

Dialyzable drug: Unknown.

⚠ *Overdose S&S:* Severe neutropenia, severe diarrhea.

PREGNANCY-LACTATION-REPRODUCTION

• May cause fetal harm. Patients of childbearing potential should avoid becoming pregnant during therapy.

• Advise patients of childbearing potential to use effective contraception during treatment and for 6 months after final dose.

• Advise male patients with partners of childbearing potential to use condoms during treatment and for 3 months after final dose.

• Drug appears in human milk. Patient shouldn't breastfeed during treatment and for 7 days after final dose.

• Drug may impair fertility.

NURSING CONSIDERATIONS

• Administer drug under supervision of a physician experienced with cancer chemotherapy.

🗵 Consider UGT1A1 genotype testing for the *28 and *6 alleles to determine UGT1A1 metabolizer status. Monitor patient with these alleles for neutropenia during and after treatment.

• Verify pregnancy before treatment.

Boxed Warning Drug may cause severe myelosuppression. ∎

Boxed Warning Drug can cause severe diarrhea. Treat diarrhea occurring within 24 hours of drug administration with 0.25 to 1 mg atropine IV, unless contraindicated. Promptly treat late diarrhea (occurring more than 24 hours after irinotecan administration) with loperamide. ∎

• Monitor patient for dehydration, electrolyte imbalances, or sepsis; treat appropriately. Institute antibiotic therapy if ileus, fever, or severe neutropenia develops. Interrupt therapy and reduce subsequent doses if severe diarrhea occurs.

• Delay subsequent doses until normal bowel function returns for at least 24 hours without an antidiarrheal.

• If neutropenic fever occurs or if ANC falls below 1,000/mm^3, temporarily stop therapy. Promptly manage febrile neutropenia with antibiotics.

• A colony-stimulating factor may be helpful in patient with significant neutropenia.

• Monitor WBC count with differential, Hb level, and platelet count before each dose.

• To decrease risk of dehydration, withhold diuretic during treatment and periods of active vomiting or diarrhea.

• Monitor patient for respiratory signs and symptoms (dyspnea, cough, fever) before and during treatment.

• *Look alike–sound alike:* Don't confuse irinotecan with irinotecan liposome or topotecan.

PATIENT TEACHING

• Inform patient about risk of diarrhea and methods to manage it; tell patient to avoid laxatives.

• Instruct patient to report all adverse reactions and to immediately contact prescriber if any of the following occur: diarrhea for first time during treatment; black or bloody stools; symptoms of dehydration (light-headedness, dizziness, faintness); inability to drink fluids due to nausea or vomiting; inability to control diarrhea within 24 hours; fever; infection; dyspnea; or cough.

• Warn patient that hair loss may occur.

• Inform patient that dizziness or visual disturbances may occur within the first 24 hours after treatment.

• Caution patient to avoid pregnancy and breastfeeding during therapy.

• Advise patient of risk of impaired infertility.

---

iron sucrose
eye-ern soo-krose

Venofer

Therapeutic class: Iron supplements
Pharmacologic class: Hematinics

AVAILABLE FORMS
Injection: 20 mg/mL of elemental iron in single-dose vials

INDICATIONS & DOSAGES

➤ **Iron deficiency anemia in patients who are hemodialysis dependent**

Adults: 100 mg (5 mL) of elemental iron IV directly in dialysis line by slow injection over 2 to 5 minutes or by infusion of 100 mg diluted in maximum of 100 mL NSS over 15 minutes per consecutive hemodialysis session. Administer early during each dialysis session. Usual total treatment course is 1,000 mg; may repeat if iron deficiency recurs.

➤ **Iron deficiency anemia in patients with CKD not on dialysis**

Adults: 200 mg by undiluted slow IV injection over 2 to 5 minutes, or as an infusion of 200 mg in maximum of 100 mL NSS over 15 minutes, on five separate occasions in a 14-day period to a total cumulative dose of 1,000 mg; may repeat if needed. Or, 500 mg diluted in maximum of 250 mL NSS infused over 3.5 to 4 hours on day 1 and day 14.

➤ **Iron deficiency anemia in patients with CKD dependent on peritoneal dialysis**

Adults: 300 mg IV infusion over 90 minutes on two separate occasions 14 days apart, followed by one 400-mg infusion over 2.5 hours 14 days later. Dilute in maximum of 250 mL NSS; may repeat if needed.

➤ **Maintenance treatment in children with hemodialysis-dependent CKD**

Children ages 2 and older: 0.5 mg/kg IV every 2 weeks for 12 weeks. Give undiluted by slow IV injection over 5 minutes or diluted in NSS to a 1 to 2 mg/mL concentration and administered over 5 to 60 minutes. May repeat if necessary. Don't give more than 100 mg/dose.

➤ **Maintenance treatment in children with non-dialysis-dependent CKD who are receiving erythropoietin or with peritoneal dialysis-dependent CKD who are receiving erythropoietin**

Children ages 2 and older: 0.5 mg/kg IV every 4 weeks for 12 weeks. Give undiluted by slow IV injection over 5 minutes or diluted in 25 mL NSS to a 1 to 2 mg/mL concentration and administered over 5 to 60 minutes. May repeat treatment if necessary. Don't give more than 100 mg per dose.

➤ **Chemotherapy-associated anemia ◆**

Adults: 200 mg IV once every 3 weeks for five doses. Or, 100 mg IV once weekly during weeks 0 to 6; then 100 mg IV every other week from weeks 8 to 14. Or, 200 mg IV once a week after each platinum-based chemotherapy cycle for up to six doses. Or, 200 mg IV after each platinum-based chemotherapy cycle for six cycles.

ADMINISTRATION

IV

▼ Inspect drug for particulate matter and discoloration before administration.

▼ For infusion, dilute 100 mg or 200 mg elemental iron in maximum of 100 mL NSS immediately before infusion, and infuse over at least 15 minutes. Dilute dose 300 mg or greater in maximum of 250 mL NSS.

▼ Store in original carton at 68° to 77° F (20° to 25° C). Don't freeze.

▼ Diluted 2 to 10 mg/mL concentrations or undiluted iron stored in a plastic syringe remains stable for 7 days at controlled room temperature or under refrigeration. IV admixture remains stable for 7 days at controlled room temperature when added to an infusion bag containing NSS (1 to 2 mg/mL concentration).

▼ **Incompatibilities:** Other IV drugs, parenteral nutrition solutions.

ACTION

Exogenous source of iron that replenishes depleted body iron stores and is essential for Hb synthesis.

Route	Onset	Peak	Duration
IV	Unknown	Unknown	Variable

Half-life: 6 hours.

ADVERSE REACTIONS

CNS: headache, asthenia, dizziness, fever, taste perversion. **CV:** *HF,* hypotension, chest pain, HTN, fluid retention, edema, graft complications, AV fistula thrombosis. **EENT:** conjunctivitis, ear pain, sinusitis, nasopharyngitis, nasal congestion. **GI:** nausea, vomiting, diarrhea, abdominal pain, peritonitis. **Metabolic:** gout, *hypoglycemia,* hyperglycemia. **Musculoskeletal:** muscle cramps, bone and muscle pain, arthralgia, back pain, limb pain. **Respiratory:** dyspnea, wheezing, cough, URI. **Skin:** rash, pruritus, infusion-site reaction, extravasation. **Other:** accidental injury, pain, *sepsis,* hypersensitivity reactions.

INTERACTIONS

Drug-drug. *Oral iron preparations:* May reduce absorption of oral iron preparations. Avoid use together.

EFFECTS ON LAB TEST RESULTS
- May increase uric acid level.
- May increase or decrease blood glucose level.

CONTRAINDICATIONS & CAUTIONS
- Contraindicated in patients with hypersensitivity to drug or its components, evidence of iron overload, or anemia not caused by iron deficiency.
- Use cautiously in older adults.

Dialyzable drug: No.

⚠ *Overdose S&S:* Accumulation of iron in storage sites, potentially leading to hemosiderosis.

PREGNANCY-LACTATION-REPRODUCTION
- Use during pregnancy only if clearly needed.
- Drug appears in human milk. Use cautiously during breastfeeding and monitor infant for constipation and diarrhea.

NURSING CONSIDERATIONS
- ⏱ *Alert:* Rare but fatal hypersensitivity reactions, characterized by anaphylactic shock, loss of consciousness, collapse, or hypotension, may occur. Monitor patient during infusion and for at least 30 minutes and until clinically stable after completing infusion. Have emergency equipment and therapies readily available.
- Mild to moderate hypersensitivity reactions, with wheezing, dyspnea, hypotension, rash, or pruritus, may occur.
- Infusing drug may reduce hypotension risk.
- Monitor patient for hypotension, dyspnea, headache, vomiting, nausea, dizziness, joint aches, paresthesia, abdominal pain, muscle pain, edema, and CV collapse, which may occur with rapid infusion or total dose administration.
- Transferrin saturation level increases rapidly after IV administration of drug. Obtain iron level at least 48 hours after IV use.
- Monitor ferritin level, transferrin saturation, Hb level, and hematocrit.
- Withhold dose in patient with signs and symptoms of iron overload.
- Keep dose selection in older adults conservative because of decreased liver, kidney, or cardiac function; other disease; and other drug therapy.

PATIENT TEACHING
- Instruct patient to report all adverse reactions and immediately notify prescriber if symptoms of overdose or allergic reaction occur.
- Inform patient that drug may temporarily discolor urine.

---

isoniazid (INH, isonicotinic acid hydrazide) ⌧
eye-soe-NYE-a-zid

Therapeutic class: Antituberculotics
Pharmacologic class: Isonicotinic acid hydrazines

AVAILABLE FORMS
Injection: 100 mg/mL
Oral solution: 50 mg/5 mL
Tablets: 100 mg, 300 mg

INDICATIONS & DOSAGES
Adjust-a-dose (for all indications): Give dose after hemodialysis.
➤ **Active TB with other antituberculotics**
Adults and children ages 15 and older: 5 mg/kg daily PO or IM in a single daily dose, up to 300 mg/day, with other antitubercu-lotic drugs, continued for 6 months to 2 years. For intermittent multiple-drug regimen, 15 mg/kg (up to 900 mg) PO or IM up to 3 times/week.
Infants and children: 10 to 15 mg/kg PO or IM in a single daily dose, up to 300 mg/day, continued long enough to prevent relapse. Give with at least one other antituberculotic. For intermittent multidrug regimen, 20 to 40 mg/kg (up to 900 mg) PO or IM two or three times weekly.
➤ **Prevention of TB**
Adults weighing more than 30 kg: 300 mg PO or IM daily in a single dose, continued for 6 months to 1 year.
Infants and children: 10 mg/kg PO or IM daily in a single dose, up to 300 mg/day, continued for up to 1 year. In situations in which adherence with daily preventive therapy can't be assured, 20 to 30 mg/kg (not to exceed 900 mg) twice weekly under direct observation of a health care worker at time of administration.

ADMINISTRATION
PO
- Don't give drug with food.

IM
• IM route may be used whenever oral route isn't possible.
• Solution may crystallize at a low temperature. Warm vial to room temperature before use to redissolve crystals.
• Inject deep IM into a large muscle mass.
• Store at room temperature.

ACTION
May inhibit cell-wall biosynthesis by interfering with lipid and DNA synthesis; bactericidal.

Route	Onset	Peak	Duration
PO, IM	Unknown	1–2 hr	Unknown

Half-life: 0.5 to 5 hours.

ADVERSE REACTIONS
CNS: peripheral neuropathy, paresthesia, *seizures, toxic encephalopathy,* memory impairment, toxic psychosis, fever. **CV:** lymphadenopathy, vasculitis. **EENT:** optic neuritis and atrophy. **GI:** epigastric distress, nausea, vomiting. **Hematologic:** *agranulocytosis, aplastic anemia, thrombocytopenia,* eosinophilia, hemolytic anemia, sideroblastic anemia. **Hepatic:** *hepatitis,* increased transaminase levels, bilirubinemia, jaundice. **Metabolic:** hyperglycemia, vitamin B3 deficiency, *metabolic acidosis.* **Skin:** irritation at injection site, rash, DRESS syndrome. **Other:** gynecomastia, hypersensitivity reactions, pyridoxine deficiency, rheumatic and lupuslike syndromes.

INTERACTIONS
Drug-drug. *Acetaminophen:* May inhibit acetaminophen metabolism. Monitor patient closely for liver toxicity.
Antacids and laxatives containing aluminum: May decrease isoniazid absorption. Give isoniazid at least 1 hour before antacid or laxative.
Benzodiazepines (diazepam, triazolam): May increase benzodiazepine level. Monitor for adverse effects.
Carbamazepine, phenytoin, valproate: May increase levels of these drugs. Closely monitor drug level, and adjust dosage as indicated.
Ketoconazole: May decrease ketoconazole level. Monitor for lack of effectiveness.
Rifampin: May increase risk of liver toxicity. Closely monitor LFT values.
Theophylline: May increase theophylline level. Closely monitor theophylline level; adjust dosage as appropriate.

Warfarin: May enhance anticoagulant activity. Monitor PT and INR.
Drug-food. *Foods containing histamines (saury, skipjack tuna, other tropical fish):* May cause headache, diaphoresis, palpitations, flushing, diarrhea, itching, wheezing, dyspnea, or hypotension. Discourage use during therapy.
Foods containing tyramine (aged cheese, beer, chocolate): May cause hypertensive crisis. Discourage use during therapy.
Drug-lifestyle. *Alcohol use:* May increase risk of drug-related hepatitis. Discourage use during therapy.

EFFECTS ON LAB TEST RESULTS
• May increase transaminase, glucose, and bilirubin levels.
• May increase eosinophil count.
• May decrease Hb and niacin level and granulocyte and platelet counts.
• May alter result of urine glucose tests that use cupric sulfate method, such as Benedict reagent and Diastix.

CONTRAINDICATIONS & CAUTIONS
Boxed Warning Contraindicated in patients with acute liver disease or isoniazid-related liver damage. Severe and sometimes fatal hepatitis associated with drug may occur even after months of treatment but usually occurs during first 3 months of treatment. Risk of developing hepatitis is age-related (increases with age), increases with daily alcohol use, and may be more common in women who are Black or Hispanic, particularly during the postpartum period. If signs or symptoms suggest liver damage, discontinue isoniazid because a more severe form of liver damage can occur. ■
Boxed Warning Defer preventative treatment in patients with acute liver disease. ■
Boxed Warning Treat patients with TB who have isoniazid-related hepatitis with alternative drugs. If isoniazid must be restarted, use only after symptoms and lab abnormalities have resolved. ■
• Use cautiously in adults over age 35, those using any medications chronically, patients with chronic non-isoniazid-related liver disease or chronic alcoholism, those with seizure disorders (especially if taking phenytoin), and those with CrCl less than 30 mL/minute.
Dialyzable drug: Yes.

⚠ *Overdose S&S:* Nausea, vomiting, dizziness, slurring of speech, blurring of vision, visual hallucinations, respiratory distress, CNS depression progressing from stupor to coma, seizures, severe metabolic acidosis, acetonuria, hyperglycemia.

PREGNANCY-LACTATION-REPRODUCTION

• Studies during pregnancy are inadequate; however, drug should be used as a treatment for active TB during pregnancy because benefit justifies fetal risk.

• Weigh benefit of preventive therapy against fetal risk. Preventive therapy generally should be started after delivery to prevent putting fetus at risk for exposure.

• Small amounts of drug in human milk don't produce toxicity in infants who are breastfed. Don't discourage breastfeeding.

NURSING CONSIDERATIONS

⚕ Drug's pharmacokinetics vary among patients because drug is metabolized in the liver by genetically controlled acetylation. Fast acetylators metabolize drug up to 5 times faster than slow acetylators. About 50% of Blacks and Whites are fast acetylators; more than 80% of patients who are of Chinese, Japanese, and Inuit descent are fast acetylators. A report suggests the risk of fatal hepatitis increases in women who are Black or Hispanic and in the postpartum period. The risk of hepatitis increases with daily alcohol use and with age.

⚕ Peripheral neuropathy is more common in patients who are slow acetylators or malnourished or have diabetes or alcoholism. Give pyridoxine to prevent peripheral neuropathy.

Boxed Warning Monitor and interview patients monthly. For patients older than age 35, also measure liver enzyme levels before and periodically throughout treatment. Elevated LFT results occur in about 15% of patients; most abnormalities are mild and transient, but some may persist throughout treatment, and progressive liver dysfunction may occur. If LFT values exceed 3 to 5 × ULN, strongly consider discontinuing treatment. ■

PATIENT TEACHING

• Instruct patient to take drug exactly as prescribed; warn against stopping drug without prescriber's consent.

• Teach about proper drug administration and handling.

Boxed Warning Tell patient to immediately notify prescriber if signs and symptoms of liver impairment occur (fatigue; malaise; appetite loss; yellowing of skin or eyes; dark urine; fever of more than 3 days' duration; abdominal tenderness, particularly of right upper quadrant). ■

• Advise patient to avoid alcoholic beverages while taking drug and to avoid certain foods (fish [such as skipjack tuna] and products containing tyramine [such as aged cheese, beer, and chocolate]) because drug has some MAO inhibitor activity.

⚕ Caution patient who is a slow acetylator or malnourished or has diabetes or alcohol use disorder to take pyridoxine, as prescribed, to prevent peripheral neuropathy.

• Encourage patient to comply fully with treatment, which may take months or years.

isosorbide dinitrate (ISDN)
eye-soe-SOR-bide

Isordil

isosorbide mononitrate (ISMN)
Imdur✦, Monoket

Therapeutic class: Antianginals
Pharmacologic class: Nitrates

AVAILABLE FORMS
isosorbide dinitrate
Tablets: 5 mg, 10 mg, 20 mg, 30 mg, 40 mg
isosorbide mononitrate
Tablets: 10 mg, 20 mg
Tablets (extended-release) ⓞⓝⓒ: 30 mg, 60 mg, 120 mg

INDICATIONS & DOSAGES
➤ **Treatment (immediate-release isosorbide mononitrate only) and prevention of angina pectoris**
Adults (dinitrate): For immediate release, 5 to 20 mg PO b.i.d. to t.i.d., titrated to maximum of 40 mg PO b.i.d. to t.i.d.
Adults (mononitrate): For immediate release, 5 to 20 mg PO b.i.d., with the two doses given 7 hours apart. For extended-release, 30 to 60 mg PO daily; titrate every 3 days to 120 mg PO daily. Rarely, 240 mg may be required.

> **HF (isosorbide dinitrate)** ◆
Adults: 20 mg immediate-release PO t.i.d.
in combination with hydralazine. Titrate
dosage every 2 to 4 weeks, as tolerated, to target dosage of 40 mg t.i.d. Maximum dosage,
120 mg daily in divided doses.

ADMINISTRATION
PO
• Tell patient taking isosorbide dinitrate to
swallow oral tablet whole on an empty stomach either 30 minutes before or 1 to 2 hours
after meals.
• Have patient swallow tablets whole; don't
crush extended-release tablets. Isosorbide
mononitrate extended-release tablets are
scored to be split.
• Don't give around the clock; allow
nitrate-free interval for at least 14 hours for
immediate-release products and longer than
18 hours for extended-release products.
⊛ **Alert:** Have patient swallow isosorbide
mononitrate extended-release tablets together
with a half-glassful of fluid.
• Store drug in a cool place, in a tightly
closed container, away from light.

ACTION
Thought to reduce cardiac oxygen demand by
decreasing preload and afterload. Drug also
may increase blood flow through the collateral coronary vessels.

Route	Onset	Peak	Duration
PO	30–45 min	30–60 min	4–8 hr
PO (extended-release)	0.5–4 hr	Unknown	6–12 hr

Half-life: Dinitrate PO, 5 to 6 hours; mononitrate,
about 5 hours.

ADVERSE REACTIONS
CNS: headache, fatigue, dizziness, transient
light-headedness, weakness, pain, emotional
lability, syncope. **CV:** orthostatic hypotension,
tachycardia, palpitations, ankle edema, flushing, chest pain, crescendo angina, rebound
HTN. **GI:** nausea, abdominal pain. **Respiratory:** URI, cough. **Skin:** rash, pruritus.
Other: hypersensitivity reaction.

INTERACTIONS
Drug-drug. *Antihypertensives:* May increase
hypotensive effects. Monitor patient closely
during initial therapy.

*PDE5 inhibitors (avanafil, sildenafil,
tadalafil, vardenafil), riociguat:* May cause
life-threatening hypotension. Use of nitrates
in any form with these drugs is contraindicated.
Drug-lifestyle. *Alcohol use:* May increase
hypotension. Discourage use together.

EFFECTS ON LAB TEST RESULTS
• May falsely reduce value in cholesterol
tests using the Zlatkis-Zak color reaction.

CONTRAINDICATIONS & CAUTIONS
• Contraindicated in patients with hypersensitivity or idiosyncrasy to nitrates and in
those with severe hypotension, increased ICP,
shock, or acute MI with low left ventricular
filling pressure.
• Nitrates may aggravate angina caused by
hypertrophic cardiomyopathy.
⊛ **Alert:** The onset of action of isosorbide
dinitrate or mononitrate isn't rapid enough
to stop an acute anginal episode.
• Rarely, methemoglobinemia can occur with
drug use.
• Use cautiously in patients with blood volume depletion (such as from diuretic therapy), mild hypotension, or suspected right
ventricular infarction.
• Safety and effectiveness in children haven't
been established.
Dialyzable drug: *Mononitrate:* Yes. *Dinitrate:*
Unknown.
⚠ **Overdose S&S:** Venous pooling, decreased cardiac output, hypotension, methemoglobinemia, headache, confusion, vertigo,
fever, palpitations, nausea, vomiting (possibly
with colic and bloody diarrhea), syncope, air
hunger, dyspnea, slow breathing, diaphoresis,
flushed skin, heart block, bradycardia, paralysis, coma.

PREGNANCY-LACTATION-REPRODUCTION
• Studies during pregnancy are inadequate.
Use during pregnancy only if clearly needed.
• It isn't known if drug appears in human
milk. Use cautiously during breastfeeding.

NURSING CONSIDERATIONS
• To prevent tolerance, a nitrate-free interval
of 10 to 14 hours per day is recommended.
The regimen for isosorbide mononitrate
(1 tablet on awakening, with second dose in
7 hours; or 1 extended-release tablet daily) is

intended to minimize nitrate tolerance by providing a substantial nitrate-free interval.
• Monitor BP, HR, and intensity and duration of drug response.
• Drug may cause headaches, especially at beginning of therapy. Dosage may be reduced temporarily, but tolerance usually develops. Treat headache with aspirin or acetaminophen.
• Monitor patient for methemoglobinemia, which has occurred with nitrate use. Signs and symptoms are those of impaired oxygen delivery despite adequate cardiac output and adequate arterial partial pressure of oxygen.
• *Look alike–sound alike:* Don't confuse Isordil with Inderal.

PATIENT TEACHING
• Caution patient to take drug as prescribed. Altering schedule to prevent headaches may be associated with loss of antianginal effect.
• *Alert:* Advise patient that abruptly stopping drug may increase angina symptoms and risk of MI.
• Explain the need for nitrate-free intervals to minimize tolerance.
• Teach about proper drug administration, handling, and storage.
• Tell patient to change to an upright position slowly, to climb stairs carefully, and to lie down at first sign of dizziness.
• Caution patient to avoid alcohol because it may worsen low BP effects.

ISOtretinoin
eye-so-TRET-i-noyn

Absorica, Absorica LD, Amnesteem, Claravis, Myorisan, Zenatane

Therapeutic class: Antiacne drugs
Pharmacologic class: Retinoic acid derivatives

AVAILABLE FORMS
Capsules: 10 mg, 20 mg, 25 mg, 30 mg, 35 mg, 40 mg
Capsules (Absorica LD): 8 mg, 16 mg, 24 mg, 32 mg

INDICATIONS & DOSAGES
➤ **Severe recalcitrant nodular acne that's unresponsive to conventional therapy**

Adults and adolescents ages 12 and older:
0.5 to 1 mg/kg/day PO in two divided doses for 15 to 20 weeks. Or, 0.4 to 0.8 mg/kg/day in two divided doses for 15 to 20 weeks (Absorica LD).
Adjust-a-dose: For adults with very severe disease and scarring or with disease primarily on trunk, increase to 2 mg/kg/day in two divided doses or 1.6 mg/kg/day in two divided doses (Absorica LD)
➤ **Moderate acne** ◆
Adults: 0.3 to 0.5 mg/kg once daily; continue until a total cumulative dose of 120 to 150 mg/kg is reached.
Children and adolescents ages 12 to 17: 0.25 to 0.4 mg/day PO for 6 to 12 months.
➤ **High-risk neuroblastoma in children, in combination with dinutuximab, sargramostim, and aldesleukin, when given after chemotherapy or hematopoietic stem cell transplantation** ◆
Children: 80 mg/m^2 every 12 hours on days 15 through 28 of a 28-day cycle for six cycles.

ADMINISTRATION
PO
• *Alert:* Hazardous drug; use safe handling and disposal precautions.
• Before use, have patient read patient information and sign consent form.
• Give drug with or shortly after meals to facilitate absorption, except Absorica or Absorica LD, which may be given without regard to meals.
• Have patient swallow capsule whole with full glass of liquid; don't crush or break tablets.
• Absorica isn't substitutable with Absorica LD due to differences in bioavailability.
• Store at room temperature.
• Protect drug from light.

ACTION
May normalize keratinization, reversibly decrease size of sebaceous glands, and make sebum less viscous and less likely to plug follicles.

Route	Onset	Peak	Duration
PO (Absorica)	Unknown	2.9–6.4 hr	Unknown
PO (Absorica LD)	Unknown	3.5–5 hr	Unknown

Half-life: 18 hours (Absorica); 24 hours (Absorica LD).

ADVERSE REACTIONS
CNS: pseudotumor cerebri, depression, *psychosis, suicidality, aggressive and violent behavior,* hallucinations, emotional instability, headache, fatigue, irritability, pain, dizziness, syncope, drowsiness, insomnia, weakness, lethargy, malaise, nervousness, paresthesia, *seizure, stroke.* **CV:** palpitations, *vascular thrombotic disease,* edema, tachycardia. **EENT:** conjunctivitis, corneal deposits, dry eyes, decreased night vision, visual disturbances, tinnitus, hearing impairment (sometimes irreversible), nasopharyngitis, epistaxis, drying of mucous membranes, dry mouth, dry nose, gum bleeding and inflammation, dry lips, lip inflammation, stye, voice alteration. **GI:** nonspecific GI symptoms, nausea, vomiting, constipation, diarrhea, abdominal pain, anorexia, *pancreatitis,* inflammatory bowel disease, esophagitis, esophageal ulceration, colitis. **GU:** abnormal menses, sexual dysfunction, hematuria, glomerulonephritis. **Hematologic:** increased erythrocyte sedimentation rate, anemia, *thrombocythemia, thrombocytopenia, neutropenia.* **Hepatic:** increased liver enzyme levels, *hepatitis.* **Metabolic:** hypertriglyceridemia, decreased HDL level, hypercholesterolemia, hyperglycemia, weight loss. **Musculoskeletal:** tendon and ligament calcification, skeletal hyperostosis, premature epiphyseal closure, decreased bone mineral density and other bone abnormalities, back pain, myalgia, arthralgia, stiffness, arthritis, tendinitis. **Respiratory:** *bronchospasm,* respiratory tract infections. **Skin:** fragility, rash, dry skin, facial skin desquamation, petechiae, pruritus, nail brittleness, hair thinning, skin infection, peeling of palms and toes, photosensitivity reaction. **Other:** hypersensitivity reaction, infection, lymphadenopathy.

INTERACTIONS
Drug-drug. *Corticosteroids:* May increase risk of osteoporosis. Use together cautiously.
Fluoride, folate, iron, minerals, multivitamins: May enhance adverse or toxic effect of retinoic acid derivatives. Avoid combination.
Medicated soaps, cleansers, and cover-ups; preparations containing alcohol; topical resorcinol peeling agents (benzoyl peroxide): May have cumulative drying effect. Use together cautiously.
Phenytoin: May increase risk of osteomalacia. Use together cautiously.

Products containing vitamin A: May increase toxic effects of isotretinoin. Avoid use together.
Tetracyclines: May increase risk of pseudotumor cerebri. Avoid use together.
Drug-lifestyle. *Alcohol use:* May increase risk of hypertriglyceridemia. Discourage use together.
Sun or UV light exposure: May increase photosensitivity reaction. Advise patient to avoid excessive sunlight or UV exposure.

EFFECTS ON LAB TEST RESULTS
- May increase AST, ALT, ALP, GGT, CK, triglyceride, LDL, LDH, glucose, and uric acid levels.
- May decrease serum HDL level.
- May increase platelet count and erythrocyte sedimentation rate.
- May increase urinary WBC and RBC counts and protein level.

CONTRAINDICATIONS & CAUTIONS
- Contraindicated in patients hypersensitive to drug or any of its components, vitamin A, or other retinoids.
- Use cautiously in patients with history of mental illness, family history of psychiatric disorders, asthma, liver disease, diabetes, heart disease, hearing impairment, hypertriglyceridemia, inflammatory bowel disease, osteoporosis, genetic predisposition for age-related osteoporosis, history of childhood osteoporosis, weak bones, anorexia nervosa, osteomalacia, or other disorders of bone metabolism.
- Drug may cause erythema multiforme and SCAR (such as SJS or TEN), which may be serious and result in hospitalization, disability, life-threatening events, or death.
- Rarely, rhabdomyolysis has been reported.
- Safety and effectiveness in children younger than age 12 haven't been established.
Dialyzable drug: Unknown.
⚠ **Overdose S&S:** Vomiting, facial flushing, abdominal pain, headache, dizziness, ataxia.

PREGNANCY-LACTATION-REPRODUCTION
Boxed Warning Contraindicated during pregnancy. Risk of severe birth defects is extremely high if isotretinoin is taken in any amount, even for short periods, during pregnancy. Any fetus exposed during pregnancy can be affected; there are no accurate means of determining whether an exposed fetus has

been affected. An increased risk of spontaneous abortion and premature births has also been reported. ∎

Boxed Warning To minimize risk of fetal exposure, drug is only available through a REMS program (iPLEDGE). ∎

⟳ Alert: Patient must have negative results from two urine or serum pregnancy tests, first performed in the office when patient is qualified for therapy and second performed during the first 5 days of the next normal menstrual period immediately preceding start of therapy. Patient must repeat, and receive negative, pregnancy test every month before each course of therapy. For patient with amenorrhea, second test should be done within 7 days after office visit and immediately preceding beginning of therapy. Patient must repeat pregnancy test every month before receiving prescription. For patient with irregular cycles or one using a contraceptive method that precludes withdrawal bleeding, second pregnancy test must be done within 7 days after office visit, immediately preceding start of therapy, and after patient has used two forms of contraception for 1 month.

• Any suspected fetal exposure during or 1 month after therapy must be immediately reported to the FDA via MedWatch at 1-800-FDA-1088 and to the iPLEDGE pregnancy registry at 1-866-495-0654 or www.ipledgeprogram.com.

Boxed Warning If pregnancy does occur during treatment, immediately discontinue drug and refer patient to an obstetrician-gynecologist experienced in reproductive toxicity. ∎

• It isn't known if drug appears in human milk. Patient should discontinue breastfeeding or discontinue drug and avoid breastfeeding for at least 8 days after last dose.

NURSING CONSIDERATIONS

• If total nodule count has been reduced by more than 70% before patient has completed 15 to 20 weeks of treatment, drug may be discontinued.

• A second course of therapy may begin 8 weeks or more after completion of first course, if necessary. Improvement may continue after completion of first course.

• Monitor baseline lipid studies, LFTs, and pregnancy test results before therapy and at monthly intervals.

• Regularly monitor glucose level.

• Monitor patient for tinnitus and hearing loss; discontinue drug and refer patient for further evaluation if these symptoms occur.

• Monitor patient for inflammatory bowel disease (abdominal pain, rectal bleeding, severe diarrhea); discontinue drug immediately if signs or symptoms occur.

• Closely watch for and report severe skin reactions. Drug may need to be discontinued.

• Most adverse reactions occur at dosages exceeding 1 mg/kg daily. Reactions are generally reversible after dosage reduction or therapy discontinuation.

⟳ Alert: If patient experiences headache, nausea and vomiting, or visual disturbances, screen for papilledema. Signs and symptoms of pseudotumor cerebri require immediately stopping drug and promptly beginning neurologic interventions.

⟳ Alert: Monitor patient for mood disturbance, psychosis, aggressive behavior, or suicidality. Drug may need to be discontinued and patient evaluated.

• Patients may be at increased risk for bone fractures or injury when participating in sports with repetitive impact.

• Spontaneous reports of osteoporosis, osteopenia, bone fractures, and delayed healing of bone fractures have occurred in patients taking drug. To decrease risk, don't exceed recommended doses and duration.

PATIENT TEACHING

⟳ Alert: Warn patient of childbearing potential that if drug is used during pregnancy, severe fetal abnormalities may occur. Patient must commit to either abstain from sex or use two reliable forms of contraception simultaneously for 1 month before, during, and for 1 month after treatment.

• Teach about proper drug administration and handling. By law, an isotretinoin medication guide must be given to patient each time isotretinoin is dispensed.

• Tell patient to immediately report visual disturbances, tinnitus, and bone, muscle, or joint pain.

• Warn patient that contact lenses may feel uncomfortable during therapy.

• Advise patient not to drive at night until effect on vision is known. Drug may decrease night vision.

• Warn patient against using abrasives, medicated soaps and cleansers, acne preparations containing peeling drugs, and topical products containing alcohol (including cosmetics, aftershave, cologne) because they may cause cumulative irritation or excessive drying of skin.

• Tell patient to avoid prolonged sun or UV light exposure and to use sunblock and wear protective clothing. Drug may have additive effect if used with other drugs that cause photosensitivity reaction.

• Inform patient that transient exacerbations may occur during therapy.

• Warn patient not to donate blood during therapy and for 1 month after stopping drug because drug could harm fetus of a pregnant recipient.

• Advise patient to consult prescriber before taking OTC medications, vitamins, or herbal supplements.

• Tell patient to immediately report adverse reactions, especially depression, suicidality, persistent headaches, visual disturbances, severe skin reactions, and persistent GI pain.

🔵 *Alert:* Advise patient to carefully read iPLEDGE and to fully understand all information before signing it.

itraconazole
eye-tra-KON-a-zole

Sporanox, Tolsura

Therapeutic class: Antifungals
Pharmacologic class: Synthetic triazoles

AVAILABLE FORMS
Capsules 🔴: 65 mg, 100 mg
Oral solution: 10 mg/mL

INDICATIONS & DOSAGES
➤ **Pulmonary and extrapulmonary blastomycosis, histoplasmosis (capsules)**
Adults: 200 mg PO daily; increase as needed and tolerated by 100 mg to maximum of 400 mg daily. Give dosages exceeding 200 mg PO daily in two divided doses. Continue treatment for at least 3 months. In life-threatening illness, give loading dosage of 200 mg PO t.i.d. for 3 days. For Tolsura, give 130 mg (two 65-mg capsules) PO daily; increase as needed and tolerated by 65 mg to maximum of 260 mg/day. Give dosages exceeding 130 mg PO daily in two divided doses. Continue treatment for at least 3 months. In life-threatening illness,

give loading dosage of 130 mg t.i.d. for 3 days.
➤ **Aspergillosis (capsules)**
Adults: 200 to 400 mg PO daily for at least 3 months. In life-threatening illness, loading dosage of 200 mg PO t.i.d. for first 3 days of treatment. For Tolsura, 130 to 260 mg PO daily. Continue treatment for at least 3 months. In life-threatening illness, loading dosage of 130 mg t.i.d. for 3 days.
➤ **Onychomycosis of the toenail (with or without fingernail involvement)**
Adults: 200 mg PO once daily for 12 consecutive weeks.
➤ **Onychomycosis of the fingernail**
Adults: 200 mg PO b.i.d. for 1 week, followed by 3 weeks drug-free. Repeat 1- week dosage.
➤ **Oropharyngeal candidiasis**
Adults: 200 mg oral solution swished in mouth vigorously and swallowed daily for 1 to 2 weeks.
➤ **Oropharyngeal candidiasis in patients unresponsive to fluconazole tablets**
Adults: 100 mg oral solution swished in mouth vigorously and swallowed b.i.d. for 2 to 4 weeks.
➤ **Esophageal candidiasis**
Adults: 100 to 200 mg oral solution swished in mouth vigorously and swallowed daily for at least 3 weeks. Treatment should continue for 2 weeks after symptoms resolve.

ADMINISTRATION
PO
• Obtain specimen for culture and other relevant lab studies before first dose. Begin therapy while awaiting results.
• Before starting therapy, confirm diagnosis of onychomycosis by sending nail specimens for testing.
• Don't interchange capsules with oral solution.
• Give capsules with a full meal.
• Give oral solution on an empty stomach, if possible.
• Have patient swallow tablets whole; don't crush or break tablets.
• Have patient vigorously swish oral solution in mouth for several seconds and then swallow.
• Store capsules at room temperature; protect from light and moisture.
• Store oral solution at or below 77° F (25° C). Don't freeze. Protect from light and moisture.

ACTION

Interferes with fungal cell-wall synthesis by inhibiting ergosterol formation and increasing cell-wall permeability, leading to osmotic instability.

Route	Onset	Peak	Duration
PO	Unknown	2–7 hr	7–14 days

Half-life: Single dose, 16 to 28 hours; repeated dosing, 34 to 42 hours.

ADVERSE REACTIONS

CNS: headache, fever, dizziness, fatigue, somnolence, malaise, asthenia, pain, tremor, abnormal dreams, anxiety, depression, insomnia, vertigo. **CV:** *HF*, HTN, chest pain, edema, orthostatic hypotension, vasculitis. **EENT:** tinnitus, rhinitis, sinusitis, pharyngitis. **GI:** nausea, vomiting, diarrhea, abdominal pain, anorexia, dyspepsia, flatulence, increased appetite, constipation, gastritis, ulcerative stomatitis, gingivitis, gastroenteritis. **GU:** albuminuria, cystitis, UTI, decreased libido, erectile dysfunction, menstrual disorder. **Hepatic:** impaired liver function. **Metabolic:** *hypokalemia*, hypertriglyceridemia, adrenal insufficiency. **Musculoskeletal:** myalgia. **Respiratory:** URI, cough, dyspnea, increased sputum, *Pneumocystis jiroveci* infection. **Skin:** rash, pruritus, diaphoresis. **Other:** gynecomastia, male breast pain, injury, herpes zoster, hypersensitivity reactions.

INTERACTIONS

⚠ *Alert:* Itraconazole has the potential for significant interactions with many drugs. Consult drug interaction resource or pharmacist for more information.

Drug-drug. *Alprazolam:* May increase and prolong drug levels, CNS depression, and psychomotor impairment. Avoid use together.

Antacids, carbamazepine, isoniazid, phenobarbital, phenytoin, rifabutin, rifampin: May decrease itraconazole level. Avoid use together.

Boxed Warning *Avanafil, cisapride, disopyramide, dofetilide, dronedarone, eplerenone, ergot alkaloids (such as dihydroergotamine, ergometrine [ergonovine], ergotamine, methylergometrine [methylergonovine]), felodipine, irinotecan, isavuconazole, ivabradine, lomitapide, lovastatin, lurasidone, methadone, naloxegol, nisoldipine, oral midazolam, pimozide, quinidine, ranolazine,* simvastatin, ticagrelor, triazolam: May increase levels of these drugs by CYP450 metabolism, causing serious CV events, including torsades de pointes, QT-interval prolongation, cardiac arrest, ventricular tachycardia, and sudden death. Use together is contraindicated. ■

Chlordiazepoxide, clonazepam, clorazepate, diazepam, estazolam, flurazepam, quazepam: May increase and prolong drug levels, CNS depression, and psychomotor impairment. Avoid use together.

Ciprofloxacin, clarithromycin, erythromycin: May increase itraconazole levels. Monitor patient for signs of itraconazole toxicity. Consider itraconazole dosage reduction.

Boxed Warning *Colchicine:* May increase colchicine level. Contraindicated in patients with kidney or liver impairment during and for 2 weeks after itraconazole treatment. Monitor therapy in all other patients and reduce colchicine dosage. ■

Cyclosporine, digoxin, tacrolimus: May increase levels of these drugs. Monitor drug levels.

Boxed Warning *Eliglustat:* May increase eliglustat level. Contraindicated in patients who are poor or intermediate metabolizers of CYP2D6 and in those taking strong or moderate CYP2D6 inhibitors. ■

Boxed Warning *Fesoterodine:* May increase fesoterodine metabolite level. Contraindicated in patients with CrCl less than 60 mL/minute or Child-Pugh class B or C liver impairment during and for 2 weeks after itraconazole treatment. Monitor all other patients for adverse reactions and limit fesoterodine dose. ■

H₂-receptor antagonists (cimetidine, famotidine): May increase or decrease itraconazole level. Refer to manufacturer's instructions.

HMG-CoA reductase inhibitors (atorvastatin, lovastatin, simvastatin), lomitapide: May increase levels and adverse effects of these drugs. Use together is contraindicated during and for 2 weeks after itraconazole treatment, except atorvastatin, which may be used at reduced dosage.

NNRTIs (efavirenz, nevirapine): May decrease itraconazole level. Use 2 weeks before and during itraconazole treatment isn't recommended.

Oral anticoagulants: May enhance anticoagulant effect. Monitor PT and INR.

Reactions in bold italics are *life-threatening*.

Oral antidiabetics: May increase risk for hypoglycemia. Monitor glucose level. Avoid use together.

PDE5 inhibitors (sildenafil, tadalafil, vardenafil): May increase levels of these drugs, increasing adverse effects. Give PDE5 inhibitors with caution and in reduced doses.

Protease inhibitors (ritonavir, saquinavir): May increase levels of these drugs; ritonavir may increase itraconazole level. Monitor patient for toxicity and reduce itraconazole dosage, if necessary.

Boxed Warning *Solifenacin:* May increase solifenacin level. Contraindicated in patients with CrCl less than 30 mL/minute or Child-Pugh class B or C liver impairment during and for 2 weeks after itraconazole treatment. Monitor all other patients for adverse effects and limit solifenacin dose. ■

EFFECTS ON LAB TEST RESULTS
• May increase ALP, ALT, AST, bilirubin, LDH, urea, glucose, triglyceride, and GGT levels.
• May decrease magnesium, calcium, and phosphate levels.
• May increase or decrease potassium level.

CONTRAINDICATIONS & CAUTIONS
Boxed Warning Contraindicated in patients taking certain drugs metabolized by CYP3A4 enzymes. Administration with itraconazole can cause elevated plasma levels and may increase or prolong pharmacologic effects of and adverse reactions to these drugs. For example, increased plasma level of some of these drugs can lead to QT-interval prolongation and ventricular tachyarrhythmias, including potentially fatal torsades de pointes. ■
• Contraindicated in patients hypersensitive to drug.
• Use cautiously in patients with hypochlorhydria (can accompany HIV infection), who may not readily absorb drug.
Boxed Warning Don't use drug to treat onychomycosis in patients with evidence of ventricular dysfunction, such as HF or history of HF. If signs or symptoms of HF occur while giving oral solution, reassess continued use. If signs or symptoms of HF occur while giving capsules, discontinue use. ■
• Use cautiously in patients receiving other highly bound drugs and in patients with kidney or liver impairment.

• Drug may cause transient or permanent hearing loss, particularly in older adults.
• Safety and effectiveness in children haven't been determined.
Dialyzable drug: No.

PREGNANCY-LACTATION-REPRODUCTION
• Don't use to treat onychomycosis in patients who are pregnant, contemplating pregnancy, or are of childbearing potential unless they are using effective contraceptive measures and they begin therapy on the second or third day after onset of menses. Effective contraception should be continued throughout therapy and for 2 months after therapy ends.
• Drug may cause maternal or fetal harm. Use to treat systemic fungal infections during pregnancy only if benefit justifies risk.
• Drug appears in human milk. Discontinue breastfeeding or discontinue drug, considering importance of drug to patient.

NURSING CONSIDERATIONS
• Perform baseline LFTs and periodically monitor results. In patient with baseline liver impairment, give drug only if patient's condition is life threatening. If liver dysfunction occurs during therapy, immediately notify prescriber.
• Monitor patient for hearing loss.
• Monitor patient for signs and symptoms of HF during treatment.
• Monitor for hypersensitivity reactions.
• Monitor for peripheral neuropathy with long-term use.
• Give with an acidic beverage, such as nondiet cola, in patient with reduced gastric acidity. Separate dosing from acid suppressive therapy to improve absorption.
• Formulations aren't interchangeable due to differences in bioavailability.

PATIENT TEACHING
• Teach patient to recognize and report signs and symptoms of HF, liver disease (anorexia, dark urine, pale stools, unusual fatigue, and jaundice), or hearing loss.
• Inform patient that dizziness and blurred or double vision can occur. Advise against driving or using machinery if these effects occur.
• Teach about proper drug administration and handling.
• Urge patient to report other drugs being taken to avoid drug interactions.

• Advise patient of childbearing potential to use an effective form of contraception during therapy and for two menstrual cycles after stopping therapy.
• Caution patient not to breastfeed during therapy.

ivabradine
eye-VAB-ra-deen

Corlanor, Lancora ✦

Therapeutic class: CV agents
Pharmacologic class: Cyclic nucleotide-gated channel blockers

AVAILABLE FORMS
Solution: 5 mg/mL
Tablets: 5 mg, 7.5 mg

INDICATIONS & DOSAGES
➤ **To reduce risk of hospitalization for worsening HF in patients with stable, symptomatic chronic HF with LVEF of 35% or less who are in sinus rhythm with resting HR of 70 beats/minute (bpm) or more and either are on maximally tolerated doses of beta blockers or have a contraindication to beta blocker use**
Adults: Initially, 5 mg PO b.i.d. After 2 weeks, adjust dosage to achieve resting HR of 50 to 60 bpm, if necessary. Maximum dosage, 7.5 mg b.i.d.
Adjust-a-dose: In patients with conduction defects or bradycardia that could lead to hemodynamic compromise, initiate therapy at 2.5 mg b.i.d. before increasing dosage based on HR. If HR is greater than 60 bpm, increase dosage by 2.5 mg b.i.d. Maximum dosage, 7.5 mg b.i.d. If HR is less than 50 bpm or patient has signs and symptoms of bradycardia, decrease dosage by 2.5 mg b.i.d.; however, if current dosage is 2.5 mg b.i.d., discontinue therapy.
➤ **Stable symptomatic HF due to dilated cardiomyopathy in patients in sinus rhythm with an elevated HR**
Children ages 6 months and older weighing more than 40 kg (tablets): 2.5 mg PO b.i.d. After 2 weeks, adjust dosage by 2.5 mg b.i.d. to a target HR reduction of at least 20% based on tolerability. Maximum dosage, 7.5 mg b.i.d. *Children ages 6 months and older weighing less than 40 kg (oral solution):* 0.05 mg/kg/dose

b.i.d. Adjust dosage at 2-week intervals by 0.05 mg/kg/dose to a target HR reduction of at least 20% based on tolerability. Maximum dosage, 0.2 mg/kg/day in children ages 6 months to 1 year. Or, 0.3 mg/kg/day to maximum of 7.5 mg b.i.d. in children ages 1 year and older.
Adjust-a-dose: In adults, if bradycardia develops, reduce dosage to previous titration dosage. If current dosage is 2.5 mg b.i.d., discontinue drug. In children, if bradycardia occurs at initial dosage, consider decrease to 0.02 mg/kg b.i.d.

ADMINISTRATION
PO
• Give drug with meals.
• For oral solution, empty entire contents of ampule(s) into medication cup; use calibrated oral syringe to measure prescribed dose from medication cup. Discard unused solution.
• Keep oral solution ampules in original foil pouches until use.
• Store tablets at room temperature.

ACTION
Reduces HR by blocking hyperpolarization-activated cyclic nucleotide-gated channel responsible for the cardiac pacemaker I_f current.

Route	Onset	Peak	Duration
PO	Rapid	1–2 hr	Unknown

Half-life: 6 hours.

ADVERSE REACTIONS
CV: *bradycardia, conduction disturbances,* HTN, atrial fibrillation. **EENT:** phosphenes, visual brightness.

INTERACTIONS
Drug-drug. *CYP3A4 inducers (barbiturates, phenytoin, rifampin):* May decrease ivabradine level. Avoid use together.
Drugs that decrease HR (amiodarone, beta blockers, digoxin): May increase risk of bradycardia. Monitor HR.
Moderate CYP3A4 inhibitors (diltiazem, verapamil): May increase ivabradine level, causing bradycardia and conduction disturbances. Avoid use together.
Strong CYP3A4 inhibitors (clarithromycin, HIV protease inhibitors [nelfinavir], itraconazole, ketoconazole, nefazodone, telithromycin): May significantly increase

ivabradine level, leading to bradycardia and conduction disturbances. Use together is contraindicated.

Drug-herb. *St. John's wort:* May decrease ivabradine level. Discourage use together.

Drug-food. *Grapefruit juice:* May increase ivabradine level, causing bradycardia and conduction disturbances. Discourage use together.

EFFECTS ON LAB TEST RESULTS
None reported.

CONTRAINDICATIONS & CAUTIONS
• Contraindicated in patients hypersensitive to drug or its components and in those with acute decompensated HF, clinically significant hypotension, sick sinus syndrome, SA block, or third-degree AV block unless a functioning demand pacemaker is present; clinically significant bradycardia; severe liver impairment; or pacemaker dependence (HR maintained exclusively by pacemaker).

• Avoid use in patients with second-degree AV block unless a functioning demand pacemaker is present.

• Use cautiously in patients with sinus node dysfunction, conduction defects (first-degree AV block, bundle-branch block), or ventricular dyssynchrony. Drug may increase risk of bradycardia, sinus arrest, and heart block.

• Not recommended in those with demand pacemakers set to rates of 60 bpm or greater.

Dialyzable drug: Unknown.

⚠ **Overdose S&S:** Severe and prolonged bradycardia.

PREGNANCY-LACTATION-REPRODUCTION
• Based on animal studies, drug may cause fetal harm. Avoid use during pregnancy; advise patients of fetal risk. Patients of childbearing potential should use effective contraception during treatment.

• If drug must be used during pregnancy, monitor patients, especially during first trimester, for destabilization of HF that could result from slowing HR. Monitor patients with HF who are in the third trimester for signs and symptoms of preterm birth. Patients who are pregnant with LVEF less than 35% on maximally tolerated doses of beta blockers may be particularly HR-dependent for augmenting cardiac output.

• Drug may appear in human milk. Patient shouldn't breastfeed during therapy.

NURSING CONSIDERATIONS
• Regularly monitor cardiac rhythm. Drug may increase risk of atrial fibrillation. Discontinue drug if atrial fibrillation develops.

• Monitor patient for bradycardia; drug may increase risk of QT-interval prolongation, which may lead to severe ventricular arrhythmias, including torsades de pointes, especially in patients with such risk factors as use of QT-prolonging drugs.

• Monitor patients for phosphenes (transient enhanced brightness in a limited area of the visual field, halos, image decomposition, colored bright lights, or multiple images), which may be triggered by sudden variations in light intensity. Onset is typically within first 2 months of treatment; phosphenes may resolve without discontinuing treatment.

PATIENT TEACHING
• Teach about proper drug administration and handling.

• Warn patient of childbearing potential that drug may cause fetal harm. Instruct patient to use effective contraception during treatment and to report pregnancy or suspected pregnancy.

• Advise patient to avoid breastfeeding during therapy because of risk of fetal harm.

• Caution patient to immediately seek medical attention for significant decreases in HR or such signs and symptoms as dizziness, fatigue, or hypotension.

• Instruct patient to report all adverse reactions and to immediately report signs and symptoms of atrial fibrillation (heart palpitations or racing, chest pressure, worsened shortness of breath).

• Warn patient about possibility of developing luminous phenomena (phosphenes), resulting in transient visual brightness. Advise patient to use caution while driving or operating machinery in situations in which sudden changes in light intensity may occur, especially at night. Explain that phosphenes may subside during treatment.

ketoconazole (oral)
kee-toe-KOE-na-zole

Therapeutic class: Antifungals
Pharmacologic class: Imidazole derivatives

AVAILABLE FORMS
Tablets: 200 mg

INDICATIONS & DOSAGES

Boxed Warning Drug should only be used when other effective antifungal therapy isn't available or tolerated and potential benefits outweigh risks. ∎

➤ **Systemic fungal infections (coccidioidomycosis, blastomycosis, histoplasmosis, chromomycosis, and paracoccidioidomycosis)**
Adults: Initially, 200 mg PO daily in a single dose; may increase dosage to 400 mg once daily in patients who don't respond. Continue until fungal infection is resolved; usual duration for systemic infection is 6 months. Maximum dosage, 400 mg daily.
Children ages 2 and older: 3.3 to 6.6 mg/kg PO daily in a single dose. Continue until fungal infection is resolved; usual duration for systemic infection is 6 months. Maximum dosage, 400 mg daily.

➤ **Prostate cancer, advanced ◆**
Adults: 400 mg PO t.i.d. (in combination with oral hydrocortisone) until disease progression occurs.

ADMINISTRATION
PO
• Give oral tablets at least 2 hours before or 1 hour after antacids, H$_2$ blockers, or PPIs to prevent decreased absorption due to high pH of gastric contents. Patients with achlorhydria should take with acidic liquid (nondiet cola or orange juice).
• A pharmacist can prepare oral suspension. Shake suspension well before giving.
• Refrigerate suspension; remains stable for 60 days.

ACTION
Interferes with fungal cell-wall synthesis by inhibiting formation of ergosterol and increasing cell-wall permeability that makes the fungus susceptible to osmotic instability.

Route	Onset	Peak	Duration
PO	Unknown	1–2 hr	Unknown

Half-life: 8 hours.

ADVERSE REACTIONS
CNS: insomnia, nervousness, dizziness, asthenia, headache, fatigue, malaise, fever, paresthesia, somnolence, taste abnormality, weakness. **CV:** orthostatic hypotension, peripheral edema. **EENT:** photophobia, epistaxis, dry mouth. **GI:** nausea, vomiting, abdominal pain, diarrhea, constipation, dyspepsia, flatulence, anorexia, increased appetite, tongue discoloration. **GU:** menstrual disorder. **Hematologic:** *thrombocytopenia.* **Hepatic:** *hepatitis,* jaundice, abnormal liver function. **Metabolic:** hyperlipidemia, alcohol intolerance. **Musculoskeletal:** myalgia. **Skin:** pruritus, rash, *erythema multiforme,* dermatitis, erythema, alopecia, urticaria, xeroderma. **Other:** *anaphylaxis,* hot flush, gynecomastia, chills.

INTERACTIONS
⊍ *Alert:* Ketoconazole can significantly interact with many drugs, especially those metabolized by CYP450 enzyme system. Consult drug interaction resource or pharmacist for additional information.
Drug-drug. *Alprazolam, eplerenone, ergot alkaloids (dihydroergotamine, ergometrine, ergotamine, methylergometrine), felodipine, irinotecan, lurasidone, oral midazolam, nisoldipine, tolvaptan, triazolam:* May increase levels of these drugs. Use together is contraindicated.
Antacids, PPIs, H$_2$ blockers: Impair ketoconazole absorption. Use together with caution, and separate dosing times.
Boxed Warning *Cisapride, disopyramide, dofetilide, dronedarone, methadone, pimozide, quinidine, ranolazine:* May increase levels of these drugs and prolong QT interval. Use together is contraindicated. ∎
Colchicine: May increase risk of adverse effects in patients with kidney or liver impairment. Use together is contraindicated.
HMG-CoA reductase inhibitors (atorvastatin, fluvastatin, lovastatin, pravastatin, simvastatin): May increase levels and adverse effects of these drugs. Use together is contraindicated. May coadminister atorvastatin with caution.
Strong CYP3A4 inducers (carbamazepine, efavirenz, isoniazid, nevirapine, rifabutin):

May decrease ketoconazole level. Use together isn't recommended. If use is unavoidable, monitor therapy.

Strong CYP3A4 inhibitors (ritonavir): May increase ketoconazole level. Use together cautiously.

Drug-lifestyle. *Alcohol use:* May cause disulfiram-like reaction (flushing, rash, peripheral edema, nausea, headache). Discourage use together.

EFFECTS ON LAB TEST RESULTS
• May increase lipid, ALP, ALT, and AST levels.
• May decrease platelet count.
• May decrease adrenal function test results.

CONTRAINDICATIONS & CAUTIONS
• Contraindicated in patients hypersensitive to drug or its components.

Boxed Warning Drug can cause serious liver toxicity that may be fatal or require liver transplantation, even in patients with no obvious risk factors for liver disease. Drug is contraindicated in patients with acute or chronic liver disease. Patients must be informed of risk. ■

Boxed Warning Because of serious adverse effects, drug isn't indicated for onychomycosis or cutaneous dermatophyte or Candida infections. ■

• Drug poorly penetrates CSF; don't use to treat fungal meningitis.
• Drug decreases adrenal corticosteroid secretions at doses of 400 mg. Don't exceed recommended dose of 400 mg.
• Safety and effectiveness in children younger than age 2 haven't been established.
Dialyzable drug: Minimal.

PREGNANCY-LACTATION-REPRODUCTION
• Based on animal studies, drug may cause fetal harm. Use in pregnancy only if benefits justify fetal risk.
• Drug may reversibly lower serum testosterone level, causing gynecomastia, impotence, and oligospermia. Testosterone levels are impaired with dosages of 800 mg daily and abolished by 1,600 mg daily.
• Drug appears in human milk. Breastfeeding isn't recommended during therapy.

NURSING CONSIDERATIONS
🖐 *Alert:* Monitor patient for signs and symptoms of liver toxicity, including elevated liver enzyme levels, nausea that doesn't subside,

vomiting, anorexia, abdominal pain, unusual fatigue, jaundice, dark urine, and pale stool.
• Assess liver function status (AST, ALT, total bilirubin, and ALP levels), PT, and INR before starting drug.
• Measure ALT level weekly for duration of treatment. If ALT level increases above ULN or 30% above baseline, or if patient develops signs and symptoms of liver toxicity, pause treatment and obtain full set of LFTs. Repeat LFTs to ensure normalization of values. If drug is restarted, monitor patient frequently.
• Monitor adrenal function in patient with adrenal insufficiency or borderline adrenal function or patient experiencing prolonged period of stress (such as major surgery).
• Review all medications patient is receiving for potential drug interactions with ketoconazole.

PATIENT TEACHING
• Teach about proper drug administration and handling.
• Review risk of drug interactions. Advise patient to report any new drugs or herbal supplements being taken.
• Make sure patient understands that treatment should continue until all tests indicate that active fungal infection has subsided. If drug is stopped too soon, infection will recur. Treatment for systemic fungal infections typically lasts 6 months.
• Review signs and symptoms of liver toxicity. Tell patient to stop drug and notify prescriber if any occur.
• Instruct patient to immediately report irregular heartbeats, palpitations, faintness, dizziness, or light-headedness.
• Caution patient to avoid alcohol consumption during treatment.
• Instruct patient to report pregnancy or plans to become pregnant or breastfeed.

ketoconazole (topical)
kee-toe-KOE-na-zole

Ketodan, Ketoderm ✦, Nizoral ◇

Therapeutic class: Antifungals
Pharmacologic class: Imidazoles

AVAILABLE FORMS
Cream: 2%
Foam: 2%
Shampoo: 1% ◇, 2%

INDICATIONS & DOSAGES

➤ **Seborrheic dermatitis**
Adults and children ages 12 and older: Apply foam to affected area b.i.d. for 4 weeks.
Adults: Apply cream to affected area b.i.d. for 4 weeks or until condition is clear.

➤ **Tinea corporis, tinea cruris, tinea pedis, tinea versicolor from susceptible organisms; cutaneous candidiasis**
Adults: Apply cream to affected and immediate surrounding area once daily for 2 weeks (6 weeks for tinea pedis). For tinea (pityriasis) versicolor, if using 2% shampoo, one application is usually sufficient.

➤ **Flaking, scaling, and itching associated with dandruff**
Adults and children ages 12 and older: Use 1% OTC shampoo every 3 to 4 days for up to 8 weeks; then apply only as needed to control dandruff.
Children younger than age 12: Consult health care provider before use.

ADMINISTRATION
Topical
• For external use only; not for ophthalmic, oral, or intravaginal use. Don't let drug contact eyes or other mucous membranes. Wash hands after application.
• When using foam, dispense into cap of can or other cool surface; don't apply directly onto hands because foam will start to melt upon contact with warm skin. If fingers are warm, rinse them in cold water and dry well; then, using fingertips, gently massage foam into affected areas until it disappears. If applicable, part hair to directly apply foam to skin.
• When using 1% OTC shampoo, apply to wet hair, lather, rinse thoroughly; repeat.
• When using 2% shampoo, apply to damp skin of affected and surrounding area, lather, leave on skin for 5 minutes, and rinse.
• Store at room temperature; protect from light. Don't expose foam containers to heat.

ACTION
Thought to alter the permeability of the cell membrane, inhibiting the growth of common dermatophytes and yeasts.

Route	Onset	Peak	Duration
Topical	Unknown	Unknown	Unknown

Half-life: Unknown.

ADVERSE REACTIONS
Skin: pruritus, application-site reaction, dry skin (with shampoo); application-site reaction, burning, photosensitivity (with foam); severe irritation, pruritus, stinging (with cream). **Other:** hypersensitivity reaction.

INTERACTIONS
None known.

EFFECTS ON LAB TEST RESULTS
None reported.

CONTRAINDICATIONS & CAUTIONS
• Contraindicated in patients with known hypersensitivity to ketoconazole or its ingredients.
• Some forms contain sulfites, which may cause allergic reactions, including anaphylaxis or asthmatic episodes.
Dialyzable drug: No.

PREGNANCY-LACTATION-REPRODUCTION
• Studies during pregnancy are inadequate. Use during pregnancy only if potential benefit justifies fetal risk.
• Drug isn't detectable in plasma with prolonged shampoo use.
• It isn't known if drug appears in human milk. Use cautiously during breastfeeding if benefit outweighs risk to infant.
• Patients shouldn't apply to breasts to avoid direct contact with infants who are breastfeeding.

NURSING CONSIDERATIONS
• Most patients show improvement soon after treatment begins.
• Treatment of tinea corporis or tinea cruris should continue for at least 2 weeks to reduce possibility of recurrence.

PATIENT TEACHING
• Teach about proper drug administration, handling, and storage.
• Tell patient to stop drug and notify prescriber if hypersensitivity reaction occurs.
• Advise patient to check with prescriber if condition worsens or fails to improve; drug may have to be stopped and diagnosis reevaluated.
• Tell patient to avoid using shampoo on scalp if skin is broken or inflamed.

Reactions in bold italics are *life-threatening*.

• Explain that foam is flammable. Instruct patient to avoid fire, flame, and smoking during and immediately after application.
• Teach patient to wash hands before and after use, unless affected areas are on hands.
• Warn patient that shampoo may cause hair discoloration, abnormal hair texture, and curl removal of permanently waved hair.
• Tell patient to continue drug for intended duration of therapy, even if signs and symptoms improve.

ketorolac tromethamine (oral, nasal, injection)
KEE-toe-role-ak

Sprix, Toradol ✤

Therapeutic class: Anti-inflammatory drugs
Pharmacologic class: NSAIDs

AVAILABLE FORMS
Injection*: 10 mg/mL ampules ✤, 15 mg/mL single-dose vials and 1-mL prefilled syringes; 30 mg/mL in single-dose vials, 1- and 2-mL prefilled syringes
Nasal spray: 15.75 mg/spray
Tablets: 10 mg

INDICATIONS & DOSAGES
Boxed Warning Adjust dosage for patients ages 65 and older, those weighing less than 50 kg, and those with serum creatinine level higher than 5 mg/dL. For these patients, don't exceed total daily dosage of 60 mg ketorolac injection or 40 mg oral ketorolac. ■
➤ **Short-term management of moderately severe, acute pain for single-dose treatment**
Adults younger than age 65 and adolescents ages 17 and older: 60 mg IM or 30 mg IV.
Adults ages 65 and older, patients weighing less than 50 kg, or patients with kidney impairment: 30 mg IM or 15 mg IV.
➤ **Short-term management of moderately severe, acute pain for multiple-dose treatment**
Adults younger than age 65 and adolescents ages 17 and older: 30 mg IM or IV every 6 hours for maximum of 5 days; maximum daily dosage, 120 mg. Or, 31.5 mg (one 15.75-mg spray in each nostril) every 6 to 8 hours; maximum daily dosage, 126 mg.
Adults ages 65 and older, patients weighing less than 50 kg, or patients with kidney

impairment: 15 mg IM or IV every 6 hours for maximum of 5 days; maximum daily dosage, 60 mg. Or, 15.75 mg (1 spray in only one nostril) every 6 to 8 hours; maximum daily dosage, 63 mg.
➤ **Short-term management of moderately severe, acute pain when switching from parenteral to oral administration**
Boxed Warning Oral therapy is indicated only as continuation of IV or IM dosing; never give as initial therapy. ■
Adults younger than age 65 and adolescents ages 17 and older: 20 mg PO as single dose; then 10 mg PO every 4 to 6 hours PRN for maximum of 5 days (combined for both parenteral and oral). Maximum daily dosage, 40 mg.
Adults ages 65 and older, patients weighing less than 50 kg, or patients with kidney impairment: 10 mg PO as single dose; then 10 mg PO every 4 to 6 hours PRN for maximum of 5 days (combined for both parenteral and oral). Maximum daily dosage, 40 mg.

ADMINISTRATION
Boxed Warning Total treatment duration for combined formulations shouldn't exceed 5 days. ■
PO
• Give drug with food if GI upset occurs.
IV
▼ Give injection over at least 15 seconds.
▼ Protect from light.
▼ Store at room temperature.
▼ **Incompatibilities:** Precipitation occurs when mixed in a small volume with hydroxyzine, meperidine, morphine sulfate, and promethazine.
IM
• When appropriate, give slowly by deep IM injection.
• Patient may feel pain at injection site.
Intranasal
• Discard nasal spray within 24 hours of first dose, even if bottle still contains medication.
• Each 1.7-g bottle contains eight sprays.
• Activate pump before first use by pumping five times.
• Have patient gently blow nose before use, sit upright or stand, and tilt head slightly forward.
• Insert tip into nostril, point away from septum, and spray once while patient holds breath. For 2-spray dose, repeat in other nostril.

K

ACTION

May inhibit prostaglandin synthesis to produce anti-inflammatory, analgesic, and antipyretic effects.

Route	Onset	Peak	Duration
PO	30–60 min	2–3 hr	4–6 hr
IV, IM	About 30 min	≤2–3 hr	4–6 hr
Intranasal	20 min	45 min	Unknown

Half-life: PO, 2 to 9 hours; IV, 5 to 6 hours; IM, 5 to 6 hours; intranasal, 5 to 6 hours.

ADVERSE REACTIONS

CNS: headache, dizziness, drowsiness. **CV:** edema, HTN. **EENT:** tinnitus. **Nasal spray only:** increased lacrimation, rhinalgia, nasal discomfort, rhinitis, throat irritation. **GI:** abdominal pain, dyspepsia, heartburn, nausea, constipation, diarrhea, flatulence, GI fullness, *GI perforation,* peptic ulceration, stomatitis, vomiting, *GI hemorrhage.* **GU:** kidney impairment. **Hematologic:** anemia, prolonged bleeding time, purpura. **Hepatic:** increased liver enzyme levels. **Skin:** rash, diaphoresis, pruritus. **Other:** injection site pain.

INTERACTIONS

Drug-drug. *ACE inhibitors, ARBs:* May cause kidney impairment, particularly with volume depletion. May decrease antihypertensive effect. Use together cautiously.
Alprazolam, fluoxetine, thiothixene: May cause hallucinations. Monitor patient closely.
Anticoagulants (warfarin): May increase anticoagulant level in blood. Use together with extreme caution, and monitor patient closely.
Beta-blockers: May decrease antihypertensive effect. Use together cautiously.
Digoxin: May increase digoxin level and prolong its half-life. Monitor digoxin level.
Diuretics: May increase risk of kidney toxicity. May decrease effectiveness of these drugs. Monitor patient closely.
Carbamazepine, phenytoin: May increase risk of seizures. Monitor patient closely.
Cyclosporine: May increase risk of kidney toxicity. Monitor kidney function.
Lithium: May increase lithium level. Monitor patient closely for lithium toxicity.
Methotrexate: May decrease methotrexate clearance and increase toxicity. Avoid use together.
Boxed Warning *NSAIDs, salicylates:* May increase risk of NSAID-related adverse effects. Use together is contraindicated. ■

Pemetrexed: May increase pemetrexed adverse effects. Refer to pemetrexed prescribing information.
Pentoxifylline: May increase risk of bleeding. Avoid use together.
Probenecid: May increase level and toxicity of ketorolac. Use together is contraindicated.
SSRIs: May increase risk of GI bleeding. Use together cautiously.
Drug-herb. *Dong quai, feverfew, garlic, ginger, horse chestnut, red clover:* May cause bleeding. Discourage use together.
White willow: Herb and drug contain similar components. Discourage use together.
Drug-lifestyle. *Alcohol use:* May increase risk of GI bleeding. Warn patient to use together with caution.
Smoking: May increase risk of GI bleeding. Encourage smoking cessation.

EFFECTS ON LAB TEST RESULTS

- May increase ALT and AST levels.
- May decrease Hb level and hematocrit.
- May increase bleeding time.
- May lead to false-positive aldosterone/renin ratio.

CONTRAINDICATIONS & CAUTIONS

Boxed Warning Contraindicated in patients hypersensitive to ketorolac, aspirin, or other NSAIDs. Hypersensitivity reactions, ranging from bronchospasm to anaphylactic shock, have occurred and appropriate counteractive measures must be available when first dose of ketorolac injection is given. ■
- Use cautiously in patients with asthma because they may have aspirin-sensitive asthma, which increases the risk of severe, potentially fatal, bronchospasm.
Boxed Warning Contraindicated in children younger than age 17, as prophylactic analgesic before major surgery, intra-operatively when hemostasis is critical, in patients with advanced kidney impairment, and in those at risk for KF from volume depletion. ■
Boxed Warning Contraindicated in patients with suspected or confirmed cerebrovascular bleeding, hemorrhagic diathesis, or incomplete hemostasis and in those at high risk for bleeding because drug inhibits platelet function. ■
Boxed Warning Drug isn't indicated for minor or chronic pain. ■
Boxed Warning NSAIDs can cause peptic ulcers, GI bleeding, and perforation of

*Reactions in bold italics are **life-threatening**.*

stomach or intestines, which can be fatal. These events can occur at any time during therapy and without warning. Drug is contraindicated in patients with active peptic ulcer disease, recent GI bleeding or perforation, and history of peptic ulcer disease or GI bleeding. Older adults are at greater risk for serious GI events. ∎

Boxed Warning Drug is contraindicated for treatment of perioperative pain in patients requiring CABG surgery. ∎

Boxed Warning NSAIDs increase risk of serious CV thrombotic events, including MI and stroke. Risk can occur early in treatment and increase with duration of use. ∎

Boxed Warning Contraindicated for epidural or intrathecal administration because of its alcohol content. ∎

🜂 *Alert:* NSAIDs increase the risk of HF.

• Use cautiously in older adults and patients with liver or kidney impairment or cardiac decompensation.

• May cause SCARs (DRESS, exfoliative dermatitis, SJS, TEN), which may be fatal.

Dialyzable drug: Unlikely.

⚠ *Overdose S&S:* Abdominal pain, GI bleeding, nausea, vomiting, peptic ulcers, kidney dysfunction, HTN, drowsiness, lethargy, coma, respiratory depression, anaphylaxis.

PREGNANCY-LACTATION-REPRODUCTION

Boxed Warning Contraindicated during labor and delivery because drug may adversely affect fetal circulation and inhibit uterine contractions. ∎

🜂 *Alert:* Use of NSAIDs at 20 weeks or later in pregnancy may cause fetal kidney dysfunction; use at 30 weeks or later may increase risk of premature closure of ductus arteriosus. Avoid use starting at 20 weeks' gestation. If potential benefit justifies fetal risk, use lowest effective dose for shortest duration. Consider ultrasound monitoring of amniotic fluid if NSAID therapy lasts longer than 48 hours. Discontinue if oligohydramnios occurs.

• Prolonged use of NSAIDs in patients of childbearing potential may be associated with infertility that's reversible upon drug discontinuation.

• Low concentrations of drug appear in human milk. Use cautiously during breastfeeding.

NURSING CONSIDERATIONS

Boxed Warning Doses higher than label recommendations won't improve efficacy and increase the risk of serious adverse events. ∎

• Use lowest effective dose for shortest period consistent with patient's treatment goals.

• Correct hypovolemia before giving drug.

🜂 *Alert:* Watch for and immediately evaluate signs and symptoms of MI (chest pain, shortness of breath, trouble breathing) or stroke (weakness in one part or side of the body, slurred speech).

• Carefully observe patients with coagulopathies and those taking anticoagulants. Drug inhibits platelet aggregation and can prolong bleeding time.

• NSAIDs may mask signs and symptoms of infection because of their antipyretic and anti-inflammatory actions.

• *Look alike–sound alike:* Don't confuse ketorolac with ketamine or Ketalar.

PATIENT TEACHING

• Teach about proper drug administration and handling.

• Warn patient using nasal spray that transient, mild to moderate nasal irritation may occur.

• Teach patient to read package insert and full directions for use of nasal spray bottle.

• Warn patient not to take ketorolac with other NSAIDs.

🜂 *Alert:* Review signs and symptoms of stroke and MI. Advise patient to seek immediate medical attention if any occur.

• Advise patient to maintain adequate fluid intake.

• Tell patient to promptly report edema, weight gain, or shortness of breath.

• Teach patient the warning signs and symptoms of liver toxicity (nausea, fatigue, lethargy, pruritus, jaundice, right upper quadrant abdominal tenderness, flulike symptoms). Advise patient to stop drug and seek immediate medical help if any occur.

• Instruct patient to stop medication and contact prescriber for rash or fever.

• Teach patient the signs and symptoms of anaphylaxis (difficulty breathing; swelling of face or throat), and stress the importance reporting them immediately.

• Instruct patient to immediately report pregnancy.

🜂 *Alert:* Warn patient of risk of NSAID use during pregnancy.

K

• Warn patient receiving drug IM that pain may occur at injection site.
• Teach signs and symptoms of GI bleeding and ulcers (epigastric pain, dyspepsia, melena, hematemesis). Instruct patient to immediately notify prescriber if any occur.
• Advise patient to take oral medication with food to prevent GI upset.
• Tell patient not to take drug for more than 5 days in a row.

SAFETY ALERT!

labetalol hydrochloride
la-BET-ah-loll

Trandate✲

Therapeutic class: Antihypertensives
Pharmacologic class: Alpha–beta blockers

AVAILABLE FORMS
Injection: 5 mg/mL in multiple-dose vials and prefilled syringes
Premixed IV solution: 1 mg/mL in 100 mL, 200 mL, 300 mL single-dose bags
Tablets: 100 mg, 200 mg, 300 mg

INDICATIONS & DOSAGES
➤ **HTN**
Adults (inpatients after IV therapy): Once supine diastolic BP begins to rise, 200 mg PO, followed by 200 to 400 mg PO in 6 to 12 hours, depending on BP response. May increase from 200 mg PO b.i.d. to 400 mg b.i.d., then to 800 mg b.i.d., then to 1,200 mg b.i.d. at 1-day intervals to achieve desired response.
Adults (outpatients): 100 mg PO b.i.d. with or without a diuretic. If needed, increase dosage to 200 mg b.i.d. after 2 to 3 days. Further increases may be made every 2 to 3 days until optimal response is reached. Usual maintenance dosage is 200 to 400 mg b.i.d. Maximum daily dosage, 2.4 g in two divided doses given alone or with a diuretic.
Adjust-a-dose: Usual maintenance dosage for older adults is 100 to 200 mg b.i.d.
➤ **Severe HTN, hypertensive emergencies**
Adults: 2 mg/minute IV infusion until satisfactory response is obtained; then infusion is stopped. Maximum dose, 300 mg. Or, give by repeated IV injection; initially, 0.25 mg/kg up to maximum of 20 mg IV over 2 minutes. Repeat injections of 40 to 80 mg every 10 minutes to maximum dose of 300 mg, as needed.

ADMINISTRATION
PO
• If dizziness occurs, give dose at bedtime or give smaller doses t.i.d.
• Food increases bioavailability of drug; give in consistent manner with regard to meals.
IV
▼ Give by slow, direct IV injection over 2 minutes at 10-minute intervals.
▼ For IV infusion, prepare by diluting with D₅W, NSS, or other compatible IV solution according to manufacturer's instructions to yield 1 mg/mL (if total volume is 200 mL) or 2 mg/3 mL (if total volume is 250 mL). Infuse at 2 mg/minute.
▼ Don't further dilute ready-to-use bags.
▼ Give labetalol infusion with an infusion-control device.
▼ Monitor BP during and after completion of infusion or IV injections.
▼ Patient should remain supine during and for 3 hours after infusion. When given IV for hypertensive emergencies, drug produces a rapid, predictable fall in BP within 5 to 10 minutes.
▼ Store at room temperature.
▼ Protect from light.
▼ **Incompatibilities:** Alkali solutions, furosemide.

ACTION
May be related to reduced peripheral vascular resistance, as a result of alpha and beta blockade.

Route	Onset	Peak	Duration
PO	20–120 min	2–4 hr	8–12 hr
IV	2–5 min	5–15 min	16–18 hr

Half-life: IV, about 5.5 hours; oral, 6 to 8 hours.

ADVERSE REACTIONS
CNS: asthenia, dizziness, fatigue, headache, vertigo, paresthesia, transient scalp tingling, taste distortion. **CV:** edema, orthostatic hypotension, flushing. **EENT:** abnormal vision, nasal congestion. **GI:** dyspepsia, nausea, vomiting. **GU:** increased BUN and creatinine, sexual dysfunction. **Hepatic:** increased transaminases. **Respiratory:** dyspnea, wheezing. **Skin:** rash, diaphoresis, pruritus.

INTERACTIONS
Drug-drug. *Beta agonists:* May blunt bronchodilator effect of these drugs in patients

with bronchospasm. May need to increase dosages of these drugs.

Beta blockers, cardiac glycosides: May increase risk of bradycardia. Monitor therapy.

Calcium channel blockers (verapamil): May increase hypotensive effects. IV coadministration is contraindicated. Use PO forms together cautiously.

Cimetidine: May enhance labetalol's effect. Use together cautiously.

CV drugs, diuretics: May increase hypotensive effects. Monitor BP.

Halothane: May increase hypotensive effect. Monitor BP closely.

Insulin, oral antidiabetics: May alter dosage requirements in previously stabilized patient with diabetes. Monitor patient closely.

Nitroglycerin: May blunt reflex tachycardia produced by nitroglycerin but not the hypotension. Monitor BP if used together.

NSAIDs: May decrease antihypertensive effects. Monitor BP.

TCAs: May increase incidence of tremor. Monitor patient for tremor.

Drug-herb. *Ma huang:* May decrease antihypertensive effects. Discourage use together.

EFFECTS ON LAB TEST RESULTS
• May increase transaminase, creatinine, and urea levels.
• May cause false-positive increase of urine free and total catecholamine levels when measured by a nonspecific trihydroxyindole fluorometric method.
• May cause false-positive test result for amphetamines when screening urine for drugs.

CONTRAINDICATIONS & CAUTIONS
• Contraindicated in patients hypersensitive to drug or its components and in those with bronchial asthma (history of obstructive airway disease), overt HF, greater than first-degree heart block (except in patients with a functioning pacemaker), cardiogenic shock, severe bradycardia, and other conditions that may cause severe and prolonged hypotension.
• Use cautiously in patients with HF, ischemic heart disease, impaired liver function, chronic bronchitis, emphysema, diabetes, PVD, and pheochromocytoma.
• Inform ophthalmologist of drug use before surgery because drug may cause intraoperative floppy iris syndrome.
• Safety and effectiveness in children haven't been established.

Dialyzable drug: No.

⚠ **Overdose S&S:** Orthostatic hypotension, bradycardia, HF, bronchospasm, seizures.

PREGNANCY-LACTATION-REPRODUCTION
• Studies during pregnancy are inadequate. Use during pregnancy only if potential benefit justifies fetal risk.
• Low amounts of drug appear in human milk and can be detected in serum of infants who are breastfed. Use cautiously during breastfeeding.

NURSING CONSIDERATIONS
• Frequently monitor BP. Drug masks common signs and symptoms of shock.
• Monitor heart rate and rhythm in patient receiving IV injection.
• Keep patient supine while patient is receiving IV therapy and for up to 3 hours after infusion ends. Closely monitor BP before allowing patient to ambulate.
• In patient with diabetes, closely monitor glucose level because beta blockers may mask certain signs and symptoms of hypoglycemia.
• Monitor patient for HF.
• Abrupt withdrawal may cause or worsen angina.
• Monitor patient for bronchospasm; discontinue drug if it occurs.
• Don't routinely withdraw long-term beta-blocker therapy before surgery.
• Rare occurrences of severe liver injury have been reported. Monitor LFT values. Use cautiously in patients with impaired liver function; drug metabolism may be decreased.
• Monitor for hypersensitivity reactions.

PATIENT TEACHING
🔵 **Alert:** Tell patient that abruptly stopping drug can worsen chest pain and trigger a heart attack.
• Caution patient to take drug in a consistent manner with regard to meals.
• Explain that dizziness is the most common adverse reaction and tends to occur in early stages of treatment, in those taking diuretics, and with higher dosages. Advise patient to minimize dizziness by rising slowly and avoiding sudden position changes.
• Warn patient that occasional, harmless scalp tingling may occur, especially when therapy begins.

lacosamide
lah-COSS-ah-mide

Motpoly XR, Vimpat

Therapeutic class: Anticonvulsants
Pharmacologic class: Functionalized
amino acids
Controlled substance schedule: V

AVAILABLE FORMS
Capsules (extended-release) ⓞⓝⓒ*:* 100 mg,
150 mg, 200 mg
Injection: 200 mg/20 mL vials
Oral solution: 10 mg/mL
Tablets ⓞⓝⓒ*:* 50 mg, 100 mg, 150 mg, 200 mg

INDICATIONS & DOSAGES
Adjust-a-dose (for all indications): In patients
with Child-Pugh class A or B liver impairment or CrCl of 30 mL/minute or less, reduce
maximum recommended daily dosage by
25%. Withhold drug in patients with Child-
Pugh class C liver impairment. Dosage supplementation of up to 50% should be considered following a 4-hour hemodialysis treatment. Reduce dosage as needed in patients
with liver or kidney impairment who are taking strong CYP3A4 and CYP2C9 inhibitors
because of increased lacosamide exposure.
➤ **Adjunctive therapy for partial-onset
seizures and primary generalized tonic-
clonic seizures**
Adults and adolescents ages 17 and older:
Initially, 50 mg PO b.i.d.; increase by 50 mg
b.i.d. at weekly intervals to recommended
daily dosage of 100 to 200 mg PO b.i.d. Or,
initially 200 mg PO as a single loading dose,
followed 12 hours later by 100 mg PO b.i.d.
for 1 week; then increase by 50 mg b.i.d. as
needed based on patient response and tolerance up to recommended maintenance dosage
of 200 mg b.i.d.
*Children ages 4 to younger than 17 weighing
50 kg or more:* Initially, 50 mg PO b.i.d.; increase as needed by 50 mg b.i.d. at weekly intervals to recommended maintenance dosage
of 100 to 200 mg PO b.i.d.
*Children ages 4 to younger than 17 weigh-
ing 30 to less than 50 kg:* Initially, 1 mg/kg
PO b.i.d.; increase as needed by 1 mg/kg b.i.d.
at weekly intervals to recommended maintenance dosage of 2 to 4 mg/kg PO b.i.d.

*Children ages 4 to younger than 17 weigh-
ing 11 to less than 30 kg:* Initially, 1 mg/kg
PO b.i.d.; increase as needed by 1 mg/kg b.i.d.
at weekly intervals to recommended maintenance dosage of 3 to 6 mg/kg PO b.i.d.
  May give IV at equivalent daily dose and
frequency when oral administration isn't feasible.
➤ **Monotherapy for partial-onset seizures**
Adults and adolescents ages 17 and older:
Initially, 100 mg PO b.i.d.; increase at weekly
intervals by 50 mg b.i.d. to recommended
daily dosage of 150 to 200 mg PO b.i.d. Or,
initially 200 mg PO as a single loading dose,
followed approximately 12 hours later by
100 mg PO b.i.d. for 1 week; then increase
by 50 mg b.i.d. as needed based on patient
response and tolerance up to recommended
maintenance dosage of 150 to 200 mg PO
b.i.d. When converting from another single
antiepileptic, titrate lacosamide to therapeutic
dosage of 150 to 200 mg PO b.i.d. and maintain for at least 3 days before initiating withdrawal of concomitant drug. Gradually withdraw concomitant drug over at least 6 weeks.
Children ages 4 to younger than 17: In patients weighing 50 kg or more, same dosing
as adults. In those weighing 30 to less than
50 kg, initially, 1 mg/kg b.i.d.; increase as
needed by 1 mg/kg b.i.d. at weekly intervals
to recommended daily dosage of 2 to 4 mg/kg
PO b.i.d. In those weighing 11 to less than
30 kg, initially, 1 mg/kg PO b.i.d.; increase as
needed by 1 mg/kg b.i.d. at weekly intervals
to recommended daily dosage of 3 to 6 mg/kg
PO b.i.d.
*Children ages 1 month to younger than
17 years:* In patients weighing 50 kg or more,
same dosing as adults. In those weighing 30
to less than 50 kg, initially, 1 mg/kg PO b.i.d.;
increase as needed by 1 mg/kg b.i.d. at weekly
intervals to recommended daily dosage of 2
to 4 mg/kg PO b.i.d. In those weighing 11 to
less than 30 kg, initially, 1 mg/kg PO b.i.d.;
increase as needed by 1 mg/kg b.i.d. at weekly
intervals to recommended daily dosage of 3 to
6 mg/kg PO b.i.d.
*Children ages 1 month and older weighing 6
to less than 11 kg:* Initially, 1 mg/kg PO b.i.d.;
increase as needed by 1 mg/kg b.i.d. at weekly
intervals to recommended daily dosage of 3 to
6 mg/kg PO b.i.d.
*Children ages 1 month and older weighing
less than 6 kg:* Initially, 0.66 mg/kg IV t.i.d.;
then increase as needed by 0.66 mg/kg IV

Reactions in bold italics are *life-threatening*.

t.i.d. at weekly intervals to recommended daily dosage of 2.5 to 5 mg/kg IV t.i.d. Or initially, 1 mg/kg PO b.i.d.; then increase by 1 mg/kg PO b.i.d. at weekly intervals to recommended PO dosage of 3.75 to 7.5 mg/kg b.i.d. *Adjust-a-dose:* May give IV at equivalent daily dose and frequency to patients weighing 6 kg or more when oral administration isn't feasible.

➤ **Partial-onset seizures (extended-release capsules)**
Adults and adolescents ages 17 and older: Initially, 200 mg PO once daily as monotherapy or 100 mg PO once daily as adjunctive therapy. Increase by 100 mg daily at weekly intervals to recommended daily dosage of 300 to 400 mg. Maximum daily dosage, 400 mg.
Children weighing at least 50 kg: Initially, 100 mg PO once daily. Increase by 100 mg daily at weekly intervals based on clinical response and tolerability. Recommended daily dosage is 300 to 400 mg daily for monotherapy and 200 to 400 mg daily for adjunctive therapy. Maximum daily dosage, 400 mg.

ADMINISTRATION
PO
• Give drug with or without food.
• Use calibrated measuring device to administer oral solution.
• May also give oral solution by NG or gastrostomy tube.
• Discard unused oral solution remaining after 6 months of first opening bottle.
• Have patient swallow tablets and capsules whole; don't crush or break tablets; don't open or crush capsules.

IV
▼ May give solution for injection without further dilution or diluted.
▼ For diluted IV infusion, dilute with NSS, D_5W, or lactated Ringer solution. Discard solution if discolored or if particulate matter is present. Diluted solution is stable for 4 hours at room temperature. May administer without further dilution.
▼ Infuse over 30 to 60 minutes. Rapid infusion over 15 minutes can be given in adults, if required.
▼ Discard unused solution in vial.
▼ IV use hasn't been studied past 5 days of consecutive treatment.
▼ **Incompatibilities:** None listed by manufacturer. Consult drug compatibility reference for more information.

ACTION
May selectively enhance slow inactivation of sodium channels, stabilizing hyperexcitable neuronal membranes and inhibiting repetitive neuronal firing.

Route	Onset	Peak	Duration
PO	Unknown	1–4 hr	Unknown
PO (extended-release)	Unknown	7 hr	Unknown
IV	Unknown	30–60 min	Unknown

Half-life: About 13 hours.

ADVERSE REACTIONS
CNS: asthenia, ataxia, balance disorder, abnormal coordination, depression, fatigue, dizziness, gait disturbance, headache, memory impairment, somnolence, syncope, paresthesia, oral paresthesia or hypoesthesia, tremor. **EENT:** blurred vision, diplopia, nystagmus, vertigo. **GI:** diarrhea, nausea, vomiting. **Skin:** pruritus, skin laceration, injection-site pain or discomfort, bruise.

INTERACTIONS
Drug-drug. *CNS depressants (buprenorphine, cannabinoid products):* May have additive depressive effects and other cognitive or neuropsychiatric adverse reactions. Use together cautiously.
Drugs that prolong PR interval (beta blockers, calcium channel blockers, sodium channel blocking AEDs): May increase risk of bradycardia or AV block. Monitor patient closely, especially with IV formulation.
Strong CYP2C9 and CYP3A4 inhibitors (clarithromycin, ketoconazole, ritonavir): May increase lacosamide level in patients with kidney or liver impairment. Consider dosage reductions.
Drug-lifestyle. *Alcohol use:* May cause additive drowsiness. Discourage use together.

EFFECTS ON LAB TEST RESULTS
• May increase LFT values.
• May decrease Hb level and neutrophil count.

CONTRAINDICATIONS & CAUTIONS
• Not recommended for patients with Child-Pugh class C liver impairment.
• Use cautiously in patients with known cardiac conduction problems, depression, myocardial ischemia structural heart disease, HF, or history of suicidality.

• Drug may predispose patients to atrial fibrillation or flutter, especially patients with diabetic neuropathy or CV disease.
• Use cautiously in patients with phenylketonuria because oral solution contains aspartame, a source of phenylalanine.
Dialyzable drug: 50%.

⚠ **Overdose S&S:** Coma, dizziness, nausea, seizures, cardiac conduction disorders, confusion, decreased LOC, cardiogenic shock, cardiac arrest, death.

PREGNANCY-LACTATION-REPRODUCTION
• Studies during pregnancy are inadequate. Use during pregnancy only if potential benefit justifies fetal risk.
• Patients who are pregnant should enroll in North American Antiepileptic Drug Pregnancy Registry (1-888-233-2334 or www.aedpregnancyregistry.org).
• It isn't known if drug appears in human milk. Weigh risk versus benefit of breastfeeding. Monitor exposed infants for excess sedation.

NURSING CONSIDERATIONS
⚡ **Alert:** Give loading dose under medical supervision because of increased risk of CNS adverse reactions.
⚡ **Alert:** Monitor patient for syncopal episodes; drug may increase risk of syncope, especially in patients with cardiac disease and in those receiving drugs that slow AV conduction.
• Obtain ECG at baseline and after titrating to maintenance dosage in patient with known conduction problems (marked first-degree AV block, second- or third-degree AV block, or sick sinus syndrome without pacemaker), sodium channelopathies (Brugada syndrome), concomitant use of drugs that prolong PR interval, or severe cardiac disease (MI, HF, structural heart disease). Also closely monitor such a patient when giving IV lacosamide.
• Monitor patient for signs and symptoms of DRESS syndrome (fever, rash, eosinophilia, hepatitis, nephritis, lymphadenopathy, myocarditis). If reaction is suspected, discontinue drug and begin alternative treatment.
• Titrate dosage carefully in patient with kidney or liver impairment.
⚡ **Alert:** Withdraw drug gradually over at least 1 week to minimize potential for increased seizure activity.
• When converting patient already on a single AED to lacosamide, continue the other AED until therapeutic dosage of lacosamide has been given for at least 3 days for tablets or IV form or 4 days for capsules. Then gradually withdraw the other AED over at least 6 weeks.
⚡ **Alert:** Drug may increase risk of suicidality. Monitor patient closely for worsening depression, suicidality, and unusual changes in mood or behavior.

PATIENT TEACHING
• Teach about proper drug administration and handling.
⚡ **Alert:** Tell patient, family, and caregivers to immediately report mood changes or suicidality.
• Warn patient to avoid driving and operating heavy machinery until drug's CNS effects are known; drug may cause dizziness and ataxia.
• Advise patient of childbearing potential to report suspected pregnancy or plans to become pregnant or breastfeed.
• Warn patient not to stop drug abruptly.
• Tell patient to avoid alcohol while taking drug.
• Inform patient with phenylketonuria that a 200-mg dose of oral solution contains 0.32 mg of phenylalanine.
• Advise patient to report blurred vision, dizziness, double vision, nausea, uncoordinated movement, or vertigo.

lamiVUDine (3TC)
lam-ah-VEW-den

Epivir, Epivir-HBV

Therapeutic class: Antiretrovirals
Pharmacologic class: Nucleoside–nucleotide reverse transcriptase inhibitors

AVAILABLE FORMS
lamivudine
Oral solution: 10 mg/mL*
Tablets: 150 mg (scored), 300 mg
lamivudine (HBV)
Oral solution: 5 mg/mL
Tablets: 100 mg

INDICATIONS & DOSAGES
Boxed Warning Lamivudine tablets and oral solution used to treat HIV-1 infection contain higher dose of active ingredient than lamivudine tablets and oral solution used to treat chronic HBV infection. Patients infected

with HIV-1 should receive only dosing forms appropriate for HIV-1 treatment. ■

➤ **HIV infection, with other antiretrovirals**

Adults: 300 mg Epivir PO once daily or 150 mg PO b.i.d.

Children ages 3 months and older: 5 mg/kg Epivir solution PO b.i.d. or 10 mg/kg PO once daily. Maximum dosage, 300 mg daily.

Children weighing 14 kg or more who can reliably swallow tablets: For 14 to less than 20 kg, 1 tablet (150 mg) PO once daily or ½ tablet (75 mg) PO b.i.d.; for 20 kg to less than 25 kg, 1½ tablets (225 mg) PO once daily or ½ tablet (75 mg) PO in morning and 1 tablet (150 mg) PO in evening; for 25 kg or more, 2 tablets (300 mg) PO once daily or 150 mg PO b.i.d.

Adjust-a-dose: For adults and adolescents weighing 25 kg or more infected with HIV and CrCl of 30 to 49 mL/minute, give 150 mg Epivir PO daily. If CrCl is 15 to 29 mL/minute, give 150 mg PO on day 1 and then 100 mg daily; if CrCl is 5 to 14 mL/minute, give 150 mg on day 1 and then 50 mg daily; if CrCl is less than 5 mL/minute, give 50 mg on day 1 and then 25 mg daily. Although data are insufficient to recommend a specific dosage adjustment in children with kidney impairment, consider dosage reduction or increase in dosing interval. No additional dosing is needed after routine hemodialysis or peritoneal dialysis.

➤ **Chronic HBV infection with evidence of HBV replication and active liver inflammation**

Adults: 100 mg PO once daily.

Children ages 2 to 17: 3 mg/kg PO once daily, up to maximum dosage of 100 mg daily. Use oral solution for doses less than 100 mg and in patients unable to swallow tablets. Optimum treatment duration isn't known.

Adjust-a-dose: For adults with chronic HBV infection and CrCl of 30 to 49 mL/minute, give first dose of 100 mg lamivudine for HBV; then give 50 mg PO once daily. If CrCl is 15 to 29 mL/minute, give first dose of 100 mg; then give 25 mg PO once daily. If CrCl is 5 to 14 mL/minute, give first dose of 35 mg; then give 15 mg PO once daily. If CrCl is less than 5 mL/minute, give first dose of 35 mg; then give 10 mg PO once daily. Data are insufficient to recommend a specific dosage in children with kidney impairment. No additional dosing is needed after routine hemodialysis or peritoneal dialysis.

ADMINISTRATION

PO
● Give drug without regard to food.
● Give missed dose as soon as possible; don't double next dose or give more than prescribed.

ACTION

A synthetic nucleoside analogue that inhibits HIV and HBV reverse transcription via viral DNA chain termination. Inhibits RNA- and DNA-dependent DNA polymerase activities.

Route	Onset	Peak	Duration
PO	Unknown	1–3 hr	Unknown

Half-life: Adults, 5 to 7 hours; children, 2 hours.

ADVERSE REACTIONS

Adverse reactions may pertain to the combination HIV therapy of lamivudine and zidovudine.

CNS: dizziness, fatigue, fever, headache, insomnia and other sleep disorders, malaise, neuropathy, depressive disorders, paresthesia. **EENT:** nasal symptoms, infections, sore throat. **GI:** anorexia, diarrhea, nausea, vomiting, abdominal pain or cramps, *pancreatitis,* dyspepsia, stomatitis. **Hematologic:** *neutropenia, thrombocytopenia,* anemia. **Hepatic:** enlarged liver (children), increased transaminase levels, hyperbilirubinemia. **Metabolic:** increased lipase, amylase, CK, ALT levels. **Musculoskeletal:** musculoskeletal pain, arthralgia, myalgia. **Respiratory:** cough, abnormal breath sounds (children). **Skin:** rash. **Other:** chills, splenomegaly, lymphadenopathy.

INTERACTIONS

Drug-drug. *Sorbitol:* May decrease lamivudine level. Avoid use together when possible.
Trimethoprim-containing drugs: May increase lamivudine level because of decreased clearance of drug. Monitor patient for toxicity.

EFFECTS ON LAB TEST RESULTS

● May increase ALT, bilirubin, and serum lipase and CK levels.
● May decrease Hb level and neutrophil and platelet counts.

CONTRAINDICATIONS & CAUTIONS

🚫 *Alert:* Lactic acidosis and severe liver enlargement with steatosis, including fatal cases, have been reported.

L

• Contraindicated in patients hypersensitive to drug.
• Use cautiously in patients with kidney impairment.
• Don't use with other combination drugs containing lamivudine or emtricitabine.
• Safety and effectiveness of lamivudine haven't been established for treatment of chronic HBV infection in patients dually infected with HIV-1 and HBV. Emergence of HBV variants associated with resistance to lamivudine has also been reported in patients infected with HIV-1 who have received lamivudine-containing antiretroviral regimens in the presence of concurrent HBV infection.
• Use lamivudine for HBV only when an alternative antiviral with a higher genetic barrier to resistance isn't available or appropriate. Drug hasn't been evaluated in patients infected with HBV/HIV-1, HCV, or hepatitis delta virus; in patients with chronic HBV infection with decompensated liver disease; or in recipients of liver transplant.
• Drug may increase risk of immune reconstitution syndrome when used in combination antiretroviral therapy.
⚠ Alert: Use drug cautiously, if at all, in children with history of pancreatitis or other significant risk factors for development of pancreatitis.
Dialyzable drug: Unknown.

PREGNANCY-LACTATION-REPRODUCTION
• Use during pregnancy only if potential benefit justifies fetal risk.
• Lamivudine is commonly used to treat HIV infection during pregnancy.
• The Antiretroviral Pregnancy Registry monitors maternal-fetal outcomes with exposure to lamivudine. To register, call 1-800-258-4263.
• Lamivudine appears in human milk. Use cautiously during breastfeeding.

NURSING CONSIDERATIONS
Boxed Warning Severe acute exacerbations of HBV have been reported in patients who have HBV alone or who are infected with both HBV and HIV-1 and have discontinued drug. Monitor liver function closely in patients who discontinue drug. If appropriate, initiate anti-hepatitis B therapy. ∎

Boxed Warning Provide HIV counseling and test patients for HIV before and during therapy because form and dosage of lamivudine for HBV infection aren't appropriate for those infected with both HBV and HIV. If giving lamivudine to patients with HBV and HIV, use the higher dosage indicated for HIV as part of an appropriate combination regimen. If treatment is prescribed for chronic HBV infection in patients with unrecognized or untreated HIV infection, HIV resistance is likely. ∎
⚠ Alert: Immediately stop treatment and notify prescriber if signs, symptoms, or lab abnormalities suggest pancreatitis. Monitor amylase level.
⚠ Alert: Lactic acidosis and liver toxicity have been reported. Notify prescriber if signs of lactic acidosis or liver toxicity occur.
• Scored tablets are preferred formulation for children infected with HIV-1 who weigh at least 14 kg and for whom a solid dosage form is appropriate because oral solution has lower rates of virologic suppression and lower plasma lamivudine exposure, and patients developed viral resistance more frequently. Monitor HIV-1 viral load more frequently when using oral solution.
• Monitor CBC, platelet count, LFT values, and kidney function results.
• To reduce risk of resistance in patients receiving HBV monotherapy, consider switching to an alternative regimen if serum HBV DNA remains detectable after 24 weeks of treatment. Guide optimal therapy by resistance testing.
• Monitor patient for infection.

PATIENT TEACHING
• Inform patient that long-term effects of drug aren't known.
• Stress importance of taking drug exactly as prescribed.
Boxed Warning Offer HIV counseling and testing to all patients before beginning treatment with lamivudine for HBV and periodically during treatment. ∎
• Inform patient that drug doesn't cure HIV infection, that opportunistic infections and other complications of HIV infection may still occur, and that transmission of HIV to others through sexual contact or blood contamination is still possible.
• Teach parents or guardians signs and symptoms of pancreatitis. Advise them to report

signs and symptoms (abdominal pain, which may radiate to back; fever; increased heart rate; nausea; vomiting) immediately.
• Instruct patient to report pregnancy or plans to become pregnant or breastfeed.

lamoTRIgine
la-MO-tri-geen

LaMICtal, Subvenite

Therapeutic class: Anticonvulsants
Pharmacologic class: Phenyltriazines

AVAILABLE FORMS

Tablets 🔲: 25 mg, 100 mg, 150 mg, 200 mg
Tablets (chewable dispersible): 2 mg, 5 mg, 25 mg
Tablets (extended-release) 🔲: 25 mg, 50 mg, 100 mg, 200 mg, 250 mg, 300 mg
Tablets (ODTs): 25 mg, 50 mg, 100 mg, 200 mg

INDICATIONS & DOSAGES

🔹 *Alert:* Extended-release formula isn't for use as initial monotherapy or for conversion to monotherapy from two or more concomitant AEDs.
Adjust-a-dose (for all indications): Generally, reduce initial, escalation, and maintenance doses by approximately 25% in patients with Child-Pugh class B or C liver impairment without ascites and 50% in patients with Child-Pugh class C liver impairment with ascites. May adjust escalation and maintenance doses according to clinical response. In patients with kidney impairment, base initial doses on patients' concomitant medications; reduced maintenance doses may be effective for patients with significant kidney impairment.
➤ **Conversion to monotherapy using extended-release formula in patients with partial seizures who are receiving treatment with a single enzyme-inducing AED (except valproate)**
Adults and children ages 13 and older: Add 50 mg extended-release tablet PO daily to current drug regimen for 2 weeks, followed by 100 mg PO daily for 2 weeks. Then increase by 100 mg every week to dosage of 400 to 600 mg PO daily. The concomitant enzyme-inducing AED can then be gradually reduced by 20% decrements each week

over a 4-week period. Two weeks after completing withdrawal of enzyme-inducing AED, decrease lamotrigine (extended-release tablet) no faster than 100 mg/day each week to achieve monotherapy maintenance dosage of 250 to 300 mg/day.
➤ **Conversion to monotherapy using extended-release formula in patients with partial seizures who are receiving adjunctive treatment with valproate**
Adults and children ages 13 and older: Add 25 mg extended-release PO every other day for 2 weeks. Then increase to 25 mg PO daily for weeks 3 and 4; 50 mg PO daily for week 5; 100 mg PO daily for week 6, and 150 mg PO daily for week 7. Maintain dosage at 150 mg PO daily while decreasing valproate dosage by no more than 500 mg/day each week until 500 mg/day is achieved; maintain for 1 week. Then simultaneously increase extended-release tablet to 200 mg/day while decreasing valproate to 250 mg/day; maintain for 1 week. Increase to 250 or 300 mg PO daily as maintenance dosage and discontinue valproate.
➤ **Conversion to monotherapy using extended-release formula in patients with partial seizures who are receiving treatment with a single drug other than an enzyme-inducing AED or valproate**
Adults and children ages 13 and older: Add 25 mg extended-release PO daily for 2 weeks; then increase to 50 mg PO daily for weeks 3 and 4 and 100 mg PO daily for week 5. Starting with week 6, continue increasing dosage each week by 50 mg PO daily until dosage of 250 to 300 mg PO daily is achieved; then withdraw concomitant AED therapy by 20% decrements each week over a 4-week period. No additional lamotrigine (extended-release tablet) adjustment is needed.
➤ **Adjunctive treatment of partial seizures or primary generalized tonic-clonic seizures caused by epilepsy or generalized seizures of Lennox-Gastaut syndrome**
Adults and children older than age 12 taking valproate: 25 mg immediate-release PO every other day for 2 weeks; then 25 mg PO daily for 2 weeks. Continue to increase, as needed, by 25 to 50 mg daily every 1 to 2 weeks until an effective maintenance dosage of 100 to 400 mg daily given in one or two divided doses is reached. When added to valproate alone, usual daily maintenance dosage is 100 to 200 mg.

L

Adults and children ages 13 and older taking valproate: 25 mg extended-release PO every other day for 2 weeks; then 25 mg PO daily for 2 weeks, 50 mg PO daily for 1 week, 100 mg PO daily for 1 week, and 150 mg PO daily for 1 week. Daily maintenance dosage is 200 to 250 mg.

Adults and children ages 13 and older not taking carbamazepine, phenytoin, phenobarbital, primidone, or valproate: 25 mg extended-release PO daily for 2 weeks; then 50 mg PO daily for 2 weeks, 100 mg PO daily for 1 week, 150 mg PO daily for 1 week, and 200 mg PO daily for 1 week. Daily maintenance dosage is 300 to 400 mg.

Adults and children older than age 12 taking anticonvulsant drugs but not carbamazepine, phenytoin, phenobarbital, primidone, or valproate: 25 mg immediate-release PO daily for 1 to 2 weeks; then 50 mg PO daily for another 2 weeks. Continue to increase by 50 mg/day every 1 to 2 weeks until an effective maintenance dose is reached. Daily maintenance dosage is 225 to 375 mg PO daily in two divided doses.

Adults and children older than age 12 taking carbamazepine, phenytoin, phenobarbital, or primidone but not valproate: 50 mg immediate-release PO daily for 2 weeks; then 100 mg PO daily in two divided doses for 2 weeks. Increase, as needed, by 100 mg daily every 1 to 2 weeks. Usual maintenance dosage is 300 to 500 mg PO daily in two divided doses.

Adults and children ages 13 and older taking carbamazepine, phenytoin, phenobarbital, or primidone but not valproate: 50 mg extended-release PO daily for 2 weeks; then 100 mg PO daily for 2 weeks, 200 mg PO daily for 1 week, 300 mg PO daily for 1 week, and 400 mg PO daily for 1 week. Daily maintenance dosage is 400 to 600 mg.

Children ages 2 to 12 weighing 6.7 to 40 kg taking valproate: 0.15 mg/kg immediate-release PO daily in one or two divided doses (rounded down to nearest whole tablet) for 2 weeks. Increase to 0.3 mg/kg daily in one or two divided doses for 2 weeks; then increase daily dose every 1 or 2 weeks by additional 0.3 mg/kg daily in one or two divided doses. Thereafter, usual maintenance dosage is 1 to 5 mg/kg daily (maximum dosage, 200 mg daily in one or two divided doses). In patients weighing less than 30 kg, maintenance dosage may need to be increased

by as much as 50% based on clinical response.

Children ages 2 to 12 weighing 6.7 to 40 kg taking anticonvulsant drugs but not carbamazepine, phenytoin, phenobarbital, primidone, or valproate: 0.3 mg/kg immediate-release PO daily in one or two divided doses (rounded down to nearest whole tablet) for 2 weeks; then 0.6 mg/kg PO daily in two divided doses for another 2 weeks; then increase daily dose every 1 to 2 weeks with additional 0.6 mg/kg PO daily in two divided doses. Thereafter, usual maintenance dose is 4.5 to 7.5 mg/kg PO daily. Maximum dosage, 300 mg daily in two divided doses. In patients weighing less than 30 kg, maintenance dosage may need to be increased by as much as 50% based on clinical response.

Children ages 2 to 12 weighing 6.7 to 40 kg taking carbamazepine, phenytoin, phenobarbital, or primidone but not valproate: 0.6 mg/kg immediate-release PO daily in two divided doses (rounded down to nearest whole tablet) for 2 weeks. Increase to 1.2 mg/kg PO daily in two divided doses for 2 weeks; then increase daily dose every 1 to 2 weeks with additional 1.2 mg/kg daily in two divided doses. Usual maintenance dosage is 5 to 15 mg/kg PO daily (maximum dosage, 400 mg daily in two divided doses). In patients weighing less than 30 kg, maintenance dosage may need to be increased by as much as 50% based on clinical response.

➤ **To convert patients from therapy with an enzyme-inducing AED alone to lamotrigine therapy**

Adults and children ages 16 and older: Add 50 mg immediate-release PO once daily to current drug regimen for 2 weeks, followed by 100 mg PO daily in two divided doses for 2 weeks. Then increase daily dosage by 100 mg every 1 to 2 weeks to maintenance dose of 500 mg daily in two divided doses. Then gradually reduce concomitant liver enzyme-inducing AED by 20% decrements weekly for 4 weeks.

➤ **To convert patients with partial seizures from adjunctive therapy with valproate to therapy with lamotrigine alone**

Adults and children ages 16 and older: Add immediate-release form until 200 mg daily is achieved; then gradually decrease valproate to 500 mg daily by decrements of no more than 500 mg daily per week. Maintain these dosages for 1 week, then increase lamotrigine to 300 mg daily while decreasing valproate to 250 mg daily. Maintain these dosages for 1 week, then stop valproate completely while increasing lamotrigine by 100 mg daily every week until a dosage of 500 mg daily is reached.

➤ **Bipolar disorder for maintenance treatment to delay time to occurrence of mood episodes (depression, mania, hypomania, mixed episodes) in patients treated for acute mood episodes with standard therapy**

Adults: Initially, 25 mg immediate-release PO once daily for 2 weeks; then 50 mg PO once daily for 2 weeks. Dosage may then be doubled at weekly intervals, to maintenance dosage of 200 mg daily.

Adults taking carbamazepine or other enzyme-inducing drugs without valproate: Initially, 50 mg immediate-release PO once daily for 2 weeks; then 100 mg daily in two divided doses for 2 weeks. Dosage is then increased by 100 mg weekly to maintenance dosage of 400 mg daily, given in two divided doses.

Adults taking valproate: Initially, 25 mg immediate-release PO every other day for 2 weeks; then 25 mg PO once daily for 2 weeks. Dosage may then be doubled at weekly intervals to maintenance dosage of 100 mg daily.

ADMINISTRATION
PO
• Starter and titration kits are available to provide doses consistent with recommended titration schedule for the first 5 weeks of treatment.
• Patient may swallow chewable dispersible tablets whole, chew them, or disperse them in a small amount of water or diluted fruit juice.
• If tablets are chewed, give a small amount of water or diluted fruit juice to aid in swallowing.
• Place ODTs on the tongue and have patient move them around in mouth.
• Patient may swallow ODTs with or without water and without regard to food.
• Give extended-release tablets once daily with or without food.
• Have patient swallow extended-release tablets whole; don't crush or cut tablets. Only use whole immediate-release tablets, ODTs, or tablets or suspension for dosing.

ACTION
Inhibits release of glutamate (an excitatory neurotransmitter) in the brain via action at voltage-sensitive sodium channels. Is a weak inhibitor of the 5-HT$_3$ receptor.

Route	Onset	Peak	Duration
PO (immediate-release)	Unknown	1–5 hr	Unknown
PO (extended-release)	Unknown	4–11 hr	Unknown

Half-life: 7 to 148 hours, depending on age, dosage schedule, use of other anticonvulsants, and other medical conditions.

ADVERSE REACTIONS
CNS: ataxia, dizziness, drowsiness, headache, migraine, somnolence, fatigue, anxiety, abnormal thinking, amnesia, decreased or increased reflexes, depression, confusion, dysarthria, emotional lability, fever, incoordination, insomnia, irritability, hypoesthesia, dream abnormality, malaise, mania, pain, asthenia, speech disorder, concentration disturbance, *seizure exacerbation, suicidality,* tremor, vertigo. **CV:** palpitations, chest pain, edema, *hemorrhage.* **EENT:** blurred vision, diplopia, vision abnormality, nystagmus, rhinitis, epistaxis, dry mouth, pharyngitis, sinusitis. **GI:** nausea, vomiting, abdominal pain, anorexia, constipation, diarrhea, dyspepsia, flatulence, *rectal hemorrhage,* peptic ulcer. **GU:** amenorrhea, dysmenorrhea, urinary frequency, vaginitis, UTI, increased libido. **Hematologic:** lymphadenopathy. **Metabolic:** weight loss or gain. **Musculoskeletal:** arthralgia, back pain, muscle spasm, neck pain, weakness. **Respiratory:** cough, dyspnea, bronchitis, *bronchospasm.* **Skin:** rash, eczema, pruritus, dermatitis, dry skin, diaphoresis, photosensitivity. **Other:** infection, accidental injury, flulike syndrome.

INTERACTIONS
Drug-drug. *Acetaminophen:* May decrease therapeutic effects of lamotrigine. Monitor patient.
Atazanavir–ritonavir, ethosuximide, lopinavir–ritonavir, oxcarbazepine, phenobarbital, phenytoin, primidone, rifampin: May decrease lamotrigine level. Monitor patient closely, and adjust lamotrigine dosage.
Carbamazepine: May decrease effects of lamotrigine while increasing toxicity of carbamazepine. Consider alternative therapy. Adjust dosages and monitor patient.

Hormonal contraceptives containing estrogen: May decrease lamotrigine level. Adjust dosage based on individual hormonal product used. By end of "pill-free" week, lamotrigine level may double.

Organic cation transporter 2 substrates (dofetilide): May increase lamotrigine or dofetilide plasma level. Avoid use together.

Valproate: May increase lamotrigine level and decrease valproate level. Monitor patient for toxicity. Reduce lamotrigine dosage if added to a multidrug regimen that includes valproic acid.

Drug-lifestyle. *Sun exposure:* May cause photosensitivity reactions. Advise patient to avoid excessive sun exposure.

EFFECTS ON LAB TEST RESULTS

• May result in false-positive readings in rapid urine drug screens, particularly for phencyclidine.

CONTRAINDICATIONS & CAUTIONS

• Contraindicated in patients hypersensitive to drug or its components.

⚕ *Alert:* Rare, multiorgan hypersensitivity reactions (DRESS) that can be fatal have occurred. Fever and lymphadenopathy may be present early without rash.

⚕ *Alert:* Drug may cause hemophagocytic lymphohistiocytosis (HLH), a rare and life-threatening immune system reaction.

• Use cautiously in patients with kidney, liver, or cardiac impairment.

• Drug isn't recommended for treatment of acute manic or mixed episodes of bipolar disorder because effectiveness hasn't been established.

⚕ *Alert:* Use cautiously in patients with structural and functional heart disorders, including HF, valvular heart disease, congenital heart disease, conduction system disease, ventricular arrhythmias, cardiac channelopathies, ischemic heart disease, or multiple risk factors for CAD, especially when used in combination with sodium channel blockers (carbamazepine, phenytoin, topiramate); drug may increase risk of serious or life-threatening arrhythmias. Assess whether potential benefits of lamotrigine outweigh risk of arrhythmia for each patient.

Boxed Warning Extended-release form isn't approved for children younger than age 13. ∎

Dialyzable drug: 20%.

⚠ *Overdose S&S:* Ataxia, nystagmus, increased seizures, decreased level of consciousness, coma, intraventricular conduction delay.

PREGNANCY-LACTATION-REPRODUCTION

• Drug may increase risk of congenital malformations in the first trimester. Use during pregnancy only if potential benefit justifies fetal risk.

• Patients who are pregnant should enroll in North American Antiepileptic Drug Pregnancy Registry (1-888-233-2334 or www.aedpregnancyregistry.org).

• Drug appears in human milk. Use cautiously during breastfeeding. Discontinue breastfeeding if infant develops drug toxicity.

NURSING CONSIDERATIONS

⚕ *Alert:* Closely monitor all patients taking or starting AEDs for changes in behavior indicating worsening of suicidality or depression. Symptoms such as anxiety, agitation, hostility, mania, and hypomania may be precursors to emerging suicidality.

• Don't stop drug abruptly because doing so may increase seizure frequency. Instead, taper drug over at least 2 weeks.

Boxed Warning Serious rashes, including SJS and TEN, and rash-related death have been reported. Serious rash occurs more frequently in children than in adults, when administered with valproate, or when initial recommended dose or escalation dose is exceeded. Stop drug at first sign of rash, unless rash is clearly not drug-related. ∎

Boxed Warning Benign rashes may occur; predicting whether rash will become serious or life-threatening is impossible. Stopping treatment may not prevent rash from becoming life-threatening or permanently disabling or disfiguring. ∎

⚕ *Alert:* Drug may cause aseptic meningitis. Monitor patient for symptoms such as headache, fever, neck stiffness, nausea, vomiting, rash, and photophobia. Discontinue drug if no other cause of meningitis is found.

• Evaluate patient for changes in seizure activity. Check adjunct anticonvulsant level.

⚕ *Alert:* Monitor patient for HLH (persistent fever; rash; liver and spleen enlargement; lymphadenopathy; abnormal bleeding, liver function, or coagulation; cytopenias; high serum ferritin level; jaundice; abdominal pain or swelling; seizures; vision changes; trouble walking). Promptly evaluate patient with fever or rash; discontinue drug if HLH or another serious immune-related reaction is suspected or an alternative cause can't be identified.

• *Look alike–sound alike:* Don't confuse lamotrigine with lamivudine or levothyroxine. Don't confuse Lamictal with Lamisil, labetalol, or Lomotil.

PATIENT TEACHING

❸ *Alert:* Counsel family member or caregivers to monitor patient for changes in behavior and to immediately report suicidality.

• Instruct patient or caregiver to report worsening of seizures.

• Inform patient that drug may cause rash, especially if administered with valproic acid. Tell patient to promptly report rash or signs or symptoms of hypersensitivity to prescriber; drug may need to be stopped.

• Strongly advise patient to inspect tablets with each prescription refill to verify tablets are correct and avoid medication errors.

• Caution patient to report all medications being taken or changes to medications, especially oral contraceptives or other hormone products.

• Warn patient not to engage in hazardous activity until drug's CNS effects are known.

• Advise patient to seek immediate medical attention for signs or symptoms of HLH.

• Teach patient or caregiver to immediately report headache, fever, mouth ulcers, bruising or petechiae, signs of infection (fever, cough, dyspnea), neck stiffness, nausea, vomiting, rash, drowsiness, confusion, or light sensitivity.

• Warn that drug may trigger sensitivity to sun. Instruct patient to take precautions until tolerance is determined.

• Warn patient not to stop drug abruptly.

❸ *Alert:* Advise patient of childbearing potential to discuss drug therapy with prescriber if considering pregnancy.

❸ *Alert:* Caution patient to seek immediate medical attention for such signs or symptoms as racing heartbeat, skipped or slow heartbeat, shortness of breath, dizziness, or fainting.

lansoprazole
lanz-AH-pray-zol

Prevacid ◇

Therapeutic class: Antiulcer drugs
Pharmacologic class: PPIs

AVAILABLE FORMS
Capsules (delayed-release) ⓄⓉⒸ: 15 mg ◇, 30 mg
Tablets (ODT delayed-release) ⓄⓉⒸ: 15 mg ◇, 30 mg

INDICATIONS & DOSAGES
Adjust-a-dose (for all indications): Recommended dosage in patients with Child-Pugh class C liver impairment is 15 mg PO daily.
➤ **Short-term treatment of active duodenal ulcer**
Adults: 15 mg PO daily before eating for 4 weeks.
➤ **Maintenance of healed duodenal ulcers**
Adults: 15 mg PO daily.
➤ **Short-term treatment of active benign gastric ulcer**
Adults: 30 mg PO once daily for up to 8 weeks.
➤ **Short-term treatment of erosive esophagitis**
Adults: 30 mg PO daily before eating for up to 8 weeks. If healing doesn't occur, 8 more weeks of therapy may be given. Maintenance dosage for healing is 15 mg PO daily.
Children ages 12 to 17: 30 mg PO once daily for up to 8 weeks.
Children ages 1 to 11 weighing more than 30 kg: 30 mg PO once daily for up to 12 weeks.
Children ages 1 to 11 weighing 30 kg or less: 15 mg PO once daily for up to 12 weeks.
➤ **Long-term treatment of pathologic hypersecretory conditions, including Zollinger-Ellison syndrome**
Adults: Initially, 60 mg PO once daily. Increase dosage, as needed. Give amounts above 120 mg/day in evenly divided doses.
➤ *Helicobacter pylori* **eradication to reduce risk of duodenal ulcer recurrence**
Adults: For patients receiving dual therapy, 30 mg PO lansoprazole with 1 g PO amoxicillin, each given t.i.d. for 14 days. For patients receiving triple therapy, 30 mg PO lansoprazole with 1 g PO amoxicillin and 500 mg PO clarithromycin, all given b.i.d. for 10 to 14 days.

➤ **Short-term treatment of symptomatic GERD**

Adults: 15 mg PO once daily for up to 8 weeks.

Children ages 12 to 17: 15 mg PO once daily for up to 8 weeks.

Children ages 1 to 11 weighing more than 30 kg: 30 mg PO once daily for up to 12 weeks.

Children ages 1 to 11 weighing 30 kg or less: 15 mg PO once daily for up to 12 weeks.

➤ **NSAID-related ulcer in patients who continue NSAID use**

Adults: 30 mg PO daily for 8 weeks.

➤ **To reduce risk of NSAID-related ulcer in patients with history of gastric ulcer who need NSAIDs**

Adults: 15 mg PO daily for up to 12 weeks.

➤ **Heartburn (OTC)**

Adults: 15 mg PO once daily for up to 14 days; may repeat 14-day course every 4 months or as directed by practitioner.

ADMINISTRATION

PO

• Give drug before a meal.

• Have patient swallow capsules whole; don't crush capsules.

• For patients who have difficulty swallowing capsules, capsules can be opened and intact granules sprinkled on 1 tablespoon of applesauce, Ensure pudding, cottage cheese, yogurt, or strained pears and swallowed immediately. Or, capsule contents may be emptied into small volume (60 mL) of apple, orange, or tomato juice and swallowed.

• Capsule contents can be mixed with 40 mL of apple juice in a syringe and given within 3 to 5 minutes via NG or nasojejunal tube. Flush with additional apple juice to give entire dose and maintain tube patency.

• Don't break or cut ODTs; allow tablet to disintegrate.

• Place ODT on patient's tongue and allow it to disintegrate with or without water until particles can be swallowed.

• To give ODTs using oral syringe, dissolve 15-mg tablet in 4 mL water or 30-mg tablet in 10 mL water and give within 15 minutes. Refill syringe with about 2 mL (15-mg tablet) or 5 mL (30-mg tablet) of water, shake gently, and give remaining contents.

• To give ODTs through 8 French or larger NG tube, dissolve 15-mg tablet in 4 mL water or 30-mg tablet in 10 mL water and give within 15 minutes. Refill syringe with about 5 mL of water, shake gently, and flush NG tube.

• ODTs contain 2.5 mg phenylalanine/15-mg tablet and 5.1 mg phenylalanine/30-mg tablet.

ACTION

Reduces acid secretion in gastric parietal cells through inhibition of (H^+, K^+)-ATPase enzyme system, inhibiting the final step in gastric acid production.

Route	Onset	Peak	Duration
PO	1–3 hr	1.7 hr	24 hr

Half-life: Less than 2 hours.

ADVERSE REACTIONS

CNS: headache, dizziness. **GI:** abdominal pain, constipation, diarrhea, nausea. **GU:** hematuria.

INTERACTIONS

Drug-drug. *Amoxicillin, clarithromycin:* May increase risk of adverse effects. Monitor patient.

Atazanavir, nelfinavir: May reduce antiviral GI absorption and activity. Avoid use with nelfinavir. Refer to antiretroviral prescribing information.

Cefuroxime: May reduce cefuroxime absorption. Avoid use together.

Clopidogrel: May decrease clopidogrel level. Monitor therapy or consider H_2 receptor antagonist (famotidine).

Digoxin: May increase digoxin level. Monitor digoxin level and adjust dosage as needed.

Erlotinib, iron salts, ketoconazole, mycophenolate mofetil: May inhibit absorption of these drugs. Monitor patient closely.

Methotrexate: May increase methotrexate level. Monitor methotrexate level and adjust dosage as needed.

Rilpivirine: May decrease rilpivirine level. Use together is contraindicated.

Saquinavir: May increase saquinavir level. Refer to saquinavir prescribing information. Monitor patient for toxicity.

Strong CYP2C19 or CYP3A inducers (ritonavir): May decrease lansoprazole level. Monitor therapy.

Strong CYP2C19 or CYP3A4 inhibitors (voriconazole): May increase lansoprazole level. Use together cautiously.

Sucralfate: May cause delayed lansoprazole absorption. Give lansoprazole at least 30 minutes before sucralfate.

Tacrolimus: May increase tacrolimus level, especially in patients with a transplant who are intermediate or poor metabolizers of CYP2C19. Monitor tacrolimus level.

Theophylline: May increase theophylline clearance. Adjust theophylline dosage when lansoprazole is started or stopped. Use together cautiously.

Warfarin: May increase bleeding time. Monitor INR and PT.

Drug-herb. *St. John's wort:* May increase risk of sun sensitivity. Advise patient to avoid excessive sunlight exposure.

Drug-food. *Any food:* May decrease rate and extent of GI absorption. Advise patient to take before meals.

EFFECTS ON LAB TEST RESULTS

• May increase LFT values and creatinine, BUN, potassium, lipid, serum urea, gastrin, globulin, and LDH levels.
• May increase or decrease cholesterol and electrolyte levels.
• May decrease Hb level.
• May increase or decrease WBC and platelet counts.
• May cause abnormal RBC count.
• May increase urinary albumin and glucose levels.
• May cause urine crystals.
• May cause positive fecal occult blood result.
• May cause false-positive results in diagnostic investigations for neuroendocrine tumors, urine screening tests for tetrahydrocannabinol, and gastrin secretion in response to secretin stimulation test.

CONTRAINDICATIONS & CAUTIONS

• Contraindicated in patients hypersensitive to drug or its components. Reactions may include anaphylaxis, angioedema, acute interstitial nephritis, and urticaria.
• *Alert:* Prolonged use of PPIs or use with medications such as digoxin or drugs that may cause hypomagnesemia (diuretics) may require magnesium supplementation and possible discontinuation of drug. Monitor magnesium level before starting treatment and periodically thereafter.
• *Alert:* Drug may increase risk of hip, wrist, and spine fractures with long-term and multiple daily dose use.
• Acute interstitial nephritis has been observed in patients taking PPIs and may occur

at any point during therapy. Discontinue drug if condition develops.
• Prolonged treatment (2 years or more) may cause vitamin B_{12} malabsorption due to hypochlorhydria or achlorhydria.
• Use oral solution cautiously in patients with phenylketonuria.
• Prolonged PPI use beyond 1 year may increase risk of fundic gland polyps. Use shortest duration of PPI therapy appropriate for condition being treated.

Dialyzable drug: No.

PREGNANCY-LACTATION-REPRODUCTION

• Studies during pregnancy are inadequate. Use during pregnancy only if clearly needed.
• It isn't known if drug appears in human milk. Discontinue breastfeeding or discontinue drug, considering importance of drug to patient.

NURSING CONSIDERATIONS

• *Alert:* Monitor for signs and symptoms of low magnesium level (abnormal HR or rhythm, palpitations, muscle spasms, tremor, seizures). In children, abnormal HR may present as fatigue, upset stomach, dizziness, and light-headedness.
• New onset and exacerbation of existing cutaneous lupus erythematosus and SLE have been reported in patients taking PPIs, including lansoprazole. Avoid administering PPIs for longer than medically indicated. Discontinue drug and refer patient to appropriate specialist for evaluation, if indicated.
• *Alert:* May increase risk of CDAD. Evaluate for CDAD in patient who develops diarrhea that doesn't improve.
• Patients with severe liver disease may need dosage adjustment, but don't adjust dosage for older adults or patients with kidney insufficiency.
• Even if symptoms respond to therapy, gastric malignancy shouldn't be ruled out.
• Monitor patient for hypersensitivity reactions, including SCARs (SJS, TEN, DRESS syndrome, acute generalized exanthematous pustulosis).
• Monitor for vitamin B_{12} deficiency (extreme fatigue, weakness, paresthesia, sore mouth or tongue, muscle weakness, vision changes, depression, confusion).
• *Look alike–sound alike:* Don't confuse Prevacid with Pepcid or Prilosec.

L

PATIENT TEACHING

• Teach about proper drug administration and handling.

• Inform patient with phenylketonuria that ODTs contain 2.5 mg phenylalanine/15-mg tablet and 5.1 mg phenylalanine/30-mg tablet.

• Advise patient to recognize and report all adverse reactions, especially hypersensitivity reactions, diarrhea that doesn't improve, and signs and symptoms of low magnesium level or SLE.

ledipasvir–sofosbuvir ⚕

LED-i-pas-vir/soe-FOS-bue-vir

Harvoni

Therapeutic class: Antivirals
Pharmacologic class: Antivirals

AVAILABLE FORMS

Pellets: 33.75 mg ledipasvir/150 mg sofosbuvir, 45 mg ledipasvir/200 mg sofosbuvir
Tablets: 45 mg ledipasvir/200 mg sofosbuvir, 90 mg ledipasvir/400 mg sofosbuvir

INDICATIONS & DOSAGES

➤ **Chronic HCV genotype 1 infection in patients who are treatment naive without cirrhosis or with compensated cirrhosis or in patients who are treatment experienced without cirrhosis** ⚕

Adults and children ages 3 and older weighing at least 35 kg: One 90 mg/400 mg tablet PO daily for 12 weeks. If pretreatment HCV-RNA is less than 6 million international units/mL in adults without cirrhosis who are treatment naive, consider treatment course of 8 weeks.

Children ages 3 and older weighing 17 to less than 35 kg: 45 mg/200 mg (tablets/pellets) PO once daily for 12 weeks.

Children ages 3 and older weighing less than 17 kg: 33.75 mg/150 mg pellets PO once daily for 12 weeks.

➤ **Chronic HCV genotype 1 infection in patients who are treatment experienced with compensated cirrhosis**

Adults and children ages 3 and older weighing at least 35 kg: One 90 mg/400 mg tablet PO once daily for 24 weeks.

Children ages 3 and older weighing 17 to less than 35 kg: 45 mg/200 mg (tablets/pellets) PO once daily for 24 weeks.

Children ages 3 and older weighing less than 17 kg: 33.75 mg/150 mg pellets PO once daily for 24 weeks.

➤ **Chronic HCV genotype 1 infection in patients who are treatment naive or treatment experienced with decompensated cirrhosis, in combination with ribavirin; chronic HCV genotype 1 or 4 infection in patients who are treatment naive or treatment experienced and received a liver transplant without cirrhosis or with compensated cirrhosis, in combination with ribavirin** ⚕

Adults and children ages 3 and older weighing at least 35 kg: One 90 mg/400 mg tablet PO once daily with ribavirin for 12 weeks.

Children ages 3 and older weighing 17 to less than 35 kg: 45 mg/200 mg (tablets/pellets) PO once daily with ribavirin for 12 weeks.

Children ages 3 and older weighing less than 17 kg: 33.75 mg/150 mg pellets PO once daily with ribavirin for 12 weeks.

Adjust-a-dose: Refer to ribavirin manufacturer's information for recommended weight-based dosing schedule and kidney impairment dosage.

➤ **Chronic HCV genotype 4, 5, or 6 infection in patients who are treatment naive or treatment experienced without cirrhosis or with compensated cirrhosis** ⚕

Adults and children ages 3 and older weighing at least 35 kg: One 90 mg/400 mg tablet PO once daily for 12 weeks.

Children ages 3 and older weighing 17 to less than 35 kg: 45 mg/200 mg (tablets/pellets) PO once daily for 12 weeks.

Children ages 3 and older weighing less than 17 kg: 33.75 mg/150 mg pellets PO once daily for 12 weeks.

ADMINISTRATION
PO

• Give drug without regard to food.

• Store at room temperature in original container.

• If giving pellets with food, sprinkle on one or more spoonfuls of nonacidic, soft food (pudding, chocolate syrup, mashed potatoes, ice cream) at or below room temperature.

• Give pellets within 30 minutes of mixing with food. Patient shouldn't chew pellets, to avoid bitter taste.

• Give missed dose within calendar day as soon as possible. If calendar day when dose is usually given has passed, omit missed dose and resume usual dosing schedule.

ACTION

Ledipasvir and sofosbuvir are direct-acting antivirals against HCV. Ledipasvir inhibits the NS5A protein, and sofosbuvir inhibits the NS5B RNA polymerase, both of which are required for viral replication.

Route	Onset	Peak	Duration
PO (ledipasvir)	Unknown	4–4.5 hr	Unknown
PO (sofosbuvir)	Unknown	0.8–1 hr	Unknown

Half-life: Ledipasvir, 47 hours; sofosbuvir, 0.5 hour.

ADVERSE REACTIONS

CNS: fatigue, asthenia, headache, insomnia, irritability, dizziness, depression. **GI:** nausea, diarrhea. **Hepatic:** hyperbilirubinemia. **Metabolic:** increased lipase level. **Musculoskeletal:** myalgia. **Respiratory:** cough, dyspnea.

INTERACTIONS

Drug-drug. 🚫 *Alert: Amiodarone:* May increase risk of symptomatic bradycardia. Avoid use together. If use together can't be avoided, advise patient of risk and monitor patient carefully.

Antacids (aluminum hydroxide, magnesium hydroxide): May decrease ledipasvir level. Separate administration of antacids and ledipasvir–sofosbuvir by 4 hours.

Anticonvulsants (carbamazepine, oxcarbazepine, phenobarbital, phenytoin), antimycobacterials (rifabutin, rifampin, rifapentine): May decrease ledipasvir–sofosbuvir levels. Use together isn't recommended.

Atorvastatin: May increase atorvastatin level; may be associated with increased risk of myopathy. Monitor patient closely.

Digoxin: May increase digoxin level. Monitor digoxin level.

H₂-receptor antagonists (famotidine): May decrease ledipasvir level. Separate administration by 12 hours or administer simultaneously if H₂-receptor antagonist dose doesn't exceed equivalent of famotidine 40 mg b.i.d.

HIV antiretroviral regimen containing tenofovir disoproxil fumarate (DF), an HIV protease inhibitor (atazanavir, darunavir, lopinavir), and ritonavir: May increase tenofovir-associated adverse reactions. Safety of use together hasn't been established. Consider alternative HCV or antiretroviral therapy or monitor patient closely for tenofovir-associated adverse reactions.

HIV antiretroviral regimen containing tenofovir DF, cobicistat, elvitegravir, and emtricitabine: May increase tenofovir level. Safety of use together hasn't been established; therefore, not recommended.

HIV antiretroviral regimen containing tenofovir DF, efavirenz, and emtricitabine or tenofovir DF without an HIV protease inhibitor, ritonavir, or cobicistat: May increase tenofovir level and risk of toxicity. Monitor patient for tenofovir-associated adverse reactions.

HIV antiretroviral regimen containing tipranavir and ritonavir: May decrease ledipasvir–sofosbuvir levels and effectiveness. Use together isn't recommended.

HMG-CoA reductase inhibitors (rosuvastatin): May increase level of reductase inhibitor and increase risk of myopathy, including rhabdomyolysis. Use together isn't recommended.

Other products containing sofosbuvir: Duplicates therapy. Use together is contraindicated.

PPIs (omeprazole): May decrease ledipasvir level. May give PPI doses equivalent to 20 mg or less of omeprazole simultaneously with ledipasvir–sofosbuvir on an empty stomach.

Simeprevir: May increase ledipasvir–sofosbuvir levels. Use together isn't recommended.

Drug-herb. *St. John's wort:* May significantly decrease drug levels and reduce effectiveness. Discourage use together.

EFFECTS ON LAB TEST RESULTS

• May increase bilirubin, lipase, and CK levels.

CONTRAINDICATIONS & CAUTIONS

• Contraindicated in patients hypersensitive to either drug or their components.

Boxed Warning Reactivation of HBV may occur in patients infected with HCV and result in fulminant hepatitis, liver failure, and death. ■

🚫 *Alert:* Symptomatic bradycardia, including fatal cardiac arrest and cases requiring pacemaker intervention, have been reported when drug is given with amiodarone. Patients taking amiodarone who are also taking beta blockers or have underlying cardiac comorbidities or advanced liver disease may be at increased risk. Symptoms may occur within hours to up to 2 weeks after start of treatment of HCV infection.

Dialyzable drug: Ledipasvir, unlikely; sofosbuvir, 18%.

PREGNANCY-LACTATION-REPRODUCTION
• Studies during pregnancy are inadequate. Use cautiously and only if benefits outweigh risk to fetus.
• If giving drug with ribavirin, combination regimen is contraindicated in patients who are pregnant and males whose partners are pregnant. Refer to ribavirin prescribing information for details about pregnancy testing, contraception, and infertility.
• It isn't known if drug appears in human milk. Use cautiously during breastfeeding and only if benefits outweigh fetal risk.

NURSING CONSIDERATIONS
Boxed Warning Test all patients for current or prior HBV infection before starting treatment. Monitor patients with HCV and HBV coinfection for hepatitis flare or HBV reactivation with lab testing, and watch for signs and symptoms of liver injury during active treatment and treatment follow-up. ■
⬥ *Alert:* Test all patients for evidence of current or prior HBV infection by measuring HBsAg and hepatitis B core antibody (anti-HBc) before initiating HCV treatment.
⬥ *Alert:* Monitor patients who are taking, have recently discontinued, or must start amiodarone for signs and symptoms of bradycardia (near-fainting or fainting, dizziness, light-headedness, malaise, weakness, excessive fatigue, shortness of breath, chest pain, confusion, memory problems). Utilize inpatient cardiac monitoring for first 48 hours; continue outpatient or self-monitoring of HR for bradycardia daily through at least first 2 weeks of treatment. Discontinue HCV treatment if signs or symptoms of bradycardia occur.
• Monitor bilirubin, liver enzyme, and serum creatinine levels at baseline and periodically when clinically indicated.
• Monitor serum HCV-RNA level at baseline, during treatment, at end of treatment, during treatment follow-up, and when clinically indicated.

PATIENT TEACHING
Boxed Warning Warn patient of risk of HBV reactivation. Instruct patient to immediately report signs and symptoms of liver injury (fatigue, weakness, loss of appetite, nausea, vomiting, yellow skin or eyes, light-colored stool). ■
• Teach about proper drug administration and handling.

⬥ *Alert:* Caution patient also taking amiodarone to seek immediate medical attention for signs and symptoms of bradycardia.
• Explain that effect of treatment on HCV transmission isn't known. Instruct patient to follow precautions to prevent transmission.
• Advise patient to report to prescriber all other prescription drugs, OTC medications, vitamins, and herbal supplements being taken because drug interactions are possible.
• Caution patient not to stop drug without first discussing with prescriber.
• Tell patient to report signs and symptoms of adverse reactions (fatigue, nausea, headache).
• Advise patient to immediately report signs and symptoms of hypersensitivity reactions (wheezing; chest tightness; fever; itching; swelling of the face, lips, tongue, or throat).
• Instruct patient to report pregnancy or plans to become pregnant or breastfeed.
• Counsel patient also taking ribavirin on reproductive risks.

leflunomide
le-FLOO-noh-mide

Arava

Therapeutic class: Antiarthritics
Pharmacologic class: Pyrimidine synthesis inhibitors

AVAILABLE FORMS
Tablets: 10 mg, 20 mg, 100 mg

INDICATIONS & DOSAGES
➤ **Active RA**
Adults: 100 mg PO loading dose every 24 hours for 3 days; then 20 mg (maximum daily dose) PO every 24 hours.
Adjust-a-dose: Eliminating loading dose may decrease risk of adverse reactions, especially in patients at risk for hematologic (concurrent immunosuppressant use) or liver toxicity (concurrent methotrexate). Dosage may be decreased to 10 mg daily if higher dosage isn't well tolerated.

ADMINISTRATION
PO
⬥ *Alert:* Hazardous drug; use safe handling and disposal precautions.
• Give drug without regard to food.

Reactions in bold italics are *life-threatening*.

ACTION

An immunomodulatory drug that inhibits dihydroorotate dehydrogenase, an enzyme involved in pyrimidine synthesis that has antiproliferative activity and anti-inflammatory effects.

Route	Onset	Peak	Duration
PO	Unknown	6–12 hr	Unknown

Half-life: Teriflunomide (active metabolite), 18 to 19 days.

ADVERSE REACTIONS

CNS: dizziness, headache, asthenia, somnolence, malaise. **CV:** HTN, chest pain, palpitations, thrombophlebitis, varicose veins. **EENT:** blurred vision, eye disorder, papilledema, retinal disorder, retinal hemorrhage, rhinitis, sore throat, dry mouth, enlarged salivary glands, oral ulcer. **GI:** diarrhea, abdominal pain, anorexia, flatulence, nausea, vomiting. **GU:** vaginal moniliasis. **Hematologic:** leukocytosis, *thrombocytopenia.* **Hepatic:** elevated liver enzyme levels, bilirubinemia, *liver toxicity.* **Musculoskeletal:** back pain, tenosynovitis. **Respiratory:** bronchitis, dyspnea. **Skin:** alopecia, rash, pruritus. **Other:** abscess, *anaphylaxis,* hypersensitivity reaction, flulike syndrome.

INTERACTIONS

Drug-drug. *Charcoal, cholestyramine:* May decrease leflunomide level. Sometimes used for this effect in leflunomide toxicity.
CYP1A2 substrates (alosetron, duloxetine, theophylline, tizanidine), CYP2C8 substrates (paclitaxel, pioglitazone, repaglinide, rosiglitazone), oral contraceptives (ethinyl estradiol, levonorgestrel): May increase levels of these drugs. Monitor patient for adverse effects.
HMG-CoA reductase inhibitors (atorvastatin, pravastatin, rosuvastatin, simvastatin): May increase levels of these drugs. Consider dosage reduction. Rosuvastatin doses shouldn't be greater than 10 mg once daily when given together with leflunomide.
Methotrexate, other liver toxic drugs: May increase risk of liver toxicity. Monitor liver enzyme levels.
NSAIDs (diclofenac, ibuprofen): May increase NSAID level. Monitor patient.
Organic anion transporter 3 (OAT3) substrates (cefaclor, cimetidine, ciprofloxacin, penicillin, furosemide): May increase

substrate level. Monitor patient, and adjust OAT3 dosage if needed.
Rifampin: May increase active leflunomide metabolite level. Use together cautiously.
Tacrolimus: May increase toxic effects of immunosuppressants. Avoid combination.
Teriflunomide: Teriflunomide is an active metabolite of leflunomide. Use together is contraindicated.
Vaccines (live-virus): May increase vaccine-related toxic effects. Vaccination with live-virus vaccines isn't recommended. Consider long half-life of drug before giving a live-virus vaccine after stopping drug.
Warfarin: May decrease INR. Monitor therapy.

EFFECTS ON LAB TEST RESULTS

- May increase AST, ALT, GGT, bilirubin and CK levels.
- May increase WBC count.
- May decrease platelet count.

CONTRAINDICATIONS & CAUTIONS

- Contraindicated in patients hypersensitive to drug or its components, in patients with Child-Pugh class C liver impairment, and in those taking teriflunomide.
- Not recommended for patients with evidence of HBV or HCV infection, severe immunodeficiency, bone marrow dysplasia, or severe uncontrolled infections.

Boxed Warning Rare cases of severe and fatal liver injury have occurred during leflunomide therapy. Drug isn't recommended in patients with risk factors for liver toxicity, including those taking other drugs that can cause liver damage, those with preexisting acute or chronic liver disease, and those with ALT more than 2 × ULN. ■

- Use cautiously in patients with kidney insufficiency.
- Severe infections (including sepsis, which may be fatal) have been reported in patients receiving leflunomide, especially *Pneumocystis jiroveci* pneumonia, TB, and aspergillosis. Most reported cases were confounded by concomitant immunosuppressive therapy or comorbid illness that, in addition to RA, predisposes patients to infection.
- Risk of malignancy, particularly lymphoproliferative disorders, increases with use of some immunosuppressants, including leflunomide.

L

• Drug isn't recommended in patients younger than age 18.
Dialyzable drug: No.
⚠ *Overdose S&S:* Diarrhea, abdominal pain, leukopenia, anemia, elevated LFT results.

PREGNANCY-LACTATION-REPRODUCTION
Boxed Warning Contraindicated during pregnancy and in patients of childbearing potential who aren't using reliable contraception because of potential for fetal harm. Exclude pregnancy before start of therapy. Stop drug and use accelerated drug elimination procedure if patient becomes pregnant. ■
• It isn't known if drug appears in human milk. Patient should discontinue breastfeeding or discontinue drug, considering importance of drug to patient.
• Patient should avoid pregnancy after drug administration until serum drug level is undetectable (less than 0.02 mg/L), accomplished by use of recommended leflunomide removal protocol.

NURSING CONSIDERATIONS
• Before starting leflunomide, evaluate patient for active TB; screen for latent TB infection; check BP; obtain blood for lab tests, including serum ALT and Hb levels, hematocrit, and WBC and platelet counts; and verify pregnancy status.
Boxed Warning Monitor liver enzyme levels at least monthly for 6 months after beginning therapy and every 6 to 8 weeks thereafter. If ALT level rises to more than $3 \times$ ULN, interrupt therapy. If drug is cause, start accelerated drug elimination procedure according to manufacturer's instructions. ■
• Drug elimination procedures include performing cholestyramine washout (8 g PO t.i.d. for 11 days), using activated charcoal powder (50 g PO suspension every 12 hours for 11 days), monitoring teriflunomide level, and monitoring LFTs weekly until normal.
• Without use of accelerated drug elimination procedure, undetectable plasma levels of teriflunomide (active metabolite of leflunomide) may take up to 2 years to reach after drug discontinuation.
• Stop drug and start cholestyramine or charcoal therapy if bone marrow suppression occurs.
⟳ *Alert:* Continue monitoring AST, ALT, and serum albumin levels monthly if treatment

includes methotrexate or other potential immunosuppressants.
• Monitor platelet and WBC counts and Hb level or hematocrit at baseline, monthly for 6 months after starting therapy, and every 6 to 8 weeks thereafter.
• Monitor patient for peripheral neuropathy; drug may need to be stopped.
• Watch for overlapping hematologic toxicity when switching to another antirheumatic.
• Carefully monitor patient after dosage reduction. Because active metabolite of leflunomide has prolonged half-life, level may take several weeks to decline.
• Rarely, SJS, TEN, and DRESS syndrome have been reported in patients receiving leflunomide. If patient develops any of these conditions, stop drug and perform accelerated drug elimination procedure.
• ILD and worsening of preexisting ILD have been reported and can be fatal. Risk increases in patients with history of ILD. If new-onset or worsening pulmonary symptoms (cough, dyspnea) with or without fever occur, discontinue drug and investigate etiology of symptoms, as appropriate.
• Monitor BP.

PATIENT TEACHING
• Explain need for and frequency of required blood tests and monitoring.
Boxed Warning Instruct patient to use birth control during treatment and until tests determine that drug is no longer active. ■
• Warn patient to notify prescriber if signs or symptoms of pregnancy (late menstrual periods, breast tenderness) occur because of risk of fetal birth defects.
• Advise patient to stop breastfeeding.
• Instruct patient to report all adverse reactions and to immediately report rash or mucous membrane lesions, unusual tiredness, abdominal pain, jaundice, easy bruising, bleeding, fever, recurrent infections, or pallor, which may be warnings of infrequent but serious adverse reactions.
• Explain that patient may continue to take aspirin, other NSAIDs, and low-dose corticosteroids during treatment.
• Tell patient that it may take 4 weeks to begin to see improvement from therapy.
• Teach about proper and safe drug administration and handling.

lemborexant
lem-boe-REX-ant

Dayvigo

Therapeutic class: Hypnotics
Pharmacologic class: Orexin receptor antagonists
Controlled substance schedule: IV

AVAILABLE FORMS
Tablets: 5 mg, 10 mg

INDICATIONS & DOSAGES
➤ **Insomnia, characterized by difficulties with sleep onset or sleep maintenance**
Adults: 5 mg PO nightly, immediately before bedtime; increase to 10 mg if needed. Maximum dosage, 10 mg once daily.
Adjust-a-dose: In patients with Child-Pugh class B liver impairment or when used together with weak CYP3A inhibitors, initial and maximum recommended dosage is 5 mg PO once nightly.

ADMINISTRATION
PO
• Give immediately before bedtime; ensure at least 7 hours remain before planned time of awakening.
• May delay sleep onset if drug is given with or soon after a meal.
• Store tablets at room temperature.

ACTION
Blocks orexin receptors, suppressing the system responsible for promoting wakefulness.

Route	Onset	Peak	Duration
PO	Unknown	1–3 hr	Unknown

Half-life: 17 to 19 hours.

ADVERSE REACTIONS
CNS: somnolence, fatigue, headache, nightmares, abnormal dreams, sleep paralysis.

INTERACTIONS
Drug-drug. *CNS depressants (benzodiazepines, opioids, TCAs):* May increase risk of CNS depression. Adjust lemborexant or CNS depressant dosage to limit additive effects.
CYP2B6 substrates (bupropion, methadone): May decrease efficacy of 2B6 substrate.

Monitor for efficacy; consider increased 2B6 substrate dosage, if needed.
Other sleep aids: May increase risk of CNS depression. Avoid use together.
Strong or moderate CYP3A inducers (bosentan, carbamazepine, efavirenz, etravirine, modafinil, rifampin): May decrease lemborexant level. Avoid use together.
Strong or moderate CYP3A inhibitors (clarithromycin, fluconazole, itraconazole, verapamil): May increase lemborexant level. Avoid use together.
Weak CYP3A inhibitors (chlorzoxazone, ranitidine): May increase lemborexant level. Don't exceed 5 mg nightly.
Drug-herb. *St. John's wort:* May decrease lemborexant level. Discourage use together.
Drug-food. *High-caloric, high-fat meals:* May delay drug's effect. Patient should avoid ingesting with or soon after a meal.
Drug-lifestyle. *Alcohol use:* May increase CNS depression. Discourage use together.

EFFECTS ON LAB TEST RESULTS
None reported.

CONTRAINDICATIONS & CAUTIONS
• Contraindicated in patients with narcolepsy.
• Use cautiously in patients with Child-Pugh class B liver impairment. Not recommended in patients with Child-Pugh class C liver impairment.
⚠ **Alert:** Use of alcohol or other CNS depressants increases risk of complex sleep behaviors.
• Use cautiously in patients with impaired respiratory function, including sleep apnea and COPD.
⚠ **Alert:** May worsen depression and increase risk of suicidality. Immediately evaluate patients who report suicidality or exhibit new behavioral changes.
• Use cautiously in patients with history of substance abuse or dependence.
• Use cautiously in patients with CrCl less than 30 mL/minute due to increased risk of somnolence.
• Safety and effectiveness in children haven't been established.
• Use cautiously in older adults.
Dialyzable drug: No.
⚠ **Overdose S&S:** Increased somnolence.

PREGNANCY-LACTATION-REPRODUCTION
• Studies during pregnancy are inadequate.

L

• Enroll patients taking drug during pregnancy in pregnancy exposure registry (1-888-274-2378).
• Low levels of drug were found in human milk. Weigh benefit to patient against risk to infant. Monitor infant exposed to drug for excessive somnolence.

NURSING CONSIDERATIONS

• Evaluate patient for medical or psychiatric causes of insomnia before drug is prescribed. If insomnia persists for more than 7 to 10 days, reevaluate patient.
• Monitor patient for complex sleep behaviors (preparing and eating food, making phone calls, sleep-walking, sleep-driving while not fully awake); discontinue drug if any occur.
• Monitor patient for daytime somnolence and fall risk, especially older adults.
• Monitor patient for sleep paralysis (inability to move or speak during sleep-wake transitions), hypnagogic/hypnopompic hallucinations (including vivid and disturbing perceptions), and leg weakness.
• Monitor patient for development of dependence on or abuse of drug.
• **Alert:** Be alert for signs and symptoms of depression, suicidality, or behavioral changes.
• **Look alike–sound alike:** Don't confuse Dayvigo with Daypro, Daysee, or Daytrana.

PATIENT TEACHING

• **Alert:** Caution patient, family, or caregiver to immediately report suicidality or new behavioral signs or symptoms.
• Teach about proper drug administration and handling.
• Warn patient that risk of daytime somnolence increases if drug is taken with less than a full night's sleep. Caution patient against driving and other activities requiring complete mental alertness.
• Explain that CNS depressant effects may persist for several days after discontinuing drug.
• Caution patient that increased drowsiness may increase risk of falls.
• Inform patient and family that drug may cause sleep paralysis, hallucinations, and leg weakness.
• Instruct patient and family to notify prescriber and discontinue drug if complex sleep behaviors occur.
• Advise patient to avoid alcohol and other CNS depressants while taking drug.

• Tell patient not to increase dosage without first consulting prescriber.
• Warn patient and family to watch for development of abuse and dependence.
• Tell patient to contact prescriber if insomnia persists for more than 7 to 10 days.
• Advise patient to report pregnancy or plans to become pregnant or breastfeed.

SAFETY ALERT!

letrozole
LET-roe-zole

Femara

Therapeutic class: Antineoplastics
Pharmacologic class: Aromatase inhibitors

AVAILABLE FORMS
Tablets: 2.5 mg

INDICATIONS & DOSAGES
Adjust-a-dose (for all indications): In patients with cirrhosis or Child-Pugh class C liver impairment, give 2.5 mg every other day.
➤ **First-line treatment of hormone receptor-positive or hormone receptor-unknown, locally advanced, or metastatic breast cancer; advanced breast cancer with disease progression after anti-estrogen therapy (such as tamoxifen)**
Patients who are postmenopausal: 2.5 mg PO once daily until tumor progression is evident.
➤ **Adjuvant treatment of hormone-positive early breast cancer**
Patients who are postmenopausal: 2.5 mg PO daily. Optimal duration of treatment is unknown.
➤ **Extended adjuvant treatment of early breast cancer following 5 years of adjuvant tamoxifen therapy**
Patients who are postmenopausal: 2.5 mg PO once daily for 5 years.

ADMINISTRATION
PO
• **Alert:** Hazardous drug; use safe handling and disposal precautions.
• Give drug without regard to meals.

ACTION
Inhibits conversion of androgens to estrogens, which decreases tumor mass or delays progression of tumor growth in some patients.

Route	Onset	Peak	Duration
PO	Unknown	2–6 wk (steady-state plasma)	Unknown

Half-life: About 2 days.

ADVERSE REACTIONS

CNS: *stroke,* headache, somnolence, insomnia, dizziness, fatigue, asthenia, mood changes, depression. **CV:** flushing, *MI, thromboembolism,* angina, *HF,* chest pain, edema, HTN. **EENT:** cataract. **GI:** nausea, vomiting, constipation, diarrhea, abdominal pain, anorexia, dyspepsia. **GU:** vaginal bleeding, vaginal irritation, vulvovaginal dryness, UTI. **Hepatic:** hyperbilirubinemia, jaundice. **Metabolic:** hypercholesterolemia, weight gain or loss. **Musculoskeletal:** bone pain, limb pain, back pain, arthralgia, fractures, osteopenia, osteoporosis, myalgia. **Respiratory:** dyspnea, cough, pleural effusion. **Skin:** rash, pruritus, alopecia, diaphoresis, night sweats. **Other:** fall, viral infections, breast pain, hot flashes, *secondary malignancies.*

INTERACTIONS

Drug-drug. *Estrogens:* May produce antagonistic effects with letrozole. Use together isn't recommended.
Methadone: May increase methadone serum level. Monitor therapy.
Tamoxifen: May reduce letrozole level. Monitor therapy.

EFFECTS ON LAB TEST RESULTS

• May increase cholesterol level.
• May decrease lymphocyte count.

CONTRAINDICATIONS & CAUTIONS

• Contraindicated in patients hypersensitive to drug or its components.
• Use drug only in patients who are postmenopausal.
• Use cautiously in patients with cirrhosis or Child-Pugh class C liver impairment; dosage adjustment isn't needed in those with Child-Pugh class A or B liver impairment.
Dialyzable drug: Unknown.

PREGNANCY-LACTATION-REPRODUCTION

• May cause fetal harm. Contraindicated in patients who are or may become pregnant.
• Patients of childbearing potential should use effective contraception during therapy and for at least 3 weeks after final dose.

• It isn't known if drug appears in human milk. Patient shouldn't breastfeed during therapy and for 3 weeks after final dose.

NURSING CONSIDERATIONS

• Verify pregnancy status before treatment.
• Dosage adjustment isn't needed in patients with CrCl of 10 mL/minute or more.
• Monitor bone density results.
• Monitor cholesterol levels.
• *Look alike–sound alike:* Don't confuse Femara with FemHRT.

PATIENT TEACHING

• Teach about proper drug administration and handling. Instruct patient to take drug exactly as prescribed.
• Review potential adverse effects and instruct patient to report them.
• Advise patient to use caution performing tasks that require alertness, coordination, or dexterity, such as driving, until drug effects are known.
• Inform patient who is recently menopausal of the need for adequate contraception until postmenopausal status is clinically well established.

SAFETY ALERT!

leuprolide acetate
loo-PROE-lide

Eligard, Fensolvi, Lupron Depot, Lupron Depot-Ped

leuprolide mesylate
Camcevi

Therapeutic class: Antineoplastics
Pharmacologic class: GnRH analogues

AVAILABLE FORMS
leuprolide acetate
Depot injection: 3.75 mg, 7.5 mg, 11.25 mg, 15 mg, 22.5 mg, 30 mg, 45 mg
Injection: 1 mg/0.2 mL
leuprolide mesylate
Emulsion injection: 42-mg prefilled syringe

INDICATIONS & DOSAGES
➤ **Advanced prostate cancer**
Adults: 1 mg subcut daily. Or, 7.5 mg IM depot injection monthly, 22.5 mg IM depot injection every 3 months, 30 mg IM depot

injection every 4 months, or 45 mg IM depot injection every 6 months. Or, 7.5 mg subcut Eligard once monthly, 22.5 mg subcut Eligard every 3 months, 30 mg subcut Eligard every 4 months, or 45 mg subcut Eligard every 6 months. Or, 42 mg subcut Camcevi emulsion every 6 months.

➤ **Central precocious puberty**

Children ages 2 and older (Lupron Depot-Ped, Fensolvi): Initially, for child weighing 25 kg or less, 7.5 mg IM once monthly; for child weighing between 25 and 37.5 kg, 11.25 mg IM once monthly; for child weighing more than 37.5 kg, 15 mg IM once monthly. If clinical suppression isn't achieved with starting dose of Lupron Depot-Ped, increase to next available higher dose in 3.75-mg increments. For IM formulation, 11.25 or 30 mg IM once every 3 months. For 6-month formulation, 45 mg subcut every 6 months. Discontinue drug at appropriate age of puberty onset.

➤ **Endometriosis**

Adults: 3.75 mg IM depot injection as single injection monthly for up to 6 months with or without norethindrone acetate. Or, 11.25 mg IM every 3 months for up to 6 months with or without norethindrone acetate.

Adjust-a-dose: May repeat treatment for an additional 6 months in combination with norethindrone acetate.

➤ **Anemia related to uterine fibroids (with iron therapy)**

Adults: 3.75 mg IM depot injection once monthly for up to 3 consecutive months. Or 11.25 mg IM depot injection for 1 dose.

➤ **Premenopausal ovarian suppression in patients with breast cancer ◆**

Adults: 3.75 mg depot IM every 28 days for up to 24 months. Or, 11.25 mg depot IM every 3 months for up to 24 months.

ADMINISTRATION

● Products have specific mixing and administration instructions. Read manufacturer's directions closely.

● *Alert:* Hazardous drug; use safe handling and disposal precautions.

● *Alert:* A fractional dose of drug formulated to give every 3, 4, or 6 months isn't equivalent to same dose of once-a-month formulation. Combined depot formulations can't be used to achieve a particular dose because release characteristics differ.

● Store leuprolide acetate powder (depot) and diluent at room temperature. Refrigerate

unopened vials or syringes of leuprolide acetate or mesylate injection, and protect injection from heat and light.

● Allow refrigerated solution to come to room temperature before use.

IM

● Never give by IV injection.

● Give depot injections under medical supervision.

● Use supplied diluent to reconstitute drug (extra diluent is provided; discard remainder).

● Inject into vial; shake well. Suspension will appear milky. Use immediately.

● Draw appropriate amount into syringe with 22G needle.

● For Lupron Depot and Lupron Depot-Ped, use within 2 hours of preparation.

● When using prefilled dual-chamber syringes, prepare for injection according to manufacturer's instructions.

● Gently shake syringe to form a uniform milky suspension. If particles adhere to stopper, tap syringe against finger.

● Remove needle guard and advance plunger to expel air from syringe. Inject entire contents IM, as with a normal injection.

Subcutaneous

● Drug must be administered by a health care provider.

● For two-syringe mixing system, connect syringes and inject liquid contents according to manufacturer's instructions.

● Mix product by pushing contents back and forth between syringes for about 45 seconds; shaking syringes won't adequately mix contents.

● Attach needle provided in kit and inject subcut.

● Suspension settles very quickly. Remix if settling occurs. Give within 30 minutes.

● Never give by IV injection.

ACTION

Stimulates and then inhibits release of FSH and LH, which suppresses testosterone and estrogen levels.

Route	Onset	Peak	Duration
IM, subcut	Variable	2–6 hr	60–90 days

Half-life: 3 hours.

ADVERSE REACTIONS

CNS: dizziness, depression, headache, migraine, sleep disorder, vertigo, pain, insomnia, paresthesia, asthenia, emotional lability, fatigue, lethargy, anxiety, fever, psychiatric events. **CV:** *arrhythmias,* angina, chest pain, *MI,* peripheral edema, ECG changes, hypotension, HTN, murmur, flushing, vasodilation, *hemorrhage.* **EENT:** nasopharyngitis, sinus congestion. **GI:** nausea, vomiting, anorexia, constipation, diarrhea, abdominal pain. **GU:** impotence, vaginitis, vaginal bleeding or discharge, urinary frequency, hematuria, UTI, amenorrhea, decreased libido, testicular atrophy. **Hematologic:** anemia. **Metabolic:** weight gain or loss, increased cholesterol levels, increased triglyceride levels. **Musculoskeletal:** transient bone pain during first week of treatment, joint disorder, myalgia, neuromuscular disorder, bone loss, back pain, arthralgia, limb pain, ligament sprain, fracture. **Respiratory:** dyspnea, URI, cough, *pulmonary fibrosis.* **Skin:** injection-site reactions, abscess, or pain; diaphoresis; dermatitis; acne; rash; pruritus. **Other:** gynecomastia, breast tenderness, androgen-like effects, hot flashes, flulike symptoms.

INTERACTIONS
None reported by manufacturer.

EFFECTS ON LAB TEST RESULTS
• May increase bilirubin, cholesterol, triglyceride, BUN, calcium, creatinine, glucose, LDH, phosphorus, AST, ALT, GGT, and uric acid levels.
• May decrease albumin, protein, and potassium levels.
• May decrease Hb level and hematocrit.
• May increase or decrease WBC and platelet counts.
• May prolong PT and PTT.
• May alter results of pituitary-gonadal system tests during therapy and for 12 weeks after.

CONTRAINDICATIONS & CAUTIONS
• Contraindicated in patients hypersensitive to drug or other GnRH analogues and in patients with undiagnosed vaginal bleeding.
• Androgen deprivation therapy may prolong QT/QTc interval. Consider if benefits of therapy outweigh risks in patients with congenital long QT syndrome, HF, or frequent electrolyte abnormalities and in patients taking drugs known to prolong QT interval.
• Seizures have been reported in patients taking leuprolide, including those with and without history of seizures, epilepsy, cerebrovascular disorders, or CNS anomalies or tumors

and in patients taking concomitant medications associated with seizures.
Dialyzable drug: Unknown.

PREGNANCY-LACTATION-REPRODUCTION
• May cause fetal harm. Contraindicated during pregnancy.
• Patients of childbearing potential should use nonhormonal contraception during treatment.
• It isn't known if drug appears in human milk. Patient should discontinue breastfeeding or discontinue drug, considering importance of drug to patient.
• May impair fertility in patients of reproductive potential.

NURSING CONSIDERATIONS
• Correct electrolyte abnormalities before starting drug; consider periodic monitoring of ECGs and electrolyte levels.
• Verify pregnancy status before use.
• In treatment of precocious puberty, increased clinical signs and symptoms of puberty, including vaginal bleeding, may occur during first weeks of therapy or after subsequent doses.
• After starting treatment for central precocious puberty, monitor patient response every 1 to 2 months with GnRH stimulation test and sex corticosteroid level determinations. Measure bone age for advancement every 6 to 12 months.
• Monitor patient for development or worsening of psychiatric symptoms (emotional lability, anger, aggression, crying, impatience) during treatment.
• Monitor child for pseudotumor cerebri (headache, papilledema, vision changes, eye pain, tinnitus, dizziness, nausea).
❸ *Alert:* During first few weeks of treatment for prostate cancer, signs and symptoms of disease may temporarily worsen or additional signs and symptoms may occur.
• In patient treated with GnRH analogues for prostate cancer, treatment is usually continued upon development of metastatic castration-resistant prostate cancer.
• May increase risk of diabetes and CV events. Monitor patient closely.
• *Look alike–sound alike:* Don't confuse Lupron Depot with Lupron Depot-Ped.

PATIENT TEACHING
• Before starting child on treatment for central precocious puberty, make sure parents understand importance of continuous therapy.

L

• Carefully instruct patient who will self-administer injection about proper technique. Advise patient to use only syringes provided by manufacturer.

• Inform patient with history of undesirable effects from other endocrine therapies that leuprolide is easier to tolerate. Advise patient to report all adverse effects.

• Explain that symptoms may worsen at first.

• Advise patient that drug may increase bone density loss, emotional lability, and depression and increase risk of MI, diabetes, hyperglycemia, seizures, stroke, and death.

• Counsel patient on drug's effect on reproductive potential.

• Advise patient of childbearing potential to use nonhormonal form of contraception during treatment.

levalbuterol hydrochloride
lev-al-BYOO-ter-ol

Xopenex

levalbuterol tartrate
Xopenex HFA

Therapeutic class: Bronchodilators
Pharmacologic class: Beta$_2$ agonists

AVAILABLE FORMS
Inhalation aerosol: 45 mcg per actuation
Solution for inhalation: 0.31 mg, 0.63 mg, or 1.25 mg in 3-mL vials; 1.25 mg/0.5 mL in vials (concentrate)

INDICATIONS & DOSAGES
➤ **To prevent or treat bronchospasm in patients with reversible obstructive airway disease**
Adults and adolescents ages 12 and older: 0.63 mg by oral inhalation via nebulizer t.i.d. every 6 to 8 hours. Patients with more severe asthma who don't respond adequately to 0.63 mg t.i.d. may benefit from 1.25 mg t.i.d.
Children ages 6 to 11: 0.31 mg by oral inhalation via nebulizer t.i.d. Routine dosage shouldn't exceed 0.63 mg t.i.d.
Adults and children ages 4 and older: 2 inhalations (90 mcg) every 4 to 6 hours. In some patients, 1 inhalation (45 mcg) every 4 hours is sufficient.

ADMINISTRATION
Inhalational
• Keep unopened vials of regular solution in foil pouch and use within 2 weeks of opening pouch. Use vials removed from pouch within 1 week and protect from light.

• Use vials of concentrated solution immediately after opening pouch.

• Dilute concentrated solution (1.25 mg/0.5 mL) with sterile NSS before administration by nebulizer connected to air compressor. Treatment takes about 5 to 15 minutes. Stop treatment when mist is no longer visible.

• Discard vial if solution isn't colorless.

• Release four test sprays before first use of inhaler or after inhaler has not been used for more than 3 days.

• Shake canister well before use.

• Avoid spraying in the eyes.

• Use a spacer device to improve inhalation, as appropriate.

• Wash actuator with warm water and air-dry thoroughly at least once a week.

• Clean nebulizer according to manufacturer's instructions.

• The compatibility of levalbuterol mixed with other drugs in a nebulizer hasn't been established.

ACTION
Relaxes bronchial smooth muscle by stimulating beta$_2$ receptors; also inhibits release of mediators from mast cells in the airways.

Route	Onset	Peak	Duration
Inhalation	5–15 min	1 hr	3–4 hr

Half-life: 3.25 to 4 hours.

ADVERSE REACTIONS
CNS: dizziness, migraine, nervousness, pain, tremor, anxiety, asthenia, fever, headache, insomnia. **CV:** tachycardia. **EENT:** rhinitis, sinusitis, turbinate edema, pharyngitis. **GI:** dyspepsia, abdominal pain, diarrhea, vomiting. **Musculoskeletal:** leg cramps, myalgia. **Respiratory:** increased cough, asthma, bronchitis. **Skin:** urticaria, rash. **Other:** lymphadenopathy, flulike syndrome, viral infection, accidental injury.

INTERACTIONS
Drug-drug. *Beta blockers:* May block pulmonary effect of drug and cause severe bronchospasm. Avoid use together, if possible. If

---

Reactions in bold italics are *life-threatening*.

use together is unavoidable, consider a cardioselective beta blocker, but use cautiously.
Digoxin: May decrease digoxin level. Monitor digoxin level.
Loop or thiazide diuretics: May cause ECG changes and hypokalemia. Use together cautiously.
MAO inhibitors, TCAs: May potentiate action of levalbuterol on vascular system. Avoid using within 2 weeks of MAO inhibitor or TCA therapy.
Other short-acting sympathomimetic aerosol bronchodilators, epinephrine: May increase adrenergic adverse effects. Avoid use together.

EFFECTS ON LAB TEST RESULTS
• May increase glucose level.
• May decrease potassium level.

CONTRAINDICATIONS & CAUTIONS
• Contraindicated in patients hypersensitive to drug or to racemic albuterol.
• Use cautiously in older adults; in patients with CV disorders (especially coronary insufficiency, HTN, and arrhythmias), seizure disorders, hyperthyroidism, or diabetes; and in those who are unusually responsive to sympathomimetic amines.
Dialyzable drug: Unknown.
⚠ *Overdose S&S:* Exaggeration of adverse reactions, hypokalemia, seizures, angina, HTN, hypotension, arrhythmias, muscle cramps, dry mouth, palpitations, nausea, insomnia, cardiac arrest, sudden death.

PREGNANCY-LACTATION-REPRODUCTION
• Studies during pregnancy are inadequate. Use during pregnancy only if potential benefit justifies fetal risk.
• Drug may interfere with uterine contractility. Use to treat bronchospasm during labor only if clearly needed.
• Patients should enroll in MotherToBaby Asthma & Pregnancy Study (1-866-626-6847 or www.mothertobaby.org/ongoing-study/asthma).
• It isn't known if drug appears in human milk. Use cautiously during breastfeeding.

NURSING CONSIDERATIONS
🔵 *Alert:* As with other inhaled beta agonists, drug can produce paradoxical bronchospasm or life-threatening CV effects. If this occurs, immediately stop drug and notify prescriber.
• Drug may worsen diabetes and ketoacidosis.

• Monitor potassium level, as drug may temporarily decrease potassium level.

PATIENT TEACHING
• Teach about proper drug administration and handling.
• Tell patient not to increase dosage or use drug more frequently without consulting prescriber.
• Urge patient or caregiver to seek immediate medical attention if levalbuterol becomes less effective, if signs and symptoms worsen, or if patient is using drug more frequently than usual.
• Tell patient that effects of levalbuterol may last up to 8 hours.
• Advise patient to use other inhalational drugs and antiasthmatics only as directed while taking levalbuterol.
• Inform patient that common adverse reactions include palpitations, rapid HR, headache, dizziness, tremor, and nervousness.
• Tell patient to discard inhaler when dose indicator display window shows "0."
• Encourage patient of childbearing potential to report pregnancy or breastfeeding.

levETIRAcetam
lee-vah-tih-RACE-ah-tam

Elepsia XR, Keppra, Keppra XR, Spritam

Therapeutic class: Anticonvulsants
Pharmacologic class: Pyrrolidine derivatives

AVAILABLE FORMS
Injection (concentrate): 500 mg/5 mL single-use vials
Injection (premixed in sodium chloride): 250 mg/50 mL, 500 mg/100 mL, 1,000 mg/100 mL, 1,500 mg/100 mL bags
Oral solution: 100 mg/mL
Tablets 🔴*:* 250 mg, 500 mg, 750 mg, 1,000 mg
Tablets (extended-release) 🔴*:* 500 mg, 750 mg, 1,000 mg, 1,500 mg
Tablets for oral suspension: 250 mg, 500 mg, 750 mg, 1,000 mg

INDICATIONS & DOSAGES
Adjust-a-dose (for all indications): For IV, immediate-release, and oral solution, in adults with CrCl of 50 to 80 mL/minute, give

500 to 1,000 mg every 12 hours; if CrCl is 30 to 50 mL/minute, give 250 to 750 mg every 12 hours; if CrCl is less than 30 mL/minute, give 250 to 500 mg every 12 hours. For patients on CKRT, give 500 to 1,000 mg every 24 hours. Give a 250- to 500-mg supplemental dose after dialysis.

Adjust-a-dose: For extended-release tablets, if CrCl is 50 to 80 mL/minute, give 1,000 to 2,000 mg every 24 hours. If CrCl is 30 to 50 mL/minute, give 500 to 1,500 mg every 24 hours. If CrCl is less than 30 mL/minute, give 500 to 1,000 mg every 24 hours.

➤ **Adjunctive therapy for myoclonic seizures of juvenile myoclonic epilepsy**
Adults and adolescents ages 12 and older: Initially, 500 mg PO or IV b.i.d., increased by 1,000 mg/day every 2 weeks to recommended dosage of 1,500 mg PO or IV b.i.d. Or, 500 mg tablets for suspension PO b.i.d., increased as needed and tolerated by 500 mg PO b.i.d. every 2 weeks to recommended dosage of 1,500 mg b.i.d.

➤ **Adjunctive therapy for primary generalized tonic-clonic seizures**
Adults and adolescents ages 16 and older: Initially, 500 mg PO or IV b.i.d. Increase by 500 mg b.i.d. every 2 weeks to recommended dosage of 1,500 mg b.i.d.
Children ages 6 to younger than 16: Initially, 10 mg/kg PO or IV b.i.d. Increase by 10 mg/kg b.i.d. at 2-week intervals to recommended dosage of 30 mg/kg b.i.d.

➤ **Adjunctive therapy for primary generalized tonic-clonic seizures (Spritam)**
Adults and children ages 6 and older weighing more than 40 kg: 500 mg PO b.i.d. Increase as needed and tolerated by 500 mg PO b.i.d. every 2 weeks to maximum recommended dosage of 1,500 mg b.i.d.
Children ages 6 and older weighing 20 to 40 kg: 250 mg PO b.i.d. Increase by 250 mg PO b.i.d. every 2 weeks to maximum of 750 mg b.i.d.

➤ **Adjunctive treatment or monotherapy for partial-onset seizures in patients with epilepsy**
Adults and adolescents ages 16 and older: Initially, 500 mg PO or IV b.i.d. Increase by 500 mg b.i.d., as needed, for seizure control at 2-week intervals to recommended dosage of 1,500 mg b.i.d.
Children ages 4 to younger than 16: Initially, 10 mg/kg PO or IV b.i.d. Increase by 10 mg/kg b.i.d. at 2-week intervals to

recommended dosage of 30 mg/kg b.i.d. If patient can't tolerate this dosage, reduce it.
Children ages 6 months to younger than 4 years: Initially, 10 mg/kg PO or IV b.i.d. Increase by 10 mg/kg b.i.d. at 2-week intervals to recommended dosage of 25 mg/kg b.i.d. Reduce dosage if patient can't tolerate total daily dosage of 50 mg/kg.
Children ages 1 month to 6 months: Initially, 7 mg/kg PO or IV b.i.d. Increase by 7 mg/kg b.i.d. at 2-week intervals to recommended dosage of 21 mg/kg b.i.d.

➤ **Adjunctive treatment for partial-onset seizures in patients with epilepsy (extended-release)**
Adults and children ages 12 and older: Initially, 1,000 mg PO once daily. May adjust dosage in increments of 1,000 mg every 2 weeks to maximum of 3,000 mg daily.

➤ **Adjunctive treatment or monotherapy for partial-onset seizures in patients with epilepsy (Spritam)**
Adults and children ages 4 and older weighing more than 40 kg: 500 mg PO b.i.d. Increase as needed and tolerated by 500 mg PO b.i.d. every 2 weeks to recommended dosage of 1,500 mg b.i.d.
Children ages 4 and older weighing 20 to 40 kg: 250 mg PO b.i.d. Increase by 250 mg PO b.i.d. every 2 weeks to maximum of 750 mg b.i.d.

ADMINISTRATION
PO
● Give drug without regard to food.
● Oral and IV forms are bioequivalent.
● Have patient swallow tablets whole; don't crush or break tablets.
● Tablets for oral solution are intended to disintegrate in mouth. Place tablet on tongue with dry hand. Follow with sip of liquid and have patient swallow only after tablet disintegrates; patient shouldn't swallow tablet intact. Or, add whole tablet to small volume of liquid in a cup (1 tablespoon or enough to cover tablet); allow tablet to disperse; then have patient immediately consume entire contents. Don't give partial tablets.
● Don't push tablets for oral solution through foil; peel foil from blister by bending up and lifting peel tab around blister seal.
● For children weighing more than 20 kg, use either tablets or oral solution. For children weighing 20 kg or less, use oral solution.

IV

▼ Dilute vials before giving. Don't further dilute premixed bags.

▼ For adults and adolescents receiving adult dosages of concentrate, dilute 500-mg, 1,000-mg, or 1,500-mg dose in 100 mL NSS, D₅W, or lactated Ringer solution to maximum levetiracetam concentration of 15 mg/mL of diluted solution. Infuse within 4 hours after mixing over 15 minutes.

▼ For children and patients requiring a smaller volume, calculate amount of diluent to not exceed a maximum levetiracetam concentration of 15 mg/mL of diluted solution. Infuse within 4 hours after mixing over 15 minutes.

▼ Be aware that premixed bags come in various sodium chloride concentrations for injection, including 0.54%, 0.75%, and 0.82%.

▼ Drug is compatible with diazepam, lorazepam, and valproate sodium for 4 hours at controlled room temperature.

▼ Store premixed solution for infusion at 68° to 77° F (20° to 25° C); don't dilute.

▼ Store vials for injection at 77° F (25° C).

▼ **Incompatibilities:** Unknown with other drugs or antiepileptics besides diazepam, lorazepam, and valproate sodium. Consult drug compatibility reference for more information.

ACTION

May inhibit simultaneous neuronal firing that leads to seizure activity.

Route	Onset	Peak	Duration
PO (immediate-release), IV	1 hr	1 hr	12 hr
PO (extended-release)	Unknown	4 hr	Unknown

Half-life: About 6 to 8 hours.

ADVERSE REACTIONS

CNS: asthenia, headache, somnolence, amnesia, anxiety, ataxia, depression, dizziness, emotional lability, hostility, aggression, abnormal behavior, irritability, agitation, nervousness, paresthesia, pain, vertigo, hypersomnia, insomnia, irritability, confusion, lethargy, sedation, abnormal gait, incoordination. **EENT:** diplopia, ear pain, conjunctivitis, rhinitis, sinusitis, sore throat, nasal congestion, pharyngitis. **GI:** anorexia, vomiting, upper abdominal pain, diarrhea, constipation, gastroenteritis. **Hematologic:** *leukopenia,*

neutropenia. **Musculoskeletal:** neck pain, joint sprain. **Respiratory:** cough. **Skin:** contusion. **Other:** infection, head injury, flulike symptoms, falls.

INTERACTIONS

Drug-drug. *Antihistamines, benzodiazepines, opioids, other drugs that cause drowsiness, TCAs:* May lead to severe sedation. Avoid use together.

Drug-lifestyle. *Alcohol use:* May lead to severe sedation. Discourage use together.

EFFECTS ON LAB TEST RESULTS

• May increase LFT and kidney function test results.

• May decrease sodium level.

• May increase eosinophil count.

• May decrease Hb level, hematocrit, and WBC, RBC, platelet, and neutrophil counts.

CONTRAINDICATIONS & CAUTIONS

• Contraindicated in patients hypersensitive to drug.

• Don't use extended-release form in patients on CKRT.

• Anaphylaxis and angioedema may occur after first dose or at any time during treatment.

• Use cautiously in patients with history of psychiatric symptoms, especially psychotic symptoms and behaviors.

• Serious skin reactions, including TEN and SJS, have been reported. Recurrence after a rechallenge is possible.

• Don't abruptly discontinue drug because withdrawal seizures may occur.

• Drug may cause hematologic abnormalities (decreased RBC, WBC, platelet, and neutrophil counts; decreased Hb level and hematocrit; increased eosinophil count). Cases of agranulocytosis have been reported.

Dialyzable drug: 50%.

⚠ *Overdose S&S:* Drowsiness, aggression, agitation, coma, depressed level of consciousness, respiratory depression, somnolence.

PREGNANCY-LACTATION-REPRODUCTION

• Studies during pregnancy are inadequate. Use during pregnancy only if potential benefit justifies fetal risk.

• Patients who are pregnant should enroll in North American Antiepileptic Drug

Pregnancy Registry (1-888-233-2334 or www.aedpregnancyregistry.org).
• Drug appears in human milk. Use cautiously during breastfeeding.

NURSING CONSIDERATIONS
• Seizures can occur with abrupt drug stoppage. Tapering is recommended.
• Monitor for somnolence and fatigue.
• Monitor closely for such adverse reactions as dizziness, which may lead to falls.
• Discontinue drug and notify prescriber of signs and symptoms of anaphylaxis (hypotension, hives, rash, respiratory distress), angioedema (swelling of face, lips, mouth, eyes, tongue, throat, feet), and serious dermatologic reaction.
• Monitor kidney function; AKI has been reported.
• Monitor patients ages 1 month to younger than 4 years for increased diastolic BP.
• *Alert:* Closely monitor all patients taking or starting AEDs for behavior changes indicating psychosis or worsening of suicidality or depression. Such symptoms as anxiety, agitation, hostility, hypomania, and mania may be precursors to emerging suicidality.
• *Look alike–sound alike:* Don't confuse levetiracetam with levofloxacin. Don't confuse Keppra with Kaletra.

PATIENT TEACHING
• *Alert:* Tell patient or caregiver to seek medical attention for emerging or worsening depression, suicidality, or unusual changes in mood or behavior.
• Teach about proper drug administration and handling.
• Warn patient to use extra care when sitting or standing to avoid falling.
• Advise patient to seek immediate medical attention for signs and symptoms of anaphylaxis or angioedema.
• Counsel patient not to stop drug abruptly because seizure activity may increase.
• Caution patient to call prescriber and not stop drug suddenly if adverse reactions occur.
• Warn that drug may cause dizziness and somnolence. Instruct patient to avoid driving, operating heavy machinery, bike riding, and other hazardous activities until drug's effects are known.

---

levocetirizine dihydrochloride
LEE-voe-se-TIR-a-zeen

Xyzal Allergy 24HR ◇

Therapeutic class: Antihistamines
Pharmacologic class: H₁-receptor antagonists

AVAILABLE FORMS
Oral solution: 2.5 mg/5 mL
Tablets (scored): 5 mg

INDICATIONS & DOSAGES
➤ **Seasonal allergic rhinitis (OTC only)**
Adults and children ages 12 and older: 5 mg PO once daily in evening; 2.5 mg PO once daily in evening may be adequate for some patients.
Children ages 6 to 11: 2.5 mg PO once daily in evening. Don't exceed 2.5 mg in 24 hours.
Children ages 2 to 5: 1.25 mg (2.5 mL) solution only PO once daily in evening. Don't exceed 1.25 mg in 24 hours.
Adjust-a-dose: Use in the presence of kidney impairment isn't recommended.
➤ **Perennial allergic rhinitis**
Children ages 6 months to 2 years: 1.25 mg (2.5 mL) PO daily in evening. Don't exceed this dosage.
Adjust-a-dose: Use in children with kidney impairment is contraindicated.
➤ **Chronic idiopathic urticaria**
Adults and children ages 12 and older: 5 mg once daily in evening; some patients with less severe symptoms may experience symptom relief with 2.5 mg once daily.
Children ages 6 to 11: 2.5 mg once daily in evening. Maximum dosage, 2.5 mg/day.
Children ages 6 months to 5 years: 1.25 mg (2.5 mL) once daily in evening. Maximum dosage, 1.25 mg/day.
Adjust-a-dose: For patients ages 12 and older with CrCl of 50 to 80 mL/minute, give 2.5 mg PO once daily; with CrCl of 30 to 50 mL/minute, give 2.5 mg PO every other day; with CrCl of 10 to 30 mL/minute, give 2.5 mg PO twice weekly (once every 3 to 4 days). Use in patients with CrCl less than 10 mL/minute, those undergoing CKRT, and children younger than age 12 with any kidney impairment is contraindicated. Adjust dosage in patients with both liver and kidney impairment.

ADMINISTRATION
PO
• Give drug in evening without regard to food.
• Use calibrated dosing device for oral solution.

ACTION
H_1-receptor inhibition creates antihistamine effect, relieving allergy symptoms.

Route	Onset	Peak	Duration
PO	1 hr	0.5–1 hr	24 hr

Half-life: Adults, 8 to 9 hours; children, 6 hours.

ADVERSE REACTIONS
CNS: asthenia, fatigue, fever, somnolence. **EENT:** otitis media, epistaxis, dry mouth, nasopharyngitis, pharyngitis. **GI:** diarrhea, vomiting, constipation. **Respiratory:** cough.

INTERACTIONS
Drug-drug. *CNS depressants:* May have additive effects when taken together. Avoid use together.
Ritonavir: May increase level and half-life of levocetirizine. Use together cautiously.
Theophylline: May decrease clearance of levocetirizine. Use together cautiously.
Drug-lifestyle. *Alcohol use:* May have additive effect when taken with levocetirizine. Discourage use together.

EFFECTS ON LAB TEST RESULTS
• May cause transient increases in bilirubin and transaminase levels.
• May prevent, reduce, or mask positive result skin wheal in diagnostic skin test.

CONTRAINDICATIONS & CAUTIONS
• Contraindicated in patients hypersensitive to drug or to cetirizine.
• Contraindicated in patients with CrCl of less than 10 mL/minute, in patients younger than age 12 with impaired kidney function, and in those undergoing hemodialysis.
• Use cautiously in older adults.
• Use cautiously in patients with predisposing factors for urine retention, such as spinal cord lesion or prostatic hyperplasia. Discontinue drug if urine retention occurs.
• Safety and effectiveness in patients younger than age 6 months haven't been established.
Dialyzable drug: Less than 10%.
⚠ *Overdose S&S:* Drowsiness; initial agitation and restlessness, then drowsiness (in children).

PREGNANCY-LACTATION-REPRODUCTION
• Studies during pregnancy are inadequate. Use only if clearly needed.
• Drug may appear in human milk. Consider benefits of breastfeeding and patient's clinical need for drug. Use only if benefits outweigh risks.

NURSING CONSIDERATIONS
• Monitor kidney function in patient with or at risk for kidney impairment.

PATIENT TEACHING
• Warn patient not to perform hazardous tasks or those requiring alertness and coordination until CNS effects are known.
• Advise patient to avoid use of alcohol and other CNS depressants while taking drug.
• Caution patient not to take more than recommended dose because of increased risk of somnolence at higher doses.

levodopa–carbidopa
lee-voe-DOE-pa/kar-bih-DOE-pa

Dhivy, Duodopa✿, Duopa, Rytary, Sinemet

Therapeutic class: Antiparkinsonian drugs
Pharmacologic class: Decarboxylase inhibitors–dopamine precursors

AVAILABLE FORMS
Capsules (extended-release) ⓄⓃⒸ: 95 mg levodopa with 23.75 mg carbidopa, 145 mg levodopa with 36.25 mg carbidopa, 195 mg levodopa with 48.75 mg carbidopa, 245 mg levodopa with 61.25 mg carbidopa
Enteral gel: levodopa 20 mg/mL with 5 mg/mL carbidopa in single-use cassettes✿
Enteral suspension: levodopa 20 mg/mL with 4.63 mg/mL carbidopa
Tablets (extended-release) ⓄⓃⒸ: 100 mg levodopa with 25 mg carbidopa, 200 mg levodopa with 50 mg carbidopa
Tablets (immediate-release): 100 mg levodopa with 10 mg carbidopa, 100 mg levodopa with 25 mg carbidopa, 250 mg levodopa with 25 mg carbidopa
Tablets (ODTs): 100 mg levodopa with 10 mg carbidopa, 100 mg levodopa with 25 mg carbidopa, 250 mg levodopa with 25 mg carbidopa

INDICATIONS & DOSAGES

➤ **Idiopathic Parkinson disease, postencephalitic parkinsonism, and symptomatic parkinsonism resulting from carbon monoxide or manganese intoxication**

Adults: 1 immediate-release tablet of 100 mg levodopa with 25 mg carbidopa PO t.i.d., increased by 1 tablet daily or every other day, as needed, to maximum daily dosage of 8 tablets. May use 250 mg levodopa with 25 mg carbidopa or 100 mg levodopa with 10 mg carbidopa tablets, as directed, to obtain maximal response. Optimum daily dosage must be determined by careful adjustment for each patient. Or, 1 extended-release capsule of 95 mg levodopa with 23.75 mg carbidopa t.i.d. for 3 days; on day 4, increase to 145 mg levodopa with 36.25 mg carbidopa t.i.d. Adjust dosage as needed; may increase up to 390 mg levodopa with 97.5 mg carbidopa t.i.d. May increase frequency of dosing to maximum of five times daily, if needed and tolerated. Maximum recommended daily dosage is 2,450 mg levodopa with 612.5 mg carbidopa. Or, 1 extended-release tablet of 200 mg levodopa with 50 mg carbidopa b.i.d. at intervals of 6 hours or more. Increase or decrease doses and dosing intervals based on response. Most patients have been adequately treated with a dosage that provides 400 to 1,600 mg of levodopa per day (divided doses) at intervals of 4 to 8 hours while awake. Allow at least a 3-day interval between dosage adjustments.

Refer to manufacturer's instructions to convert from immediate-release to extended-release formulations.

➤ **Motor fluctuations in patients with advanced Parkinson disease (Duodopa, Duopa)**

❸ *Alert:* Before initiating enteral therapy, convert patient from all other forms of levodopa to oral immediate-release levodopa–carbidopa tablets (1:4 ratio).

Adults: Total daily dosage (expressed in terms of levodopa) consists of a morning dose, a continuous dose, and extra doses, which can be used to manage acute "off" symptoms not controlled by morning and continuous doses. Refer to manufacturer's labeling for morning dose and continuous dose calculations and titration instructions. Maximum for morning and continuous doses is 2,000 mg of levodopa component over 16 hours. Maximum of extra doses is one extra dose every 2 hours. Give patient's routine nighttime dosage of oral immediate-release levodopa–carbidopa after discontinuation of daily infusion.

Adjust-a-dose: For dyskinesias or levodopa-related adverse reactions within 1 hour of morning dose on preceding day, decrease morning dose by 1 mL. For dyskinesias or adverse reactions lasting 1 hour or more on preceding day, decrease continuous dose by 0.3 mL/hour. For dyskinesias or adverse reactions lasting for two or more periods of 1 hour or more on preceding day, decrease continuous dose by 0.6 mL/hour.

ADMINISTRATION

PO

● Give drug with food to decrease GI upset, but avoid giving with high-protein meals, which can impair absorption and reduce effectiveness.

● Have patient swallow tablets whole; don't crush or break tablets.

● Give ODT immediately after removing from bottle. Place tablet on patient's tongue, where it will dissolve in seconds and be swallowed with saliva. No additional fluid is needed.

● For patients with difficulty swallowing, capsules may be opened and entire contents sprinkled on small amount of applesauce (1 to 2 tablespoons) and then consumed immediately (don't store for future use).

Enteral

● Before use, fully thaw in refrigerator. To ensure controlled thawing, take cartons containing the seven individual cassettes out of the transport box and separate cartons from each other.

● Assign a 12-week, use-by date based on the time the cartons are put into refrigerator to thaw (may take up to 96 hours to thaw).

● Once thawed, individual cartons may be packed in a closer configuration within refrigerator.

● Remove one cassette from refrigerator 20 minutes before administration (failure to use at room temperature may result in inaccurate dosage).

● Administer through either nasojejunal tube (temporary administration) or percutaneous endoscopic gastrostomy-jejunostomy tube (long-term administration) connected to CADD-Legacy 1400 pump.

● Disconnect tube from pump at end of infusion and flush tube with room temperature drinking water with a syringe.

• Cassettes are for single use only and should be discarded daily after infusion. Don't reuse opened cassettes.

ACTION

Levodopa, a dopamine precursor, relieves parkinsonian symptoms by being converted to dopamine in the brain. Carbidopa inhibits the decarboxylation of peripheral levodopa, which allows more intact levodopa to travel to the brain.

Route	Onset	Peak	Duration
PO	Unknown	30–120 min	Unknown
Enteral	Unknown	2.5 hr	Unknown

Half-life: 1.5 to 2 hours.

ADVERSE REACTIONS

CNS: syncope, agitation, bradykinetic episodes, dyskinesia, anxiety, confusion, dementia, *suicidality,* dizziness, dream abnormalities, sleep disorder, delusions, hallucinations, depression, headache, fever, insomnia, paresthesia, psychotic episodes, paranoid ideation, somnolence, fatigue, asthenia, taste alterations. **CV:** cardiac irregularities, chest pain, HTN, hypotension, orthostatic hypotension, edema, palpitations, phlebitis, *MI.* **EENT:** oropharyngeal pain, dark saliva, dry mouth. **GI:** anorexia, constipation, duodenal ulcer, diarrhea, dyspepsia, abdominal pain, *GI bleeding,* nausea, vomiting. **GU:** dark urine, urinary frequency, UTI. **Hematologic:** *agranulocytosis,* hemolytic and nonhemolytic anemia, *leukopenia, thrombocytopenia.* **Hepatic:** increased LFT values. **Metabolic:** weight gain or loss. **Musculoskeletal:** back pain, leg pain, muscle cramps, shoulder pain. **Respiratory:** dyspnea, URI, atelectasis. **Skin:** alopecia, rash, diaphoresis, dark sweat, urticaria, pruritus, purpura, bullous lesions. **Other:** increased libido, hypersensitivity, complications of enteral device insertion.

INTERACTIONS

Drug-drug. *Antihypertensives:* May cause additive hypotensive effects. Use together cautiously.

Antipsychotics (butyrophenones, phenothiazines, risperidone): May decrease levodopa activity. Monitor patient closely.

Dopamine-depleting drugs (reserpine, tetrabenazine): May decrease effects of carbidopa. Avoid use together.

Iron salts (oral): May reduce bioavailability of levodopa–carbidopa. Give iron 2 hours before or after oral levodopa–carbidopa.

Isoniazid: May antagonize antiparkinsonian actions. Use together cautiously. Therapy modification may be necessary.

MAO inhibitors (nonselective [isocarboxazid, phenelzine, tranylcypromine]): May increase risk of severe HTN. Use together is contraindicated. Discontinue MAO inhibitor 2 weeks before start of levodopa–carbidopa.

MAO inhibitors (selective [rasagiline, safinamide, selegiline]): May increase risk of orthostatic hypotension. Monitor patient closely.

Metoclopramide: May decrease therapeutic effects of levodopa–carbidopa. Monitor therapeutic effects.

Papaverine, phenytoin: May antagonize antiparkinsonian actions. Avoid use together.

Sapropterin: May increase risk of levodopa-related adverse effects. Monitor patient carefully.

TCAs: May cause increased BP and dyskinesia. Use together cautiously.

Drug-herb. *Kava:* May decrease action of drug. Discourage kava use altogether.

Drug-food. *Foods high in protein:* May decrease levodopa absorption. Don't give levodopa with high-protein foods.

EFFECTS ON LAB TEST RESULTS

• May increase BUN, creatinine, uric acid, ALT, AST, ALP, LDH, glucose, and bilirubin levels.

• May decrease Hb level and hematocrit and WBC, granulocyte, and platelet counts.

• May falsely increase urinary catecholamine level and serum and urinary uric acid levels in colorimetric tests.

• May falsely decrease urinary vanillylmandelic acid level.

• May cause false-positive results in urine ketone tests using sodium nitroprusside reagent and in urine glucose tests using cupric sulfate reagent.

• May cause false-negative urine glucose or false-positive urine acetone results in tests using glucose oxidase.

• May alter results of urine screening tests for phenylketonuria.

• May cause positive Coombs test.

CONTRAINDICATIONS & CAUTIONS

• Contraindicated in patients hypersensitive to drug. Some formulations are also

---

contraindicated in patients with angle-closure glaucoma, melanoma, or undiagnosed skin lesions.

• Use cautiously in patients with severe CV, kidney, liver, endocrine, or pulmonary disorders; orthostatic hypotension; history of peptic ulcer; psychiatric illness; MI with residual arrhythmias; bronchial asthma; emphysema; or glaucoma.

• Potentially fatal GI complications (bezoar; ileus; implant-site erosion or ulcer; intestinal hemorrhage, ischemia, obstruction, or perforation; pancreatitis; peritonitis; pneumoperitoneum; postoperative wound infection) may occur in patients receiving enteral therapy.

• May increase risk of impulse-control disorders, dyskinesia, melanoma, orthostatic hypotension, and sudden somnolence.

Dialyzable drug: Unknown.

⚠ *Overdose S&S:* Muscle twitching, blepharospasm.

PREGNANCY-LACTATION-REPRODUCTION

• Studies during pregnancy are inadequate. Use during pregnancy only if potential benefit justifies fetal risk.

• Drug appears in human milk. Use cautiously during breastfeeding.

NURSING CONSIDERATIONS

• Optimum daily dosage is determined by careful titration in each patient. Therapy should be individualized and adjusted according to desired therapeutic response.

• Observe patient and monitor vital signs, BP, when changing positions and adjusting dosage. Report significant changes.

• Monitor patient for CV signs and symptoms (chest pain, irregular HR) and neuropathy.

⚓ *Alert:* Because of risk of precipitating a symptom complex resembling NMS (fever, muscular rigidity, altered consciousness, autonomic instability), observe patient closely if levodopa dosage is abruptly reduced or stopped.

• Hallucinations or dyskinesias may require dosage reduction or drug withdrawal.

• Regularly test patients receiving long-term therapy for diabetes and acromegaly. Periodically test liver, kidney, and hematopoietic function.

• Advise patient to see a dermatologist for regular skin cancer screening.

⚓ *Alert:* Monitor patient for depression and suicidality.

PATIENT TEACHING

• Teach about proper drug administration and handling.

• Warn patient and caregivers not to increase or decrease dosage without prescriber's orders.

⚓ *Alert:* Advise family or caregivers to monitor patient for changes in behavior and to immediately report suicidality.

• Advise patient to have skin checks for appearance of melanoma.

• Caution patient about possible dizziness when standing up quickly, especially at start of therapy. Tell patient to change positions slowly and dangle legs before getting out of bed.

• Instruct patient to report adverse reactions (such as somnolence, loss of impulse control) and therapeutic effects.

• Advise patient receiving enteral therapy to immediately report abdominal pain, prolonged constipation, nausea, vomiting, fever, or melena.

• Inform patient that pyridoxine (vitamin B_6) doesn't reverse beneficial effects of levodopa–carbidopa. Multivitamins (without iron) can be taken without reversing levodopa's effects.

levodopa–carbidopa–entacapone

lee-voe-DOE-pa/kar-bih-DOE-pa/en-ta-KAP-own

Stalevo

Therapeutic class: Antiparkinsonian drugs
Pharmacologic class: Dopamine precursors–decarboxylase inhibitors–catecholamine-*O*-methyltransferase inhibitors

AVAILABLE FORMS

Tablets (film-coated) ⓄⓇⒸ: 50 mg levodopa, 12.5 mg carbidopa, and 200 mg entacapone; 75 mg levodopa, 18.75 mg carbidopa, and 200 mg entacapone; 100 mg levodopa, 25 mg carbidopa, and 200 mg entacapone; 125 mg levodopa, 31.25 mg carbidopa, and 200 mg entacapone; 150 mg levodopa, 37.5 mg carbidopa, and 200 mg entacapone; 200 mg levodopa, 50 mg carbidopa, and 200 mg entacapone

INDICATIONS & DOSAGES

➤ **Idiopathic Parkinson disease, to replace individual components at equivalent strengths; or to replace immediate-release levodopa–carbidopa for patient who has end-of-dose "wearing off," is taking total daily levodopa dosage of 600 mg or less, and has no dyskinesia**

Adults: 1 tablet PO; determine dose and interval by therapeutic response. Maximum, 8 tablets/24 hours for all strengths except levodopa 200 mg, carbidopa 50 mg, and entacapone 200 mg; for these strengths, maximum, 6 tablets/24 hours.

ADMINISTRATION

PO
- Have patient swallow tablets whole; don't crush or break tablets.
- Give only 1 tablet at each dosing interval.
- Give drug with or without food, but avoid giving with high-fat, high-calorie meal by about 2 hours to prevent decreased absorption.

ACTION

Levodopa, a dopamine precursor, relieves parkinsonian symptoms by converting to dopamine in the brain. Carbidopa inhibits the decarboxylation of peripheral levodopa, which allows more intact levodopa to travel to the brain. Entacapone is a reversible catecholamine-*O*-methyltransferase (COMT) inhibitor that increases levodopa level.

Route	Onset	Peak	Duration
PO	Unknown	1–3.5 hr	Unknown

Half-life: Carbidopa, 1.5 to 2 hours; levodopa, 1 to 3.25 hours; entacapone, 0.75 to 1 hour.

ADVERSE REACTIONS

⚠️ *Alert:* Reactions listed are those that occur more frequently with the addition of entacapone than with levodopa–carbidopa alone. Refer to levodopa–carbidopa monograph for less frequent adverse reactions.

CNS: dyskinesia, hyperkinesia, hypokinesia, agitation, anxiety, asthenia, dizziness, fatigue, dysgeusia, somnolence. **EENT:** dry mouth. **GI:** diarrhea, nausea, abdominal pain, constipation, dyspepsia, flatulence, gastritis, vomiting. **GU:** urine discoloration. **Musculoskeletal:** back pain. **Respiratory:** dyspnea. **Skin:** diaphoresis, purpura. **Other:** bacterial infection.

INTERACTIONS

Drug-drug. *Ampicillin, chloramphenicol, cholestyramine, erythromycin, probenecid, rifampin:* May interfere with entacapone excretion. Use together cautiously.
Antihypertensives: May cause orthostatic hypotension. Adjust antihypertensive dosage as needed.
CNS depressants: Additive effects. Use together cautiously.
Dopamine (D2) receptor antagonists (butyrophenones, metoclopramide, phenothiazines, risperidone), isoniazid, phenytoin: May decrease levodopa, carbidopa, and entacapone effects. Monitor patient for effectiveness.
Drugs metabolized by COMT (apomorphine, dobutamine, dopamine, epinephrine, isoetharine, isoproterenol, methyldopa, norepinephrine): May cause increased HR, arrhythmias, and excessive BP changes. Use together cautiously.
Iron salts (oral): May reduce bioavailability of levodopa–carbidopa–entacapone. Separate drugs by 2 or more hours; monitor therapy.
MAO inhibitors (nonselective [isocarboxazid, phenelzine, tranylcypromine]): May increase risk of severe HTN. Use together is contraindicated. Discontinue MAO inhibitor 2 weeks before start of levodopa–carbidopa–entacapone.
MAO inhibitors (selective [rasagiline, safinamide, selegiline]): May increase risk of orthostatic hypotension. Monitor patient closely.
Papaverine: May increase hypotensive effect and decrease therapeutic effect of levodopa. Monitor therapy. Increase levodopa–carbidopa–entacapone dosage as needed.
Selegiline: May cause severe hypotension. Use together cautiously, and monitor BP.
TCAs: May increase risk of HTN and dyskinesia. Monitor patient closely.
Warfarin: May increase risk of bleeding. Monitor INR.
Drug-food. *Foods high in protein:* May decrease levodopa absorption. Discourage taking with high-protein foods.
Drug-herb. *Kava:* May decrease action of drug. Discourage kava use altogether.
Drug-lifestyle. *Alcohol use:* May enhance CNS depressant effects. Discourage use together.

EFFECTS ON LAB TEST RESULTS
● May increase ALP, AST, ALT, LDH, glucose, BUN, and bilirubin levels.
● May decrease Hb level, hematocrit, and platelet and WBC counts.
● May cause false-positive reaction for urinary ketone bodies on a test tape.
● May cause false-negative result for glycosuria with glucose oxidase testing methods.
● May cause abnormal catecholamine and Coombs test.

CONTRAINDICATIONS & CAUTIONS
● Contraindicated in patients hypersensitive to drug or its components and in patients with angle-closure glaucoma.
● Use cautiously in patients with suspicious undiagnosed skin lesions or history of melanoma.
● Use cautiously in patients with past or current psychosis and in patients with severe pulmonary disease; bronchial asthma; biliary obstruction; peptic ulcer; chronic open-angle glaucoma; or kidney, liver, or endocrine disease.
● Drug may increase risk of impulse-control disorders, dyskinesia, melanoma, orthostatic hypotension, and sudden somnolence.
Dialyzable drug: Unlikely.
⚠ *Overdose S&S:* CNS disturbances, hypotension, tachycardia, rhabdomyolysis, transient kidney insufficiency, abdominal pain, loose stools.

PREGNANCY-LACTATION-REPRODUCTION
● Studies during pregnancy are inadequate. Use only if potential benefit justifies fetal risk.
● It isn't known if drug appears in human milk. Use cautiously during breastfeeding.

NURSING CONSIDERATIONS
● Certain CNS effects, such as dyskinesia, may occur at lower dosages and sooner with levodopa–carbidopa–entacapone than with levodopa alone. Dyskinesia may require a reduced dosage.
● Monitor patient for orthostatic hypotension, especially during dosage escalation.
● NMS-like symptoms may develop when levodopa and carbidopa are reduced or stopped, especially in patients taking antipsychotic drugs. Watch patient carefully for fever, hyperthermia, muscle rigidity, involuntary movements, altered consciousness, mental status changes, and autonomic dysfunction.

● During extended therapy, periodically monitor liver, hematopoietic, CV, and kidney function.
● Diarrhea is common; it usually develops 4 to 12 weeks after treatment starts but may appear as early as the first week or as late as many months after treatment starts.
◐ *Alert:* Monitor patient for hallucinations, depression, and suicidality.

PATIENT TEACHING
● Teach about proper drug administration and handling.
● Teach patient to report "wearing-off" effect, which may occur at end of dosing interval.
● Tell patient that urine, sweat, and saliva may turn dark (red, brown, or black) during treatment.
● Advise patient to notify prescriber if voluntary movement problems increase.
● Tell patient that diarrhea is common.
● Warn that hallucinations may occur.
● Urge patient to immediately report depression, suicidality, or loss of impulse control.
● Explain that patient may become dizzy if rising quickly. Urge patient to use caution when rising.
● Tell patient that excessive acidity, iron salts, or a high-fat, high-calorie, or high-protein diet may reduce drug's effectiveness.
● Urge patient to avoid hazardous activities until CNS effects of drug are known.
● Advise patient to see a dermatologist for regular skin cancer screening.
● Instruct patient of childbearing potential to report pregnancy.

levoFLOXacin
lee-voe-FLOX-a-sin

Therapeutic class: Antibiotics
Pharmacologic class: Fluoroquinolones

AVAILABLE FORMS
Infusion (premixed in D_5W): 250 mg in 50 mL, 500 mg in 100 mL, 750 mg in 150 mL
Ophthalmic solution: 0.5%, 1.5%
Oral solution: 25 mg/mL
Single-use vials: 500 mg, 750 mg
Tablets: 250 mg, 500 mg, 750 mg

INDICATIONS & DOSAGES
Boxed Warning Use in patients with acute bacterial sinusitis, acute bacterial

exacerbation of chronic bronchitis, and uncomplicated UTI isn't recommended because of risk of serious adverse effects. Use in these patients only when they have no other treatment options. ■

Adjust-a-dose (for all indications): For patients with CrCl of less than 50 mL/minute, adjust oral or IV dosage regimen according to manufacturer's instructions.

➤ **Acute bacterial sinusitis caused by susceptible strains of** *Streptococcus pneumoniae, Moraxella catarrhalis,* **or** *Haemophilus influenzae*
Adults: 500 mg PO or IV infusion over 60 minutes every 24 hours for 10 to 14 days or 750 mg PO or IV over 90 minutes every 24 hours for 5 days.

➤ **Mild to moderate skin and skin-structure infections caused by** *Staphylococcus aureus* **or** *Streptococcus pyogenes*
Adults: 500 mg PO or IV infusion every 24 hours for 7 to 10 days.

➤ **Acute bacterial worsening of chronic bronchitis caused by** *S. aureus, S. pneumoniae, M. catarrhalis, H. influenzae,* **or** *Haemophilus parainfluenzae*
Adults: 500 mg PO or IV infusion every 24 hours for 7 days.

➤ **To prevent inhalation anthrax after confirmed or suspected exposure to** *Bacillus anthracis*
Adults and children ages 6 months and older weighing at least 50 kg: 500 mg PO or IV infusion every 24 hours for 60 days.
Children ages 6 months and older weighing 30 to less than 50 kg: 250 mg PO or 8 mg/kg (not to exceed 250 mg/dose) oral solution or by slow IV infusion every 12 hours for 60 days.

➤ **Chronic bacterial prostatitis caused by** *Escherichia coli, Enterococcus faecalis,* **or** *Staphylococcus epidermidis*
Adults: 500 mg PO or IV infusion every 24 hours for 28 days.

➤ **Community-acquired pneumonia from** *S. pneumoniae* **(excluding multidrug-resistant strains),** *H. influenzae, H. parainfluenzae, Mycoplasma pneumoniae,* **or** *Chlamydia pneumoniae*
Adults: 750 mg PO or IV infusion every 24 hours for 5 days.

➤ **Community-acquired pneumonia caused by methicillin-susceptible** *S. aureus, S. pneumoniae, H. influenzae, H. parainfluenzae, Klebsiella pneumoniae,* *M. catarrhalis, C. pneumoniae, Legionella pneumophila,* **or** *M. pneumoniae*
Adults: 500 mg PO or IV infusion every 24 hours for 7 to 14 days.

➤ **Complicated skin and skin-structure infections caused by methicillin-sensitive** *S. aureus, E. faecalis, S. pyogenes,* **or** *Proteus mirabilis*
Adults: 750 mg PO or IV infusion every 24 hours for 7 to 14 days.

➤ **Health care–acquired pneumonia caused by methicillin-susceptible** *S. aureus, Pseudomonas aeruginosa, Serratia marcescens, E. coli, K. pneumoniae, H. influenzae,* **or** *S. pneumoniae*
Adults: 750 mg PO or IV infusion every 24 hours for 7 to 14 days.

➤ **Complicated UTI caused by** *E. faecalis, Enterobacter cloacae, E. coli, K. pneumoniae, P. mirabilis,* **or** *P. aeruginosa;* **acute pyelonephritis caused by** *E. coli*
Adults: 250 mg PO or IV infusion every 24 hours for 10 days.

➤ **Complicated UTI caused by** *E. coli, K. pneumoniae,* **or** *P. mirabilis;* **acute pyelonephritis caused by** *E. coli*
Adults: 750 mg PO or IV infusion daily for 5 days.

➤ **Mild to moderate uncomplicated UTI caused by** *E. coli, K. pneumoniae,* **or** *Staphylococcus saprophyticus*
Adults: 250 mg PO daily for 3 days.

➤ **Prophylaxis or treatment of pneumonic and septicemic plague** *(Yersinia pestis)*
Adults or children ages 6 months and older weighing 50 kg or more: 500 mg PO or IV infusion every 24 hours for 10 to 14 days.
Children ages 6 months and older weighing 30 to less than 50 kg: 250 mg PO or 8 mg/kg (not to exceed 250 mg/dose) oral solution or by slow IV infusion every 12 hours for 10 to 14 days.

➤ **Bacterial conjunctivitis**
Adults and children ages 6 and older: On days 1 through 2, instill 1 to 2 drops in affected eye(s) every 2 hours while patient is awake, up to 8 times daily. On days 3 through 7, instill 1 to 2 drops in affected eye(s) every 4 hours while patient is awake, up to 4 times daily.

➤ **Corneal ulceration caused by** *Corynebacterium* **species,** *S. aureus, S. epidermidis, S. pneumoniae, Viridans* **group streptococci,** *P. aeruginosa, S. marcescens*

L

Adults and children ages 6 and older: Instill 1 to 2 drops into affected eye every 30 minutes to 2 hours while awake and 4 to 6 hours after retiring, for 3 days. Then instill 1 to 2 drops into affected eye every 1 to 4 hours while awake on day 4 until end of treatment based on complete reepithelialization.

➤ **Neutropenia (chemotherapy-induced), antibacterial prophylaxis ♦**
Adults: 500 mg or 750 mg PO once daily. Some clinicians provide antibacterial prophylaxis if ANC is anticipated to be less than 500/mm³ for more than 7 days. For hematopoietic cell transplant recipients, begin at time of stem cell infusion and continue until recovery of neutropenia or until initiation of empirical antibiotic therapy for neutropenic fever.

ADMINISTRATION
PO
• Obtain specimen for culture and sensitivity tests before therapy and as needed to determine if bacterial resistance has occurred.
• Give drug with plenty of fluids to prevent crystalluria.
• Give 2 hours before or 2 hours after antacids, sucralfate, and products containing magnesium, aluminum, iron, or multivitamins with zinc.
• Give oral solution 1 hour before or 2 hours after a meal.
• Give missed dose right away if it's 8 hours or more until next scheduled dose; if less than 8 hours, omit dose.
IV
▼ Obtain specimen for culture and sensitivity tests before therapy and as needed to determine if bacterial resistance has occurred.
▼ Give IV form only by infusion.
▼ Dilute drug in single-use vials according to manufacturer's instructions, with D_5W or NSS for injection, to a final concentration of 5 mg/mL.
▼ Infuse doses of 500 mg or less over at least 60 minutes and doses of 750 mg over at least 90 minutes.
▼ Reconstituted solution should be clear, slightly yellow, and free of particulate matter.
▼ Reconstituted drug is stable for 72 hours at room temperature, for 14 days when refrigerated in plastic containers, and for 6 months when frozen.
▼ Thaw at room temperature or in refrigerator.

▼ **Incompatibilities:** Manufacturer recommends not mixing or infusing other drugs with levofloxacin.
Ophthalmic
• Avoid touching applicator tip to eye or other surfaces.

ACTION
Inhibits bacterial DNA gyrase and prevents DNA replication, transcription, repair, and recombination in susceptible bacteria.

Route	Onset	Peak	Duration
PO, IV	Unknown	1–2 hr	Unknown
Ophthalmic	Unknown	Unknown	Unknown

Half-life: About 6 to 8 hours.

ADVERSE REACTIONS
CNS: dizziness, headache, fever, insomnia, dysgeusia (ophthalmic). **CV:** edema, chest pain. **EENT:** foreign body or burning sensation in eye, eye pain, blurred vision, vision loss, ocular infection, photophobia (ophthalmic). **GI:** abdominal pain, diarrhea, constipation, dyspepsia, nausea, vomiting. **GU:** vaginitis. **Metabolic:** *hypoglycemia.* **Musculoskeletal:** back pain, tendon rupture. **Respiratory:** allergic pneumonitis, dyspnea. **Skin:** photosensitivity, pruritus, rash, injection-site reaction. **Other:** moniliasis, infection, hypersensitivity reactions.

INTERACTIONS
Drug-drug. *Aluminum hydroxide, aluminum–magnesium hydroxide, calcium carbonate, didanosine, iron salts, magnesium hydroxide, products containing zinc, sucralfate:* May interfere with GI absorption of levofloxacin. Give levofloxacin 2 hours before or 2 hours after these products.
Antiarrhythmics (Class IA [procainamide, quinidine] or Class III [amiodarone, dofetilide]), chlorpromazine, erythromycin, fluconazole, haloperidol, imipramine, ondansetron, ziprasidone: May increase risk of life-threatening cardiac arrhythmias. Avoid use together.
Antidiabetics: May alter glucose level. Closely monitor glucose level.
NSAIDs: May increase CNS stimulation. Monitor patient for seizure activity.
Steroids: May increase risk of tendinitis and tendon rupture. Monitor patient for tendon pain or inflammation.

Reactions in bold italics are *life-threatening*.

Theophylline: May decrease clearance of theophylline. Monitor theophylline level.
Warfarin: May increase effect of oral anticoagulant. Monitor PT and INR.
Drug-lifestyle. *Sun exposure:* May cause photosensitivity reactions. Advise patient to avoid excessive sunlight exposure.

EFFECTS ON LAB TEST RESULTS

- May increase CK and potassium levels and kidney function and LFT values.
- May increase or decrease glucose level.
- May increase eosinophil count.
- May decrease Hb level and platelet and WBC counts.
- May prolong PT and increase INR.
- May produce false-positive opioid assay results.

CONTRAINDICATIONS & CAUTIONS

Boxed Warning Drug may cause disabling and potentially irreversible adverse reactions, including tendinitis and tendon rupture, peripheral neuropathy, and CNS effects (hallucinations, anxiety, depression, insomnia, severe headaches, confusion). Discontinue drug with first signs or symptoms of these reactions. ■

- Risk of tendinitis and tendon rupture increases in patients older than age 60, in patients taking corticosteroids, and in those with heart, kidney, or lung transplants.

Boxed Warning Drug may exacerbate muscle weakness in patients with myasthenia gravis. Avoid use in patients with history of myasthenia gravis. ■

❸ *Alert:* Drug is associated with increased incidence of musculoskeletal disorders (arthralgia, arthritis, tendinopathy, gait abnormality) in children.

❸ *Alert:* Drug may increase risk of aortic dissection or rupture when used systemically. Avoid use in patients with known aortic aneurysm and in patients at risk for aortic aneurysm, including those with peripheral atherosclerotic vascular diseases, HTN, certain genetic conditions (Marfan syndrome, Ehlers-Danlos syndrome), and older adults. Drug should only be used in these patients if no other treatment options are available.

- Contraindicated in patients hypersensitive to drug, its components, or other fluoroquinolones.

❸ *Alert:* Patients receiving systemic drug have increased risk of hyperglycemia and hypoglycemia. Hypoglycemia is more common in older adults and patients with diabetes.

- Use cautiously in patients with history of seizure disorders or other CNS diseases, such as cerebral arteriosclerosis.
- Use cautiously in patients with personal or family history of QT-interval prolongation, hypokalemia, bradycardia, or recent MI and in those currently taking antiarrhythmics.
- Use cautiously and adjust dosage in patients with kidney impairment.
- Drug may increase risk of hypersensitivity reactions, including SCARs, and allergic pneumonitis.
- Drug may rarely cause serious adverse reactions, including vasculitis, arthralgia, myalgia, serum sickness, interstitial nephritis, AKI or KF, and blood dyscrasias.
- Drug may cause severe liver toxicity. Immediately discontinue drug if patient develops signs or symptoms of hepatitis.
- Drug is indicated in children age 6 months and older only for postexposure inhalational anthrax prevention and for plague.
Dialyzable drug: No.

PREGNANCY-LACTATION-REPRODUCTION

- Studies during pregnancy are inadequate. Use during pregnancy only if potential benefit justifies fetal risk.
- Drug likely appears in human milk. Patient should discontinue breastfeeding or discontinue systemic drug, considering importance of drug to patient. May use eye drops cautiously.

NURSING CONSIDERATIONS

❸ *Alert:* Monitor patient for signs and symptoms of aortic aneurysm, dissection, and rupture (sudden, severe, and constant pain in stomach, chest, or back; throbbing in stomach area, deep pain in back or side of stomach; steady, gnawing pain in stomach that lasts for hours or days; pain in chest, jaw, neck, or back; hoarseness; coughing; shortness of breath; trouble swallowing). Discontinue drug immediately if any of these aortic disorders are suspected.

- Patient with acute hypersensitivity reactions may need treatment with epinephrine, oxygen, IV fluids, antihistamines, corticosteroids, pressor amines, and airway management.
- Ensure patient is adequately hydrated to prevent highly concentrated urine, kidney casts, and crystalluria.
- Monitor patient for signs and symptoms of peripheral neuropathy (pain, burning,

tingling, numbness, weakness, or change in sensation to light touch, pain, temperature, or sense of body position).

• Most antibacterials can cause pseudomembranous colitis or CDAD. If diarrhea occurs, notify prescriber; drug may be stopped.

• Drug may cause abnormal ECG.

• **Alert:** Monitor patient receiving systemic drug for symptoms of hypoglycemia (confusion, pounding or rapid heartbeat, dizziness, pale skin, shakiness, diaphoresis, unusual hunger, trembling, headache, weakness, irritability, unusual anxiety). Immediately discontinue drug for blood glucose disturbances, and switch to nonfluoroquinolone antibiotic, if possible.

• Monitor patient receiving systemic drug for psychiatric adverse reactions (agitation, disturbances in attention, disorientation, nervousness, memory impairment, delirium). Discontinue drug for CNS adverse effects, including psychiatric adverse reactions.

• If *P. aeruginosa* is a confirmed or suspected pathogen, use with a beta-lactam.

• Monitor glucose level and results of kidney function tests, LFTs, and blood counts.

• *Look alike–sound alike:* Don't confuse levofloxacin with levetiracetam.

PATIENT TEACHING

Boxed Warning Warn patient to immediately notify prescriber for signs and symptoms of serious adverse reactions, including unusual joint or tendon pain, muscle weakness, "pins and needles" tingling or prickling sensation, numbness in arms or legs, confusion, or hallucinations. ■

• **Alert:** Warn patient to seek immediate medical attention for signs and symptoms of aortic aneurysm, dissection, or rupture.

• Instruct patient to report all adverse reactions.

• Tell patient to take drug as prescribed, even if signs and symptoms disappear.

• Teach about proper drug administration and handling.

• Advise patient to take drug with plenty of fluids to prevent crystalluria and to space antacids, sucralfate, multivitamins with zinc, and products containing magnesium, aluminum, or iron by at least 12 hours before or after oral drug administration.

• Warn patient to avoid hazardous tasks until adverse effects of drug are known.

• Advise patient to avoid excessive sunlight and UV light exposure.

• Tell patient to stop drug and notify prescriber if rash or other signs or symptoms of hypersensitivity develop.

• Instruct patient to notify prescriber of all adverse reactions, including loose stools or diarrhea.

• Instruct patient not to use contact lenses during treatment for bacterial conjunctivitis or corneal ulceration.

• **Alert:** Caution patient that significant low blood sugar level can occur. Instruct patient how to manage symptoms and to immediately report any occurrence.

• Advise patient with diabetes that more frequent monitoring of blood glucose level may be necessary during therapy.

• **Alert:** Instruct patient to immediately report psychiatric adverse reactions. Explain that they can occur after just one dose.

• Instruct patient to report diarrhea because of risk of CDAD during and for 2 months or more after treatment.

levothyroxine sodium (T₄, L-thyroxine sodium)

lee-voe-thye-ROX-een

Eltroxin♦, Ermeza, Euthyrox, Levo-T, Levoxyl, Synthroid, Thyquidity, Tirosint, Tirosint-Sol, Unithroid

Therapeutic class: Thyroid hormone replacements
Pharmacologic class: Thyroid hormones

AVAILABLE FORMS

Capsules ⊙*:* 13 mcg, 25 mcg, 37.5 mcg, 44 mcg, 50 mcg, 62.5 mcg, 75 mcg, 88 mcg, 100 mcg, 112 mcg, 125 mcg, 137 mcg, 150 mcg, 175 mcg, 200 mcg
Oral solution: 13 mcg/mL, 25 mcg/mL, 30 mcg/mL, 37.5 mcg/mL, 44 mcg/mL, 50 mcg/mL, 62.5 mcg/mL, 75 mcg/mL, 88 mcg/mL, 100 mcg/mL, 112 mcg/mL, 125 mcg/mL, 137 mcg/mL, 150 mcg/mL, 175 mcg/mL, 200 mcg/mL
Powder for injection: 100 mcg, 200 mcg, 500 mcg
Solution for injection: 20 mcg/mL, 40 mcg/mL, 100 mcg/mL
Tablets: 25 mcg, 50 mcg, 75 mcg, 88 mcg, 100 mcg, 112 mcg, 125 mcg, 137 mcg, 150 mcg, 175 mcg, 200 mcg, 300 mcg

INDICATIONS & DOSAGES

➤ **Thyroid hormone replacement**

Adults ages 60 and younger: In otherwise healthy individuals with newly diagnosed hypothyroidism, initiate at approximately 1.6 mcg/kg PO once daily. (See individual manufacturer's instructions.) Monitor TSH level and adjust dosage every 4 to 6 weeks in 12.5- to 25-mcg increments until normal thyroid function returns and TSH is normal.

Older adults and patients with underlying cardiac disease: Initiate dosage at 12.5 to 25 mcg PO daily. Adjust dosage every 6 to 8 weeks, if needed, until patient is euthyroid and TSH level normalizes.

Children in whom growth and puberty are complete: 1.6 mcg/kg PO once daily. (See individual manufacturer's instructions.)

Children older than age 12 in whom growth and puberty are incomplete: 2 to 3 mcg/kg PO daily.

Children ages 6 to 12: 4 to 5 mcg/kg PO daily.

Children ages 1 to 5: 5 to 6 mcg/kg PO daily.

Children ages 6 months to 1 year: 6 to 8 mcg/kg PO daily.

Children ages 3 to 6 months: 8 to 10 mcg/kg PO daily.

Infants and neonates birth to age 3 months: 10 to 15 mcg/kg PO daily. In neonates at risk for cardiac failure, consider lower initial dosage and increase every 4 to 6 weeks as needed.

Children at risk for hyperactivity: Initiate at one-fourth recommended full replacement dose, and increase weekly by one-fourth full recommended replacement dose until full recommended replacement dose is reached.

Adjust-a-dose: For children, adjust dosage based on clinical response and lab parameters.

➤ **Severe, long-standing hypothyroidism**

Adults and adolescents in whom growth and puberty are complete: 12.5 to 25 mcg PO daily. Increase in increments of 12.5 to 25 mcg every 2 to 4 weeks as needed.

➤ **Myxedema coma**

Adults: Initially, 300 to 500 mcg (0.3 to 0.5 mg) IV; then 50 to 100 mcg IV once daily until patient can tolerate oral administration. Consider smaller doses in patients with CV disease and in older adults.

➤ **TSH suppression in well-differentiated thyroid cancer**

Adults: Dosage is highly individualized. Generally, TSH is suppressed to below 0.1 milli-international units/L, which usually requires a dosage greater than 2 mcg/kg/day. However, in patients with high-risk tumors, target level for TSH suppression may be lower.

ADMINISTRATION

PO

• Have patient swallow capsules whole; don't crush or break capsules.

• Give drug at same time each day on an empty stomach, preferably ½ to 1 hour before breakfast.

• Give drug at least 4 hours before or after drugs known to interfere with levothyroxine.

• Give tablets with a full glass of water to prevent difficulty swallowing.

• If necessary, crush tablets and suspend in small amount of formula (except soy, which may decrease absorption), human milk, or water, and give by spoon or dropper.

• Give solution directly into mouth using calibrated oral syringe.

IV

▼ Reconstitute powder by adding 5 mL NSS injection only.

▼ Shake vial.

▼ Use immediately after reconstitution.

▼ Give at a rate not to exceed 100 mcg/minute.

▼ Discard any unused portion.

▼ **Incompatibilities:** Don't mix or give with anything other than NSS injection.

ACTION

Synthetic form of thyroxine that affects tissue growth, energy expenditure, and turnover of all substrates.

Route	Onset	Peak	Duration
PO	3–5 days	2–4 hr	Unknown
IV	6–8 hr	Unknown	Unknown

Half-life: 6 to 7 days in euthyroidism; 3 to 4 days in hyperthyroidism; 9 to 10 days in hypothyroidism.

ADVERSE REACTIONS

Note: Adverse reactions are primarily related to hyperthyroidism due to therapeutic overdosage.

CNS: insomnia, tremor, headache, fever, fatigue, anxiety, emotional lability. **CV:** tachycardia, palpitations, *arrhythmias,* angina pectoris, HTN, *HF.* **GI:** diarrhea, vomiting, abdominal cramps, increased appetite. **GU:** menstrual irregularities, impaired fertility. **Metabolic:** weight loss. **Musculoskeletal:** decreased bone density, muscle weakness, tremors. **Respiratory:** dyspnea.

Skin: allergic skin reactions, diaphoresis, hair loss. **Other:** heat intolerance, hypersensitivity reaction.

INTERACTIONS

Drug-drug. *Amiodarone, iodide (including iodine-containing radiographic contrast agents), lithium:* May reduce thyroid hormone secretion. Monitor thyroid function studies if used together.

Antacids (aluminum-, magnesium-containing), orlistat, PPIs, sevelamer, simethicone, sucralfate: May decrease levothyroxine level. Monitor therapy.

Colesevelam, cholestyramine, colestipol, sodium polystyrene sulfonate: May impair levothyroxine absorption. Separate doses by 4 to 5 hours and monitor therapy.

Beta blockers: May reduce beta-blocker effects. Monitor patient.

Carbamazepine, phenobarbital, rifampin: May increase metabolism of levothyroxine, resulting in hypothyroidism. Monitor patient.

Clofibrate, estrogens, 5-flourouracil, methadone, mitotane, tamoxifen: May decrease therapeutic effect of levothyroxine. Monitor therapy.

Digoxin: May decrease cardiac glycoside effects. Monitor patient for clinical effect.

Fosphenytoin, phenytoin: May release free thyroid hormone but total and free thyroxine levels may decrease. Monitor thyroxine level.

Insulin, oral antidiabetics: May alter glucose level. Monitor glucose level. Dosage adjustment may be needed.

Ketamine: May produce marked HTN and tachycardia. Use together cautiously.

SSRIs: May increase levothyroxine requirements. Adjust dosage as needed.

Sympathomimetics (epinephrine): May increase risk of coronary insufficiency. Monitor patient closely.

TCAs, tetracyclic antidepressants: May increase therapeutic effects and toxicity of both drugs. Monitor patient closely.

Tyrosine kinase inhibitors (dasatinib, imatinib): May decrease levothyroxine level. Monitor therapy.

Warfarin: May increase anticoagulant effects. Monitor patient for bleeding, and check PT and INR closely. Warfarin dosage adjustment may be needed.

Drug-herb. *Horseradish:* May cause abnormal thyroid function. Discourage use in patients undergoing thyroid function tests.

Lemon balm: May have antithyroid effects; may inhibit TSH. Discourage use together.

Drug-food. *Cottonseed meal, dietary fiber, soybean flour, walnuts:* May decrease drug absorption. Dosage adjustments may be needed. *Grapefruit juice:* May delay drug absorption. Tell patient to avoid use together.

EFFECTS ON LAB TEST RESULTS

• May increase calcium and phosphorous levels and LFT values.
• May decrease parathyroid hormone levels.
• May decrease thyroid function test results.
• May alter results of liothyronine, protein-bound iodine, and radioactive ^{131}I uptake studies.

CONTRAINDICATIONS & CAUTIONS

• Contraindicated in patients hypersensitive to drug or glycerol (Tirosint oral solution) and those with uncorrected adrenal insufficiency.

Boxed Warning Don't use either alone or with other therapeutic agents for treatment of obesity or for weight loss. ∎

Boxed Warning Doses beyond the range of daily hormonal requirements may produce serious or even life-threatening toxicities, especially if given with sympathomimetic amines. ∎

• Use cautiously in older adults and in patients with angina pectoris, HTN, other CV disorders, kidney insufficiency, or ischemia.
• Use cautiously in patients with diabetes, diabetes insipidus, or myxedema and during rapid replacement in those with arteriosclerosis.

Dialyzable drug: No.

⚠ *Overdose S&S:* Signs and symptoms of hyperthyroidism, confusion, disorientation, cerebral embolism, shock, coma, seizures, death.

PREGNANCY-LACTATION-REPRODUCTION

• Drug is safe to use and shouldn't be discontinued during pregnancy.
• Dosage may need to be increased in pregnancy. Measure serum TSH and free T_4 levels as soon as pregnancy is confirmed and, at minimum, during each trimester of pregnancy. Reduce dosage to prepregnancy levels immediately after delivery and measure serum TSH level 4 to 8 weeks postpartum.
• For new-onset hypothyroidism during pregnancy, normalize thyroid function as rapidly as possible. In patients with moderate to

---

Reactions in bold italics are *life-threatening*.

severe signs and symptoms, start drug at 1.6 mcg/kg daily. In patients with mild hypothyroidism, start drug at 1 mcg/kg daily. Evaluate serum TSH level every 4 weeks and adjust dosage as indicated.
• Don't use drug for infertility (unless associated with hypothyroidism).
• Drug appears minimally in human milk. Adequate replacement doses of levothyroxine are generally needed to maintain normal lactation in patients with hypothyroidism and should be continued during breastfeeding.

NURSING CONSIDERATIONS
• Monitor for loss of glycemic control in patient with diabetes. Antidiabetic doses may need to be increased when starting thyroid hormone replacement.
• In patient with CAD who must receive thyroid hormone, observe carefully for possible coronary insufficiency.
• Patients with adult hypothyroidism are unusually sensitive to thyroid hormone. Start at lowest dosage, and adjust to higher dosages according to patient's symptoms and lab data until euthyroid state is reached.
• Long-term therapy causes bone loss during premenopause. Consider basal bone density measurement, and closely monitor patient for osteoporosis.
• Patients taking levothyroxine who need to have ^{131}I uptake studies performed must stop drug 4 weeks before test.
• Patients taking anticoagulants may need their dosage modified and require careful monitoring of coagulation status.
• *Look alike–sound alike:* Don't confuse levothyroxine with lamotrigine, liothyronine, or Lanoxin.

PATIENT TEACHING
• Teach patient importance of consistently taking drug at same time each day to maintain constant hormone levels.
• Teach about proper drug administration and handling.
• Make sure patient understands that replacement therapy is usually for life. Drug should never be stopped unless directed by prescriber.
• Warn patient (especially older adult) to immediately report chest pain, palpitations, diaphoresis, nervousness, shortness of breath, or other signals of overdose or aggravated CV disease.

• Tell patient to report unusual bleeding and bruising or any other adverse reaction.
• Caution patient to tell prescriber about all medications, both OTC and prescription, and herbal products being taken.
• Instruct patient with diabetes to closely monitor glucose level and report changes.
• Tell patient who plans to have surgery to notify physician or dentist about taking levothyroxine.
• Advise patient to report pregnancy to prescriber because dosage may need adjustment.

SAFETY ALERT!

lidocaine hydrochloride (IV)
LYE-doe-kane

Xylocard✦

Therapeutic class: Antiarrhythmics
Pharmacologic class: Amide derivatives

AVAILABLE FORMS
Infusion (premixed): 0.2% (2 mg/mL), 0.4% (4 mg/mL), 0.8% (8 mg/mL)
Injection (for direct IV use): 0.5% (5 mg/mL), 1% (10 mg/mL), 2% (20 mg/mL)
Injection (for IV admixtures): 4% (40 mg/mL)

INDICATIONS & DOSAGES
➤ **Ventricular arrhythmias caused by MI, cardiac manipulation, or cardiac glycosides**
Adults: 50 to 100 mg by IV bolus at 25 to 50 mg/minute. Repeat bolus dose every 5 minutes until arrhythmia subsides or adverse reactions develop. Don't exceed 300-mg total bolus during 1-hour period. Simultaneously, begin infusion of 20 to 50 mcg/kg/minute (1 to 4 mg/minute). If single bolus has been given, smaller bolus dose may be repeated 15 to 20 minutes after start of infusion to maintain therapeutic level.
Adjust-a-dose: Reduce dosage and rate of infusion in older adults.
➤ **Ventricular arrhythmias; shock-refractory ventricular fibrillation; pulseless ventricular tachycardia ◆**
Children: 1 mg/kg by IV or intraosseous bolus. May repeat infusion, starting more than 15 minutes from first bolus. Start infusion at 20 to 50 mcg/kg/minute.
Adjust-a-dose: Reduce dosage in patients who have HF or kidney or liver disease and those who weigh less than 50 kg.

L

ADMINISTRATION

IV

▼ Give IV bolus at 25 to 50 mg/minute.

▼ Injections (additive syringes and single-use vials) containing 40 to 200 mg/mL are for the preparation of IV infusion solutions only and must be diluted before use.

▼ Prepare IV infusion by adding 1 g (using 25 mL of 4%) to 1 L of D₅W injection to provide a solution containing 1 mg/mL.

▼ Use a more concentrated solution of up to 8 mg/mL in patients with fluid restrictions.

▼ Continuously monitor cardiac rhythm in patients receiving infusions. Use infusion control device to give infusion precisely. Don't exceed 4 mg/minute; faster rate greatly increases risk of toxicity.

▼ Avoid giving injections containing preservatives.

▼ **Incompatibilities:** None listed by manufacturer. Consult drug compatibility reference for more information.

ACTION

A class IB antiarrhythmic that decreases depolarization, automaticity, and excitability in the ventricles during the diastolic phase by direct action on the tissues, especially the Purkinje network.

Route	Onset	Peak	Duration
IV	Rapid	Unknown	15–20 min

Half-life: 1.5 to 2 hours (may be prolonged in patients with HF or liver disease).

ADVERSE REACTIONS

CNS: apprehension, confusion, dizziness, drowsiness, tremor, stupor, restlessness, light-headedness, *seizures,* unconsciousness, lethargy, somnolence, anxiety, euphoria, hallucinations, nervousness, paresthesia, muscle twitching, sensation of cold, heat, or numbness. **CV:** hypotension, *bradycardia, new or worsened arrhythmias, cardiac arrest.* **EENT:** blurred or double vision, tinnitus. **GI:** vomiting. **Hematologic:** *methemoglobinemia.* **Respiratory:** *respiratory depression and arrest.* **Skin:** soreness at injection site.

INTERACTIONS

Drug-drug. *Atenolol, metoprolol, nadolol, pindolol, propranolol:* May increase lidocaine level, increasing risk of toxicity. Give bolus doses of lidocaine at slower rate. Closely monitor lidocaine level and patient.

Cimetidine: May decrease clearance of lidocaine, increasing risk of toxicity. Consider a different H₂-receptor antagonist, if possible. Closely monitor lidocaine level.

Ergot-type oxytocic drugs: May cause severe, persistent HTN or stroke. Avoid use together.

Mexiletine: May increase pharmacologic effects. Avoid use together.

Phenytoin, procainamide, propranolol, quinidine: May increase cardiac depressant effects. Monitor patient closely.

Succinylcholine: May prolong neuromuscular blockade. Monitor patient closely.

EFFECTS ON LAB TEST RESULTS

None reported.

CONTRAINDICATIONS & CAUTIONS

● Contraindicated in patients hypersensitive to amide-type local anesthetics.

● Contraindicated in those with Adams-Stokes syndrome, Wolff-Parkinson-White syndrome, and severe degrees of SA, AV, or intraventricular block in the absence of an artificial pacemaker.

● Use cautiously and at reduced dosages in patients with complete or second-degree heart block or sinus bradycardia, older adults, those with HF or kidney or liver disease, and those weighing less than 50 kg.

Dialyzable drug: No.

⚠ *Overdose S&S:* Circulatory depression, change in level of consciousness, seizures, hypoventilation.

PREGNANCY-LACTATION-REPRODUCTION

● Studies with IV lidocaine during pregnancy are inadequate. Use cautiously if clearly needed, especially during early pregnancy.

● Drug appears in human milk. Use cautiously during breastfeeding.

NURSING CONSIDERATIONS

● Monitor drug level. Therapeutic levels are 1.5 to 5 mcg/mL.

⚠ *Alert:* Monitor patient for toxicity. In many patients who are severely ill, seizures may be the first sign of toxicity, but severe reactions are usually preceded by somnolence, confusion, tremors, and paresthesia. If signs of toxicity occur, immediately stop drug and notify prescriber. Continuing could lead to seizures and coma. Give oxygen through a nasal cannula, if not contraindicated. Keep oxygen and CPR equipment available.

• Continuously monitor ECG with IV use.
• Monitor patient's response, especially BP and electrolyte, BUN, and creatinine levels.
• Correct electrolyte disturbances, especially hypokalemia or hypomagnesemia.
• If arrhythmias worsen or ECG changes occur (for example, QRS complex widens or PR interval substantially prolongs), stop infusion and notify prescriber.
• Discontinue infusion when patient's cardiac rhythm stabilizes or at earliest signs of toxicity. If indicated, begin oral antiarrhythmic maintenance therapy.

PATIENT TEACHING

• Tell patient to promptly report adverse reactions, such as palpitations, dyspnea, confusion, anxiety, vision changes, dizziness, tinnitus, nausea, and vomiting, because toxicity can occur.

SAFETY ALERT!

linagliptin
lin-a-GLIP-tin

Tradjenta

Therapeutic class: Antidiabetics
Pharmacologic class: DPP-4 inhibitors

AVAILABLE FORMS
Tablets: 5 mg

INDICATIONS & DOSAGES
➤ **Adjunct to diet and exercise to improve glycemic control in adults with type 2 diabetes as monotherapy or as combination therapy with an insulin secretagogue (such as a sulfonylurea) or insulin**
Adults: 5 mg PO daily.
Adjust-a-dose: When used in combination with an insulin secretagogue or insulin, use lower dosages of those drugs to decrease risk of hypoglycemia.

ADMINISTRATION
PO
• Give drug without regard to food.
• If dose is missed, give as soon as possible. Don't double dose.
• Store tablets at 77° F (25° C).

ACTION
Inhibits DPP-4, an enzyme that rapidly inactivates incretin hormones, which play a part in the body's regulation of glucose.

Route	Onset	Peak	Duration
PO	Rapid	1.5 hr	Unknown

Half-life: About 12 hours (accumulation).

ADVERSE REACTIONS
CNS: headache. **EENT:** nasopharyngitis. **GI:** diarrhea, constipation. **GU:** UTI. **Metabolic:** hyperlipidemia, weight gain, increased uric acid level, increased amylase level, increased lipase level, *hypoglycemia.* **Musculoskeletal:** arthralgia, back pain, myalgia. **Respiratory:** cough, URI.

INTERACTIONS
Drug-drug. *CYP3A4 or P-gp inducers (rifampin):* May decrease linagliptin level. Avoid use together.
Ritonavir: May increase linagliptin effects and risk of adverse effects. Use with caution; monitor response, and adjust dosage as necessary.
Sulfonylureas (glyburide), insulin: May increase risk of hypoglycemia. Carefully monitor glucose level, and adjust sulfonylurea or insulin dosage as necessary.
Drug-herb. *St. John's wort:* May decrease linagliptin level. Discourage use together.

EFFECTS ON LAB TEST RESULTS
• May increase lipase, amylase, triglycerides, and uric acid levels.
• May decrease glucose level.

CONTRAINDICATIONS & CAUTIONS
• Contraindicated in patients hypersensitive to drug.
• Drug not for use in patients with type 1 diabetes or for treatment of diabetic ketoacidosis.
• Use cautiously in patients at risk for HF.
• Acute pancreatitis, including fatal cases, has occurred in patients taking linagliptin. It's unknown whether patients with history of pancreatitis are at increased risk for development of pancreatitis while using linagliptin.
• Drug may cause joint pain that can be severe and disabling. Onset can range from days to years.
• Safety in children hasn't been established.
Dialyzable drug: Unlikely.

L

PREGNANCY-LACTATION-REPRODUCTION
• Studies during pregnancy are inadequate. Use during pregnancy only if clearly needed.
• It isn't known if drug appears in human milk. Use cautiously during breastfeeding.

NURSING CONSIDERATIONS
• Periodically monitor HbA$_{1c}$ and fasting blood glucose levels.
• Monitor patient for signs and symptoms of hypoglycemia (anxiety, confusion, diaphoresis, tachycardia, paresthesia) and hyperglycemia (excess thirst, urination).
• Insulin and insulin secretagogues are known to cause hypoglycemia; risk increases with linagliptin use.
• Monitor patient for signs and symptoms of pancreatitis (persistent, severe abdominal pain, which may radiate to back, and vomiting). If pancreatitis is suspected, promptly discontinue linagliptin and initiate appropriate management.
• Monitor patient for signs and symptoms of HF, especially patient with history of HF or kidney failure.
• Postmarketing cases of bullous pemphigoid requiring hospitalization have been reported in patients taking DPP-4 inhibitors. Monitor for signs and symptoms, including blisters or erosions. If bullous pemphigoid is suspected, discontinue linagliptin and refer patient to dermatologist for diagnosis and appropriate treatment.
• Monitor for hypersensitivity reactions, including anaphylaxis and SCARs.
• **Look alike–sound alike:** Don't confuse linagliptin with linaclotide.

PATIENT TEACHING
• Inform patient of risks and benefits of linagliptin and alternative modes of therapy.
• Instruct patient to take drug only as prescribed.
• Explain importance of proper diet, regular physical activity, and periodic blood glucose monitoring.
• Teach patient to recognize and manage hypoglycemia and hyperglycemia.
• Advise patient to promptly notify health care provider of periods of stress (fever, trauma, infection, surgery) because medication requirements may change.
• Review signs and symptoms of pancreatitis. Instruct patient to immediately contact prescriber if any occur.

• Advise patient to report blisters or erosions, severe joint pain, or signs and symptoms of HF (shortness of breath, edema, weight gain).

linezolid
lih-NEH-zoe-lid

Zyvox

Therapeutic class: Antibiotics
Pharmacologic class: Oxazolidinones

AVAILABLE FORMS
Injection: 200 mg/100 mL, 600 mg/300 mL ready-to-use bags
Powder for oral suspension: 100 mg/5 mL when reconstituted
Tablets: 600 mg

INDICATIONS & DOSAGES
➤ **Vancomycin-resistant *Enterococcus faecium* infections, including those with concurrent bacteremia**
Adults and children ages 12 and older: 600 mg IV or PO every 12 hours for 14 to 28 days.
Full-term neonates, infants, and children through age 11: 10 mg/kg IV or PO every 8 hours for 14 to 28 days.
Preterm neonates younger than age 7 days (gestational age less than 34 weeks):
10 mg/kg IV or PO every 12 hours for 14 to 28 days. Increase to 10 mg/kg every 8 hours when patient is 7 days old. Consider this dosage increase if neonate has inadequate response.
➤ **Hospital-acquired pneumonia caused by *Staphylococcus aureus* (methicillin-susceptible [MSSA] and MRSA strains) or *Streptococcus pneumoniae;* complicated skin and skin-structure infections, including diabetic foot infections without osteomyelitis caused by *S. aureus* (MSSA and MRSA), *Streptococcus pyogenes*, or *Streptococcus agalactiae;* community-acquired pneumonia caused by *S. pneumoniae*, including those with concurrent bacteremia, or *S. aureus* (MSSA only)**
Adults and children ages 12 and older: 600 mg IV or PO every 12 hours for 10 to 14 days.
Full-term neonates, infants, and children through age 11: 10 mg/kg IV or PO every 8 hours for 10 to 14 days.
Preterm neonates younger than age 7 days (gestational age less than 34 weeks):

10 mg/kg IV or PO every 12 hours for 10 to 14 days. Increase to 10 mg/kg every 8 hours when patient is 7 days old. Consider this dosage increase if neonate has inadequate response.

➤ **Uncomplicated skin and skin-structure infections caused by *S. aureus* (MSSA only) or *S. pyogenes***

Adults: 400 mg PO every 12 hours for 10 to 14 days.

Children ages 12 to 18: 600 mg PO every 12 hours for 10 to 14 days.

Children ages 5 to 11: 10 mg/kg PO every 12 hours for 10 to 14 days.

Full-term neonates, infants, and children younger than age 5: 10 mg/kg PO every 8 hours for 10 to 14 days.

Preterm neonates younger than age 7 days (gestational age less than 34 weeks): 10 mg/kg PO every 12 hours for 10 to 14 days. Increase to 10 mg/kg every 8 hours when patient is 7 days old. Consider this dosage increase if neonate has inadequate response.

ADMINISTRATION
PO

• Give tablets and suspension without regard to meals.

• Give one of twice-daily doses after hemodialysis on dialysis days.

• Reconstitute suspension according to manufacturer's instructions.

• Store reconstituted suspension at room temperature and use within 21 days.

IV

▼ Inspect solution for particulate matter and leaks.

▼ Don't inject additives into infusion bag. Give other IV drugs separately or via a separate IV line to avoid incompatibilities. If single IV line is used, flush line before and after infusion with a compatible solution.

▼ Infuse over 30 minutes to 2 hours. Don't infuse drug in a series connection.

▼ Give after hemodialysis on dialysis days.

▼ Store drug at room temperature in its protective overwrap. Solution may turn yellow over time, but this doesn't affect drug's potency.

▼ **Incompatibilities:** Amphotericin B, ceftriaxone, chlorpromazine hydrochloride, diazepam, erythromycin lactobionate, pentamidine isethionate, phenytoin, trimethoprim–sulfamethoxazole.

ACTION

Prevents bacterial protein synthesis by interfering with DNA translation in ribosomes. Also prevents formation of a functional 70S ribosomal subunit by binding to a site on the bacterial 50S ribosomal subunit; this limits bacterial reproduction.

Route	Onset	Peak	Duration
PO	Unknown	1–2 hr	Unknown
IV	Unknown	30 min	Unknown

Half-life: Adults, 4 to 5 hours; children ages 1 week to 11 years, 1.5 to 3 hours.

ADVERSE REACTIONS

CNS: headache, dizziness, fever, altered taste, insomnia; vertigo (children). **EENT:** oral candidiasis, tongue discoloration. **GI:** diarrhea, nausea, constipation, vomiting, abdominal pain. **GU:** vaginal candidiasis. **Hepatic:** increased LFT values. **Hematologic:** *leukopenia, myelosuppression, neutropenia, thrombocytopenia,* eosinophilia, anemia. **Skin:** rash, pruritus. **Other:** fungal infection.

INTERACTIONS

Drug-drug. *Adrenergic drugs (dopamine, epinephrine, pseudoephedrine):* May cause HTN. Monitor BP and HR; start continuous infusions of dopamine and epinephrine at lower doses and titrate to response.

Insulin, oral antidiabetics: May cause symptomatic hypoglycemia. Monitor patient closely.

MAO inhibitors (isocarboxazid, phenelzine): May increase risk of hypertensive crisis or serotonin syndrome. Use within 14 days of MAO inhibitor is contraindicated.

Serotonergic drugs (bupropion, buspirone, opioids, SSNRIs, SSRIs, TCAs, triptans): May cause serotonin syndrome or NMS-like reactions. Avoid use together.

Drug-food. *Foods and beverages high in tyramine (aged cheeses, air-dried meats, red wines, sauerkraut, soy sauce, tap beers):* May increase BP. Provide a list of foods that contain tyramine and advise that tyramine content of meals shouldn't exceed 100 mg.

EFFECTS ON LAB TEST RESULTS

• May increase ALT, AST, bilirubin, ALP, BUN, creatinine, amylase, lipase, and LDH levels.

• May decrease glucose level.

• May decrease Hb level and WBC, neutrophil, and platelet counts.

CONTRAINDICATIONS & CAUTIONS
• Contraindicated in patients hypersensitive to drug or its components.
• Drug isn't recommended in patients with carcinoid syndrome.
• Use cautiously while monitoring BP in patients with uncontrolled HTN, pheochromocytoma, or thyrotoxicosis and in patients taking sympathomimetics, vasopressors, or dopaminergics.
• Use cautiously in patients with history of or risk factors for seizures and diabetes.
⚠ *Alert:* Concomitant use with psychiatric drugs or within 2 weeks of taking psychiatric drugs that work through serotonin system of brain (SSRIs, SSNRIs, TCAs, MAO inhibitors, and others) can cause serotonin syndrome. Use linezolid with these drugs only for life-threatening or urgent conditions when potential benefits outweigh toxicity risk.
Dialyzable drug: 30%.

PREGNANCY-LACTATION-REPRODUCTION
• Studies during pregnancy are inadequate. Use during pregnancy only if potential benefit justifies fetal risk.
• Drug may appear in human milk. Use cautiously during breastfeeding.

NURSING CONSIDERATIONS
• No dosage adjustment is needed when switching from IV to oral forms.
⚠ *Alert:* Before giving linezolid, stop any serotonergic drug and monitor patient for serotonin toxicity for 2 weeks (5 weeks if fluoxetine was taken) or until 24 hours after last dose of linezolid, whichever comes first. May resume serotonergic psychiatric drugs 24 hours after last dose of linezolid.
⚠ *Alert:* Nausea and vomiting may be symptoms of lactic acidosis. Monitor patient for unexplained acidosis or low bicarbonate level, and immediately notify prescriber if they occur.
• Monitor platelet count in patients at increased risk for bleeding, those with existing thrombocytopenia, those taking other drugs that may cause thrombocytopenia, and those receiving linezolid for longer than 14 days.
• Drug may lead to myelosuppression. Monitor CBC weekly.

⚠ *Alert:* Prolonged use can cause superinfection, including CDAD, which can occur more than 2 months after treatment ends. Consider these diagnoses and take appropriate measures in patients with persistent diarrhea or secondary infections.
• Drug may cause symptomatic hypoglycemia in patients taking insulin or oral antidiabetics. Monitor patient closely.
• Inappropriate use of antibiotics may lead to development of resistant organisms; carefully consider other drugs before starting therapy, especially in outpatient setting.
• Peripheral and optic neuropathies can occur, especially in patients treated for longer-than-recommended duration. If these neuropathies occur, drug may need to be discontinued. Patients with vision changes should receive prompt ophthalmic evaluation.
• Monitor for seizures.
• Monitor for hyponatremia confusion, somnolence, weakness and, in severe cases, respiratory failure and death.
• *Look alike–sound alike:* Don't confuse Zyvox with Zovirax.

PATIENT TEACHING
• Teach about proper drug administration and handling.
• Stress importance of completing entire course of therapy, even if patient feels better.
• Tell patient to promptly report all adverse reactions.
• Caution patient to report high BP; use of cough or cold preparations, insulin, or oral antidiabetics; or treatment with SSRIs or other antidepressants.
⚠ *Alert:* Teach patient to recognize and immediately report signs and symptoms of serotonin toxicity (fever, mental status changes, muscle twitching, diaphoresis, shivering or shaking, diarrhea, loss of coordination).
• Advise patient taking prescribed psychiatric drugs that these drugs may need to be stopped during linezolid therapy but not to stop them without first speaking to prescriber.
• Teach patient to avoid eating large quantities of tyramine-containing foods (aged cheeses, soy sauce, tap beers, red wine) during therapy.
• Inform patient with phenylketonuria that each 5 mL of oral suspension contains 20 mg of phenylalanine. Tablets and injection don't contain phenylalanine.

Reactions in bold italics are *life-threatening*.

liraglutide
leer-ah-GLOO-tide

Saxenda, Victoza

Therapeutic class: Antidiabetics
Pharmacologic class: Glucagon-like
peptide-1 receptor agonists

AVAILABLE FORMS
Injection: 6-mg/mL prefilled multidose pens
that deliver doses of 0.6 mg, 1.2 mg, 1.8 mg,
2.4 mg, or 3 mg (Saxenda) or 0.6 mg, 1.2 mg,
or 1.8 mg (Victoza)

INDICATIONS & DOSAGES
➤ **Adjunct to diet and exercise to improve
glycemic control in patients with type 2 diabetes (Victoza)**
Adults and children older than age 10: Initially, 0.6 mg subcut daily; after 1 week, increase dosage to 1.2 mg subcut daily. May
increase dosage to 1.8 mg subcut daily if
needed to achieve glycemic control.
➤ **To reduce risk of major adverse CV
events in patients with type 2 diabetes and
established CV disease (Victoza)**
Adults: Initially, 0.6 mg subcut daily; after
1 week, increase dosage to 1.2 mg daily. May
increase dosage to 1.8 mg subcut daily if
needed to achieve glycemic control.
➤ **Adjunct to diet and exercise for long-
term weight management in adults with
initial BMI of 30 kg/m² or greater (obese)
or 27 kg/m² or greater (overweight) in the
presence of at least one weight-related comorbid condition (HTN, type 2 diabetes, or
dyslipidemia) (Saxenda)**
Adults: Initially, 0.6 mg subcut once daily
for 1 week. Increase by 0.6 mg/day subcut at
weekly intervals to a target dosage of 3 mg
once daily. If patient can't tolerate increased
dose during titration period, consider delaying dosage escalation for 1 week. Discontinue
drug if 3-mg dose isn't tolerated; effectiveness at lower doses hasn't been established.
➤ **Adjunct to diet and exercise for long-
term weight management in children
weighing more than 60 kg with initial BMI
corresponding to 30 kg/m² or greater for
adults (obese) by international cut-offs
(Saxenda)**

Refer to manufacturer's prescribing information for international cut-offs (Cole criteria).
Children ages 12 and older: Initially, 0.6 mg
subcut once daily for 1 week. Increase by
0.6 mg/day subcut at weekly intervals to target dose of 3 mg once daily. If increased dose
isn't tolerated, may lower dose to previous
level. Dose escalation for children may take
up to 8 weeks.
Adjust-a-dose: For children who don't tolerate
Saxenda 3 mg daily, may reduce dosage to
2.4 mg daily; discontinue if 2.4 mg daily isn't
tolerated.

ADMINISTRATION
Subcutaneous
⊘ *Alert:* Hazardous drug; use safe handling
and disposal precautions.
• Give drug once daily at any time of day, independently of meals. Inject into abdomen,
thigh, or upper arm. Rotate injection sites
within same region. Injection site and timing
can change without dosage adjustment.
• Don't mix drug with insulin for injection or
inject liraglutide and insulin in adjacent areas
at the same time.
• If dose is missed, don't increase subsequent
dose. Resume once-daily regimen with next
scheduled dose. If more than 3 days have
elapsed, initiate dose at 0.6 mg daily and, for
Victoza, increase as directed by prescriber
or, for Saxenda, increase weekly per titration
schedule to limit GI adverse reactions.
• Inspect solution before each injection. Use
solution only if it is clear, colorless, and contains no particles.
⊘ *Alert:* Multidose pens are for single-patient
use only. Never share pens (even if needle is changed). Clearly label with patient-
identifying information where it won't obstruct dosing window, warning, or other product information.
• Before first use, store drug in refrigerator
between 36° and 46° F (2° and 8° C). Discard
if pen freezes.
• After initial use, store liraglutide pen for
30 days at room temperature (59° to 86° F
[15° to 30° C]) or in refrigerator (36° to
46° F). Keep pen cap on when not in use.
Discard pen after 30 days.

ACTION
Stimulates insulin secretion and reduces
glucagon secretion; delays gastric emptying.

Route	Onset	Peak	Duration
Subcut	Unknown	8–12 hr	Unknown

Half-life: 13 hours.

ADVERSE REACTIONS

CNS: headache, dizziness, fatigue, fever, insomnia, anxiety, weakness, asthenia, depression. **CV:** increased HR, tachycardia. **EENT:** dry mouth, nasopharyngitis. **GI:** constipation, diarrhea, dyspepsia, nausea, vomiting, abdominal distention or pain, decreased appetite, flatulence, GERD, gastroenteritis. **GU:** UTI. **Hepatic:** cholelithiasis. **Metabolic:** increased lipase level, dyslipidemia, increased CK level, *hypoglycemia.* **Musculoskeletal:** limb pain, back pain. **Respiratory:** URI, cough. **Skin:** injection-site reactions, rash. **Other:** anti-liraglutide antibody formation.

INTERACTIONS

Drug-drug. *GLP-receptor agonists (liraglutide):* Duplicates treatment. Don't combine with other GLP-1 receptor agonists or other liraglutide-containing products.
Insulin, insulin secretagogues (sulfonylureas): May increase risk of hypoglycemia. Reduce insulin or secretagogue dosage before beginning Victoza and as needed. Saxenda hasn't been studied in patients taking insulin; don't use together.
Oral medications: May impair absorption of oral drugs because of delayed gastric emptying. Use together cautiously.

EFFECTS ON LAB TEST RESULTS

• May increase bilirubin, AST, ALT, amylase, lipase, and calcitonin levels.
• May decrease blood glucose level.

CONTRAINDICATIONS & CAUTIONS

Boxed Warning Drug causes dose-dependent and treatment duration-dependent thyroid C-cell tumors at clinically relevant exposures in both sexes of rats and mice. Unknown if drug causes thyroid C-cell tumors, including medullary thyroid carcinoma (MTC), in humans, as the human relevance of liraglutide-induced rodent thyroid C-cell tumors hasn't been determined. ■
Boxed Warning Contraindicated in patients with personal or family history of MTC and in patients with multiple endocrine neoplasia syndrome type 2. ■

• Contraindicated in patients with prior serious hypersensitivity reaction to liraglutide or its components.
• Avoid Saxenda use in patients with a history of or active suicidality.
• Use cautiously in patients with kidney or liver impairment and in those with history of pancreatitis or gallbladder disease.
• **Alert:** Acute pancreatitis, including fatal pancreatitis and nonfatal hemorrhagic or necrotizing pancreatitis, has occurred in patients taking liraglutide.
• Victoza isn't a substitute for insulin; don't use for treatment of diabetic ketoacidosis or type 1 diabetes.
• Victoza hasn't been studied in combination with prandial insulin.
• Saxenda isn't indicated for treatment of type 2 diabetes.
• Saxenda and Victoza contain same active ingredient and shouldn't be used together.
• Safety and effectiveness of Saxenda in combination with other products intended for weight loss haven't been established.
• Older adults may be more sensitive to drug. Use cautiously.
Dialyzable drug: Unknown.
Overdose S&S: Nausea, vomiting, hypoglycemia.

PREGNANCY-LACTATION-REPRODUCTION

• Studies of Victoza during pregnancy are inadequate. Use during pregnancy only if potential benefit justifies fetal risk.
• Saxenda is contraindicated during pregnancy because weight loss offers no potential benefit to patient who is pregnant and may result in fetal harm.
• It isn't known if drug appears in human milk. Drug appeared in milk of lactating rats. Weigh benefits of therapy against risks.

NURSING CONSIDERATIONS

• Evaluate change in body weight 16 weeks after start of therapy; discontinue Saxenda if body weight loss of at least 4% of baseline hasn't been achieved.
• For child taking Saxenda, evaluate change in body weight 12 weeks after start of therapy; discontinue drug if weight loss of at least 1% of baseline hasn't been achieved.
• Monitor patient closely for signs and symptoms of pancreatitis. Promptly discontinue drug if pancreatitis is suspected. Don't restart if pancreatitis is confirmed.

Reactions in bold italics are *life-threatening*.

• *Alert:* Patients with thyroid nodules found on exam or neck imaging and patients with elevated serum calcitonin level should be evaluated by an endocrinologist.

• Drug may increase risk of gallbladder and bile duct disease. If cholelithiasis is suspected, gallbladder studies and appropriate clinical follow-up are indicated.

• *Alert:* Monitor patient for emergence or worsening of depression, suicidality, and unusual changes in mood or behavior. Discontinue drug in patient who experiences suicidality.

• Drug isn't recommended for first-line therapy in patients who have inadequate glycemic control with diet and exercise.

• Monitor blood glucose and HbA_{1c} levels. Consider decreasing insulin and insulin secretagogue (such as sulfonylurea) dosage when initiating liraglutide.

• Monitor patient for signs and symptoms of hypoglycemia (tachycardia, palpitations, anxiety, hunger, nausea, diaphoresis, tremors, pallor, restlessness, headache, speech and motor dysfunction).

• Monitor GI status; drug slows gastric emptying.

• Monitor HR and assess for palpitations. Discontinue Saxenda for sustained increased resting heart rate.

PATIENT TEACHING

Boxed Warning Counsel patient regarding risk of MTC and describe signs and symptoms of thyroid tumors (neck mass, dysphagia, dyspnea, persistent hoarseness). ▊

• *Alert:* Counsel patient, family member, or caregivers to monitor patent for changes in behavior and to immediately report suicidality.

• Advise patient to report signs and symptoms of acute gallbladder disease or cholelithiasis (sudden, rapidly intensifying pain in upper right portion of abdomen or in center of abdomen, just below breastbone; back pain between shoulder blades; pain in right shoulder; nausea; vomiting).

• Caution patient to stop drug and report signs and symptoms of pancreatitis (persistent, severe abdominal pain that may radiate to back and may or may not be accompanied by vomiting).

• *Alert:* Warn patient not to share multidose pen with other people (even if needle is changed) because of risk of infection, including HIV and hepatitis.

• Emphasize to patient importance of adhering to diet and exercise program and monitoring glucose and HbA_{1c} levels.

• Advise patient of risk of dehydration; encourage hydration.

• Instruct patient to report palpitations or racing heartbeat.

• Warn patient of risk of hypersensitivity reactions and advise patient to report any reactions that occur.

• Teach patient how to give subcut injection; instruct patient to rotate sites to prevent injection-site reactions.

• Instruct patient to report pregnancy or plans to become pregnant or breastfeed.

lisdexamfetamine dimesylate
lis-DEX-am-FET-a-meen

Vyvanse

Therapeutic class: CNS stimulants
Pharmacologic class: Amphetamines
Controlled substance schedule: II

AVAILABLE FORMS
Capsules ◍: 10 mg, 20 mg, 30 mg, 40 mg, 50 mg, 60 mg, 70 mg
Tablets (chewable): 10 mg, 20 mg, 30 mg, 40 mg, 50 mg, 60 mg

INDICATIONS & DOSAGES
Adjust-a-dose (for all indications): For patients with GFR of 15 mL to less than 30 mL/minute/1.73 m², maximum dosage is 50 mg/day. For those with GFR less than 15 mL/minute/1.73 m², maximum dosage is 30 mg/day.

➤ **ADHD**
Adults and children ages 6 to 17: Initially, 30 mg PO once daily in the morning. Increase by 10 or 20 mg at weekly intervals to target dose of 30 to 70 mg/day. Maximum dosage, 70 mg/day.

➤ **Moderate to severe binge eating disorder (BED)**
Adults: Initially, 30 mg PO once daily in the morning. Increase by 20 mg at weekly intervals to target dosage of 50 to 70 mg/day. Maximum dosage, 70 mg/day.

ADMINISTRATION
PO
• Give drug in the morning to prevent insomnia.
• Give drug without regard to meals.

L

• Have patient swallow capsules whole, or open capsule, mix contents in yogurt, water, or orange juice, dissolve completely, and have patient take immediately; don't store.
• For chewable tablets, make sure patient chews tablets thoroughly before swallowing.
• Capsules can be substituted with chewable tablets on a unit/mg basis.
• Don't divide the dose of a single capsule or chewable tablet or give less than one capsule or chewable tablet per day.

ACTION

Increases the release of norepinephrine and dopamine from nerve terminals and blocks their reuptake into the presynaptic neuron.

Route	Onset	Peak	Duration
PO	Rapid	1 hr	8–14 hr

Half-life: Lisdexamfetamine, less than 1 hour; dextroamphetamine, 10 to 13 hours.

ADVERSE REACTIONS

CNS: dizziness, anxiety, fever, irritability, jitteriness, agitation, emotional lability, drowsiness, nightmares, paresthesia, insomnia, restlessness, tics, tremor. **CV:** tachycardia, palpitations, increased BP. **EENT:** mydriasis, diplopia, dry mouth, oropharyngeal pain. **GI:** constipation, vomiting, decreased appetite, anorexia, diarrhea, nausea, upper abdominal pain, gastroenteritis. **GU:** libido changes, erectile dysfunction, UTI. **Metabolic:** weight loss. **Respiratory:** dyspnea. **Skin:** rash, excessive sweating, pruritus.

INTERACTIONS

Drug-drug. *Antihistamines:* May inhibit sedative effects of antihistamines. Monitor patient.
Antihypertensives: May inhibit effects of antihypertensive drugs. If use together can't be avoided, closely monitor BP when lisdexamfetamine is started or stopped, and adjust antihypertensive dosage as needed.
Buspirone, fentanyl, linezolid, lithium, SSNRIs, SSRIs, tramadol, triptans, tryptophan: May increase risk of serotonin syndrome. Start lisdexamfetamine treatment with lower doses and monitor patient for signs and symptoms of serotonin syndrome, particularly during lisdexamfetamine initiation and dosage increases.
CYP2D6 inhibitors (fluoxetine, paroxetine, quinidine, ritonavir): May increase exposure of dextroamphetamine and increase risk of serotonin syndrome. Start lisdexamfetamine treatment with lower doses and monitor patient during lisdexamfetamine initiation and dosage increases.
Ethosuximide: May delay ethosuximide absorption. Monitor patient closely.
Lithium: May inhibit anorectic and CNS stimulant effects of amphetamine. Monitor patient closely.
MAO inhibitors: May cause severe HTN or hypertensive crisis. Use is contraindicated within 14 days of MAO inhibitor therapy.
Norepinephrine: May increase adrenergic effects of norepinephrine. Monitor patient closely.
Phenobarbital, phenytoin: May decrease serum level of these drugs. Monitor patient closely.
TCAs: May cause adverse CV effects and increase risk of serotonin syndrome. Avoid use together, or monitor patient closely.
Urine acidifiers (ammonium chloride, sodium acid phosphate), methenamine: May decrease serum level due to increased excretion of amphetamine. Monitor patient for decreased drug effects.
Urine alkalinizers (sodium bicarbonate): May increase lisdexamfetamine serum level because of decreased excretion of amphetamine. Monitor patient for increased drug effects and adjust dosage accordingly.
Drug-herb. *St. John's wort:* May increase risk of serotonin syndrome. Avoid use together.
Drug-food. *Caffeine:* May increase CNS stimulation. Discourage use together.
Drug-lifestyle. *Alcohol use:* May increase CNS depression. Discourage use together.

EFFECTS ON LAB TEST RESULTS

• May increase corticosteroid level.
• May interfere with urinary steroid test.

CONTRAINDICATIONS & CAUTIONS

Boxed Warning Stimulants carry a high risk of abuse and misuse, which can lead to substance use disorder, including addiction, which can lead to overdose and death. The risk increases with high doses or unapproved administration methods, such as snorting or injection. ■
• Contraindicated in patients hypersensitive to sympathomimetic amines and in those with idiosyncratic reactions to them, in patients who are agitated, and in those with history of drug abuse.

Reactions in bold italics are *life-threatening*.

• Anaphylactic reactions, SJS, angioedema, and urticaria have been noted.

• Drug may cause tolerance, requiring higher dosage to produce same effect a lower dosage once provided.

🔔 *Alert:* Drug isn't indicated or recommended for weight loss.

• Avoid use in patients with advanced arteriosclerosis, hyperthyroidism, symptomatic CV disease, structural cardiac abnormalities, cardiomyopathy, serious heart arrhythmia, moderate to severe HTN, or glaucoma and in those intolerant of changes in HR or BP.

• Use cautiously in patients with history of arrhythmias, MI, stroke, or seizures.

• Use cautiously in patients with preexisting psychosis, depression, Tourette syndrome or bipolar disorder, or family history of suicide, bipolar disorder, or depression.

• Drug isn't approved for ADHD in children younger than age 6.

• Safety and effectiveness in children with BED haven't been established.

Dialyzable drug: No.

⚠ *Overdose S&S:* Assaultiveness, psychomotor agitation, confusion, hallucinations, serotonin syndrome, life-threatening hyperthermia, hyperreflexia, panic states, rapid respiration, restlessness, rhabdomyolysis, tremor, fatigue, depression, tachyarrhythmias, circulatory collapse, HTN, hypotension, vasospasm, MI, aortic dissection, cardiomyopathy, abdominal cramps, diarrhea, nausea, vomiting, seizures, coma, death.

PREGNANCY-LACTATION-REPRODUCTION

• Studies during pregnancy are inadequate. Use during pregnancy only if potential benefit justifies fetal risk.

• Encourage patient to register in National Pregnancy Registry for ADHD Medications (1-866-961-2388 or https://womensmentalhealth.org/clinical-and researchprograms/pregnancyregistry/adhd-medications).

• Drug appears in human milk. Use during breastfeeding isn't recommended.

NURSING CONSIDERATIONS

• Diagnosis of ADHD must be based on complete history and evaluation of the child with consultation of psychological, educational, and social resources.

• Assess patient for cardiac disease, including a careful history, family history of sudden death or ventricular arrhythmia, and physical exam, before starting therapy.

• Evaluate for bipolar disorder before initiating therapy.

• Give lowest effective dose in the morning. Afternoon doses may cause insomnia.

Boxed Warning Assess patient's risk of abuse, misuse, and addiction before therapy. Reassess risk during therapy. Monitor for signs and symptoms of drug abuse, misuse, and addiction (increased HR, respiratory rate, or BP; sweating; dilated pupils; hyperactivity; restlessness; insomnia; decreased appetite; loss of coordination; tremors; flushing; vomiting; abdominal pain). Anxiety, psychosis, hostility, aggression, suicidality, and homicidal ideation may also occur. ∎

• Abrupt drug stoppage or dose reduction may cause withdrawal symptoms (dysphoria, depression, fatigue, vivid and unpleasant dreams, insomnia or hypersomnia, increased appetite, psychomotor retardation or agitation) in patient with physical dependence.

🔔 *Alert:* Periodically monitor patient for changes in HR or BP.

• Monitor patient closely for adverse CV effects, vision problems, and seizures.

• Use cautiously in patient taking other drugs that increase risk of serotonin syndrome. Monitor closely and consider an alternative nonserotonergic drug.

• Carefully observe patient for digital changes because stimulants used to treat ADHD are associated with peripheral vasculopathy, including Raynaud phenomenon.

• Effectiveness of this drug when taken for longer than 4 weeks isn't known. Periodically interrupt therapy to determine whether continuation is necessary.

• Growth may be suppressed with long-term stimulant use. Monitor child for growth and weight gain. Stop treatment if growth is suppressed or if weight gain is lower than expected.

• Drug may exacerbate tics or Tourette syndrome. Monitor patient, especially at start of therapy.

• Monitor for appearance or worsening of aggressive behavior or hostility, especially at start of therapy.

• May cause psychotic or manic episodes in patient with no prior history or exacerbation of signs and symptoms in patient with preexisting psychosis.

PATIENT TEACHING
• Teach about proper drug administration and handling.
• Advise patient and caregiver to read the medication guide.

Boxed Warning Teach patient and caregiver about risk of abuse, misuse, and addiction, which can lead to overdose and death. Advise patient to store drug in a safe (preferably locked) place. Teach about proper disposal of unused drug. Instruct patient not to give drug to anyone else. ■

❸ Alert: Instruct patient to immediately report chest pain, shortness of breath, or fainting.
• Tell patient or caregiver that abruptly stopping drug can cause severe fatigue, depression, or general withdrawal reaction.
• Caution patient to avoid activities that require alertness or good psychomotor coordination until CNS effects of drug are known.
• Advise patient taking other drugs that increase risk of serotonin syndrome to immediately report signs and symptoms of serotonin syndrome (confusion, agitation, fever, rapid heartbeat, loss of muscle coordination, vomiting, diaphoresis).
• Warn patient with seizure disorder that drug may decrease seizure threshold. Urge patient to notify prescriber if a seizure occurs.
• Instruct patient or caregiver to report palpitations, visual disturbances, worsening aggression, hallucinations, delusions, or mania.
• Advise patient or caregiver that drug may slow growth and cause weight loss.
• Instruct patient to immediately report numbness, pain, coolness, skin color change, temperature sensitivity, or unexplained wounds on fingers or toes.
• Advise patient to avoid caffeine and alcohol consumption while taking drug.
• Instruct patient to report pregnancy or plans to become pregnant or breastfeed.

---

lisinopril ⚕
lye-SIN-oh-pril

Qbrelis, Zestril

Therapeutic class: Antihypertensives
Pharmacologic class: ACE inhibitors

AVAILABLE FORMS
Oral solution: 1 mg/mL

Tablets: 2.5 mg, 5 mg, 10 mg, 20 mg, 30 mg, 40 mg

INDICATIONS & DOSAGES
➤ **HTN**
Adults: Initially, 10 mg PO, increased as needed to maximum daily dosage of 40 mg. For patients taking diuretic, initially, 5 mg PO daily.
Children ages 6 and older: Initially, 0.07 mg/kg (up to 5 mg) PO once daily. Increase dosage based on patient response and tolerance. Maximum dosage, 0.61 mg/kg (don't exceed 40 mg). Don't use in children with GFR less than 30 mL/minute/1.73 m^2.
Adjust-a-dose: In adults, if CrCl is 10 to 30 mL/minute, give 5 mg PO daily; if CrCl is less than 10 mL/minute, give 2.5 mg PO daily. May titrate dosage up to 40 mg/day.
➤ **Adjunctive treatment (with diuretics and cardiac glycosides) for HF**
Adults: Initially, 5 mg PO daily; increase as needed to maximum of 40 mg.
Adjust-a-dose: If sodium level is less than 130 mEq/L, serum creatinine level greater than 3 mg/dL, or CrCl less than 30 mL/minute, start treatment at 2.5 mg daily.
➤ **Within 24 hours of acute MI to improve survival in patients who are hemodynamically stable**
Adults: Initially, 5 mg PO; then 5 mg after 24 hours; then 10 mg once daily for at least 6 weeks.
Adjust-a-dose: For patients with systolic BP of 120 mm Hg or less during first 3 days after an infarct, decrease dosage to 2.5 mg PO. If systolic BP drops to 100 mm Hg or less, reduce daily maintenance dosage of 5 mg to 2.5 mg, if needed. If prolonged systolic BP stays under 90 mm Hg for longer than 1 hour, withdraw drug.

If CrCl is 10 to 30 mL/minute, reduce initial dosage to 2.5 mg PO daily and titrate as tolerated to maximum dosage of 40 mg daily. If patient is on hemodialysis or CrCl is less than 10 mL/minute, start treatment at 2.5 mg PO daily.

ADMINISTRATION
PO
• Give drug without regard to food.
• Oral solution is bioequivalent to lisinopril tablets.
• Store oral solution at room temperature in a tightly closed container. Protect from freezing and excessive heat.

• If tablets are made into a suspension by pharmacist, store at or below 77° F (25° C) for up to 4 weeks; shake before each use.

ACTION

Causes decreased production of angiotensin II and suppression of the RAAS.

Route	Onset	Peak	Duration
PO	1 hr	7 hr	24 hr

Half-life: 12 hours.

ADVERSE REACTIONS

CNS: dizziness, headache, fatigue, asthenia, paresthesia, syncope, vertigo, taste or smell disturbance. **CV:** orthostatic hypotension, hypotension, chest pain, flushing. **EENT:** vision changes, tinnitus, nasal congestion, dry mouth. **GI:** diarrhea, constipation, flatulence, nausea, dyspepsia, *pancreatitis.* **GU:** impaired kidney function, impotence. **Metabolic:** *hyperkalemia,* diabetes, gout, SIADH. **Respiratory:** dyspnea; dry, persistent, tickling, nonproductive cough. **Skin:** rash, diaphoresis, erythema, alopecia, pruritus, photosensitivity, *SJS, TEN,* urticaria.

INTERACTIONS

Drug-drug. *Aliskiren; ACE inhibitors, ARBs (dual therapy):* May increase risk of kidney impairment, hypotension, and hyperkalemia. Concomitant use of aliskiren is contraindicated in patients with diabetes. Avoid use together.

Allopurinol: May cause hypersensitivity reaction. Use together cautiously.

Azathioprine: May increase risk of anemia or leukopenia. Monitor hematologic studies if used together.

COX-2 inhibitors, indomethacin, NSAIDs: May increase risk of kidney dysfunction. May reduce hypotensive effects of drug. Adjust dosage as needed.

Diuretics, thiazide diuretics: May cause excessive hypotension with diuretics. Monitor BP closely.

Insulin, oral antidiabetics: May cause hypoglycemia, especially at start of lisinopril therapy. Monitor glucose level.

Lithium: May cause lithium toxicity. Monitor lithium level.

mTOR inhibitors (everolimus, sirolimus, temsirolimus): May increase risk of angioedema. Monitor patient closely.

Neprilysin inhibitors (sacubitril): May increase risk of angioedema. Use together is contraindicated. Don't give lisinopril within 36 hours of switching to or from sacubitril–valsartan (Entresto).

Phenothiazines: May increase hypotensive effects. Monitor BP closely.

Potassium-sparing diuretics, potassium supplements: May cause hyperkalemia. Monitor lab values.

Tizanidine: May cause severe hypotension. Monitor patient.

Drug-herb. *Ma huang:* May decrease antihypertensive effects. Discourage use together.

Drug-food. *Potassium-containing salt substitutes:* May cause hyperkalemia. Monitor lab values.

EFFECTS ON LAB TEST RESULTS

• May increase BUN, creatinine, potassium, and bilirubin levels and LFT values.
• May decrease Hb level and hematocrit.

CONTRAINDICATIONS & CAUTIONS

• Contraindicated in patients hypersensitive to ACE inhibitors and in those with history of angioedema related to previous treatment with ACE inhibitor.
• Use cautiously in patients with impaired kidney function; adjust dosage.
• Use cautiously in patients at risk for hyperkalemia or hypotension and in those with aortic stenosis or hypertrophic cardiomyopathy. Safety and effectiveness of lisinopril on BP control in children younger than age 6 and children with GFR less than 30 mL/minute/1.73 m² haven't been established.

 Although rare, angioedema, which can be fatal, may occur at any time during treatment, including after first dose; it may involve head and neck (potentially compromising airway) or intestine (presenting with abdominal pain). Patients who are Black and patients with idiopathic or hereditary angioedema may be at increased risk. Patients concurrently receiving mTOR inhibitor therapy (temsirolimus, sirolimus, everolimus) also may be at increased risk.

Dialyzable drug: Yes.

⚠ *Overdose S&S:* Hypotension.

PREGNANCY-LACTATION-REPRODUCTION

Boxed Warning Drug acts directly on the RAAS and can cause injury and death to a

developing fetus. When pregnancy is detected, stop drug as soon as possible. ■
• It isn't known if drug appears in human milk. Patient should discontinue breastfeeding or discontinue drug, considering importance of drug to patient.

NURSING CONSIDERATIONS

⚠ Although ACE inhibitors reduce BP in all races, BP reduction is less in patients who are Black taking an ACE inhibitor alone. Patients who are Black should take drug with a thiazide diuretic for a more favorable response.
• Frequently monitor BP. If drug doesn't adequately control BP, may add diuretics.
• Monitor WBC with differential counts before therapy, every 2 weeks for first 3 months of therapy, and periodically thereafter.
• Periodically monitor serum potassium level.
• Monitor patient for jaundice or significantly increased liver enzyme levels. ACE inhibitors have been associated with liver failure.
• *Look alike–sound alike:* Don't confuse lisinopril with fosinopril or Lioresal. Don't confuse Zestril with Zostrix, Zetia, or Zyrtec.

PATIENT TEACHING

🟦 *Alert:* Rarely, facial and throat swelling (including swelling of larynx) or intestinal swelling may occur, especially after first dose. Advise patient to report abdominal pain, breathing problems, or swelling of face, eyes, lips, or tongue.
• Warn that light-headedness can occur, especially during first few days of therapy. Tell patient to rise slowly to minimize this effect and to report symptoms to prescriber. If fainting occurs, advise patient to immediately stop drug and call prescriber.
• If unpleasant adverse reactions occur, tell patient not to stop drug suddenly but to notify prescriber.
• Advise patient to report signs and symptoms of infection (fever, sore throat).
• Tell patient of childbearing potential to notify prescriber if pregnancy occurs. Drug will need to be stopped.
• Advise patient to report signs and symptoms of hyperkalemia (muscle fatigue, weakness, nausea, abnormal heart rhythm).
• Instruct patient not to use salt substitutes that contain potassium without first consulting prescriber.
• Inform patient that a dry, nonproductive cough may develop during therapy.

---

lithium carbonate
LITH-ee-um

Carbolith✹, Lithane✹, Lithmax✹, Lithobid

Therapeutic class: Antimanics
Pharmacologic class: Alkali metals

AVAILABLE FORMS
Capsules: 150 mg, 300 mg, 600 mg
Tablets: 300 mg
Tablets (extended-release) ⓞⓝⓒ: 300 mg, 450 mg

INDICATIONS & DOSAGES

Adjust-a-dose (for all indications): In older adults and patients with CrCl of 30 to 89 mL/minute, start at lower doses. Immediate-release lithium isn't recommended in patients with CrCl of less than 30 mL/minute.

➤ **Acute mania in bipolar disorder**
Adults and children ages 7 and older weighing more than 30 kg: Initially, 300 mg PO t.i.d. Increase by 300 mg every 3 days to a goal of 600 mg PO b.i.d. or t.i.d.
Children ages 7 and older weighing 20 to 30 kg: 300 mg (immediate-release tablets or capsules) PO b.i.d. Increase by 300 mg weekly to a goal of 600 to 1,500 mg PO in divided doses daily.
Adults and children ages 12 and older (extended-release tablets): 900 mg PO b.i.d. or 600 mg PO t.i.d.
Adjust-a-dose: Individualize dosage according to serum levels and clinical response. Titrate to serum lithium level of 0.8 to 1.2 mEq/L.

➤ **Long-term control in bipolar disorder**
Adults and children ages 7 and older weighing more than 30 kg: Usual dosage, 300 to 600 mg (immediate-release tablets or capsules) PO b.i.d. or t.i.d.
Children ages 7 and older weighing 20 to 30 kg: Usual dosage, 600 to 1,200 mg (immediate-release tablets or capsules) PO in divided doses daily.
Adults and children ages 12 and older (extended-release tablets): 900 to 1,200 mg/day in divided doses. Usual dosage, 600 mg PO b.i.d.
Adjust-a-dose: Individualize dosage according to serum level and clinical response. Titrate immediate-release formulations to serum lithium level of 0.6 to 1 mEq/L

or extended-release formulation to serum lithium level of 0.6 to 1.2 mEq/L.

ADMINISTRATION
PO
• Give drug with food and plenty of water to minimize GI upset.
• Have patient swallow extended-release tablets whole; don't crush or break tablets.

ACTION
May alter chemical transmitters in the CNS, possibly by interfering with ionic pump mechanisms in brain cells, and may compete with or replace sodium ions.

Route	Onset	Peak	Duration
PO (immediate-release)	Unknown	30 min–3 hr	Unknown
PO (extended-release)	Unknown	2–6 hr	Unknown

Half-life: 18 to 36 hours.

ADVERSE REACTIONS
CNS: fatigue, lethargy, *coma, seizures,* tics, tremors, drowsiness, headache, confusion, disorientation, stupor, tongue movements, restlessness, dizziness, vertigo, psychomotor retardation, blackouts, EEG changes, ataxia, worsened organic mental syndrome, impaired speech, incoordination, fever, hypertonicity, choreoathetotic movements, extrapyramidal symptoms, hallucinations, poor memory, dysgeusia. **CV:** *arrhythmias (including Brugada syndrome), bradycardia,* reversible ECG changes, hypotension, SA node dysfunction, edema, chest tightness, peripheral vasculopathy. **EENT:** blurred vision, exophthalmos, nystagmus, tinnitus, dry mouth, salivary gland swelling, hypersalivation, dental caries. **GI:** vomiting, anorexia, diarrhea, thirst, nausea, gastritis, abdominal pain, flatulence, indigestion, fecal incontinence. **GU:** polyuria including enuresis, *kidney toxicity (with long-term use),* oliguria, glycosuria, decreased CrCl, albuminuria, urinary incontinence, sexual dysfunction. **Hematologic:** leukocytosis. **Metabolic:** dehydration, transient hyperglycemia, goiter, hypothyroidism, hyponatremia, weight gain or loss. **Musculoskeletal:** muscle weakness, muscle hyperirritability, polyarthralgia. **Skin:** pruritus, rash, diminished or absent sensation, drying and thinning of hair, acne, psoriasis, alopecia, folliculitis. **Other:** hypersensitivity reactions.

INTERACTIONS
Drug-drug. *ACE inhibitors, ARBs:* May increase lithium level. Monitor lithium level; adjust lithium dosage, as needed.
Antiarrhythmics and other drugs that prolong QT interval: May increase risk of life-threatening arrhythmias. Avoid use together.
Antipsychotics (clozapine, haloperidol, risperidone, thioridazine): May increase risk of neurotoxic reactions. Monitor patient closely.
Calcium channel blockers (verapamil): May decrease lithium level and may increase risk of neurotoxicity. Use together cautiously.
Carbamazepine, fluoxetine, methyldopa, NSAIDs, phenytoin, probenecid: May increase lithium level. Monitor patient for lithium toxicity.
Iodide-containing preparations (potassium iodide): May increase risk of hypothyroidism. Monitor thyroid levels.
Metronidazole, other nitroimidazole antibiotics: May cause lithium toxicity due to reduced lithium clearance. Monitor lithium level.
Neuromuscular blockers (succinylcholine): May cause prolonged paralysis or weakness. Monitor patient closely.
Serotonergic drugs (linezolid, MAO inhibitors, SSNRIs, SSRIs): May increase risk of serotonin syndrome. Monitor for serotonin syndrome.
Sodium bicarbonate, theophylline, urine alkalinizers: May increase lithium excretion. Patient should avoid excessive salt. Monitor lithium level.
Sodium-glucose cotransporter 2 inhibitors (canagliflozin, dapagliflozin, empagliflozin): May decrease lithium level. Monitor level more frequently during inhibitor initiation and dosage changes.
Thiazide diuretics: May increase lithium level, with possible toxic effect. Use with caution, and monitor lithium and electrolyte levels (especially sodium).
Drug-food. *Caffeine:* May decrease lithium level and drug effect. Advise patient who ingests large amounts of caffeine to tell prescriber before stopping caffeine. Adjust lithium dosage, as needed.
Sodium (salt): May change elimination of drug if sodium intake changes. Avoid major changes in sodium intake.
Drug-herb. *St. John's Wort:* May increase risk of serotonin syndrome. Discourage use together.

L

EFFECTS ON LAB TEST RESULTS
• May increase glucose, creatinine, and TSH levels.
• May decrease sodium, T_3, T_4, calcium, parathyroid hormone, and protein-bound iodine levels.
• May increase WBC and neutrophil counts.
• May increase ^{131}I uptake.

CONTRAINDICATIONS & CAUTIONS
• Contraindicated in patients hypersensitive to drug or if therapy can't be closely monitored.
• Use extreme caution in patients receiving neuromuscular blockers and diuretics; in older adults or patients who are debilitated; and in patients with thyroid disease, seizure disorder, infection, kidney or CV disease, dehydration, or sodium depletion.
• Patients with Brugada syndrome (abnormal ECG with increased risk of sudden death) or with risk factors for this condition shouldn't take lithium.
• Safety and effectiveness in children younger than age 7 haven't been established.
Dialyzable drug: Yes.
⚠ *Overdose S&S:* Diarrhea, vomiting, drowsiness, muscular weakness, lack of coordination, giddiness, ataxia, blurred vision, confusion, tinnitus, large output of dilute urine, slurred speech, loss of consciousness, myoclonic limb movements, agitation, urinary or fecal incontinence, seizures, arrhythmias, hypotension, peripheral vascular collapse, coma.

PREGNANCY-LACTATION-REPRODUCTION
• Drug may cause fetal harm if used during pregnancy. Inform patient of potential hazard to fetus.
• If patient decides to continue lithium during pregnancy, monitor serum lithium level and adjust dosage if indicated. Two to three days before delivery, decrease lithium dosage or discontinue drug to reduce risk of maternal and neonatal toxicity. Monitor neonate and provide supportive care until lithium is excreted and toxic signs and symptoms disappear, which may take up to 14 days. Consider fetal echocardiography between 16 and 20 weeks' gestation in patient with first-trimester lithium exposure, due to risk of cardiac malformations.
• Drug appears in human milk. Use during breastfeeding isn't recommended. If patient chooses to breastfeed, monitor infant's lithium level.

NURSING CONSIDERATIONS
Boxed Warning Lithium toxicity is closely related to serum lithium level and can occur at dosages close to therapeutic levels. Facilities for prompt and accurate serum lithium determinations should be available before initiation of therapy. ∎
• Monitor patient and discontinue drug if signs and symptoms of lithium toxicity (ataxia, drowsiness, weakness, tremor, vomiting) occur.
• Obtain baseline ECG, thyroid studies, kidney function studies, and electrolyte levels, including calcium.
• Check fluid intake and output, especially when surgery is scheduled.
• Weigh patient daily; monitor for edema or sudden weight gain.
• Adjust fluid and salt ingestion to compensate if excessive loss occurs from protracted diaphoresis or diarrhea. Under normal conditions, fluid intake should be 2½ to 3 L daily, and patient should follow a balanced diet with adequate salt intake.
• Monitor urine specific gravity and report level below 1.005, which may indicate diabetes insipidus.
• Drug alters glucose tolerance in patients with diabetes. Monitor glucose level closely.
• Perform outpatient follow-up of thyroid and kidney function every 2 to 3 months during 6 months of treatment, then as clinically indicated. Monitor CBC and ECG (patients older than age 40) before therapy and as needed.
• Monitor lithium level twice weekly, 12 hours after the last oral dose, until patient and levels are stable, then every 1 to 2 months or as needed.
• Monitor for encephalopathic syndrome (weakness, lethargy, fever, tremors, confusion, extrapyramidal symptoms, leukocytosis, increased BUN and fasting glucose levels) in patient also taking an antipsychotic.
• Monitor for serotonin syndrome (loss of coordination, restlessness, hallucinations, seizures, rapid heartbeat, rapid changes in BP, increased body temperature, tremors, diaphoresis, rigidity, hyperreflexia, nausea, vomiting, diarrhea). Immediately discontinue lithium and serotonergic agents if symptoms occur; begin supportive treatment.
• Palpate thyroid to check for enlargement. Monitor weight before and during therapy.
• Periodically monitor cognitive function.
• *Look alike–sound alike:* Don't confuse lithium carbonate with lanthanum carbonate.

Reactions in bold italics are *life-threatening*.

PATIENT TEACHING
• Tell patient to take drug with plenty of water and with food to minimize GI upset.
• Explain the importance of having regular blood tests to determine drug levels and to monitor therapy; even slightly high values can be dangerous.
• Warn patient and caregivers to expect transient nausea, large amounts of urine, thirst, and discomfort during first few days and to watch for evidence of toxicity.
• Instruct patient to withhold one dose and immediately call prescriber if signs and symptoms of toxicity appear, but not to stop drug abruptly.
• Warn patient to avoid hazardous activities that require alertness and good psychomotor coordination until CNS effects are known.
• Tell patient not to switch brands or take other prescription or OTC drugs without prescriber's guidance.
• Advise patient to seek immediate emergency assistance if fainting, light-headedness, abnormal heartbeat, or shortness of breath occurs because these signs and symptoms are associated with a potentially life-threatening heart disorder known as Brugada syndrome.
• Tell patient to always wear or carry medical identification.
• Instruct patient to report pregnancy or plans to become pregnant or breastfeed.

lofexidine hydrochloride ☒
loe-FEX-i-deen

Lucemyra

Therapeutic class: Opioid cessation drugs
Pharmacologic class: Alpha₂-adrenergic receptor agonists

AVAILABLE FORMS
Tablets: 0.18 mg

INDICATIONS & DOSAGES
➤ **Mitigation of opioid withdrawal symptoms to facilitate abrupt opioid discontinuation**
Adults: Initially, three 0.18-mg tablets PO q.i.d. during the peak withdrawal period (generally 5 to 7 days after last opioid dose). Allow 5 to 6 hours between doses and continue for up to 14 days, with dosing guided by symptoms. Maximum daily dosage is

2.88 mg (16 tablets); maximum single dose is 0.72 mg (4 tablets). Discontinue treatment gradually over 2 to 4 days, reducing by 1 tablet per dose every 1 to 2 days.
Adjust-a-dose: For patients with Child-Pugh class A liver impairment, give 3 tablets q.i.d. (2.16 mg/day); for those with Child-Pugh class B liver impairment, give 2 tablets q.i.d. (1.44 mg/day); for those with Child-Pugh class C liver impairment, give 1 tablet q.i.d. (0.72 mg/day). For patients with eGFR of 30 to 89.9 mL/minute/1.73 m², give 2 tablets q.i.d. (1.44 mg/day); for those with eGFR of less than 30 mL/minute/1.73 m², give 1 tablet q.i.d. (0.72 mg/day).

ADMINISTRATION
PO
• Give drug without regard to food.
• Store at room temperature.
• Protect from excess moisture and heat.
• Don't remove desiccant pack from bottle.

ACTION
A central alpha₂-adrenergic agonist that binds to receptors on adrenergic neurons. It inhibits the release of norepinephrine in the central and peripheral nervous systems, reducing the signs and symptoms of opioid withdrawal.

Route	Onset	Peak	Duration
PO	Unknown	3–5 hr	Unknown

Half-life: 11 to 13 hours (first dose); 17 to 22 hours (at steady-state).

ADVERSE REACTIONS
CNS: insomnia, dizziness, somnolence, sedation, syncope. **CV:** orthostatic hypotension, *bradycardia*, hypotension. **EENT:** tinnitus, dry mouth.

INTERACTIONS
Drug-drug. *CNS depressants (barbiturates, benzodiazepines):* May enhance CNS depressant effects. Avoid use together.
CYP2D6 inhibitors (paroxetine): May increase lofexidine level. Use together cautiously. Monitor patient for orthostatic hypotension and bradycardia.
Drugs that decrease HR: May increase risk of excessive bradycardia. Avoid use together.
Drugs that increase QT interval (methadone): May further increase QT interval. Use together cautiously and monitor ECGs.

Drugs that lower BP: May increase hypotensive effects. Avoid use together.

Naltrexone (oral route only): May decrease effectiveness of oral naltrexone if given within 2 hours of lofexidine. Monitor therapy and separate dosing times of drugs by 2 hours.

Drug-lifestyle. *Alcohol use:* May increase CNS depressive effects. Discourage use together.

EFFECTS ON LAB TEST RESULTS
None reported.

CONTRAINDICATIONS & CAUTIONS
• Avoid use in patients with severe coronary insufficiency, recent MI, cerebrovascular disease, CKD, and marked bradycardia. If drug must be used, monitor ECG, especially in patients with these conditions and electrolyte disturbances.

☯ *Alert:* Drug causes QT-interval prolongation, especially in patients with kidney impairment; prolonged QT interval increases risk of ventricular arrhythmias. Avoid use in patients with congenital long QT syndrome.

• Use cautiously in patients with HF, bradyarrhythmias, and liver or kidney impairment.

• Use cautiously in outpatient setting. Patients should be capable of self-monitoring for adverse effects.

• Drug may decrease tolerance to opioids and increase risk of fatal opioid overdose if patient resumes opioid use.

• Use drug for opioid use disorder only with a comprehensive treatment and management program.

☯ *Alert:* Drug may increase risk of discontinuation symptoms. Don't stop medication abruptly as it can increase BP, diarrhea, insomnia, chills, hyperhidrosis, and extremity pain.

☒ Use cautiously in patients who are CYP2D6 poor metabolizers. Monitor for orthostatic hypotension and bradycardia.

• Safety and effectiveness in children haven't been established.

• Use cautiously in older adults.

Dialyzable drug: Minimal.

⚠ *Overdose S&S:* Hypotension, bradycardia, sedation.

PREGNANCY-LACTATION-REPRODUCTION
• Studies during pregnancy are inadequate. Use only if benefits outweigh fetal risk.

• It isn't known if drug appears in human milk or how drug affects milk production or infants who are breastfed. Use cautiously during breastfeeding.

NURSING CONSIDERATIONS
• Monitor vital signs and watch for bradycardia and hypotension before dosing. Reduce dosage or delay or skip next dose for clinically significant hypotension or bradycardia.

• Monitor ECG in patients with HF, bradycardia, or liver or kidney impairment and in those taking medications that prolong QT interval, especially if electrolyte disturbances are present.

• Monitor electrolyte levels and correct abnormalities (hypokalemia, hypomagnesemia) before administering drug; monitor ECG when starting drug.

• Monitor patient for drug discontinuation signs and symptoms; manage by resuming previous dose, followed by gradual tapering if signs and symptoms occur.

PATIENT TEACHING
• Review signs and symptoms of hypotension. Teach patient to rise slowly from seated or lying position.

• Caution patient to stay hydrated.

• Instruct patient to withhold dose and immediately contact prescriber if signs or symptoms of low BP or slow HR occur (dizziness, light-headedness, faintness at rest or when standing up).

• Caution patient to avoid driving and operating heavy machinery until drug's effects are known.

• Advise patient not to abruptly stop drug and to follow instructions for gradual drug discontinuation.

☯ *Alert:* Inform patient and caregivers of increased risk of overdose if opioids are resumed.

• Instruct patient to report pregnancy or plans to become pregnant or breastfeed.

---

lopinavir–ritonavir ☒
low-PIN-ah-ver/ri-TON-ah-veer

Kaletra*

Therapeutic class: Antiretrovirals
Pharmacologic class: Protease inhibitors

AVAILABLE FORMS
Solution: lopinavir 400 mg and ritonavir 100 mg/5 mL (80 mg/mL and 20 mg/mL)*

Tablets ⬤: lopinavir 100 mg and ritonavir 25 mg; lopinavir 200 mg and ritonavir 50 mg

INDICATIONS & DOSAGES

➤ **HIV infection, with other antiretrovirals except efavirenz, nevirapine, or nelfinavir**
Adults: 800 mg lopinavir and 200 mg ritonavir PO once daily (only in patients with less than three lopinavir resistance-associated substitutions) or in two evenly divided doses.
Children older than 6 months to 18 years: 230 mg lopinavir and 57.5 mg/m² ritonavir (oral solution) PO b.i.d. with food. Or, if patient weighs more than 35 kg, four tablets of lopinavir 100 mg and ritonavir 25 mg PO b.i.d. If patient weighs more than 25 to 35 kg, three tablets of lopinavir 100 mg and ritonavir 25 mg PO b.i.d. If patient weighs 15 to 25 kg, two tablets of lopinavir 100 mg and ritonavir 25 mg PO b.i.d. Maximum dosage, lopinavir 400 mg and ritonavir 100 mg PO b.i.d.
Children ages 14 days to 6 months: 16 mg lopinavir and 4 mg ritonavir/kg oral solution PO b.i.d. Or, lopinavir 300 mg and ritonavir 75 mg/m² PO b.i.d.
Adjust-a-dose: In patients who are pregnant with no documented lopinavir resistance-associated substitutions, give 400 mg lopinavir and 100 mg ritonavir tablets b.i.d.; avoid oral solution due to ethanol content. Once-daily dosing isn't recommended. Data are insufficient to recommend dosing in patients who are pregnant with documented lopinavir resistance-associated substitutions. No dosage adjustment is required during postpartum period.

➤ **HIV infection, in combination with antiretrovirals efavirenz, nevirapine, or nelfinavir**
Adults: 500 mg lopinavir and 125 mg ritonavir (tablets) PO b.i.d., or 520 mg lopinavir and 130 mg ritonavir (oral solution) PO b.i.d.
Children older than 6 months to 18 years: 300 mg lopinavir and 75 mg/m² ritonavir (oral solution) PO b.i.d. Maximum dosage, lopinavir 533 mg and ritonavir 133 mg (oral solution) PO b.i.d.

Or, if patient weighs more than 45 kg, five tablets of lopinavir 100 mg and ritonavir 25 mg PO b.i.d. If patient weighs more than 30 to 45 kg, four tablets of lopinavir 100 mg and ritonavir 25 mg PO b.i.d. If patient weighs more than 20 to 30 kg, three tablets of lopinavir 100 mg and ritonavir 25 mg PO b.i.d. If patient weighs 15 to 20 kg, two tablets

of lopinavir 100 mg and ritonavir 25 mg PO b.i.d. Maximum dosage is lopinavir 500 mg and ritonavir 125 mg (tablets) PO b.i.d.

ADMINISTRATION

PO
❸ *Alert:* Many drug interactions are possible. Review all drugs patient is taking.
• Give oral solution with food. Give tablets without regard to food.
• Calculate children's doses based on either body weight or BSA.
• Have patient swallow tablets whole; don't crush or break tablets.
• Use calibrated syringe or measuring cup to administer oral solution.
• Don't use oral solution with polyurethane feeding tubes because of potential incompatibility with ethanol and propylene glycol. Feeding tubes that are compatible with ethanol and propylene glycol, such as silicone and polyvinyl chloride feeding tubes, can be used.
• Refrigerated solution remains stable until expiration date on package. If stored at room temperature, use drug within 2 months.

ACTION

Lopinavir is an HIV protease inhibitor, which produces immature, noninfectious viral particles. Ritonavir, also an HIV protease inhibitor, slows lopinavir metabolism, thereby increasing lopinavir level.

Route	Onset	Peak	Duration
PO	Unknown	4 hr	Unknown

Half-life: About 5 to 6 hours.

ADVERSE REACTIONS

CNS: anxiety, fatigue, dizziness, fever, headache, insomnia, malaise, nervousness, neuropathy, pain, paresthesia, peripheral neuritis, somnolence, tremors, dysgeusia. **CV:** edema, HTN, palpitations. **GI:** *colitis, pancreatitis,* diarrhea, nausea, abdominal pain, anorexia, cholecystitis, constipation, dyspepsia, dysphagia, enterocolitis, esophagitis, flatulence, abdominal distention, gastroenteritis, GERD, hemorrhoids, vomiting. **GU:** erectile dysfunction, menstrual disorder, increased CrCl. **Hematologic:** *leukopenia, neutropenia, thrombocytopenia in children,* anemia. **Hepatic:** *hepatitis,* increased transaminase levels, hyperbilirubinemia. **Metabolic:** decreased glucose tolerance;

🍁Canada   ◇OTC   ◆Off-label use   ⬤Do not crush   *Liquid contains alcohol   ⌘Genetic

hypertriglyceridemia; hyperglycemia; hypercholesterolemia; hyperuricemia; hyponatremia in children; hypothyroidism; weight loss; increased amylase, lipase, CK levels. **Musculoskeletal:** arthralgia, back pain, myalgia. **Respiratory:** lower or upper respiratory tract infections, bronchitis, dyspnea, lung edema. **Skin:** dry skin, dermatitis, skin infections, pruritus, rash, night sweats, lipodystrophy. **Other:** hypersensitivity reactions, chills, facial edema, flulike symptoms, gynecomastia, lymphadenopathy, viral infection.

INTERACTIONS

❸ *Alert:* Drug significantly interacts with many drugs. Consult drug compatibility reference or pharmacist for more information.
Drug-drug. *Alfuzosin:* Increases hypotension risk. Use together is contraindicated.
Amiodarone, bepridil, lidocaine, quinidine: May increase antiarrhythmic level. Use together cautiously. Monitor levels of these drugs, if possible.
Antiarrhythmics (dronedarone, flecainide, propafenone), pimozide: May increase risk of cardiac arrhythmias. Avoid use together. Dronedarone is contraindicated.
Anticancer agents (ibrutinib, vincristine): May decrease antiviral effects. Refer to prescribing information of individual agent.
Aripiprazole: May enhance adverse effects of ritonavir. Modify therapy.
Atorvastatin: May increase level of this drug and risk of myopathy and rhabdomyolysis. Use lowest possible dose and monitor patient carefully.
Atovaquone, methadone: May decrease levels of these drugs. Consider increasing dosages of these drugs.
Avanafil, sildenafil, tadalafil, vardenafil: May increase levels of these drugs and adverse effects, such as hypotension and prolonged erection. Monitor patient and adjust dosages according to manufacturer's instructions. Use with sildenafil in PAH treatment is contraindicated.
Bosentan: May increase bosentan level. Consider decreasing bosentan dosage.
Bupropion: May decrease bupropion level and antidepressant effect. Monitor patient for adequate clinical response and adjust bupropion dosage as needed.
Calcium channel blockers (felodipine, nicardipine, nifedipine): May increase levels of these drugs. Use together cautiously.

Carbamazepine, phenobarbital, phenytoin: May decrease lopinavir level. Use together cautiously. Don't use once-daily lopinavir–ritonavir. Consider therapy modification.
Clarithromycin: May increase clarithromycin level in patients with kidney impairment. Adjust clarithromycin dosage.
Cobicistat: May enhance therapeutic effects of ritonavir. Avoid use together.
Colchicine: May increase colchicine level. Contraindicated in patients with kidney or liver impairment. Decrease colchicine dosage if used together in patient with normal kidney or liver function.
Corticosteroids: May decrease lopinavir level and increase steroid level. Refer to individual product for alternative dosing or alternative product.
Cyclosporine, rapamycin, tacrolimus: May increase levels of these drugs. Monitor therapeutic levels.
Dasatinib, nilotinib: May increase levels of these drugs and risk of adverse events. Adjust dasatinib and nilotinib dosages as needed.
Delavirdine: May increase lopinavir level. Avoid use together.
Didanosine: May decrease absorption of didanosine because lopinavir–ritonavir combination is taken with food. Give didanosine 1 hour before or 2 hours after lopinavir–ritonavir combination.
Disulfiram, metronidazole: May cause disulfiram-like reaction in patients using oral solution (contains alcohol). Avoid use together.
Drugs that prolong PR interval (atazanavir, beta blockers, calcium channel blockers, digoxin): May further prolong PR interval. Use together cautiously.
Drugs that prolong QT interval (amiodarone, flecainide, propafenone): May further prolong QT interval and increase risk of ventricular arrhythmias. Avoid use together.
Efavirenz, nelfinavir, nevirapine: May decrease lopinavir level. Consider increasing lopinavir–ritonavir combination dose. Don't use a once-daily regimen of lopinavir–ritonavir combination with these drugs.
Elvitegravir: May increase elvitegravir level. Reduce dosages of both drugs and consider modifying therapy.
Ergot derivatives (dihydroergotamine, ergotamine, methylergonovine): May increase risk of ergot toxicity, characterized by peripheral vasospasm and ischemia. Use together is contraindicated.

Fentanyl: May increase or prolong sedation or cause respiratory depression. Monitor patient carefully.

Fosamprenavir with ritonavir: May increase rate of adverse reactions. Appropriate doses of combinations with respect to safety and effectiveness haven't been established.

Hepatitis C antivirals (boceprevir, dasabuvir, elbasvir—grazoprevir, glecaprevir, ombitasvir, paritaprevir, pibrentasvir, simeprevir, sofosbuvir, velpatasvir, voxilaprevir): May increase or decrease drug levels. Use together not recommended.

Hormonal contraceptives (ethinyl estradiol): May decrease effectiveness of contraceptives. Recommend nonhormonal contraceptives.

Itraconazole, ketoconazole: May increase levels of these drugs. Don't give more than 200 mg/day of these drugs.

Lamotrigine, valproic acid: May decrease levels of these drugs. Consider dosage increase of lamotrigine or valproic acid.

Lomitapide: Increases lomitapide exposure, raising liver toxicity risk. Use together is contraindicated.

Lovastatin, simvastatin: May increase risk of adverse reactions, such as myopathy and rhabdomyolysis. Use together is contraindicated.

Lurasidone, pimozide, ranolazine: Increases risk of life-threatening reactions. Use together is contraindicated.

Maraviroc: May increase maraviroc blood level. Adjust maraviroc dosage according to its prescribing information.

Methadone: May decrease methadone level. Monitor clinical response and increase methadone dosage as needed.

Midazolam (oral), triazolam: Increases exposure of these drugs and risk of severe sedation or respiratory depression. Use together is contraindicated.

Pitavastatin, pravastatin: May increase statin level and risk of myopathy and rhabdomyolysis. Use together cautiously.

Quetiapine: May increase quetiapine level. Consider another antiretroviral or decrease quetiapine dosage to one-sixth of current dose. Monitor patient for adverse effects.

Rifabutin: May increase rifabutin level. Decrease rifabutin dosage by at least 75% or maximum of 150 mg every other day or three times a week. Monitor patient carefully and adjust dosage as needed.

Rifampin: May decrease effectiveness of Kaletra. Avoid use together.

Rivaroxaban: May increase bleeding risk. Avoid use together.

Rosuvastatin: May increase statin level and risk of myopathy and rhabdomyolysis. Rosuvastatin dosage shouldn't exceed 10 mg daily.

Salmeterol: May increase salmeterol level and risk of CV adverse reactions. Use together isn't recommended.

Saquinavir: May increase level and QT-prolonging effect of saquinavir. Use cautiously together.

Trazodone: May increase trazodone level and risk of adverse reactions. Consider lower dosage of trazodone.

Voriconazole: May decrease voriconazole level. Avoid use together.

Warfarin: May affect warfarin level. Frequently monitor INR.

Drug-herb. *Garlic supplements:* May decrease level of protease inhibitors. Concurrent use isn't recommended. If combination is used, monitor patient closely for signs or symptoms of therapeutic failure.

St. John's wort: May cause loss of virologic response and possible resistance to drug. Discourage use together.

Drug-food. *Any food:* May increase absorption of oral solution. Tell patient to take with food.

EFFECTS ON LAB TEST RESULTS
- May increase glucose, amylase, lipase, cholesterol, CK, bilirubin, sodium, uric acid, and triglyceride levels and LFT values.
- May decrease Hb level and hematocrit and RBC, WBC, neutrophil, and platelet counts.

CONTRAINDICATIONS & CAUTIONS
- Contraindicated in patients hypersensitive to drug or its components.
- Concomitant use with certain other drugs may result in known or potentially significant drug interactions. Consult full prescribing information before and during treatment for potential drug interactions.
- ⚛ Genetic or phenotype testing and treatment history should guide use of drug. The number of baseline lopinavir resistance-associated substitutions affects drug's virologic response.
- Avoid use in patients with congenital long QT syndrome or hypokalemia and in those taking drugs that prolong QT interval. Correct potassium abnormalities before starting therapy.

• Use cautiously in patients with history of pancreatitis, liver impairment, HBV or HCV infection, marked elevations in liver enzyme levels, or hemophilia.

• Use cautiously in patients with cardiac conduction abnormalities or underlying cardiac disease.

• Use cautiously in older adults.

• New-onset diabetes, exacerbation of preexisting diabetes, and hyperglycemia have been reported in patients infected with HIV-1 receiving protease inhibitor therapy.

• Oral solution contains 42.4% (volume/volume) alcohol and 15.3% (weight/volume) propylene glycol; use with care, especially in infants and young children. Consider total amounts of alcohol and propylene glycol from all drugs given to children ages 14 days to 6 months to avoid toxicity.

🔸 *Alert:* Safety and effectiveness in neonates younger than age 14 days haven't been established. Use only if benefit outweighs risk. Monitor neonates for toxicity, such as hyperosmolality with or without lactic acidosis, kidney toxicity, CNS depression (stupor, coma, apnea), seizures, hypotonia, cardiac arrhythmias, ECG changes, and hemolysis. Toxicity in preterm neonates can be severe or fatal.

Dialyzable drug: Unlikely.

⚠ *Overdose S&S:* Alcohol-related toxicity.

PREGNANCY-LACTATION-REPRODUCTION

• Drug is recommended with dosage adjustments for patients who are pregnant and infected with HIV.

• Avoid use of oral solution during pregnancy because it contains alcohol.

🔹 Once-daily dosing isn't recommended in patients who are pregnant with any documented lopinavir resistance-associated amino acid substitutions.

• Encourage patient to enroll in the Antiretroviral Pregnancy Registry (1-800-258-4263 or www.apregistry.com).

• The CDC recommends that patients with HIV not breastfeed to avoid HIV transmission to the infant.

NURSING CONSIDERATIONS

• Don't administer tablets or oral solution as once-daily dosing regimen when combined with efavirenz, nevirapine, or nelfinavir.

• Avoid once-daily dosing in child younger than age 18.

• Calculate appropriate dose for each child based on body weight or BSA to avoid underdosing or exceeding recommended adult dose.

• Assess child's ability to swallow intact tablets before drug is prescribed; use oral solution if child is unable to reliably swallow tablet.

• During initial phase of treatment, patient responding to antiretroviral therapy may develop inflammatory response to indolent or residual opportunistic infections (CMV, MAC, *Pneumocystis jiroveci* pneumonia, TB), which may necessitate further evaluation and treatment. Autoimmune disorders (Graves disease, polymyositis, Guillain-Barré syndrome) have also been reported in the setting of immune reconstitution; however, onset time varies, and onset can occur many months after antiretroviral treatment initiation.

• Monitor patient for signs of fat redistribution (central obesity, buffalo hump, peripheral wasting, breast enlargement, cushingoid appearance).

• Monitor glucose, total cholesterol, and triglyceride levels before starting therapy and periodically thereafter.

• Monitor for signs and symptoms of pancreatitis (nausea, vomiting, abdominal pain, increased lipase and amylase values).

• Monitor patient for signs and symptoms of bleeding (hypotension, rapid HR).

• Consider potential for drug interactions before and during therapy. Review concomitant medications and monitor patient for adverse reactions associated with the concomitant medications.

• *Look alike–sound alike:* Don't confuse Kaletra with Keppra.

PATIENT TEACHING

• Teach about proper drug administration and handling.

• Advise patient to report all side effects to prescriber.

• Review signs and symptoms of acute pancreatitis. Instruct patient to seek emergency medical treatment if any occur.

• Tell patient to report all adverse reactions and to immediately report severe nausea, vomiting, or abdominal pain.

• Inform patient that drug doesn't cure HIV infection, that opportunistic infections and other complications of HIV infection may still occur, and that transmission of HIV to others through sexual contact or blood contamination remains possible.

Reactions in bold italics are *life-threatening*.

• Advise patient taking an erectile dysfunction drug of increased risk of adverse effects, including low BP, visual changes, and painful erections. Instruct patient to promptly report any symptoms to prescriber. Tell patient not to take more often than directed.
• Advise patient to immediately report pregnancy or plans to become pregnant.
• Warn patient to tell prescriber about other prescription or OTC drugs being taken, including herbal supplements.

SAFETY ALERT!

LORazepam
lor-AZ-e-pam

Ativan, Lorazepam Intensol, Loreev XR

Therapeutic class: Anxiolytics
Pharmacologic class: Benzodiazepines
Controlled substance schedule: IV

AVAILABLE FORMS
Capsules (extended-release) ⬛: 1 mg, 1.5 mg, 2 mg, 3 mg
Injection: 2 mg/mL, 4 mg/mL
Oral solution: 2 mg/mL
Tablets: 0.5 mg, 1 mg, 2 mg

INDICATIONS & DOSAGES
➤ **Anxiety**
Adults: 2 to 6 mg PO daily in divided doses, with largest dose taken before bedtime. Maximum dosage, 10 mg daily. Or extended-release capsule at dose equal to total daily dose of immediate-release tablets PO daily in the morning.
Adjust-a-dose: If response to extended-release form is inadequate, switch to immediate-release tablets to further titrate dosage; then resume extended-release form. If UGT inhibitor is started during use of extended-release capsules, switch to lorazepam tablets to reduce dosage.
Older adults: 1 to 2 mg PO daily in divided doses. Maximum dosage, 10 mg daily.
➤ **Insomnia from anxiety or transient situational stress**
Adults: 2 to 4 mg PO at bedtime.
➤ **Preoperative sedation**
Adults: 2 mg IV total or 0.044 mg/kg IV, whichever is smaller, 15 to 20 minutes before anticipated operative procedure. Larger doses up to 0.05 mg/kg IV, to total of 4 mg, may be needed. Or, 0.05 mg/kg IM 2 hours before procedure. Total dose shouldn't exceed 4 mg.
➤ **Status epilepticus**
Adults: 4 mg IV at rate of 2 mg/minute. If seizures continue or recur after 10 to 15 minutes, additional 4-mg dose may be given. Drug may be given IM if IV access isn't available.

ADMINISTRATION
PO
• Give extended-release capsule in morning without regard to food.
• Have patient swallow extended-release capsule whole; don't crush capsules.
• May open capsule and sprinkle entire contents over tablespoon of applesauce; then have patient swallow without chewing and follow with a drink of water. Use within 2 hours of mixing; don't store for later use.
• Use only calibrated dropper provided for oral solution.
• Mix oral solution with liquid or semisolid food (water, juice, carbonated beverage, applesauce, pudding). Gently stir liquid or food for a few seconds and have patient immediately consume entire mixture.
IV
▼ Keep emergency resuscitation equipment and oxygen available.
▼ Give slowly at no more than 2 mg/minute.
▼ Monitor respirations every 5 to 15 minutes and before each IV dose.
▼ Contains benzyl alcohol. Avoid use in neonates.
▼ Refrigerate intact vials and protect from light.
▼ **Incompatibilities:** None listed by manufacturer. Consult drug compatibility reference for more information.
IM
• For status epilepticus, may give IM if IV access isn't available.
• For IM use, inject deeply into a muscle. Don't dilute.
• Refrigerate parenteral form to prolong shelf life.

ACTION
Potentiates the effects of GABA, depresses the CNS, and suppresses the spread of seizure activity.

Route	Onset	Peak	Duration
PO	1 hr	2 hr	12–24 hr
IV	5 min	60–90 min	6–8 hr
IM	15–30 min	60–90 min	6–8 hr

Half-life: 10 to 20 hours.

ADVERSE REACTIONS

CNS: drowsiness, sedation, amnesia, hallucinations, confusion, crying, delirium, insomnia, agitation, dizziness, weakness, unsteadiness, depression, asthenia, headache, somnolence, stupor, *coma (injection).* **CV:** hypotension. **EENT:** visual disturbances. **GI:** abdominal discomfort, nausea, change in appetite. **Respiratory:** *apnea, respiratory failure, respiratory depression.* **Skin:** injection site reaction.

INTERACTIONS

Drug-drug. *CNS depressants (clozapine):* May cause delirium, sedation, excessive salivation, and ataxia. Don't start simultaneously.
Boxed Warning *Opioids:* May cause slow or difficult breathing, sedation, and death. Avoid use together. If use together is necessary, limit dosage and duration of each drug to the minimum necessary for desired effect. ∎
Oral hormonal contraceptives: May decrease lorazepam level. Monitor closely; lorazepam dosage may need to be increased.
Probenecid: May result in prolonged lorazepam half-life and a decrease in its total clearance. Reduce lorazepam dosage by 50% when coadministered.
Scopolamine: May increase sedation, hallucinations, and irrational behavior with lorazepam injection as preanesthetic. Avoid use together.
Sodium oxybate: May result in additive effects, including increased sleep duration and CNS depression. Use together is contraindicated.
UGT inhibitors (diclofenac, quinidine, ritonavir): May increase lorazepam level. Avoid use with extended-release capsules; switch to immediate-release tablets, if needed. Monitor patient.
Valproate: May increase lorazepam level. Reduce lorazepam dosage by 50% of normal adult dose when used together.
Drug-herb. *Kava:* May enhance adverse or toxic effects of CNS depressants. Monitor therapy.

Yohimbe: May diminish therapeutic effect of antianxiety agents. Monitor therapy.
Drug-lifestyle. *Alcohol use:* May cause additive CNS effects. Discourage use together.
Cannabis: May enhance CNS depressant effect of CNS depressants. Monitor therapy.

EFFECTS ON LAB TEST RESULTS

• May increase LDH level and LFT values.
• May decrease sodium level.
• May decrease WBC count.

CONTRAINDICATIONS & CAUTIONS

• Contraindicated in patients hypersensitive to drug, other benzodiazepines, or the vehicle (including polyethylene glycol, propylene glycol, benzyl alcohol) used in parenteral dosage form and in patients with acute angle-closure glaucoma. IV administration is contraindicated in patients with sleep apnea and in patients with severe respiratory insufficiency, except those who are mechanically ventilated.
• Contraindicated for intra-arterial administration.
• Extended-release formulation isn't recommended in patients with primary depressive disorder or psychosis. Preexisting depression may emerge or worsen.
Boxed Warning *Opioid class warning:* Opioids should only be prescribed with benzodiazepines or other CNS depressants to patients for whom alternative treatment options are inadequate. ∎
Boxed Warning Benzodiazepine use exposes patient to risks of abuse, misuse, and addiction, which can lead to overdose or death. Assess each patient's risk of abuse, misuse, and addiction before prescribing and periodically during therapy. ∎
⊙ Alert: Repeated or lengthy use of general anesthetic and sedation drugs during surgeries or procedures in children younger than age 3 or during the third trimester may affect brain development in children. Weigh benefits of appropriate anesthesia against risks in young children and patients who are pregnant.
• Use cautiously in patients with pulmonary, kidney, or liver impairment or history of substance abuse.
• Use cautiously in older adults and in patients who are acutely ill or debilitated.
• Capsules contain FD&C Yellow No. 5 (tartrazine), which may cause allergic reactions.
Dialyzable drug: Unknown.

Reactions in bold italics are *life-threatening*.

⚠ *Overdose S&S:* Drowsiness, confusion lethargy, ataxia, hypotonia, hypotension, hypnotic state, stage 1 to 3 coma, death.

PREGNANCY-LACTATION-REPRODUCTION
• May cause fetal harm, including neonatal withdrawal symptoms. Avoid use during pregnancy except in life-threatening situations (status epilepticus) when safer drugs can't be used.
• Monitor neonate exposed to drug late in pregnancy for sedation (respiratory depression, lethargy, hypotonia) and withdrawal symptoms (hyperreflexia, irritability, restlessness, tremors, inconsolable crying, feeding difficulties).
• Drug appears in human milk. Use during breastfeeding isn't recommended. Infants exposed through human milk should be monitored for sedation, poor feeding, and poor weight gain.

NURSING CONSIDERATIONS
• Periodically monitor liver, kidney, and hematopoietic function in patient receiving repeated or prolonged therapy.
Boxed Warning Abrupt discontinuation or rapid dosage reduction of benzodiazepines after continued use may precipitate acute withdrawal reactions, which can be life-threatening. To reduce risk of withdrawal reactions, gradually taper drug to discontinue or reduce dosage. ∎
• Paradoxical reactions (agitation, irritability, impulsivity, violent behavior, confusion, restlessness, excitement, talkativeness) have been reported, especially in children and older adults. Discontinue drug if reactions occur.
🔔 *Alert:* Monitor patient with preexisting depression for suicidality.
• *Look alike–sound alike:* Don't confuse lorazepam with alprazolam or clonazepam.

PATIENT TEACHING
Boxed Warning *Opioid class warning:* Caution patient or caregiver of patient taking an opioid with a benzodiazepine, CNS depressant, or alcohol to seek immediate medical attention for dizziness, light-headedness, extreme sleepiness, slowed or difficult breathing, or unresponsiveness. ∎
Boxed Warning Caution patient that benzodiazepines, even at recommended doses, increase risk of abuse, misuse, and addiction, which can lead to overdose and death, especially when used in combination with other drugs (opioid analgesics), alcohol, or illicit substances. ∎
• Inform patient about proper disposal of unused drug.
• Teach patient and caregiver signs and symptoms of benzodiazepine abuse, misuse, and addiction (abdominal pain, amnesia, anorexia, anxiety, aggression, ataxia, blurred vision, confusion, depression, disinhibition, disorientation, dizziness, euphoria, impaired concentration and memory, indigestion, irritability, muscle pain, slurred speech, tremors, vertigo, delirium, paranoia, suicidality, seizures, difficulty breathing, coma). Advise patient to seek emergency medical help if signs and symptoms occur. Advise patient not to take drug at a higher dose, more frequently, or for longer than prescribed.
Boxed Warning Tell patient that continued use of drug for several days to weeks may lead to physical dependence and that abrupt discontinuation or rapid dosage reduction may precipitate acute withdrawal reactions (unusual movements, responses, or expressions; seizures; sudden and severe mental or nervous system changes; depression; seeing or hearing things that others don't; homicidal thoughts; extreme increase in activity or talking; losing touch with reality; suicidality), which can be life-threatening. Instruct patient that drug discontinuation or dosage reduction may require a slow taper. ∎
Boxed Warning Advise patient about possibility of developing protracted withdrawal syndrome (anxiety; trouble remembering, learning, or concentrating; depression; problems sleeping; sensation of insects crawling under skin; weakness; shaking; muscle twitching; burning or prickling feeling in hands, arms, legs, or feet; ringing in ears), with symptoms lasting weeks to more than 12 months. ∎
🔔 *Alert:* Discuss with patient who is pregnant the benefits, risks, and appropriate timing of surgery or procedures requiring anesthetic and sedation drugs.
• When used before surgery, drug causes substantial preoperative amnesia. Patient teaching requires extra care to ensure adequate recall. Provide written materials or inform a family member, if possible.
• Warn patient to avoid hazardous activities that require alertness or good coordination until effects of drug are known.

L

- Tell patient to avoid use of alcohol while taking drug.
- Notify patient that smoking may decrease drug's effectiveness.
- Instruct patient to report pregnancy or plans to become pregnant or breastfeed.

losartan potassium ⊠
low-SAR-tan

Cozaar

Therapeutic class: Antihypertensives
Pharmacologic class: ARBs

AVAILABLE FORMS
Tablets: 25 mg, 50 mg, 100 mg

INDICATIONS & DOSAGES
Adjust-a-dose (for all indications): In adults with Child-Pugh class A or B liver impairment, starting dose is 25 mg once daily.
➤ **HTN**
Adults: Initially, 50 mg PO daily. Maximum daily dosage, 100 mg.
Children ages 6 and older: 0.7 mg/kg (up to 50 mg) PO daily, adjusted as needed up to 1.4 mg/kg/day (maximum, 100 mg).
Adjust-a-dose: For adults with intravascular volume depletion (such as those taking diuretics), initially, 25 mg. Don't use in children with eGFR less than 30 mL/minute/1.73 m^2.
➤ **Nephropathy in patients with type 2 diabetes**
Adults: 50 mg PO once daily. Increase dosage to 100 mg once daily based on BP response.
➤ **To reduce risk of stroke in patients with HTN and left ventricular hypertrophy**
Adults: Initially, 50 mg PO once daily. Adjust dosage based on BP response, adding hydrochlorothiazide 12.5 mg once daily, increasing losartan to 100 mg daily, or both. If further adjustments are required, may increase daily dosage of hydrochlorothiazide to 25 mg.

ADMINISTRATION
PO
- Give drug without regard to meals.
- If made into suspension by pharmacist, store in refrigerator for up to 4 weeks and shake well before each use.

ACTION
Inhibits vasoconstrictive and aldosterone-secreting action of angiotensin II by blocking angiotensin II receptor on the surface of vascular smooth muscle and other tissue cells.

Route	Onset	Peak	Duration
PO	6 hr	1–2 hr	Unknown

Half-life: Parent drug, about 1.5 to 3 hours; active metabolite, about 4.5 to 10 hours.

ADVERSE REACTIONS
CNS: dizziness, asthenia, fatigue, headache. **CV:** edema, chest pain, palpitations, orthostatic hypotension, hypotension. **EENT:** nasal congestion. **GI:** abdominal pain, constipation, nausea, diarrhea. **GU:** UTI. **Hematologic:** anemia. **Metabolic:** *hyperkalemia, hypoglycemia.* **Musculoskeletal:** muscle weakness, myalgia, back pain. **Respiratory:** cough, URI.

INTERACTIONS
Drug-drug. *Aliskiren; ACE inhibitors, ARBs:* May increase risk of kidney impairment, hypotension, and hyperkalemia. Concomitant use with aliskiren is contraindicated in patients with diabetes. Avoid use together in patients with GFR less than 60 mL/minute; if use together is necessary, monitor patient closely.
Amphetamines: May diminish antihypertensive effect. Monitor therapy.
Antipsychotics (atypical): May enhance hypotensive effect of these agents. Monitor therapy.
Lithium: May increase lithium level. Monitor lithium level and patient for toxicity.
NSAIDs: May decrease antihypertensive effects. Monitor BP and kidney function.
Potassium-sparing diuretics, potassium supplements: May cause hyperkalemia. Monitor patient closely.
Drug-herb. *Ma huang:* May decrease antihypertensive effects. Discourage use together.
Drug-food. *Salt substitutes containing potassium:* May cause hyperkalemia. Monitor patient closely.

EFFECTS ON LAB TEST RESULTS
- May increase potassium level.
- May decrease glucose and sodium level.
- May decrease Hb level and platelet count.

Reactions in bold italics are *life-threatening*.

CONTRAINDICATIONS & CAUTIONS
• Contraindicated in patients hypersensitive to drug.
• Use cautiously in patients with impaired kidney or liver function.
• Safety and effectiveness in children younger than age 6 haven't been established.
Dialyzable drug: No.
⚠ *Overdose S&S:* Hypotension, tachycardia, bradycardia.

PREGNANCY-LACTATION-REPRODUCTION
Boxed Warning Drugs that act directly on the RAAS can cause fetal injury and death. If pregnancy is suspected, notify prescriber because drug should be stopped as soon as possible. ▆
• It isn't known if drug appears in human milk. Patient should discontinue breastfeeding or discontinue drug, considering importance of drug to patient.

NURSING CONSIDERATIONS
• Drug can be used alone or with other antihypertensives.
• Correct fluid volume and sodium depletion before treatment.
⚕ Closely monitor patient's BP to evaluate effectiveness of therapy. When used alone, drug has less of an effect on BP in patients who are Black than in patients of other races.
• Monitor patient who is also taking diuretics for symptomatic hypotension.
• Regularly assess patient's kidney function (creatinine and BUN levels).
• Patients with severe HF whose kidney function depends on the angiotensin-aldosterone system may develop AKI during therapy. Closely monitor patient's BP, kidney function, and potassium level, especially during first few weeks of therapy and after dosage adjustments.
• *Look alike–sound alike:* Don't confuse Cozaar with Zocor or Colace.

PATIENT TEACHING
• Tell patient to avoid salt substitutes; these products may contain potassium, which can cause high potassium level in patients taking losartan.
• Advise patient to report all adverse reactions and to immediately report difficulty breathing or swelling of face, eyes, lips, or tongue

• Inform patient of childbearing potential about consequences of taking drug while pregnant. Instruct patient to immediately report suspected pregnancy.
• Advise patient not to breastfeed while taking drug.

lovastatin (mevinolin) ⚕
loe-va-STA-tin

Altoprev

Therapeutic class: Antilipemics
Pharmacologic class: HMG-CoA reductase inhibitors

AVAILABLE FORMS
Tablets: 10 mg, 20 mg, 40 mg
Tablets (extended-release) ⓓⓝⓒ: 20 mg, 40 mg, 60 mg

INDICATIONS & DOSAGES
Adjust-a-dose (for all indications): Avoid use of lovastatin with fibrates or niacin at dosages greater than 1 g daily. For patients also taking danazol, diltiazem, dronedarone, or verapamil, start lovastatin at 10 mg (immediate-release) and don't exceed 20 mg daily. For patients also taking amiodarone, lovastatin dosage shouldn't exceed 40 mg daily unless clinical benefit is likely to outweigh increased risk of myopathy or rhabdomyolysis. For older adults or patients with CrCl of less than 30 mL/minute, carefully consider dosage increase greater than 20 mg daily and implement cautiously if necessary. For patients requiring smaller reductions in cholesterol levels, use immediate-release lovastatin.
➤ **To prevent and treat CAD; hyperlipidemia**
Adults: Initially, 20 mg (immediate-release) PO once daily with evening meal. Recommended range is 10 to 80 mg as a single dose or in two divided doses; maximum daily recommended dosage, 80 mg. Or, 20 to 60 mg extended-release tablets PO at bedtime. Make dosage adjustments at intervals of 4 weeks or more.
➤ **Heterozygous familial hypercholesterolemia in adolescents** ⚕
Adolescents ages 10 to 17: Give 10 to 40 mg (immediate-release) PO daily with evening meal. Patients requiring reductions in LDL-C level of 20% or more should start with 20 mg

L

❦Canada   ◇OTC   ♦Off-label use   ⓓDo not crush   *Liquid contains alcohol   ⚕Genetic

daily. Maximum daily dosage, 40 mg. Make dosage adjustments at intervals of 4 weeks or more.

ADMINISTRATION

PO

• Give immediate-release drug with evening meal, which improves absorption and cholesterol biosynthesis. Give extended-release drug at bedtime.

• Have patient swallow extended-release tablets whole; don't crush or break tablets.

ACTION

Inhibits HMG-CoA reductase, an early (and rate-limiting) step in cholesterol biosynthesis.

Route	Onset	Peak	Duration
PO	Unknown	2–4 hr	Unknown
PO (extended-release)	3 days	12–14 hr	Unknown

Half-life: 1.1 to 1.7 hours.

ADVERSE REACTIONS

CNS: headache, dizziness, asthenia, pain. **EENT:** blurred vision, sinusitis. **GI:** abdominal pain or cramps, constipation, diarrhea, dyspepsia, flatulence, nausea, vomiting. **GU:** UTI. **Hepatic:** increased transaminase levels. **Metabolic:** increased CK level. **Musculoskeletal:** muscle cramps, back pain, arthralgia, myalgia. **Skin:** rash. **Other:** flulike syndrome, pain, infection, accidental injury.

INTERACTIONS

Drug-drug. *Amiodarone:* May decrease metabolism of lovastatin. Avoid combining lovastatin at dosages exceeding 40 mg daily with amiodarone unless clinical benefit is likely to outweigh increased risk of myopathy.

Colchicine: May increase risk of myopathy or rhabdomyolysis. If use together can't be avoided, monitor patient for unexplained muscle pain, tenderness, or weakness.

Cyclosporine, gemfibrozil: May cause severe myopathy and rhabdomyolysis. Avoid use together.

Danazol, diltiazem, verapamil: May cause myopathy and rhabdomyolysis. Don't exceed 20 mg lovastatin daily.

Dronedarone: May increase lovastatin level. Limit lovastatin to maximum of 20 mg/day (in adults). Increase monitoring for signs and symptoms of lovastatin toxicity (such as

myopathy and rhabdomyolysis). Consider therapy modification.

Erythromycin, protease inhibitors (atazanavir, darunavir, fosamprenavir, nefazodone, nelfinavir, ritonavir, saquinavir, tipranavir), strong CYP3A inhibitors (clarithromycin, itraconazole, ketoconazole, posaconazole, voriconazole): Increases risk of myopathy and rhabdomyolysis. Use together is contraindicated.

Macrolides (azithromycin, clarithromycin), nefazodone: May decrease metabolism of HMG-CoA reductase inhibitor, increasing toxicity. Monitor patient for adverse effects and report unexplained muscle pain.

Niacin, other fibrates: May increase risk of adverse and toxic effects of lovastatin. Avoid use of lovastatin with fibrates or niacin at dosages greater than 1 g daily.

Oral anticoagulants: May increase anticoagulant effect. Monitor patient closely.

Ranolazine: May increase risk of myopathy and rhabdomyolysis. Consider lovastatin dosage adjustment.

Drug-herb. *Eucalyptus, kava:* May increase risk of liver toxicity. Discourage use together. *Red yeast rice:* May increase risk of adverse reactions because herb contains compounds like those in drug. Discourage use together. *St. John's wort:* May increase metabolism of HMG-CoA reductase inhibitors, leading to decreased effectiveness of drug's cholesterol-lowering abilities. Consider therapy modification.

Drug-food. *Grapefruit juice:* May increase drug level, increasing risk of adverse effects. Discourage use together.

Drug-lifestyle. *Alcohol use:* May increase risk of liver toxicity. Discourage use together.

EFFECTS ON LAB TEST RESULTS

• May increase ALT, AST, bilirubin, CK, glucose, and HbA_{1c} levels.

• May cause thyroid function test abnormalities.

CONTRAINDICATIONS & CAUTIONS

• Contraindicated in patients hypersensitive to drug and in those with active liver disease or unexplained persistently increased transaminase levels.

• Use cautiously in patients who consume substantial quantities of alcohol or have a history of liver disease or kidney impairment.

Reactions in bold italics are ***life-threatening***.

• Drug may increase risk of rare immune-mediated necrotizing myopathy. Treatment with immunosuppressants may be required. *Dialyzable drug:* Unknown.

PREGNANCY-LACTATION-REPRODUCTION
• Drug may cause fetal harm and is contraindicated in most patients who are pregnant or may become pregnant. If patient becomes pregnant during therapy, discontinue drug and apprise patient of potential hazard to the fetus.
• May consider using in patients at high risk for CV events during pregnancy (homozygous familial hypercholesterolemia, established CV disease) on an individual basis.
• It isn't known if drug appears in human milk. Use during breastfeeding is contraindicated.

NURSING CONSIDERATIONS
• Have patient follow a diet restricted in saturated fat and cholesterol during therapy.
• Obtain LFT results at start of therapy; then monitor results periodically.
▨ Heterozygous familial hypercholesterolemia can be diagnosed in adolescent males and in females who are at least 1 year postmenarche and are 10 to 17 years old if, after adequate trial of diet therapy, LDL-C level remains over 189 mg/dL or LDL-C is over 160 mg/dL and patient has a positive family history of premature CV disease or two or more other CV disease risk factors.
• Obtain CK level in patient with unexplained muscle pain.
• Immediately discontinue lovastatin if markedly elevated CK level occurs or myopathy is diagnosed or suspected. Predisposing factors for skeletal muscle effects include advanced age (65 and older), female sex, uncontrolled hypothyroidism, and kidney impairment.
• *Look alike–sound alike:* Don't confuse lovastatin with Lotensin.

PATIENT TEACHING
• Teach about proper drug administration and handling.
• Teach about proper dietary management of cholesterol and triglycerides. When appropriate, recommend weight control, exercise, and smoking cessation programs.
• Warn of risk of myopathy and rhabdomyolysis. Instruct patient to promptly report

unexplained muscle pain, tenderness, or weakness, particularly when accompanied by malaise or fever.
• Teach patient about substances that shouldn't be taken with lovastatin and to inform other health care providers about taking lovastatin, especially if a new medication is being prescribed.
• Caution patient to avoid grapefruit juice while taking drug.
🕦 *Alert:* Tell patient of childbearing potential to immediately stop drug and report pregnancy, suspected pregnancy, or breastfeeding.

lurasidone hydrochloride
loo-RAS-i-dohne

Latuda

Therapeutic class: Antipsychotics
Pharmacologic class: Dopamine–serotonin receptor antagonists

AVAILABLE FORMS
Tablets: 20 mg, 40 mg, 60 mg, 80 mg, 120 mg

INDICATIONS & DOSAGES
Adjust-a-dose (for all indications): For patients with CrCl of 50 mL/minute or less or those concomitantly taking a moderate CYP3A4 inhibitor, recommended starting dose is 20 mg and maximum recommended dose is 80 mg. For patients with Child-Pugh class B or C liver impairment, recommended starting dose is 20 mg. Maximum recommended dose is 80 mg for patients with Child-Pugh class B impairment and 40 mg for those with Child-Pugh class C impairment. If moderate CYP3A4 inducer is used concomitantly, it may be necessary to increase lurasidone dosage.
➤ **Schizophrenia**
Adults: Initially, 40 mg PO once daily. May increase to maximum dosage of 160 mg daily.
Adolescents ages 13 to 17: 40 mg PO once daily. May increase to maximum dosage of 80 mg daily.
➤ **Depressive episodes associated with bipolar I disorder as monotherapy or as adjunctive therapy with lithium or valproate**
Adults: Initially, 20 mg PO once daily. May increase to maximum dosage of 120 mg daily.

➤ **Depressive episodes associated with bipolar I disorder (monotherapy)**
Children ages 10 to 17: 20 mg PO once daily. May increase after 1 week to maximum dosage of 80 mg daily.

ADMINISTRATION
PO
• Give drug with food containing at least 350 calories to increase absorption.
• Have patient swallow tablets whole; don't crush or break tablets.

ACTION
Exact mechanism is unknown. Drug's efficacy is mediated through antagonism at dopamine type 2 and serotonin type 2 receptors.

Route	Onset	Peak	Duration
PO	Unknown	1–3 hr	Unknown

Half-life: 18 to 40 hours.

ADVERSE REACTIONS
CNS: somnolence, akathisia, extrapyramidal symptoms, agitation, dystonia, dizziness, insomnia, abnormal dreams, anxiety, restlessness, fatigue. **CV:** tachycardia, HTN. **EENT:** blurred vision, nasopharyngitis, rhinitis, oropharyngeal pain, dry mouth, increased salivation. **GI:** nausea, vomiting, dyspepsia, abdominal pain, diarrhea, dysphagia, increased appetite. **GU:** UTI, increased creatinine level. **Metabolic:** dyslipidemia, hyperglycemia, weight gain, increased CK level. **Musculoskeletal:** back pain. **Respiratory:** URI. **Skin:** rash, pruritus. **Other:** flulike symptoms.

INTERACTIONS
Drug-drug. *Antihypertensives:* May increase risk of hypotension. Monitor orthostatic vital signs and adjust antihypertensive dosage as needed.
Centrally acting drugs: May increase risk of adverse effects (increased cognitive impairment). Avoid use together.
Moderate CYP3A4 inducers (bosentan, efavirenz, etravirine, modafinil, nafcillin): May decrease lurasidone level. Consider increasing lurasidone dosage.
Moderate inhibitors of CYP3A4 (atazanavir, diltiazem, erythromycin, fluconazole, verapamil): May increase lurasidone level. Use together cautiously and reduce lurasidone

dosage by 50%. Initial recommended lurasidone dosage is 20 mg daily. Maximum daily dosage, 80 mg.
🜂 *Alert: Opioids:* May increase CNS depression. Avoid use together. If use together can't be avoided, limit dosage and duration of each drug to minimum necessary for desired effect.
Strong inducers of CYP3A4 (carbamazepine, phenytoin, rifampin): May significantly reduce lurasidone level. Don't use together.
Strong inhibitors of CYP3A4 (clarithromycin, ketoconazole, ritonavir, voriconazole): May significantly increase lurasidone level. Use together is contraindicated.
Drug-herb. *Kava:* May enhance adverse or toxic effect of CNS depressants. Monitor therapy.
St. John's wort: May significantly reduce lurasidone level. Don't use together.
Drug-food. *Grapefruit, grapefruit juice:* May increase lurasidone level. Discourage use during therapy.
Drug-lifestyle. *Alcohol use, cannabidiol, cannabis:* May increase CNS depressant effect and risk of adverse effects (such as increased cognitive impairment). Discourage use together.

EFFECTS ON LAB TEST RESULTS
• May increase prolactin, total cholesterol, triglyceride, glucose, serum creatinine, and CK levels.
• May decrease WBC, neutrophil, and granulocyte counts.

CONTRAINDICATIONS & CAUTIONS
• Contraindicated in patients hypersensitive to drug or its components.
Boxed Warning Older adults with dementia-related psychosis treated with atypical or conventional antipsychotics are at increased risk for death. Antipsychotics aren't approved for treatment of dementia-related psychosis. ■
• Use cautiously in patients with hyperlipidemia, liver or kidney impairment, diabetes or risk factors for diabetes (family history, obesity), seizures or conditions that lower the seizure threshold (Alzheimer dementia), body temperature dysregulation, major depressive disorder, suicidality, dysphagia, or concomitant illness.
• Use cautiously in patients with known CV disease, cerebrovascular disease, and

---

Reactions in bold italics are *life-threatening*.

conditions that cause hypotension (dehydration, hypovolemia, antihypertensive use) and in patients who are antipsychotic-naive because of increased risk of dizziness, tachycardia or bradycardia, and syncope.
• Use cautiously in patients with preexisting low WBC count or history of drug-induced neutropenia or leukopenia.
• Use cautiously in patients at risk for falls, including those with diseases or conditions or who are taking medications that may cause somnolence, orthostatic hypotension, or motor or sensory instability.
• Safety and effectiveness in children with depression haven't been established.
Dialyzable drug: Unknown.

PREGNANCY-LACTATION-REPRODUCTION
• Studies during pregnancy are inadequate. Use during pregnancy only if clearly needed and potential benefit justifies fetal risk. Drug may cause abnormal muscle movements (extrapyramidal symptoms) or withdrawal symptoms in newborns.
• Enroll patients exposed to lurasidone during pregnancy in National Pregnancy Registry for Atypical Antipsychotics (1-866-961-2388 or https://womensmentalhealth.org/research/pregnancyregistry/atypicalantipsychotic).
• It isn't known if drug appears in human milk. Patient should discontinue breastfeeding or discontinue drug considering importance of drug to patient.

NURSING CONSIDERATIONS
Boxed Warning Antidepressants increase risk of suicidality in children, adolescents, and young adults. Monitor all patients for worsening of depression or emergence of suicidality. ∎
• Monitor patient for tardive dyskinesia. Risk increases in older adults and women and with long-term administration. Use lowest dose for shortest time possible to minimize risk. Discontinue drug if symptoms occur.
• Monitor patient for extrapyramidal symptoms (bradykinesia, cogwheel rigidity, drooling, extrapyramidal disorder, tremor, hypokinesia, muscle rigidity, psychomotor retardation).
• Monitor for orthostatic hypotension, syncope, and excessive sedation.
• Assess patient's fall risk at start of therapy and regularly during long-term therapy,

especially if patient is taking other medications or has disease or condition that increased risk of falls.
• Monitor for NMS (fever, diaphoresis, muscle rigidity, altered mental status, AKI, irregular pulse or BP, arrhythmias, increased CK level, rhabdomyolysis). Immediately discontinue drug if NMS occurs.
• Periodically monitor CBC, kidney function, and prolactin level; discontinue drug if severe neutropenia develops.
• Monitor patient for metabolic changes (weight gain; elevated blood glucose, triglyceride, and cholesterol levels); treat appropriately.

PATIENT TEACHING
• *Opioid class warning:* Caution patient or caregiver of patient taking an opioid with a benzodiazepine, CNS depressant, or alcohol to seek immediate medical attention for dizziness, light-headedness, extreme sleepiness, slowed or difficult breathing, or unresponsiveness.
Boxed Warning Advise family or caregivers to observe patient closely for worsening of depression or suicidality. Encourage them to immediately report such behaviors to health care provider. ∎
• Advise patient to take drug on a regular basis and not skip doses.
• Inform patient that periodic blood tests will be needed to monitor tolerance to drug.
• Tell patient to avoid overheating and to maintain adequate hydration.
• Teach patient to monitor weight and maintain a healthy diet because drug may increase weight and blood glucose and cholesterol levels.
• Instruct patient to report all adverse reactions and to immediately report sudden changes in temperature or BP, irregular HR, or severe muscle rigidity.
• Counsel patient of childbearing potential to report pregnancy or breastfeeding before taking drug.
• Tell patient to avoid alcohol and grapefruit products during therapy.
• Warn patient to avoid driving or operating hazardous machinery until drug's effects are known.

L

magnesium sulfate (injection)

Therapeutic class: Electrolyte replacements
Pharmacologic class: Minerals

AVAILABLE FORMS

Injectable: 4%, 8%, 50% in 2-, 10-, 20-, and 50-mL ampules, vials, and prefilled syringes
Injection solution: 1 g, 2 g, 4 g, 20 g, 40 g in premixed single-dose containers

INDICATIONS & DOSAGES

Adjust-a-dose (for all indications): If CrCl is less than 30 mL/minute, reduce dosage and obtain frequent serum magnesium levels. Dosing recommendations vary by manufacturer and clinical guidelines. *Note:* 1 g = 8.12 mEq of magnesium.

➤ **Mild hypomagnesemia**
Adults: 1 g IM every 6 hours for four doses, or 1 to 2 g IV over 1 to 2 hours depending on magnesium level.

➤ **Symptomatic severe hypomagnesemia, with magnesium level of 1 mg/dL or less**
Adults: 5 g IV in 1 L of D_5W or NSS over 3 hours or 4 to 8 g IV over 4 to 24 hours. Or, 250 mg/kg IM in divided doses within a period of 4 hours. Base subsequent doses on magnesium level.

➤ **Magnesium supplementation in TPN**
Adults: 8 to 24 mEq/day IV added to TPN solution.
Infants: 2 to 10 mEq/day IV added to TPN solution.

➤ **Seizures in preeclampsia or eclampsia**
Adults: Total initial dose, 10 to 14 g IV.
Give 4 to 5 g IV in 250 mL of solution over 15 to 30 minutes and simultaneously give up to 10 g IM (5 g of undiluted 50% solution in each buttock). Or, initial dose of 4 to 6 g IV over 15 minutes. Or, dilute 50% solution to 10% to 20% concentration and give initial dose of 4 g IV over 3 to 4 minutes. Subsequently, give 4 to 5 g (8 to 10 mL of the 50% solution) IM into alternate buttocks every 4 hours as needed.

After initial IV dose, 1 to 2 g/hour by IV infusion. Base subsequent doses on magnesium level; serum magnesium level of 6 mg/100 mL is considered optimal for seizure control. Don't exceed 40 g in a 24-hour period. Maximum dose in patients with CrCl less than 30 mL/minute is 20 g/48 hours. Administration beyond 7 days isn't recommended.

ADMINISTRATION

● Store between 68° and 77° F (20° and 25° C). Protect from freezing.
● Discard unused portion.

IV

▼ Dilute solution for IV infusion to a concentration of 20% or less.
▼ Visually inspect solution for particulate matter and discoloration; don't give unless solution is clear and colorless to slightly yellow.
▼ Rate of injection by IV push generally shouldn't exceed 150 mg/minute.
▼ Use infusion pump for continuous infusion to avoid respiratory or cardiac arrest.
▼ For severe hypomagnesemia, watch for respiratory depression and evidence of heart block. Ensure respiratory rate is higher than 16 breaths/minute before giving dose.
▼ **Incompatibilities:** Magnesium salt precipitate may occur when combined with multiple solutions. Consult drug compatibility reference for more information.

IM

● Undiluted 50% solutions may be given by deep IM injection to adults. Dilute solutions to 20% or less for use in infants and children.

ACTION

Replaces magnesium and maintains magnesium level; as an anticonvulsant, reduces muscle contractions by interfering with release of acetylcholine at myoneural junction.

Route	Onset	Peak	Duration
IV	Immediate	Unknown	30 min
IM	1 hr	Unknown	3–4 hr

Half-life: 4 to 5 hours in women with preeclampsia.

ADVERSE REACTIONS

CNS: *CNS depression,* weak or absent deep tendon reflexes, paralysis, drowsiness, lethargy, stupor. **CV:** *bradycardia, arrhythmias, hypotension, circulatory collapse,* flushing. **EENT:** visual disturbances. **GI:** diarrhea. **Metabolic:** *hypocalcemia,* hypermagnesemia. **Respiratory:** *respiratory distress, pulmonary edema,* decreased respiratory

Reactions in bold italics are ***life-threatening***.

rate. **Skin:** diaphoresis. **Other:** hypothermia, myasthenia crisis, tetany.

INTERACTIONS
Drug-drug. *Calcium channel blockers (amlodipine, nifedipine):* May increase magnesium-related adverse effects. Monitor therapy.
Cardiac glycosides (digoxin): May cause serious cardiac conduction changes. Use together cautiously.
CNS depressants (propofol, opioids): May increase CNS depression. Use together cautiously.
Drugs that induce magnesium loss (amphotericin B, cisplatin, cyclosporine, loop diuretics, thiazide diuretics): May reduce effectiveness of magnesium replacement. Closely monitor magnesium level.
Neuromuscular blockers (succinylcholine, atracurium): May increase neuromuscular blockage. Use together cautiously. Closely monitor clinical response.
Drug-lifestyle. *Alcohol use:* May decrease magnesium level. Discourage use together.

EFFECTS ON LAB TEST RESULTS
• May decrease calcium level.

CONTRAINDICATIONS & CAUTIONS
• Contraindicated in patients with myasthenia gravis, myocardial damage, heart block, or diabetic coma.
• Use cautiously in patients with impaired kidney function.
🔵 *Alert:* Using magnesium sulfate to stop preterm labor isn't an FDA-approved use of drug; safety and effectiveness of drug for this indication haven't been established.
Dialyzable drug: Yes.
⚠ *Overdose S&S:* Hypotension, facial flushing, feeling of warmth, thirst, nausea, vomiting, lethargy, dysarthria, drowsiness, diminished deep tendon reflexes, shallow respirations, apnea, coma, cardiac arrest, respiratory paralysis, disappearance of patellar reflex.

PREGNANCY-LACTATION-REPRODUCTION
🔵 *Alert:* Drug can cause fetal abnormalities (fetal hypocalcemia, bone abnormalities), especially when given beyond 5 to 7 days to patients who are pregnant. Use during pregnancy only if clearly needed, and inform patient of potential fetal harm.

• When drug is administered by continuous IV infusion (especially for more than 24 hours preceding delivery) to control seizures in patient with eclampsia, the neonate may show signs of magnesium toxicity, including neuromuscular or respiratory depression.
• Drug appears in human milk. Use cautiously during breastfeeding.

NURSING CONSIDERATIONS
• Keep IV calcium available to reverse magnesium intoxication.
• If appropriate, test knee-jerk and patellar reflexes before each additional dose. If absent, notify prescriber and give no more magnesium until reflexes return; otherwise, patient may develop temporary respiratory failure and need cardiopulmonary resuscitation or IV calcium administration.
• Check magnesium level after repeated doses. Monitor level hourly in patient with severe hypomagnesemia. Normal plasma magnesium level is 1.8 to 2.6 mg/dL (SI, 0.74 to 1.07 mmol/L).
• Monitor fluid intake and output. Output should be 100 mL or more during 4-hour period before dose.
• Monitor kidney function.
• Drug may contain aluminum. Premature neonates are at higher risk for aluminum toxicity due to immature kidney function. Aluminum exposure of more than 4 to 5 mcg/kg/day is associated with CNS and bone toxicity.
• Patients with prolonged exposure to magnesium sulfate who have impaired kidney function are at risk for aluminum toxicity.
• *Look alike–sound alike:* Don't confuse magnesium sulfate with manganese sulfate.

PATIENT TEACHING
• Teach about proper drug administration and handling.
• Emphasize importance of keeping lab appointments.
• Review warning signs of high or low magnesium level. Encourage patient to report all adverse effects.
• Instruct patient to report pregnancy or plans to become pregnant during therapy.

M

mannitol
MAN-i-tole

Osmitrol

Therapeutic class: Diuretics
Pharmacologic class: Osmotic diuretics

AVAILABLE FORMS
Injection: 5%, 10%, 15%, 20%, 25%

INDICATIONS & DOSAGES
⚫ *Alert:* Dosage, concentration, and rate of administration depend on patient's age, weight, and condition, including fluid requirement, urine output, and concomitant therapy. The following indications are only general guides to therapy.

➤ **To reduce IOP**
Adults and children: 1.5 to 2 g/kg as a 15% or 20% single-dose solution IV over at least 30 minutes. For maximum IOP reduction before surgery, give 60 to 90 minutes preoperatively.

➤ **To reduce ICP and treat cerebral edema**
Adults and children: Usually a maximum reduction in ICP in adults can be achieved with a dose of 0.25 g/kg IV over 30 minutes; may repeat every 6 to 8 hours.

Adjust-a-dose: Monitor fluid and electrolyte levels, serum osmolarity, and kidney, cardiac, and pulmonary function during and after infusion. Discontinue if kidney, cardiac, or pulmonary status worsens or CNS toxicity develops.

ADMINISTRATION
● Don't give IM or subcut.
IV
▼ IV infusion through a central venous catheter is preferable.
▼ To redissolve crystallized solution (crystallization occurs at low temperatures or in concentrations higher than 15%), warm containers according to manufacturer's instructions with occasional shaking. Cool to body temperature before giving. Don't use solution with undissolved crystals.
▼ Give as intermittent or continuous infusion at prescribed rate, using inline filter and infusion pump. Don't give as direct injection. Don't use polyvinyl chloride bags in series connections.
▼ Give through filtered administration set; use blood filter set to avoid infusing crystals.

▼ Check patency at infusion site before and during administration.
▼ Monitor for signs and symptoms of infiltration; if any occur, watch for inflammation, edema, and necrosis.
▼ Turn off pump before container runs dry.
▼ Discard unused portion.
▼ Store at room temperature; don't freeze.
▼ **Incompatibilities:** Blood products and other drugs.

ACTION
Increases osmotic pressure of glomerular filtrate, thus inhibiting tubular reabsorption of water and electrolytes. Elevates plasma osmolality and increases urine output.

Route	Onset	Peak	Duration
IV	0.5–3 hr	20–40 min	3–6 hr

Half-life: 0.5 to 2.5 hours.

ADVERSE REACTIONS
CNS: *seizures,* dizziness, confusion, headache, *coma,* lethargy, malaise, asthenia, fever, *rebound increased ICP.* **CV:** edema, thrombophlebitis, hypotension, HTN, *HF,* tachycardia, palpitations, angina pectoris, *cardiac arrest.* **EENT:** blurred vision, dry mouth, rhinitis. **GI:** thirst, nausea, vomiting, diarrhea. **GU:** *AKI,* urine retention, *anuria,* oliguria, hematuria, osmotic nephrosis, azotemia, polyuria. **Metabolic:** dehydration, hypovolemia, hypervolemia, fluid and electrolyte imbalances, *metabolic acidosis,* metabolic alkalosis. **Musculoskeletal:** arm pain, myalgia, rigidity. **Respiratory:** *pulmonary edema,* cough. **Skin:** local pain, urticaria, injection-site reaction (erythema, infection), diaphoresis. **Other:** chills, hypersensitivity reactions.

INTERACTIONS
Drug-drug. *Diuretics (furosemide):* May increase risk of kidney toxicity. Avoid use together.
Kidney-toxic drugs (aminoglycosides, cyclosporine): May increase risk of toxicity and kidney failure. Avoid use together.
Lithium: May increase urinary excretion of lithium. Closely monitor lithium level.
Neurotoxic drugs (aminoglycosides): May increase risk of CNS toxicity. Avoid use together.

Reactions in bold italics are *life-threatening*.

Opioid analgesics: May increase diuretic-related adverse effects and diminish diuretic therapeutic effects. Monitor therapy.

Sodium phosphates: May enhance kidney-toxic effect of sodium phosphates. Consider therapy modification.

Tobramycin: Mannitol (systemic) may enhance kidney-toxic effect of tobramycin (oral inhalation). Avoid use together.

EFFECTS ON LAB TEST RESULTS
• May increase or decrease sodium, potassium, and other electrolyte levels.
• May interfere with tests for inorganic phosphorus or ethylene glycol level.

CONTRAINDICATIONS & CAUTIONS
• Contraindicated in patients hypersensitive to drug.
• Contraindicated in patients with anuria, severe pulmonary congestion, pulmonary edema, active intracranial bleeding (except during craniotomy), or severe hypovolemia.
• Approved for use in children for reduction of ICP and IOP. Studies haven't defined optimal dose in children. Safety profile for use in children is similar to that of adults. However, children younger than age 2, particularly preterm and term neonates, may be at higher risk for fluid and electrolyte abnormalities due to decreased GFR and limited ability to concentrate urine.
• Mannitol may increase risk of postoperative bleeding after neurosurgical procedure or traumatic brain injury due to increased cerebral blood flow.
• Use cautiously in older adults and patients with kidney impairment.

Dialyzable drug: Yes.

⚠ *Overdose S&S:* KF, increased electrolyte excretion, orthostatic tachycardia or hypotension, decreased central venous pressure, CNS toxicity (coma, seizures), impaired neuromuscular function, intestinal dilation and ileus, HF, hypovolemia, hypervolemia, pulmonary edema or water intoxication if urine output is inadequate.

PREGNANCY-LACTATION-REPRODUCTION
• Studies during pregnancy are inadequate. Use during pregnancy only if potential benefit justifies fetal risk.
• It isn't known if drug appears in human milk. Use cautiously during breastfeeding.

NURSING CONSIDERATIONS
• Monitor vital signs, central venous pressure, and fluid intake and output, hourly. Report increasing oliguria. Check weight, kidney function, fluid balance, and serum and urine sodium and potassium levels daily.
• When treating elevated ICP, also monitor serum osmolarity, electrolyte levels, acid-base balance, osmol gap, and kidney, cardiac, and pulmonary function.
• Use urinary catheter in patient with urinary incontinence or coma because therapy requires strict evaluation of fluid intake and output. If patient has urinary catheter, use an hourly urometer collection system to accurately evaluate output.
• Monitor for infusion site reactions.
• Closely monitor IV site for infiltration and extravasation; drug is vesicant at concentrations greater than 5%. Extravasation must be treated with hyaluronidase.
• Don't give drug with blood products or through same administration set to avoid pseudoagglutination or hemolysis. If drug must be given simultaneously with blood products, add at least 20 mEq of sodium chloride to each liter of drug solution to prevent pseudoagglutination.
• *Look alike–sound alike:* Don't confuse Osmitrol with esmolol.

PATIENT TEACHING
• Tell patient that thirstiness and dry mouth may occur; emphasize importance of drinking only the amount of fluids ordered.
• Instruct patient to promptly report adverse reactions and discomfort at IV site.

---

maraviroc
mahr-AY-vih-rok

Celsentri ✦, Selzentry

Therapeutic class: Antiretrovirals
Pharmacologic class: CCR5 co-receptor antagonists

AVAILABLE FORMS
Oral solution: 20 mg/mL
Tablets ⊕: 25 mg, 75 mg, 150 mg, 300 mg

INDICATIONS & DOSAGES

➤ **CCR5-tropic HIV-1 infection combined with strong CYP3A4 inhibitors with or without a strong CYP3A inducer**

Adults and children ages 2 and older weighing more than 40 kg: 150 mg PO b.i.d.

Children ages 2 and older weighing 30 to less than 40 kg: 100 mg PO b.i.d.

Children ages 2 and older weighing 20 to less than 30 kg: 75 mg (tablets) or 80 mg (oral solution) PO b.i.d.

Children ages 2 and older weighing 10 to less than 20 kg: 50 mg PO b.i.d.

Adjust-a-dose: For adults with CrCl of 30 mL/minute or more, no adjustment is needed. Drug is contraindicated in patients with CrCl of less than 30 mL/minute and in those with CKD treated with dialysis.

➤ **CCR5-tropic HIV-1 infection in combination with noninteracting concomitant medications (all medications that aren't strong CYP3A inhibitors or inducers), including all NRTIs, dolutegravir, tipranavir–ritonavir, nevirapine, raltegravir, or enfuvirtide**

Adults and children ages 2 and older weighing 30 kg or more: 300 mg PO b.i.d.

Children weighing 14 to less than 30 kg: 200 mg PO b.i.d.

Children weighing 10 to less than 14 kg: 150 mg PO b.i.d.

Children weighing 6 to less than 10 kg: 100 mg (5 mL) oral solution PO b.i.d.

Children weighing 4 to less than 6 kg: 40 mg (2 mL) oral solution PO b.i.d.

Children weighing 2 to less than 4 kg: 30 mg (1.5 mL) oral solution PO b.i.d.

Adjust-a-dose: For adults with kidney impairment, no dosage adjustment is needed. If patient with CrCl less than 30 mL/minute or on hemodialysis experiences orthostatic hypotension, reduce dosage to 150 mg PO b.i.d.

➤ **CCR5-tropic HIV-1 infection in combination with strong CYP3A and moderate inducers (without a potent CYP3A inhibitor)**

Adults: 600 mg PO b.i.d.

Adjust-a-dose: Use is contraindicated in patients with CrCl of less than 30 mL/minute or on regular hemodialysis. Use isn't recommended in children.

ADMINISTRATION
PO

• Give drug without regard to food.

• Have patient swallow tablets whole; don't crush or break tablets. Use of oral solution is preferred to crushing tablets to maintain stable levels.

• Use oral solution in patients who can't swallow tablets.

• Use oral dosing syringe for oral solution.

• Give missed dose as soon as possible; don't double next dose or give more than prescribed dose.

ACTION

Blocks viral entry into cells by binding to chemokine receptor type 5 co-receptor and preventing initiation of the HIV replication cycle.

Route	Onset	Peak	Duration
PO	Unknown	30 min–4 hr	Unknown

Half-life: 14 to 18 hours.

ADVERSE REACTIONS

CNS: anxiety, dizziness, paresthesia, sensory abnormalities, peripheral neuropathy, sleep disturbances, depressive disorders, fever, pain, memory loss, tremors, facial palsy, disturbances in consciousness, *stroke, seizure.* **CV:** unstable angina, *acute cardiac failure,* CAD, endocarditis, *MI,* myocardial ischemia, vascular hypertensive disorders, edema. **EENT:** conjunctivitis, hemianopia, visual field defect, ocular infections, otitis media, ear disorders, nasal congestion, paranasal sinus disorders, sinusitis, rhinitis, esophageal candidiasis. **GI:** abdominal pain, constipation, appetite disorders, dyspepsia, stomatitis, diarrhea, flatulence, bloating, abdominal distention, GI atonic and hypomotility disorders, vomiting. **GU:** urinary tract signs and symptoms, erection and ejaculation disorders. **Hematologic:** anemia, *neutropenia.* **Hepatic:** *cirrhosis, liver failure, portal vein thrombosis,* cholestatic jaundice, increased transaminase levels, hyperbilirubinemia. **Metabolic:** lipodystrophies, increased lipase level. **Musculoskeletal:** muscle pain, joint pain, osteonecrosis, *rhabdomyolysis,* myositis. **Respiratory:** URI, lower respiratory infection, bronchitis, cough, pneumonia, breathing abnormalities. **Skin:** rash, folliculitis, pruritus, apocrine and eccrine gland disorders, lithodystrophy, erythema, benign skin neoplasms, nail changes, acne, alopecia, anogenital warts. **Other:** herpes infection, bacterial infection, tinea infection, viral

---

Reactions in bold italics are *life-threatening*.

infection, immune reconstitution syndrome, influenza.

INTERACTIONS
Drug-drug. *Antihypertensives, other drugs known to lower BP (diuretics, antidepressants, opioids):* May increase risk of hypotension. Use together cautiously.
Moderate and strong CYP3A inducers (carbamazepine, efavirenz, etravirine, phenobarbital, phenytoin, rifampin): May decrease maraviroc level. Increase maraviroc dosage as needed.
Strong CYP3A inhibitors (protease inhibitors [except tipranavir–ritonavir], clarithromycin, cobicistat, elvitegravir–ritonavir, itraconazole, ketoconazole, nefazodone): May increase maraviroc level. Decrease maraviroc dosage as needed.
Drug-herb. *St. John's wort:* May decrease maraviroc level. Discourage use together.

EFFECTS ON LAB TEST RESULTS
• May increase AST, ALT, bilirubin, amylase, lipase, and CK levels.
• May decrease ANC and Hb level.

CONTRAINDICATIONS & CAUTIONS
• Contraindicated in patients hypersensitive to drug or its components.
• Contraindicated in patients with CrCl of less than 30 mL/minute who are taking potent CYP3A inhibitors or inducers.
⚠️ *Alert:* Before starting drug, test for CCR5 tropism. Outgrowth of preexisting low-level CXCR4- or dual/mixed-tropic HIV-1 not detected by tropism testing at screening has been associated with virologic failure.
• Severe and potentially life-threatening skin and hypersensitivity reactions, including SJS, TEN, and DRESS syndrome, have been reported. Discontinue drug if signs or symptoms of hypersensitivity occur.
• Use cautiously in patients with preexisting liver dysfunction or patients who are infected with HBV or HCV.
• Use cautiously in patients with risk factors for CV events, a history of cardiac disease, or risk factors for orthostatic hypotension and in those taking another medication known to lower BP.
• During initial phase of treatment, patients treated with combination antiretroviral therapy may develop an inflammatory response to indolent or residual opportunistic infections

(CMV, MAC, *Pneumocystis jiroveci* pneumonia, TB), which may necessitate further evaluation and treatment. Autoimmune disorders (such as Graves disease, polymyositis, and Guillain-Barré syndrome) have also been reported in the setting of immune reconstitution; however, time to onset is more variable, and onset can occur many months after initiation of antiretroviral treatment.
• Because of immune suppression, risk of malignancy may increase.
• Safety and effectiveness in children younger than age 2 and in children with kidney impairment haven't been established.
Dialyzable drug: Minimal.

PREGNANCY-LACTATION-REPRODUCTION
• Studies during pregnancy are inadequate. Use during pregnancy only if potential benefit justifies fetal risk.
• Register patients exposed to drug during pregnancy in the Antiretroviral Pregnancy Registry (1-800-258-4263 or https://www.apregistry.com).
• The CDC recommends that patients with HIV-1 infection be counseled on risk of postnatal transmission of HIV-1. Maintaining viral suppression through antiretroviral therapy during pregnancy, delivery, and postpartum period decreases risk to less than 1%.

NURSING CONSIDERATIONS
Boxed Warning Liver toxicity has been reported with maraviroc use. Severe rash or evidence of a systemic allergic reaction (fever, eosinophilia, elevated IgE level) may occur before the development of liver toxicity. Immediately evaluate patients with signs or symptoms of hepatitis or allergic reaction after drug use. ■
• Monitor patient closely for signs and symptoms of infection, liver and kidney impairment, CV events, and skin and hypersensitivity reactions.
• Monitor patient for malignancy with long-term use.
• Assess viral load, CD4 count, and LFT values before and periodically during treatment.
• Monitor BP for hypotension.

PATIENT TEACHING
• Instruct patient to immediately report signs or symptoms of hepatitis or allergic reaction (rash, yellow eyes or skin, dark urine, vomiting, and abdominal pain).

• Caution patient that drug doesn't cure HIV infection and that patient may still develop HIV-related illness, including opportunistic infections.

• Warn patient that drug doesn't reduce risk of transmission of HIV to others.

• Instruct patient who feels dizzy while taking drug to avoid driving or operating machinery.

• Instruct patient to inform provider of pregnancy or plans to become pregnant while taking drug.

• Counsel patient not to breastfeed during therapy.

• Advise patient to take drug every day as prescribed with other antiretrovirals. Tell patient not to change dose or dosing schedule or stop any antiretroviral without consulting prescriber. Inform patient that missed doses may increase risk of resistance.

mavacamten ☒
mav-a-KAM-ten

Camzyos

Therapeutic class: HF drugs
Pharmacologic class: Cardiac myosin inhibitors

AVAILABLE FORMS
Capsules ᴳᴹᶜ: 2.5 mg, 5 mg, 10 mg, 15 mg

INDICATIONS & DOSAGES
➤ **Symptomatic NYHA Class II to III obstructive hypertrophic cardiomyopathy to improve functional capacity and symptoms**
Adults: Initially, 5 mg PO daily. Individualize dose based on patient's clinical status and echocardiographic assessment. Subsequent doses after titration may be 2.5, 5, 10, or 15 mg once daily. See manufacturer's instructions for initiation and maintenance dose algorithms based on LVEF and Valsalva left ventricular outflow tract assessments.
Adjust-a-dose: For patients on stable therapy with a weak CYP2C19 or moderate CYP3A4 inhibitor, start mavacamten at 5 mg PO once daily. For patients starting a weak CYP2C19 or moderate CYP3A4 inhibitor during therapy, reduce mavacamten dose by one level (15 mg to 10 mg, 10 mg to 5 mg, or 5 mg to 2.5 mg). Don't initiate concomitant weak CYP2C19 or moderate CYP3A4 inhibitors

in patients on stable mavacamten 2.5 mg daily because a lower mavacamten dose isn't available.

ADMINISTRATION
PO
• Give without regard to food.
• Have patient swallow capsules whole; don't break, crush, or open capsules.
• Give missed dose as soon as possible that day; then give next dose at usual time on the following day. Don't give two doses in the same day.
• Store at 38° to 77° F (20° to 25° C).

ACTION
Inhibits cardiac myosin, reduces dynamic left ventricular outflow tract obstruction, and improves cardiac filling pressures.

Route	Onset	Peak	Duration
PO	Unknown	1 hr	Unknown

Half-life: 6 to 9 days (normal CYP2C19 metabolizers) to 23 days (poor CYP2C19 metabolizers).

ADVERSE REACTIONS
CNS: dizziness, syncope. **CV:** *HF,* reduced LVEF.

INTERACTIONS
Drug-drug. *Cimetidine:* May increase mavacamten level. Use together cautiously.
CYP2C8 (repaglinide), CYP2C9 (tolbutamide), CYP2C19 (omeprazole), CYP3A4 (midazolam, repaglinide) substrates: May reduce substrate levels. Monitor substrate levels.
Diltiazem with a beta blocker; disopyramide; ranolazine; verapamil with a beta blocker: Use with mavacamten hasn't been studied. Avoid use together.
Disopyramide with verapamil or diltiazem: May cause left ventricular dysfunction and HF in patients with obstructive hypertrophic cardiomyopathy. Avoid use together.
Hormonal contraceptives (ethinyl estradiol, progestin): May decrease ethinyl estradiol and progestin levels, leading to contraceptive failure or breakthrough bleeding. Patient should use contraceptive method unaffected by CYP450 enzyme induction (intrauterine system) or add nonhormonal contraceptives (condoms) during therapy and for 4 months after final dose.
Boxed Warning *Moderate to strong CYP2C19 or CYP3A4 inducers (rifampin):*

---

*Reactions in bold italics are **life-threatening**.*

May decrease mavacamten level and efficacy. Use together is contraindicated. ■

Boxed Warning *Moderate to strong CYP2C19 inhibitors (amitriptyline, fluconazole, imipramine) or strong CYP3A4 inhibitors (ketoconazole):* May increase mavacamten level and risk of HF due to systolic dysfunction. Use together is contraindicated. ■

Negative inotropes (beta blockers, diltiazem, verapamil): May have additive effects. If concomitant use is unavoidable, closely monitor LVEF when initiating or increasing negative inotrope dosage until stable doses and clinical response are achieved.

Weak CYP2C19 inhibitors (esomeprazole, omeprazole), moderate CYP3A4 inhibitors (ciprofloxacin, cyclosporine): May increase mavacamten level. Adjust mavacamten dosage.

Drug-herb. *St. John's wort:* May decrease mavacamten level and effectiveness. Discourage use together.

Drug-food. *Grapefruit juice:* May increase mavacamten level and drug adverse effects. Discourage use together.

EFFECTS ON LAB TEST RESULTS
None reported.

CONTRAINDICATIONS & CAUTIONS
• Contraindicated in patients hypersensitive to drug or its components.

Boxed Warning Drug can cause HF due to systolic dysfunction. ■

Boxed Warning Echocardiogram assessments of LVEF are required before and during mavacamten use. Initiation in patients with LVEF less than 55% isn't recommended. Interrupt therapy if LVEF falls below 50% or if clinical status worsens. ■

• Consider interrupting therapy in patients with intercurrent illness because of possible exacerbation of cardiac symptoms.

• Safety and effectiveness in children haven't been established.

• Use cautiously in older adults.

Boxed Warning Because of risk of systolic dysfunction and HF, drug is only available through Camzyos REMS program. ■

Dialyzable drug: Unlikely.

⚠ *Overdose S&S:* Vasovagal reaction, hypotension, asystole, systolic dysfunction (dyspnea, edema, fatigue, dizziness, cough, wheezing).

PREGNANCY-LACTATION-REPRODUCTION
• Based on animal studies, drug may cause fetal harm.

• Patients of childbearing potential must use effective contraception during therapy and for 4 months after final dose.

• Patients using hormonal contraceptives should use additional or alternative contraceptive methods.

• Report pregnancies that occur during therapy to the Bristol Myers Squibb pregnancy outcomes study (1-800-721-5072 or www.bms.com).

• It isn't known if drug appears in human milk or how drug affects milk production or infants who are breastfed. Consider patient's clinical need and risk to the infant.

NURSING CONSIDERATIONS
• Verify pregnancy status before start of therapy.

• Daily dosing takes weeks to reach steady-state drug levels and therapeutic effects.

• Assess patient's clinical status and LVEF at baseline and at 4, 8, and 12 weeks during initiation phase, every 12 weeks during maintenance phase, and as clinically indicated. Adjust dosage according to manufacturer's algorithms.

• Schedule echocardiogram and clinical assessments 4 weeks after initiation of a CYP inhibitor; don't titrate up mavacamten dose until 12 weeks after inhibitor initiation.

• Closely monitor patient for serious intercurrent illness (serious infection) or arrhythmia (atrial fibrillation or other uncontrolled tachyarrhythmia) due to risk of developing systolic dysfunction and HF.

• Monitor for new or worsening arrhythmia, dyspnea, chest pain, fatigue, palpitations, leg edema, or elevations in N-terminal pro B-type natriuretic peptide as these signs and symptoms may indicate HF and require prompt evaluation of cardiac function.

▨ Consider pharmacogenomic evaluation to determine CYP2C19 poor metabolizers, as concentrations of drug may significantly increase.

PATIENT TEACHING
🔵 *Alert:* Advise patient of potential for drug interactions. Tell patient to report all prescription and OTC medications, herbal supplements, and vitamins taken before or during therapy.

M

• Tell patient that cardiac function assessment and echocardiography will be performed to monitor for HF. Tell patient to immediately report signs or symptoms of HF. **Boxed Warning** Inform patient of the need to enroll in drug's REMS program and importance of adhering to monitoring requirements. ■
• Inform patient of childbearing potential to report known or suspected pregnancy.
• Advise patient of childbearing potential in safe use of effective contraception during therapy and for 4 months after final dose.

medroxyPROGESTERone acetate
me-DROKS-ee-proe-JES-te-rone

Depo-Provera, Depo-subQ Provera 104, Provera

Therapeutic class: Hormones, contraceptives
Pharmacologic class: Progestins

AVAILABLE FORMS
Injection (suspension): 104 mg/0.65 mL prefilled syringes, 150 mg/mL vials and prefilled syringes
Tablets: 2.5 mg, 5 mg, 10 mg

INDICATIONS & DOSAGES
➤ **Abnormal uterine bleeding caused by hormonal imbalance**
Adults: 5 to 10 mg PO daily for 5 to 10 days, beginning day 16 or 21 of menstrual cycle. If patient has also received estrogen, give 10 mg PO daily for 10 days, beginning on day 16 of cycle.
➤ **Secondary amenorrhea**
Adults: 5 to 10 mg PO daily for 5 to 10 days. Start at any time during menstrual cycle (usually during latter half of cycle).
➤ **Endometrial hyperplasia prevention**
Patients who are postmenopausal (intact uterus) receiving conjugated estrogen 0.625 mg: 5 or 10 mg PO daily for 12 to 14 consecutive days per month, beginning day 1 or day 16 of cycle.
➤ **Pregnancy prevention**
Females who are postmenarche: 150 mg (Depo-Provera) IM once every 3 months. Or, 104 mg Depo-subQ Provera subcut once every 12 to 14 weeks. First dose during first 5 days of normal menstrual period; only

within first 5 days postpartum if patient isn't breastfeeding; and, if patient is exclusively breastfeeding, only at 6th postpartum week. Refer to manufacturer's instructions when switching from another method of contraception.
➤ **Endometriosis-associated pain**
Adults: 104 mg subcut every 12 to 14 weeks.

ADMINISTRATION
⚠ *Alert:* Hazardous drug; use safe handling and disposal precautions.
• Store at room temperature.
PO
• Give with food to increase bioavailability.
IM
• Only health care professional should inject drug.
• Shake vigorously before use.
• Give by deep IM injection in gluteal or deltoid muscle. Rotate injection sites to prevent muscle atrophy.
• IM injection may be painful. Monitor sites for evidence of sterile abscess.
Subcutaneous
• Only health care professional should inject drug.
• Shake vigorously for at least 1 minute before use.
• Give subcut injection over 5 to 7 seconds into upper anterior thigh or abdomen.
• Rotate injection sites.
• Don't rub injection area.

ACTION
Suppresses ovulation, possibly by inhibiting pituitary gonadotropin secretion, thus preventing follicular maturation and causing endometrial thinning.

Route	Onset	Peak	Duration
PO	Rapid	2–4 hr	3–5 days
IM	Slow	3 wk	3–4 mo
Subcut	Unknown	1 wk	Unknown

Half-life: Oral, 12 to 17 hours; IM, 50 days; subcut, 43 days.

ADVERSE REACTIONS
CNS: anxiety, depression, fatigue, asthenia, insomnia, somnolence, pain, dizziness, headache, nervousness, irritability. **CV:** edema, *thromboembolism.* **EENT:** neuro-ocular lesions. **GI:** bloating, abdominal pain, nausea, diarrhea. **GU:** breakthrough bleeding, dysmenorrhea, amenorrhea, cervical

erosion, abnormal secretions, decreased libido, vaginitis, vulvovaginal candidiasis, UTI. **Hepatic:** cholestatic jaundice. **Metabolic:** weight gain or loss, decreased glucose tolerance. **Musculoskeletal:** osteoporosis, arthralgia, back pain, leg cramps. **Skin:** rash, induration, sterile abscesses, acne, pruritus, melasma, alopecia, hirsutism, injection-site reaction. **Other:** breast tenderness, enlargement, or secretion; hot flashes.

INTERACTIONS

Drug-drug. *Anticonvulsants, corticosteroids:* May increase risk of bone mass. Monitor patient.

Antidiabetics: May diminish antidiabetic therapeutic effects. Monitor therapy.

NNRTIs, protease inhibitors: May increase progestin level. Monitor for progestin toxicity.

Strong or moderate CYP3A inducers (carbamazepine, phenobarbital, phenytoin, rifabutin, rifampin, rifapentine): May decrease progestin effects. Avoid use together.

Strong CYP3A inhibitors (clarithromycin, itraconazole, ketoconazole, nefazodone, ritonavir, telithromycin, voriconazole): May increase progestin effects. Monitor therapy.

Drug-herb. *St. John's wort:* May decrease progestin effects. Avoid use together.

Drug-food. *Grapefruit:* May increase progestin effects. Monitor therapy.

Drug-lifestyle. *Smoking:* May increase risk of adverse CV effects and bone loss. Recommend smoking cessation or alternative therapy.

EFFECTS ON LAB TEST RESULTS

- May increase LFT, glucose or thyroid-binding globulin, and prothrombin levels as well as coagulation factor VII, VIII, IX, and X values.
- May decrease plasma and urinary steroid levels, gonadotropin level, and sex hormone–binding globulin concentrations.
- May increase or decrease total cholesterol, triglyceride, LDL-C, and HDL-C levels.

CONTRAINDICATIONS & CAUTIONS

Boxed Warning Estrogens with progestins increase risk of dementia in patients ages 65 and older; risk of DVT, PE, stroke, and MI in patients after menopause; and risk of invasive breast cancer in all. Give estrogens with progestins at lowest effective doses and for shortest duration consistent with treatment goals and risks for the individual patient. ∎

- Contraindicated in patients hypersensitive to drug and in those with history of or active thromboembolic disorders (cerebrovascular disease, stroke, MI, DVT, PE), known or suspected breast cancer, history of breast cancer, known or suspected estrogen- or progesterone-dependent neoplasia, known or suspected pregnancy, undiagnosed abnormal vaginal bleeding, missed abortion, or liver dysfunction.

Boxed Warning Injectable drug shouldn't be used for long-term birth control (more than 2 years) unless other forms of birth control are inadequate. Loss of bone mineral density can occur and may not be reversible. Effects of use during adolescence or early adulthood on the risk of osteoporotic fracture later in life are unknown. ∎

- Use cautiously in patients with diabetes, seizures, migraine, cardiac or kidney disease, strong family history of breast cancer, asthma, depression, porphyria, SLE, hypoparathyroidism, liver hemangiomas, or breast nodules.
- Hormonal contraceptives may increase risk of breast cancer.

Dialyzable drug: Unknown.

⚠ *Overdose S&S:* Nausea, vomiting, dizziness, breast tenderness, abdominal pain, drowsiness, fatigue, withdrawal bleeding.

PREGNANCY-LACTATION-REPRODUCTION

- Drug is contraindicated in pregnancy or suspected pregnancy and as a diagnostic test for pregnancy.
- Be alert to possibility of ectopic pregnancy in patients using medroxyprogesterone contraceptive injection who become pregnant or complain of severe abdominal pain.
- Drug appears in human milk. Tablets aren't recommended for use during breastfeeding. The manufacturer recommends using the injectable form with caution during breastfeeding.
- Ovulation and fertility are likely to be delayed after stopping drug.

NURSING CONSIDERATIONS

- Verify pregnancy status prior to therapy and if interval between IM injections is more than 13 weeks or subcut injections is more than 14 weeks.
- Monitor for pain, swelling, warmth, or redness in calves; sudden, severe headaches; visual disturbances; signs of depression;

numbness in extremities; hypersensitivity re-actions; and signs and symptoms of liver dys-function (abdominal pain, dark urine, jaun-dice).

• Monitor BP regularly during treatment.

• Monitor patients sensitive to fluid re-tention, including those with epilepsy, migraines, asthma, and cardiac or kidney dysfunction.

• Due to risk of CV disorders, stop drug at least 4 to 6 weeks before any surgery asso-ciated with an increased risk of thromboem-bolism or during periods of prolonged immo-bilization.

• Drug may decrease glucose tolerance; care-fully monitor patient with diabetes.

PATIENT TEACHING

• According to FDA regulations, patient must read package insert explaining possible ad-verse effects of progestins before receiving first dose. Also, give patient verbal explana-tion.

• Warn that drug doesn't protect against HIV or other sexually transmitted diseases.

🚯 Alert: Instruct patient to immediately report adverse effects, including breast abnormali-ties, vaginal bleeding, swelling, yellowing of skin or eyes, dark urine, clay-colored stools, shortness of breath, coughing up blood, chest pain, weakness on one side of the body, trou-ble speaking, facial drooping, migraine, vi-sion changes, change in color or pain in ex-tremity, or pregnancy.

• Advise patient of importance of routine BP monitoring and annual physical exam, includ-ing breasts, abdomen, and pelvic organs.

• Teach patient how to perform routine breast self-exam.

• Advise patient that injection must be given every 3 months to maintain adequate contra-ceptive effects and that use of injections may be limited to 2 years.

• Explain that, because drug is a long-acting method of birth control, fertility may take some time to return after last injection.

• Inform patient that prolonged use may cause amenorrhea.

• Encourage adequate intake of calcium and vitamin D.

• Inform patient that drug may cause intoler-ance to contact lenses.

mefloquine hydrochloride
ME-floe-kwin

Therapeutic class: Antimalarials
Pharmacologic class: Quinine derivatives

AVAILABLE FORMS
Tablets: 250 mg

INDICATIONS & DOSAGES

➤ **Mild to moderate acute malaria in-fections caused by mefloquine-sensitive strains of *Plasmodium falciparum* or *Plasmodium vivax***

Adults: 1,250 mg (five tablets) PO as a single dose.

Children ages 6 months and older: 20 to 25 mg/kg PO as a single dose (or divided into two doses given 6 to 8 hours apart to reduce incidence and severity of adverse effects). Maximum dose, 1,250 mg.

➤ **To prevent malaria due to *P. falciparum* or *P. vivax***

Adults and children ages 6 months and older weighing more than 45 kg: 250 mg or approx-imately 5 mg/kg PO once weekly. Preventive therapy should start 1 week before entering endemic area and continue for 4 weeks after returning. Give subsequent doses on same day of each week, preferably after main meal.

Children ages 6 months and older weigh-ing 30 to 45 kg: 187.5 mg (three-quarters of 250-mg tablet) PO once weekly.

Children ages 6 months and older weighing 20 to less than 30 kg: 125 mg (one-half of 250-mg tablet) PO once weekly.

ADMINISTRATION
PO

• Give drug with food and at least 240 mL of water.

• May crush tablets and suspend in a small amount of water, milk, or other beverage when giving to small children and other pa-tients unable to swallow tablets whole.

• If patient vomits within 30 minutes of re-ceiving dose, repeat full dose; if within 30 to 60 minutes, give a half dose.

ACTION
Exact mechanism of action unknown.

Route	Onset	Peak	Duration
PO	Unknown	6–24 hr	Unknown

Half-life: 2 to 4 weeks.

ADVERSE REACTIONS

CNS: fever, dizziness, syncope, headache, fatigue, abnormal dreams, insomnia. **EENT:** tinnitus. **GI:** vomiting, nausea, diarrhea, abdominal discomfort or pain, loss of appetite. **Musculoskeletal:** myalgia. **Skin:** rash. **Other:** chills.

INTERACTIONS

Drug-drug. *Antiarrhythmics, beta blockers, antihistamines, H_1-blockers, calcium channel blockers, phenothiazines, TCAs:* May prolong QTc interval and increase risk of life-threatening cardiac arrhythmias. Coadminister with caution.

Carbamazepine, phenobarbital, phenytoin, valproic acid: May decrease drug levels and loss of seizure control at start of mefloquine therapy. Monitor anticonvulsant level.

Chloroquine, quinidine, quinine: May increase risk of seizures and ECG abnormalities. Give mefloquine at least 12 hours after last dose.

CYP3A4 inducers (rifampin): May decrease mefloquine level and reduce drug's effect. Use together cautiously.

CYP3A4 inhibitors: May increase mefloquine level and risk of adverse reactions. Use together cautiously.

Halofantrine, ketoconazole: May cause fatal prolongation of QTc interval if given with or within 15 weeks of last mefloquine dose. Avoid use together.

Live-virus vaccines: May decrease immunization result. Complete vaccination at least 3 days before start of mefloquine.

EFFECTS ON LAB TEST RESULTS

• May increase transaminase levels.
• May decrease hematocrit and WBC and platelet counts.

CONTRAINDICATIONS & CAUTIONS

• Contraindicated in patients hypersensitive to mefloquine or related compounds, in those with history of seizures, and in patients with active or recent history of depression, generalized anxiety disorder, psychosis, schizophrenia, or other major psychiatric disorders.
• Other IV antimalarials should be used to initially treat life-threatening or serious malarial infections. Mefloquine may be used after IV treatment is completed.

Boxed Warning Drug may cause neuropsychiatric adverse reactions that can persist after therapy ends. Drug shouldn't be prescribed for prophylaxis in patients with major psychiatric disorders. ■

• Use cautiously when treating patients with cardiac disease.
• Agranulocytosis and aplastic anemia have been reported in patients taking mefloquine.
• Use cautiously in patients with liver impairment.

Dialyzable drug: No.

PREGNANCY-LACTATION-REPRODUCTION

• Studies during pregnancy have shown no increase in risk of teratogenic effects after mefloquine use; however, risk to developing fetus can't be ruled out. Use only if clearly needed.
• Drug appears in human milk in small amounts. Use cautiously during breast-feeding.

NURSING CONSIDERATIONS

• Patient with *P. vivax* infection is at high risk for relapse because drug doesn't eliminate hepatic-phase exoerythrocytic parasites. Give follow-up therapy with primaquine or other 8-aminoquinolines to avoid relapse after treatment of initial infection.
• Periodically monitor LFT results.
• **Alert:** Monitor for neurologic signs and symptoms (dizziness, vertigo, tinnitus, seizures, insomnia) or psychiatric signs and symptoms (anxiety, paranoia, hallucinations, depression, restlessness, confusion, behavior changes). Be aware that signs and symptoms may be more difficult to detect in children.

Boxed Warning During prophylactic use, if psychiatric or neurologic signs and symptoms occur, drug should be discontinued and an alternative drug prescribed. ■

• In certain cases, such as when a traveler takes other medications, it may be desirable to start prophylaxis 2 to 3 weeks before departure, to assess drug combination tolerance.

PATIENT TEACHING

• Encourage patient to wear protective clothing and to use insect repellents and bednets in addition to medication for maximum protection.
• Teach about proper drug administration and handling. Instruct patient to read medication guide and to always carry information wallet card during therapy.
• Advise patient to use caution when performing activities that require alertness and

M

coordination because dizziness, disturbed sense of balance, and neuropsychiatric reactions may occur.

🕚 *Alert:* Inform patient that dizziness, vertigo, and tinnitus can occur during treatment, may continue for months or years after treatment, or may be permanent.

🕚 *Alert:* Warn patient to immediately report neurologic or psychiatric signs or symptoms and not to stop drug until discussing with prescriber.

• Counsel patient undergoing long-term therapy to have periodic ophthalmic exams because drug may cause ocular lesions.

• Instruct patient to report pregnancy or plans to become pregnant or breastfeed.

SAFETY ALERT!

megestrol acetate
me-JES-trole

Therapeutic class: Antineoplastics, hormones
Pharmacologic class: Progestins

AVAILABLE FORMS
Oral suspension: 40 mg/mL
Oral suspension (concentrated): 125 mg/mL
Tablets: 20 mg, 40 mg, 160 mg❦

INDICATIONS & DOSAGES
➤ **Breast cancer (palliative treatment)**
Adults: 40 mg PO q.i.d. for at least 2 months. Use tablets only.
➤ **Endometrial cancer (palliative treatment)**
Adults: 40 to 320 mg PO daily in divided doses for at least 2 months. Use tablets only.
➤ **Anorexia, cachexia, or unexplained significant weight loss in patients with AIDS**
Adults: 400 to 800 mg PO (10 to 20 mL regular oral suspension) or 625 mg PO (5 mL concentrated oral suspension) once daily.
➤ **Cancer-related cachexia ◆**
Adults: 200 to 600 mg PO once daily.

ADMINISTRATION
PO
🕚 *Alert:* Hazardous drug; use safe handling and disposal precautions.
• Give drug without regard to meals.
• Shake suspension well before pouring.
• Don't substitute 125-mg/mL and 40-mg/mL strengths for each other. Ensure use of correct product for dose.

• Protect tablets and oral suspension from heat; protect tablets from light.

ACTION
Inhibits hormone-dependent tumor growth by inhibiting pituitary and adrenal steroidogenesis. May also have direct cytotoxicity; appetite-stimulating mechanism is unknown.

Route	Onset	Peak	Duration
PO	Unknown	5 hr (suspension); 1–3 hr (tablets)	Unknown

Half-life: Suspension: 20 to 50 hours. Tablets: mean, 34.2 hours.

ADVERSE REACTIONS
CNS: confusion, *seizures,* depression, headache, neuropathy, insomnia, abnormal thinking, mood changes, fever, asthenia, malaise, pain, paresthesia, hypesthesia. **CV:** HTN, *cardiomyopathy,* palpitations, chest pain, edema. **EENT:** amblyopia, oral moniliasis, pharyngitis, increased salivation. **GI:** nausea, vomiting, diarrhea, flatulence, constipation, dry mouth, increased appetite, abdominal pain, dyspepsia. **GU:** breakthrough menstrual bleeding, impotence, decreased libido, UTI, urinary incontinence, urinary frequency. **Hematologic:** anemia, *leukopenia.* **Hepatic:** liver enlargement. **Metabolic:** hyperglycemia, weight gain. **Musculoskeletal:** carpal tunnel syndrome. **Respiratory:** dyspnea, pneumonia, cough, lung disorder. **Skin:** alopecia, rash, pruritus, diaphoresis, herpes lesions. **Other:** tumor flare, gynecomastia, hot flushes, infection.

INTERACTIONS
Drug-drug. *Antidiabetics:* May diminish therapeutic effect of antidiabetics. Monitor therapy.
Dofetilide: May increase dofetilide plasma level, increasing risk of life-threatening cardiac arrhythmias, including torsades de pointes. Avoid use together.
Warfarin: May increase INR. Closely monitor PT and INR.
Drug-herb. *Bloodroot, yucca:* May enhance adverse effects of progestins. Monitor therapy.

EFFECTS ON LAB TEST RESULTS
• May increase serum glucose, LDH, and urine albumin levels.
• May decrease WBC count.

Reactions in bold italics are *life-threatening*.

CONTRAINDICATIONS & CAUTIONS
• Contraindicated in patients hypersensitive to drug.
• Use cautiously in patients with history of thrombophlebitis or thromboembolism.
• Safety and effectiveness in children haven't been established.
• Use cautiously in older adults.
Dialyzable drug: Unlikely.

PREGNANCY-LACTATION-REPRODUCTION
• Drug may cause fetal harm. Oral solution is contraindicated in pregnancy. If used during pregnancy or if pregnancy occurs during therapy, apprise patient of potential fetal risk. Patient should avoid pregnancy.
• Drug appears in human milk. Patient shouldn't breastfeed during therapy.

NURSING CONSIDERATIONS
• Verify pregnancy status before start of treatment.
• May increase glucose level in patient with diabetes.
• Drug isn't intended for prophylactic use to avoid weight loss. Start treatment with megestrol acetate oral suspension only after treatable causes of weight loss are sought and addressed.
• Two months is an adequate trial period in patient with cancer.
⚠️ *Alert:* Drug may cause adrenal insufficiency, which can be fatal. Monitor for signs and symptoms (hypotension, nausea, vomiting, dizziness, weakness). Glucocorticoid therapy may be needed especially during stress or serious illness (surgery, infection).

PATIENT TEACHING
• Teach about proper drug administration and handling.
• Inform patient that therapeutic response isn't immediate. Drug must be taken for at least 2 months to determine effectiveness.
⚠️ *Alert:* Tell patient that the ES oral suspension is more concentrated than the regular oral suspension, so a smaller amount is needed if prescription is changed.
• Advise patient to stop breastfeeding during therapy because of risk of toxicity to infant.
• Caution patient of childbearing potential to use an effective form of contraception while receiving drug.

• Tell patient to report all adverse reactions, especially signs and symptoms of adrenal insufficiency.

memantine hydrochloride
me-MAN-teen

Ebixa✦, Namenda, Namenda XR

Therapeutic class: Anti-Alzheimer drugs
Pharmacologic class: N-methyl-D-aspartate receptor antagonists

AVAILABLE FORMS
Capsules (extended-release) ⬛: 7 mg, 14 mg, 21 mg, 28 mg
Oral solution: 2 mg/mL
Tablets: 5 mg, 10 mg

INDICATIONS & DOSAGES
➤ **Moderate to severe Alzheimer dementia**
Adults: Initially, 5 mg PO once daily. Increase by 5 mg/day every week until target dose is reached. Maximum, 10 mg PO b.i.d. Give doses greater than 5 mg in two divided doses.

For extended-release capsules, initially 7 mg PO once daily. Increase as tolerated by 7-mg increments each week to target dosage of 28 mg PO once daily.
To convert from immediate-release to extended-release form: Patients taking immediate-release 10 mg b.i.d. may switch to extended-release 28 mg once daily the day following the last immediate-release tablet. Patients with CrCl of 5 to 29 mL/minute taking immediate-release 5 mg b.i.d. may switch to extended-release 14 mg once daily the day following the last immediate-release tablet.
Adjust-a-dose: For patients with CrCl of 5 to 29 mL/minute, recommended immediate-release target dosage is 5 mg b.i.d. and extended-release target dosage is 14 mg/day.

ADMINISTRATION
PO
• Give drug without regard to food.
• Have patient take capsules whole or open capsules, sprinkle on applesauce, and then swallow. Don't divide or crush capsules.
• Use dosing device provided with oral solution to withdraw correct dose volume.

✦Canada   ◇OTC   ◆Off-label use   ⬛Do not crush   *Liquid contains alcohol   ⬚Genetic

Slowly squirt dose into corner of patient's mouth.
• Don't mix oral solution with any other liquid.
• If a single dose is missed, omit it. If several days are missed, may need to resume dosing at a lower dose and retitrate.
• Store at room temperature.

ACTION

Antagonizes N-methyl-D-aspartate receptors, the persistent activation of which seems to increase Alzheimer symptoms.

Route	Onset	Peak	Duration
PO (tablets, solution)	Unknown	3–7 hr	Unknown
PO (capsules)	Unknown	9–12 hr	Unknown

Half-life: 60 to 80 hours.

ADVERSE REACTIONS

CNS: aggression, agitation, anxiety, confusion, depression, dizziness, fatigue, hallucinations, headache, pain, somnolence, drowsiness. **CV:** HTN, hypotension. **GI:** constipation, diarrhea, vomiting, abdominal pain. **GU:** incontinence. **Metabolic:** weight gain. **Musculoskeletal:** back pain. **Respiratory:** cough, dyspnea. **Other:** flulike symptoms.

INTERACTIONS

Drug-drug. *NMDA antagonists (amantadine, dextromethorphan, ketamine):* Effects of combined use unknown. Use together cautiously.
Urine alkalinizers (carbonic anhydrase inhibitors, sodium bicarbonate): May decrease memantine clearance. Monitor patient for adverse effects.
Drug-food. *Foods that alkalinize urine:* May increase drug level and adverse effects. Use together cautiously.
Drug-lifestyle. *Nicotine:* May alter levels of drug and nicotine. Discourage use together.

EFFECTS ON LAB TEST RESULTS

None reported.

CONTRAINDICATIONS & CAUTIONS

• Contraindicated in patients allergic to drug or its components.
• Use cautiously in patients with seizures, CV disease, CrCl of 5 to 29 mL/minute, or Child-Pugh class C liver impairment.

• Use cautiously in patients who may have increased urine pH (from drugs, diet, kidney tubular acidosis, or severe UTI).
• Use cautiously in patients with corneal disease; condition may worsen. Periodic ophthalmic exams are recommended.
Dialyzable drug: Unknown.
⚠ **Overdose S&S:** Restlessness, psychosis, visual hallucinations, somnolence, stupor, loss of consciousness, agitation, asthenia, bradycardia, confusion, coma, dizziness, ECG changes, HTN, lethargy, unsteady gait, vertigo, vomiting, weakness.

PREGNANCY-LACTATION-REPRODUCTION

• Studies during pregnancy are inadequate. Use during pregnancy only if potential benefit justifies fetal risk.
• It isn't known if drug appears in human milk. Use cautiously during breastfeeding.

NURSING CONSIDERATIONS

• Monitor carefully for adverse reactions as patient may not be able to recognize changes or communicate effectively.
• Monitor cognitive and functional status.

PATIENT TEACHING

• Explain that drug doesn't cure Alzheimer disease but may slow progression and help patient to maintain function longer.
• Teach about proper drug administration and handling, including missed doses.
• Tell patient or caregiver to report adverse effects.
• To avoid possible interactions, advise patient not to take herbal or OTC products without consulting prescriber and to report all current medicines.

SAFETY ALERT!

meperidine hydrochloride (pethidine hydrochloride)
me-PER-i-deen

Demerol

Therapeutic class: Opioid analgesics
Pharmacologic class: Opioids
Controlled substance schedule: II

AVAILABLE FORMS

Injection: 25 mg/mL, 50 mg/mL, 75 mg/mL, 100 mg/mL

---

*Reactions in bold italics are **life-threatening**.*

Solution: 50 mg/5 mL
Tablets: 50 mg, 100 mg

INDICATIONS & DOSAGES

Adjust-a-dose (for all indications): Reduce meperidine dosage by 25% to 50% when administered with phenothiazines or other tranquilizers. Use cautiously and initiate at lower end of dosage range in older adults and patients with liver or kidney impairment; if needed, titrate dosage slowly.

➤ **Moderate to severe pain that requires an opioid analgesic and for which alternative treatments are inadequate**

Adults: 50 to 150 mg PO, IM, or subcut every 3 to 4 hours PRN.

Children: 1.1 to 1.8 mg/kg PO, IM, or subcut every 3 to 4 hours PRN. Maximum, 50 to 150 mg every 4 hours PRN.

Adjust-a-dose: For pain uncontrolled with total daily dosage of 600 mg PO, titrate drug off and switch to another analgesic. If necessary, may give IV very slowly and preferably as a diluted solution.

➤ **Preoperative analgesia**

Adults: 50 to 100 mg IM or subcut 30 to 90 minutes before beginning of anesthesia.

Children: 1.1 to 2.2 mg/kg IM or subcut up to adult dose 30 to 90 minutes before anesthesia.

➤ **Adjunct to anesthesia**

Adults: Repeated slow IV injections of fractional doses. Or, continuous IV infusion of more-dilute solution (1 mg/mL) titrated to patient's needs.

➤ **Obstetric analgesia**

Adults: 50 to 100 mg IM or subcut when pain becomes regular; may repeat at 1- to 3-hour intervals.

ADMINISTRATION

PO

• Solution has local anesthetic effect on mucous membranes if not diluted. Give with a half glass of water.

• Oral dose is less than half as effective as parenteral dose. Give IM, if possible. When changing from parenteral to oral route, increase dosage.

Boxed Warning Ensure accuracy when administering solution form. Dosing errors due to confusion between mg and mL can lead to fatal outcomes. ∎

IV

▼ Keep opioid antagonist (naloxone) available.

▼ Only give IV if ability to assist or control respirations are immediately available.

▼ Give drug by direct injection over 2 to 5 minutes using diluted solution.

▼ Drug may also be given by slow continuous infusion. Drug is compatible with most infusion solutions, including D_5W, NSS, and Ringer or lactated Ringer solutions.

▼ Store at room temperature.

▼ **Incompatibilities:** Aminophyllines, barbiturates, iodide, morphine, phenytoin, sodium bicarbonate.

IM

• Inject deep into large muscle mass.

Subcutaneous

• Subcut injection isn't recommended because it's very painful, but it may be suitable for occasional use. Monitor for pain at injection site, local tissue irritation, and induration after subcut injection.

ACTION

Unknown. Binds with opioid receptors in the CNS, altering perception of and emotional response to pain.

Route	Onset	Peak	Duration
PO	10–15 min	60–120 min	2–4 hr
IV	5 min	5–7 min	2–3 hr
IM, subcut	10–15 min	30–50 min	2–4 hr

Half-life: Oral, 3 to 8 hours; injectable, 2 to 5 hours.

ADVERSE REACTIONS

CNS: agitation, incoordination, dizziness, dysphoria, euphoria, delirium, lightheadedness, sedation, somnolence, *seizures,* hallucinations, headache, physical tremors, dependence, confusion, disorientation, syncope, weakness. **CV:** *bradycardia, circulatory depression, cardiac arrest, shock,* hypotension, tachycardia, palpitations, flushing, phlebitis after IV injection. **EENT:** visual disturbances, dry mouth. **GI:** biliary tract spasms, constipation, ileus, nausea, vomiting. **GU:** urine retention. **Musculoskeletal:** muscle twitching. **Respiratory:** *respiratory arrest, respiratory depression (central sleep apnea, sleep-related hypoxemia).* **Skin:** urticaria, diaphoresis, pruritus. **Other:** induration, local tissue irritation, pain at injection site, hypersensitivity reactions, *anaphylaxis.*

M

INTERACTIONS

Drug-drug. *Acyclovir:* Increases meperidine level and risk of adverse reactions. Use together cautiously.

Anticholinergics (benztropine, darifenacin, oxybutynin): May increase risk of urine retention, constipation, or paralytic ileus. Monitor patient closely.

Boxed Warning *Benzodiazepines, CNS depressants (sedatives, hypnotics, anxiolytics, tranquilizers, muscle relaxants, general anesthetics, antipsychotics, other opioids):* May cause slow or difficult breathing, sedation, and death. Avoid use together. If use together can't be avoided, limit dosage and duration of each drug to the minimum necessary for desired effect. ■

Cimetidine: May increase respiratory and CNS depression. Monitor patient closely.

Boxed Warning *CYP3A4 or CYP2B6 inducers (carbamazepine, phenytoin, rifampin):* May increase meperidine level and increase risk of toxicity if inducers are discontinued. Monitor patient closely when discontinuing an inducer. ■

Boxed Warning *CYP3A4 or CYP2B6 inhibitors (erythromycin, ketoconazole, ritonavir):* May increase meperidine level, which could increase or prolong adverse reactions; may cause fatal respiratory depression. Monitor patient closely. ■

Diuretics: May reduce efficacy of diuretics. Monitor therapy.

Boxed Warning *MAO inhibitors (linezolid, phenelzine):* May increase CNS and respiratory depression and hypotension that can be severe or fatal. Use of meperidine within 14 days of an MAO inhibitor is contraindicated. ■

Mixed agonist/antagonist and partial agonist opioid analgesics (butorphanol, nalbuphine, pentazocine, buprenorphine): May decrease analgesic effect and cause withdrawal symptoms. Avoid use together.

Oxybate salts (calcium, magnesium, potassium, sodium): May increase CNS depression and sleep duration. Avoid use together. If necessary, use together cautiously and monitor patient closely.

⚕ *Alert:* *Serotonergic drugs (amoxapine, antiemetics [dolasetron, granisetron, ondansetron, palonosetron], antimigraine drugs, buspirone, cyclobenzaprine, dextromethorphan, linezolid, lithium, maprotiline, methylene blue, mirtazapine, nefazodone, SNRIs, SSRIs, TCAs, trazodone, tryptophan, vilazodone):* May increase risk of serotonin syndrome. Avoid use together. If necessary, use together cautiously and monitor patient for serotonin syndrome.

Drug-herb. *Kava:* May enhance adverse effects of CNS depressants. Monitor therapy.

⚕ *Alert:* *St. John's wort:* May increase risk of serotonin syndrome. Use together cautiously and monitor patient for serotonin syndrome.

Drug-lifestyle. **Boxed Warning** *Alcohol use:* May cause slow or difficult breathing, sedation, and death. Discourage use together. ■

EFFECTS ON LAB TEST RESULTS

• May increase amylase level.
• May decrease adrenocorticotropic hormone, cortisol, and LH levels.
• May stimulate prolactin, growth hormone, and pancreatic secretion of insulin and glucagon.

CONTRAINDICATIONS & CAUTIONS

• Contraindicated in patients hypersensitive to drug and in those with significant respiratory depression, acute or severe bronchial asthma in an unmonitored setting or in the absence of resuscitative equipment, or known or suspected GI obstruction, including paralytic ileus.

Boxed Warning Use exposes patient and others to risk of opioid addiction, abuse, and misuse, which can lead to overdose and death. These effects can occur at any dose or duration. Assess patient risk before prescribing and regularly reassess patient for these behaviors and conditions. ■

Boxed Warning Prescribers are strongly encouraged to complete a REMS-compliant education program. Drug should be prescribed only by prescribers with knowledge of opioid use and ways to reduce associated risks. ■

⚕ *Alert:* Use lowest effective dose for shortest period consistent with patient's treatment goals.

⚕ *Alert:* Because risk of overdose increases as opioid dose increases, reserve titration to higher doses for patients in whom lower doses are ineffective and in whom expected benefits of higher opioid dose outweigh risks.

Boxed Warning Opioids should only be prescribed with benzodiazepines or other CNS depressants when alternative treatment options are inadequate, aren't expected to provide adequate analgesia, haven't been tolerated, or aren't expected to be tolerated. ■

🟢 *Alert:* Immediate-release formulations shouldn't be used for an extended period unless pain remains severe enough to require an opioid analgesic and alternative treatment options are inadequate to treat pain.

Boxed Warning Accidental ingestion of even one dose of an opioid, especially by children, can result in a fatal overdose. ■

🟢 *Alert:* Drug may lead to a rare but serious decrease in adrenal gland cortisol production.

• Drug may cause decreased sex hormone levels with long-term use.

🟢 *Alert:* Patients are at increased risk for oversedation and respiratory depression if they snore or have a history of sleep apnea, haven't used opioids recently or are first-time opioid users, have increased opioid dosage requirements or opioid habituation, have received general anesthesia for longer lengths of time or received other sedating drugs, have preexisting pulmonary or cardiac disease, or have thoracic or other surgical incisions that may impair breathing. Monitor patients carefully.

• Use cautiously in older adults or patients who are debilitated and in those with increased ICP, head injury, asthma and other respiratory conditions, supraventricular tachycardias, seizures, abdominal conditions, decreased bowel motility conditions, liver or kidney disease, hypothyroidism, Addison disease, urethral stricture, and prostatic hyperplasia.

• Drug may increase HTN in patients with pheochromocytoma.

Dialyzable drug: Unknown.

⚠ *Overdose S&S:* Respiratory depression, somnolence progressing to stupor, coma, bradycardia, hypotension, hypothermia, delirium, skeletal muscle flaccidity, circulatory collapse, death.

PREGNANCY-LACTATION-REPRODUCTION

Boxed Warning Prolonged use of drug during pregnancy can result in neonatal opioid withdrawal syndrome, which may be life-threatening. It requires management with expert neonatology protocols. If prolonged use is needed, advise patient of risks and ensure availability of proper treatment. ■

• Don't use before labor unless physician determines potential benefits outweigh risks; safe use before labor hasn't been established

relative to possible adverse effects on fetal development.

• Drug appears in human milk. Patient should discontinue breastfeeding or discontinue drug.

NURSING CONSIDERATIONS

Boxed Warning Regularly monitor patients for opioid addiction, abuse, and misuse, which can lead to overdose and death.

Boxed Warning May cause life-threatening or fatal respiratory depression at any time during therapy. Monitor patient closely, especially when starting or increasing doses. Proper dosing and titration are essential to reduce risk. ■

🟢 *Alert:* Drug may cause opioid-induced hyperalgesia (OIH). Symptoms include increased pain level with opioid dose increase, decreased pain level with opioid dose reduction, pain from ordinarily nonpainful stimuli without underlying disease progression, opioid tolerance or withdrawal, and addictive behavior. For suspected OIH, decrease opioid dose or switch patient to alternative opioid.

• In older adults, patients using meperidine for longer than 48 hours, those with preexisting kidney or CNS disease, and those taking more than 600 mg/day PO, the active metabolite may accumulate, causing increased adverse CNS reactions, including seizures. Avoid prolonged use.

• Monitor patient with biliary tract disease, including acute pancreatitis, for worsening signs and symptoms.

🟢 *Alert:* Carefully monitor vital signs, pain level, respiratory status, and sedation level in all patients receiving opioids, especially those receiving IV drugs, even those given postoperatively.

🟢 *Alert:* If patient is taking opioids with serotonergic drugs, watch for signs and symptoms of serotonin syndrome (agitation, hallucinations, rapid HR, fever, diaphoresis, shivering or shaking, muscle twitching or stiffness, trouble with coordination, nausea, vomiting, diarrhea), especially when starting treatment or increasing dosages. Signs and symptoms may occur within several hours of coadministration but may also occur later, especially after dosage increase. Discontinue opioid, serotonergic drug, or both if serotonin syndrome is suspected.

🟢 *Alert:* Monitor for signs and symptoms of adrenal insufficiency (nausea, vomiting, loss of appetite, fatigue, weakness, dizziness, low BP). Perform diagnostic testing if adrenal insufficiency is suspected. For confirmed adrenal insufficiency, treat with corticosteroids and wean patient off opioid, if appropriate. Discontinue corticosteroids when clinically appropriate.

- Monitor patient for signs and symptoms of decreased sex hormone levels (low libido, erectile dysfunction, amenorrhea, infertility). If signs and symptoms occur, evaluate patient and obtain specimens for lab testing.
- When giving drug parenterally, make sure patient is lying down. IV administration increases risk of adverse reactions, including severe respiratory depression, apnea, hypotension, peripheral circulatory collapse, and cardiac arrest.
- Drug may be used in some patients who are allergic to morphine.
- Reassess patient's level of pain at least 15 and 30 minutes after administration.
- Carefully monitor respiratory and CV status. Don't give if respirations are below 12 breaths/minute, respiratory rate or depth is decreased, or change in pupils is noted.
- Monitor bladder function after surgical procedures.
- Monitor bowel function. Patient may need a stimulant laxative and stool softener.

Alert: Don't stop drug abruptly; withdraw slowly and individualize gradual taper plan to prevent signs and symptoms of withdrawal, worsening pain, and psychological distress in patients who are physically dependent. Refer to manufacturer's label for specific tapering instructions.

Alert: When tapering opioids, monitor patient closely for signs and symptoms of opioid withdrawal (restlessness, lacrimation, rhinorrhea, yawning, perspiration, chills, myalgia, mydriasis, irritability, anxiety, insomnia, backache, joint pain, weakness, abdominal cramps, anorexia, nausea, vomiting, diarrhea, increased BP or HR, increased respiratory rate), which may indicate a need to taper more slowly. Also monitor patient for suicidality, use of other substances, or changes in mood.

PATIENT TEACHING

Boxed Warning Counsel patient and caregiver on serious risks, safe use, and importance of reading the medication guide with each prescription. ■

- Advise patient to take drug exactly as prescribed and to use lowest dose possible for shortest time needed.
- Inform patient that, for acute pain, drug may only be needed for a few days. Teach patient about safe disposal of unused drug.
- Caution patient that drug isn't intended for long-term use.
- Instruct patient to contact health care provider if prescribed dosage isn't controlling pain.

Alert: Warn patient to withhold drug and inform prescriber if pain level worsens, pain sensitivity increases, or new pain occurs after taking drug.

Alert: Explain assessment and monitoring process to patient and family. Instruct them to immediately report difficulty breathing or other signs or symptoms of an adverse opioid-related reaction.

Alert: Encourage patient to report all medications being taken, including prescription and OTC medications and supplements.

Alert: Caution patient to immediately report signs and symptoms of serotonin syndrome, adrenal insufficiency, and decreased sex hormone levels.

- Encourage patient who has had a surgical procedure to turn, cough, and deep-breathe to prevent lung problems.
- Caution patient who is ambulatory about getting out of bed or walking. Warn outpatient to avoid driving and other potentially hazardous activities that require mental alertness until drug's CNS effects are known.
- Teach patient that naloxone may be prescribed with the opioid when beginning and renewing therapy to reduce risk of opioid overdose and death.

Alert: Counsel patient who has been regularly taking drug not to discontinue without first discussing the need for gradual tapering with prescriber.

- Caution patient to report to prescriber pregnancy or plan to become pregnant.

meropenem

mare-oh-PEN-em

Therapeutic class: Antibiotics
Pharmacologic class: Carbapenems

AVAILABLE FORMS

Powder for injection: 500 mg, 1 g vials

Solution for injection (after reconstitution):
500 mg/mL, 1g/50 mL dual-chamber container

INDICATIONS & DOSAGES
Adjust-a-dose (for all indications): For adults with CrCl of 26 to 50 mL/minute, give usual dose every 12 hours. If CrCl is 10 to 25 mL/minute, give half usual dose every 12 hours; if CrCl is less than 10 mL/minute, give half usual dose every 24 hours.

➤ **Complicated skin and skin-structure infections from *Staphylococcus aureus* (methicillin-susceptible isolates only), *Streptococcus pyogenes, Streptococcus agalactiae*, viridans group streptococci, *Enterococcus faecalis* (excluding vancomycin-resistant isolates), *Escherichia coli, Proteus mirabilis, Bacteroides fragilis*, or *Peptostreptococcus* species**
Adults and children weighing more than 50 kg: 500 mg IV every 8 hours.
Children ages 3 months and older weighing 50 kg or less: 10 mg/kg IV every 8 hours.
Maximum dosage, 500 mg IV every 8 hours.

➤ **Complicated skin and skin-structure infections caused by *Pseudomonas aeruginosa***
Adults and children weighing more than 50 kg: 1 g IV every 8 hours.
Children ages 3 months and older weighing 50 kg or less: 20 mg/kg IV every 8 hours.
Maximum dosage, 1 g IV every 8 hours.

➤ **Complicated intra-abdominal infections (including appendicitis and peritonitis) caused by viridans group streptococci, *E. coli, Klebsiella pneumoniae, P. aeruginosa, B. fragilis, Bacteroides thetaiotaomicron*, or *Peptostreptococcus* species**
Adults and children weighing more than 50 kg: 1 g IV every 8 hours.
Children ages 3 months and older weighing 50 kg or less: 20 mg/kg IV every 8 hours. Maximum dosage, 1 g IV every 8 hours.
Children 32 weeks' or more gestational age (GA) and 14 days or more postnatal age (PNA): 30 mg/kg IV every 8 hours over 30 minutes.
Children 32 weeks' or more GA and less than 14 days PNA: 20 mg/kg IV every 8 hours.
Children less than 32 weeks' GA and 14 days or more PNA: 20 mg/kg IV every 8 hours.
Children less than 32 weeks' GA and less than 14 days PNA: 20 mg/kg IV every 12 hours.

➤ **Bacterial meningitis**
Children weighing more than 50 kg: 2 g IV every 8 hours.
Children ages 3 months and older weighing 50 kg or less: 40 mg/kg IV every 8 hours. Maximum dosage, 2 g IV every 8 hours.

ADMINISTRATION
IV
▼ Obtain specimen for culture and sensitivity tests before giving first dose. Begin therapy while awaiting results.
❸ *Alert:* Serious hypersensitivity reactions may occur in patients receiving beta-lactams. Before therapy begins, determine if patient has had previous hypersensitivity reactions to penicillins, cephalosporins, beta-lactams, or other allergens. If allergic reaction occurs, stop drug and notify prescriber. Serious anaphylactic reactions require emergency treatment.
▼ Use freshly prepared solutions of drug immediately whenever possible. Stability of drug varies with form of drug used (injection vial, infusion vial, or dual-chamber containers).
▼ For bolus, add 10 mL of sterile water for injection to 500-mg vial or 20 mL to 1-g vial. Shake to dissolve, and let stand until clear. Give over 3 to 5 minutes. May store for up to 3 hours at up to 77° F (25° C) or for 13 hours at up to 41° F (5° C).
▼ For infusion, an infusion vial (500 mg/100 mL or 1 g/100 mL) may be directly reconstituted with a compatible infusion fluid. Or, an injection vial may be reconstituted and the resulting solution added to an IV container and further diluted with an appropriate infusion fluid. Don't use ADD-Vantage vials for this purpose. Administer over 15 to 30 minutes.
▼ May store solutions prepared with NSS at 1 to 20 mg/mL for 1 hour at up to 77° F (25° C) or 15 hours at up to 41° F (5° C); use solutions prepared with D₅W immediately.
▼ Follow manufacturer's guidelines closely when using dual-chamber containers.
▼ Don't use dual-chamber containers in series connections.
▼ **Incompatibilities:** Compatibility with other drugs hasn't been established. Don't mix with or physically add to solutions containing other drugs.

ACTION

Inhibits cell-wall synthesis in bacteria.
Readily penetrates cell wall of most gram-
positive and gram-negative bacteria to reach
penicillin-binding protein targets.

Route	Onset	Peak	Duration
IV	Unknown	1 hr	6 to 8 hours

Half-life: 1 to 1.5 hours.

ADVERSE REACTIONS

CNS: headache, pain, *seizure.* **CV:** peripheral vascular disorder, *shock.* **EENT:** oral candidiasis, glossitis, pharyngitis. **GI:** *CDAD,*
GI disorder, constipation, diarrhea, nausea,
vomiting. **Hematologic:** anemia. **Hepatic:**
increased LFT results. **Metabolic:** *hypoglycemia.* **Respiratory:** *apnea,* pneumonia.
Skin: injection-site inflammation, pruritus,
rash. **Other:** *sepsis,* hypersensitivity reactions, accidental injury.

INTERACTIONS

Drug-drug. *Probenecid:* May decrease kidney excretion of meropenem. Avoid use together.
Valproic acid: May decrease valproic acid
level, increasing risk of seizures. Monitor levels frequently, and observe for seizure activity. Consider alternative antibiotic or supplemental anticonvulsant therapy.

EFFECTS ON LAB TEST RESULTS

• May increase ALT, AST, bilirubin, ALP,
LDH, creatinine, and BUN levels.
• May increase eosinophil count.
• May decrease Hb level, hematocrit, and
WBC count.
• May increase or decrease INR and platelet
count.
• May prolong or shorten PT and PTT.
• May produce a positive Coombs test.

CONTRAINDICATIONS & CAUTIONS

• Contraindicated in patients hypersensitive
to components of drug or other drugs in same
class and in patients who have had anaphylactic reactions to beta-lactams.
• Use cautiously in older adults and in patients with history of brain lesions, seizure
disorders, or impaired kidney function.
• Some formulations contain significant
sodium content and should be avoided in

patients with HF, older adults, and patients
who require restricted sodium intake.
• SCARs and CDAD have been reported with
meropenem use.
Dialyzable drug: Yes.
⚠ *Overdose S&S:* Exaggerated adverse reactions.

PREGNANCY-LACTATION-REPRODUCTION

• Studies during pregnancy are inadequate.
Use during pregnancy only if clearly
needed.
• Drug appears in human milk. Use cautiously during breastfeeding.

NURSING CONSIDERATIONS

• In patient with CNS disorder, bacterial
meningitis, or compromised kidney function,
drug may cause seizures and other CNS adverse reactions.
• If seizures occur during therapy, stop infusion and notify prescriber. Dosage adjustment
may be needed.
• Monitor patient for signs and symptoms of
superinfection. Drug may cause overgrowth
of nonsusceptible bacteria or fungi.
• Periodically assess organ system functions,
including kidney, liver, and hematopoietic
function, during prolonged therapy.
• Carefully monitor patient's fluid balance
and weight.
• If patient develops signs and symptoms
suggestive of SCAR, stop drug immediately
and consider alternative treatment.
• CDAD may occur up to months after last
dose and range from mild diarrhea to fatal colitis. If CDAD occurs, drug will need
to be stopped and appropriate treatment
begun.

PATIENT TEACHING

• Instruct patient to report adverse reactions
and signs and symptoms of superinfection.
• Advise patient to report diarrhea to prescriber for evaluation of CDAD.
ⓘ *Alert:* Advise patient to report rash, peeling skin, trouble swallowing or breathing,
or other signs and symptoms of allergic
reaction.
• Caution patient that drug can interfere with
mental alertness. Caution patient not to operate motorized vehicles or machinery until
drug effects are known.

Reactions in bold italics are *life-threatening*.

mesalamine (mesalazine)
me-SAL-a-meen

Apriso, Canasa, Delzicol, Lialda, Mezavant✦, Mezera✦, Octasa✦, Pentasa, Rowasa, Salofalk✦, sfRowasa

Therapeutic class: Anti-inflammatory drugs
Pharmacologic class: Salicylates

AVAILABLE FORMS
Capsules (controlled-release) 🞁: 250 mg, 375 mg, 500 mg
Capsules (delayed-release) 🞁: 400 mg, 500 mg✦
Rectal foam: 1 g/actuation✦, 800 mg
Rectal suspension: 2 g/60 mL✦, 4 g/60 mL, 1 g/100 mL✦, 4 g/100 mL✦
Suppositories: 500 mg✦, 1,000 mg
Tablets (delayed-release) 🞁: 400 mg✦, 800 mg✦, 1.2 g, 1.6 g✦
Tablets (extended-release) 🞁: 500 mg✦, 1,000 mg✦

INDICATIONS & DOSAGES
➤ **Active mild to moderate distal ulcerative colitis, proctitis, or proctosigmoiditis**
Adults: 1,000 mg suppository PR once daily at bedtime for 3 to 6 weeks. Or, 2,000 mg (2 actuations) foam PR once daily at bedtime for at least 6 weeks. Or, 4 g retention enema PR once daily (preferably at bedtime) for 3 to 6 weeks.
➤ **Remission-induction of active, mild to moderate ulcerative colitis in adults**
Adults: 800 mg t.i.d. (2.4 g) Delzicol capsules PO for 6 weeks. Or, two to four 1.2-g Lialda tablets (2.4 to 4.8 g) PO once daily for up to 8 weeks. Or, two 500-mg Mezera tablets (1 g) PO t.i.d. for 8 weeks.

Or two to three 1.6-g Octasa tablets (3.2 to 4.8 g) PO once daily for up to 8 weeks. Or, 1 g Pentasa capsules PO q.i.d. for a total dose of 4 g for up to 8 weeks.
Children ages 5 and older weighing 54 to 90 kg (Delzicol): 27 to 44 mg/kg/day PO in two divided doses daily for 6 weeks. Maximum dosage, 2.4 g/day.
Children weighing more than 50 kg (Lialda): Four 1.2-g tablets (4.8 g) PO once daily for 8 weeks.

Children weighing more than 35 to 50 kg (Lialda): Three 1.2-g tablets (3.6 g) PO once daily for 8 weeks.
Children ages 5 and older weighing 33 to less than 54 kg (Delzicol): 37 to 61 mg/kg/day PO in two divided doses daily for 6 weeks. Maximum dosage, 2 g/day.
Children weighing 24 to 35 kg (Lialda): Two 1.2-g tablets (2.4 g) PO once daily for 8 weeks.
Children ages 5 and older weighing 17 to less than 33 kg (Delzicol): 36 to 71 mg/kg/day PO in two divided doses daily for 6 weeks. Maximum dosage, 1.2 g/day.
➤ **Moderate ulcerative colitis**
Adults: Two 800-mg tablets (1.6 g) t.i.d. for 6 weeks. Or six 600-mg Octasa tablets (4.8 g) PO once daily or in divided doses for 10 weeks.
➤ **Maintenance of remission of ulcerative colitis in adults**
Adults: 1.5 g Apriso PO once daily in morning. Or, two 1.2-g Lialda tablets PO once daily. Or, 500 mg or 1 g Pentasa PO q.i.d. Or, 1.6 g Delzicol PO in two to four divided doses.
➤ **Maintenance of remission of ulcerative colitis in children (Lialda)**
Children weighing more than 35 kg: Two 1.2-g tablets (2.4 g) PO once daily.
Children weighing 24 to 35 kg: One 1.2-g tablet (1.2 g) PO once daily.

ADMINISTRATION
PO
• Give Lialda with food.
• Give Apriso without regard to food. Don't give with antacids.
• Don't crush or cut delayed-release or controlled-release forms.
• Intact or partially intact tablets may be present in stool. Notify prescriber if this occurs repeatedly.
• Give Delzicol without regard to food. If patient is unable to swallow Delzicol, the capsules can be opened and the contents swallowed whole.
• If patient can't swallow Pentasa capsules whole, they may be opened and the contents sprinkled on applesauce or yogurt and consumed immediately.
Rectal
• Patient should retain rectal enema dosage form overnight (for about 8 hours). Usual course of therapy for rectal form ranges from 3 to 6 weeks.

M

• Shake suspension well before each use and remove sheath before inserting into rectum.

• Results are best if bowels are evacuated prior to insertion of suppository or foam.

• Patient should retain suppository for 1 to 3 hours or longer, if possible.

• Attach applicator and shake foam canister for about 20 seconds before use. Hold applicator in position for 10 to 15 seconds before withdrawing from rectum.

• Give missed foam or suppository as soon as possible unless it is almost time for the next dose. Don't give 2 doses at same time.

• Don't cut or break Canasa suppository. Be aware that Canasa suppositories can stain fabric and other surfaces.

ACTION

An active metabolite of sulfasalazine; probably acts topically by inhibiting prostaglandin production in the colon.

Route	Onset	Peak	Duration
PO, PR	Unknown	3–12 hr	Unknown

Half-life: Usually about 25 hours but varies from 1.5 to 296 hours.

ADVERSE REACTIONS

CNS: headache, dizziness, fever, fatigue, paresthesia, pain, vertigo, anxiety. **CV:** HTN. **EENT:** visual disturbance, tinnitus, nasopharyngitis, rhinitis, sinusitis. **GI:** abdominal pain, cramps, discomfort, flatulence, diarrhea, bloody diarrhea, rectal pain, bloating, nausea, vomiting, dyspepsia, constipation, belching, exacerbation of ulcerative colitis, gastroenteritis, hemorrhoids, *pancreatitis,* tenesmus, *rectal hemorrhage,* sclerosing cholangitis (children), *hemorrhage.* **GU:** interstitial kidney inflammation, hematuria, urinary frequency, nephropathy, *kidney toxicity.* **Hematologic:** anemia. **Hepatic:** *cholestatic hepatitis,* liver insufficiency, increased transaminase levels. **Metabolic:** weight loss (children), increased triglyceride levels. **Musculoskeletal:** arthralgia, arthropathy, myalgia, back pain, lower extremity pain. **Respiratory:** cough, dyspnea. **Skin:** rash, acne, urticaria, hair loss. **Other:** chills, pain, flulike symptoms, infection.

INTERACTIONS

Drug-drug. *Antacids, H₂ antagonists, PPIs:* May cause premature release of oral delayed- or extended-release products. Avoid use together. Consider therapy modification.

Azathioprine, mercaptopurine: May cause blood disorders. Monitor blood cell counts and adjust therapy as needed.

Iron supplements: Delzicol contains iron. Use cautiously in patients at risk for iron overload.

NSAIDs, other kidney-toxic agents: May enhance kidney-toxic effects. Monitor kidney function and adverse reactions.

Varicella virus vaccines: May enhance adverse effect of varicella virus-containing vaccines, causing Reye syndrome. Consider therapy modification.

Drug-lifestyle. *Sunlight, UV light exposure:* May cause photosensitivity reactions. Advise patient to use skin protection and avoid prolonged exposure to sunlight and UV light.

EFFECTS ON LAB TEST RESULTS

• May increase bilirubin, BUN, creatinine, AST, ALT, ALP, LDH, amylase, triglyceride, and lipase levels.

• May decrease CrCl.

• May decrease Hb level and hematocrit and RBC and WBC counts.

• May falsely elevate urine normetanephrine results obtained by liquid chromatography with electrochemical detection.

CONTRAINDICATIONS & CAUTIONS

• Contraindicated in patients allergic to mesalamine, sulfites (including sulfasalazine), any salicylates, or any component of the preparation.

• Avoid use of tablets in patients at risk for upper GI obstruction (pyloric stenosis, upper GI functional disorders) due to delayed release of drug in colon.

• Use cautiously in patients predisposed to pericarditis and myocarditis due to mesalamine-induced cardiac hypersensitivity reactions.

• Use cautiously in older adults, in patients with kidney or liver impairment, and in those taking kidney-toxic drugs.

Dialyzable drug: Unknown.

⚠ *Overdose S&S:* Salicylate toxicity (confusion, diarrhea, headache, hyperventilation, diaphoresis, tinnitus, vertigo, nausea, vomiting, abdominal pain, hyperpnea, dizziness, seizure, electrolyte imbalances, kidney and liver involvement).

Reactions in bold italics are *life-threatening.*

PREGNANCY-LACTATION-REPRODUCTION
• Studies during pregnancy are inadequate. Drug crosses the placental barrier. Use during pregnancy only if clearly needed.
• Drug appears in human milk. Use cautiously during breastfeeding.
• Drug may cause decreased sperm count, which resolves with drug discontinuation.

NURSING CONSIDERATIONS
• Assess kidney function before therapy.
• Periodically monitor kidney and liver function studies and blood cell counts in patient on long-term therapy.
• Ensure patient is well hydrated during therapy; mesalamine kidney stones have been reported.
• Monitor patient for hypersensitivity reactions, including those involving organs (hepatitis, myocarditis, pericarditis, kidney inflammation, hematologic abnormalities, pneumonitis) and SCARs.
• Because mesalamine rectal suspension contains potassium metabisulfite, it may cause hypersensitivity reactions in patient sensitive to sulfites.
• Drug may be associated with acute intolerance syndrome, in which signs and symptoms (abdominal pain, cramping, bloody diarrhea, headache, fever, rash) may be similar to ulcerative colitis exacerbation. If acute intolerance syndrome is suspected, discontinue drug.
• Apriso contains phenylalanine.
• *Look alike–sound alike:* Don't confuse mesalamine with mecamylamine, megestrol, memantine, metaxalone, or methenamine; Apriso with Apri; or Lialda with Aldara.

PATIENT TEACHING
• Instruct patient to carefully follow instructions supplied with drug for safe drug administration.
• Tell patient not to take drug with antacids.
• Advise patient to drink adequate fluids.
• Explain that intact or partially intact tablet shells have been reported in stool. Instruct patient to contact health care provider if this occurs repeatedly.
• Advise patient to report all adverse reactions and to stop drug if fever or rash occurs.
• Tell patient to remove foil wrapper from suppositories before inserting into rectum.
• Teach patient about proper use of retention enema.

• Caution patient to wear protective clothing and broad-spectrum sunscreen when exposed to sunlight or UV light and to avoid prolonged exposure.

SAFETY ALERT!

metFORMIN hydrochloride
met-FOR-min

Fortamet, Glumetza, Riomet

Therapeutic class: Antidiabetics
Pharmacologic class: Biguanides

AVAILABLE FORMS
Oral solution: 500 mg/5 mL
Tablets: 500 mg, 625 mg, 750 mg, 850 mg, 1,000 mg
Tablets (extended-release) ⓘⓝⓒ: 500 mg, 750 mg, 1,000 mg

INDICATIONS & DOSAGES
Adjust-a-dose (for all indications): Contraindicated in patients with eGFR below 30 mL/minute/1.73 m^2. Starting drug in patients with eGFR between 30 and 45 mL/minute/1.73 m^2 isn't recommended. If eGFR falls below 45 mL/minute/1.73 m^2 in patients taking drug, assess benefits and risks of continuing treatment. Discontinue if eGFR falls below 30 mL/minute/1.73 m^2. For older adults or patients who are debilitated, use conservative initial and maintenance dosage because of potential decrease in kidney function.
➤ **Adjunct to diet to lower glucose level in patients with type 2 diabetes**
Adults: If using immediate-release tablets or oral solution, initially 500 mg PO b.i.d. with morning and evening meals or 850 mg PO once daily with morning meal. Titrate immediate-release forms in increments of 500 mg weekly or 850 mg every other week to maximum dosage of 2,550 mg PO daily in divided doses. If using extended-release formulation, start at 500 mg PO once daily with evening meal. May increase dose weekly (every 1 to 2 weeks for Glumetza) as tolerated in increments of 500 mg daily, to maximum dosage of 2,000 mg once daily. If higher doses are required, consider trial of 1,000 mg b.i.d. or use regular-release formulation up to maximum dosage.

M

Children ages 10 and older: 500 mg PO b.i.d. using immediate-release formulation only. Increase in increments of 500 mg weekly, to maximum dosage of 2,000 mg daily in divided doses.

➤ **Prevention of type 2 diabetes in patients with prediabetes, especially those with BMI of more than 35 kg/m^2, those younger than age 60, and patients with prior history of gestational diabetes ♦**

Adults: 850 mg immediate-release tablets PO once daily for 1 month; then increase to 850 mg b.i.d., unless GI adverse effects warrant a longer titration period.

ADMINISTRATION
PO
• Give drug with meals. Maximum doses may be better tolerated if given in three divided doses with meals (immediate-release tablets only).
• Have patient swallow extended-release tablets whole; don't crush or break tablets.
• Oral solution should be clear and given with graduated dosing cup.

ACTION
Decreases liver glucose production and intestinal absorption of glucose and improves insulin sensitivity (increases peripheral glucose uptake and use).

Route	Onset	Peak	Duration
PO (conventional)	Unknown	2–3 hr	Unknown
PO (extended-release)	Unknown	4–8 hr	Unknown
PO (solution)	Unknown	2.5 hr	Unknown

Half-life: About 4 to 9 hours.

ADVERSE REACTIONS
CNS: asthenia, headache, dizziness, chills, light-headedness, taste disorder. **CV:** chest discomfort, palpitations, flushing. **GI:** diarrhea, nausea, vomiting, indigestion, abdominal bloating, abdominal discomfort, flatulence, abnormal stools, constipation, dyspepsia, weight loss. **Metabolic:** vitamin B$_{12}$ deficiency, *hypoglycemia.* **Musculoskeletal:** myalgia. **Respiratory:** URI, dyspnea. **Skin:** nail disorder, rash, diaphoresis. **Other:** accidental injury, infection, flulike syndrome.

INTERACTIONS
Drug-drug. *Beta blockers:* Hypoglycemia may be difficult to recognize in patients

using beta blockers. Monitor patient and blood glucose level.

Calcium channel blockers, corticosteroids, estrogens, fosphenytoin, hormonal contraceptives, isoniazid, nicotinic acid, phenothiazines, phenytoin, sympathomimetics, thiazide and other diuretics, thyroid drugs: May produce hyperglycemia. Monitor patient's glycemic control. Metformin dosage may need to be increased.

Boxed Warning *Carbonic anhydrase inhibitors (acetazolamide, topiramate):* May increase risk of lactic acidosis. Monitor patient closely. ∎

Cationic drugs (amiloride, cimetidine, digoxin, morphine, procainamide, quinidine, quinine, triamterene, trimethoprim, vancomycin): May compete for common kidney tubular transport systems, which may increase metformin level. Monitor glucose level.

Dolutegravir: Increases metformin exposure. Use alternative drug or limit total daily dose of metformin. Closely monitor response to metformin.

Insulin, insulin secretagogues (sulfonylureas): May increase risk of hypoglycemia. Monitor patient closely and adjust insulin or insulin secretagogue dosage as needed.

Boxed Warning *Radiologic contrast dye:* May cause AKI or lactic acidosis. Withhold metformin at time of or before procedure and 48 hours after procedure. Restart drug only if kidney function returns to normal. ∎

Drug-herb. *Guar gum:* May decrease hypoglycemic effect. Discourage use together.

Drug-lifestyle. **Boxed Warning** *Alcohol use:* May increase drug effects and potentiate metformin's effect on lactate metabolism. Discourage use together. ∎

EFFECTS ON LAB TEST RESULTS
• May decrease vitamin B$_{12}$ and Hb levels.

CONTRAINDICATIONS & CAUTIONS
• Contraindicated in patients hypersensitive to drug and in those with liver disease or metabolic acidosis or lactic acidosis, including diabetic ketoacidosis with or without coma.
• Contraindicated in patients with eGFR below 30 mL/minute/1.73 m^2. Not recommended in patients with eGFR between 30 and 45 mL/minute/1.73 m^2.

Reactions in bold italics are ***life-threatening***.

Boxed Warning Metformin decreases liver uptake of lactate, increasing lactate blood levels and risk of lactic acidosis, especially in patients at risk. Risk factors for metformin-associated lactic acidosis include kidney impairment, concomitant use of certain drugs, age 65 or older, radiologic study with contrast, surgery and other procedures, hypoxic states, excessive alcohol intake, and liver impairment. ∎

Boxed Warning See manufacturer's instructions for steps to reduce risk and manage lactic acidosis in groups at high risk. ∎

• Discontinue drug in patients with acute HF (particularly when accompanied by hypoperfusion and hypoxemia), CV collapse (shock), acute MI, sepsis, and other conditions associated with hypoxemia that have been linked to lactic acidosis and may cause elevated BUN and creatinine due to decreased blood flow to kidneys.

• Not indicated for use in patients with type 1 diabetes.

• Use cautiously in older adults and in patients who are debilitated or malnourished.
Dialyzable drug: Yes.

⚠ *Overdose S&S:* Hypoglycemia, lactic acidosis.

PREGNANCY-LACTATION-REPRODUCTION

• Abnormal blood glucose level during pregnancy may cause fetal harm. Most experts recommend using insulin during pregnancy to maintain blood glucose level as close to normal as possible. Use metformin during pregnancy only if clearly needed.

• Drug appears in human milk. Patient should discontinue breastfeeding or discontinue drug, considering importance of drug to patient and risk of hypoglycemia in infant. Consider insulin therapy.

• Metformin increases risk of unintended pregnancy during premenopause because it may cause ovulation in some anovulatory patients.

NURSING CONSIDERATIONS

• Before therapy begins and at least annually thereafter, assess patient's kidney function. Assess more frequently in patient at risk for kidney impairment.

Boxed Warning Metformin-associated lactic acidosis has resulted in hypothermia, hypotension, resistant bradyarrhythmias, and death. Onset includes nonspecific symptoms

(malaise, myalgia, respiratory distress, somnolence, abdominal pain). It's characterized by elevated blood lactate level (greater than 5 mmol/L), anion gap acidosis (without evidence of ketonuria or ketonemia), increased lactate/pyruvate ratio, and metformin plasma level generally above 5 mcg/mL. ∎

Boxed Warning For suspected metformin-associated lactic acidosis, immediately discontinue drug and promptly institute supportive measures in a hospital setting. Prompt hemodialysis is recommended. ∎

• Consider more frequent monitoring of patient taking drug that increases risk of metformin-associated lactic acidosis, including drugs that impair kidney function, result in significant hemodynamic change, interfere with acid-base balance, or increase metformin accumulation.

• Regularly monitor patient's glucose level to evaluate effectiveness of therapy. Notify prescriber if glucose level increases despite therapy.

• If patient hasn't responded to 4 weeks of therapy with maximum dosage, an oral sulfonylurea can be added while keeping metformin at maximum dosage. If patient still doesn't respond after several months of therapy with both drugs at maximum dosage, prescriber may stop both and start insulin therapy.

• Monitor patient closely during times of increased stress (infection, fever, surgery, trauma). Insulin therapy may be needed in these situations.

• Stop drug at time of, or before, an iodinated contrast imaging procedure in patient with eGFR between 30 and 60 mL/minute/1.73 m^2; in patient with history of liver impairment, alcoholism, or HF; or in patient who will receive intra-arterial iodinated contrast. Reevaluate eGFR 48 hours after imaging procedure; restart drug if kidney function stabilizes.

• Temporarily discontinue drug in patient with restricted food and fluid intake due to surgery or other procedures because of increased risk of volume depletion, hypotension, and kidney impairment.

• Monitor patient for evidence of anemia annually. Monitor vitamin B$_{12}$ level every 2 to 3 years. Patients with inadequate vitamin B$_{12}$ or calcium intake or absorption may be predisposed to subnormal vitamin B$_{12}$ level.

• *Look alike–sound alike:* Don't confuse metformin with metronidazole.

M

PATIENT TEACHING

• Teach patient about diabetes and importance of adhering to therapeutic regimen, following a specific diet, losing weight, getting exercise, practicing good personal hygiene, and avoiding infection. Explain how and when to monitor glucose level. Teach evidence of low and high glucose levels. Explain emergency measures.

Boxed Warning Instruct patient to stop drug and immediately notify prescriber about unexplained hyperventilation, muscle pain, malaise, dizziness, light-headedness, unusual sleepiness, unexplained stomach pain, feeling of coldness, slow or irregular HR, or other nonspecific symptoms of early lactic acidosis. ∎

Boxed Warning Warn patient against excessive alcohol intake while taking drug. ∎

• Teach about proper drug administration and handling.

• Tell patient not to change drug dosage without prescriber's knowledge.

• Encourage patient to report abnormal glucose level test results.

• Inform patient that inactive ingredients may be eliminated in stool as soft mass resembling the original tablet.

• Advise patient not to take other drugs, including OTC drugs, without first checking with prescriber.

• Instruct patient to carry medical identification at all times.

• Tell patient to report all adverse reactions. Explain that diarrhea, nausea, and upset stomach generally subside over time.

• Discuss risk of unintended pregnancy with patient experiencing premenopause.

• Advise patient to discontinue breastfeeding or discontinue drug.

SAFETY ALERT!

methadone hydrochloride
METH-a-done

Metadol ✽ , Metadol-D ✽ , Methadose

Therapeutic class: Opioid analgesics
Pharmacologic class: Opioid agonists
Controlled substance schedule: II

AVAILABLE FORMS

Dispersible tablets and diskets (for methadone maintenance therapy) ⓝ*:* 40 mg
Injection: 10 mg/mL

Oral solution: 5 mg/5 mL, 10 mg/5 mL, 10 mg/mL (concentrate)
Tablets: 1 mg✽, 5 mg, 10 mg, 25 mg✽

INDICATIONS & DOSAGES

Adjust-a-dose (for all indications): For older adults and patients with kidney or liver impairment, reduce initial dose. Refer to manufacturer's instruction for conversion between methadone formulations or between methadone and other opioids.

➤ **Severe chronic pain for which alternative treatment options are inadequate**
Adults: Initiate dosing regimen for each patient individually, taking into account patient's prior analgesic treatment experience and risk factors for addiction, abuse, and misuse. Discontinue all other around-the-clock opioid drugs. Initially, 2.5 mg PO every 8 to 12 hours, or 2.5 to 10 mg IM, IV, or subcut every 8 to 12 hours. Titrate slowly, no more frequently than every 3 to 5 days, and increase dosage as needed or use rescue drug as needed to maintain analgesia.

➤ **Opioid detoxification; maintenance treatment of opioid addiction**
Adults: Initially, 20 to 30 mg PO daily to suppress withdrawal symptoms (highly individualized; some patients require higher dosage). Initial dose shouldn't exceed 30 mg. Maintenance dosage, 80 to 120 mg PO daily. Adjust dosage as needed.

ADMINISTRATION

• Store all forms at room temperature.
PO
• Oral form is legally required in maintenance programs.
• Completely dissolve dispersible tablets, disket, or oral solution in 4 oz (120 mL) of water, orange juice, or other acidic fruit beverage. Patient shouldn't chew or swallow tablets before they are dispersed in liquid.
• Dispersible tablets are cross-scored to allow breaking into two 20-mg doses or four 10-mg doses.
IV
▼ Protect from light.
▼ Rate of IV administration not defined by manufacturer.
▼ **Incompatibilities:** None listed by manufacturer. Consult drug compatibility reference for more information.

IM
- For parenteral use, IM injection is preferred. Rotate injection sites. Monitor site, as local tissue reactions may occur.
- Protect drug from light.

Subcutaneous
- Monitor for pain at injection site, tissue irritation, and induration after injection.
- Protect drug from light.

ACTION
Binds with opioid receptors in the CNS, altering perception of and emotional response to pain.

Route	Onset	Peak	Duration
PO	30–60 min	1–7.5 hr	4–8 hr
IV	Unknown	Unknown	4–8 hr
IM, subcut	10–20 min	1–2 hr	4–8 hr

Half-life: 8 to 59 hours.

ADVERSE REACTIONS
CNS: clouded sensorium, disorientation, dysphoria, hallucinations, dizziness, light-headedness, sedation, somnolence, *seizures,* agitation, euphoria, asthenia, headache, insomnia, syncope. **CV:** *arrhythmias, bradycardia, prolonged QT interval, shock, cardiac arrest, cardiomyopathy, HF, ECG abnormalities,* flushing, phlebitis, edema, hypotension, palpitations, tachycardia, T-wave inversion. **EENT:** visual disturbances, dry mouth, congenital oculomotor disorders (nystagmus, strabismus), glossitis. **GI:** nausea, vomiting, abdominal pain, anorexia, biliary tract spasm, constipation, ileus. **GU:** decreased libido, urine retention, amenorrhea, sperm abnormalities, reduced seminal vesicle and prostate secretions, hypogonadism. **Metabolic:** *hypokalemia, hypomagnesemia, hypoglycemia,* weight gain. **Respiratory:** *respiratory arrest, respiratory depression, pulmonary edema.* **Skin:** diaphoresis, pruritus, pain at injection site, induration, urticaria, rash. **Other:** physical dependence, tissue irritation, hypersensitivity reaction.

INTERACTIONS
Drug-drug. *Ammonium chloride, other urine acidifiers:* May reduce methadone effect. Watch for decreased pain control.
Anticholinergics (benztropine mesylate, darifenacin, fesoterodine): May increase risk of urine retention or severe constipation. Monitor patient closely.

Boxed Warning *Benzodiazepines, other CNS depressants (antipsychotics, anxiolytics, general anesthetics, hypnotics, MAO inhibitors, muscle relaxants, TCAs, tranquilizers):* May cause slow or difficult breathing, sedation, and death. Avoid use together. If use together can't be avoided, limit dose and duration of each drug to the minimum needed for desired effect. ■

Boxed Warning *CYP2B6, CYP2C9, CYP2C19, CYP2D6, or CYP3A4 inhibitors (all); CYP2B6, CYP2C9, CYP2C19, or CYP3A4 inducers:* Concomitant use of inhibitors and discontinuation of inducers may cause increased methadone level, resulting in potentially fatal respiratory depression. Monitor patient closely and reduce methadone dosage, if necessary. ■

Boxed Warning *CYP2B6, CYP2C9, CYP2C19, or CYP3A4 inducers; CYP2B6, CYP2C9, CYP2C19, CYP2D6, or CYP3A4 inhibitors:* Adding inducers concomitantly with methadone or stopping inhibitors may decrease methadone effect and precipitate a withdrawal syndrome. Monitor patient closely. ■

Didanosine, stavudine: May decrease levels of these drugs. Monitor therapy.
Diuretics, laxatives, mineralocorticoid hormones: May cause electrolyte disturbances and increase risk of arrhythmias. Monitor patient closely.
MAO inhibitors (linezolid, phenelzine): May increase risk of serotonin syndrome or opioid toxicity. Use within 14 days of MAO inhibitor isn't recommended.
NNRTIs (delavirdine, efavirenz, nevirapine), protease inhibitors (lopinavir–ritonavir, ritonavir), rifamycins: May increase methadone metabolism, causing opioid withdrawal symptoms. Monitor patient and adjust dose as needed.

Boxed Warning *Opioids:* May cause slow or difficult breathing, sedation, and death. Avoid use together. If use together is necessary, limit dosage and duration of each drug to the minimum necessary for desired effect. ■

Protease inhibitors, cimetidine, fluvoxamine: May increase respiratory and CNS depression. Monitor patient closely.

◊ *Alert:* Serotonergic drugs (amoxapine, antiemetics [dolasetron, granisetron, ondansetron, palonosetron], antimigraine drugs, buspirone, cyclobenzaprine, dextromethorphan, lithium, maprotiline,

M

methylene blue, mirtazapine, nefazodone, SNRIs, SSRIs, TCAs, trazodone, tryptophan, vilazodone): May increase risk of serotonin syndrome. Use together cautiously and monitor patient for serotonin syndrome.

Boxed Warning *QT interval-prolonging drugs (antiarrhythmics, chlorpromazine, citalopram, dolasetron):* May increase risk of QT-interval prolongation and ventricular arrhythmias. Use with extreme caution. ■

Zidovudine: May increase level of zidovudine. Monitor patient.

Drug-herb. ❂ *Alert: St. John's wort:* May reduce methadone effect and precipitate a withdrawal syndrome. May increase risk of serotonin syndrome. Use together cautiously and monitor patient closely.

Drug-lifestyle. **Boxed Warning** *Alcohol use:* May cause slow or difficult breathing, sedation, and death. Discourage use together. ■

EFFECTS ON LAB TEST RESULTS
• May increase amylase level.
• May decrease testosterone, potassium, magnesium, and glucose levels.

CONTRAINDICATIONS & CAUTIONS
• Contraindicated in patients hypersensitive to drug and in those with significant respiratory depression, acute or severe bronchial asthma in an unmonitored setting or in the absence of resuscitative equipment, or known or suspected GI obstruction, including paralytic ileus.

Boxed Warning Use exposes patient and others to risk of opioid addiction, abuse, and misuse, which can lead to overdose and death. These effects can occur at any dose or duration. Assess patient risk before prescribing and regularly reassess patient for these behaviors and conditions. ■

Boxed Warning Prescribers are strongly encouraged to complete a REMS-compliant education program. Drug should be prescribed only by prescribers with knowledge of opioid use and ways to reduce associated risks. ■

❂ *Alert:* Use lowest effective dose for shortest period consistent with patient's treatment goals.

❂ *Alert:* Because risk of overdose increases as opioid dose increases, reserve titration to higher doses for patients in whom lower doses are ineffective and in whom expected benefits of higher opioid dose outweigh risks.

Boxed Warning Accidental ingestion of methadone can result in a fatal overdose, especially in children. ■

Boxed Warning Prolonged QT interval and serious arrhythmias (torsades de pointes) have occurred during methadone treatment. Most cases involve patients being treated for pain with large, multiple daily doses, although cases have been reported in patients receiving doses commonly used for maintenance treatment of opioid addiction. ■

Boxed Warning *Opioid class warning:* Opioids should only be prescribed with benzodiazepines or other CNS depressants when alternative treatment options are inadequate, aren't expected to provide adequate analgesia, haven't been tolerated, or aren't expected to be tolerated. ■

❂ *Alert:* Immediate release formulations shouldn't be used for an extended period unless pain remains severe enough to require an opioid analgesic and alternative treatment options are inadequate to treat pain.

❂ *Alert:* Drug may lead to a rare but serious decrease in adrenal gland cortisol production.

❂ *Alert:* The combined use of medication-assisted treatment (MAT) drugs methadone or buprenorphine with benzodiazepines or other CNS depressants increases the risk of serious adverse effects; however, the harm caused by untreated opioid addiction may outweigh these risks. Patients may require MAT for opioid addiction indefinitely; its use should continue for as long as patients are benefiting and the drug is contributing to the intended treatment goals.

• Use cautiously in older adults or patients who are debilitated and in those with severe liver or kidney impairment, hypothyroidism, Addison disease, prostatic hyperplasia, urethral stricture, head injury, increased ICP, and respiratory conditions.

❂ *Alert:* Patients are at increased risk for oversedation and respiratory depression if they snore or have a history of sleep apnea, haven't used opioids recently or are first-time opioid users, have increased opioid dosage requirements or opioid habituation, have received general anesthesia for longer lengths of time or received other sedating drugs, have preexisting pulmonary or cardiac disease, or have thoracic or other surgical incisions that may impair breathing. Monitor patients carefully.

Reactions in bold italics are *life-threatening*.

⟲ Alert: Drug isn't indicated as a PRN analgesic.

Dialyzable drug: No.

⚠ Overdose S&S: Miosis; somnolence; respiratory depression; coma; cool, clammy skin; skeletal muscle flaccidity; apnea; bradycardia; hypotension; noncardiac pulmonary edema; death.

PREGNANCY-LACTATION-REPRODUCTION

• Use drug during pregnancy only if potential benefit justifies fetal risk. Methadone clearance may increase during pregnancy, particularly during second and third trimesters. Dosage may need to be increased or dosing interval decreased. Use lowest possible dosage.

Boxed Warning Prolonged use during pregnancy can cause neonatal opioid withdrawal syndrome, which can be life-threatening. It requires management with expert neonatology protocols. If prolonged use is needed, advise patient of risks and ensure availability of proper treatment. ∎

• Drug appears in human milk. Sedation and respiratory depression may occur in infants who are breastfeeding. Monitor for sedation and respiratory depression, and slowly wean to prevent withdrawal symptoms.

• When methadone is used to treat opioid addiction during breastfeeding, and if additional illicit substances are being abused, patient should express and discard human milk until sobriety is established.

• Long-term opioid use may cause secondary hypogonadism, which may lead to sexual dysfunction or infertility.

• Amenorrhea secondary to substance abuse may resolve after initiation of methadone maintenance treatment. Provide contraception counseling to prevent unplanned pregnancies.

NURSING CONSIDERATIONS

Boxed Warning May cause life-threatening or fatal respiratory depression at any time during therapy. Monitor patient closely, especially when starting or increasing doses. Proper dosing and titration are essential to reduce risk. ∎

Boxed Warning Regularly monitor all patients for opioid addiction, abuse, and misuse, which can lead to overdose and death. ∎

Boxed Warning QT-interval prolongation, and torsades de pointes have been observed during treatment. Be vigilant during treatment initiation and dosage titration. ∎

⟲ Alert: Drug may cause opioid-induced hyperalgesia (OIH). Symptoms include increased pain level with opioid dose increase, decreased pain level with opioid dose reduction, pain from ordinarily nonpainful stimuli without underlying disease progression, opioid tolerance or withdrawal, and addictive behavior. For suspected OIH, decrease opioid dose or switch patient to alternative opioid.

⟲ Alert: If patient is taking opioids with serotonergic drugs, watch for signs and symptoms of serotonin syndrome (agitation, hallucinations, rapid HR, fever, diaphoresis, shivering or shaking, muscle twitching or stiffness, trouble with coordination, nausea, vomiting, diarrhea), especially when starting treatment or increasing dosages. Signs and symptoms may occur within several hours of coadministration but may also occur later, especially after dosage increase. Discontinue opioid, serotonergic drug, or both if serotonin syndrome is suspected.

⟲ Alert: Work with patient to develop strategies to manage the use of prescribed or illicit benzodiazepines or other CNS depressants when starting MAT. Taper benzodiazepine or CNS depressant to discontinuation, if possible.

⟲ Alert: If patient is receiving prescribed benzodiazepines or other CNS depressants for anxiety or insomnia, verify diagnosis and consider other treatment options for these conditions, if possible.

⟲ Alert: Coordinate care to ensure other prescribers are aware of patient's MAT.

⟲ Alert: Monitor patient for illicit drug use, including urine or blood screening.

⟲ Alert: Monitor for signs and symptoms of adrenal insufficiency (nausea, vomiting, loss of appetite, fatigue, weakness, dizziness, low BP). Perform diagnostic testing if adrenal insufficiency is suspected. For confirmed adrenal insufficiency, treat with corticosteroids and wean patient off opioids, if appropriate. Discontinue corticosteroids when clinically appropriate.

• Monitor patient for signs and symptoms of decreased sex hormone levels (low libido, erectile dysfunction, amenorrhea, infertility). If signs and symptoms occur, evaluate patient and obtain specimens for lab testing.

• Reassess patient's level of pain at least 15 and 30 minutes after parenteral

M

administration and 30 minutes after oral administration.

Boxed Warning When used for detoxification and maintenance of opioid dependence, treatment products in oral form shall be dispensed only by opioid treatment programs. Administer in accordance with treatment standards cited in 42 CFR (Code of Federal Regulations) Section 8, including limitations on unsupervised administration. Dispensing hospitals and pharmacies are approved by FDA and designated state authorities. ■

• Use an around-the-clock regimen to manage severe, chronic pain.

• Give an additional analgesic to patient being treated in a methadone maintenance program, if needed to control pain.

• Monitor patient closely because drug has cumulative effect; marked sedation can occur after repeated doses.

• Monitor circulatory status and bladder and bowel function. Patient may need a stool softener and stimulant laxative.

⊕ *Alert:* Respiratory depressant effects may last longer than analgesic effects. Closely monitor patient's respiratory status.

• When used as adjunct in treatment of opioid addiction (maintenance), withdrawal is usually delayed and mild.

⊕ *Alert:* Use caution when dosing. Confusion has occurred between milliliter and milligram doses.

⊕ *Alert:* Don't stop drug abruptly; withdraw slowly and individualize gradual taper plan to prevent signs and symptoms of withdrawal, worsening pain, and psychological distress in patients who are physically dependent. Refer to manufacturer's label for specific tapering instructions.

⊕ *Alert:* When tapering opioids, monitor closely for signs and symptoms of opioid withdrawal (restlessness, lacrimation, rhinorrhea, yawning, perspiration, chills, myalgia, mydriasis, irritability, anxiety, insomnia, backache, joint pain, weakness, abdominal cramps, anorexia, nausea, vomiting, diarrhea, increased BP or HR, increased respiratory rate), which may indicate a need to taper more slowly. Also monitor patient for suicidality, use of other substances, or changes in mood.

• *Look alike–sound alike:* Don't confuse methadone with methylphenidate or dexmethylphenidate.

PATIENT TEACHING

Boxed Warning Counsel patient and caregiver on serious risks, safe use, and importance of reading the medication guide with each prescription. ■

⊕ *Alert:* Explain assessment and monitoring process to patient and family. Instruct them to immediately report difficulty breathing or other signs or symptoms of a potential adverse opioid-related reaction.

• Advise patient to take drug exactly as prescribed and to use lowest dose possible for shortest time needed.

• Warn patient that methadone isn't for use on an "as needed" basis.

⊕ *Alert:* Counsel patient who has been regularly taking drug not to discontinue without first discussing the need for gradual tapering with prescriber.

⊕ *Alert:* Warn patient to withhold drug and inform prescriber if pain level worsens, pain sensitivity increases, or new pain occurs after taking drug.

⊕ *Alert:* Encourage patient to report all medications being taken, including prescription and OTC medications and supplements.

⊕ *Alert:* Caution patient to immediately report signs and symptoms of serotonin syndrome, adrenal insufficiency, and decreased sex hormone levels.

⊕ *Alert:* Teach patient not to take nonprescribed benzodiazepines, sedatives, or alcohol when taking MAT due to increased risk of overdose and death.

⊕ *Alert:* Advise patient to notify all prescribers of MAT and not to stop MAT or other prescribed drugs without first consulting prescriber.

• Caution patient who is ambulatory about getting out of bed or walking. Warn outpatient to avoid hazardous activities that require mental alertness until drug's CNS effects are known.

• Instruct patient to increase fluid and fiber in diet, if not contraindicated, to combat constipation.

• Caution patient to report to prescriber pregnancy or plan to become pregnant.

• Teach patient who is breastfeeding to monitor infant for respiratory depression and sedation; advise patient when to contact health care provider for emergency care.

• Inform patient that prolonged opioid use may reduce fertility; it isn't known if effects

---

are reversible. Advise patient about contraceptive use, if needed.

• Teach patient that naloxone may be prescribed with the opioid when beginning and renewing therapy to reduce risk of opioid overdose and death.

methIMAzole ⚮
meth-IM-a-zole

Tapazole✿

Therapeutic class: Antihyperthyroid drugs
Pharmacologic class: Thyroid hormone antagonists

AVAILABLE FORMS
Tablets: 5 mg, 10 mg, 20 mg✿

INDICATIONS & DOSAGES
➤ **Hyperthyroidism**
Adults: If mild, 15 mg PO daily in three divided doses given at 8-hour intervals. If moderately severe, 30 to 40 mg daily in three divided doses given at 8-hour intervals. If severe, 60 mg daily in three divided doses given at 8-hour intervals. Maintenance dosage ranges, 5 to 15 mg daily.
Children: 0.4 mg/kg/day PO in three divided doses given at 8-hour intervals. Usual maintenance dosage is 0.2 mg/kg/day in three divided doses daily.

ADMINISTRATION
PO
⚈ *Alert:* Hazardous drug; use safe handling and disposal precautions.
• Use gloves to administer intact tablets.
• May give without regard to food.
• Omit a missed dose and give next scheduled dose as usual.
• Store at room temperature.

ACTION
Inhibits synthesis of thyroid hormones.

Route	Onset	Peak	Duration
PO	Rapid	1–2 hr	36–72 hr

Half-life: 4 to 6 hours.

ADVERSE REACTIONS
CNS: headache, drowsiness, vertigo, paresthesia, neuritis, CNS stimulation, loss of taste, fever. **CV:** edema, periarteritis. **GI:** nausea, vomiting, salivary gland enlargement, epigastric distress. **Hematologic:** *agranulocytosis, leukopenia, thrombocytepenia, aplastic anemia, hypoprothrombinemia.* **Hepatic:** jaundice, liver dysfunction, *hepatitis.* **Metabolic:** hypothyroidism, insulin autoimmune syndrome. **Musculoskeletal:** arthralgia, myalgia. **Skin:** rash, urticaria, discoloration, pruritus, lupuslike syndrome, abnormal hair loss. **Other:** lymphadenopathy.

INTERACTIONS
Drug-drug. *Beta blockers:* Beta-blocker clearance may be enhanced by hyperthyroidism. Dosage of beta blocker may need to be reduced when patient becomes euthyroid.
Cardiac glycosides (digoxin): May increase cardiac glycoside level. Cardiac glycoside dosage may need to be reduced.
Theophylline: May decrease theophylline clearance. Dosage adjustment may be needed.
Warfarin: May alter dosage requirements. Monitor PT and INR, and adjust warfarin dosage as needed.

EFFECTS ON LAB TEST RESULTS
• May increase LFT values and PT.
• May decrease prothrombin level.
• May decrease Hb level and granulocyte, WBC, and platelet counts.
• May alter thyroid uptake of ^{123}I or ^{131}I.

CONTRAINDICATIONS & CAUTIONS
• Contraindicated in patients hypersensitive to drug and in those with history of acute pancreatitis after methimazole use.
• Drug may cause hypoprothrombinemia and bleeding.
• Drug may rarely cause vasculitis, including cutaneous vasculitis, CNS vasculitis, glomerulonephritis, pulmonary hemorrhage, and neuropathy.
⚮ Patients with hereditary galactose intolerance, Lapp lactase deficiency, or glucose-galactose malabsorption shouldn't receive methimazole formulations that contain lactose.
Dialyzable drug: No.
⚠ *Overdose S&S:* Nausea, vomiting, epigastric distress, headache, fever, joint pain, pruritus, edema, aplastic anemia, agranulocytosis, hepatitis, nephrotic syndrome, exfoliative dermatitis, neuropathies, CNS stimulation or depression.

M

PREGNANCY-LACTATION-REPRODUCTION
• Drug may cause fetal harm, particularly in first trimester; consider other agents during this time. Drug crosses placental barrier and can cause goiter and hypothyroidism in fetus. Use cautiously during pregnancy.
• If drug is used during pregnancy or if patient becomes pregnant during therapy, apprise patient of fetal risk.
• Patients who are pregnant may need lower doses as pregnancy progresses, and drug may be stopped during last few weeks of pregnancy. Closely monitor thyroid function studies.
• Drug appears in human milk. Use cautiously and administer after breastfeeding and in divided doses.

NURSING CONSIDERATIONS
• Periodically monitor CBC to detect impending leukopenia, thrombocytopenia, aplastic anemia, and agranulocytosis.
• Monitor liver function. Stop drug if liver abnormality occurs.
• *Alert:* Drug may increase risk of agranulocytosis, which can be life-threatening. Monitor patient for sore throat, fever, and general malaise; promptly report symptoms.
• Monitor for bleeding and PT changes.
• Monitor thyroid function tests and watch for evidence of hypothyroidism (mental depression; cold intolerance; hard, nonpitting edema); notify prescriber because patient may need dosage adjustment.
• *Look alike–sound alike:* Don't confuse methimazole with methazolamide, metolazone, or metronidazole.

PATIENT TEACHING
• Teach about proper drug administration, handling, and storage.
• Warn patient to report fever, sore throat, mouth sores, rash, anorexia, itching, right upper quadrant pain, yellow skin or eyes, blood in urine, decreased urine output, shortness of breath, or coughing up blood.
• Tell patient to ask prescriber about eating iodine-rich foods, including iodized salt, bread, dairy products, and shellfish, because the iodine in these foods may make drug less effective.
• Warn patient that drug may cause drowsiness; advise patient to use caution when operating machinery or a vehicle.
• Teach patient to watch for evidence of hypothyroidism (unexplained weight gain, fatigue, cold intolerance) and to notify prescriber if it arises.
• Caution patient to report pregnancy or plans to become pregnant during therapy.

SAFETY ALERT!

methotrexate (amethopterin)
meth-oh-TREKS-ate

Otrexup, Rasuvo, RediTrex, Xatmep

methotrexate sodium
Trexall, Methofill ✦, Metoject ✦

Therapeutic class: Antineoplastics
Pharmacologic class: Folate antagonists

AVAILABLE FORMS
Injection (autoinjector, prefilled syringe):
7.5 mg, 10 mg, 12.5 mg, 15 mg, 17.5 mg, 20 mg, 22.5 mg, 25 mg, 30 mg
Injection: 10 mg/1 mL ✦, 25 mg/mL preservative-free vials; 25 mg/mL vials*
Lyophilized powder: 1,000-mg preservative-free vials
Oral solution: 2.5 mg/mL
Tablets: 2.5 mg, 5 mg, 7.5 mg, 10 mg, 15 mg

INDICATIONS & DOSAGES
Adjust-a-dose (for all indications): Reduce dosage in patients with impaired kidney function.
➤ **Trophoblastic tumors (choriocarcinoma, hydatidiform mole)**
Adults: 15 to 30 mg PO or IM daily for 5 days. Repeat after 1 or more weeks, based on response or toxicity. Number of courses is three to maximum of five.
➤ **Low risk gestational trophoblastic neoplasia (GTN)**
Adults: 30 to 200 mg/m² or 0.4 to 1 mg/kg IV or IM.
➤ **High risk GTN**
Adults: 300 mg/m² IV infusion over 12 hours as part of multidrug regimen.
➤ **Acute lymphocytic leukemia**
Adults and children: For induction, 3.3 mg/m² daily PO (tablets), IV, or IM with 60 mg/m² prednisone daily for 4 to 6 weeks or until remission occurs; then 30 mg/m² PO or IM weekly in two divided doses or 2.5 mg/kg IV every 14 days. Or, 10 to 5,000 mg/m² IV as part of multidrug regimen. Or, 20 to

30 mg/m^2/week IM as part of multidose regimen. Or, 20 mg/m^2 Trexall PO once weekly. Or, for oral solution use in children, 20 mg/m^2 once weekly.
Adjust-a-dose: Individualize dose and schedule of IV or IM injection based on disease state, patient risk category, other drugs used, phase of treatment, and treatment response.
➤ **Meningeal leukemia**
Adults and children ages 9 and older: 12 to 15 mg intrathecally every 2 days or more, up to twice weekly.
Children ages 3 to younger than 9: 12 mg intrathecally every 2 days or more, up to twice weekly.
Children ages 2 to younger than 3: 10 mg intrathecally every 2 days or more, up to twice weekly.
Children ages 1 to younger than 2: 8 mg intrathecally every 2 days or more, up to twice weekly.
Children younger than age 1: 6 mg intrathecally every 2 days or more, up to twice weekly.
Adjust-a-dose: Administration interval of less than 1 week may increase toxicity. Continue treatment until CSF cell count falls within normal range.
➤ **Lymphoma (Burkitt tumor stage I, II)**
Adults: 10 to 25 mg PO daily for 4 to 8 days, with 7- to 10-day rest intervals; commonly given with other agents.
➤ **Lymphosarcoma (stage III)**
Adults: 0.625 to 2.5 mg/kg daily PO, IM, or IV; commonly given with other agents.
➤ **Non-Hodgkin lymphoma**
Adults: Varies from 10 to 8,000 mg/m^2 IV based on treatment regimen. Single-agent use may be 8,000 mg/m^2 IV for CNS direct therapy infused over 4 hours, or 5 to 75 mg IV for cutaneous forms of lymphoma.

Combination therapy dosage is 1,000 to 3,000 mg/m^2 IV followed by leucovorin rescue. Or, 2.5 mg Trexall PO two to four times a week (maximum 10 mg/week) as part of metronomic combination chemotherapy.
➤ **Osteosarcoma**
Adults: Typically, 12 g/m^2 IV (maximum dose, 20 g) as 4-hour infusion as part of combination chemotherapy regimen. Give with leucovorin rescue regimen.
➤ **Mycosis fungoides (cutaneous T-cell lymphoma)**
Adults: 5 to 50 mg PO or IM once weekly; if poor response, may increase to 15 to

37.5 mg IM twice weekly. Or, 25 to 75 mg Trexall PO once weekly as monotherapy or 10 mg/m^2 PO twice weekly as part of combination chemotherapy.
Adjust-a-dose: Guide dosage reductions or cessation by patient response and hematologic monitoring.
➤ **Breast cancer**
Adults: 40 mg/m^2 IV as component of cyclophosphamide and 5-FU-based regimen.
➤ **Squamous cell carcinoma of head and neck**
Adults: 40 to 60 mg/m^2 IV once weekly.
➤ **Bladder cancer** ◆
Adults: 30 mg/m^2 IV every 2 weeks or days 1 and 8 every 3 weeks for 3 cycles as part of combination therapy.
➤ **GVHD prevention** ◆
Adults: 15 mg/m^2 IV on day 1 after allogeneic transplant; then 10 mg/m^2 IV days 3 and 6 or days 3, 6, and 11 as part of combination therapy.
➤ **Psoriasis**
Adults: 10 to 25 mg PO, IM, IV, or subcut as single weekly dose; or 2.5 to 5 mg PO every 12 hours for three doses weekly. Maximum dosage, 30 mg/week.
➤ **RA**
Adults: Initially, 7.5 mg PO, IM, or subcut weekly, either in single dose or divided as 2.5 mg PO every 12 hours for three doses once weekly. Dosage may be gradually increased to maximum of 20 mg weekly.
➤ **Polyarticular course, juvenile RA**
Children and adolescents ages 2 to 16: 10 mg/m^2 PO, IM, or subcut once weekly. Or, 20 to 30 mg/m^2/week IM or subcut.
➤ **Moderate to severe Crohn disease** ◆
Adults: Initially, 12.5 to 15 mg IM or subcut once weekly. May gradually increase to maximum of 25 mg IM or subcut once weekly; may reduce to 15 mg once weekly if steroid-free remission is maintained for 4 months.
➤ **SLE (moderate to severe)** ◆
Adults: 5 to 15 mg once weekly; may increase by 2.5-mg increments every 4 weeks to maximum of 25 mg once weekly, in combination with folic acid.

ADMINISTRATION
🛈 *Alert:* Hazardous drug; use safe handling and disposal precautions.
PO
● Give drug on an empty stomach.

- Use an accurate measuring device to measure oral solution.
- May store oral solution at room temperature for up to 60 days or refrigerate. Don't freeze.

IV

▼ Dilution of drug depends on product, and infusion guidelines vary depending on dose.

▼ For IV slow push, give at 10 mg/minute.

Boxed Warning Don't use formulations with benzyl alcohol for high-dose regimens unless immediate treatment is required and preservative-free formulation isn't available. ■

▼ For methotrexate therapy with leucovorin rescue, patients should be well hydrated. Administer 1 L/m^2 of IV fluids over 6 hours before initiation of methotrexate infusion. Continue hydration at 125 mL/m^2/hour during the methotrexate infusion and for 2 days after infusion has been completed.

▼ May use IV formulations containing benzyl alcohol IV, IM, or subcut. Use preservative-free formulation for intrathecal use and for treatment of neonates or low-birth-weight infants.

▼ **Incompatibilities:** None listed by manufacturer. Consult drug compatibility reference for more information.

IM

- Rotate administration sites.

Subcutaneous

- Administer subcutaneously in abdomen or thigh only.
- Methofill, Metoject, Otrexup, RediTrex, and Rasuvo are single-dose syringes for once-weekly subcut use only and are available in specific dosage strengths. Use another formulation for dosing by other routes, doses less than 7.5 mg/week, doses more than 25 or 30 mg/week, high-dose regimens, or dosage adjustments between the available doses.

Intrathecal

- Preparing and giving parenteral drug may be mutagenic, teratogenic, or carcinogenic. Follow facility protocol to reduce risks.

Boxed Warning Use preservative-free form for intrathecal administration. ■

- Reconstitute to 1 mg/mL concentration with preservative-free NSS.

ACTION

Reversibly binds to dihydrofolate reductase, blocking reduction of folic acid to tetrahydrofolate, a cofactor necessary for purine, protein, and DNA synthesis.

Route	Onset	Peak	Duration
PO	Unknown	45 min–6 hr	Unknown
IV	Immediate	Immediate	Unknown
IM	Unknown	30 min–1 hr	Unknown
Subcut	Unknown	1–2 hr	Unknown
Intrathecal	Unknown	Unknown	Unknown

Half-life: For doses below 30 mg/m^2, about 3 to 10 hours (adults), 0.7 to 5.8 hours (children); for doses of 30 mg/m^2 and above, 8 to 15 hours.

ADVERSE REACTIONS

CNS: malaise, fatigue, dizziness, headache, aphasia, hemiparesis, fever. **CV:** *thromboembolic events,* chest pain, hypotension, pericardial effusion, pericarditis. **EENT:** blurred vision, pharyngitis. **GI:** gingivitis, stomatitis, diarrhea, GI ulceration, *GI bleeding,* enteritis, nausea, vomiting. **GU:** nephropathy, tubular necrosis, *kidney failure,* menstrual dysfunction, abortion, cystitis. **Hematologic:** *leukopenia, pancytopenia, anemia, neutropenia, thrombocytopenia.* **Hepatic:** *acute toxicity, chronic toxicity, liver fibrosis,* increased liver enzyme levels. **Metabolic:** weight loss, hyperuricemia. **Musculoskeletal:** arthralgia, myalgia, osteoporosis in children on long-term therapy. **Respiratory:** *interstitial pneumonitis,* cough. **Skin:** urticaria, pruritus, dermatitis, hyperpigmentation, erythematous rashes, ecchymoses, rash, photosensitivity reactions, alopecia, acne, psoriatic lesions aggravated by exposure to sun. **Other:** chills, reduced resistance to infection, lymphadenopathy, *sepsis.*

INTERACTIONS

Drug-drug. *Acitretin (vitamin A derivative):* May increase risk of hepatitis. Avoid use together.

Folic acid derivatives: Antagonizes methotrexate effect. Avoid use together, except for leucovorin rescue with high-dose methotrexate therapy.

Fosphenytoin, phenytoin: May decrease phenytoin and fosphenytoin levels. Closely monitor drug levels.

Liver-toxic drugs (azathioprine, retinoids, sulfasalazine): May increase risk of liver toxicity. Monitor patient closely.

Nitrous oxide: Potentiates effect of methotrexate, increasing risk of methotrexate adverse reactions. Avoid use together.

Boxed Warning *NSAIDs, salicylates:* May increase methotrexate toxicity. Avoid use together. ■

Reactions in bold italics are *life-threatening*.

Oral antibiotics (tetracycline): May decrease absorption of methotrexate. Monitor therapy.
Penicillins, sulfonamides, trimethoprim: May increase methotrexate level. Monitor patient for methotrexate toxicity.
Probenecid: May impair excretion of methotrexate, causing increased level, effect, and toxicity. Monitor methotrexate level closely and adjust dosage accordingly.
PPIs (omeprazole): May cause methotrexate toxicity, especially with high doses of methotrexate. Use cautiously.
Theophylline: May increase theophylline level. Closely monitor theophylline level.
Thiopurines (mercaptopurine): May increase thiopurine level. Monitor patient closely.
Vaccines: May make immunizations ineffective; may cause risk of disseminated infection with live-virus vaccines. Postpone immunization, if possible.
Drug-food. *Any food:* May delay absorption and reduce peak level of methotrexate. Instruct patient to take drug on an empty stomach.
Drug-lifestyle. *Alcohol use:* May increase liver toxicity. Discourage use together.
Sun exposure: May cause photosensitivity reactions. Advise patient to avoid excessive sunlight exposure.

EFFECTS ON LAB TEST RESULTS
• May increase uric acid level and LFT values.
• May decrease Hb level and WBC, RBC, and platelet counts.
• May alter results of lab assay for folate, interfering with detection of folic acid deficiency.

CONTRAINDICATIONS & CAUTIONS
Boxed Warning Contraindicated in patients hypersensitive to drug. ∎
• Contraindicated in patients with psoriasis or RA who also have alcohol use disorder, alcoholic liver, chronic liver disease, blood dyscrasias, or immunodeficiency syndromes.
Boxed Warning Use drug only in patients with life-threatening neoplastic diseases and in those with severe psoriasis or RA not adequately responsive to other therapy; deaths have occurred. Closely monitor patients for bone marrow, liver, lung, and kidney toxicities. ∎
Boxed Warning Methotrexate given with radiotherapy may increase the risk of soft-tissue necrosis and osteonecrosis. ∎

Boxed Warning Unexpectedly severe (sometimes fatal) bone marrow suppression, aplastic anemia, and GI toxicity have been reported with concomitant administration of methotrexate (usually in high dosage) with some NSAIDs. ∎
Boxed Warning Use cautiously and at modified dosages in patients with impaired liver or kidney function, ascites, pleural effusions, bone marrow suppression, aplasia, leukopenia, thrombocytopenia, or anemia. ∎
• Use cautiously in very young patients, older adults, patients who are debilitated, and patients with infection, peptic ulceration, or ulcerative colitis.
Dialyzable drug: Yes (using a high-flux dialyzer).
⚠ *Overdose S&S:* Leukopenia, thrombocytopenia, anemia, pancytopenia, bone marrow suppression, mucositis, stomatitis, oral ulceration, nausea, vomiting, GI ulceration, GI bleeding, sepsis or septic shock, KF, aplastic anemia, headache, seizures, acute toxic encephalopathy, cerebellar herniation associated with increased ICP, death.

PREGNANCY-LACTATION-REPRODUCTION
Boxed Warning Contraindicated during pregnancy for nonneoplastic disease. Don't use in patients of childbearing potential with neoplasms unless benefit outweighs risk. ∎
• Contraindicated during breastfeeding.
Boxed Warning If either partner is receiving methotrexate, they should avoid conception during and for a minimum of 3 months after therapy for males and during and for 6 months after therapy for females. ∎
• Drug has been reported to cause impaired fertility, oligospermia, and menstrual dysfunction during therapy and for a short period after therapy ends.

NURSING CONSIDERATIONS
Boxed Warning Methotrexate should be used only by health care providers whose knowledge and experience include the use of antimetabolite therapy. ∎
• Verify pregnancy status prior to therapy.
Boxed Warning Use preservative-free formulation of methotrexate and diluents for intrathecal use or high-dose therapy and for neonates and low-birth-weight infants. ∎
Boxed Warning Drug can cause severe and fatal toxicities. Modify dosage or discontinue drug for bone marrow suppression,

M

infection, or kidney, GI, pulmonary, or dermatologic toxicity or hypersensitivity. ■

Boxed Warning Methotrexate-induced lung disease, including acute or chronic interstitial pneumonitis, is a potentially dangerous lesion that may occur at any time during therapy and isn't always fully reversible. Pulmonary symptoms (especially dry, nonproductive cough) may require interruption of treatment and careful investigation. ■

Boxed Warning Diarrhea and ulcerative stomatitis require interruption of therapy; hemorrhagic enteritis and death from intestinal perforation may occur. ■

Boxed Warning Malignant lymphomas may occur in patients receiving low-dose methotrexate and may regress upon discontinuing drug. ■

Boxed Warning Methotrexate may induce TLS in patients with rapidly growing tumors. ■

Boxed Warning Severe, occasionally fatal skin reactions have been reported following single or multiple doses of methotrexate. Reactions have occurred within days of methotrexate administration. Recovery has been reported with discontinuation of therapy. ■

Boxed Warning Potentially fatal opportunistic infections, especially *Pneumocystis jiroveci* pneumonia, may occur with methotrexate therapy. ■

Boxed Warning High-dose regimens for osteosarcoma require meticulous care. ■

🕭 *Alert:* Drug may be given daily or once weekly, depending on the disease. To avoid administration errors, know patient's dosing schedule.

● Periodically monitor pulmonary function tests.

● Monitor fluid intake and output daily. Encourage fluid intake of 2 to 3 L daily.

● Delayed drug elimination may occur with impaired kidney function, third space effusion (ascites), or other disorders, increasing systemic level and risk of toxicity.

🕭 *Alert:* Alkalinize urine by giving sodium bicarbonate tablets or fluids to prevent precipitation of drug, especially at high doses. Maintain urine pH above 7.

Boxed Warning Periodic monitoring of CBC with differential, platelet count, and liver and kidney function is essential. Watch for increases in AST, ALT, and ALP levels, which may signal liver dysfunction. Periodic

liver biopsies are recommended for patients with psoriasis who are receiving long-term treatment. Monitor patients at risk for impaired drug elimination (kidney dysfunction, pleural effusions, ascites) more frequently. ■

● WBC and platelet count nadirs usually occur on day 7.

● Watch for signs and symptoms of bleeding (especially GI) and infection.

● To prevent bleeding, avoid all IM injections when platelet count is below $50,000/mm^3$.

● Give blood transfusions for cumulative anemia. Patient may receive injections of RBC colony-stimulating factors to promote RBC production and decrease need for blood transfusions.

● Leucovorin rescue is needed with doses of more than 100 mg and starts 24 hours after therapy starts. Continue leucovorin until methotrexate level falls below 5×10^{-8} M. Consult specialized references for specific recommendations for leucovorin dosage. Monitor methotrexate level and adjust leucovorin dose.

● Monitor patient for neurotoxicity with intrathecal administration. Acute chemical arachnoiditis causes headache, back pain, nuchal rigidity, and fever. Paraparesis or paraplegia is present with subacute myelopathy.

● Transient acute stroke-like syndrome can occur with high-dose infusions (confusion, hemiparesis, transient blindness, seizure, coma).

PATIENT TEACHING

● Advise patient to watch for signs and symptoms of infection (fever, sore throat, fatigue) and bleeding (easy bruising, nosebleeds, bleeding gums, melena). Tell patient to take temperature daily.

Boxed Warning Fully inform patient of risks involved with methotrexate therapy. ■

● Tell patient of childbearing potential of fetal risk. Instruct patient to inform prescriber of known or suspected pregnancy.

● Counsel patient of childbearing potential to use effective contraception during treatment and for 6 months after final dose.

● Advise male patient of reproductive potential to use effective contraception during treatment and for 3 months after final dose.

● Caution patient to stop breastfeeding during therapy.

● Teach and encourage diligent mouth care to reduce risk of superinfection in mouth.

• Caution to always use accurate measuring device when administering oral solution.
• Instruct patient how to take leucovorin. Stress importance of taking as directed.
• Tell patient to use highly protective sunblock and wear protective clothing when exposed to sunlight.

SAFETY ALERT!

methyldopa
meth-il-DOE-pa

Therapeutic class: Antihypertensives
Pharmacologic class: Centrally acting antiadrenergics

AVAILABLE FORMS
Tablets: 250 mg, 500 mg

INDICATIONS & DOSAGES
➤ **HTN**
Adults: Initially, 250 mg PO b.i.d. to t.i.d. in first 48 hours. Limit initial daily dose to 500 mg/day when given with antihypertensives other than thiazide diuretics. Adjust dosage at no less than 48-hour intervals. Maintenance dosage, 500 mg to 2 g daily in two to four divided doses. Maximum recommended PO daily dosage, 3 g.
Children: Initially, 10 mg/kg/day PO daily in two to four divided doses. Maximum daily dosage, 65 mg/kg or 3 g, whichever is less.
Adjust-a-dose: Adjust dosage if other antihypertensives are added to or deleted from therapy.

ADMINISTRATION
PO
• Increase dosage in the evening to minimize sedation.
• Store pharmacy-made suspension in refrigerator or in the dark at room temperature for up to 14 days; shake well before each use.
• Store tablets at room temperature; protect from light.

ACTION
May inhibit the central vasomotor centers, decreasing sympathetic outflow to the heart, kidneys, and peripheral vasculature.

Route	Onset	Peak	Duration
PO	Unknown	2 to 4 hr	12–48 hr

Half-life: About 105 minutes.

ADVERSE REACTIONS
CNS: decreased mental acuity, sedation, headache, weakness, asthenia, dizziness, paresthesia, parkinsonism, Bell's palsy, involuntary choreoathetoid movements, psychic disturbances, depression, nightmares. **CV:** orthostatic hypotension, edema, *bradycardia, HF, myocarditis,* aggravated angina, carotid sinus hypersensitivity. **EENT:** nasal congestion, salivary gland inflammation, sore or "black" tongue, dry mouth. **GI:** *pancreatitis,* nausea, vomiting, diarrhea, constipation, flatus, abdominal distention, colitis. **GU:** amenorrhea, impotence, decreased libido. **Hematologic:** *thrombocytopenia, leukopenia, bone marrow depression,* hemolytic anemia. **Hepatic:** *hepatitis,* jaundice. **Metabolic:** hyperprolactinemia, weight gain. **Musculoskeletal:** arthralgia, myalgia. **Skin:** *TEN,* rash. **Other:** drug-induced fever, breast enlargement, gynecomastia, lactation.

INTERACTIONS
Drug-drug. *Amphetamines, pseudoephedrine, SNRIs, TCAs:* May decrease antihypertensive effects. Monitor patient closely.
Anesthetics: May need lower doses of anesthetics. Use together cautiously.
Antihypertensives: May increase risk of hypotension. Use cautiously.
Barbiturates: May increase risk of hypotension. Monitor patient closely.
Ferrous sulfate or gluconate: May decrease bioavailability of methyldopa. Separate doses.
Levodopa: May increase hypotensive effects, which may increase adverse CNS reactions. Monitor patient closely.
Lithium: May increase lithium level. Watch for increased lithium level and signs and symptoms of toxicity.
MAO inhibitors: May increase adverse effects of methyldopa. Use together is contraindicated.

EFFECTS ON LAB TEST RESULTS
• May increase BUN level and LFT values.
• May decrease Hb level, hematocrit, and platelet and WBC counts.
• May interfere with results of urinary uric acid testing, serum creatinine test, and AST test.
• May cause positive Coombs test result.
• May falsely increase urine catecholamine level, interfering with diagnosis of pheochromocytoma.

M

CONTRAINDICATIONS & CAUTIONS
• Contraindicated in patients hypersensitive to drug and in those with active liver disease (such as acute hepatitis or active cirrhosis).
• Contraindicated in those whose previous methyldopa therapy caused liver problems and in those taking MAO inhibitors.
• Use cautiously in older adults and patients with history of impaired liver function or sulfite sensitivity.
Dialyzable drug: Yes.
⚠ *Overdose S&S:* Sedation, weakness, acute hypotension, bradycardia, dizziness, constipation, abdominal distention, flatus, diarrhea, nausea, vomiting, light-headedness.

PREGNANCY-LACTATION-REPRODUCTION
• Studies during first trimester are inadequate. Use during pregnancy only if clearly needed. Available data show use during pregnancy doesn't cause fetal harm and may improve fetal outcomes compared to untreated HTN.
• Drug appears in human milk. Use cautiously during breastfeeding.

NURSING CONSIDERATIONS
• Monitor BP regularly. Older adults are more likely to experience hypotension, syncope, and sedation.
• Occasionally, tolerance may occur, usually between the second and third months of therapy. Adding a diuretic or adjusting dosage may be needed. If patient's response changes significantly, notify prescriber.
• After dialysis, monitor patient for HTN and notify prescriber, if needed. Patient may need an extra dose of drug.
• Monitor CBC with differential counts before therapy and periodically thereafter.
• Periodically monitor LFT values during first 12 weeks or if jaundice (with or without fever) occurs.
• Patient who needs blood transfusions should have direct and indirect Coombs tests to prevent cross-matching problems.
• Monitor Coombs test results before therapy and at 6 and 12 months after start of therapy. In patient who has received drug for several months, positive reaction to direct Coombs test may indicate hemolytic anemia.
• Monitor patient for involuntary twitching or writhing (choreoathetoid) movements; discontinue drug if any occur.

PATIENT TEACHING
• If unpleasant adverse reactions occur, advise patient not to suddenly stop taking drug but to notify prescriber.
• Instruct patient to report signs and symptoms of infection, yellowing of skin, flulike symptoms, and muscle aches.
• Sodium and water retention may occur but can be relieved with diuretics.
• Warn patient that, particularly at the start of therapy, drug may impair ability to perform tasks that require mental alertness.
• Inform patient to rise slowly and avoid sudden position changes to minimize low BP and dizziness upon rising and to chew gum or suck on hard candy or ice chips to relieve dry mouth.
• Tell patient that urine may turn dark if left sitting in toilet bowl or if toilet bowl has been treated with bleach.
• Instruct patient to report pregnancy or plans to become pregnant or breastfeed.

methylnaltrexone bromide
meth-il-nal-TREKS-one

Relistor

Therapeutic class: GI drugs
Pharmacologic class: Opioid antagonists

AVAILABLE FORMS
Injection: 8 mg/0.4 mL, 12 mg/0.6 mL prefilled syringe; 12 mg/0.6 mL in single-use vial
Tablets: 150 mg

INDICATIONS & DOSAGES
Adjust-a-dose (for all indications): Discontinue maintenance laxative therapy before starting drug. May resume laxative after patient has taken methylnaltrexone for 3 days if opioid-induced constipation (OIC) symptoms persist. Reevaluate need for drug when opioid regimen changes. For patients with Child-Pugh class C liver impairment weighing more than 114 kg, give 0.075 mg/kg subcut; 62 to 114 kg, give 6 mg subcut; 38 to less than 62 kg, give 4 mg subcut; less than 38 kg, give 0.075 mg/kg subcut.
➤ **OIC in patients receiving palliative care for advanced illness when response to laxatives is insufficient**
Adults weighing more than 114 kg: 0.15 mg/kg subcut every other day as needed.

Adults weighing 62 to 114 kg: 12 mg subcut every other day as needed.
Adults weighing 38 to less than 62 kg: 8 mg subcut every other day as needed.
Adults weighing less than 38 kg: 0.15 mg/kg subcut every other day as needed.
Adjust-a-dose: In patients with CrCl less than 60 mL/minute weighing more than 114 kg, give 0.075 mg/kg; 62 to 114 kg, give 6 mg; 38 to less than 62 kg, give 4 mg; less than 38 kg, give 0.075 mg/kg subcut every other day.
➤ **OIC in patients with chronic noncancer pain**
Adults: 450 mg PO or 12 mg subcut once daily.
Adjust-a-dose: In patients with CrCl less than 60 mL/minute, give 150 mg PO once daily or 6 mg subcut once daily. In patients with Child-Pugh class B or C liver impairment, give 150 mg PO once daily.

ADMINISTRATION
PO
• Give tablets with water on empty stomach at least 30 minutes before first meal of day.
Subcutaneous
• Inspect solution; don't give if particulate matter or discoloration is present.
• Give no more than one dose within 24 hours.
• Store at room temperature, away from light.
• After being drawn into syringe as directed, drug is stable at room temperature for 24 hours. Vials are for single use only.
• Give injection subcutaneously into abdomen, thigh, or upper arm; rotate injection sites. Don't inject into bruised, tender, red, or hard areas.

ACTION
Antagonizes GI mu-opioid receptors, preventing opioid-induced slowing of GI motility and transit time.

Route	Onset	Peak	Duration
PO	Unknown	1.5 hr	Unknown
Subcut	Unknown	30 min	Unknown

Half-life: PO, 15 hours.

ADVERSE REACTIONS
CNS: dizziness, tremors, headache, anxiety. **EENT:** rhinorrhea. **GI:** abdominal pain, abdominal distention, flatulence, nausea, diarrhea, vomiting. **Musculoskeletal:** muscle spasms. **Skin:** excessive sweating. **Other:** chills, hot flushes.

INTERACTIONS
Drug-drug. *Opioid antagonists (naloxone, naltrexone):* May increase risk of opioid withdrawal. Avoid combination.

EFFECTS ON LAB TEST RESULTS
None reported.

CONTRAINDICATIONS & CAUTIONS
⚠ *Alert:* Contraindicated in patients hypersensitive to drug, in those with known or suspected GI obstruction, and in those at increased risk for recurrent obstruction because of increased risk of GI perforation.
⚠ *Alert:* Use cautiously in patients with peptic ulcer disease, Ogilvie syndrome, diverticular disease, infiltrative GI tract malignancies, peritoneal metastases, or Crohn disease because of increased risk of GI perforation.
• Patients with disruptions to blood-brain barrier may be at increased risk for opioid withdrawal or reduced analgesia. Consider overall risk-benefit profile.
• Drug hasn't been studied in patients on KRT.
• Safety and effectiveness in children haven't been established.
Dialyzable drug: Unknown.
⚠ *Overdose S&S:* Orthostatic hypotension, signs and symptoms of opioid withdrawal.

PREGNANCY-LACTATION-REPRODUCTION
• Studies during pregnancy are inadequate.
• Don't use during pregnancy unless benefit outweighs fetal risk. Use during pregnancy may cause opioid withdrawal in fetus.
• It isn't known if drug appears in human milk. Patient should discontinue breastfeeding or discontinue drug, considering importance of drug to patient.

NURSING CONSIDERATIONS
⚠ *Alert:* Watch for symptoms of perforation (severe, persistent, or worsening abdominal pain). If symptoms occur, stop drug and evaluate patient.
• Monitor patient for opioid withdrawal and analgesia effectiveness during coadministration.
• Discontinue drug if treatment with the opioid pain medication is also discontinued.

PATIENT TEACHING
• Caution patient to discontinue all maintenance laxative therapy before starting methylnaltrexone.

• Explain that drug may be effective within a few minutes to a few hours after administration. Advise patient to remain near toilet facilities after receiving drug.

• Instruct patient to discontinue drug and notify prescriber if severe, persistent, or worsening abdominal pain, diarrhea, or rash occurs.

• Teach safe PO or subcut drug administration and syringe disposal.

• Inform patient that vial is for single-use.

• Advise patient to report loss of analgesia or signs and symptoms of opioid withdrawal (hyperhidrosis, chills, diarrhea, abdominal pain, anxiety, yawning).

• Warn patient to report all adverse reactions; to immediately report severe, worsening, or persistent abdominal pain; and to discontinue drug for severe or persistent diarrhea.

methylphenidate hydrochloride
meth-il-FEN-i-date

Aptensio XR, Biphentin✦, Concerta, Cotempla XR-ODT, Jornay PM, Methylin, QuilliChew ER, Quillivant XR, Relexxii, Ritalin, Ritalin LA

methylphenidate transdermal system
Daytrana

Therapeutic class: CNS stimulants
Pharmacologic class: Piperidine derivatives
Controlled substance schedule: II

AVAILABLE FORMS
Oral solution: 5 mg/5 mL, 10 mg/5 mL
Tablets (chewable): 2.5 mg, 5 mg, 10 mg
Tablets: 5 mg, 10 mg, 20 mg
Extended-release
Capsules ⬤: 10 mg, 15 mg, 20 mg, 25 mg, 30 mg, 35 mg, 40 mg, 50 mg, 60 mg, 80 mg, 100 mg
Oral suspension: 25 mg/5 mL
Tablets ⬤: 10 mg, 18 mg, 20 mg, 27 mg, 36 mg, 54 mg, 72 mg
Tablets (chewable) ⬤: 20 mg, 30 mg, 40 mg
Tablets (ODTs) ⬤: 8.6 mg, 17.3 mg, 25.9 mg
Transdermal system
Patch: 10 mg/9 hours, 15 mg/9 hours, 20 mg/ 9 hours, 30 mg/9 hours

INDICATIONS & DOSAGES
➤ **ADHD (immediate release)**
Adults (immediate-release): 20 to 30 mg PO b.i.d. or t.i.d. Dosage varies; maximum dosage, 60 mg daily.
Children ages 6 and older (immediate-release): Initially, 5 mg PO b.i.d. before breakfast and lunch, increasing by 5 to 10 mg at weekly intervals, as needed, until an optimum daily dose of 2 mg/kg is reached, not to exceed 60 mg/day.
➤ **ADHD (extended release)**
Adults ages 18 to 65 not currently taking methylphenidate or patients taking other stimulants (Concerta, Relexxii): Initially, 18 or 36 mg PO daily. May increase dosage in 18-mg increments at weekly intervals to maximum of 72 mg daily.
Adolescents ages 13 to 17 not currently taking methylphenidate or patients taking other stimulants (Concerta, Relexxii): 18 mg PO once daily in morning. Adjust dosage by 18 mg at weekly intervals to a maximum of 72 mg PO once daily in morning.
Adults and adolescents ages 13 to 17 currently taking methylphenidate (Concerta, Relexxii): If previous methylphenidate dosage was 5 mg b.i.d. or t.i.d., 18 mg PO every morning. If previous dosage was 10 mg b.i.d. or t.i.d., 36 mg PO every morning. If previous dosage was 15 mg b.i.d. or t.i.d., 54 mg every morning. If previous dosage was 20 mg b.i.d. or t.i.d., 72 mg PO every morning.
Children ages 6 to 12 not currently taking methylphenidate or patients taking other stimulants (Concerta, Relexxii): 18 mg PO once daily every morning. Adjust dosage by 18 mg at weekly intervals to a maximum of 54 mg daily every morning.
Children ages 6 to 12 currently taking methylphenidate (Concerta, Relexxii): If previous methylphenidate dosage was 5 mg b.i.d. or t.i.d., 18 mg PO every morning. If previous dosage was 10 mg b.i.d. or t.i.d., 36 mg PO every morning. If previous dosage was 15 mg b.i.d. or t.i.d., 54 mg PO every morning. Maximum conversion daily dose, 54 mg.
Adults ages 18 to 65 and children ages 6 and older (Biphentin): Initially, 10 to 20 mg PO daily in morning. Increase dosage weekly in increments of 10 mg to maximum of 60 mg daily for children and 80 mg daily for adults.
Adults and children ages 6 and older (Aptensio XR): Initially, 10 mg PO daily in morning.

Increase dosage weekly in increments of 10 mg to maximum of 60 mg daily.

Adults and children ages 6 and older (Jornay PM): Initially, 20 mg extended-release capsule PO once daily in evening. May adjust timing of administration between 6:30 p.m. and 9:30 p.m. May titrate weekly in dosages of 20 mg. Maximum dose, 100 mg daily.

Adults and children ages 6 and older (extended-release capsules): Initially, 25 mg PO once daily in morning. May titrate dosages of 10 to 15 mg in intervals of at least 5 days. Maximum dose, 85 mg daily in adults and 70 mg in children.

Children ages 6 and older (Ritalin LA): Initially, 10 to 20 mg PO once daily. Increase by 10 mg at weekly intervals to a maximum of 60 mg daily. To replace immediate-release Ritalin dosage, give total daily dose PO once daily. For example, if previous dosage was 10 mg b.i.d., give 20 mg Ritalin LA PO once daily. To replace other methylphenidate products, discontinue that treatment and titrate with Ritalin LA using the titration schedule.

Adults and children ages 6 and older (Quillivant XR, QuilliChew ER): Initially, 20 mg PO once daily in morning. Titrate dose up or down weekly in increments of 10 mg to 20 mg. Maximum, 60 mg daily.

Children ages 6 and older (Cotempla XR-ODT): Initially, 17.3 mg PO daily in morning. May increase dosage weekly in increments of 8.6 to 17.3 mg per day. Maximum, 51.8 mg daily.

➤ **ADHD (transdermal patch)**
Adults and children ages 6 and older: Initially, one 10-mg transdermal patch daily. Apply 2 hours before desired effect and remove 9 hours later. Increase dosage weekly by 5 mg as needed to maximum of 30 mg daily. Base final dose and wear time on patient response.

➤ **Narcolepsy**
Adults: 10 mg immediate-release PO b.i.d. or t.i.d. 30 to 45 minutes before meals. Dosage varies. Maximum, 60 mg/day.

Children ages 6 and older: Initially, 5 mg immediate-release PO b.i.d. (before breakfast and lunch). Increase dosage, if needed, by 5 to 10 mg weekly. Maximum dose is 60 mg daily.

Adjust-a-dose: May substitute intermediate-acting extended-release form in place of immediate-release when the total 8-hour immediate-release dosage corresponds to an extended-release strength.

ADMINISTRATION
PO
- Give chewable tablets with at least 240 mL of water or other liquid.
- Give immediate-release tablets, chewable tablets, and oral solution in divided doses b.i.d. or t.i.d., preferably 30 to 45 minutes before meals. Give last daily dose before 6 p.m. to prevent insomnia (except for Jornay PM).
- Give Jornay PM between 6:30 p.m. and 9:30 p.m. Give consistently with or without food.
- Aptensio XR, Biphentin, Jornay PM, or Ritalin LA capsules may be swallowed whole or contents of capsule may be sprinkled onto small amount of cool applesauce and taken immediately. Give with or without food.
- Extended-release tablets must be swallowed whole and never crushed, chewed, or divided.
- Concerta and Relexxii tablets may be taken with or without food and must be swallowed whole. Have patient swallow tablets whole; don't crush or break tablets.
- Vigorously shake oral suspension bottle for 10 seconds before administering dose. Use oral dosing dispenser to measure dose. May give with or without food. Suspension remains stable for up to 4 months after reconstitution.
- For ODT, remove tablet with dry hands from blister pack and immediately place on patient's tongue. Allow it to disintegrate and be swallowed without chewing or crushing; no liquid is needed. Give consistently with or without food.

Transdermal
- Apply to clean, dry, nonirritated skin on the hip. Avoid placing patch on waistline or where tight clothing may rub it off. If possible, alternate sides of the body daily.
- Don't cut patches.
- Press patch firmly in place with palm of hand for about 30 seconds to ensure good contact. Don't apply with dressing or tape.
- If patch doesn't fully adhere or partially or fully detaches, replace with a new patch at a different site; ensure total wear time doesn't exceed 9 hours.
- Upon removal, fold patch in half, sticking adhesive sides together; then flush patch down toilet or place in appropriate lidded container.

M

ACTION
Releases nerve terminal stores of norepinephrine, promoting nerve impulse transmission. At high doses, effects are mediated by dopamine.

Route	Onset	Peak	Duration
PO (Methylin, Ritalin)	Unknown	2 hr	Unknown
PO (Aptensio XR)	Unknown	2 hr; 8 hr	Unknown
PO (Biphentin)	Unknown	1–3 hr	Unknown
PO (Ritalin LA)	Unknown	1–3 hr; 4–7 hr	Unknown
PO (Jornay PM)	Unknown	14 hr	Unknown
PO (Concerta, Relexxii)	Unknown	6–10 hr	Unknown
PO (QuilliChew XR, Quillivant XR)	Unknown	5 hr	Unknown
PO (Cotempla XR-ODT)	Unknown	4.5–5 hr	Unknown
Transdermal	2 hr	8–10 hr	Unknown

Half-life: Conventional, 3 to 6 hours; Concerta, Ritalin LA, 3.5 hours; Aptensio XR, 5 hours; Biphentin, 2.1 to 2.4 hours; Jornay PM, 5.9 hours; Quillivant XR, 6 hours; QuilliChew XR, 5 hours; Relexxii, 3.6 hours; Cotempla XR-ODT, 3.5 to 5.5 hours; transdermal, 4 to 5 hours.

ADVERSE REACTIONS
CNS: nervousness, headache, *seizures,* tics, dizziness, akathisia, dyskinesia, drowsiness, fatigue, insomnia, mood swings, anxiety, irritability, restlessness, depression, tremors, vertigo, confusion, sedation, fever, agitation, psychosis (sometimes with visual and tactile hallucinations), mania, migraine, cerebral arteritis. **CV:** palpitations, tachycardia, increased BP, *arrhythmias,* angina, *MI, bradycardia,* Raynaud phenomenon, peripheral coldness. **EENT:** blurred vision, diplopia, vision changes, pupil dilation, eye pain, nasopharyngitis, sinusitis, bruxism, dry mouth, oropharyngeal pain, sore throat. **GI:** nausea, abdominal pain, anorexia, vomiting, constipation, dyspepsia, diarrhea. **GU:** decreased libido, dysmenorrhea, hematuria, priapism. **Hematologic:** *leukopenia, thrombocytopenia,* anemia, *pancytopenia.* **Hepatic:** abnormal LFTs. **Metabolic:** weight loss. **Musculoskeletal:** back pain, arthralgia, cramps, rhabdomyolysis, myalgia, muscle twitching. **Respiratory:** cough, URI. **Skin:** rash, pruritis, urticaria, dermatitis, hair loss, excoriation, application-site irritation (redness, swelling, papules), excessive sweating, bruising.

Other: motion sickness, hypersensitivity reactions, pediatric growth suppression, gynecomastia.

INTERACTIONS
Drug-drug. *Antacids, H₂ antagonists, PPIs:* May interfere with normal release of extended-release forms. Monitor therapy.
Anticonvulsants (phenobarbital, phenytoin, primidone), SSRIs, TCAs (clomipramine, desipramine, imipramine), warfarin: May increase levels of these drugs and risk of adverse effects. Monitor patient, and decrease dose of these drugs as needed. Monitor drug levels (or coagulation times if patient is also taking warfarin).
Antihypertensives: May decrease antihypertensive effect. Monitor BP.
Centrally acting alpha₂ agonists, clonidine: May cause serious adverse events. Avoid use together.
Halogenated anesthetics (desflurane, enflurane, halothane, isoflurane): May suddenly increase BP and HR during surgery. Avoid use of methamphetamine on day of surgery.
MAO inhibitors (linezolid, selegiline): May cause severe HTN or hypertensive crisis. Use together is contraindicated. Avoid using within 14 days of MAO inhibitor therapy.
Risperidone: May increase risk of extrapyramidal symptoms. Monitor patient closely.
Drug-food. *Caffeine:* May increase amphetamine and related amine effects. Discourage use together.
Drug-lifestyle. *Alcohol use:* May increase methylphenidate level, causing toxicity. Discourage use together.

EFFECTS ON LAB TEST RESULTS
• May increase transaminase levels.
• May decrease Hb level and hematocrit and platelet and WBC counts.
• May cause false-positive urine detection of amphetamines/methamphetamines.

CONTRAINDICATIONS & CAUTIONS
• Contraindicated in patients hypersensitive to drug. Some formulations are contraindicated in patients with glaucoma, motor tics, family history or diagnosis of Tourette syndrome, or history of marked anxiety, tension, or agitation. Refer to individual manufacturer's instructions.

Reactions in bold italics are *life-threatening.*

• Avoid use in patients with structural cardiac abnormalities, cardiomyopathy, CAD, and serious arrhythmias.

🔸 *Alert:* Drug may increase risk of prolonged, painful erection (priapism) in males of any age, with or without sexual stimulation. Incidence is rare, but if not treated immediately, priapism may lead to permanent damage to penis.

• Because they don't dissolve, Concerta and Relexxii aren't recommended in patients with history of peritonitis or severe GI narrowing (such as cystic fibrosis, small-bowel inflammatory disease, short-gut syndrome caused by adhesions or decreased transit time, chronic intestinal pseudoobstruction, or Meckel diverticulum).

• Use cautiously in patients with history of emotional disorder, preexisting psychosis or bipolar disorder, seizures, EEG abnormalities, or HTN and in patients whose underlying medical conditions might be compromised by increases in BP or HR, such as those with preexisting HTN, HF, recent MI, or hyperthyroidism.

Boxed Warning Stimulants carry a high risk of abuse and misuse, which can lead to substance use disorder, including addiction, which can lead to overdose and death. The risk increases with high doses or unapproved administration methods (snorting, injection). ■

• Drug may cause tolerance, requiring higher dose to produce same effect a lower dose once provided.

• Chewable tablets contain phenylalanine.

• Transdermal patch may cause irreversible chemical leukoderma (loss of skin color) at patch application site and other areas. Although not harmful, if hypopigmentation occurs, consider alternative treatments.

Dialyzable drug: Unknown.

⚠ *Overdose S&S:* Psychomotor agitation, tachyarrhythmias, confusion, seizures, delirium, dryness of mucous membranes, euphoria, flushing, hallucinations, headache, hyperreflexia, HTN or hypotension, coma, vasospasm, MI, stroke, aortic dissection, cardiomyopathy, muscle twitching, tremors, mydriasis, palpitations, diaphoresis, life-threatening hyperthermia, vomiting, serotonin syndrome, rhabdomyolysis, death.

PREGNANCY-LACTATION-REPRODUCTION
• Studies during pregnancy are inadequate. Use during pregnancy only if potential benefit justifies fetal risk.

• Stimulants cause vasoconstriction and decrease placental perfusion. Premature delivery and low birth weight in infants have been reported.

• Prescribers are encouraged to register patients in the National Pregnancy Registry for ADHD Medications (1-866-961-2388 or https://womensmentalhealth.org/research/pregnancyregistry/adhd-medications/).

• Drug appears in human milk. Use cautiously during breastfeeding and monitor infant closely for agitation, anorexia, and reduced weight gain.

NURSING CONSIDERATIONS
• Don't use drug to prevent fatigue or treat severe depression.

• Before starting drug, assess for presence of cardiac disease by performing a careful history, family history of sudden death or ventricular arrhythmia, and physical exam.

Boxed Warning Assess patient's risk of abuse, misuse, and addiction before therapy. Reassess risk during therapy. Monitor for signs and symptoms of drug abuse, misuse, and addiction (increased HR, respiratory rate, or BP; sweating; dilated pupils; hyperactivity; restlessness; insomnia; decreased appetite; loss of coordination; tremors; flushing; vomiting; abdominal pain). Anxiety, psychosis, hostility, aggression, suicidality, and homicidal ideation may also occur. ■

• Periodically reevaluate need for use.

• Drug may trigger tics and Tourette syndrome in children. Evaluate patient prior to therapy and monitor during therapy.

• Observe patient for signs of excessive stimulation. Monitor BP.

• Check CBC, differential, and platelet count with long-term use, particularly if patient shows signs or symptoms of hematologic toxicity (fever, sore throat, easy bruising).

• Monitor height and weight in child on long-term therapy. Drug may delay growth spurt, but child will attain normal height when drug is stopped.

• Carefully observe patient for digital changes; stimulants used to treat ADHD are associated with peripheral vasculopathy, including Raynaud phenomenon.

M

• If ADHD doesn't improve after 1-month at appropriate dose, prescriber may discontinue drug.

• Monitor patient using patch for chemical leukoderma. Report skin changes to prescriber.

• Monitor for vision changes.

• Abrupt drug stoppage or dose reduction may cause withdrawal symptoms (dysphoria, depression, fatigue, vivid and unpleasant dreams, insomnia or hypersomnia, increased appetite, psychomotor impairment or agitation) in patient with physical dependence.

• *Look alike–sound alike:* Don't confuse methylphenidate with methadone. Don't confuse Ritalin with ritodrine or Rifadin.

PATIENT TEACHING

• Advise patient and caregiver to read the medication guide.

Boxed Warning Teach patient and caregiver about risk of abuse, misuse, and addiction, which can lead to overdose and death. Advise patient to store drug in a safe (preferably locked) place. Teach about proper disposal of unused drug. Instruct patient not to give drug to anyone else. ▪

• Teach about proper administration, storage, and handling of prescribed formulation.

• Advise patient to avoid alcohol and caffeine during therapy.

• Caution patient with phenylketonuria that chewable tablets contain phenylalanine.

• *Alert:* Inform male patient of any age and caregivers of the rare but possible risk of priapism. Caution patient to seek medical attention if priapism (erection lasting longer than 4 hours) occurs.

• Instruct patient and caregiver to watch for signs of chemical leukoderma, especially under skin patch site, and to report any skin changes to prescriber. Warn not to stop treatment without first consulting prescriber.

• Caution patient to avoid activities that require alertness or good psychomotor coordination until CNS effects of drug are known.

• Warn patient with seizure disorder that drug may decrease seizure threshold. Tell patient to notify prescriber if seizure occurs.

• If applied patch is missing, have caregiver ask child when or how patch came off. Teach child not to share or remove patch.

• Encourage caregiver to use the application chart provided with patch carton to keep track of application and removal.

• Teach caregiver to apply patch 2 hours before the desired effect.

• Tell caregiver to remove patch sooner than 9 hours if the child has decreased evening appetite or difficulty sleeping.

• Explain that the effects of patch last for several hours after its removal.

• Warn patient and caregiver to avoid exposing patch to direct external heat sources, such as heating pads, electric blankets, and heated water beds.

• Tell caregiver to notify prescriber if the child develops bumps, swelling, or blistering at patch application site or experiences blurred vision or other serious side effects.

methylPREDNISolone
meth-il-pred-NIS-oh-lone

Medrol

methylPREDNISolone acetate
Depo-Medrol

methylPREDNISolone sodium succinate
Solu-Medrol

Therapeutic class: Corticosteroids
Pharmacologic class: Glucocorticoids

AVAILABLE FORMS
methylprednisolone
Tablets: 2 mg, 4 mg, 8 mg, 16 mg, 32 mg
methylprednisolone acetate
Injection (suspension): 20 mg/mL, 40 mg/mL, 80 mg/mL
methylprednisolone sodium succinate
Injection*: 40 mg, 125 mg, 500 mg, 1,000 mg, 2,000 mg vials

INDICATIONS & DOSAGES
➤ **Severe inflammation or immunosuppression**
Adults and children: 4 to 48 mg PO daily, depending on the disease treated. After favorable response, determine maintenance dosage by decreasing until lowest dosage that will maintain adequate clinical response is achieved. Or, 4 to 120 mg acetate IM daily, or 10 to 40 mg succinate IM or IV, with subsequent doses dictated by patient's clinical response and condition. Or, 4 to 10 mg

acetate into small joints, 10 to 40 mg acetate into medium joints, or 20 to 80 mg acetate into larger joints. Intralesional use is usually 20 to 60 mg acetate. Repeat intralesional and intra-articular injections every 1 to 5 weeks.

Children: 0.11 to 1.6 mg/kg/day PO, IM, or IV in three to four divided doses (sodium succinate).

Adjust-a-dose: Higher doses may be necessary in certain overwhelming, acute, or life-threatening situations. Alternate-day therapy (twice usual daily dose given every other day) may be appropriate for patients on long-term oral therapy.

ADMINISTRATION
PO
• Give drug with milk or food when possible. Patients who are critically ill may need to take drug with an antacid or H_2-receptor antagonist.
• Give once daily dose in morning.
IV
▼ Use only methylprednisolone sodium succinate, never acetate form.

▼ Reconstitute according to manufacturer's directions using supplied diluent, or use bacteriostatic water for injection with benzyl alcohol.

◔ *Alert:* Don't use formulations containing benzyl alcohol in neonates, which can cause potentially fatal toxicity.

▼ Compatible solutions include D_5W, NSS, and dextrose 5% in NSS.

▼ For direct injection of doses of up to 250 mg, inject diluted drug into vein or free-flowing compatible IV solution over at least 5 minutes.

▼ For intermittent IV infusion, dilute solution according to manufacturer's instructions and give over prescribed duration.

▼ For doses greater than 250 mg, give IV over at least 30 to 60 minutes to prevent arrhythmias and circulatory collapse.

▼ Discard reconstituted solution after 48 hours.

▼ **Incompatibilities:** Don't dilute or mix with other solutions. Consult drug compatibility reference for more information.
IM
• Give injection deeply into gluteal muscle. Avoid injection into deltoid muscle. Avoid subcut injection because atrophy and sterile abscesses may occur.

• Dermal atrophy may occur with large doses of acetate form. Use several small injections

rather than a single large dose, and rotate injection sites.
Intra-articular
• Don't dilute or mix methylprednisolone acetate with other solutions.
• Exclude septic joint process before injection.
• Avoid injection or leakage into dermis.

ACTION
Not clearly defined. Decreases inflammation, mainly by stabilizing leukocyte lysosomal membranes; suppresses immune response; stimulates bone marrow; and influences protein, fat, and carbohydrate metabolism.

Route	Onset	Peak	Duration
PO	Rapid	2–3 hr	30–36 hr
IV	1 hr	Immediate	12 hr
IM	6–48 hr	4–8 days	4–8 days
Intra-articular	1 wk	Unknown	1–5 wk

Half-life: ¼ hour (IV succinate); 1.3 to 3.7 hours (PO).

ADVERSE REACTIONS
CNS: euphoria, insomnia, psychotic behavior, *pseudotumor cerebri,* vertigo, headache, depression, personality changes, paresthesia, *seizures,* malaise, emotional lability, insomnia, neuritis, neuropathy, syncope. **CV:** HTN, *arrhythmias, HF, cardiomyopathy, bradycardia,* tachycardia, *myocardial rupture after MI,* edema, thrombophlebitis, *thromboembolism, fat embolism, cardiac arrest, CV collapse,* vasculitis. **EENT:** cataracts, glaucoma, increased IOP, exophthalmos, rhinitis. **GI:** peptic ulceration, GI irritation, increased appetite, *pancreatitis,* nausea, vomiting, abdominal distention, intestinal perforation, esophagitis. **GU:** menstrual irregularities, glycosuria. **Hematologic:** leukocytosis. **Hepatic:** enlarged liver, elevated liver enzymes. **Metabolic:** *hypokalemia,* hyperglycemia, diabetes, sodium and water retention, carbohydrate intolerance, hypercholesterolemia, negative nitrogen balance, *hypocalcemia.* **Musculoskeletal:** growth suppression in children, muscle weakness, osteoporosis, myopathy, vertebral compression fractures, pathologic long bone fractures, tendon rupture, aseptic necrosis; calcium deposit in soft tissue, postinjection flare (intra-articular). **Respiratory:** *pulmonary edema.* **Skin:** hirsutism, delayed wound healing, petechiae, ecchymoses, facial erythema, diaphoresis, fragile skin, acne, allergic

M

dermatitis, skin eruptions, cutaneous and subcutaneous atrophy, injection site burning or tingling, thinning scalp hair, hyperpigmentation, hypopigmentation, striae, urticaria.
Other: cushingoid state, susceptibility to infections, *acute adrenal insufficiency after increased stress or abrupt withdrawal after long-term therapy,* hypersensitivity reactions.

INTERACTIONS
Drug-drug. *Aminoglutethimide:* May decrease methylprednisolone's therapeutic effects. Monitor therapy.
Anticholinesterases: May produce severe weakness in patients with myasthenia gravis. If possible, withdraw anticholinesterase agents at least 24 hours before methylprednisolone therapy.
Antidiabetics: May increase glucose level. Antidiabetic dosage adjustment may be needed.
Aspirin, indomethacin, other NSAIDs: May increase risk of GI distress and bleeding. Use together cautiously.
Barbiturates, carbamazepine, phenytoin, rifampin: May decrease corticosteroid effect. Increase corticosteroid dosage.
Cholestyramine: May decrease methylprednisolone level. Monitor therapy.
Cyclosporine: May increase toxicity. Monitor patient closely.
Estrogens (oral contraceptives): May decrease methylprednisolone clearance. Monitor therapy.
Isoniazid: May decrease isoniazid level. Monitor therapy.
Ketoconazole and macrolide antibiotics: May decrease methylprednisolone clearance. Decreased dosage may be required.
Mifepristone: May diminish methylprednisolone's therapeutic effects. Avoid use together.
Oral anticoagulants: May alter dosage requirements. Closely monitor PT and INR.
Potassium-depleting drugs (amphotericin B, thiazide diuretics): May enhance potassium-wasting effects of methylprednisolone. Monitor potassium level.
Salicylates: May decrease salicylate level. Monitor for lack of salicylate effectiveness.
Skin-test antigens: May decrease response. Postpone skin testing until after therapy.
Toxoids, vaccines: May decrease antibody response and may increase risk of complications. Avoid use together.

Drug-herb. *Echinacea:* May decrease therapeutic effects of immunosuppressants. Discourage use together.

EFFECTS ON LAB TEST RESULTS
- May increase glucose, cholesterol, ALT, AST, ALP, sodium, and urine calcium levels.
- May decrease potassium and calcium levels.
- May suppress reactions to skin tests.

CONTRAINDICATIONS & CAUTIONS
- Contraindicated in patients hypersensitive to drug or its components; some injection formulations contain lactose.
- Contraindicated in patients with systemic fungal infections (except for intra-articular use), in premature infants (acetate and succinate forms containing benzyl alcohol), and in those receiving immunosuppressive doses together with live-virus vaccines.
- IM injections are contraindicated in patients with idiopathic thrombocytopenia purpura.
- Intrathecal use is contraindicated.
- Use cautiously in older adults and patients with GI ulceration or kidney disease, HTN, osteoporosis, diabetes, hypothyroidism, cirrhosis, diverticulitis, nonspecific ulcerative colitis, recent intestinal anastomoses, thromboembolic disorders, seizures, active hepatitis, myasthenia gravis, HF, TB, ocular herpes simplex, cataracts, glaucoma, emotional instability, and psychotic tendencies.
- Prolonged use may increase risk of infection, mask signs of infection, and activate latent infections.
Dialyzable drug: Unknown.

PREGNANCY-LACTATION-REPRODUCTION
- Studies during pregnancy are inadequate. Drug crosses placental barrier. Use during pregnancy only if potential benefit justifies fetal risk. Use lowest effective dose for shortest duration.
- Monitor infants born to mothers who received corticosteroids during pregnancy for hypoadrenalism.
- Drug appears in human milk. Patient should discontinue breastfeeding or discontinue drug, considering importance of drug to patient.

NURSING CONSIDERATIONS
⚠ *Alert:* Epidural corticosteroid injections to treat neck and back pain and radiating pain in arms and legs may result in rare but serious adverse events (loss of vision, stroke,

paralysis, death). Use of epidural corticosteroid injections isn't FDA approved.

❸ Alert: Drug may cause suppression of HPA axis, which can lead to adrenal crisis. Younger children and patients receiving high doses are at increased risk. Withdrawal from corticosteroids should be done slowly and with careful patient monitoring.

• Medrol may contain tartrazine. Watch for allergic reaction to tartrazine in patients with sensitivity to aspirin.

• Most adverse reactions to corticosteroids are dose- or duration-dependent.

❸ Alert: Different salts aren't interchangeable.

• If immediate onset of action is needed, don't use acetate form.

• Always adjust to lowest effective dose.

• Monitor weight, BP, electrolyte level, and sleep patterns. Euphoria may initially interfere with sleep, but patients typically adjust to therapy in 1 to 3 weeks.

• Monitor patient for cushingoid effects (moon facies, supraclavicular fat pad, central obesity, thinning hair, HTN, increased susceptibility to infection).

• Periodically measure growth and development in children during high-dose or prolonged treatment.

• Watch for depression and psychotic episodes, especially with high-dose therapy.

• Patient with diabetes may need increased dosage of antidiabetic agent; monitor glucose level.

• Watch for enhanced response to drug in patient with hypothyroidism or cirrhosis or decreased response in patient with hyperthyroidism.

• Unless contraindicated, give low-sodium diet that's high in potassium and protein. Give potassium supplements as needed.

• Older adults may be more susceptible to osteoporosis with prolonged use.

• Taper off dosage after long-term therapy.

• **Look alike–sound alike:** Don't confuse Solu-Medrol with Solu-Cortef. Don't confuse methylprednisolone with medroxyprogesterone or methyltestosterone.

PATIENT TEACHING
❸ Alert: Counsel patient to discuss benefits and risks and other possible treatments with health care provider before undergoing epidural corticosteroid injection.

• Tell patient not to stop drug abruptly or without prescriber's consent.

• Instruct patient to take oral form of drug with milk or food.

• Teach patient signs and symptoms of early adrenal insufficiency (fatigue, joint pain, muscle weakness, fever, anorexia, nausea, shortness of breath, dizziness, fainting).

• Instruct patient to carry or wear medical identification indicating the need for supplemental systemic glucocorticoids during stress as well as prescriber's name, name of drug, and dosage taken.

• Warn patient on long-term therapy about cushingoid effects and the need to report sudden weight gain or swelling.

• Advise patient receiving long-term therapy to consider exercise or physical therapy.

• Tell patient to ask prescriber about vitamin D or calcium supplementation.

• Instruct patient to avoid exposure to infections (chickenpox, measles) and to contact prescriber if such exposure occurs.

• Instruct patient to report pregnancy or plans to become pregnant or breastfeed.

---

methylTESTOSTERone
meth-il-tes-TOS-te-rone

Methitest

Therapeutic class: Androgens
Pharmacologic class: Androgens
Controlled substance schedule: III

AVAILABLE FORMS
Capsules: 10 mg
Tablets: 10 mg

INDICATIONS & DOSAGES
➤ **Metastatic breast cancer**
Adult females 1 to 5 years after menopause:
50 to 200 mg PO daily.
➤ **Hypogonadism; delayed puberty in carefully selected males**
Adult males and adolescent males: 10 to 50 mg PO daily. Dosages for delayed puberty are usually at the lower end of the range and limited to 4 to 6 months.

ADMINISTRATION
PO
❸ Alert: Hazardous drug; use safe handling and disposal precautions.

• Give drug without regard to food.

• Store at room temperature; protect from light, heat, and moisture.

ACTION
Stimulates target tissues to develop normally in androgen-deficient men. May have some antiestrogen properties, making it useful in treating certain estrogen-dependent breast cancers.

Route	Onset	Peak	Duration
PO	Unknown	Unknown	Unknown

Half-life: Varies from 10 to 100 minutes.

ADVERSE REACTIONS
CNS: headache, anxiety, depression, paresthesia, *stroke.* **CV:** edema, *HF, venous thromboembolism, MI.* **GI:** irritation of oral mucosa with buccal administration, nausea. **GU:** oligospermia, decreased ejaculatory volume, priapism, amenorrhea, menstrual irregularities, altered libido. **Hematologic:** *suppression of clotting factors,* polycythemia. **Hepatic:** abnormal LFT values, reversible jaundice, *cholestatic hepatitis.* **Metabolic:** hypernatremia, *hyperkalemia,* hyperphosphatemia, hypercholesterolemia, hypercalcemia. **Skin:** hirsutism, acne, male-pattern baldness. **Other:** hypersensitivity reactions, hypoestrogenic and androgenic effects in women (virilization), gynecomastia and excessive hormonal effects in men.

INTERACTIONS
Drug-drug. *Cyclosporine (systemic):* May increase cyclosporine level and associated liver toxicity. Consider therapy modification. *Insulin, oral antidiabetics:* May decrease glucose level, altering dosage requirements. Monitor glucose level in patient with diabetes. *Liver-toxic drugs:* May increase risk of liver toxicity. Monitor liver function closely. *Oxyphenbutazone:* May increase oxyphenbutazone serum level. Monitor patient. *Vitamin K antagonist (warfarin):* May increase sensitivity to oral anticoagulants, altering dosage requirements. Monitor PT and INR.
Drug-herb. *Saw palmetto:* May cause hormone-like effects. Don't use together.

EFFECTS ON LAB TEST RESULTS
• May increase sodium, potassium, chloride, phosphate, liver enzyme, lipid, and calcium levels.

• May decrease thyroxine-binding globulin and total T_4 levels.
• May increase RBC count and resin uptake of T_3 and T_4.

CONTRAINDICATIONS & CAUTIONS
• Contraindicated in men with breast or prostate cancer.
• Drug isn't indicated to enhance athletic performance.
• Use cautiously in older adults; patients with cardiac, kidney, or liver disease or diabetes; and healthy males with delayed puberty.
Dialyzable drug: Unknown.
⚠ *Overdose S&S:* Nausea, edema.

PREGNANCY-LACTATION-REPRODUCTION
• Contraindicated in patients who are or may become pregnant. Use during pregnancy may cause virilization of female fetus. If pregnancy occurs during therapy, apprise patient of potential fetal hazard.
• It isn't known if drug appears in human milk. Patient should discontinue breastfeeding or discontinue drug, considering importance of drug to patient.

NURSING CONSIDERATIONS
• In child, obtain X-rays of wrist bones before therapy begins to establish bone maturation level. During treatment, bones may mature more rapidly than they grow in length. Review X-rays every 6 months to monitor bone maturation.
• Drug is typically used only for intermittent therapy. Because of potential liver toxicity, watch closely for jaundice.
• Promptly report evidence of virilization in females.
• Watch for hypoestrogenic effects in females (flushing, diaphoresis, vaginal bleeding, nervousness, emotional lability, menstrual irregularities, and vaginitis, including itching, dryness, and burning).
• Watch for excessive hormonal effects in males. If patient is prepubertal, watch for premature epiphyseal closure, acne, priapism, growth of body and facial hair, and phallic enlargement. If patient is postpubertal, watch for testicular atrophy, oligospermia, decreased ejaculatory volume, impotence, gynecomastia, and epididymitis.
• Unless contraindicated, use with high-calorie, high-protein diet. Give small, frequent meals.

Reactions in bold italics are *life-threatening.*

• Periodically check cholesterol, calcium, and Hb levels; hematocrit; and cardiac and LFT results.

• Regularly check weight. Control edema with sodium restriction or diuretics.

• In patient with breast cancer, therapeutic response usually occurs within 3 months. If disease appears to progress, stop drug.

• Report signs of hypercalcemia. In metastatic breast cancer, hypercalcemia may indicate progression of bone metastases.

🕔 *Alert:* Drug has potential for abuse. Monitor patient for nontherapeutic uses.

• *Look alike–sound alike:* Testosterone and methyltestosterone aren't interchangeable. Don't confuse methyltestosterone with medroxyprogesterone.

PATIENT TEACHING

• Instruct patient to report pregnancy or plans to become pregnant or breastfeed.

• Review potential adverse reactions and instruct patient to report them promptly.

• Tell female patient to immediately report evidence of virilization (acne, swelling, weight gain, increased hair growth, clitoral enlargement, hoarseness, decreased breast size, deepening of voice, changes in libido, male pattern baldness, oily skin or hair).

• Teach patient signs and symptoms of hypoglycemia and method for checking glucose level; drug enhances hypoglycemia. Instruct patient to immediately report signs or symptoms of hypoglycemia.

• Advise adolescent and caregivers about potential adverse effect on bone maturation before start of therapy.

---

metoclopramide hydrochloride 🕱

met-oh-KLOE-pra-mide

Gimoti, Reglan

Therapeutic class: GI stimulants
Pharmacologic class: Dopamine antagonists

AVAILABLE FORMS

Injection: 5 mg/mL
Nasal spray: 15 mg/actuation
Oral solution: 5 mg/5 mL
Tablets: 5 mg, 10 mg
Tablets (ODTs): 5 mg, 10 mg

INDICATIONS & DOSAGES

🕱 *Adjust-a-dose (for all indications):* Refer to manufacturer's product information for dosage adjustments, if indicated, for older adults, for patients with liver or kidney impairment, in poor metabolizers of CYP2D6, and with concomitant use with strong CYP2D6 inhibitors.

➤ **To prevent or reduce nausea and vomiting from emetogenic cancer chemotherapy**
Adults: 1 to 2 mg/kg IV 30 minutes before chemotherapy; repeat every 2 hours for two doses, then every 3 hours for three doses.

➤ **To prevent or reduce postoperative nausea and vomiting**
Adults: 10 to 20 mg IM near end of surgical procedure.

➤ **To facilitate small-bowel intubation to aid in radiologic exam**
Adults and children older than age 14: 10 mg IV as single dose over 1 to 2 minutes.
Children ages 6 to 14: 2.5 to 5 mg IV as single dose slowly over 1 to 2 minutes.
Children younger than age 6: 0.1 mg/kg IV as single dose slowly over 1 to 2 minutes.

➤ **Delayed gastric emptying secondary to diabetic gastroparesis**
Adults: 10 mg PO q.i.d. for mild symptoms for 2 to 8 weeks, depending on response. Maximum daily dosage, 40 mg. Or, 1 nasal spray (15 mg) in one nostril q.i.d. for 2 to 8 weeks, depending on response. Or, 10 mg IM or by slow IV push over 1 to 2 minutes 30 minutes before each meal and at bedtime for up to 10 days for severe symptoms; then may start PO dose and continue for 2 to 8 weeks.
Adults ages 65 and older: 5 mg PO q.i.d. for 2 to 8 weeks, depending on response. Or, may switch patients on stable 10-mg dose on another form to nasal spray (15 mg) in one nostril q.i.d. for 2 to 8 weeks, depending on response.

➤ **GERD**
Adults: 10 to 15 mg PO q.i.d. continuously for up to 12 weeks. Or, up to 20 mg PO PRN before provoking situation.

ADMINISTRATION
PO

• Give drug 30 minutes before each meal and at bedtime.

• Give ODT immediately after opening sealed blister. If tablet breaks or crumbles, throw it away and obtain a new one.

M

- Place ODT on patient's tongue. Tell patient to let it melt for approximately 1 minute and then swallow.
- Don't repeat dose if inadvertently given with food.

IV

▼ Drug is compatible with D_5W, NSS for injection, dextrose 5% in half-NSS, Ringer injection, and lactated Ringer injection. NSS is preferred diluent; drug is most stable in this solution.

▼ Give doses of 10 mg or less by direct injection over 1 to 2 minutes. Dilute doses larger than 10 mg in 50 mL of compatible diluent, and infuse over at least 15 minutes. Monitor BP closely.

▼ Refer to prescribing information for additional conditional compatibilities.

▼ There is no need to protect drug from light if infusion mixture is given within 24 hours. If protected from light and refrigerated, it's stable for 48 hours.

▼ **Incompatibilities:** Cephalothin, chloramphenicol, sodium bicarbonate.

IM

- Inspect for particulate matter and discoloration. If either is present, don't use.
- Inject into a large muscle.

Intranasal

- Prime pump with 10 sprays into air before first use.
- Give 30 minutes before each meal and at bedtime.
- Have patient lean head slightly forward and aim nozzle toward back of nose; use index finger to close other nostril. Spray while patient inhales slowly. If uncertain that spray entered the nose, don't repeat dose; give next dose as scheduled.
- Omit a missed dose, and give next dose as scheduled.
- Nasal spray isn't recommended for initial therapy.
- Discard bottle 4 weeks after opening, even if bottle contains unused drug.

ACTION

Stimulates motility of upper GI tract, increases lower esophageal sphincter tone, and blocks dopamine receptors at the chemoreceptor trigger zone.

Route	Onset	Peak	Duration
PO	30–60 min	1–2 hr	1–2 hr
IV	1–3 min	Unknown	1–2 hr
IM	10–15 min	Unknown	1–2 hr
Intranasal	Unknown	0.5–3.5 hr	1–2 hr

Half-life: 4 to 6 hours; ODT, 7 hours; nasal spray, 8.1 hours.

ADVERSE REACTIONS

CNS: anxiety, depression, drowsiness, dystonic reactions, fatigue, lassitude, restlessness, *seizures, suicidality,* akathisia, confusion, dizziness, extrapyramidal symptoms, fever, hallucinations, headache, insomnia, tardive dyskinesia, NMS, taste alteration (nasal spray). **CV:** *bradycardia, supraventricular tachycardia, AV block,* hypotension, fluid retention, transient HTN, flushing, *HF.* **EENT:** visual disturbance. **GI:** bowel disorders, diarrhea, nausea. **GU:** amenorrhea, incontinence, urinary frequency, erectile dysfunction. **Hematologic:** *neutropenia, leukopenia, agranulocytosis, methemoglobinemia,* sulfhemoglobinemia, porphyria. **Hepatic:** liver toxicity. **Skin:** rash, urticaria. **Other:** loss of libido, prolactin secretion, gynecomastia, hypersensitivity reaction, including *bronchospasm.*

INTERACTIONS

Drug-drug. *Acetaminophen, tetracycline, levodopa, cyclosporine:* May increase absorption of these drugs in the small bowel. Monitor therapy.

Anticholinergics, antidiarrheals, opioid analgesics: May antagonize GI motility effects of metoclopramide. Use together cautiously.

Antiparkinsonian drugs (dopamine agonists): May decrease therapeutic effects of antiparkinsonian drugs. Monitor therapy.

Antipsychotics: May increase toxic effects of antipsychotics. Avoid use together.

CNS depressants: May cause additive CNS effects. Avoid use together.

Cyclosporine: May increase cyclosporine absorption. Monitor therapy.

CYP2D6 inhibitors (bupropion, fluoxetine, paroxetine, quinidine): May increase metoclopramide level. Adjust metoclopramide dosage as indicated. Recommended dosage adjustment: 5 mg q.i.d. before each meal and at bedtime or 10 mg t.i.d.

Digoxin: May diminish digoxin absorption. Monitor therapy.

Insulin: May increase GI motility and food delivery to intestines, increasing blood glucose level. Monitor blood glucose level.

MAO inhibitors: May increase release of catecholamines in patients with HTN. Use together cautiously.

Mivacurium, succinylcholine: Inhibits plasma cholinesterase level, leading to enhanced neuromuscular blockade. Monitor patient closely.

Phenothiazines: May increase risk of extrapyramidal effects. Monitor patient closely.

Drug-lifestyle. *Alcohol use:* May cause additive CNS effects. Discourage use together.

EFFECTS ON LAB TEST RESULTS
• May increase LFT values and aldosterone, methemogloblin, and prolactin levels.
• May decrease neutrophil and granulocyte counts.

CONTRAINDICATIONS & CAUTIONS
• Contraindicated in patients hypersensitive to drug, those with history of tardive dyskinesia or dystonic reaction to metoclopramide, and those with pheochromocytoma, other catecholamine-releasing paragangliomas, or seizure disorders.
• Contraindicated in patients for whom stimulation of GI motility might be dangerous (those with hemorrhage, obstruction, or perforation).

Boxed Warning Drug can cause irreversible tardive dyskinesia, even after drug is stopped. Risk increases with duration of therapy and total cumulative dose; there is no treatment. Discontinue drug if signs and symptoms occur. Except in rare cases, avoid treatment for longer than 12 weeks. ∎
• In addition to tardive dyskinesia, drug may cause other extrapyramidal signs and symptoms, parkinsonian symptoms, and motor restlessness.
• Metoclopramide isn't recommended for use in children due to risk of tardive dyskinesia and other extrapyramidal signs and symptoms.
• Nasal spray isn't recommended in patients with Child-Pugh class B or C liver impairment or CrCl less than 60 mL/minute and patients concurrently using strong CYP2D6 inhibitors.
• Galactorrhea, amenorrhea, gynecomastia, and impotence have been reported with prolactin-elevating drugs, including metoclopramide.

🛈 *Alert:* NMS has occurred rarely and may be fatal. If signs and symptoms develop (fever, CNS symptoms, irregular pulse, cardiac arrhythmias, or abnormal BP), discontinue drug.
• Avoid use in patients with history of depression, Parkinson disease, or HTN.
• Use cautiously in patients with cirrhosis or HF due to increased risk of fluid retention and volume overload.

Dialyzable drug: No.

⚠ *Overdose S&S:* Drowsiness, disorientation, extrapyramidal reactions; seizures, lethargy (in infants and children).

PREGNANCY-LACTATION-REPRODUCTION
• Drug crosses placental barrier and may cause extrapyramidal signs and methemoglobinemia in neonates. Use during pregnancy only if clearly needed. Monitor neonates closely.
• Drug appears in human milk. Use cautiously during breastfeeding. Monitor neonate for extrapyramidal signs and symptoms and methemoglobinemia.

NURSING CONSIDERATIONS
• Monitor bowel sounds.
• Drug may cause tardive dyskinesia, parkinsonian symptoms, and motor restlessness. Monitor patient for involuntary movements of face, tongue, and extremities, which may indicate tardive dyskinesia or other extrapyramidal adverse effects.
• Monitor patient for fever, CNS symptoms, irregular pulse, cardiac arrhythmias, or abnormal BP, which may indicate NMS.
• Monitor patient for dizziness, headache, or nervousness after stopping metoclopramide; these findings may indicate withdrawal.
• Diphenhydramine or benztropine may be used to counteract extrapyramidal adverse effects from high doses.

PATIENT TEACHING
• Teach about proper drug administration and handling for prescribed formulation.
• Tell patient to avoid activities that require alertness for 2 hours after doses.
• Urge patient to promptly report persistent or serious adverse reactions.
• Review signs and symptoms of tardive dyskinesia, other extrapyramidal signs and symptoms, and NMS. Advise patient to discontinue drug and seek immediate medical attention if such signs and symptoms occur.

M

- Advise patient not to drink alcohol during therapy.
- Instruct patient to report pregnancy or breastfeeding.

met0Lazone
me-TOLE-a-zone

Therapeutic class: Diuretics
Pharmacologic class: Thiazide-like diuretics

AVAILABLE FORMS
Tablets: 2.5 mg, 5 mg, 10 mg

INDICATIONS & DOSAGES
➤ **Edema in HF or kidney disease**
Adults: 5 to 20 mg PO once daily. Use lowest effective dose for maintenance therapy.
➤ **HTN**
Adults: 2.5 to 5 mg PO once daily. Base maintenance dosage on BP.

ADMINISTRATION
PO
- Give drug in the morning without regard to meals.

ACTION
Metolazone acts primarily to inhibit sodium reabsorption in the kidney tubule.

Route	Onset	Peak	Duration
PO	1 hr	8 hr	≥24 hr

Half-life: 6 to 20 hours.

ADVERSE REACTIONS
CNS: dizziness, headache, fatigue, vertigo, syncope, paresthesia, weakness, restlessness, drowsiness, anxiety, depression, neuropathy, nervousness. **CV:** orthostatic hypotension, palpitations, chest pain, *venous thrombosis.* **EENT:** blurred vision, dry mouth. **GI:** *pancreatitis,* anorexia, nausea, epigastric pain, vomiting, abdominal pain, diarrhea, constipation. **GU:** nocturia, polyuria, impotence. **Hematologic:** *aplastic anemia, agranulocytosis, leukopenia.* **Hepatic:** jaundice, *hepatitis.* **Metabolic:** hyperglycemia, *hypokalemia, hypomagnesemia,* hyponatremia, hypochloremia, metabolic alkalosis, hypercalcemia, volume depletion and dehydration, gout. **Musculoskeletal:** joint pain, muscle cramps. **Skin:** dermatitis, photosensitivity reactions, rash, pruritus, urticaria, skin necrosis, purpura, *SJS, TEN,* cutaneous vasculitis. **Other:** chills.

INTERACTIONS
Drug-drug. *Amphotericin B, corticosteroids:* May increase risk of hypokalemia. Closely monitor potassium level.
Anticoagulants: May decrease anticoagulant response. Monitor PT and INR.
Antidiabetics: May alter glucose level and require dosage adjustment of antidiabetics. Monitor glucose level.
Antihypertensives: May increase hypotensive effect. Monitor therapy.
Barbiturates, opioids: May increase orthostatic hypotensive effect. Monitor patient closely.
Calcium salts: May decrease calcium excretion. Monitor therapy.
Carbamazepine: May increase risk of hyponatremia. Monitor therapy.
Cholestyramine, colestipol: May decrease intestinal absorption of thiazides. Separate doses.
Diazoxide: May increase antihypertensive, hyperglycemic, and hyperuricemic effects. Use together cautiously.
Diuretics (bumetanide, ethacrynic acid, furosemide, torsemide): May cause excessive diuretic response, resulting in serious electrolyte imbalances or dehydration. Adjust dosages carefully, and monitor patient closely for signs and symptoms of excessive diuretic response.
Levodopa–carbidopa: May increase risk of hypotension. Monitor therapy.
Lithium: May decrease lithium clearance, increasing risk of lithium toxicity. Monitor lithium level.
Methenamine: May decrease effectiveness of methenamine. Monitor therapy.
NSAIDs: May increase risk of KF. May decrease diuretic and antihypertensive effects. Monitor kidney function and BP.
QT-interval-prolonging drugs: May increase risk of QT-interval prolongation and ventricular arrhythmias. Avoid use together.
Drug-herb. *Licorice:* May cause hypokalemia. Discourage use together.
Drug-lifestyle. *Alcohol use:* May increase orthostatic hypotensive effect. Discourage use together.
Sun exposure: May cause photosensitivity reaction. Advise patient to avoid excessive sunlight exposure.

Reactions in bold italics are *life-threatening*.

EFFECTS ON LAB TEST RESULTS
• May increase glucose, calcium, uric acid, cholesterol, BUN, and triglyceride levels.
• May decrease potassium, sodium, magnesium, phosphate, and chloride levels.
• May decrease Hb level and granulocyte and WBC counts.

CONTRAINDICATIONS & CAUTIONS
• Contraindicated in patients hypersensitive to thiazides, other sulfonamide-derived drugs, or metolazone and in those with anuria, hepatic coma, or precoma.
• Use cautiously in patients with impaired kidney or liver function, electrolyte imbalances, hyperuricemia, SLE, diabetes, or gout.
Dialyzable drug: Unlikely.
⚠ *Overdose S&S:* Orthostatic hypotension, dizziness, drowsiness, lethargy, syncope, CNS depression, electrolyte abnormalities, hemoconcentration, depressed respirations, GI irritation and hypermotility.

PREGNANCY-LACTATION-REPRODUCTION
• Studies during pregnancy are inadequate. Drug crosses placenta. Use during pregnancy only if clearly needed.
• Drug appears in human milk. Patient should discontinue breastfeeding or discontinue drug, considering importance of drug to patient.

NURSING CONSIDERATIONS
• Monitor fluid intake and output, weight, BP, and electrolyte levels.
• Watch for signs and symptoms of hypokalemia (muscle weakness, cramps). Drug may be used with potassium-sparing diuretic to prevent potassium loss.
• Consult dietitian about high-potassium diet.
• Monitor glucose level, especially in patient with diabetes.
• Monitor uric acid level, especially in patient with history of gout.
• Closely monitor older adults, who are especially susceptible to excessive diuresis.
• In patient with HTN, therapeutic response may be delayed several weeks.
• Monitor BP. Add another antihypertensive for inadequate response.
• Metolazone and furosemide may be used together to enhance diuretic effect.
• Unlike thiazide diuretics, metolazone is effective in patients with decreased kidney function.
• Stop thiazides and thiazide-like diuretics before parathyroid function tests.

• *Look alike–sound alike:* Don't confuse metolazone with methadone, metoprolol, metoclopramide, methimazole, or methazolamide.

PATIENT TEACHING
• Tell patient to take drug in morning to prevent need to urinate at night.
• Advise patient to avoid sudden posture changes and to rise slowly to avoid dizziness upon standing quickly.
• Instruct patient to use sunblock and protective clothing to prevent photosensitivity reactions.
• Tell patient to increase dietary intake of potassium-containing foods.
• Review adverse reactions, and instruct patient to promptly report them.
• Instruct patient to report pregnancy or plans to become pregnant or breastfeed.

metoprolol succinate
me-toe-PROE-lole

Kapspargo Sprinkle, Toprol-XL

metoprolol tartrate
Lopressor

Therapeutic class: Antihypertensives
Pharmacologic class: Selective beta-adrenergic blockers

AVAILABLE FORMS
metoprolol succinate
Capsules (extended-release): 25 mg, 50 mg, 100 mg, 200 mg
Tablets (extended-release) ⓞⓝⓒ: 25 mg, 50 mg, 100 mg, 200 mg
metoprolol tartrate
Injection: 1 mg/mL
Tablets: 25 mg, 37.5 mg, 50 mg, 75 mg, 100 mg
Tablets (sustained-release) ⓞⓝⓒ: 100 mg✦, 200 mg✦

INDICATIONS & DOSAGES
Boxed Warning Don't abruptly discontinue drug. ▪
▶**HTN**
Adults: Initially, 50 mg PO b.i.d. or 100 mg PO once daily; then up to 100 to 450 mg daily or in two or three divided doses. Or, 25 to 100 mg extended-release tablets or capsule (tartrate equivalent) PO once daily.

Adjust dosage as needed and tolerated at intervals of not less than 1 week to maximum of 400 mg (extended-release) daily or 450 mg (immediate-release) daily.

Children older than age 6 (metoprolol succinate capsule): Initially, 1 mg/kg PO once daily, not to exceed 50 mg PO daily. Adjust dosage based on BP response. Doses greater than 2 mg/kg or in excess of 200 mg/day haven't been studied.

➤ **Early intervention in acute MI**
Adults: 5 mg metoprolol tartrate IV bolus every 2 minutes for three doses. Then, starting 15 minutes after last IV dose, 25 to 50 mg PO every 6 hours for 48 hours. Maintenance dosage, 100 mg PO b.i.d.

➤ **Late intervention in acute MI**
Adults: 100 mg PO b.i.d. as soon as clinical condition allows in patients with contraindications for or intolerance to early intervention. Continue for at least 3 months.

➤ **Angina pectoris**
Adults: Initially, 100 mg PO daily as two equally divided doses, increased at weekly intervals until adequate response or pronounced decrease in HR occurs. Effects of daily dose beyond 400 mg aren't known. Or, 100 mg extended-release tablets (tartrate equivalent) once daily. Adjust dosage as needed and tolerated at intervals of not less than 1 week to maximum of 400 mg daily.

➤ **Stable symptomatic HF (NYHA Class II) resulting from ischemia, HTN, or cardiomyopathy**
Adults: 25 mg metoprolol succinate PO once daily for 2 weeks. Double dose every 2 weeks, as tolerated, to maximum of 200 mg daily.
Adjust-a-dose: In patients with more severe HF, start with 12.5 mg Toprol-XL PO once daily for 2 weeks. Kapspargo isn't suitable for doses of less than 25 mg daily.

ADMINISTRATION
PO
• Give drug with or immediately after meal.
• Extended-release tablets may be cut in half on scored line but never crushed or chewed.
• Patient may swallow extended-release capsules whole or may open capsules and sprinkle contents over soft food (applesauce, pudding, yogurt). Patient should swallow drug and food mixture within 60 minutes.
• If a dose is missed, omit missed dose and give next scheduled dose without doubling it.

IV
▼ Give drug undiluted by direct injection in intensive care setting at rate of 5 mg over 1 to 2 minutes.
▼ Store at room temperature and protect from light. Discard solution if it's discolored or contains particles.
▼ **Incompatibilities:** None listed by manufacturer. Consult drug compatibility reference for more information.

ACTION
A selective beta blocker that selectively blocks beta$_1$ receptors; decreases cardiac output, peripheral resistance, and cardiac oxygen consumption; and depresses renin secretion.

Route	Onset	Peak	Duration
PO	1 hour	1 hr	6–12 hr
PO (extended-release)	1 hour	6–12 hr	24 hr
IV	5 min	20 min	5–8 hr

Half-life: 3 to 10 hours.

ADVERSE REACTIONS
CNS: fatigue, dizziness, depression, headache, insomnia, sleep disturbance, mental confusion, nightmares, short-term memory loss, hallucinations, vertigo, *stroke.* **CV:** hypotension, *bradycardia, HF,* edema, palpitations, Raynaud syndrome, cold extremity, first-degree AV block, second- or *third-degree AV block (IV).* **EENT:** blurred vision, visual disturbances, tinnitus, rhinitis, dry mouth. **GI:** nausea, diarrhea, constipation, heartburn, flatulence, gastric pain, vomiting. **GU:** decreased libido, erectile dysfunction. **Respiratory:** dyspnea, wheezing, *bronchospasm.* **Skin:** rash, pruritus. **Other:** accidental injury.

INTERACTIONS
Drug-drug. *Amiodarone:* May increase bradycardic effects. Monitor therapy.
Barbiturates: May reduce metoprolol effect. Monitor therapy.
Calcium channel blockers: May increase hypotensive and bradycardic effects. Monitor therapy.
Cardiac glycosides: May cause excessive bradycardia and increased depressant effect on myocardium. Use together cautiously.
Catecholamine-depleting drugs (reserpine), MAO inhibitors (selegiline, isocarboxazid):

May have additive effect. Monitor patient for hypotension and bradycardia.

Clonidine: May increase risk of bradycardia. If clonidine and a beta blocker are coadministered, withdraw beta blocker several days before gradual withdrawal of clonidine to avoid rebound HTN.

CYP2D6 inhibitors (fluoxetine, paroxetine, propafenone, quinidine): May increase metoprolol level. Closely monitor vital signs if combination can't be avoided. Metoprolol dosage reduction may be needed.

Epinephrine: May blunt epinephrine effect during treatment of allergic reaction. Monitor therapy.

Hydralazine: May increase levels and effects of both drugs. Monitor patient closely. May need to adjust dosage.

Indomethacin, NSAIDs: May decrease antihypertensive effect. Monitor BP and adjust dosage.

Insulin, oral antidiabetics: May alter dosage requirements in previously stabilized patients with diabetes. Monitor patient closely.

IV lidocaine: May reduce liver metabolism of lidocaine, increasing risk of toxicity. Give bolus doses of lidocaine at a slower rate, and closely monitor lidocaine level.

Theophylline: May decrease bronchodilatory effects of theophylline. Monitor patient.

Verapamil: May increase effects of both drugs. Closely monitor cardiac function, and decrease dosages as needed.

Drug-herb. *Ma huang:* May decrease antihypertensive effects. Discourage use together.

Drug-food. *Any food:* May increase absorption. Encourage patient to take drug with food.

EFFECTS ON LAB TEST RESULTS
• May increase transaminase, ALP, and LDH levels.

CONTRAINDICATIONS & CAUTIONS
• Contraindicated in patients hypersensitive to drug or other beta blockers.
• Contraindicated in patients with sinus bradycardia, severe bradycardia, greater than first-degree heart block or sick sinus syndrome (unless permanent pacemaker is in place), cardiogenic shock, or overt HF when used to treat HTN or angina.
• When used to treat MI, drug is contraindicated in patients with HR less than 45 beats/minute, greater than first-degree heart block, PR interval of 0.24 second or longer

with first-degree heart block, systolic BP less than 100 mm Hg, or decompensated HF.
• Tartrate tablets are contraindicated in patients with severe peripheral arterial circulatory disorders.
• Use cautiously in patients with HF, diabetes, or bronchospastic or liver disease.
• Use cautiously in patients with pheochromocytoma and only after alpha blocker has been initiated to avoid paradoxical increase in BP.
• Avoid initiating high-dose, extended-release drug in patients undergoing noncardiac surgery because drug has been associated with bradycardia, hypotension, stroke, and death.
• Don't routinely withdraw long-term beta-blocker therapy before surgery.
Dialyzable drug: Yes.
⚠ **Overdose S&S:** Bradycardia, nausea, hypotension, bronchospasm, HF, cardiac arrest, coma, AV block, vomiting.

PREGNANCY-LACTATION-REPRODUCTION
• Studies during pregnancy are inadequate. Drug crosses placental barrier. Use during pregnancy only if clearly needed. Monitor fetal growth.
• Monitor neonates born to patients who received metoprolol during pregnancy for hypotension, hypoglycemia, bradycardia, and respiratory depression.
• Drug appears in human milk in very small quantities. Consider possible infant exposure with use during breastfeeding. Monitor infant for bradycardia, listlessness, and hypoglycemia.

NURSING CONSIDERATIONS
• Always check patient's apical pulse rate before giving drug. If it's slower than 60 beats/minute, withhold drug and contact prescriber immediately to verify dose.
• In patient with diabetes, closely monitor glucose level; drug masks common signs and symptoms of hypoglycemia.
• Frequently monitor BP; drug masks common signs and symptoms of shock.
• Beta blockers may mask tachycardia caused by hyperthyroidism. In patient with suspected thyrotoxicosis, taper off beta blocker to avoid thyroid storm.
Boxed Warning When stopping long-term therapy, taper dosage over 1 to 2 weeks. Abrupt discontinuation may cause

exacerbations of angina or MI. Don't discontinue therapy abruptly, even in patients treated only for HTN. Restart metoprolol, at least temporarily, if angina markedly worsens or acute coronary insufficiency occurs. ■

• Beta selectivity is lost at higher doses. Watch for peripheral side effects.

• **Look alike–sound alike:** Don't confuse metoprolol succinate with metoprolol tartrate. Don't confuse metoprolol with metaproterenol, misoprostol, or metolazone. Don't confuse Toprol-XL with Topamax, Tegretol, or Tegretol-XR.

PATIENT TEACHING

• Instruct patient to take drug exactly as prescribed and with meals.

• Caution patient to avoid driving and other tasks requiring mental alertness until response to therapy has been established.

• Advise patient to inform dentist or prescriber about use of drug before procedures or surgery.

• Tell patient to report all adverse reactions, especially weight gain and shortness of breath.

Boxed Warning Instruct patient not to stop drug suddenly but to notify prescriber about unpleasant adverse reactions. ■

---

metroNIDAZOLE (oral, injection) ⬚
met-roe-NYE-da-zole

Flagyl

metroNIDAZOLE hydrochloride ⬚

Therapeutic class: Antiprotozoals
Pharmacologic class: Nitroimidazoles

AVAILABLE FORMS

Capsules: 375 mg, 500 mg✦
Injection: 500 mg/100 mL in ready-to-use (RTU) minibags
Tablets: 250 mg, 500 mg

INDICATIONS & DOSAGES

Boxed Warning Use metronidazole only for the conditions for which it's indicated because it may be carcinogenic. Avoid unnecessary use. ■

Adjust-a-dose (for all indications): For Child-Pugh class C liver impairment, reduce dosage of tablets and IV infusion by 50%.

➤ **Amebic liver abscess**
Adults: 500 to 750 mg PO t.i.d. for 5 to 10 days.
Children: 35 to 50 mg/kg PO daily in three divided doses for 10 days.
Adjust-a-dose: For Child-Pugh class C liver impairment, reduce capsule dosage to 375 mg PO every 8 hours for 5 to 10 days.

➤ **Intestinal amebiasis**
Adults: 750 mg PO t.i.d. for 7 to 10 days.
Children: 35 to 50 mg/kg PO daily in three divided doses for 10 days. IV form may be necessary for severe infection or extraintestinal disease.
Adjust-a-dose: For Child-Pugh class C liver impairment, reduce capsule dosage to 375 mg PO every 8 hours for 5 to 10 days.

➤ **Trichomoniasis**
Adults: One 250-mg tablet PO t.i.d. for 7 days, or 2 g PO in single dose (may give the 2-g dose in two 1-g doses, both on the same day); wait 4 to 6 weeks before repeating course. Or, one 375-mg capsule PO b.i.d. for 7 days.
Adjust-a-dose: For Child-Pugh class C liver impairment, reduce capsule dosage to 375 mg PO once daily for 7 days.

➤ **Bacterial infections caused by anaerobic microorganisms**
Adults: Loading dose, 15 mg/kg IV infused over 1 hour. Maintenance dose, 7.5 mg/kg IV or 500 mg PO every 6 hours for 7 to 10 days. Infections involving bone, joint, lower respiratory tract, and endocardium may require longer treatment. Give first maintenance dose 6 hours after loading dose. Maximum dose, 4 g daily.

➤ **To prevent postoperative infection in contaminated or potentially contaminated colorectal surgery**
Adults: Infuse 15 mg/kg IV over 30 to 60 minutes and complete about 1 hour before surgery. Then infuse 7.5 mg/kg IV over 30 to 60 minutes at 6 and 12 hours after first dose.

ADMINISTRATION

• Obtain specimen for culture and sensitivity before giving first dose, if possible. Begin therapy while awaiting results.
PO
• Give tablets and capsules with food if GI upset occurs.
• Give missed dose as soon as possible unless it's close to time for next dose.

Reactions in bold italics are *life-threatening*.

IV
▼ IV RTU minibags need no preparation.
▼ Don't give by IV push. Infuse over 30 to 60 minutes.
▼ Store at room temperature. Don't remove overwrap until ready to use.
▼ **Incompatibilities:** Other IV drugs. Avoid contact of drug solution with equipment containing aluminum.

ACTION
Direct-acting trichomonacide and amebicide that works inside and outside the intestines. Thought to enter the cells of microorganisms that contain nitroreductase, forming unstable compounds that bind to DNA and inhibit synthesis, causing cell death.

Route	Onset	Peak	Duration
PO	Unknown	1–2 hr	Unknown
IV	Immediate	1 hr	Unknown

Half-life: 6 to 8 hours.

ADVERSE REACTIONS
CNS: headache, *seizures,* fever, vertigo, ataxia, dizziness, syncope, incoordination, confusion, irritability, depression, weakness, somnolence, insomnia, *encephalopathy, aseptic meningitis,* peripheral neuropathy.
CV: *prolonged QT interval,* flattened T wave, chest pain, edema, flushing, thrombophlebitis after IV infusion. **EENT:** nystagmus, optic neuropathy, rhinitis, sinusitis, nasal congestion, dry mouth, pharyngitis, furry tongue.
GI: nausea, abdominal pain, stomatitis, epigastric distress, vomiting, anorexia, diarrhea, constipation, rectal lining inflammation, metallic taste. **GU:** vaginitis, darkened urine, polyuria, dysuria, cystitis, dyspareunia, dryness of vagina and vulva, vaginal candidiasis, genital pruritus, UTI, dysmenorrhea, decreased libido. **Hematologic:** *leukopenia.*
Hepatic: jaundice, increased liver enzyme levels. **Musculoskeletal:** transient joint pains, myalgia, muscle spasms. **Respiratory:** dyspnea, URI. **Skin:** rash, pruritus, urticaria, diaphoresis, erythema. **Other:** overgrowth of nonsusceptible organisms, candidiasis, flulike symptoms, hypersensitivity reactions, including *anaphylaxis and SCARs.*

INTERACTIONS
Drug-drug. *Busulfan:* May increase busulfan toxicity. Avoid use together.

Cimetidine: May increase risk of metronidazole toxicity because of inhibited liver metabolism. Monitor for toxicity.
CYP3A4 substrates (aripiprazole, dofetilide, lomitapide, pimozide): May increase substrate level. Monitor therapy.
⊕ *Alert: Disulfiram:* May cause acute psychosis and confusion. Avoid giving metronidazole within 2 weeks of disulfiram.
5-FU: May increase 5-FU level and toxicity. Use together cautiously.
Lithium: May increase lithium level, which may cause toxicity. Monitor lithium level.
Mebendazole: May increase risk of SJS or TEN. Consider therapy modification.
Phenobarbital, phenytoin: May decrease metronidazole effectiveness; may reduce total phenytoin clearance. Monitor patient.
QT-interval-prolonging drugs (amiodarone, haloperidol): May increase risk of QT-interval prolongation and ventricular arrhythmias. Avoid use together.
Vecuronium: May potentiate neuromuscular blocking effects of vecuronium. Use together cautiously.
Warfarin, other oral anticoagulants: May increase anticoagulant effects and risk of bleeding. Closely monitor PT and INR. Reduce warfarin as needed.
Drug-lifestyle. *Alcohol use:* May cause disulfiram-like reaction, including nausea, vomiting, headache, cramps, and flushing. Warn patient to avoid alcohol during and for 3 days after completing drug therapy.

EFFECTS ON LAB TEST RESULTS
• May increase LFT values.
• May decrease WBC, platelet, and neutrophil counts.
• May interfere with ALT, AST, glucose, triglyceride, and LDH testing.

CONTRAINDICATIONS & CAUTIONS
• Contraindicated in patients hypersensitive to drug or other nitroimidazole derivatives.
▧ Contraindicated in patients with Cockayne syndrome. Irreversible liver toxicity may occur.
• Use of disulfiram within 2 weeks of metronidazole therapy and use of alcohol or propylene glycol products during treatment and for 3 days after treatment ends are contraindicated.
• Use cautiously in patients with history of blood dyscrasia, seizure disorder, or retinal or visual field changes.

M

• Use cautiously in older adults and patients who take liver-toxic drugs or have liver disease, alcohol use disorder, or kidney impairment.

• Each RTU bag contains 14 mEq of sodium.

• Prolonged use may cause superinfections, including CDAD and pseudomembranous colitis, which may occur more than 2 months after therapy ends.

Dialyzable drug: Yes.

⚠ *Overdose S&S:* Nausea, vomiting, ataxia, neurotoxicity.

PREGNANCY-LACTATION-REPRODUCTION

• Drug crosses placental barrier. Consult current guidelines for appropriate use during pregnancy.

• Drug appears in human milk. Patient should discontinue breastfeeding or discontinue drug, considering importance of drug to patient. Or, patient may express and discard human milk during metronidazole therapy and for 24 hours after final dose.

NURSING CONSIDERATIONS

• Carefully monitor LFT results in older adults and patients with liver impairment.

• Monitor closely for metronidazole-associated adverse events in patient with KF on KRT.

• Observe for edema, especially if patient is receiving corticosteroids; IV form may cause sodium retention.

• Record number and character of stools when drug is used to treat amebiasis. Give drug only after confirming *Trichomonas vaginalis* infection by wet smear or culture or identifying *Entamoeba histolytica*.

• Sexual partners of patients being treated for *T. vaginalis* infection, even if asymptomatic, must also receive treatment to avoid reinfection.

• *Look alike–sound alike:* Don't confuse metronidazole with metformin, mebendazole, meropenem, methotrexate, metoclopramide, or miconazole.

PATIENT TEACHING

• Inform patient with trichomoniasis of need for sexual partners to be treated simultaneously to avoid reinfection.

• Tell patient to avoid alcohol and alcohol-containing drugs during and for at least 3 days after treatment course.

• Alert patient that a metallic taste and dark or red-brown urine may occur.

• Tell patient to report signs and symptoms of candidal overgrowth.

• Caution patient to immediately report all adverse reactions, especially neurologic symptoms (seizures, peripheral neuropathy).

• Advise patient to report pregnancy or plans to become pregnant.

metroNIDAZOLE (topical, vaginal)

met-roe-NYE-da-zole

MetroCream, MetroGel, MetroLotion, Noritate, Nuvessa, Vandazole

Therapeutic class: Antibacterials (topical)
Pharmacologic class: Nitroimidazoles

AVAILABLE FORMS

Topical cream: 0.75%, 1%
Topical gel: 0.75%, 1%
Topical lotion: 0.75%
Vaginal gel: 0.75%, 1.3%

INDICATIONS & DOSAGES

➤ **Inflammatory papules and pustules of acne rosacea**

Adults: If using 0.75% preparation, apply thin film to affected area b.i.d., morning and evening. If using 1% preparation, apply thin film to affected area once daily. After response occurs (usually within 3 weeks), adjust frequency and duration of therapy.

➤ **Bacterial vaginosis**

Females after menarche: One applicatorful of 0.75% (approximately 37.5 mg) vaginally daily or b.i.d. for 5 days. For once-daily use, give at bedtime.

Females ages 12 and older: One applicatorful (approximately 65 mg) of 1.3% vaginal gel intravaginally once as a single dose at bedtime.

ADMINISTRATION

Topical

• Clean area thoroughly before use; then wait 15 to 20 minutes before applying drug to minimize risk of local irritation. Avoid contact with eyes.

• Cosmetics may be applied after use. Patient should wait at least 5 minutes after using lotion before applying cosmetics.

• Flush eyes immediately if inadvertent contact with drug occurs.

Vaginal
- Screw end of applicator onto tube and squeeze slowly. Plunger will stop when applicator is full.
- Insert gently into vagina as far as possible without causing discomfort.
- Wash plunger and barrel in warm, soapy water and rinse thoroughly. Dry before reassembling.

ACTION
Unknown. May cause bactericidal effect by interacting with bacterial DNA. Drug is active against many anaerobic gram-negative bacilli, anaerobic gram-positive cocci, *Gardnerella vaginalis*, and *Campylobacter fetus*.

Route	Onset	Peak	Duration
Topical	Unknown	8–12 hr	Unknown
Vaginal	Unknown	6–12 hr	Unknown

Half-life: Unknown.

ADVERSE REACTIONS
Topical form
CNS: headache. **CV:** HTN. **EENT:** nasal congestion, nasopharyngitis, sinusitis. **GU:** UTI. **Respiratory:** URI. **Skin:** transient redness, dryness, mild burning, stinging, contact dermatitis, pruritus, rash, rosacea exacerbation. **Other:** flulike symptoms.
Vaginal form
CNS: headache, dizziness, dysgeusia, depression. **EENT:** pharyngitis. **GI:** cramps, GI distress, nausea, loose stools, pain, vomiting, diarrhea, decreased appetite. **GU:** metrorrhagia, dysmenorrhea, cervicitis, vaginitis, perineal and vulvovaginal itching, vaginal burning, vaginal discharge, pelvic discomfort. **Musculoskeletal:** muscle cramps. **Skin:** transient redness, dryness, mild burning, stinging, rash, pruritus. **Other:** overgrowth of nonsusceptible organisms, breast pain.

INTERACTIONS
Drug-drug. *Disulfiram:* May cause disulfiram-like reaction when used with vaginal form of metronidazole. Don't use together, and wait 2 weeks after stopping disulfiram before starting metronidazole vaginal therapy.
Lithium: May increase lithium level in patients taking high doses of lithium. Use together cautiously. Consider monitoring lithium level.
Lopinavir: May enhance adverse and toxic effects of lopinavir and result in a disulfiram-like reaction. Monitor therapy.

Oral anticoagulants: May increase anticoagulant effect. Monitor patient for adverse reactions.
Tipranavir: May enhance adverse effect of tipranavir. Monitor therapy.
Warfarin: May increase PT. Monitor therapy.
Drug-lifestyle. *Alcohol use:* May cause disulfiram-like reaction when used with vaginal form. Don't use together or for at least 24 hours after vaginal treatment.

EFFECTS ON LAB TEST RESULTS
- May interfere with AST, ALT, LDH, triglyceride, and glucose tests.
- May decrease WBC and platelet counts.

CONTRAINDICATIONS & CAUTIONS
- Contraindicated in patients hypersensitive to drug or its ingredients, such as parabens, and other nitroimidazole derivatives.
- Use cautiously in patients with history or evidence of blood dyscrasia and in those with liver impairment.
- Use cautiously in patients with history of CNS diseases; topical products may cause peripheral neuropathy.
- Prolonged use of vaginal form can lead to fungal or bacterial superinfection.
Dialyzable drug: Yes.

PREGNANCY-LACTATION-REPRODUCTION
- Studies during pregnancy are inadequate. Drug crosses placental barrier. Use during pregnancy only if clearly needed and benefit justifies fetal risk.
- Drug may appear in human milk after vaginal or topical use because some of drug is absorbed systemically. Patient should discontinue breastfeeding or discontinue drug, considering importance of drug to patient.

NURSING CONSIDERATIONS
- Topical therapy hasn't been linked to most of the adverse effects observed with parenteral or oral therapy, but some drug may be absorbed after topical use.
- Monitor patient for worsening symptoms.
- Monitor for *Candida* vaginitis during or after treatment.

PATIENT TEACHING
- Teach about proper drug administration and handling.
- Instruct patient to avoid use of topical gel around eyes.

• If local reactions occur, advise patient to apply drug less frequently or stop using it and notify prescriber.

• Advise patient to avoid sexual intercourse and use of other vaginal products (tampons, douches) while using vaginal preparation.

• Caution patient to avoid alcohol while being treated with vaginal preparation.

micafungin sodium
mi-ka-FUN-gin

Mycamine

Therapeutic class: Antifungals
Pharmacologic class: Echinocandins

AVAILABLE FORMS
Lyophilized powder for injection: 50 mg, 100 mg in single-use vials

INDICATIONS & DOSAGES
➤ **Candidemia, acute disseminated candidiasis, and *Candida* peritonitis and abscesses**
Adults: 100 mg IV daily for 10 to 47 days (mean duration, 15 days).
Children ages 4 months and older: 2 mg/kg IV once daily. Maximum dosage, 100 mg daily.
➤ **Candidemia, acute disseminated candidiasis, *Candida* peritonitis, and abscesses without meningoencephalitis, ocular dissemination, or both**
Children younger than age 4 months: 4 mg/kg IV once daily.
➤ **Esophageal candidiasis**
Adults: 150 mg IV daily for 10 to 30 days (mean duration, 15 days).
Children ages 4 months and older weighing more than 30 kg: 2.5 mg/kg IV once daily. Maximum dosage, 150 mg daily.
Children ages 4 months and older weighing 30 kg or less: 3 mg/kg IV once daily.
➤ **To prevent candidal infection in hematopoietic stem cell transplant recipients**
Adults: 50 mg IV daily for 6 to 51 days (mean duration, 19 days).
Children ages 4 months and older: 1 mg/kg IV once daily. Maximum dosage, 50 mg daily.

ADMINISTRATION
IV
▼ Reconstitute each 50-mg or 100-mg vial with 5 mL of NSS without a bacteriostatic agent or D_5W for injection. To minimize foaming, dissolve powder by swirling vial; don't shake it. Don't use solution if precipitation or foreign matter is present.
▼ For adult, dilute dose in 100 mL of NSS or D_5W for injection.
▼ For children, add reconstituted drug to NSS or D_5W IV infusion bag or syringe. Ensure that final concentration of solution is between 0.5 and 4 mg/mL. To minimize risk of infusion reactions, administer concentrations greater than 1.5 mg/mL via central catheter.
▼ Flush line with NSS for injection before infusing drug.
▼ Infuse drug over 1 hour.
▼ May store reconstituted product and diluted infusion for up to 24 hours at room temperature.
▼ Protect diluted solution from light.
▼ Drug is preservative-free; discard partially used vials.
▼ **Incompatibilities:** Don't mix or confuse with other medications. Drug may precipitate when mixed with commonly used drugs.

ACTION
Inhibits synthesis of an essential component of fungal cell walls. Active against most *Candida* species.

Route	Onset	Peak	Duration
IV	Unknown	Unknown	Unknown

Half-life: 11 to 21 hours.

ADVERSE REACTIONS
CNS: headache, insomnia, anxiety, fever, dizziness, rigors, delirium, *intracranial hemorrhage, seizures.* **CV:** bradycardia, atrial fibrillation, cardiac disorders, HTN, hypotension, tachycardia, vascular disorders, phlebitis, *injection-site thrombosis,* edema, *cardiac arrest, MI, pericardial effusion.* **EENT:** epistaxis. **GI:** abdominal pain, abdominal distention, diarrhea, nausea, vomiting, anorexia, dyspepsia, mucositis, constipation. **GU:** decreased urine output, hematuria, *KF.* **Hematologic:** *leukopenia, neutropenia, thrombocytopenia,* anemia, *coagulopathy, pancytopenia.* **Hepatic:** elevated LFT values, liver injury, liver enlargement, hyperbilirubinemia, jaundice, *liver failure.*

Metabolic: *hypocalcemia, hypokalemia, hypomagnesemia,* hypophosphatemia, hyperglycemia, *hypoglycemia, hyperkalemia,* hypernatremia. **Respiratory:** cough, dyspnea. **Skin:** infusion-site inflammation, pruritus, rash, urticaria. **Other:** hypersensitivity reactions.

INTERACTIONS
Drug-drug. *Itraconazole, nifedipine, sirolimus:* May increase level of these drugs. Monitor patient for evidence of toxicity, and decrease dose if needed.

EFFECTS ON LAB TEST RESULTS
• May increase ALP, ALT, AST, bilirubin, BUN, creatinine, sodium, and LDH levels.
• May decrease phosphorus and potassium levels.
• May increase or decrease glucose, calcium, and magnesium levels.
• May decrease Hb level and hematocrit and neutrophil and platelet counts.

CONTRAINDICATIONS & CAUTIONS
• Contraindicated in patients hypersensitive to drug or other echinocandins.
• Drug may increase risk of liver or kidney disorder.
Dialyzable drug: No.

PREGNANCY-LACTATION-REPRODUCTION
• Based on animal studies, drug may cause fetal harm. Use during pregnancy only if potential benefit justifies fetal risk.
• It isn't known if drug appears in human milk. Use cautiously during breastfeeding.

NURSING CONSIDERATIONS
• Injection-site reactions are more common in patients receiving drug by peripheral IV.
• To reduce risk of histamine-mediated reactions, infuse drug over at least 1 hour.
🟦 *Alert:* If patient develops signs of serious hypersensitivity reaction, including shock, stop infusion and immediately notify prescriber.
• Monitor liver and kidney function during therapy.
• Monitor patient for hemolysis and hemolytic anemia.

PATIENT TEACHING
• Advise patient to report pain or redness at infusion site.

• Review adverse reactions, and instruct patient to report them immediately.
• Advise patient of childbearing potential of the risk to a fetus.
• Tell patient that lab tests will most likely be needed to monitor hematologic, kidney, and liver function.

miconazole
my-KON-a-zole

Oravig

miconazole nitrate
Desenex ◇, Fungoid Tincture ◇, Lotrimin AF ◇, Micaderm, Micatin ◇, Micozole🍁 ◇, Monistat ◇, Vagistat ◇, Zeasorb-AF ◇

Therapeutic class: Antifungals
Pharmacologic class: Imidazoles

AVAILABLE FORMS
Aerosol powder: 2% ◇
Aerosol spray: 2% ◇
Buccal tablets 🔵: 50 mg
Powder: 2% ◇
Topical ointment: 2% ◇
Topical solution: 2% ◇
Vaginal cream: 2% ◇, 4% ◇
Vaginal suppositories: 100 mg ◇, 200 mg ◇, 400 mg🍁 ◇, 1,200 mg🍁 ◇

INDICATIONS & DOSAGES
➤ **Tinea corporis, tinea cruris, tinea pedis, cutaneous candidiasis, common dermatophyte infections**
Adults and children older than age 2: Apply a thin layer b.i.d. for 2 weeks (tinea cruris) to 4 weeks (tinea pedis and corporis), or as prescribed. In children younger than age 2, use only under direction and supervision of a physician.
➤ **Vulvovaginal candidiasis**
Adults and children ages 12 and older: One applicatorful 2% or 100-mg suppository vaginally at bedtime for 7 days; repeat course, if needed. Or, one applicatorful 4% or 200-mg suppository vaginally at bedtime for 3 days. Or, one 1,200-mg suppository vaginally at bedtime for 1 day. May apply topical cream sparingly to affected area b.i.d. for 7 days or as needed for external symptoms.

➤ **Oropharyngeal candidiasis**
Adults and children ages 16 and older: One 50-mg buccal tablet to upper gum region once daily for 14 consecutive days.

ADMINISTRATION
PO
• Apply buccal tablet to the gum in the morning with dry hands after patient has brushed teeth.
• Place rounded surface of tablet against the gum just above the incisor. Apply slight pressure over upper lip for 30 seconds to ensure adhesion.
• Alternate sides of mouth for each dose.
• Patient shouldn't crush, chew, or swallow buccal tablets.
• If a buccal tablet that has been in place for at least 6 hours and dislodges or patient swallows it, don't apply a new tablet until next regularly scheduled dose.
Topical
• Clean and thoroughly dry area before application.
• Don't cover the site with an occlusive dressing.
• For tinea pedis, pay special attention to spaces between toes.
Vaginal
• Suppository is inserted high into vagina with applicator provided.
• Store drug at room temperature.

ACTION
Fungicidal; disrupts fungal cell membrane permeability.

Route	Onset	Peak	Duration
PO	Unknown	7 hr	15 hr
Topical, vaginal	Unknown	Unknown	Unknown

Half-life: 24 hours (terminal).

ADVERSE REACTIONS
CNS: headache, fatigue, pain, taste disorder, loss of ability to taste. **EENT:** dry mouth, oral discomfort, toothache. **GI:** diarrhea, nausea, upper abdominal pain, vomiting (buccal tablets), gastroenteritis. **GU:** pelvic cramps; pruritus, irritation (vaginal cream); vulvovaginal burning. **Hematologic:** anemia, *lymphopenia, neutropenia.* **Hepatic:** increased GGT level (buccal tablets). **Respiratory:** cough, URI. **Skin:** allergic contact dermatitis, burning, pain, irritation, maceration, edema.

INTERACTIONS
Drug-drug. *Fosphenytoin, phenytoin, sulfonylureas:* Buccal form may increase levels of these drugs. Monitor therapy.
Progesterone: Vaginal form of drug may diminish progesterone effects. Avoid use together.
Warfarin: May enhance anticoagulant effect. Monitor PT and INR, and observe patient for bleeding.
Drug-herb. *Saccharomyces boulardii:* Antifungals may decrease therapeutic effect. Consider alternative therapy.

EFFECTS ON LAB TEST RESULTS
• May increase GGT level.
• May decrease Hb level and lymphocyte and neutrophil counts.

CONTRAINDICATIONS & CAUTIONS
• Contraindicated in patients hypersensitive to drug or its components. Cross-sensitivity to imidazole antifungals may occur.
• Buccal tablets are contraindicated in patients hypersensitive to milk protein concentrate.
• Use buccal tablets cautiously in patients with liver impairment.
• Safety and effectiveness of buccal tablets haven't been established for children younger than age 16; don't use in younger children because of risk of choking.
Dialyzable drug: Unknown.

PREGNANCY-LACTATION-REPRODUCTION
• Based on animal studies, buccal tablets may cause fetal harm. Use buccal tablets during pregnancy only if potential benefit justifies fetal risk.
🔋 *Alert:* Use vaginal preparation during pregnancy only if recommended by prescriber.
• It isn't known if drug appears in human milk. Topical and vaginal administration should result in low systemic absorption. Use cautiously during breastfeeding.
• Vaginal forms can weaken latex condoms and diaphragms.

NURSING CONSIDERATIONS
• Carefully monitor patient with liver impairment who is taking oral form.
• Monitor patient for hypersensitivity and adverse reactions.

PATIENT TEACHING

• Advise that vaginal form is for perineal or vaginal use only. Warn patient to keep drug out of eyes.

• Caution patient that frequent or persistent yeast infections may suggest a more serious medical problem.

• Explain that vaginal forms may stain clothing.

• Warn patient to stop drug if sensitivity or chemical irritation occurs.

• Instruct patient to use drug for full treatment period prescribed and to notify prescriber if symptoms persist or worsen despite therapy.

• Advise patient to avoid tampons, douches, spermicides or other vaginal products, and sexual intercourse during vaginal treatment.

• Show patient how to properly administer prescribed formulation.

• Emphasize that patient can eat and drink with buccal tablet in place but should avoid chewing gum.

• Caution caregiver not to use OTC products in children younger than approved age, unless prescribed by health care provider.

SAFETY ALERT!

midazolam hydrochloride
MID-aye-zoe-lam

Nayzilam, Seizalam

Therapeutic class: Anxiolytics, anticonvulsants
Pharmacologic class: Benzodiazepines
Controlled substance schedule: IV

AVAILABLE FORMS

Injection: 1 mg/mL, 5 mg/mL
Injection (preservative-free): 1 mg/mL, 5 mg/mL
Nasal spray: 5 mg/0.1 mL
Syrup: 2 mg/mL

INDICATIONS & DOSAGES

➤ **Preoperative sedation (to induce sleepiness or drowsiness and relieve apprehension)**
Adults ages 60 and older: 0.02 to 0.05 mg/kg IM 30 to 60 minutes before surgery.
Adults younger than age 60: 0.07 to 0.08 mg/kg IM 30 to 60 minutes before surgery. Usual dose, 5 mg.

➤ **Moderate sedation before short diagnostic or endoscopic procedures**
Adults ages 60 and older and patients who are debilitated or chronically ill: 0.5 to 1.5 mg IV over at least 2 minutes. Incremental doses shouldn't exceed 1 mg. A total dose of up to 3.5 mg is usually sufficient.
Adults younger than age 60: Initially, small dose not to exceed 2.5 mg IV given slowly over at least 2 minutes; wait at least 2 minutes to evaluate sedative effect. Then repeat in 2 minutes PRN, in small increments of first dose over at least 2 minutes each to achieve desired effect. Total dose of up to 5 mg may be used.
Adjust-a-dose: Additional doses to maintain desired level of sedation may be given by slow titration in increments of 25% of dose used to first reach the sedative end point, if clearly needed.

➤ **To induce sleepiness and amnesia and to relieve apprehension before anesthesia or before and during procedures**
Children ages 12 to 16: Initially, no more than 2.5 mg IV given slowly; repeat in 2 minutes, if needed, in small increments of first dose over at least 2 minutes to achieve desired effect. Total dose of up to 10 mg may be used. Additional doses to maintain desired level of sedation may be given by slow titration in increments of 25% of dose used to first reach the sedative end point.
Children ages 6 to 16 who are cooperative: 0.25 to 0.5 mg/kg PO as a single dose, up to 20 mg.
Children ages 6 to 12: 0.025 to 0.05 mg/kg IV over 2 to 3 minutes. Additional doses may be given in small increments after 2 to 3 minutes. Total dose of up to 0.4 mg/kg, not to exceed 10 mg, may be used.
Children ages 6 months to 5 years: 0.05 to 0.1 mg/kg IV over 2 to 3 minutes. Additional doses may be given in small increments after 2 to 3 minutes. Total dose of up to 0.6 mg/kg, not to exceed 6 mg, may be used.
Infants and children ages 6 months to 5 years or less cooperative, older children: 0.25 to 1 mg/kg PO as a single dose, up to 20 mg.
Children: 0.1 to 0.15 mg/kg IM. Use up to 0.5 mg/kg in patients who are more anxious. May use total dose of up to 10 mg.
Adjust-a-dose: For children who are obese, base dose on ideal body weight. Children who are at high risk or debilitated and children receiving other sedatives need lower doses.

M

➤ **To induce general anesthesia**

Adults older than age 55: 0.3 mg/kg IV infusion over 20 to 30 seconds if patient hasn't received premedication, or 0.2 mg/kg IV infusion over 20 to 30 seconds if patient has received a sedative or opioid premedication. Allow 2 minutes for effect. Additional increments of 25% of first dose may be needed to complete induction.

Adults younger than age 55: 0.3 to 0.35 mg/kg IV infusion over 20 to 30 seconds if patient hasn't received premedication, or 0.25 mg/kg IV infusion over 20 to 30 seconds if patient has received a sedative or opioid premedication. Allow 2 minutes for effect. Additional increments of 25% of first dose may be needed to complete induction.

Adjust-a-dose: For patients who are debilitated, initially, 0.2 to 0.25 mg/kg. As little as 0.15 mg/kg may be needed.

➤ **As continuous infusion to sedate patients in critical care unit who are intubated**

Adults: Initially, 0.01 to 0.05 mg/kg may be given IV over several minutes, repeated at 10- to 15-minute intervals until adequate sedation is achieved. To maintain sedation, usual initial infusion rate is 0.02 to 0.1 mg/kg/hour. Higher loading dose or infusion rates may be needed in some patients. Use lowest effective rate.

Children: Initially, 0.05 to 0.2 mg/kg may be given IV over 2 to 3 minutes or longer; then continuous infusion at rate of 0.06 to 0.12 mg/kg/hour. Increase or decrease infusion to maintain desired effect.

Neonates older than 32 weeks' gestational age: Initially, 0.06 mg/kg/hour IV. Adjust rate, as needed, using lowest possible rate.

Neonates younger than 32 weeks' gestational age: Initially, 0.03 mg/kg/hour IV. Adjust rate, as needed, using lowest possible rate.

➤ **Status epilepticus (Seizalam)**

Adults: 10 mg IM once.

➤ **Acute treatment of intermittent, stereotypic episodes of frequent seizure activity (distinct from patient's usual seizure pattern) (Nayzilam)**

Adults and children older than age 12: 1 spray (5-mg dose) into one nostril; may repeat in opposite nostril after 10 minutes if no response. Don't use more than two doses per seizure cluster, no more than one episode in 3 days, and no more than five episodes in a month.

➤ **Status epilepticus** ◆

Infants, children, and adolescents: For patients weighing more than 40 kg, 10 mg IM once; for those weighing 13 to 40 kg, 5 mg IM once. Or, 0.2 mg/kg intranasally once (using parenteral solution for injection); maximum dose, 10 mg.

ADMINISTRATION

Boxed Warning Midazolam has been associated with respiratory depression and respiratory arrest, especially when used in non-critical-care settings. Restrict use to hospital and ambulatory care settings that can provide continuous monitoring of cardiac and respiratory function. Ensure availability of resuscitative drugs and equipment and personnel trained in their use and skilled in airway management. ■

PO

• Give drug without regard to food. Dispense syrup directly into mouth and don't mix with any liquid before dispensing.

• Refer to manufacturer's instructions for use of oral dispenser and press-in bottle dispenser.

IV

▼ Drug may be mixed in same syringe with morphine sulfate, meperidine, atropine, or scopolamine.

▼ When mixing infusion, use 5-mg/mL vial and dilute to 0.5 mg/mL with D_5W or NSS.

Boxed Warning Give slowly over at least 2 minutes, and wait at least 2 minutes when initiating or titrating doses to fully evaluate therapeutic effect. Initial adult dose shouldn't exceed 2.5 mg. Lower initial doses are necessary for adults ages 60 and older, for patients who are debilitated, and for those receiving concomitant opioids or other CNS depressants. ■

Boxed Warning Calculate pediatric dosages using mg/kg; titrate all dosages slowly. Initial pediatric dosage depends on child's age, procedure, and route of administration. ■

Boxed Warning Avoid rapid injection (less than 2 minutes) in neonate because rapid injection has been associated with severe hypotension and seizures, particularly when neonate has also received fentanyl. ■

▼ **Incompatibilities:** None listed by manufacturer. Consult drug compatibility reference for more information.

Reactions in bold italics are *life-threatening*.

IM
- Inject deeply into a large muscle.
- Inject Seizalam in mid-outer thigh.

Intranasal
- Don't test or prime nasal spray unit before use.
- Carefully remove nasal spray unit from blister pack. Hold nasal spray unit with thumb on plunger and middle and index fingers on each side of nozzle.
- Place tip of nozzle into one nostril until fingers on either side of nozzle touch bottom of nose; press plunger firmly to deliver dose.

ACTION
May potentiate the effects of GABA, depress the CNS, and suppress the spread of seizure activity.

Route	Onset	Peak	Duration
PO	10–20 min	45–60 min	2–6 hr
IV	90 sec–5 min	Rapid	2–6 hr
IM	15 min	15–60 min	2–6 hr
Intranasal	10 min	8–28 min	2–4 hr

Half-life: 2 to 6 hours.

ADVERSE REACTIONS
CNS: oversedation, drowsiness, amnesia, headache, *seizures,* postictal state, involuntary movements, paresthesia, hallucinations, confusion, dreaming during emergence, insomnia, nightmares, dizziness, paradoxical behavior or excitement, fever, difficulty speaking. **CV:** variations in BP and pulse rate, *arrhythmias.* **EENT:** nystagmus, increased tearing, nasal discomfort, rhinorrhea, congestion, throat irritation, excessive salivation. **GI:** nausea, retching, vomiting, hiccups. **GU:** *AKI.* **Respiratory:** *respiratory depression, apnea,* hyperventilation, shallow respirations, dyspnea, *hypoxia,* rhonchi, coughing, wheezing, *upper airway obstruction.* **Skin:** rash, injection-site reaction. **Other:** hypersensitivity reactions.

INTERACTIONS
Drug-drug. *CNS depressants:* May increase sedative effects. Use together cautiously. Adjust midazolam dosage if used with opiates or other CNS depressants.
CYP3A4 inducers (carbamazepine, phenytoin, rifampin): May decrease midazolam level. Use cautiously and adjust dosage as needed.
CYP3A4 inhibitors (calcium channel blockers, cimetidine, fluconazole, itraconazole,

ketoconazole, macrolide antibiotics [erythromycin]): May increase and prolong midazolam level, CNS depression, and psychomotor impairment. Avoid use together. If must give together, monitor patient closely.
Boxed Warning *Opioids:* May cause slow or difficult breathing, sedation, and death. Avoid use together. If use together is necessary, limit dosage and duration of each drug to minimum necessary for desired effect. ■
Protease inhibitors (ritonavir, saquinavir): May increase midazolam level and prolong sedation. Use together cautiously. Consider lower midazolam doses with combined use.
Theophylline: May antagonize sedative effect of midazolam. Use together cautiously.
Drug-herb. *Ginkgo biloba, St. John's wort:* May decrease drug level. Discourage use together.
Drug-food. *Grapefruit juice:* May increase bioavailability of oral drug. Discourage use together.
Drug-lifestyle. *Alcohol use:* May increase CNS effects. Discourage use together.

EFFECTS ON LAB TEST RESULTS
None reported.

CONTRAINDICATIONS & CAUTIONS
- Contraindicated in patients hypersensitive to drug or its components and in those with acute narrow-angle glaucoma, shock, coma, or acute alcohol intoxication.
- Intrathecal or epidural injection of parenteral forms containing benzyl alcohol is contraindicated.
- ⓘ *Alert:* Drug should only be used with individualization of the dosage.
- Use cautiously in older adults; patients who are debilitated; patients with HF, uncompensated acute illness, impaired gag reflex, or respiratory, kidney, or liver disease; and patients at risk for falls.
- Benzodiazepines are associated with paradoxical reactions (agitation, aggressive behavior, involuntary movements) and anterograde amnesia.
Boxed Warning Midazolam should only be administered by persons specifically trained in use of anesthetics and management of effects of anesthetics, including resuscitation of patients in the age-group being treated. Appropriate emergency equipment must be immediately available. ■

M

Boxed Warning Opioids should only be prescribed with benzodiazepines or other CNS depressants to patients for whom alternative treatment options are inadequate. ■

Boxed Warning Benzodiazepine use exposes patient to risks of abuse, misuse, and addiction, which can lead to overdose or death. Assess each patient's risk of abuse, misuse, and addiction before prescribing and periodically during therapy. ■

Boxed Warning Abrupt discontinuation or rapid dosage reduction of benzodiazepines after continued use may precipitate acute withdrawal reactions, which can be life-threatening. To reduce risk of withdrawal reactions, gradually taper drug to discontinue or reduce dosage. ■

• When overdose is suspected, flumazenil may be used as a reversal agent.

• Risk of suicidality is increased with intranasal form.

⊙ Alert: Repeated or lengthy use of general anesthetics and sedation drugs during surgeries or procedures in children younger than age 3 and in patients during third trimester may affect development of children's brains; weigh benefits against risks.

Dialyzable drug: Unknown.

⚠ Overdose S&S: Excessive sedation, somnolence, confusion, impaired coordination, diminished reflexes, coma, altered vital signs.

PREGNANCY-LACTATION-REPRODUCTION

• Drug crosses placental barrier. Several studies associate benzodiazepine use with increased risk of congenital malformations. Use during pregnancy isn't recommended.

• Encourage patients taking antiepileptic drugs (Seizalam or Nayzilam) during pregnancy to enroll in North American Antiepileptic Drug Pregnancy Registry (1-888-233-2334 or www.aedpregnancyregistry.org).

• Monitor neonate exposed to drug during pregnancy or labor for sedation, respiratory depression, hypotonia, and feeding problems.

• Drug appears in human milk. Use cautiously during breastfeeding.

NURSING CONSIDERATIONS

Boxed Warning A qualified individual, other than the practitioner performing the procedure, should monitor patient throughout procedure. Have oxygen and resuscitation equipment available in case of severe respiratory depression. Excessive amounts and rapid infusion have been linked to respiratory arrest. Continuously monitor patient, including children taking syrup form, for life-threatening respiratory depression. ■

• Monitor BP, HR and rhythm, respirations, airway integrity, and pulse oximetry during procedure.

• For status epilepticus, continuously monitor respiratory and cardiac function until condition stabilizes. Have airway management and resuscitation equipment available.

PATIENT TEACHING

• Teach about drug's use and potential adverse reactions; advise patient to immediately report difficulty breathing.

Boxed Warning Caution patient or caregivers of patient taking an opioid with a benzodiazepine, CNS depressant, or alcohol to seek immediate medical attention for dizziness, light-headedness, extreme sleepiness, slowed or difficult breathing, or unresponsiveness. ■

Boxed Warning Caution patient that benzodiazepines, even at recommended doses, increase the risk of abuse, misuse, and addiction, which can lead to overdose and death, especially when used in combination with other drugs (opioid analgesics), alcohol, or illicit substances. ■

Boxed Warning Review signs and symptoms of benzodiazepine abuse, misuse, and addiction (abdominal pain, amnesia, anorexia, anxiety, aggression, ataxia, blurred vision, confusion, depression, disinhibition, disorientation, dizziness, euphoria, impaired concentration and memory, indigestion, irritability, muscle pain, slurred speech, tremors, vertigo, delirium, paranoia, suicidality, seizures, difficulty breathing, coma). Instruct patient to seek emergency medical care if any occur. Explain proper disposal of unused drug. Advise patient not to take drug at higher dose, more frequently, or for longer than prescribed. ■

Boxed Warning Tell patient that continued use of drug may lead to physical dependence and that abrupt discontinuation or rapid dosage reduction may precipitate acute withdrawal reactions (unusual movements, responses, or expressions; seizures; sudden and severe mental or nervous system changes; depression; seeing or hearing things that others don't; homicidal thoughts; extreme increase in activity or talking; losing touch with reality; suicidality), which can be life-threatening. Instruct patient that discontinuation or dosage reduction may require a slow taper. ■

Boxed Warning Advise patient about possibility of developing protracted withdrawal syndrome (anxiety; trouble remembering, learning, or concentrating; depression; problems sleeping; sensation of insects crawling under skin; weakness; shaking; muscle twitching; burning or prickling feeling in hands, arms, legs, or feet; ringing in ears), with symptoms lasting weeks to more than 12 months. ■

• Because drug diminishes patient's recall of events around the time of surgery, provide written information, family member instructions, and follow-up contact.

 Alert: Discuss with caregivers of child younger than age 3 and with patient who is pregnant the benefits, risks, and appropriate timing of surgery or procedures requiring anesthetics and sedation drugs.

• Warn patient to avoid hazardous activities that require alertness or good coordination until effects of drug are known.

miglitol
MIG-li-tol

Therapeutic class: Antidiabetics
Pharmacologic class: Alpha-glucosidase inhibitors

AVAILABLE FORMS
Tablets: 25 mg, 50 mg, 100 mg

INDICATIONS & DOSAGES
➤ **Adjunct to diet in patients with type 2 diabetes, alone or with a sulfonylurea**
Adults: 25 mg PO t.i.d. May start with 25 mg PO daily and increase gradually to t.i.d. to minimize GI upset. May increase dosage after 4 to 8 weeks to 50 mg PO t.i.d.; may further increase after 3 months, based on HbA$_{1c}$ level, to maximum of 100 mg PO t.i.d.

ADMINISTRATION
PO
• Give drug with first bite of each main meal.

ACTION
Lowers glucose level by inhibiting enzymes in the small intestine, which delays the digestion of carbohydrates after a meal, resulting in a smaller increase in postprandial glucose level.

Route	Onset	Peak	Duration
PO	Unknown	2–3 hr	Unknown

Half-life: About 2 hours.

ADVERSE REACTIONS
GI: abdominal pain, diarrhea, flatulence.
Skin: rash.

INTERACTIONS
Drug-drug. *Digoxin, propranolol:* May decrease bioavailability of these drugs. Monitor clinical response and adjust dosage.
Insulin, sulfonylureas: May increase risk of hypoglycemia. Consider decreasing dosages of miglitol, insulin, and sulfonylureas.
Intestinal adsorbents (charcoal), digestive enzyme preparations (amylase, pancreatin): May reduce effect of miglitol. Avoid use together.
MAO inhibitors, salicylates, SSRIs: May enhance hypoglycemic effect. Monitor therapy.
Thiazide and thiazide-like diuretics (hydrochlorothiazide, indapamide): May decrease therapeutic effect of antidiabetics. Monitor therapy.

EFFECTS ON LAB TEST RESULTS
• May decrease iron level.

CONTRAINDICATIONS & CAUTIONS
• Contraindicated in patients hypersensitive to drug or its components; in those with diabetic ketoacidosis, inflammatory bowel disease, colonic ulceration, partial intestinal obstruction, chronic intestinal diseases with marked disorders of digestion or absorption, or conditions that may deteriorate because of increased gas formation in intestine; and in those predisposed to intestinal obstruction.
• Drug isn't recommended in patients with CrCl less than 25 mL/minute or if serum creatinine level is more than 2 mg/dL.
• Fever, trauma, infection, or surgery can cause temporary loss of blood glucose control; temporary insulin therapy may be needed.
• Safety and effectiveness in children haven't been established.

M

Dialyzable drug: Unknown.
⚠ **Overdose S&S:** Transient increases in flatulence, diarrhea, and abdominal discomfort.

PREGNANCY-LACTATION-REPRODUCTION
• Safe use in pregnancy hasn't been established. Abnormal blood glucose level during pregnancy may cause harm to fetus. Most experts recommend insulin use during pregnancy to maintain blood glucose level. Don't use miglitol during pregnancy unless clearly needed.
• Drug appears in human milk. Use during breastfeeding isn't recommended.

NURSING CONSIDERATIONS
• In patient also taking insulin or a sulfonylurea, dosage adjustment of these drugs may be needed. Monitor patient for hypoglycemia.
• Diabetes management should include diet control, an exercise program, and regular testing of urine and glucose level.
• Regularly monitor glucose level, especially during situations of increased stress (infection, fever, surgery, trauma).
• Monitor HbA$_{1c}$ level every 3 months to evaluate long-term glycemic control.
• Treat mild to moderate hypoglycemia with a ready form of sugar, such as glucose tablets or gel. Severe hypoglycemia may necessitate IV glucose or glucagon.
• Monitor patient for adverse GI effects.

PATIENT TEACHING
• Teach about proper drug administration and handling.
• Stress importance of adhering to diet, weight reduction, and exercise instructions. Urge patient to undergo regular testing of glucose and HbA$_{1c}$ levels.
• Inform patient that drug treatment relieves symptoms but doesn't cure diabetes.
• Teach patient how to recognize high and low glucose levels.
• Instruct patient to have a source of glucose readily available to treat hypoglycemia.
• Advise patient that sucrose (table sugar, cane sugar) and fruit juices shouldn't be used to treat low-glucose reactions with this drug. Oral glucose (dextrose) or glucagon is necessary to increase glucose.
• Caution patient to promptly seek medical advice during periods of stress (fever, trauma, infection, surgery) because dosage adjustment may be necessary.

• Show patient how and when to monitor glucose level.
• Advise patient that adverse GI effects are most common during first few weeks of therapy and should improve over time.
• Urge patient to carry medical identification at all times.

milnacipran hydrochloride
mil-NAY-ci-pran

Savella

Therapeutic class: Antifibromyalgia drugs
Pharmacologic class: SSNRIs

AVAILABLE FORMS
Tablets: 12.5 mg, 25 mg, 50 mg, 100 mg

INDICATIONS & DOSAGES
➤ **Fibromyalgia**
Adults: Initially, 12.5 mg PO once daily; increased to 12.5 mg b.i.d. on days 2 and 3, then 25 mg b.i.d. on days 4 to 7, then increased to 50 mg b.i.d. after day 7. May increase to 100 mg PO b.i.d. based on individual response; recommended dosage is 50 mg b.i.d.
Adjust-a-dose: For patients with CrCl of 5 to 29 mL/minute, give 25 mg b.i.d. May increase to 50 mg b.i.d. based on individual tolerance.

ADMINISTRATION
PO
• Give drug with or without food, but giving with food may improve tolerability.

ACTION
Unclear. Milnacipran is a potent inhibitor of neuronal norepinephrine and serotonin reuptake; however, it doesn't affect the uptake of dopamine or other transmitters.

Route	Onset	Peak	Duration
PO	Unknown	2–4 hr	36–48 hr

Half-life: 6 to 8 hours; active metabolite, 8 to 10 hours.

ADVERSE REACTIONS
CNS: anxiety, depression, dizziness, falls, fatigue, fever, hypoesthesia, irritability, insomnia, migraine, paresthesia, stress, somnolence, headache, tremors, taste alteration.
CV: chest discomfort, chest pain, flushing, HTN, palpitations, peripheral edema,

tachycardia. **EENT:** blurred vision, dry mouth. **GI:** abdominal distention, abdominal pain, constipation, decreased appetite, diarrhea, flatulence, GERD, dyspepsia, nausea, vomiting. **GU:** cystitis, UTI; in men— dysuria, ejaculation disorder, ejaculation failure, erectile dysfunction, libido decrease, prostatitis, scrotal pain, testicular pain, testicular swelling, urethral pain, urinary hesitation, urine retention, urine flow decrease. **Metabolic:** weight loss or gain, hypercholesterolemia. **Respiratory:** dyspnea, URI. **Skin:** hyperhidrosis, pruritus, rash. **Other:** chills, contusion, hot flush, night sweats.

INTERACTIONS

Drug-drug. *Amphetamines, antipsychotics (risperidone), buspirone, cyclobenzaprine, dopamine antagonists (metoclopramide):* May cause serotonin syndrome. If use together can't be avoided, closely monitor patient for signs and symptoms of serotonin syndrome.

⊘ Alert: *Aspirin, NSAIDs, platelet inhibitors, warfarin:* May increase risk of bleeding. Use together cautiously.

Clomipramine: May cause euphoria and orthostatic hypotension when switching from clomipramine to milnacipran. Use together may also increase risk of serotonin syndrome. Monitor patient closely.

Clonidine: May decrease antihypertensive effect of clonidine. Monitor therapy.

Digoxin: May cause orthostatic hypotension and tachycardia and digoxin-related adverse effects. Avoid use of digoxin IV; when using oral digoxin and drug together, monitor patient closely.

Epinephrine, norepinephrine: May cause paroxysmal HTN and arrhythmia. Use together cautiously.

Linezolid, methylene blue: May cause CNS toxicity and serotonin syndrome. Avoid use together.

Lithium, other serotonergic drugs (SNRIs, SSRIs, TCAs, tramadol, triptans): May cause serotonin syndrome. Avoid use together.

MAO inhibitors: May cause serotonin syndrome. Avoid using drug within 2 weeks after MAO inhibitor therapy; wait at least 5 days after stopping milnacipran or before starting MAO inhibitor.

Drug-herb. *Herbs with anticoagulant properties (alfalfa, anise, bilberry):* May increase risk of bleeding. Use together cautiously.

St. John's wort: May increase risk of serotonin syndrome. Avoid use together.

Drug-lifestyle. *Alcohol use:* May enhance psychomotor impairment and aggravate pre-existing liver disease. Don't administer to patients using alcohol or those with chronic liver disease.

EFFECTS ON LAB TEST RESULTS
- May increase transaminase levels.
- May decrease sodium level.

CONTRAINDICATIONS & CAUTIONS
- Contraindicated in patients hypersensitive to drug or its components.

⊘ Alert: Pupillary dilation that occurs after drug use may trigger an angle-closure attack in patients with anatomically narrow angles who don't have a patent iridectomy.

⊘ Alert: Serotonin syndrome, a potentially life-threatening condition, may occur, particularly with concomitant use of serotonergic drugs (including triptans and tramadol) and drugs that impair serotonin metabolism (including MAO inhibitors).

- Use cautiously in patients with history of mania, seizures, Child-Pugh class C liver impairment, or dysuria; in patients who consume substantial amounts of alcohol; and in those with HTN or controlled angle-closure glaucoma.

Boxed Warning Drug may increase risk of suicidality in children, adolescents, and young adults with major depressive disorder or other psychiatric disorder. Drug isn't approved for use in children. ■

Dialyzable drug: Unlikely.

⚠ Overdose S&S: HTN, cardiac arrest, decreased level of consciousness, confusion, dizziness, elevated LFT results.

PREGNANCY-LACTATION-REPRODUCTION
- Studies during pregnancy are inadequate. Use during pregnancy only if potential benefit justifies fetal risk. Neonates exposed to SSRIs or SNRIs late in third trimester have developed complications requiring prolonged hospitalization, respiratory support, and tube feeding.
- Manufacturer advises patients who are pregnant to enroll in Savella Pregnancy Registry (1-877-643-3010 or www.savellapregnancyregistry.com).
- Drug appears in human milk. Use cautiously during breastfeeding. Monitor infant

for agitation, irritability, poor feeding, and poor weight gain.

NURSING CONSIDERATIONS

• Monitor patient closely for worsening depression or suicidality, especially during first few months of therapy and with dosage adjustments.

• To prevent withdrawal signs and symptoms, decrease dosage gradually and watch for signs and symptoms that may arise when drug is stopped (dysphoria, irritability, agitation, dizziness, sensory disturbances, anxiety, confusion, headache, lethargy, emotional lability, insomnia, hypomania, tinnitus, seizures).

• Monitor for serotonin syndrome, including mental status changes (agitation, coma, hallucinations), autonomic instability (hyperthermia, labile BP, tachycardia), neuromuscular aberrations (hyperreflexia, incoordination), diarrhea, nausea, and vomiting.

• Carefully monitor HR and BP.

• Monitor for signs and symptoms of hyponatremia (headache, difficulty concentrating, memory impairment, confusion, weakness, unsteadiness, hallucination, syncope, seizures, coma, respiratory arrest).

• Monitor LFT values and sodium level before and during therapy.

• Monitor for dysuria, urine retention, and sexual dysfunction.

PATIENT TEACHING

Boxed Warning Warn families and caregivers to immediately report signs and symptoms of worsening depression (agitation, irritability, insomnia, hostility, impulsivity) and suicidality. ■

• Advise patient to avoid NSAIDs and aspirin while taking drug to reduce risk of bleeding.

• Tell patient to avoid alcohol while taking drug.

• Instruct patient to have frequent HR and BP monitoring.

• Tell patient to report urinary hesitation, urine retention, or signs and symptoms of sexual dysfunction. Discuss management strategies.

• Instruct patient to report pregnancy or plans to become pregnant or breastfeed.

• Warn patient not to stop drug suddenly.

• Tell patient to consult prescriber before taking other prescription or OTC drugs or herbal supplements.

• Warn patient to avoid hazardous activities that require alertness and good coordination until drug's effects are known.

• Teach about proper drug administration and handling.

SAFETY ALERT!

milrinone lactate
MIL-ri-none

Therapeutic class: Inotropes
Pharmacologic class: Bipyridine phosphodiesterase inhibitors

AVAILABLE FORMS

Injection: 1 mg/mL vial
Injection (premixed): 200 mcg/mL in D_5W

INDICATIONS & DOSAGES

➤ **Short-term treatment of acutely decompensated HF**

Adults: Give first loading dose of 50 mcg/kg IV slowly over 10 minutes; then give continuous IV infusion of 0.375 to 0.75 mcg/kg/minute (0.59 to 1.13 mg/kg/day). Titrate infusion dose based on clinical and hemodynamic responses. Maximum dosage, 1.13 mg/kg/day.

Adjust-a-dose: If CrCl is 50 mL/minute, infuse at 0.43 mcg/kg/minute; if 40 mL/minute, infuse at 0.38 mcg/kg/minute; if 30 mL/minute, infuse at 0.33 mcg/kg/minute; if 20 mL/minute, infuse at 0.28 mcg/kg/minute; if 10 mL/minute, infuse at 0.23 mcg/kg/minute; and if 5 mL/minute, infuse at 0.2 mcg/kg/minute.

ADMINISTRATION

IV

▼ Give loading dose undiluted as direct injection over 10 minutes.

▼ For continuous IV infusion, dilute vials labeled as containing 10, 20, or 50 mg of milrinone with 40, 80, or 200 mL, respectively, of ½ NSS, NSS, or D_5W to provide solutions containing approximately 200 mcg/mL of milrinone. Don't dilute 200-mcg/mL commercially available bags.

▼ Visually inspect solution. Discard if discoloration or particulate matter is present.

▼ Don't use premixed containers in series connections or administer with blood because of risk of air embolism.

▼ **Incompatibilities:** None listed by manufacturer. Consult drug compatibility reference for more information.

ACTION
Produces inotropic action by increasing cellular levels of cAMP and vasodilation by relaxing vascular smooth muscle.

Route	Onset	Peak	Duration
IV	5–15 min	Unknown	Unknown

Half-life: 2.4 hours.

ADVERSE REACTIONS
CNS: headache. **CV:** *ventricular arrhythmias,* ventricular ectopic activity, *ventricular tachycardia,* hypotension, nonsustained ventricular tachycardia, supraventricular arrhythmias, chest pain.

INTERACTIONS
None significant.

EFFECTS ON LAB TEST RESULTS
• May cause abnormal LFT results.

CONTRAINDICATIONS & CAUTIONS
• Contraindicated in patients hypersensitive to drug. Formulations containing dextrose may be contraindicated in patients with known allergy to corn or corn products.
• *Alert:* Use of milrinone for more than 48 hours in patients with HF hasn't been shown to be safe or effective.
• *Alert:* Drug has been associated with increased frequency of ventricular arrhythmias, including nonsustained ventricular tachycardia and supraventricular tachycardia and ventricular fibrillation in the high-risk population. Monitor patient closely.
• Drug isn't recommended for use in patients with severe aortic or pulmonic valvular disease in place of surgery and during acute phase after MI.
• Use cautiously in patients with atrial flutter or fibrillation because drug may increase ventricular response rate.
• Safety and effectiveness in children haven't been established.
Dialyzable drug: Unknown.
⚠ *Overdose S&S:* Hypotension.

PREGNANCY-LACTATION-REPRODUCTION
• Studies during pregnancy are inadequate. Use during pregnancy only if potential benefit justifies fetal risk.
• It isn't known if drug appears in human milk. Use cautiously during breastfeeding.

NURSING CONSIDERATIONS
• Monitor cardiac rhythm during infusion.
• In patients with atrial flutter or fibrillation, drug is typically given with digoxin and diuretics.
• Improved cardiac output may increase urine output. Reduce diuretic dosage when HF improves. Potassium loss may cause digoxin toxicity.
• Monitor fluid and electrolyte status, BP, HR, and kidney function during therapy. Excessive decrease in BP requires stopping or slowing rate of infusion.
• Correct hypoxemia and electrolyte imbalances, especially hypokalemia and hypomagnesemia, before use and throughout therapy.

PATIENT TEACHING
• Instruct patient to promptly report adverse reactions, especially angina or palpitations.
• Explain that drug may cause headaches, which can be treated with analgesics.
• Teach patient to report discomfort at IV insertion site.

---

minocycline hydrochloride
mi-noe-SYE-kleen

Minocin, Minolira, Solodyn, Ximino

Therapeutic class: Antibiotics
Pharmacologic class: Tetracyclines

AVAILABLE FORMS
Capsules ⓓⓝⓒ: 50 mg, 75 mg, 100 mg
Capsules (extended-release): 45 mg, 90 mg, 135 mg
Injection: 100-mg vial
Tablets: 50 mg, 75 mg, 100 mg
Tablets (extended-release) ⓓⓝⓒ: 45 mg, 55 mg, 65 mg, 80 mg, 90 mg, 105 mg, 115 mg, 135 mg

INDICATIONS & DOSAGES
Adjust-a-dose (for all indications): Decrease dosage or increase dosing interval in patients with kidney impairment. Don't exceed 200 mg (immediate-release) in 24 hours.

➤ **Infections caused by susceptible gram-negative and gram-positive organisms (including *Haemophilus ducreyi*, *Yersinia pestis*, and *Campylobacter fetus*), other organisms (including *Rickettsiae* species, *Mycoplasma pneumoniae*, *Chlamydia trachomatis*, and *Clostridioides* species)**

Adults: 200 mg PO or IV initially; then 100 mg PO or IV every 12 hours. May use 100 or 200 mg PO initially; then 50 mg q.i.d. Maximum dosage, 400 mg/day.

Children older than age 8: Initially, 4 mg/kg PO or IV; then 2 mg/kg PO or IV every 12 hours. Maximum, 100 mg/dose or 200 mg/dose for loading dose.

Adjust-a-dose: Duration of therapy varies with type and severity of infection.

➤ **Gonorrhea in patients allergic to penicillin**

Adults: Initially, 200 mg PO or IV; then 100 mg PO or IV every 12 hours for at least 4 days. Obtain samples for follow-up cultures within 2 to 3 days after treatment.

➤ **Syphilis in patients allergic to penicillin**

Adults: Initially, 200 mg PO or IV; then 100 mg PO or IV every 12 hours for 10 to 15 days.

➤ **Meningococcal carrier state**

Adults: 100 mg PO every 12 hours for 5 days.

➤ **Uncomplicated urethral, endocervical, or rectal infection caused by *C. trachomatis* or *Ureaplasma urealyticum***

Adults: 100 mg PO every 12 hours for at least 7 days. Or, 200 mg IV initially; then 100 mg IV every 12 hours, not to exceed 400 mg in 24 hours.

➤ **Uncomplicated gonococcal urethritis**

Adult males: 100 mg PO every 12 hours for 5 days.

➤ **Treatment of inflammatory lesions of nonnodular moderate to severe acne vulgaris**

Adults and children ages 12 and older: 1 mg/kg extended-release capsules or tablets PO once daily for 12 weeks.

➤ **Acne vulgaris**

Adults: Initially, 200 mg (immediate-release) PO; then 100 mg PO every 12 hours. Or, initially 100 to 200 mg (immediate-release) PO followed by 50 mg PO every 6 hours.

Children ages 8 and older: Initially, 4 mg/kg (immediate-release) PO followed by 2 mg/kg PO every 12 hours. Maximum, 200 mg for loading dose and 100 mg/dose for additional doses.

ADMINISTRATION

• Obtain specimen for culture and sensitivity tests before first dose. Begin therapy while awaiting results.

PO

• Give drug with full glass of water. Patient may take with food to help decrease esophageal irritation.

• Don't give drug within 1 hour of bedtime, to avoid esophageal irritation or ulceration.

• Give capsules and extended-release tablets at same time each day, with or without food.

• Have patient swallow capsules and extended-release tablets whole; don't crush or break them (except Minolira extended-release tablets, which may be split on score line).

• Don't expose drug to light, heat, or moisture.

IV

▼ Reconstitute powder with 5 mL sterile water for injection; further dilute to 100 to 1,000 mL with sodium chloride injection, dextrose injection, or dextrose and sodium chloride injection, or to 250 to 1,000 mL with Ringer injection or lactated Ringer injection. (Don't use solutions containing calcium except for lactated Ringer, because a precipitate may form.)

▼ Infuse over 60 minutes, avoid rapid administration, and don't administer with other drugs.

▼ Use parenteral therapy only when oral therapy is inadequate or isn't tolerated. Institute oral therapy as soon as possible.

▼ **Incompatibilities:** Other drugs.

ACTION

May be bacteriostatic by binding to microorganism's ribosomal subunits, inhibiting protein synthesis; may also alter the cytoplasmic membrane of susceptible microorganisms.

Route	Onset	Peak	Duration
PO	Unknown	1–4 hr	Unknown
PO (extended-release)	Unknown	3.5–4 hr	Unknown
IV	Unknown	Unknown	Unknown

Half-life: PO, 11.1 to 22.1 hours; IV, 15 to 23 hours.

ADVERSE REACTIONS

CNS: headache, light-headedness, dizziness, vertigo, mood alterations, somnolence, fatigue, *seizure,* malaise, drowsiness, fever, paresthesia, hypesthesia, sedation.

Reactions in bold italics are *life-threatening*.

CV: vasculitis, thrombophlebitis. **EENT:** tooth discoloration, tinnitus, dry mouth, oral candidiasis, glossitis. **GI:** anorexia, diarrhea, nausea, dysphagia, vomiting, dyspepsia, *pancreatitis,* stomatitis, enterocolitis, *pseudomembranous colitis.* **GU:** interstitial kidney inflammation, vulvovaginitis. **Hematologic:** *thrombocytopenia,* hemolytic anemia, *neutropenia,* eosinophilia. **Hepatic:** jaundice, *liver toxicity.* **Musculoskeletal:** arthralgia, myalgia, joint swelling, arthritis. **Respiratory:** *bronchospasm,* cough, dyspnea, *asthma exacerbation,* pneumonitis. **Skin:** maculopapular and erythematous rashes; pruritus; urticaria; hyperpigmentation of nails, skin, and mucous membranes; alopecia; injection-site reaction. **Other:** superinfection, discolored secretions, hypersensitivity reactions.

INTERACTIONS

Drug-drug. *Antacids (including sodium bicarbonate) and laxatives containing aluminum, magnesium, or calcium; antidiarrheals:* May decrease oral antibiotic absorption. Give antibiotic 1 hour before or 2 hours after these drugs.

Ergot alkaloids and their derivative: May increase risk of liver toxicity. Avoid use together.

Ferrous sulfate and other iron products, zinc: May decrease iron absorption and minocycline level. Give oral drug 2 hours before or 3 hours after iron.

Hormonal contraceptives: May decrease contraceptive effectiveness and increase risk of breakthrough bleeding. Advise patient to use second form of nonhormonal contraceptive.

Isotretinoin: May increase ICP. Don't use together.

Live-virus vaccines: May decrease vaccine effectiveness. Avoid administering together.

Methoxyflurane: May cause kidney toxicity. Avoid use together.

Oral anticoagulants: May increase anticoagulant effect. Monitor PT and INR, and adjust dosage.

Penicillins: May disrupt bactericidal action of penicillins. Avoid use together.

Retinoids (isotretinoin): May increase risk of pseudotumor cerebri. Avoid use together.

Drug-lifestyle. *Sun or UV light exposure:* May cause photosensitivity reactions. Advise patient to avoid excessive sunlight or UV exposure.

EFFECTS ON LAB TEST RESULTS

- May increase BUN and liver enzyme levels.
- May increase eosinophil count.
- May decrease Hb level and platelet and neutrophil counts.
- May falsely elevate fluorometric test results for urine catecholamines.

CONTRAINDICATIONS & CAUTIONS

- Contraindicated in patients hypersensitive to drug or other tetracyclines.

⚠ *Alert:* Severe and fatal cases of hypersensitivity reactions (including anaphylaxis and SCARs) have been reported.

- Use cautiously in patients with impaired kidney or liver function. Use IV formulations containing magnesium cautiously in patients with heart block or myocardial damage.
- Use of oral minocycline in children younger than age 8 may cause permanent discoloration of teeth, enamel defects, and bone growth retardation.
- Drug may cause superinfection, including CDAD and fungal infections. If overgrowth of nonsusceptible organisms occurs, discontinue drug and begin appropriate therapy.
- Increased ICP and pseudotumor cerebri have been reported. If visual disturbances occur, prompt ophthalmologic exam is needed.
- Drug may cause autoimmune syndromes, including drug-induced lupus-like syndrome, autoimmune hepatitis, and vasculitis with long-term acne treatment.
- Drug may cause hyperpigmentation of many organs, including nails, bone, skin, eyes, thyroid, oral mucosa, sclerae, and heart valves.

Dialyzable drug: No.

⚠ *Overdose S&S:* Dizziness, nausea, vomiting.

PREGNANCY-LACTATION-REPRODUCTION

- Studies during pregnancy are inadequate. Drug may cause fetal harm, including inhibiting bone growth and permanent tooth discoloration. Avoid use in pregnancy.
- If pregnancy occurs during therapy, stop drug immediately and apprise patient of potential fetal hazard.
- Drug appears in human milk. Patient should discontinue breastfeeding or discontinue drug, considering importance of drug to patient.
- Drug shouldn't be used to treat acne in patient attempting to conceive a child.

NURSING CONSIDERATIONS
• Monitor kidney function and LFT results.
• **Alert:** Check expiration date. Outdated or deteriorated drug may cause reversible kidney toxicity (Fanconi syndrome).
• If large doses are given, therapy is prolonged, or patient is at high risk, monitor for signs and symptoms of superinfection.
• Drug may cause mild to severe CDAD, which can occur up to 2 months after therapy ends. If diarrhea occurs, evaluate patient for CDAD. Drug may need to be discontinued and appropriate therapy begun.
• Check patient's tongue for signs of candidal infection. Stress good oral hygiene.
• Drug may discolor teeth in older children and young adults, more commonly when used long term. Watch for brown pigmentation; notify prescriber if it occurs.
• Photosensitivity reactions may occur within a few minutes to several hours after exposure. Photosensitivity lasts after therapy ends.
• Monitor patient for hypersensitivity reactions. Immediately discontinue drug if reaction occurs.
• **Look alike–sound alike:** Don't confuse Minocin with niacin or minoxidil.

PATIENT TEACHING
• Tell patient to take entire amount of drug exactly as prescribed, even if feeling better.
• Instruct patient how to properly administer prescribed formulation.
• Teach about potential adverse reactions, and instruct patient to promptly report them.
• Warn patient to avoid driving and other hazardous tasks because of possible adverse CNS effects.
• Caution patient to avoid direct sunlight and UV light, wear protective clothing, and use sunscreen.
• Warn that diarrhea may occur up to 2 months after last dose. Tell patient to report diarrhea to prescriber.
• Tell patient not to take drug if pregnant or trying to become pregnant because of potential fetal hazard.
• Warn patient that drug can decrease hormonal contraceptive effectiveness. Advise use of an additional nonhormonal method.

mirabegron
mir-a-BEG-ron

Myrbetriq

Therapeutic class: Bladder antispasmodics
Pharmacologic class: Beta$_3$-adrenergic agonists

AVAILABLE FORMS
Granules (extended-release oral suspension): 8 mg/mL (after reconstitution)
Tablets (extended-release) ⒹⓃⒸ: 25 mg, 50 mg

INDICATIONS & DOSAGES
Adjust-a-dose (for all indications): For adults with CrCl of 15 to 29 mL/minute or Child-Pugh class B liver impairment, give no more than 25 mg daily. Drug isn't recommended for patients with CrCl of less than 15 mL/minute or for patients with Child-Pugh class C liver impairment. Refer to manufacturer's instructions for recommended dosing in children ages 3 and older weighing less than 35 kg with kidney or liver impairment.
➤ **Overactive bladder with symptoms of urge incontinence, urgency, and frequency**
Adults: Initially, 25 mg PO once daily. Based on individual patient effectiveness and tolerability, may increase dosage to 50 mg once daily after 4 to 8 weeks.
➤ **Overactive bladder with symptoms of urge incontinence, urgency, and frequency in combination with solifenacin succinate**
Adults: Initially, mirabegron 25 mg PO once daily with solifenacin 5 mg PO once daily. May increase mirabegron to 50 mg PO once daily with solifenacin 5 mg PO once daily after 4 to 8 weeks if necessary.
➤ **Neurogenic detrusor overactivity**
Children ages 3 and older weighing 35 kg or more: 25 mg tablets or 6 mL (48 mg) granules PO once daily. After 4 to 8 weeks, may increase to maximum dosage of 50 mg tablets or 10 mL (80 mg) granules once daily.
Children ages 3 and older weighing 22 to less than 35 kg (extended-release granules): Initially, 4 mL (32 mg) PO once daily. After 4 to 8 weeks, may increase to maximum dosage of 8 mL (64 mg) PO once daily.
Children ages 3 and older weighing 11 to less than 22 kg (extended-release granules): Initially, 3 mL (24 mg) PO once daily. After 4 to

8 weeks, may increase to maximum dosage of 6 mL (48 mg) once daily.

ADMINISTRATION
PO
- May give tablets without regard to food.
- Patient should swallow tablets whole with water; don't crush or cut tablets.
- Give granule suspension with food.
- Granule dosing for adults hasn't been determined.
- For suspension, measure 100 mL of water and add total volume to the bottle; immediately shake vigorously for 1 minute. Let stand for 10 to 30 minutes. Shake vigorously again for 1 to 2 minutes until granules have dispersed.
- Give suspension with an appropriate dosing device.
- Store reconstituted suspension at room temperature for up to 28 days. Discard unused portion after 28 days.
- Give missed dose as soon as possible unless more than 12 hours have elapsed; then omit missed dose and give next scheduled dose.

ACTION
Relaxes the detrusor smooth muscle during storage phase of the urinary bladder fill-void cycle, increasing bladder capacity.

Route	Onset	Peak	Duration
PO	Unknown	3.5 hr	Unknown

Half-life: Adults, 50 hours; children, 26 to 31 hours.

ADVERSE REACTIONS
CNS: headache, fatigue, dizziness. **CV:** HTN, tachycardia. **EENT:** nasopharyngitis, dry mouth, sinusitis. **GI:** constipation, nausea, diarrhea, abdominal pain, gastroenteritis. **GU:** UTI, cystitis, urine retention. **Musculoskeletal:** arthralgia, back pain. **Respiratory:** URI, cough. **Other:** flulike symptoms.

INTERACTIONS
Drug-drug. *Digoxin:* May increase digoxin level. Monitor digoxin level and titrate mirabegron to lowest effective dosage.
Drugs metabolized by CYP2D6 (desipramine, flecainide, metoprolol, propafenone, thioridazine): May increase levels of these drugs. Monitor patient for adverse events; adjust dosage as needed.
Metoprolol: May decrease antihypertensive effect. Closely monitor BP.

Muscarinic antagonists (solifenacin): May increase risk of urine retention. Use together cautiously.
Warfarin: May increase warfarin level. Monitor INR; adjust warfarin dosage as necessary.

EFFECTS ON LAB TEST RESULTS
- May increase ALT, AST, GGT, and LDH levels.

CONTRAINDICATIONS & CAUTIONS
- Contraindicated in patients hypersensitive to drug or its components.
- Drug isn't recommended for use in patients with severe, uncontrolled HTN (systolic BP 180 mm Hg or higher or diastolic BP 110 mm Hg or higher) or eGFR less than 15 mL/minute/1.73 m^2 or those on KRT.
- Use cautiously in patients with HTN or bladder outlet obstruction.
- Safety and effectiveness in children younger than age 3 haven't been established.
Dialyzable drug: Unknown.
⚠ *Overdose S&S:* Palpitations, increased HR, increased BP.

PREGNANCY-LACTATION-REPRODUCTION
- Studies during pregnancy are inadequate. Use during pregnancy only if potential benefit justifies fetal risk.
- It isn't known if drug appears in human milk. Patient should discontinue breastfeeding or discontinue drug, considering importance of drug to patient.

NURSING CONSIDERATIONS
- Regularly monitor BP and pulse, especially in patient with HTN or atrial fibrillation.
- Monitor for angioedema of face, lips, tongue, or larynx, which may be life-threatening and can occur after first dose. Promptly discontinue drug if airway involvement occurs; ensure a patent airway.
- Monitor patient closely for urine retention and bladder obstruction, especially in those already taking bladder antispasmodics.
- Periodically monitor LFT values.
- Monitor patient for rash or pruritus.

PATIENT TEACHING
- Teach about proper drug administration and handling for prescribed formulation.
- Warn that drug may cause an increase in BP or pulse. Teach patient to monitor BP

and pulse at home and to report increases to health care provider.

• Explain that difficulty emptying the bladder and infrequent bladder infections may occur. Instruct patient to report concerns to health care provider.

• Tell patient to report rash or itching, which may indicate an allergy or a serious adverse reaction.

• Advise patient to immediately report signs and symptoms of a significant reaction (fast heartbeat, palpitations, back pain, bloody urine, chills, severe dizziness, passing out, severe headache, wheezing, chest tightness, fever, bad cough, blue skin, seizures, or swelling of face, lips, tongue, or throat).

• Teach patient to report pregnancy to health care provider as soon as possible.

mirtazapine
mir-TAZ-a-peen

Remeron, Remeron SolTab

Therapeutic class: Antidepressants
Pharmacologic class: Tetracyclic antidepressants

AVAILABLE FORMS
Tablets: 7.5 mg, 15 mg, 30 mg, 45 mg
Tablets (ODTs) ☐ 15 mg, 30 mg, 45 mg

INDICATIONS & DOSAGES
➤ **Major depressive disorder**
Adults: Initially, 15 mg PO at bedtime. Maintenance dose is 15 to 45 mg daily. Adjust dosage at intervals of at least 1 week.

ADMINISTRATION
PO
• Give drug without regard to food.
• Remove ODT from blister pack and immediately place on patient's tongue.
• ODT may be given with or without water. Tablet disintegrates in saliva.
• Don't split or crush ODT.

ACTION
Thought to enhance central noradrenergic and serotonergic activity.

Route	Onset	Peak	Duration
PO	Unknown	2 hr	Unknown

Half-life: About 20 to 40 hours.

ADVERSE REACTIONS
CNS: somnolence, dizziness, asthenia, abnormal dreams, abnormal thinking, tremors, confusion, drowsiness, agitation, amnesia, anxiety, apathy, depression, hypoesthesia, malaise, myasthenia, thirst, paresthesia, twitching, vertigo. **CV:** edema, peripheral edema, HTN, vasodilation. **EENT:** angle-closure glaucoma, dry mouth, sinusitis. **GI:** increased appetite, anorexia, constipation, abdominal pain, vomiting, nausea. **GU:** urinary frequency, UTI. **Metabolic:** weight gain. **Musculoskeletal:** myalgia, weakness, back pain, myasthenia, arthralgia. **Respiratory:** dyspnea, cough. **Skin:** pruritus, rash. **Other:** flulike syndrome.

INTERACTIONS
Drug-drug. *Cimetidine:* May increase mirtazapine level. Decrease mirtazapine dose if needed.

Diazepam, other CNS depressants: May cause additive CNS effects. Avoid use together.

Linezolid, methylene blue: May cause serotonin syndrome. Use together is contraindicated.

MAO inhibitors: May increase risk of serotonin syndrome. Use within 14 days of MAO inhibitor therapy is contraindicated.

QT interval-prolonging agents (antiarrhythmics, fluoroquinolones, macrolides): May cause additive QT interval-prolonging effects. Use together cautiously.

Serotonergic drugs (antidepressants, antiemetics [5-HT₃ antagonists], buspirone, fentanyl, lithium, TCAs, tramadol, triptans, tryptophan): May increase risk of serotonin syndrome. Monitor therapy.

Strong CYP3A inducers (carbamazepine, phenytoin, rifampin): May decrease mirtazapine level. Increase mirtazipine dose if needed.

Strong CYP3A inhibitors (ketoconazole, ritonavir, nefazodone): May increase mirtazapine level. Decrease mirtazapine dose if needed.

Warfarin: May increase anticoagulant effect. Closely monitor INR when mirtazapine is started or stopped, and adjust warfarin dosage as needed.

Drug-herb. *St. John's wort:* May increase risk of serotonin syndrome. Use together cautiously, and monitor patient closely for adverse reactions.

Drug-lifestyle. *Alcohol use:* May cause additive CNS effects. Discourage use together.

Reactions in bold italics are *life-threatening*.

EFFECTS ON LAB TEST RESULTS
• May increase CK, cholesterol, and triglyceride levels and LFT values.
• May decrease sodium level.
• May decrease ANC.

CONTRAINDICATIONS & CAUTIONS
• Contraindicated in patients hypersensitive to drug.
Boxed Warning Drug may increase risk of suicidality in children, adolescents, and young adults with MDD or other psychiatric disorders. Drug isn't approved for use in children. ■
• Use cautiously in patients with CV or cerebrovascular disease, seizure disorders, suicidality, liver or kidney impairment, or history of mania or hypomania.
• Use cautiously in patients with conditions that predispose them to hypotension, such as dehydration, hypovolemia, or antihypertensive therapy.
• Use may trigger angle-closure glaucoma attack due to pupil dilation in patients with anatomically narrow angles.
• Give drug cautiously to older adults; decreased clearance may occur.
• Discontinuation syndrome (dizziness, abnormal dreams, sensory disturbances, agitation, anxiety, fatigue, confusion, headache, tremors, nausea, vomiting, sweating) may occur. To prevent, gradually reduce dosage prior to stopping.
Dialyzable drug: Unknown.
⚠ *Overdose S&S:* Disorientation, drowsiness, impaired memory, tachycardia.

PREGNANCY-LACTATION-REPRODUCTION
• Studies during pregnancy are inadequate. Use during pregnancy only if clearly needed.
• Drug may appear in human milk. Use cautiously during breastfeeding.
• Encourage patients who are pregnant to enroll in the National Pregnancy Registry for Antidepressants (1-866-961-2388 or https://womensmentalhealth.org/research/pregnancyregistry/antidepressants/).

NURSING CONSIDERATIONS
🕒 *Alert:* If linezolid or methylene blue must be given, stop mirtazapine and monitor patient for serotonin toxicity for 2 weeks or until 24 hours after last dose of methylene blue or linezolid, whichever comes first. May resume mirtazapine treatment 24 hours after last dose of methylene blue or linezolid.
• Monitor for serotonin syndrome (fever, mental status changes, muscle twitching, diaphoresis, shivering or shaking, diarrhea, loss of coordination).
Boxed Warning Appropriately monitor and closely observe patients of all ages who are started on antidepressants for clinical worsening, mood changes, suicidality, or unusual changes in behavior. ■
• Monitor patient for distressing restlessness and need to move, which occurs most frequently during first few weeks of treatment.
• Although agranulocytosis rarely occurs, stop drug and monitor patient closely if sore throat, fever, stomatitis, or other signs and symptoms of infection with low WBC count develop.
• Monitor for hypersensitivity reactions, including severe skin reactions.
• Lower dosages tend to be more sedating than higher dosages.

PATIENT TEACHING
Boxed Warning Advise families and caregivers to closely observe patient for increasing suicidality. ■
🕒 *Alert:* Teach patient to recognize and immediately report signs and symptoms of serotonin toxicity.
• Caution patient to avoid hazardous activities if feeling too sleepy.
• Tell patient to report signs and symptoms of infection (fever, chills, sore throat, mucous membrane irritation, flulike syndrome).
• Instruct patient not to use alcohol or other CNS depressants while taking drug.
• Instruct patient not to take other drugs or stop drug abruptly without prescriber's approval.
• Caution patient to immediately report faintness, loss of consciousness, or palpitations.
• Tell patient of childbearing potential to immediately report suspected pregnancy and to notify prescriber if breastfeeding.
• Instruct patient how to properly administer prescribed formulation. Warn patient not to abruptly stop drug without discussing with prescriber.
• Inform patient with phenylketonuria that ODTs contain phenylalanine.

mitoXANTRONE hydrochloride
mye-toe-ZAN-trone

Therapeutic class: Antineoplastics
Pharmacologic class: DNA-reactive drugs–anthracenediones

AVAILABLE FORMS
Injection: 2 mg/mL multidose vials

INDICATIONS & DOSAGES
➤ **Combination initial therapy for acute nonlymphocytic leukemia (ANLL)**
Adults: Induction begins with 12 mg/m^2 IV daily on days 1 to 3, with 100 mg/m^2 daily of cytarabine on days 1 to 7 as a continuous 24-hour infusion. A second induction with mitoxantrone for 2 days and cytarabine for 5 days may be given if response isn't adequate. Consolidation therapy: 12 mg/m^2 IV infusion daily on days 1 and 2 and cytarabine 100 mg/m^2 for 5 days given as a continuous 24-hour infusion on days 1 through 5. First course is given approximately 6 weeks after final induction course; second is generally given 4 weeks after first. Severe myelosuppression has occurred with this regimen.
➤ **To reduce neurologic disability and frequency of relapse in chronic progressive, progressive relapsing, or worsening relapsing-remitting MS**
Adults: 12 mg/m^2 IV over 5 to 15 minutes every 3 months. Maximum cumulative lifetime dose, 140 mg/m^2.
➤ **Advanced hormone-refractory prostate cancer in combination with corticosteroids**
Adult males: 12 to 14 mg/m^2 as short IV infusion every 21 days.

ADMINISTRATION
IV
⏺ *Alert:* Hazardous drug; use safe handling and disposal precautions.
▼ Dilute dose in at least 50 mL of NSS or D$_5$W. Don't mix with other drugs. Can further dilute in D$_5$W, NSS, or D$_5$NSS; use immediately if further diluted.
Boxed Warning Give slowly into free-flowing IV infusion of NSS or D$_5$W injection over at least 3 minutes. Never give subcutaneously, intra-arterially, intramuscularly, or intrathecally. Severe local tissue damage may result if extravasation occurs. ▮
▼ Usually given as short infusion over 5 to 15 minutes.
▼ If extravasation occurs, stop infusion immediately and notify prescriber. Place ice packs over the area intermittently.
▼ Once vial is penetrated, store undiluted solution for 7 days at room temperature or 14 days in refrigerator. Don't freeze.
▼ **Incompatibilities:** Other drugs.

ACTION
Reacts with DNA, producing cytotoxic effect. Probably not specific to cell cycle.

Route	Onset	Peak	Duration
IV	Unknown	Unknown	Unknown

Half-life: Terminal half-life, 23 to 215 hours.

ADVERSE REACTIONS
CNS: fever, headache, *seizures,* asthenia, pain, fatigue, anxiety, depression. **CV:** *arrhythmias,* ECG abnormalities, *HF, ischemia,* decreased LVEF, HTN, edema, tachycardia, *hemorrhage.* **EENT:** sinusitis, conjunctivitis, blurred vision, pharyngitis, rhinitis, oral inflammation and pain. **GI:** abdominal pain, *GI hemorrhage,* diarrhea, constipation, mucositis, nausea, stomatitis, vomiting, dyspepsia, anorexia, epigastric pain. **GU:** amenorrhea, menstrual disorder, UTI, *KF,* hematuria, decreased libido, proteinuria, impotence, sterility. **Hematologic:** *myelosuppression,* anemia. **Hepatic:** jaundice, increased transaminase levels, increased GGT. **Metabolic:** hyperuricemia, *hypocalcemia, hypokalemia,* hyponatremia, hyperglycemia, weight gain or loss. **Musculoskeletal:** back pain. **Respiratory:** cough, dyspnea, URI, pneumonia. **Skin:** alopecia, ecchymoses, local irritation or phlebitis, petechiae, diaphoresis, nail bed changes. **Other:** chills, fungal infections, infection, *sepsis.*

INTERACTIONS
Drug-drug. *Clozapine:* May increase risk of neutropenia. Monitor patient closely.
Cyclosporine: May increase effects of mitoxantrone. Monitor patient closely.
Live-virus vaccines: May increase risk of vaccine-induced adverse reactions. Defer vaccination until mitoxantrone therapy has been completed.

Reactions in bold italics are *life-threatening*.

Natalizumab, tofacitinib: May increase risk of immunosuppression. Avoid use together.
Palifermin: May increase severity of oral mucositis. Don't give palifermin within 24 hours before or after mitoxantrone dose.
Pimecrolimus, tacrolimus (topical): May enhance adverse or toxic effect of mitoxantrone. Avoid use together.
Trastuzumab: May increase risk of trastuzumab-induced cardiac dysfunction. Monitor patient closely for signs and symptoms of cardiac dysfunction.

EFFECTS ON LAB TEST RESULTS
• May increase creatinine, BUN, ALT, AST, bilirubin, GGT, uric acid, and urine protein levels.
• May decrease calcium, potassium, and sodium levels.
• May decrease Hb level, hematocrit, and platelet, WBC, and granulocyte counts.

CONTRAINDICATIONS & CAUTIONS
• Contraindicated in patients hypersensitive to drug.
• Drug contains sodium metabisulfite, which may cause an allergic reaction, especially in patients with asthma.
Boxed Warning Present or history of CV disease, radiotherapy to mediastinal or pericardial area, previous therapy with other anthracyclines or anthracenediones, or use of other cardiotoxic drugs may increase risk of cardiotoxicity. ■
• Patients who have significant myelosuppression shouldn't receive drug unless benefits outweigh risks.
• Use cautiously in patients with liver impairment.
Dialyzable drug: No.
⚠ *Overdose S&S:* Severe leukopenia.

PREGNANCY-LACTATION-REPRODUCTION
• Drug may cause fetal harm. Patient should avoid pregnancy during therapy. If used during pregnancy or if pregnancy occurs during therapy, apprise patient of fetal risk.
• Patients with MS who are biologically capable of becoming pregnant even if they are using contraception should have a pregnancy test before each dose, and results should be known before drug administration.
• Drug appears in human milk. Patient should discontinue breastfeeding before starting drug.
• Drug may affect fertility.

NURSING CONSIDERATIONS
Boxed Warning Administer under the supervision of a prescriber experienced with cytotoxic chemotherapy. ■
• Closely monitor for extravasation. If extravasation occurs, initiate antidote of dexrazoxane IV or topical dimethyl sulfoxide (DMSO) as prescribed.
Boxed Warning Except when used to treat ANLL, mitoxantrone should generally not be given to patients with baseline neutrophil count less than 1,500 cells/mm^3. Frequently monitor peripheral blood cell count for all patients using drug. ■
Boxed Warning Assess all patients for cardiac signs and symptoms by history, physical exam, LVEF, and ECG before therapy. Assess patients with MS for cardiac signs and symptoms by history, physical exam, and ECG before each dose. ■
Boxed Warning Drug can cause potentially fatal HF during therapy or months to years after therapy. All patients should have baseline quantitative evaluation of LVEF. In patients with MS, evaluate LVEF before initiating treatment and before administering each dose of mitoxantrone. Patients with MS with a baseline LVEF below the lower limit of normal shouldn't receive mitoxantrone. All patients with MS who have finished treatment should undergo yearly, quantitative LVEF evaluation to detect late-occurring cardiotoxicity. Patients with MS who have experienced either a drop in LVEF to below the lower limit of normal or a clinically significant reduction in LVEF during mitoxantrone therapy shouldn't receive additional doses of mitoxantrone. ■
Boxed Warning Use of drug has been associated with cardiotoxicity; risk increases with cumulative dose of 140 mg/m^2 but can occur at any dose. Continue ongoing cardiac monitoring to detect late-occurring cardiotoxicity. ■
Boxed Warning Patients with MS shouldn't receive a cumulative mitoxantrone dose greater than 140 mg/m^2. ■
• Closely monitor hematologic and chemistry results, including LFT values. Obtain CBC and platelet counts before each course of treatment. Patient may require blood transfusion or RBC or WBC colony-stimulating factors.
• Avoid all IM injections in patient with thrombocytopenia.

M

• If severe nonhematologic toxicity occurs during first course, delay second course until patient recovers.

Boxed Warning Secondary acute myelocytic leukemia has been reported with mitoxantrone therapy. ■

• Verify pregnancy status before treatment in all patients of childbearing potential.

PATIENT TEACHING

• Advise patient to immediately report injection-site discomfort.

• Tell patient that urine may appear blue-green within 24 hours after receiving drug and that the whites of the eyes may turn blue. These effects are not harmful but may persist during therapy.

• Teach about potential adverse reactions, and tell patient to report them. Advise patient to watch for signs and symptoms of bleeding and infection.

• Advise patient of childbearing potential to use appropriate contraceptive method to avoid pregnancy during therapy.

• Inform patient of potential effects on fertility.

modafinil
moe-DAF-i-nil

Alertec✤, Provigil

Therapeutic class: CNS stimulants
Pharmacologic class: Analeptics
Controlled substance schedule: IV

AVAILABLE FORMS
Tablets: 100 mg, 200 mg

INDICATIONS & DOSAGES

➤ **To improve wakefulness in patients with excessive daytime sleepiness caused by narcolepsy, obstructive sleep apnea-hypopnea syndrome, and shift-work sleep disorder**
Adults: 200 mg PO daily, as single dose in morning. Patients with shift-work sleep disorder should take dose about 1 hour before start of shift.

Adjust-a-dose: In patients with Child-Pugh class C liver impairment, give 100 mg PO daily as single dose in the morning. Consider lower dose and close monitoring in older adults.

ADMINISTRATION
PO
• Give drug without regard to food; however, food may delay effect of drug.
• Store drug at room temperature.

ACTION
Unknown. Similar to action of sympathomimetics, including amphetamines, but drug is structurally distinct from amphetamines and doesn't alter release of dopamine or norepinephrine.

Route	Onset	Peak	Duration
PO	Unknown	2–4 hr	Unknown

Half-life: 15 hours.

ADVERSE REACTIONS
CNS: headache, nervousness, dizziness, drowsiness, insomnia, depression, anxiety, paresthesia, hypertonia, hyperkinesia, confusion, emotional lability, vertigo, tremors, dyskinesia, agitation, thirst, taste perversion. **CV:** HTN, vasodilation, chest pain, palpitations, tachycardia, edema. **EENT:** abnormal vision, epistaxis, rhinitis, dry mouth, mouth ulcer, pharyngitis. **GI:** nausea, diarrhea, anorexia, gingivitis, dyspepsia, constipation, flatulence, decreased appetite, abdominal pain. **GU:** abnormal urine. **Hematologic:** eosinophilia. **Hepatic:** abnormal LFT values. **Metabolic:** weight loss. **Musculoskeletal:** back or neck pain. **Respiratory:** *asthma.* **Skin:** diaphoresis. **Other:** chills.

INTERACTIONS
Drug-drug. *CYP2C19 substrates (diazepam, phenytoin, propranolol):* May inhibit CYP2C19, causing higher levels of drugs metabolized by this enzyme. Use together cautiously; adjust dosage as needed.
CYP3A4/5 substrates (cyclosporine, midazolam, triazolam): May decrease substrate level. Adjust substrate dosage as needed.
Dextroamphetamine, methylphenidate: May cause 1-hour delay in modafinil absorption. Separate dosing times.
Hormonal contraceptives: May reduce contraceptive effectiveness. Advise patient to use alternative or additional method of contraception during modafinil therapy and for 1 month after final dose.
MAO inhibitors: May increase risk of hypertensive crisis. Use together cautiously.

Warfarin: May increase warfarin level. Closely monitor PT and INR.
TCAs: May increase TCA level. Reduce TCA dosage.
Drug-lifestyle. *Alcohol use:* Concomitant use hasn't been studied. Avoid use together.

EFFECTS ON LAB TEST RESULTS
• May increase glucose, GGT, and ALP levels.
• May increase eosinophil count.

CONTRAINDICATIONS & CAUTIONS
• Contraindicated in patients hypersensitive to modafinil or its inactive ingredients or armodafinil.
• Drug isn't indicated for treatment of underlying respiratory obstruction as the cause of excessive sleepiness.
• Drug isn't recommended in patients with history of left ventricular hypertrophy or ischemic ECG changes, chest pain, arrhythmias, or other evidence of mitral valve prolapse linked to CNS stimulant use.
• Use cautiously in patients with recent MI or unstable angina, kidney impairment, or history of psychosis or mania.
• Use cautiously and give reduced dosage to patients with Child-Pugh class C liver impairment, with or without cirrhosis.
• Modafinil isn't approved for use in children.
Dialyzable drug: Unknown.
⚠ **Overdose S&S:** Agitation or excitation, insomnia, slight or moderate elevations in hemodynamic parameters, aggressiveness, anxiety, confusion, shortened PT, diarrhea, irritability, nausea, nervousness, palpitations, sleep disturbances, tremors, bradycardia, chest pain, HTN, tachycardia, hallucination, restlessness.

PREGNANCY-LACTATION-REPRODUCTION
• Studies during pregnancy are inadequate. Use during pregnancy only if potential benefit justifies fetal risk.
• Prescribers are encouraged to register patients who are pregnant, or patients may self-enroll, in the Provigil Pregnancy Registry (1-866-404-4106 or www.provigilpregnancyregistry.com).
• Caution patient that use of hormonal contraceptives (including depot or implantable contraceptives) with modafinil may reduce contraceptive effectiveness. Recommend an alternative method of contraception

during therapy and for 1 month after therapy ends.
• It isn't known if drug appears in human milk. Use cautiously during breastfeeding.

NURSING CONSIDERATIONS
• Life-threatening angioedema, SJS, TEN, and DRESS syndrome can occur. Monitor for rash, dysphagia, bronchospasm, fever, and organ dysfunction. Stop drug and begin appropriate treatment if any occur.
• Monitor patient for emergence or exacerbation of psychiatric signs and symptoms, persistent sleepiness, and HTN.
• *Look alike–sound alike:* Don't confuse Provigil with Nuvigil. Don't confuse Alertec with Arthrotec.

PATIENT TEACHING
🔷 *Alert:* Advise patient to stop drug and notify prescriber if rash, peeling skin, trouble swallowing or breathing, or other symptoms of allergic reaction occur.
• Caution patient to report planned, suspected, or known pregnancy or breastfeeding.
• Tell patient to avoid alcohol while taking drug.
• Warn patient to avoid activities that require alertness or good coordination until CNS effects of drug are known.

mometasone furoate
moe-MET-a-sone

Asmanex HFA, Asmanex Twisthaler, Elocon✦

mometasone furoate monohydrate
Nasonex

Therapeutic class: Anti-inflammatory drugs
Pharmacologic class: Glucocorticoids

AVAILABLE FORMS
Cream: 0.1%
Inhalation aerosol: 50 mcg/actuation, 100 mcg/actuation, 200 mcg/actuation, 400 mcg/actuation✦
Inhalation powder: 110 mcg/inhalation, 220 mcg/inhalation
Lotion: 0.1%
Nasal spray: 50 mcg/spray ◇
Ointment: 0.1%

INDICATIONS & DOSAGES
➤ **Maintenance therapy for asthma**
Adults and children ages 12 and older who previously used a bronchodilator alone or an inhaled corticosteroid: Initially, 220 mcg Asmanex Twisthaler by oral inhalation every day in evening. Maximum, 440 mcg/day.
Adults and children ages 12 and older not previously on an inhaled corticosteroid: Using Asmanex HFA 100-mcg inhaler, 2 inhalations b.i.d. (morning and evening). Maximum, 800 mcg/day.
Adults and children ages 12 and older who previously received chronic oral corticosteroid: 440 mcg Asmanex Twisthaler by oral inhalation b.i.d. Maximum, 880 mcg/day. Or, 200 mcg Asmanex HFA by oral inhalation b.i.d. (morning and evening). Maximum, 800 mcg/day.
Children ages 5 to younger than age 12 regardless of prior therapy: Using 50-mcg Asmanex HFA inhaler, 2 inhalations b.i.d. (morning and evening). Maximum, 200 mcg/day.
Children ages 4 to 11 regardless of prior therapy: 110 mcg Asmanex Twisthaler by oral inhalation once daily in evening.
Adjust-a-dose: For patients on long-term oral corticosteroid therapy, reduce oral prednisone dosage by no more than 2.5 mg/day at weekly intervals, beginning at least 1 week after starting mometasone. After stopping oral corticosteroid, reduce mometasone dosage to lowest effective amount. Carefully monitor patient for signs and symptoms of asthma instability and adrenal insufficiency.
➤ **Allergic rhinitis; nasal congestion associated with seasonal allergic rhinitis (OTC products)**
Adults and children ages 12 and older: 2 sprays (50 mcg/spray) in each nostril once daily.
Children ages 2 to 11: 1 spray (50 mcg/spray) in each nostril once daily.
➤ **Prophylaxis of seasonal allergic rhinitis**
Adults and children ages 12 and older: 2 sprays (50 mcg/spray) in each nostril once daily 2 to 4 weeks before anticipated start of pollen season.
➤ **Nasal polyps**
Adults: 2 sprays (50 mcg/spray) in each nostril once daily to b.i.d.
➤ **Dermatoses**
Adults: Apply thin film of cream or ointment to affected areas once daily. Or, apply a few drops of lotion to affected areas and massage lightly. Discontinue when control is achieved. If no improvement occurs within 2 weeks, reassess diagnosis. Elocon may be used on the scalp (lotion), face, axillae, or scrotum (cream, ointment, or lotion) for a maximum of 5 days and on the body (cream, ointment, or lotion) for a maximum of 3 days.
Children ages 12 and older: Apply a few drops of lotion to affected areas once daily and massage lightly. Discontinue when control is achieved. If no improvement occurs within 2 weeks, reassess diagnosis.
Children ages 2 and older: Apply thin film of cream or ointment to affected areas once daily. Discontinue when control is achieved. If no improvement occurs within 2 weeks, reassess diagnosis.

ADMINISTRATION
Inhalational aerosol
• Shake well before each inhalation.
• Prime before first use by releasing four test sprays into air, away from face, shaking well before each spray.
• If the inhaler hasn't been used for more than 5 days, prime inhaler again with four test sprays.
• Have patient rinse mouth with water without swallowing after administration.
Inhalational powder
• Give once-daily dosing in the evening.
• Have patient exhale fully before bringing Twisthaler up to mouth, placing between lips, and inhaling quickly and deeply.
• Patient shouldn't breathe out through inhaler but should remove inhaler and hold breath for 10 seconds, if possible.
• Have patient rinse mouth after administration.
• Discard 45 days after opening foil pouch or when dose counter reads "00."
Intranasal
• Before initial use, prime nasal spray pump 10 times or until fine spray appears.
• May store pump for 1 week without repriming. If unused for more than 1 week, reprime two times or until fine spray appears.
• Shake well before each use.
Topical
• Drug is for topical use only; not for oral, ophthalmic, or intravaginal use. Avoid use on axillae, groin, or face unless directed by prescriber.

Reactions in bold italics are *life-threatening*.

• Don't use with occlusive dressings or in diaper area if child still requires diapers or plastic pants, unless directed by prescriber.

ACTION
Unknown, although corticosteroids inhibit many cells and mediators involved in inflammation and the asthmatic response.

Route	Onset	Peak	Duration
Inhalation	Unknown	1–2.5 hr	Unknown
Intranasal	Unknown	Unknown	Unknown
Topical	8 hr	Unknown	Unknown

Half-life: Oral, 5 hours; nasal and topical, unknown.

ADVERSE REACTIONS
CNS: headache, depression, fatigue, insomnia, pain, paresthesia. **CV:** chest pain. **EENT:** increased IOP, earache, otitis media, epistaxis, nasal irritation, allergic rhinitis, pharyngitis, sinus congestion, sinusitis, dry throat, oral candidiasis, dysphonia. **GI:** abdominal pain, anorexia, dyspepsia, flatulence, gastroenteritis, nausea, vomiting, thrush. **GU:** dysmenorrhea, menstrual disorder, UTI. **Metabolic:** decreased glucocorticoid levels. **Musculoskeletal:** arthralgia, back pain, myalgia. **Respiratory:** URI, bronchitis, wheezing, respiratory disorder, cough. **Skin:** burning; pruritus; skin atrophy; furunculosis; folliculitis; taut, shiny skin; depigmentation; telangiectasia; candidiasis; bacterial infection; bruising. **Other:** flulike symptoms, infection, fever.

INTERACTIONS
Drug-drug. *Esketamine:* May decrease therapeutic effect of esketamine nasal spray. Give mometasone intranasal at least 1 hour before esketamine.
Strong CYP3A4 inhibitors (clarithromycin, cobicistat-containing products, ketoconazole, nefazodone, ritonavir, saquinavir): May increase systemic exposure to mometasone and increase risk of systemic adverse effects, especially with long-term use. Use together cautiously.
Drug-lifestyle. *Smoking:* Smoking tobacco may decrease effect of inhaled mometasone. Discourage smoking, and monitor therapy.

EFFECTS ON LAB TEST RESULTS
None reported.

CONTRAINDICATIONS & CAUTIONS
• Contraindicated in patients hypersensitive to drug or its components, in those hypersensitive to milk proteins (Asmanex Twisthaler only), and in those with status asthmaticus or other acute forms of asthma or bronchospasm (as primary treatment).
• Use cautiously in patients at high risk for decreased bone mineral content (those with family history of osteoporosis, prolonged immobilization, long-term use of drugs that reduce bone mass), patients switching from a systemic to an inhaled corticosteroid, and patients with active or dormant TB, untreated systemic infections, cataracts, glaucoma, ocular herpes simplex, diabetes, myasthenia, MI, thyroid disease, psychiatric disturbances, or immunosuppression.
• Drug may cause HPA axis suppression with potential for glucocorticosteroid insufficiency during treatment or after treatment withdrawal. Periodically evaluate patients for HPA suppression.
❂ **Alert:** Children treated with topical corticosteroids are at greater risk than adults for HPA axis suppression and Cushing syndrome. Don't use to treat diaper dermatitis.
• Discontinue drug if allergic contact dermatitis develops, usually diagnosed by failure to heal.
• If skin infections are present or develop, topical drug may need to be discontinued until infection is controlled.
Dialyzable drug: Unknown.
⚠ **Overdose S&S:** Hypercorticism with long-term overdose.

PREGNANCY-LACTATION-REPRODUCTION
• Studies during pregnancy are inadequate. Use during pregnancy only if clearly needed and benefit justifies fetal risk.
• Systemically administered corticosteroids appear in human milk and could suppress growth, interfere with endogenous corticosteroid production, or cause other untoward effects. Use cautiously during breastfeeding.

NURSING CONSIDERATIONS
❂ **Alert:** Don't use inhalation form for acute bronchospasm. Life-threatening paradoxical bronchospasm can occur after inhalation. Stop drug and use a fast-acting bronchodilator.
• Wean patient slowly from systemic corticosteroid after switching to mometasone. Monitor pulmonary function tests, betaagonist use, and asthma symptoms.

M

🔱 *Alert:* If switching from an oral corticosteroid to an inhaled form, watch patient closely for evidence of adrenal insufficiency (fatigue, lethargy, weakness, nausea, vomiting, hypotension).

• After withdrawal of oral corticosteroid, HPA function may not recover for months. Patient experiencing trauma, stress, infection, or surgery during this HPA recovery period is particularly vulnerable to adrenal insufficiency or adrenal crisis.

• Because inhaled and topical corticosteroids can be systemically absorbed, watch for cushingoid effects.

• Assess for bone loss with long-term use.

• Periodically monitor growth with long-term inhaler use in a child.

• Watch for evidence of localized mouth infections, vision changes, loss of glucose control, and immunosuppression.

• If patient has taken a corticosteroid during pregnancy, monitor neonate for hypoadrenalism.

• Monitor older adult for increased sensitivity to drug effects.

PATIENT TEACHING

• Instruct patient on proper use and routine care of the inhaler or nasal spray pump.

• Tell patient to use drug regularly as prescribed.

• Caution patient not to use inhalers for immediate relief of an asthma attack or bronchospasm. Verify prescription of a rescue inhaler.

• Instruct patient to rinse mouth after using inhaler to prevent thrush.

• Inform patient that maximal benefits of inhaler might not occur for 1 to 2 weeks or longer after therapy starts. Instruct patient to notify prescriber if condition fails to improve or worsens.

• Explain that if bronchospasm occurs after using inhaler, patient should immediately use a fast-acting bronchodilator. Urge patient to immediately contact prescriber if bronchospasm doesn't respond to the fast-acting bronchodilator.

🔱 *Alert:* Urge patient who has been weaned from an oral corticosteroid to immediately contact prescriber if an asthma attack occurs or patient experiences a period of stress. The oral corticosteroid may need to be restarted.

• Warn patient to avoid exposure to chickenpox or measles and to notify prescriber if such contact occurs.

• Long-term use of an inhaled corticosteroid may increase risk of cataracts and glaucoma; tell patient to report vision changes.

• Advise patient to write the date on a new inhaler on the day inhaler is opened and to discard inhaler after 45 days or when dose counter reads "00."

• Instruct patient not to use topical form with occlusive dressings or diapers, unless instructed by prescriber.

montelukast sodium
mon-te-LOO-kast

Singulair

Therapeutic class: Antiasthmatics
Pharmacologic class: Leukotriene-receptor antagonists

AVAILABLE FORMS
Oral granules: 4-mg packet
Tablets (chewable): 4 mg, 5 mg
Tablets (film-coated): 10 mg

INDICATIONS & DOSAGES
➤ **Asthma**
Adults and children ages 15 and older: 10 mg PO once daily in evening.
Children ages 6 to 14: 5-mg chewable tablet PO once daily in evening.
Children ages 2 to 5: 4-mg chewable tablet or 1 packet of 4-mg oral granules PO once daily in evening.
Children ages 12 to 23 months: 1 packet of 4-mg oral granules PO once daily in evening.
➤ **Seasonal allergic rhinitis, perennial allergic rhinitis**
Adults and children ages 15 and older: 10 mg PO once daily in evening.
Children ages 6 to 14: 5-mg chewable tablet PO once daily in evening.
Children ages 2 to 5: 4-mg chewable tablet or 1 packet of 4-mg oral granules PO once daily in evening.
Children ages 6 to 23 months (perennial allergic rhinitis only): 1 packet of 4-mg oral granules PO once daily in evening.
➤ **Prevention of exercise-induced bronchoconstriction**
Adults and children ages 15 and older: 10 mg PO at least 2 hours before exercise.
Children ages 6 to 14: 5 mg PO at least 2 hours before exercise (1 chewable tablet).
Adjust-a-dose: Patients already taking a daily dose shouldn't take an additional dose; an additional dose shouldn't be taken within 24 hours of a previous dose.

ADMINISTRATION
PO
- Give oral granules directly in mouth, dissolved in 5 mL of cold or room-temperature baby formula or human milk, or mixed with a spoonful of cold or room-temperature soft foods (use only applesauce, carrots, rice, or ice cream). Use within 15 minutes of opening packet.
- Give drug without regard to food.
- For patients with both asthma and allergic rhinitis, give only one dose daily in the evening.
- If dose is missed, omit dose; give next dose at regularly scheduled time.

ACTION
Reduces early and late-phase bronchoconstriction and nasal mucosa inflammation from antigen challenge.

Route	Onset	Peak	Duration
PO (chewable, granules)	Unknown	2–2.5 hr	24 hr
PO (film-coated)	Unknown	3–4 hr	24 hr

Half-life: 2.75 to 5.5 hours.

ADVERSE REACTIONS
CNS: headache, asthenia, dizziness, fatigue, fever, somnolence, weakness. **EENT:** ear pain, conjunctivitis, otitis media, rhinorrhea, nasal congestion, epistaxis, laryngitis, sinusitis, pharyngitis, rhinitis, tonsillitis, dental pain. **GI:** abdominal pain, dyspepsia, gastroenteritis, nausea, diarrhea. **GU:** pyuria. **Hematologic:** systemic eosinophilia. **Hepatic:** increased transaminase levels. **Respiratory:** URI, cough, wheezing, pneumonia, bronchitis. **Skin:** rash, dermatitis, urticaria, eczema. **Other:** flulike symptoms, trauma, varicella, viral infection.

INTERACTIONS
Drug-drug. *Gemfibrozil:* May increase montelukast level. Monitor therapy.
Lumacaftor–ivacaftor: May decrease montelukast level. Monitor therapy.

EFFECTS ON LAB TEST RESULTS
- May increase ALT and AST levels.
- May increase urinary WBC count.

CONTRAINDICATIONS & CAUTIONS
- Contraindicated in patients hypersensitive to drug or its components.
- Patients with known aspirin sensitivity should continue to avoid use of aspirin and other NSAIDs. Drug hasn't been shown to decrease the bronchoconstrictor response to aspirin and other NSAIDs in patients with asthma who are aspirin-sensitive.
- Patients with asthma may present with systemic eosinophilia that may manifest as clinical features of vasculitis consistent with Churg-Strauss syndrome. Churg-Strauss syndrome is often treated with systemic corticosteroid therapy. These reactions have sometimes been associated with reduction of oral corticosteroid dosage. Monitor patients for eosinophilia, vasculitic rash, worsening pulmonary symptoms, cardiac complications, or neuropathy.
- Use cautiously and with appropriate monitoring in patients whose dosages of systemic corticosteroids are reduced.

Boxed Warning Serious neuropsychiatric events have been reported in patients taking montelukast. Benefits may not outweigh risks of neuropsychiatric symptoms in patients with allergic rhinitis; reserve use for patients who have inadequate response or intolerance to alternative therapies. Discuss risks with patients and caregivers. ■

Boxed Warning The neuropsychiatric events reported in patients taking montelukast include, but aren't limited to, agitation, aggressive behavior or hostility, anxiousness, depression, disorientation, disturbance in attention, abnormal dreams, hallucinations, insomnia, irritability, memory impairment, restlessness, somnambulism, suicidality (including suicide), and tremors. ■

- Use cautiously in patients with liver disease, jaundice, or hepatitis.

Dialyzable drug: Unknown.

△ *Overdose S&S:* Headache, vomiting, psychomotor hyperactivity, thirst, somnolence, hyperkinesia, abdominal pain.

PREGNANCY-LACTATION-REPRODUCTION
- Studies during pregnancy are inadequate. Use during pregnancy only if clearly needed.
- Drug reportedly appears in human milk. Use cautiously during breastfeeding.

NURSING CONSIDERATIONS
- Assess patient's underlying condition. Monitor effectiveness.
- **Alert:** Don't abruptly substitute drug for inhaled or oral corticosteroids. Gradually reduce dosage of inhaled corticosteroids.
- **Alert:** Drug isn't indicated for use in patients with acute asthmatic attacks or status

M

asthmaticus, or as monotherapy for management of exercise-induced bronchospasm. Continue appropriate rescue drug for acute worsening.

Boxed Warning Monitor patients for neuropsychiatric symptoms. Immediately discontinue drug if any occur. ■

PATIENT TEACHING

• Teach about proper drug administration and handling for prescribed formulation.

• Advise patient to take drug daily, even if asymptomatic, and to contact prescriber if asthma isn't well controlled.

• Warn patient not to reduce or stop taking other prescribed antiasthmatics without prescriber's approval.

• Advise patient to seek medical attention if short-acting inhaled bronchodilators are needed more often than usual during drug therapy.

• Explain that drug isn't beneficial in acute asthma attacks or in acute exercise-induced bronchospasm. Advise patient to keep appropriate rescue drugs available.

Boxed Warning Advise patient and caregivers of risk of neuropsychiatric symptoms. Instruct them to immediately report any symptoms that occur. ■

• Advise patient with known aspirin sensitivity to continue to avoid using aspirin and NSAIDs during drug therapy.

⟲ Alert: Advise patient with phenylketonuria that chewable tablet contains phenylalanine.

SAFETY ALERT!

morphine hydrochloride
MOR-feen

Doloral✦

morphine sulfate
Duramorph PF, Infumorph, M-Eslon✦, Mitigo, MS Contin, Statex✦

Therapeutic class: Opioid analgesics
Pharmacologic class: Opioids
Controlled substance schedule: II

AVAILABLE FORMS
morphine hydrochloride
Syrup: 1 mg/mL*✦, 5 mg/mL*✦
morphine sulfate
Capsules (extended-release microgranules [M-Eslon]): ONC: 10 mg✦, 15 mg✦, 30 mg✦, 60 mg✦, 100 mg✦, 200 mg✦

Capsules (extended-release pellets) ONC:
10 mg, 20 mg, 30 mg, 45 mg, 50 mg, 60 mg, 75 mg, 80 mg, 90 mg, 100 mg, 120 mg
Injection with preservative: 0.5 mg/mL, 1 mg/mL, 2 mg/mL, 5 mg/mL, 10 mg/mL, 15 mg/mL, 50 mg/mL
Injection without preservative (Duramorph, Infumorph): 0.5 mg/mL, 1 mg/mL, 10 mg/mL, 25 mg/mL
Injection without preservative (Carpuject and prefilled syringes and vials): 2 mg/mL, 4 mg/mL, 5 mg/mL, 8 mg/mL, 10 mg/mL, 15 mg/mL
Oral solution: 10 mg/0.5 mL, 10 mg/5 mL, 20 mg/5 mL, 20 mg/mL (concentrate), 100 mg/5 mL (concentrate)
Suppositories: 5 mg, 10 mg, 20 mg, 30 mg
Tablets: 5 mg✦, 10 mg✦, 15 mg, 25 mg✦, 30 mg, 50 mg✦
Tablets (extended-release) ONC: 15 mg, 30 mg, 60 mg, 100 mg, 200 mg
Tablets (extended-release, abuse deterrent) ONC: 15 mg, 30 mg, 60 mg, 100 mg

INDICATIONS & DOSAGES
➤ **Moderate to severe pain**
Adults: Initially, 10 mg (based on 70-kg individual) IM or 0.1 to 0.2 mg/kg IV every 4 hours PRN. Or, 15 to 30 mg (immediate-release tablets) PO, or 10 to 20 mg (oral solution) PO, or 10 to 20 mg PR every 4 hours PRN.

For extended-release tablet, 15 or 30 mg PO every 8 to 12 hours.

For epidural injection, 5 mg by epidural catheter; if pain isn't adequately relieved in 1 hour, supplementary doses of 1 to 2 mg at intervals sufficient to assess effectiveness. Maximum total epidural dosage, 10 mg/24 hours.

For intrathecal injection, a single dose of 0.2 to 1 mg may provide pain relief for 24 hours (only in the lumbar area). Don't repeat injections.

➤ **Moderate to severe pain requiring continuous, around-the-clock oral opioid**
Adults: For patients receiving other oral morphine formulations, may convert to extended-release capsules by administering patient's total daily oral morphine dose as extended-release capsules once daily or by administering one-half of patient's total daily oral morphine dose b.i.d. Patient's 24-hour morphine requirement may also be divided every 8 hours and given as extended-release

---

tablets. Initial dosage in patients who are opioid-naive or opioid-nontolerant is 15 mg extended-release tablets PO every 8 or 12 hours. Don't give extended-release capsules more frequently than every 12 hours.

ADMINISTRATION
PO
Boxed Warning Take care when administering morphine oral solution to avoid dosing errors because confusion among different concentrations and between milligrams and milliliters could result in accidental overdose and death. The 20-mg/mL concentration is indicated for use only in patients who are opioid-tolerant because of risk of fatal respiratory depression in patients who are opioid-naive. It's packaged with a calibrated oral syringe for accurate dosing. ■

• Instruct patient to swallow extended-release or long-acting morphine sulfate oral formulations whole, without crushing, chewing, or dissolving, which may cause rapid, uncontrolled release and absorption of a potentially fatal dose of morphine. If necessary, extended-release capsules may be opened and entire contents poured into cool, soft foods (applesauce) and swallowed immediately without chewing.

• Give morphine sulfate without regard to food.

• May give extended-release capsules through a gastrostomy tube; flush tube with water, sprinkle contents of capsules in 10 mL of water, and flush through tube. Don't give through an NG tube.

IV
▼ For direct IV injection, give slowly over 4 to 5 minutes.

▼ For continuous infusion, mix drug with D_5W to yield 0.1 to 1 mg/mL, and give by a continuous infusion device.

▼ In adults with severe, chronic pain, maintenance IV infusion is 0.8 to 80 mg/hour; higher doses may be needed.

▼ Make sure an opioid antagonist is immediately available before IV administration.

▼ Infumorph and Duramorph are supplied in sealed ampules. Treat accidental dermal exposure to these drugs by removing contaminated clothing and rinsing affected area with water.

▼ Inspect parenteral drug products for particulate matter before opening the amber ampule and again for color after removing contents from ampule. Don't use if solution in unopened ampule contains a precipitate that doesn't disappear upon shaking. After removal, don't use solution unless it's colorless or pale yellow.

▼ **Incompatibilities:** None listed by manufacturer. Consult drug compatibility reference for more information.

IM
• Document injection site.

• Store injection solution at room temperature and protect from light.

• Solution may darken with age. Don't use if injection appears darker than pale yellow, is discolored, or contains precipitate.

Epidural or intrathecal
• Document injection site; limit to lumbar area.

• Verify proper placement of needle or catheter in intrathecal or epidural space before injecting drug.

• Inspect for particulate matter and discoloration before administration. Don't use if it's darker than pale yellow, discolored in any other way, or contains precipitate.

◑ Alert: Intrathecal dosage is usually one-tenth of epidural dosage.

• Store injection solution at room temperature until ready to use; discard unused portion.

• Protect from light; don't freeze or heat sterilize.

Rectal
• Refrigeration of rectal suppository isn't needed.

ACTION
Unknown. Binds with opioid receptors in the CNS, altering perception of and emotional response to pain.

Route	Onset	Peak	Duration
PO	30 min	1–2 hr	3–5 hr
PO (extended-release)	1–2 hr	3–4 hr	8–24 hr
IV	5–10 min	20 min	4–5 hr
IM	10–30 min	30–60 min	4–5 hr
PR	20–60 min	20–60 min	3–7 hr
Epidural	10–60 min	15–60 min	24 hr
Intrathecal	15–60 min	30–60 min	24 hr

Half-life: Immediate release, 2 to 4 hours; extended release, 11 to 24 hours; epidural, 39 to 249 minutes; intrathecal (CSF), 42 to 136 minutes; IV and IM, 1.5 to 4.5 hours.

M

ADVERSE REACTIONS

CNS: dizziness, drowsiness, headache, euphoria, light-headedness, myoclonus, nightmares, abnormal dreams, amnesia, apathy, ataxia, confusion, decreased cough reflex, sedation, hypoesthesia, paresthesia, insomnia, lethargy, somnolence, *seizures,* depression, hallucinations, nervousness, agitation, slurred speech, fever, physical dependence, vertigo, syncope, anxiety, tremors, asthenia, voice disorder, withdrawal syndrome. **CV:** *bradycardia, cardiac arrest, shock,* HTN, hypotension, tachycardia, palpitations, edema, chest pain, syncope, flushing, atrial fibrillation, vasodilation. **EENT:** miosis, blurred vision, nystagmus, conjunctivitis, diplopia, rhinitis, dry mouth. **GI:** constipation, nausea, vomiting, dry mouth, anorexia, biliary tract spasms, ileus, flatulence, abdominal pain, delayed gastric emptying, diarrhea, dysphagia, gastric atony, GERD, hiccups. **GU:** urine retention, urinary hesitancy, decreased libido, amenorrhea, impotence, prolonged labor. **Hematologic:** *thrombocytopenia, anemia, leukopenia.* **Metabolic:** hyponatremia, SIADH. **Musculoskeletal:** back pain, footdrop, ostealgia. **Respiratory:** *apnea, respiratory arrest, respiratory depression,* atelectasis, dyspnea, *hypoxia.* **Skin:** diaphoresis, pallor, rash, edema, pruritus, skin flushing, pain at injection site. **Other:** gynecomastia, flulike symptoms.

INTERACTIONS

Drug-drug. *Alvimopan:* May enhance adverse or toxic effects of alvimopan. Alvimopan is contraindicated in patients receiving therapeutic doses of opioids for more than 7 consecutive days immediately before alvimopan initiation. Consider therapy modification.
Anticholinergics (benztropine, darifenacin, oxybutynin): Increased risk of urine retention, constipation, and paralytic ileus. Use together cautiously.

Boxed Warning *Benzodiazepines, CNS depressants:* May cause slow or difficult breathing, sedation, and death. Avoid use together. If use together can't be avoided, limit dosage and duration of each drug to the minimum necessary for desired effect. ■

Diuretics: May reduce efficacy of diuretics. Monitor therapy.
General anesthetics, hypnotics, muscle relaxants, other opioid analgesics, TCAs: May cause respiratory depression, hypotension, profound sedation, or coma. Use together cautiously, reduce morphine dosage, and monitor patient response.

MAO inhibitors: May increase risk of serotonin syndrome or opioid toxicity. Don't use morphine within 14 days of MAO inhibitor. Consider use of alternative opioid with careful monitoring and small doses.

Mixed agonist/antagonist, partial agonist opioid analgesics: May reduce effect of morphine or precipitate withdrawal symptoms. Avoid use together; if use together is necessary, monitor patient closely.

P2Y12 inhibitors (clopidogrel, prasugrel, ticagrelor): May decrease absorption and peak concentration of oral inhibitors when used with IV morphine and delay onset of antiplatelet effect. Consider use of a parenteral antiplatelet agent in the setting of ACS requiring coadministration of IV morphine.

⊙ *Alert:* Serotonergic drugs (amoxapine, antiemetics [dolasetron, granisetron, ondansetron, palonosetron], antimigraine drugs, buspirone, cyclobenzaprine, dextromethorphan, linezolid, lithium, maprotiline, methylene blue, mirtazapine, nefazodone, SNRIs, SSRIs, TCAs, trazodone, tryptophan, vilazodone): May increase risk of serotonin syndrome. Use together cautiously, and monitor patient for serotonin syndrome.

Drug-herb. ⊙ *Alert: St. John's wort:* May increase risk of serotonin syndrome. Use together cautiously, and monitor patient for serotonin syndrome.

Drug-lifestyle. **Boxed Warning** *Alcohol use:* May cause slow or difficult breathing, sedation, and death. Discourage use together. ■

EFFECTS ON LAB TEST RESULTS

- May increase amylase level.
- May decrease sodium level.
- May decrease Hb level and platelet count.
- May cause abnormal LFT values.

CONTRAINDICATIONS & CAUTIONS

- Contraindicated in patients hypersensitive to drug and in those with conditions that would preclude administration of IV or neuraxial opioids (known or suspected GI obstruction, including paralytic ileus; acute or severe bronchial asthma in a setting that doesn't have resuscitative equipment).

Boxed Warning Use exposes patient and others to risk of opioid addiction, abuse, and misuse, which can lead to overdose and death.

Reactions in bold italics are *life-threatening.*

These effects can occur at any dose or duration. Assess patient risk before prescribing and regularly reassess patient for these behaviors and conditions. ▪

Boxed Warning Prescribers are strongly encouraged to complete a REMS-compliant education program. Drug should be prescribed only by prescribers with knowledge of opioid use and ways to reduce associated risks. ▪

🔸 *Alert:* Use lowest effective dose for shortest period consistent with patient's treatment goals.

🔸 *Alert:* Because risk of overdose increases as opioid dose increases, reserve titration to higher doses for patients in whom lower doses are ineffective and in whom expected benefits of higher opioid dose outweigh risks.

Boxed Warning *Opioid class warning:* Opioids should only be prescribed with benzodiazepines or other CNS depressants when alternative treatment options are inadequate, aren't expected to provide adequate analgesia, haven't been tolerated, or aren't expected to be tolerated. ▪

🔸 *Alert:* Immediate-release formulations shouldn't be used for an extended period unless pain remains severe enough to require an opioid analgesic and alternative treatment options are inadequate to treat pain.

🔸 *Alert:* Long-acting or extended-release formulations are indicated for severe, persistent pain for which extended treatment with a daily opioid is required and for which alternative treatment options are inadequate. Use isn't indicated for as-needed analgesia.

Boxed Warning Accidental ingestion of even one dose of an opioid, especially by children, can result in a fatal overdose. ▪

🔸 *Alert:* Drug may lead to a rare but serious decrease in adrenal gland cortisol production.

• Drug may cause decreased sex hormone levels with long-term use.

🔸 *Alert:* Patients are at increased risk for oversedation and respiratory depression if they snore or have a history of sleep apnea, haven't used opioids recently or are first-time opioid users, have increased opioid dosage requirements or opioid habituation, have received general anesthesia for longer lengths of time or received other sedating drugs, have preexisting pulmonary or cardiac disease, or have thoracic or other surgical incisions that may impair breathing. Monitor patients carefully.

• Contraindicated in patients with GI obstruction.

• Use with caution in older adults, patients who are debilitated, and those with head injury, increased ICP, seizures, chronic pulmonary disease, prostatic hyperplasia, Child-Pugh class C liver impairment, CrCl less than 30 mL/minute, acute abdominal conditions, hypothyroidism, Addison disease, or urethral stricture.

• Use with caution in patients with circulatory shock, biliary tract disease, CNS depression, toxic psychosis, acute alcoholism, delirium tremens, and seizure disorders.

• Morphine hydrochloride syrup isn't indicated for use in children.

Dialyzable drug: Yes.

⚠ *Overdose S&S:* Miosis, CNS depression, respiratory depression, apnea, flaccid skeletal muscles, bradycardia, hypotension, circulatory collapse, cardiac arrest, respiratory arrest, death.

PREGNANCY-LACTATION-REPRODUCTION

🔸 *Alert:* Carefully weigh risks and benefits of using drug during pregnancy. Use in pregnancy only if need for opioid analgesia clearly outweighs fetal risk.

Boxed Warning Prolonged use of opioids during pregnancy can result in neonatal opioid withdrawal syndrome, which may be life-threatening. It requires management with expert neonatology protocols. If prolonged use is needed, advise patient of risks and ensure availability of proper treatment. ▪

• Because of the potential for serious adverse reactions in breastfeeding infants (including respiratory depression, sedation, and possible withdrawal symptoms with patient's cessation of morphine), patient should discontinue breastfeeding or discontinue drug, considering importance of drug to patient.

• If morphine use is necessary in patient who is breastfeeding, use cautiously. Limit use and supplement with nonopioid agents. Monitor infant for increased sleepiness, difficulty feeding or breathing, and limpness.

• Prolonged opioid use may reduce fertility.

NURSING CONSIDERATIONS

Boxed Warning May cause life-threatening or fatal respiratory depression at any time during therapy. Monitor patient closely, especially when starting or increasing doses. Proper dosing and titration are essential to reduce risk. ▪

M

Boxed Warning Regularly monitor all patients for opioid addiction, abuse, and misuse, which can lead to overdose and death. ∎

🕓 **Alert:** Drug may cause opioid-induced hyperalgesia (OIH). Symptoms include increased pain level with opioid dose increase, decreased pain level with opioid dose reduction, pain from ordinarily nonpainful stimuli without underlying disease progression, opioid tolerance or withdrawal, and addictive behavior. For suspected OIH, decrease opioid dose or switch patient to alternative opioid.

🕓 **Alert:** If patient is taking opioids with serotonergic drugs, watch for signs and symptoms of serotonin syndrome (agitation, hallucinations, rapid HR, fever, diaphoresis, shivering or shaking, muscle twitching or stiffness, trouble with coordination, nausea, vomiting, diarrhea), especially at start of treatment and at dosage increases. Signs and symptoms may occur within several hours of coadministration but may also occur later, especially after dosage increase. Discontinue the opioid, serotonergic drug, or both if serotonin syndrome is suspected.

🕓 **Alert:** Monitor for signs and symptoms of adrenal insufficiency (nausea, vomiting, loss of appetite, fatigue, weakness, dizziness, low BP). Perform diagnostic testing if adrenal insufficiency is suspected. If adrenal insufficiency is confirmed, treat with corticosteroids and wean patient off opioids, if appropriate. Discontinue corticosteroids when clinically appropriate.

• Monitor for signs and symptoms of decreased sex hormone levels (low libido, erectile dysfunction, amenorrhea, infertility). If any occur, evaluate patient and obtain specimens for lab testing.

• Reassess patient's level of pain at least 15 and 30 minutes after giving parenterally and 30 minutes after giving orally.

🕓 **Alert:** Keep opioid antagonist (naloxone) and resuscitation equipment available.

• Carefully monitor circulatory, respiratory, bladder, and bowel function. Drug may cause hypotension, urine retention, nausea, vomiting, ileus, or altered level of consciousness regardless of route.

• If respirations drop below 12 breaths/minute, withhold dose and notify prescriber.

• Preservative-free preparations are available for epidural and intrathecal use.

• Epidural administration has been associated with less potential for immediate or late adverse effects than intrathecal administration; use epidural route whenever possible.

• Constant IV infusion of naloxone, 0.6 mg/hour, for 24 hours after intrathecal injection may reduce potential adverse effects.

Boxed Warning When epidural or intrathecal route is used, observe patients in a fully equipped and staffed environment for at least 24 hours after initial dose. ∎

• Improper or erroneous substitution of Infumorph 200 or 500 (10 or 25 mg/mL, respectively) for regular Duramorph (0.5 or 1 mg/mL) is likely to result in serious overdose, leading to seizures, respiratory depression, and possibly death.

• When drug is given epidurally, monitor closely for respiratory depression up to 24 hours after injection. Check respiratory rate and depth every 30 to 60 minutes for 24 hours. Watch for pruritus and skin flushing.

• Morphine is drug of choice for relieving MI pain but may cause transient decrease in BP.

• An around-the-clock regimen is best to manage severe, chronic pain. Verify prescription of breakthrough pain medication in addition to around-the-clock medication.

• Morphine may worsen or mask gallbladder pain.

• Constipation is commonly severe with maintenance dose. Ensure patient receives order for stool softener or stimulant laxative.

• Gradually taper morphine sulfate therapy when stopping therapy.

🕓 **Alert:** Don't stop drug abruptly; withdraw slowly and individualize gradual taper plan to prevent signs and symptoms of withdrawal, worsening pain, and psychological distress in patients who are physically dependent. Refer to manufacturer's label for specific tapering instructions.

🕓 **Alert:** When tapering opioids, monitor patient closely for signs and symptoms of opioid withdrawal (restlessness, lacrimation, rhinorrhea, yawning, perspiration, chills, myalgia, mydriasis, irritability, anxiety, insomnia, backache, joint pain, weakness, abdominal cramps, anorexia, nausea, vomiting, diarrhea, increased BP or HR, increased respiratory rate), which may indicate a need to taper more slowly. Also monitor patient for suicidality, use of other substances, and changes in mood.

• *Look alike–sound alike:* Don't confuse morphine with hydromorphone. Don't confuse MS Contin with Oxycontin.

Reactions in bold italics are *life-threatening*.

PATIENT TEACHING

Boxed Warning Counsel patient and caregiver on serious risks, safe use, and importance of reading the medication guide with each prescription. ▪

• Advise patient to take drug exactly as prescribed and to use lowest dose possible for shortest time needed.

• Inform patient that, for acute pain, drug may only be needed for a few days. Teach about safe disposal of unused drug.

• Warn patient that extended-release and long-acting formulations aren't to be taken on an "as needed" basis.

• Instruct patient to contact health care provider if prescribed dosage isn't controlling pain.

❸ *Alert:* Warn patient to withhold drug and inform prescriber if pain level worsens, pain sensitivity increases, or new pain occurs after taking drug.

❸ *Alert:* Counsel patient who has been regularly taking drug not to discontinue without first discussing the need for gradual tapering with prescriber.

❸ *Alert:* Explain assessment and monitoring process to patient and family. Instruct them to immediately report difficulty breathing or other signs or symptoms of a potential adverse opioid-related reaction.

• Encourage patient to report all medications being taken, including prescription and OTC medications and supplements.

• Warn patient that morphine can cause constipation and provide suggestions for managing it.

❸ *Alert:* Caution patient to immediately report signs and symptoms of serotonin syndrome, adrenal insufficiency, and decreased sex hormone levels.

• When using drug after surgery, encourage patient to turn, cough, and deep-breathe to prevent lung problems.

• Caution patient who is ambulatory about getting out of bed or walking. Warn outpatient to avoid driving and other potentially hazardous activities that require mental alertness until drug's adverse CNS effects are known.

Boxed Warning Drinking alcohol or taking drugs that contain alcohol while taking extended-release capsules may cause additive CNS effects and potentially fatal overdose. Warn patient to read labels on OTC drugs

carefully for alcohol content and not to use alcohol in any form. ▪

• Teach patient that naloxone may be prescribed with the opioid when beginning and renewing therapy to reduce risk of opioid overdose and death.

• Caution patient to report to prescriber pregnancy or plan to become pregnant.

moxifloxacin hydrochloride ⚇
mox-i-FLOKS-a-sin

Vigamox

Therapeutic class: Antibiotics
Pharmacologic class: Fluoroquinolones

AVAILABLE FORMS
Injection: 400 mg/250 mL
Ophthalmic solution: 0.5%
Tablets (film-coated): 400 mg

INDICATIONS & DOSAGES

Boxed Warning Use in patients with acute bacterial sinusitis or acute bacterial exacerbation of bronchitis isn't recommended due to risk of serious adverse effects. Use drug in these patients only when no other treatment options are available. ▪

➤ **Acute bacterial sinusitis caused by** *Streptococcus pneumoniae, Haemophilus influenzae,* **or** *Moraxella catarrhalis*
Adults: 400 mg PO or IV every 24 hours for 10 days.

➤ **Complicated skin and skin-structure infections caused by methicillin-susceptible** *Staphylococcus aureus, Escherichia coli, Klebsiella pneumoniae,* **or** *Enterobacter cloacae*
Adults: 400 mg PO or IV every 24 hours for 7 to 21 days.

➤ **Complicated intra-abdominal infection caused by** *E. coli, Bacteroides fragilis, Streptococcus anginosus, Streptococcus constellatus, Enterococcus faecalis, Proteus mirabilis, Clostridium perfringens, Bacteroides thetaiotaomicron,* **or** *Peptostreptococcus* **species**
Adults: 400 mg PO or IV every 24 hours for 5 to 14 days. Start with IV form; switch to PO when appropriate.

➤ **Community-acquired pneumonia from multidrug-resistant** *S. pneumoniae* **(resistant to two or more of the**

M

following antibiotics: penicillin, second-generation cephalosporins, macrolides, sulfamethoxazole–trimethoprim, tetracyclines), *S. aureus, M. catarrhalis, H. influenzae, K. pneumoniae, Chlamydia pneumoniae,* or *Mycoplasma pneumoniae*
Adults: 400 mg PO or IV every 24 hours for 7 to 14 days.

➤ **Acute bacterial exacerbation of chronic bronchitis caused by** *S. pneumoniae, H. influenzae, H. parainfluenzae, K. pneumoniae, S. aureus,* **or** *M. catarrhalis*
Adults: 400 mg PO or IV every 24 hours for 5 days.

➤ **Uncomplicated skin-structure or skin infection caused by** *S. aureus* **or** *Streptococcus pyogenes*
Adults: 400 mg PO or IV every 24 hours for 7 days.

➤ **Plague (pneumonic and septicemic) caused by susceptible isolates of** *Yersinia pestis*
Adults: For prophylaxis and treatment, 400 mg PO or IV every 24 hours for 10 to 14 days.

➤ **Bacterial conjunctivitis caused by susceptible strains of aerobic gram-positive and gram-negative organisms and** *Chlamydia trachomatis*
Adults and children: 1 drop into affected eye(s) t.i.d. for 7 days.

ADMINISTRATION
PO
• Give drug without regard to food.
• Give drug at same time each day.
• Tablets may be crushed, suspended in water, and used immediately. Crushed tablets will taste bitter.
• Store at controlled room temperature.
• If a dose is missed more than 8 hours before the next scheduled dose, give the dose. If less than 8 hours remain before next dose, omit missed dose; then continue with next scheduled dose. Don't double dose to compensate for missed dose.
IV
▼ Don't refrigerate. Product precipitates if refrigerated.
▼ Don't use if particulate matter is visible.
▼ Flush IV line with compatible solution, such as D_5W, NSS, or lactated Ringer solution, before and after use.
▼ Give only by infusion over 1 hour. Avoid rapid or bolus infusion.
▼ **Incompatibilities:** Other IV drugs.

Ophthalmic
• Place gentle pressure on lacrimal duct for 1 to 2 minutes after instilling drop.
• Don't inject solution subconjunctivally or into anterior chamber of eye.

ACTION
Interferes with action of enzymes needed for bacterial replication. Inhibits topoisomerases I (DNA gyrase) and IV, impairing bacterial DNA replication, transcription, repair, and recombination.

Route	Onset	Peak	Duration
PO, IV	Unknown	1–3 hr	Unknown
Ophthalmic	Unknown	Unknown	Unknown

Half-life: PO, 11.5 to 15.6 hours; IV, 8.2 to 15.4 hours; ophthalmic, 13 hours.

ADVERSE REACTIONS
CNS: dizziness, headache, insomnia, fever. **EENT:** conjunctivitis; dry eyes; increased lacrimation; keratitis; ocular discomfort, pain, or pruritus; reduced visual acuity; subconjunctival hemorrhage; otitis media; pharyngitis; rhinitis (with ophthalmic use). **GI:** abdominal pain, anorexia, constipation, diarrhea, dyspepsia, nausea, vomiting. **Hematologic:** anemia, neutrophilia, prolonged PT. **Hepatic:** abnormal LFT values. **Metabolic:** *hypokalemia, hypoglycemia,* hyperchloremia, hyperalbuminemia, decreased amylase level. **Respiratory:** *hypoxia.*

INTERACTIONS
Drug-drug. *Aluminum hydroxide, aluminum–magnesium hydroxide, calcium carbonate, didanosine, magnesium hydroxide, multivitamins, products containing zinc:* May interfere with GI absorption of moxifloxacin. Give moxifloxacin 4 hours before or 8 hours after these products.
Antidiabetics: May cause hyperglycemia or hypoglycemia. Monitor blood glucose control.
Class IA antiarrhythmics (procainamide, quinidine), class III antiarrhythmics (amiodarone, sotalol), drugs that prolong QT interval (antipsychotics, erythromycin, TCAs): May have additive QT-interval prolongation effect. Avoid use together.
Live-virus vaccines: May decrease effectiveness of live-virus vaccines. Don't give live-virus vaccines during therapy.

Reactions in bold italics are *life-threatening.*

NSAIDs: May increase risk of CNS stimulation and seizures. Monitor patient, and adjust treatment as needed.

Steroids: May increase risk of tendinitis and tendon rupture. Monitor patient for tendon pain or inflammation.

Sucralfate: May decrease absorption of moxifloxacin, reducing anti-infective response. If use together can't be avoided, take oral form 4 hours before or 8 hours after sucralfate.

Warfarin: May increase anticoagulant effects. Closely monitor PT and INR.

Drug-lifestyle. *Sun or UV light exposure:* May cause moderate to severe photosensitivity reactions. Advise patient to avoid excessive sunlight and UV light exposure.

EFFECTS ON LAB TEST RESULTS

- May increase ALT, ionized calcium, chloride, globulin, and albumin levels.
- May decrease potassium and amylase levels and oxygen partial pressure.
- May increase or decrease bilirubin and glucose levels.
- May increase WBC count, mean corpuscular Hb, PT, and INR.
- May decrease Hb level, hematocrit, and RBC, eosinophil, and basophil counts.
- May increase or decrease neutrophil count.

CONTRAINDICATIONS & CAUTIONS

- Contraindicated in patients hypersensitive to drug or other fluoroquinolones.

Boxed Warning Drug is associated with increased risk of tendinitis and tendon rupture, especially in patients older than age 60, patients taking corticosteroids, and those with heart, kidney, or lung transplants. ■

⚲ ❸ Alert: Drug may increase risk of aortic dissection or rupture when used systemically. Avoid use in patients with known aortic aneurysm; patients at risk for aortic aneurysm, including those with HTN, peripheral atherosclerotic vascular diseases, or certain genetic conditions (Marfan syndrome, Ehlers-Danlos syndrome); and older adults. Only use drug in these patients if no other treatment options are available.

❸ Alert: Patients receiving systemic drug are at increased risk for hypoglycemia, which can result in coma. Hypoglycemia has been reported more frequently in older adults and in patients with diabetes.

❸ Alert: Drug can prolong QT interval in some patients. Use cautiously in patients with ongoing proarrhythmic conditions, such as clinically significant bradycardia or acute myocardial ischemia.

- Seizures, increased ICP, and pseudotumor cerebri have been reported in patients taking fluoroquinolones. Drug may cause CNS events (including agitation, anxiety, confusion, depression, insomnia and, rarely, suicidality), even after first dose. Use cautiously in patients who may have CNS disorders or risk factors for seizures. Drug may need to be discontinued.

Boxed Warning Drug may exacerbate muscle weakness in patients with myasthenia gravis. Avoid use of fluoroquinolones in patients with known history of myasthenia gravis. ■

- Drug may cause CDAD, ranging in severity from mild diarrhea to fatal colitis, which can occur more than 2 months after therapy. If CDAD is suspected or confirmed, drug may need to be discontinued and appropriate therapy initiated.
- Drug may cause serious adverse reactions, including SCARs, vasculitis, serum sickness, allergic pneumonitis, AKI, interstitial kidney inflammation, hepatitis, arthralgia, myalgia, anemia, and other hematologic disorders.
- Safety and effectiveness of PO and IV formulations in children haven't been established.

Dialyzable drug: Minimal.

PREGNANCY-LACTATION-REPRODUCTION

- Studies during pregnancy are inadequate. Use during pregnancy only if potential benefit justifies fetal risk.
- Drug may appear in human milk. Patient should discontinue breastfeeding or discontinue drug, considering importance of drug to patient.

NURSING CONSIDERATIONS

Boxed Warning Monitor for tendinitis and tendon rupture, peripheral neuropathy, and CNS effects (seizures, toxic psychoses, increased ICP, pseudotumor cerebri, tremors, restlessness, anxiety, light-headedness, confusion, hallucinations, paranoia, depression, nightmares, insomnia and, rarely, suicidality). If any of these serious adverse reactions occur, immediately discontinue drug. ■

Boxed Warning Monitor for and immediately report signs and symptoms of peripheral neuropathy (pain, burning, tingling, numbness, weakness, or change in sensation to light touch, pain, or temperature, or sense of body position). ■

• Monitor patient for hypersensitivity reactions, including anaphylaxis. Discontinue drug at first sign of rash, jaundice, or other signs or symptoms of hypersensitivity.

• If diarrhea develops during therapy, send stool specimen for *Clostridioides difficile* test.

• Ensure patient with signs or symptoms of conjunctivitis doesn't wear contact lenses.

• Rupture of Achilles and other tendons is linked to fluoroquinolone use. If pain, inflammation, or tendon rupture occurs, stop drug and notify prescriber.

❸ *Alert:* Monitor for signs and symptoms of aortic aneurysm, dissection, and rupture (sudden, severe, constant pain in stomach, chest, or back; throbbing in stomach area; deep pain in back or side of stomach; steady, gnawing pain in stomach that lasts for hours or days; pain in jaw, neck, back, or chest; coughing or hoarseness; shortness of breath; trouble swallowing). Immediately discontinue drug if any of these aortic disorders is suspected.

❸ *Alert:* Monitor patient receiving systemic drug for symptoms of hypoglycemia (confusion, pounding or rapid heartbeat, dizziness, pale skin, shakiness, diaphoresis, unusual hunger, trembling, headache, weakness, irritability, unusual anxiety). Immediately discontinue drug for blood glucose disturbances, and switch to a nonfluoroquinolone antibiotic if possible.

❸ *Alert:* Monitor patient receiving systemic drug for psychiatric adverse reactions (disturbances in attention, disorientation, agitation, nervousness, memory impairment, delirium). Discontinue drug for CNS adverse effects, including psychiatric adverse reactions.

• *Look alike–sound alike:* Don't confuse Vigamox with Amoxil.

PATIENT TEACHING

Boxed Warning Warn patient to immediately report signs and symptoms of serious adverse reactions, including unusual joint or tendon pain, muscle weakness, "pins and needles" tingling or prickling sensation, numbness in arms or legs, confusion, or hallucinations. ■

❸ *Alert:* Warn patient to seek immediate medical attention for signs and symptoms of aortic aneurysm.

• Teach about proper drug administration and handling for prescribed formulation.

• Tell patient not to wear contact lenses during ophthalmic treatment.

• Instruct patient not to touch eye dropper tip to anything, including eyes and fingers.

• Tell patient to finish entire course of therapy, even if symptoms are relieved.

❸ *Alert:* Caution patient that significantly low blood glucose level can occur. Review with patient how to manage low glucose level; instruct patient on the signs and symptoms of low glucose level and to immediately report them to prescriber.

❸ *Alert:* Advise patient with diabetes to monitor blood glucose more frequently during therapy.

❸ *Alert:* Inform patient to immediately report psychiatric adverse reactions, which can occur after just one dose.

• Instruct patient to contact prescriber and stop drug if allergic reaction, rash, heart palpitations, fainting, or persistent diarrhea occurs.

• Direct patient to contact prescriber, stop drug, rest, and refrain from exercise if pain, inflammation, or tendon rupture occurs.

• Warn patient that drug may cause dizziness and light-headedness. Tell patient to avoid hazardous activities, such as driving and operating machinery, until effects of drug are known.

• Tell patient to avoid exposure to excessive sunlight and UV light and to report photosensitivity reactions to prescriber.

mupirocin
myoo-PEER-oh-sin

Therapeutic class: Antibacterials (topical)
Pharmacologic class: Antibiotics

AVAILABLE FORMS
Topical cream: 2%
Topical ointment: 2%

INDICATIONS & DOSAGES
➤ **Impetigo (topical ointment)**
Adults and children ages 2 months and older:
Apply to affected areas t.i.d. for up to 10 days. Reevaluate patient in 3 to 5 days; may cover affected area with gauze dressing, if needed.
➤ **Traumatic skin lesions infected with *Staphylococcus aureus* or *Streptococcus pyogenes* (cream)**
Adults and children ages 3 months and older:
Apply thin film with cotton swab or gauze pad

t.i.d. for 10 days; may cover with gauze dressing, if needed. Reevaluate patient if improvement doesn't occur in 3 to 5 days.

ADMINISTRATION
Topical
• Apply topical ointment and cream with gauze pad or cotton swab to avoid contamination.
• Avoid applying topical ointment or cream to eye or in nose.
• Patients should not use cosmetics and other skin products on treated areas.

ACTION
Inhibits bacterial protein synthesis by reversibly and specifically binding to bacterial isoleucyl transfer-RNA synthetase.

Route	Onset	Peak	Duration
Topical	Unknown	Unknown	Unknown

Half-life: 17 to 36 minutes.

ADVERSE REACTIONS
CNS: taste perversion, headache. **GI:** nausea. **Skin:** localized burning, erythema with topical use, pain, pruritus, rash, stinging.

INTERACTIONS
None.

EFFECTS ON LAB TEST RESULTS
None reported.

CONTRAINDICATIONS & CAUTIONS
• Contraindicated in patients hypersensitive to drug or its components.
• Use cautiously in patients with burns or large open wounds.
Dialyzable drug: Unknown.

PREGNANCY-LACTATION-REPRODUCTION
• Studies during pregnancy are inadequate. Use during pregnancy only if clearly needed.
• It isn't known if drug appears in human milk. Use cautiously during breastfeeding.

NURSING CONSIDERATIONS
• Drug isn't for ophthalmic or internal use.
• Prolonged use may cause overgrowth of nonsusceptible bacteria and fungi.
• Prolonged use may cause CDAD, ranging in severity from mild diarrhea to fatal colitis, which can occur more than 2 months after therapy ends. For suspected or confirmed CDAD, drug may need to be discontinued and appropriate therapy initiated.
• Discontinue drug if sensitization or severe local irritation occurs.

PATIENT TEACHING
• Tell patient to immediately notify prescriber if condition doesn't improve or worsens in 3 to 5 days.
• Advise patient to avoid contact with eyes and, if accidental contact occurs, to rinse well with water.
• Urge patient to immediately report diarrhea.
• Warn patient about local adverse reactions related to drug use.
• Caution patient not to use cosmetics or other skin products on treated areas.

mycophenolate mofetil
my-koe-FIN-oh-late

CellCept

mycophenolate mofetil hydrochloride
CellCept Intravenous

mycophenolic acid (mycophenolate sodium)
Myfortic

Therapeutic class: Immunosuppressants
Pharmacologic class: Mycophenolic acid derivatives

AVAILABLE FORMS
mycophenolate mofetil
Capsules 🚫: 250 mg
Powder for oral suspension: 200 mg/mL
Tablets: 500 mg
mycophenolate mofetil hydrochloride
Injection: 500 mg/vial
mycophenolic acid
Tablets (delayed-release) 🚫: 180 mg, 360 mg

INDICATIONS & DOSAGES
Adjust-a-dose (for all indications): If neutropenia develops (ANC less than $1.3 \times 10^3/\mu L$), stop drug or reduce dosage.
➤ **To prevent organ rejection in patients receiving allogeneic kidney transplants**
Adults: 1 g IV or PO (regular-release) b.i.d. with other immunosuppressants. Or, 720 mg delayed-release tablets PO b.i.d.

Children ages 5 to 16 (delayed-release): 400 mg/m^2 BSA PO b.i.d. Maximum dosage, 720 mg PO b.i.d. Or, for patients with BSA of 1.19 to 1.58 m^2, 540 mg PO b.i.d. If BSA is greater than 1.58 m^2, 720 mg PO b.i.d. Delayed-release formulation isn't recommended for BSA of less than 1.19 m^2.
Children ages 3 months to 18 years: For oral suspension, 600 mg/m^2 PO b.i.d.; maximum dosage, 1 g b.i.d. Or, for patients with BSA of 1.25 to less than 1.5 m^2, 750 mg (capsules) PO b.i.d. If BSA is 1.5 m^2 or greater, 1 g (tablets or capsules) PO b.i.d.
Adjust-a-dose: For patients with GFR less than 25 mL/minute/1.73 m^2 outside of immediate posttransplant period, avoid immediate-release dosages above 1 g b.i.d.

➤ **To prevent organ rejection in patients receiving allogeneic heart transplant, in combination with other immunosuppressants**

Adults: 1.5 g PO or IV b.i.d.
Children ages 3 months to 18 years: For oral suspension, 600 mg/m^2 PO b.i.d. If well tolerated, may increase maintenance dose to 900 mg/m^2 b.i.d. Or, for patients with BSA of 1.25 to less than 1.5 m^2, 750 mg (capsules) PO b.i.d. If BSA is 1.5 m^2 or more, 1 g (tablets or capsules) PO b.i.d.

➤ **To prevent organ rejection in patients receiving allogeneic liver transplant, in combination with other immunosuppressants**

Adults: 1 g IV b.i.d. or 1.5 g PO b.i.d.
Children ages 3 months to 18 years: For oral suspension, 600 mg/m^2 PO b.i.d. If well tolerated, may increase maintenance dose to 900 mg/m^2 b.i.d. Or, for patients with BSA of 1.25 to 1.5 m^2, 750 mg (capsules) PO b.i.d. If BSA is greater than 1.5 m^2, 1 g (tablets or capsules) PO b.i.d.

ADMINISTRATION

PO

Alert: Hazardous drug; use safe handling and disposal precautions.

- Have patient swallow tablets and capsules whole; don't crush or break tablets or open capsules.
- Give on an empty stomach (1 hour before or 2 hours after a meal). In patients who are stable after kidney transplant, may give with food if necessary.
- Avoid inhaling powder in capsule, powder for suspension, or oral suspension or having it contact skin or other mucous membranes. If contact occurs, wash skin thoroughly with soap and water, and rinse eyes with water.
- Extended-release tablets are not interchangeable with other forms.
- Suspension may be administered via NG tube with a minimum size 8 French catheter (at least 1.7-mm interior diameter).
- After reconstitution, don't mix suspension with other liquids prior to giving.
- Give a missed dose as soon as possible, unless next scheduled dose is closer than 2 hours; then omit dose and resume usual schedule.

IV

- ▼ Reconstitute using 14 mL of D_5W. Further dilute to 6 mg/1 mL: 1-g doses in 140 mL of D_5W and 1.5-g doses in 210 mL of D_5W.
- ▼ Never give by rapid or bolus IV injection. Infuse drug over at least 2 hours.
- ▼ Use within 4 hours of reconstitution and dilution.
- ▼ **Incompatibilities:** Other IV drugs and solutions.

ACTION

Inhibits proliferative response of T and B lymphocytes, suppresses antibody formation by B lymphocytes, and may inhibit recruitment of leukocytes into sites of inflammation and graft rejection.

Route	Onset	Peak	Duration
PO	Unknown	1–1.5 hr	7–18 hr
PO (extended-release)	Unknown	1.5–2.75 hr	8–17 hr
IV	Unknown	Unknown	10–17 hr

Half-life: Oral, 8 to 18 hours; IV, 17 hours.

ADVERSE REACTIONS

CNS: asthenia, fever, headache, pain, tremors, dizziness, insomnia, depression, psychosis, anxiety. **CV:** chest pain, edema, HTN, hypotension, tachycardia, phlebitis, ***thrombosis.*** **EENT:** conjunctivitis, visual disturbance, ear pain, deafness, pharyngitis. **GI:** abdominal pain, constipation, diarrhea, dyspepsia, nausea, anorexia, vomiting, oral candidiasis, flatulence. **GU:** hematuria, increased creatinine level, increased BUN level, UTI. **Hematologic:** ***leukopenia, thrombocytopenia,*** anemia, hypochromic anemia, leukocytosis. **Hepatic:** increased liver enzyme levels. **Metabolic:** hyperlipidemia, hyperglycemia, **hyperkalemia, hypokalemia, hypomagnesemia, hypocalcemia,** hyperuricemia, hypophosphatemia, increased LDH level. **Musculoskeletal:** arthralgia, back pain. **Respiratory:** cough, dyspnea, pleural effusion, bronchitis, pneumonia. **Skin:** acne, rash, alopecia, skin carcinoma, ecchymosis. **Other:** infection, *sepsis.*

INTERACTIONS
Drug-drug. *Acyclovir, ganciclovir, valacyclovir, valganciclovir, other drugs that undergo renal tubular secretion:* May increase risk of toxicity for both drugs. Monitor patient closely.

Antacids with magnesium and aluminum hydroxides: May decrease mycophenolate absorption. Give at least 2 hours after mycophenolate.

Azathioprine: May increase risk of bone marrow suppression. Don't use together.

Bile acid sequestrants, cholestyramine, cyclosporine, oral activated charcoal, trimethoprim–sulfamethoxazole, other drugs that interfere with enterohepatic recirculation: May interfere with enterohepatic recirculation, reducing mycophenolate bioavailability. Avoid use together.

Cyclosporine, drugs that alter normal GI flora (amoxicillin–clavulanate potassium, ciprofloxacin), rifamycins (rifampin): May decrease mycophenolate level. Monitor response to therapy, and increase dosage if necessary.

Drug that modulate glucuronidation (isavuconazole, telmisartan): May increase or decrease mycophenolate level. Monitor patient for efficacy and adverse reactions.

Hormonal contraceptives: May decrease effectiveness of contraceptive. Recommend addition of barrier form of contraception during treatment and for 6 weeks after treatment ends.

Immunosuppressants (sirolimus, tacrolimus): May increase immunosuppression. Monitor patient closely.

Live-virus vaccines: May decrease vaccine effectiveness. Avoid use together.

Norfloxacin and metronidazole: Combined use may decrease mycophenolate level. No effect is seen when given separately. Don't combine with mycophenolate.

Probenecid: May increase mycophenolate level. Monitor patient closely.

Sevelamer, other calcium-free phosphate binders: May decrease mycophenolate level. Avoid use together. If use together is unavoidable, give 2 hours after mycophenolate.

Drug-herb. *Cat's claw, echinacea:* May increase immunostimulation. Discourage use together.

Drug-food. *Any food:* May delay absorption of extended-release form. Advise patient to take on an empty stomach 1 hour before or 2 hours after a meal.

Drug-lifestyle. *Sunlight, UV light exposure:* May increase risk of skin cancer. Instruct patient to limit exposure to sunlight and UV light.

EFFECTS ON LAB TEST RESULTS
• May increase cholesterol, BUN, LDH, creatinine, liver enzyme, and glucose levels.
• May decrease phosphorus, calcium, and magnesium levels.
• May increase or decrease potassium level.
• May decrease Hb level and platelet count.
• May increase or decrease WBC count.

CONTRAINDICATIONS & CAUTIONS
• Contraindicated in patients hypersensitive to drug, its ingredients, or mycophenolic acid. IV formulation is contraindicated in patients sensitive to polysorbate 80.
• Use cautiously in patients with GI disorders. Bleeding and perforation may occur.
• Oral suspension contains aspartame; use cautiously in patients with phenylketonuria.
• Use cautiously in patients with CrCl less than 25 mL/minute, diabetes, or Child-Pugh class C liver impairment.

Boxed Warning Immunosuppression can increase risk of bacterial viral, fungal, and protozoal infections. ∎

Boxed Warning Immunosuppression increases the risk of lymphoma and other malignancies. ∎

⚵ Avoid use in patients with hereditary deficiencies of hypoxanthine-guanine phosphoribosyl-transferase (Lesch-Nyhan syndrome, Kelley-Seegmiller syndrome). Drug may exacerbate disease symptoms due to increased uric acid level.

Dialyzable drug: No.

⚠ **Overdose S&S:** Nausea, vomiting, diarrhea, neutropenia.

M

PREGNANCY-LACTATION-REPRODUCTION

Boxed Warning Use during pregnancy is associated with increased risk of pregnancy loss and congenital malformations. Patients of childbearing potential must receive counseling regarding pregnancy prevention and planning, including use of acceptable contraception during therapy and for 6 weeks after final dose. ■

• For patients using drug at any time during pregnancy and those becoming pregnant within 6 weeks of discontinuing therapy, prescriber should report pregnancy to the Mycophenolate Pregnancy Registry (1-800-617-8191 or www.mycophenolateREMS.com).

• It isn't known if drug appears in human milk. Breastfeeding isn't recommended during therapy.

• Sexually active male patients and their partners of childbearing potential should use effective contraception during treatment of male patient and for at least 90 days after final dose.

• Based on animal data, patients shouldn't donate semen during therapy and for 90 days after final dose.

NURSING CONSIDERATIONS

• Monitor CBC weekly during first month, twice monthly for second and third months, then monthly through first year.

Boxed Warning Drug should only be used by health care providers experienced in immunosuppressive therapy and management of patients with kidney, cardiac, or liver transplantation and in facilities equipped and staffed with adequate lab and supportive medical resources. ■

• Verify pregnancy status prior to therapy, 8 to 10 days later, and during routine follow-up visits.

• Start drug therapy within 24 hours after transplantation. Use IV form in patients unable to take oral forms.

• IV form can be given for up to 14 days; switch patient to capsules or tablets as soon as patient can tolerate oral drugs.

• Monitor liver and kidney function.

• Determine drug levels before and after immunosuppressive therapy changes or when adding or discontinuing concomitant medications.

🔵 *Alert:* Polyomavirus-associated nephropathy, PML, CMV infections, and reactivation of HBV or HCV infection have been reported in patients treated with immunosuppressants. Consider reducing immunosuppressant dosage in patients who develop evidence of new or reactivated viral infections.

🔵 *Alert:* Drugs that cause immunosuppression increase risk of opportunistic infections, including activation of latent viral infections such as BK virus-associated neuropathy, which may lead to serious outcomes, including kidney graft loss.

🔵 *Alert:* Pure red cell aplasia (PRCA) has occurred in patients treated with this drug in combination with other immunosuppressants. Patients may experience fatigue, lethargy, or pallor. PRCA may be reversible with dose reduction or stopping drug. However, this may put graft at risk.

PATIENT TEACHING

• Teach patient safe drug administration and handling for prescribed formulation.

• Stress importance of following treatment as prescribed.

• Inform patient of importance of follow-up visits and ongoing lab tests during therapy.

• Advise patient of childbearing potential about pregnancy testing requirements.

• Instruct patient in pregnancy prevention. Tell patient to immediately report suspected pregnancy.

• Caution patient not to breastfeed during therapy.

• Advise patient not to donate semen during therapy and for 90 days after final dose.

• Instruct patient not to donate blood during therapy and for at least 6 weeks after final dose because blood or blood products might be administered to a patient of childbearing potential or during pregnancy.

Boxed Warning Warn patient of increased risk of infection and lymphoma and other malignancies. ■

• Caution patient to promptly report signs and symptoms of infection (fever, cough, malaise, erythema, wound drainage, pain).

• Advise patient not to drive or operate heavy machinery if somnolence, confusion, dizziness, tremors, or hypotension occurs.

• Instruct patient with increased risk of skin cancer to limit exposure to sunlight and UV light by wearing protective clothing and using broad-spectrum sunscreen with high protection factor.

nadolol
nay-DOE-lol

Corgard

Therapeutic class: Antihypertensives, antianginals
Pharmacologic class: Nonselective beta blockers

AVAILABLE FORMS
Tablets: 20 mg, 40 mg, 80 mg, 160 mg❧

INDICATIONS & DOSAGES
Adjust-a-dose (for all indications): If CrCl is 31 to 50 mL/minute, change dosing interval to every 24 to 36 hours; if CrCl is 10 to 30 mL/minute, every 24 to 48 hours; and if CrCl is less than 10 mL/minute, every 40 to 60 hours.

Boxed Warning Abruptly stopping drug may worsen angina and cause MI. Gradually reduce dosage over 1 to 2 weeks. ▪

➤ **Angina pectoris**
Adults: 40 mg PO once daily. Increase in 40- to 80-mg increments at 3- to 7-day intervals until optimal response occurs. Usual maintenance dosage is 40 to 80 mg once daily. Doses up to 240 mg once daily may be needed.

➤ **HTN**
Adults: 40 mg PO once daily. Increase in 40- to 80-mg increments until optimal response occurs. Usual maintenance dosage is 40 to 80 mg once daily. Doses up to 320 mg daily may be needed.

ADMINISTRATION
PO
- Give drug without regard to food.
- Store at room temperature and avoid heat. Protect from light.
- Check apical pulse before giving drug. If slower than 60 beats/minute (or as directed by prescriber), withhold drug and notify prescriber.

ACTION
Reduces cardiac oxygen demand by blocking catecholamine-induced increases in HR, BP, and force of myocardial contraction. Depresses renin secretion.

Route	Onset	Peak	Duration
PO	Unknown	3–4 hr	17–24 hr

Half-life: About 20 to 24 hours.

ADVERSE REACTIONS
CNS: fatigue, dizziness, drowsiness. **CV:** *bradycardia, HF,* hypotension, rhythm and conduction disturbances, peripheral vascular insufficiency (Raynaud phenomenon).

INTERACTIONS
Drug-drug. *Acetylcholinesterase inhibitors, amiodarone, dipyridamole, ivabradine, midodrine:* May enhance bradycardic effect. Monitor HR.
Amphetamine, methylphenidate: May decrease antihypertensive effect. Monitor BP.
Antihypertensives: May increase antihypertensive effect. Closely monitor BP.
Antipsychotics (second-generation atypicals), MAO inhibitors, phenothiazines: May enhance hypotensive effect. Monitor BP.
Barbiturates, calcium channel blockers, diazoxide, duloxetine, levodopa, methoxyflurane, opioids, pentoxifylline, PDE5 inhibitors, prostacyclin analogues, quinagolide: May enhance hypotensive effect. Monitor BP.
Beta$_2$ agonists: May diminish bronchodilatory effect. Avoid use together.
Ceritinib: May increase bradycardic effect. Avoid use together. If use together is necessary, monitor BP and HR.
Cardiac glycosides: May increase bradycardic and additive AV conduction effects. Use together cautiously.
Disopyramide: May increase bradycardic and negative inotropic effects. Monitor HR and BP.
Dronedarone: May enhance bradycardic effect and increase nadolol level. Use lower initial nadolol dosage and monitor therapy.
Epinephrine: May decrease patient response to epinephrine for treatment of an allergic reaction. Monitor patient closely for decreased clinical effect.
Ergot derivatives: May increase vasoconstricting effect. Consider other therapies.
General anesthetics: May increase hypotensive effects. Consider stopping nadolol before surgery.
Insulin, oral antidiabetics: May mask symptoms of hypoglycemia (such as tachycardia) because of beta blockade. May also alter dosage requirements in patients with stable diabetes. Closely monitor glucose level, and use drug with caution in patients with diabetes.
IV lidocaine: May reduce metabolism of lidocaine, increasing risk of toxicity. Give bolus

N

doses of lidocaine at a slower rate and closely monitor lidocaine level.

NSAIDs: May decrease antihypertensive effect. Monitor BP and adjust dosage.

Prazosin: May increase risk of orthostatic hypotension in early phases of use together. Assist patient to stand slowly until effects are known.

Reserpine: May increase hypotension and bradycardia. Monitor patient for adverse effects (dizziness, syncope, orthostatic hypotension).

Verapamil: May increase effects of both drugs. Closely monitor cardiac function and decrease dosages as necessary.

Drug-herb. *Cannabis:* May increase risk of hypoglycemia. Monitor therapy.

Dong quai, ephedra, garlic, ginseng, licorice, yohimbe: May worsen HTN or affect fluid and electrolytes. Avoid use.

Drug-food. *Green tea:* May decrease nadolol level. Discourage use together.

EFFECTS ON LAB TEST RESULTS
• May lead to false-positive aldosterone/renin ratio.

CONTRAINDICATIONS & CAUTIONS
• Contraindicated in patients with bronchial asthma, sinus bradycardia and greater than first-degree heart block (except in patients with functional pacemaker), cardiogenic shock, and overt (uncompensated) HF.
• Use cautiously in patients with HF, chronic bronchitis, emphysema, kidney or liver impairment, myasthenia gravis, PVD, psoriasis, or psychiatric disease and in patients undergoing major surgery involving general anesthesia. Drug shouldn't be routinely withdrawn before major surgery.
• Generally, patients with bronchospastic disease shouldn't receive beta blockers because they may block bronchodilation.
• Use cautiously in patients with diabetes because beta blockers may mask certain signs and symptoms of hypoglycemia.
• Drug may mask certain signs and symptoms of hyperthyroidism (tachycardia) and precipitate thyroid storm with abrupt withdrawal in patients with suspected thyrotoxicosis.
• Safety and effectiveness in children haven't been determined.
Dialyzable drug: Yes.

⚠️ *Overdose S&S:* Bradycardia, cardiac failure, hypotension, bronchospasm.

PREGNANCY-LACTATION-REPRODUCTION
• Studies during pregnancy are inadequate. Use cautiously during pregnancy and only if potential benefit justifies fetal risk.
• Monitor fetal growth during pregnancy.
• Monitor neonate exposed to nadolol in utero for bradycardia, respiratory depression, and hypoglycemia.
• Drug appears in human milk. Patient should discontinue breastfeeding or discontinue drug, considering importance of drug to patient.

NURSING CONSIDERATIONS
• Frequently monitor BP and HR. If patient develops severe hypotension, immediately notify prescriber.
• Drug masks signs and symptoms of shock, hypoglycemia, and hyperthyroidism.
 Boxed Warning Abrupt withdrawal of drug may exacerbate ischemic heart disease and risk of MI. If discontinuing nadolol after long-term administration, gradually reduce dosage over 1 to 2 weeks and monitor patient closely. If angina worsens or acute coronary insufficiency develops, temporarily restart nadolol and take other measures to manage unstable angina. Because CAD is common and may be unrecognized, don't abruptly discontinue nadolol in patients treated only for HTN. ∎
• *Look alike–sound alike:* Don't confuse Corgard with Coreg.

PATIENT TEACHING
• Explain importance of taking drug as prescribed even after feeling well.
 Boxed Warning Warn patient not to stop drug suddenly. ∎
• Teach patient how to check pulse rate, and instruct patient to check it before each dose and to report pulse rate below 60 beats/minute or as directed by prescriber. Signs and symptoms of slow HR include dizziness and lightheadedness.
• Advise patient with diabetes that drug can mask normal signs or symptoms of low blood glucose level.
• Counsel patient to report pregnancy or plans to become pregnant or breastfeed.

Reactions in bold italics are *life-threatening*.

nafcillin sodium
naf-SIL-in

Therapeutic class: Antibiotics
Pharmacologic class: Penicillinase-resistant penicillins

AVAILABLE FORMS
Infusion: 1 g/50 mL, 2 g/100 mL single-dose container
Infusion or injection: 1-g, 2-g single-dose vials; 10-g multidose vials

INDICATIONS & DOSAGES
Adjust-a-dose (for all indications): Duration of therapy depends on type and severity of the infection and overall patient condition. In severe infection, continue for at least 14 days. Continue for at least 48 hours after patient is afebrile and asymptomatic and cultures are negative. Treatment of endocarditis and osteomyelitis may require a longer duration of therapy.
➤ **Systemic infection caused by penicillinase-producing staphylococci**
Adults: 500 mg IV every 4 hours or 500 mg IM every 4 to 6 hours. For severe infections, 1 g IV or IM every 4 hours.
Infants and children weighing less than 40 kg: 25 mg/kg IM b.i.d.
Neonates: 10 mg/kg IM b.i.d.

ADMINISTRATION
• Before giving drug, ensure patient isn't allergic to penicillins or cephalosporins.
• Obtain specimen for culture and sensitivity tests before giving first dose. Begin therapy while awaiting results.

IV
▼ Check container for leaks, cloudiness, or precipitate before use. Discard if present.
▼ Reconstitute and dilute drug according to manufacturer's instructions. Final concentration shouldn't exceed 40 mg/mL.
▼ Give drug by intermittent IV infusion over 30 to 60 minutes or by direct IV injection over 5 to 10 minutes.
▼ Drug is a vesicant; ensure proper needle or catheter placement before and during infusion.
▼ Reconstituted vials of 10 to 40 mg/mL are stable for 24 hours at room temperature.
▼ **Incompatibilities:** Other drugs.

IM
• Reconstitute with sterile water for injection, NSS for injection, or bacteriostatic water for injection according to manufacturer's instructions. Add 3.4 mL to 1-g vial or 6.6 mL to 2-g vial. Reconstituted vials contain 250 mg/mL.
• For neonates, use sterile water for injection or NSS for injection to avoid administration of benzyl alcohol.
• Administer clear solution by deep intragluteal IM injection immediately after reconstitution; rotate sites.
• Solutions are stable for 3 days at room temperature, for 7 days if refrigerated, and for 90 days if frozen.

ACTION
Inhibits cell-wall synthesis during bacterial multiplication.

Route	Onset	Peak	Duration
IV	Immediate	Immediate	Unknown
IM	Unknown	30–60 min	Unknown

Half-life: About 33 to 61 minutes.

ADVERSE REACTIONS
CNS: *neurotoxicity (at high doses).* **CV:** thrombophlebitis, vein irritation. **GI:** nausea, *pseudomembranous colitis,* diarrhea, vomiting, *CDAD.* **GU:** renal tubular damage, interstitial nephritis. **Hematologic:** *agranulocytosis, leukopenia, neutropenia, thrombocytopenia,* anemia, eosinophilia. **Hepatic:** cholestasis, elevated transaminase levels. **Skin:** severe tissue necrosis (with subcutaneous extravasation), injection-site pain and reactions. **Other:** hypersensitivity reactions.

INTERACTIONS
Drug-drug. *Aminoglycosides (amikacin, tobramycin, gentamicin):* May have synergistic effect; drugs are chemically and physically incompatible. Don't combine in same IV solution.
Cyclosporine: May cause subtherapeutic cyclosporine level. Monitor cyclosporine level.
CYP3A4 substrates (antivirals, clozapine, guanfacine, lurasidone): May decrease substrate level. Use with caution. Refer to substrate prescribing information.
Fentanyl, hydrocodone, methadone: May decrease levels of these drugs. Monitor pain

N

level; watch for withdrawal signs and symptoms.

Hormonal contraceptives: May decrease contraceptive effectiveness due to CYP3A4 inducer activity. Advise use of additional form of contraception during therapy.

Live-virus vaccines: May reduce effectiveness of live-virus vaccine. Don't use together.

Methotrexate: May cause methotrexate toxicity. Monitor patient closely.

Probenecid: May increase nafcillin level. Probenecid may be used for this purpose.

Ranolazine: May decrease ranolazine level. Avoid use together.

Tetracycline: May decrease nafcillin's effectiveness. Avoid use together.

Warfarin: May decrease effects of warfarin. Closely monitor PT and INR.

Zolpidem: May decrease zolpidem level. Monitor patient.

EFFECTS ON LAB TEST RESULTS
• May increase liver transaminase levels.
• May decrease potassium and Hb levels, hematocrit, and neutrophil, WBC, eosinophil, granulocyte, and platelet counts.
• May cause false-positive Coombs test and false-positive urinary and serum protein levels with sulfosalicylic acid testing, but not with dipstick testing.

CONTRAINDICATIONS & CAUTIONS
• Contraindicated in patients hypersensitive to drug or other penicillins.
• Don't use nafcillin to treat infections caused by organisms susceptible to penicillin G or to treat infections caused by methicillin-resistant *Staphylococcus* species.
• Use cautiously in patients with asthma, GI distress, combined liver and kidney dysfunction, or other drug allergies (especially to cephalosporins) because of possible cross-sensitivity.
• Use cautiously in patients with diseases that can be affected by sodium level, such as HF; drug contains sodium.
• Superinfection and CDAD can occur during therapy and for up to 2 months after therapy ends. Drug may need to be discontinued and appropriate treatment initiated.
• Drug may infrequently cause renal tubular damage and interstitial nephritis, especially with large IV doses.

• Safety and effectiveness of IV nafcillin in children haven't been determined.
Dialyzable drug: No.
⚠ *Overdose S&S:* Neurotoxic reactions.

PREGNANCY-LACTATION-REPRODUCTION
• Studies during pregnancy are inadequate. Use only if clearly needed.
• Penicillins appear in human milk. Use cautiously during breastfeeding.

NURSING CONSIDERATIONS
• Bacterial or fungal superinfection may occur with large doses or prolonged therapy, especially in older adults and patients who are debilitated or immunosuppressed.
• Serious and fatal hypersensitivity reactions can occur, including anaphylactic reactions. Obtain complete drug allergy history, and monitor patient during and after drug administration.
• Obtain samples for urinalysis and potassium, BUN, and creatinine levels before and periodically during therapy.
• Obtain LFTs before and periodically during therapy, especially when using high nafcillin doses.
• Monitor WBC count twice weekly in patient receiving drug for longer than 2 weeks. Neutropenia commonly occurs in the third week.
• Monitor patient for signs and symptoms of interstitial nephritis (abnormal urinalysis results, rash, fever, eosinophilia, hematuria, proteinuria, kidney insufficiency).
• Monitor IV site; skin sloughing from subcutaneous extravasation may occur.

PATIENT TEACHING
• Tell patient to report burning or irritation at the IV site.
• Caution patient to take drug exactly as directed. Skipping doses or not completing full course may decrease effectiveness and increase likelihood that bacteria will develop resistance.
• Advise patient to notify prescriber of all adverse reactions, especially rash or signs and symptoms of superinfection (recurring fever, chills, malaise) or CDAD (unexplained diarrhea).

Reactions in bold italics are *life-threatening*.

nalbuphine hydrochloride
NAL-byoo-feen

Nubain✤

Therapeutic class: Opioid analgesics
Pharmacologic class: Opioid agonist-
antagonists–opioid partial agonists

AVAILABLE FORMS
Injection: 10 mg/mL, 20 mg/mL

INDICATIONS & DOSAGES
Adjust-a-dose (for all indications): In patients
with kidney or liver impairment, decrease
dosage.
➤ **Moderate to severe pain (non-opioid-
tolerant patients)**
Adults: For patient weighing about 70 kg, 10
to 20 mg subcut, IM, or IV every 3 to 6 hours
PRN. Maximum, 160 mg daily. Adjust dosage
according to pain severity, physical status,
and patient's other drugs.
➤ **Adjunct to balanced anesthesia; preoperative and postoperative analgesia; obstetric analgesia during labor and delivery**
Adults: 0.3 to 3 mg/kg IV over 10 to
15 minutes; then maintenance dose of 0.25 to
0.5 mg/kg in single IV dose PRN.

ADMINISTRATION
IV
▼ Inject slowly over at least 3 to 5 minutes
into a vein or into an IV line containing a
compatible, free-flowing IV solution, such
as D₅W, NSS, or lactated Ringer solution.
Administer larger doses (0.3 to 3 mg/kg)
over 10 to 15 minutes.
▼ Respiratory depression can be reversed
with naloxone. Keep oxygen and resusci-
tation and intubation equipment available,
particularly when giving IV.
▼ Store at room temperature; protect from
excessive light.
▼ **Incompatibilities:** None listed by manu-
facturer. Consult drug compatibility reference for more information.
IM
• Document injection site.
• Store vial in carton to protect from light.
Subcutaneous
• Document injection site.
• Store vial in carton to protect from light.

ACTION
Unknown. Binds with opioid receptors in the
CNS, altering perception of and emotional
response to pain. Drug is an agonist at kappa
opioid receptors and an antagonist at mu opioid receptors.

Route	Onset	Peak	Duration
IV	2–3 min	2–3 min	3–6 hr
IM, subcut	<15 min	<15 min	3–6 hr

Half-life: 5 hours.

ADVERSE REACTIONS
CNS: dizziness, headache, sedation, vertigo.
EENT: dry mouth. **GI:** nausea, vomiting.
Skin: clamminess, diaphoresis.

INTERACTIONS
Drug-drug. *Anticholinergics (clozapine,
diphenhydramine):* May increase risk of adverse effects. Monitor patient for urine retention and constipation.
Boxed Warning *Benzodiazepines, CNS depressants:* May cause slow or difficult breathing, sedation, and death. Avoid use together.
If use together can't be avoided, limit dose
and duration of each drug to the minimum
needed for desired effect. ∎
Diuretics: May reduce efficacy of diuretics.
Monitor therapy.
*MAO inhibitors (linezolid, phenelzine, tranyl-
cypromine):* May increase risk of serotonin
syndrome or opioid toxicity. Avoid using MAO
inhibitors during treatment and don't use drug
within 14 days of MAO inhibitor therapy.
Muscle relaxants (baclofen, dantrolene): May
increase risk of respiratory depression. Monitor patient carefully.
Naltrexone: May result in opioid withdrawal
signs and symptoms and decreased opioid effectiveness. Avoid combination.
⊙ *Alert:* Serotonergic drugs (amoxapine, antiemetics [dolasetron, granisetron,
ondansetron, palonosetron], antimigraine
drugs, buspirone, cyclobenzaprine, dextromethorphan, lithium, maprotiline, methylene blue, mirtazapine, nefazodone, SNRIs,
SSRIs, TCAs, trazodone, tryptophan, vilazodone):* May increase risk of serotonin syndrome. Use together cautiously. Monitor patient for serotonin syndrome.
Drug-herb. *Cannabinoids, kava, kratom:*
May enhance CNS depressant effects.
Drug-lifestyle. **Boxed Warning** *Alcohol
use:* May cause slow or difficult breathing,

sedation, and death. Discourage use together. ■

⟳ Alert: *St. John's wort:* May increase risk of serotonin syndrome. Use together cautiously. Monitor patient for serotonin syndrome.

EFFECTS ON LAB TEST RESULTS

• May interfere with enzymatic methods for detection of opioids.

CONTRAINDICATIONS & CAUTIONS

• Contraindicated in patients hypersensitive to drug or its components and in those with significant respiratory depression, known or suspected GI obstruction (including paralytic ileus), and acute or severe asthma in an unmonitored setting or in the absence of resuscitative equipment.

Boxed Warning Use exposes patient and others to risk of opioid addiction, abuse, and misuse, which can lead to overdose and death. These effects can occur at any dose or duration. Assess patient risk before prescribing and regularly reassess patient for these behaviors and conditions. ■

⟳ Alert: Use lowest effective dose for shortest period consistent with patient's treatment goals.

⟳ Alert: Because risk of overdose increases as opioid dose increases, reserve titration to higher doses for patients in whom lower doses are ineffective and in whom expected benefits of higher opioid dose outweigh risks.

Boxed Warning *Opioid class warning:* Opioids should only be prescribed with benzodiazepines or other CNS depressants when alternative treatment options are inadequate, aren't expected to provide adequate analgesia, haven't been tolerated, or aren't expected to be tolerated. ■

⟳ Alert: Don't use immediate-release formulations for an extended period, unless pain remains severe enough to require an opioid analgesic and alternative treatment options are inadequate to treat pain.

• Use cautiously and at low doses in patients with preexisting respiratory compromise.

⟳ Alert: Drug should only be administered as a supplement to general anesthesia by those specifically trained in the use of IV anesthetics and management of respiratory effects of potent opioids. Naloxone hydrochloride and emergency resuscitative equipment should be readily available.

⟳ Alert: Patients are at increased risk for oversedation and respiratory depression if they snore or have a history of sleep apnea, haven't used opioids recently or are first-time opioid users, have increased opioid dosage requirements or opioid habituation, have received general anesthesia for longer lengths of time or received other sedating drugs, have preexisting pulmonary or cardiac disease, or have thoracic or other surgical incisions that may impair breathing. Monitor patients carefully.

⟳ Alert: Drug may lead to a rare but serious decrease in adrenal gland cortisol production.

• Drug may cause decreased sex hormone levels with long-term use.

• Use cautiously in patients with history of drug abuse, in patients with cachexia or debilitation, in older adults, and in those with emotional instability, head injury, increased ICP, impaired ventilation, MI accompanied by nausea and vomiting, upcoming biliary surgery, seizure disorders, or liver, kidney, or adrenal insufficiency.

⟳ Alert: Certain commercial preparations contain sodium metabisulfite.

Dialyzable drug: Unknown.

⚠ Overdose S&S: Sleepiness, mild dysphoria.

PREGNANCY-LACTATION-REPRODUCTION

• Studies during pregnancy are inadequate. Use only if clearly needed.

Boxed Warning Prolonged use during pregnancy can result in neonatal opioid withdrawal syndrome, which may be life-threatening. It requires management with expert neonatology protocols. If prolonged use is needed, advise patient of risks and ensure availability of proper treatment. ■

⟳ Alert: When used for pain relief during labor, fetal bradycardia can occur. Monitor fetuses and newborns for bradycardia.

• Use cautiously during breastfeeding. Monitor infant for excess sedation and respiratory depression. Withdrawal signs and symptoms can occur with stoppage of maternal opioid use or breastfeeding.

• Long-term opioid use can cause secondary hypogonadism, infertility, and sexual dysfunction.

NURSING CONSIDERATIONS

Boxed Warning Drug may cause life-threatening or fatal respiratory depression at any time during therapy. Monitor patient closely, especially when starting or increasing doses. Proper dosing and titration are essential to reduce risk. ■

• Reassess pain level at least 15 and 30 minutes after parenteral administration.

⊙ *Alert:* Carefully monitor vital signs, pain level, respiratory status, and sedation level in all patients receiving opioids, especially those receiving IV drugs, even those given postoperatively.

• Before starting drug, assess patient's risk of opioid abuse, misuse, and addiction.

Boxed Warning Regularly monitor all patients for opioid addiction, abuse, and misuse, which can lead to overdose and death. ■

⊙ *Alert:* Drug may cause opioid-induced hyperalgesia (OIH). Symptoms include increased pain level with opioid dose increase, decreased pain level with opioid dose reduction, pain from ordinarily nonpainful stimuli without underlying disease progression, opioid tolerance or withdrawal, and addictive behavior. For suspected OIH, decrease opioid dose or switch patient to alternative opioid.

⊙ *Alert:* If patient is taking opioids with serotonergic drugs, watch for signs and symptoms of serotonin syndrome (agitation, hallucinations, rapid HR, fever, diaphoresis, shivering or shaking, muscle twitching or stiffness, trouble with coordination, nausea, vomiting, diarrhea), especially at start of therapy and after dosage increase. Signs and symptoms may occur within several hours of coadministration but may also occur later, especially after dosage increase. Discontinue opioid, serotonergic drug, or both if serotonin syndrome is suspected.

⊙ *Alert:* Monitor patient for signs and symptoms of adrenal insufficiency (nausea, vomiting, loss of appetite, fatigue, low BP, weakness, dizziness). Perform diagnostic testing if adrenal insufficiency is suspected. For confirmed adrenal insufficiency, treat with corticosteroids and wean patient off opioids, if appropriate. Discontinue corticosteroids when clinically appropriate.

• Monitor patient for signs and symptoms of decreased sex hormone levels (low libido, erectile dysfunction, amenorrhea, infertility). If signs and symptoms occur, evaluate patient and obtain specimens for lab testing.

⊙ *Alert:* Don't stop drug abruptly; withdraw slowly and individualize the gradual tapering plan to prevent signs and symptoms of withdrawal, worsening pain, and psychological

distress in patients who are physically dependent. Refer to manufacturer's label for specific tapering instructions.

⊙ *Alert:* When tapering opioids, monitor patient closely for signs and symptoms of opioid withdrawal (restlessness, lacrimation, rhinorrhea, yawning, perspiration, chills, myalgia, mydriasis, irritability, anxiety, insomnia, backache, joint pain, weakness, abdominal cramps, anorexia, nausea, vomiting, diarrhea, increased BP or HR, increased respiratory rate); such symptoms may indicate a need to taper more slowly. Also monitor patient for suicidality, use of other substances, and mood changes.

• For patient who has received long-term therapy, taper dose by 25% to 50% every 2 to 4 days. If signs or symptoms of withdrawal occur, increase dosage to previous level; then taper more slowly.

• Monitor circulatory and respiratory status and bladder and bowel function. If respirations are shallow or rate is below 12 breaths/minute, withhold dose and notify prescriber.

• Severe constipation commonly occurs with maintenance therapy. Ensure patient receives order for stool softener or stimulant laxative.

• Monitor patient with history of seizures for worsening of seizure control.

• Psychological and physical dependence may occur with prolonged use.

• *Look alike–sound alike:* Don't confuse nalbuphine with naloxone.

PATIENT TEACHING

Boxed Warning Counsel patient and caregiver on serious risks, safe use, and importance of reading the medication guide with each prescription. ■

⊙ *Alert:* Encourage patient to report all medications being taken, including prescription and OTC medications and supplements.

• Inform patient that, for acute pain, drug may only be needed for a few days. Teach about safe disposal of unused drug.

• Instruct patient to contact health care provider if prescribed dosage isn't controlling pain.

⊙ *Alert:* Warn patient to inform prescriber if pain level worsens, pain sensitivity increases, or new pain occurs after taking drug.

⊙ *Alert:* Counsel patient who has been regularly taking drug not to discontinue without first discussing the need for gradual tapering with prescriber.

N

Boxed Warning Caution patient or caregiver to seek immediate medical attention for dizziness, light-headedness, extreme sleepiness, slowed or difficult breathing, or unresponsiveness. ∎

◑ *Alert:* Caution patient to immediately report signs and symptoms of serotonin syndrome.

• Caution patient who is ambulatory about getting out of bed and walking. Warn outpatient to avoid driving and other hazardous activities that require mental alertness until drug's CNS effects are known.

• Teach patient that naloxone may be prescribed with the opioid when beginning and renewing therapy to reduce risk of opioid overdose and death.

• Tell patient to report adverse effects. Review ways to manage troublesome adverse effects such as constipation.

• Instruct patient to report pregnancy or plans to become pregnant during therapy.

naloxone hydrochloride
nal-OX-one

Kloxxado, Narcan ◇, RiVive ◇, Zimhi

Therapeutic class: Antidotes
Pharmacologic class: Opioid antagonists

AVAILABLE FORMS
Injection: 0.4 mg/mL, 1 mg/mL
Injection (prefilled syringe): 5 mg/0.5 mL, 2 mg/2 mL
Nasal spray: 3 mg/ 0.1 mL ◇, 4 mg/ 0.1 mL ◇, 8 mg/0.1 mL

INDICATIONS & DOSAGES
➤ **Emergency treatment of known or suspected opioid-induced respiratory depression**
Adults: 0.4 to 2 mg IV, IM, or subcut. If desired response doesn't occur after 2 or 3 minutes, may give another dose. If still no response and additional doses are available, give every 2 or 3 minutes until emergency medical assistance arrives.
Adults and children of all ages: 5 mg/0.5 mL (Zimhi) IM or subcut. If desired response doesn't occur after 2 or 3 minutes, may give another dose. If still no response and additional doses are available, give every 2 or

3 minutes until emergency medical assistance arrives.

Or, contents of 1 nasal spray (3 mg, 4 mg or 8 mg) intranasally as a single dose; may repeat dose every 2 to 3 minutes in alternating nostrils until emergency medical assistance arrives. In neonates with known or suspected exposure to maternal opioid use, consider using another form to allow dosing according to weight and titration to effect.
Children ages 1 month and older: 0.01 mg/kg IV; second dose of 0.1 mg/kg IV, if needed. If IV route isn't available, drug may be given IM or subcut in divided doses.
Neonates: 0.01 mg/kg IV, IM, or subcut. Repeat dose every 2 to 3 minutes PRN.
Adjust-a-dose: After reversal, additional dose(s) may be needed at a later interval depending on type and duration of opioid.
➤ **Postoperative opioid depression**
Adults: 0.1 to 0.2 mg IV every 2 to 3 minutes PRN. Repeat doses may be required within 1- or 2-hour intervals depending on amount, type (short- or long-acting), and time interval since last administration. Supplemental IM doses have produced a longer-lasting effect.
Children: 0.005 to 0.01 mg IV repeated every 2 to 3 minutes PRN.
➤ **Opioid-induced pruritus** ◆
Adults: 0.25 mcg/kg/hour IV. Doses of 2 mcg/kg/hour or more are likely to reverse pain control.
Children ages 3 and older: 2 mcg/kg/hour IV; may increase to 0.5 mcg/kg/hour every few hours. Doses of 3 mcg/kg/hour or more may risk loss of pain control.

ADMINISTRATION
IV
▼ Give IV push undiluted over 30 seconds.
▼ Give continuous infusion to control adverse effects of epidural morphine.
▼ For continuous infusion, dilute 2 mg of drug in 500 mL D_5W or NSS to yield a concentration of 0.004 mg/mL; use within 24 hours.
▼ Titrate rate to patient's response.
▼ **Incompatibilities:** Alkaline solutions, amphotericin B cholesteryl sulfate, preparations containing bisulfite, sulfite, long-chain or high-molecular-weight anions.
IM
• May give IM into large muscle, such as upper arm, buttock, or thigh.

Reactions in bold italics are *life-threatening*.

- Use mixtures within 24 hours. After 24 hours, discard.
- Use prefilled syringe, if available, to administer drug into anterolateral thigh, through clothing if necessary. In children younger than age 1, pinch thigh muscle while administering.
- Refer to manufacturer's instructions for directions for specific device.

Intranasal
- Don't prime or test device before administration.
- Each container contains a single intranasal spray; don't reuse.
- To administer nasal spray, place patient in supine position and support the back of the neck to allow head to tilt back. After administration, turn patient on side.
- If repeat administration is necessary, use new container and alternate nostrils.

Subcutaneous
- May give undiluted or, if necessary, diluted in sterile water for injection to obtain weight-based dose.
- Use prefilled syringe, if available, to administer drug into anterolateral thigh, through clothing if necessary. In children younger than age 1, pinch thigh muscle while administering.

ACTION

May displace opioid analgesics from their receptors (competitive antagonism); drug has no pharmacologic activity of its own.

Route	Onset	Peak	Duration
IV	1–2 min	5–15 min	Variable
IM, subcut	2–5 min	5–15 min	Variable
Intranasal	8–13 min	20–30 min	Variable

Half-life: IV, IM, or subcut, 30 to 81 minutes in adults, 3 hours in neonates; intranasal, about 2 hours.

ADVERSE REACTIONS

CNS: *seizures,* tremors, headache, dizziness, light-headedness, asthenia, presyncope, agitation, irritability, pain, nervousness, paresthesia, restlessness, shivering, *coma,* confusion, fever, yawning, hallucination; hyperreflexia and excessive crying (in neonates). **CV:** *ventricular fibrillation, ventricular tachycardia, cardiac arrest,* increased BP, hypotension, tachycardia. **EENT:** nasal dryness, nasal irritation, edema, congestion, inflammation, rhinalgia, rhinitis, rhinorrhea, sneezing,

toothache. **GI:** nausea, vomiting, abdominal pain, constipation, abdominal cramps. **Hepatic:** elevated bilirubin level. **Musculoskeletal:** pain, muscle spasms. **Respiratory:** dyspnea, hypoxia, *pulmonary edema.* **Skin:** dry skin, diaphoresis, piloerection, injection-site pain and erythema. **Other:** hot flashes, withdrawal symptoms in patients who are opioid-dependent.

INTERACTIONS

Drug-drug. *Methylnaltrexone, naldemedine, naloxegol:* May enhance risk of opioid withdrawal. Avoid use together.

Partial opioid agonists, mixed opioid agonists-antagonists (buprenorphine, pentazocine): May cause incomplete reversal or require repeated dosing of naloxone due to long duration of action and slow binding rate of these drugs. Monitor patient for continued respiratory depression.

EFFECTS ON LAB TEST RESULTS
None reported.

CONTRAINDICATIONS & CAUTIONS
- Contraindicated in patients hypersensitive to drug.

🜂 **Alert:** Use cautiously in patients with cardiac irritability or opioid addiction. Abrupt reversal of opioid-induced CNS depression may result in sudden opioid withdrawal signs and symptoms (nausea, vomiting, diaphoresis, tachycardia, CNS excitement, increased BP).

🜂 **Alert:** In infants younger than age 4 weeks, sudden opioid withdrawal can be life-threatening. Signs and symptoms include excessive crying, increased reflexes, and seizures.

- Use cautiously in patients with history of seizures; avoid use in patients with meperidine-induced seizures.

Dialyzable drug: Unknown.

PREGNANCY-LACTATION-REPRODUCTION
- Use during pregnancy only if there's a clear indication for its use. Don't withhold drug because of fear of teratogenicity.
- Drug crosses placental barrier and may precipitate withdrawal in fetus and opioid-dependent patient. Monitor fetus for distress.
- It isn't known if drug appears in human milk. Use cautiously; however, because drug is used for opioid reversal, consider

opioid concentration in milk during breast-feeding and potential transfer of opioid to infant.

NURSING CONSIDERATIONS
• Respiratory rate increases within 1 to 2 minutes.
• Duration of action of opioid may exceed that of naloxone, and patient may relapse into respiratory depression. Monitor patient closely and repeat dose if needed.
• Abrupt postoperative reversal of opioid depression may result in adverse CV effects; monitor patient closely.
• **Alert:** Drug only reverses respiratory depression caused by opioids; it doesn't reverse other drug-induced respiratory depression, including that caused by benzodiazepines.
• Monitor patients, especially infants younger than age 4 weeks, for opioid withdrawal signs and symptoms.
• Watch for tachypnea in patient who receives drug to reverse opioid-induced respiratory depression.
• Monitor respiratory depth and rate. Provide oxygen, ventilation, and other resuscitation measures.
• Carefully observe administration site for signs and symptoms of infection after opioid emergency.
• *Look alike–sound alike:* Don't confuse naloxone with naltrexone, Lanoxin, or nalbuphine. Don't confuse Narcan with Marcaine.

PATIENT TEACHING
• Provide reassurance that patient will be closely monitored until opioid effects resolve.
• Teach about signs and symptoms of opioid toxicity emergency (unusual sleepiness or inability to awaken person, breathing problems, pinpoint pupils).
• Counsel family to give naloxone immediately for suspected overdose.
• Advise person who will be administering intranasal drug to read instructions carefully before use. Remind person that spray is single-use only
• Instruct person who will be administering drug to seek emergency help immediately after giving first dose and to give additional doses every 2 to 3 minutes if patient doesn't respond or relapses into respiratory depression before emergency assistance arrives.

• Warn that naloxone administration can precipitate acute opioid withdrawal symptoms, which can be life-threatening in neonates.

naltrexone
nal-TREX-one

Vivitrol

naltrexone hydrochloride
Revia ✽

Therapeutic class: Antidotes
Pharmacologic class: Opioid antagonists, antidotes

AVAILABLE FORMS
naltrexone
Injection: 380-mg vial dose kit
naltrexone hydrochloride
Tablets: 50 mg

INDICATIONS & DOSAGES
➤ **Adjunct for maintaining opioid-free state in patients who are detoxified**
Adults: Initially, 25 mg PO. If no withdrawal signs or symptoms occur after initiation, may start patient on 50 mg every 24 hours the following day. Or, 380 mg IM in gluteal muscle every 4 weeks or once a month.
➤ **Alcohol dependence**
Adults: 50 mg PO once daily for up to 12 weeks, or 380 mg IM in gluteal muscle every 4 weeks or once monthly.

ADMINISTRATION
• **Alert:** Don't give to patients who haven't been opioid free for at least 7 to 10 days. May consider a naloxone IV or subcut challenge test. Refer to manufacturer's instructions.
PO
• Keep container tightly closed and protect from light.
• Give without regard to meals; give with food if GI upset occurs.
IM
• Vivitrol must be prepared and administered by a health care provider.
• Use only the diluent, needles, and other components supplied with the dose kit. Don't substitute.
• Allow drug to reach room temperature before administering (about 45 minutes).

• Administer IM into gluteal muscle, alternating buttocks for each subsequent administration. Avoid giving IV, subcut, or inadvertently into fatty tissue. Monitor injection site.
• Store in refrigerator or up to 7 days at controlled room temperature. Don't freeze.
• Give missed dose as soon as possible.

ACTION

Competitive antagonist at opioid receptor sites, showing the highest affinity for mu receptors. Also modifies the hypothalamic-pituitary-adrenal axis to suppress alcohol consumption.

Route	Onset	Peak	Duration
PO	15–30 min	1 hr	24–72 hr
IM	Unknown	2 hr	>30 days

Half-life: PO, about 4 hours; IM, 5 to 10 days.

ADVERSE REACTIONS

CNS: insomnia, anxiety, nervousness, headache, depression, dizziness, fatigue, somnolence, syncope, low energy, increased energy, irritability, nervousness, suicidality, depression. **CV:** HTN. **EENT:** dry mouth, pharyngitis, toothache. **GI:** nausea, diarrhea, vomiting, abdominal pain, anorexia, constipation, increased thirst, decreased appetite. **GU:** delayed ejaculation, decreased potency. **Hepatic:** increased LFT results. **Musculoskeletal:** muscle and joint pain, muscle cramps, back pain. **Skin:** injection-site reaction, rash. **Other:** chills, flulike symptoms.

INTERACTIONS

Drug-drug. *Bremelanotide:* May decrease naltrexone's effects. Avoid use together. *Methylnaltrexone, naldemedine, naloxegol:* May enhance adverse effects; increases risk of opioid withdrawal. Avoid use together. *Products that contain opioids (including certain cough medications, antidiarrheals):* May decrease effect of opioid. Avoid use together.

EFFECTS ON LAB TEST RESULTS

• May increase GGT, AST, and ALT levels.
• May increase WBC count.
• May interfere with enzymatic methods for detecting opioids in urine.

CONTRAINDICATIONS & CAUTIONS

• Contraindicated in patients hypersensitive to drug or components of the diluent, those currently dependent on opioids, those receiving opioid analgesics, those who fail the naloxone challenge test or who have a positive urine screen for opioids, and those in acute opioid withdrawal.
• Drug may precipitate opioid withdrawal.
• Drug increases sensitivity to opioids, even at lower doses. Fatal overdose may occur if patient uses opioids at the end of a dosing interval, after missing a dose, or after discontinuing treatment. Attempts by patient to overcome blockade may also lead to fatal overdose.
• Dose-related liver injury may occur. Use cautiously in patients with Child-Pugh class A or B liver impairment or history of recent liver disease. Use in patients with Child-Pugh class C liver impairment hasn't been studied.
• Administer IM injection cautiously to patients with thrombocytopenia or coagulation disorders (hemophilia and severe liver failure).
• Suicidality and depression have been reported.
• Drug should be part of a comprehensive treatment plan that includes psychosocial support.
• Safety and effectiveness in children haven't been evaluated.
Dialyzable drug: Unknown.
⚠ *Overdose S&S:* Injection-site reaction, nausea, abdominal pain, somnolence, dizziness.

PREGNANCY-LACTATION-REPRODUCTION

• Studies during pregnancy are inadequate. Use during pregnancy only if potential benefit justifies fetal risk. Untreated opioid addiction or alcohol use can cause fetal harm.
• Drug may appear in human milk. Use cautiously during breastfeeding.

NURSING CONSIDERATIONS

⚡ *Alert:* Patient must be completely free from opioids before taking naltrexone or severe withdrawal symptoms may occur. Patients who have been addicted to short-acting opioids (heroin, meperidine) must wait at least 7 days after last opioid dose before starting drug. Patients who have been addicted to longer-acting opioids (methadone) should wait at least 10 days.
• Naloxone challenge, a test of opioid dependence, should be considered prior to treatment for opioid dependence. If signs and

symptoms of opioid withdrawal persist after naloxone challenge, don't give drug.

• In an emergency, patient may be given an opioid analgesic, but dose must be higher than usual to overcome naltrexone's effect. Watch for respiratory depression from the opioid; it may be longer and deeper.

• Discontinue drug if patient develops signs or symptoms of acute hepatitis.

☺ Alert: Monitor patient for depression and suicidality.

• Monitor for injection-site reaction (pain, tenderness, swelling, erythema, bruising, pruritus). In some cases, injection-site reaction may be very severe (induration, cellulitis, hematoma, abscess, sterile abscess, necrosis).

• Use drug only as part of a comprehensive rehabilitation program.

• **Look alike–sound alike:** Don't confuse naltrexone with naloxone or methylnaltrexone.

PATIENT TEACHING

• Advise patient to carry medical identification and to inform medical personnel about taking naltrexone.

• Tell patient that drug can block effects of opioids and opioid-like drugs, including heroin, pain medicine, antidiarrheals, and cough medicine.

☺ Alert: Warn patient that using large doses of heroin or any other opioid can cause serious injury, coma, or death.

• Advise patient who previously used opioids that sensitivity to lower doses of opioids may increase after naltrexone therapy.

• Warn patient of risk of liver injury. Instruct patient to seek medical attention if signs or symptoms of acute hepatitis occur.

☺ Alert: Tell caregiver of patient dependent on alcohol to monitor patient closely for signs of depression or suicidality and to immediately report any to prescriber.

• Provide names of nonopioid drugs that patient can continue to take for pain, diarrhea, or cough.

• Tell patient to report pain, swelling, tenderness, induration, bruising, pruritus, or redness at injection site.

• Advise patient to immediately report signs and symptoms of allergic reaction (hives, dyspnea, coughing, trouble swallowing or talking, wheezing, facial swelling).

• Counsel patient to report pregnancy or plans to become pregnant.

naproxen
na-PROX-en

EC-Naprosyn, Naprosyn

naproxen sodium
Aleve ◇, Anaprox DS, Maxidol✢ ◇, Mediproxen ◇, Motrimax✢ ◇, Naprelan

Therapeutic class: NSAIDs
Pharmacologic class: NSAIDs

AVAILABLE FORMS
naproxen
Oral suspension: 125 mg/5 mL
Tablets: 250 mg, 375 mg, 500 mg
Tablets (delayed-release) ⓞⓝⓒ: 375 mg, 500 mg
naproxen sodium
Capsules: 220 mg ◇
Tablets (extended-release) ⓞⓝⓒ: 375 mg, 500 mg, 750 mg
Tablets (film-coated) ⓞⓝⓒ: 220 mg ◇, 250 mg, 275 mg, 375 mg, 500 mg, 550 mg
Note: 220 mg of naproxen sodium contains 200 mg of naproxen

INDICATIONS & DOSAGES
Adjust-a-dose (for all indications): Consider lower dosage in older adults and patients with kidney or liver impairment. Not recommended for patients with CrCl less than 30 mL/minute.

➤ **Temporary relief of minor aches and pains; fever reduction (OTC naproxen sodium)**
Adults and children ages 12 and older: 220 mg immediate-release PO every 8 to 12 hours while symptoms last. May give 440 mg within first hour. Maximum dosage, 440 mg in any 8- to 12-hour period and 660 mg in a 24-hour period.

➤ **Acute gout**
Adults: 750 mg naproxen PO; then 250 mg every 8 hours until attack subsides. Or, 825 mg naproxen sodium PO; then 275 mg every 8 hours until attack subsides. Or, 1,000 to 1,500 mg extended-release tablets PO on day 1, followed by 1,000 mg daily until attack subsides.

➤ **Acute tendinitis, bursitis, pain, primary dysmenorrhea**
Adults: 550 mg naproxen sodium PO; then 550 mg PO every 12 hours or 275 mg every 6 to 8 hours. Initial total daily dose shouldn't exceed 1,375 mg; thereafter, total daily dose

shouldn't exceed 1,100 mg. Or, 500 mg naproxen PO; then 500 mg PO every 12 hours or 250 mg PO every 6 to 8 hours. Total daily dose shouldn't exceed 1,250 mg on day 1, or 1,000 mg thereafter. Or, 1,000 mg extended-release tablets PO once daily. May increase to 1,500 mg for limited time, then decrease to 1,000 mg daily.

➤ **Ankylosing spondylitis, osteoarthritis, RA**
Adults: 275 to 550 mg naproxen sodium PO every 12 hours. Or, 250 to 500 mg naproxen tablet or suspension every 12 hours. Or, 375 or 500 mg naproxen delayed-release tablet PO every 12 hours. Or, 750 to 1,000 mg extended-release tablets PO once daily. During long-term administration, may adjust dose up or down, depending on clinical response. In patients who tolerate lower doses well, may increase dosage to 1,500 mg/day when higher level of anti-inflammatory or analgesic activity is required.

➤ **Juvenile idiopathic arthritis**
Children ages 2 and older: 10 mg/kg PO daily in two divided doses. Maximum dosage, 15 mg/kg/day. Use naproxen tablets in children weighing 50 kg or more only.

ADMINISTRATION
PO
⏰ **Alert:** Different dosage strengths and formulations (tablets, suspension) aren't interchangeable. Consider this difference when changing strengths or formulations.
• Give drug with food, milk, or antacids to minimize GI upset. Have patient drink a full glass of water or other liquid with each dose.
• Shake suspension well.
• Have patient swallow delayed-release, extended-release, and film-coated tablets whole; doesn't crush or break them.

ACTION
May inhibit prostaglandin synthesis to produce anti-inflammatory, analgesic, and antipyretic effects.

Route	Onset	Peak	Duration
PO (immediate-release)	30–60 min	2–4 hr (naproxen) 1–2 hr (naproxen sodium)	<12 hr
PO (delayed-release)	30–60 min	4–6 hr	<12 hr
PO (suspension)	60 min	1–4 hr	<12 hr

Half-life: 12 to 17 hours.

ADVERSE REACTIONS
CNS: dizziness, drowsiness, headache, lightheadedness, vertigo, paresthesia, pain, insomnia, asthenia, fever. **CV:** edema, palpitations, chest pain, HTN. **EENT:** visual disturbances, tinnitus, hearing disturbances, pharyngitis, rhinitis, sinusitis. **GI:** nausea, abdominal pain, constipation, diarrhea, dyspepsia, dysphasia, flatulence, epigastric pain, heartburn, occult blood loss, peptic ulceration, stomatitis, thirst, vomiting, *GI bleeding.* **GU:** UTI, cystitis, abnormal kidney function. **Hematologic:** ecchymoses, increased bleeding time, anemia. **Hepatic:** elevated LFTs. **Musculoskeletal:** arthralgia, arthropathy, cramps, myalgia, tendinopathy, back pain. **Respiratory:** dyspnea, cough, bronchitis. **Skin:** diaphoresis, pruritus, purpura, rash. **Other:** flulike syndrome.

INTERACTIONS
Drug-drug. *Antacids, cholestyramine:* May delay naproxen absorption. Avoid use together.
Anticoagulants (warfarin), antiplatelets (aspirin), corticosteroids, other NSAIDs, salicylates, TCAs: May cause adverse GI reactions and bleeding. Avoid use together.
Antihypertensives (ACE inhibitors, ARBs, beta blockers), diuretics: May decrease effect of these drugs. Monitor patient.
ARBs, ACE inhibitors, tacrolimus: May cause or worsen kidney impairment. Use together cautiously.
Cyclosporine: May increase risk of kidney toxicity. Monitor kidney function; consider therapy modification.
Digoxin: May increase serum digoxin level. Monitor digoxin levels.
Lithium: May increase lithium level. Observe patient for toxicity and monitor level. Adjust lithium dosage as required.
Methotrexate: May cause toxicity. Monitor patient closely.
Oral anticoagulants, NSAIDs, SSNRIs, SSRIs, other sulfonylureas, highly protein-bound drugs: May cause toxicity. Monitor patient closely.
Pemetrexed: May result in pemetrexed toxicity (myelosuppression, kidney toxicity, GI toxicity). Consider therapy modification.
Potassium-sparing diuretics: May reduce antihypertensive effects and enhance hyperkalemic effects. Monitor patient closely.
Probenecid: May decrease elimination of naproxen. Monitor patient for toxicity.

N

Drug-herb. *Alfalfa, anise, bilberry, dong quai, feverfew, garlic, ginger, ginkgo, horse chestnut, licorice, red clover:* May cause bleeding. Discourage use together.
White willow: Herb and drug contain similar components. Discourage use together.
Drug-lifestyle. *Alcohol use, smoking:* May increase risk of GI irritation and bleeding. Discourage use together.

EFFECTS ON LAB TEST RESULTS
• May increase BUN, creatinine, ALT, AST, and potassium levels.
• May increase bleeding time.
• May interfere with urinary 5-hydroxyindoleacetic acid and 17-hydroxycorticosteroid determinations.

CONTRAINDICATIONS & CAUTIONS
• Contraindicated in patients hypersensitive to drug and in those with aspirin-sensitive asthma (chronic rhinitis, nasal polyps, bronchospasm, intolerance to aspirin and other NSAIDs).
• Drug can cause serious skin reactions (SJS, TEN). Stop drug at first sign of rash or hypersensitivity.
Boxed Warning Naproxen is contraindicated for treatment of perioperative pain after CABG. ■
• Use cautiously in older adults and in patients with HTN, hyperkalemia, kidney disease, CV disease, GI disorders, liver disease, or history of peptic ulcer disease.
• Drug may increase risk of aseptic meningitis, especially in patients with lupus and mixed connective tissue disorders.
• Drug isn't a substitute for low-dose aspirin for CV protection.
Dialyzable drug: No.
⚠ Overdose S&S: Drowsiness, heartburn, indigestion, nausea, vomiting, seizures.

PREGNANCY-LACTATION-REPRODUCTION
⊙ Alert: Use of NSAIDs at 20 weeks or later in pregnancy may cause fetal kidney dysfunction, leading to oligohydramnios and potential neonatal kidney impairment. Use at 30 weeks or later may increase risk of premature closure of ductus arteriosus. Avoid use during pregnancy starting at 20 weeks' gestation. If potential benefit justifies fetal risk, use lowest effective dose for shortest duration. Consider ultrasound monitoring of amniotic fluid when NSAID therapy exceeds 48 hours. Use of low-dose aspirin (81 mg) for certain pregnancy-related conditions under the direction of a prescriber is acceptable.
• Drug is excreted in human milk at low concentrations. Use cautiously during breastfeeding.
• NSAIDs may cause reversible infertility in women. Consider discontinuing drug in patients having difficulty conceiving.

NURSING CONSIDERATIONS
• Because NSAIDs impair synthesis of renal prostaglandins, they can decrease kidney blood flow and lead to reversible kidney impairment, especially in patients with KF, HF, or liver dysfunction; in older adults; and in those taking diuretics. Monitor these patients closely.
• Before starting therapy, correct volume status in patient with dehydration or hypovolemia.
• Monitor CBC and kidney and liver function every 4 to 6 months during long-term therapy.
• Monitor patient for neurologic effects (drowsiness, dizziness, blurred vision), which may impair physical or mental abilities.
⊙ Alert: Watch for and immediately evaluate signs and symptoms of heart attack (chest pain, shortness of breath or trouble breathing), or stroke (weakness in one part or side of the body, slurred speech).
Boxed Warning NSAIDs increase risk of serious GI adverse events, including bleeding, ulceration, and perforation of stomach or intestines, which can be fatal. Older adults are at greater risk. These events may occur at any time during therapy without warning. ■
Boxed Warning NSAIDs may increase risk of serious thrombotic events, MI, or stroke, which can be fatal. Risk may be greater with longer use or in patients with CV disease or risk factors for CV disease. ■
• Because of their antipyretic and antiinflammatory actions, NSAIDs may mask signs and symptoms of infection.
• Drug may prolong bleeding time and anemias can occur.
• *Look alike–sound alike:* Don't confuse Anaprox with Anaspaz or Avapro. Don't confuse Naprelan with Naprosyn.

PATIENT TEACHING
⊙ Alert: Drug is available without prescription (naproxen sodium, 220 mg). Instruct adult not to take more than 440 mg of naproxen sodium in any 8- to 12-hour period or 660 mg of naproxen sodium in a 24-hour period.

- Advise patient to take drug with food or milk to minimize GI upset and to drink a full glass of water or other liquid with each dose.
- Tell patient taking prescription doses for arthritis that full therapeutic effect may be delayed 2 to 4 weeks.
- Warn patient against taking naproxen and naproxen sodium at the same time.
- ⚠️ *Alert:* Advise patient to immediately seek medical attention if chest pain, shortness of breath, weakness in one part or side of the body, or slurred speech occurs.
- Review signs and symptoms of GI bleeding (blood in vomit, urine, or stool; coffee-ground vomit; melena). Instruct patient to immediately notify prescriber if any occur.
- Advise patient to immediately stop drug and contact prescriber if rash, fever, or difficulty breathing develops.
- Caution patient that use with aspirin, alcohol, other NSAIDs, or corticosteroids may increase risk of adverse GI reactions.
- Warn patient to avoid hazardous activities that require mental alertness until CNS effects are known.
- ⚠️ *Alert:* Warn patient against taking NSAIDs at 20 weeks' gestation or later unless instructed to do so by prescriber due to fetal risk. Advise patient to discuss taking OTC medications with a pharmacist or health care provider during pregnancy.

naratriptan hydrochloride
nar-ah-TRIP-tan

Therapeutic class: Antimigraine drugs
Pharmacologic class: Serotonin 5-HT₁
receptor agonists

AVAILABLE FORMS
Tablets: 1 mg, 2.5 mg

INDICATIONS & DOSAGES
➤ **Acute migraine attacks with or without aura**
Adults: 1 or 2.5 mg PO as a single dose as soon as symptoms appear. If headache returns or responds only partially, may repeat dose after 4 hours. Maximum, 5 mg in 24 hours.
Adjust-a-dose: For patients with CrCl less than 60 to 15 mL/minute or Child-Pugh class A or B liver impairment, 1 mg starting dose, not to exceed 2.5 mg in 24 hours.

ADMINISTRATION
PO
- Give drug without regard to food.
- Store pharmacy-compounded oral suspension in refrigerator; shake well before each use.

ACTION
May act as an agonist at serotonin receptors on extracerebral intracranial blood vessels, which constricts affected vessels, inhibits neuropeptide release, and reduces pain transmission in the trigeminal pathways.

Route	Onset	Peak	Duration
PO	1–2 hr	2–3 hr	Unknown

Half-life: 6 hours.

ADVERSE REACTIONS
CNS: paresthesia, dizziness, drowsiness, fatigue, vertigo, pain, sensation of pressure (chest, neck, throat, jaw). **EENT:** ear, nose, and throat infection; photophobia; pharynx constriction; dry mouth. **GI:** nausea, hyposalivation, vomiting. **Musculoskeletal:** neck pain. **Other:** sensation of warmth, cold, pressure, tightness, or heaviness.

INTERACTIONS
Drug-drug. *Antipsychotics, bromocriptine, linezolid, MAO inhibitors, methylene blue, methylphenidate, opioids, SNRIs, SSRIs, TCAs, tedizolid, tramadol:* May increase risk of serotonin syndrome. Monitor therapy.
Ergot-containing or ergot-type drugs (dihydroergotamine, methysergide), other 5-HT₁ agonists: May prolong vasospastic reactions. Use within 24 hours of naratriptan is contraindicated.
Drug-herb. *St. John's wort:* May increase serotonergic effect. Discourage use together.
Drug-lifestyle. *Smoking:* May increase naratriptan clearance. Discourage smoking.

EFFECTS ON LAB TEST RESULTS
None reported.

CONTRAINDICATIONS & CAUTIONS
- Contraindicated in patients hypersensitive to drug or its components and in those with prior or current cardiac ischemia, Wolff-Parkinson-White syndrome, vasospastic CAD, arrhythmias associated with accessory conduction pathways, cerebrovascular disease (stroke, TIA) or PVD, hemiplegic or basilar

N

---

migraines, ischemic bowel disease, or uncontrolled HTN.

• Contraindicated in older adults, patients with CrCl less than 15 mL/minute, and those with Child-Pugh class C liver impairment.

➌ Alert: Coronary artery spasm, transient ischemia, MI, ventricular tachycardia, ventricular fibrillation, and death have been reported within a few hours of administration. Discontinue drug if these occur. If signs or symptoms of angina occur after dose, evaluate patient for CAD or Prinzmetal angina before giving additional doses, and monitor ECG.

• Use cautiously in patients with risk factors for CAD, such as HTN, obesity, diabetes, hypercholesterolemia, smoking, strong family history of CAD, postmenopause, and age older than 40 (in males), unless patient is free from cardiac disease.

• Use cautiously in patients with kidney or liver impairment.

• Drug isn't indicated for prevention of migraine attacks.

• Safety and effectiveness in children younger than age 18 or when treating cluster headaches or more than four migraines in a 30-day period haven't been established.

Dialyzable drug: Unknown.

⚠ Overdose S&S: Chest pain, ischemic ECG changes, increased BP resulting in lightheadedness, neck tension, tiredness, loss of coordination.

PREGNANCY-LACTATION-REPRODUCTION

• Studies during pregnancy are inadequate. Use only if potential benefit justifies fetal risk.

• It isn't known if drug appears in human milk. Use cautiously during breastfeeding.

NURSING CONSIDERATIONS

• Patient with risk factors for CAD should undergo cardiac evaluation to rule out CAD before starting and periodically during therapy. Monitor patient closely after first dose.

• Drug can cause significant BP elevations, even in patient with no history of HTN. Monitor BP.

• Use drug only when patient has a clear diagnosis of migraine.

• Overuse of acute migraine drugs may lead to medication overuse headache, which may present as migraine-like daily headaches or as marked increase in frequency of migraine attacks.

➌ Alert: Combining drug with other serotonin-modulating drugs may cause serotonin syndrome. Symptoms include restlessness, hallucinations, rapid changes in BP, loss of coordination, fast heartbeat, increased body temperature, hyperreflexia, nausea, vomiting, and diarrhea. Serotonin syndrome is more likely to occur when starting or increasing dose of naratriptan, the SSRI, or the SNRI.

PATIENT TEACHING

• Instruct patient to take drug only as prescribed and to read the accompanying patient instruction leaflet before using drug.

• Tell patient to seek immediate medical care for chest pain, difficulty breathing, irregular heartbeat, weakness, swelling of face, rash, hives, or slurring of speech.

• Caution patient not to take other prescription or OTC drugs or herbal preparations without first consulting prescriber.

• Inform patient that drowsiness and dizziness can occur with naratriptan use. Instruct patient to evaluate ability to perform complex tasks while taking drug.

• Tell patient that drug is intended to relieve, not prevent, migraines.

• Instruct patient to take dose soon after headache starts. If no response occurs with first tablet, tell patient to seek medical approval before taking second tablet.

• Advise patient to increase fluid intake.

• Counsel patient not to use drug during known or suspected pregnancy without discussing with prescriber.

• Advise patient to notify prescriber of breastfeeding or plans to breastfeed.

• Tell patient to alert prescriber about adverse effects.

• Encourage patient to keep a headache diary record of headache frequency and medication use.

---

natalizumab
nah-tah-LIZ-yoo-mab

Tysabri

Therapeutic class: Immunomodulators
Pharmacologic class: Monoclonal antibodies

AVAILABLE FORMS
Injection: 300 mg/15 mL single-use vials

INDICATIONS & DOSAGES

➤ As monotherapy for treatment of relapsing forms of MS; to induce and maintain clinical response and remission in patients with moderately to severely active Crohn disease with evidence of inflammation who have had an inadequate response to, or are unable to tolerate, conventional therapies and inhibitors of TNF-α

Adults: 300 mg IV over 1 hour every 4 weeks.

ADMINISTRATION

IV

▼ Dilute 300 mg in 100 mL NSS to final concentration of 2.6 mg/mL.

▼ Gently invert IV bag to mix solution; don't shake.

▼ Infuse over 1 hour; don't give by IV push or bolus.

▼ Flush IV line with NSS after infusion is complete.

▼ Refrigerate solution and use within 8 hours if not used immediately. Allow to warm to room temperature before infusing.

▼ Refrigerate single-dose vials between 36° and 46° F (2° and 8° C). Don't shake or freeze; protect from light.

▼ **Incompatibilities:** Don't mix or infuse with other drugs. Don't use any diluent other than NSS.

ACTION

May block interaction between adhesion molecules on inflammatory cells and receptors on endothelial cells of vessel walls.

Route	Onset	Peak	Duration
IV	Unknown	Unknown	Unknown

Half-life: 3 to 17 days.

ADVERSE REACTIONS

CNS: depression, dysesthesia, fatigue, headache, vertigo, somnolence, tremors, syncope. **CV:** chest discomfort, peripheral edema. **EENT:** tooth infections, toothache, sinusitis, pharyngolaryngeal pain, tonsillitis. **GI:** abdominal discomfort, diarrhea, gastroenteritis, nausea, dyspepsia, constipation, flatulence, stomatitis. **GU:** UTI, vaginitis, amenorrhea, dysmenorrhea, irregular menstruation, urinary frequency, urinary urgency, urinary incontinence, ovarian cyst. **Hepatic:** abnormal LFT values, cholelithiasis. **Metabolic:** weight increase or decrease. **Musculoskeletal:** arthralgia, extremity pain,

muscle cramps, swollen joints, back pain. **Respiratory:** upper and lower respiratory tract infection, cough. **Skin:** rash, dermatitis, pruritus, dry skin, urticaria, night sweats, thermal injury, skin laceration. **Other:** hypersensitivity reaction, infusion-related reaction, herpes infection, viral infection, rigors, seasonal allergy, flulike symptoms.

INTERACTIONS

Drug-drug. *Corticosteroids, immunosuppressants, TNF inhibitors:* May increase risk of infection and PML. Avoid use together. *Live-virus vaccines:* May cause reduced effectiveness of vaccine. Defer vaccine administration until immune function has returned.

Drug-herb. *Echinacea:* May decrease effectiveness of natalizumab. Consider therapy modification.

EFFECTS ON LAB TEST RESULTS

• May increase LFT values.

• May increase lymphocyte, monocyte, eosinophil, basophil, and nucleated RBC counts.

• May decrease platelet count.

• May cause transient decrease in Hb level.

CONTRAINDICATIONS & CAUTIONS

• Contraindicated in patients hypersensitive to drug or its components and in those with current or history of PML. Use with other immunosuppressants or TNF-α inhibitors isn't recommended.

Boxed Warning Natalizumab increases risk of PML; risk increases with duration of therapy, number of infusions, prior use of immunosuppressants, and presence of anti-JC virus antibodies. Consider these factors with expected benefit when initiating and continuing treatment. ▮

• Safety and effectiveness in children haven't been established.

Dialyzable drug: Unknown.

PREGNANCY-LACTATION-REPRODUCTION

• Drug crosses placental barrier. Use in pregnancy only if benefit justifies fetal risk.

• Obtain CBC in neonates exposed to drug in utero to assess for thrombocytopenia and anemia.

• Drug appears in human milk. Effects on infants are unknown.

N

NURSING CONSIDERATIONS

Boxed Warning Drug is only available through the TOUCH Prescribing Program. ■
• Report PML and serious opportunistic and atypical infections to Biogen Idec (1-800-456-2255).
• Safety and effectiveness of natalizumab treatment beyond 2 years are unknown. When used for Crohn disease, discontinue drug after 12 weeks if patient hasn't experienced therapeutic benefit.

Boxed Warning Monitor patient for PML. Withhold drug immediately at first signs or symptoms suggestive of PML. Symptoms include clumsiness; progressive weakness; and visual, speech, and sometimes personality changes. Gadolinium-enhanced MRI and CSF analysis for JC viral DNA are recommended for diagnosis. ■
• Obtain baseline brain MRI scan before starting therapy.
⊕ **Alert:** Watch for evidence of hypersensitivity reaction during and for 1 hour after infusion (dizziness, urticaria, fever, rash, rigors, pruritus, nausea, flushing, hypotension, dyspnea, chest pain). For patient who has received 12 infusions without evidence of reaction, observe post-infusion for 13th and subsequent infusions, as clinically indicated.
• If hypersensitivity reaction occurs, stop drug and notify prescriber.
⊕ **Alert:** Drug increases risk of developing encephalitis, acute retinal necrosis, and meningitis caused by herpes simplex and varicella zoster viruses. Monitor for signs and symptoms of these conditions. Discontinue drug and initiate appropriate treatment if any occur.
• Other serious infections, including opportunistic infections, have occurred. Concurrent use of antineoplastics, immunosuppressants, or immunomodulating agents may increase the risk. Discontinue therapy until successful infection resolution.
• For patient who starts therapy while on long-term corticosteroids, begin steroid taper as soon as a therapeutic benefit has occurred. If corticosteroids can't be tapered within 6 months, discontinue drug.
• Patients who develop antibodies to drug have an increased risk of infusion-related reaction.
• Discontinue drug in patient with jaundice or other evidence of significant liver injury. Elevated liver enzymes and elevated total bilirubin level may occur as early as 6 days after first dose.
• Monitor patient for thrombocytopenia (easy bruising, abnormal bleeding, petechiae, abnormally heavy menstrual periods). Discontinue drug and immediately evaluate patient if thrombocytopenia occurs.

PATIENT TEACHING
• Inform patient that drug use requires enrollment in and adherence with TOUCH program.
• Tell patient to read the "Medication Guide for Tysabri" before each infusion.
• Urge patient to immediately report progressively worsening symptoms persisting over several days, including changes in eyesight, balance, strength, and thinking, memory, and orientation, leading to confusion and personality changes.
• Advise patient to inform all health care providers about receiving drug.
• Urge patient to immediately report rash, hives, dizziness, fever, shaking chills, or itching while drug is infusing and for up to 1 hour afterward.
• Tell patient about the potential for liver injury and low platelet count.
• Inform patient that drug may affect ability to fight infections. Instruct patient to report signs and symptoms of infection and to use caution when around people who are ill.
• Instruct patient to report pregnancy or plans to become pregnant.

SAFETY ALERT!

nateglinide ℞
na-te-GLYE-nide

Therapeutic class: Antidiabetics
Pharmacologic class: Meglitinide derivatives

AVAILABLE FORMS
Tablets: 60 mg, 120 mg

INDICATIONS & DOSAGES
➤ **Type 2 diabetes as an adjunct to diet and exercise to improve glycemic control**
Adults: 120 mg PO t.i.d. before meals. Patients near goal HbA$_{1c}$ level at start of treatment may receive 60 mg PO t.i.d.

ADMINISTRATION
PO
• Give drug 1 to 30 minutes before a meal.
• If patient plans to skip a meal, skip the dose to reduce risk of hypoglycemia.

ACTION
Lowers glucose level by stimulating insulin secretion from pancreatic beta cells.

Route	Onset	Peak	Duration
PO	20 min	1 hr	4 hr

Half-life: About 1.5 hours.

ADVERSE REACTIONS
CNS: dizziness. **GI:** diarrhea. **Metabolic: *hypoglycemia,*** hyperuricemia, weight gain. **Musculoskeletal:** back pain, arthropathy. **Respiratory:** URI, bronchitis, cough. **Other:** flulike symptoms, accidental trauma.

INTERACTIONS
Drug-drug. *Androgens, antidiabetics, glucomannan, guanethidine, MAO inhibitors, nonselective beta blockers, NSAIDs, pegvisomant, quinolones, salicylates, SSRIs, thioacetic acid:* May increase hypoglycemic action of nateglinide. Closely monitor glucose level. Consider dosage reduction.
Beta blockers, clonidine, guanethidine, reserpine: May mask signs and symptoms of hypoglycemia. Increase frequency of glucose monitoring.
Ceritinib, eltrombopag: May increase nateglinide level. Closely monitor glucose level.
Corticosteroids, rifamycins, somatostatin analogues, somatropin, sympathomimetics, thiazides, thyroid products: May decrease hypoglycemic action of nateglinide. Closely monitor glucose level. Consider dosage increase.
CYP2C9 inducers (phenytoin, rifampin): May decrease hypoglycemic action of nateglinide. Closely monitor glucose level. Consider dosage increase.
CYP2C9 inhibitors (amiodarone, fluconazole, sulfinpyrazone, voriconazole): May increase hypoglycemic action of nateglinide. Closely monitor glucose level. Consider dosage reduction.
Drug-herb. *Gymnema sylvestre:* May increase hypoglycemic action of nateglinide. Closely monitor glucose level.
St. John's wort: May decrease hypoglycemic action of nateglinide. Closely monitor glucose level.

Drug-lifestyle. *Alcohol use:* May increase hypoglycemic action of nateglinide. Closely monitor glucose level.

EFFECTS ON LAB TEST RESULTS
• May increase uric acid level.

CONTRAINDICATIONS & CAUTIONS
• Contraindicated in patients hypersensitive to drug and in those with type 1 diabetes or diabetic ketoacidosis.
• Use cautiously in patients with Child-Pugh class B or C liver impairment or adrenal or pituitary insufficiency, older adults, and patients who are malnourished.
☒ Patients known to be poor metabolizers of CYP2C9 substrates may need dosage reductions and increased glucose monitoring.
• Safety and effectiveness in children haven't been established.
Dialyzable drug: No.
⚠ **Overdose S&S:** Hypoglycemic symptoms.

PREGNANCY-LACTATION-REPRODUCTION
• It isn't known if drug causes fetal harm when administered during pregnancy. Use during pregnancy only if potential benefit justifies fetal risk.
• It isn't known if drug appears in human milk. Drug isn't recommended during breastfeeding due to risk of hypoglycemia in infant who is breastfed.

NURSING CONSIDERATIONS
• Refer to manufacturer's or FDA guidelines regarding which antidiabetics may be used together and which may not.
• Regularly monitor glucose level to evaluate drug's effectiveness.
• Observe patient for signs and symptoms of hypoglycemia. To minimize risk of hypoglycemia, make sure patient has a meal immediately after dose. If hypoglycemia occurs and patient remains conscious, give patient an oral form of glucose. If unconscious, treat patient with IV glucose.
• Risk of hypoglycemia increases with strenuous exercise, alcohol ingestion, insufficient caloric intake, changes in meal pattern, and changes to coadministered medications.
• Symptoms of hypoglycemia may be masked in patients with autonomic neuropathy and in those who use beta blockers, clonidine, or guanethidine.

N

• Insulin therapy may be needed for glycemic control in patients with fever, infection, or trauma and in those undergoing surgery.

• Closely monitor glucose level when other drugs are started or stopped to detect possible drug interactions.

• Periodically monitor HbA₁c level.

• Usually, no special dosage adjustments are necessary in older adults, but some in this age-group may have greater sensitivity to glucose-lowering effect.

PATIENT TEACHING

• Teach about proper drug administration and handling.

• Instruct patient on risk of hypoglycemia, its signs and symptoms (diaphoresis, rapid pulse, trembling, confusion, headache, irritability, nausea), and how to treat these symptoms.

• Teach patient how to monitor and log glucose level to evaluate diabetes control.

• Advise patient to notify prescriber of persistent low or high glucose level.

• Instruct patient to adhere to prescribed diet and exercise regimen.

• Explain possible long-term complications of diabetes and importance of regular preventive therapy.

• Encourage patient to wear a medical identification bracelet.

• Inform patient of potential drug-drug interactions with nateglinide.

• Advise patient to report pregnancy or plans to become pregnant.

• Caution patient that breastfeeding isn't recommended while taking drug.

SAFETY ALERT!

necitumumab
ne-si-TOOM-oo-mab

Portrazza

Therapeutic class: Antineoplastics
Pharmacologic class: Epidermal growth factor receptor antagonists

AVAILABLE FORMS
Injection: 800 mg/50 mL in single-dose vials

INDICATIONS & DOSAGES
➤ **First-line treatment of metastatic squamous cell NSCLC in combination with gemcitabine and cisplatin**

Adults: 800 mg IV infusion on days 1 and 8 of each 3-week cycle given before gemcitabine and cisplatin infusions. Continue until disease progression or unacceptable toxicity occurs.
Adjust-a-dose: **Boxed Warning** For grade 3 or 4 electrolyte abnormalities (such as hypomagnesemia, hypocalcemia, or hypokalemia), withhold drug and replace electrolytes as medically indicated. Resume subsequent cycles after electrolyte abnormalities improve to grade 2 or less. ∎

Refer to manufacturer's instructions for other toxicity-related dosage adjustments and premedication instructions.

ADMINISTRATION
IV

▼ Inspect solution for particulate matter and discoloration. If present, discard solution.

▼ Dilute to final volume of 250 mL in NSS. Don't use solutions containing dextrose.

▼ Gently invert to ensure mixing; don't shake.

▼ Store diluted infusions up to 24 hours at 36° to 46° F (2° to 8° C) or up to 4 hours at room temperature (up to 77° F [25° C]).

▼ Discard vial with any unused portion.

▼ Administer via infusion pump over 60 minutes through separate infusion line. Flush line with NSS at end of infusion.

▼ Refrigerate vials at 36° to 46° F (2° to 8° C); don't freeze. Protect from light.

▼ **Incompatibilities:** Dextrose, electrolytes, other drugs.

ACTION
A recombinant human IgG1 monoclonal antibody that binds to human epidermal growth factor receptor (EGFR) and blocks binding of EGFR to ligands, inhibiting angiogenesis and malignant progression, and allowing apoptosis.

Route	Onset	Peak	Duration
IV	Unknown	Unknown	Unknown

Half-life: 14 days.

ADVERSE REACTIONS
CNS: headache. **CV:** *cardiopulmonary arrest or sudden death, arterial thromboembolism, VTE,* phlebitis. **EENT:** oropharyngeal pain, conjunctivitis. **GI:** vomiting, diarrhea, stomatitis, dysphagia. **Metabolic:** weight loss, *hypomagnesemia, hypokalemia, hypocalcemia,* hypophosphatemia. **Musculoskeletal:** muscle spasms. **Respiratory:** hemoptysis.

Reactions in bold italics are *life-threatening*.

Skin: rash, dermatitis acneiform, acne, pruritus, dry skin, skin fissures, erythema, paronychia, skin toxicity. **Other:** infusion reaction, drug neutralizing antibody development.

INTERACTIONS
Drug-lifestyle. *Sun exposure:* May increase photosensitivity. Advise patient to avoid sun exposure.

EFFECTS ON LAB TEST RESULTS
• May decrease magnesium, potassium, calcium, and phosphorus levels.

CONTRAINDICATIONS & CAUTIONS
Boxed Warning Drug may increase risk of cardiopulmonary arrest and sudden death when used in combination with gemcitabine and cisplatin. Closely monitor electrolyte levels, including magnesium, potassium, and calcium. ■
• Drug isn't indicated for nonsquamous NSCLC.
• Drug increases risk of VTE and arterial thromboembolism (ATE), which can be fatal. Discontinue drug for serious or life-threatening VTE or ATE.
• Safety and effectiveness in children haven't been established.
• Use cautiously in older adults because of increased risk of adverse reactions.
Dialyzable drug: Unknown.

PREGNANCY-LACTATION-REPRODUCTION
• Contraindicated during pregnancy; drug may cause fetal harm. Advise patients of childbearing potential to use effective contraception during therapy and for 3 months after therapy ends.
• No data about breastfeeding exist. Patient shouldn't breastfeed during treatment and for 3 months after final dose.

NURSING CONSIDERATIONS
Boxed Warning Closely monitor electrolyte levels, including magnesium, potassium, and calcium, before each dose and for at least 8 weeks after final dose. Aggressively replace electrolytes as indicated. ■
• Monitor patient for infusion reaction.
• Monitor for skin reactions, which may be severe and usually develop within first 2 weeks of treatment. Drug may need to be withheld or discontinued or dosage reduced.
• Monitor patients for signs and symptoms of ATE (pain, pallor, pulselessness, loss of

function, coldness) and VTE (pain, swelling, erythema, dyspnea, hypotension, tachycardia).
• *Look alike–sound alike:* Don't confuse necitumumab with bevacizumab, nivolumab, pembrolizumab, or ramucirumab. Don't confuse Portrazza with Arzerra.

PATIENT TEACHING
• Review adverse reactions, and instruct the patient to immediately report them.
• Explain that drug may reduce blood levels of magnesium, calcium, and potassium and that these levels must be carefully monitored. Advise patient to take prescribed supplements.
• Advise patient that lab monitoring will be needed to monitor for adverse reactions.
• Review signs and symptoms of infusion reactions (fever, chills, difficulty breathing), and instruct patient to immediately report them.
• Warn patient of childbearing potential to use contraception during therapy and for 3 months after final dose.
• Instruct patient not to breastfeed during therapy and for 3 months after final dose.
• Caution patient to minimize sun exposure, wear protective clothing, and use sunscreen.

---

neomycin sulfate
nee-o-MYE-sin

Therapeutic class: Antibiotics
Pharmacologic class: Aminoglycosides

AVAILABLE FORMS
Tablets: 500 mg

INDICATIONS & DOSAGES
➤ **To suppress intestinal bacteria before surgery**
Adults: As part of bowel preparation regimen, 1 g neomycin PO at 1 p.m., 2 p.m., and 11 p.m. on day before 8 a.m. surgery. May give in combination with other oral and IV antibiotics.

ADMINISTRATION
PO
• For preoperative bowel preparation, provide a low-residue or clear liquid diet starting on preoperative day 3.

ACTION
Inhibits protein synthesis by binding directly to the 30S ribosomal subunit; bactericidal.

♣Canada   ◇OTC   ◆Off-label use   ⊕Do not crush   *Liquid contains alcohol   ✕Genetic

Route	Onset	Peak	Duration
PO	Unknown	1–4 hr	48–72 hr

Half-life: 2 to 3 hours.

ADVERSE REACTIONS
CNS: *neuromuscular blockade.* **EENT:** ototoxicity. **GI:** nausea, vomiting, diarrhea, malabsorption syndrome, CDAD. **GU:** *kidney toxicity.* **Respiratory:** *respiratory paralysis.*

INTERACTIONS
Drug-drug. **Boxed Warning** *Acyclovir , amphotericin B, cephalosporins, cidofovir, cisplatin, methoxyflurane, vancomycin, other aminoglycosides:* May increase kidney toxicity. Monitor kidney function test results. ■
Boxed Warning *Anesthetics, neuromuscular blockers (decamethonium, succinylcholine, tubocurarine):* May increase effects of nondepolarizing muscle relaxants, including prolonged respiratory depression and respiratory paralysis. Use together only when necessary, and expect to reduce dosage of nondepolarizing muscle relaxants. Mechanical ventilation may be needed. ■
Digoxin: May decrease digoxin absorption. Monitor digoxin level.
5-FU, methotrexate, penicillin V, vitamin B$_{12}$ (oral): May inhibit GI absorption of these drugs. Monitor therapy.
Boxed Warning *IV loop diuretics (ethacrynic acid, furosemide):* May increase ototoxicity. Monitor patient's hearing. ■
Oral anticoagulants: May inhibit vitamin K-producing bacteria; may increase anticoagulant effect. Monitor PT and INR.

EFFECTS ON LAB TEST RESULTS
• May increase BUN, creatinine, and nonprotein nitrogen levels.
• May increase urine protein, casts, and cell counts.
• May decrease urine specific gravity.

CONTRAINDICATIONS & CAUTIONS
• Contraindicated in patients hypersensitive to neomycin or other aminoglycosides and in those with intestinal obstruction or inflammatory or ulcerative GI disease.
• Use cautiously in older adults and in patients with impaired kidney function or neuromuscular disorders.
• Prolonged use can cause superinfection, including CDAD, which can occur 2 months or more after therapy ends.

• Drug's ototoxic and kidney-toxic effects limit its usefulness. Use for hepatic encephalopathy is no longer recommended.
• Safety and effectiveness of oral neomycin sulfate in patients younger than age 18 haven't been established.
Dialyzable drug: Yes.
⚠ *Overdose S&S:* Neurotoxicity, ototoxicity, kidney toxicity.

PREGNANCY-LACTATION-REPRODUCTION
• Drug may cause fetal harm. Use during pregnancy only if clearly needed.
• Other aminoglycosides are excreted in human milk. Patient should discontinue breastfeeding or discontinue drug, considering importance of drug to patient.

NURSING CONSIDERATIONS
Boxed Warning Due to increased risk of nephrotoxicity, monitor kidney function: urine output, specific gravity, urinalysis, BUN and creatinine levels, and creatinine clearance. Report evidence of declining kidney function to prescriber. ■
Boxed Warning Due to increased risk of neurotoxicity and ototoxicity, evaluate patient's hearing before and during prolonged therapy. Notify prescriber if patient has tinnitus, vertigo, or hearing loss. Deafness may start several weeks after drug is stopped. ■
Boxed Warning Don't use with other aminoglycosides or neurotoxic or kidney-toxic drugs; risk of toxicities increases. ■
• If kidney insufficiency develops during therapy, consider reducing dosage or discontinuing therapy.
• Watch for signs and symptoms of superinfection (chills, fever, diarrhea), including CDAD, which can occur more than 2 months after therapy ends.
Boxed Warning Neuromuscular blockade and respiratory paralysis have been reported after administration of aminoglycosides. Monitor patient closely. ■

PATIENT TEACHING
• Instruct patient to promptly report all adverse reactions, especially fever, chills, diarrhea, changes in hearing, changes in urine amount, or dark urine.
• Encourage patient to maintain adequate fluid intake.
• Caution patient to take drug exactly as directed. Skipping doses or not completing full

---

Reactions in bold italics are *life-threatening*.

course may decrease effectiveness and increase risk of resistant bacteria.

• Advise patient to report pregnancy or plans to become pregnant.

neratinib ⚕
ner-A-ti-nib

Nerlynx

Therapeutic class: Antineoplastics
Pharmacologic class: Tyrosine kinase inhibitors

AVAILABLE FORMS
Tablets ⓓⓝⓒ: 40 mg

INDICATIONS & DOSAGES

Adjust-a-dose (for all indications): For patients with Child-Pugh class C liver impairment, reduce dosage to 80 mg once daily. Refer to manufacturer's instructions for toxicity-related adjustments.

➤ **Extended adjuvant treatment of early-stage HER2-overexpressed or amplified breast cancer, after adjuvant trastuzumab-based therapy** ⚕

Adults: 240 mg (6 tablets) PO once daily. May initiate therapy with dosage escalation: 120 mg (3 tablets) daily week 1 (days 1 to 7), 160 mg daily (4 tablets) week 2 (days 8 to 14), then 240 mg daily day 15 and thereafter. Give continuously until disease recurrence or for up to 1 year.

➤ **Advanced or metastatic HER2-positive breast cancer in combination with capecitabine in patients who have received two or more prior anti-HER2-based regimens in the metastatic setting** ⚕

Adults: 240 mg (6 tablets) PO once daily on days 1 to 21 of a 21-day cycle plus capecitabine (750 mg/m^2 PO b.i.d.) on days 1 to 14 of a 21-day cycle. Or, initiate therapy with dosage escalation: 120 mg (3 tablets) daily week 1 (days 1 to 7), 160 mg daily (4 tablets) week 2 (days 8 to 14), then 240 mg daily day 15 and thereafter. Continue until disease progression or unacceptable toxicity occurs.

ADMINISTRATION
PO
• Give antidiarrheal prophylaxis during first two cycles of treatment; initiate with first

dose of drug. Patient should receive loperamide as follows when not using dose escalation: For weeks 1 and 2 (days 1 to 14), loperamide 4 mg t.i.d.; for weeks 3 to 8 (days 15 to 56), loperamide 4 mg b.i.d.; for weeks 9 through discontinuation of neratinib, loperamide 4 mg as needed, not to exceed 16 mg/day. Titrate dosing to achieve one to two bowel movements per day.

• If diarrhea occurs despite prophylaxis, treat with additional antidiarrheals, fluids, and electrolytes as clinically indicated. Therapy interruptions and dosage reductions may also be required to manage diarrhea.

• Give with food at the same time each day.
• Have patient swallow tablets whole; don't crush or break tablets.
• If a dose is missed, skip missed dose and resume normal schedule.
• Store at room temperature.

ACTION
A kinase inhibitor that irreversibly binds to epidermal growth factor receptor, HER2, and HER4, inhibiting their activity and causing antitumor activity.

Route	Onset	Peak	Duration
PO	Unknown	2–8 hr	Unknown

Half-life: 7 to 17 hours.

ADVERSE REACTIONS
CNS: fatigue, malaise, dizziness. **EENT:** epistaxis, dry mouth, tongue burning. **GI:** diarrhea, nausea, abdominal pain, vomiting, constipation, stomatitis, decreased appetite, mucosal inflammation, dyspepsia, abdominal distention. **GU:** UTI, dysuria, *kidney impairment.* **Hepatic:** increased ALT and AST levels, *liver toxicity.* **Metabolic:** weight loss, dehydration. **Musculoskeletal:** muscle spasms, back pain, arthralgia. **Respiratory:** URI. **Skin:** rash, dermatitis, dry skin, nail disorders, skin fissures. **Other:** flulike symptoms.

INTERACTIONS
Drug-drug. *Antacids:* May decrease neratinib level. Give neratinib 3 hours after antacids. *H_2-receptor antagonists:* May decrease neratinib level. Give neratinib at least 2 hours before or 10 hours after H_2-receptor antagonists. *Moderate and strong CYP3A4 inducers (bosentan, carbamazepine, efavirenz, phenytoin, rifampin):* May decrease neratinib level. Avoid use together.

N

Moderate and strong CYP3A4 inhibitors (aprepitant, clarithromycin, ciprofloxacin, diltiazem, ketoconazole, ritonavir): May increase neratinib level. Avoid use together.
P-gp substrates (dabigatran, digoxin, fexofenadine): May increase P-gp substrate level and increase risk of substrate-related adverse reactions. Adjust P-gp substrate dosage, if clinically indicated.
PPIs: May decrease neratinib level. Avoid use together.
Drug-herb. *St. John's wort:* May decrease neratinib level. Discourage use together.
Drug-food. *Grapefruit juice:* May increase neratinib level. Discourage use together.

EFFECTS ON LAB TEST RESULTS
● May increase creatinine, AST, and ALT levels.

CONTRAINDICATIONS & CAUTIONS
● Use cautiously in patients with severe Child-Pugh class C liver impairment.
● Safety and effectiveness in children haven't been established.
● Use cautiously in older adults because of increased severity of adverse reactions.
Dialyzable drug: Unknown.
⚠ *Overdose S&S:* Diarrhea, nausea, vomiting, dehydration.

PREGNANCY-LACTATION-REPRODUCTION
● Drug may cause fetal harm. Patients of childbearing potential should use effective contraception during treatment and for at least 1 month after final dose.
● Male patients with partners of childbearing potential should use effective contraception during treatment and for 3 months after final dose.
● Serious adverse reactions may occur in infants who are breastfed. Advise patient not to breastfeed during treatment and for at least 1 month after final dose.

NURSING CONSIDERATIONS
● Verify pregnancy status before treatment.
● Measure total bilirubin, AST, ALT, and ALP levels at baseline, monthly for the first 3 months, then every 3 months during treatment and as clinically indicated.
● Monitor for sign and symptoms of liver toxicity (worsening fatigue, nausea, vomiting, right upper quadrant tenderness, fever, rash, eosinophilia). Therapy may need to be interrupted, dosage reduced, or drug permanently discontinued.
● Monitor patient, especially older adult, for diarrhea, vomiting, and dehydration. For severe diarrhea despite prophylaxis with loperamide, administer fluid and electrolytes as needed, interrupt treatment, and reduce subsequent doses. Perform stool cultures as clinically indicated to exclude infectious causes of grade 3 or 4 diarrhea or diarrhea of any grade with complicating features (dehydration, fever, neutropenia).

PATIENT TEACHING
● Caution patient of childbearing potential that drug can cause fetal harm. Explain that pregnancy test will be performed before therapy begins.
● Counsel patient of reproductive potential about use of effective contraception.
● Advise patient not to breastfeed during therapy and for at least 1 month after final dose.
● Tell patient that lab tests will be needed during therapy.
● Stress importance of antidiarrheal prophylaxis with loperamide. Remind patient to immediately report severe episodes of diarrhea.
● Caution patient to report all adverse reactions, especially signs and symptoms of liver toxicity, such as worsening fatigue, nausea, vomiting, right upper quadrant tenderness, fever, or rash.

niCARdipine hydrochloride
nye-KAR-de-peen

Cardene IV

Therapeutic class: Antihypertensives, antianginals
Pharmacologic class: Calcium channel blockers

AVAILABLE FORMS
Capsules: 20 mg, 30 mg
Injection: 2.5 mg/mL vials; 20 mg/200 mL, 40 mg/200 mL in premixed bags

INDICATIONS & DOSAGES
➤ **Chronic stable angina (used alone or with other antianginals)**
Adults: Initially, 20 mg capsule PO t.i.d. Adjust dosage no sooner than every 3 days based on patient response. Usual range, 20 to 40 mg t.i.d.

➤ **HTN**

Adults: Initially, 20 mg capsule PO t.i.d.; range, 20 to 40 mg t.i.d. Adjust dosage every 3 days based on patient response. Or, to initiate therapy in patient who can't take oral nicardipine, 5 mg/hour IV infusion, increased by 2.5 mg/hour every 5 minutes for rapid control or every 15 minutes for gradual control to maximum of 15 mg/hour. After achieving BP goal, decrease infusion rate to 3 mg/hour. Or, as a substitute for oral nicardipine therapy, if patient takes 20 mg PO every 8 hours, 0.5 mg/hour IV infusion; if patient takes 30 mg PO every 8 hours, 1.2 mg/hour IV infusion; if patient takes 40 mg PO every 8 hours, 2.2 mg/hour IV infusion.

Adjust-a-dose: For patients with kidney impairment, use starting dose of 20 mg PO t.i.d. with slow titration. For patients with Child-Pugh class C liver impairment, use starting dose of 20 mg b.i.d. with slow titration. For patients with hypotension or tachycardia, discontinue infusion; may restart at lower dose when BP and HR stabilize.

ADMINISTRATION

PO

• Give drug with or without food, but avoid giving with high-fat meal.

IV

▼ Dilute 25-mg vial with 240 mL D₅W, dextrose 5% in NSS or half-NSS, or NSS or half-NSS to a concentration of 0.1 mg/mL. Injection remains stable in polyvinyl chloride container for 24 hours at controlled room temperature.

▼ Check premixed bags for leaks, solution clarity, and intact seal. Don't add other drugs to bag.

▼ Closely monitor BP during and after completion of infusion.

▼ Administer via central line or through large peripheral vein. To minimize risk of peripheral venous irritation, change infusion site every 12 hours.

▼ Don't combine with any product in same IV line or premixed container.

▼ Don't use plastic containers in series connections. Doing so may result in air embolism.

▼ When switching to oral form, give first dose of t.i.d. regimen 1 hour before stopping infusion. If using a different oral drug, start it when infusion ends.

▼ If solution is kept at room temperature, protect from light, and use within 24 hours.

▼ **Incompatibilities:** Sodium bicarbonate (5%) injection, lactated Ringer injection. Consult drug compatibility reference for other possible incompatibilities.

ACTION

Inhibits calcium ion influx across cardiac and smooth muscle cells but is more selective to vascular smooth muscle than cardiac muscle. Drug also dilates coronary arteries and arterioles.

Route	Onset	Peak	Duration
PO	0.5–2 hr	1–2 hr	<8 hr
IV	Immediate	45 min	<8 hr

Half-life: 8.6 (PO); 14 hours (IV).

ADVERSE REACTIONS

CNS: headache, dizziness, light-headedness, asthenia, drowsiness, paresthesia, somnolence. **CV:** increased angina, edema, palpitations, flushing, hypotension, tachycardia. **EENT:** dry mouth. **GI:** nausea, vomiting, abdominal discomfort, dyspepsia. **Musculoskeletal:** myalgia. **Skin:** rash, diaphoresis, injection-site reaction, pain at injection site.

INTERACTIONS

Drug-drug. *Antihypertensives, protease inhibitors:* May increase antihypertensive effect. Closely monitor BP.

Beta blockers (atenolol, metoprolol): May increase risk of HF. Titrate slowly.

Cimetidine: May decrease metabolism of calcium channel blockers. Monitor patient for increased pharmacologic effect.

Cyclosporine, tacrolimus: May increase plasma levels of these drugs. Monitor patient for toxicity.

Drug-food. *Grapefruit and grapefruit juice:* May increase bioavailability of nicardipine. Discourage use together.

High-fat foods: May decrease absorption of nicardipine. Discourage use together.

EFFECTS ON LAB TEST RESULTS

• May decrease phosphate level.
• May lead to false-negative aldosterone/renin ratio.

CONTRAINDICATIONS & CAUTIONS

• Contraindicated in patients hypersensitive to drug and in those with advanced aortic stenosis.

N

• Use cautiously in patients with hypotension or impaired liver or kidney function and in older adults.

• Avoid systemic hypotension when administering drug to patients who have sustained an acute cerebral infarction or hemorrhage.

• Consider lower dosages and closely monitor responses in patients with liver impairment or reduced liver blood flow.

• Titrate gradually in patients with kidney impairment.

• MI and increased angina have been noted when calcium channel blockers have been started or doses titrated, especially in the absence of concurrent beta blockade. Abrupt withdrawal can cause rebound angina in patients with CAD.

• Use cautiously in patients with HF due to increased risk of worse outcomes.

• Safety and effectiveness in patients younger than age 18 haven't been established.

Dialyzable drug: No.

⚠ *Overdose S&S:* Hypotension, bradycardia, palpitations, flushing, drowsiness, confusion, slurred speech.

PREGNANCY-LACTATION-REPRODUCTION

• Studies during pregnancy are inadequate. Use during pregnancy only if potential benefit justifies fetal risk.

• Use cautiously during breastfeeding, and monitor infant for adverse effects. Some manufacturers recommend that patient avoid breastfeeding during therapy.

NURSING CONSIDERATIONS

• Closely monitor BP and HR. Drug can cause symptomatic hypotension or tachycardia. Frequently measure BP during initial therapy.

• To reduce risk of venous thrombosis, phlebitis, and vascular impairment, don't use small veins, such as those on dorsum of the hand or wrist. Use extreme care to avoid intra-arterial administration or extravasation.

• *Look alike–sound alike:* Don't confuse nicardipine with niacinamide, nifedipine, or nimodipine. Don't confuse Cardene with Cardura, Cardizem, or codeine.

PATIENT TEACHING

• Teach about proper drug administration and handling, including taking oral form exactly as prescribed.

• Teach patient to report injection-site pain.

• Advise patient to immediately report chest pain. An increase in frequency, severity, or duration of chest pain may occur at start of therapy or during dosage adjustments.

• Caution patient to get up slowly from sitting or lying position to avoid dizziness caused by a decrease in BP.

• Instruct patient to report pregnancy or plans to become pregnant or breastfeed.

nicotine
NIK-oh-teen

Habitrol ◇, Nicoderm CQ ◇, Nicotrol, Nicotrol NS

nicotine polacrilex
Habitrol ◇, Nicorette ◇, Nicorette Mini ◇

Therapeutic class: Smoking cessation aids
Pharmacologic class: Nicotinic agonists

AVAILABLE FORMS
Gum: 2 mg ◇, 4 mg per piece
Lozenges: 2 mg ◇, 4 mg ◇
Nasal spray: 10 mg/mL (0.5 mg/actuation)
Oral inhaler: 10-mg cartridge (4 mg delivered)
Transdermal patch: 7 mg ◇, 14 mg ◇, 21 mg ◇

INDICATIONS & DOSAGES
➤ **Smoking cessation aid for the relief of nicotine withdrawal signs and symptoms as part of a comprehensive behavioral smoking cessation program**
Adults: For gum, initially, patient should slowly chew 1 piece every 1 to 2 hours weeks 1 to 6, then 1 piece every 2 to 4 hours weeks 7 to 9, then 1 piece every 4 to 8 hours weeks 10 to 12. Maximum dosage, 24 pieces/day. Patient who smokes first cigarette more than 30 minutes after waking up should use 2-mg pieces; patient who smokes first cigarette within 30 minutes of waking up should use 4-mg pieces. For best results, patient should chew at least 9 pieces per day for first 6 weeks.

For oral inhaler, patient should use 6 to 16 cartridges/day weeks 1 to 12; initially, at least 6 cartridges/day for the first 3 to 6 weeks and adjust dosage based on signs or symptoms of nicotine withdrawal or excess. After 12 weeks, taper dosage over 6 to 12 additional weeks. Use beyond 6 months isn't recommended.

For lozenge, patient who smokes within 30 minutes of waking up should use 4-mg lozenge; patient who smokes first cigarette more than 30 minutes after waking up should use 2-mg lozenge. Weeks 1 to 6, one lozenge every 1 to 2 hours; weeks 7 to 9, one lozenge every 2 to 4 hours; weeks 10 to 12, one lozenge every 4 to 8 hours. Patient should use at least 9 lozenges/day during the first 6 weeks. Maximum, 5 lozenges in 6 hours or 20 lozenges/day.

For nasal spray, initially one or two doses per hour (one dose is 1 spray in each nostril); may increase to maximum recommended dosage of 40 mg (80 sprays)/day. For best results, at least eight doses per day are recommended. Maximum, five doses per hour or 40 doses per day. Treat for 3 months. Use selected dosage for up to 8 weeks; then discontinue over next 4 to 6 weeks by using such strategies as using only one-half a dose (1 spray) at a time, using spray less frequently, tallying daily usage, skipping a dose, or setting a planned "quit date." Use beyond 6 months isn't recommended.

For transdermal patch (Habitrol) in patients who smoke more than 10 cigarettes a day, apply one 21-mg patch daily during weeks 1 to 4; during weeks 5 to 6, decrease patch strength to 14 mg; during weeks 7 to 8, decrease patch strength to 7 mg, then discontinue. If patient smokes 10 or fewer cigarettes per day, start with 14-mg patch daily for 6 weeks, then 7-mg patch for 2 weeks, then discontinue. Patient may wear patch for 24 hours.

For transdermal patch (Nicoderm CQ) in patients who smoke more than 10 cigarettes a day, apply one 21-mg patch daily during weeks 1 to 6; during weeks 7 to 8, decrease patch strength to 14 mg; during weeks 9 to 10, decrease patch strength to 7 mg; then discontinue. If patient smokes 10 or fewer cigarettes per day, start with 14-mg patch daily for 6 weeks, then 7-mg patch for 2 weeks, then discontinue. Patient may wear patch for 16 or 24 hours. If vivid dreams occur, patient should remove patch before bedtime. May move to higher dose if patient is experiencing withdrawal symptoms or lower dose if adverse effects occur.

ADMINISTRATION

🔵 *Alert:* Hazardous drug; use safe handling and disposal precautions.

Buccal (gum)
• Patient shouldn't eat or drink for 15 minutes before chewing or while chewing a piece of nicotine gum.
• Patient should chew the gum slowly until it tingles; then place it between cheek and gum. When tingle is gone, patient should begin chewing again until tingle returns. Patient should repeat this process until most of tingle is gone (about 30 minutes).
• Store at room temperature.
• Wrap used pieces of gum in paper and discard.

Buccal (lozenge)
• Patient shouldn't eat or drink 15 minutes before using lozenge or while lozenge is in mouth.
• Patient should place lozenge in mouth and allow lozenge to slowly dissolve (about 20 to 30 minutes). Patient may feel a warm or tingling sensation. Patient should minimize swallowing and not chew or swallow lozenge.
• Occasionally patient should move lozenge from one side of mouth to the other until it's completely dissolved (about 20 to 30 minutes).
• Patient shouldn't use more than one lozenge at a time or continuously use one lozenge after another because GI adverse effects may occur.
• Patient who slips and has a cigarette should continue use.
• Store at room temperature.
• Protect from light.

Inhalational
• Follow manufacturer's directions for assembling inhaler.
• Patient shouldn't inhale into lungs like a cigarette but, instead, inhale deeply into back of throat or puff in short breaths.
• Each cartridge may be used multiple times to provide a total of about 20 minutes of active puffing time. When not in use, keep mouthpiece in locked position out of reach of children and pets.
• Store mouthpiece in plastic storage case. Clean regularly with soap and water.
• Store and use at room temperature; protect from light.

Intranasal (spray)
• See manufacturer's instructions for use of device.
• Give with patient's head tilted back slightly; patient shouldn't sniff, swallow, or inhale through nose during actuation.

N

- Patient shouldn't blow nose for 2 to 3 minutes after administration.
- Avoid contact with solution. If skin, lips, mouth, eyes, or ears come in contact with nicotine solution, immediately rinse with water.

Transdermal (patch)

- Apply one new patch every 24 hours on dry, clean, and hairless skin on upper body or outer arm. Save pouch for patch disposal after use.
- Remove backing from patch and immediately press onto skin for 10 seconds. After handling patch, wash hands.
- Don't cut patch or use a patch that's damaged on opening protective pouch.
- Don't apply patch to skin that is oily, burned, broken out, cut, or irritated. Avoid using soaps, lotions, oils, or creams that contain aloe, lanolin, or glycerin moisturizers on skin where patch will be applied.
- Apply patch at the same time each day and rotate application sites. Allow at least 1 week before applying to previously used skin.
- Patient shouldn't wear more than one patch at a time or leave patch on for more than 24 hours; patches lose potency after 24 hours and increased skin irritation may occur.
- Throw away patch by folding sticky ends together, replacing in pouch, and discarding.

ACTION

Binds to nicotinic-cholinergic receptors in the adrenal medulla, neuromuscular junctions, and the brain, causing stimulation and reward effects. Replaces endogenous nicotine effects obtained from smoking or other forms of tobacco. When appropriate doses are used, reduces withdrawal symptoms, including nicotine craving associated with quitting smoking.

Route	Onset	Peak	Duration
Buccal (gum, lozenge)	Unknown	About 30 min	Unknown
Inhalation	Unknown	Within 15 min	Unknown
Intranasal	Rapid	10–20 min	Unknown
Transdermal	Unknown	2–8 hr	Unknown

Half-life: Inhaler and nasal spray, 1 to 2 hours; transdermal patch, 4 hours.

ADVERSE REACTIONS

CNS: impaired concentration, confusion, fever, headache, nervousness, pain, tremors, incoordination, increased dreaming, apathy, withdrawal signs and symptoms (dizziness, anxiety, restlessness, cravings, sleep disorder, depression, drug dependence, fatigue), paresthesia. **CV:** tachycardia, HTN, palpitations, chest discomfort or tightness, facial flushing (nasal spray). **EENT:** *Gum:* gum problems, tooth disorder, stomatitis, glossitis. *Inhaler:* mouth and throat irritation, taste disturbance, rhinitis, sinusitis, tooth disorder. *Nasal spray:* transient epistaxis, transient changes in sense of smell and taste, earache, numbness of nose or mouth, burning of nose or eyes, hoarseness, watery eyes, sneezing or runny nose, nasal mucosa irritation, ulcer, or blister. **GI:** dyspepsia, flatulence, hiccups, nausea, constipation, diarrhea, increased appetite. **GU:** menstrual disorder. **Metabolic:** weight gain. **Musculoskeletal:** back pain, arthralgia, jaw or neck pain (inhaler, gum), myalgia. **Respiratory:** cough (inhaler), bronchitis, dyspnea. **Skin:** rash, acne, application-site reaction, diaphoresis, pruritus. **Other:** allergic reaction, flulike symptoms.

INTERACTIONS

Drug-drug. *Acetaminophen, adrenergic antagonists (labetalol, prazosin), beta blockers (propranolol and others), imipramine, oxazepam, pentazocine, theophylline:* May cause deinduction of liver enzymes on smoking cessation with or without nicotine replacement. A decrease in dosages of these drugs after smoking cessation may be needed. Monitor patient closely.
Adenosine: May enhance AV-blocking and tachycardic effects of adenosine. Monitor therapy.
Adrenergic agonists (isoproterenol, phenylephrine): May decrease circulating catecholamines with smoking cessation with or without nicotine replacement. An increase in dosages of these drugs after cessation of smoking may be needed. Monitor patient.
Cimetidine: May increase nicotine level. Monitor therapy.
Insulin: May increase subcutaneous absorption of insulin. A decrease in insulin dosage after cessation of smoking may be needed. Monitor patient closely.
Nasal vasoconstrictors (xylometazoline): May delay time to onset and peak nicotine

level of nasal formulation. Advise patient of delay in nicotine effect.

Niacin: May increase flushing and dizziness. Use together cautiously.

Drug-herb. *Lobelia:* May result in additive nicotine effects. Discourage use together.

Drug-food. *Acidic foods and beverages:* May decrease absorption of lozenge. Discourage use together.

Caffeine: May increase caffeine's effects after smoking cessation. Monitor patient.

Drug-lifestyle. *Smoking:* May have additive nicotine effect and increase risk of toxicity. Discourage smoking.

EFFECTS ON LAB TEST RESULTS
None reported.

CONTRAINDICATIONS & CAUTIONS

• Contraindicated in patients with known hypersensitivity or allergy to nicotine or components of the product, including menthol (inhaler) or soy (lozenges).

• Nicotine from any source can be toxic and addictive; dependence on nicotine replacements has occurred.

• Use cautiously in patients with recent MI, serious arrhythmias, HTN, CAD, severe or worsening angina, vasospastic diseases, or PVD.

• Use oral inhaler cautiously in patients with bronchospastic disease because of potential for airway irritation. Other forms of nicotine replacement may be preferred.

• Nasal spray isn't recommended in patients with chronic allergy, rhinitis, nasal polyps, sinusitis, or severe reactive airway disease.

• Use patch cautiously in patients with skin problems and those allergic to adhesive tape.

• Use cautiously in patients with type 1 diabetes, hyperthyroidism, pheochromocytoma, CrCl less than 60 mL/minute, Child-Pugh class C liver impairment, or history of seizures.

• Use cautiously in patients with oropharyngeal inflammation, history of esophagitis, or peptic ulcer disease because healing of GI disorders may be delayed.

• Nicotine gum may cause severe occlusal stress due to its heavier viscosity compared to ordinary chewing gum. Gum may loosen inlays or fillings, damage oral mucosa and natural teeth, and stick to dentures.

• Use gum cautiously in patients receiving sodium-restricted diet.

⊍ Alert: Nicotine exposure to children and pets may cause poisoning and is potentially fatal.

• Use in children hasn't been studied.

• Use cautiously in older adults; consider initiating treatment at low end of dosage range.

Dialyzable drug: Unknown.

⚠ Overdose S&S: Lethargy, pallor, cold sweat, nausea, salivation, vomiting, abdominal pain, diarrhea, headache, dizziness, disturbed hearing and vision, tremors, mental confusion, weakness, ataxia, hypotension, seizures, arrhythmias, vascular collapse, central respiratory paralysis, coma.

PREGNANCY-LACTATION-REPRODUCTION

• Nicotine may cause fetal harm, including spontaneous abortion. Encourage patients who are pregnant to attempt smoking cessation through nonpharmacologic means. Use during pregnancy only under medical supervision and if the likelihood of smoking cessation justifies risk of nicotine use by patient who might continue to smoke during pregnancy.

• Nicotine appears in human milk; however, the amount of nicotine from nicotine replacement products in human milk isn't known. Encourage patients who are breastfeeding not to smoke. Weigh risk of exposure of infant to nicotine from nicotine replacement therapy against risks associated with patient's use of replacement therapy and continued smoking.

NURSING CONSIDERATIONS

• Connect patients who smoke with programs to assist with smoking cessation, such as government-based quit lines.

• Successful smoking cessation programs are individualized and include frequent supportive care.

• Monitor for withdrawal signs and symptoms (craving, nervousness, restlessness, irritability, mood lability, anxiety, drowsiness, sleep disturbances, impaired concentration, increased appetite, headache, myalgia, constipation, fatigue, weight gain).

• Monitor patient for tachycardia and other arrhythmias. Discontinue drug if CV signs and symptoms occur.

• Monitor for signs and symptoms of toxicity and overuse (nausea, abdominal pain, vomiting, diarrhea, diaphoresis, flushing, dizziness, disturbed hearing and vision, confusion,

N

weakness, palpitations, altered respiration, hypotension); ensure that drug is used only as directed.

• Monitor patient for temporomandibular joint dysfunction and pain due to excessive chewing of gum.

• Discontinue patch if skin redness caused by patch doesn't resolve after 4 days or if inflammation or rash occurs.

• OTC products aren't for sale to individuals younger than age 18.

• *Look alike–sound alike:* Don't confuse nicotine brand names.

PATIENT TEACHING

• Emphasize that patient should stop smoking completely while on nicotine replacement therapy to avoid additive nicotine levels higher than smoking alone.

• Teach patient how to properly apply or use products.

• Warn patient to adhere to maximum dosage ranges for these products.

• Advise patient to read all patient education material that comes with each product being used.

• Inform patient using nasal spray that nasal irritation is likely to occur but may lessen with continued use.

• Tell patient that onset of nasal spray's effect may be delayed if patient has a cold or rhinitis.

• Advise patient using gum to report jaw or tooth pain.

• Alert patient using gum that gum can stick to and damage dentures and dental work.

• Instruct patient to use hard, sugarless candy between doses of gum to help provide oral stimulation.

• Advise patient that participating in a comprehensive smoking cessation program improves success.

• Discuss benefits and risks of nicotine replacement versus smoking with patient who is or plans to become pregnant or breastfeed.

• Caution patient that smoking cessation may affect drug pharmacokinetics so dosage adjustments may be needed for other prescribed drugs.

• *Alert:* Advise patient to keep all nicotine products, including used inhaler cartridges, nasal spray bottles, and patches, out of reach of children and pets.

Reactions in bold italics are *life-threatening*.

NIFEdipine
nye-FED-i-peen

Adalat OROS✦, Adalat XL✦, Procardia XL

Therapeutic class: Antihypertensives, antianginals
Pharmacologic class: Calcium channel blockers

AVAILABLE FORMS
Capsules ⊙: 5 mg ✦, 10 mg, 20 mg
Tablets (extended-release) ⊙: 30 mg, 60 mg, 90 mg

INDICATIONS & DOSAGES
Adjust-a-dose (for all indications): For older adults and patients with kidney or liver impairment, initiate drug at low end of dosing range.

➤ **Vasospastic angina (Prinzmetal or variant angina), classic chronic stable angina pectoris**
Adults: Initially, 10 mg short-acting capsule PO t.i.d. Usual effective dosage ranges from 10 to 20 mg t.i.d. Some patients require up to 30 mg q.i.d. Maximum dosage, 180 mg/day. Adjust dosage over 7 to 14 days to evaluate response. Or, 30 to 60 mg (extended-release tablets) PO once daily. Adjust dosage over 7 to 14 days to evaluate response. Maximum dosage, 120 mg/day. Use doses of more than 90 mg cautiously and only when clinically warranted.

➤ **HTN**
Adults: Initially, 30 or 60 mg extended-release tablet PO once daily, adjusted over 7 to 14 days. Maximum dosage, 120 mg/day.

➤ **Raynaud phenomenon ◆**
Adults: Initially, 30 mg extended-release tablet PO once daily. If needed, may increase gradually, usually once every 4 weeks, but not more frequently than once every 7 to 10 days; closely monitor BP with each dosage increase. Usual effective dosage, 30 to 120 mg/day.

In hospitalized patients with severe digital ischemia, initially 10 mg immediate-release capsule PO t.i.d. May titrate in 10-mg increments based on response and tolerability up to 30 mg t.i.d. Transition to extended-release tablets for maintenance therapy.

ADMINISTRATION
PO
• May give immediate-release form without regard to food. If flushing occurs, give with a low-fat meal.

⚠ **Alert:** Don't use capsules SL to rapidly reduce severe high BP; result may be fatal.

• Have patient swallow capsules or extended-release tablets whole; don't crush or break tablets. Pharmacist can make oral suspension with liquid capsules, if needed.

• Protect capsules from direct light and moisture and store at room temperature.

ACTION
Thought to inhibit calcium ion influx across cardiac and smooth muscle cells, decreasing contractility and oxygen demand. Drug may also dilate coronary arteries and arterioles.

Route	Onset	Peak	Duration
PO	20 min	30–60 min	4–8 hr
PO (extended-release)	Unknown	2.5–5 hr	24 hr

Half-life: 2 to 5 hours.

ADVERSE REACTIONS
CNS: dizziness, fatigue, light-headedness, giddiness, headache, weakness, drowsiness, insomnia, pain, paresthesia, nervousness, mood changes, shakiness, fever, sleep disturbances, balance difficulties, tremors. **CV:** flushing, *MI, HF,* heat sensation, peripheral edema, palpitations, transient hypotension. **EENT:** blurred vision, nasal congestion, sore throat, dry mouth. **GI:** nausea, heartburn, diarrhea, constipation, cramps, flatulence, abdominal pain, dyspepsia. **GU:** impotence, polyuria. **Musculoskeletal:** muscle cramps, arthralgia, inflammation, joint stiffness. **Respiratory:** dyspnea, cough, wheezing, chest congestion, shortness of breath, pleuritic chest pain, *pulmonary edema.* **Skin:** dermatitis, pruritus, urticaria, diaphoresis, rash. **Other:** chills, sexual difficulties, inflammation.

INTERACTIONS
Drug-drug. *ACE inhibitors (benazepril):* May increase hypotensive effects. Monitor BP and adjust nifedipine dosage as needed.
Alpha$_1$ blockers (doxazosin): May increase nifedipine level. Monitor BP and adjust nifedipine dosage as needed.

Beta blockers (propranolol): May cause hypotension and HF and exacerbate angina. Use together cautiously.
Cimetidine: May increase nifedipine level. Use together cautiously.
Cyclosporine, tacrolimus: May increase serum levels of these drugs and increase risk of toxicity. Monitor serum levels and adjust dosage as needed.
CYP3A4 inhibitors (azole antifungals, erythromycin, nefazodone, ritonavir, verapamil), diltiazem: May increase effects of nifedipine. Monitor BP closely; decrease nifedipine dosage as needed.
Digoxin: May cause elevated digoxin level. Monitor digoxin level.
Diuretics, fentanyl: May increase hypotensive effects. Monitor BP.
PDE5 inhibitors (sildenafil): Increases risk of hypotension. Monitor BP and adjust nifedipine dosage if needed.
Quinidine: May decrease levels and effects of quinidine while increasing effects of nifedipine. Monitor HR and adjust nifedipine dose as needed.
Strong CYP3A4 inducers (carbamazepine, dexamethasone, phenytoin, rifabutin, rifampin): May decrease nifedipine level. Use together is contraindicated.
Vincristine: May increase risk of vincristine toxicity. Monitor therapy.
Warfarin: May prolong PT. Monitor coagulation parameters and adjust warfarin dosage as needed.
Drug-herb. *Melatonin, St. John's wort:* May interfere with antihypertensive effect. Discourage use together.
Drug-food. *Grapefruit juice:* May increase drug bioavailability. Discourage use together.
Drug-lifestyle. *Alcohol:* May increase level of drug. Limit alcohol use.

EFFECTS ON LAB TEST RESULTS
• May increase ALT, AST, ALP, CK, and LDH levels.

CONTRAINDICATIONS & CAUTIONS
• Contraindicated in patients hypersensitive to drug and in patients with cardiogenic shock, ACS, ST-segment elevation MI, or essential HTN.
• Angina exacerbation and MI have occurred at start of therapy or with dosage titration of dihydropyridine calcium channel blockers. Reflex tachycardia may occur, resulting

N

in angina or MI in patients with obstructive coronary disease, especially in the absence of concurrent beta blockade.

• BP must be lowered at a rate appropriate for patient's clinical condition to avoid symptomatic hypotension with or without syncope. Use of immediate-release nifedipine in hypertensive emergencies and urgencies isn't safe or effective. Serious adverse events (death, cerebrovascular ischemia, syncope, stroke, acute MI, fetal distress) have been reported. Don't use immediate-release nifedipine for acute BP reduction or to manage primary HTN.

• Avoid use in patients with HF; drug may worsen symptoms.

• Use with extreme caution in patients with severe aortic stenosis. Drug may reduce coronary perfusion, resulting in ischemia.

• Use cautiously in patients with hypertrophic cardiomyopathy and outflow tract obstruction because reduction in afterload may worsen symptoms.

• Use cautiously before major surgery. Cardiopulmonary bypass, intraoperative blood loss, or vasodilating anesthesia may result in severe hypotension or increased fluid requirements. Consider withdrawing nifedipine more than 36 hours before surgery if possible.

• Rare reversible elevations in BUN and serum creatinine levels have been reported in patients with preexisting CKD.

• Use cautiously in patients with liver impairment. Clearance of nifedipine is reduced in patients with cirrhosis; monitor patient and consider dosage adjustments.

🜚 **Alert:** Immediate-release drug is considered a high-risk drug for older adults because of the potential for hypotension and increased risk of precipitating myocardial ischemia in this population. Avoid use.

🜚 **Alert:** Use extended-release form cautiously because of increased risk of serious GI obstruction in patients both with and without risk factors. (Risk factors for GI obstruction include altered GI anatomy, GI hypomotility related to GERD, colon cancer, ileus, obesity, hypothyroidism, diabetes, and concomitant use of H_2 blockers, NSAIDs, laxatives, anticholinergic agents, and levothyroxine.)

• Safety and effectiveness in children haven't been established.

Dialyzable drug: Unlikely.

⚠ *Overdose S&S:* Hypotension, dizziness, palpitations, flushing, nervousness.

PREGNANCY-LACTATION-REPRODUCTION

• Drug crosses placental barrier. Oral nifedipine is preferred agent for treating chronic HTN during pregnancy. Immediate-release nifedipine is recommended for managing acute-onset, severe HTN during pregnancy and postpartum.

• Drug appears in human milk. Use during breastfeeding only if benefits outweigh risk.

NURSING CONSIDERATIONS

• Regularly monitor BP and HR, especially in patients who take beta blockers or other antihypertensives.

• Watch for signs and symptoms of HF.

• Monitor patient for peripheral edema; carefully differentiate between adverse effect and HF symptom.

• Don't give immediate-release capsules within 1 week of acute MI or in patients with ACS.

• *Look alike–sound alike:* Don't confuse nifedipine with nimodipine, nisoldipine, or nicardipine. Don't confuse Procardia XL with Cartia XT.

PATIENT TEACHING

• If patient remains on nitrate therapy during nifedipine dosage adjustment, urge continued adherence. Patient may take SL nitroglycerin, as needed, for acute chest pain.

• Tell patient that chest pain may briefly worsen as therapy starts or dosage increases.

• Teach about proper drug administration and handling.

• Tell patient not to abruptly stop drug unless directed by prescriber. Abrupt withdrawal may cause rebound angina in patient with CAD.

• Reassure patient taking extended-release tablet that the wax mold may pass in stools. Assure patient that drug has already been completely absorbed.

• Instruct patient to report pregnancy or plans to become pregnant or breastfeed.

SAFETY ALERT!

niraparib ☒
nye-RAP-a-rib

Zejula

Therapeutic class: Antineoplastics
Pharmacologic class: Poly (ADP-ribose) polymerase inhibitors

AVAILABLE FORMS

Capsules ⓞⓝⓒ: 100 mg
Tablets ⓞⓝⓒ: 100 mg, 200 mg, 300 mg

INDICATIONS & DOSAGES

Adjust-a-dose (for all indications): Refer to manufacturer's instructions for toxicity-related dosage adjustments. For patients with Child-Pugh class B liver impairment, give 200 mg/day; further reduce dosage for liver toxicity, if needed.

➤ **Maintenance treatment of deleterious or suspected deleterious germline *BRCA*-mutated (g*BRCA*mut) recurrent epithelial ovarian, fallopian tube, or primary peritoneal cancer in patients who are in complete or partial response to platinum-based chemotherapy** ☒

Adults: 300 mg PO once daily beginning no later than 8 weeks after most-recent platinum-containing regimen. Continue treatment until disease progression or unacceptable toxicity occurs.

➤ **First-line maintenance treatment of patients with advanced epithelial ovarian, fallopian tube, or primary peritoneal cancer who are in complete or partial response to first-line platinum-based chemotherapy**

Adults weighing 77 kg or more and with a platelet count of $150 \times 10^9/L$ or more: 300 mg PO once daily beginning no later than 12 weeks after most-recent platinum-containing regimen and continuing until disease progression or unacceptable toxicity occurs.

Adults weighing less than 77 kg or with a platelet count less than $150 \times 10^9/L$: 200 mg PO once daily beginning no later than 12 weeks after most-recent platinum-containing regimen and continuing until disease progression or unacceptable toxicity occurs.

ADMINISTRATION

PO

⬧ **Alert:** Hazardous drug; use safe handling and disposal precautions.

• Give without regard to food.

• Give at approximately same time each day; administer antiemetic to prevent nausea and vomiting. Bedtime administration may also help to diminish nausea.

• Have patient swallow capsules or tablets whole; don't crush or break.

• If dose is missed or vomited, don't make up dose; resume at next scheduled time.

ACTION

An inhibitor of poly (ADP-ribose) poly-merase (PARP) enzymes PARP-1 and PARP-2, which have a role in DNA repair. Inhibition of PARP enzymatic activity and increased formation of PARP-DNA complexes result in DNA damage, apoptosis, and cell death.

Route	Onset	Peak	Duration
PO	Unknown	3 hr	Unknown

Half-life: 36 hours.

ADVERSE REACTIONS

CNS: fatigue, headache, dizziness, insomnia, anxiety, taste alteration. **CV:** palpitations, HTN, tachycardia, peripheral edema. **EENT:** conjunctivitis, epistaxis, nasopharyngitis, dry mouth. **GI:** nausea, constipation, intestinal obstruction, vomiting, abdominal pain, abdominal distention, mucositis, stomatitis, diarrhea, dyspepsia, decreased appetite. **GU:** UTI, *AKI.* **Hematologic:** anemia, *neutropenia, leukopenia, thrombocytopenia.* **Hepatic:** increased liver enzyme levels. **Metabolic:** hyperglycemia, *hypomagnesemia,* weight loss. **Musculoskeletal:** myalgia, arthralgia, back pain. **Respiratory:** dyspnea, cough, bronchitis. **Skin:** rash. **Other:** *myelodysplastic syndrome (MDS), acute myeloid leukemia (AML).*

INTERACTIONS

Drug-drug. *Live-virus vaccines:* Immunosuppressants may increase adverse effects and decrease therapeutic effect of live-virus vaccines. Avoid use together.

EFFECTS ON LAB TEST RESULTS

• May increase ALP, GGT, AST, ALT, glucose, and creatinine levels.

• May decrease sodium, albumin, and magnesium levels.

• May decrease Hb level, ANC, and platelet and WBC counts.

CONTRAINDICATIONS & CAUTIONS

• Contraindicated in patients hypersensitive to drug or its components.

• Capsules contain FD&C yellow no. 5 (tartrazine), which may cause allergic-type reactions. Use cautiously in patients with aspirin hypersensitivity, who may have increased sensitivity.

N

• Drug may increase risk of bone marrow suppression, MDS, and AML. Discontinue drug if MDS or AML is confirmed.
• HTN and hypertensive crisis have occurred in patients treated with drug. Closely monitor patients with CV disorders.
• Use in patients with CrCl less than 30 mL/minute or Child-Pugh class B or C liver impairment hasn't been studied.
• Safety and effectiveness in children haven't been established.
Dialyzable drug: Unknown.

PREGNANCY-LACTATION-REPRODUCTION
• Drug may cause fetal harm. Advise patients of childbearing potential to use appropriate contraception during and for at least 6 months after final dose.
• It isn't known if drug appears in human milk. Advise against breastfeeding during treatment and for 1 month after final dose.
• Drug may impair male fertility.

NURSING CONSIDERATIONS
• Verify pregnancy status before start of treatment.
• Assess CBC before treatment; don't give drug until hematologic toxicity from previous chemotherapy has resolved.
• Monitor CBC weekly for first month, then monthly for 11 months, then periodically.
• Monitor BP and HR weekly for first 2 months, then monthly for 1 year, and then periodically thereafter. Manage HTN with medication and dosage adjustments as clinically indicated. Closely monitor patients with cardiac disorders.
• Monitor all patients for PRES (seizure, headache, visual disturbances, altered mental status, HTN). If confirmed by MRI, discontinue drug.
• *Look alike–sound alike:* Don't confuse niraparib with enasidenib, neratinib, nilotinib, nintedanib, olaparib, rucaparib, or talazoparib. Don't confuse Zejula with Zydelig or Zytiga.

PATIENT TEACHING
• Teach about proper drug administration and handling.
• Explain that lab testing will be needed to monitor treatment.
• Advise patient to report all adverse reactions.
• Teach techniques for managing nausea.

• Warn patient of risk of blood disorders. Instruct patient to report weakness, fatigue, fever, weight loss, frequent infections, bruising, bleeding easily, blood in urine or stool, and breathlessness.
• Inform patient that BP and HR will be monitored during therapy.
• Explain that pregnancy test will be needed before therapy begins and that drug can cause fetal harm. Advise patient of childbearing potential to use contraception during treatment and for 6 months after final dose.
• Inform male patient that drug may impair fertility.
• Caution patient not to breastfeed during therapy and for 1 month after final dose.

nitrofurantoin macrocrystals ⬚
nye-troh-fyoo-RAN-toyn

Furadantin, Macrodantin

nitrofurantoin monohydrate/macrocrystals ⬚
Macrobid

Therapeutic class: Antibiotics
Pharmacologic class: Nitrofurans

AVAILABLE FORMS
Capsules: 25 mg, 50 mg, 100 mg
Oral suspension: 25 mg/5 mL

INDICATIONS & DOSAGES
➤ **UTIs caused by susceptible *Escherichia coli*, *Staphylococcus aureus*, enterococci, or certain strains of *Klebsiella* and *Enterobacter* species**
Adults and children older than age 12: 50 to 100 mg PO q.i.d. with meals and at bedtime. Continue for 1 week or for at least 3 days after sterility of urine is obtained. Or, 100 mg Macrobid PO every 12 hours for 7 days.
Children ages 1 month to 12 years: 5 to 7 mg/kg PO daily in four divided doses. Continue for 1 week or for at least 3 days after sterility of urine is obtained.
➤ **UTI prophylaxis**
Adults: 50 to 100 mg PO daily at bedtime.
Children: 1 to 2 mg/kg PO daily in a single dose at bedtime or divided into two doses given every 12 hours.

ADMINISTRATION
PO
• Obtain urine specimen for culture and sensitivity tests before giving. Repeat as needed. Begin therapy while awaiting results.
• Shake suspension well before use. May mix suspension with water, milk, fruit juice, or infant formula.
• Give with food or milk to minimize GI distress and improve absorption.
• Don't open monohydrate/macrocrystals capsule; may open macrocrystals capsule and mix contents with food or juice for immediate use.
• Protect from light. Oral suspension should be dispensed in amber glass bottles.

ACTION
May interfere with bacterial enzyme systems and bacterial cell-wall formation.

Route	Onset	Peak	Duration
PO	Unknown	Unknown	Unknown

Half-life: 20 minutes to 1 hour.

ADVERSE REACTIONS
CNS: headache. **GI:** nausea, flatulence. **Hematologic:** decreased Hb level, eosinophilia. **Hepatic:** increased transaminase levels. **Metabolic:** hyperphosphatemia. **Other:** hypersensitivity reactions.

INTERACTIONS
Drug-drug. *Antacids containing magnesium trisilicate:* May decrease nitrofurantoin absorption. Avoid combination.
Dapsone (topical), nitric oxide, prilocaine, sodium nitrite, tetracaine (topical): May enhance nitrofurantoin adverse effects. Monitor therapy.
Live vaccines (BCG, cholera, typhoid): May diminish therapeutic effect of live vaccines. Avoid combination.
Probenecid, sulfinpyrazone: May inhibit excretion of nitrofurantoin, increasing drug levels and risk of toxicity. The resulting decreased urinary levels could lessen antibacterial effects. Avoid use together.
Drug-food. *Any food:* May increase absorption. Advise patient to take drug with food or milk.

EFFECTS ON LAB TEST RESULTS
• May increase AST, ALT, bilirubin, phosphorus, and ALP levels.

• May increase eosinophil count.
• May decrease Hb level and WBC, granulocyte, and platelet counts.
• May cause false-positive results in urine glucose tests using cupric sulfate (Benedict reagent, Fehling solution).

CONTRAINDICATIONS & CAUTIONS
• Contraindicated in infants ages 1 month and younger; in patients with anuria, oliguria, or CrCl less than 60 mL/minute; in patients with history of cholestatic jaundice or liver dysfunction associated with nitrofurantoin use; and in patients with known hypersensitivity to drug.
• Safety and effectiveness of Macrobid in children younger than age 12 haven't been established.
• Use cautiously in patients with kidney impairment, asthma, anemia, diabetes, electrolyte abnormalities, vitamin B deficiency, or debilitating disease. These conditions increase risk of peripheral neuropathy.
• Chronic, subacute, or acute pulmonary hypersensitivity reactions may occur. Patients on continuous treatment for 6 months or longer are at highest risk. If not recognized early, pulmonary function may be permanently impaired.
• Peripheral neuropathy, which may become severe or irreversible, has occurred.
• Optic neuritis has been reported rarely with nitrofurantoin formulations.
☒ Patients with G6PD deficiency have increased risk of developing hemolytic anemia. This deficiency is found in 10% of Blacks and a small percentage of ethnic groups of Mediterranean and Near-Eastern origin. If hemolytic anemia occurs, discontinue drug. Hemolysis ceases when drug is stopped.
Dialyzable drug: Yes.
⚠ *Overdose S&S:* Vomiting.

PREGNANCY-LACTATION-REPRODUCTION
• Contraindicated during pregnancy at 38 to 42 weeks' gestation, during labor and delivery, and when onset of labor is imminent due to possible hemolytic anemia in the neonate.
• Studies during pregnancy are inadequate. Use during pregnancy before 38 weeks for shortest effective course only if clearly needed.
• Because of possible serious adverse reactions in infants younger than age 1 month, patient should discontinue breastfeeding or

discontinue drug, considering importance of drug to patient.
• High doses may halt sperm production, which is reversible when drug is discontinued.

NURSING CONSIDERATIONS
• Carefully monitor fluid intake and output. Treatment may turn urine brown or dark yellow.
• Monitor LFT values because of risk of fatal liver reactions. Stop drug immediately if hepatitis occurs, and treat appropriately.
• Regularly monitor CBC, kidney function, and pulmonary status.
◑ *Alert:* Monitor patient for signs and symptoms of superinfection, which can occur up to 2 months after therapy ends. Use of nitrofurantoin may result in growth of nonsusceptible organisms, especially *Pseudomonas* species, or cause fungal or bacterial superinfection, such as CDAD and pseudomembranous colitis.
• Monitor patient for pulmonary sensitivity reactions (cough, chest pain, fever, chills, dyspnea, ECG changes, and pulmonary infiltration with consolidation or effusion).
• Some patients experience fewer adverse GI effects with nitrofurantoin macrocrystals.
• Dual-release capsules (25 mg nitrofurantoin macrocrystals combined with 75 mg nitrofurantoin monohydrate) enable patients to take drug only twice daily.
• *Look alike–sound alike:* Don't confuse nitrofurantoin with Neurontin.

PATIENT TEACHING
• Instruct patient to take drug for as long as prescribed, exactly as directed, even after feeling better.
• Tell patient to take drug with food or milk to minimize stomach upset.
• Instruct patient to report adverse reactions, especially peripheral neuropathy (burning sensation, numbness, tingling) and pulmonary conditions (malaise, dyspnea, cough, fever), which can become severe or irreversible.
• Advise patient to immediately report diarrhea, bloody stools with or without stomach cramps, and fever during treatment or 2 or more months after treatment ends.
• Alert patient that drug may turn urine dark yellow or brown.
• Counsel patient to report pregnancy or plans to become pregnant or breastfeed.
• Advise patient not to use antacid preparations containing magnesium trisilicate.

SAFETY ALERT!

nitroglycerin (glyceryl trinitrate)
nye-troe-GLIH-ser-in

Nitro-Bid, Nitro-Dur, Nitroject✶, Nitrolingual Pumpspray, NitroMist, Nitrostat, Rectiv, Rho-Nitro Pumpspray✶, Trinipatch✶

Therapeutic class: Vasodilators, antianginals
Pharmacologic class: Nitrates

AVAILABLE FORMS
Aerosol (translingual): 0.4 mg/metered spray
Injection: 5-mg/mL vial; 100 mcg/mL, 200 mcg/mL, 400 mcg/mL premixed in glass containers
Ointment: 2%
Rectal ointment: 0.4%
Tablets (SL) ⓄⓃⒸ*:* 0.3 mg (1/200 grain), 0.4 mg (1/150 grain), 0.6 mg (1/100 grain)
Transdermal patch: 0.1 mg/hour, 0.2 mg/hour, 0.3 mg/hour, 0.4 mg/hour, 0.6 mg/hour, 0.8 mg/hour release rate

INDICATIONS & DOSAGES
➤ **To prevent chronic anginal attacks**
Adults: For 2% ointment: Start dosage with ½ inch ointment, increasing by ½-inch increments until desired results are achieved. Range of dosage with ointment is ½ inch to 5 inches (1.25 to 12.7 cm). Usual dose is 1 to 2 inches (2.5 to 5.08 cm) applied in the morning and one dose 6 hours later. Remove ointment to provide a 10- to 12-hour nitrate-free interval. *For transdermal patch:* Starting dosage is 0.2 to 0.4 mg/hour once daily applied for 12 to 14 hours a day (with a patch-off period of 10 to 12 hours). May increase to maximum dosage of 0.8 mg/hour once daily.
➤ **Acute angina pectoris; to prevent or minimize anginal attacks before stressful events**
Adults: 1 SL tablet dissolved under tongue or in buccal pouch as soon as angina begins. Repeat every 5 minutes, if needed, to a maximum of three doses within a 15-minute period. May be used prophylactically 5 to 10 minutes before activities that might precipitate an acute angina attack.
   Or, 1 or 2 metered-dose sprays Nitrolingual Pumpspray and NitroMist into mouth,

---

preferably onto or under tongue. Repeat every 3 to 5 minutes, if needed, to a maximum of 3 sprays within a 15-minute period. May use prophylactically 5 to 10 minutes before activities that might precipitate an acute angina attack.

➤ **Perioperative HTN, HF after MI, angina pectoris in acute situations; to produce controlled hypotension during surgery**
Adults: Initially, 5 mcg/minute IV infusion, increasing as needed by 5 mcg/minute every 3 to 5 minutes until response occurs. If 20-mcg/minute rate doesn't produce a response, increase dosage by as much as 20 mcg/minute every 3 to 5 minutes. Maximum dosage, 200 mcg/minute.

➤ **Moderate to severe pain from chronic anal fissure**
Adults: 1 inch (2.5 cm) of ointment PR every 12 hours for up to 3 weeks.

ADMINISTRATION

IV

▼ Dilute with D_5W or NSS for injection. Concentration shouldn't exceed 400 mcg/mL.

▼ Always give with an infusion control device and titrate to desired response.

▼ Regular polyvinyl chloride tubing can absorb drug, making it necessary to infuse higher dosages. A special nonabsorbent polyvinyl chloride tubing is available. Always mix in glass bottles and avoid using a filter.

▼ Use the same type of infusion set when changing lines.

▼ When changing the concentration of infusion, flush the administration set with 15 to 20 mL of the new concentration before use to clear line of old drug solution.

▼ **Incompatibilities:** Other drugs.

Topical

• To apply ointment, measure prescribed amount on application paper; then place paper on any nonhairy area and tape in place. Don't rub in.

• Cover with plastic film to aid absorption and protect clothing. Remove all excess ointment from previous site before applying next dose. Avoid getting drug on fingers.

Rectal

• Cover a finger with plastic wrap, disposable surgical glove, or finger cot.

• Apply 1 inch of ointment onto covered finger.

• Gently insert ointment into anal canal using covered finger no further than first finger joint. Wash hands after use.

Transdermal

• Apply patch to any nonhairy part of skin except distal parts of arms or legs. (Absorption isn't maximal at distal sites.)

• Remove patch after 12 to 14 hours; wash skin with soap and water. Rotate patch sites.

• When stopping transdermal treatment of angina, gradually reduce dosage and frequency of application over 4 to 6 weeks.

Sublingual

• Give tablet at first sign of attack. Patient should wet tablet with saliva and place it under tongue until absorbed. Alternatively, place tablet between lip and gum above incisors or between cheek and gum and allow it to dissolve.

• Dose may be repeated every 5 minutes for a maximum of three doses. If drug doesn't provide relief, obtain prompt medical attention.

• Have patient allow whole tablets to dissolve; don't crush or break tablets, or allow patient to swallow tablets.

Translingual

• Don't shake container.

• Prime pump before use. If pump isn't used frequently, reprime before use. Follow manufacturer's instructions.

• Patients using translingual aerosol form shouldn't inhale the spray but should release it onto or under the tongue, then wait about 10 seconds before swallowing. Patient shouldn't rinse or spit for 5 to 10 minutes after a dose.

ACTION

Reduces cardiac oxygen demand by decreasing left ventricular end-diastolic pressure (preload) and, to a lesser extent, systemic vascular resistance (afterload). Also increases blood flow through the collateral coronary vessels.

Route	Onset	Peak	Duration
IV	Immediate	Immediate	3–5 min
Topical	15–30 min	1 hr	7 hr
Transdermal	30 min	2 hr	10–12 hr
SL	1–3 min	5–7 min	25 min
Buccal	3 min	Unknown	3–5 hr
Translingual	1–3 min	4–15 min	25 min
PR	Immediate	Unknown	Unknown

Half-life: About 1 to 4 minutes.

ADVERSE REACTIONS

CNS: headache, light-headedness, paresthesia, dizziness, syncope, weakness. **CV:** hypotension, bradycardia, flushing, palpitations, peripheral edema. **EENT:** pharyngitis, rhinitis, SL burning. **GI:** nausea, vomiting, abdominal pain. **Respiratory:** dyspnea, diaphoresis. **Skin:** contact dermatitis, rash. **Other:** hypersensitivity reactions.

INTERACTIONS

Drug-drug. *Antihypertensives, barbiturates:* May increase hypotensive effect. Closely monitor BP.

Aspirin: May increase nitroglycerin level and hypotensive effect. Closely monitor BP.

Avanafil, sildenafil, tadalafil, vardenafil: May cause severe hypotension. Use of nitrates in any form with these drugs is contraindicated.

Ergotamine, ergot derivatives: May diminish vasodilatory effect of nitroglycerin. Avoid use together.

Heparin: IV nitroglycerin may reduce anticoagulant effect of heparin. Monitor PTT.

Nitric oxide: May increase risk of methemoglobinemia. Monitor therapy.

Tissue plasminogen activators (alteplase, reteplase): May decrease tissue plasminogen activator antigen level. Avoid use together; if unavoidable, use lowest effective dose of nitroglycerin.

Vasodilators (rilmenidine, riociguat): May cause hypotension. Avoid use together.

Drug-lifestyle. *Alcohol use:* May increase hypotension. Discourage use together.

EFFECTS ON LAB TEST RESULTS

• IV nitroglycerin may falsely elevate triglyceride assay results with some tests.

CONTRAINDICATIONS & CAUTIONS

• Contraindicated in patients hypersensitive to nitrates.

• Contraindicated in patients with severe anemia, acute circulatory failure or shock, increased ICP, angle-closure glaucoma, orthostatic hypotension, or allergy to adhesives (transdermal).

• Avoid use in patients with early MI if hypotension (systolic BP less than 90 mm Hg or more than 30 mm Hg below baseline), marked bradycardia or tachycardia, or right ventricular infarction is present.

• IV nitroglycerin is contraindicated in patients hypersensitive to IV form and in those with cardiac tamponade, restrictive cardiomyopathy, or constrictive pericarditis.

• Use cautiously in patients with hypotension or volume depletion.

Dialyzable drug: Unknown.

⚠ *Overdose S&S:* Vasodilation, decreased cardiac output, venous pooling, severe hypotension, methemoglobinemia.

PREGNANCY-LACTATION-REPRODUCTION

• Nitroglycerin crosses placental barrier.

• Studies during pregnancy are inadequate. Use only if clearly needed.

• It isn't known if drug appears in human milk. Use cautiously during breastfeeding.

NURSING CONSIDERATIONS

• Closely monitor vital signs, particularly BP, during infusion, especially in patient with MI. Excessive hypotension can worsen ischemia.

• Monitor BP and intensity and duration of drug response.

• Drug may cause headaches, especially at beginning of therapy. Dosage may be reduced temporarily, but tolerance usually develops. Treat headache with NSAIDs or acetaminophen.

• Tolerance to drug can be minimized with a 10- to 12-hour nitrate-free interval. Check with prescriber for alterations in dosage regimen if tolerance is suspected.

• Wipe off nitroglycerin paste or remove patch before defibrillation to avoid patient burns.

• *Look alike–sound alike:* Don't confuse nitroglycerin with nitroprusside or nitrofurantoin.

PATIENT TEACHING

• Caution patient to take nitroglycerin regularly, as prescribed, and to always have it accessible.

⬥ *Alert:* Advise patient that stopping drug abruptly may cause coronary artery spasm.

• Teach about proper drug administration and handling for prescribed form of drug.

• Tell patient to take nitroglycerin at first sign of attack. If drug doesn't provide relief, patient should promptly obtain medical help.

• Advise patient who complains of a tingling sensation with SL drug to try placing tablet in cheek.

• Instruct patient to take an additional oral dose before anticipated stress or at bedtime if chest pain occurs at night.

- Urge patient using skin patches to dispose of them carefully because enough medication remains after normal use to be hazardous to children and pets.
- If patient using skin patches is scheduled for an MRI scan, advise patient to notify the facility of the patch.
- Advise patient to avoid alcohol.
- To minimize risk of falls, advise patient to rise slowly when standing up, to go up and down stairs carefully, and to lie down at first sign of dizziness.
- Instruct patient to store SL tablets in cool, dark place in tightly closed container and, if needed, to carry container in jacket pocket or purse, not in pocket close to the body.

SAFETY ALERT!

nitroprusside sodium
nye-troe-PRUSS-ide

Nipride

Therapeutic class: Antihypertensives
Pharmacologic class: Vasodilators

AVAILABLE FORMS
Injection: 25 mg/mL (concentrate) vials; 10 mg/50 mL, 20 mg/100 mL, 50 mg/100 mL ready-to-use containers

INDICATIONS & DOSAGES
➤ **To lower BP quickly in hypertensive emergencies; to produce controlled hypotension to reduce bleeding during surgery; treatment of acute HF**
Adults and children: Begin infusion at 0.3 mcg/kg/minute IV and gradually titrate every few minutes (no less than 5 minutes) until achieving desired effect or until reaching maximum dose of 10 mcg/kg/minute (whichever occurs first). BP can't be further reduced without compromising vital organ perfusion.
Adjust-a-dose: Patients also taking other antihypertensives are extremely sensitive to nitroprusside. Titrate dosage accordingly. If GFR is less than 30 mL/minute/1.73 m^2, titrate dose to less than 3 mcg/kg/minute. In patients with anuria, limit mean dose to 1 mcg/kg/minute.

ADMINISTRATION
IV
Boxed Warning Concentrated drug in vials isn't for direct injection and must be further diluted before infusion. Further dilute concentration in 250, 500, or 1,000 mL of D_5W to provide solutions with 200, 100, or 50 mcg/mL, respectively. ■
Boxed Warning Immediately discontinue infusion if adequate BP reduction doesn't occur within 10 minutes at maximum dose. ■
▼ Because drug is sensitive to light, wrap solution in foil or other opaque material; tubing need not be wrapped. Fresh solution has a faint brownish tint. Discard if solution is discolored, particulate matter is visible, or 24 hours have passed since dilution.
✪ *Alert:* Use an infusion pump. Drug is best given via piggyback through peripheral line with no other drug. Don't titrate rate of main IV line while drug is being infused. Even a small bolus can cause severe hypotension.
Boxed Warning Use drug only when available equipment and personnel allow continuous BP monitoring using either continually reinflated sphygmomanometer or (preferably) intra-arterial pressure sensor. ■
▼ When used to treat HF, guide drug titration using results of invasive hemodynamic monitoring and simultaneous urine output monitoring.
▼ Confirm drug's effect at any infusion rate after an additional 5 minutes before titrating to a higher dose to achieve desired BP.
▼ If severe hypotension occurs, stop infusion; effects of drug quickly reverse. Notify prescriber.
▼ **Incompatibilities:** Other drugs.

ACTION
Relaxes arteriolar and venous smooth muscle.

Route	Onset	Peak	Duration
IV	Immediate	1–2 min	10 min

Half-life: 2 minutes.

ADVERSE REACTIONS
CNS: headache, dizziness, *increased ICP,* loss of consciousness, apprehension, restlessness. **CV:** *bradycardia,* hypotension, tachycardia, palpitations, ECG changes, flushing, venous streaking, retrosternal discomfort. **GI:** nausea, abdominal pain, ileus. **Hematologic:** *methemoglobinemia,* decreased

N

platelet aggregation. **Metabolic:** acidosis, hypothyroidism. **Musculoskeletal:** muscle twitching. **Skin:** diaphoresis, pink color, rash. **Other:** *thiocyanate toxicity, cyanide toxicity,* irritation at IV site.

INTERACTIONS

Drug-drug. *Amphetamines, methylphenidate:* May decrease antihypertensive effect. Monitor BP.
Antipsychotics (second-generation, atypical), barbiturates, brimonidine (topical), diazoxide, duloxetine, ganglionic blockers, general anesthetics, levodopa, lormetazepam, negative inotropic drugs, pentoxifylline, prostacyclin analogues, other antihypertensives: May cause additive effects. Closely monitor BP.
Dapsone (topical), nitric oxide, prilocaine, sodium nitrite, tetracaine (topical): May enhance adverse or toxic effects. Monitor patient closely for hypoxia and cyanosis.
PDE5 inhibitors (sildenafil, vardenafil), riociguat: May increase hypotensive effects. Use together is contraindicated.

EFFECTS ON LAB TEST RESULTS

• May increase methemoglobin, cyanide, thiocyanate, and creatinine levels.

CONTRAINDICATIONS & CAUTIONS

• Contraindicated in patients hypersensitive to drug.
• Contraindicated in patients with compensatory HTN (such as those with arteriovenous shunt or coarctation of the aorta), inadequate cerebral circulation, acute HF with reduced peripheral vascular resistance (high-output HF in endotoxic sepsis), congenital optic atrophy, or tobacco-induced amblyopia and in patients who are moribund coming to emergency surgery.
• Use with extreme caution in patients with increased ICP.
• Use cautiously in patients with hypothyroidism, liver or kidney disease, hyponatremia, or low vitamin B level and in those who are poor surgical risks.
• Drug may increase methemoglobinemia risk. Evaluate and treat patients with impaired oxygenation despite adequate cardiac output and oxygen saturation level.
Dialyzable drug: Yes.
⚠ *Overdose S&S:* Hypotension, acidosis, cyanide or thiocyanate toxicity.

PREGNANCY-LACTATION-REPRODUCTION

• Studies during pregnancy are inadequate. Use only if clearly needed. Animal studies have demonstrated fetal harm. Advise patient of fetal risk.
• It isn't known if drug appears in human milk. Patient should discontinue breastfeeding or discontinue drug, considering importance of drug to patient.

NURSING CONSIDERATIONS

Boxed Warning Drug can cause severe hypotension, which can lead to ischemic injuries or death. Use drug only when available equipment and personnel allow continuous BP monitoring. Hypotension should resolve within 10 minutes after discontinuing drug. ∎
• Obtain baseline vital signs before giving drug; ascertain parameters prescriber wants to achieve. Patient receiving other antihypertensives may be more sensitive to drug.
• Keep patient in supine position when starting therapy or titrating drug.
Boxed Warning Dose-related cyanide toxicity can occur and may be lethal. Patient's ability to buffer cyanide will be exceeded in less than 1 hour at maximum rate of 10 mcg/kg/minute. Limit maximum infusion rate to as short a duration as possible. Liver dysfunction increases risk of cyanide toxicity. ∎
⚠ *Alert:* Monitor for signs and symptoms of cyanide toxicity (venous hyperoxemia with bright-red venous blood, profound hypotension, metabolic acidosis, dyspnea, bradycardia, headache, tinnitus, confusion, seizure, loss of consciousness, ataxia, or vomiting). Immediately stop drug and notify prescriber if toxicity occurs.
• Be aware that increasing dosage requirement to maintain BP control is early sign of cyanide toxicity.
Boxed Warning Although acid-base balance and venous oxygen concentration should be monitored and may indicate cyanide toxicity, these lab tests provide imperfect guidance. ∎
• *Look alike–sound alike:* Don't confuse nitroprusside with nitroglycerin.

PATIENT TEACHING

• Instruct patient to promptly report all adverse reactions, especially signs and symptoms of hypotension and cyanide toxicity.
• Tell patient to alert nurse if discomfort occurs at IV insertion site.
• Inform patient who is pregnant of fetal risk.

nivolumab ⚜
neh-VOL-you-mab

Opdivo

Therapeutic class: Antineoplastics
Pharmacologic class: Monoclonal
antibodies

AVAILABLE FORMS
Injection: 40 mg/4 mL, 100 mg/10 mL,
120 mg/12 mL, 240 mg/24 mL single-dose
vials

INDICATIONS & DOSAGES
Adjust-a-dose (for all indications): Refer to
manufacturer's instructions for dosage adjustments for adverse reactions and treatment-
related toxicities.
➤ **Unresectable or metastatic melanoma;
adjuvant treatment of melanoma with
lymph node involvement or metastatic disease in patients who have undergone complete resection**
*Adult patients and children ages 12 years
and older weighing 40 kg or more:* 240 mg
IV infusion every 2 weeks or 480 mg every
4 weeks until disease progression or unacceptable toxicity occurs.
*Children ages 12 years and older weighing
less than 40 kg:* 3 mg/kg IV infusion every
2 weeks or 6 mg/kg every 4 weeks until disease
progression or unacceptable toxicity occurs.
➤ **Unresectable or metastatic melanoma,
in combination with ipilimumab**
*Adults and children ages 12 years and older
weighing 40 kg or more:* 1 mg/kg IV infusion,
followed by ipilimumab 3 mg/kg IV infusion
on the same day, every 3 weeks for maximum
of four doses or until unacceptable toxicity
occurs; then nivolumab 240 mg IV infusion
every 2 weeks or 480 mg every 4 weeks until
disease progression or unacceptable toxicity
occurs.
*Children ages 12 years and older weighing
less than 40 kg:* 1 mg/kg IV infusion, followed by ipilimumab 3 mg/kg IV infusion on
the same day, every 3 weeks for a maximum
of four doses or until unacceptable toxicity
occurs; then nivolumab 3 mg/kg IV infusion
every 2 weeks or 6 mg/kg every 4 weeks until
disease progression or unacceptable toxicity
occurs.

➤ **Metastatic NSCLC with progression on
or after platinum-based chemotherapy** ⚜
Adults: 240 mg IV infusion every 2 weeks or
480 mg every 4 weeks until disease progression or unacceptable toxicity occurs.
➤ **First-line combination therapy for
metastatic NSCLC when tumors express
PD-L1 with no *EGFR* or *ALK* genomic
tumor aberrations**
Adults: 360 mg IV infusion every 3 weeks
followed by ipilimumab 1 mg/kg IV on the
same day every 6 weeks. Continue until disease progression or unacceptable toxicity occurs or for up to 2 years in patients without
disease progression.
➤ **First-line combination treatment of
metastatic or recurrent NSCLC with no
EGFR or *ALK* genomic aberrations** ⚜
Adults: 360 mg IV infusion every 3 weeks,
followed by ipilimumab 1 mg/kg IV on the
same day every 6 weeks and two cycles
of platinum-doublet chemotherapy every
3 weeks. Continue nivolumab and ipilimumab
until disease progression or unacceptable toxicity occurs or for up to 2 years in patients
without disease progression.
➤ **Neoadjuvant treatment of resectable
NSCLC (tumors of at least 4 cm or node-
positive), in combination with platinum-
doublet chemotherapy**
Adults: 360 mg IV infusion followed by
platinum-doublet chemotherapy on the same
day every 3 weeks for three cycles.
➤ **Advanced renal carcinoma in patients
who have received prior antiangiogenic
therapy**
Adults: 240 mg IV infusion once every 2 weeks
or 480 mg every 4 weeks until disease progression or unacceptable toxicity occurs.
➤ **Intermediate or poor risk, previously
untreated advanced renal cell carcinoma,
in combination with ipilimumab**
Adults: 3 mg/kg IV infusion followed by ipilimumab 1 mg/kg IV infusion on the same day
every 3 weeks for four doses; then nivolumab
240 mg as a single-agent IV infusion every
2 weeks or 480 mg every 4 weeks over
30 minutes until disease progression or unacceptable toxicity occurs.
➤ **Advanced renal cell carcinoma as
first-line treatment, in combination with
cabozantinib**
Adults: 240 mg IV infusion once every
2 weeks or 480 mg every 4 weeks until disease
progression or unacceptable toxicity occurs,

N

or up to 2 years with cabozantinib 40 mg PO daily without food until disease progression or unacceptable toxicity occurs.

➤ **Classical Hodgkin lymphoma that has relapsed or progressed after autologous hematopoietic stem cell transplantation (HSCT) and posttransplantation brentuximab vedotin; after three or more lines of systemic therapy that includes autologous HSCT; recurrent or metastatic squamous cell carcinoma of head and neck with disease progression on or after platinum-based therapy**

Adults: 240 mg IV infusion every 2 weeks or 480 mg every 4 weeks until disease progression or unacceptable toxicity occurs.

➤ **Locally advanced or metastatic urothelial carcinoma in patients with disease progression during or after platinum-containing chemotherapy or with disease progression within 12 months of neoadjuvant or adjuvant treatment with platinum-containing chemotherapy**

Adults: 240 mg IV infusion every 2 weeks or 480 mg every 4 weeks until disease progression or unacceptable toxicity occurs.

➤ **Adjuvant treatment of urothelial carcinoma in patients at high risk for recurrence after undergoing radical resection**

Adults: 240 mg IV infusion every 2 weeks or 480 mg IV infusion every 4 weeks until disease recurrence or unacceptable toxicity occurs, or up to 1-year treatment.

➤ **Microsatellite instability-high (MSI-H) or mismatch repair deficient (dMMR) metastatic colorectal cancer that has progressed following treatment with a fluoropyrimidine, oxaliplatin, and irinotecan**

Adults and children ages 12 and older weighing 40 kg or more: 240 mg IV infusion every 2 weeks or 480 mg every 4 weeks until disease progression or unacceptable toxicity occurs.

Adults and children ages 12 and older weighing less than 40 kg: 3 mg/kg IV infusion every 2 weeks.

➤ **MSI-H or dMMR metastatic colorectal cancer that has progressed after treatment with a fluoropyrimidine, oxaliplatin, and irinotecan in combination with ipilimumab**

Adults and children ages 12 and older weighing 40 kg or more: 3 mg/kg IV infusion over 30 minutes followed by ipilimumab 1 mg/kg IV infusion on the same day, every 3 weeks

for four doses; then nivolumab 240 mg as a single-agent IV infusion over 30 minutes every 2 weeks or 480 mg every 4 weeks until disease progression or unacceptable toxicity occurs.

Adults and children ages 12 and older weighing less than 40 kg: 3 mg/kg IV infusion followed by ipilimumab 1 mg/kg IV infusion on the same day, every 3 weeks for four doses; then nivolumab 3 mg/kg as a single-agent IV infusion over 30 minutes every 2 weeks until disease progression or unacceptable toxicity occurs.

➤ **Hepatocellular carcinoma in patients previously treated with sorafenib**

Adults: 1 mg/kg IV infusion every 3 weeks followed by ipilimumab 3 mg/kg IV infusion on the same day for four doses; then nivolumab 240 mg as a single-agent IV infusion every 2 weeks or 480 mg every 4 weeks until disease progression or unacceptable toxicity occurs.

➤ **Unresectable advanced, recurrent, or metastatic esophageal squamous cell carcinoma after prior fluoropyrimidine- and platinum-based chemotherapy**

Adults: 240 mg IV infusion every 2 weeks or 480 mg every 4 weeks until disease progression or unacceptable toxicity occurs.

➤ **Advanced or metastatic gastric cancer, gastroesophageal junction cancer, and esophageal adenocarcinoma, in combination with fluoropyrimidine- and platinum-containing chemotherapy**

Adults: 360 mg IV infusion every 3 weeks with fluoropyrimidine- and platinum-containing chemotherapy every 3 weeks; or 240 mg IV infusion every 2 weeks with fluoropyrimidine- and platinum-containing chemotherapy every 2 weeks until disease progression or unacceptable toxicity occurs, or for up to 2 years in patients without disease progression.

➤ **Adjuvant treatment of completely resected esophageal or gastroesophageal junction cancer with residual pathologic disease in patients who have received neoadjuvant chemoradiotherapy**

Adults: 240 mg IV infusion every 2 weeks or 480 mg IV infusion every 4 weeks until disease progression or unacceptable toxicity occurs, or for up to 1 year of treatment.

➤ **Unresectable advanced or metastatic esophageal squamous cell carcinoma as first-line treatment, in combination with**

fluoropyrimidine- and platinum-containing chemotherapy

Adults: 240 mg IV infusion every 2 weeks or 480 mg IV infusion every 4 weeks in combination with chemotherapy. Continue nivolumab until disease progression or unacceptable toxicity occurs, or for up to 2 years.

➤ **Unresectable advanced or metastatic esophageal squamous cell carcinoma as first-line treatment, in combination with ipilimumab**

Adults: 3 mg/kg IV infusion every 2 weeks or 360 mg IV infusion every 3 weeks with ipilimumab 1 mg/kg IV infusion every 6 weeks until disease progression or unacceptable toxicity occurs, or for up to 2 years.

➤ **Unresectable malignant pleural mesothelioma, in combination with ipilimumab**

Adults: 360 mg IV every 3 weeks followed by ipilimumab 1 mg/kg IV on the same day every 6 weeks. Continue until disease progression or unacceptable toxicity occurs, or for up to 2 years in patients without disease progression.

ADMINISTRATION

IV

▼ When administering with ipilimumab, infuse nivolumab first followed by ipilimumab on the same day. Use separate infusion bags and filters for each infusion.

▼ Refer to manufacturer's instructions for administration information of drugs used in combination therapy.

▼ Visually inspect for particulate matter and discoloration (solution should be clear to opalescent, colorless to pale yellow).

▼ Store vial refrigerated at 36° to 46° F (2° to 8° C). Don't freeze.

▼ Protect from light by storing in original package until time of use.

▼ To prepare, withdraw required volume of nivolumab, transfer to IV container, and dilute with NSS or 5% dextrose injection to yield final concentration of 1 to 10 mg/mL. Don't exceed total volume of 160 mL. For patients weighing less than 40 kg, total volume must not exceed 4 mL/kg of body weight. Mix by gentle inversion; don't shake.

▼ Discard all partially used vials.

▼ Diluted solution remains stable at room temperature for no more than 8 hours, including room temperature storage of infusion in the IV container and time for infusion administration.

▼ Diluted solution remains stable under refrigeration (36° to 46° F [2° to 8° C]) for no more than 24 hours from time of infusion preparation. Don't freeze.

▼ Give through IV line containing a sterile, nonpyrogenic, low-protein-binding inline filter (pore size, 0.2 to 1.2 microns) over 30 minutes.

▼ Flush IV line at end of infusion.

▼ **Incompatibilities:** Don't administer with other drugs through same IV line.

ACTION

A humanized monoclonal antibody that binds to the PD1 receptor found on the surface of T cells, reversing T-cell suppression and resulting in decreased tumor growth.

Route	Onset	Peak	Duration
IV	Unknown	Unknown	Unknown

Half-life: About 25 days.

ADVERSE REACTIONS

CNS: dizziness, peripheral and sensory neuropathy, fatigue, headache, neuritis, asthenia, fever. **CV:** peripheral edema, *ventricular arrhythmias,* HTN, chest pain. **EENT:** iridocyclitis. **GI:** abdominal pain, colitis, nausea, vomiting, constipation, diarrhea, stomatitis, decreased appetite. **GU:** kidney dysfunction, nephritis, kidney insufficiency. **Hematologic:** anemia, *lymphopenia, thrombocytopenia, neutropenia.* **Hepatic:** increased AST, ALT, bilirubin, and ALP levels; *hepatitis.* **Metabolic:** hyponatremia, *hyperkalemia, hypokalemia,* hyperglycemia, hypercalcemia, *hypocalcemia, hypomagnesemia,* hypothyroidism, hyperthyroidism, increased triglyceride and cholesterol levels, increased amylase level, increased lipase level, weight loss. **Musculoskeletal:** pain, arthralgia. **Respiratory:** cough, URI, dyspnea, pneumonitis, *ILD,* pleural effusion. **Skin:** rash, pruritus, erythema, exfoliative dermatitis, *erythema multiforme,* psoriasis, skin depigmentation. **Other:** infusion-related reactions, thyroiditis.

INTERACTIONS

Drug-drug. *Immunosuppressants:* May diminish therapeutic effect of nivolumab. Consider therapy modification.

EFFECTS ON LAB TEST RESULTS
• May increase creatinine, total bilirubin, amylase, lipase, ALT, AST, ALP, glucose, triglyceride, and cholesterol levels.
• May decrease sodium and magnesium levels.
• May increase or decrease thyroid function values and potassium and calcium levels.
• May decrease RBC, lymphocyte, neutrophil, and platelet counts.

CONTRAINDICATIONS & CAUTIONS
• Contraindicated in patients hypersensitive to drug or its components.
⚠ *Alert:* If nivolumab is withheld for an adverse reaction, also withhold ipilimumab.
⚠ *Alert:* Drug can cause severe immune-mediated pneumonitis or ILD (can be fatal).
• Drug can cause immune-mediated conditions (colitis, hepatitis, nephritis, kidney dysfunction, hypothyroidism, hyperthyroidism, life-threatening rash, encephalitis, other serious adverse reactions).
• Drug can cause pituitary gland inflammation and adrenal insufficiency.
• Nivolumab shouldn't be used for treatment of multiple myeloma. Use in combination with a thalidomide analogue plus dexamethasone increased risk of mortality in clinical trials. This combination isn't recommended outside the setting of a clinical trial.
• Drug hasn't been studied in patients with Child-Pugh class C liver impairment.
• Safety and effectiveness haven't been established in children younger than age 12 with melanoma, MSI-H, or dMMR metastatic colorectal cancer or in patients younger than age 18 for the other approved indications.
Dialyzable drug: Unknown.

PREGNANCY-LACTATION-REPRODUCTION
⚠ *Alert:* Drug may cause fetal harm and increase risk of abortion and premature infant death. Advise patients who are pregnant of fetal risk.
• Patients of childbearing potential should use effective contraception during treatment and for at least 5 months after final dose.
• It isn't known if drug appears in human milk. Patient should discontinue breastfeeding during treatment and for 5 months after final dose because of possible serious adverse effects in infants who are breastfed.

NURSING CONSIDERATIONS
• Verify pregnancy status before starting therapy.

• Infusion-related reactions, which can be severe or life-threatening, can occur. Discontinue drug for severe or life-threatening reactions. For mild to moderate reactions, interrupt infusion or decrease infusion rate.
• Drug can cause type 1 diabetes. Monitor glucose level and withhold drug for severe hyperglycemia until metabolic control is achieved; permanently discontinue for life-threatening hyperglycemia.
• Monitor patient for acute GVHD and liver veno-occlusive disease. Transplant-related mortality has occurred.
• Monitor for signs and symptoms of immune-mediated severe pneumonitis or ILD (fever, cough, dyspnea, chest pain) or colitis (fever, abdominal pain, diarrhea, bloody stools). Adjust dosage or discontinue drug as needed. Refer to manufacturer's instructions for corticosteroid treatment, if indicated.
• Obtain LFT values at baseline and monitor periodically during treatment because of risk of immune-mediated hepatitis. Adjust dosages or discontinue drug as needed. Refer to manufacturer's instructions for corticosteroid treatment, if indicated.
• Obtain serum creatinine level at baseline and monitor periodically during treatment because of risk of immune-mediated nephritis and kidney dysfunction. Adjust dosages or discontinue drug as needed. Refer to manufacturer's instructions for corticosteroid treatment, if indicated.
• Monitor thyroid function at baseline and periodically during treatment because of risk of immune-mediated hypothyroidism and hyperthyroidism. Administer hormone replacement therapy for hypothyroidism, or initiate medical management for control of hyperthyroidism. No recommended nivolumab dosage adjustments exist for hypothyroidism or hyperthyroidism.
• Monitor for other immune-mediated adverse reactions, which may occur during or after nivolumab discontinuation. Rule out other causes of reactions first. Based on severity of reaction, withhold drug, administer corticosteroids, or initiate hormone-replacement therapy, if appropriate.
• *Look alike–sound alike:* Don't confuse nivolumab with other monoclonal antibodies.

PATIENT TEACHING
• Instruct patient to inform prescriber if patient has known disease that affects the

immune system, lungs, liver, or kidney or has had an organ transplant.
• Educate patient and family to recognize and immediately report signs and symptoms of pneumonitis (new or worsening cough, chest pain, shortness of breath), colitis (diarrhea, bloody stools, melena, severe abdominal pain or tenderness), liver dysfunction (dark urine, yellowing of eyes, nausea, vomiting, right-sided abdominal pain, lethargy, easy bruising or bleeding), kidney dysfunction (decreased urine output, blood in urine, edema, loss of appetite), hormone gland problems (weight gain or loss, feeling hot or cold, constipation, persistent or unusual headaches, extreme fatigue, changes in mood or behavior, dizziness, hair loss, deepening voice), rash, vision changes, severe or persistent muscle or joint pains, or severe muscle weakness.
◑ *Alert:* Warn patient who is pregnant of fetal risk. Advise patient of childbearing potential to use effective contraception during and for at least 5 months after last dose.
• Advise patient to report known or suspected pregnancy to prescriber.
• Caution patient not to breastfeed while taking drug and for 5 months after last dose.
• Reinforce importance of lab tests and instruct patient to keep follow-up appointments to monitor drug's safety and effectiveness.

norelgestromin–ethinyl estradiol transdermal system
nor-el-JES-troe-min/ETH-i-nill ess-tra-DYE-ole

Evra✤, Xulane, Zafemy

Therapeutic class: Contraceptives
Pharmacologic class: Estrogen–progestin combinations

AVAILABLE FORMS
Transdermal patch: norelgestromin 4.86 mg and ethinyl estradiol 0.53 mg per patch, delivering 150 mcg norelgestromin and 35 mcg ethinyl estradiol daily; norelgestromin 6 mg and ethinyl estradiol 0.60 mg per patch delivering 200 mcg norelgestromin and 35 mcg ethinyl estradiol daily✤

INDICATIONS & DOSAGES
➤ **Pregnancy prevention**
Patients of childbearing potential with BMI less than 30 kg/m²: Apply 1 patch weekly

for 3 weeks (21 total days). Apply each new patch on the same day of the week. Week 4 is patch-free, and withdrawal bleeding is expected. On the day after week 4 ends, apply a new patch to start a new 4-week cycle. The patch-free interval between cycles should never be longer than 7 days.

ADMINISTRATION
Transdermal
◑ *Alert:* Hazardous drug; use safe handling and disposal precautions.
• Apply patch to clean, dry area of skin on buttock, abdomen, upper outer arm, or upper torso. Don't apply to breasts or to skin that is red, irritated, or cut or on the same location as the previous patch.
• Patient shouldn't apply makeup, creams, lotions, powders, or other topical products at application site.
• Press patch down firmly onto skin using palm of the hand; apply pressure for 10 seconds. Run fingers over entire surface area to smooth out any wrinkles.
• Check patch daily to ensure all edges are sticking. Don't use tape or wraps to hold patch in place.
• Don't cut, damage, or alter the patch size because doing so may impair contraception.
• If skin becomes irritated, remove patch and apply a new patch at a different site.

ACTION
Combination hormonal contraceptives act by suppressing gonadotropins. The primary mechanism of this action is ovulation inhibition. However, changes in cervical mucus increase the difficulty of sperm entry into the uterus, and endometrial changes decrease the likelihood of implantation.

Route	Onset	Peak	Duration
Transdermal	Rapid	2 days	Unknown

Half-life: Norelgestromin, 28 hours; ethinyl estradiol, about 17 hours.

ADVERSE REACTIONS
CNS: headache, migraine, emotional lability, dizziness, fatigue, insomnia, anxiety.
CV: increased BP, *PE.* **EENT:** contact lens intolerance, changes in corneal curvature.
GI: nausea, diarrhea, abdominal pain, vomiting, abdominal distention, cholestatic jaundice. **GU:** dysmenorrhea, vaginal bleeding and menstrual disorders, vulvovaginal

N

candidiasis, genital discharge, uterine spasm, vaginal dryness, vulvar dryness, premenstrual syndrome, libido changes. **Metabolic:** weight changes, fluid retention, lipid disorders. **Musculoskeletal:** muscle spasms. **Skin:** application-site reaction, melasma, pruritus, acne, dermatitis, erythema. **Other:** breast tenderness, enlargement, or secretion.

INTERACTIONS
Drug-drug. *Cyclosporine, prednisolone, theophylline, tizanidine, voriconazole:* May increase levels of these drugs. Monitor patient for adverse reactions.
CYP3A4 inducers (bosentan, carbamazepine, phenytoin, rifampin): May reduce contraceptive effectiveness, resulting in unintended pregnancy or breakthrough bleeding. Encourage backup contraception if used together.
CYP3A4 inhibitors (fluconazole, itraconazole): May increase hormone levels. Use together cautiously.
HIV protease inhibitors: May increase or decrease contraceptive level. Use together cautiously.
Lamotrigine: May decrease lamotrigine level, resulting in increased seizure risk. Dosage adjustments of lamotrigine may be necessary.
Ombitasvir, paritaprevir, ritonavir: May cause elevated ALT level when HCV combination products are used with patch. Use is contraindicated.
Sugammadex: May decrease contraceptive effectiveness. Patient should use backup contraception while using sugammadex and for 7 days after.
Thyroid hormone replacement, cortisol: May decrease thyroid hormone level. Monitor therapy and increase dosage of thyroid hormone or cortisol as necessary.
Warfarin: May increase or decrease effect of anticoagulant. Monitor patient and lab values.
Drug-herb. *St. John's wort:* May reduce effectiveness of drug. Discourage use together.
Drug-food. *Grapefruit juice:* May increase hormone level. Discourage use together.
Drug-lifestyle. **Boxed Warning** *Smoking:* May increase risk of CV adverse effects, related to age and number of cigarettes smoked daily. Urge patient not to smoke. ∎

EFFECTS ON LAB TEST RESULTS
• May increase circulating total thyroid hormone, triglyceride, other binding proteins, sex hormone-binding globulin, total circulating endogenous sex steroid, corticoid, and factor VII, VIII, IX, and X levels.
• May decrease free T_3 resin uptake and glucose tolerance.

CONTRAINDICATIONS & CAUTIONS
Boxed Warning Cigarette smoking increases the risk of serious adverse cardiac effects from hormonal contraceptive use. Risk increases with age, especially in women older than age 35, and with the number of cigarettes smoked. Hormonal contraceptives are contraindicated in women older than age 35 who smoke. ∎

⚠ *Alert:* VTE risk is greater in patients ages 15 to 44 using the norelgestromin–ethinyl estradiol transdermal system than in patients using oral contraceptives.

⚠ *Alert:* Contraceptive patch has higher steady-state level and lower peak level than oral contraceptives. Increased estrogen exposure may increase the risk of adverse events, including VTE.

Boxed Warning Contraindicated in patients with BMI of 30 kg/m^2 or more. Risk of venous thromboembolic events in these patients may be greater compared to risk in patients with BMI less than 30 kg/m^2. ∎

• Contraindicated in patients hypersensitive to drug components; in those with history of DVT or related disorder; in patients at high risk for arterial or venous thrombotic diseases or with current or history of cerebrovascular disease or CAD; in those with uncontrolled HTN and inherited or acquired hypercoagulopathies; and in those with headaches with focal neurologic conditions, migraine headaches with aura, or migraine headaches if older than age 35.

• Contraindicated in patients with past or current known or suspected breast cancer or other known or suspected estrogen- or progestin-sensitive neoplasia.

• Contraindicated in patients with thrombophlebitis, thromboembolic disorders, valvular heart disease with complications, diabetes with vascular involvement, major surgery with prolonged immobilization, undiagnosed abnormal genital bleeding, cholestatic jaundice of pregnancy or jaundice with previous hormonal contraceptive use, benign or malignant liver tumors or liver disease, or acute or chronic hepatocellular disease with abnormal liver function.

Reactions in bold italics are *life-threatening*.

• Use cautiously in patients with CV disease risk factors, conditions that might be aggravated by fluid retention, or history of depression.
• Use cautiously in patients with prediabetes or diabetes; drug may decrease glucose tolerance.
• Use cautiously in patients with personal or family history of hypertriglyceridemia; drug may increase risk of pancreatitis.
• Drug may increase lipid levels. Consider alternative drug for patient with uncontrolled dyslipidemia.
Dialyzable drug: Unknown.
⚠ *Overdose S&S:* Nausea, vomiting, withdrawal uterine bleeding.

PREGNANCY-LACTATION-REPRODUCTION
• Contraindicated with known or suspected pregnancy. Discontinue if pregnancy occurs.
• Patient should use alternative contraceptive method during breastfeeding until the infant weans completely.
• In patients who choose not to breastfeed, don't begin drug until 4 weeks after childbirth.

NURSING CONSIDERATIONS
❸ *Alert:* Patients taking combination hormonal contraceptives may be at increased risk for thrombophlebitis, venous thrombosis with or without embolism, PE, MI, cerebral hemorrhage, cerebral thrombosis, HTN, gallbladder disease, liver adenomas, benign liver tumors, mesenteric thrombosis, and retinal thrombosis.
• Increased risk of MI occurs primarily in smokers and women with HTN, morbid obesity, hypercholesterolemia, and diabetes.
• Encourage women with history of HTN or kidney disease to use different contraceptive. If drug is used, closely monitor BP and stop use if HTN occurs.
• Drug may be less effective in patients who weigh 90 kg or more.
• Risk of thromboembolic disease increases with postpartum or postabortion therapy.
• Rule out pregnancy if withdrawal bleeding fails to occur for two consecutive cycles.
• Stop drug and notify prescriber at least 4 weeks before and for 2 weeks after an elective surgery that increases the risk of thromboembolism and during and after prolonged immobilization. Teach patient about alternative methods of contraception for this time.
• Stop drug and notify prescriber if patient has headaches, vision loss, proptosis, diplopia, papilledema, retinal vascular lesions, jaundice, or depression.

PATIENT TEACHING
• Emphasize importance of having regular annual physical exams to check for adverse effects or developing contraindications.
• Warn that drug doesn't protect against HIV and other sexually transmitted diseases.
• Advise patient to immediately notify prescriber of unrelieved leg pain, sudden shortness of breath, chest pain or pressure, severe headache, weakness or numbness in arm or leg, trouble speaking, or yellowing of skin or eyes.
• Caution patient to use a backup method of contraception for the first 7 days of use.
• Tell patient switching from estrogen–progestin oral contraceptives to apply first patch on the first day of withdrawal bleeding. If no bleeding occurs within 5 days of last hormonally active pill, advise patient to obtain a pregnancy test.
• Teach about proper drug administration and handling. Instruct patient to carefully fold used patch in half so that it sticks to itself before discarding and to discard out of reach of children and pets.
• Warn patient to immediately stop use for confirmed pregnancy.
• Tell patient who wears contact lenses to report visual changes or changes in lens tolerance.
• Advise patient not to smoke while using patch.
• Counsel patient who is unsure what to do about mistakes with patch use to use a backup method of birth control and contact health care provider.
• Tell patient undergoing an MRI scan to alert facility of the transdermal patch.
• Instruct patient to report all drugs and supplements being taken because some can decrease contraceptive effectiveness; backup contraceptive method may be needed.
• Advise patient receiving thyroid hormone replacement therapy that increased doses of thyroid hormone may be needed.

N

norepinephrine bitartrate (levarterenol bitartrate, noradrenaline acid tartrate)
nor-ep-i-NEF-rin

Levophed

Therapeutic class: Vasopressors
Pharmacologic class: Alpha/beta agonists

AVAILABLE FORMS
Injection: 1 mg/mL ampule or vial; 4 mg/250 mL, 8 mg/250 mL, 16 mg/250 mL premixed container

INDICATIONS & DOSAGES
➤ **To restore BP in acute hypotension**
Adults: Initially, 8 to 12 mcg/minute IV infusion; then titrate to maintain systolic BP at 80 to 100 mm Hg in patients who were previously normotensive and 40 mm Hg below preexisting systolic BP in patients who were previously hypertensive. Average maintenance dosage is 2 to 4 mcg/minute.
Adjust-a-dose: Gradually reduce infusion rate while expanding blood volume with IV fluids when discontinuing norepinephrine.

ADMINISTRATION
IV
▼ Premixed containers require no additional dilution. Be aware there are two different concentrations.
▼ Infuse into large vein to minimize risk of extravasation. Avoid infusion into leg veins of older adults or patients with occlusive vascular disease of the legs.
▼ Add 4 mg to 1,000 mL D_5W alone or D_5W in NSS for injection. Use continuous infusion pump to regulate infusion flow rate. Avoid using a catheter tie-in technique.
▼ Never leave patient unattended during infusion. Monitor BP every 2 minutes until desired hemodynamic response is achieved; then monitor every 5 minutes.
▼ During infusion, frequently monitor ECG, cardiac output, central venous pressure, pulmonary artery occlusion pressure, pulse rate, urine output, and color and temperature of limbs. Titrate infusion rate based on findings and prescriber guidelines.
 Alert: Frequently check site for signs and symptoms of extravasation. If they appear,

immediately stop infusion and call prescriber. To prevent sloughing and necrosis, use a fine hypodermic needle to infiltrate area with 5 to 10 mg phentolamine in 10 to 15 mL of NSS as soon as possible. Immediate local hyperemic changes will occur if area is infiltrated within 12 hours. Also, check for blanching along course of infused vein, which may progress to superficial sloughing.
▼ Protect drug from light. Discard discolored solution or solution that contains precipitate. Solution will deteriorate after 24 hours.
▼ If prolonged therapy is needed, frequently change injection site.
▼ The use of NSS alone isn't recommended because of lack of oxidation protection.
▼ **Incompatibilities:** Alkalis, iron salts, oxidizers, regular insulin, thiopental.

ACTION
Stimulates alpha and beta$_1$ receptors in the sympathetic nervous system, causing vasoconstriction and cardiac stimulation.

Route	Onset	Peak	Duration
IV	Rapid	5 minutes	1–2 min after infusion

Half-life: About 2.4 min.

ADVERSE REACTIONS
CNS: headache, anxiety. **CV:** *bradycardia, severe HTN, arrhythmias, ischemic injury.* **Respiratory:** respiratory difficulties, *pulmonary edema.* **Skin:** irritation with extravasation, necrosis, and gangrene secondary to extravasation. **Other:** *anaphylaxis.*

INTERACTIONS
Drug-drug. *Alpha blockers:* May antagonize drug effects. Monitor perfusion and BP.
Antidiabetics: May decrease insulin sensitivity and increase glucose level. Monitor glucose level and adjust dosages if needed.
Antihistamines, atropine, ergot alkaloids, guanethidine, imipramine, linezolid, MAO inhibitors, methyldopa, oxytocics, TCAs: May cause severe, prolonged HTN. Use together with extreme caution.
Atomoxetine: May enhance hypertensive and tachycardic effects. Monitor BP and HR.
Inhaled anesthetics (cyclopropane, halothane): May increase risk of arrhythmias. Don't use together.

Drug-herb. *Kratom:* May enhance adverse effects of norepinephrine. Discourage use together.

EFFECTS ON LAB TEST RESULTS
None reported.

CONTRAINDICATIONS & CAUTIONS
• Avoid use in patients with mesenteric or peripheral vascular thrombosis (unless deemed necessary as a life-saving procedure), profound hypoxia, hypercarbia, or hypotension resulting from blood volume deficit (except as an emergency measure).
• Use cautiously in older adults and patients with sulfite sensitivity.
• Safety and effectiveness in children haven't been established.
Dialyzable drug: Unknown.
⚠ *Overdose S&S:* Headache, severe HTN, reflex bradycardia, increased peripheral resistance, decreased cardiac output.

PREGNANCY-LACTATION-REPRODUCTION
• Safe use during pregnancy hasn't been established. Use during pregnancy only if clearly needed.
• It isn't known if drug appears in human milk. Use cautiously during breast-feeding.

NURSING CONSIDERATIONS
• Drug isn't a substitute for blood or fluid replacement therapy. If patient has volume deficit, replace fluids before giving vasopressors.
• Keep emergency drugs on hand to reverse drug effects: atropine for reflex bradycardia, phentolamine to decrease vasopressor effects, and propranolol for arrhythmias.
• Immediately notify prescriber of decreased urine output.
• When stopping drug, gradually slow infusion rate. Continue monitoring vital signs, watching for possible severe drop in BP.
• *Alert:* Carefully monitor infusion site; extravasation can cause tissue necrosis.
• *Look alike–sound alike:* Don't confuse norepinephrine with epinephrine.

PATIENT TEACHING
• Tell patient to promptly report adverse reactions and discomfort at IV insertion site.
• Advise that vital signs will be frequently monitored.

norethindrone
nor-ETH-in-drone

Camila, Errin, Heather, Incassia, Jencycla, Lyleq, Movisse✤, Nor-QD

norethindrone acetate
Norlutate✤

Therapeutic class: Contraceptives
Pharmacologic class: Progestins

AVAILABLE FORMS
norethindrone
Tablets: 0.35 mg
norethindrone acetate
Tablets: 5 mg

INDICATIONS & DOSAGES
➤ **Amenorrhea, abnormal uterine bleeding**
Adults: 2.5 to 10 mg norethindrone acetate PO daily for 5 to 10 days, beginning in assumed latter half of menstrual cycle.
➤ **Endometriosis**
Adults: 5 mg norethindrone acetate PO daily for 14 days; then increased by 2.5 mg/day every 2 weeks, up to 15 mg daily. Therapy may continue for 6 to 9 months or until breakthrough bleeding warrants temporary termination.
➤ **Pregnancy prevention**
Patients of childbearing potential and patients who are menarchal: 0.35 mg norethindrone PO daily beginning on first day of menstruation.

ADMINISTRATION
PO
• *Alert:* Hazardous drug; use safe handling and disposal precautions.
• Give without regard to meals. May give with food if GI upset occurs.
• When used for contraception, give drug at same time every day, continuously, with no interruption between pill packs.
• Refer to prescribing information for management of missed doses.
• When drug is used to prevent pregnancy, patient should use backup method of contraception for 48 hours after a missed dose or a dose taken 3 or more hours after scheduled dose. If vomiting or diarrhea occurs soon after giving a dose, patient should use backup contraception for 48 hours.

N

ACTION

Suppresses ovulation, possibly by inhibiting pituitary gonadotropin secretion, and forms thick cervical mucus.

Route	Onset	Peak	Duration
PO	Unknown	2 hr	Unknown

Half-life: 8 to 9 hours.

ADVERSE REACTIONS

CNS: depression, headache, mood swings, dizziness, fatigue, insomnia, migraine, nervousness. **CV:** *thromboembolism*, edema. **EENT:** optic neuritis. **GI:** bloating, abdominal pain or cramping, nausea, vomiting. **GU:** breakthrough bleeding, menstrual irregularities, cervical erosion, abnormal secretions. **Hepatic:** cholestatic jaundice, *hepatitis*. **Metabolic:** weight changes. **Musculoskeletal:** limb pain. **Skin:** melasma, rash, acne, pruritus, alopecia, hirsutism, hemorrhagic skin eruptions. **Other:** *anaphylactic reactions*; breast tenderness, enlargement, or secretion; suppressed lactation; premenstrual-like syndrome.

INTERACTIONS

Drug-drug. *Barbiturates:* May decrease progestin effects. Monitor patient for diminished therapeutic response.
Cyclosporine: May increase cyclosporine level. Use together cautiously.
CYP3A4 inducers (bosentan, carbamazepine, phenobarbital, phenytoin, rifampin): May decrease effectiveness of contraceptive hormones. Consider alternative nonhormonal contraception.
CYP3A5 inhibitors (itraconazole, ketoconazole), NNRTIs (etravirine, ritonavir), protease inhibitors: May increase progestin level. Monitor therapy.
Thyroid hormone replacement: May decrease thyroid hormone level. Increase of replacement hormone may be needed.
Tranexamic acid: May enhance thrombogenic effect of tranexamic acid. Avoid use together.
Ulipristal: May decrease effectiveness of both drugs. Avoid norethindrone within 5 days of using ulipristal.
Warfarin: May increase warfarin level. Monitor PT and INR.
Drug-herb. *St. John's wort:* May decrease effectiveness of contraceptive hormones. Discourage use together.

Drug-lifestyle. *Smoking:* May increase risk of adverse CV effects. Discourage smoking. If smoking continues, may need alternative therapy.

EFFECTS ON LAB TEST RESULTS

• May increase LFT values and lipase level.
• May decrease HDL and sex hormone-binding globulin levels.
• May alter thyroid function test results and decrease metyrapone test results.

CONTRAINDICATIONS & CAUTIONS

• Contraindicated in patients hypersensitive to drug and in those with known or suspected breast cancer, undiagnosed abnormal vaginal bleeding, impaired liver function or liver disease, benign or malignant liver tumors, current or recent thromboembolic disorders (stroke, MI) or VTE, or history of these conditions.
• Use cautiously in patients with seizures, migraines, cardiac or kidney disease, asthma, and depression.
• Use cautiously in patients with risk factors for arterial vascular disease (HTN, diabetes, tobacco use, hypercholesterolemia, obesity) or VTE (personal or family history of VTE, SLE).
• Use cautiously in patients with diabetes; drug may decrease glucose tolerance, but insulin requirements generally don't change.
🛈 **Alert:** Norethindrone acetate may cause visual abnormalities due to papilledema or retinal vascular lesions. If these occur, discontinue drug.
Dialyzable drug: Unknown.

PREGNANCY-LACTATION-REPRODUCTION

• Contraindicated during pregnancy or as a diagnostic test for pregnancy; may cause fetal harm.
• Drug appears in human milk. Use cautiously during breastfeeding. Patient who breastfeeds exclusively may start progestin-only pills (POPs) 6 weeks after delivery. Patient who partially breastfeeds may start pills 3 weeks after delivery.

NURSING CONSIDERATIONS

• If switching from combined oral contraceptives to POPs, patient should take first POP the day after the last active combined pill.
• If switching from POPs to combined pills, patient should take first active combined pill

on the first day of menstruation, even if POP pack isn't finished.

❂ *Alert:* Norethindrone acetate is twice as potent as norethindrone. Norethindrone acetate shouldn't be used for contraception.

• Patients with menstrual disorders usually need preliminary estrogen treatment.

• Watch patient closely for signs of edema.

• Monitor BP.

PATIENT TEACHING
• According to FDA regulations, patient must read package insert explaining possible adverse effects before receiving first dose. Also give patient verbal explanation.

• Teach about proper drug administration and handling.

❂ *Alert:* Advise patient to immediately report unusual signs and symptoms and to stop drug and report visual disturbances, migraine, or pain or numbness in arm or leg.

• Teach patient how to perform routine breast self-exam.

• Tell patient to report suspected pregnancy to prescriber.

• Encourage patient to stop or reduce smoking because of risk of CV complications.

• Tell patient with diabetes that drug may affect glucose level. Instruct patient to closely monitor glucose level.

• Warn patient that drug doesn't protect against HIV and other sexually transmitted infections.

nortriptyline hydrochloride ⌧
nor-TRIP-ti-leen

Aventyl❦, Pamelor

Therapeutic class: Antidepressants
Pharmacologic class: TCAs

AVAILABLE FORMS
Capsules: 10 mg, 25 mg, 50 mg, 75 mg
Oral solution: 10 mg/5 mL*

INDICATIONS & DOSAGES
➤ **Depression**
Adults: 25 mg PO t.i.d. or q.i.d., gradually increased to maximum of 150 mg daily. Or, give total daily dose at bedtime.
Older adults and adolescents: 30 to 50 mg PO daily given once or in divided doses.

ADMINISTRATION
PO
• Give drug without regard to food.
• Use medication measuring device for solution.

ACTION
Unknown. Increases amount of norepinephrine, serotonin, or both in CNS by blocking reuptake by presynaptic neurons.

Route	Onset	Peak	Duration
PO	Unknown	4–9 hr	Unknown

Half-life: 14 to 51 hours.

ADVERSE REACTIONS
CNS: *stroke, seizures,* numbness, tingling, paresthesia of extremities, incoordination, ataxia, tremors, peripheral neuropathy, extrapyramidal symptoms, EEG alterations, confusional states with hallucinations, panic, delusions, disorientation, anxiety, insomnia, restlessness, agitation, nightmares, hypomania, exacerbation of psychosis, drowsiness, dizziness, weakness, fatigue, headache. **CV:** edema, hypotension, HTN, tachycardia, palpitations, *MI*, arrhythmias, *heart block,* flushing. **EENT:** blurred vision, disturbance of accommodation, mydriasis, angle-closure glaucoma, tinnitus, dry mouth. **GI:** constipation, paralytic ileus, nausea, vomiting, anorexia, epigastric distress, diarrhea, peculiar taste, stomatitis, abdominal cramps, black tongue. **GU:** urine retention, delayed micturition, dilation of urinary tract, erectile dysfunction, testicular swelling, urinary frequency, nocturia, increased or decreased libido. **Hematologic:** bone marrow depression, eosinophilia, purpura, *thrombocytopenia.* **Hepatic:** jaundice, altered liver function. **Metabolic:** weight gain or loss, SIADH. **Skin:** rash, petechiae, urticaria, itching, alopecia, photosensitivity, diaphoresis. **Other:** drug fever, gynecomastia, breast enlargement and galactorrhea (in females).

INTERACTIONS
Drug-drug. *Anticholinergics (dicyclomine, scopolamine):* May increase anticholinergic adverse effects (urine retention, constipation). Monitor patient.
Barbiturates, CNS depressants: May enhance CNS depression. Avoid use together.
Buspirone, fentanyl, lithium, SNRIs, SSRIs, TCAs, tramadol, triptans: May increase

N

risk of serotonin syndrome. Monitor patient closely.

Cimetidine, TCAs (fluoxetine, fluvoxamine, paroxetine, sertraline): May increase nortriptyline level. Monitor drug levels and patient for signs of toxicity.

Drugs that prolong QT interval (amiodarone, haloperidol): May increase risk of life-threatening cardiac arrhythmias, including torsades de pointes. Monitor patient and ECG.

Epinephrine, norepinephrine: May increase hypertensive effect. Use together cautiously.

Linezolid, methylene blue: May cause serotonin syndrome. Use extreme caution and monitor patient closely.

MAO inhibitors: May increase risk of serotonin syndrome. Concurrent use is contraindicated. Avoid using within 14 days of MAO inhibitor therapy.

Quinolones: May increase risk of life-threatening arrhythmias. Avoid use together.

Reserpine: May produce a stimulating effect in some patients. Monitor patient.

Drug-herb. *Evening primrose oil:* May cause additive or synergistic effect, lowering seizure threshold and increasing seizure risk. Discourage use together.

St. John's wort, SAM-e, yohimbe: May cause serotonin syndrome and reduced drug level. Discourage use together.

Drug-lifestyle. *Alcohol use:* May enhance CNS depression. Discourage use together.

Sun exposure: May increase risk of photosensitivity reactions. Advise patient to avoid excessive sunlight exposure.

EFFECTS ON LAB TEST RESULTS
• May increase LFT values.
• May increase or decrease glucose level.
• May increase eosinophil count.
• May decrease WBC, RBC, granulocyte, and platelet counts.

CONTRAINDICATIONS & CAUTIONS
• Contraindicated in patients hypersensitive to drug and during acute recovery phase of MI.
Boxed Warning Drug may increase risk of suicidality in children, adolescents, and young adults with major depressive disorder or other psychiatric disorder. Nortriptyline isn't approved for use in children. ∎

🕒 *Alert:* Concomitant use with linezolid or methylene blue can cause serotonin syndrome (fever, mental status changes, muscle

twitching, diaphoresis, shivering or shaking, diarrhea, loss of coordination). Use drug with linezolid or methylene blue only for life-threatening or urgent conditions when potential benefits outweigh risks of toxicity.

▨ Patients who are poor metabolizers of CYP2D6 have higher drug level when given usual doses. Approximately 7% to 10% of Whites are poor metabolizers.

• Drug isn't approved for use in patients with bipolar depression. Screen for bipolar depression before starting drug.

• Use with extreme caution in patients with glaucoma, suicidality, history of urine retention or seizures, CV disease, or hyperthyroidism and in those receiving thyroid drugs.

Dialyzable drug: No.

⚠ *Overdose S&S:* Cardiac arrhythmias, severe hypotension, shock, HF, pulmonary edema, seizures, CNS depression, coma, ECG changes, confusion, restlessness, disturbed concentration, transient visual hallucinations, dilated pupils, agitation, hyperactive reflexes, stupor, drowsiness, muscle rigidity, vomiting, hypothermia, hyperpyrexia.

PREGNANCY-LACTATION-REPRODUCTION
• Nortriptyline crosses placental barrier. Neonates may experience irritability, jitteriness, and seizures.

• Safe use during pregnancy and breastfeeding hasn't been established. Weigh potential benefits against possible risks.

• Encourage enrollment in the National Pregnancy Registry for Antidepressants (1-866-961-2388 or https://womensmentalhealth.org/research/pregnancyregistry/antidepressants/).

• Monitor for adverse reactions in patient during pregnancy and in infants who are breastfeeding.

NURSING CONSIDERATIONS
Boxed Warning Monitor all patients for clinical worsening, suicidality, or unusual changes in behavior. ∎

🕒 *Alert:* If linezolid or methylene blue must be given, stop nortriptyline and monitor patient for serotonin toxicity for 2 weeks or until 24 hours after the last dose of methylene blue or linezolid, whichever comes first. Treatment with nortriptyline may resume 24 hours after the last dose of methylene blue or linezolid.

• To withdraw drug, gradually taper dosage and monitor patient for reemerging symptoms.

Reactions in bold italics are *life-threatening*.

• Because patients using TCAs may suffer hypertensive episodes during surgery, stop drug gradually several days before surgery.

• If signs or symptoms of psychosis occur or increase, expect to reduce dosage. Record mood changes. Monitor patient for suicidality; allow patient only a minimum supply of drug.

• *Look alike–sound alike:* Don't confuse nortriptyline with amitriptyline.

PATIENT TEACHING

Boxed Warning Advise families and caregivers to closely observe patient for increased suicidality. ∎

• Teach about proper drug administration and handling.

• Teach patient to recognize and immediately report signs and symptoms of serotonin syndrome (fever, mental status changes, muscle twitching, diaphoresis, shivering or shaking, diarrhea, loss of coordination).

• Warn patient to avoid activities that require alertness and good coordination until effects of drug are known. Drowsiness and dizziness usually subside after a few weeks.

• Recommend use of sugarless hard candy or gum to relieve dry mouth. Saliva substitutes may be needed.

• Tell patient to consult prescriber before taking other prescription or OTC drugs.

• Warn patient not to stop drug suddenly.

• To prevent oversensitivity to the sun, advise patient to use sun block, wear protective clothing, and avoid prolonged exposure to strong sunlight.

• Advise patient to immediately report pregnancy or plans to become pregnant or breastfeed during treatment.

nystatin
nye-STAT-in

Nyaderm ✦, Nyamyc, Nystop

Therapeutic class: Antifungals
Pharmacologic class: Polyene macrolides

AVAILABLE FORMS
Cream: 25,000 units/g ✦, 100,000 units/g
Ointment: 100,000 units/g
Oral suspension: 100,000 units/mL
Powder: 100,000 units/g
Tablets: 500,000 units

INDICATIONS & DOSAGES
➤ **GI candidiasis**
Adults: 500,000 to 1 million units PO as tablets t.i.d. Continue for at least 48 hours after symptoms disappear to prevent relapse.
➤ **Fungal infections (cutaneous and mucocutaneous) caused by susceptible *Candida* species**
Adults and children: Apply cream or ointment and gently massage into affected areas b.i.d. Or, apply powder to lesions b.i.d. to t.i.d. until lesions have healed.
➤ **Oral candidiasis (thrush)**
Adults and children: 400,000 to 600,000 units PO as oral suspension q.i.d. for up to 14 days. Continue treatment for at least 48 hours after perioral symptoms disappear and cultures demonstrate eradication of *Candida albicans*.
Infants: 200,000 units PO as oral suspension q.i.d.

ADMINISTRATION
PO
• To treat oral candidiasis, after patient's mouth is clean of food debris, have patient hold suspension in mouth for several minutes before swallowing. When treating infants, use dropper to place one-half of dose in each side of the mouth and avoid feedings for 5 to 10 minutes after administration.
• Shake suspension well before use.
• Suspension made with bulk powder contains no preservatives. Use immediately. Don't store.
Topical
• Store at room temperature.
• For fungal infection of the feet, apply powder to feet and all footwear.

ACTION
Probably binds to sterols in fungal cell membrane, altering cell permeability and allowing leakage of intracellular components.

Route	Onset	Peak	Duration
PO, topical	24–72 hr	Unknown	Unknown

Half-life: Unknown.

ADVERSE REACTIONS
GI: nausea, vomiting, diarrhea, GI upset.
GU: irritation, sensitization. **Skin:** rash.

INTERACTIONS
Drug-drug. *Saccharomyces boulardii:* Systemic antifungal agents may diminish therapeutic effect of *Saccharomyces boulardii*. Avoid combination.

EFFECTS ON LAB TEST RESULTS
None reported.

CONTRAINDICATIONS & CAUTIONS
• Contraindicated in patients hypersensitive to drug.
• Rarely, SJS has been reported.
• Don't use topical powder for treatment of systemic, oral, intravaginal, or ophthalmic infections.
• Although approved by the FDA for treatment of intestinal candidiasis, drug isn't recommended by the Infectious Diseases Society of America.
Dialyzable drug: Unknown.
⚠ *Overdose S&S:* Nausea, GI upset.
• *Look alike–sound alike:* Don't confuse nystatin with atorvastatin, fluvastatin, or any other statins.

PREGNANCY-LACTATION-REPRODUCTION
• Use cautiously during pregnancy and only when clearly needed.
• It isn't known if drug appears in human milk; absorption is poor after oral ingestion. Use cautiously during breastfeeding.

NURSING CONSIDERATIONS
• Drug isn't effective against systemic infections.
• Monitor patient for rash.
• Avoid contact when applying topical formulations.

PATIENT TEACHING
• Advise patient to continue taking drug for at least 2 days after signs and symptoms resolve.
• Instruct patient to report redness, swelling, or irritation.
• Tell patient that overusing mouthwash or wearing poorly fitting dentures may promote infection.
• Teach patient wearing dentures to remove and clean them to avoid reinfection.
• For fungal foot infections, teach patient to dust powder freely on the feet and footwear.

ocrelizumab
oh-kre-LIZ-ue-mab

Ocrevus

Therapeutic class: MS drugs
Pharmacologic class: Monoclonal antibodies

AVAILABLE FORMS
Injection: 300 mg/10 mL preservative-free vials

INDICATIONS & DOSAGES
➤ **Relapsing or primary progressive MS**
Adults: Initially, 300 mg IV infusion on day 1, followed by 300 mg IV infusion 2 weeks later. Then 600 mg IV infusion every 6 months beginning 6 months after first 300-mg dose.

Before each infusion, premedicate with 100 mg IV methylprednisolone (or equivalent corticosteroid) 30 minutes before infusion and an antihistamine such as diphenhydramine 30 to 60 minutes before infusion. May also add an antipyretic such as acetaminophen.
Adjust-a-dose: For life-threatening or disabling infusion reactions, immediately stop infusion, provide supportive treatment, and permanently discontinue drug. For mild, moderate, and severe infusion reactions, refer to manufacturer's instructions for interrupting therapy and determining IV infusion rates.

ADMINISTRATION
🔹 *Alert:* Screen for HBV and review quantitative serum Ig test results before first dose.
IV
▼ For 300-mg dose, withdraw 10 mL of drug and dilute into infusion bag containing 250 mL NSS. For 600-mg dose, withdraw 20 mL of drug and dilute into 500 mL NSS.
▼ Use infusion solution immediately or store up to 24 hours in refrigerator at 36° to 46° F (2° to 8° C) or up to 8 hours at room temperature (up to 77° F [25° C]), including infusion time. Discard any excess solution that's not used the same day.
▼ Inspect for particulate matter or discoloration before use.
▼ Administer diluted solution through a dedicated line using an infusion set with a 0.2- or 0.22-micron in-line filter. No incompatibilities with polyvinyl chloride or

---

Reactions in bold italics are *life-threatening*.

polyolefin bags and IV administration sets have been observed.

▼ Administer infusion when solution is at room temperature.

▼ Begin 300-mg dose infusion at 30 mL/hour and increase by 30 mL/hour every 30 minutes to a maximum rate of 180 mL/hour. Duration of infusion is 2.5 hours or longer.

▼ Begin 600-mg dose infusion at 40 mL/hour and increase by 40 mL/hour every 30 minutes to maximum rate of 200 mL/hour. Duration of infusion is 3.5 hours or longer. Or, if no prior serious infusion reaction, begin 600 mg infusion at 100 mL/hour for first 15 minutes; increase to 200 mL/hour for next 15 minutes; increase to 250 mL/hour for next 30 minutes; then increase to 300 mL/hour for remaining 60 minutes. Duration of infusion is 2 hours or longer.

▼ If dose is missed, administer as soon as possible and reset dose schedule to give next dose 6 months later. Separate doses by at least 5 months.

▼ Keep vials in carton to protect from light and store in refrigerator at 36° to 46° F (2° to 8° C). Don't freeze or shake vials.

▼ **Incompatibilities:** Don't give with solutions other than NSS.

ACTION

A recombinant humanized monoclonal antibody directed against CD20-expressing B cells, which causes antibody-dependent cellular cytolysis and complement-mediated lysis.

Route	Onset	Peak	Duration
IV	14 days	Unknown	27–175 wk

Half-life: 26 days.

ADVERSE REACTIONS

CNS: depression. **CV:** peripheral edema. **GI:** diarrhea. **Musculoskeletal:** back pain, limb pain. **Respiratory:** URI, lower respiratory tract infections, cough. **Skin:** skin infections. **Other:** infusion reactions, herpes infections.

INTERACTIONS

Drug-drug. *Immunosuppressants and immune-modulating therapies (corticosteroids, daclizumab, fingolimod, mitoxantrone, natalizumab, teriflunomide):* May increase risk of immunosuppression when used in combination or when switching from listed drugs to ocrelizumab. Use together cautiously.

Other MS drugs: Use of ocrelizumab with other MS drugs hasn't been studied. Consider the potential for increased immunosuppressive effects.

Tacrolimus (topical): May enhance adverse effects of immunosuppressants. Avoid use together.

Vaccines (live-attenuated or live-virus): May decrease vaccine's effects or increase infection risk. Vaccines aren't recommended during treatment or until B-cell recovery occurs. Give all necessary live vaccine immunizations according to immunization guidelines at least 4 weeks before and all necessary nonlive vaccines at least 2 weeks before drug initiation.

Drug-herb. *Echinacea:* May decrease therapeutic effect of immunosuppressants. Discourage use together.

EFFECTS ON LAB TEST RESULTS
- May decrease total Ig level.
- May decrease neutrophil count.
- May decrease effect of *Coccidioides immitis* skin test.

CONTRAINDICATIONS & CAUTIONS
- Contraindicated in patients with history of life-threatening infusion reaction to ocrelizumab or active HBV infection.

🔷 *Alert:* Screen patient for HBV infection before therapy begins. For patients who are negative for HBsAg and positive for HB core antibody (HBcAb+) or are carriers of HBV (HBsAg+), consult a liver disease specialist before and during treatment.
- Drug may increase frequency of herpes and other infections.
- Drug may cause increased risk of malignancy, including breast cancer. Follow standard cancer screening guidelines.
- Immune-mediated colitis has been reported.
- Safety and effectiveness in children haven't been established.

Dialyzable drug: Unknown.

PREGNANCY-LACTATION-REPRODUCTION
- Studies during pregnancy are inadequate. Immunoglobulins cross placental barrier. Infants born to mothers exposed to other anti-CD20 antibodies have experienced transient peripheral B-cell depletion and lymphocytopenia.
- Patients of childbearing potential should use contraception during therapy and for 6 months after final infusion.

• Drug may appear in human milk. Risk of infant harm during breastfeeding is unknown. Consider patient's clinical need for drug and potential risks to infant.

NURSING CONSIDERATIONS

• Administer drug under supervision of an experienced health care provider with access to supportive measures to manage severe reactions.

• Before every infusion, monitor patient for signs and symptoms of infection (fever, chills, persistent cough, herpes [cold sores, shingles, genital sores]). Delay infusion until active infection resolves.

• Drug may decrease Ig level and increase risk of infection. Monitor serum Ig level during and after treatment until B-cell repletion, especially in the setting of recurrent serious infections.

• Monitor patient for infusion reactions during and for at least 1 hour after completion of infusion. Reactions include pruritus, rash, urticaria, erythema, throat irritation, bronchospasm, oropharyngeal pain, dyspnea, pharyngeal or laryngeal edema, flushing, hypotension, fever, fatigue, headache, dizziness, nausea, and tachycardia. Infusion reactions can occur up to 24 hours after infusion. If infusion reaction occurs, interrupt or discontinue infusion or decrease rate depending on severity of reaction.

• PML has occurred in patients treated with other MS drugs and can lead to severe disability or death. Monitor patient for new or worsening signs or symptoms of neurologic function changes (problems with thinking, clumsiness, vision changes, personality changes, weakness on one side of body). At first sign or symptom, withhold drug and obtain appropriate diagnostic evaluation, including MRI.

• Monitor patient for new or persistent diarrhea or other GI symptoms, and evaluate promptly if colitis is suspected.

• **Look alike–sound alike:** Don't confuse ocrelizumab with eculizumab, obiltoxaximab, obinutuzumab, ofatumumab, omalizumab, or rituximab.

PATIENT TEACHING

• Advise patient to undergo standard cancer screenings because drug may increase risk of malignancy, including breast cancer.

• Instruct patient to immediately report signs and symptoms of an infusion reaction;

explain that signs and symptoms can occur 24 hours after infusion ends.

• Tell patient to immediately report signs and symptoms of infection.

• Teach patient to immediately report signs and symptoms associated with PML.

• Advise patient of childbearing potential to use contraception during therapy and for 6 months after final infusion.

• Instruct patient to report pregnancy or breastfeeding before therapy begins.

• Inform patient that drug can cause reactivation of HBV infection, that testing for HBV will be performed before therapy begins, and that monitoring is required if patient is at risk.

• Caution patient that live-virus and live-attenuated vaccines aren't recommended during therapy. Explain that all necessary live-virus or live-attenuated vaccinations should be completed at least 4 weeks before therapy begins; nonlive vaccinations, at least 2 weeks before therapy begins.

octreotide acetate
ok-TREE-oh-tide

Mycapssa, Sandostatin, Sandostatin LAR Depot

Therapeutic class: Endocrine-metabolic agents
Pharmacologic class: Somatostatin analogues

AVAILABLE FORMS

Capsules (delayed-release) ⬛: 20 mg
Injection: 50 mcg/mL, 100 mcg/mL, 500 mcg/mL single-dose ampule, vial, or pre-filled syringe
Injection (multidose): 200 mcg/mL, 1,000 mcg/mL vials
Injection for LAR (powder for suspension): 10 mg/6 mL, 20 mg/6 mL, 30 mg/6 mL after reconstitution

INDICATIONS & DOSAGES
➤ **Flushing and diarrhea from carcinoid tumors**
Adults: 100 to 600 mcg subcut or IV daily in two to four divided doses for first 2 weeks of therapy. Usual daily dosage is 450 mcg but can range from 50 to 1,500 mcg/day. Base subsequent dosage on individual response. Or, long-acting repeatable (LAR) depot 20 mg

IM (intragluteally) at 4-week intervals for 2 months. If switching from octreotide solution, continue subcut for 2 weeks at same dosage as before the switch. After 2 months, adjust dosage based on symptoms.

➤ **Watery diarrhea from vasoactive intestinal polypeptide-secreting tumors (VIPomas)**
Adults: 200 to 300 mcg subcut or IV daily in two to four divided doses for first 2 weeks of therapy. Base subsequent dosage on individual response. Range is 150 to 750 mcg/day, but dosage usually shouldn't exceed 450 mcg daily. Or, LAR Depot 20 mg IM (intragluteally) at 4-week intervals for 2 months. If switching from octreotide solution, continue subcut for 2 weeks at same dosage as before the switch. After 2 months, adjust dosage based on symptoms.

➤ **Acromegaly**
Adults: Initially, 50 mcg subcut or IV t.i.d.; then adjust based on insulin-like growth factor 1 (IGF-1) (somatomedin C) level every 2 weeks. Or, may obtain multiple growth hormone levels at 0 to 8 hours after octreotide administration to permit more rapid dosage titration. Usual dosage is 100 mcg subcut or IV t.i.d.; some patients require up to 500 mcg t.i.d.

Or, following initial 50 mcg t.i.d. dosing with octreotide solution, begin LAR depot 20 mg IM (intragluteally) at 4-week intervals for 3 months; then adjust dosage based on growth hormone and somatomedin C levels and symptoms. See manufacturer's instructions for detailed dosing schedule and details on switching to LAR depot from octreotide solution. For depot injection, withdraw drug yearly for 4-week interval in patients who have received irradiation.

For long-term maintenance in patients who responded to and tolerated octreotide or lanreotide injections, may switch to 20-mg capsules PO b.i.d.; increase in increments of 20 mg every 2 weeks based on IGF-1 level and signs and symptoms. Maximum dosage, 80 mg daily.
Adjust-a-dose: In patients with cirrhosis of liver or KF on KRT, starting dose of LAR Depot is 10 mg IM every 4 weeks. In patients with KF, initiate capsules at 20 mg daily and titrate as tolerated.

➤ **Gastroesophageal variceal hemorrhage** ◆
Adults: 50 mcg as IV bolus, followed by continuous IV infusion of 50 mcg/hour for 2 to 5 days. May repeat bolus within first hour of treatment if hemorrhage isn't controlled.

➤ **Gastroenteropancreatic neuroendocrine tumors (metastatic)** ◆
Adults: 30 mg IM every 4 weeks until tumor progression or death. Or, initially, 20 to 30 mg IM every 28 days; titrate by 10 mg every 4 weeks or maintain same dose and reduce dosing interval to every 3 weeks if frequent supplemental subcut doses are needed. IM range is 20 to 60 mg every 28 days.

➤ **High-output gastroenteropancreatic fistula** ◆
Adults: 100 mcg subcut three times daily; discontinue and consider alternative agents if fistula output doesn't decrease after 3 to 5 days.

ADMINISTRATION
PO
• Give with a glass of water on an empty stomach at least 1 hour before or 2 hours after a meal.
• Have patient swallow capsules whole; don't crush or break capsules.
• Refrigerate unopened wallets of capsules at 36° to 46° F (2° to 8° C). After first use, may store opened wallets at room temperature for 1 month.
IV
▼ Dilute in 50 to 200 mL D₅W or NSS and infuse over 15 to 30 minutes.
▼ May be given by IV push over 3 minutes.
▼ Store solution in refrigerator between 36° and 46° F (2° and 8° C). May store at room temperature of 70° to 86° F (20° to 30° C) for up to 14 days. Discard multidose vials within 14 days after initial entry.
▼ Solution is stable for 24 hours as a parenteral admixture.
▼ Protect from light.
▼ **Incompatibilities:** TPN.
IM
• For IM route, use LAR Depot suspension only.
⊙ *Alert:* Never give injectable suspension by IV or subcut routes.
• May give as initial therapy or as alternative to prior subcut therapy.
• Don't use if particulates or discoloration is present.
• Follow mixing instructions included in packaging; give immediately after mixing.
• *For LAR Depot suspension:* Before dilution, store refrigerated between 36° and 46° F (2° and 8° C). May store at room temperature

of 68° to 77° F (20° to 25° C) for up to 10 days.

• Depot kit should remain at room temperature for 30 to 60 minutes before preparation of drug suspension.

• Rotate injection sites.

• Administer into gluteal area only; avoid deltoid muscle injections due to significant pain and discomfort at injection site.

Subcutaneous

• Use concentration with smallest volume to deliver dose.

• Bring drug to room temperature before injection.

• Don't use if particulates or discoloration is present.

• Rotate injection sites. Avoid multiple injections at same site within a short period.

• Refer to manufacturer's instructions for use of prefilled pen.

ACTION

Mimics action of naturally occurring somatostatin.

Route	Onset	Peak	Duration
IV	Rapid	Unknown	Up to 12 hr
IM (LAR)	Unknown	1 hr	Unknown
PO	Unknown	1.67–2.5 hr	Up to 48 hr
Subcut	30 min	24 min	Up to 12 hr

Half-life: 1.7 to 1.9 hours (subcut), increased in older adults and patients with cirrhosis and kidney impairment; long-acting, unknown; 2.7 hours (PO).

ADVERSE REACTIONS

CNS: confusion, dizziness, fatigue, headache, light-headedness, depression, weakness, pain. **CV:** *arrhythmias, bradycardia,* conduction abnormalities, peripheral edema, HTN. **EENT:** blurred vision, hearing loss, sinusitis, nasopharyngitis. **GI:** abdominal pain or discomfort, diarrhea, loose stools, nausea, *pancreatitis,* constipation, fat malabsorption, flatulence, abdominal distention, vomiting, dyspepsia, intestinal polyp. **GU:** urinary frequency, UTI. **Hematologic:** anemia. **Hepatic:** gallbladder abnormalities, cholelithiasis. **Metabolic:** *hypoglycemia,* hyperglycemia, hypothyroidism, suppressed secretion of growth hormone and gastroenterohepatic peptides (gastrin, VIP, insulin, glucagon, secretin, motilin, and pancreatic polypeptide). **Musculoskeletal:** backache, joint pain, osteoarthritis, myalgia. **Respiratory:** URI. **Skin:** alopecia, erythema or pain

at injection site, flushing, wheal, bruising, hair loss, pruritus, rash, diaphoresis. **Other:** cold symptoms, flulike symptoms.

INTERACTIONS

Drug-drug. *Androgens, MAO inhibitors, quinolone antibiotics, salicylates, SSRIs:* May increase risk of hypoglycemia. Monitor patient closely.

Antacids, H_2-receptor antagonists, PPIs: May decrease absorption of capsules. Increase octreotide dosage if necessary.

Beta blockers (propranolol) and other drugs that may cause bradycardia, ivabradine: May have additive effect and further lower HR. Decrease beta blocker dosage as needed.

Bromocriptine: May increase bromocriptine availability. Monitor therapy.

Codeine: May decrease codeine metabolism and decrease morphine formation. Monitor therapy.

Cyclosporine: May decrease cyclosporine level. Consider therapy modification, and monitor patient closely.

Digoxin: May increase digoxin level and bradycardic effect. Monitor level closely.

Drugs that prolong QT interval (antiarrhythmics, SSRIs, TCAs): May increase risk of life-threatening cardiac arrhythmias, including torsades de pointes. Monitor patient and ECG.

Hormonal contraceptives (levonorgestrel): May decrease level of oral contraceptive. If used together, patient should use alternative nonhormonal contraceptive or backup method.

Insulin, oral antidiabetics: May inhibit secretion of insulin and glucagon. Monitor patient and adjust dosage of antidiabetics as needed.

Lacosamide: May increase risk of AV-blocking effect of lacosamide. Monitor patient closely.

Quinidine, terfenadine, rifampin: May decrease excretion of these drugs. Use with caution and reduce dosage as needed.

Drug-food. *Any food:* May alter absorption of dietary fats. Administer injections between meals to decrease GI effects.

EFFECTS ON LAB TEST RESULTS

• May increase or decrease glucose level.

• May decrease vitamin B_{12} level.

• May alter LFT and TSH values.

• May affect Schilling test results.

Reactions in bold italics are *life-threatening*.

CONTRAINDICATIONS & CAUTIONS
• Contraindicated in patients hypersensitive to drug or its components.
• Use cautiously in older adults, who may be more sensitive to drug.
• Use cautiously in patients with pancreatitis, gallbladder or bile disorders, cardiac abnormalities, diabetes, hypothyroidism, or nutritional disorders; octreotide may cause or exacerbate these conditions.
• Use cautiously in patients with kidney or liver impairment. Dosage adjustment may be needed.
• Safety and effectiveness in children haven't been established.

Dialyzable drug: Unknown.

⚠ *Overdose S&S:* Hypoglycemia, flushing, dizziness, nausea, hypotension, arrhythmia, liver steatosis, pancreatitis, lethargy, weakness, lactic acidosis.

PREGNANCY-LACTATION-REPRODUCTION
• Drug crosses placental barrier. Use cautiously during pregnancy only if clearly needed and benefit justifies fetal risk.
• Drug may restore fertility in women with acromegaly. Patients of childbearing potential should use contraception during treatment.
• Obtain pregnancy test before LAR treatment to minimize fetal risk.
• Patients planning pregnancy should discontinue long-acting formulation approximately 2 months before planned pregnancy; patients may use short-acting formulation until conception.
• Drug appears in human milk. Use cautiously during breastfeeding.

NURSING CONSIDERATIONS
• Monitor baseline thyroid function tests.
• Monitor somatomedin C level every 2 weeks, or every 3 months for LAR depot. Dosage adjustments are based on this level.
• Periodically monitor lab tests, such as thyroid function, glucose, plasma serotonin, urine 5-hydroxyindoleacetic acid, vitamin B$_{12}$ level, and plasma substance P (for carcinoid tumors).
• Regularly monitor for gallbladder disease. Therapy may be related to development of cholelithiasis because of its effect on gallbladder motility or fat absorption.
• Monitor closely for signs and symptoms of glucose imbalance. Patients with type 1 diabetes and those receiving oral antidiabetics

or oral diazoxide may need dosage adjustments during therapy. Monitor glucose level.
• Monitor patient closely for bradycardia, arrhythmias, conduction abnormalities, and other ECG changes (prolonged QT interval).
• Drug may alter fluid and electrolyte balance. Other therapies may need adjusting.
• Monitor patient for breakthrough signs and symptoms with LAR Depot. Patient may require supplemental subcut octreotide.
• *Look alike–sound alike:* To avoid giving drug by the wrong route, don't confuse octreotide acetate injection with injectable depot suspension product. Don't confuse Sandostatin with Sandimmune, Sandostatin LAR, sargramostim, or simvastatin.

PATIENT TEACHING
• Urge patient to immediately report signs and symptoms of abdominal discomfort.
• Stress importance of adhering to treatment schedule to assure steady control and undergoing periodic lab testing during octreotide therapy.
• Advise patient to report any irregular heartbeat.
• Counsel patient to immediately report pregnancy, breastfeeding, or plans to become pregnant or breastfeed during treatment.
• Advise patient with diabetes to closely monitor blood glucose level and to discuss results with prescriber before making dosage changes.

ofloxacin (oral)
oh-FLOKS-a-sin

Therapeutic class: Antibiotics
Pharmacologic class: Fluoroquinolones

AVAILABLE FORMS
Tablets: 200 mg, 300 mg, 400 mg

INDICATIONS & DOSAGES
Boxed Warning Use in patients with acute bacterial exacerbation of bronchitis and uncomplicated UTIs isn't recommended because of risk of serious adverse effects. Use drug in these patients only when they have no other treatment options. ∎

Adjust-a-dose (for all indications): For patients with CrCl of 20 to 50 mL/minute, give first dose as recommended; then give usual maintenance dose every 24 hours. For patients with CrCl less than 20 mL/minute, give 50% of recommended dose every 24 hours. For patients with Child-Pugh class C liver impairment, don't exceed 400 mg/day.

➤ **Acute bacterial worsening of chronic bronchitis, uncomplicated skin and skin-structure infections, and community-acquired pneumonia**

Adults: 400 mg PO every 12 hours for 10 days.

➤ **Acute, uncomplicated urethral and cervical gonorrhea**

Adults: 400 mg PO as a single dose.

➤ **Mixed infection of urethra and cervix due to *Chlamydia trachomatis* and *Neisseria gonorrhoeae*; nongonococcal cervicitis or urethritis due to *C. trachomatis***

Adults: 300 mg PO every 12 hours for 7 days.

➤ **Uncomplicated cystitis caused by *Escherichia coli, Klebsiella pneumoniae,* or other organisms**

Adults: 200 mg PO every 12 hours for 3 days (*E. coli* or *K. pneumoniae*) or 200 mg PO every 12 hours for 7 days (other organisms).

➤ **Complicated UTI**

Adults: 200 mg PO every 12 hours for 10 days.

➤ **Prostatitis from *E. coli***

Adults: 300 mg PO every 12 hours for 6 weeks.

➤ **Acute pelvic inflammatory disease due to *C. trachomatis* and *N. gonorrhoeae***

Adults: 400 mg PO every 12 hours with metronidazole for 10 to 14 days.

ADMINISTRATION

PO

• Give drug without regard to food but don't give within 2 hours of antacids or vitamins.
• Give drug with plenty of fluids.
• Store tablets at room temperature.

ACTION

Interferes with DNA gyrase, which is needed for synthesis of bacterial DNA. Spectrum of action includes many gram-positive and gram-negative aerobic bacteria, including *Enterobacteriaceae* and *Pseudomonas aeruginosa.*

Route	Onset	Peak	Duration
PO	Unknown	60–120 min	Unknown

Half-life: 4 to 5 hours.

ADVERSE REACTIONS

CNS: dizziness, fatigue, fever, headache, insomnia, lethargy, nervousness, sleep disorders, somnolence, taste alteration. **CV:** chest pain, phlebitis. **EENT:** visual disturbances, pharyngitis, dry mouth. **GI:** nausea, abdominal pain or cramps, anorexia, constipation, diarrhea, flatulence, vomiting. **GU:** external genital pruritus in women, glycosuria, hematuria, proteinuria, vaginal discharge, vaginitis. **Hematologic:** *leukopenia, neutropenia,* neutrophilia, anemia, eosinophilia, leukocytosis, *thrombocytopenia, thrombocytosis,* lymphocytosis, *lymphocytopenia,* elevated erythrocyte sedimentation rate. **Musculoskeletal:** body pain, myalgia. **Skin:** pruritus, rash. **Other:** hypersensitivity reactions.

INTERACTIONS

Drug-drug. *Aluminum hydroxide, aluminum-magnesium hydroxide, calcium carbonate, magnesium hydroxide:* May decrease effects of ofloxacin. Give antacid at least 2 hours before or 2 hours after ofloxacin.

Antidiabetics: May affect glucose level, causing hypoglycemia or hyperglycemia. Monitor patient closely.

Didanosine (chewable or buffered tablets or pediatric powder for oral solution): May interfere with GI absorption of ofloxacin. Separate doses by 2 hours.

Drugs that prolong QT interval (antiarrhythmics, pimozide, ziprasidone): May increase risk of life-threatening ventricular arrhythmias. Avoid use together.

Iron salts: May decrease absorption of ofloxacin, reducing anti-infective response. Separate doses by at least 2 hours.

NSAIDs: May enhance CNS stimulation and seizure-potentiating effect of ofloxacin. Monitor therapy closely.

Sevelamer: May decrease absorption of quinolones. Give oral quinolones at least 2 hours before or 6 hours after sevelamer. Consider therapy modification.

Steroids: May increase risk of tendinitis and tendon rupture. Monitor patient for tendon pain or inflammation.

Sucralfate: May decrease absorption of ofloxacin, reducing anti-infective response. If use together can't be avoided, give ofloxacin 2 hours before or 6 hours after sucralfate.

Theophylline: May increase theophylline level. Monitor patient closely and adjust theophylline dosage as needed.

Warfarin: May prolong PT and INR. Monitor PT and INR.

Drug-lifestyle. *Sunlight or UV light exposure:* May cause photosensitivity reactions.

Reactions in bold italics are *life-threatening*.

Advise patient to avoid excessive sunlight or UV light exposure.

EFFECTS ON LAB TEST RESULTS
• May increase BUN, creatinine, and liver enzyme levels.
• May increase or decrease serum glucose level.
• May increase urinary glucose and protein levels and pH.
• May increase presence of pus and blood cells in urine.
• May decrease urine specific gravity.
• May increase erythrocyte sedimentation rate, band forms, and eosinophil count.
• May decrease Hb level, hematocrit, and neutrophil count.
• May increase or decrease WBC and platelet counts.
• May produce false-positive urine screen results for opiates.

CONTRAINDICATIONS & CAUTIONS
Boxed Warning Drug is associated with increased risk of tendinitis and tendon rupture, especially in patients older than age 60, patients taking corticosteroids, and those with heart, kidney, or lung transplants. ■
Boxed Warning Drug may exacerbate muscle weakness in patients with myasthenia gravis. Avoid use in patients with known history of myasthenia gravis. ■
• Contraindicated in patients hypersensitive to drug or other fluoroquinolones.
• Avoid use in patients with known QT-interval prolongation or uncorrected hypokalemia and those taking drugs that prolong QT interval due to risk of further QT interval prolongation and torsades de pointes.
⟳ *Alert:* Serious, even fatal, hypersensitivity reactions can occur, even after first dose. Discontinue drug at first sign of rash or hypersensitivity. Emergency treatment with epinephrine and resuscitative measures may be needed.
• Use cautiously in patients with seizure disorders, CNS diseases such as cerebral arteriosclerosis, or liver or kidney impairment.
⟳ *Alert:* Patients receiving systemic drug have an increased risk of hypoglycemia, which can result in coma. Hypoglycemia has been reported more frequently in older adults and patients with diabetes.
• Mild to life-threatening CDAD can occur during therapy and for up to 2 months after therapy ends. Monitor patient for diarrhea as

drug may need to be discontinued and other therapy begun.
⟳ *Alert:* Fluoroquinolones may increase risk of aortic dissection or rupture when used systemically. Avoid use in patients with known aortic aneurysm and patients at risk for aortic aneurysm, including those with peripheral atherosclerotic vascular diseases, HTN, certain genetic conditions (Marfan syndrome, Ehlers-Danlos syndrome), and older adults. Use drug in these patients only if no other treatment options are available.
• Safety and effectiveness in children haven't been established.
Dialyzable drug: No.
⚠ *Overdose S&S:* Nausea, vomiting, seizures, vertigo, dysgeusia, psychosis, dizziness, drowsiness, hot and cold flushes, facial swelling and numbness, slurred speech, mild to moderate disorientation.

PREGNANCY-LACTATION-REPRODUCTION
• Studies during pregnancy are inadequate. Drug crosses placental barrier. Use only if potential benefit justifies fetal risk.
• Drug appears in human milk in level similar to that found in plasma. Patient should discontinue breastfeeding or discontinue drug, considering importance of drug to patient.

NURSING CONSIDERATIONS
Boxed Warning Fluoroquinolones have been associated with disabling and potentially irreversible serious adverse reactions that have occurred together, including tendinitis and tendon rupture, peripheral neuropathy, and CNS effects (seizures, toxic psychoses, increased ICP, pseudotumor cerebri, tremors, restlessness, anxiety, light-headedness, hallucinations, confusion, paranoia, depression, nightmares, insomnia and, rarely, suicidality). If any of these serious adverse reactions occur, immediately discontinue drug. ■
Boxed Warning Monitor for signs and symptoms of peripheral neuropathy (pain, burning, tingling, numbness, weakness, or change in sensation to light touch, pain, temperature, or sense of body position) and report them immediately. Signs and symptoms can occur at any time during treatment and can last for months or years or be permanent. ■
⟳ *Alert:* Test patients treated for gonorrhea for syphilis. Drug isn't effective against syphilis, and treating gonorrhea may mask or delay syphilis symptoms.

- Periodically assess organ system functions during prolonged therapy.
- Monitor patient for overgrowth of nonsusceptible organisms.
- Monitor kidney and liver studies and CBC in patient undergoing prolonged therapy.
- Test for *Clostridioides difficile* if patient develops diarrhea.

🔔 *Alert:* Monitor patient receiving systemic drug for signs and symptoms of hypoglycemia (confusion, pounding or rapid heartbeat, dizziness, pale skin, shakiness, diaphoresis, unusual hunger, trembling, headache, weakness, irritability, unusual anxiety). Immediately discontinue drug for blood glucose disturbances and switch to a nonfluoroquinolone antibiotic, if possible.

🔔 *Alert:* Monitor patient receiving systemic drug for psychiatric adverse reactions (disturbances in attention, disorientation, agitation, nervousness, memory impairment, delirium). Discontinue drug for CNS adverse effects, including psychiatric adverse reactions.

- Monitor patient for adverse CNS effects, including dizziness, headache, seizures, or depression. Stop drug and notify prescriber if these effects occur.
- Monitor patient for hypersensitivity reactions. Stop drug and initiate supportive therapy, as indicated.

🔔 *Alert:* Monitor for signs and symptoms of aortic aneurysm, dissection, and rupture (sudden, severe, and constant pain in stomach, chest, or back; throbbing in stomach area; deep pain in back or side of stomach; steady, gnawing pain in stomach that lasts for hours or days; pain in jaw, neck, back, or chest; coughing or hoarseness; shortness of breath or trouble swallowing). Immediately discontinue drug if any of these aortic disorders are suspected.

PATIENT TEACHING
- Teach about proper drug administration and handling. Instruct patient to take drug exactly as prescribed even if feeling better.

Boxed Warning Warn patient to immediately report signs and symptoms of serious adverse reactions, including tendinitis, tendon rupture, peripheral neuropathy, and CNS effects. ∎

- Tell patient to drink plenty of fluids during drug therapy.

🔔 *Alert:* Caution patient that significantly low blood glucose level can occur. Review ways

to manage low blood glucose level, and instruct patient to immediately report such occurrences to prescriber.

🔔 *Alert:* Advise patient with diabetes that more frequent monitoring of blood glucose level may be needed during therapy.

🔔 *Alert:* Inform patient to immediately report psychiatric adverse reactions, and warn that they can occur after just one dose.

- Warn patient that dizziness and lightheadedness may occur. Advise caution when driving or operating hazardous machinery until effects of drug are known.
- Warn patient that hypersensitivity reactions may follow first dose. Advise patient to stop drug and immediately call prescriber at first sign of rash or other allergic reaction.
- Caution patient to avoid prolonged exposure to direct sunlight or UV light and to use sunscreen and protective clothing when outdoors.
- Advise patient to report severe bloody diarrhea.

🔔 *Alert:* Warn patient to seek immediate medical attention for signs and symptoms of aortic aneurysm.

OLANZapine
oh-LAN-za-peen

Zyprexa, Zyprexa Zydis

OLANZapine pamoate
Zyprexa Relprevv

Therapeutic class: Antipsychotics
Pharmacologic class: Thienobenzodiazepines

AVAILABLE FORMS
Injection: 10 mg/vial
Injection (extended-release suspension): 210 mg/vial, 300 mg/vial, 405 mg/vial
Tablets: 2.5 mg, 5 mg, 7.5 mg, 10 mg, 15 mg, 20 mg
Tablets (ODTs): 5 mg, 10 mg, 15 mg, 20 mg

INDICATIONS & DOSAGES
➤ **Schizophrenia**
Adults: Initially, 5 to 10 mg PO once daily, with goal to be at 10 mg daily within several days of starting therapy. Adjust dose in 5-mg increments at intervals of 1 week or more. Most patients respond to 10 to 15 mg daily. Safety of dosages greater than 20 mg daily

hasn't been established. Or, after establishing tolerability with oral formulation, may switch to every 2- or 4-week dosing with extended-release IM formulation according to manufacturer's conversion instructions and current oral dosing.

Children ages 13 and older: 2.5 or 5 mg PO once daily. Adjust dose as needed in increments of 2.5 or 5 mg. Maintenance dosage, 10 mg/day. Safety hasn't been established for dosages over 20 mg/day.

Adjust-a-dose: In older adults, patients who are debilitated, patients predisposed to hypotensive reactions, and patients who may metabolize olanzapine more slowly than usual (nonsmoking women older than age 65) or may be more pharmacodynamically sensitive to olanzapine, initially, give 5 mg PO or 150 mg IM every 4 weeks. Increase dosage cautiously.

➤ **Short-term treatment of acute manic episodes linked to bipolar I disorder**
Adults: Initially, 10 to 15 mg PO daily. Adjust dosage as needed in 5-mg daily increments at intervals of 24 hours or more. Maximum, 20 mg PO daily. Duration of treatment is usually 2 weeks.

Adults: 10 mg PO once daily in combination with lithium or valproate (range, 5 to 20 mg/day). Duration of treatment is 6 weeks.
Children ages 13 and older: 2.5 or 5 mg PO once daily. Adjust dose as needed in increments of 2.5 or 5 mg. Target dosage is 10 mg/day. Maximum dosage, 20 mg/day.

Adjust-a-dose: In older adults, patients who are debilitated, patients predisposed to hypotensive reactions, and patients who may metabolize olanzapine more slowly than usual (nonsmokers, females, those older than age 65) or may be more pharmacodynamically sensitive to olanzapine, initially, 5 mg PO. Increase dosage cautiously.

➤ **Maintenance treatment of bipolar I disorder**
Adults: 5 to 20 mg PO daily.
Children ages 13 and older: Continue effective dosage determined during acute response. Adjust as needed in increments of 2.5 or 5 mg to lowest dose needed to maintain remission. Maintenance dosage is usually 10 mg/day. Maximum dosage, 20 mg/day.

➤ **Agitation caused by schizophrenia and bipolar I mania**
Adults: 10 mg IM (short-acting) (range, 2.5 to 10 mg). May give subsequent doses of up to 10 mg 2 hours after first dose or 4 hours after second dose, up to 30 mg IM daily. Maximum, three 10-mg doses 2 to 4 hours apart. If maintenance therapy is required, convert patient to 5 to 20 mg PO daily.

Adjust-a-dose: In older adults, give 5 mg IM. In patients who are debilitated, in those predisposed to hypotension, and in patients sensitive to effects of drug, give 2.5 mg IM.

➤ **Depressive episodes associated with bipolar I disorder**
Adults: 5 mg PO with 20 mg fluoxetine PO once daily in the evening. Adjust dosage based on effectiveness and tolerability within ranges of 5 to 12.5 mg olanzapine and 20 to 50 mg fluoxetine.

Adjust-a-dose: If starting in combination with fluoxetine 20 mg in older adults, patients who are debilitated, patients predisposed to hypotensive reactions, and patients who may metabolize olanzapine more slowly than usual (nonsmokers, females, those older than age 65) or may be more pharmacodynamically sensitive to olanzapine, initially, 2.5 to 5 mg PO. Increase dosage cautiously.

Children ages 10 and older: 2.5 mg PO with 20 mg fluoxetine PO once daily in evening. Adjust dosage based on effectiveness and tolerability. Use of olanzapine doses above 12 mg with fluoxetine doses above 50 mg hasn't been evaluated.

➤ **Treatment-resistant depression**
Adults: 5 mg PO with 20 mg fluoxetine PO once daily in evening. Adjust dosage based on effectiveness and tolerability within ranges of 5 to 20 mg olanzapine and 20 to 50 mg fluoxetine.

Adjust-a-dose: If starting in combination with fluoxetine 20 mg in older adults, patients who are debilitated, patients predisposed to hypotensive reactions, and patients who may metabolize olanzapine more slowly than usual (nonsmokers, females, those older than age 65) or may be more pharmacodynamically sensitive to olanzapine, initially, 2.5 to 5 mg PO. Increase dosage cautiously.

➤ **Preventing chemotherapy-associated acute and delayed nausea or vomiting** ◆
Adults: 5 or 10 mg PO on day of chemotherapy (day 1), followed by 5 or 10 mg once daily on days 2 to 4 (in combination with antiemetics used for high emetic risk agents).

➤ **Chemotherapy-associated breakthrough nausea or vomiting** ◆
Adults: 5 or 10 mg PO once daily for 3 days.

O

Children ages 3 and older: 0.1 to 0.14 mg/kg/
dose ODT PO once or twice daily. Round
dose to nearest 1.25 mg.

ADMINISTRATION

PO

• Give drug without regard to food.
• Don't push tablet through foil backing; remove
foil from package and then remove tablet.
• Place ODT on patient's tongue immediately
after opening package, allow it to dissolve,
and then have patient swallow it with or without water.
• Store tablets or ODT at room temperature.
• Protect drug from light and moisture.

IM

• Be aware that there are two different IM formulations, a short-acting and a long-acting,
with different dosing schedules.
• Inspect IM solution for particulate matter
and discoloration before administration.
• To reconstitute IM injection, dissolve contents of one vial with 2.1 mL of sterile water
for injection to yield a clear yellow 5 mg/mL
solution. Store at room temperature and give
within 1 hour of reconstitution. Discard any
unused solution.
• For Zyprexa Relprevv extended-release injection, follow manufacturer's instructions for
appropriate diluent to add for each dosage.
After drug is suspended in solution, may hold
at room temperature for 24 hours.
• Olanzapine extended-release formula is intended for deep gluteal IM injection only using a 19-gauge, 1.5 inch (38 mm) needle.
⚠ *Alert:* Injection is for IM use only. Don't
administer IV or subcut.

ACTION

May block dopamine and 5-HT$_2$ receptors.

Route	Onset	Peak	Duration
PO	1–6 wk	6 hr	Unknown
IM	10–15 min	15–45 min	Unknown
IM (extended-release)	Unknown	1 wk	Months

Half-life: 21 to 54 hours; extended-release injection,
30 days.

ADVERSE REACTIONS

CNS: somnolence, insomnia, parkinsonism,
dizziness, abnormal gait, asthenia, personality disorder, auditory hallucinations, restlessness, fatigue, akathisia, headache, tremor,
articulation impairment, tardive dyskinesia,
fever, extrapyramidal events (IM), hypertonia.

CV: HTN, orthostatic hypotension, tachycardia, chest pain, ecchymosis, peripheral
edema, hypotension (IM). **EENT:** amblyopia, conjunctivitis, rhinitis, nasal congestion,
pharyngitis, sore throat. **GI:** constipation,
dry mouth, dyspepsia, increased appetite, increased salivation, vomiting, thirst, flatulence,
diarrhea, nausea. **GU:** hematuria, metrorrhagia, urinary incontinence, UTI, amenorrhea,
vaginitis, vaginal discharge. **Hematologic:**
leukopenia. **Hepatic:** increased liver enzyme
levels. **Metabolic:** hyperglycemia, dyslipidemia, weight gain. **Musculoskeletal:** joint
pain, extremity pain, back pain, neck rigidity,
twitching, muscle spasm, stiffness. **Respiratory:** increased cough, dyspnea, URI. **Skin:**
diaphoresis, ecchymosis, acne, injection-site
reaction, injection-site pain (IM). **Other:** flulike syndrome, viral infection, injury.

INTERACTIONS

Drug-drug. *Amphetamines:* May decrease
stimulatory effect of amphetamines. Monitor
therapy.
Anticholinergics (dicyclomine, scopolamine):
May increase adverse effects of anticholinergics, including severe GI hypermotility. Monitor therapy.
Antihypertensives: May potentiate hypotensive effects. Closely monitor BP.
⚠ *Alert: Benzodiazepines (diazepam, lorazepam),
opioids:* May increase CNS depression. Avoid
use together. If use together is necessary, limit
dosage and duration of each drug to minimum
necessary for desired effect.
Centrally-acting drugs: May potentiate CNS
effects. Avoid use together.
Ciprofloxacin: May increase olanzapine level.
Monitor for increased adverse effects.
*CYP1A2 inducers (carbamazepine, omepra-
zole, rifampin):* May decrease olanzapine
level. Monitor therapy.
CYP1A2 inhibitors (fluvoxamine): May increase olanzapine level. Monitor patient. May
need to reduce olanzapine dose.
Dopamine agonists, levodopa: May antago-
nize activity of these drugs. Monitor patient.
Fluoxetine: May increase olanzapine level.
Use together cautiously.
*QT-prolonging agents (antiarrhythmics, on-
dansetron, haloperidol):* May enhance QTc-
prolonging effect of QT-prolonging agents.
Consider therapy modification.
Drug-herb. *Kava:* May increase adverse or
toxic effect of olanzapine. Monitor patient.

Reactions in bold italics are *life-threatening*.

St. John's wort: May decrease drug level. Discourage use together.

Drug-lifestyle. *Alcohol use:* May increase CNS effects. Discourage use together.

Smoking: May increase drug clearance. Urge patient to quit smoking.

EFFECTS ON LAB TEST RESULTS
• May increase AST, ALT, GGT, CK, glucose, cholesterol, triglyceride, uric acid, and prolactin levels.
• May decrease protein level.
• May increase or decrease bilirubin level.
• May increase eosinophil count.
• May decrease WBC count.

CONTRAINDICATIONS & CAUTIONS
• Contraindicated in patients hypersensitive to drug.

Boxed Warning Sedation (including coma) or delirium have been reported following injections of olanzapine extended-release formula. This drug must be administered in a registered health care facility with ready access to emergency response services. Olanzapine extended-release is available only through the restricted Zyprexa Relprevv Patient Care Program. ■

Boxed Warning Drug may increase risk of CV or infection-related death in older adults with dementia. Olanzapine isn't approved to treat patients with dementia-related psychosis. ■

• Risk of severe adverse reactions (including fatalities) increases with concomitant use of anticholinergics.
• Use cautiously in patients with a current diagnosis or history of urine retention, clinically significant prostatic hypertrophy, constipation, or history of paralytic ileus or related conditions.
• Use cautiously in patients with heart disease, cerebrovascular disease, conditions that predispose patient to hypotension, history of seizures or conditions that might lower the seizure threshold, and liver impairment.
• Use cautiously in older adults, patients with history of paralytic ileus, and those at risk for aspiration pneumonia, prostatic hyperplasia, or angle-closure glaucoma.

Boxed Warning When using olanzapine and fluoxetine together, also refer to suicidality Boxed Warning section of package insert for Symbyax. ■

🔵 *Alert:* Drug may increase risk of suicidality in young adults ages 18 to 24 during first 2 months of treatment.

• Use cautiously during initiation of therapy in patients at high risk for suicide.
• Impaired core body temperature regulation may occur. Patient should be cautious of strenuous exercise, heat exposure, and dehydration.
• Safety and effectiveness of olanzapine pamoate long-acting formulation in children haven't been established.

Dialyzable drug: No.

⚠ *Overdose S&S:* Agitation, aggressiveness, dysarthria, tachycardia, extrapyramidal symptoms, reduced level of consciousness, aspiration, cardiopulmonary arrest, cardiac arrhythmias, delirium, NMS, respiratory depression or arrest, seizures, HTN, hypotension.

PREGNANCY-LACTATION-REPRODUCTION
• Studies during pregnancy are inadequate. Individualize use during pregnancy, and use only if potential benefit justifies fetal risk.
🔵 *Alert:* Neonates exposed to antipsychotics during the third trimester are at risk for developing extrapyramidal signs and symptoms (repetitive muscle movements of face and body) and withdrawal signs and symptoms (agitation, abnormally increased or decreased muscle tone, tremors, sleepiness, severe difficulty breathing, difficulty feeding) after delivery and may require intensive care support.
• Enroll patients exposed to drug during pregnancy in the National Pregnancy Registry for Atypical Antipsychotics (1-866-961-2388 or https://womensmentalhealth.org/research/pregnancyregistry/atypicalantipsychotic/).
• Drug appears in human milk. Use cautiously during breastfeeding, with close monitoring for excess sedation, irritability, poor feeding, abnormal muscle movements, and tremors.
• Drug may reversibly decrease female fertility.

NURSING CONSIDERATIONS
🔵 *Alert:* Watch for evidence of NMS (hypercongestion, muscle rigidity, altered mental status, autonomic instability), which is rare but often fatal. Immediately stop drug; monitor and treat patient as needed.
🔵 *Alert:* Drug may cause hyperglycemia. Regularly monitor patient with diabetes. In patient with risk factors for diabetes, obtain fasting blood glucose test results at baseline and periodically.
• Monitor hemodynamic response. Orthostatic hypotension associated with dizziness,

tachycardia, bradycardia, and syncope may occur, especially during initial dosage titration.

• Monitor for symptoms of metabolic syndrome (significant weight gain, increased BMI, hyperglycemia, hypercholesterolemia, HTN, hypertriglyceridemia).

• Monitor for leukopenia, neutropenia, and agranulocytosis. Monitor CBC frequently during the first few months of therapy in patient with history of low WBC count or drug-induced leukopenia or neutropenia.

✪ **Alert:** Monitor patient for DRESS syndrome (cutaneous reaction, eosinophilia, fever, or lymphadenopathy plus one or more of the following complications: hepatitis, myocarditis, pericarditis, nephritis, or pneumonia), which can be fatal. Discontinue drug immediately and provide supportive care for suspected DRESS syndrome.

• Note that ODTs contain phenylalanine.

• Monitor patient for abnormal body temperature regulation, especially if patient exercises, is exposed to extreme heat, takes anticholinergics, or is dehydrated.

• Obtain baseline and periodic LFT results.

• Monitor patient for mental status changes, sedation, coma, or delirium.

• Monitor for tardive dyskinesia, which may occur after prolonged use. It may not appear until months or years later and may disappear spontaneously or persist for life, despite stopping drug.

• Periodically reevaluate the long-term usefulness of olanzapine.

• Patient who feels dizzy or drowsy after IM injection should remain recumbent until assessment for orthostatic hypotension and bradycardia can be done. Patient should rest until feeling passes.

• Taper dosage slowly when discontinuing.

✪ **Alert:** Monitor patient receiving extended-release injection for postinjection delirium sedation syndrome (PDSS). Signs and symptoms consistent with overdose and PDSS include sedation, coma, delirium, confusion, disorientation, agitation, anxiety, and other cognitive impairment. Other possible signs and symptoms of PDSS include dysarthria, ataxia, aggression, dizziness, weakness, HTN, and seizures.

✪ **Alert:** After receiving extended-release injection and after postinjection observation period, patients must be alert, oriented, and absent of signs or symptoms of PDSS before release. Patients must be accompanied to their destination upon leaving the facility. If PDSS is suspected, patients must remain under medical supervision.

• *Look alike–sound alike:* Don't confuse olanzapine with olsalazine or quetiapine. Don't confuse Zyprexa with Zyrtec, Zestril, or Celexa. Don't confuse Zyprexa Zydis with Zelapar or zolpidem.

PATIENT TEACHING

• Teach about proper drug administration and handling for prescribed formulation.

✪ **Alert:** Caution patient or caregiver of patient taking an opioid with a benzodiazepine, CNS depressant, or alcohol to seek immediate medical attention for dizziness, lightheadedness, extreme sleepiness, slowed or difficult breathing, or unresponsiveness.

✪ **Alert:** Inform patient of risk of DRESS syndrome and importance of reporting symptoms immediately.

• Caution patient against exposure to extreme heat; drug may impair body's ability to reduce temperature.

• Inform patient of potential for weight gain.

• Advise patient to avoid alcohol.

• Tell patient to rise slowly to avoid dizziness upon standing up quickly.

• Inform patient that ODTs contain phenylalanine.

• Instruct patient with diabetes to closely monitor blood glucose level. Drug may cause hyperglycemia.

• Urge patient to report pregnancy, suspected pregnancy, or plans to become pregnant or breastfeed.

✪ **Alert:** Warn patient not to drive or operate heavy machinery for rest of day after receiving extended-release injection and to seek medical attention if signs and symptoms of PDSS occur.

SAFETY ALERT!

oliceridine ⚫
oh-li-SER-i-deen

Olinvyk

Therapeutic class: Opioid analgesics
Pharmacologic class: Opioid agonists
Controlled substance schedule: II

AVAILABLE FORMS

Injection: 1 mg/mL single-dose vials; 30 mg/30 mL single-patient-use vials for PCA

INDICATIONS & DOSAGES

❸ *Alert:* Initiate individual dosing for each patient and use lowest effective dose for shortest duration consistent with treatment goals.

➤ **Acute pain severe enough to require an IV opioid analgesic when alternative treatments are inadequate**

Adults: Initially, 1.5 mg IV, with supplemental doses of 0.75 mg beginning 1 hour after initial dose and hourly thereafter PRN. For PCA, initial dose can be followed by demand doses of 0.35 mg with 6-minute lockout; may increase to 0.5 mg. Individual single doses greater than 3 mg haven't been evaluated. Maximum daily dose, 27 mg. If maximum daily dose is met and analgesia is still required, use alternative analgesics until oliceridine can be resumed the next day.

Adjust-a-dose: For patients with Child-Pugh class A or B liver impairment, less frequent dosing may be required. For those with Child-Pugh class C liver impairment, consider reducing initial dose; administer subsequent doses after reviewing pain severity and clinical status. For patients with central sleep apnea (CSA) and sleep-related hypoxemia, consider decreasing dose.

If CYP3A4 inducers are used concomitantly, consider increased oliceridine dose. If discontinuing CYP3A4 inducer, monitor patient for respiratory depression and sedation and consider decreasing oliceridine dose.

░ Patients who are normal CYP2D6 metabolizers taking a CYP2D6 inhibitor and a strong CYP3A4 inhibitor or who are discontinuing a CYP3A4 inducer may require less frequent dosing. Patients who are known CYP2D6 poor metabolizers taking a CYP3A4 inhibitor or discontinuing a CYP3A4 inducer may require less frequent dosing.

ADMINISTRATION

IV

▼ For PCA use, transfer drug directly from vial into PCA syringe or IV bag without diluting.

▼ Inspect for particulate matter and discoloration. Don't use if particles or discoloration is present.

▼ Store at room temperature. Don't freeze.

▼ Protect from light.

▼ **Incompatibilities:** None listed by manufacturer. Consult drug compatibility reference for more information.

ACTION

Unknown. Binds with opioid receptors in the CNS, altering perception of and emotional response to pain.

Route	Onset	Peak	Duration
IV	2–5 min	Unknown	Unknown

Half-life: 1.3 to 3 hours; metabolites, 44 hours.

ADVERSE REACTIONS

CNS: anxiety, dizziness, fever, headache, insomnia, restlessness, somnolence, sedation. **CV:** flushing, HTN, hypotension, tachycardia. **EENT:** dry mouth. **GI:** constipation, diarrhea, dyspepsia, flatulence, nausea, vomiting. **Hematologic:** anemia. **Hepatic:** elevated ALT level. **Metabolic:** *hypocalcemia, hypomagnesemia, hypokalemia,* hypophosphatemia. **Musculoskeletal:** back pain, muscle spasms. **Respiratory:** cough, decreased oxygen saturation, dyspnea, *hypoxia.* **Skin:** hyperhidrosis, infusion-site extravasation, pruritus, rash.

INTERACTIONS

Drug-drug. *Anticholinergics (atropine, benztropine, hyoscyamine, solifenacin, tolterodine):* May increase risk of urine retention or severe constipation, which may lead to paralytic ileus. Monitor patient closely.

  Boxed Warning *Benzodiazepines, CNS depressants (antipsychotics, anxiolytics, general anesthetics, hypnotics, muscle relaxants, other opioids, sedatives, tranquilizers):* May cause slow or difficult breathing, sedation, and death. Avoid use together. If use together can't be avoided, limit dose and duration of each drug to the minimum needed for desired effect. ■

CNS depressants (general anesthetics, phenothiazines): May cause severe hypotension, orthostatic hypotension, and syncope. Monitor patient closely.

CYP3A4 inducers (carbamazepine, phenytoin, rifampin): May decrease oliceridine level and efficacy. Monitor patient closely for increased pain or opioid withdrawal. Consider supplemental oliceridine doses. If discontinuing CYP3A4 inducer, consider reducing oliceridine dose and monitor for respiratory depression.

Diuretics: May reduce diuretic efficacy. Monitor patient for diminished diuresis or effect on BP; increase diuretic dose as needed.

O

Mixed opioid agonist-antagonists (butorphanol, nalbuphine, pentazocine) or partial agonist (buprenorphine) analgesics: May reduce analgesic effect and precipitate withdrawal symptoms. Avoid use together.

Moderate to strong CYP2D6 inhibitors (bupropion, fluoxetine, paroxetine, quinidine) or CYP3A4 inhibitors (azole antifungals [itraconazole, ketoconazole], macrolide antibiotics [erythromycin], protease inhibitors [ritonavir, telaprevir], SSRIs): May increase oliceridine level, resulting in increased or prolonged opioid effects or adverse reactions. Patients taking a CYP2D6 inhibitor and a CYP3A4 inhibitor are at increased risk. Consider less-frequent oliceridine dosing. Monitor patient for respiratory depression and sedation. If discontinuing CYP2D6 or CYP3A4 inhibitor, may need to increase oliceridine dose. Monitor patient for opioid withdrawal.

Muscle relaxants: May enhance relaxant effect and respiratory depression. Monitor patient and decrease dose of oliceridine or muscle relaxant as necessary.

Serotonergic drugs (drugs that affect the serotonin neurotransmitter system [mirtazapine, tramadol, trazodone], 5-HT$_3$ receptor antagonists, MAO inhibitors [isocarboxazid, linezolid, methylene blue, phenelzine], muscle relaxants [cyclobenzaprine, metaxalone], SNRIs, SSRIs, TCAs, triptans): May increase risk of serotonin syndrome. Use together cautiously. Discontinue oliceridine if serotonin syndrome is suspected.

Drug-lifestyle. **Boxed Warning** *Alcohol use:* May cause slow or difficult breathing, sedation, and death. Discourage use together. ∎

EFFECTS ON LAB TEST RESULTS
- May increase ALT and amylase levels.
- May decrease calcium, magnesium, phosphate, and potassium levels.
- May decrease RBC count.

CONTRAINDICATIONS & CAUTIONS
- Contraindicated in patients hypersensitive to oliceridine and in those with significant respiratory depression, acute or severe bronchial asthma in an unmonitored setting or in the absence of resuscitative equipment, or known or suspected GI obstruction, including paralytic ileus.

Boxed Warning Use exposes patient and others to risk of opioid addiction, abuse, and misuse, which can lead to overdose and death.

These effects can occur at any dose or duration. Assess patient risk before prescribing and regularly reassess patient for these behaviors and conditions. ∎

Boxed Warning Prescribers are strongly encouraged to complete a REMS-compliant education program. Drug should be prescribed only by prescribers with knowledge of opioid use and ways to reduce associated risks. ∎

❸ *Alert:* Use lowest effective dose for shortest period consistent with patient's treatment goals.

❸ *Alert:* Because risk of overdose increases as opioid dose increases, reserve titration to higher doses for patients in whom lower doses are ineffective and in whom expected benefits of higher opioid dose outweigh risks.

Boxed Warning *Opioid class warning:* Opioids should only be prescribed with benzodiazepines or other CNS depressants when alternative treatment options are inadequate, aren't expected to provide adequate analgesia, haven't been tolerated, or aren't expected to be tolerated. ∎

- Opioids can cause sleep-related breathing disorders, including CSA and sleep-related hypoxemia; the risk increases with increased dosages. For patients with CSA, consider decreasing opioid dosage using best practices for opioid taper.
- Use cautiously in older adults, in patients who are cachectic or debilitated, and in patients with substantially decreased respiratory reserve, COPD, cor pulmonale, hypoxia, hypercapnia, or preexisting respiratory depression, due to risk of life-threatening respiratory depression. Monitor patient closely and consider use of nonopioid analgesics.
- Use cautiously in patients with increased ICP, brain tumors, head injury or impaired consciousness who are at increased risk for intracranial effects of CO_2 retention such as reduction of respiratory drive and further reduction in ICP.
- Avoid use in patients with head injury, impaired consciousness, or coma; drug may mask clinical changes.
- Use cautiously in patients with biliary tract disease or acute pancreatitis. Drug may cause increased serum amylase level and worsening of symptoms.
- Use cautiously in patients with Child-Pugh class C liver impairment, QT-interval prolongation, and adrenal insufficiency.
- Avoid total daily dose above 27 mg due to increased risk of QT-interval prolongation.

Reactions in bold italics are ***life-threatening***.

• Use cautiously in patients with seizure disorders. Drug may worsen seizure control.

• Use cautiously in patients with compromised ability to maintain BP due to reduced blood volume or use of certain CNS depressants (general anesthetics, phenothiazines). Monitor BP closely. Avoid use in patients with circulatory shock due to risk of further vasodilation.

⚱ Use cautiously in patients with decreased CYP2D6 function due to increased risk of prolonged opioid adverse reactions and exacerbated respiratory depression. Closely monitor patient for respiratory depression and sedation; consider less-frequent dosing.

• Safety of use beyond 48 hours hasn't been established.

⚠ *Alert:* Don't use immediate-release formulations for an extended period unless pain remains severe enough to require an opioid analgesic and alternative treatment options are inadequate to treat pain.

• Safety and effectiveness in children haven't been established.

Boxed Warning Accidental ingestion of even one dose of an opioid, especially by children, can result in a fatal overdose. ■

Dialyzable drug: Unlikely.

⚠ *Overdose S&S:* Respiratory depression; somnolence progressing to stupor or coma; skeletal muscle flaccidity; cold, clammy skin; constricted pupils. In some cases, marked pupil dilation (with severe hypoxia), pulmonary edema, bradycardia, hypotension, partial or complete airway obstruction, atypical snoring, death.

PREGNANCY-LACTATION-REPRODUCTION

Boxed Warning Prolonged use during pregnancy can result in neonatal opioid withdrawal syndrome, which may be life-threatening. It requires management with expert neonatology protocols. If prolonged use is needed, advise patient of risks and ensure availability of proper treatment. ■

• Oliceridine isn't recommended for use immediately before or during labor. If used, monitor infant for excess sedation and respiratory depression.

• It isn't known if drug causes major birth defects or miscarriage.

• It isn't known if drug appears in human milk. Patient deciding to breastfeed should weigh benefits of drug to risks to infant. Monitor infant who is breastfed for excess sedation

and respiratory depression. Withdrawal symptoms can occur in infants when breastfeeding is stopped or drug is discontinued.

• Prolonged opioid use may reduce fertility in patients of reproductive potential. It's unknown if effects on fertility are reversible.

NURSING CONSIDERATIONS

Boxed Warning Regularly monitor all patients for opioid addiction, abuse, and misuse, which can lead to overdose and death. ■

Boxed Warning May cause life-threatening or fatal respiratory depression at any time during therapy. Monitor patient closely, especially when starting or increasing doses. Proper dosing and titration are essential to reduce risk. ■

• If pain level increases after dosage stabilization, attempt to identify source of increased pain before increasing oliceridine dosage.

⚠ *Alert:* Drug may cause opioid-induced hyperalgesia (OIH). Symptoms include increased pain level with opioid dose increase, decreased pain level with opioid dose reduction or pain from ordinarily nonpainful stimuli without underlying disease progression, opioid tolerance or withdrawal, or addictive behavior. If OIH is suspected, decrease opioid dose or switch patient to alternative opioid.

⚠ *Alert:* Monitor patient for adrenal insufficiency (nausea, vomiting, anorexia, fatigue, weakness, dizziness, hypotension). If confirmed, wean patient off oliceridine and treat with corticosteroids until adrenal function recovers. If necessary, try other opioids.

• Monitor patient for severe hypotension, orthostatic hypotension, and syncope, especially after dosage initiation or titration.

⚠ *Alert:* Don't abruptly discontinue drug in patient physically dependent on opioids. If discontinuing drug, gradually taper dose while monitoring patient for signs and symptoms of withdrawal (restlessness; lacrimation; rhinorrhea; yawning; chills; perspiration; myalgia; mydriasis; irritability; anxiety; backache; joint pain; weakness; abdominal cramps; insomnia; diarrhea; nausea; vomiting; anorexia; increased BP, respiratory rate, HR). If withdrawal occurs, increase dosage to previous level and taper more slowly.

PATIENT TEACHING

Boxed Warning Counsel patient and caregiver on serious risks, safe use, and importance of reading the medication guide with each prescription. ■

• Instruct patient to contact provider if prescribed dosage doesn't control pain.

🌙 **Alert:** Warn patient to withhold drug and inform prescriber if pain level worsens, pain sensitivity increases, or new pain occurs after taking drug.

• Inform patient that, for acute pain, drug may only be needed for a few days.

• Teach patient that naloxone may be prescribed with the opioid when beginning and renewing therapy to reduce risk of opioid overdose and death

🌙 **Alert:** Counsel patient who has been regularly taking drug not to discontinue without first discussing the need for gradual tapering with prescriber.

🌙 **Alert:** Advise patient taking other drugs that increase risk of serotonin syndrome to immediately report signs and symptoms of serotonin syndrome (confusion, agitation, fever, rapid heartbeat, loss of muscle coordination, vomiting, diaphoresis) and seek medical attention.

• Advise patient about risk of severe constipation, including how to manage it and when to inform prescriber.

• Caution patient to report to prescriber pregnancy or plan to become pregnant.

---

olmesartan medoxomil ⚘
ol-ma-SAR-tan

Benicar, Olmetec✦

Therapeutic class: Antihypertensives
Pharmacologic class: Angiotensin II receptor antagonists

AVAILABLE FORMS
Tablets: 5 mg, 10 mg✦, 20 mg, 40 mg

INDICATIONS & DOSAGES
➤ **HTN**
Adults and children ages 6 and older weighing 35 kg or more: 20 mg PO once daily if patient has no volume depletion. May increase dosage to 40 mg PO once daily if BP isn't reduced after 2 weeks of therapy.
Children ages 6 to 16 weighing 20 to less than 35 kg: Initially, 10 mg PO daily, with maintenance dosage of 10 to 20 mg daily.

Adjust-a-dose: In patients with possible depletion of intravascular volume (those with impaired kidney function who are taking diuretics), consider a lower starting dose. Use cautiously in patients with CrCl less than 20 mL/minute.

ADMINISTRATION
PO
• Give drug without regard to food.
• Drug may be made into suspension by pharmacist if patient cannot swallow pills.
• Refrigerate suspension, which may be stored for up to 28 days.
• Shake suspension well for at least 1 minute before use.

ACTION
Blocks vasoconstrictor and aldosterone-secreting effects of angiotensin II by selectively blocking the binding of angiotensin II to the angiotensin I, or AT_1, receptor in the vascular smooth muscle.

Route	Onset	Peak	Duration
PO	Rapid	1–2 hr	24 hr

Half-life: 13 hours.

ADVERSE REACTIONS
CNS: headache, dizziness. **EENT:** rhinitis, pharyngitis, sinusitis. **GI:** diarrhea. **GU:** hematuria. **Metabolic:** hyperglycemia, hypertriglyceridemia, increased CK level. **Musculoskeletal:** back pain. **Respiratory:** bronchitis, URI. **Other:** flulike symptoms.

INTERACTIONS
Drug-drug. *ACE inhibitors:* May increase risk of hyperkalemia and decrease kidney function. Consider monotherapy; if coadministration can't be avoided, monitor kidney function and serum potassium level.

🌙 **Alert:** *Aliskiren:* May increase risk of kidney impairment, hypotension, and hyperkalemia in patients with diabetes. Use together is contraindicated in these patients. Avoid use together in patients with GFR less than 60 mL/minute.

Colesevelam: May reduce olmesartan level. Give olmesartan at least 4 hours before colesevelam.

COX-2 inhibitors, NSAIDs: May decrease antihypertensive effects of olmesartan. Coadministration in older adults, patients who are volume-depleted, and those with

---

compromised kidney function may result in deterioration of kidney function, including possible AKI. Periodically monitor BP and kidney function.

Heparin: May increase serum potassium level. Monitor serum potassium level.

Lithium: May increase serum lithium level and risk of toxicity. Closely monitor serum lithium level and adjust dosage as needed.

Potassium-sparing diuretics (amiloride, spironolactone), potassium supplements: May increase risk of hyperkalemia. Closely monitor serum potassium level; adjust therapy as needed.

Trimethoprim: May increase risk of hyperkalemia, especially in older adults. If use together can't be avoided, closely monitor potassium level.

Drug-herb. *Yohimbe:* May decrease antihypertensive effect of olmesartan. Closely monitor BP.

EFFECTS ON LAB TEST RESULTS
• May increase potassium, glucose, triglyceride, uric acid, liver enzyme, bilirubin, and CK levels.
• May decrease Hb level and hematocrit.
• May lead to false-negative aldosterone/renin ratio.

CONTRAINDICATIONS & CAUTIONS
• Contraindicated in patients hypersensitive to drug or its components and in patients with diabetes who are also taking aliskiren.
• Avoid use in patients who experienced angioedema with other ARBs and in those with kidney impairment who are also taking aliskiren.
• Use cautiously in patients who are volume- or sodium-depleted, those whose kidney function depends on the RAAS (such as patients with severe HF), those with unilateral or bilateral renal artery stenosis, and patients with diabetes.
• **Alert:** Drug can cause spruelike enteropathy (severe chronic diarrhea with substantial weight loss).
• Effectiveness in children younger than age 6 hasn't been proven.
Dialyzable drug: Unknown.
⚠ **Overdose S&S:** Hypotension, tachycardia, bradycardia.

PREGNANCY-LACTATION-REPRODUCTION
Boxed Warning Drug may cause fetal and neonatal complications and death. If patient becomes pregnant, stop drug immediately. ∎

• It isn't known if drug appears in human milk. Patient should discontinue breastfeeding or discontinue drug, considering importance of drug to patient.

NURSING CONSIDERATIONS
• Symptomatic hypotension may occur in patients who are volume- or sodium-depleted, especially those being treated with high doses of a diuretic. If hypotension occurs, place patient supine and treat until BP stabilizes. Treatment may continue once BP stabilizes.
• If BP isn't adequately controlled, a diuretic or other antihypertensives also may be prescribed.
• Closely monitor patient with HF for oliguria, azotemia, and AKI.
• Watch for signs and symptoms of angioedema.
• Monitor serum potassium level; drug can cause hyperkalemia.
• Monitor BUN and creatinine level in patient with unilateral or bilateral renal artery stenosis.
⬚ The antihypertensive effects of ACE inhibitors and ARBs are reduced in patients who are Black; use of these drugs as initial antihypertensive therapy in these patients isn't recommended.

PATIENT TEACHING
• Tell patient to take drug exactly as prescribed and not to stop taking it, even if feeling better.
• Teach about proper drug administration and handling for prescribed formulation.
• Advise patient to promptly report all adverse reactions, especially light-headedness and fainting.
• Teach patient to avoid potassium supplements and potassium-containing salt substitutes.
• Instruct patient to report signs and symptoms of angioedema (wheezing, swelling of face, lips, tongue, or throat).
• **Alert:** Tell patient to contact prescriber if severe chronic diarrhea with substantial weight loss develops, even if months to years have elapsed before symptoms occur.
• Advise patient of childbearing potential that drug can cause fetal harm. Instruct patient to immediately report pregnancy to health care provider.
• Inform patient with diabetes that glucose readings may rise and that dosage of diabetes drugs may need adjustment.
• Warn patient that inadequate fluid intake, excessive perspiration, diarrhea, or vomiting

0

may lead to an excessive drop in BP, light-headedness and, possibly, fainting.

• Instruct patient that other antihypertensives can have additive effects. Patient should inform prescriber of all medications being taken, including OTC drugs and herbal products.

olodaterol
oh-loe-DA-ter-ol

Striverdi Respimat

Therapeutic class: Bronchodilators
Pharmacologic class: Long-acting selective beta₂-adrenergic agonists

AVAILABLE FORMS
Inhalation aerosol: 2.5 mcg/actuation

INDICATIONS & DOSAGES
➤ **Long-term maintenance treatment of airway obstruction in patients with COPD, including chronic bronchitis and emphysema**
Adults: 2 inhalations once daily. Maximum dosage, 2 inhalations in 24 hours.

ADMINISTRATION
Inhalational
• Prime inhaler by spraying toward ground until aerosol cloud is seen; then repeat spray three more times before first use or if inhaler hasn't been used for more than 21 days. If not used for more than 3 days, spray once toward ground to prime.
• To administer dose, have patient breathe in slowly through the mouth and press the dose release button. Patient should then continue to breathe in slowly as long as possible and then hold breath for 10 seconds if possible. Repeat for second inhalation.
• While patient is inhaling dose, have patient hold inhaler flat; make sure patient doesn't cover air vents on the mouthpiece.
• Give at same time each day.
• Store at 68° to 77° F (20° to 25° C); avoid freezing. Discard 3 months after cartridge has been inserted into inhaler.

ACTION
Binds and activates beta₂ adrenoceptors in the lungs, resulting in relaxation of smooth muscle cells and bronchodilation.

Route	Onset	Peak	Duration
Inhalation	5 min	10–20 min	24 hr

Half-life: 7.5 hours.

ADVERSE REACTIONS
CNS: fever, dizziness. **EENT:** nasopharyngitis. **GI:** constipation, diarrhea. **GU:** UTI. **Musculoskeletal:** back pain, arthralgia. **Respiratory:** URI, bronchitis, pneumonia, cough. **Skin:** rash.

INTERACTIONS
Drug-drug. *Beta blockers:* May diminish effect of both drugs and increase risk of bronchospasm. Avoid use together, if possible.
Cannabinoid-containing products: May increase tachycardic effect of olodaterol. Monitor therapy closely.
Corticosteroids, non-potassium-sparing diuretics, xanthine derivatives (theophylline): May increase risk of hypokalemia. Monitor potassium level.
Drugs that prolong QT interval (antiarrhythmics, droperidol, haloperidol, mifepristone, TCAs, thioridazine): May increase risk of life-threatening cardiac arrhythmias. Use together cautiously.
Loop diuretics, thiazide and thiazide-like diuretics: May increase hypokalemic effect of diuretics. Monitor potassium level.
MAO inhibitors: May increase CV effects. Use together cautiously.
Other LABAs: May have additive risk of toxic adverse effects. Use together is contraindicated.
Tedizolid: May increase hypertensive and tachycardic effects of olodaterol. Monitor therapy closely.
Drug-food. *Caffeine:* May increase risk of hypokalemia. Discourage use together.

EFFECTS ON LAB TEST RESULTS
• May increase glucose level.
• May decrease potassium level.

CONTRAINDICATIONS & CAUTIONS
• Use of a LABA, including olodaterol, without an inhaled corticosteroid is contraindicated in patients with asthma. Drug isn't indicated for use in asthma.
🛈 **Alert:** Rare, paradoxical, life-threatening bronchospasm has been reported. Discontinue drug immediately and treat emergently.
• Discontinue drug if hypersensitivity reactions such as angioedema occur.

Reactions in bold italics are ***life-threatening***.

• Don't initiate drug in patients with acute deterioration of COPD.

• Contraindicated as rescue therapy for acute symptoms.

• Use cautiously in patients with extreme sensitivity to other sympathomimetics, CV conditions (coronary insufficiency, cardiac arrhythmias, HTN, hypertrophic obstructive cardiomyopathy), seizure disorders, diabetes, or thyrotoxicosis.

• Use cautiously in patients with known or suspected prolongation of QT interval.

• Safety and effectiveness in children haven't been established.

Dialyzable drug: Unknown.

⚠ *Overdose S&S:* CV toxicity, HTN or hypotension, tachycardia, arrhythmias, palpitations, dizziness, nervousness, insomnia, anxiety, headache, tremor, dry mouth, muscle spasms, nausea, fatigue, malaise, hypokalemia, hyperglycemia, metabolic acidosis.

PREGNANCY-LACTATION-REPRODUCTION

• Studies during pregnancy are inadequate. Use during pregnancy only if potential benefit justifies fetal risk.

• It isn't known if drug appears in human milk. Use cautiously during breastfeeding.

NURSING CONSIDERATIONS

• Patient must also be prescribed a short-acting inhaled beta$_2$ agonist to provide symptomatic relief.

• Monitor patient for increased use of inhaled beta$_2$ agonist and decreased control of symptoms of bronchospasm. Evaluate for deterioration of disease.

• Monitor FEV$_1$, FVC, and other pulmonary function tests; serum potassium and glucose levels; BP; and HR.

🔔 *Alert:* Excessive use of drug by using more frequently, increasing the number of inhalations, or using in combination with other medications containing LABAs may cause CV effects and death.

• Monitor patient for hypokalemia (which may increase risk of cardiac arrhythmias) and hyperglycemia.

• *Look alike–sound alike:* Don't confuse olodaterol with olopatadine. Don't confuse Striverdi Respimat with Combivent Respimat.

PATIENT TEACHING

• Warn patient that drug isn't approved for treatment of asthma. Advise that using a LABA, including olodaterol, without an inhaled corticosteroid is contraindicated in patients with asthma.

• Teach patient how to use inhaler device; then ask patient to demonstrate its use.

• Advise patient to take medication at same time each day.

• Explain that drug has a long-acting effect and should never be used as "rescue medication" to relieve acute symptoms. Advise patient to always carry a rescue inhaler.

• Instruct patient to report worsening signs or symptoms of COPD, increased frequency of rescue medication use, and decreased effectiveness of rescue medication.

• Warn patient not to use drug with other LABAs and not to regularly use short-acting beta$_2$ agonists. Short-acting beta$_2$ agonists should only be used for acute symptoms.

• Instruct patient to report URI; palpitations; chest pain; rapid heartbeat; muscle spasms; weakness; tremor; nervousness; confusion; flushed, dry skin; or excessive thirst, urination, or hunger.

• Teach patient to seek emergency medical care for serious allergic reactions (breathing problems, rash, hives, or swelling of face, mouth, or tongue).

• Caution patient not to stop drug without first discussing with prescriber.

• Instruct patient to consult prescriber before starting new prescription or OTC medications or herbal or nutritional supplements.

• Advise patient to report pregnancy, plans to become pregnant, or breastfeeding.

omadacycline
oh-MAD-a-sye-kleen

Nuzyra

Therapeutic class: Antibiotics
Pharmacologic class: Tetracyclines

AVAILABLE FORMS
Injection: 100-mg single-dose vial
Tablets: 150-mg base

INDICATIONS & DOSAGES
➤ **Community-acquired bacterial pneumonia (CABP)** caused by *Streptococcus pneumoniae, Staphylococcus aureus* **(methicillin-susceptible isolates),** *Haemophilus influenzae, Haemophilus*

parainfluenzae, Klebsiella pneumoniae, Legionella pneumophila, Mycoplasma pneumoniae, **and** *Chlamydophila pneumoniae*
Adults: Initially, 200 mg IV infusion over 60 minutes once or 100 mg IV infusion over 30 minutes b.i.d. on day 1; then 100 mg IV infusion over 30 minutes once daily or 300 mg PO once daily. Or, initially, 300 mg PO b.i.d. on day 1; then 300 mg PO once daily. Treat for 7 to 14 days.

➤ **Acute bacterial skin and skin-structure infections caused by** *S. aureus* **(methicillin-susceptible and methicillin-resistant isolates),** *Staphylococcus lugdunensis, Streptococcus pyogenes, Streptococcus anginosus* **group (includes** *S. anginosus, S. intermedius, S. constellatus),* **Enterococcus faecalis, Enterobacter cloacae,** **and** *K. pneumoniae*
Adults: Initially, 200 mg IV infusion over 60 minutes once or 100 mg IV infusion over 30 minutes b.i.d. on day 1; then 100 mg IV infusion over 30 minutes once daily. Or, initially, 450 mg PO once daily on days 1 and 2; then 300 mg PO once daily beginning on day 3. Or, 300 mg PO once daily. Treat for 7 to 14 days.

ADMINISTRATION
PO
• Patient should fast for at least 4 hours before dose; then take drug with water.
• Patient shouldn't eat or drink (except water) for 2 hours after dose or ingest dairy products, antacids, or multivitamins for 4 hours after dose.

IV
▼ Reconstitute each 100-mg vial with 5 mL sterile water, NSS, or D_5W for injection.
▼ Gently swirl contents and let stand until drug cake dissolves completely and foam disperses. Don't shake.
▼ Reconstituted solution should be yellow to dark orange; if not, discard it. Visually inspect vial for particulate matter and discoloration before further dilution and administration. If necessary, invert vial to dissolve remaining powder and swirl gently to prevent foaming.
▼ Within 1 hour of reconstitution, withdraw 5 mL or 10 mL of solution and further dilute in 100-mL bag of NSS or D_5W, for final concentration of either 1 mg/mL or 2 mg/mL. Discard unused portion of solution.

▼ Infuse diluted solution within 24 hours if kept at room temperature or within 7 days when refrigerated. Don't freeze.
▼ Remove solution from refrigerator and warm to room temperature before use.
▼ Administer through a dedicated line or Y-site. If same IV line is used for infusion of other drugs, flush line with NSS or D_5W before and after infusion of omadacycline.
▼ Administer infusion over 60 minutes for 200-mg dose or 30 minutes for 100-mg dose.
▼ Store vials at room temperature.
▼ **Incompatibilities:** Don't administer solutions containing multivalent cations (calcium, magnesium) through the same IV line. Infusion with other medications and solutions other than NSS or D_5W hasn't been studied.

ACTION
A tetracycline antibiotic that exerts its bacteriostatic effect by inhibiting bacterial protein synthesis.

Route	Onset	Peak	Duration
PO	Unknown	2.5 hr	Unknown
IV	Unknown	30 min	Unknown

Half-life: 15 to 17 hours.

ADVERSE REACTIONS
CNS: insomnia, headache, fatigue, lethargy, vertigo. **CV:** HTN, tachycardia, atrial fibrillation. **EENT:** oral candidiasis, oropharyngeal pain. **GI:** vomiting, constipation, nausea, diarrhea, abdominal pain, dyspepsia, dysgeusia. **GU:** vulvovaginal mycotic infection. **Hematologic:** thrombocytosis, anemia. **Hepatic:** elevated LFT values. **Skin:** pruritus, erythema, sweating, urticaria. **Other:** infusion-site reaction, hypersensitivity.

INTERACTIONS
Drug-drug. *Antacids containing aluminum, calcium, magnesium, bismuth subsalicylate; iron-containing preparations; iron supplements:* May decrease omadacycline absorption. Separate doses by at least 4 hours before and 4 hours after omadacycline.
Anticoagulants (warfarin): May increase anticoagulant effects. Monitor patient closely and decrease anticoagulant dosage if needed.
Drug-food. *Dairy products:* May decrease omadacycline absorption. Separate dairy

product use by at least 4 hours before and 4 hours after omadacycline.

Food, nondairy drinks (except water): May decrease omadacycline absorption. Avoid for at least 4 hours before and 2 hours after omadacycline.

Drug-lifestyle. *Sun exposure:* May cause photosensitivity. Advise patient to avoid sun exposure and to wear sun-protective clothing and sunscreen.

EFFECTS ON LAB TEST RESULTS
• May increase ALT, AST, GGT, CK, bilirubin, ALP, and lipase levels.
• May decrease Hb level and platelet count.

CONTRAINDICATIONS & CAUTIONS
• Contraindicated in patients hypersensitive to drug or its components or tetracycline class drugs.
• Use only to treat or prevent infections proven or strongly suspected to be caused by susceptible bacteria to reduce development of drug resistance.
• **Alert:** In clinical trials of patients with CABP, mortality rate was higher for treatment with omadacycline than with moxifloxacin. All deaths occurred in patients older than age 65 and most had multiple comorbid conditions. The cause of the mortality imbalance isn't known.
• **Alert:** CDAD has been reported and may range from mild diarrhea to fatal colitis.
• Use of tetracycline class drugs during the second and third trimester of pregnancy, during infancy, and in children younger than age 8 may cause permanent yellow-gray-brown discoloration of teeth, tooth enamel hypoplasia, and reversible inhibition of bone growth.
• Use cautiously in older adults.
• Safety and effectiveness in patients younger than age 18 haven't been established. Use in children younger than age 8 isn't recommended.
Dialyzable drug: 7.9%.

PREGNANCY-LACTATION-REPRODUCTION
• Drug may cause fetal harm. Advise patients of childbearing potential to use contraception during therapy.
• Tetracyclines appear in human milk. Breastfeeding isn't recommended during treatment and for 4 days after final dose.
• Based on animal studies, drug may affect fertility.

NURSING CONSIDERATIONS
• Confirm that patient doesn't have an allergy to any tetracycline class drug before starting therapy.
• Monitor patient for hypersensitivity reactions, including anaphylaxis.
• Monitor patient for signs and symptoms of CDAD (watery or bloody stools [with or without stomach cramps or fever]) during and for several months after treatment with antibacterial drugs. If CDAD is suspected or confirmed, antibiotic use other than for treatment of *Clostridioides difficile* may need to be discontinued. Initiate appropriate treatment.
• Monitor for tetracycline class adverse reactions, including photosensitivity, pseudotumor cerebri, and antianabolic activity (increased BUN level, azotemia, acidosis, hyperphosphatemia, pancreatitis, abnormal LFT values). Discontinue drug if any of these reactions are suspected.
• *Look alike–sound alike:* Don't confuse omadacycline with omacetaxine.

PATIENT TEACHING
• Warn patient that antibacterial drugs should only be used to treat bacterial infections and shouldn't be used to treat viral infections such as the common cold.
• Advise patient to report all adverse reactions.
• Caution patient to seek immediate medical attention for serious allergic reactions.
• Teach about proper drug administration and handling.
• Caution patient to take drug exactly as directed, even if feeling better. Stress importance of not skipping doses and completing therapy as prescribed.
• Warn that nonadherence may decrease treatment effectiveness and risk that the bacteria will develop resistance and not be treatable by antibacterial drugs in the future.
• *Alert:* Instruct patient to immediately report watery or bloody stools (with or without stomach cramps or fever) as these findings may indicate CDAD.
• Warn that drug can cause photosensitivity. Advise patient to avoid sun exposure and wear sun-protective clothing and sunscreen during treatment.
• Inform patient of childbearing potential of fetal risk of drug use during pregnancy. Caution patient to use contraceptives during treatment and to immediately report suspected pregnancy.

0

• Teach patient that breastfeeding isn't recommended during treatment and for 4 days after final dose.

omalizumab
oh-mah-lye-ZOO-mab

Xolair

Therapeutic class: Antiasthmatics
Pharmacologic class: Monoclonal antibodies

AVAILABLE FORMS
Powder for injection: 150 mg in single-dose vials
Prefilled syringe: 75 mg/0.5 mL (0.5 mL), 150 mg/mL (1 mL)

INDICATIONS & DOSAGES
➤ **Moderate to severe persistent asthma in patients with positive skin test or in vitro reactivity to perennial aeroallergen and whose symptoms aren't adequately controlled by inhaled corticosteroids**
Adults and children ages 6 and older: 75 to 375 mg subcut every 2 or 4 weeks. Dose and frequency vary with pretreatment IgE level (international units/mL) and patient weight. (Refer to manufacturer's instructions.)
➤ **Chronic rhinosinusitis with nasal polyps as add-on maintenance treatment in patients with inadequate response to nasal corticosteroids**
Adults: 75 to 600 mg subcut every 2 or 4 weeks. Dosage and frequency vary with pretreatment IgE level (international units/mL) and patient weight. (Refer to manufacturer's instructions.)
➤ **Chronic spontaneous urticaria in patients who are symptomatic despite H$_1$ antihistamine treatment**
Adults and adolescents ages 12 and older: 150 to 300 mg subcut every 4 weeks. (Dosing isn't dependent on serum IgE level or body weight.) Periodically reassess need for continued therapy; treatment duration hasn't been evaluated.

ADMINISTRATION
Subcutaneous
• Visually inspect contents of prefilled syringe for particulate matter and discoloration before use. Don't use unless solution is clear and colorless to pale brownish yellow.

• Reconstitute with 1.4 mL of sterile water for injection only. Swirl gently; don't shake. Continue to swirl for 5 to 10 seconds approximately every 5 minutes until no visible gel-like particles appear in solution.
• The lyophilized product takes 15 to 20 minutes to dissolve completely. Don't use if vial's contents don't dissolve completely by 40 minutes.
• Fully reconstituted product appears clear or slightly opalescent and may have a few small bubbles or foam around edge of vial.
• Use 18G needle to draw medication into syringe, then replace with a 25G needle for administration.
• Because solution is slightly viscous, it may take 5 to 10 seconds to administer.
• Give at least first three doses in a health care setting under the guidance of a health care provider.
• Divide doses of more than 150 mg between two or more injection sites.
• Don't give more than one injection per site. Choose a different injection site for each new injection that's at least 1 inch from other injection sites.
• Use reconstituted solution within 4 hours if at room temperature or within 8 hours if refrigerated. Protect from sunlight.
• Recommended injection sites are upper arm, stomach, and front and middle of thighs for lyophilized powder or upper arm and front and middle of thighs for prefilled syringe.
• Don't inject into moles, scars, bruises, tender areas, or broken skin or within 2 inches of navel.
• Store vials before reconstitution and prefilled syringes under refrigeration at 36° to 46° F (2° to 8° C).

ACTION
Inhibits binding of IgE to high-affinity receptor on surface of mast cells and basophils, which limits release of allergic response mediators.

Route	Onset	Peak	Duration
Subcut	Slow	7–8 days	Unknown

Half-life: About 24 to 26 days.

ADVERSE REACTIONS
CNS: anxiety, headache, dizziness, fatigue, pain, migraine, fever. **CV:** *MI, thrombosis, PE,* angina pectoris, peripheral edema. **EENT:** otitis media, earache, sinusitis,

nasopharyngitis. **GI:** abdominal pain, gastroenteritis, toothache. **GU:** UTI. **Musculoskeletal:** limb pain, arthralgia, fracture. **Respiratory:** URI, cough, asthma. **Skin:** dermatitis, pruritus, injection-site reaction (bruising, bleeding, burning, redness, pain, inflammation, stinging, swelling, warmth). **Other:** viral and fungal infections, alopecia.

INTERACTIONS
Drug-drug. *Loxapine (inhalation only):* May enhance adverse or toxic effect of loxapine. Avoid use together.

EFFECTS ON LAB TEST RESULTS
• May increase IgE level, which may remain elevated for up to 1 year after treatment ends.
• May increase eosinophil count.

CONTRAINDICATIONS & CAUTIONS
• Contraindicated in patients severely hypersensitive to drug or its ingredients.
Boxed Warning Anaphylaxis presenting as bronchospasm, hypotension, syncope, urticaria, or angioedema of throat or tongue has been reported after administration as early as first dose and even after 1 year of treatment. ■
Boxed Warning Initiate therapy in a health care setting because of anaphylaxis risk. After deeming therapy safe, prescriber may determine that patient or caregiver can safely administer drug using a prefilled syringe. ■
⊕ *Alert:* Drug isn't indicated for other allergic conditions or other forms of urticaria.
• Rarely, malignancies have been observed during therapy.
• Safety and effectiveness in children younger than age 6 haven't been established.
Dialyzable drug: Unknown.

PREGNANCY-LACTATION-REPRODUCTION
• Drug may increase risk of low birth weight in infants. Poorly or moderately controlled asthma also carries risks during pregnancy. Use only if clearly needed.
• It isn't known if drug appears in human milk. Use cautiously during breastfeeding.

NURSING CONSIDERATIONS
⊕ *Alert:* Don't use this drug to treat acute bronchospasm or status asthmaticus.
• Monitor patient for eosinophilia, vasculitic rash, worsening pulmonary symptoms, cardiac complications, and neuropathy, especially after reducing oral corticosteroid dosage.

• Monitor patient for fever, arthralgia, and rash. Stop therapy if patient develops these symptoms of serum sickness.
• Don't abruptly stop systemic or inhaled corticosteroid when omalizumab therapy starts; gradually taper dosage under supervision.
• Injection-site reactions (bruising, redness, warmth, burning, stinging, itching, hives, pain, induration, inflammation) may occur, usually within 1 hour after injection. These reactions last fewer than 8 days and decrease in frequency with subsequent injections.
Boxed Warning Observe patient for an appropriate time period after injection, and keep drugs available to respond to anaphylactic reactions (bronchospasm, hypotension, syncope, urticaria, angioedema of throat or tongue). These reactions usually occur within 2 hours of subcut injection; however, delayed reactions may occur up to 24 hours after administration. Anaphylaxis has also occurred beyond 1 year after beginning regularly administered treatment. If patient has a severe hypersensitivity reaction, stop treatment. ■
• After therapy has been safely established, prescriber may determine whether self-administration by patient or caregiver is appropriate based on risk assessment. See manufacturer's information for selection criteria of patients for self-administration.
⊕ *Alert:* Drug may slightly increase risk of CV and cerebrovascular events (TIA, MI, chest pain, pulmonary HTN, DVT, PE). Periodically reassess the need for continued therapy based on disease severity and asthma control.
• Drug increases IgE level, so it can't be used to determine appropriate dosage during therapy or for 1 year after therapy ends.
• Monitor pulmonary function test results for signs of infection.
• The needle cover on the prefilled syringe contains dry natural rubber (a derivative of latex), which may cause allergic reactions in individuals sensitive to latex.
• Monitor patients at high risk for parasitic (geohelminth) infection.
• *Look alike–sound alike:* Don't confuse omalizumab with obinutuzumab or ofatumumab.

PATIENT TEACHING
• Advise patient to review medication guide with each dose.
• Tell patient not to stop or reduce dosage of other asthma drugs, unless directed by prescriber.

O

• Explain that patient may not notice an immediate improvement in asthma after therapy starts.

• Show adult, adolescent age 12 or older (with adult supervision), or caregiver how to administer the subcut prefilled syringe, and assess ability to inject subcut to ensure proper administration. Discuss proper syringe disposal.

Boxed Warning Teach patient signs and symptoms of anaphylaxis, and emphasize need to seek immediate medical care if symptoms occur. ■

omega-3–fatty acids
oh-MEG-a-three/FAT-tee-AS-ids

Lovaza, Vascepa

Therapeutic class: Antilipemics
Pharmacologic class: Fatty acids

AVAILABLE FORMS
Capsules ⓄⓉⒸ: 0.5 g, 1 g

INDICATIONS & DOSAGES
➤ **Adjunct to diet to reduce triglyceride levels of 500 mg/dL or higher**
Adults: 4 g PO once daily (Lovaza only) or divided as 2 g PO b.i.d.
➤ **Adjunct to maximally tolerated statin therapy to reduce risk of MI, stroke, coronary revascularization, and unstable angina requiring hospitalization in adults with elevated triglyceride levels (150 mg/dL or higher) and established CV disease or diabetes and two or more additional risk factors for CV disease (Vascepa)**
Adults: 2 g PO b.i.d.

ADMINISTRATION
PO
• Give drug with meals.
• Have patient swallow capsules whole; don't crush, dissolve, or extract contents of capsule.
• If dose is missed, give missed dose as soon as possible; don't double dose.

ACTION
May reduce liver formation of triglycerides because two components of drug are poor substrates for the necessary enzymes. These components also block formation of other fatty acids.

Route	Onset	Peak	Duration
PO	Unknown	5–9 hr	Unknown

Half-life: Eicosapentaenoic acid, about 37 to 89 hours; docosahexaenoic acid, about 46 hours.

ADVERSE REACTIONS
CNS: altered taste. **CV:** peripheral edema, atrial fibrillation, atrial flutter. **EENT:** oropharyngeal pain. **GI:** abdominal pain, belching, constipation, dyspepsia, diarrhea, nausea. **Metabolic:** gout. **Musculoskeletal:** arthralgia, back pain. **Skin:** rash.

INTERACTIONS
Drug-drug. *Anticoagulants, antiplatelet drugs:* May prolong bleeding time. Monitor patient.
Ibrutinib: May enhance antiplatelet effect of ibrutinib. Monitor therapy.

EFFECTS ON LAB TEST RESULTS
• May increase bleeding time.
• May increase ALT, AST, triglyceride, and LDL-C levels.

CONTRAINDICATIONS & CAUTIONS
• Contraindicated in patients hypersensitive to drug or its components.
• Use cautiously in patients with known hypersensitivity to fish or shellfish.
• Use cautiously in patients with coagulopathy and in those receiving therapeutic anticoagulation or antiplatelet therapy because of risk of prolonged bleeding time.
• Effect of drug on risk of pancreatitis hasn't been determined.
• May increase risk of atrial fibrillation or atrial flutter.
• Safety and effectiveness in children haven't been established.
Dialyzable drug: Unknown.

PREGNANCY-LACTATION-REPRODUCTION
• Studies during pregnancy are inadequate. Use cautiously and only if benefit justifies fetal risk.
• Drug may appear in human milk. Use cautiously during breastfeeding.

NURSING CONSIDERATIONS
• Assess for conditions that contribute to increased triglycerides (such as diabetes and hypothyroidism) before treatment.

Reactions in bold italics are *life-threatening*.

- Evaluate patient's current drug regimen for any drugs known to sharply increase triglyceride levels, including estrogen therapy, thiazide diuretics, and beta blockers. Stopping these drugs, if appropriate, may negate the need for drug.
- Continue diet and lifestyle modifications during treatment.
- Obtain baseline triglyceride levels to confirm that they're consistently abnormal before therapy; then recheck periodically during treatment. If patient has inadequate response after 2 months, stop drug.
- Monitor LDL level to make sure it doesn't increase excessively during treatment.
- Periodically monitor transaminase levels in patient with liver impairment.
- *Look alike–sound alike:* Don't confuse Lovaza with lorazepam or lovastatin.

PATIENT TEACHING
- Explain that taking drug doesn't reduce importance of following the recommended diet and exercise plan.
- Remind patient of the need for follow-up blood work to evaluate progress.
- Teach about proper drug administration and handling for prescribed formulation.
- Advise patient to notify prescriber about bothersome side effects.
- Tell patient to report planned or suspected pregnancy.

omeprazole ⊠
oh-MEP-ra-zole

Losec✤

omeprazole magnesium
Losec✤, Nexium ◇, Prilosec ◇, Prilosec Packets

Therapeutic class: Antiulcer drugs
Pharmacologic class: PPIs

AVAILABLE FORMS
Capsules (delayed-release) ⓓⓝⓒ: 10 mg, 20 mg, 40 mg
Powder (for delayed-release oral suspension): 2.5 mg/packet, 10 mg/packet
Suspension: 2 mg/mL
Tablets (delayed-release) ⓓⓝⓒ: 20 mg ◇
Tablets (delayed-release, ODT) ⓓⓝⓒ: 20 mg ◇

INDICATIONS & DOSAGES
➤ **Symptomatic GERD without esophageal lesions**
Adults: 20 mg PO, as delayed-release form or oral suspension, daily for 4 weeks for patients who respond poorly to customary medical treatment, usually including an adequate course of H_2-receptor antagonists.
Children ages 1 to 16 weighing 20 kg or more: 20 mg PO daily for up to 4 weeks.
Children ages 1 to 16 weighing 10 to less than 20 kg: 10 mg PO daily for up to 4 weeks.
Children ages 1 to 16 weighing 5 to less than 10 kg: 5 mg PO daily for up to 4 weeks.
➤ **Erosive esophagitis (EE) due to acid-mediated GERD** ⊠
Adults: 20 mg PO daily for 4 to 8 weeks. If no response after 8 weeks, may give for an additional 4 weeks. If EE or GERD symptoms recur, consider additional 4- to 8-week courses. For maintenance of healing EE, may treat for up to 12 months.
Adjust-a-dose: When drug is used for maintenance of healing EE, dosage reduction to 10 mg once daily is recommended for patients with Child-Pugh class A, B, or C liver impairment and patients of Asian descent.
Children ages 1 to 16 weighing 20 kg or more: 20 mg PO daily for 4 to 8 weeks; continue for up to 12 months for maintenance of healing.
Children ages 1 to 16 weighing 10 to less than 20 kg: 10 mg PO daily for 4 to 8 weeks; continue for up to 12 months for maintenance of healing.
Children ages 1 to 16 weighing 5 to less than 10 kg: 5 mg PO daily for 4 to 8 weeks; continue for up to 12 months for maintenance of healing.
Infants weighing 3 to less than 5 kg: 2.5 mg once daily for up to 6 weeks.
➤ **Pathologic hypersecretory conditions (such as Zollinger-Ellison syndrome)**
Adults: Initially, 60 mg PO daily; adjust dosage based on patient response. If daily dose exceeds 80 mg, give in divided doses. Dosages up to 120 mg t.i.d. have been given. Continue therapy as long as clinically indicated.
➤ **Duodenal ulcer (short-term treatment)**
Adults: 20 mg PO, as delayed-release form or oral suspension, daily for 4 weeks. Some patients may require an additional 4 weeks.

O

➤ *Helicobacter pylori* **infection and duodenal ulcer disease to eradicate** *H. pylori* **with clarithromycin (dual therapy)**

Adults: 40 mg PO every morning with clarithromycin 500 mg PO t.i.d. for 14 days. For patients with an ulcer at start of therapy, give another 14 days of omeprazole 20 mg PO once daily.

➤ *H. pylori* **infection and duodenal ulcer disease to eradicate** *H. pylori* **with clarithromycin and amoxicillin (triple therapy)**

Adults: 20 mg PO with clarithromycin 500 mg PO and amoxicillin 1,000 mg PO, each given b.i.d. for 10 days. For patients with an ulcer at start of therapy, give another 18 days of omeprazole 20 mg PO once daily.

➤ **Short-term treatment of active benign gastric ulcer**

Adults: 40 mg PO once daily for 4 to 8 weeks.

➤ **Frequent heartburn (2 or more days a week)**

Adults: 20 mg OTC PO once daily before breakfast for 14 days. May repeat 14-day course every 4 months.

➤ **Dyspepsia ◆**

Adults: 20 mg once daily for 4- to 8-week trial; may continue longer if signs and symptoms improve.

ADMINISTRATION
PO
• Give drug at least 30 to 60 minutes before meals (best before breakfast). If administering twice daily, give first dose before breakfast and second dose before evening meal.
• Have patient swallow tablets or capsules whole. For patients who have difficulty swallowing, capsules may be opened and contents mixed with 15 mL of applesauce. Follow with water to ensure complete swallowing of pellets.
• Place ODT on tongue; tablet disintegrates with or without water. Or, patient may swallow whole with water.
• For oral suspension, empty contents of 2.5-mg packet into container containing 5 mL water; empty contents of 10-mg packet into container containing 15 mL water. Stir and leave for 2 to 3 minutes to thicken. Stir and administer within 30 minutes. If material remains after drinking, add more water, stir, and give immediately.
• For patients with NG or gastric tube, add 5 mL water to catheter-tipped syringe; then add contents of 2.5-mg packet (or 15 mL water for 10-mg packet). Immediately shake syringe

and leave for 2 to 3 minutes to thicken. Shake syringe and inject through NG or gastric tube, #6 French or larger, into stomach within 30 minutes. Refill syringe with an equal amount of water. Shake and flush any remaining contents from NG or gastric tube into stomach.
• May give concomitantly with antacids.
• If dose is missed, give missed dose as soon as possible unless close to next scheduled dose. Don't give two doses to make up for missed dose.

ACTION
Inhibits proton pump activity by binding to hydrogen-potassium adenosine triphosphatase, located at the secretory surface of gastric parietal cells, to suppress gastric acid secretion.

Route	Onset	Peak	Duration
PO	1 hr	30 min–2 hr	<3 days

Half-life: 30 to 60 minutes.

ADVERSE REACTIONS
CNS: asthenia, dizziness, headache. **GI:** abdominal pain, constipation, diarrhea, flatulence, nausea, vomiting, acid regurgitation. **Musculoskeletal:** back pain, weakness. **Respiratory:** cough, URI. **Skin:** rash.

INTERACTIONS
Drug-drug. *Ampicillin esters, azole antifungals (such as ketoconazole), erlotinib, nilotinib:* May cause poor bioavailability of these drugs because they need a low gastric pH for optimal absorption. Avoid use together.
Antiretrovirals (atazanavir, nelfinavir): May decrease level of these drugs and therapeutic effect. Avoid use with atazanavir or nelfinavir. Refer to prescribing information for other antiretrovirals.
Benzodiazepines, fosphenytoin, phenytoin, warfarin: May increase levels of these drugs. Monitor drug levels or therapeutic effect.
Bisphosphonates: May decrease therapeutic effect of bisphosphonates. Monitor therapy.
Calcium salts: May decrease GI absorption of calcium salts. Closely monitor clinical response, and increase calcium dosage if needed.
Cilostazol: May increase cilostazol level. Reduce cilostazol dosage.
Citalopram: May increase risk of QT prolongation. Limit citalopram dosage to 20 mg/day.
Clopidogrel: May decrease antiplatelet activity. Avoid use together.

Reactions in bold italics are *life-threatening*.

Cyclosporine: May increase cyclosporine level. Closely monitor cyclosporine level.

Digoxin: May increase digoxin level, causing toxicity. Monitor digoxin level.

Drugs that induce CYP2C19 or CYP3A4 (rifampin): May substantially decrease omeprazole level. Avoid concomitant use.

Fluvoxamine: May increase omeprazole level. Monitor patient for increased adverse reactions.

Fosphenytoin, phenytoin: May increase levels of these drugs. Monitor therapy closely.

Iron salts: May interfere with iron absorption. Omeprazole may need to be temporarily stopped, or parenteral iron may be given as an alternative.

Methotrexate: May increase methotrexate level, causing toxicity. Monitor patient closely.

Mycophenolate: May decrease mycophenolate level and reduce formation of active metabolite for mycophenolate. Monitor therapy.

Saquinavir: May increase saquinavir level, resulting in increased toxicity. Monitor therapy.

Tacrolimus: May increase tacrolimus level. Monitor tacrolimus trough concentration when omeprazole is started and stopped.

Voriconazole: May increase levels of both drugs. Monitor therapy.

Warfarin: May increase INR and PT, leading to abnormal bleeding and death. Monitor INR and PT, and adjust warfarin dosage if needed.

Drug-herb. *St. John's wort:* May substantially decrease omeprazole level. Instruct patient to avoid use together.

Drug-food. *Vitamin B$_{12}$:* Prolonged treatment with omeprazole (3 years or longer) may lead to malabsorption of dietary vitamin B$_{12}$. Tell patient to avoid use together.

EFFECTS ON LAB TEST RESULTS
• May increase LFT values.
• May decrease magnesium, calcium, potassium, sodium, glucose, and vitamin B$_{12}$ levels.
• May falsely elevate serum chromogranin A (CgA) level.
• May cause false-positive urine screening tests for tetrahydrocannabinol.

CONTRAINDICATIONS & CAUTIONS
• Contraindicated in patients hypersensitive to drug or its components and in patients receiving rilpivirine-containing products.
• SCARs, including SJS, TEN, DRESS syndrome, and acute generalized exanthematous pustulosis, have been reported. If reaction

occurs, discontinue drug and refer patient to specialist for evaluation.
🟦 *Alert:* High-dose, long-term PPI therapy may be associated with an increased risk of hip, wrist, and spine fractures.
🧬 Bioavailability is increased in patients of Asian descent, and reduced dosages are recommended when used for healing EE.
• Use cautiously in patients with underlying hypocalcemia (hypoparathyroidism), hypokalemia, and respiratory alkalosis and in patients on a low-sodium diet.
• Risk of fundic gland polyps increases with long-term use, especially beyond 1 year.
• Use of PPIs may increase risk of CDAD. Consider CDAD diagnosis in patients with persistent diarrhea that doesn't improve.
• New onset or exacerbation of existing cutaneous and systemic lupus erythematosus may occur; discontinue therapy and refer patient to specialist for evaluation.

Dialyzable drug: Unlikely.

⚠ *Overdose S&S:* Confusion, drowsiness, blurred vision, tachycardia, nausea, vomiting, diaphoresis, flushing, headache, dry mouth.

PREGNANCY-LACTATION-REPRODUCTION
• Use during pregnancy only if potential benefit justifies fetal risk. When treating GERD during pregnancy, PPIs may be used after lifestyle modification, when needed.
• Drug appears in human milk. Use cautiously during breastfeeding.

NURSING CONSIDERATIONS
🟦 *Alert:* May increase risk of CDAD. Evaluate for CDAD in patient who develops diarrhea that doesn't improve.
🟦 *Alert:* Watch for new or worsening rash or worsening signs and symptoms of cutaneous or systemic lupus erythematosus. If suspected, discontinue drug and notify prescriber.
• False-positive results in diagnostic investigations for neuroendocrine tumors may occur due to increased CgA level. Temporarily stop omeprazole treatment at least 14 days before assessing CgA level and consider repeating test if initial CgA level is high. For serial tests, use same commercial lab for testing because reference ranges between tests may vary.
• Long-term therapy may cause vitamin B$_{12}$ absorption problems. Assess patient for signs and symptoms of cyanocobalamin

deficiency (weakness, heart palpitations, dyspnea, paresthesia, pale skin, smooth tongue, CNS changes, loss of appetite).

• Because risk of fundic gland polyps increases with long-term use, especially beyond 1 year, use drug for shortest duration appropriate for condition being treated.

• Periodically assess patient for osteoporosis.

• Monitor for signs and symptoms of acute interstitial nephritis. If suspected, discontinue drug and evaluate patient.

• Drug increases its own bioavailability with repeated doses. Drug is unstable in gastric acid; less drug is lost to hydrolysis because drug increases gastric pH.

• Gastrin level rises in most patients during first 2 weeks of therapy.

🔆 *Alert:* Prolonged use of PPIs may cause low magnesium level, which may lead to hypocalcemia or hypokalemia. Assess magnesium level before starting treatment and periodically thereafter.

🔆 *Alert:* Monitor for signs and symptoms of low magnesium level (abnormal HR or rhythm, palpitations, muscle spasms, tremors, seizures). In children, abnormal HR may present as fatigue, upset stomach, dizziness, and lightheadedness. Magnesium supplementation or drug discontinuation may be required.

• *Look alike–sound alike:* Don't confuse Prilosec OTC with Prevacid, prednisone, Pristiq, Prozac, or prilocaine. Don't confuse omeprazole with aripiprazole, esomeprazole, or fomepizole.

PATIENT TEACHING

• Teach about proper drug administration and handling.

• Advise patient to immediately report severe skin reactions with blistering, peeling, or bleeding on any part of the skin.

• Caution patient to avoid hazardous activities if dizziness occurs.

• Advise patient that Prilosec OTC isn't intended to treat infrequent heartburn (one episode of heartburn a week or less) or for those who want immediate heartburn relief.

• Explain that Prilosec OTC may take 1 to 4 days for full effect, although some patients get complete symptom relief within 24 hours.

• Teach patient to recognize and report signs and symptoms of low magnesium level after receiving drug for at least 3 months.

• Advise patient or caregiver to report diarrhea that doesn't improve.

• Instruct patient or caregiver to report fractures, especially of hip, wrist, or spine.

onabotulinumtoxinA
oh-nuh-BOT-yoo-lin-num-TOKS-in aye

Botox

onabotulinumtoxinA (cosmetic)
Botox Cosmetic

Therapeutic class: Neuromuscular transmission blockers
Pharmacologic class: Acetylcholine release inhibitors

AVAILABLE FORMS
onabotulinumtoxinA
Injection: 100 units/vial, 200 units/vial
onabotulinumtoxinA (cosmetic)
Injection: 50 units/vial, 100 units/vial

INDICATIONS & DOSAGES
Adjust-a-dose (for all indications): When adults are being treated for one or more indications, maximum cumulative dose generally shouldn't exceed 400 units in a 3-month interval.

➤ **Overactive bladder signs and symptoms (urge urinary incontinence, urgency, and frequency) in patients with inadequate response to or intolerant of anticholinergic medication (Botox)**
Adults: Recommended total dose is 100 units, given as 0.5 mL (5 units) IM across 20 sites into detrusor muscle. Give prophylactic antibiotics (except aminoglycosides) 1 to 3 days before treatment, on treatment day, and 1 to 3 days after treatment to reduce likelihood of procedure-related UTI. Discontinue antiplatelet therapy at least 3 days before administration. Consider retreatment no sooner than 12 weeks from prior injection.

➤ **Urinary incontinence due to detrusor overactivity associated with a neurologic condition, such as spinal cord injury or MS, after inadequate response to or intolerance of anticholinergic medication (Botox)**
Adults: Recommended total dose is 200 units, given as 30 injections of 1 mL (6.7 units) each (total volume of 30 mL) IM across 30 sites into detrusor muscle. For final injection, inject approximately 1 mL of sterile NSS to

ensure that remaining medication in needle is delivered to bladder. Give prophylactic antibiotics (except aminoglycosides) 1 to 3 days before treatment, on treatment day, and 1 to 3 days after treatment to reduce likelihood of procedure-related UTI. Consider retreatment no sooner than 12 weeks from prior injection. Discontinue antiplatelet therapy at least 3 days before administration.

➤ **Neurogenic detrusor overactivity in children with inadequate response to or intolerance of anticholinergics (Botox)**

Children ages 5 and older weighing 34 kg or more: 200 units given as 20 injections (each injection 0.5 mL, for total volume of 10 mL) into detrusor muscle, spaced approximately 1 cm apart. For final injection, inject approximately 1 mL of sterile NSS to ensure remaining medication in needle is delivered to bladder. Refer to manufacturer's instructions for dilution.

Children ages 5 and older weighing less than 34 kg: 6 units/kg given as 20 injections (each injection 0.5 mL, for total volume of 10 mL) into detrusor muscle, spaced approximately 1 cm apart. For final injection, inject approximately 1 mL of sterile NSS to ensure remaining medication in needle is delivered to bladder. Refer to manufacturer's instructions for dilution and dosages.

➤ **Prophylaxis of headaches in patients with chronic migraine (15 days per month or more, with headache lasting 4 hours a day or longer) (Botox)**

Adults: Recommended total dose is 155 units, given as 0.1 mL (5 units), IM divided across seven head/neck muscles every 12 weeks. Injections should be equally divided and administered bilaterally into 31 total sites. Refer to manufacturer's instructions for injection-site diagrams.

➤ **Upper limb spasticity (Botox)**

Adults: 5 to 50 units per site IM. Up to 200 units divided into four sites for biceps brachii. Use lowest recommended starting dose. Tailor dosing in initial and sequential treatment sessions to the individual based on size, number, and location of muscles involved; severity of spasticity; presence of local muscle weakness; and patient's response to previous treatment or adverse event history with onabotulinumtoxinA. Administer no more than 50 units per site. Refer to manufacturer's instructions for specific sites and dosages. Consider retreatment no sooner than 12 weeks from prior injection.

Children ages 2 and older: 3 to 6 units/kg IM divided among affected muscles to maximum of 6 units/kg or 200 units, whichever is lower. Use lowest recommended starting dose. Tailor initial dose and sequential treatments to individual based on size, number, and location of muscles involved; severity of spasticity; presence of local muscle weakness; and patient's response to previous treatment or adverse event history with onabotulinumtoxinA. Refer to manufacturer's instructions for specific sites and dosages.

➤ **Lower limb spasticity (Botox)**

Adults: 300 to 400 units IM divided among five muscles (gastrocnemius, soleus, tibialis posterior, flexor hallucis longus, and flexor digitorum longus). Use lowest recommended starting dose and administer no more than 25 units per site. Individualize dosing in initial and sequential treatment sessions based on size, number, and location of muscles involved; severity of spasticity; presence of local muscle weakness; and patient's response to previous treatment or adverse event history with onabotulinumtoxinA. Refer to manufacturer's instructions for specific sites and dosages. May repeat therapy no sooner than 12 weeks, with appropriate dosage based on clinical condition of patient at time of retreatment.

Children ages 2 and older: 4 to 8 units/kg IM divided among affected muscles to maximum of 8 units/kg or 300 units, whichever is lower. Tailor initial dose and sequential treatments to the individual based on size, number, and location of muscles involved; severity of spasticity; presence of local muscle weakness; and patient's response to previous treatment or adverse event history with onabotulinumtoxinA. Refer to manufacturer's instructions for specific sites and dosages.

➤ **Lower limb spasticity, excluding spasticity caused by cerebral palsy (Botox)**

Children ages 2 to 17: 4 to 8 units/kg body weight IM divided among four muscles (gastrocnemius medial head, gastrocnemius lateral head, soleus, and tibialis posterior). Use lowest recommended starting dose and give no more than 8 units/kg body weight or 300 units per treatment session, whichever is lower. Maximum dose in a 3-month period is 10 units/kg body weight or 340 units when treating both lower limbs or upper and lower limbs in combination.

Individualize dosing in initial and sequential treatment sessions based on size, number, and location of muscles involved; severity of spasticity; presence of local muscle weakness; and patient's response to previous treatment or adverse event history with onabotulinumtoxinA. Refer to manufacturer's instructions for specific sites and dosages. May repeat therapy no sooner than 12 weeks, with appropriate dosage based on patient's clinical condition at time of retreatment.

⚠️ *Alert:* When treating both lower limbs, or upper and lower limbs in combination, total pediatric dosage shouldn't exceed 10 units/kg or 340 units (whichever is lower) in a 3-month interval.

➤ **Cervical dystonia to reduce severity of abnormal head position and neck pain (Botox)**

Adults and children ages 16 and older: Adjust initial and subsequent dosing based on patient's head and neck position, localization of pain, muscle hypertrophy, patient response, and adverse event history. Use lower initial dose in patients who are botulinum toxin-naive. Administer no more than 50 units per site. See prescribing information for mean doses and ranges used in studies.

➤ **Severe axillary hyperhidrosis inadequately managed by topical agents (Botox)**

Adults: 50 units (2 mL) injected intradermally in 0.1- to 0.2-mL aliquots to each axilla, evenly distributed in 10 to 15 sites approximately 1 to 2 cm apart. May administer repeat injections when clinical effect of a previous injection diminishes.

➤ **Blepharospasm associated with dystonia (Botox)**

Adults and children ages 12 and older: 1.25 to 2.5 units (0.05 to 0.1 mL volume at each site) IM into medial and lateral pretarsal orbicularis oculi of upper lid and into lateral pretarsal orbicularis oculi of lower lid. Cumulative dose in 30-day period shouldn't exceed 200 units.

➤ **Strabismus (Botox)**

Adults and children ages 12 and older: Manufacturer recommends that several drops of local anesthetic and an ocular decongestant be given several minutes before injection.

For vertical muscles and for horizontal strabismus of less than 20 prism diopters: 1.25 to 2.5 units in any one muscle. For horizontal strabismus of 20 to 50 prism diopters: 2.5 to 5 units in any one muscle. Maximum

dose is 25 units for any one muscle. For re-examination and subsequent dosing, see prescribing information. For persistent cranial nerve VI palsy lasting 1 month or longer: 1.25 to 2.5 units IM in medial rectus muscle.

➤ **Temporary improvement in appearance of moderate to severe glabellar lines associated with corrugator or procerus muscle activity (Botox Cosmetic)**

Adults: Inject 4 units (0.1 mL) IM into each of five sites, two in each corrugator muscle and one in the procerus muscle, for total dose of 20 units. Administer no more frequently than every 3 to 4 months. An effective dose for facial lines is determined by gross observation of patient's ability to activate the superficial muscles injected.

➤ **Temporary improvement in appearance of moderate to severe lateral canthal lines associated with orbicularis oculi activity (Botox Cosmetic)**

Adults: Inject 4 units (0.1 mL) IM into each of three sites per side (six total injection points) in lateral orbicularis oculi muscle, for total of 24 units (0.6 mL) (12 units per side). Administer no more frequently than every 3 months. For simultaneous treatment with glabellar lines, dose is 24 units for lateral canthal lines and 20 units for glabellar lines, with total dose of 44 units.

➤ **Temporary improvement in appearance of moderate to severe forehead lines associated with frontalis muscle activity (Botox Cosmetic)**

Adults: 4 units (0.1 mL) IM into each of five forehead line sites (20 units) with 4 units (0.1 mL) IM into each of five glabellar line sites (20 units). Recommended total dose for forehead lines and glabellar lines together is 40 units. Administer no more frequently than every 3 months.

ADMINISTRATION
IM, intradermal

⚠️ *Alert:* Don't use Botox and contact Allergan (1-800-890-4345) if carton labeling doesn't contain an intact tamper-evident seal.

• Store unopened vials refrigerated at 36° to 46° F (2° to 8° C) for up to 36 months or until expiration date.

• Reconstitute each vial with sterile, non-preserved NSS for injection by drawing up proper amount of diluent in appropriate-sized syringe (see manufacturer's instructions) and slowly injecting diluent into vial.

Reactions in bold italics are *life-threatening*.

- Discard vial if a vacuum doesn't pull the diluent into the vial.
- Gently mix drug with the NSS by rotating vial.
- Administer within 24 hours after reconstitution; store in refrigerator until administration.

ACTION

Blocks neuromuscular transmission by inhibiting release of acetylcholine. IM doses chemically denervate muscle, reducing muscular activity either temporarily or permanently. Intradermal administration causes temporary chemical denervation of sweat glands, resulting in local reduction in sweating. Intradetrusor injection affects detrusor muscle activity via inhibition of acetylcholine release.

Route	Onset	Peak	Duration
IM, intradermal	Varies by site	Varies by site	Varies by site

Half-life: Unknown.

ADVERSE REACTIONS

Overactive bladder symptoms
GU: UTI, dysuria, urine retention, bacteriuria, residual urine volume, hematuria.
Other: injection-site soreness or *hemorrhage*.
Intradetrusor injection
GI: constipation. **GU:** UTI, dysuria, urine retention, hematuria, bacteriuria, urine retention. **Musculoskeletal:** weakness, muscle spasm, gait disturbance, falls. **Other:** injection-site soreness or *hemorrhage*.
Chronic migraine headache prophylaxis
CNS: headache, worsening migraine. **CV:** HTN. **EENT:** ptosis, facial paresis. **Musculoskeletal:** neck pain, weakness, stiffness, myalgia, muscle spasm. **Respiratory:** bronchitis. **Other:** injection-site pain.
Upper and lower limb spasticity
CNS: fatigue. **GI:** nausea. **Musculoskeletal:** extremity pain, weakness. **Respiratory:** bronchitis, URI. **Other:** injection-site soreness or *hemorrhage*.
Cervical dystonia
CNS: headache, dizziness, fever, speech disorder, numbness, asthenia, drowsiness. **EENT:** ptosis, diplopia, blepharoptosis, rhinitis, oral dryness. **GI:** nausea, dysphagia. **Musculoskeletal:** neck pain, back pain, stiffness, hypertonia. **Respiratory:** URI, increased cough, dyspnea. **Other:** flulike syndrome, injection-site soreness, antibody formation.

Severe axillary hyperhidrosis
CNS: headache, fever, anxiety, dizziness. **EENT:** pharyngitis. **GI:** nausea. **Musculoskeletal:** neck or back pain. **Skin:** nonaxillary sweating, pruritus. **Other:** flulike syndrome, injection-site pain or bleeding, infection.
Blepharospasm associated with dystonia
EENT: ptosis, superficial punctate keratitis, photophobia, eye dryness, irritation, tearing, lagophthalmos, ectropion, keratitis, diplopia, entropion, local swelling of eyelid skin. **Skin:** diffuse rash. **Other:** injection-site soreness or *hemorrhage*.
Strabismus
EENT: vertical deviation due to effect on adjacent extraocular muscles, ptosis. **Other:** injection-site soreness or *hemorrhage*.
Persistent cranial nerve VI palsy
Other: injection-site soreness or *hemorrhage*.
Glabellar lines
CNS: facial paresis. **EENT:** eyelid ptosis. **Musculoskeletal:** muscular weakness. **Other:** facial pain.
Lateral canthal lines
EENT: eyelid edema.
Forehead lines
CNS: headache. **EENT:** eyelid ptosis. **Skin:** brow ptosis, skin tightness.

INTERACTIONS

Drug-drug. *Aminoglycosides, neuromuscular blockers (curare or curare-like compounds):* May increase effect of toxin and risk of respiratory depression. Use together cautiously.
Anticholinergics (benztropine, dicyclomine): May increase systemic anticholinergic effects. Avoid use together.
Anticoagulants, antiplatelet drugs: May increase risk of bleeding. Discontinue antiplatelet therapy at least 3 days before injection procedure; carefully monitor patients on anticoagulant therapy.
Muscle relaxants, other botulinum neurotoxin products: May cause excessive neuromuscular weakness. Avoid use together.

EFFECTS ON LAB TEST RESULTS

- May increase urinary RBC, leukocyte, and bacteria counts.

CONTRAINDICATIONS & CAUTIONS

Boxed Warning The effects of onabotulinumtoxinA and all botulinum toxin products may spread from injection area to produce signs and symptoms consistent with botulinum toxin effects. These may include asthenia, generalized muscle weakness, diplopia, ptosis, dysphagia, dysphonia, dysarthria, urinary incontinence, and breathing difficulties, which have reportedly occurred hours to weeks after injection. Swallowing and breathing difficulties can be life-threatening; deaths have been reported. Risk of symptoms developing is probably greatest in children treated for spasticity, but symptoms can also occur in adults treated for spasticity and other conditions, particularly in those with an underlying condition that predisposes them to these symptoms. In unapproved uses and in approved indications, cases of spread of effect have been reported at doses comparable to those used to treat cervical dystonia and at lower doses. ∎

☉ Alert: If overdose occurs, antitoxin against botulinum toxin is available from the CDC but won't reverse botulinum toxin-induced effects already apparent by the time of antitoxin administration. In the event of suspected or actual cases of botulinum toxin poisoning, contact local or state health department to process a request for antitoxin through the CDC. If you don't receive a response within 30 minutes, contact the CDC directly at 1-770-488-7100.

• Contraindicated in patients with known hypersensitivity to botulinum toxin and those with infection at injection sites.

• Contraindicated in patients being treated for overactive bladder with UTI and in patients with overactive bladder or detrusor overactivity associated with a neurologic condition who have postvoid residual urine volume greater than 200 mL but don't routinely self-catheterize.

• Use cautiously in patients with bleeding disorders and in those receiving anticoagulation therapy.

• Use cautiously in patients with inflammation at proposed injection site or when excessive weakness or atrophy presents in the target muscle.

• Use cautiously in patients with preexisting neuromuscular disorders, compromised respiratory function, or corneal exposure and ulceration due to reduced blinking.

Dialyzable drug: Unknown.

⚠ Overdose S&S: Neuromuscular weakness, aspiration pneumonia, respiratory muscle paralysis, respiratory failure, death.

PREGNANCY-LACTATION-REPRODUCTION

• Studies during pregnancy are inadequate. Use only if benefits justify fetal risk.

• It isn't known if drug appears in human milk. Use cautiously during breastfeeding.

NURSING CONSIDERATIONS

☉ Alert: Signs and symptoms of overdose usually don't occur immediately after injection. If accidental injection or oral ingestion occurs or overdose is suspected, patient should be medically supervised for several weeks for signs and symptoms of systemic muscular weakness, which could be local or distant from the injection.

Boxed Warning Monitor patient for swallowing and breathing difficulties, which can lead to death. ∎

• Prescribers administering drug must understand the relevant neuromuscular or orbital anatomy and any alterations to that anatomy due to prior surgical procedures.

• Treatment of strabismus and upper limb spasticity requires an understanding of standard electromyographic techniques and may be useful when treating cervical dystonia.

• Botox and Botox Cosmetic contain the same active ingredient in the same formulation but aren't interchangeable.

• Drug isn't interchangeable with other preparations of botulinum toxin products and can't be converted into units of other botulinum toxin products.

• When giving bladder injections, give prophylactic antibiotics (except aminoglycosides) 1 to 3 days before treatment, on the day of treatment, and 1 to 3 days after treatment to reduce likelihood of procedure-related UTI. Or, for patient receiving general anesthesia or conscious sedation, give one dose of IV prophylactic antibiotics (except aminoglycosides) before injections on the day of treatment.

• Start treatment at lowest recommended dosage.

• Watch for bronchitis and URI in patients being treated for upper limb spasticity.

• Discontinue antiplatelet therapy at least 3 days before the injection procedure; patients on anticoagulant therapy need to be managed appropriately to decrease bleeding risk.

• Repeat treatment may be administered when effect of previous injection has diminished, but generally no sooner than 12 weeks after previous injection.

• Degree or pattern of muscle spasticity at time of reinjection may necessitate alterations in dosage and location.

• To prepare eye for injection, instill several drops of local anesthetic and an ocular decongestant several minutes before injection.

• Monitor patient for retrobulbar hemorrhages and compromised retinal circulation after eye injections.

PATIENT TEACHING

Boxed Warning Caution patient to seek immediate medical attention if serious side effects occur, such as difficulty swallowing, speaking, or breathing. These side effects can occur hours, days, or even weeks after injection and can be fatal. ■

• Teach patient to report signs and symptoms of botulism toxicity (loss of strength or muscle weakness, double or blurred vision, drooping eyelids, hoarseness, change in or loss of voice, trouble speaking clearly, loss of bladder control). Inform patient to not drive a car, operate machinery, or perform other dangerous activities if these effects occur.

• Warn that onabotulinumtoxinA injections may cause reduced blinking or reduced effectiveness of blinking. Instruct patient to seek immediate medical attention if eye pain or irritation occurs after treatment.

• Instruct patient to report voiding difficulties after bladder injections for urinary incontinence.

ondansetron
on-DAN-sah-tron

ondansetron hydrochloride

Therapeutic class: Antiemetics
Pharmacologic class: Selective serotonin (5-HT$_3$) receptor antagonists

AVAILABLE FORMS

Injection: 2 mg/mL
Oral solution: 4 mg/5 mL
Tablets: 4 mg, 8 mg, 24 mg
Tablets (ODTs): 4 mg, 8 mg

INDICATIONS & DOSAGES

Adjust-a-dose (for all indications): For patients with Child-Pugh class C liver impairment, total daily dose shouldn't exceed 8 mg.

➤ **To prevent nausea and vomiting from highly emetogenic chemotherapy**

Adults: 24 mg PO as a single dose 30 minutes before chemotherapy.

Adults and children ages 6 months to 18 years: 0.15 mg/kg IV over 15 minutes beginning 30 minutes before chemotherapy, second 0.15-mg/kg IV dose 4 hours later, then third 0.15-mg/kg IV dose 8 hours after first dose. Maximum, 16 mg/dose.

➤ **To prevent nausea and vomiting from moderately emetogenic chemotherapy**

Adults and children ages 12 and older: 8 mg PO 30 minutes before chemotherapy, 8 mg PO 8 hours after first dose, and then 8 mg PO every 12 hours for 1 to 2 days after completion of chemotherapy.

Adults and children ages 6 months and older: 0.15 mg/kg IV beginning 30 minutes before chemotherapy, second 0.15-mg/kg IV dose 4 hours later, then third 0.15-mg/kg IV dose 8 hours after first dose. Maximum single IV dose, 16 mg.

Children ages 4 to 11: 4 mg PO 30 minutes before chemotherapy, 4 mg PO 4 and 8 hours after first dose, and then 4 mg PO every 8 hours for 1 to 2 days after completion of chemotherapy.

➤ **To prevent postoperative nausea and vomiting**

Adults: 16 mg PO as a single dose 1 hour before induction of anesthesia.

Adults and children older than age 12: 4 mg undiluted solution for injection IM or IV.

Children ages 1 month to 12 years weighing more than 40 kg: 4 mg IV as a single dose over 2 to 5 minutes.

Children ages 1 month to 12 years weighing 40 kg or less: 0.1 mg/kg IV as a single dose over 2 to 5 minutes. Maximum dose, 4 mg.

Adjust-a-dose: IV and IM forms may be given immediately before induction of anesthesia or postoperatively if patient didn't receive prophylactic antiemetics and experiences nausea or vomiting within 2 hours after surgery.

➤ **To prevent nausea and vomiting from radiation therapy in patients receiving total body irradiation, single high-dose fraction radiation therapy to abdomen, or daily fractionated radiation therapy to abdomen**

Adults: For patients receiving total body irradiation, 8 mg PO 1 to 2 hours before each fraction of radiation therapy each day. For patients receiving single high-dose fraction radiation therapy to the abdomen, 8 mg PO 1 to 2 hours before therapy, then every 8 hours for 1 to 2 days after completion of therapy.

O

For patients receiving daily fractionated radiation therapy, 8 mg PO 1 to 2 hours before therapy, then every 8 hours for each day therapy is given.

ADMINISTRATION

PO
- Open blister of ODT just before use by peeling off backing. Don't push ODT through foil blister.
- Place ODT on top of tongue to dissolve; then instruct patient to swallow with saliva (additional liquid isn't needed).
- Protect 4-mg tablets and oral solution from light.
- Store at room temperature.

IV
⊘ Alert: No single IV dose should exceed 16 mg due to risk of QT-interval prolongation.
- ▼ If precipitate is noted in vial, shake vigorously until dissolved.
- ▼ Dilute drug in 50 mL of D_5W injection or NSS for injection.
- ▼ Don't use diluted solution beyond 24 hours; diluents typically don't contain preservatives.
- ▼ Infuse over 15 minutes.
- ▼ Store vials at room temperature or refrigerate at 36° to 46° F (2° to 8° C).
- ▼ Protect vials from light.
- ▼ **Incompatibilities:** Alkaline solutions.

IM
- Document injection site.
- If precipitate is noted in vial, shake vigorously until dissolved.
- Give IM injection undiluted.

ACTION

May block 5-HT₃ in the CNS in the chemoreceptor trigger zone and in the peripheral nervous system on nerve terminals of the vagus nerve.

Route	Onset	Peak	Duration
PO	30 min	1–2 hr	Unknown
IV	Immediate	Unknown	Unknown
IM	Unknown	Unknown	Unknown

Half-life: About 3 to 6 hours.

ADVERSE REACTIONS

CNS: cold sensation, dizziness, fatigue, headache, malaise, sedation, fever, agitation, anxiety, pain, paresthesia. **CV:** chest pain. **GI:** constipation, diarrhea. **GU:** gynecologic disorders, urine retention. **Hepatic:** increased transaminase levels. **Respiratory:** *hypoxia.*

Skin: pruritus, rash, injection-site reaction.
Other: chills.

INTERACTIONS

Drug-drug. ⊘ Alert: *Apomorphine:* May cause profound hypotension and loss of consciousness. Use together is contraindicated.
Drugs (such as cimetidine) that alter liver drug-metabolizing enzymes, phenobarbital, rifampin: May change pharmacokinetics of ondansetron, but clinical data suggest no need to adjust dosage.
Drugs that prolong QTc interval (antiarrhythmics, antipsychotics, antidepressants): May result in ventricular arrhythmias. Use cautiously and avoid combination with drugs at highest risk for QTc-interval prolongation.
SNRIs, SSRIs: May result in serotonin syndrome. Use cautiously and monitor patient.
Tramadol: May decrease tramadol effects. Monitor patient to ensure effective pain control.
Drug-herb. *Horehound:* May enhance serotonergic effects. Discourage use together.
St. John's wort: May decrease ondansetron level. Discourage use together.

EFFECTS ON LAB TEST RESULTS
- May increase ALT and AST levels.

CONTRAINDICATIONS & CAUTIONS
- Use is contraindicated in patients hypersensitive to drug.
- ECG changes, including prolonged QT interval and torsades de pointes, have been reported. Avoid use in patients with congenital long QT syndrome.
- Use cautiously in patients with liver impairment.

Dialyzable drug: Unlikely.

⚠ Overdose S&S: Sudden transient blindness, severe constipation, hypotension, faintness, heart block, serotonin syndrome in young children (somnolence, agitation, tachycardia, tachypnea, HTN, flushing, mydriasis, diaphoresis, myoclonic movements, horizontal nystagmus, hyperreflexia, seizure).

PREGNANCY-LACTATION-REPRODUCTION
- Studies during pregnancy are inadequate. Drug crosses placental barrier during first trimester. Use only if clearly needed.
- It isn't known if drug appears in human milk. Use cautiously during breastfeeding.

Reactions in bold italics are *life-threatening.*

NURSING CONSIDERATIONS

🜂 *Alert:* Drug may increase risk of prolonged QT interval and torsades de pointes. Monitor ECG in patients with congenital long QT syndrome, in those with HF or bradyarrhythmias, and in those taking other medications that prolong QT interval.

🜂 *Alert:* Correct electrolyte abnormalities (hypokalemia, hypomagnesemia) before infusing drug.

• Monitor for decreased bowel activity, especially if patient is at risk for GI obstruction. Drug may mask progressive ileus or gastric distention.

🜂 *Alert:* Monitor for signs and symptoms of myocardial ischemia during and immediately after IV administration. Don't exceed recommended infusion rate.

• Monitor LFT results.

• Monitor for signs and symptoms of serotonin syndrome (restlessness, seizures, hallucinations, loss of coordination, fast heartbeat, rapid BP changes, increased body temperature, hyperreflexia, nausea, vomiting, diarrhea, diaphoresis, flushing, nausea, vomiting, tremors, muscle rigidity).

• Monitor for hypersensitivity reactions, including bronchospasm and anaphylaxis.

• May give drug in combination with a neurokinin-1 receptor antagonist, dexamethasone, and olanzapine, according to chemotherapy antiemetic treatment guidelines.

• *Look alike–sound alike:* Don't confuse ondansetron with dolasetron, granisetron, or palonosetron.

PATIENT TEACHING

• Teach about proper drug administration and handling.

🜂 *Alert:* Caution patient to immediately report a syncopal episode (fainting, loss of consciousness) or signs and symptoms of abnormal HR or rhythm (palpitations, dyspnea, dizziness, light-headedness).

• Tell patient that an ECG may be necessary to monitor HR and rhythm.

• Instruct patient to immediately report difficulty breathing after drug administration.

• Tell patient receiving drug IV to report discomfort at insertion site.

• Inform patient that drug may mask signs and symptoms of bowel obstruction. Instruct patient to report decreased bowel activity.

opicapone
oh-PIK-a-pone

Ongentys

Therapeutic class: Antiparkinsonians
Pharmacologic class: Catechol-O-methyltransferase inhibitors

AVAILABLE FORMS
Capsules: 25 mg, 50 mg

INDICATIONS & DOSAGES
➤ **Adjunctive treatment to levodopa–carbidopa in patients with Parkinson disease experiencing "off" episodes**
Adults: 50 mg PO daily at bedtime.
Adjust-a-dose: For patients with Child-Pugh class B liver impairment, reduce dose to 25 mg PO at bedtime. Avoid use in patients with Child-Pugh class C liver impairment.

ADMINISTRATION
PO
• Give 1 hour before and at least 1 hour after food.
• If dose is missed, resume scheduled dosing the next day; don't double dose.
• Store capsules below 86° F (30° C).

ACTION
Inhibits catechol-O-methyltransferase (COMT), a metabolizing enzyme of levodopa, resulting in higher levels of levodopa.

Route	Onset	Peak	Duration
PO	Unknown	1–4 hr	5+ days

Half-life: 1 to 2 hours.

ADVERSE REACTIONS
CNS: dyskinesia, dizziness, hallucinations, insomnia, impulse control disorder, syncope.
CV: hypotension, HTN. **EENT:** dry mouth.
GI: constipation. **Metabolic:** increased CK level, weight loss.

INTERACTIONS
Drug-drug. *Drugs metabolized by COMT (dobutamine, dopamine, epinephrine, isoproterenol, norepinephrine):* May increase risk of arrhythmias, increase HR, and cause excessive changes in BP. Use together cautiously.
Levodopa: Potentiates effects of levodopa, causing dyskinesia or exacerbating preexisting

dyskinesia. Reduce dosage of levodopa or other dopaminergic drugs as indicated.

⚡ *Alert:* *Nonselective MAO inhibitors (isocarboxazid, phenelzine, tranylcypromine):* May increase risk of arrhythmias, increase HR, or cause excessive changes in BP due to increased levels of catecholamines. Use together is contraindicated.

EFFECTS ON LAB TEST RESULTS
• May increase CK level.

CONTRAINDICATIONS & CAUTIONS
• Contraindicated in patients with history of pheochromocytoma, paraganglioma, or other catecholamine-secreting neoplasms.
• Avoid use in patients with Child-Pugh class C liver impairment.
• Avoid use in patients with major psychotic disorders because of risk of psychosis exacerbation.
• Use cautiously in patients with suspected or diagnosed dopamine dysregulation syndrome. Consider stopping drug, as indicated.
• Safety and effectiveness in children haven't been established.

Dialyzable drug: Unlikely.

PREGNANCY-LACTATION-REPRODUCTION
• Studies during pregnancy are inadequate. Use only if benefits outweigh fetal risk.
• It isn't known if drug appears in human milk or how drug affects milk production or infants who are breastfed. Weigh benefits to patient against possible risk to infant.

NURSING CONSIDERATIONS
⚡ *Alert:* Monitor patient treated with opicapone and drugs metabolized by COMT for arrhythmias, increased HR, and excessive changes in BP regardless of route of administration, including inhalation, of concomitant drug.

⚡ *Alert:* Before starting drug, assess patient for factors that increase risk of somnolence with dopaminergic therapy (concomitant sedating medications, sleep disorders).
• Monitor patient for daytime somnolence during activities that require full attention (driving, conversation, eating). If daytime somnolence occurs, consider discontinuing drug or adjusting dosage of other dopaminergic or sedating drugs.
• Monitor for development of impulse control or compulsive disorders (intense urge

to gamble or spend money, increased sexual urge, binge eating, inability to control these urges). Reevaluate current therapy for Parkinson disease and consider stopping drug if these signs or symptoms develop.
• Monitor patient for hypotension (orthostatic and nonorthostatic); if it occurs, discontinue drug or adjust dosage of other drugs that lower BP.
• Observe patient for development of dyskinesia or exacerbation of preexisting dyskinesia. Consider reducing daily levodopa dose or other dopaminergic drug if dyskinesia occurs.
• Monitor patient for hallucinations (auditory, visual, mixed); delusions; agitation; or aggressive behavior. Consider stopping drug if hallucinations or psychotic-like behaviors develop.
• When discontinuing drug, monitor patient for a symptom complex resembling NMS (elevated temperature, muscular rigidity, altered consciousness, autonomic instability). Adjust other dopaminergic agents as needed.
• *Look alike–sound alike:* Don't confuse opicapone with entacapone or tolcapone. Don't confuse Ongentys with Onglyza.

PATIENT TEACHING
⚡ *Alert:* Warn patient and caregiver about daytime somnolence. Caution patient not to operate hazardous machinery, including motor vehicles, if daytime somnolence occurs while taking drug.
• Counsel patient to report dizziness, lightheadedness, or fainting.
• Teach about proper drug administration and handling.
• Warn that drug may cause dyskinesia (sudden, uncontrolled movements) or exacerbate preexisting dyskinesia. Contact prescriber if dyskinesia occurs.
• Advise patient to report hallucinations, delusions, or aggressive behavior.
• Counsel patient to report intense uncontrollable urges to gamble, spend money, or binge eat or if increased sexual or other intense urges occur.
• Advise patient to consult prescriber before stopping drug and to inform prescriber if fever, confusion, or severe muscle stiffness develops after stopping drug.

oritavancin diphosphate
or-it-a-VAN-sin

Kimyrsa, Orbactiv

Therapeutic class: Antibiotics
Pharmacologic class: Lipoglycopeptides

AVAILABLE FORMS
Powder for injection: 400-mg, 1,200-mg vial

INDICATIONS & DOSAGES
➤ **Acute bacterial skin and skin-structure infections caused or suspected to be caused by susceptible gram-positive bacteria, including** *Staphylococcus aureus* **(methicillin-sensitive and methicillin-resistant);** *Streptococcus* **species, including** *S. pyogenes, S. agalactiae, S. dysgalactiae, S. anginosus, S. intermedius,* **and** *S. constellatus***; and vancomycin-susceptible** *Enterococcus faecalis*
Adults: 1,200 mg IV as a single dose.

ADMINISTRATION
IV
▼ Obtain specimen for culture and sensitivity testing before giving drug.
▼ The two oritavancin products differ in dose strength, duration of infusion, and preparation instructions.
▼ Prepare three 400-mg Orbactiv vials for a single 1,200-mg IV dose.
▼ Reconstitute each 400 mg Orbactiv vial with 40 mL of sterile water for injection to provide a solution containing 10 mg/mL/vial. Reconstitute each 1,200-mg Kimyrsa vial with 40 mL sterile water for injection to provide a solution containing 30 mg/mL/vial.
▼ Gently swirl vial to avoid foaming and ensure that all powder is completely reconstituted in solution. Inspect for particulate matter. Solution should be clear and colorless to pale yellow (Orbactiv) or pink (Kimyrsa).
▼ For infusion, further dilute Orbactiv in 1,000 mL D₅W; withdraw and discard 120 mL from 1,000-mL D₅W bag and add 120 mL Orbactiv reconstituted solution. Or, further dilute Kimyrsa in 250 mL NSS or D₅W; withdraw and discard 40 mL from a 250-mL IV bag and add 40 mL Kimyrsa reconstituted solution.

▼ Infuse Orbactiv over 3 hours or infuse Kimyrsa over 1 hour. If IV line is also used to infuse other drugs, flush it with D₅W before and after each infusion.
▼ Refrigerate solution after reconstitution and use within 12 hours, 6 hours (Orbactiv), or 4 hours (Kimyrsa), including infusion time, when stored at room temperature.
▼ **Incompatibilities:** NSS (Orbactiv), basic or neutral pH drugs.

ACTION
Disrupts bacterial cell-wall synthesis and bacterial membrane integrity.

Route	Onset	Peak	Duration
IV	Unknown	Unknown	Unknown

Half-life: 245 hours.

ADVERSE REACTIONS
CNS: headache, dizziness, fever. **CV:** tachycardia, peripheral edema, injection-site phlebitis, *leukocytoclastic vasculitis.* **GI:** nausea, vomiting, diarrhea. **Hematologic:** anemia, eosinophilia. **Hepatic:** elevated ALT, AST, and bilirubin levels. **Metabolic:** *hypoglycemia,* hyperuricemia. **Musculoskeletal:** tenosynovitis, osteomyelitis, myalgia. **Respiratory:** *bronchospasm,* wheezing. **Skin:** infusion-site erythema, extravasation, induration, pruritus, limb and subcutaneous abscesses, rash, urticaria, *erythema multiforme,* cellulitis. **Other:** chills, infusion reaction, hypersensitivity, *angioedema.*

INTERACTIONS
Drug-drug. *Dextromethorphan, midazolam:* May decrease levels of these drugs. Monitor patient for effectiveness.
Omeprazole: May increase omeprazole level. Monitor patient for omeprazole toxicity.
Unfractionated heparin sodium (IV): May falsely elevate PTT test results for up to 120 hours (5 days). Heparin use is contraindicated for 120 hours after oritavancin administration.
Warfarin: May prolong PT and increase INR and risk of bleeding. Monitor PT and INR, and monitor patient for bleeding.

EFFECTS ON LAB TEST RESULTS
• May increase AST, ALT, uric acid, and total bilirubin levels.
• May decrease glucose level.
• May artificially prolong PTT for up to 120 hours, prolong PT and increase INR for

up to 12 hours, and prolong activated clotting time for up to 24 hours after dose is given.
• May elevate D-dimer for up to 72 hours after dose is given.
• May cause positive indirect and direct antiglobulin tests. Positive indirect test may interfere with cross-matching for blood transfusions.

CONTRAINDICATIONS & CAUTIONS
• Contraindicated in patients hypersensitive to drug or its components.
• Drug falsely elevates PTT. Use of unfractionated heparin IV is contraindicated for 120 hours after oritavancin administration.
• Use cautiously in patients with history of hypersensitivity to glycopeptides (vancomycin, telavancin, dalbavancin); serious hypersensitivity reactions have been reported. If acute reaction occurs, discontinue drug and treat immediately.
• Drug can cause superinfection, including CDAD and pseudomembranous colitis, which can occur more than 2 months after therapy ends.
• Drug may increase risk of osteomyelitis; alternative antibacterial therapy may be needed.
• Drug hasn't been studied in patients with CrCl less than 30 mL/minute or Child-Pugh class C liver impairment.
• Safety and effectiveness in children haven't been established.
Dialyzable drug: No.

PREGNANCY-LACTATION-REPRODUCTION
• Studies during pregnancy are inadequate. Use only if potential benefits justify fetal risk.
• It isn't known if drug appears in human milk. Use cautiously during breastfeeding.

NURSING CONSIDERATIONS
• Monitor patient for signs and symptoms of CDAD (frequent, watery stools) and osteomyelitis (fever, erythema, edema, pain) during and for several months after treatment.
• Monitor for infusion-related reactions (pruritus, rash, urticaria, flushing, chest pain, back pain, chills, tremor). Slow rate or interrupt infusion if a reaction develops.
• Monitor for bleeding in patient who is also receiving warfarin.
• If patient needs anticoagulation, consider using anticoagulants that don't require PTT or INR monitoring.

• *Look alike–sound alike:* Don't confuse oritavancin with telavancin or dalbavancin. Don't confuse Orbactiv with Activase or Vibativ.

PATIENT TEACHING
• Explain that antibiotics can change normal intestinal flora and that patient should report severe watery or bloody diarrhea, which may indicate a serious intestinal infection.
• Counsel patient on appropriate antibiotic use.
• Instruct patient to report discomfort at IV insertion site.
• Warn patient that allergic reactions, including serious allergic reactions, can occur and require immediate treatment.

oseltamivir phosphate
oh-sel-TAM-i-ver

Tamiflu

Therapeutic class: Antivirals
Pharmacologic class: Selective neuraminidase inhibitors

AVAILABLE FORMS
Capsules: 30 mg, 45 mg, 75 mg
Oral suspension: 6 mg/mL after reconstitution

INDICATIONS & DOSAGES
Adjust-a-dose (for all indications): Refer to manufacturer's prescribing information for dosage adjustments for adults with kidney impairment.
➤ **To prevent influenza A and B within 48 hours of exposure**
Adults and adolescents ages 13 and older: 75 mg PO (capsule or 12.5 mL suspension) once daily for at least 10 days or up to 6 weeks during a community outbreak.
Children ages 1 to 12 weighing 40.1 kg or more: 75 mg (12.5 mL suspension) PO once daily for 10 days or up to 6 weeks during a community outbreak.
Children ages 1 to 12 weighing 23.1 to 40 kg: 60 mg (10 mL suspension) PO once daily for 10 days or up to 6 weeks during a community outbreak.
Children ages 1 to 12 weighing 15.1 to 23 kg: 45 mg (7.5 mL suspension) PO once daily for 10 days or up to 6 weeks during a community outbreak.
Children ages 1 to 12 weighing 15 kg or less: 30 mg (5 mL suspension) PO once daily for

10 days or up to 6 weeks during a community outbreak.

Adjust-a-dose: In patients who are immuno-compromised, may continue drug for up to 12 weeks. CDC recommendations for length of treatment may vary.

▶ **To treat influenza in patients who have been symptomatic for no more than 48 hours**

Adults and adolescents ages 13 and older: 75 mg PO b.i.d. (capsule or 12.5 mL suspension) for 5 days.

Children ages 1 to 12 weighing 40.1 kg or more: 75 mg (12.5 mL suspension) PO b.i.d. for 5 days.

Children ages 1 to 12 weighing 23.1 to 40 kg: 60 mg (10 mL) PO b.i.d. for 5 days.

Children ages 1 to 12 weighing 15.1 to 23 kg: 45 mg (7.5 mL) PO b.i.d. for 5 days.

Children ages 1 to 12 weighing 15 kg or less: 30 mg (5 mL) PO b.i.d. for 5 days.

Children ages 2 weeks to younger than 1 year: 3 mg/kg PO b.i.d. for 5 days. Begin treatment within 2 days of influenza onset.

ADMINISTRATION
PO

• May give without regard to food. Give with food to lessen GI adverse effects, if present.

• Store at room temperature (59° to 86° F [15° to 30° C]).

• May open capsules and mix contents with sweetened liquids, such as regular or sugar-free chocolate syrup, corn syrup, caramel topping, or light brown sugar (dissolved in water).

• Oral suspension is preferred for patients who can't swallow capsules.

• Shake oral suspension well before use and give with calibrated oral syringe or dosing cup.

• May give via NG or orogastric tube. Dissolve powder from capsule in 20 mL sterile water and inject in tube; follow with 10-mL sterile water flush.

• Once reconstituted, store oral suspension in refrigerator at 36° to 46° F (2° to 8° C) or at room temperature. Use within 10 days of preparation if stored at room temperature or within 17 days of preparation if stored under refrigeration.

• If dose is missed, give missed dose as soon as possible. If next dose is due within 2 hours, skip missed dose and give next dose on schedule.

ACTION
Inhibits influenza A and B virus enzyme neuraminidase, which is thought to play a role in viral particle aggregation and release from the host cell and appears to interfere with viral replication.

Route	Onset	Peak	Duration
PO	Unknown	Unknown	Unknown

Half-life: 1 to 10 hours.

ADVERSE REACTIONS
CNS: headache, pain. **GI:** nausea, vomiting, diarrhea (infants). **Skin:** diaper rash (infants).

INTERACTIONS
Drug-drug. *Live attenuated influenza virus vaccine:* May decrease effect of live attenuated influenza virus vaccine. Avoid giving vaccination within 2 weeks before or 48 hours after oseltamivir.

EFFECTS ON LAB TEST RESULTS
None reported.

CONTRAINDICATIONS & CAUTIONS
• Contraindicated in patients hypersensitive to drug or its components.

▨ Oral suspension contains 2 g of sorbitol, which is above the maximum limit for patients with hereditary fructose intolerance and may cause dyspepsia and diarrhea.

• Use cautiously in patients with KF, chronic cardiac or respiratory diseases, or any medical condition that may require imminent hospitalization.

• Safety and effectiveness of repeated treatment courses haven't been established.

Dialyzable drug: Yes.

⚠ *Overdose S&S:* Nausea, vomiting.

PREGNANCY-LACTATION-REPRODUCTION
• Drug is recommended to treat or prevent influenza during pregnancy. Don't use as a substitute for vaccination during pregnancy.

• Drug appears in human milk in small amounts. According to CDC, patient may continue oseltamivir while breastfeeding.

NURSING CONSIDERATIONS
• Drug must be given within 2 days of onset of symptoms.

• Initiate postexposure prophylaxis within 48 hours after close contact with an infected individual. Initiate seasonal prophylaxis during a community outbreak.

🜂 *Alert:* Closely monitor patients with influenza for neuropsychiatric symptoms (hallucinations, delirium, abnormal behavior). Evaluate risks and benefits of continuing drug.

• Monitor patient for secondary bacterial infections. Drug is only effective against influenza viruses.

• Monitor for hypersensitivity reactions, including anaphylaxis and SCARs. Discontinue drug if reactions occur.

• Monitor for confusion or abnormal behavior early in illness. Drug may increase risk of neuropsychiatric events.

• *Look alike–sound alike:* Don't confuse Tamiflu with Thera-Flu.

PATIENT TEACHING

• Instruct patient to begin treatment as soon as possible after appearance of flu symptoms.

• Teach about proper drug administration and handling.

• Advise patient to complete full course of treatment, even if symptoms resolve.

• Alert patient that drug isn't a replacement for annual influenza vaccination. Patients for whom vaccine is indicated should continue to receive the vaccine each fall.

• Teach about risk of neuropsychiatric events. Instruct patient or caregivers to report confusion or abnormal behavior.

• Warn of risk of severe allergic reactions. Instruct patient or caregivers to stop drug and seek immediate medical attention if a reaction occurs or is suspected.

🜲 Inform patient with hereditary fructose intolerance that oral suspension contains sorbitol in an amount above the daily maximum limit of sorbitol and may cause dyspepsia and diarrhea.

osilodrostat
oh-sil-oh-DROE-stat

Isturisa

Therapeutic class: Endocrine-metabolic agents
Pharmacologic class: Cortisol synthesis inhibitors

AVAILABLE FORMS
Tablets: 1 mg, 5 mg, 10 mg

INDICATIONS & DOSAGES

➤ **Cushing disease in patients for whom pituitary surgery isn't an option or hasn't been curative**

Adults: Initially, 2 mg PO b.i.d. Increase by 1 to 2 mg PO b.i.d. every 2 weeks based on cortisol change, tolerability, and clinical response. If treatment is interrupted, restart drug at lower dose. Refer to manufacturer's instructions for dosage titration and modification. Usual maintenance dose is 2 to 7 mg PO b.i.d. Maximum dosage, 30 mg PO b.i.d.

Adjust-a-dose: For patients with moderate Child-Pugh class B liver impairment, start at 1 mg PO b.i.d. For patients with Child-Pugh class C liver impairment, start at 1 mg PO once daily in the evening.

ADMINISTRATION
PO
• Give drug without regard to meals.
• If dose is missed, give at next scheduled time.
• Store tablets at 68° to 77° F (20° to 25° C).

ACTION
Inhibits the enzyme responsible for cortisol biosynthesis in the adrenal gland.

Route	Onset	Peak	Duration
PO	Unknown	1 hr	Unknown

Half-life: 4 hours.

ADVERSE REACTIONS
CNS: fatigue, headache, dizziness, fever, insomnia, anxiety, depression, malaise, syncope. **CV:** *prolonged QT interval,* edema, hypotension, HTN, tachycardia. **EENT:** nasopharyngitis. **GI:** nausea, vomiting, diarrhea, abdominal pain, decreased appetite, dyspepsia, gastroenteritis. **GU:** UTI. **Hematologic:** anemia, decreased ANC. **Hepatic:** elevated transaminase levels. **Metabolic:** hypocortisolism, *adrenal insufficiency, hypokalemia,* altered pituitary corticotroph tumor volume, increased testosterone level. **Musculoskeletal:** arthralgia, back pain, myalgia. **Respiratory:** cough. **Skin:** rash, hirsutism, acne, alopecia. **Other:** flulike symptoms.

INTERACTIONS
Drug-drug. *CYP1A2, CYP2C19 substrates with narrow therapeutic index (theophylline, tizanidine):* May increase substrate levels. Use together cautiously.

Drugs that prolong QT interval (antiarrhythmics, antipsychotics, macrolides, fluoroquinolones): May further prolong QT interval, increasing risk of cardiac arrhythmia. Avoid use together.

Strong CYP2B6, CYP3A4 inducers (carbamazepine, phenobarbital, rifampin): May decrease osilodrostat level and reduce its efficacy. Osilodrostat dosage increase may be necessary. When inducers are discontinued, reduce osilodrostat dosage as needed.

Strong CYP3A4 inhibitors (clarithromycin, itraconazole): May increase osilodrostat level and adverse reactions. Reduce osilodrostat dosage by 50%.

EFFECTS ON LAB TEST RESULTS
- May increase AST, ALT, androgen, cortisol and aldosterone precursors (11-deoxycortisol, 11-deoxycorticosterone), corticotropin, and testosterone levels.
- May decrease potassium and cortisol levels.
- May decrease ANC and RBC count.

CONTRAINDICATIONS & CAUTIONS
- Drug may increase risk of hypocortisolism, leading to life-threatening adrenal insufficiency.
- Drug may cause dose-dependent prolonged QT interval and cardiac arrhythmias. Use cautiously in patients with risk factors (congenital long QT syndrome, HF, bradyarrhythmia, uncorrected electrolyte abnormalities, concomitant use of drugs that prolong QT interval).
- Use caution when interpreting urine free cortisol levels in patients with CrCL less than 60 mL/minute due to reduced urine free cortisol excretion.
- Safety and effectiveness in children haven't been established.

Dialyzable drug: Unknown.

⚠ *Overdose S&S:* Hypocortisolism (nausea, vomiting, fatigue, hypotension, abdominal pain, loss of appetite, dizziness, syncope).

PREGNANCY-LACTATION-REPRODUCTION
- Information is insufficient to recommend use during pregnancy. Active Cushing syndrome during pregnancy is associated with increased maternal and fetal morbidity and mortality.
- It isn't known if drug appears in human milk. Patient shouldn't breastfeed during therapy and for 1 week after final dose.

NURSING CONSIDERATIONS
- Obtain baseline QTc interval before initiating therapy and repeat within 1 week. Thereafter, periodically monitor ECG; consider more frequent monitoring in patients at risk for prolonged QTc interval. Consider temporary discontinuation of drug if QTc interval is greater than 480 msec.
- Obtain baseline potassium and magnesium levels, and correct abnormalities before initiating drug, if necessary. Periodically monitor levels thereafter.
- Give oral or IV potassium supplement to patient with hypokalemia. If hypokalemia persists, osilodrostat reduction or discontinuation or administration of mineralocorticoid antagonists may be necessary.
- Monitor patient for worsening HTN, edema, and signs and symptoms of hypocortisolism (nausea, vomiting, fatigue, abdominal pain, loss of appetite). Also evaluate for precipitating causes of hypocortisolism (infection, physical stress).
- Monitor cortisol levels every 1 to 2 months once maintenance dose is achieved. Patients with liver impairment may require more frequent monitoring during dosage titration.
- Decrease dosage or temporarily discontinue drug if urine free cortisol level decreases below target range, cortisol level rapidly decreases, or patient reports signs and symptoms of hypocortisolism.
- Stop drug and administer glucocorticoid replacement therapy if serum or plasma cortisol levels are below target range and patient has signs and symptoms of adrenal insufficiency (hypotension, hypoglycemia, abnormal electrolyte levels).
- When urine cortisol and serum or plasma cortisol levels are within target range and signs and symptoms resolve, reinitiate drug at lower dose.
- Monitor female patient for development of signs and symptoms of hyperandrogenism (hirsutism, hypertrichosis, acne).
- *Look alike–sound alike:* Don't confuse osilodrostat with orlistat.

PATIENT TEACHING
- Teach patient signs and symptoms of hypocortisolism, and advise patient to contact prescriber if any occur.
- Advise female patient to report signs and symptoms of hyperandrogenism.

• Review the importance of lab monitoring and adherence to prescriber visits.
• Tell patient that ECG monitoring is needed before starting drug and periodically thereafter. Advise patient to immediately report signs and symptoms of QT-interval prolongation (irregular heartbeat).
• Educate patient on importance of contacting prescriber if worsening edema or HTN occurs.
• Advise patient to report pregnancy or plans to become pregnant during therapy.
• Caution patient not to breastfeed during therapy and for 1 week after final dose.
• Tell patient to report all drug changes to prescriber.

SAFETY ALERT!

osimertinib mesylate
oh-sim-ER-ti-nib

Tagrisso

Therapeutic class: Antineoplastics
Pharmacologic class: Tyrosine kinase inhibitors

AVAILABLE FORMS
Tablets ⒹⓇⒸ: 40 mg, 80 mg

INDICATIONS & DOSAGES
Adjust-a-dose (for all indications): Refer to manufacturer's instructions for toxicity-related dosage adjustments. If drug must be given with a strong CYP3A4 inducer, increase osimertinib dosage to 160 mg daily. Resume osimertinib at 80 mg daily 3 weeks after discontinuing strong CYP3A4 inducer.
➤ **Metastatic epidermal growth factor receptor (EGFR) T790M mutation-positive NSCLC in patients who have progressed on or after EGFR tyrosine kinase inhibitor therapy; first-line treatment of metastatic NSCLC in patients whose tumors have *EGFR* exon 19 deletions or exon 21 L858R mutations**
Adults: 80 mg PO once daily until disease progression or unacceptable toxicity occurs.
➤ **Adjuvant therapy after tumor resection in patients with NSCLC whose tumors have *EGFR* exon 19 deletions or exon 21 L858R mutations**
Adults: 80 mg PO once daily until disease recurs or unacceptable toxicity develops, or for up to 3 years.

ADMINISTRATION
PO
❶ *Alert:* Hazardous drug; use safe handling and disposal precautions. Use single gloves to administer intact tablets. Avoid exposure to crushed tablets. Prepare oral liquid in controlled device using double gloves and protective gown.
• Give drug without regard to food.
• If patient is unable to swallow solids, disperse tablet in approximately 60 mL of noncarbonated water. Stir until tablet is completely dispersed into small pieces (drug won't completely dissolve) and have patient swallow immediately. Rinse container with 120 to 240 mL of water and give to patient immediately.
• To give through NG tube, disperse tablet in 15 mL noncarbonated water and use an additional 15 mL of water to transfer any residual to the syringe. Give through NG tube, followed by 30-mL water flush.
• If dose is missed, omit missed dose and give next dose at the scheduled time.
• Store at room temperature.

ACTION
A kinase inhibitor of EGFR that binds irreversibly to select mutant forms of *EGFR*, including T790M, L858R, and exon 19 deletion. In vitro, drug also inhibits the activity of HER2, HER3, HER4, ACK1, and BLK at clinically relevant concentrations.

Route	Onset	Peak	Duration
PO	Unknown	6 hr	Unknown

Half-life: 48 hours.

ADVERSE REACTIONS
CNS: headache, fever, fatigue, dizziness. **CV:** *prolonged QTc interval,* reduced LVEF, *cardiomyopathy.* **EENT:** epistaxis, nasopharyngitis, keratitis. **GI:** diarrhea, nausea, decreased appetite, constipation, stomatitis, vomiting, abdominal pain. **GU:** UTI, increased BUN level. **Hematologic:** *lymphopenia, thrombocytopenia,* anemia, *neutropenia, leukopenia.* **Hepatic:** increased AST, ALT, and bilirubin levels. **Metabolic:** hypermagnesemia, hyponatremia, *hypokalemia,* hyperglycemia. **Musculoskeletal:** musculoskeletal pain. **Respiratory:** cough, pneumonia, URI, interstitial pneumonitis, *PE.* **Skin:** rash, dry skin,

---

Reactions in bold italics are *life-threatening*.

pruritus, urticaria, hand-foot syndrome, alopecia, nail toxicity.

INTERACTIONS

Drug-drug. *BCRP substrates (rosuvastatin, sulfasalazine, topotecan), P-gp substrates (cyclosporine, sirolimus):* Use together may increase exposure to BCRP or substrate and risk of exposure-related toxicity. Monitor patient for adverse reactions.

Drugs that prolong QT interval (amiodarone, chlorpromazine, disopyramide, moxifloxacin, procainamide, quinidine, sotalol, thioridazine, ziprasidone): May cause additive QT-interval prolongation and increased risk of cardiac arrhythmia. Avoid use together. Periodically monitor ECG if use together can't be avoided.

Strong CYP3A inducers (carbamazepine, phenytoin, rifampin): May decrease osimertinib level. Avoid use together.

Drug-herb. *St. John's wort:* May decrease osimertinib level. Discourage use together.

EFFECTS ON LAB TEST RESULTS

• May increase AST, ALT, bilirubin, magnesium, and blood glucose levels.
• May decrease sodium and potassium levels.
• May decrease Hb level and lymphocyte, leukocyte, platelet, and neutrophil counts.

CONTRAINDICATIONS & CAUTIONS

• Use cautiously in patients with congenital long QTc syndrome, HF, or electrolyte abnormalities and in those taking medications known to prolong QTc interval.
• ILD and cardiomyopathy (cardiac failure, pulmonary edema, decreased ejection fraction, stress cardiomyopathy) may occur with treatment.
• SCARs, keratitis, and cutaneous vasculitis have been reported during therapy.
• Safety and effectiveness in children haven't been established.
Dialyzable drug: Unknown.

PREGNANCY-LACTATION-REPRODUCTION

• Based on animal studies, drug may cause fetal harm. Advise patients of childbearing potential of fetal risk and instruct them to use effective contraception during therapy and for up to 6 weeks after last dose.
• Males with partners of childbearing potential should use contraception during therapy and for up to 4 months after last dose.

• It isn't known if drug appears in human milk. Because of potential for adverse effects in infants, patients shouldn't breastfeed during therapy and for 2 weeks after final dose.
• Drug may impair fertility in patients of reproductive potential. It isn't known if the effects are reversible.

NURSING CONSIDERATIONS

🧬 Confirm T790M, exon 19 deletions, or exon 21 L858R *EGFR* mutations in tumor or plasma specimens, as appropriate, before initiation of treatment.
• Verify pregnancy status before starting drug.
• Assess LVEF by echocardiogram or MUGA before therapy begins and every 3 months during therapy.
• Monitor ECG and electrolyte levels in patients with congenital long QTc syndrome, HF, or electrolyte abnormalities and in those taking medications known to prolong QTc interval.
• Monitor patient for signs and symptoms of ILD (dyspnea, cough, fever, worsening respiratory symptoms). Interrupt treatment and promptly evaluate for ILD. Discontinue drug if ILD is confirmed.
• Monitor patient for signs and symptoms of keratitis (eye inflammation, light sensitivity, lacrimation, vision changes, pain); if any occur, refer patient to ophthalmologist for evaluation.
• Monitor patient for skin toxicity (rash, nail changes, dry skin, itching); drug may increase risk of erythema multiforme, cutaneous vasculitis, and SJS.
• Monitor CBC at baseline, periodically during treatment, and as clinically indicated.
• *Look alike–sound alike:* Don't confuse osimertinib with olaparib or ospemifene. Don't confuse Tagrisso with Targretin or Tasigna.

PATIENT TEACHING

• Teach about proper drug administration and handling.
• Tell patient to promptly report all adverse reactions, especially new or worsening cough, trouble breathing, shortness of breath, fever, and symptoms of keratitis.
• Advise patient to seek medical attention for rapid heartbeat, heart pounding, swollen feet or ankles, dizziness, light-headedness, or faintness.
• Inform patient of risks of ILD, including pneumonitis. Instruct patient to immediately

report new or worsening respiratory signs or symptoms.

• Instruct patient to report signs and symptoms of QTc-interval prolongation (dizziness, light-headedness, syncope).

• Warn of risk of cardiomyopathy. Instruct patient to immediately report signs or symptoms of HF.

• Advise patient to immediately report signs or symptoms of keratitis (eye inflammation, lacrimation, light sensitivity, eye pain, red eye, vision changes).

• Warn of risk of SJS, cutaneous vasculitis, and erythema multiforme. Instruct patient to immediately report development of target lesions or severe blistering or skin peeling.

• Teach patient to report signs or symptoms of aplastic anemia (fever, bruising, bleeding, pallor, infection, tiredness, weakness).

• Advise patient not to breastfeed during therapy and for up to 2 weeks after therapy ends.

• Counsel patient of reproductive potential about fetal risk and contraception recommendations.

• Caution patient to report pregnancy or suspected pregnancy during treatment.

ospemifene
os-PEM-i-feen

Osphena

Therapeutic class: Selective estrogen receptor modulators
Pharmacologic class: Selective estrogen agonists-antagonists

AVAILABLE FORMS
Tablets: 60 mg

INDICATIONS & DOSAGES
➤ **Moderate to severe dyspareunia or vaginal dryness due to vulvar and vaginal atrophy of menopause**
Adults: 60 mg PO once daily.

ADMINISTRATION
PO
🕑 *Alert:* Hazardous drug; use safe handling and disposal precautions, including single gloving for administration.

• Give drug with food.

• Store medication at room temperature.

ACTION
Binds to estrogen receptors, activating estrogenic pathways in some tissues (agonism) and blocking estrogenic pathways in others (antagonism).

Route	Onset	Peak	Duration
PO	12 wk	2 hr	Unknown

Half-life: 26 hours.

ADVERSE REACTIONS
CNS: headache. **CV:** hot flashes. **GU:** *vaginal hemorrhage,* vaginal discharge, endometrial hyperplasia. **Musculoskeletal:** muscle spasms. **Skin:** hyperhidrosis, night sweats.

INTERACTIONS
Drug-drug. *CYP2C9, CYP2C19, CYP3A4 inducers (rifampin):* May decrease ospemifene level, decreasing therapeutic effect. Avoid use together.
CYP2C9, CYP2C19, CYP3A4 inhibitors (fluconazole, ketoconazole, omeprazole): May increase ospemifene level, increasing risk of ospemifene-related adverse effects. Avoid use together.
Estrogen agonists-antagonists, estrogens: Safety of use together hasn't been established. Don't use together.
Highly protein-bound drugs (phenytoin, tolbutamide): May increase exposure of ospemifene or highly protein-bound drug, increasing adverse reactions. Monitor clinical response when either drug is started or stopped.
Drug-herb. *St. John's wort:* May decrease drug level and therapeutic effect. Discourage use together.

EFFECTS ON LAB TEST RESULTS
None reported.

CONTRAINDICATIONS & CAUTIONS
• Contraindicated in females hypersensitive to drug or its components, in females with undiagnosed abnormal genital bleeding or known or suspected estrogen-dependent neoplasm, and in those with active or previous VTE or active or previous arterial thromboembolic disease (stroke, MI).

Boxed Warning Estrogen-alone therapy increases the risk of stroke and DVT. Ospemifene should be prescribed for shortest duration according to treatment goals and patient's individual risk factors. ∎

• Don't use in patients with known or suspected breast cancer or in those with a history of breast cancer. Drug hasn't been studied in these populations.

• Don't use in patients with Child-Pugh class C liver impairment.

• Use cautiously in patients with risk factors for CV disorders, arterial vascular disease, or VTE (obesity, SLE, family history, personal history, diabetes, tobacco use, hypercholesterolemia).

Dialyzable drug: Unknown.

PREGNANCY-LACTATION-REPRODUCTION

• Drug may cause fetal harm and is contraindicated in patients who are or may become pregnant.

• It isn't known if drug appears in human milk. Drug isn't recommended for use during breastfeeding.

NURSING CONSIDERATIONS

Boxed Warning Drug causes increased risk of endometrial cancer in patients with a uterus who use unopposed estrogens; consider adding a progestin in these patients. Patients without a uterus don't need a progestin. Evaluate patient for uterine cancer if persistent or recurrent abnormal genital bleeding occurs. Consider random or directed endometrial sampling to rule out malignancy, if indicated. ■

• Immediately discontinue drug if VTE or thromboembolic or hemorrhagic stroke is suspected or occurs.

• Discontinue drug at least 4 to 6 weeks before surgery that's associated with an increased risk of VTE or during periods of extended immobilization.

• Monitor patient for signs and symptoms of PE or cardiac event (sudden onset of shortness of breath and chest pain).

• *Look alike–sound alike:* Don't confuse ospemifene with osimertinib, raloxifene, or toremifene.

PATIENT TEACHING

• Instruct patient to take drug with food for better absorption.

• Warn that drug may initiate or worsen hot flashes.

• Advise patient to immediately report all adverse reactions, especially hypersensitivity reactions and unusual vaginal discharge or bleeding.

• Caution patient that drug may increase risk of blood clots, stroke, or heart attack. To decrease risk, drug may need to be discontinued at least 4 to 6 weeks before elective surgery or during prolonged immobilization.

• Instruct patient to seek immediate care if weakness on one side of the body, trouble speaking or thinking, change in balance, droop on one side of the face, or blurred eyesight develops.

• Inform patient that drug is contraindicated in patients who are or may become pregnant.

oteseconazole
oh-tes-e-KON-a-zole

Vivjoa

Therapeutic class: Antifungals
Pharmacologic class: Azole antifungals

AVAILABLE FORMS
Capsules ⓞⓝⓒ: 150 mg

INDICATIONS & DOSAGES

➤ **To reduce incidence of recurrent vulvovaginal candidiasis (RVVC) in patients with a history of RVVC who aren't of childbearing potential**
Adults: 600 mg PO as single dose on day 1; followed by 450 mg as single dose on day 2; then, starting on day 14, 150 mg every 7 days for 11 weeks (weeks 2 through 12). Or, if given in combination with fluconazole, fluconazole 150 mg PO on days 1, 4, and 7; followed by oteseconazole 150 mg once daily on days 14 through 20; then, starting on day 28, oteseconazole 150 mg PO every 7 days for 11 weeks (weeks 4 through 14).

ADMINISTRATION
PO
• Give drug with food.
• Have patient swallow capsules whole; don't crush, open, or dissolve capsules.
• Store at 68° to 77° F (20° to 25° C).

ACTION
Inhibits fungal cell membrane formation and integrity.

Route	Onset	Peak	Duration
PO	Unknown	5–10 hr	Unknown

Half-life: 138 days.

ADVERSE REACTIONS
CNS: headache. **GI:** dyspepsia, nausea. **GU:** dysuria; menorrhagia; metrorrhagia; vulvo-vaginal burning, discomfort, or pain. **Other:** hot flashes.

INTERACTIONS
Drug-drug. *BCRP substrates (rosuvastatin):* May increase level and adverse effects of substrate. Use lowest possible starting dose of substrate or consider reducing substrate dosage. Monitor patient for adverse effects.

EFFECTS ON LAB TEST RESULTS
• May increase CK level.

CONTRAINDICATIONS & CAUTIONS
• Contraindicated in patients hypersensitive to drug or its components.
• Safety and effectiveness in patients who are premenarchal haven't been established.
• Contraindicated in patients with Child-Pugh class B or C liver impairment and in patients with CrCl of 29 mL/minute or less with or without CKRT.
• Use cautiously in older adults.
Dialyzable drug: Unlikely.

PREGNANCY-LACTATION-REPRODUCTION
• Based on animal studies, drug may cause fetal harm.
• Drug is contraindicated in patients of child-bearing potential and during pregnancy.
• It isn't known if drug appears in human milk or how drug affects milk production. Drug is contraindicated during breastfeeding due to potential for adverse effects.

NURSING CONSIDERATIONS
• If specimens for fungal culture are obtained before therapy, may start antifungal therapy before culture results are known and adjust therapy as needed after results.

PATIENT TEACHING
🔵 *Alert:* Explain that drug is contraindicated in patients of childbearing potential and during pregnancy and breastfeeding.
• Teach about proper drug administration and handling.
• Ensure that patient fully understands the dosing schedule for oteseconazole or oteseconazole plus fluconazole.

• Advise patient to report all OTC and prescription medications, vitamins, and herbal supplements being taken.

oxaliplatin
ox-AL-i-pla-tin

Therapeutic class: Antineoplastics
Pharmacologic class: Platinum-containing compounds

AVAILABLE FORMS
Solution for injection: 5 mg/mL

INDICATIONS & DOSAGES
Adjust-a-dose (for all indications): For patients with CrCl less than 30 mL/minute, initial recommended dose is 65 mg/m^2. Refer to manufacturer's instructions for toxicity-related dosage adjustments. Refer to manufacturer's instructions for additional information on coadministered drugs.
➤ **With 5-FU and leucovorin (5-FU/LV) for first-line treatment of advanced colorectal cancer or adjuvant treatment of stage III colon cancer in patients who have had complete resection of a primary tumor**
Adults: On day 1, 85 mg/m^2 oxaliplatin IV and leucovorin 200 mg/m^2 IV simultaneously over 120 minutes, in separate bags using Y-line, followed by 5-FU 400 mg/m^2 IV bolus over 2 to 4 minutes, followed by 600 mg/m^2 5-FU IV infusion over 22 hours.

On day 2, 200 mg/m^2 leucovorin IV infusion over 120 minutes, followed by 400 mg/m^2 5-FU IV bolus over 2 to 4 minutes, followed by 600 mg/m^2 5-FU IV infusion over 22 hours.

Repeat cycle every 2 weeks until disease progression or unacceptable toxicity occurs for advanced colorectal cancer. Repeat cycle every 2 weeks for up to 12 cycles or unacceptable toxicity for adjuvant treatment.
➤ **Esophageal cancer ◆**
Adults: For CAPOX, 130 mg/m^2 IV on day 1 every 3 weeks (in combination with capecitabine and nivolumab) until disease progression or unacceptable toxicity occurs.
Adults: For FLOT, 85 mg/m^2 IV on day 1 every 2 weeks (in combination with 5-FU, leucovorin, and docetaxel) for four preoperative and four postoperative cycles, or eight cycles in advanced or metastatic disease.

Adults: For FOLFOX4, 85 mg/m² IV on day 1 every 2 weeks (in combination with 5-FU and leucovorin and radiation) for three cycles, then without radiation for three more cycles.

Adults: For mFOLFOX, 85 mg/m² IV on day 1 every 2 weeks (in combination with 5-FU, leucovorin, and nivolumab) until disease progression or unacceptable toxicity occurs.

➤ **Gastric cancer ◆**

Adults: For CAPOX, 130 mg/m² IV on day 1 every 3 weeks (in combination with capecitabine) for eight cycles following gastrectomy, or (in combination with capecitabine and nivolumab) until disease progression or unacceptable toxicity occurs.

Adults: For FLOT, 85 mg/m² IV on day 1 every 2 weeks (in combination with 5-FU, leucovorin, and docetaxel) for four preoperative and four postoperative cycles, or for eight cycles in advanced or metastatic disease.

Adults: For mFOLFOX, 85 mg/m² IV on day 1 every 2 weeks (in combination with 5-FU, leucovorin, and nivolumab) until disease progression or unacceptable toxicity occurs.

➤ **Pancreatic cancer, adjuvant therapy ◆**

Adults: 85 mg/m² IV every 2 weeks (in combination with 5-FU, leucovorin, and irinotecan) for 24 weeks.

➤ **Pancreatic cancer, advanced or metastatic ◆**

Adults: 85 mg/m² IV every 2 weeks (in combination with 5-FU, leucovorin, and irinotecan) for up to 6 months, or 110 to 130 mg/m² IV on day 1 every 3 weeks (in combination with capecitabine) until disease progression or unacceptable toxicity occurs.

ADMINISTRATION

IV

🔆 *Alert:* Hazardous drug; use safe handling and disposal precautions.

▼ Reconstitute powder using sterile water for injection or D₅W. Add 10 mL to a 50-mg vial or 20 mL to a 100-mg vial, for a yield of 5 mg/mL. Never reconstitute with solution containing chloride.

▼ Further dilute reconstituted solutions in infusion solution of 250 to 500 mL of D₅W.

▼ Inspect bag for particulate matter and discoloration; discard if present.

▼ Don't use needles or IV administration sets that contain aluminum because it displaces the platinum, causing it to lose potency and form a black precipitate.

▼ Premedicate with an antiemetic.

▼ Give oxaliplatin and leucovorin over 2 hours at the same time in separate bags, using Y-line. Extend infusion time to 6 hours to decrease acute toxicities.

▼ When used in combination with 5-FU, infuse oxaliplatin first.

▼ Store unopened vials at room temperature. Reconstituted solutions are stable if refrigerated (36° to 46° F [2° to 8° C]) for up to 24 hours. After final dilution, solutions are stable for 6 hours at room temperature and up to 24 hours under refrigeration.

▼ **Incompatibilities:** Alkaline solutions or drugs such as 5-FU. Flush infusion line with D₅W before giving any other drugs simultaneously.

ACTION

Inhibits cell replication and transcription by forming platinum complexes that cross-link with DNA molecules. Not specific to cell cycle.

Route	Onset	Peak	Duration
IV	Unknown	Unknown	Unknown

Half-life: 392 hours (long, terminal phase).

ADVERSE REACTIONS

CNS: pain, peripheral neuropathy, fatigue, headache, dizziness, insomnia, fever, taste perversion, sensory disturbance, anxiety, depression, paresthesia, neuralgia, ataxia, somnolence. **CV:** chest pain, flushing, *thromboembolism, hemorrhage,* edema, peripheral edema, hypotension, tachycardia. **EENT:** abnormal lacrimation, epistaxis, conjunctivitis, abnormal vision, rhinitis, pharyngolaryngeal dysesthesias, pharyngitis, dry mouth. **GI:** nausea, vomiting, diarrhea, stomatitis, abdominal pain, anorexia, constipation, dyspepsia, gastroesophageal reflux, flatulence, mucositis, dysphagia. **GU:** dysuria, hematuria, urinary frequency, increased serum creatinine level, proctitis. **Hematologic:** *neutropenia,* anemia, *leukopenia, thrombocytopenia.* **Hepatic:** increased LFT levels, ascites. **Metabolic:** *hypokalemia, hypocalcemia,* hyponatremia, hyperglycemia, hypoalbuminemia, weight gain or loss, dehydration. **Musculoskeletal:** back pain, arthralgia, myalgia, muscle weakness. **Respiratory:** dyspnea, cough, URI, hiccups, hemoptysis, *pulmonary toxicity.* **Skin:** injection-site reaction, rash, alopecia, dry skin, pruritus, diaphoresis, hand-foot syndrome. **Other:** infection, rigors, *hypersensitivity reactions,* hot flashes.

INTERACTIONS

Drug-drug. *Anticoagulants:* May increase risk of hemorrhage. Monitor patient closely.

Bacillus Calmette-Guérin (BCG): May diminish therapeutic effect of BCG (intravesical). Avoid use together.

Clozapine: May increase risk of agranulocytosis. Avoid use together.

Deferiprone: May increase risk of neutropenia. Avoid use together.

Denosumab: May increase risk of serious infections. Monitor therapy.

Drugs that prolong QT interval (Class IA and III antiarrhythmics): May further prolong QT interval, increasing risk of cardiac arrhythmia. Avoid use together.

Fosphenytoin, phenytoin: May decrease level of fosphenytoin and phenytoin. Monitor therapy.

Kidney-toxic drugs (such as gentamicin): May decrease elimination of these drugs and increase gentamicin level. Monitor patient for toxicity.

Leflunomide: May increase risk of pancytopenia, agranulocytosis, or thrombocytopenia. Consider not using a leflunomide loading dose in patients receiving other immunosuppressants. Monitor for bone marrow suppression at least monthly. Consider therapy modification.

Live-virus vaccines, pimecrolimus, tacrolimus (topical): May enhance adverse or toxic effects of these drugs. Avoid use together.

Natalizumab: May enhance adverse or toxic effect of natalizumab; specifically, may increase risk of concurrent infection. Avoid use together.

Roflumilast: May enhance roflumilast's immunosuppressive effect. Consider therapy modification.

Sipuleucel-T: May diminish sipuleucel-T therapeutic effect. Monitor therapy.

Taxane derivatives: May enhance myelosuppressive effect of taxane derivatives. To limit toxicity, administer taxane derivative before platinum derivative when given as sequential infusions. Consider therapy modification.

Tofacitinib: May enhance immunosuppressive effect of tofacitinib. Avoid use together.

Topotecan: May enhance adverse or toxic effect of topotecan. Consider therapy modification.

Trastuzumab: May increase neutropenia. Monitor therapy.

Vaccines (inactivated): May diminish therapeutic effect of inactivated vaccines. Monitor therapy.

EFFECTS ON LAB TEST RESULTS

• May increase glucose, creatinine, bilirubin, ALP, AST, and ALT levels.

• May decrease potassium, albumin, calcium, and sodium levels.

• May decrease Hb level and neutrophil, WBC, and platelet counts.

CONTRAINDICATIONS & CAUTIONS

Boxed Warning Serious and fatal hypersensitivity adverse reactions, including anaphylaxis, can occur. Oxaliplatin is contraindicated in patients with hypersensitivity reactions to oxaliplatin and other platinum-based drugs. Immediately and permanently discontinue oxaliplatin for hypersensitivity reactions, and administer appropriate treatment. ▪

• Oxaliplatin may cause acute (within hours or 1 to 2 days) or persistent (greater than 14 days) peripheral sensory neuropathy.

• Oxaliplatin has been associated with rare, sometimes fatal, pulmonary fibrosis and rhabdomyolysis.

• Extravasation of oxaliplatin can cause tissue necrosis. If extravasation occurs, immediately stop infusion and notify provider.

• Severe myelosuppression with sepsis, neutropenic sepsis, and septic shock have occurred in patients receiving oxaliplatin with 5-FU and leucovorin.

• Use cautiously in patients with kidney impairment or peripheral sensory neuropathy.

• Use cautiously in patients with CV disease and avoid use in patients with congenital long QT syndrome. May cause QT-interval prolongation and ventricular arrhythmias.

Dialyzable drug: Unknown.

⚠ *Overdose S&S:* Thrombocytopenia, dyspnea, wheezing, paresthesia, vomiting, chest pain, respiratory failure, bradycardia, dysesthesia, laryngospasm, neurotoxicity, myelosuppression, nausea, diarrhea.

PREGNANCY-LACTATION-REPRODUCTION

• Drug may cause fetal harm. Inform patients of fetal risk.

• Patients of childbearing potential should use effective contraception during therapy and for at least 9 months after final dose.

• Males with partners of childbearing potential should use effective contraception during therapy and for 6 months after final dose.

• It isn't known if drug appears in human milk. Breastfeeding isn't recommended

---

during treatment and for 3 months after final dose.

• Drug may impair fertility.

NURSING CONSIDERATIONS

• Administer drug under the supervision of a physician experienced in use of cancer chemotherapeutic agents.

Boxed Warning Monitor patient for anaphylactic reactions, which may occur within minutes of administration. Immediately and permanently discontinue drug if reactions develop; manage reactions as clinically indicated. ■

• Drug doesn't require patient prehydration.

• Kidney impairment reduces drug clearance. Monitor kidney function.

• Monitor CBC, platelet count, and LFT and kidney function results before each cycle.

• Review ECG in patients with known prolonged QT interval.

• Monitor electrolyte levels. Correct abnormalities at baseline and periodically during treatment.

• Watch for injection-site reactions; extravasation with necrosis may occur. If extravasation occurs, immediately stop infusion and disconnect, gently aspirate extravasated solution, remove needle, and elevate extremity.

• Monitor patient for neuropathy. Acute neuropathy occurs within 2 days of dosing and resolves within 14 days. Persistent peripheral neuropathy occurs more than 14 days after dosing and causes paresthesia, dysesthesia, hypoesthesia, and other neurologic impairments that can interfere with daily activities (such as walking and swallowing).

• Monitor patient for pulmonary toxicity. Withhold treatment and assess unexplained respiratory signs and symptoms. Discontinue drug for confirmed ILD or pulmonary fibrosis.

• Monitor patient for PRES (headache, altered mental function, seizures, vision changes, HTN). Confirm with MRI; permanently discontinue drug if diagnosis is confirmed.

• Monitor patient for bleeding, especially when drug is used in combination with 5-FU or leucovorin.

• Monitor for signs and symptoms of rhabdomyolysis (muscle pain, weakness, fever, red-brown urine, decreased urine output). Permanently discontinue drug if any are present.

• Avoid ice and cold exposure during infusion of drug because cold temperatures can worsen acute neurologic symptoms. Cover patient with a blanket during infusion.

• Older adults are at greater risk for diarrhea, dehydration, hypokalemia, and fatigue.

• *Look alike–sound alike:* Don't confuse oxaliplatin with carboplatin or cisplatin.

PATIENT TEACHING

• Inform patient of potential serious adverse reactions and the need to promptly report them.

• Tell patient to avoid exposure to cold or cold objects (such as cold drinks and ice cubes), which can bring on or worsen acute symptoms of peripheral neuropathy. Advise patient to drink warm drinks, wear warm clothing, and cover any exposed skin (hands, face, and head).

• Inform patient of the need for frequent blood tests.

• Advise patient to immediately report trouble breathing or signs or symptoms of an allergic reaction (rash, hives, swelling of lips or tongue, sudden cough).

• Instruct patient to report fever, signs and symptoms of infection, persistent vomiting, diarrhea, or signs and symptoms of dehydration (thirst, dry mouth, light-headedness, decreased urination).

• Warn patient of risk of fetal harm if oxaliplatin is used during pregnancy. Advise use of effective contraception.

• Advise patient of reproductive potential who desires children to consider fertility preservation before therapy.

• Caution patient not to breastfeed during treatment and for 3 months after final dose.

• Advise patient that dizziness and vision abnormalities may affect patient's ability to drive and use machinery.

SAFETY ALERT!

oxazepam
oks-A-ze-pam

Therapeutic class: Anxiolytics
Pharmacologic class: Benzodiazepines
Controlled substance schedule: IV

AVAILABLE FORMS
Capsules: 10 mg, 15 mg, 30 mg

INDICATIONS & DOSAGES
➤ **Alcohol withdrawal, severe anxiety**
Adults: 15 to 30 mg PO t.i.d. or q.i.d.

➤ **Mild to moderate anxiety**
Adults and children older than age 12: 10 to 15 mg PO t.i.d. or q.i.d.
➤ **Severe anxiety syndromes, agitation, anxiety associated with depression**
Adults and children older than age 12: 15 to 30 mg PO t.i.d. or q.i.d.
➤ **Anxiety, tension, irritability, agitation**
Older adults: 10 mg PO t.i.d. May increase cautiously to 15 mg t.i.d. or q.i.d.

ADMINISTRATION
PO
• Give drug without regard to food.

ACTION
May stimulate GABA receptors in the ascending reticular activating system.

Route	Onset	Peak	Duration
PO	Unknown	3 hr	Unknown

Half-life: About 8 hours.

ADVERSE REACTIONS
CNS: drowsiness, lethargy, dizziness, vertigo, headache, syncope, tremor, slurred speech, transient amnesia. **CV:** edema. **GI:** nausea. **GU:** altered libido. **Skin:** rash.

INTERACTIONS
Drug-drug. *Clozapine:* May enhance toxic effect of clozapine. Consider decreasing oxazepam dosage.
CNS depressants: May increase CNS depression. Use together cautiously.
Melatonin: May enhance sedative effect of benzodiazepines. Use with caution.
Boxed Warning *Opioids:* May cause slow or difficult breathing, sedation, and death. Avoid use together. If use together is necessary, limit dosage and duration of each drug to minimum necessary for desired effect. ∎
Drug-herb. *Cannabinoid-containing products, kava, kratom, valerian:* May increase sedation. Discourage use together.
Yohimbe: May decrease effect of oxazepam. Discourage use together.
Drug-lifestyle. *Alcohol use:* May cause additive CNS effects. Discourage use together.

EFFECTS ON LAB TEST RESULTS
• May increase LFT values.
• May decrease WBC count.

CONTRAINDICATIONS & CAUTIONS
• Contraindicated in patients hypersensitive to drug and in those with psychoses.
Boxed Warning Opioids should only be prescribed with benzodiazepines or other CNS depressants to patients for whom alternative treatment options are inadequate. ∎
Boxed Warning Benzodiazepine use exposes patient to risks of abuse, misuse, and addiction, which can lead to overdose or death. Assess each patient's risk of abuse, misuse, and addiction before prescribing and periodically during therapy. ∎
Boxed Warning Abrupt discontinuation or rapid dosage reduction of benzodiazepines after continued use may precipitate acute withdrawal reactions, which can be life-threatening. To reduce risk of withdrawal reactions, gradually taper drug to discontinue or reduce dosage. ∎
• Use cautiously in older adults and in patients at risk for falls.
• Use cautiously in patients with respiratory disease or history of substance abuse and in patients in whom a decrease in BP might lead to cardiac problems.
• Safety and effectiveness in children younger than age 6 haven't been established. Absolute dosage for children ages 6 to 12 isn't established.
Dialyzable drug: No.
⚠ *Overdose S&S:* Drowsiness, confusion, lethargy, ataxia, hypotonia, hypotension, hypnotic state, coma, death.

PREGNANCY-LACTATION-REPRODUCTION
• Drug crosses placental barrier and may adversely affect the fetus (premature birth, low birth weight, hypoglycemia, respiratory problems), especially in first and third trimesters. Use during pregnancy should almost always be avoided.
• Drug appears in human milk. Drowsiness, lethargy, poor feeding, and weight loss may occur in breastfed infants. Breastfeeding isn't recommended.

NURSING CONSIDERATIONS
• Periodically monitor liver, kidney, and hematopoietic function in patient receiving repeated or prolonged therapy.
Boxed Warning Concomitant use of benzodiazepines and opioids may result in profound sedation, respiratory depression, coma, and death. Limit dosages and durations to the

minimum required. Monitor patients for signs and symptoms of respiratory depression and sedation. ∎

• Monitor patient closely for fall risk.

• *Look alike–sound alike:* Don't confuse oxazepam with oxaprozin, oxcarbazepine, or quazepam.

PATIENT TEACHING

Boxed Warning Caution patient or caregiver of patient taking an opioid with a benzodiazepine, CNS depressant, or alcohol to seek immediate medical attention if patient experiences dizziness, light-headedness, extreme sleepiness, slowed or difficult breathing, or unresponsiveness. ∎

Boxed Warning Caution patient that benzodiazepines, even at recommended doses, increase risk of abuse, misuse, and addiction, which can lead to overdose and death, especially when used in combination with other drugs (opioid analgesics), alcohol, or illicit substances. ∎

Boxed Warning Inform patient on proper disposal of unused drug and about signs and symptoms of benzodiazepine abuse, misuse, and addiction (abdominal pain, amnesia, anorexia, anxiety, aggression, ataxia, blurred vision, confusion, depression, disinhibition, disorientation, dizziness, euphoria, impaired concentration and memory, indigestion, irritability, muscle pain, slurred speech, tremors, vertigo, delirium, paranoia, suicidality, seizures, difficulty breathing, coma). Instruct patient to seek emergency medical help if any occur. Advise patient not to take drug at a higher dose, more frequently, or for longer than prescribed. ∎

Boxed Warning Tell patient that continued use of drug for several days to weeks may lead to physical dependence and that abrupt discontinuation or rapid dosage reduction may precipitate acute withdrawal reactions (seizures; unusual movements, responses, or expressions; sudden and severe mental or nervous system changes; depression; seeing or hearing things that others don't; homicidal thoughts; extreme increase in activity or talking; losing touch with reality; suicidality), which can be life-threatening. Instruct patient that discontinuation or dosage reduction may require a slow taper. ∎

Boxed Warning Advise patient about risk of protracted withdrawal syndrome (anxiety; depression; trouble remembering, learning,

or concentrating; problems sleeping; sensation of insects crawling under skin; weakness; shaking; muscle twitching; burning or prickling feeling in hands, arms, legs, or feet; ringing in ears), with symptoms lasting weeks to more than 12 months. ∎

• Warn patient to avoid hazardous activities, including driving and operating machinery, that require alertness or good coordination until effects of drug are known.

• Tell patient to avoid use of alcohol.

• Notify patient that smoking may decrease drug's effectiveness.

• Warn patient of childbearing potential to avoid use during pregnancy.

OXcarbazepine ✄

ox-car-BAZ-e-peen

Oxtellar XR, Trileptal

Therapeutic class: Anticonvulsants
Pharmacologic class: Carboxamide derivatives

AVAILABLE FORMS

Oral suspension: 300 mg/5 mL (60 mg/mL)
Tablets (extended-release) ⓄⓃⒸ: 150 mg, 300 mg, 600 mg
Tablets (film-coated): 150 mg, 300 mg, 600 mg

INDICATIONS & DOSAGES

Adjust-a-dose (for all indications): If CrCl is less than 30 mL/minute, start therapy at 150 mg PO b.i.d. immediate-release or 300 mg PO daily extended-release (one-half usual starting dose) and increase slowly to achieve desired response. In patients with CKD on dialysis, use immediate-release formulation instead of extended-release formulation.

➤ **Adjunctive treatment of partial seizures; monotherapy for partial-onset seizures**
Adults: Initially, 300 mg immediate-release tablets or suspension PO b.i.d.; increase by maximum of 600 mg daily (300 mg PO b.i.d.) at weekly intervals. Maximum recommended daily dosage, 1,200 mg PO in two divided doses. Or, 600 mg extended-release tablets PO daily; may increase at weekly intervals in 600-mg/day increments. Usual dosage, 1,200 to 2,400 mg daily.
Older adults: When using extended-release tablets, consider lower starting dose (300 or

---

450 mg/day). May increase at weekly intervals in increments of 300 to 450 mg/day.
Children ages 6 to 17 (extended-release): 8 to 10 mg/kg PO once daily, not to exceed 600 mg daily in first week. May increase at weekly intervals in 8- to 10-mg/kg increments once daily, not to exceed 600 mg. Target daily dosage in patients weighing more than 39 kg is 1,800 mg/day; from 29.1 to 39 kg, 1,200 mg/day; and from 20 to 29 kg, 900 mg/day.
Children ages 4 to 16 (immediate-release): Initially, 8 to 10 mg/kg PO daily in two divided doses, not to exceed 600 mg/day. Target maintenance dose depends on patient's weight and should be divided into two doses. If patient weighs between 20 and 29 kg, target maintenance dose is 900 mg daily in two divided doses. If patient weighs between 29.1 and 39 kg, target maintenance dose is 1,200 mg daily in two divided doses. If patient weighs more than 39 kg, target maintenance dose is 1,800 mg daily in two divided doses. Target doses should be achieved over 2 weeks.
Children ages 2 to younger than 4 (immediate-release, adjunctive therapy only): Initially, 8 to 10 mg/kg PO daily in two divided doses, not to exceed 600 mg/day. If patient weighs less than 20 kg, consider starting dose of 16 to 20 mg/kg. Maximum maintenance dosage should be achieved over 2 to 4 weeks and shouldn't exceed 60 mg/kg/day in two-dose divided regimen.
Adjust-a-dose: If drug is used concomitantly with strong CYP3A4 enzyme inducers or UGT inducers, which include certain antiepileptic drugs, consider initiating dosage of extended-release formulation at 900 mg once daily in adults and 12 to 15 mg/kg once daily in children. Refer to Interactions section and product insert for more information.

➤ **To change from multidrug to single-drug treatment of partial seizures**
Adults: Initially, 300 mg immediate-release tablets or suspension PO b.i.d., while reducing dose of concomitant anticonvulsant. Increase oxcarbazepine by maximum of 600 mg daily at weekly intervals over 2 to 4 weeks. Recommended daily dose is 2,400 mg PO in two divided doses. Withdraw other anticonvulsant completely over 3 to 6 weeks.
Children ages 4 to 16: Initially, 8 to 10 mg/kg immediate-release tablets or suspension PO daily in two divided doses, while reducing dose of concomitant anticonvulsant. Increase oxcarbazepine by maximum of 10 mg/kg

daily at weekly intervals to achieve recommended daily dose by weight listed in manufacturer's instructions. Withdraw other anticonvulsant completely over 3 to 6 weeks. See manufacturer's instructions for weight-based maintenance dosing with oxcarbazepine monotherapy.

ADMINISTRATION
PO
● Give immediate-release tablets and oral suspension without regard to food.
● Give extended-release tablets on an empty stomach (at least 1 hour before or 2 hours after a meal). Have patient swallow extended-release tablets whole; don't crush or break tablets.
● For ease of swallowing, use multiple lower-strength tablets for appropriate dose.
● Higher doses may be needed when converting from immediate-release to extended-release form.
● Oral tablets and suspension may be interchanged at equal doses.
● For suspension, firmly insert plastic adapter provided with bottle. Cover adapter with child-resistant cap when not in use.
● Shake bottle for at least 10 seconds, remove child-resistant cap, and insert oral dosing syringe provided to withdraw appropriate dose.
● May give dose directly from oral syringe or may mix in a small glass of water immediately before patient swallows it.
● Rinse syringe with warm water after use and allow to dry thoroughly.
● Use suspension within 7 weeks of first opening container.

ACTION
Thought to prevent seizure spread in the brain by blocking voltage-sensitive sodium channels and to produce anticonvulsant effects by increasing potassium conduction and modulating high-voltage activated calcium channels.

Route	Onset	Peak	Duration
PO	Unknown	Immediate-release: 3–13 hr (adults), 1 hr (children); extended-release: 7 hr (adults)	Unknown

Half-life: Immediate-release: About 2 hours for drug; about 9 hours for active metabolite (adults). Children ages 2 to 5, 4.8 to 6.7 hours for active metabolite; children ages 6 to 8, 7.2 to 9.3 hours for active metabolite. Extended-release: 7 to 11 hours for drug.

ADVERSE REACTIONS

CNS: abnormal gait, ataxia, dizziness, drowsiness, fatigue, headache, tremors, vertigo, *seizures,* abnormal coordination, balance disorder, agitation, amnesia, fever, anxiety, asthenia, confusion, emotional lability, feeling abnormal, hypoesthesia, impaired concentration, insomnia, falls, somnolence, nervousness, speech disorder, thirst, taste perversion, abnormal EEG. **CV:** chest pain, edema, hypotension. **EENT:** abnormal vision, diplopia, nystagmus, abnormal accommodation, ear pain, ear infection, epistaxis, rhinitis, sinusitis, toothache, dry mouth, nasopharyngitis. **GI:** abdominal pain, nausea, vomiting, anorexia, rectal hemorrhage, constipation, diarrhea, dyspepsia, gastritis. **GU:** urinary frequency, UTI, vaginitis. **Hematologic:** lymphadenopathy. **Metabolic:** hyponatremia, weight gain. **Musculoskeletal:** back pain, muscular weakness. **Respiratory:** URI, bronchitis, pulmonary infection, coughing, pneumonia. **Skin:** acne, bruising, diaphoresis, purpura, rash. **Other:** allergic reaction, infection, hot flashes.

INTERACTIONS

Drug-drug. *CYP3A4 inducers, UGT inducers (rifampin, carbamazepine, phenobarbital):* May decrease oxcarbazepine level. Monitor therapy.
CYP3A4 substrates (cyclosporine, itraconazole, rivaroxaban): May decrease substrate levels. Modify substrate dosage as needed.
Dolutegravir, elvitegravir, ledipasvir, rilpivirine, simeprevir, sofosbuvir, tenofovir, ulipristal: May decrease levels of these drugs. Avoid use together.
Hormonal contraceptives: May decrease levels of ethinyl estradiol and levonorgestrel, reducing hormonal contraceptive effectiveness. Caution patients of childbearing potential to use alternative forms of contraception.
Phenytoin: May decrease oxcarbazepine level and increase phenytoin level. Monitor patient closely.
Valproic acid: May decrease oxcarbazepine level. Monitor patient and level closely.
Drug-lifestyle. *Alcohol use:* May increase CNS depression. Discourage use together.

EFFECTS ON LAB TEST RESULTS

• May decrease sodium level.
• May decrease serum T_4 without affecting T_3 or TSH levels.

CONTRAINDICATIONS & CAUTIONS

• Contraindicated in patients hypersensitive to drug or its components or to eslicarbazepine acetate.
• Use cautiously in patients hypersensitive to carbamazepine; cross hypersensitivity reactions may occur.
⚠️ *Alert:* SCARs have been reported with oxcarbazepine use. Reactions may be life-threatening and require hospitalization. Recurrence of serious skin reactions after rechallenge with oxcarbazepine has also been reported.
▓ Screen patients of Asian ancestry for the human leukocyte antigen allele (HLA-B*1502) before therapy; these patients may be at increased risk for SJS or TEN with oxcarbazepine therapy.
• Drug may cause exacerbation of or new onset of primary generalized seizures, especially in children.
• May increase risk of suicidality.
Dializable drug: Unknown.

PREGNANCY-LACTATION-REPRODUCTION

• Studies during pregnancy are inadequate. Drug may cause fetal harm. Use cautiously during pregnancy and only if benefit justifies fetal risk.
• Encourage patients who are taking drug during pregnancy to register in the North American Antiepileptic Drug Pregnancy Registry (1-888-233-2334 or www.aedpregnancyregistry.org).
• Plasma levels of the active metabolite of oxcarbazepine may gradually decrease throughout pregnancy and increase after delivery. Monitor patient carefully during pregnancy and postpartum period.
• Drug and its active metabolite appear in human milk. Use cautiously during breastfeeding.

NURSING CONSIDERATIONS

• Patient with history of hypersensitivity reaction to carbamazepine may develop hypersensitivity to oxcarbazepine. Ask about carbamazepine hypersensitivity and stop drug immediately if signs or symptoms of hypersensitivity occur.
⚠️ *Alert:* Closely monitor all patients taking or starting antiepileptic drugs for changes in behavior indicating worsening of suicidality or depression. Symptoms such as anxiety, agitation, hostility, mania, and hypomania may be precursors to emerging suicidality.

🔆 *Alert:* Withdraw drug gradually to minimize risk of increased seizure activity.

• Watch for signs and symptoms of hyponatremia (nausea, malaise, headache, lethargy, confusion, decreased sensation).

• Monitor sodium level in patient receiving oxcarbazepine for maintenance treatment, especially if patient is receiving other therapies that may decrease sodium level.

• Oxcarbazepine use has been linked to several nervous system–related adverse reactions, including psychomotor slowing, difficulty with concentration, speech and language problems, somnolence, fatigue, and coordination abnormalities, such as ataxia and gait disturbances.

🔆 *Alert:* Rare serious and sometimes fatal dermatologic reactions can occur. If skin reactions occur, discontinue drug.

• Monitor patient for DRESS syndrome (fever; rash; lymphadenopathy; facial edema; organ system disorders, such as hepatitis, nephritis, myocarditis, myositis, hematologic abnormalities). Immediately evaluate patient and discontinue drug if alternative cause isn't determined.

• *Look alike–sound alike:* Don't confuse oxcarbazepine with carbamazepine, oxazepam, or oxaprozin. Don't confuse Trileptal with TriLipix.

PATIENT TEACHING

• Teach about proper drug administration and handling.

• Tell patient to contact prescriber before interrupting or stopping drug.

• Advise patient not to discontinue drug abruptly because of risk of increased seizure frequency.

• Instruct patient to report signs and symptoms of low sodium in blood (nausea, malaise, headache, lethargy, confusion).

🔆 *Alert:* Serious skin reactions, including DRESS syndrome, SJS, and TEN, can occur. Advise patient to immediately report rashes, fever, or swollen lymph nodes to prescriber.

• Caution patient to avoid driving and other potentially hazardous activities that require mental alertness until effects of drug are known.

• Instruct patient using hormonal contraceptives to use alternative form of contraception during therapy.

• Teach patient to report pregnancy or plans to become pregnant or breastfeed.

• Tell patient to avoid alcohol during therapy.

---

oxybutynin
oks-i-BYOO-ti-nin

Oxytrol, Oxytrol for Women ◇

oxybutynin chloride
Ditropan XL, Gelnique

Therapeutic class: Urinary antispasmodics
Pharmacologic class: Antimuscarinics

AVAILABLE FORMS
oxybutynin
Transdermal patch: 36-mg patch delivering 3.9 mg/day ◇
oxybutynin chloride
Syrup: 5 mg/5 mL
Tablets: 2.5 mg, 5 mg
Tablets (extended-release) 🔵ⁿᵍ: 5 mg, 10 mg, 15 mg
Topical gel: 10% in 1-g single-dose sachets

INDICATIONS & DOSAGES
➤ **Overactive bladder**
Adults: 5 mg (immediate-release tablet) PO b.i.d. to t.i.d.; maximum, 5 mg q.i.d. Or, 5 to 10 mg (extended-release tablet) PO once daily. Adjust dosage weekly in 5-mg increments, as needed, to maximum of 30 mg PO daily. Or, apply one patch twice weekly (every 3 to 4 days) to dry, intact skin on abdomen, hip, or buttock. Or, 1 g topical gel (10%) once daily.
Older adults: Start with lower initial dose of 2.5 mg (immediate-release) PO b.i.d. or t.i.d.
➤ **Symptoms of detrusor overactivity associated with a neurologic condition (such as spina bifida)**
Children ages 5 and older (immediate-release): 5 mg PO b.i.d. or t.i.d.
Children ages 6 and older (extended-release): 5 mg once daily; adjust in 5-mg increments at weekly intervals. Maximum dosage, 20 mg/day.

ADMINISTRATION
PO
• Give drug without regard to food.
• Have patient swallow extended-release tablets whole; don't crush or break tablets.
• Measure syrup dose with liquid medication dispenser or syringe.

Reactions in bold italics are *life-threatening*.

Topical (gel)

- Use immediately after opening sachets.
- Prime pump before initial use. One full depression of pump provides one dose. Discard after 30 doses.
- Apply to dry, intact skin on abdomen, upper arm, shoulder, or thigh.
- Don't apply to recently shaved skin.
- Rotate application sites.
- Patient shouldn't bathe, shower, or swim for 1 hour after gel application.
- Cover treated area with clothing after gel has dried to prevent transfer of medication to others.

Transdermal

- Apply immediately after removing from protective pouch.
- Apply to dry, intact skin on abdomen, hip, or buttock.
- Don't apply to areas with cuts, scrapes, or irritation.
- Avoid reapplication to same site within 7 days.
- Don't expose patch to sunlight.
- Don't cut patch.
- Contact with water while bathing, swimming, showering, or exercising won't change the effect; however, patient should avoid rubbing the patch area during these activities.

ACTION

Relaxes smooth muscle of bladder by antagonizing muscarinic receptors, relieving symptoms of overactive bladder.

Route	Onset	Peak	Duration
PO	30–60 min	60 min	6–10 hr
PO (extended-release)	Unknown	4–6 hr	24 hr
Topical (gel)	Unknown	Unknown	Unknown
Transdermal	Unknown	24–48 hr	96 hr

Half-life: Tablets or oral solution, 2 to 3 hours; extended-release tablets, 12 to 13 hours; patch, 64 hours.

ADVERSE REACTIONS

PO

CNS: dizziness, insomnia, nervousness, drowsiness, restlessness, asthenia, fatigue, fever, headache, somnolence, confusion, altered taste, thirst. **CV:** palpitations, flushing, peripheral edema, increased or decreased BP. **EENT:** blurred vision, dry eyes, eye irritation, nasopharyngitis, sinus or nasal congestion, hoarseness, dry mouth, sore throat, coated tongue, oropharyngeal pain, nasal

dryness. **GI:** nausea, vomiting, constipation, diarrhea, dyspepsia, decreased GI motility, flatulence, dysphagia, belching, abdominal pain, GERD. **GU:** dysuria, urinary hesitancy, urine retention, urinary frequency, increased residual urine volume, impotence, UTI, cystitis. **Metabolic:** fluid retention, hyperglycemia. **Musculoskeletal:** back pain, arthralgia, limb pain. **Respiratory:** URI, bronchitis, cough, *asthma.* **Skin:** rash, dry skin, pruritus. **Other:** fungal infection, falls.

Topical (gel)

CNS: dizziness, fatigue, headache. **EENT:** dry mouth, nasopharyngitis. **GI:** viral gastroenteritis, constipation. **GU:** UTI. **Metabolic:** increased serum glucose level. **Respiratory:** URI. **Skin:** application-site reaction, pruritus.

Transdermal patch

EENT: abnormal vision, dry mouth. **GI:** diarrhea, constipation. **GU:** dysuria. **Skin:** application site pruritus, erythema, vesicles, macules, rash, burning.

INTERACTIONS

Drug-drug. *Amantadine, anticholinergics (dicyclomine, scopolamine):* May increase anticholinergic effects (dry mouth, constipation, blurred vision, somnolence). Use together cautiously.

Cannabinoid-containing products: May enhance tachycardic effect of cannabinoid-containing products. Monitor therapy closely.

CNS depressants: May increase CNS effects. Use together cautiously.

CYP3A4 inhibitors (clarithromycin, erythromycin, itraconazole, ketoconazole, miconazole): May increase oxybutynin level. Use together cautiously.

Ipratropium (oral inhalation): May increase anticholinergic effects (dry mouth, constipation, blurred vision, somnolence). Avoid use together.

Opioid agonists (buprenorphine): May increase risk of constipation and urine retention. Monitor therapy closely.

Drug-lifestyle. *Alcohol use:* May increase CNS effects. Discourage use together.

Exercise, hot weather: May cause heatstroke. Advise patient to use with caution in hot weather.

EFFECTS ON LAB TEST RESULTS

- May increase glucose level.
- May suppress wheal and flare reactions to skin test antigens.

CONTRAINDICATIONS & CAUTIONS

• Contraindicated in patients hypersensitive to drug or its components and in those with conditions that decrease GI motility, uncontrolled narrow-angle glaucoma, urine or gastric retention, or obstructive uropathy.
• Angioedema may occur after single dose.
• Use cautiously in older adults and in patients with autonomic neuropathy, reflux esophagitis, myasthenia gravis, Parkinson disease, or liver or kidney disorders.
• Use cautiously in patients with preexisting dementia treated with a cholinesterase inhibitor.
• Extended-release form isn't recommended for children who can't swallow tablet whole without chewing, dividing, or crushing or for children younger than age 6.
• Use extended-release form cautiously in patients with bladder outflow obstruction, gastric obstruction, ulcerative colitis, intestinal atony, myasthenia gravis, or GERD and in those taking drugs that worsen esophagitis (such as bisphosphonates).
Dialyzable drug: Unknown.
⚠ *Overdose S&S:* Restlessness, tremors, irritability, seizures, delirium, dehydration, hallucinations, flushing, fever, cardiac arrhythmias, vomiting, urine retention, hypotension or HTN, respiratory failure, paralysis, coma.

PREGNANCY-LACTATION-REPRODUCTION

• Studies during pregnancy are inadequate.
• Use cautiously during pregnancy and only if benefit justifies fetal risk.
• It isn't known if drug appears in human milk. Use cautiously during breastfeeding.
• Lactation suppression has been reported.

NURSING CONSIDERATIONS

• Drug may aggravate symptoms of hyperthyroidism, CAD, HF, arrhythmias, tachycardia, HTN, and prostatic hyperplasia.
• Monitor patient for anticholinergic effects (confusion, constipation, dry mouth, dizziness, blurred vision, tachycardia). Consider dosage reduction or discontinuation if they occur.
• Monitor patient for episodes of incontinence and postvoid residual.
• *Look alike–sound alike:* Don't confuse oxybutynin with OxyCONTIN. Don't confuse Ditropan with Detrol, diazepam, Diprivan, or dithranol.

PATIENT TEACHING

• Teach about proper drug administration and handling for prescribed formulation.
• Warn patient to avoid hazardous activities, such as operating machinery and driving, until CNS effects of drug are known.
• Caution patient that using drug during very hot weather may cause fever or heatstroke because it suppresses sweating.
• Warn patient to only wear one patch at a time.
• Tell patient to carefully dispose of old patches in trash in a manner that prevents accidental application or ingestion by children and pets.
• Tell patient to remove patch before undergoing MRI.
• Gel contains alcohol. Caution patient to avoid open flames and smoking until gel has dried.
• Advise patient to avoid alcohol while taking drug.
• Tell patient that drug may cause dry mouth, urine retention, and constipation.
• Warn of risk of angioedema. Instruct patient to seek immediate medical attention if symptoms (swelling of tongue or throat, difficulty breathing) occur.

SAFETY ALERT!

oxyCODONE
oks-i-KOE-done

Xtampza ER

oxyCODONE hydrochloride
Oxaydo, OxyCONTIN, Oxy.IR✦, OxyNEO✦, Roxicodone, Roxybond, Supeudol✦

Therapeutic class: Opioid analgesics
Pharmacologic class: Opioids
Controlled substance schedule: II

AVAILABLE FORMS
oxycodone
Capsules (extended-release, 12-hour abuse deterrent): 9-mg base, 13.5-mg base, 18-mg base, 27-mg base, 36-mg base
oxycodone hydrochloride
Capsules: 5 mg
Oral solution: 5 mg/5 mL
Oral solution (concentrate): 20 mg/mL
Tablets (extended-release, 12-hour abuse-deterrent) ⬛: 10 mg, 15 mg, 20 mg, 30 mg, 40 mg, 60 mg, 80 mg

---

Reactions in bold italics are *life-threatening*.

Tablets (immediate-release): 5 mg, 7.5 mg, 10 mg, 15 mg, 20 mg, 30 mg

INDICATIONS & DOSAGES

➤ **Acute and chronic pain severe enough to require an opioid analgesic and for which alternative treatments are inadequate**
Adults: 5 to 15 mg immediate-release PO every 4 to 6 hours. Titrate dosage based on response. For acute pain, use PRN. For control of severe, chronic pain, give on a regularly scheduled basis every 4 to 6 hours.
➤ **Pain severe enough to require daily, around-the-clock, long-term opioid treatment and for which alternative treatment options are inadequate**
Adults who aren't opioid-tolerant: 10 mg extended-release tablets or 9 mg extended-release capsules PO every 12 hours. May increase dose every 1 to 2 days until desired pain control is achieved.
Adults who are opioid-tolerant: Refer to manufacturer's instructions for extended-release tablets or capsules or concentrated oral solution (20 mg/mL) for conversion from other formulations and drugs.
Children ages 11 and older who are opioid-tolerant (extended-release tablets): Refer to manufacturer's recommendations for conversion from other opioids.
Adjust-a-dose: For older adults, patients who are debilitated, those with liver or kidney impairment, and patients receiving CNS depressants, decrease initial starting dose by one-third to one-half.

ADMINISTRATION
PO
• To minimize GI upset, give drug after meals or with milk.
• Have patient swallow extended-release tablet whole; don't crush or break.
❸ *Alert:* The 60- and 80-mg extended-release tablets, or a single dose of more than 40 mg, or a total daily dose of more than 80 mg is limited to patients who are opioid-tolerant. Oxycodone concentrated oral solution (20-mg/mL) is indicated for use in patients who are opioid-tolerant only.
Boxed Warning Use care when administering oxycodone concentrated oral solution to avoid dosing errors due to confusion between milligram and milliliter and among other oxycodone solutions with different concentrations. Such confusion could result in accidental

overdose and death. Ensure that proper dose is communicated and dispensed. ∎
❸ *Alert:* Oxycodone extended-release capsules aren't bioequivalent to oxycodone hydrochloride extended-release tablets.

ACTION
Unknown. Binds with opioid receptors in the CNS, altering perception of and emotional response to pain.

Route	Onset	Peak	Duration
PO (immediate-release)	10–15 min	0.5–1 hr	3–6 hr
PO (extended-release)	Unknown	4–5 hr	12 hr

Half-life: 3 to 4 hours. Extended-release tablets, 4.5 hours; extended-release capsules, 5.6 hours.

ADVERSE REACTIONS
CNS: clouded sensorium, dizziness, fever, euphoria, light-headedness, physical dependence, withdrawal syndrome, sedation, somnolence, headache, asthenia, abnormal dreams, insomnia, confusion, agitation, irritability, depression, migraine, tremor. **CV:** *bradycardia,* hypotension, edema, *HF, DVT,* thrombophlebitis, flushing, HTN, vasodilation, tachycardia. **EENT:** blurred vision, pharyngitis, rhinitis, sinusitis, oropharyngeal pain, dry mouth. **GI:** constipation, nausea, vomiting, ileus, diarrhea, anorexia, gastritis, GERD, abdominal pain. **GU:** urine retention, dysuria, UTI. **Hematologic:** anemia; decreased Hb level, platelet count, and RBC count. **Hepatic:** increased ALT level. **Metabolic:** hypochloremia, hyponatremia, hyperglycemia, weight loss, gout. **Musculoskeletal:** weakness, arthralgia, myalgia, back pain, tremor. **Respiratory:** *respiratory depression,* cough, dyspnea. **Skin:** diaphoresis, pruritus. **Other:** chills, withdrawal syndrome, hypersensitivity reaction, accidental injury.

INTERACTIONS
Drug-drug. *Alvimopan:* May enhance alvimopan-related toxicity. Alvimopan is contraindicated in patients receiving opioids for more than 7 consecutive days before starting alvimopan.
Anticholinergic agents (dicyclomine, scopolamine): May increase risk of constipation and urine retention. Monitor therapy closely.
Boxed Warning *Benzodiazepines, CNS depressants:* May cause slow or difficult

breathing, sedation, and death. Avoid use together. If use together is necessary, limit dosage and duration of each drug to minimum necessary for desired effect. ∎

Boxed Warning *CYP3A4 inducers (such as carbamazepine, phenytoin, rifampin):* May increase oxycodone level and cause oxycodone-related adverse reactions if inducer is discontinued. Taper inducers cautiously, and adjust oxycodone dosage as needed. ∎

Boxed Warning *CYP3A4 and CYP2D6 inhibitors such as azole antifungals (ketoconazole), macrolide antibiotics (erythromycin), protease inhibitors (ritonavir):* May increase oxycodone level, increase or prolong adverse effects, and cause fatal respiratory depression. Carefully monitor patient over extended period and adjust oxycodone dosage as needed. ∎

Diuretics: May reduce effect of diuretic. Monitor therapy.

General anesthetics, hypnotics, MAO inhibitors, TCAs: May cause additive adverse effects (CNS or respiratory depression). Use together cautiously. Reduce oxycodone dose and monitor response.

Mixed agonist/antagonists, partial opioid analgesics (butorphanol, nalbuphine, pentazocine): May decrease analgesic effect of oxycodone. Avoid use together.

Muscle relaxants (cyclobenzaprine, metaxalone): May increase neuromuscular blockage and increase respiratory depression. Monitor patient closely, and adjust dose of either drug as necessary.

⭘ *Alert:* Serotonergic drugs (amoxapine, antiemetics [dolasetron, ondansetron], antimigraine drugs, buspirone, cyclobenzaprine, dextromethorphan, linezolid, lithium, MAO inhibitors, maprotiline, methylene blue, mirtazapine, nefazodone, SNRIs, SSRIs, TCAs, trazodone, tryptophan, vilazodone):* May increase risk of serotonin syndrome. Use together cautiously, and monitor patient for serotonin syndrome.

Drug-herb. *Cannabinoid-containing products, kava:* May enhance adverse effects of CNS depressants. Discourage use together.

⭘ *Alert:* *St. John's wort:* May increase risk of serotonin syndrome and decrease oxycodone level. Use together cautiously.

Drug-lifestyle. **Boxed Warning** *Alcohol use:* May cause slow or difficult breathing, sedation, and death. Discourage use together. ∎

EFFECTS ON LAB TEST RESULTS

- May increase blood glucose and ALT levels.
- May decrease chloride and sodium levels.
- May decrease Hb level and RBC and platelet counts.

CONTRAINDICATIONS & CAUTIONS

Boxed Warning Use exposes patient and others to risk of opioid addiction, abuse, and misuse, which can lead to overdose and death. These effects can occur at any dose or duration. Assess patient risk before prescribing and regularly reassess patient for these behaviors and conditions. ∎

Boxed Warning Prescribers are strongly encouraged to complete a REMS-compliant education program. Drug should be prescribed only by prescribers with knowledge of opioid use and ways to reduce associated risks. ∎

Boxed Warning *Opioid class warning:* Opioids should only be prescribed with benzodiazepines or other CNS depressants when alternative treatment options are inadequate, aren't expected to provide adequate analgesia, haven't been tolerated, or aren't expected to be tolerated. ∎

⭘ *Alert:* Immediate-release formulations shouldn't be used for an extended period unless pain remains severe enough to require an opioid analgesic and alternative treatment options are inadequate to treat pain.

⭘ *Alert:* Long-acting or extended-release formulations are indicated for severe, persistent pain for which extended treatment with a daily opioid analgesic is required and for which alternative treatment options are inadequate. Use isn't indicated for as-needed analgesia.

⭘ *Alert:* Patients are at increased risk for oversedation and respiratory depression if they snore or have a history of sleep apnea, haven't used opioids recently or are first-time opioid users, have increased opioid dosage requirements or opioid habituation, have received general anesthesia for longer lengths of time or received other sedating drugs, have preexisting pulmonary or cardiac disease, or have thoracic or other surgical incisions that may impair breathing. Monitor patients carefully.

- Contraindicated in patients hypersensitive to drug.
- Contraindicated in patients with known or suspected paralytic ileus, significant respiratory depression, or acute or severe bronchial asthma.

Reactions in bold italics are *life-threatening*.

• Use cautiously in older adults, in patients who are debilitated, and in those with head injury, increased ICP, brain tumor, impaired consciousness, seizures, asthma, COPD, prostatic hyperplasia, liver or kidney impairment, acute abdominal conditions, urethral stricture, hypothyroidism, Addison disease, and arrhythmias.

Boxed Warning Serious, life-threatening, or fatal respiratory depression may occur with use of extended-release oxycodone. Crushing, dissolving, or chewing extended-release tablets can cause rapid release and absorption of a potentially fatal dose of oxycodone. ■

✺ *Alert:* Use lowest effective dose for shortest period consistent with patient's treatment goals.

✺ *Alert:* Drug may lead to rare but serious decrease in adrenal gland cortisol production.

• Drug may cause decreased sex hormone levels with long-term use.

✺ *Alert:* Because risk of overdose increases as opioid dose increases, reserve titration to higher doses for patients in whom lower doses are ineffective and in whom expected benefits of higher opioid dose outweigh risks.

Boxed Warning Accidental ingestion of even one dose of drug, especially by children, can result in a fatal oxycodone overdose. ■

Dialyzable drug: Unknown.

⚠ *Overdose S&S:* CNS depression, respiratory depression, apnea, flaccid skeletal muscles, bradycardia, hypotension, circulatory collapse, cardiac arrest, respiratory arrest, death.

PREGNANCY-LACTATION-REPRODUCTION

✺ *Alert:* Carefully weigh risks and benefits of using drug during pregnancy.

Boxed Warning Prolonged use during pregnancy can result in neonatal opioid withdrawal syndrome, which may be life-threatening. It requires management with expert neonatology protocols. If prolonged use is needed, advise patient of risks and ensure availability of proper treatment. ■

• Studies during pregnancy are inadequate. Use only if potential benefit justifies fetal risk.

• Drug isn't recommended for use during or immediately before labor, as uterine contractions may be adversely affected.

• Naloxone should be available to reverse opioid-induced respiratory depression in the neonate.

• Drug appears in human milk. Breastfeeding isn't recommended.

• Long-term opioid use may cause secondary hypogonadism, which may lead to sexual dysfunction or infertility.

NURSING CONSIDERATIONS

Boxed Warning May cause life-threatening or fatal respiratory depression at any time during therapy. Monitor patient closely, especially when starting or increasing doses. Proper dosing and titration are essential to reduce risk. ■

Boxed Warning Routinely monitor all patients for opioid addiction, abuse, and misuse, which can lead to overdose and death. ■

✺ *Alert:* Carefully monitor vital signs, pain level, respiratory status, and sedation level in all patients receiving opioids, especially those receiving IV drugs (even when given postoperatively) and in patients with impaired consciousness or coma.

• Reassess patient's level of pain at least 15 and 30 minutes after administration.

• For full analgesic effect, give drug before patient has intense pain.

✺ *Alert:* Drug may cause opioid-induced hyperalgesia (OIH). Symptoms include increased pain level with opioid dose increase, decreased pain level with opioid dose reduction or pain from ordinarily nonpainful stimuli without underlying disease progression, opioid tolerance or withdrawal, or addictive behavior. If OIH is suspected, decrease opioid dose or switch patient to alternative opioid.

• Keep opioid antagonist (naloxone) and resuscitation equipment available.

✺ *Alert:* If patient is taking opioids with serotonergic drugs, watch for signs and symptoms of serotonin syndrome (agitation, hallucinations, rapid HR, fever, diaphoresis, shivering or shaking, muscle twitching or stiffness, trouble with coordination, nausea, vomiting, diarrhea), especially at start of treatment or with dosage increases. Signs and symptoms may occur within several hours of coadministration but may also occur later, especially after dosage increase. Discontinue opioid, serotonergic drug, or both if serotonin syndrome is suspected.

✺ *Alert:* Monitor for signs and symptoms of adrenal insufficiency (nausea, vomiting, loss of appetite, fatigue, weakness, dizziness, low BP). Perform diagnostic testing if adrenal insufficiency is suspected. If adrenal insufficiency is confirmed, treat with corticosteroids and wean patient off opioids, if appropriate.

Discontinue corticosteroids when clinically appropriate.

• Monitor patient for signs and symptoms of decreased sex hormone levels (low libido, erectile dysfunction, amenorrhea, infertility). If signs and symptoms occur, evaluate patient and obtain specimens for lab testing.

• Patient taking extended-release form around-the-clock may need to take immediate-release form for worsening of pain or prevention of incident or breakthrough pain.

• Single-drug oxycodone solution or tablets are especially useful for patients who shouldn't take aspirin or acetaminophen.

• Monitor patient's bladder and bowel patterns. Patient may need stimulant laxative because drug has a constipating effect.

Boxed Warning Drug is potentially addictive, even at recommended doses, especially if drug is misused. Chewing, crushing, snorting, or injecting it can lead to overdose and death. ■

• OxyCONTIN has been formulated to prevent immediate access to full-dose oxycodone by cutting, chewing, or breaking tablets. Attempts to dissolve tablets result in a gummy substance that can't be drawn up into a syringe or injected.

🚷 *Alert:* Don't stop drug abruptly; withdraw slowly and individualize gradual taper plan to prevent signs and symptoms of withdrawal, worsening of pain, and psychological distress in patient who is physically dependent. Refer to manufacturer's label for specific tapering instructions.

🚷 *Alert:* When tapering opioids, monitor patient closely for signs and symptoms of opioid withdrawal (restlessness, lacrimation, rhinorrhea, yawning, perspiration, chills, myalgia, mydriasis, irritability, anxiety, insomnia, backache, joint pain, weakness, abdominal cramps, anorexia, nausea, vomiting, diarrhea, increased BP or HR, increased respiratory rate), which may indicate a need to taper more slowly. Also monitor for suicidality, use of other substances, and mood changes.

• *Look alike–sound alike:* Don't confuse oxycodone with hydrocodone, OxyCONTIN, or oxymorphone. Don't confuse OxyCONTIN with MS Contin or oxybutynin, Roxicodone with Roxybond.

PATIENT TEACHING
Boxed Warning Counsel patient and caregiver on serious risks, safe use, and importance

of reading the medication guide with each prescription. ■

• Advise patient to take drug exactly as prescribed and to use lowest dose possible for shortest time needed.

• Inform patient that, for acute pain, drug may only be needed for a few days.

• Teach about safe disposal of unused drug.

• Warn patient that extended-release and long-acting formulations aren't to be taken on an "as needed" basis.

• Instruct patient to contact provider if prescribed dosage isn't controlling pain.

🚷 *Alert:* Warn patient to withhold drug and inform prescriber if pain level worsens, pain sensitivity increases, or new pain occurs after taking drug.

• Instruct patient to take drug before pain is intense.

• Explain assessment and monitoring process to patient and family. Instruct them to immediately report difficulty breathing or other signs or symptoms of a potential adverse opioid-related reaction.

• Tell patient to take drug with milk or after eating.

Boxed Warning Instruct patient or caregiver to keep drug out of reach of children because accidental ingestion of even one dose can result in a fatal oxycodone overdose. Advise them to immediately seek emergency medical help if accidental ingestion occurs. ■

🚷 *Alert:* Encourage patient to report all medications being taken, including prescription and OTC medications and supplements.

🚷 *Alert:* Caution patient to immediately report symptoms of serotonin syndrome, adrenal insufficiency, and decreased sex hormone levels.

• Caution patient who is ambulatory about getting out of bed or walking. Warn patient to avoid hazardous activities until drug's CNS effects are known.

• Inform patient that urine drug testing and review of state prescription drug monitoring program will be done periodically.

• Teach patient that naloxone may be prescribed with the opioid when beginning and renewing therapy to reduce risk of opioid overdose and death.

🚷 *Alert:* Counsel patient who has been regularly taking drug not to discontinue without first discussing the need for gradual tapering with prescriber.

• Caution patient to report to prescriber pregnancy or plan to become pregnant.

oxyCODONE hydrochloride–acetaminophen
oks-i-KOE-done/a-seet-a-MIN-oh-fen

Endocet, Nalocet, Percocet, Prolate

Therapeutic class: Opioid analgesics
Pharmacologic class: Opioid agonists–
para-aminophenol derivatives
Controlled substance schedule: II

AVAILABLE FORMS
Oral solution: 5 mg oxycodone hydrochloride/325 mg acetaminophen, 10 mg oxycodone hydrochloride/300 mg acetaminophen per 5 mL
Tablets: 2.5 mg oxycodone hydrochloride/300 mg acetaminophen, 2.5 mg oxycodone hydrochloride/325 mg acetaminophen, 5 mg oxycodone hydrochloride/300 mg acetaminophen, 5 mg oxycodone hydrochloride/325 mg acetaminophen, 7.5 mg oxycodone hydrochloride/300 mg acetaminophen, 7.5 mg oxycodone hydrochloride/325 mg acetaminophen, 10 mg oxycodone hydrochloride/300 mg acetaminophen, 10 mg oxycodone hydrochloride/325 mg acetaminophen

INDICATIONS & DOSAGES
➤ **Pain severe enough to require an opioid analgesic and for which alternative treatments are inadequate**
Adults: Initial dose is based on oxycodone content; maximum daily dose based on acetaminophen content. Oxycodone 2.5 to 10 mg and acetaminophen 300 or 325 mg PO every 6 hours PRN for pain. Adjust dosage based on pain severity and patient response. Maximum daily doses shouldn't exceed 60 mg oxycodone and 4 g acetaminophen.
Adjust-a-dose: Consider decreased dosage in patients with kidney or liver impairment, older adults, and patients overly sensitive to effects of opioids. Gradually taper dosage if therapy lasts for more than a few weeks.

ADMINISTRATION
PO
- Give drug without regard to food.
- Give oral solution with an accurate measuring device (calibrated oral syringe or measuring cup).
- Store at room temperature.

ACTION
Oxycodone binds with opioid receptors in the CNS, altering perception of and emotional response to pain. Acetaminophen is thought to produce analgesia by inhibiting prostaglandin and other substances that sensitize pain receptors. The combination reduces pain more effectively than acetaminophen alone.

Route	Onset	Peak	Duration
PO (aceta-minophen)	<1 hr	10–60 min	4–6 hr
PO (oxy-codone)	10–15 min	30 min–1 hr	3–6 hr

Half-life: Acetaminophen, 1.25 to 3 hours; oxycodone, 3.5 to 4 hours.

ADVERSE REACTIONS
CNS: paresthesia, hypoesthesia, dizziness, drowsiness, fatigue, headache, dysphoria, euphoria, insomnia. **CV:** peripheral edema, flushing. **EENT:** dry mouth. **GI:** nausea, vomiting, constipation, dyspepsia, diarrhea. **GU:** dysuria. **Hematologic:** *hemolytic anemia, neutropenia, pancytopenia, thrombocytopenia.* **Hepatic:** increased liver enzyme levels. **Respiratory:** cough, *apnea, respiratory depression.* **Skin:** pruritus, rash, erythema, erythematous dermatitis, excoriation.

INTERACTIONS
Drug-drug. *Anticholinergics (atropine, dicyclomine, scopolamine):* May increase risk of paralytic ileus. Monitor patient closely.
Boxed Warning *Benzodiazepines, CNS depressants:* May cause slow or difficult breathing, sedation, and death. Avoid use together. If use together is necessary, limit dosage and duration of each drug to minimum necessary for desired effect. ∎
Beta blockers (propranolol): May inhibit acetaminophen metabolism. Use together carefully.
Boxed Warning *CYP3A4 inducers (carbamazepine, phenytoin, rifampin):* May increase oxycodone level and cause oxycodone-related adverse reactions if inducer is discontinued. Taper inducers cautiously and adjust oxycodone dosage as needed. ∎
Boxed Warning *CYP3A4 inhibitors (such as azole antifungals [ketoconazole]):* May increase oxycodone level, increase or prolong adverse effects, and cause fatal respiratory depression. Carefully monitor patient over extended period and adjust oxycodone dosage as needed. ∎

Desmopressin: May increase desmopressin-related toxicity. Monitor therapy.
Diuretics: May reduce effect of diuretic. Monitor therapy.
General anesthetics, neuromuscular blockers: May increase CNS depression. Use together cautiously, decreasing dosage of one or both agents.
Lamotrigine, zidovudine: May decrease effects of these drugs. Use together cautiously.
Mixed opioid agonist-antagonist combinations: May decrease effects of oxycodone and precipitate withdrawal. Use together carefully.
Oral contraceptives: May decrease acetaminophen level and half-life. Use together cautiously.
Probenecid: May increase effectiveness of acetaminophen. Use together cautiously.
⚠ *Alert: Serotonergic drugs (amoxapine, antiemetics [dolasetron, granisetron, ondansetron, palonosetron], antimigraine drugs, buspirone, cyclobenzaprine, dextromethorphan, linezolid, lithium, MAO inhibitors, maprotiline, methylene blue, mirtazapine, nefazodone, SNRIs, SSRIs, TCAs, trazodone, tryptophan, vilazodone):* May increase risk of serotonin syndrome. Use together cautiously, and monitor patient for serotonin syndrome.
Drug-herb. *Cannabinoid-containing products, kava:* May enhance adverse effects of CNS depressants. Monitor therapy carefully.
⚠ *Alert: St. John's wort:* May increase risk of serotonin syndrome and decrease oxycodone level. Warn patient to use together cautiously.
Drug-lifestyle. **Boxed Warning** *Alcohol use:* May cause slow or difficult breathing, sedation, and death. Discourage use together. ■

EFFECTS ON LAB TEST RESULTS
• May increase potassium, amylase, bilirubin, and liver enzyme levels.
• May increase or decrease blood glucose level.
• May decrease platelet count.
• May cause cross-reactivity with urinary assays used to detect cocaine and marijuana.
• Acetaminophen may cause false-positive result for urinary 5-hydroxyindoleacetic acid.

CONTRAINDICATIONS & CAUTIONS
Boxed Warning Use exposes patient and others to risk of opioid addiction, abuse, and misuse, which can lead to overdose and death. These effects can occur at any dose or duration.

Assess patient risk before prescribing and regularly reassess patient for these behaviors and conditions. ■
Boxed Warning Prescribers are strongly encouraged to complete a REMS-compliant education program. Drug should be prescribed only by prescribers with knowledge of opioid use and ways to reduce associated risks. ■
• Contraindicated in patients hypersensitive to components of drug and in those with significant respiratory depression, acute or severe bronchial asthma, hypercarbia, or known or suspected GI obstruction, including paralytic ileus.
Boxed Warning Acetaminophen may increase risk of acute liver failure, liver transplant, and death. Liver injury is generally associated with use of acetaminophen at doses exceeding 4,000 mg/day and the use of more than one acetaminophen-containing product. ■
⚠ *Alert:* Use lowest effective dose for shortest period consistent with patient's treatment goals.
⚠ *Alert:* Because risk of overdose increases as opioid dose increases, reserve titration to higher doses for patients in whom lower doses are ineffective and in whom expected benefits of higher opioid dose outweigh risks.
Boxed Warning Accidental ingestion of even one dose of an opioid, especially by children, can result in a fatal overdose. ■
Boxed Warning *Opioid class warning:* Opioids should only be prescribed with benzodiazepines or other CNS depressants when alternative treatment options are inadequate, aren't expected to provide adequate analgesia, haven't been tolerated, or aren't expected to be tolerated. ■
⚠ *Alert:* Immediate-release formulations shouldn't be used for an extended period unless pain remains severe enough to require an opioid analgesic and alternative treatment options are inadequate to treat pain.
⚠ *Alert:* Patients are at increased risk for oversedation and respiratory depression if they snore or have a history of sleep apnea, haven't used opioids recently or are first-time opioid users, have increased opioid dosage requirements or opioid habituation, have received general anesthesia for longer lengths of time or received other sedating drugs, have preexisting pulmonary or cardiac disease, or have thoracic or other surgical incisions that may impair breathing.

Reactions in bold italics are *life-threatening*.

⟳ *Alert:* May cause serious, potentially fatal skin reactions, including SJS, TEN, and acute generalized exanthematous pustulosis. Reaction may occur with first or subsequent use of acetaminophen.

⟳ *Alert:* Drug may lead to rare but serious decrease in adrenal gland cortisol production.

• Drug may cause decreased sex hormone levels with long-term use.

• Use cautiously in patients with increased sensitivity to codeine; head injury; increased ICP; intracranial lesions; seizures; alcohol use disorder; delirium tremens; biliary disease, including pancreatitis; liver disease; COPD; preexisting respiratory impairment; or cor pulmonale.

• Use cautiously in patients with acute abdominal conditions because this drug may obscure diagnostic signs or markedly increase respiratory depression or CSF pressure.

• Use cautiously in patients who are hypotensive, in older adults, in patients who are debilitated, and in those with kidney or liver impairment, hypothyroidism, urethral stricture, or Addison disease.

• Safety and effectiveness in children haven't been established.

Dialyzable drug: Oxycodone, unknown; acetaminophen, yes.

⚠ *Overdose S&S: Oxycodone:* Pinpoint pupils; respiratory depression; loss of consciousness; somnolence; stupor; coma; skeletal muscle flaccidity; cold, clammy skin; bradycardia; hypotension; apnea; circulatory collapse; cardiac arrest; death. *Acetaminophen:* Nausea; vomiting; general malaise; diaphoresis; liver necrosis; renal tubular necrosis; hypoglycemic coma; coagulation defects.

PREGNANCY-LACTATION-REPRODUCTION

⟳ *Alert:* Opioids cross the placenta. Carefully weigh risks and benefits of using drug during pregnancy.

Boxed Warning Prolonged use during pregnancy can result in neonatal opioid withdrawal syndrome, which may be life-threatening. It requires management with expert neonatology protocols. If prolonged use is needed, advise patient of risks and ensure availability of proper treatment. ∎

• Don't use immediately before labor.

• Use during breastfeeding isn't recommended. Monitor infants exposed to drug for excess sedation and respiratory depression.

NURSING CONSIDERATIONS

Boxed Warning May cause life-threatening or fatal respiratory depression at any time during therapy. Monitor patient closely, especially when starting or increasing doses. Proper dosing and titration are essential to reduce risk. ∎

• Initiate dosing regimen for each patient individually, taking into account patient's severity of pain, patient response, prior analgesic treatment experience, and risk factors for addiction, abuse, and misuse.

Boxed Warning Regularly monitor all patients for opioid addiction, abuse, and misuse, which can lead to overdose and death. ∎

⟳ *Alert:* Carefully monitor vital signs, pain level, respiratory status, and sedation level in all patients receiving opioids, especially those receiving IV drugs, even those given postoperatively.

⟳ *Alert:* Drug may cause opioid-induced hyperalgesia (OIH). Symptoms include increased pain level with opioid dose increase, decreased pain level with opioid dose reduction or pain from ordinarily nonpainful stimuli without underlying disease progression, opioid tolerance or withdrawal, or addictive behavior. If OIH is suspected, decrease opioid dose or switch patient to alternative opioid.

• Keep opioid antagonist (naloxone) and resuscitation equipment available.

⟳ *Alert:* If patient is taking opioids with serotonergic drugs, watch for signs and symptoms of serotonin syndrome (agitation, hallucinations, rapid HR, fever, diaphoresis, shivering or shaking, muscle twitching or stiffness, trouble with coordination, nausea, vomiting, diarrhea), especially at start of treatment and at dosage increases. Signs and symptoms may occur within several hours of coadministration but may also occur later, especially after dosage increase. Discontinue opioid, serotonergic drug, or both if serotonin syndrome is suspected.

⟳ *Alert:* Monitor patient for signs and symptoms of adrenal insufficiency (nausea, vomiting, loss of appetite, fatigue, weakness, dizziness, low BP). Perform diagnostic testing if adrenal insufficiency is suspected. If adrenal insufficiency is confirmed, treat with corticosteroids and wean patient off opioids, if appropriate. Discontinue corticosteroids when clinically appropriate.

• Monitor patient for signs and symptoms of decreased sex hormone levels (low libido,

O

erectile dysfunction, amenorrhea, infertility). If signs and symptoms occur, evaluate patient and obtain specimens for lab testing.

• Monitor for reddening of skin, rash, blisters, and detachment of upper surface of skin. Stop drug immediately for suspected skin reaction.

• Monitor for orthostatic hypotension.

• Carefully monitor patient with a head injury. Oxycodone's effects on pupillary response and consciousness may mask worsening of neurologic status.

• Carefully monitor patient with an acute abdominal condition. Drug may mask signs and symptoms.

• Observe for seizures in patient with convulsive disorder.

• Monitor bowel motility postoperatively, especially after intra-abdominal surgery.

⊕ **Alert:** Don't stop drug abruptly; withdraw slowly and individualize gradual taper plan to prevent signs and symptoms of withdrawal, worsening of pain, and psychological distress in patients who are physically dependent. Refer to manufacturer's label for specific tapering instructions.

⊕ **Alert:** When tapering opioids, monitor closely for signs and symptoms of opioid withdrawal (restlessness; lacrimation; chills; perspiration; rhinorrhea; yawning; myalgia; mydriasis; irritability; anxiety; insomnia; backache; joint pain; weakness; abdominal cramps; anorexia; nausea; vomiting; diarrhea; increased BP, HR, or respiratory rate), which may indicate a need to taper more slowly. Also monitor for suicidality, use of other substances, and mood changes.

• *Look alike–sound alike:* Don't confuse oxycodone and acetaminophen with hydrocodone and acetaminophen. Don't confuse Percocet with Fioricet.

PATIENT TEACHING

Boxed Warning Counsel patient and caregiver on serious risks, safe use, and importance of reading the medication guide with each prescription. ∎

Boxed Warning Caution patient or caregiver of patient taking an opioid with a benzodiazepine, CNS depressant, or alcohol to seek immediate medical attention if patient experiences dizziness, light-headedness, extreme sleepiness, slowed or difficult breathing, or unresponsiveness. ∎

Boxed Warning Teach patient to look for acetaminophen on labels of all prescriptions and OTC medications being taken and to not use more than one product containing acetaminophen. Warn patient to seek medical attention if acetaminophen intake exceeds 4,000 mg/day, even if feeling well. ∎

• Advise patient to take drug exactly as prescribed and to use lowest dose possible for shortest time needed.

• Inform patient that, for acute pain, drug may only be needed for a few days.

• Teach about safe disposal of unused drug.

• Instruct patient to contact health care provider if prescribed dosage isn't controlling pain.

• Explain assessment and monitoring process to patient and family. Instruct them to immediately report difficulty breathing or other signs or symptoms of a potential adverse opioid-related reaction.

Boxed Warning Instruct patient or caregiver to keep drug out of reach of children because accidental ingestion of even one dose can result in a fatal oxycodone overdose. Advise them to immediately seek emergency medical help if accidental ingestion occurs. ∎

⊕ **Alert:** Warn patient to withhold drug and inform prescriber if pain level worsens, pain sensitivity increases, or new pain occurs after taking drug.

⊕ **Alert:** Encourage patient to report all medications being taken, including prescription and OTC medications and supplements.

⊕ **Alert:** Caution patient to immediately report signs and symptoms of serotonin syndrome, adrenal insufficiency, and decreased sex hormone levels.

⊕ **Alert:** Warn patient to stop drug and seek medical attention immediately if rash or reaction occurs while using acetaminophen.

• Advise patient not to drive a car or operate heavy machinery while taking this drug.

• Caution patient to report to prescriber pregnancy or plan to become pregnant.

• Warn patient who is breastfeeding not to use drug because it can cause toxicity (sleepiness, difficulty breastfeeding, breathing difficulties, limpness) in infants.

• Teach patient that naloxone may be prescribed with the opioid when beginning and renewing therapy to reduce risk of opioid overdose and death.

⊕ **Alert:** Counsel patient who has been regularly taking drug not to discontinue without first discussing the need for gradual tapering with prescriber.

Reactions in bold italics are *life-threatening*.

oxyMORphone hydrochloride
oks-i-MOR-fone

Therapeutic class: Opioid analgesics
Pharmacologic class: Opioids
Controlled substance schedule: II

AVAILABLE FORMS
Tablets (extended-release): 5 mg, 7.5 mg,
10 mg, 15 mg, 20 mg, 30 mg, 40 mg
Tablets (immediate-release): 5 mg, 10 mg

INDICATIONS & DOSAGES
Adjust-a-dose (for all indications): For
older adults and patients with Child-Pugh
Class A liver impairment or CrCl less than
50 mL/minute, start with lowest possible dose
and slowly increase as tolerated. For patients
receiving CNS depressants, begin at one-third
to one-half of usual dose.

Refer to manufacturer's product information for instructions about converting from
other formulations or opioids.

➤ **Acute pain severe enough to require an
opioid analgesic and for which alternative
treatments are inadequate**
Adults: 10 to 20 mg immediate-release PO
every 4 to 6 hours. Adjust dosage based on
pain severity, prior analgesic experience, and
patient response.

➤ **Chronic pain severe enough to require
daily, around-the-clock, long-term opioid
treatment and for which alternative treatments are inadequate**
Adults: 5 mg extended-release PO every 12 hours.
Adjust dosage based on pain severity, prior
analgesic experience and patient response.

ADMINISTRATION
PO
• Give 1 hour before or 2 hours after a meal.
Boxed Warning Have patient swallow
extended-release tablets whole to avoid ex-
posure to a potentially fatal dose of drug. ∎

ACTION
May bind with opioid receptors in the CNS,
altering perception of and emotional response
to pain.

Route	Onset	Peak	Duration
PO	Varies	Varies	Varies

Half-life: Immediate-release, 7 to 9 hours;
extended-release, 9 to 11 hours.

ADVERSE REACTIONS
CNS: dizziness, headache, sedation, fatigue,
lethargy, drowsiness, somnolence, fever, dysphoria, light-headedness, confusion, anxiety,
insomnia, depression. **CV:** HTN, hypotension, tachycardia, flushing, edema. **EENT:**
blurred vision, dry mouth. **GI:** constipation,
nausea, vomiting, diarrhea, abdominal pain,
decreased appetite, dyspepsia, flatulence,
abdominal distention. **GU:** urine retention.
Metabolic: weight loss, dehydration. **Respiratory:** *hypoxia,* dyspnea. **Skin:** diaphoresis,
pruritus.

INTERACTIONS
Drug-drug. *Anticholinergics (dicyclomine,
scopolamine):* May increase risk of urine retention or severe constipation, leading to paralytic ileus. Monitor patient for abdominal
pain or distention.
Boxed Warning *Benzodiazepines, CNS
depressants:* May cause slow or difficult
breathing, sedation, and death. Avoid use together. If use together can't be avoided, limit
dosage and duration of each drug to minimum
needed for desired effect. ∎
Cimetidine, muscle relaxants: May increase
respiratory depression. Monitor patient
closely.
Diuretics: May decrease diuretic effect. Monitor therapy.
Eluxadoline: May increase constipation.
Avoid combination.
MAO inhibitors: May cause severe opioid potentiation. Don't use opioids if patient has received MAO inhibitors within 14 days. Avoid
combination.
*Mixed agonist or antagonist, partial ago-
nist opioid analgesics (buprenorphine, nalbuphine, pentazocine):* May reduce analgesic
effect or precipitate withdrawal symptoms.
Don't use together.
Propofol: May increase bradycardia risk.
Monitor ECG closely.
⊘ Alert: *Serotonergic drugs (amoxapine,
antiemetics [dolasetron, granisetron, ondansetron, palonosetron], antimigraine
drugs, buspirone, cyclobenzaprine, dextromethorphan, linezolid, lithium, MAO inhibitors, maprotiline, methylene blue, mirtazapine, nefazodone, SNRIs, SSRIs, TCAs,
trazodone, tryptophan, vilazodone):* May increase risk of serotonin syndrome. Use together cautiously, and monitor patient for
serotonin syndrome.

Drug-herb. *Cannabinoid-containing products, kava:* May enhance adverse effects of CNS depressants. Monitor therapy closely.

⚠ *Alert: St. John's wort:* May increase risk of serotonin syndrome. Warn patient to use together cautiously, and monitor patient for serotonin syndrome.

Drug-lifestyle. **Boxed Warning** *Alcohol use:* May cause slow or difficult breathing, sedation, and death. Discourage use together. ∎

EFFECTS ON LAB TEST RESULTS
• May increase amylase and prolactin levels.

CONTRAINDICATIONS & CAUTIONS
Boxed Warning Prescribers are strongly encouraged to complete a REMS-compliant education program. Drug should be prescribed only by prescribers with knowledge of opioid use and ways to reduce associated risks. ∎

• Contraindicated in patients hypersensitive to drug; in those with acute or severe bronchial asthma in an unmonitored setting or in the absence of resuscitative equipment, severe respiratory depression, upper airway obstruction, or GI obstruction, including paralytic ileus; and in those with Child-Pugh class B or C liver impairment.

Boxed Warning Use exposes patient and others to risk of opioid addiction, abuse, and misuse, which can lead to overdose and death. These effects can occur at any dose or duration. Assess patient risk before prescribing and regularly reassess patient for these behaviors and conditions. ∎

⚠ *Alert:* Use lowest effective dose for shortest period consistent with patient's treatment goals.

⚠ *Alert:* Because risk of overdose increases as opioid dose increases, reserve titration to higher doses for patients in whom lower doses are ineffective and in whom expected benefits of higher opioid dose outweigh risks.

Boxed Warning *Opioid class warning:* Opioids should only be prescribed with benzodiazepines or other CNS depressants when alternative treatment options are inadequate, aren't expected to provide adequate analgesia, haven't been tolerated, or aren't expected to be tolerated. ∎

⚠ *Alert:* Immediate-release formulations shouldn't be used for an extended period unless pain remains severe enough to require an opioid analgesic and alternative treatment options are inadequate to treat pain.

⚠ *Alert:* Long-acting and extended-release formulations are indicated for severe, persistent pain for which extended treatment with a daily opioid analgesic is required and for which alternative treatment options are inadequate. Use isn't indicated for as-needed analgesia.

Boxed Warning Accidental ingestion of even one dose of an opioid, especially by children, can result in a fatal overdose. ∎

⚠ *Alert:* Drug may lead to rare but serious decrease in adrenal gland cortisol production.

• Drug may cause decreased sex hormone levels with long-term use.

⚠ *Alert:* Patients are at increased risk for oversedation and respiratory depression if they snore or have a history of sleep apnea, haven't used opioids recently or are first-time opioid users, have increased opioid dosage requirements or opioid habituation, have received general anesthesia for longer lengths of time or received other sedating drugs, have preexisting pulmonary or cardiac disease, or have thoracic or other surgical incisions that may impair breathing. Monitor patients carefully.

• Use cautiously in older adults, in patients who are debilitated, and in those with head injury, increased ICP, seizures, asthma, COPD, acute abdominal conditions, biliary tract disease (including pancreatitis), acute alcoholism, delirium tremens, prostatic hyperplasia, kidney or liver impairment, urethral stricture, respiratory depression, hypothyroidism, Addison disease, or arrhythmias.

Dialyzable drug: Unknown.

⚠ *Overdose S&S:* Miosis, CNS depression, respiratory depression, apnea, flaccid skeletal muscles, bradycardia, hypotension, circulatory collapse, cardiac arrest, respiratory arrest, death.

PREGNANCY-LACTATION-REPRODUCTION
• Opioids cross the placental barrier. During pregnancy, use minimum effective dose and only if benefit justifies fetal risk.

• Use cautiously during labor as drug may affect uterine contractions and fetal HR.

Boxed Warning Prolonged use during pregnancy can result in neonatal opioid withdrawal syndrome, which may be life-threatening. It requires management with expert neonatology protocols. If prolonged use is needed, advise patient of risks and ensure availability of proper treatment. ∎

Reactions in bold italics are *life-threatening*.

❸ *Alert:* Closely monitor neonate whose mother received opioid analgesics during labor for signs and symptoms of respiratory depression. A specific opioid antagonist, such as naloxone or nalmefene, should be available for reversal of opioid-induced respiratory depression in a neonate.

• Use cautiously during breastfeeding. Use lowest dose for shortest duration. Monitor infants for apnea and sedation.

• Chronic use may increase risk of infertility.

NURSING CONSIDERATIONS

• Keep opioid antagonist (naloxone) and resuscitation equipment available.

Boxed Warning May cause life-threatening or fatal respiratory depression at any time during therapy. Monitor patient closely, especially when starting or increasing doses. Proper dosing and titration are essential to reduce risk. ■

Boxed Warning Regularly monitor all patients for opioid addiction, abuse, and misuse, which can lead to overdose and death. ■

❸ *Alert:* Drug may cause opioid-induced hyperalgesia (OIH). Symptoms include increased pain level with opioid dose increase, decreased pain level with opioid dose reduction or pain from ordinarily nonpainful stimuli without underlying disease progression, opioid tolerance or withdrawal, or addictive behavior. If OIH is suspected, decrease opioid dose or switch patient to alternative opioid.

❸ *Alert:* If patient is taking opioids with serotonergic drugs, watch for signs and symptoms of serotonin syndrome (agitation, hallucinations, rapid HR, fever, diaphoresis, shivering or shaking, muscle twitching or stiffness, trouble with coordination, nausea, vomiting, diarrhea), especially at start of treatment or after dosage increases. Signs and symptoms may occur within several hours of coadministration but may also occur later, especially after dosage increase. Discontinue opioid, serotonergic drug, or both if serotonin syndrome is suspected.

❸ *Alert:* Monitor for signs and symptoms of adrenal insufficiency (nausea, vomiting, loss of appetite, fatigue, weakness, dizziness, low BP). Perform diagnostic testing if adrenal insufficiency is suspected. If adrenal insufficiency is confirmed, treat with corticosteroids and wean patient off opioids, if appropriate. Discontinue corticosteroids when clinically appropriate.

• Monitor patient for signs and symptoms of decreased sex hormone levels (low libido, erectile dysfunction, amenorrhea, infertility). If signs and symptoms occur, evaluate patient and obtain specimens for lab testing.

• Use of drug may worsen gallbladder pain.

• Monitor bladder and bowel function. Administer a stimulant laxative as ordered.

❸ *Alert:* Don't stop drug abruptly; individualize slow taper plan to prevent signs and symptoms of withdrawal, worsening of pain, and psychological distress in patients who are physically dependent. Refer to manufacturer's label for specific tapering instructions.

❸ *Alert:* When tapering opioids, monitor patients closely for signs and symptoms of opioid withdrawal (restlessness; lacrimation; rhinorrhea; yawning; perspiration; chills; myalgia; mydriasis; irritability; anxiety; insomnia; backache; joint pain; weakness; abdominal cramps; anorexia; nausea; vomiting; diarrhea; increased BP, HR, or respiratory rate), which may indicate a need to taper more slowly. Also monitor for suicidality, use of other substances, and mood changes.

• *Look alike–sound alike:* Don't confuse oxymorphone with hydromorphone, oxymetholone, or oxycodone.

PATIENT TEACHING

Boxed Warning Counsel patient and caregiver on serious risks, safe use, and importance of reading the medication guide with each prescription. ■

• Encourage patient to report all medications being taken, including prescription and OTC medications and supplements.

• Advise patient to take drug exactly as prescribed and to use lowest dose possible for shortest time needed.

• Inform patient that, for acute pain, drug may only be needed for a few days.

• Teach about safe disposal of unused drug.

• Warn patient that extended-release formulations aren't to be taken on an "as needed" basis.

• Instruct patient to contact health care provider if prescribed dosage isn't controlling pain.

❸ *Alert:* Caution patient to immediately report signs and symptoms of serotonin syndrome, adrenal insufficiency, and decreased sex hormone levels.

❸ *Alert:* Warn patient to withhold drug and inform prescriber if pain level worsens, pain

---

♣Canada   ◇OTC   ◆Off-label use   ⊕Do not crush   *Liquid contains alcohol   ⅜Genetic sensitivity increases, or new pain occurs after taking drug.

• Instruct patient to ask for drug before pain is intense.

• Explain the assessment and monitoring process to patient and family. Instruct them to immediately report difficulty breathing or other signs of a potential adverse opioid-related reaction.

• Instruct patient not to share oxymorphone with others and to take steps to protect oxymorphone from theft or misuse.

• Caution patient who is ambulatory about getting out of bed or walking. Warn outpatient to avoid driving and other hazardous activities that require mental alertness until CNS effects are known.

Boxed Warning Instruct patient to keep tablets in a child-resistant container in a safe place out of reach of children. Accidental ingestion of even one dose by a child can result in death. In case of accidental ingestion, immediately seek emergency medical help. ■

• Teach patient that naloxone may be prescribed with the opioid when beginning and renewing therapy to reduce risk of opioid overdose and death.

• Caution patient to report to prescriber pregnancy or plan to become pregnant.

🔵 *Alert:* Counsel patient who has been regularly taking drug not to discontinue without first discussing the need for gradual tapering with prescriber.

SAFETY ALERT!

oxytocin (synthetic injection)
oks-i-TOE-sin

Pitocin

Therapeutic class: Oxytocics
Pharmacologic class: Exogenous hormones

AVAILABLE FORMS
Injection: 10 units/mL

INDICATIONS & DOSAGES
➤ **To induce or stimulate labor**
Adults: Initially, 0.5 to 1 milliunit/minute IV infusion. Increase rate by 1 to 2 milliunits/minute at 30- to 60-minute intervals until normal contraction pattern is established. Decrease rate when labor is

firmly established. Rates exceeding 9 to 10 milliunits/minute are rarely required.
➤ **To reduce postpartum bleeding after expulsion of placenta**
Adults: 10 to 40 units IV infused at rate needed to sustain uterine contraction and control uterine atony. Or, 10 units IM after delivery of placenta.
➤ **Incomplete, inevitable, or elective abortion**
Adults: 10 units IV infusion at 10 to 20 milliunits (20 to 40 drops)/minute. Don't exceed 30 units in 12 hours.

ADMINISTRATION
IV
▼ Never give drug simultaneously by more than one route.
▼ To induce or stimulate labor, dilute drug by adding 10 units to 1 L of NSS or lactated Ringer solution.
▼ To produce intense uterine contractions and reduce postpartum bleeding, dilute drug by adding 10 to 40 units to 1,000 mL of NSS or lactated Ringer solution.
▼ To treat abortion, add 10 units to 500 mL NSS or D₅W.
▼ Don't give bolus injection; use an infusion pump. Give drug only by piggyback infusion so that it may be stopped without interrupting IV line.
▼ **Incompatibilities:** None listed by manufacturer. Consult drug compatibility reference for more information.
IM
• Drug isn't recommended for routine IM use, but 10 units may be given IM after delivery of placenta to control postpartum uterine bleeding.
• Never give drug simultaneously by more than one route.

ACTION
Causes potent and selective stimulation of uterine and mammary gland smooth muscle.

Route	Onset	Peak	Duration
IV	1 min	Unknown	1 hr
IM	3–5 min	Unknown	2–3 hr

Half-life: 1 to 6 minutes.

ADVERSE REACTIONS
Maternal
CNS: *subarachnoid hemorrhage, seizures, coma.* **CV:** *arrhythmias,* HTN, PVCs,

---

Reactions in bold italics are *life-threatening*.

hypotension, tachycardia. **GI:** nausea, vomiting. **GU:** *abruptio placentae,* tetanic uterine contractions, *postpartum hemorrhage, uterine rupture,* impaired uterine blood flow, pelvic hematoma, increased uterine motility. **Hematologic:** *afibrinogenemia, possibly related to postpartum bleeding; pelvic hematoma.* **Other:** *anaphylaxis, death from oxytocin-induced water intoxication,* hypersensitivity reactions.

Fetal or neonatal

CNS: *brain damage, seizures.* **CV:** *bradycardia, arrhythmias,* PVCs. **EENT:** neonatal retinal hemorrhage. **Hepatic:** jaundice. **Other:** *low Apgar score at 5 minutes, death.*

INTERACTIONS
Drug-drug. *Carboprost tromethamine:* May enhance adverse effect of oxytocin. Avoid use together.

Cyclopropane anesthetics: May cause bradycardia and hypotension. Use together cautiously.

Dinoprostone: May enhance oxytocic effects of oxytocin. Use together isn't recommended. If used sequentially, closely monitor uterine activity. Administer oxytocin 30 minutes after removing dinoprostone vaginal insert and 6 to 12 hours after application of dinoprostone gel.

Drugs that prolong QT interval (azithromycin, clofazimine, ondansetron): May increase risk of life-threatening cardiac arrhythmias, including torsades de pointes. Use together cautiously.

Misoprostol: May increase oxytocin adverse effects. Avoid use together.

Vasoconstrictors: May cause severe HTN if oxytocin is given within 3 to 4 hours of vasoconstrictor in patient receiving caudal block anesthetic. Avoid use together.

EFFECTS ON LAB TEST RESULTS
None reported.

CONTRAINDICATIONS & CAUTIONS
• Contraindicated in patients hypersensitive to drug.

• Contraindicated when vaginal delivery isn't advised (placenta previa, vasa previa, invasive cervical carcinoma, genital herpes, prolapsed cord), when cephalopelvic disproportion is present, or when delivery requires conversion, as in transverse lie.

• Contraindicated in fetal distress when delivery isn't imminent, in prematurity, in other

obstetric emergencies, and in patients with severe toxemia or hypertonic uterine patterns.

• Use cautiously, if at all, in patients with invasive cervical cancer and in those with previous cervical or uterine surgery (including cesarean section), grand multiparity, uterine sepsis, traumatic delivery, or overdistended uterus.

🚫 *Alert:* May cause antidiuretic effect and risk of severe water intoxication, seizures, or death, particularly with large doses or when given by slow infusion over 24 hours and if patient is receiving fluids by mouth.

Dialyzable drug: Unknown.

⚠ *Overdose S&S:* Uterine hypersensitivity, tumultuous labor, uterine rupture, cervical and vaginal lacerations, postpartum hemorrhage, uteroplacental hypoperfusion, variable deceleration of fetal HR, fetal hypoxia, hypercapnia, perinatal liver necrosis, water intoxication, seizures, death.

PREGNANCY-LACTATION-REPRODUCTION
Boxed Warning Drug is only indicated for medical, rather than elective, induction of labor. ■

• Use cautiously during first and second stages of labor because tetanic contraction, uterine hypertonicity, cervical laceration, uterine rupture, and maternal and fetal death have been reported.

• Drug isn't expected to cause fetal abnormalities when used as indicated. Use cautiously during pregnancy and breastfeeding. Administration of exogenous oxytocin may disrupt initiation of breastfeeding.

NURSING CONSIDERATIONS
🚫 *Alert:* All patients receiving oxytocin IV must be under continuous observation by trained personnel who have a thorough knowledge of the drug and are qualified to identify complications.

🚫 *Alert:* Immediately discontinue oxytocin infusion if uterine hyperactivity or fetal distress occurs. Administer oxygen to patient. Patient and fetus must be evaluated by the responsible physician.

• Use drug to induce or reinforce labor only when pelvis is known to be adequate, when vaginal delivery is indicated, when fetal maturity is assured, and when fetal position is favorable. Use drug only in hospital where critical care facilities and prescriber are immediately available.

- Monitor fluid intake and output. Antidiuretic effect may lead to fluid overload, seizures, and coma from water intoxication.
- Monitor and record uterine contractions, HR, BP, intrauterine pressure, fetal HR, and blood loss at least every 15 minutes.

PATIENT TEACHING
- Teach about proper drug administration and handling.
- Instruct patient to promptly report adverse reactions (site irritation, nausea, bleeding, blurred vision, difficulty speaking, itching, wheezing, swelling, heartbeat that doesn't feel normal, trouble passing urine, bad belly pain, or weakness on one side of body).

SAFETY ALERT!

PACLitaxel (conventional)
pac-li-TAKS-el

Therapeutic class: Antineoplastics
Pharmacologic class: Taxoids

AVAILABLE FORMS
Injection: 30 mg/5 mL, 100 mg/16.7 mL, 300 mg/50 mL vials

INDICATIONS & DOSAGES
Adjust-a-dose (for all indications): Refer to manufacturer's instructions for toxicity-related and liver impairment dosage adjustments and management. Treatment isn't recommended if transaminase levels are $10 \times$ ULN or greater or bilirubin levels are greater than $5 \times$ ULN for 3-hour infusion, or if transaminase levels are $10 \times$ ULN or greater or bilirubin levels are greater than 7.5 mg/dL for 24-hour infusion.
➤ **AIDS-related Kaposi sarcoma**
Adults: 135 mg/m² IV over 3 hours every 3 weeks, or 100 mg/m² IV over 3 hours every 2 weeks.
Adjust-a-dose: Reduce dexamethasone dose for premedication to 10 mg PO.
➤ **First-line and subsequent therapy for advanced ovarian cancer**
Adults (previously untreated): 175 mg/m² IV over 3 hours every 3 weeks, followed by cisplatin 75 mg/m²; or 135 mg/m² IV over 24 hours every 3 weeks, followed by cisplatin 75 mg/m² every 3 weeks.

Adults (previously treated): 135 or 175 mg/m² IV over 3 hours every 3 weeks.
➤ **Metastatic or relapsed breast cancer**
Adults: 175 mg/m² IV over 3 hours every 3 weeks.
➤ **Adjuvant treatment of node-positive breast cancer**
Adults: 175 mg/m² IV over 3 hours every 3 weeks for four cycles given after completion of a doxorubicin-containing combination chemotherapy.
➤ **First treatment of advanced NSCLC in patients who aren't candidates for curative surgery or radiation**
Adults: 135 mg/m² IV infusion over 24 hours, followed by cisplatin 75 mg/m². Repeat cycle every 3 weeks.

ADMINISTRATION
IV
⚕ *Alert:* Hazardous drug; use safe handling and disposal precautions.
Boxed Warning To reduce risk or severity of hypersensitivity, patients must receive pretreatment with diphenhydramine, H_2-receptor antagonists, and corticosteroids. Fatal reactions have occurred despite premedication. ∎
▼ Prepare and store infusion solutions in glass containers or polypropylene bottles, or use polypropylene or polyolefin bags. Undiluted concentrate shouldn't contact polyvinyl chloride IV bags or tubing.
▼ Dilute concentrate before infusion. Compatible solutions include NSS for injection, D_5W, 5% dextrose in NSS for injection, and 5% dextrose in lactated Ringer injection. Dilute to yield 0.3 to 1.2 mg/mL. Diluted solutions are stable for 27 hours at room temperature. Prepared solution may appear hazy.
▼ Give through polyethylene-lined administration sets, and use an in-line 0.22-micron filter.
⚕ *Alert:* Watch for irritation and infiltration; extravasation can cause tissue damage and necrosis. Administration of hyaluronidase may be needed.
▼ Closely monitor patient and vital signs during infusion, especially during first hour.
⚕ *Alert:* When indicated, cisplatin dose should follow paclitaxel dose.
▼ **Incompatibilities:** Y-site incompatibilities: amiodarone, amphotericin B cholesteryl sulfate, amphotericin conventional, amphotericin B liposomal, chlorpromazine,

diazepam, digoxin, gemtuzumab ozogamicin, hydroxyzine, idarubicin, indomethacin, labetalol, methylprednisolone sodium succinate, phenytoin, propranolol. Consult a drug incompatibility reference for additional information.

ACTION

Prevents depolymerization of cellular microtubules, inhibiting normal reorganization of microtubule network needed for mitosis and other vital cellular functions.

Route	Onset	Peak	Duration
IV	Unknown	Unknown	Unknown

Half-life: 13.1 to 52.7 hours.

ADVERSE REACTIONS

CNS: peripheral neuropathy, asthenia, fever. **CV:** *bradycardia,* tachycardia, HTN, hypotension, edema, flushing, abnormal ECG, *arrhythmias,* syncope, *venous thrombosis.* **GI:** nausea, vomiting, diarrhea, mucositis. **Hematologic:** *neutropenia, leukopenia, thrombocytopenia,* anemia, *bleeding.* **Hepatic:** elevated LFT values. **Musculoskeletal:** myalgia, arthralgia. **Respiratory:** dyspnea. **Skin:** alopecia, diaphoresis, rash, injection-site reaction, nail changes. **Other:** hypersensitivity reactions, *anaphylaxis,* infections.

INTERACTIONS

Drug-drug. *Cisplatin:* May cause additive myelosuppressive effects. Give paclitaxel before cisplatin to increase paclitaxel clearance. *CYP2C8 and CYP3A4 inducers (carbamazepine, phenobarbital):* May decrease paclitaxel level. Monitor therapy.
CYP2C8 and CYP3A4 inhibitors (clarithromycin, cyclosporine, dexamethasone, diazepam, etoposide, felodipine, ketoconazole, quinidine, retinoic acid, teniposide, testosterone, verapamil, vincristine): May increase paclitaxel level. Monitor patient for toxicity.
Doxorubicin: May increase plasma levels of doxorubicin and its active metabolite, doxorubicinol. Use together cautiously.
Live-virus vaccines: May increase risk of vaccine-induced adverse reactions. Use together isn't recommended. Patients with malignancies who are in remission can receive live-virus vaccines 3 months after completion of chemotherapy.

EFFECTS ON LAB TEST RESULTS

• May increase ALP, ALT, AST, and bilirubin levels.
• May decrease Hb level and neutrophil, WBC, and platelet counts.

CONTRAINDICATIONS & CAUTIONS

• Contraindicated in patients hypersensitive to drug or other drugs formulated with polyoxyethylated castor oil.
Boxed Warning Anaphylaxis and severe hypersensitivity reactions can occur. Permanently discontinue drug if such hypersensitivity reactions occur. ∎
Boxed Warning Contraindicated in those with solid tumors with baseline neutrophil counts below 1,500/mm^3, or in those with AIDS-related Kaposi sarcoma with baseline neutrophil counts below 1,000/mm^3. ∎
• Use cautiously in patients with liver impairment.
• Use cautiously in older adults, who may be at higher risk for severe adverse effects.
• Safety and effectiveness in children haven't been determined.
Dialyzable drug: No.
⚠ *Overdose S&S:* Bone marrow suppression, sensory neurotoxicity, mucositis, acute ethanol toxicity (in children), CNS toxicity (in children).

PREGNANCY-LACTATION-REPRODUCTION

• Drug may cause fetal harm. Patients should avoid pregnancy and male patients shouldn't father a child during therapy.
• Drug may appear in human milk. Patient should discontinue breastfeeding or discontinue drug, considering importance of drug to patient.
• Drug may affect fertility.

NURSING CONSIDERATIONS

Boxed Warning Administer drug under supervision of prescriber experienced with cancer chemotherapeutic agents and when adequate diagnostic and treatment facilities are readily available to manage complications. ∎
• Patient may experience peripheral neuropathies, which may be cumulative and dose related. Patients with severe symptoms may need dosage reduction.
Boxed Warning Monitor blood counts before and during therapy. Bone marrow toxicity is the most common and dose-limiting

toxicity. Institute bleeding precautions, as indicated. ■
• Monitor vital signs closely during infusion, especially during the first hour.
• Monitor infusion site for extravasation.
• If patient develops significant cardiac conduction abnormalities, use indicated therapy and continuous cardiac monitoring during therapy and subsequent infusions.
• *Look alike–sound alike:* Don't confuse paclitaxel with paroxetine or with paclitaxel protein-bound particles.

PATIENT TEACHING
• Advise patient to report any pain or burning at site of injection.
• Urge patient to report fever, sore throat, fatigue, easy bruising, nosebleeds, bleeding gums, or melena. Tell patient to take temperature daily.
• Instruct patient to immediately report trouble breathing; swelling of face, lips, tongue, or throat; trouble swallowing; hives; or rash.
• Teach patient to report tingling or burning sensation or numbness in limbs immediately.
• Warn patient that reversible hair loss will probably occur.
• Caution patient of childbearing potential to avoid pregnancy or breastfeeding during therapy. Recommend consulting prescriber before becoming pregnant.
• Counsel male patient not to father a child during therapy.

SAFETY ALERT!

PACLitaxel protein-bound particles
pac-li-TAKS-el

Abraxane

Therapeutic class: Antineoplastics
Pharmacologic class: Taxoids

AVAILABLE FORMS
Lyophilized powder for injection: 100 mg in single-use vials

INDICATIONS & DOSAGES
Adjust-a-dose (for all indications): Don't give to patients with serum bilirubin level more than 5 × ULN or AST level more than 10 × ULN. Refer to manufacturer's instructions for toxicity-related dosage adjustments.

➤ **Metastatic breast cancer after failure of combination chemotherapy or relapse within 6 months of adjuvant chemotherapy (previous therapy should have included an anthracycline unless clinically contraindicated)**
Adults: 260 mg/m² IV over 30 minutes every 3 weeks.
Adjust-a-dose: For patients with serum bilirubin level greater than 1.5 to 5 × ULN and AST level less than 10 × ULN, recommended dosage is 200 mg/m²/dose initially; may increase dosage to 260 mg/m²/dose in subsequent courses if patient tolerates reduced dosage for two cycles.
➤ **NSCLC as first-line treatment in combination with carboplatin in patients who aren't candidates for curative surgery or radiation therapy**
Adults: 100 mg/m² IV over 30 minutes on days 1, 8, and 15 of each 21-day cycle. Give carboplatin immediately after paclitaxel protein-bound particles dose on day 1 of each 21-day cycle. Refer to manufacturer's instructions for carboplatin dosage.
Adjust-a-dose: For patients with serum bilirubin level greater than 1.5 to 5 × ULN and AST level less than 10 × ULN, recommended dosage is 80 mg/m²/dose; may increase dosage to 100 mg/m²/dose in subsequent courses if patient tolerates reduced dosage for two cycles.
➤ **Metastatic pancreatic adenocarcinoma as first-line treatment in combination with gemcitabine**
Adults: 125 mg/m² IV over 30 to 40 minutes on days 1, 8, and 15 of each 28-day cycle. Give gemcitabine IV immediately after each dose of paclitaxel protein-bound particles. Refer to manufacturer's instructions for gemcitabine dosage.
Adjust-a-dose: Drug isn't recommended for patients with serum bilirubin level greater than 1.5 and AST level less than 10 × ULN; or with serum bilirubin level more than 5 × ULN or AST level more than 10 × ULN.

ADMINISTRATION
IV
⊕ *Alert:* Hazardous drug; use safe handling and disposal precautions.
▼ Reconstitute the vial with 20 mL of NSS to yield 5 mg/mL of drug. Direct the stream slowly, over at least 1 minute, onto the inside wall of the vial to avoid foaming. Let the

---

*Reactions in bold italics are **life-threatening**.*

vial sit for 5 minutes to ensure proper wetting of the powder. Gently swirl or turn the vial for at least 2 minutes until completely dissolved. If foaming occurs, let the solution stand for 15 minutes for the foam to subside. If particles are visible, gently invert the vial again to ensure complete resuspension. The solution should appear milky and uniform. Inject the correct dose into an empty polyvinyl chloride-type IV bag and use immediately.

▼ Visually inspect reconstituted suspension in IV bag for proteinaceous strands, particulate matter, or discoloration before administration; discard suspension if present.

▼ Give drug over 30 minutes (breast cancer and NSCLC) or over 30 to 40 minutes (pancreatic adenocarcinoma).

▼ The suspension for infusion, when prepared in an infusion bag, can be stored at 36° to 46° F (2° to 8° C), protected from bright light, for up to 24 hours.

▼ Store unopened vials at room temperature in the original package. Store reconstituted vials at 36° to 46° F (2° to 8° C) for up to 24 hours, protected from light.

▼ The total combined refrigerated storage time of reconstituted solution in vial and infusion bag is 24 hours. This may be followed by storage in infusion bag at ambient temperature and lighting conditions for a maximum of 4 hours.

▼ **Incompatibilities:** None listed by manufacturer. Consult a drug compatibility reference for more information.

ACTION
Prevents depolymerization of cellular microtubules, inhibiting reorganization of the microtubule network and disrupting mitosis and other vital cell functions.

Route	Onset	Peak	Duration
IV	Unknown	Unknown	Unknown

Half-life: 13 to 27 hours.

ADVERSE REACTIONS
CNS: asthenia, depression, peripheral neuropathy, headache, fatigue, sensory neuropathy, fever, dysgeusia. **CV:** abnormal ECG, edema, HTN, hypotension, *severe CV event, bleeding.* **EENT:** visual disturbances, epistaxis, macular edema. **GI:** anorexia, diarrhea, nausea, constipation, oral candidiasis, vomiting, mucositis. **GU:** increased

creatinine level, UTI. **Hematologic:** anemia, *neutropenia, thrombocytopenia, myelosuppression.* **Hepatic:** increased liver enzyme levels. **Metabolic:** dehydration, *hypokalemia.* **Musculoskeletal:** arthralgia, myalgia. **Respiratory:** cough, dyspnea, pneumonia, respiratory tract infection, pneumonitis. **Skin:** alopecia, rash, injection-site reactions. **Other:** infections, hypersensitivity reactions, *sepsis.*

INTERACTIONS
Drug-drug. *Clozapine:* May increase risk of agranulocytosis. Avoid use together.
CYP2C8 and CYP3A4 inducers (carbamazepine, phenobarbital): May decrease paclitaxel level. Use cautiously together.
CYP2C8 and CYP3A4 inhibitors (clarithromycin, cyclosporine, dexamethasone, ketoconazole, verapamil): May increase paclitaxel level. Use cautiously together.
Live-virus vaccines: May increase vaccine-related adverse effects. Avoid use together. Don't give vaccines for at least 3 months after immunosuppressants.
Vaccines (inactivated): May diminish vaccine effectiveness. Monitor therapy.

EFFECTS ON LAB TEST RESULTS
• May increase ALP, AST, bilirubin, creatinine, and GGT levels.
• May decrease Hb level and neutrophil and platelet counts.

CONTRAINDICATIONS & CAUTIONS
Boxed Warning Contraindicated in patients with baseline neutrophil count of less than 1,500/mm³. ■
• Contraindicated in patients hypersensitive to drug or its components; severe and sometimes fatal hypersensitivity reactions can occur. Don't rechallenge patients who experience a hypersensitivity reaction.
• Use cautiously in patients hypersensitive to other taxanes; cross-hypersensitivity can occur.
• Use cautiously in patients with liver impairment; increased exposure and toxicity can occur.
• Use isn't recommended in patients with metastatic pancreatic adenocarcinoma who have total bilirubin greater than 1.5 × ULN and AST of 10 × ULN or more.
• Use hasn't been studied in patients with creatinine level less than 30 mL/minute.

P

• Drug contains human albumin; although rare, viruses and Creutzfeldt-Jakob disease may be transmitted.

• Safety and effectiveness in children haven't been established.

Dialyzable drug: Unknown.

⚠ **Overdose S&S:** Bone marrow suppression, sensory neurotoxicity, mucositis.

PREGNANCY-LACTATION-REPRODUCTION

• Drug may cause fetal harm. Patients of childbearing potential should avoid pregnancy during therapy and for at least 6 months after final dose. Males shouldn't father a child during therapy and for at least 3 months after final dose.

• Drug may impair fertility.

• Drug appears in human milk. Patient shouldn't breastfeed during therapy and for 2 weeks after final dose.

NURSING CONSIDERATIONS

◑ *Alert:* Give only under supervision of practitioner experienced in using chemotherapy in a facility that can manage associated complications.

◑ *Alert:* Don't substitute Abraxane for other forms of paclitaxel.

Boxed Warning Monitor CBC frequently to evaluate for neutropenia, which may be severe and may result in infection. ■

• Don't repeat dose until neutrophil count recovers to more than 1,500/mm³ and platelet count recovers to more than 100,000/mm³.

• Obtain CBC before dosing on day 1 for metastatic breast cancer and before days 1, 8, and 15 for NSCLC or pancreatic cancer.

• If patient becomes febrile regardless of ANC, initiate treatment with broad-spectrum antibiotics.

• Watch for pneumonitis in patients receiving drug in combination with gemcitabine. Interrupt treatment for suspected pneumonitis (sudden onset of dry, persistent cough; dyspnea). For confirmed pneumonitis, permanently discontinue treatment with paclitaxel and gemcitabine.

• Assess for severe hematologic, neurologic, cutaneous, or GI toxicities, which may require dosage reductions or drug discontinuation.

• Monitor patient for hypersensitivity reactions; don't rechallenge patients with severe reactions.

• Assess patient for symptoms of sensory neuropathy and severe neutropenia.

• Monitor LFT and kidney function test results.

• Monitor infusion site closely for extravasation and infiltration.

• Verify pregnancy status before treatment.

PATIENT TEACHING

• Warn patient that alopecia commonly occurs but is reversible after therapy.

• Teach patient to recognize signs of neuropathy, such as tingling, burning, and numbness in arms and legs.

• Tell patient to report signs and symptoms of infection, pneumonitis, hypersensitivity reactions, severe abdominal pain, or severe diarrhea.

• Advise patient to contact prescriber if nausea and vomiting persist or interfere with adequate nutrition. Reassure patient that an antiemetic can be prescribed.

• Explain that many patients experience weakness and fatigue, so it's important to rest.

• To reduce or prevent mouth sores, remind patient to perform proper oral hygiene.

• Tell patient to avoid pregnancy during therapy and for at least 6 months after final dose and not to breastfeed during therapy and for 2 weeks after final dose.

• Advise male patient to avoid fathering a child during therapy and for at least 3 months after final dose.

• Inform patient of reproductive potential that drug may impair fertility.

SAFETY ALERT!

palbociclib ⚕
pal-boe-SYE-klib

Ibrance

Therapeutic class: Antineoplastics
Pharmacologic class: Kinase inhibitors

AVAILABLE FORMS
Capsules ⦿: 75 mg, 100 mg, 125 mg
Tablets ⦿: 75 mg, 100 mg, 125 mg

INDICATIONS & DOSAGES
➤ **Hormone receptor (HR)-positive, HER2-negative advanced or metastatic breast cancer, as initial endocrine-based therapy, in combination with an aromatase inhibitor, or in combination with**

fulvestrant in patients with disease progression after endocrine therapy ⚕

Adult males or adult females who are postmenopausal: 125 mg PO daily for 21 consecutive days followed by 7 days off to complete a cycle of 28 days.

When given with an aromatase inhibitor, refer to prescribing information for the inhibitor being used. For males treated in combination with an aromatase inhibitor, consider treatment with a luteinizing hormone-releasing hormone (LHRH) agonist.

When given with fulvestrant, recommended dosage of fulvestrant is 500 mg PO on days 1, 15, and 29, and once monthly thereafter; refer to full prescribing information for fulvestrant. Patients who are premenopausal and perimenopausal treated with the combination of palbociclib and fulvestrant should be treated with LHRH agonist according to current standards.

Adjust-a-dose: For patients with Child-Pugh class C liver impairment, decrease dosage to 75 mg PO daily. If concomitant use of strong CYP3A inhibitors is unavoidable, decrease palbociclib dosage to 75 mg daily. If strong inhibitor is discontinued, increase palbociclib dosage after three to five half-lives have passed from CYP3A inhibitor dose. Refer to manufacturer's instructions for toxicity-related dosage adjustments.

ADMINISTRATION

PO

🛑 *Alert:* Hazardous drug; use safe handling and disposal precautions.

• Give tablets without regard to food.
• Give capsules whole with food.
• Have patients swallow capsules and tablets whole; don't crush, break, or open before they are swallowed. Capsules or tablets shouldn't be ingested if they are broken, cracked, or otherwise not intact.
• If patient vomits after taking a dose or misses a dose, give the next prescribed dose at usual time.

ACTION

Inhibits cyclin-dependent kinase 4 and 6. Reduces cellular proliferation of ER-positive breast cancer cell line by blocking progression of cell from G_1 to S phase of cell cycle, resulting in decreased phosphorylation and decreased tumor growth.

Route	Onset	Peak	Duration
PO	N/A	4–12 hr	N/A

Half-life: 24 to 34 hours.

ADVERSE REACTIONS

CNS: asthenia, fatigue, fever, taste alteration. **EENT:** blurred vision, dry eyes, increased tearing, epistaxis. **GI:** decreased appetite, stomatitis, nausea, diarrhea, vomiting. **Hematologic:** *neutropenia, leukopenia,* anemia, *thrombocytopenia.* **Hepatic:** increased transaminase levels. **Skin:** alopecia, rash, dry skin. **Other:** infections.

INTERACTIONS

Drug-drug. *Alfentanil, cyclosporine, dihydroergotamine, ergotamine, everolimus, fentanyl, midazolam, pimozide, quinidine, sirolimus, tacrolimus:* May increase levels of these drugs. Dosages of these drugs may need to be decreased.

Strong or moderate CYP3A inducers (carbamazepine, rifampin, phenytoin): May decrease palbociclib level. Avoid concurrent use.

Strong CYP3A inhibitors (clarithromycin, itraconazole, ritonavir): May increase palbociclib level. Avoid use together; if unavoidable, decrease palbociclib dosage.

Drug-herb. *St. John's wort:* May decrease palbociclib level. Discourage use together.

Drug-food. *Grapefruit, grapefruit juice:* May increase palbociclib level. Discourage use together.

EFFECTS ON LAB TEST RESULTS

• May increase ALT and AST levels.
• May decrease Hb level and WBC, neutrophil, lymphocyte, and platelet counts.

CONTRAINDICATIONS & CAUTIONS

• Contraindicated in patients hypersensitive to drug or its components.

🛑 *Alert:* May cause severe or fatal ILD and pneumonitis.

• May cause neutropenia and increase risk of infection.
• Drug hasn't been studied in children.
• Use cautiously in older adults, who may have greater sensitivity to drug's effects.

Dialyzable drug: Unknown.

P

PREGNANCY-LACTATION-REPRODUCTION
- Drug can cause fetal harm. Patients of childbearing potential should use effective contraception during treatment and for at least 3 weeks after final dose.
- Patients shouldn't breastfeed during treatment and for 3 weeks after final dose.
- Male patients with partners of childbearing potential should use effective contraception during treatment and for 3 months after final dose.
- Drug may cause infertility in males. Patients should consider sperm preservation before treatment.

NURSING CONSIDERATIONS
- Monitor CBC before start of therapy, at beginning of each cycle, on day 15 of first two cycles, and as clinically indicated. Interrupt therapy and adjust dosage as necessary.
- Monitor patient for myelosuppression or infection; treat appropriately.
- Verify pregnancy status before treatment.
- ❸ *Alert:* Monitor patients for new or worsening pulmonary symptoms; if they occur, interrupt therapy immediately and evaluate patient. If infection, neoplasm, and other causes are excluded, permanently discontinue treatment in patients with severe ILD or pneumonitis.

PATIENT TEACHING
- ❸ *Alert:* Warn patient to immediately report difficulty or discomfort with breathing or shortness of breath while at rest or with low activity; these may be symptoms of ILD or pneumonitis.
- Instruct patient in safe drug administration and handling.
- Teach patient to report signs and symptoms of decreased bone marrow function and infection (fever, chills, shortness of breath, weakness, abnormal bleeding or bruising).
- Instruct patient to tell prescriber of all medications being taken, including prescription and OTC drugs and herbal products.
- Caution patient to avoid grapefruit and grapefruit juice.
- Advise patient of fetal risk and to use effect contraception.
- Inform male patient of reproductive potential of infertility risk.

paliperidone
pal-ee-PER-i-done

Invega

paliperidone palmitate
Invega Hafyera, Invega Sustenna, Invega Trinza

Therapeutic class: Antipsychotics
Pharmacologic class: Benzisoxazole derivatives

AVAILABLE FORMS
Injection: 39 mg/0.25 mL, 78 mg/0.5 mL, 117 mg/0.75 mL, 156 mg/mL, 234 mg/1.5 mL, 273 mg/0.88 mL, 410 mg/1.32 mL, 546 mg/1.75 mL, 819 mg/2.63 mL, 1,092 mg/3.5 mL; 1,560 mg/5 mL single-dose prefilled syringe
Tablets (extended-release) ⒹⒼ: 1.5 mg, 3 mg, 6 mg, 9 mg

INDICATIONS & DOSAGES
Adjust-a-dose (for all indications): In patients with CrCl of 50 to less than 80 mL/minute, initial dosage is 3 mg PO once daily and maximum dosage is 6 mg once daily; in patients with CrCl of 10 to 49 mL/minute, initial dosage is 1.5 mg PO once daily and maximum dosage is 3 mg once daily; in patients with CrCl less than 10 mL/minute, use isn't recommended. If using injectable form (Invega Sustenna) and CrCl is 50 to less than 80 mL/minute, give 156 mg IM on day 1 and 117 mg IM on day 8, followed by monthly injections of 78 mg IM. If using injectable 3-month form (Invega Trinza) and CrCl is 50 to less than 80 mL/minute, adjust dosage and stabilize patient using the monthly IM injection, then transition to the 3-month IM injection. Invega Trinza isn't recommended in patients with CrCl of less than 50 mL/minute. Invega Hafyera isn't recommended in patients with CrCl less than 90 mL/minute.
➤ **Schizophrenia and schizoaffective disorder**
Adults: 6 mg PO once daily in the morning; may increase or decrease dose in 3-mg increments not sooner than every 4 days in schizoaffective disorder or every 5 days in schizophrenia to a range of 3 to 12 mg daily; maximum dose is 12 mg/day. Or, 234 mg IM on treatment day 1 and 156 mg IM on day 8,

both administered in deltoid muscle. Recommended maintenance dosage for schizophrenia is 117 mg IM monthly. Adjustments may be made monthly based on tolerability and efficacy using available strengths. Maximum recommended monthly dose, 234 mg. See manufacturer's instructions for missed dosage schedules.

➤ **Schizophrenia**

Adults: Use 3-month IM paliperidone (Invega Trinza) only after monthly IM paliperidone (Invega Sustenna) has been established as adequate treatment for at least 4 months. The last two doses of monthly IM paliperidone should be the same dosage strength before starting 3-month IM paliperidone. Initiate 3-month IM paliperidone with next scheduled monthly IM paliperidone. Base 3-month dose on the previous monthly dose, using the equivalent 3.5 times higher dose. May adjust dosage of 3-month paliperidone every 3 months in increments ranging from 273 to 819 mg based on response and tolerability.

Use 6-month IM paliperidone (Invega Hafyera) only after monthly IM paliperidone (Invega Sustenna) has been established as adequate treatment for at least 4 months and at same dosage for at least 2 months, or after 3-month IM paliperidone (Invega Trinza) has been established as adequate treatment for at least one 3-month cycle. Initiate with the next scheduled once-a-month injection, or up to 1 week before or after, or with the next scheduled every-3-month injection, or up to 2 weeks before or after. Base dosage on dosage of previous product. If last dose of once-a-month product was 156 mg, give 1,092 mg of 6-month product; if last dose of once-a-month product was 234 mg, give 1,560 mg of 6-month product. If last dose of 3-month product was 546 mg, give 1,092 mg of 6-month product; if last dose of 3-month product was 819 mg, give 1,560 mg of 6-month product.

Because of long-acting nature of Invega Trinza and Invega Hafyera, patient's response to adjusted dose may not be apparent for several months. See manufacturer's instructions for missed dosage schedules.

Adolescents ages 12 to 17: Initially, 3 mg PO daily. May increase dosage by 3 mg/day every 5 days based on clinical response. Maximum dose is 12 mg/day for patients weighing 51 kg or more and 6 mg/day for patients weighing less than 51 kg.

ADMINISTRATION
PO
• Have patient swallow tablets whole; don't crush or break tablets.
• May be given without regard for food.
IM
• Inspect for particulate matter and discoloration.
• Don't give IV or subcut.
• For Invega Sustenna, shake syringe vigorously for at least 10 seconds to ensure a homogenous suspension before administration. Only use needle provided in kit.
• For Invega Trinza, shake syringe vigorously for at least 15 seconds within 5 minutes of administration.
• For Invega Hafyera, shake syringe vigorously for at least 15 seconds, rest briefly, then shake again for 15 seconds within 5 minutes of administration.
• For Invega Trinza or Invega Hafyera, use the thin-wall needles provided. Don't use needles from the 1-month pack or other commercially available needles, to reduce the risk of blockage.
• Inject slowly and deeply into deltoid or gluteal muscle.
• Injection is for single use only. Don't administer dose in divided injections.
• Administer first two doses of Invega Sustenna into deltoid muscle. After second dose, can give monthly maintenance doses in deltoid or gluteal muscle.
• If incomplete administration occurs, don't reinject the dose remaining in the syringe. Don't administer another dose.
• Alternate injection sites at each administration.
• May give monthly or 3-month IM paliperidone maintenance doses within 7 days before or after next monthly dose date.
• Refer to manufacturer's instructions for missed dose management and switching from other antipsychotics.
• Store at room temperature.

ACTION
Exact mechanism remains unclear. May antagonize both central dopamine (D_2) and serotonin type 2 receptors, as well as alpha$_1$, alpha$_2$, and H_1 receptors. Drug is a major active metabolite of risperidone.

P

Route	Onset	Peak	Duration
PO	Unknown	24 hr	Unknown
IM (Sustenna)	1 day	13 days	126 days
IM (Trinza)	1 day	30–33 days	Up to 18 months
IM (Hafyera)	1 day	29–32 days	Up to 18 months

Half-life: 23 hours (oral); 25 to 49 days (IM, monthly, Sustenna), 84 to 139 days (IM, 3-monthly, Trinza); 148 to 159 days (IM, Hafyera).

ADVERSE REACTIONS

CNS: headache, somnolence, agitation, anxiety, asthenia, dizziness, dystonia, extrapyramidal symptoms, fatigue, lethargy, nightmares, psychosis, fever, sedation, sleep disorder, insomnia. **CV:** HTN, orthostatic hypotension, edema, palpitations, sinus arrhythmia, *bradycardia,* tachycardia, *AV block,* bundle-branch block. **EENT:** blurred vision, eye movement disorder, epistaxis, nasopharyngitis, rhinitis, dry mouth, sialorrhea, sore throat, tongue paralysis, swollen tongue. **GI:** abdominal pain, dyspepsia, nausea, vomiting, diarrhea, constipation, increased or decreased appetite. **GU:** amenorrhea, irregular menses, decreased libido, erectile dysfunction, UTI. **Metabolic:** blood insulin increases, hyperprolactinemia, weight gain. **Musculoskeletal:** back pain, pain, musculoskeletal stiffness; muscle spasms of head, neck, and spine. **Respiratory:** cough, URI. **Skin:** pruritus, rash, injection-site reaction. **Other:** breast tenderness, gynecomastia, galactorrhea, hypersensitivity reactions.

INTERACTIONS

❶ *Alert:* Paliperidone can significantly interact with many drugs. Consult a drug interaction resource or pharmacist for additional information.
Drug-drug. *Antihypertensives, drugs that induce hypotension:* May worsen orthostatic hypotension. Monitor patient closely.
Centrally acting drugs: May worsen CNS adverse effects. Use cautiously together.
Divalproex sodium, valproate: Increases paliperidone level. Consider paliperidone dosage reduction.
Drugs that prolong QTc interval, such as antiarrhythmics (amiodarone, procainamide, quinidine, sotalol), antipsychotics (chlorpromazine, thioridazine), quinolone antibiotics (moxifloxacin): May further prolong QTc interval. Avoid using together.

Levodopa, other dopamine agonists: May antagonize effects of these drugs. Use cautiously together.
Opioid agonists: Opioids may cause slow or difficult breathing, sedation, and death. Avoid use together. If use together is necessary, limit dosage and duration of each drug to minimum necessary for desired effect.
Risperidone: May increase toxic effects of paliperidone. Avoid use together.
Serotonin modulators: May increase risk of NMS and serotonin syndrome. Monitor therapy.
Strong CYP3A and P-gp inducers (carbamazepine, rifampin): May decrease paliperidone level. Dosage may need to be increased or decreased depending on use. Avoid using inducers with extended-release IM formulation, if possible. If inducer is necessary, consider using paliperidone extended-release tablets.
Drug-herb. *St. John's wort:* May decrease serum level of paliperidone. Consider therapy modification.
Drug-lifestyle. *Alcohol use:* May worsen CNS side effects. Discourage use together.

EFFECTS ON LAB TEST RESULTS

• May increase blood glucose, blood insulin, lipid, and prolactin levels.
• May decrease HDL level.
• May decrease WBC count.

CONTRAINDICATIONS & CAUTIONS

• Contraindicated in patients hypersensitive to paliperidone or risperidone.
Boxed Warning Older adults with dementia-related psychosis treated with atypical or conventional antipsychotics are at increased risk for death. Antipsychotics aren't approved for treatment of dementia-related psychosis. ▮
• Avoid use in patients with congenital long QT syndrome or history of cardiac arrhythmias.
• Oral drug isn't recommended in patients with preexisting severe GI narrowing.
• Use cautiously in patients with history of seizures, conditions that lower seizure threshold, or Parkinson disease; in those at risk for aspiration pneumonia or impaired temperature regulation; and in those with bradycardia, hypokalemia, hypomagnesemia, CV disease, cerebrovascular disease, dehydration, or hypovolemia; and in older adults.
• Use cautiously in patients with diabetes or risk factors for diabetes (obesity, family history of diabetes).

Reactions in bold italics are *life-threatening*.

- Use cautiously in patients with history of suicidality.
- Somnolence, orthostatic hypotension, and motor and sensory instability may lead to falls and fall-related injuries.
- Rare cases of priapism (requiring surgery) have been reported.

Dialyzable drug: Unknown.

⚠ *Overdose S&S:* Extrapyramidal symptoms, unsteady gait, drowsiness, sedation, tachycardia, hypotension, prolonged QT interval.

PREGNANCY-LACTATION-REPRODUCTION
- Use in pregnancy only if potential benefit justifies fetal risk.
- Patients exposed to drug during pregnancy should enroll in the National Pregnancy Registry for Atypical Antipsychotics (1-866-961-2388 or online at https://womensmentalhealth.org/research/pregnancyregistry/atypicalantipsychotic/).
- *Alert:* Neonates exposed to antipsychotics during the third trimester are at increased risk for developing extrapyramidal signs and symptoms and withdrawal signs and symptoms after delivery.
- Drug appears in human milk. The known benefits of breastfeeding should outweigh the unknown risks of infant's exposure to paliperidone. Monitor infants exposed to drug for sedation, failure to thrive, jitteriness, tremors, and abnormal muscle movements.
- Drug may inhibit reproductive function because it increases prolactin levels.

NURSING CONSIDERATIONS
- Establish tolerability with oral paliperidone or oral risperidone before treating with paliperidone injection.
- *Alert:* Monitor patient for atypical ventricular tachycardia, such as torsades de pointes, and ECG changes, particularly lengthening of the QT interval.
- Obtain baseline BP before starting therapy, and monitor BP regularly. Watch for orthostatic hypotension.
- *Alert:* Watch for evidence of NMS, a rare but deadly complication.
- Monitor patient for tardive dyskinesia; it may disappear spontaneously or persist for life despite discontinuing drug. Seek smallest dosage and shortest duration of treatment that produce a clinical response.
- *Alert:* Drug may cause hyperglycemia, dyslipidemia, weight gain, and other metabolic changes. Monitor patient with diabetes regularly. In patient at risk for diabetes, obtain fasting blood glucose results at baseline and periodically.
- Monitor patient for seizure activity.
- Assess patient for dysphagia.
- Monitor patient for abnormal body temperature regulation, especially if patient exercises, is exposed to extreme heat, takes anticholinergics, or becomes dehydrated.
- Monitor patient for somnolence and sedation. Antipsychotics, including paliperidone, have the potential to impair judgment, thinking, or motor skills.
- Assess fall risk at start of treatment and recurrently during long-term therapy.
- Dispense lowest appropriate quantity of drug, to reduce risk of overdose.

PATIENT TEACHING
- Teach patient safe drug administration.
- Advise patient to seek immediate medical care for signs and symptoms of NMS (fever, muscle rigidity, altered mental status, irregular pulse or BP, tachycardia, diaphoresis, or cardiac arrhythmia).
- Caution patient or caregiver of patient taking an opioid with a benzodiazepine, CNS depressant, or alcohol to seek immediate medical attention if patient experiences dizziness, light-headedness, extreme sleepiness, slowed or difficult breathing, or unresponsiveness.
- Advise patient to avoid alcohol during therapy.
- Tell patient that remains of the tablet coating may appear in feces.
- Instruct patient not to perform activities that require mental alertness until effects of drug are known.
- Advise patient that drug may cause somnolence, orthostatic hypotension, and motor and sensory instability, which may lead to falls and fall-related injuries.
- Warn patient to use caution in performing excessively strenuous activities because body temperature may be disrupted.
- Advise patient that drug may lower BP and to change positions slowly.
- Inform patient with a preexisting low WBC count or a history of drug-induced leukopenia or neutropenia that CBC monitoring will be needed during therapy.
- Instruct patient to seek medical attention for amenorrhea, galactorrhea, erectile dysfunction, or gynecomastia.

• Advise patient to seek medical attention for an erection lasting more than 4 hours.
• Caution patient to contact prescriber before taking other drugs, to avoid potential interactions.
• Advise patient to report pregnancy or plans to breastfeed.

palonosetron hydrochloride
pal-oh-NOE-se-tron

Aloxi ✤

Therapeutic class: Antiemetics
Pharmacologic class: Selective serotonin (5-HT$_3$) receptor antagonists

AVAILABLE FORMS
Injection: 0.25 mg/2 mL, 0.25 mg/5 mL single-use vials; 0.25 mg/5-mL prefilled syringe

INDICATIONS & DOSAGES
➤ **Prevention of chemotherapy-induced nausea and vomiting (moderate and highly emetogenic regimens)**
Adults: 0.25 mg given IV over 30 seconds, 30 minutes before chemotherapy starts.
➤ **Prevention of chemotherapy-induced nausea and vomiting (including highly emetogenic chemotherapy)**
Children ages 1 month to younger than 17 years: Infuse 20 mcg/kg IV over 15 minutes beginning about 30 minutes before chemotherapy starts. Maximum dosage, 1.5 mg.
➤ **Prevention of postoperative nausea and vomiting (PONV) for up to 24 hours after surgery**
Adults: 0.075 mg IV over 10 seconds immediately before anesthesia induction.

ADMINISTRATION
IV
▼ Flush with NSS before and after injection.
▼ Inspect for particulate matter and discoloration; solution should be clear and colorless.
▼ Give by rapid IV injection through a peripheral or central IV line.
▼ Don't use prefilled syringe to give dose of less than 0.25 mg.
▼ Discard unused portion.
▼ Store at room temperature. Protect from light.
▼ **Incompatibilities:** Don't mix with other drugs.

ACTION
Antagonizes 5-HT$_3$ receptors in the GI tract and brain, which inhibits emesis caused by chemotherapy.

Route	Onset	Peak	Duration
IV	30 min	Unknown	5 days

Half-life: 40 hours (adults); 20 to 30 hours (children).

ADVERSE REACTIONS
CNS: dizziness, headache, weakness. **CV:** *bradycardia, prolonged QT interval (PONV).* **GI:** constipation, diarrhea. **GU:** urine retention.

INTERACTIONS
Drug-drug. *Antiarrhythmics or other drugs that prolong the QTc interval, diuretics that induce electrolyte abnormalities, high-dose anthracycline:* May increase risk of prolonged QTc interval. Use together cautiously.
Apomorphine: May cause profound hypotension and loss of consciousness. Use together is contraindicated.
Fentanyl, 5-HT$_3$ receptor antagonists, IV methylene blue, lithium, MAO inhibitors, mirtazapine, SNRIs, SSRIs, tramadol: May increase risk of serotonin syndrome. Avoid use together.

EFFECTS ON LAB TEST RESULTS
• May increase glucose, ALT, AST, and bilirubin levels.
• May increase or decrease potassium level.

CONTRAINDICATIONS & CAUTIONS
• Contraindicated in patients hypersensitive to palonosetron or its ingredients.
• Use cautiously in patients hypersensitive to other 5-HT$_3$ antagonists, in those taking drugs that affect cardiac conduction, and in those with cardiac conduction abnormalities, hypokalemia, or hypomagnesemia.
Dialyzable drug: Unlikely.

PREGNANCY-LACTATION-REPRODUCTION
• Studies during pregnancy are inadequate.
• Use in pregnancy only if clearly needed.
• It isn't known if drug appears in human milk. Consider risk of infant exposure when deciding to discontinue breastfeeding during therapy.

NURSING CONSIDERATIONS
• Before giving this drug, check patient's potassium level.

Reactions in bold italics are *life-threatening*.

• Consider adding corticosteroids to the antiemetic regimen, particularly for patients receiving highly emetogenic chemotherapy.
• Monitor patient for hypersensitivity reactions.
• Make sure patient has additional antiemetics for breakthrough nausea or vomiting.
• If patient has cardiac conduction abnormalities, assess ECG before giving drug.
• Monitor patient for serotonin syndrome (restlessness, hallucinations, loss of coordination, seizures, fast heartbeat, rapid changes in BP, increased body temperature, hyperreflexia, nausea, vomiting, diarrhea).

PATIENT TEACHING

• Instruct patient to seek immediate medical attention for signs or symptoms of hypersensitivity reaction.
• Advise patient to take a different antiemetic for breakthrough nausea or vomiting at the first sign of nausea rather than waiting until symptoms become severe.
• Inform patient of risk of serotonin syndrome and to seek immediate medical attention if signs or symptoms occur.
• Urge patient with a history of cardiac conduction abnormalities to report any changes in drug regimen, such as adding or stopping an antiarrhythmic.
• Instruct patient to report pregnancy or plans to become pregnant or to breastfeed.

pamidronate disodium
pa-mi-DROE-nate

Therapeutic class: Antiosteoporotics
Pharmacologic class: Bisphosphonates

AVAILABLE FORMS
Solution for injection: 3 mg/mL, 6 mg/mL, 9 mg/mL in 10-mL vials

INDICATIONS & DOSAGES
➤ **Moderate to severe hypercalcemia from cancer (with or without bone metastases)**
Adults: Dosage depends on severity of hypercalcemia. Correct calcium level for albumin. Corrected calcium (CCa) level is calculated using this formula:

$$\text{CCa} \atop (\text{mg/dL}) = \text{serum} \atop \text{calcium} \atop (\text{mg/dL}) + \text{0.8 (4 − serum} \atop \text{albumin)} \atop (\text{g/dL})$$

Give patients with CCa levels of 12 to 13.5 mg/dL 60 to 90 mg by IV infusion as a single dose over 2 to 24 hours. Give patients with CCa levels greater than 13.5 mg/dL 90 mg by IV infusion over 2 to 24 hours. Allow at least 7 days before retreatment to permit full response to first dose.
➤ **Moderate to severe Paget disease**
Adults: 30 mg IV as a 4-hour infusion on 3 consecutive days for total dose of 90 mg. Repeat cycle as needed.
➤ **Osteolytic bone metastases of breast cancer with standard antineoplastic therapy**
Adults: 90 mg IV infusion over 2 hours every 3 to 4 weeks.
Adjust-a-dose: Withhold treatment for creatinine 10% or more above baseline.
➤ **Osteolytic bone lesions of multiple myeloma**
Adults: 90 mg IV over 4 hours once monthly.
Adjust-a-dose: Withhold treatment for creatinine 10% or more above baseline.

ADMINISTRATION
IV
⚠ *Alert:* Hazardous drug; use safe handling and disposal precautions.
▼ Dilute solution in 250 mL (2-hour infusion), 500 mL (4-hour infusion), or 1,000 mL (up to 24-hour infusion) of half-NSS or NSS or D₅W for injection.
▼ Inspect solution for precipitate before use.
▼ Give drug only by IV infusion. Injecting a bolus may cause kidney toxicity.
▼ Infusions longer than 2 hours may reduce the risk of kidney toxicity, particularly in patients with preexisting kidney insufficiency.
▼ Diluted solution remains stable for 24 hours at room temperature.
▼ **Incompatibilities:** Calcium-containing infusion solutions, such as Ringer injection. Give in a line separate from all other drugs.

ACTION
An antihypercalcemic that inhibits resorption of bone but apparently not bone formation. Adsorbs to hydroxyapatite crystals in bone and may directly block calcium phosphate dissolution and mature osteoclast formation.

Route	Onset	Peak	Duration
IV	Unknown	Unknown	Unknown

Half-life: 21 to 35 hours.

ADVERSE REACTIONS

CNS: asthenia, fatigue, somnolence, fever, headache, psychosis, anxiety, insomnia, drowsiness, syncope, pain. **CV:** atrial fibrillation/flutter, tachycardia, HTN, edema, fluid overload, *HF.* **EENT:** sinusitis, rhinitis. **GI:** abdominal pain, anorexia, dyspepsia, constipation, diarrhea, nausea, stomatitis, vomiting, *GI hemorrhage.* **GU:** kidney dysfunction, UTI, uremia. **Hematologic:** *leukopenia, neutropenia, thrombocytopenia,* anemia. **Metabolic:** hypothyroidism, hypophosphatemia, *hypokalemia, hypomagnesemia, hypocalcemia.* **Musculoskeletal:** arthralgia, back pain, myalgia, skeletal pain, weakness. **Respiratory:** cough, dyspnea, pleural effusions, URI. **Skin:** infusion-site reaction, infusion-site pain. **Other:** metastases, candidiasis.

INTERACTIONS

Kidney-toxic drugs, thalidomide: May increase risk of kidney dysfunction. Use with caution.

EFFECTS ON LAB TEST RESULTS

- May increase creatinine level.
- May decrease phosphate, potassium, magnesium, and calcium levels.
- May decrease Hb level and WBC and platelet counts.
- May interfere with technetium-99m diphosphonate imaging agents.

CONTRAINDICATIONS & CAUTIONS

- Contraindicated in patients hypersensitive to drug or other bisphosphonates.
- ☉ *Alert:* Increased risk of atypical fractures of thigh and osteonecrosis of jaw possible in patients treated with bisphosphonates.
- Use cautiously in patients with kidney impairment.

Dialyzable drug: Yes.

⚠ *Overdose S&S:* High fever, hypotension, taste perversion, hypocalcemia.

PREGNANCY-LACTATION-REPRODUCTION

- Drug may cause fetal harm. Use during pregnancy isn't recommended.
- It isn't known if drug appears in human milk. Patient should discontinue breastfeeding or discontinue drug, considering importance of drug to patient.

NURSING CONSIDERATIONS

- Assess hydration before treatment. Use drug only after patient has been vigorously hydrated with NSS. In patients with mild to moderate hypercalcemia, hydration alone may be sufficient.
- Because drug can cause electrolyte imbalances, monitor electrolyte levels, especially calcium, phosphate, and magnesium. Short-term use of calcium may be needed in patients with severe hypocalcemia.
- Monitor CBC and differential count, creatinine and Hb levels, and hematocrit.
- Carefully monitor patients with preexisting anemia, leukopenia, or thrombocytopenia during first 2 weeks of therapy.
- Monitor patient's temperature. Patient may experience a slight temperature elevation for 24 to 48 hours after therapy.
- ☉ *Alert:* Because kidney dysfunction may lead to KF, single doses shouldn't exceed 90 mg.
- Assess creatinine level at baseline and before each treatment.
- In patients treated for bone metastases who have kidney dysfunction, withhold dose until kidney function returns to baseline. Treating bone metastases in patients with severe kidney disease isn't recommended. For other indications, determine whether the potential benefit outweighs the risk.
- Severe musculoskeletal pain may occur within several days to several months of start of therapy. Symptoms may resolve partially or completely with drug stoppage.
- Bisphosphonates can interfere with bone-imaging agents.
- Patients should have a dental exam with appropriate preventive dentistry before taking drug, especially those with risk factors, including cancer, chemotherapy, corticosteroid therapy, and poor oral hygiene. These patients should avoid dental procedures, if possible, during therapy.

PATIENT TEACHING

- Explain use and administration of drug to patient and family.
- Instruct patient to report adverse reactions promptly.
- Tell patient to immediately report groin or thigh pain.
- Instruct patient to take vitamin D and calcium supplements as prescribed.
- Caution patient to maintain good oral hygiene and have regular dental checkups.

Reactions in bold italics are *life-threatening*.

• Advise patient to report pregnancy or breastfeeding.

---

pancrelipase
pan-kre-LYE-pase

Creon, Pancreaze, Pertzye, Viokace, Zenpep

Therapeutic class: Digestive enzymes
Pharmacologic class: Pancreatic enzymes

AVAILABLE FORMS
Creon
Capsules (delayed-release) ⊙**◎**: 3,000 units lipase, 9,500 units protease, 15,000 units amylase; 6,000 units lipase, 19,000 units protease, 30,000 units amylase; 12,000 units lipase, 38,000 units protease, 60,000 units amylase; 24,000 units lipase, 76,000 units protease, 120,000 units amylase; 36,000 units lipase, 114,000 units protease, 180,000 units amylase

Pancreaze
Capsules (delayed-release) ⊙**◎**: 2,600 units lipase, 8,800 units protease, 15,200 units amylase; 4,200 units lipase, 14,200 units protease, 24,600 units amylase; 10,500 units lipase, 35,500 units protease, 61,550 units amylase; 16,800 units lipase, 56,800 units protease, 98,400 units amylase; 21,000 units lipase, 54,700 units protease, 83,900 units amylase; 37,000 units lipase, 97,300 units protease, 149,900 units amylase

Pertzye
Capsules (delayed-release) ⊙**◎**: 4,000 units lipase, 14,375 units protease, 15,125 units amylase; 8,000 units lipase, 28,750 units protease, 30,250 units amylase; 16,000 units lipase, 57,500 units protease, 60,500 units amylase; 24,000 units lipase, 86,250 units protease, 90,750 units amylase

Viokace
Tablets ⊙**◎**: 10,440 units lipase, 39,150 units protease, 39,150 units amylase; 20,880 units lipase, 78,300 units protease, 78,300 units amylase

Zenpep
Capsules (enteric-coated beads) ⊙**◎**: 3,000 units lipase, 10,000 units protease, 14,000 units amylase; 5,000 units lipase, 17,000 units protease, 24,000 units amylase; 10,000 units lipase, 32,000 units protease, 42,000 units amylase; 15,000 units lipase, 47,000 units protease, 63,000 units amylase; 20,000 units lipase, 63,000 units protease, 84,000 units amylase; 25,000 units lipase, 79,000 units protease, 105,000 units amylase; 40,000 units lipase, 126,000 units protease, 168,000 units amylase

INDICATIONS & DOSAGES
➤ **Pancreatic insufficiency due to cystic fibrosis and other conditions**
Adults and children older than age 4: 500 lipase units/kg PO per meal to a maximum of 2,500 lipase units/kg per meal (or 10,000 lipase units/kg per day) or less than 4,000 lipase units/g fat ingested per day.
Children older than age 12 months to 4 years: 1,000 lipase units/kg PO per meal up to maximum dose of 2,500 lipase units/kg per meal, 10,000 lipase units/kg daily, or 4,000 lipase units/g of fat ingested daily.
Infants up to age 12 months: 2,000 to 4,000 lipase units PO per 120 mL of formula or per breastfeeding.
➤ **Exocrine pancreatic insufficiency due to chronic pancreatitis or pancreatectomy (Creon)**
Adults: 72,000 lipase units PO per meal while consuming at least 100 g of fat per day. Or, 500 lipase units/kg per meal. Adjust dosage to patient's response. Give half of full meal dose with each snack.
➤ **Exocrine pancreatic insufficiency due to chronic pancreatitis or pancreatectomy, with a PPI (Viokace)**
Adults: 500 lipase units/kg PO per meal to a maximum of 2,500 lipase units/kg per meal (or 10,000 lipase units/kg/day) or less than 4,000 lipase units/g fat ingested per day. Adjust dosage to patient's response. Give half of full meal dose with each snack.

ADMINISTRATION
PO
• Give drug before or with meals and snacks.
• Have patient swallow capsules or tablets whole; don't crush or break capsules or tablets. May open capsules containing enteric-coated microspheres and sprinkle capsule contents on a small quantity of soft food at room temperature. Have patient swallow immediately, without chewing, and follow dose with glass of water or juice to avoid mucosal irritation.
• For infants, mix capsule contents with applesauce and give within 15 minutes of each

P

feeding. Follow with 120 mL of formula or human milk. Don't mix directly with formula or human milk. Capsule contents may be administered directly into infant's mouth before feeding. Avoid contact with or inhalation of powder because it may be highly irritating. Older children may swallow capsules with food.

• Viokace tablets aren't enteric-coated; therefore, patient should take with a PPI. Ensure patient swallows entire tablet with sufficient fluid; mucosal irritation could result from retained drug.

• Consult manufacturer's guidance on gastrostomy tube administration.

• Give half the prescribed dose at start of a meal and the second half in the middle of the meal.

• Total daily dose should reflect about three meals plus two or three snacks per day.

• If a dose is missed, omit the missed dose and give next dose with the next meal or snack. Don't double dose.

ACTION
Replaces endogenous exocrine pancreatic enzymes and aids digestion of starches, fats, and proteins.

Route	Onset	Peak	Duration
PO	Variable	Variable	Variable

Half-life: Unknown.

ADVERSE REACTIONS
CNS: headache, dizziness. **CV:** edema. **EENT:** nasopharyngitis. **GI:** abdominal pain, abnormal feces, nausea, frequent bowel movements, diarrhea (with high doses), dyspepsia, vomiting, weight loss, flatulence, anal pruritus, early satiety. **GU:** kidney cyst. **Hematologic:** anemia, lymphadenopathy. **Hepatic:** ascites, biliary tract stones, acute gallbladder distension. **Metabolic:** weight loss, hyperglycemia, *hypoglycemia.* **Respiratory:** cough. **Skin:** contusion, rash. **Other:** infection.

INTERACTIONS
Drug-drug. *Oral iron supplement:* May decrease iron response. Monitor patient for decreased effectiveness.

EFFECTS ON LAB TEST RESULTS
• May increase uric acid and LFT levels.
• May decrease Hb level.

CONTRAINDICATIONS & CAUTIONS
• Use cautiously in patients with a known allergy to proteins of porcine origin.
• Use cautiously in patients with gout, kidney impairment, or hyperuricemia.
🔵 *Alert:* Use of high-dose pancreatic enzymes has been associated with fibrosing colonopathy. Use cautiously when doses exceed 2,500 lipase units/kg/meal (or are greater than 10,000 lipase units/kg/day).
Dialyzable drug: Unknown.
⚠ *Overdose S&S:* Transient intestinal upset, diarrhea.

PREGNANCY-LACTATION-REPRODUCTION
• Use cautiously during pregnancy and only if clearly needed. Nutrition should be optimized during pregnancy.
• It isn't known if drug appears in human milk; however, it's unlikely since drug isn't absorbed systemically. Use cautiously during breastfeeding.

NURSING CONSIDERATIONS
🔵 *Alert:* Use drug only for confirmed exocrine pancreatic insufficiency. It isn't effective in GI disorders unrelated to enzyme deficiency.
• Monitor patient's stools. Adequate replacement decreases number of bowel movements and improves stool consistency.
• Individual products aren't bioequivalent and shouldn't be interchanged without prescriber supervision.
• Dosage varies with degree of maldigestion and malabsorption, amount of fat in diet, and enzyme activity of individual preparations.

PATIENT TEACHING
• Instruct patient or caregiver in safe drug administration.
• Advise patient to take drug with food and generous amounts of liquid.
• Instruct patient to consult prescriber before changing brands.
• Advise patient to report unusual or severe stomach area pain, bloating, trouble passing stool, nausea, vomiting, or diarrhea, which may indicate fibrosing colonopathy.
• Instruct patient to report pregnancy or plans to become pregnant.

Reactions in bold italics are *life-threatening*.

pancuronium bromide
pan-kyoo-ROE-nee-um

Therapeutic class: Skeletal muscle relaxants
Pharmacologic class: Nondepolarizing
neuromuscular blockers

AVAILABLE FORMS
Injection: 1 mg/mL

INDICATIONS & DOSAGES
➤ **Adjunct to anesthesia to relax skeletal muscle, facilitate intubation, and assist with mechanical ventilation**
Adults and children ages 1 month and older:
Initially, 0.04 to 0.1 mg/kg IV; then 0.01 mg/kg IV every 25 to 60 minutes. For ET intubation, a bolus dose of 0.06 to 0.1 mg/kg IV is recommended. Conditions for intubation are often present within 2 to 3 minutes.
Neonates: Individualize dosage. It's recommended that a test dose of 0.02 mg/kg IV be given first to measure responsiveness.

ADMINISTRATION
IV
Boxed Warning This drug should be administered by adequately trained individuals familiar with its actions, characteristics, and hazards. ■
▼ Only staff skilled in airway management should use drug.
▼ Drug has no known effect on consciousness, pain threshold, or cerebration. To avoid patient distress, don't induce neuromuscular blockade before unconsciousness.
▼ Keep ET equipment, ventilator, oxygen, atropine, edrophonium, epinephrine, and neostigmine immediately available.
▼ Store in refrigerator. The 10-mL vial will maintain full clinical potency for up to 6 months at room temperature.
▼ Compatible in solution with NSS, dextrose 5%, dextrose 5% and sodium chloride, and lactated Ringer solution.
▼ When mixed with approved solutions in glass or plastic containers, drug will remain stable in solution for 48 hours with no alteration in potency or pH.
▼ May administer undiluted by rapid IV injection.
▼ **Incompatibilities:** Alkaline solutions, barbiturates, diazepam, thiopental sodium.

Consult a drug compatibility reference for additional information.

ACTION
Prevents acetylcholine from binding to receptors on the motor end plate, blocking neuromuscular transmission.

Route	Onset	Peak	Duration
IV	30–45 sec	3–4.5 min	35–65 min

Half-life: 89 to 161 minutes.

ADVERSE REACTIONS
CV: tachycardia, increased BP, flushing.
EENT: excessive salivation. **Musculoskeletal:** residual muscle paralysis or weakness.
Respiratory: *prolonged respiratory insufficiency or apnea.* **Skin:** transient rashes.
Other: allergic or idiosyncratic hypersensitivity reactions.

INTERACTIONS
Drug-drug. *Aminoglycosides (amikacin, gentamicin, neomycin, streptomycin, tobramycin), tetracyclines, bacitracin:* May increase the effects of pancuronium, including prolonged respiratory depression. Use together only when necessary. Dose of pancuronium may need to be reduced.
Azathioprine: May decrease neuromuscular blockade induced by pancuronium. Monitor patient.
Calcium channel blockers, clindamycin, general anesthetics (enflurane, halothane, isoflurane), ketamine, lincomycin, magnesium salts, polymyxin antibiotics (colistin, polymyxin B sulfate), procainamide, quinine: May enhance neuromuscular blockade, increasing skeletal muscle relaxation and prolonging effect of pancuronium. Use together cautiously during and after surgery.
Carbamazepine, phenytoin: May decrease effects of pancuronium. May need to increase pancuronium dose.
Diuretics: May cause electrolyte imbalance or alter neuromuscular blockade. Monitor electrolytes before giving drug.
Lithium, opioid analgesics: May enhance neuromuscular blockade, increasing skeletal muscle relaxation and possibly causing respiratory paralysis. Use cautiously, and reduce dose of pancuronium.
Muscle relaxants (vecuronium, atracurium): May have additive effect. Don't use together.

Quinidine: May cause recurrent paralysis if quinidine is given during recovery. Monitor patient closely.

Succinylcholine: May increase intensity and duration of neuromuscular blockade. Allow effects of succinylcholine to subside before giving pancuronium.

Theophylline: May produce a dose-dependent reversal of neuromuscular blocking effects. Monitor patient for clinical effect.

EFFECTS ON LAB TEST RESULTS
None reported.

CONTRAINDICATIONS & CAUTIONS
• Contraindicated in patients hypersensitive to pancuronium, bromides, or components of the formulation.
• Use cautiously in patients with previous anaphylactic reactions to neuromuscular blocking agents. Cross-sensitivity has been reported.
• Use cautiously in older adults or patients who are debilitated; in patients with kidney, liver, or pulmonary impairment; and in those with respiratory depression, myasthenia gravis, myasthenic syndrome related to lung cancer, dehydration, thyroid disorders, CV disease, collagen diseases, porphyria, electrolyte disturbances, hyperthermia, severe obesity, and toxemic states. Also, use large doses cautiously in patients undergoing cesarean section.
• Long-term use in the ICU has been associated with prolonged paralysis or skeletal muscle weakness, especially when used with other drugs that enhance neuromuscular blocking agents, such as antibiotics and opioids.
• **Alert:** Some formulations contain benzyl alcohol, which has been associated with fatal gasping syndrome in premature neonates.
Dialyzable drug: Unknown.
Overdose S&S: Residual neuromuscular blockade (skeletal muscle weakness, decreased respiratory reserve, low tidal volume, apnea).

PREGNANCY-LACTATION-REPRODUCTION
• It isn't known if drug can cause fetal harm. Use during pregnancy only if benefit justifies fetal risk.
• There is no information on the use of drug during breastfeeding.

NURSING CONSIDERATIONS
• Dosage depends on anesthetic used, individual needs, and response. Dosages are representative and must be adjusted.
• Allow succinylcholine effects to subside before giving this drug.
• Monitor baseline electrolyte levels (electrolyte imbalance can increase neuromuscular effects) and vital signs, especially respirations and HR.
• Measure fluid intake and output; kidney dysfunction may prolong duration of action because 25% of drug is excreted unchanged in the urine.
• A peripheral nerve stimulator (PNS) and train-of-four monitoring are recommended. Make sure there's some evidence of spontaneous recovery before attempting pharmacologic reversal with neostigmine.
• Monitoring with a PNS may prevent excess dosing.
• Monitor respirations closely until patient recovers fully from neuromuscular blockade, as indicated by tests of muscle strength (hand grip, head lift, ability to cough).
• After spontaneous recovery starts, neuromuscular blockade may be reversed with an anticholinesterase (such as neostigmine or edrophonium), which is usually given with an anticholinergic (such as atropine).
• Drug doesn't cause histamine release or hypotension, but it may raise HR and BP.
• Give analgesics for pain.
• **Alert:** Careful dosage calculation is essential. Always verify dosage with another health care professional.

PATIENT TEACHING
• Explain all events and procedures to patient because patient can still hear.

pantoprazole sodium
pan-TOE-pray-zol

Pantoloc✦, Protonix, Protonix IV, Tecta✦

Therapeutic class: Antiulcer drugs
Pharmacologic class: PPIs

AVAILABLE FORMS
Granules for delayed-release suspension :
40 mg/packet
Injection: 40 mg/vial

Tablets (delayed-release) ⓓⓝⓖ: 20 mg, 40 mg
Tablets (enteric-coated) ⓓⓝⓖ: 20 mg✽, 40 mg✽

INDICATIONS & DOSAGES

➤ **Short-term treatment of erosive esophagitis associated with GERD**
Adults: 40 mg PO once daily for up to 8 weeks. For patients who haven't healed after 8 weeks of treatment, another 8-week course may be considered. Or, 40 mg IV once daily for 7 to 10 days. Switch to PO form when patient can take orally.
Children ages 5 and older weighing 40 kg or more: 40 mg PO once daily for up to 8 weeks.
Children ages 5 and older weighing 15 to less than 40 kg: 20 mg PO once daily for up to 8 weeks.

▨ *Adjust-a-dose:* Consider dosage reduction in children who are poor CYP2C19 metabolizers.

➤ **Long-term maintenance of healing erosive esophagitis and reduction in relapse rates of daytime and nighttime heartburn symptoms in patients with GERD**
Adults: 40 mg PO once daily.

➤ **Treatment of pathologic hypersecretion conditions, including Zollinger-Ellison syndrome**
Adults: Individualize dosage. Usual dosage is 40 mg PO b.i.d. Usual IV dose is 80 mg IV every 12 hours for no more than 6 days. For those needing a higher dose, 80 mg every 8 hours is expected to maintain acid output below 10 mEq/hour. Maximum daily dose, 240 mg/day. When converting from IV to PO form, ensure continuity of suppression of acid secretion.

➤ **Functional dyspepsia ◆**
Adults: 20 to 40 mg PO once daily for 4 to 8 weeks. May continue longer in patients with symptom improvement.

➤ **Uncomplicated peptic ulcer ◆**
Adults: 40 mg PO once daily for 4 to 8 weeks. In patients with refractory or recurrent disease, may increase dosage to 40 mg PO b.i.d.

➤ **Acute upper GI bleeding ◆**
Adults: 40 mg IV b.i.d. for at least 72 hours before transitioning to oral dosing. After 14 days, decrease to 40 mg PO once daily.

ADMINISTRATION
PO
• Give tablets without regard for food and make sure patient swallows them whole.
• May give with antacids.

• Have patient swallow tablets whole; don't crush or break tablets. Don't allow patient to chew granules for delayed-release oral suspension.
• Give 30 to 60 minutes before a meal. For twice-daily dosing, give first dose before breakfast and second dose before dinner.
• Give delayed-release granules for oral suspension in 1 tsp applesauce or 1 tsp (5 mL) apple juice 30 minutes before a meal by mouth. To give via NG tube, mix with 10 mL apple juice; then flush tube twice with 10 mL apple juice. Don't give in water or other liquids or foods.
• Delayed-release granule packets can't be divided to make a smaller dose.

IV
▼ Safety and effectiveness of the IV form for GERD and in patients with a history of erosive esophagitis for more than 10 days are unknown.
▼ Reconstitute each vial with 10 mL of NSS.
▼ Compatible diluents for infusion include NSS, D₅W, and lactated Ringer solution for injection.
▼ For patients with GERD, further dilute with 100 mL of diluent to yield 0.4 mg/mL.
▼ For patients with hypersecretion, combine two reconstituted vials and further dilute with 80 mL of diluent to a total volume of 100 mL, to yield 0.8 mg/mL.
▼ Infuse diluted solutions over 15 minutes at a rate of about 7 mL/minute.
▼ For a 2-minute infusion, give the reconstituted vials (final yield of about 4 mg/mL) over at least 2 minutes.
▼ Reconstituted 15-minute infusion (0.4 mg/mL) may be stored for up to 6 hours and the diluted solutions for up to 24 hours at room temperature.
▼ Reconstituted 2-minute solution (4 mg/mL) may be stored for up to 24 hours at room temperature before infusion.
▼ **Incompatibilities:** Midazolam, zinc-containing products or solutions. Don't give another infusion simultaneously through the same line.

ACTION
Inhibits proton pump activity by binding to hydrogen-potassium adenosine triphosphatase, located at secretory surface of gastric parietal cells, to suppress gastric acid secretion.

Route	Onset	Peak	Duration
PO	Unknown	2.5 hr	>24 hr
IV	15–30 min	Unknown	24 hr

Half-life: 1 hour.

ADVERSE REACTIONS

CNS: asthenia, dizziness, headache, depression, vertigo, fever. **CV:** edema, thrombophlebitis (IV). **EENT:** blurred vision, otitis media, pharyngitis, rhinitis, sinusitis, dry mouth. **GI:** abdominal pain, constipation, diarrhea, flatulence, nausea, vomiting. **Hematologic:** *leukopenia, thrombocytopenia.* **Hepatic:** elevated liver enzyme levels. **Metabolic:** hyperglycemia, hypertriglyceridemia, increased CK level. **Musculoskeletal:** arthralgia, myalgia, back pain, hypertonia, neck pain. **Respiratory:** URI. **Skin:** rash, pruritus, urticaria. **Other:** flulike syndrome, infection, injection-site reaction, photosensitivity reactions, hypersensitivity reaction.

INTERACTIONS

Drug-drug. *Ampicillin esters, dasatinib, erlotinib, iron salts, mycophenolate, nilotinib:* May decrease absorption of these drugs. Monitor patient closely and separate doses.
Atazanavir, nelfinavir: May reduce antiviral activity of these drugs. Adjust dosage as needed; coadministration not recommended.
Azole antifungals (itraconazole, ketoconazole): May decrease plasma levels of these drugs. Avoid combination if possible.
Methotrexate: May increase methotrexate level and risk of toxicity. Closely monitor methotrexate level, and watch for signs and symptoms of methotrexate toxicity. Consider temporarily stopping pantoprazole with high-dose methotrexate therapy.
Rilpivirine: May decrease antiviral effect and increase risk of drug resistance. Concomitant use is contraindicated.
Saquinavir: May increase saquinavir level. Monitor for toxicity.
Warfarin: May increase INR and prolong PT. Monitor patient and lab values.
Drug-lifestyle. *Sun exposure:* May increase risk of sunburn. Advise patient to avoid excessive sunlight exposure.

EFFECTS ON LAB TEST RESULTS

• May increase glucose, CK, and triglyceride levels.

• May decrease vitamin B_{12} and magnesium levels.
• May increase LFT values.
• May decrease WBC and platelet counts.
• May cause false-positive urine screen test for tetrahydrocannabinol.
• May increase serum chromogranin A level, causing a false-positive result in diagnostic investigation for neuroendocrine tumors.

CONTRAINDICATIONS & CAUTIONS

• Contraindicated in patients hypersensitive to components of the formulation.
• PPI therapy may be associated with an increased risk of osteoporosis-related fractures. Use lowest dose and shortest duration of therapy appropriate to condition being treated.
• May increase risk of acute tubulointerstitial nephritis (TIN), which may occur at any point during PPI therapy.
• PPI use is associated with increased risk of fundic gland polyps that increases with long-term use, especially beyond 1 year.
• Cutaneous lupus erythematosus (CLE) and SLE have been reported, occurring as both new onset and an exacerbation of existing autoimmune disease in patients of all ages within weeks to years after continuous drug therapy.
• IV formulation contains edetate disodium, a chelator of zinc. Consider zinc supplements in patients at risk for zinc deficiency.
• Prolonged oral use (over 3 years) may lead to vitamin B_{12} deficiency.
Dializable drug: No.

PREGNANCY-LACTATION-REPRODUCTION

• There are no adequate studies during pregnancy. Use cautiously and only if clearly needed.
• Drug appears in human milk in limited amount. Use cautiously during breastfeeding.

NURSING CONSIDERATIONS

• Symptomatic response to therapy doesn't preclude the presence of gastric malignancy.
⚠ *Alert:* Prolonged use of PPIs may cause low magnesium levels. Monitor magnesium levels before start of treatment and periodically thereafter.
⚠ *Alert:* Monitor patient for signs and symptoms of low magnesium level, such as abnormal HR or rhythm, palpitations, muscle spasms, tremor, or seizures. In children, abnormal HR may present as fatigue, upset

stomach, dizziness, and light-headedness. Magnesium supplementation or drug discontinuation may be required.

⚠️ *Alert:* May increase risk of CDAD. Evaluate for CDAD in patients who develop diarrhea that doesn't improve.

• If signs or symptoms consistent with CLE or SLE are noted, discontinue drug and refer patient to the appropriate specialist for evaluation. Most patients improve with discontinuation of the PPI in 4 to 12 weeks.

• Monitor patient for TIN (symptomatic hypersensitivity reactions, nonspecific symptoms of decreased kidney function [malaise, nausea, anorexia]). Discontinue drug and evaluate patient with suspected acute TIN.

• Monitor patient for hypersensitivity reactions, including SCARs; discontinue drug if present.

• *Look alike–sound alike:* Don't confuse Protonix with Prilosec, Prozac, or Prevacid. Don't confuse pantoprazole with aripiprazole.

PATIENT TEACHING

• Teach patient or caregiver safe drug administration.

• Instruct patient to take exactly as prescribed and at the same time every day.

• Tell patient that antacids don't affect drug absorption.

• Advise patient to immediately report diarrhea that doesn't improve.

• Instruct patient to report fractures, especially of the hip, wrist, or spine.

• Teach patient to report all adverse reactions and to recognize and report signs and symptoms of low magnesium level.

• Advise patient of childbearing potential to report known or suspected pregnancy.

PARoxetine hydrochloride
pa-ROKS-e-teen

Paxil, Paxil CR

PARoxetine mesylate

Therapeutic class: Antidepressants
Pharmacologic class: SSRIs

AVAILABLE FORMS
paroxetine hydrochloride
Suspension: 10 mg/5 mL
Tablets ⓄⓃⒸ: 10 mg, 20 mg, 30 mg, 40 mg

Tablets (controlled-release) ⓄⓃⒸ: 12.5 mg, 25 mg, 37.5 mg
paroxetine mesylate
Capsules: 7.5 mg

INDICATIONS & DOSAGES

Adjust-a-dose (for all indications): For older adults and patients who are debilitated and those with kidney or liver impairment taking immediate-release form, initially, 10 mg PO daily, preferably in morning. If patient doesn't respond after full antidepressant effect has occurred, increase dose in 10-mg/day increments at intervals of at least 1 week to a maximum of 40 mg daily. If using controlled-release form, start therapy at 12.5 mg daily. Don't exceed 50 mg daily for MDD or panic disorder, or 37.5 mg daily for social anxiety disorder.

➤ **MDD (excluding capsules)**
Adults: Initially, 20 mg PO daily, preferably in morning. If patient doesn't improve, increase dose by 10 mg daily at intervals of at least 1 week to a maximum of 50 mg daily. If using controlled-release form, initially, 25 mg PO daily. Increase dose in 12.5-mg/day increments at intervals of at least 1 week to a maximum of 62.5 mg daily.

➤ **OCD (Paxil only)**
Adults: Initially, 20 mg PO daily, preferably in morning. Increase dose in 10-mg day increments at intervals of at least 1 week. Maximum daily dose, 60 mg.

➤ **Panic disorder (excluding capsules)**
Adults: Initially, 10 mg PO daily. Increase dose in 10-mg/day increments at intervals of at least 1 week, up to a maximum of 60 mg daily. Or, 12.5 mg Paxil CR PO as a single daily dose. Increase dose in 12.5-mg/day increments at intervals of at least 1 week, up to a maximum of 75 mg daily.

➤ **Social anxiety disorder (Paxil and Paxil CR only)**
Adults: Initially, 20 mg PO daily. Dosage range is 20 to 60 mg daily. Adjust dosage to maintain patient on lowest effective dose. Or, 12.5 mg Paxil CR PO as a single daily dose. Increase dose in 12.5-mg/day increments at intervals of at least 1 week, up to a maximum of 37.5 mg daily.

➤ **Generalized anxiety disorder (Paxil only)**
Adults: 20 mg PO daily initially. Increase dose in 10-mg/day increments at intervals of at least 1 week, up to a maximum of 50 mg

---

daily. Doses greater than 20 mg/day don't appear to have an added benefit.

➤ **PTSD (Paxil only)**
Adults: Initially, 20 mg PO daily. Increase dose in 10-mg/day increments at intervals of at least 1 week. Maximum daily dose, 50 mg PO.

➤ **Premenstrual dysphoric disorder (PMDD) (Paxil CR only)**
Adults: Initially, 12.5 mg Paxil CR PO as a single daily dose. May be given daily throughout menstrual cycle or daily during the luteal phase of menstrual cycle. Dose changes should occur at intervals of at least 1 week. Maximum daily dose, 25 mg PO.

➤ **Moderate to severe vasomotor symptoms associated with menopause (capsules only)**
Adults: 7.5 mg capsule PO daily at bedtime.

ADMINISTRATION
PO
• Give drug in the morning without regard for food (excluding capsules). Give capsules at bedtime.
• Have patient swallow controlled-release tablets whole; don't crush or break tablets.
• Shake oral suspension well before each use. Measure with oral syringe or calibrated measuring device.

ACTION
Thought to be linked to drug's inhibition of CNS neuronal uptake of serotonin.

Route	Onset	Peak	Duration
PO	Unknown	3–8 hr	Unknown
PO (controlled-release)	Unknown	6–10 hr	Unknown

Half-life: Paroxetine, 21 hours; controlled-release, 15 to 20 hours; paroxetine mesylate, 33.2 hours.

ADVERSE REACTIONS
CNS: amnesia, asthenia, depersonalization, dizziness, drugged feeling, fatigue, headache, insomnia, abnormal dreams, impaired concentration, somnolence, tremor, twitching, nervousness, anxiety, paresthesia, confusion, agitation, taste perversion. **CV:** palpitations, vasodilation, HTN, tachycardia, chest pain. **EENT:** blurred vision, tinnitus, lump or tightness in throat, dry mouth, pharyngitis, rhinitis, sinusitis. **GI:** nausea, constipation, diarrhea, flatulence, vomiting, dyspepsia, decreased appetite, abdominal pain. **GU:** ejaculatory disturbances, sexual dysfunction,

decreased libido, urinary frequency, other urinary disorders, dysmenorrhea, female genital disorders. **Metabolic:** weight gain. **Musculoskeletal:** myopathy, myalgia, myasthenia, back pain. **Respiratory:** dyspnea. **Skin:** diaphoresis, rash, pruritus. **Other:** yawning, infection.

INTERACTIONS
Drug-drug. *Anticoagulants, platelet inhibitors:* May impair platelet aggregation and increase risk of bleeding. Monitor patient for signs and symptoms of bleeding.
Atomoxetine: May alter atomoxetine level. Initiate atomoxetine at a reduced dosage.
Cimetidine: May increase paroxetine level and risk of adverse reactions. Dosage adjustments may be needed.
Drugs metabolized by CYP2D6 (desipramine, dextromethorphan, flecainide, metoprolol, propafenone): May increase CYP2D6 substrate level. Adjust substrate dosage.
Drugs that prolong QT interval (antiarrhythmics [amiodarone, disopyramide, dofetilide, procainamide, quinidine, sotalol], chlorpromazine, cisapride, dolasetron, droperidol, mefloquine, mesoridazine, moxifloxacin, pentamidine, pimozide, tacrolimus, ziprasidone): May increase risk of life-threatening cardiac arrhythmias, including torsades de pointes. Monitor patient closely.
Fosamprenavir, ritonavir: May decrease paroxetine plasma level. Adjust dosage as needed.
Galantamine: May alter oral bioavailability of galantamine. Use together cautiously.
Linezolid, methylene blue: May cause serotonin syndrome. Allow at least 2 weeks after stopping linezolid before giving paroxetine.
MAO inhibitors (phenelzine, selegiline, tranylcypromine): May cause serotonin syndrome and signs and symptoms resembling NMS. Avoid using within 14 days of MAO inhibitor therapy.
NSAIDs: May increase risk of GI bleeding. If possible, avoid concurrent use. If coadministration can't be avoided, consider shortening NSAID treatment duration, decreasing dosage, or switching to acetaminophen or a TCA.
Pimozide, thioridazine: May increase levels of these drugs. Avoid using together.
Risperidone: May increase risperidone level, increasing risk of adverse reactions, including serotonin syndrome. Use together cautiously.

---

*Reactions in bold italics are **life-threatening**.*

Serotonergic agents (amphetamines, buspirone, lithium, SNRIs, SSRIs, tramadol, triptans): May increase risk of serotonin syndrome. Monitor patient closely.
Sympathomimetics (dopamine, dobutamine, epinephrine): May increase effect of sympathomimetics and increase risk of serotonin syndrome. Monitor patient.
Tamoxifen: May reduce level of active tamoxifen metabolite. Avoid combination.
TCAs: May increase level and elimination half-life of TCAs. TCA dosage reduction may be needed.
Warfarin: May increase anticoagulant effect. Monitor therapy.
Drug-herb. *SAM-e:* May increase risk of serotonin syndrome. Avoid use together.
St. John's wort: May increase sedative-hypnotic effects and risk of serotonin syndrome. Discourage use together.
Drug-lifestyle. *Alcohol use:* May alter psychomotor function. Discourage use together.

EFFECTS ON LAB TEST RESULTS
● May increase LFT values.
● May decrease sodium level.
● May decrease Hb level.

CONTRAINDICATIONS & CAUTIONS
● Contraindicated in patients hypersensitive to drug or its components; some formulations contain polysorbate 80.
Boxed Warning Antidepressants increase the risk of suicidality in children, adolescents, and young adults with depression and other psychiatric disorders. Providers should balance this risk with clinical needs; paroxetine not approved for use in children. ■
❸ Alert: Use with linezolid or methylene blue can cause serotonin syndrome. Use with linezolid or methylene blue only for life-threatening or urgent conditions when potential benefits outweigh risks of toxicity.
● Angle-closure glaucoma has occurred in patients with untreated anatomically narrow angles.
● Liver or kidney impairment increases plasma levels; use cautiously and reduce dosage if needed.
● Use cautiously in patients with history of seizure disorders or mania and in those with other severe, systemic illness.
● Use cautiously in patients at risk for volume depletion and monitor them appropriately.
Dialyzable drug: Unlikely.

⚠ Overdose S&S: Coma, confusion, dizziness, nausea, somnolence, tachycardia, tremor, vomiting, AKI, aggressive reactions, bradycardia, dystonia, liver necrosis, HTN, hypotension, jaundice, manic reactions, mydriasis, myoclonus, rhabdomyolysis, seizures, serotonin syndrome, stupor, liver impairment, syncope, urine retention, ventricular arrhythmias.

PREGNANCY-LACTATION-REPRODUCTION
● Drug can cause fetal harm, especially if taken in the first trimester. Manufacturer suggests discontinuing drug or switching to another antidepressant unless benefits justify continuing treatment. Consider other treatment options for patients planning pregnancy.
● Contraindicated for treatment of vasomotor symptoms during pregnancy.
● Drug appears in human milk. Use during breastfeeding only if benefit of treating postpartum depression with this drug outweighs risk. Monitor infants for growth.

NURSING CONSIDERATIONS
● Patients taking Paxil CR for PMDD should be periodically reassessed to determine the need for continued treatment.
● If signs or symptoms of psychosis occur or increase, expect prescriber to reduce dosage. Record mood changes. Monitor patient for suicidality, and allow only a minimum supply of drug.
Boxed Warning Monitor all patients starting antidepressant therapy for clinical worsening, suicidality, or unusual changes in behavior. ■
❸ Alert: If linezolid or methylene blue must be given, stop paroxetine and monitor patient for serotonin toxicity for 2 weeks or until 24 hours after the last dose of methylene blue or linezolid, whichever comes first. Treatment with paroxetine may be resumed 24 hours after the last dose of methylene blue or linezolid.
● Monitor patient for complaints of sexual dysfunction. In males, they include anorgasmia, erectile difficulties, and delayed ejaculation or orgasm; in females, they include anorgasmia or difficulty with orgasm.
❸ Alert: Don't stop drug abruptly. Withdrawal syndrome (headache, myalgia, lethargy, flu-like symptoms) may occur with abrupt withdrawal. Taper over 1 to 2 weeks.
❸ Alert: Combining triptans with an SSRI or an SNRI may cause serotonin syndrome

or NMS-like reactions. Signs and symptoms of serotonin syndrome may include restlessness, hallucinations, loss of coordination, fast heartbeat, rapid changes in BP, increased body temperature, overactive reflexes, nausea, vomiting, and diarrhea. Serotonin syndrome may be more likely to occur when starting or increasing the dose of triptan, SSRI, or SNRI.

• *Look alike–sound alike:* Don't confuse paroxetine with fluoxetine or paclitaxel. Don't confuse Paxil with Doxil, paclitaxel, or Plavix.

PATIENT TEACHING

Boxed Warning Advise families and caregivers to closely observe patient for increased suicidality. ∎

⊕ *Alert:* Teach patient to recognize and immediately report signs and symptoms of serotonin toxicity.

• Teach patient safe drug administration.

• Warn patient to avoid activities that require alertness and good coordination until effects of drug are known.

• Advise patient to report sexual dysfunction and to consult prescriber for management strategies.

• Instruct patient to report pregnancy or plans to become pregnant or to breastfeed.

• Tell patient to avoid alcohol and to consult prescriber before taking other prescription or OTC drugs or herbal medicines.

• Instruct patient not to stop taking drug abruptly.

SAFETY ALERT!
BIOSIMILAR DRUG

pegfilgrastim
peg-fil-GRA-stim

Neulasta, Neulasta Onpro Kit

pegfilgrastim-apgf
Nyvepria

pegfilgrastim-bmez
Ziextenzo

pegfilgrastim-cbqv
Udenyca

pegfilgrastim-fpgk
Stimufend

pegfilgrastim-jmdb
Fulphila

pegfilgrastim-pbbk
Fylnetra

Therapeutic class: Colony-stimulating factors
Pharmacologic class: Hematopoietics

AVAILABLE FORMS
Injection: 6 mg/0.6 mL prefilled syringe

INDICATIONS & DOSAGES

➤ **To reduce incidence of infection in patients with nonmyeloid malignancies receiving myelosuppressive chemotherapy that may cause febrile neutropenia**
Adults and children weighing more than 45 kg: 6 mg subcut once per chemotherapy cycle. Don't give in period between 14 days before and 24 hours after administration of cytotoxic chemotherapy.
Children: Give once per chemotherapy cycle, beginning 24 hours after completion of chemotherapy. Children weighing 31 to 44 kg, give 4 mg subcut. Children weighing 21 to 30 kg, give 2.5 mg subcut. Children weighing 10 to 20 kg, give 1.5 mg subcut. Children weighing less than 10 kg, give 0.1 mg/kg subcut.

➤ **To increase survival in patients acutely exposed to myelosuppressive doses of radiation (Neulasta)**
Adults and children weighing 45 kg or more: 6 mg subcut as soon as possible after suspected or confirmed exposure. Repeat 1 week after first dose.
Children: Give as soon as possible after suspected or confirmed exposure. Repeat 1 week after first dose. Children weighing 31 to 44 kg, give 4 mg subcut. Children weighing 21 to 30 kg, give 2.5 mg subcut. Children weighing 10 to 20 kg, give 1.5 mg subcut. Children weighing less than 10 kg, give 0.1 mg/kg subcut.

ADMINISTRATION
Subcutaneous
⊕ *Alert:* Don't use prefilled syringe for patients requiring less than 6 mg (0.6 mL), as syringe doesn't have graduated markings for smaller doses. Transfer drug to appropriately marked syringe to measure dose of less than 0.6 mL.

● Alert: Needle cap contains dry natural rubber derived from latex; persons with latex allergies shouldn't administer the drug.
• Allow drug to come to room temperature as directed by manufacturer before giving; protect from light.
• Don't shake.
• Don't use if visible discoloration or particulate matter is present.
• Refer to manufacturer's instructions for storage and stability information; requirements vary by product.
• Refer to manufacturer's instructions for administering drug using the Neulasta Onpro Kit with sterile on-body injector (OBI) and for its removal and disposal.
• After a missed dose due to failure or leakage of OBI for Neulasta, give a new dose manually by single-dose prefilled syringe as soon as possible.

ACTION

Binds cell receptors to stimulate proliferation, differentiation, commitment, and end-cell function of neutrophils.

Route	Onset	Peak	Duration
Subcut	Unknown	Unknown	Unknown

Half-life: 15 to 80 hours, adults; 20 to 38 hours, children.

ADVERSE REACTIONS

Musculoskeletal: bone pain, extremity pain.

INTERACTIONS

Drug-drug. *Belotecan:* May increase neutropenic effect of belotecan. Don't give G-CSF for at least 24 hours after belotecan; monitor patient closely.
Bleomycin, topotecan: May increase pulmonary toxicity of these drugs. Monitor therapy.
Tisagenlecleucel: May increase risk of tisagenlecleucel adverse effects. Avoid combination.

EFFECTS ON LAB TEST RESULTS

• May increase granulocyte count.
• May decrease platelet count.
• May cause transient positive bone imaging changes.

CONTRAINDICATIONS & CAUTIONS

• Contraindicated in patients hypersensitive to filgrastim or components of the drug.

• Drug isn't indicated for peripheral blood progenitor cell mobilization in hematopoietic stem cell transplantation.
• Myelodysplastic syndrome (MDS) and acute myeloid leukemia (AML) have been associated with the use of pegfilgrastim products in conjunction with chemotherapy or radiotherapy in patients with breast and lung cancer. Monitor patients for signs and symptoms of MDS and AML in these settings.
• G-CSF drugs may act as growth factor for any tumor type.
• Use cautiously in patients with sickle cell disease, those receiving chemotherapy causing delayed myelosuppression, and those receiving radiation therapy.
• Neulasta OBI isn't recommended for acute radiation exposure or for use in children.
• Neulasta OBI uses acrylic adhesive; use cautiously in patients with reactions to acrylic adhesive.

Dialyzable drug: Unknown.

⚠ Overdose S&S: Leukocytosis, bone pain, edema, dyspnea, pleural effusions.

PREGNANCY-LACTATION-REPRODUCTION

• There are no adequate studies during pregnancy. Use only if potential benefit justifies fetal risk.
• It isn't known if drug appears in human milk. Use cautiously during breastfeeding.

NURSING CONSIDERATIONS

● Alert: Splenic rupture may occur rarely. Assess patient who experiences signs or symptoms of left upper abdominal or shoulder pain for an enlarged spleen or splenic rupture.
• Obtain CBC and platelet count before therapy and monitor during therapy.
• Monitor patient for allergic-type reactions, including anaphylaxis, rash, and urticaria, which can occur anytime during treatment.
• Evaluate patient with fever, lung infiltrates, or respiratory distress for ARDS. Notify prescriber if respiratory status worsens.
• Keep patient with sickle cell disease well hydrated, and monitor for symptoms of sickle cell crisis. Discontinue use if sickle cell crisis occurs.
• Monitor patient for capillary leak syndrome (hypotension, hypoalbuminemia, edema, hemoconcentration) and manage with symptomatic treatment, if necessary.

❸ *Alert:* After acute radiation exposure, obtain a baseline CBC but don't delay drug administration if a CBC isn't readily available. Estimate patient's absorbed radiation dose (level of radiation exposure) based on information from public health authorities, biodosimetry if available, or clinical findings, such as time to onset of vomiting or lymphocyte depletion kinetics.

• Monitor patient for aortitis (fever, abdominal pain, malaise, back pain, increased C-reactive protein and WBC count), which may occur as early as the first week of treatment. Discontinue drug if aortitis is suspected.

• Monitor patient for signs and symptoms of glomerulonephritis (azotemia, hematuria, proteinuria).

• *Look alike–sound alike:* Don't confuse pegfilgrastim with filgrastim. Don't confuse Neulasta with Neupogen or Lunesta.

PATIENT TEACHING

• Advise patient to report all adverse reactions.

• Tell patient to report signs and symptoms of allergic reactions, fever, or breathing problems.

❸ *Alert:* Inform patient that, rarely, splenic rupture may occur. Advise patient to immediately report upper left abdominal or shoulder tip pain.

• Tell patient with sickle cell disease to keep drinking fluids and report signs or symptoms of sickle cell crisis.

• Instruct patient or caregiver how to give drug if it's to be given at home, including danger of reusing syringes and proper syringe disposal.

• Instruct patient using OBI not to expose injector to oxygen-rich environments (hyperbaric chamber), MRI, X-ray (including airport X-ray), CT scan, or ultrasound (may damage injector system).

• Instruct patient to keep OBI at least 4 inches (10 cm) away from electrical equipment, including cell phones, cordless phones, microwaves, and other common appliances (injector may not work properly).

• Advise patient to avoid activities, such as traveling, driving, or operating machinery, for 26 to 29 hours after using OBI.

• Caution patient to report OBI device failure immediately to determine need for replacement dose.

---

peginterferon alfa-2a ℞
peg-in-ter-FEER-on

Pegasys

Therapeutic class: Antivirals
Pharmacologic class: Interferons

AVAILABLE FORMS

Injection*: 180 mcg/1 mL single-dose vial; 180 mcg/0.5 mL prefilled syringe

INDICATIONS & DOSAGES

Adjust-a-dose (for all indications): Refer to manufacturer's instructions for toxicity-related dosage adjustments. In adults with CrCl less than 30 mL/minute, including patients on hemodialysis, decrease dosage to 135 mcg once weekly. There are no recommendations for children with kidney impairment.

➤ **Chronic HCV infection with compensated liver disease in patients not previously treated with interferon alfa, in combination with other HCV antiviral drugs** ℞
Adults with HCV genotype 1 or 4: 180 mcg subcut once weekly as monotherapy or combination therapy with ribavirin for 48 weeks. Refer to prescribing information of the other HCV antiviral for duration of entire treatment regimen. If used with ribavirin with or without other HCV antivirals, treatment duration is 48 weeks.

Adults with HCV genotype 2 or 3: 180 mcg subcut once weekly. Refer to prescribing information of the other HCV antiviral for duration of entire treatment regimen. If used with ribavirin with or without other HCV antivirals, treatment duration is 24 weeks.

Children ages 5 and older: 180 mcg/1.73 m^2 × BSA subcut once weekly in combination with ribavirin. Treat children with genotype 2 or 3 for 24 weeks, and with other genotypes for 48 weeks. Maximum dose, 180 mcg once weekly. Patients who turn age 18 during therapy should continue pediatric dosage for treatment duration.

➤ **Chronic HCV infection (regardless of genotype) in patients with HIV-1 infection who haven't previously been treated with interferon alfa**
Adults: 180 mcg subcut once weekly. When used with ribavirin, treatment duration is

48 weeks. When used with other HCV antivirals, refer to prescribing information of the other HCV antiviral for treatment duration.

➤ **Chronic HBV infection in patients with compensated liver disease and evidence of viral replication and liver inflammation**
Adults: 180 mcg subcut once weekly for 48 weeks.

➤ **Hepatitis B e-antigen (HBeAg)-positive chronic HBV infection in noncirrhotic children who have evidence of viral replication and elevation in serum ALT level**
Children ages 3 and older: 180 mcg/1.73 m² × BSA subcut once weekly. Maximum recommended dosage, 180 mcg weekly; recommended duration of therapy, 48 weeks. Patients who turn age 18 during therapy should maintain pediatric dosage through completion of therapy.

ADMINISTRATION
Subcutaneous
• Vials and prefilled syringes are for single use only. Discard unused portion.
• Don't shake. Allow to reach room temperature before use, but don't leave out of refrigerator for more than 24 hours. Don't freeze.
• Protect from light.
• For children, use 180-mcg/mL vial to withdraw appropriate dose and give using a 1-mL tuberculin syringe. Use of a prefilled syringe isn't recommended.
• Visually inspect drug for particulate matter and discoloration before administration; don't use if particulate matter is visible or product is discolored.
• Give in abdomen or thigh; rotate injection site.
• Give on same day and at approximately same time each week.

ACTION
Causes reversible decreases in leukocyte and platelet counts, partially through stimulation of production of effector proteins in vitro. Inhibits HCV RNA replication.

Route	Onset	Peak	Duration
Subcut	Unknown	3–4 days	<1 wk

Half-life: 160 hours (range, 84 to 353 hours).

ADVERSE REACTIONS
CNS: depression, dizziness, headache, insomnia, irritability, fever, anxiety, asthenia, impaired concentration, memory impairment, mood alteration, nervousness, rigors, pain. **EENT:** blurred vision, epistaxis, nasopharyngitis, dry mouth. **GI:** abdominal pain, anorexia, diarrhea, nausea, vomiting. **Hematologic:** *neutropenia, thrombocytopenia,* anemia, *lymphopenia.* **Hepatic:** increased transaminase levels. **Metabolic:** hypothyroidism, weight loss. **Musculoskeletal:** arthralgia, myalgia, back pain. **Respiratory:** cough, dyspnea, URI. **Skin:** alopecia, pruritus, dermatitis, diaphoresis, rash, dry skin, eczema, injection-site reaction. **Other:** flu-like syndrome, growth inhibition.

INTERACTIONS
Drug-drug. *Methadone:* May increase methadone level. Monitor patient closely and decrease methadone dosage as needed.
NRTIs (emtricitabine, tenofovir, abacavir): May cause severe and potentially fatal liver decompensation. If used together in patients coinfected with HIV who are taking NRTIs, monitor for toxicities.
Ribavirin: May cause additive hematologic toxicity. Monitor hematologic function.
Telbivudine: May increase risk of peripheral neuropathy. Avoid use together.
Theophylline, other drugs metabolized by CYP1A2: May increase theophylline level and interact with other drugs metabolized by this enzyme system. Monitor theophylline level; adjust dosage as needed.
Zidovudine: May enhance adverse or toxic effect of zidovudine; may decrease zidovudine metabolism. Monitor therapy.

EFFECTS ON LAB TEST RESULTS
• May increase triglyceride, AST, and ALT levels.
• May decrease Hb level, hematocrit, ANC, and WBC and platelet counts.
• May increase or decrease thyroid function test values.

CONTRAINDICATIONS & CAUTIONS
• Contraindicated in patients hypersensitive to interferon alfa-2a or any components of formulation.
• Contraindicated in patients with autoimmune hepatitis or Child-Pugh class B and C liver impairment.
• Contraindicated in neonates and infants due to benzyl alcohol content.
• Use cautiously in patients with a history of depression.

• Use cautiously in patients with baseline neutrophil counts less than 1,500/mm³, baseline platelet counts less than 90,000/mm³, or baseline Hb level less than 10 g/dL.

• Use cautiously in patients with CrCl less than 50 mL/minute.

• Use cautiously in patients with cardiac disease or HTN, thyroid disease, autoimmune disorders, pulmonary disorders, colitis, pancreatitis, and ophthalmologic disorders.

• Use cautiously in older adults because they may be at increased risk for adverse reactions.

⚠ *Alert:* Use cautiously in patients also taking ribavirin. Ribavirin is also known to cause hemolytic anemia, which may worsen cardiac disease.

• Drug may inhibit growth in children.

• Safety and effectiveness haven't been established in patients who have failed to respond to other interferon alfa treatments, in solid organ transplant recipients, in patients with HBV infection also infected with HCV or HIV, or in patients with hepatitis C also infected with HBV or HIV with a CD4+ cell count less than 100 cells/mm³.

Dialyzable drug: No.

⚠ *Overdose S&S:* Fatigue, elevated liver enzyme levels, neutropenia, thrombocytopenia.

PREGNANCY-LACTATION-REPRODUCTION

• There are no adequate studies of drug used as monotherapy during pregnancy. Use drug as monotherapy only if potential benefit justifies fetal risk and only in patients of childbearing potential when they are using effective contraception. Some professional guidelines discourage use during pregnancy.

• Combination therapy with ribavirin may cause fetal birth defects or death and is contraindicated during pregnancy. Refer to ribavirin prescribing information for current pregnancy testing and contraception recommendations.

• It isn't known if drug appears in human milk. Patient should discontinue breastfeeding or discontinue drug, considering importance of drug to patient.

• Drug may disrupt the menstrual cycle. It isn't known if drug impairs fertility.

NURSING CONSIDERATIONS

Boxed Warning Alpha interferons may cause or aggravate fatal or life-threatening neuropsychiatric (aggressive behavior, psychoses, hallucinations, bipolar disorders,

mania), autoimmune (hepatitis, ITP, RA, interstitial nephritis, SLE), ischemic, and infectious disorders. Monitor patients closely with periodic clinical and lab evaluations. Withdraw patients with persistently severe or worsening signs or symptoms of these conditions from therapy. ■

• Obtain CBC before treatment and monitor counts routinely during therapy. Stop drug in patients who develop severe decrease in neutrophil or platelet counts.

• Monitor patient for hypersensitivity reactions (including angioedema and anaphylaxis) and severe skin reactions (including SJS and exfoliative dermatitis).

• Stop drug if uncontrollable thyroid disease, hyperglycemia, hypoglycemia, or diabetes occurs during treatment.

• If persistent or unexplained pulmonary infiltrates or pulmonary dysfunction occur, stop drug.

• Stop drug if signs and symptoms of colitis (abdominal pain, bloody diarrhea, fever) occur. Symptoms should resolve within 1 to 3 weeks.

• Stop drug if signs and symptoms of pancreatitis (fever, malaise, abdominal pain) occur.

• Obtain baseline eye exam and periodically monitor eye exams during treatment. Stop drug if new or worsening disorders occur.

• Monitor kidney function, liver function, and uric acid and TSH levels.

• *Look alike–sound alike:* Don't confuse peginterferon alfa-2a with interferon alfa-2a, interferon alfa-2b, or interferon alfa-n3.

PATIENT TEACHING

• Advise patient to read medication guide that comes with drug.

• Teach patient proper way to give drug and dispose of needles and syringes, if appropriate.

• Instruct patient to immediately report depression or suicidality.

• Tell patient to report signs and symptoms of pancreatitis, colitis, eye disorders, or respiratory disorders.

• Advise patient who feels dizzy, tired, confused, or sleepy to avoid driving or operating machinery.

• Caution patient not to switch to another brand of interferon without consulting health care provider.

• Tell patient that flulike symptoms commonly occur. Inform patient that injecting in the evening may lessen symptoms.

• Advise patient of childbearing potential that drug may alter menstrual cycles and impair fertility.

⚠ *Alert:* When drug is used with ribavirin, tell patient and partners to take extreme care to avoid pregnancy following ribavirin prescribing information.

SAFETY ALERT!

pembrolizumab ⚠
pem-broe-LIZ-ue-mab

Keytruda

Therapeutic class: Antineoplastics
Pharmacologic class: Monoclonal antibodies

AVAILABLE FORMS
Injection: 25 mg/mL (4 mL) solution in single-use vial

INDICATIONS & DOSAGES
⚠ *Alert:* Refer to manufacturer's instructions for additional treatment criteria by diagnosis, dosing information of drugs used in combination therapy regimens, and treatment duration.

Adjust-a-dose (for all indications): Refer to manufacturer's instructions for toxicity-related dosage adjustments.

➤ **Unresectable or metastatic melanoma**
Adults: 200-mg IV infusion every 3 weeks or 400-mg IV infusion every 6 weeks.

➤ **Adjuvant treatment of melanoma with lymph node involvement after complete resection**
Adults: 200-mg IV infusion every 3 weeks or 400-mg IV infusion every 6 weeks.
Children ages 12 and older: 2 mg/kg IV over every 3 weeks up to maximum dose of 200 mg.

➤ **Head and neck squamous cell carcinoma**
Adults: 200-mg IV infusion every 3 weeks or 400-mg IV infusion every 6 weeks.

➤ **NSCLC** ⚠
Adults: 200-mg IV infusion every 3 weeks or 400-mg IV infusion every 6 weeks.

➤ **Classical Hodgkin lymphoma**
Adults: 200-mg IV infusion every 3 weeks or 400-mg IV infusion every 6 weeks.
Children age 12 and older: 2 mg/kg IV over 30 minutes every 3 weeks up to maximum dose of 200 mg.

➤ **Primary mediastinal large B-cell lymphoma (PMBCL)**
Adults: 200-mg IV infusion every 3 weeks or 400-mg IV infusion every 6 weeks.
Children ages 12 and older: 2 mg/kg IV over 30 minutes every 3 weeks up to maximum dose of 200 mg.

➤ **Urothelial carcinoma**
Adults: 200-mg IV infusion every 3 weeks or 400-mg IV infusion every 6 weeks.

➤ **Microsatellite instability-high (MSI-H) or mismatch repair deficient solid tumors** ⚠
Adults: 200-mg IV infusion every 3 weeks or 400-mg IV infusion every 6 weeks.
Children ages 2 and older: 2 mg/kg IV infusion every 3 weeks up to maximum dose of 200 mg.

➤ **MSI-H or mismatch repair deficient colorectal cancer** ⚠
Adults: 200-mg IV infusion every 3 weeks or 400-mg IV infusion every 6 weeks.

➤ **MSI-H or mismatch repair deficient endometrial carcinoma** ⚠
Adults: 200-mg IV infusion every 3 weeks or 400-mg IV infusion every 6 weeks.

➤ **Gastric cancer**
Adults: 200-mg IV infusion every 3 weeks or 400-mg IV infusion every 6 weeks.

➤ **Esophageal carcinoma**
Adults: 200-mg IV infusion every 3 weeks or 400-mg IV infusion every 6 weeks.

➤ **Cervical cancer**
Adults: 200-mg IV infusion every 3 weeks or 400-mg IV infusion every 6 weeks.

➤ **Hepatocellular carcinoma**
Adults: 200-mg IV infusion every 3 weeks or 400-mg IV infusion every 6 weeks.

➤ **Recurrent locally advanced or metastatic Merkel cell carcinoma (MCC)**
Adults: 200-mg IV infusion every 3 weeks or 400-mg IV infusion every 6 weeks.
Children: 2 mg/kg IV infusion every 3 weeks up to maximum dose of 200 mg.

➤ **Advanced renal cell carcinoma, in combination with axitinib or lenvatinib**
Adults: 200-mg IV infusion every 3 weeks, or 400-mg IV infusion every 6 weeks, in combination with 5 mg axitinib PO b.i.d. or lenvatinib 20 mg PO daily.

➤ **Endometrial carcinoma that isn't MSI-H or mismatch repair deficient, in combination with lenvatinib** ⚠
Adults: 200-mg IV infusion every 3 weeks, or 400-mg IV infusion every 6 weeks, in combination with lenvatinib 20 mg PO once daily.

P

➤ **Tumor mutational burden-high (TMB-H) solid tumors** ⚠

Adults: 200-mg IV infusion every 3 weeks, or 400-mg IV infusion every 6 weeks.

Children ages 2 and older: 2 mg/kg IV infusion every 3 weeks up to maximum dose of 200 mg.

➤ **Cutaneous squamous cell carcinoma**

Adults: 200-mg IV infusion every 3 weeks or 400-mg IV infusion every 6 weeks.

➤ **Triple-negative breast cancer (TNBC), in combination with chemotherapy (neoadjuvant and adjuvant)**

Adults: Neoadjuvant treatment in combination with chemotherapy for 24 weeks (eight doses of 200-mg IV infusion every 3 weeks or four doses of 400-mg IV infusion every 6 weeks), followed by adjuvant treatment as a single agent for up to 27 weeks (nine doses of 200-mg IV infusion every 3 weeks or five doses of 400-mg IV infusion every 6 weeks).

➤ **Locally recurrent unresectable or metastatic TNBC that expresses PD-L1, in combination with chemotherapy** ⚠

Adults: 200-mg IV infusion every 3 weeks or 400-mg IV infusion every 6 weeks. Give before chemotherapy when given on same day.

✳ *NEW INDICATION:* **Adjuvant treatment following resection and platinum-based chemotherapy for patients with stage IB, II, or IIIA NSCLC**

Adults: 200-mg IV infusion every 3 weeks or 400-mg IV infusion every 6 weeks until disease recurrence or unacceptable toxicity occurs, or up to 12 months in patients without disease recurrence.

ADMINISTRATION

IV

▼ Don't give as IV push or bolus.

▼ Visually inspect solution for particulate matter and discoloration. Solution appears clear to slightly opalescent, colorless to slightly yellow. Discard if particles are visible.

▼ Dilute to yield 1 to 10 mg/mL in bag of NSS or D₅W. Gently invert bag to mix solution.

▼ Discard unused portion left in vial.

▼ Administer infusion over 30 minutes using an IV line with a nonpyrogenic, low-protein-binding 0.2- to 5-micron filter.

▼ Diluted solution remains stable for 96 hours if refrigerated and for 6 hours at room temperature. Don't freeze.

▼ **Incompatibilities:** Don't infuse other drugs through same infusion line.

ACTION

A humanized monoclonal antibody that binds to the PD1 receptor found on the surface of T cells, reversing T-cell suppression and resulting in decreased tumor growth.

Route	Onset	Peak	Duration
IV	Unknown	Unknown	Unknown

Half-life: 22 days.

ADVERSE REACTIONS

CNS: asthenia, fatigue, fever, confusion, peripheral neuropathy, weakness, headache, dizziness, insomnia. **CV:** peripheral edema, HTN, pericarditis, *MI, arrhythmia, cardiac tamponade,* pericardial effusion. **EENT:** uveitis, nasopharyngitis. **GI:** anorexia, nausea, constipation, diarrhea, vomiting, abdominal pain, colitis, stomatitis. **GU:** *KF,* nephritis, UTI. **Hematologic:** anemia, *lymphocytopenia, thrombocytopenia, neutropenia, increased INR.* **Hepatic:** *hepatitis,* increased AST, ALT, and ALP levels. **Metabolic:** hyperthyroidism, hypothyroidism, hyperglycemia, *hyponatremia, hyperkalemia, hypokalemia, hypomagnesemia,* hypoalbuminemia, hypertriglyceridemia, hypercholesterolemia, hypophosphatemia, decreased serum bicarbonate level, hypercalcemia, *hypocalcemia.* **Musculoskeletal:** arthralgia, back pain, musculoskeletal pain, myalgia, myositis, immune-mediated arthritis. **Respiratory:** cough, dyspnea, URI, pneumonitis, pneumonia, pleural effusion, *respiratory failure.* **Skin:** pruritus, rash, immune-mediated rash, vitiligo. **Other:** antibody development, flulike symptoms, hypophysitis, infection, chills, *sepsis.*

INTERACTIONS

Drug-drug. *Thalidomide:* May increase mortality in patients with multiple myeloma when used with pembrolizumab and dexamethasone. This combination isn't recommended.

EFFECTS ON LAB TEST RESULTS

• May increase glucose, triglyceride, cholesterol, creatinine, ALP, ALT, and AST levels.

• May decrease bicarbonate, sodium, magnesium, and albumin levels.

• May increase or decrease potassium, calcium, and thyroid hormone levels.

• May decrease Hb level and lymphocyte, platelet, and WBC counts.

CONTRAINDICATIONS & CAUTIONS

• Contraindicated in patients hypersensitive to drug or its components.

☒ ☉ Alert: Patients with *EGFR* or *ALK* genomic tumor aberrations should have disease progression on FDA-approved therapy before receiving pembrolizumab.

☉ Alert: Drug can cause immune-mediated reactions (pneumonitis, pericarditis, myelitis, hepatitis, endocrinopathies, colitis, nephritis, kidney dysfunction); drug may need to be withheld or permanently discontinued.

• Severe, life-threatening infusion-related reactions have occurred in patients receiving drug.

• Use cautiously in patients who receive allogeneic hematopoietic stem cell transplantation before or after treatment with a PD-1/PD-L1 blocking antibody. Serious or fatal complications have occurred, including GVHD, hepatic veno-occlusive disease, and steroid-requiring febrile syndrome. Monitor patient closely if benefits outweigh risks.

• Use hasn't been studied in patients with Child-Pugh class B or C liver impairment.

• Safety and effectiveness have been established in children younger than age 18 with cHL, PMBCL, MCC, MSI-H cancer, and TMB-H cancer, or in children ages 12 to 17 for adjuvant treatment of melanoma. Safety and effectiveness in children haven't been established in the other approved indications.

Dialyzable drug: Unknown.

PREGNANCY-LACTATION-REPRODUCTION

• Drug may cause fetal harm. Don't use during pregnancy. Patients of childbearing potential should use highly effective contraception during therapy and for 4 months after final dose.

• It isn't known if drug appears in human milk. Patient shouldn't breastfeed during therapy and for 4 months after final dose.

NURSING CONSIDERATIONS

• Verify pregnancy status in patients of childbearing potential before initiation.

• Monitor patient closely for signs and symptoms of hypersensitivity or infusion reactions. Stop infusion and have drugs, such as epinephrine, antihistamines, and corticosteroids, available for immediate treatment of such a reaction.

• Assess for signs and symptoms of immune-mediated reactions. Thyroid disorders, liver toxicity, and hypophysitis typically occur early

in treatment. Pulmonary, kidney, and GI toxicity may develop after 6 months of treatment.

• Monitor patient for immune-mediated pneumonitis (shortness of breath, chest pain, new or worsening cough). Evaluate radiographically, give corticosteroids if clinically indicated, and withhold or discontinue drug based on grade.

• Monitor patient for signs and symptoms of immune-mediated colitis (increased frequency of bowel movements or diarrhea; abdominal pain or tenderness; melena). or immune-mediated hepatitis (elevated liver enzyme levels, jaundice, tea-colored urine, nausea, vomiting, anorexia, right upper quadrant abdominal pain, abnormal bleeding or bruising). Give corticosteroids as clinically indicated and withhold or discontinue drug based on toxicity grade.

• Monitor patient for signs and symptoms of hypophysitis, immune-mediated inflammation of pituitary gland (persistent or unusual headaches, extreme weakness, dizziness, fainting, vision changes). Give corticosteroids and hormone replacement as clinically indicated and withhold or discontinue drug based on toxicity grade.

• Monitor patient for signs and symptoms of immune-mediated endocrine disorders (hypothyroidism, hyperthyroidism, adrenal insufficiency), which may include tachycardia, weight loss or gain, edema, and hair loss. Assess hormone levels at baseline, periodically during treatment, and as clinically indicated. Give corticosteroids and hormone replacement as clinically indicated, and withhold or discontinue drug based on toxicity grade.

• Be aware of potential for less common immune-mediated adverse reactions, such as exfoliative dermatitis, uveitis, arthritis, myositis, pancreatitis, hemolytic anemia, and partial seizures in patients with inflammatory foci in the brain. Based on severity of adverse reaction, withhold drug and administer corticosteroids.

PATIENT TEACHING

• Caution patient about the risk of immune-mediated adverse effects that may require corticosteroid treatment and interruption of therapy or discontinuation of drug.

• Teach patient signs and symptoms of lung problems (dyspnea, chest pain, cough), colitis (diarrhea, melena, abdominal pain), liver problems (yellowing of the skin or eyes, dark

---

urine, nausea or vomiting, decreased appetite, abdominal pain, bleeding or bruising), hormone gland problems (rapid heartbeat, weight loss, diaphoresis, weight gain, hair loss, feeling cold), kidney problems (changes in the amount or color of urine), and other problems (rash, vision changes, muscle or joint pain, muscle weakness) and to report them to prescriber.
• Advise patient to report pregnancy and plans to become pregnant or to breastfeed.
• Teach patient of childbearing potential of potential hazard to fetus and to use contraception during therapy and for 4 months after final dose.
• Advise patient to stop breastfeeding during therapy and for 4 months after final dose.
• Instruct patient to keep lab test appointments as requested by prescriber to monitor drug's safety and effectiveness.

SAFETY ALERT!

PEMEtrexed disodium ☒
pem-e-TREKS-ed

Alimta, Pemfexy, Pemrydi RTU

Therapeutic class: Antineoplastics
Pharmacologic class: Folate antagonists

AVAILABLE FORMS

Injection (lyophilized powder for solution):
100 mg, 500 mg, 750 mg, 1,000 mg in single-use vials
Solution for injection: 100 mg, 500 mg, 800 mg, 1,000 mg (25 mg/mL) multidose vial
Solution (ready to use): 100 mg/10 mL, 500 mg/50 mL, 1,000 mg/100 mL single-use vials

INDICATIONS & DOSAGES

Adjust-a-dose (for all indications): Refer to manufacturer's instructions for toxicity-related dosage adjustments for patients with CrCl of 45 mL/minute or more.

➤ **Malignant pleural mesothelioma in patients whose disease is unresectable or who aren't candidates for curative surgery, in combination with cisplatin**
Adults: 500 mg/m² IV infusion on day 1 of each 21-day cycle before cisplatin. Refer to full prescribing information for cisplatin.
➤ **Locally advanced or metastatic NSCLC after prior chemotherapy; as single-agent maintenance therapy for patients whose**

disease hasn't progressed after four cycles of platinum-based first-line chemotherapy
Adults: 500 mg/m² IV infusion on day 1 of each 21-day cycle.
➤ **Locally advanced or metastatic, non-squamous NSCLC as initial treatment in combination with cisplatin**
Adults: 500 mg/m² IV infusion administered before cisplatin on day 1 of each 21-day cycle for up to six cycles in the absence of disease progression or unacceptable toxicity. Refer to full prescribing information for cisplatin.
➤ **Initial treatment of metastatic nonsquamous NSCLC with no *EGFR* or *ALK* genomic tumor aberrations, in combination with pembrolizumab and platinum chemotherapy** ☒
Adults: 500 mg/m² IV infusion administered after pembrolizumab and before carboplatin or cisplatin on day 1 of each 21-day cycle for four cycles. After completion of platinum-based therapy, may give pemetrexed as maintenance therapy, alone or with pembrolizumab, until disease progression or unacceptable toxicity occurs. Refer to the full prescribing information for pembrolizumab and carboplatin or cisplatin.

ADMINISTRATION

IV
⚠ *Alert:* Hazardous drug; use safe handling and disposal precautions.
▼ Premedicate with folic acid 400 to 1,000 mcg PO once daily beginning 7 days before first dose of drug and continue during therapy and for 21 days after last dose.
▼ Premedicate with vitamin B₁₂ 1 mg IM 1 week before first dose of pemetrexed and every three cycles thereafter. Don't substitute PO vitamin B₁₂ for IM. After the first cycle, may give vitamin B₁₂ injections on the first day of the cycle.
▼ Premedicate with dexamethasone 4 mg PO b.i.d. the day before, the day of, and the day after pemetrexed administration.
▼ Transfer calculated dose of ready-to-use solution (Pemrydi RTU) to empty IV bag; don't further dilute.
▼ Reconstitute 100-mg vial with 4.2 mL or 500-mg vial with 20 mL of preservative-free NSS to yield 25 mg/mL.
▼ Swirl vial gently until powder is completely dissolved. Solution should be clear and colorless to yellow or yellow-green. If particulate matter is observed, discard vial.

▼ Calculate appropriate dose, and further dilute with NSS so total volume of solution is 100 mL.

▼ Give over 10 minutes.

▼ Reconstituted solution and dilution are stable for 24 hours refrigerated.

▼ Dilute Pemfexy solution with D_5W to a total volume of 100 mL. Don't use diluents other than D_5W.

▼ **Incompatibilities:** Calcium-containing diluents, including Ringer or lactated Ringer for injection; other drugs or diluents. Consult a compatibility reference for full details.

ACTION

Disturbs cell replication by inhibiting several folate-dependent enzymes involved in nucleotide synthesis.

Route	Onset	Peak	Duration
IV	Unknown	Unknown	Unknown

Half-life: 3.5 hours.

ADVERSE REACTIONS

CNS: depression, fatigue, fever, neuropathy, taste disturbance. **CV:** edema, HTN, *thrombosis,* chest pain. **EENT:** conjunctivitis, increased tearing, pharyngitis. **GI:** anorexia, constipation, diarrhea, dyspepsia, nausea, stomatitis, vomiting. **GU:** elevated creatinine level, *KF.* **Hematologic:** anemia, *leukopenia, neutropenia, thrombocytopenia.* **Hepatic:** increased transaminase levels, increased ALP level. **Metabolic:** dehydration, hyperglycemia, hypoalbuminemia, *hyponatremia,* hypophosphatemia, *hypocalcemia, hyperkalemia, hypokalemia.* **Musculoskeletal:** arthralgia, myalgia. **Respiratory:** cough, dyspnea. **Skin:** alopecia, rash, pruritus, urticaria, *erythema multiforme.* **Other:** allergic reaction, infection.

INTERACTIONS

Drug-drug. *Ibuprofen:* May decrease pemetrexed clearance in patients with CrCl between 45 and 79 mL/minute. Avoid ibuprofen for 2 days before, during, and 2 days after pemetrexed therapy. Monitor patient for myelosuppression and assess kidney and GI toxicity status more frequently if ibuprofen use can't be avoided.
Kidney-toxic drugs, probenecid: May delay pemetrexed clearance. Monitor patient.
Vaccines, inactivated: May decrease vaccine effectiveness. Complete age-appropriate vaccinations at least 2 weeks before start of drug therapy or, if vaccine is given within 2 weeks, revaccinate at least 3 months after drug is discontinued.
Vaccines, live: May increase adverse effects and decrease effectiveness of vaccine. Avoid use during and for 3 months after drug therapy.

EFFECTS ON LAB TEST RESULTS

• May increase glucose, ALT, AST, ALP, GGT, and creatinine levels.
• May decrease albumin, sodium, phosphate, and calcium levels.
• May increase or decrease potassium level.
• May decrease Hb level, hematocrit, ANC, and platelet and WBC counts.

CONTRAINDICATIONS & CAUTIONS

• Contraindicated in patients with a history of severe hypersensitivity reaction to drug.
• Drug can cause KF. Don't use in patients with CrCl of less than 45 mL/minute.
• Drug can cause severe myelosuppression requiring transfusions, which may lead to neutropenic infection, serious interstitial pneumonitis (including fatal cases), and radiation recall in patients who received radiation weeks to years previously.
• Safety and effectiveness in children haven't been established.
Dialyzable drug: Unknown.
⚠ **Overdose S&S:** Neutropenia, anemia, thrombocytopenia, mucositis, rash, infection with or without fever, diarrhea.

PREGNANCY-LACTATION-REPRODUCTION

• Drug can cause fetal harm. Avoid use during pregnancy. Patients of childbearing potential should use effective contraception during therapy and for 6 months after final dose. Males with partners of childbearing potential should use contraception during treatment and for 3 months after final dose.
• If used during pregnancy or if patient becomes pregnant during therapy, inform patient that drug may harm fetus.
• It isn't known if drug appears in human milk. Patient shouldn't breastfeed during and for 1 week after treatment.
• Drug may impair male fertility. It's unknown if effects are reversible.

NURSING CONSIDERATIONS

• Patient shouldn't start a new cycle of treatment unless ANC is 1,500/mm^3 or more, platelet count is 100,000/mm^3 or more, and CrCl is 45 mL/minute or more.
• Verify pregnancy status before treatment.
• Monitor patient for hypersensitivity reactions.
• Monitor patient for new-onset or worsening of pulmonary symptoms (dyspnea, cough, fever). Evaluate patient for pneumonitis if they occur.
• Monitor kidney function, CBC, platelet count, Hb level, hematocrit, and LFT values.
• Assess patient for neurotoxicity, mucositis, and diarrhea. Severe symptoms may warrant dosage adjustment.
• Monitor patient for infections and skin toxicity (SJS, TEN).
• To reduce the risk and severity of pemetrexed toxicity, give a corticosteroid, such as dexamethasone 4 mg PO b.i.d., the day before, the day of, and the day after giving this drug.
• **Alert:** To reduce toxicity, patient should take folic acid daily and receive IM vitamin B$_{12}$.
• **Look alike–sound alike:** Don't confuse pemetrexed with methotrexate or pralatrexate.

PATIENT TEACHING

• Stress importance of taking prescribed premedications to reduce risk of treatment-related toxicity.
• Inform patient that blood cell counts may drop during therapy. Instruct patient to report infection, fever, bleeding, or signs and symptoms of anemia (fatigue, shortness of breath, cold hands and feet, pallor).
• Tell patient who has received prior radiation about the risk of radiation recall. Advise patient to immediately report inflammation or blisters in a previously irradiated area.
• Urge patient to report adverse effects, especially fever, sore throat, infection, diarrhea, fatigue, bleeding, cough, shortness of breath, and limb pain.
• Advise patient of childbearing potential and male patient with partners of childbearing potential of fetal risk and the need for effective contraception.
• Caution patient not to breastfeed during treatment and for 1 week after final dose.

penicillin G benzathine (benzathine benzylpenicillin)

pen-i-SILL-in

Bicillin L-A

Therapeutic class: Antibiotics
Pharmacologic class: Natural penicillins

AVAILABLE FORMS

Injection: 600,000 units/syringe (1 mL);
1,200,000 units/syringe (2 mL);
2,400,000 units/syringe (4 mL)

INDICATIONS & DOSAGES

➤ **Group A streptococcal URIs**
Adults: 1.2 million units IM as a single injection.
Children weighing 27 kg or more:
900,000 units IM as a single injection.
Infants and children weighing less than 27 kg:
300,000 to 600,000 units IM as a single injection.
➤ **To prevent poststreptococcal rheumatic fever and glomerulonephritis**
Adults and children weighing 27 kg or more: 1.2 million units IM once monthly or 600,000 units IM every 2 weeks.
➤ **Congenital syphilis**
Children ages 2 to 12: Follow CDC guidelines.
Children younger than age 2: 50,000 units/kg to maximum of 2.4 million units IM as a single dose.
➤ **Syphilis (primary, secondary, and latent)**
Adults: 2.4 million units IM as a single dose.
➤ **Syphilis (tertiary and neurosyphilis)**
Adults: 2.4 million units IM once every 7 days for 3 doses.
➤ **Yaws, bejel, and pinta**
Adults: 1.2 million units IM as a single injection.

ADMINISTRATION

IM
Boxed Warning Inadvertent IV use may cause cardiac arrest and death. Don't give IV or mix with other IV solutions. ■
• Before giving drug, ask patient about allergic reactions to penicillin.
• Obtain specimen for culture and sensitivity tests before giving first dose. Begin therapy while awaiting results.
• Warm to room temperature before giving to lessen injection-site pain.

- Inspect visually for particulate matter and discoloration before administration.
- Inject deep into upper outer quadrant of buttocks or ventrogluteal site in adults and in midlateral thigh in infants and small children. Rotate injection sites. Avoid injection into or near major nerves or blood vessels to prevent permanent neurovascular damage.
- Inject at a slow, steady rate to prevent needle occlusion.
- Injection may be painful, but ice applied to the site may ease discomfort.
- Store in refrigerator at 36° to 46° F (2° to 8° C); don't freeze.

ACTION
Inhibits cell-wall synthesis during bacterial multiplication.

Route	Onset	Peak	Duration
IM	Unknown	12–24 hr	1–4 wk

Half-life: Unknown.

ADVERSE REACTIONS
CNS: neuropathy, headache. **GI:** *pseudomembranous colitis,* enterocolitis, nausea, vomiting, bloody stools, *CDAD.* **GU:** kidney dysfunction. **Hematologic:** *agranulocytosis, leukopenia, thrombocytopenia,* eosinophilia, hemolytic anemia. **Skin:** hypersensitivity reactions, sterile abscess at injection site. **Other:** *anaphylaxis,* hypersensitivity reactions.

INTERACTIONS
Drug-drug. *Aminoglycosides (amikacin, gentamicin, tobramycin):* May decrease aminoglycoside level. Monitor therapy.
Live-virus vaccines: May decrease effectiveness of live-virus vaccines. Avoid concurrent use.
Methotrexate: May increase risk of methotrexate toxicity. Monitor patient closely.
Probenecid: May increase penicillin level. Probenecid may be used for this purpose.
Tetracycline: May antagonize penicillin G benzathine effects. Avoid using together.
Warfarin: May increase anticoagulant effects. Monitor therapy.

EFFECTS ON LAB TEST RESULTS
- May increase BUN, creatinine, and AST levels.
- May increase urine myoglobin and protein levels.
- May decrease Hb level and platelet, WBC, and granulocyte counts.

- May cause positive Coombs test results.
- May cause false-positive CSF protein test results.
- May alter urine glucose testing using cupric sulfate (Benedict reagent).

CONTRAINDICATIONS & CAUTIONS
- Contraindicated in patients hypersensitive to drug or other penicillins.
- **Alert:** Intravascular administration, including direct intra-arterial injection or injection immediately adjacent to arteries, has resulted in severe neurovascular damage, including transverse myelitis with permanent paralysis, gangrene requiring amputation of digits and more proximal portions of extremities, and necrosis and sloughing at and surrounding the injection site.
- Use cautiously in patients allergic to other drugs, especially to cephalosporins, because of possible cross-sensitivity.
- Use cautiously in older adults and patients with a history of significant allergies or asthma.
- Drug may cause CDAD ranging in severity from mild diarrhea to fatal colitis. For suspected or confirmed CDAD, discontinue drug and start CDAD treatment.
- Drug may cause SCARs, including SJS, DRESS syndrome, and TEN. Monitor patient closely.
Dialyzable drug: Yes.
Overdose S&S: Neuromuscular hyperexcitability, seizures.

PREGNANCY-LACTATION-REPRODUCTION
- There are no adequate studies during pregnancy; fetal adverse effects haven't been reported. Use only if clearly needed.
- Drug appears in human milk. Use cautiously during breastfeeding.

NURSING CONSIDERATIONS
- **Alert:** Bicillin L-A is the only penicillin G benzathine product indicated for sexually transmitted infections. Don't substitute penicillin G benzathine and penicillin G procaine (Bicillin C-R) because it may not be effective.
- Monitor for diarrhea and severe skin reactions. Drug may need to be stopped.
- Drug's extremely slow absorption time makes allergic reactions difficult to treat.
- Large doses or prolonged therapy may cause bacterial or fungal superinfection, especially in older adults or patients who are debilitated or immunosuppressed.

• Monitor patients with syphilis for Jarisch-Herxheimer reactions (fever, chills, myalgia, headache, exacerbation of skin lesions, tachycardia, hyperventilation, flushing, mild hypotension). Reactions occur 1 to 2 hours after initial treatment and resolve within 12 to 24 hours.

• *Look alike–sound alike:* Don't confuse penicillin G benzathine with penicillamine or the various other types of penicillin.

PATIENT TEACHING
• Tell patient to report adverse reactions promptly.
• Advise patient that watery and bloody stools with or without stomach cramps and fever may occur during and up to 2 months or more after antibiotic use. Instruct the patient to report these symptoms as soon as possible.
• Warn patient that IM injection may be painful but that ice applied to the site may ease discomfort.
• Tell patient that entire drug course must be completed exactly as prescribed, even if feeling better, to increase effectiveness of treatment and decrease risk of bacterial resistance.

penicillin G potassium (benzylpenicillin potassium)
pen-i-SILL-in

Pfizerpen

Therapeutic class: Antibiotics
Pharmacologic class: Natural penicillins

AVAILABLE FORMS
Injection: 1 million units, 5 million units, 20 million units/vial
Premixed injection: 1 million units/50 mL, 2 million units/50 mL, 3 million units/50 mL

INDICATIONS & DOSAGES
Adjust-a-dose (for all indications): For patients who are uremic with CrCl greater than 10 mL/minute/1.73 m^2, give full loading dose followed by one-half of loading dose every 4 to 5 hours. If CrCl is less than 10 mL/minute/1.73 m^2, give full loading dose followed by one-half of loading dose every 8 to 10 hours. Make additional dosage modification in patients with both liver disease and kidney impairment.

➤ **Actinomycosis**
Adults: For cervicofacial infections, 1 to 6 million units/day in divided doses IM or IV

every 4 to 6 hours. For thoracic or abdominal infections, 10 to 20 million units/day in divided doses IM or IV every 4 to 6 hours or by continuous IV infusion.

➤ **Anthrax**
Adults: 8 million units/day in divided doses IM or IV every 6 hours; higher doses may be required depending on susceptibility of the organism.

➤ **Clostridial infections (botulism, gas gangrene, tetanus)**
Adults: 20 million units/day in divided doses IM or IV every 4 to 6 hours.

➤ **Diphtheria**
Adults: 2 to 3 million units/day in divided doses IM or IV every 4 to 6 hours for 10 to 12 days.
Children: 150,000 to 250,000 units/kg/day in equal doses IM or IV every 6 hours for 7 to 10 days.

➤ **Disseminated gonococcal infections**
Adults: 10 million units/day in divided doses IM or IV every 4 to 6 hours. Duration depends on type of infection.
Children weighing 45 kg or more with arthritis, endocarditis, or meningitis: 10 million units/day in four equally divided doses IM or IV, with duration of therapy depending on type of infection.
Children weighing less than 45 kg with arthritis: 100,000 units/kg/day in four equally divided doses IM or IV for 7 to 10 days.
Children weighing less than 45 kg with endocarditis: 250,000 units/kg/day in equal doses IM or IV every 4 hours for 4 weeks.
Children weighing less than 45 kg with meningitis: 250,000 units/kg/day in equal doses IM or IV every 4 hours for 10 to 14 days.

➤ **Erysipelothrix endocarditis**
Adults: 12 to 20 million units/day in divided doses IM or IV every 4 to 6 hours for 4 to 6 weeks.

➤ **Fusospirochetosis**
Adults: 5 to 10 million units/day in divided doses IM or IV every 4 to 6 hours.

➤ **Haverhill fever; rat bite fever**
Adults: 12 to 20 million units/day in divided doses IM or IV every 4 to 6 hours for 3 to 4 weeks.

➤ **Haverhill fever (with endocarditis caused by *Streptobacillus moniliformis*); rat bite fever**
Children: 150,000 to 250,000 units/kg/day in equal doses every 4 hours for 4 weeks.

➤ *Listeria monocytogenes* endocarditis or meningitis
Adults: 15 to 20 million units/day in divided doses IM or IV every 4 to 6 hours. Treat for 2 weeks for meningitis and 4 weeks for endocarditis.

➤ **Meningococcal meningitis or septicemia**
Adults: 24 million units/day as 2 million units IM or IV every 2 hours.

➤ **Meningitis caused by susceptible strains of pneumococcus and meningococcus**
Children: 250,000 units/kg/day in equal doses IM or IV every 4 hours for 7 to 14 days, depending on infecting organism. Maximum dosage, 12 to 20 million units/day.

➤ **Neurosyphilis**
Adults: 12 to 24 million units/day (2 to 4 million units every 4 hours) IM or IV for 10 to 14 days. Many experts recommend penicillin G benzathine 2.4 million units IM weekly for 3 weeks following completion of this regimen.

➤ **Syphilis (congenital and neurosyphilis) after newborn period**
Children: 200,000 to 300,000 units/kg/day (given as 50,000 units/kg IV every 4 to 6 hours) for 10 to 14 days.

➤ *Pasteurella multocida* bacteremia or meningitis
Adults: 4 to 6 million units/day in divided doses IM or IV every 4 to 6 hours for 2 weeks.

➤ **Serious staphylococcal infections**
Adults: 5 to 24 million units/day in equally divided doses IM or IV every 4 to 6 hours.

➤ **Serious streptococcal infections**
Adults: 12 to 24 million units/day in equally divided doses IM or IV every 4 to 6 hours.

➤ **Serious streptococcal infections, such as pneumonia and endocarditis (*Streptococcus pneumoniae*), and meningococcal infections**
Children: 150,000 to 300,000 units/kg/day in equal doses IM or IV every 4 to 6 hours. Duration of therapy depends on infecting organism and type of infection.

➤ **Leptospirosis ◆**
Adults: 1.5 million units IV every 6 hours for 7 days.

ADMINISTRATION
• Obtain specimen for culture and sensitivity tests before giving first dose. Begin therapy while awaiting results.
• Before giving, ask patient about allergic reactions to penicillin.

• May give IM or by continuous IV infusion for dosages of 500,000, 1 million, or 5 million units. Drug is also suitable for intrapleural, intra-articular, intrathecal, and other local instillations.
• Administer 20 million unit dosage form by IV infusion only.
🛈 *Alert:* Don't use in children requiring less than 1 million units/dose.

IV
▼ Reconstitute drug with sterile water for injection or NSS for injection. Volume of diluent varies with manufacturer.
▼ Reconstituted solution may be stored in refrigerator for up to 7 days.
▼ For continuous infusion, add reconstituted drug to 1 to 2 L of compatible solution. Determine how much fluid is needed and what the rate should be for a 24-hour period; then, add the drug to this fluid.
▼ Don't administer premixed solutions to patients requiring less than 1 million units per dose.
▼ Intermittent IV infusions are usually administered over 15 to 30 minutes.
▼ Thaw frozen bags at room temperature. May keep at room temperature for 24 hours or under refrigeration for 14 days. Don't refreeze thawed antibiotics.
▼ **Incompatibilities:** None listed by manufacturer. Consult a drug incompatibility reference for more information.

IM
• Vials containing 20 million units aren't intended for IM use.
• IM is the preferred route. Keep total volume of injection small.
• Give deep into large muscle; injection may be extremely painful.
• IM injection may be painful, but ice applied to the site may help alleviate discomfort.

ACTION
Inhibits cell-wall synthesis during bacterial multiplication.

Route	Onset	Peak	Duration
IV	Immediate	Immediate	Unknown
IM	Unknown	15–30 min	Unknown

Half-life: 31 to 50 minutes.

ADVERSE REACTIONS
CNS: agitation, anxiety, confusion, depresssion, dizziness, fatigue, hallucinations, lethargy, neuropathy; hyperreflexia, myoclonic

twitches, *seizures, coma* (high doses). **CV:** local thrombophlebitis or phlebitis. **EENT:** black or hairy tongue. **GI:** *pseudomembranous colitis,* enterocolitis, nausea, vomiting, *CDAD.* **GU:** interstitial nephritis (high doses), kidney dysfunction. **Hematologic:** *agranulocytosis, leukopenia, thrombocytopenia,* anemia, eosinophilia, hemolytic anemia. **Metabolic:** *hyperkalemia* (high doses). **Musculoskeletal:** arthralgia, myalgia. **Skin:** exfoliative dermatitis, maculopapular rash, pain at injection site. **Other:** *anaphylaxis,* hypersensitivity reactions, overgrowth of non-susceptible organisms.

INTERACTIONS

Drug-drug. *Aminoglycosides (amikacin, gentamicin, tobramycin):* May decrease aminoglycoside level. Monitor therapy.
Aspirin, furosemide, indomethacin, sulfonamides, thiazide diuretics: May compete with penicillin for kidney tubular secretion, prolonging penicillin half-life. Monitor patient.
Bacteriostatic antibacterial agents (chloramphenicol, macrolide antibiotics, sulfonamides, tetracyclines): May decrease bactericidal effect of penicillin. Avoid use together.
Live-virus vaccines: May decrease effectiveness of live-virus vaccines. Don't use together.
Methotrexate: May increase risk of methotrexate toxicity. Monitor patient closely.
Potassium-sparing diuretics: May increase risk of hyperkalemia. Avoid using together.
Probenecid: May increase penicillin level. Probenecid may be used for this purpose.
Warfarin: May increase or decrease anticoagulant effects. Monitor PT and INR.

EFFECTS ON LAB TEST RESULTS

• May increase potassium level.
• May decrease Hb level and platelet, WBC, and granulocyte counts.
• May cause positive Coombs test result.
• May cause false-positive CSF protein test result.
• May alter urine glucose testing using cupric sulfate (Benedict reagent, Fehling solution, or Clinitest tablet).

CONTRAINDICATIONS & CAUTIONS

• Contraindicated in patients hypersensitive to drug or other penicillins.
• Use cautiously in patients with other drug allergies, especially to cephalosporins, because of possible cross-sensitivity.

• Use cautiously in older adults and patients with kidney impairment, significant allergies, or asthma.
• Drug may cause CDAD ranging in severity from mild diarrhea to fatal colitis. If CDAD is suspected or confirmed, drug may need to be discontinued and treatment initiated.
• SCARs (SJS, TEN, DRESS syndrome, acute generalized exanthematous pustulosis) have been reported.
Dialyzable drug: Yes.
⚠ *Overdose S&S:* Agitation, confusion, asterixis, hallucinations, stupor, coma, multifocal myoclonus, seizures, encephalopathy, hyperkalemia.

PREGNANCY-LACTATION-REPRODUCTION

• There are no adequate studies during pregnancy. Use only if clearly needed.
• Penicillins appear in human milk. Use cautiously during breastfeeding.

NURSING CONSIDERATIONS

• Monitor IV site for phlebitis.
• Monitor kidney function closely. Patients with poor kidney function may have increased levels of penicillin and are at increased risk for adverse effects.
• Due to increased risk of electrolyte imbalances, monitor potassium and sodium levels closely in patients receiving more than 10 million units IV daily.
• Monitor liver function and CBC periodically during therapy.
• Observe patient closely. With large doses and prolonged therapy, bacterial or fungal superinfection may occur, especially in older adults or patients who are debilitated or immunosuppressed.
• For most acute infections, continue treatment for at least 48 to 72 hours after patient becomes asymptomatic. For group A beta-hemolytic streptococcal infections, maintain treatment for at least 10 days to reduce risk of rheumatic fever.
• Monitor patients with syphilis or other spirochetal infections (Lyme disease, relapsing fever) for Jarisch-Herxheimer reactions (fever, chills, myalgia, headache, exacerbation of skin lesions, tachycardia, hyperventilation, flushing, mild hypotension). Reactions occur 1 to 2 hours after initial treatment and resolve within 12 to 24 hours.
• *Look alike–sound alike:* Don't confuse penicillin G potassium with Polycillin,

penicillamine, or the various other types of penicillin.

PATIENT TEACHING

• Tell patient to notify prescriber if rash, fever, or chills develop. A rash is the most common allergic reaction.

• Warn patient that IM injection may be painful but that ice applied to the site may help alleviate discomfort.

• Advise patient that watery and bloody stools with or without stomach cramps and fever may occur during and for up to 2 months or more after antibiotic use. Instruct patient to report these symptoms as soon as possible.

• Tell patient that entire course of drug must be completed exactly as prescribed, even if feeling better, to increase effectiveness of treatment and decrease risk of bacterial resistance.

penicillin G procaine (benzylpenicillin procaine)
pen-i-SILL-in

Therapeutic class: Antibiotics
Pharmacologic class: Natural penicillins

AVAILABLE FORMS
Injection: 600,000 units/mL in 1-mL and 2-mL syringes

INDICATIONS & DOSAGES
➤ **Cutaneous anthrax**
Adults: 600,000 to 1 million units/day IM.
➤ **Inhalational anthrax (postexposure)**
Adults: 1.2 million units IM every 12 hours. Available safety data for penicillin G procaine at this dose would best support a duration of therapy of 2 weeks or less.
Children: 25,000 units/kg (maximum, 1.2 million units) IM every 12 hours.
Note: Treatment of inhalational anthrax (postexposure) must be continued for a total of 60 days. Consider risks and benefits of continuing administration of penicillin G procaine for more than 2 weeks or switching to an effective alternative treatment.
➤ **Bacterial endocarditis (group A streptococci), only in extremely sensitive infections**
Adults: 600,000 to 1 million units/day IM.
➤ **Adjunctive therapy for diphtheria with antitoxin**
Adults: 300,000 to 600,000 units/day IM for 14 days.

➤ **Diphtheria carrier state**
Adults: 300,000 units/day IM for 10 days.
➤ **Erysipeloid**
Adults: 600,000 to 1 million units/day IM.
➤ **Fusospirochetosis (Vincent infection)**
Adults: 600,000 to 1 million units/day IM.
➤ **Pneumonia (pneumococcal), moderately severe (uncomplicated)**
Adults: 600,000 to 1 million units/day IM for a minimum of 10 days.
➤ **Rat bite fever (*Streptobacillus moniliformis* and *Spirillum minus*)**
Adults: 600,000 to 1 million units/day IM.
➤ **Staphylococcal infections, moderately severe to severe**
Adults: 600,000 to 1 million units/day IM for a minimum of 10 days.
➤ **Streptococcal infections (group A), including moderately severe to severe tonsillitis, erysipelas, scarlet fever, URI, and skin and soft-tissue infections**
Adults: 600,000 to 1 million units/day IM for minimum of 10 days.
➤ **Syphilis (primary, secondary, and latent syphilis with negative spinal fluid exam)**
Adults and children older than age 12: 600,000 units/day IM for 8 days; total, 4.8 million units.
➤ **Late syphilis (tertiary syphilis, neurosyphilis, and latent syphilis with positive spinal fluid exam or no spinal fluid exam)**
Adults: 600,000 units/day IM for 10 to 15 days; total, 6 to 9 million units.
➤ **Congenital syphilis**
Children weighing less than 31.7 kg: 50,000 units/kg/day IM for 10 days. Maximum dosage, 2.4 million units/day.
➤ **Yaws, bejel, pinta**
Adults: Treatment as for syphilis in the corresponding stage of disease.

ADMINISTRATION
IM
• Before giving drug, ask patient about allergic reactions to penicillin.
• Obtain specimen for culture and sensitivity tests before giving first dose. Begin therapy while awaiting results.
• Give deep in upper outer quadrant of buttocks or ventrogluteal site in adults and in midlateral thigh in neonates, infants, and small children. Rotate injection sites. Don't give subcut. Don't massage injection site.

• Inject at a slow, steady rate to avoid needle blockage caused by high concentration of suspended material in product.

🔵 *Alert:* Inadvertent IV, intravascular, or intra-arterial administration may cause severe or permanent vascular damage. Injection into or near major nerves may cause permanent nerve damage.

• IM injection may be painful, but ice applied to the site may help alleviate discomfort.

• Inspect for particulate matter and discoloration before administration.

• Store at 36° to 46° F (2° to 8° C); don't freeze.

ACTION

Inhibits cell-wall synthesis during bacterial multiplication.

Route	Onset	Peak	Duration
IM	Unknown	1–4 hr	15–24 hr

Half-life: Unknown.

ADVERSE REACTIONS

CNS: depression, dizziness, fatigue, lethargy, fever. **CV:** edema. **GI:** *pseudomembranous colitis.* **Musculoskeletal:** arthralgia. **Skin:** rash, urticaria, *SCARs.* **Other:** *anaphylaxis,* hypersensitivity reactions, chills, overgrowth of nonsusceptible organisms.

INTERACTIONS

Drug-drug. *Aminoglycosides (amikacin, gentamicin, tobramycin):* May decrease aminoglycoside level. Monitor therapy.
Live-virus vaccines: May decrease vaccine effectiveness. Avoid concurrent use.
Methotrexate: May increase risk of methotrexate toxicity. Monitor patient closely.
Probenecid: May increase penicillin level. Probenecid may be used for this purpose.
Tetracycline: May decrease bactericidal effect of penicillin. Avoid use together.
Warfarin: May increase effects of warfarin. Monitor coagulation status and adjust warfarin dosage as needed.

EFFECTS ON LAB TEST RESULTS

• May decrease Hb level and platelet, WBC, and granulocyte counts.

CONTRAINDICATIONS & CAUTIONS

• Contraindicated in patients hypersensitive to drug, other penicillins, or any of its components.

• Drug is no longer indicated for treatment of gonorrhea.

• Use cautiously in patients with other drug allergies, especially to cephalosporins, because of possible cross-sensitivity.

• In patients with a history of hypersensitivity to procaine, administer intradermal test with 0.1 mL of 1% or 2% procaine solution and observe for wheal, flare, or eruption. If these occur, don't use drug and treat sensitivity supportively.

🔬 Use cautiously in patients with G6PD deficiency, congenital or idiopathic methemoglobinemia, cardiac or pulmonary compromise, or exposure to oxidizing agents and in infants younger than age 6 months due to increased risk of methemoglobinemia related to procaine.

• Drug may cause CDAD ranging in severity from mild diarrhea to fatal colitis. If CDAD is suspected or confirmed, drug may need to be discontinued and treatment initiated.

Dialyzable drug: Yes.

⚠ *Overdose S&S:* Neuromuscular hyperexcitability, seizures.

PREGNANCY-LACTATION-REPRODUCTION

• Penicillin G crosses the placental barrier; however, there are no adequate studies during pregnancy and no human evidence of adverse effects on the fetus if used during pregnancy. Use only when clearly needed.

• Drug appears in human milk. Use cautiously during breastfeeding.

NURSING CONSIDERATIONS

🔵 *Alert:* Continue postexposure treatment for inhalation anthrax for 60 days. Prescriber should consider the risk-benefit ratio of continuing penicillin longer than 2 weeks, compared with switching to another drug.

• Monitor patient for diarrhea and initiate therapeutic measures as needed. Drug may need to be stopped.

• Allergic reactions are hard to treat because of drug's slow absorption rate.

• Monitor patient for SCARs. Stop drug immediately if SCARs are suspected.

• Monitor patients for procaine neuropsychiatric reaction (anxiety, confusion, agitation, depression, weakness, seizure, hallucination, combativeness, expressed "fear of impending death"), especially after a large single dose. Reactions are transient and last 15 to 30 minutes.

- Monitor patients at risk for methemoglobinemia (cyanosis, headache, tachycardia, shortness of breath, light-headedness, fatigue). Signs and symptoms may occur immediately after exposure or hours later.
- Monitor kidney and hematopoietic function periodically with prolonged use.
- Monitor patients for fibrosis and atrophy from repeated IM injections.
- Monitor patients with syphilis for Jarisch-Herxheimer reactions (fever, chills, myalgia, headache, exacerbation of skin lesions, tachycardia, hyperventilation, flushing, mild hypotension). Reactions occur 1 to 2 hours after initial treatment and resolve within 12 to 24 hours.
- If large doses are given or if therapy is prolonged, bacterial or fungal superinfection may occur, especially in older adults and patients who are debilitated or immunosuppressed.
- Treatment duration depends on site and cause of infection.
- *Look alike–sound alike:* Don't confuse penicillin G procaine with penicillamine or the various other types of penicillin.

PATIENT TEACHING

- Tell patient to report adverse reactions promptly. A rash is the most common allergic reaction.
- Warn patient that IM injection may be painful but that ice applied to the site may help alleviate discomfort.
- Advise patient that watery and bloody stools with or without stomach cramps and fever may occur during and for up to 2 months or more after antibiotic use. Instruct patient to report these symptoms as soon as possible.
- Tell patient that entire drug course must be completed exactly as prescribed, even if feeling better, to increase effectiveness of treatment and decrease risk of bacterial resistance.

penicillin G sodium (benzylpenicillin sodium)

pen-i-SILL-in

Therapeutic class: Antibiotics
Pharmacologic class: Natural penicillins

AVAILABLE FORMS

Injection: 5 million-unit vial

INDICATIONS & DOSAGES

Adjust-a-dose (for all indications): If CrCl is less than 10 mL/minute, give the full loading dose followed by 50% of the loading dose every 8 to 10 hours. If patient is uremic and CrCl is more than 10 mL/minute, give full loading dose; then give half the loading dose every 4 to 5 hours for additional doses. Make additional dosage adjustments in patients with both liver and kidney impairment.

➤ **Actinomycosis**
Adults: For cervicofacial infections, 1 to 6 million units/day IM or IV in divided doses every 4 to 6 hours. For thoracic or abdominal infections, 10 to 20 million units/day in divided doses every 4 to 6 hours.

➤ **Anthrax**
Adults: 8 million units/day IM or IV in divided doses every 6 hours; higher dosages may be required depending on susceptibility of the organism.

➤ **Clostridial infections (botulism, gas gangrene, tetanus)**
Adults: 20 million units/day IM or IV in divided doses every 4 to 6 hours.

➤ **Diphtheria**
Adults: 2 to 3 million units/day IM or IV in divided doses every 4 to 6 hours for 10 to 12 days.
Children: 150,00 to 250,00 units/kg/day IM or IV in equally divided doses every 6 hours for 7 to 10 days.

➤ **Disseminated gonococcal infections**
Adults and children weighing 45 kg or more with arthritis, meningitis, or endocarditis: 10 million units/day IM or IV in equally divided doses every 4 to 6 hours; duration of therapy depends on the type of infection.
Children weighing less than 45 kg with arthritis: 100,000 units /kg/day IM or IV in equally divided doses every 6 hours for 7 to 10 days.
Children weighing less than 45 kg with meningitis: 250,000 units/kg/day IM or IV in equal doses every 4 hours for 10 to 14 days.
Children weighing less than 45 kg with endocarditis: 250,000 units/kg/day IM or IV in equal doses every 4 hours for 4 weeks.

➤ *Erysipelothrix* **endocarditis**
Adults: 12 to 20 million units/day IM or IV in divided doses every 4 to 6 hours for 4 to 6 weeks.

➤ **Fusospirochetosis**
Adults: 5 to 10 million units/day IM or IV in divided doses every 4 to 6 hours.

P

➤ **Haverhill fever; rat bite fever**
Adults: 12 to 20 million units/day IM or IV in divided doses every 4 to 6 hours for 3 to 4 weeks.
Children: 150,00 to 250,00 units/kg/day IM or IV in equally divided doses every 4 hours for 4 weeks.

➤ ***Listeria monocytogenes* infections, including endocarditis or meningitis**
Adults: 15 to 20 million units/day IM or IV in divided doses every 4 to 6 hours. Treat for 2 weeks for meningitis and 4 weeks for endocarditis.

➤ **Meningococcal meningitis or septicemia**
Adults: 24 million units/day as 2 million units IM or IV every 2 hours.

➤ **Meningitis caused by susceptible strains of pneumococcus or meningococcus**
Children: 250,000 units/kg/day IM or IV in divided doses every 4 hours for 7 to 14 days, depending on the infecting organism. Maximum dosage, 12 to 20 million units/day.

➤ **Neurosyphilis**
Adults: 12 to 24 million units/day (2 to 4 million units IM or IV every 4 hours) for 10 to 14 days. Many experts recommend benzathine penicillin G 2.4 million units IM weekly for 3 weeks following completion of this regimen.

➤ **Neurosyphilis; congenital syphilis**
Children after the newborn period: 200,000 to 300,000 units/kg/day IM or IV (administered as 50,000 units/kg every 4 to 6 hours) for 10 to 14 days.

➤ ***Pasteurella multocida* infections, including bacteremia or meningitis**
Adults: 4 to 6 million units/day IM or IV in divided doses every 4 to 6 hours for 2 weeks.

➤ **Serious staphylococcal and streptococcal infections**
Adults: 5 to 24 million units/day IM or IV in equally divided doses every 4 to 6 hours.

➤ **Serious infections due to susceptible strains of streptococci or meningococcus (such as pneumonia or endocarditis)**
Children: 150,000 units/kg/day IM or IV in equally divided doses every 4 to 6 hours. Duration depends on infecting organism and type of infection.

ADMINISTRATION

⚡ *Alert:* Don't use in patients requiring less than 1 million units/dose.
• Obtain specimen for culture and sensitivity tests before giving first dose. Begin therapy while awaiting results.

• Before giving, ask patient about allergic reactions to penicillin.
• Reconstitute drug with sterile water for injection, NSS for injection, or D₅W. Check manufacturer's instructions for volume of diluent necessary to produce desired drug level.
• May refrigerate reconstituted solution for 3 days.

IV
▼ Give by intermittent infusion. Dilute drug in 50 to 100 mL, and give over 30 minutes to 2 hours every 4 to 6 hours.
▼ Sterile reconstituted solution may be kept in refrigerator for up to 3 days.
▼ **Incompatibilities:** None listed by manufacturer. Consult a drug incompatibility reference for more information.

IM
• IM is the preferred route.
• Injection may be painful, but ice applied to site may help alleviate discomfort.
• Give deep in upper outer quadrant of buttocks in adults and in midlateral thigh in small children. Rotate injection sites. Don't give subcut.

ACTION

Inhibits cell-wall synthesis during bacterial multiplication.

Route	Onset	Peak	Duration
IV	Immediate	Immediate	Unknown
IM	Unknown	15–30 min	Unknown

Half-life: 31 to 50 minutes.

ADVERSE REACTIONS

CNS: neuropathy. **CV:** phlebitis or thrombophlebitis (IV form), *HF*. **EENT:** black or hairy tongue. **GI:** enterocolitis, *ischemic colitis*, nausea, vomiting, stomatitis, *pseudomembranous colitis, CDAD*. **GU:** kidney tubular damage, *interstitial nephritis*. **Hematologic:** hemolytic anemia, *agranulocytosis, leukopenia, thrombocytopenia*, anemia, eosinophilia. **Metabolic:** electrolyte disturbances. **Musculoskeletal:** arthralgia. **Skin:** injection-site pain. **Other:** hypersensitivity reactions, *anaphylaxis*, overgrowth of nonsusceptible organisms.

INTERACTIONS

Drug-drug. *Aminoglycosides (amikacin, gentamicin, tobramycin):* May decrease aminoglycoside level. Monitor therapy.

Reactions in bold italics are *life-threatening*.

Aspirin, furosemide, indomethacin, sulfon-amides, thiazide diuretics: May compete with penicillin for kidney tubular secretion, pro-longing the half-life of penicillin. Monitor patient.

Bacteriostatic antibacterial agents (chloram-phenicol, macrolide antibiotics, sulfonamides, tetracyclines): May decrease bactericidal ef-fect of penicillin. Avoid concomitant use.

Live-virus vaccines: May decrease effective-ness of live-virus vaccines. Avoid concurrent use.

Methotrexate: May increase risk of methotrexate toxicity. Monitor patient closely.

Probenecid: May increase penicillin level. Probenecid may be used for this purpose.

Tetracyclines: May interfere with bactericidal action of penicillins. Avoid coadministration.

Warfarin: May increase or decrease anticoag-ulant effects. Monitor PT and INR.

EFFECTS ON LAB TEST RESULTS
- May decrease Hb level and platelet, WBC, granulocyte, and RBC counts.
- May cause positive Coombs test result.
- May cause false-positive CSF protein test result.
- May alter urine glucose testing using cupric sulfate (Benedict reagent, Fehling solution, or Clinitest tablet).

CONTRAINDICATIONS & CAUTIONS
- Contraindicated in patients hypersensitive to drug or other penicillins.
- Use cautiously in patients with kidney im-pairment.
- Drug may cause CDAD ranging in severity from mild diarrhea to fatal colitis. If CDAD is suspected or confirmed, drug may need to be discontinued and treatment initiated.
- Use cautiously in patients with other drug allergies, especially to cephalosporins, be-cause of possible cross-sensitivity.
- Use cautiously in patients on sodium-restricted diets. Sodium content is 1.68 mEq per million units of penicillin G.
- Drug may cause kidney tubular damage, interstitial nephritis, HF, and electrolyte im-balance when given in high doses.
Dialyzable drug: Yes.
⚠ **Overdose S&S:** Neuromuscular hyperex-citability, agitation, confusion, hallucinations, stupor, coma, encephalopathy, hypernatremia, seizures.

PREGNANCY-LACTATION-REPRODUCTION
- There are no adequate studies during preg-nancy. Use only if clearly needed.
- Drug appears in human milk. Use cau-tiously during breastfeeding.

NURSING CONSIDERATIONS
- Drug may alter normal colon flora. Moni-tor patient for diarrhea, and initiate therapeu-tic measures as needed. Drug may need to be stopped.
- Observe patient closely. With large doses and prolonged therapy, bacterial or fungal overgrowth of nonsusceptible organisms (su-perinfection) may occur, especially in older adults or patients who are debilitated or im-munosuppressed.
- For most acute infections, continue treat-ment for at least 48 to 72 hours after patient becomes asymptomatic. Maintain antibiotic therapy for group A beta-hemolytic strepto-coccal infections for at least 10 days to reduce risk of rheumatic fever.
- Give high doses (above 10 million units) by IV slowly because of the potential ad-verse effects of electrolyte imbalance from the sodium content.
- Monitor patients for kidney tubular dam-age and interstitial nephritis (fever, rash, eosinophilia, proteinuria, eosinophiluria, hematuria, increased BUN level).
- Monitor patients with syphilis or other spirochetal infections (Lyme disease, relaps-ing fever) for Jarisch-Herxheimer reactions (fever, chills, myalgia, headache, exacerba-tion of skin lesions, tachycardia, hyperventi-lation, flushing, mild hypotension). Reactions occur 1 to 2 hours after initial treatment and resolve within 12 to 24 hours.
- ***Look alike–sound alike:*** Don't confuse peni-cillin G sodium with penicillamine or the var-ious other types of penicillin.

PATIENT TEACHING
- Tell patient to report adverse reactions promptly, especially hypersensitivity reac-tions and diarrhea.
- Instruct patient to report discomfort at IV site.
- Warn patient receiving IM injection that the injection may be painful but that ice applied to site may help alleviate discomfort.
- Advise patient that watery and bloody stools with or without stomach cramps and fever may occur during and for up to 2 months or more after antibiotic use. Instruct

P

patient to report these symptoms as soon as possible.

penicillin V potassium (phenoxymethyl penicillin potassium)
pen-i-SIL-in

Therapeutic class: Antibiotics
Pharmacologic class: Natural penicillins

AVAILABLE FORMS
Oral suspension: 125 mg/5 mL, 250 mg/5 mL (after reconstitution)
Tablets: 250 mg, 500 mg

INDICATIONS & DOSAGES
➤ **Fusospirochetosis (Vincent infection) of the oropharynx and staphylococcal infections**
Adults and children ages 12 and older: 250 to 500 mg PO every 6 to 8 hours.
➤ **Pneumococcal infections**
Adults and children ages 12 and older: 250 to 500 mg PO every 6 hours until patient has been afebrile for at least 2 days.
➤ **Streptococcal infections**
Adults and children ages 12 and older: 125 to 250 mg PO every 6 to 8 hours for 10 days.
➤ **Group A beta-hemolytic streptococcal pharyngitis**
Adults and children ages 12 and older: 500 mg PO b.i.d. to t.i.d., or 250 mg PO q.i.d. for 10 days.
➤ **To prevent recurrent rheumatic fever or chorea**
Adults and children ages 12 and older: 125 to 250 mg PO b.i.d.
➤ **Bacterial endocarditis prophylaxis in patients with congenital heart disease or rheumatic or other acquired valvular heart disease**
Adults and children ages 12 and older weighing more than 27.2 kg: 2 g PO 1 hour before dental or upper respiratory tract surgical procedure, followed by 1 g 6 hours later.
Children ages 12 and older weighing less than 27.2 kg: 1 g PO 1 hour before dental or upper respiratory tract surgical procedure, followed by 500 mg 6 hours later.

ADMINISTRATION
PO
• Before giving drug, ask patient about allergic reactions to penicillins.

• Obtain specimen for culture and sensitivity tests before giving first dose. Begin therapy while awaiting results.
• Give on an empty stomach 1 hour before or 2 hours after meals, to enhance absorption.
• Give drug with food if patient has stomach upset.
• Store oral solution in refrigerator. Discard any portion after 14 days.

ACTION
Inhibits cell-wall synthesis during bacterial multiplication.

Route	Onset	Peak	Duration
PO	Unknown	30–60 min	Unknown

Half-life: 30 minutes.

ADVERSE REACTIONS
CNS: fever. **EENT:** black hairy tongue. **GI:** epigastric distress, nausea, diarrhea, oral candidiasis, vomiting. **Hematologic:** *leukopenia, thrombocytopenia,* eosinophilia, hemolytic anemia. **Skin:** skin eruptions, urticaria. **Other:** *anaphylaxis,* hypersensitivity reactions, overgrowth of nonsusceptible organisms.

INTERACTIONS
Drug-drug. *Aminoglycosides (amikacin, gentamicin, tobramycin):* May decrease aminoglycoside level. Monitor therapy.
Live-virus vaccines: May decrease live-virus vaccine effects. Avoid concurrent use.
Methotrexate: May increase risk of methotrexate toxicity. Monitor patient closely.
Probenecid: May increase penicillin level. Probenecid may be used for this purpose.
Tetracyclines: May impair bactericidal effects of penicillin V. Avoid use together.
Warfarin: May increase anticoagulant effects. Monitor therapy.

EFFECTS ON LAB TEST RESULTS
• May increase eosinophil count.
• May decrease Hb level and platelet, WBC, and granulocyte counts.
• May alter results of turbidimetric test methods using sulfosalicylic acid, acetic acid, trichloroacetic acid, and nitric acid.

CONTRAINDICATIONS & CAUTIONS
• Contraindicated in patients hypersensitive to drug or other penicillins.
• Drug may cause CDAD ranging in severity from mild diarrhea to fatal colitis. If CDAD is

suspected or confirmed, drug may need to be discontinued and treatment initiated.

• Use cautiously in patients with GI disturbances, seizure disorder, or kidney impairment and in those with other drug allergies, especially to cephalosporins, because of possible cross-sensitivity.

Dialyzable drug: Unknown.

⚠ *Overdose S&S:* Neuromuscular hyperexcitability, seizures.

PREGNANCY-LACTATION-REPRODUCTION

• May use cautiously during pregnancy.
• Drug appears in human milk. Use cautiously during breastfeeding.

NURSING CONSIDERATIONS

• Drug may alter normal colon flora. Monitor patient for diarrhea, and initiate therapeutic measures as needed. Drug may need to be stopped.
• Periodically assess kidney function and CBC in patients receiving long-term therapy.
• If large doses are given or if therapy is prolonged, bacterial or fungal superinfection may occur, especially in older adults and patients who are debilitated or immunosuppressed.
• After treatment for streptococcal infections, reculture patient to determine whether streptococci have been eradicated.
• Amoxicillin is preferred over other antibiotics for endocarditis prophylaxis; however, penicillin V can be used as an alternative, if necessary.
• *Look alike–sound alike:* Don't confuse penicillin V potassium with penicillamine or the various other types of penicillin.

PATIENT TEACHING

• Instruct patient to take entire quantity of drug exactly as prescribed, even after feeling better.
• Tell patient to take drug with food if stomach upset occurs.
• Advise patient that watery and bloody stools with or without stomach cramps and fever may occur during and up to 2 months or more after antibiotic use. Instruct patient to report these symptoms as soon as possible.
• Instruct patient to discard any unused reconstituted suspension after 14 days.
• Advise patient to notify prescriber if rash, fever, or chills develop. A rash is the most common allergic reaction.

pentamidine isethionate
pen-TAM-i-deen

NebuPent, Pentam

Therapeutic class: Antiprotozoals
Pharmacologic class: Diamidine derivatives

AVAILABLE FORMS
Aerosol, powder for solution: 300-mg vial
Injection: 300-mg vial

INDICATIONS & DOSAGES

➤ *Pneumocystis jiroveci* **pneumonia (Pentam)**
Adults and children age 4 months and older: 4 mg/kg IV or IM once daily for 14 to 21 days.

➤ **To prevent** *P. jiroveci* **pneumonia in patients at high risk (NebuPent)**
Adults: 300 mg by inhalation using a Respirgard II nebulizer once every 4 weeks.

ADMINISTRATION
IV
▼ Reconstitute drug with 3 to 5 mL sterile water for injection or D₅W.
▼ Dilute reconstituted drug in 50 to 250 mL D₅W. Reconstituted solution is stable for 48 hours.
▼ Infuse over 60 to 120 minutes.
▼ IV infusion solutions prepared in D₅W are stable at room temperature for up to 24 hours.
▼ To minimize risk of hypotension, infuse drug slowly with patient lying down. Closely monitor BP.
⊙ **Alert:** Closely monitor infusion. Extravasation may cause ulceration, tissue necrosis, or sloughing and may require surgical debridement and skin grafting. If extravasation occurs, discontinue infusion immediately and manage symptoms.
▼ **Incompatibilities:** None listed by manufacturer. Consult a drug incompatibility reference for more information.
IM
• Reconstitute drug with 3 mL sterile water for a solution containing 100 mg/mL.
• Give deep into muscle.
• Rotate injection sites.
• Solution is stable for 48 hours after reconstitution. Store at room temperature to avoid crystallization.

🍁 Canada   ◇ OTC   ◆ Off-label use   ⓓⓞⓝ Do not crush   *Liquid contains alcohol   ▒ Genetic

P

Inhalational

🔶 *Alert:* Hazardous drug; use safe handling and disposal precautions.

• Give aerosol form only by Respirgard II nebulizer. Dosage recommendations are based on particle size and delivery rate of this device. Deliver dose until nebulizer chamber is empty (about 30 to 45 minutes).

• To give aerosol, mix contents of one vial in 6 mL sterile water for injection. Don't use NSS. Don't mix with other drugs.

• Don't use the Respirgard II to administer a bronchodilator because there may be an incompatibility between pentamidine and the bronchodilator.

• Don't use low-pressure (less than 20 pounds per square inch [PSI]) compressors. The flow rate should be 5 to 7 L/minute from 40- to 50-PSI air or oxygen source.

• Solution remains stable for 48 hours after reconstitution when kept in original vial at room temperature, protected from light.

ACTION

May interfere with biosynthesis of DNA, RNA, phospholipids, and proteins in susceptible organisms.

Route	Onset	Peak	Duration
IV, IM, inhalation	Unknown	Unknown	Unknown

Half-life: IV, about 5 to 8 hours; IM, 7 to 11 hours; inhalation, unknown.

ADVERSE REACTIONS

CNS: confusion, hallucinations, headache, fatigue, dizziness, fever, metallic or bad taste. **CV:** chest pain, hypotension. **EENT:** pharyngitis, sinusitis. **GI:** nausea, diarrhea, anorexia. **GU:** azotemia, impaired kidney function. **Hematologic:** *leukopenia, thrombocytopenia,* anemia. **Hepatic:** elevated LFT results. **Metabolic:** *hypoglycemia.* **Respiratory:** cough, wheezing, dyspnea, bronchitis, URI, *bronchospasm.* **Skin:** night sweats, rash; sterile abscess or necrosis, pain, or induration at site of IM injection. **Other:** infection.

INTERACTIONS

Drug-drug. *Amphotericin B, capreomycin, cisplatin, methoxyflurane, polymyxin B, vancomycin:* May increase risk of kidney toxicity. Monitor kidney function test results closely. *Antidiabetics:* May initially cause hypoglycemia, then hyperglycemia, because pentamidine may

harm pancreatic cells. Monitor blood glucose levels and adjust dosages when needed.
Antineoplastics: May cause additive bone marrow suppression. Use together cautiously; monitor hematologic study results.
Drugs that prolong the QT interval (antipsychotics; antiarrhythmics, such as amiodarone, disopyramide, procainamide, quinidine, sotalol; fluoroquinolones; macrolides; TCAs): May cause additive effect. Use together cautiously; monitor patient for adverse cardiac effects.

EFFECTS ON LAB TEST RESULTS

• May increase BUN, creatinine, and potassium levels and LFT values.

• May increase or decrease glucose level.

• May decrease Hb level, hematocrit, and WBC and platelet counts.

CONTRAINDICATIONS & CAUTIONS

• Contraindicated in patients with history of anaphylactic reaction or hypersensitivity to inhaled or parenteral pentamidine.

• Fatalities due to severe hypotension, hypoglycemia, acute pancreatitis, and cardiac arrhythmias have been reported.

• Use cautiously in patients with HTN, hypotension, ventricular tachycardia, hypoglycemia, hyperglycemia, hypocalcemia, leukopenia, thrombocytopenia, anemia, diabetes, pancreatitis, SJS, or liver or kidney dysfunction.

• Use inhalation formulation cautiously in patients with asthma or a history of smoking.

🔶 *Alert:* Severe hypotension may occur after a single IV or IM dose, and is more likely with rapid IV administration. Monitor patients closely.

Dialyzable drug: No.

⚠️ *Overdose S&S:* Kidney and liver impairment, hypotension, cardiopulmonary arrest.

PREGNANCY-LACTATION-REPRODUCTION

• It isn't known if drug causes fetal harm. Use during pregnancy only if potential benefits justify unknown risks and only if clearly needed.

• It isn't known if drug appears in human milk. Use cautiously during breastfeeding and only if potential benefits justify unknown risks.

NURSING CONSIDERATIONS

🔶 *Alert:* Monitor glucose, creatinine, and BUN levels daily. After parenteral

---

Reactions in bold italics are *life-threatening*.

administration, glucose level may decrease initially; hypoglycemia may be severe in 5% to 10% of patients. After several months of therapy, this may be followed by hyperglycemia and type 1 diabetes, which may be permanent.

• Monitor CBC with platelet count, kidney function, LFT results, calcium level, and ECG before, during, and after therapy.

♦ Alert: Monitor BP during and after infusion because of increased risk of severe hypotension with IV or IM administration.

• Extravasation can lead to ulceration, tissue necrosis, or sloughing at injection site. Monitor IV site closely.

• Inhalation drug may cause bronchospasm or cough, especially in patients with a history of asthma or smoking. Use of an inhaled bronchodilator before each inhaled pentamidine dose may minimize symptom recurrence.

• Use of aerosolized drug has been associated with acute pancreatitis. Discontinue drug if signs or symptoms of acute pancreatitis occur.

• In patients with AIDS, drug may produce less severe adverse reactions than sulfamethoxazole–trimethoprim.

PATIENT TEACHING

• Instruct patient to use the aerosol device until the chamber is empty, which may take up to 45 minutes.

• Warn patient that IM injection is painful.

• Instruct patient to complete the full course, even if feeling better.

• Tell patient to report signs and symptoms of pulmonary infection, such as shortness of breath, fever, or cough.

• Instruct patient to report pregnancy or plans to become pregnant or to breastfeed.

SAFETY ALERT!

pertuzumab ⍟
per-TU-zoo-mab

Perjeta

Therapeutic class: Antineoplastics
Pharmacologic class: Monoclonal antibodies

AVAILABLE FORMS

Injection: 420 mg/14 mL (30 mg/mL) in single-use vials

INDICATIONS & DOSAGES

Adjust-a-dose (for all indications): Refer to manufacturer's information for adjustments related to missed or delayed doses and for complete information on drugs used in combination with pertuzumab.

➤ **HER2-positive metastatic breast cancer with trastuzumab and docetaxel in patients who haven't received prior anti-HER2 therapy or chemotherapy for metastatic disease** ⍟

Adults: Initial loading dose of 840 mg IV as a 60-minute infusion in combination with trastuzumab 8 mg/kg and docetaxel 75 mg/m². Administer a maintenance regimen every 3 weeks with pertuzumab 420 mg IV as a 30- to 60-minute infusion in combination with trastuzumab 6 mg/kg or trastuzumab hyaluronidase-oysk (600 mg trastuzumab/10,000 units hyaluronidase) subcut over 2 to 5 minutes and docetaxel (may increase docetaxel dose to 100 mg/m² if initial dose is tolerated).

➤ **Neoadjuvant treatment of HER2-positive, locally advanced, inflammatory, or early-stage breast cancer in combination with other drugs** ⍟

Adults: Initial loading dose of 840 mg IV as a 60-minute infusion, then a maintenance regimen every 3 weeks with pertuzumab 420 mg IV as a 30- to 60-minute infusion in combination with either four preoperative cycles with trastuzumab or trastuzumab hyaluronidase-oysk and docetaxel followed by three postoperative cycles of 5-FU, epirubicin, and cyclophosphamide (FEC); or three or four preoperative cycles of FEC alone followed by three or four preoperative cycles of pertuzumab in combination with docetaxel and trastuzumab or trastuzumab hyaluronidase-oysk; or six preoperative cycles of pertuzumab in combination with docetaxel, carboplatin, and trastuzumab (TCH) or trastuzumab hyaluronidase-oysk; or four preoperative cycles of dose-dense doxorubicin and cyclophosphamide (ddAC) alone followed by four preoperative cycles of pertuzumab in combination with paclitaxel and trastuzumab or trastuzumab hyaluronidase-oysk. After surgery, continue trastuzumab or trastuzumab hyaluronidase-oysk to complete 1 year of treatment, up to 18 cycles.

➤ **Adjuvant treatment of patients with HER2-positive early breast cancer at high risk for recurrence as part of a complete**

regimen for breast cancer, including anthracycline or taxane-based chemotherapy
Adults: Initial loading dose, 840 mg IV as a 60-minute infusion in combination with trastuzumab 8 mg/kg or trastuzumab hyaluronidase-oysk (600 mg trastuzumab/ 10,000 units hyaluronidase) subcut over 2 to 5 minutes starting day 1 of first taxane-containing cycle. Administer a maintenance regimen every 3 weeks with pertuzumab 420 mg IV as a 30- to 60-minute infusion in combination with trastuzumab 6 mg/kg. Continue maintenance regimen for a total of 1 year (up to 18 cycles) or until disease recurrence or unmanageable toxicity, whichever occurs first. Withhold or discontinue pertuzumab if trastuzumab or trastuzumab hyaluronidase-oysk is withheld or discontinued.

ADMINISTRATION
IV
⚠ *Alert:* Hazardous drug; use safe handling and disposal precautions.
▼ Don't administer as IV push or bolus.
▼ Inspect solution for particulates and discoloration. Solution should be clear to slightly opalescent and colorless to pale brown.
▼ Withdraw appropriate amount of pertuzumab and dilute in 250 mL NSS in a PVC or non-PVC polyolefin infusion bag.
▼ Invert bag gently to mix solution; don't shake.
▼ Administer immediately or may refrigerate diluted solution for up to 24 hours.
▼ Administer pertuzumab sequentially. Pertuzumab and trastuzumab or trastuzumab hyaluronidase-oysk can be given in any order. Give docetaxel after pertuzumab and trastuzumab or trastuzumab hyaluronidase-oysk. Observe patient for 30 to 60 minutes after infusing pertuzumab before administering the other drugs.
▼ Refrigerate vials. Store in outer carton to protect from light.
▼ **Incompatibilities:** Other drugs. Only mix with NSS.

ACTION
Binds to HER2 protein receptor, causing inhibition of signaling pathways, which results in cell growth arrest and apoptosis.

Route	Onset	Peak	Duration
IV	Unknown	Unknown	Unknown

Half-life: 18 days.

ADVERSE REACTIONS
CNS: fatigue, asthenia, fever, peripheral neuropathy, headache, dizziness, insomnia, taste alteration. **CV:** peripheral edema, *left ventricular dysfunction.* **EENT:** increased tearing, nasopharyngitis, oropharyngeal pain. **GI:** diarrhea, nausea, vomiting, constipation, stomatitis, decreased appetite, abdominal pain. **Hematologic:** *neutropenia,* anemia, *leukopenia, thrombocytopenia.* **Hepatic:** elevated liver enzyme levels. **Metabolic:** *hypokalemia,* hyperuricemia, hyperphosphatemia. **Musculoskeletal:** myalgia, arthralgia. **Respiratory:** URI, dyspnea, cough, pleural effusion. **Skin:** alopecia, hand-foot syndrome, rash, pruritus, dry skin, paronychia, nail disorder, infusion-site reaction. **Other:** mucosal inflammation, infusion-related hypersensitivity, immunogenicity.

INTERACTIONS
None reported.

EFFECTS ON LAB TEST RESULTS
• May increase liver enzyme, phosphate, and uric acid levels.
• May decrease potassium level.
• May decrease platelet, WBC, and RBC counts.

CONTRAINDICATIONS & CAUTIONS
Boxed Warning Pertuzumab can cause subclinical and clinical cardiac failure. Evaluate LVEF in all patients before and during treatment. Discontinue drug for a confirmed clinically significant decrease in left ventricular function. ■
• Contraindicated in patients hypersensitive to drug or its components.
• Drug hasn't been studied in patients with a history of HF or reduced LVEF, uncontrolled HTN, recent MI, serious cardiac arrhythmia, cumulative prior anthracycline exposure of greater than 360 mg/m^2 of doxorubicin or its equivalent, and in those with CrCl less than 30 mL/minute. Prior exposure to radiotherapy may increase risk of left ventricular dysfunction.
Dialyzable drug: Unknown.

PREGNANCY-LACTATION-REPRODUCTION
Boxed Warning Exposure to drug during pregnancy can result in embryo or fetal death, delayed kidney development, and other birth defects. Verify pregnancy status before

Reactions in bold italics are *life-threatening*.

starting drug. Advise patients of risks and the need for effective contraception during therapy and for 7 months after therapy ends. ■

• If patient becomes pregnant during therapy, monitor closely. If oligohydramnios occurs, perform fetal testing.

• Contact Genetech at 1-888-835-2555 if drug is given during pregnancy or if patient becomes pregnant during or within 7 months after the last dose when given in combination with trastuzumab.

• It isn't known if drug appears in human milk. Patient should discontinue breastfeeding or discontinue drug, considering importance of drug to patient. Consider drug's extended half-life when making breastfeeding decisions after therapy ends.

NURSING CONSIDERATIONS

Boxed Warning Assess LVEF before starting treatment and at regular intervals about every 12 weeks during treatment. ■

• Withhold or discontinue pertuzumab if trastuzumab is withheld or discontinued. If docetaxel is discontinued, treatment with pertuzumab and trastuzumab may continue.

• Monitor patient for hypersensitivity or infusion reactions for 60 minutes after first infusion and for 30 minutes after subsequent infusions. For significant infusion-related reactions, slow or interrupt infusion and treat symptoms. If severe reactions occur, consider permanently discontinuing drug.

• Monitor CBC regularly.

• Monitor patients for fever or infection.

▨ An increased incidence of febrile neutropenia has occurred in patients of Asian descent.

• Verify pregnancy status before starting drug.

PATIENT TEACHING

Boxed Warning Inform patient of childbearing potential that drug may cause fetal harm. Counsel patient to use reliable birth control methods while taking this drug and for 7 months after therapy ends. ■

• Teach patient that hair loss (alopecia) and skin and nail adverse reactions are common during treatment.

• Instruct patient to immediately report fever or other signs and symptoms of infection.

• Caution patient to immediately report shortness of breath, unusual edema, weight gain, or excessive fatigue.

• Advise patient to immediately report signs or symptoms of LVEF dysfunction,

including worsening shortness of breath, cough, palpitations, weight gain of more than 5 lb in 24 hours, dizziness or loss of consciousness, swelling of the ankles, legs, or face.

• Tell patient that regular monitoring of cardiac function will be needed.

phentermine hydrochloride
FEN-ter-meen

Adipex-P, Lomaira

Therapeutic class: Anorexiants
Pharmacologic class: Sympathomimetic amines
Controlled substance schedule: IV

AVAILABLE FORMS
Capsules: 15 mg, 30 mg, 37.5 mg
Tablets: 8 mg, 37.5 mg
Tablets (ODTs): 15 mg, 30 mg, 37.5 mg

INDICATIONS & DOSAGES
➤ **Short-term adjunct in exogenous obesity for patients with an initial BMI of 30 kg/m^2 or more, or of 27 kg/m^2 or more in the presence of other risk factors (controlled HTN, diabetes, hyperlipidemia)**
Adults and children ages 16 and older: 15 to 37.5 mg PO daily as a single dose or two divided doses. Or, 15 to 37.5 mg ODT PO daily.
Adults (Lomaira): 8 mg PO t.i.d. 30 minutes before meals.
Adjust-a-dose: Individualize dosage to obtain adequate response with lowest effective dose. Maximum dose of Adipex-P is 15 mg daily for patients with eGFR of 15 to 29 mL/minute/1.73 m^2.

ADMINISTRATION
PO
• Tablets are scored and may be split to achieve lower dose.

• Give Adipex-P before breakfast or 1 to 2 hours after breakfast. Give Lomaira 30 minutes before meals. Give ODT in the morning with or without food.

• Avoid giving in the late evening, to prevent insomnia.

• Using dry hands, immediately place ODT on top of the tongue to dissolve; then have patient swallow with or without water.

P

ACTION

Unknown. Phentermine is a sympathomimetic amine with pharmacologic properties similar to amphetamines. The mechanism of action in reducing appetite may be secondary to CNS effects, including stimulation of the hypothalamus to release norepinephrine.

Route	Onset	Peak	Duration
PO	Unknown	3–4.4 hr	Unknown

Half-life: About 20 hours.

ADVERSE REACTIONS

CNS: insomnia, overstimulation, headache, restlessness, euphoria, dysphoria, dizziness, tremor, psychosis, taste alteration. **CV:** palpitations, tachycardia, ischemic events, increased BP, *primary pulmonary HTN,* valvular heart disease. **GI:** dry mouth, constipation, diarrhea, other GI disturbances. **GU:** erectile dysfunction, altered libido. **Skin:** urticaria.

INTERACTIONS

Drug-drug. *Acetazolamide, antacids, sodium bicarbonate:* May increase kidney reabsorption. Monitor patient for enhanced effects.
Adrenergic neuron blockers: May reduce hypotensive effect. Monitor patient for cardiac changes.
Ammonium chloride, ascorbic acid: May decrease level and increase excretion of phentermine. Monitor patient for decreased phentermine effects.
Dexfenfluramine, fenfluramine: May increase risk of primary pulmonary HTN and valvular heart disease. Monitor patient closely.
Insulin, oral antidiabetics: May alter antidiabetic requirements. Monitor glucose level.
MAO inhibitors: May cause severe HTN or hypertensive crisis. Contraindicated within 14 days of MAO inhibitor therapy.
Other products for weight loss: Effects of coadministration are unknown. Use together isn't recommended.
SSRIs (fluoxetine, fluvoxamine, paroxetine, sertraline): May increase risk of serotonin syndrome. Use together isn't recommended.
Drug-food. *Alcohol use:* May increase risk of adverse drug reactions. Discourage use together.
Caffeine: May increase CNS stimulation. Discourage use together.

EFFECTS ON LAB TEST RESULTS

None reported.

CONTRAINDICATIONS & CAUTIONS

• Contraindicated in patients hypersensitive to sympathomimetic amines, in those with idiosyncratic reactions to them, in patients who are agitated, and within 14 days after taking an MAO inhibitor.
• Contraindicated in patients with history of drug abuse, hyperthyroidism, CV disease (heart disease, stroke, CAD, HF, arrhythmias, moderate to severe or uncontrolled HTN, advanced arteriosclerosis), or glaucoma.
• Rare cases of valvular heart disease have been reported in patients who have taken phentermine alone.
• Avoid Adipex-P in patients with eGFR less than 15 mL/minute/1.73 m^2 or those requiring dialysis.
• Use cautiously in older adults and patients with HTN (even mild HTN), kidney impairment, or seizure disorders.
• Safety and effectiveness in children younger than age 16 haven't been determined.
Dialyzable drug: Unknown.
⚠ **Overdose S&S:** Restlessness, tremor, hyperreflexia, rapid respiration, confusion, assaultiveness, hallucinations, panic states, fatigue, depression, arrhythmias, HTN, hypotension, circulatory collapse, nausea, vomiting, diarrhea, abdominal cramps, seizures, coma.

PREGNANCY-LACTATION-REPRODUCTION

• Contraindicated during pregnancy and breastfeeding.

NURSING CONSIDERATIONS

• Use drug with a weight-reduction program.
• Monitor patient for tolerance, dependence, or potential abuse. Drug is chemically related to amphetamines, which carry a high abuse potential.
• Monitor BP.
• Don't stop drug abruptly; taper dosage.
• *Look alike–sound alike:* Don't confuse phentermine with phentolamine or phenytoin.

PATIENT TEACHING

• Counsel patient in use of effective contraception and to immediately report pregnancy.
• Instruct patient to immediately report shortness of breath or dyspnea, which could be an early sign of a serious adverse effect such as primary pulmonary HTN.
• Advise patient to avoid products that contain caffeine and to report evidence of excessive stimulation.

Reactions in bold italics are *life-threatening*.

• Warn patient that fatigue may result as drug effects wear off and that patient will need more rest.

• Caution patient to avoid operating hazardous machinery, including automobiles, until drug's effects are known.

• Warn patient that drug may lose its effectiveness over time.

• Advise patient not to stop drug abruptly. Remind patient that drug is for short-term use (usually a few weeks).

⚠️ *Alert:* Caution patient to keep drug in a safe place and protect it from theft.

⚠️ *Alert:* Advise patient never to give drug to anyone else because it can cause harm or death.

• Stress importance of eating healthy and other healthy lifestyle choices.

phentermine hydrochloride–topiramate
FEN-ter-meen/toe-PIE-rah-mate

Qsymia

Therapeutic class: Anorexiants-anticonvulsants
Pharmacologic class: Sympathomimetic amines-sulfamate-substituted monosaccharides
Controlled substance schedule: IV

AVAILABLE FORMS
Capsules (extended-release) 🚫*:* 3.75 mg phentermine/23 mg topiramate, 7.5 mg phentermine/46 mg topiramate, 11.25 mg phentermine/69 mg topiramate, 15 mg phentermine/92 mg topiramate

INDICATIONS & DOSAGES
Adjust-a-dose (for all indications): For patients with CrCl less than 50 mL/minute, or Child-Pugh class B liver impairment, don't exceed 7.5 mg phentermine/46 mg topiramate once daily.

➤ **Chronic weight management, as an adjunct to diet and increased physical activity in patients with initial BMI of 30 kg/m² or greater (obese) or 27 kg/m² or greater (overweight) and at least one weight-related comorbidity, such as HTN, type 2 diabetes, or dyslipidemia**
Adults: Initially, 3.75 mg phentermine/23 mg topiramate PO every morning for 14 days;

then increase to 7.5 mg phentermine/46 mg topiramate every morning. Evaluate weight loss after 12 weeks of treatment. If patient hasn't lost at least 3% of baseline body weight escalate dosage to 11.25 mg phentermine/69 mg topiramate every morning for 14 days, followed by 15 mg phentermine/92 mg topiramate every morning. Evaluate weight loss 12 weeks after dosage escalation. If patient hasn't lost at least 5% of baseline body weight, discontinue drug by decreasing dosage to every other day for at least 1 week before stopping treatment altogether.

➤ **Chronic weight management, as an adjunct to diet and increased physical activity in children with BMI in the 95th percentile or more standardized for age and sex**
Children ages 12 and older: Initially, 3.75 mg phentermine/23 mg topiramate PO every morning for 14 days; then increase to 7.5 mg phentermine/46 mg topiramate every morning. Evaluate weight loss after 12 weeks of therapy. If child hasn't lost at least 3% of baseline BMI, escalate dosage to 11.25 mg phentermine/69 mg topiramate every morning for 14 days, followed by 15 mg phentermine/92 mg topiramate every morning. Evaluate BMI 12 weeks after dosage escalation. If patient hasn't lost at least 5% of baseline BMI, discontinue drug by decreasing dose to every other day for at least 1 week before stopping therapy.

Adjust-a-dose: If child's weight loss exceeds 0.9 kg/week, consider dosage reduction.

ADMINISTRATION
PO
• Give drug in morning with or without food. Don't give in evening due to risk of insomnia.

• Have patient swallow capsules whole; don't open, crush, or break capsules.

ACTION
Phentermine: Unknown. Drug is a sympathomimetic amine with pharmacologic properties similar to amphetamines. Mechanism of action in reducing appetite may be secondary to CNS effects, including stimulation of the hypothalamus to release norepinephrine. Topiramate: Unknown in weight management. May involve appetite suppression and satiety enhancement via neurotransmitter or enzymatic effects.

Route	Onset	Peak	Duration
PO	Unknown	6 hr (phentermine); 9 hr (topiramate)	Unknown

Half-life: Phentermine, 20 hours; topiramate, 65 hours.

ADVERSE REACTIONS

CNS: paresthesia, headache, dizziness, taste alteration, hypoesthesia, disturbance in attention or memory, cognitive impairment, insomnia, depression, anxiety, fatigue, fever, irritability, thirst. **CV:** palpitations, chest discomfort, increased HR. **EENT:** blurred vision, eye pain, dry eyes, otitis, nasal congestion, nasopharyngitis, sinusitis, sinus congestion, oral paresthesia, pharyngolaryngeal pain, dry mouth. **GI:** constipation, nausea, diarrhea, dyspepsia, GERD, gastroenteritis, decreased appetite, abdominal pain. **GU:** UTI, dysmenorrhea, increased creatinine level. **Metabolic:** hyperammonemia, *hypokalemia, metabolic acidosis, hypoglycemia.* **Musculoskeletal:** arthralgia, back pain, extremity pain, muscle spasms, musculoskeletal pain, neck pain, ligament sprain, decreased bone mineral density (children), slowed height growth (children). **Respiratory:** cough, bronchitis, URI. **Skin:** alopecia, rash. **Other:** procedural pain, flulike symptoms.

INTERACTIONS

Drug-drug. *Amitriptyline:* May increase amitriptyline level. Monitor therapy.
Anticholinergics (atropine, benztropine): May increase risk of heat-related disorders, such as decreased sweating and increased body temperature. Use together cautiously.
Antihypertensive (ACE inhibitors, ARBs, beta blockers): May increase risk of hypotension and related symptoms. Monitor BP.
Carbamazepine, phenytoin: May decrease topiramate level. Use together cautiously.
Carbonic anhydrase inhibitors (acetazolamide, methazolamide, zonisamide): May increase risk of metabolic acidosis and kidney stones. May also increase risk of heat-related disorders, such as decreased sweating and increased body temperature. Avoid concurrent use.
CNS depressants (barbiturates, benzodiazepines, sleep medications): May increase CNS depressant effects. Avoid use together. If use together is necessary, consider dosage reduction of phentermine–topiramate.

Diltiazem: May decrease diltiazem level and increase topiramate level. Use together cautiously.
Lithium: High topiramate dosage may increase lithium level. Monitor lithium level.
MAO inhibitors: May increase risk of hypertensive crisis. Use is contraindicated during or within 14 days of MAO inhibitor administration.
Non-potassium-sparing diuretics (loop and thiazide diuretics): May increase risk of hypokalemia. Monitor potassium level.
Oral antidiabetics, insulin: May increase risk of hypoglycemia. Monitor glucose level closely.
Oral contraceptives: May decrease estrogen level and increase progestin level, thereby increasing irregular bleeding. Use together isn't expected to increase risk of pregnancy. Consider therapy modification and adding an additional, nonhormonal contraceptive method.
Other weight-loss drugs: Use with other weight-loss drugs hasn't been studied. Avoid use together.
Pioglitazone: May decrease pioglitazone level. Monitor glucose level closely.
SSRIs (fluoxetine, fluvoxamine, paroxetine, sertraline): May increase risk of serotonin syndrome. Use together cautiously.
Valproic acid: May increase risk of hyperammonemia and encephalopathy. Monitor patient and measure blood ammonia level if symptoms develop.
Drug-herb. *Weight-loss supplements:* Use with other weight-loss products hasn't been studied. Avoid use together.
Drug-food. *Ketogenic diet (high-protein, low-carbohydrate):* May increase risk of kidney stones. Use together cautiously.
Drug-lifestyle. *Alcohol use:* May increase CNS depressant effects. Discourage use together.

EFFECTS ON LAB TEST RESULTS

• May increase creatinine and ammonium levels.
• May decrease sodium bicarbonate, potassium, and glucose levels.

CONTRAINDICATIONS & CAUTIONS

• Contraindicated in patients hypersensitive to drug or its components or with idiosyncrasy to the sympathomimetic amines, in those with glaucoma or hyperthyroidism, and during or within 14 days after administration of MAO inhibitors.

Reactions in bold italics are *life-threatening.*

• Avoid use in patients with Child-Pugh class C liver impairment or KFRT and in those with a history of or active suicidality or suicide attempts.

• Use cautiously in patients with increased resting HR, especially those with cardiac or cerebrovascular disease (history of MI or stroke in the past 6 months, life-threatening arrhythmias, HF); in patients with history of or active depression; in older adults; and in those at risk for development of metabolic acidosis or kidney stones.

⊕ **Alert:** Drug is a controlled substance because it can be abused, leading to drug dependence.

• Drug is only available through a REMS program and certified pharmacies that are enrolled in the Qsymia certified pharmacy network.

Dialyzable drug: Phentermine, no; topiramate, yes.

⚠ **Overdose S&S:** Phentermine: Restlessness, tremor, rapid respiration, confusion, hallucinations, arrhythmias, changes in BP, nausea, vomiting, diarrhea. Topiramate: Metabolic acidosis, seizures, drowsiness, speech disturbance, blurred vision, hypotension, abdominal pain, agitation, dizziness, depression.

PREGNANCY-LACTATION-REPRODUCTION

• Contraindicated during pregnancy due to risk for major congenital malformations, including cleft lip or cleft palate, and being small for gestational age.

• Assess for pregnancy before and monthly during treatment. Patients of childbearing potential should use effective contraception during therapy.

• Prescribers and patients should report pregnancies that occur during therapy to the Qsymia Pregnancy Surveillance Program (1-888-998-4887).

• Drug is present in human milk. Use isn't recommended during breastfeeding due to risk to infant.

• For patients taking combined oral contraceptives (COCs), use of drug may cause irregular bleeding. Patients should continue taking the COC and contact health care provider.

NURSING CONSIDERATIONS

• Verify pregnancy status of patients of childbearing potential before and monthly during therapy.

• Gradually decrease dosage when discontinuing drug to lower risk of seizures. If it's

necessary to stop drug immediately, monitor patient closely.

• Monitor patient for mood disorders and insomnia; if present, decrease dosage or discontinue drug.

• Monitor patient for emergence or worsening of depression, suicidality, or unusual changes in mood or behavior. Discontinue drug in patients who experience suicidality.

• Monitor resting HR. If sustained tachycardia occurs, decrease dosage or stop drug.

• Assess electrolyte, glucose, and bicarbonate levels before and periodically during treatment.

• Drug causes decreased sweating, which can predispose patients to heat-related disorders. Monitor fluid loss, especially in hot weather.

• Monitor BP regularly, especially in patients with history of HTN.

• Monitor patient for ocular changes (acute myopia, severe and persistent eye pain, vision changes, anterior chamber shallowing, redness, increased IOP, mydriasis). Discontinue drug immediately if any of these symptoms occur.

• Monitor patient for potential abuse of drug. Phentermine has a known potential for abuse.

• Phentermine is related chemically and pharmacologically to amphetamines.

PATIENT TEACHING

• Advise patient to take drug once daily in the morning and to avoid nighttime dosing because of insomnia.

• Inform patient that drug is only available through certified pharmacies that are enrolled in the Qsymia certified pharmacy network.

⊕ **Alert:** Tell patient to keep drug in a safe place and protect it from theft. Advise patient never to give drug to anyone else because it can cause harm or death and is against the law.

• Warn patient not to increase dosage without first discussing with prescriber.

• Advise patient of childbearing potential of fetal risk and that pregnancy testing will be done before start of therapy and monthly during therapy.

• Counsel patient to use effective contraception and to immediately report pregnancy.

• Instruct patient to tell all health care providers about all medications, nutritional supplements, and vitamins (including weight-loss products) that are being taken or may be taken during therapy.

• Caution patient to report sustained periods of heart pounding or racing while at rest; mood changes, depression, or suicidality;

prolonged diarrhea; scheduled surgery; occurrence or history of seizures; or use of a high-protein, low-carbohydrate diet.

• Teach patient to immediately report severe and persistent eye pain or significant vision changes.

• Instruct patient to report changes in attention, concentration, memory, or difficulty finding words.

• Tell patient to avoid operating hazardous machinery, including automobiles, until effects of drug are known.

• Advise patient with diabetes to monitor glucose level closely and to report episodes of hypoglycemia. Medication regimen may need adjustment.

• Caution patient to watch for decreased sweating or increased body temperature during physical activity, especially during hot weather.

• Warn patient not to stop drug abruptly as seizures may result.

• Advise patient to increase fluid intake to prevent kidney stones and to report severe side or back pain or blood in urine.

phenytoin (diphenylhydantoin) ⚮
FEN-i-toe-in

Dilantin-125, Dilantin Infatabs

phenytoin sodium
Dilantin, Phenytek

Therapeutic class: Anticonvulsants
Pharmacologic class: Hydantoin derivatives

AVAILABLE FORMS
phenytoin
Oral suspension: 125 mg/5 mL*
Tablets (chewable): 50 mg
phenytoin sodium
Injection: 50 mg/mL
phenytoin sodium (extended)
Capsules (extended-release): 30 mg, 100 mg, 200 mg, 300 mg

INDICATIONS & DOSAGES
➤ **To control tonic-clonic (grand mal) and psychomotor (temporal lobe) seizures**
Adults: Highly individualized. Initially, 100 mg (immediate-release, extended-release) PO t.i.d. Adjust dosage at no less than

7- to 10-day intervals until desired response is obtained. Usual range, 300 to 600 mg daily. If patient is stabilized on 100-mg extended-release capsules t.i.d., once-daily dosing with 300-mg extended-release capsules is an alternative. Or, 125 mg oral solution t.i.d. in patients without previous treatment. May increase to 625 mg daily.
Children: 5 mg/kg/day in two to three equally divided doses. Adjust dosage at no less than 7- to 10-day intervals. Usual maintenance dose range is 4 to 8 mg/kg daily. Maximum dose is 300 mg/day.
➤ **To control tonic-clonic (grand mal) and psychomotor (temporal lobe) seizures in patients requiring a loading dose**
Adults: Initially, 1 g (extended-release) PO divided into three doses (400 mg, 300 mg, 300 mg), given at 2-hour intervals with careful monitoring. Begin maintenance dosage of 100 mg (extended-release) PO t.i.d. to q.i.d. 24 hours after loading dose.
➤ **Generalized tonic-clonic status epilepticus; prevention and treatment of seizures during neurosurgery**
Adults: Loading dose of 10 to 15 mg/kg IV (1 to 1.5 g may be needed) at a rate not exceeding 50 mg/minute; then maintenance dosage of 100 mg PO or IV every 6 to 8 hours.
Children: Loading dose of 15 to 20 mg/kg IV, at a rate not exceeding 1 to 3 mg/kg/minute or 50 mg/minute, whichever is slower; then highly individualized maintenance dosages.

ADMINISTRATION
⊕ *Alert:* Hazardous drug; use safe handling and disposal precautions.
PO
• Give divided doses with or after meals to decrease adverse GI reactions.
• If daily dose can't be divided equally, give larger dose before bedtime.
• For chewable tablets, patient may chew thoroughly before swallowing or may swallow whole.
• Shake suspension well before use. Administer dose using a calibrated oral dosing syringe.
• Different oral forms aren't interchangeable.
• Have patient swallow extended-release capsules whole; don't crush or cut.
• For oral suspension, withhold enteral feedings for 1 to 2 hours before and 1 to 2 hours after giving drug, if possible, to improve absorption.

IV

▼ Clear tubing with NSS. Use only clear solution for injection. A slight yellow color is acceptable.

▼ To give as an infusion, dilute in NSS to a final concentration of phenytoin sodium in the solution of no less than 5 mg/mL. Begin infusion immediately after mixture has been prepared; infusion should run through an 0.22- to 0.55-micron in-line filter. Infusion must be completed within 4 hours.

▼ Check patency of catheter before giving. Monitor site for extravasation because it can cause severe tissue damage.

Boxed Warning Drug must be administered slowly to reduce the risk of severe hypotension and cardiac arrhythmias. In adults, don't exceed 50 mg/minute IV. In children, administer drug at a rate not exceeding 1 to 3 mg/kg/minute or 50 mg/minute, whichever is slower. Continuous monitoring of BP and ECG during IV administration is essential. ■

▼ Follow each injection with injection of sterile NSS through the same needle or catheter.

▼ If possible, don't give by IV push into veins on back of hand to avoid purple glove syndrome. Inject into larger veins or central venous catheter, if available.

▼ Discard 4 hours after preparation. Don't refrigerate.

▼ **Incompatibilities:** Amikacin, aminophylline, amphotericin B, cephapirin, ciprofloxacin, D_5W, diltiazem, dobutamine, enalaprilat, fat emulsions, hydromorphone, insulin (regular), levorphanol, lidocaine, lincomycin, meperidine, morphine sulfate, nitroglycerin, norepinephrine, other IV drugs or infusion solutions, pentobarbital sodium, potassium chloride, procaine, propofol, streptomycin, sufentanil citrate, theophylline, vitamin B complex with C. If giving as infusion, don't mix drug with D_5W because it will precipitate. Consult a compatibility drug reference for additional details.

IM

• Give IM only if dosage adjustments are made; IM dose is 50% greater than oral dose.

• Be aware that drug isn't ordinarily given IM because drug may precipitate at injection site; cause pain, necrosis, or abscess formation; and be absorbed erratically.

• Don't give by IM route for treatment of status epilepticus as peak plasma levels may not be attained for up to 24 hours.

ACTION

May stabilize neuronal membranes and limit seizure activity either by increasing efflux or decreasing influx of sodium ions across cell membranes in the motor cortex during generation of nerve impulses.

Route	Onset	Peak	Duration
PO	Unknown	1.5–3 hr	Unknown
PO (extended-release)	Unknown	4–12 hr	Unknown
IV	Immediate	1–2 hr	Unknown
IM	Unknown	Unknown	Unknown

Half-life: Varies with dose, formulation, and concentration changes.

ADVERSE REACTIONS

CNS: ataxia, decreased coordination, confusion, slurred speech, dizziness, headache, insomnia, somnolence, nervousness, twitching, paresthesia, peripheral neuropathy, vertigo, taste alteration. **CV:** *bradycardia,* periarteritis nodosa, hypotension, *CV arrest.* **EENT:** diplopia, nystagmus, blurred vision, gingival hyperplasia, lip enlargement. **GI:** nausea, vomiting, constipation. **GU:** Peyronie disease. **Hematologic:** *agranulocytosis, leukopenia, pancytopenia, thrombocytopenia,* macrocythemia, megaloblastic anemia. **Hepatic:** *toxic hepatitis, acute liver failure,* increased ALP or GGT levels. **Metabolic:** hyperglycemia. **Musculoskeletal:** osteomalacia. **Skin:** bullous or purpuric dermatitis, discoloration of skin if given by IV push in back of hand, exfoliative dermatitis, hypertrichosis, inflammation at injection site, necrosis, pain, photosensitivity reactions, scarlatiniform or morbilliform rash. **Other:** hypersensitivity reactions, lymphadenopathy, SLE, thickening of facial features.

INTERACTIONS

✪ *Alert:* Phenytoin can significantly interact with many drugs. Consult a drug interaction resource or pharmacist for additional information.

Drug-drug. *Acetaminophen:* May decrease the therapeutic effects of acetaminophen and increase the incidence of liver toxicity. Monitor for toxicity.

P

Amiodarone, antihistamines, chloramphenicol, cimetidine, cycloserine, fluconazole, isoniazid, metronidazole, omeprazole, phenylbutazone, salicylates, sulfonamides, ticlopidine: May increase phenytoin activity and toxicity. Monitor patient for toxicity and adjust dosage as needed.

Antacids: May decrease phenytoin absorption. Separate dosing times.

Anticoagulants (apixaban, dabigatran), ticagrelor: May decrease phenytoin level.

Atracurium, cisatracurium, pancuronium, rocuronium, vecuronium: May decrease the effects of nondepolarizing muscle relaxant. May need to increase the nondepolarizing muscle relaxant dose.

Barbiturates, carbamazepine, dexamethasone, diazepam, diazoxide, folic acid, rifampin, theophylline, vigabatrin: May decrease phenytoin activity. Monitor phenytoin level.

Carbamazepine, digoxin, doxycycline, quinidine, theophylline: May decrease effects of these drugs. Monitor patient.

Colesevelam: May impair phenytoin absorption. Administer phenytoin 4 hours prior to colesevelam.

Corticosteroids: May decrease phenytoin level and corticosteroid effects. Measure phenytoin level and adjust phenytoin and corticosteroid dosages as needed.

Cyclosporine: May decrease cyclosporine levels, risking organ rejection. Monitor cyclosporine levels closely and adjust dosage as needed.

CYP2C9 substrates: May increase serum drug level. Use cautiously in patients who are intermediate or poor metabolizers of CYP2C9 substrates. Monitor patient for toxicity and decrease dosage as appropriate.

Disulfiram: May increase toxic effects of phenytoin. Monitor phenytoin level closely and adjust dosage as needed.

Efavirenz: May increase phenytoin level and decrease efavirenz level. Monitor patient and adjust dosages of either or both drugs if needed.

Erlotinib: May increase phenytoin level and decrease erlotinib level. Monitor patient response.

Hormonal contraceptives: May increase phenytoin level and decrease contraceptive effectiveness. Monitor phenytoin level and adjust dosage if needed. Alternative form of contraception is recommended during therapy.

Isoniazid: May increase phenytoin level. Monitor phenytoin level and patient for toxicity.

Lithium: May increase toxicity of lithium, despite normal lithium levels. Monitor patient for adverse effects.

Methylphenidate: May increase phenytoin level. Monitor phenytoin level and adjust phenytoin dosage as needed.

NNRTIs (delavirdine, efavirenz, rilpivirine): May cause loss of virologic response. Use with delavirdine is contraindicated. Monitor patient closely.

Phenobarbital, valproate: May increase or decrease phenytoin level and worsen valproate-associated hyperammonemia. Monitor therapy.

Protease inhibitors (fosamprenavir, lopinavir–ritonavir): May decrease levels of both drugs. Measure phenytoin level and adjust dosage of phenytoin or protease inhibitor as needed.

Warfarin: May increase effects of warfarin and increase phenytoin level. Monitor patient for bleeding.

Drug-herb. *St. John's wort:* May decrease phenytoin level. Monitor phenytoin level.

Drug-food. *Enteral tube feedings:* May interfere with absorption of oral drug. Monitor serum drug level more frequently.

Drug-lifestyle. *Alcohol use (acute):* May increase phenytoin level. Discourage use together.

Alcohol use (long-term): May decrease drug's activity. Strongly discourage use together.

EFFECTS ON LAB TEST RESULTS
- May increase TSH, ALP, GGT, and glucose levels.
- May decrease T_3 and T_4 levels.
- May decrease Hb level, hematocrit, and platelet, WBC, RBC, and granulocyte counts.
- May falsely reduce protein-bound iodine or free T_4 level test results.
- May cause lower than normal dexamethasone and metyrapone test results.

CONTRAINDICATIONS & CAUTIONS
- Contraindicated in patients hypersensitive to hydantoins and in those with a history of prior acute liver toxicity attributable to phenytoin. Parenteral phenytoin is also contraindicated in patients with sinus bradycardia, SA block, second- or third-degree AV block, or Adams-Stokes syndrome.

Reactions in bold italics are *life-threatening*.

• Use cautiously in patients with liver or kidney dysfunction, hypotension, hypoalbuminemia, myocardial insufficiency, diabetes, porphyria, or respiratory depresssion; in older adults or patients who are debilitated; and in those receiving other hydantoin derivatives.

• Older adults tend to metabolize drug slowly and may need reduced dosages.

Dialyzable drug: Yes.

⚠ *Overdose S&S:* Ataxia, dysarthria, nystagmus, hyperreflexia, lethargy, nausea, slurred speech, tremor, vomiting, coma, hypotension, circulatory and respiratory depression.

PREGNANCY-LACTATION-REPRODUCTION

• Drug may cause fetal harm. Prenatal exposure may increase risk of congenital malformations and other adverse outcomes. Avoid use during pregnancy when possible; if necessary, use as monotherapy. Dosage adjustments may be needed to maintain clinical response because therapeutic dose needs usually increase during pregnancy.

• A potentially life-threatening bleeding disorder related to decreased levels of vitamin K-dependent clotting factors that may occur in neonates exposed to phenytoin in utero can be prevented with vitamin K administration to the mother before delivery and to the neonate after birth.

• Drug may interact with hormone-containing contraceptives; use of nonhormonal contraceptives is recommended.

• Patients exposed to drug during pregnancy should enroll in the North American AED Pregnancy Registry (1-888-233-2334 or https://www.aedpregnancyregistry.org/).

• Drug appears in human milk. Breastfeeding isn't recommended.

NURSING CONSIDERATIONS

Boxed Warning Carefully monitor cardiac status during and after IV administration. CV toxicity may increase with infusion rates above those recommended. Toxicity has also been reported at or below the recommended infusion rate. Reduction in infusion rate or discontinuation of IV administration may be needed. ▪

▓ Patients of Asian descent who have tested positive for the allele HLA-B*1502 have an increased risk of SCARs, including SJS and TEN. Monitor these patients carefully.

• If rash appears, stop drug. If rash is scarlatiniform or morbilliform, resume drug after

rash clears. If rash reappears, stop therapy. If rash is exfoliative, purpuric, or bullous, don't resume drug.

• Monitor patient for hypersensitivity reactions, including angioedema.

• Don't stop drug suddenly because this may worsen seizures. Call prescriber immediately if adverse reactions develop.

• Monitor drug level. Total phenytoin therapeutic level ranges from 10 to 20 mcg/mL in adults and children and 8 to 15 mcg/mL in neonates. Free phenytoin therapeutic level ranges from 1 to 2 mcg/mL.

• Monitor the unbound fraction of phenytoin in patients with kidney or liver impairment or hypoalbuminemia. The fraction of unbound phenytoin increases in these patients.

• Long-term use may decrease bone mineral density. Vitamin D and calcium supplements may be needed.

• Because of the risks of cardiac and local toxicity with parenteral phenytoin, use oral form when possible.

• Monitor CBC and calcium level every 6 months, and periodically monitor liver function. Prescriber may prescribe folic acid and vitamin B_{12} for evident megaloblastic anemia.

• Maintain seizure precautions, as needed.

🔵 *Alert:* Closely monitor all patients for changes in behavior that may indicate worsening suicidality or depression.

• Watch for gingival hyperplasia, especially in children.

• After seizures become controlled with divided doses, once-daily dosing may be considered.

• *Look alike–sound alike:* Don't confuse phenytoin with mephenytoin, fosphenytoin, phenelzine, phentermine, or phenobarbital. Don't confuse Dilantin with Dilaudid, diltiazem, or Dipentum.

PATIENT TEACHING

• Tell patient to report all adverse reactions and to notify prescriber if rash develops.

• Advise patient and caregivers to immediately report changes in behavior that may indicate worsening suicidality or depression.

• Caution patient to avoid driving and other potentially hazardous activities that require mental alertness until drug's CNS effects are known.

- Advise patient not to change brands or dosage forms once stabilized on therapy.
- Tell patient not to use capsules that are discolored.
- Advise patient to avoid alcohol.
- Warn patient and parents not to stop drug abruptly.
- Stress importance of good oral hygiene and regular dental exams. Surgical removal of excess gum tissue may be needed periodically if dental hygiene is poor.
- Advise patient of childbearing potential who isn't planning a pregnancy to use effective contraception; warn patient about potential for decreased hormonal contraceptive efficacy.
- Instruct patient to report pregnancy, plans to become pregnant, breastfeeding, or plans to breastfeed during therapy.
- Advise patient that drug may cause an increase in blood glucose levels.

pilocarpine hydrochloride (oral)
pye-loe-KAR-peen

Salagen

Therapeutic class: Cholinergic agonists
Pharmacologic class: Cholinergic agonists

AVAILABLE FORMS
Tablets: 5 mg, 7.5 mg

INDICATIONS & DOSAGES
Adjust-a-dose (for all indications): For patients with Child-Pugh class B liver impairment, initial dose is 5 mg PO b.i.d. Adjust dosage based on tolerance.
➤ **Xerostomia from salivary gland hypofunction caused by radiotherapy for cancer of head and neck**
Adults: 5 mg PO t.i.d.; may increase to 10 mg PO t.i.d. as needed.
➤ **Dry mouth in patients with Sjögren syndrome**
Adults: 5 mg PO q.i.d.

ADMINISTRATION
PO
- Don't give drug with a high-fat meal.
- Store at room temperature.

ACTION
Cholinergic parasympathomimetic that increases secretion of salivary glands, eliminating dryness.

Route	Onset	Peak	Duration
PO	20 min	1 hr	3–5 hr

Half-life: 45 minutes to 1.35 hours.

ADVERSE REACTIONS
CNS: asthenia, dizziness, fever, headache, tremor, pain, somnolence, taste perversion. **CV:** flushing, HTN, tachycardia, edema, palpitations. **EENT:** abnormal vision, lacrimation, amblyopia, conjunctivitis, tinnitus, epistaxis, rhinitis, sinusitis, pharyngitis, voice alteration, increased salivation, glossitis. **GI:** nausea, dyspepsia, diarrhea, constipation, abdominal pain, flatulence, stomatitis, vomiting, dysphagia. **GU:** urinary frequency, urinary incontinence, UTI, vaginitis. **Musculoskeletal:** myalgia, weakness, back pain. **Skin:** diaphoresis, rash, pruritus. **Other:** chills, flu-like syndrome, infection, hypersensitivity reaction.

INTERACTIONS
Drug-drug. *Beta blockers:* May increase risk of conduction disturbances. Use together cautiously.
Drugs with anticholinergic effects (atropine, inhaled ipratropium): May decrease anticholinergic effects. Use together cautiously.
Drugs with parasympathomimetic effects: May result in additive pharmacologic effects. Monitor patient closely.
Drug-food. *High-fat meals:* May reduce drug absorption. Discourage patient from eating high-fat meals.

EFFECTS ON LAB TEST RESULTS
None reported.

CONTRAINDICATIONS & CAUTIONS
- Contraindicated in patients hypersensitive to pilocarpine, in those with uncontrolled asthma, and in those for whom miosis is undesirable, as in acute iritis or angle-closure glaucoma.
- Use in Child-Pugh class C liver impairment isn't recommended.
- Use cautiously in patients with CV disease, controlled asthma, chronic bronchitis, COPD, cholelithiasis, biliary tract disease, nephrolithiasis, Child-Pugh class B liver

---

impairment, or cognitive or psychiatric disturbances.
• Safety and effectiveness in children haven't been established.
Dialyzable drug: Unknown.
⚠ *Overdose S&S:* Exaggerated parasympathetic effects, CV depression, bronchoconstriction, death.

PREGNANCY-LACTATION-REPRODUCTION
• There are no adequate studies during pregnancy. Use only if potential benefit justifies fetal risk.
• It isn't known if drug appears in human milk. Patient should discontinue breastfeeding or discontinue drug, considering importance of rug to patient.

NURSING CONSIDERATIONS
• Monitor patient for signs and symptoms of toxicity: headache, visual disturbance, lacrimation, diaphoresis, respiratory distress, GI spasm, nausea, vomiting, diarrhea, AV block, tachycardia, bradycardia, hypotension, HTN, shock, mental confusion, arrhythmia, and tremors. Immediately report suspected toxicity.
• Monitor patient for dehydration from diaphoresis and poor fluid intake.
• Patients with head and neck cancer may need at least 12 weeks of uninterrupted therapy to assess benefits of continuing therapy after early improvement. In patients with Sjögren syndrome, efficacy is seen by 6 weeks.
• *Look alike–sound alike:* Don't confuse Salagen with selegiline.

PATIENT TEACHING
• Warn patient that driving ability may be impaired, especially at night, by drug-induced visual disturbances.
• Advise patient to drink plenty of fluids to prevent dehydration.
• Tell older adults with Sjögren syndrome that this age-group may be especially prone to urinary frequency, diarrhea, and dizziness.
• Advise patient not to take drug with a high-fat meal.
• Instruct patient to report changes in eyesight and eye pain or irritation.

pioglitazone hydrochloride
pye-oh-GLI-ta-zone

Actos

Therapeutic class: Antidiabetics
Pharmacologic class: Thiazolidinediones

AVAILABLE FORMS
Tablets: 15 mg, 30 mg, 45 mg

INDICATIONS & DOSAGES
➤ **Type 2 diabetes, alone or with a sulfonylurea, metformin, or insulin as an adjunct to diet and exercise to improve glycemic control**
Adults: Initially, 15 or 30 mg PO once daily. Titrate in 15-mg increments to maximum of 45 mg daily based on HbA_{1c}.
Adjust-a-dose: For patients taking pioglitazone with insulin, reduce insulin by 10% to 25% if hypoglycemia occurs. For patients taking insulin secretagogue, decrease secretagogue if hypoglycemia occurs. Maximum recommended dose of pioglitazone is 15 mg when used with gemfibrozil or other strong CYP2C8 inhibitors. Start with 15 mg in patients with NYHA Class I or II HF.

ADMINISTRATION
PO
• Give drug without regard for meals.
• For missed dose, skip missed dose and resume regular schedule the following day; don't double dose.

ACTION
Lowers glucose level by decreasing insulin resistance and liver glucose production. Improves sensitivity of insulin in muscle and adipose tissue.

Route	Onset	Peak	Duration
PO	30 min	≤2 hr	Unknown

Half-life: 3 to 7 hours.

ADVERSE REACTIONS
CNS: headache, dizziness. **CV:** edema, *HF,* HTN, chest pain. **EENT:** macular edema, sinusitis, pharyngitis, tooth disorder. **GI:** diarrhea, flatulence. **GU:** UTI. **Hematologic:** anemia. **Metabolic:** *hypoglycemia,* weight gain. **Musculoskeletal:** myalgia, fractures, back pain. **Respiratory:** URI.

P

INTERACTIONS

Drug-drug. *CYP2C8 inducers (rifampin):* May decrease pioglitazone level. Don't exceed maximum recommended pioglitazone dose of 45 mg.

Insulin: May increase incidence of edema and HF and may cause additive or synergistic pharmacologic effects. If hypoglycemia occurs, decrease insulin dosage. If edema or HF occurs, decrease pioglitazone dosage.

Ketoconazole: May increase pioglitazone level. Monitor glucose level more frequently.

Strong CYP2C8 inhibitors (gemfibrozil): May increase pioglitazone level. Monitor patient and glucose level. Maximum pioglitazone dose is 15 mg.

Sulfonylureas: May increase risk of hypoglycemia. If hypoglycemia occurs, reduce sulfonylurea dosage.

Topiramate: May decrease pioglitazone level. Monitor glycemic control.

Drug-herb. *Eucalyptus:* May increase hypoglycemic effects. Discourage use together.

Drug-lifestyle. *Alcohol use:* May alter glycemic control and increase risk of hypoglycemia. Discourage use together.

EFFECTS ON LAB TEST RESULTS

• May increase LFT values and CK, HDL, and total cholesterol levels.

• May decrease glucose and triglyceride levels.

• May decrease Hb level and hematocrit.

CONTRAINDICATIONS & CAUTIONS

Boxed Warning Contraindicated in patients with NYHA Class III or IV HF; not recommended in those with symptomatic HF. ■

• Contraindicated in patients hypersensitive to drug or its components and in those with active bladder cancer.

• Don't use in patients with type 1 diabetes and diabetic ketoacidosis; use cautiously in those with active liver disease.

• Safety and effectiveness in children haven't been established.

Dialyzable drug: Unknown.

PREGNANCY-LACTATION-REPRODUCTION

• Use during pregnancy only if benefit justifies fetal risk. Insulin is preferred antidiabetic during pregnancy.

• It isn't known if drug appears in human milk. Patient should discontinue breastfeeding or discontinue drug, considering importance of drug to patient.

NURSING CONSIDERATIONS

❸ *Alert:* Measure liver enzyme levels before start of therapy. In patients with liver disorder, monitor LFT values periodically during treatment. Obtain LFT results in patients who develop signs and symptoms of liver dysfunction, such as nausea, vomiting, abdominal pain, fatigue, anorexia, or dark urine. Stop drug if patient develops jaundice or if LFT results show ALT level greater than 3 × ULN with bilirubin level greater than 2 × ULN.

Boxed Warning Drug can cause fluid retention, leading to or worsening HF. Observe patients carefully for signs and symptoms of HF (excessive, rapid weight gain; dyspnea; edema). If these signs and symptoms develop, the HF should be managed according to the current standards of care. Also, stopping or reducing dose of pioglitazone must be considered. ■

• Hb level and hematocrit may drop, usually during first 4 to 12 weeks of therapy.

• Management of type 2 diabetes should include diet control. Because caloric restrictions, weight loss, and exercise help improve insulin sensitivity and help make drug therapy effective, these measures are essential for proper diabetes management.

❸ *Alert:* Watch for hypoglycemia, especially in patients receiving combination therapy. Dosage adjustments of these drugs may be needed.

• Monitor glucose level regularly, especially during situations of increased stress, such as infection, fever, surgery, and trauma.

❸ *Alert:* Drug may be associated with an increased risk of bladder cancer when used for more than 1 year. Monitor patients for signs and symptoms of bladder cancer (blood in urine, abdominal pain). If considering use in patients with a history of bladder cancer, weigh benefits of blood glucose control with drug against unknown risks of cancer recurrence.

• Monitor patient for blurred vision or decreased visual acuity. Refer patient with symptoms to an ophthalmologist for macular edema evaluation.

• Long-term treatment increases risk of fractures (forearm, hand, wrist, foot, ankle, fibula, and tibia) in females. Give only if risk outweighs benefits.

• *Look alike–sound alike:* Don't confuse pioglitazone with rosiglitazone. Don't confuse Actos with Actonel.

Reactions in bold italics are *life-threatening*.

PATIENT TEACHING
• Instruct patient in safe drug administration.
• Caution patient to adhere to dietary instructions and to have glucose and HbA$_{1c}$ levels tested regularly.
• Teach patient taking pioglitazone with insulin or oral antidiabetics the signs and symptoms of hypoglycemia.
• Advise patient to notify prescriber during periods of stress, such as fever, trauma, infection, or surgery, because dosage may need adjustment.
• Instruct patient how and when to monitor glucose level.
• Notify patient that blood tests of liver function will be performed before therapy starts and, if appropriate, periodically thereafter.
• Tell patient to immediately report all adverse reactions, especially unexplained nausea, vomiting, abdominal pain, fatigue, anorexia, and dark urine, because these symptoms may indicate liver problems.
• Warn patient to report signs or symptoms of HF (unusually rapid weight gain, swelling, or shortness of breath).
• Advise patient with insulin resistance who is anovulatory and premenopausal that therapy may cause resumption of ovulation; recommend using contraception.
• Tell patient to have regular eye exams and to report any visual changes immediately.
• Advise patient to report blood in the urine, red-colored urine, new or worsening urge to urinate, or pain when urinating; these symptoms may indicate bladder cancer.

---

piperacillin sodium–tazobactam sodium
pi-PER-a-sil-in/ta-zoe-BAK-tam

Zosyn

Therapeutic class: Antibiotics
Pharmacologic class: Extended-spectrum penicillins-beta-lactamase inhibitors

AVAILABLE FORMS
Powder for injection: 2 g piperacillin and 0.25 g tazobactam per vial, 3 g piperacillin and 0.375 g tazobactam per vial, 4 g piperacillin and 0.5 g tazobactam per vial
Premixed, frozen solution for injection: 2 g piperacillin and 0.25 g tazobactam per 50-mL container, 3 g piperacillin and

0.375 g tazobactam per 50-mL container, 4 g piperacillin and 0.5 g tazobactam per 100-mL container

INDICATIONS & DOSAGES
➤ **Moderate to severe infections from piperacillin-resistant, piperacillin-tazobactam-susceptible, beta-lactamase-producing strains of microorganisms in appendicitis (complicated by rupture or abscess) and peritonitis caused by *Escherichia coli, Bacteroides fragilis, B. ovatus, B. thetaiotaomicron*, or *B. vulgatus;* skin and skin-structure infections caused by *Staphylococcus aureus;* postpartum endometritis or pelvic inflammatory disease caused by *E. coli;* moderately severe community-acquired pneumonia caused by *Haemophilus influenzae***
Adults: 3.375 g (3 g piperacillin/0.375 g tazobactam) every 6 hours by IV infusion for 7 to 10 days.
➤ **Appendicitis, peritonitis**
Children weighing more than 40 kg with normal kidney function: 3.375 g (3 g piperacillin/0.375 g tazobactam) every 6 hours by IV infusion for 7 to 10 days.
Children ages 9 months and older weighing 40 kg or less with normal kidney function: 100 mg piperacillin/12.5 mg tazobactam per kg of body weight every 8 hours by IV infusion for 7 to 10 days.
Children ages 2 to 9 months with normal kidney function: 80 mg piperacillin/10 mg tazobactam per kg of body weight every 8 hours by IV infusion for 7 to 10 days.
➤ **Moderate to severe health care-associated pneumonia caused by piperacillin-resistant, beta-lactamase-producing strains of *S. aureus* or by piperacillin-tazobactam-susceptible *Acinetobacter baumannii, H. influenzae, Klebsiella pneumoniae*, and *Pseudomonas aeruginosa***
Adults and children weighing more than 40 kg with normal kidney function: 4.5 g (4 g piperacillin/0.5 g tazobactam) IV every 6 hours with aminoglycoside. Patients with *P. aeruginosa* should continue aminoglycoside or antipseudomonal fluoroquinolone treatment; if *P. aeruginosa* isn't isolated, aminoglycoside or fluoroquinolone treatment may be stopped. Duration of treatment is usually 7 to 14 days.
Children older than 9 months weighing 40 kg or less with normal kidney function: 100 mg

piperacillin/12.5 mg tazobactam per kg of body weight every 6 hours by IV infusion for 7 to 10 days.

Children ages 2 to 9 months with normal kidney function: 80 mg piperacillin/10 mg tazobactam per kg of body weight every 6 hours by IV infusion for 7 to 10 days.

Adjust-a-dose: In adults, if CrCl is 20 to 40 mL/minute, give 3.375 g (3 g piperacillin/0.375 g tazobactam) every 6 hours; if CrCl is less than 20 mL/minute, give 2.25 g (2 g piperacillin/0.25 g tazobactam) every 6 hours. In patients on hemodialysis or continuous ambulatory peritoneal dialysis, give 2.25 g (2 g piperacillin/0.25 g tazobactam) every 8 hours. In patients on hemodialysis, give a supplemental dose of 0.75 g (0.67 g piperacillin/0.08 g tazobactam) after each session. Dosage adjustments for children with kidney impairment haven't been established.

ADMINISTRATION

IV

▼ Before giving drug, ask patient about allergic reactions to penicillins, cephalosporins, or beta-lactamase inhibitors.

▼ Obtain specimen for culture and sensitivity tests before giving first dose. Therapy may begin while awaiting results.

▼ Reconstitute each gram (based on piperacillin content) with 5 mL of diluent, such as sterile or bacteriostatic water for injection, NSS for injection, bacteriostatic NSS for injection, D_5W, dextrose 5% in NSS for injection, or dextran 6% in NSS for injection.

▼ Shake until dissolved.

▼ Further dilute to 50 to 150 mL before infusion.

▼ Use drug immediately after reconstitution.

▼ Stop any primary infusion during administration, if possible.

▼ Infuse over at least 30 minutes.

▼ Discard unused drug in single-dose vials after 24 hours if stored at room temperature or 48 hours if refrigerated.

▼ Diluted drug remains stable in IV bags for 24 hours at room temperature or for 1 week refrigerated.

▼ Store premixed, frozen solution containers at or below –4° F (–20° C).

▼ Thaw frozen container at room temperature or under refrigeration. Don't force-thaw by immersion in water baths or by microwave irradiation.

▼ Check for minute leaks by squeezing container firmly. If leaks are detected, discard solution as sterility may be impaired.

▼ Visually inspect solution, which may precipitate while frozen but will dissolve upon reaching room temperature with little or no agitation. If, after visual inspection, solution remains cloudy, an insoluble precipitate is noted, or if any seals or outlet ports aren't intact, discard container.

▼ Don't use plastic containers in series connections.

▼ **Incompatibilities:** Other drugs.

ACTION

Inhibits cell-wall synthesis during bacterial multiplication.

Route	Onset	Peak	Duration
IV	Immediate	Immediate	Unknown

Half-life: About 0.7 to 1.2 hours.

ADVERSE REACTIONS

CNS: headache, insomnia, fever, agitation, anxiety, dizziness, pain. **CV:** chest pain, edema, HTN, hypotension, tachycardia, phlebitis at IV site, thrombophlebitis. **EENT:** rhinitis, oral candidiasis. **GI:** diarrhea, constipation, nausea, abdominal pain, dyspepsia, stool changes, vomiting. **GU:** *KF,* interstitial nephritis, increased BUN and creatinine levels. **Hematologic:** *thrombocythemia.* **Hepatic:** abnormal LFT values. **Skin:** pruritus, rash. **Other:** candidiasis, hypersensitivity reactions, inflammation.

INTERACTIONS

Drug-drug. *Aminoglycosides (amikacin, gentamicin, streptomycin, tobramycin):* Penicillins may decrease level of aminoglycosides. Consider therapy modification.

Anticoagulants (warfarin, heparin): May affect coagulation effect or thrombocyte function. Monitor clotting times closely.

Live-virus vaccines: May decrease vaccine effectiveness. Don't use together.

Methotrexate: May increase risk of methotrexate toxicity. Monitor closely.

Probenecid: May increase piperacillin level. Probenecid may be used for this purpose.

Vancomycin: May increase kidney toxicity. Monitor therapy.

Vecuronium: May prolong neuromuscular blockade. Monitor patient closely.

EFFECTS ON LAB TEST RESULTS

• May increase serum sodium level because of sodium content in drug.
• May increase BUN, creatinine, ALP, ALT, and AST levels.
• May increase eosinophil count.
• May decrease Hb level and neutrophil and WBC counts.
• May increase or decrease platelet count.
• May prolong PTT and PT.
• May cause false-positive result for urine glucose tests using copper reduction method such as Clinitest.
• May cause false-positive test for *Aspergillus*.

CONTRAINDICATIONS & CAUTIONS

• Contraindicated in patients hypersensitive to drug, other penicillins, cephalosporins, or beta-lactamase inhibitors.
• Drug can cause CDAD. Consider possibility of CDAD in all patients who present with diarrhea after antibiotic use.
• Use cautiously in patients with kidney impairment or seizure disorders. Penicillins can cause neuromuscular excitability or seizures.
• Use cautiously in patients who are critically ill and in patients with bleeding tendencies, uremia, hypokalemia, and allergies to other drugs.
Dialyzable drug: Yes.
△ *Overdose S&S:* Neuromuscular hyperexcitability, seizures.

PREGNANCY-LACTATION-REPRODUCTION

• There are no adequate studies during pregnancy. Piperacillin and tazobactam cross the placental barrier in humans. Use only if clearly needed.
• Drug appears in low concentrations in human milk. Use cautiously if breastfeeding.

NURSING CONSIDERATIONS

❶ *Alert:* Drug may cause CDAD ranging in severity from mild diarrhea to fatal colitis. Monitor patient for diarrhea and initiate therapeutic measures as needed. Drug may need to be stopped.
• Studies have shown that drug is an independent risk factor for KF and delayed recovery of kidney function in patients who are critically ill. Alternative treatments should be considered; if such options are inadequate or unavailable, monitor kidney function during therapy.

• SCARs can occur. If rash develops, monitor patient closely and discontinue drug if lesion progresses.
• Hemodialysis removes 30% to 40% of a dose in 4 hours. Additional doses may be needed after each dialysis period.
• If large doses are given or if therapy is prolonged, bacterial or fungal superinfection may occur, especially in older adults or patients who are debilitated or immunosuppressed.
• Drug contains 2.84 mEq (65 mg) sodium per gram of piperacillin. Monitor sodium intake and electrolyte levels.
• Monitor CBC and coagulation parameters.
❶ *Alert:* Monitor patient for hemophagocytic lymphohistiocytosis (fever, rash, lymphadenopathy, enlarged liver and spleen, cytopenia), a life-threatening excessive immune activation syndrome that occurs most often in infants younger than age 18 months. Discontinue drug immediately for such signs or symptoms.
• Monitor patient with cystic fibrosis for fever and rash.
• *Look alike–sound alike:* Don't confuse Zosyn with Zyvox.

PATIENT TEACHING

• Tell patient to report allergic and other adverse reactions promptly.
• Instruct patient to report discomfort at IV site.
• Advise patient that watery and bloody stools with or without stomach cramps and fever may occur during and for up to 2 months or more after antibiotic use. Instruct patient to report these symptoms as soon as possible.

---

pitavastatin calcium ▨
pih-tav-a-STAT-in

Livalo

pitavastatin magnesium
Zypitamag

Therapeutic class: Antilipemics
Pharmacologic class: HMG-CoA reductase inhibitors

AVAILABLE FORMS

Tablets (calcium): 1 mg, 2 mg, 4 mg
Tablets (magnesium): 2 mg, 4 mg

INDICATIONS & DOSAGES

Adjust-a-dose (for all indications): For adults with GFR of 15 to 59 mL/minute/1.73 m² and those with KFRT, start with 1 mg PO daily; maximum dosage is 2 mg daily.

➤ **Primary hyperlipidemia or mixed dyslipidemia as adjunctive therapy with diet to decrease total cholesterol (TC), LDL cholesterol (LDL-C), and apolipo-protein B (apo B) triglyceride levels, and to increase HDL cholesterol level (Zypitamag)**

Adults: Initially, 2 mg PO daily. May increase dosage as needed, to maximum of 4 mg PO daily.

➤ **Primary hyperlipidemia (Livalo)**

Adults: Initially, 2 mg PO daily. May increase as needed, to maximum of 4 mg daily.

➤ **Heterozygous familial hypercholesterolemia (HeFH) (Livalo)** ⬚

Adults and children ages 8 and older: Initially, 2 mg PO daily. May increase as needed, to maximum of 4 mg daily.

ADMINISTRATION

PO

• May give without regard to food at same time each day.

ACTION

Inhibits HMG-CoA reductase, a liver enzyme that's needed for cholesterol biosynthesis.

Route	Onset	Peak	Duration
PO	Unknown	1 hr	Unknown

Half-life: 12 hours.

ADVERSE REACTIONS

CNS: headache. **EENT:** nasopharyngitis. **GI:** constipation, diarrhea. **Musculoskeletal:** back pain, myalgia, extremity pain. **Other:** flulike symptoms, hypersensitivity reactions.

INTERACTIONS

Drug-drug. *Colchicine:* May cause myopathy, including rhabdomyolysis. Use cautiously together.
Cyclosporine: May increase pitavastatin level. Use together is contraindicated.
Erythromycin: May increase pitavastatin levels. Don't exceed 1 mg pitavastatin daily.
Fibrates (gemfibrozil), niacin: May increase risk of myopathy. Use together cautiously; consider reducing pitavastatin dosage when combined with niacin.

Rifampin: May increase pitavastatin levels. Don't exceed 2 mg pitavastatin daily.
Vitamin K antagonists (warfarin): May enhance anticoagulant effect. Monitor therapy.
Drug-herb. *Herbal cholesterol-lowering products:* May increase pitavastatin levels. Discourage using together.

EFFECTS ON LAB TEST RESULTS

• May increase AST, ALT, CK, bilirubin, HbA₁c, and glucose levels.

CONTRAINDICATIONS & CAUTIONS

• Contraindicated in patients hypersensitive to drug or its components and in those with active liver disease, which may include unexplained persistent elevations of transaminase levels.

• Use cautiously in older adults and in patients with kidney impairment, inadequately treated hypothyroidism, a history of myopathy or rhabdomyolysis, or a history of substantial alcohol consumption.

• Statin therapy should be interrupted if patient shows signs of serious liver injury, hyperbilirubinemia, or jaundice. The drug shouldn't be restarted if another cause can't be found.

• Drug hasn't been studied in Fredrickson Type I, III, and V dyslipidemias.

• Safety and effectiveness of Livalo in children younger than age 8 with HeFH or in children with other types of hyperlipidemia haven't been established. Safety and effectiveness of Zypitamag in children haven't been established.

Dialyzable drug: Unlikely.

PREGNANCY-LACTATION-REPRODUCTION

• May cause fetal harm. Use during pregnancy is contraindicated unless benefits to patient outweigh fetal risk. Patients of childbearing potential should use effective contraception during treatment.

• The FDA has determined that statin use in patients at high risk for CV events during pregnancy may be considered on an individual basis.

• Drug should be discontinued before conception. If pregnancy occurs during therapy, apprise patient of fetal risks with continued use.

• Drug is contraindicated during breastfeeding.

---

*Reactions in bold italics are **life-threatening**.*

NURSING CONSIDERATIONS
• Start pitavastatin only after diet and other nondrug therapies have proved ineffective.
• Monitor LFT results and CK levels before therapy, 12 weeks after therapy initiation, after a dosage change, and periodically thereafter.
• Monitor lipid levels at baseline, 4 weeks after start of therapy, and after titration; adjust dosage accordingly.
• Discontinue drug if myopathy develops or if CK level markedly increases. Doses greater than 4 mg once daily were associated with an increased risk of severe myopathy in premarketing clinical studies. Don't exceed 4 mg once daily.
• Temporarily withhold drug if patient develops sepsis; hypotension; dehydration; severe metabolic, endocrine, or electrolyte disorders; uncontrolled seizures; or trauma or if patient requires major surgery. These conditions may predispose patient to myopathy or rhabdomyolysis.
• *Look alike–sound alike:* Don't confuse pitavastatin with atorvastatin, fluvastatin, lovastatin, nystatin, pravastatin, rosuvastatin, or simvastatin.

PATIENT TEACHING
• Instruct patient in safe drug administration.
• Explain the importance of controlling serum lipid levels. Teach appropriate dietary management (restricting saturated fat and cholesterol intake), weight control, and exercise.
• Advise patient of childbearing potential to use contraception during therapy and to discuss future pregnancy and breastfeeding plans with health care provider.
• Warn patient to report unexplained muscle pain, tenderness, or weakness, especially if accompanied by fever or malaise.
• Teach patient that blood tests to check liver enzyme levels will be needed after start of therapy, after a dosage increase, and periodically thereafter.
• Tell patient that drug may increase blood glucose level; however, the CV benefits are thought to outweigh blood glucose level increase.

plecanatide
ple-KAN-a-tide

Trulance

Therapeutic class: Laxatives
Pharmacologic class: Guanylate cyclase-C agonists

AVAILABLE FORMS
Tablets: 3 mg

INDICATIONS & DOSAGES
➤ **Chronic idiopathic constipation or IBS with constipation**
Adults: 3 mg PO daily.

ADMINISTRATION
PO
• May give with or without food.
• Patient should swallow tablets whole, if possible.
• For patients with swallowing difficulties, may crush tablet and mix with 1 tsp of room temperature applesauce; give immediately.
• May dissolve tablet by placing whole tablet in a cup and adding 30 mL of room temperature water; swirl for at least 10 seconds. Give mixture immediately. To give any portion left in cup, add an additional 30 mL of water and swirl for at least 10 seconds. Give immediately; don't store mixture.
• If giving dissolved tablet by NG or gastric feeding tube, place tablet in 30 mL of water and swirl for at least 15 seconds. Draw up mixture using an appropriate syringe and administer. Flush tube with 30 mL of water before and at least 10 mL of water after administration.
• Skip a missed dose and give next dose at regularly scheduled time. Don't double dose.
• Store in dry place at room temperature. Keep drug in its original bottle with supplied desiccant.

ACTION
Plecanatide and its active metabolite bind to guanylate cyclase-C and act locally on the luminal surface of the intestinal epithelium, resulting in increased secretion of chloride and bicarbonate into the intestinal lumen, resulting in increased intestinal fluid and accelerated transit.

Route	Onset	Peak	Duration
PO	Unknown	Unknown	Unknown

Half-life: Unknown due to negligible systemic absorption.

ADVERSE REACTIONS
CNS: dizziness. **EENT:** sinusitis, nasopharyngitis. **GI:** diarrhea, abdominal distention, flatulence, abdominal tenderness, nausea. **GU:** UTI. **Hepatic:** elevated liver enzyme levels. **Respiratory:** URI.

INTERACTIONS
None reported.

EFFECTS ON LAB TEST RESULTS
• May increase AST and ALT levels.

CONTRAINDICATIONS & CAUTIONS
Boxed Warning Contraindicated in patients younger than age 6 because of risk of serious dehydration. ∎
Boxed Warning Safety and effectiveness in patients younger than age 18 haven't been established. Avoid use in patients age 6 to younger than age 18. ∎
• Contraindicated in patients with known or suspected mechanical GI obstruction.
• Don't administered to patients with severe diarrhea. Diarrhea is the most common adverse effect of plecanatide.
• Use cautiously in older adults.
Dialyzable drug: Unlikely.

PREGNANCY-LACTATION-REPRODUCTION
• Drug isn't absorbed systemically; use during pregnancy isn't expected to result in fetal exposure.
• Drug isn't expected to appear in human milk because it isn't absorbed systemically. Use cautiously during breastfeeding.

NURSING CONSIDERATIONS
• Monitor patient for diarrhea. If severe diarrhea occurs, withhold drug and rehydrate patient.
• *Look alike–sound alike:* Don't confuse Trulance with Trulicity.

PATIENT TEACHING
• Teach patient safe drug administration.
• Instruct patient to stop taking drug if severe diarrhea occurs and to contact prescriber.
• *Alert:* Warn patient to securely store drug away from children. Accidental ingestion may cause severe diarrhea and dehydration.

ponesimod
poe-NES-i-mod

Ponvory

Therapeutic class: MS drugs
Pharmacologic class: Sphingosine 1-phosphate receptor modulators

AVAILABLE FORMS
Tablets ⓄⓃⒸ: 2 mg, 3 mg, 4 mg, 5 mg, 6 mg, 7 mg, 8 mg, 9 mg, 10 mg, 20 mg

INDICATIONS & DOSAGES
➤ **Relapsing forms of MS, including clinically isolated syndrome, relapsing-remitting disease, and active secondary progressive disease**
Adults: Initially, 1 tablet PO daily from starter pack for days 1 to 14: days 1 and 2, give 2 mg; days 3 and 4, give 3 mg; days 5 and 6, give 4 mg; day 7, give 5 mg; day 8, give 6 mg; day 9, give 7 mg; day 10, give 8 mg; day 11, give 9 mg; days 12 to 14, give 10 mg; then begin maintenance dose, 20 mg PO daily starting on day 15.

ADMINISTRATION
PO
• *Alert:* Hazardous drug; use safe handling and disposal precautions.
• Give without regard to food.
• Have patient swallow tablets whole; don't crush or break tablets.
• Give first dose in appropriate setting with resources to manage symptomatic bradycardia.
• If patient has missed fewer than four consecutive titration doses, resume treatment with first missed titration dose and continue titration schedule.
• If patient has missed fewer than four consecutive maintenance doses, resume treatment with maintenance dose.
• If patient has missed four or more consecutive daily doses during titration or maintenance, reinitiate with day 1 of titration regimen with a new starter pack and complete first-dose monitoring in patients for whom it's recommended.
• Store tablets at 68° to 77° F (20° to 25° C) in original package; protect from moisture.

ACTION
Decreases ability of lymphocytes to leave the lymph nodes, reducing number of

lymphocytes in peripheral blood that migrate into the CNS.

Route	Onset	Peak	Duration
PO	Unknown	2–4 hr	Unknown

Half-life: 33 hours.

ADVERSE REACTIONS
CNS: depression, dizziness, fatigue, fever, insomnia, migraine, somnolence, vertigo, *seizures.* **CV:** AV conduction delay, *brady-cardia,* chest discomfort, HTN, peripheral edema. **EENT:** macular edema, rhinitis, sinusitis, dry mouth. **GI:** dyspepsia. **GU:** UTI. **Hematologic:** elevated C-reactive protein level, *lymphopenia.* **Hepatic:** increased LFT values. **Metabolic:** hypercholesterolemia, *hyperkalemia.* **Musculoskeletal:** back pain, extremity pain, joint swelling. **Respiratory:** cough, dyspnea, pneumonia, URI. **Other:** infection, herpes zoster.

INTERACTIONS
Drug-drug. *Alemtuzumab:* May prolong effects of alemtuzumab and have additive immunosuppressive effects. Don't initiate ponesimod therapy after alemtuzumab.
Immunemodulating, immunosuppressive, or antineoplastic therapies: May have additive immunosuppressive effects. Use together cautiously. When switching from drugs with prolonged immune effects, consider their half-life and mode of action.
Beta blockers (atenolol, carvedilol, labetalol, metoprolol): May have additive HR-lowering effects. Use cautiously together; beta blocker dose interruption may be necessary. May initiate beta blockers in patients on stable doses of ponesimod.
Beta interferon, glatiramer acetate: May have additive immunosuppressive effects. May start ponesimod immediately after discontinuation of these drugs.
⚠ *Alert:* Drugs that prolong QT interval (Class IA [procainamide, quinidine] and Class III [amiodarone, sotalol] antiarrhythmics), diltiazem, verapamil, other drugs that may decrease HR (digoxin): May have additive effects on HR. Consult cardiologist before use together.
Drugs that slow HR or AV conduction: May have additive effects. Monitor patient closely; consult cardiologist as appropriate.
Strong CYP3A4 and UGT1A1 inducers (carbamazepine, phenytoin, rifampin):

May decrease ponesimod level. Avoid use together.
Vaccines: May decrease effectiveness of vaccine during therapy and for 2 weeks after final dose of ponesimod. Live attenuated vaccines may increase risk of infection; administer at least 1 month before starting ponesimod. Avoid live vaccines during ponesimod therapy and for 2 weeks after final dose.
Drug-lifestyle. *Sun exposure:* May increase risk of skin cancer. Limit exposure to sunlight and UV light.

EFFECTS ON LAB TEST RESULTS
• May increase transaminase, bilirubin, C-reactive protein, cholesterol, and potassium levels.
• May decrease lymphocyte count.

CONTRAINDICATIONS & CAUTIONS
• Contraindicated in patients with history of MI, unstable angina, stroke, TIA, decompensated HF requiring hospitalization, or Class III or IV HF during last 6 months.
• Contraindicated in patients with Mobitz type II second- or third-degree AV block or sick sinus syndrome, or SA block, unless patient has a functioning pacemaker.
• Avoid use in patients with Child-Pugh class B or C liver impairment.
• Use cautiously in patients with preexisting heart and cerebrovascular conditions, HTN, arrhythmias, prolonged QTc interval, risk of prolonged QTc interval, or concomitant drug therapy that slows HR or AV conduction or prolongs QTc interval after consulting cardiologist on monitoring strategy.
• Use cautiously in patients with sinus bradycardia (HR less than 55 beats/minute) or first- or second-degree (Mobitz type I) AV block, or in patients in stable condition with history of MI or HF with onset more than 6 months before drug initiation. Consult cardiologist and perform first-dose monitoring in these patients.
• Use cautiously in patients with pulmonary fibrosis, asthma, and COPD. Dose-dependent reductions in respiratory function were seen in patients treated with drug.
• Use cautiously in patients with macular edema and in those at increased risk for macular edema (diabetes, uveitis).
• Avoid use in patients receiving concomitant phototherapy (UV-B radiation or PUVA-photochemotherapy).

• Drug increases risk of life-threatening and fatal infections.

• Drug may cause severe exacerbation of MS, including disease rebound, after discontinuation.

• Safety and effectiveness in children haven't been established.

• Use cautiously in older adults.

Dialyzable drug: No.

⚠ *Overdose S&S:* Bradycardia, AV conduction block.

PREGNANCY-LACTATION-REPRODUCTION

• Based on animal studies, drug may cause fetal harm. Advise patients who are pregnant of the fetal risk.

• Patients of childbearing potential should use effective contraception during therapy and for 1 week after final dose.

• It isn't known if drug appears in human milk or how drug affects milk production or infants who are breastfed. Consider benefits and risk before use during breastfeeding.

NURSING CONSIDERATIONS

• Obtain baseline ECG for preexisting conduction abnormalities. If present, consult cardiologist.

• Administer first dose in a setting where resources to appropriately manage symptomatic bradycardia are available for patients at risk. After first dose, monitor patient for 4 hours for bradycardia with hourly HR and BP measurement. Obtain ECG before dose and after 4-hour observation period. If abnormalities occur, follow prescribing instructions to determine additional required monitoring.

• Review CBC within 6 months of starting drug. Delay therapy in patients with active infection until it resolves.

• Obtain transaminase and bilirubin levels within 6 months of starting therapy. If liver dysfunction is suspected during therapy, recheck transaminase and bilirubin levels. Discontinue drug for confirmed liver injury.

• Obtain ophthalmic evaluation of the fundus, including macula, at baseline, with a reported vision change, and periodically in patients at increased risk.

• Obtain antibody test for varicella zoster virus (VZV) in patient without confirmed history of varicella or without documentation of a full course of vaccination against VZV before therapy. Give varicella vaccine in patient who is antibody-negative and delay start of ponesimod for 4 weeks.

• Monitor patient for active infection. Consider interrupting therapy for serious infection.

• Monitor patient for signs and symptoms of cryptococcal meningitis (headache, fever, neck pain, nausea, vomiting, sensitivity to light, confusion) and disseminated cryptococcal infections (fever, cough, hemoptysis, chest pain, night sweats, weight loss). If infection is diagnosed, suspend therapy and begin appropriate treatment.

🔷 *Alert:* Monitor patient for signs and symptoms or MRI findings suggestive of PML (progressive weakness on one side of body or clumsiness of limbs; vision disturbances; changes in thinking, memory, and orientation leading to confusion and personality changes). If suspected, suspend therapy; if confirmed, discontinue drug.

🔷 *Alert:* Monitor patient for signs and symptoms of PRES (cognitive deficits, behavioral changes, severe headache, visual disturbances, seizure; increased ICP, accelerated neurologic deterioration). Promptly perform a physical and neurologic exam and consider MRI. Delay in diagnosis and treatment may lead to permanent neurologic deficit. If PRES is suspected, discontinue drug.

• Obtain spirometric evaluation of respiratory function in patient with pulmonary fibrosis, asthma, and COPD during therapy as clinically indicated.

• Monitor BP periodically during therapy. Treat elevations appropriately.

• Obtain periodic skin exams for malignancies.

• Monitor patient for infection during therapy and for 2 weeks after stopping drug. Give other immunosuppressants cautiously during this time.

• Monitor patient for exacerbation of MS, including disease rebound after drug is stopped. Initiate appropriate treatment as indicated.

PATIENT TEACHING

• Teach patient about safe drug administration and handling, reporting a missed dose, and not to discontinue drug without first discussing with prescriber.

• Tell patient about increased risk of infection during therapy and for 2 weeks after stopping drug. Advise patient to report signs and symptoms of infection (fever, fatigue, body aches, chills, nausea, vomiting, headache with neck stiffness, light sensitivity, confusion).

• Advise patient to avoid vaccines 1 month before starting drug, during therapy, and for 2 weeks after stopping drug.

• Inform patient that use of other drugs to suppress the immune system may increase risk of infection.

• Counsel patient that drug initiation may cause transient bradycardia. Inform patient with certain cardiac conditions that a cardiology consult is necessary with monitoring after first dose of drug and after dose interruption or drug discontinuation.

• Instruct patient to report signs and symptoms of bradycardia (dizziness, lightheadedness, palpitations, shortness of breath, confusion, chest pain, tiredness).

• Tell patient to report new-onset or worsening breathing difficulties.

• Instruct patient to report unexplained nausea, vomiting, abdominal pain, fatigue, anorexia, jaundice, or dark urine.

• Inform patient that drug may increase risk of skin cancer. Tell patient to limit exposure to sunlight and UV light by wearing protective clothing and using sunscreen with high protection factor, and to report suspicious skin lesions.

• Advise patient of childbearing potential to use effective contraception during therapy and for 1 week after final dose.

• Tell patient to report blurriness, shadows or blind spot in the center of vision, light sensitivity, or unusually colored vision.

• Instruct patient to immediately report signs and symptoms of PRES. Emphasize that delayed treatment could lead to permanent neurologic sequelae.

• Advise patient to report worsening MS symptoms after stopping drug.

---

posaconazole ⚚
poe-sa-KON-a-zole

Noxafil, Posanol ♣

Therapeutic class: Antifungals
Pharmacologic class: Triazole antifungals

AVAILABLE FORMS
Injection: 300 mg (18 mg/mL) single-dose vial
Oral suspension: 40 mg/mL
Powder for oral suspension (delayed-release): 300 mg
Tablets (delayed-release) ⓓⓝⓒ: 100 mg

INDICATIONS & DOSAGES
➤ **Prevention of invasive *Aspergillus* and *Candida* infections in patients who are immunocompromised and at high risk until recovered from neutropenia or immunosuppression**
Adults: 200 mg (5 mL) oral suspension PO t.i.d. Or, 300 mg IV or delayed-release tablet PO b.i.d. on first day, then 300 mg once daily.
Children ages 2 to younger than 18 weighing more than 40 kg: 6 mg/kg to maximum of 300 mg IV infusion b.i.d. on first day, then 6 mg/kg to maximum of 300 mg once daily. Or, 300 mg delayed-release tablet PO b.i.d. on first day, then 300 mg once daily.
Children ages 2 to younger than 18 weighing 40 kg or less: 6 mg/kg up to maximum of 300 mg IV infusion b.i.d. on first day, then 6 mg/kg to maximum of 300 mg once daily.
➤ **Oropharyngeal candidiasis**
Adults and children ages 13 and older: 100 mg (2.5 mL) PO oral suspension b.i.d. on first day, then 100 mg (2.5 mL) once daily for 13 days.
➤ **Oropharyngeal candidiasis resistant to itraconazole or fluconazole treatment**
Adults and children ages 13 and older: 400 mg (10 mL) PO oral suspension b.i.d.; duration of treatment is based on severity of underlying disease and patient response.
➤ **Treatment of invasive aspergillosis**
Adults and children ages 13 and older: 300 mg delayed-release tablet PO or IV b.i.d. on first day, then 300 mg PO or IV once daily for 6 to 12 weeks. May switch between IV and delayed-release tablets; no loading dose is required when switching between formulations.

ADMINISTRATION
PO
• Delayed-release tablets and oral suspension shouldn't be used interchangeably because of differences in dosing of each formulation.
PO (suspension)
• Give with a full meal, liquid nutritional supplement, or an acidic carbonated beverage (ginger ale).
• Shake well before giving it.
• Measure doses using calibrated spoon provided with the drug, which has two markings, one for 2.5 mL and one for 5 mL. After patient takes dose, fill spoon with water and have patient drink it to ensure a full dose.
• Store at room temperature.
PO (delayed-release tablets)
• Administer with or without food.

P

• Patient should swallow tablets whole; don't divide or crush tablets.
• Delayed-release oral formulation is preferred for prophylaxis due to higher plasma drug exposures.

IV

▼ Bring refrigerated vial to room temperature.
▼ To prepare, transfer one vial of drug to IV bag or bottle of half-NSS, NSS, D_5W, D_5W half-NSS, D_5W NSS, or D_5W with 20 mEq potassium chloride to achieve a final concentration that's between 1 and 2 mg/mL. Solution may be colorless to yellow.
▼ Use mixture immediately after preparation, or it can be stored up to 24 hours refrigerated (36° to 46° F [2° to 8° C]).
❸ *Alert:* When multiple dosing is required, administer via central venous catheter (CVC). Infuse over 90 minutes. Don't give by IV push or bolus.
▼ If a CVC isn't available, administer only once through peripheral venous catheter over 30 minutes in advance of CVC insertion or to bridge during CVC replacement or use for another IV treatment; multiple peripheral infusions given through the same vein may result in infusion-site reactions.
▼ An in-line filter (0.22-micron polyethersulfone or polyvinylidene difluoride) must be used during infusion.
▼ **Incompatibilities:** Diluents, including lactated Ringer solution, 5% dextrose with lactated Ringer solution, 4.2% sodium bicarbonate. Consult a drug incompatibility reference for more information.

ACTION

Blocks the synthesis of ergosterol, a vital component of the fungal cell membrane.

Route	Onset	Peak	Duration
PO (suspension)	Unknown	3–5 hr	Unknown
PO (tablets)	Unknown	4–5 hr	Unknown
IV	Unknown	Unknown	Unknown

Half-life: Suspension, 20 to 66 hours; tablets, 26 to 31 hours; injection, 27 hours.

ADVERSE REACTIONS

CNS: dizziness, fatigue, fever, headache, insomnia, weakness, paresthesia. **CV:** edema, HTN, hypotension, tachycardia, thrombophlebitis at IV site, *PE.* **EENT:** blurred vision, epistaxis, pharyngitis. **GI:** abdominal pain, anorexia, constipation, stomatitis, oral candidiasis, diarrhea, dyspepsia, mucositis, nausea, vomiting, *pancreatitis.* **GU:** *vaginal hemorrhage, AKI.* **Hematologic:** anemia, *neutropenia, thrombocytopenia, hemolytic-uremic syndrome.* **Hepatic:** bilirubinemia, *liver insufficiency,* increased liver enzyme levels, jaundice, *hepatitis.* **Metabolic:** hyperglycemia, *hypokalemia, hypomagnesemia, hypocalcemia, adrenocortical insufficiency,* weight loss, dehydration. **Musculoskeletal:** arthralgia, back pain, musculoskeletal pain. **Respiratory:** cough, dyspnea, URI, pneumonia. **Skin:** petechiae, pruritus, rash, diaphoresis. **Other:** bacteremia, CMV infection, herpes simplex, rigors, chills, hypersensitivity reaction.

INTERACTIONS

Drug-drug. *Atazanavir, ritonavir:* May increase level of these drugs. Frequently monitor for adverse effects and toxicity during coadministration.
Calcium channel blockers, phenytoin: May increase levels of these drugs. Reduce dosages, increase monitoring of levels, and observe patient for adverse effects.
Cimetidine, phenytoin: May decrease level and effectiveness of posaconazole. Avoid using together.
Cyclosporine: May increase cyclosporine level. Reduce cyclosporine dosage to about three-fourths original dose at start of posaconazole therapy and monitor cyclosporine level. Adjust cyclosporine dosage at end of posaconazole therapy.
CYP3A4 substrates (astemizole, cisapride, halofantrine, pimozide, quinidine, terfenadine): May lead to QT-interval prolongation and torsades de pointes. Use together is contraindicated.
Digoxin: May increase digoxin level. Monitor digoxin level.
Efavirenz: May significantly decrease posaconazole level. Avoid use together unless benefit outweighs risks.
Ergot alkaloids (dihydroergotamine, ergotamine): May increase ergot level. Use together is contraindicated.
Fosamprenavir: May decrease posaconazole level. Monitor patient closely for breakthrough fungal infection.
Glipizide: May enhance hypoglycemic effect. Monitor glucose level.
HMG-CoA reductase inhibitors metabolized through CYP3A4 (simvastatin): May increase

Reactions in bold italics are *life-threatening*.

levels of these drugs. Use together is contraindicated.

Metoclopramide: May decrease posaconazole level when used with posaconazole suspension. Monitor patient for breakthrough fungal infections.

Midazolam: May significantly increase midazolam level and potentiate or prolong sedative or hypnotic effects. Reversal agents should be readily available.

PPIs: May decrease posaconazole level. Consider therapy modification.

QTc interval-prolonging drugs: May enhance prolongation of QTc interval. When used with moderate QTc interval-prolonging drugs, monitor therapy. Avoid use with high-risk QTc interval-prolonging drugs; unavoidable, monitor QTc interval and cardiac rhythm closely.

Rifabutin: May decrease level and effectiveness of posaconazole while increasing rifabutin level and risk of toxicity. Avoid using together. If unavoidable, monitor patient for uveitis, leukopenia, and other adverse effects.

Sirolimus: May increase sirolimus level, resulting in sirolimus toxicity. Use together is contraindicated.

Tacrolimus: May increase tacrolimus level. Reduce tacrolimus dosage to about one-third original dose when starting posaconazole and monitor tacrolimus trough level. Adjust tacrolimus dosage accordingly at end of posaconazole therapy.

Venetoclax: May increase venetoclax level and risk of toxicity. Coadministration during initiation and ramp-up phase is contraindicated in patients with chronic lymphocytic leukemia or small lymphocytic lymphoma due to risk of TLS.

Vinca alkaloids (vincristine, vinblastine): May increase levels of vinca alkaloids, leading to neurotoxicity and other serious adverse reactions. Don't use together unless there are no alternative antifungal treatment options.

Drug-food. *Any food, liquid nutritional supplements:* May greatly enhance absorption of drug. Always give drug with liquid supplement or food.

Drug-lifestyle. *Alcohol:* May interfere with delayed-release of powder for oral suspension. Discourage use together.

EFFECTS ON LAB TEST RESULTS
• May increase AST, ALT, bilirubin, creatinine, ALP, and glucose levels.

• May decrease potassium, magnesium, and calcium levels.

• May decrease WBC, RBC, and platelet counts.

CONTRAINDICATIONS & CAUTIONS
• Contraindicated in patients hypersensitive to drug or its components, or other azole antifungals.

⚠ Powder for delayed-release oral suspension is contraindicated in patients with known or suspected hereditary fructose intolerance (HFI).

• Use cautiously in patients with potentially proarrhythmic conditions or liver or kidney insufficiency.

• May cause electrolyte disturbances.

🕐 *Alert:* Drug may prolong QT interval and increase risk of torsades de pointes.

Dialyzable drug: No.

PREGNANCY-LACTATION-REPRODUCTION
• There are no adequate studies during pregnancy. Drug may cause fetal harm. Avoid use during pregnancy. Use only if potential benefit outweighs fetal risk.

• It isn't known if drug appears in human milk. Patient should discontinue breastfeeding or discontinue drug, considering importance of drug to patient.

NURSING CONSIDERATIONS
• Use IV route only when oral administration isn't possible.

• Avoid IV route in patients with eGFR less than 50 mL/minute, unless benefit vs. risk to patient justifies its use. Closely monitor serum creatinine level; if increases occur, consider changing to oral therapy.

⚠ Assess for history of HFI (nausea, vomiting, abdominal pain with ingestion of sorbitol, fructose, or sucrose). Monitor children receiving oral suspension closely; HFI may have not yet been diagnosed.

• Correct electrolyte imbalances, especially potassium, magnesium, and calcium imbalances, before therapy.

• Monitor patient for signs and symptoms of electrolyte imbalance (slow, weak, or irregular pulse; ECG change; nausea; neuromuscular irritability; tetany).

• Obtain baseline LFTs, including bilirubin level, before therapy and periodically during treatment. Notify prescriber if patient develops signs or symptoms of liver dysfunction.

P

• Monitor patient weighing more than 120 kg closely for breakthrough fungal infections because of lower plasma drug exposure.

• Monitor patient with severe vomiting or diarrhea for breakthrough fungal infection.

• *Look alike–sound alike:* Don't confuse posaconazole with fluconazole, ketoconazole, itraconazole, or voriconazole. Don't confuse Noxafil with minoxidil.

PATIENT TEACHING

• Instruct patient in safe drug administration. Tell patient or caregiver to measure doses of suspension using dosing spoon or syringe provided with drug. Household spoons vary in size and may yield an incorrect dose.

• Instruct patient who can't take a liquid supplement or eat a full meal with immediate-release suspension to notify prescriber. A different anti-infective may be needed, or monitoring may need to be increased.

• Tell patient to report irregular heartbeat, fainting, or severe diarrhea or vomiting.

• Explain the signs and symptoms of liver dysfunction (abdominal pain, yellowing skin or eyes, pale stools, dark urine).

• Urge patient to contact prescriber or pharmacist before taking other prescription or OTC drugs, herbal supplements, or dietary supplements.

• Tell patient of childbearing potential that drug may cause fetal harm.

⚕ Inform patient and caregivers that Noxafil PowderMix for delayed-release oral suspension contains sorbitol and can be life-threatening in patients with HFI.

potassium acetate

Therapeutic class: Potassium supplements
Pharmacologic class: Potassium salts

AVAILABLE FORMS

Injection: 2 mEq/mL in 20-mL, 50-mL, and 100-mL vials

INDICATIONS & DOSAGES

➤ **To correct or prevent hypokalemia**
Adults: Individualize dosage and give by IV infusion; normal daily requirements are 40 to 80 mEq/24 hours.
Children: Individualize dosage and give by IV infusion; normal daily requirements are

2 to 3 mEq/kg/24 hours. For newborns, normal daily requirement is 2 to 6 mEq/kg/24 hours.

ADMINISTRATION

IV

▼ Use only when oral replacement isn't feasible.

▼ Don't give undiluted potassium. Maximum infusion rate is 1 mEq/kg/hour.

▼ Don't add potassium to a hanging bag. Mix well to avoid layering.

▼ To prevent pain, use largest peripheral vein and a well-placed small-bore needle.

▼ Give only by infusion, never IV push or IM. Watch for pain and redness at infusion site.

▼ Give slowly as diluted solution; rapid infusion may cause fatal hyperkalemia.

▼ May give by intraosseous infusion if necessary.

▼ **Incompatibilities:** None listed by manufacturer. Consult a drug incompatibility reference for more information.

ACTION

Replaces potassium and maintains potassium level.

Route	Onset	Peak	Duration
IV	Immediate	Immediate	Unknown

Half-life: Unknown.

ADVERSE REACTIONS

CNS: paresthesia of limbs, listlessness, confusion, weakness or heaviness of legs, flaccid paralysis. **CV:** *arrhythmias, cardiac arrest, heart block,* abnormal ECG, hypotension. **Metabolic:** *hyperkalemia.* **Skin:** redness at infusion site.

INTERACTIONS

Drug-drug. *ACE inhibitors, aldosterone blockers, ARBs, potassium-sparing diuretics:* May increase hyperkalemia risk. Use together with caution.
Eplerenone: May increase hyperkalemia risk. Use together is contraindicated when eplerenone is used to treat HTN.
Heparin: May enhance hyperkalemic effects of potassium salts. Monitor therapy.
Drug-food. *Potassium-containing salt substitutes:* May increase risk of hyperkalemia. Use together cautiously.

Reactions in bold italics are *life-threatening*.

EFFECTS ON LAB TEST RESULTS
• May increase potassium and bicarbonate levels.

CONTRAINDICATIONS & CAUTIONS
• Contraindicated in patients with CrCl less than 30 mL/minute with oliguria, anuria, or azotemia.
• Contraindicated in patients with adrenal insufficiency and in those with diseases that cause high potassium levels.
• Use cautiously in patients with cardiac disease, Child-Pugh class C liver insufficiency, or kidney impairment.
⚠ Alert: Product contains aluminum and may reach toxic levels with prolonged parenteral administration in patients with kidney impairment. Premature neonates are particularly at risk.
Dialyzable drug: Yes
⚠ Overdose S&S: Paresthesia, flaccid paralysis, listlessness, confusion, weakness and heaviness of legs, hypotension, cardiac arrhythmias, heart block, ECG changes, cardiac arrest.

PREGNANCY-LACTATION-REPRODUCTION
• There are no adequate studies during pregnancy. Use only if benefit justifies fetal risk.
• It isn't known if drug appears in human milk. Use cautiously during breastfeeding.

NURSING CONSIDERATIONS
• During therapy, monitor ECG, fluid intake and output, and potassium, creatinine, and BUN levels. Never give potassium postoperatively until urine flow is established.
• Monitor patient for adverse reactions due to hyperkalemia, including muscle weakness or paralysis, and cardiac conduction abnormalities (heart block, ventricular arrhythmias, asystole).
• Monitor IV site carefully for extravasation.
⚠ Alert: Consider a separate storage area for concentrated IV potassium. Fatal outcomes are possible if concentrated potassium is administered by IV push.
• Carefully give solutions containing acetate ions to patients with metabolic or respiratory alkalosis and to those with conditions such as liver, in which acetate levels may be increased or utilization of the ion may be impaired.
• **Look alike–sound alike:** Potassium preparations aren't interchangeable; verify preparation before use.

PATIENT TEACHING
• Explain use and administration to patient and family.

• Tell patient to report adverse effects, especially pain at insertion site.
• Advise patient to immediately report signs and symptoms of hyperkalemia (arrhythmia, bradycardia, weakness).

SAFETY ALERT!

potassium chloride
Klor-Con, Klor-Con 10, Klor-Con M10, Klor-Con M15, Klor-Con M20, Klor-Con Sprinkle, K-Tab

Therapeutic class: Potassium supplements
Pharmacologic class: Potassium salts

AVAILABLE FORMS
Capsules (extended-release) 🚫: 8 mEq, 10 mEq
Injection concentrate: 2 mEq/mL
Injection for IV infusion: 10 mEq, 20 mEq, 30 mEq, 40 mEq in various solutions and volumes
Oral liquid: 20 mEq/15 mL, 40 mEq/15 mL
Powder for oral administration: 20 mEq/packet
Tablets (extended-release) 🚫: 8 mEq, 10 mEq, 15 mEq, 20 mEq

INDICATIONS & DOSAGES
➤ **To prevent hypokalemia**
Adults: Initially, 20 mEq of potassium supplement PO daily. Adjust dosage, as needed, based on potassium levels. Patient should take no more than 20 mEq at a single dose; divide dose if patient requires more than 20 mEq/day.
Children birth to age 16 years: 1 mEq/kg/day oral liquid. Adjust dosage, as needed, based on potassium levels. Don't exceed 3 mEq/kg/day.
➤ **Hypokalemia**
Adults: 40 to 100 mEq PO in two to five divided doses daily. Patient should take no more than 20 mEq at a single dose. Maximum dose of diluted IV potassium chloride is 40 mEq/L at 10 mEq/hour. Don't exceed 200 mEq daily. Further doses are based on potassium levels and blood pH. Give IV potassium replacement only with monitoring of ECG and potassium level.
Children birth to age 16 years: 2 to 4 mEq/kg/day oral liquid in divided doses. Don't exceed 1 mEq/kg or 40 mEq as a single dose. Don't exceed 100 mEq/day.

➤ **Severe hypokalemia**
Adults: For serum potassium greater than 2.5 mEq/L, give up to 40 mEq/L IV. Don't exceed 10 mEq/L.

For serum potassium level less than 2 mEq/L or threat of severe hypokalemia, cautiously give IV at a rate not to exceed 40 mEq/hour. Continuously monitor ECG during infusion, and frequently monitor serum potassium levels. Don't exceed 400 mEq IV daily.

ADMINISTRATION

PO
- Give with meals and a full glass of water or other liquid to minimize GI irritation.
- Enteric-coated tablets are not recommended because of increased risk of GI bleeding and small-bowel ulcerations.
- Tablets in wax matrix may lodge in the esophagus and cause ulceration in patients with esophageal compression from an enlarged left atrium. Use sugar-free liquid form in these patients and in those with esophageal stasis or obstruction. Have patient sip slowly to minimize GI irritation.
- Don't crush extended-release forms.
- For patients with difficulty swallowing whole tablets, may break some extended-release tablets (Klor-Con M) in half. Or, place a whole tablet in 120 mL water and allow to disintegrate over 2 minutes, then stir for 30 seconds to create a suspension and have patient drink it immediately. Add 30 mL water to glass, swirl, and have patient drink immediately; repeat to ensure entire dose is consumed.
- For extended-release capsules, may open capsules, sprinkle contents on a spoonful of applesauce or pudding, and. have patient swallow immediately without chewing; follow with a full glass of water or juice. Don't add to hot foods or save mixture for later.
- Completely dissolve powder for oral solution in at least 120 mL cold water or other beverage Increase dilution if GI irritation occurs.

IV
▼ Use only when oral replacement isn't feasible or when hypokalemia is life-threatening.
▼ Give by infusion only, never IV push or IM. Give slowly as dilute solution; rapid infusion may cause fatal hyperkalemia.
▼ Administer high concentrations (200 to 400 mEq/L) exclusively via a central route and infusion pump at maximum rate of 40 mEq/hour.

▼ If burning occurs during infusion, decrease rate.
▼ Drug is a vesicant/irritant (at concentrations greater than 0.1 mEq/mL); ensure proper needle or catheter placement before and during infusion. Avoid extravasation.
▼ **Incompatibilities:** None listed by manufacturer. Consult a drug incompatibility reference for more information.

ACTION
Replaces potassium and maintains potassium level.

Route	Onset	Peak	Duration
PO	Unknown	Unknown	Unknown
IV	Immediate	Immediate	Unknown

Half-life: Unknown.

ADVERSE REACTIONS
CNS: paresthesia of limbs, listlessness, confusion, weakness or heaviness of limbs, flaccid paralysis. **CV:** *arrhythmias, HF, heart block, cardiac arrest,* ECG changes, hypotension, phlebitis or venous thrombosis at injection site. **GI:** nausea, vomiting, abdominal pain, diarrhea, flatulence. **Metabolic:** hypovolemia, hyponatremia, *hyperkalemia, metabolic acidosis.* **Respiratory:** dyspnea. **Skin:** injection-site reactions, extravasation. **Other:** infusion reaction (febrile response).

INTERACTIONS
Drug-drug. *ACE inhibitors, ARBs, digoxin, heparins, potassium-sparing diuretics:* May cause hyperkalemia. Use together with extreme caution. Monitor potassium level.
Eplerenone: May increase hyperkalemia risk. Use together is contraindicated when eplerenone is used to treat HTN.
NSAIDs: May cause potassium retention. Closely monitor potassium level in patients taking NSAIDs.

EFFECTS ON LAB TEST RESULTS
- May increase potassium and chloride levels.
- May decrease sodium level.

CONTRAINDICATIONS & CAUTIONS
- Contraindicated in patients hypersensitive to potassium chloride or components of the formulation, in patients with KF, and in those with conditions in which potassium retention is present.

Reactions in bold italics are *life-threatening*.

• Use cautiously in patients with cardiac disease, HF, kidney impairment, and acid-base disorders.

Dialyzable drug: Yes.

⚠️ *Overdose S&S:* ECG changes, weakness, flaccidity, respiratory paralysis, cardiac arrhythmias, death.

PREGNANCY-LACTATION-REPRODUCTION

• It isn't known if drug causes fetal harm. Use only if clearly needed.

• It isn't known if drug appears in human milk. Use cautiously during breastfeeding.

NURSING CONSIDERATIONS

• Patients at increased risk for GI lesions when taking oral potassium include those with scleroderma, diabetes, mitral valve replacement, cardiomegaly, or esophageal strictures, and older adults or patients who are immobile.

• Drug is commonly used orally with potassium-wasting diuretics to maintain potassium levels.

• Monitor continuous ECG and electrolyte levels during therapy.

• Monitor kidney function. After surgery, don't give drug until urine flow is established.

• Monitor patient for hyperkalemia (palpitations, shortness of breath, chest pain, nausea, vomiting).

• Patient may be sensitive to tartrazine in some of these products.

❂ *Alert:* Consider a separate storage area for concentrated IV potassium. Fatal outcomes are possible if concentrated potassium is administered by IV push.

• *Look alike–sound alike:* Potassium preparations aren't interchangeable; verify preparation before use and don't switch products. Don't confuse KCl with HCl.

PATIENT TEACHING

• Teach patient safe drug administration.

• Inform patient of signs and symptoms of hyperkalemia, and tell patient to notify prescriber if they occur.

• Tell patient to report discomfort at IV insertion site.

• Warn patient not to use potassium-containing salt substitutes concurrently, except with prescriber's permission.

• Tell patient not to be concerned if wax matrix appears in stool because the drug has already been absorbed.

pramipexole dihydrochloride
pram-ah-PEX-ole

Mirapex ER

Therapeutic class: Antiparkinsonian drugs
Pharmacologic class: Nonergot dopamine agonists

AVAILABLE FORMS

Tablets: 0.125 mg, 0.25 mg, 0.5 mg, 0.75 mg, 1 mg, 1.5 mg

Tablets (extended-release) 🞰: 0.375 mg, 0.75 mg, 1.5 mg, 2.25 mg, 3 mg, 3.75 mg, 4.5 mg

INDICATIONS & DOSAGES

➤ **Parkinson disease**

Adults: Initially, 0.125 mg immediate-release tablets PO t.i.d. Adjust doses slowly (not more often than every 5 to 7 days) over several weeks until desired therapeutic effect is achieved. Maintenance dosage is 1.5 to 4.5 mg daily in three divided doses. Or, 0.375 mg (extended-release form) PO once daily. May titrate dosage gradually (not more often than every 5 days), first to 0.75 mg PO daily, then by 0.75-mg increments to maximum recommended dosage of 4.5 mg/day.

Adjust-a-dose: For patients with CrCl over 50 mL/minute, first dosage of immediate-release tablets is 0.125 mg PO t.i.d., titrated up to 1.5 mg t.i.d. For those with CrCl of 30 to 50 mL/minute, first dosage is 0.125 mg PO b.i.d., titrated up to 0.75 mg t.i.d. For those with CrCl of 15 mL/minute to less than 30 mL/minute, first dosage is 0.125 mg PO daily, titrated up to 1.5 mg daily. If using extended-release tablets, in patients with CrCl of 30 to 50 mL/minute, initially give dose every other day. Use caution and assess response and tolerability before increasing to daily dosing after 1 week and before titration. Titrate dosage in 0.375-mg increments up to 2.25 mg/day, no more frequently than at weekly intervals. Don't use extended-release tablets in patients with CrCl of less than 30 mL/minute or in patients on hemodialysis. To discontinue treatment, taper at a rate of 0.75 mg/day until a daily dose of 0.75 mg has been reached, then reduce by 0.375 mg/day.

➤ **Moderate to severe primary restless legs syndrome (immediate-release only)**

Adults: 0.125 mg PO daily. May increase after 4 to 7 days to 0.25 mg PO daily, as needed.

May increase again after 4 to 7 days to 0.5 mg PO daily, if needed.

Adjust-a-dose: For patients with CrCl of 20 to 60 mL/minute, increase the duration between titration steps to 14 days.

ADMINISTRATION
PO
- Give drug with or without food; giving with food may reduce nausea.
- Have patient swallow extended-release tablets whole; don't crush or break tablets.
- If a significant interruption in therapy occurs, retitration may be warranted.
- For restless legs syndrome, give 2 to 3 hours before bedtime.
- Give a missed dose as soon as possible, but no later than 12 hours after regularly scheduled time. After 12 hours, skip missed dose and give next dose on the following day at regularly scheduled time.

ACTION
Exact action is unknown; thought to stimulate dopamine receptors.

Route	Onset	Peak	Duration
PO	Rapid	2 hr	Unknown
PO (extended-release)	Unknown	6 hr	Unknown

Half-life: About 8 to 12 hours.

ADVERSE REACTIONS
CNS: amnesia, asthenia, confusion, dizziness, abnormal dreams, new or worsening dyskinesia, extrapyramidal syndrome, hallucinations, headache, insomnia, somnolence, akathisia, drowsiness, delusions, dystonia, abnormal gait, hypoesthesia, hypertonia, tremor, myoclonus, paranoid reaction, malaise, sleep disorders, thinking abnormalities, depression, vertigo, fever, equilibrium disturbance, impulse control disorders, fatigue. **CV:** orthostatic hypotension, chest pain, edema. **EENT:** accommodation abnormalities, diplopia, abnormal vision, rhinitis, nasal congestion, increased salivation, dry mouth. **GI:** constipation, diarrhea, nausea, anorexia, increased appetite, dysphagia, vomiting, abdominal pain or discomfort, dyspepsia. **GU:** erectile dysfunction, decreased libido, urinary frequency, UTI, urinary incontinence. **Metabolic:** weight loss. **Musculoskeletal:** arthritis, bursitis, myasthenia, twitching, extremity pain, muscle spasm. **Respiratory:** dyspnea, cough, pneumonia. **Skin:** skin disorders. **Other:** accidental injury, flulike symptoms.

INTERACTIONS
Drug-drug. *Antipsychotics (typical [fluphenazine, haloperidol, thioridazine]):* May diminish therapeutic effects of pramipexole. Avoid use together if possible; if unavoidable, monitor therapy carefully. *Cimetidine, diltiazem, quinidine, quinine, triamterene, verapamil:* May increase pramipexole level. Adjust dosage as needed. *Dopamine antagonists (metoclopramide, prochlorperazine, promethazine):* May reduce pramipexole effectiveness. Monitor patient closely.
Drug-lifestyle. *Alcohol use:* May increase sedative effects. Avoid use together.

EFFECTS ON LAB TEST RESULTS
- May increase CK level.

CONTRAINDICATIONS & CAUTIONS
- Contraindicated in patients hypersensitive to drug or its components.
- Use cautiously in patients with kidney impairment or hypotension and in older adults.
- Use cautiously in patients with a known major psychotic disorder due to risk of exacerbating psychosis.
- Drug may cause or exacerbate dyskinesia.
- Drug may cause postural deformities, including antecollis (forward head and neck flexion), bent spine syndrome (forward trunk flexion), and Pisa syndrome (lateral trunk flexion). Dosage reduction or drug discontinuation may be necessary.
Dialyzable drug: Unknown.

PREGNANCY-LACTATION-REPRODUCTION
- There are no studies during pregnancy. Use only if benefit clearly justifies fetal risk.
- It isn't known if drug appears in human milk. Drug inhibits prolactin secretion and may inhibit lactation. Patient should discontinue breastfeeding or discontinue drug, considering importance of drug to patient.

NURSING CONSIDERATIONS
- Drug may cause orthostatic hypotension, especially during dosage increases. Monitor patient closely.
- Drug may cause impaired impulse control and compulsive behaviors. Monitor patient

---

Reactions in bold italics are *life-threatening*.

for problems with impulse control (gambling urges, intense sexual urges, binge eating).
• Adjust dosage gradually to achieve maximal therapeutic effect, balanced against the main adverse effects of dyskinesia, hallucinations, somnolence, and dry mouth.
• Assess patients for preexisting sleep disorder and monitor for daytime sleepiness and for episodes of falling asleep without warning. Drug may need to be discontinued.
• Monitor patients for hallucinations (visual, auditory, or mixed) and new or worsening psychotic-like behaviors (paranoia, delusions, agitation, disorientation, aggressive behavior, agitation, delirium). Drug may need to be discontinued.
• Monitor patients for rhabdomyolysis and postural deformity.
• *Look alike–sound alike:* Don't confuse Mirapex with Hiprex, Mifeprex, or MiraLax.

PATIENT TEACHING
• Teach patient safe drug administration.
• Instruct patient not to rise rapidly after sitting or lying down because of risk of dizziness.
• Tell patient about potential for daytime sleepiness and falling asleep without warning and to report episodes to prescriber. Caution patient to avoid hazardous activities until CNS response to drug is known.
• Advise patient to use caution before taking drug with other CNS depressants.
• Tell patient (especially older adults) to immediately report hallucinations and changes in impulse control behaviors.
• Instruct patient to take drug with food if nausea develops.
• Caution patient to report pregnancy or plans to become pregnant or to breastfeed.
• Inform patient that it may take 4 weeks for effects of drug to be noticed because of slow adjustment schedule.
• Instruct patient that drug should be tapered gradually and not stopped abruptly.
• Advise patient to report problems with muscle control (dyskinesias).
• Inform patient that residue resembling a swollen tablet or pieces of original tablet may appear in stool.
• Alert patient and caregivers that patient may have intense urges to spend money or to gamble, increased sexual urges, binge eating, or other intense urges that may be uncontrollable.

---

pramlintide acetate
PRAM-lin-tide

SymlinPen 60, SymlinPen 120

Therapeutic class: Antidiabetics
Pharmacologic class: Human amylin analogues

AVAILABLE FORMS
Injection: 1,000 mcg/mL in 1.5-mL and 2.7-mL multidose pen injectors

INDICATIONS & DOSAGES
➤ **Adjunct to insulin in patients with type 1 diabetes**
Adults: Initially, 15 mcg subcut before major meals. Reduce mealtime insulin doses, including premixed insulins, by 50%. Increase pramlintide dose by 15-mcg increments every 3 days if no nausea occurs, to a maintenance dose of 30 to 60 mcg. Adjust insulin dose as needed.
Adjust-a-dose: If significant nausea at 45 or 60 mcg persists, decrease to 30 mcg. If nausea persists at 30 mcg, consider stopping.
➤ **Adjunct to insulin in patients with type 2 diabetes**
Adults: Initially, 60 mcg subcut immediately before major meals. Reduce mealtime insulin doses, including premixed insulins, by 50%. Increase pramlintide dose to 120 mcg if no significant nausea occurs for at least 3 days. Adjust insulin dose as needed.
Adjust-a-dose: If significant nausea persists at 120 mcg, decrease to 60 mcg.

ADMINISTRATION
Subcutaneous
• Allow medication to reach room temperature before injecting.
• Give each dose subcut into abdomen or thigh. Rotate injection sites.
• Administer immediately before each major meal consisting of 250 kcal or more or containing 30 g or more of carbohydrates.
• Always administer pramlintide and insulin as separate injections. The injection site for pramlintide should be distinct from the site for concomitant insulin injection.
• Don't transfer drug to syringe for administration. Don't mix with insulin.
• **Alert:** Multidose pens are for single-patient use only. Pens should never be shared, even

if the needle is changed. Clearly label with patient identifying information where it won't obstruct the dosing window, warning, or other product information.

• For a missed dose, wait until the next scheduled dose time and give usual amount.

• Use 1.5-mL injector for 15-, 30-, 45-, or 60-mcg doses. Use 2.7-mL injector for 60- or 120-mcg doses.

• After initial use, may keep refrigerated or at room temperature (36° to 86° F [2° to 30° C]).

• Discard after 30 days; protect from light.

ACTION

Slows rate at which food leaves stomach, reducing initial postprandial increase in glucose level. Decreases hyperglycemia by reducing postprandial glucagon level; reduces total caloric intake by reducing appetite.

Route	Onset	Peak	Duration
Subcut	Unknown	19–21 min	3 hr

Half-life: Parent drug and metabolite, about 48 minutes each.

ADVERSE REACTIONS

CNS: dizziness, fatigue, headache. **EENT:** pharyngitis. **GI:** abdominal pain, anorexia, nausea, vomiting. **Metabolic:** *hypoglycemia.* **Musculoskeletal:** arthralgia. **Respiratory:** cough. **Skin:** injection-site reaction. **Other:** allergic reaction, accidental injury.

INTERACTIONS

Drug-drug. *ACE inhibitors, disopyramide, fibrates, fluoxetine, MAO inhibitors, oral antidiabetics, pentoxifylline, propoxyphene, salicylates, sulfonamides:* May increase risk of hypoglycemia. Monitor glucose level closely.

Alpha-glucosidase inhibitors (acarbose), anticholinergics (atropine, benztropine, TCAs): May alter GI motility and slow intestinal absorption. Avoid using together.

Beta blockers, clonidine, guanethidine, reserpine: May mask signs of hypoglycemia. Monitor glucose level closely.

Oral drugs dependent on rapid onset of action (such as analgesics, antibiotics, oral contraceptives): May delay absorption because of slowed gastric emptying. If rapid effect is needed, give oral drug 1 hour before or 2 hours after pramlintide.

EFFECTS ON LAB TEST RESULTS

None reported.

CONTRAINDICATIONS & CAUTIONS

• Contraindicated in patients hypersensitive to drug or its components, including metacresol, and in patients with gastroparesis or hypoglycemia unawareness.

• Don't use in patients nonadherent with current insulin and glucose monitoring regimen, patients with an HbA$_{1c}$ level greater than 9%, patients with recurrent severe hypoglycemia during the previous 6 months, and patients who take drugs that stimulate GI motility.

• Use cautiously in patients with visual or dexterity impairment.

• Pramlintide alone doesn't cause hypoglycemia. May increase risk of hypoglycemia when used with insulin or other antidiabetics, such as a sulfonylurea or metformin. Closely monitor patient and adjust insulin dosages, as needed to reduce risk.

• Safe use in children hasn't been established.

• Use cautiously in older adults.

Dialyzable drug: Unknown.

⚠ *Overdose S&S:* Severe nausea, vomiting, diarrhea, vasodilation, dizziness.

PREGNANCY-LACTATION-REPRODUCTION

• There are no adequate studies during pregnancy. Use only if potential benefit justifies fetal risk. Other agents are currently preferred to treat diabetes in patients who are pregnant.

• It isn't known if drug appears in human milk. Use during breastfeeding only if benefit clearly outweighs risk to infant.

NURSING CONSIDERATIONS

• Before starting drug, review patient's HbA$_{1c}$ level, recent blood glucose monitoring data, hypoglycemic episodes, current insulin regimen, and body weight.

Boxed Warning When used with insulin, the risk of severe hypoglycemia is highest within first 3 hours after pramlintide injection. Serious injuries may occur if severe hypoglycemia develops while patient is operating a motor vehicle or heavy machinery or engaging in other high-risk activities. ■

Boxed Warning Appropriate patient selection, careful patient instruction, and insulin dosage adjustments are critical to reducing hypoglycemia risk. ■

• Symptoms of hypoglycemia may be masked in patients with a long history of diabetes,

Reactions in bold italics are *life-threatening*.

diabetic nerve disease, or intensified diabetes control.

• Notify prescriber of severe nausea and vomiting. A reduced dose may be needed.

• If patient has persistent nausea or recurrent, unexplained hypoglycemia that requires medical assistance, stop drug.

• Monitor patient for local reaction at injection site (erythema, edema, pruritus). Minor reactions usually resolve in a few days to weeks.

• If patient doesn't adhere to glucose monitoring or drug dosage adjustments, drug will need to be stopped.

PATIENT TEACHING

• Instruct patient in safe drug administration and storage.

• Teach patient how to take drug exactly as prescribed, at mealtimes. Explain that it doesn't replace daily insulin but may lower the amount of insulin needed.

• Explain that a meal is considered more than 250 calories or 30 g of carbohydrates.

• Caution patient not to change doses of pramlintide or insulin without consulting prescriber.

🕒 **Alert:** Warn patient not to share multidose pen with other people, even if the needle is changed, because of risk of transmission of bloodborne pathogens, including HIV and hepatitis virus.

Boxed Warning Tell patient to refrain from driving, operating heavy machinery, or performing other risky activities that may cause harm to patient or others until drug's effects on glucose level are known. ■

Boxed Warning Caution patient about possibility of severe hypoglycemia, particularly within 3 hours after injection. ■

• Teach patient and family members the signs and symptoms of hypoglycemia (hunger, headache, diaphoresis, tremor, irritability, difficulty concentrating).

• Instruct patient and family members what to do if patient develops hypoglycemia.

• Tell patient to report severe nausea and vomiting to prescriber.

• Advise patient of childbearing potential to report known or suspected pregnancy or plans to become pregnant.

• Teach patient how to handle unplanned situations, such as illness or stress, low or forgotten insulin dose, accidental use of too much insulin or drug, not enough food, or missed meals.

prasugrel hydrochloride
PRA-soo-grel

Effient

Therapeutic class: Antiplatelet drugs
Pharmacologic class: Adenosine diphosphate-induced platelet aggregation inhibitors

AVAILABLE FORMS
Tablets: 5 mg, 10 mg

INDICATIONS & DOSAGES

➤ **To reduce thrombotic CV events in patients with ACS (unstable angina and non-ST-elevation MI) managed with PCI; to reduce thrombotic CV events in patients with ACS (ST-elevation MI) managed with primary or delayed PCI**

Adults: Initially, single 60-mg loading dose; then 10 mg PO once daily. Patient should also take aspirin 75 to 325 mg PO daily.

Adjust-a-dose: For adults weighing less than 60 kg, consider reducing dosage to 5 mg PO once daily.

ADMINISTRATION
PO

• May give drug with or without food.

• Don't break tablets. In an emergent primary PCI setting, crushing tablets (using a commercially available syringe crusher) and mixing with 25 mL water led to faster absorption and a quicker, more potent antiplatelet effect (as early as 30 minutes).

• Tablets may be chewed and swallowed (bitter to taste) or crushed and mixed in food or liquid (applesauce, juice, water) and given immediately by mouth or gastric tube.

• Administration via an enteral tube that bypasses the acidic environment of the stomach may result in reduced bioavailability of prasugrel.

ACTION

Inhibits platelet activation and aggregation through irreversible binding of its active metabolite to the P2Y$_{12}$ class of ADP receptors on platelets.

Route	Onset	Peak	Duration
PO	Rapid	30 min	5–9 days

Half-life: 7 hours (range, 2 to 15 hours).

🍁 Canada   ◇ OTC   ◆ Off-label use   ⊜ Do not crush   *Liquid contains alcohol   ⚥ Genetic

ADVERSE REACTIONS
CNS: dizziness, fatigue, headache, fever. **CV:** atrial fibrillation, ***bradycardia,*** HTN or hypotension, peripheral edema, ***hemorrhage.*** **EENT:** epistaxis. **GI:** ***GI bleeding,*** nausea, diarrhea. **Hematologic:** anemia, ***leukopenia.*** **Metabolic:** hyperlipidemia. **Musculoskeletal:** back pain, extremity pain, noncardiac chest pain. **Respiratory:** cough, dyspnea. **Skin:** rash.

INTERACTIONS
Drug-drug. *Direct factor Xa inhibitors (rivaroxaban), direct thrombin inhibitors (dabigatran, desirudin), fibrinolytics (tenecteplase), heparin, low-molecular-weight heparin, NSAIDs (long-term use), platelet inhibitors, warfarin:* May increase the risk of bleeding. Use together cautiously.
Opioids: Delay absorption of prasugrel due to slowed gastric emptying. Consider therapy modification.
Vitamin E (systemic): May enhance antiplatelet effect. Monitor therapy.
Drug-herb. *Fish oil, garlic, ginger, ginkgo, omega-3 fatty acids:* Inhibit platelet aggregation. Use cautiously together; monitor patient for bleeding.

EFFECTS ON LAB TEST RESULTS
- May increase lipid levels.
- May increase Hb level.
- May decrease WBC and platelet counts.

CONTRAINDICATIONS & CAUTIONS
Boxed Warning Contraindicated in patients with pathologic bleeding (such as peptic ulcer or intracranial hemorrhage) and in those with a history of TIA or stroke. ■
Boxed Warning Drug isn't recommended in patients age 75 and older because of the increased risk of intracranial and fatal bleeding and uncertain benefit, except in high-risk situations (patients with diabetes or a history of prior MI). In these situations, drug's effect appears to be greater; its use may be considered. ■
Boxed Warning Don't start drug in patients likely to undergo urgent CABG. ■
Boxed Warning Use cautiously in patients who weigh less than 60 kg and in those with a propensity to bleed or who are using drugs that increase bleeding risk (warfarin, heparin, fibrinolytic therapy, long-term NSAID use) because of increased risk of bleeding. ■

- Contraindicated in patients with hypersensitivity to prasugrel, its components, or other thienopyridines. Angioedema can occur.
- Use cautiously in patients at risk for increased bleeding from trauma, surgery, or other pathologic conditions and in those with Child-Pugh class C liver impairment.
Dialyzable drug: Unlikely.
⚠ ***Overdose S&S:*** Bleeding due to impaired clotting ability.

PREGNANCY-LACTATION-REPRODUCTION
- There are no adequate studies during pregnancy. Use during pregnancy and breastfeeding only if maternal benefit justifies fetal risk.

NURSING CONSIDERATIONS
Boxed Warning Drug may cause significant, sometimes fatal, bleeding. Suspect bleeding in patient who is hypotensive and has recently undergone PCI, CABG, or other surgical procedure. Manage bleeding without stopping drug, if possible. Stopping drug within first few weeks after ACS occurrence increases the risk of further CV events. ■
- Monitor patient for unusual bleeding or bruising and hypersensitivity reactions.
Boxed Warning If possible, discontinue drug 7 days before CABG or any surgery. ■
- Bleeding associated with CABG may be treated with transfusion of blood products, such as RBCs and platelets; however, platelets may be ineffective if given within 6 hours of loading dose or within 4 hours of maintenance dose.
⟳ *Alert:* Drug may cause fatal thrombotic thrombocytopenic purpura (thrombocytopenia, hemolytic anemia, neurologic signs and symptoms, kidney dysfunction, and fever) that requires urgent treatment, including plasmapheresis.
- ***Look alike–sound alike:*** Don't confuse prasugrel with pravastatin or propranolol.

PATIENT TEACHING
- Instruct patient in safe drug administration.
- Inform patient that bruising will occur more easily and that it may take longer than usual to stop bleeding.
- Teach patient to report prolonged or excessive bleeding, bruising, blood in the stool or urine, fever, fatigue, low urine output, or neurologic signs and symptoms.
- Advise patient to inform health care providers, including dentists, of prasugrel

use before scheduling surgery or taking new drugs.

• Inform patient that duration of therapy may be determined by the type of stent used and not to discontinue drug without first consulting prescriber.

pravastatin sodium (eptastatin) ▧
prah-va-STA-tin

Therapeutic class: Antilipemics
Pharmacologic class: HMG-CoA reductase inhibitors

AVAILABLE FORMS
Tablets: 10 mg, 20 mg, 40 mg, 80 mg

INDICATIONS & DOSAGES
Adjust-a-dose (for all indications): In patients with CrCl less than 30 mg/mL, start with 10 mg PO daily; maximum daily dose, 40 mg. In patients taking cyclosporine, begin with 10 mg PO and adjust to higher dosages with caution; maximum daily dose, 20 mg. In patients taking clarithromycin or erythromycin, limit dose to 40 mg once daily.

➤ **Primary and secondary prevention of coronary events; hyperlipidemia; primary dysbetalipoproteinemia; hypertriglyceridemia**
Adults: Initially, 40 mg PO once daily at the same time each day, with or without food. Adjust dosage every 4 weeks or more, based on patient tolerance and response; maximum daily dose, 80 mg. Dosage range, 10 to 80 mg daily.

➤ **Heterozygous familial hypercholesterolemia** ▧
Adolescents ages 14 to 18: 40 mg PO once daily. Maximum dose, 40 mg daily.
Children ages 8 to 13: 20 mg PO once daily. Maximum dose, 20 mg daily.

ADMINISTRATION
PO
• Give drug without regard for meals.
• If patient is also taking a bile acid resin (cholestyramine, colestipol, colesevelam), administer pravastatin 1 hour before or 4 hours after the resin.

ACTION
Inhibits HMG-CoA reductase, an early (and rate-limiting) step in cholesterol biosynthesis.

Route	Onset	Peak	Duration
PO	Unknown	60–90 min	Unknown

Half-life: 1.8 hours.

ADVERSE REACTIONS
CNS: dizziness, fatigue, headache, fever. **CV:** chest pain, angina, edema. **EENT:** sinus abnormality. **GI:** nausea constipation, diarrhea, vomiting. **Hepatic:** elevated liver enzyme levels. **Metabolic:** increased CK level. **Musculoskeletal:** pain, muscle cramp, myalgia, injury. **Respiratory:** URI, cough. **Skin:** rash. **Other:** flulike symptoms.

INTERACTIONS
Drug-drug. *Cholestyramine, colestipol:* May decrease pravastatin level. Give pravastatin 1 hour before or 4 hours after these drugs.
Clarithromycin, erythromycin: May increase pravastatin level. Limit pravastatin to 40 mg once daily.
Colchicine: May increase risk of myopathy or rhabdomyolysis. Consider therapy modification.
Cyclosporine: May increase pravastatin level and pravastatin-related adverse reactions. If concomitant use can't be avoided, limit pravastatin to 20 mg daily.
⊘ *Alert:* *Darunavir, lopinavir:* May increase pravastatin level and risk of myopathy and rhabdomyolysis. Use together cautiously.
Fibrates (fenofibrate): May increase risk of muscle pain and weakness. Avoid combination unless there are no other options.
Gemfibrozil: May increase risk of myopathy or rhabdomyolysis. Avoid use together.
Liver-toxic drugs: May increase risk of liver toxicity. Avoid using together.
Niacin: May increase risk of myopathy and rhabdomyolysis. Use cautiously together. Monitor patient closely, especially during titration.
Protease inhibitors (ritonavir, saquinavir): May reduce pravastatin level. Monitor clinical response.
Rifampin: May decrease pravastatin levels. Carefully monitor clinical response.
Warfarin: May increase anticoagulant effect of warfarin. Monitor therapy.
Drug-herb. *Kava kava:* May increase risk of liver toxicity. Discourage use together.
Red yeast rice: May increase risk of adverse reactions; herb contains compounds similar to those in drug. Discourage use together.

P

Drug-food. *Oat bran:* May decrease effectiveness of pravastatin. Separate administration times as much as possible.
Drug-lifestyle. *Alcohol use:* May increase risk of liver toxicity. Discourage use together.

EFFECTS ON LAB TEST RESULTS
• May increase ALT, AST, CK, ALP, HbA_{1c}, fasting glucose, and bilirubin levels.
• May alter thyroid function test values.

CONTRAINDICATIONS & CAUTIONS
• Contraindicated in patients hypersensitive to drug and in those with acute or decompensated cirrhosis or conditions that cause unexplained, persistent elevations of transaminase levels.
• Use cautiously in patients who consume large quantities of alcohol or have a history of liver disease or KF.
• Interrupt statin therapy if patient shows signs of serious liver injury, hyperbilirubinemia, or jaundice. Don't restart drug if another cause can't be found.
• Statins may rarely cause rhabdomyolysis with AKI and immune-mediated necrotizing myopathy.
• Statins may alter blunt adrenal or gonadal steroid hormone levels.
• Safety and effectiveness in children younger than age 8 haven't been established.
Dialyzable drug: Unknown.

PREGNANCY-LACTATION-REPRODUCTION
• May cause fetal harm. Use during pregnancy is contraindicated unless benefits to patient outweigh fetal risk. Discontinue drug before conception. If pregnancy occurs during therapy, apprise patient of fetal risks with continued use.
• The FDA has determined that statin use in patients at high risk for CV events during pregnancy may be considered on an individual basis.
• Drug appears in human milk. Contraindicated during breastfeeding.

NURSING CONSIDERATIONS
• Patient should follow a diet restricted in saturated fat and cholesterol during therapy.
▧ Use in children with heterozygous familial hypercholesterolemia if LDL cholesterol level is at least 190 mg/dL, or if LDL cholesterol is at least 160 mg/dL and patient has either a positive family history of premature CV disease or two or more other CV disease risk factors.
• Obtain LFT results at start of therapy and periodically. A liver biopsy may be performed if elevated liver enzyme levels persist.
• Monitor patient for fatigue and severe signs or symptoms affecting muscles. Evaluate patient for conditions that increase risk of muscle problems and obtain CK and creatinine levels and urinalysis for myoglobinuria. Drug may need to be withheld or discontinued.
• Withhold drug temporarily for acute or serious conditions predisposing patient to KF secondary to rhabdomyolysis, including sepsis, hypotension, major surgery, trauma, uncontrolled epilepsy, or severe metabolic, endocrine, or electrolyte disorder.
• *Look alike–sound alike:* Don't confuse pravastatin with nystatin, pitavastatin, or prasugrel.

PATIENT TEACHING
• Instruct patient in safe drug administration.
• Tell patient to report adverse reactions.
• Inform patient that LFTs will be performed before and periodically throughout treatment.
• Tell patient to promptly report signs and symptoms of liver injury, including fatigue, anorexia, right upper quadrant discomfort, dark urine, or jaundice.
• Teach patient to promptly report any unexplained muscle pain, tenderness, or weakness, especially if accompanied by malaise or fever or if symptoms persist after discontinuing drug.
• Inform patient that drug may increase blood sugar levels; CV benefits are thought to outweigh the slight increase in risk.
• Teach patient about proper dietary management of cholesterol and triglycerides. When appropriate, recommend weight control, exercise, and smoking cessation programs.
• Inform patient that it may take up to 4 weeks to achieve full therapeutic effect.
◑ *Alert:* Tell patient of childbearing potential to stop drug and immediately report known or suspected pregnancy or breastfeeding.

Reactions in bold italics are *life-threatening*.

prazosin hydrochloride
PRA-zoh-sin

Minipress

Therapeutic class: Antihypertensives
Pharmacologic class: Alpha blockers

AVAILABLE FORMS
Capsules: 1 mg, 2 mg, 5 mg

INDICATIONS & DOSAGES
➤ **HTN**
Adults: Initially, 1 mg PO b.i.d. or t.i.d. Increase dosages slowly to maintenance of 6 to 15 mg daily in divided doses. Maximum daily dose, 20 mg. Some patients need larger dosages (up to 40 mg daily in divided doses).
Adjust-a-dose: If other antihypertensives or diuretics are added to therapy, decrease prazosin dosage to 1 to 2 mg t.i.d. and retitrate to maintenance dosage.

ADMINISTRATION
PO
• Give drug without regard for meals.

ACTION
Unknown. Thought to act by blocking alpha-adrenergic receptors.

Route	Onset	Peak	Duration
PO	30–90 min	2–4 hr	10–24 hr

Half-life: 2 to 3 hours.

ADVERSE REACTIONS
CNS: dizziness, syncope, headache, drowsiness, nervousness, weakness, depression, vertigo, lack of energy. **CV:** orthostatic hypotension, palpitations, edema. **EENT:** blurred vision, reddened sclera, epistaxis, nasal congestion, dry mouth. **GI:** vomiting, diarrhea, nausea, constipation. **GU:** urinary frequency. **Respiratory:** dyspnea. **Skin:** rash.

INTERACTIONS
Drug-drug. *Antihypertensives, diuretics:* May increase hypotension. Reduce prazosin dosage to 1 or 2 mg t.i.d.; retitrate as needed. *PDE5 inhibitors (avanafil, sildenafil, tadalafil, vardenafil):* May increase frequency of hypotensive effect or syncope with loss of consciousness. Initiate PDE5 inhibitor at the lowest dose.

Drug-herb. *Ma huang:* May decrease antihypertensive effects. Discourage use together. *Yohimbe:* May reduce prazosin effect. Discourage use together.

EFFECTS ON LAB TEST RESULTS
• May increase LFT values.
• May cause positive ANA titer.
• May alter results of screening tests for pheochromocytoma by increasing urinary metabolite of norepinephrine and vanillylmandelic acid.

CONTRAINDICATIONS & CAUTIONS
• Contraindicated in patients hypersensitive to drug or its components, or quinazolines.
• Use cautiously in patients receiving other antihypertensives.
• Not approved for use in children.
• Intraoperative floppy iris syndrome has been observed during cataract surgery in some patients treated with alpha$_1$ blockers.
• May cause syncope with sudden loss of consciousness.
• Prolonged erections and priapism have been reported with alpha-1 blockers.
Dialyzable drug: No.
⚠ *Overdose S&S:* Profound drowsiness, depressed reflexes, hypotension.

PREGNANCY-LACTATION-REPRODUCTION
• There are no adequate studies during pregnancy. Use only if maternal benefits justify maternal and fetal risk.
• Drug appears in small amounts in human milk. Use cautiously during breastfeeding.

NURSING CONSIDERATIONS
• Monitor BP and pulse rate frequently.
• Older adults may be more sensitive to drug's hypotensive effects.
• Adherence might be improved with twice-daily dosing. Discuss dosing change with prescriber if adherence problems are suspected.
⚠ *Alert:* If first dose is more than 1 mg, first-dose syncope may occur.
• *Look alike–sound alike:* Don't confuse prazosin with prednisone.

PATIENT TEACHING
• Warn patient that dizziness may occur with first dose. If dizziness occurs, tell patient to sit or lie down. Reassure patient that this effect disappears with continued dosing. Dizziness may also occur with alcohol use,

prolonged standing, exercise, or during hot weather.

• Caution patient to avoid driving or performing hazardous tasks for the first 24 hours after starting drug or increasing dose.

• Tell patient not to suddenly stop taking drug, but to notify prescriber if unpleasant adverse reactions occur.

• Advise patient to minimize low BP and dizziness upon standing by rising slowly and avoiding sudden position changes.

• Priapism may occur. Advise patient to seek emergency treatment for erections lasting longer than 4 hours.

• Advise patient of childbearing potential to report pregnancy, plans to become pregnant, or breastfeeding.

prednisoLONE
pred-NISS-oh-lone

prednisoLONE sodium phosphate
Orapred ODT, Pediapred

Therapeutic class: Corticosteroids
Pharmacologic class: Glucocorticoids-mineralocorticoids

AVAILABLE FORMS
prednisolone
Syrup: 15 mg/5 mL
Tablets: 5 mg
prednisolone sodium phosphate
Oral solution: 5 mg/5 mL, 10 mg/5 mL, 15 mg/5 mL, 20 mg/5 mL, 25 mg/5 mL
Tablets (ODTs) ⓞ: 10 mg, 15 mg, 30 mg

INDICATIONS & DOSAGES
➤ **Severe inflammation, disorders requiring immunosuppression**
Adults: 5 to 60 mg PO daily.
Children: 0.14 to 2 mg/kg/day PO in three or four divided doses (4 to 60 mg/m²/day).
Adjust-a-dose: Dosage requirements vary; individualize based on disease process and patient response.
➤ **Uncontrolled asthma in those taking inhaled corticosteroids and long-acting bronchodilators**
Children: 1 to 2 mg/kg/day prednisolone sodium phosphate in single or divided doses. Continue short course (or "burst" therapy)

until child achieves a peak expiratory flow rate of 80% of personal best, or until symptoms resolve. This usually requires 3 to 10 days of treatment but can take longer. Tapering the dose after improvement doesn't necessarily prevent relapse.
➤ **Acute exacerbations of MS**
Adults and children: 200 mg/day prednisolone sodium phosphate PO as single or divided dose for 7 days; then 80 mg every other day for 1 month.
➤ **Nephrotic syndrome**
Children: 60 mg/m² prednisolone sodium phosphate PO in three divided doses daily for 4 weeks, followed by 4 weeks of single-dose alternate-day therapy at 40 mg/m²/day.

ADMINISTRATION
PO
• Give drug with food or milk to reduce GI irritation. Patient may need another drug to prevent GI irritation.
• Don't cut or crush ODTs.
• Don't remove ODTs from blister pack until right before dosing.
• Patient may swallow ODT whole or allow to dissolve in mouth with or without water.

ACTION
Not clearly defined. Decreases inflammation, mainly by stabilizing leukocyte lysosomal membranes; suppresses immune response; stimulates bone marrow; and influences protein, fat, and carbohydrate metabolism.

Route	Onset	Peak	Duration
PO	Rapid	1–2 hr	18–36 hr

Half-life: 2 to 4 hours.

ADVERSE REACTIONS
CNS: euphoria, insomnia, *increased ICP, seizures,* psychotic behavior, vertigo, headache, paresthesia, mood swings, neuropathy, neuritis, paraparesis, paresthesia, personality change, sensory disturbance. **CV:** *arrhythmias, bradycardia, cardiac enlargement, circulatory collapse, fat embolism, HF, thromboembolism,* HTN, edema, *pulmonary edema,* syncope, tachycardia, thrombophlebitis, vasculitis. **EENT:** cataracts, glaucoma, exophthalmos, increased IOP. **GI:** peptic ulceration, ulcerative esophagitis, *pancreatitis,* abdominal distention, GI irritation, increased appetite, nausea, vomiting. **GU:** menstrual irregularities, altered motility and

number of sperm, increased urine calcium level. **Hepatic:** elevated liver enzyme levels, liver enlargement. **Metabolic:** *hypokalemia,* metabolic alkalosis, hyperglycemia, hypernatremia, carbohydrate intolerance, hypercholesterolemia, *hypocalcemia,* latent diabetes, weight gain, protein catabolism (negative nitrogen balance). **Musculoskeletal:** growth suppression in children, muscle weakness, osteoporosis, aseptic necrosis of femoral and humeral heads, loss of muscle mass, pathologic long bone fractures, myopathy, tendon rupture, vertebral compression fractures. **Skin:** diaphoresis, dry scalp, ecchymoses, petechiae, pigmentation changes, striae, thin fragile skin, facial erythema, hirsutism, delayed wound healing, acne, skin eruptions. **Other:** hypersensitivity reactions; after increased stress—*acute adrenal insufficiency,* susceptibility to infections, cushingoid state; withdrawal symptoms (rebound inflammation, fatigue, weakness, arthralgia, fever, dizziness, depression, fainting, orthostatic hypotension, dyspnea, nausea, anorexia, *hypoglycemia*).

INTERACTIONS

Drug-drug. *Anticholinesterase agents (donepezil, rivastigmine):* May cause severe weakness in patients with myasthenia gravis. If possible, withdraw anticholinesterase agent at least 24 hours before corticosteroid therapy.
Antidiabetics: May increase glucose level. Adjust antidiabetic dosage as necessary.
Aspirin, indomethacin, other NSAIDs: May increase risk of GI distress and bleeding. Use together cautiously.
Cyclosporine: May increase toxicity and risk of seizures. Monitor patient closely.
CYP3A4 inducers (barbiturates, carbamazepine, fosphenytoin, phenytoin, rifampin): May decrease corticosteroid effect. Increase corticosteroid dosage.
CYP3A4 inhibitors (azole antifungals, macrolide antibiotics): May decrease corticosteroid metabolism and increase risk of toxicity. Reduce steroid dosage as needed.
Drugs that deplete potassium (thiazide diuretics, amphotericin B): May increase risk of hypokalemia. Monitor potassium level.
Estrogens: May increase pharmacologic and toxic effects of prednisolone. Monitor patient closely.
Isoniazid: May decrease isoniazid level. Monitor therapy.

Oral anticoagulants (warfarin): May alter anticoagulant dosage requirements. Monitor PT and INR closely.
Salicylates: May decrease salicylate level and effectiveness. Monitor patient.
Skin-test antigens: May decrease response. Postpone skin testing until after therapy.
Toxoids, vaccines: May decrease antibody response and may increase risk of organism replication in some live attenuated vaccines. Avoid using together.

EFFECTS ON LAB TEST RESULTS

• May increase glucose, sodium, and cholesterol levels and LFT values.
• May decrease T_3, T_4, potassium, and calcium levels.
• May decrease ^{131}I uptake and protein-bound iodine levels in thyroid function tests.
• May alter skin test results.
• May cause false-negative results in nitroblue tetrazolium test for systemic bacterial infections.

CONTRAINDICATIONS & CAUTIONS

• Contraindicated in patients hypersensitive to drug or its ingredients, in those with systemic fungal infections or cerebral malaria, and in those receiving immunosuppressive doses together with live-virus vaccines.
• Use cautiously in patients with recent MI, GI ulcer, kidney disease, HTN, osteoporosis, diabetes, hypothyroidism, cirrhosis, active hepatitis, diverticulitis, nonspecific ulcerative colitis, recent intestinal anastomoses, thromboembolic disorders, seizures, myasthenia gravis, HF, TB, ocular herpes simplex, emotional instability, and psychotic tendencies.
• **Alert:** Prolonged use can increase incidence of secondary infection, activate latent infections, prolong viral infections, and mask infections.
• Drug can suppress HPA axis, which can lead to adrenal crisis. Always withdraw drug slowly and carefully.
• Drug may increase risk of Kaposi sarcoma. Discontinuing drug may result in clinical improvement.
Dialyzable drug: Unknown.
⚠ *Overdose S&S:* Abnormal fat deposits, accentuated menopausal symptoms, acne, adrenal insufficiency, decreased glucose tolerance, decreased resistance to infection, dry scaly skin, ecchymosis, excessive appetite, fluid retention, fractures, headache, hypertrichosis,

hypokalemia, increased BP, diaphoresis, menstrual disorder, mental symptoms, moon face, negative nitrogen balance with delayed bone and wound healing, neuropathy, osteoporosis, peptic ulcer, pigmentation, striae, tachycardia, thinning scalp hair, thrombophlebitis, weakness, weight gain; liver enlargement, abdominal distention (in children).

PREGNANCY-LACTATION-REPRODUCTION
• Drug can cause fetal harm. If drug is used during pregnancy, or if patient becomes pregnant during therapy, advise patient about fetal risk.
• Observe infants born to mothers who have received corticosteroids during pregnancy for signs and symptoms of hypoadrenalism.
• Drug appears in human milk and could suppress growth, interfere with endogenous corticosteroid production, or cause other untoward effects in the infant. Use cautiously during breastfeeding. Refer to manufacturer's instructions for each product.

NURSING CONSIDERATIONS
• Determine whether patient is hypersensitive to other corticosteroids.
• Always adjust to lowest effective dose.
• Most adverse reactions to corticosteroids are dose- or duration-dependent.
• Monitor patient's weight, BP, and electrolyte levels.
• Monitor patient for cushingoid effects, including moon face, buffalo hump, central obesity, thinning hair, HTN, and increased susceptibility to infection.
• Watch for depression or psychotic episodes, especially during high-dose therapy.
• Patients with certain GI conditions (abscess, other infections, diverticulitis, peptic ulcers, recent anastomosis) may be at risk for GI perforation. The drug may mask the signs.
• Patients with diabetes may need increased antidiabetic dosage; monitor glucose level.
• Give patient low-sodium diet that's high in potassium and protein. Give potassium supplements as needed.
• Monitor bone density in older adults and patients who are postmenopausal who may be more susceptible to osteoporosis with long-term use.
• Monitor patient for acute myopathy with high-dose therapy; monitor CK level.
• Gradually reduce dosage after long-term therapy to prevent withdrawal symptoms.

• **Look alike–sound alike:** Don't confuse prednisolone with prednisone.

PATIENT TEACHING
• Instruct patient in safe drug administration and to take drug exactly as prescribed.
• Tell patient not to stop drug abruptly or without prescriber's consent.
• Teach patient signs and symptoms of early adrenal insufficiency: fatigue, muscle weakness, joint pain, fever, anorexia, nausea, shortness of breath, dizziness, and fainting.
• Instruct patient to carry medical identification that includes prescriber's name and name and dosage of drug, and teach patient the need for supplemental systemic glucocorticoids during stress.
• Warn patient on long-term therapy about cushingoid effects and the need to notify prescriber about sudden weight gain or swelling.
• Tell patient to report slow healing.
• Advise patient receiving long-term therapy to consider exercise or physical therapy and to ask prescriber about vitamin D or calcium supplement.
• Instruct patient to avoid exposure to infections and to notify prescriber if exposure occurs.
• Tell patient to avoid immunizations while taking drug.
• Advise patient of childbearing potential to report pregnancy, plans to become pregnant, or breastfeeding.

predniSONE
PRED-ni-sone

Prednisone Intensol*, Rayos, Winpred ✦

Therapeutic class: Corticosteroids
Pharmacologic class: Adrenocorticoids

AVAILABLE FORMS
Oral solution: 5 mg/5 mL*, 5 mg/mL (concentrate)*
Tablets: 1 mg, 2.5 mg, 5 mg, 10 mg, 20 mg, 50 mg
Tablets (delayed-release) ⦿: 1 mg, 2 mg, 5 mg

INDICATIONS & DOSAGES
➤ **Severe inflammation, disorders requiring immunosuppression, endocrine deficiency disorders (immediate-release, delayed-release)**

Adults and children: Initially, 5 to 60 mg PO daily in single dose or two to four divided doses. Maintenance dosage is given daily or every other day (immediate-release only). Use lowest dose that will maintain adequate clinical response. Dosage must be individualized, and constant monitoring is needed.

➤ **Acute exacerbations of MS (immediate-release)**
Adults: 200 mg PO daily for 7 days; then 80 mg PO every other day for 1 month.

ADMINISTRATION
PO
• Unless contraindicated, give drug with food to reduce GI irritation. Patient may need another drug to prevent GI irritation.
• May dilute solution in juice or other flavored diluent or semisolid food such as applesauce before using.
• Have patient swallow delayed-release tablets whole; don't break or crush them.
• Discard opened bottle of solution after 90 days. Administer only using the provided calibrated dropper.

ACTION
Not clearly defined. Decreases inflammation, mainly by stabilizing leukocyte lysosomal membranes; suppresses immune response; stimulates bone marrow; and influences protein, fat, and carbohydrate metabolism.

Route	Onset	Peak	Duration
PO (immediate-release)	Variable	2 hr	Variable
PO (delayed-release)	4 hr	6–6.5 hr	Unknown

Half-life: 2 to 3 hours.

ADVERSE REACTIONS
CNS: depression, euphoria, malaise, fever, insomnia, psychotic behavior, behavior and mood changes, personality change, *increased ICP,* meningitis, neuritis, vertigo, syncope, headache, paresthesia, abnormal sensory symptoms, arachnoiditis, neuropathy, paraplegia, *seizures.* **CV:** *HF, pulmonary edema,* HTN, edema, *arrhythmias, bradycardia, cardiac arrest, circulatory collapse, myocardial rupture after recent MI,* tachycardia, thrombophlebitis, *fat embolism, thromboembolism,* cardiac enlargement, vasculitis. **EENT:** cataracts, exophthalmos, glaucoma, increased IOP, blurred vision, oral

candidiasis. **GI:** peptic ulceration, ulcerative esophagitis, perforation of the intestine, *pancreatitis,* GI irritation, increased appetite, nausea, vomiting, constipation, diarrhea, abdominal distention. **GU:** menstrual irregularities, increased urine calcium level. **Hematologic:** anemia, *neutropenia.* **Hepatic:** liver enlargement, increased liver enzymes. **Metabolic:** *hypokalemia,* hypernatremia, hyperglycemia, carbohydrate and glucose intolerance, diabetes, hypercholesterolemia, *hypocalcemia,* weight gain, metabolic alkalosis, protein catabolism (negative nitrogen balance), fluid retention. **Musculoskeletal:** growth suppression in children, muscle mass loss, muscle weakness, steroid myopathy, osteopenia, osteoporosis, arthralgia, aseptic necrosis of femoral and humeral head, pathologic long bone fracture, tendon rupture, vertebral compression fractures. **Respiratory:** hiccups. **Skin:** hirsutism, delayed wound healing, acne, allergic dermatitis, cutaneous and subcutaneous atrophy, dry scalp, petechiae, ecchymoses, various skin eruptions, diaphoresis, thin fragile skin, thinning hair, striae, facial erythema, pigmentation changes, urticaria. **Other:** cushingoid state, abnormal fat deposits, susceptibility to infections, hypersensitivity reaction; *acute adrenal insufficiency* after increased stress or abrupt withdrawal after long-term therapy, withdrawal symptoms (rebound inflammation, fatigue, weakness, arthralgia, fever, dizziness, lethargy, depression, fainting, orthostatic hypotension, dyspnea, anorexia, *hypoglycemia*).

INTERACTIONS
Drug-drug. *Aminoglutethimide:* May lead to loss of corticosteroid-induced adrenal suppression. Use cautiously together.
Antidiabetics: May increase blood glucose level. Adjust antidiabetic dosage as necessary.
Aspirin, indomethacin, other NSAIDs: May increase risk of GI distress and bleeding. Use together cautiously.
Cardiac glycosides (digoxin): May increase risk of arrhythmias due to hypokalemia. Monitor patient closely.
Cholestyramine: May decrease prednisone level. Monitor therapy.
Cyclosporine: May increase toxicity and cause seizures. Monitor patient closely.
CYP3A4 inducers (barbiturates, carbamazepine, fosphenytoin, phenobarbital,

P

phenytoin, rifampin): May decrease effect of prednisone. Increase prednisone dosage.

CYP3A4 inhibitors (ketoconazole, macrolides, troleandomycin): May increase prednisone level. Titrate prednisone dosage to avoid toxicity.

Isoniazid: May decrease isoniazid level. Monitor therapy.

Oral anticoagulants (warfarin): May alter dosage requirements. Monitor PT and INR closely.

Potassium-depleting drugs (thiazide diuretics, amphotericin B): May enhance potassium-wasting effects of prednisone. Monitor potassium level.

Salicylates: May decrease salicylate level. Monitor patient for lack of salicylate effectiveness.

Skin-test antigens: May decrease response. Postpone skin testing until after therapy.

Toxoids, live or attenuated vaccines: May decrease antibody response and may increase risk of neurologic complications. Avoid using together.

EFFECTS ON LAB TEST RESULTS

• May increase glucose, sodium, and cholesterol levels.

• May decrease T_3, T_4, potassium, and calcium levels.

• May decrease ^{131}I uptake and protein-bound iodine values in thyroid function tests.

• May cause false-negative results in nitroblue tetrazolium test for systemic bacterial infections.

• May alter reactions to skin tests.

CONTRAINDICATIONS & CAUTIONS

• Contraindicated in patients hypersensitive to drug or its components; in those with systemic fungal infections (immediate-release only), cerebral malaria, or active ocular herpes simplex; and in those receiving immunosuppressive doses together with live-virus vaccines.

• Use cautiously in patients with recent MI, GI ulcer, kidney disease, HTN, osteoporosis, diabetes, seizures, hypothyroidism, cirrhosis, active hepatitis, diverticulitis, nonspecific ulcerative colitis, recent intestinal anastomoses, thromboembolic disorders, myasthenia gravis, HF, TB, ocular herpes simplex, and psychiatric disturbances.

• **Alert:** Patients are more susceptible to infections (from mild to fatal) during therapy.

Drug can also mask signs and symptoms of infection.

• Drug can cause cataracts or glaucoma.

• **Alert:** High-dose therapy is associated with acute myopathy that often occurs in patients receiving neuromuscular drugs or in those with diseases such as myasthenia gravis.

Dializable drug: Unknown.

PREGNANCY-LACTATION-REPRODUCTION

• May cause fetal harm. Use only if potential benefits justify fetal risk.

• Monitor infants born to mothers who received substantial amounts of drug during pregnancy for signs and symptoms of hypoadrenalism.

• Drug appears in human milk. Patient should discontinue breastfeeding or discontinue drug, considering importance of drug to patient.

• Drug may increase or decrease motility and number of sperm.

NURSING CONSIDERATIONS

• Determine if patient is hypersensitive to other corticosteroids.

• Immediate-release drug may be used for alternate-day therapy.

• Always adjust to lowest effective dose.

• Most adverse reactions to corticosteroids are dose- or duration-dependent.

• For better results and less toxicity, give a once-daily dose in the morning.

• Monitor BP, sleep patterns, and potassium level.

• If therapy lasts 6 weeks or more, monitor IOP.

• Weigh patient daily; report sudden weight gain to prescriber.

• Drug can cause HPA axis suppression and result in corticosteroid insufficiency if withdrawn. Reduce dosage gradually and reinstitute corticosteroid therapy if needed.

• Monitor patient for HPA axis suppression and cushingoid effects (moon face, buffalo hump, central obesity, thinning hair, HTN, increased susceptibility to infection).

• Watch for depression or psychosis, especially during high-dose therapy.

• Patient with diabetes may need increased insulin; monitor glucose level.

- Patients with thyroid status changes may need dosage adjustment.
- Drug can cause osteoporosis at any age. Monitor bone density in patients on long-term therapy and bone growth in children. Institute bone-loss prevention measures if therapy is expected to last 3 months or more.
- Older adults and patients who are post-menopausal may be more susceptible to osteoporosis with long-term use.
- Monitor growth in children on long-term therapy.
- Monitor patient for signs and symptoms of infection. Drug may mask or worsen infections, including latent amebiasis.
- Unless contraindicated, give low-sodium diet that's high in potassium and protein. Give potassium supplements as needed.
- Gradually reduce dosage after long-term therapy.
- *Look alike–sound alike:* Don't confuse prednisone with prednisolone or primidone.

PATIENT TEACHING
- Instruct patient in safe drug administration.
- Tell patient not to stop drug abruptly or without prescriber's consent.
- Advise patient to report all adverse reactions.
- Teach patient signs and symptoms of early adrenal insufficiency: fatigue, muscle weakness, joint pain, fever, anorexia, nausea, shortness of breath, dizziness, and fainting.
- Instruct patient to carry or wear medical identification indicating the need for supplemental systemic glucocorticoids during stress. It should include prescriber's name and name and dosage of drug.
- Warn patient on long-term therapy about cushingoid effects (moon face, buffalo hump) and the need to notify prescriber about sudden weight gain or swelling.
- Advise patient receiving long-term therapy to consider exercise or physical therapy. Also, tell patient to ask prescriber about vitamin D or calcium supplement.
- Tell patient to report slow healing.
- Advise patient receiving long-term therapy to have periodic eye exams.
- Instruct patient to report infection, to avoid exposure to infections, and to contact prescriber if exposure occurs.
- Counsel patient to report pregnancy or plans to become pregnant or to breastfeed.

pregabalin
pre-GAB-a-lin

Lyrica, Lyrica CR

Therapeutic class: Anticonvulsants
Pharmacologic class: CNS drugs
Controlled substance schedule: V

AVAILABLE FORMS
Capsules: 25 mg, 50 mg, 75 mg, 100 mg, 150 mg, 200 mg, 225 mg, 300 mg
Oral solution: 20 mg/mL
Tablets (extended-release): 82.5 mg, 165 mg, 330 mg

INDICATIONS & DOSAGES
Adjust-a-dose (for all indications): Refer to specific product information for guidelines regarding dosing in patients with kidney impairment.
➤ **Fibromyalgia**
Adults (immediate-release and oral solution): 75 mg PO b.i.d. (150 mg/day). May increase to 150 mg b.i.d. (300 mg/day) within 1 week, based on patient response. If pain relief insufficient with 300 mg/day, increase to 225 mg b.i.d. (450 mg/day).
➤ **Diabetic peripheral neuropathy**
Adults: Initially, 50 mg PO t.i.d. May increase to 100 mg PO t.i.d. within 1 week based on patient response. Maximum dose, 300 mg/day. Or, initially 165 mg (extended-release) PO once daily after an evening meal. Increase to 330 mg within 1 week, based on patient response. Maximum dose, 330 mg once daily.
➤ **Neuropathic pain associated with spinal cord injury**
Adults: Initially, 75 mg PO b.i.d. (150 mg/day). May increase to 150 mg b.i.d. (300 mg/day) within 1 week based on patient response. If pain relief is insufficient after 2 to 3 weeks, increase to 300 mg b.i.d. Maximum dose, 600 mg/day.
➤ **Postherpetic neuralgia**
Adults: Initially, 75 mg PO b.i.d. or 50 mg PO t.i.d. May increase to 300 mg/day in two or three equally divided doses within 1 week based on patient response. If pain relief insufficient after 2 to 4 weeks, may increase to 300 mg b.i.d. or 200 mg t.i.d. Maximum dose, 600 mg/day. Or, initially 165 mg (extended-release) PO once daily after an evening meal.

Increase to 330 mg within 1 week, based on patient response. If pain relief is insufficient after 2 to 4 weeks and patient tolerates drug, may increase up to 660 mg. Maximum dose, 660 mg once daily.

➤ **Partial-onset seizures (adjunctive therapy)**
Adults: Initially, 75 mg PO b.i.d. or 50 mg PO t.i.d. Dosage may be increased to maximum 600 mg/day based on patient response and tolerability.
Children ages 4 to 16 weighing 30 kg or more: 2.5 mg/kg/day PO in two or three divided doses. May increase weekly up to 10 mg/kg/day (maximum, 600 mg/day).
Children ages 4 to 16 weighing less than 30 kg: 3.5 mg/kg/day PO in two or three divided doses. May increase to 14 mg/kg/day.
Children ages 1 month to younger than 4 years: 3.5 mg/kg/day PO in three divided doses. May increase to 14 mg/kg/day.

ADMINISTRATION
PO
- Give immediate-release form without regard for food.
- Give extended-release form after an evening meal.
- Have patient swallow extended-release tablets whole; don't crush or split.
- Give a missed immediate-release dose as soon as possible unless it's almost time for the next dose; then skip missed dose and give next dose as regularly scheduled.
- If an extended-release dose is missed after evening meal, give before bedtime after a snack. If dose is missed before bedtime, give in morning with a meal. If dose is missed in morning, wait until evening meal to give next scheduled dose.
- Don't stop drug abruptly. Instead, taper gradually over at least 1 week.
- Follow manufacturer's instructions when switching from immediate-release to extended-release form.
- Store Lyrica CR in original container.

ACTION
May contribute to analgesic and anticonvulsant effects by binding to sites in CNS.

Route	Onset	Peak	Duration
PO (immediate-release)	Unknown	0.7–1.5 hr	Unknown
PO (extended-release)	Unknown	5–12 hr	Unknown

Half-life: Adults, 6.3 hours. Children up to age 6, 3 to 4 hours; children ages 7 up to 17, 4 to 6 hours.

ADVERSE REACTIONS
CNS: ataxia, dizziness, somnolence, tremor, abnormal gait, abnormal thinking, amnesia, anxiety, asthenia, balance disorder, confusion, fatigue, fever, depersonalization, euphoria, headache, hyperesthesia, hypertonia, incoordination, myoclonus, nervousness, nystagmus, pain, paresthesia, stupor, twitching, vertigo. **CV:** edema, chest pain, HTN, hypotension. **EENT:** blurred or abnormal vision, conjunctivitis, diplopia, eye disorder, otitis media, tinnitus, dry mouth, nasopharyngitis, sinusitis. **GI:** abdominal pain, constipation, diarrhea, flatulence, gastroenteritis, increased appetite, vomiting, nausea. **GU:** anorgasmia, erectile dysfunction, decreased libido, urinary incontinence, urinary frequency, UTI. **Hematologic:** *thrombocytopenia.* **Hepatic:** increased transaminase levels. **Metabolic:** *hypoglycemia,* weight gain, increased or decreased appetite. **Musculoskeletal:** arthralgia, back and chest pain, leg cramps, myalgia, myasthenia, neuropathy. **Respiratory:** bronchitis, dyspnea, cough. **Skin:** ecchymosis, pruritus, contact dermatitis. **Other:** accidental injury, viral infection, flulike syndrome, hypersensitivity reaction.

INTERACTIONS
Drug-drug. *ACE inhibitors:* May increase risk of angioedema with concomitant use. Monitor patient.
CNS depressants: May have additive CNS effects, including respiratory depression and cognitive and gross motor function effects. Use lowest effective dose of pregabalin and monitor patient response.
Pioglitazone, rosiglitazone: May cause additive fluid retention and weight gain. Monitor patient closely.
Drug-lifestyle. ⚠ *Alert: Alcohol use:* May increase risk of CNS depression and respiratory difficulties. Discourage use together.

EFFECTS ON LAB TEST RESULTS
- May increase CK, ALK, and AST levels.
- May decrease platelet count.

CONTRAINDICATIONS & CAUTIONS
• Contraindicated in patients hypersensitive to drug or its components.
• Use cautiously in patients with NYHA Class III or IV HF.
☻ *Alert:* May cause life-threatening and fatal respiratory depression in older adults and in patients with respiratory risk factors (CNS depressant or opioid use, COPD). Begin treatment at lowest dose and monitor patient closely.
☻ *Alert:* Use cautiously in patients with depression. Drug may increase risk of suicidality.
☻ *Alert:* Use cautiously in patients with history of substance abuse. Drug may cause physical and psychological dependence.
• Drug may prolong QT interval; however, clinical trial data didn't show an increase in related adverse effects.
Dialyzable drug: Yes.
⚠ *Overdose S&S:* Exaggerated adverse effects.

PREGNANCY-LACTATION-REPRODUCTION
• There are no adequate studies during pregnancy. Drug may cause fetal harm. Use in pregnancy only if potential benefit clearly justifies fetal risk.
• Patients exposed to drug during pregnancy should enroll in the North American AED Pregnancy Registry (1-888-233-2334 or https://www.aedpregnancyregistry.org/).
• Drug appears in human milk. Patient should discontinue breastfeeding or discontinue drug, taking into consideration importance of drug to patient.
• Drug may decrease sperm count.

NURSING CONSIDERATIONS
☻ *Alert:* Monitor patient for signs and symptoms of hypersensitivity reactions (hives, rash, dyspnea, wheezing, angioedema). Signs and symptoms of angioedema include swelling of the face, mouth, and neck, which may compromise breathing. Discontinue drug immediately if angioedema occurs.
☻ *Alert:* Monitor patient for worsening depression, suicidality, or unusual mood or behavior changes.
• Monitor patient's weight and fluid status, especially if patient has HF.
• Check for changes in vision.
• Withdraw drug gradually over 1 week, especially in patients with seizure disorder.

☻ *Alert:* Watch for signs of rhabdomyolysis, such as dark, red, or cola-colored urine; muscle tenderness; generalized weakness; or muscle stiffness or aching.
• *Look alike–sound alike:* Don't confuse Lyrica with Lopressor or Hydrea.

PATIENT TEACHING
• Instruct patient in safe drug administration.
• Warn patient not to stop drug abruptly and to instead taper it over at least 1 week.
☻ *Alert:* Caution patient or caregiver to seek immediate medical attention for confusion or disorientation; unusual dizziness or lightheadedness; lethargy; extreme sleepiness; slow, shallow, or difficult breathing; unresponsiveness; or cyanosis of the lips, fingers, or toes.
• Advise patient that drug may cause angioedema, with swelling of the face, mouth (lip, gum, and tongue), and neck (larynx and pharynx), that can lead to life-threatening respiratory compromise. Instruct patient to discontinue drug and immediately seek medical care if these symptoms occur.
• Tell patient to seek immediate medical care for a hypersensitivity reaction, such as blisters, dyspnea, hives, rash, or wheezing.
☻ *Alert:* Counsel patient, caregiver, and family about risk of suicidality. Advise them of the need to be alert for the emergence or worsening of symptoms of depression, unusual changes in mood or behavior, or the emergence of suicidality or thoughts about self-harm and to immediately report behaviors of concern to health care provider.
• Caution patient to avoid hazardous activities until drug's effects are known.
• Instruct patient to watch for weight changes and water retention.
• Advise patient to report vision changes and malaise or fever accompanied by muscle pain, tenderness, or weakness.
• Tell male patient taking pregabalin who plans to father a child to consult prescriber about fetal risk because of male-mediated teratogenicity.
• Advise patient of childbearing potential to report pregnancy, plans to become pregnant, or breastfeeding.
• Urge patient with diabetes to inspect skin closely for ulcer formation.
• Advise patient to avoid alcohol.

procainamide hydrochloride
proe-KANE-a-myed

Therapeutic class: Antiarrhythmics
Pharmacologic class: Procaine derivatives

AVAILABLE FORMS
Injection: 100 mg/mL, 500 mg/mL

INDICATIONS & DOSAGES
➤ **Life-threatening ventricular arrhythmias**
Adults: Loading dose: 100 mg every 5 minutes by slow IV push, no faster than 50 mg/minute, until arrhythmias disappear, adverse effects develop, or 500 mg has been given. Or, give a loading dose of 500 to 600 mg IV infusion over 25 to 30 minutes. Maximum total dose given by repeated bolus injections or loading infusion is 1 g. Maintenance infusion: To maintain therapeutic levels, give continuous infusion of 2 to 6 mg/minute based on clinical response and patient condition; monitor closely.

For patients with less-threatening arrhythmias but who are nauseated, vomiting, or are ordered to receive nothing by mouth, give 50 mg/kg IM divided into fractional doses of one-eighth to one-fourth every 3 to 6 hours. If more than three injections are given, assess patient factors, such as age and kidney function, clinical response and, if available, blood levels of procainamide and *N*-acetylprocainamide (NAPA) in adjusting further dosages for that patient. For arrhythmias occurring during surgery, give 100 to 500 mg IM.

Adjust-a-dose: For older adults or patients with kidney or liver dysfunction, decrease dosage or increase dosing interval, as needed.

ADMINISTRATION
IV
▼ Vials for IV injection contain 1 g of drug: 100 mg/mL (10 mL) or 500 mg/mL (2 mL).
▼ Direct injection into a vein or into tubing of an established IV line should be done slowly at a rate not to exceed 50 mg/minute.
▼ For loading dose infusion, dilute with compatible IV solution, such as D₅W injection (1 g diluted to 50 mL), and give with patient supine at a rate not exceeding 25 to 50 mg/minute. Keep patient supine during IV administration.

▼ For IV infusion to maintain therapeutic levels, dilute 1 g procainamide in 500 or 250 mL D₅W and administer at 2 to 6 mg/minute based on response and clinical condition.
▼ Monitor patient receiving infusion at all times. Use an infusion-control device to give infusion precisely.
⊙ *Alert:* Monitor BP and ECG continuously during IV administration. Watch for prolonged QTc intervals and widening of the QRS complexes, heart block, or increased arrhythmias. If such reactions occur, withhold drug, obtain rhythm strip, and notify prescriber immediately. Hypotension can occur with rapid administration. Watch closely for adverse reactions during infusion, and notify prescriber if they occur.
▼ Solution may turn slightly yellow upon standing. Discard solutions that are slightly darker than yellow or discolored in any other way.
▼ **Incompatibilities:** 5% dextrose in normal saline, esmolol, milrinone, phenytoin sodium.
IM
● Use IM route only if IV route isn't feasible. IM injection may be painful and can increase CK level.

ACTION
Decreases excitability, conduction velocity, automaticity, and membrane responsiveness with prolonged refractory period. Larger than usual doses may induce AV block.

Route	Onset	Peak	Duration
IV	Immediate	Immediate	Unknown
IM	10–30 min	15–60 min	Unknown

Half-life: About 3 to 4 hours.

ADVERSE REACTIONS
CNS: psychosis with hallucinations, giddiness, confusion, depression, dizziness, weakness, bitter taste. **CV:** flushing, hypotension, *bradycardia, AV block, ventricular fibrillation, ventricular asystole.* **GI:** abdominal pain, nausea, vomiting, anorexia, diarrhea. **Skin:** maculopapular rash, urticaria, pruritus. **Other:** lupuslike syndrome, *angiodema.*

INTERACTIONS
Drug-drug. *Amiodarone:* May increase procainamide level and toxicity and have additive effects on QTc interval and QRS complex. Avoid using together.

Reactions in bold italics are *life-threatening*.

Antiarrhythmics: May enhance antiarrhythmic and hypotensive effects. Avoid using together.

Anticholinergics (atropine, benztropine, glycopyrrolate): May increase antivagal effects. Monitor patient closely.

Cimetidine: May increase procainamide level. Avoid using together if possible. Monitor procainamide level closely and adjust the dosage as necessary.

Macrolides and related antibiotics (azithromycin, clarithromycin, erythromycin, telithromycin): May prolong the QT interval. Avoid use together.

Neuromuscular blockers (succinylcholine, rocuronium): May increase skeletal muscle relaxant effect. May need to decrease dosage of neuromuscular blocker.

Quinolones (ciprofloxacin): Life-threatening arrhythmias, including torsades de pointes, can occur. Avoid using together; sparfloxacin use is contraindicated.

Thioridazine, ziprasidone: May prolong QTc interval. Avoid using together.

Trimethoprim: May increase procainamide level. Watch for toxicity.

Drug-herb. *Licorice:* May prolong QTc interval. Urge caution.

EFFECTS ON LAB TEST RESULTS

• May increase ALT, AST, ALP, LDH, and bilirubin levels.
• May decrease Hb level, hematocrit, and WBC and platelet counts.
• May cause positive ANA titers and positive direct antiglobulin (Coombs) tests.

CONTRAINDICATIONS & CAUTIONS

Boxed Warning Because of its proarrhythmic effects, reserve procainamide for patients with life-threatening ventricular arrhythmias. ■

• Contraindicated in patients hypersensitive to this drug and related drugs.
• Drug contains sulfite, which can cause allergic-type reactions, including anaphylaxis. Sensitivity to sulfites may be more frequent in patients with asthma.
• Contraindicated in patients with complete heart block in the absence of an artificial pacemaker. Also contraindicated in those with SLE or atypical ventricular tachycardia (torsades de pointes).
• Use with extreme caution in patients with ventricular tachycardia during coronary occlusion.

• Use cautiously in patients with HF or other conduction disturbances, such as bundle-branch heart block, first-degree heart block, sinus bradycardia, or digoxin intoxication, and in those with liver or kidney insufficiency.
• Avoid use in patients with second-degree heart block or some types of hemiblock unless ventricular rate is controlled by a pacemaker.
• Use cautiously in patients with myasthenia gravis; drug may worsen symptoms.
Boxed Warning Use cautiously in patients with blood dyscrasias or bone marrow suppression. ■

Dialyzable drug: Procainamide, 20 to 50%; metabolite NAPA, less than 5%.

⚠ *Overdose S&S:* Progressive widening of QRS complex, prolonged QT and PR intervals, lowered R and T waves, increasing AV block, ventricular ectopy, ventricular tachycardia, hypotension, CNS depression, tremor, respiratory depression.

PREGNANCY-LACTATION-REPRODUCTION

• Use during pregnancy only if clearly needed. Not known if drug can harm fetus.
• Procainamide and metabolite NAPA appear in human milk. Patient should discontinue breastfeeding or discontinue drug, considering importance of drug to patient.

NURSING CONSIDERATIONS

• Digitalize or cardiovert patients with atrial flutter or fibrillation before therapy with procainamide to prevent ventricular rate acceleration in patient.
• Monitor level of drug and its active metabolite NAPA.
• Monitor ECG closely. If QRS widens more than 25% or marked prolongation of the QTc interval occurs, check for overdosage.
• Hypokalemia predisposes patient to arrhythmias. Monitor electrolytes, especially potassium level.
• Monitor BP carefully. Older adults may be more likely to develop hypotension.
Boxed Warning Agranulocytosis, bone marrow depression, neutropenia, hypoplastic anemia, and thrombocytopenia have been noted in patients during the first 12 weeks of therapy. Monitor CBC at weekly intervals for the first 3 months of therapy and periodically thereafter. ■
Boxed Warning Check CBC promptly if patient develops signs of infection, bruising,

or bleeding. Discontinue drug for identified hematologic disorder. CBC usually returns to normal within 1 month of discontinuation. ■

Boxed Warning Positive ANA titer is common in about 60% of patients who don't have symptoms of lupuslike syndrome. This response seems to be related to prolonged use, not dosage. If positive ANA titer develops, assess the benefits and risks of continued therapy. ■

• Discontinue IV therapy for persistent conduction disturbances or hypotension. As soon as cardiac rhythm stabilizes, start oral antiarrhythmic maintenance therapy 3 to 4 hours after last IV dose.

PATIENT TEACHING
• Instruct patient to report all adverse reactions and to immediately report fever, rash, muscle pain, diarrhea, bleeding, bruises, pleuritic chest pain, or signs and symptoms of infection.
• Advise patient to report sulfite sensitivity before receiving drug.

---

prochlorperazine
proe-klor-PER-a-zeen

Compro

prochlorperazine edisylate

prochlorperazine maleate
Prochlorazine ✤

Therapeutic class: Antiemetics
Pharmacologic class: Dopamine antagonists

AVAILABLE FORMS
prochlorperazine
Suppositories: 25 mg
prochlorperazine edisylate
Injection: 5 mg/mL
prochlorperazine maleate
Tablets: 5 mg, 10 mg

INDICATIONS & DOSAGES
➤ **To control preoperative nausea**
Adults: 5 to 10 mg IM 1 to 2 hours before induction of anesthesia; repeat once in 30 minutes, if needed. Or, 5 to 10 mg IV at no more than 5 mg/minute 15 to 30 minutes before induction of anesthesia; repeat once, if needed. Maximum IM and IV dose, 40 mg/day.

➤ **Severe nausea and vomiting**
Adults: 5 to 10 mg PO t.i.d. or q.i.d.; 25 mg PR b.i.d.; or 5 to 10 mg IM, repeated every 3 to 4 hours, as needed. Maximum IM dose, 40 mg daily. Or, 2.5 to 10 mg IV at no more than 5 mg/minute. Maximum IV dose, 40 mg daily.
Children weighing 18 to 39 kg: 2.5 mg PO t.i.d.; or 5 mg PO b.i.d. Maximum, 15 mg daily. Or, 0.132 mg/kg by deep IM injection t.i.d. to q.i.d. Control is usually achieved with one dose.
Children weighing 14 to 17 kg: 2.5 mg PO b.i.d. or t.i.d. Maximum, 10 mg daily. Or, 0.132 mg/kg by deep IM injection t.i.d. to q.i.d. Control is usually achieved with one dose.
Children weighing 9 to 13 kg: 2.5 mg PO once daily or b.i.d. Maximum, 7.5 mg daily. Or, 0.132 mg/kg by deep IM injection t.i.d. to q.i.d. Control is usually achieved with one dose.

➤ **Schizophrenia**
Adults: Treatment guidelines may not include drug as recommended therapy for this indication. According to prescribing information, for mild conditions, 5 or 10 mg PO t.i.d. or q.i.d. For moderate to severe conditions, start with 10 mg PO t.i.d. or q.i.d.; increase by small increments every 2 or 3 days until symptoms are controlled or adverse reactions become bothersome. Patients may respond on 50 to 75 mg/day in divided doses. For severe conditions, 100 to 150 mg PO daily. Or, for severe symptoms, 10 to 20 mg by deep IM injection. Repeat the initial IM dose every 2 to 4 hours (or, in resistant cases, every hour) to gain control of patient, as necessary. More than three or four IM doses are seldom necessary. If, in rare cases, parenteral therapy is needed for a prolonged period, give 10 to 20 mg IM every 4 to 6 hours. After control is achieved, switch patient to an oral form of drug at same dosage level or higher.
Children ages 2 to 12: Initially, 2.5 mg PO b.i.d. or t.i.d., not to exceed 10 mg on the first day. Increase dosage according to patient response. Maximum dose, 20 mg/day (ages 2 to 5) or 25 mg/day (ages 6 to 12). Or, 0.132 mg/kg IM as a single dose. Don't exceed 10 mg/day on first day of therapy.

➤ **Nonpsychotic anxiety**
Adults: Treatment guidelines may not include drug as recommended therapy for this indication. According to prescribing information,

give 5 mg PO t.i.d. or q.i.d. Maximum dose is 20 mg/day for no longer than 12 weeks.

ADMINISTRATION
PO
• Administer without regard to meals.
IV
▼ Give undiluted or diluted in isotonic solution by slow IV injection or infusion at a rate not to exceed 5 mg/minute. Don't exceed 10 mg in a single dose or total IV dose of 40 mg/day.
▼ Don't give by bolus injection.
▼ To prevent contact dermatitis, avoid getting injection solution on hands or clothing.
▼ Store at room temperature and protect from light.
▼ **Incompatibilities:** Other IV drugs.
IM
• For IM use, inject deeply into upper outer quadrant of gluteal region.
• Don't give by subcut route or mix in syringe with another drug.
• To prevent contact dermatitis, avoid getting injection solution on hands or clothing.
• Store in light-resistant container. Slight yellowing doesn't affect potency; discard extremely discolored solutions.
Rectal
• Don't remove from wrapper until ready to use.
• Moisten suppository with water before insertion.
• If suppository is too soft because of warm storage, chill in refrigerator for 30 minutes or run cold water over it before removing wrapper.

ACTION
Acts on the chemoreceptor trigger zone to inhibit nausea and vomiting; in larger doses, it partially depresses vomiting center.

Route	Onset	Peak	Duration
PO	30–60 min	Unknown	3–4 hr
IV	Unknown	Unknown	Unknown
IM	10–20 min	Unknown	3–4 hr
PR	1 hr	Unknown	3–12 hr

Half-life: PO, 6 to 10 hours (single dose); 14 to 22 hours (repeated dosing). IV, 6 to 10 hours.

ADVERSE REACTIONS
CNS: agitation, cognitive impairment, decreased cough reflex, temperature dysregulation, extrapyramidal reactions, dizziness, EEG changes, fever, headache, insomnia, pseudoparkinsonism, sedation, drowsiness, motor dysfunction, motor restlessness, dystonia, tardive dyskinesia. **CV:** orthostatic hypotension, ECG changes, tachycardia, edema. **EENT:** blurred vision, ocular changes, dry mouth, nasal congestion. **GI:** constipation, obstipation, increased appetite, intestinal obstruction, nausea, vomiting. **GU:** urine retention, dark urine, ejaculation disorder, priapism, menstrual irregularities. **Hematologic:** *agranulocytosis, transient leukopenia,* hemolytic anemia, eosinophilia. **Hepatic:** cholestasis, cholestatic jaundice. **Metabolic:** *hypoglycemia,* hyperglycemia, weight gain. **Skin:** mild photosensitivity reactions, allergic reactions, exfoliative dermatitis, contact dermatitis, urticaria, eczema, skin pigmentation. **Other:** hypersensitivity reactions, gynecomastia, hyperprolactinemia, lupus-like syndrome.

INTERACTIONS
Drug-drug. *Antacids:* May inhibit absorption of oral phenothiazines. Separate antacid and phenothiazine doses by at least 2 hours.
Anticholinergics, including antidepressants and antiparkinsonian drugs: May increase anticholinergic activity and may aggravate parkinsonian symptoms. Use together cautiously.
Anticoagulants: May decrease anticoagulant effects. Monitor PT and INR, and adjust dosage as needed.
Anticonvulsants: May lower seizure threshold; dosage adjustments of anticonvulsants may be needed. May increase phenytoin level and risk of toxicity. Monitor patient closely.
Barbiturates: May decrease phenothiazine effect. Monitor patient for decreased antiemetic effect.
CNS depressants (anesthetics, opioids): May intensify or prolong action of these drugs. Monitor patient. Contraindicated with high doses of CNS depressants.
Loop diuretics, thiazides: May add to orthostatic hypotension caused by prochlorperazine. Monitor BP.
Nitroglycerin: May impair absorption of SL nitroglycerin tablets. Monitor therapy.
Propranolol: May increase plasma levels of both drugs. Observe for increased adverse effects.
Drug-herb. *Kava kava:* May increase risk of dystonic reactions. Discourage use together.

P

Drug-lifestyle. *Alcohol use:* May increase CNS depression, particularly psychomotor skills. Strongly discourage use together.

EFFECTS ON LAB TEST RESULTS
• May increase LFT values.
• May decrease platelet, RBC, WBC, and granulocyte counts.
• May cause false-positive results for phenylketonuria and pregnancy tests.

CONTRAINDICATIONS & CAUTIONS
• Contraindicated in patients hypersensitive to phenothiazines and in patients with CNS depression, including those in a coma.
• Contraindicated during pediatric surgery and in children younger than age 2 or weighing less than 9 kg.
Boxed Warning Drug isn't approved for treatment of older adults with dementia-related psychosis due to increased risk of death. ■
• Use cautiously in patients with impaired CV function, glaucoma, seizure disorders, and Parkinson disease; in those who have been exposed to extreme heat or who are debilitated or appear emaciated; and in children with acute illness.
• *Alert:* Potentially irreversible tardive dyskinesia and potentially fatal NMS have been reported with antipsychotic use.
Dialyzable drug: No.
⚠ *Overdose S&S:* Dystonic reactions, CNS depression, agitation, restlessness, seizures, ECG changes, cardiac arrhythmias, fever, hypotension, dry mouth, ileus.

PREGNANCY-LACTATION-REPRODUCTION
• Safe use during pregnancy hasn't been established. Use only if potential benefit justifies fetal risk.
• *Alert:* Neonates exposed to antipsychotics in the third trimester are at risk for extrapyramidal or withdrawal symptoms after delivery that may range in severity from mild to severe and may require intensive care support.
• Drug may appear in human milk. Use cautiously during breastfeeding.

NURSING CONSIDERATIONS
• Watch for orthostatic hypotension, especially when giving drug IV.
• To reduce hypotension risk, patients receiving IV drug must remain supine and be observed for at least 30 minutes after administration.

• Monitor CBC, electrolyte levels, fasting glucose level, lipid panel, and LFT values during long-term therapy.
• *Alert:* Use drug only when vomiting can't be controlled by other measures or when only a few doses are needed. If more than four doses are needed in 24 hours, notify prescriber.
• Monitor for decreased GI motility and urine retention.
• Immediately report signs and symptoms of tardive dyskinesia (involuntary rhythmic movements of the face, tongue, or jaw) as drug may need to be discontinued.
• Immediately report signs and symptoms of NMS (high fever, confusion, muscle rigidity, unstable vital signs); drug should be discontinued and supportive therapy begun.
• *Look alike–sound alike:* Don't confuse prochlorperazine with chlorpromazine.

PATIENT TEACHING
• Advise patient to report all adverse reactions and to immediately report signs and symptoms of tardive dyskinesia and NMS.
• Tell patient to avoid extreme heat because drug may interfere with the body's thermoregulatory mechanisms.
• Advise patient to avoid alcohol while taking drug because of increased CNS depression.
• Tell patient to call prescriber if more than prescribed doses are needed within 24 hours.
• Instruct patient to report pregnancy or plans to become pregnant or to breastfeed.

SAFETY ALERT!

promethazine hydrochloride
proe-METH-a-zeen

Histantil ✤ , Phenergan, Promethegan

Therapeutic class: Antiemetics
Pharmacologic class: Phenothiazines

AVAILABLE FORMS
Injection: 25 mg/mL, 50 mg/mL
Suppositories: 12.5 mg, 25 mg, 50 mg
Syrup: 6.25 mg/5 mL*
Tablets: 12.5 mg, 25 mg, 50 mg

INDICATIONS & DOSAGES
➤ **Motion sickness**
Adults: 25 mg PO or PR taken 30 minutes to 1 hour before departure. May repeat dose 8 to 12 hours later PRN. Then, 25 mg PO b.i.d.

on successive travel days on rising and again before the evening meal.

Children ages 2 and older: 12.5 to 25 mg PO or PR 30 minutes to 1 hour before departure. May repeat dose 8 to 12 hours later PRN.

➤ **Nausea and vomiting**

Adults: 12.5 to 25 mg PO, IM, IV, or PR every 4 to 6 hours PRN.

Children ages 2 and older: 0.25 to 1 mg/kg PO or PR every 4 to 6 hours PRN, or 0.25 to 0.5 mg/kg IM or IV every 4 to 6 hours PRN.

Adjust-a-dose: Don't use antiemetics to treat vomiting of unknown etiology in children and adolescents.

➤ **Rhinitis, allergy symptoms**

Adults: 25 mg PO or PR at bedtime, or 12.5 mg PO or PR t.i.d. and at bedtime. Or, 25 mg deep IM or IV. May repeat dose within 2 hours if needed. Use oral dosing as soon as possible.

Children ages 2 and older: Maximum dose is 25 mg PO or PR at bedtime, or 6.25 to 12.5 mg PO or PR t.i.d. Use lowest effective dose and avoid other respiratory depressants.

➤ **Nighttime sedation**

Adults: 25 to 50 mg PO, IM, or PR at bedtime. Or, 25 mg IV at bedtime.

Children ages 2 and older: 0.5 to 1.1 mg/kg/ dose (maximum, 25 mg) PO or PR at bedtime. Manufacturer doesn't provide exact dosage of parenteral promethazine. Use lowest possible effective dose.

➤ **Adjunct to analgesics for routine preoperative or postoperative sedation**

Adults: 25 to 50 mg IM, PO, or PR. Or, 25 mg IV in combination with an appropriately reduced dose of opioid or barbiturate and the required amount of a belladonna alkaloid.

Children ages 2 and older: 0.5 to 1.1 mg/kg PO, IM, IV, or PR in combination with an appropriately reduced dose of opioid or barbiturate and the appropriate dose of an atropine-like drug.

➤ **Obstetric sedation**

Adults: 25 to 50 mg deep IM or IV in the early stages of labor. When labor is definitely established, may give 25 to 75 mg IM or IV with an appropriately reduced dose of desired opioid. If necessary, may repeat once or twice at 4-hour intervals. Maximum dose, 100 mg/24 hours.

ADMINISTRATION

PO

• Reduce GI distress by giving drug with food or milk.

IV

▼ If solution is discolored or contains a precipitate, discard.

▼ Give injection through a free-flowing IV line; consider giving over 10 to 15 minutes to minimize risk of phlebitis.

Boxed Warning Be alert for extravasation. Severe chemical irritation and damage can result. ■

🛈 *Alert:* Don't give at a concentration above 25 mg/mL or a rate above 25 mg/minute.

Boxed Warning Don't give IV solution subcutaneously or intra-arterially. ■

▼ **Incompatibilities:** None listed by manufacturer. Consult a drug incompatibility reference for more information.

IM

Boxed Warning IM injection is the preferred parenteral route. Inject deep IM into large muscle mass. ■

• Rotate injection sites.

Rectal

• If suppository is too soft, place wrapped in refrigerator for 15 minutes or run under cold water.

• Store in refrigerator between 36° and 46° F (2° and 8° C).

ACTION

Phenothiazine derivative that competes with histamine for H_1-receptor sites on effector cells. Prevents, but doesn't reverse, histamine-mediated responses. At high doses, drug also has local anesthetic effects.

Route	Onset	Peak	Duration
PO	15–60 min	Unknown	<12 hr
IV	3–5 min	Unknown	<12 hr
IM, PR	20 min	Unknown	<12 hr

Half-life: Approximately 9 to 19 hours depending on route and formulation.

ADVERSE REACTIONS

CNS: drowsiness, sedation, confusion, dizziness, faintness, disorientation, extrapyramidal symptoms, insomnia, nightmares, agitation, lassitude, incoordination, fatigue, tremors, *seizures,* catatoniclike state, hysteria. **CV:** hypotension, HTN, *bradycardia,* tachycardia; injection-related thrombophlebitis, *venous thrombosis.* **EENT:** blurred vision, diplopia, tinnitus, nasal congestion, dry mouth, tongue protrusion. **GI:** nausea, vomiting. **GU:** urine retention. **Hematologic:** *leukopenia, thrombocytopenia, agranulocytosis.* **Hepatic:**

jaundice. **Metabolic:** hyperglycemia. **Respiratory:** *asthma, respiratory depression, apnea.* **Skin:** photosensitivity, rash, urticaria, injectionsite reaction, dermatitis, severe tissue injury (abscess, tissue necrosis, gangrene), extravasation. **Other:** *angioedema.*

INTERACTIONS

Drug-drug. *Anticholinergics, TCAs:* May increase anticholinergic effects. Avoid using together.

Antipsychotics: May increase risk of NMS. Monitor patient; discontinue promethazine if interaction is suspected.

CNS depressants: May increase sedation. Use together cautiously. If used together, reduce CNS depressant dosage.

Epinephrine: May block or reverse effects of epinephrine. Use other pressor drugs instead.

MAO inhibitors: May increase extrapyramidal effects. Avoid using together.

Drug-lifestyle. *Alcohol use:* May increase sedation. Discourage use together.

Sun exposure: May cause photosensitivity reactions. Advise patient to avoid extensive sunlight exposure and to use sun block.

EFFECTS ON LAB TEST RESULTS
• May increase blood glucose level.
• May decrease WBC, platelet, and granulocyte counts.
• May prevent, reduce, or mask positive result in diagnostic skin test.
• May cause false-positive or false-negative pregnancy test result.
• May cause false-positive or false-negative result with urine detection of amphetamine and methamphetamine.

CONTRAINDICATIONS & CAUTIONS
• Contraindicated in patients hypersensitive to drug, in those who have experienced adverse reactions to phenothiazines, in patients who are comatose, and for antihistamine treatment of lower respiratory tract symptoms, including asthma.

Boxed Warning Contraindicated in children younger than age 2 because of the potential for fatal respiratory depression. Use the lowest effective dose in children older than age 2 and avoid administering with drugs that can cause respiratory depression. ∎

• Use cautiously in patients with a history of seizures and in those taking drugs that affect

the seizure threshold as drug can lower the seizure threshold.

• Use cautiously in patients with pulmonary, liver, or CV disease; in children who are acutely ill or dehydrated; and in those with intestinal obstruction, prostatic hyperplasia, bladder-neck obstruction, angle-closure glaucoma, seizure disorders, CNS depression, bone marrow depression, or stenosing or peptic ulcerations.

Dialyzable drug: No.

⚠ **Overdose S&S:** Hypotension, respiratory depression, ataxia, athetosis, positive Babinski reflex, unconsciousness, hyperreflexia, hypertonia, dry mouth, fixed dilated pupils, flushing, GI symptoms, seizures, sudden death; hyperexcitability, nightmares (in children).

PREGNANCY-LACTATION-REPRODUCTION
• There are no adequate studies during pregnancy. Use only if potential benefit justifies fetal risk.
• Use of drug within 2 weeks of delivery may inhibit platelet aggregation in newborn.
• It isn't known if drug appears in human milk. Patient should discontinue breastfeeding or discontinue drug, considering importance of drug to patient.

NURSING CONSIDERATIONS
Boxed Warning Perivascular extravasation, unintentional intra-arterial injection, or intraneuronal or perineuronal infiltration of the drug may result in irritation and tissue damage. Adverse reactions include burning, pain, thrombophlebitis, tissue necrosis, and gangrene. ∎
• Monitor patient for NMS (altered mental status, autonomic instability, muscle rigidity, and hyperpyrexia).
• Stop drug 4 days before diagnostic skin testing because antihistamines can prevent, reduce, or mask positive skin test response.
• Drug is used as an adjunct to analgesics, usually to increase sedation; it has no analgesic activity.
• *Look alike–sound alike:* Don't confuse promethazine with chlorpromazine or prednisone.

PATIENT TEACHING
• Teach patient safe drug administration.
• When treating motion sickness, tell patient to take first dose 30 to 60 minutes before travel; dose may be repeated in 8 to 12 hours,

if necessary. On succeeding days of travel, patient should take dose upon arising and with evening meal.

• Warn patient to avoid alcohol and hazardous activities that require alertness until CNS effects of drug are known.

• Tell patient to report all adverse reactions promptly.

• Warn patient about possible photosensitivity reactions. Advise patient to avoid sun, sunlamps, and tanning beds; use sun block; and wear protective clothing and eyewear.

• Advise patient to report discomfort at IV site immediately.

• Instruct patient to report involuntary muscle movements.

• Instruct patient to report pregnancy or plans to become pregnant or to breastfeed.

propafenone hydrochloride
proe-PAF-a-non

Rythmol SR

Therapeutic class: Antiarrhythmics
Pharmacologic class: Sodium channel antagonists

AVAILABLE FORMS
Capsules (extended-release) ⓓⓝⓒ: 225 mg, 325 mg, 425 mg
Tablets (immediate-release): 150 mg, 225 mg, 300 mg

INDICATIONS & DOSAGES
Adjust-a-dose (for all indications): Consider reducing dosage in patients with liver impairment, significant widening of the QRS complex, or second- or third-degree AV block. Reduce dosage in older adults.

➤ **To treat life-threatening ventricular arrhythmias; to prolong time to recurrence of paroxysmal supraventricular tachycardia (PSVT) and paroxysmal atrial fibrillation or flutter in patients without structural heart disease**
Adults: Initially, 150 mg immediate-release tablet PO every 8 hours. May increase every 3 or 4 days to 225 mg every 8 hours. If needed, may increase to 300 mg every 8 hours. Maximum daily dose, 900 mg.

➤ **To prolong time until recurrence of symptomatic atrial fibrillation (AF) in**

patients with episodic AF who don't have structural heart disease
Adults: Initially, 150-mg immediate-release tablet PO every 8 hours. May increase dosage after 3 to 4 days to 225- to 300-mg immediate-release tablet PO every 8 hours. Maximum dosage, 900 mg/day. Or, 225 mg extended-release capsule PO every 12 hours. May increase dose after 5 days to 325 mg PO every 12 hours. May increase dose to 425 mg every 12 hours.

ADMINISTRATION
PO
• Give without regard to food.
• Have patient swallow capsules whole; don't crush or open capsules.
• Skip a missed dose. Don't double the dose but give next dose at the usual time.

ACTION
Reduces inward sodium current in cardiac cells, prolongs refractory period in AV node, and decreases excitability, conduction velocity, and automaticity in cardiac tissue.

Route	Onset	Peak	Duration
PO (immediate-release)	Unknown	3.5 hr	Unknown
PO (extended-release)	Unknown	3–8 hr	Unknown

Half-life: 2 to 10 hours.

ADVERSE REACTIONS
CNS: depression, dizziness, anxiety, asthenia, ataxia, drowsiness, fatigue, headache, insomnia, syncope, tremor, weakness, unusual taste.
CV: *HF, bradycardia, arrhythmias, ventricular tachycardia,* PVCs, *ventricular fibrillation,* AF, bundle-branch block, angina, chest pain, edema, first-degree AV block, hypotension, prolonged QRS complex, intraventricular conduction delay, palpitations, murmur.
EENT: blurred vision, dry mouth. **GI:** nausea, vomiting, constipation, diarrhea, dyspepsia, anorexia, flatulence. **GU:** hematuria. **Hepatic:** increased ALP level. **Respiratory:** dyspnea, crackles, URI, wheezing. **Skin:** rash, diaphoresis, ecchymosis.

INTERACTIONS
Drug-drug. *Antiarrhythmics (amiodarone), fluoxetine, paroxetine, sertraline:* May increase risk of prolonged QTc interval and arrhythmias. Avoid use together.

P

Beta blockers (metoprolol, propranolol): May increase level of these drugs. Adjust dosage of beta blocker as needed and monitor therapy.
Cardiac glycosides (digoxin): May increase glycoside level. Reduce glycoside dosage and monitor patient closely.
Cimetidine: May increase propafenone levels. Monitor patient for adverse effects and toxicity.
Cyclosporine: May increase cyclosporine level, causing toxicity. Monitor patient closely; dosage adjustment may be necessary.
CYP2D6 inhibitors (paroxetine, ritonavir, sertraline) and CYP3A4 inhibitors (erythromycin, ketoconazole, saquinavir): May increase propafenone level with combined inhibitor use. Avoid use together.
Desipramine, imipramine, venlafaxine: May decrease metabolism of these drugs. Monitor patient closely.
Lidocaine: May decrease lidocaine metabolism. Monitor patient for increased CNS adverse effects and lidocaine toxicity.
Local anesthetics: May increase risk of CNS toxicity. Monitor patient closely.
Mexiletine: May decrease mexiletine metabolism, increasing level and adverse reactions. Monitor mexiletine level and patient closely.
Orlistat: May reduce absorption of propafenone. Abrupt discontinuation of orlistat can result in severe adverse events. Use together with caution.
QTc interval-prolonging drugs (haloperidol, quinidine, TCAs): Use together may enhance QTc-interval prolongation and risk of ventricular arrhythmias. Monitor patient closely and consider therapy modification.
Ritonavir: May increase propafenone level, causing life-threatening arrhythmias. Avoid using together.
Theophylline: May increase theophylline level. Monitor theophylline level and ECG closely.
Warfarin: May increase warfarin level. Monitor PT and INR closely, and adjust warfarin dose as needed.
Drug-food. *Grapefruit, grapefruit juice:* May increase drug level. Discourage use together.
Drug-lifestyle. *Smoking:* May increase propafenone level and risk of cardiac arrhythmias.

EFFECTS ON LAB TEST RESULTS
• May increase urine ketone, glucose, LDH, uric acid, ALP, ALT, and AST levels.

• May decrease potassium level.
• May cause positive ANA titers.

CONTRAINDICATIONS & CAUTIONS
• Contraindicated in patients hypersensitive to drug and in those with HF; cardiogenic shock; SA, AV, or intraventricular disorders of impulse conduction without a pacemaker; bradycardia; Brugada syndrome; marked hypotension; bronchospastic disorders and severe obstructive pulmonary disease; or electrolyte imbalances.
Boxed Warning Class IC antiarrhythmics, including propafenone, may significantly increase risk of adverse effects in patients with structural heart disease. ■
Boxed Warning Because of propafenone's proarrhythmic effects, reserve its use for patients with life-threatening ventricular arrhythmias. ■
• Drug has caused new or worsened arrhythmias. Monitor ECG before and during therapy.
• Drug may cause overt HF.
• Use cautiously in patients taking other cardiac depressants and in those with liver or kidney impairment.
• Use cautiously in patients with myasthenia gravis; may cause exacerbation.
Dialyzable drug: Unlikely.
⚠ *Overdose S&S:* Hypotension, somnolence, bradycardia, intra-atrial and intraventricular conduction disturbance.

PREGNANCY-LACTATION-REPRODUCTION
• There are no adequate studies during pregnancy. Use only if potential benefit justifies fetal risk.
• Drug appears in human milk. Use drug cautiously during breastfeeding if clearly needed.
• Drug may transiently impair spermatogenesis.

NURSING CONSIDERATIONS
◑ *Alert:* Perform continuous cardiac monitoring at start of therapy and during dosage adjustments. If PR interval or QRS complex increases by more than 25%, reduce dosage.
• Monitor HR and BP.
• Monitor electrolyte levels and correct abnormalities before and during therapy.
• If using with digoxin, frequently monitor ECG and digoxin level.
• Pacing and sensing thresholds of artificial pacemakers may change; monitor pacemaker function.

Reactions in bold italics are *life-threatening*.

• Agranulocytosis may develop during first 2 to 3 months of therapy. If patient has an unexplained fever, monitor leukocyte count. WBC count usually normalizes 14 days after drug is discontinued.

PATIENT TEACHING
• Instruct patient in safe drug administration. Stress importance of taking drug exactly as prescribed.
• Advise patient to report all adverse reactions promptly, including fever, sore throat, chills, and other signs and symptoms of infection.
• Tell patient to report palpitations, dizziness, passing out, swelling in arms or legs, trouble breathing, or sudden weight gain.
• Caution patient to report prolonged diarrhea, diaphoresis, vomiting, or loss of appetite or thirst, any of which may cause an electrolyte imbalance.
• Instruct patient to report changes in OTC, prescription, and supplement use.
• Advise patient to report pregnancy or plans to become pregnant or to breastfeed.

SAFETY ALERT!

propofol
PROE-po-fole

Diprivan

Therapeutic class: Sedative-hypnotics
Pharmacologic class: Phenol derivatives

AVAILABLE FORMS
Injection: 10 mg/mL*

INDICATIONS & DOSAGES
➤ **To induce general anesthesia**
Adults younger than age 55 classified as American Society of Anesthesiologists (ASA) Physical Status (PS) category I or II: 2 to 2.5 mg/kg IV. Give in 40-mg boluses every 10 seconds until desired response.
Children ages 3 to 16 classified as ASA PS I or II: 2.5 to 3.5 mg/kg IV over 20 to 30 seconds.
Adjust-a-dose: In older adults and patients who are debilitated, hypovolemic, or classified as ASA PS III or IV, give 1 to 1.5 mg/kg, in 20-mg boluses, every 10 seconds. For cardiac anesthesia, give 20 mg (0.5 to 1.5 mg/kg) every 10 seconds until desired response is

achieved. For patients undergoing neurosurgery, give 20 mg (1 to 2 mg/kg) every 10 seconds until desired response is achieved.
➤ **To maintain anesthesia**
Healthy adults younger than age 55: 0.1 to 0.2 mg/kg/minute (6 to 12 mg/kg/hour) IV. Or, 25- to 50-mg intermittent boluses PRN.
Healthy children ages 2 months to 16 years: Initially, 200 to 300 mcg/kg/minute for 30 minutes, then 125 to 150 mcg/kg/minute (7.5 to 9 mg/kg/hour) IV titrated to achieve desired clinical effect. Younger children may require higher maintenance infusion rates than older children.
Adjust-a-dose: In older adults and patients who are debilitated, hypovolemic, or classified as ASA PS III or IV, give half the usual maintenance dose (0.05 to 0.1 mg/kg/minute or 3 to 6 mg/kg/hour). For cardiac anesthesia with secondary opioid, 100 to 150 mcg/kg/minute; low dose with primary opioid, 50 to 100 mcg/kg/minute. For patients undergoing neurosurgery, give 100 to 200 mcg/kg/minute (6 to 12 mg/kg/hour).
➤ **Monitored anesthesia care**
Healthy adults younger than age 55: Initially, 100 to 150 mcg/kg/minute (6 to 9 mg/kg/hour) IV for 3 to 5 minutes or a slow injection of 0.5 mg/kg over 3 to 5 minutes. For maintenance dose, give infusion of 25 to 75 mcg/kg/minute (1.5 to 4.5 mg/kg/hour) for first 10 to 15 minutes, then reduce dosage to 25 to 50 mcg/kg/minute or incremental 10- or 20-mg boluses.
Adjust-a-dose: In older adults and patients who are debilitated or classified as ASA PS III or IV, give 80% of usual adult maintenance dose. Don't use rapid bolus.
➤ **To sedate patients in the ICU who are intubated**
Adults: Initially, 5 mcg/kg/minute (0.3 mg/kg/hour) IV for 5 minutes. Increments of 5 to 10 mcg/kg/minute (0.3 to 0.6 mg/kg/hour) over 5 to 10 minutes may be used until desired sedation is achieved. Maintenance rate, 5 to 50 mcg/kg/minute (0.3 to 3 mg/kg/hour). Maximum dosage, 4 mg/kg/hour unless benefits outweigh risks.

ADMINISTRATION
IV
⚠ *Alert:* Maintain strict aseptic technique when handling solution. Drug can support growth of microorganisms; don't use if solution might be contaminated. Don't

P

access vial more than once or use for multiple patients.

▼ Shake well.

▼ Don't use if emulsion shows evidence of separation.

▼ Titrate drug daily to maintain minimum effective level. Allow 3 to 5 minutes between dosage adjustments to assess effects.

▼ Discard tubing and unused portions of drug after 12 hours.

▼ Store between 40° and 77° F (4° and 25° C); don't freeze.

▼ **Incompatibilities:** Other IV drugs, blood and plasma.

ACTION
Unknown. Rapid-acting IV sedative-hypnotic.

Route	Onset	Peak	Duration
IV	<40 sec	Unknown	10–15 min

Half-life: Initial, 40 minutes; terminal, 4 to 7 hours and up to 3 days after 10-day infusion.

ADVERSE REACTIONS
CNS: dystonic or choreiform movement.
CV: *bradycardia, arrhythmia,* hypotension, HTN, decreased cardiac output, tachycardia.
Metabolic: hyperlipidemia. **Respiratory:** *apnea, respiratory acidosis.* **Skin:** rash, pruritus. **Other:** burning or stinging at injection site.

INTERACTIONS
Drug-drug. *Inhaled anesthetics (enflurane, halothane, isoflurane), opioids (alfentanil, fentanyl, meperidine, morphine), sedatives (barbiturates, benzodiazepines, chloral hydrate, droperidol):* May increase anesthetic and sedative effects and further decrease BP and cardiac output. Monitor patient closely.
Valproate: May increase propofol level. Reduce propofol dosage and monitor patient closely.

EFFECTS ON LAB TEST RESULTS
• May increase serum triglyceride levels.

CONTRAINDICATIONS & CAUTIONS
• Contraindicated in patients hypersensitive to drug or its components (soybean oil, glycerol, egg lecithin, disodium edetate, sodium hydroxide); in patients with allergies to eggs, egg products, soybeans, or soy products; and in those unable to undergo general anesthesia or sedation.

🔸 *Alert:* Repeated or lengthy use of general anesthetic and sedation drugs during surgeries or procedures in children younger than age 3 or in patients during the third trimester may affect the development of children's brains. Weigh benefits of appropriate anesthesia in young children and patients who are pregnant against risks.

• Use cautiously in older adults, patients who are hemodynamically unstable or who have seizures, and in those with respiratory disease, disorders of lipid metabolism, or increased ICP.

Dialyzable drug: Unknown.

⚠ *Overdose S&S:* Cardiorespiratory depression.

PREGNANCY-LACTATION-REPRODUCTION
• There are no adequate studies during pregnancy. Use only if clearly needed.
• Drug isn't recommended for obstetric uses, including cesarean deliveries, as it may cause neonatal CNS and respiratory depression.
• Drug appears in human milk. Avoid use during breastfeeding.

NURSING CONSIDERATIONS
• If drug is used for prolonged sedation in ICU, urine may turn green.
• For general anesthesia or monitored anesthesia care sedation, trained staff not involved in the surgical or diagnostic procedure should give drug. For ICU sedation, persons skilled in managing patients who are critically ill and trained in cardiopulmonary resuscitation and airway management should give drug.
• Continuously monitor vital signs.
• Monitor patient at risk for hyperlipidemia for elevated triglyceride levels.
• Drug contains 0.1 g of fat (1.1 kcal)/mL. Reduce other lipid products if given together.
• Some formulations contain ethylenediaminetetraacetic acid, a strong metal chelator. Consider supplemental zinc during prolonged therapy and in patients predisposed to zinc deficiency (those with burns, sepsis, or diarrhea).
• Some formulations contain sodium metabisulfite, which may cause allergic-type reactions, including anaphylactic signs and symptoms and life-threatening or less severe asthmatic episodes, in susceptible people.
• When giving drug in the ICU, assess patient's CNS function daily to determine minimum dose needed.

Reactions in bold italics are *life-threatening*.

• Stop drug gradually to prevent abrupt awakening and increased agitation.
• Drug may be misused. Manage drug to prevent risk of diversion.

PATIENT TEACHING

• Advise patient that performance of activities requiring mental alertness may be impaired for some time after drug use.
• Tell patient that abnormal dreams or anesthesia awareness may occur.
⟲ Alert: Discuss with parents or caregivers of child younger than age 3 and with patients who are pregnant the benefits, risks, and appropriate timing of surgery or procedures requiring anesthetic and sedation drugs.

SAFETY ALERT!

propranolol hydrochloride ✂
proe-PRAN-oh-lol

Hemangeol, Inderal LA, Inderal XL, InnoPran XL

Therapeutic class: Antihypertensives
Pharmacologic class: Nonselective beta blockers

AVAILABLE FORMS

Capsules (extended-release) ⒹⓃⒸ: 60 mg, 80 mg, 120 mg, 160 mg
Injection: 1 mg/mL
Oral solution: 4 mg/mL, 4.28 mg/mL, 8 mg/mL
Tablets: 10 mg, 20 mg, 40 mg, 60 mg, 80 mg

INDICATIONS & DOSAGES

➤ **Angina pectoris**
Adults: Total doses of 80 to 320 mg/day (immediate-release) PO in two to four divided doses. Or, one 80-mg extended-release capsule daily. Increase dosage at 3- to 7-day intervals until optimal response is obtained or a maximum of 320 mg PO daily has been given.

➤ **To decrease risk of death after MI**
Adults: Initially, 40 mg PO t.i.d. After 1 month, titrate to 60 to 80 mg t.i.d. as tolerated. Maintenance dose is 180 to 240 mg/day in divided doses b.i.d., t.i.d., or q.i.d.

➤ **Supraventricular, ventricular, and atrial arrhythmias; tachyarrhythmias caused by digoxin intoxication, excessive catecholamine action during anesthesia, or hyperthyroidism**
Adults: 1 to 3 mg by slow IV push, not to exceed 1 mg/minute. After 3 mg have been given, another dose may be given in 2 minutes; subsequent doses, no sooner than every 4 hours. Transfer to oral therapy as soon as possible. Usual maintenance dose is 10 to 30 mg PO t.i.d. or q.i.d.

➤ **HTN**
Adults: Initially, 80 mg PO daily in two divided doses or extended-release form once daily. Increase at 3- to 7-day intervals to maximum daily dose of 640 mg (immediate-release or LA extended-release). Usual maintenance dose is 120 to 240 mg daily or 120 to 160 mg daily as extended-release. For Inderal XL or InnoPran XL, dose is 80 mg PO once daily at bedtime. Give consistently with or without food. Adjust to maximum of 120 mg daily if needed. Full effects are seen in about 2 to 3 weeks.

➤ **Essential tremor**
Adults: 40 mg (tablets or oral solution) PO b.i.d. Usual maintenance dose is 120 to 320 mg daily in three divided doses.

➤ **Hypertrophic subaortic stenosis**
Adults: 20 to 40 mg PO t.i.d. or q.i.d. before meals and at bedtime, or 80 to 160 mg LA extended-release capsules once daily.

➤ **Adjunctive therapy in pheochromocytoma**
Adults: 60 mg PO daily in divided doses with an alpha blocker 3 days before surgery. For inoperable tumors, 30 mg PO daily in divided doses with an alpha blocker.

➤ **Prevention of migraine**
Adults: Initially, 80 mg PO in divided doses (immediate-release) or daily (LA extended-release). May increase to 160 to 240 mg/day.

➤ **Proliferating infantile hemangioma requiring systemic therapy (Hemangeol)**
Infants ages 5 weeks to 5 months: Initially, 0.6 mg/kg PO b.i.d. for 1 week, then increase to 1.1 mg/kg PO b.i.d. Increase to maintenance dose of 1.7 mg/kg PO b.i.d. after 2 weeks of treatment and maintain for 6 months. Administer doses at least 9 hours apart during or after feeding.
Adjust-a-dose: Readjust dosage periodically for changes in child's weight.

ADMINISTRATION
PO
• Give immediate-release tablets on an empty stomach. Give extended-release capsules consistently with or without food. Food may increase absorption of propranolol.

P

- Have patient swallow extended-release capsules whole; don't crush or open capsules.
- Adherence may be improved by giving drug twice daily or as extended-release capsules. Check with prescriber.
- Check BP and apical pulse before giving drug. If hypotension or extremes in pulse rate occur, withhold drug and notify prescriber.
- Monitor HR and BP for 2 hours after first dose and when increasing Hemangeol dosage.
- Give Hemangeol during or right after a feeding. Skip dose if child isn't eating or is vomiting. Don't shake before use.
- Give Hemangeol directly into child's mouth using the oral dosing syringe. If needed, may dilute with a small quantity of milk or fruit juice and give in baby's bottle.
- Don't substitute extended-release form for immediate-release on a milligram-for-milligram basis. Retitration may be necessary.

IV

▼ For direct injection, give into a large vessel or into the tubing of a free-flowing, compatible IV solution; don't give by continuous IV infusion.

▼ Drug is compatible with D_5W, half-NSS, NSS, and lactated Ringer solution.

▼ Infusion rate shouldn't exceed 1 mg/minute.

▼ Double-check dose and route. IV doses are much smaller than oral doses.

▼ Monitor BP, ECG, central venous pressure, and HR and rhythm frequently, especially during IV administration. If patient develops severe hypotension, notify prescriber; a vasopressor may be prescribed.

▼ For overdose, give IV isoproterenol, IV atropine, or glucagon; refractory cases may require a pacemaker.

▼ **Incompatibilities:** None.

ACTION

Reduces cardiac oxygen demand by blocking catecholamine-induced increases in HR, BP, and force of myocardial contraction. Drug depresses renin secretion and prevents vasodilation of cerebral arteries.

Route	Onset	Peak	Duration
PO	30 min	1–4 hr	12 hr
PO (Hemangeol)	Rapid	1–4 hr	Unknown
PO (extended-release)	Unknown	6–14 hr	24 hr
IV	Immediate	1 min	5 min

Half-life: About 3 to 6 hours; 8 hours for InnoPran XL; 3 to 6 hours for Hemangeol.

ADVERSE REACTIONS

CNS: fatigue, lethargy, nightmares, agitation, irritability, dizziness. **CV:** hypotension, ***bradycardia.*** **GI:** abdominal cramping, constipation, diarrhea, decreased appetite, nausea, vomiting. **Respiratory:** bronchitis, bronchiolitis (infants). **Skin:** rash, alopecia. **Other:** hypersensitivity reactions.

INTERACTIONS

Drug-drug. *ACE inhibitors, alpha blockers, antiarrhythmics (amiodarone), calcium channel blockers (diltiazem, verapamil):* May increase risk of hypotension and other cardiac adverse effects. Use together cautiously.

Adrenergic blockers (clonidine): May decrease effect of clonidine. Rebound HTN may occur if clonidine is withdrawn abruptly. Withdraw propranolol several days before stopping clonidine.

Cholestyramine, colestipol: May decrease propranolol level if given together. Give propranolol at least 1 hour before or 4 hours after these drugs.

CYP1A2 (phenytoin, montelukast) or CYP2C19 (rifampin) inducers: May decrease propranolol level. Monitor therapy.

CYP2D6 (buproprion, quinidine), CYP1A2 (ciprofloxacin), or CYP2C19 (fluconazole, ticlopidine) inhibitors: May increase propranolol level. Monitor for bradycardia and hypotension.

Dobutamine, isoproterenol: May decrease effects of these drugs. Monitor therapy.

Epinephrine: May cause severe vasoconstriction. Monitor BP and observe patient carefully.

Glucagon: May antagonize propranolol effect. May be used therapeutically and in emergencies.

Insulin, oral antidiabetics: May alter requirements for these drugs in previously stabilized diabetics. Monitor patient for hypoglycemia.

Lidocaine: May increase lidocaine level. Monitor lidocaine level closely.

MAO inhibitors, TCAs: May increase hypotensive effect. Monitor therapy.

NSAIDs: May blunt antihypertensive effect. Monitor therapy.

Phenothiazines (chlorpromazine, thioridazine): May increase risk of serious adverse reactions to either drug. Use with thioridazine is contraindicated. If chlorpromazine must be used, monitor pulse rate and BP and decrease propranolol dosage as needed.

*Reactions in bold italics are **life-threatening**.*

Propafenone: May increase propranolol level. Monitor for bradycardia and hypotension, and adjust propranolol dose as needed.

Reserpine: May increase risk of hypotension, bradycardia, vertigo, or syncope. Monitor therapy.

Theophylline: May decrease theophylline clearance by 30% to 52% and diminish bronchodilatory effect. Consider therapy modification.

Warfarin: May increase warfarin level. Monitor PT and INR.

Drug-herb. *Ma huang:* May decrease antihypertensive effects. Discourage use together.

Drug-lifestyle. *Alcohol use:* May increase or decrease propranolol level. Discourage alcohol use.

Smoking: May decrease propranolol level. Monitor clinical response and adjust dosage as needed. Discourage smoking.

EFFECTS ON LAB TEST RESULTS
• May increase T_4, BUN, transaminases, ALP, potassium, and LDH levels.
• May decrease T_3 level.
• May decrease granulocyte count.

CONTRAINDICATIONS & CAUTIONS
◐ **Alert:** Abrupt withdrawal of drug may cause exacerbation of angina or MI. To discontinue drug, gradually reduce dosage over 1 to 2 weeks. If angina worsens or acute coronary insufficiency develops, resume therapy at least temporarily. Because CAD may be unrecognized, don't discontinue drug abruptly, even when taken for other indications.

• Contraindicated in patients with known hypersensitivity to drug, bronchial asthma, sinus bradycardia and heart block greater than first-degree, cardiogenic shock, and overt and decompensated HF (unless heart failure is secondary to a tachyarrhythmia that can be treated with propranolol).

• Hemangeol is contraindicated in infants weighing less than 2 kg, premature infants with corrected age younger than 5 weeks, infants with HR less than 80 beats/minute or BP lower than 50/30 mm Hg, and in infants with greater than first-degree heart block, decompensated HF, asthma, pheochromocytoma, or history of bronchospasm.

• Use cautiously in patients with liver or kidney impairment, Wolff-Parkinson-White syndrome, or nonallergic bronchospastic diseases, and in those taking other antihypertensives.

• Use cautiously in patients who have diabetes because drug masks some symptoms of hypoglycemia.

• Use cautiously in patients with kidney insufficiency due to increased risk of hypoglycemia.

• In patients with thyrotoxicosis, use drug cautiously because it may mask the signs and symptoms. Abrupt withdrawal may exacerbate symptoms of hyperthyroidism, including thyroid storm.

• Older adults may experience enhanced adverse reactions and may need dosage adjustment.

Dialyzable drug: No.

⚠ **Overdose S&S:** Bradycardia, hypotension.

PREGNANCY-LACTATION-REPRODUCTION
• There are no adequate studies during pregnancy. Use only if potential benefit justifies fetal risk.

• Drug is associated with fetal intrauterine growth retardation and neonatal bradycardia, hypoglycemia, and respiratory depression. If drug is used during pregnancy, ensure adequate monitoring of infants is available at birth.

• Drug appears in human milk. Use cautiously during breastfeeding. Monitor infants for signs and symptoms of beta blockade and hypoglycemia.

NURSING CONSIDERATIONS
• Drug masks common signs and symptoms of shock and hypoglycemia.
• Monitor HR and BP.
▣ Some antihypertensives are less effective in lowering BP when used as monotherapy in patients who are Black. Monitor these patients for expected therapeutic effects; dosage and therapy adjustments may be necessary.

◐ **Alert:** Don't stop drug before surgery for pheochromocytoma. Before any surgical procedure, tell anesthesiologist that patient is receiving propranolol.

• **Look alike–sound alike:** Don't confuse propranolol with prasugrel. Don't confuse Inderal with Isordil, Adderall, or Imuran.

PATIENT TEACHING
• Instruct patient in safe drug administration.
• Caution patient to continue taking drug as prescribed, even if feeling well, and to promptly report adverse reactions.

- Advise patient that propranolol may interfere with glaucoma screening because it can reduce IOP.
- Teach caregiver to skip Hemangeol dose if child isn't eating or is vomiting.
- **Alert:** Caution patient not to stop drug without advice from prescriber because abruptly stopping drug can worsen chest pain or cause an MI.
- Advise patient to avoid smoking and alcohol.
- Inform patient or caregivers of risk of hypoglycemia, especially in children with prolonged physical exertion.

pyridostigmine bromide
peer-id-oh-STIG-meen

Mestinon*, Regonol*

Therapeutic class: Muscle stimulants
Pharmacologic class: Cholinesterase inhibitors

AVAILABLE FORMS
Injection: 5 mg/mL
Syrup: 60 mg/5 mL*
Tablets: 30 mg, 60 mg
Tablets (extended-release) ONC: 180 mg

INDICATIONS & DOSAGES
Adjust-a-dose (for all indications): Smaller doses may be required in patients with kidney disease. Adjust dosage to achieve desired effect.
➤ **Antidote for nondepolarizing neuromuscular blockers (Regonol)**
Adults: 0.1 to 0.25 mg/kg IV. Immediately before or with dose, also give atropine sulfate 0.6 to 1.2 mg IV or an equipotent dose of glycopyrrolate.
➤ **Myasthenia gravis (Mestinon)**
Adults: 60 to 120 mg immediate-release PO every 3 or 4 hours. Average dosage is 600 mg daily, but dosages up to 1,500 mg daily may be needed. Or, 180 to 540 mg extended-release tablets PO daily or b.i.d., with at least 6 hours between doses.
Adjust-a-dose: Adjust dosage for each patient, based on response and tolerance.

ADMINISTRATION
PO
- Have patient swallow extended-release capsules whole; don't crush or break.

- If patient has trouble swallowing, give syrup form. If patient can't tolerate sweet flavor, give over ice chips.
IV
- **Alert:** Drug should only be administered by individuals familiar with its actions, characteristics, and hazards.
▼ Don't use solution if it contains particulate matter or appears discolored.
▼ Position patient to ease breathing. Keep atropine injection available, and be prepared to give it immediately.
▼ Monitor vital signs frequently, especially respirations. Provide respiratory support as needed.
▼ Give injection no faster than 1 mg/minute. Rapid infusion may cause bradycardia and seizures.
▼ **Incompatibilities:** Alkaline solutions.

ACTION
Inhibits acetylcholinesterase, blocking destruction of acetylcholine from the parasympathetic and somatic efferent nerves. Acetylcholine accumulates, promoting increased stimulation of the receptors.

Route	Onset	Peak	Duration
PO	20–30 min	2 hr	3–4 hr
PO (extended-release)	30–60 min	1–2 hr	6–12 hr
IV	2–5 min	Unknown	2–3 hr

Half-life: 1 to 3 hours depending on route.

ADVERSE REACTIONS
CNS: headache with high doses, weakness, syncope, hyperesthesia. **CV:** *bradycardia,* hypotension, thrombophlebitis at IV site. **EENT:** miosis, amblyopia, epistaxis, rhinorrhea, increased salivation. **GI:** nausea, vomiting, abdominal cramps, diarrhea, increased peristalsis. **GU:** urinary frequency, urinary urgency, dysmenorrhea. **Musculoskeletal:** muscle cramps, muscle fasciculations, muscle weakness, tingling in extremities, myalgia, neck pain. **Respiratory:** *bronchospasm, bronchoconstriction,* increased bronchial secretions. **Skin:** rash, diaphoresis, dry skin.

INTERACTIONS
Drug-drug. *Antibiotics (aminoglycosides [streptomycin, gentamicin], bacitracin, polymyxin B, tetracyclines):* May increase or prolong neuromuscular blockade. Monitor IV pyridostigmine effect closely.

Reactions in bold italics are *life-threatening*.

Anticholinergics (scopolamine, dicyclomine):
May decrease effect of anticholinergic. Monitor therapy.
Bradycardia-causing agents (beta blockers):
May increase bradycardia risk. Monitor therapy.
Corticosteroids: May increase risk of pyridostigmine adverse effects (muscle weakness). Monitor therapy.
Magnesium: May enhance neuromuscular blockade. Monitor therapy.
Quinidine: May cause recurrent paralysis during recovery. Monitor therapy.
Succinylcholine: May enhance neuromuscular blockade of succinylcholine. Monitor therapy.

EFFECTS ON LAB TEST RESULTS
None reported.

CONTRAINDICATIONS & CAUTIONS
• Contraindicated in patients hypersensitive to anticholinesterases or bromides and in those with mechanical obstruction of the intestinal or urinary tract.
• Use cautiously in patients with bronchospastic disease, COPD, asthma, bradycardia, arrhythmias, epilepsy, recent coronary occlusion, vagotonia, kidney impairment, hyperthyroidism, glaucoma, or peptic ulcer.
• Safety and effectiveness in children haven't been established. Some formulations contain benzyl alcohol; drug isn't indicated for use in neonates.
Dialyzable drug: Unknown.

PREGNANCY-LACTATION-REPRODUCTION
• Drug may cross placental barrier. Use during pregnancy only if potential benefits justify maternal and fetal hazards.
• Drug appears in human milk. Use cautiously during breastfeeding.

NURSING CONSIDERATIONS
• Stop all other cholinergics before giving this drug.
• Monitor and document patient's response after each dose. Optimum dosage is difficult to judge.
• Monitor ECG, BP, and HR, especially when giving drug IV.
• Monitor patient for cholinergic reactions (nausea, vomiting, diarrhea, increased salivation). Use atropine immediately to treat cholinergic crisis (life-threatening increase in muscle weakness involving the muscles of respiration).

• Mestinon syrup contains 5% alcohol.
• ***Look alike–sound alike:*** Don't confuse pyridostigmine with physostigmine. Don't confuse Regonol with Reglan.

PATIENT TEACHING
• Advise patient to report all adverse reactions.
• When giving drug for myasthenia gravis, stress importance of taking exactly as prescribed, on time, in evenly spaced doses.
• Explain that patient may have to take drug for life.
• Advise patient to wear or carry medical identification that indicates patient has myasthenia gravis.
• Instruct patient to report pregnancy or plans to become pregnant or to breastfeed.

QUEtiapine fumarate
kwe-TYE-a-peen

Seroquel, Seroquel XR

Therapeutic class: Antipsychotics
Pharmacologic class: Dibenzothiazepine derivatives

AVAILABLE FORMS
Tablets: 25 mg, 50 mg, 100 mg, 150 mg, 200 mg, 300 mg, 400 mg
Tablets (extended-release) ⬛: 50 mg, 150 mg, 200 mg, 300 mg, 400 mg

INDICATIONS & DOSAGES
Adjust-a-dose (for all indications): Titrate slower and use lower target doses in older adults and patients who are debilitated or who are predisposed to hypotension. Begin older adults on 50 mg/day (immediate-release or extended-release) and increase by 50 mg/day as needed depending on clinical response and tolerability. Patients with liver impairment should begin immediate-release with 25 mg/day and increase by 25 to 50 mg/day to an effective dose, or begin extended-release with 50 mg/day and increase by 50 mg/day to an effective dose, depending on clinical response and tolerability.
  Adjust dosage when drug is used in combination with CYP3A4 inducers and inhibitors.
➤ **Schizophrenia**
Adults: Initially, 25 mg (immediate-release) PO b.i.d., increased in increments of 25 to 50 mg b.i.d. or t.i.d. on days 2 and 3, as

tolerated. Target range is 300 to 400 mg daily divided into two or three doses by day 4. Further dosage adjustments, if indicated, should occur at intervals of not less than 2 days. Dosage can be increased or decreased by 25 to 50 mg b.i.d. Effect generally occurs at 150 to 750 mg daily. Maximum dosage: 750 mg/day for acute therapy and 800 mg/day for maintenance treatment.

Or, initially, 300 mg/day (extended-release) PO once daily, preferably in the evening. Titrate within a dosage range of 400 to 800 mg/day, depending on individual response and tolerance. Increase at intervals as short as 1 day and in increments of up to 300 mg/day. Maximum dosage, 800 mg/day.

Adolescents ages 13 to 17: Initially, 25 mg (immediate-release) PO b.i.d. on day 1; 50 mg b.i.d. on day 2; 100 mg b.i.d. on day 3; 150 mg b.i.d. on day 4; and 200 mg b.i.d. on day 5. Adjust dosage by no more than 100 mg/day. Usual dosage is 400 to 800 mg/day, divided into two or three doses depending on response and tolerability; maximum dosage, 800 mg/day. Or initially, 50 mg/day (extended-release) PO on day 1; 100 mg/day on day 2; 200 mg/day on day 3; 300 mg/day on day 4; and 400 mg/day on day 5. Make adjustments in increments of no greater than 100 mg/day. Usual extended-release dosage is 400 to 800 mg/day; maximum dosage, 800 mg/day.

➤ **Monotherapy and adjunctive therapy with lithium or divalproex for the short-term treatment of acute manic episodes associated with bipolar I disorder; adjunctive maintenance therapy with lithium or divalproex**

Adults: Initially, 50 mg (immediate-release) PO b.i.d. on day 1; 100 mg b.i.d. on day 2; 150 mg b.i.d. on day 3; and 200 mg b.i.d. on day 4. Further dosage adjustments after day 4 should be no greater than 200 mg daily to a maximum daily dose of 800 mg. Usual dose is 400 to 800 mg daily. For maintenance therapy with lithium or divalproex, continue treatment at the dosage required to maintain symptom remission.

Or, start with 300 mg (extended-release) PO on day 1 and 600 mg PO on day 2 once daily in the evening. Dosage may be adjusted based on response and tolerability to maximum dosage of 800 mg/day.

➤ **Bipolar I disorder, acute manic episodes**

Children and adolescents ages 10 to 17: Total daily dosage is 50 mg PO on day 1; 100 mg

on day 2; 200 mg on day 3; 300 mg on day 4; and 400 mg on day 5, given in divided doses b.i.d. or t.i.d. (immediate-release) or daily (extended-release). After day 5, adjust dosage in increments of no more than 100 mg/day within the recommended range of 400 to 600 mg/day. Maximum dosage, 600 mg/day.

➤ **Bipolar depression**

Adults: Initially, 50 mg PO once daily at bedtime; increase on day 2 to 100 mg; on day 3 to 200 mg; and on day 4 to maintenance dose of 300 mg/day. Maximum dosage, 300 mg/day (immediate- or extended-release).

➤ **Major depressive disorder, adjunctive therapy with antidepressants**

Adults: 50 mg PO (extended-release) once daily in the evening on days 1 and 2. On day 3, may increase dosage to 150 mg PO once daily in the evening. Dosages ranging from 150 to 300 mg/day have proved effective.

ADMINISTRATION
PO
• Have patients swallow extended-release tablets whole; don't crush or break.
• Give immediate-release tablets without regard for food; give extended-release tablets without food or with a light meal (about 300 calories), preferably in the evening.
• Patients being treated with divided doses of immediate-release form may be switched to extended-release tablets at equivalent total daily dose taken once daily. Individual dosage adjustments may be necessary.

ACTION
Blocks dopamine type 2 (D_2) and serotonin type 2A ($5\text{-}HT_{2A}$) receptors. Its action may be mediated through this antagonism.

Route	Onset	Peak	Duration
PO	Unknown	1.5 hr	Unknown
PO (extended-release)	Unknown	6 hr	Unknown

Half-life: 6 hours; extended-release, 7 to 12 hours.

ADVERSE REACTIONS
CNS: dyskinesia, akathisia, dizziness, headache, drowsiness, somnolence, hypertonia, dysarthria, asthenia, agitation, extrapyramidal reactions, parkinsonism, fatigue, lethargy, hypersomnia, pain, change in dreams, anxiety, schizophrenia, paresthesia, irritability, restlessness, migraine, ataxia, balance disorder, confusion, disorientation,

fever, depression, attention disturbance, speech disorder, syncope, thirst, tremor, twitching, weakness. **CV:** orthostatic hypotension, tachycardia, palpitations, peripheral edema, hypotension, HTN. **EENT:** blurred vision, amblyopia, ear pain, epistaxis, nasal congestion, pharyngitis, rhinitis, sinusitis, dry mouth, toothache, tooth abscess. **GI:** dyspepsia, abdominal pain, constipation, nausea, vomiting, increased or decreased appetite, diarrhea, gastroenteritis, dysphagia, GERD. **GU:** UTI, decreased libido, hyperprolactinemia, urinary frequency. **Hematologic:** *leukopenia, neutropenia, agranulocytosis.* **Metabolic:** weight gain, hyperglycemia, hyperlipidemia, hypothyroidism, increased transaminase levels. **Musculoskeletal:** back pain, neck pain, arthralgia, myalgia, restless leg syndrome, muscle rigidity, stiffness, muscle spasms. **Respiratory:** cough, dyspnea. **Skin:** rash, diaphoresis, pallor, acne. **Other:** flulike syndrome, *accidental overdose.*

INTERACTIONS

Drug-drug. *Anticholinergics:* May increase anticholinergic effects. Use together cautiously; monitor patient for urine retention.
Antihypertensives: May increase effects of antihypertensives. Monitor BP.
CNS depressants: May increase CNS effects. Use together cautiously.
Dopamine agonists, levodopa: May decrease the effects of these drugs. Monitor patient.
Lorazepam: May increase lorazepam level and increase CNS depression. Monitor patient for increased CNS effects.
Opioids: May increase CNS depression. Avoid use together if possible. If use together is necessary, limit dosage and duration of each drug to minimum necessary for desired effect. Consider therapy modification.
QTc interval-prolonging drugs: May enhance QTc-interval prolongation and risk of ventricular arrhythmias. Avoid use in patients at highest risk; monitor therapy for those at lower risk.
Strong CYP3A4 inducers (carbamazepine, phenobarbital, phenytoin, rifampin, thioridazine): May decrease quetiapine level. Increase quetiapine dosage up to fivefold of original dose when used in combination with prolonged treatment (more than 7 to 14 days); titrate based on clinical response and tolerability. When CYP3A4 inducer is

discontinued, reduce quetiapine dosage to original level within 7 to 14 days.
Strong CYP3A4 inhibitors (erythromycin, fluconazole, itraconazole, ketoconazole, nefazodone, ritonavir): May increase quetiapine level. Reduce quetiapine dosage to one-sixth of original dose when used together. When the CYP3A4 inhibitor is discontinued, increase quetiapine dosage by sixfold.
Drug-herb. *St. John's wort:* May increase risk of serotonin syndrome and decrease quetiapine serum concentration. Consider therapy modification.
Drug-lifestyle. *Alcohol use, cannabis, cannabidiol:* May increase CNS effects. Discourage use together.

EFFECTS ON LAB TEST RESULTS

• May increase liver enzyme values, and prolactin, TSH, cholesterol, LDL-C, triglyceride, and glucose levels.
• May decrease T_4 and HDL-C levels.
• May decrease WBC count.
• May cause false-positive results in urine enzyme immunoassays for methadone and TCAs.

CONTRAINDICATIONS & CAUTIONS

• Contraindicated in patients hypersensitive to drug or its ingredients.
Boxed Warning The risk of cerebrovascular adverse events (stroke, transient ischemic attack) and death is increased in older adults with dementia-related psychosis. Quetiapine isn't approved to treat dementia-related psychosis. ∎
Boxed Warning Suicidality may occur in children, adolescents, and young adults (younger than age 24) who are taking quetiapine. Watch for clinical worsening and suicidality in patients of all ages who are started on antidepressant therapy. Quetiapine isn't approved for use in children younger than age 10. ∎
• Avoid use when risk of torsades de pointes or sudden death may be increased, including in patients with a history of cardiac arrhythmias such as bradycardia, hypokalemia, or hypomagnesemia. Also avoid use with other drugs that prolong the QTc interval and in patients with congenital prolongation of the QT interval.
• Use cautiously in patients with increased risk of QT-interval prolongation, such as those with CV disease, family history of

Q

QT-interval prolongation, HF, or heart hypertrophy, and in older adults.

• Use cautiously in patients at risk for falls, including those with diseases, conditions, or who are taking medications that may cause somnolence, orthostatic hypotension, or motor or sensory instability.

• Use cautiously in patients with CV disease, cerebrovascular disease, conditions that predispose to hypotension, a history of seizures or conditions that lower the seizure threshold, urine retention, clinically significant prostatic hypertrophy, or constipation, and conditions in which core body temperature may be elevated.

• Use cautiously in patients with kidney disease; experience is limited.

• Use cautiously in patients at risk for aspiration pneumonia.

• Use cautiously in patients with preexisting low WBC count or history of drug-induced leukopenia or neutropenia. Drug may cause leukopenia, neutropenia, and agranulocytosis, including fatal cases.

Dialyzable drug: Unknown.

⚠ *Overdose S&S:* Drowsiness, hypotension, sedation, tachycardia, hypokalemia, delirium, QTc-interval prolongation, first-degree heart block.

PREGNANCY-LACTATION-REPRODUCTION

↻ *Alert:* Neonates exposed to antipsychotics during third trimester are at risk for developing extrapyramidal signs and symptoms (repetitive muscle movements of face and body) and withdrawal signs and symptoms (agitation, abnormally increased or decreased muscle tone, tremors, sleepiness, severe difficulty breathing, difficulty feeding) after delivery. Use in pregnancy only if potential benefit justifies fetal risk.

• Enroll patients exposed to drug during pregnancy in the National Pregnancy Registry for Atypical Antipsychotics (1-866-961-2388 or www.womensmentalhealth.org/research/pregnancy registry).

• Drug appears in human milk. Breastfeeding isn't recommended.

• Drug may reversibly decrease fertility.

NURSING CONSIDERATIONS

↻ *Alert:* Watch for evidence of NMS (extrapyramidal effects, hyperthermia, autonomic disturbance), which is rare but deadly.

• Assess fall risk before and during long-term antipsychotic treatment, especially in those with conditions or who are taking other drugs that increase fall risk.

• Monitor patient for tardive dyskinesia, which may occur after prolonged use. It may not appear until months or years later and may disappear spontaneously or persist for life, despite ending drug. Antipsychotic treatment may suppress signs and symptoms of tardive dyskinesia and may mask the underlying process. Consider discontinuing therapy if tardive dyskinesia occurs.

• Hyperglycemia may occur in patients taking drug. Monitor patients with diabetes regularly. Monitor all patients for signs and symptoms of hyperglycemia. If present, check fasting blood glucose level.

• Monitor BP before and periodically during therapy. Hypotension can occur in all patients and HTN in children and adolescents.

• Monitor CBC frequently during first few months; discontinue therapy at first sign of decline in WBC count.

• Monitor patient with signs and symptoms of infection for neutropenia. Treat promptly if signs and symptoms of neutropenia occur; discontinue drug for ANC less than 1,000/mm^3.

• Check waist circumference and BMI to monitor for weight gain.

↻ *Alert:* Monitor patient for symptoms of metabolic syndrome (significant weight gain and increased BMI, HTN, hyperglycemia, hypercholesterolemia, and hypertriglyceridemia).

• Monitor patient for hyperprolactinemia (galactorrhea, amenorrhea, gynecomastia, impotence, decreased bone density).

• Drug use may cause cataract formation with long-term use. Obtain baseline ophthalmologic exam and reassess every 6 months.

• Gradually reduce dosage when discontinuing drug and monitor patient for withdrawal signs and symptoms (insomnia, nausea, vomiting, headache, dizziness, irritability).

PATIENT TEACHING

Boxed Warning Suicidality may occur in children, adolescents, and young adults (younger than age 24) taking quetiapine. Advise families and caregivers of need for close observation and communication with prescriber if suicidality occurs. ∎

• Instruct patient in proper drug administration.

- Advise patient and caregiver to use caution when quetiapine is being taken with other centrally acting drugs because of the risk of increased CNS effects.
- Caution patient to avoid alcohol, cannabis, and cannabidiol while taking drug.
- Tell patient to report other prescription or OTC drugs being taken.
- Warn patient about risk of dizziness when standing up quickly. The risk is greatest during the 3- to 5-day period of first dosage adjustment, when resuming treatment, and when increasing dosages.
- Tell patient to avoid becoming overheated or dehydrated.
- Advise patient to report signs and symptoms of hyperglycemia (excessive thirst, excessive urination, excessive hunger or weakness).
- Warn patient to avoid activities that require mental alertness until effects of drug are known, especially during first dosage adjustment or dosage increases.
- Remind patient to have an eye exam at start of therapy and every 6 months during therapy to check for cataracts.
- Tell patient of childbearing potential to report planned, suspected, or known pregnancy.
- Advise patient not to breastfeed during therapy.
- Tell patient and caregivers to report all adverse reactions and to be alert for fever, muscle rigidity, repetitive muscle movements of the face, anxiety, agitation, panic attacks, insomnia, irritability, hostility, aggressiveness, impulsivity, motor restlessness, hypomania, mania, other unusual changes in behavior, worsening of depression, and suicidality.
- Advise patient that drug may cause somnolence, orthostatic hypotension, and motor and sensory instability, which may lead to falls, fractures, or other injuries.
- Tell patient not to stop medication abruptly.

quinapril hydrochloride 🕱
KWIN-a-pril

Accupril

Therapeutic class: Antihypertensives
Pharmacologic class: ACE inhibitors

AVAILABLE FORMS
Tablets: 5 mg, 10 mg, 20 mg, 40 mg

INDICATIONS & DOSAGES
➤ **HTN**
Adults: Initially, 10 to 20 mg PO daily. May adjust dosage based on patient response at intervals of at least 2 weeks. Most patients are controlled at 20 to 80 mg daily as a single dose or in two equally divided doses. If patient is taking a diuretic, start therapy with 5 mg daily.
Older adults: For patients age 65 and older, start therapy at 10 mg PO daily and titrate to optimal response.
Adjust-a-dose: For adults with CrCl over 60 mL/minute, give 10 mg once daily initially; for CrCl of 30 to 60 mL/minute, 5 mg PO daily initially; for CrCl of 10 to 30 mL/minute, 2.5 mg PO daily initially.
➤ **HF**
Adults: 5 mg PO b.i.d. initially. Dosage may be increased at weekly intervals. Usual effective dose is 20 to 40 mg daily in two equally divided doses.
Adjust-a-dose: For patients with CrCl over 30 mL/minute, first dose is 5 mg PO daily; and if CrCl is 10 to 30 mL/minute, first dose is 2.5 mg PO daily. If tolerated, increase to b.i.d. dosing the next day. Adjust dosage at weekly intervals thereafter.

ADMINISTRATION
PO
- Don't give drug with a high-fat meal because this may decrease absorption of drug.
- Store at room temperature.

ACTION
Prevents conversion of angiotensin I to angiotensin II, a potent vasoconstrictor. Less angiotensin II decreases peripheral arterial resistance, decreasing aldosterone secretion, which reduces sodium and water retention and lowers BP.

Route	Onset	Peak	Duration
PO	1 hr	1–4 hr	24 hr

Half-life: Quinapril, 0.8 hour; quinaprilat, 3 hours.

ADVERSE REACTIONS
CNS: headache, dizziness, fatigue. **CV:** hypotension, chest pain. **GI:** abdominal pain, vomiting, nausea, diarrhea. **Metabolic:** elevated creatinine and BUN levels, *hyperkalemia.* **Musculoskeletal:** back pain, myalgia. **Respiratory:** cough, dyspnea. **Skin:** rash.

Q

INTERACTIONS

Drug-drug. ❸ *Alert: Aliskiren:* May increase risk of kidney impairment, hypotension, and hyperkalemia in patients with diabetes and those with GFR less than 60 mL/minute. Concomitant use is contraindicated in patients with diabetes. Avoid concomitant use in patients with kidney impairment.

Diuretics, other antihypertensives: May cause excessive hypotension. Stop diuretic or reduce dose of quinapril, as needed.

Gold: May increase nitritoid reactions (facial flushing, nausea, vomiting, hypotension). Monitor therapy.

Lithium: May increase lithium level and lithium toxicity. Monitor lithium level.

mTOR inhibitor (temsirolimus), neprilysin inhibitors (sacubitril, sacubitril–valsartan): May increase risk of angioedema. Use together is contraindicated; do not use within 36 hours of neprilysin inhibitor.

NSAIDs: May decrease antihypertensive effects. Monitor BP. Combination may result in significant decrease in kidney function. Monitor kidney function.

Potassium-sparing diuretics, potassium supplements: May increase risk of hyperkalemia. Monitor patient closely.

Tetracycline and other drugs that interact with magnesium: May decrease absorption if taken with quinapril. Separate dosing times by at least 2 hours if used together. Consider therapy modification.

Drug-herb. *Yohimbe:* May decrease antihypertensive effects. Discourage use together.

Drug-food. *Salt substitutes containing potassium:* May cause hyperkalemia. Discourage use together.

EFFECTS ON LAB TEST RESULTS

- May increase potassium, BUN, and creatinine levels, and LFT values.
- May decrease sodium level.
- May decrease granulocyte and platelet counts.
- May lead to false-negative aldosterone/renin ratio.

CONTRAINDICATIONS & CAUTIONS

- Contraindicated in patients hypersensitive to ACE inhibitors and in those with a history of angioedema related to treatment with an ACE inhibitor.

- Use cautiously in patients with impaired kidney function.
- AKI and hypertensive crisis have been reported.
- Safety and effectiveness in children haven't been established.

Dializable drug: No.

⚠ **Overdose S&S:** Severe hypotension.

PREGNANCY-LACTATION-REPRODUCTION

Boxed Warning Use of drugs that act directly on the RAAS can cause injury and death to a developing fetus. Stop drug as soon as possible for confirmed pregnancy. ∎

- Drug appears in human milk. Use cautiously during breastfeeding.

NURSING CONSIDERATIONS

- Monitor patient for angioedema, including of head, neck, and extremities (stridor, edema of face, tongue, glottis) and of intestines (abdominal pain with or without nausea or vomiting). If there is airway involvement, treat emergently, including epinephrine 1:1,000 (0.3 to 0.5 mL) if necessary.
- Assess kidney and liver function before and periodically throughout therapy.
- Monitor BP for effectiveness of therapy. When adjusting dosage, measure BP before giving dose (trough) and 2 to 6 hours after dosing (peak).
- Monitor potassium level. Risk factors for hyperkalemia include kidney insufficiency, diabetes, and concomitant use of drugs that raise potassium level.
- ⚕ Although ACE inhibitors reduce BP in all races, they reduce it less in Blacks taking an ACE inhibitor alone. These patients should use drug in combination therapy for a more favorable response.
- ⚕ ACE inhibitors appear to increase risk of angioedema in patients who are Black.
- Other ACE inhibitors have caused agranulocytosis and neutropenia. Monitor CBC with differential counts before therapy and periodically thereafter.

PATIENT TEACHING

- Advise patient to report signs of infection, such as fever and sore throat.
- ❸ *Alert:* Advise patient to report signs or symptoms of breathing difficulty or swelling of face, eyes, lips, or tongue, which may occur especially after the first dose.

Reactions in bold italics are *life-threatening*.

- Tell patient to rise slowly to minimize light-headedness and to report signs and symptoms to prescriber. If fainting occurs, patient should stop taking drug and call prescriber immediately.
- Inform patient that inadequate fluid intake, vomiting, diarrhea, and excessive perspiration can increase risk for light-headedness and fainting. Tell patient to use caution in hot weather and during exercise.
- Tell patient to avoid salt substitutes. These products may contain potassium, which can cause high potassium level in patients taking quinapril.
- Advise patient of childbearing potential about potential fetal hazards and to immediately report pregnancy. Drug will need to be stopped.
- Tell patient to avoid taking with a high-fat meal because this may decrease absorption of drug.

RABEprazole sodium
ra-BEP-ra-zole

Aciphex

Therapeutic class: Antiulcer drugs
Pharmacologic class: PPIs

AVAILABLE FORMS
Tablets (delayed-release) ⓄⓃⒸ: 20 mg

INDICATIONS & DOSAGES
➤ **Healing of erosive or ulcerative GERD**
Adults: 20 mg PO daily for 4 to 8 weeks. Additional 8-week course may be considered, if needed.
➤ **Maintenance of healing of erosive or ulcerative GERD**
Adults: 20 mg PO daily for up to 12 months.
➤ **Healing of duodenal ulcers**
Adults: 20 mg PO daily after morning meal for up to 4 weeks.
➤ **Pathologic hypersecretory conditions, including Zollinger-Ellison syndrome**
Adults: Initially, 60 mg PO daily; may increase, as needed, to 100 mg PO daily or 60 mg PO b.i.d. for as long as clinically indicated.
➤ **Symptomatic GERD, including daytime and nighttime heartburn**
Adults: 20 mg PO daily for 4 weeks. May consider additional 4-week course, if needed.

Children age 12 and older: 20 mg PO daily for up to 8 weeks.
➤ *Helicobacter pylori* **eradication, to reduce risk of duodenal ulcer recurrence**
Adults: 20 mg PO b.i.d., combined with amoxicillin 1,000 mg PO b.i.d. and clarithromycin 500 mg PO b.i.d., for 7 days with morning and evening meals.

ADMINISTRATION
PO
- Have patient swallow tablets whole; don't crush or cut tablets.
- Give tablets without regard for food but if used for treatment of duodenal ulcers, give after a meal; when used for *H. pylori* eradication, give with food.
- Give a missed dose as soon as possible or skip dose if it's almost time for next dose.

ACTION
Blocks proton pump activity and gastric acid secretion by inhibiting gastric hydrogen-potassium adenosine triphosphatase (an enzyme) at secretory surface of gastric parietal cells.

Route	Onset	Peak	Duration
PO	<1 hr	2–5 hr	24 hr

Half-life: 1 to 2 hours.

ADVERSE REACTIONS
CNS: headache, pain, dizziness, taste perversion. **CV:** peripheral edema. **EENT:** dry mouth, pharyngitis. **GI:** abdominal pain, constipation, diarrhea, flatulence, nausea, vomiting. **Hepatic:** elevated liver enzyme levels, *hepatitis, hepatic encephalopathy.* **Musculoskeletal:** arthralgia, myalgia. **Other:** infection.

INTERACTIONS
Drug-drug. *Antiretrovirals (atazanavir, nelfinavir, saquinavir):* May increase or decrease exposure of antiretrovirals. Refer to antiretroviral prescribing information.
Clarithromycin: May increase rabeprazole level. Monitor patient closely.
Cyclosporine: May inhibit cyclosporine metabolism. Use together cautiously.
Digoxin: May increase digoxin level. Monitor digoxin levels.
Drugs dependent on gastric pH for absorption (ketoconazole, iron salts, dasatinib): May reduce absorption of these drugs

R

---

because of rabeprazole's effect on reducing intragastric acidity. Monitor patient closely.
Methotrexate: May increase methotrexate level and risk of toxicity. Closely monitor methotrexate level, and watch for signs and symptoms of methotrexate toxicity. Rabeprazole may need to be suspended or stopped in patients taking high-dose methotrexate.
Rilpivirine-containing products: May reduce antiviral effect and promote drug resistance. Use together is contraindicated.
Tacrolimus: May increase tacrolimus level. Monitor tacrolimus level; adjust dosage as indicated.
Warfarin: May increase warfarin level. Monitor PT and INR.

EFFECTS ON LAB TEST RESULTS

• May decrease magnesium and vitamin B_{12} levels.
• Can cause false-positive in the diagnosis of neuroendocrine tumors and gastrinoma.
• Can cause false-positive for tetrahydro-cannabinol urine screening tests.

CONTRAINDICATIONS & CAUTIONS

• Contraindicated in patients hypersensitive to drug, other benzimidazoles (lansoprazole, omeprazole), or components of these formulations.
• For *H. pylori* eradication, refer to manufacturer's instructions for contraindications to clarithromycin and amoxicillin and other administration information.
• Avoid use in patients with Child-Pugh class C liver impairment. If necessary, monitor for adverse reactions.
• Long-term (1 year or more) and multiple daily-dose rabeprazole therapy may be associated with increased risk of osteoporosis-related fractures of hip, wrist, or spine. Use lowest dosage and shortest duration of therapy appropriate to condition being treated. May consider vitamin D and calcium supplementation and following appropriate guidelines to reduce risk of fractures in patients at risk.
• Acute tubulointerstitial nephritis has been observed in patients taking rabeprazole and may occur at any point during therapy. Discontinue drug if this condition develops.
• Vitamin B_{12} malabsorption and deficiency have been reported in patients receiving prolonged daily treatment (longer than 3 years) with acid suppressants.

• Cutaneous lupus erythematosus (CLE) and SLE have been reported, occurring as both new onset and an exacerbation of existing autoimmune disease in patients of all ages within weeks to years after continuous drug therapy.
• Long-term use (1 year or more) may increase risk of fundic gland polyps. Use lowest dosage and shortest duration of therapy appropriate to condition being treated.
• SCARs, including SJS, TEN, and DRESS, have been reported with the use of PPIs. Discontinue rabeprazole at first signs or symptoms of these reactions; consider further evaluation.
Dialyzable drug: No.

PREGNANCY-LACTATION-REPRODUCTION

• There are no adequate studies during pregnancy. Use only if potential benefit justifies fetal risk.
• It isn't known if drug appears in human milk. Use cautiously during breastfeeding.

NURSING CONSIDERATIONS

• Consider additional courses of therapy if duodenal ulcer or GERD isn't healed after first course of therapy.
• If *H. pylori* eradication is unsuccessful, do susceptibility testing. If patient is resistant to clarithromycin or susceptibility testing isn't possible, expect to start therapy using a different antimicrobial.
🔵 *Alert:* PPI use lasting longer than 3 months may cause low magnesium levels, especially with concurrent magnesium-lowering drug (digoxin, diuretics) use. Monitor magnesium levels before and during treatment.
🔵 *Alert:* Monitor patients for signs and symptoms of low magnesium level (abnormal HR or rhythm, palpitations, muscle spasms, tremor, seizures). In children, abnormal HR may present as fatigue, upset stomach, dizziness, and light-headedness. Magnesium supplementation or drug discontinuation may be needed.
• Symptomatic response to therapy doesn't preclude presence of gastric malignancy.
🔵 *Alert:* Patients treated for *H. pylori* eradication have developed pseudomembranous colitis with nearly all antibiotics, including clarithromycin and amoxicillin. Monitor patient closely.
🔵 *Alert:* May increase CDAD. Evaluate for CDAD in patients who develop diarrhea

---

Reactions in bold italics are *life-threatening*.

that doesn't improve. Use lowest dosage and shortest duration appropriate to condition being treated.

• If signs or symptoms of CLE or SLE appear, discontinue drug and refer patient to the appropriate specialist for evaluation. Most patients improve with discontinuation of the PPI alone in 4 to 12 weeks.

• Temporarily stop treatment at least 14 days before diagnostic testing for neuroendocrine tumors and gastrinoma.

• *Look alike–sound alike:* Don't confuse Aciphex with Accupril or Aricept. Don't confuse rabeprazole with aripiprazole.

PATIENT TEACHING

• Instruct patient in safe drug administration. Explain importance of taking drug exactly as prescribed.

• Inform patient of risks associated with long-term use.

• Teach patient to recognize and report signs and symptoms of low magnesium levels.

raloxifene hydrochloride
ral-OKS-i-feen

Evista

Therapeutic class: Antiosteoporotics
Pharmacologic class: Selective estrogen receptor modulators

AVAILABLE FORMS
Tablets: 60 mg

INDICATIONS & DOSAGES

➤ **To prevent or treat osteoporosis; to reduce risk of invasive breast cancer in patients who have osteoporosis or are at high risk for invasive breast cancer**
Adult females after menopause: 60 mg PO once daily.

ADMINISTRATION
PO

• Give drug without regard for food.

• Stop drug at least 72 hours before prolonged immobilization and resume only after patient is fully mobilized.

ACTION
Reduces resorption of bone and decreases overall bone turnover. Also has estrogen antagonist activity to block some estrogen effects in breast and uterine tissues.

Route	Onset	Peak	Duration
PO	Unknown	Unknown	Unknown

Half-life: 27.7 to 32.5 hours.

ADVERSE REACTIONS
CNS: depression, insomnia, fever, migraine, headache, vertigo, neuralgia, hyperesthesia, syncope. **CV:** chest pain, peripheral edema, varicose veins, *thromboembolism.* **EENT:** conjunctivitis, sinusitis, rhinitis, pharyngitis, laryngitis. **GI:** nausea, diarrhea, dyspepsia, vomiting, flatulence, gastroenteritis, GI disorder, abdominal pain. **GU:** vaginitis, UTI, cystitis, leukorrhea, uterine disorder, endometrial disorder, *vaginal hemorrhage,* urinary tract disorder. **Metabolic:** weight gain. **Musculoskeletal:** arthralgia, myalgia, arthritis, tendon disorder, leg cramps, muscle spasms. **Respiratory:** cough, pneumonia, bronchitis. **Skin:** rash, diaphoresis. **Other:** infection, flulike syndrome, hot flashes, breast pain.

INTERACTIONS
Drug-drug. *Bile acid sequestrants (cholestyramine):* May cause significant decrease in raloxifene level. Avoid using together.
Highly protein-bound drugs (clofibrate, diazepam, diazoxide, ibuprofen, lidocaine, naproxen): May interfere with binding sites. Use together cautiously.
Levothyroxine: May decrease levothyroxine absorption. Consider therapy modification.
Ospemifene: May increase adverse toxic effects of both drugs. Avoid combination.
Systemic estrogens: Safety of concomitant use hasn't been established. Use together isn't recommended.
Warfarin: May decrease PT. Monitor PT and INR closely.

EFFECTS ON LAB TEST RESULTS
• May increase triglyceride level.

CONTRAINDICATIONS & CAUTIONS
Boxed Warning Increased risk of VTE and death from stroke. Contraindicated in patients with a history of, or active VTE, including deep vein thrombosis and PE, and retinal vein thrombosis. Consider risk-benefit balance in patients at risk for stroke, including those with documented CAD or

who are at increased risk for major coronary events. ■

• Raloxifene shouldn't be used for primary or secondary prevention of CV disease.

• Use cautiously in patients liver impairment or CrCl less than 60 mL/minute.

• Safety and effectiveness of drug in adult males haven't been evaluated.

• Safety of use with systemic estrogens and in patients who are premenopausal haven't been established. Use isn't recommended.

• Drug hasn't been studied adequately in patients with a history of breast cancer.

Dialyzable drug: Unknown.

⚠ *Overdose S&S:* Leg cramps, dizziness, ataxia, flushing, rash, tremors, vomiting, elevated ALP level.

PREGNANCY-LACTATION-REPRODUCTION

• Contraindicated during pregnancy. Drug isn't indicated for use in patients who may become pregnant; drug may cause fetal harm. If drug is used during pregnancy or if pregnancy occurs during therapy, apprise patient of fetal risk.

• Contraindicated during breastfeeding.

NURSING CONSIDERATIONS

• Watch for signs of blood clots. Greatest risk of thromboembolic events occurs during first 4 months of treatment.

• Evaluate breast abnormalities; drug doesn't eliminate risk of breast cancer.

• Conduct breast exams and obtain mammograms before starting and regularly during therapy.

• Monitor bone mineral density at baseline and every 1 to 3 years thereafter. Effect on bone mineral density beyond 2 years of drug treatment isn't known.

• Measure height and weight annually.

• Monitor serum calcium and vitamin D levels.

• For osteoporosis treatment, add supplemental calcium (average of 1,500 mg daily) and vitamin D (400 to 800 units daily) to the diet if daily intake is inadequate.

• Monitor triglyceride level if previous treatment with estrogen caused elevation.

PATIENT TEACHING

• Teach patient safe drug administration.

• Advise patient to avoid long periods of restricted movement (such as during traveling) because of increased risk of VTE.

• Inform patient that hot flashes or flushing may occur and that drug doesn't aid in reducing them.

• Instruct patient to practice other bone loss-prevention measures, including taking supplemental calcium and vitamin D if dietary intake is inadequate, performing weight-bearing exercises, and stopping alcohol consumption and smoking.

• Advise patient to report unexplained uterine bleeding or breast abnormalities during therapy.

• Explain adverse reactions and instruct patient to read patient information insert before starting therapy and each time prescription is renewed.

raltegravir potassium
ral-TEG-ra-vir

Isentress, Isentress HD

Therapeutic class: Antiretrovirals
Pharmacologic class: HIV integrase strand transfer inhibitors

AVAILABLE FORMS
Powder for oral suspension: 100-mg packets
Tablets (chewable): 25 mg, 100 mg
Tablets (film-coated) ⦿: 400 mg, 600 mg

INDICATIONS & DOSAGES
➤ **HIV-1 infection, with other antiretrovirals**
Adults and children weighing 40 kg or more who are treatment-naive or virologically suppressed on an initial regimen of raltegravir 400-mg tablet b.i.d.: 1,200 mg (two 600-mg tablets) PO once daily or 400-mg tablet PO b.i.d. or 300 mg chewable tablets b.i.d. if child can't swallow a tablet.
Adults who are treatment-experienced: 400-mg tablet PO b.i.d.
Adults: When administered concomitantly with rifampin, 800 mg (two 400-mg tablets) PO b.i.d.
Children weighing 28 to less than 40 kg: 400-mg tablet b.i.d. or 200 mg chewable tablets PO b.i.d. if child can't swallow a tablet.
Children weighing 25 to less than 28 kg: 400-mg tablet b.i.d. or 150 mg chewable tablets PO b.i.d. if child can't swallow a tablet.
Children at least age 4 weeks weighing 20 to less than 25 kg: 150 mg chewable tablets PO b.i.d.

Children at least age 4 weeks weighing 14 to less than 20 kg: 100 mg chewable tablets or 100 mg oral suspension (10 mL) PO b.i.d.
Children at least age 4 weeks weighing 10 to less than 14 kg: 75 mg chewable tablets or 80 mg oral suspension (8 mL) PO b.i.d.
Children at least age 4 weeks weighing 8 to less than 10 kg: 50 mg chewable tablets or 60 mg oral suspension (6 mL) PO b.i.d.
Children at least age 4 weeks weighing 6 to less than 8 kg: 50 mg chewable tablets or 40 mg oral suspension (4 mL) PO b.i.d.
Children at least age 4 weeks weighing 4 to less than 6 kg: 25 mg chewable tablet or 30 mg oral suspension (3 mL) PO b.i.d.
Children at least age 4 weeks weighing 3 to less than 4 kg: 25 mg chewable tablet or 25 mg oral suspension (2.5 mL) PO b.i.d.
Full-term neonate (birth to 28 days): Refer to manufacturer's instructions for dosage based on weight and age.

ADMINISTRATION
PO
- Don't substitute chewable tablets or oral suspension for film-coated tablets.
- Give drug without regard for meals.
- If a dose is missed, give missed dose as soon as possible; don't double next dose.

Tablets and chewable tablets
- Maximum dosage of chewable tablets is 300 mg b.i.d.
- Have patient swallow film-coated tablets whole; don't crush or cut.
- The 100-mg chewable tablet can be broken into two equal halves.
- Chewable tablets can be chewed or swallowed whole.

Oral suspension
- Maximum dosage of oral suspension is 100 mg b.i.d.
- Patients can continue oral suspension as long as weight remains below 20 kg.
- To administer, open foil packet. Measure 10 mL of water in provided mixing cup. Pour packet contents into the water, close lid, and swirl for 45 seconds. Don't shake or turn mixing cup upside down. Final concentration, 10 mg/mL.
- When mixed, measure recommended suspension dose into the oral dosing syringe.
- Give within 30 minutes of mixing. Discard any remaining suspension in the trash.
- If patient received drug 2 to 24 hours before delivery, give neonate's first dose between 24 and 48 hours after birth.

- See detailed "Instructions for Use" that comes with the oral suspension.

ACTION
Inhibits HIV-1 integrase, an enzyme required for HIV-1 replication.

Route	Onset	Peak	Duration
PO	Rapid	1.5–3 hr	Unknown

Half-life: About 9 hours.

ADVERSE REACTIONS
CNS: headache, fatigue, dizziness, insomnia, asthenia, abnormal dreams, depression, nightmares. **GI:** nausea, abdominal pain, vomiting, diarrhea, flatulence, decreased appetite. **Hematologic:** anemia, *neutropenia, thrombocytopenia.* **Hepatic:** increased LFT values. **Metabolic:** hyperglycemia, increased lipase level, increased CK level, increased lipid levels. **Musculoskeletal:** myopathy, *rhabdomyolysis.* **Skin:** rash.

INTERACTIONS
Drug-drug. *Antacids containing aluminum, magnesium, or calcium carbonate:* Ingestion with raltegravir may significantly decrease raltegravir plasma level. Coadministration or staggered administration isn't recommended.
Etravirine, tipranavir with ritonavir: May decrease level of raltegravir HD. Coadministration isn't recommended.
Fibric acid derivatives, HMG-CoA reductase inhibitors: May increase risk of rhabdomyolysis. Monitor therapy.
Strong inducers of drug-metabolizing enzymes (carbamazepine, phenobarbital, phenytoin): May affect raltegravir metabolism. Coadministration isn't recommended.
UGT1A1 inducers (rifampin): May decrease raltegravir level. Adjust raltegravir dosage to 800 mg b.i.d. when giving with rifampin. Use with 600-mg tablets isn't recommended. Use together in children hasn't been studied.

EFFECTS ON LAB TEST RESULTS
- May increase serum creatinine, bilirubin, AST, ALT, ALP, amylase, lipase, glucose, cholesterol, triglyceride, and CK levels.
- May decrease Hb level and neutrophil and platelet counts.

CONTRAINDICATIONS & CAUTIONS
🜲 *Alert:* Severe, potentially life-threatening and fatal skin reactions have been reported,

R

including SJS and TEN. Hypersensitivity reactions, including rash; organ dysfunction, including liver failure; and general malaise, muscle or joint aches, edema, conjunctivitis, facial edema, angioedema, oral blisters, and eosinophilia have also been reported. Discontinue drug immediately if signs or symptoms of SCARs or hypersensitivity reactions occur.

⚠ Alert: Use cautiously in older adults, especially those with liver, kidney, and cardiac insufficiency.

Dialyzable drug: Unknown.

PREGNANCY-LACTATION-REPRODUCTION

● Based on data from the Antiretroviral Pregnancy Registry, the risk for birth defects isn't increased with exposure to raltegravir during pregnancy. Once-daily dosing isn't recommended due to limited available data.

● Enroll patients who are pregnant and exposed to drug in the Antiretroviral Pregnancy Registry (1-800-258-4263 or https://www.apregistry.com/).

● The CDC recommends that patients with HIV infection not breastfeed to avoid HIV transmission to the infant.

NURSING CONSIDERATIONS

● Obtain lab tests, including viral load, CD4 count, CBC, platelet count, and LFTs, before therapy and regularly throughout therapy.

● Use drug with at least one other antiretroviral.

● Watch for signs and symptoms of myopathy or rash.

● Monitor patient for signs and symptoms of depression and suicidality.

● Monitor patient for immune reconstitution syndrome (inflammatory response to indolent or residual opportunistic infections [CMV, MAC, *Pneumocystis jiroveci* pneumonia, TB]), which may necessitate further evaluation and treatment.

● Autoimmune disorders (such as Graves disease, polymyositis, and Guillain-Barré syndrome) have been reported in the setting of immune reconstitution; time to onset varies, and can occur many months after initiation treatment.

● Avoid dosing before a dialysis session because the extent to which drug may be dialyzable is unknown.

PATIENT TEACHING

● Inform patient that drug doesn't cure HIV infection, that patient may continue to develop opportunistic infections and other complications of HIV infection, and transmit HIV to others through sexual contact or blood contamination.

● Advise patient to use barrier protection during sexual intercourse.

● Tell patient that breastfeeding isn't recommended.

● Instruct patient in safe drug preparation and administration.

● Advise patient to immediately report worsening symptoms or unexplained muscle pain, tenderness, or weakness while taking the drug.

● Instruct patient to avoid missing any doses to decrease the risk of developing resistance.

● Caution patient to immediately stop taking raltegravir and seek medical attention if a rash associated with any of the following signs or symptoms develops: fever; generally ill feeling; extreme tiredness; muscle or joint aches; blisters; oral lesions; eye inflammation; facial swelling; swelling of the eyes, lips, or mouth; breathing difficulty; or signs and symptoms of liver problems (yellowing of skin or whites of eyes, dark or tea-colored urine, pale-colored stools or bowel movements, nausea, vomiting, loss of appetite, pain, aching or sensitivity on right side below ribs).

● Inform patient with phenylketonuria that the chewable tablets contain phenylalanine.

● Advise patient to report use of other drugs, including OTC drugs because of risk of interaction.

ramelteon
ra-MEL-tee-on

Rozerem

Therapeutic class: Hypnotics
Pharmacologic class: Melatonin receptor agonists

AVAILABLE FORMS
Tablets ⊘*:* 8 mg

INDICATIONS & DOSAGES

➤ **Insomnia characterized by trouble falling asleep**
Adults: 8 mg PO within 30 minutes of bedtime. Maximum dose is 8 mg daily.

Reactions in bold italics are *life-threatening*.

ADMINISTRATION
PO
• Don't give drug with or immediately after a high-fat meal.
• Have patient swallow tablet whole; don't break or crush.

ACTION
Acts on receptors believed to maintain the circadian rhythm underlying the normal sleep-wake cycle.

Route	Onset	Peak	Duration
PO	Rapid	0.5–1.5 hr	Unknown

Half-life: Parent compound, 1 to 2.6 hours; metabolite M-II, 2 to 5 hours.

ADVERSE REACTIONS
CNS: worsened depression, dizziness, fatigue, headache, somnolence, worsened insomnia. **GI:** nausea.

INTERACTIONS
Drug-drug. *CNS depressants:* May cause excessive CNS depression. Use together cautiously.
Donepezil, doxepin: May increase ramelteon level. Monitor patient closely.
🔴 *Alert: Opioids:* May cause slow or difficult breathing, sedation, and death. Avoid use together. If use together is necessary, limit dosage and duration of each drug to minimum necessary for desired effect.
Strong CYP enzyme inducer (rifampin): May decrease ramelteon level. Monitor patient for lack of effect.
Strong CYP1A2 inhibitor (fluvoxamine): May increase ramelteon level. Use together is contraindicated.
Strong CYP2C9 inhibitor (fluconazole), strong CYP3A4 inhibitor (ketoconazole), weak CYP1A2 inhibitors: May increase ramelteon level. Use together cautiously.
Drug-food. *Food (especially high-fat meals):* May delay time to peak drug effect. Tell patient to take drug on an empty stomach.
Drug-lifestyle. *Alcohol use:* May cause excessive CNS depression. Discourage alcohol use.

EFFECTS ON LAB TEST RESULTS
• May increase prolactin level.
• May decrease testosterone level.

CONTRAINDICATIONS & CAUTIONS
• Contraindicated in patients hypersensitive to drug or its components. Don't use in patients with Child-Pugh class C liver impairment, severe sleep apnea, or severe COPD.
• Use cautiously in patients with depression or Child-Pugh class B liver impairment.
• Drug is associated with abnormal thinking and behavior changes, including worsening depression, hallucinations, aggression, bizarre behavior, agitation, mania, amnesia, anxiety, and other neuropsychiatric symptoms, which may occur unpredictably.
• Safety and effectiveness in children haven't been established.
Dialyzable drug: No.

PREGNANCY-LACTATION-REPRODUCTION
• There are no adequate studies during pregnancy. Drug may cause fetal harm. Use only if clearly needed and potential benefit justifies fetal risk.
• Drug appears in human milk. Use cautiously during breastfeeding. Monitor infants exposed to drug for somnolence and feeding problems.
• Drug has been associated with decreased testosterone levels and increased prolactin levels. Effects on reproduction are unknown.

NURSING CONSIDERATIONS
🔴 *Alert:* Anaphylaxis and angioedema may occur as early as the first dose. Monitor patient closely. Emergency treatment may be needed.
• Thoroughly evaluate the cause of insomnia before starting drug.
• Assess patient for behavioral or cognitive disorders.
• Failure of insomnia to resolve after 7 to 10 days of treatment may indicate presence of a primary psychiatric or medical illness that should be evaluated.
🔴 *Alert:* Monitor patient for signs and symptoms of depression, worsening of depression, and suicidality.
• Drug doesn't cause physical dependence.
• *Look alike–sound alike:* Don't confuse Rozerem with Remeron. Don't confuse ramelteon with Remeron.

PATIENT TEACHING
• Instruct patient in safe drug administration.
• Caution patient or caregiver of patient taking an opioid with a benzodiazepine, CNS

R

depressant, or alcohol to seek immediate medical attention for dizziness, lightheadedness, extreme sleepiness, slowed or difficult breathing, or unresponsiveness. Advise patient to avoid alcohol while taking drug.

🔹 *Alert:* Warn patient that drug may cause allergic reactions, facial swelling, and complex sleep-related behaviors, such as driving, eating, and making phone calls while asleep. Advise patient to report these adverse effects.

• Advise patient and caregiver to report signs and symptoms of depression, worsening of depression, suicidality, nightmares, or hallucinations.

• Caution against performing activities that require mental alertness or physical coordination after taking drug.

• Tell patient to consult prescriber if insomnia worsens or behavior changes.

• Urge patient to consult prescriber if menses stops, libido decreases, or galactorrhea or fertility problems develop.

ramipril 🔞
RA-mi-pril

Altace

Therapeutic class: Antihypertensives
Pharmacologic class: ACE inhibitors

AVAILABLE FORMS
Capsules 🔞: 1.25 mg, 2.5 mg, 5 mg, 10 mg

INDICATIONS & DOSAGES
➤ **HTN**
Adults: Initially, 2.5 mg PO once daily for patients not taking a diuretic and 1.25 mg PO once daily for patients taking a diuretic. Increase dosage, if needed, based on patient response. Maintenance dose, 2.5 to 20 mg daily as a single dose or in divided doses.
Adjust-a-dose: For patients with CrCl less than 40 mL/minute, give 1.25 mg PO daily. Adjust dosage gradually based on response. Maximum daily dose, 5 mg.
➤ **HF after MI**
Adults: Initially, 2.5 mg PO b.i.d. If hypotension occurs, decrease dosage to 1.25 mg PO b.i.d. Adjust as tolerated, with dosage increase at 1 week and subsequent increases about 3 weeks apart, to target dosage of 5 mg PO b.i.d.

Adjust-a-dose: For patients with CrCl less than 40 mL/minute, give 1.25 mg PO daily. Adjust dosage gradually based on response. Maximum dosage is 2.5 mg b.i.d.
➤ **To reduce risk of MI, stroke, and death from CV causes**
Adults ages 55 and older: 2.5 mg PO once daily for 1 week, then 5 mg PO once daily for 3 weeks. Increase as tolerated to a maintenance dose of 10 mg PO once daily.
Adjust-a-dose: In patients who are hypertensive or who have recently had an MI, daily dose may be divided.

ADMINISTRATION
PO
• Give drug without regard for meals.
• Have patient swallow capsules whole; don't crush.
• If patient can't swallow capsules, open capsule and sprinkle contents on a small amount of applesauce (4 oz) or mix with 120 mL of water or apple juice. May store for up to 24 hours at room temperature or up to 48 hours under refrigeration if not given immediately.

ACTION
Prevents conversion of angiotensin I to angiotensin II, a potent vasoconstrictor. Less angiotensin II decreases peripheral arterial resistance, decreasing aldosterone secretion, which reduces sodium and water retention and lowers BP.

Route	Onset	Peak	Duration
PO	1–2 hr	2–4 hr	24 hr

Half-life: 13 to 17 hours.

ADVERSE REACTIONS
CNS: headache, dizziness, fatigue, vertigo, syncope. **CV:** hypotension, angina pectoris. **GI:** nausea, vomiting, diarrhea. **GU:** abnormal kidney function. **Metabolic:** *hyperkalemia.* **Respiratory:** cough.

INTERACTIONS
Drug-drug. 🔹 *Alert: ACE inhibitors, ARBs, aliskiren:* May increase risk of kidney impairment, hypotension, and hyperkalemia. Aliskiren used together with ramipril is contraindicated in patients with diabetes and should be avoided in patients with GFR less than 60 mL/minute.

Reactions in bold italics are *life-threatening*.

Diuretics: May cause excessive hypotension, especially at start of therapy. Decrease or discontinue diuretic, increase sodium intake, or reduce starting dose of ramipril.

Insulin, oral antidiabetics: May cause hypoglycemia, especially at start of ramipril therapy. Monitor glucose level closely.

Iron dextran: May increase risk of anaphylactic-type reaction. Monitor patient closely.

Lanthanum: May decrease ramipril level. Give ramipril at least 2 hours before or after lanthanum.

Lithium: May increase lithium level. Use together cautiously and monitor lithium level.

mTOR inhibitors (temsirolimus): May increase risk of angioedema. Monitor therapy.

Neprilysin inhibitors (sacubitril): May increase risk of angioedema. Use together is contraindicated. Allow 36 hours between drugs.

NSAIDs (salicylates): May decrease antihypertensive effects and increase risk of kidney impairment. Monitor BP and kidney function.

Potassium-sparing diuretics, potassium supplements: May cause hyperkalemia; ramipril attenuates potassium loss. Monitor potassium level closely.

Telmisartan: May increase risk of kidney impairment. Avoid use together.

Drug-herb. *Capsaicin:* May cause cough. Discourage use together.

Grass pollen allergen extract (5 grass extract): May increase risk of severe allergic reaction to 5 grass extract. Don't use together.

Ma huang: May decrease antihypertensive effects. Discourage use together.

Drug-food. *Salt substitutes containing potassium:* May cause hyperkalemia; ramipril attenuates potassium loss. Discourage use of salt substitutes during therapy.

EFFECTS ON LAB TEST RESULTS
• May increase BUN, creatinine, bilirubin, liver enzyme, glucose, and potassium levels.
• May decrease Hb level and hematocrit.
• May decrease RBC and platelet counts.

CONTRAINDICATIONS & CAUTIONS
• Contraindicated in patients hypersensitive to ACE inhibitors and in those with a history of angioedema related to ACE inhibitor use.
• Use cautiously in patients with a history of angioedema unrelated to ACE inhibitors.
• Use cautiously in patients with kidney or liver impairment.

• Anaphylactoid reactions have been reported in patients dialyzed with high-flux membranes and also treated with ACE inhibitors and in those undergoing LDL apheresis with dextran sulfate absorption.

Dialyzable drug: Unknown.

⚠ *Overdose S&S:* Hypotension.

PREGNANCY-LACTATION-REPRODUCTION
Boxed Warning Use during pregnancy can cause injury and death to the developing fetus. Stop drug as soon as pregnancy is detected. ■
• Drug may appear in human milk. Use during breastfeeding isn't recommended.

NURSING CONSIDERATIONS
• Monitor BP regularly for drug effectiveness.
• Correct fluid and electrolyte imbalances before starting therapy.
• Closely assess kidney function in patients during first few weeks of therapy, then regularly thereafter. Dosage reduction or drug stoppage may be necessary.
▨ Although ACE inhibitors reduce BP in all races, they reduce it less in patients who are Black taking the ACE inhibitor alone. These patients should use drug in combination therapy for a more favorable response.
▨ ACE inhibitors appear to increase risk of angioedema in patients who are Black.
• Discontinue drug if patient develops jaundice or significant liver enzyme elevation (rare).
• Monitor CBC with differential counts before therapy and periodically thereafter.
• Drug may reduce Hb and WBC, RBC, and platelet counts, especially in patients with impaired kidney function or collagen vascular diseases (SLE or scleroderma).
• Monitor potassium level. Risk factors for hyperkalemia include kidney impairment, diabetes, and concomitant use of drugs that raise potassium level.
• *Look alike–sound alike:* Don't confuse ramipril with enalapril. Don't confuse Altace with alteplase.

PATIENT TEACHING
• Teach patient safe drug administration.
• Tell patient to report adverse reactions. Dosage adjustment or discontinuation may be needed.
⊘ *Alert:* Instruct patient to immediately report signs or symptoms of angioedema (breathing

R

difficulty or swelling of face, eyes, lips, or tongue).
• Inform patient that light-headedness can occur, especially during first few days of therapy. Tell patient to rise slowly to minimize this effect and to report light-headedness to prescriber. If fainting occurs, advise patient to stop drug and call prescriber immediately.
• Advise patient to report signs and symptoms of infection, such as fever and sore throat.
• Tell patient to avoid potassium salt substitutes.
Boxed Warning Tell patient of childbearing potential to report pregnancy. Drug will need to be stopped. ∎

SAFETY ALERT!

ramucirumab ⚥
ra-mue-SIR-ue-mab

Cyramza

Therapeutic class: Antineoplastics
Pharmacologic class: Monoclonal antibodies

AVAILABLE FORMS
Injection: 10 mg/mL single-dose vial

INDICATIONS & DOSAGES
Adjust-a-dose (for all indications): Refer to manufacturer's instructions for toxicity-related dosage.

➤ **Advanced gastric cancer or gastroesophageal junction adenocarcinoma, as a single agent or in combination with paclitaxel, after prior fluoropyrimidine- or platinum-containing chemotherapy**
Adults: 8 mg/kg IV every 2 weeks. Continue until disease progression or unacceptable toxicity. When given in combination, administer ramucirumab before paclitaxel.

➤ **Metastatic NSCLC in combination with docetaxel in patients with disease progression on or after platinum-based chemotherapy. (Patients with *EGFR* or *ALK* genomic tumor aberrations should have shown disease progression after treatment for these aberrations.)** ⚥
Adults: 10 mg/kg IV on day 1 of a 21-day cycle before docetaxel infusion. Continue until disease progression or unacceptable toxicity.

➤ **First-line treatment, in combination with erlotinib, for metastatic NSCLC with *EGFR* exon 19 deletions or exon 21 (L858R) mutations** ⚥
Adults: 10 mg/kg IV infusion every 2 weeks. Continue until disease progression or unacceptable toxicity occurs. Refer to manufacturer's instructions for erlotinib prescribing information.

➤ **Colorectal cancer in combination with FOLFIRI (irinotecan, folinic acid, and 5-FU) in patients with disease progression on or after therapy with bevacizumab, oxaliplatin, and a fluoropyrimidine**
Adults: 8 mg/kg IV every 2 weeks before FOLFIRI administration. Continue until disease progression or unacceptable toxicity.

➤ **Hepatocellular carcinoma in patients who have an alpha-fetoprotein of at least 400 ng/mL and have been treated with sorafenib**
Adults: 8 mg/kg IV infusion every 2 weeks. Continue until disease progression or unacceptable toxicity.

ADMINISTRATION
IV
⊙ *Alert:* Hazardous drug; use safe handling and disposal precautions.
▼ Administer the first infusion over 60 minutes. If tolerated, may administer subsequent infusions over 30 minutes.
▼ For each infusion, premedicate with IV histamine (H₁) antagonist (diphenhydramine). For patients with prior grade 1 or 2 infusion-related reaction, also premedicate with dexamethasone or equivalent and acetaminophen before each infusion.
▼ Dilute drug with NSS to final volume of 250 mL. Diluted solution remains stable for 24 hours if refrigerated or 4 hours at room temperature. Gently invert container; don't shake.
▼ Inspect solution for particles and discoloration before administration.
▼ Give infusion through separate infusion line using a protein-sparing 0.22-micron filter. Flush line with NSS at end of infusion.
▼ Store vials in refrigerator at 36° to 46° F (2° to 8° C) until ready to use. Keep vial in outer carton to protect from light. Don't freeze vial.
▼ **Incompatibilities:** Dextrose solutions, electrolytes, other medications.

Reactions in bold italics are *life-threatening*.

ACTION
A vascular endothelial growth factor receptor 2 antagonist that inhibits proliferation and migration of human endothelial cells, angiogenesis, and tumor growth.

Route	Onset	Peak	Duration
IV	Unknown	Unknown	Unknown

Half-life: 14 days.

ADVERSE REACTIONS
CNS: headache, fatigue, insomnia, fever. **CV:** HTN, peripheral edema, *arterial thromboembolic events, hemorrhage.* **EENT:** increased tearing, epistaxis, gum hemorrhage. **GI:** diarrhea, intestinal obstruction, stomatitis, *GI hemorrhage, GI perforation,* decreased appetite, abdominal pain, ascites, nausea, vomiting. **GU:** proteinuria. **Hematologic:** anemia, *neutropenia, thrombocytopenia.* **Hepatic:** increased LFT values. **Metabolic:** hyponatremia, hypoalbuminemia, hypothyroidism, *hypokalemia, hypocalcemia.* **Musculoskeletal:** back pain. **Skin:** rash, alopecia, hand-foot syndrome. **Other:** *sepsis,* infections, antibody development, infusion-related reaction.

INTERACTIONS
None reported.

EFFECTS ON LAB TEST RESULTS
• May increase LFT values and TSH and urine protein levels.
• May decrease sodium, calcium, potassium, and albumin levels.
• May decrease Hb level and RBC, neutrophil, and platelet counts.

CONTRAINDICATIONS & CAUTIONS
• Drug increases risk of hemorrhage, including severe and sometimes fatal hemorrhagic events. Permanently discontinue drug in patients who experience severe bleeding.
• Withhold drug 28 days before surgery. Resume at least 2 weeks after the surgical intervention based on clinical judgment of adequate wound healing. If patient develops wound-healing complications during therapy, discontinue drug until wound is fully healed.
• Permanently discontinue drug in patients who experience GI perforation, a potentially fatal event.
• Use cautiously in patients with Child-Pugh class B or C liver impairment if potential benefits outweigh risks.

⚠ *Alert:* Rare and sometimes fatal PRES has been reported.
• Safety and effectiveness in children haven't been established.
Dialyzable drug: Unknown.

PREGNANCY-LACTATION-REPRODUCTION
• Drug may cause fetal harm. Patients of childbearing potential should use effective contraception during and for at least 3 months after last ramucirumab dose.
• It isn't known if drug appears in human milk. Because of the risk of serious adverse reactions in infants who are breastfed, breastfeeding isn't recommended during treatment.
• Based on animal data, drug may impair fertility in adult females.

NURSING CONSIDERATIONS
⚠ *Alert:* Serious, sometimes fatal, arterial thromboembolic events, including MI, cardiac arrest, stroke, and cerebral ischemia, have occurred. Monitor patient closely, and permanently discontinue drug in patients who experience a severe embolic event.
• Assess BP every 2 weeks or more frequently as clinically indicated. Control HTN before start of therapy. If severe HTN occurs, withhold drug until controlled. Discontinue drug permanently if HTN can't be controlled, in hypertensive crisis, or in hypertensive encephalopathy.
• Premedicate before each infusion, and monitor patient for infusion-related reactions.
⚠ *Alert:* Assess patient for signs and symptoms of GI perforation (severe abdominal pain, nausea, vomiting, fever).
⚠ *Alert:* Monitor recent wounds for complications during therapy.
• Monitor patients with Child-Pugh class B or C liver impairment for new-onset or worsening encephalopathy, ascites, or hepatorenal syndrome.
• Monitor patient for signs and symptoms of PRES (HTN, headache, visual disturbances, altered consciousness, seizures). Confirm diagnosis with MRI; discontinue drug and provide supportive care.
• Monitor thyroid function.
• Monitor for proteinuria. Withhold drug for protein levels of 2 g or more per 24 hours. Permanently discontinue for protein levels greater than 3 g per 24 hours or nephrotic syndrome.

R

• *Look alike–sound alike:* Don't confuse Cyramza with Cimzia.

PATIENT TEACHING

❂ *Alert:* Inform patient that drug can cause severe bleeding. Advise patient to contact prescriber for bleeding or symptoms of bleeding, including light-headedness.

• Warn patient of increased risk of embolic events.

• Advise patient to undergo routine BP monitoring and to contact health care provider if BP is elevated or if signs and symptoms of HTN (severe headache, light-headedness, or neurologic symptoms) occur.

❂ *Alert:* Caution patient to notify health care provider for severe diarrhea, vomiting, or severe abdominal pain.

❂ *Alert:* Warn patient that drug may impair wound healing. Instruct patient not to undergo surgery without first discussing risk with health care provider.

• Teach patient about risk of maintaining pregnancy, risk to fetus, and risk to postnatal infant development during and after treatment with ramucirumab. Discuss need to avoid pregnancy, including use of adequate contraception, for at least 3 months after last dose.

• Advise patient of childbearing potential that drug may impair fertility.

• Counsel patient on the need to discontinue breastfeeding during treatment.

ranolazine
ra-NOE-la-zeen

Aspruzyo Sprinkle

Therapeutic class: Antianginals
Pharmacologic class: CV drugs

AVAILABLE FORMS

Granules (extended-release) ⓄⓃⒸ: 500 mg, 1,000 mg
Tablets (extended-release) ⓄⓃⒸ: 500 mg, 1,000 mg

INDICATIONS & DOSAGES
➤ **Chronic angina**
Adults: Initially, 500 mg PO b.i.d. Increase, if needed, to maximum of 1,000 mg b.i.d.
Adjust-a-dose: Limit maximum dose to 500 mg b.i.d. in patients on moderate CYP3A inhibitors.

ADMINISTRATION
PO
• Give without regard for meals.
• Have patient swallow tablets whole; don't crush or cut tablets. Granules shouldn't be crushed or chewed.
• Sprinkle granules on 1 tablespoon of soft food and have patient consume immediately.
• To give through NG or gastrostomy (G) tube, add granules to catheter tip syringe with 50 mL water for NG tube or 30 mL water for G tube. Gently shake for 15 seconds, then promptly deliver through a #12 French or larger NG or G tube. Rinse syringe with additional water to ensure all granules were given.
• If a dose is missed, give at next scheduled time; don't double a dose.

ACTION
May result from increased efficiency of myocardial oxygen use when myocardial metabolism is shifted away from fatty acid oxidation toward glucose oxidation. Antianginal and anti-ischemic properties don't decrease HR or BP and don't increase myocardial work.

Route	Onset	Peak	Duration
PO	Rapid	2–5 hr	Unknown

Half-life: 7 hours.

ADVERSE REACTIONS
CNS: dizziness, headache, syncope, vertigo, confusion. **CV:** palpitations, *bradycardia,* peripheral edema, hypotension. **EENT:** blurred vision, tinnitus, dry mouth. **GI:** abdominal pain, constipation, nausea, vomiting, dyspepsia, anorexia. **GU:** hematuria. **Respiratory:** dyspnea. **Skin:** excessive sweating.

INTERACTIONS
Drug-drug. *CYP2D6 substrates (antipsychotics, TCAs):* May increase levels of these drugs. Substrate dosage reduction may be needed.
CYP3A inducers (carbamazepine, phenobarbital, phenytoin, rifabutin, rifampin, rifapentine): May reduce ranolazine level to subtherapeutic levels. Use together is contraindicated.
Digoxin: May increase digoxin level. Monitor digoxin level periodically; digoxin dosage may need to be reduced.
Drugs that prolong QT interval (antiarrhythmics [dofetilide, quinidine,

Reactions in bold italics are *life-threatening*.

sotalol], antipsychotics [chlorpromazine, ziprasidone]): May increase risk of prolonged QT interval and ventricular arrhythmia. Use cautiously together.

Metformin: May increase metformin level when given with ranolazine 1,000 mg b.i.d. Limit metformin dosage to 1,700 mg/day and monitor blood glucose level.

Moderate CYP3A inhibitors (diltiazem, erythromycin, verapamil): May increase ranolazine level. Limit maximum ranolazine dosage to 500 mg b.i.d.

P-gp inhibitors (amiloride, atorvastatin, cyclosporine, felodipine): May increase ranolazine level. Use cautiously together and titrate ranolazine dosage based on clinical response.

Simvastatin: May increase simvastatin level. Limit simvastatin dosage to 20 mg once daily, and monitor patient for adverse effects.

Strong CYP3A inhibitors (clarithromycin, ketoconazole, nefazodone, ritonavir, saquinavir): May increase ranolazine level. Use together is contraindicated.

Drug-herb. *St. John's wort:* May reduce ranolazine level to subtherapeutic levels. Discourage use together.

Drug-food. *Grapefruit products:* May increase drug level and prolong QT interval. Discourage use together.

Drug-lifestyle. *Alcohol:* May cause rapid release of ranolazine from granules. Discourage alcohol use with sprinkle form.

EFFECTS ON LAB TEST RESULTS
• May increase potassium, creatinine, and BUN levels.

CONTRAINDICATIONS & CAUTIONS
• Contraindicated in patients with liver cirrhosis.
• Use cautiously in patients with kidney impairment. Discontinue drug if AKI develops.
⚠ *Alert:* Drug prolongs QT interval according to dose. Use cautiously in patients taking QT interval-prolonging drugs and in those with family history of long QT syndrome, congenital long QT syndrome, or acquired QT-interval prolongation. Clinical studies didn't show an increased risk of proarrhythmia or sudden death.
• Drug isn't indicated for ACS.
Dialyzable drug: Unlikely.

PREGNANCY-LACTATION-REPRODUCTION
• Studies during pregnancy are inadeqate. Use only if potential benefit justifies fetal risk.

• It isn't known if drug appears in human milk. Patient should discontinue breastfeeding or discontinue drug, considering importance of drug to patient.

NURSING CONSIDERATIONS
• Obtain baseline ECG and monitor subsequent ECG for prolonged QT interval. Measure QTc interval regularly.
• Monitor kidney function at baseline and periodically during treatment in patients with CrCl less than 60 mL/min.
• Monitor electrolyte levels, especially potassium, and correct abnormalities.

PATIENT TEACHING
• Teach patient about drug's potential to affect heart rhythm. Advise patient to immediately report palpitations or fainting.
• Urge patient to report all other prescription or OTC drugs or herbal supplements being taken.
• Tell patient to keep taking other drugs prescribed for angina.
• Teach patient safe drug administration.
• Explain that drug won't stop a sudden anginal attack. Advise patient to keep other treatments, such as SL nitroglycerin, readily available.
• Tell patient to avoid activities that require mental alertness until drug's effects are known.

rasagiline mesylate
ra-SA-ji-leen

Azilect

Therapeutic class: Antiparkinsonians
Pharmacologic class: Irreversible, selective MAO inhibitors type B

AVAILABLE FORMS
Tablets: 0.5 mg, 1 mg

INDICATIONS & DOSAGES
➤ **Parkinson disease**
Adults: As monotherapy, 1 mg PO once daily. As adjunct to levodopa, initial dose is 0.5 mg PO once daily. May increase to 1 mg PO once daily based on tolerance and clinical response.
Adjust-a-dose: If patient has Child-Pugh class A liver impairment or takes a CYP1A2 inhibitor, give 0.5 mg once daily.

R

ADMINISTRATION
PO
- Give drug without regard to meals.
- If a dose is missed, omit the missed dose and give next dose as scheduled; don't double dose.

ACTION
Unknown. May increase extracellular dopamine level in the CNS, improving neurotransmission and relieving signs and symptoms of Parkinson disease.

Route	Onset	Peak	Duration
PO	Variable	1 hr	1 wk

Half-life: 3 hours.

ADVERSE REACTIONS
Monotherapy
CNS: headache, depression, fever, hallucinations, malaise, paresthesia, vertigo. **EENT:** conjunctivitis, rhinitis. **GI:** dyspepsia, gastroenteritis. **Musculoskeletal:** arthralgia, arthritis, neck pain. **Skin:** ecchymosis. **Other:** falls, flulike syndrome.
Adjunctive therapy
CNS: insomnia, dizziness, headache, abnormal dreams, ataxia, dyskinesia, dystonia, hallucinations, paresthesia, somnolence. **CV:** peripheral edema, orthostatic hypotension, *hemorrhage.* **EENT:** dry mouth, gingivitis. **GI:** nausea, abdominal pain, anorexia, constipation, diarrhea, dyspepsia, vomiting, *GI hemorrhage.* **Metabolic:** weight loss. **Musculoskeletal:** arthralgia, back pain, hernia, myasthenia, neck pain, tenosynovitis. **Respiratory:** dyspnea, cough, URI. **Skin:** ecchymosis, rash, diaphoresis. **Other:** infection, accidental injury, falls.

INTERACTIONS
Drug-drug. *Ciprofloxacin and other CYP1A2 inhibitors:* May double rasagiline level. Decrease rasagiline dosage to 0.5 mg daily.
Cyclobenzaprine: May enhance serotonergic effects. Concomitant use is contraindicated.
Dextromethorphan: May cause episodes of psychosis or bizarre behavior. Use together is contraindicated.
Dopamine antagonists (antipsychotics, metoclopramide): May decrease effectiveness of rasagiline. Avoid use together.
Levodopa: May increase rasagiline level. Watch for dyskinesia, dystonia, hallucinations, and hypotension, and reduce levodopa dosage if needed.

MAO inhibitors: May cause serotonin syndrome. Contraindicated with or within 14 days of other MAO inhibitors.
Opiate agonists (fentanyl, meperidine, methadone, tramadol): May cause severe, sometimes fatal, serotonin syndrome. Concomitant use is contraindicated.
SNRIs, SSRIs, TCAs, tetracyclic antidepressants, triazolopyridine antidepressants: May cause serotonin syndrome. Stop rasagiline for at least 14 days before starting an antidepressant. Stop fluoxetine for 5 weeks before starting rasagiline.
Sympathomimetics (decongestants): May cause severe hypertensive reaction. Use together cautiously.
Drug-herb. *St. John's wort:* May cause severe reaction. Use together is contraindicated.
Drug-food. *Foods with very high levels of tyramine (more than 150 mg), such as aged cheeses, cured meats, fava beans:* May cause hypertensive reaction. Urge patient to avoid foods high in tyramine.

EFFECTS ON LAB TEST RESULTS
None reported.

CONTRAINDICATIONS & CAUTIONS
- Exacerbation of HTN may occur during treatment, which may require medication adjustment if sustained.
- Somnolence and falling asleep without prior warning while engaged in ADLs (including operating motor vehicles) have been reported in some patients. Evaluate patient for factors that may increase these risks.
- Use cautiously in patients with Child-Pugh class A liver impairment. Use in patients with Child-Pugh class B or C liver impairment isn't recommended.
Dialyzable drug: Unknown.
⚠ **Overdose S&S:** Drowsiness, dizziness, faintness, irritability, hyperactivity, agitation, severe headache, hallucinations, trismus, opisthotonos, seizures, coma, rapid and irregular pulse, HTN, hypotension and vascular collapse, precordial pain, respiratory depression and failure, hyperpyrexia, diaphoresis, cool and clammy skin.

PREGNANCY-LACTATION-REPRODUCTION
- There are no adequate studies during pregnancy. Use only if potential benefit justifies fetal risk.

Reactions in bold italics are *life-threatening*.

• It isn't known if drug appears in human milk. Use cautiously during breastfeeding.

NURSING CONSIDERATIONS

• Orthostatic hypotension occurs most frequently during first 2 months of therapy; help patient to rise from a reclining position.

• Monitor patient for new-onset HTN or HTN that isn't adequately controlled after starting drug.

• Monitor patient for serotonin syndrome (restlessness, hallucinations, loss of coordination, seizures, fast heartbeat, rapid BP changes, elevated body temperature, hyperreflexia, nausea, vomiting, diarrhea).

• Monitor patient for drowsiness, significant daytime sleepiness, or episodes of falling asleep during activities that require active participation. Discontinue drug if these symptoms occur.

• Ask patient or caregiver about new or worsening impulsive or compulsive behaviors, such as new or increased gambling urges, sexual urges, uncontrolled spending, or other urges; patient may not recognize these behaviors as abnormal.

• Monitor patient for dyskinesia and dopaminergic adverse effects when drug is used as an adjunct to levodopa. Drug may also exacerbate preexisting dyskinesia.

• Screen patient's skin periodically for melanoma; patients with Parkinson disease have a higher skin cancer risk.

• Monitor patient for withdrawal-related signs and symptoms (elevated temperature, muscle rigidity, altered level of consciousness, autonomic instability), especially after rapid dosage reduction or withdrawal or change in drugs.

• Notify prescriber if patient is having elective surgery; drug may need to be stopped or MAO-safe anesthetics used.

• *Look alike–sound alike:* Don't confuse Azilect with Aricept.

PATIENT TEACHING

• Instruct patient in safe drug administration.

• Explain the risk of hypertensive crisis if patient ingests foods containing high levels of tyramine while taking rasagiline. Give patient a list of these foods.

• Advise patient to rise slowly after prolonged sitting or lying down.

• Review signs and symptoms of serotonin syndrome and tell patient to report them immediately.

• Advise patient that drug may cause patient to fall asleep during activities that require active participation and to report if drowsiness, significant daytime sleepiness, or episodes of falling asleep during such activities occur.

• Tell patient to report difficulty controlling impulsive or compulsive behaviors.

• Urge patient to watch for skin changes that could suggest melanoma and to have periodic skin exams.

• Tell patient to report plans to become pregnant or to breastfeed.

• Advise patient to contact prescriber before discontinuing rasagiline.

relugolix
re-loo-GOE-lix

Orgovyx

Therapeutic class: Endocrine drugs
Pharmacologic class: GnRH receptor antagonists

AVAILABLE FORMS
Tablets ⓄⓃⒸ: 120 mg

INDICATIONS & DOSAGES
➤ **Advanced prostate cancer**
Adults: 360 mg PO on day 1, then 120 mg PO once daily.
Adjust-a-dose: If use with combined P-gp and strong CYP3A inducers can't be avoided, increase relugolix dosage to 240 mg once daily. After discontinuing the combined P-gp and strong CYP3A inducer, resume 120 mg daily relugolix dosage.

ADMINISTRATION
PO
• Give without regard to food and at same time each day.
• Have patient swallow tablets whole; don't crush or cut tablets.
• Give missed dose as soon as possible. If more than 12 hours has elapsed since the missed dose, skip the dose and resume regular schedule the next day.
• If therapy is interrupted beyond 7 days, restart drug at 360 mg on day 1, then continue with 120 mg once daily.
• Store at room temperature. Don't store above 86° F (30° C).

R

ACTION
Reduces release of LH, FSH, and testosterone by binding to pituitary GnRH receptors.

Route	Onset	Peak	Duration
PO	Unknown	2.25 hr	Unknown

Half-life: 60.8 hours.

ADVERSE REACTIONS
CNS: fatigue. **GI:** constipation, diarrhea. **Hematologic:** anemia. **Hepatic:** elevated AST and ALT levels. **Metabolic:** hyperglycemia, hypertriglyceridemia. **Musculoskeletal:** musculoskeletal pain. **Other:** hot flushes, hypersensitivity reactions.

INTERACTIONS
Drug-drug. *Combined P-gp and strong CYP3A inducers (carbamazepine, dexamethasone, rifampin):* May decrease relugolix level and effectiveness. Avoid use together. If unable to avoid use together, increase relugolix dosage.
Drugs that prolong QTc interval (ciprofloxacin, haloperidol, lithium, methadone, procainamide, SSRIs, TCAs): May increase risk of prolonged QTc interval. Monitor patient closely.
Oral P-gp inhibitors (amiodarone, erythromycin, ketoconazole, saquinavir): May increase relugolix level. Avoid use together. If unable to avoid use together, give inhibitor at least 6 hours after relugolix and monitor patient frequently for adverse reactions. May interrupt relugolix therapy for up to 2 weeks if a short course of P-gp inhibitor therapy is required.
Drug-herb. *St John's wort:* May decrease relugolix level and effectiveness. Discourage use together.

EFFECTS ON LAB TEST RESULTS
• May increase glucose, triglyceride, ALT, and AST levels.
• May decrease Hb, PSA, and testosterone levels.

CONTRAINDICATIONS & CAUTIONS
• Contraindicated in patients with severe hypersensitivity to drug or any of its components. Pharyngeal edema and angioedema have been reported.
• Androgen deprivation therapy may prolong QT interval. Weigh benefits of therapy against risk in patients with congenital long QT

syndrome, HF, or frequent electrolyte abnormalities, and in patients taking drugs known to prolong QT interval.
• Safety and effectiveness in females and children haven't been established.
Dialyzable drug: Unknown.

PREGNANCY-LACTATION-REPRODUCTION
• Drug may cause fetal harm and loss of pregnancy.
• It isn't known if drug appears in human milk or how drug affects milk production or infants who are breastfed.
• Male patients with partners of child-bearing potential should use effective contraception during therapy and for 2 weeks after final dose.
• Drug may impair fertility in male patients of reproductive potential.

NURSING CONSIDERATIONS
• Monitor patient for signs and symptoms of prolonged QT interval.
• Obtain ECG and electrolyte levels at baseline and periodically during therapy. Correct electrolyte abnormalities, as necessary.
• Monitor PSA level periodically. If PSA level increases, obtain serum testosterone level.
• Monitor patient for signs and symptoms of hyperglycemia.
• Obtain LFT values at baseline and periodically during therapy.
• Monitor patient for signs and symptoms of anemia.
• Monitor for hypersensitivity reactions; discontinue drug if serious reactions occur.

PATIENT TEACHING
• Teach patient how to properly take and store drug.
• Advise patients to seek immediate medical care for severe hypersensitivity reactions.
• Instruct patient about signs and symptoms of prolonged QT interval (palpitations, chest pain, dizziness, fainting) and to immediately report if they occur.
• Inform patient about adverse reactions related to androgen deprivation therapy, including hot flushes, increased weight, decreased sex drive, and difficulties with erectile function.
• Advise male patient with partner of childbearing potential to use effective

---

Reactions in bold italics are *life-threatening*.

contraception during therapy and for 2 weeks after final dose.
• Inform male patient that drug may cause infertility.

relugolix–estradiol–norethindrone acetate
re-loo-GOE-lix/ess-tra-DYE-ole/ nor-ETH-in-drone

Myfembree

Therapeutic class: Hormones
Pharmacologic class: GnRH receptor antagonists-estrogens-progestins

AVAILABLE FORMS
Tablets: relugolix 40 mg, estradiol 1 mg, norethindrone acetate 0.5 mg

INDICATIONS & DOSAGES
Adjust-a-dose (all indications): If use with oral P-gp inhibitors can't be avoided, give Myfembree first and separate dosing by at least 6 hours.
➤ **Management of heavy menstrual bleeding associated with uterine leiomyomas (fibroids); management of moderate to severe pain associated with endometriosis**
Adults who are premenopausal: 1 tablet PO daily for up to 24 months.

ADMINISTRATION
PO
• Give at approximately same time each day, without regard to meals.
• Start drug after onset of menses but no later than 7 days after onset.
• If a dose is missed, give missed dose as soon as possible the same day and resume regular schedule the next day at usual time.
• Store tablets at room temperature.

ACTION
Nonpeptide GnRH receptor antagonist that binds to pituitary GnRH receptors, reduces release of LH and FSH, decreases serum levels of estradiol and progesterone, and reduces bleeding associated with uterine fibroids and pain associated with endometriosis. Estradiol may reduce bone loss that can occur with relugolix, and norethindrone may protect uterus from the adverse effects of unopposed estrogen.

Route	Onset	Peak	Duration
PO	Unknown	1–7 hr	Unknown

Half-life: 10.9 to 61.5 hours.

ADVERSE REACTIONS
CNS: headache, anxiety, depression, dizziness, fatigue, irritability, mood disorders. **CV:** HTN, edema. **EENT:** toothache. **GI:** dyspepsia, diarrhea. **GU:** abnormal uterine bleeding, decreased libido, vulvovaginal dryness. **Metabolic:** increased lipid levels. **Musculoskeletal:** bone loss, back pain, arthralgia. **Skin:** alopecia, hyperhidrosis, night sweats. **Other:** hot flush, breast cyst, hypersensitivity reactions.

INTERACTIONS
Drug-drug. *Combined P-gp and strong CYP3A inducers (rifampin):* May decrease relugolix, estradiol, or norethindrone level. Avoid use together.
Estrogen-containing contraceptives: May increase estrogen level and risk of estrogen-associated adverse events. May decrease efficacy of relugolix, estradiol, and norethindrone. Avoid use together.
P-gp inhibitors (erythromycin): May increase relugolix level. Avoid use together. If use is unavoidable, separate doses by 6 hours and monitor for adverse reactions.
Drug-herb. *St. John's wort:* May decrease drug levels. Discourage use together.
Drug-lifestyle. <u>Boxed Warning</u> *Smoking:* May increase risk of CV events, especially in patients older than age 35. Use together is contraindicated. ∎

EFFECTS ON LAB TEST RESULTS
• May increase liver transaminase, binding protein (thyroid-binding globulin, corticosteroid-binding globulin), angiotensinogenrenin substrate, alpha-1 antitrypsin, ceruloplasmin, glucose, total cholesterol, LDL, and triglyceride levels.
• May decrease free thyroid, corticosteroid hormone, and free testosterone levels.
• May increase platelet count, fibrinogen plasminogen antigen, and clotting factor.
• May increase bleeding times.
• May decrease antithrombin III and antifactor Xa levels.

R

CONTRAINDICATIONS & CAUTIONS

Boxed Warning Estrogen and progestin combination increases risk of thrombotic or thromboembolic disorders (VTE, stroke, and MI), especially in patients at increased risk for these events. ■

Boxed Warning Contraindicated in patients with current or history of thrombotic or thromboembolic disorders, in patients older than age 35 who smoke, and in patients with uncontrolled HTN, dyslipidemia, vascular disease, or obesity. ■

• Contraindicated in patients at high risk for arterial, venous thrombotic, or thromboembolic disorder (cerebrovascular disease, CAD, PVD, thrombogenic valvular or thrombogenic rhythm diseases of heart, inherited or acquired hypercoagulopathies, or headaches with focal neurologic symptoms or migraine headaches with aura if older than age 35).

• Contraindicated in patients hypersensitive to drug or its components.

• Contraindicated in patients with known osteoporosis, current or history of breast cancer or other hormone-sensitive malignancies, increased risk of hormone-sensitive malignancies, known liver impairment or disease, or undiagnosed abnormal uterine bleeding.

• Stop drug immediately if arterial or venous thrombotic, CV, or cerebrovascular event occurs or if hormone-sensitive malignancy is diagnosed.

• Stop drug if sudden unexplained partial or complete vision loss, proptosis, diplopia, papilledema, or retinal vascular lesions occur. Evaluate patient immediately for retinal vein thrombosis.

• Limit therapy to 24 months. Drug may reduce bone mineral density (BMD) that may not be completely reversible. Baseline and periodic BMD assessments are recommended. Assess risks and benefits for patients with other risk factors for bone loss.

• Use cautiously in patients with well-controlled HTN.

• Use cautiously in patients with history of cholestatic jaundice related to past estrogen use or pregnancy.

• Use cautiously in patients with prediabetes, diabetes, or hypertriglyceridemia. Drug may decrease glucose tolerance and increase cholesterol and triglyceride levels.

• Drug may cause uterine fibroid prolapse or expulsion.

• Safety and effectiveness in children haven't been established.

Dialyzable drug: Unknown.

⚠ *Overdose S&S:* Nausea, vomiting, breast tenderness, abdominal pain, drowsiness, fatigue, withdrawal bleeding.

PREGNANCY-LACTATION-REPRODUCTION

• Drug is contraindicated during pregnancy and may cause early pregnancy loss. Exclude pregnancy before starting therapy.

• Drug may delay ability to recognize pregnancy because it alters menstrual bleeding. If pregnancy is suspected, perform testing; stop drug if pregnancy is confirmed.

• Enroll patients exposed to drug during pregnancy in Myfembree Pregnancy Exposure Registry (1-855-428-0707).

• Patients of childbearing potential should use effective nonhormonal contraception during therapy and for 1 week after final dose. Avoid use with hormonal contraceptives.

• Drug may appear in human milk. Weigh benefits against risk to infant.

NURSING CONSIDERATIONS

• Verify pregnancy status before start of therapy. Monitor patient for pregnancy.

• Monitor patient for hypersensitivity reaction; immediately stop drug if reaction occurs.

• Monitor patient for signs and symptoms of liver impairment or gallbladder disease. Periodically obtain LFTs.

• Monitor patient for development of impaired glucose tolerance or hyperlipidemia.

• Monitor patient for thromboembolic disorders.

🔵 *Alert:* Assess patient for mood changes, depression, and suicidal ideation during therapy. Reevaluate benefits and risk of continued therapy if changes occur. Refer patient with new or worsening signs or symptoms to a mental health professional, as appropriate.

• Monitor patient's BP and stop drug if BP rises significantly.

• Obtain dual-energy X-ray absorptiometry at baseline and periodically during therapy.

• Monitor standard of care surveillance breast exams and mammography.

• Monitor patient for severe uterine bleeding and cramping.

• Stop drug 4 to 6 weeks before surgery that's associated with an increased risk of thromboembolism, or during periods of prolonged immobilization.

Reactions in bold italics are *life-threatening*.

PATIENT TEACHING

• Instruct patient to start drug as soon as possible after onset of menses but no later than 7 days after start of menses.

• Advise patient that using estrogen and progestin combinations may increase risk of venous and arterial thrombotic or thromboembolic events.

• Tell patient to seek medical attention for severe uterine bleeding because drug may cause uterine fibroid prolapse or expulsion.

• Inform patient about risk of bone loss and that calcium and vitamin D supplements may be beneficial if dietary intake isn't adequate. Advise patient to take oral iron supplements at least 2 hours apart from calcium and vitamin D.

• Tell patient that depression, mood disorders, and suicidality may occur while taking drug and to promptly seek medical attention for new-onset or worsening depression, anxiety, or other mood changes.

• Advise patient to promptly seek medical attention for signs or symptoms of liver injury (jaundice, right upper abdominal pain).

• Advise patient that drug may delay recognition of pregnancy because it may reduce duration and amount of menstrual bleeding. Tell patient to use effective nonhormonal contraception during therapy and to stop drug if pregnancy is confirmed.

• Inform patient that alopecia, hair loss, and hair thinning may occur during therapy, and may not reverse after stopping drug. Advise patient to contact provider about concerns or changes regarding hair.

• Advise patient to report use of other prescription or OTC drugs or dietary supplements; concomitant use may decrease drug's therapeutic effects.

---

remdesivir
rem-DE-si-vir

Veklury

Therapeutic class: Antivirals
Pharmacologic class: SARS-CoV-2 nucleotide analogue RNA polymerase inhibitors

AVAILABLE FORMS

Injection: 100 mg/20 mL single-dose vial
Powder for injection: 100 mg single-dose vial

INDICATIONS & DOSAGES

Adjust-a-dose (for all indications): Consider discontinuing drug if ALT level increases to greater than 10 times the ULN. Discontinue drug if signs or symptoms of liver inflammation accompany ALT elevation.

➤ **Coronavirus disease 2019 (COVID-19) requiring hospitalization**
Adults and children age 12 and older weighing 40 kg or more: 200 mg IV infusion on day 1 followed by maintenance dose of 100 mg IV infusion once daily starting on day 2 for 5 days in patients not requiring invasive mechanical ventilation or extracorporeal membrane oxygenation (ECMO); if no clinical improvement, may extend therapy 5 additional days. Therapy duration for patients requiring invasive mechanical ventilation or ECMO is 10 days.
Children ages 28 days and older weighing 3 to less than 40 kg: Initiate therapy as soon as possible after diagnosis with 5 mg/kg IV infusion on day 1, followed by maintenance dose of 2.5 mg/kg IV infusion once daily on day 2 for 5 days in patients not requiring invasive mechanical ventilation or ECMO; if no clinical improvement, may extend therapy 5 additional days. Give for 10 days to patients requiring invasive mechanical ventilation or ECMO.

➤ **Nonhospitalized patients with mild to moderate COVID-19 at high risk for progression to severe COVID-19, including hospitalization or death**
Adults and children ages 12 and older weighing 40 kg or more: Initiate therapy as soon as possible after diagnosis and within 7 days of symptom onset with 200 mg IV infusion on day 1, followed by 100 mg IV infusion once daily on days 2 and 3.
Children ages 28 days and older weighing 3 to less than 40 kg: Initiate therapy as soon as possible and within 7 days of symptom onset with 5 mg/kg IV infusion on day 1, followed by 2.5 mg/kg IV infusion once daily on days 2 and 3.

ADMINISTRATION

IV
▼ Remdesivir lyophilized powder is the only form approved for use in children weighing less than 40 kg.
▼ Prepare diluted solution on same day as administration.

R

▼ Let single-dose solution vial reach room temperature (68° to 77° F [20° to 25° C]). Sealed vials can remain at room temperature for up to 12 hours before dilution.

▼ Reconstitute powder with 19 mL sterile water for injection. Immediately shake for 30 seconds; allow contents to settle for 2 to 3 minutes. If contents aren't dissolved, repeat as necessary. Shake until dissolution. Discard vial if contents don't dissolve completely.

▼ Inspect solution for particulates and discoloration. Discard vial if the reconstituted powder or solution contains particulate matter or discoloration. Before dilution, solution should be clear or slightly yellow.

▼ For patients weighing at least 40 kg: Immediately further dilute reconstituted powder in 100 or 250 mL NSS or dilute the solution in 250 mL NSS. From NSS infusion bag, withdraw (and discard) 40 mL for 200-mg dose or 20 mL for 100-mg dose. Inject desired dose of drug into infusion bag and gently invert bag 20 times to mix solution. Don't shake.

▼ For children weighing 3 to less than 40 kg: Immediately further dilute 100 mg/20 mL reconstituted solution to a concentration of 1.25 mg/mL in NSS with the volume required based on weight-based dose. A syringe and syringe pump should be used for infusion volumes less than 50 mL.

▼ Give infusion over 30 to 120 minutes.

▼ Drug may be given without regard to the timing of dialysis.

▼ Prepared solution is stable for 24 hours at room temperature or 48 hours refrigerated.

▼ Store vials of powder below 86° F (30° C). Refrigerate vials of solution at 36° to 46° F (2° to 8° C).

▼ **Incompatibilities:** Other medications or solutions; use only NSS for the final dilution.

ACTION
Inhibits viral replication.

Route	Onset	Peak	Duration
IV	Unknown	40 min	Unknown

Half-life: 1 hour.

ADVERSE REACTIONS
GI: nausea. **GU:** *AKI,* decreased GFR, proteinuria, glycosuria. **Hematologic:** decreased Hb, prolonged PT, *lymphocytopenia.*

*Reactions in bold italics are **life-threatening**.*

Hepatic: elevated transaminase levels, hyperbilirubinemia. **Metabolic:** hyperglycemia, hypernatremia, hypercalcemia, increased lipase, hypoalbuminemia, increased uric acid, *hypokalemia.* **Skin:** extravasation, injection-site erythema, rash. **Other:** hypersensitivity reactions, infusion reaction.

INTERACTIONS
Drug-drug. *Chloroquine phosphate, hydroxychloroquine:* May decrease antiviral activity. Don't use together.
Other drugs: Interaction studies with concomitant medications haven't been conducted in humans. Monitor patient closely.

EFFECTS ON LAB TEST RESULTS
• May increase ALT, AST, bilirubin, glucose, lipase, uric acid, sodium, and calcium levels.
• May decrease potassium and albumin levels, CrCl, and eGFR.
• May increase creatinine level.
• May prolong PT and PTT.
• May increase urinary glucose and protein levels.
• May decrease Hb level and lymphocyte count.

CONTRAINDICATIONS & CAUTIONS
• Contraindicated in patients with clinically significant hypersensitivity reactions to drug or its components.
• Hypersensitivity, including infusion-related and anaphylactic reactions, has been observed during and after administration.
• Use cautiously in older adults.
Dialyzable drug: Unknown.

PREGNANCY-LACTATION-REPRODUCTION
• Studies during pregnancy are ongoing. Available data hasn't identified any major drug-associated risks with second- or third-trimester exposure. Use only if potential benefit justifies risk.
• A remsdesivir pregnancy exposure registry is available at https://covid-pr.pregistry.com or 1-800-616-3791.
• Drug appears in human milk. Use cautiously during breastfeeding.
• Patients with COVID-19 should follow clinical guidelines to avoid exposing infant to virus.

NURSING CONSIDERATIONS
• Drug should only be administered in a setting capable of providing acute care for severe

infusion or hypersensitivity reactions and to activate the emergency medical system, as necessary.

• Monitor patient for hypersensitivity reactions (hypotension, HTN, tachycardia, bradycardia, hypoxia, fever, dyspnea, wheezing, angioedema, rash, nausea, diaphoresis, shivering). Consider slower infusion time (up to 120 minutes) to prevent hypersensitivity reaction. If significant hypersensitivity reaction occurs, immediately discontinue drug and initiate appropriate treatment.

• Obtain baseline eGFR and monitor kidney function as needed during therapy.

• Monitor LFT values and PT before and during therapy.

PATIENT TEACHING

• Advise patient that hypersensitivity reaction may occur and to report changes in HR, fever, shortness of breath, wheezing, rash, nausea, diaphoresis, shivering, or swelling of lips, face, or throat.

• Caution patient that drug may increase risk of kidney and liver dysfunction. Advise patient to immediately report signs or symptoms of liver inflammation (dark urine, fatigue, upset stomach or stomach pain, light-colored stools, vomiting, or jaundice).

• Instruct patient to immediately report pregnancy or breastfeeding.

SAFETY ALERT!

repaglinide
re-PAG-li-nide

Therapeutic class: Antidiabetics
Pharmacologic class: Meglitinides

AVAILABLE FORMS
Tablets: 0.5 mg, 1 mg, 2 mg

INDICATIONS & DOSAGES
➤ **Type 2 diabetes, as adjunct to diet and exercise**
Adults: For patients whose HbA$_{1c}$ level is below 8%, starting dose is 0.5 mg PO before each meal. For patients whose HbA$_{1c}$ is 8% or more, first dose is 1 to 2 mg PO before each meal. Recommended dosage range is 0.5 to 4 mg before meals b.i.d., t.i.d., or q.i.d. Maximum daily dose is 16 mg.

Determine dosage by glucose response. May double dosage up to 4 mg before each

meal until satisfactory glucose response is achieved. At least 1 week should elapse between dosage adjustments to assess response to each dose.

Adjust-a-dose: In patients with CrCl of 20 to 40 mL/minute, starting dosage is 0.5 mg. Gradually titrate dosage, if needed, to achieve glycemic control. Use cautiously in patients with impaired liver function and allow longer intervals between dosage adjustments to allow full assessment of response. Dosage adjustment is recommended with concomitant use of strong CYP3A4 or CYP2C8 inhibitors or inducers.

ADMINISTRATION
PO
• Give drug within 30 minutes before meals.
• If patient skips a meal, skip the scheduled dose to reduce the risk of hypoglycemia.

ACTION
Stimulates insulin release from beta cells in the pancreas by closing adenosine triphosphate (ATP)-dependent potassium channels in beta cell membranes, which causes calcium channels to open. Increased calcium influx induces insulin secretion; the overall effect is to lower glucose level.

Route	Onset	Peak	Duration
PO	15–60 min	1 hr	6 hr

Half-life: 1 hour.

ADVERSE REACTIONS
CNS: headache, paresthesia. **CV:** chest pain. **EENT:** rhinitis, sinusitis, tooth disorder. **GI:** constipation, diarrhea, dyspepsia, nausea, vomiting. **GU:** UTI. **Metabolic:** *hypoglycemia,* hyperglycemia. **Musculoskeletal:** arthralgia, back pain. **Respiratory:** bronchitis, URI. **Other:** hypersentivity reaction.

INTERACTIONS
Drug-drug. *Antidiabetic agents, ACE inhibitors, ARBs, chloramphenicol, coumarin derivatives, MAO inhibitors, NSAIDs, other highly-protein-bound drugs, probenecid, salicylates, sulfonamides:* May increase risk of hypoglycemia. Monitor glucose level. *Beta blockers, clonidine, guanethidine, reserpine:* May blunt signs and symptoms of hypoglycemia. Closely monitor glucose level. *Calcium channel blockers, corticosteroids, estrogens, fosphenytoin, hormonal*

R

contraceptives, isoniazid, nicotinic acid, phenothiazines, phenytoin, sympathomimetics, thiazides and other diuretics, thyroid products: May produce hyperglycemia, resulting in loss of glycemic control. Monitor glucose level.

Clarithromycin: May increase repaglinide levels. Adjust repaglinide dosage.

Clopidogrel: May increase repaglinide level. Start repaglinide at 0.5 mg before each meal. Maximum dosage is 4 mg/day. Avoid use together if possible.

Cyclosporine: May increase repaglinide level. Don't exceed repaglinide dosage of 6 mg/day; monitor glucose level closely.

CYP2C8 and CYP3A4 inducers (rifampin, barbiturates, carbamezapine): May decrease repaglinide level. Monitor glucose level and increase repaglinide dosage as necessary.

CYP2C8 and CYP3A4 inhibitors (ketoconazole, itraconazole, erythromycin, trimethoprim, montelukast): May increase repaglinide level. Monitor glucose level and reduce repaglinide dosage as necessary.

Gemfibrozil: Significantly increases repaglinide level. Use together is contraindicated.

Statins (atorvastatin, simvastatin): May increase repaglinide level. Monitor glucose level.

Thiazolidinediones (pioglitazone, rosiglitazone): May increase risk of hypoglycemia, edema, and weight gain. Monitor patient.

Drug-herb. *Burdock:* May increase hypoglycemic effects. Discourage use together.
St. John's wort: May decrease repaglinide level and its therapeutic effect. Don't use together.

Drug-food. *Grapefruit juice:* May increase level of drug. Discourage use together.

Drug-lifestyle. *Alcohol use:* May alter glycemic control, most commonly causing hypoglycemia. Discourage use together.

EFFECTS ON LAB TEST RESULTS
● May increase or decrease glucose level.

CONTRAINDICATIONS & CAUTIONS
● Contraindicated in patients hypersensitive to drug or its inactive ingredients and in those with type 1 diabetes or diabetic ketoacidosis with or without coma.
● Drug isn't indicated for use in combination with NPH insulin due to risk of serious CV adverse events.

● Use cautiously in older adults and in patients with liver or kidney insufficiency.
Dialyzable drug: Unknown.
⚠ *Overdose S&S:* Hypoglycemia, severe hypoglycemic reactions (coma, seizures, neurologic impairment).

PREGNANCY-LACTATION-REPRODUCTION
● Safety during pregnancy hasn't been established. Use only if clearly needed.
● Abnormal blood glucose levels during pregnancy may cause fetal harm. Most experts recommend insulin during pregnancy to maintain blood glucose levels as close to normal as possible.
● Drug is present in animal milk. It isn't known if drug appears in human milk. Use during breastfeeding isn't recommended.

NURSING CONSIDERATIONS
● Increase dosage carefully in patients with kidney dysfunction.
● Monitor glucose and HbA_{1c} levels for loss of glycemic control, especially during stress, such as fever, trauma, infection, or surgery.
● Hypoglycemia may be difficult to recognize in patients with longstanding diabetes or diabetic nerve disease, in older adults, and in patients taking beta blockers.
● When switching to a different oral antidiabetic, begin new drug on day after last dose of repaglinide.

PATIENT TEACHING
● Stress importance of diet and exercise with drug therapy.
● Discuss symptoms of hypoglycemia with patient and family.
● Encourage patient to keep regular appointments and have HbA_{1c} level checked every 3 months to determine long-term glucose control.
● Teach patient safe drug administration.
● Instruct patient to monitor glucose level carefully. Teach patient what to do when ill, undergoing surgery, or under added stress.
● Advise patient planning pregnancy to first consult prescriber. Insulin may be needed during pregnancy and breastfeeding.
● Teach patient to carry candy or other simple sugars to treat mild hypoglycemia episodes. Patient experiencing severe episode may need emergency treatment.
● Advise patient to avoid alcohol, which lowers glucose level.

Reactions in bold italics are *life-threatening*.

reslizumab
res-LIZ-ue-mab

Cinqair

Therapeutic class: Immunomodulators
Pharmacologic class: Interleukin-5
antagonist monoclonal antibodies

AVAILABLE FORMS
Injection: 100 mg/10 mL single-use vial

INDICATIONS & DOSAGES
➤ **Add-on maintenance treatment of patients with severe asthma with an eosinophilic phenotype**
Adults: 3 mg/kg IV infusion once every 4 weeks.

ADMINISTRATION
IV
▼ Don't give as IV push or bolus.
▼ Visually inspect for particulate matter and discoloration. Solution should be clear to slightly hazy, opalescent, colorless to slightly yellow. Particles that appear as translucent-to-white and amorphous may be present. Discard if solution appears discolored or if particulates are present.
▼ Discard any unused portion. Drug doesn't contain preservative.
▼ To minimize foaming, slowly inject required volume into a 50-mL NSS infusion bag of polyvinyl chloride or polyolefin. Gently invert bag. Don't shake. Don't mix or dilute with other drugs.
▼ Time between preparation and administration shouldn't exceed 16 hours. If not used immediately, store diluted reslizumab solution in refrigerator at 36° to 46° F (2° to 8° C) or at room temperature, protected from light, for up to 16 hours.
▼ If refrigerated, allow diluted solution to warm to room temperature before infusion.
▼ Use an infusion set with an in-line, low-protein-binding, 0.2-micron polyether-sulfone, polyvinylidene fluoride, nylon, or cellulose acetate in-line infusion filter.
▼ Infuse over 20 to 50 minutes (depending on the volume to be infused based on patient weight); then flush IV administration set with NSS to ensure that all reslizumab has been administered.

▼ **Incompatibilities:** Physical and biochemical compatibility studies haven't been conducted. Don't infuse with other drugs or solutions other than NSS.

ACTION
Binds to interleukin-5, reducing production and survival of eosinophils, which limits inflammation, a component of the pathogenesis of asthma; however, its exact mechanism in asthma hasn't been established.

Route	Onset	Peak	Duration
IV	Unknown	Unknown	Unknown

Half-life: 24 days.

ADVERSE REACTIONS
EENT: oropharyngeal pain. **Musculoskeletal:** myalgia, musculoskeletal chest pain, neck pain, muscle spasm, extremity pain, muscle fatigue, bone and muscle pain. **Other:** antibody development.

INTERACTIONS
None reported.

EFFECTS ON LAB TEST RESULTS
• May increase CK level.
• May decrease blood eosinophil count.

CONTRAINDICATIONS & CAUTIONS
Boxed Warning Anaphylaxis has occurred in patients receiving reslizumab. Give only in a health care setting prepared to manage anaphylactic reactions. Discontinue if patient experiences anaphylaxis. ■
• Contraindicated in patients hypersensitive to drug or its components.
• Drug isn't indicated for status asthmaticus, acute bronchospasm, or acute asthma exacerbations.
• Drug isn't indicated for eosinophilic conditions other than severe asthma with an eosinophilic phenotype.
• Safety and effectiveness in children haven't been established.
Dialyzable drug: Unlikely.

PREGNANCY-LACTATION-REPRODUCTION
• Studies during pregnancy are inadequate. Weigh risks to fetus against risks of the patient's poorly controlled asthma.
• Monoclonal antibodies such as reslizumab are known to cross placental barrier. Risk appears to be greater during second and third

R

trimesters. Closely monitor patients who are pregnant; adjust reslizumab dosage as necessary to maintain optimal asthma control.

• It isn't known if reslizumab appears in human milk; however, human IgG is known to appear in human milk. Use cautiously during breastfeeding.

NURSING CONSIDERATIONS

Boxed Warning Monitor patient for signs and symptoms of anaphylaxis (dyspnea, decreased oxygen saturation, wheezing, vomiting, urticaria) during infusion and for an appropriate amount of time after infusion has been completed. Discontinue drug immediately if severe systemic reaction occurs. ∎

• If patient has preexisting parasitic infection, treat infection before initiating drug. If patient becomes infected with parasites while receiving drug and doesn't respond to antiparasitic treatment, discontinue drug until infection resolves.

• Don't abruptly discontinue systemic or inhaled corticosteroids upon initiation of reslizumab. If appropriate, decrease corticosteroid dosage gradually.

• *Look alike–sound alike:* Don't confuse reslizumab with infliximab, ixekizumab, or rituximab.

PATIENT TEACHING

Boxed Warning Teach patient signs and symptoms of anaphylaxis (mucosal swelling, airway compromise, reduced BP, rash, hives, itching). Instruct patient to immediately report signs and symptoms of an allergic reaction that occur during or after receiving a reslizumab infusion. ∎

• Explain to patient that reslizumab doesn't treat acute asthma symptoms or exacerbations. Advise patient to seek medical attention if asthma remains uncontrolled or worsens after initiation of reslizumab.

• Inform patient that there is a small risk of malignancy associated with reslizumab therapy.

• Warn patient not to discontinue systemic or inhaled corticosteroids except under medical supervision. Inform patient that reducing corticosteroid dosage may be associated with signs and symptoms of systemic withdrawal or may unmask conditions previously suppressed by corticosteroid therapy.

• Tell patient to notify provider of existing or developing parasitic infection.

• Teach patient to report all adverse reactions to prescriber.

• Advise patient to discuss pregnancy or breastfeeding with prescriber.

ribavirin
rye-ba-VYE-rin

Virazole

Therapeutic class: Antivirals
Pharmacologic class: Nucleosides–nucleotides

AVAILABLE FORMS
Capsules ⓄⓉⒸ: 200 mg
Powder for inhalation solution: 6 g in 100-mL glass vial
Tablets: 200 mg

INDICATIONS & DOSAGES
Adjust-a-dose (for all indications): Refer to manufacturer's instructions for each formulation for dosage adjustments in patients with impaired kidney function or hematologic toxicity. Some formulations are contraindicated in patients with CrCl less than 50 mL/minute or in patients with Child-Pugh class B and C liver impairment.

➤ **Hospitalized infants and young children with RSV infection**
Infants and young children: Solution in concentration of 20 mg/mL delivered via a Small Particle Aerosol Generator (SPAG-2) and mechanical ventilator, oxygen hood, oxygen tent, or face mask. Treatment is given for 12 to 18 hours/day for 3 to 7 days.

➤ **Chronic HCV monoinfection in combination with interferon alfa-2b (capsules)**
Adults weighing more than 105 kg: 1,400 mg PO daily in two divided doses, 600 mg in the morning and 800 mg in the evening.
Adults weighing more than 81 to 105 kg: 1,200 mg PO daily in two divided doses, 600 mg in the morning and 600 mg in the evening.
Adults weighing 66 to 80 kg: 1,000 mg PO daily in two divided doses, 400 mg in the morning and 600 mg in the evening.
Adults weighing less than 66 kg: 800 mg PO daily in two divided doses, 400 mg in the morning and 400 mg in the evening.
Adjust-a-dose: Individualize adult therapy duration for 24 or 48 weeks based on genotype or prior treatment failure.

Children ages 3 and older weighing more than 73 kg: 1,200 mg PO daily in two divided doses, 600 mg in the morning and 600 mg in the evening.

Children ages 3 and older weighing 60 to 73 kg: 1,000 mg PO daily in two divided doses, 400 mg in the morning and 600 mg in the evening.

Children ages 3 and older weighing 47 to 59 kg: 800 mg PO daily in two divided doses, 400 mg in the morning and 400 mg in the evening.

Adjust-a-dose: For children with HCV genotypes 2 or 3, recommended therapy duration is 24 weeks; for genotype 1, therapy duration is 48 weeks

➤ **Chronic HCV monoinfection in combination with peginterferon alfa-2a (tablets)**

Adults with genotype 1 or 4 weighing 75 kg or more: 1,200 mg PO daily in two divided doses for 48 weeks.

Adults with genotype 1 or 4 weighing less than 75 kg: 1,000 mg daily in two divided doses for 48 weeks.

Adults with genotype 2 or 3: 800 mg PO daily in two divided doses for 24 weeks.

Adolescents and children ages 5 and older weighing 75 kg or more: 1,200 mg PO daily in two divided doses, 600 mg in the morning and 600 mg in the evening.

Adolescents and children ages 5 and older weighing 60 to 74 kg: 1,000 mg PO daily in two divided doses, 400 mg in the morning and 600 mg in the evening.

Adolescents and children ages 5 and older weighing 47 to 59 kg: 800 mg PO daily in two divided doses, 400 mg in the morning and 400 mg in the evening.

Adolescents and children ages 5 and older weighing 34 to 46 kg: 600 mg PO daily in two divided doses, 200 mg in the morning and 400 mg in the evening.

Adolescents and children ages 5 and older who weigh 23 to 33 kg: 400 mg PO daily in two divided doses, 200 mg in the morning and 200 mg in the evening.

Adjust-a-dose: Treatment duration for children and adolescents with genotype 2 or 3 is 24 weeks and for all other genotypes is 48 weeks

➤ **Chronic HCV infection (regardless of genotype) in patients with HIV infection, in combination with peginterferon alfa-2a**

Adults: 800 mg (tablets) PO daily in two divided doses for 48 weeks.

ADMINISTRATION

❸ *Alert:* Hazardous drug; use safe handling and disposal precautions.

Inhalational

• Give by a SPAG-2 only. Don't use any other aerosol-generating device.

• Administer in a well-ventilated room with at least six air changes/hour.

• Use sterile USP water for injection, not bacteriostatic water. Water used to reconstitute this drug must not contain any antimicrobial product. Follow manufacturer's instructions for preparation.

• Discard solutions placed in the SPAG-2 unit at least every 24 hours before adding newly reconstituted solution.

• Don't give with other aerosolized medications.

• Store reconstituted solutions at room temperature for 24 hours.

PO

• Give drug with food and at the same time every day.

❸ *Alert:* Have patient swallow capsules whole; don't open, crush, or break.

ACTION

Inhibits viral activity by an unknown mechanism, possibly by inhibiting RNA and DNA synthesis by depleting intracellular nucleotide pools.

Route	Onset	Peak	Duration
Inhalation	Unknown	Unknown	Unknown
PO	Unknown	2 hr	Unknown

Half-life: After multiple doses (capsules), 12 days, (inhalation), 40 days; after a single dose (tablets), 120 to 170 hours.

ADVERSE REACTIONS

CNS: fatigue, anxiety, depression, dizziness, headache, insomnia, agitation, emotional lability, lack of concentration, memory impairment, pain, asthenia, taste perversion, irritability, nervousness, fever, malaise, aggressive or hostile behaviors, *suicidality.* **CV:** chest pain, flushing; hypotension, digoxin toxicity, tachycardia, *bradycardia, cardiac arrest (inhalation).* **EENT:** blurred vision, conjunctivitis, rhinitis, sinusitis, pharyngitis, dry mouth. **GI:** anorexia, diarrhea, nausea, vomiting, abdominal pain, dyspepsia, constipation. **GU:** menstrual disorder. **Hematologic:** anemia, hemolytic anemia, *leukopenia, neutropenia, thrombocytopenia,*

R

reticulocytosis. **Hepatic:** hyperbilirubinemia, liver enlargement, *liver decompensation.* **Metabolic:** hyperuricemia, hypothyroidism. **Musculoskeletal:** myalgia, arthralgia, back pain, extremity pain. **Respiratory:** dyspnea, URI, cough; worsening of pulmonary status, *bronchospasm, pulmonary edema,* hypoventilation, pneumonia, *pneumothorax, apnea,* atelectasis, ventilator dependence (inhalation). **Skin:** alopecia, dermatitis, eczema, dermatologic disorder, pruritus, rash, dry skin, diaphoresis. **Other:** viral infection, flulike illness, bacterial infection, pediatric growth suppression (height and weight), rigors, chills.

INTERACTIONS
Drug-drug. *Azathioprine:* May induce severe pancytopenia and increase risk of myelotoxicity (neutropenia, thrombocytopenia, anemia). Monitor closely for signs of myelosuppression. Consider an alternative agent if possible.
Didanosine: May increase toxicity. Coadministration is contraindicated.
Influenza vaccine (live): May decrease therapeutic effect of vaccine. Avoid giving antiviral 48 hours before and up to 2 weeks after vaccination.
Lamivudine, stavudine, zidovudine: May decrease antiviral activity of these drugs. Use together cautiously; consider therapy modification.
NRTIs (abacavir, emtricitabine, lamivudine, tenofovir): May increase risk of liver impairment and anemia. Consider discontinuing NRTI. Reduce dosage or discontinue interferon, ribavirin, or both for worsening clinical toxicity.
Warfarin: May decrease anticoagulation effect. Monitor PT and INR.

EFFECTS ON LAB TEST RESULTS
• May increase TSH, uric acid, ALT, AST, and bilirubin levels.
• May increase reticulocyte count.
• May decrease Hb level and WBC and platelet counts.

CONTRAINDICATIONS & CAUTIONS
Boxed Warning Monotherapy is ineffective for treatment of chronic HCV infection; drug shouldn't be used alone for this indication. ∎
Boxed Warning Aerosol form isn't indicated for use in adults. ∎

Boxed Warning Ribavirin may cause hemolytic anemia and worsen cardiac disease, leading to potentially fatal MI. Patients with a history of significant or unstable cardiac disease shouldn't be treated with ribavirin. ∎
• Aerosol form is contraindicated in patients hypersensitive to drug.
• Oral form is contraindicated in patients with known hypersensitivity to ribavirin or its components, autoimmune hepatitis, or hemoglobinopathies.
• Capsules are contraindicated in patients with CrCl of less than 50 mL/minute.
• Ribavirin tablets and peginterferon alfa-2a combination therapy is contraindicated in patients with Child-Pugh class B and C liver impairment; and in patients with Child-Pugh class A, B, and C liver impairment and chronic HCV infection coinfected with HIV before treatment.
Boxed Warning In infants, aerosolized ribavirin has been associated with sudden deterioration of respiratory function. Monitor respiratory function carefully and stop treatment if sudden respiratory deterioration occurs. Reinstitute only with extreme caution, continuous monitoring, and consideration of concomitant administration of bronchodilators. ∎
• Use cautiously in older adults and patients with liver or kidney insufficiency.
• Maintain pediatric dosing throughout therapy in those who start treatment before their 18th birthday.
Dialyzable drug: 50%.
⚠ *Overdose S&S:* Increased severity of adverse reactions.

PREGNANCY-LACTATION-REPRODUCTION
Boxed Warning Contraindicated in patients who are pregnant and in men whose partners are pregnant; significant teratogenic and embryocidal effects have occurred in all animal species exposed to ribavirin. ∎
Boxed Warning Adult females receiving ribavirin and adult males receiving ribavirin who have partners of childbearing potential should use extreme care to avoid pregnancy during therapy and should use at least two reliable forms of effective contraception during therapy and during 6-month (tablets) and 9-month (capsules) posttreatment follow-up. ∎
• If pregnancy occurs during therapy or during the 6 months (tablets) or 9 months (capsules) after therapy ends, advise patient of teratogenic fetal risk.

Reactions in bold italics are *life-threatening.*

• Patients of childbearing potential must have a negative pregnancy test immediately before start of therapy. Pregnancy tests must be performed monthly during therapy and for 6 months after therapy ends.

• Advise health care workers who are pregnant to avoid unnecessary exposure to aerosol form.

• It isn't known if drug appears in human milk. Patient should discontinue breastfeeding or discontinue drug, considering importance of drug to patient.

NURSING CONSIDERATIONS
Aerosol form
❸ Alert: The long-term and cumulative effects in health care personnel exposed to this form aren't known. Eye irritation and headache may occur.

Boxed Warning Use in patients on ventilators should only be undertaken by health care providers and staff familiar with this mode of administration and the specific ventilator used. Experienced providers and staff should use procedures that minimize accumulation of drug precipitate, which can result in ventilator dysfunction and increases in pulmonary pressures. ∎

• Inhalation form is indicated only for severe lower respiratory tract infection caused by RSV. Begin treatment while awaiting test results.

• Because RSV infection is commonly mild and self-limiting, most children with RSV infection don't require treatment with antivirals. Premature infants or those with cardiopulmonary disease benefit most from treatment with ribavirin aerosol.

Oral form
• Don't start therapy until a negative pregnancy test is confirmed in patient or partner of patient; pregnancy test is required every month during therapy and for 6 to 9 months afterward.

• Monitor hematologic status, liver and kidney function, and TSH level at baseline and throughout therapy.

• Combination therapy has been observed to inhibit growth in children ages 5 to 17. Monitor child's height and weight during therapy.

❸ Alert: Monitor patient for suicidality, severe depression, hemolytic anemia, bone marrow suppression, autoimmune and infective disorders, ophthalmic disorders, CV disorders, pulmonary dysfunction, pancreatitis, and diabetes.

• Stop drug if pulmonary infiltrates, severe pulmonary impairment, or pancreatitis occurs.

• In patients receiving azathioprine with ribavirin, monitor CBC, including platelet counts, weekly for first month, twice monthly for second and third months, then monthly or more frequently if dosage or other therapy changes are necessary.

• Monitor HCV-RNA level. If patients who have been previously treated have a detectable HCV-RNA level at week 12 or 24 of treatment, sustained virologic response is unlikely; consider therapy discontinuation.

PATIENT TEACHING
• Inform parents or caregivers of need for drug, and answer any questions.

• Teach patient safe drug administration and handling.

• Advise patient and caregivers to seek immediate medical attention if suicidality and worsening of depression occur.

• Encourage parents or caregivers to immediately report any subtle change in child.

• Warn patient of childbearing potential that drug may harm a fetus, and provide contraception counseling. Advise patient that extreme care must be taken to avoid pregnancy during therapy and for 6 to 9 months after completion of treatment.

• Advise patient to immediately report a pregnancy.

• Caution patient to be well hydrated, especially during initial stages of treatment.

SAFETY ALERT!

ribociclib ✄
RYE-boe-sye-klib

Kisqali

Therapeutic class: Antineoplastics
Pharmacologic class: Cyclin-dependent kinase inhibitors

AVAILABLE FORMS
Tablets ⊙: 200 mg

INDICATIONS & DOSAGES
Adjust-a-dose (all indications): Refer to manufacturer's instructions for toxicity-related dosage adjustment. For patients with Child-Pugh class B or C liver impairment, reduce starting dose to 400 mg once

daily. For patients with eGFR 15 to less than 30 mL/minute/1.73m², reduce starting dose to 200 mg PO once daily. If use with a strong CYP3A inhibitor can't be avoided, reduce ribociclib dose to 400 mg once daily; allow 5 half-lives of the inhibitor after discontinuation of the inhibitor before returning to the initial ribociclib dose.

➤ **Initial endocrine-based therapy for treatment of hormone receptor-positive, HER2-negative advanced or metastatic breast cancer, in combination with aromatase inhibitor**

Adults: 600 mg (three 200-mg tablets) PO once daily for 21 consecutive days followed by 7 days off therapy. Letrozole 2.5 mg once daily is given throughout 28-day cycle. For dosing and administration with other aromatase inhibitors, refer to the respective prescribing information.

Also treat adult males or females who are premenopausal or perimenopausal with a luteinizing hormone-releasing hormone (LHRH) agonist, according to current clinical practice standards.

➤ **Hormone receptor-positive, HER-2 negative advanced or metastatic breast cancer in combination with fulvestrant as initial endocrine-based therapy or after disease progression on endocrine therapy in adult males and females who are postmenopausal** ▨

Adults: 600 mg (three 200-mg tablets) PO once daily for 21 consecutive days followed by 7 days off therapy. Give 500 mg fulvestrant PO on days 1, 15, and once monthly thereafter. Refer to full fulvestrant prescribing information.

Adult males should also be treated with an LHRH agonist, according to current clinical practice standards.

ADMINISTRATION
PO
✪ *Alert:* Hazardous drug; use safe handling and disposal precautions.
• May give without regard for food.
• Have patient swallow tablets whole; don't crush or cut them before swallowing. Don't use cracked, broken, or damaged tablets.
• Give medication at same time each day, preferably in morning.
• Skip a missed dose or a dose lost due to vomiting after intake. Give next dose at its usual time.

ACTION
A cyclin-dependent kinase inhibitor that prevents progression through cell cycle, resulting in arrest in G1 phase. The combination of ribociclib and an aromatase inhibitor causes increased inhibition of tumor growth compared to each agent alone. The combination of ribociclib and fulvestrant results in tumor growth inhibition in estrogen receptor-positive breast cancer models.

Route	Onset	Peak	Duration
PO	Unknown	1–4 hr	Unknown

Half-life: 30 to 55 hours.

ADVERSE REACTIONS
CNS: headache, insomnia, fatigue, dizziness, vertigo, fever. **CV:** peripheral edema, *prolonged QT interval,* syncope. **GI:** nausea, diarrhea, vomiting, constipation, stomatitis, abdominal pain, decreased appetite. **GU:** UTI, increased creatinine. **Hematologic:** *neutropenia, leukopenia, lymphopenia, thrombocytopenia,* anemia. **Hepatic:** abnormal LFT values. **Metabolic:** *hypoglycemia.* **Musculoskeletal:** back pain, arthralgia. **Respiratory:** cough, dyspnea, ILD, pneumonitis. **Skin:** alopecia, rash, pruritus. **Other:** infections.

INTERACTIONS
Drug-drug. *CYP3A substrates with narrow therapeutic index (alfentanil, cyclosporine, ergotamine, everolimus, fentanyl, midazolam, pimozide, quinidine, sirolimus, tacrolimus):* May increase exposure to these drugs. Decrease substrate dosage when concomitant use with ribociclib is necessary.
Drugs that prolong QT interval (amiodarone, bepridil, chloroquine, clarithromycin, disopyramide, haloperidol, methadone, moxifloxacin, ondansetron, pimozide, procainamide, quinidine, sotalol): May increase risk of prolonged QT interval and ventricular arrhythmias. Avoid use together.
Strong CYP3A4 inducers (carbamazepine, phenytoin, rifampin): May decrease ribociclib level. Avoid use together.
Strong CYP3A4 inhibitors (clarithromycin, conivaptan, ketoconazole, lopinavir–ritonavir, nefazodone, nelfinavir, posaconazole, ritonavir, saquinavir): May increase ribociclib level. Avoid use together. If coadministration is unavoidable, decrease ribociclib dosage. If strong inhibitor is discontinued,

resume prior ribociclib dosage after at least five half-lives of the CYP3A inhibitor.
Tamoxifen: May increase tamoxifen level and prolong QT interval. Use together isn't indicated.

Drug-herb. *St. John's wort:* May decrease ribociclib level. Discourage use together.
Drug-food. *Grapefruit or grapefruit juice, pomegranates or pomegranate juice:* May increase ribociclib level. Don't use together.

EFFECTS ON LAB TEST RESULTS
• May increase ALT, AST, GGT, and serum creatinine levels.
• May decrease phosphorus, glucose, albumin, and potassium levels.
• May decrease Hb level and leukocyte, neutrophil, lymphocyte, and platelet counts.

CONTRAINDICATIONS & CAUTIONS
◑ *Alert:* Ribociclib may cause rare but severe or fatal ILD and pneumonitis.
• Drug may prolong QT interval. Avoid use in patients with long QT syndrome, uncontrolled or significant cardiac disease (recent MI, HF, unstable angina, bradyarrhythmias), or electrolyte abnormalities and in those taking drugs known to prolong the QTc interval.
• Drug may increase risk of hepatobiliary toxicity, SCARs, and neutropenia.
Dialyzable drug: Unknown.

PREGNANCY-LACTATION-REPRODUCTION
• Drug may cause fetal harm; avoid use during pregnancy. Obtain a pregnancy test before start of therapy. Patients of childbearing potential should use effective contraception during therapy and for at least 3 weeks after final dose.
• Unknown if drug appears in human milk. Patients shouldn't breastfeed during therapy and for at least 3 weeks after final dose.
• Drug may impair fertility in males.

NURSING CONSIDERATIONS
◑ *Alert:* Monitor patients for new or worsening pulmonary symptoms (hypoxia, cough, dyspnea, interstitial infiltrates on radiologic images); if they occur, interrupt therapy immediately and evaluate the patient. If infection, neoplasm, and other causes are excluded, permanently discontinue treatment in patients with severe ILD or pneumonitis.
• Monitor LFTs before start of therapy, every 2 weeks for the first two cycles, then at

beginning of each subsequent four cycles, and as clinically indicated because of the risk of hepatobiliary toxicity. Interrupt therapy, reduce dosage, or discontinue drug based on LFT values.
• Monitor electrolyte levels (potassium, calcium, phosphorus, magnesium) before start of therapy, at beginning of first six cycles, and as clinically indicated. Correct electrolyte abnormalities before therapy begins.
• Assess baseline ECG. Initiate treatment only in patients with a baseline QTcF (QT interval corrected for HR via Fridericia's method) of less than 450 msec. Repeat ECG on day 14 of the first cycle, before the second cycle, and as clinically indicated. Interrupt, reduce, or discontinue therapy based on QT-interval prolongation.
• Assess CBC before start of therapy, every 2 weeks for first two cycles, at beginning of subsequent four cycles, then as clinically indicated. Interrupt, reduce, or discontinue therapy based on CBC results.
• Monitor patient closely for hepatobiliary toxicity and neutropenia.
• Monitor patient for SCARs (SJS, TEN, drug-induced hypersensitivity syndrome, and DRESS syndrome). Withhold treatment and consult a dermatologist if signs and symptoms occur.
• Verify pregnancy status before treatment.

PATIENT TEACHING
◑ *Alert:* Warn patient to immediately report difficulty or discomfort with breathing or shortness of breath while at rest or with low activity; these may be symptoms of ILD or pneumonitis.
• Teach patient to immediately report signs and symptoms related to QT-interval prolongation (fast or irregular heartbeat, dizziness, syncope).
• Advise patient to immediately report signs and symptoms of liver dysfunction (jaundice, dark or brown urine, fatigue, loss of appetite, upper abdominal pain, bleeding or bruising more easily than usual), skin reactions, and infection (fever, chills, pain, malaise).
• Inform patient of childbearing potential of fetal risk and to use effective contraception during therapy and for at least 3 weeks after final dose.
• Advise patient not to breastfeed during therapy and for at least 3 weeks after final dose.

R

rifAMPin (rifampicin)
rif-AM-pin

Rifadin, Rofact✚

Therapeutic class: Antituberculotics
Pharmacologic class: Semisynthetic rifamycins

AVAILABLE FORMS
Capsules: 150 mg, 300 mg
Powder for injection: 600 mg/vial

INDICATIONS & DOSAGES
➤ **Pulmonary TB, with other antituberculotics**
Adults: 10 mg/kg PO or IV daily in single dose. Maximum daily dose is 600 mg.
Children: 10 to 20 mg/kg PO or IV daily in single dose. Maximum daily dose is 600 mg.
➤ **Meningococcal carriers**
Adults: 600 mg PO or IV every 12 hours for 2 days.
Children ages 1 month and older: 10 mg/kg PO or IV every 12 hours for 2 days, not to exceed 600 mg/day.
Neonates: 5 mg/kg PO or IV every 12 hours for 2 days.
➤ **Cholestatic pruritus** ♦
Adults: 150 to 300 mg PO b.i.d.

ADMINISTRATION
PO
• For pulmonary TB, give drug with other antituberculotics.
• For best absorption, give capsules 1 hour before or 2 hours after a meal with a full glass of water.
• For patients who can't tolerate capsules on an empty stomach or those who have difficulty swallowing capsules or when lower doses are needed, consult pharmacist for preparation of an oral suspension.
IV
▼ Reconstitute drug with 10 mL of sterile water for injection to yield 60 mg/mL.
▼ Add to 100 mL of D_5W and infuse over 30 minutes, or add to 500 mL of D_5W and infuse over 3 hours.
▼ When dextrose is contraindicated, dilute with NSS for injection. Once prepared, dilutions in D_5W remain stable for up to 8 hours and dilutions in NSS remain stable for up to 6 hours at room temperature.

▼ **Incompatibilities:** Diltiazem, other IV solutions.

ACTION
Inhibits DNA-dependent RNA polymerase, which impairs RNA synthesis; bactericidal.

Route	Onset	Peak	Duration
PO	Unknown	2–4 hr	<24 hr
IV	Unknown	Unknown	<24 hr

Half-life: 3 to 4 hours (adults). Varies with repeated administration and age.

ADVERSE REACTIONS
CNS: headache, fatigue, drowsiness, behavioral changes, dizziness, confusion, impaired concentration, generalized numbness, ataxia, fever. **CV:** flushing, *shock.* **EENT:** abnormal vision, conjunctivitis, sore mouth or tongue, tooth discoloration. **GI:** *pseudomembranous colitis,* epigastric pain, heartburn, anorexia, nausea, vomiting, abdominal cramps, diarrhea, flatulence. **GU:** menstrual disturbances, elevated BUN. **Hematologic:** anemia, *thrombocytopenia, transient leukopenia,* eosinophilia, hemolytic anemia, vitamin-K coagulation disorder. **Hepatic:** jaundice, *liver toxicity.* **Metabolic:** hyperuricemia. **Musculoskeletal:** muscular weakness, extremity pain. **Respiratory:** shortness of breath, wheezing. **Skin:** pruritus, urticaria, rash. **Other:** flulike syndrome, discoloration of body fluids, porphyria exacerbation, hypersensitivity reactions.

INTERACTIONS
⊕ *Alert:* Rifampin can significantly interact with many drugs. Consult a drug interaction resource or pharmacist for additional information.
Drug-drug. *Antithrombotics (clopidogrel, ticagrelor):* May increase or decrease antithrombotic level. Avoid use together.
Atazanavir, darunavir, fosamprenavir, saquinavir, tipranavir: May decrease antiviral levels, resulting in loss of antiviral efficacy or development of viral resistance. Use together is contraindicated.
Benzodiazepines, beta blockers, chloramphenicol, citalopram, corticosteroids, cyclosporine, dapsone, digoxin, disopyramide, doxycycline, enalapril, losartan, methadone, mexiletine, nifedipine, ondansetron, opioid analgesics, phenytoin, propafenone, quinidine, ritonavir, rosiglitazone, sulfonylureas,

---

Reactions in bold italics are *life-threatening*.

tacrolimus, TCAs, theophylline, tocainide, triazolam, verapamil, zolpidem: May decrease effectiveness of these drugs. Monitor effectiveness.

Daclatasvir, simeprevir, sofosbuvir, telaprevir: May decrease levels of these hepatitis C antivirals. Avoid use together.

Efavirenz, zidovudine: May decrease levels of these antiretrovirals. Avoid use together.

Halothane: May increase risk of liver toxicity. Monitor LFT results.

Hormonal contraceptives (estrogens, progestins): May decrease hormone exposure. Patient should use nonhormonal contraceptives during rifampin therapy.

Isoniazid: May increase risk of liver toxicity. Monitor LFT results.

Ketoconazole, para-aminosalicylate sodium: May interfere with absorption of rifampin. Separate doses by 8 to 12 hours.

Macrolide antibiotics, protease inhibitors: May increase rifampin level and decrease level of other drug. Monitor patient for clinical and adverse effects.

Praziquantel: May decrease praziquantel level. Use together is contraindicated.

Probenecid: May increase rifampin levels. Use together cautiously.

Saquinavir: May increase risk of severe liver toxicity. Use together is contraindicated.

Voriconazole: May decrease voriconazole's therapeutic effects while increasing the risk of rifampin adverse effects. Use together is contraindicated.

Warfarin: May increase requirements for anticoagulant. Monitor PT and INR closely, and adjust dosage of anticoagulants.

Drug-lifestyle. *Alcohol use:* May increase risk of liver toxicity. Discourage use together.

EFFECTS ON LAB TEST RESULTS
● May increase ALT, AST, ALP, bilirubin, BUN, and uric acid levels.
● May increase eosinophil count.
● May decrease Hb level and platelet and WBC counts.
● May increase urine RBC count.
● May alter standard folate and vitamin B_{12} assay results.

CONTRAINDICATIONS & CAUTIONS
● Contraindicated in patients hypersensitive to rifampin or related drugs.

● Drug isn't indicated for treatment of meningococcal disease, only for short-term treatment of asymptomatic carrier states.
● Use cautiously in patients with liver disease or diabetes.
● Paradoxical drug reactions (recurrence or appearance of new symptoms) have been reported.
● Hypersensitivity reactions, including erythema multiforme, SJS, TEN, and DRESS syndrome, have occurred. Discontinue drug for SCAR signs or symptoms.
Dialyzable drug: Poorly.
⚠ **Overdose S&S:** Nausea; vomiting; abdominal pain; pruritus; headache; increasing lethargy; unconsciousness; transient increases in liver enzyme or bilirubin levels; brownish red or orange discoloration of skin, urine, sweat, saliva, tears, and feces; facial or periorbital edema; hypotension; tachycardia; ventricular arrhythmias; seizures; cardiac arrest; liver enlargement; jaundice.

PREGNANCY-LACTATION-REPRODUCTION
● There are no adequate human studies during pregnancy. Drug may cross placental barrier and cause fetal harm. Use only if clearly needed and potential benefit justifies fetal risk.
● Drug can cause postnatal hemorrhages in the mother and infant when given during last few weeks of pregnancy; treatment with vitamin K may be indicated.
● Drug appears in human milk. Patient should discontinue breastfeeding or discontinue drug, considering importance of drug to patient.

NURSING CONSIDERATIONS
● Monitor liver function, blood counts, coagulation tests, and uric acid level. In patients with existing impaired liver function, monitor LFT values, especially AST and ALT, before therapy, then every 2 to 4 weeks during therapy.
● Watch for and report signs and symptoms of liver impairment.
● Monitor for pulmonary toxicity (respiratory failure, pulmonary fibrosis, acute respiratory distress). Discontinue drug if toxicity occurs.
● Monitor for thrombotic microangiopathy (TMA). Discontinue drug if symptoms and blood test results suggest TMA (unexplained thrombocytopenia, anemia).
● Monitor patients on intermittent therapy for adherence.
● Monitor for hypersensitivity reactions.

R

- *Look alike–sound alike:* Don't confuse rifampin with rifabutin, rifaximin, or rifapentine.

PATIENT TEACHING
- Instruct patient on safe drug administration.
- Warn patient that drowsiness may occur and that drug can turn body fluids red-orange and permanently stain contact lenses.
- Advise patient to use nonhormonal contraception.
- Caution patient to report fever, loss of appetite, malaise, nausea, vomiting, dark urine, or yellowing of eyes or skin.
- Advise patient to avoid alcohol during drug therapy.
- Instruct patient on importance of not missing any doses and completing full course of therapy.

rifapentine
rif-a-PEN-teen

Priftin

Therapeutic class: Antituberculotics
Pharmacologic class: Synthetic rifamycins

AVAILABLE FORMS
Tablets (film-coated): 150 mg

INDICATIONS & DOSAGES
- **❸** *Alert:* Give drug as directly observed therapy for all indications.
- ➤ **Pulmonary TB, with at least one other antituberculotic to which the isolate is susceptible**
Adults and children age 12 and older: During initial phase of short-course therapy, 600 mg PO twice weekly for 2 months, with an interval between doses of at least 3 days (72 hours). During continuation phase of short-course therapy, 600 mg PO once weekly for 4 months, combined with isoniazid or other appropriate agent.
Older adults: Begin therapy at low end of dosing range.
- ➤ **Latent TB infection caused by *Mycobacterium tuberculosis*, in combination with isoniazid, in patients at high risk for progression to TB disease**
Adults and children ages 2 and older: Base rifapentine dosage on patient's weight and administer PO once weekly for 12 weeks. If patient weighs more than 50 kg, give 900 mg;

if patient weighs 32.1 to 50 kg, give 750 mg; if patient weighs 25.1 to 32 kg, give 600 mg; if patient weighs 14.1 to 25 kg, give 450 mg; if patient weighs 10 to 14 kg, give 300 mg. Maximum dosage, 900 mg once weekly.
Adjust-a-dose: Recommended isoniazid dose in adults and children 12 and older is 15 mg/kg (rounded to nearest 50 or 100 mg) up to maximum of 900 mg once weekly for 12 weeks. Recommended isoniazid dose in children ages 2 to 11 is 25 mg/kg (rounded to nearest 50 or 100 mg) up to maximum of 900 mg for 12 weeks.

ADMINISTRATION
PO
- Give drug with meals to increase bioavailability and possibly reduce the incidence of GI upset, nausea, and vomiting.
- For patients who can't swallow tablets whole, tablets may be crushed and added to small amount of semisolid food and consumed immediately.
- **❸** *Alert:* Give drug with appropriate daily companion drugs. Compliance with all drug regimens, especially with daily companion drugs on the days when rifapentine isn't given, is crucial for early sputum conversion and protection from relapse of TB.

ACTION
Inhibits DNA-dependent RNA polymerase in susceptible strains of *M. tuberculosis*. Demonstrates bactericidal activity against the organism both intracellularly and extracellularly.

Route	Onset	Peak	Duration
PO	Unknown	3–10 hr	Unknown

Half-life: 17 hours.

ADVERSE REACTIONS
CNS: headache, dizziness, fever. **CV:** chest pain. **EENT:** conjunctivitis. **GI:** anorexia, nausea, vomiting, dyspepsia, diarrhea, abdominal pain. **GU:** uremia, proteinuria, hematuria, urinary casts, elevated BUN. **Hematologic:** *leukopenia, leukocytosis, neutropenia,* anemia, *thrombocythemia, thrombocytopenia,* lymphadenopathy. **Hepatic:** increased transaminase levels, *hepatitis.* **Musculoskeletal:** arthralgia, back pain. **Respiratory:** hemoptysis, cough. **Skin:** diaphoresis, rash, pruritus, maculopapular rash. **Other:** hypersensitivity reactions.

Reactions in bold italics are *life-threatening*.

INTERACTIONS

🜊 *Alert:* Rifapentine may significantly interact with many drugs. Consult a drug interaction resource or pharmacist for more information.

Drug-drug. *Antiarrhythmics (disopyramide, mexiletine, quinidine, tocainide), antibiotics (chloramphenicol, clarithromycin, dapsone, doxycycline, fluoroquinolones), anticonvulsants (phenytoin), antifungals (fluconazole, itraconazole, ketoconazole), barbiturates, benzodiazepines (diazepam), beta blockers, calcium channel blockers (diltiazem, nifedipine, verapamil), cardiac glycosides, clofibrate, corticosteroids, haloperidol, HIV protease inhibitors (nelfinavir, ritonavir, saquinavir), immunosuppressants (cyclosporine, tacrolimus), levothyroxine, opioid analgesics (methadone), oral anticoagulants (warfarin), oral antidiabetics (sulfonylureas), progestins, quinine, reverse transcriptase inhibitors (delavirdine, zidovudine), sildenafil, TCAs (amitriptyline, nortriptyline), theophylline:* May decrease activity of these drugs because of cytochrome P-450 enzyme metabolism. May need to adjust dosage of these drugs.

Hormonal contraceptives: May reduce effectiveness of contraceptive. Patient should use nonhormonal contraceptives during therapy.

EFFECTS ON LAB TEST RESULTS

- May increase uric acid, ALT, and AST levels.
- May decrease blood glucose level.
- May increase platelet count.
- May decrease Hb level and neutrophil and WBC counts.
- May alter folate and vitamin B_{12} assay results.

CONTRAINDICATIONS & CAUTIONS

- Contraindicated in patients hypersensitive to rifamycins (rifapentine, rifampin, or rifabutin).
- Patients with abnormal LFT values or liver disease and those initiating treatment for active pulmonary TB should receive rifapentine only when necessary and under strict medical supervision.
- For patients with active pulmonary TB who are infected with HIV, don't use drug once weekly in the continuation phase regimen in combination with isoniazid because of a

higher rate of failure or relapse with rifampin-resistant organisms. Rifapentine hasn't been studied as part of the initial phase treatment regimen in this population.

- Rule out active TB disease before starting treatment for latent TB infection.
- Patients considered at high risk for progression to TB disease include those in close contact with patients with active TB or recent conversion to a positive result on tuberculin skin test, patients with pulmonary fibrosis on X-ray, and patients with HIV infection.
- Rifapentine in combination with isoniazid isn't recommended for patients presumed to be exposed to rifamycin- or isoniazid-resistant *M. tuberculosis.*
- Use cautiously in patients with cavitary pulmonary lesions or positive sputum cultures after initial treatment phase and in patients with bilateral pulmonary disease; higher relapse rates may occur in these patients.
- CDAD has been reported, ranging from mild diarrhea to fatal colitis, and can occur more than 2 months after therapy ends. Drug may need to be discontinued and appropriate measures initiated.
- Avoid using drug in patients with porphyria.

Dialyzable drug: Unlikely.

⚠ *Overdose S&S:* Hematuria, neutropenia, hyperglycemia, hyperuricemia, arthritis, increased ALT level, pruritus.

PREGNANCY-LACTATION-REPRODUCTION

- There are no adequate studies during pregnancy. Drug may cause fetal harm. Use only if potential benefit justifies fetal risk.
- Drug may cause postnatal hemorrhages in the patient and infant when another rifamycin is given during last few weeks of pregnancy. Monitor PT in patients who are pregnant and neonates exposed to rifapentine during last few weeks of pregnancy. Treatment with vitamin K may be indicated.
- It isn't known if drug appears in human milk. Use cautiously during breastfeeding. If used, monitor infant for liver toxicity.

NURSING CONSIDERATIONS

- Monitor patient for signs and symptoms of hypersensitivity reaction (flulike illness, hypotension, urticaria, angioedema, bronchospasm, conjunctivitis, thrombocytopenia, neutropenia). Stop drug and notify prescriber if hypersensitivity reaction occurs.

- Monitor for SCARs, including SJS and DRESS syndrome. Discontinue drug at first appearance of rash, mucosal lesions, or other signs and symptoms of hypersensitivity.
- Rifamycin antibiotics may cause liver toxicity. In patients with abnormal LFT values or liver disease and patients starting treatment for active pulmonary TB, obtain serum transaminase levels before start of therapy and every 2 to 4 weeks during therapy. Discontinue drug if evidence of liver injury occurs.
- Monitor patient for CDAD.
- *Look alike–sound alike:* Don't confuse rifapentine with rifabutin or rifampin.

PATIENT TEACHING

- Teach patient safe drug administration and storage.
- Stress importance of strict adherence to this drug regimen and that of daily companion drugs, as well as needed follow-up visits and lab tests.
- Advise patient of childbearing potential to use nonhormonal contraceptives.
- Caution mother of infant exposed to rifapentine through human milk to watch for signs and symptoms of liver toxicity (irritability, prolonged unexplained crying, jaundice, loss of appetite, vomiting, darkened urine, lightened stool).
- Instruct patient to report all adverse reactions, especially fever, appetite loss, malaise, nausea, vomiting, darkened urine, yellowish skin and eyes, joint pain or swelling, skin or mucosal lesions, or excessive loose stools or diarrhea.
- Tell patient that drug may turn body fluids red-orange and permanently stain dentures or contact lenses. Instruct patient to remove soft contact lenses during therapy.

rifAXIMin
rif-AX-i-min

Xifaxan

Therapeutic class: Antibiotics
Pharmacologic class: Rifamycin antibacterials

AVAILABLE FORMS
Tablets: 200 mg, 550 mg

INDICATIONS & DOSAGES
➤ **Traveler's diarrhea from noninvasive strains of** *Escherichia coli*
Adults and children ages 12 and older: 200 mg PO t.i.d. for 3 days.
➤ **To reduce risk of overt hepatic encephalopathy recurrence**
Adults: 550 mg PO b.i.d.
➤ **IBS with diarrhea**
Adults: 550 mg PO t.i.d. for 14 days. May repeat regimen twice if symptoms recur.

ADMINISTRATION
PO
- Give drug without regard for food.

ACTION
Binds to the beta-subunit of bacterial DNA-dependent RNA polymerase, which inhibits bacterial RNA synthesis and kills *E. coli.*

Route	Onset	Peak	Duration
PO	Unknown	1 hr	Unknown

Half-life: 5.6 to 6 hours.

ADVERSE REACTIONS
CNS: depression, dizziness, fatigue, fever, headache. **CV:** peripheral edema. **EENT:** nasopharyngitis. **GI:** ascites, abdominal pain, nausea, *CDAD.* **Hematologic:** anemia. **Hepatic:** increased ALT level. **Musculoskeletal:** arthralgia, muscle spasms, myalgia. **Respiratory:** dyspnea. **Skin:** rash, pruritus.

INTERACTIONS
Drug-drug. *P-gp inhibitors (cyclosporine, diltiazem, ketoconazole, PPIs, saquinavir):* May increase systemic exposure of rifaximin. Use together cautiously.
Warfarin: May interfere with effect on INR. Monitor INR and PT closely.

EFFECTS ON LAB TEST RESULTS
- May increase CK and ALT levels.
- May decrease Hb level.

CONTRAINDICATIONS & CAUTIONS
- Contraindicated in patients hypersensitive to rifaximin or its components, rifamycin, or other antimicrobial agents.
- Hypersensitivity reactions, including exfoliative dermatitis, angioneurotic edema, and anaphylaxis, have occurred.
- Use of drug for traveler's diarrhea without proven or strongly suspected bacterial

infection or as prophylaxis isn't likely to be beneficial and increases risk of development of drug-resistant bacteria.

• Use with caution in patients with Child-Pugh class C liver impairment.

• Safety and effectiveness in children younger than age 12 with traveler's diarrhea and younger than age 18 with liver encephalopathy or IBS haven't been established.

Dialyzable drug: Unknown.

PREGNANCY-LACTATION-REPRODUCTION

• Studies during pregnancy are inadequate.

• Some animal studies have demonstrated adverse events. Because of limited absorption of rifaximin in patients with normal liver function, fetal exposure to drug is expected to be low.

• It isn't known if drug appears in human milk. Use cautiously during breastfeeding.

NURSING CONSIDERATIONS

• Don't use drug in patients whose illness may be caused by *Campylobacter jejuni, Shigella,* or *Salmonella.*

🔵 *Alert:* Don't use drug in patients with blood in the stool, diarrhea with fever, or diarrhea from pathogens other than *E. coli.*

• Stop drug if diarrhea worsens or lasts longer than 24 to 48 hours. Patient may need a different antibiotic.

• Patients who have diarrhea after antibiotic therapy may have CDAD, which may range from mild to life-threatening.

• Monitor patient for overgrowth of nonsusceptible organisms.

• *Look alike–sound alike:* Don't confuse rifaximin with rifampin or rifapentine.

PATIENT TEACHING

• Teach patient safe drug administration.

• Tell patient to take all the prescribed drug, even if feeling better before drug is finished.

• Advise patient to notify prescriber if diarrhea worsens or lasts longer than 1 or 2 days after starting treatment. A different treatment may be needed.

• Caution patient that CDAD (watery and bloody stools with or without stomach cramps and fever) may occur as late as 2 or more months after the last dose of antibiotic. Advise patient to report signs or symptoms of CDAD as soon as possible.

• Explain that this drug is only for treating diarrhea caused by contaminated foods or

beverages while traveling and not for any other type of infection.

• Caution patient not to share drug with others.

rilpivirine hydrochloride
ril-pi-VIR-een

Edurant

Therapeutic class: Antiretrovirals
Pharmacologic class: NNRTIs

AVAILABLE FORMS
Tablets: 25 mg

INDICATIONS & DOSAGES

➤ **HIV-1 infection in patients who are antiretroviral-naive with HIV-1 RNA 100,000 copies/mL or less at start of therapy, in combination with other antiretrovirals**

Adults and adolescents ages 12 and older weighing at least 35 kg: 25 mg PO once daily.

Adjust-a-dose: For patients concomitantly receiving rifabutin, increase rilpivirine dosage to 50 mg once daily. When rifabutin is stopped, decrease rilpivirine to 25 mg once daily. For patients who are pregnant and were already on a stable rilpivirine regimen before pregnancy and who are virologically suppressed (HIV-1 RNA less than 50 copies/mL), recommended dosage is 25 mg once daily.

➤ **In combination with cabotegravir for short-term treatment of HIV-1 infection in patients who are virologically suppressed (HIV-1 RNA less than 50 copies/mL) on a stable regimen as an oral lead-in to assess tolerability of rilpivirine before use of cabotegravir–rilpivirine (Cabenuva) extended-release injectable suspensions**

Adults and adolescents ages 12 and older weighing at least 35 kg: 25 mg PO once daily in combination with cabotegravir 30 mg PO once daily. Use oral lead-in dose for at least 28 days.

➤ **In combination with cabotegravir for short-term treatment of HIV-1 infection in patients with HIV-1 RNA less than 50 copies/mL who are on a stable oral therapy regimen but who will miss scheduled injections with cabotegravir–rilpivirine (Cabenuva) extended-release injectable suspensions by more than 7 days to up to 2 consecutive months**

R

Adults and adolescents ages 12 and older weighing at least 35 kg: One 25-mg tablet PO once daily in combination with cabotegravir 30 mg PO once daily at approximately the same time each day with a meal, starting the same time as planned missed injection and continuing until the day injection dosing is restarted. Refer to Cabenuva prescribing information for dosing instructions.

Adjust-a-dose: For oral therapy with rilpivirine and cabotegravir lasting more than 2 months, an alternative oral regimen, which may include rilpivirine, is recommended.

ADMINISTRATION
PO
● Give drug with a normal to high-calorie meal.
● Have patient swallow tablets whole with water.
● Don't give a missed dose if next scheduled dose is within 12 hours.
● Store tablets at room temperature and in the original bottle to protect from light.

ACTION
Inhibits HIV-1 replication by noncompetitive inhibition of HIV-1 reverse transcriptase but doesn't inhibit the human cellular DNA polymerases alpha, beta, and gamma.

Route	Onset	Peak	Duration
PO	Rapid	4–5 hr	Unknown

Half-life: 50 hours.

ADVERSE REACTIONS
CNS: abnormal dreams, dizziness, fatigue, headache, insomnia, depressive disorders. **GI:** nausea, vomiting, abdominal pain. **GU:** increased creatinine level. **Hepatic:** increased transaminase levels, hyperbilirubinemia. **Metabolic:** hyperlipidemia. **Skin:** rash.

INTERACTIONS
Drug-drug. *Antacids (aluminum or magnesium hydroxide, calcium carbonate):* May significantly decrease rilpivirine level. Give antacids either 2 hours before or at least 4 hours after rilpivirine.
Anticonvulsants (carbamazepine, oxcarbazepine, phenobarbital, phenytoin): May decrease rilpivirine level, decrease response, and increase risk of resistance to NNRTIs. Use together is contraindicated.
Azole antifungals (fluconazole, itraconazole, ketoconazole, voriconazole): May increase

rilpivirine level and decrease antifungal level. Monitor effectiveness of antifungal.
Delavirdine: May increase rilpivirine level. Don't use together.
Drugs that prolong QT interval: May increase risk of torsades de pointes. Use together cautiously.
H_2-receptor antagonists (cimetidine, famotidine): May significantly decrease rilpivirine level. Give H_2-receptor antagonists at least 12 hours before or 4 hours after rilpivirine.
Macrolide antibiotics (clarithromycin, erythromycin): May increase rilpivirine level and risk of torsades de pointes. When possible, consider an alternative such as azithromycin.
Methadone: May decrease levels of both drugs. Monitor effectiveness of methadone and adjust methadone dosage as needed.
Other NNRTIs (efavirenz, etravirine, nevirapine): May decrease rilpivirine level. Don't use together.
PPIs (esomeprazole, lansoprazole, pantoprazole, rabeprazole): May decrease rilpivirine level and virologic response, and increase risk of resistance to NNRTIs. Use together is contraindicated.
Rifabutin: May decrease rilpivirine level. Increase rilpivirine dose to 50 mg once daily during coadministration. Use with cabotegravir–rilpivirine injections is contraindicated.
Rifampin, rifapentine: May decrease rilpivirine level and virologic response, and increase risk of resistance to NNRTIs. Use together is contraindicated.
Systemic glucocorticoids (dexamethasone): May decrease rilpivirine level and virologic response, and increase risk of resistance to NNRTIs. Use together is contraindicated.
Drug-herb. *St. John's wort:* May decrease rilpivirine level and virologic response, and increase risk of resistance to NNRTIs. Use together is contraindicated.
Drug-food. *Grapefruit products:* May inhibit metabolism of rilpivirine. Avoid use during therapy.

EFFECTS ON LAB TEST RESULTS
● May increase AST, ALT, bilirubin, creatinine, total cholesterol, HDL, LDL, and triglyceride levels.
● May decrease cortisol level.

CONTRAINDICATIONS & CAUTIONS
● Contraindicated in patients hypersensitive to drug or its components.

Reactions in bold italics are *life-threatening*.

- Use cautiously when administering with drugs known to prolong QT interval, in older adults, and in patients with CrCl less than 30 mL/minute or liver disease.
- Adverse liver events have been reported. Patients with underlying HBV or HCV infection or marked elevations in transaminase levels before treatment may be at increased risk for worsening or development of transaminase elevations.
- Severe skin and hypersensitivity reactions have been reported, including severe rash or rash accompanied by fever, blisters, mucosal involvement, conjunctivitis, facial edema, angioedema, hepatitis, eosinophilia, or DRESS syndrome. Most rashes occurred within first 4 to 6 weeks of therapy.
- Use in combination with cabotegravir only in patients with no history of treatment failure and no known or suspected resistance to either cabotegravir or rilpivirine.
- Safety and effectiveness in children younger than age 12 or weighing less than 35 kg haven't been established.

Dialyzable drug: Unlikely.

PREGNANCY-LACTATION-REPRODUCTION
- Enroll patients exposed to drug during pregnancy in the Antiretroviral Pregnancy Registry (1-800-258-4263 or https://www.apregistry.com/Contact.aspx).
- Use cautiously during pregnancy. Monitor viral load closely.
- It isn't known if drug appears in human milk. Counsel patient with HIV infection on current CDC recommendations on transmission of HIV through breastfeeding.

NURSING CONSIDERATIONS
- Patients should take drug with a regular meal and not with a protein drink; taking drug with a protein-rich drink may lower rilpivirine exposure by 50%.
- Always use rilpivirine in combination with other antiretrovirals.
- Drug isn't a cure for HIV infection. Patients must stay on continuous antiretroviral therapy to control HIV infection and decrease HIV-related illnesses.
- Monitor patient for severe rash or rash accompanied by fever, blisters, mucosal involvement, conjunctivitis, facial edema, angioedema, hepatitis, eosinophilia, or DRESS syndrome. Discontinue drug if hypersensitivity

reaction or rash develops; initiate appropriate therapy.
- Monitor patients for reemergence of infections, such as *Mycobacterium avium*, cytomegalovirus, *Pneumocystis jiroveci* pneumonia, and TB, during initial combination treatment. Treat infections appropriately.
- Monitor patients for autoimmune disorders (Graves disease, polymyositis, Guillain-Barré syndrome, autoimmune hepatitis) that have also been reported to occur with immune reconstitution; however, the time to onset varies and can occur many months after initiation of treatment.
- Monitor patients for depressive disorders (depressed mood, dysphoria, negative thoughts, suicidality). Weigh risks of continued therapy against benefits of treatment.
- Monitor liver enzyme levels before and during treatment for patients with underlying liver disease. Consider monitoring liver enzyme levels for patients without preexisting liver dysfunction or other risk factors. Monitor patients with CrCl less than 30 mL/minute for adverse reactions during treatment.

PATIENT TEACHING
- Advise patient that rilpivirine isn't a cure for HIV infection or AIDS and that patient must stay on continuous antiretroviral therapy to control HIV infection.
- Tell patient to report all medications and supplements being taken because many of them may interact with rilpivirine.
- Instruct patient in safe drug administration.
- Warn patient that rilpivirine may cause depressed or altered mood and to report mood changes or symptoms of depression immediately.
- Advise patient to immediately report hypersensitivity reaction or rash.
- Tell patient to report pregnancy immediately.

risankizumab-rzaa
RIS-an-KIZ-ue-mab

Skyrizi

Therapeutic class: Immunomodulators
Pharmacologic class: Interleukin-23 receptor antagonists

AVAILABLE FORMS
Injection (IV): 600 mg/10 mL vial

Injection (subcut): 75 mg/0.83 mL, 90 mg/mL, 150 mg/mL prefilled syringes; 150 mg/mL prefilled pen; 180 mg/1.2 mL, 360 mg/2.4 mL prefilled cartridges with on-body injector

INDICATIONS & DOSAGES
➤ **Moderate to severe plaque psoriasis in patients who are candidates for systemic therapy or phototherapy**
Adults: 150 mg subcut at week 0, week 4, and every 12 weeks thereafter.
➤ **Active psoriatic arthritis**
Adults: 150 mg subcut at week 0, week 4, and every 12 weeks thereafter, alone or in combination with nonbiologic DMARDs.
➤ **Moderate to severe Crohn disease**
Adults: 600 mg IV infusion over at least 1 hour at weeks 0, 4, and 8, then 180 mg or 360 mg subcut at week 12 and every 8 weeks thereafter. Use the lowest effective dosage.

ADMINISTRATION
IV
▼ Withdraw 10 mL of solution from vial and inject into 100, 250, or 500 mL IV bag or glass bottle of D₅W for final concentration of 1.2 to 6 mg/mL.
▼ Don't shake vial or diluted solution.
▼ Allow diluted solution to warm to room temperature if stored in refrigerator before start of infusion.
▼ Infuse over at least 1 hour. Complete infusion within 8 hours of dilution if stored at room temperature.
▼ Refrigerate diluted solution for up to 20 hours at 36° to 46° F (2° to 8° C).
▼ Store vials at 36° to 46° F (2° to 8° C), protected from light.
▼ **Incompatibilities:** Don't infuse in same IV line with other drugs.
Subcutaneous
• Give injections in thighs, abdomen, or upper outer arm.
• Except for arm injection sites, patients may self-inject after proper training. The 90 mg/mL should be prepared and administered by a healthcare professional.
• Don't inject into areas where skin is tender, bruised, erythematous, indurated, or affected by psoriasis.
• If more than one injection is required for a single dose, give each in different anatomic locations.
• Keep in original carton to protect from light until use.

• Allow solution to warm to room temperature out of direct sunlight in the carton for 15 to 30 minutes for prefilled syringes, 30 to 90 minutes for prefilled pens, and 45 to 90 minutes for prefilled cartridge before use.
• Inspect solution for particulate matter and discoloration before use. Don't administer if solution contains large particles or is cloudy or discolored.
• Don't use if the syringe has been shaken, dropped, or damaged or if the tray seal is broken or missing.
• Give a missed dose as soon as possible; then resume dosing at the regular scheduled time.
• Store refrigerated at 36° to 46° F (2° to 8° C). Don't use if the liquid has been frozen.

ACTION
An IgG1 monoclonal antibody that selectively binds to the p19 subunit of IL-23, thereby inhibiting its interaction with the IL-23 receptor, which inhibits the release of proinflammatory cytokines and chemokines.

Route	Onset	Peak	Duration
IV	Unknown	Unknown	Unknown
Subcut	Unknown	3–14 days	Unknown

Half-life: About 28 days (plaque psoriasis, psoriatic arthritis); 21 days (Crohn disease).

ADVERSE REACTIONS
CNS: headache, fatigue, fever. **GI:** abdominal pain. **GU:** UTI. **Hematologic:** anemia. **Hepatic:** increased LFTs. **Musculoskeletal:** arthralgia, back pain, arthropathy. **Respiratory:** URI. **Skin:** injection site reactions, tinea infections. **Other:** infection, antibody development.

INTERACTIONS
Drug-drug. *Live vaccines:* Unknown if drug affects response to live or inactive vaccines. Avoid use together.

EFFECTS ON LAB TEST RESULTS
• May increase LFTs.
• May decrease RBC count.

CONTRAINDICATIONS & CAUTIONS
• Contraindicated in patients with prior serious hypersensitivity reaction to risankizumab-rzaa.
• Drug may increase risk of infection. Don't start drug in patients with clinically active

infection until the infection resolves or is adequately treated.

• Use cautiously in patients with chronic infection or a history of recurrent infections.

• Evaluate patients for TB before initiating treatment. Don't give to patients with active TB. Consider anti-TB therapy in patients with a history of latent or active TB in whom adequate treatment can't be confirmed.

• Drug may increase risk of liver injury in patients with Crohn disease. Consider other treatment options in patients with liver cirrhosis.

• Safety and effectiveness in children haven't been established.

Dialyzable drug: Unknown.

PREGNANCY-LACTATION-REPRODUCTION

• Studies during pregnancy are inadequate. Human IgG crosses the placental barrier and drug may be transferred to the developing fetus.

• Consider delaying live-virus immunizations at least 5 months in infants exposed in utero.

• Encourage patients who are pregnant to enroll in the Pregnancy Exposure Registry by calling 1-877-302-2161 or visiting https://glowpregnancyregistry.com.

• It isn't known if drug appears in human milk. Maternal IgG is present in human milk. Before use in a patient who is breastfeeding, consider the benefits of breastfeeding along with risk to the infant.

NURSING CONSIDERATIONS

• Evaluate patients for TB before, during, and after therapy. Anti-TB therapy may be required.

• Complete all age-appropriate immunizations according to current guidelines and schedules before therapy.

• Obtain baseline LFT values in patients with Crohn disease and monitor values during induction, for at least up to 12 weeks of treatment, and periodically thereafter.

• Monitor patients for signs and symptoms of infection (fever, diaphoresis, chills, cough, dyspnea, bloody phlegm, muscle aches, weight loss, diarrhea or stomach pain, frequent urination, burning pain with urination; warm, red, or painful skin sores that aren't psoriasis). If infection occurs or isn't responding to therapy, withhold drug until infection resolves.

PATIENT TEACHING

• Tell patient to report all adverse reactions.

• Instruct patient and caregivers on proper injection technique and needle and syringe disposal; supervise initial self-injection.

• Warn patient that drug may lower the ability of the immune system to fight infections. Stress importance of reporting history of infections to prescriber and of immediately reporting signs and symptoms of infection.

• Teach patient with a history of TB or active TB that treatment for TB may be needed before therapy begins.

• Instruct patient to seek immediate medical attention for signs and symptoms of liver dysfunction (rash, nausea, vomiting, abdominal pain, fatigue, anorexia, jaundice, dark urine).

• Counsel patient to become up-to-date with appropriate vaccines before therapy begins.

• Advise patient to report pregnancy, plans to become pregnant, breastfeeding, or plans to breastfeed before therapy begins.

risedronate sodium
ris-ED-roe-nate

Actonel, Atelvia

Therapeutic class: Antiosteoporotics
Pharmacologic class: Bisphosphonates

AVAILABLE FORMS
Tablets ⒹⓃⒸ: 5 mg, 30 mg, 35 mg, 75 mg, 150 mg
Tablets (delayed-release) ⒹⓃⒸ: 35 mg

INDICATIONS & DOSAGES
➤ **To prevent and treat postmenopausal osteoporosis**
Adult females: 5-mg immediate-release tablet PO once daily. Or, 35-mg immediate-release tablet PO once weekly. Or, 75 mg immediate-release tablet PO on 2 consecutive days for a total of 150 mg each month. Or, one 150-mg immediate-release tablet PO once monthly.

➤ **To treat postmenopausal osteoporosis**
Adult females: 35-mg delayed-release tablet PO once weekly.

➤ **To increase bone mass in males with osteoporosis**
Adult males: 35-mg immediate-release tablet PO once weekly.

➤ **To prevent or treat glucocorticoid-induced osteoporosis in patients taking**

R

7.5 mg or more of prednisone or equivalent glucocorticoid daily
Adults: 5-mg immediate-release tablet PO daily.
➤ **Paget disease**
Adults: 30-mg immediate-release tablet PO daily for 2 months. If relapse occurs or ALP level doesn't normalize, may repeat treatment course 2 months or more after completing first treatment course.

ADMINISTRATION
PO
● Give immediate-release tablets at least 30 minutes before the first food, drink, or medication of the day, other than water. Give with 8 oz of plain water.
● Patient shouldn't eat or drink anything except plain water or take other medications for at least 30 minutes after taking immediate-release risedronate.
● Give delayed-release tablet in the morning immediately after breakfast and not under fasting conditions because of a higher risk of abdominal pain if taken when fasting. Give with 8 oz of plain water.
● Warn patient against lying down for 30 minutes after taking drug.
● Have patient swallow tablets whole; don't crush or cut tablets.
● Refer to manufacturer's instructions for missed doses.

ACTION
Reverses loss of bone mineral density by reducing bone turnover and bone resorption. In patients with Paget disease, drug causes bone turnover to return to normal.

Route	Onset	Peak	Duration
PO	Unknown	1 hr	Unknown
PO (delayed-release)	Unknown	3 hr	Unknown

Half-life: 561 hours.

ADVERSE REACTIONS
CNS: asthenia, headache, depression, dizziness, insomnia, pain. **CV:** HTN, *arrhythmia,* chest pain, peripheral edema. **EENT:** cataract, pharyngitis, rhinitis, sinusitis. **GI:** nausea, diarrhea, abdominal pain, vomiting, dyspepsia, gastritis, GERD, constipation. **GU:** UTI, BPH, kidney stones. **Musculoskeletal:** arthralgia, arthritis, neck pain, back pain, limb pain, myalgia, bone pain, traumatic fracture, joint disorder. **Respiratory:** URI,

bronchitis, cough. **Skin:** rash. **Other:** infection, flulike symptoms, hypersensitivity reaction.

INTERACTIONS
Drug-drug. *Aspirin, NSAIDs:* May increase risk of upper GI adverse events. Use cautiously together.
Calcium supplements; antacids that contain calcium, magnesium, or aluminum: May interfere with risedronate absorption. Advise patient to separate dosing times.
H₂-receptor antagonists, PPIs: May affect enteric coating on delayed-release tablets, increasing bioavailability. Use together isn't recommended.
Drug-food. *Any food:* May interfere with absorption of drug. Advise patient to take immediate-release tablets at least 30 minutes before first food or drink of the day (other than water).

EFFECTS ON LAB TEST RESULTS
● May increase parathyroid hormone level.
● May decrease calcium and phosphorus levels.

CONTRAINDICATIONS & CAUTIONS
● Contraindicated in patients hypersensitive to components of the product, in patients with hypocalcemia or conditions that delay esophageal emptying, and in those who can't stand or sit upright for 30 minutes after administration.
● Use cautiously in patients with kidney impairment. Drug isn't recommended for use in patients with CrCl less than 30 mL/minute.
● Hypersensitivity and skin reactions have been reported, including angioedema, generalized rash, bullous skin reactions, SJS, and TEN.
⚠ *Alert:* Drug may increase risk of thigh fractures.
● Drug increases risk of osteonecrosis of the jaw, which can occur spontaneously. For patients requiring invasive dental procedures, discontinuing bisphosphonate treatment may reduce risk.
● Use cautiously in patients with upper GI disorders, such as dysphagia, esophagitis, and esophageal or gastric ulcers.
● Treat hypocalcemia and other disturbances of bone and mineral metabolism before starting treatment.
● Immediate-release and delayed-release formulations contain the same active ingredient and must not be given together.

Reactions in bold italics are *life-threatening.*

Dialyzable drug: Unknown.

⚠ *Overdose S&S:* Hypocalcemia, hypophosphatemia.

PREGNANCY-LACTATION-REPRODUCTION
• There are no adequate studies during pregnancy but fetal exposure to drug is likely. Discontinue drug for confirmed pregnancy.
• It isn't known if drug appears in human milk. Patient should discontinue breastfeeding or discontinue drug, considering importance of drug to patient.

NURSING CONSIDERATIONS
• Assess sex steroid hormonal status of all patients with glucocorticoid-induced osteoporosis; hormone replacement may be appropriate.
• Monitor patient for osteonecrosis of the jaw. Associated risk factors include invasive dental procedures, cancer diagnosis, concomitant treatment such as chemotherapy and steroids, poor oral hygiene, and preexisting dental disease. If signs or symptoms occur, stop drug and refer patient to oral surgeon.
• *Alert:* Drug may cause dysphagia, esophagitis, and esophageal or gastric ulcers. Monitor patient for symptoms of esophageal disease.
• Severe musculoskeletal pain has been associated with bisphosphonate use and may occur within days, months, or years of start of therapy. When drug is stopped, symptoms may resolve partially or completely.
• Give supplemental calcium and vitamin D if dietary intake is inadequate. Because calcium supplements and drugs containing calcium, aluminum, or magnesium may interfere with risedronate absorption, separate dosing times.
• Periodically evaluate need for continued therapy in all patients. Consider discontinuation of therapy in patients at low risk for fracture after 3 to 5 years of use.
• Periodically evaluate risk of fracture in patients who discontinue therapy.
• Monitor patient for eye inflammation. Refer patient for ophthalmologic evaluation if inflammation occurs.
• Bisphosphonates can interfere with bone-imaging agents.
• *Look alike–sound alike:* Don't confuse Actonel with Actos.

PATIENT TEACHING
• Explain that drug may reverse bone loss by stopping more bone loss and increasing bone strength.
• Stress importance of adhering to special dosing instructions, including staying in an upright position for 30 minutes after taking drug with plain water and to avoid taking other medications for at least 30 minutes after a risedronate dose.
• Tell patient not to chew, cut, crush, or suck the tablet because doing so may irritate the mouth.
• Advise patient to immediately report GI discomfort (such as difficulty or pain when swallowing, retrosternal pain, or severe heartburn).
• Tell patient that Actonel and Atelvia contain the same active ingredient and must not be taken together.
• Advise patient to take calcium and vitamin D if dietary intake is inadequate, but to take them at a different time than risedronate.
• Counsel patient to stop smoking and drinking alcohol, as appropriate. Also, advise patient to perform weight-bearing exercise.

risperiDONE
ris-PEER-i-dohn

Perseris, RisperDAL, RisperDAL Consta, Rykindo, Uzedy

Therapeutic class: Antipsychotics
Pharmacologic class: Benzisoxazole derivatives

AVAILABLE FORMS
Injection (IM): 12.5 mg, 25 mg, 37.5 mg, 50 mg
Injection (subcut): 50 mg/0.14 mL, 75 mg/0.21 mL, 100 mg/0.28 mL, 125 mg/0.35 mL, 150 mg/0.42 mL, 200 mg/0.56 mL, 250 mg/0.7 mL prefilled syringes
Injection kit (subcut): 90 mg/0.6 mL, 120 mg/0.8 mL prefilled powder syringes with liquid syringes to mix for administration
Oral solution: 1 mg/mL
Tablets: 0.25 mg, 0.5 mg, 1 mg, 2 mg, 3 mg, 4 mg
Tablets (ODTs): 0.25 mg, 0.5 mg, 1 mg, 2 mg, 3 mg, 4 mg

R

INDICATIONS & DOSAGES

Adjust-a-dose (for all indications): Refer to prescribing information for dosage adjustment for appropriate formulation when administered with a CYP3A4 inducer (increase risperidone dosage; decrease dosage when enzyme inducer is discontinued) or with a CYP2D6 inhibitor (reduce risperidone dosage; increase dosage as needed when enzyme inhibitor is discontinued).

➤ **Schizophrenia**

Adults: May give drug PO once daily or b.i.d. Initial dosing is generally 2 mg PO daily. Increase dosage at intervals not less than 24 hours, in increments of 1 to 2 mg/day, as tolerated, to recommended dose of 4 to 8 mg/day. Periodically reassess to determine need for maintenance treatment with an appropriate dose. Maximum dose, 16 mg/day.

Adjust-a-dose: In older adults, patients with hypotension, and those with CrCl of less than 30 mL/minute or Child-Pugh class C liver impairment, use lower starting dosage of 0.5 mg PO b.i.d. May increase in increments of 0.5 mg or less b.i.d. Increase to dosages above 1.5 mg b.i.d. at intervals of at least 1 week.

Adolescents ages 13 to 17: Start treatment with 0.5 mg PO once daily, given as a single daily dose in either morning or evening. Adjust dose, if indicated, at intervals of not less than 24 hours, in increments of 0.5 or 1 mg/day, as tolerated, to a recommended dosage of 3 mg/day. Reassess periodically to determine need for maintenance treatment with an appropriate dose. Maximum dose, 6 mg/day.

➤ **Parenteral maintenance therapy for schizophrenia or bipolar I disorder (as monotherapy or as combination therapy with lithium or valproate)**

Adults: Establish tolerance to oral risperidone before giving IM. Give 25 mg deep IM every 2 weeks.

Adjust dose no sooner than every 4 weeks. Maximum, 50 mg IM every 2 weeks. Continue oral antipsychotic for 3 weeks with Risperdal Consta or 7 days with Rykindo after first IM injection, then stop oral therapy. Continue therapy at lowest dose needed. Periodically reevaluate long-term risks and benefits of drug for individual patient. For adults switching from every 2 week IM formulation (Risperdal Consta) to Rykindo, the same dose should be continued beginning 4 weeks (no later than 5) after last IM injection of previous

therapy. Oral risperidone supplementation not recommended.

For subcut dosing, inject 90 or 120 mg once monthly (Perseris 90 mg corresponds to 3 mg/day oral risperidone and Perseris 120 mg corresponds to 4 mg/day oral risperidone). Subcut Uzedy dose is based on previous PO dose, beginning the day after last PO dose (2 mg/day PO risperdone corresponds to Uzedy 50 mg once monthly or 100 mg once every 2 months; 3 mg/day PO risperidone corresponds to Uzedy 75 mg once monthly or 150 mg once every 2 months; 4 mg/day PO risperidone corresponds to Uzedy 100 mg once monthly or 200 mg once every 2 months; 5 mg/day PO risperidone corresponds to 125 mg once monthly or 250 mg once every 2 months). No oral supplementation is recommended.

Adjust-a-dose: In patients with liver or kidney impairment, titrate slowly to 2 mg PO daily for 1 week. If tolerated, give 25 mg IM every 2 weeks, or may consider initial dose of 12.5 mg IM. Continue oral form of risperidone (or another antipsychotic) for 3 weeks after first injection of Risperdal Consta or 7 days after first injection of Rykindo to maintain therapeutic drug level.

➤ **Monotherapy or combination therapy with lithium or valproate for maintenance treatment of acute manic or mixed episodes from bipolar I disorder**

Adults: Initially, 2 to 3 mg PO once daily. Adjust dose by 1 mg daily. Dosage range, 1 to 6 mg daily. Or, after tolerability with oral risperidone has been established, 25 mg IM every 2 weeks. Some patients may benefit from a higher dose of 37.5 or 50 mg. Continue oral form of risperidone for 3 weeks after first injection of Risperdal Consta or 7 days after first injection of Rykindo to maintain therapeutic drug level.

Adjust-a-dose: In older adults, patients with hypotension, and those with CrCl less than 30 mL/min or Child-Pugh class C liver impairment, start with 0.5 mg PO b.i.d. May increase dosage to 1 mg b.i.d or 2 mg PO daily after at least 1 week. If total daily dose is at least 2 mg PO, may switch to 25 mg IM every 2 weeks. Oral supplementation should continue for 3 weeks after first injection.

Children and adolescents ages 10 to 17: 0.5 mg PO as a single daily dose in either morning or evening. Adjust dose, if indicated, at intervals not less than 24 hours, in increments of 0.5 or 1 mg/day, as tolerated, to a recommended dose of 2.5 mg/day.

➤ **Irritability, including aggression, self-injury, and temper tantrums, associated with an autistic disorder**
Adolescents and children ages 5 to 17 weighing 20 kg or more: Initially, 0.5 mg PO once daily or in two divided doses. After 4 days, may increase dose to 1 mg/day. Increase dosage further in 0.5-mg increments as needed at intervals of at least 2 weeks up to 3 mg/day.
Children ages 5 to 17 weighing more than 15 and less than 20 kg: Initially, 0.25 mg PO once daily or in two divided doses. After 4 days, may increase dosage to 0.5 mg/day. Increase dosage further in 0.25-mg increments as needed at intervals of at least 2 weeks up to 3 mg/day.

ADMINISTRATION
PO
• Give drug without regard for meals.
• Oral solution isn't compatible with cola or tea.
• Open package for ODTs immediately before giving by peeling off foil backing with dry hands. Don't push tablets through the foil. ODTs can be swallowed with or without liquid.
IM
• Drug should be administered by a health care professional.
• Continue oral therapy for first 3 weeks of Riperdal Consta or 7 weeks of Rykindo IM injection therapy until injections take effect, then stop oral therapy.
• Bring injection to room temperature for at least 30 minutes before preparation (don't warm any other way).
• To reconstitute IM injection, inject premeasured diluent into vial and shake vigorously for at least 10 seconds (Risperdal Consta) or 30 seconds (Rykindo). Suspension appears uniform, thick, and milky; particles are visible, but no dry particles remain. Use drug immediately after reconstitution. Just before injection, shake vigorously again. See manufacturer's package insert for more detailed instructions.
• Use Risperdal Consta injection kit with 1-inch needle for deltoid muscle injection and kit with 2-inch needle for gluteal muscle injection. Rykindo should be only be injected into gluteal muscle.

• Inject deep IM into gluteal or deltoid muscle, alternating injections.
• Refrigerate IM injection kit and protect it from light. Drug can be stored at less than 77° F (25° C) for no more than 7 days before administration.
Subcutaneous
• Subcut injection are given in abdomen or back of upper arm only. Don't give by any other route.
• Only a health care professional should administer drug.
• Allow package to come to room temperature for at least 15 minutes (Perseris) or 30 minutes (Udezy) before preparation.
• Prepare medication immediately before administration according to manufacturers instructions.
• Give a missed dose as soon as possible.

ACTION
Blocks dopamine, 5-HT$_2$, alpha$_1$ and alpha$_2$ adrenergic, and H$_1$ histaminergic receptors in the brain.

Route	Onset	Peak	Duration
PO	Unknown	1 hr	Unknown
IM	3 wk	4–6 wk	7 wk
Subcut	Unknown	4–6 hr	4 wk

Half-life: PO, 20 hours; IM, 3 to 6 days; subcut (Perseris), 9 to 11 days; subcut (Udezy), 14 to 22 days.

ADVERSE REACTIONS
CNS: akathisia, asthenia, sedation, somnolence, dystonia, headache, insomnia, agitation, anxiety, pain, parkinsonism, abnormal gait, ataxia, dizziness, fever, hallucinations, manic symptoms, impaired concentration, abnormal thinking and dreaming, tremor, hypoesthesia, fatigue, depression, nervousness, vertigo, syncope. **CV:** tachycardia, *bradycardia,* bundle-branch block, ECG changes, chest pain, hypotension, edema, palpitations, HTN. **EENT:** abnormal vision, conjunctivitis, decreased visual acuity, ear disorder (IM), rhinorrhea, nasal congestion, epistaxis, rhinitis, sinusitis, nasopharyngitis, dry mouth, increased saliva, toothache, sore throat. **GI:** constipation, nausea, vomiting, dyspepsia, abdominal pain, anorexia, increased appetite, diarrhea. **GU:** urinary incontinence, increased urination, abnormal orgasm, decreased libido, vaginal dryness, amenorrhea, menstrual disorder, cystitis, erectile dysfunction,

R

UTI. **Metabolic:** weight gain or loss, hyperglycemia. **Musculoskeletal:** arthralgia, back pain, limb pain, myalgia, muscle rigidity, muscle spasm. **Respiratory:** cough, dyspnea, bronchitis, pneumonia, URI. **Skin:** rash, eczema, pruritus, dry skin, photosensitivity reactions, acne; injection-site pain, reaction, or infection (IM, subcut). **Other:** increased thirst, galactorrhea, gynecomastia, hypersensitivity reaction, viral infection, falls, injury.

INTERACTIONS

Drug-drug. *Antihypertensives, drugs with hypotensive effects:* May enhance hypotensive effects. Monitor BP.

Clozapine: May decrease risperidone clearance, increasing adverse reactions (GI hypomotility). Monitor patient closely.

CNS depressants: May cause additive CNS depression. Use together cautiously.

CYP2D6 inhibitors (fluoxetine, paroxetine): May increase risk of risperidone's adverse effects, including serotonin syndrome. Monitor patient closely and decrease risperidone dose as needed.

CYP3A4 inducers (carbamazepine, phenobarbital, phenytoin, rifampin): May increase risperidone clearance and decrease effectiveness. Monitor patient closely.

Dopamine agonists, levodopa: May antagonize effects of these drugs. Use together cautiously and monitor patient.

Methylphenidate: May increase risk of extrapyramidal symptoms with change in dosage of either medication. Monitor patient closely.

❶ **Alert:** *Opioids:* May increase CNS depression. Avoid use together. If use together is necessary, limit dosage and duration of each drug to minimum necessary for desired effect.

QTc interval-prolonging drugs (dofetilide, procainamide, sotalol): May increase risk of QTc-interval prolongation and risk of life-threatening ventricular arrhythmias. Use together cautiously unless contraindicated.

Drug-lifestyle. *Alcohol use:* May cause additive CNS depression. Discourage use together.

EFFECTS ON LAB TEST RESULTS

• May increase AST, ALT, blood glucose, cholesterol, triglyceride, GGT, and prolactin levels.

• May decrease Hb level, hematocrit, and WBC count.

CONTRAINDICATIONS & CAUTIONS

• Contraindicated in patients hypersensitive to risperidone or paliperidone.

Boxed Warning Older adults with dementia-related psychosis treated with antipsychotics are at increased risk for death. Drug isn't approved to treat older adults with dementia-related psychosis. ∎

• Use cautiously in patients with CV disease, cerebrovascular disease, dehydration, hypovolemia, history of seizures, or conditions that could affect metabolism or hemodynamic responses.

• Use cautiously in patients exposed to extreme heat.

• Use caution in patients at risk for aspiration pneumonia.

• Use IM or subcut injection cautiously in patients with liver or kidney impairment.

• Somnolence, orthostatic hypotension, and motor and sensory instability have been reported, which may lead to falls and fall-related injuries.

Dialyzable drug: Unknown.

⚠ *Overdose S&S:* Drowsiness, sedation, tachycardia, hypotension, extrapyramidal symptoms, QT-interval prolongation, seizures, torsades de pointes.

PREGNANCY-LACTATION-REPRODUCTION

❶ **Alert:** Neonates exposed to antipsychotics during the third trimester are at risk for developing extrapyramidal signs and symptoms (repetitive muscle movements of the face and body) and withdrawal signs and symptoms (agitation, abnormally increased or decreased muscle tone, tremors, sleepiness, severe difficulty breathing, difficulty feeding) after delivery. Use in patients who are pregnant only if potential benefit justifies fetal risk.

• Enroll patients exposed to drug during pregnancy in the National Pregnancy Registry for Atypical Antipsychotics (1-866-961-2388 or https://womensmentalhealth.org/research/pregnancyregistry/atypicalantipsychotic/).

• Drug appears in human milk. Patient should discontinue breastfeeding or discontinue drug, considering importance of drug to patient.

• Drug may cause hyperprolactinemia, which may decrease reproductive function in both males and females.

NURSING CONSIDERATIONS

❶ **Alert:** Obtain baseline BP measurements before starting therapy, and monitor BP regularly. Watch for orthostatic hypotension, especially during first dosage adjustment.

• Monitor patient for tardive dyskinesia, which may occur after prolonged use. It may not appear until months or years later and may disappear spontaneously or persist for life, despite stopping drug.

❸ *Alert:* Watch for evidence of NMS (extrapyramidal effects, hyperthermia, autonomic disturbance), which is rare but can be fatal.

❸ *Alert:* Life-threatening hyperglycemia may occur in patients taking atypical antipsychotics. Monitor patients with diabetes regularly.

• Monitor patient for symptoms of metabolic syndrome (significant weight gain and increased BMI, HTN, hyperglycemia, hypercholesterolemia, and hypertriglyceridemia).

• Periodically reevaluate drug's risks and benefits, especially during prolonged use.

• Patients experiencing persistent somnolence may benefit from administering half the daily PO dose b.i.d.

• Monitor CBC in patients with preexisting low WBC count or history of drug-induced leukopenia or neutropenia.

• Assess fall risk when initiating treatment and recurrently for patients on long-term therapy, especially for older adults and patients with diseases, conditions, or other drug regimens that could increase fall risk.

• *Look alike–sound alike:* Don't confuse risperidone with reserpine or ropinirole. Don't confuse Risperdal with Restoril.

PATIENT TEACHING

• Instruct patient in safe drug administration.

• Warn patient to avoid activities that require alertness until effects of drug are known.

• Caution patient or caregiver of patient taking an opioid with a benzodiazepine, CNS depressant, or alcohol to seek immediate medical attention for dizziness, light-headedness, extreme sleepiness, slowed or difficult breathing, or unresponsiveness.

• Warn patient to rise slowly and use precautions to avoid fainting when starting therapy.

• Advise patient that drug may increase fall risk due to somnolence, orthostatic hypotension, and motor and sensory instability.

• Warn patient to use caution in hot weather to prevent heatstroke.

• Inform male patient of possibility of prolonged or painful penile erections, and to seek immediate medical attention if they occur.

• Inform patient with phenylketonuria that ODT contains phenylalanine.

• Advise patient to avoid alcohol during therapy.

• Caution patient to report pregnancy or breastfeeding to provider.

ritonavir
ri-TOE-na-veer

Norvir

Therapeutic class: Antiretrovirals
Pharmacologic class: Protease inhibitors

AVAILABLE FORMS
Oral powder: 100-mg packet
Tablets ⓄⓃⒸ: 100 mg

INDICATIONS & DOSAGES
➤ **HIV infection, with other antiretrovirals**
Adults: 600 mg PO b.i.d. To reduce adverse GI effects, begin with 300 mg PO b.i.d. and increase by 100 mg b.i.d. at 2- to 3-day intervals.

Children older than age 1 month: 350 to 400 mg/m^2 PO b.i.d.; don't exceed 600 mg PO b.i.d. Initially, start with 250 mg/m^2 b.i.d. and increase by 50 mg/m^2 PO b.i.d. at 2- to 3-day intervals. If children can't reach b.i.d. doses of 400 mg/m^2 because of adverse effects, consider alternative therapy.

Adjust-a-dose: Dosage reduction is necessary when drug is used with other protease inhibitors: atazanavir, darunavir, fosamprenavir, saquinavir, and tipranavir. Consult full prescribing information for dosage modification.

ADMINISTRATION
PO
• Give drug with meals.

• Don't use oral powder for doses less than 100 mg or for incremental doses between 100-mg intervals.

• Mix oral powder with soft food, such as applesauce or vanilla pudding, or with liquid, such as water, chocolate milk, or infant formula, to lessen bitter aftertaste. Give within 2 hours of preparation; discard and prepare new dose if more than 2 hours have elapsed since preparation.

• Oral powder can be mixed with water and administered via a feeding tube.

R

• Have patient swallow tablets whole; don't break or crush tablets.

• Give a missed dose as soon as possible; then return to normal schedule. Don't double next dose.

ACTION

An HIV-1 protease inhibitor. Drug binds to the protease-active site and inhibits activity of the enzyme, preventing cleavage of the viral polyproteins and causing formation of immature, noninfectious viral particles.

Route	Onset	Peak	Duration
PO	Unknown	2–4 hr	Unknown

Half-life: 3 to 5 hours.

ADVERSE REACTIONS

CNS: anxiety, paresthesia, confusion, depression, disturbance in attention, dizziness, fatigue, headache, pain, peripheral neuropathy, somnolence, syncope, taste perversion. **CV:** HTN, hypotension, edema, flushing. **EENT:** blurred vision, oropharyngeal pain. **GI:** diarrhea, nausea, vomiting, *pancreatitis,* abdominal pain, GERD, *GI hemorrhage,* dyspepsia, flatulence. **GU:** urinary frequency. **Hematologic:** anemia, *neutropenia, thrombocytopenia.* **Hepatic:** increased LFT values, *hepatitis.* **Metabolic:** electrolyte imbalance due to severe diarrhea, gout, hyperglycemia, lipid disorders. **Musculoskeletal:** arthralgia, myalgia, myopathy. **Respiratory:** cough. **Skin:** pruritus, rash, acne, lipodystrophy. **Other:** hypersensitivity reactions.

INTERACTIONS

⊖ *Alert:* Ritonavir can significantly interact with many drugs. Consult a drug interaction resource or pharmacist for more information.

Drug-drug. *Antiarrhythmics (amiodarone, dronedarone, flecainide, propafenone, quinidine):* May cause cardiac arrhythmias. Use together is contraindicated.

Apixaban: May increase apixaban level. Refer to manufacturer's instructions for possible dosage reductions.

Atovaquone, divalproex, lamotrigine, phenytoin: May decrease levels of these drugs. Use together cautiously and monitor drug levels closely.

Beta blockers, calcium channel blockers, digoxin, disopyramide, fluoxetine, lidocaine, mexiletine, nefazodone: May increase levels

of these drugs, causing cardiac and neurologic events. Use together cautiously.

Buspirone, carbamazepine, clonazepam, clorazepate, cyclosporine, desipramine, dexamethasone, diazepam, dronabinol, estazolam, ethosuximide, methamphetamine, perphenazine, prednisone, quinine, risperidone, sirolimus, SSRIs, tacrolimus, TCAs, thioridazine, timolol, tramadol, zolpidem: May increase levels of these drugs. Use cautiously together and consider decreasing dosage of these drugs by 50%. Monitor therapeutic levels.

Clarithromycin: May increase clarithromycin level. If CrCl ranges from 30 to 60 mL/minute, reduce clarithromycin dosage by 50%. If CrCl is less than 30 mL/minute, reduce clarithromycin dosage by 75%.

Colchicine: May increase risk of serious or life-threatening reactions in patients with kidney or liver impairment. Use together is contraindicated.

Delavirdine: May increase ritonavir level. Adjusted dose recommendations aren't established. Use together cautiously.

Drugs that prolong QT interval (antiarrhythmics, encorafenib, ivosidenib, levofloxacin): May have additive QT-interval prolonging effect. Use cautiously together.

Edoxaban: May increase edoxaban level. Consider dosage adjustment if using for venous thromboembolism. (Dosage adjustment isn't needed for atrial fibrillation.)

Ethinyl estradiol: May decrease ethinyl estradiol level. Use an alternative or additional method of birth control.

Fluticasone: May significantly increase fluticasone level, causing systemic corticosteroid effects (including Cushing syndrome). Don't use together, if possible.

⊖ *Alert: HMG-CoA reductase inhibitors (atorvastatin, pitavastatin, pravastatin, rosuvastatin):* May increase statin level and risk of myopathy and rhabdomyolysis. Use together cautiously at recommended dosage for the statin given in combination with ritonavir. Refer to prescribing information for statin dosage limitations.

Itraconazole, ketoconazole: May increase levels of these drugs. Don't exceed 200 mg/day of these drugs.

⊖ *Alert: Lovastatin, simvastatin:* May increase statin level and risk of myopathy and rhabdomyolysis. Use together is contraindicated.

Reactions in bold italics are *life-threatening*.

Meperidine: May increase meperidine metabolite level. Dosage increases and long-term use together aren't recommended because of CNS effects. Use cautiously together.
Methadone: May decrease methadone levels. Consider increasing methadone dosage.
PDE5 inhibitors (sildenafil, tadalafil, vardenafil): May increase levels of PDE5 inhibitor, causing hypotension, syncope, visual changes, or prolonged erection. Monitor for adverse reactions. Tell patient not to exceed 25 mg of sildenafil in a 48-hour period, 10 mg of tadalafil in a 72-hour period, or 2.5 mg of vardenafil in a 72-hour period.
Protease inhibitors (atazanavir, darunavir, fosamprenavir, saquinavir, tipranavir): May increase other protease inhibitor levels. Decrease ritonavir dosage. Consult prescribing information for combined use.
Quinine: May increase quinine level. Consider decreased quinine dosage when used together.
Rifabutin: May increase rifabutin levels. Monitor patient and reduce rifabutin daily dosage by at least 75% of usual dose.
Rifampin, rifapentine: May decrease ritonavir levels. Consider using rifabutin.
Rivaroxaban: May increase risk of bleeding. Avoid use together.
Theophylline: May decrease theophylline levels. Increase dose based on blood levels.
Trazodone: May increase trazodone level, causing nausea, dizziness, hypotension, and syncope. Avoid using together. If unavoidable, use cautiously and lower trazodone dose.
Voriconazole: Decreases voriconazole level and reduces antifungal response. Voriconazole is contraindicated with ritonavir doses of 400 mg every 12 hours or greater.
Warfarin: May affect INR. Monitor patient frequently after initiating coadministration and adjust warfarin dosage as needed.
Drug-herb. *St. John's wort:* May substantially reduce drug levels. Use together is contraindicated.
Drug-lifestyle. *Smoking:* May decrease drug levels. Discourage smoking.

EFFECTS ON LAB TEST RESULTS
• May increase ALT, AST, GGT, amylase, bilirubin, glucose, triglyceride, lipid, CK, and uric acid levels.
• May decrease Hb level, hematocrit, and WBC, RBC, platelet, and neutrophil counts.

CONTRAINDICATIONS & CAUTIONS
Boxed Warning Administration with sedative-hypnotics, antiarrhythmics, or ergot alkaloid preparations may result in potentially serious or life-threatening adverse events because of possible effects on the liver metabolism of certain drugs. Review medications taken by patients before administering ritonavir or when administering other medications to patients already taking ritonavir. ▪
• Contraindicated in patients hypersensitive to drug or its components.
• Use cautiously in patients with liver disease, liver enzyme abnormalities, or hepatitis and in those with signs or symptoms of pancreatitis.
❂ *Alert:* Patients with advanced HIV infection may have increased risk of elevated triglyceride levels and, in some cases, fatal pancreatitis.
• Hyperglycemia requiring treatment has been reported in patients receiving protease inhibitors. Use cautiously with diabetes.
• Use cautiously in patients with hemophilia A or B. Drug may increase risk of bleeding. Additional factor VIII may be needed.
• Safety and effectiveness in children younger than age 1 month haven't been established.
Dialyzable drug: Unlikely.
⚠ *Overdose S&S:* Paresthesia, KF with eosinophilia.

PREGNANCY-LACTATION-REPRODUCTION
• There are no adequate studies during pregnancy. Use only if potential benefit justifies fetal risk.
• Enroll patients who are pregnant and exposed to drug in the Antiretroviral Pregnancy Registry (1-800-258-4263 or https://www.apregistry.com/).

NURSING CONSIDERATIONS
• Monitor patient for immune reconstitution syndrome. During initial phase of treatment, patients responding to antiretroviral therapy may develop an inflammatory response to indolent or residual opportunistic infections (CMV, MAC, *Pneumocystis jiroveci* pneumonia, TB), which may necessitate further evaluation and treatment. Autoimmune disorders (Graves disease, polymyositis, Guillain-Barré syndrome) have also been reported in the setting of immune reconstitution; however, time

to onset is more variable, and can occur many months after initiation of antiretroviral treatment.

• Monitor for hypersensitivity reactions (rash, bronchospasm, angioedema, SCARs).

• Patients beginning regimens with ritonavir and nucleosides may improve GI tolerance by starting ritonavir alone and then adding nucleosides before completing 2 weeks of ritonavir.

• In patients with liver disease, monitor liver enzyme and triglyceride levels frequently, especially during first 3 months of treatment.

• Monitor for pancreatitis (nausea, vomiting, abdominal pain, increased lipase or amylase levels).

• Monitor lipid levels before and periodically during therapy.

• Monitor for hyperglycemia, new onset diabetes, or exacerbation of diabetes.

• Monitor patient for redistribution or accumulation of body fat, which has been observed with antiretroviral therapy.

• *Look alike–sound alike:* Don't confuse ritonavir with Retrovir. Don't confuse Norvir with Norvasc.

PATIENT TEACHING

• Explain that drug doesn't cure HIV infection and that opportunistic infections and other complications of HIV infection may continue to develop. Drug hasn't been shown to reduce the risk of transmitting HIV to others through sexual contact or blood contamination.

• Teach patient safe drug administration.

• Caution patient to take drug as prescribed and not to adjust dosage or stop therapy without first consulting prescriber.

• Instruct patient using hormonal contraceptives to use an alternative contraceptive or an additional barrier method during therapy.

• Caution patient to report signs and symptoms of pancreatitis immediately.

• Counsel patient that ritonavir must always be taken in combination with other antiretrovirals.

• Advise patient to report use of other drugs, including OTC drugs; this drug interacts with many drugs.

• Caution patient to report pregnancy or breastfeeding to prescriber.

Reactions in bold italics are *life-threatening*.

SAFETY ALERT!
BIOSIMILAR DRUG

riTUXimab
ri-TUK-si-mab

Rituxan

riTUXimab-abbs
Truxima

riTUXimab-arrx
Riabni

riTUXimab-pvvr
Ruxience

Therapeutic class: Antineoplastics
Pharmacologic class: Monoclonal antibodies

AVAILABLE FORMS
Injection: 10 mg/mL in 10-mL and 50-mL single-use, sterile vials

INDICATIONS & DOSAGES
➤ **Previously untreated, follicular CD20-positive, B-cell non-Hodgkin lymphoma (NHL) with cyclophosphamide-vincristine-prednisolone (CVP) chemotherapy regimen**
Adults: 375 mg/m^2 IV on day 1 of each CVP cycle, for up to 8 doses.
➤ **Maintenance therapy for patients with previously untreated follicular, CD20-positive, B-cell NHL who achieved complete or partial response to rituximab in combination with chemotherapy**
Adults: 375 mg/m^2 IV as single agent every 8 weeks for 12 doses beginning 8 weeks after completion of combination therapy.
➤ **Previously untreated low-grade, CD20-positive, B-cell NHL following first-line treatment with CVP chemotherapy**
Adults: For patients who fail to progress after 6 to 8 cycles of CVP chemotherapy, give 375 mg/m^2 IV once weekly for 4 doses every 6 months for up to 16 doses.
➤ **Relapsed or refractory low-grade or follicular, CD20-positive, B-cell NHL**
Adults: Initially, 375 mg/m^2 IV once weekly for 4 or 8 doses. Retreatment for patients with progressive disease, 375 mg/m^2 IV infusion once weekly for 4 doses.

➤ **With ibritumomab tiuxetan (Zevalin) for relapsed or refractory low-grade, follicular or transformed B-cell NHL**
Adults: 250 mg/m² IV 4 hours before indium-111 Zevalin infusion. Repeat in 7 to 9 days, 4 hours before yttrium-90 Zevalin infusion. Refer to ibritumomab prescribing information.

➤ **Diffuse large B-cell, CD20-positive NHL, given with cyclophosphamide-Adriamycin (doxorubicin)-Oncovin (vincristine)-prednisone (CHOP) chemotherapy regimen or other anthracycline-based chemotherapy regimens**
Adults: 375 mg/m² IV on day 1 of each chemotherapy cycle for up to 8 infusions.

➤ **CD20-positive chronic lymphocytic leukemia (CLL) in combination with fludarabine and cyclophosphamide**
Adults: 375 mg/m² IV given day before combination treatment. Then give 500 mg/m² IV on day 1 of cycles two through six in combination with fludarabine and cyclophosphamide (every 28 days).

➤ **With methotrexate to reduce signs and symptoms of moderate to severely active RA in patients who have had an inadequate response to one or more TNF antagonists**
Adults: Two 1,000-mg IV infusions 2 weeks apart. To reduce incidence and severity of infusion reactions, give methylprednisolone 100 mg IV or its equivalent 30 minutes before each infusion. May give additional courses every 24 weeks or based on clinical evaluation but no sooner than every 16 weeks.

➤ **Wegener granulomatosis (WG); microscopic polyangiitis (MPA) in combination with glucocorticoids**
Adults: 375 mg/m² IV once weekly for 4 weeks. Give methylprednisolone 1,000 mg/day IV for 1 to 3 days followed by oral prednisone 1 mg/kg/day (not to exceed 80 mg/day and tapered per clinical need) to treat severe vasculitis symptoms. This regimen should begin within 14 days before or with initiation of rituximab and may continue during and after 4-week course of rituximab treatment.
Children ages 2 to 17: 375 mg/m² IV once weekly for 4 weeks. Give IV methylprednisolone 30 mg/kg (not to exceed 1 g/day) once daily for 3 days. Refer to manufacturer's instructions for follow-up treatment dosing for adults and children.

➤ **Moderate to severe pemphigus vulgaris (Rituxan only)**
Adults: Initially, give two 1,000-mg IV infusions separated by 2 weeks in combination with a tapering course of glucocorticoids; then use a maintenance schedule of rituximab 500-mg IV infusion at month 12 and every 6 months thereafter or based on clinical evaluation. If patient relapses, give rituximab 1,000-mg IV infusion; consider resuming or increasing dosage of the glucocorticoid based on clinical evaluation. Allow at least 16 weeks between rituximab infusions. Methylprednisolone 100 mg IV or equivalent glucocorticoid is recommended 30 minutes before each rituximab infusion.

➤ **Previously untreated, advanced stage, CD20-positive, diffuse large B-cell lymphoma, Burkitt lymphoma, Burkitt-like lymphoma, or mature B-cell acute leukemia (AL), in combination with chemotherapy (Rituxan only)**
Children ages 6 months and older: 375 mg/m² IV infusion in combination with systemic Lymphome Malin de Burkitt (LMB) chemotherapy. Give 2 doses (48 hours apart) during each of the 2 induction courses, and on day 1 of each of the 2 consolidation courses. Give prednisone component of regimen before rituximab. Refer to manufacturer's instructions for additional dosing information.

➤ **Burkitt lymphoma ♦**
Adults: 375 mg/m² IV on days 1 and 11 of cycles one and three and days 2 and 8 of cycles two and four. Or, 375 mg/m² IV at start of each chemotherapy cycle, followed by two additional doses 3 and 6 weeks after completion of chemotherapy. Or, 50 mg/m² IV on day 8 and 375 mg/m² IV on days 10 and 12 of cycle two, followed by 375 mg/m² IV on day 8 of cycles three to seven.

ADMINISTRATION

IV

▼ Premedicate with acetaminophen and an antihistamine before each infusion.
▼ Protect vials from direct sunlight.
▼ Dilute to yield 1 to 4 mg/mL in bag of D₅W or NSS. Gently invert bag to mix solution.
▼ Give as an infusion; don't give as IV push or bolus.
▼ Begin infusion at rate of 50 mg/hour. If no hypersensitivity or infusion-related events occur, increase rate by 50 mg/hour every 30 minutes, to maximum of 400 mg/hour. Start subsequent infusions at 100 mg/hour and increase by 100 mg/hour every

30 minutes, to maximum of 400 mg/hour as tolerated.

▼ For children with mature B-cell NHL or AL, begin infusion at 0.5 mg/kg/hour (50 mg/hour maximum); may increase rate by 0.5 mg/kg/hour every 30 minutes, to a maximum of 400 mg/hour.

▼ For previously untreated follicular NHL and diffuse large B-cell NHL, patients may receive a 90-minute infusion in cycle two with a glucocorticoid-containing chemotherapy regimen if they didn't experience a grade 3 or 4 infusion-related adverse event during cycle one. Refer to manufacturer's instructions.

▼ Discard unused portion left in vial.

▼ Store diluted solutions in refrigerator at 36° to 46° F (2° to 8° C) for 24 hours because they don't contain a preservative.

▼ **Incompatibilities:** Other IV drugs.

ACTION
A murine and human monoclonal antibody directed against CD20 antigen found on surface of normal and malignant B lymphocytes. Binding to this antigen mediates lysis of B cells.

Route	Onset	Peak	Duration
IV	Variable	Variable	6–12 mo

Half-life: Varies widely, possibly because of differences in tumor burden among patients and changes in CD20-positive B-cell populations on repeated therapy.

ADVERSE REACTIONS
CNS: asthenia, fever, headache, agitation, dizziness, fatigue, hypesthesia, hypertonia, insomnia, malaise, anxiety, pain, paresthesia, peripheral neuropathy, taste perversion. **CV:** hypotension, chest pain, edema, flushing, HTN, peripheral edema, *serious CV event.* **EENT:** conjunctivitis, epistaxis, rhinitis, sinusitis, throat irritation, oral candidiasis. **GI:** nausea, abdominal pain or enlargement, anorexia, diarrhea, dyspepsia, vomiting. **GU:** UTI. **Hematologic:** *leukopenia, neutropenia, thrombocytopenia, lymphopenia,* anemia. **Hepatic:** hepatobiliary disease, increased transaminase levels. **Metabolic:** hyperglycemia, hyperuricemia, increased LDH level, hypophosphatemia, *hypocalcemia,* weight gain. **Musculoskeletal:** back pain, myalgia, arthralgia, muscle spasms. **Respiratory:** *bronchospasm,* bronchitis, URI, cough increase, dyspnea, *pulmonary toxicity.* **Skin:** pruritus, rash, pain at injection site,

urticaria, night sweats. **Other:** chills, rigors, *angioedema, infusion reaction,* infection, antibody development.

INTERACTIONS
Drug-drug. *Certolizumab, denosumab, tocilizumab:* May increase risk of serious infection. Avoid use together.
Cisplatin: May cause kidney toxicity. Monitor kidney function tests.
Leflunomide: May increase risk of hematologic toxicity. Monitor patient for bone marrow suppression at least monthly if both medications are needed.
❸ *Alert:* *Live-virus vaccines:* Virus replication may occur. Avoid vaccination with live-virus vaccines within 4 weeks before or during treatment.

EFFECTS ON LAB TEST RESULTS
• May increase glucose, potassium, uric acid, ALT, and LDH levels.
• May decrease calcium level.
• May increase or decrease phosphate level.
• May decrease Hb level and WBC, platelet, and neutrophil counts.

CONTRAINDICATIONS & CAUTIONS
Boxed Warning HBV reactivation, including fulminant hepatitis, liver failure, and death, may occur in patients treated with rituximab. ■
❸ *Alert:* Consult hepatitis expert when screening identifies patients at risk for HBV reactivation due to prior HBV infection.
• Use cautiously in patients with a history of arrhythmia or angina.
• Drug isn't recommended for use in patients with severe, active infections.
Dialyzable drug: Unknown.

PREGNANCY-LACTATION-REPRODUCTION
• Verify pregnancy status before treatment.
• Based on human data, drug can cause adverse developmental outcomes, including B-cell lymphocytopenia, in infants exposed to drug in utero. Advise patients who are pregnant of the fetal risk. Monitor exposed newborns and infants for infection.
• Patients of childbearing potential should use effective contraception during therapy and for 12 months after therapy ends.
• It isn't known if drug appears in human milk. Patient should discontinue breastfeeding during and for 6 months after treatment.

Reactions in bold italics are *life-threatening*.

NURSING CONSIDERATIONS

Boxed Warning Deaths from infusion reactions have occurred; most fatal reactions are associated with the first infusion. Closely monitor patient. Discontinue rituximab infusion for severe reactions and administer medical treatment for grade 3 or 4 infusion reactions. ■

• Monitor patient for infusion-related reactions (urticaria, hypotension, bronchospasm, angioedema, hypoxia, pulmonary infiltrates, ARDS, MI, cardiogenic shock). Depending on severity of the reaction, interrupt infusion or slow infusion rate and institute medical management. If symptoms resolve, continue infusion at no more than one-half the previous rate.

• Monitor BP closely during infusion.

• If serious or life-threatening arrhythmias occur, stop infusion. If patient develops significant arrhythmias, monitor cardiac function during and after subsequent infusions.

• *Pneumocystis jiroveci* pneumonia and antiherpetic viral prophylaxis is recommended for patients with CLL during and for up to 12 months after treatment ends; with WG and MPA during and for up to 6 months after treatment; and should be considered for pemphigus vulgaris during and after treatment.

Boxed Warning Screen all patients for HBV infection before treatment by measuring HbsAg and hepatitis B core antibody. Monitor patients with evidence of current or prior HBV infection during and for several months after therapy. If HBV reactivation occurs, discontinue rituximab and concomitant chemotherapy and begin appropriate treatment. ■

• Monitor patients for bacterial, fungal, and new or reactivated viral infections.

• Monitor patients with WG and MPA carefully for signs and symptoms of infection (fever, pain, cold or flu symptoms, erythema) if biological agents or DMARDs are used concomitantly.

• Ensure patient is up-to-date with all immunizations in agreement with current immunization guidelines before starting drug, if possible. Give non-live vaccines at least 4 weeks before a course of rituximab.

Boxed Warning Severe mucocutaneous reactions (TEN, SJS, paraneoplastic pemphigus, lichenoid or vesiculobullous dermatitis) may occur, with variable onset. Avoid further infusions and promptly start treatment of the skin reaction. ■

• Infusion-related reactions are most severe with first infusion. Subsequent infusions are generally well tolerated.

⊘ Alert: AKF requiring dialysis has been reported in the setting of TLS after treatment of patients with NHL.

• Patients at high risk for TLS may receive prophylactic allopurinol and hydration to correct hyperuricemia. Monitor kidney function and fluid balance, and correct electrolyte abnormalities.

Boxed Warning JC virus infection resulting in PML has been reported in patients within 12 months of their last rituximab infusion. Monitor patient for new-onset neurologic manifestations. ■

• Obtain CBC at regular intervals, more frequently in patients in whom cytopenias develop.

• Monitor patient for abdominal pain. Bowel obstruction and perforation have occurred with chemotherapy.

• *Look alike–sound alike:* Don't confuse rituximab with infliximab.

PATIENT TEACHING

• Provide patient with medication guide to read before each treatment session.

• Tell patient to report signs and symptoms of hypersensitivity, such as itching, rash, chills, or rigor, during and after infusion.

• Urge patient to report all adverse reactions, especially fever, sore throat, fatigue, easy bruising, nosebleeds, bleeding gums, abdominal pain, or melena, and to take temperature daily.

• Advise patient of childbearing potential to use effective contraception during therapy and for 12 months after final dose.

• Counsel patient to avoid breastfeeding during and for 6 months after therapy ends.

R

SAFETY ALERT!

rivaroxaban 〖
riv-a-ROX-a-ban

Xarelto

Therapeutic class: Anticoagulants
Pharmacologic class: Factor Xa inhibitors

AVAILABLE FORMS
Granules for oral suspension: 1 mg/mL after reconstitution
Tablets: 2.5 mg, 10 mg, 15 mg, 20 mg

INDICATIONS & DOSAGES

➤ **Prophylaxis of DVT that may lead to PE in patients undergoing knee or hip replacement surgery**

Adults: 10 mg PO once daily, 6 to 10 hours after surgery once hemostasis has been established. Treat for 35 days after hip replacement surgery and 12 days after knee replacement surgery.

Adjust-a-dose: If CrCl is less than 15 mL/minute, avoid use.

➤ **Treatment of DVT or PE**

Adults: 15 mg PO b.i.d. for 21 days; then 20 mg PO once daily for remainder of treatment.

Adjust-a-dose: If CrCl is less than 15 mL/minute, avoid use.

➤ **To decrease risk of recurrent DVT or PE after initial 6 months of treatment**

Adults: 10 mg PO once daily.

Adjust-a-dose: If CrCl is less than 15 mL/minute, avoid use.

➤ **VTE prophylaxis in patients who are acutely ill and at risk for thromboembolic complications but aren't at high risk for bleeding**

Adults: 10 mg PO once daily for total duration of 31 to 39 days.

Adjust-a-dose: If CrCl is less than 15 mL/minute, avoid use.

➤ **Stroke and systemic embolism risk reduction in patients with nonvalvular atrial fibrillation**

Adults: 20 mg once daily.

Adjust-a-dose: In patients with CrCl of 15 to 50 mL/minute, reduce dosage to 15 mg once daily.

➤ **To reduce risk of major CV events in patients with chronic CAD**

Adults: 2.5 mg PO b.i.d. in combination with aspirin (75 to 100 mg) once daily.

➤ **To reduce risk of major thrombotic vascular events in patients with PAD, including patients after recent lower extremity revascularization due to symptomatic PAD once hemostasis is established**

Adults: 2.5 mg PO b.i.d. in combination with aspirin (75 to 100 mg) once daily.

➤ **VTE and to reduce risk of recurrent VTE after at least 5 days of initial parenteral anticoagulant therapy**

Children from birth to younger than age 18, weighing 50 kg or more: 20 mg oral suspension or tablets PO daily.

Children from birth to younger than age 18 weighing 30 to 49.9 kg: 15 mg oral suspension or tablets PO daily.

Children from birth to younger than age 18 weighing 12 to 29.9 kg: 5 mg oral suspension PO b.i.d.

Children from birth to younger than age 18 weighing 10 to 11.9 kg: 3 mg oral suspension PO t.i.d.

Children from birth to younger than age 18 weighing 9 to 9.9 kg: 2.8 mg oral suspension PO t.i.d.

Children from birth to younger than age 18 weighing 8 to 8.9 kg: 2.4 mg oral suspension PO t.i.d.

Children from birth to younger than age 18 weighing 7 to 7.9 kg: 1.8 mg oral suspension PO t.i.d.

Children from birth to younger than age 18 weighing 5 to 6.9 kg: 1.6 mg oral suspension PO t.i.d.

Children from birth to less than age 18 weighing 4 to 4.9 kg: 1.4 mg oral suspension PO t.i.d.

Children from birth to younger than age 18 weighing 3 to 3.9 kg: 0.9 mg oral suspension PO t.i.d.

Children from birth to younger than age 18 weighing 2.6 to 2.9 kg: 0.8 mg oral suspension PO t.i.d.

Adjust-a-dose: Children younger than age 6 months should have been at least 37 weeks of gestation at birth, have had at least 10 days of oral feeding, and weigh 2.6 kg or more at time of dosing. Continue therapy for at least 3 months and up to 12 months, when necessary. In children younger than age 2 with catheter-related thrombosis, continue therapy for at least 1 month and up to 3 months, when necessary. Avoid use in children age 1 and older with eGFR less than 50 mL/minute/1.72 m^2. Refer to manufacturer's instructions for kidney impairment in children younger than age 1 and for recommendations for switching to and from other anticoagulants.

➤ **Thromboprophylaxis in patients with congenital heart disease after Fontan procedure**

Children ages 2 and older weighing 50 kg or more: 10 mg oral suspension or tablets PO daily.

Children ages 2 and older weighing 30 to 49.9 kg: 7.5 mg oral suspension PO daily.

Children ages 2 and older weighing 20 to 29.9 kg: 2.5 mg oral suspension PO b.i.d.

Children ages 2 and older weighing 12 to 19.9 kg: 2 mg oral suspension PO b.i.d.

Children ages 2 and older weighing 10 to 11.9 kg: 1.7 mg oral suspension PO b.i.d.
Children ages 2 and older, weighing 8 to 9.9 kg: 1.6 mg oral suspension PO b.i.d.
Children ages 2 and older weighing 7 to 7.9 kg: 1.1 mg oral suspension PO b.i.d.
Adjust-a-dose: Avoid use in children ages 1 and older with eGFR less than 50 mL/minute/1.73m². Refer to manufacturer's instructions for kidney impairment in children younger than age 1 and for recommendations for switching to and from other anticoagulants.

ADMINISTRATION
PO
• Give 2.5- or 10-mg tablets without regard for food. Give 15- and 20-mg tablets with food. For nonvalvular atrial fibrillation, give with evening meal.
• For patients unable to swallow tablets whole, crush tablet and mix with applesauce immediately before use; administer orally. Immediately follow administration of a crushed 15- or 20-mg tablet with food.
• For administration via NG or gastric feeding tube, crush tablet and suspend in 50 mL of water; confirm gastric placement and administer within 4 hours. Delivery of drug into the small intestine will result in reduced absorption. Immediately follow administration of a crushed 15- or 20-mg tablet with an enteral feeding.
• May give suspension via NG or gastric feeding tube. Flush tube with water after administration. For children with recurrent VTE, immediately follow with enteral feeding to increase absorption.
• Oral suspensions should be prepared by a pharmacist, stored at room temperature, and used within 60 days of preparation.
• For adults, if 2.5-mg b.i.d. dose is missed, give single dose at next scheduled time. If 15-mg b.i.d. dose is missed, give dose immediately to ensure intake of 30 mg/day; may give two 15-mg tablets at once. If daily 10-mg, 15-mg, or 20-mg dose is missed, give the missed dose immediately; don't double dose within the same day to make up for a missed dose.
• For children, give a missed daily dose as soon as possible but only on the same day. If not possible, skip the missed dose and continue the next day as prescribed. Give a missed morning dose of b.i.d. dosing as soon as possible; may give together with evening dose. Give a missed evening dose only in the

same evening. Skip a missed t.i.d. dose and resume regular dosing at the next scheduled time without compensating for the missed dose.
• If child vomits or spits up within 30 minutes after receiving a dose, give a new dose. If more than 30 minutes elapse, don't give a new dose; give the next dose as scheduled. Contact preciber if child vomits repeatedly.

ACTION
Selectively blocks the active site of factor Xa, which is necessary for coagulation.

Route	Onset	Peak	Duration
PO	Unknown	2–4 hr	Unknown

Half-life: 5 to 9 hours.

ADVERSE REACTIONS
CNS: syncope, fatigue, dizziness, anxiety, depression, insomnia. **EENT:** epistaxis, oropharyngeal pain, sinusitis. **GI:** abdominal pain, dyspepsia, gastroenteritis, vomiting. **GU:** UTI. **Hematologic:** *bleeding events (including hemorrhage, intracranial hemorrhage).* **Musculoskeletal:** extremity pain, muscle spasm, back pain. **Respiratory:** cough. **Skin:** wound secretion, pruritus, blister.

INTERACTIONS
Drug-drug. *Anticoagulants (warfarin), antithrombotic agents, aspirin, fibrinolytics, NSAIDs, P2Y₁₂ platelet aggregation inhibitors, thienopyridines, SNRIs, SSRIs:* May increase bleeding risk. Avoid use together. Monitor patient carefully for bleeding if drugs must be given together.
Combined P-gp and strong CYP3A4 inducers (carbamazepine, phenytoin, rifampin): May significantly decrease rivaroxaban level. Avoid use together.
Combined P-gp and strong CYP3A4 inhibitors (conivaptan, itraconazole, ketoconazole, lopinavir–ritonavir, ritonavir): May significantly increase rivaroxaban level. Avoid use together.
Combined P-gp and weak or moderate CYP3A4 inhibitors (amiodarone, azithromycin, diltiazem, dronedarone, erythromycin, felodipine, quinidine, ranolazine, verapamil): May increase rivaroxaban level. Use together only if benefit outweighs risk. Avoid use in patients with CrCl 15 to less than 80 mL/minute.
Mifepristone: May increase risk of bleeding. Avoid use together.

R

Drug-herb. *Herbs with anticoagulant or antiplatelet properties (alfalfa, anise, bilberry):* May enhance adverse effects of anticoagulants; bleeding may occur. Avoid use together. *St. John's wort:* May significantly decrease rivaroxaban level. Avoid use together.

EFFECTS ON LAB TEST RESULTS
• May decrease granulocyte and platelet counts.

CONTRAINDICATIONS & CAUTIONS
Boxed Warning There is an increased risk of epidural or spinal hematomas, possibly resulting in long-term or permanent paralysis, in patients who have received anticoagulants and are receiving neuraxial anesthesia or undergoing spinal puncture. Patients at increased risk include those with indwelling epidural catheters; concomitant use of other drugs that affect hemostasis, such as NSAIDs, platelet inhibitors, and other anticoagulants; history of traumatic or repeated epidural or spinal punctures; and history of spinal deformity or spinal surgery. Consider risks and benefits before neuraxial intervention in patients anticoagulated or to be anticoagulated for thromboprophylaxis. Optimal timing between rivaroxaban administration and neuraxial procedures isn't known. ■

Boxed Warning Discontinuing rivaroxaban prematurely places patients at increased risk for thrombotic events. If rivaroxaban must be discontinued for a reason other than pathological bleeding or completion of a course of therapy, consider another anticoagulant. ■

• Contraindicated in patients hypersensitive to drug and in those with active major bleeding.

🕒 **Alert:** Patients who are acutely ill and with the following conditions are at increased risk for bleeding with the use of rivaroxaban for primary VTE prophylaxis: history of bronchiectasis, pulmonary cavitation, or pulmonary hemorrhage; active cancer (undergoing acute, in-hospital cancer treatment); active gastroduodenal ulcer in the 3 months before treatment; history of bleeding in the 3 months before treatment; or dual antiplatelet therapy. Rivaroxaban isn't used for primary VTE prophylaxis in these hospitalized patients who are acutely ill and at high risk for bleeding.

• Use isn't recommended in patients with prosthetic heart valves.

• Don't use in patients with triple positive antiphospholipid syndrome due to increased risk of recurrent thrombotic events compared to vitamin K antagonist therapy.

• Use cautiously in conditions associated with increased risk of hemorrhage, and in older adults.

• Avoid use in patients with CrCl of less than 15 mL/minute who are taking drug for PE or DVT treatment or recurrence prophylaxis or prophylaxis of DVT after hip or knee replacement surgery.

• Avoid use in patients with Child-Pugh class B or C liver impairment and in those with liver disease associated with coagulopathy.

🏮 Use cautiously in patients of Japanese descent because drug exposure in these patients may be increased up to 40% when compared to other ethnicities, but differences are reduced when values are corrected for body weight.

Dialyzable drug: No.

⚠ *Overdose S&S:* Hemorrhage.

PREGNANCY-LACTATION-REPRODUCTION
• There are no adequate studies during pregnancy. Use cautiously and only if potential benefit justifies fetal risk because of the potential for pregnancy-related hemorrhage or emergent delivery with use of an anticoagulant that isn't readily reversible.

• Drug appears in human milk; however, the effects on infants who are breastfed are unknown.

NURSING CONSIDERATIONS
Boxed Warning Monitor patient frequently for signs and symptoms of neurologic impairment after neuraxial anesthesia or spinal puncture. Urgent treatment is necessary for neurologic compromise. ■

• Don't remove an epidural catheter earlier than 18 hours after last administration of drug, and don't give next dose until 6 hours after catheter removal unless traumatic puncture occurred; if puncture has occurred, wait 24 hours before giving next dose.

• Monitor patient carefully for bleeding, which can occur at any site during therapy.

• If an anticoagulant must be discontinued to reduce risk of bleeding with surgical or other procedures, stop drug at least 24 hours before procedure. When deciding whether to delay a procedure until 24 hours after last dose, weigh increased risk of bleeding against the urgency of intervention. Restart drug after procedure when adequate hemostasis has been established, as time to onset of therapeutic effect is short.

🔸 **Alert:** Watch for signs and symptoms of blood loss. Search for a bleeding site if an unexplained fall in hematocrit or BP occurs. Patients with CrCl less than 50 mL/minute are at increased risk.

PATIENT TEACHING

• Instruct patient to take drug only as directed and not to discontinue drug without consulting prescriber.
• Tell patient how to manage a missed dose.
🔸 **Alert:** If patient has had neuraxial anesthesia or spinal puncture, especially if taking concomitant NSAIDs or platelet inhibitors, advise patient to watch for signs and symptoms of spinal or epidural hematoma (midline back pain, tingling, numbness of the limbs, muscular weakness, bowel or bladder dysfunction). If any of these signs and symptoms occur, advise patient to contact prescriber immediately.
• Advise patient to watch for bleeding risks, especially if patient had a spinal catheter or is currently taking drugs or supplements that increase bleeding risk.
• Instruct patient to report pregnancy and plans to become pregnant or to breastfeed.
• Caution patient to report changes in medications or herbal supplements or unusual bleeding or bruising.
• Instruct patient to inform all health care providers that patient is taking rivaroxaban before scheduling invasive procedures (including dental procedures).

rivastigmine
ri-va-STIG-meen

Exelon Patch

rivastigmine tartrate

Therapeutic class: Anti-Alzheimer drugs
Pharmacologic class: Cholinesterase inhibitors

AVAILABLE FORMS

Capsules 🔵: 1.5 mg, 3 mg, 4.5 mg, 6 mg
Transdermal patch: 4.6 mg/24 hours, 9.5 mg/24 hours, 13.3 mg/24 hours

INDICATIONS & DOSAGES

Adjust-a-dose (for all indications): Patients with GFR less than 50 mL/min or Child-Pugh class A or B liver impairment may be able to only tolerate lower doses of oral drug. For patients with Child-Pugh class A or B liver impairment, consider using 4.6 mg/24 hours transdermal patch for both initial and maintenance dose. For patients weighing less than 50 kg, watch for toxicities (nausea, vomiting) and if they occur, consider reducing maintenance dose; reduce dose of transdermal patch to 4.6 mg/24 hours.

➤ **Mild to moderate Alzheimer dementia**
Adults: Initially, 1.5 mg PO b.i.d. If tolerated, may increase to 3 mg b.i.d. then to 4.5 mg b.i.d. and finally to 6 mg b.i.d., as tolerated, with at least 2 weeks at each dose. Effective dosage range is 6 to 12 mg daily; maximum, 12 mg daily. Or, 4.6 mg/24 hours transdermal patch once daily. After 4 weeks, if tolerated, increase to 9.5 mg/24 hours transdermal patch for as long as therapeutic benefit persists; if needed after at least 4 weeks, increase to 13.3 mg/24 hours transdermal patch. Maximum dose, 13.3 mg/24 hours.

➤ **Severe Alzheimer dementia (transdermal patch only)**
Adults: Initially, 4.6 mg/24 hours transdermal patch once daily. After 4 weeks, if tolerated, increase to 9.5 mg/24 hours transdermal patch; then, if tolerated after an additional 4 weeks, increase to 13.3 mg/24 hours transdermal patch.

➤ **Mild to moderate dementia associated with Parkinson disease**
Adults: Initially, 1.5 mg PO b.i.d. May increase, as tolerated, to 3 mg b.i.d., then to 4.5 mg b.i.d., and finally to 6 mg b.i.d. after at least 4 weeks at each dose; maximum dose, 12 mg daily.

Or, 4.6 mg/24 hours transdermal patch once daily. After 4 weeks, if tolerated, increase to 9.5 mg/24 hours transdermal patch for as long as therapeutic benefit persists; if needed after at least 4 weeks, increase to 13.3 mg/24 hours transdermal patch. Maximum dose, 13.3 mg/24 hours.

➤ **Neuropsychiatric symptoms associated with Lewy body dementia ◆**
Adults: Initially, 1.5 mg PO b.i.d.; increase as tolerated by 1.5 mg b.i.d. every 2 weeks to a maximum of 6 mg b.i.d.

R

ADMINISTRATION
PO
• Give drug with food in morning and evening.
• Have patient swallow capsule whole; don't open or crush.
• If therapy is interrupted for more than 3 days, restart with 1.5 mg b.i.d. and retitrate.
Transdermal
• Apply patch once daily to clean, dry, hairless skin on the upper or lower back, upper arm, or chest, in a place not rubbed by tight clothing. Press firmly for 30 seconds until edges stick well.
• Change the site daily, and don't use the same site within 14 days. Avoid exposing patch to external heat sources (sauna, excess sunlight).
• Avoid eye contact; wash hands with soap and water after removing patch. In case of contact with eyes or if eyes become red after handling patch, rinse immediately with plenty of water. Seek medical advice if symptoms don't resolve.

ACTION
Thought to increase acetylcholine level by inhibiting cholinesterase enzyme, which causes acetylcholine hydrolysis.

Route	Onset	Peak	Duration
PO	Rapid	1 hr	8–10 hr
Transdermal	30–60 min	8–16 hr	24 hr

Half-life: Oral, 1.5 hours; transdermal, 3 hours.

ADVERSE REACTIONS
CNS: anxiety, headache, dizziness, syncope, fatigue, asthenia, malaise, somnolence, tremor, insomnia, confusion, depression, anxiety, hallucinations, aggression, psychomotor hyperactivity, hypokinesia, bradykinesia, dyskinesia, cogwheel rigidity, vertigo, agitation, nervousness, gait disturbance. **CV:** HTN. **EENT:** excess salivation. **GI:** nausea, vomiting, diarrhea, anorexia, abdominal pain, dyspepsia. **GU:** UTI, incontinence. **Metabolic:** dehydration, weight loss. **Skin:** diaphoresis, rash, application-site pruritus or erythema. **Other:** falls.

INTERACTIONS
Drug-drug. *Anticholinergics (scopolamine, diphenhydramine, dicyclomine):* May decrease effect of both drugs. Avoid use together.

Beta blockers, bradycardia-inducing drugs: May worsen bradycardia. Use together isn't recommended.
Cholinergic antagonists (bethanechol, pilocarpine, succinylcholine): May increase effects of these drugs. Monitor patient closely.
Metoclopramide: May enhance risk of extrapyramidal reactions. Use together isn't recommended.
Neuromuscular blockers (rocuronium): May decrease neuromuscular blocking effect. Monitor patient closely.
NSAIDs: May increase risk of peptic ulcer disease due to increased acid. Monitor patient for symptoms of active or occult GI bleeding.
Drug-lifestyle. *Smoking:* May increase drug clearance. Discourage smoking.

EFFECTS ON LAB TEST RESULTS
None reported.

CONTRAINDICATIONS & CAUTIONS
• Contraindicated in patients hypersensitive to drug, other carbamate derivatives, or other components of drug.
• Isolated cases of generalized skin reactions have been reported with oral or transdermal formulations. Discontinue drug if allergic dermatitis occurs.
• Contraindicated in patients with history of transdermal patch application-site reaction suggestive of allergic contact dermatitis.
• Use cautiously in patients with history of CV disease, GI bleeding, seizure disorder, GU conditions, asthma, or obstructive pulmonary disease.
Dialyzable drug: No.
⚠ **Overdose S&S:** Nausea, vomiting, excessive salivation, diaphoresis, bradycardia, hypotension, respiratory depression, syncope, seizures, muscle weakness.

PREGNANCY-LACTATION-REPRODUCTION
• There are no adequate studies during pregnancy. Use only if clearly needed.
• It isn't known if drug appears in human milk. Patient should discontinue breastfeeding or discontinue drug, considering importance of drug to patient.

NURSING CONSIDERATIONS
• Expect significant GI adverse effects (nausea, vomiting, anorexia, weight loss), which may lead to dehydration. These effects are less common during maintenance doses.

Reactions in bold italics are *life-threatening*.

• Monitor patient for evidence of active or occult GI bleeding.

• Dramatic memory improvement is unlikely. As disease progresses, the benefits of drug may decline.

• Carefully monitor patient with a history of GI bleeding, NSAID use, arrhythmias, seizures, or pulmonary conditions for adverse effects.

• If adverse reactions, such as diarrhea, loss of appetite, nausea, or vomiting, occur with transdermal patch, stop use for several days, then restart at the same or lower dose. If treatment is interrupted for more than 3 days, restart patch at the lowest dose and retitrate.

• Patients weighing less than 50 kg may experience more adverse reactions when using the transdermal patch.

• Application-site reactions may occur with the transdermal patch. Discontinue treatment if application-site reaction spreads beyond the patch size, if there's evidence of a more intense local reaction (increasing erythema, edema, papules, vesicles), and if symptoms don't significantly improve within 48 hours after patch removal.

• When switching from oral form to the transdermal patch, patients on a total daily dose of less than 6 mg can be switched to 4.6 mg/24 hours. Patients taking 6 to 12 mg PO can switch to the 9.5 mg/24 hour patch. The patch should be applied on the day after the last oral dose.

PATIENT TEACHING

• Teach patient and caregiver safe drug administration.

• Advise patient that memory improvement may be subtle and that drug more likely slows future memory loss.

• Tell patient to report nausea, vomiting, or diarrhea.

• Advise patient to consult prescriber before using OTC drugs.

• Advise patient to remove used patch, place in previously saved pouch and discard in trash (away from pets or children), and then wash hands with soap and water. In case of contact with eyes or if eyes become red after handling patch, tell patient to rinse immediately with plenty of water and seek medical advice if symptoms don't resolve.

roflumilast
roe-FLUE-mi-last

Daliresp, Zoryve

Therapeutic class: Miscellaneous respiratory drugs; antipsoriatic
Pharmacologic class: Selective phosphodiesterase inhibitors

AVAILABLE FORMS
Cream: 0.3%
Tablets: 250 mcg, 500 mcg

INDICATIONS & DOSAGES

➤ **To reduce risk of COPD exacerbations in patients with severe COPD associated with chronic bronchitis and a history of exacerbations**
Adults: Initially, 250 mcg once daily for 4 weeks; then increase to maintenance dosage of 500 mcg PO daily.

➤ **Plaque psoriasis, including intertriginous areas**
Adults and children age 12 and older: 0.3% cream applied to affected areas once daily.

ADMINISTRATION
PO
• Give drug without regard to food.
Topical
• Rub in completely. Unless treatment is for the hands, wash hands after application.
• Not for ophthalmic, oral, or intravaginal use.

ACTION
Selectively inhibits phosphodiesterase-4 (PDE_4), a cAMP-metabolizing enzyme in lung tissue. Inhibition of PDE_4 leads to accumulation of intracellular cAMP. Effects of drug are thought to be related to increased intracellular cAMP in lung cells. Mechanism by which roflumilast exerts its therapeutic action in psoriasis isn't well defined.

Route	Onset	Peak	Duration
PO	Unknown	1–2 hr	Unknown
Topical	Unknown	Unknown	Unknown

Half-life: Tablet: 17 hours; N-oxide metabolite, 30 hours. Cream: 4 days; N-oxide metabolite, 4.6 days.

ADVERSE REACTIONS
CNS: anxiety, depression, headache, insomnia, dizziness, tremor. **EENT:** rhinitis, sinusitis.

R

GI: abdominal pain, diarrhea, dyspepsia, gastritis, nausea, vomiting, decreased appetite. **GU:** UTI. **Metabolic:** weight loss. **Musculoskeletal:** back pain, muscle spasms. **Respiratory:** URI. **Skin:** application-site pain. **Other:** flulike symptoms.

INTERACTIONS
Drug-drug. *Ciprofloxacin (systemic):* May increase roflumilast level. Monitor therapy.
CYP450 inducers (carbamazepine, phenobarbital, phenytoin, rifampin): May decrease the effectiveness of roflumilast. Avoid use together.
CYP450 inhibitors (cimetidine, erythromycin, fluvoxamine, ketoconazole): May increase roflumilast level and risk of adverse reactions. Use together cautiously.
Immunosuppressants (except short-term corticosteroids, beclomethasone [oral inhalation], cytarabine [liposomal], fluticasone [oral inhalation]): May enhance immunosuppressive effect. Consider therapy modification.
Oral contraceptives containing gestodene and ethinyl estradiol: May increase roflumilast exposure and risk of adverse effects. Use cautiously together.

EFFECTS ON LAB TEST RESULTS
None reported.

CONTRAINDICATIONS & CAUTIONS
• Contraindicated in patients with Child-Pugh class B or C liver impairment.
• Use cautiously in patients with history of depression or suicidality.
Dialyzable drug: Unlikely.

PREGNANCY-LACTATION-REPRODUCTION
• There are no adequate studies during pregnancy. Use only if potential benefit justifies fetal risk.
• Don't use during labor and delivery.
• Drug may appear in human milk. Patient should discontinue breastfeeding or discontinue drug, considering importance of drug to patient.
• If topical use is necessary while breastfeeding, avoid applying cream to nipple and areola to prevent direct infant exposure.

NURSING CONSIDERATIONS
• Drug isn't a bronchodilator and isn't indicated for relief of acute bronchospasm.

• Monitor patients for signs and symptoms of psychiatric adverse events, including insomnia, anxiety, depression, suicidality, and suicide attempts. If events occur, evaluate the risks versus benefits of continuing drug.
• Monitor weight regularly; if unexplained or significant weight loss occurs, evaluate cause and consider stopping drug.

PATIENT TEACHING
• Teach patient that drug isn't a bronchodilator and shouldn't be used for relief of acute bronchospasm.
• Instruct patient in safe drug administration.
• Advise patient, family, and caregivers to watch for signs and symptoms of psychiatric adverse events, including insomnia, anxiety, depression, suicidality, and suicide attempts, and to report any occurrences to the health care provider.
• Tell patient to report unexplained or significant weight loss.

rolapitant hydrochloride
roe-LA-pi-tant

Varubi

Therapeutic class: Antiemetics
Pharmacologic class: Substance P and neurokinin-1 receptor antagonists

AVAILABLE FORMS
Tablets: 90 mg

INDICATIONS & DOSAGES
➤ **Prevention of delayed nausea and vomiting associated with cisplatin-based highly emetogenic chemotherapy (in combination with other antiemetics)**
Adults: 180 mg PO. Administer within 2 hours of chemotherapy on day 1. Give 20 mg dexamethasone on day 1, 30 minutes before chemotherapy and then 8 mg PO b.i.d. on days 2, 3, and 4. Also give a 5-HT₃ receptor antagonist on day 1. Refer to dexamethasone and 5-HT₃ receptor antagonist manufacturers' instructions for more information.
➤ **Prevention of delayed nausea and vomiting associated with anthracycline and cyclophosphamide-based or moderately emetogenic chemotherapy, in combination with other antiemetics**

Adults: 180 mg PO. Administer within 2 hours of chemotherapy on day 1. Give 20 mg PO dexamethasone 30 minutes before chemotherapy on day 1. Also give a 5-HT₃ receptor antagonist on day 1. Refer to dexamethasone and 5-HT₃ receptor antagonist manufacturers' instructions for more information.

ADMINISTRATION
PO
• Give drug before each scheduled chemotherapy cycle.
• Give no more frequently than every 2 weeks.
• Give without regard to meals.
• Store at room temperature.

ACTION
A selective and competitive antagonist of human substance P/neurokinin-1 receptors in brain. Appears to be synergistic with 5-HT₃ antagonists and corticosteroids.

Route	Onset	Peak	Duration
PO	30 min	4 hr	Unknown

Half-life: About 7 days.

ADVERSE REACTIONS
CNS: dizziness. **GI:** abdominal pain, decreased appetite, dyspepsia, stomatitis. **GU:** UTI. **Hematologic:** *neutropenia,* anemia. **Respiratory:** hiccups.

INTERACTIONS
Drug-drug. *BCRP substrates with a narrow therapeutic index (irinotecan, methotrexate, rosuvastatin, topotecan):* May increase BCRP substrate level and risk of adverse reactions. Monitor patient. Use lowest effective rosuvastatin dose.
CYP2D6 substrates (dextromethorphan, TCAs): May increase CYP2D6 substrate level for at least 28 days after rolapitant dose. Monitor patient closely for increased adverse effects.
CYP2D6 substrates with a narrow therapeutic index (pimozide, thioridazine): May increase substrate level and risk of QT-interval prolongation. Use is contraindicated.
Dabigatran, edoxaban: May increase anticoagulant level. Consider therapy modification.
P-gp substrates with a narrow therapeutic index (digoxin): May increase substrate level. Monitor drug levels; watch for increased adverse reactions if concomitant use can't be avoided.

Strong CYP3A4 inducers (rifampin): May decrease rolapitant level. Avoid concomitant use, if possible.
Warfarin: May increase warfarin level. Monitor INR and PTT; adjust doses as needed to maintain target INR.

EFFECTS ON LAB TEST RESULTS
• May decrease Hb level and neutrophil count.

CONTRAINDICATIONS & CAUTIONS
• Drug hasn't been studied in patients with Child-Pugh class C liver impairment; avoid use. Monitor closely for adverse reactions if use can't be avoided.
• Safety and effectiveness in children haven't been established; studies showed irreversible infertility and impaired sexual development in rats. Don't use for children younger than age 2.
Dialyzable drug: Unlikely.

PREGNANCY-LACTATION-REPRODUCTION
• There are no data regarding use during pregnancy. Use only if benefits outweigh fetal risk.
• It isn't known if drug appears in human milk. Give only if benefits outweigh risks to infant who is breastfed.
• May reversibly impair fertility in adult females.

NURSING CONSIDERATIONS
⦿ *Alert:* Before giving drug, assess patient's current drug list for potential drug-drug interactions.
• Drug is used to prevent, not treat, nausea and vomiting.
• Always use drug in combination with a corticosteroid and a 5-HT₃ inhibitor.
• *Look alike–sound alike:* Don't confuse rolapitant with aprepitant or fosaprepitant. Don't confuse Varubi with valrubicin.

PATIENT TEACHING
• Remind patient that rolapitant is taken in combination with a corticosteroid and a 5-HT₃ inhibitor.
• Inform patient that rolapitant prevents nausea and vomiting; it doesn't treat them. Advise patient to take other antiemetics for breakthrough nausea and vomiting.
• Instruct patient to take drug 1 to 2 hours before scheduled chemotherapy.
• Inform patient that rolapitant is associated with drug-drug interactions and that it's

R

important to report all medications being taken, including OTC drugs and supplements, before starting therapy.

• Advise patient to inform prescriber and pharmacist of dosage changes or new prescription drug therapy because drug interactions can be delayed after rolapitant is discontinued.

• Counsel patient to report pregnancy, plans to become pregnant, or breastfeeding.

rOPINIRole hydrochloride
roe-PIN-i-role

Therapeutic class: Antiparkinsonian drugs
Pharmacologic class: Nonergot dopamine agonists

AVAILABLE FORMS
Tablets: 0.25 mg, 0.5 mg, 1 mg, 2 mg, 3 mg, 4 mg, 5 mg
Tablets (extended-release) ⓞⓝⓒ: 2 mg, 4 mg, 6 mg, 8 mg, 12 mg

INDICATIONS & DOSAGES
Adjust-a-dose (for all indications): For patients with CKD on KRT using immediate-release formula, give 0.25 mg PO t.i.d. for Parkinson disease and 0.25 mg PO daily for restless legs syndrome. Base further dosage escalations on tolerability and need for efficacy. Recommended maximum total daily dose in patients receiving regular KRT is 18 mg/day for Parkinson disease and 3 mg daily for restless legs syndrome. Supplemental doses after dialysis aren't required. No dosage adjustment is necessary in patients with CrCl of 30 to 50 mL/min.

For patients with CKD on KRT using extended-release formula, give 2 mg once daily initially; titrate upward to maximum dose of 18 mg/day if needed. Supplemental doses after dialysis aren't required.

▶ **Parkinson disease**
Adults: Initially, 0.25 mg PO t.i.d. Increase dosage by 0.25 mg t.i.d. at weekly intervals for 4 weeks. After week 4, daily dosage may be increased by 1.5 mg/day on a weekly basis up to a dosage of 9 mg/day, and then by up to 3 mg/day weekly to a total maximum dosage of 24 mg/day (8 mg t.i.d.). For extended-release formula, starting dosage is 2 mg PO once daily for 1 to 2 weeks. May increase extended-release tablets by 2 mg/day at 1-week or longer intervals to maximum

dosage of 24 mg/day. To switch from immediate-release to extended-release tablets, refer to manufacturer's instructions.
▶ **Moderate to severe restless legs syndrome (immediate-release)**
Adults: Initially, 0.25 mg PO 1 to 3 hours before bedtime. May increase dose as needed and tolerated after 2 days to 0.5 mg, then to 1 mg by end of first week. May further increase dose as needed and tolerated as follows: Week 2, give 1 mg once daily. Week 3, give 1.5 mg once daily. Week 4, give 2 mg once daily. Week 5, give 2.5 mg once daily. Week 6, give 3 mg once daily. Week 7, give 4 mg once daily. Maximum dosage, 4 mg/day. Patient should take all doses 1 to 3 hours before bedtime.

ADMINISTRATION
PO
• Give drug with food if nausea occurs.
• Have patient swallow extended-release tablets whole; don't crushed or cut.
• Don't double dose after a missed dose.

ACTION
Thought to stimulate dopamine (D_2) receptors.

Route	Onset	Peak	Duration
PO (immediate-release)	Unknown	1–2 hr	6 hr
PO (extended-release)	Unknown	6–10 hr	Unknown

Half-life: 6 hours.

ADVERSE REACTIONS
Early Parkinson disease (without levodopa)
CNS: dizziness, fatigue, somnolence, syncope, hallucinations, aggravated Parkinson disease, headache, confusion, hyperkinesia, hypesthesia, vertigo, amnesia, impaired concentration, malaise, asthenia, pain. **CV:** orthostatic hypotension, orthostatic symptoms, HTN, edema, chest pain, extrasystoles, atrial fibrillation, palpitations, tachycardia, flushing. **EENT:** abnormal vision, eye abnormality, xerophthalmia, dry mouth, pharyngitis, rhinitis, sinusitis. **GI:** nausea, vomiting, dyspepsia, flatulence, abdominal pain, anorexia, constipation. **GU:** UTI, erectile dysfunction. **Musculoskeletal:** back pain. **Respiratory:** bronchitis, dyspnea, yawning. **Skin:** diaphoresis. **Other:** viral infection, peripheral ischemia.
Advanced Parkinson disease (with levodopa)
CNS: dizziness, somnolence, headache, hallucinations, aggravated parkinsonism, insomnia,

abnormal dreaming, confusion, tremor, anxiety, nervousness, amnesia, paresis, paresthesia, syncope, pain. **CV:** hypotension, HTN. **EENT:** dry mouth, diplopia. **GI:** nausea, abdominal pain, vomiting, constipation, diarrhea, dysphagia, flatulence, increased saliva. **GU:** UTI, pyuria, urinary incontinence. **Hematologic:** anemia. **Metabolic:** weight decrease, suppressed prolactin. **Musculoskeletal:** dyskinesia, arthralgia, arthritis, hypokinesia, back pain. **Respiratory:** URI, dyspnea. **Skin:** diaphoresis. **Other:** falls, injury, viral infection.

Restless legs syndrome
CNS: fatigue, somnolence, dizziness, vertigo, paresthesia. **CV:** peripheral edema. **EENT:** nasopharyngitis, nasal congestion, dry mouth. **GI:** nausea, vomiting, diarrhea, dyspepsia. **Musculoskeletal:** arthralgia, muscle cramps, extremity pain, back pain. **Respiratory:** cough. **Skin:** diaphoresis. **Other:** flu-like symptoms.

INTERACTIONS
Drug-drug. *BP-lowering agents:* May enhance hypotensive effect. Monitor BP carefully.
CNS depressants: May increase CNS effects. Use together cautiously.
CYP1A2 inducers (cimetidine, omeprazole): May decrease ropinirole level. Monitor therapy.
CYP1A2 inhibitors (ciprofloxacin): May increase ropinirole level. Monitor therapy.
Dopamine antagonists (phenothiazines), metoclopramide: May decrease ropinirole effects. Monitor therapy.
Estrogens: May increase ropinirole level. Adjust ropinirole dosage if estrogen therapy is started or stopped during treatment.
Drug-lifestyle. *Alcohol use:* May increase sedative effect. Discourage use together.
Smoking: May increase drug clearance. Discourage use together.

EFFECTS ON LAB TEST RESULTS
• May increase ALP level.
• May decrease Hb level.

CONTRAINDICATIONS & CAUTIONS
• Contraindicated in patients hypersensitive to drug.
• Ropinirole hasn't been studied in patients with CrCl less than 30 mL/minute or Child-Pugh class C liver impairment. Use cautiously.
• No benefit was shown in patients with advanced Parkinson disease taking daily dosages of extended-release tablets greater than 8 mg/day, or with early Parkinson disease taking daily dosages greater than 12 mg/day.

Dialyzable drug: Unlikely.
⚠ *Overdose S&S:* Nausea, dizziness, visual hallucinations, hyperhidrosis, claustrophobia, chorea, palpitations, asthenia, nightmares, vomiting, increased coughing, fatigue, syncope, vasovagal syncope, dyskinesia, agitation, chest pain, orthostatic hypotension, somnolence, confusion.

PREGNANCY-LACTATION-REPRODUCTION
• There are no adequate studies during pregnancy. Use only if potential benefit justifies fetal risk.
• Drug inhibits prolactin secretion and could inhibit lactation. It isn't known if drug appears in human milk. Use cautiously during breastfeeding.

NURSING CONSIDERATIONS
🛈 *Alert:* Monitor patient carefully for orthostatic hypotension, especially during dosage increases.
• Although not reported with ropinirole, other adverse reactions reported with dopaminergic therapy include hyperpyrexia, fibrotic complications, and confusion, which may occur with rapid dosage reduction or withdrawal of drug.
• Patient may have syncope, with or without bradycardia. Monitor patient carefully, especially for 4 weeks after start of therapy and with dosage increases.
• Rapid dosage reduction or withdrawal of drug can cause signs and symptoms resembling NMS (elevated temperature, muscular rigidity, altered consciousness, autonomic instability). When used for Parkinson disease, withdraw drug gradually over 7 days. For immediate-release form, reduce frequency from t.i.d. to b.i.d. for 4 days; then, for next 3 days, reduce frequency to once daily before complete withdrawal.
• Withdraw extended-release form gradually over 7 days.
• When used for restless legs syndrome, gradual reduction of the daily dose is recommended.
• Drug can cause somnolence and sudden episodes of falling asleep. Continually reassess patient for drowsiness or sleepiness and for factors that could contribute to sleepiness.

• Avoid use in patients with major psychotic disorders. Drug may cause changes in or worsening of mental status, abnormal thinking, and behavioral changes, which may be severe and include paranoid ideation, delusions, hallucinations, confusion, psychotic-like behavior, disorientation, aggressive behavior, agitation, and delirium.

• Augmentation (an increase in symptoms or earlier onset of symptoms in evening or even afternoon, or spread of symptoms to other extremities) and early-morning rebound symptoms (onset of symptoms in early morning) were observed in a post-marketing trial in restless legs syndrome. Adjust dosage or discontinue treatment if augmentation or early-morning rebound symptoms occur.

• Ask patient about development or worsening of impulsive or compulsive behaviors (new or increased gambling urges, sexual urges, uncontrolled spending, other urges), because patient may not recognize these behaviors as abnormal.

• Patients with Parkinson disease have an increased risk of melanoma. Monitor patient for melanoma development during periodic dermatologic screenings.

• *Look alike–sound alike:* Don't confuse ropinirole with risperidone.

PATIENT TEACHING

• Teach patient about safe drug administration.
• Advise patient to inform prescriber if starting or stopping medications, OTC drugs or herbs, or smoking.
• Tell patient (especially older adult) to contact prescriber if paranoid ideation, delusions, hallucinations, confusion, psychotic-like behavior, disorientation, aggressive behavior, agitation, or delirium occurs.
• Instruct patient not to rise rapidly after sitting or lying down because of risk of dizziness, which may occur more frequently early in therapy or when dosage increases.
• Sleepiness and sudden episodes of falling asleep can occur, sometimes without warning. Tell patient to minimize hazardous activities until CNS effects of drug are known.
• Tell patient to contact prescriber if experiencing difficulty controlling impulsive or compulsive behaviors.
• Advise patient to avoid alcohol.
• Tell patient to notify prescriber about planned, suspected, or known pregnancy or breastfeeding.

rosuvastatin calcium ⚕
roe-SOO-va-STAT-tin

Crestor, Ezallor Sprinkle

Therapeutic class: Antilipemics
Pharmacologic class: HMG-CoA reductase inhibitors

AVAILABLE FORMS
Capsules ⓞⓝⓒ: 5 mg, 10 mg, 20 mg, 40 mg
Tablets: 5 mg, 10 mg, 20 mg, 40 mg

INDICATIONS & DOSAGES
Adjust-a-dose (for all indications): May titrate dosage every 4 weeks or more based on lipid levels. If CrCl is less than 30 mL/minute in patient not on KRT initially, give 5 mg once daily; don't exceed 10 mg once daily.
⚕ For patients of Asian descent, initial dose is 5 mg.

➤ **Risk reduction in patients without clinical evidence of CAD but with multiple risk factors**
Adults: Usual starting dosage, 10 to 20 mg PO once daily. Recommended dosage, 5 to 40 mg tablets PO once daily.

➤ **Heterozygous familial hypercholesterolemia** ⚕
Adults: 5 to 40 mg tablets PO daily.
Children ages 10 to 17: 5 to 20 mg tablets PO daily.
Children ages 8 to younger than 10: 5 to 10 mg tablets PO daily.

➤ **Homozygous familial hypercholesterolemia** ⚕
Adults: Usual starting dosage, 10 to 20 mg PO once daily. Recommended dosage, 5 to 40 mg PO once daily either alone or with other lipid-lowering treatments.
Children ages 7 to 17: 20 mg tablets PO once daily either alone or with other lipid-lowering treatments.

➤ **Adjunct to diet to reduce LDL-C in patients with primary hyperlipidemia, or to reduce LDL-C and slow the progresssion of atherosclerosis**
Adults: Usual starting dosage, 10 to 20 mg PO once daily. Reommended dosage, 5 to 40 mg tablets PO once daily.

➤ **Adjunct to diet to treat primary dysbetalipoproteinemia (type III hyperlipoproteinemia)** ⚕

Adults: Initially, 10 to 20 mg PO once daily. Dosage range, 5 to 40 mg PO once daily.

➤ **Adjunct to diet to treat hypertriglyceridemia**

Adults: Initially, 10 to 20 mg tablets or capsules PO once daily. Dosage range, 5 to 40 mg PO once daily.

ADMINISTRATION
PO
• Give drug without regard for meals.
• Have patient swallow tablets and capsules whole; don't crush tablets or capsules, or cut tablets.
• May open capsules and sprinkle contents on a teaspoon of soft food, such as applesauce or pudding. Give within 60 minutes of preparation. Patient shouldn't chew mixtures.
• For NG administration, empty contents of capsule into a 60-mL catheter-tipped syringe, add 40 mL water, replace plunger, and shake syringe vigorously for 15 seconds. Immediately attach syringe to NG tube and administer contents. Flush NG tube with additional 20 mL water.

ACTION
Inhibits HMG-CoA reductase, increases LDL receptors on liver cells, and inhibits liver synthesis of very-low-density lipoprotein.

Route	Onset	Peak	Duration
PO	1 wk	3–5 hr	Unknown

Half-life: About 19 hours.

ADVERSE REACTIONS
CNS: asthenia, dizziness, headache. **GI:** abdominal pain, constipation, diarrhea, nausea. **Hepatic:** elevated ALT level. **Metabolic:** diabetes, increased CK. **Musculoskeletal:** arthralgia, myalgia.

INTERACTIONS
Drug-drug. *Antacids:* May decrease rosuvastatin level. Give antacids at least 2 hours after rosuvastatin.

Atazanavir, atazanavir–ritonavir, lopinavir–ritonavir, simeprevir, capmatinib, teriflunomide, regorafenib: May increase rosuvastatin level and risk of myopathy and rhabdomyolysis. Don't exceed 10 mg rosuvastatin daily.

Colchicine: May increase risk of myopathy and rhabdomyolysis. Avoid use together. If use together is necessary, monitor patient

closely and assess CK level during use and after dosage increases.

Cyclosporine, darolutamide: May increase rosuvastatin level and risk of myopathy or rhabdomyolysis. Don't exceed 5 mg of rosuvastatin daily. Monitor patient.

Daptomycin: May increase risk of rhabdomyolysis. Withhold rosuvastatin temporarily or monitor patient and CK level closely during coadministration.

Eltrombopag: May increase rosuvastatin level and risk of toxicity. Consider reducing rosuvastatin dosage.

Fenofibrates: May increase rosuvastatin level and risk of myopathy or rhabdomyolysis. Use together cautiously.

Fostamatinib: May increase rosuvastatin level and risk of myopathy and rhabdomyolysis. Don't exceed 20 mg rosuvastatin daily.

Gemfibrozil: May significantly increase rosuvastatin level and risk of myopathy or rhabdomyolysis. Avoid use together. If used together, don't exceed 10 mg/day of rosuvastatin.

Hormonal contraceptives: May increase ethinyl estradiol and norgestrel levels. Watch for adverse effects.

Niacin: May increase risk of myopathy or rhabdomyolysis. Monitor patient closely.

Sofosbuvir/velpatasvir/voxilaprevir, ledispasivir/sofosbuvir: May increase risk of myopathy and rhabdomyolysis. Avoid use together.

Warfarin: May prolong INR. Achieve stable INR before starting drug; monitor INR frequently.

Drug-herb. *Red yeast rice:* May enhance adverse or toxic effects of HMG-CoA reductase inhibitors (statins). Discourage use together.

Drug-lifestyle. *Alcohol use:* May increase risk of liver toxicity. Discourage use together.

EFFECTS ON LAB TEST RESULTS
• May increase HbA_{1c}, fasting blood sugar, CK, ALT, AST, glucose, glutamyl transpeptidase, ALP, and bilirubin levels.
• May cause thyroid function abnormalities, dipstick-positive proteinuria, and microscopic hematuria.

CONTRAINDICATIONS & CAUTIONS
• Contraindicated in patients hypersensitive to rosuvastatin or its components, patients with active liver disease, and those with unexplained persistently increased transaminase levels.

• Use cautiously in patients with substantial alcohol intake or history of liver disease, and in those at increased risk for myopathies, such as those with kidney impairment, advanced age, or hypothyroidism.

⅀ Use cautiously in patients of Asian descent because they have a greater risk of elevated drug levels.

• Rare postmarketing reports of cognitive impairment (memory loss, forgetfulness, amnesia, memory impairment, confusion) have been associated with statin use. These reported symptoms are generally reversible upon discontinuation, with variable times to symptom onset (1 day to years) and symptom resolution (median of 3 weeks).

• Immune-mediated necrotizing myopathy, although rare, has been reported with statin use.

• Ezallor capsules aren't approved for use in children.

Dialyzable drug: No.

⚠ *Overdose S&S:* Unexplained muscle pain, tenderness, or weakness, especially with malaise or fever.

PREGNANCY-LACTATION-REPRODUCTION

• May cause fetal harm. Use during pregnancy contraindicated unless benefits outweigh fetal risk. Discontinue drug before conception. If pregnancy occurs during therapy, apprise patient of potential fetal risks with continued use during pregnancy.

• According to the FDA, statin use may be considered during pregnancy in patients at high risk for CV events. Base decision on individual needs.

• Advise patients of childbearing potential to use effective contraception during therapy.

• Drug may appear in human milk. Use while breastfeeding is contraindicated.

NURSING CONSIDERATIONS

• Before therapy starts, assess patient for underlying causes of hypercholesterolemia, including poorly controlled diabetes, hypothyroidism, nephrotic syndrome, dyslipoproteinemias, obstructive liver disease, drug interaction, and alcoholism.

• Before therapy starts, advise patient to control hypercholesterolemia with diet, exercise, and weight reduction.

• Interrupt statin therapy if patient shows signs or symptoms of serious liver injury,

hyperbilirubinemia, or jaundice. Don't restart drug if another cause can't be found.

• Monitor LFTs at baseline and with any indication of liver toxicity.

⊘ *Alert:* Rarely, rhabdomyolysis with AKI has developed in patients taking drugs in this class, including rosuvastatin.

• Monitor lipid panel at baseline and a fasting lipid profile within 4 to 12 weeks after initiation or dosage adjustment and every 3 to 12 months thereafter.

• Patients who are age 65 or older, have hypothyroidism, or have kidney impairment may be at a greater risk for developing myopathy while receiving a statin.

• Notify prescriber if CK level becomes markedly elevated, myopathy is suspected, or if routine urinalysis shows persistent proteinuria and patient is taking 40 mg daily.

• Withhold drug temporarily if patient becomes predisposed to myopathy or rhabdomyolysis because of sepsis, hypotension, major surgery, trauma, uncontrolled seizures, or severe metabolic, endocrine, or electrolyte disorders.

• Monitor for immune-mediated necrotizing myopathy (proximal muscle weakness and elevated CK, despite discontinuation of statin). Discontinue drug if suspected.

PATIENT TEACHING

• Instruct patient to take drug exactly as prescribed.

• Teach patient about diet, exercise, and weight control.

• Inform patient that rare instances of memory loss and confusion have occurred with statin use. These reported events were generally not serious and resolved when drug was discontinued.

• Advise patient that drug may increase blood glucose level but that CV benefits are thought to outweigh slight increase in risk.

• Tell patient to immediately report unexplained muscle pain, tenderness, or weakness (especially if accompanied by malaise or fever) and loss of appetite, upper abdominal pain, dark-colored urine, or yellowing of skin or eyes.

• Instruct patient to take drug at least 2 hours before aluminum- or magnesium-containing antacids.

• Tell patient to immediately report known or suspected pregnancy or if breastfeeding.

rucaparib camsylate ░
roo-KAP-a-rib

Rubraca

Therapeutic class: Antineoplastics
Pharmacologic class: Poly (ADP-ribose)
polymerase (PARP) inhibitors

AVAILABLE FORMS
Tablets: 200 mg, 250 mg, 300 mg

INDICATIONS & DOSAGES
Adjust-a-dose (for all indications): To manage any adverse reaction, interrupt therapy
or consider dosage reduction. First dosage
reduction, 500 mg b.i.d.; second dosage reduction, 400 mg b.i.d.; third dosage reduction,
300 mg b.i.d. For prolonged hematologic toxicities, interrupt therapy and monitor blood
counts weekly until recovery. If levels haven't
recovered to grade 1 or less after 4 weeks, refer patient to hematologist for further investigation.

➤ **Maintenance treatment of patients with**
***BRCA*-mutated recurrent epithelial ovar-**
ian, fallopian tube, or primary peritoneal
cancer who are in a complete or partial re-
sponse to platinum-based chemotherapy
Adults: 600 mg PO b.i.d. Continue treatment
until disease progression or unacceptable toxicity occurs.

➤ **Deleterious *BRCA* mutation (germline**
or somatic)-associated metastatic
castration-resistant prostate cancer in pa-
tients who have been treated with androgen
receptor-directed therapy and a taxane-
based chemotherapy ░
Adults: 600 mg (two 300-mg tablets) PO
b.i.d., for a total daily dose of 1,200 mg. Patient should also receive a GnRH analogue
concurrently or should have had bilateral orchiectomy. Continue treatment until disease
progression or unacceptable toxicity occurs.

ADMINISTRATION
PO
• May give without regard for food.
• Omit a missed dose and give next dose at
its scheduled time. Don't replace vomited
doses.
• Store at 68° to 77° F (20° to 25° C).

ACTION
Induces cytotoxicity by inhibiting PARP enzyme activity and increased formation of
PARP-DNA complexes, resulting in DNA
damage, apoptosis, and cell death.

Route	Onset	Peak	Duration
PO	Unknown	1.9 hr	Unknown

Half-life: 26 hours.

ADVERSE REACTIONS
CNS: fatigue, dizziness, fever, depression,
insomnia, taste alteration. **CV:** peripheral
edema. **EENT:** nasopharyngitis. **GI:** nausea,
vomiting, constipation, decreased appetite,
diarrhea, abdominal pain or distention, dyspepsia, stomatitis. **GU:** increased creatinine
level. **Hematologic:** anemia, *thrombocy-*
topenia, neutropenia, leukopenia, lympho-
cytopenia. **Hepatic:** increased LFT values.
Metabolic: increased cholesterol level, increased triglyceride levels, hyponatremia.
Respiratory: URI, dyspnea. **Skin:** rash,
photosensitivity reaction, pruritus, hand-foot
syndrome.

INTERACTIONS
Drug-drug. *CYP450 substrates:* May increase systemic substrate exposure and toxicity risk. Dosage adjustments may be needed.
Warfarin: May increase warfarin level. Monitor PT and INR.
Drug-lifestyle. *Sun exposure:* May cause
photosensitivity. Patient should use appropriate sun protection to avoid sunburn.

EFFECTS ON LAB TEST RESULTS
• May increase creatinine, ALT, AST, ALP,
triglyceride, and cholesterol levels.
• May decrease sodium level.
• May decrease Hb level, ANC, and lympho-
cyte, WBC, and platelet counts.

CONTRAINDICATIONS & CAUTIONS
• Use cautiously in patients with CrCl between 30 and 89 mL/minute or Child-Pugh
class A or B liver impairment. Use in patients
with CrCl of less than 30 mL/ minute, for
those on KRT, or for patients with Child-Pugh
class C liver impairment hasn't been studied.
• Drug may increase risk of myelodysplastic
syndrome (MDS) or acute myeloid leukemia
(AML). For confirmed MDS or AML, discontinue drug.

R

• Safety and effectiveness in children haven't been established.
• Use cautiously in older adults.
Dialyzable drug: Unknown.

PREGNANCY-LACTATION-REPRODUCTION
• Drug can cause fetal harm. Patients of childbearing potential should use effective contraception during therapy and for 6 months after final dose.
• Male patients with partners of child-bearing potential or who are pregnant should use effective contraception during treatment and for 3 months after final dose.
• Advise patients not to breastfeed during therapy and for 2 weeks after final dose.
• Male patients shouldn't donate sperm during therapy and for 3 months after final dose.

NURSING CONSIDERATIONS
Patients should be tested for *BRCA* mutation (germline or somatic) before treatment. Information on tests may be found at https://www.fda.gov/medical-devices/vitro-diagnostics/list-cleared-or-approved-companion-diagnostic-devices-vitro-and-imaging-tools.
• Monitor CBC at baseline and monthly thereafter. Don't start therapy until patient has recovered from hematologic toxicity caused by prior chemotherapy (grade 1 or less).
• Verify pregnancy status before therapy.

PATIENT TEACHING
• Instruct patient in safe drug administration and handling.
• Advise patients of reproductive potential in effective contraception use. Tell patient that pregnancy testing will be performed before treatment begins.
• Caution patient not to breastfeed during treatment and for 2 weeks after final dose.
• Warn patient that drug may cause photosensitivity and to use appropriate sun protection.
• Advise patient to report all adverse reactions, especially weakness, fatigue, fever, weight loss, frequent infections, bruising, easy bleeding, dyspnea, blood in urine or stool, nausea, and vomiting.

sacubitril–valsartan
sak-UE-bi-tril/val-SAR-tan

Entresto

Therapeutic class: Antihypertensives
Pharmacologic class: Neprilysin inhibitors–ARBs

AVAILABLE FORMS
Tablets: 24 mg sacubitril/26 mg valsartan, 49 mg sacubitril/51 mg valsartan, 97 mg sacubitril/103 mg valsartan

INDICATIONS & DOSAGES
Adjust-a-dose (for all indications): For patients not currently taking an ACE inhibitor or ARB, or previously taking a low dose of these agents, and patients with estimated GFR less than 30 mL/minute/1.73 m^2 or Child-Pugh class B liver impairment, reduce initial dose to half the usual starting dose, then follow the recommended dosage escalation. Initiate patients weighing 40 to 50 kg who meet these criteria at 0.8 mg/kg PO b.i.d.

➤ **To reduce risk of CV death and hospitalization for HF in patients with chronic HF**
Adults: Initially, 49 mg sacubitril/51 mg valsartan PO b.i.d. Increase after 2 to 4 weeks to target maintenance dose of 97 mg sacubitril/103 mg valsartan, as tolerated.

➤ **Symptomatic HF in children with systemic left ventricular systolic dysfunction**
Children ages 1 year and older weighing at least 50 kg: Initially, 49 mg sacubitril/51 mg valsartan PO b.i.d. If tolerated, may increase to 72 mg sacubitril/78 mg valsartan after 2 weeks, then increase to 97 mg sacubitril/103 mg valsartan after 2 additional weeks.
Children ages 1 year and older weighing at least 40 kg to less than 50 kg: Initially, 24 mg sacubitril/26 mg valsartan PO b.i.d. If tolerated, may increase to 49 mg sacubitril/51 mg valsartan after 2 weeks, then increase to 72 mg sacubitril/78 mg valsartan after 2 additional weeks.
Children ages 1 year and older weighing less than 40 kg: Initially, 1.6 mg/kg PO b.i.d. If tolerated, may increase to 2.3 mg/kg after 2 weeks, then increase to 3.1 mg/kg after 2 additional weeks.

ADMINISTRATION
PO
• If patient is switching to or from an ACE inhibitor, allow a washout period of 36 hours between giving the two drugs.
• May give without regard for food.
• Give a missed dose as soon as possible on the same day; then resume twice-daily dosing. Omit missed dose if close to the scheduled next dose.
• An oral suspension may be prepared by a pharmacist for patients unable to swallow tablets. Suspension can be stored for up to 15 days, but not above 77° F (25° C); don't refrigerate. Shake before use.

ACTION
Sacubitril inhibits neprilysin and valsartan inhibits the effects of angiotensin II, enhancing the protective neurohormonal systems of the heart (natriuretic peptide system) while suppressing the harmful RAAS.

Route	Onset	Peak	Duration
PO	Unknown	0.5–2 hr	Unknown

Half-life: Sacubitril, 1.4 hours; valsartan, 9.9 hours.

ADVERSE REACTIONS
CNS: dizziness. **CV:** hypotension. **GU:** *AKI, KF.* **Hematologic:** anemia. **Metabolic:** *hyperkalemia.* **Respiratory:** cough. **Other:** falls.

INTERACTIONS
Drug-drug. *ACE inhibitors:* May increase risk of angioedema. Use together is contraindicated. Don't give sacubitril–valsartan within 36 hours of switching from or to an ACE inhibitor.
Aliskiren: May increase risk of KF. Contraindicated for use together in patients with diabetes. Avoid use in patients with GFR less than 60 mL/minute/1.73 m^2.
ARBs: Will cause dual blockade of the RAAS as product contains valsartan. Avoid concurrent use.
Canagliflozin: May enhance hyperkalemic and hypotensive effects. Monitor potassium level and BP carefully.
Cyclooxygenase-2 inhibitors, NSAIDs: May increase risk of KF. Monitor kidney function closely.
Lithium: May increase lithium level and toxicity risk. Monitor serum lithium level.

Potassium-sparing diuretics (amiloride, spironolactone, triamterene), potassium supplements: May increase serum potassium level. Use cautiously and monitor patient closely.
Sodium phosphates: May enhance risk of acute phosphate nephropathy. Seek alternative bowel preparations.

EFFECTS ON LAB TEST RESULTS
• May increase serum creatinine and potassium levels.
• May decrease Hb level and hematocrit.

CONTRAINDICATIONS & CAUTIONS
• Contraindicated in patients with a history of angioedema related to previous ACE or ARB therapy and in patients hypersensitive to components of drug.
• Use in patients with Child-Pugh class C liver impairment isn't recommended.
 Drug may cause angioedema requiring emergency treatment and which can be fatal. Risk is greater in patients who are Black than in patients of other ethnicities.
• Drug lowers BP and may cause symptomatic hypotension.
• ACE inhibitors and ARBs have been associated with oliguria, progressive azotemia, AKI, hyperkalemia, and death. Monitor patient closely.
Dialyzable drug: Unlikely.
△ Overdose S&S: Hypotension.

PREGNANCY-LACTATION-REPRODUCTION
Boxed Warning Use during pregnancy can cause injury and death to developing fetus from effects on the RAAS. Stop drug as soon as pregnancy is detected. ■
• Use during pregnancy only if there is no appropriate alternative therapy and drug is considered lifesaving for patient. Advise patients who are pregnant of fetal risk.
• It isn't known if drug appears in human milk. Because of potential for serious reactions in infant, patient shouldn't breastfeed during therapy.

NURSING CONSIDERATIONS
• Drug is usually given with other HF therapies, in place of an ACE inhibitor or other ARB.
• Monitor patients for hypotension. Patients who are volume- or salt-depleted, such as those on high-dose diuretics, may be at

S

increased risk. Correct volume or salt depletion before start of therapy. Consider dosage adjustment of diuretics and concomitant antihypertensives. Reduce dosage or temporarily discontinue sacubitril–valsartan for persistent hypotension.

⚸ Monitor all patients, especially patients who are Black, for angioedema (swelling of the face, tongue, throat, and lips; airway compromise; dyspnea). Discontinue drug and treat emergently.

• Monitor kidney function and reduce dosage or temporarily interrupt therapy in patients who develop clinically significant decreased kidney function.

• Monitor serum potassium level periodically; treat appropriately. Patients with CKD, diabetes, hypoaldosteronism, or a high-potassium diet may be at increased risk for hyperkalemia. Reduce dosage or interrupt therapy as clinically indicated.

PATIENT TEACHING

• Advise patient to report all adverse reactions, especially signs and symptoms of angioedema and allergic reaction (swelling of the face, lips, tongue, or throat; trouble breathing). Advise patient to seek immediate emergency medical help if they occur.

• Instruct patient to take drug exactly as prescribed and not to take within 36 hours of an ACE inhibitor.

• Tell patient to report pregnancy as drug can cause fetal harm. Caution patient not to breastfeed during therapy.

• Caution patient to report dizziness, lightheadedness, or extreme fatigue.

safinamide mesylate
sa-FIN-a-mide

Xadago

Therapeutic class: Antiparkinsonian drugs
Pharmacologic class: MAO-B inhibitors

AVAILABLE FORMS
Tablets: 50 mg, 100 mg

INDICATIONS & DOSAGES
➤ **Parkinson disease in patients experiencing "off" episodes as adjunctive treatment to levodopa–carbidopa**

Adults: 50 mg PO once daily. After 2 weeks, may increase to 100 mg daily based on individual need and tolerability.

Adjust-a-dose: For patients with Child-Pugh class B liver impairment, maximum recommended dosage is 50 mg once daily. If patient progresses to Child-Pugh class C liver impairment, discontinue drug. When discontinuing, first taper 100-mg dosage to 50 mg for 1 week.

ADMINISTRATION
PO
• May give without regard for food.
• Give at same time each day.
• If a dose is missed, patient should take the next dose at same time the next day.
• Store at room temperature.

ACTION
An inhibitor of MAO-B. Blockade of MAO-B is thought to result in an increase in dopamine levels by blocking the catabolism of dopamine, which then increases dopaminergic activity in brain.

Route	Onset	Peak	Duration
PO	Unknown	2–3 hr	Unknown

Half-life: 20 to 26 hours.

ADVERSE REACTIONS
CNS: dyskinesia, insomnia, anxiety. **CV:** orthostatic hypotension, HTN. **GI:** nausea, dyspepsia. **Respiratory:** cough. **Other:** fall.

INTERACTIONS
Drug-drug. *Cold remedies; nasal, oral, and ophthalmic decongestants; sympathomimetic medications (amphetamine, methylphenidate):* May increase risk of hypertensive crisis. Use together is contraindicated.

Dextromethorphan: May cause episodes of psychosis or bizarre behavior. Use together is contraindicated.

Dopamine antagonists (antipsychotics, metoclopramide): May decrease effectiveness of safinamide and exacerbate Parkinson symptoms. Monitor therapy.

Isoniazid: Isoniazid has some MAO-inhibiting activity. Watch for HTN and reaction to dietary tyramine in patients taking both drugs.

MAO inhibitors (linezolid, MAO-B inhibitors), opioids (meperidine, methadone, tramadol), SNRIs, TCAs, mirtazapine, maprotiline, trazodone: May increase risk of serotonin syndrome. Use together is contraindicated. Allow at least 14 days to lapse after discontinuing safinamide and starting these drugs.

SSRIs: May cause serotonin syndrome. Monitor patient for signs and symptoms of serotonin syndrome; use lowest effective dosage of SSRI with safinamide.

Drug-herb. *St John's wort:* May increase risk of serotonin syndrome. Discourage use together. Allow 14 days to lapse between discontinuing safinamide and starting St. John's wort.

Drug-food. *Tyramine-containing foods (aged, fermented, cured, pickled, or smoked food):* May increase risk of HTN. Discourage intake of these types of food.

Drug-lifestyle. *Alcohol use:* May increase sedative effects. Discourage use together.

EFFECTS ON LAB TEST RESULTS
• May increase ALT and AST levels.

CONTRAINDICATIONS & CAUTIONS
• Contraindicated in patients hypersensitive to drug or its components and in patients with Child-Pugh class C liver impairment.
• Use cautiously in patients with Child-Pugh class B liver impairment.
• Use cautiously in patients with major psychotic disorder; drug may exacerbate psychosis. Consider dosage reduction or drug discontinuation if patient develops hallucinations or psychotic-like behaviors.
• Safinamide isn't effective alone for the treatment of Parkinson disease. Patients should also take levodopa–carbidopa.
• Safety and effectiveness in children haven't been established.
Dialyzable drug: Unknown.

PREGNANCY-LACTATION-REPRODUCTION
• There are no adequate studies during pregnancy. Developmental toxicity and teratogenic effects were observed in animal studies. Other Parkinson disease agents may be preferred. Use only if benefits outweigh fetal risk.
• It isn't known if drug appears in human milk. Use cautiously during breastfeeding if benefits outweigh risk of infant exposure.

NURSING CONSIDERATIONS
• Monitor patients for hypersensitivity reactions, including dyspnea and swelling of the tongue and oral mucosa.
• Monitor patients for new-onset HTN or uncontrolled HTN.
• Monitor patients for serotonin syndrome (mental status changes [agitation, hallucinations, delirium, coma], tachycardia, labile BP, dizziness, diaphoresis, flushing, hyperthermia, rigidity, monoclonus, hyperreflexia, incoordination, seizures, nausea, vomiting, diarrhea).
• Monitor LFT values and discontinue drug if patient develops Child-Pugh class C liver impairment.
• Patients may experience excessive drowsiness and fall asleep suddenly without warning. Monitor patients for daytime sleepiness or falling asleep during activities (driving, talking, eating). Drug may need to be discontinued.
• Monitor patients for new-onset or exacerbated dyskinesia. Reducing levodopa or other dopaminergic drug dosage may be needed.
• A withdrawal syndrome (elevated temperature, muscular rigidity, confusion, altered consciousness, autonomic instability) resembling NMS may occur with rapid dosage reduction, drug withdrawal, or changes in drug regimen that increase central dopaminergic tone. Adjust dosage carefully and taper dosage before discontinuation.
• Monitor for hallucinations or psychotic-like behaviors. If signs and symptoms occur, dosage reduction or drug discontinuation may be needed.
• Drug may cause impulse control or compulsive behaviors. Monitor patients for new or increased gambling urges, sexual urges, uncontrolled spending, binge eating, or other intense urges and the inability to control these urges. If signs or symptoms occur, dosage reduction or drug discontinuation may be needed.
• Periodically monitor for visual changes in patients with a history of retinal or macular degeneration, uveitis, personal or family history of retinal disease, albinism, retinitis pigmentosa, diabetic retinopathy, or other retinopathy.

PATIENT TEACHING
• Tell patient to report all adverse reactions to prescriber.

S

- Inform patient that drug may elevate BP. Advise patient to monitor BP and report elevations.
- Teach patient signs and symptoms of serotonin syndrome and to report them should they occur.
- Explain that drug can cause sleepiness and patient can fall asleep suddenly during daily activities. Caution patient not to drive, operate heavy machinery, work in high places, or engage in other dangerous activities until drug's effects are known.
- Advise patient to avoid foods that contain large amounts of tyramine (aged, fermented, cured, smoked, or pickled foods) because of the potential for substantial increases in BP.
- Warn patient not to discontinue drug rapidly; drug should be tapered to avoid withdrawal.
- Explain that drug may cause retinal changes. Tell patient to notify prescriber if visual changes occur.
- Advise patient to immediately report hallucinations, psychotic behavior, compulsive behaviors, or problems with impulse control (gambling, spending money, sexual urges, binge eating).
- Caution patient to immediately report pregnancy, plans to become pregnant, breastfeeding, or plans to breastfeed during treatment.

salmeterol xinafoate
sal-ME-te-role

Serevent Diskus

Therapeutic class: Bronchodilators
Pharmacologic class: Long-acting selective beta$_2$ agonists

AVAILABLE FORMS
Inhalation powder: 50 mcg/dose

INDICATIONS & DOSAGES
➤ **Asthma; to prevent bronchospasm only as combined therapy with an inhaled corticosteroid (ICS) in patients with reversible obstructive airway disease, including nocturnal asthma**
Adults and children ages 4 and older: 1 inhalation (50 mcg) b.i.d. in the morning and evening, about 12 hours apart.
➤ **To prevent exercise-induced bronchospasm**

Adults and children ages 4 and older: 1 inhalation (50 mcg) at least 30 minutes before exercise. Additional doses shouldn't be taken for at least 12 hours.
➤ **COPD, including emphysema and chronic bronchitis**
Adults: 1 inhalation (50 mcg) b.i.d. in the morning and evening, about 12 hours apart.

ADMINISTRATION
Inhalational
- Inhaler must be used in a level, flat position.
- Patient should hold breath for about 10 seconds after inhaling, then breathe out fully.
- Don't use a spacer device with this drug.
- Don't wash the inhaler and always keep it in a dry place.
- Discard inhaler 6 weeks after opening foil pouch or when counter reads "0."
- Omit a missed dose and give next dose at the usual time.

ACTION
Unclear. Selectively activates beta$_2$ receptors, which results in bronchodilation; also, blocks the release of allergic mediators from mast cells lining the respiratory tract.

Route	Onset	Peak	Duration
Inhalation	30–120 min	20 min	12 hr

Half-life: 5.5 hours.

ADVERSE REACTIONS
CNS: anxiety, headache, migraine, dizziness, tremor, nervousness, paresthesia, sleep disturbance, fever, pain. **CV:** tachycardia, palpitations, HTN, edema. **EENT:** conjunctivitis, keratitis, nasal congestion, sinusitis, rhinitis, pharyngitis, candidiasis of mouth or throat, hyposalivation, throat irritation, dental discomfort, tracheitis, ear signs and symptoms. **GI:** nausea, vomiting, dyspepsia, GI infections. **Metabolic:** hyperglycemia. **Musculoskeletal:** joint and back pain, myalgia, muscle cramps, muscle stiffness, arthralgia, articular rheumatism. **Respiratory:** bronchitis, URI, cough, viral respiratory infection, *asthma.* **Skin:** rash, urticaria, photodermatitis. **Other:** hypersensitivity reactions, flulike symptoms.

INTERACTIONS
Drug-drug. *Antiarrhythmics (amiodarone, disopyramide, sotalol), chlorpromazine, dolasetron, droperidol, moxifloxacin,*

pentamidine, pimozide, tacrolimus, thiori-dazine, ziprasidone: May prolong QT interval and increase risk of life-threatening arrhythmias. Monitor QT interval closely.

Beta agonists, other methylxanthines, theophylline: May cause adverse cardiac effects with excessive use. Monitor patient.

Beta blockers (nonselective): May diminish bronchodilatory effects. Use cardioselective beta blockers if therapy is indicated.

CYP3A4 inhibitors (atazanavir, clarithromycin, ketoconazole, ritonavir): May increase CV effects. Avoid use together.

Diuretics (non-potassium-sparing): May worsen hypokalemia and ECG changes. Use cautiously together.

MAO inhibitors (phenelzine, selegiline), TCAs (doxepin, imipramine): May increase risk of adverse CV effects. Avoid use together within 14 days.

EFFECTS ON LAB TEST RESULTS
• May decrease potassium and glucose levels.

CONTRAINDICATIONS & CAUTIONS
• Contraindicated in patients hypersensitive to drug, its ingredients, or milk proteins.

🔹 *Alert:* Contraindicated as primary treatment for acute asthma or COPD.

Boxed Warning Contraindicated for treatment of asthma without an ICS. Using without an ICS may increase the risk of asthma-related death. ▪

Boxed Warning Only use salmeterol as additional therapy for patients whose condition isn't adequately controlled on other medications or patients whose disease severity warrants initiation of treatment with two maintenance therapies. Don't use salmeterol for patients whose asthma is adequately controlled on low- or medium-dose ICS. ▪

• Clinical trial data don't suggest an increased risk of death with the use of salmeterol in patients with COPD.

• Paradoxical bronchospasm that may be life-threatening may occur; distinguish from inadequate response. Discontinue salmeterol and start alternative treatment if paradoxical bronchospasm occurs.

🔹 *Alert:* Don't use drug with other medications containing LABAs.

• Use cautiously in patients unusually responsive to sympathomimetics and those with coronary insufficiency, arrhythmias, HTN,

other CV disorders, thyrotoxicosis, liver impairment, diabetes, or seizure disorders.

Dialyzable drug: Unknown.

⚠ *Overdose S&S:* Exaggeration of adverse reactions, hypokalemia, seizures, angina, HTN, hypotension, dry mouth, muscle cramps, dizziness, fatigue, insomnia, tachycardia, ventricular arrhythmias, cardiac arrest, sudden death.

PREGNANCY-LACTATION-REPRODUCTION
• There are no adequate studies during pregnancy. Use cautiously during pregnancy.

• Providers and patients are encourage to enroll exposed patients in the MotherToBaby Pregnancy Studies at https://mothertobaby.org/ongoing-study/asthma/ or 866-626-6847.

• Drug may interfere with uterine contractility during labor. Use only if benefits outweigh risks.

• It isn't known if drug appears in human milk. Use cautiously during breastfeeding.

NURSING CONSIDERATIONS
Boxed Warning LABAs may increase risk of asthmarelated hospitalization in children and adolescents. For children and adolescents with asthma who require addition of a LABA to an ICS, a fixed-dose combination product should be used to ensure adherence with both drugs. ▪

• Drug isn't indicated for acute bronchospasm.

🔹 *Alert:* Monitor patient for rash and urticaria, which may signal a hypersensitivity reaction.

• Monitor patient for hypokalemia and hyperglycemia.

PATIENT TEACHING
Boxed Warning Teach parents of child or adolescent who requires the use of a separate ICS and a LABA that appropriate steps must be taken to ensure adherence with both treatment components, because of the increased risk of asthma-related death. ▪

• Instruct patient in safe drug administration.

• Remind patient to take drug at about 12-hour intervals for optimal effect and to take drug even when feeling better.

• Advise patient that immediate hypersensitivity reactions (such as urticaria, angioedema, rash, bronchospasm, and hypotension, including anaphylaxis) may occur after

S

administration of this drug and to seek immediate medical attention if such reactions occur.

🔵 *Alert:* Tell patient drug shouldn't be used to treat acute bronchospasm. Patient must use a short-acting beta₂ agonist, such as albuterol, to treat worsening symptoms.

• Tell patient to contact prescriber if the short-acting agonist no longer provides sufficient relief or if patient needs more than 4 inhalations daily. This may be a sign that the asthma symptoms are worsening. Tell patient not to increase the dosage of salmeterol.

• If patient takes an ICS, patient should continue to use it regularly. Warn patient not to take other drugs without prescriber's consent.

• Advise patient to report pregnancy during therapy.

SAFETY ALERT!

sargramostim (GM-CSF; granulocyte-macrophage colony-stimulating factor)
sar-GRAM-oh-stim

Leukine

Therapeutic class: Hematopoietics
Pharmacologic class: Colony-stimulating factors

AVAILABLE FORMS
Powder for injection: 250 mcg

INDICATIONS & DOSAGES
➤ **To accelerate hematopoietic reconstitution after autologous or allogeneic bone marrow transplantation in patients with non-Hodgkin lymphoma or acute lymphoblastic leukemia or in patients with Hodgkin lymphoma**
Adults and children ages 2 and older:
250 mcg/m² daily as 2-hour IV infusion beginning 2 to 4 hours after bone marrow transplantation and not less than 24 hours after last dose of chemotherapy or radiotherapy. Don't give until post-marrow infusion ANC falls below 500 cells/mm³. Continue until ANC exceeds 1,500 cells/mm³ for 3 consecutive days.
Adjust-a-dose: For allogeneic transplantation, discontinue immediately if blast cells appear or disease progression occurs. Temporarily discontinue or reduce dosage by 50% if a

severe adverse reaction occurs. Interrupt therapy or reduce dosage by 50% if ANC exceeds 20,000 cells/mm³ or WBC count exceeds 50,000 cells/mm³.
➤ **Neutrophil recovery after induction chemotherapy in acute myelogenous leukemia (AML)**
Adults ages 55 and older: Initially, 250 mcg/m² IV once daily over 4 hours beginning day 11 or 4 days after completion of induction therapy; initiate only if bone marrow is hypoplastic with less than 5% blasts on day 10. If a second induction cycle is needed, begin sargramostim 4 days after completing chemotherapy and only if bone marrow is hypoplastic with less than 5% blasts. Continue until the ANC exceeds 1,500 cells/mm³ for 3 consecutive days or for a maximum of 42 days.
Adjust-a-dose: Discontinue immediately if leukemic regrowth occurs. Reduce dosage by 50% or temporarily discontinue if a severe adverse reaction occurs. Interrupt therapy or reduce dosage by 50% if ANC exceeds 20,000 cells/mm³.
➤ **Mobilization of peripheral blood progenitor cells (PBPCs)**
Adults: 250 mcg/m² by continuous IV infusion over 24 hours or by subcut injection once daily. Continue through PBPC collection.
Adjust-a-dose: If WBC count exceeds 50,000 cells/mm³, reduce dosage by 50%. If adequate numbers of cells aren't collected, consider other mobilization therapy.
➤ **Post-PBPC transplantation**
Adults: 250 mcg/m² by continuous IV infusion over 24 hours or by subcut injection once daily beginning immediately after PBPC infusion; continue until ANC exceeds 1,500 cells/mm³ for 3 consecutive days.
➤ **Bone marrow transplantation failure or engraftment delay**
Adults and children ages 2 and older:
250 mcg/m² as a 2-hour IV infusion daily for 14 days. This course of therapy may be repeated after 7 days of no therapy. If engraftment still hasn't occurred, a third course of 500 mcg/m² daily IV for 14 days may be attempted after another therapy-free 7 days.
Adjust-a-dose: Stimulation of marrow precursors may result in rapid rise of WBC count. If blast cells appear or if the underlying disease progresses, stop therapy. If WBC count exceeds 50,000 cells/mm³ or ANC exceeds

20,000 cells/mm³, temporarily stop drug or reduce dose by 50%.

➤ **To increase survival in patients acutely exposed to myelosuppressive doses of radiation (hematopoietic syndrome of acute radiation syndrome) given as soon as possible after suspected or confirmed exposure to radiation doses greater than 2 gray**

Adults and children weighing more than 40 kg: 7 mcg/kg subcut once daily. Continue until ANC remains more than 1,000 cells/mm³ for three consecutive CBCs obtained every third day, or exceeds 10,000 cells/mm³ after a radiation-induced nadir.

Children weighing 15 to 40 kg: 10 mcg/kg subcut once daily. Continue until ANC remains more than 1,000 cells/mm³ for three consecutive CBCs obtained every third day, or exceeds 10,000 cells/mm³ after a radiation-induced nadir.

Children weighing less than 15 kg: 12 mcg/kg subcut once daily. Continue until ANC remains more than 1,000 cells/mm³ for three consecutive CBCs obtained every third day, or exceeds 10,000 cells/mm³ after a radiation-induced nadir.

➤ **Neuroblastoma in children at high risk ◆**

Children and adolescents: 250 mcg/m² subcut or IV once daily for 14 days, beginning 3 days before administration of dinutuximab (each cycle is 28 days); sargramostim is administered during cycles 1, 3, and 5 (regimen also includes dinutuximab, isotretinoin, and aldesleukin).

ADMINISTRATION

IV

▼ Reconstitute powder for injection with 1 mL of sterile or bacteriostatic water for injection. Direct stream of sterile water against side of vial and gently swirl contents to minimize foaming. Avoid excessive or vigorous agitation or shaking.

▼ Further dilute in NSS. If drug yield falls below 10 mcg/mL, add human albumin to NSS at final concentration of 0.1% before adding sargramostim to prevent adsorption to components of the delivery system. To yield 0.1% human albumin, add 1 mg human albumin to each milliliter of NSS (dilute 1 mL of 5% human albumin in 50 mL of NSS).

▼ Don't use in-line filter.

▼ Give as soon as possible after mixing and no later than 6 hours after reconstituting.

▼ **Incompatibilities:** Other IV drugs, unless specific compatibility data are available.

Subcutaneous

● Reconstitute powder for injection with 1 mL sterile or bacteriostatic water for injection; use sterile water without preservatives to reconstitute drug when administering to neonates or infants to avoid benzyl alcohol exposure. Direct stream of sterile or bacteriostatic water against side of vial and gently swirl contents to minimize foaming. Avoid excessive or vigorous agitation or shaking.

● May refrigerate solution reconstituted with sterile water for up to 24 hours; may refrigerate solution reconstituted with bacteriostatic water preserved with benzyl alcohol for up to 20 days.

ACTION

Induces cellular responses by binding to specific receptors on surfaces of target cells.

Route	Onset	Peak	Duration
IV	15 min	Immediate	Unknown
Subcut	15 min	2.5–4 hr	Unknown

Half-life: IV, about 1 hour; subcut, about 4 hours.

ADVERSE REACTIONS

CNS: asthenia, CNS disorders, fever, headache, malaise, anxiety, insomnia, pain, paresthesia. **CV:** *hemorrhage,* edema, peripheral edema, HTN, hypotension, supraventricular arrhythmias, chest pain, pericardial effusion, tachycardia. **EENT:** retinal hemorrhage, epistaxis, pharyngitis, rhinitis. **GI:** anorexia, diarrhea, dysphagia, abdominal pain, GI disorders, nausea, stomatitis, vomiting, *GI hemorrhage.* **GU:** urinary tract disorder, abnormal kidney function, increased creatinine level, elevated BUN. **Hematologic:** blood dyscrasias, anemia, *thrombocytopenia, leukopenia.* **Hepatic:** liver damage, bilirubinemia, increased ALT level. **Metabolic:** hyperglycemia, decreased albumin level, *hypomagnesemia,* weight loss. **Musculoskeletal:** arthralgia, bone pain. **Respiratory:** dyspnea, lung disorders, pleural effusion. **Skin:** alopecia, pruritus, rash. **Other:** hypersensitivity reaction, mucous membrane disorder, chills, infection, *sepsis,* antisargramostim antibodies.

S

INTERACTIONS

Drug-drug. *Bleomycin, cyclophosphamide:* May enhance risk of pulmonary toxicity. Monitor patient closely.

Corticosteroids, lithium: May increase myeloproliferative effects of sargramostim. Use cautiously together.

EFFECTS ON LAB TEST RESULTS

• May increase BUN, creatinine, AST, ALT, ALP, bilirubin, and glucose levels.
• May decrease Hb, calcium, magnesium, and albumin levels.
• May decrease leukocyte and platelet counts.

CONTRAINDICATIONS & CAUTIONS

• Contraindicated in patients hypersensitive to drug or its components or to yeast-derived products.
• Infusion-related reactions (respiratory distress, hypoxia, flushing, hypotension, syncope, tachycardia) may occur after administration of the first dose.
• Lyophilized powder reconstituted with bacteriostatic water contains benzyl alcohol, which can cause fatal neonatal gasping syndrome. Avoid use in neonates.
• Use cautiously in patients with cardiac disease, hypoxia, fluid retention, pulmonary infiltrates, HF, or impaired kidney or liver function because these conditions may worsen.
• Drug may interfere with bone imaging studies; increased hematopoietic activity of the bone marrow may appear as transient positive bone imaging changes.
• Safety and effectiveness haven't been established in children younger than age 2 or for neutrophil recovery after induction chemotherapy for AML or autologous PBPC mobilization and collection.
Dialyzable drug: Unknown.

⚠ *Overdose S&S:* Dyspnea, malaise, nausea, fever, rash, sinus tachycardia, headache, chills.

PREGNANCY-LACTATION-REPRODUCTION

• There are no adequate studies during pregnancy. Use only if clearly needed; if needed, use only lyophilized powder reconstituted with preservative-free sterile water to avoid risk posed by benzyl alcohol.
• It isn't known if drug appears in human milk. Tell patient to avoid breastfeeding during treatment and for at least 2 weeks after final dose.

NURSING CONSIDERATIONS

• If severe adverse reactions occur, reduce dose by 50% or temporarily stop drug and notify prescriber. Resume therapy when reactions decrease. Transient rash and local reactions at injection site may occur.
• Monitor patient for infusion-related reactions (respiratory distress, hypoxia, flushing, hypotension, syncope, tachycardia), which may occur after administration of the first dose. If patient exhibits signs of dyspnea, reduce infusion rate by 50%; if symptoms persist or worsen, discontinue infusion.
• Rapidly dividing progenitor cells may be sensitive to cytotoxic therapies, rendering drug ineffective; don't give within 24 hours of cytotoxic chemotherapy or prior to radiotherapy.
• Monitor CBC with differential, including exam for presence of blast cells, biweekly.
• Monitor body weight and hydration status; drug may increase risk of effusions and capillary leak syndrome.
• Monitor patients, especially those with preexisting cardiac disease, for supraventricular arrhythmias.
• Drug accelerates myeloid recovery in patients receiving bone marrow that is either unpurged or purged by anti-B cell monoclonal antibodies more than in those who receive chemically purged bone marrow.
• Drug may produce a limited response in patients with transplants who have received extensive radiotherapy or other myelotoxic drugs.
• Drug can act as a growth factor for any tumor type, particularly myeloid malignant disease.

PATIENT TEACHING

• Review administration schedule with patient and caregivers, and address their concerns.
• Urge patient to report all adverse reactions promptly.
• Instruct patient who will self-administer drug in injection technique, drug storage, and needle disposal.
• Caution patient to report pregnancy or breastfeeding to prescriber.

Reactions in bold italics are *life-threatening*.

sarilumab
sar-IL-ue-mab

Kevzara

Therapeutic class: Antirheumatics
Pharmacologic class: Monoclonal
antibodies

AVAILABLE FORMS
Injection: 150 mg/1.14 mL, 200 mg/1.14 mL
single-dose prefilled syringes and pens

INDICATIONS & DOSAGES
➤ **Moderately to severely active RA in
patients who have had an inadequate
response or intolerance to one or more
DMARDs, as monotherapy or in combination with methotrexate or other conventional DMARDs**
Adults: 200 mg subcut once every 2 weeks.
Adjust-a-dose: Reduce dosage to 150 mg every 2 weeks for management of neutropenia,
thrombocytopenia, and elevated liver enzyme
levels. Refer to manufacturer's instructions
for specific toxicity-related dosage adjustments.
✳ *NEW INDICATION:* **Polymyalgia rheumatica in patients who have had an inadequate
response to corticosteroids or who can't
tolerate corticosteroid taper**
Adults: 200 mg subcut once every 2 weeks in
combination with a tapering course of corticosteroids or as monotherapy following corticosteroid discontinuation.
Adjust-a-dose: Discontinue drug for ANC
below 1,000/mm³, platelet count below
100,000 mm³, or AST or ALT levels above
3 times the ULN. Withhold treatment until infection is controlled if serious or opportunistic infection occurs.

ADMINISTRATION
Subcutaneous
• Allow prefilled syringe to sit at room temperature for 30 minutes or prefilled pen to
sit at room temperature for 60 minutes before subcut injection; don't warm in any other
way.
• Inspect solution before use. Don't use if solution is cloudy, discolored, or contains particles, or if any part of prefilled syringe appears
to be damaged.
• Inject the full amount in syringe or pen.

• Rotate injection sites. Don't inject
into bruises, scars, or tender or damaged
skin.
• Keep unused syringes or pens in original
carton to protect from light and store in refrigerator between 36° and 46° F (2° and
8° C); don't freeze, heat, or shake.
• May store drug at room temperature up to
77° F (25° C) for up to 14 days in carton. Use
within 14 days after refrigeration.

ACTION
An interleukin 6 (IL-6) receptor antagonist
that binds to both soluble and membrane-
bound IL-6 receptors causing an anti-
inflammatory effect that leads to a reduction
in C-reactive protein levels.

Route	Onset	Peak	Duration
Subcut	Unknown	2–4 days	28 days (150-mg dose), 43 days (200-mg dose)

Half-life: 150-mg dose, 8 days; 200-mg dose,
10 days.

ADVERSE REACTIONS
CNS: fatigue. **EENT:** nasopharyngitis, oral
herpes simplex. **GI:** constipation. **GU:** UTI.
Hematologic: *neutropenia, leukopenia,
thrombocytopenia.* **Hepatic:** increased ALT
and AST levels. **Metabolic:** hyperlipidemia.
Musculoskeletal: myalgia. **Respiratory:**
URI. **Skin:** injection-site reaction. **Other:**
infection, *malignancy,* immunosuppression,
antibody development.

INTERACTIONS
Drug-drug. *Biological DMARDs (anti-CD20
monoclonal antibodies, IL-1R antagonists,
selective costimulation modulators, TNF antagonists):* May increase risk of immunosuppression and infection. Avoid use together.
Corticosteroids: May increase risk of immunosuppression and infection. Monitor patient closely.
Corticosteroids, NSAIDs: May increase risk
of GI perforation. Avoid concurrent use.
*CYP450 substrates (atorvastatin, lovas-
tatin, oral contraceptives, theophylline,
warfarin):* May alter substrate levels. Use
cautiously together. Monitor substrate levels if possible and adjust substrate dosage as
needed.
Live-virus vaccines: May increase risk of
infection. Avoid use together.

S

EFFECTS ON LAB TEST RESULTS
• May increase AST, ALT, LDL, HDL, cholesterol, and triglyceride levels.
• May decrease ANC and neutrophil and platelet counts.

CONTRAINDICATIONS & CAUTIONS
• Contraindicated in patients with hypersensitivity to drug or its components.
Boxed Warning Serious infections leading to hospitalization or death, including bacterial, viral, invasive fungal, TB, and other opportunistic infections, can occur. Avoid use in patients with an active infection. Consider risks and benefits of use in patients with chronic or recurrent infection. ■
• Older adults and patients with a history of serious or opportunistic infections, exposure to TB, or a history of living or traveling to areas of endemic TB or mycoses may be at increased risk of infections.
• Risk of GI perforation may increase in patients with concurrent diverticulitis.
• Drug isn't recommended in patients with active liver disease, ALT or AST level more than $1.5 \times$ ULN, ANC less than 2,000 cells/mm^3, or platelet count less than 150,000 cells/mm^3.
• Drug may increase risk of viral reactivation, including herpes zoster.
• Drug may increase risk of malignancies.
• Drug use hasn't been studied in patients with liver impairment or CrCl less than 30 mL/minute.
• Safety and effectiveness in children haven't been established.
Dialyzable drug: Unknown.

PREGNANCY-LACTATION-REPRODUCTION
• Effect of drug on a fetus is unknown; however, monoclonal antibodies cross the placental barrier in the third trimester and may affect immune response in infants exposed in utero. Use in pregnancy only if potential benefit justifies fetal risk.
• It isn't known if drug appears in human milk. Consider benefits and risks of drug before patient starts breastfeeding.

NURSING CONSIDERATIONS
Boxed Warning Monitor patients for infection during treatment. Interrupt treatment if serious or opportunistic infection occurs; don't restart drug until infection is controlled. ■

• Perform prompt and complete testing to evaluate a new infection during treatment and initiate appropriate antimicrobial therapy while closely monitoring patient.
Boxed Warning Assess patient for TB risk factors and test for latent TB before drug initiation. If positive, start treatment for TB before beginning therapy. Consider anti-TB therapy for patients with a history of TB in whom an adequate course of treatment can't be confirmed and in patients who test negatively for latent TB but have risk factors for TB. ■
• Monitor neutrophil and platelet counts before therapy, 4 to 8 weeks after start of therapy, and every 3 months thereafter.
• Monitor ALT and AST levels before therapy, 4 to 8 weeks after start of therapy, and every 3 months thereafter. Assess bilirubin level or other LFT values as clinically indicated.
• Monitor lipid parameters (LDL, HDL, triglycerides) 4 to 8 weeks after start of therapy and every 6 months thereafter.
• Monitor patients for hypersensitivity reactions (injection-site rash, generalized rash, urticaria). If anaphylaxis or other severe hypersensitivity reaction occurs, stop drug immediately.
• Monitor patients with concurrent diverticulitis and those who are taking corticosteroids or NSAIDs for GI perforation. Promptly evaluate acute abdominal signs and symptoms.
• *Look alike–sound alike:* Don't confuse sarilumab with sirolimus. Don't confuse Kevzara with Keppra.

PATIENT TEACHING
Boxed Warning Warn patient that drug may lower resistance to infection and to contact prescriber immediately if signs and symptoms of infection appear, to ensure rapid evaluation and appropriate treatment. ■
• Assess patient for ability to self-administer drug. Instruct patient or caregivers in injection technique, drug storage, and syringe disposal.
• Advise patient to seek immediate medical attention for serious allergic reactions (shortness of breath, chest pain, dizziness, moderate or severe stomach pain or vomiting, or swelling of lips, tongue, or face).
• Caution patient (especially if taking NSAIDs or steroids or with a history of GI perforation) of increased risk of GI perforation. Instruct patient to seek medical attention

immediately for severe, persistent abdominal pain.
• Tell patient to discuss plans for surgery or a medical procedure with prescriber.
• Instruct patient to keep carton in an insulated bag with an ice pack when traveling.
• Caution patient to immediately report pregnancy that occurs during treatment.

sAXagliptin
sax-a-GLIP-tin

Onglyza

Therapeutic class: Antidiabetics
Pharmacologic class: DPP-4 enzyme inhibitors

AVAILABLE FORMS
Tablets ⓘ: 2.5 mg, 5 mg

INDICATIONS & DOSAGES
➤ **Adjunct to diet and exercise to improve glycemic control in type 2 diabetes**
Adults: 2.5 or 5 mg PO once daily.
Adjust-a-dose: For patient with eGFR of 45 mL/minute/1.73 m^2 or less or if patient is taking strong CYP3A4/5 inhibitors, give 2.5 mg PO once daily. If patient requires hemodialysis, give 2.5 mg once daily after treatment.

ADMINISTRATION
PO
• Give drug without regard for food.
• Have patient swallow tablets whole; don't crush or cut tablets.

ACTION
Inhibits DPP-4, an enzyme that rapidly inactivates incretin hormones, which play a part in body's regulation of glucose. By increasing active incretin levels, drug helps to increase insulin release and decrease circulating glucose.

Route	Onset	Peak	Duration
PO	Unknown	2 hr	24 hr

Half-life: 2.5 hours.

ADVERSE REACTIONS
CNS: headache. **CV:** peripheral edema. **GU:** UTI, increased creatinine level, *AKI, KF.* **Metabolic:** *hypoglycemia.* **Respiratory:** URI. **Other:** hypersensitivity reaction.

INTERACTIONS
Drug-drug. *Insulin, sulfonylureas (glimepiride, glipizide, glyburide):* May increase risk of hypoglycemia. Decrease dosage of insulin or sulfonylurea if used together.
Strong CYP3A4/5 inhibitors (atazanavir, clarithromycin, itraconazole, ketoconazole, nefazodone, nelfinavir, ritonavir, saquinavir): May increase saxagliptin level. Reduce dosage to 2.5 mg PO daily.

EFFECTS ON LAB TEST RESULTS
• May increase creatinine level.
• May decrease glucose level.
• May decrease lymphocyte count.

CONTRAINDICATIONS & CAUTIONS
• Contraindicated in patients hypersensitive to drug or its components.
• Hypersensitivity reactions (anaphylaxis, angioedema, xfoliative skin conditions such as bullous pemphigoid) have occurred within first 3 months of therapy initiation. Discontinue drug for suspected hypersensitivity.
• Use cautiously in patients with a history of angioedema to another DPP-4 inhibitor because it's unknown if such patients will be predisposed to angioedema with saxagliptin.
• **Alert:** Use cautiously in patients with a history of HF or kidney disease. Drug may increase risk of HF in these patients.
• Rare cases of acute pancreatitis have been reported. Discontinue drug for suspected pancreatitis.
• Drug isn't indicated to treat type 1 diabetes or diabetic ketoacidosis.
• Safety and effectiveness in children haven't been established.
• Use cautiously in older adults.
Dialyzable drug: 23%.

PREGNANCY-LACTATION-REPRODUCTION
• There are no adequate studies during pregnancy. Use only if clearly needed.
• It isn't known if drug appears in human milk. Use cautiously during breastfeeding.

NURSING CONSIDERATIONS
• **Alert:** Drug may cause joint pain that can be severe and disabling. Report severe, persistent joint pain to prescriber; drug may need to be discontinued.
• **Alert:** Monitor patient for signs and symptoms of HF (dyspnea, orthopnea, tiredness, weakness, fatigue, weight gain, peripheral

S

or abdominal edema). Drug may need to be discontinued; other antidiabetics may be required.

• Monitor blood glucose level and watch for signs and symptoms of hypoglycemia.

• Monitor HbA_{1c} level periodically to assess long-term glycemic control.

• Assess kidney function before starting drug and periodically thereafter.

• Monitor patient for hypersensitivity reactions, including skin blistering or erosions. Discontinue drug for suspected bullous pemphigoid and consider referral to a dermatologist.

• Include diet control and exercise in the patient's type 2 diabetes management plan because calorie restriction, weight loss, and exercise help improve insulin sensitivity and the effects of drug therapy.

• *Look alike–sound alike:* Don't confuse saxagliptin with sitagliptin.

PATIENT TEACHING
• Instruct patient in safe drug administration.
• Tell patient to stop drug and seek immediate medical attention for signs and symptoms of hypersensitivity (rash, flaking or peeling skin, itching, or swelling of the skin, face, lips, tongue, or throat).

◊ *Alert:* Instruct patient to immediately report signs and symptoms of HF to prescriber. Patient shouldn't stop drug without first discussing with prescriber.

◊ *Alert:* Instruct patient to report severe and persistent joint pain to prescriber as drug may need to be discontinued.

• Advise patient that drug isn't a substitute for diet and exercise and that it's important to follow a prescribed dietary and physical activity routine and to monitor glucose levels.

• Inform patient and family members of the signs and symptoms of hypoglycemia and hyperglycemia and the steps to take should these occur.

• Tell patient to notify prescriber during periods of stress (fever, infection, or surgery) because dosage may need adjustment.

• Teach patient to stop drug if signs and symptoms of pancreatitis (persistent severe abdominal pain, sometimes radiating to the back; vomiting) occur.

• Advise patient to immediately report skin blisters or erosions.

• Caution patient to report pregnancy or breastfeeding to prescriber.

---

scopolamine
skoe-POL-a-meen

Transderm Scop

Therapeutic class: Antiemetics
Pharmacologic class: Belladonna alkaloids–antimuscarinics

AVAILABLE FORMS
Transdermal patch: 1 mg/3 days

INDICATIONS & DOSAGES
➤ **To prevent postoperative nausea and vomiting**
Adults: Apply 1 transdermal patch to skin behind the ear the evening before surgery. To minimize exposure of a newborn to drug, apply patch 1 hour before cesarean birth. Keep patch in place for 24 hours after surgery; then remove and discard.

➤ **To prevent nausea and vomiting from motion sickness**
Adults: Apply 1 transdermal patch to skin behind the ear at least 4 hours before antiemetic is needed. Remove and place a new patch behind other ear if needed for longer than 3 days.

ADMINISTRATION
Transdermal
• Keep in foil wrapper until ready to use.
• Wear gloves to apply or remove patch.
• Apply patch to skin behind ear on clean, dry, hairless area.
• If patch dislodges, replace with a new one.
• Don't cut patch in any way.
• Don't apply more than one patch at a time.
• After patch removal, wash application site thoroughly.
• Fold patch in half after removal to avoid accidental contact with drug; then discard.

ACTION
Inhibits muscarinic actions of acetylcholine on autonomic effectors innervated by postganglionic cholinergic neurons. May affect neural pathways originating in the inner ear to inhibit nausea and vomiting.

Route	Onset	Peak	Duration
Transdermal	4 hr	24 hr	72 hr

Half-life: 9.5 hours.

ADVERSE REACTIONS

CNS: dizziness, drowsiness, agitation, confusion. **EENT:** dilated pupils, visual impairment, dry mouth, pharyngitis. **Skin:** contact dermatitis.

INTERACTIONS

Drug-drug. *Amantadine, antihistamines, antiparkinsonian drugs, disopyramide, hypnotics (zolpidem), anxiolytics (alprazolam), opioids (meperidine), muscle relaxants, phenothiazines, procainamide, quinidine, TCAs:* May increase risk of adverse CNS reactions. Avoid using together. If use can't be avoided, monitor patient closely.

Anticholinergics (benztropine, cyclopentolate, darifenacin): May increase risk of intestinal obstruction, urine retention, or other CNS adverse reactions. Monitor patient closely.

Glucagon: May enhance adverse effects of glucagon, especially GI effects. Use together cautiously.

Glycopyrrolate (oral inhalation): May enhance adverse and anticholinergic effects. Avoid concurrent use.

Drug-lifestyle. *Alcohol use:* May increase risk of CNS depression. Discourage use together.

EFFECTS ON LAB TEST RESULTS

• May interfere with gastric secretion test.

CONTRAINDICATIONS & CAUTIONS

• Contraindicated in patients hypersensitive to scopolamine, other belladonna alkaloids, or components in the formulation or delivery system and in patients with angle-closure glaucoma.

• Use cautiously in patients with open-angle glaucoma, history of seizures, risk factors for seizures or psychosis, pyloric obstruction, urinary bladder neck obstruction, impaired kidney or liver function, and patients suspected of having intestinal obstruction.

• Use cautiously in patients taking oral medications; absorption of oral medications may be decreased due to decreased gastric motility and delayed gastric emptying.

• Drug isn't recommended for use in children because a safe and effective dose hasn't been established and children are particularly susceptible to the adverse effects of drug.

• Use cautiously in older adults because of the increased likelihood of CNS effects, such as hallucinations, confusion, and dizziness.

• Use cautiously in patients in hot or humid environments; drug can increase risk of heatstroke.

Dialyzable drug: Unknown.

⚠ **Overdose S&S:** Lethargy, somnolence, coma, confusion, agitation, hallucinations, leukocytosis, seizures, visual disturbances, dry flushed skin, dry mouth, decreased bowel sounds, urine retention, tachycardia, HTN, supraventricular arrhythmias, circulatory or respiratory collapse, death.

PREGNANCY-LACTATION-REPRODUCTION

• Use during pregnancy only if potential benefit justifies risk to mother and fetus.

• Eclamptic seizures have been reported during pregnancy, with severe preeclampsia soon after injection of IV and IM scopolamine. Avoid use of transdermal scopolamine in patients with severe preeclampsia.

• Drug appears in human milk. Use cautiously during breastfeeding.

NURSING CONSIDERATIONS

• Monitor patient because some patients become temporarily excited or disoriented and some develop amnesia or become drowsy. Reorient patient as needed.

• Monitor patient for new or worsening psychiatric signs or symptoms (acute psychosis, agitation, speech disorder, hallucinations, paranoia, delusion).

• Monitor patient for decreased GI motility and urine retention.

• Stop drug if patient experiences signs and symptoms of angle-closure glaucoma or has difficulty urinating.

• Monitor patient for withdrawal signs and symptoms (dizziness, nausea, vomiting, abdominal cramps, diaphoresis, headache, confusion, weakness, bradycardia, hypotension) when drug is discontinued after several days of use. Withdrawal signs and symptoms usually present 24 hours or more after patch removal.

• Tolerance may develop with prolonged therapy.

• Atropine-like toxicity may cause dose-related adverse reactions. Individual tolerance varies greatly.

🔵 *Alert:* Overdose may cause curare-like effects such as respiratory paralysis. Keep emergency equipment available.

• Remove patch before MRI to prevent skin burns.

PATIENT TEACHING
• Instruct patient in safe drug administration, including to wash and dry hands thoroughly before and after applying transdermal patch and before touching the eye to avoid temporary pupil dilation and blurred vision.
• Advise patient that the transdermal method releases a controlled therapeutic amount of drug. Transderm Scop is effective if applied at least 4 hours before experiencing motion.
• Remind patient to remove one patch before applying another and to not apply more than one patch at a time.
• Alert patient to possible withdrawal signs and symptoms with use beyond 72 hours.
• Advise patient that eyes may be more sensitive to light while wearing patch. Advise patient to wear sunglasses for comfort.
• Warn patient to avoid activities that require alertness until CNS effects of drug are known.
• Instruct patient to read brochure that comes with transdermal product.
• Instruct patient requiring an MRI to inform facility about transdermal patch use.
• Urge patient to report urinary hesitancy or urine retention.
• Caution patient to report pregnancy or breastfeeding to prescriber.

---

selegiline
se-LE-ji-leen

Emsam

selegiline hydrochloride
(L-deprenyl hydrochloride)
Zelapar

Therapeutic class: Antiparkinsonian drugs
Pharmacologic class: MAO inhibitors

AVAILABLE FORMS
selegiline
Transdermal system: 6 mg/24 hours, 9 mg/24 hours, 12 mg/24 hours
selegiline hydrochloride
Capsules: 5 mg
Tablets: 5 mg
Tablets (ODTs): 1.25 mg

INDICATIONS & DOSAGES
➤ **Adjunctive treatment with levodopa–carbidopa in managing signs and symptoms of Parkinson disease**

Adults: For capsules and tablets, 10 mg PO daily divided as 5 mg at breakfast and 5 mg at lunch. After 2 or 3 days, may gradually decrease levodopa–carbidopa dosage. Or, if using ODTs, start with 1.25 mg PO once daily. Increase to 2.5 mg daily after at least 6 weeks, if tolerated and needed. Maximum dose is 10 mg/day for tablets and capsules and 2.5 mg once daily for ODTs.
Adjust-a-dose: For adults with Child Pugh class A or B liver impairment, reduce the ODT dose to 1.25 mg once daily depending on clinical response and tolerability.
➤ **Major depressive disorder (Emsam)**
Adults: Apply one patch daily. Initially, use 6 mg/day. Increase, if needed, in increments of 3 mg/day at intervals of 2 or more weeks. Maximum daily dose, 12 mg.
Adults ages 65 and older: 6 mg transdermal patch daily.

ADMINISTRATION
PO
• Don't give food or liquids for 5 minutes before and after giving ODTs.
• Don't push ODTs through foil backing; peel backing off and gently remove tablet.
• Place tablet on top of tongue.
Transdermal
• Apply patch to dry, intact skin on the upper torso, upper thigh, or outer surface of the upper arm once every 24 hours.
• Apply at the same time each day and rotate application sites.
• Don't cut transdermal patch into smaller pieces.
• Don't apply heat to patch; it may increase drug level.

ACTION
May inhibit MAO type B (mainly found in the brain) and dopamine metabolism. At higher-than-recommended doses, drug nonselectively inhibits MAO, including MAO type A (mainly found in the intestine). May also directly increase dopaminergic activity by decreasing reuptake of dopamine into nerve cells.

Route	Onset	Peak	Duration
PO (tablet, capsule)	Unknown	40–90 min	Unknown
PO (ODT)	5 min	10–15 min	Unknown
Transdermal	Unknown	Unknown	24 hr

Half-life: Selegiline, 2 to 10 hours; N-desmethyl deprenyl, 2 hours; L-amphetamine, 17.75 hours; L-methamphetamine, 20.5 hours.

Reactions in bold italics are *life-threatening*.

ADVERSE REACTIONS
Oral form

CNS: anxiety, dizziness, loss of balance, depression, increased bradykinesia, dyskinesia, headache, confusion, hallucinations, vivid dreams, insomnia, lethargy, somnolence, tremor, ataxia, pain. **CV:** HTN, palpitations, chest pain. **EENT:** dysphagia, pharyngitis, rhinitis, dry mouth, tooth disorder. **GI:** constipation, nausea, abdominal pain, diarrhea, stomatitis, dyspepsia, vomiting, flatulence. **GU:** urine retention. **Metabolic:** weight loss, *hypokalemia.* **Musculoskeletal:** aches, leg cramps, myalgia, back pain. **Respiratory:** dyspnea. **Skin:** rash, ecchymosis, skin disorders.

Transdermal form

CNS: headache, insomnia. **CV:** orthostatic hypotension. **EENT:** sinusitis, dry mouth, pharyngitis. **GI:** diarrhea, dyspepsia. **GU:** abnormal ejaculation. **Metabolic:** weight gain or loss. **Skin:** application-site reaction, rash.

INTERACTIONS
Drug-drug. *Bupropion, cyclobenzaprine, mirtazapine, MAO inhibitors, sympathomimetic amines (including amphetamines, cold products, and weight-loss preparations containing vasoconstrictors):* May cause hypertensive crisis. Separate use by at least 14 days.
Dextromethorphan: May increase risk of psychosis or bizarre behavior. Use together is contraindicated.
Linezolid, methylene blue: May cause serotonin syndrome. Don't administer within 14 days of each other.
Opioids (meperidine, methadone, tramadol): May increase risk of serotonin syndrome. Separate use by at least 14 days.
SSRIs (citalopram, fluoxetine, fluvoxamine), SNRIs (duloxetine, venlafaxine), TCAs (amitriptyline, doxepin), MAO-B inhibitors (olanzapine, rasagiline): May cause serotonin syndrome. Separate use by at least 2 weeks (5 weeks if switching to or from fluoxetine).
Drug-herb. *St. John's wort:* May cause increased serotonergic effects. Warn against using together.
Drug-food. ⚡ *Alert:* Foods high in tyramine (aged cheese or meats, fava beans, herring, sauerkraut, unpasteurized beer): May cause hypertensive crisis, especially at increased doses. Provide patient with a list of foods to avoid beginning on first day of transdermal

daily dose of 9 mg or 12 mg and for 2 weeks after dosage reduction to 6 mg daily, or after discontinuation of 9- or 12-mg daily dose.
Drug-lifestyle. *Alcohol use:* May increase risk of adverse effects. Discourage use together.

EFFECTS ON LAB TEST RESULTS
• May cause positive result for amphetamine on urine drug screen.

CONTRAINDICATIONS & CAUTIONS
• Contraindicated in patients hypersensitive to drug, and in patients with pheochromocytoma (transdermal patch).

Boxed Warning Transdermal patch is contraindicated in patients younger than age 12 because of risk of hypertensive crisis. ■

⚡ *Alert:* Concomitant use with linezolid or methylene blue can cause serotonin syndrome (fever, mental status changes, muscle twitching, diaphoresis, shivering or shaking, diarrhea, loss of coordination). Use drug with linezolid or methylene blue only for life-threatening or urgent conditions when benefits outweigh risks of toxicity.

• Don't use oral drug with transdermal system.

• ODTs aren't recommended in patients with Child-Pugh class C liver impairment or CrCl less than 30 mL/minute.

• ODT contains phenylalanine; use with caution in patients with phenylketonuria.

• Orthostatic hypotension may occur during first 2 months of therapy or after dosage increases, especially in older adults.

• Somnolence and falling asleep without warning while engaged in ADLs (including operating motor vehicles) have been reported in some patients. Evaluate patients for factors that may increase these risks, such as older adults with sleep disorders and patients taking sedatives.

• Avoid use in patients with major psychotic disorders. Drug may cause changes in or worsening of mental status, abnormal thinking, and behavioral changes, which may be severe and include paranoid ideation, delusions, hallucinations, confusion, psychotic-like behavior, disorientation, aggressive behavior, agitation, and delirium. Drug isn't approved for bipolar depression.

• Reevaluate patients receiving transdermal patch for extended periods for continued effectiveness.

S

🍁Canada   ◇OTC   ◆Off-label use   ⊕Do not crush   *Liquid contains alcohol   ⬚Genetic

• Hypertensive reactions have been reported in patients who ingested tyramine-containing foods while receiving oral selegiline.

Dialyzable drug: Unknown.

⚠ *Overdose S&S:* Drowsiness, dizziness, faintness, irritability, hyperactivity, agitation, severe headache, hallucinations, trismus, opisthotonos, seizures, coma, rapid and irregular pulse, HTN, hypotension and vascular collapse, precordial pain, respiratory depression and failure, hyperpyrexia, diaphoresis, cool and clammy skin.

PREGNANCY-LACTATION-REPRODUCTION
• There are no adequate studies during pregnancy. Use only if potential benefit justifies fetal risk.
• It isn't known if drug appears in human milk. Because of risk of serious adverse reactions, including hypertensive reactions, patient shouldn't breastfeed during and for 7 days after final oral dose or 5 days after final patch dose.

NURSING CONSIDERATIONS
⚙ **Alert:** Some patients experience new or increased adverse reactions to levodopa, such as dyskinesia, when used with selegiline. Reduce dosage of levodopa–carbidopa by 10% to 30%.

Boxed Warning Transdermal system used to treat depression may increase risk of suicidality in children, adolescents, and young adults ages 18 to 24, especially during first few months of treatment, especially in those with major depressive or other psychiatric disorder. ■

⚙ **Alert:** If linezolid or methylene blue must be given, stop selegiline and monitor patient for serotonin toxicity for 2 weeks, or until 24 hours after last dose of methylene blue or linezolid, whichever comes first. May resume selegiline 24 hours after last dose of methylene blue or linezolid.
• Monitor patients with major depressive disorder for worsening of symptoms and of suicidality, especially during the first few weeks of treatment and during dosage changes.

⚙ **Alert:** Monitor patient carefully for orthostatic hypotension, especially during first 2 months of treatment and after dosage increases. Help patient rise from a reclining position.
• Monitor patient for new-onset HTN or HTN that isn't adequately controlled after starting drug.

• Monitor patient taking antidepressants and selegiline concomitantly for serotonin syndrome (restlessness, hallucinations, loss of coordination, seizures, tachycardia, rapid BP changes, increased body temperature, hyperreflexia, nausea, vomiting, diarrhea). Discontinue serotonergic drugs immediately if signs and symptoms occur.
• Monitor patient for drowsiness, significant daytime sleepiness, or episodes of falling asleep during activities that require active participation. Discontinue drug if present.
• Monitor patient for psychotic-like behavior, changes in mental status, abnormal thinking, and behavioral changes.
• Ask patient about development or worsening of impulsive or compulsive behaviors (new or increased gambling urges, sexual urges, binge eating, uncontrolled spending, or other urges) because patient may not recognize these behaviors as abnormal.
• Examine patient's skin periodically for possible melanoma, because of risk of skin cancer associated with drug and with Parkinson disease.
• Examine patient's mouth for irritation or ulceration; be aware of patient complaints of swallowing or mouth pain when taking ODTs.

PATIENT TEACHING
• Instruct patient in safe drug administration.
⚙ **Alert:** Teach patient to recognize and immediately report signs and symptoms of serotonin toxicity. Patients taking certain antidepressants are at increased risk.
• Advise patient not to take drug in evening because doing so may cause insomnia.
⚙ **Alert:** Warn patient about the many drugs, including OTC drugs, that may interact with this drug and about the need to consult a pharmacist or prescriber before using them.
• Explain risk of hypertensive crisis if patient ingests foods or beverages containing tyramine during therapy; if using a 9-mg/day or higher transdermal system, patient should avoid these products altogether. Give patient a list of tyramine-containing foods and products.
• Teach patient and family signs and symptoms of hypertensive crisis: severe headache, sore or stiff neck, nausea, vomiting, diaphoresis, rapid heartbeat, dilated pupils, and photophobia.
• Instruct patient not to rise rapidly after sitting or lying down because of risk of dizziness, which may occur more frequently early in therapy or after dosage increases.

Reactions in bold italics are *life-threatening*.

• Explain that drug may cause patient to fall asleep during activities that require active participation. Advise patient to contact prescriber if drowsiness, significant daytime sleepiness, or episodes of falling asleep during such activities occur.

• Tell patient to report paranoid ideation, delusions, hallucinations, confusion, psychotic-like behavior, disorientation, aggressive behavior, agitation, or delirium.

• Advise patient to contact prescriber if having trouble controlling impulsive or compulsive behaviors (new or increased gambling urges, sexual urges, binge eating, uncontrolled spending, or other urges).

• Urge patient to watch for skin changes that could suggest melanoma and to have periodic skin exams by a provider.

• Advise patient taking ODTs to report mouth pain, pain when swallowing, or ulcerations.

• Caution patient to contact prescriber before discontinuing selegiline.

• Tell patient that each ODT contains 1.25 mg phenylalanine.

Boxed Warning Advise family members of patient using transdermal system to watch for and immediately report new or worsening suicidality. ■

• Tell patient to avoid exposing transdermal system to direct external heat sources, such as heating pads, electric blankets, hot tubs, heated water beds, and prolonged sunlight.

• Inform patient that MAO inhibitors may need to be stopped 10 days before surgery requiring general anesthesia and to discuss MAO inhibitor use with surgeon.

• Advise patient planning pregnancy or breastfeeding to first contact prescriber.

---

semaglutide
sem-a-GLOO-tide

Ozempic, Rybelsus, Wegovy

Therapeutic class: Antidiabetics
Pharmacologic class: Human glucagon-like peptide-1 receptor agonists

AVAILABLE FORMS
Injection: prefilled pen injectors delivering 0.25 mg, 0.5 mg, 1 mg, 1.7 mg, 2 mg, 2.4 mg per injection
Tablets <small>ONC</small>: 3 mg, 7 mg, 14 mg

INDICATIONS & DOSAGES
➤ **Adjunct to diet and exercise to improve glycemic control in patients with type 2 diabetes; to reduce risk of major adverse CV events (CV death, nonfatal MI or nonfatal stroke) in patients with type 2 diabetes and established CV disease (Ozempic only)**
Adults: Initially, 0.25 mg subcut once weekly for 4 weeks; then increase to 0.5 mg once weekly. After 4 weeks, if needed, may increase to 1 mg once weekly. After 4 weeks, if needed, increase to 2 mg once weekly. Maximum dose, 2 mg once weekly.

Or, initially, 3 mg PO once daily for 30 days. After 30 days, increase to 7 mg PO once daily. After 30 days, if needed, may increase to 14 mg PO once daily.

➤ **Adjunct to diet and exercise for long-term weight management in adults with initial BMI of at least 30 kg/m^2, or at least 27 kg/m^2 and at least one weight-related comorbid condition (HTN, type 2 diabetes, or dyslipidemia), or in children with an initial BMI at the 95th percentile or greater for age and sex assigned at birth (Wegovy only)**
Adults and children ages 12 and older: Initially, 0.25 mg subcut once weekly for 4 weeks, then increase to 0.5 mg for 4 weeks, then 1 mg for 4 weeks, then 1.7 mg for 4 weeks, then to 2.4 mg weekly maintenance dose.

Adjust-a-dose: If any dose isn't initially tolerated, delay dose escalation for 4 weeks. If 2.4-mg dose isn't tolerated, temporarily decrease to 1.7 mg for 4 weeks, then reescalate. If 2.4 mg isn't tolerated after reescalation, discontinue drug.

ADMINISTRATION
PO
• Patient should take on an empty stomach at least 30 minutes before first food, beverage, or other oral medications of the day with no more than 4 oz (120 mL) of water only.

• Have patient swallow tablets whole; don't crush or cut them.

• Use 3-mg dose for initiating treatment. It isn't effective for glycemic control.

• Giving two 7-mg tablets to achieve a 14-mg dose isn't recommended.

• If a dose is missed, skip missed dose and give next dose the following day.

• Patients on 0.5 mg weekly of subcut form can be transitioned to oral form 7 mg or 14 mg. Patients can start oral semaglutide up to

S

7 days after the last subcut injection. There is no equivalent oral dose for 1 mg subcut semaglutide.

• Patients taking 14 mg PO daily can be transitioned to subcut form at a dose of 0.5 mg once weekly. Patients can start the subcut injection the day after last oral dose.

Subcutaneous

• Semaglutide solution appears clear and colorless. Don't use if particulate matter or coloration is seen.

• Use 0.25-mg dose for initiating treatment only. It isn't effective for glycemic control.

• Give drug once weekly on same day each week at any time of day, without regard to meals.

• Administer subcut in abdomen, thigh, or upper arm. Rotate injection sites.

• Administer insulin as a separate injection; never mix the products. May inject semaglutide and insulin in same body region but not in sites adjacent to one another.

• May change the day of weekly administration if time between doses is at least 48 hours.

• Give a missed Ozempic dose as soon as possible within 5 days after missed dose. If more than 5 days have passed, skip missed dose and give next dose on the regularly scheduled day.

• Give a missed Wegovy dose as soon as possible if more than 48 hours before next scheduled dose. Omit missed dose if less than 48 hours until next scheduled dose.

🔆 *Alert:* Device is for single patient use. Never share this device with others, even if the needle has been changed, since it could transmit blood-borne pathogens.

• Store pen capped without a needle attached. Use a new needle for each use. After each use, remove and safely discard needle.

• Before first use, refrigerate Ozempic and Wegovy pens between 36° and 46° F (2° and 8° C). Don't store in freezer or directly adjacent to the refrigerator cooling element.

• After first use, store Ozempic pen for up to 56 days at room temperature (59° to 86° F [15° to 30° C]) or refrigerated (36° to 46° F [2° to 8° C]); don't freeze. Protect from excessive heat and sunlight.

• May keep Wegovy pen at 46° to 86° F (8° to 30° C) for up to 28 days before cap removal, if needed.

ACTION

Stimulates release of insulin and lowers glucagon secretion in presence of elevated glucose levels. Also causes a minor delay in gastric emptying in the early postprandial phase.

Route	Onset	Peak	Duration
PO	Unknown	1 hr	Unknown
Subcut	Unknown	1–3 days	Unknown

Half-life: About 1 week.

ADVERSE REACTIONS

CNS: headache, fatigue, dizziness. **CV:** increased HR, hypotension. **EENT:** diabetic retinopathy complications. **GI:** nausea, vomiting, diarrhea, abdominal pain, constipation, dyspepsia, belching, flatulence, GERD, gastritis, gastroenteritis, cholelithiasis, decreased appetite (PO), abdominal distension. **Hematologic:** *hypoglycemia.* **Metabolic:** increased amylase level, increased lipase level. **Skin:** hair loss, injection-site reaction. **Other:** immunogenicity.

INTERACTIONS

Drug-drug. *Insulin, insulin secretagogues (glipizide, repaglinide):* May increase risk of hypoglycemia. A reduced insulin or insulin secretagogue dosage may be required.
Oral medications: May change therapeutic effect of oral drugs because semaglutide delays gastric emptying. Monitor patient closely.
Other weight loss drugs: Safety and effectiveness of coadministration are unknown. Use together isn't recommended.
Drug-herb. *Herbal products for weight loss:* Safety and effectiveness of coadministration are unknown. Discourage use together.

EFFECTS ON LAB TEST RESULTS

• May increase amylase and lipase levels.

CONTRAINDICATIONS & CAUTIONS

• Contraindicated in patients hypersensitive to drug or its components.

• Drug isn't indicated for type 1 diabetes or the treatment of diabetic ketoacidosis, or as a substitute for insulin.

Boxed Warning Semaglutide caused thyroid adenomas and carcinomas after lifetime exposure in rodents. It isn't known whether drug causes thyroid C-cell tumors, including medullary thyroid carcinoma (MTC). ■

Boxed Warning Contraindicated in patients with a personal or family history of MTC and in patients with multiple endocrine neoplasia syndrome type 2 (MEN 2). ■

• Use cautiously in patients with a history of diabetic retinopathy. Rapid improvement in glucose control has been associated with temporary worsening of diabetic retinopathy. The effect of long-term improved glucose control using this drug and diabetic retinopathy hasn't been studied.

• Use cautiously in patients with a history of CKD; worsening of kidney function has been reported, particularly in patients who experienced nausea, vomiting, and diarrhea.

• Cases of pancreatitis have occurred. For suspected pancreatitis, discontinue drug and treat appropriately. For confirmed pancreatitis, don't restart drug.

• Use in patients with a history of pancreatitis hasn't been studied. Consider use of other antidiabetics.

• Avoid Wegovy in patients with a history of suicide attempts or active suicidality. Suicidality has been reported with other weight management products.

• Safety and effectiveness in children haven't been determined.

Dialyzable drug: Unknown.

PREGNANCY-LACTATION-REPRODUCTION

• Based on animal studies, drug may adversely affect fetus. Poorly controlled diabetes, especially in patients who are pregnant, carries many risks. Use of glucagon-like peptide-1 receptor agonists isn't recommended for patients with type 2 diabetes planning pregnancy.

• Appropriate weight gain during pregnancy, even in patients who are overweight or obese, is recommended.

• Patients planning pregnancy should discontinue drug at least 2 months before conception.

• Register patients exposed to Wegovy during pregnancy at 1-800-727-6500.

• Drug is likely to appear in human milk based on animal studies. Breastfeeding isn't recommended during treatment with oral semaglutide. Consider mother's clinical need and risks to infant during treatment with subcut semaglutide.

NURSING CONSIDERATIONS

Boxed Warning Monitor patients for MTC or MEN 2. It isn't known if routine monitoring of serum calcitonin level or thyroid ultrasound can detect these cancers early. Further evaluate patients with elevated serum calcitonin level or thyroid nodules on physical exam or neck imaging. ■

🜲 *Alert:* Monitor patients for hypersensitivity reactions, including anaphylaxis and angioedema. Discontinue drug and treat appropriately if reaction occurs. Use cautiously in patients with a history of hypersensitivity to another glucagon-like peptide-1 agonist.

• Monitor patients for pancreatitis (persistent severe abdominal pain that may radiate to the back or be accompanied by vomiting). For suspected pancreatitis, discontinue drug.

• Monitor patients for acute gallbladder disease. Rapid or substantial weight loss can increase the risk.

• Monitor patients with a history of diabetic retinopathy for disease progression.

• Monitor patients for AKI. Assess kidney function at baseline and during dosage adjustments. Assess for nausea, vomiting, diarrhea, or dehydration, which are associated with worsening of kidney function.

• Monitor glucose level and HbA$_{1c}$.

• Monitor glucose level before and periodically during treatment for weight loss in patients with type 2 diabetes.

• Monitor patients for signs and symptoms of hypoglycemia (confusion, irritability, shakiness, diaphoresis, hunger, palpitations, pallor, speech and motor dysfunction).

• Monitor HR periodically; drug may need to be discontinued for sustained increase in resting HR.

• Monitor patients taking drug for weight management for new or worsening depression, suicidality, or unusual changes in mood or behavior.

• *Look alike–sound alike:* Don't confuse semaglutide with sitagliptin.

PATIENT TEACHING

• Instruct patient to report all adverse reactions.

• Teach patient proper drug administration, storage, and disposal of pens, if applicable.

• Tell patient how to manage missed doses.

🜲 *Alert:* Caution patient never to share injection pen with another person, even if the needle is changed, due to risk of bloodborne pathogen transmission.

Boxed Warning Counsel patient on risk of MTC and MEN 2 and to report signs and symptoms of thyroid tumors (neck mass, dysphagia, dyspnea, persistent hoarseness). ■

• Caution patient to discontinue drug and seek immediate medical attention for

hypersensitivity reactions (difficulty breathing, throat or tongue swelling).
- Advise patient taking Wegovy to report new or worsening depression, suicidality, and other unusual changes in mood or behavior and to discontinue drug.
- Instruct patient taking Wegovy to report palpitations or racing heartbeat at rest.
- Caution patient to immediately report signs and symptoms of pancreatitis and to discontinue drug.
- Instruct patient to report vision changes.
- Inform patient of the risk of kidney injury. Risk increases with risk of dehydration due to GI adverse effects. Instruct patient to take precautions to avoid fluid depletion and to report nausea, vomiting, diarrhea, or dehydration to prescriber. Advise patient that worsening kidney impairment may require dialysis.
- Caution patient about the use of drug during pregnancy and while breastfeeding. Advise patient not to breastfeed while taking oral semaglutide. Encourage patient to discuss drug with prescriber before a planned pregnancy.
- Stress importance of adhering to proper diet and regular physical activity and that glucose and HbA_{1c} levels and other lab tests will be monitored during therapy.
- Teach patient to recognize and manage hypoglycemia. Caution patient who is also taking insulin or insulin secretagogues about the increased risk of hypoglycemia.
- Advise patient to immediately report stresses to the body (fever, surgery, trauma, infection) because drug requirements may change.
- Tell patient that nausea, vomiting, and diarrhea are common at start of therapy but decrease over time for most patients.

---

serdexmethylphenidate–dexmethylphenidate

ser-dex-meth-il-FEN-i-date/
dex-meth-il-FEN-i-date

Azstarys

Therapeutic class: CNS stimulants
Pharmacologic class: Norepinephrine and dopamine reuptake inhibitors
Controlled substance schedule: II

AVAILABLE FORMS
Capsules: serdexmethylphenidate/dexmethylphenidate: 26.1 mg/5.2 mg, 39.2 mg/7.8 mg, 52.3 mg/10.4 mg

INDICATIONS & DOSAGES
➤ **ADHD**
Adults and children age 13 and older: Initially, serdexmethylphenidate 39.2 mg/dexmethylphenidate 7.8 mg PO once daily in the morning. May increase after 1 week to maximum dosage of serdexmethylphenidate 52.3 mg/dexmethylphenidate 10.4 mg PO daily.
Children ages 6 to 12: Initially, serdexmethylphenidate 39.2 mg/dexmethylphenidate 7.8 mg PO once daily in the morning. May increase dosage after 1 week, serdexmethylphenidate 52.3 mg/dexmethylphenidate 10.4 mg PO once daily, or decrease dosage, serdexmethylphenidate 26.1 mg/dexmethylphenidate 5.2 mg PO daily, depending on response and tolerability. Maximum dosage, serdexmethylphenidate 52.3 mg/dexmethylphenidate 10.4 mg PO daily.
Adjust-a-dose: Reduce dosage or discontinue drug if paradoxical aggravation of ADHD symptoms or other adverse reactions occur. Periodically discontinue drug to assess child's condition. If no improvement after dosage adjustment over 1 month, discontinue drug.

ADMINISTRATION
PO
- Give without regard to meals.
- Have patient swallow capsule whole or mix capsule contents in 50 mL water or 2 tablespoons applesauce. Give entire mixture within 10 minutes. Don't store.
- If switching from another methylphenidate drug, discontinue that drug and initiate this drug using the dosage schedule above.
- Store at room temperature.

ACTION
Exact mechanism unknown.

Route	Onset	Peak	Duration
PO	Unknown	2–4.5 hr	Unknown

Half-life: Serdexmethylphenidate, 5.7 hours; dexmethylphenidate, 11.7 hours.

ADVERSE REACTIONS
CNS: anxiety, dizziness, dyskinesia, emotional lability, fever, insomnia, irritability.
CV: increased BP, palpitations, tachycardia.

GI: abdominal pain, anorexia, dyspepsia, nausea, vomiting. **Metabolic:** weight loss. **Musculoskeletal:** growth suppression. **Other:** hypersensitivity reactions.

INTERACTIONS

Drug-drug. *Antihypertensives (ACE inhibitors, ARBs, beta blockers, calcium channel blockers, centrally acting alpha-2 receptor agonists, potassium-sparing and thiazide diuretics):* May decrease effectiveness of antihypertensives. Monitor BP and adjust antihypertensive dosage as needed.

MAO inhibitors (isocarboxazid, linezolid, methylene blue, phenelzine, selegiline, tranylcypromine): May cause hypertensive crisis. Avoid use together or within 14 days of discontinuing MAO inhibitor.

Halogenated anesthetics (desflurane, enflurane, halothane, isoflurane, sevoflurane): May increase risk of sudden HTN and tachycardia during surgery. Avoid use on day of surgery.

Risperidone: May increase risk of extrapyramidal reaction with drug dosage changes. Monitor patient for extrapyramidal reaction.

Serotonergic drugs (opioids, SNRIs, SSRIs, TCAs): May increase risk of serotonin syndrome. Use together cautiously.

EFFECTS ON LAB TEST RESULTS

- May increase ALP, bilirubin, and liver enzyme levels.
- May decrease platelet count.
- May increase or decrease WBC count.

CONTRAINDICATIONS & CAUTIONS

Boxed Warning Stimulants carry a high risk of abuse and misuse, which can lead to substance use disorder, including addiction, which can lead to overdose and death. The risk increases with high doses or unapproved administration methods, such as snorting or injection. ■

- Drug may cause tolerance, requiring a higher dose to produce the same effect a lower dose once provided.
- Contraindicated in patients hypersensitive to serdexmethylphenidate, methylphenidate, or its components.
- Avoid use in patients with structural cardiac abnormalities, cardiomyopathy, heart rhythm abnormalities, CAD, or other serious heart problems. Sudden death, stroke, and MI have been reported with CNS stimulants.

- Drug may cause peripheral vasculopathy, including Raynaud phenomenon. May need to reduce dosage or discontinue drug.
- Drug may exacerbate signs and symptoms of behavior disturbance and thought disorder in patients with a preexisting psychotic disorder. Use cautiously.
- Drug may induce manic or mixed mood episode in patients with bipolar disorder. Use cautiously.
- Drug may cause psychotic or manic signs or symptoms in patients with no history of psychotic disorder. If signs or symptoms occur, consider discontinuing drug.
- Drug may increase risk of prolonged and painful erection (priapism), sometimes requiring surgical intervention.
- Drug may cause weight loss and slowed growth rates in children. Interrupt or discontinue therapy if these occur.
- Don't substitute drug for other methylphenidate products.
- Long-term efficacy of methylphenidate use in children hasn't been established.
- Safety and effectiveness in children younger than age 6 haven't been established.
- Drug hasn't been studied in patients age 65 and older.

Dialyzable drug: Unknown.

⚠ **Overdose S&S:** Nausea, vomiting, diarrhea, restlessness, anxiety, agitation, tremors, hyperreflexia, muscle twitching, seizures (may be followed by coma), stroke, life-threatening hyperthermia, euphoria, psychomotor agitation, confusion, hallucinations, delirium, sweating, flushing, headache, tachyarrhythmias, palpitations, cardiac arrhythmias, HTN or hypotension, vasospasm, MI, aortic dissection, cardiomyopathy, tachypnea, mydriasis, dryness of mucous membranes, serotonin syndrome, rhabdomyolysis, death.

PREGNANCY-LACTATION-REPRODUCTION

- There are no adequate studies of use during pregnancy. It isn't known if drug increases risk of major birth defects, miscarriage, or adverse maternal or fetal outcomes.
- Use of CNS stimulants during pregnancy can cause vasoconstriction and decreased placental perfusion. Premature delivery and low birth weight have been reported in amphetamine-dependent patients.
- Enroll patients exposed to drug during pregnancy in the National Pregnancy Registry for Psychostimulants (1-866-961-2388).

• Unknown if drug appears in human milk, or how drug affects milk production. Before use during breastfeeding, consider benefits of therapy and risks to infant, and monitor breastfed infant for adverse effects.

NURSING CONSIDERATIONS

Boxed Warning Assess patient's risk of abuse, misuse, and addiction before therapy. Reassess risk during therapy. Monitor for signs and symptoms of drug abuse, misuse, and addiction (increased HR, respiratory rate, or BP; sweating; dilated pupils; hyperactivity; restlessness; insomnia; decreased appetite; loss of coordination; tremors; flushing; vomiting; abdominal pain). Anxiety, psychosis, hostility, aggression, suicidality, and homicidal ideation may also occur. ■

• Abrupt drug stoppage or dose reduction may cause withdrawal symptoms (dysphoria, depression, fatigue, vivid and unpleasant dreams, insomnia or hypersomnia, increased appetite, psychomotor retardation or agitation) in patient with physical dependence.

• Assess patient for cardiac abnormalities (family history of sudden death, ventricular arrythmia, cardiomyopathy).

• Screen patient for history of depressive symptoms, depression, bipolar disorder, and family history of suicide.

• Monitor patient for tolerance to drug.

• Monitor patient for HTN and tachycardia.

• Monitor patient for exertional chest pain, unexplained syncope, or arrhythmias.

• Carefully observe patient for digital changes and signs and symptoms of peripheral vasculopathy, including Raynaud phenomenon. Refer patient to rheumatologist if indicated.

• Monitor height and weight in children.

PATIENT TEACHING

Boxed Warning Teach patient and caregiver about risk of abuse, misuse, and addiction, which can lead to overdose and death. Advise patient to store drug in a safe (preferably locked) place. Teach about proper disposal of unused drug. Instruct patient not to give drug to anyone else. ■

• Advise patient and caregiver to read the medication guide.

• Instruct patient on proper drug administration and storage.

• Caution patient and caregiver to dispose of remaining, unused, or expired drug in accordance with local requirements or drug take-back programs.

• Advise patient and caregiver about serious CV risks (sudden death, MI, stroke) and to immediately report exertional chest pain or unexplained syncope.

• Inform patient about risk of increased HR and BP and need for frequent monitoring during therapy.

• Tell patient about risk of peripheral vasculopathy, including Raynaud phenomenon, and to report new numbness, pain, skin color change, sensitivity to temperature in fingers or toes, or unexplained wounds on fingers or toes.

• Inform patient and caregiver that at recommended doses, drug can cause psychotic or manic symptoms, even in patients with no history of psychotic disorders or mania. Tell patient to report new or worsening symptoms, such as mania, hearing voices, or seeing or believing things that aren't real.

• Inform male patient and caregiver of risk of priapism and to seek immediate medical attention if this occurs.

• Advise child and caregiver of risk of weight loss and slow growth rate.

• Instruct patient of childbearing potential to report pregnancy or plans to become pregnant during therapy.

• Tell patient who is breastfeeding to monitor infant for agitation, poor feeding, and reduced weight gain.

• Inform patient and caregiver that therapy may be stopped periodically to assess ADHD symptoms.

sertraline hydrochloride
SIR-trah-leen

Zoloft

Therapeutic class: Antidepressants
Pharmacologic class: SSRIs

AVAILABLE FORMS
Capsules ⓄⓃⒸ: 150 mg, 200 mg
Oral concentrate: 20 mg/mL *
Tablets: 25 mg, 50 mg, 100 mg

INDICATIONS & DOSAGES
Adjust-a-dose (for all indications): If dosage changes are needed, increase by 25 to 50 mg (except when used for premenstrual dysmorphic disorder) at intervals of no less than

1 week. For patients with Child-Pugh class A liver impairment, both recommended starting dosage and therapeutic range are half recommended daily dosage.

➤ **MDD**

Adults: 50 mg PO daily. Adjust dosage weekly as needed and tolerated; dosage ranges from 50 to 200 mg daily. May switch to capsule form when dosage is 150 or 200 mg daily.

➤ **OCD**

Adults and adolescents ages 13 to 17: 50 mg PO once daily. If patient doesn't improve, increase dosage weekly, up to 200 mg daily. May switch to capsule form when dosage is 150 or 200 mg daily.

Children ages 6 to 12: Initially, 25 mg PO daily. Increase dosage weekly, as needed, up to 200 mg daily. May switch to capsule form when dosage is 150 or 200 mg daily.

➤ **Panic disorder, PTSD, social anxiety disorder**

Adults: Initially, 25 mg PO daily for 1 week; increase by 25 or 50 mg PO daily once a week to achieve an adequate response. Maximum, 200 mg daily, as tolerated.

➤ **Premenstrual dysphoric disorder**

Adults: Initially, 50 mg PO daily either continuously or only during luteal phase of menstrual cycle. If no response, may increase dose 50 mg per menstrual cycle, up to 150 mg daily for continuous use or up to 100 mg daily for luteal phase doses. If a 100-mg daily dosage has been established with luteal phase dosing, give 50 mg daily for 2 to 3 days at the beginning of each luteal phase before increasing to 100 mg.

➤ **Generalized anxiety disorder ◆**

Adults: Initially, 25 mg once daily. May increase based on response and tolerability in increments of 25 to 50 mg at intervals of 1 to 2 weeks or more. Usual dosage, 50 to 150 mg/day. Maximum dosage, 200 mg/day.

ADMINISTRATION

PO

• Give drug without regard for food.

• Don't use oral concentrate dropper, which is made of rubber, for patient with latex allergy.

• Dilute oral concentrate before administration. Mix oral concentrate with 4 oz (120 mL) of water, ginger ale, lemon-lime soda, lemonade, or orange juice only, and give immediately.

• Have patient swallow capsules whole. Don't crush or open capsules.

ACTION

Thought to be linked to drug's inhibition of CNS neuronal reuptake of serotonin.

Route	Onset	Peak	Duration
PO	1 wk	4–8 hr	Unknown

Half-life: 62 to 104 hours.

ADVERSE REACTIONS

CNS: fatigue, headache, tremor, dizziness, insomnia, somnolence, anxiety, agitation, hyperkinesia, aggression. **CV:** palpitations. **EENT:** visual disturbances, blurred vision, mydriasis, dry mouth, epistaxis. **GI:** nausea, diarrhea, dyspepsia, vomiting, constipation, thirst, flatulence, anorexia, abdominal pain, decreased appetite. **GU:** male sexual dysfunction, decreased libido, urinary incontinence. **Metabolic:** weight loss. **Musculoskeletal:** myalgia, arthralgia, muscle twitching. **Skin:** rash, pruritus, diaphoresis, alopecia, purpura.

INTERACTIONS

Drug-drug. *Agents with antiplatelet properties (NSAIDs, P2Y12 inhibitors, SSRIs), aspirin, clopidogrel, heparin:* May enhance antiplatelet effect and bleeding risk. Monitor therapy.

Amphetamines (fluoxetine, selegiline), buspirone, dextromethorphan, dihydroergotamine, lithium salts, other SSRIs (sumatriptan, trazodone) or SNRIs (duloxetine, venlafaxine), TCAs (amitriptyline, imipramine), opioids (tramadol, meperidine), ʟ-tryptophan: May increase the risk of serotonin syndrome. Avoid combinations of drugs that increase the availability of serotonin in CNS; monitor patient closely if used together.

Apixaban, dabigatran, edoxaban, rivaroxaban: May increase bleeding risk. Monitor patient carefully.

CYP2D6 substrates (atomoxetine, desipramine, dextromethorphan, flecainide, metoprolol, nebivolol, perphenazine, propafenone, thioridazine, tolterodine, venlafaxine): May increase exposure of substrate. If concurrent use is needed, decrease substrate dosage. If sertraline is discontinued, an increased substrate dosage may be needed.

Disulfiram: Oral concentrate contains alcohol, which may react with drug. Use together is contraindicated.

Diuretics: May increase risk of hyponatremia. Monitor patient closely.

S

Drugs that prolong QTc interval (amiodarone, droperidol, erythromycin, methadone, moxifloxacin, procainamide, sotalol, tacrolimus, ziprasidone): May increase risk of QTc-interval prolongation or ventricular arrhythmias, including torsades de pointes. Avoid use together.

Fosphenytoin, phenytoin: May increase phenytoin level. Monitor phenytoin level and reduce phenytoin dosage if needed.

Linezolid, methylene blue: May cause serotonin syndrome. Use extreme caution and monitor patient closely. If treatment is necessary, discontinue sertraline before treatment with linezolid or methylene blue.

MAO inhibitors (phenelzine, selegiline, tranylcypromine): May cause serotonin syndrome or signs and symptoms resembling NMS. Use of sertraline with or within 2 weeks of an MAO inhibitor is contraindicated.

Pimozide: May increase risk of QT-interval prolongation and ventricular arrhythmias. Use together is contraindicated.

Triptans: May cause serotonin syndrome (restlessness, hallucinations, loss of coordination, fast heartbeat, rapid changes in BP, increased body temperature, hyperreflexia, nausea, vomiting, and diarrhea) or NMS-like reactions. Use cautiously, with close monitoring, especially at the start of treatment and during dosage adjustments.

Warfarin, other highly protein-bound drugs: May increase level of sertraline or other highly protein-bound drug. May prolong PT or increase INR. Monitor patient closely; monitor PT and INR.

Drug-herb. *Alfalfa, anise, bilberry:* May increase risk of bleeding. Consider alternative agents.

St. John's wort: May cause additive effects and serotonin syndrome. Discourage use together.

Drug-lifestyle. *Alcohol use:* May increase psychomotor impairment. Discourage use together.

EFFECTS ON LAB TEST RESULTS
- May increase cholesterol, TSH, ALT, and AST levels.
- May decrease sodium level.
- May increase or decrease glucose level.
- May show false-positive urine immunoassay screening tests for benzodiazepines.

CONTRAINDICATIONS & CAUTIONS
- Contraindicated in patients hypersensitive to drug or its components.
- Use cautiously in patients at risk for suicide and in those with seizure disorders, major affective disorder, or diseases or conditions that affect metabolism or hemodynamic responses.
- Screen patients for bipolar disorder; drug may activate manic or hypomanic states.
- Use cautiously in older adults and patients who are volume-depleted. Drug may increase risk of hyponatremia.
- Avoid use in patients with angle-closure glaucoma.
- Use cautiously in patients at risk for QT-interval prolongation.
- ⚠️ *Alert:* Sertraline isn't approved for use in children except those with OCD.
- ⚠️ *Alert:* Drug may increase risk of bleeding, especially with concomitant use of aspirin, NSAIDs, other antiplatelet drugs, warfarin, and other anticoagulants.

Dialyzable drug: Unknown.

⚠️ *Overdose S&S:* Somnolence, vomiting, tachycardia, nausea, dizziness, agitation, tremor, bradycardia, bundle-branch block, coma, seizures, delirium, hallucinations, HTN, hypotension, manic reactions, pancreatitis, prolonged QT interval, serotonin syndrome, stupor, syncope.

PREGNANCY-LACTATION-REPRODUCTION
- There are no adequate studies during pregnancy. Use only if potential benefit justifies fetal risk.
- Neonates exposed to sertraline and other SSRIs or SNRIs late in third trimester have developed complications requiring prolonged hospitalization, respiratory support, and tube feeding.
- Neonates exposed to SSRIs during pregnancy may be at increased risk for persistent pulmonary HTN of the newborn.
- Oral concentrate contains 12% alcohol and isn't recommended during pregnancy.
- Enroll patients exposed to drug during pregnancy in the National Pregnancy Registry for Antidepressants (1-866-961-2388 or https://womensmentalhealth.org/research/pregnancyregistry/antidepressants/).
- It isn't known if drug appears in human milk. Use cautiously during breastfeeding.

Reactions in bold italics are *life-threatening*.

NURSING CONSIDERATIONS

• Record mood changes. Monitor patient for suicidality, and allow only a minimum supply of drug.

Boxed Warning Drug may increase risk of suicidality in children, adolescents, and young adults with MDD or other psychiatric disorder. ∎

Boxed Warning Closely monitor all patients being treated with antidepressants for clinical worsening, suicidality, and unusual changes in behavior, especially during initial few months of treatment or at times of dosage increases or decreases. ∎

• Assess patients for sexual dysfunction at baseline and periodically during treatment. SSRIs may cause sexual dysfunction that patients may not spontaneously.

• Monitor patients for hyponatremia (headache, difficulty concentrating, memory impairment, confusion, weakness, unsteadiness, falls, hallucinations, seizure, respiratory arrest).

⚠ *Alert:* If linezolid or methylene blue must be given, stop sertraline and monitor patient for serotonin toxicity for 2 weeks, or until 24 hours after the last dose of methylene blue or linezolid, whichever comes first. May resume sertraline 24 hours after last dose of methylene blue or linezolid.

⚠ *Alert:* Combining triptans with an SSRI or SNRI may cause serotonin syndrome (restlessness, hallucinations, loss of coordination, tachycardia, rapid changes in BP, increased body temperature, overactive reflexes, nausea, vomiting, diarrhea) or NMS-like reactions. Serotonin syndrome may be more likely to occur when starting or increasing the dose of triptan, SSRI, or SNRI.

• Gradual dosage reduction is recommended when stopping treatment. Monitor patient for discontinuation syndrome (nausea, diaphoresis, dysphoric mood, agitation, dizziness, paresthesia, tremor, insomnia, tinnitus, seizures, lethargy, confusion), especially after abrupt end of treatment.

• *Look alike–sound alike:* Don't confuse sertraline with cetirizine.

PATIENT TEACHING

Boxed Warning Advise families and caregivers to closely observe patient for increased suicidality. ∎

• Instruct patient in safe drug administration.

⚠ *Alert:* Teach patient to recognize and immediately report signs and symptoms of serotonin syndrome.

• Advise patient to use caution when performing hazardous tasks that require alertness.

• Tell patient to avoid alcohol and to consult prescriber before taking OTC drugs.

• Advise patient to avoid stopping drug abruptly and to discuss a gradual taper plan with prescriber.

• Caution patient to report pregnancy or breastfeeding to prescriber.

• Inform patient that drug may cause sexual dysfunction and to discuss changes and management with health care provider.

---

sevelamer carbonate
se-VEL-a-mer

Renvela

sevelamer hydrochloride
Renagel

Therapeutic class: Hypophosphatemics
Pharmacologic class: Polymeric phosphate binders

AVAILABLE FORMS
sevelamer carbonate
Oral suspension: 0.8-g, 2.4-g packets
Tablets (film-coated) 🚫: 800 mg
sevelamer hydrochloride
Tablets (film-coated) 🚫: 400 mg, 800 mg

INDICATIONS & DOSAGES
➤ **To control phosphorus level in patients with CKD on dialysis**
Adults not taking a phosphate binder: Initially, 800 to 1,600 mg PO with each meal, based on phosphorus level. If phosphorus level is greater than 5.5 mg/dL and less than 7.5 mg/dL, start with 800 mg t.i.d. with meals. If phosphorus level is 7.5 mg/dL or greater, start with 1,600 mg t.i.d., with meals.
Adults switching from calcium acetate: Initially, if taking one 667-mg calcium acetate tablet per meal, start with 800 mg PO per meal. If taking two 667-mg calcium acetate tablets per meal, start with 1,600 mg per meal. If taking three 667-mg calcium acetate tablets per meal, start with 2,400 mg per meal.

S

Adjust-a-dose: If phosphorus level is greater than 5.5 mg/dL, increase by 800 mg per meal at 2-week intervals. If phosphorus level is 3.5 to 5.5 mg/dL, maintain current dose. If phosphorus level is less than 3.5 mg/dL, decrease by 300 mg per meal.

Children ages 6 and older not taking a phosphate binder (Renvela only): Initially, 800 to 1,600 mg PO t.i.d. with meals, based on BSA. For BSA of 0.75 m² to less than 1.2 m², give 800 mg per meal or snack. Increase or decrease by 400 mg/dose at 2-week intervals as needed to achieve target levels. For BSA of 1.2 m² or greater, give 1,600 mg per meal or snack. Increase or decrease by 800 mg/dose at 2-week intervals as needed to achieve target levels.

ADMINISTRATION
PO
• Have patient swallow tablet whole; don't cut or crush tablets.
• Mix powder packets with appropriate amount of water as directed. Stir mixture vigorously immediately before giving (it doesn't dissolve) and have patient drink entire preparation within 30 minutes.
• May also premix entire contents of powder packet with a small amount of food or beverage and have patient consume within 30 minutes as part of a meal. Don't heat or add to heated foods or liquids.
• Give drug with meals.
• Drug may bind to other drugs and decrease their bioavailability. Give other drugs 1 hour before or 3 hours after this drug.

ACTION
Inhibits intestinal phosphate absorption and decreases phosphorus levels.

Route	Onset	Peak	Duration
PO	Unknown	Unknown	Unknown

Half-life: Unknown.

ADVERSE REACTIONS
GI: diarrhea, dyspepsia, vomiting, nausea, constipation, flatulence, abdominal pain; peritonitis (patients on peritoneal dialysis).

INTERACTIONS
Drug-drug. *Ciprofloxacin, other quinolones:* May bind with quinolones. Give quinolones either 2 hours before or 6 hours after sevelamer.

Mycophenolate: May decrease mycophenolic acid level, decreasing effectiveness. Administer sevelamer 2 hours after mycophenolate.
Drug where decreased bioavailability significantly affects safety or efficacy (levothyroxine, cyclosporine, tacrolimus): May decrease effectiveness or increase adverse effects. Separate administration times by at least several hours. Consider therapy modification.

EFFECTS ON LAB TEST RESULTS
• May decrease phosphorus, folic acid, and vitamins D, E, and K levels.

CONTRAINDICATIONS & CAUTIONS
• Contraindicated in patients hypersensitive to drug or its components and in those with hypophosphatemia or bowel obstruction.
• Use cautiously in patient with dysphagia, swallowing disorders, severe GI motility disorders, or major GI tract surgery.
• May reduce absorption of folic acid and vitamins D, E, and K.
Dialyzable drug: Unknown.

PREGNANCY-LACTATION-REPRODUCTION
• There are no adequate studies during pregnancy. Use cautiously during pregnancy. Drug isn't absorbed systemically.
• Drug may decrease serum levels of fat-soluble vitamins and folic acid in patients who are pregnant. Consider supplementation if clinically indicated.
• Drug isn't absorbed systemically; breast-feeding isn't expected to result in exposure of the child.

NURSING CONSIDERATIONS
• Monitor serum chemistries, including phosphorus, calcium, and bicarbonate levels.
• Monitor parathyroid hormone level.
• *Look alike–sound alike:* Don't confuse Renvela with Renagel.

PATIENT TEACHING
• Instruct patient to take with meals and to adhere to prescribed diet.
• **Alert:** Inform patient that tablets must be taken whole because contents expand in water. Warn patient not to cut, crush, or chew tablets.
• Advise patient to take reconstituted oral suspension within 30 minutes.
• Tell patient to check with pharmacist before taking other drugs at same time as sevelamer.

Reactions in bold italics are *life-threatening*.

• Inform patient about common adverse reactions, including constipation that, if left untreated, may lead to severe complications.

sildenafil citrate
sil-DEN-a-fill

Revatio, Viagra

Therapeutic class: Erectile dysfunction drugs
Pharmacologic class: PDE5 inhibitors

AVAILABLE FORMS
Injection: 10 mg/12.5 mL single-use vials
Oral suspension (Revatio): 10 mg/mL
Tablets (Revatio): 20 mg
Tablets (Viagra): 25 mg, 50 mg, 100 mg

INDICATIONS & DOSAGES
➤ **Erectile dysfunction (Viagra only)**
Adult men younger than age 65: 50 mg PO, as needed, 30 minutes to 4 hours (usually about 1 hour) before sexual activity. Dosage range is 25 to 100 mg based on effectiveness and tolerance. Maximum is one dose daily.
Adult men ages 65 and older: 25 mg PO, as needed, about 1 hour before sexual activity. Dosage may be adjusted based on patient response.
Adjust-a-dose: For adults with liver impairment or CrCl less than 30 mL/minute, decrease starting dose to 25 mg PO. May adjust dosage based on patient response.
➤ **To improve exercise ability and delay clinical worsening in patients with WHO Group 1 PAH (Revatio only)**
Adults: 20 mg PO t.i.d., 4 to 6 hours apart. May titrate to maximum dosage of 80 mg t.i.d. based on symptoms and tolerability. Or 10 mg IV bolus t.i.d.
Children ages 1 to 17 years weighing more than 45 kg: 20 mg PO t.i.d. Dose may be titrated to a maximum dose of 40 mg t.i.d. based on symptoms and tolerability.
Children ages 1 to 17 years weighing more than 20 to 45 kg: 20 mg PO t.i.d.
Children ages 1 to 17 years weighing 20 kg or less: 10 mg PO t.i.d.

ADMINISTRATION
🕙 *Alert:* Don't substitute Viagra for Revatio because there isn't an equivalent dose.

PO
• Give without regard for food.
• Don't give to patients taking nitrates.
• Follow manufacturer's directions for reconstitution of powder for oral suspension.
• Shake suspension for at least 10 seconds before use; don't mix with other medications.
• Label Revatio suspension with expiration date that's 60 days from reconstitution date.
IV
▼ Inspect solution visually for particulate matter and discoloration before administering.
▼ Don't give to patients taking nitrates.
▼ The 10-mg IV dose is equivalent to 20-mg oral dose (Revatio).
▼ **Incompatibilities:** None listed by manufacturer. Consult a drug incompatibility reference for more information.

ACTION
When sexual stimulation causes local release of nitric oxide, inhibition of PDE5 by sildenafil causes increased levels of cyclic guanosine monophosphate (cGMP) in the corpus cavernosum, resulting in smooth muscle relaxation and inflow of blood to the corpus cavernosum. In PAH, drug increases cGMP level by preventing its breakdown by phosphodiesterase, prolonging smooth muscle relaxation of the pulmonary vasculature, which leads to vasodilation.

Route	Onset	Peak	Duration
PO	15–30 min	30–120 min	4 hr
IV	Unknown	Unknown	Unknown

Half-life: 4 hours.

ADVERSE REACTIONS
CNS: headache, dizziness. **CV:** flushing.
EENT: visual disturbance (temporary vision loss, diplopia, photophobia, altered color perception, blurred vision), nasal congestion, epistaxis. **GI:** dyspepsia, diarrhea, gastritis, nausea. **GU:** UTI. **Musculoskeletal:** back pain, myalgia, limb pain. **Skin:** erythema, rash.

INTERACTIONS
Drug-drug. *Alpha blockers (doxazosin, prazosin):* May cause symptomatic hypotension. Consider dosage reduction.
Amyl nitrate: May increase vasodilatory effects. Don't use together.
Antihypertensives: May increase hypotension. Use cautiously.

S

CYP3A inducers (bosentan): May decrease sildenafil level and increase bosentan level. Monitor patient closely for bosentan adverse reactions. Increase Revatio dosage as indicated.
CYP3A inhibitors (erythromycin, itraconazole, ketoconazole, protease inhibitors, ritonavir, saquinavir): May increase sildenafil level and risk of adverse events. Reduce Viagra starting dose to 25 mg when used with moderate inhibitors. When used with strong inhibitors, maximum Viagra dosage is 25 mg in a 48-hour period. Use of strong inhibitors with Revatio isn't recommended.
Guanylate cyclase (GC) stimulators (riociguat): May potentiate hypotensive effects of GC stimulators. Use together is contraindicated.
Isosorbide, nitroglycerin: May cause severe hypotension. Use of nitrates in any form with sildenafil is contraindicated.
Other PDE5 inhibitors: May increase risk of hypotension. Don't use together.
Vitamin K antagonists: May increase risk of bleeding (primarily epistaxis). Monitor patient.
Drug-herb. *St. John's wort:* May decrease sildenafil level. Don't use together.
Drug-food. *Grapefruit:* May increase drug level, while delaying absorption. Advise patient to avoid using together.
Drug-lifestyle. *Alcohol use:* Excessive alcohol intake may increase risk of hypotension. Advise patient to avoid or limit alcohol consumption.

EFFECTS ON LAB TEST RESULTS
• May increase sodium, uric acid, and liver enzyme levels.
• May increase or decrease glucose level.

CONTRAINDICATIONS & CAUTIONS
• Contraindicated in patients hypersensitive to drug or its components.
• Use cautiously in patients ages 65 and older; in patients with liver impairment or CrCl less than 30 mL/minute, retinitis pigmentosa, bleeding disorders, or active peptic ulcer disease; in those who have suffered an MI, stroke, or life-threatening arrhythmia within past 6 months; in those with history of HF, CAD, uncontrolled BP, or anatomic deformation of the penis (angulation, cavernosal fibrosis, or Peyronie disease); and in those with conditions that may predispose them to priapism (sickle cell anemia, multiple myeloma, or leukemia).

• Vision loss, including permanent loss of vision, has been reported in patients taking drug for erectile dysfunction and may be a sign of nonarteritic anterior ischemic optic neuropathy (NAION). Risk may increase with history of vision loss. Other risk factors for NAION include low cup-to-disk ratio, CAD, diabetes, HTN, hyperlipidemia, smoking, and age older than 50.
• Pulmonary vasodilators used to treat PAH can worsen the CV status of patients with pulmonary veno-occlusive disease (PVOD). Use in patients with PVOD isn't recommended. If pulmonary edema occurs after drug is given for PAH, consider possibility of PVOD.
• Safe and effective use of drug to treat PAH in patients with sickle cell anemia hasn't been established. Drug may increase risk of vaso-occlusive crises requiring hospitalization.
• Safe use of drug to treat PAH in children hasn't been established. Use isn't recommended, particularly prolonged use, due to increased mortality.
• Hearing loss with or without tinnitus and dizziness have been reported. Obtain prompt medical attention for hearing loss.
Dialyzable drug: Unlikely.

PREGNANCY-LACTATION-REPRODUCTION
• Viagra isn't indicated for use in adult females. There are no adequate studies during pregnancy or breastfeeding.
• Information regarding use of drug to treat PAH during pregnancy is limited. Current guidelines recommend that patients with PAH use effective contraception and avoid pregnancy.
• Drug is excreted in human milk; effects on infant are unknown. If used during breastfeeding, monitor infant closely.

NURSING CONSIDERATIONS
⚠ *Alert:* Systemic vasodilatory properties cause transient decreases in supine BP and cardiac output (about 2 hours after ingestion).
• The serious CV events linked to this drug's use in erectile dysfunction mainly involve patients with underlying CV disease who are at increased risk for cardiac effects related to sexual activity.
• Patients with PAH caused by connective tissue disease are more prone to epistaxis during therapy than those with primary pulmonary HTN.
• IV use is for patients with PAH temporarily unable to take oral medications.

Reactions in bold italics are *life-threatening*.

- *Look alike–sound alike:* Don't confuse Viagra with Allegra.

PATIENT TEACHING
- Instruct patient in safe drug administration.
- Caution patient to take drug only as prescribed.
- Advise patient that drug shouldn't be used with nitrates or GC stimulators under any circumstances. Revatio and Viagra or other PDE5 inhibitors used for erectile dysfunction shouldn't be used together.
- Advise patient of potential cardiac risk of sexual activity, especially in presence of CV risk factors. Instruct patient to notify prescriber and refrain from further activity if such symptoms as chest pain, dizziness, or nausea occur when starting sexual activity.
- Warn patient that erections lasting longer than 4 hours and priapism (painful erections lasting longer than 6 hours) may occur; tell patient to seek immediate medical attention if either of these occurs. Penile tissue damage and permanent loss of potency may result if priapism isn't treated immediately.
- Inform patient that drug used for erectile dysfunction doesn't protect against sexually transmitted diseases; advise patient to use protective measures such as condoms.
- Advise patient receiving HIV medications of the increased risk of sildenafil adverse events, including low BP, visual changes, and priapism, and to promptly report such symptoms to prescriber. Tell patient not to exceed 25 mg of sildenafil.
- Inform patient that maximum benefit can be expected less than 2 hours after ingestion.
- Caution patient that impairment of color discrimination (blue, green) may occur and to avoid hazardous activities that rely on color discrimination.
- Instruct patient to immediately report vision or hearing changes.

silodosin
SI-lo-doe-sin

Rapaflo

Therapeutic class: BPH drugs
Pharmacologic class: Alpha₁ blockers

AVAILABLE FORMS
Capsules ⓞ: 4 mg, 8 mg

INDICATIONS & DOSAGES
➤ **To improve symptoms of BPH**
Adult males: 8 mg PO once daily.
Adjust-a-dose: For patients with CrCl of 30 to 50 mL/minute, give 4 mg PO once daily.

ADMINISTRATION
PO
- Give drug once daily with a meal.
- For patients who can't swallow capsules, contents of capsule may be sprinkled on a tablespoonful of cool applesauce, swallowed within 5 minutes without chewing, and followed with 8 oz (240 mL) of cool water to ensure complete swallowing of the powder. Don't subdivide capsule contents or store for future use.

ACTION
Causes relaxation of smooth muscles in prostate and bladder tissues by antagonizing postsynaptic alpha₁ adrenoreceptors, thereby improving urine flow and reducing signs and symptoms of BPH.

Route	Onset	Peak	Duration
PO	Unknown	3 hr	Unknown

Half-life: About 13 hours.

ADVERSE REACTIONS
CNS: asthenia, dizziness, headache, insomnia. **CV:** orthostatic hypotension. **EENT:** nasal congestion, nasopharyngitis, rhinorrhea, sinusitis. **GI:** abdominal pain, diarrhea. **GU:** retrograde ejaculation, increased PSA level.

INTERACTIONS
Drug-drug. *Alpha blockers (doxazosin, prazosin):* May increase risk of symptomatic hypotension. Avoid use together.
Antihypertensives: May cause dizziness and orthostatic hypotension. Use together cautiously and monitor patient for adverse reactions.
Moderate CYP3A4 inhibitors (diltiazem, erythromycin, verapamil): May increase silodosin level. Use together cautiously.
PDE5 inhibitors (sildenafil, tadalafil): May cause symptomatic hypotension. Monitor patient closely.
Strong CYP3A4 inhibitors (clarithromycin, itraconazole, ketoconazole, ritonavir): May increase silodosin level. Use together is contraindicated.

Strong P-gp/ABCB1 inhibitors (cyclosporine, ketoconazole, ritonavir, verapamil): May increase silodosin level. Use together isn't recommended.

Drug-herb. *St. John's wort:* May decrease silodosin level and its effects. Consider modifying therapy.

EFFECTS ON LAB TEST RESULTS
• May increase PSA level.

CONTRAINDICATIONS & CAUTIONS
• Contraindicated in patients hypersensitive to drug or its components and in those with CrCl less than 30 mL/minute or Child-Pugh class C liver impairment.
• Drug isn't indicated to treat HTN.
• Safety and effectiveness in children haven't been established.
Dialyzable drug: Unlikely.
⚠ **Overdose S&S:** Orthostatic hypotension.

PREGNANCY-LACTATION-REPRODUCTION
• Drug isn't approved for use in females.
• Drug may cause reversible decrease in male fertility based on animal studies.

NURSING CONSIDERATIONS
• Because BPH and prostate cancer cause similar signs and symptoms, prostate cancer should be ruled out before the start of silodosin therapy.
• Monitor patient for orthostatic hypotension. Carefully monitor older adults for hypotension; risk of orthostatic hypotension increases with age.
• Current or previous use of an alpha blocker may predispose patient to floppy iris syndrome during cataract surgery.

PATIENT TEACHING
• Instruct patient in safe drug administration.
• Warn patient about possible hypotension and instruct that it may cause dizziness.
• Caution patient against driving or operating hazardous machinery until drug's effects are known.
• Advise patient who needs cataract surgery to inform ophthalmologist about taking silodosin.
• Inform patient about the possibility of retrograde ejaculation, which is reversible upon drug discontinuation and doesn't pose a safety concern.

simvastatin ▧
sim-va-STAT-in

FloLipid, Zocor

Therapeutic class: Antilipemics
Pharmacologic class: HMG-CoA reductase inhibitors

AVAILABLE FORMS
Oral suspension: 20 mg/5 mL, 40 mg/5 mL
Tablets: 5 mg, 10 mg, 20 mg, 40 mg, 80 mg

INDICATIONS & DOSAGES
Adjust-a-dose (for all indications): In patients with CrCl less than 30 mL/minute, start with 5 mg PO daily.
➤ **To reduce risk of death from CV disease and CV events in patients at high risk for coronary events; to reduce total cholesterol and LDL-C, apolipoprotein B, and triglyceride levels and increase HDL-C level in patients with primary hyperlipidemia and mixed dyslipidemia; to reduce triglyceride levels; to reduce triglyceride and VLDL cholesterol levels in patients with dysbetalipoproteinemia**
Adults: Initially, 10 to 20 mg PO daily in evening. In patients at high risk for a CAD event due to existing CAD, diabetes, PVD, or history of stroke, recommended initial dose is 40 mg PO daily. Adjust dosage every 4 weeks based on patient tolerance and response. Patients unable to achieve their LDL-C goals utilizing simvastatin 40 mg shouldn't be titrated to 80-mg dose but should be placed on alternative LDL-C lowering treatment.
➤ **To reduce total cholesterol and LDL-C levels in patients with homozygous familial hypercholesterolemia in combination with other therapies** ▧
Adults: 40 mg PO daily in evening.
➤ **Heterozygous familial hypercholesterolemia in children** ▧
Males and postmenarchal females ages 10 to 17: Give 10 mg PO once daily in the evening. Maximum, 40 mg daily.

ADMINISTRATION
PO
• Give drug in the evening.
• Give oral suspension in the evening on an empty stomach. Shake bottle well for 20 seconds before using.

Reactions in bold italics are *life-threatening*.

ACTION

Inhibits HMG-CoA reductase, an early (and rate-limiting) step in cholesterol biosynthesis.

Route	Onset	Peak	Duration
PO	Unknown	1–2 hr	Unknown

Half-life: Unknown.

ADVERSE REACTIONS

CNS: headache, insomnia, vertigo. **CV:** edema, atrial fibrillation. **EENT:** sinusitis. **GI:** abdominal pain, constipation, gastritis, nausea. **GU:** UTI. **Metabolic:** diabetes. **Hepatic:** increased transaminase levels. **Musculoskeletal:** myalgia. **Respiratory:** URI, bronchitis. **Skin:** eczema.

INTERACTIONS

Drug-drug. *Amiodarone, amlodipine, ranolazine:* May increase risk of myopathy and rhabdomyolysis. Don't exceed 20 mg simvastatin daily.

Azole antifungals (fluconazole, itraconazole, ketoconazole), daptomycin, macrolides (azithromycin, clarithromycin, erythromycin): May increase simvastatin level and adverse effects. Avoid using together or, if it can't be avoided, suspend simvastatin therapy for course of treatment.

Bile acid sequestrants (cholestyramine, colestipol): May decrease GI absorption of simvastatin. Separate administration times by at least 4 hours.

Colchicine: May increase risk of myopathy and rhabdomyolysis. Monitor patient closely.

Cyclosporine, danazol, gemfibrozil: May increase risk of myopathy and rhabdomyolysis. Use together is contraindicated.

Digoxin: May slightly increase digoxin level. Closely monitor digoxin levels at the start of simvastatin therapy.

Diltiazem, dronedarone, verapamil: May increase risk of myopathy and rhabdomyolysis. Don't exceed 10 mg simvastatin daily.

Efavirenz, rifampin: May decrease simvastatin level. Monitor effectiveness.

Fibrates (other than gemfibrozil): Increase risk of myopathy. Use cautiously together.

Liver-toxic drugs: May increase risk for liver toxicity. Avoid using together.

Lomitapide: May increase risk of myopathy or rhabdomyolysis. Reduce simvastatin dosage by 50% when starting lomitapide; don't exceed simvastatin 20 mg/day (or 40 mg/day for patients who previously

tolerated simvastatin 80 mg/day for 1 year or more without muscle toxicity).

▨ *Niacin:* May increase risk of myopathy and rhabdomyolysis with niacin dose of 1 g/day or more. Patients of Chinese descent and possibly others of Asian descent shouldn't receive simvastatin with lipid-modifying dose of niacin products.

Strong CYP3A4 inhibitors (nefazodone, protease inhibitors [amprenavir, atazanavir, darunavir, nelfinavir, ritonavir, saquinavir]): May inhibit metabolism of simvastatin and increase risk of adverse effects, including rhabdomyolysis. Use together is contraindicated.

Warfarin: May slightly enhance anticoagulant effect. Monitor PT and INR when therapy starts or dose is adjusted.

Drug-herb. *Eucalyptus, kava kava:* May increase risk of liver toxicity. Discourage use together.

Red yeast rice: May increase risk of rhabdomyolysis. Discourage use together.

St. John's wort: May decrease simvastatin level. Discourage use together.

Drug-food. *Grapefruit juice:* Large amounts (greater than 1 quart/day [1 L/day]) may increase drug levels, increasing risk of adverse effects, including myopathy and rhabdomyolysis. Discourage use together.

Drug-lifestyle. *Alcohol use:* May increase risk of liver toxicity. Discourage use together.

EFFECTS ON LAB TEST RESULTS

• May increase HbA_{1c}, fasting blood glucose, ALT, AST, ALP, GGT, and CK levels.

CONTRAINDICATIONS & CAUTIONS

• Simvastatin occasionally causes myopathy manifested as muscle pain, tenderness, or weakness, with CK level more than 10 × ULN. Myopathy may take the form of rhabdomyolysis with or without AKI secondary to myoglobinuria, and rare fatalities have occurred. The risk of myopathy is dose related. Predisposing factors for myopathy include age 65 and older, female sex, uncontrolled hypothyroidism, and kidney impairment.

• Contraindicated in patients hypersensitive to drug and in those with active liver disease or conditions that cause unexplained persistent elevations of transaminase levels.

• Contraindicated for use at its highest dosage (80 mg/day) in patients not previously prescribed simvastatin or in patients who have

S

had prior muscle toxicity. Patients who can't reach their goal LDL-C level on 40-mg dose should be switched to an alternative agent. Only patients who have tolerated the 80-mg dose without muscle toxicity for more than 12 months should continue taking 80 mg daily.
• Immune-mediated necrotizing myopathy (IMNM) (proximal muscle weakness, persistent CK elevation even after statin is stopped, positive anti-HMG CoA reductase antibody, biopsy positive for necrotizing myopathy) has been reported rarely with statin use. Treat IMNM with immunosuppressants.
• Use cautiously in older adults and patients who consume large amounts of alcohol or have a history of liver disease.
• Rare reports of cognitive impairment (memory loss, forgetfulness, amnesia, memory impairment, confusion) have been associated with statin use. These reported symptoms are generally not serious and are reversible upon statin discontinuation, with variable times to symptom onset (1 day to years) and symptom resolution (median of 3 weeks).
• Safety and effectiveness in children younger than age 10 or in premenarchal females haven't been established.
Dialyzable drug: Unknown.

PREGNANCY-LACTATION-REPRODUCTION
• May cause fetal harm. Use during pregnancy is contraindicated unless benefits outweigh fetal risk. Discontinue drug before conception.
• If pregnancy occurs during therapy, apprise patient of fetal risks with continued use during pregnancy.
• Contraindicated during breastfeeding.

NURSING CONSIDERATIONS
• Obtain LFT results before initiation of treatment and thereafter when clinically indicated. Obtain lipid determinations after 4 weeks of therapy and periodically thereafter.
• Monitor all patients for myopathy (unexplained muscle pain, weakness, or tenderness). Periodic CK determinations may be considered in patients starting therapy or in patients whose dosage is being increased, but there's no assurance that such monitoring will prevent myopathy.
• Interrupt statin therapy if patient shows signs or symptoms of serious liver injury, hyperbilirubinemia, or jaundice. Don't restart drug if another cause can't be found.

• A daily dose of 40 mg significantly reduces risk of death from CAD, nonfatal MI, stroke, and revascularization procedures.
• ***Look alike–sound alike:*** Don't confuse Zocor with Cozaar.

PATIENT TEACHING
• Instruct patient in safe drug administration.
• Teach patient about proper dietary management of cholesterol and triglycerides. When appropriate, recommend weight control, exercise, and smoking cessation programs.
• Inform patient that rare instances of memory loss and confusion have occurred with statin use. These reported events were generally not serious and resolved when drug was discontinued.
• Tell patient that drug may increase blood glucose level, but CV outweigh increased risk.
• Caution patient to immediately report unexplained muscle pain, tenderness, or weakness (especially if accompanied by malaise or fever) and loss of appetite, upper abdominal pain, dark-colored urine, or yellowing of skin or eyes.
• *Alert:* Tell patient to stop drug and immediately report pregnancy or breastfeeding.

SAFETY ALERT!

sirolimus
sir-OH-li-mus

Rapamune

Therapeutic class: Immunosuppressants
Pharmacologic class: MTOR inhibitors

AVAILABLE FORMS
Oral solution: 1 mg/mL
Tablets ⒸⓃⒸ: 0.5 mg, 1 mg, 2 mg

INDICATIONS & DOSAGES
➤ **With cyclosporine and corticosteroids, to prevent organ rejection in patients receiving kidney transplants**
Adults and children ages 13 and older with low-to-moderate immunogenic risk: Initially, 6 mg PO for patients with low-to-moderate immunologic risk weighing 40 kg or more or 3 mg/m^2 for patients weighing less than 40 kg as one-time dose as soon as possible after transplantation but 4 hours after administration of cyclosporine; then maintenance dose of 2 mg PO once daily for patients

weighing 40 kg or more or 1 mg/m^2 PO once daily for patients weighing less than 40 kg.
Adults with high immunogenic risk: May give up to 15 mg PO on day 1 after transplantation, then 5 mg/day PO beginning on day 2 after transplantation. Obtain trough level between days 5 and 7 and adjust dosage as needed.

Maximum daily dose shouldn't exceed 40 mg. If a loading dose requires more than 40 mg, give that loading dose over 2 days. Monitor trough levels at least 3 to 4 days after a loading dose.

Adjust-a-dose: When adjusting maintenance dosage, continue patient on new dosage for at least 7 to 14 days before further adjustments; drug has a long half-life.

For patients with Child-Pugh class A or B liver impairment, reduce maintenance dose by about one-third; for those with Child-Pugh class C liver impairment, by about one-half. It isn't necessary to reduce loading dose. From 2 to 4 months after transplant in patients with low-to-moderate risk of graft rejection, taper off cyclosporine over 4 to 8 weeks and adjust sirolimus dose every 1 to 2 weeks to obtain levels between 16 and 24 nanograms/mL. Base dosage adjustments on clinical status, tissue biopsies, and lab findings. Refer to manufacturer's instructions for more information.

➤ **Lymphangioleiomyomatosis**
Adults: Initially, 2 mg PO daily consistently with or without food at same time each day. Measure trough level in 10 to 20 days and adjust dosage to achieve sirolimus trough level of between 5 and 15 nanograms/mL, allowing at least 7 to 14 days at new dosage level before further dosage adjustment. After achieving a stable dosage, monitor drug levels at least every 3 months.

ADMINISTRATION
PO
🔹 *Alert:* Drug is a hazardous agent; use safe handling and disposal precautions.
• Give drug consistently either with or without food.
• Have patients swallow tablets whole. Don't crush or cut tablets.
• Dilute oral solution before use. After dilution, use immediately and discard oral solution syringe.
• When diluting oral solution, empty correct amount into glass or plastic container holding at least 2 oz (60 mL) of water or orange juice. Don't use grapefruit juice or any other liquid.

Stir vigorously and have patient drink immediately. Refill container with at least 4 oz (120 mL) of water or orange juice, stir again, and have patient drink all contents.
• Oral solution may develop a slight haze during refrigeration, which doesn't affect potency of drug. If haze develops, bring to room temperature and shake until haze disappears.
• Store oral solution away from light, and refrigerate at 36° to 46° F (2° to 8° C). After opening bottle, use contents within 1 month. If needed, store bottles and pouches at room temperature (up to 77° F [25° C]) for several days. Oral solution may be kept in oral amber syringe for 24 hours at room temperature.
• Store tablets between 68° and 77° F (20° and 25° C). Protect from light.

ACTION
Inhibits T-cell activation and proliferation that occurs in response to antigenic and cytokine stimulation. Also inhibits antibody formation.

Route	Onset	Peak	Duration
PO	Unknown	1–3 hr (solution); 1–6 hr (tablet)	Unknown

Half-life: Adults, about 46 to 78 hours; children, 13.7 ± 6.2 hours.

ADVERSE REACTIONS
CNS: fever, headache, pain, dizziness. **CV:** chest pain, edema, HTN, tachycardia, *VTE.* **EENT:** epistaxis. **GI:** abdominal pain, constipation, diarrhea, nausea, ascites, stomatitis, *pancreatitis.* **GU:** UTI, pyelonephritis, nephrotic syndrome, menstrual disorder, ovarian cysts, increased creatinine level. **Hematologic:** anemia, lymphadenopathy, *thrombocytopenia, leukopenia, thrombotic thrombocytopenic purpura, hemolytic-uremic syndrome.* **Hepatic:** *liver toxicity.* **Metabolic:** hyperlipidemia, *hypokalemia, hypoglycemia,* diabetes. **Musculoskeletal:** arthralgia, bone necrosis, myalgia. **Respiratory:** URI, pneumonia. **Skin:** acne, rash, fungal dermatitis, pruritus, *melanoma, squamous cell carcinoma, basal cell carcinoma.* **Other:** *sepsis,* abnormal healing, infection, lymphocele, herpes simplex, herpes zoster, mycobacterial infections, *malignancy.*

INTERACTIONS
Drug-drug. *ACE inhibitors (captopril, enalapril, lisinopril):* May increase risk of angioedema. Use together cautiously.

S

Aminoglycosides, amphotericin B, other kidney-toxic drugs: May increase risk of kidney toxicity. Use with caution.

Calcineurin inhibitors (CNI) (cyclosporine, pimecrolimus, tacrolimus): May increase risk of CNI-induced hemolyticuremic syndrome, thrombotic thrombocytopenic purpura, or thrombotic microangiopathy. Monitor patient closely.

Cannabidiol: May increase sirolimus level and risk of adverse reactions. Consider sirolimus dose reduction.

Cyclosporine: May increase sirolimus level and toxicity. Give sirolimus 4 hours after cyclosporine. If cyclosporine is stopped, higher doses of sirolimus are needed; monitor level and adjust dosage as needed.

HMG-CoA reductase inhibitors or fibrates: May increase risk of rhabdomyolysis with the combination of sirolimus and cyclosporine. Monitor patient closely.

Ketoconazole: May increase rate and extent of sirolimus absorption. Avoid using together.

Live-virus vaccines: May reduce vaccine effectiveness. Avoid using together.

Rifampin: May decrease sirolimus level. Alternative to rifampin should be prescribed.

Strong CYP3A4 inducers (rifampin, rifabutin): May decrease sirolimus level. Avoid use together. Consider alternative agents.

Strong CYP3A4 inhibitors (ketoconazole, itraconazole, erythromycin, clarithromycin): May increase sirolimus level. Avoid use together. Consider alternative agents.

Verapamil: May increase verapamil level. Use together cautiously.

Weak and moderate CYP3A4 inducers (carbamazepine, phenobarbital, phenytoin, rifapentine): May decrease sirolimus level. Monitor patient closely.

Weak and moderate CYP3A4 and P-gp inhibitors (cimetidine, diltiazem, fluconazole, ritonavir, indinavir): May increase sirolimus level. Use cautiously together.

Drug-herb. *St. John's wort:* May decrease sirolimus levels. Discourage use together.

Drug-food. *Grapefruit juice:* May decrease drug metabolism. Discourage use together.

Drug-lifestyle. *Sun exposure:* May increase risk of skin cancer. Advise patient to avoid sunlight exposure.

EFFECTS ON LAB TEST RESULTS

• May increase urine protein, creatinine, glucose, LDH, liver enzyme, cholesterol, triglyceride, and other lipid levels.

• May decrease phosphate and potassium levels.
• May increase RBC count.
• May decrease platelet count.
• May increase or decrease WBC count.

CONTRAINDICATIONS & CAUTIONS

• Contraindicated in patients hypersensitive to active drug, its derivatives, or components of product.

• Use cautiously in patients with hyperlipidemia and impaired liver or kidney function.

• Cases of ILD, including pneumonitis, bronchiolitis obliterans organizing pneumonia, and pulmonary fibrosis (some fatal), have occurred. ILD may be associated with pulmonary HTN; risk may increase with higher trough levels. ILD may resolve with reduced doses or with drug discontinuation.

Boxed Warning Fatal bronchial anastomotic dehiscence has been reported in patients with lung transplants when sirolimus has been used as part of an immunosuppressive regimen. Safety and effectiveness of sirolimus as immunosuppressive therapy haven't been established in patients with liver or lung transplants. Use in these patients isn't recommended. ∎

Boxed Warning Using this drug with tacrolimus or cyclosporine may cause hepatic artery thrombosis, leading to graft loss and death in patients with liver transplants. ∎

Boxed Warning Patients taking drug are more susceptible to infection, lymphoma, and other malignancies. ∎

Dialyzable drug: No.

⚠ *Overdose S&S:* Exaggerated adverse effects.

PREGNANCY-LACTATION-REPRODUCTION

• There are no adequate studies during pregnancy; drug may cause fetal harm. Patient of childbearing potential must use effective contraception before and during therapy and for 12 weeks after therapy ends.

• It isn't known if drug appears in human milk. Patient should discontinue breastfeeding or discontinue drug, considering importance of drug to patient.

• Drug affects male and female fertility. In most cases, azoospermia has been reversible when drug is discontinued.

NURSING CONSIDERATIONS

Boxed Warning Only those experienced in immunosuppressive therapy and management of patients with kidney transplants should prescribe drug. Manage patients receiving drug in facilities equipped and staffed with adequate lab and supportive medical resources. ■

❻ **Alert:** Drugs causing immunosuppression increase risk of opportunistic infections, including activation of latent viral infections such as BK virus-associated neuropathy, which may lead to serious outcomes, including kidney graft loss.

❻ **Alert:** Drug has been associated with hypersensitivity reactions, including anaphylactic reactions, angioedema, exfoliative dermatitis, and hypersensitivity vasculitis. Monitor patient closely.

• Use drug in regimen with cyclosporine and corticosteroids. After 2 to 4 months of combined therapy in patients who are at low-to-moderate risk, wean off cyclosporine as cyclosporine inhibits the metabolism and transport of sirolimus. Sirolimus levels may decrease when cyclosporine is discontinued unless the sirolimus dosage is increased.

⚗ Cyclosporine withdrawal in patients with high risk of graft rejection isn't recommended. This includes patients with Banff grade III acute rejection or vascular rejection before cyclosporine withdrawal, those who are dialysis dependent, those with serum creatinine level greater than 4.5 mg/dL, patients who are Black, patients with retransplants or multiorgan transplants, and patients with high panel of reactive antibodies.

• After transplantation, give antimicrobial prophylaxis for *Pneumocystis jiroveci* for 1 year and for CMV for 3 months.

• Monitor kidney function tests, including urine protein levels. Adjustment of immunosuppressive regimen may be needed.

• Monitor cholesterol and triglyceride levels. Treat with lipid-lowering drugs (as indicated), diet, and exercise.

• Assess for rhabdomyolysis.

• Monitor drug levels closely in patients ages 13 and older who weigh less than 40 kg, patients with liver impairment, those also receiving strong CYP3A4 inducers or inhibitors, after dosage change, and after cyclosporine dosing is markedly reduced or stopped.

• Monitor patient for impaired or delayed wound healing (including wound dehiscence), fluid accumulation (including edema, lymphedema, pleural effusion, ascites, pericardial effusion), and malignancies (including skin carcinoma).

PATIENT TEACHING

• Teach patient how to properly store, dilute, and give drug.

• Advise patient to report adverse effects and that drug may increase risk of infections and certain cancers.

• Alert patient of childbearing potential about risks during pregnancy and to use effective contraception before and during therapy and for 12 weeks after final dose.

• Inform patient that drug may impair fertility.

• Caution patient to wash area with soap and water if drug solution touches skin or mucous membranes.

• Advise patient to limit UV light and sun exposure because of the increased risk of skin cancer.

SITagliptin phosphate
sit-a-GLIP-tin

Januvia

Therapeutic class: Antidiabetics
Pharmacologic class: DPP-4 enzyme inhibitors

AVAILABLE FORMS
Tablets: 25 mg, 50 mg, 100 mg

INDICATIONS & DOSAGES

➤ **To improve glycemic control in addition to diet and exercise in patients with type 2 diabetes, alone or in combination therapy**
Adults: 100 mg PO once daily.

Adjust-a-dose: For patients with eGFR of 30 to less than 45 mL/minute/1.73 m^2, give 50 mg once daily; for patients with eGFR less than 30 mL/minute/1.73 m^2, give 25 mg once daily. Give without regard to timing of dialysis session.

ADMINISTRATION
PO
• Give drug without regard for food.

ACTION
Inhibits DPP-4, an enzyme that rapidly inactivates incretin hormones, which play a part in the body's regulation of glucose. By increasing and prolonging active incretin levels, the drug helps to increase insulin release and decrease circulating glucose.

S

Route	Onset	Peak	Duration
PO	Rapid	1–4 hr	Unknown

Half-life: About 12.5 hours.

ADVERSE REACTIONS
CNS: headache. **CV:** edema. **EENT:** nasopharyngitis. **GI:** abdominal pain, nausea, diarrhea. **Metabolic:** *hypoglycemia.* **Respiratory:** URI.

INTERACTIONS
Drug-drug. *Insulin, insulin secretagogues:* May increase risk of hypoglycemia. Dosage adjustment of these drugs may be required.

EFFECTS ON LAB TEST RESULTS
• May increase creatinine level.
• May increase WBC count.

CONTRAINDICATIONS & CAUTIONS
• Contraindicated in patients with type 1 diabetes or diabetic ketoacidosis.
• Consider risk and benefits before initiating drug in patients at risk for HF.
• Contraindicated in patients with history of hypersensitivity to sitagliptin. Angioedema, anaphylaxis, and exfoliative skin conditions such as SJS have been reported, some after first dose or up to 3 months after drug initiation.
• Bullous pemphigoid has been reported in patients taking DPP-4 inhibitors.
• Use cautiously in older adults, in patients with kidney insufficiency, and in those taking other antidiabetics.
• Drug may increase risk of pancreatitis. Safe use in patients with a history of pancreatitis hasn't been evaluated.
• Safety and effectiveness in children haven't been evaluated.
Dializable drug: 13.5%.

PREGNANCY-LACTATION-REPRODUCTION
• There are no adequate studies during pregnancy. Agents other than sitagliptin are recommended. Use only if clearly needed.
• Report prenatal exposure to the Januvia Pregnancy Registry (1-800-986-8999).
• It isn't known if drug appears in human milk. Use cautiously during breastfeeding.

NURSING CONSIDERATIONS
• Assess kidney function before start of therapy and periodically thereafter.

• Monitor HbA$_{1c}$ level periodically to assess long-term glycemic control.
• Management of type 2 diabetes should include diet control. Because caloric restrictions, weight loss, and exercise help improve insulin sensitivity and help make drug therapy effective, these measures are essential for proper diabetes management.
• Watch for hypoglycemia, especially in patients receiving combination therapy.
• Monitor patient for pancreatitis. Discontinue drug for suspected pancreatitis.
• Monitor patient for skin blistering or erosions. Discontinue drug for suspected bullous pemphigoid and consider referral to a dermatologist.
• Drug may cause joint pain that can be severe and disabling. Report severe and persistent joint pain to prescriber; drug may need to be discontinued.
• ***Look alike–sound alike:*** Don't confuse sitagliptin with saxagliptin.

PATIENT TEACHING
• Tell patient that drug isn't a substitute for diet and exercise and that it's important to follow a prescribed dietary and physical activity routine and to monitor glucose level.
• Instruct patient to immediately report signs and symptoms of pancreatitis (persistent, severe abdominal pain that may radiate to the back, with or without vomiting).
• Inform patient and family members of signs and symptoms of hyperglycemia and hypoglycemia and steps to take if these symptoms occur.
• Advise patient to report all adverse reactions, and to immediately report signs and symptoms of hypersensitivity (rash, swelling of the face).
• Teach patient to notify prescriber if signs or symptoms of HF develop (shortness of breath, rapid weight increase, or swelling of the feet).
• Instruct patient that during periods of stress (fever, trauma, infection, or surgery), medication requirements may change and dosage adjustments may be needed. Advise patient to seek medical advice promptly.
• Advise patient to immediately report new or worsening joint pain that's severe and persistent because drug may need to be discontinued.
• Provide patient with information on complications associated with diabetes and ways to assess for them.

- Tell patient drug may be taken without regard for food.
- Caution patient to immediately report pregnancy, plans to become pregnant, breastfeeding, or intent to breastfeed during treatment.

sodium ferric gluconate complex
Ferrlecit

Therapeutic class: Iron supplements
Pharmacologic class: Macromolecular iron complexes–hematinics

AVAILABLE FORMS
Injection: 62.5 mg elemental iron (12.5 mg/mL) in 5-mL vials*

INDICATIONS & DOSAGES
➤ **Iron deficiency anemia in patients with CKD receiving long-term hemodialysis and supplemental erythropoietin**
Adults and children older than age 15: 10 mL (125 mg elemental iron) IV per dialysis session. Most patients need minimum cumulative dose of 1 g elemental iron given over more than eight sequential dialysis treatments to achieve a favorable Hb or hematocrit response.
Children ages 6 to 15: 1.5 mg/kg of elemental iron (maximum 125 mg/dose) IV over 1 hour per dialysis session. Maximum dosage, 125 mg per dose.

ADMINISTRATION
IV
▼ Drug contains benzyl alcohol. Don't use in neonates.
▼ For adults, dilute in 100 mL NSS; for children, dilute in 25 mL NSS. Give immediately over 1 hour.
▼ Alternatively, give to adults undiluted at a rate not to exceed 1 mL/minute (12.5 mg of elemental iron/minute) per dialysis session.
▼ **Incompatibilities:** Other IV drugs. Don't add drug to parenteral nutrition solutions for infusion.

ACTION
Restores total body iron content, which is critical for normal Hb synthesis and oxygen transport.

Route	Onset	Peak	Duration
IV	Unknown	Varies	Unknown

Half-life: 1 hour in healthy, iron-deficient adults.

ADVERSE REACTIONS
CNS: asthenia, headache, fatigue, malaise, dizziness, paresthesia, agitation, somnolence, syncope, pain, fever, light-headedness, weakness, decreased level of consciousness. **CV:** hypotension, HTN, tachycardia, *bradycardia,* angina, chest pain, *MI,* edema, vasodilation, *thrombosis.* **EENT:** conjunctivitis, abnormal vision, rhinitis, pharyngitis, deafness, eye disorders. **GI:** anorexia, nausea, vomiting, diarrhea, rectal disorder, dyspepsia, belching, flatulence, *melena,* abdominal pain. **GU:** UTI, menorrhagia. **Hematologic:** anemia, abnormal erythrocytes, leukocytosis. **Metabolic:** *hyperkalemia, hypoglycemia, hypokalemia,* hypervolemia. **Musculoskeletal:** myalgia, arthralgia, back pain, arm pain, cramps. **Respiratory:** dyspnea, cough, URI, pneumonia, pulmonary edema. **Skin:** pruritus, diaphoresis, rash, injection-site reaction. **Other:** infection, chills, rigors, flulike syndrome, *sepsis, carcinoma,* lymphadenopathy.

INTERACTIONS
Drug-drug. *ACE inhibitors:* May increase risk of ferric gluconate adverse effects, including sensitivity reactions. Monitor patient closely.
Oral iron preparations: May reduce absorption of oral iron preparations. Avoid using together.

EFFECTS ON LAB TEST RESULTS
- May increase serum ferritin level and transferrin saturation.
- May decrease glucose level.
- May increase or decrease potassium level.
- May increase Hb level and hematocrit.
- May increase leukocyte count.

CONTRAINDICATIONS & CAUTIONS
- Contraindicated in patients hypersensitive to drug or its components (such as benzyl alcohol) and in those with iron overload or anemias not related to iron deficiency.
- Avoid use in patients with iron overload, which often occurs in hemoglobinopathies and other refractory anemias.
- Use cautiously in older adults.
- Safety and effectiveness in children younger than age 6 haven't been established.
⟳ **Alert:** Drug contains benzyl alcohol, which is associated with adverse events and death in

S

neonates and infants, including fatal gasping syndrome.

Dialyzable drug: No.

PREGNANCY-LACTATION-REPRODUCTION

• There are no adequate studies during pregnancy. Drug may increase fetal risk due to hypersensitivity reactions and benzyl alcohol exposure. Use only if clearly needed.

• It isn't known if drug appears in human milk and drug contains benzyl alcohol. Use alternative iron replacement therapy during breastfeeding.

NURSING CONSIDERATIONS

❂ *Alert:* Dosage is expressed in milligrams of elemental iron.

❂ *Alert:* Before administering, assess patients for history of reactions to iron products.

❂ *Alert:* Life-threatening hypersensitivity reactions, such as CV collapse, cardiac arrest, bronchospasm, oral or pharyngeal edema, dyspnea, angioedema, urticaria, and pruritus (sometimes linked to pain and muscle spasm of the chest or back) may occur during infusion. Monitor patients closely during infusion and for at least 30 minutes after infusion until clinically stable. Ensure that emergency measures to treat anaphylaxis are immediately available.

❂ *Alert:* Closely monitor patients during and after drug administration for profound hypotension with flushing, light-headedness, malaise, fatigue, weakness, or severe chest, back, flank, or groin pain; these symptoms may be associated with hypersensitivity reactions and usually resolve within 2 hours.

• Monitor ferritin level, iron saturation, Hb level, and hematocrit.

• Check with patient about other potential sources of iron, such as OTC iron preparations and iron-containing multiple vitamins with minerals.

PATIENT TEACHING

• Teach patient to immediately report all adverse reactions, especially those occurring during and after the infusion.

• Abdominal pain, diarrhea, vomiting, drowsiness, and rapid breathing may indicate iron poisoning. Urge patient to notify prescriber immediately.

sodium zirconium cyclosilicate

SOE-dee-um zir-KOE-nee-um SYE-kloe-sil-i-kate

Lokelma

Therapeutic class: Antidotes
Pharmacologic class: Potassium binders

AVAILABLE FORMS

Powder for oral suspension: 5-g, 10-g packets

INDICATIONS & DOSAGES

➤ **Hyperkalemia**

Adults: Initially, 10 g PO t.i.d. for up to 48 hours. For maintenance treatment, give 10 g PO once daily.

Adjust-a-dose: Monitor serum potassium level and adjust dosage based on target potassium level range. During maintenance treatment, titrate dosage based on potassium level at intervals of 1 week or longer, in increments of 5 g. Decrease dosage or stop drug if potassium level falls below desired target range.

Adults on KRT: Initially, 5 g PO once daily on nondialysis days. For potassium level greater than 6.5 mEq/L, start at 10 mg PO on non-dialysis days.

Adjust-a-dose: Monitor serum potassium level and adjust dosage based on predialysis serum potassium value after the long interdialytic interval and desired target range. During initiation and after a dosage adjustment, assess serum potassium level after 1 week. Recommended maintenance dosage ranges from 5 to 15 g once daily on non-dialysis days. Discontinue drug or decrease dosage if serum potassium level falls below desired target range based on the predialysis value after the long interdialytic interval, or patient develops clinically significant hypokalemia.

ADMINISTRATION

PO

• Empty entire contents of packet(s) into a glass containing at least 3 tablespoons of water or more if desired, stir well, and have patient drink immediately. If powder remains in the glass, add water, stir, and have patient drink immediately. Repeat until no powder remains.

- Give other oral medications at least 2 hours before or 2 hours after giving sodium zirconium cyclosilicate.
- Store at 59° to 86° F (15° to 30° C).

ACTION

A potassium binder that preferentially exchanges potassium for hydrogen and sodium. Increases fecal potassium excretion through binding potassium in lumen of GI tract; reduces concentration of free potassium in GI lumen and lowers serum potassium levels.

Route	Onset	Peak	Duration
PO	1 hr	Unknown	Unknown

Half-life: Unknown.

ADVERSE REACTIONS

CV: edema. **Metabolic:** *hypokalemia.*

INTERACTIONS

Drug-drug. *Drugs with pH-dependent solubility (atorvastatin, clopidogrel, dabigatran, furosemide):* May increase or decrease efficacy of coadministered drugs with pH-dependent solubility. Separate drug administration from other oral medications by at least 2 hours.

EFFECTS ON LAB TEST RESULTS

- May increase bicarbonate level.
- May decrease potassium level.

CONTRAINDICATIONS & CAUTIONS

- **⚠ Alert:** Drug shouldn't be used as emergency treatment for life-threatening hyperkalemia because of its delayed onset of action.
- Drug hasn't been studied in patients with GI motility disorders (severe constipation, bowel obstruction or impaction, postoperative bowel motility disorders). Avoid use in these patients as drug may worsen GI conditions.
- Safety and effectiveness in children haven't been established.

Dialyzable drug: No.

⚠ Overdose S&S: Hypokalemia.

PREGNANCY-LACTATION-REPRODUCTION

- Drug isn't absorbed systemically and isn't expected to result in fetal exposure.
- Breastfeeding isn't expected to result in exposure of infant to drug.

NURSING CONSIDERATIONS

- Monitor potassium level; adjust dosage based on serum potassium level and desired target range.
- Monitor patient for signs and symptoms of edema, especially in patients who should restrict sodium intake or are prone to fluid overload (HF, kidney disease). Each 5-g dose contains 400 mg of sodium. Adjust dietary sodium, if appropriate, and increase diuretic dosage as needed.
- Drug has radioopaque properties and may appear like an imaging agent during abdominal X-ray procedures.

PATIENT TEACHING

- Teach patient to report all adverse reactions.
- Stress importance of drinking the entire dose.
- Advise patient taking other oral medications to separate dosing of drug by at least 2 hours (before or after).
- Instruct patient to adjust dietary sodium, if appropriate.

---

sofosbuvir ⚕
soe-FOS-bue-vir

Sovaldi

Therapeutic class: Antivirals
Pharmacologic class: Nucleotide analogue NS5B polymerase inhibitors

AVAILABLE FORMS

Oral pellets: 150 mg, 200 mg
Tablets: 200 mg, 400 mg

INDICATIONS & DOSAGES

Adjust-a-dose (for all indications): Sofosbuvir dosage reduction isn't recommended. Discontinue sofosbuvir if concomitant antivirals are stopped. Adjust concomitant ribavirin or peginterferon alfa dosage if GFR is less than 50 mL/minute or liver decompensation or adverse reactions occur. Refer to manufacturer's instructions for ribavirin or peginterferon alfa dosage adjustments.

➤ **Chronic HCV infection (genotype 1 or 4), as component of combination antiviral regimen in patients who are treatment-naive without cirrhosis or with compensated cirrhosis (Child-Pugh class A)** ⚕
Adults: 400 mg PO daily with peginterferon alfa and ribavirin for 12 weeks. For patients

with HCV genotype 1 who can't receive interferon, give 400 mg PO daily with ribavirin for 24 weeks.

➤ **Chronic HCV infection (genotype 2), as part of combination antiviral regimen in patients who are treatment-naive or treatment-experienced without cirrhosis or with compensated cirrhosis (Child-Pugh class A)** ⊗

Adults and children ages 3 and older weighing at least 35 kg: 400 mg PO daily with ribavirin for 12 weeks.

Children ages 3 and older weighing 17 to less than 35 kg: 200 mg PO daily with ribavirin for 12 weeks.

Children ages 3 and older weighing less than 17 kg: 150 mg PO daily with ribavirin for 12 weeks.

➤ **Chronic HCV infection (genotype 3), as part of combination antiviral regimen in patients who are treatment-naive or treatment-experienced without cirrhosis or with compensated cirrhosis (Child-Pugh class A)** ⊗

Adults and children ages 3 and older weighing at least 35 kg: 400 mg PO daily with ribavirin for 24 weeks.

Children ages 3 and older weighing 17 to less than 35 kg: 200 mg PO daily with ribavirin for 24 weeks.

Children ages 3 and older weighing less than 17 kg: 150 mg PO daily with ribavirin for 24 weeks.

➤ **Chronic HCV infection with hepatocellular carcinoma in patients awaiting liver transplant**

Adults and children ages 3 and older: 400 mg PO daily with ribavirin for 48 weeks or until liver transplant.

ADMINISTRATION
PO

• Give without regard for food.
• Children unable to swallow tablets can use the pellet formulation.
• Patients shouldn't chew oral pellets. If giving without food, pour entire contents of packet directly in the mouth. Patients may drink water after swallowing pellets if needed. If giving with food, sprinkle pellets on one or more spoonfuls of nonacidic food (pudding, chocolate syrup, mashed potatoes, ice cream) at or below room temperature. Gently mix and give within 30 minutes. Patients should swallow entire contents without chewing to avoid a bitter aftertaste.

ACTION
Inhibits HCV NS5B RNA polymerase, inhibiting viral replication.

Route	Onset	Peak	Duration
PO	Unknown	0.5–2 hr	Unknown

Half-life: 0.4 hour.

ADVERSE REACTIONS
CNS: headache, insomnia, asthenia, fever, fatigue, irritability. **GI:** nausea, diarrhea, decreased appetite. **Hematologic:** anemia, **_neutropenia, thrombocytopenia._** **Hepatic:** hyperbilirubinemia. **Metabolic:** increased CK level. **Musculoskeletal:** myalgia. **Skin:** pruritus, rash. **Other:** flulike illness, chills.

INTERACTIONS
Drug-drug. ⊙ *Alert: Amiodarone:* May increase risk of symptomatic bradycardia, including cardiac arrest and cases requiring pacemaker intervention. Avoid use together. If use together can't be avoided, advise patient of risk and monitor carefully.
Anticonvulsants (carbamazepine, oxcarbazepine, phenobarbital, phenytoin, primidone), antimycobacterials (rifabutin, rifampin, rifapentine), HIV protease inhibitors (tipranavir, ritonavir): May decrease sofosbuvir level. Avoid use together.
Drug-herb. *St. John's wort:* May decrease sofosbuvir level. Discourage use together.

EFFECTS ON LAB TEST RESULTS
• May increase CK, bilirubin, and lipase levels.
• May decrease Hb level and neutrophil and platelet counts.

CONTRAINDICATIONS & CAUTIONS
• Contraindicated in patients hypersensitive to drug or its components.
• Refer to prescribing information for peginterferon alfa and ribavirin for contraindications when drug is given in these combination regimens.
Boxed Warning Reactivation of HBV may occur in patients coinfected with HCV and result in fulminant hepatitis, liver failure, and death. Screen all patients for current or prior HBV infection before treatment by measuring HBsAg and anti-HBc; if patient is positive for HBV infection, assess baseline HBV DNA. ∎

◆ *Alert:* Symptomatic bradycardia, including fatal cardiac arrest and cases requiring pacemaker intervention, has been reported when sofosbuvir is administered with amiodarone. Patients taking amiodarone who are also taking beta blockers or who have underlying cardiac comorbidities or advanced liver disease may be at increased risk. Signs and symptoms may occur within hours to up to 2 weeks after start of HCV therapy.

• Safety and effectiveness of drug haven't been studied in patients with eGFR of less than 30 mL/minute, or decompensated cirrhosis.

• Using in combination with other products containing sofosbuvir isn't recommended.

• Safety and effectiveness in children younger than age 3 with HCV genotype 2 or 3 and children with genotype 1 or 4 haven't been established.

Dialyzable drug: 18%.

PREGNANCY-LACTATION-REPRODUCTION

• Combination therapy with ribavirin is contraindicated in patients who are pregnant and in males whose partners are pregnant. Obtain baseline negative pregnancy test before start of therapy.

• Patients of childbearing potential and male patients with partners of childbearing potential must use two forms of effective nonhormonal contraception while receiving treatment regimens that include ribavirin and for 9 months for female patients or 6 months for male patients after therapy ends.

• Patients who are pregnant, are coinfected with HCV/HIV-1, and are taking concomitant antiretrovirals should enroll in the Antiretroviral Pregnancy Registry (1-800-258-4263).

• Combination therapy with ribavirin is contraindicated with breastfeeding. Patients must discontinue breastfeeding or discontinue drug.

NURSING CONSIDERATIONS

• Sofosbuvir isn't recommended as monotherapy. Always use as part of combination regimen.

• Refer to ribavirin or peginterferon alfa prescribing information for complete guidance on their concomitant use.

Boxed Warning Monitor patient with current or prior HBV infection for hepatitis flare or HBV reactivation with lab testing; watch for signs and symptoms of liver injury during active and posttreatment follow-up. ∎

◆ *Alert:* Monitor patients who must take amiodarone or who recently discontinued amiodarone for signs and symptoms of bradycardia (near-fainting or fainting, dizziness, light-headedness, malaise, weakness, excessive fatigue, shortness of breath, chest pain, confusion or memory problems). Inpatient cardiac monitoring should be utilized for first 48 hours, then outpatient monitoring for bradycardia should continue daily through at least first 2 weeks of treatment. Discontinue HCV treatment if signs or symptoms occur.

• Monitor blood counts and bilirubin, liver enzyme, and serum creatinine levels at baseline and periodically when clinically indicated.

• Monitor serum HCV-RNA level at baseline, during treatment, at end of treatment, during treatment follow-up, and when clinically indicated.

• Treatment response varies based on patient and viral factors. Monitor patient carefully.

PATIENT TEACHING

• Advise patient that using drug as single agent isn't recommended. Sofosbuvir must always be used in a combination regimen with ribavirin or peginterferon and ribavirin.

Boxed Warning Warn patient to immediately report signs and symptoms of liver injury (fatigue, weakness, loss of appetite, nausea, vomiting, yellowing of skin or eyes, light-colored stool). ∎

• Teach patient to immediately report signs and symptoms of hypersensitivity reaction (wheezing, chest tightness, fever, itching, heavy cough, blue-colored skin, seizures, or swelling of face, lips, tongue, or throat) and to seek medical attention.

◆ *Alert:* Caution patient to seek immediate medical attention for signs and symptoms of bradycardia.

• Explain to patient and partner the risk of birth defects, contraception requirements, and pregnancy testing related to therapy.

• Teach patient to report all signs and symptoms of adverse reactions, such as headache, dyspepsia, and insomnia.

• Caution patient not to use other medications while taking this drug without first notifying prescriber.

• Teach patient to keep drug in original container.

• Advise patient to report liver problems (other than HCV infection), history of liver transplant, severe kidney problems or dialysis, positive HIV status, or other medical conditions.

• Warn patient not to breastfeed while taking drug.

• Instruct patient not to discontinue drug without first discussing with prescriber.

sofosbuvir–velpatasvir
soe-FOS-bue-vir/vel-PAT-as-vir

Epclusa

Therapeutic class: Antivirals
Pharmacologic class: Nucleotide analogue NS5B polymerase inhibitors/HCV NS5A inhibitors

AVAILABLE FORMS
Oral pellets: 150 mg sofosbuvir and 37.5 mg velpatasvir, 200 mg sofosbuvir and 50 mg velpatasvir
Tablets: 200 mg sofosbuvir and 50 mg velpatasvir, 400 mg sofosbuvir and 100 mg velpatasvir

INDICATIONS & DOSAGES
➤ **Chronic HCV genotype 1, 2, 3, 4, 5, or 6 infection without cirrhosis or with compensated cirrhosis (Child-Pugh class A) or with decompensated cirrhosis (Child-Pugh class B or C) in combination with ribavirin**
Adults and children ages 3 and older weighing at least 30 kg: 400 mg sofosbuvir and 100 mg velpatasvir PO once daily for 12 weeks. Refer to manufacturer's instructions for ribavirin dosing, if prescribed.
Children ages 3 and older weighing 17 to less than 30 kg: 200 mg sofosbuvir and 50 mg velpatasvir PO once daily for 12 weeks. Refer to manufacturer's instructions for ribavirin dosing, if prescribed.
Children ages 3 and older weighing less than 17 kg: 150 mg sofosbuvir and 37.5 mg velpatasvir PO once daily for 12 weeks. Refer to manufacturer's instructions for ribavirin dosing, if prescribed.

ADMINISTRATION
PO
• Keep tablets in original container.
• May give without regard for food.

• Oral pellets can be taken directly in the mouth or given with food to increase palatability.
• Sprinkle oral pellets on one or more spoonfuls of nonacidic soft food (pudding, chocolate syrup, ice cream) at or below room temperature and give within 15 minutes of gently mixing.
• To avoid bitter aftertaste, patient shouldn't chew pellets.
• Store below 86° F (30° C).

ACTION
Sofosbuvir and velpatasvir are direct-acting antivirals that inhibit viral replication of HCV.

Route	Onset	Peak	Duration
PO (sofosbuvir)	Unknown	0.5–1 hr	Unknown
PO (velpatasvir)	Unknown	3 hr	Unknown

Half-life: Sofosbuvir, 0.5 hour; velpatasvir, 15 hours.

ADVERSE REACTIONS
CNS: headache, fatigue, asthenia, insomnia, irritability, depression. **GI:** nausea, vomiting, diarrhea. **Hematologic:** anemia. **Metabolic:** CK elevations, increased lipase level. **Skin:** rash.

INTERACTIONS
⊘ *Alert:* Sofosbuvir–velpatasvir interacts significantly with many drugs. Consult a drug interaction resource or pharmacist for more information.
Drug-drug. *Antacids (aluminum hydroxide, magnesium hydroxide):* May decrease velpatasvir level. Separate antacid and drug administration by 4 hours.
⊘ *Alert: Amiodarone:* May result in serious symptomatic bradycardia. Use together isn't recommended; if coadministration is necessary, monitor cardiac function.
Anticonvulsants (carbamazepine, oxcarbazepine, phenobarbital, phenytoin), antimycobacterial drugs (rifabutin, rifampin, rifapentine): May decrease levels of both antivirals. Avoid use together.
Atorvastatin, rosuvastatin: May significantly increase statin level and risk of rhabdomyolysis. Use together cautiously and monitor patient closely. Don't exceed a 10-mg dose of rosuvastatin.
Digoxin: May increase digoxin level. Monitor level and adjust digoxin dosage as needed.
Efavirenz: May decrease velpatasvir level. Use together isn't recommended.

H₂-receptor antagonists (famotidine): May decrease velpatasvir level. Give H₂-receptor antagonist simultaneously or 12 hours apart from drug at a dose that doesn't exceed an equivalent of famotidine 40 mg b.i.d.

Moderate to potent CYP2B6, CYP2C8, or CYP3A4 inducers (carbamazepine), P-gp inducers: May significantly decrease sofosbuvir or velpatasvir level, reducing therapeutic effect. Use together isn't recommended.

PPIs (omeprazole): May decrease velpatasvir level. Avoid use together, but if coadministration is necessary, give drug 4 hours before omeprazole 20 mg.

Substrates of P-gp, BCRP and OATP inhibitors (clarithromycin, cyclosporine, tacrolimus): May increase substrate level. Monitor therapy.

Tenofovir: May increase tenofovir level. Monitor patient for tenofovir-associated adverse reactions.

Tipranavir/ritonavir: May decrease levels of both antivirals. Avoid use together.

Topotecan: May increase topotecan level. Avoid use together.

Drug-herb. *St. John's wort:* May decrease antiviral levels and therapeutic effects. Discourage use together.

EFFECTS ON LAB TEST RESULTS
• May increase lipase, CK, and indirect bilirubin levels.
• May decrease Hb level.

CONTRAINDICATIONS & CAUTIONS
• Combination regimen with ribavirin is contraindicated in patients for whom ribavirin is contraindicated. Refer to ribavirin manufacturer's instructions for contraindications, warnings, and precautions.

Boxed Warning Reactivation of HBV infection may occur in patients coinfected with HCV, resulting in fulminant hepatitis, liver failure, and death. Screen all patients for current or prior HBV infection: measure HBsAg and anti-hepatitis B core antibody (anti-HBc) before treatment and, if positive for HBV infection, assess baseline HBV DNA level. ∎

🔵 *Alert:* Serious symptomatic bradycardia may occur in patients taking amiodarone, particularly in patients also taking beta blockers, in those with underlying cardiac comorbidities and in patients with advanced liver disease.

• Safety and effectiveness in children younger than age 3 haven't been established.

Dialyzable drug: Sofosbuvir active metabolite, 53%; velpatasvir, unlikely.

PREGNANCY-LACTATION-REPRODUCTION
• Use of sofosbuvir and velpatasvir in pregnancy hasn't been adequately studied. Use during pregnancy isn't recommended.
• Combination regimen with ribavirin is contraindicated in patients who are pregnant and in males whose partners are pregnant.
• Patients should be treated for HCV prior to considering pregnancy to optimize health of patient and fetus.
• Patients using combination treatment with ribavirin should use two effective forms of contraception during treatment and for 6 months (males) or 9 months (females) after therapy ends. Refer to ribavirin manufacturer's instructions for pregnancy testing before, during, and after therapy and for information about breastfeeding.
• It isn't known if sofosbuvir and velpatasvir and their metabolites appear in human milk or how they affect human milk production. Use cautiously, weighing benefits and risks.

NURSING CONSIDERATIONS
Boxed Warning Monitor patient with current or prior HBV infection for hepatitis flare or HBV reactivation with lab testing. Watch for signs and symptoms of liver injury during active therapy and posttreatment follow-up. ∎

🔵 *Alert:* For patients taking amiodarone (with or without beta blockers) who begin Epclusa, those who begin amiodarone while taking Epclusa, and those who discontinue amiodarone just before starting Epclusa, cardiac monitoring in an inpatient setting for first 48 hours of coadministration is recommended, followed by outpatient or self-monitoring of HR daily for at least 2 weeks.
• Monitor patient for bradycardia (near-fainting, syncope, dizziness, light-headedness, malaise, weakness, excessive fatigue, shortness of breath, chest pain, confusion, memory problems) and report immediately.
• Clinical and LFT monitoring, including direct bilirubin, is recommended for patients with decompensated cirrhosis taking Epclusa plus ribavirin.
• Monitor patient for anemia.

PATIENT TEACHING
Boxed Warning Warn patient to immediately report signs and symptoms of liver injury

(fatigue, weakness, loss of appetite, nausea, vomiting, yellowing of skin or eyes, and light-colored stool). ■

• Advise patient to report other prescription or OTC medications or herbal products being taken, including St. John's wort.

• Inform patient that it's important not to miss or skip doses and to take this medication for as long as prescriber recommends.

• Advise patient to avoid pregnancy during combination treatment with ribavirin and to contact prescriber immediately if pregnancy occurs.

۞ Alert: Counsel patient who is also taking amiodarone about the risk of symptomatic bradycardia. Teach patient to self-monitor HR. Caution patient to seek medical attention for signs and symptoms of bradycardia.

sofosbuvir–velpatasvir–voxilaprevir ۞

soe-FOS-bue-vir/vel-PAT-as-vir/ vox-i-LA-pre-vir

Vosevi

Therapeutic class: Antivirals
Pharmacologic class: Nucleotide analogue HCV NS5B polymerase inhibitors-NS5A inhibitors-NS3/4A protease inhibitors

AVAILABLE FORMS
Tablets: 400 mg sofosbuvir/100 mg velpatasvir/100 mg voxilaprevir

INDICATIONS & DOSAGES
➤ **Chronic HCV infection without cirrhosis or with compensated cirrhosis (Child-Pugh class A) in patients with genotype 1, 2, 3, 4, 5, or 6 infection who have previously been treated with an HCV regimen containing an NS5A inhibitor, or in patients with genotype 1a or 3 infection who have previously been treated with an HCV regimen containing sofosbuvir without an NS5A inhibitor** ۞
Adults: 1 tablet PO daily for 12 weeks.

ADMINISTRATION
PO
• Give with food to increase drug absorption.
• Store below 86° F (30° C) in original container.

ACTION
Sofosbuvir inhibits HCV NS5B RNA-dependent RNA polymerase, velpatasvir inhibits HCV NS5A protein, and voxilaprevir inhibits NS3/4A protease. All three work together to halt HCV viral replication.

Route	Onset	Peak	Duration
PO	Unknown	2 hr (sofosbuvir); 4 hr (velpatasvir, voxilaprevir)	Unknown

Half-life: Sofosbuvir, 0.5 hour; velpatasvir, 17 hours; voxilaprevir, 33 hours.

ADVERSE REACTIONS
CNS: headache, insomnia, asthenia, depression, fatigue. **GI:** diarrhea, nausea. **Hepatic:** hyperbilirubinemia. **Metabolic:** lipase elevation, CK elevation. **Skin:** rash.

INTERACTIONS
۞ Alert: Sofosbuvir–velpatasvir–voxilaprevir may interact significantly with many drugs. Consult a drug interaction resource or pharmacist for more information.

Drug-drug. ۞ Alert: *Amiodarone:* May increase risk of symptomatic bradycardia, including cardiac arrest and cases requiring pacemaker intervention. Avoid use together. If administration can't be avoided, advise patient of risk and monitor carefully.

Antacids: May decrease velpatasvir level. Separate antacids and drug by 4 hours.

Atazanavir, cyclosporine, lopinavir: May increase voxilaprevir level. Use together isn't recommended.

Atorvastatin, fluvastatin, lovastatin, simvastatin: May increase statin level. Avoid use together. If necessary, give lowest necessary statin dose based on risks and benefits.

Dabigatran: May increase dabigatran level, especially in patient with CrCl less than 45 mL/minute. Use cautiously together, monitor patient closely, and refer to dabigatran prescribing information for dosage adjustments.

Digoxin: May increase digoxin level. Use cautiously together and monitor digoxin level.

Efavirenz: May decrease velpatasvir and voxilaprevir levels. Use together isn't recommended.

H2-receptor antagonists (famotidine): May decrease velpatasvir level. Limit concurrent H2-receptor antagonist to equivalent of famotidine 40 mg b.i.d.

Moderate to potent CYP2B6, CYP2C8, or CYP3A4 inducers (carbamazepine, oxcarbazepine, phenobarbital, phenytoin, rifabutin, rifapentine), P-gp inducers: May significantly decrease sofosbuvir–velpatasvir–voxilaprevir level. Avoid use together.

Pitavastatin, rosuvastatin: May increase rosuvastatin and pitavastatin levels and risk of myopathy and rhabdomyolysis. Avoid use together.

PPIs (omeprazole): May decrease velpatasvir level. Limit omeprazole to a dose of 20 mg. Other PPIs haven't been studied.

Pravastatin: May increase pravastatin level and risk of myopathy and rhabdomyolysis. Limit pravastatin dose to 40 mg.

Rifampin: May decrease sofosbuvir–velpatasvir–voxilaprevir levels. Use together is contraindicated.

Substrates of BCRP, OATP1B1, OATP1B3, OATP2B1, P-gp (imatinib, irinotecan, lapatinib, methotrexate, mitoxantrone, sulfasalazine, topotecan): May decrease levels of these substrates. Avoid use together.

Tenofovir disoproxil fumarate: May increase tenofovir level, especially in patients with kidney impairment. Monitor patient for tenofovir-associated adverse reactions; refer to tenofovir prescribing information for dosage adjustments.

Tipranavir/ritonavir: May decrease sofosbuvir and velpatasvir levels. Avoid use together.

Drug-herb. *St. John's wort:* May significantly decrease sofosbuvir, velpatasvir, or voxilaprevir level. Discourage use together.

Drug-food. *Any food:* Increases drug levels. Give concurrently with food.

EFFECTS ON LAB TEST RESULTS

• May increase lipase, CK, and total bilirubin levels.

CONTRAINDICATIONS & CAUTIONS

Boxed Warning HBV reactivation has been reported, in some cases resulting in fulminant hepatitis, liver failure, and death. Test all patients for evidence of current or prior HBV infection before initiation of HCV treatment. ∎

❸ *Alert:* Use cautiously in patients with risk factors for liver failure (hepatocellular carcinoma, alcohol abuse).

❸ *Alert:* Symptomatic bradycardia, including fatal cardiac arrest and cases requiring pacemaker intervention, has been reported when amiodarone has been administered with a sofosbuvir-containing regimen. Patients taking amiodarone who are also taking beta

blockers or who have underlying cardiac co-morbidities or advanced liver disease may be at increased risk. Signs and symptoms may occur within hours or up to 2 weeks after start of HCV therapy.

• Drug isn't recommended in patients with Child-Pugh class B or C liver impairment.

• Dosage adjustment isn't recommended in patients with kidney impairment, including patients on dialysis.

• Safety and effectiveness in children haven't been established.

Dialyzable drug: Sofosbuvir metabolite, yes; velpatasvir and voxilaprevir, unlikely.

PREGNANCY-LACTATION-REPRODUCTION

• Drug hasn't been adequately studied during pregnancy. Use during pregnancy isn't recommended.

• Treatment of HCV infection should be completed prior to pregnancy to optimize health of patient and fetus.

• It isn't known if drug or its metabolites appear in human milk or affect milk production. Consider benefits and risks before use during breastfeeding.

NURSING CONSIDERATIONS

Boxed Warning Before initiating HCV treatment, test all patients for current or prior HBV infection by measuring HBsAg and hepatitis B core antibody (anti-HBc). ∎

Boxed Warning Monitor patients coinfected with HCV or HBV for HBV reactivation and hepatitis flare during HCV treatment and posttreatment follow-up. Manage HBV infection as clinically indicated. ∎

❸ *Alert:* Monitor closely for liver failure and discontinue drug in patients who develop signs and symptoms of decompensation.

❸ *Alert:* Administration with amiodarone isn't recommended. If these drugs must be used together or if amiodarone has been discontinued just before beginning HCV therapy, monitor patient for signs and symptoms of bradycardia (near-fainting, fainting, dizziness, light-headedness, malaise, weakness, excessive fatigue, shortness of breath, chest pain, confusion, or memory problems). Utilize inpatient cardiac monitoring for first 48 hours; outpatient monitoring of HR should continue daily for at least first 2 weeks of treatment. Discontinue drug if signs or symptoms of bradycardia occur.

• *Look alike–sound alike:* Don't confuse sofosbuvir–velpatasvir combination with sofosbuvir–velpatasvir–voxilaprevir combination.

PATIENT TEACHING
• Advise patient to report a history of HBV infection before therapy begins.

Boxed Warning Warn patient that therapy can increase risk of HBV reactivation and that lab testing for HBV exposure will be needed before therapy begins. ∎
• Explain that for therapy to be effective, patient needs to take drug exactly as prescribed for the entire duration.
• Caution patient not to stop treatment without first discussing with prescriber.
• *Alert:* Caution patient to seek immediate medical attention for signs and symptoms of bradycardia.
• *Alert:* Warn patient to immediately report signs and symptoms of liver injury (fatigue, weakness, loss of appetite, nausea, vomiting, yellowing of skin or eyes, light-colored stool).
• Caution patient to immediately report pregnancy or breastfeeding to prescriber.

solifenacin succinate
sole-ah-FEN-ah-sin

VESIcare, VESIcare LS

Therapeutic class: Urinary antispasmodics
Pharmacologic class: Antimuscarinics

AVAILABLE FORMS
Oral suspension: 1 mg/mL
Tablets (film-coated): 5 mg, 10 mg

INDICATIONS & DOSAGES
➤ **Overactive bladder with urinary urgency, frequency, and urge incontinence**
Adults: 5 mg PO once daily. If well-tolerated, may increase to 10 mg once daily.
Adjust-a-dose: For patients with CrCl less than 30 mL/minute or Child-Pugh class B liver impairment, or if drug is taken concurrently with CYP3A4 inhibitors, maximum dose is 5 mg.
➤ **Neurogenic detrusor overactivity (oral suspension)**
Children ages 2 and older weighing 60 kg or more: Initially, 5 mg PO once daily. May

titrate to lowest effective dose; maximum daily dose, 10 mg.
Children ages 2 and older weighing more than 45 to 60 kg: Initially, 4 mg PO once daily. May titrate to lowest effective dose; maximum daily dose, 8 mg.
Children ages 2 and older weighing more than 30 to 45 kg: Initially, 3 mg PO once daily. May titrate to lowest effective dose; maximum daily dose, 6 mg.
Children ages 2 and older weighing more than 15 to 30 kg: Initially, 3 mg PO once daily. May titrate to lowest effective dose; maximum daily dose, 5 mg.
Children ages 2 and older weighing 9 to 15 kg: Initially, 2 mg PO once daily. May titrate to lowest effective dose; maximum daily dose, 4 mg.
Adjust-a-dose: Don't exceed recommended initial dose in children with CrCl less than 30 mL/minute or Child-Pugh class B liver impairment, or in those taking concomitant CYP3A4 inhibitors.

ADMINISTRATION
PO
• Give drug without regard for food.
• Patient should swallow tablet whole with water.
• Follow oral suspension dose with liquid, such as water or milk.
• Omit a missed tablet dose; give the next dose as scheduled.
• Give a missed dose of oral solution as soon as possible within 12 hours of missed dose. If more than 12 hours elapse, skip missed dose.

ACTION
Relaxes smooth muscle of bladder by antagonizing muscarinic receptors, relieving symptoms of overactive bladder.

Route	Onset	Peak	Duration
PO	Unknown	3–8 hr (tablets); 2–6 hr (oral suspension)	Unknown

Half-life: Tablets, 45 to 68 hours; oral suspension, 26 hours.

ADVERSE REACTIONS
CNS: depression, dizziness, fatigue. **CV:** HTN, leg swelling. **EENT:** blurred vision, dry eyes, dry mouth, pharyngitis. **GI:** constipation, dyspepsia, nausea, upper abdominal pain, vomiting. **GU:** urine retention, UTI. **Respiratory:** cough. **Other:** influenza.

INTERACTIONS

Drug-drug. *Drugs that prolong QT interval (amiodarone, haloperidol, macrolides, fluoroquinolones):* May increase risk of serious cardiac arrhythmias. Use together isn't recommended.

Other anticholinergic drugs (dicyclomine, scopolamine, diphenhydramine): May increase risk of adverse effects. Monitor therapy.

Potassium chloride (solid oral dosage forms only): May increase ulcer risk. Avoid using solid oral dosage forms of potassium chloride.

Strong CYP3A4 inducers (carbamazepine, phenobarbital, phenytoin): May decrease solifenacin level. Monitor therapy.

Strong CYP3A4 inhibitors (ketoconazole): May increase solifenacin level. Don't exceed solifenacin starting dose when used together.

EFFECTS ON LAB TEST RESULTS

None reported.

CONTRAINDICATIONS & CAUTIONS

• Contraindicated in patients hypersensitive to drug or its components and in patients with urine or gastric retention or uncontrolled narrow-angle glaucoma.

• Drug isn't recommended for use in patients with Child-Pugh class C liver impairment.

• Angioedema has been reported, including after first dose.

• Use cautiously in older adults and in patients with a history of prolonged QT interval, those being treated for angle-closure glaucoma, and those with bladder outflow obstruction, decreased GI motility, kidney insufficiency, or Child-Pugh class B liver impairment.

Dialyzable drug: Unknown.

⚠ **Overdose S&S:** Anticholinergic effects (fixed and dilated pupils, blurred vision, failure of heel-to-toe exam, tremors, dry skin).

PREGNANCY-LACTATION-REPRODUCTION

• There are no adequate studies during pregnancy. Use only if potential benefit justifies fetal risk.

• It isn't known if drug appears in human milk. Use cautiously during breastfeeding after considering risks to the infant.

NURSING CONSIDERATIONS

• Assess bladder function, and monitor drug effects.

• Watch for urine retention in patient with bladder outlet obstruction.

• Monitor patient for decreased gastric motility and constipation.

• Monitor patient for signs and symptoms of anticholinergic CNS effects (including headache, confusion, hallucinations, and somnolence), particularly after beginning treatment or increasing dosage. If patient experiences CNS effects, consider dosage reduction or drug discontinuation.

PATIENT TEACHING

• Explain that drug may cause blurred vision and drowsiness. Tell patient not to drive, operate heavy machinery, or perform hazardous activities or tasks until effects of the drug are known.

• Discourage use of other drugs that may cause dry mouth, constipation, urine retention, or blurred vision.

• Teach patient safe drug administration.

• Urge patient to report all adverse reactions, especially swelling in the face, lips, or tongue or abdominal pain or constipation that lasts 3 days or longer.

• Tell patient that drug decreases the ability to sweat normally, and advise cautious use in hot environments or during strenuous activity.

---

somatropin ⚛
soe-ma-TROE-pin

Genotropin, Humatrope, Norditropin, Nutropin AQ, Omnitrope, Saizen, Serostim, Zomacton, Zorbtive

Therapeutic class: Growth hormones
Pharmacologic class: Anterior pituitary hormones

AVAILABLE FORMS

Genotropin injection: 5 mg and 12 mg in two-chamber pen cartridges

Genotropin MiniQuick injection (preservative-free): 0.2 mg, 0.4 mg, 0.6 mg, 0.8 mg, 1 mg, 1.2 mg, 1.4 mg, 1.6 mg, 1.8 mg, 2 mg in two-chamber pen cartridges

Humatrope injection: 5 mg vial; 6 mg, 12 mg, 24 mg pen cartridges

Norditropin injection: 5 mg/1.5 mL, 10 mg/1.5 mL, 15 mg/1.5 mL, 30 mg/3 mL prefilled pens

Nutropin AQ injection: 5 mg/2-mL device, 10 mg/2-mL device or pen, 20 mg/2-mL device or pen

Omnitrope injection: 5.8 mg/vial; 5 mg/ 1.5 mL, 10 mg/1.5 mL pen cartridge

Saizen injection: 5 mg, 8.8 mg vials

Serostim injection: 5 mg, 6 mg single-dose vials; 4 mg multidose vial

Zomacton injection: 5 mg*, 10 mg vials

Zorbtive injection: 8.8 mg vials

INDICATIONS & DOSAGES

➤ **Long-term treatment of growth failure in children with inadequate secretion of endogenous growth hormone (GH)**

Children: 0.18 to 0.3 mg/kg/week Humatrope subcut, divided into equal doses given six to seven times weekly. Or, up to 0.3 mg/kg Nutropin AQ subcut weekly in daily divided doses; in patients who are pubertal, a weekly dosage of up to 0.7 mg/kg (Nutropin AQ) in daily divided doses may be used. Or, Saizen 0.18 mg/kg/week subcut divided into equal doses given on 3 alternate days six times per week or daily. Or, Norditropin 0.024 to 0.034 mg/kg/day subcut given on 6 or 7 days each week. Or, 0.16 to 0.24 mg/kg Genotropin or Omnitrope subcut weekly divided into six or seven doses. Or, 0.18 to 0.3 mg/kg/week Zomacton divided into equal doses given 3, 6, or 7 days per week.

➤ **Replacement of endogenous GH in adults with GH deficiency**

Adults: Initially, not more than 0.006 mg/kg Humatrope or Zomacton subcut daily. May increase to maximum of 0.0125 mg/kg Humatrope or Zomacton daily. Or, initially 0.004 mg/kg Norditropin subcut daily. May increase Norditropin to maximum of 0.016 mg/kg daily after about 6 weeks.

Or, initially, not more than 0.006 mg/kg Nutropin AQ subcut daily. May increase dosage to maximum of 0.025 mg/kg daily in patients younger than age 35 or 0.0125 mg/kg daily in patients older than age 35. Or, starting dosages not exceeding 0.04 mg/kg Genotropin or Omnitrope subcut weekly divided into six or seven equal doses; may increase at 4- to 8-week intervals to a maximum dose of 0.08 mg/kg subcut weekly divided into six or seven equal doses. Or, initially, not more than 0.005 mg/kg Saizen subcut daily. May increase after 4 weeks to a maximum dose of 0.01 mg/kg daily based on patient tolerance and clinical response.

Or, non-weight-based dosing: Initially, 0.2 mg Genotropin, Humatrope, Norditropin, Nutropin, Saizen or Zomacton subcut daily (range 0.15 to 0.3 mg/day); may increase by 0.1 to 0.2 mg/day every 1 to 2 months based on clinical response and insulin-like growth factor-1 level.

➤ **Growth failure from CKD up to time of kidney transplantation**

Children: Up to 0.35 mg/kg/week Nutropin AQ subcut divided into daily doses.

➤ **Long-term treatment of short stature from Turner syndrome**

Children: Up to 0.375 mg/kg/week Humatrope or Nutropin AQ subcut, divided into equal doses given three to seven times weekly. Or, up to 0.375 mg/kg/week Zomacton subcut divided into equal doses given three, six, or seven times weekly. Or, up to 0.067 mg/ kg/day Norditropin subcut given on 6 or 7 days each week. Or, 0.33 mg/kg/week Genotropin or Omnitrope divided into six or seven once-daily subcut injections per week.

➤ **Short stature in children with Noonan syndrome (Norditropin only)**

Children: Up to 0.46 mg/kg subcut weekly, divided into six or seven equal daily doses.

➤ **Long-term treatment of growth failure in children with Prader-Willi syndrome diagnosed by genetic testing**

Children: 0.24 mg/kg Genotropin, Norditropin, or Omnitrope subcut weekly divided into six or seven equal daily doses. Individualize dosage based on growth response.

➤ **Long-term treatment of growth failure in children born small for gestational age (SGA) who don't catch up by age 2**

Children: 0.48 mg/kg Genotropin or Omnitrope subcut weekly divided into six or seven doses.

➤ **Short stature in children born SGA who don't catch up by age 2 to 4**

Children: Up to 0.067 mg/kg/day Norditropin or Humatrope subcut given on 6 or 7 days each week. Or, up to 0.47 mg/kg/week Zomacton divided into three, six, or seven equal doses.

➤ **Idiopathic short stature**

Children: Up to 0.37 mg/kg Humatrope subcut weekly divided into six or seven equal doses or Zomacton divided into three, six, or seven equal doses. Or, up to 0.47 mg/kg/week Genotropin, Omnitrope, or Norditropin subcut divided into six or seven equal doses. Or, up to 0.3 mg/kg/week Nutropin AQ subcut divided into equal daily doses.

➤ **Short stature or growth failure in children with short stature homeobox-containing (SHOX) gene deficiency** ⚥
Children: 0.35 mg/kg Humatrope subcut weekly divided into six or seven equal doses or Zomacton divided into three, six, or seven equal doses.

➤ **Short bowel syndrome (Zorbtive only)**
Adults: 0.1 mg/kg/day subcut daily for 4 weeks. Maximum dosage, 8 mg/day.

Adjust-a-dose: For moderate toxicity, treat symptomatically with analgesics or reduce dosage to 0.05 mg/kg/day; maximum dosage, 4 mg/day).

➤ **HIV wasting or cachexia (Serostim only)**
Adults and children weighing more than 55 kg: 6 mg subcut daily at bedtime.
Adults and children weighing 45 to 55 kg: 5 mg subcut daily at bedtime.
Adults and children weighing 35 to 45 kg: 4 mg subcut daily at bedtime.
Adults and children weighing less than 35 kg: 0.1 mg/kg/day subcut daily at bedtime.

ADMINISTRATION

• Refer to product insert for brand-specific reconstitution and preparation instructions.

Subcutaneous

⚠ *Alert:* Don't use products containing benzyl alcohol in neonates or if patient has a known benzyl alcohol sensitivity.

⚠ *Alert:* When administering to newborn, reconstitute with sterile water for injection.

• After reconstitution, make sure solution is clear. Don't inject solution if it's cloudy or contains particles.

• For patients on hemodialysis, give drug before bedtime or at least 3 to 4 hours after dialysis. For long-term cycling peritoneal dialysis, give drug in the morning after completion of dialysis. For long-term ambulatory peritoneal dialysis, give drug in the evening at the time of the overnight exchange.

• Rotate injection sites to avoid tissue atrophy.

• Store reconstituted drug in refrigerator; use within manufacturer's recommended time frame for each drug. Preservative-free preparations should be used immediately and unused portion discarded.

• If patient develops sensitivity to diluent, reconstitute drug with sterile water for injection. When drug is reconstituted in this way, use only one reconstituted dose per vial,

refrigerate solution if it isn't used immediately after reconstitution, use reconstituted dose within 24 hours, and discard unused portion.

ACTION

Purified GH of recombinant DNA origin that stimulates skeletal, linear, muscle, and organ growth.

Route	Onset	Peak	Duration
Subcut	Unknown	Varies by brand	18–20 hr

Half-life: Varies by brand. Refer to manufacturer's drug label.

ADVERSE REACTIONS

CNS: headache, pain, hypoesthesia, paresthesia, fatigue, fever, depression, insomnia. **CV:** edema, chest pain, HTN. **EENT:** periorbital edema, otitis media, pharyngitis, rhinitis, sinusitis, tonsillitis. **GI:** nausea, vomiting, flatulence, abdominal pain, gastritis. **GU:** UTI. **Hematologic:** eosinophilia, anemia. **Hepatic:** increased transaminase level. **Metabolic:** mild hyperglycemia, hypothyroidism, impaired glucose tolerance, hyperlipidemia, new or worsening diabetes. **Musculoskeletal:** arthralgia, carpal tunnel syndrome, myalgia, new or exacerbated scoliosis, limb pain, bone pain, limb stiffness, abnormal bone growth. **Respiratory:** URI, bronchitis, dyspnea. **Skin:** injection-site pain or reaction, diaphoresis, hematoma, rash, acne. **Other:** antibodies to GH, infection, flulike syndrome, gynecomastia, hypersensitivity reaction.

INTERACTIONS

Drug-drug. *Corticotropin, corticosteroids:* Long-term use may inhibit growth response to GH and reduce cortisol level. Monitor patient for lack of effect and hypoadrenalism.
CYP450 substrates (alprazolam, cyclosporine, erythromycin, warfarin): May alter substrate level. Monitor therapy.
Estrogen replacement: May decrease somatropin level. Increase somatropin dosage as necessary.
Insulin, oral antidiabetics: Somatropin may decrease insulin sensitivity. Antidiabetic dosage may need adjustment.

EFFECTS ON LAB TEST RESULTS

• May increase cholesterol, triglyceride, phosphorus, AST, ALT, ALP, HbA$_{1c}$, IGF-1, TSH, and parathyroid hormone levels.

S

- May increase or decrease glucose level.
- May decrease eosinophil count.

CONTRAINDICATIONS & CAUTIONS
- Contraindicated in patients with hypersensitivity to somatropin or its excipients.
- Contraindicated in patients with closed epiphyses and in those with active proliferative or severe nonproliferative diabetic retinopathy.
- Contraindicated in patients with active malignancy. An increased risk of second neoplasm has been reported in childhood cancer survivors treated with somatropin. Patients with HIV and children with short stature (genetic cause) have increased baseline risk of developing malignancies. Consider risk and benefits before initiating therapy; monitor these patients carefully.
- Contraindicated in patients with Prader-Willi syndrome who are severely obese, have a history of upper airway obstruction or sleep apnea, or have severe respiratory impairment.
- Contraindicated in patients with acute critical illness due to complications following open heart or abdominal surgery, trauma, or acute respiratory failure. Safety of continuing somatropin treatment in patients receiving replacement doses for approved indications who concurrently develop acute critical illnesses hasn't been established. Weigh potential benefit of treatment continuation against risks.
- Serious systemic hypersensitivity reactions, including anaphylactic reactions and angioedema, have been reported.
- For patients hypersensitive to either metacresol or glycerin, don't use supplied diluent to reconstitute Humatrope.
- Use cautiously in children with hypothyroidism and in those with GH deficiency caused by intracranial lesion.
- Use cautiously in patients with diabetes.
- May increase risk of pancreatitis, especially in female children with Turner syndrome.
- Patients receiving somatropin who have or are at risk for pituitary hormone deficiency may be at risk for reduced serum cortisol levels or unmasking of central (secondary) hypoadrenalism. Also, patients treated with glucocorticoid replacement for previously diagnosed hypoadrenalism may require an increase in maintenance or stress doses once somatropin therapy begins.
- *Dialyzable drug:* Unknown.

⚠ *Overdose S&S:* Fluid retention, hypoglycemia followed by hyperglycemia, glucose intolerance, gigantism, acromegaly.

PREGNANCY-LACTATION-REPRODUCTION
- There are no adequate studies during pregnancy. Use only if clearly needed.
- It isn't known if drug appears in human milk. Use cautiously during breastfeeding.

NURSING CONSIDERATIONS
- Frequently examine children with hypothyroidism and those whose GH deficiency is caused by an intracranial lesion for progression or recurrence of underlying disease.
- Obtain hip X-rays to check for slipped capital femoral epiphysis or femoral avascular necrosis before starting somatropin in patients with growth failure secondary to CKD.
- Watch for slipped capital femoral epiphysis (limb, hip, or knee pain) or progression of scoliosis in patients with rapid growth.
- *Alert:* Assess patients with Prader-Willi syndrome for sleep apnea and upper airway obstruction before treatment. Interrupt treatment if signs of upper airway obstruction occur.
- Monitor patient with Prader-Willi syndrome for signs of respiratory infection.
- Monitor child's height regularly. Regular checkups, including monitoring of blood and radiologic studies, are also needed.
- Monitor patient's glucose level regularly because GH may induce a state of insulin resistance or new-onset diabetes.
- Transient fluid retention may occur in adults, including arthralgia, myalgia, or nerve compression syndromes such as carpal tunnel syndrome, in addition to edema.
- Excessive glucocorticoid therapy inhibits somatropin's growth-promoting effect. Patients with coexisting corticotropin deficiency should have their glucocorticoid replacement dosage carefully adjusted to avoid growth inhibition.
- Monitor results of periodic thyroid function tests for hypothyroidism; condition may need thyroid hormone treatment.
- Patient should have ophthalmic exams to assess for intracranial hypertension (IH) before and periodically during therapy. Monitor patient for signs and symptoms of IH (papilledema, visual changes, headache, nausea, vomiting). Patients with Turner syndrome may be at increased risk.

- Monitor patients with preexisting tumors or growth failure secondary to an intracranial lesion for recurrence or progression of underlying disease; discontinue therapy with evidence of recurrence.
- Monitor all patients for increased growth, or potential malignant changes, of skin lesions.
- Monitor patients for signs and symptoms of serious systemic hypersensitivity reactions.
- Monitor patient for pancreatitis (abdominal pain with or without vomiting).
- Only adults with GH deficiency alone or together with multiple hormone deficiencies from pituitary or hypothalamic disease, surgery, radiation, or trauma or those who were GH deficient as children and have been confirmed GH deficient as adults can take Saizen.
- *Look alike–sound alike:* Don't confuse somatropin with somatrem or sumatriptan

PATIENT TEACHING

- Inform parents that child with endocrine disorders (including GH deficiency) may have an increased risk of slipped capital epiphyses. Tell parents to notify prescriber if they notice their child limping.
- Advise parents to be alert for limping or complaints of hip or knee pain in children.
- Instruct patient with diabetes to monitor glucose level closely and report changes to prescriber.
- Instruct patient or parents in appropriate injection technique and needle disposal. Tell them to rotate injection sites.
- Advise patient or parents that serious systemic hypersensitivity reactions, including anaphylaxis and angioedema, can occur and to seek immediate medical attention if an allergic reaction occurs.
- Stress importance of close follow-up care and of reporting all adverse reactions.

---

sotalol hydrochloride
SOE-ta-lole

Betapace, Betapace AF, Sorine, Sotylize

Therapeutic class: Antiarrhythmics
Pharmacologic class: Nonselective beta blockers

AVAILABLE FORMS
Oral solution: 5 mg/mL
Solution for injection: 15 mg/mL
Tablets: 80 mg, 120 mg, 160 mg, 240 mg
Tablets (AF): 80 mg, 120 mg, 160 mg

INDICATIONS & DOSAGES

Boxed Warning Calculate CrCl before dosing; adjust dosing interval based on CrCl. Don't initiate therapy with IV sotalol or oral solution if baseline QTc exceeds 450 msec. ∎

Boxed Warning *Adjust-a-dose (for all indications):* If QT interval prolongs to 500 msec or greater, reduce dosage, lengthen dosing interval, or discontinue drug. ∎

➤ **Life-threatening ventricular arrhythmias**
Adults: Initially, 80 mg PO b.i.d. Increase dosage in increments of 80 mg/day every 3 days as needed and tolerated. Most patients respond to 160 to 320 mg/day, although some patients with refractory arrhythmias need up to 640 mg/day. Or, IV loading dose infused over 1 hour based on target oral dose and CrCl. Refer to manufacturer's instructions. May substitute IV for PO sotalol maintenance doses using the same dosing frequency and infusing over 5 hours. If oral dose is 80 mg, give 75 mg IV; if oral dose is 120 mg, give 112.5 mg IV; if oral dose is 160 mg, give 150 mg IV.

Children ages 2 and older with normal kidney function: Initially, 1.2 mg/kg PO t.i.d. Titrate dosage to a maximum of 2.4 mg/kg PO (equivalent to 360 mg total daily dose for adults). Guide titration by clinical response, HR, and QTc interval. Allow at least 36 hours between dose increments.

Children younger than age 2 with normal kidney function: Calculate dosage according to age factor plotted on the logarithmic scale found in manufacturer's instructions.

Adjust-a-dose: Adults: If CrCl is 30 to 60 mL/minute, increase dosage interval to every 24 hours; if CrCl is 10 to 29 mL/minute, increase interval to every 36 to 48 hours; and if CrCl is less than 10 mL/minute, individualize dosage.

Children: Use in any age-group with decreased kidney function should be at lower dosages or at increased intervals between doses. Use of sotalol in children with kidney impairment hasn't been investigated.

➤ **To maintain normal sinus rhythm or to delay recurrence of atrial fibrillation or atrial flutter (AFIB or AFL) in patients**

S

with symptomatic AFIB or AFL who are currently in sinus rhythm

Adults: 80 mg PO b.i.d. (Don't use if baseline QT interval exceeds 450 msec.) Increase dosage as needed to 120 mg PO b.i.d. after 3 days if QTc interval is less than 500 msec. Maximum dosage, 160 mg PO b.i.d. Or, IV loading dose infused over 1 hour based on target oral dose and CrCl. Refer to manufacturer's instructions. May substitute IV for PO sotalol maintenance doses using the same dosing frequency and infusing over 5 hours. If oral dose is 80 mg, give 75 mg IV; if oral dose is 120 mg, give 112.5 mg IV; if oral dose is 160 mg, give 150 mg IV.

Children ages 2 and older with normal kidney function: Initially, 1.2 mg/kg PO t.i.d. Titrate dosage to a maximum of 2.4 mg/kg (equivalent to 360 mg total daily dose for adults). Guide titration by clinical response, HR, and QTc interval. Allow at least 36 hours between dose increments.

Children younger than age 2 with normal kidney function: Calculate dosage according to age factor plotted on the logarithmic scale found in manufacturer's instructions.

Adjust-a-dose: Adults: If CrCl is 40 to 60 mL/minute, increase dosage interval to every 24 hours; if CrCl is less than 40 mL/minute, use is contraindicated. *Children:* Use in any age-group with decreased kidney function should be at lower dosages or at increased intervals between doses. Use of sotalol in children with kidney impairment hasn't been investigated.

ADMINISTRATION
PO
• May give without regard for food, but patient should take the same way each time.

• Skip a missed dose and give next dose at the usual time. Don't double the dose or shorten dosing interval.

IV
▼ Dilute drug with NSS, D₅W, or lactated Ringer solution in a volume of 120 to 250 mL to compensate for dead space in the infusion set.

▼ Give loading dose over 1 hour.

▼ Use an infusion pump to administer drug at a constant rate over 5 hours when substituting for PO.

▼ IV sotalol hasn't been studied in children.

▼ **Incompatibilities:** None listed by manufacturer. Consult a drug incompatibility reference for more information.

ACTION
Depresses sinus HR, slows AV conduction, decreases cardiac output, and lowers systolic and diastolic BP. Drug also has class III antiarrhythmic properties and can prolong duration of the cardiac action potential.

Route	Onset	Peak	Duration
PO	1–2 hr	2–4 hr	Unknown
IV	5–10 min	Unknown	Unknown

Half-life: Adults, 12 hours; children, 9.5 hours.

ADVERSE REACTIONS
CNS: asthenia, headache, dizziness, weakness, fatigue, light-headedness, sleep disorder. **CV:** chest pain, palpitations, *bradycardia, AV block, prolonged QT interval, proarrhythmic events (polymorphic ventricular tachycardia, PVCs, ventricular fibrillation),* edema, ECG abnormalities, hypotension, vasodilation. **EENT:** visual disturbance. **GI:** nausea, vomiting, diarrhea, abdominal pain. **Musculoskeletal:** pain. **Respiratory:** dyspnea, URI. **Skin:** excessive sweating.

INTERACTIONS
Drug-drug. *Antacids containing aluminum oxide and magnesium hydroxide:* May reduce bradycardic effect. Avoid sotalol administration within 2 hours of antacid.

Antihypertensives: May increase hypotensive effects or cause marked bradycardia. Monitor BP and pulse closely.

Beta₂-agonists (albuterol, isoproterenol, terbutaline), theophylline: May diminish the bronchodilatory effect. Monitor therapy.

Clonidine: Increased risk of bradycardia and AV block. May enhance rebound effect after withdrawal of clonidine. Stop sotalol several days before withdrawing clonidine.

Drugs that prolong QT interval (Class I and III antiarrhythmics, macrolide antibiotics, phenothiazines, quinolones, TCAs): May cause excessive QT prolongation. Avoid use together.

General anesthetics: May increase myocardial depression. Monitor patient closely.

Insulin, oral antidiabetics: May enhance hypoglycemic effect and mask signs and symptoms of hypoglycemia. Adjust antidiabetic dosage accordingly.

Reactions in bold italics are *life-threatening*.

Negative chronotropes (beta blockers [metoprolol], calcium channel blockers [diltiazem, verapamil], digoxin): May increase risk of bradycardia and hypotension. Monitor patient closely.

Prazosin: May increase the risk of orthostatic hypotension. Assist patient to stand slowly until effects are known.

EFFECTS ON LAB TEST RESULTS
• May increase glucose level.
• May cause false-positive catecholamine level.

CONTRAINDICATIONS & CAUTIONS
• Contraindicated in patients hypersensitive to drug.
• Contraindicated in those with severe sinus node dysfunction, sinus bradycardia, second- and third-degree AV block unless patient has a pacemaker, congenital or acquired long QT-interval syndrome, cardiogenic shock, uncontrolled HF, and bronchial asthma. For treatment of AFIB or AFL, drug is contraindicated if QT interval exceeds 450 msec.
• Contraindicated in patients with hypokalemia (less than 4 mEq/L) or hypomagnesemia before correction of imbalance.
• Use of beta blockers in patients with bronchospastic diseases (chronic bronchitis, emphysema) isn't recommended. If used, give smallest effective dose.

Boxed Warning Sotalol can cause life-threatening ventricular tachycardia associated with QT-interval prolongation. ▮

• Use cautiously in patients with kidney impairment, hypothyroidism, or diabetes.
• Use cautiously in patients with a history of allergic reactions, including anaphylaxis. Patients taking beta blockers may have more severe reactions and be less responsive to epinephrine.
• Use of beta blockers may increase risk of general anesthesia and surgical procedures; however, beta blockers shouldn't routinely be withheld before major surgery.
Dialyzable drug: Yes.

⚠ *Overdose S&S:* Bradycardia, bronchospasm, HF, hypoglycemia, hypotension, asystole, QT-interval prolongation, torsades de pointes, ventricular tachycardia, death.

PREGNANCY-LACTATION-REPRODUCTION
• Use only if potential benefit justifies fetal risk. Drug crosses placental barrier and appears in amniotic fluid. Adverse effects may include growth restriction, fetal bradycardia, hyperbilirubinemia, hypoglycemia, uterine contractions, and intrauterine death.
• Drug appears in human milk. Use during breastfeeding isn't recommended due to potential for serious adverse effects.

NURSING CONSIDERATIONS
Boxed Warning Because proarrhythmic events may occur at start of therapy and during dosage adjustments, patients should be hospitalized for a minimum of 3 days in a facility that can provide calculations of CrCl, continuous ECG monitoring, and cardiac resuscitation. Calculate CrCl before dosing; adjust dosing interval based on CrCl. ▮

Boxed Warning Baseline QTc interval must be less than or equal to 450 msec before starting sotalol IV or oral suspension. If QT interval prolongs to 500 msec or more, decrease dosage or frequency or discontinue drug. ▮

• Assess patient for new or worsened symptoms of HF.
• Monitor BP closely.
• Although patients receiving IV lidocaine may start sotalol therapy without ill effects, withdraw other antiarrhythmics before therapy begins. Sotalol therapy typically is delayed until two or three half-lives of the withdrawn drug have elapsed. After withdrawing amiodarone, give sotalol only after QT interval normalizes.
• Adjust dosage slowly, allowing 3 days between dosage increments for adequate monitoring of QT intervals and for drug levels to reach a steady-state level.
• Monitor electrolytes regularly, especially if patient is receiving diuretics. Electrolyte imbalances, such as hypokalemia or hypomagnesemia, may enhance QT-interval prolongation and increase the risk of serious arrhythmias such as torsades de pointes.
• Abrupt withdrawal of beta blockers may exacerbate angina and increase risk of MI. Gradually reduce dosage over 1 to 2 weeks after long-term use. Monitor patient closely.
• Beta blockers may mask signs and symptoms of hyperthyroidism (tachycardia). Abrupt withdrawal of beta blockers in patients with thyroid disease may exacerbate signs and symptoms of hyperthyroidism, including thyroid storm.
• *Look alike–sound alike:* Don't confuse sotalol with Sudafed. Don't confuse Betapace with Betapace AF.

S

PATIENT TEACHING

• Explain that patient will need to be hospitalized for initiation of drug therapy.
• Instruct patient in safe drug administration.
• Warn patient to report all adverse reactions and to immediately report fast, irregular heartbeat; light-headedness; or fainting.
• Encourage patient to report severe diarrhea, unusual sweating, vomiting, anorexia, or excessive thirst; these conditions could lead to electrolyte changes.
• Stress need to take drug as prescribed, even when feeling well. Caution patient against stopping drug suddenly.
• Caution patient against using OTC drugs and decongestants while taking drug.
• Advise patient to report pregnancy or plans to become pregnant or to breastfeed.

spironolactone

speer-on-oh-LAK-tone

Aldactone, CaroSpir

Therapeutic class: Diuretics
Pharmacologic class: Potassium-sparing diuretics-aldosterone receptor antagonists

AVAILABLE FORMS

Oral suspension: 25 mg/5 mL
Tablets: 25 mg, 50 mg, 100 mg

INDICATIONS & DOSAGES

➤ **Edema, cirrhosis, or nephrotic syndrome (except CaroSpir)**
Adults: Initially, 100 mg PO (tablets) daily as a single dose or in divided doses. When used as the only agent for diuresis, give drug for at least 5 days before increasing to desired dose. Usual dosage ranges from 25 to 200 mg PO daily. When given for cirrhosis, initiate drug in a hospital setting and titrate slowly.
➤ **Edema from cirrhosis (CaroSpir)**
Adults: Initially, 75 mg suspension PO daily in single or divided doses. Initiate therapy in a hospital setting and slowly titrate. When used as the only agent for diuresis, give for at least 5 days before increasing dosage. If patient requires more than 100 mg, use another formulation.
➤ **HTN**
Adults: Initially, 25 to 100 mg (tablets) PO daily or in divided doses. Or, 20 to 75 mg suspension PO daily in single or divided

doses. May titrate dosage at 2-week intervals. Dosages higher than 75 (suspension) or 100 (tablets) mg/day generally don't provide additional BP reductions.
➤ **To manage primary hyperaldosteronism (except CaroSpir)**
Adults: 100 to 400 mg (tablets) PO daily. Use lowest effective dose.
➤ **Severe HF (class III or IV), usually as adjunct to other HF therapies (except CaroSpir)**
Adults: 25 mg (tablets) PO daily in patients with serum potassium level of 5.0 mEq/L or less and eGFR greater than 50 mL/minute/1.73 m². May increase to 50 mg (tablets) PO daily as clinically indicated.
Adjust-a-dose: Patients who develop hyperkalemia on 25 mg daily may have dosage decreased to every other day. In patients with eGFR between 30 and 50 mL/minute/1.73 m², consider initiating at 25 mg every other day.
➤ **NYHA HF (class III or IV) with other HF therapies (except CaroSpir)**
Adults: Initially, 20 mg suspension PO once daily in patients with serum potassium level of 5.0 mEq/L or less and eGFR greater than 50 mL/minute/1.73 m². May increase dosage to 37.5 mg if 20-mg dose is tolerated.
Adjust-a-dose: In patients with eGFR between 30 and 50 mL/minute/1.73 m², consider initial dose of 10 mg, because of risk of hyperkalemia. If patient develops hyperkalemia on 20-mg once-daily therapy, may reduce dosage to 20 mg every other day.

ADMINISTRATION

PO
⚠ *Alert:* Hazardous agent; use safe handling and disposal precautions.
• CaroSpir suspension isn't therapeutically equivalent to Aldactone tablets.
• May give tablets or suspension with or without food but give consistently with respect to food.

ACTION

Antagonizes aldosterone in the distal tubules, increasing sodium and water excretion.

Route	Onset	Peak	Duration
PO (tablets)	Unknown	3–4 hr	2–3 days
PO (suspension)	Unknown	2.5–5 hr	Unknown

Half-life: Tablets, 1.25 hours; suspension, 1 to 2 hours.

ADVERSE REACTIONS

CNS: headache, drowsiness, lethargy, confusion, ataxia, fever. **CV:** vasculitis. **GI:** diarrhea, *gastric bleeding*, ulceration, cramping, gastritis, nausea, vomiting. **GU:** *KF*, erectile dysfunction, menstrual disturbances, postmenopausal bleeding, decreased libido.
Hematologic: *agranulocytosis, thrombocytopenia.* **Hepatic:** *liver toxicity.* **Metabolic:** *hyperkalemia,* hypovolemia, hyponatremia, mild acidosis, hyperuricemia. **Musculoskeletal:** leg cramps. **Skin:** chloasma, alopecia, urticaria, hirsutism, maculopapular eruptions, *DRESS syndrome, SJS, TEN.* **Other:** *anaphylaxis,* gynecomastia, breast soreness.

INTERACTIONS

Drug-drug. *ACE inhibitors, ARBs, heparin, low-molecular-weight heparins, trimethoprim:* May increase risk of hyperkalemia. Use together with caution and monitor potassium levels.
Cholestyramine: May increase risk of metabolic acidosis and hyperkalemia. Monitor therapy.
Digoxin: May alter digoxin clearance, increasing risk of toxicity. Monitor digoxin level.
🔆 *Alert:* **Eplerenone:** May increase risk of severe hyperkalemia. Use together is contraindicated.
Lithium: May reduce lithium clearance and increase risk of lithium toxicity. Monitor patient closely.
NSAIDs: May decrease diuretic effect and increase potassium level. Monitor patient closely.
Potassium-sparing diuretics, potassium supplements: May result in hyperkalemia. Don't use together.
Warfarin: May decrease anticoagulant effect. Monitor PT and INR, especially with dosage change.
Drug-herb. *Licorice:* May block ulcer-healing and aldosterone-like effects of herb; may increase risk of hypokalemia. Discourage use together.
Drug-food. *Potassium-rich foods, such as citrus fruits and tomatoes, salt substitutes containing potassium:* May increase risk of hyperkalemia. Urge caution.

EFFECTS ON LAB TEST RESULTS

• May increase glucose, uric acid, BUN, and potassium levels.

• May decrease sodium, magnesium, and calcium levels.
• May decrease granulocyte count.
• May cause hypochloremic alkalosis.
• May alter fluorometric determinations of plasma and urinary 17-hydroxycorticosteroid levels.

CONTRAINDICATIONS & CAUTIONS

• Drug has been shown to be tumorigenic in long-term toxicity studies in rats.
• Contraindicated in patients hypersensitive to drug and in those with Addison disease or hyperkalemia.
• Use cautiously in patients with fluid or electrolyte imbalances and in those with impaired kidney or liver function.
• Drug isn't recommended for primary treatment of HTN.
• Drug should be initiated in a hospital setting for patients with liver disease with cirrhosis and ascites. Drug can cause fluid and electrolyte disturbances, impair neurologic function, and worsen hepatic encephalopathy and coma.
• Safety and effectiveness in children haven't been established.
⚠ **Overdose S&S:** Drowsiness, confusion, rash, nausea, vomiting, dizziness, diarrhea, hyperkalemia.

PREGNANCY-LACTATION-REPRODUCTION

• Use of diuretics to treat edema during normal pregnancies isn't appropriate. Drug may cause fetal harm because of its antiandrogenic activity; avoid use during pregnancy.
• A major metabolite of drug appears in human milk. Use cautiously during breastfeeding, considering importance of drug to patient.

NURSING CONSIDERATIONS

• Drug increases serum potassium level and may be useful for treating edema when use of other diuretics has caused hypokalemia.
• Monitor electrolyte levels (especially potassium), kidney function, fluid intake and output, weight, and BP closely.
• Monitor older adults closely as this age-group is more susceptible to excessive diuresis.
• Inform lab that patient is taking spironolactone because drug may interfere with tests that measure digoxin level.
• Drug is less potent than thiazide and loop diuretics and is useful as an adjunct to other

diuretic therapy. Diuretic effect is delayed 2 to 3 days when used alone.

• Maximum antihypertensive response may be delayed for up to 2 weeks.

• Watch for hyperchloremic metabolic acidosis, especially in patients with cirrhosis.

PATIENT TEACHING

• Instruct patient in safe drug administration and handling.

• Tell patient to report all adverse reactions.

◆ **Alert:** To prevent serious hyperkalemia, warn patient to avoid excessive ingestion of potassium-rich foods (citrus fruits, tomatoes, bananas, dates, apricots), salt substitutes containing potassium, and potassium supplements.

• Caution patient not to perform hazardous activities if adverse CNS reactions occur.

• Advise patient about possible breast tenderness or enlargement.

• Instruct patient to immediately report pregnancy, plans to become pregnant, breastfeeding, or plans to breastfeed during treatment.

SAFETY ALERT!

succinylcholine chloride (suxamethonium chloride)
suks-in-il-KOE-leen

Anectine, Quelicin

Therapeutic class: Skeletal muscle relaxants
Pharmacologic class: Depolarizing neuromuscular blockers

AVAILABLE FORMS

Injection: 20 mg/mL single-dose vial; 100 mg/mL multidose vial

INDICATIONS & DOSAGES

➤ **Adjunct to anesthesia; to facilitate tracheal intubation; to provide skeletal muscle relaxation during surgery or mechanical ventilation**

Adults: 0.6 mg/kg IV given over 10 to 30 seconds. Dosage ranges, 0.3 to 1.1 mg/kg. For longer response, give 1 mg/mL solution as a continuous infusion at 0.5 to 10 mg/minute, or give an initial IV injection of 0.3 to 1.1 mg/kg followed by further injections of 0.04 to 0.07 mg/kg, as needed, to maintain relaxation. Or, 3 to 4 mg/kg IM. Maximum IM dose, 150 mg.

Children: 1 to 2 mg/kg IV or 3 to 4 mg/kg IM. Maximum IM dose, 150 mg.

ADMINISTRATION

IV

▼ Only staff skilled in airway management should use drug.

▼ A test dose of 5 to 10 mg may be given to evaluate sensitivity to drug. If no respiratory depression occurs or transient depression lasts for up to 5 minutes, then patient can metabolize drug, and it is safe to continue. Don't give if patient develops respiratory paralysis sufficient to need ET intubation.

▼ Use within 24 hours after reconstitution.

▼ Store injectable form in refrigerator.

▼ **Incompatibilities:** Alkaline solutions, barbiturates, nafcillin, sodium bicarbonate, solutions with pH above 8.5, thiopental sodium.

IM

• Inject deeply, preferably high into deltoid muscle. Use IM route only when IV access isn't available.

• Store injectable form in refrigerator.

ACTION

Binds with a high affinity to cholinergic receptors, prolonging depolarization of the motor end plate and ultimately producing muscle paralysis.

Route	Onset	Peak	Duration
IV	30–60 sec	1–2 min	4–6 min
IM	2–3 min	Unknown	10–30 min

Half-life: Unknown.

ADVERSE REACTIONS

CV: *arrhythmias, bradycardia, cardiac arrest,* tachycardia, HTN, hypotension.
EENT: increased IOP, excessive salivation.
Metabolic: *hyperkalemia.* **Musculoskeletal:** postoperative muscle pain, muscle fasciculation, jaw rigidity, *rhabdomyolysis with AKI.* **Respiratory:** *apnea, bronchoconstriction, prolonged respiratory depression.* **Skin:** rash. **Other:** allergic or idiosyncratic hypersensitivity reactions, *anaphylaxis, malignant hyperthermia.*

INTERACTIONS

Drug-drug. *Aminoglycosides, anticholinesterases (echothiophate, edrophonium, neostigmine, physostigmine, pyridostigmine), aprotinin, general anesthetics (enflurane, halothane,*

isoflurane), glucocorticoids, hormonal contraceptives, lidocaine, lithium, magnesium, metoclopramide, oxytocin, polymyxin antibiotics (colistin, polymyxin B sulfate), procainamide, quinidine: May enhance neuromuscular blockade, increasing skeletal muscle relaxation and potentiating effect. Use together cautiously during and after surgery.
Cardiac glycosides: May increase risk of arrhythmias. Use together cautiously.
Cyclophosphamide, lithium, MAO inhibitors: May enhance neuromuscular blockade and prolong apnea. Use together cautiously.
Opioid analgesics: May enhance neuromuscular blockade, increasing skeletal muscle relaxation and possibly causing respiratory paralysis. Use together cautiously.
Parenteral magnesium sulfate: May enhance neuromuscular blockade, may increase skeletal muscle relaxation, and may cause respiratory paralysis. Use together cautiously, preferably at reduced doses.

EFFECTS ON LAB TEST RESULTS
• May increase CK, myoglobin, and potassium levels.

CONTRAINDICATIONS & CAUTIONS
✂ Contraindicated in patients hypersensitive to drug and in those with personal or family history of malignant hyperthermia.
• Contraindicated in patients with skeletal muscle myopathies and after the acute phase of injury following acute major burns, multiple trauma, skeletal muscle denervation, or upper motor neuron injury.
• Drug increases IOP. Use only when potential benefit outweighs risk when an increase in IOP is undesirable, such as in narrow-angle glaucoma or penetrating eye injury.
✂ Use carefully in patients with reduced plasma cholinesterase activity due to risk of prolonged neuromuscular block. Plasma cholinesterase activity may be diminished in the presence of genetic abnormalities of plasma cholinesterase, pregnancy, severe liver or kidney disease, malignant tumors, infections, burns, anemia, decompensated heart disease, peptic ulcer, myxedema, and certain drugs and chemicals.
• Use cautiously in older adults or patients who are debilitated; in patients with liver, kidney, or pulmonary impairment; and in those with respiratory depression, severe burns or trauma, electrolyte imbalances,

hyperkalemia, paraplegia, spinal CNS injury, stroke, degenerative or dystrophic neuromuscular disease, myasthenia gravis, myasthenic syndrome related to lung cancer, dehydration, thyroid disorders, collagen diseases, porphyria, fractures, muscle spasms, dislocations, eye surgery, and pheochromocytoma.
Dialyzable drug: Unknown.
⚠ **Overdose S&S:** Prolonged neuromuscular blockade (skeletal muscle weakness, decreased respiratory reserve, low tidal volume, apnea).

PREGNANCY-LACTATION-REPRODUCTION
• There are no adequate studies during pregnancy. Use only if clearly needed.
• Use large doses cautiously in patients undergoing cesarean section; monitor patient and neonate for apnea and neonate for flaccidity.
• It isn't known if drug appears in human milk. Use cautiously during breastfeeding.

NURSING CONSIDERATIONS
• Drug has no known effect on consciousness, pain threshold, or cerebration. To avoid patient distress, don't induce neuromuscular blockade before unconsciousness.
• Dosage depends on anesthetic used, individual needs, and response. Recommended dosages must be individually adjusted. Drug should only be administered by experienced personnel trained in its use.
Boxed Warning Drug may cause acute rhabdomyolysis with hyperkalemia followed by ventricular arrhythmias, cardiac arrest, and death after administration to apparently healthy children who have undiagnosed skeletal muscle myopathy, most frequently Duchenne muscular dystrophy. Institute treatment for hyperkalemia when a healthy-appearing child develops cardiac arrest soon after administration of succinylcholine. In children, drug should be reserved for use in emergency intubation, for instances when securing the airway is necessary, or for IM use when a suitable vein is inaccessible. ■
✂ Assess patients for personal or family history of malignant hyperthermia as drug is contraindicated in these patients.
• Children may be less sensitive to drug than adults.
• May cause a transient increase in ICP and may increase intragastric pressure, which could result in regurgitation and possible aspiration of stomach contents.

- Monitor baseline electrolyte levels and vital signs. Check respirations every 5 to 10 minutes during infusion.
- Monitor respirations closely until tests of muscle strength (hand grip, head lift, ability to cough) indicate full recovery from neuromuscular blockade.
- **⟳ Alert:** Don't use reversing drugs. Unlike nondepolarizing drugs, neostigmine or edrophonium may worsen neuromuscular blockade if given before succinylcholine is metabolized by cholinesterase.
- Repeated or continuous infusions aren't advisable; they may cause reduced response or prolonged muscle relaxation and apnea.
- Give analgesics for pain.
- Keep airway clear. Have emergency respiratory support equipment (ET equipment, ventilator, oxygen, atropine, and epinephrine) immediately available.
- **⟳ Alert:** Carefully calculate dosage and always verify dosage with another health care professional.

PATIENT TEACHING
- Explain all events and procedures to patient because patient can still hear.
- Reassure patient that postoperative stiffness is normal and will soon subside.

---

sucralfate
soo-KRAL-fayt

Carafate

Therapeutic class: Antiulcer drugs
Pharmacologic class: GI protectants

AVAILABLE FORMS
Suspension: 1 g/10 mL
Tablets: 1 g

INDICATIONS & DOSAGES
Adjust-a-dose (for all indications): Use caution when selecting starting dose for older adults, starting at the low end of the dosing range.
➤ **Short-term treatment of duodenal ulcer**
Adults: 1 g PO q.i.d. 1 hour before meals and at bedtime. Continue for 4 to 8 weeks unless healing has been demonstrated by X-ray or endoscopic exam.
➤ **Maintenance therapy for duodenal ulcer (tablets only)**
Adults: 1 g PO b.i.d.

ADMINISTRATION
PO
- Shake suspension well before pouring.
- Give suspension with an accurate measuring device (calibrated oral syringe or measuring cup).
- After administration, flush NG tube with water to ensure passage into stomach.
- Give drug on an empty stomach 1 hour before meals.

ACTION
Selectively forms a coating that acts locally to protect the gastric lining against peptic acid, pepsin, and bile salts.

Route	Onset	Peak	Duration
PO	Unknown	Unknown	6 hr

Half-life: Unknown.

ADVERSE REACTIONS
GI: constipation.

INTERACTIONS
Drug-drug. *Aluminum-containing drugs (some antacids):* May increase total body burden of aluminum. Use cautiously in patients with CKD.
Antacids: May decrease binding of drug to gastroduodenal mucosa, impairing effectiveness. Separate doses by 30 minutes.
Cimetidine, digoxin, fosphenytoin, furosemide (oral), ketoconazole, phenytoin, quinidine, tetracycline, theophylline: May decrease absorption of these drugs. Separate doses by at least 2 hours.
Ciprofloxacin, levofloxacin, moxifloxacin, ofloxacin: May decrease absorption of these drugs, reducing anti-infective response. If use together can't be avoided, give 2 hours before sucralfate.
Warfarin: May decrease anticoagulant effect. Monitor effectiveness and adjust dosage as necessary.

EFFECTS ON LAB TEST RESULTS
- May increase glucose level.

CONTRAINDICATIONS & CAUTIONS
- Contraindicated in patients with known hypersensitivity reactions to the active substance or to the components.
- Use cautiously in patients with CKD; toxic reactions may be greater in patients with impaired kidney function.

Reactions in bold italics are *life-threatening*.

• Safety and effectiveness in children haven't been established.
Dialyzable drug: Unknown.
⚠ *Overdose S&S:* Dyspepsia, abdominal pain, nausea, vomiting.

PREGNANCY-LACTATION-REPRODUCTION

• There are no adequate studies during pregnancy. Use only if clearly needed.
• It isn't known if drug appears in human milk. Use cautiously during breastfeeding.

NURSING CONSIDERATIONS

• Drug causes few adverse reactions because it's minimally absorbed.
• Monitor patient for severe, persistent constipation.
• Drug is as effective as cimetidine in healing duodenal ulcer.
• Drug contains aluminum but isn't classified as an antacid. Monitor patient with kidney insufficiency for aluminum toxicity.
• Hyperglycemia has been reported in patients with diabetes who are taking suspension. Closely monitor blood glucose level and adjust dosage of antidiabetics if indicated.

PATIENT TEACHING

• Teach patient safe medication administration.
• Instruct patient to continue prescribed regimen to ensure complete healing. Pain and other ulcer signs and symptoms may subside within first few weeks of therapy.
• Urge patient to avoid cigarette smoking, which may increase gastric acid secretion and worsen disease.

SAFETY ALERT!

SUFentanil
soo-FEN-ta-nil

Dsuvia

Therapeutic class: Opioid analgesics
Pharmacologic class: Opioid agonists
Controlled substance schedule: II

AVAILABLE FORMS
Tablets (SL): 30 mcg

INDICATIONS & DOSAGES
➤ **Management of acute pain severe enough to require an opioid analgesic and**
for which alternative treatments are inadequate
Adults: 30 mcg SL PRN with a minimum of 1 hour between doses. Maximum cumulative dose, 360 mcg/day (12 tablets). Don't use for more than 72 hours.

ADMINISTRATION
Sublingual
Boxed Warning Drug is only to be administered by a health care professional in a medically certified health care setting. ■
• Drug is packaged as a single-use product. Don't reuse. Don't use if pouch is broken or single-dose applicator (SDA) is damaged.
🛈 *Alert:* Wear gloves when administering drug and dispose of SDA in biohazard waste.
• Follow manufacturer's instructions for use of delivery applicator.
• If patient has excessively dry mouth, provide ice chips before giving drug.
• Patient should allow drug to dissolve under the tongue and not chew or swallow the tablet.
• Patient should minimize talking and not eat or drink for 10 minutes after each dose.
• Visually confirm SL tablet placement.
• Store at 68° to 77° F (20° to 25° C) in a secure, limited-access location in accordance with institutional procedures for Schedule II products.

ACTION
An opioid agonist that is relatively selective for the mu-opioid receptor, although it can bind to other opioid receptors at higher doses. The analgesia and sedation effects are thought to be mediated through opioid-specific receptors throughout the CNS, with no ceiling effect to analgesia.

Route	Onset	Peak	Duration
SL	Unknown	1 hr	Unknown

Half-life: 13.4 hours.

ADVERSE REACTIONS
CNS: dizziness, headache. **CV:** hypotension. **GI:** nausea, vomiting. **Respiratory:** *respiratory depression,* decreased oxygen saturation.

INTERACTIONS
Drug-drug. *Anticholinergics (scopolamine, dicyclomine):* May increase risk of urine retention or severe constipation, which may lead to paralytic ileus. Monitor patient for

signs and symptoms of urine retention or reduced gastric motility.

Boxed Warning *Benzodiazepines, CNS depressants:* May cause slow or difficult breathing, sedation, and death. Avoid use together. If use together can't be avoided, limit dose and duration of each drug to minimum needed for desired effect. ∎

Boxed Warning *CYP3A4 inducers (carbamazepine, phenytoin, rifampin):* May decrease sufentanil level and lead to decreased efficacy or withdrawal symptoms in patients who have developed physical dependence. If use together is necessary, consider an alternative medication that permits dosage titration. Monitor patient for opioid withdrawal. If the CYP3A4 inducer is discontinued, consider decreasing sufentanil dosage and monitor patient for signs and symptoms of respiratory depression. ∎

Boxed Warning *CYP3A4 inhibitors (erythromycin, ketoconazole, ritonavir):* May increase sufentanil level, leading to increased or prolonged opioid effects. Monitor patient for respiratory depression and sedation. If use together is necessary, consider an alternative medication that permits dosage titration. If the CYP3A4 inhibitor is discontinued, consider increasing sufentanil dosage until stable drug effects are achieved and monitor patient for opioid withdrawal symptoms. ∎

Diuretics: May decrease effects of diuretics by inducing release of ADH. Monitor patients for signs and symptoms of diminished diuresis or effects on BP and increase diuretic dosage as needed.

MAO inhibitors (linezolid, phenelzine, tranylcypromine): May increase risk of serotonin syndrome or opioid toxicity. Use of sufentanil isn't recommended for patients taking MAO inhibitors or within 14 days of stopping MAO inhibitor treatment.

Mixed agonist/antagonist and partial opioid analgesics (buprenorphine, butorphanol, nalbuphine): May reduce analgesic effect of sufentanil or precipitate withdrawal symptoms. Avoid use together.

Muscle relaxants: May enhance neuromuscular blocking action of skeletal muscle relaxants and produce increased respiratory depression. Monitor patient for signs and symptoms of respiratory depression; decrease dosage of skeletal muscle relaxant or consider discontinuing sufentanil.

Serotonergic drugs (mirtazapine, SNRIs, SSRIs, TCAs, tramadol, trazodone, triptans): May increase risk of serotonin syndrome. If use together is necessary, monitor patient closely, especially during treatment initiation and dosage adjustment. Discontinue sufentanil if serotonin syndrome is suspected.

Drug-lifestyle. **Boxed Warning** *Alcohol use:* May cause slow or difficult breathing, sedation, and death. Discourage use together. ∎

EFFECTS ON LAB TEST RESULTS
● May increase amylase, liver enzyme, and creatinine levels.

CONTRAINDICATIONS & CAUTIONS
● Contraindicated in patients with significant respiratory depression, acute or severe bronchial asthma in an unmonitored setting or in the absence of resuscitative equipment, known or suspected GI obstruction (including paralytic ileus), or known hypersensitivity to sufentanil or its components.

Boxed Warning Accidental ingestion of even one dose of an opioid, especially by children, can result in a fatal overdose. ∎

Boxed Warning Prescribers are strongly encouraged to complete a REMS-compliant education program. Drug should be prescribed only by prescribers with knowledge of opioid use and ways to reduce associated risks. ∎

● *Alert:* Use lowest effective dose for shortest period consistent with patient's treatment goals.

● *Alert:* Because risk of overdose increases as opioid dose increases, reserve titration to higher doses for patients in whom lower doses are ineffective and in whom expected benefits of higher opioid dose outweigh risks.

Boxed Warning *Opioid class warning:* Opioids should only be prescribed with benzodiazepines or other CNS depressants when alternative options are inadequate, not expected to provide adequate analgesia, haven't been tolerated, or aren't expected to be tolerated. ∎

Boxed Warning Use exposes patient and others to risk of opioid addiction, abuse, and misuse, which can lead to overdose and death. These effects can occur at any dose or duration. Assess patient risk before prescribing and regularly reassess patient for these behaviors and conditions. ∎

● *Alert:* Immediate-release formulations shouldn't be used for an extended period unless pain remains severe enough to require an opioid analgesic and alternative treatments are inadequate to treat pain.

• Opioids can cause sleep-related breathing disorders, including central sleep apnea (CSA) and sleep-related hypoxemia. Opioid use increases risk of CSA in a dose-dependent fashion. In patients with CSA, consider minimizing sufentanil use; monitor patients for signs or symptoms of respiratory depression.

• Use cautiously in patients with chronic pulmonary disease, in older adults, and in patients who are cachectic or debilitated, as they are at increased risk for respiratory depression, even at recommended doses. Consider nonopioid analgesics whenever possible.

• Drug may cause severe hypotension, including orthostatic hypotension and syncope in patients who are ambulatory. Use cautiously in patients with hypovolemia or CV disease and in those taking drugs that may exaggerate hypotensive effects. Avoid use in patients with circulatory shock.

• Avoid use in patients with impaired consciousness or coma. Sufentanil isn't suitable for use in patients who aren't alert and able to follow directions.

• Drug may mask clinical changes in patients with head injury.

• Drug may increase frequency of seizures in patients with seizure disorders and may increase risk of seizures occurring in other clinical settings.

• Use cautiously in patients with bradyarrhythmias; drug may lower HR.

• Drug isn't approved for use in children, for use long-term, or for home use.

Dialyzable drug: Unknown.

⚠ *Overdose S&S:* Respiratory depression, somnolence, stupor, coma, skeletal muscle flaccidity, cold and clammy skin, constricted pupils, pulmonary edema, bradycardia, hypotension, partial or complete airway obstruction, atypical snoring, marked hypoxia-related mydriasis, death.

PREGNANCY-LACTATION-REPRODUCTION
Boxed Warning Prolonged use during pregnancy can result in neonatal opioid withdrawal syndrome, which may be life-threatening. It requires management with expert neonatology protocols. If prolonged use is needed, advise patient of risks and ensure availability of proper treatment. ■

• Opioids cross the placental barrier and may produce respiratory depression and psychophysiologic effects in neonates. Sufentanil shouldn't be used during or immediately before labor when other analgesics are more appropriate.

• Infants exposed to sufentanil through human milk should be monitored for excess sedation and respiratory depression. Withdrawal symptoms can occur in infants who are breastfed when opioid analgesic administration or breastfeeding is stopped.

• Long-term use of opioids may reduce fertility in females and males of reproductive potential. It isn't known if these effects on fertility are reversible.

NURSING CONSIDERATIONS
Boxed Warning May cause life-threatening or fatal respiratory depression at any time during therapy. Monitor patient closely, especially when starting or increasing doses. Proper dosing and titration are essential to reduce risk. ■

Boxed Warning Regularly monitor all patients for opioid addiction, abuse, and misuse, which can lead to overdose and death. ■

🔵 *Alert:* Drug may cause opioid-induced hyperalgesia (OIH). Symptoms include increased pain level with opioid dose increase, decreased pain level with opioid dose reduction, pain from ordinarily nonpainful stimuli without underlying disease progression, opioid tolerance or withdrawal, and addictive behavior. For suspected OIH, decrease opioid dose or switch patient to alternative opioid.

• Watch for serotonin syndrome in patient who is taking concomitant serotonergic drugs. Assess for mental status changes (agitation, hallucinations, coma), autonomic instability (tachycardia, labile BP, hyperthermia), neuromuscular abnormalities (hyperreflexia, loss of coordination, rigidity), and GI signs and symptoms (nausea, vomiting, diarrhea). Discontinue sufentanil for suspected serotonin syndrome.

• Use cautiously in patients with liver impairment and CrCl less than 30 mL/minute; monitor patients closely for respiratory depression, sedation, and hypotension.

• Monitor patients with a history of seizure disorders for worsened seizure control.

• Monitor patients for adrenal insufficiency (nausea, vomiting, anorexia, fatigue, weakness, dizziness, hypotension). If adrenal

S

insufficiency is diagnosed, treat with physiologic replacement of corticosteroids, and wean patient from the opioid.
• Monitor patients for hypotension, especially for changes in HR, particularly when initiating therapy.
• Monitor patients with biliary tract disease (acute pancreatitis) for worsening symptoms.
• Use cautiously in patients susceptible to the intracranial effects of carbon dioxide retention, such as those with brain tumors or increased ICP. Drug may decrease respiratory drive. Monitor patients for sedation and respiratory depression.
• Monitor neonates exposed to opioids during labor for excess sedation and respiratory depression. Monitor neonates with prolonged exposure in utero for opioid withdrawal syndrome (irritability, hyperactivity, abnormal sleep pattern, high-pitched cry, tremor, vomiting, diarrhea, failure to gain weight).
Boxed Warning Drug must be discontinued before patient leaves the certified medically supervised setting. Don't use for more than 72 hours. ∎
• *Look alike–sound alike:* Don't confuse Dsuvia with Duavee.

PATIENT TEACHING
Boxed Warning Counsel patient and caregiver on serious risks, safe use, and importance of reading the medication guide with each prescription. ∎
• Instruct patient to inform health care provider if prescribed dosage isn't controlling pain.
🔸 *Alert:* Counsel patient who has been regularly taking drug not to discontinue without first discussing the need for gradual tapering with prescriber.
🔸 *Alert:* Warn patient to inform prescriber if pain level worsens, pain sensitivity increases, or new pain occurs after taking drug.
• Teach patient to report all adverse reactions.
• Warn patient that hypersensitivity reactions, including anaphylaxis, have been reported. Advise patient to immediately report signs and symptoms of hypersensitivity reactions.
• Caution patient that sufentanil may cause orthostatic hypotension and syncope. Teach patient how to recognize signs and symptoms of low BP and how to reduce risk of serious consequences of hypotension.
• Inform patient that opioids can cause adrenal insufficiency, and to report signs and symptoms of adrenal insufficiency if they occur.

• Warn patient with a history of seizure disorder that drug can increase risk of seizures.
• Caution patient to report to prescriber pregnancy or plan to become pregnant.
• Advise patient who is breastfeeding to monitor infant for increased sleepiness (more than usual), breathing difficulties, or limpness. Instruct patient to seek immediate medical care if these signs or symptoms occur.

---

sulfamethoxazole–trimethoprim ⚥
sul-fa-meth-OX-a-zole/tri-meth-O-prim

Bactrim, Bactrim DS, Sulfatrim*

Therapeutic class: Antibiotics
Pharmacologic class: Sulfonamides-folate antagonists

AVAILABLE FORMS
Injection: sulfamethoxazole 80 mg/mL and trimethoprim 16 mg/mL in 5-mL vials*
Oral suspension: sulfamethoxazole 200 mg and trimethoprim 40 mg/5 mL*
Tablets (double-strength): sulfamethoxazole 800 mg and trimethoprim 160 mg
Tablets (single-strength): sulfamethoxazole 400 mg and trimethoprim 80 mg

INDICATIONS & DOSAGES
Adjust-a-dose (for all indications): For patients with CrCl of 15 to 30 mL/minute, reduce daily dose by 50%. Don't give to those with CrCl less than 15 mL/minute.
➤ **Shigellosis, or UTIs caused by susceptible strains of *Escherichia coli*, *Proteus*, *Klebsiella*, *Morganella morganii*, or *Enterobacter* species**
Adults: 800 mg sulfamethoxazole/160 mg trimethoprim PO every 12 hours for 10 to 14 days in UTIs and for 5 days in shigellosis. If indicated, give 8 to 10 mg/kg/day IV, based on trimethoprim component, in two to four divided doses every 6, 8, or 12 hours for 5 days for shigellosis or up to 14 days for severe UTIs. Maximum daily dose, 60 mL trimethoprim.
Children ages 2 months and older: 8 mg/kg/day PO, based on trimethoprim component, in two divided doses every 12 hours for 10 days for UTIs and 5 days for shigellosis. If indicated, give 8 to 10 mg/kg/day IV, based on trimethoprim component, in two to four divided doses every 6, 8, or 12 hours for up to

---

14 days for severe UTIs and 5 days for shigellosis. Don't exceed adult dose.

➤ **Otitis media in patients with penicillin allergy or penicillin-resistant infection**
Children ages 2 months and older: 8 mg/kg/day PO, based on trimethoprim component, in two divided doses every 12 hours for 10 days.

➤ **Acute exacerbation of chronic bronchitis due to susceptible strains of *Streptococcus pneumoniae* or *Haemophilus influenzae***
Adults: 800 mg sulfamethoxazole/160 mg trimethoprim PO every 12 hours for 14 days.

➤ **Traveler's diarrhea**
Adults: 800 mg sulfamethoxazole/160 mg trimethoprim PO b.i.d. for 5 days.

➤ *Pneumocystis jiroveci* **pneumonia**
Adults and children older than age 2 months: 15 to 20 mg/kg/day IV or PO, based on trimethoprim component, in equally divided doses every 6 hours (PO) or in divided doses every 6 to 8 hours (IV) for 14 days. Some guidelines recommend treatment duration of 21 days.

➤ *P. jiroveci* **pneumonia prophylaxis in patients who are immunosuppressed**
Adults: 800 mg sulfamethoxazole/160 mg trimethoprim every 24 hours.
Children older than age 2 months: 750 mg/m² sulfamethoxazole with trimethoprim 150 mg/m² daily in equally divided doses b.i.d., on 3 consecutive days per week. Maximum daily dose, 1,600 mg/sulfamethoxazole and 320 mg trimethoprim.

ADMINISTRATION

- Before giving drug, ask if patient is allergic to sulfa drugs.
- Obtain specimen for culture and sensitivity tests before giving. Begin therapy while awaiting results.

PO
- Give without regard to meals.
- Give drug with 8 oz (240 mL) of water.
- Shake suspension well before using.

IV
▼ Don't give by rapid infusion or bolus injection.
▼ Dilute each 5 mL of concentrate in 75 to 125 mL of D₅W. Don't mix with other drugs or solutions.
▼ Infuse slowly over 60 to 90 minutes.
▼ Don't refrigerate; use within 6 hours if diluted in 125 mL, within 4 hours if diluted in 100 mL, and within 2 hours if diluted in 75 mL.

▼ Discard solution if it's cloudy or crystallized.
▼ Never give drug IM.
▼ **Incompatibilities:** None listed by manufacturer. Consult a drug incompatibility reference for more information.

ACTION

Sulfamethoxazole inhibits formation of dihydrofolic acid from PABA; trimethoprim inhibits dihydrofolate reductase formation. Both decrease bacterial folic acid synthesis and are bactericidal.

Route	Onset	Peak	Duration
PO	Unknown	1–4 hr	Unknown
IV	Immediate	Unknown	Unknown

Half-life: Sulfamethoxazole, 9 to 12 hours; trimethoprim, 6 to 11 hours.

ADVERSE REACTIONS

CNS: *seizures,* apathy, aseptic meningitis, ataxia, depression, fatigue, hallucinations, headache, insomnia, nervousness, peripheral neuritis, vertigo. **CV:** thrombophlebitis, polyarteritis nodosa. **EENT:** tinnitus, conjunctival and scleral injection, glossitis. **GI:** *pancreatitis, pseudomembranous colitis,* diarrhea, nausea, vomiting, abdominal pain, anorexia, stomatitis. **GU:** *kidney toxicity,* crystalluria, hematuria, interstitial nephritis, *KF.* **Hematologic:** *agranulocytosis, aplastic anemia,* eosinophilia, *leukopenia, neutropenia, thrombocytopenia,* hemolytic anemia, megaloblastic anemia, ITP, *methemoglobinemia.* **Hepatic:** *liver toxicity,* jaundice. **Metabolic:** *hyperkalemia, hypoglycemia,* hyponatremia. **Musculoskeletal:** arthralgia, muscle weakness, myalgia, *rhabdomyolysis.* **Respiratory:** pulmonary infiltrates, cough, shortness of breath, interstitial lung disease. **Skin:** generalized skin eruption, exfoliative dermatitis, photosensitivity reactions, pruritus, urticaria, rash, *SCARs.* **Other:** *anaphylaxis,* hypersensitivity reactions.

INTERACTIONS

Drug-drug. *Antiarrhythmics (amiodarone, disopyramide, quinidine, sotalol), arsenic trioxide, chlorpromazine, dolasetron, droperidol, mefloquine, moxifloxacin, pentamidine, pimozide, tacrolimus, thioridazine, ziprasidone, other drugs that prolong QT interval:* May prolong QT interval and increase risk

S

of life-threatening cardiac arrhythmias, including torsades de pointes. Use together with caution unless contraindicated. Consult pharmacist as necessary.

Cyclosporine: May decrease cyclosporine level and increase kidney toxicity risk. Avoid using together.

Digoxin: May increase digoxin level. Monitor digoxin level.

Diuretics: May increase incidence of thrombocytopenia with purpura in older adults receiving certain diuretics, mainly thiazides. Avoid concomitant use.

Dofetilide: May increase dofetilide level and effects. May increase risk of prolonged QT-interval syndrome and fatal ventricular arrhythmias. Contraindicated for use together.

Indomethacin: May increase sulfamethoxazole blood level. Avoid concomitant use.

Leucovorin: May increase risk of treatment failure and mortality during treatment of HIV-positive patients with *P. jiroveci* pneumonia. Avoid use together.

Methotrexate: May increase methotrexate level. Monitor methotrexate level.

Oral antidiabetics: May increase hypoglycemic effect. Monitor glucose level.

Phenytoin: May inhibit metabolism of phenytoin. Monitor phenytoin level.

Procainamide: May prolong QT interval. Closely monitor patient for clinical and ECG signs of toxicity.

Pyrimethamine: May increase risk of megaloblastic anemia. Avoid use together.

TCAs: May decrease efficacy of TCAs. Monitor therapeutic response to TCAs and adjust dosage accordingly.

Warfarin: May increase anticoagulant effect. Monitor patient for bleeding; monitor PT and INR.

Zidovudine: May cause hematologic abnormalities and increase risk of myelotoxicity. Monitor patient closely.

Drug-herb. *St. John's wort:* May decrease drug level. Discourage use together.

Drug-lifestyle. *Sun exposure:* May increase risk of photosensitivity reactions. Advise patient to avoid excessive sunlight exposure.

EFFECTS ON LAB TEST RESULTS
• May increase aminotransferase, bilirubin, potassium, BUN, and creatinine levels.
• May decrease sodium and glucose levels.
• May decrease Hb level and granulocyte, platelet, and WBC counts.

CONTRAINDICATIONS & CAUTIONS
• Contraindicated in patients hypersensitive to trimethoprim or sulfonamides and in patients with a history of trimethoprim or sulfonamide drug-induced immune thrombocytopenia.
• Severe, life-threatening, and fatal cases of thrombocytopenia have been reported and may be immune-mediated. Thrombocytopenia usually resolves within 1 week of drug discontinuation.
• Contraindicated in those with CrCl less than 15 mL/minute, porphyria, megaloblastic anemia from folate deficiency, or marked liver damage.
• Contraindicated in infants younger than age 2 months.
• Avoid use in patients with liver or kidney impairment, in those with possible folate deficiency (older adults, chronic alcohol abuse, malnutrition, malabsorption syndrome, severe allergies, bronchial asthma, and patients on anticonvulsive therapy). Drug may increase risk of folic acid deficiency.
• Some forms may contain benzyl alcohol, which, in newborn infants, has been associated with an increased incidence of neurologic and other complications that are sometimes fatal. Avoid use in neonates.
• Use cautiously and in reduced dosages in patients with CrCl of 15 to 30 mL/minute, severe allergy or bronchial asthma, or blood dyscrasia.
🖉 Use cautiously in patients with G6PD deficiency as hemolytic anemia can result.
• May cause CDAD ranging from mild diarrhea to fatal colitis.
Dialyzable drug: Moderately.
⚠ *Overdose S&S:* Headache, drowsiness, unconsciousness, fever, depression, confusion, anorexia, colic, nausea, vomiting, diarrhea, hematuria, crystalluria; blood dyscrasias and jaundice (late signs).

PREGNANCY-LACTATION-REPRODUCTION
• There are no adequate studies during pregnancy; drug may cause fetal harm. Use only if potential benefit justifies fetal risk.
• Contraindicated during breastfeeding because of risk of bilirubin displacement and kernicterus.

NURSING CONSIDERATIONS
🕙 *Alert:* Double-check dosage, which may be written as trimethoprim component.

Reactions in bold italics are *life-threatening*.

❸ *Alert:* "DS" product means "double strength."

• Monitor kidney function, CBC, potassium level, and LFT results.

• Promptly report rash, sore throat, fever, cough, mouth sores, or iris lesions—early signs and symptoms of erythema multiforme, which may progress to life-threatening SJS, or blood dyscrasias.

• Watch for signs and symptoms of superinfection, such as fever, chills, and increased pulse.

❸ *Alert:* Adverse reactions, especially hypersensitivity reactions, rash, and fever, occur more frequently in patients with AIDS.

• Monitor patient for CDAD, which can occur 2 months or more after therapy ends. Discontinue drug and provide supportive treatment for suspected or confirmed CDAD.

PATIENT TEACHING

• Instruct patient in safe drug administration.
• Tell patient to take drug as prescribed, even if feeling better.
• Encourage patient to drink plenty of fluids to prevent crystalluria and kidney stone formation.
• Tell patient to report adverse reactions promptly, especially diarrhea, fever, rash, bruising, bleeding, and throat or other pain.
• Instruct patient receiving drug IV to report discomfort at IV insertion site.
• Advise patient to avoid prolonged sun exposure, wear protective clothing, and use sunscreen.
• Caution patient to report pregnancy or breastfeeding to prescriber.

sulfaSALAzine (salazosulfapyridine, sulphasalazine) ▨

sul-fuh-SAL-uh-zeen

Azulfidine, Azulfidine EN-tabs, Salazopyrin✦, Salazopyrin EN-Tabs✦

Therapeutic class: Anti-inflammatory drugs
Pharmacologic class: Sulfonamide salicylates

AVAILABLE FORMS
Tablets: 500 mg
Tablets (delayed-release) ⓄⓃⒼ: 500 mg

INDICATIONS & DOSAGES

➤ **Mild to moderate ulcerative colitis, adjunctive therapy in severe ulcerative colitis, prolongation of remission period between acute ulcerative colitis attacks**

Adults: Initially, 3 to 4 g PO daily in evenly divided doses not exceeding 8 hours apart; may start with 1 to 2 g, with gradual increase to minimize adverse effects. Usual maintenance dose is 2 g PO daily.

Children ages 6 and older: Initially, 40 to 60 mg/kg PO daily, divided into three to six doses; may start at lower dose if GI intolerance occurs. Maintenance dose is 30 mg/kg in each 24-hour period, divided into four doses.

➤ **RA in patients who have responded inadequately to salicylates or NSAIDs**

Adults (delayed-release tablets): 2 g PO daily in two evenly divided doses. To reduce possible GI intolerance, start at 0.5 to 1 g daily. May increase to 3 g PO daily if clinical response after 12 weeks is inadequate.

➤ **Polyarticular-course juvenile RA in patients who have responded inadequately to salicylates or other NSAIDs**

Children ages 6 and older (delayed-release tablets): 30 to 50 mg/kg PO daily in two evenly divided doses. Maximum dose, 2 g daily. To reduce possible GI intolerance, start with one-quarter to one-third of planned maintenance dose and increase weekly until reaching maintenance dose at 1 month.

ADMINISTRATION
PO

• Give drug with food to decrease GI irritation.
• Have patient swallow delayed-release tablets whole; don't crush or cut them.
• An oral suspension may be made by a pharmacist. Shake well before use.

ACTION
May be related to observed anti-inflammatory or immunomodulatory properties.

Route	Onset	Peak	Duration
PO	Unknown	3–12 hr	Unknown

Half-life: 4 to 11 hours.

ADVERSE REACTIONS
CNS: *seizures,* dizziness, headache, depression, hallucinations, fever. **GI:** nausea, vomiting, abdominal pain, gastric distress, anorexia, stomatitis, dyspepsia.

S

GU: oligospermia, infertility. **Hematologic:** *agranulocytosis, leukopenia, thrombocytopenia, hemolytic anemia.* **Hepatic:** abnormal LFT values. **Skin:** rash, urticaria, pruritus, cyanosis.

INTERACTIONS

Drug-drug. *Digoxin:* May reduce absorption of digoxin. Monitor patient closely.

Folic acid: May decrease absorption of folic acid. Monitor patient.

Methotrexate: May enhance liver toxic effect of methotrexate. Monitor patient for hematologic toxicity and adverse GI events, especially nausea.

Prilocaine: May increase risk of significant methemoglobinemia. Monitor patient. Avoid lidocaine and prilocaine in infants receiving such agents.

Thiopurines (azathioprine, mercaptopurine): May increase leukopenia. Monitor WBC count closely.

Warfarin: May alter anticoagulant effect. Monitor therapy.

Drug-herb. *Dong quai, St. John's wort:* May also cause photosensitization. Discourage use together.

EFFECTS ON LAB TEST RESULTS

• May increase ALT and AST levels.
• May decrease Hb level and granulocyte, platelet, and WBC counts.
• May interfere with measurements, by liquid chromatography, of urinary normetanephrine and cause false-positive test results in patients exposed to sulfasalazine or its metabolite.

CONTRAINDICATIONS & CAUTIONS

• Contraindicated in patients hypersensitive to drug, its metabolites, sulfonamides, or salicylates and in those with porphyria or intestinal and urinary obstruction.
• Use cautiously and in reduced doses in patients with impaired hematologic, liver, or kidney function; severe allergy; or bronchial asthma.
※ Use cautiously in patients with G6PD deficiency as hemolytic anemia can result.
• SCARs, some fatal, including DRESS syndrome, exfoliative dermatitis, SJS, and TEN, have been reported. Patients are at highest risk for SCARs early in therapy, with most events occurring within first month of treatment. Discontinue drug at first appearance of rash or mucosal lesions.

• Serious CNS reactions can occur, including seizures, meningitis, spinal cord disorders, peripheral neuropathy, hearing loss, ataxia, and hallucinations.

Dialyzable drug: Yes.

⚠ *Overdose S&S:* Nausea, gastric distress, abdominal pain, drowsiness, seizures.

PREGNANCY-LACTATION-REPRODUCTION

• There are no adequate studies during pregnancy. Use only if clearly needed.
• Drug and its active metabolite appear in human milk. Use cautiously during breastfeeding; monitor infant for kernicterus and diarrhea or bloody stools.
• Oligospermia and infertility have been observed in men treated with drug; stopping drug may reverse these effects.

NURSING CONSIDERATIONS

• Therapeutic response in patients with RA may occur as soon as 4 weeks after starting therapy, but may take up to 12 weeks in others.
• Drug may cause urine discoloration.
⚕ *Alert:* Stop drug immediately and notify prescriber if patient shows signs and symptoms of hypersensitivity.
• Maintain adequate fluid intake to prevent crystalluria and stone formation.
• Obtain CBCs, including differential WBC count and LFT values, before start of treatment and every second week during first 3 months of therapy, monthly during the second 3 months, once every 3 months thereafter, and as clinically indicated.
• Obtain a urinalysis with careful microscopic exam and an assessment of kidney function periodically during treatment.
• Serum sulfapyridine levels greater than 50 mcg/mL appear to be associated with an increased incidence of adverse reactions.
• *Look alike–sound alike:* Don't confuse sulfasalazine with sulfadiazine.

PATIENT TEACHING

• Instruct patient in safe drug administration and to drink plenty of water.
• Advise patient that drug may produce an orange-yellow discoloration of skin and urine and may cause contact lenses to turn yellow.
• Teach patient about adverse reactions and to report them. Advise patient of the need for careful medical supervision. A sore throat,

Reactions in bold italics are *life-threatening.*

fever, pallor, purpura, or jaundice may indicate a serious blood disorder.
- Advise patient that blood and urine tests will be needed to monitor treatment and that it's important to keep lab and health care provider appointments.
- Caution patient to report pregnancy or breastfeeding to prescriber.

SUMAtriptan succinate
sue-mah-TRIP-tan

Imitrex, Imitrex STATdose, Onzetra Xsail, Tosymra, Zembrace SymTouch

Therapeutic class: Antimigraine drugs
Pharmacologic class: Serotonin 5-HT$_1$ receptor agonists

AVAILABLE FORMS
Injection: 3 mg/0.5 mL, 4 mg/0.5 mL, 6 mg/0.5 mL single-dose autoinjector; 6 mg/0.5 mL vials
Nasal powder: 11 mg/disposable nosepiece
Nasal solution: 5 mg, 10 mg, 20 mg per actuation
Tablets 🞕: 25 mg, 50 mg, 100 mg

INDICATIONS & DOSAGES
➤ **Acute migraine attacks (with or without aura)**
Adults: 1 to 6 mg subcut depending on product; maximum dose is 12 mg in 24 hours, separated by at least 1 hour. Or 25 to 100 mg PO, initially. If desired response isn't achieved in 2 hours, may give second dose of 25 to 100 mg. Additional doses may be used in at least 2-hour intervals. Maximum daily oral dose, 200 mg.

For nasal spray, give 5 mg, 10 mg, or 20 mg once in one nostril; may repeat once after 2 hours, for maximum daily dose of 40 mg. Or, Tosymra 10 mg given as a single spray in one nostril. Maximum recommended dose within 24 hours is 30 mg, with doses separated by at least 1 hour. May also give at least 1 hour after another sumatriptan product.

For nasal powder, one 11-mg nasal dose in each nostril (22 mg total), using the Xsail breath-powered delivery device. If desired response isn't achieved in 2 hours, or migraine returns after transient improvement,

may give second 22-mg nasal dose. Maximum recommended dose within 24 hours, two nasal doses (44 mg) or one nasal dose of 22 mg and one dose of another sumatriptan product, separated by at least 2 hours.

Adjust-a-dose: In patients with Child-Pugh class A or B liver impairment, the maximum single oral dose shouldn't exceed 50 mg.

➤ **Cluster headache (subcut except Zembrace)**
Adults: 6 mg subcut. Maximum recommended dose is two 6-mg injections in 24 hours, separated by at least 1 hour.

ADMINISTRATION
PO
- Give drug without regard for food.
- Have patient swallow tablet whole; don't crush or break tablet.
Subcutaneous
- Redness or pain at injection site should subside within 1 hour after injection.
- Use injection site with adequate skin and subcutaneous tissue thickness to accommodate length of needle.
Intranasal spray
- Have patient blow nose before use.
- Give medication for inhalation in one nostril, while blocking the other nostril.
- Patient should keep head upright and breathe gently for 10 to 20 seconds after administration.
Intranasal powder
- Use with the Xsail device only; insert disposable nosepiece into the device body.
- Pierce capsule inside nosepiece by pressing and releasing the white piercing button one time on the device body.
- Insert nosepiece into one nostril, ensuring a tight seal; rotate device, place mouthpiece into mouth, and blow forcefully through mouthpiece for 2 to 3 seconds to deliver powder into the nasal cavity.
- Remove and discard nosepiece; repeat in other nostril, using a second nosepiece.

ACTION
May act as agonist at serotonin receptors on extracerebral intracranial blood vessels, which constricts affected vessels, inhibits neuropeptide release, and reduces pain transmission in trigeminal pathways.

S

Route	Onset	Peak	Duration
PO	30 min	2–2.5 hr	Unknown
Subcut	10 min	12 min	Unknown
Intranasal spray	15–30 min	5–23 min	Unknown
Intranasal powder	Unknown	45 min	Unknown

Half-life: About 2 hours; intranasal, about 3 hours.

ADVERSE REACTIONS

CNS: dizziness, vertigo, drowsiness, headache, malaise, fatigue, pain, paresthesia, tingling, warm or hot sensation, burning sensation; heaviness, pressure, or tightness; strange feeling, tight feeling in head, cold sensation, numbness, taste alteration, unusual or bad taste (nasal spray), weakness. **CV:** flushing, pressure or tightness in chest. **EENT:** altered vision; discomfort of throat, nasal cavity or sinus, mouth, jaw, or tongue; rhinorrhea; rhinitis; pharyngeal edema. **GI:** abdominal discomfort, dysphagia, diarrhea, nausea, vomiting. **Musculoskeletal:** myalgia, muscle cramps, neck pain. **Respiratory:** **bronchospasm,** upper respiratory tract inflammation and dyspnea (PO). **Skin:** injection site reaction, diaphoresis.

INTERACTIONS

Drug-drug. *Ergot and ergot derivatives, other 5-HT$_1$ agonists (triptans):* May prolong vasospastic effects. Don't use within 24 hours of sumatriptan therapy.
MAO inhibitors: May reduce sumatriptan clearance. Use within 2 weeks of MAO inhibitor is contraindicated.
Serotonergic drugs (methylene blue, SNRIs, SSRIs, TCAs): May cause serotonin syndrome. Monitor patient closely if use together can't be avoided.
Drug-herb. *St. John's wort:* May increase serotonin levels. Use together cautiously.

EFFECTS ON LAB TEST RESULTS

• May increase liver enzyme levels.

CONTRAINDICATIONS & CAUTIONS

• Contraindicated in patients with hypersensitivity to drug or its components and in those with history, symptoms, or signs of ischemic cardiac, cerebrovascular (such as stroke or TIA), or peripheral vascular disease; hemiplegic or basilar migraine; significant underlying CV diseases, including angina pectoris, MI, and silent myocardial ischemia;

Wolff-Parkinson-White syndrome or arrhythmias associated with other cardiac accessory conduction pathway disorders; uncontrolled HTN; or Child-Pugh class C liver impairment.

• Use cautiously in patients with risk factors for CAD, such as patients who are postmenopausal, males older than age 40, or patients with HTN, hypercholesterolemia, obesity, diabetes, smoking, or family history of CAD.

• Noncoronary vasospastic reactions may occur with use of 5-HT$_1$ agonists, including peripheral vascular ischemia, GI ischemia and infarction (abdominal pain, bloody diarrhea), splenic infarction, Raynaud syndrome, or transient or permanent blindness.

• Before use, exclude other neurologic conditions in patients not previously diagnosed with migraine or cluster headaches and in those with atypical symptoms.

• Safety and effectiveness in children haven't been established.
Dialyzable drug: Unknown.

PREGNANCY-LACTATION-REPRODUCTION

• There are no adequate studies during pregnancy. Use only if potential benefit justifies fetal risk.

• Drug appears in human milk after subcut administration. Refer to individual manufacturer's instructions regarding breastfeeding.

NURSING CONSIDERATIONS

⚠️ *Alert:* When giving drug to patient at risk for CAD, give first dose in presence of other medical personnel. Rarely, serious adverse cardiac effects can follow administration.
⚠️ *Alert:* Combining drug with serotonergic drugs may cause serotonin syndrome (restlessness, hallucinations, loss of coordination, fast heartbeat, rapid changes in BP, increased body temperature, hyperreflexia, nausea, vomiting, diarrhea). Serotonin syndrome may occur when starting or increasing dose of drug or serotonergic drugs.

• Monitor BP; significant BP elevations have occurred even in patients without a history of HTN.

• Monitor patient for seizures. Seizures have been reported in patients with and without a history of seizures.

• After subcut injection, most patients experience relief in 1 to 2 hours.

• *Look alike–sound alike:* Don't confuse sumatriptan with somatropin.

PATIENT TEACHING

• Inform patient that drug is intended only to treat migraine attacks, not to prevent them or reduce their occurrence.

• Teach safe drug administration.

• Advise patient to take drug only as prescribed. Medication overuse headaches or increased frequency of migraine attacks may occur.

• Caution patient who is pregnant or may become pregnant not to use drug but to discuss with prescriber risks and benefits of using drug during pregnancy.

• Tell patient that drug may be taken at any time during a migraine attack, as soon as signs or symptoms appear.

🕔 *Alert:* Tell patient to report all adverse reactions and to immediately report persistent or severe chest pain. Warn patient to stop using drug and to call prescriber if pain or tightness in the throat, wheezing, heart throbbing, rash, lumps, hives, or swollen eyelids, face, or lips develop.

SAFETY ALERT!

SUNItinib malate
su-NIT-e-nib

Sutent

Therapeutic class: Antineoplastics
Pharmacologic class: Protein-tyrosine kinase inhibitors

AVAILABLE FORMS
Capsules: 12.5 mg, 25 mg, 37.5 mg, 50 mg

INDICATIONS & DOSAGES

Adjust-a-dose (for all indications): Refer to manufacturer's instructions for toxicity-related dosage adjustments.

➤ **GI stromal tumor after disease progression on or intolerance to imatinib; advanced renal cell carcinoma**

Adults: 50 mg PO once daily for 4 weeks, followed by 2 weeks off the drug. Repeat cycle until disease progression or unacceptable toxicity.

Adjust-a-dose: Increase or decrease dosage in 12.5-mg increments based on individual safety and tolerability. If drug must be

administered with a strong CYP3A4 inhibitor, reduce dosage to a minimum of 37.5 mg/day. If drug must be administered with a CYP3A4 inducer, consider increasing dosage to 87.5 mg daily; carefully monitor patient for toxicity.

➤ **Progressive, well-differentiated pancreatic neuroendocrine tumors in patients with unresectable locally advanced or metastatic disease**

Adults: 37.5 mg PO once daily given continuously without a scheduled off-treatment period. Maximum recommended dosage, 50 mg daily. Continue until disease progression or unacceptable toxicity.

Adjust-a-dose: Increase or decrease in 12.5-mg increments based on patient tolerance and safety. If drug must be administered with a strong CYP3A4 inhibitor, consider decreasing dosage to 25 mg daily. If drug must be administered with a CYP3A4 inducer, consider increasing dosage to 62.5 mg daily and carefully monitor patient for toxicity.

➤ **Adjuvant treatment of patients at high risk for recurrent renal cell carcinoma (RCC) after nephrectomy**

Adults: 50 mg PO once daily, on a schedule of 4 weeks on treatment followed by 2 weeks off treatment for a maximum of nine 6-week cycles.

Adjust-a-dose: Increase or decrease dosage in 12.5-mg increments based on individual safety and tolerability. If drug must be administered with a strong CYP3A4 inhibitor, reduce dosage to a minimum of 37.5 mg/day. If drug must be administered with a CYP3A4 inducer, consider increasing dosage to 87.5 mg daily; carefully monitor patient for toxicity.

ADMINISTRATION
PO

🕔 *Alert:* Hazardous agent; use safe handling and disposal. Avoid contact with broken capsules.

• Give drug without regard for meals.

• If a dose is missed by less than 12 hours, give missed dose right away. If a dose is missed by more than 12 hours, skip missed dose and give next scheduled dose at its regular time.

S

ACTION
A multi-kinase inhibitor targeting several receptor tyrosine kinases, which are involved in tumor growth, pathologic angiogenesis, and metastatic progression of cancer.

Route	Onset	Peak	Duration
PO	Unknown	6–12 hr	Unknown

Half-life: 40 to 60 hours; primary metabolite, 80 to 110 hours.

ADVERSE REACTIONS
CNS: altered taste, asthenia, dizziness, fatigue, fever, headache, insomnia, depression. **CV:** *decreased LVEF,* HTN, peripheral edema, chest pain. **EENT:** dry mouth, nasopharyngitis, oral pain. **GI:** abdominal pain, anorexia, GERD, constipation, diarrhea, dyspepsia, flatulence, mucositis, nausea, stomatitis, vomiting, hemorrhoids. **GU:** increased creatinine level. **Hematologic:** *bleeding, lymphopenia, neutropenia, thrombocytopenia,* anemia. **Hepatic:** elevated LFT values. **Metabolic:** hypernatremia, hyperuricemia, *hypokalemia, hyperkalemia,* hyponatremia, hypercalcemia, *hypocalcemia, hypomagnesemia,* hypophosphatemia, hypothyroidism, increased lipase level, increased amylase level, hyperbilirubinemia, weight loss. **Musculoskeletal:** arthralgia, back pain, limb pain, myalgia. **Respiratory:** cough, dyspnea, URI. **Skin:** alopecia, dry skin, hair color changes, hand-foot syndrome, rash, erythema, pruritus, skin discoloration. **Other:** flulike symptoms, chills.

INTERACTIONS
Drug-drug. *Bevacizumab:* May enhance hypertensive effect of sunitinib and increase risk of microangiopathic hemolytic anemia. Avoid use together.
QTc interval-prolonging drugs (antiarrhythmics [amiodarone, disopyramide, dofetilide, procainamide, quinidine, sotalol], arsenic trioxide, chlorpromazine, cisapride, dolasetron, droperidol, mefloquine, mesoridazine, moxifloxacin, pentamidine, pimozide, tacrolimus, thioridazine, ziprasidone): May increase risk of QTc-interval prolongation and ventricular arrhythmias. Carefully monitor ECG and QT interval. Consider therapy modification.
Strong CYP3A4 inducers (carbamazepine, dexamethasone, phenobarbital, phenytoin, rifabutin, rifampin, rifapentine): May decrease

sunitinib level and effects. If use together can't be avoided, increase sunitinib dosage.
Strong CYP3A4 inhibitors (atazanavir, clarithromycin, itraconazole, ketoconazole, nefazodone, nelfinavir, ritonavir, saquinavir, voriconazole): May increase sunitinib level and toxicity. If use together can't be avoided, decrease sunitinib dosage.
Drug-herb. *Echinacea, St. John's wort:* May cause an unpredictable decrease in drug level. Discourage use together.
Drug-food. *Grapefruit:* May increase drug level. Discourage use together.

EFFECTS ON LAB TEST RESULTS
• May increase AST, ALT, ALP, total and indirect bilirubin, amylase, lipase, creatinine, uric acid, and TSH levels.
• May decrease phosphorus, magnesium, and albumin levels.
• May increase or decrease potassium, calcium, glucose, and sodium levels.
• May decrease Hb level, hematocrit, and RBC, neutrophil, lymphocyte, WBC, and platelet counts.

CONTRAINDICATIONS & CAUTIONS
• Contraindicated in patients hypersensitive to drug or its components.
• Use cautiously in patients with electrolyte imbalance or a history of HTN, QT-interval prolongation, concurrent antiarrhythmic use, bradycardia, MI, angina, CABG, symptomatic HF, stroke, TIA, or PE.
• Thrombotic microangiopathy (TMA), including thrombotic thrombocytopenic purpura and hemolytic uremic syndrome, sometimes leading to kidney failure or a fatal outcome, has been reported. Discontinue if TMA develops.
• Proteinuria and nephrotic syndrome have been reported, and some cases have resulted in kidney failure and fatal outcomes. Monitor patient for development or worsening of proteinuria.
• SCARs (erythema multiforme, SJS, and TEN), have been reported, some of which were fatal. If patient develops signs or symptoms of a progressive rash, often with blisters or mucosal lesions, discontinue drug. If a diagnosis of SJS or TEN is suspected, don't restart drug.
• Necrotizing fasciitis, including of the perineum and secondary to fistula formation,

---

Reactions in bold italics are *life-threatening*.

sometimes fatal, has been reported. Discontinue drug if necrotizing fasciitis develops.
• Drug has been associated with symptomatic hypoglycemia, which may result in loss of consciousness or require hospitalization. Blood glucose level reductions may be worse in patients with diabetes. Check blood glucose levels regularly during and after discontinuation of treatment. Assess if antidiabetic dosage needs adjustment to minimize risk of hypoglycemia.
Dialyzable drug: No.

PREGNANCY-LACTATION-REPRODUCTION
• Drug can cause fetal harm when used during pregnancy. If used during pregnancy, or if patient becomes pregnant while taking drug, apprise patient of fetal risk.
• Patients of childbearing potential should use effective contraception during treatment and for at least 4 weeks after final dose.
• Male patients with partners of childbearing potential should use effective contraception during treatment and for 7 weeks after final dose.
• It isn't known if drug appears in human milk. Patient should discontinue breastfeeding or discontinue drug, considering importance of drug to patient.
• Sunitinib treatment may compromise male and female fertility.

NURSING CONSIDERATIONS
Boxed Warning Drug may cause severe, sometimes fatal, liver toxicity. Monitor liver function before and during each cycle of therapy. ∎
• Obtain LFT values at baseline, before each treatment cycle, and when clinically indicated.
• Verify pregnancy status before treatment.
⚠ Alert: Drug may cause CV events, including HF, myocardial disorders, and cardiomyopathy, which may be fatal. Monitor CV status closely.
• Obtain baseline evaluation of LVEF in all patients before treatment. If patient had a cardiac event in the year before treatment, check LVEF periodically.
• Interrupt therapy or decrease dosage in patients with LVEF less than 50% and more than 20% below baseline.
• Monitor patient's BP closely. If severe HTN occurs, notify prescriber. Drug may need to be withheld until BP is controlled.

• Monitor patient for signs and symptoms of HF, especially if there is a history of heart disease.
• Obtain CBC with platelet count and serum phosphate, magnesium, and calcium levels before each treatment cycle.
• Obtain urinalysis at baseline and periodically during treatment, with follow-up measurement of 24-hour urine protein as clinically indicated to evaluate patient for nephrotic syndrome.
• Check blood glucose level regularly during and after discontinuation of treatment. Assess if antidiabetic dosage needs adjustment to minimize risk of hypoglycemia.
• Thyroid dysfunction (hypothyroidism, hyperthyroidism, thyroiditis) may occur. Monitor thyroid function at baseline and closely monitor patients for signs and symptoms suggestive of thyroid dysfunction.
• For patients with CKD on hemodialysis, no starting dosage adjustment is recommended. However, given the decreased exposure compared to patients with normal kidney function, may increase subsequent doses gradually up to twofold based on safety and tolerability.
• Patient who has seizures may have reversible posterior leukoencephalopathy syndrome. Signs and symptoms include HTN, headache, decreased alertness, altered mental functioning, and vision loss. Stop treatment temporarily.
• Impaired wound healing has been reported during therapy. Temporarily interrupt therapy in patients undergoing major surgical procedures. May resume drug when provider determines patient has recovered.
• Provide antiemetics or antidiarrheals as needed for adverse GI effects.
• Monitor patient with RCC or GI stromal tumor with high tumor burden closely and treat as clinically indicated because of the risk of TLS. Correct dehydration and high uric acid levels before treatment.
• Osteonecrosis of the jaw has been reported. Consider preventive dentistry before treatment with sunitinib. If possible, avoid invasive dental procedures, particularly in patients receiving IV bisphosphonate therapy.
⚠ Alert: Drug may cause bleeding in GI tract, urinary tract, respiratory tract, and brain, which may be fatal. Monitor patient and CBC closely.

• Drug may cause GI perforation in patients with intraabdominal malignancies. Monitor patient closely.

PATIENT TEACHING

• Advise patient to keep appointments for blood tests and periodic heart function evaluations.

• Teach patient safe drug administration and handling.

• Tell patient about common adverse effects, such as diarrhea, nausea, vomiting, fatigue, mouth pain, and taste disturbance, and to report all adverse reactions.

• Advise patient that severe hypoglycemia can occur. Inform patient of the signs, symptoms, and risks associated with hypoglycemia.

• Inform patient about changes that may occur in skin and hair, including color changes and dry, red, blistering skin of the hands and feet.

• Urge patient to tell prescriber about all prescribed and OTC drugs or herbal supplements.

• Warn patient not to consume grapefruit products during therapy.

• Tell patient to notify prescriber about unusual bleeding, trouble breathing, fainting, light-headedness, heart palpitations, wheezing, severe or prolonged diarrhea or vomiting, or swelling of the hands or lower legs.

• Advise patient of reproductive potential on effective contraception use.

suvorexant
soo-voe-REX-ant

Belsomra

Therapeutic class: Hypnotics
Pharmacologic class: Orexin receptor antagonists
Controlled substance schedule: IV

AVAILABLE FORMS
Tablets: 5 mg, 10 mg, 15 mg, 20 mg

INDICATIONS & DOSAGES
➤ **Insomnia characterized by difficulties with sleep onset or sleep maintenance**
Adults: 10 mg PO daily within 30 minutes of going to bed. If 10-mg dose is tolerated

but not effective, increase to a maximum of 20 mg PO daily. Don't exceed more than one dose per night.

Adjust-a-dose: For patients taking concomitant moderate CYP3A4 inhibitors, give 5 mg PO daily at night. Maximum dose, 10 mg daily.

ADMINISTRATION
PO
• Give drug within 30 minutes of bedtime and ensure at least 7 hours remain before planned time of awakening.

• May give without regard to food; however, the time to drug's effect is delayed if drug is taken with or soon after a meal.

ACTION
Blocks orexin receptors, suppressing the system responsible for promoting wakefulness.

Route	Onset	Peak	Duration
PO	30 min	2 hr	Unknown

Half-life: 12 hours.

ADVERSE REACTIONS
CNS: somnolence, headache, dizziness, abnormal dreams. **EENT:** dry mouth. **GI:** diarrhea. **Respiratory:** cough, URI.

INTERACTIONS
Drug-drug. ❶ *Alert: Benzodiazepines, opioids:* May cause slow or difficult breathing, sedation, and death. Avoid use together. If use together is necessary, limit dosage and duration of each drug to minimum necessary for desired effect.

CNS depressants, including other drugs that treat insomnia: May cause excessive CNS depression. Use together isn't recommended.
Digoxin: May decrease digoxin metabolism. Monitor digoxin level.
Moderate CYP3A4 inhibitors (amprenavir, aprepitant, atazanavir, ciprofloxacin, diltiazem, erythromycin, fluconazole, fosamprenavir, imatinib, verapamil): May decrease suvorexant metabolism. Decrease initial suvorexant daily dose to 5 mg; don't exceed a dose of 10 mg.
Strong CYP3A4 inducers (carbamazepine, phenytoin, rifampin): May decrease clinical effect of suvorexant. Monitor patient for reduced therapeutic effect.
Strong CYP3A4 inhibitors (clarithromycin, conivaptan, itraconazole, ketoconazole,

Reactions in bold italics are *life-threatening.*

nefazodone, nelfinavir, posaconazole, ritonavir, saquinavir, telaprevir): May increase risk of additive toxicity. Avoid use together.

Drug-food. *Grapefruit juice:* May decrease drug metabolism and increase drug level. Decrease suvorexant dosage.

Drug-lifestyle. *Alcohol use:* May cause excessive CNS depression. Discourage use together.

EFFECTS ON LAB TEST RESULTS
• May increase cholesterol level.

CONTRAINDICATIONS & CAUTIONS
• Contraindicated in patients hypersensitive to drug or its components and in those with narcolepsy.
• Not recommended for use in patients with Child-Pugh class C liver impairment.
• **Alert:** Drug may increase risk of suicidality. Immediately evaluate patients who report suicidality or exhibit new behavioral signs or symptoms.
• Use cautiously in patients with compromised respiratory status (obstructive sleep apnea, COPD) or a history of drug abuse or dependence.
• Drug can cause drowsiness. Patients, especially older adults, are at higher risk for falls.
• Safety and effectiveness in children haven't been studied.
Dialyzable drug: Unknown.
Overdose S&S: Increased frequency and duration of somnolence.

PREGNANCY-LACTATION-REPRODUCTION
• Drug hasn't been studied in pregnancy. Use cautiously during pregnancy and only if benefits outweigh fetal risk.
• It isn't known if drug appears in human milk. Use cautiously during breastfeeding.

NURSING CONSIDERATIONS
• Use the smallest effective dosage in all patients. Lower dosages may be necessary in obese or female patients.
• Complex sleep behaviors, such as sleepwalking, "sleep driving" (driving while not fully awake), preparing and eating food, making phone calls, or having sex with subsequent amnesia of the event, have been reported. These behaviors may occur after the first or any subsequent use of the drug,

with or without concomitant use of alcohol or CNS depressants, which increase the risk. Discontinue drug for complex sleep behavior.
• Monitor patient for daytime somnolence.
• Carefully evaluate patient for physical or psychiatric causes of sleep disturbances before drug is prescribed. If insomnia persists for more than 7 to 10 days, reevaluate patient.
• Monitor patients for sleep paralysis (inability to move or speak during sleep-wake transitions), hallucinations, and mild cataplexy signs and symptoms (periods of leg weakness).
• **Alert:** Worsening of depression or suicidality may occur. Be alert for signs and symptoms of depression or behavioral changes.

PATIENT TEACHING
• Teach patient safe drug administration.
• Instruct patient not to increase dosage without first consulting prescriber.
• Advise patient to avoid alcohol and other drugs that cause sleepiness while taking suvorexant.
• Caution patient that increased drowsiness may increase the risk of falls in some patients, especially older adults.
• Tell patient to notify prescriber if abnormal thoughts and behavior, symptoms of depression (changes in mood, excessive tiredness), or insomnia that persists for more than 7 to 10 days occurs.
• **Alert:** Caution patient to immediately report suicidality or new behavioral signs or symptoms.
• Inform patient that sleep paralysis (inability to move or speak during sleep-wake transitions), vivid and disturbing perceptions, and temporary leg weakness can occur.
• Advise patient that daytime somnolence can occur and to avoid performing activities that require mental alertness or physical coordination (such as driving) until fully awake.
• Warn patient of the risk of performing complex behaviors, such as driving, eating, and making phone calls, while asleep and to report if these symptoms occur.
• Advise patient to report pregnancy, plans to become pregnant, or to breastfeed.

tacrolimus (topical)
tack-ROW-lim-us

Protopic

Therapeutic class: Immunomodulators
Pharmacologic class: Calcineurin inhibitors

AVAILABLE FORMS
Ointment: 0.03%, 0.1%

INDICATIONS & DOSAGES
➤ **Moderate to severe atopic dermatitis in patients unresponsive to other therapies or unable to use other therapies**
Adults and children ages 16 and older: Apply a thin layer of 0.03% or 0.1% strength to affected areas b.i.d. and rub in completely.
Children ages 2 to 15: Apply a thin layer of 0.03% strength to affected areas b.i.d. and rub in completely.

ADMINISTRATION
Topical
⊙ *Alert:* Hazardous drug; use safe handling and disposal precautions.
• In patients with infected atopic dermatitis, clear infection at treatment site before using drug.
• Don't use with occlusive dressings.
• Stop drug when signs and symptoms resolve.
• If signs and symptoms of atopic dermatitis don't improve within 6 weeks, refer patient to health care provider to confirm diagnosis.

ACTION
Unknown. Probably acts as an immune system modulator in the skin by inhibiting T-lymphocyte activation, which causes immunosuppression. Also inhibits the release of mediators from mast cells and basophils in skin.

Route	Onset	Peak	Duration
Topical	Unknown	Unknown	Unknown

Half-life: Unknown.

ADVERSE REACTIONS
CNS: headache, hyperesthesia, asthenia, insomnia, fever, depression, paresthesia, pain.
CV: peripheral edema, HTN, facial edema.
EENT: conjunctivitis, otitis media, ear pain, pharyngitis, rhinitis, sinusitis, periodontal abscess, tooth disorder. **GI:** diarrhea, vomiting, nausea, abdominal pain, gastroenteritis,

dyspepsia. **GU:** UTI, dysmenorrhea. **Musculoskeletal:** back pain, arthralgia, myalgia. **Respiratory:** increased cough, *asthma,* pneumonia, bronchitis. **Skin:** alopecia, burning, cellulitis, pruritus, erythema, infection, herpes simplex, eczema herpeticum, pustular rash, folliculitis, acne, urticaria, maculopapular rash, fungal dermatitis, sunburn, tingling, benign skin neoplasm, vesiculobullous rash, dry skin, varicella zoster, herpes zoster, eczema, exfoliative dermatitis, contact dermatitis. **Other:** flulike symptoms, accidental injury, infection, alcohol intolerance, cyst, allergic reaction, lack of drug effect.

INTERACTIONS
Drug-drug. *CYP3A4 inhibitors (calcium channel blockers, cimetidine, erythromycin, ketoconazole, protease inhibitors):* May increase tacrolimus level if systemic absorption occurs. Use together cautiously.
Immunosuppressants: May enhance adverse effects of other immunosuppressants. Avoid use together.
Tacrolimus (systemic): May increase toxicity. Use together cautiously and decrease dosage as needed.
Drug-lifestyle. *Alcohol use:* May cause flushing. Discourage use together.
Sun exposure: May cause phototoxicity. Advise patient to avoid excessive sunlight and artificial UV light exposure.

EFFECTS ON LAB TEST RESULTS
None reported.

CONTRAINDICATIONS & CAUTIONS
• Contraindicated in patients hypersensitive to drug.
   Boxed Warning Although a causal relationship hasn't been established, rare cases of skin malignancy and lymphoma have been reported in patients treated with topical calcineurin inhibitors. Avoid long-term use and don't use in children younger than age 2. Only use 0.03% ointment for children ages 2 to 15. ∎
• Don't use in patients who are immunocompromised or in patients with skin conditions with a skin barrier defect (Netherton syndrome, generalized erythroderma) that increase the risk of systemic absorption.
• Safety hasn't been established beyond 1 year of noncontinuous use.
• Kidney insufficiency has been reported in patients who were prescribed ointment for

application to large BSAs. Use cautiously in patients at risk for kidney impairment.
☻ **Alert:** Use only after other therapies have failed or aren't advisable.
Dialyzable drug: Unknown.

PREGNANCY-LACTATION-REPRODUCTION
• Studies on topical tacrolimus use during pregnancy are inadequate. Drug crosses placental barrier with systemic use. Use only if potential benefit justifies fetal risk.
• Drug appears in human milk. Patient should discontinue breastfeeding or discontinue drug, considering importance of drug to patient.

NURSING CONSIDERATIONS
• Ensure treatment area bacterial or viral skin infections have resolved before starting tacrolimus.
• Use of drug may increase risk of varicella zoster, herpes simplex virus, and eczema herpeticum.
• Consider stopping drug in patient with lymphadenopathy of unknown cause or diagnosed acute mononucleosis.
• Monitor all cases of lymphadenopathy until resolution.
• Local adverse effects are most common during the first few days of treatment.
• Avoid use on areas of skin affected by premalignant and malignant skin conditions.

PATIENT TEACHING
• Teach about proper drug administration, storage, and handling.
• Tell patient to wash hands before and after applying drug and to avoid applying drug to wet skin.
• Urge patient not to use bandages or other occlusive dressings over treatment area.
• Tell patient not to bathe, shower, or swim immediately after application because doing so could wash off the ointment.
• Explain that patient can apply a moisturizer after topical tacrolimus.
• Tell patient to stop treatment when signs and symptoms resolve.
• Instruct patient to report symptoms that worsen or fail to improve.
• Advise patient to avoid or minimize exposure to natural and artificial sunlight.
• Caution patient not to use drug for any disorder other than that for which it was prescribed.
• Encourage patient to report adverse reactions.

tadalafil ✖
tah-DAL-ah-fill

Adcirca, Alyq, Cialis, Tadliq

Therapeutic class: Erectile dysfunction drugs
Pharmacologic class: PDE5 inhibitors

AVAILABLE FORMS
Oral suspension: 20 mg/5 mL
Tablets (film-coated): 2.5 mg, 5 mg, 10 mg, 20 mg

INDICATIONS & DOSAGES
➤ **Erectile dysfunction (Cialis)**
Adults: 10 mg PO as a single dose, PRN, at least 30 minutes before sexual activity. Base range of 5 to 20 mg on effectiveness and tolerance. Maximum, one dose daily. Or, 2.5 mg PO once daily without regard to timing of sexual activity; may increase to 5 mg PO daily.
Adjust-a-dose: If CrCl ranges from 30 to 50 mL/minute, begin 5 mg once daily; maximum dosage is 10 mg once every 48 hours. If CrCl falls below 30 mL/minute or patient requires hemodialysis, maximum is 5 mg once every 72 hours as needed; daily use isn't recommended. Use cautiously in patients with Child-Pugh class A or B liver impairment; don't exceed 10 mg daily. Patients taking strong CYP3A4 inhibitors shouldn't exceed one 10-mg dose every 72 hours if taken as needed; the once-daily dose shouldn't exceed 2.5 mg.
➤ **BPH (Cialis)**
Adults: 5 mg PO once daily taken at approximately the same time every day. When used with finasteride, 5 mg once daily taken at approximately the same time every day for up to 26 weeks.
Adjust-a-dose: In patients with CrCl of 30 to 50 mL/minute, starting dose is 2.5 mg PO daily. May increase to 5 mg PO daily based on individual response. Not recommended for patients with CrCl less than 30 mL/minute or in patients on hemodialysis.
➤ **BPH and erectile dysfunction (Cialis)**
Adults: 5 mg PO once daily taken at approximately the same time every day, without regard to timing of sexual activity.
Adjust-a-dose: In patients with CrCl of 30 to 50 mL/minute, starting dosage is 2.5 mg PO

T

daily. May increase to 5 mg PO daily based on individual response. Not recommended for patients with CrCl less than 30 mL/minute or in patients on hemodialysis.

➤ **PAH (Adcirca, Alyq, Tadliq)**
Adults: 40 mg (solution or two 20-mg tablets) PO once daily.
Adjust-a-dose: For patients with CrCl of 31 to 80 mL/minute, start with 20 mg PO once daily. Increase to 40 mg once daily as tolerated. Avoid use in patients with CrCl of 30 mL/minute or less and in those on hemodialysis. Consider starting dose of 20 mg PO once daily in patients with Child-Pugh class A or B liver impairment.

In patients receiving ritonavir for at least 1 week, start at 20 mg PO once daily and increase to 40 mg as tolerated. Don't use drug when starting ritonavir; stop drug at least 24 hours before starting ritonavir. After at least 1 week, may resume drug at 20 mg PO once daily and increase to 40 mg as tolerated.

ADMINISTRATION
PO
• Give drug without regard to food.
• Don't split Cialis tablets. Give entire dose as prescribed.
• Dividing 40-mg PAH dose over the course of the day isn't recommended.

ACTION
Inhibits PDE5 enzyme, which leads to increased cyclic guanosine monophosphate levels, prolonged smooth muscle relaxation, and increased blood flow into the corpus cavernosum and pulmonary arteries. Also affects the smooth muscle of the prostate and bladder and their vascular supply.

Route	Onset	Peak	Duration
PO	Within 1 hr	0.5–6 hr	Up to 36 hr

Half-life: 15 to 17.5 hours; PAH (in patients not receiving bosentan), 35 hours.

ADVERSE REACTIONS
CNS: dizziness, headache. **CV:** flushing, HTN. **EENT:** nasal congestion, nasopharyngitis. **GI:** dyspepsia, abdominal pain, diarrhea, GERD, gastroenteritis, nausea. **GU:** UTI. **Musculoskeletal:** back pain, limb pain, myalgia. **Respiratory:** cough, respiratory tract infection.

INTERACTIONS
Drug-drug. *Alpha blockers (doxazosin, alfuzosin):* May increase risk of hypotension. For erectile dysfunction, patient should be on stable dose before starting tadalafil at lowest recommended dosage. Use with tadalafil for BPH treatment isn't recommended; stop alpha blocker at least 1 day before starting tadalafil.
Antihypertensives (amlodipine, ARBs, enalapril, metoprolol): May increase hypotensive effect. Monitor patient closely.
Guanylate cyclase stimulators (riociguat): May increase hypotension. Use together is contraindicated.
Nitrates: May enhance hypotensive effects. Use together is contraindicated. If patient requires nitrates, wait at least 48 hours after last tadalafil dose.
Other PDE5 inhibitors (sildenafil, vardenafil): Use together hasn't been studied. Discourage use together.
Rifampin, other CYP3A inducers: May decrease tadalafil level. Avoid use together for PAH. For erectile dysfunction or BPH, monitor patient closely.
Strong CYP3A4 inhibitors (ketoconazole, protease inhibitors, ritonavir): May increase tadalafil level. For erectile dysfunction, don't exceed a 10-mg dose of Cialis every 72 hours if taken PRN or 2.5 mg once-daily dose. For PAH, avoid use together.
Drug-food. *Grapefruit, grapefruit juice:* May increase drug level. Discourage use together.
Drug-lifestyle. *Alcohol use:* May increase risk of headache, dizziness, orthostatic hypotension, and increased HR. Discourage use together.
Inhaled street drugs ("poppers," amyl nitrate, butyl nitrate, nitrite): May enhance hypotensive effects, causing dizziness, syncope, MI, or stroke. Use together is contraindicated.

EFFECTS ON LAB TEST RESULTS
None reported.

CONTRAINDICATIONS & CAUTIONS
• Contraindicated in patients hypersensitive to drug or its components.
• Use cautiously in patients with Child-Pugh class A or B liver impairment.
• Drug isn't recommended for patients with Child-Pugh class C liver impairment, CrCl less than 30 mL/minute, unstable angina, angina that occurs during sexual intercourse,

---

*Reactions in bold italics are **life-threatening**.*

NYHA Class II or greater HF within past 6 months, uncontrolled arrhythmias, hypotension (lower than 90/50 mm Hg), uncontrolled HTN, stroke within past 6 months, or MI within past 90 days.
• Use cautiously in patients with left ventricular outflow obstruction or autonomic dysfunction. Use in patients with pulmonary veno-occlusive disease isn't recommended.
⚵ Drug isn't recommended for patients whose cardiac status makes sexual activity inadvisable or for those with known hereditary degenerative retinal disorders.
• Nonarteritic anterior ischemic optic neuropathy (NAION), a rare cause of decreased vision, including permanent vision loss, has been reported with all PDE5 inhibitors; a causal relationship hasn't been established. Most, but not all, patients had underlying risk factors for NAION.
• Use cautiously in patients with bleeding disorders, significant peptic ulceration, or kidney impairment.
• Use cautiously in patients with conditions that predispose them to priapism (sickle cell anemia, multiple myeloma, leukemia) and in those with anatomic penis abnormalities.
• Safety and effectiveness in children with PAH haven't been established.
• Use cautiously in older adults.
Dialyzable drug: No.

PREGNANCY-LACTATION-REPRODUCTION
• Studies during pregnancy are inadequate. Tadalafil crosses the placental barrier. Untreated PAH during pregnancy increases risk of HF, stroke, preterm delivery, and maternal and fetal death.
• It isn't known if drug appears in human milk. Use cautiously during breastfeeding if tadalafil is required for PAH.

NURSING CONSIDERATIONS
❶ *Alert:* Sexual activity may increase cardiac risk. Evaluate patient's cardiac risk before starting drug.
• Before drug initiation, assess patient for underlying causes of erectile dysfunction.
• Transient decreases in supine BP may occur. Monitor for orthostatic hypotension.
• Prolonged erections and priapism may occur.
• Monitor patient for (rare) vision or hearing loss. Report immediately.

• *Look alike–sound alike:* Don't confuse tadalafil with sildenafil or vardenafil. Don't confuse Alyq with Alli.

PATIENT TEACHING
• Warn patient that taking drug with nitrates or guanylate cyclase stimulators could cause a serious drop in BP, which increases the risk of heart attack and stroke.
• Tell patient to seek immediate medical attention if chest pain develops after taking drug.
• Explain that drug doesn't protect against sexually transmitted infections and patient should use protective measures.
• Urge patient to seek emergency medical care for an erection lasting more than 4 hours.
• Tell patient to take drug about 30 to 60 minutes before anticipated sexual activity, if using as needed. Explain that drug has no effect without sexual stimulation.
• Warn patient not to change dosage unless directed by prescriber.
• Caution patient against drinking large amounts of alcohol while taking drug.
• Instruct patient to report vision or hearing changes, especially sudden loss of vision in one or both eyes.

SAFETY ALERT!

tamoxifen citrate
ta-MOX-i-fen

Soltamox

Therapeutic class: Antineoplastics
Pharmacologic class: Nonsteroidal antiestrogens

AVAILABLE FORMS
Oral solution: 10 mg/5 mL*
Tablets: 10 mg, 20 mg

INDICATIONS & DOSAGES
➤ **Estrogen receptor-positive metastatic breast cancer**
Adults: 20 to 40 mg PO daily; divide doses of more than 20 mg/day into two doses.
➤ **Adjuvant treatment of early-stage estrogen receptor-positive breast cancer; to reduce occurrence of contralateral breast cancer**
Adults: 20 mg PO daily for 5 to 10 years.
➤ **To reduce breast cancer occurrence**
High-risk adults: 20 mg PO daily for 5 years.

T

➤ **Ductal carcinoma in situ (DCIS) after breast surgery and radiation to reduce risk of invasive breast cancer**
Adults: 20 mg PO daily for 5 years.
➤ **Prevention or treatment of antiandrogen-associated gynecomastia in patients with prostate cancer ◆**
Adults: 20 mg PO daily for up to 12 months.

ADMINISTRATION
PO
⊕ *Alert:* Hazardous drug; use safe-handling and disposal precautions.
• Give drug without regard to food.
• Use supplied dosing cup for oral solution.
• Store drug at room temperature. Protect from light and excessive heat.
• Don't freeze or refrigerate oral solution; use within 3 months of opening.

ACTION
Competes with estrogen for estrogen receptor-positive breast cancer cells, thereby preventing their growth.

Route	Onset	Peak	Duration
PO	Unknown	5 hr	Several wk

Half-life: Terminal phase, 5 to 7 days for tamoxifen and 14 days for the metabolite.

ADVERSE REACTIONS
CNS: sleepiness, headache, fatigue, depression, insomnia, dizziness, anxiety, mood changes, paresthesia, pain, *ischemic cerebrovascular event.* **CV:** fluid retention, chest pain, HTN, edema, flushing, ischemic heart disease, lymphedema, vasodilation, *thromboembolism.* **EENT:** corneal changes, cataracts, retinopathy, pharyngitis, sinusitis. **GI:** nausea, vomiting, diarrhea, constipation, dyspepsia, GI disorder, abdominal cramps, abdominal pain, anorexia. **GU:** amenorrhea, irregular menses, vaginal discharge, vaginal dryness, vaginitis, vulvovaginitis, ovarian cysts, vaginal bleeding, increased creatinine level, UTI. **Hematologic:** *leukopenia, thrombocytopenia,* anemia. **Hepatic:** elevated liver enzyme levels. **Metabolic:** weight gain or loss, hypercholesterolemia. **Musculoskeletal:** bone pain, arthralgia, arthritis, osteoporosis, fracture, arthrosis, myalgia. **Respiratory:** *PE,* cough, dyspnea, bronchitis. **Skin:** skin changes, rash, diaphoresis, alopecia. **Other:** accidental injury, tumor pain, hot flashes,
infection, flulike syndrome, *neoplasm,* breast pain.

INTERACTIONS
Drug-drug. *Aromatase inhibitors (anastrozole, letrozole):* May decrease aromatase inhibitor level. Avoid use together.
Cytotoxic drugs: May increase risk of thromboembolic events. Monitor patient.
Drugs that prolong QTc interval: May increase risk of life-threatening cardiac arrhythmias. Use together cautiously.
Strong CYP2D6 inhibitors (fluoxetine, paroxetine, sertraline): May decrease serum level of active metabolites of tamoxifen and decrease tamoxifen's therapeutic effects. Avoid use together.
Strong CYP3A4 inducers (rifampin): May decrease tamoxifen level. Monitor patient for clinical effects.
Warfarin: May significantly increase anticoagulant effect. Closely monitor patient, PT, and INR.
Drug-herb. *St. John's wort:* May decrease tamoxifen level. Discourage use together.
Drug-food. *Grapefruit, grapefruit juice:* May decrease tamoxifen metabolism. Discourage use together.

EFFECTS ON LAB TEST RESULTS
• May increase serum creatinine, calcium, T_4, cholesterol, bilirubin, lipid, and liver enzyme levels.
• May decrease WBC and platelet counts.

CONTRAINDICATIONS & CAUTIONS
• Contraindicated in patients hypersensitive to drug.
• Contraindicated as therapy to reduce risk of breast cancer in high-risk patients and patients with DCIS who concurrently are taking coumarin-type anticoagulants or in patients with history of VTE.
Boxed Warning Serious and life-threatening events associated with tamoxifen include uterine malignancies, stroke, and PE. Discuss potential benefits and risks with patients at high risk for breast cancer and patients with DCIS who are considering tamoxifen to reduce the risk of developing breast cancer. Benefits of drug outweigh its risks in most patients already diagnosed with breast cancer. ∎
• Use cautiously in patients with leukopenia, thrombocytopenia, or bone marrow suppression.

Reactions in bold italics are *life-threatening*.

• Drug increases risk of endometrial changes, including hyperplasia, polyps, endometrial cancer, and uterine cancer.
• Drug may increase risk of fatty liver, cholestasis, hepatitis, liver necrosis, and liver cancer.
Dialyzable drug: No.
⚠ *Overdose S&S:* Tremors, hyperreflexia, unsteady gait, dizziness, seizures, prolonged QT interval.

PREGNANCY-LACTATION-REPRODUCTION
• May cause fetal harm when used during pregnancy. Fetal risks include the potential long-term risk of a diethylstilbestrol (DES)-like syndrome. Patients of childbearing potential should use barrier or nonhormonal contraceptives during treatment and for 2 months after final dose.
• Drug may cause infertility in females.
• Breastfeeding is contraindicated during therapy and for 3 months after final dose.

NURSING CONSIDERATIONS
• Verify pregnancy status before treatment.
• Monitor lipid levels during long-term therapy in patient with hyperlipidemia.
• Monitor calcium level. At start of therapy, drug may compound hypercalcemia related to bone metastases.
• Monitor patient for signs and symptoms of venous thromboembolism.
• Monitor bone mineral density in patient who is premenopausal.
• Ensure patient has baseline and periodic gynecologic exams because of a slight increased risk of endometrial cancer.
• Ensure patient has periodic eye exams because of increased risk of cataracts, retinal vein thrombosis, and retinopathy.
• Closely monitor CBC in patient with leukopenia or thrombocytopenia.
• Monitor liver function periodically.
• Patient may initially experience worsening symptoms.
• Karyopyknotic index of vaginal smears and estrogen effect of Papanicolaou smears may vary in patients after menopause.
• *Look alike–sound alike:* Don't confuse tamoxifen with tamsulosin.

PATIENT TEACHING
• Teach about proper drug administration and handling.

• Reassure patient that acute worsening of bone pain during therapy usually indicates drug will produce good response. Give analgesics to relieve pain.
• Strongly encourage patient who is taking or has taken drug to have regular gynecologic exams because drug may increase risk of uterine cancer.
• Encourage patient to have mammograms and breast exams as recommended.
• Advise patient to use a barrier form of contraception because short-term therapy induces ovulation in patients who are premenopausal.
• Instruct patient to report vaginal bleeding or changes in menstrual cycle.
• Caution patient to use effective nonhormonal contraception during treatment and for 2 months after final dose. Advise patient to consult prescriber before becoming pregnant.
• Tell patient to report all adverse reactions, especially signs and symptoms of stroke (headache; vision changes; confusion; difficulty speaking; weakness of face, arm, or leg, especially on one side of the body), PE (chest pain, difficulty breathing, rapid breathing, diaphoresis, fainting), and DVT (leg swelling, tenderness).
• Advise patient to report vision changes.

tamsulosin hydrochloride
tam-soo-LOE-sin

Flomax, Flomax CR✦

Therapeutic class: BPH drugs
Pharmacologic class: Alpha blockers

AVAILABLE FORMS
Capsules ⬤: 0.4 mg

INDICATIONS & DOSAGES
➤ **BPH**
Adults: 0.4 mg PO once daily. If no response after 2 to 4 weeks, increase dosage to 0.8 mg PO once daily.
➤ **Ureteral stone expulsion** ◆
Adults: 0.4 mg PO daily until expulsion of stones or for up to 4 weeks for medical expulsive therapy of stones at least 5 to 10 mm. Or, 0.4 mg daily starting immediately after lithotripsy for 2 weeks to 3 months.

T

ADMINISTRATION

PO

• Have patient swallow capsules whole; don't crush or open capsules.

• Give drug about 30 minutes after same meal each day.

• If a dose is missed, give missed dose as soon as possible. If 1 day elapses without a dose, continue with next regularly scheduled dose. If dose is missed for several days, consult prescriber.

• If treatment is interrupted for several days, restart with 0.4 mg daily.

ACTION

Selectively blocks alpha receptors in the prostate, leading to relaxation of smooth muscles in the bladder neck and prostate, improving urine flow and reducing symptoms of BPH.

Route	Onset	Peak	Duration
PO	Unknown	4–7 hr	9–15 hr

Half-life: 9 to 13 hours.

ADVERSE REACTIONS

CNS: dizziness, headache, asthenia, insomnia, somnolence, syncope, vertigo. **CV:** chest pain, orthostatic hypotension. **EENT:** rhinitis, pharyngitis, sinusitis, tooth disorder. **GI:** diarrhea, nausea. **GU:** decreased libido, abnormal ejaculation. **Musculoskeletal:** back pain. **Respiratory:** increased cough. **Other:** infection.

INTERACTIONS

Drug-drug. *Alpha blockers (doxazosin, prazosin):* May interact with tamsulosin. Avoid use together.

Cimetidine: May increase tamsulosin level. Use together cautiously.

Moderate CYP3A4 inhibitors (erythromycin): May increase tamsulosin level. Use cautiously and monitor therapy.

Moderate and strong CYP2D6 inhibitors (paroxetine, terbinafine): May increase tamsulosin level. Monitor therapy.

PDE5 inhibitors: May cause symptomatic hypotension. Use together cautiously.

Strong CYP3A4 inhibitors (ketoconazole): May increase tamsulosin level. Avoid use together.

Warfarin: Studies are limited and inconclusive. Use together cautiously.

Drug-herb. *St. John's wort:* May decrease tamsulosin level. Discourage use together.

EFFECTS ON LAB TEST RESULTS

None reported.

CONTRAINDICATIONS & CAUTIONS

• Contraindicated in patients hypersensitive to drug or its components.

• Use cautiously in patients with serious or life-threatening sulfa allergy.

• Intraoperative floppy iris syndrome has been observed during cataract and glaucoma surgery in some patients who are taking or had previously taken alpha₁ blockers, including tamsulosin, which may increase risk of eye complications during and after surgery. Avoid initiating therapy in patients scheduled for cataract or glaucoma surgery.

• Drug is not indicated for use in children.

Dialyzable drug: Unlikely.

⚠ *Overdose S&S:* Severe headache, hypotension.

PREGNANCY-LACTATION-REPRODUCTION

• Drug isn't indicated for use in females.

• Don't use drug for off-label indication during pregnancy or breastfeeding.

NURSING CONSIDERATIONS

• Monitor patient for decreases in BP. Drug may cause orthostatic hypotension and syncope, especially with first dose.

• Symptoms of BPH and prostate cancer are similar; screen for prostate cancer before starting therapy and at regular intervals during therapy.

• Rare but serious priapism can occur and must be treated urgently.

• *Look alike–sound alike:* Don't confuse Flomax with Fosamax, Flonase, or Flovent.

PATIENT TEACHING

• Teach about proper drug administration and handling.

• Advise patient that drug may cause sudden drop in BP, especially after first dose or when changing doses. Tell patient to rise slowly from a chair or bed when starting therapy and to avoid situations in which injury could result from fainting.

• Instruct patient not to drive or perform hazardous tasks for 12 hours after first dose or changes in dose until response can be monitored.

• Warn that, although rare, priapism can occur. Tell patient to report it immediately.

---

*Reactions in bold italics are **life-threatening**.*

• Advise patient considering cataract or glaucoma surgery to inform the ophthalmologist about taking drug.

tapinarof
ta-PIN-ar-of

Vtama

Therapeutic class: Aryl hydrocarbon receptor agonists
Pharmacologic class: Antipsoriatics

AVAILABLE FORMS
Cream: 1%

INDICATIONS & DOSAGES
➤ **Plaque psoriasis**
Adults: Thin layer applied to psoriatic skin lesions once daily.

ADMINISTRATION
Topical
• Avoid applying to unaffected areas of skin.
• Not for oral, ophthalmic, or intravaginal use.
• Store drug at 68° to 77° F (20° to 25° C).

ACTION
Exact mechanism unknown.

Route	Onset	Peak	Duration
Topical	Unknown	Unknown	Unknown

Half-life: Unknown.

ADVERSE REACTIONS
CNS: headache. **EENT:** nasopharyngitis.
Skin: contact dermatitis, folliculitis, pruritus.
Other: flulike syndrome.

INTERACTIONS
None reported.

EFFECTS ON LAB TEST RESULTS
None reported.

CONTRAINDICATIONS & CAUTIONS
• Safety and effectiveness in children haven't been established.
Dialyzable drug: Unlikely.

PREGNANCY-LACTATION-REPRODUCTION
• Studies during pregnancy are inadequate. Use during pregnancy only if potential benefit justifies fetal risk.

• It isn't known if drug appears in human milk or how drug affects milk production or infants who are breastfed. Consider patient's clinical need and risk to infant.

NURSING CONSIDERATIONS
• Monitor patient's skin for signs and symptoms of adverse skin reactions (itching, redness, burning, peeling).

PATIENT TEACHING
• Teach about proper drug administration and handling, including the need to wash hands after application, unless treatment area is the hands.
• Instruct patient to report side effects.
• Advise patient to report pregnancy or plans to become pregnant or breastfeed during therapy.

tasimelteon
TAS-i-MEL-tee-on

Hetlioz, Hetlioz LQ

Therapeutic class: Hypnotics
Pharmacologic class: Melatonin receptor agonists

AVAILABLE FORMS
Capsules ⓞⓝⓒ: 20 mg
Oral suspension: 4 mg/mL

INDICATIONS & DOSAGES
➤ **Non-24-hour sleep-wake disorder**
Adults: 20 mg PO at same time each night before bedtime.
➤ **Nighttime sleep disturbances in Smith-Magenis syndrome**
Adults and children ages 16 and older: 20 mg PO 1 hour before bedtime.
Children ages 3 to 15 weighing more than 28 kg: 20 mg oral suspension PO 1 hour before bedtime.
Children ages 3 to 15 weighing 28 kg or less: 0.7 mg/kg oral suspension PO 1 hour before bedtime.

ADMINISTRATION
PO
• Give drug without food.
• Have patient swallow capsules whole; don't crush or open capsules.

• Prior to first use, place press-in bottle adapter into bottle neck.
• Shake oral suspension for at least 30 seconds before administration. Turn bottle upside down and withdraw prescribed amount from bottle.
• Give at same time each night. If patient can't take dose at approximately the same time on a given night, skip that dose.
• After administration, patient should limit activities to prepare for sleep.
• Do not substitute capsules and oral suspension for each other.
• Store capsules at room temperature.
• Refrigerate oral suspension. After opening, discard 48-mL bottle after 5 weeks and 158-mL bottle after 8 weeks.

ACTION

Binds to melatonin receptors in the brain, resulting in regulation of sleep-wake cycle.

Route	Onset	Peak	Duration
PO (capsules)	Unknown	0.5–3 hr	Unknown
PO (suspension)	Unknown	15–30 min	Unknown

Half-life: 1 to 2 hours.

ADVERSE REACTIONS

CNS: headache, nightmares, abnormal dreams. **GU:** UTI. **Hepatic:** elevated ALT level. **Respiratory:** URI.

INTERACTIONS

Drug-drug. *Beta blockers (acebutolol, metoprolol):* May reduce tasimelteon efficacy when beta blocker is given at night. Monitor therapy.
Strong CYP3A4 inducers (carbamazepine, primidone, rifampin): May decrease tasimelteon level, resulting in decreased efficacy. Avoid use together.
Strong CYP1A2 inhibitors (fluvoxamine): May increase tasimelteon level and risk of adverse events. Avoid use together.
Drug-herb. *St. John's wort:* May decrease drug level and decrease effectiveness. Discourage use together.
Drug-food. *Alcohol use:* May cause additive effect of tasimelteon. Discourage use together.
Drug-lifestyle. *Smoking:* May decrease tasimelteon exposure by 40% compared to nonsmokers. Discourage use together.

EFFECTS ON LAB TEST RESULTS

• May increase ALT level.

CONTRAINDICATIONS & CAUTIONS

• Contraindicated in patients hypersensitive to drug or its components.
• Use in patients with Child-Pugh class C liver impairment isn't recommended.
• Use cautiously in older adults. Drug may have up to twofold increase in exposure, increasing risk of adverse events in these patients.
Dialyzable drug: Yes.

PREGNANCY-LACTATION-REPRODUCTION

• Studies during pregnancy are inadequate. Use only if benefits outweigh fetal risk.
• It isn't known if drug appears in human milk. Use cautiously during breastfeeding.

NURSING CONSIDERATIONS

• Drug levels after administration are 20% to 30% greater in females than males.
• Drug's effects may not occur for weeks or months because of individual differences in circadian rhythms.

PATIENT TEACHING

• Teach about proper drug administration and handling.
• Explain that, after taking drug, patient should limit activity to preparing for bed. Drug decreases mental alertness and can impair ability to perform other activities.
• Advise patient that drug may take several weeks or months to become effective.
• Caution patient to avoid alcohol because of additive effects.
• Inform patient that smoking decreases effects of drug and should be avoided.

telavancin
tell-uh-VAN-sin

Vibativ

Therapeutic class: Antibiotics
Pharmacologic class: Lipoglycopeptides

AVAILABLE FORMS

Lyophilized powder for injection: 750-mg single-use vials

INDICATIONS & DOSAGES

Adjust-a-dose (for all indications): For patients with CrCl of 30 to 50 mL/minute, give 7.5 mg/kg every 24 hours. For patients with CrCl of 10 to 29 mL/minute, give 10 mg/kg every 48 hours.

➤ **Complicated skin and skin-structure infections caused by susceptible gram-positive organisms, such as MRSA,** *Staphylococcus aureus, Streptococcus pyogenes, Streptococcus agalactiae, Streptococcus anginosus* **group, or** *Enterococcus faecalis* **(vancomycin-susceptible isolates only)**

Adults: 10 mg/kg IV infusion once every 24 hours for 7 to 14 days.

➤ **Hospital-acquired or ventilator-associated bacterial pneumonia (HABP or VABP) caused by susceptible isolates of** *S. aureus* **(including methicillin-susceptible and methicillin-resistant isolates)**

Adults: 10 mg/kg IV once every 24 hours for 7 to 21 days.

ADMINISTRATION

IV

▼ Reconstitute 750-mg vial with 45 mL sterile water, D_5W, or NSS for injection. Mix thoroughly but don't shake; reconstitution may take up to 20 minutes. Resultant solution has a concentration of 15 mg/mL.

▼ Further dilute doses of 150 to 800 mg in 100 to 250 mL of D_5W, NSS, or lactated Ringer solution before infusion. Further dilute doses less than 150 mg or greater than 800 mg to a final concentration of 0.6 to 8 mg/mL.

▼ Inspect for particulate matter before infusion.

▼ Infuse drug over 60 minutes.

▼ Reconstituted solution remains stable for 12 hours at room temperature or 7 days if refrigerated.

▼ Diluted IV solution remains stable for 12 hours at room temperature or 7 days if refrigerated, including reconstituted time. Diluted solution in the infusion bag may be frozen for up to 32 days.

▼ **Incompatibilities:** Other IV drugs. If line is used for other IV drugs, flush with D_5W, NSS, or lactated Ringer solution before and after infusion.

ACTION

Inhibits bacterial cell-wall synthesis by binding to the bacterial cell membrane and disrupting its function.

Route	Onset	Peak	Duration
IV	Unknown	Unknown	Unknown

Half-life: About 6.6 to 9.6 hours.

ADVERSE REACTIONS

CNS: taste disturbance, dizziness. **GI:** abdominal pain, decreased appetite, diarrhea, nausea, vomiting. **GU:** *AKI,* foamy urine, new-onset or worsening kidney impairment. **Skin:** generalized pruritus, infusion-site pain, infusion-site reaction, localized erythema, rash. **Other:** rigors.

INTERACTIONS

Drug-drug. *Drugs that affect kidney function (NSAIDs, ACE inhibitors, loop diuretics):* May increase risk of kidney impairment. Monitor kidney function.

Drugs that prolong QTc interval (erythromycin, sotalol, thioridazine): May enhance QTc-prolonging effect. Avoid use together when possible. Closely monitor for evidence of QT prolongation and other cardiac rhythm alterations.

Heparin: May artificially prolong PTT, which could lead to incorrect decrease of heparin dosage. Concomitant use with IV unfractionated heparin is contraindicated.

Vaccines (cholera, live attenuated Ty21a strain of typhoid): May diminish vaccine's effect. Avoid cholera vaccine within 14 days of oral or parenteral antibiotics; don't give typhoid vaccine until at least 3 days after final antibiotic dose.

EFFECTS ON LAB TEST RESULTS

• May increase factor Xa level, INR, and creatinine level.

• May falsely prolong PT, PTT, and activated clotting time.

• May falsely affect urine qualitative dipstick protein assays and quantitative dye methods, such as pyrogallol red-molybdate.

CONTRAINDICATIONS & CAUTIONS

🔵 *Alert:* Reserve drug for treatment of pneumonia when alternative treatments aren't suitable.

🔵 *Alert:* Contraindicated in patients hypersensitive to drug or its components. Serious and potentially fatal hypersensitivity reactions, including anaphylactic reactions, may occur after first or subsequent doses. Use

T

cautiously in patients with known hypersensitivity to vancomycin.

⚠️ **Alert:** Concomitant use of IV unfractionated heparin sodium is contraindicated because PTT test results may be artificially prolonged for 0 to 18 hours after administration.

• Avoid use in patients with prolonged QTc interval, uncompensated HF, or severe left ventricular hypertrophy.

Boxed Warning Patients with preexisting CrCl of 50 mL/minute or less treated with telavancin for HABP or VABP have demonstrated higher mortality than those treated with vancomycin. Use drug in such patients only when anticipated benefit outweighs risk. ■

Boxed Warning New-onset and worsening kidney impairment has been reported. Monitor kidney function. ■

• Use cautiously in patients at risk for kidney impairment, including those with diabetes, HF, or HTN.

• When used to treat skin and skin-structure infections, drug is less effective in patients with CrCl of 50 mL/minute or less. Consider alternative therapy.

• Older adults are more likely to have reduced kidney function; use cautiously and base dosage on kidney function.

• Safety and effectiveness in children haven't been established.

Dialyzable drug: 5.9%.

PREGNANCY-LACTATION-REPRODUCTION
Boxed Warning May cause fetal harm. Adverse outcomes have been observed in animal studies. ■

Boxed Warning Verify pregnancy status before starting drug in patients of childbearing potential. Advise patients who are pregnant of fetal risk. Patients of childbearing potential should use effective contraception during treatment and for 2 days after final dose. ■

• It isn't known if drug appears in human milk. Use cautiously during breastfeeding.

• Drug may impair male fertility.

NURSING CONSIDERATIONS
Boxed Warning Monitor kidney function at baseline and during therapy. ■

⚠️ **Alert:** Rapid IV infusion may cause "redman syndrome" (flushing of upper body; urticaria; pruritus; rash on face, neck, trunk, and upper extremities). Infuse over at least 60 minutes.

• If diarrhea develops, evaluate patient for CDAD, which can be fatal and can occur more than 2 months after final dose.

• Watch for signs and symptoms of superinfection, such as continued fever, chills, and increased pulse rate.

• Obtain blood samples for PT, INR, PTT, activated clotting time, and coagulation-based factor X activity as close as possible to next telavancin dose.

• Monitor patient for hypersensitivity reactions, including anaphylaxis, which may occur at any time during therapy. Stop drug at first sign of hypersensitivity reaction.

• *Look alike–sound alike:* Don't confuse telavancin with telithromycin.

PATIENT TEACHING
Boxed Warning Advise patients of childbearing potential to use an effective method of contraception during therapy and for 2 days after final dose. ■

• Tell patient to report a history of kidney problems, heart problems (including QTc-interval prolongation), or diabetes before starting drug.

• Instruct patient to report all adverse reactions, especially diarrhea that develops during treatment or within 2 months of completing treatment.

---

telmisartan
tell-mah-SAR-tan

Micardis

Therapeutic class: Antihypertensives
Pharmacologic class: ARBs

AVAILABLE FORMS
Tablets: 20 mg, 40 mg, 80 mg

INDICATIONS & DOSAGES
Adjust-a-dose (for all indications): In patients with biliary obstructive disorders or liver insufficiency, initiate at low dose and slowly titrate up.

➤ **HTN**
Adults: 40 mg PO once daily. Adjust to 20 to 80 mg once daily based on BP response.

➤ **CV risk reduction in patients at high risk and unable to take ACE inhibitors**
Adults ages 55 and older: 80 mg PO once daily.

ADMINISTRATION
PO
- Give drug without regard to food.
- Remove tablet from blister pack immediately before administration.
- Give a missed dose as soon as possible. If almost time for next dose, omit missed dose and give next dose at its regular time.

ACTION
Blocks vasoconstricting and aldosterone-secreting effects of angiotensin II by preventing angiotensin II from binding to the angiotensin I receptor.

Route	Onset	Peak	Duration
PO	3 hr	30–60 min	24 hr

Half-life: 24 hours.

ADVERSE REACTIONS
CNS: dizziness, pain, fatigue, headache. **CV:** chest pain, HTN, peripheral edema, intermittent claudication. **EENT:** sinusitis, pharyngitis. **GI:** nausea, abdominal pain, diarrhea, dyspepsia. **GU:** UTI. **Musculoskeletal:** back pain, myalgia. **Respiratory:** cough, URI. **Skin:** ulceration. **Other:** flulike symptoms.

INTERACTIONS
Drug-drug. *ACE inhibitors:* May affect kidney function and cause AKI. Consider therapy modification.
Aliskiren: Increases risk of kidney impairment, hypotension, and hyperkalemia. Use together is contraindicated in patients with diabetes. Avoid coadministration in patients with GFR less than 60 mL/minute.
COX-2 inhibitors, NSAIDs: May result in worsening kidney function. May decrease antihypertensive effect. Periodically monitor BP and kidney function.
Digoxin: May increase digoxin level. Closely monitor digoxin level.
Lithium: May cause reversible increase in lithium level and toxicity. Monitor lithium level, and adjust lithium dosage as needed.
Potassium-sparing diuretics, potassium supplements: May increase risk of hyperkalemia. Monitor potassium level.
Ramipril, ramiprilat: May increase levels of these drugs and decrease telmisartan level. Avoid use together.
Drug-food. *Salt substitutes containing potassium:* May cause hyperkalemia. Discourage use together.

EFFECTS ON LAB TEST RESULTS
- May increase BUN, potassium, serum creatinine, and liver enzyme levels.
- May decrease Hb level.

CONTRAINDICATIONS & CAUTIONS
- Contraindicated in patients hypersensitive to drug or its components.
- Use cautiously in patients with biliary obstruction disorders, hypotension, or kidney or liver insufficiency and in those with an activated RAAS, such as patients who are volume- or sodium-depleted (for example, those being treated with high doses of diuretics).
- Safety and effectiveness in children haven't been established.
Dialyzable drug: No.
⚠ *Overdose S&S:* Hypotension, dizziness, tachycardia, bradycardia.

PREGNANCY-LACTATION-REPRODUCTION
Boxed Warning Use during pregnancy can cause injury and death to a developing fetus because drug acts directly on the RAAS. Stop drug as soon possible after detecting pregnancy. ∎
- It isn't known if drug appears in human milk. Patient shouldn't breastfeed during therapy.

NURSING CONSIDERATIONS
- Monitor patient for hypotension after starting drug. Place patient supine if hypotension occurs, and give IV NSS, if needed.
- If possible, correct volume and sodium depletion before first dose.
- Monitor potassium level periodically during therapy.
- Most of antihypertensive effect occurs within 2 weeks. Maximal BP reduction usually occurs after 4 weeks. Diuretic may be added if BP isn't controlled by drug alone.
🕙 *Alert:* In patient whose kidney function may depend on activity of the RAAS (such as patient with severe HF), drug may cause oliguria or progressive azotemia and (rarely) AKI or death.
- Drug isn't removed by hemodialysis. Patient undergoing dialysis may develop orthostatic hypotension. Closely monitor BP.
- Carefully monitor patient with impaired liver function or biliary obstruction.
- Monitor patient for hypersensitivity reactions. Angioedema has been reported

T

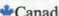

rarely. If signs or symptoms of angioedema (swelling of head and neck) occur, immediately discontinue drug.

• Although rare, rhabdomyolysis has been reported. Monitor patient for myalgia, stiffness, and muscle weakness.

PATIENT TEACHING

• Teach about proper drug administration and handling.

• Inform patient of childbearing potential of consequences of second- and third-trimester exposure to drug. Instruct patient to immediately report pregnancy.

• Advise patient not to breastfeed during therapy.

• Explain that, if dizziness or low BP occurs on standing, patient should lie down, rise slowly from a lying to standing position, and climb stairs slowly.

• Advise patient to report all adverse reactions.

• Caution patient not to use salt substitutes that contain potassium.

SAFETY ALERT!

temazepam
te-MAZ-e-pam

Restoril

Therapeutic class: Hypnotics
Pharmacologic class: Benzodiazepines
Controlled substance schedule: IV

AVAILABLE FORMS
Capsules: 7.5 mg, 15 mg, 22.5 mg, 30 mg

INDICATIONS & DOSAGES
➤ **Short-term treatment (7 to 10 days) of insomnia**
Adults: 7.5 to 30 mg PO at bedtime.
Older adults and patients who are debilitated: Initially, 7.5 mg PO at bedtime until individualized response is determined.

ADMINISTRATION
PO
• Give drug without regard to food.

ACTION
Potentiates GABA neuronal inhibition in the CNS.

Route	Onset	Peak	Duration
PO	10–20 min	1.5 hr	Unknown

Half-life: Terminal, 3.5 to 18.4 hours.

ADVERSE REACTIONS
CNS: drowsiness, dizziness, hangover effect, lethargy, disturbed coordination, daytime sedation, confusion, nightmares, vertigo, euphoria, weakness, headache, fatigue, nervousness, anxiety, depression. **EENT:** blurred vision, dry mouth. **GI:** abdominal discomfort, diarrhea, nausea.

INTERACTIONS
Drug-drug. *CNS depressants (barbiturates, antipsychotics, sedatives, anxiolytics, antidepressants, sedative antihistamines, anticonvulsants, aesthetics):* May increase CNS depression. Use together cautiously.

Boxed Warning *Opioids:* May cause slow or difficult breathing, sedation, and death. Avoid use together. If use together is necessary, limit dosage and duration of each drug to minimum necessary for desired effect. ∎

Drug-herb. *Calendula, kava, lemon balm, passion flower, skullcap, valerian:* May enhance sedation. Discourage use together.

Drug-lifestyle. *Alcohol use:* May cause additive CNS depressant effects. Discourage use together.

EFFECTS ON LAB TEST RESULTS
• May increase LFT values.

CONTRAINDICATIONS & CAUTIONS
• Contraindicated in patients hypersensitive to drug or other benzodiazepines.

Boxed Warning Opioids should only be prescribed with benzodiazepines or other CNS depressants to patients for whom alternative treatment options are inadequate. ∎

Boxed Warning Benzodiazepine use exposes patient to risks of abuse, misuse, and addiction, which can lead to overdose or death. Assess patient's risk of abuse, misuse, and addiction before and periodically during therapy. ∎

Boxed Warning Abrupt discontinuation or rapid dosage reduction of benzodiazepines after continued use may precipitate acute withdrawal reactions, which can be life-threatening. To reduce risk of withdrawal reactions, gradually taper drug to discontinue or reduce dosage. ∎

Reactions in bold italics are *life-threatening*.

• Use cautiously in patients with chronic pulmonary insufficiency, impaired liver or kidney function, severe or latent depression, suicidality, and history of substance use disorder.

• Use cautiously in patients who are debilitated, those ages 65 and older, and others at increased risk for oversedation, dizziness, confusion, ataxia, and falls.

⚠ *Alert:* Drug may cause rare but serious injury, including death, due to complex sleep behaviors, such as sleepwalking, sleep driving, and engaging in other activities while not fully awake. These behaviors can occur even at the lowest recommended dosages and after just one dose.

Dialyzable drug: Unknown.

⚠ *Overdose S&S:* Somnolence, impaired coordination, slurred speech, confusion, coma, decreased reflexes, hypotension, seizures, respiratory depression, apnea.

PREGNANCY-LACTATION-REPRODUCTION

• Use in patients who are or may become pregnant isn't recommended; drug may cause fetal harm. If used during pregnancy or if patient becomes pregnant during therapy, apprise patient of fetal risk.

• Encourage patient to enroll in the National Pregnancy Registry for Sedative-Hypnotics and Other Sleep Medications (1-866-961-2388 or https://womensmentalhealth.org/research/pregnancyregistry/sleep-medications).

• It isn't known if drug appears in human milk. Use cautiously during breastfeeding; monitor infant for drowsiness, lethargy, and weight loss.

NURSING CONSIDERATIONS

⚠ *Alert:* Monitor patient closely for hypersensitivity reactions. Anaphylaxis and angioedema may occur as early as the first dose (rare).

• Assess mental status before starting therapy and reduce dosages in older adults, who may be more sensitive to drug's adverse CNS effects.

• Take precautions to prevent drug hoarding by patient who is depressed, suicidal, or drug-dependent or has history of drug abuse.

• To discontinue drug, follow gradual dosage-tapering schedule and monitor for withdrawal signs and symptoms (cramps, seizures, tremor, diaphoresis).

• *Look alike–sound alike:* Don't confuse Restoril with Risperdal or Vistaril. Don't confuse temazepam with flurazepam.

PATIENT TEACHING

⚠ *Alert:* Warn patient that drug may cause allergic reactions (rare), facial swelling (rare), and complex sleep-related behaviors, such as driving, eating, and making phone calls while asleep. Advise patient to report these adverse effects.

Boxed Warning Caution patient or caregiver of patient taking an opioid with a benzodiazepine, CNS depressant, or alcohol to seek immediate medical attention if patient experiences dizziness, light-headedness, extreme sleepiness, slowed or difficult breathing, or unresponsiveness. ∎

Boxed Warning Caution patient that benzodiazepines, even at recommended doses, increase risk of abuse, misuse, and addiction, which can lead to overdose and death, especially when used in combination with other drugs (opioid analgesics), alcohol, or illicit substances. ∎

• Tell patient to avoid alcohol.

• Teach about proper drug administration and handling, including proper disposal of unused drug.

• Advise patient not to take drug at a higher dose, more frequently, or for longer than prescribed.

Boxed Warning Tell patient that continued use of drug for several days to weeks may lead to physical dependence and that abrupt discontinuation or rapid dosage reduction may precipitate acute withdrawal reactions, which can be life-threatening. Instruct patient that discontinuation or dosage reduction may require a slow taper. ∎

• Advise patient about possibility of developing protracted withdrawal syndrome (anxiety; trouble remembering, learning, or concentrating; depression; problems sleeping; feeling like insects are crawling under skin; weakness; shaking; muscle twitching; burning or prickling feeling in hands, arms, legs, or feet; ringing in ears), with symptoms lasting weeks to more than 12 months.

• Explain that drug increases risk of falls. Caution patient to avoid performing activities that require mental alertness or physical coordination.

⚠ *Alert:* Warn patient of risk of injury or death related to complex sleep behaviors.

Direct patient to stop drug and immediately report an episode of complex sleep behavior or failure to remember activities performed while taking drug.

• Caution patient to report pregnancy or breastfeeding to prescriber.

• Tell patient to not take drug unless patient can stay in bed a full night (7 to 8 hours) before becoming active again.

SAFETY ALERT!

tenecteplase
teh-NEK-ti-plaze

TNKase

Therapeutic class: Thrombolytics
Pharmacologic class: Recombinant tissue plasminogen activators

AVAILABLE FORMS
Injection: 50 mg/vial

INDICATIONS & DOSAGES
➤ **To reduce risk of death from acute ST-elevation MI**
Adults weighing 90 kg or more: 50 mg (10 mL) by IV bolus over 5 seconds.
Adults weighing 80 to less than 90 kg: 45 mg (9 mL) by IV bolus over 5 seconds.
Adults weighing 70 to less than 80 kg: 40 mg (8 mL) by IV bolus over 5 seconds.
Adults weighing 60 to less than 70 kg: 35 mg (7 mL) by IV bolus over 5 seconds.
Adults weighing less than 60 kg: 30 mg (6 mL) by IV bolus over 5 seconds. Maximum dose, 50 mg.

ADMINISTRATION
IV
▼ Give IV only. Don't give IM or subcut.
▼ Drug is copackaged with 10-mL syringe with dual cannula device and 10-mL vial of sterile water for injection.
▼ Fill supplied syringe with 10 mL supplied sterile water for injection, and inject entire contents into drug vial. Gently swirl solution once mixed. Don't shake. Visually inspect product for particulate matter before administration.
▼ Draw up appropriate dose needed from reconstituted vial; discard any unused portion. Give drug immediately, or refrigerate at 36° to 46° F (2° to 8° C) and use within 8 hours.

▼ Give drug in a designated line. Flush dextrose-containing lines with NSS before administration.
▼ Give drug rapidly over 5 seconds.
▼ Store vial in refrigerator at 36° to 46° F (2° to 8° C).
▼ **Incompatibilities:** Solutions containing dextrose, other IV drugs.

ACTION
Promotes fibrinolysis by binding to fibrin and converting plasminogen to plasmin.

Route	Onset	Peak	Duration
IV	Immediate	Immediate	Unknown

Half-life: 90 to 130 minutes.

ADVERSE REACTIONS
CV: *bleeding, thromboembolic events, reperfusion arrhythmias.* **Other:** bleeding at puncture site, hypersensitivity reaction.

INTERACTIONS
Drug-drug. *Anticoagulants (direct thrombin inhibitors, heparin, vitamin K antagonists), drugs that alter platelet function (aspirin, dipyridamole, glycoprotein IIb/IIIa inhibitors [eptifibatide, tirofiban], NSAIDs, P2Y12 inhibitors, SSRIs):* May increase risk of bleeding when used before, during, or after tenecteplase use. Use together cautiously.
Drug-herb. *Alfalfa, anise, bilberry:* May increase bleeding risk. Consider therapy modification.

EFFECTS ON LAB TEST RESULTS
• May prolong PTT.
• May interfere with coagulation test results or fibrinolytic activity measurements.

CONTRAINDICATIONS & CAUTIONS
• Contraindicated in patients with hypersensitivity to drug; active internal bleeding; history of stroke; intracranial or intraspinal surgery or trauma during previous 2 months; intracranial neoplasm, aneurysm, or arteriovenous malformation; severe uncontrolled HTN; or bleeding diathesis.
• Use cautiously in patients who have had recent major surgery, organ biopsy, obstetric delivery, or previous puncture of noncompressible vessels.
• Use cautiously in patients ages 75 and older and patients with recent trauma, recent GI or GU bleeding, high risk of left ventricular

---

Reactions in bold italics are *life-threatening*.

thrombus, acute pericarditis, systolic BP 180 mm Hg or higher or diastolic BP 110 mm Hg or higher, Child-Pugh class C liver impairment, hemostatic defects, subacute bacterial endocarditis, septic thrombophlebitis, occluded AV cannula at seriously infected site, diabetic hemorrhagic retinopathy, or cerebrovascular disease.

• Safety and effectiveness in children haven't been established.
Dialyzable drug: Unknown.

PREGNANCY-LACTATION-REPRODUCTION

• Studies during pregnancy are inadequate. Use only if potential benefit justifies fetal risk.

• It isn't known if drug appears in human milk. Use cautiously during breastfeeding.

NURSING CONSIDERATIONS

• Begin therapy as soon as possible after onset of MI symptoms.

• Avoid noncompressible arterial punctures and internal jugular and subclavian venous punctures. Minimize all arterial and venous punctures during treatment.

• Avoid IM injections and nonessential patient handling for first few hours after treatment.

• Give heparin as prescribed but not in the same IV line.

• Monitor patient for bleeding. If serious bleeding occurs, immediately stop heparin and antiplatelet drugs.

🕒 *Alert:* Use exact patient weight for dosage. Overestimation of patient weight can lead to significant increase in bleeding or intracerebral hemorrhage.

• Monitor ECG for reperfusion arrhythmias.

• Life-threatening cholesterol embolism has been rarely reported in patients treated with thrombolytics. Signs and symptoms include livedo reticularis (purple toe syndrome), AKI, gangrenous digits, HTN, pancreatitis, MI, cerebral infarction, spinal cord infarction, retinal artery occlusion, bowel infarction, and rhabdomyolysis.

• *Look alike–sound alike:* Don't confuse tenecteplase with alteplase or reteplase. Don't confuse TNKase with Activase.

PATIENT TEACHING

• Tell patient to immediately report all adverse reactions, including bleeding.

• Explain use of drug to patient and family.

tenofovir alafenamide
te-NOE-fo-veer

Vemlidy

tenofovir disoproxil fumarate
Viread

Therapeutic class: Antiretrovirals
Pharmacologic class: NRTIs

AVAILABLE FORMS
tenofovir alafenamide
Tablets: 25 mg
tenofovir disoproxil fumarate
Oral powder: 40 mg/scoopful
Tablets: 150 mg, 200 mg, 250 mg, 300 mg

INDICATIONS & DOSAGES
➤ **Chronic HBV infection in patients with Child-Pugh class A liver impairment (tenofovir alafenamide)**
Adults and children ages 12 and older: 25 mg PO daily.
➤ **HIV-1 infection, with other antiretrovirals; chronic HBV infection (tenofovir disoproxil fumarate)**
Adults and children ages 2 and older weighing 35 kg or more: 300 mg PO once daily.
Adults and children ages 2 and older weighing 17 to less than 35 kg and able to swallow intact tablet: 8 mg/kg PO once daily. Maximum dosage, 300 mg/day. See product insert for specific weight-based dosing recommendations.
Adults and children ages 2 and older weighing at least 10 kg and unable to swallow tablet: 8 mg/kg PO powder once daily. Maximum dosage, 300 mg/day. See product insert for specific weight-based dosing recommendations.
Adjust-a-dose: For adults with CrCl of 30 to 49 mL/minute, 300 mg PO every 48 hours; CrCl of 10 to 29 mL/minute, 300 mg PO every 72 to 96 hours. For patients receiving hemodialysis, 300 mg PO every 7 days or after a total of about 12 hours of hemodialysis. No recommendations exist for patients with CrCl of less than 10 mL/minute who are not receiving CKRT or for children with kidney impairment.

T

ADMINISTRATION
PO

• Give tenofovir alafenamide with food. Give tenofovir disoproxil fumarate without regard to food.

• For patients receiving dialysis, give dose after session.

• Monitor weight periodically and adjust dosage accordingly.

• For patients receiving tenofovir powder, measure only with supplied dosing scoop. One level scoop delivers tenofovir 40 mg. Mix with 2 to 4 oz of soft food not requiring chewing (such as applesauce, baby food, or yogurt). Patient should ingest entire mixture immediately to avoid bitter taste. Don't mix in liquid because powder may float on top of liquid, even after stirring.

ACTION

An antiviral that inhibits HIV replication by inhibiting viral RNA-dependent DNA polymerase and inhibits replication of HBV by inhibiting HBV polymerase.

Route	Onset	Peak	Duration
PO (alafen-amide)	Unknown	0.5 hr	Unknown
PO (disoproxil fumarate)	Unknown	36–144 min	Unknown

Half-life: Alafenamide, 0.5 hour; disoproxil fumarate, 17 hours.

ADVERSE REACTIONS
Tenofovir alafenamide

CNS: headache, fatigue. **GI:** abdominal pain, nausea, diarrhea, dyspepsia, vomiting, flatulence. **GU:** glycosuria. **Hepatic:** increased transaminase levels. **Metabolic:** increased amylase, CK, LDL-C, and triglyceride levels. **Musculoskeletal:** back pain, arthralgia, decreased bone mineral density. **Respiratory:** cough. **Skin:** rash.

Tenofovir disoproxil fumarate

CNS: asthenia, headache, pain, fever, peripheral neuropathy, insomnia, dizziness, depression, anxiety, fatigue. **CV:** chest pain. **EENT:** sinusitis, nasopharyngitis. **GI:** nausea, abdominal pain, dyspepsia, diarrhea, vomiting, anorexia, flatulence. **GU:** hematuria. **Hematologic:** *neutropenia.* **Hepatic:** increased ALP and transaminase levels. **Metabolic:** hyperglycemia; increased amylase, CK, cholesterol, and triglyceride levels; weight loss. **Musculoskeletal:** arthralgia, back pain,

myalgia, decreased bone mineral density. **Respiratory:** URI, pneumonia. **Skin:** rash, pruritus, diaphoresis. **Other:** lipodystrophy.

INTERACTIONS

Drug-drug. *Adefovir:* May diminish therapeutic effect of tenofovir; may increase level of both drugs, resulting in additive kidney toxicity. Avoid use together.

Atazanavir: May decrease atazanavir level, increasing risk of resistance. Give both drugs with ritonavir.

Atazanavir with ritonavir, darunavir with ritonavir, lopinavir–ritonavir: May increase tenofovir-associated adverse reactions. Monitor patient carefully.

Carbamazepine: May decrease tenofovir alafenamide level. Increase tenofovir alafenamide dosage to 50 mg once daily.

Didanosine: Use with tenofovir disoproxil may increase didanosine level. Monitor patient closely. Adjust didanosine dosage.

Drugs that reduce kidney function or compete for renal tubular secretion (acyclovir, aminoglycosides, cidofovir, ganciclovir, NSAIDs, valacyclovir, valganciclovir): May increase levels of tenofovir or other drugs eliminated by the kidneys. Monitor patient for adverse effects.

Ledipasvir–sofosbuvir: May increase tenofovir exposure. When given with tenofovir without an HIV-1 protease inhibitor/ritonavir or an HIV-1 protease inhibitor/cobicistat combination, monitor patient for adverse reactions associated with tenofovir. When given with tenofovir and an HIV-1 protease inhibitor/ritonavir or an HIV-1 protease inhibitor/cobicistat combination, consider modifying therapy. If use together is necessary, monitor patient for tenofovir-associated adverse effects.

Oxcarbazepine, phenobarbital, phenytoin: May decrease tenofovir alafenamide level. Avoid use together.

Rifabutin, rifampin, rifapentine: May decrease tenofovir alafenamide level. Avoid use together.

Sofosbuvir–velpatasvir: May increase tenofovir exposure. Monitor patient for tenofovir-associated adverse effects.

Drug-herb. *St. John's wort:* May decrease tenofovir alafenamide level. Discourage use together.

Drug-food. *Fatty meals:* May increase tenofovir bioavailability. Monitor patient for adverse effects.

Reactions in bold italics are *life-threatening*.

EFFECTS ON LAB TEST RESULTS
• May increase amylase, lipase, AST, ALT, ALP, CK, serum and urine glucose, creatinine, phosphate, cholesterol, and triglyceride levels.
• May decrease neutrophil count.

CONTRAINDICATIONS & CAUTIONS
• Contraindicated in patients hypersensitive to components of drug.
• Use very cautiously in patients with risk factors for liver disease or with liver impairment.
• Use cautiously in patients with kidney impairment and those at higher risk for decreased kidney function, including older adults and patients with concurrent or recent kidney-toxic therapy.
• Tenofovir alafenamide isn't recommended for use in patients with CrCl less than 15 mL/minute who aren't on CKRT or those with Child-Pugh class B or C liver impairment.
• Tenofovir disoproxil isn't recommended for use in patients with CrCl less than 10 mL/minute who aren't on CKRT.
• Immune reconstitution syndrome has been reported in patients with HIV-1 treated with combination antiretroviral therapy.
• Lactic acidosis and severe liver enlargement with steatosis, including fatal cases, have been reported with use of nucleoside analogues.
• Don't use tenofovir as monotherapy for treatment of HIV-1 infection.
• Don't use tenofovir for treatment of HIV-1 infection in combination with fixed-dose combination products that also contain tenofovir, such as Complera, Descovy, Genvoya, and Truvada.
• Don't administer tenofovir with adefovir.
Dialyzable drug: Yes.

PREGNANCY-LACTATION-REPRODUCTION
• Studies during pregnancy are inadequate. Use only if clearly needed.
• Enroll patients exposed to drug during pregnancy in the Antiretroviral Pregnancy Registry (1-800-258-4263 or www.apregistry.com).
• The CDC recommends counseling patients with HIV-1 infection on the risk of postnatal HIV-1 transmission. Maintaining viral suppression through antiretroviral therapy during pregnancy, delivery, and postpartum period decreases the risk to less than 1%.
• Tenofovir is present in human milk. Use cautiously during breastfeeding in patients with HBV infection.

NURSING CONSIDERATIONS
• Before starting drug, test patient for HBV and HIV-1 infection. Don't use tenofovir alone in patients with HIV-1 infection.
🛈 *Alert:* Monitor all patients for lactic acidosis and liver enlargement with steatosis, with or without elevated transaminase levels. Risk factors include long-term antiretroviral use, obesity, and being female.
• Assess estimated CrCl and serum creatinine, urine glucose, and urine protein levels at baseline and during therapy as clinically appropriate in all patients. In patients with CKD, also assess serum phosphorus level.
Boxed Warning Severe acute exacerbations of hepatitis have been reported in patients infected with HBV after anti-HBV therapy has stopped. Monitor liver function closely for at least several months. Resumption of therapy may be warranted. ∎
• Drug may be linked to osteomalacia and decreased bone mineral density, increased creatinine and BUN levels, and phosphaturia. Monitor patient carefully.
• Drug may lead to decreased HIV-RNA level and CD4$^+$ cell counts.
• Monitor patient for immune reconstitution syndrome, an inflammatory response to indolent or residual opportunistic infections that may require further evaluation and treatment. Autoimmune disorders have also been reported.

PATIENT TEACHING
• Teach about proper drug administration and handling.
• Inform patient that drug doesn't cure HIV infection, that opportunistic infections and other complications of HIV infection may still occur, and that transmission of HIV to others through sexual contact or blood contamination is still possible.
• Advise patient to obtain all ordered lab tests to assess safety of treatment regimen.
• Tell patient to report adverse effects, including nausea, vomiting, diarrhea, flatulence, and headache.
• Instruct patient to consult prescriber before taking OTC or other prescription medications or supplements, vitamins, or herbal supplements.
• Advise patient to discuss pregnancy and breastfeeding risks with prescriber.

🍁Canada   ◇OTC   ◆Off-label use   ⊜Do not crush   *Liquid contains alcohol   ✠Genetic

terazosin hydrochloride
ter-AY-zoe-sin

Therapeutic class: Antihypertensives
Pharmacologic class: Alpha blockers

AVAILABLE FORMS
Capsules: 1 mg, 2 mg, 5 mg, 10 mg

INDICATIONS & DOSAGES
➤ **HTN**
Adults: Initially, 1 mg PO at bedtime. May increase dosage gradually based on response. Usual dosage range, 1 to 5 mg daily. Maximum recommended dosage, 20 mg daily. If response is substantially diminished at 24 hours, consider dosage increase or use of a twice-daily regimen.
➤ **Symptomatic BPH**
Adults: Initially, 1 mg PO at bedtime. Dosage may be titrated stepwise to 2, 5, or 10 mg once daily to achieve optimal response. Most patients need 10 mg daily for optimal response. Maximum recommended dosage, 20 mg/day.

ADMINISTRATION
PO
• Give drug without regard to food.
• Give twice-daily regimen doses 12 hours apart.
• If drug is discontinued for several days or longer, restart drug with initial dosing regimen.

ACTION
Improves urine flow in patients with BPH by blocking alpha-adrenergic receptors in the bladder neck and prostate, relieving urethral pressure. Also reduces peripheral vascular resistance and BP via arterial and venous dilation.

Route	Onset	Peak	Duration
PO	15 min	1 hr	24 hr

Half-life: About 12 hours.

ADVERSE REACTIONS
CNS: anxiety, headache, dizziness, fever, insomnia, asthenia, syncope, nervousness, paresthesia, drowsiness, somnolence, vertigo. **CV:** chest pain, edema, palpitations, orthostatic hypotension, tachycardia, *arrhythmia,* vasodilation. **EENT:** blurred vision, conjunctivitis, tinnitus, nasal congestion, epistaxis, sinusitis, pharyngitis, rhinitis, dry mouth.

GI: nausea, abdominal pain, constipation, diarrhea, dyspepsia, flatulence, vomiting. **GU:** erectile dysfunction, urinary frequency, urinary incontinence, UTI. **Metabolic:** gout. **Musculoskeletal:** arthralgia, arthritis, back pain, joint disorder, limb pain, myalgia. **Respiratory:** dyspnea, cough, bronchitis. **Skin:** pruritus, rash, diaphoresis. **Other:** flulike syndrome, cold symptoms.

INTERACTIONS
Drug-drug. *Antihypertensives, antipsychotics, calcium channel blockers, PDE5 inhibitors (tadalafil, vardenafil):* May increase hypotensive effect. Use together cautiously.
Drug-herb. *Yohimbe:* May diminish antihypertensive effect of drug. Monitor therapy.

EFFECTS ON LAB TEST RESULTS
• May decrease total protein, albumin, total cholesterol, and combined LDL-C and VLDL-C levels.
• May decrease Hb level, hematocrit, and WBC and platelet counts.

CONTRAINDICATIONS & CAUTIONS
• Contraindicated in patients hypersensitive to drug.
• May cause marked lowering of BP, especially orthostatic hypotension, and syncope in association with first dose or first few days of therapy. A similar effect can be expected if therapy is interrupted for several days then restarted, dosage is rapidly increased, or another antihypertensive is introduced. Always initiate treatment with a 1-mg dose at bedtime.
• Intraoperative floppy iris syndrome has been observed during cataract and glaucoma surgery in some patients who are taking or had previously taken alpha$_1$ blockers, which may increase risk of eye complications during and after surgery. Don't initiate drug in patients scheduled for cataract or glaucoma surgery.
• May cause CNS depression and impair mental alertness.
• Rare cases of priapism have been reported.
Dialyzable drug: 10%.
⚠ *Overdose S&S:* Hypotension.

PREGNANCY-LACTATION-REPRODUCTION
• Studies during pregnancy are inadequate. Use only if potential benefit justifies fetal risk.
• It isn't known if drug appears in human milk. Use cautiously during breastfeeding.

---

*Reactions in bold italics are **life-threatening**.*

NURSING CONSIDERATIONS

• Monitor BP frequently. Evaluate patient for signs and symptoms of hypotension (dizziness, palpitations).

• Symptoms of BPH and prostate cancer are similar. Rule out prostate cancer before starting therapy.

PATIENT TEACHING

• Tell patient not to stop drug suddenly. Instruct patient to notify prescriber if adverse reactions occur.

• Review rare but serious risk of priapism. Instruct patient to report it immediately.

• Warn patient to avoid hazardous activities that require mental alertness, such as driving and operating heavy machinery, for 12 hours after first dose.

• Tell patient that light-headedness from hypotension can occur. Advise patient to rise slowly and to report signs and symptoms to prescriber.

• Advise patient considering cataract or glaucoma surgery to inform ophthalmologist about terazosin use.

terbinafine hydrochloride (oral)
ter-BIN-ah-feen

Therapeutic class: Antifungals
Pharmacologic class: Synthetic allylamine derivatives

AVAILABLE FORMS
Tablets: 250 mg

INDICATIONS & DOSAGES

➤ **Fingernail and toenail onychomycosis caused by dermatophytes (tinea unguium)**
Adults: 250 mg PO once daily for 6 weeks for fingernail infection and 12 weeks for toenail infection.

ADMINISTRATION
PO

• Confirm diagnosis with nail specimen testing (potassium hydroxide preparation, fungal culture, or nail biopsy).

• Give tablets without regard to food.

• Give missed dose as soon as possible unless it's less than 4 hours before next scheduled dose.

• Store tablets at room temperature. Protect them from light.

ACTION

Prevents biosynthesis of ergosterol, causing a deficiency of this essential component of fungal cell membranes.

Route	Onset	Peak	Duration
PO	Unknown	≤2 hr	Unknown

Half-life: Adults, 36 hours; children, 27 to 31 hours.

ADVERSE REACTIONS

CNS: headache, taste disturbances. **EENT:** vision disturbances. **GI:** diarrhea, dyspepsia, nausea, abdominal pain, flatulence. **Hematologic:** *neutropenia.* **Hepatic:** liver enzyme elevations. **Skin:** rash, pruritus, urticaria.

INTERACTIONS

Drug-drug. *Caffeine:* May decrease caffeine clearance. Use together cautiously.
Cimetidine: May increases terbinafine level. Avoid use together.
Codeine: May decrease codeine's therapeutic effect. Monitor therapy.
Cyclosporine: May decrease cyclosporine level. Monitor cyclosporine level.
CYP2C9, CYP3A4 enzyme inhibitors (amiodarone, fluconazole): May substantially increase terbinafine level. Use together cautiously.
CYP2D6 substrates (class 1C antiarrhythmics [flecainide], beta blockers, MAO inhibitors type B, SSRIs [paroxetine, venlafaxine], TCAs): May increase substrate level. Dosage adjustment may be needed. Monitor therapy.
Rifampin: Significantly decreases terbinafine level. Avoid use together.
Tamoxifen: May decrease level of tamoxifen's active metabolite. Consider alternative to terbinafine.
Tramadol: May increase tramadol level. Monitor patient closely.
Warfarin: May alter anticoagulation effect. Monitor PT.
Drug-lifestyle. *Sunlight, UV light:* May increase risk of photosensitivity reactions. Encourage patient to minimize exposure.

EFFECTS ON LAB TEST RESULTS

• May increase AST and ALT levels.

• May decrease Hb level and platelet, neutrophil, and lymphocyte counts.

CONTRAINDICATIONS & CAUTIONS

• Contraindicated in patients hypersensitive to drug or its components.

• Contraindicated in patients with chronic or active liver disease. Cases of liver failure, some leading to liver transplant or death, have occurred in patients with and without preexisting liver disease.

• Disturbances of taste and smell have been reported and may last up to 1 year or become permanent.

• Depressive signs and symptoms have occurred during postmarketing use.

• Serious skin reactions (SJS, TEN, and others) and hypersensitivity reactions have occurred.

• Thrombotic microangiopathy (TMA), including thrombotic thrombocytopenic purpura and hemolytic-uremic syndrome, can occur. Fatalities have been reported.

• New and worsened cases of cutaneous lupus erythematosus and SLE have been reported. Discontinue drug in patients with signs and symptoms of SLE.

• Safety and effectiveness in children haven't been established.

• Use cautiously in older adults.

Dialyzable drug: Unknown.

⚠ *Overdose S&S:* Abdominal pain, dizziness, frequent urination, headache, nausea, rash, vomiting.

PREGNANCY-LACTATION-REPRODUCTION
• Studies during pregnancy are inadequate. Because treatment can be postponed until after pregnancy, initiation during pregnancy isn't recommended.

• Drug appears in human milk. Use during breastfeeding isn't recommended.

NURSING CONSIDERATIONS
• Obtain liver function test results before treatment to screen for chronic or active liver disease.

• Periodically monitor LFT values during treatment. Stop drug if evidence of liver injury develops.

• Monitor CBC in patients taking drug for longer than 6 weeks, especially those with known or suspected immunodeficiency or signs or symptoms of secondary infection. Stop drug if neutrophil count is 1,000 cells/mm³ or less.

• Monitor and evaluate patients who develop unexplained thrombocytopenia and anemia for TMA. Discontinue drug if clinical signs and symptoms and lab findings consistent with TMA occur.

• Monitor patient for depression and changes in taste or smell. Discontinue drug if taste or smell disturbance occurs.

• Monitor for skin reactions. If any occur, discontinue drug.

• *Look alike–sound alike:* Don't confuse terbinafine with terbutaline.

PATIENT TEACHING
• Inform patient that successful treatment may take 12 weeks for toenail infections and 6 weeks for fingernail infections.

• Teach about proper drug administration and handling.

• Tell patient to immediately report depression; smell, taste, or vision disturbances (changes in ocular lens and retina may occur); and signs or symptoms of liver injury (persistent nausea, anorexia, fatigue, vomiting, right upper quadrant pain, jaundice, dark urine, pale stools).

• Advise patient to minimize exposure to sunlight with sunscreen and protective clothing and to avoid UV light (tanning beds, UVA or UVB treatment).

---

terconazole
ter-CONE-uh-zole

Therapeutic class: Antifungals
Pharmacologic class: Triazole derivatives

AVAILABLE FORMS
Vaginal cream: 0.4%*, 0.8%*
Vaginal suppositories: 80 mg

INDICATIONS & DOSAGES
➤ **Vulvovaginal candidiasis**
Adults: One applicatorful of cream or 1 suppository inserted into vagina at bedtime: 0.4% cream for 7 consecutive days; 0.8% cream or 80-mg suppository for 3 consecutive days. Repeat course, if needed, after reconfirmation of diagnosis by smear or culture.

ADMINISTRATION
Vaginal
• Confirm diagnosis of candidiasis by smear or culture.

• Insert drug high in vagina at bedtime.

• Use applicator supplied by manufacturer.

• Wash applicator after each use and allow it to dry thoroughly.

• Store drug at room temperature.

ACTION
May increase *Candida* cell membrane permeability.

Route	Onset	Peak	Duration
Vaginal	Unknown	5–10 hr	Unknown

Half-life: 6.4 to 8.5 hours.

ADVERSE REACTIONS
CNS: headache, fever, pain. **GI:** abdominal pain. **GU:** dysmenorrhea, vulvovaginal discomfort (burning, irritation, itching).

INTERACTIONS
None reported.

EFFECTS ON LAB TEST RESULTS
None reported.

CONTRAINDICATIONS & CAUTIONS
• Contraindicated in patients hypersensitive to drug or its inactive ingredients.
• Safety and effectiveness in children haven't been determined.
Dialyzable drug: Unknown.

PREGNANCY-LACTATION-REPRODUCTION
• Because drug is systemically absorbed, don't administer during first trimester unless prescriber considers it essential to patient's welfare.
• May use during second and third trimesters if potential benefit outweighs fetal risk.
• It isn't known if drug appears in human milk. Patient should discontinue breastfeeding or discontinue drug, considering importance of drug to patient.

NURSING CONSIDERATIONS
• Menstruation and hormonal contraceptives don't impact drug's therapeutic effect.
• Assess patient's ability to self-administer. Self-administration may be difficult for patient with arthritis or limited range of motion.
• *Look alike–sound alike:* Don't confuse terconazole with tioconazole.

PATIENT TEACHING
• Advise patient to continue treatment during menstrual period. However, instruct patient not to use tampons.
• Teach self-administration of drug; remind patient to insert drug high in vagina.
• Tell patient to use drug for full treatment period prescribed. Explain how to prevent reinfection.

• Instruct patient to notify prescriber and stop drug if fever, chills, other flulike signs and symptoms, irritation, or sensitivity develops.
• Caution patient to refrain from sexual intercourse during treatment if advised by prescriber.
• Tell patient that suppository formulation may react with latex or rubber, weakening condoms and diaphragms. Use of condoms or diaphragms during treatment isn't recommended.
• Advise patient that male partner also may need treatment if symptomatic (penile itching, redness, or discomfort).
• Inform patient of pregnancy and breastfeeding risks.

testosterone
tes-TOS-te-rone

Natesto, Testopel

testosterone cypionate
Depo-Testosterone

testosterone enanthate
Xyosted

testosterone undecanoate
Aveed, Jatenzo, Kyzatrex, Tlando

Therapeutic class: Androgens
Pharmacologic class: Androgens
Controlled substance schedule: III

AVAILABLE FORMS
testosterone
Nasal gel (metered): 5.5 mg/actuation
Pellets (subcut implant): 12.5 mg, 25 mg, 37.5 mg, 50 mg, 75 mg, 100 mg, 200 mg
testosterone cypionate
Injection (in oil): 100 mg/mL*, 200 mg/mL*
testosterone enanthate
Autoinjector: 50 mg/0.5 mL, 75 mg/0.5 mL, 100 mg/0.5 mL
Injection (in oil): 200 mg/mL
testosterone undecanoate
Capsules: 100 mg, 112.5 mg, 150 mg, 158 mg, 198 mg, 200 mg, 237 mg
Injection (in oil): 250 mg/mL

INDICATIONS & DOSAGES
➤ **Hypogonadism**
Men: 50 to 400 mg cypionate or enanthate in oil IM every 2 to 4 weeks. Or, 75 mg

enanthate autoinjector subcut in abdominal region once a week. Or, initially, 750 mg undecanoate in oil IM and 4 weeks later; then 750 mg IM every 10 weeks thereafter. Or, initially, 200 to 237 mg undecanoate capsules PO b.i.d. Or, 150 to 450 mg (2 to 6 pellets) implanted subcut every 3 to 6 months. Or, 11 mg (2 pump actuations; 1 actuation per nostril) intranasally t.i.d., once in the morning, once in the afternoon, and once in the evening (6 to 8 hours apart), preferably at same time each day for a total daily dose of 33 mg.

Adjust-a-dose: When total testosterone level consistently exceeds 1,050 ng/dL, discontinue nasal spray therapy. If total testosterone level is consistently below 300 ng/dL, consider alternative treatment. Adjust dosage based on serum testosterone level. Consult product inserts for specific dosage adjustments.

➤ **Delayed puberty**
Men and boys: 50 to 200 mg enanthate IM every 2 to 4 weeks for 4 to 6 months. Or, 150 to 450 mg pellets implanted subcut every 3 to 6 months for a limited duration, such as 4 to 6 months.

➤ **Metastatic breast cancer**
Patients 1 to 5 years after menopause: 200 to 400 mg enanthate IM every 2 to 4 weeks.

ADMINISTRATION

🜀 *Alert:* Hazardous drug; use safe handling and disposal precautions.
PO
• Give drug with food.
IM
• Store IM preparations at room temperature. If crystals appear, warm and shake bottle to disperse them.
• Inject drug deep into upper outer quadrant of gluteal muscle.
• Rotate injection sites. Report soreness at site.
Subcutaneous
• In most men, pellets are implanted in area on anterior abdominal wall.
• Number of pellets implanted depends on required dose.
• Enanthate autoinjector isn't for IM or IV administration.
• Don't use autoinjector if liquid is cloudy, visible particles are present, or seal is broken.
• Don't use autoinjector within 2 inches of navel; where skin is tender, bruised, red, scaly, or hard; or in areas with scars, tattoos, or stretch marks.

Intranasal
• Prime pump before first use by inverting and then depressing pump 10 times (discard this portion of product into sink).
• Have patient blow nose before application.
• To administer, insert actuator into nostril until pump reaches base of nose; tilt so tip is in contact with lateral wall of nostril. Depress slowly until pump stops; then remove from nose while wiping tip to transfer gel to lateral side of nostril.
• After administration, press on nostrils just below bridge of nose and lightly massage.
• Make sure patient refrains from blowing nose or sniffing for 1 hour after administration.
• If gel gets on hands, wash with warm soap and water.

ACTION

Stimulates target tissues to develop normally in androgen-deficient men. May have some antiestrogen properties, making it useful in treating certain estrogen-dependent breast cancers.

Route	Onset	Peak	Duration
PO	Unknown	2–4 hr	Unknown
IM	Unknown	4–42 days	2–10 wk
Subcut (implant)	Unknown	Unknown	3–6 mo
Subcut (enanthate)	Unknown	6–168 hr	Unknown
Intranasal	Unknown	40 min	Unknown

Half-life: 10 to 100 minutes; cypionate, about 8 days.

ADVERSE REACTIONS

Refer to manufacturer's prescribing information for each product, including abuse-related adverse reactions.
CNS: headache, anxiety, depression, paresthesia, sleep apnea, mood swings, aggressive behavior, irritability, bitter taste. **CV:** edema, HTN, increased HR. **EENT:** nasal discomfort, dryness, or congestion; nasopharyngitis; epistaxis; rhinorrhea; parosmia; nasal scabbing; gum or mouth irritation; gum pain, tenderness, or edema. **GI:** nausea, diarrhea. **GU:** amenorrhea, oligospermia, erection disorder, ejaculatory disorder, increased or decreased libido, priapism, prostatitis, increased PSA level. **Hematologic:** polycythemia, *suppression of clotting factors*. **Hepatic:** altered LFT values, reversible jaundice, *cholestatic hepatitis*. **Metabolic:** hypercholesterolemia, *hyperkalemia,* hypercalcemia, weight gain, hyperphosphatemia, hypernatremia.

Musculoskeletal: back pain, arthralgia.
Respiratory: cough, URI. **Skin:** pain, implantation- or injection-site reaction, induration at injection site, implantation site infection, pellet extrusion, local edema, acne, hyperhidrosis, hirsutism, male pattern baldness. **Other:** androgenic effects in females, gynecomastia, hypersensitivity reactions, hypoestrogenic effects in females, excessive hormonal effects in males.

INTERACTIONS
Drug-drug. *Corticosteroids:* May increase risk of edema. Use together cautiously, especially in patients with cardiac, liver, or kidney disease.
Cyclosporine: Androgens may enhance liver-toxic effects. Consider therapy modification.
Drugs that increase BP (NSAIDs, pseudoephedrine): May increase risk of HTN. Monitor therapy.
Liver-toxic drugs: May increase risk of liver toxicity. Closely monitor liver function.
Insulin, oral antidiabetics: May decrease glucose level and alter dosage requirements. Monitor glucose level in patients with diabetes.
Oral anticoagulants (warfarin): May increase sensitivity; may alter dosage requirements. Monitor PT and INR; decrease anticoagulant dose if necessary.
Drug-food. *Licorice:* May decrease testosterone level. Discourage use together.

EFFECTS ON LAB TEST RESULTS
• May increase LFT values and sodium, potassium, phosphate, cholesterol, calcium, creatinine, CK, and serum PSA levels.
• May increase resin uptake of T_3 and T_4.
• May increase Hb level, hematocrit, and RBC count.
• May decrease thyroxine-binding globulin, total T_4, and 17-ketosteroid levels.
• May decrease leukocyte count.
• May cause abnormal glucose tolerance test results.

CONTRAINDICATIONS & CAUTIONS
• Contraindicated in patients hypersensitive to drug or its components and in those with hypercalcemia or cardiac, liver, or kidney decompensation.
• Contraindicated in men with breast cancer or known or suspected prostate cancer.
• VTEs have been reported in patients using testosterone products.

Boxed Warning Serious pulmonary oil microembolism reactions (involving urge to cough, dyspnea, throat tightening, chest pain, dizziness, and syncope) and episodes of anaphylaxis, including life-threatening reactions, have been reported to occur during or immediately after administration of testosterone undecanoate injection. These reactions can occur after any injection during therapy, including after first dose. Observe patients for 30 minutes after each dose. Drug is available only through the Aveed REMS program. ∎

Boxed Warning Oral and subcutaneous testosterone products can increase BP, increasing the risk of major adverse CV events, including nonfatal MI, nonfatal stroke, and CV death. These forms are only indicated for hypogonadal conditions with structural or genetic causes. Before initiating drug, consider evaluating patient's baseline CV risk and ensure adequate BP control. ∎

⊕ Alert: Drug has potential for abuse, usually at doses higher than those prescribed and usually in conjunction with other anabolic androgenic steroids (AASs). Abuse is associated with serious safety risks, such as MI, HF, stroke, depression, hostility, aggression, liver toxicity, and male infertility. Withdrawal signs and symptoms (depression, fatigue, irritability, loss of appetite, decreased libido, and insomnia) can occur in patients abusing high testosterone doses.

⊕ Alert: Contraindicated in men with age-related low testosterone signs and symptoms only. Testosterone replacement therapy is only approved for men with primary or secondary hypogonadism resulting from certain medical conditions and with low testosterone levels confirmed by lab testing.

• Prolonged use of high doses of androgens has been associated with peliosis hepatis and liver neoplasms, including hepatocellular carcinoma.
• Use cautiously in older adults.
• Intranasal form isn't recommended for use with nasally administered drugs other than sympathomimetic decongestants or for use in patients with mucosal inflammatory disorders, sinus disease or history of nasal disorders, nasal or sinus surgery, nasal fracture within previous 6 months, or nasal fracture that caused a deviated anterior nasal septum.
• Use cautiously in patients with sleep apnea or those with risk factors for sleep apnea (obesity, chronic lung disease).

T

Dialyzable drug: Unknown.
⚠ *Overdose S&S:* Stroke (with enanthate injection).

PREGNANCY-LACTATION-REPRODUCTION
• Drug is teratogenic and may cause fetal harm. Use is contraindicated during pregnancy. If pregnancy occurs during therapy, apprise patient of fetal risk.
• Contraindicated during breastfeeding because of potential for virilization in infants who are breastfed.
• Large doses may suppress spermatogenesis and cause irreversible infertility in males.

NURSING CONSIDERATIONS
• Verify pregnancy status before treatment.
• Cypionate, enanthate, and undecanoate are long-acting solutions.
⚠ *Alert:* If testosterone abuse is suspected, check that serum testosterone level is within therapeutic range. Consider possibility of testosterone and AAS abuse in patient who presents with serious CV or psychiatric adverse events.

Boxed Warning Starting about 6 weeks after initiating subcut therapy or 3 weeks after initiating PO therapy, periodically monitor patient for and treat new-onset or worsening HTN. Reevaluate whether benefits of drug outweigh risks in patients who develop CV risk factors or CV disease during treatment. Use subcut and PO testosterone only for treatment of men with hypogonadal conditions associated with structural or genetic conditions. ∎

• If patient experiences severe rhinitis, temporarily discontinue intranasal therapy until signs and symptoms resolve. If signs and symptoms persist, replace with alternative testosterone replacement therapy.
• Periodically monitor patient's liver function, and check PSA, cholesterol, HDL-C, and Hb levels and hematocrit.
⚠ *Alert:* Confirm low testosterone level on at least two mornings before initiating therapy. Avoid measuring testosterone level later in day, when levels can be low, even in patients who don't have hypogonadism.
• Monitor testosterone level after initial dosage titration and periodically, as described in prescribing information for each product. Adjust dosage if needed.
• Evaluate for DVT if patient reports pain, edema, or warmth and erythema in lower

extremity; evaluate for PE if patient presents with acute shortness of breath. For suspected VTE, discontinue drug and initiate appropriate workup and management.
• In patient with metastatic breast cancer, hypercalcemia usually indicates progression of bone metastases. Report signs and symptoms of hypercalcemia.
• Report evidence of virilization in adult females. Androgenic effects include acne, edema, weight gain, increased hair growth, hoarseness, clitoral enlargement, decreased breast size, changes in libido, male pattern baldness, and oily skin or hair.
• Watch for hypoestrogenic effects in adult females (flushing; diaphoresis; vaginitis, including itching, drying, and burning; vaginal bleeding; menstrual irregularities).
• Watch for excessive hormonal effects in adult males and male children. During prepuberty, watch for premature epiphyseal closure, acne, priapism, growth of body and facial hair, and phallic enlargement. After puberty, watch for testicular atrophy, oligospermia, decreased ejaculatory volume, impotence, gynecomastia, and epididymitis.
• Drug may increase risk of depression and suicidality. Evaluate patient with new-onset or worsening depression, anxiety, mood changes, or suicidality.
• Routinely monitor patient's weight and BP.
• Monitor prepubertal male by X-ray for rate of bone maturation.
• Using testosterone esters to treat males with hypogonadism may potentiate sleep apnea. Monitor patient with risk factors (obesity, chronic lung disease).
⚠ *Alert:* Therapeutic response in breast cancer is usually apparent within 3 months. If disease progresses, stop drug.
• Androgens may alter results of lab studies during therapy and for 2 to 3 weeks after therapy ends.
⚠ *Alert:* Testosterone salts aren't interchangeable.
• *Look alike–sound alike:* Don't confuse testosterone with testolactone.

PATIENT TEACHING
• Make sure patient understands importance of using effective contraception during therapy.
• Teach about proper drug administration and handling.
• Instruct patient to report suspected pregnancy and to stop drug immediately.

• Advise patient to wear cotton underwear and to wash after intercourse to decrease risk of vaginitis.

❸ Alert: Warn patient to seek immediate medical attention for signs and symptoms of heart attack (chest pain, shortness of breath, trouble breathing) or stroke (weakness in one part or side of the body, slurred speech).

• Advise patient and caregiver to seek medical attention for manifestations of new-onset or worsening depression, suicidality, anxiety, or other mood changes.

• Review signs and symptoms of virilization. Instruct patient to notify prescriber if any occur.

• Instruct male patient to report priapism, reduced ejaculatory volume, or gynecomastia.

• Warn patient with diabetes to be alert for hypoglycemia and to notify prescriber if it occurs.

• Instruct patient using testosterone for delayed puberty to have hand and wrist X-rays every 6 months, as prescribed.

• Tell patient to report sudden weight gain.

• Warn patient that drug shouldn't be used to enhance athletic performance.

testosterone transdermal
tes-TOS-te-rone

Androderm, AndroGel, Fortesta, Testim, Vogelxo

Therapeutic class: Androgens
Pharmacologic class: Androgens

AVAILABLE FORMS
1% gel*: 25 mg, 50 mg per unit dose; 12.5 mg per pump actuation
1.62% gel*: 20.25 mg, 40.5 mg per unit dose; 20.25 mg per pump actuation
Transdermal cream: 0.2%, 0.4%, 10%, 20%
2% gel: 10 mg per pump actuation
Transdermal solution*: 30 mg per metered-dose pump
Transdermal system: 2 mg/day, 4 mg/day

INDICATIONS & DOSAGES
➤ **Primary or hypogonadotropic hypogonadism**
Adult males: One Androderm 4 mg/day system (don't use two 2-mg/day patches) applied to back, abdomen, upper arm, or thigh nightly. After 2 weeks, may increase dosage to 6 mg

once daily or decrease to 2 mg once daily, depending on morning serum testosterone level.

Or, initially, 50 mg of 1% gel (two 25-mg packets, four 12.5-mg pumps, or one 50-mg packet) applied every morning to shoulders, upper arms, or abdomen. Check testosterone level after about 2 weeks. If response is inadequate, may increase to 75 mg daily. Then adjust to 100 mg if needed.

Or, initially, 40.5 mg of 1.62% gel (2 pumps or one 40.5-mg packet) applied once daily in morning to upper arms or shoulders. May adjust dosage between minimum of 20.25 mg (1 pump or one 20.25-mg packet) and maximum of 81 mg (4 pumps or two 40.5-mg packets) titrated based on predose morning serum testosterone level at about 14 days and 28 days after starting treatment or last dosage adjustment.

Or, 50 mg of Testim (1 tube) applied once daily in morning to shoulders and upper arms (don't apply to genitals or abdomen). May increase to maximum of 100 mg/day, if needed, based on testosterone level.

Or, initially 40 mg (4 pumps) of Fortesta once daily to thighs in morning. May adjust dosage between 10 mg and maximum of 70 mg based on testosterone level drawn 2 hours after application approximately 14 days and 35 days after start of treatment and last dosage adjustment.

Or, initially 60 mg (2 pumps) of solution, one actuation to each axilla, once daily. May adjust dosage between 30 mg (1 actuation) and a maximum of 120 mg (4 actuations) based on serum testosterone level drawn 2 to 8 hours after application and at least 14 days after starting treatment or last dosage adjustment. For doses of more than 60 mg daily, alternate axillae, allowing them to dry completely before applying next actuation.

Or, 50 mg of Vogelxo once daily to shoulders or upper arms. If serum testosterone level falls below normal range, increase to maximum dosage of 100 mg/day.

ADMINISTRATION
❸ Alert: Hazardous drug; use safe handling and disposal precautions.
Transdermal
• Wear gloves when handling patches. Fold used patches with adhesive sides together to discard.
• Apply patch immediately after opening pouch and removing protective liner.

- Apply patch nightly to clean, dry, intact skin on back, abdomen, upper arms, or thighs only. Press firmly in place to ensure good contact. Rotate sites; don't reuse a site for 7 days.
- Don't apply to bony areas or parts of body subject to prolonged pressure while sleeping or sitting.
- Don't apply to oily, damaged, or irritated skin.
- Reapply patch if it falls off. If patch can't be reapplied and has been worn at least 12 hours, apply a new patch at next scheduled application time.
- Patient should avoid swimming, showering, and washing administration site for at least 3 hours after application.

Topical
- 1.62% gel, 1% gel, and topical solution aren't interchangeable.
- Fully prime pump according to manufacturer's instructions. Discard this portion of product.
- Wear gloves to apply gel to clean, dry, intact skin as directed for each product. Don't apply to the genitals or bony prominences.
- Application in the morning is preferable. Allow application sites to dry before dressing. Cover application site with clothing.
- Patient should avoid swimming and washing administration site for 2 to 5 hours after application, depending on product.
- Gel contains alcohol and is flammable. Patient should avoid fire, flames, and smoking until gel has dried.
- Apply topical solution, using applicator provided, to clean, dry, intact skin of axilla as directed. Don't use the fingers or hand to rub solution into skin.
- Patient should apply deodorant or antiperspirant (stick or roll-on) at least 2 minutes before applying the solution.

ACTION
Releases testosterone, which stimulates target tissues to develop normally in androgen-deficient males.

Route	Onset	Peak	Duration
Transdermal, topical	Unknown	4–24 hr	24 hr– 10 days

Half-life: 10 to 100 minutes.

ADVERSE REACTIONS
CNS: abnormal dreams, asthenia, depression, headache, sleep apnea, smell disorder, aggressive behavior, emotional lability, fatigue, insomnia, irritability, nervousness, taste disorder. **CV:** HTN, edema. **GI:** *GI bleeding,* diarrhea, increased appetite, vomiting. **GU:** prostatitis, prostate abnormalities, UTI, ejaculation disorder, erectile dysfunction, polyuria, decreased libido, pelvic pain, urinary incontinence, increased PSA level. **Hematologic:** increased Hb, polycythemia. **Hepatic:** abnormal LFT results, hyperbilirubinemia, reversible jaundice. **Metabolic:** hypernatremia, *hypokalemia,* hypercalcemia, hyperphosphatemia, hypercholesterolemia, weight gain. **Skin:** alopecia; application-site pruritus, blister, erythema, vesicles, burning, or induration; acne irritation; allergic contact dermatitis; hyperhidrosis. **Other:** gynecomastia, breast tenderness, flulike syndrome, hot flash.

INTERACTIONS
Drug-drug. *Corticosteroids:* May increase risk of edema. Use together cautiously, especially in patients with kidney, cardiac, or liver disease.
Cyclosporine: Androgens may enhance livertoxic effect. Consider therapy modification.
Liver-toxic drugs: May increase risk of liver toxicity. Closely monitor liver function.
Insulin, oral antidiabetics: May enhance hypoglycemic effect and alter dosage requirements of listed drugs. Monitor glucose level in patients with diabetes.
Oral anticoagulants (warfarin): May alter anticoagulant dosage requirements. Monitor PT and INR.

EFFECTS ON LAB TEST RESULTS
- May increase PSA, sodium, phosphate, cholesterol, liver enzyme, calcium, creatinine, and TSH levels.
- May decrease glucose, potassium, HDL-C, and total T_4 levels.
- May increase Hb level, hematocrit, and RBC count.
- May increase resin uptake of T_3 and T_4.

CONTRAINDICATIONS & CAUTIONS
- Contraindicated in patients hypersensitive to drug, in adult females, and in adult males with known or suspected breast or prostate cancer.
- ⚠️ *Alert:* Contraindicated in males with age-related low testosterone symptoms only. Testosterone replacement therapy is only approved for males with primary or secondary

hypogonadism resulting from certain medical conditions and with low testosterone levels confirmed by lab testing.
• Use cautiously in patients with cancer who are at risk for hypercalcemia (and associated hypercalciuria).
❸ *Alert:* Drug has potential for abuse, usually at doses higher than those prescribed and usually in conjunction with other anabolic androgenic steroids (AASs). Abuse is associated with serious safety risks, such as MI, HF, stroke, depression, hostility, aggression, liver toxicity, and male infertility. Withdrawal signs and symptoms (depression, fatigue, irritability, loss of appetite, decreased libido, and insomnia) can occur in patients abusing high testosterone doses.
❸ *Alert:* Drug may increase risk of heart attack and stroke.
• VTEs have been reported in patients using testosterone products.
• Prolonged use of high doses of androgens has been associated with development of peliosis hepatis and liver neoplasms, including hepatocellular carcinoma.
• Use cautiously in older adults.
Dialyzable drug: Unknown.

PREGNANCY-LACTATION-REPRODUCTION
• Drug isn't indicated for use in females. Apprise patients who are pregnant of risk of virilization of a female fetus with transfer of testosterone from males undergoing treatment.
• Drug is teratogenic; may cause fetal harm.
• Contraindicated in patients who are breastfeeding because of risk of virilization in infant.
• Drug may suppress spermatogenesis.

NURSING CONSIDERATIONS
Boxed Warning Virilization in children can occur after secondary exposure to transdermal application sites on patient. Children should avoid contact with unwashed or unclothed application sites. ■
• Monitor serum calcium level in patient with cancer who is at risk for hypercalcemia (and associated hypercalciuria).
❸ *Alert:* For suspected testosterone abuse, check that serum testosterone level falls within therapeutic range. Consider testosterone and anabolic androgenic steroid abuse in patient who presents with serious CV or psychiatric adverse events.

• Treatment of males who are hypogonadal with testosterone esters may increase risk of sleep apnea. Monitor patient with risk factors (obesity, chronic lung disease).
• Periodically assess LFT results, lipid profiles, Hb level, hematocrit (with long-term use), and levels of prostatic acid phosphatase and PSA.
❸ *Alert:* Confirm low testosterone level on at least two mornings before initiating therapy. Avoid measuring testosterone level later in day, when levels can be low, even in males who don't have hypogonadism. Refer to manufacturer's instructions for product-specific recommendations.
• Watch for excessive hormonal effects.
• Evaluate for DVT if patient reports pain, edema, or warmth and erythema in lower extremity; evaluate for PE if patient presents with acute shortness of breath. For suspected VTE, discontinue drug and initiate appropriate workup and management.
• Remove topical patch before MRI because patch contains aluminum.

PATIENT TEACHING
• Teach patient how to prime pump and self-administer drug according to individual manufacturer's instructions.
Boxed Warning Instruct patient to strictly adhere to recommended instructions for use to avoid secondary exposure in children. ■
• Tell patient to wash hands thoroughly after using product and to cover treated area with clothing.
• Instruct patient to thoroughly wash application site with soap and water if anticipating direct skin-to-skin contact.
• Warn patient with diabetes that drug may cause hypoglycemia.
❸ *Alert:* Warn patient to seek immediate medical attention for signs and symptoms of heart attack (chest pain, shortness of breath, trouble breathing) or stroke (weakness in one part or side of the body, slurred speech).
• Advise patient to report persistent erections, nausea, vomiting, changes in skin color, ankle swelling, or sudden weight gain to prescriber.
• Tell patient that Androderm doesn't have to be removed during sexual intercourse or while showering.
• Caution patient undergoing MRI to alert facility about transdermal patch use.

T

tetracycline hydrochloride
tet-ra-SYE-kleen

Therapeutic class: Antibiotics
Pharmacologic class: Tetracyclines

AVAILABLE FORMS
Capsules: 250 mg, 500 mg

INDICATIONS & DOSAGES
Adjust-a-dose (for all indications): Decrease recommended dosages or extend dosing intervals in patients with kidney impairment.

➤ **Infections caused by susceptible organisms, such as *Haemophilus ducreyi, Yersinia pestis, Campylobacter fetus, Rickettsiae species, Mycoplasma pneumoniae, Chlamydia psittaci, Chlamydia trachomatis, Entamoeba species, Actinomyces species, Bacillus anthracis, Vibrio cholerae, Listeria monocytogenes, Fusobacterium fusiforme, Haemophilus influenzae, Treponema species, Francisella tularensis, Clostridioides species, Escherichia coli, Enterobacter aerogenes, Shigella species, Klebsiella species, Borrelia species, Streptococcus pneumoniae, Streptococcus pyogenes,* and *Staphylococcus aureus***
Adults: 1 to 2 g/day PO in two or four divided doses, depending on the severity of infection.
Children older than age 8: 25 to 50 mg/kg PO daily in divided doses every 6 hours.

➤ **Uncomplicated urethral, endocervical, or rectal infections caused by *C. trachomatis***
Adults: 500 mg PO q.i.d. for at least 7 days.

➤ **Brucellosis**
Adults: 500 mg PO q.i.d. for 3 weeks in combination with streptomycin.

➤ **Uncomplicated gonorrhea in patients allergic to penicillin**
Adults: 500 mg PO q.i.d. for 7 days.

➤ **Syphilis in patients allergic to penicillin**
Adults and adolescents: 500 mg PO q.i.d. for 15 days. If infection has lasted 1 year or longer, treat for 30 days.

➤ **Acne (moderate to severe; long-term therapy) as adjunct to topical therapy**
Adults and adolescents: Initially, 1 g PO daily in divided doses. For maintenance, 125 to 500 mg daily. (Alternate-day or intermittent therapy may be adequate in some patients.).

ADMINISTRATION
PO
● Obtain specimen for culture and sensitivity tests before giving first dose. Begin therapy while awaiting results.
● For streptococcal infections, continue therapy for 10 days.
● Milk and other dairy products, antacids, and iron products interfere with drug absorption, reducing its effectiveness. For best drug absorption, give drug with a full glass of water on an empty stomach, at least 1 hour before or 2 hours after meals.
● Give drug with adequate amount of fluid at least 1 hour before bedtime to prevent esophageal irritation and ulceration.
● Store drug at room temperature. Protect from light.
🔆 *Alert:* Be careful not to administer outdated drug because of highly increased risk of kidney toxicity and Fanconi syndrome.

ACTION
May exert bacteriostatic effect by binding to the 30S and possibly 50S ribosomal subunits of microorganisms, thus inhibiting protein synthesis. May also alter the cytoplasmic membrane of susceptible microorganisms.

Route	Onset	Peak	Duration
PO	Unknown	2–4 hr	Unknown

Half-life: 6 to 11 hours.

ADVERSE REACTIONS
CNS: headache. **EENT:** black, hairy tongue; glossitis; oral candidiasis; sore throat. **GI:** diarrhea, epigastric distress, nausea, anorexia, dysphagia, enterocolitis, esophagitis, esophageal ulceration, vomiting. **GU:** inflammatory lesions in anogenital region (candida overgrowth). **Hematologic:** *thrombocytopenia,* hemolytic anemia, *neutropenia,* eosinophilia. **Hepatic:** *liver toxicity.* **Musculoskeletal:** bone growth retardation in children younger than age 8. **Skin:** increased pigmentation, maculopapular and erythematous rash, photosensitivity reactions, urticaria. **Other:** enamel defects, hypersensitivity reactions, permanent discoloration of teeth.

INTERACTIONS
Drug-drug. *Antacids, laxatives, and multivitamins containing aluminum, magnesium, or calcium; antidiarrheals containing bismuth subsalicylate:* May decrease antibiotic

---

Reactions in bold italics are *life-threatening*.

absorption. Give antibiotic 1 hour before or 2 hours after these drugs.

Ferrous sulfate and other iron products, sodium bicarbonate, zinc: May decrease antibiotic absorption. Give tetracycline 2 hours before or 3 hours after these products.

Isotretinoin: May increase risk of pseudotumor cerebri. Avoid use together.

🕭 *Alert: Methoxyflurane:* May cause fatal kidney toxicity. Avoid use together.

Oral anticoagulants: May increase anticoagulant effects. Monitor PT and INR, and adjust anticoagulant dosage.

Penicillins: May interfere with bactericidal action of penicillins. Avoid use together.

Drug-food. *Dairy products:* May decrease antibiotic absorption. Give antibiotic 1 hour before or 2 hours after eating or drinking dairy products.

Drug-lifestyle. *Sun exposure:* May cause photosensitivity reactions. Advise patient to avoid excessive sunlight exposure.

EFFECTS ON LAB TEST RESULTS
• May increase BUN and liver enzyme levels.
• May increase eosinophil count.
• May decrease RBC, platelet, and neutrophil counts.

CONTRAINDICATIONS & CAUTIONS
• Contraindicated in patients hypersensitive to drug or other tetracyclines.
• CDAD, ranging in severity from mild diarrhea to fatal colitis, has been reported with use of nearly all antibacterial drugs, including tetracyclines.
• Use cautiously in patients with kidney or liver impairment. Avoid use or use cautiously in children younger than age 8 because drug may cause permanent discoloration of teeth, enamel defects, and bone growth retardation.
• Drug isn't indicated for treatment of neurosyphilis.
Dialyzable drug: No.
⚠ **Overdose S&S:** Dizziness, nausea, vomiting.

PREGNANCY-LACTATION-REPRODUCTION
• Don't use during pregnancy unless absolutely necessary. May have toxic effects on developing fetus (often related to retardation of skeletal development and discoloration of teeth). If used during pregnancy or if patient becomes pregnant during therapy, apprise patient of fetal risk.

• Patients who are pregnant and have kidney disease may be more prone to developing tetracycline-associated liver failure.
• Drug appears in human milk. Patient should discontinue breastfeeding or discontinue drug, considering importance of drug to patient.

NURSING CONSIDERATIONS
• For suspected or confirmed CDAD, discontinue ongoing use of antibacterial drugs not directed at *Clostridioides difficile*. Institute appropriate fluid and electrolyte management, protein supplementation, and antibacterial treatment of *C. difficile*.
• If large doses are given, therapy is prolonged, or patient is at high risk, monitor for signs and symptoms of superinfection.
• Pseudotumor cerebri (benign intracranial HTN) has been associated with tetracycline use in adults. Monitor patient for clinical manifestations (headache, blurred vision, diplopia, vision loss; papilledema can be found on fundoscopy).
• In patient with kidney or liver impairment, monitor kidney function and LFT values.
• Assess mouth for signs of candidal infection. Emphasize good oral hygiene.
• For suspected coexistent syphilis, perform dark field exam before therapy and monitor blood serology monthly for at least 4 months.
• Photosensitivity reactions may occur within a few minutes to several hours after sun or UV light exposure. Photosensitivity lasts after therapy ends. Discontinue drug at first sign of skin erythema.

PATIENT TEACHING
• Teach about proper drug administration and handling.
• Tell patient to take drug exactly as prescribed, even after feeling better, and to take entire amount prescribed.
• Instruct patient to check drug's expiration date and not to use if outdated.
• Advise patient to promptly report all adverse reactions and to immediately report headache, blurred vision, diplopia, vision loss, watery diarrhea, abdominal cramping and pain, fever, or blood or pus in stool.
• Warn patient to avoid direct sunlight and UV light and to use sun protection.
• Caution patient to report pregnancy or breastfeeding to prescriber.

tiaGABine hydrochloride
tye-AG-ah-been

Gabitril

Therapeutic class: Anticonvulsants
Pharmacologic class: GABA enhancers

AVAILABLE FORMS
Tablets: 2 mg, 4 mg, 12 mg, 16 mg

INDICATIONS & DOSAGES
➤ **Adjunctive treatment of partial seizures**
Adults taking enzyme-inducing anticonvulsants: Initially, 4 mg PO once daily. May increase total daily dosage by 4 to 8 mg at weekly intervals until clinical response or up to 56 mg daily. Give total daily dosage in two to four divided doses.
Children ages 12 to 18 taking enzyme-inducing anticonvulsants: Initially, 4 mg PO once daily. May increase total daily dose by 4 mg at beginning of week 2 and thereafter by 4 to 8 mg per week until clinical response or up to 32 mg daily. Give total daily dose in two to four divided doses.
Adjust-a-dose: Consider dosage adjustment when there is an addition, discontinuation, or dosage change in the enzyme-inducing drug (carbamazepine, phenytoin, primidone, phenobarbital).
Adjust-a-dose: For patients with liver impairment, reduce first and maintenance doses or increase dosing intervals. For patients who are noninduced (taking only non-enzyme-inducing anticonvulsants), reduce tiagabine dosage and, if necessary, titrate slowly.

ADMINISTRATION
PO
• Give drug with food.
• If a dose is missed, don't attempt to make up for missed dose by increasing next dose. Consider retritrating drug if more than one dose has been missed.

ACTION
Unknown. May act by facilitating the effects of the inhibitory neurotransmitter GABA. May make more GABA available by binding to recognition sites linked to GABA uptake carrier.

Route	Onset	Peak	Duration
PO	Rapid	45 min (fasting)	Unknown

Half-life: 2 to 5 hours when given with enzyme inducers; 7 to 9 hours when given without enzyme inducers.

ADVERSE REACTIONS
CNS: asthenia, dizziness, nervousness, somnolence, abnormal gait, agitation, ataxia, confusion, depersonalization, depression, difficulty with concentration and attention, difficulty with memory, emotional lability, euphoria, hostility, insomnia, language problems, paresthesia, speech disorder, stupor, tremor, twitching, pain, malaise, syncope, paranoia, migraine, hallucination, vertigo. **CV:** vasodilation, chest pain, HTN, palpitations, tachycardia, lymphadenopathy, edema. **EENT:** amblyopia, nystagmus, abnormal vision, ear pain, otitis media, tinnitus, epistaxis, gingivitis, mouth ulceration, pharyngitis. **GI:** nausea, diarrhea, abdominal pain, vomiting, stomatitis, increased appetite. **GU:** UTI, dysmenorrhea, dysuria, metrorrhagia, urinary incontinence, vaginitis. **Metabolic:** weight gain or loss. **Musculoskeletal:** generalized weakness, myasthenia, neck pain, arthralgia, myalgia, hyperkinesia, hypokinesia. **Respiratory:** increased cough, bronchitis, dyspnea, pneumonia. **Skin:** pruritus, rash, dry skin, ecchymosis, alopecia, diaphoresis. **Other:** accidental injury, flulike syndrome, chills, infection, allergic reaction.

INTERACTIONS
Drug-drug. *CNS depressants (benzodiazepines, muscle relaxants, opioids, SSRIs):* May enhance CNS effects. Avoid use together if possible.
CYP3A4 inducers (carbamazepine, phenobarbital, phenytoin): May decrease tiagabine level. Monitor patient closely.
Drug-herb. *Kava:* May enhance adverse CNS effects of tiagabine. Monitor patient closely.
St. John's wort: May decrease tiagabine level. Monitor patient closely.
Drug-lifestyle. *Alcohol use:* May enhance CNS effects. Use together cautiously and monitor therapy.

EFFECTS ON LAB TEST RESULTS
None reported.

CONTRAINDICATIONS & CAUTIONS
• Contraindicated in patients hypersensitive to drug or its components.
🔵 *Alert:* Drug may cause new-onset seizures and status epilepticus in patients without a history of epilepsy. In these patients, stop drug and evaluate for underlying seizure disorder. Drug shouldn't be used for off-label uses.
• Use cautiously in patients with psychiatric symptoms and liver impairment.
• Safety and effectiveness haven't been established in children younger than age 12.
Dialyzable drug: Unlikely.
⚠ *Overdose S&S:* Somnolence, impaired consciousness, agitation, confusion, speech difficulty, hostility, depression, weakness, seizures.

PREGNANCY-LACTATION-REPRODUCTION
• Drug may cause fetal harm, but studies during pregnancy are inadequate. Use only if clearly needed.
• Encourage patients who are taking drug during pregnancy to register in the North American Antiepileptic Drug Pregnancy Registry (1-888-233-2334 or www.aedpregnancyregistry.org).
• It isn't known if drug or its metabolites appear in human milk. Use during breastfeeding only if benefit clearly outweighs risks.

NURSING CONSIDERATIONS
🔵 *Alert:* Closely monitor all patients taking or starting antiepileptic drugs for changes in behavior indicating worsening of suicidality or depression. Symptoms such as anxiety, agitation, hostility, mania, and hypomania may be precursors to emerging suicidality.
• Withdraw drug gradually unless safety concerns require a more rapid withdrawal because sudden withdrawal may cause more frequent seizures.
🔵 *Alert:* Use of anticonvulsants, including tiagabine, may cause status epilepticus and sudden unexpected death in patients with and without epilepsy.
• Monitor patient for cognitive and neuropsychiatric symptoms (impaired concentration, speech or language problems, confusion, somnolence, fatigue).
• Drug may cause moderately severe to incapacitating generalized weakness, which resolves after reducing dosage or stopping drug.

• Periodically monitor LFT values, especially in patients with liver impairment.
• Monitor tiagabine level.
• Monitor patient for serious rash, including SJS.
• *Look alike–sound alike:* Don't confuse tiagabine with tizanidine; both have 4-mg starting doses.

PATIENT TEACHING
🔵 *Alert:* Advise patient, caregivers, and family to immediately report new-onset or worsening depression, emergence of suicidality, thoughts of self-harm, or other unusual changes in mood or behavior.
• Teach about proper drug administration and handling. Caution patient to take drug only as prescribed.
• Warn patient that drug may cause dizziness, somnolence, and other signs and symptoms of CNS depression. Advise patient to avoid driving and other potentially hazardous activities that require mental alertness until drug's CNS effects are known.
• Caution patient to report pregnancy or breastfeeding to prescriber.
• Warn patient not to discontinue drug abruptly because of risk of seizures.
• Advise patient not to drink alcohol while taking drug.

SAFETY ALERT!

ticagrelor
TYE-ka-GREL-or

Brilinta

Therapeutic class: Antiplatelet drugs
Pharmacologic class: P2Y$_{12}$ platelet inhibitors

AVAILABLE FORMS
Tablets: 60 mg, 90 mg

INDICATIONS & DOSAGES
➤ **ACS or a history of MI to reduce rate of CV death, MI, and stroke; after stent placement for treatment of ACS to reduce rate of thrombosis**
Adults: Initially, 180 mg PO as loading dose; then maintenance dose of 90 mg PO b.i.d. during first year after an ACS event. After 1 year, 60 mg b.i.d. Give daily maintenance dose with aspirin (75 to 100 mg daily).

▶ **To reduce risk of a first MI or stroke in patients with CAD at high risk**
Adults: 60 mg b.i.d. in combination with aspirin (75 to 100 mg daily). Continue ticagrelor and aspirin indefinitely.

▶ **To reduce risk of stroke in patients with acute ischemic stroke (NIH Stroke Scale score of 5 or less) or high-risk TIA**
Adults: Initially, 180 mg PO as loading dose; then maintenance dose of 90 mg PO b.i.d. for up to 30 days. Use in combination with loading dose of aspirin (300 to 325 mg) and daily maintenance dose of aspirin (75 to 100 mg).

ADMINISTRATION
PO
● Give drug without regard to food.
● For patients unable to swallow tablets whole, tablets can be crushed, mixed with water, and drunk or given via NG tube.
● Omit a missed dose and give next dose at its scheduled time. Don't give extra dose to make up for missed dose.
● Store drug at room temperature in original container. Keep away from moisture and humidity.

ACTION
Inhibits platelet aggregation by reversibly interacting with the $P2Y_{12}$ ADP receptor.

Route	Onset	Peak	Duration
PO	Rapid	1–5 hr	8 hr

Half-life: 7 hours (ticagrelor), 9 hours (active metabolite).

ADVERSE REACTIONS
CNS: headache, dizziness. **CV:** *bleeding, bradyarrhythmias,* abnormal ECG. **GI:** nausea, diarrhea. **GU:** increased creatinine level. **Respiratory:** dyspnea.

INTERACTIONS
Drug-drug. *Anticoagulants, antiplatelet agents, fibrinolytics, long-term NSAIDs, omega-3 fatty acids, vitamin E:* May increase risk of bleeding. Use together cautiously.
Boxed Warning *Aspirin:* Maintenance doses of aspirin greater than 100 mg/day may decrease ticagrelor effectiveness and increase risk of bleeding. Maintenance doses of aspirin shouldn't exceed 100 mg/day. ∎
Digoxin: May increase digoxin level. Monitor digoxin level at start of treatment and with any changes to treatment.

Opioids (morphine): May decrease ticagrelor level. Consider using parenteral antiplatelet agent in patients with ACS who require coadministration of morphine or another opioid.
Other $P2Y_{12}$ platelet inhibitors: Increase risk of bleeding. Use together is contraindicated.
Statins: May increase levels of these drugs. Don't exceed 40 mg of simvastatin or lovastatin with concurrent ticagrelor use.
Strong CYP3A4 inducers (carbamazepine, dexamethasone, phenobarbital, phenytoin, rifampin): May significantly decrease ticagrelor and active metabolite levels and therapeutic effect. Avoid use together. ∎
Strong CYP3A4 inhibitors (clarithromycin, itraconazole, ketoconazole, nefazodone, ritonavir, saquinavir, telithromycin): May significantly increase ticagrelor level and risk of adverse reactions. Avoid use together. ∎
Drug-herb. *Alfalfa, anise, bilberry:* May increase risk of bleeding. Discourage use together.
St. John's wort: May increase metabolism of ticagrelor and decrease drug's effectiveness. Discourage use together.
Drug-food. *Grapefruit, grapefruit juice:* May increase ticagrelor level. Monitor therapy closely.

EFFECTS ON LAB TEST RESULTS
● May increase uric acid and creatinine levels.
● May cause false-negative functional tests for heparin-induced thrombocytopenia.

CONTRAINDICATIONS & CAUTIONS
Boxed Warning Drug can cause serious, sometimes fatal bleeding. Contraindicated in patients with history of intracranial hemorrhage or active pathologic bleeding (including peptic ulcer). ∎
Boxed Warning Don't start ticagrelor in patients who will undergo planned urgent CABG. If possible, discontinue ticagrelor at least 5 days before any surgery. ∎
● Contraindicated in patients hypersensitive to drug. Avoid use in those with Child-Pugh class C liver impairment.
● Use isn't recommended in patients with an NIH Stroke Scale score greater than 5 who are receiving thrombolysis.
● Use cautiously in patients with Child-Pugh class B liver impairment, older adults, patients with history of a bleeding disorder, and patients who have had percutaneous invasive procedures.

Reactions in bold italics are *life-threatening*.

⟳ Alert: Drug can cause ventricular pauses. Bradyarrhythmias, including AV block, have been reported. Patients with history of sick sinus syndrome, second- or third-degree AV block, or bradycardia-related syncope (without pacemakers) weren't studied.

Dialyzable drug: No.

⚠ Overdose S&S: Bleeding, nausea, vomiting, diarrhea, ventricular pauses.

PREGNANCY-LACTATION-REPRODUCTION

• Studies during pregnancy are inadequate. Use only if potential benefit justifies fetal risk.

• It isn't known if drug or its active metabolites appear in human milk. Breastfeeding isn't recommended during treatment.

NURSING CONSIDERATIONS

Boxed Warning If possible, manage bleeding without discontinuing ticagrelor; premature discontinuation of treatment increases risk of MI, stent thrombosis, and death. If drug must be temporarily stopped, restart as soon as possible. ∎

• Monitor patient for bleeding.

• Monitor for respiratory effects (dyspnea, sleep apnea, Cheyne-Stokes respiration). Rule out underlying conditions that require treatment in patient with new, prolonged, or worsened difficulty breathing.

• Dyspnea secondary to ticagrelor therapy is usually mild to moderate and often self-limiting with continued treatment. If ticagrelor is discontinued for intolerable dyspnea, prescriber should consider another antiplatelet agent.

• Ticagrelor can be given to patients with ACS who have already received a loading dose of clopidogrel.

PATIENT TEACHING

Boxed Warning Tell patient not to take more than 100 mg of aspirin per day. Warn that other OTC products may also contain aspirin. ∎

• Teach about proper drug administration and handling.

• Inform patient that bleeding and bruising may occur more easily and that bleeding will take longer to stop. Tell patient to immediately report unexpected, prolonged, or excessive bleeding or blood in urine or stool.

• Warn patient not to stop drug without consulting prescriber.

• Caution patient to notify all health care providers about taking ticagrelor before any scheduled surgery or dental appointment. Advise patient to discuss with original prescriber recommendations by other providers to stop taking ticagrelor.

• Warn that ticagrelor may cause mild to moderate shortness of breath. Tell patient to report unexpected shortness of breath, especially if it's severe.

• Advise patient to report pregnancy or plans to become pregnant before using drug.

• Warn patient taking drug not to breastfeed.

---

tiotropium bromide
tye-oh-TROH-pee-um

Spiriva HandiHaler, Spiriva Respimat

Therapeutic class: Bronchodilators
Pharmacologic class: Anticholinergics

AVAILABLE FORMS

Capsules (powder for inhalation): 18 mcg
Spray inhaler (Respimat): 1.25 mcg/actuation, 2.5 mcg/actuation

INDICATIONS & DOSAGES

➤ **To reduce COPD exacerbations; maintenance treatment of bronchospasm in COPD, including chronic bronchitis and emphysema**
Adults: 2 oral inhalations of 1 capsule (18 mcg) once daily using HandiHaler inhalation device. Or, 2 inhalations of 2.5 mcg/actuation spray once daily.

➤ **Long-term maintenance treatment of asthma (Spiriva Respimat)**
Adults and children ages 6 and older: 2 inhalations of 1.25 mcg/actuation spray once daily. Maximum benefits in lung function may take 4 to 8 weeks of dosing.

ADMINISTRATION
Inhalational
Capsules

• Give capsules only by oral inhalation with HandiHaler device. One capsule contains two inhalations.

• Open capsule blister immediately before use; don't store capsules in device.

• Capsules aren't for oral ingestion.

T

Respimat spray inhaler
• Before first use, insert cartridge into inhaler.
• Prime unit before using it for first time by actuating inhaler toward ground until aerosol cloud is visible; then repeat process three more times.
• If not used for more than 3 days, actuate inhaler once to prepare it for use. If not used for more than 21 days, actuate inhaler until aerosol cloud is visible; then repeat the process three more times.
• When labeled number of actuations (28 or 60) have been dispensed from Respimat inhaler, a locking mechanism engages to prevent further actuations.

ACTION
Competitive, reversible inhibition of muscarinic receptors in smooth muscle leads to bronchodilation.

Route	Onset	Peak	Duration
Inhalation	Unknown	5–7 min	>24 hr

Half-life: COPD, 25 hours; asthma, 44 hours.

ADVERSE REACTIONS
CNS: depression, paresthesia, headache, dizziness, fever, insomnia. **CV:** *angina pectoris,* chest pain, edema, palpitations, HTN. **EENT:** cataract, epistaxis, dry mouth, sinusitis, laryngitis, dysphonia, pharyngitis, rhinitis, oropharyngeal candidiasis. **GI:** abdominal pain, constipation, dyspepsia, GERD, stomatitis, vomiting, diarrhea. **GU:** UTI. **Metabolic:** hypercholesterolemia, hyperglycemia. **Musculoskeletal:** arthritis, leg pain, myalgia, skeletal pain. **Respiratory:** URI, cough, bronchitis. **Skin:** rash, pruritus. **Other:** allergic reaction, candidiasis, flulike syndrome, herpes zoster, infections.

INTERACTIONS
Drug-drug. *Anticholinergics (dicyclomine, scopolamine):* May increase anticholinergic adverse reactions. Avoid use together.
Glucagon: May increase risk of GI adverse effects. Avoid use together.
Opioids: May increase risk of constipation and urine retention. Monitor patient closely.
Potassium chloride: May increase ulcer risk. Avoid use together.

EFFECTS ON LAB TEST RESULTS
• May increase cholesterol and glucose levels.

CONTRAINDICATIONS & CAUTIONS
• Contraindicated in patients hypersensitive to tiotropium, ipratropium, or components of the product. Use cautiously in patients hypersensitive to atropine or its derivatives.
• Immediate hypersensitivity reactions can occur, including urticaria, angioedema, rash, itching, and anaphylaxis.
• Use cautiously in patients with CrCl of less than 60 mL/minute and in patients with angle-closure glaucoma, prostatic hyperplasia, or bladder neck obstruction due to anticholinergic effects.
• Use capsule cautiously in patients with severe hypersensitivity to milk protein.
• Safety and effectiveness of capsules in children haven't been established.
Dialyzable drug: Unknown.
⚠ *Overdose S&S:* Change in mental status, tremors, abdominal pain, severe constipation.

PREGNANCY-LACTATION-REPRODUCTION
• Studies during pregnancy are inadequate. Use only if potential benefit justifies fetal risk.
• It isn't known if drug appears in human milk. Use cautiously during breastfeeding.

NURSING CONSIDERATIONS
⚡ *Alert:* Use drug for maintenance treatment of COPD or asthma, not for acute bronchospasm.
• Watch for evidence of hypersensitivity (especially angioedema) and paradoxical bronchospasm. Discontinue drug immediately.
• Monitor patient for anticholinergic effects (dry mouth, constipation, tachycardia, blurred vision, new or worsening glaucoma, dysuria, urine retention).
• *Look alike–sound alike:* Don't confuse Spiriva with Inspra.

PATIENT TEACHING
• Explain that drug is for maintenance treatment of COPD or asthma and not for immediate relief of breathing problems.
• Warn patient that capsules are for inhalation and shouldn't be swallowed.
• Instruct patient in proper drug administration and storage.
• Provide full instructions for HandiHaler device or Respimat spray inhaler. Demonstrate use and observe return demonstration from patient.

- Caution patient not to get powder or spray in eyes.
- Review signs and symptoms of hypersensitivity and paradoxical bronchospasm. Tell patient to stop drug and contact prescriber if any occur.
- Advise patient to immediately report eye pain, blurred vision, visual halos, colored images, or red eyes.

tirbanibulin
tir-ban-i-BUE-lin

Klisyri

Therapeutic class: Antineoplastics
Pharmacologic class: Microtubule inhibitors

AVAILABLE FORMS
Ointment: 1% single-dose packet

INDICATIONS & DOSAGES
➤ **Actinic keratosis on the face or scalp**
Adults: Apply ointment evenly to affected area once daily for 5 consecutive days.

ADMINISTRATION
Topical
- For topical use only; not for oral or ophthalmic use.
- Use one single-dose packet per application; discard packet and unused ointment after use.
- Don't apply to a treatment area of more than 25 cm².
- Don't apply occlusive dressings to affected area.
- Wash hands immediately with soap and water after applying drug.
- Avoid washing and touching treated area for approximately 8 hours after application; after 8 hours, may wash area with mild soap.
- Avoid getting drug near and around mouth, lips, and periocular area. If ocular exposure occurs, flush with water.
- Store drug at 68° to 77° F (20° to 25° C). Don't refrigerate or freeze.

ACTION
Unknown.

Route	Onset	Peak	Duration
Topical	Unknown	7 hr	Unknown

Half-life: Unknown.

ADVERSE REACTIONS
Skin: application-site pruritus, application-site pain, crusting, erosion, erythema, flaking, pustulation, scaling, swelling, vesiculation, ulceration.

INTERACTIONS
None reported.

EFFECTS ON LAB TEST RESULTS
None reported.

CONTRAINDICATIONS & CAUTIONS
- Safety and effectiveness in children haven't been established.
- Older adults may have greater sensitivity to drug.
Dialyzable drug: Unknown.

PREGNANCY-LACTATION-REPRODUCTION
- Drug hasn't been studied during pregnancy. It's unknown if drug increases risk of major birth defects, miscarriage, or adverse patient or fetal outcomes.
- It isn't known if drug appears in human milk or how drug affects milk production or infants who are breastfed. Consider benefits and risk to infant.

NURSING CONSIDERATIONS
- Monitor patient for local skin reactions of treated area.
- Monitor for eye irritation.
- Flush patient's eye if accidental exposure occurs, and notify prescriber.
- Don't use ointment if skin hasn't healed from previous drug, procedure, or surgical treatment.
- Avoid using occlusive dressings over treatment area.
- *Look alike–sound alike:* Don't confuse tirbanibulin with eribulin, terbinafine, or terbutaline.

PATIENT TEACHING
- Teach about proper drug administration and handling.
- Review potential adverse effects.
- Tell patient to flush eye with water and notify prescriber if accidental contact with eye occurs.
- Instruct patient to wash hands well after applying drug.

T

• Caution patient to avoid inadvertent transfer of drug to other areas of body or to another person.

tirzepatide
tir-ZEP-a-tide

Mounjaro

Therapeutic class: Antidiabetics
Pharmacologic class: Glucose-dependent insulinotropic polypeptide receptor and glucagon-like peptide-1 receptor agonists

AVAILABLE FORMS
Injection: 2.5 mg/0.5 mL, 5 mg/0.5 mL, 7.5 mg/0.5 mL, 10 mg/0.5 mL, 12.5 mg/0.5 mL, 15 mg/0.5 mL single-dose pens or vials.

INDICATIONS & DOSAGES
➤ **Adjunct to diet and exercise to improve glycemic control in adults with type 2 diabetes**
Adults: Initially, 2.5 mg subcut once weekly. After 4 weeks, increase to 5 mg subcut once weekly. If additional glycemic control is needed, increase in 2.5-mg increments after 4 weeks on current dosage, up to maximum dosage of 15 mg once weekly.

ADMINISTRATION
Subcutaneous
• Give drug at any time of day, without regard to food.
• Inspect solution before use. Solution should be clear and colorless to slightly yellow. Don't use if particulate matter or discoloration is present.
• Inject into abdomen, thigh, or upper arm.
• Rotate injection sites with each dose.
• Don't mix drug with insulin for injection. Give as separate injections in the same body region but not adjacent to each other.
• If a dose is missed, give dose as soon as possible within 4 days (96 hours) of missed dose; if more than 4 days have passed, skip missed dose and give next dose on regularly scheduled day; then resume once-weekly schedule.
• May change day of weekly administration if the time between two doses is at least 72 hours.
• Store at 36° to 46° F (2° to 8° C). May store unrefrigerated, below 86° F (30° C) for up to 21 days.

ACTION
Enhances insulin secretion and reduces glucagon levels.

Route	Onset	Peak	Duration
Subcut	Unknown	8–72 hr	Unknown

Half-life: About 5 days.

ADVERSE REACTIONS
CV: sinus tachycardia. **GI:** abdominal distention, abdominal pain, constipation, decreased appetite, diarrhea, dyspepsia, belching, flatulence, GERD, nausea, vomiting. **Metabolic:** increased amylase and lipase levels. **Skin:** injection-site reaction. **Other:** hypersensitivity, antidrug antibody development.

INTERACTIONS
Drug-drug. *Insulin, insulin secretagogues (sulfonylureas):* May increase risk of hypoglycemia. Monitor blood glucose level and reduce dosage of insulin or insulin secretagogues accordingly.
Oral contraceptives: May reduce contraceptive effectiveness due to delayed gastric emptying. Switch to nonoral contraceptive method or add barrier contraceptive method for 4 weeks after starting tirzepatide and for 4 weeks after each dosage increase.
Oral medications: May affect absorption of concomitant oral medications. Use together cautiously.

EFFECTS ON LAB TEST RESULTS
• May increase amylase and lipase levels.
• May decrease blood glucose level.

CONTRAINDICATIONS & CAUTIONS
Boxed Warning Contraindicated in patients with personal or family history of medullary thyroid carcinoma (MTC) and in those with multiple endocrine neoplasia syndrome type 2. ■
Boxed Warning Thyroid C-cell adenomas and carcinomas occurred in animal studies. It isn't known if tirzepatide causes thyroid C-cell tumors, including MTC, in humans. ■
• Contraindicated in patients with known hypersensitivity to drug or its components.
• Drug is associated with GI adverse reactions, sometimes severe. Not recommended for use in patients with severe GI disease.
• Safety and effectiveness in children haven't been established.
Dialyzable drug: Unlikely.

Reactions in bold italics are *life-threatening*.

PREGNANCY-LACTATION-REPRODUCTION
• Based on animal studies, drug may cause fetal harm. Use only if potential benefit justifies fetal risk.
• It isn't known if drug appears in human milk or how drug affects milk production or infants who are breastfed. Use cautiously during breastfeeding.

NURSING CONSIDERATIONS
• Initiation dose isn't intended for glycemic control.
• Monitor patient for signs and symptoms of pancreatitis (vomiting and persistent, severe abdominal pain, which may radiate to back); discontinue drug if suspected.
• Concomitant use with insulin or insulin secretagogue may increase risk of hypoglycemia, including severe hypoglycemia. Reduced dosage of insulin or insulin secretagogue may be necessary.
• Monitor patient for hypersensitivity reactions (rash, urticaria, wheezing); discontinue drug if suspected.
• Monitor patient for severe GI adverse reactions (nausea, vomiting, abdominal distention) and dehydration.
• Monitor kidney function in patients with impaired kidney function, especially those reporting severe adverse GI reactions and dehydration.
• Monitor for cholelithiasis (abdominal pain, nausea, vomiting, jaundice). If suspected, clinically evaluate.
• Monitor patient with history of diabetic retinopathy for disease progression. Rapid improvement in glycemic control may be associated with temporary worsening of diabetic retinopathy.

PATIENT TEACHING
• Teach about proper drug administration and handling.
Boxed Warning Inform patient that drug causes thyroid C-cell tumors in rats and that human relevance of tirzepatide-induced rodent thyroid C-cell tumors hasn't been determined. ■
• Counsel patient to report signs and symptoms of thyroid tumors (lump in neck, persistent hoarseness, dysphagia, dyspnea).
• Instruct patient to stop drug and report suspected pancreatitis.
• Caution patient about increased risk of hypoglycemia when drug is used with insulin

or an insulin secretagogue (such as a sulfonylurea).
• Educate patient on signs and symptoms of hypoglycemia (dizziness, sweating, confusion, drowsiness, headache, blurred vision, slurred speech, shakiness, jitteriness, tachycardia, anxiety, irritability, mood change, hunger, weakness).
• Advise patient to immediately report signs or symptoms of hypersensitivity and to stop drug.
• Instruct patient to report severe or persistent GI symptoms (nausea, vomiting, diarrhea).
• Inform patient about risk of dehydration. Explain precautions to avoid fluid depletion.
• Educate patient on potential risk of worsening kidney function. Explain signs and symptoms (fatigue; weakness; muscle cramps; decreased urination; edema of legs, ankles, and feet).
• Tell patient to report vision changes during therapy.
• Instruct patient to contact health care provider for clinical follow-up if gallbladder disease is suspected.
• Warn patient who is pregnant of fetal risk. Advise patient to report pregnancy or plans to become pregnant.
• Instruct patient that drug may reduce efficacy of oral contraceptives. Advise patient to switch to a nonoral contraceptive method or to add a barrier contraceptive for 4 weeks after initiation and 4 weeks after each dosage escalation.

tiZANidine hydrochloride
tis-AN-i-deen

Zanaflex

Therapeutic class: Skeletal muscle relaxants
Pharmacologic class: Centrally acting alpha$_2$-adrenergic agonists

AVAILABLE FORMS
Capsules: 2 mg, 4 mg, 6 mg
Tablets: 2 mg, 4 mg

INDICATIONS & DOSAGES
➤ **Management of spasticity**
Adults: Initially, 2 mg PO every 6 to 8 hours, to maximum of three doses in 24 hours. Dosage can be increased gradually in 2- to

4-mg increments, with 1 to 4 days between increases. Maximum, 36 mg daily.

Adjust-a-dose: Use cautiously and reduce dosage during titration in patients with liver impairment or CrCl of less than 25 mL/minute. If higher dosages are needed, increase individual doses rather than frequency.

ADMINISTRATION
PO
• Give drug consistently as either tablets or capsules and with or without food for same absorption rate and effect.

🔴 *Alert:* Capsules and tablets are bioequivalent only under fasting conditions.

ACTION
Central alpha$_2$ agonist that may reduce spasticity by increasing presynaptic inhibition of motor neurons at the level of the spinal cord.

Route	Onset	Peak	Duration
PO	Unknown	1–2 hr	3–6 hr

Half-life: 2.5 hours; metabolites, 20 to 40 hours.

ADVERSE REACTIONS
CNS: somnolence, sedation, asthenia, weakness, tiredness, dizziness, speech disorder, dyskinesia, nervousness, hallucinations, delusions. **CV:** hypotension, *bradycardia.* **EENT:** blurred vision, dry mouth, visual field defect, pharyngitis, rhinitis, sinusitis. **GI:** constipation, vomiting, dyspepsia. **GU:** UTI, urinary frequency. **Hepatic:** abnormal LFTs. **Other:** infection, flulike syndrome.

INTERACTIONS
Drug-drug. *Antihypertensives, other alpha agonists (clonidine):* May cause hypotension. Monitor patient closely. Avoid use with other alpha agonists.

Baclofen, benzodiazepines, cannabis, dronabinol, magnesium sulfate, other CNS depressants: May have additive CNS depressant effects. Avoid use together.

CYP1A2 inhibitors (amiodarone, acyclovir, cimetidine, famotidine, fluoroquinolones, mexiletine, propafenone, ticlopidine, verapamil, zileuton): May significantly increase tizanidine level. Avoid use together. If use together is unavoidable, reduce tizanidine dosage.

Drugs that prolong QTc interval (procainamide, clarithromycin, levofloxacin): May increase QTc interval and risk of ventricular arrhythmias. Monitor therapy.

🔴 *Alert: Opioids:* May increase risk of CNS depression. Avoid use together. If use together is necessary, limit dosage and duration of each drug to minimum necessary for desired effect.

Oral contraceptives: May increase tizanidine level. Avoid use together. If use is necessary, reduce tizanidine dosage.

Strong CYP1A2 inhibitors (ciprofloxacin, fluvoxamine): May increase tizanidine level and risk of adverse effects. Use together is contraindicated.

Drug-herb. *Kava:* May enhance adverse CNS effects. Monitor patient closely.

Drug-lifestyle. *Alcohol use:* May increase CNS depression. Discourage use together.

EFFECTS ON LAB TEST RESULTS
• May increase AST and ALT levels.

CONTRAINDICATIONS & CAUTIONS
• Contraindicated in patients hypersensitive to drug.
• Use cautiously in patients with CrCl less than 25 L/minute or any liver impairment and in older adults.
• May cause sedation, which may interfere with everyday activities.
• Safety and effectiveness in children haven't been established.

Dialyzable drug: Unlikely.

⚠ *Overdose S&S:* Lethargy, somnolence, confusion, coma, bradycardia, hypotension, respiratory depression, depressed cardiac function.

PREGNANCY-LACTATION-REPRODUCTION
• Drug hasn't been studied during pregnancy. Animal data suggest fetal risk. Use only if potential benefit justifies fetal risk.
• It isn't known if drug appears in human milk. Use cautiously during breastfeeding.
• Based on animal studies, drug may impair fertility.

NURSING CONSIDERATIONS
• Due to its short duration of therapeutic effect, reserve drug for daily activities and times when relief of spasticity is most important.
• Obtain LFT results before treatment, 1 month after maximum dose is achieved, and if liver injury is suspected.

Reactions in bold italics are *life-threatening*.

- Monitor kidney function, especially in an older adult or patient with kidney insufficiency.
- Monitor for signs and symptoms of excess sedation if patient is taking drug along with another CNS depressant.
- Consider discontinuing drug in patient who develops hallucinations.
- **Alert:** Stop drug gradually, especially in patients taking high doses (20 to 28 mg daily) for a prolonged period (9 weeks or more) and in those taking concomitant opioids. Decrease dosage slowly by 2 to 4 mg/day to minimize the potential for rebound HTN, tachycardia, and hypertonia.
- *Look alike–sound alike:* Don't confuse tizanidine with tiagabine. Don't confuse Zanaflex with Xiaflex.

PATIENT TEACHING

- Caution patient to avoid alcohol and activities that require alertness, such as driving and operating machinery, until drug's effects are known. Drug may cause drowsiness.
- Inform patient that dizziness upon standing quickly can be minimized by rising slowly.
- **Alert:** Explain that tizanidine absorption varies depending on whether drug is taken with or without food. Advise patient that drug should always be taken the same way to reduce risk of changes in efficacy and adverse reactions.
- Instruct patient to inform the health care provider and pharmacist when medications are added or removed from patient's regimen.
- Advise patient not to suddenly stop taking medication.

tobramycin
toe-bra-MYE-sin

Tobrex

tobramycin sulfate
Bethkis, Kitabis Pak, TOBI, TOBI Podhaler

Therapeutic class: Antibiotics
Pharmacologic class: Aminoglycosides

AVAILABLE FORMS
Inhalation powder: 28-mg capsules
Injection: 10 mg/mL (pediatric), 40 mg/mL multidose vials
Nebulizer solution (for inhalation): 300 mg/ 4 mL, 300 mg/5 mL

Ophthalmic ointment: 0.3%
Ophthalmic solution: 0.3%
Powder for injection: 1.2-g vial

INDICATIONS & DOSAGES
➤ **Serious infection caused by sensitive strains of *Escherichia coli, Proteus, Klebsiella, Enterobacter, Serratia, Staphylococcus aureus, Citrobacter, Pseudomonas*, or *Providencia***
Adults: 3 mg/kg/day IM or IV in three equal doses every 8 hours. For life-threatening infections, up to 5 mg/kg/day in divided doses every 6 to 8 hours; reduce to 3 mg/kg daily as soon as clinically indicated.
Children older than age 1 week: 6 to 7.5 mg/kg/day IM or IV in three or four divided doses.
Neonates younger than age 1 week or preterm infants: Up to 4 mg/kg/day IV or IM in two equal doses every 12 hours.
Adjust-a-dose: For patients with kidney impairment, give loading dose of 1 mg/kg; then give decreased doses at 8-hour intervals or same dose at prolonged intervals. For patients on hemodialysis, adjust dosage based on dialysis method, filter type, and flow rate; give after dialysis and adjust according to serum concentrations. For patients with severe cystic fibrosis, initially give 10 mg/kg/day IV or IM in four divided doses. For patients with obesity, calculate dose using estimated lean body weight plus 40% of excess weight.
➤ **To manage patients with cystic fibrosis and *Pseudomonas aeruginosa* infection**
Adults and children ages 6 and older: 300 mg via nebulizer every 12 hours for 28 days. Or, using TOBI Podhaler device, have patient inhale contents of four 28-mg (112 mg) capsules every 12 hours for 28 days. Stop therapy for 28 days; then repeat and continue cycles of 28 days on drug and 28 days off.
➤ **External ocular infections by susceptible bacteria**
Adults and children ages 2 months and older: In mild to moderate infections, instill 1 or 2 drops into affected eye(s) every 4 hours, or apply ½-inch (1.27-cm) ribbon of ointment every 8 to 12 hours. In severe infections, instill 2 drops into infected eye(s) every 60 minutes until condition improves; then reduce frequency. Or, apply ½-inch ribbon of ointment every 3 to 4 hours until condition improves; then reduce frequency to b.i.d. to t.i.d.

T

ADMINISTRATION

• For IV, IM, and inhalational use, obtain specimen for culture and sensitivity tests before giving. Begin therapy while awaiting results.

IV

▼ For adults, dilute in 50 to 100 mL of NSS or D₅W; use a smaller volume for children.

▼ Keep reconstituted solution in refrigerator and use within 96 hours or keep at room temperature for 24 hours.

▼ Infuse over 20 to 60 minutes.

▼ After infusion, flush line with NSS or D₅W.

▼ **Incompatibilities:** Don't mix with other drugs; administer separately.

IM

• Withdraw appropriate dose directly from vial.

Inhalational

• Capsules aren't for oral ingestion.

• Give nebulizer solution over 15 minutes using handheld Pari LC Plus reusable nebulizer. Refer to manufacturer's instructions for recommended compressor.

• Give capsules only by oral inhalation using Podhaler device. A new Podhaler device is supplied with each weekly pack of capsules. Use only for 7 days; then discard.

• Store capsules in blister packs at room temperature and remove immediately before use.

• Give doses as close to 12 hours apart as possible. Don't give doses less than 6 hours apart.

• If several inhaled medications and chest physiotherapy have been prescribed, follow prescriber's recommendations for when to administer them in relation to each other; guidelines recommend giving Podhaler last.

• Don't dilute or mix with other drugs, including dornase alfa, in a nebulizer.

• Unrefrigerated inhalation solution normally appears slightly yellow but may darken with age (doesn't affect quality).

• Store solution in refrigerator until expiration date or at room temperature for up to 28 days. Protect from light.

Ophthalmic

🢒 *Alert:* Tobramycin ophthalmic solution isn't for injection.

• When administering two different ophthalmic solutions, allow at least 10 minutes between instillations.

• Apply light finger pressure on lacrimal sac for 1 minute after instilling drops.

• Apply ointment to conjunctiva. Don't let tube touch eye.

ACTION

Generally bactericidal. Inhibits protein synthesis by binding directly to the 30S ribosomal subunit.

Route	Onset	Peak	Duration
IV	Immediate	30 min	8 hr
IM	Unknown	30–60 min	8 hr
Inhalation	Unknown	60 min	Unknown
Ophthalmic	Unknown	Unknown	Unknown

Half-life: For IV: Adults, 2 to 3 hours; adults with impaired kidney function, 5 to 70 hours. Neonates weighing 1,200 g or less, 11 hours; neonates weighing more than 1,200 g, 2 to 9 hours. Infants, 3 to 5 hours. Children and adolescents, 0.5 to 3 hours. *For inhalational:* Adults, 3 to 4.4 hours.

ADVERSE REACTIONS

CNS: headache, lethargy, confusion, disorientation, fever, dizziness, malaise, vertigo; taste perversion (inhalation). **EENT:** hearing loss, tinnitus, ototoxicity; blurred vision (ophthalmic); voice disorder, epistaxis, laryngitis, oropharyngeal pain, pharyngitis, rhinitis, tonsillitis (inhalation). **GI:** vomiting, nausea, diarrhea. **GU:** *kidney toxicity,* possible increase in urinary excretion of casts. **Hematologic:** anemia, eosinophilia, *leukopenia, agranulocytosis, thrombocytopenia.* **Metabolic:** electrolyte imbalances, hyperglycemia. **Musculoskeletal:** muscle twitching, myalgia, chest discomfort. **Respiratory:** cough, dyspnea, bronchitis, decreased forced expiratory volume, hemoptysis, rales, wheezing, increased sputum (inhalation). **Skin:** rash, urticaria, pruritus, dermatitis, injection site pain.

INTERACTIONS

Drug-drug. ▐ Boxed Warning ▐ *Acyclovir, amphotericin B, cephalosporins, cidofovir, cisplatin, colistin, methoxyflurane, polymyxin B, vancomycin, other aminoglycosides:* May increase kidney toxicity or neurotoxicity when used with injectable tobramycin formulation. Avoid use together. Monitor kidney function. ▐

▐ Boxed Warning ▐ *Cyclosporine, foscarnet, NSAIDs:* May increase risk of kidney toxicity. Avoid use together. ▐

General anesthetics: May increase neuromuscular blockade. Monitor patient for increased clinical effects.

▐ Boxed Warning ▐ *IV loop diuretics (ethacrynic acid, furosemide):* May increase ototoxicity when used with injectable tobramycin. Monitor patient's hearing. ▐

Reactions in bold italics are *life-threatening*.

Neuromuscular blocking agents (atracurium, pancuronium, vecuronium): May increase effects of nondepolarizing muscle relaxants, including prolonged respiratory depression. Use together only when necessary, and expect to reduce dosage of nondepolarizing muscle relaxant.

Parenteral penicillins: May decrease tobramycin level. Monitor therapy.

EFFECTS ON LAB TEST RESULTS

• May increase AST, ALT, LDH, bilirubin, BUN, creatinine, nonprotein nitrogen, glucose, and urine urea levels.
• May decrease calcium, magnesium, sodium, and potassium levels.
• May increase eosinophil count, Ig levels, and RBC sedimentation rate (inhalation).
• May decrease Hb level, hematocrit, and platelet count.
• May increase or decrease WBC count.

CONTRAINDICATIONS & CAUTIONS

• Contraindicated in patients hypersensitive to drug or other aminoglycosides.
Boxed Warning Use tobramycin injection cautiously in premature infants and neonates because of their kidney immaturity and resulting prolongation of drug's serum half-life. ■
Boxed Warning For injectable tobramycin, neurotoxicity can occur. Auditory changes are irreversible, are usually bilateral, and may be partial or total. Other manifestations of neurotoxicity may include numbness, skin tingling, muscle twitching, and seizures. Risk of hearing loss increases with degree of exposure to either high peak or high trough levels; other factors that may increase patient risk are advanced age and dehydration. Patients who develop cochlear damage may not have symptoms during therapy to warn them of eighth-nerve toxicity, and partial or total irreversible bilateral deafness may continue to develop after drug discontinuation. ■
🔵 **Alert:** Avoid concurrent or sequential use with other drugs with neurotoxic, kidney toxic, or ototoxic potential.
• Use cautiously in patients with impaired kidney function or neuromuscular disorders and in older adults.
Boxed Warning For injectable tobramycin, neuromuscular blockade can occur. Closely monitor patients at high risk, including patients with underlying neuromuscular disorders (myasthenia gravis) and those

concomitantly receiving neuromuscular blockers. Neuromuscular blockade is reversible but may require treatment. ■
Dialyzable drug: Yes.
⚠ **Overdose S&S:** Kidney toxicity, dizziness, tinnitus, vertigo, loss of high-tone hearing acuity, neuromuscular blockade, respiratory failure, respiratory paralysis (systemic); punctate keratitis, erythema, tearing, edema, eyelid itching (ophthalmic).

PREGNANCY-LACTATION-REPRODUCTION

Boxed Warning Aminoglycosides can cause fetal harm when given during pregnancy. ■
• Studies during pregnancy are inadequate. If used during pregnancy or if patient becomes pregnant during therapy, apprise patient of fetal risk.
• Amount of drug that appears in human milk isn't known. Because of the potential for adverse effects in the infant, patient should discontinue breastfeeding or discontinue drug, considering importance of drug to patient.

NURSING CONSIDERATIONS

• Dosage should be determined by appropriate pharmacokinetic methods and patient-specific parameters.
• Monitor peak and trough levels to determine dosage in patient with burns or cystic fibrosis, in whom drug levels may be reduced. Reserve higher peak levels for patient with cystic fibrosis, who needs greater lung penetration.
• Don't obtain blood samples by fingerstick to monitor tobramycin level; skin contaminated with drug may falsely elevate drug level.
• Follow facility protocol for obtaining peak and trough levels. Guidelines recommend obtaining blood samples for peak level 30 minutes after IV infusion or 1 hour after IM injection; trough level at 8 hours or just before next scheduled dose.
Boxed Warning Peak levels over 12 mcg/mL and trough levels over 2 mcg/mL may increase risk of toxicity. Periodically monitor peak and trough serum levels. ■
• If ophthalmic tobramycin is given with systemic tobramycin, carefully monitor levels.
• Weigh patient and review kidney function studies before therapy.
Boxed Warning Monitor patient for signs and symptoms of neurotoxicity, including numbness, skin tingling, muscle twitching, and seizures. ■

T

Boxed Warning Closely monitor patient for ototoxicity and kidney toxicity. ■

🔵 *Alert:* Notify prescriber if patient complains of tinnitus, vertigo, or hearing loss.

Boxed Warning If possible, obtain serial audiograms in patient old enough to be tested, particularly patient at high risk. Evidence of impaired kidney, vestibular, or auditory function requires drug discontinuation or dosage adjustment. ■

Boxed Warning Monitor kidney function: urine output, specific gravity, urinalysis, serum creatinine, CrCl, and BUN. Notify prescriber about signs and symptoms of decreasing kidney function. Advanced age and dehydration may increase risk of kidney toxicity. ■

• Watch for signs and symptoms of superinfection (continued fever, chills, increased pulse rate).

• Monitor electrolyte levels.

• If no response occurs in 3 to 5 days, therapy may be stopped and new specimens obtained for culture and sensitivity testing.

• *Look alike–sound alike:* Don't confuse Tobrex with TobraDex.

PATIENT TEACHING

🔵 *Alert:* Explain that capsules are for inhalation only and shouldn't be swallowed.

• Provide full instructions on inhalation or ophthalmic drug administration and storage.

• Advise patient not to wear contact lenses during treatment of ophthalmic infections.

• Teach patient how to use and maintain nebulizer and compressor.

• Instruct patient to promptly report all adverse reactions.

• Caution patient not to perform hazardous activities if adverse CNS reactions occur.

• Encourage patient to maintain adequate fluid intake.

tocilizumab ⊠
toe-sih-LIZ-oo-mab

Actemra

Therapeutic class: Antiarthritics
Pharmacologic class: Interleukin-6 receptor inhibitors

AVAILABLE FORMS

Injection (for IV use): 80 mg/4 mL, 200 mg/10 mL, 400 mg/20 mL in single-use vials

Injection (for subcut use): 162 mg/0.9 mL in prefilled syringe or autoinjector

INDICATIONS & DOSAGES

Adjust-a-dose (for all indications): Refer to manufacturer's instructions for toxicity-related dosage adjustments.

➤ **Systemic juvenile idiopathic arthritis (SJIA) alone or in combination with methotrexate** ⊠

Children ages 2 and older weighing 30 kg or more: 8 mg/kg IV infusion once every 2 weeks. Or, 162 mg subcut once each week. *Children ages 2 and older weighing less than 30 kg:* 12 mg/kg IV infusion once every 2 weeks. Or, 162 mg subcut once every 2 weeks.

Adjust-a-dose: If appropriate, concomitant methotrexate or other medications should be dose-modified or stopped and tocilizumab dosage adjusted until the clinical situation has been evaluated. In SJIA, the decision to discontinue tocilizumab for a lab abnormality should be based on medical assessment of the individual patient.

➤ **As monotherapy or with methotrexate or other nonbiologic DMARDs for moderately to severely active RA when response to one or more DMARDs is inadequate**

Adults: Initially, 4 mg/kg IV infusion every 4 weeks. May increase dosage to 8 mg/kg every 4 weeks based on clinical response. Maximum dose, 800 mg per infusion. Or, for patients weighing 100 kg or more, 162 mg subcut once each week. Or, for patients weighing less than 100 kg, 162 mg subcut every other week, followed by an increase to every week based on clinical response.

➤ **Polyarticular juvenile idiopathic arthritis (PJIA) alone or in combination with methotrexate** ⊠

Children ages 2 and older weighing 30 kg or more: 8 mg/kg IV infusion once every 4 weeks. Or, 162 mg subcut once every 2 weeks. *Children ages 2 and older weighing less than 30 kg:* 10 mg/kg IV infusion once every 4 weeks. Or, 162 mg subcut once every 3 weeks.

Adjust-a-dose: Don't change dose based on a single-visit weight because weight may fluctuate. If appropriate, concomitant methotrexate or other medications should be dose-modified or stopped and tocilizumab dosage adjusted until the clinical situation has been evaluated. In PJIA, the decision to discontinue tocilizumab for a lab abnormality should be based on medical assessment of the individual patient.

➤ **Giant cell arteritis (GCA)** ☒
Adults: 6 mg/kg IV infusion every 4 weeks in combination with a tapering course of glucocorticoids. Maximum dose, 600 mg per infusion. Or, 162 mg subcut once each week in combination with a tapering course of glucocorticoids. Or, 162 mg subcut once every other week in combination with a tapering course of glucocorticoids as clinically indicated. May continue tocilizumab after glucocorticoids are stopped.

➤ **Chimeric antigen receptor (CAR) T cell-induced severe or life-threatening cytokine release syndrome (CRS), alone or in combination with corticosteroids**
Adults and children ages 2 and older weighing 30 kg or more: 8 mg/kg IV infusion. May repeat infusion up to three more doses at least 8 hours apart if no clinical improvement in signs and symptoms of CRS. Maximum dose, 800 mg per infusion.
Adults and children ages 2 and older weighing less than 30 kg: 12 mg/kg IV. May repeat infusion up to three more doses at least 8 hours apart if no clinical improvement in signs and symptoms of CRS. Maximum dose, 800 mg per infusion.

➤ **To slow decline in pulmonary function in patients with systemic sclerosis-associated interstitial lung disease (SSc-ILD)**
Adults: 162 mg subcut once each week. Subcut administration with prefilled autoinjector hasn't been studied for this indication.

✱ *NEW INDICATION:* **COVID-19 in hospitalized patients receiving systemic corticosteroids who require supplemental oxygen, noninvasive or invasive mechanical ventilation, or extracorporeal membrane oxygenation**
Adults: 8 mg/kg IV infusion over 60 minutes.

If clinical signs or symptoms worsen or don't improve after first dose, one additional dose may be given at least 8 hours after initial infusion. Maximum dose, 800 mg/infusion.
Adjust-a-dose: Don't initiate in patients with ANC below 1,000/mm^3, platelet count below 50,000/mm^3, or ALT or AST above 10 times ULN.

ADMINISTRATION
IV
▼ Check body weight before calculating each dose. For patients weighing 30 kg or more, dilute to 100 mL in NSS or half-NSS for IV infusion following manufacturer's instructions. For patients weighing less than 30 kg, dilute to 50 mL in NSS or half-NSS for IV infusion following manufacturer's instructions. Allow diluted solutions to reach room temperature before infusing.
▼ Don't use solution if it's discolored or contains particulate matter.
▼ Store NSS infusion solutions at 36° to 46° F (2° to 8° C) or at room temperature for up to 24 hours. Store half-NSS infusion solutions at 36° to 46° F for up to 24 hours or at room temperature for up to 4 hours. Protect all solutions from light.
▼ Administer infusion over 60 minutes. Don't administer as IV push or bolus.
▼ **Incompatibilities:** Don't infuse in same line with other IV drugs.
Subcutaneous
• When transitioning from IV therapy to subcut administration, administer the first subcut dose instead of the next scheduled IV dose.
• Dosing interruption or reduction in administration frequency of subcut dose from every week to every other week is recommended for management of certain dose-related lab changes, including elevated liver enzyme levels, neutropenia, and thrombocytopenia.
• Remove prefilled syringe from refrigerator 30 minutes before use. Remove autoinjector 45 minutes before use. Don't warm in any other way.
• Don't use if product contains particulate matter, is cloudy, or is discolored or if any part of syringe or autoinjector is damaged.
• Inject full amount in syringe or autoinjector (0.9 mL).
• Rotate injection sites with each injection. Never give into moles, scars, or areas where skin is tender, bruised, red, hard, or not intact.
• Don't rub injection site.

ACTION
Inhibits interleukin-6-mediated inflammatory processes by decreasing inflammatory markers, such as C-reactive protein level, rheumatoid factor, and erythrocyte sedimentation rate.

Route	Onset	Peak	Duration
IV	Unknown	Unknown	Unknown
Subcut	Unknown	3–4.5 days	Unknown

Half-life: IV, 11 to 13 days; subcut, 5 to 13 days.

ADVERSE REACTIONS

CNS: dizziness, headache, anxiety, insomnia. **CV:** HTN, peripheral edema. **EENT:** nasopharyngitis, oral mucosa ulcer. **GI:** gastritis, stomatitis, upper abdominal pain, gastric ulcer, nausea, diarrhea, constipation. **GU:** UTI. **Hematologic:** *thrombocytopenia, neutropenia.* **Hepatic:** elevated LFT values. **Metabolic:** elevated lipid levels, weight gain, *hypokalemia.* **Respiratory:** bronchitis, URI. **Skin:** rash, pruritus, urticaria, injection-site reactions. **Other:** infection, anti-tocilizumab antibody development, infusion-related reactions.

INTERACTIONS

Drug-drug. *Biological DMARDs (anti-CD20 monoclonal antibodies, interleukin-1 receptor antagonists, selective costimulation modulators, TNF antagonists):* May increase risk of serious infection. Don't use together.
Cyclosporine, theophylline, warfarin: May decrease drug levels. Closely monitor levels, and adjust dosage as needed.
CYP3A4 substrates (atorvastatin, lovastatin, omeprazole, simvastatin): May decrease levels of these drugs. Avoid use together.
Hormonal contraceptives: May decrease effects of contraceptives. Consider nonhormonal alternatives for contraception.
Live-virus vaccines: No data are available on secondary transmission of infection from live-virus vaccine. Avoid use together.
Drug-herb. *Echinacea:* May decrease effect of immunosuppressants. Discourage use together.

EFFECTS ON LAB TEST RESULTS

• May increase bilirubin, ALT, AST, and lipid levels.
• May decrease potassium level.
• May decrease leukocyte, platelet, and neutrophil counts.

CONTRAINDICATIONS & CAUTIONS

Boxed Warning Risks and benefits of treatment with tocilizumab should be carefully considered before start of therapy in patients with chronic or recurrent infection. ■
Boxed Warning Patients treated with tocilizumab are at increased risk for developing serious infections (active pulmonary or extrapulmonary TB; invasive fungal infections [candidiasis, aspergillosis, pneumocystis]; or bacterial, viral, and

other infections caused by opportunistic pathogens) that may lead to hospitalization or death. Most patients who developed these infections were taking concomitant immunosuppressants, such as methotrexate or corticosteroids. ■
• Contraindicated in patients hypersensitive to drug or its components.
• Months to years after treatment, serious cases of liver injury have been observed in patients taking drug IV or subcut, some cases resulting in liver transplant or death. Avoid use in patients with active liver disease or liver impairment.
• Don't initiate drug in patients with ANC less than 2,000/mm³ or platelet count less than 100,000/mm³ or in those with ALT or AST level more than 1.5 × ULN.
Alert: Use cautiously in patients who have been exposed to TB or have history of chronic or recurrent infection, serious or opportunistic infection, or underlying conditions that increase risk of infection. Use cautiously in those who have resided or traveled in areas with endemic TB or mycosis.
Alert: Patients with severe or life-threatening CRS frequently have cytopenias or elevated ALT or AST level due to chemotherapy or CRS. Before start of therapy, consider the potential benefit of treating CRS versus risks of short-term treatment with tocilizumab.
• Use cautiously in patients at risk for GI perforation.
• Use cautiously in patients with preexisting CNS demyelinating disorders such as MS.
• Drug may increase risk of malignancy.
• For patients older than age 65 being treated with tocilizumab, give drug cautiously because serious infections are more common in this population.
Dialyzable drug: Unknown.

PREGNANCY-LACTATION-REPRODUCTION

• Based on animal data, drug may pose a risk to the fetus. Use during pregnancy only if benefit outweighs fetal risk.
• It isn't known if drug appears in human milk. Patient should discontinue breastfeeding or discontinue drug.

NURSING CONSIDERATIONS

Boxed Warning Monitor patient closely for signs and symptoms of infection during and after treatment. Drug may need to be discontinued if infection occurs during treatment. ■

Boxed Warning Patient should be evaluated and treated, if necessary, for latent TB before start of therapy. Monitor patient for possible TB development during therapy, even if patient tested negative before therapy. ■

• Before starting drug, screen patient for prior HBV infection due to risk of viral reactivation.

• Monitor patient for hypersensitivity reactions, including anaphylaxis. Ensure supportive measures are available to treat hypersensitivity reactions.

• Suspect GI perforation in patient with new-onset abdominal symptoms.

• Monitor lipid levels and neutrophil and platelet counts at baseline and every 4 to 8 weeks during therapy.

• For patients with RA, GCA, and SSc-ILD, obtain LFTs before starting drug, every 4 to 8 weeks after start of therapy for first 6 months of treatment, and every 3 months thereafter. Monitor neutrophil and platelet counts before starting drug, every 4 to 8 weeks after start of therapy, and every 3 months thereafter. Monitor lipid levels at baseline and 4 to 8 weeks after starting therapy. Check subsequent levels according to clinical guidelines.

• For patients with PJIA and SJIA, monitor LFTs at the time of second administration and thereafter every 4 to 8 weeks for patients with PJIA and every 2 to 4 weeks for patients with SJIA.

• Promptly measure LFT values in patients with signs and symptoms of liver injury (fatigue, anorexia, right upper abdominal discomfort, dark urine, jaundice).

• Monitor patient closely for signs and symptoms of demyelinating disorders.

• Ensure recommended immunizations (except live-virus vaccines) are up-to-date before beginning therapy.

• Subcut injection is intended for use under the guidance of a health care practitioner. After proper training, patient may self-inject drug or patient's caregiver may administer drug if health care practitioner deems appropriate. Assess suitability of patient for subcut home use.

PATIENT TEACHING

🔵 **Alert:** Warn patient to seek immediate medical attention for abdominal pain, fatigue, anorexia, dark urine, jaundice, or signs and

symptoms of infection (fever, chills, muscle aches) or hypersensitivity reaction (rash; shortness of breath; swelling of lips, tongue, or face; chest pain; faintness; abdominal pain; vomiting).

• Inform patient that prescriber will order blood tests before and during therapy.

• Teach patient or caregiver proper subcut injection technique and instruct them to follow manufacturer's instructions. Caution patient to inform prescriber before administering next dose if signs or symptoms of allergic reaction occur.

• Instruct patient that TB and hepatitis B screening are needed before therapy begins.

• Advise patient to report pregnancy or plans to become pregnant or breastfeed.

• Tell patient to avoid exposure to infections.

• Remind patient to contact prescriber before scheduling surgery.

• Caution patient to avoid live-virus vaccines during therapy.

• Recommend that patient use nonhormonal contraception during therapy.

tofacitinib citrate ⬛
toe-fa-SYE-ti-nib

Xeljanz, Xeljanz XR

Therapeutic class: Antirheumatics
Pharmacologic class: Janus kinase inhibitors

AVAILABLE FORMS
Oral solution: 1 mg/mL
Tablets: 5 mg, 10 mg
Tablets (extended-release) ⬛: 11 mg, 22 mg

INDICATIONS & DOSAGES
Adjust-a-dose (for all indications): Refer to manufacturer's instructions for toxicity-related dosage adjustments.

➤ **Moderately to severely active RA after inadequate response or intolerance to one or more TNF blockers; active psoriatic arthritis after inadequate response or intolerance to one or more TNF blockers, in combination with nonbiologic DMARDs; ankylosing spondylitis after inadequate response or intolerance to one or more TNF blocker**
Adults: 5 mg (immediate-release) PO b.i.d. Or, 11 mg (extended-release) once daily.

Adjust-a-dose: Reduce dosage to 5 mg (immediate-release) once daily in patients with CrCl less than 60 mL/minute or Child-Pugh class B liver impairment, in those receiving concurrent strong CYP3A4 inhibitors, and in those receiving a moderate CYP3A4 inhibitor with a strong CYP2C19 inhibitor.

➤ **Moderately to severely active ulcerative colitis after inadequate response or intolerance to one or more TNF blockers**
Adults: 10 mg (immediate-release) PO b.i.d. or 22 mg (extended-release) for at least 8 weeks; then 5 or 10 mg (immediate-release) b.i.d. or 11 or 22 mg (extended-release) once daily depending on therapeutic response. Use lowest effective dose to maintain response. Discontinue after 16 weeks of treatment with 10 mg b.i.d. (immediate-release) or 22 mg once daily (extended-release) if adequate therapeutic benefit isn't achieved.
Adjust-a-dose: In patients with CrCl less than 60 mL/minute or Child-Pugh class B liver impairment, in those receiving concurrent strong CYP3A4 inhibitors, and in those receiving a moderate CYP3A4 inhibitor with a strong CYP2C19 inhibitor: If patient is taking 10 mg b.i.d. (immediate-release), reduce dosage to 5 mg b.i.d.; if patient is taking 5 mg b.i.d., reduce dosage to 5 mg once daily. If patient is taking 22 mg (extended-release) once daily, reduce dosage to 11 mg once daily; if patient is taking 11 mg (extended-release) once daily, reduce dosage to 5 mg (immediate-release) once daily.

➤ **Polyarticular course juvenile idiopathic arthritis (pcJIA) after inadequate response or intolerance to one or more TNF blockers**
Children ages 2 and older weighing 40 kg or more: 5 mg (tablet or 5 mL oral solution) PO b.i.d.
Children ages 2 and older weighing 20 to less than 40 kg: 4 mg (4 mL) oral solution PO b.i.d.
Children ages 2 and older weighing 10 to less than 20 kg: 3.2 mg (3.2 mL) oral solution PO b.i.d.
Adjust-a-dose: In patients receiving strong CYP3A4 inhibitors or a moderate CYP3A4 inhibitor with a strong CYP2C19 inhibitor and in those with CrCl less than 60 mL/minute or Child-Pugh class B liver impairment, reduce to once-daily dosing.

ADMINISTRATION
PO
• Give drug without regard to food.
• Have patient swallow extended-release tablets whole; don't crush or cut tablets.
• May switch patient treated with 5-mg immediate-release tablets b.i.d. to 11-mg extended-release tablets once daily the day after last 5-mg dose. May switch patient treated with 10-mg immediate-release tablets b.i.d. to 22-mg extended-release tablets once daily the day after last 10-mg dose.
• May switch patient treated with 5 mL oral solution to 5-mg immediate-release tablet.
• Give oral solution using included press-in bottle adapter and oral dosing syringe.
• For patient on hemodialysis, give dose after dialysis session. If patient took dose before dialysis, don't give supplemental dose after dialysis.
• Store drug at room temperature. Store oral solution in original bottle and carton to protect from light. Use within 60 days of opening bottle or discard.

ACTION
Inhibits activity of Janus kinases, preventing activation of certain intracellular activities that influence immune cell function.

Route	Onset	Peak	Duration
PO (immediate-release)	Unknown	0.5–1 hr	Unknown
PO (extended-release)	Unknown	4 hr	Unknown

Half-life: Immediate-release, 3 hours; extended-release, 6 to 8 hours.

ADVERSE REACTIONS
CNS: headache, paresthesia, insomnia, fever. **CV:** HTN. **EENT:** nasopharyngitis, sinus congestion. **GI:** diarrhea, gastroenteritis. **GU:** UTI, increased creatinine level. **Hematologic:** anemia. **Metabolic:** elevated lipid levels, increased CK level. **Respiratory:** URI. **Skin:** rash, erythema, pruritus, acne. **Other:** infection, herpes zoster.

INTERACTIONS
Drug-drug. *Immunosuppressants (azathioprine, cyclosporine, corticosteroids, methotrexate, tacrolimus):* May increase risk of immunosuppression and serious infection. Use together isn't recommended.

Live-virus vaccines: May increase adverse effects of vaccines. Avoid use together; don't give live-attenuated vaccines for at least 3 months after immunosuppressants.

Moderate CYP3A4 inhibitors plus strong CYP2C19 inhibitors (fluconazole), strong CYP3A4 inhibitors (ketoconazole): May increase tofacitinib plasma level. Decrease tofacitinib dosage per manufacturer's instructions.

Strong CYP3A4 inducers (rifampin): May decrease tofacitinib plasma level. Use together isn't recommended.

Drug-herb. *Echinacea:* May diminish therapeutic effect of immunosuppressants. Discourage use together.

St. John's wort: May decrease level of CYP3A4 substrates. Discourage use together.

EFFECTS ON LAB TEST RESULTS
- May increase creatinine, CK, liver enzyme, and lipid levels.
- May decrease Hb level and lymphocyte and neutrophil counts.

CONTRAINDICATIONS & CAUTIONS
- Contraindicated in patients hypersensitive to drug or its components.
- Use in patients with Child-Pugh class C liver impairment isn't recommended.

🜂 Alert: Use cautiously in patients at risk for serious infection (including those who have resided or traveled in areas with endemic TB or mycoses), those at risk for GI perforation (history of diverticulitis), and those with known malignancy.

Boxed Warning Serious infections leading to hospitalization or death, including TB and bacterial, invasive fungal, viral, and other opportunistic infections, have occurred in patients receiving tofacitinib, especially patients on concomitant immunosuppressants, such as methotrexate or corticosteroids. Evaluate risk before starting therapy in patients with chronic or recurrent infection. If a serious infection develops, interrupt therapy until infection is controlled. ∎

Boxed Warning Lymphoma and other malignancies have been observed in patients treated with tofacitinib. In patients with RA, a higher rate of malignancies was observed compared to those treated with TNF blockers. Patients who are current or past smokers are at increased risk for lymphomas and lung cancers. ∎

Boxed Warning Epstein-Barr virus-associated posttransplant lymphoproliferative disorder has been increasingly observed in patients with kidney transplant treated with tofacitinib and concomitant immunosuppressants. ∎

Boxed Warning Patients ages 50 and older with RA and at least one CV risk factor treated with tofacitinib have an increased risk of major adverse CV events (CV death, MI, stroke) and thrombosis (PE, venous, and arterial) when compared to use of other TNF blockers in patients with RA. ∎

- When treating patients with ulcerative colitis, use lowest effective dose for shortest duration needed to achieve and maintain therapeutic response.
- Patients shouldn't receive live-virus vaccines during therapy. Update immunizations according to current guidelines before starting drug.
- Use cautiously when giving extended-release formulation to patients with preexisting severe GI narrowing. Although rare, obstructive signs and symptoms have been reported in patients with known strictures who have ingested other drugs that use a nondeformable extended-release formulation.
- Consider risks and benefits of treatment before initiating therapy in patients with a known malignancy other than a successfully treated nonmelanoma skin cancer or when considering continuing tofacitinib in patients who develop a malignancy.
- Safety and efficacy of oral solution in children for indications other than pcJIA or of extended-release tablets in children haven't been established.
- Effectiveness of tofacitinib as monotherapy hasn't been studied in patients with psoriatic arthritis.
- Use cautiously in patients with history of chronic lung disease, patients who develop ILD, patients with diabetes, and patients older than age 65 because of increased risk of serious infection.

Dialyzable drug: Unknown.

PREGNANCY-LACTATION-REPRODUCTION
- Studies during pregnancy are inadequate, but drug may cause fetal harm. Use only if potential benefit justifies fetal risk.
- It isn't known if drug appears in human milk. Patient shouldn't breastfeed while taking drug and for at least 18 hours after final

dose of immediate-release form or 36 hours after final dose of extended-release form.

• Based on animal studies, drug may reduce fertility in patients of childbearing potential. It isn't known if this effect is reversible.

NURSING CONSIDERATIONS

Boxed Warning Before therapy, test patient for latent TB. If test is positive, begin TB treatment before starting tofacitinib therapy. Monitor all patients for active TB during treatment, even if initial latent TB test is negative. ■

Boxed Warning Monitor patient for thrombosis, including PE, DVT, and arterial thrombosis. Promptly evaluate patient if signs or symptoms occur and discontinue drug. ■

▧ Drug may reactivate viral infections such as herpes zoster. Risk of reactivation of herpes zoster appears to be higher in patients treated in Japan and Korea.

• Impact of drug on chronic viral hepatitis reactivation is unknown. Screen for viral hepatitis in accordance with clinical guidelines before starting therapy.

• Monitor patient during and after treatment for signs and symptoms of infection. Interrupt treatment if serious infection occurs; don't restart until infection is resolved.

• Monitor lymphocyte count at baseline and every 3 months thereafter.

• Monitor neutrophil count, platelet, and Hb level at baseline; after 4 to 8 weeks of treatment; and every 3 months thereafter.

• Don't initiate therapy if lymphocyte count falls below 500/mm³, ANC falls below 1,000/mm³, or Hb level falls below 9 g/dL.

• Regularly monitor LFT results, especially in patient with history of taking DMARDs such as methotrexate. For suspected drug-induced liver injury, stop drug until drug cause is ruled out.

• Assess lipid levels 4 to 8 weeks after drug initiation and then periodically; manage appropriately as needed.

• Monitor patient for GI perforation. Promptly evaluate sudden new-onset abdominal pain or other GI signs and symptoms, especially if patient is also taking NSAIDs.

• Perform periodic skin exams of patient who is at increased risk for skin cancer.

• May cause HTN; monitor BP.

PATIENT TEACHING

Boxed Warning Inform patient that drug may increase risk of major CV events, including MI, stroke, and CV death. ■

Boxed Warning Warn patient to stop drug and immediately report signs and symptoms of thrombosis (sudden shortness of breath, chest pain that worsens with breathing, swelling of leg or arm, leg pain or tenderness, red or discolored skin in affected extremity). ■

• Advise patient to inform prescriber of all adverse reactions, especially signs and symptoms of infection, abdominal pain, or illness.

• Caution patient to regularly undergo lab testing (CBC, liver enzymes, lipids) as directed.

• Instruct patient to report pregnancy or plans to become pregnant.

• Warn patient to avoid live-virus vaccines.

• Inform patient that inert extended-release tablet shell may pass in stool but active medication will have already been absorbed.

---

tolterodine tartrate ▧
toll-TEAR-oh-deen

Detrol, Detrol LA

Therapeutic class: Urinary antispasmodics
Pharmacologic class: Antimuscarinics

AVAILABLE FORMS

Capsules (extended-release) ⒪ⓃⒸ: 2 mg, 4 mg
Tablets: 1 mg, 2 mg

INDICATIONS & DOSAGES

➤ **Overactive bladder in patients with symptoms of urinary frequency, urgency, or urge incontinence**
Adults: 2-mg tablet PO b.i.d. or 4-mg extended-release capsule PO once daily. Dose may be reduced to 1-mg tablet PO b.i.d. or 2-mg extended-release capsule PO once daily, based on patient response and tolerance.
Adjust-a-dose: For patients with CrCl of 10 to 30 mL/minute and those taking a strong CYP3A4 inhibitor, give 1-mg tablet PO b.i.d. or 2-mg extended-release capsule PO daily. For patients with Child-Pugh class A or B liver impairment, give 2-mg extended-release capsule PO daily. For patients with Child-Pugh class C liver impairment, give 1-mg tablet PO b.i.d.

ADMINISTRATION
PO
• Have patient swallow extended-release capsules whole; don't crush or open capsules.
• Give drug without regard to meals.

ACTION
Relaxes smooth muscle of bladder by antagonizing muscarinic receptors, relieving symptoms of overactive bladder.

Route	Onset	Peak	Duration
PO	Unknown	1–2 hr	Unknown
PO (extended-release)	Unknown	2–6 hr	Unknown

Half-life: Immediate-release tablet, 2 to 11 hours; extended-release capsule, about 18 hours.

ADVERSE REACTIONS
CNS: headache, fatigue, vertigo, dizziness, somnolence, drowsiness, anxiety. **CV:** chest pain. **EENT:** abnormal vision, dry eyes, sinusitis, dry mouth. **GI:** abdominal pain, constipation, diarrhea, dyspepsia. **GU:** dysuria, urine retention. **Metabolic:** weight gain. **Musculoskeletal:** arthralgia. **Respiratory:** bronchitis. **Skin:** dry skin. **Other:** flulike syndrome, infection.

INTERACTIONS
Drug-drug. *Anticholinergics (ipratropium, tiotropium):* Coadministration may increase frequency or severity of anticholinergic adverse reactions (blurred vision, constipation, dry mouth, somnolence). Monitor patient closely.
CYP3A4 inhibitors (clarithromycin, erythromycin, itraconazole, ketoconazole, miconazole): May increase tolterodine level. Don't give more than 1-mg tablet b.i.d. or 2-mg extended-release capsule once daily of tolterodine if used together.
Class IA (procainamide, quinidine), Class III (amiodarone, sotalol) antiarrhythmics; CYP2D6 or CYP3A4 inhibitors (fluoxetine, ketoconazole): May increase risk of QT-interval prolongation. Use together cautiously.
Drug-food. *Grapefruit, grapefruit juice:* May increase drug level. Monitor patient.

EFFECTS ON LAB TEST RESULTS
None reported.

CONTRAINDICATIONS & CAUTIONS
• Contraindicated in patients hypersensitive to drug or its components or to fesoterodine fumarate extended-release tablets and in those with uncontrolled angle-closure glaucoma or urine or gastric retention.
• Use cautiously in patients with significant bladder outflow obstruction, GI obstructive disorders (pyloric stenosis), controlled angle-closure glaucoma, myasthenia gravis, and liver or kidney impairment.
• An additive effect of tolterodine with other drugs that prolong QT interval cannot be excluded, which increases risk of life-threatening cardiac arrhythmias. Consider this when tolterodine is prescribed to patients with known history of QT-interval prolongation or those who are taking other drugs that prolong QT interval, such as Class IA or Class III antiarrhythmics.
 May increase risk of QT-interval prolongation in poor CYP2D6 metabolizers.
• Extended-release capsules aren't recommended for use in patients with Child-Pugh class C liver impairment or those with CrCl of less than 10 mL/minute.
• Effectiveness in children hasn't been established.

Dialyzable drug: Unknown.

⚠ Overdose S&S: Dry mouth, severe central anticholinergic effects, QT-interval prolongation.

PREGNANCY-LACTATION-REPRODUCTION
• Studies during pregnancy are inadequate. Use only if potential benefit justifies fetal risk.
• It isn't known if drug appears in human milk. Use cautiously during breastfeeding.

NURSING CONSIDERATIONS
• Assess baseline bladder function and GI motility. Monitor therapeutic effects.
• Monitor patient for residual urine after voiding.
• Monitor relevant lab values in patient with liver or kidney impairment.
• Monitor for hypersensitivity reactions, including anaphylaxis and angioedema. Discontinue drug and promptly initiate appropriate therapy if difficulty breathing, upper airway obstruction, or decreased BP occurs.
• *Look alike–sound alike:* Don't confuse tolterodine with fesoterodine. Don't confuse Detrol with Ditropan.

PATIENT TEACHING

• Advise patient to avoid driving and other potentially hazardous activities until effects of drug are known.

• Instruct patient to immediately report all adverse reactions and signs and symptoms of infection, urine retention, GI problems, or difficulty breathing.

• Teach about proper drug administration and handling.

• Caution patient to immediately report pregnancy or plans to become pregnant or breast-feed during treatment.

tolvaptan ℞
tol-VAP-tan

Jinarc✦, Jynarque, Samsca

Therapeutic class: Vasopressin antagonists
Pharmacologic class: Selective vasopressin receptor antagonists

AVAILABLE FORMS
Tablets: 15 mg, 30 mg, 45 mg, 60 mg, 90 mg

INDICATIONS & DOSAGES

➤ **Hypervolemic and euvolemic hyponatremia (serum sodium level less than 125 mEq/L or symptomatic hyponatremia that has resisted correction with fluid restriction), including patients with HF and SIADH (Samsca only)**

Adults: Initially, 15 mg PO once daily. After at least 24 hours, may increase to 30 mg PO once daily to maximum dosage of 60 mg PO once daily for no more than 30 days. Titrate dosage at 24-hour intervals to desired serum sodium level.

➤ **To slow kidney function decline in patients at risk for rapidly progressing autosomal dominant polycystic kidney disease (ADPKD) (Jynarque only)** ℞

Adults: Initially, 60 mg PO daily, as 45 mg taken on waking and 15 mg taken 8 hours later. Titrate to 60 mg plus 30 mg, then to 90 mg plus 30 mg per day if tolerated, with at least weekly intervals between titrations. May be down-titrated based on tolerability.

Adjust-a-dose: When administered with a moderate CYP3A inhibitor, reduce Jynarque dosage per manufacturer's instructions. Use with a strong CYP3A inhibitors is contraindicated.

ADMINISTRATION
PO

• Give drug without regard to food.

• For patients with hyponatremia, avoid fluid restriction during first 24 hours of therapy.

• Make sure patient drinks water when thirsty and throughout the day and night if awake.

• Give a missed Samsca dose as soon as possible, unless it's almost time for the next scheduled dose; then skip the missed dose and give the next scheduled dose.

• Skip a missed Jynarque dose and give the next dose at its scheduled time.

ACTION

Antagonizes the effect of vasopressin, causing an increase in urine excretion, which results in an increase in free water clearance, a decrease in urine osmolality, and ultimately an increase in serum sodium level.

Route	Onset	Peak	Duration
PO	2–4 hr	2–4 hr	Unknown

Half-life: Dose-dependent, 3 to 12 hours.

ADVERSE REACTIONS

CNS: asthenia, fatigue, dizziness, fever, *stroke,* thirst. **CV:** *intracardiac thrombus, PE, ventricular fibrillation, DVT,* palpitations. **EENT:** dry mouth. **GI:** anorexia, constipation, nausea, *GI bleeding,* abdominal distention, *ischemic colitis,* diarrhea, dyspepsia. **GU:** polyuria, urinary frequency or urgency, *urethral hemorrhage, vaginal hemorrhage,* nocturia. **Hematologic:** *DIC.* **Metabolic:** fluid imbalance, hyperglycemia, hyperuricemia, *diabetic ketoacidosis.* **Musculoskeletal:** *rhabdomyolysis.* **Respiratory:** *respiratory failure.* **Skin:** dry skin, rash.

INTERACTIONS

Drug-drug. *ACE inhibitors, ARBs, potassium-sparing diuretics:* May increase hyperkalemic effect of these drugs. Closely monitor potassium level.

CYP3A inducers (barbiturates, carbamazepine, phenytoin, rifabutin, rifampin, rifapentine): May decrease tolvaptan level. Avoid concomitant use with strong inducers, if possible. Monitor patient response, and adjust dosage as needed.

Digoxin: May increase digoxin level. Monitor patient, and adjust digoxin dosage as needed.

Reactions in bold italics are *life-threatening*.

Hypertonic sodium chloride solution: May increase risk of too-rapid increase in serum sodium level. Avoid use together.

Moderate CYP3A inhibitors (aprepitant, conivaptan, diltiazem, erythromycin, fluconazole, verapamil): May increase tolvaptan level. Adjust tolvaptan dosage when used with Jynarque. Avoid use with Samsca.

Strong CYP3A inhibitors (ketoconazole): May significantly increase tolvaptan level. Use together is contraindicated.

V₂-agonists (desmopressin): May decrease therapeutic effect of desmopressin. Avoid use together.

Drug-herb. *St John's wort:* May decrease drug level. Discourage use together.

Drug-food. *Grapefruit, grapefruit juice:* May increase drug level. Discourage use together.

EFFECTS ON LAB TEST RESULTS
• May increase glucose, potassium, uric acid, ALT, AST, and bilirubin levels.
• May prolong PT.

CONTRAINDICATIONS & CAUTIONS
Boxed Warning Tolvaptan can cause serious and potentially fatal liver injury. Acute liver failure requiring liver transplantation has been reported. ∎

▧ **Boxed Warning** Samsca is contraindicated for use in ADPKD outside of the FDA-approved REMS program. Tolvaptan can cause serious and potentially fatal liver injury and shouldn't be prescribed or used outside of the FDA-approved REMS program. Jynarque is available only through the Jynarque REMS program. In Canada, Jinarc is available only through a controlled liver safety monitoring and distribution program. ∎

Boxed Warning Samsca should be initiated and reinitiated only in a hospital setting where serum sodium level can be closely monitored. ∎

• Contraindicated in patients hypersensitive to drug or its components.
• Contraindicated in patients who require urgent rise in serum sodium level, are anuric, or are unable to sense or appropriately respond to thirst.
• Samsca is contraindicated in patients with hypovolemic hyponatremia.
• Jynarque and Jinarc are contraindicated in patients with history or signs or symptoms of significant liver impairment or injury (doesn't

apply to uncomplicated polycystic liver disease) or hypovolemia.
• Jynarque is contraindicated in patients with uncorrected abnormal serum sodium level or uncorrected urinary outflow obstruction.
▧ Jinarc is contraindicated in patients with hypernatremia, galactose intolerance, Lapp lactase deficiency, or glucose-galactose malabsorption.
• Use cautiously in patients with dehydration; avoid use in those receiving hypertonic saline solution.
• Avoid use in patients with underlying liver disease, including cirrhosis, because the ability to recover from liver injury may be impaired. Use isn't recommended in patients with CrCl less than 10 mL/minute.
Dialyzable drug: Unlikely.
⚠ **Overdose S&S:** Polyuria, thirst, dehydration, hypovolemia, hypernatremia.

PREGNANCY-LACTATION-REPRODUCTION
• Studies during pregnancy are inadequate. Use only if potential benefit justifies fetal risk.
• It isn't known if drug appears in human milk. Patient shouldn't breastfeed during therapy due to potential for serious adverse reactions in infant.

NURSING CONSIDERATIONS
Boxed Warning Don't correct hyponatremia (for example, more than 12 mEq/L/24 hours) too rapidly; doing so may cause osmotic demyelination, resulting in dysarthria, mutism, dysphagia, lethargy, affective changes, spastic quadriparesis, seizures, coma, and death. Slower correction may be necessary in patients who are susceptible, including those with severe malnutrition, alcoholism, or advanced liver disease. ∎

Boxed Warning To reduce risk of significant or irreversible liver injury, perform ALT, AST, and bilirubin blood testing before start of ADPKD treatment, at 2 and 4 weeks after initiation, monthly for 18 months, and every 3 months thereafter. Monitor patient for concurrent signs and symptoms that may indicate liver injury. Prompt action in response to lab abnormalities or signs and symptoms indicative of liver injury can mitigate, but not eliminate, risk of serious liver toxicity. ∎

🔆 **Alert:** Monitor LFT values and promptly assess liver function in patients reporting fatigue, anorexia, right upper abdominal discomfort, dark urine, or jaundice. For

suspected liver injury, immediately stop drug, initiate treatment, and investigate cause. Don't reinitiate drug unless cause of liver injury is definitively unrelated to tolvaptan therapy.
• Immediately discontinue Jynarque for signs or symptoms consistent with liver injury or if ALT, AST, or bilirubin level increases to greater than $2 \times$ ULN. Obtain repeat tests within 48 to 72 hours, and continue testing as appropriate. If lab abnormalities stabilize or resolve, restart drug with more frequent monitoring if ALT and AST levels remain below $3 \times$ ULN. Don't restart drug in patient who experiences signs or symptoms consistent with liver injury or whose ALT or AST level exceeds $3 \times$ ULN at any time during treatment unless there's another explanation for liver injury and the injury has resolved.
• In patient taking Jynarque who has a stable, low baseline AST or ALT level, an increase above $2 \times$ baseline, even if less than $2 \times$ ULN, may indicate early liver injury. Such elevations may warrant treatment suspension and prompt (48 to 72 hours) reevaluation of LFT trends before reinitiation of therapy with more frequent monitoring.
• During Jynarque therapy, if serum sodium level increases above normal range or patient becomes hypovolemic or dehydrated and fluid intake can't be increased, suspend drug until serum sodium level, hydration status, and volume status are within normal range.
• Monitor serum electrolyte levels, volume status, and neurologic status when therapy is begun, during dosage titration, and regularly during therapy.
• Monitor potassium level in patient with potassium level greater than 5 mEq/L and in those who are taking drugs known to increase potassium level.
• After treatment for hyponatremia has ended, patient should resume fluid restriction. Monitor for changes in serum sodium level and volume status.
• Monitor patient for weight loss, tachycardia, and hypotension, which may signal dehydration.

PATIENT TEACHING
• Teach about proper drug administration and handling.
• Advise patient to promptly report all adverse reactions, especially difficulty speaking or swallowing, drowsiness, fatigue, mood changes, trouble controlling body movement,

seizures, anorexia, right upper abdominal discomfort, dark urine, or jaundice.
• Teach patient to inform prescriber of all drugs, herbs, and supplements being taken because of the potential for interactions.
• Advise patient to continue ingestion of fluid in response to thirst during therapy and to resume previous fluid restriction after tolvaptan is discontinued.
• Caution patient to prevent dehydration.
• Tell patient not to stop or restart drug without first consulting prescriber; Samsca should only be restarted in the hospital where sodium level can be closely monitored.
• Inform patient that Samsca should be stopped after 30 days to decrease risk of liver injury.
• Caution patient to report pregnancy or plans to become pregnant.
• Advise patient not to breastfeed.

topiramate ⚠
toe-PIE-rah-mate

Eprontia, Qudexy XR, Topamax, Trokendi XR

Therapeutic class: Anticonvulsants
Pharmacologic class: Sulfamate-substituted monosaccharides

AVAILABLE FORMS
Capsules, sprinkles: 15 mg, 25 mg
Capsules (extended-release) ⓓⓝⓖ: 25 mg, 50 mg, 100 mg, 150 mg, 200 mg
Oral solution: 25 mg/mL
Tablets ⓓⓝⓖ: 25 mg, 50 mg, 100 mg, 200 mg

INDICATIONS & DOSAGES
Adjust-a-dose (for all indications): For adults, if CrCl is less than 70 mL/minute/1.73 m², reduce dosage by 50%. For patients at high risk for kidney insufficiency, obtain an estimated CrCl before dosing. For patients on hemodialysis, supplemental doses may be needed to avoid rapid drops in drug level during prolonged dialysis treatment.
➤ **Initial monotherapy for partial-onset or primary generalized tonic-clonic seizures**
Adults and children ages 10 and older: Recommended daily dosage is 400 mg (immediate-release) PO in two divided doses (morning and evening). To achieve this dosage, adjust as follows: first week, 25 mg

PO b.i.d.; second week, 50 mg PO b.i.d.; third week, 75 mg PO b.i.d.; fourth week, 100 mg PO b.i.d.; fifth week, 150 mg PO b.i.d.; and sixth week, 200 mg PO b.i.d. Or, using extended-release capsules, initially 50 mg PO once daily. Increase dosage weekly by increments of 50 mg for first 4 weeks, then 100 mg for weeks 5 and 6 to recommended 400 mg once daily.

Children ages 2 to younger than 10 (immediate-release, Qudexy XR extended-release) or children ages 6 to younger than 10 (Trokendi XR extended-release): During titration period, initially 25 mg/day (immediate-release or extended-release) PO nightly for first week. Based on tolerability, can increase to 50 mg/day (once daily for extended-release or 25 mg PO b.i.d. for immediate-release) in the second week. Can increase by 25 to 50 mg/day each subsequent week as tolerated. Attempt titration to minimum maintenance dosage over 5 to 7 weeks of total titration period. Based on tolerability and seizure control, can attempt additional titration to higher dosage (up to maximum maintenance dosage) at 25 to 50 mg/day in weekly increments. Total daily dosage shouldn't exceed maximum maintenance dosage for each range of body weight.

Give maintenance doses of extended-release form once daily; give maintenance doses of immediate-release form in two equally divided PO doses daily. If patient weighs up to 11 kg, maintenance dosage range is 150 mg/day to maximum of 250 mg/day. If patient weighs 12 to 22 kg, maintenance dosage range is 200 mg/day to maximum of 300 mg/day. If patient weighs 23 to 31 kg, maintenance dosage range is 200 mg/day to maximum of 350 mg/day. If patient weighs 32 to 38 kg, maintenance dosage range is 250 mg/day to maximum of 350 mg/day. If patient weighs more than 38 kg, maintenance dosage range is 250 mg/day to maximum of 400 mg/day.

➤ **Adjunctive treatment for partial-onset or primary generalized tonic-clonic seizures or Lennox-Gastaut syndrome**
Adults and children ages 17 and older: Initially, 25 to 50 mg PO daily; increase gradually by 25 to 50 mg/week until an effective daily dose is reached. Adjust to recommended daily dose of 200 to 400 mg PO in two divided doses of immediate-release or once daily of extended-release for adults with

partial-onset seizures or Lennox-Gastaut syndrome, or 400 mg PO in two divided doses of immediate-release or once daily of extended-release for adults with primary generalized tonic-clonic seizures.

Children ages 6 to 16 (Trokendi XR) or ages 2 to 16 (Qudexy XR): Initially, 25 mg PO daily at bedtime (based on range of 1 to 3 mg/kg once daily) for first week. Increase dosage at 1- or 2-week intervals by increments of 1 to 3 mg/kg daily. Guide dosage titration by clinical outcome. Recommended daily dosage is 5 to 9 mg/kg once daily.

Children ages 2 to 16 (immediate-release): Initially, 25 mg/day (or less, based on range of 1 to 3 mg/kg/day) PO given at bedtime for 1 week. Increase at 1- or 2-week intervals by 1 to 3 mg/kg daily (given in two divided doses) to achieve optimal response. Guide titration by clinical outcome. Recommended daily dosage is 5 to 9 mg/kg, in two divided doses. Maximum, 400 mg/day.

➤ **To prevent migraine headache**
Adults and adolescents ages 12 and older: For immediate-release, initially, 25 mg PO daily in evening for first week; 25 mg PO b.i.d. in morning and evening for second week; 25 mg PO in morning and 50 mg PO in evening for third week; and 50 mg PO b.i.d. in morning and evening for fourth week. Recommended total daily dose is 100 mg.

For extended-release, initially, 25 mg PO once daily. After 1 week, increase to 50 mg daily, then weekly by 25 mg daily to recommended daily dose of 100 mg. Guide dosage and titration rate according to clinical outcome. Allow longer intervals between dosage adjustments, if needed.

ADMINISTRATION
PO
• Give drug without regard to food.
• Immediate-release and Qudexy XR capsules may be opened and contents sprinkled on a teaspoon of soft food. Patient should swallow immediately without chewing.
• Have patient swallow Trokendi XR capsules whole and intact. Don't sprinkle capsule contents on food or crush capsules; doing so may disrupt the triphasic release properties.
• Don't break tablets, due to bitter taste.
• Use a calibrated measuring device for the oral solution.
• Discard unused portion of oral solution after 60 days.

ACTION

Unknown. May block a sodium channel and potentiate the activity of GABA while inhibiting glutamate and carbonic anhydrase.

Route	Onset	Peak	Duration
PO (immediate-release)	Unknown	0.5–2 hr	Unknown
PO (extended-release)	Unknown	About 20 hr (Qudexy XR); 24 hr (Trokendi XR)	Unknown

Half-life: Immediate-release, 21 hours; extended-release, 31 to 56 hours.

ADVERSE REACTIONS

CNS: anxiety; asthenia; ataxia; confusion; dizziness; fatigue; insomnia; nervousness; paresthesia; psychomotor slowing; somnolence; speech tremor; abnormal coordination; gait abnormality; aggressive reaction; agitation; depression; emotional lability; fever; hyperkinesia; hypertonia; hypoesthesia; personality disorder; vertigo; taste perversion; difficulty with concentration, memory, attention, mood, or language. **CV:** chest pain, flushing. **EENT:** abnormal vision, diplopia, nystagmus, conjunctivitis, secondary angle-closure glaucoma, epistaxis, pharyngitis, sinusitis, rhinitis, dry mouth, increased salivation. **GI:** anorexia, nausea, constipation, diarrhea, abdominal pain, dyspepsia, gastroenteritis, gingivitis, vomiting, gastritis. **GU:** decreased libido, hematuria, impotence, intermenstrual bleeding, menstrual disorder, menorrhagia, urinary frequency, kidney stones, urinary incontinence, UTI, vaginitis, *vaginal hemorrhage,* cystitis. **Hematologic:** anemia. **Hepatic:** increased GGT level. **Metabolic:** weight gain or loss, metabolic acidosis. **Musculoskeletal:** arthralgia, back or leg pain, cramps, muscle weakness, myalgia. **Respiratory:** URI, bronchitis, coughing, dyspnea, pneumonia. **Skin:** acne, alopecia, decreased sweating, pruritus, rash. **Other:** breast pain, flulike syndrome, hot flashes, infection, hyperthermia.

INTERACTIONS

Drug-drug. *Amitriptyline:* May increase amitriptyline level. Monitor response and adjust amitriptyline dosage as needed.
Cannabidiol, cannabis: May enhance CNS depressant effect of topiramate. Monitor therapy.
Carbamazepine: May decrease topiramate level. Monitor patient.

Carbonic anhydrase inhibitors (acetazolamide, dichlorphenamide): May increase risk of metabolic acidosis and kidney stone formation. Avoid use together.
CNS depressants (benzodiazepines, opioids), magnesium sulfate: May cause CNS depression and other adverse cognitive and neuropsychiatric events. Use together cautiously.
Fosphenytoin, phenytoin: May decrease topiramate level and increase phenytoin level. Monitor levels.
Hormonal contraceptives: May decrease effectiveness. Report changes in menstrual patterns. Advise patient to use another contraceptive method.
Hydrochlorothiazide: May increase topiramate level. Monitor patient and decrease topiramate dosage as needed.
Lithium: May increase serum lithium level. Monitor patient and lithium level closely.
Pioglitazone: May increase pioglitazone level. Monitor patient closely.
Salicylates: May enhance toxicity of both agents. Avoid use together.
Valproic acid: May decrease valproic acid and topiramate level. May increase risk of hypothermia and hyperammonemia. Monitor patient.
Warfarin: May decrease anticoagulation effect. Monitor PT and INR.
Drug-herb. *Kava:* May increase CNS depressant effects. Discourage use together.
Drug-food. *Ketogenic diet:* May increase possibility of acidosis or kidney stones. Monitor patient for adverse effects.
Drug-lifestyle. *Alcohol use:* May cause CNS depression and other adverse cognitive and neuropsychiatric events. Discourage use together. Trokendi is contraindicated within 6 hours of alcohol use.

EFFECTS ON LAB TEST RESULTS

- May increase liver enzyme and ammonia levels.
- May decrease bicarbonate level.
- May decrease Hb level and hematocrit.

CONTRAINDICATIONS & CAUTIONS

- Contraindicated in patients hypersensitive to drug or its components.
- Use cautiously in patients with liver or kidney impairment.
- Bioequivalence hasn't been demonstrated between Trokendi XR and Qudexy XR.

Reactions in bold italics are *life-threatening*.

• Acute myopia associated with secondary angle-closure glaucoma has been reported in adults and children receiving topiramate. Such symptoms as acute-onset decreased visual acuity and ocular pain typically occur within 1 month of therapy initiation.

• Serious skin reactions (SJS, TEN) have been reported. Discontinue drug at first sign of rash, unless not drug related.

• Use cautiously with other drugs that predispose patients to heat-related disorders, including other carbonic anhydrase inhibitors and anticholinergics.

▧ Use cautiously in patients with inborn errors of metabolism or reduced liver mitochondrial activity, which may increase risk of hyperammonemia with or without encephalopathy. Risk increases with coadministration of valproic acid.

Dialyzable drug: Yes.

⚠ *Overdose S&S:* Abdominal pain, abnormal coordination, agitation, blurred vision, seizures, depression, diplopia, dizziness, drowsiness, hypotension, lethargy, impaired mentation, speech disturbance, stupor, severe metabolic acidosis.

PREGNANCY-LACTATION-REPRODUCTION

🚫 *Alert:* Drug may cause fetal harm, including birth defects. Use during pregnancy only if potential benefit outweighs fetal risk. Consider alternative medications with a lower risk of adverse outcomes during pregnancy. Patients of childbearing potential who aren't planning pregnancy should use effective contraception while taking this drug.

• Encourage patients who become pregnant during therapy to register in the North American Antiepileptic Drug Pregnancy Registry (1-888-233-2334 or www.aedpregnancyregistry.org).

• Although drug's effects on labor and delivery haven't been established, development of topiramate-induced metabolic acidosis in the mother or fetus may result in adverse effects and fetal death.

• Tell patients of childbearing potential that drug may decrease the effectiveness of hormonal contraceptives. Advise patients using hormonal contraceptives to report change in menstrual patterns.

• Drug appears in human milk, but effect of exposure in infants isn't known. Use cautiously during breastfeeding.

NURSING CONSIDERATIONS

🚫 *Alert:* Closely monitor all patients taking or starting AEDs for changes in behavior indicating worsening of suicidality or depression. Symptoms such as anxiety, agitation, hostility, mania, and hypomania may be precursors to emerging suicidality.

• Monitor patient for cognitive and neuropsychiatric adverse reactions, including behavior disturbances, somnolence, fatigue, confusion, psychomotor slowing, and difficulty with concentration, memory, speech, or language.

• If needed, withdraw anticonvulsant (including topiramate) gradually to minimize risk of increased seizure activity.

• Monitoring topiramate level isn't necessary.

• Monitor patient for hyperammonemia (unexplained lethargy, vomiting, mental status changes), especially patient taking valproic acid.

• Drug may infrequently cause decreased sweating and hyperthermia, mainly in children. Monitor patient closely, especially in hot weather.

• Drug may cause metabolic acidosis from renal bicarbonate loss. Factors that may predispose patients to acidosis, such as kidney disease, severe respiratory disorders, status epilepticus, diarrhea, surgery, ketogenic diet, or drugs, may add to topiramate's bicarbonate-lowering effects.

• Measure baseline and periodic bicarbonate levels. Monitor for signs and symptoms of metabolic acidosis (hyperventilation, fatigue, anorexia, cardiac arrhythmias, stupor). If metabolic acidosis develops and persists, consider reducing dosage, gradually stopping drug, or offering alkali treatment.

• Drug increases risk of kidney stones. Encourage fluid intake to lower risk.

• Monitor kidney function, electrolyte and ammonia levels, and weight.

• Monitor patient for SCARs, including SJS and TEN. Discontinue drug at first sign of rash, unless clearly not drug related.

• Drug is rapidly cleared by dialysis. A prolonged period of dialysis may cause low drug level and seizures. A supplemental dose may be needed.

• Discontinue drug as rapidly as possible, according to judgment of health care provider, if patient experiences acute myopia and secondary angle-closure glaucoma.

• *Look alike–sound alike:* Don't confuse Topamax with Toprol-XL, Tegretol, or Tegretol-XR.

PATIENT TEACHING

• Teach about proper drug administration and handling.

• Tell patient not to consume alcohol within 6 hours before or 6 hours after taking Trokendi XR form.

• Instruct patient to report all adverse reactions and to immediately seek medical attention if blurred vision, visual disturbances, or eye pain occurs to reduce risk of permanent vision loss.

• Advise patient to immediately report high or persistent fever or decreased sweating.

• Tell patient to use appropriate caution when engaging in activities in which loss of consciousness could result in danger to patient or others nearby. Some patients with epilepsy continue to have unpredictable seizures and may need to avoid such activities entirely.

• Caution patient to drink plenty of fluids during therapy to minimize risk of forming kidney stones.

• Teach patient that a ketogenic diet may increase kidney stone or acidosis risk.

• Advise patient not to drive or operate hazardous machinery until CNS effects of drug are known. Drug can cause sleepiness, dizziness, confusion, and concentration problems.

• **Alert:** Teach patient of childbearing potential to use effective contraception during treatment, and explain the drug's effect on fetal development. Tell patient to report pregnancy or plans to become pregnant during therapy.

• Caution patient not to stop drug abruptly to prevent onset of seizures.

SAFETY ALERT!

topotecan hydrochloride
toh-poh-TEE-ken

Hycamtin

Therapeutic class: Antineoplastics
Pharmacologic class: DNA topoisomerase inhibitors

AVAILABLE FORMS

Capsules ⓞⓝⓒ: 0.25 mg, 1 mg
Injection (lyophilized powder): 4-mg single-dose vial
Injection (solution): 1 mg/mL, 4 mg/4 mL vial

INDICATIONS & DOSAGES

Adjust-a-dose (for all indications): Refer to manufacturer's instructions for toxicity-related dosage adjustments.

➤ **Relapsed small-cell lung cancer (SCLC) in patients with a prior complete or partial response who are at least 45 days from end of first-line chemotherapy**

Adults: 2.3 mg/m^2/day PO or 1.5 mg/m^2 IV once daily for 5 consecutive days, starting on day 1 of a 21-day cycle. Repeat cycle every 21 days. Round calculated dose to nearest 0.25 mg.

Adjust-a-dose: For patients with CrCl of 30 to 49 mL/minute, give 1.5 mg/m^2/day; CrCl less than 30 mL/minute, 0.6 mg/m^2/day.

➤ **SCLC in patients with platinum-sensitive disease who progressed at least 60 days after initiation of first-line chemotherapy; metastatic ovarian cancer after failure of first or subsequent chemotherapy**

Adults: 1.5 mg/m^2 IV infusion daily for 5 consecutive days, starting on day 1 of a 21-day cycle. Maximum recommended dosage, 4 mg. For ovarian cancer, continue until disease progression or unacceptable toxicity occurs.

Adjust-a-dose: For patients with CrCl of 20 to 39 mL/minute, decrease dosage to 0.75 mg/m^2.

➤ **With cisplatin, stage IV-B, recurrent, or persistent cervical cancer unresponsive to surgery or radiation**

Adults: 0.75 mg/m^2 by IV infusion on days 1, 2, and 3, followed by 50 mg/m^2 cisplatin by IV infusion on day 1. Maximum recommended topotecan dosage, 4 mg. Repeat cycle every 21 days. Adjust subsequent doses of drug based on hematologic toxicities.

ADMINISTRATION

• **Alert:** Verify dosage using BSA before administration. Calculate CrCl with Cockcroft-Gault method using ideal body weight.

PO

• **Alert:** Hazardous drug; use safe handling and disposal precautions.

• Give drug without regard to food.

• Have patient swallow capsules whole; don't crush or cut capsules.

• If patient misses a dose or vomits after taking a dose, don't give replacement dose.

IV

• **Alert:** Hazardous drug; use safe handling and disposal precautions.

▼ Reconstitute each 4-mg vial of lyophilized powder with 4 mL sterile water for injection.

▼ Further dilute appropriate volume of solution or reconstituted solution in either NSS or D₅W before administration.

▼ Lyophilized form contains no antibacterial preservative; use reconstituted product immediately. Discard any unused portion.

▼ Infuse over 30 minutes and monitor insertion site during infusion. If extravasation occurs, immediately discontinue infusion and notify prescriber.

▼ When giving topotecan with cisplatin, always give topotecan first.

▼ If stored at 68° to 77° F (20° to 25° C) and exposed to normal lighting, reconstituted drug remains stable for 24 hours. Protect unopened vials from light.

▼ **Incompatibilities:** Many drugs are incompatible with topotecan. Consult drug compatibility reference for information.

ACTION

Interacts with topoisomerase I, inducing reversible single-strand DNA breaks. Drug binds to the topoisomerase I-DNA complex and prevents repair of these single-strand breaks.

Route	Onset	Peak	Duration
PO	Unknown	1–2 hr	Unknown
IV	Unknown	Unknown	Unknown

Half-life: Oral, 3 to 6 hours; IV, 2 to 3 hours.

ADVERSE REACTIONS

CNS: asthenia, fatigue, fever, pain. **EENT:** pharyngitis. **GI:** abdominal pain, anorexia, constipation, diarrhea, nausea, intestinal obstruction, stomatitis, vomiting. **Hematologic:** anemia, *leukopenia, neutropenia, thrombocytopenia.* **Hepatic:** hyperbilirubinemia, elevated liver enzyme levels. **Metabolic:** weight gain or loss. **Musculoskeletal:** weakness. **Respiratory:** coughing, dyspnea, pneumonia. **Skin:** alopecia, diaphoresis, rash. **Other:** chills, infection, *sepsis.*

INTERACTIONS

Drug-drug. *BCRP inhibitors (cyclosporine, eltrombopag), P-gp inhibitors (cyclosporine, ketoconazole, ritonavir):* May increase systemic exposure to oral topotecan. Avoid concomitant use.

Cisplatin, cytotoxic agents: May increase severity of myelosuppression. Use together with extreme caution. Dosage reductions may be needed.

Fosphenytoin, phenytoin: May decrease topotecan level. Consider using alternative agent to phenytoin.

G-CSF: May increase myelosuppression and risk of ILD. If G-CSF is to be used, don't start it until 24 hours after last dose of IV topotecan treatment each cycle.

Drug-herb. *Echinacea:* May diminish therapeutic effect of topotecan. Avoid use together.

EFFECTS ON LAB TEST RESULTS

• May increase ALT, AST, and bilirubin levels.
• May decrease Hb level and WBC, platelet, and neutrophil counts.

CONTRAINDICATIONS & CAUTIONS

⊗ *Alert:* Administer drug under the supervision of a health care provider experienced in the use of chemotherapeutic agents. Ensure that appropriate diagnostic and treatment facilities are readily available.

• Contraindicated in patients hypersensitive to drug or its components.

• Use cautiously in patients with kidney impairment and in patients with history of ILD, pulmonary fibrosis, lung cancer, thoracic radiation, and use of drugs that cause lung toxicity.

• Safety and effectiveness in children haven't been established.

Dialyzable drug: Unknown.

⚠ *Overdose S&S:* Bone marrow suppression.

PREGNANCY-LACTATION-REPRODUCTION

• Drug can cause fetal harm. If used during pregnancy or if patient becomes pregnant during therapy, apprise patient of potential hazard to fetus.

• Patients of childbearing potential should use highly effective contraception during treatment and for at least 6 months after final dose.

• Drug may damage spermatozoa, possibly resulting in genetic and fetal abnormalities. Advise males with partners of childbearing potential to use effective contraception during and for 3 months after final dose.

• It isn't known if drug appears in human milk. Advise patient not to breastfeed during treatment and for 1 week after final dose.

• Drug may have both acute and long-term adverse effects on male and female fertility. Patient should seek counseling on fertility and family planning options before starting treatment.

NURSING CONSIDERATIONS

• Verify pregnancy status of patient of childbearing potential before therapy.

Boxed Warning Before starting first course of therapy, patient must have baseline neutrophil count of 1,500/mm³ or more and platelet count of 100,000/mm³ or more. Perform peripheral blood counts frequently to monitor patient for bone marrow suppression, primarily neutropenia, which may be severe and result in infection and death. ∎

• Don't give subsequent courses until neutrophil count recovers to more than 1,000/mm³, platelet count recovers to more than 100,000/mm³, and Hb level recovers to 9 g/dL (with transfusion, if needed).

• G-CSF may be used to promote cell growth and decrease risk of infection, starting no sooner than 24 hours after last dose of topotecan.

❸ *Alert:* Fatalities due to neutropenic colitis have been reported. Consider possibility of neutropenic colitis in patients presenting with fever, neutropenia, and a compatible pattern of abdominal pain.

❸ *Alert:* Drug may cause ILD, which may be fatal. Monitor for cough, fever, dyspnea, and hypoxia; stop drug if they occur.

• Monitor CBC with differential and platelet count, kidney function tests, and bilirubin level before each infusion and regularly during therapy.

• If extravasation occurs, immediately discontinue infusion and manage appropriately. Ensure proper needle and catheter placement before and during infusion.

• Monitor patient taking oral topotecan for diarrhea; manage with antidiarrheals at first sign of diarrhea. Withhold drug and reduce dosage based on severity.

• *Look alike–sound alike:* Don't confuse topotecan with irinotecan. Don't confuse Hycamtin with Mycamine.

PATIENT TEACHING

• Teach about proper drug administration and handling, especially for capsules.

• Urge patient to promptly report all adverse reactions, especially sore throat, fever, chills, and unusual bleeding or bruising.

• Advise patient that although diarrhea is common, it may become severe and should be reported to health care provider.

• Caution patient to avoid contact with people with infections.

• Warn of potential hazard to fetus if drug is used during pregnancy or if patient becomes pregnant while taking drug.

• Counsel patient of reproductive potential on effective contraception use.

• Caution patient to avoid breastfeeding during therapy and for 1 week after final dose.

• Teach patient and family about drug's adverse reactions and need for frequent monitoring of blood counts.

torsemide ⌷

TOR-seh-mide

Soaanz

Therapeutic class: Diuretics
Pharmacologic class: Loop diuretics

AVAILABLE FORMS

Tablets: 5 mg, 10 mg, 20 mg, 40 mg, 60 mg, 100 mg

INDICATIONS & DOSAGES

➤ **Edema in patients with HF**

Adults: Initially, 10 to 20 mg PO once daily. If response is inadequate, double dose until desired effect is achieved. Maximum, 200 mg daily.

➤ **Edema in patients with CKD**

Adults: Initially, 20 mg PO once daily. If response is inadequate, double dose until response is obtained. Maximum, 200 mg daily.

➤ **Edema in patients with cirrhosis (except Soaanz)**

Adults: Initially, 5 to 10 mg PO once daily with an aldosterone antagonist or a potassium-sparing diuretic. If response is inadequate, double dose until desired effect is achieved. Maximum, 40 mg daily.

➤ **HTN (except Soaanz)**

Adults: Initially, 5 mg PO daily. Increase to 10 mg if needed and tolerated after 4 to 6 weeks. Add another antihypertensive if response is still inadequate.

ADMINISTRATION
PO

• Give drug without regard to food.

• To prevent nocturia, give drug in the morning.

ACTION

Enhances excretion of sodium, chloride, and water by acting on the ascending loop of Henle.

Route	Onset	Peak	Duration
PO	1 hr	1–2 hr	6–8 hr

Half-life: 3.5 hours.

ADVERSE REACTIONS
CV: ECG abnormalities, chest pain, edema, orthostatic hypotension. **GU:** polyuria. **Metabolic:** *hypokalemia,* hypercholesterolemia, hypertriglyceridemia, hyperglycemia.

INTERACTIONS
Drug-drug. *ACE inhibitors, ARBs:* May increase risk of hypotension and kidney impairment. Use together cautiously.

Aminoglycoside antibiotics (gentamycin), cisplatin, ethacrynic acid: May increase ototoxicity. Avoid use together if possible.

Amphotericin B, corticosteroids, metolazone: May increase risk of hypokalemia. Monitor potassium level.

Antidiabetics: May decrease hypoglycemic effect, resulting in higher glucose level. Monitor glucose level.

Chlorothiazide, chlorthalidone, hydrochlorothiazide, indapamide, metolazone: May cause excessive diuretic response, resulting in serious electrolyte abnormalities or dehydration. Adjust doses carefully, and monitor patient closely for signs and symptoms of excessive diuretic response.

Cholestyramine: May decrease absorption of torsemide. Give torsemide at least 1 hour before or 4 to 6 hours after cholestyramine.

CYP2C9 inducers (rifampin): May decrease torsemide level. Monitor patient closely and adjust torsemide dosage if indicated.

CYP2C9 inhibitors (amiodarone, fluconazole, miconazole, oxandrolone): May increase torsemide level. Monitor patient closely and adjust torsemide dosage if indicated.

CYP2C9 substrates (sensitive ones, such as celecoxib, and those with narrow therapeutic range, such as warfarin or phenytoin): May affect efficacy and safety of substrate. Monitor patient and adjust dosages if necessary.

Digoxin: Electrolyte imbalance caused by diuretic may lead to digoxin-induced arrhythmia. Use together cautiously.

Lithium: May increase lithium level and cause toxicity. Use together cautiously and monitor lithium level.

Methotrexate: May increase methotrexate level; may diminish therapeutic effects of torsemide. Consider therapy modification.

NSAIDs: May decrease effects of loop diuretics and increase risk of AKI. Use together cautiously.

Probenecid: May decrease diuretic effect. Monitor therapy.

Radiocontrast agents: May increase risk of kidney toxicity. Use together cautiously.

Salicylates: May increase salicylate level, possibly leading to toxicity, and decrease diuretic effect. Use together cautiously.

Drug-herb. *Licorice:* May cause unexpected rapid potassium loss. Discourage use together.

Yohimbe: May decrease antihypertensive effect of torsemide. Monitor therapy closely.

EFFECTS ON LAB TEST RESULTS
• May increase BUN, creatinine, cholesterol, glucose, AST, ALT, GGT, triglyceride, and uric acid levels.
• May decrease vitamin B_1, calcium, chloride, sodium, potassium, and magnesium levels.
• May decrease RBC, WBC, and platelet counts.
• Can cause false-negative aldosterone/renin ratios.

CONTRAINDICATIONS & CAUTIONS
• Contraindicated in patients hypersensitive to drug, other sulfonamide derivatives, or povidone and in those with anuria or hepatic coma.
• Use cautiously in patients with liver disease and related cirrhosis and ascites; sudden changes in fluid and electrolyte balance may precipitate hepatic coma in these patients.
• SCARs (including SJS and TEN), leukopenia, thrombocytopenia, pancreatitis, tinnitus, and ototoxicity have been reported with torsemide use.
▨ The antihypertensive effects of torsemide are, on average, greater in patients who are Black than in other patients.
• Safety and effectiveness in children haven't been determined.
Dialyzable drug: No.
⚠ **Overdose S&S:** Dehydration, hypovolemia, hypotension, hypokalemia, hypochloremic alkalosis, hemoconcentration.

PREGNANCY-LACTATION-REPRODUCTION
• Studies during pregnancy are inadequate. Use only if clearly needed.
• It isn't known if drug appears in human milk. Diuretics can suppress lactation. Use cautiously during breastfeeding.

♥Canada ◇OTC ◆Off-label use ☁Do not crush *Liquid contains alcohol ▨ Genetic

NURSING CONSIDERATIONS

• Monitor fluid intake and output, kidney function, electrolyte levels, BP, weight, and pulse rate during rapid diuresis and routinely with long-term use. Drug can cause profound diuresis and water and electrolyte depletion.
• Watch for signs of hypokalemia, such as muscle weakness and cramps.
• Periodically monitor glucose level.
• Consult prescriber and dietitian about providing a high-potassium diet or potassium supplement.
• Monitor older adults, who are especially susceptible to excessive diuresis with potential for circulatory collapse and thromboembolic complications.
• Monitor patient for tinnitus and hearing loss, which are usually reversible. Higher than recommended doses, kidney impairment, and hypoproteinemia may increase risk.
• *Look alike–sound alike:* Don't confuse torsemide with furosemide.

PATIENT TEACHING

• Tell patient to take drug in morning to prevent the need to urinate at night.
• Advise patient to change positions slowly to prevent dizziness and to limit alcohol intake and strenuous exercise in hot weather to prevent dizziness.
• Instruct patient to immediately report ringing in ears because it may indicate toxicity.
• Tell patient to report weakness, cramping, nausea, and dizziness.
• Advise patient to check with prescriber or pharmacist before taking OTC drugs.

traMADol hydrochloride
TRAM-uh-dohl

ConZip, Durela✦, Qdolo, Ralivia✦, Tridural✦, Zytram XL✦

Therapeutic class: Centrally-acting synthetic opioid
Pharmacologic class: Synthetic centrally active analgesics
Controlled substance schedule: IV

AVAILABLE FORMS

Capsules (extended-release) ⒹⓃⒸ: 100 mg, 200 mg, 300 mg
Solution: 5 mg/mL
Tablets: 50 mg, 100 mg

Tablets (extended-release) ⒹⓃⒸ: 75 mg✦, 100 mg, 150 mg✦, 200 mg, 300 mg, 400 mg✦

INDICATIONS & DOSAGES

🔔 *Alert:* Initiate dosing regimen for each patient individually, considering patient's severity of pain, response, prior analgesic treatment experience, and risk factors for addiction, abuse, and misuse. Use lowest effective dosage for shortest duration consistent with individual patient treatment goals.

➤ **Moderate to moderately severe pain severe enough to require an opioid**
Adults: Initially, 25 mg (immediate-release) PO in the morning. Adjust by 25 mg every 3 days to 100 mg/day (25 mg q.i.d.). Thereafter, adjust by 50 mg every 3 days to reach 200 mg/day (50 mg q.i.d.). Thereafter, give 50 to 100 mg PO every 4 to 6 hours PRN. Maximum, 400 mg daily.

➤ **Pain severe enough to require daily, around-the-clock, long-term opioid treatment**
Adults ages 18 and older not taking immediate-release tablets: 100 mg extended-release form PO once daily. Titrate by 100 mg every 5 days to relieve pain. Do not exceed 300 mg/day.
Adults ages 18 and older currently taking immediate-release tablets: Calculate the 24-hour tramadol immediate-release dose and initiate a total daily dose of extended-release product rounded down to the next lowest 100-mg increment. Subsequently, individualize according to patient need. Maximum dosage, 300 mg daily.
Adjust-a-dose: For immediate-release form, if CrCl is less than 30 mL/minute, increase dose interval to every 12 hours; maximum, 200 mg daily. For patients with Child-Pugh class C liver impairment, give 50 mg (immediate-release) every 12 hours. For patients older than age 75, maximum is 300 mg (immediate-release) daily in divided doses. Don't use extended-release form in patients with Child-Pugh class C liver impairment or CrCl less than 30 mL/minute.

ADMINISTRATION
PO
• Give drug without regard to meals in a consistent manner.
• Have patient swallow extended-release capsules or tablets whole; don't crush or break capsules or tablets.

Reactions in bold italics are *life-threatening*.

Boxed Warning Avoid dosing errors when giving oral solution; don't confuse "mg" and "mL," which could result in accidental overdose and death. ∎

• Use an oral dosing device or calibrated syringe for solution to correctly measure prescribed amount.

• Patient undergoing dialysis can receive the regular dose on the day of dialysis.

ACTION

Unknown. Thought to bind to opioid receptors and inhibit reuptake of norepinephrine and serotonin.

Route	Onset	Peak	Duration
PO	1 hr	2–3 hr	Unknown
PO (extended-release)	Unknown	10–12 hr	Unknown

Half-life: 7.6 hours; extended-release, 8 to 10 hours.

ADVERSE REACTIONS

CNS: dizziness, headache, somnolence, drowsiness, vertigo, anxiety, asthenia, hypoesthesia, lethargy, CNS stimulation, confusion, coordination disturbance, ataxia, depersonalization, euphoria, malaise, nervousness, sleep disorder, insomnia, fever, paresthesia, tremor, hypertonia, depression, agitation, apathy, pain, restlessness. **CV:** vasodilation, flushing, chest pain, orthostatic hypotension, HTN, peripheral edema. **EENT:** visual disturbances, dry mouth, sore throat, nasal or sinus congestion, rhinorrhea, nasopharyngitis, pharyngitis, rhinitis, sinusitis. **GI:** constipation, nausea, vomiting, abdominal pain, anorexia, diarrhea, dyspepsia, flatulence, viral gastroenteritis. **GU:** menopausal symptoms, urinary frequency, urine retention, pelvic pain, UTI, prostate disorder. **Metabolic:** weight loss, hyperglycemia. **Musculoskeletal:** arthralgia, neck pain, back pain, limb pain, myalgia. **Respiratory:** bronchitis, URI. **Skin:** rash, diaphoresis, dermatitis, pruritus. **Other:** chills, hot flash, withdrawal syndrome, accidental injury, falls, flulike symptoms.

INTERACTIONS

Drug-drug. *Anticholinergics (atropine, benztropine, cyclopentolate):* May increase risk of urine retention or severe constipation and paralytic ileus. Monitor patient closely.

Boxed Warning *Benzodiazepines, CNS depressants:* May cause slow or difficult breathing, sedation, and death. Avoid use together. If use together is necessary, limit dosage and duration of each drug to minimum necessary for desired effect. ∎

Carbamazepine: May decrease tramadol level, decrease effect of carbamazepine, and increase CNS depression. Avoid use together.

Cyclobenzaprine, neuroleptics, other opioids, SSNRIs, SSRIs, TCAs: May increase risk of seizures. Monitor patient closely.

Boxed Warning *CYP2D6 inhibitors (bupropion, fluoxetine, quinidine):* May decrease therapeutic effect of tramadol. Monitor patient closely for withdrawal signs and symptoms, seizures, and serotonin syndrome. If inhibitor is discontinued, monitor patient for opioid toxicity, including respiratory depression. ∎

Boxed Warning *CYP3A4 inducers:* May decrease tramadol level. Monitor therapy closely. If inducer is discontinued, consider decreasing tramadol dosage and monitor patient for seizures, serotonin syndrome, sedation, and respiratory depression. ∎

Boxed Warning *CYP3A4 inhibitors:* May increase tramadol level. Monitor therapy closely. If inhibitor is discontinued, consider increasing tramadol dosage and monitor patient for opioid withdrawal. ∎

Digoxin: May increase risk of digoxin toxicity. Monitor therapy.

Diuretics: May decrease effectiveness of diuretic. Monitor therapy.

MAO inhibitors: May increase risk of serotonin syndrome. Concomitant use or use with 14 days of MAO inhibitor therapy is contraindicated.

Mixed agonist/antagonist and partial agonist opioid analgesics (buprenorphine, butorphanol, nalbuphine, pentazocine): May reduce analgesic effect of tramadol and precipitate withdrawal symptoms. Avoid use together.

Serotonergic drugs (amoxapine, antiemetics [dolasetron, granisetron, ondansetron, palonosetron], antimigraine drugs, buspirone, cyclobenzaprine, dextromethorphan, linezolid, lithium, maprotiline, methylene blue, mirtazapine, nefazodone, SSNRIs, SSRIs, TCAs, trazodone, tryptophan, vilazodone): May increase risk of serotonin syndrome. Use together cautiously and monitor patient for serotonin syndrome.

Warfarin: May increase anticoagulant effects. Monitor therapy closely.

T

Drug-herb. *Kava:* May increase CNS depression. Discourage use together.

🌢 *Alert:* *St. John's wort:* May increase risk of serotonin syndrome. Use together cautiously and monitor patient for serotonin syndrome.

Drug-lifestyle. **Boxed Warning** *Alcohol use:* May cause slow or difficult breathing, sedation, and death. Discourage use together. ■

EFFECTS ON LAB TEST RESULTS
• May increase BUN, creatinine, GGT, and liver enzyme levels.
• May decrease Hb, sodium, and glucose levels.

CONTRAINDICATIONS & CAUTIONS
Boxed Warning Prescribers are strongly encouraged to complete a REMS-compliant education program. Drug should be prescribed only by prescribers with knowledge of opioid use and ways to reduce associated risks. ■

• Contraindicated in patients hypersensitive to drug or opioids, in patients with Child-Pugh class C liver impairment, in patients who are suicidal, and in those with acute intoxication from alcohol, hypnotics, centrally acting analgesics, opioids, or psychotropic drugs.

• Contraindicated in patients with GI obstruction, including paralytic ileus.

• Contraindicated in patients with significant respiratory depression or acute or severe bronchial asthma or hypercapnia in unmonitored settings or where resuscitative equipment isn't available.

• Extended-release forms aren't recommended in patients with CrCl less than 30 mL/minute.

Boxed Warning Use exposes patient and others to risk of opioid addiction, abuse, and misuse, which can lead to overdose and death. These effects can occur at any dose or duration. Assess patient risk before prescribing and regularly reassess patient for these behaviors and conditions. ■

🌢 *Alert:* Use lowest effective dose for shortest period consistent with patient's treatment goals.

🌢 *Alert:* Because risk of overdose increases as opioid dose increases, reserve titration to higher doses for patients in whom lower doses are ineffective and in whom expected benefits of higher opioid dose outweigh risks.

🌢 *Alert:* Immediate-release formulations shouldn't be used for an extended period unless pain remains severe enough to require an opioid analgesic and alternative treatment options are inadequate to treat pain.

🌢 *Alert:* Long-acting or extended-release formulations are indicated for severe, persistent pain for which extended treatment with a daily opioid analgesic is required and for which alternative treatment options are inadequate. Use isn't indicated for as-needed analgesia.

Boxed Warning The effects of concomitant use or discontinuation of CYP3A4 inducers or inhibitors or CYP2D6 inhibitors with tramadol are complex and require careful consideration of the effects on tramadol and the active metabolite, M1. ■

Boxed Warning *Opioid class warning:* Opioids should only be prescribed with benzodiazepines or other CNS depressants when alternative treatment options are inadequate, not expected to provide adequate analgesia, haven't been tolerated, or aren't expected to be tolerated. ■

🌢 *Alert:* Serious hypersensitivity reactions can occur, usually after the first dose. Patients with history of anaphylactic reaction to codeine and opioids may be at increased risk.

🌢 *Alert:* Patients are at increased risk for oversedation and respiratory depression if they snore or have a history of sleep apnea, haven't used opioids recently or are first-time opioid users, have increased opioid dosage requirements or opioid habituation, have received general anesthesia for longer lengths of time or received other sedating drugs, have preexisting pulmonary or cardiac disease, or have thoracic or other surgical incisions that may impair breathing. Monitor patients carefully.

• Use cautiously in patients at risk for seizures or respiratory depression; in patients with increased ICP or head injury, acute abdominal conditions, or kidney or liver impairment; and in patients with physical dependence on opioids. Withdrawal symptoms may occur if drug is abruptly discontinued.

🌢 *Alert:* Drug can cause life-threatening serotonin syndrome.

🌢 *Alert:* Use cautiously in patients who are experiencing depression or emotional disturbance because of increased risk of suicide.

🌢 *Alert:* Drug may lead to rare but serious decrease in adrenal gland cortisol production.

• Drug may cause decreased sex hormone levels with long-term use.

Reactions in bold italics are *life-threatening*.

▧ **Boxed Warning** Life-threatening respiratory depression and death have occurred in children who received drug, mostly after tonsillectomy or adenoidectomy in children who have CYP2D6 polymorphism. Drug is contraindicated in children younger than age 12 and in children younger than age 18 after tonsillectomy or adenoidectomy. Avoid using drug in patients ages 12 to 18 who have risk factors that increase the risk of respiratory depression (postoperative status, obstructive sleep apnea, obesity, severe pulmonary disease, neuromuscular disease, use of other respiratory depressants). ■

Boxed Warning Accidental ingestion of even one dose of an opioid, especially by children, can result in a fatal overdose. ■

• Use with extreme caution in older adults and in patients with cachexia or debilitation.
Dialyzable drug: 7%.

⚠ *Overdose S&S:* Lethargy; somnolence; stupor; coma; seizures; skeletal muscle flaccidity; respiratory depression; cool, clammy skin; miosis; bradycardia; hypotension; cardiac arrest; death.

PREGNANCY-LACTATION-REPRODUCTION
• Safe use during pregnancy hasn't been established. Use only if potential benefit justifies fetal risk.

Boxed Warning Prolonged use during pregnancy can result in neonatal opioid withdrawal syndrome, which may be life-threatening. It requires management with expert neonatology protocols. If prolonged use is needed, advise patient of risks and ensure availability of proper treatment. ■

• Use during breastfeeding isn't recommended due to risk of serious adverse reactions in breastfed infants, such as excess sleepiness, difficulty breastfeeding, or serious breathing problems that could result in death.

NURSING CONSIDERATIONS
Boxed Warning May cause life-threatening or fatal respiratory depression at any time during therapy. Monitor patient closely, especially when starting or increasing doses. Proper dosing and titration are essential to reduce risk. ■

Boxed Warning Regularly monitor all patients for opioid addiction, abuse, and misuse, which can lead to overdose and death. ■

• Reassess patient's level of pain after administration.

🔹 *Alert:* Carefully monitor vital signs, pain level, respiratory status, and sedation level in all patients receiving opioids, especially those receiving IV drugs, even those given postoperatively.

• Monitor bowel and bladder function. Anticipate need for stimulant laxative.

• For better analgesic effect, give drug before onset of intense pain.

• Monitor patient at risk for seizures. Drug may reduce seizure threshold.

🔹 *Alert:* Drug may cause opioid-induced hyperalgesia (OIH). Symptoms include increased pain level with opioid dose increase, decreased pain level with opioid dose reduction, pain from ordinarily nonpainful stimuli without underlying disease progression, opioid tolerance or withdrawal, or addictive behavior. If OIH is suspected, decrease opioid dose or switch patient to alternative opioid.

• In case of an overdose, naloxone may also increase risk of seizures. Assess potential need for access to naloxone.

• Monitor patient for drug dependence. Drug can produce dependence like that of codeine and thus has risk of abuse.

• Monitor patient for hyponatremia (confusion, disorientation), especially when initiating therapy. Females older than age 65 may be at higher risk.

• Monitor patient, especially patient with predisposing risk factors for hypoglycemia (diabetes). Monitor blood glucose level and discontinue drug if appropriate.

🔹 *Alert:* Don't stop drug abruptly; withdraw slowly and individualize the gradual tapering plan to prevent signs and symptoms of withdrawal, worsening pain, and psychological distress in patients who are physically dependent. Refer to manufacturer's label for specific tapering instructions.

🔹 *Alert:* When tapering opioids, monitor patient closely for signs and symptoms of opioid withdrawal (restlessness, lacrimation, rhinorrhea, yawning, perspiration, chills, myalgia, mydriasis, irritability, anxiety, insomnia, backache, joint pain, weakness, abdominal cramps, anorexia, nausea, vomiting, diarrhea, increased BP or HR, increased respiratory rate). Such signs and symptoms may indicate a need to taper more slowly. Also monitor patient for suicidality, use of other substances, and mood changes.

🔹 *Alert:* If patient is taking opioids with serotonergic drugs, watch for signs and symptoms

T

of serotonin syndrome (agitation, hallucinations, rapid HR, fever, diaphoresis, shivering or shaking, muscle twitching or stiffness, trouble with coordination, nausea, vomiting, diarrhea), especially when starting treatment or increasing dosages. Signs and symptoms may occur within several hours of coadministration but may also occur later, especially after dosage increase. Discontinue the opioid, serotonergic drug, or both if serotonin syndrome is suspected.

● *Alert:* Monitor patient for signs and symptoms of adrenal insufficiency (nausea, vomiting, loss of appetite, fatigue, weakness, dizziness, low BP). Perform diagnostic testing if adrenal insufficiency is suspected. If adrenal insufficiency is confirmed, treat with corticosteroid and wean patient off opioid, if appropriate. Discontinue corticosteroid when clinically appropriate.

● Monitor patient for signs and symptoms of decreased sex hormone levels (low libido, erectile dysfunction, amenorrhea, infertility). If signs and symptoms occur, further evaluate patient.

● *Look alike–sound alike:* Don't confuse tramadol with trazodone or trandolapril.

PATIENT TEACHING

Boxed Warning Counsel patient and caregiver on serious risks, safe use, and importance of reading the medication guide with each prescription. ∎

● Advise patient to take drug exactly as prescribed and to use lowest dose possible for shortest time needed.

● Inform patient that, for acute pain, drug may only be needed for a few days. Teach patient about safe disposal of unused drug.

● Warn patient that extended-release and long-acting formulations aren't to be taken on an "as needed" basis.

● *Alert:* Counsel patient who has been regularly taking drug not to discontinue without first discussing the need for gradual tapering with prescriber.

● *Alert:* Warn patient to withhold drug and inform prescriber if pain level worsens, pain sensitivity increases, or new pain occurs after taking drug.

Boxed Warning Advise patient that crushing, chewing, or dissolving extended-release form can cause rapid release of the drug and a potentially fatal dose. ∎

Boxed Warning Tell patient to keep drug away from children. Accidental ingestion of even one dose of tramadol, especially in children, can result in fatal overdose. ∎

● Teach patient that naloxone may be prescribed with the opioid when beginning and renewing therapy to reduce risk of opioid overdose and death.

● Explain assessment and monitoring process to patient and family. Instruct them to immediately report difficulty breathing or other signs or symptoms of a potential adverse opioid-related reaction.

● Tell patient to take drug as prescribed and not to increase dose or dosage interval unless ordered by prescriber.

● Caution patient who is ambulatory to be careful when rising and walking. Warn outpatient to avoid driving and other potentially hazardous activities that require mental alertness until drug's CNS effects are known.

● Advise patient to check with prescriber before taking OTC drugs because drug interactions can occur.

● *Alert:* Encourage patient to report all medications being taken, including prescription and OTC medications and supplements because drug interactions can occur.

● Advise patient that drug may cause constipation.

● *Alert:* Caution patient to immediately report signs and symptoms of serotonin syndrome, adrenal insufficiency, and decreased sex hormone levels.

● Caution patient to report to prescriber pregnancy or plan to become pregnant.

SAFETY ALERT!
BIOSIMILAR DRUG

trastuzumab ▨
trass-too-ZOO-mab

Herceptin

trastuzumab-anns
Kanjinti

trastuzumab-dkst
Ogivri

trastuzumab-dttb
Ontruzant

Reactions in bold italics are *life-threatening*.

trastuzumab-pkrb
Herzuma

trastuzumab-qyyp
Trazimera

Therapeutic class: Antineoplastics
Pharmacologic class: Monoclonal antibodies

AVAILABLE FORMS
Lyophilized powder for injection: 150-mg single-dose vial, 420-mg multiple-dose vial

INDICATIONS & DOSAGES
Adjust-a-dose (for all indications): If LVEF decreased 16% or more from baseline or if LVEF is below normal limits with a 10% or more decrease from baseline, withhold treatment for at least 4 weeks and repeat LVEF every 4 weeks. May resume treatment if LVEF returns to normal within 4 to 8 weeks and remains at 15% or less decrease from baseline. Discontinue drug permanently for persistent (more than 8 weeks) LVEF decline or for more than three incidents of treatment interruptions for cardiomyopathy.

➤ **HER2-overexpressing metastatic gastric or gastroesophageal junction adenocarcinoma in patients not previously treated for metastatic disease in combination with cisplatin and capecitabine or 5-FU** ☒
Adults: Initially, 8 mg/kg IV infusion; then 6 mg/kg IV every 3 weeks until disease progression or intolerable toxicity occurs.

➤ **Metastatic breast cancer in patients whose tumors overexpress HER2 protein** ☒
Adults: Loading dose of 4 mg/kg IV infusion. If tolerated, continue with 2 mg/kg IV infusion weekly. If patient hasn't previously received one or more chemotherapy regimens for their metastatic disease, drug is given with paclitaxel. Continue until disease progression occurs.

➤ **After surgical resection of HER2-overexpressing node-positive, node-negative (ER/PR negative or with one high-risk feature) breast cancer** ☒
Adults: During treatment with paclitaxel, docetaxel, or docetaxel–carboplatin, give loading dose of 4 mg/kg IV infusion. Then 2 mg/kg IV weekly during chemotherapy for the first 12 weeks (paclitaxel or docetaxel) or 18 weeks (docetaxel–carboplatin). One week after the last weekly dose, continue trastuzumab 6 mg/kg IV every 3 weeks for up to a total of 52 weeks.

➤ **As single agent after surgical resection of HER2-overexpressing breast cancer within 3 weeks of completion of multimodality, anthracycline-based chemotherapy** ☒
Adults: Initial dose, 8 mg/kg IV infusion. Then 6 mg/kg IV every 3 weeks for up to a total of 52 weeks.

➤ **Neoadjuvant treatment of HER2-positive locally advanced, inflammatory, or early breast cancer** ☒ ◆
Adults: Initially, 8 mg/kg IV (cycle 1), followed by 6 mg/kg IV every 3 weeks for a total of four neoadjuvant cycles; postoperatively, three cycles of adjuvant FEC (5-FU, epirubicin, and cyclophosphamide) chemotherapy and continue trastuzumab to complete 1 year of treatment.

➤ **HER2-positive metastatic breast cancer (in combination with pertuzumab and docetaxel) in patients without prior anti-HER2 therapy or chemotherapy to treat metastatic disease** ☒ ◆
Adults: Initially, 8 mg/kg IV. Then maintenance dosage of 6 mg/kg IV every 3 weeks until disease progression or unacceptable toxicity occurs.

➤ **HER2-positive metastatic breast cancer (in combination with either docetaxel or vinorelbine)** ☒ ◆
Adults: Initially, 8 mg/kg IV. Then maintenance dosage of 6 mg/kg IV every 3 weeks until disease progression or unacceptable toxicity occurs (in combination with docetaxel or vinorelbine). Or, 4 mg/kg IV loading dose, followed by maintenance dosage of 2 mg/kg IV weekly until disease progression occurs (in combination with docetaxel).

➤ **HER2-positive, hormone receptor-positive metastatic breast cancer (in combination with an aromatase inhibitor) when chemotherapy isn't immediately indicated** ☒ ◆
Adults: Initially, 4 mg/kg IV. Then maintenance dosage of 2 mg/kg IV weekly until disease progression occurs (in combination with anastrozole).

➤ **HER2-overexpressing metastatic breast cancer (in combination with lapatinib) that had progressed on prior trastuzumab-containing therapy** ☒ ◆

T

Adults: Initially, 4 mg/kg IV. Then maintenance dosage of 2 mg/kg IV every week.

ADMINISTRATION

IV

✪ *Alert:* Hazardous drug; use safe handling and disposal precautions.

▼ Reconstitute drug with bacteriostatic water for injection, according to manufacturer's instructions for vial size, to yield a multidose solution containing 21 mg/mL. Don't shake vial during reconstitution. Make sure reconstituted preparation appears colorless to pale yellow and free of particulates.

▼ After reconstitution, use single-dose solution without preservative immediately or label multidose vial containing benzyl alcohol with expiration 28 days from date of reconstitution and refrigerate at 36° to 46° F (2° to 8° C).

▼ Discard unused portion in single-dose vial. Avoid use of other reconstitution diluents.

▼ Determine dose and calculate volume of 21-mg/mL solution needed. Withdraw this amount from vial and add it to an infusion bag containing 250 mL of NSS. Don't use D_5W or dextrose-containing solutions. Gently invert bag to mix solution. Store diluted solution in infusion bag containing NSS at 36° to 46° F (2° to 8° C) for no more than 24 hours before use. Don't freeze.

▼ If using 150-mg vial, reconstitute with 7.4 mL of sterile water for injection to yield a concentration of 21 mg/mL; add to 250-mL NSS infusion bag. Use immediately or refrigerate at 36° to 46° F (2° to 8° C) for no more than 24 hours.

▼ Don't give as IV push or bolus.

▼ Infuse loading dose over 90 minutes. If well tolerated, infuse maintenance doses over 30 to 90 minutes.

▼ If patient misses a dose by 1 week or less, give usual maintenance dose as soon as possible; don't wait until next planned cycle. Give subsequent maintenance doses 7 or 21 days later according to weekly or 3-weekly schedules, respectively. If patient misses a dose by more than 1 week, give a reloading dose as soon as possible, followed by maintenance dose 7 or 21 days later, according to weekly or 3-weekly schedules.

▼ Before reconstitution, store vials in refrigerator at 36° to 46° F (2° to 8° C).

▼ **Incompatibilities:** Other IV drugs or dextrose solutions.

ACTION

A recombinant DNA-derived monoclonal antibody that selectively binds to HER2, inhibiting proliferation of tumor cells that overexpress HER2.

Route	Onset	Peak	Duration
IV	Unknown	Unknown	Unknown

Half-life: Unknown.

ADVERSE REACTIONS

CNS: asthenia, dizziness, fever, headache, insomnia, pain, depression, neuropathy, paresthesia, peripheral neuritis, fatigue, altered taste. **CV:** peripheral edema, edema, *HF,* HTN, *arrhythmias,* tachycardia, decreased LVEF, palpitations. **EENT:** epistaxis, dysphagia, pharyngitis, rhinitis, sinusitis, nasopharyngitis, sore throat. **GI:** abdominal pain, anorexia, diarrhea, nausea, vomiting, constipation, dyspepsia, mucosal inflammation stomatitis. **GU:** UTI, *KF.* **Hematologic:** *leukopenia, neutropenia, thrombocytopenia,* anemia. **Metabolic:** weight loss, *hypokalemia.* **Musculoskeletal:** back pain, weakness, arthralgia, bone pain, muscle spasm, myalgia. **Respiratory:** dyspnea, cough, URI. **Skin:** rash, acne, nail disorder, pruritus. **Other:** *anaphylaxis,* chills, flulike syndrome, herpes simplex, infection, allergic reaction, infusion-related reaction, accidental injury.

INTERACTIONS

Drug-drug. `Boxed Warning` *Anthracyclines (daunorubicin, doxorubicin):* May increase risk of cardiac dysfunction. Avoid anthracycline-based therapy for up to 7 months after stopping trastuzumab–hyaluronidase. If used together, carefully monitor patient's cardiac function. ∎

Myelosuppressive chemotherapy: May increase neutropenic effect of myelosuppressant. Monitor therapy closely.

EFFECTS ON LAB TEST RESULTS

● May decrease potassium level.
● May decrease Hb level and platelet and WBC counts.

Reactions in bold italics are *life-threatening*.

CONTRAINDICATIONS & CAUTIONS

• Contraindicated in patients hypersensitive to drug.

• Use cautiously in older adults and in patients with cardiac dysfunction.

Boxed Warning Drug can cause serious and fatal infusion reactions and pulmonary toxicity. ■

• Use with extreme caution in patients with pulmonary compromise, symptomatic intrinsic pulmonary disease (asthma, COPD), or extensive tumor involvement of the lungs.

Boxed Warning Drug can cause subclinical and clinical HF, with greatest risk when administered concurrently with anthracyclines. ■

• Safety and effectiveness in children haven't been established.

Dialyzable drug: Unknown.

PREGNANCY-LACTATION-REPRODUCTION

Boxed Warning Exposure to drug during pregnancy can result in oligohydramnios, in some cases complicated by pulmonary hypoplasia, skeletal abnormalities, and neonatal death. Advise patient of these risks and the need for effective contraception. ■

• Advise patient of childbearing potential to use effective contraception during treatment and for 7 months after final dose.

• If drug is used during pregnancy or if patient becomes pregnant during therapy or within 7 months after final dose, fetal harm can occur. Immediately report Herceptin exposure to the Genentech Adverse Event Line (1-888-835-2555).

• It isn't known if drug appears in human milk. Patient should discontinue breastfeeding or discontinue drug, considering importance of drug to patient and the 7-month wash-out period after treatment.

NURSING CONSIDERATIONS

• Verify pregnancy status before start of therapy.

Boxed Warning Evaluate LVEF before and during treatment. Discontinue drug in patients receiving adjuvant therapy and withhold drug in those with metastatic disease for clinically significant decreases in LVEF. ■

• Assess LVEF by echocardiogram or MUGA scan before therapy, every 3 months during therapy, and when therapy ends.

• Repeat LVEF measurement at 4-week intervals if drug is withheld for significant left ventricular cardiac dysfunction.

• Assess LVEF every 6 months for 2 years after therapy ends when drug is used in adjuvant therapy.

• Monitor patient receiving both drug and chemotherapy closely for cardiac dysfunction or failure, anemia, kidney toxicity, leukopenia, diarrhea, and infection.

▩ Drug is only indicated in tumors with HER2 protein overexpression or HER2 gene amplification. Assessment of tumor specimens should be performed using FDA-approved tests specific for breast or gastric cancers by labs with demonstrated proficiency to obtain reliable results.

Boxed Warning Signs and symptoms of serious infusion reactions and pulmonary toxicity usually occur during or within 24 hours of infusion. Interrupt infusion if patient experiences dyspnea or clinically significant hypotension and monitor patient until signs and symptoms completely resolve. Discontinue drug for anaphylaxis, angioedema, interstitial pneumonitis, or ARDS. ■

• Assess for first-infusion symptom complex, commonly consisting of chills or fever. Other signs and symptoms include nausea, vomiting, pain, rigors, headache, dizziness, dyspnea, hypotension, rash, and asthenia and occur infrequently with subsequent infusions.

• For mild to moderate infusion reaction, decrease infusion rate. For dyspnea and hypotension, interrupt infusion. For severe infusion reaction, discontinue drug.

• *Look alike–sound alike:* Don't confuse trastuzumab with ado-trastuzumab emtansine or fam-trastuzumab deruxtecan. Don't confuse Herceptin with Herceptin Hylecta.

PATIENT TEACHING

• Warn about risk of first-dose infusion-related adverse reactions. Instruct patient to report all adverse reactions to prescriber.

• Urge patient to immediately notify prescriber if signs or symptoms of heart problems occur (shortness of breath, increased cough, swelling in arms or legs). Tell patient that these effects can occur after therapy ends.

• Caution patient to discuss breastfeeding during therapy with prescriber.

Boxed Warning Advise patient of the fetal risks of drug exposure and the need for effective contraception. ■

• Tell patient to avoid pregnancy during therapy and for 7 months after last dose and to immediately notify prescriber if pregnancy occurs during this time.

trastuzumab–hyaluronidase-oysk ⌧

tras-TOOZ-ue-mab/hye-al-ur-ON-i-dase

Herceptin Hylecta

Therapeutic class: Antineoplastics
Pharmacologic class: Monoclonal antibodies–endoglycosidases

AVAILABLE FORMS

Injection: 600 mg trastuzumab and 10,000 units hyaluronidase/5 mL in single-dose vial

INDICATIONS & DOSAGES

Adjust-a-dose (for all indications): Withhold drug for at least 4 weeks if a 16% or more absolute decrease in LVEF from pretreatment values occurs or if LVEF is below institutional limits of normal and a 10% or more absolute decrease in LVEF from pretreatment values occurs. May resume therapy within 4 to 8 weeks if LVEF returns to normal limits and the absolute decrease in LVEF from baseline is 15% or less. Permanently discontinue therapy for a persistent (more than 8 weeks) LVEF decline or for suspension of therapy on more than three occasions for cardiomyopathy.

➤ **Adjuvant treatment of HER2 overexpressing node-positive or node-negative (ER/PR-negative or with one high-risk feature) breast cancer as part of a treatment regimen with doxorubicin, cyclophosphamide, and either paclitaxel or docetaxel; as part of a treatment regimen with docetaxel and carboplatin; or as a single agent after multimodality anthracycline-based therapy** ⌧
Adults: 600 mg trastuzumab/10,000 units hyaluronidase subcut once every 3 weeks for 52 weeks or until disease recurrence. Extending treatment in adjuvant breast cancer beyond 1 year isn't recommended.

➤ **First-line treatment of HER2-overexpressing metastatic breast cancer in combination with paclitaxel or as a single agent for treatment of HER2-overexpressing breast cancer in patients** who have received one or more chemotherapy regimens for metastatic disease ⌧
Adults: 600 mg trastuzumab/10,000 units hyaluronidase subcut once every 3 weeks until disease progression occurs.

ADMINISTRATION
Subcutaneous

⊘ *Alert:* Hazardous drug; use safe handling and disposal precautions.

• Don't administer intravenously.

• Drug isn't interchangeable with conventional trastuzumab products, ado-trastuzumab emtansine, or fam-trastuzumab deruxtecan.

• Drug should be administered by a health care professional.

• Inspect visually for particulate matter and discoloration before administration; don't use vial if abnormalities are present.

• Discard any unused portion remaining in vial; vial is for single use only.

• To avoid needle clogging, attach hypodermic injection needle to syringe immediately before administration. Drug is compatible with syringes made with polypropylene and polycarbonate and with stainless steel transfer and injection needles.

• Withdraw solution from vial and into syringe; replace transfer needle with syringe closing cap. Label syringe with peel-off sticker.

• Alternate injection site between left and right thigh.

• Give new injections at least 1 inch (2.5 cm) from previous site on healthy skin and never into area where skin is red, bruised, tender, or hard or with moles or scars.

• Administer dose subcut over approximately 2 to 5 minutes.

• Can store prepared syringe in refrigerator at 36° to 46° F (2° to 8° C) for up to 24 hours and subsequently at 68° to 77° F (20° to 25° C) for up to 4 hours. Protect from light. Don't shake or freeze.

• If one dose is missed, give next dose as soon as possible. The interval between doses shouldn't be less than 3 weeks.

ACTION

Trastuzumab is a HER2/neu receptor antagonist that inhibits the proliferation of human tumor cells that overexpress HER2. Hyaluronidase is an enzyme shown to increase the absorption rate of a trastuzumab product into the systemic circulation.

Route	Onset	Peak	Duration
Subcut (trastuzumab)	Unknown	3 days	Unknown
Subcut (hyaluronidase)	Unknown	Unknown	24–48 hr

Half-life: trastuzumab, unknown; hyaluronan, 0.5 day.

ADVERSE REACTIONS

CNS: asthenia, fatigue, headache, fever, chills, dizziness, altered taste, insomnia, neuropathy, peripheral neuritis, paresthesia, pain, depression. **CV:** HTN, left ventricular dysfunction, decreased LVEF, *HF,* flushing, *arrhythmia,* tachycardia, edema. **EENT:** epistaxis, nasal inflammation or discomfort, sinusitis, pharyngitis, rhinitis. **GI:** nausea, diarrhea, vomiting, stomatitis, constipation, abdominal pain, dyspepsia, decreased appetite. **GU:** UTI, irregular menstruation, amenorrhea. **Hematologic:** *neutropenia,* anemia, *leukopenia, granulocytopenia, febrile neutropenia.* **Hepatic:** abnormal LFT values. **Musculoskeletal:** myalgia, arthralgia, back pain, limb pain, bone pain. **Respiratory:** cough, dyspnea, URI, bronchitis. **Skin:** alopecia, rash, radiation skin injury, incision-site pain and complications, cellulitis, nail disorder, pruritus, skin discoloration, acne, injection-site reactions, erythema. **Other:** accidental injury, hypersensitivity reactions, herpes simplex, viral infection, infection, flu-like syndrome, mucosal inflammation.

INTERACTIONS

Drug-drug. **Boxed Warning** *Anthracyclines (daunorubicin, doxorubicin):* May increase risk of cardiac dysfunction. Avoid anthracycline-based therapy for up to 7 months after stopping trastuzumab–hyaluronidase. If used together, carefully monitor patient's cardiac function. ■
Myelosuppressive chemotherapy: May increase neutropenic effect of myelosuppressants. Monitor therapy closely.

EFFECTS ON LAB TEST RESULTS
• May increase ALT level.
• May decrease WBC and RBC counts.

CONTRAINDICATIONS & CAUTIONS
Boxed Warning Drug can cause subclinical and clinical HF, with greatest risk when administered concurrently with anthracyclines. ■

Boxed Warning Drug can cause serious and fatal pulmonary toxicity, including dyspnea, interstitial pneumonitis, pulmonary infiltrates, pleural effusions, noncardiogenic pulmonary edema, pulmonary insufficiency and hypoxia, ARDS, and pulmonary fibrosis. Patients with symptomatic intrinsic lung disease or with extensive tumor involvement of lungs, resulting in dyspnea at rest, appear to have more-severe toxicity. ■
• May exacerbate chemotherapy-induced neutropenia.
• Severe administration-related reactions, including hypersensitivity and anaphylaxis, have been reported. Patients experiencing dyspnea at rest due to complications of advanced malignancy and comorbidities may be at increased risk for a severe or fatal administration-related reaction.
• Safety and effectiveness in children haven't been studied.
• Patients ages 65 and older are at increased risk for cardiac dysfunction.
Dialyzable drug: Unknown.

PREGNANCY-LACTATION-REPRODUCTION
Boxed Warning Drug can cause fetal harm (oligohydramnios and pulmonary hypoplasia, skeletal abnormalities) and neonatal death. Verify pregnancy status before start of treatment. Apprise patients who are pregnant and patients of childbearing potential that exposure to these drugs during pregnancy or within 7 months before conception can result in fetal harm. ■
Boxed Warning Patients of childbearing potential should use effective contraception during treatment and for 7 months after final dose. ■
• If drug is administered during pregnancy, or if patient becomes pregnant while receiving drug or within 7 months after the final dose, health care providers and patient should immediately report exposure to Genentech pregnancy pharmacovigilance program (1-888-835-2555).
• No information is available regarding the presence of trastuzumab or hyaluronidase in human milk. Discontinue drug or discontinue breastfeeding, considering importance of drug to patient and the 7-month wash-out period after treatment.

NURSING CONSIDERATIONS

• Verify pregnancy status before start of treatment.

Boxed Warning Monitor patient for pulmonary toxicity, which usually occurs during or within 24 hours of administration. Discontinue drug for anaphylaxis, angioedema, interstitial pneumonitis, or ARDS and monitor patient until symptoms completely resolve. Keep medications and emergency equipment immediately available. ∎

Boxed Warning Evaluate LVEF before and during treatment. Discontinue drug in patient receiving adjuvant therapy; withhold drug in patient with metastatic disease for clinically significant decreases in LVEF. ∎

• Obtain thorough baseline cardiac assessment, including history, physical exam, and determination of LVEF by echocardiogram or MUGA scan. Obtain baseline LVEF measurement immediately before initiation of therapy, then every 3 months during and upon completion of therapy. Repeat LVEF measurement at 4-week intervals if therapy is withheld for significant left ventricular cardiac dysfunction. Obtain LVEF measurements every 6 months for at least 2 years after completion of therapy as a component of adjuvant therapy.

• *Look alike–sound alike:* Don't confuse trastuzumab–hyaluronidase-oysk with ado-trastuzumab emtansine, fam-trastuzumab deruxtecan, or intravenous trastuzumab.

PATIENT TEACHING

Boxed Warning Advise patient to immediately report signs and symptoms of cardiotoxicity, including new-onset or worsening shortness of breath, cough, swelling of ankles or legs, swelling of face, palpitations, weight gain of more than 5 lb in 24 hours, dizziness, or loss of consciousness. ∎

Boxed Warning Warn patient who is pregnant or patient of childbearing potential of fetal risk from exposure to drug during pregnancy or within 7 months before conception. Caution patient of childbearing potential to use effective contraception during treatment and for 7 months after the final dose. ∎

• Explain that pregnancy testing is required before therapy begins. Instruct patient to immediately report known or suspected pregnancy.

• Advise patient to immediately report signs and symptoms of hypersensitivity and administration-related reactions (dizziness, nausea, chills, fever, vomiting, diarrhea, urticaria, angioedema, breathing problems, chest pain).

---

traZODone hydrochloride
TRAYZ-oh-dohn

Therapeutic class: Antidepressants
Pharmacologic class: Serotonin reuptake inhibitor

AVAILABLE FORMS
Tablets ⓘ: 50 mg, 100 mg, 150 mg, 300 mg

INDICATIONS & DOSAGES
➤ **Major depressive disorder**
Adults: Initially, 150 mg PO daily in divided doses; then increased by 50 mg daily every 3 to 4 days, as needed. Dosages range from 150 to 400 mg daily. Maximum, 600 mg daily for inpatients and 400 mg daily for outpatients.
Adjust-a-dose: After achieving an adequate response, gradually reduce dosage as needed depending on therapeutic response.

ADMINISTRATION
PO
• Give drug shortly after meals or a light snack to obtain optimal absorption and decrease risk of dizziness.
• If drowsiness occurs, consider giving a large portion of the dose at bedtime.
• Have patient swallows tablets whole or break them along the score lines. Don't crush tablets.

ACTION
Unknown. Inhibits CNS neuronal uptake of serotonin; not a tricyclic derivative.

Route	Onset	Peak	Duration
PO	Unknown	1–2 hr	Unknown

Half-life: 5 to 9 hours.

ADVERSE REACTIONS
CNS: drowsiness, dizziness, nervousness, fatigue, confusion, decreased concentration, malaise, tremor, headache, insomnia, syncope, disorientation, incoordination. **CV:** hypotension, HTN, edema. **EENT:** blurred vision, red or itchy eyes, tinnitus, dry mouth, nasal congestion. **GI:** constipation, nausea, vomiting, diarrhea. **Metabolic:** weight gain or loss. **Musculoskeletal:** aches, pains.

Reactions in bold italics are *life-threatening*.

INTERACTIONS
Drug-drug. *Amphetamines, antipsychotics, buspirone, dextromethorphan, dihydroer-gotamine, lithium salts, meperidine, opioid analgesics, SSRIs or SSNRIs (duloxetine, venlafaxine), sumatriptan (and other 5-HT₃ antagonists), TCAs, tramadol, tryptophan:* May increase the risk of serotonin syndrome. Avoid combining drugs that increase the availability of serotonin in the CNS; monitor patient closely if used together.
Anticoagulants (aspirin, clopidogrel, dabi-gatran, NSAIDs, rivaroxaban), antiplatelet agents: May increase risk of bleeding. Monitor patient closely.
Antihypertensives: May increase hypotensive effect of trazodone. Antihypertensive dosage may need to be decreased.
Clonidine, CNS depressants: May enhance CNS depression. Avoid use together.
CYP3A4 inducers (carbamazepine, pheny-toin, rifampin): May reduce trazodone level. Monitor patient closely; may need to increase trazodone dosage.
CYP3A4 inhibitors (clarithromycin, coni-vaptan, ketoconazole): May increase tra-zodone level. May cause nausea, hypotension, and fainting. Consider decreasing trazodone dosage. Avoid combination with conivaptan.
Digoxin, fosphenytoin, phenytoin: May increase levels of these drugs. Watch for toxicity.
Drugs that prolong QTc interval (antiar-rhythmics [amiodarone, disopyramide, pro-cainamide, quinidine, sotalol], chlorpro-mazine, gatifloxacin, thioridazine, ziprasi-done): May increase QTc-interval prolong-ing effect and risk of ventricular arrhythmias. Consider therapy modification.
Linezolid, methylene blue: May cause sero-tonin syndrome. Don't use together.
Alert: *MAO inhibitors (isocarboxazid, selegiline):* May increase risk of serotonin syndrome. Allow at least 14 days between discontinuing an MAO inhibitor and starting trazodone and at least 14 days after stopping trazodone before starting an MAO inhibitor.
Protease inhibitors (amprenavir, atazanavir, fosamprenavir, lopinavir–ritonavir, nelfin-avir, ritonavir, saquinavir): May increase trazodone levels and adverse effects. Monitor patient and adjust trazodone dose, as needed.
Warfarin: May increase risk of bleeding. Closely monitor INR.
Drug-herb. *Ginkgo biloba:* May cause seda-tion. Discourage use together.

St. John's wort: May cause serotonin syn-drome. Discourage use together.
Drug-lifestyle. *Alcohol use:* May enhance CNS depression. Discourage use together.

EFFECTS ON LAB TEST RESULTS
• May increase amylase, bilirubin, ALT, and AST levels.
• May decrease sodium level.
• May decrease Hb level.
• May increase WBC count.
• May cause false-positive urine test for amphetamine/methamphetamine.

CONTRAINDICATIONS & CAUTIONS
Boxed Warning Drug may increase risk of suicidality in children, adolescents, and young adults ages 18 to 24, especially during the first few months of treatment, especially those with major depressive disorder or other psychiatric disorder. Drug isn't approved for use in children. ■
• Contraindicated in patients hypersensitive to drug.
• Avoid use in patients with history of ar-rhythmias, symptomatic bradycardia, hy-pokalemia, hypomagnesemia, or known QT-interval prolongation; in combination with drugs that prolong QT interval; or during initial recovery phase of MI. Drug may in-crease risk of arrhythmias and prolong QTc interval.
Alert: Concomitant use with linezolid or methylene blue can cause serotonin syn-drome. Use drug with linezolid or methylene blue only for life-threatening or urgent condi-tions when potential benefit outweighs risk of toxicity.
• Use cautiously in patients at risk for sui-cide, in patients with kidney or liver impair-ment, in those with history of seizures, and with medications that may lower seizure threshold.
• Drug may increase risk of mixed-manic episodes. Screen patients for personal or fam-ily history of bipolar disorder, mania, or hy-pomania before starting therapy.
• May cause mild pupillary dilation, which may trigger an angle-closure attack in patients with anatomically narrow angles who don't have a patent iridectomy.
Dialyzable drug: Unlikely.
Overdose S&S: Priapism, respiratory arrest, seizures, ECG changes, drowsiness, vomiting.

PREGNANCY-LACTATION-REPRODUCTION

• Studies during pregnancy are inadequate. Use only if clearly needed and potential benefit justifies fetal risk.

• Encourage patients exposed to antidepressants during pregnancy to enroll in the National Pregnancy Registry for Antidepressants (866-961-2388 or https://womensmentalhealth.org/research/pregnancyregistry/antidepressants).

• Drug may appear in human milk. Use cautiously during breastfeeding.

NURSING CONSIDERATIONS

• Monitor patient for signs and symptoms of serotonin syndrome (mental status changes, tachycardia, labile BP, hyperreflexia, incoordination, nausea, vomiting, diarrhea) or NMS (hyperthermia, muscle rigidity, rapidly fluctuating vital signs, mental status change). If these signs and symptoms occur, immediately discontinue trazodone and any other serotonergic, antidopaminergic, or antipsychotic drugs.

• Monitor patient for hypotension.

• Using trazodone for depression in a patient who is bipolar can trigger a mixed-manic episode. If patient develops manic symptoms, withhold trazodone and initiate appropriate therapy.

⚠ *Alert:* If linezolid or methylene blue must be given, stop trazodone and monitor patient for serotonin toxicity for 2 weeks, or until 24 hours after last dose of methylene blue or linezolid, whichever comes first. May resume trazodone 24 hours after last dose of methylene blue or linezolid.

• Record mood changes. Monitor patient for suicidality and allow only minimum supply of drug.

• Consider evaluating patient who hasn't had an iridectomy for narrow-angle glaucoma risk factors.

• *Look alike–sound alike:* Don't confuse trazodone hydrochloride with tramadol hydrochloride. Don't confuse trazodone with ziprasidone.

PATIENT TEACHING

• Teach about proper drug administration and handling.

• Tell patient to report a persistent, painful erection (priapism); immediate intervention may be needed.

⚠ *Alert:* Advise patient to immediately report signs and symptoms of serotonin toxicity and NMS.

• Warn patient to avoid activities that require alertness and good coordination until effects of drug are known.

Boxed Warning Teach caregivers to recognize and report suicidality. ■

• Tell patient that it might take up to 6 weeks to see therapeutic effect if used for depression.

• Advise patient not to stop drug abruptly to avoid withdrawal symptoms.

• Caution patient to avoid alcohol because it will increase sedation.

• Advise patient to report pregnancy or plans to become pregnant or breastfeed during therapy.

tretinoin (retinoic acid, vitamin A acid)
TRET-i-noyn

Altreno, Atralin, Avita, Renova, Retin-A, Retin-A Micro, StieVA-A❋

Therapeutic class: Antiacne drugs
Pharmacologic class: Retinoids

AVAILABLE FORMS
Cream: 0.01%❋, 0.02%, 0.025%, 0.05%, 0.1%
Gel: 0.01%, 0.025%, 0.04%, 0.05%
Lotion: 0.05%
Microsphere gel: 0.04%, 0.06%, 0.08%, 0.1%

INDICATIONS & DOSAGES
➤ **Acne vulgaris (except Renova)**
Adults: Clean affected area and lightly apply once daily at bedtime.
Children ages 12 and older (Retin-A, Retin-A Micro, StieVA-A): Clean affected area and lightly apply once daily at bedtime.
Children ages 10 and older (Atralin): Clean affected area and lightly apply once daily at bedtime.
Children ages 9 and older (Altreno): Apply a thin layer to affected areas once daily.
➤ **Adjunctive use in the mitigation of fine facial wrinkles in patients who use comprehensive skin care and sunlight avoidance programs (Renova)**
Adults: Apply small, pea-size amount (¼ inch or 5 mm in diameter) to cover the entire face lightly, once daily in the evening.

---

*Reactions in bold italics are **life-threatening**.*

ADMINISTRATION
Topical
- 🜂 *Alert:* Hazardous drug; use safe handling and disposal precautions.
- Clean area thoroughly before application, and avoid getting drug in eyes, mouth, paranasal creases, or mucous membranes.
- Patients using Renova should gently wash face with mild soap, pat skin dry, and wait 20 to 30 minutes before applying medication.

ACTION
Modifies epithelial growth and differentiation. In acne, inhibits comedones by increasing epidermal cell mitosis and turnover.

Route	Onset	Peak	Duration
Topical	Unknown	Unknown	Unknown

Half-life: Unknown.

ADVERSE REACTIONS
Skin: dry skin, feeling of warmth, slight stinging, local erythema, pruritus, local skin exfoliation or desquamation, application-site pain, swelling, blistering, crusting, temporary hyperpigmentation or hypopigmentation, burning sensation, skin irritation, dermatitis, photosensitivity.

INTERACTIONS
Drug-drug. *Multivitamins:* May increase adverse effects of retinoic acid. Avoid use together.
Topical drugs containing benzoyl peroxide, resorcinol, salicylic acid, or sulfur: May increase risk of skin irritation. Avoid use together.
Topical minoxidil or photosensitizing drugs (fluoroquinolones, phenothiazines, sulfonamides, tetracyclines, thiazides): May increase risk of skin irritation. Avoid use together.
Drug-food. *Vitamin A:* Vitamin A supplementation can cause toxicity. Discourage excessive intake of vitamin A (cod liver oil, halibut fish oil).
Drug-lifestyle. *Abrasive cleansers, cream depilatories, medicated cosmetics, skin preparations containing alcohol, waxes:* May increase risk of skin irritation. Discourage use together.
Sun exposure, tanning lamps: May increase photosensitivity reaction. Advise patient to avoid excessive exposure.

EFFECTS ON LAB TEST RESULTS
None reported.

CONTRAINDICATIONS & CAUTIONS
- Contraindicated in patients hypersensitive to drug or its components and in those with sunburn.
- Use cautiously in patients with eczema.
- Use Atralin gel and Altreno lotion with caution in patients with known sensitivities or allergies to fish because gel contains soluble fish proteins.
- Use cautiously in patients with significant sun exposure (such as occupation-related) and in those inherently sensitive to sunlight.
Dialyzable drug: Unknown.
⚠ *Overdose S&S:* Marked redness, skin peeling, skin discomfort.

PREGNANCY-LACTATION-REPRODUCTION
- 🜂 *Alert:* Don't use if patient is pregnant, attempting to become pregnant, or at high risk for pregnancy.
- Studies during pregnancy are inadequate. Use of other agents is preferred.
- It isn't known if drug appears in human milk. Use cautiously during breastfeeding.

NURSING CONSIDERATIONS
- Initially, drug may be applied every 2 to 3 days using a lower concentration to reduce irritation.
- After satisfactory response, consider less-frequent applications or use of other formulations.
- *Look alike–sound alike:* Don't confuse tretinoin with trientine, triamcinolone, or isotretinoin.

PATIENT TEACHING
- Teach about proper drug administration and handling.
- Teach patient to wash hands after application.
- Warn patient against using strong or medicated cosmetics, soaps, or other skin cleansers. Also advise patient to avoid topical products containing alcohol, astringents, spices, and lime because they may interfere with drug's actions.
- Caution patient not to apply to sunburned skin.
- Tell patient using drug for treatment of fine wrinkles to avoid washing face or applying

T

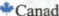

another skin product or cosmetic for 1 hour after application. Advise patient to apply skin moisturizer at least every morning to protect treated areas from dryness.

• Inform patient that normal use of cosmetics is allowed.

• Advise patient not to stop drug if temporary worsening of inflammatory lesions occurs. If severe local irritation develops, advise patient to stop drug temporarily and notify prescriber. Dosage will be readjusted when application is resumed. Some redness and scaling are normal reactions.

• Warn patient that increased sensitivity to wind or cold temperatures may occur.

• Instruct patient to minimize exposure to sunlight or UV rays during treatment. If sunburn develops, advise patient to delay therapy until sunburn subsides. Tell patient who can't avoid exposure to sunlight to use SPF-15 sunblock and to wear protective clothing.

• Warn patient that a temporary increase in lesions may occur, which will improve in 2 to 3 weeks.

• Tell patient not to use drug if pregnant or trying to become pregnant. Advise patient to stop drug and report suspected pregnancy.

---

triamcinolone acetonide (injection)

trye-am-SIN-oh-lone

Kenalog-10*, Kenalog-40*, Kenalog-80*, Triesence, Xipere, Zilretta

Therapeutic class: Corticosteroids
Pharmacologic class: Glucocorticoids

AVAILABLE FORMS

Injection (intra-articular, extended-release powder): 32 mg per vial
Injection (suspension): 10 mg/mL, 40 mg/mL, 80 mg/mL
Injection (intravitreal): 40 mg/mL
Injection (suprachoroidal): 40 mg/mL

INDICATIONS & DOSAGES

➤ **Severe inflammation, immunosuppression**

Adults: 60 mg IM; then 20 to 100 mg IM as needed every 6 weeks, if possible. Or, individualize initial intralesional dose depending on specific disease and lesion. For maintenance, use lowest dosage and time intervals to maintain adequate clinical response. Or, initially, 2.5 to 15 mg into joints (depending on joint size) or soft tissue; then may increase to 10 mg for smaller areas and 40 mg for larger areas. Maximum dose (several joints at one time), 80 mg.

Children: Dosage varies depending on specific disease. Initial dose range, 0.11 to 1.6 mg/kg/day IM in three or four divided doses (3.2 to 48 mg/m² BSA/day). Or, 2.5 to 5 mg for smaller joints or 5 to 15 mg for larger joints, depending on specific disease.

➤ **Management of osteoarthritis pain of the knee (Zilretta extended-release)**

Adults: 32 mg (5 mL) as single intra-articular injection. Drug isn't intended for repeat administration.

➤ **Ophthalmic diseases (sympathetic ophthalmia, temporal arteritis, uveitis, ocular inflammatory conditions unresponsive to topical corticosteroids)**

Adults and children: 4 mg (100 mcL of 40 mg/mL suspension) injected intravitreally, with subsequent doses as needed during treatment.

➤ **Visualization during vitrectomy**

Adults and children: 1 to 4 mg (25 to 100 mcL of 40 mg/mL suspension) injected intravitreally.

➤ **Macular edema associated with uveitis (Xipere only)**

Adults: 4 mg as single suprachoroidal injection.

ADMINISTRATION

IM (Kenalog-40 or Kenalog-80)

• Give deep into gluteal muscle. Rotate injection sites to prevent muscle atrophy.

• Don't use 10 mg/mL strength for this route.

• Shake well before use and ensure there's no clumping.

• Administer immediately after withdrawal to prevent settling in the syringe.

• Don't administer IV or via epidural or intrathecal route.

Intra-articular

• Prepare extended-release product only using diluent supplied in kit. Refer to manufacturer labeling for preparation instructions and administration techniques.

• Promptly inject after preparation.

Reactions in bold italics are *life-threatening*.

• If needed, may store in vial for up to 4 hours at ambient conditions. Gently swirl vial to resuspend any settled microspheres before preparing syringe for injection.

• Extended-release form isn't interchangeable with other formulations of injectable triamcinolone acetonide.

• Strict aseptic technique is mandatory.

• Drug is commonly administered with a local anesthetic.

• Refrigerate extended-release product before use. If unable to refrigerate, store sealed, unopened kits at or below 77° F (25° C) for up to 6 weeks; then discard.

Intralesional (Kenalog-10)

• Strict aseptic technique is mandatory.

• Inject directly into lesion intradermally or subcutaneously.

• Use of a tuberculin syringe and small-bore needle (23G to 25G) is preferable.

Intravitreal

• Before injecting, give adequate anesthesia and broad-spectrum microbicide.

• Shake vial vigorously for 10 seconds to ensure uniform suspension. Inspect suspension for clumping or granules. If present, don't use.

• Inject drug without delay under controlled aseptic conditions.

• Each vial is for treatment of a single eye only.

• Protect from light. Don't freeze. Store between 39° and 77° F (4° and 25° C).

Suprachoroidal

• Before injecting, give adequate anesthesia and broad-spectrum microbicide.

• Shake vial vigorously for 10 seconds to ensure uniform suspension. Inspect suspension for clumping or granules. If present, don't use.

• Inject only using SCS Microinjector under aseptic conditions. Administer injection without delay to prevent settling.

• Each vial is for treatment of a single eye.

• Protect from light. Don't freeze. Store between 59° and 77° F (15° and 25° C).

ACTION

Not clearly defined. Decreases inflammation, mainly by stabilizing leukocyte lysosomal membranes; suppresses immune response; stimulates bone marrow; influences protein, fat, and carbohydrate metabolism; and suppresses adrenal function at high doses.

Route	Onset	Peak	Duration
IM, intra-articular, intralesional	12–48 hr	Unknown	30–42 days
Intra-articular (extended-release)	Unknown	7 hr	Unknown
Intravitreal, supra-choroidal	Unknown	Unknown	Unknown

Half-life: 300 minutes; intravitreal, 13 to 24 days.

ADVERSE REACTIONS

⚠ **Alert:** Systemic reactions associated with corticosteroid therapy are possible. Refer to manufacturer's prescribing information for additional information.

CNS: euphoria, insomnia, *pseudotumor cerebri, seizures,* headache, paresthesia, psychotic behavior, vertigo, *stroke.* **CV:** *arrhythmias, HF, thromboembolism,* HTN, edema, thrombophlebitis. **EENT:** cataracts, dry eye, photophobia, vitreous floaters, uveitis, punctate keratitis, conjunctival edema, eyelid ptosis, glaucoma, increased IOP, eye pain and inflammation, reduced visual acuity, conjunctival hemorrhage, sinusitis, injection-site reactions (ophthalmic injections). **GI:** *pancreatitis,* GI irritation, peptic ulceration, increased appetite, nausea, vomiting. **GU:** menstrual irregularities, increased urine calcium level. **Metabolic:** *hypokalemia,* hyperglycemia, carbohydrate intolerance, hypercholesterolemia, hypocalcemia. **Musculoskeletal:** growth suppression in children, muscle weakness, osteoporosis, acute myopathy, joint swelling. **Respiratory:** cough. **Skin:** hirsutism, delayed wound healing, acne, various skin eruptions, contusions. **Other:** *acute adrenal insufficiency,* cushingoid state, susceptibility to infections after increased stress or abrupt withdrawal after long-term therapy.

INTERACTIONS

Drug-drug. *Anticholinesterase drugs (ambenonium, neostigmine):* May cause severe weakness in patients with myasthenia gravis. Withdraw anticholinesterase drug at least 24 hours before corticosteroid therapy, if possible.

Antidiabetics: May increase blood glucose level. Adjust dosage of antidiabetics as needed.

Aspirin, indomethacin, other NSAIDs: May increase risk of GI distress and bleeding. Use together cautiously.

T

Barbiturates, carbamazepine, fosphenytoin, phenytoin, rifampin: May decrease corticosteroid effect. Increase corticosteroid dosage.

Cyclosporine: May increase toxicity and seizures. Monitor patient closely.

CYP3A4 inhibitors (clarithromycin, ketoconazole, nefazodone, ritonavir), macrolide antibiotics: May increase corticosteroid adverse effects. Use together cautiously and monitor patient for adverse effects.

Digoxin: May increase risk of hypokalemia-related arrhythmias. Monitor patient.

Estrogens, hormonal contraceptives: May decrease metabolism of some corticosteroids. Monitor therapy.

Isoniazid: May decrease isoniazid level and antituberculin effect. Monitor therapy.

Oral anticoagulants: May alter dosage requirements. Closely monitor PT and INR.

Potassium-depleting drugs (thiazide and loop diuretics, amphotericin B): May enhance potassium-wasting effects of triamcinolone. Monitor potassium level.

Salicylates: May decrease salicylate level. Monitor for lack of salicylate effectiveness.

Skin-test antigens: May decrease response. Postpone skin testing until after therapy.

Toxoids, vaccines: May decrease antibody response and increase risk of neurologic complications. Defer routine administration of vaccines or toxoids until corticosteroid therapy is discontinued, if possible.

Drug-herb. *Echinacea:* May decrease therapeutic effect of immunosuppressants. Discourage use together.

EFFECTS ON LAB TEST RESULTS
* May increase sodium and glucose levels.
* May decrease potassium and calcium levels.
* May alter reactions to skin tests.

CONTRAINDICATIONS & CAUTIONS
* Contraindicated in patients hypersensitive to drug or its ingredients, in patients with cerebral malaria, in those with systemic fungal infections, and in those receiving immunosuppressive doses together with live-virus vaccines.
* IM injections are contraindicated in patients with ITP.
* Intravitreal injections are contraindicated in patients with active ocular herpes simplex virus.
* Suprachoroidal injections are contraindicated in patients with active or suspected

ocular or periocular infections, including most viral diseases of cornea and conjunctiva, active epithelial herpes simplex keratitis, vaccinia, varicella, mycobacterial infections, and fungal diseases.
* Extended-release form is for intra-articular use only for osteoarthritis pain of knee as one-time injection; repeat dosing hasn't been studied.
* Safety and effectiveness of extended-release and suprachoroidal forms in children haven't been established.
* Use cautiously in patients with recent MI, GI ulcer, kidney disease, HTN, osteoporosis, diabetes, hypothyroidism, cirrhosis, diverticulitis, nonspecific ulcerative colitis, recent intestinal anastomoses, seizures, thromboembolic disorders, myasthenia gravis, active hepatitis, lactation, HF, TB, ocular herpes simplex, emotional instability, or psychotic tendencies.
* **Alert:** Use of corticosteroids increases risk of cataracts.

Dialyzable drug: Unknown.

PREGNANCY-LACTATION-REPRODUCTION
* Some manufacturers report that human studies show that triamcinolone acetonide can cause fetal harm. Use only if potential benefit justifies fetal risk.
* Carefully observe infants born to patients who have received corticosteroids during pregnancy for signs and symptoms of hypoadrenalism.
* Drug appears in human milk and could suppress infant growth, interfere with endogenous corticosteroid production, or cause other untoward effects. Use cautiously during breastfeeding.

NURSING CONSIDERATIONS
* Determine whether patient is sensitive to other corticosteroids.
* Always adjust to lowest effective dose.
* Most adverse reactions to corticosteroids are dose- or duration-dependent.
* Monitor patient's weight, BP, and glucose and electrolyte levels. If used for more than 6 weeks, monitor IOP.
* Monitor for cushingoid effects (moon face, buffalo hump, central obesity, thinning hair, HTN, increased susceptibility to infection).
* Watch for depression or psychotic episodes, especially during high-dose therapy.

Reactions in bold italics are *life-threatening*.

• For patient with diabetes, monitor glucose level. Increased insulin dosage may be needed.

• Drug may mask or worsen infections, including latent amebiasis.

• Older adults may be more susceptible to osteoporosis with long-term use.

• Unless contraindicated, give low-sodium diet that's high in potassium and protein. Give potassium supplements as needed.

• Gradually reduce dosage after long-term (more than 10 to 14 days) therapy.

🔋 *Alert:* Ophthalmic injections must be performed under mandatory aseptic technique, which includes use of sterile gloves, sterile drape, and sterile eyelid speculum.

🔋 *Alert:* Monitor patient receiving ophthalmic injections for increased IOP, which can lead to glaucoma and damage to optic nerve.

• Intra-articular injection may be complicated by joint infection. Increased pain accompanied by local swelling, further restriction of joint motion, fever, and malaise suggest septic arthritis. For confirmed septic arthritis, institute appropriate antimicrobial therapy.

• *Look alike–sound alike:* Don't confuse triamcinolone with Triaminic. Don't confuse Kenalog with Ketalar.

PATIENT TEACHING

• Tell patient not to stop drug abruptly or without prescriber's consent.

• Review signs and symptoms of early adrenal insufficiency (fever, fatigue, muscle weakness, joint pain, anorexia, nausea, shortness of breath, dizziness, fainting).

• Instruct patient to carry medical identification that includes prescriber's name and drug's name and dosage and indicates patient's need for supplemental systemic glucocorticoids during stress.

• Warn patient on long-term therapy about cushingoid effects (moon face, buffalo hump) and the need to notify prescriber about sudden weight gain and swelling.

• Tell patient to report slow wound healing.

• Advise patient receiving long-term therapy to consider exercise or physical therapy. Also, tell patient to ask prescriber about vitamin D or calcium supplement.

• Instruct patient to avoid exposure to infections and to notify prescriber if exposure occurs.

• Tell patient to report ophthalmic signs and symptoms (eye pain, redness, sensitivity to light, vision loss or disturbance) to prescriber and to seek immediate care from an ophthalmologist if any occur.

• Caution patient to report pregnancy or breastfeeding to prescriber.

triamcinolone acetonide (intranasal)
trye-am-SIN-oh-lone

Nasacort Allergy 24 Hour ◊,
Nasacort AQ ◊🍁

Therapeutic class: Corticosteroids
Pharmacologic class: Corticosteroids

AVAILABLE FORMS
Nasal spray: 55 mcg/spray ◊

INDICATIONS & DOSAGES
➤ **Nasal symptoms of seasonal and perennial allergic rhinitis**
Adults and children ages 12 and older: 2 sprays in each nostril once daily while sniffing gently; may decrease to 1 spray in each nostril once daily after symptom control. Adjust to minimum effective dosage.
Children ages 6 to 11: 1 spray in each nostril once daily while sniffing gently. Maximum, 2 sprays in each nostril once daily. Adjust to minimum effective dosage.
Children ages 2 to 5: 1 spray in each nostril once daily while sniffing gently.
Adjust-a-dose: Start older adults at lower end of dosing range.

ADMINISTRATION
Intranasal
• Shake well before each use.
• Release 5 sprays into air to prime before first use. Reprime with 1 spray if not used for 2 weeks or more.
• Instruct patient to gently blow nose to clear nostrils.
• Insert nozzle into nostril, pointing away from septum. Hold other nostril closed and have patient sniff gently while spraying.
• Instruct patient not to blow nose for 15 minutes after use.

ACTION
Controls the rate of protein synthesis, depresses migration of polymorphonuclear leukocytes and fibroblasts, reverses capillary

T

permeability, and stabilizes lysosomal membranes at the cellular level.

Route	Onset	Peak	Duration
Intranasal	Unknown	1.5–4 hr	Unknown

Half-life: About 3 hours.

ADVERSE REACTIONS

CNS: headache, bitter taste. **EENT:** nasal irritation, burning, epistaxis, nasal and sinus congestion, rhinitis, nasopharyngitis, oral candidiasis, sinusitis, sneezing, stinging, throat pain, rhinorrhea, excoriation, tooth disorder, nasal dryness. **GI:** dyspepsia, nausea, vomiting, upper abdominal pain, diarrhea. **Respiratory:** *asthma symptoms,* cough, bronchitis. **Skin:** rash. **Other:** flulike syndrome.

INTERACTIONS
None reported.

EFFECTS ON LAB TEST RESULTS
None reported.

CONTRAINDICATIONS & CAUTIONS
• Contraindicated in patients hypersensitive to drug or its components and in those with untreated mucosal infection.
• Use with caution, if at all, in patients with active or quiescent tuberculous infection of respiratory tract, glaucoma, cataracts, increased IOP, ocular herpes simplex, eye infection, or untreated fungal, bacterial, or systemic viral infection.
• Use cautiously in patients already receiving systemic corticosteroids because of increased likelihood of HPA axis suppression.
• Use cautiously in patients with recent nasal septal ulcers, nasal surgery, or trauma because drug may inhibit wound healing.
• Use cautiously in patients with severe or recurrent nosebleeds.
• Drug isn't indicated for use in children younger than age 2 when used for self-medication.
Dialyzable drug: Unknown.
⚠ *Overdose S&S:* GI upset, nasal irritation, headache.

PREGNANCY-LACTATION-REPRODUCTION
• Studies during pregnancy are inadequate. Other agents may be preferred during pregnancy. Use only if potential benefit justifies fetal risk.

• It isn't known if drug appears in human milk. Use cautiously during breastfeeding.

NURSING CONSIDERATIONS
❸ *Alert:* Excessive doses may cause signs and symptoms of hyperadrenocorticism and adrenal axis suppression; stop drug slowly.
• To decrease risk of adverse effects, individualize drug dosage and titrate to minimum effective dosage.
• Monitor growth rate in children, which may be slower while using this product, especially if child needs to use spray for longer than 2 months a year.
• Discontinue drug if symptom relief hasn't occurred after 1 week of treatment.
• *Look alike–sound alike:* Don't confuse triamcinolone with Triaminic.

PATIENT TEACHING
• Teach patient how to use nasal spray, including how to prime pump.
• Instruct patient to avoid getting aerosol in eyes or mouth. If this occurs, tell patient to rinse with copious amounts of cool tap water.
• Tell patient not to blow nose for 15 minutes after use.
• Stress importance of using drug on a regular schedule because its effectiveness depends on regular use. Warn patient not to exceed prescribed dosage.
• Tell patient to notify prescriber if signs and symptoms don't diminish or if condition worsens in 1 week.
• Warn patient to avoid exposure to chickenpox or measles and, if exposed, to notify prescriber.
• Instruct patient to watch for and report signs and symptoms of nasal infection. Drug may need to be stopped.

triamcinolone acetonide (topical)
trye-am-SIN-oh-lone

Aristocort✹, Kenalog, Oracort✹, Oralone, Triderm, Tritocin

Therapeutic class: Corticosteroids
Pharmacologic class: Corticosteroids

AVAILABLE FORMS
Aerosol*: 0.2 mg/2-second spray (0.147 mg/g)
Cream: 0.025%, 0.1%, 0.5%

Reactions in bold italics are *life-threatening*.

Dental paste: 0.1%
Lotion: 0.025%, 0.1%
Ointment: 0.025%, 0.05%, 0.1%, 0.5%

INDICATIONS & DOSAGES
➤ **Inflammation and pruritus from corticosteroid-responsive dermatoses**
Adults and children: Clean area; apply aerosol, cream, lotion, or ointment sparingly b.i.d. to q.i.d. Rub in lightly. Or, 3 or 4 applications of spray daily.
➤ **Symptom relief from oral inflammatory and ulcerative oral lesions**
Adults and children: Apply paste at bedtime and, if needed, b.i.d. to q.i.d., preferably after meals.

ADMINISTRATION
Topical
● Gently wash skin before applying. To avoid skin damage, rub in gently, leaving a thin coat. When treating hairy sites, part hair and apply directly to lesions.
● Don't apply near eyes or in ear canal.
● When using aerosol near face, cover patient's eyes and warn against inhaling spray. Aerosol contains alcohol and may cause irritation or burning when used on open lesions. Spray at 3 to 6 inches (7.6 to 15.25 cm) from affected area.
● Occlusive dressings may be used in severe or resistant dermatoses.
● Apply small amount of dental paste to oral lesion without rubbing; press to lesion until thin film develops.
● Instruct patient not to rinse after using dental paste and to avoid eating or drinking for 30 minutes after application.

ACTION
Unclear. Diffuses across cell membranes to form complexes with cytoplasmic receptors, showing anti-inflammatory, antipruritic, vasoconstrictive, and antiproliferative activity.

Route	Onset	Peak	Duration
Topical	Several hr	Unknown	1 wk

Half-life: Biologic, 18 to 36 hours.

ADVERSE REACTIONS
EENT: oral mucosa changes; oral burning, itching, irritation, dryness, maceration, atrophy, blistering, or peeling. **GU:** glycosuria. **Metabolic:** hyperglycemia. **Skin:** burning, pruritus, irritation, dryness, erythema,

folliculitis, hypertrichosis, hypopigmentation, acneiform eruptions, perioral dermatitis, allergic contact dermatitis, maceration, desquamation, atrophy, striae, miliaria. **Other:** *HPA axis suppression,* Cushing syndrome, secondary infection.

INTERACTIONS
Drug-drug. *Aldesleukin:* Corticosteroids may decrease antineoplastic effect. Avoid combination.

EFFECTS ON LAB TEST RESULTS
● May increase glucose level.

CONTRAINDICATIONS & CAUTIONS
● Contraindicated in patients hypersensitive to drug or its components.
● Contraindicated in the presence of fungal, viral, or bacterial infections of the mouth or throat (paste).
● Don't use as monotherapy in primary bacterial infections (impetigo, paronychia, erysipelas, cellulitis, angular cheilitis), treatment of rosacea, perioral dermatitis, or acne.
● Considered a medium-potency (0.025% and 0.1% cream, ointment, lotion) and high-potency (0.5% cream, ointment) drug, according to vasoconstrictive properties.
● Don't use very-high-potency or high-potency agents on face, groin, or axilla areas.
● Drug isn't for ophthalmic use.
● Prolonged corticosteroid therapy may interfere with growth and development in children.
● Use cautiously in older adults because of age-related changes in skin integrity and risks associated with systemic absorption.
Dialyzable drug: Unknown.
⚠ **Overdose S&S:** Systemic effects, including reversible HPA axis suppression, Cushing syndrome, hyperglycemia, glycosuria.

PREGNANCY-LACTATION-REPRODUCTION
● Studies during pregnancy are inadequate. Use only if potential benefit justifies fetal risk. Don't use in large amounts or for prolonged periods during pregnancy.
● It isn't known if drug appears in human milk. Use cautiously during breastfeeding.

NURSING CONSIDERATIONS
● Monitor for and report occurrence of skin infection, striae, or atrophy.

T

- If antifungal or antibiotic combined with corticosteroid fails to provide prompt improvement, stop corticosteroid until infection is controlled.
- Systemic absorption is more likely with use of occlusive dressings, prolonged treatment, or extensive body surface treatment.
- Avoid using plastic pants or tight-fitting diapers on treated areas in young children. Children may absorb larger amounts of drug and be more susceptible to systemic toxicity.
- Monitor skin integrity.
- If used for prolonged time and on large skin areas, monitor patient for HPA axis suppression and fungal or bacterial superinfection.
- When used in oral cavity, reevaluate if no improvement occurs in 7 days.
- When using aerosol solution, reevaluate if no improvement occurs in 2 weeks.

PATIENT TEACHING
- Teach about proper drug administration and handling.
- Advise patient not to use an occlusive dressing unless instructed to. If an occlusive dressing is ordered, advise patient to leave it in place for no longer than 12 hours each day and not to use the dressing on infected or weeping lesions.
- Caution patient that aerosol is flammable. Patient should avoid heat, flames, and smoking when applying aerosol.
- Tell patient to stop drug and report signs of systemic absorption, skin irritation or ulceration, hypersensitivity, infection, or lack of improvement.

triamterene–hydroCHLOROthiazide
try-AM-tur-een/hye-droe-klor-oh-THYE-a-zide

Maxzide, Maxzide-25

Therapeutic class: Antihypertensives-diuretics
Pharmacologic class: Thiazide diuretics-potassium-sparing diuretics

AVAILABLE FORMS
Capsules: triamterene 37.5 mg/hydrochlorothiazide 25 mg
Tablets: triamterene 37.5 mg/hydrochlorothiazide 25 mg, triamterene 75 mg/hydrochlorothiazide 50 mg

INDICATIONS & DOSAGES
➤ **HTN or edema in patients who develop hypokalemia on hydrochlorothiazide alone or who require a thiazide diuretic and in whom development of hypokalemia can't be risked**
Adults: Triamterene 37.5 mg/hydrochlorothiazide 25 mg PO one or two tablets or capsules daily as a single dose. Or, triamterene 75 mg/hydrochlorothiazide 50 mg PO daily.

ADMINISTRATION
PO
- May give drug without regard to meals, but can give with food to minimize GI upset.
- To prevent nocturia, give drug in the morning.
- Giving two tablets or capsules in divided doses may increase risk of electrolyte imbalance and kidney dysfunction; give as single dose once daily.

ACTION
Triamterene works on distal tubule and collecting duct to inhibit reabsorption of sodium in exchange for potassium and hydrogen. Hydrochlorothiazide increases excretion of sodium, chloride, potassium, hydrogen, and water by inhibiting reabsorption in distal segment of the nephron.

Route	Onset	Peak	Duration
PO (triamterene)	2–4 hr	1 hr	7–9 hr
PO (hydrochlorothiazide)	2 hr	4 hr	6–12 hr

Half-life: Triamterene, 1.5 to 2.5 hours; hydrochlorothiazide, 6 to 15 hours.

ADVERSE REACTIONS
CNS: weakness, fatigue, dizziness, fever, headache, drowsiness, insomnia, depression, anxiety, vertigo, restlessness, paresthesia, taste alteration. **CV:** *arrhythmia,* orthostatic hypotension, chest pain, tachycardia. **EENT:** yellow vision, transient blurred vision, dry mouth, inflamed salivary gland. **GI:** diarrhea, nausea, vomiting, constipation, abdominal pain, *pancreatitis,* change in appetite, gastric irritation, cramping. **GU:** erectile dysfunction, *AKI,* glycosuria, interstitial nephritis, kidney stones, urine discoloration. **Hematologic:** *leukopenia, thrombocytopenia,* purpura, anemia, *agranulocytosis.* **Hepatic:** jaundice, altered LFT results.

Reactions in bold italics are *life-threatening*.

Metabolic: *hyperkalemia, hypokalemia,* hyperglycemia, diabetes, hyperuricemia, hyponatremia, *metabolic acidosis,* hypochloremia, hypercalcemia, *hypomagnesemia.* **Musculoskeletal:** muscle cramps. **Respiratory:** shortness of breath, *pulmonary edema.* **Skin:** rash, urticaria, photosensitivity. **Other:** hypersensitivity.

INTERACTIONS

Drug-drug. *ACE inhibitors and ARBs, potassium-containing medications (penicillin G potassium):* May increase risk of hyperkalemia. Use together cautiously.

Adrenocorticotropic hormone, amphotericin B, beta$_2$-agonists, corticosteroids: May increase electrolyte depletion, particularly potassium. Use together carefully.

Amiloride, spironolactone, triamterene-containing agents: May increase risk of hyperkalemia. Use together is contraindicated.

Antidiabetics (oral agents and insulin): May increase or decrease blood glucose level. Dosage adjustment of antidiabetic may be required.

Antigout drugs: May increase uric acid level. Increase dosage of antigout medication, if indicated.

Barbiturates, opioids: May increase risk of orthostatic hypotension. Use together cautiously.

Bile acid sequestrants: May decrease absorption of thiazide diuretics. Consider therapy modification.

Calcium salts, multivitamins: May decrease calcium excretion. Monitor therapy closely.

Dofetilide: May increase QTc interval-prolonging effect of dofetilide. Avoid use together.

Lithium: May increase lithium level, especially in patients with kidney insufficiency. Avoid use together.

NSAIDs: May diminish antihypertensive effects and increase risk of AKI. Use together cautiously.

Neuromuscular blocking agents, nondepolarizing (tubocurarine): May increase responsiveness to muscle relaxant. Avoid use together.

Other antihypertensives: May increase risk of hypotension. Use together carefully and adjust dosage as appropriate.

Polystyrene, other exchange resins: May reduce potassium level, increase sodium retention, and increase edema. Avoid use together except in presence of hyperkalemia.

Potassium supplements: May increase risk of hyperkalemia. Avoid use together.

Vitamin D analogues (calcipotriene, calcitriol, ergocalciferol, paricalcitol): May increase hypercalcemic effect of vitamin D. Monitor therapy closely.

Drug-herb. *Yohimbe:* May decrease antihypertensive effect of hydrochlorothiazide. Monitor therapy closely.

Drug-food. *Salt substitutes with potassium:* May increase risk of hyperkalemia. Discourage use together.

Drug-lifestyle. *Alcohol use:* May increase risk of orthostatic hypotension. Discourage use together.

Sun exposure: May increase risk of photosensitivity. Discourage sun exposure.

EFFECTS ON LAB TEST RESULTS

• May increase BUN, creatinine, liver enzyme, calcium, uric acid, cholesterol, and triglyceride levels.
• May increase urine glucose level.
• May decrease folic acid, sodium, chloride, magnesium, and phosphate levels.
• May increase or decrease potassium level and blood glucose level.
• May decrease protein-bound iodine level without signs of thyroid imbalance.
• May decrease leukocyte and platelet counts.
• May interfere with quinidine assays and parathyroid function tests.

CONTRAINDICATIONS & CAUTIONS

Boxed Warning Abnormal elevation of serum potassium level (5.5 mEq/L or more) can occur and is more likely in patients with kidney impairment or diabetes (even without concurrent kidney impairment), in older adults, and in patients with severe illness. ■
• Contraindicated in patients hypersensitive to either drug or to sulfonamides and in those with preexisting hyperkalemia, anuria, AKI, and CKD.
• Don't use fixed-dose combinations for initial therapy, except in patients in whom hyperkalemia can't be risked (patients taking cardiac glycosides and those with history of cardiac arrhythmias).
• Use cautiously in patients with impaired liver function, electrolyte imbalances, or lupus and in those with history of kidney stones or gout.

• Use cautiously in patients at risk for metabolic or respiratory acidosis. Closely monitor acid-base balance and electrolyte levels.

• Safety and effectiveness in children haven't been established.

Dialyzable drug: Unlikely.

⚠ *Overdose S&S:* Hyperkalemia or hypokalemia, dehydration, nausea, vomiting, weakness, hypotension, lethargy, GI irritation, coma.

PREGNANCY-LACTATION-REPRODUCTION

• Studies during pregnancy are inadequate. Use only if potential benefit justifies fetal risk.

• Hydrochlorothiazide is present in human milk; excretion of triamterene isn't known. Patient should discontinue breastfeeding or discontinue drug, considering importance of drug to patient.

NURSING CONSIDERATIONS

Boxed Warning Monitor potassium level at initiation of therapy, with dosage changes, and with any illness that may influence kidney function. ■

• Watch for warning signs and symptoms of hyperkalemia (paresthesia, muscular weakness, fatigue, flaccid paralysis, bradycardia, shock). For suspected hyperkalemia, obtain potassium level and ECG.

• If hyperkalemia is present, stop combination and use thiazide alone.

• For potassium level greater than 6.5 mEq/L, consider IV calcium chloride, sodium bicarbonate, glucose, or sodium polystyrene sulfonate; consider dialysis if no improvement occurs.

• Monitor patient for infection (sore throat, fever), which could be a sign of leukopenia, or for bruising, which could be a sign of thrombocytopenia.

• Monitor for acute myopia and secondary angle-closure glaucoma (acute vision changes, ocular pain usually within hours to weeks of drug ingestion), especially in patient with history of possible sulfonamide or penicillin allergy. Discontinue drug as soon as possible if symptoms occur.

• Monitor for hyperuricemia or acute gout. Antigout drug dosages may need adjustment.

• Thiazides may alter calcium and phosphate levels. Discontinue drug before testing parathyroid function.

• Monitor patient with diabetes for changes in antidiabetic or insulin requirements. Patients with latent diabetes may become fully diabetic during therapy.

• Monitor BP, fluid balance, LFT values, and electrolyte levels.

PATIENT TEACHING

• Teach patient to report light-headedness, especially during first few days of therapy. Warn patient to discontinue drug and notify prescriber if syncope occurs.

• Caution patient to notify prescriber if fluid loss occurs from excessive perspiration, dehydration, vomiting, or diarrhea.

• Advise patient not to use salt substitutes that contain potassium.

• Instruct patient to promptly report signs and symptoms of infection or bruising.

• Explain that, to be effective, drug must be taken daily as prescribed. Instruct patient to continue to take drug even if feeling well.

• Advise patient to avoid taking drug at bedtime to prevent nighttime diuresis.

• Review warning signs and symptoms of fluid and electrolyte imbalances (decreased urine production; drowsiness; dry mouth; fast HR; fatigue; low BP; muscle fatigue, pain, or cramps; restlessness; stomach disturbances; thirst; weakness).

• Advise patient to keep follow-up appointments to monitor electrolyte levels.

• Warn patient to avoid sun exposure.

• Caution patient to avoid alcohol to decrease risk of sudden drop in BP.

• Instruct patient to consult prescriber before taking other prescription or OTC medications, herbal products, or vitamin and mineral supplements.

SAFETY ALERT!

triazolam
trye-AY-zoe-lam

Halcion

Therapeutic class: Hypnotics
Pharmacologic class: Benzodiazepines
Controlled substance schedule: IV

AVAILABLE FORMS
Tablets: 0.125 mg, 0.25 mg

Reactions in bold italics are *life-threatening*.

INDICATIONS & DOSAGES
➤ **Short-term treatment (7 to 10 days) of insomnia**
Adults: 0.25 mg PO at bedtime. May increase to maximum of 0.5 mg if response to lower dose is inadequate.
Adjust-a-dose: Older adults, patients with low body weight, and patients who are debilitated: 0.125 mg PO at bedtime. Maximum dose, 0.25 mg.

ADMINISTRATION
PO
• Don't give drug with or right after a meal.
• Give immediately before bedtime; onset is rapid.

ACTION
Unknown. Probably acts on the limbic system, thalamus, and hypothalamus of the CNS to produce hypnotic effects by increasing levels of the inhibitory neurotransmitter GABA.

Route	Onset	Peak	Duration
PO	15–30 min	<2 hr	6–7 hr

Half-life: 1.5 to 5.5 hours.

ADVERSE REACTIONS
CNS: drowsiness, ataxia, dizziness, headache, nervousness, light-headedness. **GI:** nausea, vomiting.

INTERACTIONS
Drug-drug. *Anticonvulsants, antihistamines, CNS depressants, dronabinol, magnesium sulfate, psychotropics:* May cause excessive CNS depression. Use together cautiously.
Cimetidine, fluvoxamine, isoniazid, macrolide antibiotics (clarithromycin, erythromycin), oral contraceptives, ranitidine: May increase triazolam level. Monitor patient closely and consider triazolam dosage reduction.
CYP3A4 inducers (dexamethasone, phenytoin, rifampin): May decrease triazolam level. Consider alternative drug (strong inducers) or monitor therapy closely (moderate inducers).
Moderate or weak CYP3A inhibitors (diltiazem): May increase CNS depression and prolong effects of triazolam. Reduce triazolam dosage.
Boxed Warning *Opioids:* May cause slow or difficult breathing, sedation, coma, and death. Avoid use together. If use together is necessary, limit dosage and duration of each drug to minimum necessary for desired effect. ■

Strong CYP3A inhibitors (azole antifungals [ketoconazole, miconazole], lopinavir, nefazodone, ritonavir, saquinavir): May increase and prolong triazolam level. Use together is contraindicated.
Drug-herb. *Calendula, hops, kava, lemon balm, passion flower, skullcap, valerian:* May enhance sedative effect of drug. Discourage use together.
St. John's wort: May decrease triazolam level. Discourage use together.
Yohimbe: May decrease effect of antianxiety agents. Monitor therapy closely.
Drug-food. *Grapefruit, grapefruit juice:* May delay onset and increase drug effects. Discourage use together.
Drug-lifestyle. ◑ *Alert:* Alcohol use: May cause additive CNS effects. Discourage use together.

EFFECTS ON LAB TEST RESULTS
• May increase LFT values.

CONTRAINDICATIONS & CAUTIONS
• Contraindicated in patients hypersensitive to drug or other benzodiazepines.
Boxed Warning Benzodiazepine use exposes patient to risk of abuse, misuse, and addiction, which can lead to overdose or death. Assess each patient's risk of abuse, misuse, and addiction before prescribing and periodically during therapy. ■
• Prescription should be written for short-term use of 7 to 10 days, with quantities limited to a 1-month supply.
Boxed Warning Abrupt discontinuation or rapid dosage reduction of benzodiazepines after continued use may precipitate acute withdrawal reactions, which can be life-threatening. To reduce risk of withdrawal reactions, gradually taper drug to discontinue or reduce dosage. ■
Boxed Warning Opioids should only be prescribed with benzodiazepines to patients for whom alternative treatment options are inadequate. ■
• Use cautiously in patients with impaired liver or kidney function, chronic pulmonary insufficiency, sleep apnea, mental depression, suicidality, or history of drug abuse.
• Minor changes in EEG patterns (usually low-voltage fast activity) may occur during and after therapy.

T

Dialyzable drug: Unlikely.

⚠ *Overdose S&S:* Somnolence, impaired co-ordination, slurred speech, confusion, coma, decreased reflexes, hypotension, seizures, respiratory depression, apnea, death.

PREGNANCY-LACTATION-REPRODUCTION

• Drug may cause fetal harm. Patient should stop drug before becoming pregnant. If patient becomes pregnant, apprise patient of fetal risk.

• Data collection on pregnancy exposure is ongoing at the National Pregnancy Registry for Psychiatric Medications (1-866-961-2388 or https://womensmentalhealth.org/pregnancyregistry).

• Monitor infants exposed to drug during pregnancy for respiratory depression, sedation, withdrawal, and feeding problems.

• Drug may appear in human milk. Use during breastfeeding isn't recommended.

NURSING CONSIDERATIONS

❸ *Alert:* Anaphylaxis and angioedema may occur as early as first dose; monitor patient closely.

• Assess mental status before starting therapy, and reduce dosages in older adult.

• Use lowest effective dose; significant dose-related adverse reactions can occur.

• Use of drug for more than 3 weeks requires patient evaluation for primary psychiatric or medical conditions, which may be causing insomnia.

• Monitor for abnormal thinking and behavior changes (aggressiveness, extroversion, bizarre behavior, agitation, hallucinations, depersonalization, worsening depression).

• Take precautions to prevent hoarding or overdosing by patient who is depressed, suicidal, or drug-dependent or who has history of drug abuse.

• Monitor patient for increased daytime anxiety.

• *Look alike–sound alike:* Don't confuse triazolam with alprazolam. Don't confuse Halcion with Haldol or halcinonide.

PATIENT TEACHING

Boxed Warning Caution patient or caregiver of patient taking an opioid with a benzodiazepine, CNS depressant, or alcohol to seek immediate medical attention if patient experiences dizziness, light-headedness, extreme sleepiness, slowed or difficult breathing, or unresponsiveness. ■

Boxed Warning Caution patient that benzodiazepines, even at recommended dosages, increase risk of abuse, misuse, and addiction, which can lead to overdose and death, especially when used in combination with other drugs (opioid analgesics), alcohol, or illicit substances. ■

Boxed Warning Warn about signs and symptoms of benzodiazepine abuse, misuse, and addiction (abdominal pain, amnesia, anorexia, anxiety, aggression, ataxia, blurred vision, confusion, depression, disinhibition, disorientation, dizziness, euphoria, impaired concentration and memory, indigestion, irritability, muscle pain, slurred speech, tremors, vertigo, delirium, paranoia, suicidality, seizures, difficulty breathing, coma). Instruct patient and caregiver to seek emergency medical help if any occur. Review proper disposal of unused drug. ■

• Advise patient not to take drug at higher dose, more frequently, or for longer than prescribed.

Boxed Warning Tell patient that continued use of drug for several days to weeks may lead to physical dependence and that abrupt discontinuation or rapid dosage reduction may precipitate acute withdrawal reactions (unusual movements, responses, or expressions; seizures; sudden and severe mental or nervous system changes; depression; seeing or hearing things that others don't; homicidal thoughts; extreme increase in activity or talking; losing touch with reality; suicidality), which can be life-threatening. Instruct patient that discontinuation or dosage reduction may require a slow taper. ■

Boxed Warning Advise patient about possibility of developing protracted withdrawal syndrome (anxiety; trouble remembering, learning, or concentrating; depression; problems sleeping; feeling like insects are crawling under skin; weakness; shaking; muscle twitching; burning or prickling feeling in hands, arms, legs, or feet; ringing in ears), with symptoms lasting weeks to more than 12 months. ■

❸ *Alert:* Warn patient that drug may cause allergic reactions, facial swelling, and complex sleep-related behaviors (driving, eating, and making phone calls while asleep). Advise patient to report these effects.

• Warn patient not to take more than prescribed amount; overdose can occur at total

daily dose of 2 mg (or four times highest recommended amount).
- Tell patient to avoid alcohol use while taking drug.
- Caution patient to avoid performing activities that require mental alertness or physical coordination.
- Inform patient that drug doesn't tend to cause morning drowsiness.
- Tell patient that rebound insomnia may occur for 1 or 2 nights after stopping therapy.
- Caution patient to avoid pregnancy and breastfeeding while taking drug.
- Advise patient to take drug immediately before bedtime and not with, or immediately after, a meal.
- Instruct patient to consult prescriber before taking other prescription or OTC medications or herbal products.

trospium chloride
TROZ-pee-um

Trosec✦

Therapeutic class: Urinary antispasmodics
Pharmacologic class: Antimuscarinics

AVAILABLE FORMS
Capsules (extended-release): 60 mg
Tablets: 20 mg

INDICATIONS & DOSAGES
➤ **Overactive bladder (urinary urge incontinence, urgency, frequency)**
Adults: 20 mg (immediate-release) tablet PO b.i.d. Or, 60 mg extended-release capsule PO once daily in the morning.
Adjust-a-dose: For adults ages 75 and older, reduce dosage to 20 mg (immediate-release) PO once daily based on patient tolerance. For CrCl of less than 30 mL/minute, give 20 mg (immediate-release) PO once daily at bedtime. Extended-release form isn't recommended if CrCl falls below 30 mL/minute.

ADMINISTRATION
PO
- Give tablets at least 1 hour before meals or on an empty stomach.
- Give extended-release form in the morning with water on an empty stomach at least 1 hour before meal.

ACTION
Relaxes smooth muscle of the bladder by antagonizing muscarinic receptors, relieving symptoms of overactive bladder.

Route	Onset	Peak	Duration
PO	Unknown	5–6 hr	Unknown

Half-life: About 20 hours (immediate-release); 35 hours (extended-release).

ADVERSE REACTIONS
CNS: fatigue, headache. **CV:** tachycardia. **EENT:** dry eyes, mouth, and nose; nasopharyngitis. **GI:** constipation, abdominal pain and distention, dyspepsia, flatulence, nausea. **GU:** urine retention, UTI. **Skin:** rash. **Other:** flulike symptoms.

INTERACTIONS
Drug-drug. *Anticholinergics (scopolamine, hyoscyamine):* May increase dry mouth, constipation, and other adverse effects. Monitor patient.
Metformin: May decrease trospium level. Monitor patient closely.
Opioid analgesics: May increase risk of constipation and urine retention. Monitor therapy closely.
Prokinetic GI agents (metoclopramide): May decrease therapeutic effect of GI prokinetic agents. Monitor therapy closely.
Drug-food. *High-fat foods:* May significantly decrease absorption. Give drug at least 1 hour before meals or on an empty stomach.
Drug-lifestyle. *Alcohol use:* May increase drowsiness. Use of alcoholic beverages within 2 hours of taking extended-release capsules isn't recommended. Discourage use together.

EFFECTS ON LAB TEST RESULTS
None reported.

CONTRAINDICATIONS & CAUTIONS
- Contraindicated in patients hypersensitive to drug or any of its ingredients and in those with or at risk for urine retention, gastric retention, or uncontrolled narrow-angle glaucoma.
- Use cautiously in patients with significant bladder outflow obstruction, obstructive GI disorders, ulcerative colitis, intestinal atony, myasthenia gravis, kidney insufficiency, Child-Pugh class B or C liver impairment, or controlled narrow-angle glaucoma.
- Safety and effectiveness in children haven't been determined.

Dialyzable drug: Unknown.
⚠ *Overdose S&S:* Severe anticholinergic effects, tachycardia, mydriasis.

PREGNANCY-LACTATION-REPRODUCTION
● Studies during pregnancy are inadequate. Use only if potential benefit justifies fetal risk.
● It isn't known if drug appears in human milk. Use during breastfeeding only if potential benefit justifies risk to infant.

NURSING CONSIDERATIONS
● Assess patient to determine baseline bladder function, and monitor patient for therapeutic effects.
● Angioedema of face, lips, tongue, or larynx, which may be life-threatening, can occur after first dose. Discontinue drug and promptly provide treatment to ensure a patent airway.
● Various CNS anticholinergic effects have been reported, including dizziness, confusion, hallucinations, and somnolence. Monitor patient for anticholinergic CNS effects, particularly after beginning treatment or increasing dosage. Dosage may need to be reduced or drug discontinued.
● If patient has bladder outflow obstruction, watch for evidence of urine retention.
● Monitor patient for decreased gastric motility and constipation.
● Periodically monitor kidney and liver function during therapy.

PATIENT TEACHING
● Teach about proper drug administration and handling.
● Caution patient about risk of angioedema. Instruct patient to seek immediate medical care for difficulty breathing or swelling of tongue or throat.
● Discourage use of other drugs that may cause dry mouth, constipation, blurred vision, or urine retention.
● Tell patient that alcohol use may increase drowsiness and fatigue. Discourage alcohol consumption. Advise patient not to use alcohol within 2 hours of taking extended-release capsules.
● Explain that drug may decrease sweating and increase risk of heatstroke when used in hot environments or during strenuous activities.
● Urge patient to avoid activities that are hazardous or require mental alertness until drug's effects are known.

● Advise patient to report pregnancy or plans to become pregnant or breastfeed during therapy.

---

uliPRIStal acetate ⚠
UE-li-PRIS-tal

Ella

Therapeutic class: Contraceptives
Pharmacologic class: Progesterone agonists-antagonists

AVAILABLE FORMS
Tablets: 30 mg

INDICATIONS & DOSAGES
➤ **Prevention of pregnancy following unprotected intercourse or known or suspected contraceptive failure**
Adult females and postmenarchal adolescents: 30 mg (1 tablet) PO as soon as possible within 120 hours (5 days) after unprotected intercourse or known or suspected contraceptive failure.

ADMINISTRATION
PO
🔵 *Alert:* Hazardous drug; use safe-handling and disposal precautions.
● Give drug without regard to food.
● If vomiting occurs within 3 hours of tablet ingestion, may repeat dose.
● May give at any time during menstrual cycle.

ACTION
Inhibits or delays ovulation and alters the endometrium to avoid egg implantation; prevents progestin from binding to progesterone receptor.

Route	Onset	Peak	Duration
PO	Unknown	1 hr	Unknown

Half-life: 26 to 38 hours.

ADVERSE REACTIONS
CNS: headache, fatigue, dizziness. **GI:** nausea, abdominal pain. **GU:** dysmenorrhea, intermenstrual bleeding, irregular menses.

INTERACTIONS
Drug-drug. *CYP3A4 inducers (barbiturates, bosentan, carbamazepine, efavirenz, felbamate, griseofulvin, oxcarbazepine, phenytoin,*

---

rifampin, topiramate): May decrease effectiveness of contraceptive. Avoid use together.
CYP3A4 inhibitors (itraconazole, ketoconazole): May increase serum ulipristal level and risk of adverse reactions. Monitor patient.
Hormonal contraceptives (progestin): May impair ability of ulipristal to delay ovulation or decrease effectiveness of regular hormonal contraceptives. Hormonal contraceptives shouldn't be resumed until 5 days after patient takes ulipristal. Patient should use reliable barrier method of contraception until next menstrual period.
Drug-herb. *St. John's wort:* May decrease effectiveness of contraceptive. Avoid use together.

EFFECTS ON LAB TEST RESULTS
None reported.

CONTRAINDICATIONS & CAUTIONS
• Contraindicated for termination of existing pregnancy or as routine contraception.
• Contraindicated in females who are prepubescent or postmenopausal.
• Safety and effectiveness of repeated use within same menstrual cycle aren't known; repeat use isn't recommended.
⊠ Drug exposure in patients of South Asian descent may exceed that in patients who are White or Black; however, no difference in effectiveness and safety was observed.
Dialyzable drug: Unknown.

PREGNANCY-LACTATION-REPRODUCTION
• Studies during pregnancy are inadequate. Drug is contraindicated during pregnancy.
• Drug appears in human milk. Effect of drug exposure on newborns and infants hasn't been studied; risk to infants who are breastfed can't be excluded.

NURSING CONSIDERATIONS
• Rule out pregnancy before use.
• Perform follow-up physical and pelvic exam if patient's health or pregnancy status is a concern after drug administration.
• Exclude ectopic pregnancy in patient who becomes pregnant or complains of lower abdominal pain 3 to 5 weeks after ulipristal use.
• Fertility returns rapidly after drug administration; patient should initiate or continue routine contraceptives as soon as possible but not sooner than 5 days after emergency contraception.

• Drug may reduce effectiveness of regular hormonal contraceptives; additional use of a barrier method is recommended for subsequent intercourse during same menstrual cycle.
• After drug administration, menses can occur a few days earlier or later than usual. For menses delayed beyond 1 week, rule out pregnancy.
• Drug doesn't protect against HIV infection or other STIs.
• *Look alike–sound alike:* Don't confuse ulipristal with ursodiol.

PATIENT TEACHING
• Teach patient that drug isn't intended for routine use as a contraceptive and should only be used once per menstrual cycle.
• Advise patient not to take additional levonorgestrel emergency contraceptive pills within 5 days of ulipristal acetate.
• Instruct patient to take as soon as possible and not more than 120 hours (5 days) after unprotected intercourse or known or suspected contraceptive failure.
• Warn patient not to use ulipristal during pregnancy or to breastfeed for 24 hours after taking drug.
• Tell patient to contact prescriber if vomiting occurred within 3 hours of taking drug.
• Advise patient to immediately report lower abdominal pain.
• Instruct patient to resume routine contraceptives no sooner than 5 days after ulipristal and to use a barrier method during same menstrual cycle.
• Advise patient that after drug administration, menses can occur a few days earlier or later than usual. Tell patient to report late menses beyond 1 week because testing will be necessary to rule out pregnancy.
• Warn patient that drug doesn't protect against HIV infection or other STIs.

U

ursodiol
ur-soe-DYE-ol

Reltone, Urso Forte, Urso 250

Therapeutic class: Miscellaneous GI drugs
Pharmacologic class: Bile acids

AVAILABLE FORMS
Capsules: 200 mg, 300 mg, 400 mg
Tablets: 250 mg, 500 mg

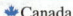

INDICATIONS & DOSAGES
➤ **Gallstone dissolution (capsules only)**
Adults: 8 to 10 mg/kg daily PO in two or three divided doses.
➤ **Gallstone prevention in patients undergoing rapid weight loss (capsules only)**
Adults: 600 mg PO daily or 300 mg PO b.i.d.
➤ **Primary biliary cholangitis (PBC) (tablets only)**
Adults: 13 to 15 mg/kg PO daily in two to four divided doses.

ADMINISTRATION
PO
• Give capsules without regard to food.
• Give tablets with food.
• May break scored tablets in half to achieve recommended dose. Don't use tablet segments that break incorrectly.
• Due to bitter taste, store halved tablets separately from whole tablets.
• Store at room temperature.

ACTION
Decreases secretion of cholesterol from the liver, reabsorbs cholesterol by the intestine, and subsequently decreases the cholesterol content of bile stones. Increases bile acid level and displaces toxic levels of endogenous hydrophobic bile acids that accumulate in cholestatic liver disease.

Route	Onset	Peak	Duration
PO	Unknown	3 wk	Unknown

Half-life: Unknown.

ADVERSE REACTIONS
CNS: dizziness, fatigue, headache, insomnia. **CV:** chest pain. **EENT:** allergy, pharyngitis, rhinitis, sinusitis. **GI:** abdominal pain, constipation, diarrhea, dyspepsia, flatulence, GI disorder, nausea, peptic ulcer, vomiting. **GU:** increased creatinine level, UTI, dysmenorrhea. **Hematologic:** *leukopenia, thrombocytopenia.* **Hepatic:** cholecystitis. **Metabolic:** increased glucose level. **Musculoskeletal:** arthralgia, arthritis, back pain, musculoskeletal pain, myalgia. **Respiratory:** bronchitis, cough, URI. **Skin:** alopecia, rash. **Other:** flu-like symptoms, viral infection.

INTERACTIONS
Drug-drug. *Aluminum-based antacids:* May reduce ursodiol absorption. Give antacid 2 hours after ursodiol or consider therapy modification.
Bile acid sequestrants (cholestyramine, colestipol): May reduce ursodiol absorption. Give ursodiol 1 hour before or at least 4 to 5 hours after sequestrant. Monitor therapy.
Clofibrate, estrogens, oral contraceptives: May counteract effect of ursodiol. Avoid use together.

EFFECTS ON LAB TEST RESULTS
• May increase LFT values and glucose and creatinine levels.
• May decrease WBC and platelet counts.

CONTRAINDICATIONS & CAUTIONS
• Capsules are contraindicated in patients with calcified cholesterol stones, radiopaque stones, and radiolucent bile pigment stones, which ursodiol can't dissolve.
• Capsules are contraindicated in patients with compelling reasons for cholecystectomy, including unremitting acute cholecystitis, cholangitis, biliary obstruction, gallstone pancreatitis, or biliary GI fistula.
• Tablets are contraindicated in patients with biliary obstruction.
• Contraindicated in patients with hypersensitivity or intolerance to ursodiol or bile acids.
• Use cautiously for gallstone indications in patients with chronic liver disease and in patients with a nonvisualized gallbladder.
• Patients with variceal bleeding, hepatic encephalopathy, or ascites and those in need of an urgent liver transplant should receive appropriate specific treatment.
• Patients treated for PBC who present with GI obstruction symptoms should be evaluated for enteroliths (bozoars). Patients with intestinal stenosis or stasis (Crohn disease, surgical enteroanastomoses) may be at increased risk.
• Safety and effectiveness in children haven't been established.
• Use cautiously in older adults.
Dialyzable drug: Unlikely.

PREGNANCY-LACTATION-REPRODUCTION
• Studies during pregnancy are inadequate. Routine use during pregnancy isn't recommended.
• Available data show drug may be used cautiously during pregnancy for intrahepatic cholestasis, especially during second and third trimesters.

• Drug may appear in human milk. Use cautiously during breastfeeding.

NURSING CONSIDERATIONS
• Monitor LFTs at baseline, every month for 3 months, and then every 6 months in patients with PBC.
• Monitor AST and ALT levels at baseline and as clinically indicated in patient receiving drug for gallstones.
• Obtain gallbladder ultrasounds every 6 months for first year of therapy to monitor gallstone response. If gallstones have dissolved, continue therapy, and obtain repeat ultrasound within 1 to 3 months to confirm dissolution. If partial stone dissolution doesn't occur by 12 months of therapy, likelihood of success is greatly reduced.

PATIENT TEACHING
• Teach about proper drug administration and handling.
• Advise patient that gallstone dissolution requires months of therapy, complete dissolution doesn't occur in all patients, and recurrence of stones within 5 years has been observed in 50% of patients.
• Inform patient that gallbladder ultrasounds will be obtained to monitor therapy.
• Explain that most patients who achieve complete stone dissolution showed complete or partial dissolution on the first treatment evaluation.

ustekinumab
us-te-KIN-ue-mab

Stelara

Therapeutic class: Immunomodulators
Pharmacologic class: Monoclonal antibodies

AVAILABLE FORMS
Injection: 45 mg/0.5 mL, 90 mg/mL prefilled syringes; 45 mg/0.5 mL in single-dose vials
IV infusion: 130 mg/26 mL in single-dose vials

INDICATIONS & DOSAGES
➤ **Moderate to severe plaque psoriasis in patients who are candidates for phototherapy or systemic therapy**
Adults and children ages 6 and older weighing more than 100 kg: Initially, 90 mg subcut,

with repeat dose in 4 weeks. Then maintenance dosage of 90 mg subcut every 12 weeks.
Adults weighing 100 kg or less and children ages 6 and older weighing 60 to 100 kg: Initially, 45 mg subcut, with repeat dose in 4 weeks. Then maintenance dosage of 45 mg subcut every 12 weeks.
Children ages 6 and older weighing less than 60 kg: Initially, 0.75 mg/kg subcut, with repeat dose in 4 weeks. Then maintenance dosage of 0.75 mg/kg subcut every 12 weeks.
➤ **Psoriatic arthritis as monotherapy or in combination with methotrexate**
Adults and children ages 6 and older weighing 60 kg or more: Initially, 45 mg subcut; repeat in 4 weeks. Then maintenance dosage of 45 mg subcut every 12 weeks.
Children ages 6 and older weighing less than 60 kg: Initially, 0.75 mg/kg subcut, with repeat dose in 4 weeks. Then maintenance dosage of 0.75 mg/kg subcut every 12 weeks.
➤ **Psoriatic arthritis with coexistent moderate to severe plaque psoriasis as monotherapy or in combination with methotrexate**
Adults and children ages 6 and older weighing more than 100 kg: Initially, 90 mg subcut; repeat dose in 4 weeks. Then maintenance dosage of 90 mg subcut every 12 weeks.
➤ **Moderately to severely active ulcerative colitis or Crohn disease**
Adults weighing more than 85 kg: Initially, 520 mg IV infusion; after 8 weeks, begin maintenance dosage of 90 mg subcut every 8 weeks.
Adults weighing from 55 to 85 kg: Initially, 390 mg IV infusion; after 8 weeks, begin maintenance dosage of 90 mg subcut every 8 weeks.
Adults weighing 55 kg or less: Initially, 260 mg IV infusion; after 8 weeks, begin maintenance dosage of 90 mg subcut every 8 weeks.

ADMINISTRATION
• Refrigerate vials (upright) and syringes at 36° to 46° F (2° to 8° C) and protected from light. Don't freeze or shake.

IV
▼ After calculating dosage and volume, withdraw an equal amount of fluid from 250-mL bag of NSS or 0.45% NSS and discard. Add drug to NSS bag or 0.45% NSS and gently mix.

U

▼ Each vial is for single use only. Discard any remaining solution.

▼ May store diluted solution for up to 8 hours at room temperature.

▼ Inspect diluted solution before infusion; don't use if particulate matter or discoloration is present.

▼ Infuse over at least 1 hour using an in-line 0.2-micron, low-protein-binding filter.

▼ **Incompatibilities:** Don't infuse in same IV line with other drugs.

Subcutaneous

• May store prefilled syringes at room temperature for 30 days or less in original container protected from light. Once syringes are at room temperature, don't put back into refrigerator. Discard within 30 days if not used.

• Discard any unused portion.

• Before administration, inspect for particulate matter, cloudiness, and discoloration; don't use if present. Drug should appear colorless to light yellow and may contain a few small translucent or white particles.

🔁 *Alert:* Needle cover on prefilled syringe contains a latex derivative. People sensitive to latex shouldn't handle needle cover.

• Give each subcut injection at a different anatomic location than previous injection; sites include upper arms, gluteal regions, tops of thighs, and any quadrant of abdomen. Don't administer into areas with psoriasis or where skin is tender, bruised, erythematous, or indurated.

• Only administer drug under guidance and supervision of a health care provider and to patients who will be closely monitored and have regular follow-up visits with a health care provider.

ACTION

Antagonizes interleukin 12 and 23 cytokines by binding to an interleukin-specific P40 protein subunit that disrupts interleukin-based inflammatory and immune responses.

Route	Onset	Peak	Duration
Subcut	Unknown	7–13.5 days	Unknown
IV	Unknown	Unknown	Unknown

Half-life: 10 to 126 days (psoriasis); 19 days (ulcerative colitis or Crohn disease).

ADVERSE REACTIONS

CNS: depression, dizziness, fatigue, headache, asthenia, fever. **EENT:** nasopharyngitis, pharyngolaryngeal pain, sinusitis, dental infection. **GI:** diarrhea, nausea, vomiting, abdominal pain. **GU:** vulvovaginal candidiasis or mycotic infection, UTI. **Musculoskeletal:** back pain, myalgia, arthralgia. **Respiratory:** URI, bronchitis. **Skin:** injection-site erythema, pruritus, acne. **Other:** *malignancies,* antibody development, flulike symptoms, infection.

INTERACTIONS

Drug-drug. *Allergen immunotherapy:* May increase risk of allergic reaction. Use together cautiously.

CYP450 substrates (cyclosporine, warfarin): May alter drug levels. Monitor patient for clinical effects, and adjust dosage as needed.

Inactivated vaccines: May not elicit an immune response sufficient to prevent disease. Revaccination may be required.

Live-virus vaccines: May transmit infection. Use together is contraindicated.

Pimecrolimus, tacrolimus (topical): May enhance adverse effect of ustekinumab. Avoid use together.

Drug-herb. *Echinacea:* May decrease therapeutic effect of ustekinumab. Discourage use together.

EFFECTS ON LAB TEST RESULTS

None reported.

CONTRAINDICATIONS & CAUTIONS

• Contraindicated in patients with clinically significant hypersensitivity to drug or its components. Hypersensitivity reactions, including anaphylaxis and angioedema, have been reported.

• Drug may increase risk of infections and reactivation of latent infections, including serious bacterial, fungal, and viral infections.

• Drug is contraindicated in patients with a clinically important active infection. Don't administer ustekinumab until the infection resolves or is adequately treated. Exercise caution when considering use of ustekinumab in patients with a chronic infection or history of recurrent infection.

• Don't administer to patients with active TB. Initiate treatment of latent TB before administering ustekinumab. Consider anti-TB therapy before initiation of ustekinumab in patients with history of latent or active TB in which an adequate course of treatment can't be confirmed.

• Drug may increase risk of malignancy. Safety of ustekinumab hasn't been evaluated in patients with history of malignancy or known malignancy.

• Safety of use in combination with other immunosuppressants or phototherapy hasn't been evaluated in psoriasis studies.

• Drug may decrease protective effect of allergen immunotherapy, which may increase risk of allergic reaction to dose of allergen immunotherapy. Use cautiously in patients receiving or who have received allergen immunotherapy, particularly for anaphylaxis.

• Cases of interstitial pneumonia, eosinophilic pneumonia, and cryptogenic organizing pneumonia have been reported with serious outcomes, including respiratory failure and prolonged hospitalization.

Dialyzable drug: Unknown.

PREGNANCY-LACTATION-REPRODUCTION

• Studies during pregnancy are inadequate. Use only if potential benefit outweighs fetal risk.

• Drug may appear in human milk. Use cautiously during breastfeeding.

NURSING CONSIDERATIONS

• Evaluate patient for TB before initiating drug.

• Closely monitor patient for signs and symptoms of active TB (fever, cough, night sweats, fatigue, unexplained weight loss) during and after treatment.

• Ensure patient receives all immunizations appropriate for age as recommended by current immunization guidelines before starting treatment. Ensure patient being treated with ustekinumab doesn't receive live-virus vaccines. Don't give bacillus Calmette-Guérin vaccines for 1 year before initiating treatment, during treatment, or for 1 year after discontinuation of treatment.

• For children, manufacturer recommends that drug be administered by a health care provider. If prescriber deems appropriate, patient may self-inject or a caregiver may inject after proper training.

• Use caution when administering live-virus vaccines to household contacts of patient receiving drug because of risk of shedding, which could lead to transmission to patient.

• Monitor patient for signs and symptoms of infection (fever, fatigue, sore throat, erythema, pain, cough). If infection develops, withhold drug and treat infection.

• Monitor patient for signs and symptoms of PRES (headache, seizures, confusion, visual disturbances).

• Monitor for nonmelanoma skin cancer. Closely follow patients who are older than age 60, have a medical history of prolonged immunosuppressive therapy, or have history of psoralen-UVA treatment.

• Monitor patient for cough, dyspnea, and interstitial infiltrates after one to three doses. For confirmed noninfectious pneumonia, discontinue drug and institute appropriate treatment.

• *Look alike–sound alike:* Don't confuse ustekinumab with infliximab or rituximab.

PATIENT TEACHING

• Caution patient to immediately report signs and symptoms of PRES or pneumonia.

• Inform patient that drug may lower ability of immune system to fight infections. Stress importance of communicating any history of infections to health care provider and reporting signs and symptoms of infection.

• Advise patient to seek immediate medical attention if signs or symptoms of serious allergic reactions (wheezing, chest tightness, fever, itching, cough, blue skin color, seizures, facial swelling) occur.

• Instruct patient or caregiver in injection techniques. Assess ability to inject subcutaneously to ensure proper administration. Ensure first self-injection is performed under supervision of a qualified health care professional.

• Tell patient or caregiver to follow directions provided in the medication guide.

• Advise patient that needle cover on prefilled syringe contains a latex derivative, which may cause allergic reactions in latex-sensitive individuals.

• Instruct patient or caregiver in proper technique for syringe and needle disposal. Advise patient not to reuse or share needles or syringes.

• Caution patient to avoid live-virus vaccines during and after therapy.

• Warn patient that drug may increase risk of malignancy.

• Advise patient of childbearing potential to report pregnancy or plans to become pregnant or breastfeed.

U

---

valACYclovir hydrochloride
val-ah-SYE-kloe-vir

Valtrex

Therapeutic class: Antivirals
Pharmacologic class: Nucleoside analogue
DNA polymerase inhibitor

AVAILABLE FORMS
Tablets: 500 mg, 1 g

INDICATIONS & DOSAGES
➤ **Herpes zoster infection (shingles)**
Adults: 1 g PO t.i.d. for 7 days.
Adjust-a-dose: For patients with CrCl of
30 to 49 mL/minute, give 1 g PO every
12 hours; if CrCl is 10 to 29 mL/minute, give
1 g PO every 24 hours; if CrCl is less than
10 mL/minute, give 500 mg PO every 24 hours.
➤ **First episode of genital herpes**
Adults: 1 g PO b.i.d. for 10 days.
Adjust-a-dose: For patients with CrCl of 10 to
29 mL/minute, give 1 g PO every 24 hours; if
CrCl is less than 10 mL/minute, give 500 mg
PO every 24 hours.
➤ **Recurrent episode of genital herpes**
Adults: 500 mg PO b.i.d. for 3 days, given at
first sign or symptom of an episode.
Adjust-a-dose: For patients with CrCl of
29 mL/minute or less, give 500 mg PO every
24 hours.
➤ **Long-term suppression of recurrent
genital herpes in patients who are immuno-
competent**
Adults: 1 g PO once daily. In patients with
history of nine or less recurrences per
year, use alternative dose of 500 mg once
daily.
Adjust-a-dose: For patients with CrCl of
29 mL/minute or less, give 500 mg PO every
24 hours (every 48 hours if patient has nine or
less occurrences per year).
➤ **Long-term suppression of recurrent
genital herpes in patients with HIV and
CD4$^+$ cell count of 100/mm^3 or greater**
Adults: 500 mg PO b.i.d.
Adjust-a-dose: For patients with CrCl of
29 mL/minute or less, give 500 mg PO every
24 hours.
➤ **To reduce transmission of genital herpes in patients with history of nine or fewer
occurrences per year**
Adults: 500 mg PO daily for source partner.

➤ **Cold sores (herpes labialis)**
Adults and children ages 12 and older: 2 g PO
b.i.d. for 1 day taken 12 hours apart.
Adjust-a-dose: For patients with CrCl of 30
to 49 mL/minute, give 1 g every 12 hours
for two doses; if CrCl is 10 to 29 mL/minute,
give 500 mg every 12 hours for two doses; if
CrCl is less than 10 mL/minute, give 500 mg
as a single dose.
➤ **Chickenpox**
Children ages 2 to younger than 18: 20 mg/kg
PO t.i.d. for 5 days. Maximum, 1 g t.i.d.

ADMINISTRATION
PO
• Give drug without regard to meals.
• An oral suspension may be compounded by
a pharmacist if needed.
• Suspension must be refrigerated then
shaken before each dose.
• Discard unused portion after 28 days.
• Give after hemodialysis on dialysis
days.

ACTION
Rapidly converts to acyclovir, which in
turn becomes incorporated into viral DNA,
thereby terminating growth of the DNA
chain; inhibits viral DNA polymerase, causing inhibition of viral replication.

Route	Onset	Peak	Duration
PO	30 min	1.4–2.6 hr	Unknown

Half-life: 2.5 to 3.25 hours.

ADVERSE REACTIONS
CNS: headache, depression, dizziness, fatigue, fever. **EENT:** nasopharyngitis, rhinorrhea. **GI:** nausea, abdominal pain, diarrhea,
vomiting. **GU:** dysmenorrhea. **Hematologic:** *thrombocytopenia, neutropenia.* **Hepatic:** increased ALP, ALT, and AST levels.
Metabolic: dehydration. **Musculoskeletal:**
arthralgia. **Respiratory:** URI. **Skin:** rash.
Other: herpes simplex.

INTERACTIONS
Drug-drug. *kidney-toxic drugs (aminoglycosides, contrast dye, cyclosporine, lithium):*
May increase risk of AKI. Use together cautiously.

EFFECTS ON LAB TEST RESULTS
• May increase ALP, ALT, AST, and creatinine levels.

- May decrease Hb level.
- May decrease platelet and WBC counts.

CONTRAINDICATIONS & CAUTIONS
- Contraindicated in patients hypersensitive to valacyclovir, acyclovir, or components of the formulation.
- **Alert:** Thrombotic thrombocytopenic purpura (TTP) and hemolytic-uremic syndrome (HUS) may occur in allogeneic bone marrow or kidney transplant recipients and patients with advanced HIV at doses of 8 g/day. Discontinue drug if signs or symptoms or lab findings of TTP or HUS occur.
- **Alert:** Use cautiously in older adults or patients with dehydration, in those with kidney impairment, and in those receiving other kidney toxic drugs. CNS effects, such as agitation, hallucinations, confusion, delirium, seizures, and encephalopathy, can occur in patients with normal or abnormal kidney function.
- Safety and effectiveness of therapy beyond 12 months (beyond 6 months in patients infected with HIV-1) for suppressive therapy or beyond 8 months in reduction of transmission of genital herpes haven't been established.
- Safety and effectiveness in prepubertal children haven't been established, except for chickenpox.
Dialyzable drug: 33%.

PREGNANCY-LACTATION-REPRODUCTION
- Studies during pregnancy are inadequate. Use only if potential benefit outweighs fetal risk.
- Drug appears in human milk. Use cautiously during breastfeeding.

NURSING CONSIDERATIONS
- Start treatment for herpes zoster infection at earliest signs or symptoms. It's most effective when started within 48 hours of onset of rash.
- Monitor kidney function; give appropriate dose adjusted for kidney status.
- If kidney failure and anuria occur, hemodialysis may be beneficial until kidney function returns.
- Monitor patient for CNS changes (agitation, hallucinations, confusion, delirium, seizures, encephalopathy). Discontinue drug if changes occur.
- **Look alike–sound alike:** Don't confuse valacyclovir with valganciclovir or acyclovir. Don't confuse Valtrex with Keflex, Valcyte, or Zovirax.

PATIENT TEACHING
- Teach about proper drug administration and handling.
- Review signs and symptoms of herpes infection (rash, tingling, itching, pain), and instruct patient to immediately notify prescriber if any occur. Treatment should begin as soon as possible after symptoms appear, preferably within 48 hours of onset of zoster rash.
- Caution patient to immediately report CNS changes, kidney problems, and any adverse reactions.
- Tell patient that drug isn't a cure for herpes but may decrease length and severity of symptoms.
- Advise patient with genital herpes to use safer sex practices in combination with suppressive therapy, even if no symptoms appear.
- Caution patient to maintain adequate hydration.
- Advise patient to report pregnancy or plans to become pregnant or breastfeed.

valproate sodium ⚕
val-PROH-ayt

valproic acid

divalproex sodium
Depakote, Depakote ER, Depakote Sprinkle, Epival ✦

Therapeutic class: Anticonvulsants
Pharmacologic class: Carboxylic acid derivatives

AVAILABLE FORMS
The strengths of valproate sodium and divalproex sodium are expressed in terms of valproic acid.
valproate sodium
Injection: 100 mg/mL
valproic acid
Capsules ⓄⓃⒸ: 250 mg
Solution: 250 mg/5 mL
divalproex sodium
Capsules (delayed-release sprinkle) ⓄⓃⒸ: 125 mg
Tablets (delayed-release) ⓄⓃⒸ: 125 mg, 250 mg, 500 mg
Tablets (extended-release) ⓄⓃⒸ: 250 mg, 500 mg

INDICATIONS & DOSAGES
Adjust-a-dose (for all indications): For older adults, start at lower dosage. Increase dosage

more slowly and with regular monitoring of fluid and nutritional intake. Watch for dehydration, somnolence, and other adverse reactions.

➤ **Simple and complex absence seizures, mixed seizure types (including absence seizures)**
Adults and children ages 2 and older: Initially, 10 to 15 mg/kg valproic acid PO or valproate sodium IV daily, or 15 mg/kg PO divalproex sodium PO daily; then increase by 5 to 10 mg/kg daily at weekly intervals up to maximum of 60 mg/kg daily.

➤ **Complex partial seizures**
Adults and children ages 10 and older: 10 to 15 mg/kg PO or valproate sodium IV daily; then increase by 5 to 10 mg/kg daily at weekly intervals up to 60 mg/kg daily.

➤ **Mania**
Adults: Initially, 750 mg delayed-release PO daily in divided doses, or 25 mg/kg extended-release PO once daily. Adjust dosage based on patient's response. Maximum dosage for either form, 60 mg/kg daily.

➤ **To prevent migraine headache**
Adults: Initially, 250 mg delayed-release divalproex sodium PO b.i.d. Some patients may need up to 1,000 mg daily. Or, 500 mg extended-release PO daily for 1 week; then 1,000 mg PO daily.

ADMINISTRATION

🜂 *Alert:* Hazardous agent; use safe-handling and disposal precautions.

PO
• Have patient swallow delayed- or extended-release tablets whole; don't crush or cut tablets.
• Give drug with food or milk to reduce adverse GI effects.
• Don't give syrup to patients who need sodium restriction. Check with prescriber.
• Sprinkle capsules may be swallowed whole or opened and contents sprinkled on a teaspoonful of soft food. Patient should swallow immediately without chewing.
• Give a missed dose as soon as possible, unless it's almost time for the next scheduled dose.

IV
▼ IV use is indicated only in patients who can't take drug orally. Switch patient to oral form as soon as feasible; effects of IV use for longer than 14 days are unknown.
▼ Dilute valproate sodium injection with at least 50 mL of a compatible diluent. It's

physically compatible and chemically stable in D_5W, NSS, and lactated Ringer solution for 24 hours at room temperature. Discard unused portion left in vial.
▼ Infuse drug over 60 minutes at no more than 20 mg/minute and at same frequency as oral dosage.
▼ Monitor drug level, and adjust dosage as needed.
▼ **Incompatibilities:** None listed by manufacturer. Consult drug compatibility reference for more information.

ACTION

Hasn't been established. Activity in epilepsy is thought to be related to increased brain concentrations of GABA.

Route	Onset	Peak	Duration
PO	Unknown	Variable	Unknown
IV	Unknown	1 hr	Unknown

Half-life: Adults, 9 to 16 hours; children, 3.5 to 67 hours, based on age.

ADVERSE REACTIONS

CNS: asthenia, dizziness, headache, insomnia, pain, paresthesia, tardive dyskinesia, nervousness, somnolence, vertigo, tremor, agitation, abnormal gait, dysarthria, hallucinations, hypertonia, abnormal thinking, amnesia, ataxia, depression, emotional lability, catatonic reactions, malaise, confusion, fever, abnormal dreams, personality disorder, psychosis, speech disorder, taste alteration. **CV:** *arrhythmia,* chest pain, edema, HTN, hypotension, vasodilation, tachycardia, palpitations. **EENT:** blurred vision, diplopia, dry eyes, photophobia, eye pain, conjunctivitis, nystagmus, deafness, ear pain, tinnitus, epistaxis, rhinitis, dry mouth, gum hemorrhage, oral ulcerations, pharyngitis, periodontal abscess. **GI:** abdominal pain, anorexia, diarrhea, fecal incontinence, flatulence, gastroenteritis, glossitis, stomatitis, dyspepsia, nausea, vomiting, hematemesis, eructation, *pancreatitis,* constipation, increased appetite. **GU:** vaginitis, dysmenorrhea, dysuria, cystitis, urinary frequency, urinary incontinence. **Hematologic:** *hemorrhage, leukopenia, thrombocytopenia,* anemia. **Hepatic:** increased transaminase levels. **Metabolic:** hypoproteinemia, weight gain or loss. **Musculoskeletal:** back and neck pain, arthralgia, twitching, myasthenia, leg cramps. **Respiratory:** bronchitis, cough, dyspnea, hiccups, pneumonia.

Skin: dry skin; alopecia; diaphoresis; ecchymosis; petechiae; discoid lupus erythematosus; furunculosis; seborrhea; rash; pruritus; injection-site pain, inflammation, or reaction.
Other: flulike syndrome, infection, chills, accidental injury.

INTERACTIONS
⚠️ *Alert:* Drug can significantly interact with many drugs. Consult a drug interaction resource or pharmacist for additional information.
Drug-drug. *Aspirin, erythromycin, felbamate:* May cause valproic acid toxicity. Use together cautiously, and monitor drug level.
Benzodiazepines, other CNS depressants: May cause excessive CNS depression. Avoid use together.
Carbamazepine: May cause carbamazepine CNS toxicity, decrease valproic acid level, and cause loss of seizure control. Use together cautiously, if at all. Monitor patient for seizure activity and toxicity during therapy and for at least 1 month after stopping either drug.
Carbapenem antibiotics (ertapenem, imipenem, meropenem): May decrease valproic acid level and cause loss of seizure control. Consider alternative antimicrobial agent. Monitor levels closely.
Clonazepam: May increase risk of absence seizures in patients with history of absence seizures. Monitor patient closely.
Estrogen-containing hormonal contraceptives: May decrease valproate level and increase seizure frequency. Monitor valproate level and clinical response.
Ethosuximide: May increase ethosuximide level. Monitor patient closely.
Fosphenytoin, phenytoin: May increase or decrease phenytoin level; may decrease valproate level. Monitor patient closely.
Lamotrigine: May increase lamotrigine level and decrease valproate level; serious skin reactions may occur. Monitor levels closely.
Methotrexate: May decrease valproate level. Monitor valproate level and clinical response.
Phenobarbital: May increase phenobarbital level and increase clearance of valproate. Monitor patient closely.
Propofol: May increase propofol level. Reduce propofol dosage.
Rifampin: May decrease valproate level. Monitor level of valproate.

Rufinamide: May increase rufinamide level. Begin valproate therapy at low dosage, and titrate to clinically effective dosage.
TCAs (amitriptyline, nortriptyline): May increase TCA level. Monitor drug level.
Topiramate: May cause hyperammonemia with and without encephalopathy. Concomitant use has been associated with hypothermia. Check blood ammonia levels in patients reporting hypothermia.
Warfarin: May displace warfarin from binding sites. Monitor PT and INR.
Zidovudine: May increase zidovudine level. Monitor therapy.
Drug-lifestyle. *Alcohol use:* May cause excessive CNS depression. Discourage use together.

EFFECTS ON LAB TEST RESULTS
● May increase ammonia, ALT, and AST levels.
● May increase eosinophil count and bleeding time.
● May decrease platelet, RBC, and WBC counts.
● May cause false-positive results for urine ketone levels.
● May alter thyroid function test results.

CONTRAINDICATIONS & CAUTIONS
● Contraindicated in patients hypersensitive to drug, in those with liver disease or significant liver dysfunction, and in those with a urea cycle disorder (UCD).
▧ **Boxed Warning** Patients with hereditary neurometabolic syndromes caused by DNA mutations of the mitochondrial DNA polymerase gamma (*POLG*) gene, such as Alpers-Huttenlocher syndrome, are at high risk for acute liver failure and fatalities. Drug is contraindicated in patients known to have mitochondrial disorders caused by *POLG* mutations and in children younger than age 2 who are suspected of having a mitochondrial disorder. In patients older than age 2 who are clinically suspected of having a hereditary mitochondrial disease, use only after other anticonvulsants have failed. ▪
Boxed Warning Liver failure resulting in fatalities has occurred, usually during the first 6 months of treatment. In patients with epilepsy, loss of seizure control may also occur. ▪
Boxed Warning Patients at high risk for fatal liver toxicity include those with congenital

V

metabolic disorders, intellectual disability, or organic brain disease; those taking multiple anticonvulsants; and children younger than age 2. In children younger than age 2, use with extreme caution and as a sole agent, weighing benefits of therapy against risks. ■

Boxed Warning Life-threatening pancreatitis has been reported in children and adults receiving valproate shortly after initial use as well as after several years of use. ■

• Safety and effectiveness of Depakote ER in children younger than age 10 haven't been established.

Dialyzable drug: 20%.

⚠ *Overdose S&S:* Somnolence, heart block, deep coma, hypernatremia.

PREGNANCY-LACTATION-REPRODUCTION

Boxed Warning Valproate can cause neural tube defects and other organ system malformations. It also increases the risk of lower cognitive test scores. Avoid use in patients who may become pregnant, unless other medications have failed to provide adequate symptom control or aren't tolerated. Patients of childbearing potential should use effective contraception when drug use can't be avoided. ■

Boxed Warning Drug is contraindicated for prevention of migraines during pregnancy. ■

Boxed Warning Use during pregnancy in patients with epilepsy or bipolar disorder only if other drugs have failed to control symptoms. Drug is contraindicated for use in pregnancy for reversible conditions not associated with permanent injury or death. ■

• To prevent major seizures, patients with epilepsy who are pregnant shouldn't abruptly discontinue drug.

• Patients taking valproate during pregnancy may develop liver failure or clotting abnormalities, including thrombocytopenia, hypofibrinogenemia, or decrease in other coagulation factors, which may result in hemorrhagic complications in the neonate, including death.

• Hypoglycemia in neonates and fatal cases of liver failure in infants after maternal use during pregnancy have been reported.

• Male infertility has been reported.

• Patients who are pregnant should enroll in the North American Antiepileptic Drug Pregnancy Registry (1-888-233-2334 or www.aedpregnancyregistry.org).

• Drug appears in human milk. Use cautiously during breastfeeding.

• Monitor infants who are breastfed for liver damage (jaundice, unusual bruising, bleeding).

NURSING CONSIDERATIONS

Boxed Warning During treatment, closely monitor patient older than age 2 who is suspected of having a mitochondrial disorder for development of acute liver injury; perform regular clinical assessments and LFTs. Perform *POLG* mutation screening in accordance with current clinical practice. ■

Boxed Warning Fatal liver toxicity may follow nonspecific signs and symptoms, such as malaise, fever, anorexia, facial edema, vomiting, weakness, and lethargy. If these signs and symptoms occur during therapy, immediately notify prescriber because patient might be developing liver dysfunction and must stop drug. Monitor LFT values before therapy and at frequent intervals, especially during first 6 months. ■

🕃 *Alert:* Closely monitor all patients taking or starting AEDs for changes in behavior indicating worsening of suicidality or depression. Symptoms such as anxiety, agitation, hostility, mania, and hypomania may be precursors to emerging suicidality.

🕃 *Alert:* Dose-related thrombocytopenia can occur. Monitor CBC, platelet count, PT, and INR before starting therapy and at frequent intervals. Decrease dose or discontinue drug if hemorrhage, bruising, or coagulation disorder occurs.

🕃 *Alert:* Monitor for and immediately report symptoms of DRESS syndrome (rash, fever, swollen glands). Discontinue drug for suspected DRESS syndrome.

• Monitor valproate and concomitant drug levels closely when introducing or withdrawing enzyme-inducing drugs.

• Be aware that adverse reactions may not be caused by valproic acid alone because it's usually used with other anticonvulsants.

• When converting adults and children ages 10 and older with seizures from Depakote to Depakote ER, make sure extended-release dose is 8% to 20% higher than regular dose taken previously. See manufacturer's package insert for more details.

• Never withdraw drug suddenly because sudden withdrawal may worsen seizures. Call prescriber at once if adverse reactions develop.

- Notify prescriber if tremors occur; dosage reduction may be needed.
- Monitor drug level. Therapeutic level ranges from 50 to 100 mcg/mL for seizure control and 50 to 125 mcg/mL for mania.
- When converting patient from brand-name drug to generic drug, use caution because breakthrough seizures may occur.

⚠️ **Alert:** Sometimes fatal, hyperammonemic encephalopathy may occur when starting valproate therapy in patient with UCD. Evaluate patient with UCD risk factors before starting valproate therapy. Patient who develops symptoms of unexplained hyperammonemic encephalopathy during valproate therapy should stop drug, undergo prompt appropriate treatment, and undergo evaluation for underlying UCD.

- **Look alike–sound alike:** Don't confuse Depakote with Depakote ER.

PATIENT TEACHING

⚠️ **Alert:** Explain that drug may increase risk of suicidality. Tell patient and caregivers to immediately report emergence or worsening of depression, unusual changes in mood or behavior, emergence of suicidality, or thoughts about self-harm.
- Teach about proper drug administration and handling.
- Advise patient and caregivers to keep drug out of children's reach.
- Warn patient and caregivers not to stop drug therapy abruptly.

⚠️ **Alert:** Tell patient to immediately report rash (with or without blisters), fever, swollen lymph nodes, mouth ulcers, or skin shedding.

Boxed Warning Warn patients and caregivers that abdominal pain, nausea, vomiting, and anorexia can be symptoms of pancreatitis that require prompt medical evaluation. ■

Boxed Warning Caution patients and caregivers to report signs and symptoms of liver toxicity. Explain the need for routine blood testing. ■

- Advise patient to avoid driving and other potentially hazardous activities that require mental alertness until drug's CNS effects are known.
- Instruct patient or parents to call prescriber if malaise, weakness, lethargy, facial swelling, loss of appetite, or vomiting occurs.
- Tell patient to report pregnancy or plans to become pregnant or breastfeed during therapy.

valsartan
val-SAR-tan

Diovan

Therapeutic class: Antihypertensives
Pharmacologic class: ARBs

AVAILABLE FORMS
Solution: 4 mg/mL
Tablets: 40 mg, 80 mg, 160 mg, 320 mg

INDICATIONS & DOSAGES
➤ **HTN (used alone or with other antihypertensives)**
Adults: Initially, 80 or 160 mg tablets PO once daily or 40 to 80 mg oral solution b.i.d. Expect reduction in BP in 2 to 4 weeks. If additional antihypertensive effect is needed, may increase to 160 or 320 mg daily. Usual dosage range, 80 to 320 mg daily.
Children ages 6 to 16: Initially, 0.65 mg/kg oral solution b.i.d. (up to 40 mg total). Adjust dosage according to patient response and tolerability, up to 1.35 mg/kg b.i.d. or 160 mg daily.
Children ages 1 to 16: Initially, 1 mg/kg tablet or suspension prepared from tablets PO once daily (up to 40 mg total). Consider starting dose of 2 mg/kg in select patients when greater BP reduction is needed. Adjust dosage according to patient response and tolerability, up to 4 mg/kg or 160 mg daily.
➤ **NYHA Class II to IV HF**
Adults: Initially, 40 mg PO b.i.d.; increase as tolerated to 80 mg b.i.d., and then to target dose of 160 mg b.i.d. or highest dose tolerated.
➤ **To reduce CV death in patients with left ventricular failure or dysfunction who are stable after MI**
Adults: 20 mg PO b.i.d. Initial dose may be given as soon as 12 hours after MI. Increase dose to 40 mg b.i.d. within 7 days. Increase subsequent doses, as tolerated, to target dose of 160 mg b.i.d. or highest dose tolerated.
Adjust-a-dose: Consider dosage reduction in patients with symptomatic hypotension or kidney dysfunction.

ADMINISTRATION
PO
- Give drug without regard to food.
- Tablets aren't recommended for patients younger than age 6.

V

- Pharmacists may prepare a suspension from tablets for children ages 1 to 5, patients older than age 5 who are unable to swallow pills, and children for whom the calculated dose doesn't correspond to an available tablet strength.
- Shake suspension at least 10 seconds before pouring. Store suspension at room temperature for 30 days or in refrigerator for 75 days.
- Oral solution and suspension aren't therapeutically equivalent to tablet formulation; peak level is higher. When switching between formulations, expect to adjust valsartan dosage.
- Give a missed dose as soon as possible. If almost time for next dose, don't give missed dose; give next dose at scheduled time.

ACTION

Blocks the binding of angiotensin II to receptor sites in vascular smooth muscle and the adrenal gland, which inhibits the pressor effects of the RAAS.

Route	Onset	Peak	Duration
PO (solution)	Unknown	0.7–3.7 hr	24 hr
PO (tablets)	2 hr	2–4 hr	24 hr

Half-life: 6 hours.

ADVERSE REACTIONS

CNS: dizziness, headache, fatigue, vertigo, syncope. **CV:** edema, hypotension, orthostatic hypotension. **EENT:** blurred vision, rhinitis, sinusitis, pharyngitis. **GI:** abdominal pain, diarrhea, nausea. **GU:** kidney impairment. **Hematologic:** *neutropenia.* **Metabolic:** *hyperkalemia.* **Musculoskeletal:** arthralgia, back pain. **Respiratory:** URI, cough. **Other:** viral infection.

INTERACTIONS

Drug-drug. *ACE inhibitors:* May increase risk of kidney dysfunction, hypotension, and hyperkalemia. Avoid use together but, if necessary, closely monitor BP, serum potassium level, and kidney function.
Aliskiren: May increase risk of kidney impairment, hypotension, and hyperkalemia in patients with diabetes and in those with GFR less than 60 mL/minute. Concomitant use is contraindicated in patients with diabetes. Avoid concomitant use in those with GFR less than 60 mL/minute.
Antihepaciviral combination products (ledipasvir–sofosbuvir, glecaprevir–pibrentasvir): May increase valsartan level.

Consider therapy modification or decrease valsartan dosage and monitor patient for hypotension and worsening kidney function.
Lithium: May increase lithium level. Monitor lithium level and patient for toxicity.
NSAIDs: May result in deterioration of kidney function in older adults, patients who are volume-depleted, and those with compromised kidney function. Monitor kidney function. May also decrease antihypertensive effect. Monitor BP.
Potassium supplements, potassium-sparing diuretics, other angiotensin II blockers: May increase potassium level. May also increase creatinine level in patients with HF. Avoid use together.
Trimethoprim: May increase risk of hyperkalemia, especially in older adults. Closely monitor serum potassium level.
Drug-food. *Salt substitutes containing potassium:* May increase potassium level. May also increase creatinine level in patients with HF. Discourage use together.

EFFECTS ON LAB TEST RESULTS

- May increase potassium, BUN, and creatinine levels.
- May decrease neutrophil count.

CONTRAINDICATIONS & CAUTIONS

- Contraindicated in patients hypersensitive to drug or its components.
- ⏺ *Alert:* Angioedema, a rare life-threatening reaction, has been reported. Discontinue drug immediately and treat emergently if angioedema occurs.
- Use cautiously in patients with kidney impairment. Patients with kidney function dependent in part on RAAS (such as those with renal artery stenosis, CKD, severe HF, or volume depletion) are at increased risk for AKI.
- Use cautiously in patients with Child-Pugh class C liver impairment.
- Safety and effectiveness haven't been established in children younger than age 6 and in children of any age with GFR less than 30 mL/minute/1.73 m^2.
Dialyzable drug: No.
⚠ *Overdose S&S:* Hypotension, tachycardia, bradycardia, decreased level of consciousness, circulatory collapse, shock.

PREGNANCY-LACTATION-REPRODUCTION

Boxed Warning Drugs that act directly on the RAAS can cause injury and death to a

---

*Reactions in bold italics are **life-threatening**.*

developing fetus. When pregnancy is detected, stop drug as soon as possible. ■
• It isn't known if drug appears in human milk. Patient should discontinue breastfeeding or discontinue drug, considering importance of drug to patient.

NURSING CONSIDERATIONS
• Monitor BP and watch for hypotension. Excessive hypotension can occur when drug is given with high doses of diuretics.
• Correct volume and sodium depletions before starting drug.
• Monitor serum BUN, creatinine, and potassium levels.

PATIENT TEACHING
• Teach about proper drug administration and handling.
• Advise patient to report all adverse effects, especially dizziness upon standing or other signs and symptoms of hypotension.
• Tell patient of childbearing potential to report pregnancy. Drug will need to be stopped.

vancomycin hydrochloride
van-koh-MYE-sin

Firvanq Kit, Vancocin

Therapeutic class: Antibiotics
Pharmacologic class: Glycopeptides

AVAILABLE FORMS
Capsules: 125 mg, 250 mg
Powder for injection: 500-mg, 750-mg, 1-g, 1.25-g, 1.5-g. 5-g, 10-g vials
Powder for oral solution: 25 mg/mL, 50 mg/mL concentration after dilution
Premixed for injection: 500 mg, 750 mg, 1 g, 1.25 g, 1.5 g, 1.75 g, 2 g

INDICATIONS & DOSAGES
Adjust-a-dose (for all indications): In kidney insufficiency, adjust dosage based on degree of kidney impairment, drug level, severity of infection, and susceptibility of causative organism. Initially, give 15 mg/kg, and adjust subsequent doses as needed. In patients who lack kidney function, follow initial dose of 15 mg/kg with dosage of 1.9 mg/kg/24 hours.
➤ **Serious or severe infections when other antibiotics are ineffective or contraindicated, including those caused by MRSA,**

Staphylococcus epidermidis, **or diphtheroid organisms**
Adults: 500 mg IV every 6 hours or 1 g IV every 12 hours.
Children ages 1 month and older: 10 mg/kg IV every 6 hours.
Neonates younger than age 1 month: 15 mg/kg IV loading dose; then 10 mg/kg IV every 12 hours if child is younger than age 1 week or 10 mg/kg IV every 8 hours if older than 1 week but younger than 1 month.
Older adults: 15 mg/kg IV loading dose. Subsequent doses are based on kidney function and drug levels.
➤ **CDAD**
Adults: 125 mg PO every 6 hours for 10 days.
Children: 40 mg/kg/day PO in three or four divided doses for 7 to 10 days. Maximum daily dosage, 2 g.
➤ **Staphylococcal enterocolitis**
Adults: 500 mg to 2 g PO in three or four divided doses daily for 7 to 10 days.
Children: 40 mg/kg/day PO in three or four divided doses for 7 to 10 days. Maximum daily dosage, 2 g.

ADMINISTRATION
❸ *Alert:* Obtain specimen for culture and sensitivity tests before administration. Because of emergence of vancomycin-resistant enterococci, reserve use for treatment of serious infections caused by gram-positive bacteria resistant to beta-lactam anti-infectives.
PO
• Powder for oral solution must be reconstituted by pharmacist before use.
❸ *Alert:* Oral form is ineffective for systemic infections.
IV
▼ IV route is ineffective for CDAD and staphylococcal enterocolitis.
▼ Reconstitute with sterile water for injection to provide a solution containing 50 mg/mL.
▼ Refrigerate solution after reconstitution, and use within 96 hours.
▼ For infusion, further dilute with NSS for injection or D_5W to a final concentration of no more than 5 mg/mL and infuse as soon as possible at no faster than 30 minutes for every 500 mg or over at least 60 minutes, whichever is longer.
▼ Drug is an irritant; give by secure IV route and ensure proper needle or catheter placement before and during infusion. Pain,

tenderness, and necrosis may occur with extravasation. Can minimize frequency and severity of thrombophlebitis by slow infusion of drug and rotation of venous access sites.

▼ Drug is available premixed in NSS or D₅W solution in a variety of volumes.

▼ Thawed, premixed solution remains stable for 72 hours at room temperature or for 30 days in refrigerator. Don't refreeze.

⊘ *Alert:* Rapid infusion (over several minutes) has been associated with hypotension, shock and, rarely, cardiac arrest.

▼ Check site daily for phlebitis and irritation. Severe irritation and necrosis can result from extravasation.

▼ **Incompatibilities:** Beta-lactam antibiotics, many other drugs (vancomycin has a low pH). Consult drug compatibility reference for more information.

ACTION

Hinders bacterial cell-wall synthesis, damaging the bacterial plasma membrane and making the cell more vulnerable to osmotic pressure. Also interferes with RNA synthesis.

Route	Onset	Peak	Duration
PO	Unknown	Unknown	Unknown
IV	Immediate	Immediate	Unknown

Half-life: 4 to 6 hours.

ADVERSE REACTIONS

CNS: fever, pain, headache, fatigue, dizziness, malaise, vertigo, depression, insomnia. **CV:** hypotension, chest pain, edema, flushing, phlebitis at injection site. **EENT:** ototoxicity, tinnitus. **GI:** nausea, abdominal pain, vomiting, diarrhea, constipation, flatulence. **GU:** *kidney toxicity,* interstitial nephritis, renal tubular necrosis, UTI. **Hematologic:** *neutropenia,* eosinophilia, *thrombocytopenia,* anemia. **Metabolic:** *hypokalemia (PO).* **Musculoskeletal:** myalgia, back pain. **Respiratory:** dyspnea, wheezing. **Skin:** dermatitis, erythema, injection-site reaction or pain. **Other:** hypersensitivity reaction, chills, superinfection.

INTERACTIONS

Drug-drug. *Anesthetics:* May cause erythema, histamine-like flushing, and anaphylactoid reaction. Monitor patient closely. *Kidney-toxic drugs (aminoglycosides, amphotericin B, bacitracin, cisplatin, colistin,* *piperacillin, polymyxin B, viomycin), neurotoxic drugs:* May increase risk of kidney toxicity or ototoxicity. Monitor kidney function and hearing function test results.

Nondepolarizing muscle relaxants: May enhance neuromuscular blockade. Monitor patient closely.

NSAIDs: May increase vancomycin level. Monitor therapy.

EFFECTS ON LAB TEST RESULTS

- May increase BUN and creatinine levels.
- May decrease potassium level.
- May increase eosinophil count.
- May decrease neutrophil and WBC counts.

CONTRAINDICATIONS & CAUTIONS

- Contraindicated in patients hypersensitive to drug or its components.
- Use cautiously in patients receiving other neurotoxic, kidney-toxic, or ototoxic drugs; in patients older than age 60; and in those with impaired liver or kidney function, hearing loss, or allergies to other antibiotics.

Dialyzable drug: Poorly dialyzable.

PREGNANCY-LACTATION-REPRODUCTION

- It isn't known if drug causes fetal harm. Use during pregnancy only if clearly needed. **Boxed Warning** Verify pregnancy status before using IV formulations containing polyethylene glycol and N-acetyl-D-alanine. Fetal malformations have occurred in animal studies using these formulations. If vancomycin is needed during first or second trimester, use other available formulations. ■
- Drug appears in human milk. Patient should discontinue breastfeeding or discontinue drug, considering importance of drug to patient.

NURSING CONSIDERATIONS

- Obtain hearing evaluation before and during prolonged therapy.
- Monitor patient's fluid balance, and watch for oliguria and cloudy urine.
- Monitor patient carefully for vancomycin flushing syndrome (red-man syndrome), which can occur with rapid drug infusion. Signs and symptoms include maculopapular rash on face, neck, trunk, and limbs and pruritus and hypotension caused by histamine release. If wheezing, urticaria, or pain and muscle spasms of chest and back occur, stop infusion and notify prescriber.

Reactions in bold italics are *life-threatening*.

• Assess kidney function (BUN, creatinine level and CrCl, urinalysis, and urine output) before and during therapy.
• Carefully monitor vancomycin level to adjust IV dosage requirements.
• Monitor patient for hypersensitivity reactions, including skin reactions.
• Monitor IV site for irritation, phlebitis, and extravasation.
• Periodically monitor leukocyte count during IV therapy.
• Monitor patient for signs and symptoms of superinfection. CDAD can occur more than 2 months after therapy ends.
• *Look alike–sound alike:* Don't confuse vancomycin with clindamycin, gentamicin, or Vibramycin.

PATIENT TEACHING
• Advise patient to take entire amount of drug exactly as directed, even after feeling better.
• Instruct patient receiving drug IV to report discomfort at IV insertion site.
• Tell patient to report ringing in ears.
• Advise patient to immediately report adverse reactions to prescriber.
• Caution patient to immediately report pregnancy or plans to become pregnant or breastfeed during therapy.

vardenafil hydrochloride
var-DEN-ah-fill

Therapeutic class: Erectile dysfunction drugs
Pharmacologic class: PDE5 inhibitors

AVAILABLE FORMS
Tablets (film-coated): 2.5 mg, 5 mg, 10 mg, 20 mg
Tablets (ODTs) ⓄⓃⒸ: 10 mg

INDICATIONS & DOSAGES
➤ **Erectile dysfunction**
Adults: 10 mg PO as single dose, as needed, 1 hour before sexual activity. Dosage range is 5 to 20 mg for film-coated tablets based on effectiveness and tolerance. Maximum, 10 mg/day for ODT or 20 mg once daily for tablets.
Adjust-a-dose: For patients with Child-Pugh class B liver impairment and patients ages 65 and older, first dose of film-coated tablets is 5 mg daily, as needed. Don't exceed 10 mg daily in patients with liver impairment.

Dosage adjustment may be needed in patients taking potent CYP3A4 inhibitors. Consult manufacturer's instructions for drug-interaction dosage adjustments.

ADMINISTRATION
PO
• Tablets and ODTs aren't interchangeable.
• Give drug without regard to food.
• Don't split or crush ODTs.
• Place ODT on tongue to disintegrate. Have patient take without water or other liquid.
• Don't remove ODT from blister pack until ready to use.

ACTION
Increases cyclic guanosine monophosphate levels, prolongs smooth muscle relaxation, and promotes blood flow into the corpus cavernosum by inhibiting PDE5.

Route	Onset	Peak	Duration
PO	60 min	30–120 min	Unknown

Half-life: 4 to 6 hours.

ADVERSE REACTIONS
CNS: headache, dizziness. **CV:** flushing, hypotension, tachycardia. **EENT:** rhinitis, sinusitis, nasal congestion. **GI:** dyspepsia, nausea. **Metabolic:** increased CK level. **Musculoskeletal:** back pain. **Other:** flulike syndrome, accidental injury.

INTERACTIONS
Drug-drug. *Alpha blockers:* May enhance hypotensive effects. Start concomitant treatment at reduced dosage only if patient is stable on alpha-blocker therapy.
Antiarrhythmics (Class IA [quinidine, procainamide], Class III [amiodarone, sotalol]): May prolong QTc interval. Avoid use together.
Antihypertensives (ACE inhibitors, calcium channel blockers, beta blockers, thiazide diuretics): May increase hypotensive effects. Use together cautiously.
Guanylate cyclase (GC) stimulators (riociguat), nitrates: May enhance hypotensive effects. Use together is contraindicated.
Strong and moderate CYP3A4 inhibitors (erythromycin, itraconazole, ketoconazole, ritonavir): May increase vardenafil level. Reduce vardenafil dosage and extend dosing interval according to manufacturer's instructions. Use with ODTs is contraindicated.

V

Drug-food. *Grapefruit, grapefruit juice:* May increase vardenafil level. Discourage use together.
High-fat meals: May reduce peak level of drug. Discourage use with high-fat meal.
Drug-lifestyle. *Alcohol use:* May increase risk of hypotension and orthostasis. Discourage use together.

EFFECTS ON LAB TEST RESULTS
• May increase CK and liver transaminase levels.

CONTRAINDICATIONS & CAUTIONS
• Contraindicated in patients hypersensitive to drug or its components.
• Not recommended in patients with unstable angina, hypotension (systolic less than 90 mm Hg), uncontrolled HTN (over 170/110 mm Hg), stroke, life-threatening arrhythmia, MI within past 6 months, severe cardiac failure, Child-Pugh class C liver impairment, KFRT, congenital QTc-interval prolongation, or hereditary degenerative retinal disorders.
• Don't use ODTs in patients with Child-Pugh class B or C liver impairment or in those who require dialysis.
• Use cautiously in patients with left ventricular outflow obstruction (aortic stenosis, idiopathic hypertrophic subaortic stenosis) who can be sensitive to vasodilation effect.
• Use cautiously in patients with bleeding disorders or significant peptic ulceration.
• Use cautiously in those with anatomic penis abnormalities or conditions that predispose patient to priapism (sickle cell anemia, multiple myeloma, leukemia).
• May cause vision loss and visual disturbances. Use cautiously in patients with or at increased risk for nonarteritic ischemic optic neuropathy ("crowded optic disc").
• May cause sudden decreased or loss of hearing, tinnitus, and dizziness.
Dialyzable drug: Unlikely.
⚠ *Overdose S&S:* Back pain or myalgia, abnormal vision.

PREGNANCY-LACTATION-REPRODUCTION
• Drug isn't indicated for use in females.

NURSING CONSIDERATIONS
⊎ *Alert:* Sexual activity may increase cardiac risk. Evaluate patient's cardiac risk before start of therapy.

• Before patient starts drug, assess for underlying cause of erectile dysfunction.
• Transient decreases in supine BP may occur.
• Prolonged erections and priapism may occur.

PATIENT TEACHING
• Teach about proper drug administration and handling.
• Explain that drug doesn't protect against STIs. Tell patient to use protective measures.
• Urge patient to seek immediate medical care if erection lasts more than 4 hours.
• Explain that drug has no effect without sexual stimulation.
• Warn patient not to change dose unless directed by prescriber.
• Tell patient to stop drug and seek medical attention for sudden vision loss in one or both eyes or sudden decrease in or loss of hearing.

varenicline tartrate
vah-RENN-ih-kleen

Therapeutic class: Smoking cessation aids
Pharmacologic class: Nicotinic acetylcholine receptor partial agonists

AVAILABLE FORMS
Tablets: 0.5 mg, 1 mg

INDICATIONS & DOSAGES
➤ **Smoking cessation**
Adults: Start dosing 1 week before patient stops smoking. Or, patient can begin dosing, then stop smoking between days 8 and 35 of treatment. Give 0.5 mg PO once daily on days 1 through 3. Days 4 through 7, give 0.5 mg PO b.i.d. Day 8 through end of week 12, give 1 mg PO b.i.d. If patient successfully stops smoking, give an additional 12-week course to help with long-term success.

Or, for patients who are sure they aren't able or willing to quit abruptly, consider a gradual approach by initiating drug and reducing smoking simultaneously until complete abstinence by 12 weeks. Then continue drug for additional 12 weeks.
Adjust-a-dose: Consider dosage reduction in patients who can't tolerate adverse effects. In patients with CrCL less than 30 mL/minute, give 0.5 mg PO once daily. Adjust as needed to maximum of 0.5 mg b.i.d. In patients with KFRT, give 0.5 mg once daily.

ADMINISTRATION
PO
- Give drug with full glass of water after a meal.

ACTION
Blocks the effects of nicotine by binding at alpha$_4$ beta$_2$ neuronal nicotinic acetylcholine receptors. Drug also increases dopamine activity, decreasing cravings and withdrawal symptoms.

Route	Onset	Peak	Duration
PO	4 days	3–4 hr	24 hr

Half-life: 24 hours.

ADVERSE REACTIONS
CNS: abnormal dreams, headache, insomnia, altered attention or emotions, asthenia, depression, drowsiness, fatigue, irritability, lethargy, anxiety, agitation, tension, hostility, malaise, nightmares, sleep disorder, somnolence, altered taste. **CV:** angina, chest pain, edema, hot flush, HTN. **EENT:** epistaxis, rhinorrhea, dry mouth. **GI:** nausea, abdominal pain, constipation, diarrhea, dyspepsia, flatulence, GERD, vomiting, increased or decreased appetite. **Respiratory:** dyspnea, URI. **Skin:** rash, hyperhidrosis, pruritis. **Other:** flulike symptoms.

INTERACTIONS
Drug-drug. *Nicotine-replacement therapy:* May increase nausea, vomiting, dizziness, dyspepsia, and fatigue. Monitor patient closely.
Insulin, theophylline, warfarin: Smoking cessation may alter action of these drugs. Monitor therapy and adjust dosage as necessary.
Drug-lifestyle. ☻ *Alert: Alcohol use:* May decrease alcohol tolerance, with symptoms of increased drunkenness, unusual or aggressive behavior, or amnesia. Advise patient to reduce alcohol consumption until alcohol tolerance is known.

EFFECTS ON LAB TEST RESULTS
- May increase LFT values.

CONTRAINDICATIONS & CAUTIONS
- Contraindicated in patients hypersensitive to drug or its components.
- Consider risks versus benefits before use. Drug increases likelihood of abstinence from smoking for as long as 1 year. Health benefits of quitting smoking are immediate and substantial.
☻ *Alert:* Serious neuropsychiatric events (depression, hostility, mania, psychosis, hallucinations, paranoia, delusions, homicidal ideation, aggression, agitation, anxiety, panic, suicidality) have been reported with use of this drug. Carefully weigh risks versus benefits of smoking cessation. Somnambulism has been reported.
☻ *Alert:* Drug may be associated with increased risk of CV events (stroke, angina, MI, need for coronary revascularization, new diagnosis of PVD, or admission for a procedure to treat PVD) in patients who have CV disease. Risks and benefits should be considered before prescribing.
☻ *Alert:* Drug may increase risk of seizures. Use cautiously in patients who have history of seizures or are at increased risk for seizures.
- Hypersensitivity reactions (angioedema, SJS, erythema multiforme) have been reported. Stop drug at first sign or symptom of hypersensitivity reaction.
- Use cautiously in older adults and in patients with CrCl less than 30 mL/minute or preexisting psychiatric illness.
- Not recommended for use in children ages 16 and younger.
Dialyzable drug: Yes.

PREGNANCY-LACTATION-REPRODUCTION
- Studies during pregnancy are inadequate. Use only if potential benefit justifies fetal risk.
- It isn't known if drug appears in human milk. Use cautiously during breastfeeding and monitor exposed infant for seizures and vomiting.

NURSING CONSIDERATIONS
- Assess patient's readiness and motivation to stop smoking.
- Encourage patient who is motivated to quit but didn't succeed during prior therapy or who relapsed after treatment to make another attempt after identifying and addressing contributing factors to failed attempt.
☻ *Alert:* Monitor for changes in behavior, agitation, depressed mood, hostility, suicidality, and worsening of preexisting psychiatric illness; report immediately.
- Notify prescriber if patient develops intolerable adverse reactions, such as nausea; dosage reduction may be needed.

V

• Monitor patient for hypersensitivity reactions. Discontinue drug if such signs and symptoms as swelling of face, mouth, neck, or extremities or a rash with mucosal lesions occurs.

• Temporarily monitor drug levels of theophylline, warfarin, and insulin (if applicable) after patient stops smoking to ensure they're within therapeutic range.

PATIENT TEACHING

• Teach about proper drug administration and handling. Caution patient to take drug as directed.

• Provide patient with educational materials and needed counseling.

• Sleepwalking has been reported in patients taking drug. Some patients have described harmful behavior to self, others, or property. Instruct patient to discontinue drug and notify prescriber if such behaviors occur.

❸ *Alert:* Caution patient that drug can affect reaction to alcohol. Advise patient to reduce alcohol consumption until alcohol tolerance is known.

❸ *Alert:* Warn patient to stop drug and seek medical attention if seizures occur.

• Advise patient to discontinue drug and seek immediate medical care if swelling of face, mouth, extremities, and neck or a rash with mucosal lesions develops.

• Explain that nausea and insomnia are common and usually temporary. Urge patient to contact prescriber if adverse effects are persistently troubling; dosage reduction may help.

• Urge patient to continue trying to abstain from smoking if early lapses occur after successfully quitting.

• Tell patient that dosages of other drugs may need adjustment when patient stops smoking.

• Advise patient to use caution when driving or operating machinery until effects of drug are known.

❸ *Alert:* Instruct patient and family to monitor patient for changes in behavior and mood, including agitation, depression, hostility, suicidality, and worsening of preexisting psychiatric illness. Tell them to immediately stop drug and report these changes to health care provider.

• If patient plans to become pregnant or to breastfeed, explain risks of smoking and risks and benefits of taking drug to aid smoking cessation.

SAFETY ALERT!

vasopressin
vay-soe-PRESS-in

Vasostrict

Therapeutic class: Antidiuretic hormones
Pharmacologic class: Posterior pituitary hormones

AVAILABLE FORMS

Injection (ready to use): 20 units/100 mL, 40 units/100 mL, 60 units/100 mL single-dose vials
Injection (solution for dilution): 20 units/mL single-dose vials; 200 units/10 mL multiple-dose vials

INDICATIONS & DOSAGES

➤ **Vasodilatory shock in patients who remain hypotensive despite fluids and catecholamines**
Adults: For postcardiotomy shock, begin IV infusion at 0.03 unit/minute; for septic shock begin IV infusion at 0.01 unit/minute. If target BP isn't achieved, titrate dosage up by 0.005 unit/minute at 10- to 15-minute intervals. After target BP has been maintained for 8 hours (without use of catecholamines), taper drug by 0.005 unit/minute every hour as tolerated to maintain BP. Maximum dosage for postcardiotomy shock, 0.1 unit/minute; for septic shock, 0.07 unit/minute.

ADMINISTRATION

IV

▼ For IV infusion with solution for dilution, dilute in NSS or D_5W to concentration of 0.1 to 1 unit/mL. For patients with fluid restrictions, mix 5 mL (100 units) in 100 mL; for patients with no fluid restrictions, mix 2.5 mL (50 units) in 500 mL.

▼ Inspect for particulate matter and discoloration before use.

▼ Titrate to lowest dosage compatible with a clinically acceptable response. Monitor BP every 10 to 15 minutes.

▼ Administer by CVAD if possible, using an infusion pump.

▼ Store intact vials at 68° to 77° F (20° to 25° C) for up to 12 months or refrigerate until manufacturer's original expiration date.

▼ Discard unused diluted solution after 18 hours at room temperature or 24 hours

---

*Reactions in bold italics are **life-threatening**.*

under refrigeration. Discard vials 48 hours after first entry.

▼ **Incompatibilities:** None listed by manufacturer. Consult drug compatibility reference for more information.

ACTION

Causes contraction of smooth muscle in the vascular bed and increases systemic vascular resistance and mean arterial BP. Tends to decrease HR and cardiac output.

Route	Onset	Peak	Duration
IV	Rapid	15 min	20 min

Half-life: Less than 10 minutes.

ADVERSE REACTIONS

CV: *hemorrhagic shock, HF,* atrial fibrillation, *bradycardia, myocardial ischemia, decreased cardiac output, distal limb ischemia, intractable bleeding.* **GI:** *mesenteric ischemia.* **GU:** **AKI.** **Hematologic:** *thrombocytopenia.* **Hepatic:** hyperbilirubinemia. **Metabolic:** *hyponatremia.* **Skin:** ischemic lesions.

INTERACTIONS

Drug-drug. *Catecholamines:* Causes additive effect on mean arterial pressure and other hemodynamic parameters. Adjust vasopressin dosage as needed.
Drugs suspected of causing diabetes insipidus (clozapine, demeclocycline, foscarnet, lithium): May decrease pressor and antidiuretic effects. Adjust vasopressin dosage as needed.
Drugs suspected of causing SIADH (chlorpropamide, cyclophosphamide, enalapril, felbamate, haloperidol, ifosfamide, methyldopa, pentamidine, SSRIs, TCAs, vincristine): May increase pressor and antidiuretic effects. Adjust vasopressin dosage as needed.
Ganglionic blockers (pentolinium, trimetaphan): May increase sensitivity to pressor effects. Monitor patient and BP. Adjust vasopressin dosage as needed.
Indomethacin: May prolong effect on cardiac index and systemic vascular resistance. Adjust vasopressin dosage as needed.

EFFECTS ON LAB TEST RESULTS

• May increase bilirubin level.
• May decrease sodium level.
• May decrease platelet count.

CONTRAINDICATIONS & CAUTIONS

• Contraindicated in patients allergic or hypersensitive to 8-arginine vasopressin. Multidose vial is also contraindicated in patients allergic to chlorobutanol.
• Use in patients with impaired cardiac response may worsen cardiac output.
• Reversible diabetes insipidus, manifested by development of polyuria, diluted urine, and hypernatremia, may occur after cessation of treatment. Some patients may require readministration of vasopressin or administration of desmopressin to correct fluid and electrolyte shifts.
• Use cautiously in older adults.
• Safety and effectiveness in children haven't been established.
Dialyzable drug: Unknown.
⚠ *Overdose S&S:* Hyponatremia; ventricular arrhythmias; rhabdomyolysis; nonspecific GI symptoms; peripheral, mesenteric, or coronary ischemia.

PREGNANCY-LACTATION-REPRODUCTION

• Studies during pregnancy are inadequate, and it isn't known whether drug can cause fetal harm. Drug may produce tonic uterine contractions that could threaten continuation of pregnancy.
• Because of increased clearance during second and third trimesters, increased dosage may be needed.
• It isn't known if drug appears in human milk.

NURSING CONSIDERATIONS

🕓 *Alert:* Extravasation may result in severe tissue damage. Ensure proper IV catheter placement before and during infusion, and monitor patient closely.
• Monitor patient for hypersensitivity reactions.
• Monitor BP and hemodynamic parameters every 10 to 15 minutes during therapy.
• Monitor urine specific gravity and fluid intake and output to aid evaluation of drug effectiveness.
• Monitor serum electrolyte levels, fluid status, and urine output during and after therapy.
• Monitor ECG.
• Monitor for bleeding, palpitations, and signs and symptoms of ischemia (chest pain, limb peripheral pain, paresthesia, coldness, decreased or absent pulses, abdominal pain, nausea, vomiting).

V

• *Look alike–sound alike:* Don't confuse vasopressin with desmopressin.

PATIENT TEACHING

• Instruct patient to immediately report all adverse reactions, especially bleeding, chest pain, palpitations, limb pain, limb coldness and pallor, paresthesia, nausea, vomiting, or abdominal pain.

• Advise patient to immediately report signs or symptoms of hypersensitivity reactions (breathing difficulty, wheezing, hives, nausea, vomiting, or swelling of face, lips, or tongue).

• Tell patient to immediately report infusion-site symptoms.

venlafaxine besylate
ven-la-FAX-een

venlafaxine hydrochloride
Effexor XR

Therapeutic class: Antidepressants
Pharmacologic class: SSNRIs

AVAILABLE FORMS

Capsules (extended-release) ⓞⓝⓒ: 37.5 mg, 75 mg, 150 mg
Tablets: 25 mg, 37.5 mg, 50 mg, 75 mg, 100 mg
Tablets (extended-release) ⓞⓝⓒ: 112.5 mg (besylate); 37.5 mg, 75 mg, 150 mg, 225 mg (hydrochloride)

INDICATIONS & DOSAGES

Adjust-a-dose (for all indications): For patients with CrCl 30 to 89 mL/minute, reduce daily amount by 25% in patients taking immediate-release tablets. Reduce by 25% to 50% in those taking extended-release form. For those with CrCl less than 30 mL/minute or on hemodialysis, reduce total daily dosage by 50% or more and withhold dose until dialysis is completed. For patients with Child-Pugh class A or B liver impairment, reduce daily dosage by 50%. For patients with Child-Pugh class C liver impairment, reduce total daily dosage by 50% or more.

➤ **Major depressive disorder**
Adults: Initially, 75 mg PO daily in two or three divided doses with food. For some patients, may be desirable to start at 37.5 mg/day for 4 to 7 days. Increase as tolerated and

needed by 75 mg daily every 4 days. For outpatients with moderate depression, usual maximum is 225 mg daily; in certain patients with severe depression, dose may be as high as 375 mg daily.

For extended-release capsules or tablets, 75 mg PO daily in single dose. For some patients, may be desirable to start at 37.5 mg PO daily for 4 to 7 days before increasing to 75 mg daily. Dosage may be increased by 75 mg daily every 4 days to maximum of 225 mg daily.

May switch immediate-release formulation to extended-release formulation by using nearest equivalent dose in mg/day. (For example, switch 37.5 mg immediate-release b.i.d. to 75 mg extended-release daily.)

➤ **Generalized anxiety disorder**
Adults: Initially, 75 mg extended-release capsule PO daily in single dose. For some patients, may be desirable to start at 37.5 mg PO daily for 4 to 7 days before increasing to 75 mg daily. Dosage may be increased by 75 mg daily every 4 days to maximum of 225 mg daily.

➤ **Panic disorder**
Adults: Initially, 37.5 mg extended-release capsule PO daily for 1 week; then increase dosage to 75 mg daily. If patient doesn't respond, may increase dosage by up to 75 mg/day in no less than weekly intervals, as needed, to maximum of 225 mg daily.

➤ **Social anxiety disorder (except besylate)**
Adults: Initially, 75 mg extended-release capsule or tablet PO daily as single dose. Maximum dosage, 75 mg/day.

➤ **Vasomotor signs and symptoms of menopause ◆**
Adults: Initially, 37.5 mg once daily; may increase after 1 week based on response and tolerability to 75 mg once daily for extended-release form or 75 mg/day in two to three divided doses for immediate-release form.

ADMINISTRATION
PO

• Give drug with food and a full glass of water at approximately the same time each day.

• For extended-release capsules and tablets, have patient swallow whole; don't crush, break, or place in water.

• May give pellet-filled capsules by carefully opening capsule and sprinkling pellets on spoonful of applesauce. Patient should swallow applesauce immediately without chewing, then follow with a glass of water to ensure that all pellets are swallowed.

• Give a missed dose as soon as possible, unless it's almost time for the next scheduled dose. Don't give two doses at the same time.

ACTION
Potent and selective inhibitor of neuronal serotonin and norepinephrine reuptake and weak inhibitor of dopamine reuptake.

Route	Onset	Peak	Duration
PO (immediate-release)	Unknown	2 hr	Unknown
PO (extended-release)	Unknown	5.5 hr	Unknown

Half-life: Immediate-release, 3 to 7 hours; extended-release, 7.5 to 14 hours.

ADVERSE REACTIONS
CNS: asthenia, headache, migraine, somnolence, dizziness, nervousness, insomnia, anxiety, tremor, abnormal dreams, paresthesia, agitation, twitching, weakness, syncope, taste alteration, amnesia, depersonalization, hypesthesia, vertigo, apathy, confusion, fever. **CV:** HTN, hypotension, tachycardia, vasodilation, palpitations, chest pain, edema. **EENT:** blurred vision, mydriasis, visual disturbance, tinnitus, dry mouth, sinusitis, trismus. **GI:** nausea, vomiting, constipation, anorexia, diarrhea, dyspepsia, flatulence, abdominal pain, bruxism. **GU:** abnormal ejaculation, erectile dysfunction, anorgasmia, urinary frequency, impaired urination, heavy menstrual bleeding, decreased libido, albuminuria. **Metabolic:** weight gain, weight loss, increased appetite, hypercholesterolemia, hypertriglyceridemia. **Musculoskeletal:** neck pain. **Respiratory:** yawning, cough, dyspnea. **Skin:** diaphoresis, alopecia, pruritus, photosensitivity, urticaria, ecchymosis, rash. **Other:** chills, accidental injury, flulike symptoms.

INTERACTIONS
Drug-drug. *Anticoagulants, aspirin, NSAIDs:* May increase antiplatelet effect of aspirin and NSAIDs and anticoagulant effect of anticoagulants. Monitor patient for increased risk of bleeding.
Antipsychotics (clozapine, risperidone): May increase risk of antipsychotic adverse reactions, including NMS. Monitor patient closely.

Cimetidine: May increase levels of both drugs. Use together cautiously.
Linezolid, methylene blue (IV): May cause serotonin syndrome. Use together is contraindicated.
MAO inhibitors (phenelzine, selegiline, tranylcypromine): May cause serotonin syndrome. Use within 14 days of MAO inhibitor therapy is contraindicated.
Serotonergic drugs (5-HT$_3$ antagonists, fentanyl, lithium, meperidine, tramadol, trazodone, triptans): May cause serotonin syndrome. Monitor patient closely.
Warfarin: May increase PT or INR. Monitor patient closely.
Drug-herb. *St. John's wort:* May cause serotonin syndrome. Monitor patient closely. Discourage use together.
Drug-lifestyle. *Alcohol use:* May increase mental and psychomotor impairment. Discourage alcohol use.

EFFECTS ON LAB TEST RESULTS
• May increase cholesterol and triglyceride levels.
• May decrease sodium level.
• May cause false-positive urine immunoassay screening tests for phencyclidine and amphetamine.

CONTRAINDICATIONS & CAUTIONS
• Contraindicated in patients hypersensitive to drug or any of its components.
Boxed Warning Antidepressants may increase risk of suicidality in children and young adults. Venlafaxine isn't approved for use in children. ■
❸ Alert: Concomitant use with serotonergic drugs, linezolid, or methylene blue can cause serotonin syndrome. Concomitant use of these drugs and venlafaxine is recommended only for life-threatening or urgent conditions when potential benefit outweighs risk of toxicity.
• Use cautiously in patients with kidney impairment, HTN, or diseases or conditions that could affect hemodynamic responses or metabolism and in those with history of mania or seizures.
• Carefully evaluate patients for history of drug abuse and follow such patients closely, observing for signs and symptoms of venlafaxine misuse or abuse (tolerance, dose incrementation, drug-seeking behavior).

V

• May trigger angle-closure attack. Use cautiously in patients at risk for acute narrow-angle glaucoma.

• Hyponatremia can occur, which may be a result of SIADH. Older adults, patients who are volume-depleted, and those taking diuretics are at increased risk. Discontinue drug if symptomatic hyponatremia develops.

Dialyzable drug: Unlikely.

⚠ *Overdose S&S:* Altered level of consciousness, somnolence, paresthesia of all four limbs, tachycardia, bradycardia, mydriasis, seizures, vomiting, ECG changes, hypotension, liver necrosis, rhabdomyolysis, serotonin syndrome, vertigo, death.

PREGNANCY-LACTATION-REPRODUCTION

• Use only if clearly needed and potential benefit justifies fetal risk. Use in middle to late pregnancy may increase risk of preeclampsia. Exposure to SNRIs near delivery may increase risk of postpartum hemorrhage.

❸ *Alert:* Neonates exposed to drug during late third trimester have developed complications (sometimes immediately upon delivery) that require respiratory support, tube feedings, and prolonged hospitalization.

• Encourage patients who are pregnant to enroll in the National Pregnancy Registry for Antidepressants (1-866-961-2388 or https://womensmentalhealth.org/research/pregnancyregistry/antidepressants)

• Drug may appear in human milk. Patient should discontinue breastfeeding or discontinue drug, considering importance of drug to patient.

NURSING CONSIDERATIONS

❸ *Alert:* Closely monitor all patients for signs and symptoms of clinical worsening and suicidality, especially at the beginning of therapy and with dosage adjustments. Signs and symptoms may include agitation, insomnia, anxiety, aggressiveness, or panic attacks.

❸ *Alert:* Sudden discontinuation or abrupt decrease in venlafaxine dose can lead to serotonin withdrawal (agitation, confusion, flu-like symptoms, sensory disturbances, tremor). Reduce dosage gradually and watch for symptoms. Discontinuation may take several months in some patients.

❸ *Alert:* If linezolid or methylene blue must be given, stop venlafaxine and monitor patient for serotonin toxicity for 2 weeks or until 24 hours after last dose of methylene blue or linezolid, whichever comes first. May resume serotonergic psychiatric drugs 24 hours after last dose of methylene blue or linezolid.

• Carefully monitor BP. Drug therapy may cause sustained, dose-dependent increases in BP.

• Monitor for signs and symptoms of hyponatremia (headache, difficulty concentrating, memory impairment, confusion, weakness, unsteadiness and, in severe cases, hallucinations, syncope, seizure, respiratory arrest, coma, death).

• Monitor weight, particularly in patient with depression who is underweight.

❸ *Alert:* Monitor for signs and symptoms of serotonin syndrome (restlessness, hallucinations, loss of coordination, tachycardia, rapid BP changes, increased body temperature, overactive reflexes, nausea, vomiting, diarrhea). Serotonin syndrome may be more likely to occur when starting or increasing dosage of triptan, SSRI, or SSNRI.

• SSNRIs may cause sexual dysfunction. Monitor patient for signs and symptoms and exclude other causes, such as underlying psychiatric disorder. Inquire specifically about changes; patient may not report spontaneously.

PATIENT TEACHING

• Teach about proper drug administration and handling.

• Inform patient that if drug needs to be stopped, it should be tapered gradually by the prescriber and not stopped abruptly.

❸ *Alert:* Warn caregivers to closely monitor patient for signs and symptoms of worsening condition or suicidality.

• Caution patient to avoid hazardous activities that require alertness and good coordination until effects of drug are known.

• Tell patient to avoid alcohol and to consult prescriber before taking other prescription or OTC drugs or supplements.

• Teach patient to recognize and immediately report signs and symptoms of serotonin toxicity (fever, mental status changes, muscle twitching, diaphoresis, shivering or shaking, diarrhea, loss of coordination).

• Advise patient to report pregnancy or plans to become pregnant or breastfeed during therapy.

Reactions in bold italics are *life-threatening*.

verapamil hydrochloride
ver-AP-a-mill

Calan SR, Isoptin SR ♣, Verelan, Verelan PM

Therapeutic class: Antihypertensives
Pharmacologic class: Calcium channel blockers

AVAILABLE FORMS
Capsules (extended-release) ⓄⓃⒸ: 100 mg, 120 mg, 180 mg, 200 mg, 240 mg, 300 mg, 360 mg
Injection: 2.5 mg/mL
Tablets: 40 mg, 80 mg, 120 mg
Tablets (extended-release) ⓄⓃⒸ: 120 mg, 180 mg, 240 mg

INDICATIONS & DOSAGES
Adjust-a-dose (for all indications): In patients with severe liver dysfunction, give 30% of dose.
➤ **Vasospastic angina (Prinzmetal or variant angina); unstable angina; classic chronic, stable angina pectoris**
Adults: Initially, 80 to 120 mg (immediate-release) PO t.i.d. Increase dosage at daily or weekly intervals as needed. Some patients may require up to 480 mg daily. Maximum, 480 mg/day.
Adjust-a-dose: In patients with kidney or liver impairment, older adults, and patients with low weight, reduce initial dosage to 40 mg t.i.d.
➤ **To prevent paroxysmal supraventricular tachycardia**
Adults: 240 to 480 mg (immediate-release) PO daily in three or four divided doses. Maximum, 480 mg/day.
➤ **Atrial flutter or atrial fibrillation with rapid ventricular rate; supraventricular arrhythmias**
Adults: 0.075 to 0.15 mg/kg (5 to 10 mg) by IV push with ECG and BP monitoring. Repeat dose of 0.15 mg/kg (10 mg) in 30 minutes if inadequate response.
Children ages 1 to 15: Give 0.1 to 0.3 mg/kg as IV bolus; not to exceed 5 mg. Repeat dose in 30 minutes if inadequate response. Don't exceed 10 mg as single dose.
Children younger than age 1: Give 0.1 to 0.2 mg/kg as IV bolus with continuous ECG

monitoring. Repeat dose in 30 minutes if inadequate response.
➤ **Chronic atrial fibrillation or flutter in patients who have been receiving digoxin**
Adults: 240 to 320 mg (immediate-release) PO daily in three or four divided doses.
➤ **HTN**
Adults: Initially, 80 mg immediate-release tablet PO t.i.d. May increase weekly based on therapeutic effect to maximum of 480 mg/day. Or, initially, 240 mg extended-release capsules (Verelan) PO once daily in the morning; if inadequate response, may increase by 120 mg daily to maximum of 480 mg. If using Verelan PM, 200 mg PO daily at bedtime; may increase to 300 mg at bedtime if inadequate response. Maximum dose, 400 mg. If using extended-release tablets (Calan SR), 180 mg PO in the morning. Evaluate weekly and approximately 24 hours after previous dose. May increase as follows: 240 mg each morning; 180 mg each morning plus 180 mg each evening, or 240 mg each morning plus 120 mg each evening; 240 mg every 12 hours.
Adjust-a-dose: In patients with kidney or liver impairment, older adults, and patients of small stature, reduce initial dosage to 40 mg t.i.d. for immediate-release tablets, 120 mg once daily for Verelan or Calan SR, or 100 mg once daily for Verelan PM.

ADMINISTRATION
PO
● Pellet-filled capsules may be given by carefully opening capsule and sprinkling pellets on a spoonful of applesauce. Patient should immediately swallow without chewing, followed by a glass of cool water to ensure that all pellets are swallowed.
● Oral suspension may be compounded by a pharmacist, if needed.
● Have patient swallow long-acting forms of drug whole; don't crush or break tablets.
IV
▼ IV form is contraindicated in patients receiving IV beta blockers and in those with ventricular tachycardia.
▼ Inject directly into vein or into tubing of free-flowing, compatible solution, such as D₅W, half-NSS, NSS, Ringer solution, or lactated Ringer solution.
▼ Give doses over at least 2 minutes (3 minutes in older adults) to minimize risk of adverse reactions.
▼ Continuously monitor ECG and BP.

V

▼ **Incompatibilities:** Albumin, amphotericin B, hydralazine, solutions with a pH greater than 6, sulfamethoxazole–trimethoprim. Consult drug compatibility reference for more information.

ACTION

A calcium channel blocker that inhibits calcium ion influx across cardiac and smooth-muscle cells, thus decreasing myocardial contractility and oxygen demand; also dilates coronary arteries and arterioles.

Route	Onset	Peak	Duration
PO	1–2 hr	1–2 hr	8–10 hr
PO (extended-release)	30 min	5–9 hr	24 hr
IV	Immediate	1–5 min	0.5–6 hr

Half-life: 2.8 to 12 hours (varies by product).

ADVERSE REACTIONS

CNS: dizziness, headache, fatigue, sleep disturbances, pain, lethargy. **CV:** transient hypotension, *HF, bradycardia, AV block, ventricular asystole, ventricular fibrillation,* edema, flushing, HTN, tachycardia. **EENT:** gingival hyperplasia, pharyngitis, sinusitis. **GI:** constipation, nausea, diarrhea, dyspepsia. **Musculoskeletal:** myalgia. **Respiratory:** dyspnea. **Skin:** rash. **Other:** flulike syndrome, infection, accidental injury.

INTERACTIONS

Drug-drug. *Amiodarone:* May cause bradycardia and decrease cardiac output. Monitor patient closely.

Antihypertensives (ACE inhibitors, beta blockers, diuretics, vasodilators), quinidine: May cause hypotension. Monitor BP.

Barbiturates (phenobarbital): May increase verapamil clearance. Monitor response and adjust verapamil dose as needed.

Beta blockers: May have additive effects on HR, AV conduction, or cardiac contractility. Use together cautiously.

Carbamazepine: May increase level of carbamazepine. Monitor patient for toxicity, and adjust dosage as needed.

Clonidine: May increase risk of bradycardia and need for pacemaker insertion. Monitor HR closely.

Cyclosporine: May increase cyclosporine level. Monitor cyclosporine level.

CYP3A4 inducers (dexamethasone, phenytoin, dabrafenib, modafinil, nafcillin): May decrease verapamil level. Monitor for verapamil effect; adjust dosage as needed.

Digoxin: May increase digoxin level and risk of toxicity. Closely monitor digoxin level and cardiac function, and decrease dosages as needed.

Disopyramide: May cause HF. Avoid use 48 hours before or 24 hours after verapamil.

Dofetilide: May increase dofetilide level. Avoid use together.

Flecainide: May enhance negative inotropic effect and prolongation of AV conduction. Use together cautiously.

HMG-CoA reductase inhibitors that are substrates of CYP3A4 (atorvastatin, lovastatin, simvastatin): May elevate plasma levels of these drugs and risk of myopathy. If coadministration can't be avoided, limit dose of HMG-CoA reductase inhibitor. Don't give doses greater than 10 mg daily of simvastatin or greater than 40 mg daily of lovastatin. Closely monitor drug level, and adjust dosage as needed.

Inhalation anesthetics (enflurane): May potentiate cardiac effects. Titrate doses carefully to avoid excessive CV depression.

Ivabradine: May increase ivabradine level and risk of bradycardia and conduction disturbances. Avoid use together.

Lithium: May decrease or increase lithium level. Monitor lithium level.

Macrolide antibiotics (clarithromycin, erythromycin): May increase macrolide and verapamil levels. Closely monitor cardiac function, and adjust dosage as needed.

Moderate and strong CYP3A4 inhibitors (ketoconazole, ritonavir): May increase verapamil level. Monitor therapy closely.

mTOR inhibitors (everolimus, sirolimus, tacrolimus): May increase levels of these drugs. Monitor drug level closely, and adjust dosage as needed.

Neuromuscular blockers: May potentiate activity of these drugs. Monitor neuromuscular function, and adjust dosage of either drug as needed.

Quinidine: May increase risk of bradycardia in patients with hypertrophic cardiomyopathy. Avoid use together in these patients.

Rifampin: May decrease oral bioavailability of verapamil. Monitor for lack of effect.

Theophylline: May decrease clearance of theophylline. Monitor for signs of theophylline toxicity.

Reactions in bold italics are *life-threatening*.

Drug-herb. *St. John's wort:* May decrease drug level and effect. Discourage use together.

Drug-food. *Grapefruit juice:* May increase drug level. Discourage use together.

Drug-lifestyle. *Alcohol use:* May increase alcohol level. Discourage use together.

EFFECTS ON LAB TEST RESULTS

• May increase ALT, AST, ALP, and bilirubin levels.

• May cause false-positive urine detection of methadone.

CONTRAINDICATIONS & CAUTIONS

• Contraindicated in patients hypersensitive to drug and in those with severe left ventricular dysfunction, cardiogenic shock, secondor third-degree AV block, or sick sinus syndrome, except in presence of functioning pacemaker, atrial flutter or fibrillation associated with accessory bypass tract syndrome, severe HF (unless secondary to therapy), and severe hypotension.

• IV form is contraindicated in patients receiving IV beta blockers and in those with wide-complex ventricular tachycardia (QRS complex of 0.12 second or more).

• Use cautiously in older adults, children, and patients with increased ICP, hypertrophic cardiomyopathy, or liver or kidney disease.

• Use cautiously in patients with Duchenne muscular dystrophy; drug may precipitate respiratory muscle failure.

Dialyzable drug: No.

⚠ **Overdose S&S:** Hypotension, bradycardia, arrhythmias, hyperglycemia, depressed mental status, noncardiogenic pulmonary edema, increasing AV block.

PREGNANCY-LACTATION-REPRODUCTION

• Studies during pregnancy are inadequate. Drug crosses placental barrier. Use only if clearly needed. Fetal monitoring is recommended.

• Drug appears in human milk. Some manufacturers recommend that patients stop breastfeeding.

NURSING CONSIDERATIONS

• Frequently monitor PR interval.

• Monitor BP at start of therapy, during dosage adjustments, and routinely during therapy. Assist patient with walking because dizziness may occur.

• Notify prescriber if signs and symptoms of HF occur (swelling of hands and feet, shortness of breath).

• Monitor kidney function test and LFT results during prolonged treatment.

• **Look alike–sound alike:** Don't confuse Verelan with Vivarin or Voltaren.

PATIENT TEACHING

• Tell patient to report all adverse reactions, especially palpitations, slow heartbeat, dizziness, dyspnea, or swelling.

• Teach about proper drug administration and handling. Instruct patient to take drug exactly as prescribed.

• Caution patient against abruptly stopping drug.

• If patient continues nitrate therapy during oral verapamil dosage adjustment, urge continued adherence. SL nitroglycerin may be taken, as needed, for acute chest pain.

• Drug significantly inhibits alcohol elimination. Advise patient to avoid or severely limit alcohol use.

vericiguat
ver-i-SIG-ue-at

Verquvo

Therapeutic class: Pulmonary vasodilators
Pharmacologic class: Soluble guanylate cyclase stimulators

AVAILABLE FORMS

Tablets: 2.5 mg, 5 mg, 10 mg

INDICATIONS & DOSAGES

➤ **Reduces risk of CV death and HF rehospitalization after a hospitalization for HF or need for outpatient IV diuretics in patients with symptomatic chronic HF and ejection fraction less than 45%**

Adults: 2.5 mg PO once daily. Double dosage approximately every 2 weeks up to target maintenance dosage of 10 mg once daily, as tolerated.

ADMINISTRATION

PO

• Give drug with food.

• May crush and mix with water immediately before giving.

- If a dose is missed, give as soon as possible on the same day of missed dose; don't give two doses on the same day.
- Store tablets at room temperature.

ACTION
Directly stimulates soluble guanylate cyclase independently of and synergistically with nitric oxide, causing increased levels of intracellular cyclic guanosine monophosphate, leading to smooth muscle relaxation and vasodilation.

Route	Onset	Peak	Duration
PO	Unknown	4 hr (with food)	Unknown

Half-life: 30 hours.

ADVERSE REACTIONS
CV: hypotension. **Hematologic:** anemia.

INTERACTIONS
Drug-drug. *Other soluble guanylate cyclase stimulators (riociguat):* May increase risk of adverse effects. Use together is contraindicated.
PDE5 inhibitors (avanafil, sildenafil, vardenafil): May increase risk of hypotension. Avoid use together.

EFFECTS ON LAB TEST RESULTS
- May decrease RBC count.

CONTRAINDICATIONS & CAUTIONS
- Drug hasn't been studied in patients with Child-Pugh class C liver impairment, those with eGFR less than 15 mL/minute/1.73 m², or those who require dialysis.
- Safety and effectiveness in children haven't been established.
- Use cautiously in older adults.
Dialyzable drug: Unlikely.

PREGNANCY-LACTATION-REPRODUCTION
Boxed Warning Exclude pregnancy before starting therapy. Drug may cause fetal harm and is contraindicated in patients who are pregnant. ■
Boxed Warning Patients of childbearing potential must use effective forms of contraception during therapy and for 1 month after final dose. ■
- Notify manufacturer of patients exposed to drug during pregnancy (1-877-888-4231 or https://pregnancyreporting.verquvo-us.com).

- It isn't known if drug appears in human milk or how drug affects milk production or infants who are breastfed. Advise patients not to breastfeed during therapy.

NURSING CONSIDERATIONS
- Verify pregnancy status before starting drug.
- Monitor patient for hypotension.
- Monitor patient for anemia.

PATIENT TEACHING
- Instruct patient on proper self-administration.
Boxed Warning Advise patient to report pregnancy or plans to become pregnant during therapy. ■
Boxed Warning Tell patient of childbearing potential to use effective contraception during therapy and for 1 month after final dose. ■
- Inform patient not to breastfeed during therapy.

vibegron
vye-BEG-ron

Gemtesa

Therapeutic class: Bladder antispasmodics
Pharmacologic class: Beta-3 adrenergic agonists

AVAILABLE FORMS
Tablets: 75 mg

INDICATIONS & DOSAGES
➤ **Overactive bladder with symptoms of urge urinary incontinence, urgency, and urinary frequency**
Adults: 75 mg PO once daily.

ADMINISTRATION
PO
- Give drug without regard to food.
- Have patient swallow tablets whole with a glass of water.
- May crush tablets and mix with approximately 15 mL of applesauce; give immediately and follow with a glass of water.
- Store tablets at room temperature.

ACTION
Relaxes detrusor smooth muscle and increases bladder capacity during bladder filling.

Route	Onset	Peak	Duration
PO	Unknown	1–3 hr	Unknown

Half-life: 30.8 hours.

ADVERSE REACTIONS
CNS: headache. **EENT:** dry mouth, nasopharyngitis. **GI:** constipation, diarrhea, nausea. **GU:** UTI, urine retention. **Respiratory:** bronchitis, URI. **Other:** hot flushes.

INTERACTIONS
Drug-drug. *Digoxin:* May increase digoxin level. Monitor digoxin level.

EFFECTS ON LAB TEST RESULTS
None reported.

CONTRAINDICATIONS & CAUTIONS
• Contraindicated in patients hypersensitive to drug or its components.
• Drug may increase risk of urine retention. Use cautiously in patients with bladder outlet obstruction.
• Avoid use in patients with eGFR less than 15 mL/minute/1.73 m^2 (with or without hemodialysis) and in those with Child-Pugh class C liver impairment.
• Safety and effectiveness in children haven't been established.
Dialyzable drug: Unknown.

PREGNANCY-LACTATION-REPRODUCTION
• Studies during pregnancy are inadequate. Use only if benefit outweighs fetal risk.
• It isn't known if drug appears in human milk; drug was detected in animal milk studies. Consider benefits and possible risk to infant.

NURSING CONSIDERATIONS
• Monitor patient for urine retention. Discontinue drug if urine retention occurs.
• If patient is taking digoxin, monitor digoxin level before and during therapy and adjust digoxin dosage as needed. Continue monitoring upon discontinuation of therapy, and adjust digoxin dosage as needed.
• *Look alike–sound alike:* Don't confuse vibegron with vigabatrin or Vigadrone.

PATIENT TEACHING
• Teach about proper drug administration and handling.

• Explain that drug may cause urine retention. Instruct patient to report urinary hesitancy or urine retention.
• Advise patient to report pregnancy or plans to become pregnant or breastfeed during therapy.

vigabatrin
veye-gah-BA-trin

Sabril, Vigadrone

Therapeutic class: Anticonvulsants
Pharmacologic class: GABA transaminase inhibitors

AVAILABLE FORMS
Powder for oral solution: 500 mg
Tablets: 500 mg

INDICATIONS & DOSAGES
Adjust-a-dose (for all indications): For patients with CrCl of 51 to 80 mL/minute, reduce dosage by 25%; CrCl of 31 to 50 mL/minute, reduce dosage by 50%; CrCl of 11 to 30 mL/minute, reduce dosage by 75%.
➤ **Refractory complex partial seizures in patients with inadequate response to several alternative treatments**
Adults and children ages 17 and older and children weighing more than 60 kg: Initially, 500 mg PO b.i.d. May increase dosage weekly in 500-mg/day increments to maximum of 1,500 mg PO b.i.d.
Children ages 2 to 16 weighing 25 to 60 kg: Initially, 250 mg b.i.d. PO. Increase in weekly intervals to maximum of 1,000 mg b.i.d., depending on response.
Children ages 2 to 16 weighing more than 20 to 25 kg: Initially, 250 mg b.i.d. PO. Increase in weekly intervals to maximum of 750 mg b.i.d., depending on response.
Children ages 2 to 16 weighing more than 15 to 20 kg: Initially, 225 mg b.i.d. PO. Increase in weekly intervals to maximum maintenance of 650 mg b.i.d., depending on response.
Children ages 2 to 16 weighing 10 to 15 kg: Initially, 175 mg b.i.d. PO. Increase in weekly intervals to maximum maintenance of 525 mg b.i.d., depending on response.
➤ **Infantile spasms**
Infants and children ages 1 month to 2 years: 50 mg/kg/day PO in two divided doses. Titrate in 25- to 50-mg/kg/day increments

V

every 3 days as needed. Maximum dosage, 150 mg/kg/day (75 mg/kg b.i.d.).

ADMINISTRATION
PO
🕕 *Alert:* Hazardous drug; use safe handling and disposal precautions.
• Give drug without regard to food.
• Empty entire contents of appropriate number of packets (500 mg/packet) of powder into cup, and dissolve in 10 mL of cold or room-temperature water per packet. Use oral syringe supplied with medication to measure water and give solution. Concentration of final solution is 50 mg/mL. Use immediately after reconstitution, and discard any unused portion.
• Discard solution if it isn't clear, colorless, and free of particles.

ACTION
Precise mechanism unknown. Thought to control seizures by inhibiting GABA transaminase, the enzyme responsible for metabolizing the inhibitory neurotransmitter GABA, thereby increasing GABA levels in the CNS.

Route	Onset	Peak	Duration
PO	Unknown	1–2.5 hr	Unknown

Half-life: 5.5 to 10.5 hours.

ADVERSE REACTIONS
CNS: abnormal behavior, abnormal coordination, abnormal dreams, abnormal thinking, anxiety, asthenia, attention disturbance, confusion, *seizures,* depression, dizziness, dysarthria, expressive language disorder, fatigue, drowsiness, fever, gait disorder, headache, hyperreflexia, hypoesthesia, hyporeflexia, ataxia, insomnia, irritability, lethargy, malaise, memory impairment, nervousness, paresthesia, peripheral neuropathy, postictal state, sedation, impaired consciousness, sensory disturbance, sensory loss, somnolence, *status epilepticus,* thirst, tremor, vertigo, dystonia, hypotonia, hypertonia. **CV:** chest pain, peripheral edema. **EENT:** asthenopia, blurred vision, diplopia, nystagmus, eye pain, strabismus, conjunctivitis, visual field defect, tinnitus, otitis media, sinus headache, nasal congestion, nasopharyngitis, pharyngolaryngeal pain, sinusitis, toothache. **GI:** abdominal distention, constipation, diarrhea, dyspepsia, increased or decreased

appetite, nausea, stomach discomfort, abdominal pain, vomiting, gastroenteritis. **GU:** dysmenorrhea, erectile dysfunction, UTI. **Hematologic:** anemia. **Metabolic:** weight gain. **Musculoskeletal:** arthralgia, back pain, contusion, extremity pain, joint sprain, myalgia, muscle spasm, muscle strain, muscle twitching. **Respiratory:** bronchitis, cough, pulmonary congestion, URI, pneumonia, infectious croup. **Skin:** rash, wound secretion. **Other:** flulike syndrome, infection.

INTERACTIONS
Drug-drug. *Cannabidiol, cannabis, clonazepam:* May enhance CNS depression. Monitor therapy.
Boxed Warning *Drugs associated with serious adverse ophthalmic effects, such as retinopathy (hydroxychloroquine) or glaucoma (corticosteroids, TCAs):* May increase risk of serious adverse ophthalmic effects. Avoid coadministration unless benefits clearly outweigh risks. ∎
Fosphenytoin, phenytoin: May decrease phenytoin level, especially when drug is started or stopped. Monitor drug levels.
Drug-lifestyle. *Alcohol use:* May increase CNS depression. Advise patient to avoid alcohol.

EFFECTS ON LAB TEST RESULTS
• May decrease ALT and AST levels.
• May decrease Hb level, hematocrit, and RBC count.
• May increase amino acid levels in urine and lead to false-positive tests for genetic metabolic disorders.

CONTRAINDICATIONS & CAUTIONS
• Contraindicated in patients hypersensitive to drug or its components and as first-line therapy for complex partial seizures.
🕕 *Alert:* Use drug only when potential benefits outweigh risk of vision loss.
Boxed Warning Drug may cause progressive and permanent bilateral concentric visual field constriction and may reduce visual acuity; onset is unpredictable and can occur anytime during therapy. Risk of visual impairment increases with increasing dosage and cumulative exposure, but no dosage or exposure is known to be free of risk of vision loss, which may continue after drug is discontinued. Because of risk of permanent vision loss, drug is available only through the Vigabatrin

REMS program. Patients should undergo visual exams before, every 3 months during, and 3 to 6 months after therapy. ■

Boxed Warning Due to risk of vision loss, withdraw drug in patients who don't show substantial benefit within 3 months of initiation for refractory complex partial seizures and within 2 to 4 weeks of initiation in patients with infantile spasms, or sooner if treatment failure becomes obvious. Periodically reassess patients' response to and continued need for drug. Use drug at lowest dosage with shortest exposure time as clinically necessary. ■

Boxed Warning Don't use drug in patients who have or are at high risk for other types of irreversible vision loss, unless benefits clearly outweigh risks. ■

• Drug may cause MRI abnormalities or neurotoxicity (intramyelinic edema) and increase risk of peripheral neuropathy in adults.
• Use cautiously in patients with history of depression, suicidality, or anemia.
Dialyzable drug: 40% to 60%.
⚠ *Overdose S&S:* Unconsciousness, coma, drowsiness, vertigo, psychosis, apnea, respiratory depression, bradycardia, agitation, irritability, confusion, headache, hypotension, abnormal behavior, increased seizure activity, status epilepticus, speech disorder.

PREGNANCY-LACTATION-REPRODUCTION
• Studies during pregnancy are inadequate; animal studies suggest drug may cause fetal harm. Use only if potential benefit justifies fetal risk.
• Patients taking drug during pregnancy should enroll in the North American Antiepileptic Drug Pregnancy Registry (1-888-233-2334 or www.aedpregnancyregistry.org).
• Drug appears in human milk. Patient should discontinue breastfeeding or discontinue drug, considering importance of drug to patient.

NURSING CONSIDERATIONS
⬩ *Alert:* Closely monitor all patients taking or starting therapy with antiepileptics for changes in behavior indicating worsening suicidality or depression. Symptoms such as anxiety, agitation, hostility, mania, and hypomania may be precursors to emerging suicidality.
• Discontinue drug if patient fails to comply with therapy.

⬩ *Alert:* Don't withdraw drug suddenly. For adult, taper by decreasing dose by 1,000 mg/day weekly until discontinued. For child with complex partial seizures, taper daily dose by one-third every week for 3 weeks. For infantile spasms, decrease daily dose at rate of 25 to 50 mg/kg every 3 to 4 days.
• Monitor patient closely for such adverse effects as dizziness, which may lead to falls.
• Monitor patient closely for anemia, somnolence, fatigue, peripheral neuropathy, peripheral edema, and weight gain.
• Monitor ALT and AST levels. Drug decreases levels, making these measurements unreliable for detecting early liver injury.

PATIENT TEACHING
• Teach about proper drug administration and handling.
• Advise patient to read manufacturer's medication guide before starting treatment and before each prescription refill.
• Warn that drug may cause dizziness and somnolence. Instruct patient to avoid driving and other hazardous activities until drug's effects are known.

Boxed Warning Inform patient that drug may cause vision loss. Explain importance of regular eye exams and need to immediately report vision changes. Counsel patient that vision loss may be severe before it's detected. ■

• Advise patient to call prescriber and not to stop drug suddenly if adverse reactions occur.
• Tell patient to report pregnancy or plans to become pregnant during therapy.
• Inform patient that drug appears in human milk. Instruct patient to avoid breastfeeding.

---

vilazodone hydrochloride
vil-AZ-oh-dohne

Viibryd

Therapeutic class: Antidepressants
Pharmacologic class: SSRIs–partial 5-HT$_{1A}$ receptor agonists

AVAILABLE FORMS
Tablets: 10 mg, 20 mg, 40 mg

INDICATIONS & DOSAGES
➤ **Major depressive disorder**
Adults: Initially, 10 mg PO daily for 7 days; then 20 mg PO daily. After 7 days, may

V

increase to 40 mg PO daily. Recommended range, 20 to 40 mg.

Adjust-a-dose: Don't exceed 20 mg once daily when used in combination with a strong CYP3A4 inhibitor. Based on clinical response, consider increasing dosage twofold, up to maximum of 80 mg once daily, over 1 to 2 weeks in patients taking strong CYP3A4 inducers for more than 14 days.

ADMINISTRATION
PO
• Give drug with food.
• Give a missed dose as soon as possible. If it's almost time for the next dose, skip missed dose and give next dose at regular time. Don't double dose.

ACTION
Binds to serotonin reuptake sites and 5-HT$_{1A}$ receptors; is a partial agonist at serotonergic 5-HT$_{1A}$ receptors.

Route	Onset	Peak	Duration
PO	Unknown	4–5 hr	Unknown

Half-life: 25 hours.

ADVERSE REACTIONS
CNS: dizziness, headache, somnolence, paresthesia, insomnia, abnormal dreams, restlessness, fatigue, sedation, tremor. **CV:** palpitations. **EENT:** dry mouth. **GI:** abdominal distention, abdominal pain, diarrhea, nausea, vomiting, dyspepsia, flatulence, gastroenteritis, increased appetite. **GU:** delayed ejaculation, erectile dysfunction, sexual dysfunction, abnormal orgasm, decreased libido. **Metabolic:** weight gain. **Musculoskeletal:** arthralgia.

INTERACTIONS
Drug-drug. *Anticoagulants (apixaban, aspirin, heparin, NSAIDs, warfarin), antiplatelet agents:* May increase risk of bleeding. Monitor patient closely. Adjust dosages of these drugs, or discontinue them.
Antipsychotics (olanzapine, risperidone): May increase risk of antipsychotic adverse effects, including NMS. Monitor patient closely.
CNS drugs: May cause additive effects. Use together cautiously.
Digoxin: May increase digoxin level. Monitor level before and during use with vilazodone. Reduce digoxin dose as necessary.

MAO inhibitors, linezolid, methylene blue: May increase risk of serious or fatal adverse effects. Don't use concurrently with MAO inhibitor or within 14 days of starting or discontinuing an MAO inhibitor.
Serotonergics (buspirone, SSNRIs, SSRIs, tramadol, triptans): May cause serotonin syndrome. Use together with extreme caution.
Strong CYP3A4 inducers (carbamazepine, phenytoin, rifampin): May decrease vilazodone level. Monitor effectiveness, and adjust vilazodone dosage as needed.
Strong CYP3A4 inhibitors (clarithromycin, itraconazole, voriconazole): May increase vilazodone level. Reduce vilazodone dosage to 20 mg daily.
Drug-herb. *Herbs with anticoagulant or antiplatelet properties (alfalfa, anise, bilberry):* May increase bleeding risk. Discourage use together.
St. John's wort: May increase risk of serotonin syndrome. Discourage use together.
Drug-lifestyle. *Alcohol use:* May increase psychomotor impairment. Discourage use together.

EFFECTS ON LAB TEST RESULTS
• May decrease sodium level.

CONTRAINDICATIONS & CAUTIONS
Boxed Warning Drug may increase risk of suicidality in children, adolescents, and young adults with major depressive disorder or other psychiatric disorders. Drug isn't approved for use in children. ■
❸ *Alert:* Life-threatening serotonin syndrome (fever, mental status changes, muscle twitching, diaphoresis, shivering or shaking, diarrhea, loss of coordination) has been reported with antidepressant use. Risk increases when antidepressants are used with other serotonergic drugs and with drugs that impair serotonin metabolism.
❸ *Alert:* Concomitant use with methylene blue or linezolid can cause serotonin syndrome. Don't initiate drug in patients receiving linezolid or methylene blue.
• Contraindicated in patients hypersensitive to drug or its inactive components.
• Use cautiously in patients with personal or family history of depression, hypomania, Child-Pugh class C liver impairment, seizure disorder, or untreated angle-closure glaucoma.

Reactions in bold italics are *life-threatening*.

• Hyponatremia and SIADH, which may be life-threatening, have resulted from treatment with other SSRIs and SSNRIs, especially in older adults and patients who take diuretics or are otherwise volume-depleted.
Dialyzable drug: Unlikely.
⚠ *Overdose S&S:* Serotonin syndrome, lethargy, restlessness, hallucinations, disorientation.

PREGNANCY-LACTATION-REPRODUCTION
• Neonates born to patients who used drug in third trimester can develop complications (including persistent pulmonary HTN of newborn) upon delivery, requiring prolonged hospitalization, respiratory support, and enteral feedings. Use drug during pregnancy only if potential benefits outweigh fetal risk.
• Patients taking drug during pregnancy should enroll in the North American Antiepileptic Drug Pregnancy Registry (1-888-233-2334 or www.aedpregnancyregistry.org).
• Drug may appear in human milk. Use only if benefit outweighs risk to infant.

NURSING CONSIDERATIONS
• Evaluate patient for major depressive disorder.
• Screen patient for risk of bipolar disorder. Vilazodone isn't approved for treatment of bipolar depression. Use of an antidepressant in patient with bipolar disorder may precipitate mixed or manic episodes.
• Evaluate patient for history of drug abuse, and watch closely for signs and symptoms of misuse or abuse (increased tolerance, drug-seeking behavior, requests for dosage increase).
• *Alert:* If linezolid or methylene blue must be given concurrently with vilazodone (or other serotonergic drug), stop serotonergic drug and monitor patient for serotonin toxicity for 2 weeks (5 weeks if fluoxetine was taken) or until 24 hours after last dose of methylene blue or linezolid, whichever comes first. May resume vilazodone 24 hours after last dose of methylene blue or linezolid.
• Closely monitor patient who has recently taken an MAO inhibitor for tremors, myoclonus, diaphoresis, nausea, vomiting, flushing, dizziness, and hyperthermia.

• Monitor patient taking anticoagulant or antiplatelet agent for signs and symptoms of bleeding.
• When discontinuing vilazodone, avoid abrupt discontinuation. Gradually reduce dosage and monitor for adverse events. If withdrawal symptoms become intolerable, consider resuming previous prescribed dosage and decreasing dosage at a more gradual rate.
• Monitor for signs and symptoms of hyponatremia (headache, difficulty concentrating, memory impairment, confusion, weakness, unsteadiness, hallucinations, syncope, seizures, coma, respiratory arrest). Discontinue vilazodone in patient with symptomatic hyponatremia, and treat appropriately.
• Monitor patient for acute-angle glaucoma.

PATIENT TEACHING
Boxed Warning Advise family or caregiver to closely observe patient for increased suicidality. ■
• Teach about proper drug administration and handling.
• *Alert:* Teach patient to recognize and immediately report signs and symptoms of serotonin toxicity (fever, mental status changes, muscle twitching, diaphoresis, shivering, shaking, diarrhea, loss of coordination).
• Warn patient not to stop drug abruptly.
• Instruct patient to inform prescriber of all other medicines being taken to avoid dangerous interactions.
• Tell patient to immediately seek medical attention if fever, rigidity, rapid changes in pulse rate or BP, diaphoresis, or confusion occurs.
• Counsel patient to keep all appointments for monitoring blood work and for follow-up care.
• Advise patient to use caution when driving or operating hazardous equipment until effects of drug are known. Drug may impair judgment, thinking, and motor skills.
• Caution patient and caregivers to watch for signs and symptoms of onset of manic or hypomanic episodes.
• Warn patient to avoid alcohol during drug therapy.
• Advise patient to report pregnancy or plans to become pregnant or breastfeed during therapy.

V

viloxazine
vye-LOX-a-zeen

Qelbree

Therapeutic class: ADHD drugs
Pharmacologic class: Selective norepinephrine reuptake inhibitors

AVAILABLE FORMS
Capsules (extended-release) ⓄⓃⒸ*:* 100 mg, 150 mg, 200 mg

INDICATIONS & DOSAGES
➤ **ADHD**
Adults: Initially, 200 mg PO once daily. May titrate by 200-mg increments weekly to maximum dosage of 600 mg once daily, depending on response and tolerability.
Children ages 12 to 17: Initially, 200 mg PO once daily. After 1 week, may titrate by 200-mg increments to maximum dosage of 400 mg daily, depending on response and tolerability.
Children ages 6 to 11: Initially, 100 mg PO once daily. May titrate by 100-mg increments weekly to maximum dosage of 400 mg daily, depending on response and tolerability.
Adjust-a-dose: For eGFR less than 30 mL/minute/1.73 m^2, starting dosage is 100 mg once daily. May titrate weekly by 50- to 100-mg increments once daily to maximum dose of 200 mg once daily.

ADMINISTRATION
PO
• Give drug without regard to food.
• Have patient swallow capsules whole; don't crush or cut capsules.
• If patient can't swallow capsules whole, open capsule and sprinkle contents over a teaspoon of applesauce; have patient consume without chewing (within 2 hours). Don't store.
• Store drug at 68° to 77° F (20° to 25° C).

ACTION
Exact mechanism unknown. Believed to inhibit reuptake of norepinephrine.

Route	Onset	Peak	Duration
PO	Unknown	5 hr	Unknown

Half-life: 7 hours.

ADVERSE REACTIONS
CNS: fatigue, fever, headache, insomnia, irritability, lethargy, sedation, somnolence, dizziness. **CV:** increased diastolic BP, tachycardia. **EENT:** dry mouth. **GI:** abdominal discomfort or pain, decreased appetite, nausea, vomiting, constipation, GERD. **Respiratory:** URI.

INTERACTIONS
Drug-drug. *CYP2D6 substrates (atomoxetine, desipramine, dextromethorphan, nortriptyline, metoprolol, perphenazine, risperidone, tolterodine, venlafaxine); CYP3A4 substrates (avanafil, buspirone, conivaptan, darifenacin, darunavir, ebastine, everolimus, ibrutinib, lomitapide, lovastatin, lurasidone, midazolam, naloxegol, nisoldipine, saquinavir, simvastatin, sirolimus, tipranavir, triazolam, vardenafil):* May increase substrate level and risk of adverse reactions. Monitor patient closely and adjust substrate dosage as clinically indicated.
MAO inhibitors (isocarboxazid, phenelzine, rasagiline, safinamide, selegiline, tranylcypromine): May increase risk of hypertensive crisis with concomitant use or within 14 days after discontinuing MAO inhibitor. Use during this time frame is contraindicated.
Moderately sensitive CYP1A2 substrates (clozapine, pirfenidone): May increase substrate level and risk of adverse reactions. Avoid use together. If concomitant use is unavoidable, reduce substrate dosage.
Sensitive CYP1A2 substrates, CYP1A2 substrates with narrow therapeutic range (alosetron, duloxetine, ramelteon, tasimelteon, theophylline, tizanidine): May increase substrate level and risk of adverse reactions. Use together is contraindicated.

EFFECTS ON LAB TEST RESULTS
None reported.

CONTRAINDICATIONS & CAUTIONS
Boxed Warning Drug increases risk of suicidality. Monitor patients closely. ∎
• Drug may induce mania or mixed episodes in patients with bipolar disorder. Screen patients for bipolar disorder before drug initiation.
• Use cautiously in patients with CrCl less than 30 mL/minute.
• Safety and effectiveness in children younger than age 6 haven't been established.
Dialyzable drug: Unknown.

---

*Reactions in bold italics are **life-threatening**.*

⚠ **Overdose S&S:** Drowsiness, impaired consciousness, diminished reflexes, increased HR.

PREGNANCY-LACTATION-REPRODUCTION
• Based on animal studies, drug may cause patient and fetal harm. Discontinue drug if pregnancy occurs.
• Enroll patients exposed to drug during pregnancy in the National Pregnancy Registry for ADHD Medications (1-866-961-2388 or https://womensmentalhealth.org/research/pregnancyregistry/adhd-medications).
• It isn't known if drug appears in human milk or how drug affects milk production or infants who are breastfed. Weigh patient's clinical need and risk to infant against benefits of breastfeeding.

NURSING CONSIDERATIONS
Boxed Warning Monitor patient for clinical worsening or emergence of suicidality, especially during drug initiation and dosage changes. If signs or symptoms occur, consider discontinuing drug. ■
• Assess patient for personal or family history of suicide, bipolar disorder, or depression before drug initiation.
• Assess HR and BP at baseline, after dosage increase, and periodically during therapy.
• Periodically assess need for drug and dosage adjustments in patient taking drug long term.
• Monitor patient for mania or hypomania and excessive fatigue or somnolence.
• **Look alike–sound alike:** Don't confuse viloxazine with vilazodone.

PATIENT TEACHING
Boxed Warning Caution patient or caregiver to immediately report suicidality or new behavioral signs or symptoms. ■
• Teach about proper drug administration and handling.
• Tell patient or caregiver to report signs and symptoms of mania and hypomania (extreme increase in activity and talking, racing thoughts, severe insomnia, reckless behavior, excessive happiness or irritability).
• Caution patient that drug may cause fatigue or somnolence. Warn patient not to perform hazardous tasks or tasks requiring mental alertness until effects of drug are known.
• Inform patient that changes in BP and HR will be monitored while during therapy.

• Explain that drug may affect body weight, and weight will be monitored for changes.
• Instruct patient to report pregnancy or plans to become pregnant during therapy.

SAFETY ALERT!

vinBLAStine sulfate (VLB)
vin-BLAS-teen

Therapeutic class: Antineoplastics
Pharmacologic class: Vinca alkaloids

AVAILABLE FORMS
Injection: 1 mg/mL in 10-mL vials

INDICATIONS & DOSAGES
⚠ **Alert:** Manufacturer's labeling may not reflect current clinical practice. Dosing and frequency may vary by treatment protocol or phase.
Adjust-a-dose (for all indications): For patients with bilirubin level above 3 mg/dL, give 50% of usual dose. Refer to manufacturer's instructions for dose adjustments.
➤ **Hodgkin lymphoma**
Adults: 3.7 mg/m^2 IV in combination with other chemotherapeutic drugs.
Children: 6 mg/m^2 IV in combination with other chemotherapeutic drugs.
Adjust-a-dose: Adjust dose based on WBC response. Frequency and duration of treatment vary based on concomitant drugs and hematologic response.
➤ **Non-Hodgkin lymphomas; Kaposi sarcoma**
Adults: 3.7 mg/m^2 IV in combination with other chemotherapeutic drugs.
Adjust-a-dose: Adjust dose based on WBC response. Frequency and duration of treatment vary based on concomitant drugs and hematologic response.
➤ **Letterer-Siwe disease (histiocytosis X)**
Children: 6.5 mg/m^2 IV as a single agent.
➤ **Testicular germ-cell carcinomas**
Adults: 3.7 mg/m^2 IV in combination with other chemotherapeutic drugs.
Children: 3 mg/m^2/day IV on days 1 through 5 of each cycle in combination with other chemotherapeutic drugs.
➤ **Bladder cancer ◆**
Adults: 3 mg/m^2 IV on day 2 every 14 days in combination with other chemotherapeutic drugs.

ADMINISTRATION

IV

⚫ *Alert:* Hazardous drug; use safe handling and disposal precautions.

Boxed Warning Drug is for IV use only; fatal if given by other routes. ∎

⚫ *Alert:* When drug is dispensed in anything other than the original container, it must be packaged in provided overwrap and labeled, using provided auxiliary sticker and must state "Do not remove covering until moment of injection. For intravenous use only. Fatal if given by other routes."

⚫ *Alert:* To prevent inadvertent intrathecal use, The Joint Commission, WHO, Institute for Safe Medication Practices, and National Comprehensive Cancer Network recommend dispensing vinblastine in a 25 to 50 mL minibag (*not* in a syringe).

▼ Infuse minibag over no more than 30 minutes. Longer infusion times increase risk of vein irritation and extravasation.

▼ If minibag use isn't possible, inject drug directly into tubing of running IV line over 1 minute.

Boxed Warning Make sure catheter is properly positioned in vein. Drug is a vesicant; if extravasation occurs, immediately stop infusion and notify prescriber. Moderate heat applied to area of leakage and local injection of hyaluronidase may help disperse drug. ∎

▼ **Incompatibilities:** Cefepime, furosemide, pantoprazole.

ACTION

Arrests mitosis in metaphase, blocking cell division.

Route	Onset	Peak	Duration
IV	Unknown	Unknown	Unknown

Half-life: Initial phase, 3.7 minutes; second phase, 1.6 hours; terminal phase, 25 hours.

ADVERSE REACTIONS

CNS: loss of deep tendon reflexes, numbness, paresthesia, peripheral neuropathy and neuritis, *seizures,* depression, dizziness, headache, malaise. **CV:** HTN. **EENT:** pharyngitis, oral vesiculation. **GI:** anorexia, constipation, ileus, nausea, stomatitis, vomiting, abdominal pain, *bleeding ulcer, rectal bleeding,* diarrhea, *hemorrhagic enterocolitis.* **Hematologic:** anemia, *leukopenia, thrombocytopenia.* **Musculoskeletal:** muscle pain and weakness, bone pain, jaw pain. **Respiratory:** *acute bronchospasm,* shortness of breath. **Skin:** irritation, phlebitis, cellulitis, reversible alopecia, vesiculation and necrosis with extravasation. **Other:** pain at tumor site.

INTERACTIONS

Drug-drug. *CYP450 inhibitors (azole antifungals, erythromycin):* May increase vinblastine toxicity. Avoid combination if possible. Monitor patient closely for toxicity.
Mitomycin: May increase risk of bronchospasm and shortness of breath. Monitor patient's respiratory status.
Ototoxic drugs (platinum-containing antineoplastics): May cause temporary or permanent hearing impairment. Monitor hearing function.
Phenytoin: May decrease plasma phenytoin level. Monitor phenytoin level closely.
Vaccines (inactivated): May diminish therapeutic effect of vaccines. Complete all age-appropriate vaccinations at least 2 weeks before starting vinblastine. If patient is vaccinated during therapy, revaccinate at least 3 months after drug is stopped.
Vaccines (live): May enhance adverse or toxic effect of live-virus vaccines and diminish their therapeutic effect. Avoid use with vinblastine; don't vaccinate for at least 3 months after therapy ends.
Drug-herb. *St. John's wort:* May decrease vinblastine level. Discourage use together.

EFFECTS ON LAB TEST RESULTS

● May decrease Hb level and WBC and platelet counts.

CONTRAINDICATIONS & CAUTIONS

● Contraindicated in patients hypersensitive to drug and in those with bacterial infection or significant granulocytopenia unless it's a result of the disease being treated.

● Avoid use in older adults with cachexia or ulcerated skin due to increased leukopenic response.

● Use cautiously in patients with liver dysfunction, pulmonary dysfunction, or CV disease.

Dialyzable drug: No.

⚠ *Overdose S&S:* Exaggerated effects, neurotoxicity.

PREGNANCY-LACTATION-REPRODUCTION

● Drug can cause fetal harm. If drug is used during pregnancy or if patient becomes

pregnant during therapy, inform patient of potential fetal hazard. Patients of childbearing potential should avoid pregnancy during therapy.
• It isn't known if drug appears in human milk. Patient should discontinue breastfeeding or discontinue drug, considering importance of drug to patient.

NURSING CONSIDERATIONS
Boxed Warning Drug should be administered by personnel experienced in vinblastine sulfate administration. ∎
• To reduce nausea, give antiemetic before drug.
• Don't give drug into limb with compromised circulation.
• Monitor infusion site closely to prevent extravasation.
↻ Alert: After giving drug, monitor patient for life-threatening acute bronchospasm. If it occurs, immediately notify prescriber. Reaction is most likely to occur in patients also receiving mitomycin.
• Monitor patient for stomatitis. If it occurs, stop drug and notify prescriber.
• Assess bowel activity. Give laxatives as indicated. Stool softeners may be used prophylactically.
• Don't repeat dosage more frequently than every 7 days or severe leukopenia will occur. Nadir occurs on days 5 to 10. WBC count recovers rapidly, usually within another 7 to 14 days.
• Assess patient for numbness and tingling in hands and feet. Assess gait for early evidence of footdrop.
• Drug is less neurotoxic than vincristine.
• **Look alike–sound alike:** Don't confuse vinblastine with vincristine or vinorelbine.

PATIENT TEACHING
• Tell patient to report evidence of infection (fever, sore throat, fatigue) and bleeding (easy bruising, nosebleeds, bleeding gums, melena). Tell patient to take temperature daily.
• Urge patient to report pain, swelling, burning, or any unusual feeling at injection site during infusion.
• Warn patient that hair loss may occur but is usually temporary.
• Caution patient to avoid pregnancy during therapy.
• Tell patient that pain may occur in jaw and in the organ with the tumor.

vinCRIStine sulfate
vin-KRIS-teen

Vincasar PFS

Therapeutic class: Antineoplastics
Pharmacologic class: Vinca alkaloids

AVAILABLE FORMS
Injection: 1 mg/mL in 1-mL, 2-mL preservative-free vials

INDICATIONS & DOSAGES
↻ Alert: Manufacturer's labeling may not reflect current clinical practice. Dosage, frequency, and duration of treatment vary by treatment protocol or phase.
➤ **Acute lymphoblastic and other leukemias, Hodgkin lymphoma, malignant lymphoma, neuroblastoma, rhabdomyosarcoma, Wilms tumor**
Adults: 1.4 mg/m² IV weekly.
Children weighing more than 10 kg: 1.5 to 2 mg/m² IV weekly.
Children weighing 10 kg and less or with BSA less than 1 m²: Initially, 0.05 mg/kg IV weekly. Titrate as tolerated, up to 2 mg/dose.
Adjust-a-dose: For patients with direct bilirubin level above 3 mg/dL, reduce dosage by 50%.

ADMINISTRATION
IV
↻ Alert: Hazardous drug; use safe handling and disposal precautions.
Boxed Warning Administer by IV route only; fatal if given by other routes. ∎
▼ Inject slowly over 1 minute directly into tube of running IV line of NSS or D₅W only.
↻ Alert: To prevent inadvertent intrathecal administration, The Joint Commission, WHO, National Comprehensive Cancer Network, and Institute for Safe Medication Practices recommend dispensing vincristine in a minibag (*not* in a syringe).
Boxed Warning Make sure catheter is positioned correctly in vein. Drug is a vesicant; if extravasation occurs, immediately stop infusion and notify prescriber. Local injection of hyaluronidase and application of moderate heat to area of leakage may help disperse drug. ∎
▼ Give as a short 5- to 10-minute infusion in 25 to 50 mL of NSS or D₅W.

V

▼ All vials contain 1 mg/mL solution; refrigerate vials.

▼ **Incompatibilities:** Cefepime, furosemide, idarubicin, pantoprazole, phenytoin, sodium bicarbonate. Consult drug compatibility reference for more information.

ACTION

Arrests mitosis in metaphase, blocking cell division.

Route	Onset	Peak	Duration
IV	Unknown	Unknown	Unknown

Half-life: Initial phase, 5 minutes; second phase, 2.25 hours; terminal phase, 6.5 days.

ADVERSE REACTIONS

CNS: loss of deep tendon reflexes, paresthesia, peripheral neuropathy, ataxia, foot drop, cranial nerve palsies, fever, headache, sensory loss, neuritic pain, abnormal gait, dizziness, vertigo. **CV:** HTN, hypotension. **EENT:** blindness, diplopia, optic and extraocular neuropathy, photophobia, ptosis, visual disturbances, nystagmus, temporary or permanent deafness, vocal cord paralysis, hoarseness, oral ulceration. **GI:** constipation, cramps, nausea, stomatitis, vomiting, *intestinal necrosis,* anorexia, diarrhea, dysphagia, ileus. **GU:** dysuria, polyuria, urine retention. **Hematologic:** *thrombocytopenia, leukopenia,* anemia. **Hepatic:** *hepatic veno-occlusive disease.* **Metabolic:** weight loss, dehydration, hyperuricemia. **Musculoskeletal:** cramps, jaw pain, myalgia, muscle weakness, muscle wasting. **Respiratory:** *acute bronchospasm,* dyspnea. **Skin:** phlebitis, cellulitis at injection site, rash, reversible alopecia, severe local reaction following extravasation. **Other:** hypersensitivity reactions.

INTERACTIONS

Drug-drug. *Anticholinergics, antidepressants, antipsychotics, opioids, and other drugs that may cause urinary retention:* May worsen urinary retention. If possible, avoid use of these drugs for first few days after vincristine administration, especially in older adults.
Fosphenytoin, phenytoin: May reduce levels of these drugs. Monitor levels closely.
HIV protease inhibitors (atazanavir, ritonavir): May increase pharmacologic effects of vincristine. Monitor patient for profound neutropenia and severe neuropathy.

Temporarily suspend HIV protease inhibitor or reduce vincristine dosage if significant hematologic or GI toxicity occurs.
Mitomycin: May increase frequency of bronchospasm and acute pulmonary reactions. Monitor patient's respiratory status.
Moderate CYP3A4 inhibitors (erythromycin, verapamil): May increase vincristine level. Use together cautiously.
Ototoxic drugs: May potentiate loss of hearing. Use together with caution.
Strong CYP3A4 inducers (phenobarbital, rifampin): May decrease vincristine level. Use together cautiously.
Strong CYP3A4 inhibitors (clarithromycin, ketoconazole): May increase vincristine level and risk of toxicity. Consider alternative to inhibitor therapy.
Triazole antifungals (itraconazole, posaconazole, voriconazole): Concomitant use may increase risk of neurotoxicity. Consider therapy modification.
Vaccines (inactivated): May diminish therapeutic effect of vaccines. Complete all age-appropriate vaccinations at least 2 weeks before starting vincristine. If patient is vaccinated during therapy, revaccinate at least 3 months after drug is stopped.
Vaccines (live): May enhance adverse or toxic effect of live-virus vaccines and diminish their therapeutic effect. Avoid use with vincristine; don't vaccinate for at least 3 months after drug is stopped.
Warfarin: May increase anticoagulant effects. Monitor INR and adjust warfarin dose as needed.
Drug-herb. *Echinacea, St. John's wort:* May decrease vincristine level. Discourage use together.

EFFECTS ON LAB TEST RESULTS

- May increase uric acid level.
- May decrease sodium level.
- May decrease Hb level and WBC and platelet counts.

CONTRAINDICATIONS & CAUTIONS

- Contraindicated in patients hypersensitive to drug and in those with demyelinating form of Charcot-Marie-Tooth syndrome.
- Don't give to patients who are receiving radiation therapy through ports that include the liver.
- Use cautiously in patients with liver impairment, neuromuscular disease, or infection.

Reactions in bold italics are *life-threatening*.

Dialyzable drug: No.
⚠ *Overdose S&S:* Exaggerated effects, death.

PREGNANCY-LACTATION-REPRODUCTION
• Drug may cause fetal harm. If used during pregnancy or if patient becomes pregnant during therapy, inform patient of potential fetal hazard. Patients of childbearing potential should use effective contraception during therapy.
• It isn't known if drug appears in human milk. Patient should discontinue breastfeeding or discontinue drug, considering importance of drug to patient.
• Drug may impair fertility.

NURSING CONSIDERATIONS
Boxed Warning Drug should be administered by personnel experienced in administration of vincristine sulfate. ∎
• Watch for hyperuricemia, especially in patient with leukemia or lymphoma. Maintain hydration and give allopurinol to prevent uric acid nephropathy. Watch for toxicity.
• If SIADH (rare) develops, restrict fluids, if needed. Monitor fluid intake and output.
• Because of risk of neurotoxicity, don't give drug more often than once weekly. Children are more resistant to neurotoxicity than adults. Neurotoxicity is dose related and usually reversible.
• Older adults and patients with underlying neurologic disease may be more susceptible to neurotoxic effects.
• Monitor for depression of Achilles tendon reflex, numbness, tingling, footdrop or wristdrop, difficulty walking, ataxia, and slapping gait. Monitor patient's ability to walk on heels. Support patient while walking.
• Monitor bowel function. Constipation may be an early sign of neurotoxicity.
• *Look alike–sound alike:* Don't confuse vincristine with vincristine liposomal, vinblastine, or vinorelbine.

PATIENT TEACHING
• Advise patient to report all adverse reactions, especially pain or burning at injection site during or after administration.
• Instruct patient to report increased shortness of breath and evidence of infection (fever, sore throat, fatigue) and bleeding (easy bruising, nosebleeds, bleeding gums, melena). Tell patient to take temperature daily.

• Teach patient to follow a prophylactic bowel management plan and to report constipation.
• Warn patient that hair loss may occur, but explain that it's usually temporary.
• Caution patient not to breastfeed, to avoid becoming pregnant during therapy, and to consult prescriber before becoming pregnant.

vonoprazan–amoxicillin
von-OH-pra-zan/am-ox-i-SILL-in

Voquezna Dual Pak

Therapeutic class: Antacids–anti-infectives
Pharmacologic class: Potassium-competitive acid blockers–antibacterials

AVAILABLE FORMS
Copackage containing:
Capsules: amoxicillin 500 mg
Tablets: vonoprazan 20 mg

INDICATIONS & DOSAGES
➤ *Helicobacter pylori* infection
Adults: Vonoprazan 20 mg PO b.i.d. plus amoxicillin 1,000 mg PO t.i.d. for 14 days.

ADMINISTRATION
PO
• Give drug without regard to food.
• If a dose is missed, give within 4 hours of scheduled dose. If more than 4 hours have elapsed, skip dose and give next dose at regularly scheduled time. Continue normal dosing schedule until medication is completed.
• Store drug at room temperature and protect from light.

ACTION
Vonoprazan is a proton pump inhibitor that blocks acid secretion. Amoxicillin inhibits bacterial cell-wall synthesis by binding to penicillin-binding proteins.

Route	Onset	Peak	Duration
PO (vonoprazan)	2–3 hr	2.5–3 hr	Unknown
PO (amoxicillin)	Unknown	1–2 hr	Unknown

Half-life: Vonoprazan, 7 hours; amoxicillin: 1 hour.

ADVERSE REACTIONS
CNS: dysgeusia, headache. **CV:** HTN. **EENT:** nasopharyngitis. **GI:** abdominal pain, diarrhea.

V

GU: vulvovaginal candidiasis. **Other:** hypersensitivity reaction.

INTERACTIONS

Drug-drug. *Allopurinol:* May increase incidence of rash. Discontinue allopurinol at first sign of rash.

Atazanavir: May alter absorption of atazanavir. Avoid use together.

Clopidogrel: May reduce clopidogrel level and platelet inhibition. Carefully monitor efficacy of clopidogrel or use alternative antiplatelet therapy.

CYP2C19 substrates (cilostazol, citalopram): May increase substrate level. Monitor patient for adverse reactions.

CYP3A4 substrates (cyclosporine, tacrolimus): May increase substrate level and risk of adverse reactions of substrate. Monitor substrate level and watch for adverse effects.

Drugs dependent on gastric pH for absorption (antiretrovirals, dasatinib, erlotinib, iron salts, itraconazole, ketoconazole, mycophenolate mofetil, nilotinib): May decrease absorption and effectiveness of these drugs. If used concomitantly, refer to prescribing information for individual drugs.

Nelfinavir: May alter nelfinavir absorption. Avoid use together.

Oral anticoagulants: May increase PT and INR. Monitor patient closely and adjust oral anticoagulant dosage as necessary.

Probenecid: May increase amoxicillin exposure and adverse reactions. Monitor patient for adverse reactions.

Rilpivirine: May alter rilpivirine absorption. Avoid use together.

Strong or moderate CYP3A inducers (efavirenz, rifampin): May decrease vonoprazan effectiveness. Avoid use together.

EFFECTS ON LAB TEST RESULTS

• May cause false-positive urine glucose test based on Benedict copper reduction reaction. Use test based on enzymatic glucose oxidase reactions when testing patients treated with drug.

• May cause false-positive serum chromogranin A (CgA) test for neuroendocrine tumors.

CONTRAINDICATIONS & CAUTIONS

• Contraindicated in patients hypersensitive to vonoprazan, amoxicillin, or other betalactams (penicillins or cephalosporins).

• Avoid use in patients with eGFR less than 30 mL/minute or Child-Pugh class B or C liver impairment.

• Avoid use in patients with mononucleosis; drug may increase risk of erythematous rash.

• Serious and fatal hypersensitivity reactions, including anaphylaxis, have been reported. If hypersensitivity reactions occur, discontinue therapy and initiate immediate supportive care.

• SCARs have occurred. Discontinue at first sign or symptom of SCARs or other signs or symptoms of hypersensitivity and consider further evaluation.

• CDAD has been reported with use of acid-suppressing therapies and nearly all antibacterial agents.

• Safety and effectiveness in children haven't been established.

• Use cautiously in older adults.

Dialyzable drug: Vonoprazan, no. Amoxicillin, yes.

⚠ *Overdose S&S:* Amoxicillin: interstitial nephritis, crystalluria, reversible kidney impairment.

PREGNANCY-LACTATION-REPRODUCTION

• Studies during pregnancy are inadequate. Use with caution during pregnancy.

• It isn't known if drug appears in human milk or how drug affects infants who are breastfed or milk production. Patient who is breastfeeding should pump and discard milk during therapy and for 2 days after final dose and feed infant stored human milk (collected before therapy) or formula.

NURSING CONSIDERATIONS

• Monitor patient for hypersensitivity reactions. If reactions occur, discontinue drug and begin immediate supportive care.

• Monitor patient for SCARs. Discontinue drug at first sign or symptom and evaluate further.

• Monitor patient for diarrhea during and after therapy. If CDAD is confirmed, discontinue drug and manage patient as clinically indicated.

• If CgA testing is needed, assess CgA level 14 days after therapy ends and retest if CgA level is high.

• *Look alike–sound alike:* Don't confuse vonoprazan with voriconazole.

Reactions in bold italics are *life-threatening*.

PATIENT TEACHING
- Teach about proper drug administration and handling.
- Advise patient to take drug as directed and to complete full course of therapy, even if feeling better. Explain that skipping doses and not completing full course may decrease treatment effectiveness and increase likelihood of bacterial resistance.
- Counsel patient that treatment of *H. pylori* infection is important due to its association with stomach ulcers, atrophic gastritis, and increased risk of gastric cancer.
- Advise patient that hypersensitivity reactions can occur. Tell patient to immediately report a new rash, urticaria, drug eruptions, facial swelling, or difficulty breathing.
- Teach patient about risk of serious skin reactions. Tell patient to stop drug immediately and report signs or symptoms of rash, mucosal lesions, or other signs or symptoms of reaction.
- Inform patient that diarrhea may occur and that, rarely, watery and bloody stools (with or without stomach cramps and fever) may develop 2 months or more after the final dose. Tell patient experiencing watery and bloody stools to notify health care provider as soon as possible.
- Instruct patient who is breastfeeding to pump and discard milk during therapy and for 2 days after final dose.

---

vorapaxar sulfate
VOR-a-PAX-ar

Zontivity

Therapeutic class: Antiplatelet drugs
Pharmacologic class: Platelet aggregation inhibitors

AVAILABLE FORMS
Tablets: 2.08 mg

INDICATIONS & DOSAGES
➤ **To reduce thrombotic CV events in patients with history of MI or peripheral arterial disease, in combination with aspirin or clopidogrel**
Adults: 1 tablet (2.08 mg) PO once daily.

ADMINISTRATION
PO
- Give drug without regard to food.
- Store tablets in original package at room temperature. Keep desiccant packet in bottle to protect drug from moisture.

ACTION
A reversible antagonist of the protease-activated receptor-1 expressed on platelets, thereby inhibiting platelet aggregation.

Route	Onset	Peak	Duration
PO	Unknown	1–2 hr	Unknown

Half-life: 5 to 13 days.

ADVERSE REACTIONS
CNS: depression. **EENT:** retinopathy, retinal disorders, diplopia. **GI:** *GI bleeding.* **Hematologic:** *hemorrhage,* anemia, iron deficiency. **Skin:** rash, eruption, exanthemas.

INTERACTIONS
Drug-drug. *Anticoagulants (apixaban, rivaroxaban, warfarin):* May increase risk of bleeding. Avoid use together.
Drugs known to cause bleeding (fibrinolytics, NSAIDs [long-term], SSNRIs, SSRIs): Increase risk of bleeding. Use together cautiously. Avoid use with urokinase.
Strong CYP3A inducers (carbamazepine, phenytoin, rifampin): May decrease vorapaxar level. Avoid use together.
Strong CYP3A inhibitors (boceprevir, clarithromycin, conivaptan, ketoconazole, nefazodone, nelfinavir, ritonavir, saquinavir, telithromycin): May increase vorapaxar level. Avoid use together.
Drug-herb. *Herbs with anticoagulant or antiplatelet properties (alfalfa, anise, bilberry):* May increase bleeding risk. Discourage use together.
St. John's wort: May decrease vorapaxar level. Discourage use together.

EFFECTS ON LAB TEST RESULTS
- May decrease RBC count.

CONTRAINDICATIONS & CAUTIONS
Boxed Warning Don't use in patients with history of intracranial hemorrhage, stroke, TIA, or active pathologic bleeding. Antiplatelet drugs, including vorapaxar, increase risk of bleeding, including intracranial hemorrhage and fatal bleeding. ■

V

• Drug has only been studied in combination with aspirin or clopidogrel.

• Use cautiously in patients with low body weight, reduced kidney or liver function, or history of bleeding disorder.

• Use isn't recommended in patients with Child-Pugh class C liver impairment.

• Older adults are at higher risk for bleeding. Consider patient's age before administering drug.

• Safety and effectiveness in children haven't been established.

Dialyzable drug: Unlikely.

PREGNANCY-LACTATION-REPRODUCTION

• Drug can cause serious adverse reactions, including maternal hemorrhage. Discontinue drug when pregnancy is detected and begin alternative therapy with a shorter duration of action.

• It isn't known if drug appears in human milk. Use during breastfeeding isn't recommended.

NURSING CONSIDERATIONS

🕐 **Alert:** Briefly stopping drug during an episode of acute bleeding isn't useful for managing bleeding because of drug's long half-life. There's no known treatment to reverse the antiplatelet effect; drug will significantly inhibit platelet aggregation for 4 weeks after discontinuation. Monitor patient for bleeding.

• Discontinue drug if patient experiences a stroke, TIA, or intracranial hemorrhage.

• Periodically monitor Hb level and hematocrit.

• Evaluate for possible bleeding in patient with hypotension who has recently had coronary angiography, PCI, CABG, or another surgical procedure.

PATIENT TEACHING

Boxed Warning Caution patient that drug increases risk of bleeding, including intracranial hemorrhage and fatal bleeding. ∎

• Advise patient to tell other providers about taking drug, especially before any surgery or dental procedure.

• Instruct patient to take drug exactly as prescribed in addition to aspirin or clopidogrel and not to discontinue drug without first consulting prescriber.

• Teach patient to report bruising or severe prolonged or excessive unexplained bleeding

(blood in stool, vomit, or urine and coughing up blood or blood clots).

• Advise patient to report all prescription and OTC medications, vitamins, herbs, and other dietary supplements being taken to prescriber and pharmacist so that they're aware of other treatments that may affect bleeding risk.

• Caution patient to immediately report pregnancy or plans to become pregnant.

• Tell patient that breastfeeding isn't recommended during therapy.

voriconazole ⚥

vor-ah-KON-ah-zole

Vfend

Therapeutic class: Antifungals
Pharmacologic class: Synthetic triazoles

AVAILABLE FORMS

Oral suspension: 40 mg/mL after reconstitution
Powder for injection: 200 mg/vial
Tablets: 50 mg, 200 mg

INDICATIONS & DOSAGES

Adjust-a-dose (for all indications): For adults with Child-Pugh class A or B liver impairment, decrease maintenance dosage by 50%. In adults with CrCl of less than 50 mL/minute, use PO form instead of IV form to prevent IV mixture component accumulation.

➤ **Esophageal candidiasis**

Adults, children ages 12 to 14 weighing 50 kg or more, and children ages 15 and older regardless of body weight: 200 mg PO every 12 hours.

Adults weighing less than 40 kg: 100 or 150 mg PO every 12 hours.

Children ages 2 to younger than 12 and children ages 12 to 14 weighing less than 50 kg: Initially, 4 mg/kg IV every 12 hours. If patient can't tolerate 4-mg/kg IV dose, reduce dose by 1-mg/kg steps. If inadequate response and patient can tolerate initial IV dose, increase dose by 1-mg/kg steps. After at least 5 days of IV therapy and significant clinical improvement, consider an oral regimen of 9 mg/kg PO every 12 hours. If patient can't tolerate 9-mg/kg PO dose, reduce dose by 1-mg/kg or 50-mg steps. If inadequate response and patient can tolerate initial PO dose, increase dose by 1-mg/kg or 50-mg steps to maximum of 350 mg PO every 12 hours.

Adjust-a-dose: For all patients, treat for at least 14 days and for at least 7 days after symptoms resolve.

➤ **Invasive aspergillosis; serious infections caused by *Fusarium* species and *Scedosporium apiospermum* in patients intolerant of or refractory to other therapy**

Adults, children ages 12 to 14 weighing 50 kg or more, and children ages 15 and older regardless of body weight: Initially, 6 mg/kg IV every 12 hours for two doses; then maintenance dose of 4 mg/kg IV every 12 hours. If patient can't tolerate 4-mg/kg dose, decrease to 3 mg/kg. Continue IV therapy for at least 7 days. Switch to PO form as tolerated, using PO maintenance dosages.

Adults weighing 40 kg or more, children ages 12 to 14 weighing 50 kg or more, and children ages 15 and older regardless of body weight: 200 mg PO every 12 hours. May increase to 300 mg PO every 12 hours, if needed. If patient can't tolerate 300-mg dose, reduce dose in 50-mg decrements to a minimum of 200 mg every 12 hours.

Adults weighing less than 40 kg: 100 mg PO every 12 hours. May increase to 150 mg PO every 12 hours, if needed. If patient can't tolerate 150-mg dose, reduce dose to 100 mg every 12 hours.

Children ages 2 to younger than 12 and children ages 12 to 14 weighing less than 50 kg: Initially, 9 mg/kg IV every 12 hours for two doses; then maintenance dose of 8 mg/kg IV every 12 hours. If patient can't tolerate 8-mg/kg IV dose, reduce dose by 1-mg/kg steps. If inadequate response and patient can tolerate initial IV maintenance dose, increase dose by 1-mg/kg steps. Continue IV therapy for at least 7 days; then switch to 9 mg/kg PO every 12 hours. If patient can't tolerate 9-mg/kg PO dose, reduce dose by 1-mg/kg or 50-mg steps. If inadequate response and patient can tolerate initial PO maintenance dose, increase dose by 1-mg/kg or 50-mg steps to maximum of 350 mg PO every 12 hours.

➤ **Candidemia in patients who are non-neutropenic; *Candida* infections of the kidney, abdomen, bladder wall, or wounds and disseminated skin infections**

Adults, children ages 12 to 14 weighing 50 kg or more, and children ages 15 and older regardless of body weight: Initially, 6 mg/kg IV every 12 hours for two doses; then 3 to 4 mg/kg IV every 12 hours for maintenance, depending on severity of the infection. If patient can't tolerate 4-mg/kg dose, decrease to 3 mg/kg. Switch to PO form as tolerated, using PO maintenance dosages.

Adults weighing 40 kg or more, children ages 12 to 14 weighing 50 kg or more, and children ages 15 and older regardless of body weight: 200 mg PO every 12 hours. May increase to 300 mg PO every 12 hours, if needed. If unable to tolerate 300-mg dose, reduce dose in 50-mg decrements to a minimum of 200 mg every 12 hours.

Adults weighing less than 40 kg: 100 mg PO every 12 hours. May increase to 150 mg PO every 12 hours, if needed. If patient can't tolerate 150-mg dose, reduce dose to 100 mg every 12 hours.

Children ages 2 to younger than 12 and children ages 12 to 14 weighing less than 50 kg: Initially, 9 mg/kg IV every 12 hours for two doses; then maintenance dose of 8 mg/kg IV every 12 hours. If patient can't tolerate 8-mg/kg IV dose, reduce dose by 1-mg/kg steps. If inadequate response and patient can tolerate initial IV maintenance dose, increase dose by 1-mg/kg steps. Continue IV therapy for at least 5 days; then switch to 9 mg/kg PO every 12 hours. If patient can't tolerate 9-mg/kg PO dose, reduce dose by 1-mg/kg or 50-mg steps. If inadequate response and patient can tolerate initial PO maintenance dose, increase dose by 1-mg/kg or 50-mg steps to maximum of 350 mg PO every 12 hours.

Adjust-a-dose: Treat patients with candidemia for at least 14 days after symptoms resolve or after the last positive culture result, whichever is longer.

ADMINISTRATION

• Obtain specimens for fungal culture and other relevant lab studies (including histopathology) before starting therapy to isolate and identify causative organism(s). May start drug before study results are known. Adjust therapy, if necessary, when results become available.

⊘ Alert: Hazardous agent; use safe-handling and disposal precautions.

PO

• Give tablets or oral suspension at least 1 hour before or 1 hour after a meal or enteral tube feeding.

• For oral suspension, give only with dispenser provided in medication package.

• Don't mix oral suspension with other drugs or beverages.

• Shake suspension for 10 seconds before each use. Store at room temperature. Discard unused portion of suspension after 14 days.

IV

▼ Reconstitute powder with 19 mL of water for injection to obtain a volume of 20 mL of clear concentrate containing 10 mg/mL of drug. Discard vial if a vacuum doesn't pull the diluent into vial. Shake vial until powder completely dissolves. Use reconstituted solution immediately.

▼ Further dilute 10-mg/mL solution to 5 mg/mL or less. Follow manufacturer's instructions for diluting.

▼ Infuse over 1 to 3 hours at 5 mg/mL or less and maximum hourly rate of 3 mg/kg/hour.

⊕ *Alert:* Don't administer as IV bolus injection.

▼ Don't infuse concomitantly with any blood product or short-term infusion of concentrated electrolytes, even if the two infusions are running in separate IV lines (or cannulas).

▼ **Incompatibilities:** Blood products, electrolyte supplements, 4.2% sodium bicarbonate infusion. Consult drug compatibility reference for more information.

ACTION

Inhibits the cytochrome P-450-dependent synthesis of ergosterol, a vital component of fungal cell membranes.

Route	Onset	Peak	Duration
PO, IV	Immediate	1–2 hr	12 hr

Half-life: Variable depending on dose.

ADVERSE REACTIONS

CNS: fever, headache, hallucinations. **CV:** tachycardia, HTN, hypotension, peripheral edema. **EENT:** abnormal vision, photophobia, chromatopsia, epistaxis. **GI:** nausea, vomiting, abdominal pain, diarrhea, constipation, mucosal inflammation. **GU:** kidney dysfunction, *AKI.* **Hematologic:** *thrombocytopenia.* **Hepatic:** abnormal LFT values, cholestatic jaundice. **Metabolic:** *hypokalemia.* **Respiratory:** cough, dyspnea, URI, hemoptysis. **Skin:** rash. **Other:** chills.

INTERACTIONS

Refer to prescribing information for additional drug interaction information.

Drug-drug. *Astemizole, cisapride, ivabradine, pimozide, quinidine, terfenadine:* May increase levels of these drugs, leading to torsades de pointes and prolonged QT interval. Use together is contraindicated.

Benzodiazepines, calcium channel blockers, methadone, NSAIDs, sulfonylureas, vinca alkaloids: May increase levels of these drugs. Adjust dosages of these drugs, and monitor patient for adverse reactions.

Carbamazepine, long-acting barbiturates, rifabutin, rifampin, ritonavir (high-dose therapy): May decrease voriconazole level. Use together is contraindicated.

Cyclosporine, tacrolimus: May increase levels of these drugs. Adjust dosages, and monitor levels.

Efavirenz: May significantly decrease voriconazole level while significantly increasing efavirenz level. Adjust dosages of both drugs. Use of voriconazole when efavirenz dosage is 400 mg or more/day is contraindicated. In adults also receiving efavirenz, increase voriconazole dosage to 400 mg PO every 12 hours and decrease efavirenz dosage to 300 mg PO every 24 hours. When treatment with voriconazole is stopped, restore initial efavirenz dosage.

Ergot alkaloids (ergotamine), tolvaptan: May increase levels of these drugs. Use together is contraindicated.

Fluconazole: May increase voriconazole level. Avoid use together. Monitor patient for adverse effects 24 hours after last fluconazole dose.

HIV protease inhibitors (amprenavir, nelfinavir, saquinavir), NNRTIs (delavirdine): May increase levels of both drugs. Monitor patient for adverse reactions and toxicity.

HMG-CoA reductase inhibitors (atorvastatin, fluvastatin, lovastatin, pravastatin, rosuvastatin, simvastatin): May increase levels and adverse effects (including rhabdomyolysis) of these drugs. Monitor patient closely and reduce dosage of HMG-CoA reductase inhibitor as needed.

Letermovir: May decrease voriconazole level. Monitor effectiveness.

Lurasidone, sirolimus, tolvaptan: May significantly increase levels of these drugs. Use together is contraindicated.

Naloxegol: May increase naloxegol level and risk of opioid withdrawal symptoms. Use together is contraindicated.

Reactions in bold italics are *life-threatening*.

Omeprazole: May increase omeprazole level. When initiating voriconazole therapy in patients already receiving omeprazole doses of 40 mg or greater, reduce omeprazole dose by half.

Opioids, long-acting (fentanyl, oxycodone): May increase levels of these drugs. Adjust dosages of these drugs, and monitor patient for adverse reactions.

Oral contraceptives containing ethinyl estradiol and norethindrone: May increase voriconazole level. Monitor patient closely.

Phenytoin: May decrease voriconazole level and increase phenytoin level. Increase voriconazole maintenance dose, and monitor phenytoin level. In adults also receiving phenytoin, increase maintenance dose of voriconazole to 5 mg/kg IV every 12 hours, or increase PO dose from 100 to 200 mg (in adults weighing 40 kg or less) or from 200 to 400 mg (in adults weighing more than 40 kg).

Ritonavir: May decrease voriconazole level. Use with ritonavir dosages of 400 mg b.i.d. is contraindicated. Avoid using with low-dose ritonavir (100 mg b.i.d.) unless benefits outweigh risks.

Venetoclax: May increase risk of TLS during initiation and ramp-up phase of chronic lymphocytic leukemia or small lymphocytic lymphoma treatment. Use together is contraindicated.

Warfarin: May significantly prolong PT and increase INR. Monitor PT, INR, and bleeding.

Drug-herb. *St. John's wort:* May increase drug level. Use together is contraindicated.

Drug-lifestyle. *Sun exposure:* May cause photosensitivity. Advise patient to avoid excessive sunlight exposure.

EFFECTS ON LAB TEST RESULTS

• May increase CK, cholesterol, ALP, AST, ALT, bilirubin, creatinine, GGT, urine glucose, and urine albumin levels.
• May decrease albumin level.
• May increase or decrease glucose, calcium, magnesium, potassium, sodium, or phosphorus level.
• May decrease Hb level, hematocrit, and platelet, WBC, and RBC counts.

CONTRAINDICATIONS & CAUTIONS

• Contraindicated in patients hypersensitive to drug or its components.
▨ Tablets are contraindicated in patients with rare hereditary galactose intolerance, Lapp

lactase deficiency, or glucose-galactose malabsorption due to lactose content.
• May prolong QT interval. Rare cases of torsades de pointes, cardiac arrest, and sudden death have been reported. Use cautiously in patients with proarrhythmic conditions (congenital or acquired QT-interval prolongation, cardiomyopathy, sinus bradycardia, existing symptomatic arrhythmias) and in those taking concomitant drugs that can prolong QT interval.
• Use cautiously in patients hypersensitive to other azoles.
• Use cautiously in patients with risk factors for acute pancreatitis (recent chemotherapy, stem cell transplant).
• SCARs, including SJS, TEN, and DRESS syndrome, have been reported. Discontinue drug for exfoliative cutaneous reactions.
• IV administration is recommended in children ages 2 to 12 with malabsorption and very low body weight for age because oral bioavailability may be limited.
Dialyzable drug: Yes.
⚠ *Overdose S&S:* Photophobia.

PREGNANCY-LACTATION-REPRODUCTION

• Drug can cause fetal harm. Use during pregnancy only if benefit clearly outweighs fetal risk. If used during pregnancy, inform patient of potential hazard to fetus.
• Patient of childbearing potential should use effective contraception.
• It isn't known if drug appears in human milk. Patient should discontinue breastfeeding or discontinue drug, considering importance of drug to patient.

NURSING CONSIDERATIONS

• Correct electrolyte disturbances before initiation of and during therapy.
• Obtain ECG for patients with concomitant medications or conditions that prolong QT interval.
• Infusion reactions (flushing, fever, diaphoresis, tachycardia, chest tightness, dyspnea, faintness, nausea, pruritus, rash) may occur as soon as infusion starts. If reaction occurs, notify prescriber; infusion may need to be stopped.
• Closely monitor kidney function and serum creatinine level.
• Monitor LFT results at start of and during therapy. Monitor patient who develops abnormal LFT results for more severe liver

V

injury. If patient develops signs and symptoms of liver disease, drug may need to be stopped.

• Monitor for SCARs and photosensitivity skin reactions that could lead to melanoma or squamous cell carcinoma of the skin. Phototoxicity reactions are more common in children.

• If drug is continued despite phototoxicity-related lesion, obtain regular dermatologic evaluations. Discontinue drug if patient develops a skin lesion consistent with squamous cell carcinoma or melanoma.

• Monitor for signs and symptoms of azole-induced adrenal insufficiency (fatigue, aches, weight loss, hypotension, loss of body hair, hyperpigmentation) and, in patient taking corticosteroid, Cushing syndrome (weight gain, round face, thinning skin, diaphoresis).

• If treatment lasts longer than 28 days, vision changes may occur.

• Skeletal fluorosis and periostitis have been reported with long-term therapy. Evaluate complaints of skeletal pain and discontinue drug for radiologic findings compatible with fluorosis or periostitis.

• *Look alike–sound alike:* Don't confuse voriconazole with fluconazole, itraconazole, or posaconazole.

PATIENT TEACHING

• Teach about proper drug administration and handling.

• Advise patient to avoid driving or operating machinery while taking drug, especially at night, because vision changes (blurring, photophobia, changes in color perception) may occur.

• Tell patient to avoid strong, direct sunlight and to use sun-protective measures.

• Advise patient to avoid becoming pregnant during therapy because of risk of fetal harm.

vortioxetine hydrobromide
vor-tie-OX-e-teen

Trintellix

Therapeutic class: Antidepressants
Pharmacologic class: Multimodal antidepressants

AVAILABLE FORMS
Tablets: 5 mg, 10 mg, 20 mg

INDICATIONS & DOSAGES
➤ **Major depressive disorder**
Adults: 10 mg PO once daily. Increase as tolerated to target dosage of 20 mg once daily.
Adjust-a-dose: If 10 mg once daily isn't tolerated, decrease dosage to 5 mg once daily. If discontinuing drug when patient is taking 15 or 20 mg daily, first decrease dosage to 10 mg daily for 1 week; then stop drug to avoid adverse reactions. Reduce dosage by 50% when giving with strong CYP2D6 inhibitor. Increase dosage by up to three times original dose when giving with strong CYP inducer for more than 14 days.

⚕ For patients who are known CYP2D6 poor metabolizers, maximum recommended dosage is 10 mg daily.

ADMINISTRATION
PO
• Give drug without regard to meals.
• Store tablets at room temperature.

ACTION
Antidepressant effect of vortioxetine isn't fully understood but is thought to be related to its enhancement of serotonergic activity in the CNS through inhibition of the reuptake of serotonin (5-HT) as well as 5-HT_3 receptor antagonism and 5-HT_{1A} receptor agonism.

Route	Onset	Peak	Duration
PO	2–4 wk	7–11 hr	Unknown

Half-life: 66 hours.

ADVERSE REACTIONS
CNS: dizziness, abnormal dreams. **EENT:** dry mouth. **GI:** nausea, diarrhea, constipation, vomiting, flatulence. **GU:** sexual dysfunction. **Skin:** pruritus.

INTERACTIONS
Drug-drug. *Aspirin, clopidogrel, heparin, NSAIDs, warfarin:* May increase risk of bleeding. Use together cautiously.
Diuretics: May increase risk of hyponatremia. Monitor patient carefully.
Linezolid, methylene blue: May increase risk of serotonin syndrome. Use together is contraindicated.
MAO inhibitors (selegiline, phenelzine): May cause severe adverse effects from impaired serotonin metabolism. Concurrent use is contraindicated. Don't restart MAO inhibitor for at least 21 days after vortioxetine has been

stopped. Start vortioxetine at least 14 days after MAO inhibitor has been stopped.
Serotonergics (buspirone, fentanyl, lithium, SSNRIs, SSRIs, TCAs, tramadol, triptans, tryptophan products): May increase risk of serotonin syndrome. Monitor patient carefully.
Strong CYP inducers (carbamazepine, phenytoin, rifampin): May decrease vortioxetine level if coadministered for more than 14 days. Consider increasing vortioxetine dosage with concurrent use, to maximum of three times original dose. Decrease vortioxetine dosage to original level within 14 days when strong CYP inducer is discontinued.
Strong CYP2D6 inhibitors (bupropion, fluoxetine, paroxetine, quinidine): May increase vortioxetine level. Decrease vortioxetine dosage by half when given together. Increase vortioxetine dosage to original level when CYP2D6 inhibitor is discontinued.
Drug-herb. *Herbs with anticoagulant or antiplatelet properties (alfalfa, anise, bilberry):* May increase bleeding risk. Discourage use together.
St. John's wort: May increase risk of serotonin syndrome. Discourage use together.
Drug-lifestyle. *Alcohol use:* May increase psychomotor impairment. Discourage use together.

EFFECTS ON LAB TEST RESULTS
• May decrease sodium level.
• May cause false-positive urine enzyme immunoassays for methadone.

CONTRAINDICATIONS & CAUTIONS
• Contraindicated in patients hypersensitive to drug or its components.
Boxed Warning Drug increases risk of suicidality in children, adolescents, and young adults. Drug isn't approved for use in children. ■
• Use cautiously in patients with personal or family history of bipolar disorder, mania, or hypomania.
• Use cautiously in patients who take diuretics or are otherwise volume-depleted because of increased risk of hyponatremia.
• Drug may increase bleeding risk, particularly if used with drugs or herbs that interfere with hemostasis.
• Drug may trigger an angle-closure attack in patients with anatomically narrow angles who don't have a patent iridectomy.

Dialyzable drug: Unknown.
⚠ **Overdose S&S:** Dizziness, diarrhea, abdominal discomfort, generalized pruritus, somnolence, flushing, nausea.

PREGNANCY-LACTATION-REPRODUCTION
• Drug's effects during pregnancy are unknown. Third-trimester use may increase risk of persistent pulmonary hypertension and withdrawal in newborns. Use only if potential benefits outweigh fetal risk.
• Encourage patients who are pregnant to enroll in the National Pregnancy Registry for Antidepressants (1-866-961-2388 or https://womensmentalhealth.org/research/pregnancyregistry/antidepressants).
• It isn't known if drug appears in human milk. Patient should discontinue breastfeeding or discontinue drug, considering importance of drug to patient.

NURSING CONSIDERATIONS
Boxed Warning Monitor for signs and symptoms of worsening depression, suicidality, or unusual changes in behavior, especially during initial treatment or with dosage changes, either increases or decreases. ■
• Screen patient for bipolar disorder before drug initiation. Drug isn't approved for use in bipolar depression.
• Monitor for signs and symptoms of hyponatremia and SIADH (headache, difficulty concentrating, memory impairment, confusion, weakness, unsteadiness, hallucination, syncope, seizure, coma, respiratory arrest, death). Discontinue drug if hyponatremia occurs.
• Monitor for signs and symptoms of serotonin syndrome, including mental status changes (agitation, hallucinations, delirium, coma), autonomic instability (tachycardia, labile blood pressure, dizziness, diaphoresis, flushing, hyperthermia), neuromuscular symptoms (tremor, rigidity, myoclonus, hyperreflexia, incoordination), seizures, and severe GI symptoms (nausea, vomiting, diarrhea). Discontinue drug immediately if signs or symptoms occur.
• Drug may cause withdrawal syndrome (dysphoric mood, irritability, agitation, dizziness, sensory disturbances, anxiety, confusion, headache, lethargy, emotional lability, insomnia, hypomania, tinnitus, and seizures). To discontinue therapy, reduce dosage of 15 mg once daily or more to 10 mg once daily

for 1 week before full discontinuation to prevent withdrawal. If intolerable withdrawal signs and symptoms occur after dosage reduction or drug discontinuation, consider resuming previous dosage and then tapering more gradually.

• Serotonergic antidepressants may cause signs and symptoms of sexual dysfunction. Assess for sexual dysfunction before and during treatment.

PATIENT TEACHING

Boxed Warning Advise patient and caregivers to watch for signs and symptoms of suicidality, especially during dosage adjustment. ■

• Tell patient to report all adverse reactions to prescriber.

• Warn patient about signs and symptoms of serotonin syndrome or autonomic instability.

• Advise patient that nausea, dry mouth, dizziness, constipation, diarrhea, or sexual dysfunction may occur.

• Warn patient not to stop drug abruptly or without discussing with prescriber.

• Caution patient about operating machinery and performing tasks that require alertness while taking drug.

• Caution patient to report pregnancy or breastfeeding to prescriber.

SAFETY ALERT!

warfarin sodium 💊
WAR-far-in

Jantoven

Therapeutic class: Anticoagulants
Pharmacologic class: Vitamin K antagonists

AVAILABLE FORMS
Tablets: 1 mg, 2 mg, 2.5 mg, 3 mg, 4 mg, 5 mg, 6 mg, 7.5 mg, 10 mg

INDICATIONS & DOSAGES
➤ **Prophylaxis and treatment of venous thromboembolic disorders (DVT, PE) and embolic complications from atrial fibrillation or cardiac valve replacement; adjunct to reduce risk of stroke or systemic embolism after MI**
Adults: 2 to 5 mg PO daily for 2 to 4 days; then dosage based on daily PT and INR until stable in therapeutic range. Usual

maintenance dosage, 2 to 10 mg PO daily. Base dosages on INR target goals and other clinical factors. Individualize duration of treatment as clinically indicated.

🔻 *Adjust-a-dose:* Consider lower initiation and maintenance doses for older adults, patients who are debilitated, patients of Asian descent, and those with CYP2C9 and VKORC1 genotypes. Patients with CYP2C9 gene variant may require more time to achieve maximum INR effect. Monitor INR more frequently in patients with kidney impairment.

ADMINISTRATION
PO
• Establish baseline coagulation parameters before therapy. PT and INR determinations are essential for proper control. Recommended INR ranges from 2 to 3 for most patients. Target INR in patients with tilting disk valves and bileaflet mechanical valves in mitral position, caged ball, or caged disk valves ranges from 2.5 to 3.5.

• Give drug at same time daily.

• Give a missed dose as soon as possible on the same day; don't double dose to make up for a missed dose.

ACTION
Inhibits vitamin K-dependent activation of clotting factors II, VII, IX, and X, formed in the liver. Also inhibits anticoagulant proteins C and S.

Route	Onset	Peak	Duration
PO	Within 24 hr	4 hr	2–5 days

Half-life: 20 to 60 hours.

ADVERSE REACTIONS
CNS: taste perversion. **CV:** vasculitis. **GI:** abdominal pain, diarrhea, flatulence, bloating, nausea, vomiting. **Hematologic:** *hemorrhage.* **Hepatic:** *hepatitis,* elevated liver enzyme levels. **Respiratory:** tracheal or tracheobronchial calcification. **Skin:** alopecia, pruritus, rash, dermatitis. **Other:** chills, hypersensitivity or allergic reactions (*anaphylactic reactions,* urticaria).

INTERACTIONS
⟳ *Alert:* Consult labeling of all concurrently used drugs to obtain further information about interactions with warfarin.

Reactions in bold italics are *life-threatening*.

Drug-drug. *Acetaminophen:* May increase bleeding with long-term therapy (more than 2 weeks) at high doses (more than 2 g/day) of acetaminophen. Monitor therapy.

Allopurinol, amiodarone, anabolic steroids, anticoagulants (argatroban, bivalirudin), aspirin, azole antifungals, beta blockers (atenolol, propranolol), cephalosporins, chloramphenicol, cimetidine, corticosteroids, cyclosporine, danazol, diazoxide, diflunisal, disulfiram, erythromycin, ethacrynic acid, felbamate, fibric acids, fluoroquinolones, fluoxymesterone, furosemide, glucagon, HMG-CoA reductase inhibitors (lovastatin, simvastatin), heparin, isoniazid, lansoprazole, macrolide antibiotics (azithromycin, clarithromycin, erythromycin), meclofenamate, methimazole, methyldopa, methylphenidate, methyltestosterone, metronidazole, nalidixic acid, neomycin (oral), NSAIDs, omeprazole, oxandrolone, pentoxifylline, propafenone, propylthiouracil, quinidine, quinolones (ciprofloxacin, levofloxacin, ofloxacin), salicylates, selective cyclo-oxygenase-2 inhibitors (celecoxib), SSRIs, sulfamethoxazole–trimethoprim, sulfonamides, tamoxifen, tetracyclines, thiazides, thrombolytics, thyroid drugs, ticlopidine, tramadol, vitamin E, valproic acid, zafirlukast: May increase anticoagulant effect. Monitor patient carefully for bleeding. Reduce anticoagulant dosage as directed.

Aprepitant, ascorbic acid, barbiturates, bosentan, carbamazepine, clozapine, corticotropin, cyclosporine, dicloxacillin, griseofulvin, haloperidol, meprobamate, mercaptopurine, nafcillin, oral contraceptives containing estrogen, phenytoin, protease inhibitors (ritonavir), raloxifene, ribavirin, rifampin, spironolactone, sucralfate, thiazide diuretics, trazodone, vitamin K: May reduce PT and thereby decrease INR, which reduces the anticoagulant effect. Carefully monitor PT and INR. Increase warfarin dosage, as needed.

Sulfonylureas (oral antidiabetics): May increase hypoglycemic response. Monitor glucose level.

Drug-herb. *Coenzyme Q10, ginseng, St. John's wort:* May reduce action of warfarin. Modify therapy.

Green tea: May decrease anticoagulant effect caused by vitamin K content of green tea. Advise patient to minimize variable consumption of green tea.

Herbs with anticoagulant properties (dong quai, fenugreek, feverfew, garlic, ginger, ginkgo, willow bark): May increase risk of bleeding. Discourage use together.

Drug-food. *Cranberry juice:* May increase risk of severe bleeding. Discourage use together.

Foods, multivitamins, and other enteral products containing vitamin K: May impair anticoagulation. Tell patient to maintain consistent daily intake of foods containing vitamin K.

Drug-lifestyle. *Alcohol use:* May enhance anticoagulant effects. Tell patient to avoid large amounts of alcohol.

EFFECTS ON LAB TEST RESULTS

- May increase ALT and AST levels.
- May falsely decrease theophylline level.
- May increase INR and prolong PT and PTT.

CONTRAINDICATIONS & CAUTIONS

- Contraindicated in patients hypersensitive to drug and in those with active ulceration or bleeding from GI, GU, or respiratory tract; aneurysm; dissecting aorta; cerebrovascular hemorrhage; severe or malignant HTN; subacute bacterial endocarditis, pericarditis, or pericardial effusion; or blood dyscrasias or hemorrhagic tendencies.
- Contraindicated with recent or contemplated surgery involving large open areas, eye, brain, or spinal cord; recent prostatectomy; or major regional lumbar block anesthesia, spinal puncture, or diagnostic or therapeutic invasive procedures.
- Contraindicated in unsupervised patients with conditions that increase risk of nonadherence (dementia, alcohol use disorder, psychosis).
- Fatal and serious calciphylaxis (calcium uremic arteriolopathy) has been reported in patients with and without CKD. If calciphylaxis is diagnosed, stop drug and treat calciphylaxis. Consider alternative anticoagulation.
- Avoid using in patients with history of warfarin-induced necrosis and in situations in which lab facilities for coagulation testing are inadequate.
- Use cautiously in patients with infectious diseases or intestinal flora disturbance (sprue, antibiotic therapy), HTN, kidney disease, Child-Pugh class B or C liver disease, drainage tubes in any orifice, deficiency in protein C-mediated anticoagulant response,

W

polycythemia vera, vasculitis, diabetes, heparin-induced thrombocytopenia, or conditions that increase risk of hemorrhage. Also use cautiously in conjunction with regional or lumbar block anesthesia and during cataract surgery.

• AKI may occur in patients with altered glomerular integrity or history of kidney disease, possibly in relation to episodes of excessive anticoagulation and hematuria.

• Drug may increase release of atheromatous plaque emboli, most commonly affecting the kidneys, pancreas, spleen, and liver. Signs and symptoms depend on the site of embolization and may progress to necrosis and death.

Dialyzable drug: Unknown.

⚠ *Overdose S&S:* Blood in stools or urine, excessive bruising, persistent oozing from superficial injuries, excessive menstrual bleeding, melena, petechiae.

PREGNANCY-LACTATION-REPRODUCTION

• Drug can cause fetal harm and is contraindicated during pregnancy, except in patients with mechanical heart valves who are at high risk for thromboembolism and for whom benefits of warfarin may outweigh fetal risks.

• Drug is contraindicated in patients experiencing threatened abortion, eclampsia, and preeclampsia.

• Verify pregnancy status before starting drug.

• Patients of childbearing potential should use effective contraception during therapy and for 1 month after final dose.

• Drug hasn't been detected in human milk. Use cautiously during breastfeeding. Monitor infants for bruising or bleeding.

NURSING CONSIDERATIONS

Boxed Warning Warfarin can cause major or fatal bleeding, which is more likely to occur during starting period and with higher dose. Drugs, dietary changes, and other factors affect INR levels achieved with warfarin therapy. Regularly monitor INR in all patients. Consider more-frequent INR monitoring in those at high risk for bleeding. ∎

• At start of therapy, monitor INR daily until stabilized in therapeutic range; then monitor every 1 to 4 weeks.

• Avoid IM injections when possible.

• Regularly inspect patient for bleeding gums, bruises on arms or legs, petechiae,

nosebleeds, melena, hematuria, and hematemesis.

• Monitor patient for purple-toes syndrome due to microemboli, characterized by dark purple or mottled color of toes; may occur 3 to 10 weeks, or even later, after starting therapy.

🔵 *Alert:* Withhold drug and call prescriber at once in the event of fever or rash (signs of severe adverse reactions).

• Monitor INR more frequently in patient with compromised kidney function to maintain INR within therapeutic range.

• Effect can be neutralized by oral or parenteral vitamin K.

• Older adults, patients who are debilitated, and patients with CKD or liver failure are especially sensitive to drug's effect.

• Make sure that patient isn't taking additional anticoagulants, unless instructed by prescriber.

• *Look alike–sound alike:* Don't confuse Jantoven with Janumet or Januvia.

PATIENT TEACHING

• Stress the importance of adhering to prescribed dosage and follow-up appointments for monitoring. Tell patient to carry a card that identifies patient's increased risk of bleeding.

• Tell patient and family about measures to prevent bleeding. Instruct them to watch for signs of bleeding or abnormal bruising, and to call prescriber at once if any occur.

• Warn patient to avoid OTC products containing aspirin, other salicylates, or drugs that may interact with warfarin, unless ordered by prescriber.

• Advise patient to consult prescriber before initiating any herbal therapy because many herbs have anticoagulant, antiplatelet, or fibrinolytic properties.

• Instruct patient to report heavier than usual menstruation. Dosage adjustment may be needed.

• Advise patient to use electric razor when shaving and to use a soft toothbrush.

• Caution patient to avoid activities and sports that may result in traumatic injury.

• Instruct patient to immediately report pain, discoloration of skin, unusual symptom (for example, sudden cool, painful, purple discoloration of toes), bruising, bleeding, blood in urine, bloody or black stools, headache, dizziness, or weakness.

Reactions in bold italics are *life-threatening*.

• Inform patient that consuming foods high in vitamin K (such as green, leafy vegetables) can decrease anticoagulant effects. Tell patient to read food labels and to eat a balanced diet with consistent intake of vitamin K. Nutritional supplements and multivitamins that contain vitamin K may also impair coagulation. Advise patient to notify prescriber before making any dietary changes.

• Tell patient to inform all health care providers about taking warfarin and to inform warfarin prescriber of new medication orders and upcoming surgeries or procedures.

• Advise patient to report serious illness, severe diarrhea, infections, or fever to prescriber.

• Caution patient of childbearing potential of fetal risk. Advise patient to report pregnancy or plans to become pregnant.

---

zafirlukast
zah-FUR-luh-kast

Accolate

Therapeutic class: Antiasthmatics
Pharmacologic class: Leukotriene receptor antagonists

AVAILABLE FORMS
Tablets: 10 mg, 20 mg

INDICATIONS & DOSAGES
➤ **Prevention and long-term treatment of asthma**
Adults and children ages 12 and older: 20 mg PO b.i.d.
Children ages 5 to 11: 10 mg PO b.i.d.

ADMINISTRATION
PO
• Give drug 1 hour before or 2 hours after a meal.
• Protect drug from light and moisture.

ACTION
Selectively competes for leukotriene receptor sites, blocking inflammatory action.

Route	Onset	Peak	Duration
PO	Rapid	2–3 hr	12 hr

Half-life: 10 hours.

ADVERSE REACTIONS
CNS: headache, asthenia, dizziness, pain, fever. **GI:** abdominal pain, diarrhea, nausea, vomiting, dyspepsia. **Hepatic:** increased ALT level. **Musculoskeletal:** back pain, myalgia. **Other:** accidental injury, infection.

INTERACTIONS
Drug-drug. *Aspirin:* May increase zafirlukast level. Monitor patient for adverse effects.
Erythromycin, theophylline: May decrease zafirlukast level. Monitor patient for decreased effectiveness.
Moderate and strong CYP2C9 inhibitors (fluconazole): May increase zafirlukast level. Use together cautiously.
Warfarin: May increase warfarin level, prolonging PT. Monitor PT and INR, and adjust anticoagulant dosage as needed.
Drug-food. *Any food:* May reduce rate and extent of drug absorption. Advise patient to take drug 1 hour before or 2 hours after a meal.

EFFECTS ON LAB TEST RESULTS
• May increase ALT level.

CONTRAINDICATIONS & CAUTIONS
• Contraindicated in patients hypersensitive to drug and in those with liver impairment, including cirrhosis.
• Use cautiously in older adults.
• Safety and effectiveness in children younger than age 5 haven't been determined.
Dialyzable drug: Unknown.
⚠ **Overdose S&S:** Rash, upset stomach.

PREGNANCY-LACTATION-REPRODUCTION
• Studies during pregnancy are inadequate. Use during pregnancy only if clearly needed.
• Drug appears in human milk. Don't use during breastfeeding because of potential for tumorigenicity shown in animal studies.

NURSING CONSIDERATIONS
⚡ *Alert:* Monitor for eosinophilia, vasculitic rash, worsening pulmonary symptoms, cardiac complications, and neuropathy consistent with Churg-Strauss syndrome, usually associated with decrease or withdrawal of steroid therapy.
• Drug isn't indicated to reverse bronchospasm in acute asthma attacks, including status asthmaticus.

🜂 **Alert:** Drug may cause behavior and mood changes, including agitation, depression, insomnia, and suicidality. Monitor patient and consider discontinuing drug if neuropsychiatric symptoms develop.

🜂 **Alert:** Periodically monitor LFTs. Life-threatening liver failure has been reported. Immediately discontinue drug for suspected liver failure (right upper quadrant abdominal pain, nausea, fatigue, lethargy, pruritus, jaundice, flulike symptoms, anorexia, enlarged liver).

● *Look alike–sound alike:* Don't confuse Accolate with Accupril or Accutane.

PATIENT TEACHING

● Teach about proper drug administration and handling.

● Explain that drug is for long-term treatment of asthma. Instruct patient to keep taking drug even if symptoms resolve.

● Advise patient that drug isn't indicated for use in reversal of bronchospasm in acute asthma attacks, including status asthmaticus.

● Caution patient to continue taking other antiasthmatics, as prescribed.

● Warn that drug may cause behavior and mood changes. Instruct patient to report development of these symptoms to prescriber.

● Teach patient to report rare but serious signs and symptoms of liver dysfunction.

● Advise patient to report pregnancy or plans to become pregnant or breastfeed.

zaleplon
ZAL-e-plon

Therapeutic class: Hypnotics
Pharmacologic class: Pyrazolopyrimidines
Controlled substance schedule: IV

AVAILABLE FORMS
Capsules: 5 mg, 10 mg

INDICATIONS & DOSAGES
➤ **Short-term treatment of insomnia (up to 30 days)**
Adults: 10 mg PO daily at bedtime; may increase to 20 mg as needed. Reevaluate patient if drug is used for more than 2 to 3 weeks.
Adjust-a-dose: For older adults, low-weight adults, and patients who are debilitated, initially, give 5 mg PO daily at bedtime; doses of more than 10 mg aren't recommended. For

patients with Child-Pugh class A or B liver impairment and those also taking cimetidine, 5 mg PO daily at bedtime.

ADMINISTRATION
PO
● Give drug immediately before bed or after patient has gone to bed and has had trouble falling asleep.
● Don't give drug after a high-fat or heavy meal because onset may be delayed.

ACTION
A hypnotic with chemical structure unrelated to benzodiazepines that interacts with the GABA-benzodiazepine receptor complex in the CNS. Modulation of this complex is thought to be responsible for sedative, anxiolytic, muscle relaxant, and anticonvulsant effects of benzodiazepines.

Route	Onset	Peak	Duration
PO	Rapid	1 hr	Unknown

Half-life: 1 hour.

ADVERSE REACTIONS
CNS: amnesia, anxiety, asthenia, confusion, depersonalization, depression, difficulty concentrating, dizziness, drowsiness, fever, hallucinations, headache, hypertonia, hypoesthesia, malaise, migraine, nervousness, paresthesia, somnolence, tremor, vertigo, smell alteration, taste perversion. **CV:** chest pain, peripheral edema. **EENT:** abnormal vision, eye pain, conjunctivitis, ear pain, sound sensitivity, epistaxis, dry mouth. **GI:** abdominal pain, anorexia, colitis, constipation, dyspepsia, nausea. **GU:** dysmenorrhea. **Musculoskeletal:** arthralgia, arthritis, back pain, myalgia. **Respiratory:** bronchitis. **Skin:** photosensitivity reactions, pruritus, rash.

INTERACTIONS
Drug-drug. *Cimetidine:* May increase zaleplon bioavailability and peak level. Use initial zaleplon dose of 5 mg.
CNS depressants (imipramine, thioridazine): May cause additive CNS effects. Use together cautiously.
CYP3A4 inducers (carbamazepine, phenobarbital, phenytoin, rifampin): May reduce zaleplon bioavailability and peak level. Consider using a different hypnotic.
🜂 **Alert:** *Opioids:* May cause slow or difficult breathing, sedation, and death. Avoid

use together. If use together is necessary, limit dosage and duration of each drug to minimum necessary for desired effect.

Promethazine: May decrease zaleplon plasma level. Use together cautiously.

Drug-food. *Heavy meals, high-fat foods:* May prolong absorption, delaying peak drug level by about 2 hours; may delay sleep onset. Advise patient not to take with meals.

Drug-lifestyle. *Alcohol use:* May increase CNS effects. Discourage use together.

EFFECTS ON LAB TEST RESULTS
• May increase cholesterol level.

CONTRAINDICATIONS & CAUTIONS
• Contraindicated in patients hypersensitive to drug or its components.
• Contraindicated in patients with Child-Pugh class C liver impairment.
• If hypersensitivity reactions occur, don't rechallenge patient.
Boxed Warning Drug may cause rare but serious injury, including death, due to complex sleep behaviors, such as sleepwalking, sleep driving, and engaging in other activities while not fully awake. These behaviors can occur even at lowest recommended dosages and after just one dose. Drug is contraindicated in patients who have experienced complex sleep behaviors after taking drug in past. ▪
• Avoid use in patients with sensitivity to tartrazine (FD&C Yellow No. 5), which is contained in capsules. Reactions may be more common in patients with aspirin hypersensitivity.
• Use cautiously in older adults; in patients with depression or debilitation; in patients with history of drug dependence, benzodiazepine abuse, or benzodiazepine-like hypnotic abuse; and in patients with compromised respiratory function.
• Use cautiously in patients with diseases or conditions that affect metabolism or hemodynamic responses.
• Drug may cause changes in behavior and thinking, including out-of-character extroversion or aggressive behavior, loss of personal identity, confusion, strange behavior, agitation, hallucinations, worsening of depression, or suicidality.
Dialyzable drug: Unknown.

⚠ *Overdose S&S:* Drowsiness, confusion, lethargy, ataxia, hypotension, respiratory depression, coma, death.

PREGNANCY-LACTATION-REPRODUCTION
• Studies during pregnancy are inadequate. Use during pregnancy isn't recommended.
• Drug appears in human milk in a small amount. Use during breastfeeding isn't recommended.

NURSING CONSIDERATIONS
• Closely monitor patients who have compromised respiratory function caused by illness, older adults, and patients who are debilitated because they are more sensitive to respiratory depression.
• Start treatment only after carefully evaluating patient because sleep disturbances may be a symptom of an underlying physical or psychiatric disorder. Failure of drug to relieve insomnia after 7 to 10 days requires further evaluation.
• Adverse reactions are usually dose-related. Consult prescriber about dose reduction if adverse reactions occur.
• *Look alike–sound alike:* Don't confuse zaleplon with Zelapar, Zemplar, or zolpidem.

PATIENT TEACHING
Boxed Warning Warn patient of risk of injury or death related to complex sleep behaviors. Direct patient to stop drug and immediately report complex sleep behavior or inability to remember activities performed while taking drug. ▪
⚠ *Alert:* Warn patient that drug may cause allergic reactions. Advise patient to report these adverse effects.
• Advise patient that drug works rapidly and should only be taken immediately before bedtime or after going to bed when patient has had trouble falling asleep.
• Tell patient not to take drug after a high-fat or heavy meal.
• Inform patient that risk of next-day psychomotor impairment increases if drug is taken with less than 7 to 8 hours sleep or is taken with other CNS depressants, including alcohol, or at higher-than-recommended dosage.
• Caution patient that drowsiness, dizziness, light-headedness, and coordination problems occur most often within 1 hour after taking drug.

Z

• Advise patient to avoid alcohol use while taking drug and to notify prescriber before taking other prescription or OTC drugs.
• Instruct patient to report sleep problems that continue despite use of drug.
• Notify patient that dependence can occur and that drug is recommended for short-term use only.
• Warn patient not to abruptly stop drug because of risk of withdrawal symptoms, including unpleasant feelings, stomach and muscle cramps, vomiting, diaphoresis, shakiness, and seizures.
• Notify patient that insomnia may recur for a few nights after stopping drug but should resolve on its own.
• Warn that drug may cause changes in behavior and thinking (complex behaviors, out-of-character extroversion or aggressive behavior, loss of personal identity, confusion, strange behavior, agitation, hallucinations, worsening of depression, suicidality). Tell patient to immediately notify prescriber if any of these changes occur; drug may need to be discontinued.
• Advise patient to report pregnancy or plans to become pregnant or breastfeed.

zidovudine
zid-oh-VEW-den

Retrovir

Therapeutic class: Antiretrovirals
Pharmacologic class: Nucleoside-nucleotide reverse transcriptase inhibitors

AVAILABLE FORMS
Capsules ⒪: 100 mg
Injection: 10 mg/mL
Syrup: 50 mg/5 mL
Tablets ⒪: 300 mg

INDICATIONS & DOSAGES
Adjust-a-dose (for all indications): In patients with significant anemia (Hb level less than 7.5 g/dL or more than 25% below baseline) or significant neutropenia (granulocyte count less than 750/mm³ or more than 50% below baseline), interrupt therapy until evidence of bone marrow recovery. In patients receiving dialysis or with CrCl less than 15 mL/minute, give 100 mg PO or 1 mg/kg IV every 6 to 8 hours. For patients with Child-Pugh class A

or B liver impairment or cirrhosis, daily dosage may need to be reduced.
➤ **HIV infection, with other antiretrovirals**
Adults: 300 mg PO b.i.d. If patient can't tolerate oral drug, 1 mg/kg IV infused over 1 hour every 4 hours until patient can receive PO form.
Children ages 4 weeks to less than 18 years: Do not exceed recommended adult dosage. For children weighing 30 kg or more, 300 mg PO b.i.d. or 200 mg PO t.i.d. For children weighing 9 to less than 30 kg, 9 mg/kg PO b.i.d. or 6 mg/kg PO t.i.d. For children weighing 4 to less than 9 kg, 12 mg/kg PO b.i.d. or 8 mg/kg PO t.i.d.
➤ **To prevent maternal-fetal transmission of HIV**
Patients who are pregnant and at more than 14 weeks' gestation: 100 mg PO five times daily until start of labor. Then 2 mg/kg (total body weight) IV over 1 hour, followed by continuous IV infusion of 1 mg/kg/hour until umbilical cord is clamped.
Neonates: 2 mg/kg PO every 6 hours, starting within 12 hours after birth and continuing until 6 weeks old. Or, 1.5 mg/kg via IV infusion over 30 minutes every 6 hours.

ADMINISTRATION
⚠ *Alert:* Hazardous drug; use safe-handling and disposal precautions.
PO
• Give drug without regard to meals.
• Use calibrated measuring device to accurately measure oral liquid dose.
• Protect capsules from heat and moisture.
• Give a missed dose as soon as possible, unless it's close to the next scheduled dose.
IV
▼ Give by IV route only until patient can tolerate oral drug.
⚠ *Alert:* Vial stoppers contain natural rubber latex, which may cause allergic reactions in latex-sensitive individuals.
▼ Remove calculated dose from vial; add to D_5W to achieve a concentration no greater than 4 mg/mL.
▼ Infuse drug over 1 hour (adults) or 30 minutes (neonates) at constant rate. Avoid rapid infusion and bolus injection.
▼ Don't give by IM injection.
▼ Protect undiluted vials from light.
▼ After dilution, solution remains stable for 24 hours at room temperature and for 48 hours if refrigerated at 36° to 46° F

Reactions in bold italics are *life-threatening*.

(2° to 8° C). Administer diluted solution within 8 hours if stored at 77° F (25° C) or within 24 hours if refrigerated at 36° to 46° F.

▼ **Incompatibilities:** None listed by manufacturer. Consult drug compatibility reference for more information.

ACTION
NRTI that inhibits replication of HIV by blocking DNA synthesis.

Route	Onset	Peak	Duration
PO, IV	Unknown	30–90 min	Unknown

Half-life: 0.5 to 3 hours.

ADVERSE REACTIONS
CNS: asthenia, dizziness, fever, fatigue, headache, malaise, neuropathy, insomnia, paresthesia, somnolence, decreased reflexes, irritability. **CV:** lymphadenopathy, *HF*, ECG abnormality, left ventricular dilation, edema. **EENT:** ear symptoms, nasal discharge or congestion. **GI:** anorexia, nausea, vomiting, abdominal pain, cramps, constipation, diarrhea, dyspepsia, stomatitis. **GU:** hematuria. **Hematologic:** *neutropenia, agranulocytosis, severe bone marrow suppression, thrombocytopenia,* anemia. **Hepatic:** altered LFT values, liver enlargement. **Metabolic:** increased lipase and amylase levels, weight loss. **Musculoskeletal:** arthralgia, myalgia, myopathy. **Respiratory:** cough, wheezing. **Skin:** rash. **Other:** chills, splenomegaly.

INTERACTIONS
Drug-drug. *Atovaquone, fluconazole, methadone, probenecid, trimethoprim, valproic acid:* May increase zidovudine level. May need to adjust dosage.
Clarithromycin: May enhance myelosuppressive effect of zidovudine and decrease zidovudine level. Closely monitor response to zidovudine and consider staggering zidovudine and clarithromycin doses when possible to minimize potential for interaction. Consider therapy modification.
Doxorubicin, ribavirin, stavudine: May have antagonistic effects. Avoid use together.
Ganciclovir, other bone marrow suppressive or cytotoxic drugs: May increase hematologic toxicity of zidovudine. Use together cautiously.
Interferon alfa: May increase risk of toxicity, including liver decompensation, neutropenia,

and anemia. Monitor patient closely. Discontinue zidovudine or adjust or discontinue interferon alfa, as appropriate. Refer to interferon alfa prescribing information.
Orlistat: May decrease level of antiretrovirals. Monitor therapy.
Ribavirin: May increase risk of anemia. Avoid use together.

EFFECTS ON LAB TEST RESULTS
• May increase lipase, amylase, bilirubin, ALT, AST, ALP, and LDH levels.
• May decrease Hb level and RBC, WBC, granulocyte, neutrophil, and platelet counts.

CONTRAINDICATIONS & CAUTIONS
• Contraindicated in patients who have had a potentially life-threatening hypersensitivity reaction to drug or its components. Reactions, such as anaphylaxis and SJS, can occur.
Boxed Warning Use cautiously and with close monitoring in patients with advanced symptomatic HIV infection and those with severe bone marrow depression. Use of drug has been associated with hematologic toxicity, including neutropenia and severe anemia. ■
• Use cautiously in patients with liver enlargement, hepatitis, or other risk factors for liver disease and in those with kidney insufficiency.
• Use cautiously in patients with granulocyte count less than 1,000 cells/mm³ or Hb level less than 9.5 g/dL.
Boxed Warning Prolonged use has been associated with myopathy. ■
Dialyzable drug: Unlikely.
⚠ *Overdose S&S:* Fatigue, headache, vomiting, hematologic disturbances.

PREGNANCY-LACTATION-REPRODUCTION
• U.S. Department of Health and Human Services perinatal HIV guidelines consider zidovudine in combination with lamivudine to be an alternative regimen for use during pregnancy in patients who are antiretroviral-naive.
• Administer zidovudine IV near delivery regardless of antepartum regimen or mode of delivery in patients with HIV RNA greater than 1,000 copies/mL or unknown HIV RNA status.
• Register patients exposed to zidovudine during pregnancy in the Antiretroviral Pregnancy Registry (1-800-258-4263 or www.apregistry.com).

Z

• The CDC recommends counseling patients with HIV-1 infection on the risk of postnatal HIV-1 transmission. Maintaining viral suppression through antiretroviral therapy during pregnancy, delivery, and postpartum period decreases the risk to less than 1%.

• In couples who want to conceive, partner with HIV infection should attain maximum viral suppression before conception.

NURSING CONSIDERATIONS

Boxed Warning Although rare, lactic acidosis without hypoxemia and severe liver enlargement with steatosis may occur. Notify prescriber if patient develops unexplained tachypnea, dyspnea, or decrease in bicarbonate level. Therapy may need to be suspended until lactic acidosis is ruled out. ■

• Frequently monitor blood studies to detect anemia, agranulocytosis, or liver decompensation. Patients may need to reduce dosage or temporarily stop therapy.

• Monitor for signs and symptoms of immune reconstitution syndrome (fever, pain, erythema, wound drainage, swollen lymph nodes, rash) and autoimmune disorders, which have been reported in patients treated with combination antiretroviral therapy.

• Monitor for signs of lipoatrophy (localized fatty tissue loss) during therapy. If feasible, switch to an alternative regimen if lipoatrophy is suspected.

• Drug may temporarily decrease morbidity and mortality in certain patients with AIDS.

• Health care providers caring for patients infected with HIV and their infants may call the Perinatal HIV Hotline for clinical consultations (888-448-8765).

• *Look alike–sound alike:* Don't confuse Retrovir with ritonavir.

PATIENT TEACHING

• Teach about proper drug administration, storage, and handling.

• Tell patient to take drug exactly as directed and not to share it with others.

• Remind patient to comply with the dosage schedule. Suggest ways to avoid missing doses, perhaps by using an alarm clock.

• Explain that dosages vary among patients. Instruct patient not to change dosing instructions unless directed by prescriber.

• Warn patient not to take other drugs for AIDS unless approved by prescriber.

• Advise patient that monotherapy isn't recommended. Encourage patient to discuss any questions with prescriber.

• Stress importance of complying with frequent lab testing because drug-related anemia may occur, requiring blood transfusion.

• Advise patient who is pregnant and infected with HIV-1 that drug therapy only reduces risk of HIV transmission to newborn. Long-term risks to infants are unknown.

• Inform patient who is pregnant and considering use of zidovudine for prevention of HIV-1 transmission to infant that transmission may still occur, despite therapy.

• Advise patient who is pregnant and infected with HIV-1 of the risk of postnatal transmission of HIV through breastfeeding.

• Instruct patient to report loss of subcutaneous fat, most evident in face, limbs, and buttocks, which may be only partially reversible over months to years if therapy is changed to a non-zidovudine-containing regimen.

• Advise patient to report signs and symptoms of lactic acidosis (nausea, vomiting, shortness of breath, weakness).

• Warn that potentially life-threatening hypersensitivity reactions can occur. Instruct patient to immediately report any rash.

ziprasidone hydrochloride
zih-PRAZ-i-done

Geodon, Zeldox✦

ziprasidone mesylate
Geodon

Therapeutic class: Antipsychotics
Pharmacologic class: Benzisoxazole derivatives

AVAILABLE FORMS
Capsules ⒪: 20 mg, 40 mg, 60 mg, 80 mg
IM injection: 20 mg/mL single-dose vials

INDICATIONS & DOSAGES
➤ **Schizophrenia**
Adults: Initially, 20 mg PO b.i.d. Dosages are highly individualized. Adjust dosage, if necessary, no more frequently than every 2 days; to allow for lowest possible dosage, allow interval of several weeks to assess symptom response.

Effective dosage range is usually 20 to 100 mg b.i.d., but dosage greater than 80 mg b.i.d. generally isn't recommended.

➤ **Rapid control of acute agitation in patients with schizophrenia**

Adults: 10 to 20 mg IM as needed, up to maximum dosage of 40 mg daily. May give doses of 10 mg every 2 hours; may give doses of 20 mg every 4 hours, up to maximum dosage of 40 mg/day. If long-term therapy is indicated, replace with oral ziprasidone as soon as possible.

➤ **Acute bipolar I mania, including manic and mixed episodes, as monotherapy; maintenance treatment of bipolar I disorder as an adjunct to lithium or valproate**

Adults: 40 mg PO b.i.d. on day 1. Increase to 60 to 80 mg PO b.i.d. on day 2; then adjust dosage based on patient response from 40 to 80 mg b.i.d.

ADMINISTRATION

🛈 *Alert:* Hazardous drug; use safe handling and disposal precautions.

PO
• Always give drug with food.
• Have patient swallow capsules whole; don't crush or cut capsules.

IM
• To prepare IM ziprasidone, add 1.2 mL of sterile water for injection to vial and shake vigorously until drug is completely dissolved. Reconstituted solution contains 20 mg/mL ziprasidone.
• Don't mix injection with other medicinal products or solvents other than sterile water for injection.
• Inspect parenteral drug products for particulate matter and discoloration before administration. Discard unused portion of reconstituted solution.
• Effects of giving drug IM for more than 3 consecutive days are unknown. If long-term therapy is necessary, switch to PO form as soon as possible.
• Store injection at room temperature, and protect it from light. After reconstitution, store away from light for up to 24 hours at 59° to 86° F (15° to 30° C) or up to 7 days refrigerated (36° to 46° F [2° to 8° C]).

ACTION

May inhibit dopamine and serotonin-2 receptors, causing reduction in schizophrenia symptoms.

Route	Onset	Peak	Duration
PO	Unknown	6–8 hr	12 hr
IM	Unknown	1 hr	Unknown

Half-life: PO, about 7 hours; IM, 2 to 5 hours.

ADVERSE REACTIONS

CNS: confusion, headache, somnolence, akathisia, dizziness, extrapyramidal symptoms (hypertonia, dystonia, dyskinesia, hypokinesia, tremor, paralysis, twitching), vertigo, abnormal gait, asthenia, hostility, tremors, fever, hypesthesia, ataxia, amnesia, delirium, akinesia, dysarthria, neuropathy, choreoathetosis, incoordination, anxiety, insomnia, hypertonia, agitation, cogwheel rigidity, paresthesia, personality disorder, psychosis, speech disorder, withdrawal syndrome. **CV:** *bradycardia,* orthostatic hypotension, tachycardia, chest pain, HTN, vasodilation. **EENT:** abnormal vision, rhinitis, dry mouth, facial edema, dysphagia, tongue edema, increased salivation, tooth disorder, pharyngitis. **GI:** nausea, diarrhea, constipation, dyspepsia, anorexia, abdominal pain, *rectal hemorrhage,* vomiting. **GU:** dysmenorrhea, priapism. **Metabolic:** hyperglycemia. **Musculoskeletal:** myalgia, flank pain, back pain. **Respiratory:** cough, dyspnea, infection. **Skin:** rash, injection-site pain, furunculosis, fungal dermatitis, diaphoresis, photosensitivity reaction. **Other:** accidental injury, flulike syndrome, chills.

INTERACTIONS

Drug-drug. *Antihypertensives:* May enhance hypotensive effects. Monitor BP.
Carbamazepine: May decrease ziprasidone level. May need to increase ziprasidone dose to achieve desired effect.
CNS depressants (benzodiazepines, hypnotics), magnesium sulfate: May increase CNS depression. Monitor therapy.
CYP3A4 inhibitors (itraconazole, ketoconazole): May increase ziprasidone level. Ziprasidone dosage reduction may be needed to achieve desired effect.
Drugs that decrease potassium or magnesium, such as diuretics: May increase risk of arrhythmias. Monitor potassium and magnesium levels if using these drugs together.
Levodopa, dopamine agonists (ropinirole, rotigotine): May decrease effect of these drugs. Avoid use together.

Z

🔷 **Alert:** *Opioids:* May cause slow or difficult breathing, sedation, and death. Avoid use together. If use together is necessary, limit dosage and duration of each drug to minimum necessary for desired effect.

QT interval-prolonging drugs (antiarrhythmics [amiodarone, disopyramide, dofetilide, procainamide, quinidine, sotalol], arsenic trioxide, dolasetron, droperidol, mefloquine, pentamidine, phenothiazines, pimozide, quinolones, tacrolimus): May increase risk of life-threatening arrhythmias. Use together is contraindicated.

Serotonin modulators (nefazodone, trazodone, vilazodone, vortioxetine): May increase risk of serotonin syndrome and NMS. Monitor therapy.

Drug-lifestyle. *Alcohol use:* May increase dizziness, drowsiness, confusion, and difficulty concentrating. Discourage use together.

EFFECTS ON LAB TEST RESULTS
● May increase glucose and lipid levels.
● May decrease WBC count.

CONTRAINDICATIONS & CAUTIONS
● Contraindicated in patients hypersensitive to drug and in those with recent MI or uncompensated HF.
● Contraindicated in patients with history of prolonged QT interval or congenital long QT syndrome and in those taking other drugs that prolong QT interval.

Boxed Warning Older adults with dementia-related psychosis treated with antipsychotics are at increased risk for death. Drug isn't approved for treatment of dementia-related psychosis. ▮

🔷 **Alert:** Rarely, drug is associated with SCARs (SJS, DRESS syndrome).
● Use cautiously in patients with history of seizures, bradycardia, hypokalemia, or hypomagnesemia; in those with acute diarrhea; and in those with conditions that may lower seizure threshold (such as Alzheimer dementia).
● Use cautiously in patients at risk for aspiration pneumonia.
● Use cautiously in patients at risk for falls, including older adults and those who have diseases or conditions or are taking medications that may cause somnolence, orthostatic hypotension, or motor or sensory instability.
● Use cautiously in patients with known CV disease (history of MI or ischemic heart disease, HF, conduction abnormalities),

cerebrovascular disease, or conditions that predispose patient to hypotension (dehydration, hypovolemia, use of antihypertensives).
● Drug may elevate prolactin level and occurrence of galactorrhea, amenorrhea, gynecomastia, and erectile dysfunction. Long-term hyperprolactinemia with hypogonadism may lead to decreased bone density.
● Don't use IM form in patients with schizophrenia who are already taking oral ziprasidone.
● Use cautiously in older adults and in patients with kidney or liver impairment.
Dialyzable drug: No.

⚠ **Overdose S&S:** Sedation, slurred speech, transitory HTN, anxiety, extrapyramidal symptoms, somnolence, tremor.

PREGNANCY-LACTATION-REPRODUCTION
● Studies during pregnancy are inadequate. Use only if potential benefit justifies fetal risk.
● Due to risk of hyperprolactinemia, which can cause reversible reduction of reproductive function, use of an agent other than ziprasidone may be preferred in patients who are planning pregnancy.
🔷 **Alert:** Neonates exposed to antipsychotics during third trimester are at risk for developing extrapyramidal signs and symptoms (repetitive movements of face and body) and withdrawal symptoms (agitation, abnormally increased or decreased muscle tone, tremors, sleepiness, severe difficulty breathing, difficulty feeding) after delivery.
● Enroll patients exposed to drug during pregnancy in the National Pregnancy Registry for Atypical Antipsychotics (1-866-961-2388 or https://womensmentalhealth.org/research/pregnancyregistry/atypicalantipsychotic).
● It isn't known if drug or its metabolites appear in human milk. Breastfeeding isn't recommended.

NURSING CONSIDERATIONS
🔷 **Alert:** Monitor for and immediately report signs and symptoms of DRESS syndrome (rash, fever, swollen glands) or other SCARs. Discontinue drug for suspected SCARs.
🔷 **Alert:** Hyperglycemia may occur. Regularly monitor patient with diabetes. Patient with risk factors for diabetes should undergo fasting blood glucose testing at baseline and periodically. Monitor all patients for symptoms of hyperglycemia (excessive hunger or thirst, frequent urination, weakness).

Reactions in bold italics are *life-threatening*.

Hyperglycemia may be reversible when drug is stopped.

❸ *Alert:* Monitor for symptoms of metabolic syndrome (significant weight gain and increased BMI, HTN, hyperglycemia, hypercholesterolemia, and hypertriglyceridemia).

• Stop drug in patient with a QTc interval longer than 500 msec.

• Dizziness, palpitations, and syncope may be symptoms of a life-threatening arrhythmia, such as torsades de pointes. Provide CV evaluation and monitoring in patient who experiences these symptoms.

• Don't give to patient with electrolyte disturbances, such as hypokalemia or hypomagnesemia, because these conditions increase the risk of arrhythmias. Assess serum electrolyte levels at baseline and periodically during therapy; correct abnormalities.

❸ *Alert:* Patient taking an antipsychotic may develop life-threatening NMS (hyperpyrexia, muscle rigidity, altered mental status, autonomic instability) or tardive dyskinesia. Assess abnormal involuntary movement before starting therapy, at dosage changes, and periodically thereafter to monitor for tardive dyskinesia.

• Monitor for abnormal body temperature regulation, especially if patient is exercising strenuously, is exposed to extreme heat, is also receiving anticholinergics, or is at risk for dehydration.

• Assess fall risk when initiating treatment and recurrently for patients on long-term therapy, especially older adults and patients who have diseases or conditions or are taking other drugs that increase fall risk.

• Closely monitor patient at risk for suicide.

• *Look alike–sound alike:* Don't confuse ziprasidone with trazodone, zafirlukast, zidovudine, zonisamide, or Zyprexa.

PATIENT TEACHING

• Teach about proper drug administration and handling.

• Tell patient to immediately report signs or symptoms of dizziness, fainting, irregular heartbeat, or relevant heart problems.

• Advise patient to report recent episodes of diarrhea, abnormal movements, sudden fever, muscle rigidity, or change in mental status.

❸ *Alert:* Tell patient to immediately report rash (with or without blisters), fever, swollen lymph nodes, mouth ulcers, skin shedding, or targetlike spots in skin.

• Advise patient to report pregnancy or plans to become pregnant.

• Tell patient that breastfeeding isn't recommended during therapy.

• Warn that drug can cause sleepiness. Advise patient to use care when operating machinery or driving a motor vehicle.

• Inform patient that drug may cause somnolence, orthostatic hypotension, and motor and sensory instability, which can lead to falls and, consequently, fractures or other injuries.

• Advise patient that symptoms may not improve for 4 to 6 weeks.

zoledronic acid
zoh-leh-DROH-nik

Reclast

Therapeutic class: Antiosteoporotics
Pharmacologic class: Bisphosphonates

AVAILABLE FORMS
Injection as ready-to-infuse solution: 4 mg/ 100 mL, 5 mg/100 mL
Injection: 4 mg/5 mL vial

INDICATIONS & DOSAGES

➤ **Hypercalcemia caused by malignancy**
Adults: 4 mg by IV infusion. If albumin-corrected calcium level doesn't return to normal, may repeat 4 mg. Let at least 7 days pass before retreatment to allow full response to first dose.

Adjust-a-dose: Assess serum creatinine level before each treatment or retreatment. Dosage adjustments aren't necessary for patients presenting with serum creatinine level less than 4.5 mg/dL before initiation of therapy.

➤ **Multiple myeloma; bone metastases of solid tumors in conjunction with standard antineoplastics**
Adults: 4 mg IV infusion every 3 to 4 weeks. Treatment duration depends on type of cancer. Use for prostate cancer only after it has progressed after treatment with at least one course of hormonal therapy. Give patients an oral calcium supplement of 500 mg and a multiple vitamin containing 400 international units of vitamin D daily.

Adjust-a-dose: For patients with CrCl of 50 to 60 mL/minute, give 3.5 mg; 40 to 49 mL/ minute, 3.3 mg; 30 to 39 mL/minute, 3 mg. For patients with normal baseline creatinine level but an increase of 0.5 mg/dL and in those with abnormal baseline creatinine level who have an increase of 1 mg/dL, withhold drug. Resume treatment at same dose as that before treatment interruption only when creatinine level has returned to within 10% of baseline value. If CrCl falls below 30 mL/minute, don't give drug.

➤ **Paget disease of bone (osteitis deformans)**
Adults: 5 mg by IV infusion. May repeat if relapse occurs. Patient also needs 750 mg b.i.d. or 500 mg t.i.d. elemental calcium and 800 international units vitamin D daily, especially during the 2 weeks after dosing.

➤ **Treatment of osteoporosis in males and females who are postmenopausal; to treat and prevent glucocorticoid-induced osteoporosis in patients taking a daily dosage equivalent to 7.5 mg or greater of prednisone and who are expected to remain on glucocorticoids for at least 12 months**
Adults: 5 mg by IV infusion once a year.

➤ **Prevention of osteoporosis**
Adults who are postmenopausal: 5 mg by IV infusion once every 2 years.

➤ **Prevention of osteopenia secondary to androgen-deprivation therapy in prostate cancer ◆**
Adults: 4 mg IV every 6 months, or 4 mg or 5 mg once every 12 months for up to 3 years.

➤ **Prevention of osteopenia associated with aromatase inhibitor therapy in females with breast cancer ◆**
Adults: 4 mg IV every 6 months, or 5 mg IV once every 12 months for 3 to 5 years.

ADMINISTRATION

IV

▼ Further dilute concentrate by withdrawing 5 mL to obtain 4 mg of drug and mix in 100 mL of NSS or D_5W. For ready-to-use bottles or bags, if reduced doses are needed for patients with kidney impairment, withdraw appropriate volume of solution and label with final drug content and final volume. Refer to manufacturer's instructions.

▼ If drug isn't used immediately after reconstitution, refrigerate solution and give within 24 hours.

▼ If refrigerated, allow refrigerated solution to reach room temperature before administration.

▼ Infuse over no less than 15 minutes at a constant infusion rate to adequately hydrated patient. Give as single IV solution through separate infusion line.

▼ Flush IV line with 10 mL NSS after infusion.

▼ After opening, solution remains stable for 24 hours at 36° to 46° F (2° to 8° C).

▼ May store vials, bags, and bottles at room temperature.

▼ **Incompatibilities:** Solutions containing calcium (such as lactated Ringer solution) and other IV drugs.

ACTION

Inhibits bone resorption, probably by inhibiting osteoclast activity and osteoclastic resorption of mineralized bone and cartilage. Decreases calcium release induced by the stimulatory factors produced by tumors.

Route	Onset	Peak	Duration
IV	Unknown	Unknown	Unknown

Half-life: Triphasic with terminal half-life, 146 hours.

ADVERSE REACTIONS

CNS: headache, anxiety, somnolence, insomnia, confusion, agitation, depression, paresthesia, hypoesthesia, fatigue, weakness, dizziness, fever, asthenia, malaise, vertigo, lethargy. **CV:** hypotension, HTN, atrial fibrillation, palpitations, leg edema, chest pain. **EENT:** eye pain, sore throat. **GI:** nausea, constipation, diarrhea, abdominal pain, vomiting, anorexia, dysphagia, decreased appetite, dyspepsia, abdominal distention, stomatitis. **GU:** increased creatinine level, UTI. **Hematologic:** anemia, *granulocytopenia, neutropenia, thrombocytopenia, pancytopenia.* **Metabolic:** dehydration, weight decrease, hypophosphatemia, hypocalcemia, *hypokalemia, hypomagnesemia.* **Musculoskeletal:** arthralgia, myalgia, back pain, osteonecrosis of the jaw, osteoarthritis, muscle spasms, bone pain, neck pain, shoulder pain, extremity pain. **Respiratory:** dyspnea, cough. **Skin:** alopecia, dermatitis, rash, pruritus, hyperhidrosis. **Other:** *progression of cancer,* rigors, infection, candidiasis, flulike symptoms.

INTERACTIONS

Drug-drug. *Aminoglycosides, calcitonin, loop diuretics:* May have additive effects that lower calcium level. Use together cautiously, and monitor calcium level.

Kidney-toxic drugs, such as NSAIDs: May increase risk of kidney toxicity. Monitor serum creatinine level before each dose.

EFFECTS ON LAB TEST RESULTS
- May increase creatinine level.
- May decrease calcium, phosphorus, magnesium, and potassium levels.
- May decrease Hb level and hematocrit and RBC, WBC, and platelet counts.

CONTRAINDICATIONS & CAUTIONS
- Contraindicated in patients hypersensitive to drug, other bisphosphonates, or drug's ingredients. Reclast (5-mg dose) is contraindicated in patients with hypocalcemia, CrCl of less than 35 mL/minute, or evidence of AKI. Use of 4-mg dose in patients with severe kidney impairment isn't recommended.
- 🜂 **Alert:** Reclast may increase risk of KF, especially in patients with underlying kidney impairment, dehydration, and advanced age. Screen patients before use and monitor them carefully.
- 🜂 **Alert:** Patients treated with bisphosphonates may be at increased risk for fractures of the thigh.
- Patients must be adequately supplemented with calcium and vitamin D.
- Use cautiously in older adults and patients with aspirin-sensitive asthma because other bisphosphonates have been linked to bronchoconstriction in aspirin-sensitive patients with asthma.
- Optimal duration of use for osteoporosis hasn't been determined. Consider patients at low risk for fracture for drug discontinuation after 3 to 5 years of use, and periodically reevaluate their fracture risk.
- Osteonecrosis of neck and jaw has been reported with bisphosphonate use. Risk increases with duration of exposure. Patients should receive preventive dental exams before starting therapy and avoid invasive dental procedures.
- *Dialyzable drug:* Unknown.
- ⚠ **Overdose S&S:** Hypocalcemia, hypophosphatemia, hypomagnesemia, kidney impairment.

PREGNANCY-LACTATION-REPRODUCTION
- Drug shouldn't be used during pregnancy. Patients should avoid pregnancy during therapy. Discontinue drug when pregnancy is recognized.
- Drug may cause fetal harm if used during pregnancy or if patient becomes pregnant after completing therapy because drug binds to bone long term and may be released over weeks to years. Inform patient of potential fetal hazard.
- It isn't known if drug appears in human milk. Patient should discontinue breastfeeding or discontinue drug, considering importance of drug to patient.

NURSING CONSIDERATIONS
- Adequately hydrate patient before giving drug; urine output should be about 2 L daily.
- Carefully monitor calcium, phosphate, magnesium, and creatinine levels. Monitor creatinine level before each dose. Correct decreased calcium, phosphorus, and magnesium levels using IV calcium gluconate, potassium and sodium phosphate, and magnesium sulfate.
- Closely monitor kidney function. Patients with kidney impairment may be at a greater risk for adverse reactions.
- Patients, especially those who have cancer or poor oral hygiene or are receiving chemotherapy or corticosteroids, should have dental exams with appropriate preventive dentistry before therapy and avoid invasive dental procedures.
- Osteonecrosis of the jaw has been reported rarely in patients after menopause who have osteoporosis treated with bisphosphonates, including zoledronic acid. All patients should have routine oral exams before treatment and should be monitored during therapy.
- Severe incapacitating bone, joint, and muscle pain may occur. Withhold future doses if severe symptoms occur. Symptoms may resolve partially or completely with drug stoppage.
- Adequately supplement patients with calcium and vitamin D.
- Administration of acetaminophen after administration may reduce the incidence of acute-phase reaction symptoms.

PATIENT TEACHING
- Teach about proper drug administration and handling.
- Instruct patient to promptly report adverse effects (fever, flulike symptoms, myalgia, arthralgia, headache, muscle cramps, numbness, tingling, difficulty swallowing, palpitations, jaw pain, thigh and bone pain, edema).
- Explain the importance of periodic lab tests to monitor therapy and kidney function.

Z

• On day of treatment, instruct patient to drink at least two glasses of fluid, such as water, within a few hours before infusion. Advise patient of importance of calcium and vitamin D supplementation.

• Advise patient to report persistent pain or nonhealing sore of the mouth or jaw and to maintain good oral hygiene and receive routine dental checkups.

• Advise patient to consult prescriber before becoming pregnant or breastfeeding.

ZOLMitriptan
zohl-mah-TRIP-tan

Zomig

Therapeutic class: Antimigraine drugs
Pharmacologic class: Serotonin 5-HT₁ receptor agonists

AVAILABLE FORMS
Nasal spray: 2.5 mg, 5 mg
Tablets (immediate-release): 2.5 mg, 5 mg
Tablets (ODTs) ᴼᵀᶜ: 2.5 mg, 5 mg

INDICATIONS & DOSAGES
➤ **Acute migraine headaches**
Adults: Initially, 1.25 or 2.5 mg. Increase to 5 mg per dose, as needed. If using ODTs, initially, 2.5 mg PO. If headache returns after first dose, give second dose no sooner than 2 hours after first dose. Maximum dosage, 10 mg in 24 hours.
Adjust-a-dose: In patients with Child-Pugh class B or C liver impairment, give 1.25 mg. Limit total daily dose in patients with Child-Pugh class C liver impairment to no more than 5 mg/day. In patients taking cimetidine, limit maximum single dose to 2.5 mg, not to exceed 5 mg in any 24-hour period.
Adults and children ages 12 and older: Initially, 1 spray (2.5 mg) into nostril; may increase to maximum 5-mg single dose if needed. If headache returns after first dose, give second dose no sooner than 2 hours after first dose. Maximum dosage, 10 mg in 24 hours.
Adjust-a-dose: Nasal spray isn't recommended in patients with Child-Pugh class B or C liver impairment. In patients taking cimetidine, limit maximum single dose to 2.5 mg, not to exceed 5 mg in any 24-hour period.

ADMINISTRATION
PO
• If patient needs a 1.25-mg dose, break a 2.5-mg immediate-release tablet in half.
• Give ODT immediately after opening.
• Don't break or crush ODT.
• Have patient dissolve ODT on the tongue and swallow with saliva, not fluid.
Intranasal
• Patient should gently blow nose before use.
• Remove cap and insert device into nostril while blocking the opposite nostril.
• Press plunger device while patient gently breathes in through the nose. Patient should then breathe gently through the mouth for 5 to 10 seconds.
• Don't test or prime spray before use; nasal sprayer contains only one dose.
• Discard after use.

ACTION
May act as an agonist at serotonin receptors on extracerebral intracranial blood vessels, which constricts affected vessels, inhibits neuropeptide release, and reduces pain transmission in the trigeminal pathways.

Route	Onset	Peak	Duration
PO	Unknown	1.5–3 hr	Unknown
Intranasal	5 min	3 hr	Unknown

Half-life: 3 hours.

ADVERSE REACTIONS
CNS: dizziness, somnolence, vertigo, paresthesia, asthenia, pain, drowsiness, depersonalization, headache, dysgeusia, hyperesthesia, warm or cold sensations. **CV:** palpitations; chest pain, pressure, tightness, or heaviness; facial edema. **EENT:** pain, tightness, or pressure in the neck, throat, or jaw; nasal irritation; dry mouth. **GI:** dyspepsia, dysphagia, nausea, abdominal pain, vomiting. **Musculoskeletal:** arthralgia, myalgia. **Skin:** diaphoresis. **Other:** chills, hypersensitivity reaction.

INTERACTIONS
Drug-drug. *Cimetidine:* May double half-life of zolmitriptan. Limit maximum single dose of zolmitriptan to 2.5 mg, not to exceed 5 mg in any 24-hour period. Monitor patient closely.
Ergot-containing drugs, other triptans: May exacerbate headaches and increase

---

vasoconstricting effects. Avoid using within 24 hours of zolmitriptan.

MAO inhibitors: May increase zolmitriptan level. Avoid using within 2 weeks of MAO inhibitor.

Methylene blue: May enhance serotonergic effect and result in serotonin syndrome. Avoid use together.

SSRIs, tramadol: May cause additive serotonin effects, resulting in weakness, hyperreflexia, or incoordination. Monitor patient closely.

EFFECTS ON LAB TEST RESULTS
None reported.

CONTRAINDICATIONS & CAUTIONS
• Contraindicated in patients hypersensitive to drug or its components and in patients with uncontrolled HTN, hemiplegic or basilar migraine, stroke history, TIA history, PVD, ischemic bowel disease, Wolff-Parkinson-White syndrome or arrhythmias associated with other cardiac accessory conduction pathway disorders, ischemic heart disease (angina pectoris, history of MI or documented silent ischemia), symptoms of ischemic heart disease (coronary artery vasospasm, including Prinzmetal variant angina), or other significant heart disease.
• 5-HT₁ agonists may increase risk of serious cardiac, cerebrovascular, and other vasospastic adverse events (arrhythmias, MI, cerebral hemorrhage, subarachnoid hemorrhage, stroke, GI ischemia, splenic infarct).
• Use cautiously in patients with liver disease and in those with risk factors for CAD (those with HTN, obesity, diabetes, hypercholesterolemia, smoking, or family history; patients who are postmenopausal; and males older than age 40).
• Partial vision loss and blindness, both transient and permanent, have been reported with use of 5-HT₁ agonists.
Dialyzable drug: Unknown.
⚠ *Overdose S&S:* Sedation.

PREGNANCY-LACTATION-REPRODUCTION
• Drug has caused fetal harm in animal studies, but human studies during pregnancy are inadequate. Use only if clearly needed and potential benefit justifies fetal risk.
• Drug appears in human milk. Use cautiously during breastfeeding. Withholding

breastfeeding for 24 hours after ingestion minimizes infant exposure.

NURSING CONSIDERATIONS
• Drug isn't indicated to prevent migraines or treat hemiplegic or basilar migraines.
• Safety of drug hasn't been established for cluster headaches or for treatment of an average of more than three headaches (oral formulation) or four headaches (intranasal formulation) in a 30-day period.
• Perform CV exam in patient who is triptan-naive and has multiple CV risk factors (increased age, diabetes, HTN, smoking, obesity, strong family history of CAD). Consider initiating therapy in a medically supervised setting with ECG monitoring. Patient with negative CV exam should have periodic exams during therapy.
• Discontinue drug if arrhythmias occur.
• Monitor for medication overuse headaches. Patients taking ergotamine, triptans, opioids, or a combination of drugs for 10 or more days a month may experience exacerbation of headaches and require detoxification, including withdrawal of overused drugs and treatment of withdrawal symptoms.
⊙ *Alert:* Combining drug with an SSRI or an SSNRI may cause serotonin syndrome. Signs and symptoms include restlessness, hallucinations, loss of coordination, fast heartbeat, rapid changes in BP, increased body temperature, overactive reflexes, nausea, vomiting, and diarrhea. Serotonin syndrome may be more likely to occur when starting or increasing the dose of drug, SSRI, or SSNRI.
• Zomig ODT tablets contain phenylalanine, which can be harmful to patients with phenylketonuria.
• *Look alike–sound alike:* Don't confuse zolmitriptan with rizatriptan, sumatriptan, or zolpidem. Don't confuse Zomig with Zoloft or Zonegran.

PATIENT TEACHING
• Tell patient that drug is intended to relieve, not prevent, signs and symptoms of migraine; it isn't used to treat other types of headaches; and misuse of drug to treat more than 10 headaches per month may lead to worsening of headaches.
• Teach about proper drug administration and handling. Stress that patient should take drug as prescribed.

Z

• Caution patient to immediately report pain or tightness in chest or throat, heart throbbing, shortness of breath, slurred speech, rash, skin lumps, or swelling of face, lips, or eyelids.

• Advise patient to report pregnancy or plans to become pregnant or breastfeed during therapy.

• Warn that serotonin syndrome may occur if drug is used with other drugs that increase serotonin level (SSRIs, SSNRIs).

SAFETY ALERT!

zolpidem tartrate ☒
ZOL-pih-dem

Ambien, Ambien CR, Edluar, Sublinox✦

Therapeutic class: Hypnotics
Pharmacologic class: Imidazopyridines
Controlled substance schedule: IV

AVAILABLE FORMS
Capsules: 7.5 mg
Tablets: 5 mg, 10 mg
Tablets (extended-release) ⓞ: 6.25 mg, 12.5 mg
Tablets (ODTs) ⓞ: 1.75 mg, 3.5 mg, 5 mg, 10 mg

INDICATIONS & DOSAGES
➤ **Short-term management of insomnia**
Adults: 5 or 10 mg (males) or 5 mg (females) immediate-release or 6.25 or 12.5 mg (men) or 6.25 mg (women) extended-release PO immediately before bedtime. Or, 5 or 10 mg (males) or 5 mg (females) SL once per night immediately before bedtime. At time of dose, at least 7 to 8 hours should remain before planned time of awakening. May increase to 10 mg as needed.
Adjust-a-dose: For older adults, patients who are debilitated, and patients with Child-Pugh class A or B liver insufficiency, 5 mg PO or SL immediately before bedtime. Or, 6.25 mg of extended-release form. Maximum daily dosage, 10 mg immediate-release and 12.5 mg extended-release.
➤ **Sleep maintenance in insomnia (SL tablets)**
Adults: 3.5 mg (males) or 1.75 mg (females) SL once per night as needed for middle-of-the-night awakening with at least

4 hours of bedtime remaining before planned waking.
Adjust-a-dose: For older adults, patients with liver impairment, or patients taking concomitant CNS depressant, 1.75 mg SL is recommended.

ADMINISTRATION
PO
• For rapid sleep onset, don't allow patient to take drug with or immediately after meals.

• Have patient swallow extended-release tablets whole; don't crush or break.

• Place SL tablet under tongue to disintegrate. Don't allow patient to swallow tablet whole or take with water.

• Capsules are only available in 7.5 mg strength. Use another immediate-release product for 5- or 10-mg dose.

ACTION
Although drug interacts with one of three identified GABA-benzodiazepine receptor complexes, it isn't a benzodiazepine. It exhibits hypnotic activity and minimal muscle relaxant and anticonvulsant properties.

Route	Onset	Peak	Duration
PO	30 min	30–120 min	6–8 hr

Half-life: 1.5 to 8.5 hours.

ADVERSE REACTIONS
CNS: headache, amnesia, abnormal dreams, balance disorder, asthenia, attention disturbance, anxiety, fever, hallucinations, disorientation, feeling intoxicated, ataxia, drowsiness, depression, dizziness, hypoesthesia, vertigo, confusion, disinhibition, lethargy, light-headedness, nervousness, sleep disorder, euphoria, mood swings, memory disorder, paresthesia. **CV:** palpitations, chest pain. **EENT:** diplopia, eye redness, abnormal vision, eye symptoms, tinnitus, pharyngitis, sinusitis, dry mouth, labyrinthitis, throat irritation. **GI:** abdominal pain, abdominal distress, abdominal tenderness, change in appetite, gastroenteritis, GERD, vomiting, diarrhea, constipation, hiccups, dyspepsia, nausea. **GU:** dysuria, UTI, menstrual disorder. **Musculoskeletal:** arthralgia, myalgia, back pain. **Respiratory:** respiratory tract infection, bronchitis, cough, dyspnea. **Skin:** rash, urticaria, bruising. **Other:** flulike syndrome, hypersensitivity reactions.

INTERACTIONS

Drug-drug. *Chlorpromazine, imipramine:* May cause additive effect of decreased alertness. Monitor patient closely.

CNS depressants (benzodiazepines, TCAs): May cause excessive CNS depression. Use together cautiously.

CYP3A4 inducers (rifampin): May decrease effects of zolpidem. Avoid use together.

CYP3A4 inhibitors (ketoconazole, verapamil): May increase zolpidem level. Use low zolpidem dosage and monitor therapy.

❸ *Alert: Opioids:* May cause slow or difficult breathing, sedation, and death. Avoid use together. If use together is necessary, limit dosage and duration of each drug to minimum necessary for desired effect.

Sertraline: May increase zolpidem level. Use together cautiously.

Drug-herb. *Calendula, chamomile, gotu kola, kava, valerian:* May increase risk of CNS depression. Discourage use together.

St. John's wort: May decrease zolpidem level and effects. Discourage use together.

Drug-food. *Grapefruit, grapefruit juice:* May decrease zolpidem metabolism. Discourage use together.

Drug-lifestyle. *Alcohol use:* May cause excessive CNS depression. Discourage use together.

EFFECTS ON LAB TEST RESULTS

• May increase ALT, AST, and bilirubin levels.

• May decrease radioactive iodine uptake.

CONTRAINDICATIONS & CAUTIONS

• Contraindicated in patients hypersensitive to drug or its components.

Boxed Warning Drug may cause rare but serious injury, including death, due to complex sleep behaviors, such as sleepwalking, sleep driving, and engaging in other activities while not fully awake. These behaviors can occur even at the lowest recommended dosages and after just one dose. Drug is contraindicated in patients who have experienced complex sleep behaviors after taking the drug in past. ■

• Avoid use in patients with Child-Pugh class C liver impairment because it may contribute to encephalopathy.

• Use cautiously in patients with compromised respiratory status, Child-Pugh class A or B liver impairment, myasthenia gravis, or history of depression or worsening depression.

❸ *Alert:* Drug level may remain elevated the day after drug use, impairing mental alertness. Risk increases if patient sleeps for less than 7 hours; takes drug with other CNS depressants, including alcohol; or takes higher-than-recommended dosage.

❸ *Alert:* Patients taking extended-release formulation shouldn't drive or engage in other activities that require complete mental alertness the day after taking drug because drug level can remain high enough to impair these activities.

❸ *Alert:* Drug can cause drowsiness and decreased level of consciousness, which may lead to falls and severe injuries, such as hip fractures and intracranial hemorrhage.

• Abnormal thinking and behavior changes have been reported in patients treated with zolpidem. Some of these changes included decreased inhibition (aggressiveness and extroversion that seemed out of character), bizarre behavior, agitation, and depersonalization. Visual and auditory hallucinations have been reported. Immediately evaluate signs or symptoms of new behaviors.

▧ Females have a lower zolpidem clearance than men; therefore, lower initial doses are recommended.

Dialyzable drug: No.

⚠ *Overdose S&S:* Impaired consciousness, somnolence, coma, CV or respiratory compromise, death.

PREGNANCY-LACTATION-REPRODUCTION

• Drug crosses placental barrier. Use during pregnancy only if potential benefit outweighs fetal risk.

• Monitor neonates exposed to zolpidem during pregnancy and labor for excess sedation, hypotonia, and respiratory depression; manage accordingly.

• Drug appears in human milk. Use cautiously during breastfeeding.

• Monitor infants exposed to zolpidem through human milk for excess sedation, hypotonia, and respiratory depression. Patient may consider expressing and discarding milk during treatment and for 23 hours after zolpidem administration to minimize infant's drug exposure.

NURSING CONSIDERATIONS

🟢 *Alert:* Anaphylaxis and angioedema may occur as early as the first dose. Monitor patient closely. Discontinue drug and don't restart if these effects occur.

• Use drug only for short-term management of insomnia, usually 7 to 10 days. Reevaluate patient if insomnia persists.

• Use smallest effective dose for each patient.

• Take precautions to prevent hoarding by patient who is depressed, suicidal, or drug-dependent or has history of drug abuse.

• Monitor patient for withdrawal signs and symptoms after rapid dosage reduction or abrupt drug discontinuation.

• *Look alike–sound alike:* Don't confuse zolpidem with lorazepam, zaleplon, or zolmitriptan. Don't confuse Ambien with Abilify or Ativan.

PATIENT TEACHING

Boxed Warning Warn patient of risk of injury or death related to complex sleep behaviors. Direct patient to immediately stop drug and report complex sleep behavior or inability to remember activities performed while taking drug. ■

• Teach about proper drug administration and handling for prescribed formulation.

• Instruct patient to take drug immediately before going to bed. Caution that onset of action is rapid. For rapid sleep onset, instruct patient not to take drug with or immediately after meals.

🟢 *Alert:* Warn that drug may cause allergic reactions, facial swelling, and respiratory depression. Advise patient to immediately report these adverse effects.

🟢 *Alert:* Tell patient that drug has the potential to cause next-day impairment and that this risk increases if patient doesn't carefully follow dosing instructions. Tell patient to wait for at least 8 hours after dosing before driving or engaging in other activities requiring full mental alertness. Inform patient that impairment can be present even if patient feels fully awake.

🟢 *Alert:* Tell patient that drug can cause drowsiness and decreased level of consciousness, which may lead to falls and severe injuries.

• Tell patient to avoid alcohol use while taking drug.

• Caution patient to avoid performing activities that require mental alertness or physical coordination during therapy.

zonisamide
zoh-NISS-a-mide

Zonegran, Zonisade

Therapeutic class: Anticonvulsants
Pharmacologic class: Sulfonamides

AVAILABLE FORMS
Capsules 🔴: 25 mg, 50 mg, 100 mg
Oral suspension: 100 mg/5 mL

INDICATIONS & DOSAGES
➤ **Adjunctive therapy for partial seizures in patients with epilepsy**
Adults and children older than age 16: Initially, 100 mg PO daily for 2 weeks. May increase dosage by 100 mg PO daily, with dose stable for at least 2 weeks to achieve steady state at each level. Maximum recommended dosage, 600 mg daily; however, no evidence of increased response with doses above 400 mg/day.
Adjust-a-dose: For patients with kidney or liver impairment, titrate dosages more slowly and monitor more frequently.

ADMINISTRATION
PO
🟢 *Alert:* Hazardous drug; use safe-handling and disposal precautions.

• Give drug without regard to food.

• Have patient swallow capsules whole; don't crush or open capsules.

• May give solution once or twice daily.

• Shake solution well before giving.

• Measure and give solution using an accurate measuring device.

• Discard unused solution 30 days after opening bottle.

ACTION
May stabilize neuronal membranes and suppress neuronal hypersynchronization at sodium and calcium channels, which prevents seizures.

Route	Onset	Peak	Duration
PO (capsules)	Unknown	2–6 hr	Unknown
PO (solution)	Unknown	0.5–5 hr	Unknown

Half-life: 63 hours.

ADVERSE REACTIONS

CNS: dizziness, headache, somnolence, *status epilepticus,* abnormal gait, agitation or irritability, anxiety, asthenia, ataxia, confusion, depression, difficulties in concentration or memory, difficulties in verbal expression, fatigue, hyperesthesia, incoordination, insomnia, mental slowing, nervousness, paresthesia, schizophrenic or schizophreniform behavior, speech disorders, tremors, taste perversion. **EENT:** amblyopia, diplopia, nystagmus, tinnitus, pharyngitis, rhinitis, dry mouth. **GI:** anorexia, abdominal pain, constipation, diarrhea, dyspepsia, nausea, vomiting. **GU:** kidney stones. **Metabolic:** weight loss. **Respiratory:** cough. **Skin:** pruritus, rash, ecchymosis. **Other:** accidental injury, flulike syndrome.

INTERACTIONS

Drug-drug. *Other carbonic anhydrase inhibitors (acetazolamide, dichlorphenamide, topiramate):* May increase severity of metabolic acidosis and increase risk of kidney stone formation. Monitor patient for development or worsening of metabolic acidosis. *Other CNS depressants:* May cause CNS depression and other cognitive or neuropsychiatric adverse events. Use together cautiously. *Strong CYP3A4 inducers (carbamazepine, phenobarbital, phenytoin, valproate):* May decrease zonisamide level. Monitor patient closely.
Drug-herb. *Kava:* May enhance adverse or toxic effects of zonisamide. Monitor therapy.
Drug-lifestyle. *Alcohol use:* May cause CNS depression and other cognitive or neuropsychiatric adverse events. Discourage use together.

EFFECTS ON LAB TEST RESULTS

- May increase chloride, ALP, BUN, and creatinine levels.
- May decrease serum bicarbonate, phosphorus, calcium, and albumin levels.

CONTRAINDICATIONS & CAUTIONS

- Contraindicated in patients hypersensitive to drug or other sulfonamides.
- Use cautiously in patients with kidney or liver impairment or kidney stones. Avoid use in patients with eGFR less than 50 mL/minute.
- Use cautiously in patients with history of psychiatric symptoms.

- Use cautiously with other drugs that predispose patients to heat-related disorders, including but not limited to carbonic anhydrase inhibitors and drugs with anticholinergic activity.
- Drug may increase risk of SCARs.
- Safety and effectiveness in children younger than age 16 haven't been established; children are at increased risk for oligohidrosis and hyperthermia.
Dialyzable drug: Yes.
⚠ *Overdose S&S:* CNS symptoms, coma, bradycardia, hypotension, respiratory depression.

PREGNANCY-LACTATION-REPRODUCTION

- Drug may cause fetal harm. Use during pregnancy only if potential benefit justifies fetal risk.
- Patients of childbearing potential should use effective contraception during therapy and for 1 month after final dose.
- Monitor neonates of patients treated with zonisamide during pregnancy for metabolic acidosis; transient metabolic acidosis may occur after birth.
- Encourage patients taking drug during pregnancy to enroll in the North American Antiepileptic Drug Pregnancy Registry (1-888-233-2334 or www.aedpregnancyregistry.org).
- Drug appears in human milk. Patient should discontinue breastfeeding or discontinue drug, considering importance of drug to patient.

NURSING CONSIDERATIONS

🕙 *Alert:* Monitor patient for signs and symptoms of hypersensitivity.
🕙 *Alert:* Rarely, patients receiving sulfonamides have died because of severe reactions, such as SJS, fulminant liver necrosis, aplastic anemia, otherwise unexplained rashes, and agranulocytosis. If signs and symptoms of hypersensitivity or other serious reactions occur, immediately stop drug and notify prescriber.
🕙 *Alert:* Closely monitor all patients taking or starting AEDs for changes in behavior indicating worsening suicidality or depression. Symptoms such as anxiety, agitation, hostility, mania, and hypomania may be precursors to emerging suicidality.
- If patient develops AKI or a significant sustained increase in creatinine or BUN level, stop drug and notify prescriber. Periodically monitor kidney function.

• Drug can cause metabolic acidosis, especially in patients with predisposing conditions or therapies. The risk is more common and severe in younger patients. Measure serum bicarbonate level before starting treatment and periodically during treatment, even in the absence of symptoms.

• Reduce dosage or stop drug gradually because abrupt discontinuation may increase seizures or cause status epilepticus.

• Increase fluid intake and urine output to help prevent kidney stones, especially in patient with predisposing factors.

• Monitor patient for cognitive and neuropsychiatric adverse reactions, including psychomotor slowing, difficulty with concentration, speech or language problems (especially word-finding difficulties), somnolence or fatigue, depression, and psychosis.

PATIENT TEACHING

• Teach about proper drug administration and handling.

• Advise patient to immediately call prescriber if rash develops or seizures worsen.

🔋 *Alert:* Warn patient and family that drug increases risk of suicidality. Instruct them to watch for and immediately report to prescriber new or worsening symptoms of depression, unusual changes in mood or behavior, or emergence of suicidality.

• Tell patient to immediately report sudden back or abdominal pain, pain when urinating, bloody or dark urine, fever, sore throat, mouth sores or easy bruising, decreased sweating, fever, depression, or speech or language problems.

• Advise patient to avoid dehydration and to maintain adequate fluid intake.

• Warn that drug can cause drowsiness. Caution patient not to drive or operate dangerous machinery until drug's effects are known.

• Advise patient not to stop taking drug without prescriber's approval because abrupt withdrawal can cause seizures.

• Advise patient to report pregnancy or plans to become pregnant or breastfeed during therapy. Instruct patient of childbearing potential to use contraception during therapy.

Reactions in bold italics are *life-threatening*.

adagrasib
a-DA-gra-sib

Krazati

Therapeutic class: Antineoplastics
Pharmacologic class: KRAS inhibitors

AVAILABLE FORMS
Tablets ⬤*:* 200 mg

INDICATIONS & DOSAGES
➤ **KRAS G12C-mutated locally advanced or metastatic NSCLC in patients who have received at least one prior systemic therapy**
Adults: 600 mg P.O. b.i.d. until disease progresses or unacceptable toxicity occurs.
Adjust-a-dose: Refer to manufacturer's instructions for toxicity-related dosage adjustments. First dosage reduction for adverse reactions is 400 mg P.O. b.i.d.; second dosage reduction is 600 mg P.O. daily. Permanently discontinue drug if patient can't tolerate 600 mg/day.

ADMINISTRATION
PO
- Give at same time each day without regard to food.
- Have patient swallow tablets whole; don't crush or cut tablets.
- If patient vomits after taking dose, give additional dose and then resume regular dosing at next scheduled time.
- If a dose is missed by more than 4 hours, skip missed dose and give next dose at its scheduled time.
- Don't remove desiccant from container.
- Store tablets at room temperature (68° to 77° F [20° to 25° C]).

ACTION
Irreversibly inhibits KRAS protein, which inhibits tumor cell growth and results in tumor regression.

Route	Onset	Peak	Duration
PO	Unknown	6 hr	Unknown

Half-life: 23 hours.

ADVERSE REACTIONS
CNS: dizziness, fatigue, fever, mental status changes. **CV:** edema, *HF,* hypotension, *PE, prolonged QT interval.* **GI:** abdominal pain, constipation, decreased appetite, diarrhea, *GI bleeding,* GI obstruction, nausea, vomiting. **GU:** kidney impairment. **Hematologic:** anemia, *leukopenia, lymphopenia, neutropenia, thrombocytopenia.* **Hepatic:** decreased albumin, *liver toxicity,* increased liver enzymes. **Metabolic:** decreased weight, dehydration, *hypokalemia, hypomagnesemia,* hyponatremia, increased amylase, increased lipase.

Musculoskeletal: muscular weakness, musculoskeletal pain. **Respiratory:** cough, dyspnea, *hypoxia,* ILD, interstitial pneumonitis, pleural effusion, pneumonia, *pulmonary hemorrhage, respiratory failure.* **Other:** *sepsis, sudden death.*

INTERACTIONS
Drug-drug. *Drugs that prolong QT interval (amiodarone, fluoxetine, haloperidol, levofloxacin, methadone):* May prolong the QT interval. Avoid use together.
Sensitive CYP2C9 or CYP2D6 substrates or P-gp substrates (digoxin, dextromethorphan, warfarin): May increase substrate level. Avoid use together when minimal concentration changes may lead to serious adverse reactions.
Sensitive CYP3A4 substrates (midazolam): May increase substrate level. Avoid use together.
Strong CYP3A4 inducers (rifampin): May reduce adagrasib level. Avoid use together.
Strong CYP3A4 inhibitors (itraconazole): May increase adagrasib level. Avoid concomitant use until adagrasib level has reached steady state (after approximately 8 days).
Drug-herb. *St. John's wort:* May reduce adagrasib level. Discourage use together.

EFFECTS ON LAB TEST RESULTS
- May decrease sodium, magnesium, potassium, albumin, and Hb levels.
- May increase AST, ALT, creatinine, lipase, and amylase levels.
- May decrease lymphocyte, leukocyte, neutrophil, and platelet counts.

CONTRAINDICATIONS & CAUTIONS
- Drug may increase risk of prolonged QTc interval, tachyarrhythmias, torsades de pointes, and sudden death. Avoid use in patients with congenital QT syndrome.
- Use cautiously in patients with HF, bradyarrhythmias, or electrolyte abnormalities and patients unable to avoid taking medication known to prolong QT interval.
- Safety and effectiveness in children haven't been established.
Dializable drug: Unlikely.

PREGNANCY-LACTATION-REPRODUCTION
- Studies during pregnancy are inadequate.
- It isn't known if drug appears in human milk or how drug affects milk production or infants who are breastfed. Due to potential for adverse reactions in infant who is breastfed, patient shouldn't breastfeed during therapy and for 1 week after final dose.
- Drug may impair fertility.

NURSING CONSIDERATIONS
- Monitor for development or worsening of GI adverse reactions (nausea, diarrhea, vomiting, GI bleeding, GI obstruction, ileus). Provide supportive

NEW DRUGS

 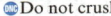

care as needed. Withhold, reduce dose, or permanently discontinue drug based on severity.
• Obtain ECGs and electrolyte levels at baseline, periodically during therapy, and as clinically indicated in patient at risk for prolonged QT interval.
• Obtain AST, ALT, ALP, and total bilirubin levels at baseline, monthly for 3 months, and as clinically indicated. Monitor more frequently if patient develops increased transaminase levels. Withhold, reduce dose, or permanently discontinue drug based on severity.
• Monitor for development of signs and symptoms of ILD or pneumonitis (dyspnea, cough, fever). Withhold drug if ILD or pneumonitis is suspected and permanently discontinue drug if no other cause is identified.
• *Look alike–sound alike:* Don't confuse adagrasib with afatinib, axitinib, or sotorasib.

PATIENT TEACHING
• Teach about proper drug administration and handling.
• Warn that drug can cause severe GI adverse reactions. Instruct patient to report severe or persistent signs and symptoms.
• Warn that drug can cause prolonged QTc interval. Instruct patient to report signs and symptoms of arrhythmias.
• Inform patient about risk of liver toxicity. Explain that blood levels will be monitored during therapy.
• Caution patient to immediately report signs and symptoms of liver dysfunction (stomach pain, nausea, vomiting, fatigue, dark-colored urine, light-colored bowel movements, jaundice [yellow skin or eyes], loss of appetite, fever).
• Inform patient of risk of ILD and pneumonitis. Instruct patient to immediately report new or worsening respiratory symptoms.
• Tell patient not to breastfeed during therapy and for 1 week after final dose.
• Inform patient that drug may cause infertility.

bexagliflozin
bex-a-gli-FLOE-zin

Brenzavvy

Therapeutic class: Antidiabetics
Pharmacologic class: Sodium-glucose co-transporter 2 (SGLT2) inhibitors

AVAILABLE FORMS
Tablets: 20 mg

INDICATIONS & DOSAGES
➤ **Adjunct to diet and exercise to improve glycemic control in patients with type 2 diabetes**
Adults: 20 mg PO once daily in the morning.

ADMINISTRATION
PO
• Give drug without regard to food.
• Have patient swallow tablets whole; don't crush or cut tablets.
• Give a missed dose as soon as possible. Don't double the next dose.
• Store at room temperature.

ACTION
Reduces renal reabsorption of filtered glucose, lowers the renal threshold for glucose, and increases urinary glucose excretion.

Route	Onset	Peak	Duration
PO	Unknown	2 to 4 hr	Unknown

Half-life: 12 hours.

ADVERSE REACTIONS
GI: thirst. **GU:** decreased eGFR, genital mycotic infection, increased creatinine level, increased urination, UTI, vaginal pruritus. **Metabolic:** *hypoglycemia,* volume depletion. **Musculoskeletal:** lower limb amputation. **Skin:** rash. **Other:** *sepsis.*

INTERACTIONS
Drug-drug. *Insulin and insulin secretagogues (glimepiride, glyburide, sulfonylurea agents):* Increases risk of hypoglycemia. When used together, decrease insulin or insulin secretagogue dose as needed.
Lithium: May decrease lithium level. Monitor lithium level more frequently upon initiation and discontinuation of bexagliflozin.
Uridine glucuronosyltransferase enzyme inducers (phenobarbital, rifampicin): May decrease bexagliflozin level and its efficacy. Consider adding another antihyperglycemic agent, if necessary.

EFFECTS ON LAB TEST RESULTS
• May increase Hb, creatinine, and LDL-C levels and hematocrit.
• May decrease eGFR.
• Causes positive urine glucose test results.
• May cause unreliable 1,5-AG assay results.

CONTRAINDICATIONS & CAUTIONS
• Contraindicated in patients hypersensitive to drug or its components and in patients on dialysis.
• Drug isn't recommended in patients with eGFR less than 30 mL/minute/1.73 m² or type 1 diabetes.
• Drug hasn't been studied in patients with Child-Pugh class C liver impairment.
• Drug may increase risk of ketoacidosis. Use cautiously in patients with pancreatic insulin deficiency, caloric restriction, or alcohol use disorder.
• Use cautiously in patients with history of amputation, PVD, neuropathy, or diabetic foot ulcers (studies show increased risk of lower limb amputation with another SGLT2 inhibitor).
• Drug may decrease intravascular volume and cause symptomatic hypotension or acute transient

NEW DRUGS

changes in creatinine. Older adults, patients with impaired kidney function (eGFR less than 60 mL/minute/1.73 m²) or low systolic BP, and patients taking loop diuretics may be at increased risk. AKI, sometimes requiring hospitalization and dialysis, has been reported in patients receiving SGLT2 inhibitors.
• Drug may increase risk of UTI, including urosepsis and pyelonephritis.
• Fournier gangrene (rare but serious necrotizing fasciitis of the perineum that requires urgent surgical intervention) has been reported in patients receiving SGLT2 inhibitors.
• Drug may increase risk of genital mycotic infection. Patients who have history of genital mycotic infection or are uncircumcised are at greater risk.
• Safety and effectiveness in children haven't been established.
Dialyzable drug: Unknown.

PREGNANCY-LACTATION-REPRODUCTION
• Based on animal data, use during pregnancy isn't recommended during second and third trimesters.
• It isn't known if drug appears in human milk or how drug affects milk production or infants who are breastfed. Studies indicate that drug is present in animal milk. Patient shouldn't breastfeed during therapy.

NURSING CONSIDERATIONS
• Assess kidney function before starting therapy and periodically thereafter. Patients with kidney impairment may be more likely to experience adverse reactions, including genital mycotic infection, increased urination, thirst, volume depletion, and AKI.
• Correct volume depletion before initiating drug. Monitor patient for signs and symptoms of volume depletion (orthostatic hypotension, dizziness, weakness).
• Monitor blood glucose level.
🔵 *Alert:* Monitoring glycemic control with urine glucose tests isn't recommended. Use an alternative monitoring method.
• Monitor for signs and symptoms of ketoacidosis (dehydration, vomiting, abdominal pain, malaise, shortness of breath). Insulin, fluid, and carbohydrate replacement may be required.
• Monitor patient more closely and consider temporarily withholding drug with prolonged fasting due to acute illness or after surgery.
• Monitor patient for hypersensitivity reactions. Anaphylaxis and angioedema may occur with SGLT2 inhibitors.
• Monitor for signs and symptoms of lower limb infection (including osteomyelitis), new pain or tenderness, sores, and ulcers. Discontinue drug if any occur.
• Monitor for signs and symptoms of UTI and treat promptly.
🔵 *Alert:* Watch for and immediately report signs and symptoms of necrotizing fasciitis of the perineum (temperature above 100.4° F [38° C];

general feeling of unwellness; tenderness, redness, or swelling of area from genitals to anus). Signs and symptoms can quickly worsen. Immediately discontinue drug, closely monitor blood glucose level, and prepare to administer broad-spectrum antibiotics.
• Monitor for signs and symptoms of genital mycotic infection and treat appropriately.
• ***Look alike-sound alike:*** Don't confuse bexagliflozin with bexarotene or other SGLT2 inhibitors.

PATIENT TEACHING
• Teach about proper drug administration and handling.
• Counsel patient to perform routine preventative foot care and to immediately report new pain, tenderness, sores, ulcers, or infections of leg or foot. Warn patient of increased risk of lower limb amputation.
🔵 *Alert:* Instruct patient to stop drug and immediately seek medical attention if signs and symptoms of ketoacidosis (nausea, vomiting, abdominal pain, tiredness, labored breathing) occur.
🔵 *Alert:* Counsel patient to promptly seek medical attention if pain, tenderness, redness or swelling of area from genitals to anus, malaise, or fever above 100.4° F (38° C) develops.
• Explain that urine will test positive for glucose during therapy.
• Advise patient to maintain adequate fluid intake. Explain that symptomatic hypotension may occur due to dehydration. Instruct patient to report symptoms to prescriber.
• Teach about potential for UTI. Instruct patient to report symptoms to prescriber.
• Inform patient that hypoglycemic episodes may increase if drug is taken with insulin or an insulin secretagogue, requiring lower dose of insulin or insulin secretagogue.
• Alert patient to watch for signs and symptoms of yeast infection of vagina (vaginal odor, white or yellow discharge, itching) or penis (rash or redness of glans or foreskin, itching, swelling, foul-smelling discharge, pain). Instruct patient to report these signs or symptoms to prescriber as soon as possible.
• Advise pregnant patient or female of childbearing potential of fetal risk. Tell patient to report pregnancy or plans to become pregnant.
• Instruct patient not to breastfeed during therapy.

daprodustat
dap-roe-DOO-stat

Jesduvroq

Therapeutic class: Hematopoietics
Pharmacologic class: Hypoxia-inducible factor prolyl hydroxylase (HIF PH) inhibitors

AVAILABLE FORMS
Tablets 🔵: 1 mg, 2 mg, 4 mg, 6 mg, 8 mg

NEW DRUGS

INDICATIONS & DOSAGES

➤ **Anemia due to CKD in patients who have been receiving dialysis for at least 4 months**

Adults not being treated with an erythropoiesis-stimulating agent (ESA): If pretreatment Hb level is less than 9 g/dL, 4 mg PO once daily. If pretreatment Hb level is 9 to 10 g/dL, 2 mg PO once daily. If pretreatment Hb level is greater than 10 g/dL, 1 mg PO once daily.

Adults being switched from an ESA: For patients switching from epoetin alfa, darbepoetin alfa, or ethoxy PEG-epoetin beta, refer to manufacturer's instructions for daprodustat dosing instructions based on current ESA drug and dosage.

Adjust-a-dose: Increase or decrease dose by one dose level at a time. Dose levels are 1 mg, 2 mg, 4 mg, 6 mg, 8 mg, 12 mg, 16 mg, and 24 mg. Decrease dose if Hb level rapidly increases by more than 1 g/dL over 2 weeks or 2 g/dL over 4 weeks, or if Hb level exceeds 11 g/dL. Don't increase dose more frequently than every 4 weeks. If Hb level exceeds 12 g/dL, interrupt therapy. Restart at one dose level lower when Hb level drops to target range. Maximum, 24 mg once daily. Reduce daprodustat starting dose by half in patients on clopidogrel or a moderate CYP2C8 inhibitor or with Child-Pugh class B liver impairment, except in patients whose starting dose is already 1 mg. Discontinue therapy if clinically meaningful Hb level increase isn't achieved by 24 weeks.

ADMINISTRATION

PO

• Give without regard to food or concomitant administration of iron or phosphate binders.
• Have patient swallow tablets whole; don't crush or cut tablets.
• Give without regard to timing or type of dialysis.
• Give a missed dose as soon as possible, unless it is the same day as the next dose. In this case, skip missed dose and give next dose at the usual time. Don't double a dose to make-up a missed dose.

ACTION

Reversible inhibitor of HIF-PH1, HIF-PH2, and HIF-PH3 that increases transcription of HIF-responsive genes, including erythropoietin.

Route	Onset	Peak	Duration
PO	6–8 hr	1–4 hr	Unknown

Half-life: 1 to 4 hours.

ADVERSE REACTIONS

CNS: dizziness, *stroke.* **CV:** *HF,* HTN, *thrombotic vascular events (MI, DVT, PE, vascular access thrombosis).* **GI:** abdominal pain, gastric and esophageal erosion. **Other:** hypersensitivity.

INTERACTIONS

Drug-drug. *CYP2C8 inducers (rifampin):* May decrease daprodustat level and efficacy. Monitor Hb level and adjust daprodustat dose when initiating or discontinuing CYP2C8 inducers.

Moderate CYP2C8 inhibitors (clopidogrel): May increase daprodustat level. Reduce daprodustat starting dose when initiating therapy, unless starting dose is already 1 mg. Monitor Hb level and adjust daprodustat dose when initiating or discontinuing CYP2C8 inhibitors.

Strong CYP2C8 inhibitors (gemfibrozil): May increase daprodustat level. Avoid use together.

Drug-lifestyle. *Alcohol use:* May increase risk of gastric or esophageal erosion. Discourage use together.

Tobacco smoking: May increase risk of gastric or esophageal erosion. Discourage use together.

EFFECTS ON LAB TEST RESULTS

• May increase Hb level.

CONTRAINDICATIONS & CAUTIONS

Boxed Warning Daprodustat increases risk of potentially fatal thrombotic vascular events (MI, stroke, VTE, vascular access thrombosis). Patients with CV or cerebrovascular disease are at increased risk for these events. ■

⊙ *Alert:* Avoid use in patients with history of MI, cerebrovascular event, or ACS within 3 months before starting drug. Hb level rise of greater than 1 g/dL over 2 weeks may contribute to these risks.

Boxed Warning Targeting Hb level greater than 11 g/dL is expected to further increase risk of death and arterial and venous thrombotic events, as occurs with ESAs, which also increase erythropoietin level. No trial has identified a Hb target, daprodustat dose, or dosing strategy that doesn't increase these risks. Use lowest dose sufficient to reduce need for RBC transfusion. ■

⊙ *Alert:* Contraindicated in patients with uncontrolled HTN. Hypertensive crisis, including hypertensive encephalopathy and seizures, has been reported.

• Drug indicated for use only in patients on dialysis; others may be at greater risk for CV mortality, stroke, VTE, serious AKI, hospitalization for HF, and serious GI erosion.
• Use in patients with Child-Pugh Class C liver impairment isn't recommended.
• Patients with history of HF are at increased risk for hospitalization for HF.
• Gastric or esophageal erosion, including GI bleeding and need for RBC transfusion, may occur. Use cautiously in patients at increased risk (history of GI erosion or peptic ulcer disease, concomitant use of medications that increase risk of GI erosion, current tobacco smoking, current alcohol use).
• Use isn't recommended in patients with active malignancies. Increased hypoxia-inducible factor levels may be associated with unfavorable effects on cancer growth.
• Drug hasn't been shown to improve quality of life, fatigue, or patient well-being.

• Drug isn't a substitute for transfusion in patients who require immediate correction of anemia.
• Safety and effectiveness in children haven't been established.
• Drug abuse may occur in athletes for the effects on erythropoiesis.
Dialyzable drug: No.
⚠ *Overdose S&S:* GI adverse reactions, headache.

PREGNANCY-LACTATION-REPRODUCTION
• Based on animal studies, drug may cause fetal harm. Advise patients who are pregnant of risk to fetus.
• It isn't known if drug appears in human milk or how drug affects milk production or infants who are breastfed.
• Due to serious adverse drug reactions, patient shouldn't breastfeed during therapy and for 1 week after final dose.

NURSING CONSIDERATIONS
• Before initiating therapy, correct and exclude other causes of anemia (vitamin deficiency, metabolic or chronic inflammatory conditions, bleeding).
• Evaluate iron status before and during therapy. Give supplemental iron when serum ferritin level is less than 100 mcg/mL or transferrin saturation is less than 20%. Most patients require supplemental iron.
• Assess ALT, AST, ALP, and total bilirubin levels at baseline. Repeat if patient develops signs or symptoms of liver disease during therapy.
• After start of therapy and each dose adjustment, monitor Hb level every 2 weeks for the first month and every 4 weeks thereafter.
• Monitor BP; initiate or adjust antihypertensive therapy as needed.
• Monitor for signs and symptoms of GI erosion (abdominal discomfort or pain; nausea; vomiting; blood in vomit or stools; black, tarry stools; dysphagia; throat or chest pain).
• *Look alike–sound alike:* Don't confuse daprodustat with dapsone.

PATIENT TEACHING
• Teach about proper drug administration and handling.
• *Alert:* Inform patient of increased risk of death, MI, stroke, VTE, and thrombosis of vascular access. Tell patient to seek immediate medical attention if signs or symptoms of these conditions occur.
• Explain the need for regular laboratory tests to check Hb level.
• Review signs and symptoms of HF. Tell patient to report symptom worsening to health care provider.
• Instruct patient to seek prompt medical care if signs or symptoms of gastric or esophageal erosion or GI bleeding occur.
• Tell patient about risk of HTN and importance of undergoing regular BP checks and adhering to prescribed antihypertensive regimen.

• Counsel patient to report known or suspected pregnancy.
• Instruct patient not to breastfeed during therapy and for 1 week after final dose.

deucravacitinib
due-krav-a-SYE-ti-nib

Sotyktu

Therapeutic class: Antipsoriatics
Pharmacologic class: Janus kinase (JAK) inhibitors

AVAILABLE FORMS
Tablets ⒼⓃⒸ: 6 mg

INDICATIONS & DOSAGES
➤ **Moderate-to-severe plaque psoriasis in patients who are candidates for systemic therapy or phototherapy**
Adults: 6 mg PO once daily.

ADMINISTRATION
PO
• Give drug without regard to food.
• Have patient swallow tablets whole; don't crush or cut tablets.
• Store tablets at 68° to 77° F (20° to 25° C).

ACTION
Precise mechanism unknown; inhibits tyrosine kinase 2, resulting in immunosuppression.

Route	Onset	Peak	Duration
PO	Unknown	2–3 hr	Unknown

Half-life: 10 hours.

ADVERSE REACTIONS
EENT: mouth ulcers. **Hepatic:** increased liver enzyme levels. **Metabolic:** increased CK level. **Musculoskeletal:** rhabdomyolysis. **Respiratory:** URI. **Skin:** acne, folliculitis. **Other:** infection (bacterial and viral), malignancy.

INTERACTIONS
Drug-drug. *Live vaccines:* May increase risk of infection. Avoid use together.
Potent immunosuppressants: May increase immunosuppression. Avoid use together.

EFFECTS ON LAB TEST RESULTS
• May increase GFR.
• May increase triglyceride, liver enzyme, and CK levels.

CONTRAINDICATIONS & CAUTIONS
• Contraindicated in patients hypersensitive to drug or its components. Hypersensitivity reactions, including angioedema, have been reported.

NEW DRUGS

• Use cautiously in patients with known or suspected liver disease. Drug isn't recommended in patients with Child-Pugh class C liver impairment.

• Drug isn't recommended for use in patients with active HBV or HCV.

• Drug may increase risk of infection, including herpesvirus infection. Avoid use in patients with active or serious infection.

• Use cautiously in patients who have been exposed to TB and in those with history of chronic or recurrent infection, serious or opportunistic infection, or underlying conditions that increase risk of infection.

• Evaluate for active or latent TB before initiating drug. Don't administer to patients with active TB. Note that drug may reactivate latent TB. Initiate treatment of latent TB before giving drug. Consider anti-TB therapy in patients with history of latent or active TB when adequate course of treatment can't be confirmed.

• Use cautiously in patients with known malignancy and in patients who develop malignancy during therapy. Malignancies, including lymphomas, were observed in clinical trials.

• Drug isn't approved for use in patients with RA. Higher rates of all-cause mortality, including sudden CV death, major adverse CV events (MI, stroke), thrombosis (DVT, PE), and malignancies (excluding non-melanoma skin cancer), have occurred in patients with RA treated with JAK inhibitors than in patients treated with TNF blockers.

• Safety and effectiveness in children haven't been established.

• Use cautiously in older adults due to increased risk of adverse reactions.

Dialyzable drug: 5.4%.

PREGNANCY-LACTATION-REPRODUCTION

• Studies during pregnancy are inadequate. It isn't known if drug causes fetal harm.

• Report patient exposed to drug during pregnancy to Bristol-Myers Squibb's adverse event system (1-800-721-5072).

• It isn't known if drug appears in human milk or how drug affects milk production or infants who are breastfed. Weigh benefit to patient against possible risk to infant.

NURSING CONSIDERATIONS

• Evaluate patient for latent TB before start of therapy. Initiate treatment of latent TB before giving drug.

• Monitor for hypersensitivity reactions.

• Monitor for infection. If new infection occurs, evaluate patient, initiate appropriate antimicrobial therapy, and withhold drug until infection resolves.

• Review malignancy history with patient, and monitor for possible development.

• Monitor for rhabdomyolysis and elevated CK level. Stop drug if marked CK elevation occurs or myopathy is suspected or diagnosed.

• Monitor triglyceride level at baseline and periodically thereafter. Manage patient according to hyperlipidemia guidelines.

• Monitor LFT values at baseline and periodically thereafter, especially in patients with known or suspected liver disease. If treatment-related increases in LFTs occur and liver injury is suspected, interrupt therapy until liver injury is excluded.

• Ensure immunizations are up-to-date according to current immunization guidelines.

PATIENT TEACHING

• Advise patient to discontinue drug and seek immediate medical attention if symptoms of hypersensitivity reaction occur.

• Inform patient that drug may lower immune system's ability to fight infection. Advise patient to immediately report signs or symptoms of infection.

• Alert patient that herpesvirus infection, which may be serious, can occur with use of drug.

• Inform patient of risk of malignancies, including lymphomas. Tell patient to report any history of cancer.

• Counsel patient that drug may increase risk of rhabdomyolysis. Advise patient to immediately report unexplained muscle pain, tenderness, or weakness, particularly if accompanied by malaise or fever.

• Explain that blood tests may be necessary before and during therapy.

• Caution patient that vaccination with live vaccines isn't recommended during therapy due to risk of infection. Instruct patient to report use of drug before any vaccination.

• Tell patient to report pregnancy to health care provider and drug manufacturer (1-800-721-5072).

elacestrant ☒
el-a-KES-trant

Orserdu

Therapeutic class: Antineoplastics
Pharmacologic class: Estrogen receptor antagonists

AVAILABLE FORMS
Tablets ⓒ: 86 mg, 345 mg

INDICATIONS & DOSAGES
➤ **Estrogen receptor–positive, HER2-negative, ESR1-mutated advanced or metastatic breast cancer with disease progression following at least one line of endocrine therapy** ☒

Postmenopausal females and adult males: 345 mg PO once daily until disease progresses or unacceptable toxicity occurs.

Adjust-a-dose: Refer to manufacturer's instructions for toxicity-related dosage adjustments. Reduce dosage to 258 mg once daily for patients with

Child-Pugh class B liver impairment. Avoid use in patients with Child-Pugh class C liver impairment. Avoid concomitant use with strong or moderate CYP3A4 inducers and inhibitors.

ADMINISTRATION
PO
• Give at approximately the same time each day with food to reduce nausea and vomiting.
• Have patient swallow tablets whole; don't crush or cut tablets.
• Don't give broken, cracked, or damaged tablets.
• If a dose is missed beyond 6 hours or if vomiting occurs, skip dose and give next dose the following day at the regularly scheduled time.
• Store at controlled room temperature.

ACTION
Binds to estrogen receptor alpha to inhibit cell proliferation.

Route	Onset	Peak	Duration
PO	Unknown	1–4 hr	Unknown

Half-life: 30 to 50 hours.

ADVERSE REACTIONS
CNS: dizziness, fatigue, headache, insomnia. **EENT:** stomatitis. **GI:** abdominal pain, constipation, decreased appetite, diarrhea, dyspepsia, GERD, nausea, vomiting. **Hematologic:** decreased Hb. **Hepatic:** altered LFTs. **Metabolic:** hyponatremia, increased cholesterol, increased creatinine, increased triglycerides. **Musculoskeletal:** musculoskeletal pain. **Respiratory:** cough, dyspnea. **Skin:** rash. **Other:** hot flushing.

INTERACTIONS
Drug-drug. *BCRP substrates (rosuvastatin), P-gp substrates (digoxin):* May increase substrate level and risk of adverse reactions. Refer to substrate product label and reduce substrate dosage.
Strong and moderate CYP3A4 inducers (efavirenz, rifampin): May increase elacestrant level and its effectiveness. Avoid use together.
Strong and moderate CYP3A4 inhibitors (fluconazole, itraconazole): May increase elacestrant level and risk of adverse reactions. Avoid use together.

EFFECTS ON LAB TEST RESULTS
• May increase ALT, AST, creatinine, cholesterol, and triglyceride levels.
• May decrease sodium and Hb levels.

CONTRAINDICATIONS & CAUTIONS
• Avoid use in patients with Child-Pugh class C liver impairment.
• Safety and effectiveness in children haven't been established.
Dialyzable drug: Unknown.

PREGNANCY-LACTATION-REPRODUCTION
• Based on animal studies, drug may cause fetal harm. Advise patient who is pregnant of risk to fetus.
• Females of childbearing potential and males with female partners of childbearing potential should use effective contraception during therapy and for 1 week after final dose.
• It isn't known if drug appears in human milk or how drug affects milk production or infants who are breastfed. Patient shouldn't breastfeed during therapy and for 1 week after final dose.
• Based on animal studies, drug may impair fertility.

NURSING CONSIDERATIONS
• Monitor lipid levels before initiating drug and periodically during therapy.
• Verify pregnancy status in patient of childbearing potential before drug initiation.
• *Look alike-sound alike:* Don't confuse elacestrant with fulvestrant.

PATIENT TEACHING
• Teach about proper drug administration and handling.
• Advise patient that lipid levels will be monitored before and during therapy.
• Warn patient of risk to a fetus.
• Direct a female of childbearing potential and male patient with female partner of childbearing potential to use effective contraception during therapy and for 1 week after final dose.
• Instruct patient to not breastfeed during therapy and for 1 week after final dose.
• Warn patient that drug may impair fertility.

SAFETY ALERT!

fezolinetant
fez-oh-LIN-e-tant

Veozah

Therapeutic class: Menopause drugs
Pharmacologic class: Neurokinin 3 receptor antagonists

AVAILABLE FORMS
Tablets ⓓⓝⓒ: 45 mg

INDICATIONS & DOSAGES
➤ **Moderate to severe vasomotor symptoms due to menopause**
Adults: 45 mg PO once daily.

ADMINISTRATION
PO
• Give drug without regard to food; give with liquid at same time each day.
• Have patient swallow tablets whole; don't crush or break tablets.

- Don't give a missed dose less than 12 hours before the next dose. Resume regular schedule the next day.
- Store drug at 68° to 77° F (20° to 25° C).

ACTION
Modulates neuronal activity in the thermoregulatory center.

Route	Onset	Peak	Duration
PO	Unknown	1–4 hr	Unknown

Half-life: 9.6 hours.

ADVERSE REACTIONS
CNS: insomnia. **GI:** abdominal pain, diarrhea. **Hepatic:** increased transaminase levels. **Musculoskeletal:** back pain. **Other:** hot flashes.

INTERACTIONS
Drug-drug. *CYP1A2 inhibitors (cimetidine, ciprofloxacin, fluvoxamine):* May increase fezolinetant level. Avoid use together.

EFFECTS ON LAB TEST RESULTS
- May increase transaminase levels.

CONTRAINDICATIONS & CAUTIONS
- Contraindicated in patients with known cirrhosis, severe kidney impairment, or KFRT.
- Safety and effectiveness in children haven't been established.

Dialyzable drug: Unknown.

PREGNANCY-LACTATION-REPRODUCTION
- Studies during pregnancy are inadequate. It isn't known if drug causes fetal harm.
- It isn't known if drug appears in human milk or how drug affects milk production or infants who are breastfed.

NURSING CONSIDERATIONS
- Monitor LFT results at baseline; at 3, 6, and 9 months after start of therapy; and as clinically indicated.
- Monitor for signs and symptoms of liver toxicity (nausea, vomiting, jaundice).
- Monitor patient's menopause symptoms to determine drug's efficacy.

PATIENT TEACHING
- Teach about proper drug administration and handling.
- Tell patient to report signs or symptoms of liver toxicity.
- Explain that blood tests are needed before and during therapy to monitor liver function.
- Advise patient to report use of all medications, including OTC medications and supplements.

lecanemab-irmb ℞
lek-AN-e-mab

Leqembi

Therapeutic class: Anti-Alzheimer drugs
Pharmacologic class: Amyloid beta-directed antibodies

AVAILABLE FORMS
Injection: 200 mg/2 mL (100 mg/mL), 500 mg/5 mL (100 mg/mL) single-use vials

INDICATIONS & DOSAGES
➤ **Mild cognitive impairment or mild dementia stage of Alzheimer disease**
Adults: 10 mg/kg IV infusion over 1 hour once every 2 weeks.
Adjust-a-dose: See manufacturer's instructions for dosage reductions in patients with amyloid-related imaging abnormalities-edema (ARIA-E) or amyloid-related imaging abnormalities-hemosiderin deposition (ARIA-H), which vary based on symptom severity and MRI findings.

ADMINISTRATION
IV
▼ Inspect vial and diluted solution for particulate matter and discoloration; don't use if present. Solution should be clear to opalescent and colorless to pale yellow.
▼ Withdraw required volume of drug from vial(s) and add to one 250 mL bag of NSS. Discard unused portion from vial.
▼ Gently invert bag to mix solution. Don't shake.
▼ Use prepared solution immediately or store refrigerated at 36° to 46° F (2° to 8° C) for up to 4 hours or at room temperature for up to 4 hours. Don't freeze.
▼ Before infusion, allow refrigerated solution to reach room temperature.
▼ Infuse solution through an IV line containing a low-protein-binding 0.2 micron in-line filter. Flush line after infusion.
▼ Give missed dose as soon as possible.
▼ Protect vials from light and store at 36° F to 46° F (2° C to 8° C). Don't freeze or shake.
▼ **Incompatibilities:** None listed by manufacturer. Consult drug compatibility reference for more information.

ACTION
Humanized immunoglobulin gamma 1 monoclonal antibody directed at reducing amyloid beta plaques.

Route	Onset	Peak	Duration
IV	Unknown	Unknown	Unknown

Half-life: 5–7 days.

NEW DRUGS

ADVERSE REACTIONS
CNS: *ARIA-E,* headache. **CV:** atrial fibrillation.
EENT: cough. **GI:** diarrhea. **Hematologic:**
lymphopenia. **Other:** infusion-related reactions.

INTERACTIONS
Drug-drug. *Antithrombotics, thrombolytic agents,
antiplatelets, anticoagulants:* May increase risk of
bleeding. Use together cautiously. Consider temporarily withholding lecanemab-irmb if anticoagulant
must be used for 4 weeks or less.

EFFECTS ON LAB TEST RESULTS
• May decrease lymphocyte count.

CONTRAINDICATIONS & CAUTIONS
⚠ *Alert:* ARIA, which is usually asymptomatic but
can include seizures and status epilepticus (rare),
may develop. Closely monitor patients during first
14 weeks of therapy. ARIA-E appears as brain
edema or sulcal effusions. ARIA-H causes micro-
hemorrhage and superficial siderosis and usually
occurs with ARIA-E.
✻ Although ARIA can occur in any patient treated
with this drug, risk is increased in patients who are
ApoE ε4 homozygote positive. Consider testing for
APOE ε4 status before initiating drug.
• Use clinical judgment when considering whether to
continue dosing in patients with recurrent ARIA-E.
⚠ *Alert:* Intracerebral hemorrhage may occur
(rare). Use cautiously in patients with history of
cerebral hemorrhage greater than 1 cm in greatest
diameter, more than four microhemorrhages,
superficial siderosis, evidence of vasogenic edema,
evidence of cerebral contusion, aneurysm, vascular
malformation, infective lesions, multiple lacunar in-
farcts or stroke involving a major vascular territory,
or severe small vessel or white matter disease.
• Safety and effectiveness in children haven't been
established.
Dialyzable drug: Unknown.

PREGNANCY-LACTATION-REPRODUCTION
• Studies during pregnancy are inadequate.
• It isn't known if drug appears in human milk or
how drug affects milk production or infants who
are breastfed. Weigh benefit to patient against possible risk to infant.

NURSING CONSIDERATIONS
• Confirm presence of amyloid beta pathology
before initiating therapy.
• Ensure baseline brain MRI (obtained within
1 year) is available before initiating therapy.
• Obtain MRI results before 5th, 7th, and 14th infusions for comparison against baseline MRI results.
• Monitor patient for ARIA symptoms (headache,
confusion, vision changes, dizziness, aphasia,
weakness, nausea, gait difficulty, seizure and focal
neurologic deficits). If any occur, ensure patient
undergoes clinical evaluation and MRI imaging

(if indicated). ARIA symptoms usually resolve
over time.
• Monitor patient for infusion-related reactions, including flulike symptoms, nausea, vomiting, HTN,
and oxygen desaturation. If any occur, reduce
infusion rate or discontinue infusion, and treat as
clinically indicated. At subsequent infusions, consider premedication with antihistamines, NSAIDs,
or corticosteroids.
• Alzheimer's Network for Treatment and Diag-
nostics (ALZ-NET) is a voluntary provider-
enrolled patient registry that collects information
on treatments for patients with Alzheimer disease.
Information is available at http://www.alz-net.org.

PATIENT TEACHING
• Advise patient that drug may cause ARIA and
that some people experience symptoms. Instruct
patient to report symptoms to health care provider.
✻ Inform patient that, although ARIA can occur in
any patient treated with this drug, risk is increased
in patients who are ApoE ε4 homozygote positive.
Explain that testing can determine the presence of
ApoE ε4 genotype.
• Tell patient that the ALZ-NET registry collects
information on treatments for patients with Alzheimer disease. Discuss registry enrollment.
• Warn patient of risk of infusion-related reactions.

lenacapavir
len-a-KAP-a-veer

Sunlenca

Therapeutic class: Antiretrovirals
Pharmacologic class: Capsid inhibitors

AVAILABLE FORMS
Injection: 463.5 mg/1.5 mL single-dose vial
Tablets: 300 mg

INDICATIONS & DOSAGES
➤ **HIV-1 infection, given in combination with other
antiretrovirals in heavily treatment-experienced patients with multidrug-resistant HIV-1 infection who
are failing their current antiretroviral regimen due to
resistance, intolerance, or safety considerations**
Adults: For initiation option 1: 927 mg subcut and
600 mg PO once on day 1; 600 mg PO once on day
2; then maintenance regimen. For initiation option
2: 600 mg PO once on days 1 and 2; 300 mg PO
once on day 8; 927 mg subcut once on day 15; then
maintenance regimen. For maintenance regimen:
927 mg subcut every 6 months (26 weeks) from date
of last injection. May give within 2 weeks before or
after 6-month target date.

ADMINISTRATION
PO
• Give drug without regard to food.

NEW DRUGS

- Store in original blister pack at room temperature.

Subcutaneous
- Two 1.5-mL injections are required for a complete dose.
- Drug is provided in a kit with vials, vial access device, needles, and syringes.
- Inspect solution for particulate matter and discoloration; solution should be yellow in color without particles. Vial stoppers don't contain natural rubber latex.
- After withdrawing solution from vials, give as soon as possible into abdomen at two separate sites at least 2 inches (5 cm) away from naval.
- During maintenance period, if more than 28 weeks have elapsed since last injection and if clinically appropriate to continue treatment, restart initiation dose regimen from day 1, using either Option 1 or Option 2.
- Solution is preservative-free. Discard unused solution.
- Store at room temperature.
- Protect vials from light in original carton until just before preparing injections.

ACTION

Inhibits HIV-1 replication by interfering with multiple essential steps of the viral lifecycle, including capsid-mediated nuclear uptake of HIV-1 proviral DNA, virus assembly and release, and capsid core formation.

Route	Onset	Peak	Duration
PO	Unknown	4 hr	Unknown
Subcut	Unknown	77–84 days	Unknown

Half-life: Oral 10–12 days; subcut 8–12 weeks.

ADVERSE REACTIONS

GI: nausea. **GU:** glycosuria, increased creatinine level, proteinuria. **Hepatic:** increased AST, ALT, and direct bilirubin levels. **Metabolic:** hyperglycemia. **Skin:** injection site reactions (discomfort, edema, erythema, extravasation, hematoma, induration, edema, mass, nodule, pain, pruritus, swelling, ulcer).

INTERACTIONS

⬧ Alert: Lenacapavir has the potential for significant interactions with many drugs. Consult a drug interaction resource for additional information.
Drug-drug. ⬧ Alert: *Anticonvulsants (carbamazepine, oxcarbazepine, phenobarbital, phenytoin):* May decrease lenacapavir level and increase risk of resistance. Avoid use together. Consider alternative anticonvulsant.
⬧ Alert: *Antimycobacterials (rifabutin, rifampin, rifapentine):* May decrease lenacapavir level and increase risk of resistance. Avoid use together.
Antiretrovirals (atazanavir/cobicistat, atazanavir–ritonavir, efavirenz, nevirapine, tipranavir–ritonavir): May alter lenacapavir level. Use with efavirenz,

nevirapine, or tipranavir–ritonavir may decrease lenacapavir level and increase risk of resistance. Use with atazanavir–cobicistat or atazanavir–ritonavir may increase lenacapavir level. Avoid use together with any of these agents.
Combined P-gp, UGT1A1, and strong CYP3A inhibitors (atazanavir, cobicistat): May significantly increase lenacapavir level. Avoid use together.
Corticosteroids, systemic (dexamethasone, hydrocortisone, cortisone): May increase systemic corticosteroid level, increasing risk of Cushing syndrome and adrenal suppression. Initiate with lowest starting dose and titrate carefully while monitoring for safety.
CYP3A substrates: Lenacapavir may increase exposure of drugs primarily metabolized by CYP3A initiated within 9 months after the last subcutaneous dose of lenacapavir, increasing risk of adverse reactions. See prescribing information of sensitive CYP3A substrate for dosing with moderate CYP3A inhibitors.
Digoxin: May increase digoxin level. Use cautiously and monitor digoxin therapeutic level.
Direct oral anticoagulants (dabigatran, edoxaban, rivaroxaban): May increase direct oral anticoagulant level. Refer to anticoagulant prescribing information for concomitant use with combined moderate CYP3A and P-gp inhibitors.
Ergot derivatives (dihydroergotamine, ergotamine, methylergonovine): May increase ergot derivative level. Avoid use together.
HMG-CoA reductase inhibitors (lovastatin, simvastatin): May increase reductase inhibitor level. Initiate reductase inhibitor at lowest starting dose and titrate carefully while monitoring for safety.
Midazolam (oral), triazolam: May increase level of these drugs. Use cautiously.
Moderate CYP3A inducers (efavirenz): May significantly decrease lenacapavir level and increase risk of resistance. Avoid use together.
Naloxegol: May increase naloxegol level. Avoid use together. If use together is unavoidable, decrease naloxegol dosage and monitor for adverse reactions.
Opioid analgesic for treatment of opioid dependence (buprenorphine, methadone): Effects of these opioid analgesics are unknown. Carefully titrate buprenorphine or methadone dose to desired effect; use lowest possible initial or maintenance dose. In patients currently taking buprenorphine or methadone, dosage adjustment may be needed when starting lenacapavir. Monitor clinical signs and symptoms.
Opioid analgesics metabolized by CYP3A (fentanyl, oxycodone): May increase level of these opioids. Monitor closely for effect and adverse reactions.
PDE5 inhibitors (sildenafil, tadalafil, vardenafil): When used for PAH, use of lenacapavir and tadalafil isn't recommended. When used for erectile dysfunction, refer to prescribing information for PDE5 inhibitor for dosage recommendations.

NEW DRUGS

Strong CYP3A inducers (rifampin): May significantly decrease lenacapavir level and increase risk of resistance. Avoid use together.
Tramadol: May increase tramadol level. Consider decreasing tramadol dosage.
Drug-herb. *St. John's wort:* May decrease lenacapavir level. Discourage use together.

EFFECTS ON LAB TEST RESULTS
• May increase creatinine, glucose, AST, ALT, and direct bilirubin levels.

CONTRAINDICATIONS & CAUTIONS
• Use cautiously in patients with severe liver impairment or KFRT.
• Immune reconstitution syndrome may occur in patients treated with combination antiretroviral therapy. Autoimmune disorders (Graves disease, polymyositis, Guillain-Barré syndrome, autoimmune hepatitis) may occur with immune reconstitution syndrome.
• Nonadherence to medication regimen could lead to loss of virologic response and development of resistance.
• Safety and effectiveness in children haven't been established.
Dialyzable drug: Unlikely.

PREGNANCY-LACTATION-REPRODUCTION
• Studies during pregnancy are inadequate.
• Enroll patient exposed to drug during pregnancy in the Antiretroviral Pregnancy Registry (1-800-258-4263 or www.apregistry.com).
• It isn't known if drug appears in human milk or how drug affects milk production or infants who are breastfed. Patient shouldn't breastfeed during therapy.

NURSING CONSIDERATIONS
• Monitor patient for immune reconstitution syndrome (inflammatory response to indolent or residual opportunistic infections, such as *Mycobacterium avium* infection, cytomegalovirus, *Pneumocystis jirovecii* pneumonia, or tuberculosis). Immediately evaluate signs and symptoms of infection and treat as clinically indicated.
◐ *Alert:* Residual concentrations of drug may remain in systemic circulation for 12 months or longer.
• If drug is discontinued, begin an alternative, fully suppressive antiretroviral regimen, if possible, no later than 28 weeks after final injection of lenacapavir.
• If virologic failure occurs, begin an alternative regimen, if possible.
• Monitor patient for persistent injection site reactions (swelling, pain, erythema, nodule, induration, pruritus, extravasation, mass).
• *Look alike-sound alike:* Don't confuse lenacapavir with letermovir.

PATIENT TEACHING
• Teach about proper drug administration and handling.
• Advise patient to report all prescription and OTC drugs and herbal supplements being taken before, during, and for up to 9 months after taking lenacapavir.
◐ *Alert:* Teach patient about dosing schedule and importance of adherence to avoid risk of development of resistance and loss of virologic response. Tell patient to immediately report abrupt discontinuation of lenacapavir or any other drug in patient's antiretroviral regimen.
◐ *Alert:* Advise patient to immediately report any signs or symptoms of infection.
• Instruct patient to report injection site reactions. Explain that nodules and indurations at injection site may take longer to resolve than other injection site reactions.
• Inform patient about antiretroviral pregnancy registry, which monitors fetal outcomes of pregnant patients exposed to drug.
◐ *Alert:* Warn patient not to breastfeed.

leniolisib ✕
len-i-oh-LIS-ib

Joenja

Therapeutic class: Immunomodulators
Pharmacologic class: Kinase inhibitors

AVAILABLE FORMS
Tablets: 70 mg

INDICATIONS & DOSAGES
➤ **Activated phosphoinositide 3-kinase delta syndrome** ✕
Adults and children ages 12 and older weighing at least 45 kg: 70 mg PO b.i.d. 12 hours apart.

ADMINISTRATION
PO
• Give drug without regard to food.
• If a dose is missed by more than 6 hours, skip missed dose and give next dose at its scheduled time.
• If vomiting occurs within 1 hour after dose, give drug again as soon as possible.
• If vomiting occurs more than 1 hour after dose, wait and give dose at next scheduled time.
• Store at room temperature.

ACTION
Inhibits phosphoinositide 3-kinase delta by blocking active binding sites and inhibiting pathways that increase production of PIP and dysregulates B and T cells.

Route	Onset	Peak	Duration
PO	Unknown	1 hr	Unknown

Half-life: 10 hours.

ADVERSE REACTIONS
CNS: fatigue, fever, headache. **CV:** tachycardia. **EENT:** sinusitis. **GI:** diarrhea. **Hematologic:** *neutropenia.* **Musculoskeletal:** back pain, neck pain. **Skin:** alopecia, atopic dermatitis.

INTERACTIONS
Drug-drug. *BCRP, OATP1B1, OATP1B3 substrates (methotrexate, pravastatin, prazosin, rosuvastatin):* May increase substrate level. Avoid use together.
CYP1A2 substrates with narrow therapeutic index (theophylline): May increase substrate level. Avoid use together.
Live vaccines: May decrease vaccine effectiveness. Avoid use together.
Moderate and strong CYP3A4 inducers (efavirenz, phenytoin, rifampin): May decrease leniolisib level. Avoid use together.
Strong CYP3A4 inhibitors (clarithromycin, itraconazole, ketoconazole, ritonavir): May increase leniolisib level. Avoid use together.
Drug-herb. *St. John's wort:* May decrease leniolisib level. Discourage use together.
Drug-food. *Grapefruit, grapefruit juice:* May increase leniolisib level. Discourage use together.

EFFECTS ON LAB TEST RESULTS
• May decrease ANC.

CONTRAINDICATIONS & CAUTIONS
• Use in patients with Child-Pugh class B or C liver impairment hasn't been established and isn't recommended.
• Safety and effectiveness in children younger than age 12 or weighing less than 45 kg haven't been established.
Dialyzable drug: Unlikely.

PREGNANCY-LACTATION-REPRODUCTION
• Based on animal studies, drug may cause fetal harm.
• Patients of childbearing potential should use effective contraception during therapy and for 1 week after final dose.
• It isn't known if drug appears in human milk or how drug affects milk production or infants who are breastfed. Patient shouldn't breastfeed during therapy and for 1 week after final dose.

NURSING CONSIDERATIONS
• Verify pregnancy status before start of therapy.
• Obtain current medication and supplement list to check for potential drug interactions.
• Tablet contains lactose.
• *Look alike–sound alike:* Don't confuse leniolisib with lenvatinib.

PATIENT TEACHING
• Teach about proper drug administration and handling.

• Advise patient and caregiver to immediately report adverse effects.
• Inform lactose-intolerant patient that drug contains lactose.
• Counsel patient of childbearing potential to use effective contraception during therapy and for 1 week after final dose.
• Advise patient to report pregnancy or plans to become pregnant or breastfeed during therapy.

lotilaner
loe-ti-LAN-er

Xdemvy

Therapeutic class: Antiparasitics
Pharmacologic class: Ectoparasiticides

AVAILABLE FORMS
Ophthalmic solution: 0.25%

INDICATIONS & DOSAGES
➤ *Demodex* blepharitis
Adults: 1 drop in each eye b.i.d. (approximately 12 hours apart) for 6 weeks.

ADMINISTRATION
Ophthalmic
• Instruct patient to remove contact lenses before instillation. Wait at least 15 minutes after instillation before reinserting contact lenses.
• Don't touch tip of dropper to eye or surrounding tissue.
• If patient is using additional ophthalmic medications, allow at least 5 minutes between each product.
• If a dose is missed, skip missed dose and give next dose at its scheduled time.
• After opening, drug may be used until expiration date on bottle.
• Store drug at 59° to 77° F (15° to 25° C).

ACTION
Causes a fatal paralytic action in *Demodex* mites.

Route	Onset	Peak	Duration
Ophthalmic	Unknown	2 hr	Unknown

Half-life: 11 days.

ADVERSE REACTIONS
EENT: bacterial eyelid infection, corneal inflammation, eyelid cyst, stinging and burning at instillation site.

INTERACTIONS
• None reported.

EFFECTS ON LAB TEST RESULTS
• None reported.

NEW DRUGS

CONTRAINDICATIONS & CAUTIONS
• Safety and effectiveness in children haven't been established.
Dialyzable drug: Unknown.

PREGNANCY-LACTATION-REPRODUCTION
• Studies during pregnancy are inadequate. Systemic exposure by ophthalmic route is low.
• It isn't known if drug appears in human milk. Use cautiously during breastfeeding.

NURSING CONSIDERATIONS
• Monitor patient for eye irritation and signs and symptoms of infection (redness, swelling, discharge).

PATIENT TEACHING
• Teach about proper drug administration and handling.
• Advise patient that stinging and burning at instillation site can occur.
• Inform patient that damage to eye and subsequent vision loss may result from use of contaminated solution.
• Instruct patient to immediately report a new ocular condition (such as trauma or infection), ocular surgery, or any ocular reactions, particularly conjunctivitis or eyelid reactions, during therapy.
• Caution patient that drug contains potassium sorbate, which may discolor soft contact lenses. Tell patient to remove contact lenses before use and reinsert them 15 minutes or more after instillation.

SAFETY ALERT!

nirmatrelvir–ritonavir
nir-ma-TREL-vir/ri-TOE-na-veer

Paxlovid

Therapeutic class: Antivirals
Pharmacologic class: Protease inhibitors

AVAILABLE FORMS
Tablets ⓄⓃⒸ: 150 mg nirmatrelvir copackaged with 100 mg ritonavir

INDICATIONS & DOSAGES
➤ **Mild to moderate COVID-19 in patients at high risk for progression to severe COVID-19, including hospitalization or death**
Adults: 300 mg nirmatrelvir with 100 mg ritonavir PO b.i.d. for 5 days.
Adjust-a-dose: For patients with eGFR of 30 to 59 mL/minute, give 150 mg nirmatrelvir with 100 mg ritonavir PO b.i.d. for 5 days.

ADMINISTRATION
PO
• Nirmatrelvir must be given with ritonavir to achieve desired therapeutic effect.

• Ensure prescription specifies dosages in mg of nirmatrelvir and ritonavir.
• Remove tablets from blister card immediately before administration. Give all tablets at the same time.
• Give drugs without regard to food.
• Have patient swallow tablets whole; don't crush or break tablets.
• If a dose is missed within 8 hours of the usual time, give as soon as possible and then resume normal dosing schedule. If a dose is missed by more than 8 hours, skip missed dose and give next dose at its scheduled time.
• Store drugs at room temperature.

ACTION
Nirmatrelvir prevents viral replication. Ritonavir inhibits CYP3A-mediated metabolism of nirmatrelvir, resulting in increased nirmatrelvir level; it isn't active against SARS-CoV-2 M^{pro}.

Route	Onset	Peak	Duration
PO	Unknown	3 hr (nirmatrelvir) 4 hr (ritonavir)	Unknown

Half-life: 6 hours (nirmatrelvir); 6 hours (ritonavir).

ADVERSE REACTIONS
CNS: altered taste, headache, malaise. **CV:** HTN. **GI:** abdominal pain, diarrhea, nausea, vomiting. **Hepatic:** *hepatitis,* increased transaminase levels, jaundice. **Skin:** *SJS, TEN.* **Other:** *anaphylaxis,* hypersensitivity reactions.

INTERACTIONS
⚠ *Alert:* Combination nirmatrelvir and ritonavir has the potential to significantly interact with many other drugs. Consult a pharmacist or drug interaction resource for additional information.
Drug-drug. *Alpha-1-adrenoreceptor antagonists (alfuzosin, tamsulosin):* May increase alpha-1-adrenoreceptor antagonist level and risk of hypotension. Avoid use together. Use with alfuzosin is contraindicated.
Antiarrhythmics (amiodarone, disopyramide, dronedarone, flecainide, lidocaine [systemic], propafenone, quinidine): May increase antiarrhythmic level. Use together cautiously with disopyramide or lidocaine, and monitor therapeutic level, if available. Use with amiodarone, dronedarone, flecainide, propafenone, or quinidine is contraindicated.
Antibacterials (clarithromycin, erythromycin): May increase antibacterial level. Refer to antibacterial prescribing information.
Anticancer drugs (abemaciclib, ceritinib, dasatinib, encorafenib, ibrutinib, ivosidenib, neratinib, nilotinib, venetoclax, vinblastine, vincristine): May increase anticancer drug level. Avoid use with encorafenib or ivosidenib due to risk of serious adverse events, including prolonged QT interval. Avoid use with ibrutinib, neratinib, or venetoclax. Coadministration with vincristine or vinblastine may lead to significant hematologic or GI adverse effects.

NEW DRUGS

♣ Canada   ◇ OTC   ♦ Off-label use   ⓄⓃⒸ Do not crush   *Liquid contains alcohol   ⌘ Genetic

Anticoagulants (apixaban, dabigatran, rivaroxaban, warfarin): May increase risk of bleeding and anticoagulant level. May increase or decrease warfarin level. Closely monitor INR when used with warfarin. Avoid use with rivaroxaban. Reduce dosage of apixaban or dabigatran, or avoid use together. Refer to anticoagulant prescribing information.

Anticonvulsants (carbamazepine, phenobarbital, primidone, phenytoin): May cause loss of virologic response and possible resistance. Avoid use together.

Antifungals (isavuconazonium, itraconazole, ketoconazole, voriconazole): May increase isavuconazonium, itraconazole, ketoconazole, and nirmatrelvir/ritonavir levels. Refer to antifungal prescribing information. May decrease voriconazole level; avoid use with voriconazole.

Anti-HIV agents (bictegravir–emtricitabine–tenofovir, efavirenz, maraviroc, nevirapine, zidovudine): May alter anti-HIV agent level. Refer to anti-HIV agent prescribing information.

Anti-HIV protease inhibitors (atazanavir, darunavir, tipranavir): May increase protease inhibitor level. Refer to protease inhibitor prescribing information. Patients on ritonavir- or cobicistat-containing HIV regimens should continue treatment as indicated. Monitor for increased adverse events.

Antimigraine medications (eletriptan, rimegepant, ubrogepant): May increase antimigraine medication level. Avoid use of eletriptan within 72 hours of nirmatrelvir–ritonavir due to risk of serious adverse reactions, including CV and cerebrovascular events. Avoid use with ubrogepant due to risk of serious adverse reactions. Avoid use with rimegepant.

Antimycobacterial (bedaquiline, rifabutin): May increase antimycobacterial level. Refer to antimycobacterial prescribing information.

Antipsychotics (clozapine, lurasidone, pimozide, quetiapine): May increase antipsychotic level. Refer to antipsychotic prescribing information.

Apalutamide: May decrease nirmatrelvir or ritonavir level. Avoid use together.

Bosentan: May increase bosentan level and decrease nirmatrelvir or ritonavir level. Discontinue bosentan at least 36 hours before initiating nirmatrelvir–ritonavir.

Bupropion: May decrease bupropion level. Monitor for adequate antidepressant response.

Calcium channel blockers (amlodipine, diltiazem, felodipine, nicardipine, nifedipine, verapamil): May increase calcium channel blocker level. Monitor closely and consider decreasing calcium channel blocker dosage.

Cilostazol: May increase cilostazol level. Decrease cilostazol dosage.

Clonazepam: May increase clonazepam level. Decrease clonazepam dosage as indicated, and monitor therapy.

Clopidogrel: May decrease clopidogrel level. Use together cautiously.

Colchicine: May increase colchicine level and risk of serious reactions. Use together is contraindicated in patients with kidney or liver impairment.

Corticosteroids metabolized by CYP3A (betamethasone, budesonide, ciclesonide, dexamethasone, fluticasone, methylprednisolone, mometasone, triamcinolone): May increase corticosteroid level. Consider alternative corticosteroid (beclomethasone, prednisone, prednisolone).

CV agents (aliskiren, ticagrelor, vorapaxar): May increase CV agent level. Avoid use together.

Cystic fibrosis transmembrane conductance regulator potentiators (ivacaftor, elexacaftor–tezacaftor–ivacaftor, tezacaftor–ivacaftor): May increase cystic fibrosis drug level. Refer to individual product prescribing information for dosage adjustment.

Darifenacin: May increase darifenacin level. Ensure darifenacin dosage doesn't exceed 7.5 mg daily. Refer to darifenacin prescribing information.

Digoxin: May increase digoxin level. Monitor digoxin level.

Eplerenone, ivabradine: May increase eplerenone or ivabradine level. Use together is contraindicated.

Ergot derivatives (dihydroergotamine, ergotamine, methylergonovine): May increase ergot derivative level and risk of toxicity. Use together is contraindicated.

Ethinyl estradiol: May decrease hormone level. Consider using additional, nonhormonal contraceptive during therapy and until 1 menstrual cycle after stopping nirmatrelvir–ritonavir.

Finerenone: May increase finerenone level. Use together is contraindicated.

Flibanserin: May increase flibanserin level and risk of hypotension, syncope, and CNS depression. Use together is contraindicated.

Hepatitis C direct-acting antivirals (elbasvir–grazoprevir, glecaprevir–pibrentasvir, ombitasvir–paritaprevir–ritonavir–dasabuvir, sofosbuvir–velpatasvir–voxilaprevir): May increase antiviral drug level. Avoid use with glecaprevir–pibrentasvir. Patients on ritonavir-containing HCV regimens should continue treatment as indicated. Monitor for increased drug adverse events with use together. Refer to HCV antiviral prescribing information.

HMG-CoA reductase inhibitors (atorvastatin, rosuvastatin): May increase statin level. Consider temporary discontinuation of these statins during therapy but no need to withhold them before or after nirmatrelvir–ritonavir therapy.

HMG-CoA reductase inhibitors (lovastatin, simvastatin): May increase statin level and risk of myopathy. Use of nirmatrelvir–ritonavir with these statins is contraindicated.

Immunosuppressants (cyclosporine, tacrolimus): May increase immunosuppressant level. Avoid use together when close monitoring of immunosuppressant level isn't feasible. If coadministered, adjust immunosuppressant dosage, closely monitor immunosuppressant level, and assess for adverse reactions.

Reactions in bold italics are *life-threatening.*

Immunosuppressants (voclosporin): May increase voclosporin level. Use together is contraindicated due to risk of kidney toxicity.

Ivabradine: May increase ivabradine level and risk of bradycardia or conduction disturbances. Use together is contraindicated.

Janus kinase (JAK) inhibitors (tofacitinib, upadacitinib): May increase JAK inhibitor level. Adjust tofacitinib dosage. Dosage adjustment for concomitant upadacitinib depends on upadacitinib indication. Refer to JAK inhibitor prescribing information.

Lomitapide: May increase risk of liver toxicity and GI adverse reactions. Use together is contraindicated.

Lumacaftor–ivacaftor: May decrease level of nirmatrelvir or ritonavir. Use together is contraindicated.

Methadone: May decrease methadone level. Monitor methadone-maintained patient closely for withdrawal, and adjust methadone dosage accordingly.

mTOR inhibitors (everolimus, sirolimus): May increase mTOR inhibitor level. Avoid use together.

Neuropsychiatric agents (aripiprazole, brexpiprazole, cariprazine, iloperidone, lumateperone, pimavanserin, suvorexant): May increase neuropsychiatric drug level. Avoid use with suvorexant. Adjust dosage of aripiprazole, brexpiprazole, cariprazine, iloperidone, lumateperone, or pimavanserin.

Opioid analgesics (fentanyl, hydrocodone, oxycodone, meperidine): May increase opioid level. Closely monitor for therapeutic and adverse opioid effects, including potentially fatal respiratory depression. Consider decreasing opioid dosage.

Opioid antagonists (naloxegol): May increase naloxegol level. Use together is contraindicated due to risk of opioid withdrawal.

PDE5 inhibitors for erectile dysfunction (avanafil, sildenafil, tadalafil, vardenafil): May increase PDE5 inhibitor level. Avoid use with avanafil. Adjust dosage of sildenafil, tadalafil, or vardenafil. Refer to PDE5 inhibitor prescribing information.

PDE5 inhibitors for pulmonary HTN (sildenafil, tadalafil): May increase PDE5 inhibitor level. Use of sildenafil is contraindicated for pulmonary HTN due to risk of sildenafil-associated adverse events. Avoid use with tadalafil for pulmonary HTN.

sGC stimulator (riociguat): May increase riociguat level. Adjust riociguat dosage when used for pulmonary HTN.

Ranolazine: May increase ranolazine level. Use is contraindicated due to risk of serious or life-threatening reactions.

Salmeterol: May increase salmeterol level and risk of CV adverse events (prolonged QT interval, palpitations, sinus tachycardia). Avoid use together.

Saxagliptin: May increase saxagliptin level. Decrease saxagliptin dosage. Refer to saxagliptin prescribing information.

Sedative-hypnotics (buspirone, clorazepate, diazepam, flurazepam, parenteral midazolam, zolpidem): May increase sedative-hypnotic level. Consider dosage decrease, and monitor for adverse events. Ensure parenteral midazolam is given in a setting with monitoring and appropriate medical management.

Sedative-hypnotics (oral midazolam, triazolam): May increase sedative-hypnotic level. Use together is contraindicated.

Silodosin: May increase silodosin level and risk of postural hypotension. Use together is contraindicated.

Tolvaptan: May increase tolvaptan level and risk of dehydration, hypovolemia, and hyperkalemia. Use together is contraindicated.

Trazodone: May increase trazodone level and its adverse reactions (nausea, dizziness, hypotension, syncope). Consider decreasing trazodone dosage.

Drug-herb. *St. John's wort:* May decrease drug level and loss of virologic response. Discourage use together.

EFFECTS ON LAB TEST RESULTS
- May increase transaminase levels.

CONTRAINDICATIONS & CAUTIONS
- Contraindicated with drugs primarily metabolized by CYP3A and for which elevated levels are associated with serious or life-threatening reactions.
- Contraindicated with drugs that are strong CYP3A inducers in patients in whom significantly reduced nirmatrelvir or ritonavir level may be associated with loss of virologic response and possible resistance.

Boxed Warning Consider benefit of therapy in reducing hospitalization and death as well as whether risk of potential drug-drug interactions for an individual patient can be appropriately managed. ∎

- Nirmatrelvir–ritonavir isn't approved for preexposure or postexposure prevention of COVID-19.
- Contraindicated in patients with history of hypersensitivity reactions (TEN, SJS) to drug or its components. Anaphylaxis, SCARs, and other hypersensitivity reactions have been reported.
- Transaminase level elevations, hepatitis, and jaundice have occurred in patients receiving ritonavir. Use cautiously in patients with preexisting liver disease, liver enzyme abnormalities, or hepatitis. Drug isn't recommended in patients with Child-Pugh class C liver impairment.
- Drug isn't recommended in patients with eGFR less than 30 mL/minute or patients with KFRT.
- Drug may increase risk of developing resistance to HIV protease inhibitors in patients with uncontrolled or undiagnosed HIV-1 infection.
- Use cautiously in older adults.
- Safety and effectiveness in children haven't been established.

Dialyzable drug: Unknown.

PREGNANCY-LACTATION-REPRODUCTION
- Studies during pregnancy are inadequate. It isn't known if drug causes fetal harm. Use cautiously during pregnancy.

NEW DRUGS

• It isn't known if nirmatrelvir is present in human milk; ritonavir is present in human milk. Use cautiously during pregnancy.
• Ritonavir may reduce efficacy of combined hormonal contraceptives. Patients should use effective alternative contraceptive or an additional barrier method of contraception during therapy.

NURSING CONSIDERATIONS

Boxed Warning Ritonavir, a strong CYP3A inhibitor, may interact with some concomitant medications and result in potentially severe, life-threatening, or fatal events. Before giving drug, review all medications for potential drug-drug interactions and assess need for dosage adjustment, interruption, and additional monitoring. ■
• Start therapy as soon as possible after diagnosis of COVID-19 and within 5 days of symptom onset, even if baseline symptoms are mild.
• Immediately discontinue drug and initiate appropriate medications and supportive care if patient experiences anaphylaxis or hypersensitivity reaction.
• Completion of 5-day treatment course and continued isolation in accordance with public health recommendations are important to maximize viral clearance and minimize SARS-CoV-2 transmission.

PATIENT TEACHING

🕲 *Alert:* Warn patient that nirmatrelvir–ritonavir may interact with or be contraindicated for use with certain drugs. Advise patient to report use of prescription and OTC medications and supplements.
• Teach about proper drug administration and handling.
• Emphasize importance of completing 5-day treatment course and continuing isolation in accordance with public health recommendations.
• Caution patient that anaphylaxis, serious skin reactions, and other hypersensitivity reactions may occur, even after a single dose. Tell patient to immediately stop drug and report first sign of skin rash, hives, or other skin reactions; difficulty swallowing or breathing; any symptom that suggests angioedema (swelling of lips, tongue, or face; tightness of throat; hoarseness); or other symptoms of allergic reaction.
• Teach patient to report all adverse effects.
• Advise patient to report pregnancy or plans to become pregnant or breastfeed during therapy.

SAFETY ALERT!

olutasidenib 🔏
oh-loo-ta-SID-e-nib

Rezlidhia

Therapeutic class: Antineoplastics
Pharmacologic class: Isocitrate
dehydrogenase-1 (IDH1) inhibitors

AVAILABLE FORMS
Capsules ⓞⓝⓒ: 150 mg

INDICATIONS & DOSAGES

➤ **Relapsed or refractory acute myeloid leukemia with a susceptible IDH1 mutation**
Adults: 150 mg PO b.i.d. until disease progresses or unacceptable toxicity occurs. If no disease progression or unacceptable toxicity occurs, treat for a minimum of 6 months to allow time for clinical response.
Adjust-a-dose: Refer to manufacturer's instruction for toxicity-related dosage adjustments.

ADMINISTRATION
PO
• Give drug at the same time each day.
• Don't give two doses within 8 hours.
• Give on an empty stomach at least 1 hour before or 2 hours after meal.
• Have patient swallow capsules whole; don't break or open capsules.
• Don't give additional dose if vomiting occurs; continue with dosing schedule.
• If a dose is missed, give dose as soon as possible and at least 8 hours before next scheduled dose. Resume normal schedule the next day.
• Store at 68° to 77° F (20° to 25° C).

ACTION
Inhibits mutated IDH1, which decreases the level of 2-hydroxyglutarate in leukemia cells and restores normal cell differentiation.

Route	Onset	Peak	Duration
PO	Unknown	4 hr	Unknown

Half-life: 67 hours.

ADVERSE REACTIONS
CNS: fatigue, fever, headache, malaise. **CV:** edema, HTN. **GI:** abdominal pain, constipation, decreased appetite, diarrhea, gallbladder disorders, mucositis, nausea, vomiting. **GU:** increased creatinine. **Hematologic:** increased lymphocytes, leukocytosis. **Hepatic:** *liver toxicity,* increased ALP, increased bilirubin, increased transaminase. **Metabolic:** *hypokalemia,* hyponatremia, hypophosphatemia, increased lipase, increased uric acid. **Musculoskeletal:** arthralgia. **Respiratory:** cough, dyspnea. **Skin:** rash. **Other:** *differentiation syndrome.*

INTERACTIONS
Drug-drug. *Moderate or strong CYP3A inducers (dexamethasone, phenytoin, rifampin):* May decrease olutasidenib level. Avoid use together.
Sensitive CYP3A substrates (digoxin, sirolimus): May decrease substrate level. Avoid use together. If concomitant use can't be avoided, monitor for loss of therapeutic effect of substrate.

EFFECTS ON LAB TEST RESULTS
• May increase WBC and lymphocyte counts.
• May increase transaminase, ALP, creatinine, uric acid, lipase, and bilirubin levels.

Reactions in bold italics are *life-threatening.*

- May decrease potassium, sodium, and phosphorus levels.

CONTRAINDICATIONS & CAUTIONS
- Drug may increase risk of liver toxicity. Use cautiously in patients with Child-Pugh class A or B liver impairment. Use in patients with Child-Pugh class C liver impairment hasn't been established.
- Safety and effectiveness in children haven't been established.
- Older adults are at increased risk for liver toxicity and HTN.
Dialyzable drug: Unknown.

PREGNANCY-LACTATION-REPRODUCTION
- Drug may cause fetal harm.
- It isn't known if drug appears in human milk or how drug affects milk production or infants who are breastfed.
- Patient shouldn't breastfeed during therapy and for 2 weeks after final dose.

NURSING CONSIDERATIONS
- Ensure that FDA-approved testing has confirmed the presence of mutated IDH1 in blood or bone marrow before starting drug.
- **Alert:** Monitor blood counts and blood chemistry results, including LFTs, before therapy, once weekly for first 2 months; once every other week for 3rd month; once for 4th month, and once every other month for the duration of therapy. Correct any abnormalities as clinically indicated.
- Monitor for signs and symptoms of liver dysfunction (fatigue, anorexia, abdominal discomfort, dark urine, jaundice).
- **Boxed Warning** Differentiation syndrome, which can be fatal, can occur. Monitor patient for signs and symptoms (leukocytosis, dyspnea, pulmonary infiltrates, pleuropericardial effusion, kidney injury, fever, edema, weight gain). If differentiation syndrome is suspected, withhold drug and initiate corticosteroids and hemodynamic monitoring until symptoms resolve. ∎
- **Alert:** If leukocytosis occurs with differentiation syndrome, initiate treatment with hydroxyurea, as clinically indicated. Taper corticosteroids and hydroxyurea after symptoms resolve.
- **Alert:** Differentiation syndrome may recur with premature discontinuation of corticosteroids or hydroxyurea treatment. Institute supportive measures and hemodynamic monitoring until improvement occurs; withhold dose of olutasidenib and consider dosage reduction based on recurrence.

PATIENT TEACHING
Boxed Warning Advise patient of risk of differentiation syndrome, which can occur as early as 1 day after starting drug and up to 18 months after. Instruct patient to immediately report fever, cough, difficulty breathing, decreased urinary output, low blood pressure, weight gain, or swelling of arms or legs. ∎

- Teach about proper drug administration and handling.
- Warn that drug may cause fetal harm. Advise pregnant patient of potential risk to fetus.
- Tell patient not to breastfeed during therapy and for 2 weeks after final dose.
- Instruct patient to report GI reactions (nausea, constipation, diarrhea, vomiting, abdominal pain, mucositis).
- Instruct patient to immediately report signs and symptoms of liver impairment (right upper abdominal discomfort, dark urine, jaundice, anorexia, fatigue).

SAFETY ALERT!

omaveloxolone ▧
oh-ma-vel-OX-oh-lone

Skyclarys

Therapeutic class: Miscellaneous CNS drugs
Pharmacologic class: Nuclear factor (erythroid-derived 2) activators

AVAILABLE FORMS
Capsules ⊙NC: 50 mg

INDICATIONS & DOSAGES
➤ **Friedreich ataxia** ▧
Adults and adolescents ages 16 and older: 150 mg PO once daily.
Adjust-a-dose: If given with strong CYP3A4 inhibitor, reduce omaveloxolone dosage to 50 mg once daily. If given with moderate CYP3A4 inhibitor and for patients with Child-Pugh class B liver impairment, reduce omaveloxolone dosage to 100 mg once daily. If adverse reactions occur, further decrease dosage to 50 mg once daily. Discontinue if adverse reactions occur at 50-mg dose.

ADMINISTRATION
PO
- Give drug on an empty stomach 1 hour before a meal.
- Have patient swallow capsules whole; don't break or open capsules.
- If a dose is missed, give next dose as scheduled the following day. Don't make up for a missed dose.
- Store drug at room temperature.

ACTION
Exact mechanism unknown. Thought to activate the nuclear factor (erythroid-derived 2)-like pathway, which is involved in the cellular response to oxidative stress.

Route	Onset	Peak	Duration
PO	Unknown	7–14 hr	Unknown

Half-life: 57 hours.

NEW DRUGS

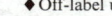

ADVERSE REACTIONS

CNS: fatigue, headache. **CV:** increased B-type natriuretic peptide (BNP) level. **EENT:** oropharyngeal pain. **GI:** abdominal pain, decreased appetite, diarrhea, nausea, vomiting. **Hepatic:** increased liver enzyme levels. **Metabolic:** increased LDL-level, decreased HDL-level. **Musculoskeletal:** back pain, musculoskeletal pain, spasms. **Skin:** rash. **Other:** flulike syndrome.

INTERACTIONS

Drug-drug. *BCRP and OATP1B1 substrates (rosuvastatin), CYP2C8 substrates (repaglinide), CYP3A4 substrates (midazolam):* May decrease substrate level and effectiveness.
Hormonal contraceptives (pill, patch, ring, implant, and progestin-only pill): May decrease contraceptive effectiveness. Avoid use together.
Strong or moderate CYP3A4 inducers: May decrease omaveloxolone level and effectiveness. Avoid use together.
Strong or moderate CYP3A4 inhibitors: May increase omaveloxolone level. Avoid use together. If use together can't be avoided, reduce omaveloxolone dose.
Drug-herb. *St. John's wort:* May decrease omaveloxolone level. Discourage use together.
Drug-food. *Grapefruit, grapefruit juice:* May increase omaveloxolone level. Discourage use together.

EFFECTS ON LAB TEST RESULTS

• May increase ALT, AST, bilirubin, BNP, and LDL-C levels.
• May decrease HDL-C level.

CONTRAINDICATIONS & CAUTIONS

• May worsen cardiac function. Use cautiously in patients with HF or cardiac disease.
• Avoid use in patients with Child-Pugh class C liver impairment.
• Safety and effectiveness in children younger than age 16 haven't been established.
Dialyzable drug: Unknown.

PREGNANCY-LACTATION-REPRODUCTION

• Based on animal studies, drug may cause fetal harm. Avoid use during pregnancy.
• It isn't known if drug appears in human milk or how drug affects milk production or infants who are breastfed. Use only if benefits to patient outweigh risk to infant.
• May decrease efficacy of hormonal contraceptives. Patient of childbearing potential should use an alternative contraceptive method or additional nonhormonal contraceptive (condoms) during therapy and for 28 days after final dose.

NURSING CONSIDERATIONS

• Obtain baseline ALT, AST, and total bilirubin levels. Monitor monthly for first 3 months and periodically thereafter. If transaminase levels

increase to greater than 5 times ULN, or greater than 3 times ULN with evidence of liver dysfunction (elevated bilirubin level), immediately discontinue drug and repeat LFTs as soon as possible. If transaminase levels stabilize or resolve, drug may be restarted with appropriate monitoring.
• Obtain baseline BNP level. Monitor patient for signs and symptoms of fluid overload. If signs and symptoms develop, worsen, or require hospitalization, evaluate BNP and cardiac function and manage appropriately.
• Assess lipid levels at baseline and periodically during therapy. Manage lipid abnormalities as clinically indicated.
• *Look alike-sound alike:* Don't confuse omaveloxolone with oxandrolone. Don't confuse Skyclarys with Skyrizi.

PATIENT TEACHING

• Teach about proper drug administration and handling.
• Inform patient that blood tests will be needed periodically during therapy.
• Advise patient to report signs and symptoms of fluid overload (weight gain of 3 lb [1.4 kg] or more in 1 day or 5 lb [2.3 kg] or more in 1 week, peripheral edema, palpitations, shortness of breath).
• Counsel patient that increases in LDL-C and decreases in HDL-C can occur and may require treatment.
• Tell patient to report use of all prescription and OTC medications, herbal products, and supplements.
• Advise patient to report pregnancy or plans to become pregnant or breastfeed during therapy.
• Instruct patient of childbearing potential to use nonhormonal contraceptive during therapy and for 28 days after final dose.

omidenepag isopropyl
oh-mi-DEN-e-pag

Omlonti

Therapeutic class: Anti-glaucoma drugs–antihypertensives
Pharmacologic class: Selective prostaglandin E2 receptor agonists

AVAILABLE FORMS

Ophthalmic solution: 0.002% (0.02 mg/mL)

INDICATIONS & DOSAGES

➤ **Reduction of elevated IOP in patients with open-angle glaucoma or ocular HTN**
Adults: Instill 1 drop in affected eye(s) once daily in the evening.

ADMINISTRATION

Ophthalmic
• Gently shake the bottle.

Reactions in bold italics are *life-threatening.*

• Separate dose by at least 5 minutes from other topical ophthalmic drugs.
• Have patient remove contact lenses before dose; may reinsert 15 minutes after dose.
• Don't touch tip of dropper to any surface, including eye.
• Refrigerate drug at 36° to 46° F (2° to 8° C) before use. Once opened, store at room temperature for up to 31 days.

ACTION
Unknown. A prostaglandin receptor agonist that decreases IOP.

Route	Onset	Peak	Duration
Ophthalmic	Unknown	10–15 min	Unknown

Half-life: Unknown.

ADVERSE REACTIONS
CNS: headache. **EENT:** blurred vision, conjunctival hyperemia, dry eye, eye irritation, eye pain, instillation site pain, ocular hyperemia, photophobia, punctate keratitis, visual impairment.

INTERACTIONS
None reported.

EFFECTS ON LAB TEST RESULTS
None reported.

CONTRAINDICATIONS & CAUTIONS
• Drug may cause irreversible increase in brown pigmentation of iris. This effect may not be noticeable for months to years.
• Drug may gradually change eyelashes and vellus hair in treated eye (increased length, thickness, and number of lashes or hairs). These effects are usually reversible on discontinuation.
• Ocular inflammation has been reported. Use with caution in patients with active ocular inflammation, including iritis or uveitis.
• Macular edema has been reported. Use with caution in patients with aphakic or pseudophakic glaucoma and in patients with risk factors for macular edema.
Dialyzable drug: Not likely.

PREGNANCY-LACTATION-REPRODUCTION
• Studies during pregnancy are inadequate. Use cautiously during pregnancy.
• It isn't known if drug appears in human milk or how drug affects milk production or infants who are breastfed. Systemic exposure to omidenepag after topical ocular administration is low.

NURSING CONSIDERATIONS
• Monitor patient for changes in eyelashes, vellus hair, and pigmentation of iris and eyelid of treated eye.
• Monitor patient for ocular inflammation.
• Monitor patient for macular edema.

PATIENT TEACHING
• Teach about proper drug administration and handling.
• Advise patient not to touch tip of dropper to eye or surrounding tissue because doing so may contaminate the solution.
• Inform patient about potential for increased brown pigmentation of iris and eyelid.
• Alert patient to possibility of eyelash and vellus hair changes in treated eye, which can result in differences between eyes in eyelash and vellus hair length, thickness, and number and direction of eyelash growth. Explain that eyelash changes usually reverse after stopping drug.
• Tell patient to immediately report a new ocular condition (trauma, infection, inflammation), sudden decrease in visual acuity, ocular surgery, or any ocular reactions, particularly conjunctivitis or eyelid reactions.

SAFETY ALERT!

perfluorohexyloctane
per-floor-oh-hex-il-OK-tane

Miebo

Therapeutic class: Miscellaneous ophthalmic drugs
Pharmacologic class: Semifluorinated alkanes

AVAILABLE FORMS
Ophthalmic solution: 100% multidose bottles

INDICATIONS & DOSAGES
➤ **Dry eye disease**
Adults: Instill 1 drop q.i.d. into affected eye(s).

ADMINISTRATION
Ophthalmic
• Instruct patient to remove contact lenses before instilling drug. Wait at least 30 minutes after administration before reinserting contact lenses.
• Remove cap from dropper bottle, hold bottle upright, and gently squeeze.
• While squeezing, turn bottle upside down and release pressure (drawing air into bottle). Squeeze again to release a drop into eye.
• Repeat for other affected eye, if applicable.
• Don't touch tip of bottle to eye or surrounding tissue.
• After opening, drug may be used until expiration date on bottle.
• Don't use drug if solution is discolored or cloudy.
• Store drug at 68° to 77° F (20° to 25° C).

ACTION
Exact mechanism is unknown. Forms a monolayer at the air-liquid interface of tear film, which may reduce evaporation.

NEW DRUGS

Route	Onset	Peak	Duration
Ophthalmic	Unknown	Unknown	Unknown

Half-life: Unknown.

ADVERSE REACTIONS
EENT: blurred vision, conjunctival redness.

INTERACTIONS
• None reported.

CONTRAINDICATIONS & CAUTIONS
• Safety and effectiveness in children haven't been established.
Dialyzable drug: Unknown.

PREGNANCY-LACTATION-REPRODUCTION
• Studies during pregnancy are inadequate. Use cautiously during pregnancy.
• It isn't known if drug appears in human milk or how drug affects milk production or infants who are breastfed. Use cautiously during breastfeeding.

NURSING CONSIDERATIONS
• Monitor patient for conjunctival irritation and blurred vision.

PATIENT TEACHING
• Teach about proper drug administration and handling.
• Inform patient that blurred vision may occur after instilling drops.

SAFETY ALERT!

pirtobrutinib
pir-toe-BROO-ti-nib

Jaypirca

Therapeutic class: Antineoplastics
Pharmacologic class: Kinase inhibitors

AVAILABLE FORMS
Tablets 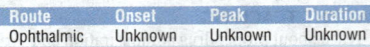: 50 mg, 100 mg

INDICATIONS & DOSAGES
➤ **Relapsed or refractory mantle cell lymphoma after at least two lines of systemic therapy, including Bruton tyrosine kinase (BTK) inhibitor**
Adults: 200 mg PO once daily until disease progresses or unacceptable toxicity occurs.
Adjust-a-dose: Refer to manufacturer's instructions for toxicity-related dosage adjustments. If severe kidney impairment occurs (eGFR 15 to 29 mL/minute) and current dosage is 200 mg once daily, reduce to 100 mg once daily; otherwise reduce dosage by 50 mg. If current dose is 50 mg once daily, discontinue drug. If concomitant use of a strong CYP3A inhibitor is unavoidable, reduce pirtobrutinib dose by 50 mg. If current dose is 50 mg once

daily, interrupt pirtobrutinib therapy for duration of strong CYP3A inhibitor use. After discontinuation of strong CYP3A inhibitor for five half-lives, resume pirtobrutinib dosage taken before initiating inhibitor. If concomitant use with a moderate CYP3A inducer is unavoidable and current dosage of pirtobrutinib is 200 mg once daily, increase to 300 mg once daily. If current pirtobrutinib dosage is 50 mg or 100 mg once daily, increase by 50 mg.

ADMINISTRATION
PO
• Give at approximately the same time each day without regard to food.
• Have patient swallow tablets whole with water; don't open or cut tablets.
• If a dose is missed by more than 12 hours, don't make up the dose. Give next dose as scheduled.
• Store at room temperature.

ACTION
Inhibits BTK activity and results in decreased B-cell proliferation.

Route	Onset	Peak	Duration
PO	Unknown	2 hr	Unknown

Half-life: 19 hours.

ADVERSE REACTIONS
CNS: dizziness, fatigue, fever, peripheral neuropathy. **CV:** atrial fibrillation, atrial flutter, edema, *hemorrhage.* **GI:** abdominal pain, constipation, diarrhea, nausea. **GU:** increased creatinine. **Hematologic:** anemia, bruising, *lymphocytopenia, neutropenia, thrombocytopenia,* transient lymphocytosis. **Hepatic:** increased transaminase, increased ALP. **Metabolic:** *hyperkalemia, hypocalcemia, hypokalemia,* hyponatremia, increased lipase. **Musculoskeletal:** arthralgia, arthritis, musculoskeletal pain. **Respiratory:** cough, dyspnea, pleural effusion, pneumonia, URI. **Skin:** rash. **Other:** infection, *second primary malignancy, sepsis.*

INTERACTIONS
Drug-drug. *Antithrombotic agents (apixaban, heparin, warfarin):* May increase risk of bleeding. Use together cautiously.
Sensitive CYP2C8 (repaglinide), CYP2C19 (omeprazole), CYP3A (midazolam), P-gp (digoxin), or BCRP (rosuvastatin) substrates: May increase sensitive substrate level and risk of substrate-related adverse reactions. Refer to sensitive substrate product label for additional information.
Strong CYP3A inhibitors (itraconazole): May increase pirtobrutinib level and risk of adverse reactions. Avoid use together. If concomitant use is unavoidable, reduce pirtobrutinib dose.
Strong or moderate CYP3A inducers (bosentan, efavirenz, rifampin): May decrease pirtobrutinib level and efficacy. Avoid use together. If concomitant use is unavoidable, increase pirtobrutinib dose.

Drug-lifestyle. *Sunlight:* May increase risk of new skin cancer or other cancers. Advise patient to use sun protection.

EFFECTS ON LAB TEST RESULTS
- May increase creatinine, ALT, AST, ALP, lipase, and calcium levels.
- May increase or decrease potassium level.
- May decrease Hb and sodium levels.
- May decrease platelet and neutrophil counts.
- May increase or decrease lymphocyte count.

CONTRAINDICATIONS & CAUTIONS
⚠ *Alert:* Fatal and serious bacterial, viral, fungal, and opportunistic infections have occurred. Consider prophylaxis (vaccinations, antimicrobials) in patients at increased risk for infections.
⚠ *Alert:* Drug may cause fatal and serious hemorrhage. Consider withholding drug for 3 to 7 days before and after surgery, depending on type of surgery and risk of bleeding.
- Use cautiously in patients with cardiac risk factors (HTN, previous arrhythmias). Drug may increase risk of developing atrial fibrillation or flutter.
- Use cautiously in older adults.
- Safety and effectiveness in children haven't been established.
Dialyzable drug: Unlikely.

PREGNANCY-LACTATION-REPRODUCTION
- Based on animal studies, drug can cause fetal harm.
- Females of childbearing potential should use effective contraception during therapy and for 1 week after final dose.
- It isn't known if drug appears in human milk or how drug affects milk production or infants who are breastfed. Patient shouldn't breastfeed during therapy and for 1 week after final dose.

NURSING CONSIDERATIONS
- Monitor for signs and symptoms of infection.
- Monitor for signs and symptoms of bleeding.
- Regularly monitor CBC during therapy.
- Monitor for signs and symptoms of arrhythmias (palpitations, dizziness, syncope, chest discomfort, dyspnea).
- Monitor for development of second primary malignancies.
- Verify pregnancy status in patient of childbearing potential before initiating drug.
- *Look alike-sound alike:* Don't confuse pirtobrutinib with acalabrutinib, ibrutinib, or zanubrutinib. Don't confuse Jaypirca with Jakafi.

PATIENT TEACHING
- Teach about proper drug administration and handling.
- Explain risk of fatal and serious hemorrhage. Instruct patient to watch for signs of bleeding (bleeding gums, nosebleeds).

- Tell patient that drug may need to be interrupted for major surgeries.
- Advise patient of need for periodic monitoring of blood counts during therapy.
- Counsel patient to report signs and symptoms of arrhythmias.
⚠ *Alert:* Warn patient that other malignancies (including skin cancer other solid tumors) have occurred in patients treated with drug. Tell patient to use sun protection and to monitor for development of other cancers.
- Advise patient of childbearing potential of fetal risk. Tell patient to use effective contraception during therapy and for 1 week after final dose.
- Warn patient not to breastfeed during therapy and for 1 week after final dose.

ritlecitinib
rit-le-SYE-ti-nib

Litfulo

Therapeutic class: Immunosuppressants
Pharmacologic class: Janus kinase (JAK) inhibitors

AVAILABLE FORMS
Tablets ⓄⓃⒸ: 50 mg

INDICATIONS & DOSAGES
➤ **Severe alopecia areata**
Adults and children ages 12 and older: 50 mg PO once daily.
Adjust-a-dose: Discontinue drug if platelet count is less than 50,000/mm³ or absolute lymphocyte count (ALC) is less than 500 cells/mm³. May restart once ALC returns above this value.

ADMINISTRATION
PO
- Give drug without regard to food.
- Have patient swallow capsules whole; don't crush or break capsules.
- Give a missed dose as soon as possible unless next dose is less than 8 hours away; then skip missed dose and give next dose at its scheduled time.
- Store drug at 68° to 77° F (20° to 25° C).

ACTION
Irreversibly inhibits JAK 3 and tyrosine kinase. Also inhibits signaling of immune receptors.

Route	Onset	Peak	Duration
PO	Unknown	1 hr	Unknown

Half-life: 1.3 to 2.3 hours.

ADVERSE REACTIONS
CNS: dizziness, fever, headache. **GI:** diarrhea, stomatitis. **Hematologic:** decreased RBC count. **Metabolic:** increased CK level. **Skin:** acne, atopic

NEW DRUGS

dermatitis, folliculitis, rash, urticaria. **Other:** herpes zoster, infection.

INTERACTIONS
Drug-drug. *CYP1A2 substrates (clozapine, theophylline, zolpidem), CYP3A substrates (midazolam):* Increases substrate level and risk of adverse reactions. Monitor substrate closely, and adjust substrate dosage as needed.
CYP3A inducers (rifampin): May decrease ritlecitinib level. Avoid use together.
JAK inhibitors, biologic immunomodulators, potent immunosuppressants (cyclosporine): May enhance adverse reactions of immunosuppressants. Avoid use together.
Live-virus vaccines: May increase risk of vaccine-associated infection and diminish vaccine's effect. Avoid live vaccines just before and during therapy.
Drug-food. *Caffeine*: May increase risk of adverse reactions to caffeine. Advise patient to avoid or minimize use of caffeine.

EFFECTS ON LAB TEST RESULTS
• May increase CK, ALT, and AST levels.
• May decrease RBC, lymphocyte, and platelet counts.

CONTRAINDICATIONS & CAUTIONS
• Contraindicated in patients with known hypersensitivity to drug or its components. Hypersensitivity reactions (anaphylaxis, urticaria, rash) have been reported.
Boxed Warning Drug increases risk of bacterial, fungal, viral, and opportunistic infections, which can lead to hospitalization and death. Interrupt therapy for serious infection until infection is controlled. ■
Boxed Warning Drug shouldn't be given to patients with active TB. Avoid use in patients with active, serious infections. ■
• Use cautiously in patients who have chronic or recurrent infections, have been exposed to TB, have history of serious infection or opportunistic infection, have resided in or traveled to areas with endemic TB or mycoses, or have underlying conditions that may predispose them to infection.
• Viral reactivation, including herpes zoster, has occurred.
Boxed Warning Research shows that, in patients with RA, the risk of all-cause mortality, including sudden CV death and major adverse CV events (MI, stroke), was higher in patients treated with another JAK inhibitor than in those treated with TNF blockers. Drug isn't approved for use in patients with RA. ■
• Use cautiously in patients who are current or former smokers and those with other CV risk factors.
Boxed Warning Malignancies have occurred in patients treated with drug. In patients with RA, rates of lymphoma and lung cancer were higher in patients treated with another JAK inhibitor than in those treated with TNF blockers. ■

• Nonmelanoma skin cancer has occurred. Use cautiously in patients with known malignancy other than successfully treated nonmelanoma skin cancer or cervical cancer. Patients who currently smoke or previously smoked may be at increased risk for malignancy.
Boxed Warning Thrombosis has occurred in patients treated with drug. The incidence of PE and venous and arterial thrombosis was higher in patients treated with another JAK inhibitor than in those treated with TNF blockers. Avoid use in patients who are at increased risk for thrombosis. ■
• Use of drug isn't recommended in patients with Child-Pugh class C liver impairment, hepatitis B, or hepatitis C.
• Safety and effectiveness in children younger than age 12 haven't been established.
• Use cautiously in older adults.
Dialyzable drug: Unknown.
⚠ *Overdose S&S:* Extension of immunosuppressive and adverse effects.

PREGNANCY-LACTATION-REPRODUCTION
• Studies during pregnancy are inadequate. It isn't known if drug causes fetal harm.
• Report patients who are exposed to drug during pregnancy to Pfizer's pregnancy exposure registry (1-877-390-2940).
• It isn't known if drug appears in human milk, but drug is present in animal milk. Advise patient to avoid breastfeeding during therapy and for 14 hours after final dose.

NURSING CONSIDERATIONS
Boxed Warning Test patient for latent TB before and during therapy; treat latent TB before initiating drug. Monitor all patients for active TB during therapy, even patients with initial negative latent TB test. ■
• Obtain ALC and platelet counts before therapy, at 4 weeks, and routinely during therapy.
• Screen patient for viral hepatitis before therapy.
• Monitor LFT results at baseline and routinely during therapy. If drug-induced liver injury is suspected, interrupt drug until diagnosis is excluded.
• Monitor for development of thrombosis and embolism. If signs or symptoms occur, interrupt therapy and treat as clinically appropriate.
• Discontinue drug in patients who experience stroke or MI.
• Evaluate infection risk before therapy, and monitor for signs and symptoms of infection during therapy. If patient develops infection, interrupt therapy and evaluate for immunocompromised state.
• Perform periodic skin exams in patient at increased risk for skin cancer.
• Ensure that patient's immunizations, including prophylactic herpes zoster, are current before starting drug.
• Monitor patient for hypersensitivity reaction. Discontinue drug if reaction occurs.

• *Look alike-sound alike:* Don't confuse ritleci-tinib with other kinase inhibitors or other drugs that end in "-nib."

PATIENT TEACHING

◊ *Alert:* Instruct patient to report signs or symptoms of infection. Review increased risk of herpes zoster during therapy.

◊ *Alert:* Warn that drug may cause blood clots in lungs and eyes. Instruct patient to seek immediate medical attention if vision changes or shortness of breath occurs.

◊ *Alert:* Inform patient that drug may increase risk of major adverse CV events, including MI, stroke, and CV death.

◊ *Alert:* Warn that drug may increase risk of certain cancers, including skin cancer. Tell patient to obtain periodic skin exams during therapy.

◊ *Alert:* Instruct patient to stop drug and seek immediate medical attention if signs or symptoms of allergic reaction (rash, hives, difficulty breathing, throat tightness) occur.

• Teach about proper drug administration and handling.

• Inform patient that blood tests are required before and during therapy.

• Counsel patient to avoid live-virus vaccines before and during therapy. Instruct patient to alert all health care providers about current therapy with ritlecitinib.

• Advise patient to report pregnancy or plans to become pregnant or breastfeed during therapy.

• Advise patient not to breastfeed during therapy and for 14 hours after final dose.

• Counsel patient that temporary drug interruption (less than 6 weeks) isn't expected to result in significant loss of regrown scalp hair.

sodium phenylbutyrate–taurursodiol
SOE-dee-um fen-il-BYOO-ti-rate–taur-ur-so-DYE-ol

Albrioza✤, Relyvrio

Therapeutic class: Miscellaneous CNS drugs
Pharmacologic class: Histone deacetylase inhibitors, hydrophilic bile acids

AVAILABLE FORMS
Oral suspension: 3 g sodium phenylbutyrate and 1 g taurursodiol in single-dose packet

INDICATIONS & DOSAGES
➤ **ALS**
Adults: Initially, 1 packet PO daily for 3 weeks. Then increase to maintenance dosage, 1 packet b.i.d.

ADMINISTRATION
PO
• Give drug before snack or meal.
• Empty contents of 1 packet into 8 oz of room temperature water and stir vigorously.
• Give PO within 1 hour of preparation. Alternatively, give via feeding tube.
• Discard unused suspension after 1 hour.
• Store at room temperature. Protect from moisture.

ACTION
Unknown.

Route	Onset	Peak	Duration
PO sodium phenylbutyrate	Unknown	0.5 hr	Unknown
PO taurursodiol	Unknown	4.5 hr	Unknown

Half-life: Sodium phenylbutyrate: 0.46 hour; taurursodiol: 4.34 hours.

ADVERSE REACTIONS
CNS: dizziness, fatigue. **EENT:** salivary hypersecretion. **GI:** abdominal pain, diarrhea, nausea. **Respiratory:** URI.

INTERACTIONS
Drug-drug. *Aluminum-based antacids:* May interfere with taurursodiol absorption. Avoid use together; consider other acid-lowering agents.
Bile acid sequestering agents (cholestyramine, colesevelam, colestipol): May decrease taurursodiol absorption. Avoid use together. Consider alternative cholesterol-lowering agents.
CYP1A2, CYP2B6, CYP3A4 substrates (aminophylline, bupropion, ramelteon): May decrease substrate level. Avoid use together when a small change in substrate plasma level may lead to serious toxicities or loss of efficacy.
CYP2B6 and CYP2C8 substrates (repaglinide): May increase substrate level. Avoid use together when a small change in substrate plasma level may lead to serious toxicities or loss of efficacy.
Histone deacetylase (HDAC) inhibitor (phenylbutyrate): May increase risk of adverse effects. Avoid use of other HDAC inhibitors due to additive effects.
Inhibitors of bile acid transporters (cyclosporine): May exacerbate accumulation of conjugated bile salts in liver and result in clinical symptoms. Avoid use together; if concomitant use is necessary, use caution and monitor serum transaminase and bilirubin levels.
OAT1 substrates (adefovir, statins, tenofovir): May increase substrate level. Avoid use together.
OATP1B3 inhibitors (pioglitazone, rifampicin): May increase taurursodiol level. Avoid use together.
P-gP and BCRP substrates (digoxin, methotrexate, rosuvastatin): May increase substrate level. Avoid use together when a small change in substrate level may lead to serious toxicities or loss of efficacy.
Probenecid: May affect kidney excretion of sodium phenylbutyrate metabolites. Avoid use together.

NEW DRUGS

Strong CYP3A4 inducers (phenytoin, rifampin): May decrease taurursodiol level. Monitor use together.

EFFECTS ON LAB TEST RESULTS
May increase sodium level.

CONTRAINDICATIONS & CAUTIONS
• Avoid use in patients with moderate or severe kidney or liver impairment.
• Use cautiously in patients with disorders that interfere with bile acid circulation, disorders of enterohepatic circulation (biliary infection, active cholecystitis), severe pancreatic disorders (pancreatitis), and intestinal disorders that may alter concentrations of bile acids (ileal resection, regional ileitis).
• Use cautiously in patients with conditions sensitive to sodium intake, such HF, kidney disease or kidney failure, and other conditions associated with sodium retention.
• Safety and effectiveness in children haven't been established.
Dialyzable drug: Unknown.

PREGNANCY-LACTATION-REPRODUCTION
Studies during pregnancy are inadequate.
It isn't known if drug appears in human milk or how drug affects milk production or infants who are breastfed. Weigh benefit to patient against possible risk to infant.

NURSING CONSIDERATIONS
• Consult specialist for patient with a disorder that interferes with bile acid circulation.
• Monitor patient for new or worsening diarrhea.
• In patient who is sensitive to high sodium intake, consider total daily sodium intake and monitor patient appropriately. Each packet contains 464 mg of sodium.

PATIENT TEACHING
• Teach about proper drug administration and handling.
• Advise patient to report new or worsening diarrhea.
• Caution patient who is sensitive to sodium to limit sodium intake while taking drug.
• Advise patient to report pregnancy or plans to become pregnant or breastfeed during therapy.

SAFETY ALERT!

sotagliflozin
soe-ta-gli-FLOE-zin

Inpefa

Therapeutic class: Antidiabetics
Pharmacologic class: Sodium-glucose
cotransporter (SGLT) 2 inhibitors

AVAILABLE FORMS
Tablets ⬤⬤⬤: 200 mg, 400 mg

INDICATIONS & DOSAGES
➤ **Reduction of risk of CV death, hospitalization for HF, and urgent visits in patients with HF or type 2 diabetes, CKD, and other CV risk factors**
Adults: 200 mg PO daily. After 2 weeks, may increase to 400 mg PO once daily, as tolerated.
Adjust-a-dose: Decrease to 200 mg PO daily as necessary based on tolerance.

ADMINISTRATION
PO
• Give drug within 1 hour before first meal of the day.
• Have patient swallow tablets whole; don't crush or cut tablets.
• If a dose is missed by more than 6 hours, skip missed dose and resume normal schedule the next day.
• Store drug at 68° to 77° F (20° to 25° C).

ACTION
An inhibitor of SGLT2 that reduces kidney reabsorption of glucose and sodium to lower cardiac preload and afterload and down-regulate sympathetic activity. An inhibitor of SGLT1 that reduces intestinal absorption of glucose and sodium.

Route	Onset	Peak	Duration
PO	Unknown	1.25 to 4 hr	Unknown

Half-life: 21 to 35 hours.

ADVERSE REACTIONS
CNS: dizziness. **GI:** diarrhea. **GU:** genital mycotic infection, UTI. **Metabolic:** *diabetic ketoacidosis (DKA),* hypoglycemia, volume depletion.

INTERACTIONS
Drug-drug. *Digoxin:* May increase digoxin level. Monitor digoxin level.
Insulin, insulin secretagogues: May increase risk of hypoglycemia. Monitor glucose level, and reduce insulin or insulin secretagogue dosage as needed.
Lithium: May decrease lithium level. Frequently monitor lithium level during initiation of sotagliflozin and with changes in therapy.
Loop diuretics (furosemide, torsemide): May increase risk of volume depletion. Use together cautiously.
Rifampin: May decrease sotagliflozin level. Monitor for clinical effect.
Drug-food. *All food:* May increase sotagliflozin level. Instruct patient to take drug no more than 1 hour before first meal of the day.

EFFECTS ON LAB TEST RESULTS
• May decrease eGFR.
• May increase creatinine level.
• May increase urine glucose level.
• Interferes with 1,5-AG assay for monitoring glucose level.

NEW DRUGS

CONTRAINDICATIONS & CAUTIONS

• Contraindicated in patients with history of serious hypersensitivity reaction to drug or its components.

• Use of drug isn't recommended in patients with Child-Pugh class B or C liver impairment.

• Use cautiously in patients with risk factors for ketoacidosis (history of pancreatitis, pancreatic surgery, acute febrile illness, reduced caloric intake, ketogenic diet, surgery, insulin dose reduction, volume depletion, or alcohol abuse).

• Patients with eGFR less than 60 mL/minute/ 1.73 m², older adults, and patients taking loop diuretics may be at increased risk for volume depletion (may manifest as symptomatic hypotension or acute transient changes in creatinine).

• Drug may increase risk of DKA. Blood glucose level may be lower than typically expected for DKA (less than 250 mg/dL).

• Drug may increase risk of serious UTIs, including pyelonephritis and urosepsis, and Fournier gangrene (rare but serious necrotizing fasciitis of the perineum).

• Safety and effectiveness in patients with eGFR less than 25 mL/minute/1.73 m² and those on dialysis haven't been established.

• Safety and effectiveness in children younger than 18 years haven't been established.

Dialyzable drug: Unknown.

PREGNANCY-LACTATION-REPRODUCTION

• Studies during pregnancy are inadequate. Based on animal studies, use of drug isn't recommended during second and third trimesters.

• It isn't known if drug appears in human milk or how drug affects milk production or infants who are breastfed. Breastfeeding during therapy isn't recommended.

NURSING CONSIDERATIONS

• Assess volume status and correct volume depletion before start of therapy.

• Assess kidney function at baseline and as indicated. Monitor for signs and symptoms of hypotension. Changes in creatinine and eGFR generally occur within 4 weeks of starting therapy and then stabilize. Evaluate changes that don't fit this pattern.

• For patient with decompensated HF, begin dosing as soon as patient is hemodynamically stable.

• Consider ketone monitoring in patient with type 1 diabetes and in patient at risk for ketoacidosis.

• Assess for ketoacidosis regardless of blood glucose level in patient with signs and symptoms of severe metabolic acidosis (nausea, vomiting, abdominal pain, malaise, shortness of breath, glycosuria, hyperglycemia). If ketoacidosis is suspected, discontinue drug and treat as clinically indicated. Ensure ketoacidosis resolves before restarting drug.

• Withhold drug, if possible, in situations that could predispose patient to ketoacidosis. Restart when patient is clinically stable and has resumed oral intake.

• Withhold drug for at least 3 days, if possible, before major surgery or procedures associated with prolonged fasting. Restart when patient is clinically stable and has resumed oral intake.

• Monitor patient for signs and symptoms of UTI and genital mycotic infections. Treat as clinically indicated.

• Assess patient with pain, tenderness, erythema, swelling in genital or perineal area, fever, or malaise for necrotizing fasciitis. If suspected, treat with broad-spectrum antibiotics and, if necessary, surgical debridement. Discontinue drug, monitor blood glucose level, and provide appropriate alternative therapy for HF.

• *Look alike–sound alike:* Don't confuse sotagliflozin with sotalol or other drugs that end in "-flozin."

PATIENT TEACHING

• Teach about proper drug administration and handling.

• **Alert:** Inform patient that drug can increase risk of life-threatening DKA. Review precipitating factors and signs and symptoms of ketoacidosis.

• Explain that blood glucose level may be normal even in presence of ketoacidosis and that monitoring for ketones may be necessary. Instruct patient to stop drug and seek medical attention if signs or symptoms of ketoacidosis occur.

• Inform patient that urine will test positive for glucose during therapy.

• Review importance of diet, exercise, and monitoring of blood glucose and HbA₁c levels.

• Teach about signs and symptoms of hypoglycemia and hyperglycemia, their management, and importance of monitoring for diabetes complications.

• Advise patient to seek medical advice during periods of stress (fever, trauma, infection, surgery) because medication requirements may change.

• Tell patient to report symptoms of hypotension to health care provider.

• Explain that dehydration may increase the risk of hypotension. Encourage patient to maintain adequate fluid intake.

• Teach about risk of UTI. Advise patient to seek medical attention if signs or symptoms occur.

• Explain that the risk of hypoglycemia increases when drug is used with insulin and that a lower insulin dosage may be required.

• Warn that necrotizing fasciitis of the perineum has occurred in patients with diabetes. Instruct patient to promptly seek medical attention if fever above 100.4° F (38° C); malaise; or pain, tenderness, redness, or swelling of area from genitals to rectum occurs.

• Alert patient to watch for signs and symptoms of yeast infection of vagina (vaginal odor, white or yellow discharge, itching) or penis (rash or redness of glans or foreskin, itching, swelling, foul-smelling

NEW DRUGS

discharge, pain). Instruct patient to report these signs or symptoms to prescriber as soon as possible.
• Warn that hypersensitivity reactions (urticaria, anaphylactic reactions, angioedema) may occur. Instruct patient to report signs or symptoms and stop drug until seen by health care provider.
• Advise patient of fetal risk. Advise patient to report pregnancy or plans to become pregnant during therapy.
• Instruct patient not to breastfeed during therapy.

sparsentan
spar-SEN-tan

Filspari

Therapeutic class: Miscellaneous GU drugs
Pharmacologic class: Endothelin and angiotensin II receptor antagonists

AVAILABLE FORMS
Tablets ⒹⓉⒸ: 200 mg, 400 mg

INDICATIONS & DOSAGES
➤ **Reduction of proteinuria in patients with primary immunoglobulin A nephropathy (IgAN) at risk for rapid disease progression**
Adults: 200 mg PO once daily. After 14 days, increase to 400 mg PO once daily, as tolerated. Consider repeating titration when resuming drug after an interruption.
Adjust-a-dose: Refer to manufacturer's instructions for dosage adjustment and monitoring in patients with transaminase elevations of more than $3 \times$ ULN. If therapy is withheld, don't resume in patients with symptoms of liver toxicity or liver enzyme and bilirubin levels that haven't returned to pretreatment levels. Stop drug permanently if ALT or AST is greater than $8 \times$ ULN without another cause.

ADMINISTRATION
PO
• Before starting drug, discontinue RAAS inhibitors, endothelin receptor antagonists, and aliskiren.
• Patient should swallow tablets whole with water before morning or evening meal. Maintain same dosing pattern in relationship to meals.
• If a dose is missed, skip missed dose and give next dose at its scheduled time.
• Store at 68° to 77° F (20° to 25° C). Store in original container.

ACTION
Antagonizes endothelin type A and angiotensin II receptors that are thought to contribute to the pathogenesis of IgAN.

Route	Onset	Peak	Duration
PO	Unknown	3 hr	Unknown

Half-life: 9.6 hours.

ADVERSE REACTIONS
CNS: dizziness. **CV:** hypotension, orthostatic hypotension, peripheral edema. **GU:** *AKI.* **Hematologic:** anemia. **Hepatic:** increased transaminase levels. **Metabolic:** *hyperkalemia.*

INTERACTIONS
Drug-drug. *Antacids and acid-reducing agents (H₂ antagonists, PPIs):* May decrease sparsentan level. Give sparsentan 2 hours before or after antacids. Avoid use together with H₂ antagonists and PPIs.
CYP2B6, 2C9, 2C19 substrates (bupropion): May decrease substrate level. Monitor for substrate efficacy and consider dosage adjustment.
Drugs that increase serum potassium (potassium-sparing diuretics, potassium supplements): May increase risk of hyperkalemia. Monitor potassium level.
Moderate CYP3A inhibitors (cyclosporine): May increase sparsentan level and risk of adverse reactions. Monitor BP, edema, potassium level, and kidney function.
NSAIDs (COX-2 inhibitors): May worsen kidney function. Monitor for signs and symptoms of worsening kidney function.
P-gp substrates (digoxin, fexofenadine) and BCRP substrates (cimetidine, glyburide, rosuvastatin): May increase substrate level and substrate-related adverse reactions. Avoid use together.
❶ *Alert:* *RAAS inhibitors (ACE inhibitors, ARBs), endothelin receptor antagonists (ambrisentan, bosentan), aliskiren:* May increase risk of hypotension, syncope, hyperkalemia, and decreased kidney function. Avoid use together.
Strong CYP3A inducers (rifampin): May decrease sparsentan level. Avoid use together.
Strong CYP3A inhibitors (itraconazole): May increase sparsentan level. Avoid use together. If use can't be avoided, interrupt sparsentan.
Drug-food. *Potassium-containing salt substitutes:* May cause hyperkalemia. Monitor potassium level.

EFFECTS ON LAB TEST RESULTS
• May increase transaminase and potassium levels.
• May decrease RBC count.
• May cause initial small decrease in eGFR that stabilizes within 4 weeks.

CONTRAINDICATIONS & CAUTIONS
Boxed Warning Drug is only available through a REMS program due to risks (elevated aminotransferase levels, liver toxicity, liver failure, major birth defects). Prescribers, patients, and pharmacies must enroll. ■
❶ *Alert:* Avoid use in patients with any degree of liver impairment (Child-Pugh classes A to C), including those with aminotransferases levels greater than $3 \times$ ULN at baseline.
• Drug inhibits RAAS and may increase risk of AKI.
• Use cautiously in patients with fluid retention, risk of hypotension, and advanced kidney disease.

Reactions in bold italics are *life-threatening.*

- Use in patients with HF hasn't been established.
- Safety and effectiveness in children haven't been established.
Dialyzable drug: Unlikely.

PREGNANCY-LACTATION-REPRODUCTION
Boxed Warning Drug is contraindicated during pregnancy; may cause major birth defects and fetal death. Verify negative pregnancy status before, monthly during, and for 1 month after stopping drug. ∎
- Patient of childbearing potential should use effective contraception before, during, and for 1 month after final dose.
- It isn't known if drug appears in human milk or how drug affects milk production or infants who are breastfed. Patient shouldn't breastfeed during therapy.

NURSING CONSIDERATIONS
Boxed Warning Measure transaminase and bilirubin levels before starting drug, monthly for 12 months, and then every 3 months during therapy. Interrupt therapy for aminotransferase elevations greater than 3 × ULN, and monitor patient closely. Consider restarting drug in patient without symptoms of liver toxicity when liver enzyme and bilirubin levels return to pretreatment values. ∎
- Monitor for signs and symptoms of liver toxicity (nausea, vomiting, right upper quadrant pain, fatigue, anorexia, jaundice, dark urine, fever, itching).
- Monitor BP. Eliminating or adjusting other antihypertensive drugs, maintaining appropriate volume status, and reducing dosage or interrupting administration of sparsentan may be necessary. A transient hypotensive response isn't a contraindication to further sparsentan dosing once BP has stabilized.
- Periodically monitor kidney function. Patients whose kidney function may depend in part on RAAS activity (patients with renal artery stenosis, CKD, severe HF, or volume depletion) may be at risk for developing AKI. Consider withholding or stopping therapy in patients who experience a clinically significant decrease in kidney function.
- Periodically monitor potassium level; treat hyperkalemia appropriately. Consider dosage reduction or discontinuation of drug.
- Monitor for fluid retention. Diuretic therapy, fluid management, or dosage modification of drug may be necessary.
- *Look alike-sound alike:* Don't confuse sparsentan with bosentan or losartan.

PATIENT TEACHING
- Teach about proper drug administration and handling.
Boxed Warning Inform patient that enrollment in REMS program is necessary to ensure compliance with monitoring requirements. ∎

Boxed Warning Tell patient to immediately stop drug and seek medical attention if symptoms of liver toxicity occur. ∎
Boxed Warning Alert patient of childbearing potential of need for pregnancy testing before, monthly during, and 1 month after stopping drug. Review effective contraceptive options, as outlined in prescribing information. ∎
- Advise patient not to breastfeed during therapy.
- Caution patient about risk of hypotension and importance of staying hydrated.
- Warn that fluid retention may occur. Instruct patient to immediately report unusual weight gain or lower extremity swelling.
- Counsel patient to report use of all prescription and OTC medications (antihypertensives, potassium supplements, antacids, pain products), vitamins, supplements, herbal products, and salt substitutes that contain potassium.

SAFETY ALERT!

sulbactam–durlobactam
suhl-BAK-tam/DUR-loe-BAK-tam

Xacduro

Therapeutic class: Antibiotics
Pharmacologic class: Beta-lactam antibacterials/beta lactamase inhibitors

AVAILABLE FORMS
Powder for injection: sulbactam 1-g single-dose vial packaged with two durlobactam 0.5-g single-dose vials

INDICATIONS & DOSAGES
➤ **Hospital-acquired bacterial pneumonia and ventilator-associated bacterial pneumonia (HABP/VABP) caused by susceptible isolates of *Acinetobacter baumannii-calcoaceticus* complex**
Adults ages 18 and older: 1 g sulbactam and 1 g of durlobactam every 6 hours IV for 7 to 14 days based on patient's condition.
Adjust-a-dose: For patients with CrCl of 130 mL/minute or more, give every 4 hours; CrCl of 30 to 44 mL/minute, every 8 hours; CrCl of 15 to 29 mL/minute, every 12 hours; CrCl less than 15 mL/minute, every 12 hours for 3 doses, then every 24 hours after third dose. For patients whose CrCl declines to less than 15 mL/minute during therapy, give every 24 hours.

ADMINISTRATION
IV
- Obtain specimen for culture and sensitivity tests before administration. Begin therapy while awaiting results.
- Reconstitute sulbactam 1-g vial with 5 mL of sterile water for injection. Gently shake to dissolve into clear, colorless to slightly yellow solution.

NEW DRUGS

• Reconstitute durlobactam 0.5-g vial with 2.5 mL of sterile water for injection. Gently shake to dissolve into clear, light yellow to orange solution.
• Inspect for particulate matter and discoloration before use. Don't use if solution is cloudy or contains particulates.
• Reconstituted solutions aren't for direct injection and must be diluted within 1 hour of reconstitution.
• Withdraw 5 mL of sulbactam and 5 mL (2.5 mL from each vial) of durlobactam and add to 100 mL bag of NSS. Discard unused portion.
• Refrigerate solution at 36° to 46° F (2° to 8° C) until administration. Don't freeze.
• Allow solution to reach room temperature (15 to 30 minutes) before infusion.
• Give by IV infusion over 3 hours.
• Time from start of reconstitution to end of infusion shouldn't exceed 24 hours.
• For patients on hemodialysis, give after dialysis session is complete.
• Refrigerate vials at 36° to 46° F (2° to 8° C). Don't freeze.
• Incompatibilities: Don't mix with other drugs or add to solutions containing other drugs.

ACTION
Sulbactam inhibits penicillin-binding protein enzymes required for bacterial cell wall synthesis. Durlobactam protects sulbactam from degradation by beta-lactamases; durlobactam alone doesn't have antibacterial activity against *Acinetobacter baumannii-calcoaceticus* complex.

Route	Onset	Peak	Duration
IV (sulbactam)	Unknown	3.2 hr	Unknown
IV (durlobactam)	Unknown	3.1 hr	Unknown

Half-life: 0.99 to 3.31 hours (sulbactam); 1.75 to 3.29 hours (durlobactam).

ADVERSE REACTIONS
CV: *arrhythmias.* **GI:** constipation, diarrhea. **GU:** *AKI.* **Hematologic:** anemia, *thrombocytopenia.* **Hepatic:** liver test abnormalities. **Metabolic:** *hypokalemia.*

INTERACTIONS
Drug-drug. *OAT1 inhibitors (probenecid):* May increase sulbactam level. Avoid use together.

EFFECTS ON LAB TEST RESULTS
• May increase ALT, AST, and creatinine levels.
• May decrease potassium level.

CONTRAINDICATIONS & CAUTIONS
• Contraindicated in patients with history of hypersensitivity to sulbactam, durlobactam, or other beta-lactam antibacterial drugs.
• Use cautiously in patients with kidney impairment and older adults, who are more likely to have kidney impairment.

• Not indicated for treatment of HABP/VABP caused by pathogens other than susceptible isolates of *Acinetobacter baumannii-calcoaceticus* complex.
• To reduce development of drug-resistant bacteria, only use drug to treat or prevent infections that are proven or strongly suspected to be caused by susceptible bacteria.
• CDAD, ranging in severity from mild diarrhea to fatal colitis, has been reported with nearly all antibacterial agents. If CDAD is suspected or confirmed, consider the risks of continuing therapy.
• Safety and effectiveness in children haven't been established.
Dialyzable drug: 41% (sulbactam), 33% (durlobactam).

PREGNANCY-LACTATION-REPRODUCTION
• Studies during pregnancy are inadequate. Use cautiously during pregnancy.
• Sulbactam is present in human milk in low levels. Use cautiously during breastfeeding.

NURSING CONSIDERATIONS
• Monitor patient for hypersensitivity reactions, including anaphylaxis and serious skin reactions. Discontinue drug if reaction occurs.
• Monitor patient's kidney function at baseline and regularly during therapy, especially if patient is receiving hemodialysis or is seriously ill and receiving IV fluid resuscitation. Adjust dosage accordingly.
• Monitor patient for CDAD. Start appropriate treatment as indicated (fluid and electrolytes, protein supplementation, antibacterial drug treatment of *C. difficile*, and surgical evaluation).
• *Look alike–sound alike:* Don't confuse sulbactam or durlobactam with other bactam agents.

PATIENT TEACHING
❸ *Alert:* Advise patient that serious allergic reactions may occur and require immediate treatment.
• Explain that antibiotics can change normal intestinal flora and that patient should report frequent watery or bloody diarrhea (even 2 months or more after therapy), which may indicate a serious intestinal infection.

terlipressin
ter-li-PRES-in

Terlivaz

Therapeutic class: Vasoconstrictors
Pharmacologic class: Posterior pituitary hormones

AVAILABLE FORMS
Powder for injection: 0.85 mg single-dose vial

NEW DRUGS

INDICATIONS & DOSAGES

➤ **Improved kidney function in patients with hepatorenal syndrome with rapid reduction in kidney function**
Adults: 0.85 mg (1 vial) IV bolus over 2 minutes every 6 hours on days 1 to 3. On day 4, compare serum creatinine (SCr) level to baseline. If SCr has decreased by 30% or more, continue 0.85 mg IV bolus every 6 hours. If SCr has decreased by less than 30%, increase dose to 1.7 mg (2 vials) IV bolus every 6 hours. If SCr is at or above baseline, discontinue drug. Continue for 24 hours after two consecutive SCr values at least 2 hours apart of less than 1.5 mg/dL have been achieved or for a maximum of 14 days.

ADMINISTRATION
IV
• Reconstitute each vial with 5 mL NSS. Inspect vial for particulate matter and discoloration.
• May give drug through peripheral IV or CVAD. A dedicated CVAD isn't required. Flush line after administration.
• Give each vial by IV bolus over 2 minutes.
• May store at 36° to 46° F (2° to 8° C) for up to 48 hours, if not given immediately. Don't freeze. Reconstituted vials don't need protection from light.
• Store unopened vials at 36° to 46° F (2° to 8° C) in original carton to protect from light.

ACTION
Thought to increase renal blood flow by reducing portal HTN and blood circulation in portal vessels and increasing effective arterial volume and mean arterial pressure.

Route	Onset	Peak	Duration
IV	5 min	1.2–2 hr	6 hr

Half-life: 0.9 hour (parent drug), 3 hours (lysine-vasopressin metabolite).

ADVERSE REACTIONS
CV: *bradycardia.* **GI:** abdominal pain, diarrhea, nausea. **Metabolic:** fluid overload. **Respiratory:** dyspnea, pleural effusion, *respiratory failure.* **Other:** *ischemia-related events, sepsis.*

INTERACTIONS
None reported.

EFFECTS ON LAB TEST RESULTS
• None reported.

CONTRAINDICATIONS & CAUTIONS
Boxed Warning Drug may cause serious or fatal respiratory failure. Patients with volume overload or acute-on-chronic liver failure (ACLF) grade 3 are at increased risk. ∎
• Contraindicated in patients experiencing hypoxia or worsening respiratory symptoms and in patients with ongoing coronary, peripheral, or mesenteric ischemia.

• Avoid use in patients with ACLF grade 3.
• Drug-related adverse reactions may make patients ineligible for liver transplantation. In patients with high priority for liver transplantation, drug benefits may not outweigh risks.
• Drug can cause ischemic events (cardiac, cerebrovascular, peripheral, or mesenteric). Avoid use in patients with history of CV, cerebrovascular, or ischemic disease. Discontinue use in patients who experience signs or symptoms of ischemia.
• Patients with SCr greater than 5 mg/dL are unlikely to benefit from drug.
• Safety and effectiveness in children haven't been established.
• Use cautiously in older adults because greater sensitivity to drug is possible.
Dialyzable drug: Unknown.

PREGNANCY-LACTATION-REPRODUCTION
• Drug may cause fetal harm because it induces uterine contractions and endometrial ischemia. Advise patients who are pregnant of potential risk to fetus.
• It isn't known if drug appears in human milk or how drug affects milk production or infants who are breastfed. Weigh benefit to patient against possible risk to infant.

NURSING CONSIDERATIONS
Boxed Warning Assess oxygenation saturation (SpO_2) before initiating drug. Don't initiate in a patient experiencing hypoxia (SpO_2 less than 90%) until SpO_2 improves. Monitor patient for hypoxia using continuous pulse oximetry during therapy and discontinue drug if SpO_2 decreases below 90%. ∎
• Monitor patient for changes in respiratory status.
• Monitor patient's kidney function.
• Monitor for signs and symptoms of ischemic adverse reactions (cyanosis, abdominal pain).

PATIENT TEACHING
• Advise patient to report all adverse events.
• Counsel patient that side effects may decrease chances of getting liver transplant.
• Inform fertile patient that drug may cause fetal harm. Instruct patient to report known or suspected pregnancy.

SAFETY ALERT!

trofinetide ⌧
troe-FIN-e-tide

Daybue

Therapeutic class: Miscellaneous CNS drugs
Pharmacologic class: Glycine-proline-glutamate analogs

AVAILABLE FORMS
Oral solution: 200 mg/mL

NEW DRUGS

INDICATIONS & DOSAGES

➤ **Rett syndrome**

Adults and children ages 2 and older weighing 50 kg or more: 12,000 mg (60 mL) PO b.i.d.

Adults and children ages 2 and older weighing 35 kg to less than 50 kg: 10,000 mg (50 mL) PO b.i.d.

Adults and children ages 2 and older weighing 20 to less than 35 kg: 8,000 mg (40 mL) PO b.i.d.

Adults and children ages 2 and older weighing 12 to less than 20 kg: 6,000 mg (30 mL) PO b.i.d.

Adults and children ages 2 and older weighing 9 to less than 12 kg: 5,000 mg (25 mL) PO b.i.d.

Adjust-a-dose: Interrupt drug, reduce dosage, or discontinue drug for severe diarrhea, suspected dehydration, or significant weight loss.

ADMINISTRATION

PO

- Give drug without regard to food.
- When giving through gastrojejunal tube, give through G-port.
- Use calibrated measuring device (oral syringe, dosing cup) to accurately measure and deliver dose.
- If dose is missed, skip missed dose and give next dose as scheduled.
- If vomiting occurs after dose, don't repeat dose. Instead, continue with next scheduled dose.
- Discard unused solution after 14 days of opening bottle.
- Store upright and refrigerated at 36° to 46° F (2° to 8° C). Don't freeze.

ACTION

Exact mechanism unknown.

Route	Onset	Peak	Duration
PO	Unknown	2–3 hr	Unknown

Half-life: 1.5 hours.

ADVERSE REACTIONS

CNS: anxiety, fatigue, fever, *seizures.* **EENT:** nasopharyngitis. **GI:** decreased appetite, diarrhea, vomiting. **Metabolic:** weight loss.

INTERACTIONS

Drug-drug. *CYP3A4 substrates (carbamazepine, midazolam):* May increase substrate level. Monitor substrate with a narrow therapeutic index.
OATP1B1, OATP1B3 substrates (methotrexate, valproic acid): May increase substrate level. Avoid use together with substrates that have a narrow therapeutic index.

EFFECTS ON LAB TEST RESULTS

- None reported.

CONTRAINDICATIONS & CAUTIONS

- Use in patients with moderate or severe kidney impairment isn't recommended.

- Safety and effectiveness in children younger than age 2 haven't been established.
Dialyzable drug: Unlikely.

PREGNANCY-LACTATION-REPRODUCTION

- Studies during pregnancy are inadequate. It isn't known if drug causes fetal harm. Use during pregnancy only if benefit outweighs fetal risk.
- It isn't known if drug appears in human milk. Use cautiously during breastfeeding.

NURSING CONSIDERATIONS

- Ensure patient stops laxatives before initiating drug.
- Consider starting antidiarrheal treatment if diarrhea occurs.
- Monitor hydration, and increase oral fluids if needed.
- Monitor patient's weight.
- *Look alike-sound alike:* Don't confuse trofinetide with dofetilide. Don't confuse Daybue with Daypro.

PATIENT TEACHING

- Teach about proper drug administration and handling.
- Warn that drug can cause vomiting. Instruct patient and caregiver not to repeat dose if patient vomits.
- Tell patient and caregiver to report patient weight loss to prescriber.
- Explain that drug can cause diarrhea. Advise patient to stop laxatives before starting therapy. Instruct patient to report diarrhea, and explain how to manage it and prevent dehydration.
- Advise patient to report pregnancy or plans to become pregnant or breastfeed during therapy.

SAFETY ALERT!

zavegepant
za-VE-je-pant

Zavzpret

Therapeutic class: Antimigraine drugs
Pharmacologic class: Calcitonin gene-related peptide receptor antagonists

AVAILABLE FORMS

Nasal spray: 10 mg per unit-dose device

INDICATIONS & DOSAGES

➤ **Acute treatment of migraine with or without aura**
Adults: One spray (10 mg) into 1 nostril, as needed. Maximum, 10 mg in 24 hours.

ADMINISTRATION

Intranasal

- Have patient gently blow nose before use.
- Don't test spray, prime, or press plunger before dosing.

Reactions in bold italics are *life-threatening.*

- Remove cap and insert device into patient's nostril while blocking opposite nostril.
- Don't allow patient to lay down or tilt head during dose delivery.
- Press plunger device while patient gently breathes in through nose. Patient should then breathe gently through mouth for 5 to 10 seconds. Spray only one time into one nostril.
- Remove device and keep patient's head level for 20 seconds while patient breathes in through nose and out through mouth.
- If patient feels drip from nose, have patient gently sniff to retain dose.
- Store at room temperature.
- Keep device in sealed blister package until time of use.

ACTION
Unknown.

Route	Onset	Peak	Duration
Intranasal	Within 2 hr	30 min	Unknown

Half-life: 6.55 hours.

ADVERSE REACTIONS
CNS: taste disorder. **EENT:** nasal discomfort. **GI:** nausea, vomiting.

INTERACTIONS
Drug-drug. *Intranasal decongestants (azelastine, oxymetazoline):* May decrease absorption of zavegepant. Avoid use together. If use together can't be avoided, give decongestants at least 1 hour after zavegepant.
OATP1B3 inducers (clotrimazole, progesterone), sodium taurocholate co-transporting polypeptide (NTCP) inducers: May decrease zavegepant level. Avoid use together.
OATP1B3 inhibitors (clarithromycin, rifampin), NTCP inhibitors (rifampin): May increase zavegepant level. Avoid use together.

CONTRAINDICATIONS & CAUTIONS
- Contraindicated in patients with history of hypersensitivity to drug or any of its components.
- Hypersensitivity reactions, including facial swelling and urticaria, have occurred.
- Avoid use in patients with CrCl less than 30 mL/minute or Child-Pugh class C liver impairment.
- Safety of treating more than 8 migraines in a 30-day period hasn't been established.
- Safety and effectiveness in children haven't been established.
Dialyzable drug: Unknown.

PREGNANCY-LACTATION-REPRODUCTION
- Studies during pregnancy are inadequate. Use only if potential benefit justifies fetal risk.

- It isn't known if drug appears in human milk or how drug affects milk production or infants who are breastfed. Use cautiously in patients who are breastfeeding.

NURSING CONSIDERATIONS
- Monitor for hypersensitivity reactions (facial swelling, urticaria). Stop drug and initiate treatment if any occur.

PATIENT TEACHING
⚠ Alert: Instruct patient to take only 1 dose in 24 hours.
- Teach about proper drug administration and handling.
- Warn patient that safety of treating more than 8 migraines in a 30-day period hasn't been established.
- Advise patient that use with intranasal decongestants should be avoided. Explain that, if use together is unavoidable, patient should use intranasal decongestant at least 1 hour after zavegepant.
- Tell patient to report hypersensitivity reactions and stop drug if any occur.

NEW DRUGS

Appendices

Antacids: Indications and dosages

Refer to manufacturer's instructions for complete prescribing and safety information.

aluminum hydroxide
a-LOO-mi-num

Therapeutic class: Antacids
Pharmacologic class: Aluminum salts

AVAILABLE FORMS
Oral suspension: 320 mg/5 mL ◇

INDICATIONS & DOSAGES
➤ **Acid indigestion, heartburn, GI upset, dyspepsia**
Adults: 640 mg PO five to six times daily after meals and at bedtime. Maximum, 3,840 mg/day.

aluminum hydroxide–magnesium carbonate
a-LOO-mi-num

Acid Gone ◇ , Gaviscon ◇

Therapeutic class: Antacids
Pharmacologic class: Aluminum salts

AVAILABLE FORMS
Tablets (chewable): 160 mg aluminum hydroxide/105 mg magnesium carbonate ◇
Oral suspension: 95 mg aluminum hydroxide/358 mg magnesium carbonate/15 mL; 254 mg aluminum hydroxide/237.5 mg magnesium carbonate/5 mL ◇

INDICATIONS & DOSAGES
➤ **Acid indigestion, heartburn, GI upset**
Adults and children ages 12 and older: 2 to 4 chewable tablets PO q.i.d.; maximum, 16 tablets/24 hours. Or, 15 to 30 mL (95 mg aluminum hydroxide/358 mg magnesium carbonate) PO q.i.d.; maximum, 120 mL/24 hours. Or, 10 to 20 mL (254 mg aluminum hydroxide/237.5 mg magnesium carbonate) PO q.i.d.; maximum, 80 mL/24 hours.

calcium carbonate
KAL-see-um

Alka-Seltzer Heartburn ◇ ,
Cal-Gest ◇ , Maalox ◇ ,
Maalox Children's ◇ , TC Max ◇ ,
Titralac ◇ , Tums ◇

Therapeutic class: Antacids
Pharmacologic class: Calcium salts

AVAILABLE FORMS
1 g calcium carbonate is equal to 400 mg of elemental calcium.
Oral suspension: 1,250 mg/5 mL ◇
Powder for oral solution: 800 mg/2 g ◇ , 4,000 mg/unit dose packet ◇
Tablets: 648 mg ◇ , 1,250 mg ◇ , 1,500 mg ◇
Tablets (chewable): 260 mg ◇ , 400 mg ◇ ,
420 mg ◇ , 500 mg ◇ , 600 mg ◇ , 750 mg ◇ ,
1,000 mg ◇ , 1,177 mg ◇ , 1,250 mg ◇

INDICATIONS & DOSAGES
➤ **Acid indigestion, heartburn**
Adults: 1 to 4 tablets, 5 to 10 mL oral suspension, or 1.3 to 2 g powder PO PRN according to package directions or as directed by prescriber. Maximum, 8,000 mg daily for up to 2 weeks.
Children ages 12 and older: 1,000 to 3,000 mg when symptomatic. Maximum, 7,500 mg daily for up to 2 weeks.
Children ages 6 to 11: 800 mg PO when symptomatic. Maximum, 2,400 mg daily for up to 2 weeks.
Children ages 2 to 5, weighing more than 10.9 kg: 400 mg PO when symptomatic. Maximum, 1,200 mg daily for up to 2 weeks.
➤ **Calcium supplement**
Adults: 500 mg to 4 g PO daily in one to three divided doses.

magnesium oxide
mag-NEE-see-um

Mag-200 ◇ , Mag-Ox 400 ◇ ,
Maox ◇

Therapeutic class: Antacids
Pharmacologic class: Magnesium salts

AVAILABLE FORMS
Tablets: 100 mg ◇ , 200 mg ◇ , 400 mg ◇ , 420 mg ◇ ,
500 mg ◇

INDICATIONS & DOSAGES
➤ **Acid indigestion**
Adults: 400 mg PO once daily or b.i.d. according to the package directions or as directed by prescriber. Maximum, 800 mg/day for up to 2 weeks.
➤ **Dietary supplement**
Adults: 400 to 800 mg PO daily or as directed by prescriber. Maximum, 800 mg/day.

Antidiarrheals: Indications and dosages

Refer to manufacturer's instructions for complete prescribing and safety information.

bismuth subsalicylate
BIZ-muth SUB-sa-LIS-i-late

Bismatrol ◇, Kaopectate ◇,
Pepto-Bismol ◇

Therapeutic class: Antidiarrheals
Pharmacologic class: Adsorbents

AVAILABLE FORMS
Caplets ⓄⓉⒸ: 262 mg ◇
Capsules ⓄⓉⒸ: 262 mg ◇
Oral suspension: 262 mg/15 mL (regular strength) ◇,
525 mg/15 mL (maximum strength) ◇
Tablets (chewable): 262 mg ◇

INDICATIONS & DOSAGES
➤ **Diarrhea, gas, travelers' diarrhea**
Adults and children ages 12 and older: 525 mg PO every 30 to 60 minutes or 1,050 mg PO every 60 minutes PRN for up to 2 days. Maximum, 4,200 mg/24 hours.
➤ **Indigestion, heartburn, nausea**
Adults and children ages 12 and older: 525 mg PO every 30 to 60 minutes. Maximum, 4,200 mg/24 hours.

crofelemer
kro-FEL-e-mer

Mytesi

Therapeutic class: Antidiarrheals
Pharmacologic class: Antidiarrheals

AVAILABLE FORMS
Tablets (delayed-release) ⓄⓉⒸ: 125 mg

INDICATIONS & DOSAGES
➤ **Noninfectious diarrhea in patients with HIV/AIDS on antiretroviral therapy**
Adults: 125 mg PO b.i.d.

diphenoxylate hydrochloride–atropine sulfate
dye-fen-OKS-ul-ate/AT-roe-peen

Lomotil*

Therapeutic class: Antidiarrheals
Pharmacologic class: Opioids-anticholinergics
Controlled substance schedule: V

AVAILABLE FORMS
Oral solution: 2.5 mg diphenoxylate and 0.025 mg atropine/5 mL
Tablets: 2.5 mg diphenoxylate and 0.025 mg atropine

INDICATIONS & DOSAGES
➤ **Acute, nonspecific diarrhea**
Adults and children ages 13 and older: Initially, 5 mg PO q.i.d.; reduce dosage with initial control of symptoms. Maximum, 20 mg/day.

loperamide hydrochloride
loe-PER-a-mide

Diamode ◇, Imodium A-D ◇

Therapeutic class: Antidiarrheals
Pharmacologic class: Piperidine derivatives

AVAILABLE FORMS
Capsules: 2 mg
Oral liquid: 1 mg/7.5 mL ◇
Tablets: 2 mg ◇

INDICATIONS & DOSAGES
Boxed Warning Don't exceed recommended dosages due to risk of torsades de pointes, cardiac arrest, and death. Use is contraindicated in children younger than age 2. ∎
➤ **Acute, nonspecific diarrhea (including travelers' diarrhea)**
Adults and children ages 13 and older (prescription): Initially, 4 mg PO; then 2 mg after each loose stool. Maximum, 16 mg/day. Limit use to 48 hours.
Adults and children ages 12 and older (OTC): Initially, 4 mg PO; then 2 mg after each loose stool. Maximum, 8 mg/day. Limit use to 48 hours.
Children ages 9 to 11 weighing 27.1 to 43 kg: 2 mg PO; then 1 mg after each loose stool. Maximum, 6 mg daily. Don't give OTC capsules.
Children ages 6 to 8 weighing 21 to 27 kg: 2 mg PO; then 1 mg after each loose stool. Maximum, 4 mg daily. Don't give OTC capsules.
Children ages 2 to 5 weighing 13 to less than 21 kg (oral liquid only): 1 mg PO; then 1 mg after each loose stool. Maximum, 3 mg/day.
➤ **Chronic diarrhea associated with inflammatory bowel disease**
Adults (prescription): Initially, 4 mg PO; then 2 mg after each loose stool until diarrhea subsides, for up to 10 days. Adjust dosage to individual response. Maximum, 16 mg/day.
➤ **Reduced discharge volume from ileostomy**
Adults (prescription): Initially, 2 mg PO 2 to 3 times per day. May increase by 2 mg/day as needed to maximum dosage of 16 mg/day.

telotristat ethyl
tel-OH-tri-stat

Xermelo

Therapeutic class: Antidiarrheals
Pharmacologic class: Tryptophan hydroxylase inhibitors

AVAILABLE FORMS
Tablets: 250 mg

INDICATIONS & DOSAGES
➤ **Carcinoid syndrome diarrhea in combination with somatostatin analogue (SSA) therapy in patients inadequately controlled by SSA therapy**
Adults: 250 mg PO t.i.d.

Laxatives: Indications and dosages

Refer to manufacturer's instructions for complete prescribing and safety information.

bisacodyl
bis-a-KOE-dil

Biscolax ◇ , Carter's Little Pills ❦ ◇ , Codulax ❦ ◇ , Dulcolax ◇ , Ex-Lax Ultra ◇ , Fleet Bisacodyl ◇ , Silver Bullet ❦ ◇ , The Magic Bullet ◇ , Woman's Laxative ◇

Therapeutic class: Laxatives
Pharmacologic class: Diphenylmethane derivatives

AVAILABLE FORMS
Enema: 10 mg/30 mL ◇
Suppositories: 10 mg ◇
Tablets (delayed-release): **OTC:** 5 mg ◇

INDICATIONS & DOSAGES
➤ **Constipation**
Adults and children ages 12 and older: 5 to 15 mg PO as single daily dose PRN. Or, 10-mg suppository or enema PR daily PRN.
Children ages 6 to 11: 5 mg PO PRN; oral dose isn't recommended if child can't swallow tablet whole. Or, ½ suppository once daily PRN; don't give enema in children younger than age 12.
➤ **Bowel cleansing prior to rectal exam**
Adults and children ages 12 and older: 10 mg enema as single daily dose.

calcium polycarbophil
FiberCon ◇ , Fiber-Lax ◇

Therapeutic class: Laxatives
Pharmacologic class: Hydrophilic drugs

AVAILABLE FORMS
Tablets: 625 mg ◇

INDICATIONS & DOSAGES
➤ **Constipation**
Adults and children ages 12 and older: 2 tablets (1,250 mg) PO once daily to q.i.d. PRN. Maximum, 8 tablets (5 g) in 24 hours.

docusate calcium (dioctyl calcium sulfosuccinate)
DOK-yoo-sayt

Kao-Tin Capsule ◇ , Surfak ◇

docusate sodium (dioctyl sodium sulfosuccinate)
Colace ◇ , Correctol Extra Gentle ◇ , DocuSol Kids Enema ◇ , DOK ◇ , Dulcolax Stool Softener ◇ , Enemeez Mini ◇ , Pedia-Lax Liquid Stool Softener ◇ , Phillips Stool Softener ◇ , Selax ❦

Therapeutic class: Laxatives
Pharmacologic class: Surfactants

AVAILABLE FORMS
docusate calcium
Capsules: 240 mg ◇
docusate sodium
Capsules: 100 mg ◇ , 250 mg ◇
Oral liquid: 50 mg/5 mL ◇ , 50 mg/15 mL ◇ , 100 mg/10 mL ◇
Rectal suspension: 100 mg/5 mL ◇ , 283 mg/5 mL ◇
Syrup: 60 mg/15 mL ◇
Tablets: 100 mg ◇

INDICATIONS & DOSAGES
➤ **Constipation (stool softener)**
Adults and children ages 12 and older: 50 to 300 mg docusate sodium PO daily as single dose or divided doses or 240 mg docusate calcium PO daily PRN for up to 1 week, or as directed. Or, 283-mg enema PR one to three times daily for up to 1 week.
Children ages 2 to 11: 100 mg docusate sodium PO daily as single dose or divided doses, or as directed. Maximum, 150 mg/24 hours. Or, 100-mg enema PR once daily for up to 1 week.

glycerin
GLI-ser-in

Fleet ◇ , Pedia-Lax ◇

Therapeutic class: Laxatives
Pharmacologic class: Trihydric alcohols

AVAILABLE FORMS
Enema: 5.4 g ◇
Liquid suppository: 2.8 g ◇
Suppositories: 1 g (child) ◇ , 2 g (adult) ◇

INDICATIONS & DOSAGES
➤ **Constipation**

Adults and children ages 6 and older: One 2-g suppository or enema/day PRN.
Children ages 2 to younger than age 6: One 1-g or 2.8-g suppository/day PRN.

lactulose
LAK-tyoo-lose

Constulose, Enulose, Kristalose

Therapeutic class: Laxatives
Pharmacologic class: Disaccharides

AVAILABLE FORMS
Oral solution: 10 g/15 mL
Packets: 10 g, 20 g
Rectal solution: 10 g/15 mL

INDICATIONS & DOSAGES
➤ **Constipation**

Adults: 10 to 20 g PO daily, increased to 40 g daily, if needed.
➤ **Prevention and treatment of hepatic encephalopathy, including stages of precoma and coma**
Adults: Initially, 20 to 30 g PO every 1 to 2 hours to produce two soft stools daily; then reduce frequency to t.i.d. or q.i.d. to produce two or three soft stools daily. Usual dose is 60 to 100 g daily in divided doses. Or, 200 g (300 mL) diluted with 700 mL of water or NSS and given as retention enema PR every 4 to 6 hours, as needed.
Older children and adolescents: Initially, 26.7 to 60 g/day (40 to 90 mL/day) PO in divided doses to produce two or three soft stools daily; then adjust dosage to maintain stool output.
Infants: Initially, 1.7 to 6.7 g/day (2.5 to 10 mL/day) PO in divided doses to produce two or three soft stools daily; then adjust dosage to maintain stool output.

linaclotide
LIN-a-KLOE-tide

Constella✦, Linzess

Therapeutic class: Laxatives
Pharmacologic class: Guanylate cyclase-C agonists

AVAILABLE FORMS
Capsules ⓄⓃⒸ: 72 mcg, 145 mcg, 290 mcg

INDICATIONS & DOSAGES
Boxed Warning Contraindicated in children younger than age 2 due to risk of serious dehydration. ◼
➤ **IBS with constipation**
Adults: 290 mcg PO once daily.

➤ **Chronic idiopathic constipation**
Adults: 72 to 145 mcg PO once daily.
✳ *NEW INDICATION:* **Functional constipation**
Children ages 6 to 17: 72 mcg PO once daily.

lubiprostone
loo-bi-PROS-tone

Amitiza

Therapeutic class: Laxatives
Pharmacologic class: Chloride channel activators

AVAILABLE FORMS
Capsules ⓄⓃⒸ: 8 mcg, 24 mcg

INDICATIONS & DOSAGES
➤ **Chronic idiopathic constipation; opioid-induced constipation in patients with chronic, noncancer pain**
Adults: 24 mcg PO b.i.d.
Adjust-a-dose: For patients with Child-Pugh class B liver impairment, starting dose is 16 mcg b.i.d.; for those with Child-Pugh class C liver impairment, starting dose is 8 mcg b.i.d. If adequate response isn't obtained, may increase to full dose as tolerated.
➤ **IBS with constipation**
Adult females ages 18 and older: 8 mcg PO b.i.d.
Adjust-a-dose: For patients with Child-Pugh class C liver impairment, starting dose is 8 mcg once daily. If adequate response isn't obtained, may increase to full dose as tolerated.

magnesium citrate
(citrate of magnesia)
Citroma ◇

magnesium hydroxide
(milk of magnesia)
Dulcolax ◇, Milk of Magnesia ◇,
Pedia-Lax Chewable ◇,
Phillips' Milk of Magnesia ◇

magnesium sulfate
(Epsom salts) ◇
Therapeutic class: Laxatives
Pharmacologic class: Magnesium salts

AVAILABLE FORMS
magnesium citrate
Oral solution: 1.75 g/30 mL ◇
magnesium hydroxide
Chewable tablets: 400 mg ◇, 600 mg ◇, 1,200 mg ◇
Oral suspension: 400 mg/5 mL ◇, 800 mg/5 mL ◇, 1,200 mg/15 mL ◇, 2,400 mg/10 mL ◇
magnesium sulfate
Granules: About 40 mEq magnesium/5 g ◇

INDICATIONS & DOSAGES
➤ **Constipation**
Adults and children ages 12 and older: 195 to 300 mL
magnesium citrate PO daily as single dose or divided
doses. Or, 2,400 to 4,800 mg magnesium hydroxide
chewable tablets PO as single daily dose or divided
doses. Or, 30 to 60 mL magnesium hydroxide liquid
(400 mg/5 mL) PO daily as single dose or divided
doses. Or, 15 to 30 mL magnesium hydroxide liquid
(800 mg/5 mL) PO daily as single dose or divided
doses. Or, 10 to 20 mL magnesium hydroxide
(1,200 mg/5 mL) PO daily as single dose or divided
doses. Or, 10 to 20 g magnesium sulfate granules
dissolved in 8 fluid oz water PO as single dose; may
repeat after 4 hours PRN.
Children ages 6 to 11: 90 to 210 mL magnesium
citrate PO daily as single dose or divided doses. Or,
1,200 to 2,400 mg magnesium hydroxide chewable
tablets PO daily as single dose or divided doses. Or,
15 to 30 mL magnesium hydroxide liquid (400 mg/
5 mL) daily as single dose or divided doses. Or, 7.5 to
15 mL magnesium hydroxide liquid (800 mg/5 mL)
PO daily as single dose at bedtime or divided doses.
Or, 5 to 10 mL magnesium hydroxide liquid
(1,200 mg/5 mL) PO daily as single dose or divided
doses. Or, 5 to 10 g magnesium sulfate dissolved in
8 fluid oz water PO daily as single dose; may repeat
after 4 hours PRN.
Children ages 2 to 5: 60 to 90 mL magnesium
citrate PO daily as single dose or divided doses. 1 to
3 magnesium hydroxide chewable (400-mg) tablets
PO daily as single dose or divided doses. Or, 5 to
15 mL magnesium hydroxide liquid (400 mg/5 mL)
PO daily as single dose or divided doses.

polyethylene glycol 3350 (PEG)
pol-ee-ETH-ih-leen

Clearlax✦◇, GaviLAX◇,
GlycoLax◇, Lax-A-Day✦◇,
MiraLax◇, Relaxa✦◇

Therapeutic class: Laxatives
Pharmacologic class: Osmotic drugs

AVAILABLE FORMS
Powder for solution: 17 g/dose

INDICATIONS & DOSAGES
➤ **Constipation**
Adults and children ages 17 and older: 17 g PO dissolved in 120 to 240 mL beverage once daily for up
to 7 days.

polyethylene glycol–electrolyte solution (PEG-ES)
pol-ee-ETH-ih-leen

GoLYTELY, MoviPrep, NuLYTELY,
Plenvu, Suflave

Therapeutic class: Laxatives
Pharmacologic class: Osmotic laxatives

AVAILABLE FORMS
Powder for oral solution: Strength and dose of
PEG-ES vary by manufacturer.

INDICATIONS & DOSAGES
➤ **Bowel preparation**
Adults: 240 mL PO every 10 minutes or via NG tube
at a rate of 1.2 to 1.8 L/hour until 4 L consumed or
rectal effluent is clear. For MoviPrep, Plenvu, or
Suflave, refer to package instructions for split-dose
or full-dose regimen.
Children ages 6 months and older (Nulytely): 25 mL/
kg/hour PO or via NG tube until rectal effluent is clear
and free of solid matter.

sodium phosphate monobasic monohydrate–sodium phosphate dibasic anhydrous

Therapeutic class: Laxatives
Pharmacologic class: Osmotic laxatives

AVAILABLE FORMS
Tablets: 1.5 g sodium phosphate (1.102 g monobasic
sodium phosphate and 0.398 g dibasic sodium phosphate)

INDICATIONS & DOSAGES
Boxed Warning Acute phosphate kidney impairment has been reported. Patients should follow the
recommended split dosing regimen. ▪
➤ **Bowel cleansing before colonoscopy**
Adults: 32 tablets taken in the following manner:
The evening before the procedure, 4 tablets PO with
240 mL of clear liquid every 15 minutes for a total of
20 tablets (five doses); 3 to 5 hours before the procedure, 4 tablets PO with 240 mL of clear liquid every
15 minutes for a total of 12 tablets (three doses). A
minimum of 7 days should elapse before repeating
usage.

sodium phosphates
Fleet Enema ◇, Fleet Enema
Extra ◇, Fleet for Children ◇,
Pedia-Lax ◇

Therapeutic class: Laxatives
Pharmacologic class: Acid salts

AVAILABLE FORMS
Enema solution: 19 g monobasic sodium phosphate
and 7 g dibasic sodium phosphate in 118-mL, 133-mL,
or 197-mL bottles ◇
Enema solution (pediatric use): 9.5 g monobasic sodium phosphate and 3.5 g dibasic sodium phosphate in
59-mL or 66-mL bottles ◇

INDICATIONS & DOSAGES
➤ **Constipation**
Adults and children ages 12 and older: 1 bottle enema
PR once in 24 hours PRN.
Children ages 5 to 11: 1 bottle enema for pediatric use
PR once in 24 hours PRN.
Children ages 2 to younger than 5: One-half bottle
enema for pediatric use PR once in 24 hours PRN.

sodium picosulfate–
magnesium oxide–anhydrous
citric acid
Clenpiq

Therapeutic class: Laxatives
Pharmacologic class: Peristaltic
stimulants–osmotic agents

AVAILABLE FORMS
Oral solution: 10 mg sodium picosulfate, 3.5 g magnesium oxide, and 12 g anhydrous citric acid/175 mL
bottle

INDICATIONS & DOSAGES
➤ **Colon cleansing before colonoscopy**
Adults and children ages 9 and older: Two separate
doses are required as a split dose regimen. Give first
bottle during the evening before colonoscopy (5 p.m.
to 9 p.m.), followed by at least five 240-mL drinks
of clear liquids within 5 hours. Give second bottle
next day during the morning, approximately 5 hours
before colonoscopy. Follow dose with at least four
240-mL drinks of clear liquids up to 2 hours before
colonoscopy.

Vitamins and minerals: Indications and dosages

Refer to manufacturer's instructions for complete prescribing and safety information.

ascorbic acid (vitamin C)
AS-kor-bik AS-id

Ascor, C-Caps ◇, Halls Defense Vitamin C Drops ◇, Nature's Way ◇

Therapeutic class: Vitamin C supplements
Pharmacologic class: Vitamins

AVAILABLE FORMS
Capsules: 500 mg ◇
Capsules (timed-release): 500 mg ◇
Crystals: 1,000 mg/½ tsp
Injection: 500 mg/mL
Lozenges: 60 mg ◇
Oral solution: 100 mg/mL ◇, 500 mg/15 mL ◇
Powder: 60 mg/¼ tsp ◇, 1,000 mg/tsp ◇, 1,060 mg/¼ tsp ◇
Tablets: 250 mg ◇, 500 mg ◇, 1,000 mg ◇, 1,500 mg ◇
Tablets (chewable): 100 mg ◇, 250 mg ◇, 400 mg ◇, 500 mg ◇
Tablets (timed-release): 500 mg ◇
Wafer: 500 mg ◇

INDICATIONS & DOSAGES
➤ **RDA**
Males ages 19 and older: 90 mg.
Females ages 19 and older: 75 mg.
Males ages 14 to 18: 75 mg.
Females ages 14 to 18: 65 mg.
Children ages 9 to 13: 45 mg.
Children ages 4 to 8: 25 mg.
Children ages 1 to 3: 15 mg.
Infants ages 7 months to 1 year: 50 mg.
Neonates and infants up to age 6 months: 40 mg.
Females ages 19 and older who are pregnant: 85 mg.
Females ages 14 to 18 who are pregnant: 80 mg.
Females ages 19 and older who are breastfeeding: 120 mg.
Females ages 14 to 18 who are breastfeeding: 115 mg.
Adult smokers: Increase RDA by 35 mg daily.
➤ **Frank and subclinical scurvy**
Adults: Depending on severity, 100 to 300 mg PO or 200 mg IV daily.
Children ages 11 and older: 200 mg IV or IM daily.
Children ages 1 to younger than 11: 100 mg IV daily.
Infants ages 5 to younger than 12 months: 50 mg IV daily.
➤ **Wound healing**
Adults and children: 300 to 500 mg IV once daily for 1 week to 10 days.

cholecalciferol (vitamin D₃)
kole-e-kal-SI-fer-ole

Bio-D-Mulsion ◇, Decara ◇, Dialyvite Vitamin D3 Max ◇, Osteo-Vit3 ◇, VitaMelts ◇

ergocalciferol (vitamin D₂)
Calcidol ◇, Drisdol

Therapeutic class: Vitamin D supplements
Pharmacologic class: Vitamins

AVAILABLE FORMS
cholecalciferol
Capsules: 25 mcg (1,000 international units), 50 mcg (2,000 international units), 125 mcg (5,000 international units), 250 mcg (10,000 international units), 625 mcg (25,000 international units), 1.25 mg (50,000 international units)
Liquid: 400 international units/mL ◇, 400 international units/0.03 mL ◇, 2,000 international units/0.03 mL ◇, 4,000 international units/2 drops, 5,000 international units/mL ◇
Tablets: 10 mcg (400 international units) ◇, 20 mcg (800 international units) ◇, 25 mcg (1,000 international units) ◇, 50 mcg (2,000 international units) ◇, 75 mcg (3,000 international units) ◇, 125 mcg (5,000 international units) ◇, 1,250 mcg (50,000 international units) ◇
Tablets (chewable): 10 mcg (400 international units) ◇, 25 mcg (1,000 international units) ◇, 50 mcg (2,000 international units) ◇
ergocalciferol
Capsules: 1.25 mg (50,000 international units)
Oral liquid: 200 mcg (8,000 international units)/mL in 60-mL dropper bottle ◇
Tablets: 10 mcg (400 international units) ◇, 50 mcg (2,000 international units) ◇

INDICATIONS & DOSAGES
➤ **RDA**
Adults older than age 70: 20 mcg (800 international units).
Adults to age 70 and children ages 1 and older: 15 mcg (600 international units).
Children from birth to less than 12 months: 10 mcg (400 international units).
Females who are pregnant or breastfeeding: 15 mcg (600 international units).
➤ **Rickets and other vitamin-D-deficiency diseases**
Adults and children: Individualize cholecalciferol dosage based on age and serum 25-hydroxyvitamin D level. For vitamin D-resistant rickets, give 12,000 to 500,000 international units ergocalciferol PO daily. After correction of deficiency, maintenance includes adequate diet and RDA supplements.

➤ **Hypoparathyroidism**
Adults and children: 1.25 to 5 mg (50,000 to 200,000 international units) ergocalciferol PO daily with calcium supplement.

coenzyme Q10 (ubidecarenone)
CoQ10◇, Mega CoQ10◇, Vitaline CoQ10◇

Therapeutic class: Coenzymes
Pharmacologic class: Antioxidants

AVAILABLE FORMS
Capsules: 10 mg◇, 30 mg◇, 50 mg◇, 60 mg◇, 75 mg◇, 100 mg◇, 120 mg◇, 125 mg◇, 150 mg◇, 200 mg◇, 400 mg◇
Capsules (extended-release): 100 mg◇
Liquid (liposomal): 2.5 mg/drop◇, 100 mg/mL◇
Oral liquid: 6 mg/mL◇
Syrup: 10 mg/mL◇
Tablets: 50 mg◇, 60 mg◇, 100 mg◇
Tablets (chewable): 30 mg◇, 100 mg◇
Wafers: 60 mg◇, 100 mg◇, 300 mg◇, 400 mg◇, 600 mg◇

INDICATIONS & DOSAGES
➤ **Dietary supplement for conditions associated with coenzyme Q10 deficiency**
Adults: 10 to 400 mg/day PO in one dose or up to three divided doses. Higher doses (up to 3,000 mg/day) have been used.

cyanocobalamin (vitamin B₁₂)
Dodex, Nascobal, Vitamin Deficiency System-B12, Vibisone

hydroxocobalamin (vitamin B₁₂)
Cyanokit

Therapeutic class: Vitamin B₁₂ supplements
Pharmacologic class: Corrinoids

AVAILABLE FORMS
cyanocobalamin
Injection*: 1,000 mcg/mL, 2,000 mcg/mL
Intranasal spray: 500 mcg/spray
Liquid (SL): 3,000 mcg◇
Lozenges: 50 mcg◇, 100 mcg◇, 250 mcg◇, 500 mcg◇
Tablets: 100 mcg◇, 250 mcg◇, 500 mcg◇, 1,000 mcg◇
Tablets (extended-release): 1,000 mcg◇
Tablets (SL): 2,500 mcg◇
hydroxocobalamin
Injection: 1,000 mcg/mL, 5 g/vial

INDICATIONS & DOSAGES
➤ **RDA for cyanocobalamin**
Adults and children ages 14 and older: 2.4 mcg.
Children ages 9 to 13: 1.8 mcg.
Children ages 4 to 8: 1.2 mcg.
Children ages 1 to 3: 0.9 mcg.
Infants ages 7 months to 1 year: 0.5 mcg.
Neonates and infants ages 6 months and younger: 0.4 mcg.
Females who are pregnant: 2.6 mcg.
Females who are breastfeeding: 2.8 mcg.
➤ **Vitamin B₁₂ deficiency from inadequate diet, subtotal gastrectomy, or other condition, disorder, or disease, except malabsorption related to pernicious anemia or other GI disease**
Adults and children (cyanocobalamin): 100 mcg IM or deep subcut daily for 6 to 7 days. If improvement occurs, 100 mcg on alternate days for seven doses, then every 3 to 4 days for 2 to 3 weeks. Maintenance dose, 100 mcg IM or deep subcut monthly.
Adults (hydroxocobalamin): 30 mcg IM daily for 5 to 10 days. Maintenance dose, 100 to 200 mcg IM monthly.
Children (hydroxocobalamin): 1 to 5 mg in single doses of 100 mcg IM over 2 or more weeks, depending on severity of deficiency. Maintenance dose, 30 to 50 mcg IM every 4 weeks.
➤ **Pernicious anemia or vitamin B₁₂ malabsorption**
Adults: Initially, 100 mcg cyanocobalamin IM or deep subcut daily for 6 to 7 days. With observed response, 100 mcg IM or deep subcut every other day for 7 doses, then 100 mcg every 3 to 4 days for 2 to 3 weeks, and then 100 mcg IM or deep subcut once monthly.
➤ **Maintenance therapy for remission of pernicious anemia after IM vitamin B₁₂ therapy in patients without nervous system involvement; dietary deficiency; malabsorption disorders; inadequate secretion of intrinsic factor**
Adults: Initially, 1 spray in one nostril once weekly (Nascobal), given at least 1 hour before or after hot foods or liquids.
➤ **Schilling test flushing dose**
Adults and children: 1,000 mcg hydroxocobalamin IM as single dose.
➤ **Cyanide poisoning**
Adults: Initially, 5 g hydroxocobalamin IV over 15 minutes. Based on patient's condition, may repeat 5 g dose IV over 15 minutes to 2 hours.

doxercalciferol (vitamin D analogue)
dox-er-kal-SIF-er-ol

Hectorol

Therapeutic class: Vitamin D supplements
Pharmacologic class: Vitamin D analogues

AVAILABLE FORMS
Capsules: 0.5 mcg, 1 mcg, 2.5 mcg
Injection: 2 mcg/mL in 1-mL, 2-mL vials

INDICATIONS & DOSAGES
➤ **Secondary hyperparathyroidism in patients requiring dialysis for CKD**
Adults: Initially, 10 mcg PO three times weekly at dialysis. Adjust dosage as needed to lower intact parathyroid hormone (iPTH) level to 150 to 300 picograms (pg)/mL. Increase dose by 2.5 mcg after 8 weeks and at 8-week intervals thereafter if iPTH level doesn't decrease by 50% and fails to reach target range. Maximum, 20 mcg PO three times weekly. If iPTH level falls below 100 pg/mL, suspend drug for 1 week; then give at dose that's at least 2.5 mcg less than last dose.

Or, 4 mcg IV bolus three times a week at the end of dialysis, no more frequently than every other day. Adjust dosage as needed to lower iPTH level to 150 to 300 pg/mL. May increase dose given three times weekly by 1 to 2 mcg at 8-week intervals if iPTH level doesn't decrease by 50% and fails to reach target range. Maximum, 18 mcg weekly. If iPTH level falls below 100 pg/mL, suspend drug for 1 week; then give at dose that's at least 1 mcg lower than last dose.
➤ **Secondary hyperparathyroidism in patients with stage 3 or 4 CKD who require dialysis**
Adults: 1 mcg PO daily. Adjust dosage as needed to lower iPTH level to 35 to 70 pg/mL for stage 3 or 70 to 110 pg/mL for stage 4. Increase dosage at 2-week intervals by 0.5 mcg if level is above 70 pg/mL for stage 3 or above 110 pg/mL for stage 4. If level falls below 35 pg/mL for stage 3 or 70 pg/mL for stage 4, suspend treatment for 1 week; then give at dose at least 0.5 mcg lower than last dose. Maximum, 3.5 mcg daily.

---

ferrous fumarate
FAIR-us FUE-ma-rate

Ferretts ◇ , Ferrimin ◇ , Ferrocite ◇

Therapeutic class: Iron supplements
Pharmacologic class: Hematinics

AVAILABLE FORMS
Each 100 mg of ferrous fumarate provides 33 mg of elemental iron.
Tablets ⓄⓃⒸ: 29 mg ◇ , 106 mg ◇ , 150 mg ◇ elemental iron

INDICATIONS & DOSAGES
➤ **Iron deficiency**
Adults: 29 to 150 mg of elemental iron PO once daily, every other day, or as directed by prescriber. Daily dosing may decrease absorption.
Children: 3 to 6 mg/kg/day of elemental iron PO in one to three divided doses up to maximum of 120 mg/day.

---

ferrous gluconate
FAIR-us GLUE-koe-nate

Ferate ◇ , Fergon ◇

Therapeutic class: Iron supplements
Pharmacologic class: Hematinics

AVAILABLE FORMS
Each 100 mg of ferrous gluconate provides 11.6 mg of elemental iron.
Tablets ⓄⓃⒸ: 27 mg ◇ , 38 mg ◇ elemental iron

INDICATIONS & DOSAGES
➤ **Iron deficiency**
Adults: 27 to 38 mg of elemental iron PO once daily, every other day, or as directed by prescriber. Daily dosing may decrease absorption.
Children: 3 to 6 mg/kg/day of elemental iron PO in one to three divided doses.

---

ferrous sulfate
FAIR-us SUL-fate

FeroSol ◇*, Fer-In-Sol ◇ ,
Fe-Vit Iron ◇

ferrous sulfate (dried)
Feosol ◇ , Slow FE ◇ ,
Slow Release Iron ◇

Therapeutic class: Iron supplements
Pharmacologic class: Hematinics

AVAILABLE FORMS
Each 100 mg of ferrous sulfate provides 20 mg of elemental iron or 30 mg of elemental iron in ferrous sulfate dried products.
Elixir: 44 mg/5 mL ◇* elemental iron
Liquid: 15 mg/mL ◇ , 60 mg/5 mL ◇ elemental iron
Tablets: 65 mg ◇ elemental iron
Tablets (extended-release) ⓄⓃⒸ: 45 mg ◇ , 50 mg (dried) ◇ , 65 mg ◇ elemental iron

INDICATIONS & DOSAGES
➤ **Iron deficiency**
Adults, children, and infants: Refer to individual manufacturer's dosage instructions or take as directed by prescriber. Immediate-release products are usually given in divided doses daily. Extended-release formulations are given once daily. Lower daily doses may cause less GI adverse events in older adults. Daily dosing may decrease absorption.

---

folic acid (vitamin B₉)
FA-8 ◇

Therapeutic class: Vitamin B₉ supplements
Pharmacologic class: Vitamins

AVAILABLE FORMS
Capsules: 0.8 mg ◇, 5 mg ◇, 20 mg ◇
Injection: 10-mL vials (5 mg/mL)*
Tablets: 0.4 mg ◇, 0.8 mg ◇, 1 mg

INDICATIONS & DOSAGES
➤ **RDA**
Adults and children ages 14 and older: 400 mcg.
Children ages 9 to 13: 300 mcg.
Children ages 4 to 8: 200 mcg.
Children ages 1 to 3: 150 mcg.
Infants ages 7 months to 1 year: 80 mcg.
Neonates and infants younger than age 6 months: 65 mcg.
Females who are pregnant: 600 mcg.
Females who are breastfeeding: 500 mcg.
➤ **Megaloblastic or macrocytic anemia from folic acid or other nutritional deficiency, liver disease, alcoholism, intestinal obstruction, or excessive hemolysis**
Adults and children: Initially, up to 1 mg PO, IM, IV, or subcut daily until anemia resolves; then proper diet and RDA supplements to prevent recurrence.
Adults and children ages 4 and older: Maintenance dose up to 0.4 mg PO, IM, IV, or subcut daily.
Children younger than age 4: Maintenance dose up to 0.3 mg PO, IM, or subcut daily.
Infants: Maintenance dose 0.1 mg PO, IM, IV, or subcut daily.
Females who are pregnant or breastfeeding: Maintenance dose 0.8 mg PO, IM, IV, or subcut daily.

iron dextran
EYE-ern DEKS-tran

INFeD

Therapeutic class: Iron supplements
Pharmacologic class: Hematinics

AVAILABLE FORMS
1 mL iron dextran provides 50 mg elemental iron.
Injection: 50 mg elemental iron/mL in 2-mL single-dose vials

INDICATIONS & DOSAGES
Boxed Warning Anaphylactic-type reactions have occurred. Have emergency equipment and trained personnel readily available. Give a test dose prior to first injection. Observe patient for anaphylaxis. Use only in patients who need IV therapy. ∎

➤ **Iron deficiency anemia**
Adults and children weighing more than 15 kg: IV or IM test dose is required. (See manufacturer's instructions.) Total treatment dosage may be calculated using dosage table in manufacturer's instructions or by using this formula:
Dose (mL) = 0.0442 (desired Hb – observed Hb) × LBW + (0.26 × LBW).
Note: LBW = lean body weight in kg. For males, LBW = 50 kg + 2.3 kg for each inch of patient's height over 5 feet. For females, LBW = 45.5 kg + 2.3 kg for each inch of patient's height over 5 feet.
Children weighing 5 to 15 kg: Use dosage table in package insert or calculate dosage as follows:
Dose (mL) = 0.0442 (desired Hb – observed Hb) × weight in kg + (0.26 × weight in kg).
➤ **Iron replacement for blood loss**
Adults and children older than age 4 months: Replacement iron (in mg) = (Blood loss [in mL] × hematocrit) ÷ 50 mg/mL.
Note: This formula is based on the approximation that 1 mL of normocytic, normochromic red cells contains 1 mg of elemental iron.

leucovorin calcium (citrovorum factor, folinic acid)
loo-kuh-VAW-ruhn

Therapeutic class: Folic acid analogues
Pharmacologic class: Antidotes

AVAILABLE FORMS
Injection: 50-mg, 100-mg, 200-mg, 350-mg, 500-mg vials for reconstitution (contains no preservatives)
Solution for injection: 100 mg/10-mL vials
Tablets: 5 mg, 10 mg, 15 mg, 25 mg

INDICATIONS & DOSAGES
➤ **Leucovorin rescue after high-dose methotrexate therapy**
Adults: 15 mg (approximately 10 mg/m²) PO, IM, or IV every 6 hours for 10 doses starting 24 hours after start of methotrexate infusion. Continue until methotrexate level falls below 5×10^{-8} M. See manufacturer's instructions for dosage adjustment guidelines for methotrexate toxicity.
➤ **Impaired methotrexate elimination or inadvertent overdose**
Adults: 10 mg/m² PO, IM, or IV every 6 hours until serum methotrexate level is less than 10^{-8} M. If 24-hour serum creatinine level increases 50% over baseline or if 24-hour methotrexate level is greater than 5×10^{-6} M or 48-hour level is greater than 9×10^{-7} M, increase dosage to 100 mg/m² IV every 3 hours until methotrexate level is less than 10^{-8} M.
➤ **Folic acid antagonist overdose (trimethoprim, pyrimethamine)**
Adults and children: 5 to 15 mg PO daily.

► **Folate-deficient megaloblastic anemia**
Adults and children: Up to 1 mg IM or IV daily.
► **Palliative treatment of advanced colorectal cancer**
Adults: 20 mg/m^2 IV followed by 5-FU 425 mg/m^2 IV. Or, 200 mg/m^2 IV over 3 minutes or longer followed by 5-FU 370 mg/m^2. Repeat daily for 5 consecutive days. May repeat at 4-week intervals for two additional courses; then at intervals of 4 to 5 weeks, if tolerated. Give 5-FU and leucovorin separately to avoid precipitate formation.

niacin (nicotinic acid, vitamin B$_3$)
NAI-uh-sin

Endur-Acin ◇ , Niacor, Slo-Niacin ◇

niacinamide ◊ (nicotinamide ◊)

Therapeutic class: Vitamin B$_3$ supplements
Pharmacologic class: Antilipemics

AVAILABLE FORMS
niacin
Capsules (extended-release): 250 mg ◇ , 500 mg
Tablets: 50 mg ◇ , 100 mg ◇ , 250 mg ◇ , 500 mg
Tablets (extended-release): 250 mg ◇ , 500 mg ◇ , 750 mg ◇ , 1,000 mg ◇
niacinamide
Tablets: 100 mg ◇ , 500 mg ◇

INDICATIONS & DOSAGES
► **RDA**
Males ages 14 and older: 16 mg.
Females ages 14 and older: 14 mg.
Children ages 9 to 13: 12 mg.
Children ages 4 to 8: 8 mg.
Children ages 1 to 3: 6 mg.
Infants ages 7 months to 1 year: 4 mg.
Neonates and infants younger than age 6 months: 2 mg.
Females who are pregnant: 18 mg.
Females who are breastfeeding: 17 mg.
► **Niacin deficiency**
Adults: 50 mg twice daily or 100 to 250 mg once daily.
► **Dyslipidemia in patients who can't achieve desired response or are intolerant to other therapies**
Adults: Initially, 250 mg Niacor PO daily after evening meal; increase at 4- to 7-day intervals up to 1 to 2 g PO daily in two or three divided doses. Maximum, 6 g daily. Or, initially, 500 mg extended-release tablets daily at bedtime with low-fat snack; increase at 4-week intervals by 500 mg daily to maximum of 2 g daily.

paricalcitol
par-rih-KAL-sih-tol

Zemplar

Therapeutic class: Vitamin D supplements
Pharmacologic class: Vitamin D analogues

AVAILABLE FORMS
Capsules: 1 mcg, 2 mcg, 4 mcg
Injection: 2 mcg/mL, 5 mcg/mL

INDICATIONS & DOSAGES
► **To prevent or treat secondary hyperparathyroidism in patients with stage 3 or 4 CKD**
Adults: Initial dosage based on baseline intact parathyroid hormone (iPTH) levels. If iPTH is less than or equal to 500 picograms (pg)/mL, 1 mcg PO daily or 2 mcg PO three times weekly, no more often than every other day. If iPTH is greater than 500 pg/mL, 2 mcg PO daily or 4 mcg PO three times weekly, no more often than every other day. Adjust dosage at 2- to 4-week intervals based on iPTH level.
Children ages 10 to 16: Initially, 1 mcg PO three times weekly, no more frequently than every other day. As indicated, increase each dose by 1 mcg every 4 weeks or decrease each dose by 1 mcg at any time based on iPTH, serum calcium, and phosphorus levels.
► **To prevent or treat secondary hyperparathyroidism in patients with stage 5 CKD on dialysis**
Adults: 0.04 to 0.1 mcg/kg (2.8 to 7 mcg) IV no more often than every other day during dialysis. May safely give doses as high as 0.24 mcg/kg. If satisfactory response isn't observed, increase dosage by 2 to 4 mcg at 2- to 4-week intervals. Or, calculate initial PO dose in mcg, based on baseline iPTH level divided by 80 and administered three times weekly, no more frequently than every other day. Initiate only after baseline serum calcium level has been adjusted to 9.5 mg/dL or less. Titrate as indicated by using most recent iPTH level divided by 80. Decrease dosage by 2 to 4 mcg if serum calcium level is elevated.
Children ages 10 to 16: Calculate initial PO dosage in mcg, rounded down to nearest whole number, based on baseline iPTH level divided by 120 and administered three times weekly, no more frequently than every other day. As indicated, increase each dose every 4 weeks or decrease each dose at any time to maintain iPTH within target range.

phytonadione (vitamin K$_1$)
fye-toe-na-DYE-one

K1-1000 ◇

Therapeutic class: Vitamin K supplements
Pharmacologic class: Vitamin K analogues

AVAILABLE FORMS
Injection (emulsion): 2 mg/mL, 10 mg/mL
Tablets: 100 mcg ◇, 5 mg

INDICATIONS & DOSAGES
Boxed Warning Administration using IV or
IM route is associated with a risk of severe and
possibly even fatal hypersensitivity reactions. Re-
strict use of these routes to situations in which
the subcut route isn't feasible and the serious risk
is justified. ∎
➤ **RDA**
Males ages 19 and older: 120 mcg.
*Females ages 19 and older, including those who are
pregnant or breastfeeding:* 90 mcg.
Children ages 14 to 18: 75 mcg.
Children ages 9 to 13: 60 mcg.
Children ages 4 to 8: 55 mcg.
Children ages 1 to 3: 30 mcg.
Infants ages 7 months to 1 year: 2.5 mcg.
Neonates and infants younger than age 6 months:
2 mcg.
*Females ages 14 to 18 who are pregnant or breast-
feeding:* 75 mcg.
➤ **Hypoprothrombinemia caused by vitamin K
malabsorption, drug therapy, or excessive
vitamin A dosage**
Adults: Depending on severity, 2.5 to 25 mg PO, IM,
subcut, or if unavoidable, IV (at a rate of no more than
1 mg/minute); may repeat in 6 to 8 hours. Maximum
single dose, 50 mg.
➤ **Hypoprothrombinemia caused by effect of oral
anticoagulants**
Adults: 2.5 to 10 mg PO based on PT and INR. May
repeat in 12 to 48 hours. Or, 2.5 to 10 mg subcut, IM,
or IV (at a rate of no more than 1 mg/minute) based on
INR and severity of bleeding. May repeat after 6 to
8 hours as needed. Maximum single dose, 50 mg.
➤ **Prevention of vitamin K-deficiency-related
bleeding in neonates**
Neonates: 0.5 to 1 mg IM within 1 hour after birth.
➤ **Vitamin K-deficiency-related bleeding in
neonates**
Neonates: 1 mg subcut or IM. Higher dose as needed
if mother has been receiving oral anticoagulant.

pyridoxine hydrochloride (vitamin B₆)
peer-i-DOKS-een hye-droe-KLOR-ide

B-natal ◇

Therapeutic class: Vitamin B6 supplements
Pharmacologic class: Vitamins

AVAILABLE FORMS
Capsules: 250 mg ◇
Injection: 100 mg/mL

Tablets: 25 mg ◇, 50 mg ◇, 100 mg ◇, 250 mg ◇,
500 mg ◇
Tablets (extended-release): 200 mg ◇

INDICATIONS & DOSAGES
➤ **RDA**
Adults ages 19 to 50: 1.3 mg.
Males ages 51 and older: 1.7 mg.
Females ages 51 and older: 1.5 mg.
Males ages 14 to 18: 1.3 mg.
Females ages 14 to 18: 1.2 mg.
Children ages 9 to 13: 1 mg.
Children ages 4 to 8: 0.6 mg.
Children ages 1 to 3: 0.5 mg.
Infants ages 7 months to 1 year: 0.3 mg (0.03 mg/kg).
Neonates and infants younger than age 6 months:
0.1 mg (0.01 mg/kg).
Females who are pregnant: 1.9 mg.
Females who are breastfeeding: 2 mg.
➤ **Dietary vitamin B₆ deficiency**
Adults: 10 to 20 mg IM or IV daily for 3 weeks; then
maintenance dose of 2 to 5 mg PO daily for several
weeks.

sodium fluoride
SOE-dee-um FLOR-ide

sodium fluoride, topical
ACT ◇, Fluoridex, Gel-Tin ◇,
Just For Kids ◇, Listerine Total
Care ◇, Periomed ◇, Prevident,
SF 5000 Plus

Therapeutic class: Fluoride supplements
Pharmacologic class: Minerals and
electrolytes

AVAILABLE FORMS
sodium fluoride
Lozenges: 1 mg
Solution: 0.125 mg/drop, 0.25 mg/drop, 0.2 mg/mL,
0.5 mg/mL
Tablets (chewable): 0.25 mg, 0.5 mg, 1 mg
sodium fluoride, topical
Cream: 1.1%
Gel: 0.4% ◇, 1.1%
Paste: 0.454% ◇, 1.1%
Rinse: 0.02% ◇, 0.04% ◇, 0.05%, 0.2%

INDICATIONS & DOSAGES
➤ **Prevention of dental caries**
Adults and children older than age 6: 5 to 10 mL of
rinse once daily or b.i.d. (see product instructions) for
1 minute. Or, thin ribbon or pea-sized amount of paste
or cream applied to teeth with toothbrush once daily
or b.i.d. Or, thin ribbon of gel applied to teeth with
toothbrush once daily after brushing. Patient shouldn't
eat, drink, or rinse for 30 minutes after use.
Adults: 1 lozenge PO once daily.

➤ **Prevention of dental caries if fluoride ion level in drinking water is less than 0.3 parts/million (ppm)**
Children ages 6 to 16: 1 mg PO daily.
Children ages 3 to 5: 0.5 mg PO daily.
Infants and children ages 6 months to 2 years: 0.25 mg PO daily.
➤ **Prevention of dental caries if fluoride ion level in drinking water is 0.3 to 0.6 ppm**
Children ages 6 to 16: 0.5 mg PO daily.
Children ages 3 to 5: 0.25 mg PO daily.

thiamine hydrochloride (vitamin B₁)
THIGH-a-min

Thiamiject ✚

Therapeutic class: Vitamin B₁ supplements
Pharmacologic class: Vitamins

AVAILABLE FORMS
Capsules: 50 mg ◇, 100 mg ◇
Injection: 100 mg/mL
Tablets: 50 mg ◇, 100 mg ◇, 250 mg ◇

INDICATIONS & DOSAGES
➤ **RDA**
Males ages 14 and older: 1.2 mg.
Females ages 19 and older: 1.1 mg.
Females ages 14 to 18: 1 mg.
Children ages 9 to 13: 0.9 mg.
Children ages 4 to 8: 0.6 mg.
Children ages 1 to 3: 0.5 mg.
Infants ages 7 months to 1 year: 0.3 mg.
Neonates and infants younger than age 6 months: 0.2 mg.
Females who are pregnant: 1.4 mg.
Females who are breastfeeding: 1.4 mg.
➤ **Beriberi**
Adults: Depending on severity, 10 to 20 mg IM t.i.d. for up to 2 weeks; then dietary correction and PO multivitamin supplement containing 5 to 10 mg thiamine daily for 1 month.
Children: 25 mg IV daily if infantile beriberi isn't responsive to oral therapy.
➤ **Wet beriberi with myocardial failure**
Adults and children: 10 to 20 mg IV t.i.d. given slowly.
➤ **Thiamine deficiency**
Adults: Up to 100 mg/L IV by rapid infusion. Then daily parenteral doses at RDA if GI disturbances prevent adequate oral absorption. Or, 1 tablet or capsule PO daily.
➤ **Neuritis of pregnancy in patients unable to take adequate oral therapy due to vomiting**
Adults: 5 to 10 mg IM daily.
➤ **Wernicke encephalopathy**
Adults: Initially, 100 mg IV; then 50 to 100 mg IM daily until patient consumes a regular balanced diet.

tocopherols (vitamin E)
tow-KUH-feh-ruhlz

Natural Vitamin E ◇, SoluVita-E ◇

Therapeutic class: Vitamin E supplements
Pharmacologic class: Antioxidants

AVAILABLE FORMS
Capsules 🅞🅝🅒: 100 international units ◇, 200 international units ◇, 400 international units ◇, 1,000 international units ◇
Liquid: 15 international units/0.3 mL ◇
Tablets: 100 international units ◇, 200 international units ◇, 400 international units ◇

INDICATIONS & DOSAGES
Note: RDAs for vitamin E have been converted to α-tocopherol equivalents (α-TE). One α-TE equals 1 mg of D-α tocopherol, or 1.49 international units.
➤ **RDA**
Adults and children ages 14 to 18: 15 mg.
Children ages 9 to 13: 11 mg.
Children ages 4 to 8: 7 mg.
Children ages 1 to 3: 6 mg.
Infants ages 7 months to 1 year: 5 mg.
Neonates and infants younger than age 6 months: 4 mg.
Females who are pregnant: 15 mg.
Females who are breastfeeding: 19 mg.
➤ **Dietary supplement**
Adults: For tablets or capsules, 100 to 1,000 mg PO daily (dosages vary by product). Or, 30 units (0.6 mL of 15 units/0.3 mL drops) PO daily.
Children ages 4 and older (using 15 units/0.3 mL drops): 30 units (0.6 mL) PO daily.
Children ages 1 to 3 (using 15 units/0.3 mL drops): 10 units (0.2 mL) PO daily.
Children younger than age 1 (using 15 units/0.3 mL drops): 5 units (0.1 mL) PO daily.

vitamin A
Vitamin A Fish ◇

vitamin A palmitate

Therapeutic class: Vitamin A supplements
Pharmacologic class: Antioxidants

AVAILABLE FORMS
Note: Each international unit is equivalent to 0.3 mcg retinol equivalent (RE).
Capsules: 7,500 international units ◇, 8,000 international units ◇, 10,000 international units ◇, 25,000 international units
Injection: 50,000 international units/mL in 2-mL vials
Tablets: 10,000 international units ◇, 15,000 international units ◇

✚ Canada   ◇ OTC   ◆ Off-label use   🅞🅝🅒 Do not crush   *Liquid contains alcohol.

INDICATIONS & DOSAGES
➤ RDA
Males older than age 14: 900 mcg RE.
Females older than age 14: 700 mcg RE.
Children ages 9 to 13: 600 mcg RE.
Children ages 4 to 8: 400 mcg RE.
Children ages 1 to 3: 300 mcg RE.
Infants ages 7 to 12 months: 500 mcg RE.
Neonates and infants younger than age 6 months: 400 mcg RE.
Females ages 19 to 50 who are pregnant: 770 mcg RE.
Females ages 14 to 18 who are pregnant: 750 mcg RE.
Females ages 19 to 50 who are breastfeeding: 1,300 mcg RE.
Females ages 14 to 18 who are breastfeeding: 1,200 mcg RE.

➤ Severe vitamin A deficiency
Adults and children older than age 8: 100,000 international units IM or PO for 3 days; then 50,000 international units PO or IM daily for 2 weeks; then adequate dietary nutrition and RE vitamin A supplements.
Children ages 1 to 8: 17,500 to 35,000 international units IM daily for 10 days.
Infants: 7,500 to 15,000 international units IM daily for 10 days.

➤ Prevention of recurrent vitamin A deficiency
Adults and children older than age 8: 10,000 to 20,000 international units PO daily for 2 months; then adequate dietary nutrition and RE vitamin A supplements.
Infants and children up to age 8: 5,000 to 10,000 international units PO daily for 2 months; then adequate dietary nutrition and RE vitamin A supplements.

Additional OTC drugs: Indications and dosages

Refer to manufacturer's instructions for complete prescribing and safety information.

benzocaine
ben-ZOH-cane

HurriCaine ◇ , Ora-film ◇ ,
Zilactin Baby ◇

Therapeutic class: Dermatologic agents
Pharmacologic class: Topical anesthetics

AVAILABLE FORMS
Gel: 7.5% ◇ , 10% ◇ , 20% ◇
Liquid: 20% ◇
Lozenge: 15 mg ◇
Ointment, cream: 5% ◇ , 7.5% ◇ , 10% ◇ , 20% ◇
Spray (external aerosol): 2% ◇ , 5% ◇ , 20% ◇
Spray (oral): 20% ◇

INDICATIONS & DOSAGES
Refer to individual manufacturer's instructions for use.
➤ **Sore throat**
Adults and children ages 5 and older: Allow 1 lozenge to dissolve slowly in mouth. May repeat every 2 hours PRN.
Adults and children ages 2 and older: 1 spray to affected area or throat up to q.i.d. PRN.
➤ **Mouth and gum irritation**
Adults: 1 spray or thin layer of gel, liquid, cream, or ointment to affected area up to q.i.d. PRN.
Children ages 2 and older: Apply thin layer of gel, liquid, cream, or ointment to affected area up to q.i.d. PRN.
➤ **Dermal irritation**
Adults and children ages 2 and older: Apply ointment or spray to affected area up to q.i.d. PRN.
➤ **Hemorrhoids**
Adults: Apply ointment to affected area up to six times a day or liquid up to t.i.d. PRN.

cetirizine hydrochloride
seh-TI-rah-zeen

Reactine ✽ ◇ , Zyrtec ◇

Therapeutic class: Antihistamines
Pharmacologic class: Piperazine derivatives

AVAILABLE FORMS
Capsules: 10 mg ◇
Syrup: 5 mg/5 mL ◇
Tablets: 5 mg ◇ , 10 mg ◇ , 20 mg ✽

Tablets (chewable): 2.5 mg ◇ , 5 mg ◇ , 10 mg ◇
Tablets (ODTs): 10 mg ◇

INDICATIONS & DOSAGES
Adjust-a-dose (for all indications): For adults and children ages 6 and older receiving hemodialysis, those with liver impairment, those with CrCl less than 31 mL/minute, and patients ages 65 and older, give 5 mg PO daily. Don't use in children younger than age 6 with kidney or liver impairment.
➤ **Seasonal allergic rhinitis**
Adults and children ages 6 and older: 5 to 10 mg PO once daily.
Children ages 2 to 5: 2.5 mg PO once daily. May increase to 2.5 mg b.i.d. or 5 mg daily. Maximum, 5 mg/day.
➤ **Perennial allergic rhinitis; chronic urticaria**
Adults and children ages 6 and older: 5 to 10 mg PO once daily.
Children ages 2 to 5 years: 2.5 mg PO once daily; may increase to maximum of 5 mg once daily or 2.5 mg b.i.d.
Children ages 12 to 23 months: 2.5 mg PO once daily; may increase to 2.5 mg b.i.d.
Children ages 6 to 11 months: 2.5 mg PO once daily.

chlorpheniramine maleate
KLOR-fen-EER-a-meen

Allergy Relief ◇ , Chlor-Trimeton ◇ ,
Clorrelief ◇ , Diabetic Tussin
Allergy ◇ , Pharbechlor ◇

Therapeutic class: Antihistamines
Pharmacologic class: Alkylamines

AVAILABLE FORMS
Liquid: 2 mg/mL ◇
Oral spray: 0.5% ◇
Syrup: 2 mg/5 mL ◇ *
Tablets: 4 mg ◇
Tablets (extended-release) ⓞⓝⓒ: 12 mg ◇

INDICATIONS & DOSAGES
➤ **Allergic rhinitis**
Adults and children ages 12 and older: 4 mg PO every 4 to 6 hours, not to exceed 24 mg daily. Or, 12 mg extended-release PO every 12 hours, not to exceed 24 mg daily. Or, 4 sprays every 4 to 6 hours, not to exceed 6 applications in 24 hours.
Children ages 6 to 11: 2 mg PO every 4 to 6 hours, not to exceed 12 mg daily. Or, 2 sprays every 4 to 6 hours, not to exceed 3 applications in 24 hours.

dextromethorphan hydrobromide
dex-troe-meth-OR-fan

Buckley's Cough ◇, Delsym ◇, Robitussin ◇, Scot-Tussin Diabetes ◇, Triaminic Long Acting Cough ◇*

Therapeutic class: Antitussives
Pharmacologic class: Levorphanol derivatives

AVAILABLE FORMS
Capsules: 15 mg ◇
Liquid (extended-release): 30 mg/5 mL ◇
Lozenges: 5 mg ◇
Solution: 7.5 mg/5 mL ◇, 10 mg/5 mL ◇*,
12.5 mg/5 mL ◇, 15 mg/5 mL ◇*
Strips (orally disintegrating): 7.5 mg ◇*
Syrup: 7.5 mg/5 mL ◇, 10 mg/5 mL ◇,
20 mg/15 mL ◇
Tablets: 15 mg ◇

INDICATIONS & DOSAGES
➤ **Cough suppressant**
Adults and children ages 12 and older: 10 to 20 mg PO every 4 hours, or 20 to 30 mg every 6 to 8 hours. Or, 60 mg extended-release liquid PO b.i.d. Or, 5 to 15 mg lozenges PO every 4 hours. Maximum, 120 mg/day.
Children ages 6 to 11: 5 to 10 mg PO every 4 hours, or 15 mg every 6 to 8 hours. Or, 30 mg extended-release liquid PO b.i.d. Maximum, 60 mg/day. Or 5 to 10 mg lozenges PO every 4 hours, up to 60 mg/day.
Children ages 4 and 5: 2.5 to 5 mg PO every 4 hours, or 7.5 mg every 6 to 8 hours. Or, 15 mg extended-release liquid PO b.i.d. Maximum, 30 mg daily.

fexofenadine hydrochloride
fecks-oh-FEN-ah-deen

Allegra ◇, Allegra Hives ◇

Therapeutic class: Antihistamines
Pharmacologic class: Piperidines

AVAILABLE FORMS
Oral suspension: 30 mg/5 mL ◇
Tablets (12 hour): 60 mg ◇
Tablets (24 hour): 120 mg ✤ ◇, 180 mg ◇
Tablets (ODTs): 30 mg ◇

INDICATIONS & DOSAGES
Adjust-a-dose (for all indications): Use with caution in patients with kidney impairment; dosage adjustment may be needed.

➤ **Seasonal allergies/hay fever**
Adults and children ages 12 and older: 60 mg PO b.i.d., or 120 or 180 mg PO once daily.
Children ages 2 to 11: 30 mg PO every 12 hours. Maximum, 60 mg daily.
➤ **Chronic idiopathic urticaria**
Adults 180 mg PO once daily.

guaiFENesin (glyceryl guaiacolate)
gwye-FEN-ah-sin

Altarussin ◇, Balminil DM ✤ ◇, Diabetic Tussin ◇, Geri-Tussin ◇, Mucinex ◇, Mucus Relief ◇, Refenesen 400 ◇, Tussin ◇

Therapeutic class: Expectorants
Pharmacologic class: Propanediol derivatives

AVAILABLE FORMS
Granules: 100 mg ◇
Liquid: 100 mg/5 mL ◇*, 200 mg/10 mL ◇,
300 mg/15 mL ◇, 400 mg/20 mL ◇
Syrup: 100 mg/5 mL ◇
Tablets: 200 mg ◇, 400 mg ◇
Tablets (extended-release) ⓓⓝⓒ*:* 600 mg ◇,
1,200 mg ◇

INDICATIONS & DOSAGES
➤ **Expectorant**
Adults and children ages 12 and older: 200 to 400 mg PO every 4 hours, or 600 to 1,200 mg (extended-release tablets) PO every 12 hours. Maximum, 2,400 mg daily.
Children ages 6 to 11: 100 to 200 mg PO every 4 hours. Maximum, 1,200 mg daily.
Children ages 4 to 5: 50 to 100 mg granules, syrup, or liquid every 4 hours as needed. Maximum, 600 mg daily.

loratadine
lor-AT-ah-deen

Claritin ◇, Claritin RediTabs ◇

Therapeutic class: Antihistamines
Pharmacologic class: Piperidines

AVAILABLE FORMS
Capsules: 10 mg ◇
Syrup: 5 mg/5 mL ◇
Tablets: 10 mg ◇
Tablets (chewable): 5 mg ◇
Tablets (ODTs): 5 mg ◇, 10 mg ◇

INDICATIONS & DOSAGES
➤ **Allergic rhinitis**
Adults and children ages 6 and older: 10 mg PO daily.

✤ Canada   ◇ OTC   ◆ Off-label use   ⓓⓝⓒ Do not crush   *Liquid contains alcohol.

Children ages 2 to 5: 5 mg chewable tablets or syrup PO daily.
➤ **To relieve itching due to hives (urticaria)**
Adults and children ages 6 and older: 10 mg PO daily.

meclizine hydrochloride (meclozine hydrochloride)
MEK-lih-zeen

Antivert, Bonine ◇, Motion-Time ◇, Travel-Ease ◇

Therapeutic class: Antivertigo drugs
Pharmacologic class: Anticholinergics

AVAILABLE FORMS
Tablets ⬛ⁿᶜ: 12.5 mg ◇, 25 mg ◇, 50 mg ◇
Tablets (chewable): 25 mg ◇

INDICATIONS & DOSAGES
➤ **Vertigo**
Adults and children ages 12 and older: 25 to 100 mg PO daily in divided doses. Dosage varies with response.
➤ **Motion sickness**
Adults and children ages 12 and older: 25 to 50 mg PO 1 hour before travel; then once daily for duration of trip.

minoxidil (topical)
mi-NOX-i-dill

Men's Rogaine ◇, Women's Rogaine ◇

Therapeutic class: Hair-growth stimulants
Pharmacologic class: Direct-acting vasodilators

AVAILABLE FORMS
Topical foam: 5% ◇
Topical solution: 2% ◇, 5% ◇

INDICATIONS & DOSAGES
➤ **Androgenetic alopecia**
Adults: 1 mL of solution to affected area b.i.d. or half capful of foam applied to affected area b.i.d. (males) or daily (females). Maximum, 2 mL of solution daily.

oxymetazoline hydrochloride (intranasal)
ox-ee-met-AZ-oh-leen

Afrin 12 Hour ◇, Dristan ◇

Therapeutic class: Decongestants
Pharmacologic class: Sympathomimetics

AVAILABLE FORMS
Nasal solution: 0.05% ◇

INDICATIONS & DOSAGES
➤ **Nasal congestion**
Adults and children ages 6 and older: 2 to 3 sprays of 0.05% solution in each nostril b.i.d. Don't use for more than 3 days.

phenylephrine hydrochloride (intranasal)
fen-ill-EF-rin

4-Way Fast Acting ◇, 4-Way Menthol ◇, Nasal Four ◇, Neo-Synephrine Mild ◇, Neo-Synephrine Maximum ◇

Therapeutic class: Vasoconstrictors
Pharmacologic class: Adrenergics

AVAILABLE FORMS
Nasal solution: 0.25% ◇, 0.5% ◇, 1% ◇

INDICATIONS & DOSAGES
➤ **Nasal congestion**
Adults and children ages 12 and older: 2 to 3 drops or 2 to 3 sprays of 0.25% to 1% solution in each nostril every 4 hours PRN. Don't use for longer than 3 (children) or 5 (adults) days.
Children ages 6 to 11: 2 to 3 drops or 2 to 3 sprays of 0.25% solution in each nostril every 4 hours PRN. Don't use for longer than 3 days.

pseudoephedrine hydrochloride
soo-dow-eh-FED-rin

Sudafed ◇, SudoGest ◇, Zephrex-D ◇

Therapeutic class: Decongestants
Pharmacologic class: Adrenergics

AVAILABLE FORMS
Oral solution: 15 mg/5 mL ◇
Syrup: 15 mg/5 mL ◇
Tablets: 30 mg ◇, 60 mg ◇
Tablets (abuse-deterrent) ⬛ⁿᶜ: 30 mg ◇
Tablets (extended-release) ⬛ⁿᶜ: 120 mg ◇, 240 mg ◇

INDICATIONS & DOSAGES
⟳ *Alert:* Don't use drug with an MAO inhibitor or within 2 weeks of stopping an MAO inhibitor.
➤ **Nasal decongestant**
Adults and children ages 12 and older: 60 mg PO every 4 to 6 hours; 120 mg extended-release tablet PO every 12 hours; or 240 mg extended-release tablet PO once daily. Maximum, 240 mg daily.

Children ages 6 to 11 (immediate-release products only): 30 mg PO every 4 to 6 hours. Maximum, 120 mg daily.
Children ages 4 to 5 (immediate-release products only): 15 mg PO every 4 to 6 hours or 1 mg/kg/dose every 6 hours. Maximum, 60 mg daily.

pyrethrins–piperonyl butoxide
pye-RETH-rinz/pi-PER-oh-nil

LiceMD ◇, Lice Killing Shampoo ◇, VanaLice ◇

Therapeutic class: Pediculicides
Pharmacologic class: Pyrethrins

AVAILABLE FORMS
Gel: pyrethrins 0.3% and piperonyl butoxide 3.5%
Shampoo: pyrethrins 0.33% and piperonyl butoxide 4% ◇

INDICATIONS & DOSAGES
➤ ***Pediculus humanus* infestations**
Adults and children ages 2 years and older: Apply to hair, scalp, or other infested areas until entirely wet. Allow to remain for 10 minutes but no longer. Wash thoroughly with warm water and soap or shampoo. Remove dead lice and eggs with fine-toothed comb. Repeat treatment in 7 to 10 days to kill newly hatched lice.

simethicone
sye-METH-ih-kone

Gas Relief ◇, Gas-X ◇, Infacol ✽ ◇, Mylanta Gas Minis ◇, Mylicon ◇, Pediacol ✽ ◇, Phazyme ◇

Therapeutic class: Antiflatulents
Pharmacologic class: Polydimethylsiloxanes

AVAILABLE FORMS
Capsules: 125 mg ◇, 180 mg ◇, 250 mg ◇
Drops: 40 mg/0.6 mL ◇, 40 mg/mL ✽
Liquid: 20 mg/0.3 mL ◇
Strips (orally disintegrating): 40 mg ◇, 62.5 mg ◇
Tablets (chewable): 80 mg ◇, 125 mg ◇

INDICATIONS & DOSAGES
➤ **GI gas retention**
Adults and children older than age 12: 40 to 125 mg PO q.i.d. as needed after each meal and at bedtime; may give single doses of up to 160 to 500 mg after meals or at bedtime, up to 500 mg daily. For drops, 40 to 80 mg PO as needed after each meal and at bedtime, up to 500 mg daily.

Children ages 2 to 12 or weighing more than 11 kg: 40 mg PO q.i.d. as needed after meals and at bedtime, up to 480 mg daily.
Children younger than age 2 or weighing less than 11 kg: 20 mg PO q.i.d. as needed after meals and at bedtime, up to 240 mg daily.

terbinafine hydrochloride (topical)
ter-BIN-ah-fin

Lamisil ◇, Lamisil AT ◇

Therapeutic class: Antifungals
Pharmacologic class: Allylamine derivatives

AVAILABLE FORMS
Cream: 1% ◇

INDICATIONS & DOSAGES
➤ **Athlete's foot**
Adults and children ages 12 and older: For athlete's foot between toes, apply b.i.d. (morning and night) for 1 week or as directed by prescriber. For athlete's foot on bottom or sides of foot, apply b.i.d. (morning and night) for 2 weeks or as directed by prescriber.
➤ **Jock itch, ringworm**
Adults and children ages 12 and older: Apply once daily for 1 week or as directed by prescriber.

witch hazel
wich HAY-zel

Dickinsons Witch Hazel ◇, Preparation H Wipes ◇

Therapeutic class: Dermatologic agents
Pharmacologic class: Astringents

AVAILABLE FORMS
External pads: 20% ◇, 50% ◇
External solution: 86% ◇

INDICATIONS & DOSAGES
➤ **Anal or vaginal irritation, hemorrhoids**
Adults and children ages 12 and older: Apply to affected area up to six times daily or after each bowel movement.
➤ **Minor skin irritation**
Adults and children ages 12 and older: Apply to affected area PRN.

Common combination drugs: Indications and dosages

Refer to manufacturer's instructions for complete prescribing and safety information.

Analgesics

butalbital–acetaminophen–caffeine– codeine phosphate ⊠

Fioricet with Codeine

Controlled substance schedule: III

AVAILABLE FORMS

Capsules: 50 mg butalbital, 300 mg acetaminophen, 40 mg caffeine, and 30 mg codeine phosphate

INDICATIONS & DOSAGES

Boxed Warning Acetaminophen has been associated with acute liver failure and death. ■

⊠ **Boxed Warning** Opioid use increases risk of addiction, abuse, and misuse. Opioids can cause fatal respiratory depression. Opioids can cause respiratory depression and death in children with ingestion of even one dose, particularly with ultra-rapid metabolizers. Opioids combined with benzodiazepines or CNS depressants can cause death. Use during pregnancy can cause neonatal opioid withdrawal syndrome. Effects of concomitant use or discontinuation of CYP3A4 inducers or inhibitors or 2D6 inhibitors with codeine are complex; use cautiously together. ■

➤ **Tension headache**

Adults: 1 to 2 capsules PO every 4 hours PRN. Maximum, 6 capsules in 24 hours.

butalbital–aspirin–caffeine–codeine phosphate

Ascomp with Codeine

Controlled substance schedule: III

AVAILABLE FORMS

Capsules: 50 mg butalbital, 325 mg aspirin, 40 mg caffeine, and 30 mg codeine phosphate

INDICATIONS & DOSAGES

Boxed Warning Opioid use increases risk of addiction, abuse, and misuse. Opioids can cause fatal respiratory depression. Opioids can cause respiratory depression and death in children with ingestion of even one dose, particularly with ultra-rapid metabolizers. Opioids combined with benzodiazepines or CNS depressants can cause death. Use during pregnancy can cause neonatal opioid withdrawal syndrome. Effects of concomitant use or discontinuation of CYP3A4 inducers or inhibitors or 2D6 inhibitors with codeine are complex; use cautiously together. ■

➤ **Tension headache**

Adults: 1 to 2 capsules PO every 4 hours PRN. Maximum dosage, 6 capsules in 24 hours.

hydrocodone bitartrate–ibuprofen

Controlled substance schedule: II

AVAILABLE FORMS

Tablets: 5 mg hydrocodone bitartrate and 200 mg ibuprofen, 7.5 mg hydrocodone bitartrate and 200 mg ibuprofen, 10 mg hydrocodone bitartrate and 200 mg ibuprofen

INDICATIONS & DOSAGES

Boxed Warning Opioid use increases risk of addiction, abuse, and misuse. Opioids can cause fatal respiratory depression. Opioids can cause respiratory depression and death in children with ingestion of even one dose. Opioids combined with benzodiazepines or CNS depressants can cause death. Use during pregnancy can cause neonatal opioid withdrawal syndrome. ■

➤ **Acute pain (short-term)**

Adults and children ages 16 and older: 1 tablet PO every 4 to 6 hours PRN. Maximum, 5 tablets in 24 hours.

ibuprofen–famotidine

Duexis

AVAILABLE FORMS

Tablets ⊙: 800 mg ibuprofen and 26.6 mg famotidine

INDICATIONS & DOSAGES

Boxed Warning Contraindicated for the treatment of perioperative pain after CABG surgery. NSAIDs can increase risk of serious heart attack or stroke and GI adverse reactions (bleeding, ulceration, and perforation), which can be fatal. ■

➤ **RA and osteoarthritis**

Adults: 1 tablet PO t.i.d.

Adjust-a-dose: Older adults may need reduced dosages. Use not recommended in patients with CrCl less than 50 mL/minute.

naproxen–esomeprazole

Vimovo

AVAILABLE FORMS

Tablets ⊙: 375 mg naproxen and 20 mg esomeprazole, 500 mg naproxen and 20 mg esomeprazole

INDICATIONS & DOSAGES

Boxed Warning Contraindicated for the treatment of perioperative pain after CABG surgery. NSAIDs can increase risk of serious heart attack or stroke and GI adverse reactions (bleeding, ulceration, and perforation), which can be fatal. ■

➤ **Osteoarthritis, RA, or ankylosing spondylitis in patients at risk for gastric ulcer development**

Adults: 1 tablet PO b.i.d.

➤ **Juvenile idiopathic arthritis in patients at risk for gastric ulcer development**

Adults and adolescents ages 12 and older weighing more than 50 kg: 1 tablet PO b.i.d.

Adolescents ages 12 and older weighing 38 to less than 50 kg: 1 tablet (375 naproxen/20 mg esomeprazole) PO b.i.d.

pentazocine–naloxone hydrochloride

Controlled substance schedule: IV

AVAILABLE FORMS

Tablets: 50 mg pentazocine and 0.5 mg naloxone hydrochloride

INDICATIONS & DOSAGES

Boxed Warning Opioid use increases risk of addiction, abuse, and misuse. Opioids can cause fatal respiratory depression. Opioids can cause respiratory depression and death in children with ingestion of even one dose. Opioids combined with benzodiazepines or CNS depressants can cause death. Use during pregnancy can cause neonatal opioid withdrawal syndrome. ■

➤ **Moderate to severe pain**
Adults and children ages 12 and older: 1 tablet PO every 3 to 4 hours. May increase to 2 tablets if necessary. Maximum, 12 tablets in 24 hours.

tramadol hydrochloride–acetaminophen
Controlled substance schedule: IV
AVAILABLE FORMS
Tablets: 37.5 mg tramadol hydrochloride and 325 mg acetaminophen
INDICATIONS & DOSAGES
Boxed Warning Acetaminophen has been associated with acute liver failure and death. ■
Boxed Warning Opioid use increases risk of addiction, abuse, and misuse. Opioids can cause fatal respiratory depression. Opioids can cause respiratory depression and death in children with ingestion of even one dose. Opioids combined with benzodiazepines or CNS depressants can cause death. Use during pregnancy can cause neonatal opioid withdrawal syndrome. ■

➤ **Acute pain**
Adults: 2 tablets PO every 4 to 6 hours PRN for up to 5 days. Maximum, 8 tablets in 24 hours.
Adjust-a-dose: Patients with CrCl less than 30 mL/minute shouldn't exceed 2 tablets every 12 hours.

Antiacne drugs

benzoyl peroxide–adapalene
Epiduo, Epiduo Forte
AVAILABLE FORMS
Topical gel: 2.5% benzoyl peroxide and 0.1% adapalene, 2.5% benzoyl peroxide and 0.3% adapalene
INDICATIONS & DOSAGES
➤ **Acne vulgaris**
Adults and children ages 9 and older (Epiduo): Apply thin film to affected area(s) of face or trunk once daily after washing.
Adults and children ages 12 and older (Epiduo Forte): Apply thin film to affected area(s) of face or trunk once daily after washing.

clindamycin phosphate–tretinoin
Veltin, Ziana
AVAILABLE FORMS
Topical gel: 1.2% clindamycin phosphate and 0.025% tretinoin
INDICATIONS & DOSAGES
➤ **Acne vulgaris**
Adults and children ages 12 and older: Apply pea-size amount to cover entire affected area once daily in the evening or at bedtime. Avoid eyes, lips, and mucous membranes.

Antidiabetics

alogliptin benzoate–metFORMIN hydrochloride
Kazano
AVAILABLE FORMS
Tablets: 12.5 mg alogliptin benzoate and 500 mg metformin, 12.5 mg alogliptin benzoate and 1,000 mg metformin
INDICATIONS & DOSAGES
Boxed Warning Metformin can cause serious and sometimes fatal lactic acidosis; prompt hemodialysis is recommended. ■
➤ **Adjunct to diet and exercise to improve glycemic control in patients with type 2 diabetes**
Adults: 1 tablet PO b.i.d. with food. Adjust dosage based on effectiveness and tolerability. Maximum 25 mg alogliptin and 2,000 mg metformin daily.
Adjust-a-dose: Discontinue drug if eGFR falls below 30 mL/minute/1.73 m^2.

alogliptin benzoate–pioglitazone hydrochloride
Oseni
AVAILABLE FORMS
Tablets: 12.5 mg alogliptin benzoate and 15 mg pioglitazone hydrochloride, 12.5 mg alogliptin benzoate and 30 mg pioglitazone hydrochloride, 12.5 mg alogliptin benzoate and 45 mg pioglitazone hydrochloride, 25 mg alogliptin benzoate and 15 mg pioglitazone hydrochloride, 25 mg alogliptin benzoate and 30 mg pioglitazone hydrochloride, 25 mg alogliptin benzoate and 45 mg pioglitazone hydrochloride
INDICATIONS & DOSAGES
Boxed Warning Pioglitazone can cause or exacerbate HF. Drug isn't recommended in patients with symptomatic HF and is contraindicated in patients with NYHA Class III or IV HF. ■
➤ **Adjunct to diet and exercise to improve glycemic control in patients with type 2 diabetes**
Adults inadequately controlled on diet and exercise, inadequately controlled on metformin monotherapy, or in need of additional glycemic control on alogliptin: Alogliptin 25 mg/pioglitazone 15 mg or alogliptin 25 mg/pioglitazone 30 mg PO once daily. May titrate to a maximum of alogliptin 25 mg/pioglitazone 45 mg once daily based on glycemic response as determined by HbA$_{1c}$.
Adults who require additional glycemic control on pioglitazone: Alogliptin 25 mg/pioglitazone 15 mg, alogliptin 25 mg/pioglitazone 30 mg, or alogliptin 25 mg/pioglitazone 45 mg PO once daily as appropriate based on current therapy. May titrate to a maximum of alogliptin 25 mg/pioglitazone 45 mg once daily based on glycemic response as determined by HbA$_{1c}$.
Adults switching from alogliptin administered with pioglitazone: Initiate at dosage of alogliptin and pioglitazone based on current therapy. May titrate to maximum of alogliptin 25 mg/pioglitazone 45 mg once daily based on glycemic response as determined by HbA$_{1c}$.

Adults with HF (NYHA Class I or II): Alogliptin 25 mg/pioglitazone 15 mg PO once daily. May titrate to a maximum of alogliptin 25 mg/pioglitazone 45 mg once daily based on glycemic response as determined by HbA$_{1c}$.

Adjust-a-dose: For patients with CrCl of 30 mL/min to less than 60 mL/min, 12.5 mg/15 mg, 12.5 mg/ 30 mg, or 12.5 mg/45 mg PO once daily.

canagliflozin–metFORMIN hydrochloride
Invokamet, Invokamet XR
AVAILABLE FORMS
Tablets (immediate-release): 50 mg canagliflozin and 500 mg metformin, 50 mg canagliflozin and 1,000 mg metformin, 150 mg canagliflozin and 500 mg metformin, 150 mg canagliflozin and 1,000 mg metformin
Tablets (extended-release) ⓓ: 50 mg canagliflozin and 500 mg extended-release metformin, 50 mg canagliflozin and 1,000 mg extended-release metformin, 150 mg canagliflozin and 500 mg extended-release metformin, 150 mg canagliflozin and 1,000 mg extended-release metformin
INDICATIONS & DOSAGES
Boxed Warning Metformin can cause serious and sometimes fatal lactic acidosis; prompt hemodialysis is recommended. ∎
➤ **Adjunct to diet and exercise to improve glycemic control in patients with type 2 diabetes; to reduce risk of major adverse CV events in patients with type 2 diabetes and established CV disease; to reduce risk of KF, doubling of serum creatinine level, CV death, and hospitalization for HF in patients with type 2 diabetes and diabetic nephropathy with albuminuria greater than 300 mg/day**
Adults not on canagliflozin or metformin: Initiate therapy with 50 mg canagliflozin and 500 mg metformin PO b.i.d. with meals. Or, 2 extended-release tablets, each containing 50 mg canagliflozin and 500 mg metformin, once daily with morning meal. May increase dosage gradually if needed to reduce metformin's GI adverse effects. Don't exceed maximum daily dosage of 2,000 mg of metformin and 300 mg of canagliflozin.
Adults already on metformin: 50 mg canagliflozin plus previously prescribed dose of metformin PO b.i.d. with meals. Or, extended-release tablets containing 100 mg canagliflozin plus previously prescribed dose of metformin PO once daily with morning meal. May increase dosage gradually if needed to reduce metformin's GI adverse effects. Don't exceed maximum daily dosage of 2,000 mg of metformin and 300 mg of canagliflozin.
Adults already on canagliflozin: 500 mg metformin plus previously prescribed dose of canagliflozin PO b.i.d. with meals. Or, extended-release tablets containing 1,000 mg metformin plus previously prescribed dose of canagliflozin PO once daily with morning meal. May increase dosage gradually if needed to reduce metformin's GI adverse effects. Don't exceed maximum daily dosage of 2,000 mg of metformin and 300 mg of canagliflozin.

Adults already on canagliflozin and metformin: Switch to the same total daily doses of each component PO b.i.d. with meals. Or, extended-release product at same prescribed doses once daily with morning meal. May increase dosage gradually if needed to reduce metformin's GI adverse effects. Don't exceed maximum daily dosage of 2,000 mg of metformin and 300 mg of canagliflozin.
Adjust-a-dose: Limit dosage of canagliflozin to 50 mg b.i.d. or 100 mg daily in patients with eGFR of 45 to less than 60 mL/minute/1.73 m². Discontinue canagliflozin-metformin if eGFR falls below 30 mL/ minute/1.73 m². If used with UDP-glucuronosyl-transferase enzyme inhibitor, refer to manufacturer's instructions for dosing adjustments based on kidney function.

dapagliflozin–sAXagliptin
Qtern
AVAILABLE FORMS
Tablets ⓓ: 5 mg dapagliflozin and 5 mg saxagliptin, 10 mg dapagliflozin and 5 mg saxagliptin
INDICATIONS & DOSAGES
➤ **Adjunct to diet and exercise to improve glycemic control in patients with type 2 diabetes**
Adults: 1 tablet daily in the morning.
Adults not on dapagliflozin: Initially, 5 mg dapagliflozin/5 mg saxagliptin PO once daily in the morning. May increase to 10 mg dapagliflozin/5 mg saxagliptin daily.

glipiZIDE–metFORMIN hydrochloride
AVAILABLE FORMS
Tablets: 2.5 mg glipizide and 250 mg metformin hydrochloride, 2.5 mg glipizide and 500 mg metformin hydrochloride, 5 mg glipizide and 500 mg metformin hydrochloride
INDICATIONS & DOSAGES
Boxed Warning Metformin can cause serious and sometimes fatal lactic acidosis; prompt hemodialysis is recommended. ∎
Adjust-a-dose (for all indications): Discontinue drug if eGFR falls below 30 mL/minute/1.73 m².
➤ **Initial adjunctive therapy to diet and exercise to improve glycemic control in patients with type 2 diabetes**
Adults: Initially, glipizide 2.5 mg/metformin 250 mg once a day with a meal. In patients with fasting glucose level of 280 to 320 mg/dL, consider initiating therapy with glipizide 2.5 mg/metformin 500 mg b.i.d. May increase dosage every 2 weeks based on glycemic response to maximum daily dosage of 10 mg glipizide with 2,000 mg metformin in divided doses.
➤ **Second-line therapy when diet, exercise, and initial treatment with a sulfonylurea or metformin don't achieve glycemic control**
Adults: Initially, 2.5 mg glipizide/500 mg metformin or 5 mg glipizide/500 mg metformin PO b.i.d. with morning and evening meals. Increase dosage in increments of no more than glipizide 5 mg/metformin 500 mg up to maximum daily dosage of glipizide 20 mg/metformin 2,000 mg.

glyBURIDE–metFORMIN hydrochloride

AVAILABLE FORMS
Tablets: 1.25 mg glyburide and 250 mg metformin hydrochloride, 2.5 mg glyburide and 500 mg metformin hydrochloride, 5 mg glyburide and 500 mg metformin hydrochloride

INDICATIONS & DOSAGES
Boxed Warning Metformin can cause serious and sometimes fatal lactic acidosis; prompt hemodialysis is recommended. ∎

➤ **Adjunctive therapy to diet and exercise to improve glycemic control in patients with type 2 diabetes**
Adults: Initially, 1.25 mg glyburide/250 mg metformin PO daily or b.i.d. with meals.
Adults inadequately controlled on metformin, glyburide, or another sulfonyluric monotherapy: 2.5 mg glyburide/500 mg metformin or 5 mg glyburide/500 mg metformin PO b.i.d. with meals.
Adults currently on metformin and glyburide or other sulfonyluric: Switch to same total daily doses.
Adjust-a-dose: Gradually increase dosage according to glycemic control and tolerability up to maximum dosage of 20 mg glyburide and 2,000 mg metformin daily. Discontinue drug if eGFR falls below 30 mL/minute/1.73 m^2.

linagliptin–metFORMIN hydrochloride

Jentadueto, Jentadueto XR

AVAILABLE FORMS
Tablets: 2.5 mg linagliptin and 500 mg metformin hydrochloride, 2.5 mg linagliptin and 850 mg metformin hydrochloride, 2.5 mg linagliptin and 1,000 mg metformin hydrochloride
Tablets (extended-release) ⓓⓝⓒ*:* 2.5 mg linagliptin and 1,000 mg metformin hydrochloride, 5 mg linagliptin and 1,000 mg metformin hydrochloride

INDICATIONS & DOSAGES
Boxed Warning Metformin can cause serious and sometimes fatal lactic acidosis; prompt hemodialysis is recommended. ∎

➤ **Adjunct to diet and exercise to improve glycemic control in adults with type 2 diabetes**
Adults already on metformin: 2.5 mg linagliptin PO b.i.d. or 5 mg linagliptin extended-release PO once daily plus previously prescribed dosage of metformin.
Adults not on metformin: 2.5 mg linagliptin/500 mg metformin PO b.i.d. or 5 mg linagliptin/1,000 mg metformin extended-release PO once daily.
Adults currently on linagliptin and metformin: Switch to same total daily dose for immediate release. For extended-release, switch to 5 mg linagliptin and a similar metformin dosage.
Adjust-a-dose: Gradually titrate dosage to achieve glycemic control. Maximum 5 mg linagliptin and 2,000 mg metformin daily. Discontinue drug if eGFR falls below 30 mL/minute/1.73 m^2.

pioglitazone hydrochloride–metFORMIN hydrochloride

ActoPlus Met

AVAILABLE FORMS
Tablets: 15 mg pioglitazone and 500 mg metformin hydrochloride, 15 mg pioglitazone and 850 mg metformin hydrochloride

INDICATIONS & DOSAGES
Boxed Warning Pioglitazone can cause or exacerbate HF. Drug isn't recommended in patients with symptomatic HF and is contraindicated in patients with NYHA Class III or IV HF. ∎

Boxed Warning Metformin can cause serious and sometimes fatal lactic acidosis; prompt hemodialysis is recommended. ∎

➤ **Adjunct to diet and exercise to improve glycemic control in patients with type 2 diabetes**
Adults already on metformin: 15 mg pioglitazone/500 mg metformin PO b.i.d. or 15 mg pioglitazone/850 mg metformin PO once daily or b.i.d. with food based on current metformin dosage.
Adults already on pioglitazone: 15 mg pioglitazone/500 mg metformin PO b.i.d. or 15 mg pioglitazone/850 mg metformin PO once daily.
Adults with HF (NYHA Class I or II): 15 mg pioglitazone/500 mg metformin or 15 mg pioglitazone/850 mg metformin PO once daily.
Adults already on metformin and pioglitazone: Switch to same total daily dosages of each component.
Adjust-a-dose: Gradually titrate dosage to achieve glycemic control. Maximum, 45 mg pioglitazone and 2,550 mg metformin daily. Discontinue drug if eGFR falls below 30 mL/minute/1.73 m^2.

sitagliptin phosphate–metFORMIN hydrochloride

Janumet, Janumet XR

AVAILABLE FORMS
Tablets: 50 mg sitagliptin phosphate and 500 mg metformin hydrochloride, 50 mg sitagliptin phosphate and 850 mg metformin hydrochloride ✦, 50 mg sitagliptin phosphate and 1,000 mg metformin hydrochloride
Tablets (extended-release) ⓓⓝⓒ*:* 50 mg sitagliptin phosphate and 500 mg extended-release metformin hydrochloride, 50 mg sitagliptin phosphate and 1,000 mg extended-release metformin hydrochloride, 100 mg sitagliptin phosphate and 1,000 mg extended-release metformin hydrochloride

INDICATIONS & DOSAGES
Boxed Warning Metformin can cause serious and sometimes fatal lactic acidosis; prompt hemodialysis is recommended. ∎

➤ **Adjunct to diet and exercise to improve glycemic control in patients with type 2 diabetes**
Adults already on metformin (immediate-release): 50 mg sitagliptin PO b.i.d. plus previously prescribed dosage of metformin. If necessary for patients taking 850 mg metformin PO b.i.d., recommended starting

dosage is 50 mg sitagliptin/1,000 mg metformin PO b.i.d.

Adults already on metformin (extended-release): 100 mg/day sitagliptin plus previously prescribed dosage of metformin. For patients taking 850 mg immediate-release metformin PO b.i.d. or 1,000 mg metformin PO b.i.d., recommended starting dosage is 100 mg sitagliptin/2,000 mg extended-release metformin PO once daily.

Adults not on metformin: 50 mg sitagliptin/500 mg metformin PO b.i.d. or 100 mg sitagliptin/1,000 mg extended-release metformin PO once daily.

Adjust-a-dose: Gradually titrate dosage to achieve glycemic control. Maximum, 100 mg sitagliptin and 2,000 mg metformin daily. Discontinue drug if eGFR falls below 30 mL/minute/1.73 m².

Antigout drugs

probenecid–colchicine

AVAILABLE FORMS

Tablets: 500 mg probenecid and 0.5 mg colchicine

INDICATIONS & DOSAGES

➤ **Chronic gouty arthritis**

Adults: 1 tablet PO daily for 1 week; then 1 tablet PO b.i.d. If necessary, increase daily dosage by 1 tablet every 4 weeks within tolerance (usually not above 4 tablets daily) if symptoms aren't controlled or 24-hour uric acid excretion isn't above 700 mg.

Antihypertensives

amLODIPine besylate–benazepril hydrochloride

Lotrel

AVAILABLE FORMS

Capsules: 2.5 mg amlodipine besylate and 10 mg benazepril hydrochloride, 5 mg amlodipine besylate and 10 mg benazepril hydrochloride, 5 mg amlodipine besylate and 20 mg benazepril hydrochloride, 5 mg amlodipine besylate and 40 mg benazepril hydrochloride, 10 mg amlodipine besylate and 20 mg benazepril hydrochloride, 10 mg amlodipine besylate and 40 mg benazepril hydrochloride

INDICATIONS & DOSAGES

Boxed Warning Drugs that act directly on the RAAS can cause fetal harm; when pregnancy is detected, discontinue drug as soon as possible. ∎

➤ **HTN**

Adults: Initially, 2.5 mg amlodipine/10 mg benazepril PO daily in the morning. Titrate dosage based on BP response. Maximum, 10 mg amlodipine and 40 mg benazepril daily. Or substitute at same dosage for individual components.

Adjust-a-dose: Consider lower initial doses for older adults and patients with liver impairment. Drug isn't recommended in patients with CrCl of 30 mL/minute or less.

amLODIPine besylate–hydroCHLOROthiazide–olmesartan medoxomil

Tribenzor

AVAILABLE FORMS

Tablets: 5 mg amlodipine besylate, 12.5 mg hydrochlorothiazide, and 20 mg olmesartan medoxomil; 5 mg amlodipine besylate, 12.5 mg hydrochlorothiazide, and 40 mg olmesartan medoxomil; 5 mg amlodipine besylate, 25 mg hydrochlorothiazide, and 40 mg olmesartan medoxomil; 10 mg amlodipine besylate, 12.5 mg hydrochlorothiazide, and 40 mg olmesartan medoxomil; 10 mg amlodipine besylate, 25 mg hydrochlorothiazide, and 40 mg olmesartan medoxomil

INDICATIONS & DOSAGES

Boxed Warning Drugs that act directly on the RAAS can cause fetal harm; when pregnancy is detected, discontinue drug as soon as possible. ∎

➤ **HTN**

Adults: Adjust dosages of individual products; then switch to appropriate combination product. One tablet PO daily. May increase dosage after 2 weeks. Maximum recommended, 10 mg amlodipine/25 mg hydrochlorothiazide/40 mg olmesartan daily.

Adjust-a-dose: Drug isn't recommended in patients with CrCl of 30 mL/minute or less.

amLODIPine besylate–olmesartan medoxomil

Azor

AVAILABLE FORMS

Tablets: 5 mg amlodipine besylate and 20 mg olmesartan medoxomil, 5 mg amlodipine besylate and 40 mg olmesartan medoxomil, 10 mg amlodipine besylate and 20 mg olmesartan medoxomil, 10 mg amlodipine besylate and 40 mg olmesartan medoxomil

INDICATIONS & DOSAGES

Boxed Warning Drugs that act directly on the RAAS can cause fetal harm; when pregnancy is detected, discontinue drug as soon as possible. ∎

➤ **HTN**

Adults: Initially, 5 mg amlodipine/20 mg olmesartan PO once daily. Titrate as needed every 1 to 2 weeks up to maximum of 10 mg amlodipine/40 mg olmesartan once daily.

amLODIPine besylate–telmisartan

AVAILABLE FORMS

Tablets: 5 mg amlodipine besylate and 40 mg telmisartan, 5 mg amlodipine besylate and 80 mg telmisartan, 10 mg amlodipine besylate and 40 mg telmisartan, 10 mg amlodipine besylate and 80 mg telmisartan

INDICATIONS & DOSAGES

Boxed Warning Drugs that act directly on the RAAS can cause fetal harm; when pregnancy is detected, discontinue drug as soon as possible. ∎

➤ **HTN**

Adults: 1 tablet PO daily. Substitute for its individually titrated components or initiate therapy with 5 mg amlodipine/40 mg telmisartan or 5 mg amlodipine/80 mg telmisartan. May increase dosage after at least

2 weeks. Maximum, 10 mg amlodipine/80 mg telmisartan daily.

amLODIPine besylate–valsartan
Exforge
AVAILABLE FORMS

Tablets: 5 mg amlodipine besylate and 160 mg valsartan, 5 mg amlodipine besylate and 320 mg valsartan, 10 mg amlodipine besylate and 160 mg valsartan, 10 mg amlodipine besylate and 320 mg valsartan
INDICATIONS & DOSAGES
Boxed Warning Drugs that act directly on the RAAS can cause fetal harm; when pregnancy is detected, discontinue drug as soon as possible. ■
➤ **HTN**
Adults: Substitute for its individually titrated components or initiate therapy with 5 mg amlodipine/160 mg valsartan PO once daily if patient isn't volume depleted. Increase after 1 to 2 weeks to desired effect or maximum of 10 mg amlodipine/320 mg valsartan daily.

amLODIPine besylate–valsartan–hydroCHLOROthiazide
Exforge HCT
AVAILABLE FORMS

Tablets: 5 mg amlodipine besylate, 160 mg valsartan, and 12.5 mg hydrochlorothiazide; 10 mg amlodipine besylate, 160 mg valsartan, and 12.5 mg hydrochlorothiazide; 5 mg amlodipine besylate, 160 mg valsartan, and 25 mg hydrochlorothiazide; 10 mg amlodipine besylate, 160 mg valsartan, and 25 mg hydrochlorothiazide; 10 mg amlodipine besylate, 320 mg valsartan, and 25 mg hydrochlorothiazide
INDICATIONS & DOSAGES
Boxed Warning Drugs that act directly on the RAAS can cause fetal harm; when pregnancy is detected, discontinue drug as soon as possible. ■
➤ **HTN**
Adults: 1 tablet PO once daily as substitute for the individually titrated components. Or, initiate in patients not adequately controlled on any two of the following antihypertensive classes: calcium channel blockers, ARBs, and diuretics. May increase dosage after 2 weeks. Maximum recommended dose, 10 mg amlodipine/320 mg valsartan/25 mg hydrochlorothiazide.
Adjust-a-dose: In older adults and patients with liver impairment, use lower doses and titrate cautiously.

atenolol–chlorthalidone
Tenoretic
AVAILABLE FORMS

Tablets: 50 mg atenolol and 25 mg chlorthalidone, 100 mg atenolol and 25 mg chlorthalidone
INDICATIONS & DOSAGES
➤ **HTN**
Adults: Initially, 50 mg atenolol/25 mg chlorthalidone PO daily. May increase to 100 mg atenolol/25 mg chlorthalidone if needed.

Adjust-a-dose: If CrCl is 15 to 35 mL/minute/1.73 m^2, maximum dosage is 50 mg atenolol/25 mg chlorthalidone daily. If CrCl is less than 15 mL/minute/1.73 m^2, maximum dosage is 50 mg atenolol/25 mg chlorthalidone every other day.

benazepril hydrochloride–hydroCHLOROthiazide
Lotensin HCT
AVAILABLE FORMS

Tablets: 5 mg benazepril and 6.25 mg hydrochlorothiazide, 10 mg benazepril and 12.5 mg hydrochlorothiazide, 20 mg benazepril and 12.5 mg hydrochlorothiazide, 20 mg benazepril and 25 mg hydrochlorothiazide
INDICATIONS & DOSAGES
Boxed Warning Drugs that act directly on the RAAS can cause fetal harm; when pregnancy is detected, discontinue drug as soon as possible. ■
➤ **HTN**
Adults: 1 tablet PO daily in the morning. Initially, 10 mg benazepril and 12.5 mg hydrochlorothiazide in patients not adequately controlled on individual component as monotherapy. Or substitute for individually titrated components. Wait 2 to 3 weeks before increasing hydrochlorothiazide dosage. Maximum dosage, 20 mg benazepril and 25 mg hydrochlorothiazide daily.
Adjust-a-dose: Drug isn't recommended in patients with CrCl of 30 mL/minute/1.73 m^2 or less.

bisoprolol fumarate–hydroCHLOROthiazide
Ziac
AVAILABLE FORMS

Tablets: 2.5 mg bisoprolol fumarate and 6.25 mg hydrochlorothiazide, 5 mg bisoprolol fumarate and 6.25 mg hydrochlorothiazide, 10 mg bisoprolol fumarate and 6.25 mg hydrochlorothiazide
INDICATIONS & DOSAGES
➤ **HTN**
Adults: Initially, 2.5 mg bisoprolol/6.25 mg hydrochlorothiazide PO daily. Increase dosage in 14-day intervals; optimal antihypertensive effect may require 2 to 3 weeks. Or, substitute for previously titrated individual components. Maximum, 20 mg bisoprolol and 12.5 mg hydrochlorothiazide daily.
Adjust-a-dose: Use caution when titrating drug in patients with kidney or liver impairment.

candesartan cilexetil–hydroCHLOROthiazide
Atacand HCT
AVAILABLE FORMS

Tablets: 16 mg candesartan cilexetil and 12.5 mg hydrochlorothiazide, 32 mg candesartan cilexetil and 12.5 mg hydrochlorothiazide, 32 mg candesartan cilexetil and 25 mg hydrochlorothiazide
INDICATIONS & DOSAGES
Boxed Warning Drugs that act directly on the RAAS can cause fetal harm; when pregnancy is detected, discontinue drug as soon as possible. ■

➤ **HTN**
Adults: Initially, 16 mg candesartan/12.5 mg hydro-chlorothiazide PO daily in one or two divided doses in patients who aren't controlled on monotherapy with individual product or aren't volume-depleted. Titrate dosage to clinical effect. Expect maximum effect within 4 weeks of drug initiation or dosage change. Or, substitute for previously titrated individual components.

enalapril maleate–hydroCHLOROthiazide
Vaseretic
AVAILABLE FORMS
Tablets: 5 mg enalapril maleate and 12.5 mg hydrochlorothiazide, 10 mg enalapril maleate and 25 mg hydrochlorothiazide
INDICATIONS & DOSAGES
Boxed Warning Drugs that act directly on the RAAS can cause fetal harm; when pregnancy is detected, discontinue drug as soon as possible. ■
➤ **HTN**
Adults: Initially, 5 mg enalapril maleate/12.5 mg hydrochlorothiazide or 10 mg enalapril/25 mg hydrochlorothiazide PO daily in patients not adequately controlled with either enalapril or hydrochlorothiazide monotherapy. Increase dosage based on response after 2 to 3 weeks. Or, substitute for previously titrated individual components. Maximum, 20 mg enalapril and 50 mg hydrochlorothiazide daily.
Adjust-a-dose: Drug isn't recommended in patients with CrCl of 30 mL/minute/1.73 m² or less.

fosinopril–hydroCHLOROthiazide
AVAILABLE FORMS
Tablets: 10 mg fosinopril sodium and 12.5 mg hydrochlorothiazide, 20 mg fosinopril sodium and 12.5 mg hydrochlorothiazide
INDICATIONS & DOSAGES
Boxed Warning Drugs that act directly on the RAAS can cause fetal harm; when pregnancy is detected, discontinue drug as soon as possible. ■
➤ **HTN**
Adults: 1 tablet PO per day in the morning in patients not adequately controlled on either fosinopril or hydrochlorothiazide monotherapy. Titrate based on clinical effect. Or, substitute for previously titrated individual components.
Adjust-a-dose: Drug isn't recommended in patients with CrCl of 30 mL/minute/1.73 m² or less.

irbesartan–hydroCHLOROthiazide
Avalide
AVAILABLE FORMS
Tablets: 150 mg irbesartan and 12.5 mg hydrochlorothiazide, 300 mg irbesartan and 12.5 mg hydrochlorothiazide
INDICATIONS & DOSAGES
Boxed Warning Drugs that act directly on the RAAS can cause fetal harm; when pregnancy is detected, discontinue drug as soon as possible. ■
➤ **HTN**
Adults: Initially, 150 mg irbesartan/12.5 mg hydrochlorothiazide PO daily in patients not adequately

controlled on either irbesartan or hydrochlorothiazide monotherapy or as initial therapy. Titrate based on clinical effect; can increase dosage after 1 to 2 weeks. Or, substitute for previously titrated individual components. Maximum, 300 mg irbesartan and 25 mg hydrochlorothiazide daily.
Adjust-a-dose: Drug isn't recommended in patients with CrCl of 30 mL/minute/1.73 m² or less.

lisinopril–hydroCHLOROthiazide ⬚
Zestoretic
AVAILABLE FORMS
Tablets: 10 mg lisinopril and 12.5 mg hydrochlorothiazide, 20 mg lisinopril and 12.5 mg hydrochlorothiazide, 20 mg lisinopril and 25 mg hydrochlorothiazide
INDICATIONS & DOSAGES
➤ **HTN in patients not adequately controlled on lisinopril or hydrochlorothiazide monotherapy**
Adults: Initially, 10 mg lisinopril and 12.5 mg hydrochlorothiazide or 20 mg lisinopril and 12.5 mg hydrochlorothiazide PO once daily; titrate based on clinical response. Don't increase hydrochlorothiazide component until 2 to 3 weeks have elapsed. In patients on adequate pressure control on single-agent hydrochlorothiazide 25 mg PO daily but with significant potassium loss, switch to 10 mg lisinopril and 12.5 mg hydrochlorothiazide tablets. Maximum, 80 mg lisinopril and 50 mg hydrochlorothiazide PO once daily.
Adjust-a-dose: Not for use in patients with CrCl of less than 30 mL/minute/1.73 m². For older adults, dosage should be at low end of dosing range.

losartan potassium–hydroCHLOROthiazide
Hyzaar
AVAILABLE FORMS
Tablets: 50 mg losartan potassium and 12.5 mg hydrochlorothiazide, 100 mg losartan potassium and 12.5 mg hydrochlorothiazide, 100 mg losartan potassium and 25 mg hydrochlorothiazide
INDICATIONS & DOSAGES
Boxed Warning Drugs that act directly on the RAAS can cause fetal harm; when pregnancy is detected, discontinue drug as soon as possible. ■
➤ **HTN; risk reduction for stroke in patients with HTN and left ventricular hypertrophy**
Adults: 1 tablet PO daily as a substitute for individual titrated components or in patients not adequately controlled with monotherapy with either of the component products. May use as initial therapy in those with severe HTN when benefits outweigh risks. Titrate after 3 weeks. Maximum, losartan 100 mg and hydrochlorothiazide 25 mg once daily.

metoprolol tartrate–hydroCHLOROthiazide
AVAILABLE FORMS
Tablets: 50 mg metoprolol tartrate and 25 mg hydrochlorothiazide, 100 mg metoprolol tartrate and 25 mg hydrochlorothiazide, 100 mg metoprolol tartrate and 50 mg hydrochlorothiazide

INDICATIONS & DOSAGES
➤ **HTN**

Adults: Adjust dosage using individual products; then switch to appropriate combination product. Usual dosage is 100 to 200 mg metoprolol/25 to 50 mg hydrochlorothiazide PO once daily or 50 to 100 mg metoprolol/12.5 to 25 mg hydrochlorothiazide PO b.i.d.

olmesartan medoxomil–hydroCHLOROthiazide
Benicar HCT
AVAILABLE FORMS

Tablets: 20 mg olmesartan medoxomil and 12.5 mg hydrochlorothiazide, 40 mg olmesartan medoxomil and 12.5 mg hydrochlorothiazide, 40 mg olmesartan medoxomil and 25 mg hydrochlorothiazide

INDICATIONS & DOSAGES

Boxed Warning Drugs that act directly on the RAAS can cause fetal harm; when pregnancy is detected, discontinue drug as soon as possible. ■
➤ **HTN**

Adults: Initially in patients not controlled on olmesartan monotherapy, 40 mg olmesartan/12.5 mg hydrochlorothiazide PO daily. Initially in patients not controlled on hydrochlorothiazide monotherapy, 20 mg olmesartan/12.5 mg hydrochlorothiazide PO daily. May titrate dosage at 2- to 4-week intervals. Or, substitute for previously titrated individual components. Maximum, 40 mg olmesartan and 25 mg hydrochlorothiazide daily.

quinapril hydrochloride–hydroCHLOROthiazide
Accuretic
AVAILABLE FORMS

Tablets: 10 mg quinapril hydrochloride and 12.5 mg hydrochlorothiazide, 20 mg quinapril hydrochloride and 12.5 mg hydrochlorothiazide, 20 mg quinapril hydrochloride and 25 mg hydrochlorothiazide

INDICATIONS & DOSAGES

Boxed Warning Drugs that act directly on the RAAS can cause fetal harm; when pregnancy is detected, discontinue drug as soon as possible. ■
➤ **HTN**

Adults: Initially, 10 mg quinapril/12.5 mg hydrochlorothiazide or 20 mg quinapril/12.5 mg hydrochlorothiazide PO daily in patients not adequately controlled on quinapril monotherapy or who are controlled on 25 mg hydrochlorothiazide daily but experience significant potassium loss. May titrate dosage at 2- to 3-week intervals. Or, substitute for previously titrated individual components.

Adjust-a-dose: Discontinue drug if eGFR falls below 30 mL/minute/1.73 m^2 or serum creatinine level is more than 3 mg/dL.

telmisartan–hydroCHLOROthiazide
Micardis HCT
AVAILABLE FORMS

Tablets: 40 mg telmisartan and 12.5 mg hydrochlorothiazide, 80 mg telmisartan and 12.5 mg hydrochlorothiazide, 80 mg telmisartan and 25 mg hydrochlorothiazide

INDICATIONS & DOSAGES

Boxed Warning Drugs that act directly on the RAAS can cause fetal harm; when pregnancy is detected, discontinue drug as soon as possible. ■
➤ **HTN**

Adults: Initially, 80 mg telmisartan/12.5 mg hydrochlorothiazide PO per day in patients without adequate control with monotherapy on either of the component drugs or who are controlled on 25 mg hydrochlorothiazide daily but experience significant potassium loss. May adjust up to 160 mg telmisartan and 25 mg hydrochlorothiazide, based on patient's response after 2 to 4 weeks of therapy. Or, substitute for previously titrated individual components. Not for use as initial therapy.

Adjust-a-dose: In patients with Child-Pugh class A or B liver impairment or biliary obstructive disorders, begin therapy with 40 mg telmisartan/12.5 mg hydrochlorothiazide PO once daily. Don't use in patients with Child-Pugh class C liver impairment. Drug isn't recommended in patients with CrCl of 30 mL/minute/1.73 m^2 or less.

trandolapril–verapamil hydrochloride
AVAILABLE FORMS

Tablets (extended-release): 1 mg trandolapril and 240 mg verapamil hydrochloride, 2 mg trandolapril and 180 mg verapamil hydrochloride, 2 mg trandolapril and 240 mg verapamil hydrochloride, 4 mg trandolapril and 240 mg verapamil hydrochloride

INDICATIONS & DOSAGES

Boxed Warning Drugs that act directly on the RAAS can cause fetal harm; when pregnancy is detected, discontinue drug as soon as possible. ■
➤ **HTN**

Adults: 1 tablet PO per day with food. Adjust dosage using individual products; then switch to appropriate combination product.

Adjust-a-dose: In patients with liver impairment or CrCl of less than 30 mL/minute, lower dosages are recommended.

valsartan–hydroCHLOROthiazide
Diovan HCT
AVAILABLE FORMS

Tablets: 80 mg valsartan and 12.5 mg hydrochlorothiazide, 160 mg valsartan and 12.5 mg hydrochlorothiazide, 160 mg valsartan and 25 mg hydrochlorothiazide, 320 mg valsartan and 12.5 mg hydrochlorothiazide, 320 mg valsartan and 25 mg hydrochlorothiazide

INDICATIONS & DOSAGES

Boxed Warning Drugs that act directly on the RAAS can cause fetal harm; when pregnancy is detected, discontinue drug as soon as possible. ■
➤ **HTN**

Adults: Initially, 160 mg valsartan/12.5 mg hydrochlorothiazide PO daily. Titrate to desired effect after 1 to 2 weeks. Or, substitute for previously titrated individual components. Maximum, 320 mg valsartan and 25 mg hydrochlorothiazide daily.

Antilipemics

ezetimibe–simvastatin
Vytorin ☒

AVAILABLE FORMS

Tablets: 10 mg ezetimibe and 10 mg simvastatin, 10 mg ezetimibe and 20 mg simvastatin, 10 mg ezetimibe and 40 mg simvastatin, 10 mg ezetimibe and 80 mg simvastatin

INDICATIONS & DOSAGES

➤ **Homozygous familial hypercholesterolemia; primary (heterozygous familial or nonfamilial) hyperlipidemia or mixed hyperlipidemia** ☒

Adults: 1 tablet PO daily in the evening in combination with cholesterol-lowering diet and exercise. May adjust dosage of simvastatin in combination based on patient response. Usual dosing range is 10 mg ezetimibe/10 mg simvastatin to 10 mg ezetimibe/40 mg simvastatin daily.

Only use 10 mg ezetimibe/80 mg simvastatin in patients who have been taking drug long-term without evidence of muscle toxicity. In patients unable to achieve LDL-C goal using 10 mg ezetimibe/40 mg simvastatin, don't titrate to 10 mg ezetimibe/80 mg simvastatin dose; use alternative therapy.

If giving with a bile acid sequestrant, give drug at least 2 hours before or 4 hours after the bile acid sequestrant.

Adjust-a-dose: For patients with GFR less than 60 mL/minute, give 10 mg ezetimibe/20 mg simvastatin once daily in the evening. Refer to manufacturer's instructions for dosage adjustments when used with concomitant drugs. Use with niacin doses of 1,000 mg or more isn't recommended when treating patients who are Chinese because of increased risk of myopathy. ☒

Antimigraine drugs

ergotamine tartrate–caffeine
Migergot

AVAILABLE FORMS

Tablets: 1 mg ergotamine tartrate and 100 mg caffeine

Suppositories: 2 mg ergotamine tartrate and 100 mg caffeine

INDICATIONS & DOSAGES

Boxed Warning Use with potent CYP3A4 inhibitors, including protease inhibitors and macrolide antibiotics, can cause serious vasospasm and is contraindicated. ∎

➤ **Prevention and treatment of vascular headache**

Adults: 2 tablets PO at first sign of attack. Follow with 1 tablet every 30 minutes, if needed. Maximum, 6 tablets per attack; 10 tablets per week. Or, 1 suppository PR at first sign of attack; follow with second dose after 1 hour, if needed. Maximum, 2 suppositories per attack; 5 suppositories per week.

SUMAtriptan succinate–naproxen sodium
Treximet

AVAILABLE FORMS

Tablets 🌀: 10 mg sumatriptan and 60 mg naproxen, 85 mg sumatriptan and 500 mg naproxen

INDICATIONS & DOSAGES

Boxed Warning NSAIDs may cause an increased risk of serious and sometimes fatal CV thrombotic events, MI, stroke, and GI adverse reactions. Contraindicated after CABG surgery. ∎

➤ **Migraine headache**

Adults: One 85 mg sumatriptan/500 mg naproxen tablet PO at first sign of migraine. May follow with second dose 2 hours later. Maximum, 2 tablets in 24 hours. Limit use to 5 migraine headaches in 30-day period.

Children ages 12 and older: One 10 mg sumatriptan/ 60 mg naproxen PO at first sign of migraine. Maximum, 1 tablet in 24 hours. Limit use to 2 migraine headaches in 30-day period.

Adjust-a-dose: If Child-Pugh class A or B liver impairment, one 10 mg sumatriptan/ 60 mg naproxen in 24 hours.

Antiplatelet drugs

dipyridamole–aspirin

AVAILABLE FORMS

Capsules 🌀: 200 mg dipyridamole and 25 mg aspirin

INDICATIONS & DOSAGES

➤ **Reduction of stroke risk in patients with transient ischemia of the brain or ischemic stroke due to thrombosis**

Adults: 1 capsule PO b.i.d. in the morning and evening. Not interchangeable with individual components of aspirin and dipyridamole tablets.

Antiretrovirals

abacavir sulfate–lamiVUDine
Epzicom

AVAILABLE FORMS

Tablets: 600 mg abacavir and 300 mg lamivudine

INDICATIONS & DOSAGES

☒ **Boxed Warning** Contraindicated in patients with prior hypersensitivity reaction to abacavir and in patients who are positive for HLA-B*5701; screen for HLA-B*5701 allele before starting drug. Never restart drug in patients who have had a hypersensitivity reaction to abacavir; severe signs and symptoms, including death, can occur within hours. Severe acute exacerbations of HBV infection have been reported in patients infected with both HBV and HIV who have discontinued lamivudine. Monitor patients closely and begin HBV treatment if appropriate. ∎

➤ **HIV infection**

Adults and children weighing 25 kg or more: 1 tablet PO daily in combination with other antiretrovirals.

Adjust-a-dose: Use isn't recommended in patients with CrCl less than 30 mL/minute or Child-Pugh class B or C liver impairment.

---

abacavir sulfate–lamiVUDine–zidovudine ⚭

Trizivir

AVAILABLE FORMS

Tablets: 300 mg abacavir sulfate, 150 mg lamivudine, and 300 mg zidovudine

INDICATIONS & DOSAGES

⚭ **Boxed Warning** Contraindicated in patients with prior hypersensitivity reaction to abacavir and in patients positive for HLA-B*5701; screen for the HLA-B*5701 allele before starting drug. Never restart drug in patients who have had a hypersensitivity reaction to abacavir; severe signs and symptoms, including death, can occur within hours. Hematologic toxicity, myopathy, lactic acidosis, and severe liver enlargement with steatosis, including fatal cases, have been reported. Severe acute exacerbations of HBV infection have been reported in patients infected with both HBV and HIV who have discontinued lamivudine. Monitor patients closely and begin anti-HBV treatment if appropriate. ∎

➤ **HIV infection**

Adults and children weighing 40 kg or more: 1 tablet PO b.i.d., alone or with other antiretrovirals.

Adjust-a-dose: Use isn't recommended in patients with CrCl less than 50 mL/minute or Child-Pugh class A liver impairment. Use is contraindicated in patients with Child-Pugh class B or C liver impairment.

bictegravir–emtricitabine–tenofovir alafenamide

Biktarvy

AVAILABLE FORMS

Tablets: 30 mg bictegravir, 120 mg emtricitabine, and 15 mg tenofovir alafenamide; 50 mg bictegravir, 200 mg emtricitabine, and 25 mg tenofovir alafenamide

INDICATIONS & DOSAGES

Boxed Warning Severe, acute reactivations of HBV infection have been reported in patients infected with both HIV and HBV who have discontinued emtricitabine or tenofovir. Close monitoring over several months is recommended. If appropriate, initiate anti-hepatitis B therapy. ∎

➤ **HIV-1 infection in patients who have no antiretroviral treatment history or to replace current antiretroviral regimen in patients who are virologically suppressed (HIV-1 RNA less than 50 copies/mL) on a stable antiretroviral regimen with no history of treatment failure and no known substitutions associated with resistance to the individual components**

Adults and children weighing at least 25 kg: 1 tablet of 50 mg bictegravir, 200 mg emtricitabine, and 25 mg tenofovir alafenamide PO daily.

Children weighing 14 to less than 25 kg: 1 tablet of 30 mg bictegravir, 120 mg emtricitabine, and 15 mg tenofovir alafenamide PO daily.

Adjust-a-dose: Use isn't recommended in patients with CrCl less than 15 to 30 mL/minute, CrCl below 15 mL/minute not on hemodialysis, or below 15 mL/minute on hemodialysis with no antiretroviral

treatment history. Use isn't recommended in patients with Child-Pugh class C liver impairment.

efavirenz–emtricitabine–tenofovir disoproxil fumarate

AVAILABLE FORMS

Tablets: 600 mg efavirenz, 200 mg emtricitabine, and 300 mg tenofovir disoproxil fumarate

INDICATIONS & DOSAGES

Boxed Warning Severe, acute reactivations of HBV infection have been reported in patients infected with both HIV and HBV who have discontinued emtricitabine or tenofovir. Close monitoring over several months is recommended. If appropriate, initiate anti-hepatitis B therapy. ∎

➤ **HIV infection**

Adults and children weighing at least 40 kg: 1 tablet PO daily on empty stomach. Dosing at bedtime may improve tolerability of nervous system symptoms.

Adjust-a-dose: If given with rifampin in patients weighing 50 kg or more, give additional 200 mg of efavirenz per day. Use isn't recommended in patients with CrCl less than 50 mL/minute or Child-Pugh class B or C liver impairment.

emtricitabine–rilpivirine–tenofovir disoproxil fumarate

Complera

AVAILABLE FORMS

Tablets: 200 mg emtricitabine, 25 mg rilpivirine, and 300 mg tenofovir disoproxil fumarate

INDICATIONS & DOSAGES

Boxed Warning Severe, acute reactivations of HBV infection have been reported in patients infected with both HIV and HBV who have discontinued emtricitabine or tenofovir. Close monitoring over several months is recommended. If appropriate, initiate anti-hepatitis B therapy. ∎

➤ **HIV infection**

Adults and children weighing 35 kg or more: 1 tablet PO once daily with food.

Adjust-a-dose: Use isn't recommended in patients with CrCl less than 50 mL/minute. If taken with rifabutin, give an additional 25 mg of rilpivirine.

emtricitabine–tenofovir disoproxil fumarate

Truvada

AVAILABLE FORMS

Tablets: 100 mg emtricitabine and 150 mg tenofovir disoproxil fumarate, 133 mg emtricitabine and 200 mg tenofovir disoproxil fumarate, 167 mg emtricitabine and 250 mg tenofovir disoproxil fumarate, 200 mg emtricitabine and 300 mg tenofovir disoproxil fumarate

INDICATIONS & DOSAGES

Boxed Warning For preexposure prophylaxis, confirm that patients are HIV-negative immediately before initiating and periodically (at least every 3 months) during use to decrease risk of drug resistance. Severe acute exacerbations of

HBV infection have been reported in HBV-infected patients who have discontinued drug. Monitor patients closely and begin anti-HBV therapy if appropriate. ■

➤ **Preexposure prophylaxis (adults and adolescents weighing at least 35 kg); treatment of HIV infection in combination with other retrovirals**

Adults and adolescents (preexposure prophylaxis and treatment) and children weighing 35 kg or more (treatment): 200 mg emtricitabine/300 mg tenofovir disoproxil fumarate PO daily.

Children weighing 28 to less than 35 kg: 167 mg emtricitabine/250 mg tenofovir disoproxil fumarate PO daily.

Children weighing 22 to less than 28 kg: 133 mg emtricitabine/200 mg tenofovir disoproxil fumarate PO daily.

Children weighing 17 to less than 22 kg: 100 mg emtricitabine/150 mg tenofovir disoproxil fumarate PO daily.

Adjust-a-dose: For adults with CrCl of 30 to 49 mL/minute, give dose every 48 hours; withhold drug for CrCl of less than 30 mL/minute. There are no dosage recommendations for children with kidney impairment. Drug isn't recommended for preexposure prophylaxis in individuals with estimated CrCl below 60 mL/minute.

lamiVUDine–zidovudine
Combivir
AVAILABLE FORMS
Tablets: 150 mg lamivudine and 300 mg zidovudine
INDICATIONS & DOSAGES
Boxed Warning Hematologic toxicity, myopathy, lactic acidosis, severe liver enlargement (including fatal cases), and exacerbations of HBV infection have been reported. ■

➤ **HIV infection**
Adults and children weighing 30 kg or more: 1 tablet PO b.i.d.
Adjust-a-dose: Use isn't recommended in patients with CrCl less than 50 mL/minute or liver impairment.

Antiulcer drugs
bismuth subcitrate potassium–metroNIDAZOLE–tetracycline
Pylera
AVAILABLE FORMS
Capsules: 140 mg bismuth subcitrate potassium, 125 mg metronidazole, and 125 mg tetracycline hydrochloride
INDICATIONS & DOSAGES
Boxed Warning Metronidazole has been shown to be carcinogenic in mice and rats. It's unknown if it's carcinogenic in humans. ■

➤ **Eradication of *Helicobacter pylori* infection; active duodenal ulcers associated with *H. pylori* infection**
Adults: Give each dose (which includes all 3 capsules) PO q.i.d. after meals and at bedtime for 10 days with

omeprazole 20 mg PO b.i.d. (after morning and evening meals) for 10 days.

lansoprazole–amoxicillin–clarithromycin
AVAILABLE FORMS
Daily administration pack: Two 30-mg lansoprazole capsules, four 500-mg amoxicillin capsules, and two 500-mg clarithromycin tablets
INDICATIONS & DOSAGES
➤ **Eradication of *Helicobacter pylori* infection in patients with duodenal ulcer disease**
Adults: 30 mg lansoprazole, 1 g amoxicillin, and 500 mg clarithromycin PO b.i.d. before eating (morning and evening) for 10 to 14 days.
⚠ *Alert:* Clarithromycin may increase risk of altered cardiac conduction. Avoid use in patients at high risk.

Benign prostatic hyperplasia drug
dutasteride–tamsulosin hydrochloride
Jalyn
AVAILABLE FORMS
Capsules ⓓⓝⓒ: 0.5 mg dutasteride and 0.4 mg tamsulosin hydrochloride
INDICATIONS & DOSAGES
➤ **Symptomatic BPH**
Adult males: 1 capsule PO daily 30 minutes after same meal each day.

Contraceptives
segesterone acetate–ethinyl estradiol
Annovera
AVAILABLE FORMS
Vaginal ring: 103 mg segesterone acetate and 17.4 mg ethinyl estradiol, delivering average of 0.15 mg segesterone acetate and 0.013 mg ethinyl estradiol daily
INDICATIONS & DOSAGES
Boxed Warning Cigarette smoking increases risk of serious CV events from combination hormonal contraceptives; avoid use in patients older than age 35 who smoke. ■
➤ **Contraception**
Patients of childbearing potential: 1 vaginal ring inserted into vagina and left in place continuously for 21 days, followed by 7-day vaginal ring-free interval. One vaginal ring provides 13 cycles of contraception for approximately 1 year.

Diuretics
aMILoride hydrochloride–hydroCHLOROthiazide
AVAILABLE FORMS
Tablets: 5 mg amiloride hydrochloride and 50 mg hydrochlorothiazide
INDICATIONS & DOSAGES
Boxed Warning May cause potentially fatal hyperkalemia; carefully monitor serum potassium level. ■
➤ **HF or HTN**
Adults: 1 to 2 tablets PO per day as single daily dose or in divided doses with food.

spironolactone–hydroCHLOROthiazide
Aldactazide
AVAILABLE FORMS
Tablets: 25 mg spironolactone and 25 mg hydrochlorothiazide, 50 mg spironolactone and 50 mg hydrochlorothiazide
INDICATIONS & DOSAGES
Adjust-a-dose (all indications): In older adults, initiate with lowest available dose. Avoid spironolactone dosages of more than 25 mg/day in older adults with HF or kidney impairment.
➤ **Edema**
Adults: 25 to 200 mg spironolactone/25 to 200 mg hydrochlorothiazide PO in single or divided doses daily.
➤ **HTN**
Adults: 50 to 100 mg spironolactone/50 to 100 mg hydrochlorothiazide PO in single or divided doses daily.

Heart failure drugs

isosorbide dinitrate–hydrALAZINE hydrochloride
BiDil
AVAILABLE FORMS
Tablets: 20 mg isosorbide dinitrate and 37.5 mg hydralazine
INDICATIONS & DOSAGES
➤ **Adjunct to standard HF therapy in patients who self-identify as Black**
Adults: 1 to 2 tablets PO t.i.d. Maximum, 2 tablets PO t.i.d.

Menopause drugs

conjugated estrogens–bazedoxifene acetate
Duavee
AVAILABLE FORMS
Tablets: 0.45 mg conjugated estrogens and 20 mg bazedoxifene acetate
INDICATIONS & DOSAGES
Boxed Warning Product may increase risk of endometrial cancer. Product isn't for use for preventing CV disease or dementia. Product shouldn't be used with additional estrogens; use at lowest effective doses, for shortest duration, consistent with treatment goals and risks for the individual patient. ■
➤ **Vasomotor symptoms associated with menopause; postmenopausal osteoporosis prevention**
Adults: 1 tablet PO once daily.

conjugated estrogens/conjugated estrogens–medroxyPROGESTERone acetate
Premphase
AVAILABLE FORMS
Tablets: 0.625 mg conjugated estrogens, 0.625 mg conjugated estrogens and 5 mg medroxyprogesterone acetate
INDICATIONS & DOSAGES
Boxed Warning Product may increase risk of endometrial and breast cancer and CV disease. Product isn't for use for preventing dementia or CV disease. Use at lowest effective doses, for the shortest duration, consistent with treatment goals and risks for the individual patient. ■
➤ **Moderate to severe symptoms (vasomotor, vulvar, and vaginal atrophy) of menopause; prevention of postmenopausal osteoporosis**
Patients with intact uterus: 1 tablet PO per day. Use estrogen (maroon tablet) alone on days 1 to 14 and estrogen–medroxyprogesterone acetate (light blue tablet) on days 15 to 28.

conjugated estrogens–medroxyPROGESTERone acetate
Prempro
AVAILABLE FORMS
Tablets: 0.3 mg conjugated estrogens and 1.5 mg medroxyprogesterone, 0.45 mg conjugated estrogens and 1.5 mg medroxyprogesterone; 0.625 mg conjugated estrogens and 2.5 mg medroxyprogesterone, 0.625 mg conjugated estrogens and 5 mg medroxyprogesterone
INDICATIONS & DOSAGES
Boxed Warning Product may increase risk of endometrial and breast cancers and CV disease. Product isn't for use for preventing dementia. Use at lowest effective doses, for the shortest duration, consistent with treatment goals and risks for the individual patient. ■
➤ **Symptoms of menopause (vasomotor, vulvar, and vaginal atrophy); prevention of postmenopausal osteoporosis**
Patients with intact uterus: 1 tablet PO per day.

Miscellaneous cardiac drugs

amLODIPine besylate–atorvastatin calcium
Caduet
AVAILABLE FORMS
Tablets: 2.5 mg amlodipine besylate and 10 mg atorvastatin calcium, 2.5 mg amlodipine besylate and 20 mg atorvastatin calcium, 2.5 mg amlodipine besylate and 40 mg atorvastatin calcium, 5 mg amlodipine besylate and 10 mg atorvastatin calcium, 5 mg amlodipine besylate and 20 mg atorvastatin calcium, 5 mg amlodipine besylate and 40 mg atorvastatin calcium, 5 mg amlodipine besylate and 80 mg atorvastatin calcium, 10 mg amlodipine besylate and 10 mg atorvastatin calcium, 10 mg amlodipine besylate and 20 mg atorvastatin calcium, 10 mg amlodipine besylate and 40 mg atorvastatin calcium, 10 mg amlodipine besylate and 80 mg atorvastatin calcium
INDICATIONS & DOSAGES
Adjust-a-dose (all indications): For small or fragile patients, older adults, children older than age 6, and patients with liver insufficiency, initially, 2.5 mg amlodipine once daily. Atorvastatin is contraindicated in patients with active liver disease or unexplained LFT elevations. Refer to manufacturer's instructions for dosage adjustments when used with other drugs.

➤ **HTN, CAD (amlodipine); prevention of CV disease, hyperlipidemia (atorvastatin)**
Adults and children older than age 6 : Determine most effective dose for each component; then select most appropriate combination product. When titrating amlodipine, wait 7 to 14 days between titration steps. When titrating atorvastatin, adjust dosage at intervals of 4 weeks or more. Or, substitute for individually titrated components. Maximum, amlodipine 10 mg and atorvastatin 80 mg daily.

aspirin–omeprazole
Yosprala
AVAILABLE FORMS
Tablets (delayed-release) ⓪Nℂ*:* 81 mg delayed-release aspirin and 40 mg immediate-release omeprazole; 325 mg delayed-release aspirin and 40 mg immediate-release omeprazole
INDICATIONS & DOSAGES
➤ **To reduce risk of aspirin-associated gastric ulcers in patients who require aspirin for secondary prevention of CV and cerebrovascular events**
Adults: 1 tablet PO once daily 60 minutes before a meal.

Opioid agonists

buprenorphine hydrochloride–naloxone hydrochloride
Suboxone, Zubsolv
Controlled substance schedule: III
AVAILABLE FORMS
SL film (Suboxone): 2 mg buprenorphine and 0.5 mg naloxone, 4 mg buprenorphine and 1 mg naloxone, 8 mg buprenorphine and 2 mg naloxone, 12 mg buprenorphine and 3 mg naloxone
SL tablets: 2 mg buprenorphine and 0.5 mg naloxone, 8 mg buprenorphine and 2 mg naloxone
SL tablets (Zubsolv): 0.7 mg buprenorphine and 0.18 mg naloxone, 1.4 mg buprenorphine and 0.36 mg naloxone 2.9 mg, buprenorphine and 0.71 mg naloxone, 5.7 mg buprenorphine and 1.4 mg naloxone, 8.6 mg buprenorphine and 2.1 mg naloxone, 11.4 mg buprenorphine and 2.9 mg naloxone
INDICATIONS & DOSAGES
➤ **Induction of opioid dependence treatment**
Refer to manufacturer's instructions for specific product and drug dependency.
➤ **Opioid dependence**
Adults: Maintenance dose is based on buprenorphine. Refer to manufacturer's instructions for specific product.

Psychotherapeutics

chlordiazePOXIDE–amitriptyline
Controlled substance schedule: IV
AVAILABLE FORMS
Tablets: 5 mg chlordiazepoxide and 12.5 mg amitriptyline, 10 mg chlordiazepoxide and 25 mg amitriptyline

INDICATIONS & DOSAGES
▐ Boxed Warning ▐ Product is not approved for use in children because of increased suicide risk. Monitor patients on antidepressants for appearance or worsening of suicidality. Benzodiazepine use with opioids can cause sedation and fatal respiratory depression. Use of product increases risk of addiction, abuse, and misuse. ▐
➤ **Severe depression with anxiety**
Adults: 10 mg chlordiazepoxide/25 mg amitriptyline PO t.i.d. to up to six times daily. For patients who don't tolerate higher doses, 5 mg chlordiazepoxide/ 12.5 mg amitriptyline PO t.i.d. to q.i.d. Reduce dosage after initial response.
Adjust-a-dose: Older adults may need lower dosages. Gradually taper dosage to discontinue therapy.

OLANZapine–FLUoxetine hydrochloride
Symbyax
AVAILABLE FORMS
Capsules: 3 mg olanzapine and 25 mg fluoxetine, 6 mg olanzapine and 25 mg fluoxetine, 6 mg olanzapine and 50 mg fluoxetine, 12 mg olanzapine and 25 mg fluoxetine, 12 mg olanzapine and 50 mg fluoxetine
INDICATIONS & DOSAGES
▐ Boxed Warning ▐ Drug increases risk of suicidality. Not approved for use in children younger than age 10 because of suicide risk or in patients with dementia-related psychosis because of increased risk of death. ▐
➤ **Bipolar I disorder or treatment resistant depression**
Adults: 1 capsule PO daily in the evening. Initially, 6 mg olanzapine/25 mg fluoxetine capsule, adjusted according to effectiveness and tolerability.
Children ages 10 and older with bipolar depression: Initially, 3 mg olanzapine/25 mg fluoxetine PO daily in the evening, adjusted according to effectiveness and tolerability.

perphenazine–amitriptyline hydrochloride
AVAILABLE FORMS
Tablets: 2 mg perphenazine and 10 mg amitriptyline hydrochloride, 2 mg perphenazine and 25 mg amitriptyline hydrochloride, 4 mg perphenazine and 10 mg amitriptyline hydrochloride, 4 mg perphenazine and 25 mg amitriptyline hydrochloride, 4 mg perphenazine and 50 mg amitriptyline hydrochloride
INDICATIONS & DOSAGES
▐ Boxed Warning ▐ Drug increases risk of suicidality. Not approved for use in children because of suicide risk or in patients with dementia-related psychosis because of increased risk of death. ▐
➤ **Anxiety, agitation, or depression**
Adults: 2 to 4 mg perphenazine/10 to 25 mg amitriptyline PO t.i.d. to q.i.d. or 4 mg perphenazine/50 mg amitriptyline PO b.i.d. Reduce dosage after initial response. In severely ill patients with schizophrenia, initial dose of 2 tablets (4 mg perphenazine/25 mg

amitriptyline) PO t.i.d.; if needed, add fourth dose at bedtime.

Respiratory tract drugs

budesonide–formoterol fumarate dihydrate

Breyna, Symbicort

AVAILABLE FORMS

Aerosol inhalation: 80 mcg budesonide and 4.5 mcg formoterol fumarate dihydrate per actuation, 160 mcg budesonide and 4.5 mcg formoterol fumarate dihydrate per actuation

INDICATIONS & DOSAGES

➤ **Asthma, COPD**

Adults and children ages 12 and older: Initially, 2 inhalations b.i.d. approximately 12 hours apart. For COPD, use only 160 mcg budesonide and 4.5 mcg formoterol fumarate dihydrate.

Children ages 6 to younger than 12: 2 inhalations of 80 mcg budesonide and 4.5 mcg formoterol fumarate dihydrate b.i.d.

chlorpheniramine polistirex–HYDROcodone polistirex

Controlled substance schedule: II

AVAILABLE FORMS

Oral solution (extended-release): 8 mg chlorpheniramine polistirex and 10 mg hydrocodone polistirex (equivalent to 10 mg hydrocodone bitartrate)/5 mL

INDICATIONS & DOSAGES

Boxed Warning Opioid use increases risk of addiction, abuse, and misuse. Opioids can cause fatal respiratory depression. Opioids can cause respiratory depression and death in children with ingestion of even one dose. Opioids combined with benzodiazepines or CNS depressants can cause death. Use during pregnancy can cause neonatal opioid withdrawal syndrome. Avoid use in patients taking CYP3A4 inhibitors or inducers. ■

➤ **Cough and upper respiratory signs and symptoms associated with allergy or cold**

Adults: 5 mL PO every 12 hours. Maximum, 16 mg chlorpheniramine polistirex and 20 mg hydrocodone polistirex in 24 hours.

ipratropium bromide–albuterol sulfate

Combivent Respimat

AVAILABLE FORMS

Metered-dose inhaler: 20 mcg ipratropium bromide and 100 mcg albuterol sulfate

Nebulizer solution: 0.5 mg ipratropium bromide and 2.5 mg albuterol sulfate/3 mL

INDICATIONS & DOSAGES

➤ **COPD in patients who require more than a single bronchodilator**

Adults: 1 inhalation q.i.d.; may give additional doses as needed up to maximum of 6 total inhalations in 24 hours. Or, 1 nebulization every 6 hours; may give up to 6 nebulizations in 24 hours.

loratadine–pseudoephedrine sulfate

Alavert Allergy/Sinus ◇, Claritin-D ◇, Claritin-D 24 Hour ◇

AVAILABLE FORMS

Tablets (extended-release) ⊙: 5 mg loratadine and 120 mg pseudoephedrine, 10 mg loratadine and 240 mg pseudoephedrine

INDICATIONS & DOSAGES

➤ **Cold; allergy symptoms**

Adults and children ages 12 and older: 5 mg loratadine/120 mg pseudoephedrine PO b.i.d. or 10 mg loratadine/240 mg pseudoephedrine PO daily. Maximum, 10 mg loratadine/240 mg pseudoephedrine daily.

mometasone furoate–formoterol fumarate dihydrate

Dulera

AVAILABLE FORMS

Oral inhalation: 50 mcg mometasone furoate and 5 mcg formoterol fumarate dihydrate, 100 mcg mometasone furoate and 5 mcg formoterol fumarate dihydrate, 200 mcg mometasone furoate and 5 mcg formoterol fumarate dihydrate

INDICATIONS & DOSAGES

➤ **Asthma**

Adults and children older than age 12: 2 inhalations b.i.d. Base starting dose on prior therapy with inhaled corticosteroids.

Children ages 5 to younger than 12: Using a 50-mcg mometasone furoate/5 mcg formoterol fumarate dihydrate inhaler, 2 inhalations b.i.d. (morning and evening). Maximum, 200 mcg mometasone furoate/20 mcg formoterol fumarate dihydrate daily.

Adjust-a-dose: Titrate to the lowest effective dose after 2 to 3 months when asthma becomes well controlled.

Antidotes: Indications and dosages

Refer to manufacturer's instructions for complete prescribing and safety information.

activated charcoal
Actidose-Aqua, Actidose with Sorbitol, Char-Flo with Sorbitol, EZ Char, Insta-Char Aqueous, Insta-Char in Sorbitol

Therapeutic class: Antidotes
Pharmacologic class: Adsorbents

AVAILABLE FORMS
Liquid: 15 g◇*, 25 g◇*, 50 g◇*
Oral suspension: 25 g◇
Powder for reconstitution: 25 g◇

INDICATIONS & DOSAGES
➤ **Emergency use to adsorb swallowed poisons**
Adjust-a-dose (all indications): Follow instructions for product use and dosing as directed by prescriber, including poison control center. Dosing may vary depending on poison ingested, age, weight, and formulation used.
Adults and children ages 12 and older weighing more than 32 kg: 50 to 100 g PO (aqueous base); may repeat every 4 to 6 hours. Or, 50 to 100 g or 1 to 2 g/kg PO (sorbitol base) as single dose; may give additional dose with aqueous base formulation.
Children ages 1 to 12 weighing 16 to 32 kg: 25 to 50 g PO; may repeat every 4 to 6 hours. Or, 15 to 30 g or 1 to 2 g/kg PO (sorbitol base) as single dose; may give additional dose with aqueous base formulation.
Children younger than age 1 (aqueous only): 1 g/kg. May repeat every 4 to 6 hours.
Adults and children (EZ Char): For patients weighing 22 kg or more, give entire amount of reconstituted liquid (25 g); for those weighing 11 to less than 22 kg, give 60 to 120 mL (4 to 8 tablespoons) of reconstituted liquid; for those weighing 5.5 to less than 11 kg, give 30 to 60 mL (2 to 4 tablespoons) of reconstituted liquid; for those weighing 2.7 to less than 5.5 kg, give 15 to 30 mL (1 to 2 tablespoons) of reconstituted liquid. Repeat dose immediately, if necessary.

amifostine
am-i-FOS-steen

Ethyol

Therapeutic class: Cytoprotective drugs
Pharmacologic class: Organic thiophosphates

AVAILABLE FORMS
Injection: 500 mg in single-use vials

INDICATIONS & DOSAGES
Adjust-a-dose (all indications): Refer to manufacturer's instructions for interrupting therapy if hypotension occurs.
➤ **Reduction of cumulative kidney toxicity associated with repeated administration of cisplatin in patients with advanced ovarian cancer**
Adults: 910 mg/m^2 once daily as 15-minute IV infusion, starting 30 minutes before chemotherapy. Premedication with antiemetics, including dexamethasone 20 mg IV and a serotonin 5-HT$_3$ receptor antagonist, are recommended.
➤ **Moderate to severe xerostomia in patients undergoing postoperative radiation treatment for head and neck cancer, when the radiation port includes a substantial portion of the parotid glands**
Adults: 200 mg/m^2 once daily as 3-minute IV infusion, starting 15 to 30 minutes before standard fraction radiation therapy. Premedication with oral 5-HT$_3$ receptor antagonists, alone or in combination with other antiemetics, is recommended.

deferasirox
de-FER-a-sir-ox

Exjade, Jadenu, Jadenu Sprinkle

Therapeutic class: Chelating agents
Pharmacologic class: Heavy metal antagonists

AVAILABLE FORMS
Sprinkles: 90 mg, 180 mg, 360 mg
Tablets: 90 mg, 180 mg, 360 mg
Tablets for oral suspension ⓄⓃⒸ: 125 mg, 250 mg, 500 mg

INDICATIONS & DOSAGES
Boxed Warning Drug can cause fatal liver failure, KF, and GI hemorrhage. Monitor patient carefully. ■

Adjust-a-dose (for all indications): When converting therapy from Exjade to Jadenu, the dose of Jadenu should be approximately 30% lower (rounded to the nearest whole tablet) than the current dose of Exjade. Contraindicated in patients with platelet count less than 50,000/mm^3. Discontinue drug if eGFR is less than 40 mL/minute/1.73 m^2. Start older adults at low end of dosing range. Reduce starting dosage by 50% in patients with Child-Pugh class B liver impairment. Closely monitor all patients with Child-Pugh class A or B liver impairment for effectiveness and adverse reactions. Reduce starting dosage by 50% in patients with eGFR of 40 to 60 mL/minute/1.73 m^2. Use cautiously in children with eGFR between 40 and 60 mL/minute/1.73 m^2. If treatment is needed, use minimum effective dosage and frequently monitor kidney function.

Adjust-a-dose: For unavoidable use with a bile acid sequestrant or UDP-glucuronosyltransferase (UGT) inducer, increase deferasirox dosage by 50% and monitor ferritin level.

➤ **Chronic iron overload caused by blood transfusions (transfusional hemosiderosis)**
Adults and children ages 2 and older with eGFR greater than 60 mL/minute/1.73 m²: Exjade oral suspension: Initially, 20 mg/kg PO daily on an empty stomach 30 minutes before eating. Monitor serum ferritin level monthly, and adjust dosage every 3 to 6 months by 5 or 10 mg/kg based on ferritin trends. Maximum, 40 mg/kg daily. Interrupt therapy and continue monthly monitoring if serum ferritin level drops below 500 mcg/L.

Jadenu: Initially, 14 mg/kg PO once daily on an empty stomach or with a light meal. Monitor serum ferritin level monthly, and adjust dosage every 3 to 6 months by increments of 3.5 or 7 mg/kg, based on serum ferritin trends. Maximum, 428 mg/kg daily. If serum ferritin level falls below 1,000 mcg/L at two consecutive visits, consider dosage reduction, especially if dosage is greater than 17.5 mg/kg/day. Interrupt therapy if serum ferritin level drops below 500 mcg/L and continue monthly monitoring.
Adjust-a-dose: Interrupt therapy for children with acute illnesses that can cause volume depletion and monitor more frequently. Resume therapy as appropriate.

For adults: If serum creatinine level increases by 33% or more above the average baseline measurement, repeat serum creatinine within 1 week and, if still elevated by 33% or more, reduce Exjade dose by 10 mg/kg or Jadenu dose by 7 mg/kg.

For children ages 2 to 17: Reduce Exjade dose by 10 mg/kg/day or Jadenu dose by 7 mg/kg if eGFR decreases by greater than 33% below the average baseline measurement; retest eGFR within 1 week.

➤ **Chronic iron overload in patients with non-transfusion-dependent thalassemia syndromes and with liver iron (Fe) concentration (LIC) of at least 5 mg Fe per gram of dry weight (dw) and serum ferritin level greater than 300 mcg/L**
Adults and children ages 10 and older with eGFR greater than 60 mL/minute/1.73 m²: Exjade oral suspension: Initially, 10 mg/kg PO once daily 30 minutes before food. If baseline LIC is greater than 15 mg Fe/g dw, may increase to 20 mg/kg/day after 4 weeks. Interrupt treatment when serum ferritin level is less than 300 mcg/L, and obtain LIC to determine if LIC is less than 3 mg Fe/g dw. If LIC remains greater than 7 mg Fe/g dw after 6 months of therapy, increase dosage to maximum of 20 mg/kg/day. If LIC is 3 to 7 mg Fe/g dw after 6 months, continue treatment at maximum of 10 mg/kg/day. If LIC is less than 3 mg Fe/g dw, stop treatment. Continue to monitor LIC, and restart treatment when LIC rises again to more than 5 mg Fe/g dw.

Jadenu: Initially, 7 mg/kg PO once daily on an empty stomach or with a light meal. If baseline LIC is greater than 15 mg Fe/g dw, may increase to 14 mg/kg/day after 4 weeks. Interrupt treatment when serum ferritin level is less than 300 mcg/L, and obtain LIC to determine if LIC is less than 3 mg Fe/g dw. If LIC remains greater than 7 mg Fe/g dw after 6 months of therapy, increase dosage to maximum of 14 mg/kg/day. If LIC is 3 to 7 mg Fe/g dw after 6 months, continue treatment at maximum of 7 mg/kg/day. If LIC is less than 3 mg Fe/g dw, stop treatment. Continue to monitor LIC and restart treatment when LIC rises again to more than 5 mg Fe/g dw.
Adjust-a-dose: Increase monitoring frequency and consider dose interruption for children who have acute illness that can cause volume depletion.

For adults: If serum creatinine level increases by 33% or more above the average baseline measurement, repeat serum creatinine within 1 week and, if still elevated by 33% or more, interrupt Exjade therapy if dose is 5 mg/kg or reduce by 50% if dose is 10 or 20 mg/kg; interrupt Jadenu therapy if dose is 3.5 mg/kg or reduce by 50% if dose is 7 or 14 mg/kg.

For children ages 10 to 17: Reduce Exjade dose by 5 mg/kg/day or Jadenu dose by 3.5 mg/kg if eGFR decreases by greater than 33% below the average baseline measurement; retest eGFR within 1 week.

deferiprone
de-FER-i-prone

Ferriprox

Therapeutic class: Chelating drugs
Pharmacologic class: Heavy metal antagonists

AVAILABLE FORMS
Solution: 100 mg/mL
Tablets: 500 mg, 1 g (for t.i.d. dosing); 1g (for b.i.d. dosing)

INDICATIONS & DOSAGES
Boxed Warning Drug can cause agranulocytosis, which can lead to serious infections and death. Measure ANC before therapy and weekly during therapy. Interrupt therapy for neutropenia or infection. Advise patients to immediately report signs or symptoms of infection. ■
Adjust-a-dose (for all indications): To minimize GI upset when initiating therapy, may start at 45 mg/kg/day and increase weekly by 15 mg/kg/day. If serum ferritin level falls consistently below 500 mcg/L, consider temporary therapy interruption. For ANC less than 1,500/mm³, immediately interrupt therapy and monitor until recovery; don't rechallenge unless potential benefit outweighs risk. For ANC less than 500/mm³, consider hospitalization and other clinically appropriate management; don't resume unless potential benefits outweigh risks.
➤ **Transfusional iron overload due to thalassemia syndromes, sickle cell disease, or other anemias**
Adults and children ages 8 and older: Initially, 75 mg/kg/day PO in divided doses (t.i.d. tablets or b.i.d.

tablets). May titrate to maximum dosage of 99 mg/kg/day based on patient response and therapeutic goals. Round dose to nearest 500 mg (one-half 1-g tablet) or 250 mg (one-half 500-mg tablet).

Adults and children ages 3 and older: Initially, 25 mg/kg oral solution PO t.i.d., for total of 75 mg/kg/day. May titrate to maximum dosage of 99 mg/kg/day based on patient response and therapeutic goals. Round dose to nearest 2.5 mL of oral solution.

digoxin immune Fab (ovine)
di-JOX-in

DigiFab

Therapeutic class: Antidotes
Pharmacologic class: Antibody fragments

AVAILABLE FORMS
Injection: 40-mg vial

INDICATIONS & DOSAGES
➤ **Life-threatening digoxin toxicity**
Adults and children: Base dosage on ingested amount or level of digoxin. When calculating antidote amount, round up to nearest whole number. Each vial of digoxin immune Fab binds to about 0.5 mg of digoxin. For digoxin tablets, calculate number of antidote vials as follows: multiply ingested amount by 0.8; then divide answer by 0.5. For example, if patient takes 25 tablets of 0.25 mg digoxin, the ingested amount is 6.25 mg; multiply 6.25 mg by 0.8 and divide answer by 0.5 to obtain 10 vials of antidote. If digoxin level is known, determine the number of antidote vials as follows: multiply the digoxin level in nanograms per milliliter by patient's weight in kilograms; then divide by 100.
➤ **Acute toxicity or if estimated ingested amount or digoxin level is unknown**
Adults and children: Consider giving 10 vials of digoxin immune Fab and observing patient's response. Follow with another 10 vials, if indicated. Dosage should be effective in most life-threatening cases in adults and children but may cause volume overload in young children.
➤ **Toxicity during prolonged therapy if digoxin level is unknown**
Adults and children: 6 vials of antidote for patients weighing 20 kg or more or 1 vial of antidote for patients weighing less than 20 kg.

dimercaprol
dye-mer-KAP-role

BAL in Oil

Therapeutic class: Chelating drugs
Pharmacologic class: Heavy metal antagonists

AVAILABLE FORMS
Injection: 100 mg/mL

INDICATIONS & DOSAGES
➤ **Severe arsenic or gold poisoning**
Adults and children: 3 mg/kg deep IM every 4 hours for 2 days, q.i.d. on third day, and then b.i.d. for 10 days.
➤ **Mild arsenic or gold poisoning**
Adults and children: 2.5 mg/kg deep IM q.i.d. for 2 days, b.i.d. on third day, and then once daily for 10 days.
➤ **Mercury poisoning**
Adults and children: Initially, 5 mg/kg deep IM; then 2.5 mg/kg daily or b.i.d. for 10 days.
➤ **Acute lead encephalopathy**
Adults and children: 4 mg/kg given alone by deep IM; then every 4 hours with edetate calcium disodium administered at a separate site for 2 to 7 days. For less-severe poisoning, reduce to 3 mg/kg after first dose.

doxapram hydrochloride
DOKS-a-pram

Dopram

Therapeutic class: CNS stimulants
Pharmacologic class: Analeptics

AVAILABLE FORMS
Injection: 20 mg/mL*

INDICATIONS & DOSAGES
➤ **Postanesthesia respiratory stimulation**
Adults and children ages 12 and older: 0.5 to 1 mg/kg as single IV injection (not to exceed 1.5 mg/kg) or as multiple injections every 5 minutes. Maximum, 2 mg/kg or 3 g daily. Or, 250 mg in 250 mL of NSS, D_5W, or $D_{10}W$ infused at initial rate of 5 mg/minute IV until response is satisfactory. Maintain at 1 to 3 mg/minute. Maximum total infusion, 4 mg/kg or 3 g daily.
➤ **Drug-induced CNS depression**
Adults and children ages 12 and older: For injection, priming dose of 1 to 2 mg/kg IV, repeated in 5 minutes and again every 1 to 2 hours until patient awakens (and if relapse occurs). Maximum daily dosage, 3 g.

For intermittent infusion, priming dose of 1 to 2 mg/kg IV, repeated in 5 minutes and again in 1 to 2 hours, if needed. If response occurs, give IV infusion (1 mg/mL) at 1 to 3 mg/minute until patient awakens. Don't infuse for longer than 2 hours or give more than 3 g/day. May resume IV infusion after rest period of 30 minutes to 2 hours, if needed.
➤ **COPD related to acute hypercapnia**
Adults: 1 to 2 mg/minute by IV infusion using 2 mg/mL solution. Maximum, 3 mg/minute. Don't infuse for longer than 2 hours. Discontinue infusion if blood gas levels deteriorate.

edetate calcium disodium
ED-e-tate

Therapeutic class: Chelating drugs
Pharmacologic class: Heavy metal antagonists

AVAILABLE FORMS
Injection: 200 mg/mL

INDICATIONS & DOSAGES

Boxed Warning Toxic effects of drug can be fatal. Use with extreme caution in patients with lead encephalopathy and cerebral edema. Never exceed recommended daily dosage, and avoid rapid IV infusion. ■

➤ **Acute lead encephalopathy or lead level greater than 70 mcg/dL**
Adults and children: Use in conjunction with dimercaprol. Consult published protocols and specialized references for dosage recommendations.

➤ **Lead poisoning without encephalopathy or asymptomatic with lead level less than 70 mcg/dL but greater than 20 mcg/dL**
Adults and children: 1 g/m^2/day IV infused over 8 to 12 hours once daily or 1 g/m^2 IM daily in divided doses spaced 8 to 12 hours apart for 5 days.
For adults with lead nephropathy: If serum creatinine level is 2 to 3 mg/dL, 500 mg/m^2 every 24 hours for 5 days; if serum creatinine level is 3 to 4 mg/dL, 500 mg/m^2 every 48 hours for three doses; if serum creatinine level is more than 4 mg/dL, 500 mg/m^2 once weekly. May repeat these regimens at 1-month intervals.

glucarpidase
gloo-KAR-pid-ase

Voraxaze

Therapeutic class: Antidotes
Pharmacologic class: Recombinant bacterial enzymes

AVAILABLE FORMS
Powder for injection: 1,000 units/vial

INDICATIONS & DOSAGES

➤ **Methotrexate toxicity (more than 1 micromole/L) in patients with impaired kidney function**
Adults and children ages 1 month and older: 50 units/kg as single IV injection over 5 minutes.

lanthanum carbonate
LAN-thah-num

Fosrenol

Therapeutic class: Antihyperphosphatemics
Pharmacologic class: Non-calcium, non-aluminum phosphate binders

AVAILABLE FORMS
Oral powder: 750 mg, 1 g
Tablets (chewable): 500 mg, 750 mg, 1 g

INDICATIONS & DOSAGES

➤ **Reduction of serum phosphate level in patients with KF**
Adults: Initially, 500 mg PO t.i.d. with meals. Adjust every 2 to 3 weeks by 750 mg daily until reaching desired phosphate level. Reducing phosphate level to less than 6 mg/dL usually requires 1,500 to 3,000 mg daily. Maximum daily dosage, 4,500 mg.

🜨 Alert: Drug has the potential to bind to other orally administered drugs. Consider separating the administration of other oral medications by at least 2 hours.

mesna
MEZ-nuh

Mesnex

Therapeutic class: Cytoprotective drugs
Pharmacologic class: Antidotes

AVAILABLE FORMS
Injection: 100 mg/mL*
Tablets: 400 mg

INDICATIONS & DOSAGES

➤ **Prophylaxis of ifosfamide-induced hemorrhagic cystitis**
Adults (IV only regimen): Total daily mesna dose is 60% of ifosfamide dose. Give 20% of ifosfamide dose weight by weight (w/w) IV bolus injection at time of ifosfamide administration and then at 4 and 8 hours after ifosfamide dose. For example, if ifosfamide dose is 1.2 g/m^2, mesna dose is 240 mg/m^2 given at same time as ifosfamide and then 4 hours and 8 hours after ifosfamide. Repeat dosing schedule each day ifosfamide is given.
Adults (IV and PO dosing regimen): Total daily mesna dose is 100% of ifosfamide dose. Give 20% of ifosfamide dose (w/w) IV bolus injection at same time as ifosfamide administration. Then give 40% of ifosfamide dose (w/w) as PO tablets at 2 hours and 6 hours after ifosfamide dose. Repeat dosing each day ifosfamide is given. This ratio of IV and oral dosing hasn't been established as effective for daily ifosfamide doses higher than 2 g/m^2.

Adjust-a-dose: If ifosfamide dosage increases or decreases, modify mesna dosage to maintain mesna-to-ifosfamide ratio.

➤ **Prevention of cyclophosphamide-induced hemorrhagic cystitis (with high-dose cyclophosphamide)** ◆

Adults younger than age 40: 2,100 mg/m²/day continuous IV infusion (mesna dose equivalent to cyclophosphamide dose) for 2 days with cyclophosphamide infusion during cycles 1, 2, 3, and 6.

naloxegol oxalate
nal-OX-ee-gol

Movantik

Therapeutic class: Antidotes
Pharmacologic class: Opioid antagonists

AVAILABLE FORMS
Tablets: 12.5 mg, 25 mg

INDICATIONS & DOSAGES
➤ **Opioid-induced constipation in patients with chronic noncancer pain, including patients with chronic pain related to prior cancer or its treatment who don't require frequent opioid dosage escalation**
Adults: 25 mg PO once daily in the morning at least 1 hour before or 2 hours after first meal of the day. If 25 mg isn't tolerated, reduce to 12.5 mg once daily.
Adjust-a-dose: For CrCl less than 60 mL/minute, decrease starting dose to 12.5 mg; if tolerated, may increase to 25 mg as needed. If use with a moderate CYP3A4 inhibitor is necessary, decrease dosage to 12.5 mg daily.

phentolamine mesylate
fen-TOLE-a-meen

OraVerse

Therapeutic class: Antidotes
Pharmacologic class: Alpha blockers

AVAILABLE FORMS
Injection: 0.4 mg/1.7 mL, 5 mg/mL

INDICATIONS & DOSAGES
➤ **Prevention of dermal necrosis from norepinephrine extravasation (excluding OraVerse)**
Adults: Add 10 mg of phentolamine to each liter of solution containing norepinephrine; pressor effect of norepinephrine is unaffected.
➤ **Dermal necrosis and sloughing after IV extravasation of norepinephrine or dopamine (excluding OraVerse)**
Adults: Infiltrate area with 5 to 10 mg phentolamine in 10 mL of NSS within 12 hours of extravasation.
➤ **Reversal of soft-tissue anesthesia (OraVerse only)**
Dosage depends on amount of anesthetic used. Refer to manufacturer's instructions.

➤ **Diagnosis of pheochromocytoma, control or prevention of HTN before or during pheochromocytomectomy (excluding OraVerse)**
Adults: For diagnosis, 5 mg IV or IM, with close BP monitoring. For pheochromocytomectomy, 5 mg IV or IM 1 to 2 hours before surgical removal of tumor; during surgery, may give additional 5 mg IV as needed.
Children: For diagnosis, 1 mg IV or 3 mg IM, with close BP monitoring. For pheochromocytomectomy, 1 mg IV or IM 1 to 2 hours before surgical removal of tumor; during surgery, may give additional 1 mg IV as needed.

pralidoxime chloride (2-PAM chloride, 2-pyridine-aldoxime methochloride)
pra-li-DOKS-eem

Protopam Chloride

Therapeutic class: Antidotes
Pharmacologic class: Quaternary ammonium oximes

AVAILABLE FORMS
Injection: 1 g/20 mL vial

INDICATIONS & DOSAGES
➤ **Antidote for organophosphate poisoning in combination with atropine**
Adults: 1 to 2 g in 100 mL of NSS by IV infusion over 15 to 30 minutes. If not practical or if pulmonary edema is present, 1 g in 20 mL of sterile water by slow IV push over at least 5 minutes. Repeat in 1 hour if muscle weakness persists. May give additional doses cautiously. May use IM or subcut injection if IV route isn't feasible.
Adults and children weighing 40 kg or more with mild symptoms: 600 mg (2 mL) IM. Wait 15 minutes and, if symptoms persist, give second dose; after an additional 15 minutes, may give third dose as needed. If patient develops severe symptoms any time after first dose, give two additional 600-mg doses IM in rapid succession for a total cumulative dose of 1,800 mg.
Adults and children weighing 40 kg or more with severe symptoms: Three 600-mg doses (three doses of 2 mL each) IM in rapid succession. If symptoms persist after complete 1,800-mg regimen, may repeat series beginning approximately 1 hour after last injection.
Children ages 16 and younger (IV dosing): Loading dose of 20 to 50 mg/kg (maximum 2 g) IV over 15 to 30 minutes, followed by 10 to 20 mg/kg/hour by continuous IV infusion. Or, initial dose of 20 to 50 mg/kg IV over 15 to 30 minutes, followed by second dose of 20 to 50 mg/kg IV in 1 hour if muscle weakness persists. May repeat dose every 10 to 12 hours PRN. Maximum, 2 g/dose. Or, if pulmonary edema is present or giving intermittent or continuous IV infusions isn't practical, 20 to 50 mg/kg as 50-mg/mL solution in water by IV push slowly over 5 minutes. If muscle

weakness persists, may give additional doses every 10 to 12 hours.

Children ages 16 and younger who weigh less than 40 kg (IM dosing): For mild symptoms, 15 mg/kg IM in anterolateral thigh. If symptoms persist after 15 minutes, give second dose of 15 mg/kg IM. If symptoms persist after second dose, give third dose of 15 mg/kg IM. If patient develops severe symptoms any time after first dose, give second and third doses in rapid succession. For severe symptoms, give all three doses of 15 mg/kg IM each in rapid succession. Maximum combined dose for three injections is 45 mg/kg.

➤ **Control of overdose of anticholinesterase drugs used in treatment of myasthenia gravis**
Adults: 1 to 2 g IV; then 250 mg IV every 5 minutes PRN.

protamine sulfate
PROE-ta-meen

Therapeutic class: Antidotes
Pharmacologic class: Heparin antagonists

AVAILABLE FORMS
Injection: 10 mg/mL

INDICATIONS & DOSAGES
Boxed Warning Drug can cause severe hypotension, CV collapse, noncardiogenic pulmonary edema, catastrophic pulmonary vasoconstriction, and pulmonary HTN. Keep vasopressors and resuscitation equipment immediately available. Don't give when bleeding occurs without prior heparin use. ■

➤ **Heparin overdose**
Adults: Dosage should be guided by blood coagulation studies. 1 mg of protamine sulfate neutralizes not less than 100 USP heparin units. Give by slow IV injection over 10 minutes in doses not to exceed 50 mg.

rasburicase ⌧
ras-BUR-ih-kase

Elitek

Therapeutic class: Replacement enzymes
Pharmacologic class: Recombinant urate-oxidases

AVAILABLE FORMS
Injection: 1.5 mg, 7.5 mg in single-dose vials with diluent

INDICATIONS & DOSAGES
Boxed Warning Drug can cause serious and fatal hypersensitivity reactions. Don't give to patients with G6PD deficiency due to risk of hemolysis; screen those at higher risk before starting therapy. Drug can cause methemoglobinemia. Immediately and permanently discontinue drug if a

serious hypersensitivity reaction, hemolysis, or methemoglobinemia occurs. Drug interferes with uric acid in blood sample measurements. Follow sampling guidelines. ■

➤ **Initial management of plasma uric acid level in patients with leukemia, lymphoma, or solid tumor malignancies who are receiving chemotherapy that's expected to result in tumor lysis and subsequent elevation of plasma uric acid level**
Adults and children: 0.2 mg/kg IV infusion over 30 minutes daily for up to 5 days. Drug is only indicated for a single course of treatment.

sodium polystyrene sulfonate
pol-ee-STYE-reen

Kayexalate ✥, SPS

Therapeutic class: Potassium-removing resins
Pharmacologic class: Cation-exchange resins

AVAILABLE FORMS
Powder: approximately 15 g/4 tsp
Suspension: 15 g/60 mL*

INDICATIONS & DOSAGES
➤ **Hyperkalemia**
Adults: 15 g PO daily to q.i.d. in water or syrup (3 to 4 mL/g of resin). Or, mix powder with appropriate medium (aqueous suspension or diet appropriate for KF) and instill through NG tube. Or, 30 to 50 g as a suspension or in 100 mL of an aqueous vehicle every 6 hours as warm emulsion (at body temperature) deep into sigmoid colon (20 cm). Following retention period, irrigate colon to remove resin.
Children: 1 g/kg/dose PO or by NG tube every 6 hours.
Infants and small children: 1 mEq potassium/g of resin PO or by NG tube daily to q.i.d.
Neonates: 0.5 to 1 g/kg as rectal suspension. Use minimum effective dosage. Following retention, irrigate colon to remove resin.

succimer
SUX-i-mer

Chemet

Therapeutic class: Chelating drugs
Pharmacologic class: Heavy metal chelators

AVAILABLE FORMS
Capsules: 100 mg

INDICATIONS & DOSAGES
➤ **Lead poisoning in children with lead levels greater than 45 mcg/dL**
Children ages 12 months and older: Initially, 10 mg/kg or 350 mg/m² PO every 8 hours for 5 days. Then reduce to 10 mg/kg or 350 mg/m² PO every 12 hours for additional 14 days. Maximum, 500 mg/dose.

sugammadex sodium
soo-GAM-ma-dex

Bridion

Therapeutic class: Antidotes
Pharmacologic class: Modified gamma cyclodextrins

AVAILABLE FORMS
Injection: 200 mg/2 mL, 500 mg/5 mL in single-dose vials

INDICATIONS & DOSAGES
➤ **Reversal of neuromuscular blockade induced by rocuronium bromide and vecuronium bromide in patients undergoing surgery**
Adults and children ages 2 and older (routine reversal of rocuronium- and vecuronium-induced neuromuscular blockade): Base doses and timing of drug administration on monitoring for twitch responses and extent of spontaneous recovery that has occurred. Give 4 mg/kg IV bolus over 10 seconds if recovery of the twitch response has reached one to two posttetanic counts (PTC) and there are no twitch responses to train-of-four (TOF) stimulation. Give 2 mg/kg IV over 10 seconds if spontaneous recovery has reached the reappearance of the second twitch (T_2) in response to TOF stimulation.
Adults (immediate reversal of rocuronium-induced neuromuscular blockade): If there is a clinical need to reverse neuromuscular blockade (approximately 3 minutes) after administration of a single 1.2-mg/kg dose of rocuronium, give sugammadex 16 mg/kg IV over 10 seconds.

Selected ophthalmic drugs: Indications and dosages

Refer to manufacturer's instructions for complete prescribing and safety information.

aflibercept
a-FLIB-er-sept

Eylea, Eylea HD

Therapeutic class: Vascular endothelial growth factor inhibitors
Pharmacologic class: Antiangiogenetic drugs

AVAILABLE FORMS
Intravitreal injection: 2 mg in 0.05-mL single-use vial and prefilled syringe; 8 mg in 0.07 mL single-use vial

INDICATIONS & DOSAGES
➤ **Neovascular (wet) age-related macular degeneration**
Adults: 2 mg (0.05 mL) intravitreal injection every 4 weeks for first 12 weeks; then 2 mg (0.05 mL) once every 8 weeks. Some patients may need every-4-week dosing after first 12 weeks and may be treated with one dose every 12 weeks after 1 year of effective therapy. Or, 8 mg (0.07 mL HD) intravitreal injection every 4 weeks for 3 doses; then 8 mg once every 8 to 16 weeks.
➤ **Macular edema following retinal vein occlusion (Eylea only)**
Adults: 2 mg (0.05 mL) intravitreal injection once every 4 weeks.
➤ **Diabetic macular edema (DME); diabetic retinopathy (DR)**
Adults: 2 mg (0.05 mL) intravitreal injection every 4 weeks for first 5 injections; then 2 mg (0.05 mL) every 8 weeks. Some patients may need every-4-week dosing after first five injections. Or, 8 mg (0.07 mL HD) intravitreal injection every 4 weeks for 3 doses; then 8 mg once every 8 to 16 weeks for DME or every 8 to 12 weeks for DR.
✳ *NEW INDICATION:* **Retinopathy of prematurity (Eylea only)**
Preterm infants: 0.4 mg (0.01 mL) intravitreal injection; may be given bilaterally on the same day. May repeat injection in each eye. Interval between doses injected into the same eye should be at least 10 days.

alcaftadine
al-CAFF-tuh-deen

Lastacaft ◇

Therapeutic class: Antihistamines
Pharmacologic class: Histamine$_1$-receptor antagonists

AVAILABLE FORMS
Ophthalmic solution: 0.25% (2.5 mg/mL) ◇

INDICATIONS & DOSAGES
➤ **Itching associated with allergic conjunctivitis**
Adults and children ages 2 and older: 1 drop in each eye once daily.

bepotastine besilate
beh-POT-uh-steen

Bepreve

Therapeutic class: Antihistamines (ophthalmic)
Pharmacologic class: Histamine$_1$-receptor antagonists

AVAILABLE FORMS
Ophthalmic solution: 1.5%

INDICATIONS & DOSAGES
➤ **Itching associated with allergic conjunctivitis**
Adults and children ages 2 and older: 1 drop in affected eye(s) b.i.d.

besifloxacin hydrochloride
beh-sih-FLOX-ah-sin

Besivance

Therapeutic class: Antibiotics
Pharmacologic class: Fluoroquinolones

AVAILABLE FORMS
Ophthalmic suspension: 0.6%

INDICATIONS & DOSAGES
➤ **Conjunctivitis caused by CDC coryneform group G,** *Aerococcus viridans, Corynebacterium pseudodiphtheriticum, C. striatum, Haemophilus influenzae, Moraxella catarrhalis, M. lacunata, Pseudomonas aeruginosa, Staphylococcus aureus, S. epidermidis, S. hominis, S. lugdunensis, S. warneri, Streptococcus mitis* **group,** *S. oralis, S. pneumoniae,* **or** *S. salivarius*

Adults and children ages 1 and older: 1 drop in affected eye t.i.d., 4 to 12 hours apart, for 7 days.

bimatoprost
by-MAT-oh-prost

Durysta, Latisse, Lumigan, Vistitan ✚

Therapeutic class: Antiglaucoma drugs
Pharmacologic class: Prostaglandin analogues

AVAILABLE FORMS
Intraocular implant: 10 mcg
Ophthalmic solution: 0.01%, 0.03%
Topical ophthalmic solution: 0.03%

INDICATIONS & DOSAGES
➤ **Increased IOP in patients with open-angle glaucoma or ocular HTN**
Adults and adolescents ages 16 and older: 1 drop ophthalmic solution in conjunctival sac of affected eye(s) once daily in the evening.
Adults: 1 implant inserted in anterior chamber of affected eye. Don't exceed 1 implant per eye.
➤ **Hypotrichosis of eyelashes (Latisse)**
Adults and children ages 5 and older: 1 drop topical ophthalmic solution nightly applied directly to skin of upper eyelid margin at base of eyelashes with single-use applicator; use second applicator for second eye (if needed).

brinzolamide–brimonidine tartrate
brin-ZOL-ah-mide/brih-MOE-neh-deen

Simbrinza

Therapeutic class: Antiglaucoma drugs
Pharmacologic class: Carbonic anhydrase inhibitors–alpha$_2$ adrenergic receptor agonists

AVAILABLE FORMS
Ophthalmic suspension: brinzolamide 1% and brimonidine 0.2%

INDICATIONS & DOSAGES
➤ **Reduction of IOP in patients with open-angle glaucoma or ocular HTN**
Adults and children ages 2 and older: 1 drop in affected eye(s) t.i.d.
Adjust-a-dose: Use isn't recommended if eGFR falls below 30 mL/minute/1.73 m².

brolucizumab-dbll
broe-lue-SIZ-ue-mab

Beovu

Therapeutic class: Immunomodulators
Pharmacologic class: Vascular endothelial growth factor inhibitors

AVAILABLE FORMS
Solution for intravitreal injection: 6 mg/0.05 mL in single-use vial or prefilled syringe

INDICATIONS & DOSAGES
➤ **Neovascular (wet) age-related macular degeneration**
Adults: 6 mg intravitreal injection monthly (every 25 to 31 days) for three doses; then every 8 to 12 weeks thereafter.
➤ **Diabetic macular edema**
Adults: 6 mg intravitreal injection every 6 weeks (every 39 to 45 days) for five doses; then every 8 to 12 weeks thereafter.

bromfenac sodium
BROM-fen-ak

BromSite, Prolensa

Therapeutic class: Anti-inflammatory drugs (ophthalmic)
Pharmacologic class: NSAIDs

AVAILABLE FORMS
Ophthalmic solution: 0.07%, 0.075%, 0.09%

INDICATIONS & DOSAGES
➤ **Inflammation and pain after cataract surgery**
Adults: For 0.07% solution and 0.09% solution, 1 drop in affected eye(s) once daily beginning 1 day before surgery, continued on day of surgery and for first 14 days after surgery. For 0.075% solution, 1 drop in affected eye(s) b.i.d. (morning and evening) beginning 1 day before surgery, continued on day of surgery and for first 14 days after surgery.

carteolol hydrochloride
KAR-tee-oh-lol

Therapeutic class: Antiglaucoma drugs
Pharmacologic class: Nonselective beta blockers

AVAILABLE FORMS
Ophthalmic solution: 1%

INDICATIONS & DOSAGES
➤ **Reduction of IOP in patients with open-angle glaucoma or intraocular HTN**
Adults: 1 drop in each affected eye(s) b.i.d.

cenegermin-bkbj
sen-EH-jer-min bkbj

Oxervate

Therapeutic class: Growth factors
Pharmacologic class: Human nerve growth factors

AVAILABLE FORMS
Ophthalmic solution: 0.002% (20 mcg/mL) multi-dose vial

INDICATIONS & DOSAGES
➤ **Neurotrophic keratitis**
Adults and children ages 2 and older: 1 drop in affected eye(s) every 2 hours six times a day for 8 weeks.

ciprofloxacin hydrochloride
si-proe-FLOX-a-sin

Ciloxan

Therapeutic class: Antibiotics
Pharmacologic class: Fluoroquinolones

AVAILABLE FORMS
Ophthalmic ointment: 0.3%
Ophthalmic solution: 0.3%

INDICATIONS & DOSAGES
➤ **Corneal ulcers caused by *Pseudomonas aeruginosa, Staphylococcus aureus, S. epidermidis, Streptococcus pneumoniae, Serratia marcescens,* or *Streptococcus* viridans group**
Adults, children, and neonates: 2 drops in affected eye(s) every 15 minutes for first 6 hours; then 2 drops every 30 minutes for remainder of first day. On second day, 2 drops hourly. On days 3 to 14, 2 drops every 4 hours. Treatment may be continued after day 14 if reepithelialization hasn't occurred.
➤ **Bacterial conjunctivitis caused by *Haemophilus influenzae, Staphylococcus aureus, S. epidermidis, Streptococcus pneumoniae,* or *S. viridans* group**
Adults and children older than age 1: 1 or 2 drops in conjunctival sac of affected eye(s) every 2 hours while awake for first 2 days; then 1 or 2 drops every 4 hours while awake for next 5 days.
Adults and children older than age 2: ½-inch (1.27-cm) ribbon of ointment into conjunctival sac t.i.d. for first 2 days; then ½-inch ribbon b.i.d. for next 5 days.

cycloSPORINE
cy-cloh-SPORE-inn

Cequa, Restasis, Verkazia

Therapeutic class: Immunomodulators
Pharmacologic class: Calcineurin inhibitors

AVAILABLE FORMS
Ophthalmic emulsion: 0.05%, 0.1%
Ophthalmic solution: 0.09%

INDICATIONS & DOSAGES
➤ **To increase tear production in patients whose tear production is presumed to be suppressed due to ocular inflammation associated with keratoconjunctivitis sicca**
Adults: 1 drop of 0.05% emulsion or 0.09% solution in each eye b.i.d. approximately 12 hours apart.
➤ **Vernal keratoconjunctivitis**
Adults and children ages 4 and older: 1 drop of 0.1% emulsion in each affected eye q.i.d. (morning, noon, afternoon, and evening).

dexamethasone
dex-a-METH-a-sone

Dextenza, Dexycu, Maxidex, Ozurdex

dexamethasone sodium phosphate

Therapeutic class: Anti-inflammatory drugs (ophthalmic)
Pharmacologic class: Corticosteroids

AVAILABLE FORMS
dexamethasone (ophthalmic)
Insert (ophthalmic): 0.4 mg
Intraocular implant: 0.7 mg
Intraocular suspension: 9%
Ophthalmic suspension: 0.1%
dexamethasone sodium phosphate
Ophthalmic solution: 0.1%

INDICATIONS & DOSAGES
➤ **Inflammatory conditions of eyelid, conjunctiva, cornea, and anterior segment of globe (allergic conjunctivitis, acne rosacea, keritinitis, iritis, cyclitis, or selective infective conjunctivitis); corneal injury from chemical or thermal burns or foreign body penetration**
Adults and children: Initially, 1 or 2 drops of solution into conjunctival sac every hour during the day and every 2 hours during the night. Decrease to 1 drop every 4 hours when favorable response is noted. As condition improves, taper to 1 drop t.i.d. or q.i.d. to control symptoms. Treatment may extend from a few days to several weeks.

Or, 1 or 2 drops of suspension into conjunctival sac up to six times daily. In severe disease, drops of suspension may be used hourly, being tapered to discontinuation as inflammation subsides.

➤ **Macular edema; posterior-segment uveitis; diabetic macular edema**
Adults: 1 implant (0.7 mg) injected intravitreally into each affected eye.

➤ **Ocular postoperative inflammation**
Adults: 0.005 mL (517 mcg) of 9% suspension injected into posterior chamber at end of ocular surgery or single 0.4-mg insert placed into the lower lacrimal canaliculus.

➤ **Ocular itching associated with allergic conjunctivitis**
Adults: Single 0.4-mg insert placed into the lower lacrimal canaliculus.

difluprednate
die-FLU-pred-nate

Durezol

Therapeutic class: Anti-inflammatory drugs (ophthalmic)
Pharmacologic class: Corticosteroids

AVAILABLE FORMS
Ophthalmic emulsion: 0.05%

INDICATIONS & DOSAGES
➤ **Inflammation and pain associated with ocular surgery**
Adults and children: 1 drop into conjunctival sac of affected eye q.i.d. for 2 weeks, beginning 24 hours after surgery; then decrease to b.i.d. for 1 week; and then taper according to response.

➤ **Endogenous anterior uveitis**
Adults: 1 drop into conjunctival sac of affected eye q.i.d. for 14 days; then taper as clinically indicated.

dorzolamide hydrochloride
dor-ZOLE-ah-mide

Trusopt

Therapeutic class: Antiglaucoma drugs
Pharmacologic class: Carbonic anhydrase inhibitors–sulfonamides

AVAILABLE FORMS
Ophthalmic solution: 2%

INDICATIONS & DOSAGES
➤ **Increased IOP in patients with ocular HTN or open-angle glaucoma**
Adults and children: 1 drop into conjunctival sac of affected eye(s) t.i.d.

epinastine hydrochloride
ep-ih-NAS-teen

Therapeutic class: Antihistamines
Pharmacologic class: H_1-receptor antagonists–mast cell stabilizers

AVAILABLE FORMS
Ophthalmic solution: 0.05%

INDICATIONS & DOSAGES
➤ **To prevent pruritus from allergic conjunctivitis**
Adults and children ages 2 and older: 1 drop in each eye b.i.d. Continue treatment as long as allergen is present, even if symptoms resolve.

fluorometholone
flur-oh-METH-oh-lone

FML, FML Forte

fluorometholone acetate
Flarex

Therapeutic class: Anti-inflammatory drugs (ophthalmic)
Pharmacologic class: Corticosteroids

AVAILABLE FORMS
fluorometholone
Ophthalmic suspension: 0.1%, 0.25%
fluorometholone acetate
Ophthalmic suspension: 0.1%

INDICATIONS & DOSAGES
➤ **Steroid responsive inflammatory conditions of cornea, conjunctiva, sclera, or anterior segment of eye**
Adults and children older than age 2: 1 drop b.i.d. to q.i.d. In severe conditions, may increase dosing frequency to every 4 hours during initial 24 to 48 hours, if needed.
Adults (fluorometholone acetate): 1 to 2 drops q.i.d.; in severe conditions, may give 2 drops and increase dosing frequency to every 2 hours during initial 24 to 48 hours, if needed.

gatifloxacin
ga-ti-FLOKS-a-sin

Zymar✦, Zymaxid

Therapeutic class: Antibiotics
Pharmacologic class: Fluoroquinolones

AVAILABLE FORMS
Solution: 0.3%✦, 0.5%

INDICATIONS & DOSAGES

➤ **Bacterial conjunctivitis caused by *Staphylococcus aureus, S. epidermidis, Streptococcus pneumoniae,* or *Haemophilus influenzae***

Adults and children ages 1 and older: 1 drop of Zymar in affected eye every 2 hours while patient is awake, up to eight times daily for 2 days; then 1 drop up to q.i.d. while patient is awake on days 3 to 7.

➤ **Bacterial conjunctivitis caused by *Streptococcus mitis* group, *S. aureus, S. epidermidis, S. oralis, S. pneumoniae,* or *Haemophilus influenzae***

Adults and children ages 1 and older: 1 drop Zymaxid in affected eye every 2 hours while patient is awake, up to eight times on day 1; then 1 drop b.i.d. to q.i.d. while patient is awake on days 2 to 7.

gentamicin sulfate
jen-ta-MYE-sin

Therapeutic class: Antibiotics
Pharmacologic class: Aminoglycosides

AVAILABLE FORMS
Ophthalmic solution: 0.3%

INDICATIONS & DOSAGES

➤ **External ocular infections (conjunctivitis, keratoconjunctivitis, corneal ulcers, blepharitis, blepharoconjunctivitis, acute meibomianitis, and dacryocystitis) caused by susceptible organisms (*Staphylococcus aureus, S. epidermidis, Streptococcus pyogenes, S. pneumoniae, Klebsiella aerogenes, K. pneumoniae, Escherichia coli, Haemophilus influenzae, Neisseria gonorrhoeae, Pseudomonas aeruginosa, Serratia marcescens*)**

Adults and children ages 1 month and older: 1 to 2 drops in affected eye every 4 hours. In severe infections, up to 2 drops every hour.

ketorolac tromethamine
KEE-toe-role-ak

Acular, Acular LS, Acuvail

Therapeutic class: Anti-inflammatory drugs (ophthalmic)
Pharmacologic class: NSAIDs

AVAILABLE FORMS
Ophthalmic solution: 0.4%, 0.45%, 0.5%

INDICATIONS & DOSAGES

➤ **Relief from ocular itching caused by seasonal allergic conjunctivitis (Acular)**

Adults and children ages 2 and older: 1 drop of 0.5% solution into conjunctival sac in each eye q.i.d.

➤ **Relief of postoperative inflammation after cataract extraction (Acular)**

Adults and children ages 2 and older: 1 drop of 0.5% solution in affected eye(s) q.i.d. beginning 24 hours after cataract surgery and continuing through first 2 weeks of postoperative period.

➤ **Reduction of ocular pain, burning, and stinging after corneal refractive surgery (Acular LS)**

Adults and children ages 3 and older: 1 drop 0.4% solution q.i.d. in affected eye(s), as needed, for up to 4 days after surgery.

➤ **Reduction of pain and inflammation after cataract surgery (Acuvail)**

Adults: 1 drop 0.45% solution b.i.d. in affected eye(s) beginning 1 day before surgery and continuing on day of surgery and through first 2 weeks after surgery.

ketotifen fumarate
kee-toe-TYE-fen

Alaway ◇, Zaditor ◇

Therapeutic class: Antihistamines (ophthalmic)
Pharmacologic class: H₁-receptor antagonists–mast cell stabilizers

AVAILABLE FORMS
Ophthalmic solution: 0.025%

INDICATIONS & DOSAGES

➤ **Temporary prevention of eye itching from allergic conjunctivitis or temporary relief of itchy eyes due to pollen, ragweed, grass, animal hair, or dander**

Adults and children ages 3 and older: 1 drop in each affected eye every 8 to 12 hours but not more than b.i.d.

latanoprost
lah-TAN-oh-prost

Xalatan, Xelpros

Therapeutic class: Antiglaucoma drugs
Pharmacologic class: Prostaglandin analogues

AVAILABLE FORMS
Ophthalmic solution: 0.005% (50 mcg/mL)

INDICATIONS & DOSAGES

➤ **Increased IOP in patients with ocular HTN or open-angle glaucoma**

Adults: 1 drop in each affected eye once daily in the evening.

levobunolol hydrochloride
LEE-voe-BYOO-no-lahl

Therapeutic class: Antiglaucoma drugs
Pharmacologic class: Nonselective beta blockers

AVAILABLE FORMS
Ophthalmic solution: 0.5%

INDICATIONS & DOSAGES
➤ **Reduction of IOP in patients with open-angle glaucoma or ocular HTN**
Adults: 1 or 2 drops 0.5% solution once daily. May give 1 drop of 0.5% solution b.i.d. for severe or uncontrolled glaucoma.

lifitegrast
LIF-i-teg-rast

Xiidra

Therapeutic class: Anti-inflammatory drugs (ophthalmic)
Pharmacologic class: Lymphocyte function-associated antigen-1 antagonists

AVAILABLE FORMS
Ophthalmic solution: 5%

INDICATIONS & DOSAGES
➤ **Dry eye disease**
Adults: 1 drop in each eye b.i.d., approximately 12 hours apart.

netarsudil
ne-TAR-soo-dil

Rhopressa

Therapeutic class: Antiglaucoma drugs
Pharmacologic class: Rho kinase inhibitors

AVAILABLE FORMS
Ophthalmic solution: 0.02%

INDICATIONS & DOSAGES
➤ **Reduction of elevated IOP in patients with open-angle glaucoma or ocular HTN**
Adults: 1 drop in affected eye(s) once daily in the evening.

netarsudil–latanoprost
ne-TAR-soo-dil/la-TAN-oh-prost

Rocklatan

Therapeutic class: Antiglaucoma drugs
Pharmacologic class: Rho kinase inhibitors–prostaglandin F2 alpha analogues

AVAILABLE FORMS
Ophthalmic solution: netarsudil 0.2 mg/mL (0.02%)/latanoprost 0.05 mg/mL (0.005%)

INDICATIONS & DOSAGES
➤ **Reduction of elevated IOP in patients with open-angle glaucoma or ocular HTN**
Adults: 1 drop into affected eye(s) once daily in the evening.

ofloxacin
oh-FLOX-a-sin

Ocuflox

Therapeutic class: Antibiotics
Pharmacologic class: Fluoroquinolones

AVAILABLE FORMS
Ophthalmic solution: 0.3%

INDICATIONS & DOSAGES
➤ **Conjunctivitis caused by *Staphylococcus aureus, S. epidermidis, Streptococcus pneumoniae, Enterobacter cloacae, Haemophilus influenzae, Proteus mirabilis,* or *Pseudomonas aeruginosa***
Adults and children older than age 1: 1 or 2 drops into conjunctival sac every 2 to 4 hours daily while patient is awake for first 2 days; then 1 or 2 drops q.i.d. on days 3 through 7.
➤ **Bacterial corneal ulcer caused by *Staphylococcus aureus, S. epidermidis, Streptococcus pneumoniae, Pseudomonas aeruginosa, Serratia marcescens,* or *Propionibacterium acnes***
Adults and children older than age 1: 1 or 2 drops every 30 minutes while patient is awake and 1 or 2 drops every 4 and 6 hours after patient goes to bed on days 1 and 2. 1 or 2 drops hourly while patient is awake on day 3; continue for 4 to 6 days. Then 1 or 2 drops q.i.d. for an additional 3 days or until cured.

phenylephrine hydrochloride
fen-ill-EF-rin

Mydfrin ✦

Therapeutic class: Mydriatics
Pharmacologic class: Sympathomimetic
amines-adrenergics

AVAILABLE FORMS
Ophthalmic solution: 2.5%, 10%

INDICATIONS & DOSAGES
➤ **Mydriasis**
Adults and children ages 1 and older: 1 drop of 2.5%
or 10% solution every 3 to 5 minutes, up to 3 drops per
eye. May repeat dose.
Children younger than age 1: 1 drop of 2.5% solution
every 3 to 5 minutes, up to 3 drops per eye.

pilocarpine hydrochloride
pie-low-KAR-peen

Vuity

Therapeutic class: Miotics
Pharmacologic class: Direct-acting
parasympathomimetics

AVAILABLE FORMS
Ophthalmic solution: 1%, 1.25%, 2%, 4%

INDICATIONS & DOSAGES
➤ **Primary open-angle glaucoma or ocular HTN**
Adults and children ages 2 and older: 1 drop of 1%,
2%, or 4% solution daily up to q.i.d.; adjust concentration and frequency to control IOP. Start pilocarpine-
naive patients on 1% concentration.
Children younger than age 2: 1 drop of 1% solution
in eye t.i.d.
➤ **Management of acute angle-closure glaucoma**
Adults and children ages 2 and older: 1 drop of 1%
or 2% solution in affected eye up to three times in a
30-minute period.
Children younger than age 2: 1 drop of 1% solution
in eye(s) t.i.d.
➤ **Prevention of postoperative elevated IOP associated with laser surgery**
Adults and children ages 2 and older: 1 drop of 1%,
2%, or 4% solution in affected eye(s) 15 to 60 minutes
before surgery. May instill 2 drops, spaced at least
5 minutes apart.
➤ **Induction of miosis**
Adults and children ages 2 and older: 1 drop of 1%,
2%, or 4% solution in eye(s). May give 2 drops,
spaced at least 5 minutes apart.
➤ **Induction of miosis before goniotomy or
trabeculotomy**

Children: 1 drop of 1% or 2% solution in eye(s) 15 to
60 minutes before surgery.
➤ **Presbyopia (Vuity)**
Adults: 1 drop of 1.25% solution in each eye(s) once
daily. May administer second dose 3 to 6 hours after
first dose.

prednisoLONE acetate
(suspension)
pred-NISS-oh-lone

Pred Forte, Pred Mild

prednisoLONE sodium
phosphate (solution)
Therapeutic class: Anti-inflammatory drugs
(ophthalmic)
Pharmacologic class: Corticosteroids

AVAILABLE FORMS
prednisolone acetate
Ophthalmic suspension: 0.12%, 1%
prednisolone sodium phosphate
Ophthalmic solution: 1%

INDICATIONS & DOSAGES
➤ **Inflammation of palpebral and bulbar conjunctiva, cornea, and anterior segment of globe**
prednisolone acetate
Adults: 1 or 2 drops into affected eye(s) b.i.d. to q.i.d.
In severe conditions, may increase dosing frequency
during initial 24 to 48 hours, if needed. If signs and
symptoms fail to improve after 2 days, reevaluate. In
chronic conditions, taper doses gradually.
prednisolone sodium phosphate
Adults: 1 or 2 drops into conjunctival sac hourly
during the day and every 2 hours at night until response is observed. May reduce to 1 drop every
4 hours, then 1 drop t.i.d. to q.i.d. as needed for adequate
response. In chronic conditions, taper doses gradually.

sulfacetamide
sul-fah-SEE-tah-mide

Therapeutic class: Antibiotics
Pharmacologic class: Sulfonamides

AVAILABLE FORMS
Ophthalmic ointment: 10%
Ophthalmic solution: 10%

INDICATIONS & DOSAGES
➤ **Conjunctivitis and other superficial ocular infections due to susceptible microorganisms**
Adults and children ages 2 months and older: 1 or
2 drops into lower conjunctival sac every 2 to 3 hours.
Increase interval as condition responds. Or, ½-inch
ribbon of 10% ointment into conjunctival sac every

3 to 4 hours and at bedtime. Ointment may be used at night along with drops during the day. Usual duration of treatment is 7 to 10 days.

➤ **Trachoma**
Adults and children ages 2 months and older: 2 drops into lower conjunctival sac every 2 hours with systemic sulfonamide therapy.

tafluprost
TA-floo-prost

Zioptan

Therapeutic class: Antiglaucoma drugs
Pharmacologic class: Prostaglandin analogues

AVAILABLE FORMS
Ophthalmic solution: 0.0015%

INDICATIONS & DOSAGES
➤ **Increased IOP in patients with open-angle glaucoma or ocular HTN**
Adults: 1 drop into conjunctival sac of affected eye once daily in the evening.

tetrahydrozoline hydrochloride
tet-rah-hi-DRAZ-oh-leen

Visine Red Eye Comfort ◇

Therapeutic class: Vasoconstrictors
Pharmacologic class: Sympathomimetics

AVAILABLE FORMS
Ophthalmic solution: 0.05% ◇

INDICATIONS & DOSAGES
➤ **Conjunctival congestion, irritation, and allergic conditions**
Adults (all products) and children ages 6 and older (Visine products): 1 or 2 drops in affected eye(s) up to q.i.d. or as directed by prescriber.

timolol
tye-MOE-lol

Betimol, Istalol, Timoptic

Therapeutic class: Antiglaucoma drugs
Pharmacologic class: Nonselective beta blockers

AVAILABLE FORMS
Ophthalmic gel-forming solution: 0.25%, 0.5%
Ophthalmic solution: 0.25%, 0.5%
Ophthalmic solution (preservative-free): 0.25%, 0.5%

INDICATIONS & DOSAGES
➤ **Reduction of IOP in ocular HTN or open-angle glaucoma**
Adults: Initially, 1 drop of 0.25% solution in each affected eye b.i.d. If no response, then 1 drop of 0.5% solution in each affected eye b.i.d. If IOP is controlled, reduce dosage to 1 drop daily. Or, 1 drop of gel-forming solution (0.25% or 0.5%) in each affected eye once daily. Or, for Istalol, initially, 1 drop of 0.5% solution in each affected eye once daily in the morning. If response is unsatisfactory, concomitant therapy may be considered.
Children ages 2 and older: Initially, 1 drop of 0.25% Timoptic or timolol generic solution in each affected eye b.i.d. If no response, increase to 1 drop of 0.5% solution in each affected eye b.i.d. If IOP is controlled, reduce dosage to 1 drop daily. Or, 1 drop of gel-forming solution into each affected eye once daily.

travoprost
TRA-voe-prost

Izba ✦, Travatan Z

Therapeutic class: Antiglaucoma drugs
Pharmacologic class: Prostaglandin analogues

AVAILABLE FORMS
Ophthalmic solution: 0.003% ✦, 0.004%

INDICATIONS & DOSAGES
➤ **Reduction of IOP in patients with open-angle glaucoma or ocular HTN**
Adults and children ages 16 and older: 1 drop in each affected eye once daily in the evening.
Adults (Izba): 1 drop in each affected eye once daily in the evening.

voretigene neparvovec-rzyl ⌧
vor-RET-i-jeen ne-PAR-voe-vek

Luxturna

Therapeutic class: Ophthalmic gene therapies
Pharmacologic class: Adeno-associated virus gene therapies

AVAILABLE FORMS
Injection: 0.5 mL single-use vial with two vials of diluent

INDICATIONS & DOSAGES
➤ **Confirmed biallelic *RPE65* mutation-associated retinal dystrophy ⌧**
Adults younger than age 65 and children ages 1 and older: Subretinal injection of 0.3 mL (1.5×10^{11} vector genomes [vg]) to each eye on separate days within a close interval, but no fewer than 6 days apart.

Selected biologicals and blood derivatives: Indications and dosages

albumin 5%
al-BYOO-min

Albuked-5, Albuminex 5%, AlbuRx 5%, Albutein 5%, Flexbumin 5%, Plasbumin-5

albumin 25%
Albuked-25, Albuminex 25%, Albutein 25%, Flexbumin 25%, Human Albumin Grifols 25%, Kedbumin, Plasbumin-25

Therapeutic class: Plasma volume expanders
Pharmacologic class: Blood derivatives

AVAILABLE FORMS
albumin 5%
Injection: 50 mg/mL in 50-mL, 100-mL, 250-mL, 500-mL vials
albumin 25%
Injection: 250 mg/mL in 20-mL, 50-mL, 100-mL vials

INDICATIONS & DOSAGES
➤ **Hypovolemic shock**
Adults: Initially, 12.5 to 25 g (250 to 500 mL) of 5% solution by IV infusion, repeated every 15 to 30 minutes, as needed. As plasma volume approaches normal, rate of infusion of 5% solution shouldn't exceed 2 to 4 mL/minute. Dosage of 25% solution varies with patient's condition and response. As plasma volume approaches normal, rate of infusion of 25% solution shouldn't exceed 1 mL/minute.
Older children and adolescents: Initially, 12.5 to 25 g IV (250 to 500 mL) of albumin 5%; repeat in 30-minute intervals as needed.
Infants and younger children: Initially, 0.5 to 1 g/kg/dose IV (10 to 20 mL/kg/dose of albumin 5%); repeat at 30-minute intervals as needed.
➤ **ARDS**
Adults: 25 g of 25% solution by IV infusion over 30 minutes; may repeat at 8-hour intervals for 3 days if necessary. Titrate to fluid loss and normalization of serum total protein.
➤ **Burns**
Adults: 25% solution infused no faster than 2 to 3 mL/minute (for Flexbumin, 1 mL/minute) to maintain plasma albumin concentration at approximately 2.5 ± 0.5 g/100 mL with a plasma oncotic pressure of 20 mm Hg (equal to a total plasma protein concentration of 5.2 g/100 mL). Duration of therapy is determined by loss of protein from burned areas and in urine.

➤ **Hypoalbuminemia**
Adults: 200 to 300 mL of 25% albumin. Dosage varies with patient's condition and response. Usual daily dosage is 50 to 75 g. Rate of infusion shouldn't exceed 2 to 3 mL/minute.
Children: Usual daily dosage is 25 g of 25% albumin. Rate of infusion shouldn't exceed 2 mL/minute.
➤ **Prevention of central volume depletion after paracentesis due to cirrhotic ascites**
Adults: 6 to 8 g of 25% solution IV infusion for every 1 L of ascitic fluid removed or 50 g total for paracentesis volumes of 5 L or more.
➤ **Ovarian hyperstimulation syndrome**
Adults: 50 to 100 g of 25% solution IV infusion over 4 hours; may repeat at 4- to 12-hour intervals as necessary.
➤ **Acute nephrosis**
Adults: 100 mL of 25% albumin daily for 7 to 10 days in combination with diuretic.
➤ **Hemolytic disease of the newborn**
Children: 1 g/kg body weight of 25% albumin IV before or during exchange transfusion.

anti-inhibitor coagulant complex (human)
Feiba, Feiba NF✹

Therapeutic class: Clotting factors
Pharmacologic class: Plasma proteins

AVAILABLE FORMS
Injection: Number of units of factor VIII correctional activity indicated on label of vial

INDICATIONS & DOSAGES
Boxed Warning Thrombotic and thromboembolic events have been reported. Monitor patient closely. ▪
➤ **Prevention or control of hemorrhagic episodes in patients with hemophilia A and B with inhibitors**
Adults and children ages 31 days and older: For joint hemorrhage, 50 to 100 units/kg IV every 12 hours until pain and acute disabilities improve. For mucous membrane hemorrhage, 50 to 100 units/kg IV every 6 hours for at least 1 day or until bleeding resolves. For soft-tissue hemorrhage, 100 units/kg IV every 12 hours until bleeding resolves. For other severe hemorrhage, 100 units/kg IV every 6 to 12 hours until bleeding resolves. For all indications, don't exceed single dose of 100 units/kg body weight or daily dose of 200 units/kg body weight.
➤ **Management of perioperative bleeding in patients with hemophilia A and B with inhibitors**
Adults and children ages 31 days and older: 50 to 100 units/kg IV immediately before surgery as

one-time dose; then 50 to 100 units/kg IV every 6 to 12 hours postoperatively until bleeding resolves and healing is achieved. Don't exceed single dose of 100 units/kg body weight or daily dose of 200 units/kg body weight.

➤ **Routine prophylaxis to prevent or reduce frequency of bleeding episodes in patients with hemophilia A and B with inhibitors**
Adults and children ages 31 days and older: 85 units/kg IV every other day.

antihemophilic factor (AHF, factor VIII)
Advate, Adynovate, Afstyla, Eloctate, Esperoct, Hemofil M, Jivi, Koate, Kogenate FS, Kovaltry, Novoeight, Nuwiq, Obizur, Recombinate, Xyntha

Therapeutic class: Clotting factors
Pharmacologic class: Plasma proteins

AVAILABLE FORMS
Injection: Vials, with diluent; units specified on label

INDICATIONS & DOSAGES
➤ **Factor VIII deficiency, hemophilia A**
Drug provides hemostasis in factor VIII deficiency, hemophilia A. Specific dosage depends on patient's weight, severity of hemorrhage, and presence of inhibitors. Mild bleeding episodes require a circulating factor VIII level 20% to 40% of normal; moderate to major bleeding episodes and minor surgery, a level 30% to 60% of normal; severe bleeding or major surgery, a level 60% to 100% of normal, depending on product used. Refer to specific brand for actual dosage.

beractant
ber-AKT-ant

Survanta

Therapeutic class: Lung surfactants
Pharmacologic class: Bovine lung extracts

AVAILABLE FORMS
Suspension for intratracheal instillation: 25 mg/mL in 4- and 8-mL single-dose vials

INDICATIONS & DOSAGES
➤ **Prevention of respiratory distress syndrome (RDS) in premature neonates weighing 1,250 g or less at birth or having symptoms consistent with surfactant deficiency**
Neonates: 4 mL/kg intratracheally. Divide each dose into four quarter-doses and give each quarter-dose over 2 to 3 seconds with infant in a different position to ensure even distribution of drug; between quarter-doses, manually ventilate infant for at least

30 seconds or until stable. Give drug as soon as possible, preferably within 15 minutes of birth. Repeat in 6 hours if respiratory distress continues. Don't exceed four doses in 48 hours.

➤ **Rescue treatment of RDS in premature infants**
Neonates: 4 mL/kg intratracheally. Divide each dose into four quarter-doses and give each quarter-dose over 2 to 3 seconds with infant in a different position to ensure even distribution of drug; between quarter-doses, manually ventilate for at least 30 seconds or until stable. Give dose as soon as RDS is confirmed by X-ray, preferably within 8 hours of birth. Repeat in 6 hours if respiratory distress continues. Don't exceed four doses in 48 hours.

calfactant
kal-FAK-tant

Infasurf

Therapeutic class: Lung surfactants
Pharmacologic class: Bovine lung extracts

AVAILABLE FORMS
Intratracheal suspension: 35 mg phospholipids and 0.7 mg proteins/mL in 3-mL, 6-mL vials

INDICATIONS & DOSAGES
➤ **Prevention of respiratory distress syndrome (RDS) in premature infants younger than 29 weeks' gestational age at high risk for RDS; treatment of infants younger than age 72 hours who develop RDS (confirmed by clinical and radiologic findings) and need an endotracheal tube**
Neonates: 3 mL/kg of body weight at birth intratracheally, given in two aliquots of 1.5 mL/kg each, every 12 hours for a total of up to three doses.

caplacizumab-yhdp
kap-la-SIZ-ue-mab

Cablivi

Therapeutic class: Immunomodulators
Pharmacologic class: Anti-von Willebrand factors

AVAILABLE FORMS
Injection: 11 mg single-dose vial

INDICATIONS & DOSAGES
➤ **Acquired thrombotic thrombocytopenic purpura (aTTP), in combination with plasma exchange and immunosuppressive therapy**
Adults: On day 1 of plasma exchange therapy, 11 mg IV bolus at least 15 minutes before plasma exchange, followed by 11 mg subcut after completion of plasma exchange. On subsequent days during daily plasma exchange, 11 mg subcut once daily following plasma

exchange. Then 11 mg subcut once daily for 30 days following the last daily plasma exchange. After initial treatment course, if signs and symptoms of persistent underlying disease such as suppressed ADAMTS13 activity levels remain, may extend treatment for a maximum of 28 days. Discontinue drug if patient experiences more than two recurrences of aTTP during therapy.

coagulation factor Xa (recombinant), inactivated-zhzo
Andexxa

Therapeutic class: Antidotes
Pharmacologic class: Factor Xa proteins

AVAILABLE FORMS
Injection: 200-mg vials

INDICATIONS & DOSAGES
Boxed Warning Use of drug has been associated with thromboembolic and ischemic events, including MI, stroke, cardiac arrest, and sudden death. Monitor patient for thromboembolic events and initiate anticoagulation when appropriate. ■

➤ **Reversal of anticoagulation in patients treated with rivaroxaban or apixaban in life-threatening or uncontrolled bleeding**
Adults: Base dosing on the specific factor Xa inhibitor, dose of factor Xa inhibitor, and time since patient's last dose of factor Xa inhibitor. If last dose of rivaroxaban was 10 mg or less taken less than 8 hours or an unknown time ago, last dose of apixaban was 5 mg or less taken less than 8 hours or an unknown time ago, or either rivaroxaban or apixaban at any dose was taken 8 hours or more ago, give initial bolus dose of 400 mg IV at target rate of 30 mg/minute, followed 2 minutes later with IV infusion of 4 mg/minute for up to 120 minutes.

If last dose of rivaroxaban was greater than 10 mg or last dose is unknown and was taken less than 8 hours or an unknown time ago, or last dose of apixaban was greater than 5 mg or last dose is unknown, give initial bolus dose of 800 mg IV at target rate of 30 mg/minute, followed 2 minutes later with IV infusion of 8 mg/minute for up to 120 minutes.

emicizumab-kxwh
em-i-SIZ-ue-mab

Hemlibra

Therapeutic class: Antibodies
Pharmacologic class: Monoclonal IgG4 antibodies

AVAILABLE FORMS
Injection: 30 mg/mL, 60 mg/0.4 mL, 105 mg/0.7 mL, 150 mg/mL single-dose vials

INDICATIONS & DOSAGES
Boxed Warning Thrombotic events have been reported after average cumulative amount of more than 100 units/kg was given within 24 hours of activated prothrombin complex concentrate (aPCC). Discontinue aPCC or suspend emicizumab dose if symptoms occur. ■

➤ **Routine prophylaxis to prevent or reduce frequency of bleeding episodes in patients with hemophilia A (congenital factor VIII deficiency) with or without factor VIII inhibitors** ⚇
Adults and children: 3 mg/kg subcut once weekly for 4 weeks; then 1.5 mg/kg once weekly or 3 mg/kg subcut once every 2 weeks or 6 mg subcut once every 4 weeks.

factor IX complex
Profilnine, Profilnine SD

factor IX (human)
AlphaNine SD, Immunine VH ✽

factor IX (recombinant)
Alprolix, BeneFIX, Ixinity, Rixubis

factor IX (recombinant [glycopegylated])
Rebinyn

Therapeutic class: Clotting factors
Pharmacologic class: Plasma proteins

AVAILABLE FORMS
Injection: Vials, with diluent; international units specified on label

INDICATIONS & DOSAGES
➤ **Factor IX deficiency (hemophilia B or Christmas disease)**
Adults and children: Dosage is highly individualized, depending on degree of deficiency, level of factor IX desired, patient's weight and condition, and bleeding severity. Infusion rates vary with product and patient comfort. Refer to manufacturer's instructions for each product to calculate dosage.

hepatitis B immune globulin (human)
hep-ah-TYE-tis

HepaGam B, HyperHEP B, Nabi-HB

Therapeutic class: Prophylaxis drugs
Pharmacologic class: Immune serums

AVAILABLE FORMS
Injection: 0.5-mL neonatal single-dose syringe; 1-mL single-dose syringe; 1-mL, 5-mL vials

INDICATIONS & DOSAGES
➤ **Postexposure HBV prophylaxis**
Adults and children: 0.06 mL/kg (usual dose is 3 to 5 mL) IM as soon as possible (within 24 hours if possible) but within 7 days after exposure (within 14 days if sexual exposure). Repeat dose 28 days after exposure if patient doesn't elect to receive or doesn't respond to hepatitis B vaccine.
Infants younger than age 12 months if primary caregiver has acute HBV infection: 0.5 mL IM.
Neonates born to HBsAg-positive patients: 0.5 mL IM within 12 hours of birth. Active vaccination with hepatitis B vaccine may begin at the same time.
➤ **Prevention of HBV infection recurrence after liver transplantation in patients who are HBsAg-positive (HepaGam B only)**
Adults: 20,000 international units IV at rate of 2 mL/ minute, first dose simultaneously with grafting of transplanted liver (anhepatic phase). Then give daily on days 1 through 7, every 2 weeks from day 14 through 12 weeks and monthly from month 4 onward.
Adjust-a-dose: Adjust dose in patients who don't reach anti-HBs levels of 500 international units/L within first week after transplantation. In patients with surgical bleeding or abdominal fluid drainage of more than 500 mL and those undergoing plasmapheresis, give 10,000 international units IV every 6 hours until target level is reached.

luspatercept-aamt
lus-PAT-er-sept

Reblozyl

Therapeutic class: Hematopoietics
Pharmacologic class: Erythroid maturation agents

AVAILABLE FORMS
Injection: 25 mg, 75 mg single-use vials

INDICATIONS & DOSAGES
Adjust-a-dose (for all indications): Review Hb and transfusion record before each dose; follow manufacturer's instructions for dosage modifications if response to treatment is insufficient, if rapid rise in Hb occurs, or for predose Hb level of 11.5 g/dL or greater. For grade 3 or 4 hypersensitivity reactions, discontinue treatment. For other grade 3 or 4 adverse reactions, interrupt treatment until adverse reaction resolves to no higher than grade 1; then restart treatment at next lower dose. Discontinue treatment if dose delay continues for longer than 12 consecutive weeks.

➤ **Anemia in patients with beta-thalassemia who require regular RBC transfusions**
Adults: 1 mg/kg subcut once every 3 weeks. Titrate dose by response to maximum dose of 1.25 mg/kg.
➤ **Anemia in patients who fail an erythropoiesis-stimulating agent and require two or more RBC transfusions over 8 weeks with very low- to intermediate-risk myelodysplastic syndrome with ring sideroblasts or with myelodysplastic or myeloproliferative neoplasm with ring sideroblasts and thrombocytosis**
Adults: 1 mg/kg subcut once every 3 weeks. Titrate dose by response to maximum dose of 1.75 mg/kg.
✳ *NEW INDICATION:* **Anemia in patients with very low- to intermediate-risk myelodysplastic syndrome who may require RBC transfusions and who are erythropoiesis-stimulating-agent naive**
Adults: 1 mg/kg subcut once every 3 weeks. Maximum dose, 1.75 mg/kg.

lymphocyte immune globulin (antithymocyte globulin [equine], ATG, LIG)
Atgam

Therapeutic class: Immunosuppressants
Pharmacologic class: Immunoglobulins

AVAILABLE FORMS
Injection: 50 mg/mL in 5-mL ampules

INDICATIONS & DOSAGES
Boxed Warning   Drug can cause anaphylaxis. Only use drug in facilities with adequate laboratory and supportive medical resources. ∎
➤ **Acute renal allograft rejection**
Adults and children: 10 to 15 mg/kg IV daily for 14 days. May give additional alternate-day therapy to total of 21 doses. Start therapy when rejection is diagnosed.
➤ **Aplastic anemia**
Adults and children: 10 to 20 mg/kg IV daily for 8 to 14 days. May give additional alternate-day therapy to total of 21 doses.

plasma protein fraction
Plasmanate

Therapeutic class: Plasma volume expanders
Pharmacologic class: Plasma proteins

AVAILABLE FORMS
Injection: 5% (50 mg/mL) solution in 50-mL, 250-mL, 500-mL vials

INDICATIONS & DOSAGES
➤ **Shock**
Adults: Dosage varies with patient's condition and response. Typical minimum effective dose is 250 to 500 mL. Adjust rate according to clinical response.

SAFETY ALERT!

protein C concentrate ⚞
Ceprotin

Therapeutic class: Anticoagulants
Pharmacologic class: Protein C
replacements

AVAILABLE FORMS
Injection: 500 international units/vial, 1,000 international units/vial

INDICATIONS & DOSAGES
Adjust-a-dose (for all indications): Adjust dosage based on severity of protein C deficiency, plasma level of protein C, and patient's age and condition.
➤ **Venous thrombosis and purpura fulminans in patients with severe congenital protein C deficiency**
Adults, neonates, and children: Initially for acute episodes and short-term prophylaxis, 100 to 120 international units/kg IV; then 60 to 80 international units/kg IV every 6 hours for subsequent three doses to maintain peak protein C activity of 100%. Maintenance dosage of 45 to 60 international units/kg IV every 6 to 12 hours to maintain trough protein C activity level above 25%.
➤ **Long-term prevention of venous thrombosis and purpura fulminans**
Adults, neonates, and children: 45 to 60 international units/kg IV every 12 hours to maintain trough protein C activity level above 25%.

rabies immune globulin (human)
HyperRAB, Imogam Rabies-HT, Kedrab

Therapeutic class: Antibodies
Pharmacologic class: Immunoglobulins

AVAILABLE FORMS
Injection: 150 international units/mL in 2-mL, 10-mL vials; 300 international units/mL in 1-mL, 3-mL, 5-mL vials

INDICATIONS & DOSAGES
➤ **Rabies exposure**
Adults and children: 20 international units/kg IM at time of first dose of rabies vaccine. If anatomically feasible, use as much of full dose as possible to infiltrate wound area; give remainder IM in a different site.

Rh₀(D) immune globulin intramuscular (human) (IGIM)
HyperRHO S/D Full Dose,
HyperRHO S/D Mini-Dose,
MICRhoGAM, RhoGAM

Rh₀(D) immune globulin intravenous (human) (IGIV)
Rhophylac, WinRho SDF

Therapeutic class: Immune globulins
Pharmacologic class: Immunoglobulins

AVAILABLE FORMS
IGIM
Injection: 50-mcg syringe (250 international units, microdose), 300-mcg syringe (1,500 international units, standard dose)
IGIV
Injection: 120-mcg (600 international units), 300-mcg (1,500 international units), 500-mcg (2,500 international units), 1,000-mcg (5,000 international units), 3,000-mcg (15,000 international units) vials; 300-mcg (1,500 international units) syringe

INDICATIONS & DOSAGES
Boxed Warning Intravascular hemolysis leading to compromising anemia, multisystem organ failure, and death have been reported in patients treated for ITP with IGIV. ∎
➤ **Rh exposure after abortion, miscarriage, ectopic pregnancy, or childbirth**
Adults: Transfusion unit or blood bank determines fetal RBC volume entering patient's blood; 300 mcg IGIM is given IM if fetal RBC volume is less than 15 mL. More than one dose may be needed if severe feto-maternal hemorrhage occurs; must be given within 72 hours after delivery or miscarriage.
➤ **Prevention of Rh antibody formation after actual or threatened pregnancy termination (spontaneous or induced)**
Adults: Consult transfusion unit or blood bank. Up to and including 12 weeks' gestation, 1 IGIM microdose vial (50 mcg) IM will suppress immune reaction to 2.5 mL Rh₀(D)-positive RBCs. At 13 weeks' gestation and later, use 1 IGIM standard dose (300 mcg). Ideally, give within 3 hours, but may be given up to 72 hours after abortion or miscarriage.
➤ **Rh exposure after amniocentesis and chorionic villus sampling before 34 weeks' gestation**
Adults: 300 mg given IV or IM immediately after procedure.
➤ **Rh exposure after abortion, amniocentesis after 34 weeks' gestation, or other manipulations past 34 weeks' gestation with increased risk of Rh isoimmunization**

Adults: 120 mcg IGIV, given IV or IM within 72 hours of delivery, miscarriage, or manipulation.

➤ **Suppression of Rh isoimmunization during pregnancy**

Adults: 300 mcg IV or IM at 28 weeks' gestation. If given early in pregnancy, give additional doses at 12-week intervals to maintain adequate levels of passively acquired anti-Rh antibodies. Then, within 72 hours of delivery, give 120 mcg WinRho or 300 mcg HyperRHO, RhoGAM, or Rhophylac IM or IV. If more than 72 hours have elapsed, give drug as soon as possible, up to 28 days.

➤ **Incompatible blood transfusion**

Adults: Total dose depends on volume of RBCs or whole blood infused. Consult blood bank or transfusion unit at once; must be given within 72 hours. Give 600 mcg WinRho IV every 8 hours or 1,200 mcg IM every 12 hours until total dose has been given.

➤ **Chronic ITP in patients who are Rh₀(D) antigen-positive; ITP secondary to HIV; acute ITP in children**

Adults and children: Initially, 50 mcg/kg IV as single dose or divided into two doses on separate days. If Hb level is less than 10 g/dL, reduce first dose to 25 to 40 mcg/kg. Then give 25 to 60 mcg/kg IV as needed to elevate platelet count with specific individually determined dosage.

---

romiplostim
roh-mih-PLOH-stim

Nplate

Therapeutic class: Hematopoietics
Pharmacologic class: Thrombopoietin receptor agonists

AVAILABLE FORMS

Injection: 125-mcg, 250-mcg, 500-mcg single-use vials

INDICATIONS & DOSAGES

➤ **ITP in patients who have had an insufficient response to corticosteroids, immunoglobulins, or splenectomy**

Adults; children ages 1 and older with ITP for at least 6 months: Initially, 1 mcg/kg subcut once weekly. Adjust dosage in increments of 1 mcg/kg/week to maintain platelet count of 50 × 10⁹/L or higher, as needed, to reduce risk of bleeding. Maximum dose, 10 mcg/kg weekly. Refer to manufacturer's instructions for dosage adjustments for platelet counts. Discontinue if platelet count doesn't increase after 4 weeks at maximum dosage.

➤ **To increase survival in patients (including term neonates) acutely exposed to myelosuppressive doses of radiation**

Adults and children: 10 mcg/kg subcut as soon as possible after suspected or confirmed exposure to radiation level greater than 2 gray (Gy).

---

tetanus immune globulin (human)
HyperTET

Therapeutic class: Prophylaxis drugs
Pharmacologic class: Immunoglobulins

AVAILABLE FORMS

Injection: 250-unit vial or syringe

INDICATIONS & DOSAGES

➤ **Postexposure prevention of tetanus after injury in patients whose immunization is incomplete or unknown**

Adults and children ages 7 and older: 250 units deep IM injection.

Children younger than age 7: 250 units deep IM injection is recommended; may also give 4 units/kg.

Less commonly used drugs: Indications and dosages

Refer to manufacturer's instructions for complete prescribing and safety information.

SAFETY ALERT!

acalabrutinib
a-KAL-a-broo-ti-nib

Calquence

Therapeutic class: Antineoplastics
Pharmacologic class: Kinase inhibitors

AVAILABLE FORMS
Capsules ⬤: 100 mg
Tablets ⬤: 100 mg

INDICATIONS & DOSAGES
Adjust-a-dose (for all indications): Refer to manufacturer's instructions for toxicity-related dosage adjustments. Avoid concomitant use with CYP3A inhibitors; if a CYP3A inhibitor is necessary and will be used short term (up to 7 days), interrupt acalabrutinib therapy. If patient is taking with a moderate CYP3A inhibitor, reduce acalabrutinib dosage to 100 mg once daily. Avoid concomitant use with strong CYP3A inducers; if use together can't be avoided, increase acalabrutinib dosage to 200 mg b.i.d.
➤ **Mantle cell lymphoma in patients who have received at least one prior therapy**
Adults: 100 mg PO approximately every 12 hours until disease progresses or unacceptable toxicity occurs.
➤ **Chronic lymphocytic leukemia (CLL) or small lymphocytic lymphoma (SLL)**
Adults: 100 mg PO approximately every 12 hours; continue until disease progresses or unacceptable toxicity occurs. Or, with obinutuzumab for patients with previously untreated CLL or SLL, 100 mg PO approximately every 12 hours until disease progresses or unacceptable toxicity occurs, beginning with cycle 1 (each cycle is 28 days). Start obinutuzumab at cycle 2 for six cycles. Refer to obinutuzumab prescribing information for recommended dosing. Give acalabrutinib before obinutuzumab when given on same day.

SAFETY ALERT!

acarbose
a-KAR-boz

Therapeutic class: Antidiabetics
Pharmacologic class: Alpha-glucosidase inhibitors

AVAILABLE FORMS
Tablets: 25 mg, 50 mg, 100 mg

INDICATIONS & DOSAGES
➤ **Adjunct to diet and exercise to improve glycemic control in patients with type 2 diabetes**
Adults: Dosages individualized. Initially, 25 mg PO t.i.d. with first bite of each main meal. Adjust dosage every 4 to 8 weeks, based on 1-hour postprandial glucose level or HbA_{1c} level and tolerance. Maintenance

dosage is 50 to 100 mg PO t.i.d. For patients who weigh less than 60 kg, don't exceed 50 mg PO t.i.d. For patients who weigh more than 60 kg, don't exceed 100 mg PO t.i.d.

aclidinium bromide
a-cli-DIN-ee-um

Tudorza Genuair ✦, Tudorza Pressair

Therapeutic class: Miscellaneous respiratory drugs
Pharmacologic class: Anticholinergics

AVAILABLE FORMS
Dry powder inhaler: 400 mcg/actuation

INDICATIONS & DOSAGES
➤ **Maintenance treatment of COPD**
Adults: 400 mcg (1 inhalation) b.i.d.

alfuzosin hydrochloride
al-foo-ZOE-sin

Uroxatral

Therapeutic class: BPH drugs
Pharmacologic class: Alpha₁ blockers

AVAILABLE FORMS
Tablets (extended-release): 10 mg

INDICATIONS & DOSAGES
➤ **BPH**
Adults: 10 mg PO once daily.

alirocumab ⬡
AL-i-rok-ue-mab

Praluent

Therapeutic class: Antilipemics
Pharmacologic class: Proprotein convertase subtilisin/kexin type 9 antibody inhibitors

AVAILABLE FORMS
Injection: 75 mg/mL, 150 mg/mL in single-dose prefilled pens

INDICATIONS & DOSAGES
➤ **Adjunct to diet, alone or in combination with other LDL-C lowering therapies, to treat primary hyperlipidemia, including heterozygous familial hypercholesterolemia (HeFH) ⬡; to reduce risk of MI, stroke, and unstable angina requiring hospitalization in patients with established CV disease who require additional lowering of LDL-C level**
Adults: 75 mg subcut every 2 weeks or 300 mg subcut every 4 weeks. If LDL-C response is inadequate (within 4 to 8 weeks), may increase dosage to maximum of 150 mg every 2 weeks. Recommended dosage in patients with HeFH undergoing LDL apheresis is 150 mg subcut every 2 weeks, without regard to the timing of apheresis.

➤ **Adjunct to other LDL-C lowering therapies in patients with homozygous familial hypercholesterolemia to reduce LDL-C level** ▧
Adults: 150 mg subcut every 2 weeks.

alosetron hydrochloride
a-LOE-se-tron

Lotronex

Therapeutic class: Anti-IBS drugs
Pharmacologic class: Selective 5-HT$_3$ receptor antagonists

AVAILABLE FORMS
Tablets: 0.5 mg, 1 mg

INDICATIONS & DOSAGES
Boxed Warning Drug is only appropriate for adult females with severe diarrhea-predominant IBS who haven't responded to conventional therapy. Infrequent but serious GI adverse reactions have been reported and resulted in hospitalization and, rarely, blood transfusion, surgery, and death. If constipation or ischemic colitis symptoms develop, stop drug. ∎
➤ **Severe diarrhea-predominant IBS**
Adult females: 0.5 mg PO b.i.d. If, after 4 weeks, drug is well tolerated but doesn't adequately control IBS symptoms, increase to 1 mg b.i.d. (maximum dosage, 2 mg/day). After 4 weeks at this dosage, if symptoms aren't controlled, stop drug.

SAFETY ALERT!

alprostadil (injection)
al-PROS-ta-dill

Prostin VR Pediatric

Therapeutic class: Prostaglandins
Pharmacologic class: Prostaglandins

AVAILABLE FORMS
Injection: 500 mcg/mL ampules

INDICATIONS & DOSAGES
Boxed Warning Apnea may occur, especially in neonates weighing less than 2 kg at birth and during first hour of infusion. ∎
➤ **Palliative therapy for temporary maintenance of patency of ductus arteriosus until surgery can be performed**
Neonates: 0.05 to 0.1 mcg/kg/minute by IV infusion. When therapeutic response is achieved, reduce infusion rate to lowest dose that will maintain response. Maximum, 0.4 mcg/kg/minute. Or, give drug through umbilical artery catheter placed at ductal opening.

alprostadil (intracavernosal injection; urogenital suppository)
al-PROSS-ta-dil

Caverject, Caverject Impulse, Edex, Muse

Therapeutic class: Erectile dysfunction drugs
Pharmacologic class: Prostaglandins

AVAILABLE FORMS
Intracavernosal injection: 20 mcg/vial, 40 mcg/vial
Intracavernosal injection (injection device): 10 mcg/cartridge, 20 mcg/cartridge, 40 mcg/cartridge
Intracavernosal injection (syringe): 10 mcg/syringe, 20 mcg/syringe
Urethral suppository: 250 mcg, 500 mcg, 1,000 mcg

INDICATIONS & DOSAGES
➤ **Erectile dysfunction of vasculogenic, psychogenic, or mixed causes**
Adults (injection): Dosages highly individualized. Initially, 2.5 mcg by intracavernosal injection. If partial response occurs, give second dose of 2.5 mcg; increase by 5 to 10 mcg until patient achieves erection suitable for intercourse lasting no longer than 1 hour. If no response to first dose, increase second dose to 7.5 mcg within 1 hour; then increase by 5 to 10 mcg until patient achieves suitable erection. After initial doses, patient must remain in prescriber's office until complete detumescence occurs. Don't repeat for at least 24 hours. For Edex, 1 to 40 mcg by intracavernosal injection over 5 to 10 seconds. Use lowest effective dose no more than three times per week, with at least 24 hours between doses.
Adults (urethral suppository): Initially, 250 mcg, under supervision of prescriber. Adjust dosage PRN until response is sufficient for sexual intercourse. Maximum of two administrations in 24 hours; maximum dose 1,000 mcg.
➤ **Erectile dysfunction of neurogenic cause (spinal cord injury)**
Adults: Dosages highly individualized. Initially, 1.25 mcg by intracavernosal injection. If partial response occurs, give second dose of 1.25 mcg. Increase in increments of 2.5 mcg to dose of 5 mcg; then increase in increments of 5 mcg until patient achieves erection suitable for intercourse lasting no longer than 1 hour. If no response to first dose, give next higher dose within 1 hour. After initial doses, patient must remain in prescriber's office until complete detumescence occurs. Don't repeat procedure for at least 24 hours. For Edex, 1 to 40 mcg by intracavernosal injection over 5 to 10 seconds. Use lowest effective dose no more than three times per week with at least 24 hours between doses.

alvimopan
al-VIM-oh-pan

Entereg

Therapeutic class: Bowel restorative drugs
Pharmacologic class: Peripherally acting mu-opioid receptor antagonists

AVAILABLE FORMS
Capsules: 12 mg

INDICATIONS & DOSAGES
Boxed Warning Due to risk of MI, drug is for short-term use in hospitalized patients. Only available through a REMS program. ∎

> **Management of postoperative ileus after partial large- or small-bowel resection surgery with primary anastomosis to accelerate recovery**

Adults: 12 mg PO 30 minutes to 5 hours before surgery, followed by 12 mg PO b.i.d. beginning first day after surgery for up to 7 days or maximum of 15 in-hospital doses (180 mg).

amisulpride
am-ee-SUL-pride

Barhemsys

Therapeutic class: Antiemetics
Pharmacologic class: Dopamine antagonists

AVAILABLE FORMS
Injection: 5 mg/2 mL, 10 mg/4 mL

INDICATIONS & DOSAGES
> **Prevention of postoperative nausea and vomiting (PONV), either alone or in combination with antiemetic of a different class**

Adults: 5 mg IV as single dose over 1 to 2 minutes at time of anesthesia induction.

> **PONV in patients who have received antiemetic prophylaxis with agent of a different class or haven't received prophylaxis**

Adults: 10 mg IV as single dose infused over 1 to 2 minutes.

anakinra
ann-ACK-in-rah

Kineret

Therapeutic class: Immunomodulators
Pharmacologic class: Interleukin-1 receptor antagonists

AVAILABLE FORMS
Injection: 100 mg/0.67 mL in prefilled glass syringe

INDICATIONS & DOSAGES
Adjust-a-dose (for all indications): If CrCl is less than 30 mL/minute, consider every-other-day dosing.
> **Neonatal-onset multisystem inflammatory disease**

Adults and children: Initially, 1 to 2 mg/kg subcut once daily. May increase in 0.5- to 1-mg/kg increments to maximum of 8 mg/kg daily. May divide total daily dose into two equal doses.

> **Moderately to severely active RA after one or more failures with DMARDs, alone or combined with DMARDs other than TNF blockers**

Adults: 100 mg subcut daily at the same time each day.

> **Interleukin-1 receptor antagonist deficiency**

Adults and children: Initially, 1 to 2 mg/kg subcut once daily. May increase in 0.5- to 1-mg/kg increments to maximum of 8 mg/kg daily.

angiotensin II
an-jee-oh-TEN-sin

Giapreza

Therapeutic class: Vasoconstrictors
Pharmacologic class: Angiotensin II analogues

AVAILABLE FORMS
Injection: 0.5 mg/mL, 2.5 mg/mL in 1-mL single-dose vials

INDICATIONS & DOSAGES
> **To increase BP in patients with septic or other distributive shock**

Adults: Initially, 20 nanograms/kg/minute IV infusion. May titrate by up to 15 nanograms/kg/minute every 5 minutes as needed to achieve or maintain target BP. Don't exceed 80 nanograms/kg/minute during first 3 hours of treatment. Dosages as low as 1.25 nanograms/kg/minute may be effective. Maintenance dosages shouldn't exceed 40 nanograms/kg/minute. Once shock has sufficiently improved, wean patient by down-titrating every 5 to 15 minutes by increments of up to 15 nanograms/kg/minute.

anidulafungin
ah-nid-doo-la-FUN-jin

Eraxis

Therapeutic class: Antifungals
Pharmacologic class: Echinocandins

AVAILABLE FORMS
Powder for injection: 50 mg/vial, 100 mg/vial

INDICATIONS & DOSAGES
> **Candidemia and other *Candida* infections (intra-abdominal abscess, peritonitis)**

Adults: 200-mg loading dose by IV infusion at no more than 1.1 mg/minute on day 1; then 100 mg daily for at least 14 days after last positive culture result.
Children ages 1 month and older: 3-mg/kg loading dose (not to exceed 200 mg) by IV infusion at no more than 1.1 mg/minute on day 1; then 1.5 mg/kg (not to exceed 100 mg) daily for at least 14 days after last positive culture result.

> **Esophageal candidiasis**

Adults: 100-mg loading dose by IV infusion at no more than 1.1 mg/minute on day 1; then 50 mg daily for at least 14 days and for at least 7 days after symptoms resolve.

apomorphine hydrochloride
ah-poe-MORE-feen

Apokyn, Movapo ✦

Therapeutic class: Antiparkinsonian drugs
Pharmacologic class: Nonergot-derivative dopamine agonists

AVAILABLE FORMS
Solution for injection:* 10 mg/mL

INDICATIONS & DOSAGES

➤ **Intermittent hypomobility, "off" episodes caused by advanced Parkinson disease (given with an antiemetic)**

Adults: Initially, give a 1-mg or 2-mg subcut test dose when patient is in an "off" episode. Measure supine and standing BP before first dose and every 20 minutes for at least the first hour. If patient tolerates and responds to drug, start with the same dose needed as outpatient. Titrate dosage in 1-mg increments every few days to effect and tolerance. Don't exceed 6 mg. Separate doses by at least 2 hours.

If patient doesn't tolerate test dose or tolerates test dose but doesn't respond adequately, refer to manufacturer's instructions for further medically supervised dosing.

Treatment with concomitant antiemetic is recommended starting 3 days before drug initiation and continuing as necessary to control nausea and vomiting, generally up to 2 months.

Adjust-a-dose: In patients with CrCl of 30 to less than 90 mL/minute, give test and starting doses of 1 mg subcut.

arformoterol tartrate
arr-fohr-MOH-tur-ahl

Brovana

Therapeutic class: Bronchodilators
Pharmacologic class: Long-acting selective beta$_2$ agonists

AVAILABLE FORMS
Solution for inhalation: 15 mcg/2 mL vials

INDICATIONS & DOSAGES
➤ **Maintenance treatment of bronchoconstriction in patients with COPD**
Adults: 15 mcg inhaled via nebulizer every 12 hours. Maximum, 30 mcg daily.

armodafinil
ar-moe-DAF-i-nil

Nuvigil

Therapeutic class: Stimulants
Pharmacologic class: CNS stimulants
Controlled substance schedule: IV

AVAILABLE FORMS
Tablets: 50 mg, 150 mg, 200 mg, 250 mg

INDICATIONS & DOSAGES
➤ **To improve wakefulness in patients with excessive sleepiness caused by narcolepsy, obstructive sleep apnea (OSA), or shift-work sleep disorder**
Adults: 150 to 250 mg PO daily in morning. For OSA, dosages exceeding 150 mg daily may not be more effective. For shift-work sleep disorder, 150 mg PO daily, 1 hour before start of shift.
Adjust-a-dose: Reduce dosage in patients with Child-Pugh class C liver impairment. Consider lower doses in older adults.

atezolizumab ⬚
a-te-zoe-LIZ-ue-mab

Tecentriq

Therapeutic class: Antineoplastics
Pharmacologic class: Monoclonal antibodies

AVAILABLE FORMS
Injection: 840 mg/14 mL, 1,200 mg/20 mL single-dose vial

INDICATIONS & DOSAGES
Adjust-a-dose (for all indications): Dosage reductions aren't recommended for toxicities; drug is either withheld or permanently discontinued. Refer to manufacturer's instructions for toxicity-related dosage adjustments.

➤ **First-line treatment of extensive-stage small cell lung cancer, in combination with carboplatin and etoposide**
Adults: 840-mg IV infusion every 2 weeks, 1,200-mg IV infusion every 3 weeks, or 1,680-mg IV infusion every 4 weeks. If using with carboplatin and etoposide, give before chemotherapy when given on same day.
Adjust-a-dose: Refer to prescribing information for other chemotherapy agents for dosing information.

➤ **First-line treatment for metastatic nonsquamous NSCLC in patients with no *EGFR* or *ALK* genomic tumor aberrations, in combination with paclitaxel protein-bound particles and carboplatin or in combination with bevacizumab, paclitaxel, and carboplatin** ⬚
Adults: 840-mg IV infusion every 2 weeks, 1,200-mg IV infusion every 3 weeks, or 1,680-mg IV infusion every 4 weeks until disease progresses or unacceptable toxicity occurs. Infuse before chemotherapy and bevacizumab when given on same day.
Adjust-a-dose: Refer to prescribing information for the chemotherapy agents or bevacizumab for dosing information. After completion of four to six cycles of chemotherapy, and if bevacizumab is discontinued, atezolizumab may be continued.

➤ **Metastatic NSCLC in patients whose tumors have high PD-L1 expression, with no *EGFR* or *ALK* genomic tumor aberrations, or have disease progression during or after platinum-containing chemotherapy** ⬚
Adults: 840-mg IV infusion every 2 weeks, 1,200-mg IV infusion every 3 weeks, or 1,680-mg IV infusion every 4 weeks until disease progresses or unacceptable toxicity occurs.

➤ **Adjuvant treatment after resection and platinum-based chemotherapy for patients with stage II to IIIA NSCLC whose tumors express PD-L1**
Adults: 840-mg IV infusion every 2 weeks, 1,200-mg every 3 weeks, or 1,680-mg IV infusion every 4 weeks until disease progresses or unacceptable toxicity occurs, or up to 1 year.

➤ **Unresectable or metastatic hepatocellular carcinoma in combination with bevacizumab in patients who haven't received prior systemic therapy**

Adults: 840-mg IV infusion every 2 weeks, 1,200-mg IV infusion every 3 weeks, or 1,680-mg IV infusion every 4 weeks. Give 15 mg/kg bevacizumab after atezolizumab on same day every 3 weeks until disease progresses or unacceptable toxicity occurs. If bevacizumab is discontinued, may continue atezolizumab. Refer to manufacturer's instructions for bevacizumab prescribing information.

➤ *BRAF* **V600 mutation-positive unresectable or metastatic melanoma in combination with cobimetinib and vemurafenib** ⚥

Adults: After completion of 28-day cycle of cobimetinib and vemurafenib, give atezolizumab 840-mg IV infusion every 2 weeks, 1,200-mg IV infusion every 3 weeks, or 1,680-mg IV infusion every 4 weeks with cobimetinib 60 mg PO once daily (21 days on/7 days off) and vemurafenib 720 mg PO b.i.d. until disease progresses or unacceptable toxicity occurs. Refer to manufacturer's instructions for cobimetinib and vemurafenib prescribing information.

✷ *NEW INDICATION:* **Unresectable or metastatic alveolar soft part sarcoma**

Adults: 840-mg IV infusion every 2 weeks, 1,200-mg IV infusion every 3 weeks, or 1,680-mg IV infusion every 4 weeks until disease progresses or unacceptable toxicity occurs.

Children older than age 2 years: 15 mg/kg (1,200 mg maximum dose) every 3 weeks until disease progresses or unacceptable toxicity occurs.

SAFETY ALERT!

atracurium besylate
at-truh-KYOO-ree-um

Therapeutic class: Skeletal muscle relaxants
Pharmacologic class: Nondepolarizing neuromuscular blockers

AVAILABLE FORMS
Injection: 10 mg/mL

INDICATIONS & DOSAGES
➤ **Adjunct to general anesthesia to facilitate ET intubation and relax skeletal muscles during surgery or mechanical ventilation**

Adults and children ages 2 and older: 0.4 to 0.5 mg/kg by IV bolus. Give maintenance dose of 0.08 to 0.1 mg/kg within 20 to 45 minutes during prolonged surgery and every 15 to 25 minutes in patients receiving balanced anesthesia. For prolonged procedures, use a constant infusion at 9 to 10 mcg/kg/minute initially; then reduce to 5 to 9 mcg/kg/minute. For infusion in ICU, infusion rate of 11 to 13 mcg/kg/minute should provide adequate neuromuscular blockade.

Children ages 1 month to 2 years: First dose, 0.3 to 0.4 mg/kg IV for those under halothane anesthesia. Frequent maintenance doses may be needed.

Adjust-a-dose: In adults, adolescents, children, or infants with significant CV disease or history suggesting a greater risk of histamine release (anaphylactic

reaction, asthma), give initial dose of 0.3 to 0.4 mg/kg slowly or in divided doses over 1 minute. In adults receiving enflurane or isoflurane at the same time, reduce initial atracurium dose by 33% (0.25 to 0.35 mg/kg). In adults receiving atracurium following succinylcholine, initial dose is 0.3 to 0.4 mg/kg.

avanafil
a-VAN-a-fill

Stendra

Therapeutic class: Erectile dysfunction drugs
Pharmacologic class: PDE5 inhibitors

AVAILABLE FORMS
Tablets: 50 mg, 100 mg, 200 mg

INDICATIONS & DOSAGES
➤ **Erectile dysfunction**

Adults: 100 mg PO daily as needed 15 minutes before sexual activity. May increase to maximum of 200 mg daily 15 minutes before sexual activity or decrease to 50 mg daily 30 minutes before sexual activity. Use lowest effective dosage. Maximum, one dose daily.

Adjust-a-dose: In patients taking moderate CYP3A4 inhibitors, maximum dosage is 50 mg PO daily. Don't use in patients taking strong CYP3A4 inhibitors or any form of nitrates. In patients taking stable dose of an alpha blocker, initially give 50 mg PO daily; adjust as needed and tolerated.

SAFETY ALERT!

avatrombopag maleate
a-va-TROM-boe-PAG

Doptelet

Therapeutic class: Hematopoietics
Pharmacologic class: Thrombopoietin receptor agonists

AVAILABLE FORMS
Tablets: 20 mg

INDICATIONS & DOSAGES
➤ **Thrombocytopenia in patients with chronic liver disease scheduled to undergo a procedure**

Adults: Begin dosing 10 to 13 days before scheduled procedure. For platelet count of 40×10^9/L to less than 50×10^9/L, give 40 mg PO once daily for 5 consecutive days. For platelet count less than 40×10^9/L, give 60 mg PO once daily for 5 consecutive days. Patient should undergo procedure within 5 to 8 days after final dose.

➤ **Chronic ITP in patients who have had an insufficient response to a previous treatment**

Adults: 20 mg PO once daily. Adjust dosage or frequency of dosing to maintain platelet count of 50×10^9/L or greater. Maximum, 40 mg/day.

azaCITIDine
ay-za-SYE-ti-deen

Onureg, Vidaza

Therapeutic class: Antineoplastics
Pharmacologic class: Pyrimidine nucleoside analogues

AVAILABLE FORMS
Powder for injection: 100-mg vials
Tablets ⓒ⓪: 200 mg, 300 mg

INDICATIONS & DOSAGES
Adjust-a-dose (for all indications): Refer to manufacturer's instructions for toxicity-related dosage adjustments.
➤ **Myelodysplastic syndrome, including refractory anemia, refractory anemia with ringed sideroblasts (if patient has neutropenia or thrombocytopenia, or needs transfusions), refractory anemia with excess blasts, refractory anemia with excess blasts in transformation, or chronic myelomonocytic leukemia**
Adults: Initially, 75 mg/m² subcut or IV daily for 7 days; repeat cycle every 4 weeks. May increase to 100 mg/m² if no response occurs after two treatment cycles and nausea and vomiting are the only toxic reactions. Minimum of four treatment cycles are recommended. Continue treatment if patient continues to benefit.
➤ **Continued treatment of patients with acute myeloid leukemia who achieved first complete remission or complete remission with incomplete blood count recovery following intensive induction chemotherapy and who can't complete intensive curative therapy**
Adults: 300 mg PO once daily on days 1 through 14 of each 28-day cycle. Continue until disease progresses or unacceptable toxicity occurs. Give an antiemetic before each dose for at least the first two cycles.
➤ **Newly diagnosed juvenile myelomonocytic leukemia (JMML)**
Children ages 1 year and older weighing 10 kg or more: 75 mg/m² IV infusion daily for 7 days in a 28-day cycle. Treat for minimum of three cycles and maximum of six cycles.
Children ages 1 month to younger than 1 year or weighing less than 10 kg: 2.5 mg/kg IV infusion daily for 7 days in a 28-day cycle. Treat for minimum of three cycles and maximum of six cycles.
Adjust-a-dose: Consider treatment delays up to 14 days for nonhematologic toxicities. Hematologic toxicity is difficult to differentiate from natural course of JMML; dosage reduction for hematologic toxicity isn't recommended during first three cycles. Discontinue therapy if neutrophil count is less than 0.5×10^9/L at end of cycle 3 or on day 1 of cycles 5 or 6.
➤ **Acute myeloid leukemia** ♦
Adults: 75 mg/m²/day subcut or IV for 7 days every 4 weeks for at least six cycles. May continue treatment if

patient continues to benefit or until disease progresses or unacceptable toxicity occurs.

azelaic acid
aze-eh-LAY-ik

Azelex, Finacea

Therapeutic class: Antiacne drugs
Pharmacologic class: Dicarboxylic acids

AVAILABLE FORMS
Cream: 20%
Foam: 15%
Gel: 15%

INDICATIONS & DOSAGES
➤ **Mild to moderate inflammatory acne vulgaris**
Adults and children ages 12 and older: Apply thin film of cream gently but thoroughly massaged into affected areas b.i.d., in morning and evening. Improvement usually occurs within 4 weeks.
➤ **Mild to moderate rosacea**
Adults: Apply thin film of foam or gel gently massaged into affected areas b.i.d., in morning and evening. Reassess if no improvement in 12 weeks.

azilsartan kamedoxomil
ay-zil-SAR-tan

Edarbi

Therapeutic class: Antihypertensives
Pharmacologic class: ARBs

AVAILABLE FORMS
Tablets: 40 mg, 80 mg

INDICATIONS & DOSAGES
Boxed Warning Drugs that act directly on RAAS can cause fetal harm; when pregnancy is detected, discontinue drug as soon as possible. ∎
➤ **HTN (alone or in combination with other antihypertensives)**
Adults: 80 mg PO once daily.
Adjust-a-dose: For patients treated with high doses of diuretics, consider initiating therapy at 40 mg PO daily.

bedaquiline fumarate
bed-AK-wi-leen

Sirturo

Therapeutic class: Antituberculotics
Pharmacologic class: Diarylquinolines

AVAILABLE FORMS
Tablets: 20 mg, 100 mg

INDICATIONS & DOSAGES
Boxed Warning Due to increased risk of death, drug should be reserved for use when an effective treatment regimen can't otherwise be provided. QT-interval prolongation can occur; avoid concomitant drugs that prolong QT interval. ∎

➤ **Pulmonary multidrug-resistant TB as part of combination therapy**

Adults and children ages 5 and older weighing at least 30 kg: 400 mg PO once daily for first 2 weeks; 200 mg PO three times a week (48 hours between doses) for a total of 600 mg/week for weeks 3 to 24. *Children ages 5 and older weighing 15 to less than 30 kg:* 200 mg PO once daily for first two weeks; 100 mg PO three times a week (48 hours between doses) for a total of 300 mg/week for weeks 3 to 24. *Adjust-a-dose:* In first 2 weeks, if a dose is missed, don't make it up but continue the dosing schedule. From 3 weeks on, if a dose is missed, have patient take dose as soon as possible; then resume the three-times-a-week schedule.

SAFETY ALERT!

belinostat ⊠
be-LIN-oh-stat

Beleodaq

Therapeutic class: Antineoplastics
Pharmacologic class: Histone deacetylase inhibitors

AVAILABLE FORMS
Injection: 500-mg single-use vial

INDICATIONS & DOSAGES
➤ **Relapsed or refractory peripheral T-cell lymphoma**

Adults: 1,000 mg/m² IV infusion over 30 minutes once daily on days 1 through 5 of 21-day cycle. Repeat cycles until disease progresses or unacceptable toxicity occurs.

Adjust-a-dose: Refer to manufacturer's instructions for toxicity-related dosage adjustments. For patients homozygous for the *UGT1A1*28* allele, reduce starting dose to 750 mg/m² because drug clearance may be decreased (may affect 20% of Blacks, 10% of Whites, and 2% of Asians). ⊠

belumosudil
bel-ue-MOE-soo-dil

Rezurock

Therapeutic class: Immunomodulators
Pharmacologic class: Kinase inhibitors

AVAILABLE FORMS
Tablets ⓄⓃⒸ: 200 mg

INDICATIONS & DOSAGES
➤ **Chronic GVHD after failure of at least two prior lines of systemic therapy**

Adults and children ages 12 and older: 200 mg PO daily until progression of chronic GVHD requires new systemic therapy.

Adjust-a-dose: Refer to manufacturer's instructions for toxicity-related dosage adjustments. If drug is used concomitantly with strong CYP3A inducers or PPIs, increase dosage to 200 mg b.i.d.

bempedoic acid ⊠
bem-pe-DOE-ik

Nexletol

Therapeutic class: Antilipemics
Pharmacologic class: Adenosine triphosphate-citrate lyase inhibitors

AVAILABLE FORMS
Tablets: 180 mg

INDICATIONS & DOSAGES
➤ **Heterozygous familial hypercholesterolemia or established atherosclerotic CV disease as an adjunct to diet and maximally tolerated statin therapy in patients who require additional lowering of LDL-C** ⊠

Adults: 180 mg PO once daily.

SAFETY ALERT!

bendamustine hydrochloride
ben-dah-MOO-steen

Belrapzo, Bendeka, Treanda, Vivimusta

Therapeutic class: Antineoplastics
Pharmacologic class: Mechlorethamine derivatives

AVAILABLE FORMS
Injection solution: 100 mg/4 mL vials
Lyophilized powder for injection: 25 mg, 100 mg in single-use vials

INDICATIONS & DOSAGES
Adjust-a-dose (for all indications): Refer to manufacturer's instructions for dosage adjustments for hematologic and nonhematologic toxicities.
🔆 *Alert:* Available formulations have different concentrations; don't mix or combine. See manufacturer's instructions for preparation.
➤ **Chronic lymphocytic leukemia**

Adults: 100 mg/m² IV on days 1 and 2 of 28-day cycle, given for up to six cycles.
➤ **Indolent B-cell non-Hodgkin lymphoma that has progressed during or within 6 months of treatment with rituximab or a rituximab-containing regimen**

Adults: 120 mg/m² IV on days 1 and 2 of 21-day cycle, given for up to eight cycles.

benzonatate
ben-ZOE-na-tate

Therapeutic class: Antitussives
Pharmacologic class: Local anesthetics

AVAILABLE FORMS
Capsules ⓄⓃⒸ: 100 mg, 150 mg, 200 mg

INDICATIONS & DOSAGES
➤ **Symptomatic relief of cough**

Adults and children older than age 10: 100 to 200 mg PO t.i.d. PRN, up to 600 mg daily.

berotralstat ⬚

ber-oh-TRAL-stat

Orladeyo

Therapeutic class: Miscellaneous hematologic drugs
Pharmacologic class: Plasma kallikrein inhibitors

AVAILABLE FORMS
Capsules: 110 mg, 150 mg

INDICATIONS & DOSAGES
➤ **Prophylaxis to prevent attacks of hereditary angioedema** ⬚
Adults and children ages 12 and older: 150 mg PO once daily.
Adjust-a-dose: For patients with Child-Pugh class B or C liver impairment, concomitant use with P-gp or BCRP inhibitors, or persistent GI reactions, decrease dosage to 110 mg PO once daily.

betaxolol hydrochloride

beh-TAX-oh-lol

Betoptic S

Therapeutic class: Antiglaucoma drugs–antihypertensives
Pharmacologic class: Beta blockers

AVAILABLE FORMS
Ophthalmic solution: 0.5%
Ophthalmic suspension: 0.25%
Tablets: 10 mg, 20 mg

INDICATIONS & DOSAGES
➤ **Chronic open-angle glaucoma, ocular HTN (ophthalmic only)**
Adults: Instill 1 or 2 drops of solution or 1 drop of suspension in affected eye(s) b.i.d.
➤ **HTN**
Adults: 10 mg PO once daily. May increase dosage to 20 mg daily if desired response isn't achieved after 7 to 14 days.
Adjust-a-dose: To prevent bradycardia, reduce starting dosage to 5 mg daily older adults. In patients with CrCl less than 30 mL/minute, reduce initial dosage to 5 mg daily. May increase dosage by 5 mg/day every 2 weeks to maximum dosage of 20 mg/day. Taper dosage over 2 weeks before discontinuing drug.

bezlotoxumab

BEZ-loe-tox-ue-mab

Zinplava

Therapeutic class: Toxin binders
Pharmacologic class: Monoclonal antibodies

AVAILABLE FORMS
Injection: 1,000 mg/40 mL (25 mg/mL) in single-dose vials

INDICATIONS & DOSAGES
➤ **To reduce recurrence of *Clostridioides difficile* infection (CDI) in patients receiving antibacterial treatment for CDI and who are at high risk for CDI recurrence**
Adults and children ages 1 and older: 10 mg/kg by IV infusion over 60 minutes as a one-time dose during antibacterial treatment for CDI.

SAFETY ALERT!

bicalutamide

bye-ka-LOO-ta-mide

Casodex

Therapeutic class: Antineoplastics
Pharmacologic class: Androgen receptor inhibitors

AVAILABLE FORMS
Tablets: 50 mg

INDICATIONS & DOSAGES
➤ **Metastatic prostate cancer in combination with a luteinizing hormone-releasing hormone analogue**
Adult males: 50 mg PO once daily.

blinatumomab ⬚

blin-a-TOOM-oh-mab

Blincyto

Therapeutic class: Antineoplastics
Pharmacologic class: Monoclonal antibodies

AVAILABLE FORMS
Injection: 35-mcg single-use vial

INDICATIONS & DOSAGES
Boxed Warning Drug can cause fatal cytokine release syndrome and neurologic toxicities. ▮
⟳ Alert: Strictly follow preparation and administration instructions to minimize medication errors.
Adjust-a-dose (for all indications): If the interruption after an adverse event is no longer than 7 days, continue the same cycle to a total of 28 days of infusion inclusive of days before and after the interruption in that cycle. If an interruption due to an adverse event is longer than 7 days, start a new cycle. Refer to manufacturer's instructions for toxicity-related dosage adjustments.
➤ **Relapsed or refractory B-cell precursor acute lymphoblastic leukemia (ALL)** ⬚
Adults and children: A treatment course consists of up to two induction cycles followed by three additional consolidation cycles and up to four additional cycles of continued therapy. A single cycle of treatment induction or consolidation consists of 28 days of continuous IV infusion followed by a 14-day treatment-free interval (total 42 days). A single cycle of continued therapy consists of 28 days of continuous IV infusion followed by a 56-day treatment-free interval (total 84 days).

For patients weighing 45 kg or more, for cycle 1, initially give 9 mcg/day by continuous IV infusion on days 1 through 7, then 28 mcg/day by continuous IV infusion on days 8 through 28, followed by a 14-day treatment-free interval (total 42 days). For subsequent induction and consolidation cycles, give 28 mcg/day on days 1 through 28, each cycle followed by a 14-day treatment-free interval (total 42 days). For each cycle of continued therapy, give 28 mcg/day, followed by a 56-day treatment-free interval (total 84 days).

For patients weighing 22 to less than 45 kg, doses are calculated using patient's BSA. For cycle 1, initially give 5 mcg/m²/day (not to exceed 9 mcg/day) by continuous IV infusion on days 1 through 7, then 15 mcg/m²/day (not to exceed 28 mcg/day) by continuous IV infusion on days 8 through 28, followed by a 14-day treatment-free interval (total 42 days). For subsequent induction and consolidation cycles, give 15 mcg/m²/day (not to exceed 28 mcg/day) on days 1 through 28, each cycle followed by a 14-day treatment-free interval (total 42 days). For each cycle of continued therapy, give 15 mcg/m²/day (not to exceed 28 mcg/day), followed by a 56-day treatment-free interval (total 84 days). Drug isn't recommended for use in patients weighing less than 22 kg.

➤ **B-cell precursor ALL in first or second complete remission with minimal residual disease greater than or equal to 0.1%**
Adults and children: A treatment course consists of one induction cycle followed by up to three additional cycles for consolidation.

For patients weighing 45 kg or more, the dose for a single cycle of treatment induction or consolidation is 28 mcg/day continuous IV infusion for 28 days, followed by a 14-day treatment-free interval (total 42 days). For patients weighing 22 to less than 45 kg, the dose for a single cycle of treatment induction or consolidation, calculated using patient's BSA, is 15 mcg/m²/day (not to exceed 28 mcg/day) continuous IV infusion for 28 days, followed by a 14-day treatment-free interval (total 42 days). Drug isn't recommended for use in patients weighing less than 22 kg.

brexanolone
brex-AN-oh-lone

Zulresso

Therapeutic class: Antidepressants
Pharmacologic class: GABA_A receptor modulators
Controlled substance schedule: IV

AVAILABLE FORMS
Injection: 100 mg/20 mL single-dose vial

INDICATIONS & DOSAGES
Boxed Warning Drug can cause excessive sedation or sudden loss of consciousness. Monitoring is recommended. ∎

➤ **Postpartum depression**
Patients ages 15 and older: Give as continuous IV infusion over a total of 60 hours, titrating dosage as follows: 0 to 4 hours, 30 mcg/kg/hour; 4 to 24 hours, increase infusion rate to 60 mcg/kg/hour; 24 to 52 hours,

increase infusion rate to 90 mcg/kg/hour or consider a dosage of 60 mcg/kg/hour if higher infusion rate isn't tolerated; 52 to 56 hours, decrease infusion rate to 60 mcg/kg/hour; 56 to 60 hours, decrease infusion rate to 30 mcg/kg/hour.
Adjust-a-dose: For excessive sedation, stop infusion until symptoms resolve and resume at the same or lower infusion rate.

brivaracetam
briv-a-RA-se-tam

Briviact

Therapeutic class: Anticonvulsants
Pharmacologic class: Anticonvulsants
Controlled substance schedule: V

AVAILABLE FORMS
Injection: 50 mg/5 mL single-dose vial
Oral solution: 10 mg/mL
Tablets ⊘: 10 mg, 25 mg, 50 mg, 75 mg, 100 mg

INDICATIONS & DOSAGES
➤ **Adjunctive therapy or monotherapy for partial-onset seizures in patients with epilepsy**
Adults and children ages 16 and older: Initially, 50 mg PO or IV b.i.d. Titrate dosage to individual patient tolerability and therapeutic response to minimum of 25 mg b.i.d. and maximum of 100 mg b.i.d.
Children ages 4 and older weighing 50 kg or more: 25 to 50 mg PO or IV b.i.d. Adjust dosage based on clinical response and tolerability. Minimum, 25 mg b.i.d.; maximum, 100 mg b.i.d.
Children ages 1 month and older weighing 20 to less than 50 kg: 0.5 to 1 mg/kg PO or IV b.i.d. Adjust dosage based on clinical response and tolerability. Minimum, 0.5 mg/kg b.i.d.; maximum, 2 mg/kg b.i.d.
Children ages 1 month and older weighing 11 to less than 20 kg: 0.5 to 1.25 mg/kg PO or IV b.i.d. Adjust dosage based on clinical response and tolerability. Minimum, 0.5 mg/kg b.i.d.; maximum, 2.5 mg/kg b.i.d.
Children ages 1 month and older weighing less than 11 kg: 0.75 to 1.5 mg/kg PO or IV b.i.d. Adjust dosage based on clinical response and tolerability. Minimum, 0.75 mg/kg b.i.d.; maximum, 3 mg/kg b.i.d.
Adjust-a-dose: Refer to manufacturer's instructions for dosage adjustments in adults and children with liver impairment. In patients also taking rifampin, increase brivaracetam dosage by up to 100% (double the dose).

bromocriptine mesylate
broe-moe-KRIP-teen

Cycloset, Parlodel

Therapeutic class: Antiparkinsonian drugs
Pharmacologic class: Dopamine receptor agonists

AVAILABLE FORMS
Capsules: 5 mg
Tablets: 0.8 mg, 2.5 mg

INDICATIONS & DOSAGES

➤ **Parkinson disease (except Cycloset)**
Adults: 1.25 mg PO b.i.d. with meals. Increase dosage by 2.5 mg/day every 14 to 28 days to lowest dosage that produces an optimal therapeutic response. Maximum, 100 mg daily.

➤ **Hyperprolactinemia-associated disorders, including amenorrhea with or without galactorrhea, hypogonadism, or infertility (except Cycloset)**
Adults and adolescents ages 16 and older: 1.25 to 2.5 mg PO daily, increased by 2.5 mg daily at 2- to 7-day intervals until desired effect occurs. Usual therapeutic dosage, 2.5 to 15 mg daily.
Children ages 11 to 15: 1.25 to 2.5 mg PO daily. May increase as tolerated until therapeutic response is achieved. Range, 2.5 to 10 mg daily in children with prolactin-secreting pituitary adenomas.

➤ **Acromegaly (except Cycloset)**
Adults: 1.25 to 2.5 mg PO with bedtime snack for 3 days. May add another 1.25 to 2.5 mg every 3 to 7 days as tolerated until therapeutic benefit occurs. Maximum, 100 mg daily. Usual therapeutic dosage, 20 to 30 mg daily.

➤ **Type 2 diabetes (Cycloset only)**
Adults: Initially, 0.8 mg PO daily within 2 hours after waking in the morning. May increase by 0.8 mg weekly until maximum tolerated dosage of 1.6 to 4.8 mg daily is achieved.
Adjust-a-dose: Dosage shouldn't exceed 1.6 mg once daily during concomitant use of a moderate CYP3A4 inhibitor. Avoid use with strong CYP3A4 inhibitors.

SAFETY ALERT!

busulfan
byoo-SUL-fan

Busulfex, Myleran

Therapeutic class: Antineoplastics
Pharmacologic class: Alkyl sulfonates

AVAILABLE FORMS
Injection: 6 mg/mL
Tablets: 2 mg

INDICATIONS & DOSAGES
Boxed Warning Injection causes severe and prolonged myelosuppression at recommended dosage. Hematopoietic progenitor cell transplantation is required to prevent potentially fatal complications. Oral form can induce severe bone marrow hypoplasia. Should only be prescribed by experienced health care professionals. ∎

➤ **Hematopoietic stem-cell conditioning regimen for chronic myelocytic leukemia, in combination with cyclophosphamide**
Adults: 0.8 mg/kg (ideal or actual body weight, whichever is lower) IV over 2 hours every 6 hours for 4 days (a total of 16 doses) beginning 7 days before transplant. Give cyclophosphamide 60 mg/kg IV over 1 hour daily for 2 days beginning no sooner than 6 hours after 16th dose of IV busulfan.

➤ **Palliative treatment of chronic myelogenous (myeloid, myelocytic, granulocytic) leukemia**
Adults and children: 4 to 8 mg (60 mcg/kg or 1.8 mg/m²) PO daily until WBC count falls to 15,000/mm³. Stop drug until WBC count rises to approximately 50,000/mm³; then resume dosage as before. When remission is shorter than 3 months, may give maintenance therapy of 1 to 3 mg PO daily.

C1 esterase inhibitor subcutaneous (human) ⌀
ES-ter-ase

Berinert, Cinryze, Haegarda

Therapeutic class: Miscellaneous hematologic drugs
Pharmacologic class: Serine protease inhibitors

AVAILABLE FORMS
Injection: 500 international units (Berinert, Cinryze); 2,000 international units, 3,000 international units (Haegarda) in single-use vials packaged with sterile water for injection

INDICATIONS & DOSAGES
➤ **Routine prophylaxis to prevent hereditary angioedema (HAE) attack (except Berinert)** ⌀
Adults and adolescents ages 12 and older: 60 international units/kg Haegarda subcut twice weekly (every 3 or 4 days). Or, 1,000 international units Cinryze IV at a rate of 1 mL/minute (10 minutes) every 3 or 4 days; may consider doses up to 2,000 international units (not exceeding 80 units/kg) IV based on individual patient response.
Children ages 6 to 11: 60 international units/kg Haegarda subcut twice weekly (every 3 or 4 days). Or, 500 international units Cinryze IV at a rate of 1 mL/minute (5 minutes) every 3 or 4 days; may consider doses up to 1,000 international units IV based on individual patient response.

➤ **Treatment of HAE attack (Berinert only)** ⌀
Adults and children ages 6 and older: 20 international units/kg by slow IV injection at a rate of approximately 4 mL/minute.

SAFETY ALERT!

cabazitaxel
ka-baz-ih-TAX-el

Jevtana

Therapeutic class: Antineoplastics
Pharmacologic class: Taxoids

AVAILABLE FORMS
Injection: 60 mg/1.5 mL

INDICATIONS & DOSAGES
Boxed Warning Drug is associated with severe hypersensitivity and neutropenic deaths. Closely monitor patient and blood cell counts and provide appropriate therapy. Contraindicated for use in patients with history of severe hypersensitivity reaction to drug or drugs formulated with polysorbate 80. ∎

▶ **In combination with prednisone for metastatic castration-resistant prostate cancer previously treated with docetaxel-containing treatment regimen**

Adults: 20 mg/m² IV over 1 hour every 3 weeks. A dose of 25 mg/m² can be used in select patients at prescriber's discretion. Give oral prednisone 10 mg daily throughout cabazitaxel therapy. Premedicate at least 30 minutes before each dose of cabazitaxel with the following IV medications to reduce risk or severity of hypersensitivity: antihistamine (5 mg dexchlorpheniramine, or 25 mg diphenhydramine or equivalent antihistamine), corticosteroid (8 mg dexamethasone or equivalent steroid), and H₂ antagonist. Antiemetic prophylaxis is recommended.

Adjust-a-dose: Refer to manufacturer's instructions for toxicity-related dosage adjustments, liver impairment, and use with strong CYP3A inhibitors.

cannabidiol
kan-a-bi-DYE-ol

Epidiolex

Therapeutic class: Anticonvulsants
Pharmacologic class: Cannabinoids

AVAILABLE FORMS
Oral solution: 100 mg/mL

INDICATIONS & DOSAGES
▶ **Seizures associated with Lennox-Gastaut syndrome (LGS), Dravet syndrome (DS), or tuberous sclerosis complex (TSC)**

Adults and children ages 1 and older: Initially, 2.5 mg/kg PO b.i.d. After 1 week, increase to maintenance dosage of 5 mg/kg PO b.i.d. If necessary, may further increase dosage, as tolerated, in weekly increments of 2.5 mg/kg b.i.d. to a maximum maintenance dosage of 10 mg/kg for LGS and DS or 12.5 mg/kg b.i.d. for TSC. For patients in whom a more rapid titration is warranted, may increase dosage no more frequently than every other day.

Adjust-a-dose: For Child-Pugh class B liver impairment, initiate therapy at 1.25 mg/kg PO b.i.d. Increase to maintenance dosage of 2.5 to 5 mg/kg PO b.i.d. for LGS or DS or 6.25 mg/kg for TSC PO b.i.d. For patients with Child-Pugh class C liver impairment, initiate therapy at 0.5 mg/kg PO b.i.d. Increase to maintenance dose of 1 to 2 mg/kg PO b.i.d. for LGS or DS or 2.5 mg/kg PO b.i.d. for TSC. Discontinue drug in patients with transaminase elevations greater than 3 × ULN and bilirubin levels greater than 2 × ULN and in those with sustained transaminase elevations greater than 5 × ULN.

SAFETY ALERT!

capmatinib ⬡
kap-MA-ti-nib

Tabrecta

Therapeutic class: Antineoplastics
Pharmacologic class: Kinase inhibitors

AVAILABLE FORMS
Tablets ⬤: 150 mg, 200 mg

INDICATIONS & DOSAGES
▶ **Metastatic NSCLC in patients whose tumors have a mutation that leads to mesenchymal-epithelial transition exon 14 skipping** ⬡

Adults: 400 mg PO b.i.d.

Adjust-a-dose: If adverse reactions occur, lower dosage to 300 mg PO b.i.d. for first dosage reduction and to 200 mg PO b.i.d. for second dosage reduction. Permanently discontinue drug in patients unable to tolerate 200 mg PO b.i.d. See manufacturer's instructions for specific dosage reductions due to severity of adverse reactions.

carboprost tromethamine
KAR-boe-prost

Hemabate

Therapeutic class: Oxytocics
Pharmacologic class: Prostaglandins

AVAILABLE FORMS
Injection: 250 mcg/mL

INDICATIONS & DOSAGES
Boxed Warning Strictly adhere to recommended dosages and only use in a hospital that can provide immediate intensive and acute surgical care. ■

▶ **Termination of pregnancy between weeks 13 and 20 of gestation**

Adults: Initially, 250 mcg deep IM; optionally, may give a 100-mcg IM test dose. Give subsequent doses of 250 mcg at intervals of 1.5 to 3.5 hours, depending on uterine response. Dosage may be increased in increments to 500 mcg if contractility is inadequate after several 250-mcg doses. Total dose shouldn't exceed 12 mg or continuous administration for more than 2 days.

▶ **Refractory postpartum hemorrhage**

Adults: 250 mcg by deep IM injection. Repeat doses every 15 to 90 minutes as needed. Maximum total dose is 2 mg (eight doses).

SAFETY ALERT!

carfilzomib
car-FIL-zoe-mib

Kyprolis

Therapeutic class: Antineoplastics
Pharmacologic class: Proteasome inhibitors

AVAILABLE FORMS
Powder for injection: 10 mg, 30 mg, 60 mg in single-use vials

INDICATIONS & DOSAGES
⊕ *Alert:* See manufacturer's instructions for administration precautions. ■

▶ **Relapsed or refractory multiple myeloma**

Adults: Calculate dosage using patient's actual BSA at baseline. In patients with BSA greater than 2.2 m², calculate dosage based on BSA of 2.2 m². For monotherapy, 20 mg/m^2 IV over 10 minutes on 2 consecutive days each week for 3 weeks (days 1, 2, 8, 9, 15, and 16), followed by 12-day rest period (days 17 to 28). If tolerated, may increase to 27 mg/m^2 in cycle 1 days 8, 9, 15, and 16 and to 27 mg/m^2 for subsequent cycles. From cycle 13 on, omit day 8 and 9 doses.

Or, 20 mg/m^2 IV over 30 minutes on 2 consecutive days each week for 3 weeks (days 1, 2, 8, 9, 15, and 16), followed by 12-day rest period (days 17 to 28). If tolerated, may increase to 56 mg/m^2 in cycle 1 days 8, 9, 15, and 16 and to 56 mg/m^2 for subsequent cycles. From cycle 13 on, omit day 8 and 9 doses. Treatment may continue until disease progresses or unacceptable toxicity occurs.

For combination regimens, refer to manufacturer's instructions.

Adjust-a-dose: Refer to manufacturer's instructions for dosage adjustments based on toxicities.

carisoprodol
kar-eye-soe-PROE-dol

Soma

Therapeutic class: Skeletal muscle relaxants
Pharmacologic class: Carbamate derivatives
Controlled substance schedule: IV

AVAILABLE FORMS
Tablets: 250 mg, 350 mg

INDICATIONS & DOSAGES
➤ **Relief of discomfort associated with acute, painful musculoskeletal conditions**
Adults: 250 to 350 mg PO t.i.d. and at bedtime for a maximum of 2 to 3 weeks.

cefiderocol
sef-i-DER-oh-kol

Fetroja

Therapeutic class: Antibiotics
Pharmacologic class: Cephalosporins

AVAILABLE FORMS
Injection: 1-g vials

INDICATIONS & DOSAGES
Adjust-a-dose (for all indications): If CrCl is 120 mL/minute or greater, give 2-g IV infusion every 6 hours; if CrCl is 30 to 59 mL/minute, give 1.5-g IV infusion every 8 hours; if CrCl is 15 to 29 mL/minute, give 1-g IV infusion every 8 hours; if CrCl is less than 15 mL/minute, give 0.75-g IV infusion every 12 hours. Refer to manufacturer's instructions for patients receiving CKRT.
➤ **Complicated UTI caused by *Escherichia coli*, *Klebsiella pneumoniae*, *Proteus mirabilis*, *Pseudomonas aeruginosa*, or *Enterobacter cloacae* complex in patients with limited or no other treatment options**
Adults: 2-g IV infusion every 8 hours given over 3 hours for 7 to 14 days.

➤ **Hospital-acquired bacterial pneumonia and ventilator-associated bacterial pneumonia caused by *Acinetobacter baumannii* complex, *E. coli*, *E. cloacae* complex, *K. pneumoniae*, *P. aeruginosa*, and *Serratia marcescens***
Adults: 2-g IV infusion every 8 hours given over 3 hours for 7 to 14 days.

cefOXitin sodium
se-FOKS-i-tin

Therapeutic class: Antibiotics
Pharmacologic class: Second-generation cephalosporins

AVAILABLE FORMS
Infusion: 1 g, 2 g

INDICATIONS & DOSAGES
Adjust-a-dose (for all indications): For adults with KF, give loading dose of 1 to 2 g. For adults with CrCl of 30 to 50 mL/minute, give 1 to 2 g every 8 to 12 hours; if CrCl is 10 to 29 mL/minute, 1 to 2 g every 12 to 24 hours; if CrCl is 5 to 9 mL/minute, 0.5 to 1 g every 12 to 24 hours; and if CrCl is less than 5 mL/minute, 0.5 to 1 g every 24 to 48 hours. For patients receiving hemodialysis, give loading dose of 1 to 2 g after each hemodialysis session; then give maintenance dose based on creatinine level. For patients receiving continuous ambulatory peritoneal dialysis, give 1 g every 24 hours.
➤ **Serious infection of respiratory or GU tract; gynecologic, skin, soft-tissue, bone, or joint infection; bloodstream or intra-abdominal infection caused by susceptible organisms (such as *Escherichia coli* and other coliform bacteria, penicillinase- and non-penicillinase-producing *Staphylococcus aureus*, *Staphylococcus epidermidis*, streptococci, *Klebsiella*, *Haemophilus influenzae*, *Neisseria gonorrhoeae*, *Clostridium* species, *Peptococcus niger*, *Peptostreptococcus* species, and *Bacteroides*, including *B. fragilis***
Adults: 1 to 2 g IV every 6 to 8 hours for uncomplicated infections. May use up to 12 g daily in four to six equally divided doses for life-threatening infections.
Children older than age 3 months: 80 to 160 mg/kg daily IV in four to six equally divided doses. Maximum, 12 g daily.
➤ **Perioperative prophylaxis in patients undergoing uncontaminated GI surgery, vaginal or abdominal hysterectomy, or cesarean birth**
Adults: 2 g IV 30 to 60 minutes before initial surgical incision; then 2 g IV every 6 hours for up to 24 hours. For patients undergoing cesarean birth, 2 g IV as soon as umbilical cord is clamped; may give additional 2-g doses 4 and 8 hours after initial dose.
Children ages 3 months and older: 30 to 40 mg/kg IV 30 to 60 minutes before initial surgical incision; then 30 to 40 mg/kg every 6 hours for up to 24 hours.

ceftaroline fosamil
sef-TAR-oh-leen

Teflaro

Therapeutic class: Antibiotics
Pharmacologic class: Fifth-generation cephalosporins

AVAILABLE FORMS
Injection: 400 mg, 600 mg in single-use vials

INDICATIONS & DOSAGES
➤ **Acute bacterial skin and skin-structure infections (ABSSSI) caused by susceptible isolates of *Staphylococcus aureus*, *Streptococcus pyogenes*, *Streptococcus agalactiae*, *Escherichia coli*, *Klebsiella pneumoniae*, or *Klebsiella oxytoca*; community-acquired bacterial pneumonia (CABP) caused by susceptible isolates of *Streptococcus pneumoniae*, *S. aureus*, *Haemophilus influenzae*, *K. pneumoniae*, *K. oxytoca*, or *E. coli***
Adults: 600 mg IV over 5 to 60 minutes every 12 hours. For ABSSSI, continue treatment for 5 to 14 days; for CABP, continue treatment for 5 to 7 days.
Children older than age 2 and younger than 18 weighing more than 33 kg: 400 mg IV every 8 hours or 600 mg IV every 12 hours for 5 to 14 days.
Children older than age 2 and younger than 18 weighing 33 kg or less: 12 mg/kg IV every 8 hours for 5 to 14 days.
Children age 2 months to younger than 2 years: 8 mg/kg IV every 8 hours for 5 to 14 days.
Adjust-a-dose: For adults with CrCl of 31 to 50 mL/minute, give 400 mg IV every 12 hours; CrCl of 15 to 30 mL/minute, 300 mg IV every 12 hours; CrCl less than 15 L/minute, including those on hemodialysis, 200 mg IV every 12 hours (administer after dialysis treatment).

➤ **ABSSSI caused by susceptible isolates**
Infants with gestational age of at least 34 weeks and postnatal age of at least 12 days to less than 2 months: 6 mg/kg IV infusion over 30 to 60 minutes every 8 hours for 5 to 14 days.

cenobamate
sen-oh-BAM-ate

Xcopri

Therapeutic class: Anticonvulsants
Pharmacologic class: Anticonvulsants
Controlled substance schedule: V

AVAILABLE FORMS
Tablets ⓒⓃⓒ: 12.5 mg, 25 mg, 50 mg, 100 mg, 150 mg, 200 mg

INDICATIONS & DOSAGES
➤ **Partial-onset seizures**
Adults: Initially, 12.5 mg PO once daily on weeks 1 and 2; then 25 mg once daily weeks 3 and 4; 50 mg once daily weeks 5 and 6; 100 mg once daily weeks 7 and 8; and 150 mg once daily weeks 9 and 10. Maintenance dose of 200 mg once daily at week 11. If

necessary, may increase dosage above 200 mg by increments of 50 mg once daily every 2 weeks to maximum of 400 mg.
Adjust-a-dose: In patients with Child-Pugh class A or B liver impairment, maximum dosage is 200 mg once daily. Consider dosage reduction in patients with CrCl less than 90 mL/minute. If phenytoin is used concomitantly, gradually decrease phenytoin dosage by up to 50% as cenobamate is being increased. Avoid abrupt withdrawal; gradually reduce dosage over at least 2 weeks if discontinuing drug.

cetrorelix acetate
set-roe-REL-iks

Cetrotide

Therapeutic class: Infertility drugs
Pharmacologic class: Gonadotropin-releasing hormone antagonists

AVAILABLE FORMS
Powder for injection: 0.25 mg

INDICATIONS & DOSAGES
➤ **Inhibition of premature LH surges in patients undergoing controlled ovarian stimulation**
Adults: Start ovarian stimulation therapy with gonadotropins on cycle day 2 or 3. Give cetrorelix acetate 0.25 mg subcut on stimulation day 5 (morning or evening) or day 6 (morning), and continue once daily until day of hCG administration.

cevimeline hydrochloride
seh-vih-MEH-leen

Evoxac

Therapeutic class: Cholinergic agonists
Pharmacologic class: Cholinergic agonists

AVAILABLE FORMS
Capsules: 30 mg

INDICATIONS & DOSAGES
➤ **Dry mouth in patients with Sjögren syndrome**
Adults: 30 mg PO t.i.d.

SAFETY ALERT!

chlorambucil
klor-AM-byoo-sill

Leukeran

Therapeutic class: Antineoplastics
Pharmacologic class: Nitrogen mustards

AVAILABLE FORMS
Tablets: 2 mg

INDICATIONS & DOSAGES
Boxed Warning Drug can severely suppress bone marrow function, is a carcinogen, is probably mutagenic and teratogenic, and produces human infertility. ■
➤ **Palliation of chronic lymphocytic leukemia; malignant lymphomas, including lymphosarcoma, giant follicular lymphoma, and Hodgkin lymphoma**

Adults: For initiation of therapy or short courses of treatment, 0.1 to 0.2 mg/kg PO daily for 3 to 6 weeks (usually 4 to 10 mg daily). Adjust dosage according to patient response; reduce when WBC count falls abruptly. Or, for intermittent dosing schedule, initial single dose of 0.4 mg/kg; then doses at biweekly or monthly intervals, increasing by 0.1-mg/kg increments until lymphocytosis is controlled or toxicity occurs. Maintenance dosage, if used, shouldn't exceed 0.1 mg/kg/day and may be as low as 0.03 mg/kg/day.

Adjust-a-dose: Reduce first dose if given within 4 weeks after full course of radiation therapy or myelosuppressive drugs or if pretreatment WBC or platelet count is depressed from bone marrow disease.

chloramphenicol sodium succinate
klor-am-FEN-i-kole

Therapeutic class: Antibiotics
Pharmacologic class: Dichloroacetic acid derivatives

AVAILABLE FORMS
Injection: 1-g vials

INDICATIONS & DOSAGES
Boxed Warning Drug is associated with serious and fatal blood dyscrasias. Use alternative therapies when possible. Patient should be hospitalized during therapy to closely monitor blood lab levels. ■
➤ *Haemophilus influenzae* **meningitis, acute** *Salmonella typhi* **infection, and meningitis, bacteremia, or other severe infections caused by sensitive** *Salmonella* **species, rickettsia, lymphogranuloma, psittacosis, or various sensitive gram-negative organisms**
Adults: 50 mg/kg IV daily, divided every 6 hours. May increase dosage up to 100 mg/kg daily, if needed.
Full-term infants older than age 2 weeks with normal metabolic processes and children: Up to 50 mg/kg IV daily, divided every 6 hours. May use up to 100 mg/kg/day in four divided doses for bacteremia or meningitis; reduce to 50 mg/kg/day as soon as possible.
Neonates ages 2 weeks and younger: 25 mg/kg IV daily divided every 6 hours.
Preterm infants, and children and infants with suspected immature metabolic processes: 25 mg/kg IV once daily.

Adjust-a-dose: For patients with kidney or liver impairment, excessive blood levels may result from administration of the recommended dosage. Determine drug blood concentration at appropriate intervals and adjust dosage accordingly.

SAFETY ALERT!

chlordiazePOXIDE hydrochloride
klor-dye-az-e-POX-ide

Therapeutic class: Anxiolytics
Pharmacologic class: Benzodiazepines
Controlled substance schedule: IV

AVAILABLE FORMS
Capsules: 5 mg, 10 mg, 25 mg

INDICATIONS & DOSAGES
Boxed Warning Benzodiazepine use exposes patient to risks of abuse, misuse, and addiction, which can lead to overdose or death. Benzodiazepine use with opioids can cause sedation and fatal respiratory depression. ■
Boxed Warning Abrupt discontinuation or rapid dosage reduction of benzodiazepines after continued use may precipitate acute and life-threatening withdrawal reactions. To reduce risk, gradually taper drug to discontinue or reduce dosage. ■
Adjust-a-dose (for all indications): In older adults and patients who are debilitated, give 5 mg PO b.i.d. to q.i.d. Use smallest effective dosage to prevent oversedation or ataxia.
➤ **Mild to moderate anxiety**
Adults: 5 to 10 mg PO t.i.d. or q.i.d.
Children older than age 6: 5 mg PO b.i.d. to q.i.d. Maximum, 10 mg PO b.i.d. or t.i.d.
➤ **Severe anxiety**
Adults: 20 to 25 mg PO t.i.d. or q.i.d.
➤ **Withdrawal symptoms of acute alcoholism**
Adults: 50 to 100 mg PO. Repeat as needed, up to 300 mg daily.
➤ **Preoperative apprehension and anxiety**
Adults: 5 to 10 mg PO t.i.d. or q.i.d. on days before surgery.

chlorproMAZINE hydrochloride
klor-PROE-ma-zeen

Therapeutic class: Antipsychotics
Pharmacologic class: Phenothiazines

AVAILABLE FORMS
Injection: 25 mg/mL
Oral solution: 30 mg/mL, 100 mg/mL
Tablets: 10 mg, 25 mg, 50 mg, 100 mg, 200 mg

INDICATIONS & DOSAGES
Boxed Warning Older adults with dementia-related psychosis treated with antipsychotics are at increased risk for death. Drug isn't approved to treat these patients. ■
➤ **Acute schizophrenia, mania**
Adults and children older than age 12: For patients with acute disease who are hospitalized, 25 mg IM; may give additional 25 to 50 mg IM in 1 hour if needed. Increase over several days to 400 mg every 4 to 6 hours for severe cases. Switch to oral therapy as soon as possible. Or, 25 mg PO t.i.d. initially; then gradually increase to effective dose (usually 500 mg, or 400 mg in patients less acutely disturbed) daily in divided doses. For outpatients, 30 to 75 mg daily in two to four divided doses. Increase dosage by 20 to 50 mg twice weekly until symptoms are controlled. Gradually reduce dosage to lowest effective maintenance dosage after symptoms have been controlled for a reasonable period.

➤ **Nausea and vomiting**

Adults and children older than age 12: 10 to 25 mg PO every 4 to 6 hours PRN. Or, 25 mg IM initially. If no hypotension occurs, may give 25 to 50 mg IM every 3 to 4 hours PRN until vomiting stops. Or, during surgery, 12.5 mg IM, repeated in 30 minutes if needed, or fractional 2-mg doses IV at 2-minute intervals to maximum dose of 25 mg.

Children ages 6 months to 12 years: 0.55 mg/kg PO every 4 to 6 hours or IM every 6 to 8 hours PRN. Maximum IM dose in children younger than age 5 or weighing less than 23 kg is 40 mg. Maximum IM dose in children ages 5 to 12 or weighing 23 to 45 kg is 75 mg.

➤ **Acute intermittent porphyria, intractable hiccups**

Adults and children older than age 12: 25 to 50 mg PO t.i.d. or q.i.d. If hiccups persist for 2 to 3 days on oral therapy, give 25 to 50 mg IM. If hiccups persist, give 25 to 50 mg diluted in 500 to 1,000 mL of NSS and infused slowly with patient in supine position. For porphyria, give 25 mg IM t.i.d. or q.i.d. until patient can take oral therapy.

➤ **Tetanus**

Adults and children older than age 12: 25 to 50 mg IV or IM t.i.d. or q.i.d.

Children ages 6 months to 12 years: 0.55 mg/kg IM or IV every 6 to 8 hours. Maximum parenteral dosage in children weighing less than 23 kg is 40 mg daily; for children weighing 23 to 45 kg, may give 75 mg, except in severe cases. If giving IV, dilute to 1 mg/mL with NSS and give at a rate of 0.5 mg/minute.

➤ **Behavioral disorders, hyperactivity**

Children ages 6 months to 12 years: For outpatients, 0.55 mg/kg PO every 4 to 6 hours or IM every 6 to 8 hours as needed. For patients who are hospitalized, start with low oral doses and increase gradually. In severe behavioral disorders, 50 to 100 mg PO daily or, in older children, 200 mg/day or more PO may be necessary. Dosages beyond 500 mg/day haven't been shown to improve behavior in those with intellectual disability or severe emotional disturbance. In patients ages 5 and younger or weighing less than 23 kg who are hospitalized, don't exceed 40 mg/day IM. In children ages 5 to 12 weighing 23 to 45 kg, don't exceed 75 mg/day IM, except in unmanageable cases.

➤ **Preoperative sedation, anxiety**

Adults and children older than age 12: Preoperatively, 25 to 50 mg PO 2 to 3 hours before surgery or 12.5 to 25 mg IM 1 to 2 hours before surgery.

Children ages 6 months to 12 years: Preoperatively, 0.55 mg/kg PO 2 to 3 hours before surgery or IM 1 to 2 hours before surgery.

Older adults: Lower dosages are sufficient; dosage increments should be more gradual than in younger adults.

chlorthalidone
klor-THAL-i-done

Thalitone

Therapeutic class: Antihypertensives
Pharmacologic class: Thiazide diuretics

AVAILABLE FORMS
Tablets: 15 mg, 25 mg, 50 mg

INDICATIONS & DOSAGES
➤ **Edema**
Adults: 50 to 100 mg PO daily or 100 mg PO on alternating days (maximum, 200 mg/day).
➤ **HTN**
Adults: 15 to 25 mg PO daily.

cholestyramine
koe-LESS-tir-a-meen

Prevalite

Therapeutic class: Antilipemics
Pharmacologic class: Bile acid sequestrants

AVAILABLE FORMS
Powder for oral suspension: 4-g single-dose packets; multidose cans with each level scoop equivalent to 4 g of cholestyramine resin

INDICATIONS & DOSAGES
➤ **Primary hyperlipidemia; adjunct for reduction of increased cholesterol level in patients with primary hypercholesterolemia; pruritus caused by partial bile obstruction**
Adults: 4 g PO once daily or b.i.d. Maintenance dosage, 8 to 16 g daily in two divided doses. Maximum, 24 g daily.
Children: 240 mg/kg/day PO in two to three divided doses, not to exceed 8 g/day.

SAFETY ALERT!

cidofovir
sye-DOE-fo-veer

Therapeutic class: Antivirals
Pharmacologic class: Nucleosides-nucleotides

AVAILABLE FORMS
Injection: 75 mg/mL ■

INDICATIONS & DOSAGES
Boxed Warning Cidofovir is indicated only for the treatment of CMV retinitis in patients with AIDS. Neutropenia may occur; monitor neutrophil counts. Kidney toxicity may occur. Prehydrate with NSS and give probenecid with each cidofovir infusion. Monitor kidney function. ■
➤ **CMV retinitis in patients with AIDS**
Adults: Initially, 5 mg/kg IV infused over 1 hour once weekly for 2 consecutive weeks; then maintenance dosage of 5 mg/kg IV infused over 1 hour once every 2 weeks.

Adjust-a-dose: For patients with creatinine level of 0.3 to 0.4 mg/dL above baseline, reduce dosage to 3 mg/kg at same rate and frequency. If creatinine level reaches 0.5 mg/dL or more above baseline or patient develops 3+ or higher proteinuria, stop drug.

Don't start drug if serum creatinine level is more than 1.5 mg/dL, CrCl is 55 mL/minute or less, or urine protein level is 100 mg/dL or more (at least 2+ proteinuria).

ciprofloxacin hydrochloride (otic)
si-proe-FLOX-a-sin

Cetraxal

Therapeutic class: Antibiotics
Pharmacologic class: Fluoroquinolones

AVAILABLE FORMS
Otic solution: 0.2% (5 mg in 0.25-mL single-use container)

INDICATIONS & DOSAGES
➤ **Acute otitis externa caused by susceptible isolates of *Pseudomonas aeruginosa* or *Staphylococcus aureus***
Adults and children ages 1 and older: 0.5 mg (0.25 mL) of 0.2% solution (contents of one single-dose container) instilled into affected ear b.i.d. for 7 days.

SAFETY ALERT!

cisatracurium besylate
sis-ah-trah-KYOO-ree-hum

Nimbex

Therapeutic class: Skeletal muscle relaxants
Pharmacologic class: Nondepolarizing neuromuscular blockers

AVAILABLE FORMS
Injection: 2 mg/mL, 10 mg/mL*

INDICATIONS & DOSAGES
Adjust-a-dose (for all indications): In patients with neuromuscular disease, such as myasthenia gravis or carcinomatosis, don't exceed 0.02 mg/kg. Patients with burns may need a higher dose.
➤ **Adjunct to general anesthesia to facilitate ET intubation and relax skeletal muscles during surgery**
Adults: First dose of 0.15 to 0.2 mg/kg IV; then maintenance dose of 0.03 mg/kg IV 40 to 50 minutes after initial 0.15 mg/kg dose or 50 to 60 minutes after 0.2 mg/kg dose PRN. Adjust maintenance dose based on clinical criteria, including response to peripheral nerve stimulation.

Or, as a continuous infusion in an operating room (OR), after initial bolus dose, give maintenance infusion at 3 mcg/kg/minute and reduce to 1 to 2 mcg/kg/minute as needed. Initiate infusion only after early evidence of spontaneous recovery from initial bolus dose.
Children ages 2 to 12: 0.1 to 0.15 mg/kg IV over 5 to 10 seconds. After first dose, give maintenance infusion

of 3 mcg/kg/minute and reduce to 1 to 2 mcg/kg/minute as needed.
Children ages 1 to 23 months: 0.15 mg/kg over 5 to 10 seconds. No information is available for continuous infusion.
Adjust-a-dose: During CABG surgery (adults) with induced hypothermia, reduce infusion rate by 50%.
➤ **To maintain neuromuscular blockade during mechanical ventilation in ICU**
Adults: Principles for infusion in OR apply to use in ICU. After first dose, give 3 mcg/kg/minute by IV infusion. Range, 0.5 to 10.2 mcg/kg/minute.

SAFETY ALERT!

cladribine
KLA-dri-been

Mavenclad

Therapeutic class: Immunomodulators
Pharmacologic class: Purine antimetabolites

AVAILABLE FORMS
Injection: 10 mg (1 mg/mL) single-use vial
Tablets ⓓⓝⓒ: 10 mg

INDICATIONS & DOSAGES
Boxed Warning Drug can cause fetal harm; use is contraindicated in adults of reproductive potential who don't plan to use effective contraception. ■
Boxed Warning Drug can increase risk of malignancy; use is contraindicated in patients with current malignancy. ■
➤ **Relapsing forms of MS, including relapsing-remitting disease and active secondary progressive disease, in patients who have had inadequate response to or are unable to tolerate other MS therapies**
Adults weighing 40 kg or more: 3.5 mg/kg PO over 2 years, administered as 1.75 mg/kg each year. Divide the 1.75-mg/kg dose over two cycles, each lasting 4 to 5 consecutive days. Don't administer more than 2 tablets (20 mg) daily. For first year of treatment, start first cycle at any time. Administer second cycle 23 to 27 days after last dose of first cycle. For second year of treatment, start first cycle at least 43 weeks after last dose of first year's second cycle. Administer second cycle 23 to 27 days after last dose of second year's first cycle. Following 2 years of treatment, don't administer additional doses of drug during the next 2 years.
Adjust-a-dose: Lymphocytes must be within normal limits before start of treatment. Lymphocyte count must be at least 800 cells/mm^3 before start of second treatment course. If needed, delay second treatment course for up to 6 months to allow lymphocyte recovery to at least 800 cells/mm^3. If this recovery takes more than 6 months, discontinue treatment.
➤ **Hairy cell leukemia**
Adults: 0.09 mg/kg/day continuous infusion for 7 consecutive days.

cloBAZam ⌧

KLOE-ba-zam

Onfi, Sympazan

Therapeutic class: Anticonvulsants
Pharmacologic class: Benzodiazepines
Controlled substance schedule: IV

AVAILABLE FORMS

Oral film: 5 mg, 10 mg, 20 mg
Oral suspension: 2.5 mg/mL
Tablets: 10 mg, 20 mg

INDICATIONS & DOSAGES

Boxed Warning Benzodiazepine use exposes patient to risks of abuse, misuse, and addiction, which can lead to overdose or death. Benzodiazepine use with opioids can cause sedation and fatal respiratory depression. ∎
Boxed Warning Abrupt discontinuation or rapid dosage reduction of benzodiazepines after continued use may precipitate acute and life-threatening withdrawal reactions. To reduce risk, gradually taper drug to discontinue or reduce dosage. ∎

➤ **Adjunctive treatment of seizures associated with Lennox-Gastaut syndrome**

Adults and children ages 2 and older weighing more than 30 kg: Initially, 5 mg PO b.i.d. for 6 days. On day 7, increase to 10 mg PO b.i.d.; on day 14, titrate to 20 mg PO b.i.d. as tolerated. Dosage escalation shouldn't proceed more rapidly than weekly. Maximum, 40 mg/day.

Adults and children ages 2 and older weighing 30 kg or less: Initially, 5 mg PO once daily for 6 days. On day 7, increase to 5 mg PO b.i.d.; on day 14, titrate to 10 mg PO b.i.d. as tolerated. Dosage escalation shouldn't proceed more rapidly than weekly. Maximum, 20 mg/day.

⌧ *Adjust-a-dose:* For older adults, patients with Child-Pugh class A or B liver impairment, and those who are poor CYP2C19 metabolizers, initially 5 mg PO daily for 1 week; then titrate according to weight but at half the recommended dose, as tolerated. If necessary, may start additional titration to maximum dosage (20 or 40 mg/day depending on weight) on day 21. To discontinue, taper by decreasing dose by 5 to 10 mg/day weekly.

clomiPHENE citrate

KLOE-mi-feen

Clomid

Therapeutic class: Ovulation stimulants
Pharmacologic class: Chlorotrianisene derivatives

AVAILABLE FORMS

Tablets: 50 mg

INDICATIONS & DOSAGES

➤ **Ovulatory dysfunction**

Adults: 50 mg PO daily for 5 days, starting on day 5 of menstrual cycle (first day of menstrual flow is day 1)

if bleeding occurs or at any time if patient hasn't had recent uterine bleeding. If ovulation doesn't occur, may increase dosage to 100 mg PO daily for 5 days as soon as 30 days after first course. Repeat until conception occurs or until three ovulatory responses occur. Therapy beyond six cycles isn't recommended.

clomiPRAMINE hydrochloride

kloe-MI-pra-meen

Anafranil

Therapeutic class: Antidepressants
Pharmacologic class: TCAs

AVAILABLE FORMS

Capsules: 25 mg, 50 mg, 75 mg

INDICATIONS & DOSAGES

Boxed Warning Drug increases risk of suicidality in children, adolescents, and young adults. ∎
➤ **OCD**

Adults: Initially, 25 mg PO daily with meals, gradually increased to 100 mg/day in divided doses during first 2 weeks. Thereafter, increase every 2 to 3 weeks to maximum of 250 mg/day in divided doses, as needed. After titration, may give total daily dose at bedtime.

Children ages 10 and older and adolescents: Initially, 25 mg PO daily with meals, gradually increased over first 2 weeks to maximum of 3 mg/kg daily or 100 mg PO daily in divided doses, whichever is smaller. Maximum, 3 mg/kg or 200 mg daily, whichever is smaller; give at bedtime after titration.

Adjust-a-dose: Periodically reassess and adjust dosage to maintain patient on lowest effective dosage.

SAFETY ALERT!

cobimetinib fumarate ⌧

koe-bi-ME-ti-nib

Cotellic

Therapeutic class: Antineoplastics
Pharmacologic class: Kinase inhibitors

AVAILABLE FORMS

Tablets ⓝ*:* 20 mg

INDICATIONS & DOSAGES

➤ **Unresectable or metastatic melanoma with a *BRAF* V600E or V600K mutation in combination with vemurafenib; monotherapy for histiocytic neoplasm** ⌧

Adults: 60 mg PO once daily for first 21 days of each 28-day treatment cycle until disease progresses or unacceptable toxicity occurs.

Adjust-a-dose: Refer to manufacturer's instructions for toxicity-related dosage adjustments. If concurrent short-term (14 days or less) use of a moderate CYP3A inhibitor can't be avoided in patients taking cobimetinib 60 mg, decrease cobimetinib dosage to 20 mg daily. Resume previous dosage after inhibitor is discontinued. Use alternative to the CYP3A inhibitor in patients taking less than 60 mg.

---

colesevelam hydrochloride ⚕
koe-leh-SEVE-eh-lam

Welchol

Therapeutic class: Antilipemics
Pharmacologic class: Bile acid sequestrants

AVAILABLE FORMS
Powder for oral suspension: 3.75-g packets
Tablets: 625 mg

INDICATIONS & DOSAGES
➤ **Adjunct to diet and exercise to reduce elevated LDL-C in patients with primary hyperlipidemia; to reduce LDL-C in children who are postmenarchal with heterozygous familial hypercholesterolemia and unable to reach LDL-C target levels despite adequate trial of diet and lifestyle modification** ⚕
Adults and children ages 10 to 17: 3 tablets (1,875 mg) PO b.i.d. or 6 tablets (3,750 mg) PO once daily. Or, one 3.75-g packet PO once daily.
➤ **Adjunct to diet and exercise to improve glycemic control in patients with type 2 diabetes**
Adults: 3 tablets (1,875 mg) PO b.i.d. or 6 tablets (3,750 mg) PO once daily. Or, one 3.75-g packet PO once daily.

collagenase *Clostridium histolyticum*
kuh-LAJ-eh-nase klos-TRID-ee-um hiss-toe-LIH-teh-kum

Xiaflex

collagenase *Clostridium histolyticum*-aaes

QWO

Therapeutic class: Anticollagen drugs
Pharmacologic class: Enzymes

AVAILABLE FORMS
Powder for injection: 0.9 mg, 1.84 mg single-use vials

INDICATIONS & DOSAGES
Boxed Warning Xiaflex is associated with penile fracture and other related penile injuries, which may require surgery. ∎
➤ **Dupuytren contracture with palpable cord (Xiaflex)**
Adults: 0.58 mg injected into palpable cord with contracture of metacarpophalangeal joint or proximal interphalangeal joint. May repeat up to three times per cord at 4-week intervals. Two joints in same hand may be treated at same treatment visit.
➤ **Peyronie disease with palpable plaque and curvature deformity of at least 30 degrees at start of therapy (Xiaflex)**
Adult males: Initially, 0.58 mg injected into target plaque once; then repeat injection 1 to 3 days later. May repeat up to four treatment cycles of two injections at approximately 6-week intervals. Discontinue treatment if curvature deformity is less than 15 degrees after any cycle.

➤ **Moderate to severe cellulite in the buttocks (QWO)**
Adult females: 0.84 mg subcut per treatment area; may repeat every 21 days for a total of three treatment visits. Maximum, 12 injections (3.6 mL) in a single buttock.

conivaptan hydrochloride
kah-nih-VAP-tan

Vaprisol

Therapeutic class: Vasopressin antagonists
Pharmacologic class: Arginine vasopressin receptor antagonists

AVAILABLE FORMS
Injection (premixed): 20 mg/100 mL D₅W

INDICATIONS & DOSAGES
➤ **Euvolemic hyponatremia (such as from SIADH, hypothyroidism, adrenal insufficiency, pulmonary disorders) and hypervolemic hyponatremia in patients who are hospitalized**
Adults: Loading dose of 20 mg IV over 30 minutes followed by continuous infusion of 20 mg IV over 24 hours for 2 to 4 days. If sodium level isn't rising at desired rate, increase to maximum of 40 mg over 24 hours by continuous infusion. Total duration of infusion shouldn't exceed 4 days.
Adjust-a-dose: If sodium level rises more than 12 mEq/L in 24 hours, stop infusion. If hyponatremia persists or recurs and patient has had no adverse neurologic effects from the rapid rise in sodium level, restart infusion at reduced dose. If patient develops hypotension or hypovolemia, stop infusion. Monitor vital signs and volume status often. If hyponatremia persists once patient is no longer hypotensive and volume returns to normal, restart infusion at reduced dose. In patients with Child-Pugh class B or C liver impairment, give loading dose of 10 mg over 30 minutes followed by continuous infusion of 10 mg over 24 hours for 2 to 4 days. If serum sodium level isn't rising at desired rate, may titrate dosage upward to 20 mg over 24 hours. Don't use if CrCl is less than 30 mL/minute.

SAFETY ALERT!

copanlisib dihydrochloride
ko-PAN-li-sib

Aliqopa

Therapeutic class: Antineoplastics
Pharmacologic class: Kinase inhibitors

AVAILABLE FORMS
Injection (lyophilized, preservative-free): 60-mg single-dose vials

INDICATIONS & DOSAGES
➤ **Relapsed follicular lymphoma in patients who have received at least two prior systemic therapies**
Adults: 60 mg IV infusion over 1 hour on days 1, 8, and 15 of a 28-day treatment cycle on an intermittent

schedule (3 weeks on and 1 week off). Continue until disease progresses or unacceptable toxicity occurs.
Adjust-a-dose: Reduce dosage to 45 mg in patients with Child-Pugh class B liver impairment or to 30 mg in patients with Child-Pugh class C liver impairment. If concomitant use of a strong CYP3A inhibitor is unavoidable, reduce copanlisib dosage to 45 mg. Refer to manufacturer's instructions for toxicity-related dosage adjustments and drug discontinuation.

crizanlizumab-tmca
kriz-an-LIZ-ue-mab

Adakveo

Therapeutic class: Immunomodulators
Pharmacologic class: Monoclonal antibodies

AVAILABLE FORMS
Injection: 100 mg/10 mL single-dose vials

INDICATIONS & DOSAGES
▶ **To reduce frequency of vaso-occlusive crises in patients with sickle cell disease**
Adults and children ages 16 and older: 5 mg/kg IV infusion over 30 minutes at week 0, week 2, then every 4 weeks thereafter. Give with or without hydroxyurea.

crotamiton
kroe-TAM-ih-tuhn

Crotan

Therapeutic class: Scabicides-pediculicides
Pharmacologic class: Scabicides

AVAILABLE FORMS
Lotion: 10%

INDICATIONS & DOSAGES
▶ **Scabies eradication**
Adults: Wash entire body with soap and water. Then thoroughly massage lotion into skin from chin down to toes (with special attention to skinfolds, creases, interdigital spaces, and genital area). Put lotion under fingernails after trimming nails short. Repeat application in 24 hours. Change clothing and bed linen the next morning. Wait another 48 hours after last application; then wash off.
▶ **Itching**
Adults: Apply locally, massaging gently into affected area until completely absorbed; repeat PRN.

dalbavancin hydrochloride
dal-ba-VAN-sin

Dalvance

Therapeutic class: Antibiotics
Pharmacologic class: Lipoglycopeptides

AVAILABLE FORMS
Injection: 500-mg single-use vial

INDICATIONS & DOSAGES
▶ **Acute bacterial skin and skin-structure infections caused by susceptible strains of gram-positive microorganisms (*Staphylococcus aureus* [including

MRSA], *Streptococcus pyogenes, Streptococcus agalactiae, Streptococcus dysgalactiae, Streptococcus anginosus* group [*S. anginosus, S. intermedius, S. constellatus*], *Enterococcus faecalis* [vancomycin-susceptible strains])**
Adults: 1,500 mg IV infusion as single dose, or 1,000 mg IV infusion followed by second dose of 500 mg IV infusion 1 week later.
Children ages 6 to younger than 18: 18 mg/kg IV infusion as single dose, up to maximum of 1,500 mg.
Children from birth to younger than age 6: 22.5 mg/kg IV infusion as single dose, up to maximum of 1,500 mg.

Adjust-a-dose: For patients with CrCl of less than 30 mL/minute who aren't receiving hemodialysis, give 1,125 mg IV infusion as single dose, or 750 mg IV infusion followed by second dose of 375 mg IV infusion 1 week later. No dosage adjustment is necessary for patients on regularly scheduled hemodialysis; give without regard to hemodialysis timing. Dosage adjustment for children with CrCl less than 30 mL/minute hasn't been established.

dalfampridine
dal-FAM-prih-deen

Ampyra

Therapeutic class: MS drugs
Pharmacologic class: Potassium channel blockers

AVAILABLE FORMS
Tablets (extended-release) **DNC**: 10 mg

INDICATIONS & DOSAGES
▶ **To improve walking in patients with MS**
Adults: 10 mg PO every 12 hours. Maximum, 20 mg daily.

dantrolene sodium
DAN-troe-leen

Dantrium, Dantrium IV, Revonto, Ryanodex

Therapeutic class: Skeletal muscle relaxants
Pharmacologic class: Hydantoin derivatives

AVAILABLE FORMS
Capsules: 25 mg, 50 mg, 100 mg
Injection: 20 mg/vial, 250 mg/vial

INDICATIONS & DOSAGES
Boxed Warning Drug can cause liver toxicity; only use for indicated conditions and at lowest effective dose. Stop drug if benefits aren't evident within 45 days. ▪
▶ **Spasticity and sequelae from severe chronic disorders, such as MS, cerebral palsy, spinal cord injury, and stroke**
Adults and children ages 5 and older weighing 50 kg or more: Initially, 25 mg PO daily; then 25 mg t.i.d., 50 mg t.i.d. and, finally, 100 mg t.i.d. Maintain each dosage level for 7 days to determine response. May increase t.i.d. to q.i.d. if necessary. Maximum, 400 mg daily.

Children ages 5 and older weighing less than 50 kg:
Initially, 0.5 mg/kg PO daily; then 0.5 mg/kg t.i.d.,
1 mg/kg t.i.d. and, finally, 2 mg/kg t.i.d. Maintain each
dosage level for 7 days to determine response. May
increase t.i.d. to q.i.d. if necessary. Maximum,
100 mg q.i.d.

Adjust-a-dose: If no further benefit is observed
at next higher dose, decrease dosage to previous
lower dose.

➤ **To manage malignant hyperthermic crisis**
Adults and children: Initially, 1 mg/kg IV push.
Repeat, as needed, up to cumulative dose of 10 mg/kg.
Or, follow Malignant Hyperthermia Association of the
United States (MHAUS) recommendations.

➤ **To prevent or attenuate malignant hyperthermic crisis in susceptible patients who need surgery**
Adults and children ages 5 and older: 4 to 8 mg/kg
PO daily in three or four divided doses for 1 or
2 days before procedure. Give final dose 3 or 4 hours
before procedure. Or, 2.5 mg/kg IV about 1.25 hours
before anesthesia; infuse Dantrium or Revonto over
1 hour, or Ryanodex over at least 1 minute. Or, follow
MHAUS recommendations.

➤ **To prevent recurrent malignant hyperthermic
crisis**
Adults and children ages 5 and older: 4 to 8 mg/kg
PO daily in four divided doses for up to 3 days after
hyperthermic crisis. Or, follow MHAUS recommendations.

darunavir ethanolate ✂
dar-OO-na-veer

Prezista

Therapeutic class: Antiretrovirals
Pharmacologic class: Protease inhibitors

AVAILABLE FORMS
Oral suspension: 100 mg/mL
Tablets ⓒ: 75 mg, 150 mg, 600 mg, 800 mg

INDICATIONS & DOSAGES
➤ **HIV infection, with ritonavir and other antiretrovirals** ✂
*Adults who are treatment-experienced with at least
one darunavir resistance-associated substitution or
when genotypic testing isn't feasible (testing is recommended):* 600 mg PO b.i.d., given with 100 mg
ritonavir PO b.i.d.

*Adults who are treatment-naive or treatment-
experienced with no darunavir resistance-associated
substitutions:* 800 mg PO once daily, given with
ritonavir 100 mg PO once daily.

Patients who are pregnant: 600 mg PO b.i.d., given
with ritonavir 100 mg PO b.i.d. May consider 800 mg
PO once daily, given with ritonavir 100 mg PO once
daily only in certain patients who are pregnant and are
already on a stable 800-mg dose with ritonavir 100-mg
once-daily regimen before pregnancy, are virologically
suppressed (HIV-1 RNA less than 50 copies/mL), and
in whom a change to twice-daily darunavir 600 mg
with ritonavir 100 mg may compromise tolerability or
adherence.

*Children ages 3 to younger than 18 weighing at
least 10 kg who are treatment-naive or treatment-
experienced with no darunavir resistance-associated
substitutions:* 35 mg/kg PO once daily with ritonavir
7 mg/kg PO once daily. Don't exceed recommended
dosage for adults who are treatment-experienced. Refer
to manufacturer's prescribing information for weight-
based dosage table.

*Children ages 3 to younger than 18 weighing at least
10 kg who are treatment-experienced with at least one
darunavir resistance-associated substitution:* 20 mg/kg
PO b.i.d. with ritonavir 3 mg/kg PO b.i.d. Don't exceed
recommended dosage for adults who are treatment-
experienced. Refer to manufacturer's prescribing information for weight-based dosage table.

SAFETY ALERT!

dasatinib ✂
duh-SAH-ti-nib

Sprycel

Therapeutic class: Antineoplastics
Pharmacologic class: Protein-tyrosine kinase
inhibitors

AVAILABLE FORMS
Tablets ⓒ: 20 mg, 50 mg, 70 mg, 80 mg, 100 mg,
140 mg

INDICATIONS & DOSAGES
Adjust-a-dose (for all indications): Refer to manufacturer's instructions for dosage adjustments when
given with strong CYP3A4 inducers or inhibitors.
➤ **Chronic, accelerated, or myeloid or lymphoid
blast phase Philadelphia chromosome-positive
(Ph+) chronic myeloid leukemia (CML) with resistance or intolerance to earlier treatment, including
imatinib; Ph+ acute lymphoblastic leukemia with
resistance or intolerance to prior therapy** ✂
Adults: 140 mg PO once daily. If patient tolerates this
dose but fails to respond to treatment, increase to
180 mg PO once daily. Continue until disease
progresses or intolerable adverse effects occur.
➤ **Newly diagnosed Ph+ chronic-phase CML;
children with Ph+ CML in chronic phase** ✂
Adults: 100 mg PO daily. May increase to 140 mg
daily.
Children weighing 45 kg or more: 100 mg PO once
daily. May increase to 120 mg daily.
Children weighing 30 to less than 45 kg: 70 mg PO
once daily. May increase to 90 mg daily.
Children weighing 20 to less than 30 kg: 60 mg PO
once daily. May increase to 70 mg daily.
Children weighing 10 to less than 20 kg: 40 mg PO
once daily. May increase to 50 mg daily.
Adjust-a-dose: Recalculate pediatric dose every
3 months, or more often if necessary, based on changes
in body weight. Continue until disease progresses or
intolerable adverse effects occur.
➤ **Newly diagnosed Ph+ acute lymphoblastic
leukemia in combination with chemotherapy** ✂
Children ages 1 and older weighing 45 kg or more:
100 mg PO once daily.

Children ages 1 and older weighing 30 to less than 45 kg: 70 mg PO once daily.
Children ages 1 and older weighing 20 to less than 30 kg: 60 mg PO once daily.
Children ages 1 and older weighing 10 to less than 20 kg: 40 mg PO once daily.
Adjust-a-dose: Recalculate pediatric dose every 3 months, or more often if necessary, based on changes in body weight. Continue treatment for up to 2 years.

SAFETY ALERT!

DAUNOrubicin hydrochloride
daw-nah-ROO-buh-sin

Therapeutic class: Antineoplastics
Pharmacologic class: Anthracycline topoisomerase inhibitors

AVAILABLE FORMS
Injection: 5 mg/mL

INDICATIONS & DOSAGES
Boxed Warning Inject into rapidly flowing IV infusion; never give by IM or subcut route because severe local tissue necrosis may result. Drug may cause severe myelosuppression or myocardial toxicity in the form of potentially fatal HF, during therapy or months to years afterward. Reduce dosage in patients with kidney or liver impairment. Drug should only be used by health care professionals experienced in leukemia chemotherapy. ■

☉ Alert: Maximum adult lifetime cumulative dose is 550 mg/m², in patients who received mediastinal radiation, maximum lifetime cumulative dose is 400 mg/m². Maximum lifetime cumulative dose in children ages 2 and older is 300 mg/m². Maximum lifetime cumulative dose in children younger than 2 is 10 mg/kg.
Adjust-a-dose (for all indications): If bilirubin level is 1.2 to 3 mg/dL, give three-fourths normal dose; if bilirubin or creatinine level exceeds 3 mg/dL, give one-half normal dose. Dosages vary. Check treatment protocol with prescriber.
➤ **To induce remission in acute nonlymphocytic (myelogenous, monocytic, erythroid) leukemia**
Adults ages 60 and older: 30 mg/m²/day IV on days 1, 2, and 3 of first course and on days 1 and 2 of subsequent courses in combination with cytarabine infusions.
Adults younger than age 60: 45 mg/m²/day IV on days 1, 2, and 3 of first course and on days 1 and 2 of subsequent courses in combination with cytarabine infusions.
➤ **To induce remission in acute lymphocytic leukemia (with combination therapy)**
Adults: 45 mg/m²/day IV on days 1, 2, and 3 of first course.
Children ages 2 and older: 25 mg/m² IV on day 1 every week for up to 6 weeks..
Children younger than age 2 or with BSA less than 0.5 m²: 1 mg/kg/dose IV on day 1 every week for up to 6 weeks (dose based on body weight, not BSA). Administration frequency is specific to each combination chemotherapy regimen.

daunorubicin liposome–cytarabine liposome
daw-nah-ROO-buh-sin/sye-TARE-a-been

Vyxeos

Therapeutic class: Antineoplastics
Pharmacologic class: Anthracycline topoisomerase inhibitors–nucleoside metabolic inhibitors

AVAILABLE FORMS
Injection (liposomes as a lyophilized cake): 44 mg daunorubicin/100 mg cytarabine in single-dose vials

INDICATIONS & DOSAGES
Boxed Warning Verify drug name and dosage before preparation and administration to avoid dosing errors. ■
➤ **Newly diagnosed, therapy-related acute myeloid leukemia (t-AML) or AML with myelodysplasia-related changes (AML-MRC)**
Adults and children ages 1 and older: A full course of therapy consists of one to two induction cycles followed by up to two consolidation cycles.

For initial induction cycle, 44 mg/m² daunorubicin and 100 mg/m² cytarabine IV infusion on days 1, 3, and 5. For patients who fail to achieve a response with first induction cycle, give second induction cycle of 44 mg/m² daunorubicin and 100 mg/m² cytarabine IV infusion on days 1 and 3. May give second induction cycle 2 to 5 weeks after first induction cycle if no unacceptable toxicity occurred with previous cycle.

Give first consolidation cycle 5 to 8 weeks after start of the last induction. Recommended dose for each consolidation cycle is 29 mg/m² daunorubicin and 65 mg/m² cytarabine IV infusion on days 1 and 3. Give second consolidation cycle 5 to 8 weeks after start of first consolidation cycle in patients without disease progression or unacceptable toxicity.
Adjust-a-dose: Refer to manufacturer's instructions for toxicity-related dosage adjustments.

defibrotide sodium
dee-FIB-roe-tide

Defitelio

Therapeutic class: Thromblytics
Pharmacologic class: Thromblytics

AVAILABLE FORMS
Injection: 200 mg/2.5 mL (80 mg/mL)

INDICATIONS & DOSAGES
➤ **Hepatic veno-occlusive disease (VOD), also known as sinusoidal obstruction syndrome, with kidney or lung dysfunction after hematopoietic stem-cell transplantation**
Adults and children: 6.25 mg/kg IV given as a 2-hour infusion every 6 hours. Administer for a minimum of 21 days; if after 21 days signs and symptoms of hepatic VOD haven't resolved, continue until resolution of VOD or for a maximum of 60 days.

Adjust-a-dose: Refer to manufacturer's instructions for toxicity-related dosage interruption and discontinuation.

deflazacort
de-FLAZE-a-kort

Emflaza

Therapeutic class: Muscular dystrophy drugs
Pharmacologic class: Corticosteroids

AVAILABLE FORMS
Oral suspension*: 22.75 mg/mL
Tablets: 6 mg, 18 mg, 30 mg, 36 mg

INDICATIONS & DOSAGES
➤ **Duchenne muscular dystrophy**
Adults and children ages 2 and older: 0.9 mg/kg PO once daily.
Adjust-a-dose: Round dose up to nearest 0.1 mL when using oral suspension. Round dose up to nearest possible dose based on available tablet strengths. Decrease dosage to one-third of recommended dosage when used with moderate or strong CYP3A4 inhibitors. Discontinue gradually if given for more than a few days.

desipramine hydrochloride
des-IP-ra-meen

Norpramin

Therapeutic class: Antidepressants
Pharmacologic class: TCAs

AVAILABLE FORMS
Tablets: 10 mg, 25 mg, 50 mg, 75 mg, 100 mg, 150 mg

INDICATIONS & DOSAGES
Boxed Warning Antidepressants increase risk of suicidality in children, adolescents, and young adults with depression and other psychiatric disorders. Drug isn't approved for use in children. ■
➤ **Depression**
Adults: Initially, 25 to 50 mg PO once daily or in divided doses; increase based on tolerance and clinical response. Usual dosage, 100 to 200 mg daily in single dose or divided doses; maximum, 300 mg daily.
Adolescents and older adults: 25 to 100 mg PO once daily or in divided doses; increase gradually to maximum of 150 mg daily, if needed.

desloratadine
dess-lor-AT-a-deen

Clarinex

Therapeutic class: Antihistamines
Pharmacologic class: Piperidines

AVAILABLE FORMS
Tablets: 5 mg
Tablets (ODTs): 2.5 mg, 5 mg

INDICATIONS & DOSAGES
➤ **Seasonal allergic rhinitis (patients ages 2 and older); perennial allergic rhinitis or chronic idiopathic urticaria (patients ages 6 months and older)**
Adults and children ages 12 and older: 5 mg PO once daily.
Children ages 6 to 11: 2.5 mg ODT PO once daily.
Adjust-a-dose: In adults with liver or kidney impairment, start dosage at 5 mg PO every other day.

deutetrabenazine ✂
doo-tet-ra-BEN-a-zeen

Austedo

Therapeutic class: Antichorea drugs
Pharmacologic class: Vesicular monoamine transporter 2 inhibitors

AVAILABLE FORMS
Tablets ⓓ: 6 mg, 9 mg, 12 mg
Tablets (extended-release) ⓓ: 6 mg, 12 mg, 24 mg

INDICATIONS & DOSAGES
Boxed Warning Drug can increase risk of depression and suicidality in patients with Huntington disease. Contraindicated for use in patients who are suicidal and those with untreated or inadequately treated depression. ■
➤ **Chorea associated with Huntington disease or tardive dyskinesia**
Adults: Initially, 6 mg PO b.i.d. or 12 mg extended-release PO once daily with food in patients not being switched from tetrabenazine. Titrate up at weekly intervals by 6 mg/day to a tolerated dose that reduces chorea, up to a maximum of 48 mg/day. If total daily dose of immediate-release tablets is 12 mg or more, give in two divided doses. Can discontinue drug without tapering. To resume after treatment interruption of more than 1 week, retitrate dosage. To resume after treatment interruption of less than 1 week, resume at previous dosage without titration.

  If switching from immediate- to extended-release formulation, give the same total daily dose. If switching from tetrabenazine to deutetrabenazine, stop tetrabenazine and initiate deutetrabenazine the next day. Refer to manufacturer's prescribing information for deutetrabenazine dosage based on last tetrabenazine dose.
✂ *Adjust-a-dose:* In patients currently receiving strong CYP2D6 inhibitors or for those who are known poor CYP2D6 metabolizers, don't exceed 36 mg/day.

dexlansoprazole
deks-lan-SOE-pra-zole

Dexilant

Therapeutic class: Antiulcer drugs
Pharmacologic class: PPIs

AVAILABLE FORMS
Capsules: 30 mg, 60 mg

INDICATIONS & DOSAGES
➤ **Healing of erosive esophagitis**
Adults and children ages 12 and older: Initially, 60-mg capsule PO once daily for up to 8 weeks.
Adjust-a-dose: For patients with Child-Pugh class B liver impairment, maximum dosage is 30-mg capsule PO daily for up to 8 weeks.
➤ **Maintenance of healed erosive esophagitis; heartburn relief**
Adults and children ages 12 and older: One 30-mg capsule PO daily for up to 6 months in adults and 16 weeks in patients ages 12 to 17.
➤ **Symptomatic nonerosive GERD**
Adults and children ages 12 and older: One 30-mg capsule PO daily for 4 weeks.

SAFETY ALERT!

dexmedetomidine hydrochloride
deks-MED-e-toe-mi-deen

Igalmi, Precedex

Therapeutic class: Sedatives
Pharmacologic class: Alpha$_2$-adrenergic agonists

AVAILABLE FORMS
Injection (concentrate): 100 mcg/mL in 2-mL and 10-mL single-use vials
Injection (ready-to-use): 4 mcg/mL in 20-mL single-use vials and 50-mL, 100-mL, and 250-mL single-use bottles
SL film 🚫: 120 mcg, 180 mcg

INDICATIONS & DOSAGES
Adjust-a-dose (for all indications): In patients with Child-Pugh class A, B, or C liver impairment and in those older than age 65, consider reducing dosage.
➤ **ICU sedation**
Adults: Loading infusion of 1 mcg/kg IV over 10 minutes; then maintenance infusion of 0.2 to 0.7 mcg/kg/hour titrated to achieve desired level of sedation. Infusion not to exceed 24 hours.
Adjust-a-dose: For conversion from an alternative sedative therapy, a loading infusion may not be needed.
➤ **Procedural sedation in patients who are not intubated**
Adults: Loading infusion of 1 mcg/kg IV over 10 minutes; then maintenance infusion, generally initiated at 0.6 mcg/kg/hour and titrated to achieve desired clinical effect. Dosages range from 0.2 to 1 mcg/kg/hour.
Children ages 2 to younger than 18 years: Loading infusion of 2 mcg/kg IV over 10 minutes; then maintenance infusion initiated at 1.5 mcg/kg/hour and titrated to achieve desired clinical effect. Dosages range from 0.5 to 1.5 mcg/kg/hour.
Children ages 1 month to younger than 2 years: Loading infusion of 1.5 mcg/kg IV over 10 minutes; then maintenance infusion initiated at 1.5 mcg/kg/hour and titrated to achieve desired clinical effect. Dosages range from 0.5 to 1.5 mcg/kg/hour.
Adjust-a-dose: For less-invasive procedures, such as ophthalmic surgery in adults, a loading infusion of

0.5 mcg/kg IV given over 10 minutes may be suitable. In patients older than age 65, give a loading infusion of 0.5 mcg/kg IV over 10 minutes.
➤ **Awake fiber-optic intubation**
Adults: Initial loading infusion of 1 mcg/kg IV over 10 minutes; then maintenance infusion of 0.7 mcg/kg/hour until endotracheal tube is secured.
➤ **Acute treatment of agitation associated with schizophrenia or bipolar I or II disorder**
Adults up to age 65: 120 mcg SL or buccally for mild or moderate agitation; if agitation persists, may give up to two additional 60-mcg doses at least 2 hours apart. Or, 180 mcg SL or buccally for severe agitation; if agitation persists, may give up to two additional 90-mcg doses at least 2 hours apart.
Adults ages 65 and older: 120 mcg SL or buccally for mild, moderate, or severe agitation; if agitation persists, may give up to two additional 60-mcg doses at least 2 hours apart.
Adjust-a-dose: For patients with Child-Pugh class A or B liver impairment, give 90 mcg for mild or moderate agitation or 120 mcg for severe agitation. For Child-Pugh class C liver impairment, give 60 mcg for mild or moderate agitation or 90 mcg for severe agitation. If agitation persists in patients with liver impairment, may give up to two additional 60-mcg doses at least 2 hours apart. If systolic BP (SBP) is less than 90 mm Hg, diastolic BP (DBP) is less than 60 mm Hg, HR is less than 60 beats/minute, or postural decrease in SBP is more than 20 mm Hg or DBP is more than 10 mm Hg after prior dose, don't repeat dose.

difelikefalin
dye-fel-i-KEF-a-lin

Korsuva

Therapeutic class: Miscellaneous CNS drugs
Pharmacologic class: Kappa opioid receptor agonists

AVAILABLE FORMS
Injection: 65 mcg/1.3 mL (50 mcg/mL)

INDICATIONS & DOSAGES
➤ **Moderate to severe pruritus associated with CKD in patients on hemodialysis**
Adults: 0.5 mcg/kg IV bolus injection at end of each hemodialysis treatment.

dimenhyDRINATE
dye-men-HYE-dri-nate

Dramamine ◇, Driminate ◇, Gravol ◇, Travel Tabs ✤ ◇

Therapeutic class: Antivertigo drugs
Pharmacologic class: Anticholinergics

AVAILABLE FORMS
Caplets (long-acting): 100 mg ✤ ◇
Capsules: 50 mg ◇
Injection: 50 mg/mL
Oral solution: 15 mg/5 mL ◇
Suppositories: 25 mg ✤ ◇, 50 mg ✤ ◇, 100 mg ✤ ◇

Tablets: 15 mg✦◇, 50 mg◇
Tablets (chewable): 15 mg✦◇, 50 mg◇

INDICATIONS & DOSAGES
➤ **To prevent and treat motion sickness**
Adults and children ages 12 and older: 50 to 100 mg PO every 4 to 6 hours; 50 mg IM every 4 hours PRN; 50 mg IV diluted in 10 mL NSS for injection, injected over 2 minutes every 4 hours PRN. May give 100 mg IV every 4 hours PRN when drowsiness isn't objectionable or is even desirable. Maximum, 400 mg daily. For prevention, use drug at least 30 minutes before motion exposure.
Children ages 6 to 11: 25 to 50 mg PO every 6 to 8 hours, not to exceed 150 mg in 24 hours. Or, 1.25 mg/kg or 37.5 mg/m² IM q.i.d.
Children ages 8 and older: 25 to 50 mg PR b.i.d. to t.i.d. PRN. For prevention, use drug at least 30 minutes but preferably 1 to 2 hours before traveling.
Children ages 2 to 5: 12.5 to 25 mg PO every 6 to 8 hours, not to exceed 75 mg in 24 hours. Or, 1.25 mg/kg or 37.5 mg/m² IM q.i.d. Maximum, 300 mg daily.

dimethyl fumarate
dye-METH-il

Tecfidera

Therapeutic class: Immunomodulators
Pharmacologic class: Nuclear factor-like 2 pathway activators

AVAILABLE FORMS
Capsules (delayed-release) ⓓⓝⓒ: 120 mg, 240 mg

INDICATIONS & DOSAGES
➤ **Relapsing MS**
Adults: Initially, 120 mg PO b.i.d. for 7 days; then increase to maintenance dosage of 240 mg b.i.d.
Adjust-a-dose: Consider temporary dosage reduction to 120 mg b.i.d. for patients who can't tolerate maintenance dose. Resume recommended dose of 240 mg b.i.d. within 4 weeks; then consider discontinuing drug if patient can't tolerate return to maintenance dose.

Consider interrupting or discontinuing therapy in patients with lymphocyte count of less than 500/mm³ persisting for more than 6 months. Consider withholding drug in patients with serious infections until resolution. Individualize decisions about restarting therapy based on clinical circumstances.

dinoprostone
dye-noe-PROST-ohn

Cervidil, Prepidil

Therapeutic class: Oxytocics
Pharmacologic class: Prostaglandins

AVAILABLE FORMS
Endocervical gel: 0.5 mg/application (2.5-mL syringe)
Vaginal insert: 10 mg

INDICATIONS & DOSAGES
➤ **To ripen an unfavorable cervix at or near term in patients with a medical or obstetric need for labor induction**
Adults: Apply 0.5 mg endocervical gel intravaginally; if cervix remains unfavorable after 6 hours, repeat dose. Don't exceed 1.5 mg (three applications) within 24 hours. After obtaining desired response, wait 6 to 12 hours before giving IV oxytocin. Or, place 10-mg vaginal insert transversely in posterior vaginal fornix immediately after removing insert from foil. Take insert out when active labor begins or after 12 hours have passed, whichever occurs first. After insert removal, wait at least 30 minutes before giving oxytocin.

SAFETY ALERT!

dinutuximab
din-ue-TUX-i-mab

Unituxin

Therapeutic class: Antineoplastics
Pharmacologic class: GD2-binding monoclonal antibodies

AVAILABLE FORMS
Injection: 17.5 mg/5 mL (3.5 mg/mL) in single-use vials

INDICATIONS & DOSAGES
Boxed Warning Life-threatening infusion reactions can occur. Give required prehydration and premedication before each infusion and monitor patient for infusion reaction during and for at least 4 hours after infusion. Interrupt drug for infusion reaction and permanently discontinue for anaphylaxis. Drug causes severe neuropathic pain and requires IV opioids before, during, and after infusion. Discontinue drug for severe unresponsive pain and severe sensory or motor neuropathy.
➤ **High-risk neuroblastoma, in combination with granulocyte-macrophage colony-stimulating factor, interleukin-2, and 13-*cis*-retinoic acid, in patients who achieved at least a partial response to prior first-line multiagent, multimodality therapy**
Children: 17.5 mg/m²/day IV over 10 to 20 hours for 4 consecutive days for up to five cycles. Cycles 1, 3, and 5 are 24 days in duration, and drug is administered on days 4, 5, 6, and 7. Cycles 2 and 4 are 32 days in duration, and drug is administered on days 8, 9, 10, and 11.
Adjust-a-dose: Refer to manufacturer's instructions for toxicity-related dosage adjustments and drug discontinuation.

disulfiram
dye-SUL-fi-ram

Therapeutic class: Alcohol deterrents
Pharmacologic class: Aldehyde dehydrogenase inhibitors

AVAILABLE FORMS
Tablets: 250 mg, 500 mg

INDICATIONS & DOSAGES

Boxed Warning Never give drug to a patient who is intoxicated or without patient's full knowledge. ■

➤ **Alcohol use disorder, moderate to severe**

Adults: 250 to 500 mg PO as single dose in morning for 1 to 2 weeks (or in evening if drowsiness occurs) beginning after patient has abstained from alcohol for at least 12 hours. Maintenance dosage is 125 to 500 mg PO daily (average 250 mg) until permanent self-control is established. Treatment may continue for months or years.

dolutegravir sodium
doe-loo-TEG-ra-vir

Tivicay, Tivicay PD

Therapeutic class: Antiretrovirals
Pharmacologic class: Integrase strand transfer inhibitors

AVAILABLE FORMS

Tablets: 10 mg, 25 mg, 50 mg
Tablets for oral suspension: 5 mg

INDICATIONS & DOSAGES

❸ *Alert:* Tivicay tablets and tablets for oral suspension can't be interchanged on a milligram-per-milligram basis. Children weighing 3 to 14 kg should only receive oral suspension.

➤ **HIV-1 infection in adults who are treatment-naive or treatment-experienced and in children who are treatment-naive or treatment-experienced and are integrase strand transfer inhibitor (INSTI)-naive, in combination with other antiretrovirals**

Adults and children weighing 20 kg or more (tablet): 50 mg PO once daily.

Children weighing 14 to less than 20 kg (tablets): 40 mg PO once daily.

Children weighing 20 kg or more (suspension): 30 mg PO once daily.

Children weighing 14 to less than 20 kg (suspension): 25 mg PO once daily.

Children ages 4 weeks and older weighing 10 to less than 14 kg (suspension): 20 mg PO once daily.

Children ages 4 weeks and older weighing 6 to less than 10 kg (suspension): 15 mg PO once daily.

Children ages 4 weeks and older weighing 3 to less than 6 kg (suspension): 5 mg PO once daily.

Adjust-a-dose: If administered with the potent UGT1A/CYP3A inducers carbamazepine, efavirenz, fosamprenavir/ritonavir, tipranavir/ritonavir, or rifampin, for adults give dolutegravir 50 mg b.i.d. For children, increase the weight-based dose of dolutegravir to b.i.d.

➤ **HIV-1 infection in patients who are INSTI-experienced with certain INSTI-associated resistance substitutions or clinically suspected INSTI resistance, or in patients who are treatment-naive or treatment-experienced INSTI-naive when administered with certain UGT1A or CYP3A inducers**

Adults: 50 mg PO b.i.d.

➤ **HIV-1 infection with rilpivirine as a complete regimen to replace the current antiretroviral regimen in patients who are virologically suppressed (HIV-1 RNA less than 50 copies/mL) on a stable antiretroviral regimen for at least 6 months with no history of treatment failure or known substitutions associated with resistance to either antiretroviral**

Adults: 50 mg PO once daily with rilpivirine 25 mg PO once daily.

dolutegravir–lamivudine
doe-loo-TEG-ra-vir/la-MI-vyoo-deen

Dovato

Therapeutic class: Antiretrovirals
Pharmacologic class: Integrase strand transfer inhibitors–nucleoside analogues/reverse transcriptase inhibitors

AVAILABLE FORMS

Tablets: 50 mg dolutegravir/300 mg lamivudine

INDICATIONS & DOSAGES

Boxed Warning Screen all patients for coinfection with HBV to prevent emergence from lamivudine-resistant HBV variants and potential exacerbation of HBV infection when lamivudine is discontinued. Additional anti-HBV therapy may be necessary. ■

➤ **HIV-1 infection in patients with no antiretroviral treatment history; HIV-1 infection as replacement for a current stable antiretroviral regimen in patients who are virologically suppressed (HIV-1 RNA less than 50 copies/mL) with no history of treatment failure and no known substitutions associated with resistance to the individual components**

Adults: 1 tablet PO once daily.

Adjust-a-dose: If administered with carbamazepine or rifampin, give 1 tablet PO once daily followed by an additional dolutegravir 50-mg tablet approximately 12 hours from the combination product dose. If a dosage reduction of lamivudine is needed for patients with CrCl of less than 30 mL/minute, use individual components of this product.

droxidopa
droks-eye-DOE-pa

Northera

Therapeutic class: Vasopressors
Pharmacologic class: Norepinephrine precursors

AVAILABLE FORMS

Capsules: 100 mg, 200 mg, 300 mg

INDICATIONS & DOSAGES

Boxed Warning Increased risk of supine HTN; monitor supine BP before and during treatment and more frequently with dosage increases. Elevating head of the bed lessens risk. Reduce dosage or discontinue drug if supine HTN can't be managed with head elevation. ■

➤ **Symptomatic neurogenic orthostatic hypotension caused by primary autonomic failure (Parkinson disease, multiple system atrophy, and pure autonomic failure), dopamine beta-hydroxylase deficiency, nondiabetic autonomic neuropathy**

Adults: Initially, 100 mg PO t.i.d. in morning, at midday, and in late afternoon at least 3 hours before bedtime. Titrate to symptomatic response in increments of 100 mg t.i.d. every 24 to 48 hours. Maximum, 600 mg t.i.d. Periodically reassess treatment effectiveness.

dupilumab
doo-PIL-ue-mab

Dupixent

Therapeutic class: Immunomodulators
Pharmacologic class: Monoclonal antibodies

AVAILABLE FORMS
Injection: 100 mg/0.67 mL, 200 mg/1.14 mL, 300 mg/2 mL in single-dose prefilled syringes; 200 mg/1.14 mL, 300 mg/2 mL in single-dose prefilled pen

INDICATIONS & DOSAGES
➤ **Moderate to severe atopic dermatitis not adequately controlled with topical therapy or when other therapies aren't advisable**

Adults and children ages 6 to 17 weighing 60 kg or more: Initially, 600 mg subcut given as two 300-mg injections in different sites, followed by 300 mg subcut every other week.

Children ages 6 to 17 weighing 30 to less than 60 kg: Initially, 400 mg subcut given as two 200-mg injections in different sites, followed by 200 mg subcut every other week.

Children ages 6 to 17 weighing 15 to less than 30 kg: Initially, 600 mg subcut given as two 300-mg injections in different sites, followed by 300 mg subcut every 4 weeks.

Children ages 6 months to 5 years weighing 15 to less than 30 kg: 300 mg subcut every 4 weeks.

Children ages 6 months to 5 years weighing 5 to less than 15 kg: 200 mg subcut every 4 weeks.

➤ **Add-on maintenance treatment for inadequately controlled chronic rhinosinusitis with nasal polyposis**

Adults: 300 mg subcut every other week.

➤ **Add-on maintenance treatment in patients with moderate to severe asthma with an eosinophilic phenotype or with oral corticosteroid-dependent asthma**

Adults and children ages 12 and older: Initially, 400 mg subcut (two 200-mg injections), followed by 200 mg every other week. Or, initially 600 mg subcut (two 300-mg injections), followed by 300 mg every other week. Or, for patients requiring concomitant oral corticosteroids or with comorbid moderate to severe atopic dermatitis for which drug is indicated, initially 600 mg subcut, followed by 300 mg every other week.

Children ages 6 to 11 weighing 30 kg or more: 200 mg subcut every other week.

Children ages 6 to 11 weighing 15 to less than 30 kg: 100 mg subcut every other week or 300 mg every 4 weeks.

➤ **Eosinophilic esophagitis**

Adults and children ages 12 and older weighing at least 40 kg: 300 mg subcut once a week.

➤ **Prurigo nodularis**

Adults: Initially, 600 mg subcut given as two 300-mg injections in different sites, followed by 300 mg subcut every other week.

ecallantide ⌀
ee-KAL-lan-tide

Kalbitor

Therapeutic class: Protein inhibitors
Pharmacologic class: Human plasma kallikrein inhibitors

AVAILABLE FORMS
Injection: 10 mg/mL vials

INDICATIONS & DOSAGES
Boxed Warning Anaphylaxis has been reported after administration. ■

➤ **Acute attacks of hereditary angioedema ⌀**

Adults and adolescents ages 12 and older: 30 mg subcut given as three 10-mg injections; give additional 30-mg dose within 24 hours if attack persists.

econazole nitrate
ee-KOE-na-zole

Ecoza

Therapeutic class: Antifungals
Pharmacologic class: Imidazole derivatives

AVAILABLE FORMS
Cream: 1%
Foam: 1%

INDICATIONS & DOSAGES
➤ **Tinea corporis, tinea cruris, tinea pedis, tinea versicolor**

Adults: Rub cream into affected areas daily for at least 2 weeks (1 month for tinea pedis).

Adults and children ages 12 and older (tinea pedis only): Apply foam to affected areas daily for 4 weeks.

➤ **Cutaneous candidiasis**

Adults: Rub cream into affected areas b.i.d. (morning and evening) for 2 weeks.

SAFETY ALERT!

eculizumab
eck-u-LIZ-uh-mob

Soliris

Therapeutic class: Hemolysis inhibitors
Pharmacologic class: Monoclonal IgG antibodies

AVAILABLE FORMS
Injection: 10 mg/mL in 300-mg single-use vials

INDICATIONS & DOSAGES
Boxed Warning Life-threatening and fatal meningococcal infections have occurred. Meningococcal

vaccine is required at least 2 weeks before administration of eculizumab, unless risks of delaying treatment outweigh risks of infection. Access is restricted through a REMS program; prescribers must be enrolled. ■

➤ **Hemolysis in patients with paroxysmal nocturnal hemoglobinuria**
Adults: 600 mg IV every 7 days for 4 weeks; 900 mg 7 days later; then 900 mg every 14 days thereafter.

➤ **Atypical hemolytic-uremic syndrome**
Adults and children weighing 40 kg or more: 900 mg IV weekly for 4 weeks; 1,200 mg at week 5; then 1,200 mg every 2 weeks.
Children ages 2 months and older weighing 30 to 39 kg: 600 mg IV weekly for 2 weeks; 900 mg at week 3; then 900 mg every 2 weeks.
Children ages 2 months and older weighing 20 to 29 kg: 600 mg IV weekly for 2 weeks; 600 mg at week 3; then 600 mg every 2 weeks.
Children ages 2 months and older weighing 10 to 19 kg: 600 mg IV weekly for one dose; 300 mg at week 2; then 300 mg every 2 weeks.
Children ages 2 months and older weighing 5 to 9 kg: 300 mg IV weekly for one dose; 300 mg at week 2; then 300 mg every 3 weeks.
Adjust-a-dose: Give a supplemental dose within 60 minutes after each plasmapheresis or plasma exchange session. If most recent dose was 300 mg, give 300-mg supplemental dose. If most recent dose was 600 mg or more, give 600-mg supplemental dose. For patients receiving fresh frozen plasma, if most recent dose was 300 mg or more, give 300-mg supplemental dose 1 hour before each unit of fresh frozen plasma.

➤ **Refractory generalized myasthenia gravis in patients who are anti-acetylcholine receptor antibody-positive; neuromyelitis optica spectrum disorder in patients who are anti-aquaporin-4 antibody positive**
Adults: 900 mg IV weekly for 4 weeks; 1,200 mg at week 5; then 1,200 mg every 2 weeks.
Adjust-a-dose: Give a supplemental dose within 60 minutes after each plasmapheresis or plasma exchange session. If most recent dose was 300 mg, give 300-mg supplemental dose. If most recent dose was 600 mg or more, give 600-mg supplemental dose. For patients receiving fresh frozen plasma, if most recent dose was 300 mg or more, give 300-mg supplemental dose 1 hour before each unit of fresh frozen plasma.

edaravone
ed-a-RAV-one

Radicava

Therapeutic class: Miscellaneous CNS drugs
Pharmacologic class: Free radical scavengers

AVAILABLE FORMS
Injection: 30 mg/100 mL premixed bags
Suspension: 105 mg/5 mL

INDICATIONS & DOSAGES
➤ **ALS**
Adults: For initial treatment cycle, 60 mg IV infusion over 60 minutes daily for 14 days, followed by 14-day drug-free period. Or, for initial treatment cycle, 105 mg PO or NG in morning after overnight fasting for 14 days, followed by 14-day drug-free period. For all subsequent treatment cycles, 60 mg IV infusion daily, or 105 mg PO or NG for 10 out of 14 days, followed by 14-day drug-free period.
Adjust-a-dose: May switch patient from 60 mg IV to 105 mg PO solution daily.

elexacaftor–tezacaftor–ivacaftor and ivacaftor ⌧
el-ex-a-KAF-tor/tez-a-KAF-tor/eye-va-KAF-tor

Trikafta

Therapeutic class: Metabolic agents
Pharmacologic class: Cystic fibrosis transmembrane conductance regulator (CFTR) facilitators (elexacaftor and tezacaftor)–CFTR potentiators (ivacaftor)

AVAILABLE FORMS
Granules: 80 mg elexacaftor, 40 mg tezacaftor, 60 mg ivacaftor (fixed-dose combination) copackaged with 59.5 mg ivacaftor; 100 mg elexacaftor, 50 mg tezacaftor, ivacaftor 75 mg (fixed-dose combination), copackaged with 75 mg ivacaftor.
Tablets : 50 mg elexacaftor, 25 mg tezacaftor, 37.5 mg ivacaftor (fixed-dose combination) copackaged with 75 mg ivacaftor; 100 mg elexacaftor, 50 mg tezacaftor, 75 mg ivacaftor (fixed-dose combination) copackaged with 150 mg ivacaftor

INDICATIONS & DOSAGES
➤ **Cystic fibrosis in patients who have at least one F508del mutation in the *CFTR* gene or a *CFTR* gene mutation responsive based on *in vitro* data ⌧**
Adults and children ages 6 and older weighing 30 kg or more: 2 tablets (each containing 100 mg elexacaftor, 50 mg tezacaftor, and 75 mg ivacaftor) PO in the morning, followed by one 150-mg ivacaftor tablet in the evening about 12 hours later.
Children ages 6 to younger than 12 weighing less than 30 kg: 2 tablets (each containing 50 mg elexacaftor, 25 mg tezacaftor, and 37.5 mg ivacaftor) PO in the morning, followed by one 75-mg ivacaftor tablet in the evening about 12 hours later.
Children ages 2 to younger than 6 years weighing 14 kg or more: One packet oral granules (each containing 100 mg elexacaftor, 50 mg tezacaftor, and 75 mg ivacaftor) PO in the morning, followed by one 75-mg ivacaftor packet oral granules about 12 hours later.
Children ages 2 to younger than 6 years weighing 14 kg or less: One packet oral granules (each containing 80 mg elexacaftor, 40 mg tezacaftor, and 60 mg ivacaftor) PO in the morning, followed by one 59.5-mg ivacaftor packet oral granules about 12 hours later.
Adjust-a-dose: For patients with Child-Pugh class B liver impairment and those currently receiving

moderate and strong CYP3A inhibitors, refer to manufacturer's instructions for dosage adjustments.

eltrombopag ⚇
ell-trom-BOW-pag

Promacta, Revolade✦

Therapeutic class: Hematopoietics
Pharmacologic class: Thrombopoietin
receptor agonists

AVAILABLE FORMS
Powder for oral suspension: 12.5-mg, 25-mg packets
Tablets ⓞⓝⓒ: 12.5 mg, 25 mg, 50 mg, 75 mg

INDICATIONS & DOSAGES
Boxed Warning Drug increases risk of liver toxicity. In patients with HCV infection, use with interferon and ribavirin may increase risk of liver decompensation. Consult prescribing information for specific monitoring guidelines. ∎

➤ **Thrombocytopenia associated with chronic ITP when response to corticosteroids, immunoglobulins, or splenectomy is inadequate**
Adults and children ages 6 and older: Initially, 50 mg PO once daily.
Children ages 1 to 5: Initially, 25 mg PO once daily.
⚇ *Adjust-a-dose:* Adjust dosage as necessary to achieve and maintain platelet count at 50×10^9/L or greater; maximum dosage is 75 mg daily. For patients older than age 6 and of East Asian descent and those with Child-Pugh class A, B, or C liver impairment, reduce dosage to 25 mg once daily. For patients older than age 6 of East Asian descent and any liver impairment, reduce dosage to 12.5 mg once daily. Refer to manufacturer's instructions for dosage adjustments based on hematologic parameters.

➤ **Thrombocytopenia in patients with chronic HCV infection to allow use of interferon-based therapy**
Adults: Initially, 25 mg PO once daily. Increase by 25-mg increments every 2 weeks as necessary to achieve target platelet count required to initiate antiviral therapy. Maximum, 100 mg daily.
Adjust-a-dose: During antiviral therapy, adjust dosage to avoid peginterferon dose reduction. Refer to manufacturer's instructions for dosage adjustments based on hematologic parameters. Discontinue drug when antiviral treatment is stopped.

➤ **Severe aplastic anemia when response to immunosuppressive therapy is insufficient**
Adults: Initially, 50 mg PO once daily. Adjust dosage as necessary in 50-mg increments every 2 weeks to achieve target platelet count of 50×10^9/L or greater. Maximum, 150 mg daily.
⚇ *Adjust-a-dose:* In patients of East Asian descent and those with Child-Pugh class A, B, or C liver impairment, reduce initial dosage to 25 mg once daily. Refer to manufacturer's instructions for dosage adjustments based on hematologic parameters.

If no hematologic response has occurred after 16 weeks of therapy, or new cytogenetic abnormalities are observed, discontinue drug.

➤ **First-line treatment of severe aplastic anemia, in combination with standard immunosuppressive therapy**
Adults and children ages 12 and older: 150 mg PO once daily for 6 months.
Children ages 6 to 11: 75 mg PO once daily for 6 months.
Children ages 2 to 5: 2.5 mg/kg PO once daily for 6 months.
⚇ *Adjust-a-dose:* In patients of East Asian descent and those with Child-Pugh class A, B, or C liver impairment, reduce initial dosage by 50%. Don't initiate if baseline ALT or AST level is more than $6 \times$ ULN. Refer to manufacturer's instructions for toxicity-related dosage adjustments.

emapalumab-lzsg
em-a-PAL-ue-mab

Gamifant

Therapeutic class: Immunomodulators
Pharmacologic class: Monoclonal antibodies

AVAILABLE FORMS
Injection: 10 mg/2 mL, 50 mg/10 mL, 100 mg/20 mL single-dose (5 mg/mL) vials

INDICATIONS & DOSAGES
➤ **Primary hemophagocytic lymphohistiocytosis (HLH) in patients with refractory, recurrent, or progressive disease or intolerance to conventional HLH therapy**
Adults and children: 1 mg/kg IV infusion over 1 hour twice weekly (every 3 to 4 days) until hematopoietic stem cell transplantation or unacceptable toxicity occurs.
Adjust-a-dose: If improvement in clinical condition is unsatisfactory, may increase dose to 3 mg/kg on day 3; to 6 mg/kg from day 6 onwards; to 10 mg/kg on day 9 onwards. See manufacturer's information for specific criteria for dosage increases. After clinical condition stabilizes, decrease dosage to previous level to maintain clinical response.

entacapone
en-TA-ka-pone

Comtan

Therapeutic class: Antiparkinsonian drugs
Pharmacologic class: Catechol-O-methyltransferase inhibitors

AVAILABLE FORMS
Tablets: 200 mg

INDICATIONS & DOSAGES
➤ **Adjunct to levodopa–carbidopa for treatment of idiopathic Parkinson disease in patients with signs and symptoms of end-of-dose wearing-off**
Adults: 200 mg PO with each dose of levodopa–carbidopa, up to eight times daily. Maximum, 1,600 mg daily. May need to reduce daily levodopa dose or extend interval between levodopa doses to optimize patient's response.

✦Canada   ◇OTC   ◆Off-label use   ⓞⓝⓒDo not crush   *Liquid contains alcohol   ⚇Genetic

enzalutamide
en-za-LOO-ta-mide

Xtandi

Therapeutic class: Antineoplastics
Pharmacologic class: Androgen receptor inhibitors

AVAILABLE FORMS
Capsules 🚫: 40 mg
Tablets 🚫: 40 mg, 80 mg

INDICATIONS & DOSAGES
Adjust-a-dose (for all indications): If use with strong CYP3A4 inducers is unavoidable, increase dosage to 240 mg once daily. If use with strong CYP2C8 inhibitors is unavoidable, reduce dosage to 80 mg once daily. Refer to manufacturer's instructions for toxicity-related dosage adjustments.
➤ **Castration-resistant prostate cancer; metastatic castration-sensitive prostate cancer**
Adults: 160 mg PO once daily after a bilateral orchiectomy or with a GnRH analogue. Continue until disease progresses or unacceptable toxicity occurs.

erdafitinib ⚛
er-da-Fl-ti-nib

Balversa

Therapeutic class: Antineoplastics
Pharmacologic class: Kinase inhibitors

AVAILABLE FORMS
Tablets 🚫: 3 mg, 4 mg, 5 mg

INDICATIONS & DOSAGES
➤ **Locally advanced or metastatic urothelial carcinoma with susceptible *FGFR3* or *FGFR2* genetic alterations that has progressed during or following at least one line of prior platinum-containing chemotherapy, including within 12 months of neoadjuvant or adjuvant platinum-containing chemotherapy** ⚛
Adults: 8 mg PO once daily. May increase to 9 mg once daily if serum phosphate level is less than 5.5 mg/dL and there are no ocular disorders or grade 2 or greater adverse reactions 14 to 21 days after start of treatment. Continue treatment until disease progresses or unacceptable toxicity occurs.
Adjust-a-dose: Refer to manufacturer's instructions for toxicity-related dosage adjustments.

eslicarbazepine acetate
es-li-kar-BAZ-e-peen

Aptiom

Therapeutic class: Anticonvulsants
Pharmacologic class: Carboxamide derivatives

AVAILABLE FORMS
Tablets: 200 mg, 400 mg, 600 mg, 800 mg

INDICATIONS & DOSAGES
➤ **Partial-onset seizures**
Adults: Initially, 400 mg PO once daily; may initiate treatment at 800 mg daily if need for additional seizure reduction outweighs increased risk of adverse reactions. May increase in weekly increments of 400 to 600 mg once daily to recommended maintenance dosage of 800 to 1,600 mg once daily.

For monotherapy, consider 800-mg once-daily maintenance dose in patients unable to tolerate 1,200-mg daily dose. For adjunctive therapy, consider 1,600-mg daily dose in patients who didn't achieve a satisfactory response with 1,200-mg daily dose.
Children ages 4 to 17: Dosage is based on body weight; increase based on clinical response and tolerability, but no more frequently than once per week.

For patients weighing more than 38 kg, initially 400 mg PO once daily; titrate in 400-mg increments to 800 to 1,200 mg PO once daily. For those weighing 32 to 38 kg, initially 300 mg PO once daily; titrate in 300-mg increments to 600 to 900 mg PO once daily. For those weighing 22 to 31 kg, initially 300 mg PO once daily; titrate in 300-mg increments to 500 to 800 mg PO once daily. For those weighing 11 to 21 kg, initially 200 mg PO once daily; titrate in 200-mg increments to 400 to 600 mg PO once daily.
Adjust-a-dose: For patients with CrCl of less than 50 mL/minute, the initial, titration, and maintenance dosages should generally be reduced by 50%. Maintenance dosages may be adjusted according to clinical response. Consider adjusting dosages of both eslicarbazepine and carbamazepine if given concurrently. Consider increasing eslicarbazepine dosage if given with enzyme-inducing AEDs (such as phenobarbital, primidone, or phenytoin).

etelcalcetide
e-tel-KAL-se-tide

Parsabiv

Therapeutic class: Hyperparathyroidism drugs
Pharmacologic class: Calcimimetics

AVAILABLE FORMS
Injection: 2.5 mg/0.5 mL, 5 mg/mL, 10 mg/2 mL in single-dose vials

INDICATIONS & DOSAGES
➤ **Secondary hyperparathyroidism in patients with CKD on hemodialysis**
Adults: Initially, 5 mg IV bolus injection three times per week at end of hemodialysis treatment. Maintenance dosage is individualized and determined by titration based on parathyroid hormone (PTH) level and corrected serum calcium response. Dosage range is 2.5 to 15 mg three times weekly. Increase dosage in 2.5- or 5-mg increments based on PTH level in patients with corrected serum calcium level within normal range and PTH level above recommended target range. Increase dosage no more frequently than every 4 weeks.

Adjust-a-dose: If PTH level is below target range, decrease dosage or temporarily discontinue drug. In patients with corrected serum calcium level below lower limit of normal (LLN), but at or above 7.5 mg/dL without symptoms of hypocalcemia, consider decreasing dosage, temporarily discontinuing drug, or using concomitant therapies to increase corrected serum calcium level.

If drug is stopped, reinitiate at a lower dose when PTH level is within target range and hypocalcemia has been corrected. If corrected serum calcium level falls below LLN or signs or symptoms of hypocalcemia develop, start or increase calcium supplementation (calcium, calcium-containing phosphate binders, or vitamin D sterols or increases in dialysate calcium concentration). Etelcalcetide dosage reduction or discontinuation may be necessary.

If corrected serum calcium level falls below 7.5 mg/dL or patient reports signs and symptoms of hypocalcemia, stop drug and treat hypocalcemia; when corrected serum calcium level is within normal limits, signs and symptoms of hypocalcemia have resolved, and predisposing factors for hypocalcemia have been addressed, reinitiate at a dose 5 mg lower than last administered dose. If last administered dose was 2.5 or 5 mg, reinitiate at 2.5-mg dose.

etodolac
ee-toe-DOE-lak

Therapeutic class: Anti-inflammatory drugs
Pharmacologic class: NSAIDs

AVAILABLE FORMS
Capsules: 200 mg, 300 mg
Tablets: 400 mg, 500 mg
Tablets (extended-release): 400 mg, 500 mg, 600 mg

INDICATIONS & DOSAGES
Boxed Warning Contraindicated for the treatment of perioperative pain after CABG surgery. NSAIDs can increase risk of serious heart attack or stroke and GI adverse reactions (bleeding, ulceration, and perforation), which can be fatal. ∎

➤ **Acute pain**
Adults: 200 to 400 mg (immediate-release) PO every 6 to 8 hours, not to exceed 1,000 mg daily.

➤ **Osteoarthritis and RA**
Adults: 300 mg PO b.i.d. or t.i.d. or 400 or 500 mg (immediate-release) PO b.i.d. Maximum, 1,000 mg daily. For extended-release tablets, 400 to 1,000 mg PO daily.

➤ **Juvenile RA**
Children ages 6 to 16 weighing more than 60 kg: 1,000 mg (extended-release) PO once daily.
Children ages 6 to 16 weighing 46 to 60 kg: 800 mg (extended-release) PO once daily.
Children ages 6 to 16 weighing 31 to 45 kg: 600 mg (extended-release) PO once daily.
Children ages 6 to 16 weighing 20 to 30 kg: 400 mg (extended-release) PO once daily.

evolocumab ⌧
e-voe-LOK-ue-mab

Repatha

Therapeutic class: Antilipemics
Pharmacologic class: Proprotein convertase subtilisin kexin type 9 antibody inhibitors

AVAILABLE FORMS
Injection: 140 mg/mL solution in single-dose prefilled syringe or autoinjector
Injection (Pushtronex on-body infusor system): 420 mg/3.5 mL

INDICATIONS & DOSAGES
➤ **Adjunct to diet, alone or in combination with other LDL-C lowering therapies, in patients with primary hyperlipidemia, including heterozygous familial hypercholesterolemia (HeFH), who require additional lowering of LDL-C** ⌧
Adults: 140 mg subcut every 2 weeks or 420 mg subcut once monthly. When switching dosage regimens, give first dose of new regimen on next scheduled date of prior regimen.

➤ **Adjunct to diet and other LDL-C lowering therapies in children with HeFH to reduce LDL-C** ⌧
Children ages 10 and older: 140 mg subcut every 2 weeks or 420 mg subcut once monthly. When switching dosage regimens, give first dose of new regimen on next scheduled date of prior regimen.

➤ **Adjunct to other LDL-C lowering therapies (statins, ezetimibe, LDL apheresis) in patients with homozygous familial hypercholesterolemia in patients who require additional lowering of LDL-C** ⌧
Adults and children ages 10 and older: 420 mg subcut once monthly. May increase to 420 mg every 2 weeks if clinically meaningful response isn't achieved in 12 weeks. Patients on lipid apheresis may begin treatment with 420 mg every 2 weeks to correspond with their apheresis schedule, given after apheresis session.

➤ **To reduce risk of MI, stroke, and coronary revascularization in patients with established CV disease**
Adults: 140 mg subcut every 2 weeks or 420 mg subcut once monthly. When switching dosage regimens, give first dose of new regimen on next scheduled date of prior regimen.

SAFETY ALERT!

exemestane
ex-e-MES-tane

Aromasin

Therapeutic class: Antineoplastics
Pharmacologic class: Aromatase inhibitors

AVAILABLE FORMS
Tablets: 25 mg

INDICATIONS & DOSAGES
Adjust-a-dose (for all indications): In patients also taking strong CYP3A4 inducers, increase daily dose to 50 mg.

> **Advanced breast cancer in patients who are postmenopausal whose disease has progressed after treatment with tamoxifen**
Adults: 25 mg PO once daily after a meal.

> **Early-stage estrogen receptor-positive breast cancer in patients who are postmenopausal who have taken tamoxifen for 2 to 3 years**
Adults: 25 mg PO once daily after a meal to complete a 5-year course, unless cancer recurs or is found in the other breast.

> **First-line adjuvant treatment of estrogen receptor-positive early breast cancer in patients who are postmenopausal ◆**
Adults: 25 mg PO once daily after a meal for 5 years.

> **Adjuvant therapy for hormone receptor-positive high-risk disease, in combination with ovarian function suppression ◆**
Patients who are premenopausal: 25 mg PO once daily after a meal after completion of chemotherapy or 6 to 8 weeks after ovarian functions suppression begins.

> **To reduce risk of breast cancer ◆**
Patients ages 35 and older who are postmenopausal: 25 mg PO once daily after a meal for 5 years.

SAFETY ALERT!

fedratinib
fed-RA-ti-nib

Inrebic

Therapeutic class: Antineoplastics
Pharmacologic class: Kinase inhibitors

AVAILABLE FORMS
Capsules: 100 mg

INDICATIONS & DOSAGES
Boxed Warning Serious and fatal encephalopathy, including Wernicke, can occur. Assess thiamine level in all patients before and periodically during treatment, and as clinically indicated. Don't start fedratinib in patients with thiamine deficiency. If encephalopathy is suspected, immediately discontinue fedratinib and initiate parenteral thiamine. ■

> **Intermediate-2 or high-risk primary or secondary (post-polycythemia vera or post-essential thrombocythemia) myelofibrosis**
Adults: 400 mg PO once daily if baseline platelet count is 50×10^9/L or greater.
Adjust-a-dose: In patients with CrCl of 15 to 29 mL/minute, decrease dosage to 200 mg once daily. If administering with strong CYP3A4 inhibitors, reduce dosage to 200 mg PO once daily. When administration with a strong CYP3A4 inhibitor is discontinued, increase fedratinib dosage to 300 mg once daily during first 2 weeks after discontinuation; then increase to 400 mg once daily as tolerated. Refer to manufacturer's instructions for toxicity-related dosage adjustments.

ferumoxytol
fer-yoo-MOX-i-tol

Feraheme

Therapeutic class: Iron salts
Pharmacologic class: Iron supplements

AVAILABLE FORMS
Injection: 510 mg elemental iron per 17 mL (30 mg/mL) single-dose vial

INDICATIONS & DOSAGES
Boxed Warning Fatal and serious hypersensitivity reactions, including anaphylaxis, can occur even if drug was previously tolerated. Give as IV infusion over at least 15 minutes and only when personnel and therapies are immediately available to treat hypersensitivity reactions. ■

> **Iron-deficiency anemia (IDA) in patients intolerant of or who have had an unsatisfactory response to oral iron or who have CKD**
Adults: 510 mg IV infusion. Repeat in 3 to 8 days. If IDA persists or recurs 1 month after second infusion, may repeat the two-dose treatment course.

fesoterodine fumarate
fes-oh-TER-oh-deen

Toviaz

Therapeutic class: Antispasmodics
Pharmacologic class: Muscarinic receptor antagonists

AVAILABLE FORMS
Tablets (extended-release) 🄳🄽🄲: 4 mg, 8 mg

INDICATIONS & DOSAGES
> **Urge incontinence, urinary urgency, and urinary frequency from overactive bladder**
Adults: 4 mg PO once daily; increase to 8 mg once daily if needed.
Adjust-a-dose: Don't exceed 4 mg daily in patients with CrCl of less than 30 mL/minute and in those taking potent CYP3A4 inhibitors.

> **Neurogenic detrusor overactivity**
Children ages 6 and older weighing more than 35 kg: 4 mg PO once daily for 1 week; then increase to 8 mg once daily.
Children ages 6 and older weighing more than 25 and up to 35 kg: 4 mg PO once daily. May increase to 8 mg once daily if needed.
Adjust-a-dose: For children weighing more than 25 and up to 35 kg, drug isn't recommended if eGFR is less than 30 mL/minute/1.73 m^2. If child weighs 35 kg or more and eGFR is 15 to 29 mL/minute/1.73 m^2, recommended dosage is 4 mg daily; drug isn't recommended if eGFR is less than 15 mL/minute/1.73 m^2. If coadministering strong CYP3A4 inhibitors in child weighing more than 35 kg, maximum dosage is 4 mg daily; coadministration isn't recommended in child weighing more than 25 and up to 35 kg.

fish oil triglycerides emulsion
fish oyl try-GLYC-e-rides

Omegaven

Therapeutic class: Nutritional supplements
Pharmacologic class: Essential fatty acid supplements

AVAILABLE FORMS
Injection: 5 g/50 mL, 10 g/100 mL single-dose bottles

INDICATIONS & DOSAGES
➤ **Source of calories and fatty acids in patients with parenteral nutrition-associated cholestasis**
Children: Recommended and maximum dosage is 1 g/kg/day by IV infusion. Initially, infuse at 0.2 mL/kg/hour for first 15 to 30 minutes of infusion; if tolerated, gradually increase until reaching the required rate after 30 minutes. Maximum infusion rate shouldn't exceed 1.5 mL/kg/hour.
Adjust-a-dose: If triglyceride level is greater than 250 mg/dL in neonates and infants or greater than 400 mg/dL in older children, consider stopping drug for 4 hours and obtaining a repeat serum triglyceride level. Resume therapy based on new result, as indicated. If triglyceride level remains elevated, consider a reduced dose of 0.5 to 0.75 g/kg/day with an incremental increase to 1 g/kg/day.

flibanserin
flib-AN-ser-in

Addyi

Therapeutic class: Miscellaneous sexual dysfunction aids
Pharmacologic class: Serotonin agonist/antagonist agents

AVAILABLE FORMS
Tablets: 100 mg

INDICATIONS & DOSAGES
Boxed Warning Drug interacts with alcohol. Advise patient to wait at least 2 hours after consuming one or two standard alcoholic drinks or to skip dose after consuming three or more standard alcoholic drinks. Drug is contraindicated for use with strong or moderate CYP3A4 inhibitors and in patients with liver impairment. ∎
➤ **Acquired, generalized hypoactive sexual desire disorder in patients who are premenopausal**
Adults: 100 mg PO once daily at bedtime. If no improvement after 8 weeks, discontinue drug.

SAFETY ALERT!

fludarabine phosphate
floo-DARE-a-been

Therapeutic class: Antineoplastics
Pharmacologic class: Purine antagonists

AVAILABLE FORMS
Powder for injection: 50 mg
Solution for injection: 50 mg/2 mL

INDICATIONS & DOSAGES
Boxed Warning Drug may cause severe bone marrow suppression, neurotoxicity, and autoimmune disorders, such as hemolytic anemia, thrombocytopenia, and acquired hemophilia. Use in combination with pentostatin for treatment of refractory chronic lymphocytic leukemia (CLL) isn't recommended due to high risk of fatal pulmonary toxicity. Drug should only be given under supervision of a health care provider experienced with antineoplastic therapy. ∎
➤ **B-cell CLL in patients with no or inadequate response to at least one standard alkylating drug regimen**
Adults: 25 mg/m² IV over 30 minutes daily for 5 consecutive days. Repeat cycle every 28 days. Optimal duration of treatment hasn't been established, but it's recommended to give three additional cycles after maximal response is obtained.
Adjust-a-dose: In patients with CrCl of 30 to 70 mL/minute, reduce dose by 20%. If CrCl is less than 30 mL/minute, don't give drug.
➤ **Newly diagnosed pediatric acute myeloid leukemia as part of a multiagent chemotherapy regimen, in combination with cytarabine and idarubicin during consolidation phase of treatment ◆**
Children: 10.5 mg/m² IV over 15 minutes as single dose, followed by continuous IV infusion of 30.5 mg/m²/day for 48 hours during consolidation phase of treatment.
➤ **Allogeneic hematopoietic stem cell transplantation in older adults as a myeloablative conditioning regimen, in combination with busulfan ◆**
Adults: 40 mg/m²/day IV for 4 days (in combination with busulfan) beginning 6 days before transplantation.

fludrocortisone acetate
floo-droe-KOR-ti-sone

Therapeutic class: Mineralocorticoids
Pharmacologic class: Mineralocorticoids

AVAILABLE FORMS
Tablets: 0.1 mg

INDICATIONS & DOSAGES
➤ **Salt-losing adrenogenital syndrome (congenital adrenal hyperplasia)**
Adults: 0.1 to 0.2 mg PO daily.
➤ **Addison disease (adrenocortical insufficiency)**
Adults: 0.1 mg PO daily. Usual dosage range is 0.1 mg three times weekly to 0.2 mg daily. Decrease dosage to 0.05 mg daily if transient HTN develops.

flunisolide (intranasal)
floo-NISS-oh-lide

Therapeutic class: Corticosteroids
Pharmacologic class: Glucocorticoid

AVAILABLE FORMS
Nasal spray: 25 mcg/spray

INDICATIONS & DOSAGES
➤ **Symptoms of seasonal or perennial allergic rhinitis**
Adults and children ages 15 and older: Starting dosage, 2 sprays in each nostril b.i.d.; may increase to 2 sprays in each nostril t.i.d. as needed. Maximum total daily dosage, 8 sprays in each nostril per day.
Children ages 6 to 14: Starting dosage, 1 spray in each nostril t.i.d. or 2 sprays in each nostril b.i.d. Maximum total daily dosage, 4 sprays in each nostril per day.

fluPHENAZine decanoate
floo-FEN-a-zeen

fluPHENAZine hydrochloride
Therapeutic class: Antipsychotics
Pharmacologic class: Phenothiazines

AVAILABLE FORMS
fluphenazine decanoate
Depot injection: 25 mg/mL*
fluphenazine hydrochloride
Elixir: 2.5 mg/5 mL *
IM injection: 2.5 mg/mL
Oral concentrate: 5 mg/mL*
Tablets: 1 mg, 2.5 mg, 5 mg, 10 mg

INDICATIONS & DOSAGES
Boxed Warning Drug isn't indicated for use in older adults with dementia-related psychosis because of increased risk of death. ∎
➤ **Psychotic disorders**
Adults: Initially, 2.5 to 10 mg fluphenazine hydrochloride PO daily in divided doses every 6 to 8 hours; may increase cautiously to 20 mg/day. Maintenance dosage is 1 to 5 mg PO daily. Maximum total dosage, 40 mg/day. IM doses are one-third to one-half of PO doses. Usual initial IM dose is 1.25 mg. Give more than 10 mg daily with caution.
   Or, 12.5 to 25 mg of fluphenazine decanoate IM or subcut every 3 to 4 weeks (response may last up to 6 weeks in some patients); may increase cautiously in 12.5 mg increments. Base frequency on patient response. Maintenance dose, 25 to 100 mg.
Older adults: Initially, 1 to 2.5 mg fluphenazine hydrochloride PO daily in 1 to 4 divided doses; adjust based on patient response.

fosamprenavir calcium
foss-am-PREN-ah-ver

Lexiva

Therapeutic class: Antiretrovirals
Pharmacologic class: Protease inhibitors

AVAILABLE FORMS
Oral suspension: 50 mg/mL
Tablets: 700 mg

INDICATIONS & DOSAGES
Adjust-a-dose (for all indications, excluding adults): There are no dosing recommendations for children with liver impairment. Dosage for children

shouldn't exceed recommended adult dosage of 700 mg fosamprenavir with ritonavir 100 mg b.i.d. Drug isn't approved for once-daily dosing in children.
➤ **HIV infection, with other antiretrovirals**
Adults: In patients not previously treated, 1,400 mg PO b.i.d. (without ritonavir). Or, 1,400 mg PO once daily with ritonavir 100 to 200 mg PO once daily. Or, 700 mg PO b.i.d. with ritonavir 100 mg PO b.i.d. In patients previously treated with a protease inhibitor, 700 mg PO b.i.d. plus ritonavir 100 mg PO b.i.d.
Adjust-a-dose: If patient has Child-Pugh class A liver impairment, reduce dosage to 700 mg PO b.i.d. without ritonavir (in patients who are therapy-naive) or 700 mg b.i.d. plus ritonavir 100 mg once daily (in patients who are therapy-naive or protease inhibitor-experienced). If patient has Child-Pugh class B liver impairment, reduce dosage to 700 mg b.i.d. (in patients who are therapy-naive) without ritonavir or 450 mg b.i.d. plus ritonavir 100 mg once daily (in patients who are therapy-naive or protease inhibitor-experienced). If patient has Child-Pugh class C liver impairment, reduce dosage to 350 mg b.i.d. without ritonavir (in patients who are therapy-naive) or 300 mg b.i.d. plus ritonavir 100 mg once daily (in patients who are therapy-naive or protease inhibitor-experienced).
➤ **HIV infection with other antiretrovirals for protease inhibitor-naive children ages 4 weeks and older**
Children ages 4 weeks to 18 years weighing 20 kg or more: 18 mg/kg PO with ritonavir 3 mg/kg b.i.d.
Children ages 4 weeks to 18 years weighing 15 to less than 20 kg: 23 mg/kg PO with ritonavir 3 mg/kg b.i.d.
Children ages 4 weeks to 18 years weighing 11 to less than 15 kg: 30 mg/kg PO with ritonavir 3 mg/kg b.i.d.
Children ages 4 weeks to 18 years weighing less than 11 kg: 45 mg/kg PO with ritonavir 7 mg/kg b.i.d.
➤ **HIV infection with other antiretrovirals for protease inhibitor-experienced children ages 6 months and older**
Children ages 6 months to 18 years weighing 20 kg or more: 18 mg/kg PO with ritonavir 3 mg/kg b.i.d.
Children ages 6 months to 18 years weighing 15 to less than 20 kg: 23 mg/kg PO with ritonavir 3 mg/kg b.i.d.
Children ages 6 months to 18 years weighing 11 to less than 15 kg: 30 mg/kg PO with ritonavir 3 mg/kg b.i.d.
Children ages 6 months to 18 years weighing less than 11 kg: 45 mg/kg PO with ritonavir 7 mg/kg b.i.d.
➤ **HIV infection without ritonavir in protease inhibitor-naive children**
Children ages 2 years and older: 30 mg/kg PO b.i.d. For patients weighing at least 47 kg, may use adult regimen of fosamprenavir 1,400 mg b.i.d. Maximum, 1,400 mg b.i.d.

fostemsavir
fos-TEM-sa-vir

Rukobia

Therapeutic class: Antiretrovirals
Pharmacologic class: HIV-1 gp120
attachment inhibitors

AVAILABLE FORMS
Tablets (extended-release) ⓞⓣⓒ: 600 mg

INDICATIONS & DOSAGES
➤ **HIV-1 infection, in combination with other antiretrovirals, in patients with multidrug-resistant
HIV-1 infection who are heavily treatment-
experienced but failing their current antiretroviral
regimen due to resistance, intolerance, or safety
considerations**
Adults: 600 mg PO b.i.d.

fremanezumab-vfrm
FRE-ma-nez-ue-mab

Ajovy

Therapeutic class: Antimigraine drugs
Pharmacologic class: Calcitonin gene-related
peptide antagonists

AVAILABLE FORMS
Injection: 225 mg/1.5 mL single-dose prefilled
syringe or autoinjector

INDICATIONS & DOSAGES
➤ **Prevention of migraine headache**
Adults: 225 mg subcut once a month or 675 mg (three
consecutive injections of 225 mg each) subcut every
3 months (quarterly).

galantamine hydrobromide
gah-LAN-tah-meen

Therapeutic class: Anti-Alzheimer drugs
Pharmacologic class: Cholinesterase
inhibitors

AVAILABLE FORMS
Capsules (extended-release): 8 mg, 16 mg, 24 mg
Oral solution: 4 mg/mL
Tablets: 4 mg, 8 mg, 12 mg

INDICATIONS & DOSAGES
➤ **Mild to moderate Alzheimer dementia**
Adults: Initially, 4 mg immediate-release tablets or
solution PO b.i.d., preferably with morning and evening meals. If dose is well tolerated after minimum of
4 weeks of therapy, increase dosage to 8 mg b.i.d. A
further increase to 12 mg b.i.d. may be attempted, but
only after at least 4 weeks of therapy at the previous
dosage. Dosage range is 16 to 24 mg daily in two divided doses.

Or, 8 mg extended-release capsule PO once daily
in the morning with food. Increase to 16 mg PO once
daily after a minimum of 4 weeks. May further

increase to 24 mg once daily after a minimum of
4 weeks, based on patient response and tolerability.
Dosage range is 16 to 24 mg daily.
Adjust-a-dose: For patients with Child-Pugh class B
liver impairment or CrCl of 9 to 59 mL/minute, dosage usually shouldn't exceed 16 mg daily. Drug isn't
recommended for patients with Child-Pugh class C
liver impairment or CrCl less than 9 mL/minute.

galcanezumab-gnlm
GAL-ka-nez-ue-mab

Emgality

Therapeutic class: Antimigraine drugs
Pharmacologic class: Monoclonal antibodies

AVAILABLE FORMS
Injection: 100 mg/mL single-dose prefilled syringe;
120 mg/mL in single-dose autoinjector or prefilled
syringe

INDICATIONS & DOSAGES
➤ **Prevention of migraine headache**
Adults: Initially, 240 mg subcut (administered as two
consecutive injections of 120 mg each) once as loading dose; then 120 mg subcut once monthly.
➤ **Episodic cluster headache**
Adults: Initially, 300 mg subcut (three consecutive
injections of 100 mg) once at onset of cluster period;
then monthly until end of cluster period.

SAFETY ALERT!

gilteritinib ⓧ
GIL-te-ri-ti-nib

Xospata

Therapeutic class: Antineoplastics
Pharmacologic class: Kinase inhibitors

AVAILABLE FORMS
Tablets ⓞⓝⓒ: 40 mg

INDICATIONS & DOSAGES
Boxed Warning Drug can cause differentiation
syndrome (fever, dyspnea, hypoxia, pulmonary infiltrates, pleural or pericardial effusions, rapid weight
gain or peripheral edema, hypotension, or kidney
dysfunction), which can be fatal or life-threatening if
not treated. If differentiation syndrome is suspected,
initiate corticosteroid therapy and hemodynamic
monitoring. ■
➤ **Relapsed or refractory acute myeloid leukemia
with an *FLT3* mutation** ⓧ
Adults: 120 mg PO once daily for a minimum of
6 months.
Adjust-a-dose: See manufacturer's instructions for
toxicity-related dosage adjustments, including for
QT-interval prolongation.

♣Canada   ◇ OTC   ◆ Off-label use   ⓞⓝⓒDo not crush   *Liquid contains alcohol   ⓧ Genetic

glasdegib
glas-DEG-ib

Daurismo

Therapeutic class: Antineoplastics
Pharmacologic class: Hedgehog pathway inhibitors

AVAILABLE FORMS
Tablets: 25 mg, 100 mg

INDICATIONS & DOSAGES
Boxed Warning Drug can cause severe birth defects and fetal death. ■
➤ **Newly diagnosed acute myeloid leukemia, in combination with low-dose cytarabine, in patients who are age 75 or older or who have comorbidities that preclude use of intensive induction chemotherapy**
Adults: 100 mg PO once daily on days 1 to 28, in combination with cytarabine 20 mg subcut b.i.d. on days 1 to 10 of each 28-day cycle. Treat for a minimum of six cycles to allow time for clinical response or until unacceptable toxicity or loss of disease control occurs.
Adjust-a-dose: Refer to glasdegib manufacturer's instructions for toxicity-related dosage adjustments. Refer to cytarabine manufacturer's instructions for dosing and toxicity-related information.

glucagon
GLOO-ka-gon

Baqsimi, GlucaGen Diagnostic Kit, GlucaGen HypoKit, Gvoke

Therapeutic class: Diagnostic agents
Pharmacologic class: Antihypoglycemics

AVAILABLE FORMS
Nasal powder: 3 mg/dose
Powder for injection: 1-mg (1-unit) vials
Solution: 0.5 mg/0.1 mL, 1 mg/0.2 mL prefilled syringe or autoinjector; 1 mg/0.2 mL vial

INDICATIONS & DOSAGES
➤ **Hypoglycemia in patients with diabetes**
Adults and children weighing more than 20 kg or older than age 6: 1 mg (1 mL) IV, IM, or subcut.
Children weighing 20 kg or less: 0.5 mg (0.5 mL) or 20 to 30 mcg/kg IV, IM, or subcut. Maximum dose, 1 mg.
Adults and children weighing more than 25 kg or age 6 or older or when weight is unknown (GlucaGen): 1 mg (1 mL) IV, IM, or subcut.
Children weighing less than 25 kg or younger than age 6 when weight is unknown (GlucaGen): 0.5 mg (0.5 mL) IV, IM, or subcut.
Adults and children ages 4 and older (Baqsimi): 3 mg (1 spray) into 1 nostril.
Adults and children ages 2 and older weighing 45 kg or more (Gvoke): 1 mg subcut into lower abdomen, outer thigh, or outer upper arm.

Children ages 2 to younger than 12 weighing less than 45 kg (Gvoke): 0.5 mg subcut into lower abdomen, outer thigh, or outer upper arm.
Adjust-a-dose: If no response, may repeat dose in 15 minutes.
➤ **Diagnostic aid for radiologic exam of the GI tract**
Adults: 0.2 to 0.75 mg IV or 1 mg IM before radiologic exam. Refer to manufacturer's instruction for dosage by anatomic area.

goserelin acetate
GOE-se-rel-in

Zoladex

Therapeutic class: Antineoplastics
Pharmacologic class: Gonadotropin-releasing hormone analogues

AVAILABLE FORMS
Implants: 3.6 mg, 10.8 mg

INDICATIONS & DOSAGES
➤ **Endometriosis, including pain relief and lesion reduction**
Adults: 3.6 mg subcut every 28 days into anterior abdominal wall below navel. Maximum length of therapy is 6 months.
➤ **Endometrial thinning before endometrial ablation**
Adults: 3.6 mg subcut into anterior abdominal wall below navel. One or two implants given 4 weeks apart. When one depot is given, surgery should be performed at 4 weeks; when two depots are given, surgery should be performed within 2 to 4 weeks after second depot.
➤ **Palliative treatment of advanced breast cancer in patients who are pre perimenopausal or perimenopausal**
Adult females: 3.6 mg subcut every 28 days into anterior abdominal wall below navel.
➤ **Palliative treatment of advanced prostate cancer**
Adult males: 3.6 mg subcut every 28 days or 10.8 mg subcut every 12 weeks into anterior abdominal wall below navel.
➤ **Locally confined prostate cancer in combination with radiotherapy and flutamide**
Adult males: Start 8 weeks before initiating radiotherapy and continue during radiation therapy. 3.6 mg subcut into anterior abdominal wall below navel, followed in 28 days by 10.8 mg subcut. Or, four injections of 3.6 mg at 28-day intervals, two injections preceding and two during radiotherapy.

guanFACINE hydrochloride
GWAHN-fa-seen

Intuniv

Therapeutic class: Antihypertensives
Pharmacologic class: Centrally acting antiadrenergics

AVAILABLE FORMS

Tablets: 1 mg, 2 mg
Tablets (extended-release) ◉: 1 mg, 2 mg, 3 mg, 4 mg

INDICATIONS & DOSAGES

➤ **HTN**

Adults and children ages 12 and older: Initially, 1 mg immediate-release tablet PO once daily at bedtime. If response isn't adequate after 3 to 4 weeks, may increase dosage to 2 mg daily.

➤ **ADHD**

Children ages 6 to 17: Extended-release form only. Initially, 1 mg PO once daily in a.m. or p.m. at approximately same time each day. Adjust dosage in increments of 1 mg/week as needed. Target dosage range is 0.05 to 0.12 mg/kg PO once daily as tolerated and necessary. Doses above 4 mg/day haven't been evaluated in children ages 6 to 12 or above 7 mg/day in adolescents ages 13 to 17.

Adjust-a-dose: Refer to manufacturer's instructions for dosage adjustment for use with CYP3A4 inhibitors or inducers.

HYDROXYprogesterone caproate

hye-drox-ee-proh-JESS-te-rone

Makena

Therapeutic class: Hormones
Pharmacologic class: Progestins

AVAILABLE FORMS

Injection: 250 mg/mL in single-dose and multidose vials; 275 mg/1.1 mL autoinjector

INDICATIONS & DOSAGES

➤ **To reduce risk of preterm birth in patients with singleton pregnancy and history of singleton spontaneous preterm birth**

Adolescents and patients ages 16 and older who are pregnant: 250 mg IM in gluteus maximus (if using vial) or 275 mg subcut in back of either upper arm (if using autoinjector) once weekly starting between 16 weeks, 0 days and 20 weeks, 6 days of gestation and continuing until week 37 (through 36 weeks, 6 days) of gestation or delivery, whichever occurs first.

ibalizumab-uiyk

eye-ba-LIZ-ue-mab

Trogarzo

Therapeutic class: Antiretrovirals
Pharmacologic class: CD4-directed postattachment HIV-1 inhibitors

AVAILABLE FORMS

Injection: 200 mg/1.33 mL (150 mg/mL) single-dose vials

INDICATIONS & DOSAGES

➤ **HIV-1 infection, in combination with other antiretrovirals, in patients with multidrug-resistant HIV-1 infection who are heavily treatment-experienced and failing their current antiretroviral regimen**

Adults: 2,000 mg IV infusion loading dose, followed by 800 mg IV infusion maintenance doses every 2 weeks.

icosapent ethyl

eye-KOE-sa-pent

Vascepa

Therapeutic class: Antilipemics
Pharmacologic class: Ethyl esters

AVAILABLE FORMS

Capsules ◉: 500 mg, 1 g

INDICATIONS & DOSAGES

➤ **Adjunct to diet to reduce triglyceride levels 500 mg/dL or more**

Adults: 2 g PO b.i.d. with food.

➤ **Adjunct to maximally tolerated statin therapy to reduce risk of MI, stroke, coronary revascularization, and unstable angina requiring hospitalization in patients with elevated triglyceride level (150 mg/dL or more) and established CV disease or in patients with diabetes and two or more additional risk factors for CV disease**

Adults: 2 g PO b.i.d. with food.

SAFETY ALERT!

IDArubicin hydrochloride

eye-da-ROO-bi-sin

Idamycin PFS

Therapeutic class: Antineoplastics
Pharmacologic class: Semisynthetic anthracyclines

AVAILABLE FORMS

Injection: 1 mg/mL in 5-, 10-, and 20-mL single-dose vials

INDICATIONS & DOSAGES

Dosages vary. Check treatment protocol with prescriber.

Boxed Warning Reduce dosage in patients with liver or kidney impairment. Don't give idarubicin if bilirubin level exceeds 5 mg/dL. Severe local tissue necrosis can occur with extravasation. Give slowly into freely flowing IV infusion. Drug can cause myocardial toxicity, leading to HF, and severe myelosuppression. Drug should be given under supervision of a physician experienced in leukemia chemotherapy in a facility with appropriate lab and supportive resources. ■

➤ **Acute myeloid leukemia with other approved antileukemic drugs**

Adults: 12 mg/m² daily for 3 days by slow IV injection (over 10 to 15 minutes) with 100 mg/m² daily of cytarabine for 7 days by continuous IV infusion. Or, cytarabine as 25-mg/m² bolus; then 200 mg/m² daily for 5 days by continuous IV infusion. May give a second course, if needed.

Adjust-a-dose: If patient experiences severe mucositis, delay second course of therapy until recovery is complete; reduce dosage by 25%. Consider dosage reduction if bilirubin or creatinine level is above normal range.

➤ **Acute myeloid leukemia (newly diagnosed)** ♦
Infants, children, adolescents: Per clinical trial CCG-2961, for induction and consolidation, 5 mg/m^2/dose IV daily for 4 days on days 0 to 3 in combination with cytarabine, etoposide, thioguanine, and dexamethasone. Or, for consolidation only, 12 mg/m^2/dose IV daily for 3 days on days 0 to 2 in combination with fludarabine and cytarabine.

SAFETY ALERT!

ifosfamide
eye-FOSS-fa-mide

Ifex

Therapeutic class: Antineoplastics
Pharmacologic class: Nitrogen mustards

AVAILABLE FORMS
Powder for injection: 1-g, 3-g vials

INDICATIONS & DOSAGES
➤ **Germ cell testicular cancer as third-line chemotherapy in combination with certain other antineoplastics and mesna**
Adults: 1.2 g/m^2 IV daily for 5 consecutive days. Repeat treatment every 3 weeks or after patient recovers from hematologic toxicity. Don't repeat doses until WBC count exceeds 2,000/mm^3 and platelet count exceeds 50,000/mm^3.
➤ **Ewing sarcoma** ♦
Adults: 1,800 mg/m^2/day IV for 5 days (VAC/IE regimen; in combination with mesna and etoposide); alternate with VAC (vincristine, doxorubicin, and cyclophosphamide) every 3 weeks for a total of 17 courses.
Adults and children: 3,000 mg/m^2/day IV on days 1, 2, 22, 23, 43, and 44 for four courses (VAIA regimen; in combination with vincristine, doxorubicin, dactinomycin, and mesna).

Or, 2,000 mg/m^2/day IV for 3 days every 3 weeks for 14 courses (in combination with vincristine, doxorubicin, dactinomycin, and mesna).

Or, 3,000 mg/m^2/day IV over 1 to 3 hours for 3 days every 3 weeks for six courses (VIDE regimen; in combination with vincristine, doxorubicin, etoposide, and mesna).

Or, 1,800 mg/m^2/day IV over 1 hour for 5 days every 3 weeks for 12 cycles (IE regimen; in combination with etoposide and mesna).

Or, 1,800 mg/m^2/day IV for 5 days every 3 weeks for up to 12 cycles (ICE regimen; in combination with carboplatin and etoposide [and mesna]).
Children: 1,800 mg/m^2/day IV for 5 days (IE regimen; in combination with mesna and etoposide); alternate with VAC (vincristine, doxorubicin, and cyclophosphamide) every 3 weeks for a total of 17 courses.

Or, 1,800 mg/m^2/day IV for 5 days every 3 to 4 weeks for two courses (ICE regimen; in combination with carboplatin and etoposide [and mesna]), followed by CAV (cyclophosphamide, doxorubicin, and vincristine).

➤ **Soft tissue sarcoma** ♦
Adults: 3,000 mg/m^2/day IV over 4 hours for 3 days every 3 weeks for at least two cycles or until disease progresses.

Or, 1,500 mg/m^2/day IV for 4 days every 3 weeks until disease progresses or unacceptable toxicity occurs (EIA regimen; in combination with etoposide, doxorubicin, and regional hyperthermia).

Or, 2,000 mg/m^2/day IV continuous infusion for 3 days every 3 weeks (MAID regimen; in combination with mesna, doxorubicin, and dacarbazine).

Or, 2,500 mg/m^2/day IV continuous infusion for 3 days every 3 weeks (in combination with mesna, doxorubicin, and dacarbazine); reduce ifosfamide to 1,500 mg/m^2/day in patients with prior pelvic irradiation.

Or, 1,800 mg/m^2/day IV over 1 hour for 5 days every 3 weeks for five cycles (in combination with mesna and epirubicin).

Or, 1,500 mg/m^2/day IV over 2 hours for 4 days every 3 weeks for four to six cycles (AIM regimens; in combination with mesna and doxorubicin).

Or, 2,000 to 3,000 mg/m^2/day IV over 3 hours for 3 days (in combination with mesna and doxorubicin).

imipenem–cilastatin sodium–relebactam
im-i-PEN-em/sye-la-STAT-in/rel-e-BAK-tam

Recarbrio

Therapeutic class: Anti-infectives
Pharmacologic class: Penem antibacterials–renal dehydropeptidase inhibitors–beta-lactamase inhibitors

AVAILABLE FORMS
Injection: 1.25-g (imipenem 500 mg, cilastatin 500 mg, relebactam 250 mg) vial

INDICATIONS & DOSAGES
Adjust-a-dose (for all indications): For CrCl of 60 to 89 mL/minute, give 1 g IV every 6 hours (imipenem 400 mg, cilastatin 400 mg, relebactam 200 mg); for CrCl of 30 to 59 mL/minute, give 750 mg IV every 6 hours (imipenem 300 mg, cilastatin 300 mg, relebactam 150 mg); for CrCl of 15 to 29 mL/minute, give 500 mg IV every 6 hours (imipenem 200 mg, cilastatin 200 g, relebactam 100 mg); for CrCl less than 15 mL/minute, don't administer unless hemodialysis is instituted within 48 hours. For patients with CKD on hemodialysis, give 500 mg IV every 6 hours. Give after hemodialysis and at intervals timed from the end of that hemodialysis session.
➤ **Complicated UTIs, including pyelonephritis, caused by susceptible gram-negative microorganisms (*Enterobacter cloacae, Escherichia coli, Klebsiella aerogenes, Klebsiella pneumoniae,* and *Pseudomonas aeruginosa*) in patients with limited or no alternative treatment options**
Adults: 1.25 g by IV infusion over 30 minutes every 6 hours for 4 to 14 days guided by severity and location of the infection and clinical response.

➤ **Complicated intra-abdominal infections caused by susceptible gram-negative microorganisms** (*Bacteroides caccae, Bacteroides fragilis, Bacteroides ovatus, Bacteroides thetaiotaomicron, Bacteroides uniformis, Bacteroides vulgatus, Bifidobacterium stercoris, Citrobacter freundii, E. cloacae, E. coli, Fusobacterium nucleatum, K. aerogenes, Klebsiella oxytoca, K. pneumoniae, Parabacteroides distasonis,* and *P. aeruginosa*) **in patients with limited or no alternative treatment options**
Adults: 1.25 g by IV infusion over 30 minutes every 6 hours for 4 to 14 days guided by severity and location of the infection and clinical response.

➤ **Hospital-acquired pneumonia and ventilator-associated pneumonia caused by susceptible gram-negative organisms** (*Acinetobacter calcoaceticus-baumannii* complex, *E. cloacae, E. coli, Haemophilus influenzae, K. aerogenes, K. oxytoca, K. pneumoniae, P. aeruginosa,* and *Serratia marcescens*)
Adults: 1.25 g by IV infusion over 30 minutes every 6 hours for 4 to 14 days guided by severity and location of the infection and clinical response.

imiquimod
ih-mih-KWI-mahd

Aldara, Vyloma✤, Zyclara

Therapeutic class: Immunosuppressants (topical)
Pharmacologic class: Immune response modifiers

AVAILABLE FORMS
Cream: 2.5%, 3.75% in 30-mL pump bottles (one dose is one full actuation); 3.75%, 5 % in single-use packets

INDICATIONS & DOSAGES
➤ **External genital and perianal warts**
Adults and adolescents ages 12 and older: Apply thin layer of 3.75% cream once daily before sleep; leave on for 8 hours. Continue for up to 8 weeks. Or, apply thin layer of 5% cream three times per week before sleep; leave on for 6 to 10 hours. Continue for up to 16 weeks.

➤ **Typical, nonhyperkeratotic, nonhypertrophic actinic keratoses on face or scalp in immunocompetent adults**
Adults: Wash area with mild soap and water, and allow to dry for at least 10 minutes. Apply 2.5% or 3.75% cream once daily at bedtime for two 2-week cycles. Separate cycles by a 2-week no-treatment period.

Or, apply 5% cream to face or scalp, but not both concurrently, twice weekly at bedtime; wash off after about 8 hours. Treat for 16 weeks.

➤ **Superficial basal cell carcinoma (Aldara only)**
Adults: Wash area with mild soap and water, and allow to dry thoroughly. Apply thin layer of 5% cream to biopsy-confirmed area, including 1 cm of skin surrounding tumor, five times a week at bedtime; wash off after about 8 hours. Treat for 6 weeks.

indapamide
in-DAP-a-mide

Therapeutic class: Diuretics/antihypertensives
Pharmacologic class: Thiazide-like diuretics

AVAILABLE FORMS
Tablets: 1.25 mg, 2.5 mg

INDICATIONS & DOSAGES
➤ **Edema of HF**
Adults: Initially, 2.5 mg PO daily in the morning, increased to 5 mg daily after 1 week, if needed.
➤ **HTN**
Adults: Initially, 1.25 mg PO daily in the morning, increased to 2.5 mg daily after 4 weeks, if needed. Increased to 5 mg daily after 4 more weeks, if needed. If inadequate response, give a second antihypertensive at 50% of usual starting dose, if needed.

inotersen ▧
in-oh-TER-sen

Tegsedi

Therapeutic class: Endocrine-metabolic agents
Pharmacologic class: Antisense oligonucleotides

AVAILABLE FORMS
Injection: 284 mg/1.5 mL single-dose, prefilled syringe

INDICATIONS & DOSAGES
Boxed Warning Drug can cause glomerulonephritis that may require immunosuppressive therapy and may result in dialysis-dependent KF. Testing before and monitoring during treatment is required. ■
Boxed Warning Drug can cause sudden and unpredictable thrombocytopenia that can be life-threatening and is contraindicated with platelet count less than $100 \times 10^9/L$. Testing before and monitoring during treatment is required. ■
➤ **Polyneuropathy of hereditary transthyretin-mediated amyloidosis** ▧
Adults: 284 mg subcut once weekly on the same day every week.
Adjust-a-dose: Refer to manufacturer's instructions for monitoring and dosage adjustments based on platelet count and kidney function.

SAFETY ALERT!

inotuzumab ozogamicin
in-oh-TOOZ-ue-mab

Besponsa

Therapeutic class: Antineoplastics
Pharmacologic class: Antibody-drug conjugates

AVAILABLE FORMS
Injection (lyophilized): 0.9 mg lyophilized powder in single-dose vials

---

INDICATIONS & DOSAGES

Boxed Warning Liver toxicity, including fatal and life-threatening hepatic veno-occlusive disease, has occurred. A higher posthematopoietic stem cell transplant (HSCT) nonrelapse mortality rate occurred in patients receiving inotuzumab. ■

➤ **Relapsed or refractory B-cell precursor acute lymphoblastic leukemia**

Adults: Premedicate with a corticosteroid, antipyretic, and antihistamine. For cycle 1, total dose is 1.8 mg/m² given as three divided doses during a 21-day cycle. On day 1, give 0.8 mg/m² IV infusion; on days 8 and 15, give 0.5 mg/m² IV infusion. Cycle 1 may be extended to 28 days if patient achieves complete remission (CR) or CR with incomplete hematologic recovery (CRi) or to allow recovery from toxicity.

For subsequent cycles in patients who achieve a CR or CRi, total dose per cycle is 1.5 mg/m², given as three divided doses during a 28-day treatment cycle. On days 1, 8, and 15, give 0.5 mg/m² IV infusion.

For subsequent cycles in patients who don't achieve CR or CRi, total dose per cycle is 1.8 mg/m², given as three divided doses during a 28-day treatment cycle. On day 1, give 0.8 mg/m² IV infusion; on days 8 and 15, give 0.5 mg/m² IV infusion. Discontinue drug in patients who don't achieve CR or CRi within three cycles.

For patients proceeding to HSCT, recommended treatment duration is two cycles. May consider third cycle for those who don't achieve CR or CRi and minimal residual disease negativity after two cycles.

For patients not proceeding to HSCT, may give additional cycles of treatment, up to a maximum of six cycles.

Adjust-a-dose: Refer to manufacturer's instructions for toxicity-related dosage adjustments and drug discontinuation.

SAFETY ALERT!

interferon gamma-1b
in-ter-FEER-on

Actimmune

Therapeutic class: Immune response modifiers
Pharmacologic class: Biological response modifiers

AVAILABLE FORMS

Injection: 100 mcg (2 million international units) in 0.5-mL vials

INDICATIONS & DOSAGES

➤ **Chronic granulomatous disease in patients ages 1 year and older; severe malignant osteopetrosis in patients ages 1 month and older**

Adults and children with BSA greater than 0.5 m²: 50 mcg/m² (1 million international units/m²) subcut three times weekly, preferably at bedtime.
Adults and children with BSA of 0.5 m² or less: 1.5 mcg/kg subcut three times weekly.
Adjust-a-dose: If patient has severe reaction, decrease dosage by 50% or stop drug until reaction subsides.

isavuconazonium sulfate
eye-sa-vue-koe-na-ZOE-nee-um

Cresemba

Therapeutic class: Antifungals
Pharmacologic class: Triazole antifungals

AVAILABLE FORMS

Capsules ⓞⓣⓒ 74.5 mg (equal to isavuconazole 40 mg), 186 mg (equal to isavuconazole 100 mg)
Injection: 372 mg (equal to isavuconazole 200 mg)/vial

INDICATIONS & DOSAGES

➤ **Invasive aspergillosis; invasive mucormycosis fungal infection**

Adults: Loading doses of 372 mg IV or PO every 8 hours for six doses (48 hours); then maintenance dosage of 372 mg IV or PO once daily. Initiate maintenance dosage 12 to 24 hours after last loading dose. May switch between IV and PO formulations for maintenance dosing; no need to restart dosing with a loading dose when switching between formulations.

isoproterenol hydrochloride
eye-soe-proe-TER-e-nole

Therapeutic class: Bronchodilators, inotropes
Pharmacologic class: Nonselective beta-adrenergic agonists

AVAILABLE FORMS

Injection: 0.2 mg/mL in ampules or vials

INDICATIONS & DOSAGES

➤ **Bronchospasm during anesthesia**

Adults: Dilute 1 mL (0.2 mg) with 9 mL of NSS or D_5W. Give 0.01 to 0.02 mg IV and repeat as necessary.

➤ **Heart block; Adams-Stokes attacks, except when caused by ventricular tachycardia or fibrillation; cardiac arrest until electric shock or pacemaker therapy is available**

Adults: Initially, 0.02 to 0.06 mg IV bolus or via infusion at 5 mcg/minute IV; for subsequent bolus, 0.01 to 0.2 mg IV. Or, initially, 0.2 mg IM or subcut; then 0.02 to 1 mg IM or 0.15 to 0.2 mg subcut as needed. Or, initially, 0.02 mg intracardiac.

➤ **Shock**

Adults: 0.5 to 5 mcg/minute (0.25 to 2.5 mg) by continuous IV infusion. Usual concentration is 1 mg in 500 mL D_5W. Titrate infusion rate according to HR, central venous pressure, BP, and urine flow.

istradefylline
iz-TRA-de-FYE-leen

Nourianz

Therapeutic class: Antiparkinsonian drugs
Pharmacologic class: Adenosine receptor antagonists

AVAILABLE FORMS

Tablets: 20 mg, 40 mg

INDICATIONS & DOSAGES

➤ **Adjunct to levodopa–carbidopa in patients with Parkinson disease experiencing "off" episodes**
Adults: 20 mg PO once daily. May increase to maximum of 40 mg PO once daily based on individual need and tolerability.

Adjust-a-dose: For patients with Child-Pugh class B liver impairment or concomitant use of strong CYP3A4 inhibitors, maximum recommended dosage is 20 mg PO once daily. For patients who use tobacco in amounts of 20 or more cigarettes per day (or the equivalent of another tobacco product), recommended dosage is 40 mg PO once daily.

SAFETY ALERT!

ivosidenib ⚥
EYE-voe-SID-e-nib

Tibsovo

Therapeutic class: Antineoplastics
Pharmacologic class: Isocitrate dehydrogenase-1 inhibitors

AVAILABLE FORMS
Tablets ⓄⓃⒸ: 250 mg

INDICATIONS & DOSAGES
Boxed Warning Can cause differentiation syndrome (fever, dyspnea, hypoxia, pulmonary infiltrates, pleural and pericardial effusion, rapid weight gain, peripheral edema, hypotension, and liver, kidney, or multiorgan dysfunction), which can be fatal if not treated. If differentiation syndrome is suspected, initiate corticosteroid therapy and hemodynamic monitoring until symptom resolution. ■

Adjust-a-dose (for all indications): If use with strong CYP3A4 inhibitor can't be avoided, reduce ivosidenib dosage to 250 mg daily. If strong CYP3A4 inhibitor is discontinued, increase ivosidenib to 500 mg daily after at least five half-lives of inhibitor. Refer to manufacturer's instructions for toxicity-related dosage adjustments.

➤ **Relapsed or refractory acute myeloid leukemia (AML) with susceptible *IDH1* mutation ⚥**
Adults: 500 mg PO daily. Treat for a minimum of 6 months to allow time for clinical response or until disease progresses or unacceptable toxicity occurs.

➤ **Newly diagnosed AML with susceptible *IDH1* mutation in patients who are age 75 or older or who have comorbidities that preclude use of intensive induction chemotherapy, as monotherapy or in combination with azacitidine ⚥**
Adults ages 75 and older: 500 mg PO daily with azacitidine 75 mg/m² subcut or IV once daily on days 1 to 7 (or days 1 to 5 and 8 to 9) of each 28-day cycle until disease progresses or unacceptable toxicity occurs. Treat for a minimum of 6 months to allow time for clinical response. Refer to azacitidine manufacturer's instructions for additional dosing information.

➤ **Locally advanced or metastatic cholangiocarcinoma with *IDH1* mutation in patients who have been previously treated**

Adults: 500 mg PO daily until disease progresses or unacceptable toxicity occurs.

SAFETY ALERT!

ixabepilone
ecks-ah-BEH-pill-own

Ixempra Kit

Therapeutic class: Antineoplastics
Pharmacologic class: Microtubule inhibitors

AVAILABLE FORMS
Injection: 15-mg, 45-mg vials with diluent

INDICATIONS & DOSAGES
Boxed Warning Drug is contraindicated in patients with AST or ALT level greater than 2.5 × ULN or bilirubin level 1 × ULN when used with capecitabine due to increased toxicity and neutropenia-related death. ■

➤ **With capecitabine for metastatic or locally advanced breast cancer, after failure of anthracycline and a taxane, or in patients whose cancer is taxane-resistant and for whom further anthracycline therapy is contraindicated; or alone for metastatic or locally advanced breast cancer, after failure of anthracycline, a taxane, and capecitabine**
Adults: 40 mg/m² IV over 3 hours every 3 weeks. Dosages for patients with BSA greater than 2.2 m² should be calculated based on 2.2 m². Premedicate with an H_1-receptor antagonist, such as diphenhydramine 50 mg PO (or equivalent), and an H_2-receptor antagonist 1 hour before ixabepilone infusion. For patients who experienced a prior hypersensitivity reaction, premedicate with corticosteroids (such as dexamethasone 20 mg IV 30 minutes before infusion or PO 60 minutes before infusion) in addition to the H_1- and H_2-receptor antagonists.

Adjust-a-dose: Refer to manufacturer's instructions for monotherapy and combination therapy dosage adjustments for toxicities and liver failure.

ketoprofen
kee-toe-PROE-fen

Therapeutic class: Anti-inflammatory drugs
Pharmacologic class: NSAIDs

AVAILABLE FORMS
Capsules: 25 mg, 50 mg, 75 mg
Capsules (extended-release): 200 mg

INDICATIONS & DOSAGES
Boxed Warning Contraindicated for the treatment of perioperative pain after CABG surgery. NSAIDs can increase risk of serious heart attack or stroke and GI adverse reactions (bleeding, ulceration, and perforation), which can be fatal. ■

Adjust-a-dose (for all indications): For patients ages 75 and older, reduce dosage. For patients with mildly impaired kidney function, maximum dosage is 150 mg daily. For patients with GFR of less than 25 mL/minute/1.73 m² or impaired liver function and

---

♣Canada   ◇OTC   ♦Off-label use   ⓄⓃⒸDo not crush   *Liquid contains alcohol   ⚥Genetic

serum albumin level less than 3.5 g/dL, maximum dosage is 100 mg daily.
➤ **RA, osteoarthritis**
Adults: 75 mg PO t.i.d., 50 mg PO q.i.d., or 200 mg as an extended-release capsule once daily. Maximum, 300 mg daily; 200 mg daily for extended-release capsules.
➤ **Mild to moderate pain, dysmenorrhea**
Adults: 25 to 50 mg PO every 6 to 8 hours PRN. Maximum, 300 mg daily.

lanadelumab-flyo
LAN-a-del-ue-mab

Takhzyro

Therapeutic class: Prophylaxis drugs
Pharmacologic class: Monoclonal antibodies

AVAILABLE FORMS
Injection: 150 mg/mL, 300 mg/2 mL prefilled syringe; 300 mg/2 mL single-dose vial

INDICATIONS & DOSAGES
➤ **Prevention of hereditary angioedema attacks**
Adults and children ages 12 and older: Initially, 300 mg subcut every 2 weeks. If patient is attack-free for more than 6 months, may consider decreasing dosage to 300 mg subcut every 4 weeks.
Children ages 6 to younger than 12 years: Initially, 150 mg subcut every 2 weeks. If child is attack free for more than 6 months, may consider decreasing dosage to 150 mg subcut every 4 weeks.
Children ages 2 to younger than 6 years: 150 mg subcut every 4 weeks.

SAFETY ALERT!

lapatinib ⚶
lah-PAH-tih-nihb

Tykerb

Therapeutic class: Antineoplastics
Pharmacologic class: Kinase inhibitors

AVAILABLE FORMS
Tablets: 250 mg

INDICATIONS & DOSAGES
Boxed Warning Severe and fatal liver toxicity has been observed. ∎
Adjust-a-dose (for all indications): Refer to manufacturer's instructions for toxicity-related dosage adjustments and use with strong CYP3A4 inhibitors or inducers.
➤ **Advanced or metastatic breast cancer with capecitabine when tumors overexpress HER2 and patient has had prior therapy, including an anthracycline, a taxane, and trastuzumab** ⚶
Adults: 1,250 mg (5 tablets) PO once daily as single dose on days 1 through 21, with 2,000 mg/m²/day capecitabine given PO in two doses 12 hours apart on days 1 to 14. Repeat 21-day cycle. Continue until disease progresses or unacceptable toxicity occurs.

➤ **HER2-positive, hormone receptor-positive metastatic breast cancer in patients who are postmenopausal** ⚶
Adult females: 1,500 mg PO once daily in combination with letrozole 2.5 mg PO once daily.

SAFETY ALERT!

larotrectinib ⚶
lar-oh-TREK-ti-nib

Vitrakvi

Therapeutic class: Antineoplastics
Pharmacologic class: Kinase inhibitors

AVAILABLE FORMS
Capsules ⓓ: 25 mg, 100 mg
Oral solution: 20 mg/mL

INDICATIONS & DOSAGES
➤ **Solid tumors that have a neurotrophic receptor tyrosine kinase gene fusion without a known acquired resistance mutation, are metastatic or associated with likelihood of surgical resection resulting in severe morbidity, and have no satisfactory alternative treatments or have progressed after treatment** ⚶
Adults and children ages 1 month and older with BSA of at least 1 m²: 100 mg PO b.i.d. until disease progresses or unacceptable toxicity occurs.
Children ages 1 month and older with BSA less than 1 m²: 100 mg/m² PO b.i.d. until disease progresses or unacceptable toxicity occurs.
Adjust-a-dose: For Child-Pugh class B or C liver impairment, reduce starting dose by 50%. If administration with a strong CYP3A4 inhibitor is unavoidable, reduce larotrectinib dose by 50%. If administration with a strong CYP3A4 inducer is unavoidable, double larotrectinib dose. If CYP3A4 drug is discontinued, allow 3 to 5 elimination half-lives before resuming prior larotrectinib dose. Refer to manufacturer's instructions for toxicity-related dosage adjustments.

lasmiditan
las-MID-i-tan

Reyvow

Therapeutic class: Antimigraine drugs
Pharmacologic class: Serotonin receptor agonists
Controlled substance schedule: V

AVAILABLE FORMS
Tablets ⓓ: 50 mg, 100 mg

INDICATIONS & DOSAGES
➤ **Acute treatment of migraine with or without aura**
Adults: 50 mg, 100 mg, or 200 mg PO PRN. Maximum, one dose in 24 hours; four doses within 30 days.

lefamulin
lef-a-MUE-lin

Xenleta

Therapeutic class: Antibacterials
Pharmacologic class: Pleuromutilin anti-infectives

AVAILABLE FORMS
Injection: 150 mg/15 mL vial
Tablets ⓞⓝⓒ: 600 mg

INDICATIONS & DOSAGES
➤ **Community-acquired bacterial pneumonia caused by susceptible strains of *Streptococcus pneumoniae, Staphylococcus aureus* (methicillin-susceptible isolates), *Haemophilus influenzae, Legionella pneumophila, Mycoplasma pneumoniae,* and *Chlamydophila pneumoniae***
Adults: 150 mg IV infusion over 60 minutes every 12 hours for 5 to 7 days. Or, 600 mg PO every 12 hours for 5 days. May switch from IV form to oral form to complete treatment course.
Adjust-a-dose: For patients with Child-Pugh class C liver impairment, reduce IV dose to 150 mg infused every 24 hours. Tablets aren't recommended for patients with Child-Pugh class B or C liver impairment.

lenvatinib mesylate ⊠
len-VA-ti-nib

Lenvima

Therapeutic class: Antineoplastics
Pharmacologic class: Kinase inhibitors

AVAILABLE FORMS
Capsules: 4 mg, 10 mg

INDICATIONS & DOSAGES
Adjust-a-dose (for all indications): See manufacturer's instructions for toxicity-related dosage adjustments and management.
➤ **Locally recurrent or metastatic, progressive, radioactive iodine-refractory differentiated thyroid cancer**
Adults: 24 mg PO daily until disease progresses or unacceptable toxicity occurs.
Adjust-a-dose: For CrCl less than 30 mL/minute or Child-Pugh class C liver impairment, decrease dosage to 14 mg PO daily.
➤ **Advanced renal cell carcinoma after one prior antiangiogenic therapy, in combination with everolimus**
Adults: 18 mg PO once daily with everolimus 5 mg PO once daily until disease progresses or unacceptable toxicity occurs. Refer to everolimus prescribing information for recommended dosage information.
Adjust-a-dose: For patients with preexisting CrCl less than 30 mL/minute or Child-Pugh class C liver impairment, decrease lenvatinib dosage to 10 mg PO daily.

➤ **Advance renal cell carcinoma as first-line treatment, in combination with pembrolizumab**
Adults: 20 mg PO once daily with pembrolizumab 200 mg IV infusion over 30 minutes every 3 weeks until disease progresses or unacceptable toxicity occurs or up to 2 years. After 2 years of combined therapy, may continue lenvatinib as single agent until disease progresses or unacceptable toxicity occurs. Refer to pembrolizumab prescribing information for recommended dosage information.
Adjust-a-dose: For preexisting CrCl less than 30 mL/minute or Child-Pugh class C liver impairment, decrease lenvatinib dosage to 10 mg PO daily.
➤ **Unresectable hepatocellular carcinoma, first-line treatment**
Adults weighing 60 kg or more: 12 mg PO once daily until disease progresses or unacceptable toxicity occurs.
Adults weighing less than 60 kg: 8 mg PO once daily until disease progresses or unacceptable toxicity occurs.
➤ **Advanced endometrial carcinoma microsatellite instability-high or mismatch repair-deficient in patients who have disease progression after prior systemic therapy and aren't candidates for curative surgery or radiation, in combination with pembrolizumab** ⊠
Adults: 20 mg PO once daily with pembrolizumab 200 mg IV infusion every 3 weeks until disease progresses or unacceptable toxicity occurs. Refer to pembrolizumab prescribing information for recommended dosage information.
Adjust-a-dose: For preexisting CrCl less than 30 mL/minute or Child-Pugh class C liver impairment, decrease lenvatinib dosage to 10 mg PO daily.

letermovir
let-ER-moe-vir

Prevymis

Therapeutic class: Antivirals
Pharmacologic class: CMV DNA terminase complex inhibitors

AVAILABLE FORMS
Injection: 240 mg/12 mL, 480 mg/24 mL single-use vials
Tablets ⓞⓝⓒ: 240 mg, 480 mg

INDICATIONS & DOSAGES
Adjust-a-dose (for all indications): If drug is administered with cyclosporine, decrease dosage to 240 mg PO or IV once daily. If cyclosporine is initiated after start of letermovir, decrease following doses letermovir to 240 mg once daily, starting with the next dose. If cyclosporine is discontinued after start of letermovir, increase following doses of letermovir to 480 mg once daily, starting with the next dose. If cyclosporine dosing is interrupted due to high cyclosporine level, don't adjust letermovir dosage.

✦ Canada   ◇ OTC   ◆ Off-label use   ⓞⓝⓒ Do not crush   *Liquid contains alcohol   ⊠ Genetic

➤ **Prophylaxis of CMV infection and disease in CMV-seropositive recipients [R+] of an allogeneic hematopoietic stem cell transplant**

Adults: 480 mg PO or IV infusion over 1 hour once daily beginning between day 0 and day 28 posttransplant and continuing through 100 days posttransplant. In patient at risk for late CMV infection and disease, may continue through 200 days posttransplant.

✳ *NEW INDICATION:* **Prophylaxis of CMV disease in kidney transplant recipients at high risk (donor CMV seropositive/recipient CMV seronegative)**

Adults: 480 mg administered once daily PO or IV infusion over 1 hour beginning day 0 to 7 posttransplant and continuing through 200 days posttransplant.

levomilnacipran hydrochloride
lee-voe-mil-NAY-sih-pran

Fetzima

Therapeutic class: Antidepressants
Pharmacologic class: SSNRIs

AVAILABLE FORMS
Capsules (extended-release) 🚫: 20 mg, 40 mg, 80 mg, 120 mg

INDICATIONS & DOSAGES
Boxed Warning Antidepressants increase risk of suicidality in children, adolescents, and young adults. Drug isn't approved for use in children. ∎

➤ **Major depressive disorder**

Adults: Initially, 20 mg PO once daily for 2 days; then increase to 40 mg once daily. May increase in increments of 40 mg at intervals of 2 or more days. Maximum, 120 mg once daily.

Adjust-a-dose: For patients with CrCl of 30 to 59 mL/minute, maximum maintenance dosage is 80 mg once daily. If CrCl is 15 to 29 mL/minute, maximum maintenance dosage is 40 mg once daily. Don't use if CrCl is less than 15 mL/minute.

L-glutamine
ell-GLOO-ta-meen

Endari

Therapeutic class: Miscellaneous hematologic drugs
Pharmacologic class: Amino acids

AVAILABLE FORMS
Oral powder: 5 g per packet

INDICATIONS & DOSAGES
➤ **To reduce acute complications of sickle cell disease**

Adults and children ages 5 and older weighing more than 65 kg: 15 g (3 packets) PO b.i.d.

Adults and children ages 5 and older weighing 30 to 65 kg: 10 g (2 packets) PO b.i.d.

Children ages 5 and older weighing less than 30 kg: 5 g (1 packet) PO b.i.d.

lidocaine (intradermal, ophthalmic, topical)
LYE-doe-kane

Lidocaine, Lidoderm

lidocaine hydrochloride
Akten, AneCream ◇, AneCream 5, Glydo, Lidodan ♣ ◇, LidoPatch ◇, Maxilene ♣ ◇, RectiCare ◇, Solarcaine ◇, Xolido ◇, Xylocaine, Zingo

Therapeutic class: Analgesics
Pharmacologic class: Local anesthetics

AVAILABLE FORMS
Cream: 2% ◇, 3%, 3.88%, 4% ◇, 4.12%, 5% ◇, 10%
Gel: 2% ◇, 2.8%, 3% ◇, 4% ◇, 5% ◇
Jelly: 2%
Lotion: 1% ◇, 2.75%, 3%, 3.5%, 4%
Ointment: 4% ◇, 5%
Ophthalmic gel: 3.5%
Patch: 1.8%, 3.5% ◇, 4% ◇, 5%
Powder for injection: 0.5-mg single-use intradermal injection system
Topical solution: 2%, 4%
Topical spray: 0.5%
Viscous oral solution: 2%, 4%

INDICATIONS & DOSAGES
Boxed Warning Postmarketing cases of seizures, cardiopulmonary arrest, and death in patients younger than age 3 have been reported with use of lidocaine 2% viscous solution when it wasn't administered in strict adherence to the dosing and administration recommendations. Lidocaine 2% viscous solution isn't approved for teething pain. ∎

Adjust-a-dose (for all indications): Decrease dosage as needed based on patient's age, weight, and physical condition.

➤ **Urethra anesthesia and treatment of painful urethritis**

Male adults and children: Slowly instill 15 mL (300 mg lidocaine) 2% jelly into urethra using an easy syringelike action, until patient has a feeling of tension or until about 15 mL is instilled. Apply penile clamp for 5 to 10 minutes at the corona; then, if needed, instill an additional 15 mL as needed for adequate anesthesia. Before catheterization, 5 to 10 mL (100 to 200 mg) is usually adequate. Maximum dose for adults is 600 g in any 12-hour period. Maximum dose for children is 4.5 mg/kg.

Female adults and children: Slowly instill 3 to 5 mL (60 to 100 mg) of 2% jelly into urethra. A small amount of jelly may be applied to cotton swab and deposited into urethral opening before instillation. Allow several minutes for anesthetic effect to occur. Maximum dose for adults is 600 g in any 12-hour period. Maximum dose for children is 4.5 mg/kg.

➤ **Anesthetic lubricant for ET intubation**

Adults and children: Apply moderate amount of 2% jelly to external surface of ET tube shortly before use. Maximum dose in adults is 30 mL (600 mg) in any 12-hour period. Maximum dose in children is 4.5 mg/kg.

Or, apply up to 5 g per single application, approximately 6 inches, of 5% ointment to external surface of ET tube shortly before use. Maximum dose of 5% ointment in adults is 20 g (equivalent to lidocaine base 1,000 mg) per day. Maximum dose of 5% ointment in children is 4.5 mg/kg.

➤ **Topical anesthesia of accessible mucous membranes of oral and nasal cavities and proximal portions of digestive tract**

Adults: 15 mL 2% topical viscous solution to affected areas not more frequently than every 3 hours. Maximum, 4.5 mg/kg, not to exceed 300 mg/dose.

Adults and children ages 10 and older: 1 to 5 mL (40 to 200 mg) 4% oral topical solution to affected area as a spray, applied with cotton applicators or packs, or instilled into a cavity. Maximum, 4.5 mg/kg, not to exceed 300 mg/dose.

Children younger than age 10 who have normal lean body mass and normal body development: 4% oral topical solution to affected area as a spray, applied with cotton applicators or packs, or instilled into a cavity. May determine dose by applying one of the standard pediatric drug formulas. Maximum, 4.5 mg/kg.

➤ **Oropharynx anesthetic**

Adults and children (used in dentistry): Apply 5% ointment to previously dried oral mucosa. For use in adults with insertion of new dentures, apply to all denture surfaces with mucosal contact. Maximum for adults is 5 g/single application (equivalent to lidocaine base 250 mg or 6 inches of ointment) or 20 g of ointment (equivalent to 1,000 g lidocaine base) per day. Patient should consult a dentist at least every 48 hours throughout denture-fitting period. Maximum for children is 5 g/single application (equivalent to 250 mg lidocaine base or approximately 6 inches of ointment) or 4.5 mg/kg lidocaine base.

Adults: 15 mL 2% solution swished in mouth and spit out or gargled and swallowed no more frequently than every 3 hours. Maximum for adults is 4.5 mg/kg/dose (or 300 mg/dose); eight doses per 24 hours.

Children ages 3 and older: Don't exceed 4.5 mg/kg/dose (or 300 mg/dose) swished in the mouth and spit out no more frequently than every 3 hours (four doses in 12 hours).

Children younger than age 3: 1.2 mL 2% solution applied to immediate area with cotton-tipped applicator no more frequently than every 3 hours. Maximum is four doses in 12 hours and 1.2 mL/dose.

➤ **Skin discomfort (irritation, itching, pain)**

🔵 *Alert:* For children weighing less than 10 kg, a single application should be applied over an area no greater than 100 cm². For children weighing between 10 and 20 kg, a single application should be applied over an area no greater than 600 cm².

Adults and children (5% ointment): Apply ointment topically for adequate control of symptoms. Maximum for adults is 5 g/single application (equivalent to lidocaine base 250 mg or approximately 6 inches of ointment) or 20 g of ointment (equivalent to lidocaine base 1,000 mg)/day. Maximum for children is 5 g/single application (equivalent to lidocaine base

250 mg or approximately 6 inches of ointment) or 4.5 mg/kg lidocaine base.

Adults and children ages 2 and older (cream, gel, spray): 4% cream or 4% gel or spray to affected areas t.i.d. to q.i.d. Or, 2% gel to affected areas t.i.d. as needed.

➤ **Local analgesia for venipuncture (Zingo)**

Adults and children ages 3 and older: Apply one intradermal lidocaine (0.5 mg) device to site planned for venipuncture 1 to 3 minutes before needle insertion.

➤ **Anorectal discomfort**

Adults and children ages 12 and older: Apply 5% cream or 5% gel to affected area up to six times a day.

➤ **Postherpetic neuralgia**

Adults: Apply 5% patch to most painful area for up to 12 hours in any 24-hour period. Maximum, 3 patches in a single application.

➤ **Ocular surface anesthesia (Akten)**

Adults and children: Apply 2 drops to ocular surface in area of planned procedure. Reapply as needed to maintain anesthetic effect. ∎

---

liothyronine sodium (T₃)

lye-oh-THYE-roe-neen

Cytomel

Therapeutic class: Thyroid hormone replacements
Pharmacologic class: Thyroid hormones

AVAILABLE FORMS

Injection: 10 mcg/mL in 1-mL vials*
Tablets: 5 mcg, 25 mcg, 50 mcg

INDICATIONS & DOSAGES

Boxed Warning Drugs with thyroid hormone activity, alone or with other therapeutic agents, shouldn't be used for treatment of obesity or for weight loss. Dosage beyond daily hormonal requirements may produce serious or even life-threatening toxicity. ∎

➤ **Myxedema coma, premyxedema coma**

Adults: Initially, 10 to 20 mcg IV for patients with CV disease; 25 to 50 mcg IV for patients who don't have CV disease. Adjust dosage based on patient's condition and response. Switch patient to oral therapy as soon as possible.

➤ **Thyroid hormone replacement**

Adults: Initially, 25 mcg PO daily; increase by up to 25 mcg every 1 to 2 weeks until satisfactory response occurs. Usual maintenance dosage, 25 to 75 mcg daily.

Children: 5 mcg daily; increase by 5 mcg daily every 3 to 4 days until desired response. For maintenance, infants may require only 20 mcg daily; children ages 1 to 3 may require 50 mcg daily; and children older than age 3 may require full adult dosage.

Adjust-a-dose: For older adults and patients with CV disease, give 5 mcg once daily; may increase by 5 mcg/day every 2 weeks. Consider a lower starting dose in infants up to 3 months who are at risk for HF. For children at risk for hyperactivity, start at one-fourth the recommended full replacement dose and increase weekly by one-fourth the full dose until full recommended dose is reached.

➤ **TSH suppression in patients with well-differentiated thyroid cancer**

Adults: Adjust PO dosage based on desired therapeutic range.

➤ **T₃ suppression test to differentiate hyperthyroidism from euthyroidism**

Adults: 75 to 100 mcg PO daily for 7 days; radioactive iodine uptake is determined before and after hormone administration.

---

lomitapide mesylate ⚕
lom-i-TA-pide

Juxtapid

Therapeutic class: Antilipemics
Pharmacologic class: Microsomal triglyceride transfer protein inhibitors

AVAILABLE FORMS
Capsules ⓒ: 5 mg, 10 mg, 20 mg, 30 mg

INDICATIONS & DOSAGES
Boxed Warning Drug may cause increased transaminase levels or steatosis. Due to risk of liver toxicity, drug is only indicated in patients with clinical or laboratory diagnosis consistent with homozygous familial hypercholesterolemia (HoFH). ∎

➤ **Adjunct to low-fat diet and other lipid-lowering treatments, including LDL apheresis where available, to reduce LDL, total cholesterol, apolipoprotein B, and non-HDL cholesterol levels in patients with HoFH** ⚕

Adults: 5 mg PO once daily. May increase to 10 mg daily after at least 2 weeks; may increase at least 4 weeks later to 20 mg, then at least 4 weeks later to 40 mg, then at least 4 weeks later to 60 mg. Measure ALT, AST, ALP, and total bilirubin levels with any dosage increase. Maximum, 60 mg daily.

Adjust-a-dose: In patients with KF receiving dialysis and in patients with Child-Pugh class A liver impairment, don't exceed 40 mg PO daily. Maximum dosage is 30 mg daily with concomitant weak CYP3A4 inhibitors and 40 mg daily with concomitant oral contraceptives. Refer to manufacturer's instructions for drug-interaction and toxicity-related dosage adjustments.

SAFETY ALERT!

lomustine (CCNU)
loe-MUS-teen

Gleostine

Therapeutic class: Antineoplastics
Pharmacologic class: Nitrosoureas

AVAILABLE FORMS
Capsules: 10 mg, 40 mg, 100 mg

INDICATIONS & DOSAGES
Boxed Warning Drug can cause severe and fatal myelosuppression. Monitor blood cell counts

weekly for at least 6 weeks after a dose. Ensure that patient is prescribed and takes only a single dose every 6 weeks. Fatal toxicity occurs with overdose. ∎

➤ **Brain tumor, Hodgkin lymphoma**

Adults and children: 130 mg/m² PO as single dose every 6 weeks. Round doses to nearest 10 mg. Don't give repeat doses until WBC exceeds 4,000/mm³ and platelet count is greater than 100,000/mm³.

Adjust-a-dose: Reduce dosage to 100 mg/m² once every 6 weeks in patients with compromised bone marrow function. Refer to manufacturer's instructions for dosage adjustments for hematologic toxicity or use with other myelosuppressive drugs.

---

lumacaftor–ivacaftor ⚕
LOO-ma-kaf-tor/EYE-va-kaf-tor

Orkambi

Therapeutic class: Metabolic agents
Pharmacologic class: Cystic fibrosis transmembrane conductance regulator (CFTR) potentiators

AVAILABLE FORMS
Granules: lumacaftor 75 mg/ivacaftor 94 mg, 100 mg lumacaftor/125 mg ivacaftor, 150 mg lumacaftor/188 mg ivacaftor
Tablets: 100 mg lumacaftor/125 mg ivacaftor, 200 mg lumacaftor/125 mg ivacaftor

INDICATIONS & DOSAGES
➤ **Cystic fibrosis in patients who are homozygous for the F508del mutation in the *CFTR* gene** ⚕

Adults and children ages 12 and older: 400 mg lumacaftor/250 mg ivacaftor PO every 12 hours with fat-containing food.

Children ages 6 to 11: 200 mg lumacaftor/250 mg ivacaftor PO every 12 hours with fat-containing food.

Children ages 2 to 5 weighing 14 kg or more: 150 mg lumacaftor/188 mg ivacaftor packet of granules every 12 hours with fat-containing food.

Children ages 2 to 5 weighing less than 14 kg: 100 mg lumacaftor/125 mg ivacaftor packet of granules PO every 12 hours with fat-containing food.

Children ages 1 to 2 weighing 14 kg or more: lumacaftor 150 mg/ivacaftor 188 mg packet of granules PO every 12 hours with fat-containing food.

Children ages 1 to 2 weighing 9 to less than 14 kg: lumacaftor 100 mg/ivacaftor 125 mg packet of granules PO every 12 hours with fat-containing food.

Children ages 1 to 2 weighing 7 to less than 9 kg: lumacaftor 75 mg/ivacaftor 94 mg packet of granules PO every 12 hours with fat-containing food.

Adjust-a-dose: Refer to manufacturer's instructions for liver impairment, drug-interaction, and toxicity-related dosage adjustments.

lumasiran ☒
loo-ma-SIR-an

Oxlumo

Therapeutic class: Metabolic agents
Pharmacologic class: Hydroxyacid oxidase 1-directed small interfering RNA

AVAILABLE FORMS
Injection: 94.5 mg/0.5 mL single-dose vials

INDICATIONS & DOSAGES
➤ **Primary hyperoxaluria type 1 to lower urinary oxalate levels** ☒
Adults and children weighing 20 kg or more: 3 mg/kg subcut once monthly for 3 months; then 3 mg/kg subcut once every 3 months.
Children weighing 10 to less than 20 kg: 6 mg/kg subcut once monthly for 3 months; then 6 mg/kg subcut once every 3 months.
Children weighing less than 10 kg: 6 mg/kg subcut once monthly for 3 months; then 3 mg/kg subcut once monthly.

lumateperone
loo-ma-TE-per-one

Caplyta

Therapeutic class: Antipsychotics
Pharmacologic class: Central serotonin and dopamine receptor antagonists

AVAILABLE FORMS
Capsules: 10.5 mg, 21 mg, 42 mg

INDICATIONS & DOSAGES
Boxed Warning Antidepressants increase risk of suicidality in children, adolescents, and young adults. Drug isn't approved for use in children. ■
Boxed Warning Older adults with dementia-related psychosis treated with antipsychotics are at increased risk for death; drug isn't approved for treatment of dementia-related psychosis. ■
Adjust-a-dose (all indications): For patients who have Child-Pugh class B or C liver impairment or who take a moderate CYP3A4 inhibitor, decrease lumateperone dosage to 21 mg once daily. If administered with strong CYP3A4 inhibitor, decrease lumateperone dosage to 10.5 mg once daily.
➤ **Schizophrenia; depressive episodes associated with bipolar I or II disorder (bipolar depression) as monotherapy or as adjunctive therapy with lithium or valproate**
Adults: 42 mg PO once daily.
SAFETY ALERT!

lurbinectedin
loor-bin-EK-te-din

Zepzelca

Therapeutic class: Antineoplastics
Pharmacologic class: Alkylating agents

AVAILABLE FORMS
Injection: 4-mg single-dose vial

INDICATIONS & DOSAGES
➤ **Metastatic SCLC with disease progression on or after platinum-based chemotherapy**
Adults: 3.2 mg/m² IV infusion over 60 minutes every 21 days until disease progresses or unacceptable toxicity occurs.
Adjust-a-dose: Initiate treatment only if ANC is at least 1,500 cells/mm³ and platelet count is at least 100,000/mm³. Refer to manufacturer's instructions for use with strong CYP3A inhibitors and for toxicity-related dosage adjustments.

lusutrombopag
loo-soo-TROM-boe-pag

Mulpleta

Therapeutic class: Hematopoietics
Pharmacologic class: Thrombopoietin receptor agonists

AVAILABLE FORMS
Tablets: 3 mg

INDICATIONS & DOSAGES
➤ **Thrombocytopenia in patients with chronic liver disease scheduled to undergo a procedure**
Adults: 3 mg PO once daily for 7 days, beginning 8 to 14 days before procedure. Procedure should occur 2 to 8 days after final dose.

mecasermin ☒
meh-KAH-sur-men

Increlex

Therapeutic class: Growth factors
Pharmacologic class: Human insulin growth factors

AVAILABLE FORMS
Injection: 10 mg/mL in 4-mL vials

INDICATIONS & DOSAGES
➤ **Growth failure in children with severe primary insulin growth factor-1 deficiency or children with growth hormone gene deletion who have developed neutralizing antibodies to growth hormone** ☒
Children ages 2 and older: Initially, 0.04 to 0.08 mg/kg subcut b.i.d. If well tolerated for at least 1 week, may increase by 0.04 mg/kg per dose to maximum of 0.12 mg/kg b.i.d.

meloxicam
mel-OX-i-kam

Therapeutic class: Antirheumatics
Pharmacologic class: NSAIDs

AVAILABLE FORMS
Capsules: 5 mg, 10 mg
Oral suspension: 7.5 mg/5 mL
Tablets: 7.5 mg, 15 mg

INDICATIONS & DOSAGES

Boxed Warning Contraindicated for the treatment of perioperative pain after CABG surgery. NSAIDs can increase risk of serious heart attack or stroke and GI adverse reactions (bleeding, ulceration, and perforation), which can be fatal. ■

Adjust-a-dose (for all indications): Use isn't recommended in patients with CrCl of less than 20 mL/minute, as drug hasn't been studied in this population. If patient is receiving hemodialysis, give no more than 7.5-mg tablet or oral suspension or 5-mg capsule once daily.

➤ **To relieve signs and symptoms of osteoarthritis or RA**

Adults: 7.5 mg PO tablets or suspension once daily; may increase as needed to maximum of 15 mg daily. For osteoarthritis only, 5 mg capsule PO once daily; may increase to 10 mg in patients who require additional analgesia. Use lowest effective dosage for shortest duration consistent with individual patient treatment goals.

➤ **To relieve signs and symptoms of pauciarticular or polyarticular course juvenile RA**

Children weighing 60 kg or more: 7.5 mg PO daily.
Children ages 2 and older: 0.125 mg/kg oral suspension PO once daily, up to maximum of 7.5 mg.

---

menotropins
men-oh-TROE-pins

Menopur

Therapeutic class: Ovulation stimulants
Pharmacologic class: Gonadotropins

AVAILABLE FORMS
Injection: 75 international units of LH activity and 75 international units of FSH per vial

INDICATIONS & DOSAGES
➤ **Assisted reproductive technologies**

Adults: Initially, 225 units subcut into lower abdomen daily starting on cycle day 2 or 3. Menopur may be used in combination with urofollitropin, but total initial dose of both shouldn't exceed 225 units (150 international units of menotropins and 75 international units of urofollitropin or 75 international units of menotropins and 150 international units of urofollitropin). Adjust dosage after 5 days based on ovarian response (determined by ultrasound evaluation of follicular growth and serum estradiol level). Don't make additional adjustments more frequently than every 2 days and don't exceed 150 units per adjustment. Maximum, 450 units daily. Use for maximum of 20 days.

---

mepolizumab
me-poe-LIZ-ue-mab

Nucala

Therapeutic class: Miscellaneous respiratory drugs
Pharmacologic class: Monoclonal antibodies

AVAILABLE FORMS
Injection: 40 mg/0.4 mL, 100 mg/mL single-dose pre-filled syringe; 100 mg/mL single-dose autoinjector; 100-mg single-dose vials

INDICATIONS & DOSAGES
➤ **Add-on maintenance treatment of severe asthma in patients with an eosinophilic phenotype**
Adults and children ages 12 and older: 100 mg subcut every 4 weeks.
Children ages 6 to 11: 40 mg subcut every 4 weeks.
➤ **Eosinophilic granulomatosis with polyangiitis**
Adults: 300 mg given as three separate 100-mg subcut injections once every 4 weeks.
➤ **Hypereosinophilic syndrome persisting for 6 months or more without an identifiable nonhematologic secondary cause**
Adults and children ages 12 and older: 300 mg given as three separate 100-mg subcut injections once every 4 weeks.
➤ **Add-on maintenance treatment of chronic rhinosinusitis with nasal polyps in patients with inadequate response to nasal corticosteroids**
Adults: 100 mg subcut once every 4 weeks.

---

methylergonovine maleate
meth-il-er-goe-NOE-veen

Methergine

Therapeutic class: Oxytocics
Pharmacologic class: Ergot alkaloids

AVAILABLE FORMS
Injection: 0.2 mg/mL in 1-mL vials
Tablets: 0.2 mg

INDICATIONS & DOSAGES
➤ **Prevention and treatment of postpartum hemorrhage caused by uterine atony or subinvolution; control of uterine hemorrhage in second stage of labor**
Adults: 0.2 mg IM after delivery of anterior shoulder, after delivery of placenta, or during puerperium. May repeat every 2 to 4 hours as needed. During life-threatening emergencies, 0.2 mg IV over at least 1 minute while monitoring BP and uterine contractions. During puerperium, 0.2 mg PO every 6 to 8 hours for up to 7 days. Decrease dosage if severe cramping occurs.

SAFETY ALERT!

---

midostaurin ⚕
mi-doe-STOR-in

Rydapt

Therapeutic class: Antineoplastics
Pharmacologic class: Tyrosine kinase inhibitors

AVAILABLE FORMS
Capsules ⓄⓃⒸ: 25 mg

INDICATIONS & DOSAGES
Adjust-a-dose (for all indications): Refer to manufacturer's instructions for toxicity-related adjustments.

➤ **Newly diagnosed acute myeloid leukemia in patients with *FLT3* mutation in combination with daunorubicin and cytarabine** ⌧
Adults: 50 mg PO b.i.d. with food on days 8 to 21 of each induction cycle (in combination with daunorubicin and cytarabine) and on days 8 to 21 of each consolidation cycle (in combination with high-dose cytarabine).
➤ **Aggressive systemic mastocytosis, systemic mastocytosis with associated hematologic neoplasm, or mast cell leukemia**
Adults: 100 mg PO b.i.d. with food until disease progresses or unacceptable toxicity occurs.

migalastat hydrochloride ⌧
mi-GAL-a-stat

Galafold

Therapeutic class: Metabolic agents
Pharmacologic class: Pharmacological chaperones

AVAILABLE FORMS
Capsules ⓞⓣⓒ: 123 mg

INDICATIONS & DOSAGES
➤ **Confirmed Fabry disease with an amenable galactosidase alpha gene variant** ⌧
Adults: 123 mg PO once every other day, at the same time of day.

miSOPROStol
mye-soe-PROST-ole

Cytotec

Therapeutic class: Antiulcer drugs
Pharmacologic class: Prostaglandin E_1 analogues

AVAILABLE FORMS
Tablets: 100 mcg, 200 mcg

INDICATIONS & DOSAGES
Boxed Warning Drug can cause abortion, premature birth, birth defects, and uterine rupture and is contraindicated during pregnancy. Advise patients of the risk; warn them not to give drug to others. ■
➤ **Prevention of NSAID-induced gastric ulcer**
Adults: 200 mcg PO q.i.d. with food; if not tolerated, decrease to 100 mcg PO q.i.d. Give dosage for duration of NSAID therapy.

moexipril hydrochloride
moe-EX-eh-pril

Therapeutic class: Antihypertensives
Pharmacologic class: ACE inhibitors

AVAILABLE FORMS
Tablets: 7.5 mg, 15 mg

INDICATIONS & DOSAGES
Boxed Warning Drugs that act directly on the RAAS can cause fetal harm; when pregnancy is detected, discontinue as soon as possible. ■

➤ **HTN, alone or in combination with thiazide diuretics**
Adults: Initially, 7.5 mg PO once daily as monotherapy, given 1 hour before a meal. Or initially, 3.75 mg if diuretic therapy can't be discontinued. Increase dosage incrementally according to BP response. Recommended dosage range, 7.5 to 30 mg daily in one or two divided doses.
Adjust-a-dose: For patients currently being treated with a diuretic, if possible, stop diuretic 2 to 3 days before therapy is initiated to reduce likelihood of hypotension. If BP isn't adequately controlled with moexipril alone, may reinstitute diuretic therapy. For patients with CrCl of 40 mL/minute/1.73 m² or less, cautiously give initial dosage of 3.75 mg once daily. May titrate upward to maximum of 15 mg daily.

moxetumomab pasudotox-tdfk
MOX-e-toom-oh-mab pa-SOO-doe-tox

Lumoxiti

Therapeutic class: Antineoplastics
Pharmacologic class: Anti-CD22s

AVAILABLE FORMS
Injection (lyophilized cake or powder): 1 mg/mL single-dose vial

INDICATIONS & DOSAGES
Boxed Warning Drug can cause capillary leak syndrome and hemolytic-uremic syndrome. Monitor patient closely and delay or discontinue drug as recommended. ■
➤ **Relapsed or refractory hairy cell leukemia after at least two prior systemic therapies, including treatment with a purine nucleoside analogue**
Adults: 0.04 mg/kg IV infusion over 30 minutes on days 1, 3, and 5 of each 28-day cycle. Continue treatment for a maximum of six cycles unless disease progression or unacceptable toxicity occurs.
Adjust-a-dose: Refer to manufacturer's information for toxicity-related dosage adjustments.

nafarelin acetate ⌧
nah-FAR-eh-lin

Synarel

Therapeutic class: Endocrine-metabolic agents
Pharmacologic class: Gonadotropin-releasing hormone analogues

AVAILABLE FORMS
Nasal spray: 2 mg/mL (200 mcg/spray)

INDICATIONS & DOSAGES
➤ **Central precocious puberty** ⌧
Children ages 8 and younger (females) or ages 9 and younger (males): 2 sprays (400 mcg) into each nostril in the morning and evening, for a total of 8 sprays (1,600 mcg) per day. If necessary, may increase dosage to a total of 9 sprays (1,800 mcg) per day, administered as 3 sprays (600 mcg) into alternating nostrils

---

t.i.d. Continue treatment until resumption of puberty is desired.

➤ **Endometriosis**

Adults: Begin treatment between days 2 and 4 of menstrual cycle. Administer 1 spray (200 mcg) into one nostril in the morning and 1 spray (200 mcg) into the other nostril in the evening for a total of 2 sprays (400 mcg) per day. If persistent regular menstruation continues after 2 months of treatment, increase dose to 1 spray (200 mcg) into each nostril in the morning and 1 spray (200 mcg) into each nostril in the evening, for a total of 4 sprays (800 mcg) per day. Recommended duration of treatment is 6 months.

nefazodone hydrochloride
ne-FAZ-oh-done

Therapeutic class: Antidepressants
Pharmacologic class: Antidepressants

AVAILABLE FORMS
Tablets: 50 mg, 100 mg, 150 mg, 200 mg, 250 mg

INDICATIONS & DOSAGES
Boxed Warning Antidepressants increase risk of suicidality in children, adolescents, and young adults. Drug isn't approved for use in children. ∎
Boxed Warning Life-threatening liver failure has been reported; discontinue drug if clinical signs or symptoms suggest liver failure or hepatocellular injury. ∎

➤ **Depression**

Adults: Initially, 100 mg/day PO b.i.d. Increase dosage in increments of 100 to 200 mg/day in two divided doses at intervals of no less than 1 week. Effective dosage range is 300 to 600 mg/day.

Adjust-a-dose: In older adults and patients who are debilitated, especially women, initially 50 mg PO b.i.d. Don't start drug until 14 days after administration of an MAO inhibitor.

SAFETY ALERT!

nelarabine
neh-LAR-uh-been

Arranon, Atriance ♣

Therapeutic class: Antineoplastics
Pharmacologic class: DNA demethylation agents; prodrugs of cytotoxic deoxyguanosine

AVAILABLE FORMS
Injection: 5 mg/mL in 50-mL vials

INDICATIONS & DOSAGES
Boxed Warning Severe neurologic adverse reactions have been reported, including altered mental states, CNS effects (including seizures), and peripheral neuropathy, ranging from numbness and paresthesia to motor weakness and paralysis. ∎

➤ **Relapsed or refractory T-cell acute lymphoblastic leukemia and T-cell lymphoblastic lymphoma after treatment with at least two chemotherapy regimens**

Adults: 1,500 mg/m^2 IV over 2 hours on days 1, 3, and 5. Repeat every 21 days.

Children ages 1 year and older: 650 mg/m^2 IV over 1 hour daily for 5 consecutive days. Repeat every 21 days.

Adjust-a-dose: Continue therapy until transplant, disease progression, or unacceptable toxicity occurs or until patient no longer benefits from therapy. Refer to manufacturer's information for toxicity-related dosage adjustments.

niMODipine
nye-MOE-dih-peen

Nymalize

Therapeutic class: Vasodilators
Pharmacologic class: Calcium channel blockers

AVAILABLE FORMS
Capsules (DNC): 30 mg
Oral solution: 6 mg/mL in 5-mL and 10-mL prefilled oral syringe; 60 mg/10 mL in 237-mL bottle

INDICATIONS & DOSAGES
Boxed Warning Don't administer parenterally; may cause life-threatening reactions and death. ∎

➤ **To improve neurologic deficits after subarachnoid hemorrhage from ruptured intracranial berry aneurysm**

Adults: 60 mg PO every 4 hours, given 1 hour before or 2 hours after a meal, for 21 days. Begin therapy within 96 hours after subarachnoid hemorrhage.

Adjust-a-dose: For patients with Child-Pugh class C liver impairment, 30 mg PO every 4 hours for 21 days.

nintedanib esylate
nin-TED-a-nib

Ofev

Therapeutic class: Miscellaneous respiratory drugs
Pharmacologic class: Tyrosine kinase inhibitors

AVAILABLE FORMS
Capsules (DNC): 100 mg, 150 mg

INDICATIONS & DOSAGES
➤ **Idiopathic pulmonary fibrosis; chronic fibrosing ILD with a progressive phenotype; to slow rate of decline in pulmonary function in patients with systemic sclerosis-associated ILD**

Adults: 150 mg PO b.i.d. approximately 12 hours apart with food.

Adjust-a-dose: In patients with Child-Pugh class A liver impairment, give 100 mg b.i.d. Refer to manufacturer's instructions for toxicity-related dosage adjustments.

nisoldipine
nye-SOHL-di-peen

Sular

Therapeutic class: Antihypertensives
Pharmacologic class: Calcium channel blockers

AVAILABLE FORMS
Tablets (extended-release) ⓓ*:* 8.5 mg, 17 mg, 20 mg, 25.5 mg, 30 mg, 34 mg, 40 mg

INDICATIONS & DOSAGES
➤ **HTN**
Adults: Dosage must be adjusted to each patient's needs. Initially, 17 mg PO once daily, 1 hour before or 2 hours after a meal; increased by 8.5 mg/week or at longer intervals, as needed. Usual maintenance dosage, 17 to 34 mg daily; dosages of more than 34 mg daily aren't recommended.

Or, initially, 20 mg PO once daily, 1 hour before or 2 hours after a meal; increased by 10 mg/week or at longer intervals, as needed. Usual maintenance dosage, 20 to 40 mg daily. Dosages of more than 60 mg daily aren't recommended.
Adjust-a-dose: For patients older than age 65 or patients with liver impairment, initially 8.5 to 10 mg PO once daily; adjust dosage as for other adults.

nitazoxanide
nye-te-ZOCKS-a-nide

Alinia

Therapeutic class: Antiprotozoals
Pharmacologic class: Antiprotozoals

AVAILABLE FORMS
Oral suspension: 100 mg/5 mL
Tablets: 500 mg

INDICATIONS & DOSAGES
➤ **Diarrhea caused by *Cryptosporidium parvum* or *Giardia lamblia***
Adults and children ages 12 and older: 500 mg PO with food every 12 hours for 3 days.
Children ages 4 to 11: 200 mg (10 mL) PO with food every 12 hours for 3 days.
Children ages 1 to 3: 100 mg (5 mL) PO with food every 12 hours for 3 days.

nusinersen sodium
neu-si-NER-sen

Spinraza

Therapeutic class: Miscellaneous CNS drugs
Pharmacologic class: Antisense oligonucleotides

AVAILABLE FORMS
Injection: 12 mg/5 mL single-use vials

INDICATIONS & DOSAGES
➤ **Spinal muscular atrophy**
Adults and children: Initially, 12 mg (5 mL) intrathecally once every 14 days for three doses; then fourth dose of 12 mg intrathecally 30 days after third dose. Maintenance dose of 12 mg intrathecally once every 4 months thereafter.

obeticholic acid
oh-BET-i-kol-ik

Ocaliva

Therapeutic class: Miscellaneous GI drugs
Pharmacologic class: Farnesoid X receptor agonists

AVAILABLE FORMS
Tablets: 5 mg, 10 mg

INDICATIONS & DOSAGES
Boxed Warning Liver decompensation and failure, in some cases fatal, have been reported in patients with primary biliary cholangitis with cirrhosis. Permanently discontinue in patients with clinical evidence of liver decompensation, compensated cirrhosis with evidence of portal HTN, or clinically significant liver adverse reactions. ∎
➤ **Primary biliary cholangitis in combination with ursodeoxycholic acid (UDCA) in patients with an inadequate response to UDCA or as monotherapy in patients unable to tolerate UDCA**
Adults: 5 mg PO once daily in patients without cirrhosis or with compensated cirrhosis without portal HTN who haven't achieved an adequate biochemical response to an appropriate dosage of UDCA for at least 1 year or are intolerant to UDCA. If adequate reduction in alkaline phosphatase or total bilirubin level hasn't been achieved after 3 months and patient is tolerating drug, increase to maximum of 10 mg once daily.
Adjust-a-dose: For patients with intolerable pruritus, consider one or more of these options: Add an antihistamine or a bile-acid binding resin, decrease dosage (to 5 mg every other day for patients unable to tolerate 5 mg daily or to 5 mg once daily for patients unable to tolerate 10 mg daily), or withhold drug for up to 2 weeks and then restart at reduced dosage. Discontinue drug in patients with persistent, intolerable pruritus despite management strategies.

obiltoxaximab
oh-bil-tox-AX-i-mab

Anthim

Therapeutic class: Antibodies
Pharmacologic class: Monoclonal antibodies

AVAILABLE FORMS
Injection: 600 mg/6 mL (100 mg/mL) single-dose vials

INDICATIONS & DOSAGES

Boxed Warning Because of risk of hypersensitivity and anaphylaxis, administer drug in a setting monitored by trained personnel and equipped to manage anaphylaxis. ∎

➤ **Inhalational anthrax due to *Bacillus anthracis* in combination with appropriate antibacterial drugs; prophylaxis of inhalational anthrax due to *B. anthracis* when alternative therapies aren't available or aren't appropriate**

Adults and children weighing more than 40 kg: 16 mg/kg/dose IV over 90 minutes as single dose. *Adults weighing 40 kg or less and children weighing more than 15 to 40 kg:* 24 mg/kg/dose IV over 90 minutes as single dose. *Children weighing 15 kg or less:* 32 mg/kg/dose IV over 90 minutes as single dose.

odevixibat ✄
oh-de-VIX-i-bat

Bylvay

Therapeutic class: Miscellaneous GI drugs
Pharmacologic class: Bile acid transporter inhibitors

AVAILABLE FORMS
Capsules 🔵*:* 400 mcg, 1,200 mcg
Oral pellets: 200 mcg, 600 mcg

INDICATIONS & DOSAGES
Adjust-a-dose (all indications): Refer to manufacturer's instructions for toxicity-related dosage adjustments.

➤ **Pruritus in patients with progressive familial intrahepatic cholestasis ✄**

Adults and children ages 3 months and older: 40 mcg/kg PO daily with morning meal. If no improvement after 3 months, increase dosage in 40-mcg/kg increments up to 120 mcg/kg PO daily. Maximum, 6 mg daily.

✱ ***NEW INDICATION:*** **Cholestatic pruritus in patients with Alagille syndrome ✄**

Adults and children ages 12 months and older: 120 mg/kg PO once daily with morning meal.

ofloxacin (otic)
of-FLOKS-a-sin

Therapeutic class: Antibiotics
Pharmacologic class: Fluoroquinolones

AVAILABLE FORMS
Otic solution: 0.3%

INDICATIONS & DOSAGES
➤ **Chronic suppurative otitis media with perforated tympanic membrane**
Adults and children ages 12 and older: 10 drops into affected ear b.i.d. for 14 days.
➤ **Otitis externa**
Adults and children ages 13 and older: 10 drops into affected ear once daily for 7 days.

Children ages 6 months to younger than 13 years: 5 drops into affected ear once daily for 7 days.
➤ **Acute otitis media in children with tympanostomy tubes**
Children ages 1 to 12: 5 drops into affected ear b.i.d. for 10 days.

SAFETY ALERT!

olaparib ✄
oh-LAP-a-rib

Lynparza

Therapeutic class: Antineoplastics
Pharmacologic class: Poly ADP-ribose polymerase inhibitors

AVAILABLE FORMS
Tablets 🔵*:* 100 mg, 150 mg

INDICATIONS & DOSAGES
Adjust-a-dose (for all indications): For patients with CrCl of 31 to 50 mL/minute, reduce dosage to 200 mg PO b.i.d. Refer to manufacturer's instructions for toxicity-related dosage adjustments and drug's use with CYP3A inhibitors.

➤ **Maintenance treatment of recurrent epithelial ovarian, fallopian tube, or primary peritoneal cancer in patients who have complete or partial response to platinum-based chemotherapy**
Adults: 300 mg PO b.i.d. Continue treatment until disease progresses or unacceptable toxicity occurs.

➤ **First-line maintenance treatment (in combination with bevacizumab) of advanced epithelial ovarian, fallopian tube, or primary peritoneal cancer in adults who have complete or partial response to first-line, platinum-based chemotherapy and whose cancer is associated with homologous recombination deficiency-positive status, defined by either a deleterious or suspected deleterious *BRCA*-mutation or genomic instability ✄**
Adults: 300 mg PO b.i.d., continued until disease progresses or unacceptable toxicity occurs, or up to 2 years in patients with complete response. Give in combination with bevacizumab 15 mg/kg IV infusion every 3 weeks for a total of 15 months, including chemotherapy and maintenance doses.

➤ **Maintenance treatment of deleterious or suspected deleterious germline or somatic *BRCA*-mutated advanced epithelial ovarian, fallopian tube, or primary peritoneal cancer in patients who have complete or partial response to first-line platinum-based chemotherapy ✄**
Adults: 300 mg PO b.i.d. continued until disease progresses or unacceptable toxicity occurs, or up to 2 years in patients with complete response. Patient may continue beyond 2 years if continued treatment is beneficial.

➤ **Deleterious or suspected deleterious germline *BRCA*-mutated (*gBRCAm*), HER2-negative metastatic breast cancer in patients previously treated with chemotherapy in the neoadjuvant, adjuvant, or metastatic setting ✄**

Adults: 300 mg PO b.i.d. until disease progresses or unacceptable toxicity occurs.

➤ **Adjuvant treatment of deleterious or suspected deleterious *gBRCAm* HER2-negative, high-risk early breast cancer** ▩

Adults: 300 mg PO b.i.d. for 1 year, or until disease recurrence or unacceptable toxicity occurs.

➤ **First-line maintenance treatment of deleterious or suspected deleterious *gBRCAm* metastatic pancreatic adenocarcinoma in adults whose disease hasn't progressed on at least 16 weeks of a first-line, platinum-based chemotherapy regimen** ▩

Adults: 300 mg PO b.i.d. until disease progresses or unacceptable toxicity occurs.

➤ **Deleterious or suspected deleterious germline or somatic homologous recombination repair gene-mutated metastatic castration-resistant prostate cancer in adults who have progressed after prior enzalutamide or abiraterone treatment** ▩

Adults: 300 mg PO b.i.d. until disease progresses or unacceptable toxicity occurs. Patients should also receive a GnRH analogue or have had bilateral orchiectomy.

✴ *NEW INDICATION:* **Deleterious or suspected deleterious BRCA-mutated metastatic castration-resistant prostate cancer in combination with abiraterone and prednisone or prednisolone**

Adults: 300 mg PO b.i.d., until disease progresses or unacceptable toxicity occurs. Patients should also receive a GnRH analogue or have had bilateral orchiectomy. Recommended abiraterone dosage, 1,000 mg PO once daily in combination with prednisone or prednisolone 5 mg PO b.i.d. Refer to abiraterone prescribing information for more details.

olopatadine hydrochloride
oh-loh-PAT-ah-dine

Pataday

Therapeutic class: Antihistamines
Pharmacologic class: H_1-receptor antagonists

AVAILABLE FORMS
Nasal spray: 665 mcg/spray
Ophthalmic solution: 0.1% ◇, 0.2% ◇, 0.7% ◇

INDICATIONS & DOSAGES
➤ **Seasonal allergic rhinitis (nasal)**
Adults and children ages 12 and older: 2 sprays into each nostril b.i.d.
Children ages 6 to 11: 1 spray into each nostril b.i.d.
➤ **Allergic conjunctivitis**
Adults and children ages 2 and older: 1 drop (0.1%) in each affected eye b.i.d. at an interval of 6 to 8 hours.
Adults and children ages 2 and older: 1 drop (0.2%, 0.7%) in each affected eye once a day.

olsalazine sodium
ol-SAL-uh-zeen

Dipentum

Therapeutic class: Anti-inflammatory drugs
Pharmacologic class: Salicylates

AVAILABLE FORMS
Capsules: 250 mg

INDICATIONS & DOSAGES
➤ **Maintenance of remission of ulcerative colitis in patients intolerant of sulfasalazine**
Adults: 500 mg PO b.i.d.

onasemnogene abeparvovec-xioi ▩
on-a-SEM-noe-jeen a-be-PAR-voe-vek

Zolgensma

Therapeutic class: CNS agents
Pharmacologic class: Gene therapies

AVAILABLE FORMS
Injection: 2.0×10^{13} vector genomes (vg)/mL in vials of 5.5 mL or 8.3 mL in a kit of two to nine vials

INDICATIONS & DOSAGES
Boxed Warning Drug can cause acute liver failure with fatal outcomes. Assess liver function before infusion and monitor patient for at least 3 months after infusion. Give corticosteroids to all patients before and after drug infusion. ■
➤ **Spinal muscular atrophy with bi-allelic mutations in the survival motor neuron 1 gene** ▩
Children younger than age 2: 1.1×10^{14} vg/kg body weight as single IV infusion over 60 minutes.

orlistat
ORE-lah-stat

Alli ◇, Xenical

Therapeutic class: Antiobesity drugs
Pharmacologic class: Lipase inhibitors

AVAILABLE FORMS
Capsules: 60 mg ◇, 120 mg

INDICATIONS & DOSAGES
➤ **To manage obesity, including weight loss and weight maintenance with a reduced-calorie diet; to reduce risk of weight gain after previous weight loss**
Adults and children ages 12 and older: 120 mg PO t.i.d. with or up to 1 hour after each main meal containing fat.
➤ **Weight loss (OTC formulation)**
Adults ages 18 and older: One 60-mg capsule PO with each meal containing fat. Dosage shouldn't exceed 3 capsules a day.

❤Canada   ◇ OTC   ◆ Off-label use   ⊕Do not crush   *Liquid contains alcohol   ▩ Genetic

oxacillin sodium
oks-a-SIL-in

Therapeutic class: Antibiotics
Pharmacologic class: Penicillins

AVAILABLE FORMS
Injection: 1-g, 2-g, 10-g vials; 1 g/50 mL, 2 g/50 mL premixed solution

INDICATIONS & DOSAGES
➤ **Infections caused by penicillinase-producing staphylococci that have demonstrated susceptibility to the drug; empirical therapy in suspected cases of resistant staphylococcal infections**
Adults: For mild to moderate infections, 250 to 500 mg IV or IM every 4 to 6 hours. For severe infections, 1 g IV or IM every 4 to 6 hours.
Infants and children weighing less than 40 kg: For mild to moderate infections, 50 mg/kg/day IV or IM in equally divided doses every 6 hours. For severe infections, 100 mg/kg/day IV or IM in equally divided doses every 4 to 6 hours.
Premature infants and neonates: 25 mg/kg/day IV or IM.
Adjust-a-dose: Duration of therapy depends on type and severity of the infection and overall condition of patient. In severe infections, continue drug for at least 14 days. Continue drug for at least 48 hours after patient is afebrile and asymptomatic and cultures are negative. Treatment of endocarditis and osteomyelitis may require a longer duration of therapy. Consider dosage reduction in patients with known or suspected kidney impairment.

ozanimod
oh-ZAN-i-mod

Zeposia

Therapeutic class: MS drugs
Pharmacologic class: Sphingosine 1-phosphate receptor modulators

AVAILABLE FORMS
Capsules ⓞ: 0.23 mg, 0.46 mg, 0.92 mg

INDICATIONS & DOSAGES
➤ **Relapsing forms of MS, including clinically isolated syndrome, relapsing-remitting disease, and active secondary progressive disease; moderate to severe active ulcerative colitis**
Adults: Initially, 0.23 mg PO once daily on days 1 to 4, then 0.46 mg PO once daily on days 5 to 7, then maintenance dose of 0.92 mg PO once daily.
Adjust-a-dose: For patients with Child-Pugh class A or B liver impairment, give maintenance dosage of 0.92 mg every other day.

ozenoxacin
oz-en-OX-a-sin

Xepi

Therapeutic class: Antibiotics
Pharmacologic class: Quinolone antibiotics

AVAILABLE FORMS
Cream: 1%

INDICATIONS & DOSAGES
➤ **Impetigo due to *Staphylococcus aureus* or *Streptococcus pyogenes***
Adults and children ages 2 months and older: Apply thin layer topically to affected area b.i.d. for 5 days. Affected area may be up to 100 cm² in patients 12 years and older or 2% of BSA, not to exceed 100 cm² in patients younger than age 12 years.

SAFETY ALERT!

panitumumab ✄
pan-eh-TOO-moo-mab

Vectibix

Therapeutic class: Antineoplastics
Pharmacologic class: Monoclonal antibodies

AVAILABLE FORMS
Solution for infusion: 20 mg/mL

INDICATIONS & DOSAGES
Boxed Warning Dermatologic toxicities occur in 90%—and are severe in 15%—of patients receiving monotherapy. ■
➤ **Wild-type RAS (defined as wild-type in both KRAS and NRAS) metastatic colorectal cancer as first-line therapy in combination with FOLFOX (5-FU, leucovorin, oxaliplatin); as monotherapy following disease progression during or after fluoropyrimidine-, oxaliplatin-, and irinotecan-containing regimens ✄**
Adults: 6 mg/kg IV infusion over 60 minutes every 14 days as single agent or in combination with FOLFOX. For doses greater than 1,000 mg, infuse over 90 minutes.
Adjust-a-dose: For patients with mild or moderate (grade 1 or 2) infusion reactions, reduce infusion rate by 50%. For patients with severe infusion reactions, stop drug permanently. Refer to manufacturer's instructions for toxicity-related dosage adjustments and drug discontinuation.

parathyroid hormone
par-a-THYE-roid

Natpara

Therapeutic class: Hormone replacements
Pharmacologic class: Parathyroid hormone analogues

AVAILABLE FORMS
Injection: 25 mcg, 50 mcg, 75 mcg, 100 mcg multi-dose cartridges

INDICATIONS & DOSAGES

Boxed Warning May increase risk of osteosarcoma. Reserve use for patients for whom potential benefits outweigh this risk. ■

➤ **Adjunct to calcium and vitamin D to control hypocalcemia in patients with hypoparathyroidism who can't be well controlled on calcium supplements and active forms of vitamin D alone**

Adults: Initially, 50 mcg subcut once daily in thigh. Titrate maintenance dosage to lowest dosage that achieves a total albumin-corrected serum calcium level within lower half of normal total serum calcium range (between 8 and 9 mg/dL) without the need for active forms of vitamin D and with calcium supplementation sufficient to meet daily requirements. Maximum, 100 mcg daily.

Adjust-a-dose: If albumin-corrected serum calcium level can't be maintained above 8 mg/dL without an active form of vitamin D or oral calcium supplementation, may increase Natpara dosage in increments of 25 mcg every 4 weeks to maximum of 100 mcg daily. If total serum calcium level is repeatedly above 9 mg/dL after active form of vitamin D has been discontinued and calcium supplement has been decreased to a dosage sufficient to meet daily requirements, may decrease Natpara to 25 mcg/day.

patiromer sorbitex calcium
pa-TIR-oh-mer

Veltassa

Therapeutic class: Potassium-removing resins
Pharmacologic class: Cation exchange polymers

AVAILABLE FORMS
Oral powder: 8.4-g, 16.8-g, 25.2-g packets

INDICATIONS & DOSAGES
➤ **Nonemergency treatment of hyperkalemia**

Adults: Initially, 8.4 g PO once daily. Monitor serum potassium level and adjust dosage based on potassium level at intervals of 1 week or longer, in increments of 8.4 g, to reach desired potassium concentration. Maximum, 25.2 g once daily.

SAFETY ALERT!

PAZOPanib
paz-OH-pa-nib

Votrient

Therapeutic class: Antineoplastics
Pharmacologic class: Multi-tyrosine kinase inhibitors

AVAILABLE FORMS
Tablets ⓘ: 200 mg

INDICATIONS & DOSAGES
Boxed Warning Severe and fatal liver toxicity has been observed. ■

➤ **Advanced renal cell carcinoma; advanced soft-tissue sarcoma in patients who have received prior chemotherapy**

Adults: 800 mg PO daily at least 1 hour before or 2 hours after a meal. Continue until disease progresses or unacceptable toxicity occurs.

Adjust-a-dose: For patients with Child-Pugh class B liver impairment, give 200 mg PO daily. Drug isn't recommended for patients with Child-Pugh class C liver impairment. When coadministration of strong CYP3A4 inhibitors is necessary, decrease pazopanib dosage to 400 mg PO daily. Refer to manufacturer's instructions for toxicity-related dosage adjustments.

pegcetacoplan
peg-set-a-KOE-plan

Empaveli

Therapeutic class: Immunomodulators
Pharmacologic class: Complement inhibitors

AVAILABLE FORMS
Injection: 1,080 mg/20 mL (54 mg/mL) single-dose vial

INDICATIONS & DOSAGES
Boxed Warning Drug may increase risk of serious infections, including meningococcal infections. Comply with most current vaccine recommendations against encapsulated bacteria before treatment. ■

➤ **Paroxysmal nocturnal hemoglobinuria**

Adults: 1,080 mg subcut infusion twice weekly.

Adjust-a-dose: For LDH level greater than 2 × ULN, give 1,080 mg subcut infusion every 3 days. Monitor LDH level twice weekly for at least 4 weeks after dosage increase. To reduce risk of hemolysis with abrupt treatment discontinuation when switching from eculizumab, initiate pegcetacoplan while continuing eculizumab at current dose; after 4 weeks, discontinue eculizumab and continue pegcetacoplan. When switching from ravulizumab, initiate pegcetacoplan no more than 4 weeks after last dose of ravulizumab. Give 2 weeks of antibacterial prophylaxis to patient if drug must be started immediately and vaccines were given less than 2 weeks prior to start.

peginterferon beta-1a
peg-in-ter-FEER-on

Plegridy

Therapeutic class: Antivirals
Pharmacologic class: Biological response modifiers

AVAILABLE FORMS
Injection (IM): 125 mcg/0.5 mL in prefilled syringe
Injection (subcut): 63 mcg/0.5 mL, 94 mcg/0.5 mL, 125 mcg/0.5 mL in prefilled pen-injector or prefilled syringe

INDICATIONS & DOSAGES
➤ **Relapsing forms of MS**

Adults: 63 mcg subcut or IM on first day; 94 mcg subcut or IM on day 15; then, 125 mcg subcut or IM on day 29 and every 14 days thereafter.

pegloticase ⚛
peg-LOE-ti-kase

Krystexxa

Therapeutic class: Antigout agents
Pharmacologic class: Uric acid-specific enzymes

AVAILABLE FORMS
Injection: 8 mg/mL in 2-mL single-use vial

INDICATIONS & DOSAGES
Boxed Warning Drug can cause G6PD deficiency-associated hemolysis and methemoglobinemia. Screen patients at risk for G6PD deficiency before initiation. Due to risk of hypersensitivity and anaphylaxis, administer drug in a setting monitored by trained personnel and equipped to manage anaphylaxis, and premedicate with antihistamines and corticosteroids. Assess uric acid level before infusions and discontinue treatment if level increases above 6 mg/dL. ■

➤ **Chronic gout in patients refractory to conventional therapy**
Adults: 8 mg by IV infusion over no less than 120 minutes every 2 weeks.

pegvaliase-pqpz
peg-VAL-i-ase pqpz

Palynziq

Therapeutic class: Phenylalanine reducers
Pharmacologic class: Phenylalanine-metabolizing enzymes

AVAILABLE FORMS
Injection: 2.5 mg/0.5 mL, 10 mg/0.5 mL, 20 mg/mL in single-dose prefilled syringes

INDICATIONS & DOSAGES
Boxed Warning Due to risk of hypersensitivity and anaphylaxis, administer initial dose in a setting monitored by trained personnel and equipped to manage anaphylaxis. Instruct patient and patient's observer (if applicable) to recognize signs and symptoms of anaphylaxis if self-administering; confirm their competency. ■

➤ **To reduce blood phenylalanine concentrations in patients with phenylketonuria who have uncontrolled blood phenylalanine concentrations greater than 600 micromol/L on existing management**
Adults: Initially, 2.5 mg subcut once weekly for 4 weeks. Then titrate dosage in step-wise fashion over at least 5 weeks to achieve a dosage of 20 mg subcut once daily as follows: 2.5 mg subcut twice weekly for 1 week, then 10 mg subcut once weekly for 1 week, then 10 mg subcut twice weekly for 1 week, then 10 mg subcut four times per week for 1 week, then 10 mg subcut once daily for 1 week, then maintenance dosage of 20 mg subcut once daily for at least 24 weeks.

Consider a dosage increase to 40 mg subcut once daily in patients who have been maintained continuously on 20 mg once daily for at least 24 weeks and who haven't achieved a blood phenylalanine concentration of 600 micromol/L or less. Consider increasing to a maximum of 60 mg subcut once daily in patients who haven't achieved a response with 40 mg once daily continuous treatment for at least 16 weeks. Use lowest effective and tolerated dosage.
Adjust-a-dose: For patients with blood phenylalanine concentrations less than 30 micromol/L, may reduce dosage with or without dietary protein and phenylalanine intake modification to maintain phenylalanine level above 30 micromol/L. Discontinue drug in patients who haven't achieved a response after 16 weeks of continuous treatment with 60 mg subcut once daily.

pentoxifylline
pen-tox-IH-fi-leen

Therapeutic class: Hemorrheologic drugs
Pharmacologic class: Xanthine derivatives

AVAILABLE FORMS
Tablets (extended-release) ⊙⊙⊙*:* 400 mg

INDICATIONS & DOSAGES
➤ **Intermittent claudication from chronic occlusive vascular disease**
Adults: 400 mg PO t.i.d. with meals for at least 8 weeks.
Adjust-a-dose: For patients with CrCl less than 30 mL/minute, reduce dosage to 400 mg once daily. May decrease to 400 mg b.i.d. if GI and CNS adverse effects occur. If adverse effects persist, discontinue drug.

perampanel
per-AMP-an-ell

Fycompa

Therapeutic class: Anticonvulsants
Pharmacologic class: Noncompetitive AMPA receptor antagonists
Controlled substance schedule: III

AVAILABLE FORMS
Oral suspension: 0.5 mg/mL
Tablets: 2 mg, 4 mg, 6 mg, 8 mg, 10 mg, 12 mg

INDICATIONS & DOSAGES
Boxed Warning Serious or life-threatening psychiatric and behavioral adverse reactions are reported in patients with and without prior psychiatric history. ■
Adjust-a-dose (for all indications): In older adults and those with Child-Pugh class A or B liver impairment, don't increase dosage more frequently than every 2 weeks. In patients with Child-Pugh class A liver impairment, maximum dosage is 6 mg once daily; Child-Pugh class B liver impairment, 4 mg once daily. Refer to manufacturer's instructions for use with CYP3A4 inducers.

➤ **Monotherapy or adjunctive therapy for partial-onset seizures with or without secondarily generalized seizures in patients with epilepsy**

Adults and children ages 4 and older: Initially, 2 mg PO once daily at bedtime. Increase dosage no more frequently than weekly intervals by increments of 2 mg once daily. Base dosage increases on clinical response and tolerability. Recommended maintenance dosage, 8 to 12 mg once daily at bedtime, although some patients may respond to 4 mg once daily.

➤ **Adjunctive therapy in treatment of primary generalized tonic-clonic seizures in patients with epilepsy**

Adults and children ages 12 and older: Initially, 2 mg PO once daily at bedtime. Increase dosage no more frequently than weekly intervals by increments of 2 mg once daily. Base dosage increases on clinical response and tolerability. Recommended maintenance dose, 8 mg once daily at bedtime, although if needed, may increase to 12 mg once daily.

---

peramivir
per-AM-i-vir

Rapivab

Therapeutic class: Antivirals
Pharmacologic class: Neuraminidase inhibitors

AVAILABLE FORMS
Injection: 200 mg/20 mL (10 mg/mL) vials

INDICATIONS & DOSAGES
➤ **Acute uncomplicated influenza in patients who have been symptomatic for no more than 2 days**

Adults and adolescents ages 13 and older: 600 mg IV infusion over 15 to 30 minutes as single dose.

Adjust-a-dose: For patients with CrCl of 30 to 49 mL/minute, dose is 200 mg; for patients with CrCl of 10 to 29 mL/minute, dose is 100 mg. For patients with KF requiring dialysis, give after dialysis at a dose adjusted for kidney function.

Children ages 6 months to 12 years: 12 mg/kg (up to 600 mg) IV infusion over 15 to 30 minutes as single dose.

Adjust-a-dose: For patients with CrCl of 30 to 49 mL/minute, dose is 4 mg/kg; for patients with CrCl of 10 to 29 mL/minute, dose is 2 mg/kg. For patients with KF requiring dialysis, give after dialysis at a dose adjusted for kidney function.

No data are available to support a recommended dosage adjustment for patients ages 6 months to younger than 2 years with CrCl less than 50 mL/minute.

---

perindopril erbumine
pur-IN-doh-pril

Coversyl✽

Therapeutic class: Antihypertensives
Pharmacologic class: ACE inhibitors

AVAILABLE FORMS
Tablets: 2 mg, 4 mg, 8 mg

INDICATIONS & DOSAGES
Boxed Warning Drugs that act directly on the RAAS can cause fetal harm; when pregnancy is detected, discontinue drug as soon as possible. ∎

Adjust-a-dose (for all indications): For patients with CrCl of 30 mL/minute or greater, initially 2 mg PO daily. Maximum maintenance dosage, 8 mg daily. Not recommended for patients with CrCl of less than 30 mL/minute. For patients taking diuretics, consider reducing diuretic dose before initiating drug. If diuretic therapy can't be altered, monitor patient closely for at least 2 hours after initiating perindopril and until BP has stabilized for another hour. Adjust dosage based on patient's BP response.

➤ **To reduce risk of CV death or nonfatal MI in patients with stable CAD**

Adults ages 70 or younger: 4 mg PO once daily for 2 weeks; then increase as tolerated to 8 mg once daily.
Adults older than age 70: Initially, 2 mg PO once daily for first week; then 4 mg once daily for second week and 8 mg once daily after that, if tolerated.

➤ **Essential HTN**

Adults: Initially, 4 mg PO once daily. Increase dosage until BP is controlled or to maximum of 16 mg/day. Usual maintenance dosage is 4 to 8 mg once daily; may be given in two divided doses.
Adults older than age 65: Initially, 4 mg PO daily as one dose or in two divided doses. May increase dosage by more than 8 mg/day with careful BP monitoring.

---

permethrin
per-METH-rin

Kwellada-P✽ ◇, Nix ◇

Therapeutic class: Scabicides-pediculicides
Pharmacologic class: Pyrethroids

AVAILABLE FORMS
Cream: 5%
Crème rinse /lotion: 1% ◇
Lotion: 5%✽ ◇

INDICATIONS & DOSAGES
➤ **Infestation with *Pediculus humanus capitis* (head louse) and its nits (crème rinse/lotion)**

Adults and children ages 2 months and older: Use after hair has been washed with conditioner-free shampoo, rinsed with water, and towel dried. Apply enough (25 to 50 mL) of 1% formulation to saturate hair and scalp. Allow drug to remain on hair for 10 minutes before rinsing off with warm water. Remove remaining nits with comb. Usually only one application is needed. May repeat 7 days after first treatment if lice or nits are still present.

➤ **Infestation with *Sarcoptes scabiei* (5% cream or lotion)**

Adults and children ages 2 months and older: Thoroughly massage into skin from head to soles of feet. Treat infants on hairline, neck, scalp, temple, and forehead. Wash cream off after 8 to 14 hours. Usually, one application is needed. May retreat if living mites are observed 14 days after first treatment.

---

perphenidone
per-FEN-uh-zeen

Therapeutic class: Antipsychotics
Pharmacologic class: Phenothiazines

AVAILABLE FORMS
Tablets: 2 mg, 4 mg, 8 mg, 16 mg

INDICATIONS & DOSAGES
Boxed Warning Older adults with dementia-related psychosis treated with antipsychotics are at increased risk for death. Drug isn't approved to treat these patients. ■
➤ **Schizophrenia in patients who are nonhospitalized**
Adults: Initially, 4 to 8 mg PO t.i.d.; reduce as soon as possible to minimum effective dosage.
➤ **Schizophrenia in patients who are hospitalized**
Adults: Initially, 8 to 16 mg PO b.i.d., t.i.d., or q.i.d.; increase to 64 mg daily, as needed.
➤ **Severe nausea and vomiting**
Adults: 8 to 16 mg PO daily in divided doses to maximum of 24 mg. Reduce as soon as possible to minimum effective dosage.

pimavanserin tartrate
pim-a-VAN-ser-in

Nuplazid

Therapeutic class: Antipsychotics
Pharmacologic class: 5-HT receptor inverse agonist and antagonists

AVAILABLE FORMS
Capsules: 34 mg
Tablets: 10 mg

INDICATIONS & DOSAGES
Boxed Warning Older adults with dementia-related psychosis treated with antipsychotics are at increased risk for death. Drug isn't approved to treat these patients. ■
➤ **Hallucinations and delusions associated with Parkinson disease psychosis**
Adults: 34 mg PO once daily.
Adjust-a-dose: If drug is used with strong CYP3A4 inhibitors, reduce pimavanserin dosage to 10 mg once daily.

pirfenidone
pir-FEN-i-done

Esbriet

Therapeutic class: Miscellaneous respiratory drugs
Pharmacologic class: Antifibrotics

AVAILABLE FORMS
Capsules: 267 mg
Tablets: 267 mg, 534 mg, 801 mg

INDICATIONS & DOSAGES
➤ **Idiopathic pulmonary fibrosis**
Adults: Initially, 267 mg PO t.i.d. days 1 to 7 of therapy; then increase to 534 mg PO t.i.d. for 7 more days (days 8 to 14); then increase to 801 mg PO t.i.d. starting on day 15 of therapy. Maintenance dosage, 801 mg PO t.i.d. Maximum dosage, 2,403 mg/day.
Adjust-a-dose: If treatment is interrupted for 14 or more consecutive days, restart drug with 2-week titration period. Refer to manufacturer's instructions for toxicity-related dosage adjustments and use with CYP1A2 inhibitors.

pitolisant hydrochloride 🗶
pi-TOL-i-sant

Wakix

Therapeutic class: CNS stimulants
Pharmacologic class: Histamine-3 receptor antagonist/inverse agonists

AVAILABLE FORMS
Tablets: 4.45 mg, 17.8 mg

INDICATIONS & DOSAGES
➤ **Excessive daytime sleepiness or cataplexy in patients with narcolepsy**
Adults: Dosage ranges from 17.8 to 35.6 mg PO once daily in the morning upon wakening. Initially, 8.9 mg (two 4.45-mg tablets) PO once daily for 1 week. Week 2, increase to 17.8 mg (one 17.8-mg tablet) PO once daily. Week 3 may increase to maximum recommended dosage of 35.6 mg (two 17.8-mg tablets) PO once daily based on tolerability.
Adjust-a-dose: For patients with Child-Pugh class B liver impairment, initiate at 8.9 mg PO once daily and increase after 14 days to maximum dosage of 17.8 mg PO once daily. For patients with eGFR of 15 to 59 mL/minute/1.73 m^2 or patients known to be poor CYP2D6 metabolizers, initiate at 8.9 mg PO once daily and increase after 7 days to maximum dosage of 17.8 mg PO once daily. Refer to manufacturer's instruction for use with strong CYP2D6 inhibitors or CYP3A4 inducers.

plerixafor
pleh-RIX-uh-for

Mozobil

Therapeutic class: Hematopoietics
Pharmacologic class: CXCR4 chemokine receptor inhibitors

AVAILABLE FORMS
Injection: 24 mg/1.2 mL (20 mg/mL) in single-use vials

INDICATIONS & DOSAGES
➤ **To mobilize hematopoietic stem cells for collection and subsequent autologous transplantation in patients with non-Hodgkin lymphoma or multiple myeloma**

Adults: Initiate plerixafor after patient has received G-CSF (filgrastim) 10 mcg/kg once daily in the morning for 4 days. Give 0.24 mg/kg (actual body weight) subcut once daily or, for patients weighing 83 kg or less, give 20 mg fixed dose subcut once daily, approximately 11 hours before initiation of each apheresis. Repeat plerixafor dose for up to 4 consecutive evenings and administer G-CSF 10 mcg/kg on each day before apheresis. Don't exceed 40 mg/day.
Adjust-a-dose: For patients with CrCl of 50 mL/minute or less, give 0.16 mg/kg once daily (not to exceed 27 mg/day). For patients weighing 83 kg or less, give fixed dose of 13 mg.

potassium iodide
po-TASS-ee-um

Iosat ◇ , ThyroSafe ◇

Therapeutic class: Antihyperthyroid drugs
Pharmacologic class: Salts of stable iodine

AVAILABLE FORMS
Oral solution: 65 mg/mL ◇
Tablets: 65 mg, 130 mg

INDICATIONS & DOSAGES
➤ **Radiation protectant for thyroid gland**
Adults and children ages 12 to 18 weighing at least 68 kg: 130 mg PO every 24 hours for 10 to 14 days as directed by public health authorities. Repeat dosing in patients who are pregnant or breastfeeding as directed.
Children ages 3 to 12 and children ages 12 to 18 weighing less than 68 kg: 65 mg PO every 24 hours as directed by public health authorities.
Children older than 1 month to 3 years: 32.5 mg PO every 24 hours as directed by public health authorities.
Neonates from birth to 1 month: 16.25 mg PO every 24 hours as directed by public health authorities.

prabotulinumtoxinA-xvfs
pra-bot-ue-LYE-num-TOX-in-A

Jeuveau

Therapeutic class: Neuromuscular transmission blockers
Pharmacologic class: Acetylcholine release inhibitors

AVAILABLE FORMS
Injection: 100 units/single-dose vial

INDICATIONS & DOSAGES
Boxed Warning All botulinum toxin products can spread beyond intended injection area to produce symptoms lasting hours to weeks after injection. Drug isn't approved for treatment of spasticity. ▪
➤ **Temporary improvement in the appearance of moderate to severe glabellar lines associated with corrugator and/or procerus muscle activity**
Adults: Inject 0.1 mL (4 units) IM into each of the five sites for a total dose of 20 units. See prescribing information for diagram and complete administration instructions. Retreatment may occur no less than 3 months from prior dose. Consider cumulative dose

if other botulinum toxin agents have been used to treat other conditions.

SAFETY ALERT!

PRALAtrexate
pral-ah-TREX-ate

Folotyn

Therapeutic class: Antineoplastics
Pharmacologic class: Folate analogue metabolic inhibitors

AVAILABLE FORMS
Injection: 20 mg/mL in single-use vials

INDICATIONS & DOSAGES
➤ **Relapsed or refractory peripheral T- cell lymphoma**
Adults: 30 mg/m² IV push over 3 to 5 minutes weekly for 6 weeks in 7-week cycles until disease progresses or unacceptable toxicity occurs. Initiate supplementation with folic acid and vitamin B₁₂ before treatment.
Adjust-a-dose: Refer to manufacturer's instructions for dosage adjustments for adverse reactions.

SAFETY ALERT!

pralsetinib ☒
pral-SE-ti-nib

Gavreto

Therapeutic class: Antineoplastics
Pharmacologic class: Kinase inhibitors

AVAILABLE FORMS
Capsules: 100 mg

INDICATIONS & DOSAGES
Adjust-a-dose (for all indications): Refer to manufacturer's instructions for toxicity-related dosage adjustments and use with CYP3A inhibitors or inducers or P-gp inhibitors.
➤ **Metastatic *RET* fusion-positive NSCLC** ☒
Adults: 400 mg PO once daily. Continue until disease progresses or unacceptable toxicity occurs.
➤ **Advanced or metastatic *RET* fusion-positive thyroid cancer in patients who require systemic therapy and are radioactive iodine-refractory (if radioactive iodine is appropriate)** ☒
Adults and children ages 12 and older: 400 mg PO once daily. Continue until disease progresses or unacceptable toxicity occurs.

prasterone
PRAS-ter-one

Intrarosa

Therapeutic class: Hormone replacements
Pharmacologic class: Synthetic steroids

AVAILABLE FORMS
Vaginal insert: 6.5 mg

INDICATIONS & DOSAGES
➤ **Moderate to severe dyspareunia, a symptom of vulvar and vaginal atrophy, due to menopause**

Adults: 1 vaginal insert intravaginally once daily at bedtime.

pretomanid
pre-TOE-ma-nid

Therapeutic class: Antituberculotics
Pharmacologic class: Nitroimidazoles

AVAILABLE FORMS
Tablets ⓄⒹⒸ: 200 mg

INDICATIONS & DOSAGES
▶ **Pulmonary extensively drug-resistant, treatment-intolerant, or nonresponsive multidrug-resistant TB, in combination with bedaquiline and linezolid**
Adults: 200 mg PO once daily for 26 weeks. Give in combination with bedaquiline 400 mg PO once daily for 2 weeks followed by 200 mg 3 times per week, with at least 48 hours between doses, for 24 weeks for a total of 26 weeks and linezolid 1,200 mg daily PO for 26 weeks. May extend dosing of combination regimen beyond 26 weeks if necessary. Give regimen by directly observed therapy.
Adjust-a-dose: If AST elevations are accompanied by total bilirubin elevation greater than $2 \times ULN$, or are greater than $8 \times ULN$, or are greater than $5 \times ULN$ and persist beyond 2 weeks, interrupt treatment with the entire regimen. If myelosuppression, peripheral neuropathy, or optic neuropathy due to linezolid occurs, decrease linezolid dosage to 600 mg daily and, if necessary, further reduce dosage to 300 mg daily or interrupt dosing.

primaquine phosphate
PRIM-a-kwin

Therapeutic class: Antimalarials
Pharmacologic class: Aminoquinolines

AVAILABLE FORMS
Tablets: 26.3 mg (equivalent to 15-mg base)

INDICATIONS & DOSAGES
▶ **To prevent relapse of *Plasmodium vivax* malaria**
Adults: 1 tablet (15 mg base) PO daily for 14 days. Give concurrently with chloroquine.

primidone
PRI-mi-done

Mysoline

Therapeutic class: Anticonvulsants
Pharmacologic class: Barbiturate analogues

AVAILABLE FORMS
Tablets: 50 mg, 125 mg, 250 mg

INDICATIONS & DOSAGES
▶ **Control of grand mal, psychomotor, and focal epileptic seizures**
Adults and children ages 8 and older: Initially, 100 to 125 mg PO at bedtime on days 1 to 3; then 100 to 125 mg PO b.i.d. on days 4 to 6; then 100 to 125 mg

PO t.i.d. on days 7 to 9, followed by maintenance dosage of 250 mg PO t.i.d. May increase maintenance dosage to 250 mg q.i.d., if needed. May increase dosage to maximum of 2 g daily in divided doses. See manufacturer's instructions for beginning therapy in patients already receiving other anticonvulsants.
Children younger than age 8: Initially, 50 mg PO at bedtime for 3 days; then 50 mg PO b.i.d. for days 4 to 6; then 100 mg PO b.i.d. for days 7 to 9, followed by maintenance dosage of 125 to 250 mg PO t.i.d. or 10 to 25 mg/kg daily in divided doses.

probenecid
proe-BEN-e-sid

Therapeutic class: Uricosurics
Pharmacologic class: Sulfonamide derivatives

AVAILABLE FORMS
Tablets: 500 mg

INDICATIONS & DOSAGES
▶ **Adjunct to penicillin therapy**
Adults and children ages 15 and older weighing more than 50 kg: 500 mg PO q.i.d.
Children ages 2 to 14 or weighing 50 kg or less: Initially, 25 mg/kg or 0.7 g/m² PO; then 40 mg/kg/day or 1.2 g/m² in four divided doses daily.
▶ **Hyperuricemia of gout, gouty arthritis**
Adults: 250 mg PO b.i.d. for first week; then 500 mg b.i.d. Review maintenance dosage every 6 months and reduce daily dosage by increments of 500 mg, if indicated.

prucalopride succinate
proo-KAL-oh-pride

Motegrity

Therapeutic class: GI drugs
Pharmacologic class: Selective serotonin-4 ($5\text{-}HT_4$) receptor agonists

AVAILABLE FORMS
Tablets: 1 mg, 2 mg

INDICATIONS & DOSAGES
▶ **Chronic idiopathic constipation**
Adults: 2 mg PO once daily.
Adjust-a-dose: For patients with CrCl less than 30 mL/minute, decrease dosage to 1 mg PO once daily.

pyrazinamide
peer-a-ZIN-a-mide

Therapeutic class: Antituberculotics
Pharmacologic class: Nicotinamide analogues

AVAILABLE FORMS
Tablets: 500 mg

INDICATIONS & DOSAGES

➤ **Initial treatment of active TB with other anti-tuberculotics or after treatment failure with other primary drugs in any form of active TB**

Adults and children: 15 to 30 mg/kg PO once daily. Don't exceed 3 g/day. Or, 50 to 70 mg/kg lean body weight PO twice weekly. This dosage may exceed the recommended 3-g/day maximum dose, but an increased incidence of adverse reactions hasn't been reported. Administer pyrazinamide for first 2 months of a 6-month or longer treatment regimen for drug-susceptible TB. Treat known or suspected drug-resistant infections with individualized regimens, which may frequently include pyrazinamide.

Patients with HIV infection may need longer courses of therapy. Refer to the CDC (www.CDC.gov) for current treatment recommendations and complete drug regimens.

Adjust-a-dose: For older adults, use dosages at the low end of the dosing range.

SAFETY ALERT!

quINIDine gluconate
KWIN-i-deen

quINIDine sulfate
Therapeutic class: Antiarrhythmics
Pharmacologic class: Cinchona alkaloids

AVAILABLE FORMS
quinidine gluconate (62% quinidine base)
Tablets (extended-release) ⓄⓃⒸ: 324 mg
quinidine sulfate (83% quinidine base)
Tablets: 200 mg, 300 mg

INDICATIONS & DOSAGES
Boxed Warning Therapy for non-life-threatening arrhythmias may result in increased mortality; risk is probably greatest in patients with structural heart disease. ■

Adjust-a-dose (for all indications): In patients with liver impairment or HF, reduce dosage. Discontinue drug if QRS complex widens to 130% of pretreatment duration, QTc interval widens to 130% of pretreatment duration and is longer than 500 msec, P waves disappear, or patient develops significant tachycardia, symptomatic bradycardia, or hypotension.

➤ **Atrial flutter or fibrillation (pharmacologic conversion)**

Adults: For quinidine gluconate, 648 mg (two 324-mg tablets) PO every 8 hours if no cardioversion after three or four doses, may increase cautiously to desired effect. For quinidine sulfate, 400 mg PO every 6 hours. If no cardioversion after four or five doses, may increase cautiously to desired effect.

➤ **Paroxysmal atrial fibrillation or flutter; maintenance of sinus rhythm**

Adults: For quinidine gluconate, initially 324 mg (extended-release) every 8 to 12 hours. May increase dosage cautiously to desired effect to usual dosage range of 324 to 648 mg every 8 hours. For quinidine sulfate, initially 200 mg (immediate-release) every

6 hours. May increase dosage cautiously to desired effect.

➤ **Ventricular arrhythmias**

Note: Dosing regimens for suppression of life-threatening ventricular arrhythmias haven't been adequately studied. For patients with structural heart disease or other risk factors for toxicity, initiate or adjust dosage in a setting where continuous monitoring and resuscitation are available. Monitor patients for 2 to 3 days once the appropriate dosage has been achieved.

Adults: For quinidine gluconate, 324 mg (extended-release) every 8 to 12 hours. May increase dosage cautiously up to 648 mg every 8 to 12 hours. For quinidine sulfate, initially 200 mg (immediate-release) every 6 hours. May increase dosage cautiously up to 600 mg every 6 to 12 hours.

radioactive iodine (sodium iodide, ¹³¹I)
Hicon Sodium Iodide ¹³¹I Therapeutic

Therapeutic class: Radiopharmaceuticals
Pharmacologic class: Antithyroid drugs

AVAILABLE FORMS
All radioactivity concentrations are determined at time of calibration.
Capsules (diagnostic use): Radioactivity range, 100 mCi/capsule
Concentrated solution for preparation of capsules or oral solution: 250 mCi/0.25 mL, 500 mCi/0.5 mL, 1,000 mCi/mL vials

INDICATIONS & DOSAGES
➤ **Hyperthyroidism**
Adults: Usual dosage is 4 to 10 mCi PO. Dosage is based on estimated weight of thyroid gland and thyroid uptake.

➤ **Thyroid cancer**
Adults: Initially, 30 to 100 mCi PO, with subsequent doses of 100 to 200 mCi for metastases. Dosage is based on estimated malignant thyroid tissue and metastatic tissue as determined by total body scan. Repeat treatment according to clinical status.

➤ **Diagnostic procedures**
Adults: For thyroid function testing, 5 to 30 mCi PO 24 hours before uptake measurement. For thyroid imaging (scintigraphy), 50 to 100 mCi 16 to 24 hours before imaging.

ravulizumab-cwvz
rav-ue-LIZ-ue-mab
Ultomiris

Therapeutic class: Immunomodulators
Pharmacologic class: Complement inhibitors

AVAILABLE FORMS
Injection: 300 mg/30 mL (10 mg/mL), 300 mg/3 mL (100 mg/mL), 1,100 mg/11 mL (100 mg/mL) single-dose vials

INDICATIONS & DOSAGES

Boxed Warning Risk of life-threatening meningococcal infections and sepsis. ■

Adjust-a-dose (for all indications): Supplemental dosing is required for patients weighing 40 kg or more receiving concomitant plasma exchange (PE), plasmapheresis (PP), or intravenous immunoglobulin (IVIg). Additional dose is given within 4 hours after PE, PP, or IVIg and is based on weight, current dose, and concomitant treatment. Refer to manufacturer's instructions for ravulizumab-cwvz dosing.

➤ **Paroxysmal nocturnal hemoglobinuria; inhibition of complement-mediated thrombotic microangiopathy in patients with atypical hemolytic-uremic syndrome**

Adults and children ages 1 month and older weighing 100 kg or more: 3,000 mg IV infusion loading dose, followed by maintenance dose of 3,600 mg IV infusion in 2 weeks and once every 8 weeks thereafter.

Adults and children ages 1 month and older weighing 60 to less than 100 kg: 2,700 mg IV infusion loading dose, followed by maintenance dose of 3,300 mg IV infusion in 2 weeks and once every 8 weeks thereafter.

Adults and children ages 1 month and older weighing 40 to less than 60 kg: 2,400 mg IV infusion loading dose, followed by maintenance dose of 3,000 mg IV infusion in 2 weeks and once every 8 weeks thereafter.

Children ages 1 month and older weighing 30 to less than 40 kg: 1,200-mg IV loading dose, followed by maintenance dose of 2,700-mg IV infusion in 2 weeks and once every 8 weeks thereafter.

Children ages 1 month and older weighing 20 to less than 30 kg: 900-mg IV infusion loading dose, followed by maintenance dose of 2,100-mg IV infusion in 2 weeks and once every 8 weeks thereafter.

Children ages 1 month and older weighing 10 to less than 20 kg: 600-mg IV infusion loading dose, followed by maintenance dose of 600-mg IV infusion in 2 weeks and once every 4 weeks thereafter.

Children ages 1 month and older weighing 5 to less than 10 kg: 600-mg IV infusion loading dose, followed by maintenance dose of 300-mg IV infusion in 2 weeks and once every 4 weeks thereafter.

Patients switching from eculizumab to ravulizumab: Administer a ravulizumab loading dose 2 weeks after last eculizumab infusion; then follow maintenance dosing according to patient's weight.

➤ **Generalized myasthenia gravis in patients who are anti-acetylcholine receptor antibody-positive**

Adults weighing 100 kg or more: 3,000 mg IV infusion loading dose, followed by maintenance dose of 3,600 mg IV infusion in 2 weeks and once every 8 weeks thereafter.

Adults weighing 60 to less than 100 kg: 2,700 mg IV infusion loading dose, followed by maintenance dose of 3,300 mg IV infusion in 2 weeks and once every 8 weeks thereafter.

Adults weighing 40 to less than 60 kg: 2,400 mg IV infusion loading dose, followed by maintenance dose of 3,000 mg IV infusion in 2 weeks and once every 8 weeks thereafter.

Patients switching from eculizumab to ravulizumab: Administer a ravulizumab loading dose 2 weeks after last eculizumab infusion or 1 week after last eculizumab induction infusion; then follow maintenance dosing according to patient's weight.

SAFETY ALERT!

regorafenib ⌧

re-goe-RAF-e-nib

Stivarga

Therapeutic class: Antineoplastics
Pharmacologic class: Kinase inhibitors

AVAILABLE FORMS

Tablets: 40 mg

Boxed Warning May cause severe or fatal liver toxicity. Monitor closely. ■

Adjust-a-dose (for all indications): Refer to manufacturer's instructions for toxicity-related dosage adjustments and discontinuation.

➤ **Metastatic colorectal cancer previously treated with fluoropyrimidine-, oxaliplatin-, and irinotecan-based chemotherapy, an anti-vascular endothelial growth factor therapy and, if *KRAS* wild type, an anti-epidermal growth factor receptor therapy** ⌧

Adults: 160 mg PO once a day for first 21 days of each 28-day cycle. Continue therapy until disease progresses or unacceptable toxicity occurs.

➤ **Locally advanced, unresectable, or metastatic GI stromal tumor previously treated with imatinib mesylate and sunitinib malate**

Adults: 160 mg PO once daily for first 21 days of each 28-day cycle. Continue therapy until disease progresses or unacceptable toxicity occurs.

➤ **Hepatocellular carcinoma in patients previously treated with sorafenib**

Adults: 160 mg PO once daily for first 21 days of each 28-day cycle. Continue treatment until disease progresses or unacceptable toxicity occurs.

retapamulin

re-te-PAM-ue-lin

Altabax

Therapeutic class: Antibiotics
Pharmacologic class: Pleuromutilins

AVAILABLE FORMS

Topical ointment: 1%

INDICATIONS & DOSAGES

➤ **Impetigo due to *Staphylococcus aureus* (methicillin-susceptible isolates only) or *Streptococcus pyogenes***

Adults and children ages 9 months and older: Apply thin layer to affected area (up to 100 cm² in total BSA in adults or 2% total BSA in children) b.i.d. for 5 days.

SAFETY ALERT!

reteplase (recombinant)
RET-ah-place

Retavase Half-Kit, Retavase Kit

Therapeutic class: Thrombolytics
Pharmacologic class: Tissue plasminogen activators

AVAILABLE FORMS
Injection: 10 units/vial, in a kit with components for reconstitution of one or two single-use vials

INDICATIONS & DOSAGES
➤ **Acute ST-elevation MI (STEMI)**
Adults: Give bolus injection of 10 units as soon as possible after onset of STEMI. If complications, such as serious bleeding or anaphylactoid reaction, don't occur after first bolus, give second bolus of 10 units 30 minutes after start of first. Give each bolus IV over 2 minutes.

revefenacin
REV-e-fen-a-sin

Yupelri

Therapeutic class: Bronchodilators
Pharmacologic class: Anticholinergics

AVAILABLE FORMS
Solution for inhalation: 175 mcg/3 mL unit-dose vial

INDICATIONS & DOSAGES
➤ **Maintenance treatment of COPD**
Adults: 175 mcg oral inhalation via nebulizer once daily.

rifabutin
rif-ah-BYOO-tin

Mycobutin

Therapeutic class: Antituberculotics
Pharmacologic class: Semisynthetic ansamycins

AVAILABLE FORMS
Capsules: 150 mg

INDICATIONS & DOSAGES
➤ **To prevent disseminated *Mycobacterium avium* complex in patients with advanced HIV infection**
Adults: 300 mg PO daily as single dose. May give with food or give 150 mg b.i.d. to minimize GI distress.
Adjust-a-dose: For patients with CrCl of less than 30 mL/minute, reduce rifabutin dosage by 50%.

rifamycin
rif-a-MYE-sin

Aemcolo

Therapeutic class: Antibiotics
Pharmacologic class: Ansamycins

AVAILABLE FORMS
Tablets (delayed-release) ⓓⓝⓒ*:* 194 mg

INDICATIONS & DOSAGES
➤ **Travelers' diarrhea caused by noninvasive strains of *Escherichia coli***
Adults: 388 mg PO b.i.d. for 3 days.

riluzole
RIL-yoo-zole

Exservan, Rilutek, Tiglutik

Therapeutic class: Neuroprotectors
Pharmacologic class: Benzothiazoles

AVAILABLE FORMS
Film: 50 mg
Suspension (oral): 50 mg/10 mL
Tablets: 50 mg

INDICATIONS & DOSAGES
➤ **Amyotrophic lateral sclerosis**
Adults: 50 mg PO every 12 hours, taken on empty stomach 1 hour before or 2 hours after a meal.

rimegepant
ri-ME-je-pant

Nurtec ODT

Therapeutic class: Antimigraine drugs
Pharmacologic class: Calcitonin gene-related peptide receptor antagonists

AVAILABLE FORMS
Tablets (ODTs): 75 mg

INDICATIONS & DOSAGES
➤ **Acute migraine with or without aura**
Adults: 75 mg PO as single dose. Maximum, 75 mg in 24 hours; 18 doses in 30 days.
➤ **Prevention of episodic migraine**
Adults: 75 mg PO every other day.

riociguat
RYE-oh-sig-ue-at

Adempas

Therapeutic class: Vasodilators
Pharmacologic class: Soluble guanylate cyclase stimulators

AVAILABLE FORMS
Tablets: 0.5 mg, 1 mg, 1.5 mg, 2 mg, 2.5 mg

INDICATIONS & DOSAGES
Boxed Warning Drug may cause fetal harm. Exclude pregnancy before treatment; patient should avoid pregnancy for 1 month after treatment. For females, Adempas is available only through the Adempas REMS Program. ∎
➤ **Chronic thromboembolic pulmonary HTN (CTEPH) (WHO Group 4), after surgical treatment, or inoperable CTEPH, to improve exercise capacity and WHO functional class; pulmonary artery HTN (WHO Group 1) to improve exercise**

capacity and WHO functional class and to delay clinical worsening

Adults: Initially, 1 mg PO t.i.d. Increase dosage by 0.5 mg t.i.d. if systolic BP remains greater than 95 mm Hg and patient has no signs or symptoms of hypotension. Dosage increases should occur no less than 2 weeks apart. Titrate to highest tolerated dosage. Maximum, 2.5 mg PO t.i.d.

Adjust-a-dose: Patients unable to tolerate initial 1-mg dosage due to hypotension may start at 0.5 mg PO t.i.d. Decrease dosage by 0.5 mg PO t.i.d. in patients experiencing hypotension. Patients who smoke may need dosages titrated higher than 2.5 mg PO t.i.d. Patients who quit smoking during treatment may need a dosage decrease. Consider a starting dose of 0.5 mg PO t.i.d. for patients taking strong CYP and P-gp/BCRP inhibitors.

SAFETY ALERT!

ripretinib
rip-RE-ti-nib

Qinlock

Therapeutic class: Antineoplastics
Pharmacologic class: Tyrosine kinase inhibitors

AVAILABLE FORMS
Tablets ⬤: 50 mg

INDICATIONS & DOSAGES
➤ **Advanced GI stromal tumor in patients who have received prior treatment with three or more kinase inhibitors, including imatinib**
Adults: 150 mg PO once daily until disease progresses or unacceptable toxicity occurs.

Adjust-a-dose: For patients unable to avoid taking with a moderate CYP3A inducer, increase ripretinib dosage to 150 mg b.i.d. during coadministration. Resume once-daily ripretinib dosing 14 days after moderate CYP3A inducer is discontinued. Refer to manufacturer's instructions for toxicity-related dosage adjustments. Permanently discontinue drug if patient can't tolerate 100-mg dose.

risankizumab-rzaa
ris-an-KIZ-ue-mab

Skyrizi

Therapeutic class: Immunomodulators
Pharmacologic class: Interleukin-23 receptor antagonists

AVAILABLE FORMS
Injection (IV): 600 mg/10 mL single-dose vial
Injection (subcut): 75 mg/0.83 mL prefilled syringe, 90 mg/mL prefilled syringe; 150 mg/mL prefilled syringe or pen
Injection (subcut on-body injector): 180 mg/1.2 mL, 360 mg/2.4 mL (150 mg/mL) prefilled cartridge

INDICATIONS & DOSAGES
➤ **Moderate to severe plaque psoriasis in patients who are candidates for systemic therapy or phototherapy; active psoriatic arthritis**
Adults: 150 mg subcut at weeks 0 and 4 and every 12 weeks thereafter.
➤ **Moderately to severely active Crohn disease**
Adults: 600 mg IV infusion over at least 1 hour at weeks 0, 4, and 8; then 180 mg or 360 mg subcut at week 12 and every 8 weeks thereafter.

risdiplam ⬰
ris-DIP-lam

Evrysdi

Therapeutic class: Miscellaneous CNS drugs
Pharmacologic class: Survival of motor neuron 2-directed RNA splicing modifiers

AVAILABLE FORMS
Oral solution: 0.75 mg/mL (60-mg bottles)

INDICATIONS & DOSAGES
➤ **Spinal muscular atrophy** ⬰
Adults and children ages 2 and older weighing 20 kg or more: 5 mg PO daily.
Children ages 2 and older weighing less than 20 kg: 0.25 mg/kg PO daily.
Children ages 2 months to younger than 2 years: 0.2 mg/kg PO daily.
Children younger than 2 months: 0.15 mg/kg PO daily.

SAFETY ALERT!

romiDEPsin
roh-mih-DEP-sin

Istodax

Therapeutic class: Antineoplastics
Pharmacologic class: Histone deacetylase inhibitors

AVAILABLE FORMS
Injection: 10 mg/2 mL, 27.5 mg/5.5 mL vials
Injection (powder for solution): 10-mg vial

INDICATIONS & DOSAGES
➤ **Cutaneous T-cell lymphoma and peripheral T-cell lymphoma in patients who have received at least one prior systemic therapy**
Adults: 14 mg/m² by IV infusion over 4 hours on days 1, 8, and 15 of 28-day cycle. Repeat every 28 days if effective and well tolerated.

Adjust-a-dose: Refer to manufacturer's instructions for toxicity-related dosage adjustments and discontinuation.

romosozumab-aqqg
roe-moe-SOZ-ue-mab

Evenity

Therapeutic class: Antiosteoporotics
Pharmacologic class: Sclerostin inhibitors

AVAILABLE FORMS
Injection: 105 mg/1.17 mL single-use prefilled syringe

INDICATIONS & DOSAGES
Boxed Warning Drug can increase risk of MI, stroke, and CV death. ■
➤ **Osteoporosis in patients after menopause at high risk for fracture or in patients who have failed or are intolerant of other osteoporosis therapy**
Adults: 210 mg (two syringes) subcut once every month for 12 months.

rufinamide
roo-FIN-ah-mide

Banzel

Therapeutic class: Anticonvulsants
Pharmacologic class: Triazole derivatives

AVAILABLE FORMS
Suspension: 40 mg/mL
Tablets: 200 mg, 400 mg

INDICATIONS & DOSAGES
➤ **Adjunct treatment of seizures associated with Lennox-Gastaut syndrome**
Adults and children ages 17 and older: Initially, 400 to 800 mg PO daily in two equally divided doses. Increase dosage by 400 to 800 mg/day every 2 days to 3,200 mg PO daily in divided doses.
Children ages 1 to younger than 17: Initially, 10 mg/kg/day PO in two equally divided doses. Increase dosage by 10 mg/kg every other day to 45 mg/kg/day or 3,200 mg (whichever is less) PO daily in two divided doses.
Adjust-a-dose: Dialysis clears drug by 30%; dosage adjustment may be necessary. For patients taking valproate, start rufinamide at dosages less than 400 mg/day (adults) or less than 10 mg/kg/day (children).

SAFETY ALERT!

ruxolitinib phosphate
rux-oh-LI-ti-nib

Jakafi

Therapeutic class: Antineoplastics
Pharmacologic class: Janus-associated kinase inhibitors

AVAILABLE FORMS
Tablets: 5 mg, 10 mg, 15 mg, 20 mg, 25 mg

INDICATIONS & DOSAGES
Adjust-a-dose (for all indications): Refer to manufacturer's instructions for toxicity-related dosage adjustments, dosage modifications for kidney or liver impairment, or use with strong CYP3A4 inhibitors or fluconazole.
➤ **Intermediate or high-risk myelofibrosis, including primary myelofibrosis, post-polycythemia vera myelofibrosis, and post-essential thrombocythemia myelofibrosis**
Adults: Initially, 20 mg PO b.i.d. if platelet count is greater than 200×10^9/L, 15 mg PO b.i.d. if platelet count is 100 to 200×10^9/L, or 5 mg PO b.i.d. if platelet count is 50 to less than 100×10^9/L. May increase in 5-mg increments b.i.d. to maximum of 25 mg b.i.d. Don't increase during first 4 weeks of therapy and not more frequently than every 2 weeks.

Consider dosage increases in patients who meet all the following conditions: failure to achieve either a 50% reduction from pretreatment baseline in palpable spleen length or a 35% reduction in spleen volume as measured by CT scan or MRI; platelet count greater than 125×10^9/L at 4 weeks and never below 100×10^9/L; and ANC greater than 0.75×10^9/L.

Long-term maintenance at 5-mg b.i.d. dosage hasn't shown response; limit continued use at this dosage to patients in whom benefits outweigh risks.

Discontinue drug after 6 months if no spleen reduction or symptom improvement occurs. If drug must be stopped for any reason except thrombocytopenia, taper gradually by 5 mg b.i.d. each week.
➤ **Polycythemia vera in patients who have an inadequate response to or are intolerant of hydroxyurea**
Adults: Initially, 10 mg PO b.i.d. If response is inadequate and platelet count is 140×10^9 or greater, Hb level is 12 g/dL or greater, and ANC is 1.5×10^9/L or greater, may increase dosage by 5 mg b.i.d. to maximum of 25 mg b.i.d. (Maximum, 50 mg/day.) Dosage shouldn't be increased during first 4 weeks of therapy or more frequently than every 2 weeks. Inadequate response is defined as one of the following: continued need for phlebotomy, WBC count higher than ULN, platelet count greater than ULN, or palpable spleen that's reduced by less than 25% from baseline.
➤ **Steroid-refractory acute GVHD**
Adults and children ages 12 and older: Initially, 5 mg PO b.i.d. May increase to 10 mg b.i.d. after at least 3 days of treatment if ANC and platelet counts aren't decreased by 50% or more from first day of dosing.
Adjust-a-dose: After 6 months of treatment in patients who have discontinued corticosteroids, taper drug by one dose level every 8 weeks (10 mg b.i.d. to 5 mg b.i.d. to 5 mg once daily). Consider retreatment if acute GVHD recurs during or after taper.
➤ **Chronic GVHD after failure of one or two lines of systemic therapy**
Adults and children ages 12 and older: 10 mg PO b.i.d.
Adjust-a-dose: After 6 months of treatment in patients who have discontinued corticosteroids, taper drug by one dose level every 8 weeks (10 mg b.i.d. to 5 mg b.i.d. to 5 mg once daily). Consider retreatment if GVHD recurs during or after taper.

sarecycline

sar-e-SYE-kleen

Seysara

Therapeutic class: Antibiotics
Pharmacologic class: Tetracyclines

AVAILABLE FORMS
Tablets: 60 mg, 100 mg, 150 mg

INDICATIONS & DOSAGES
➤ **Inflammatory lesions of nonnodular moderate to severe acne vulgaris**
Adults and children ages 9 and older weighing 85 to 136 kg: 150 mg PO once daily.
Adults and children ages 9 and older weighing 55 to 84 kg: 100 mg PO once daily.
Adults and children ages 9 and older weighing 33 to 54 kg: 60 mg PO once daily.
Adjust-a-dose: If no improvement after 12 weeks, reassess treatment with sarecycline.

secnidazole

sek-NID-a-zole

Solosec

Therapeutic class: Antibiotics
Pharmacologic class: Nitroimidazoles

AVAILABLE FORMS
Oral granules: 2 g/packet

INDICATIONS & DOSAGES
➤ **Bacterial vaginosis**
Patients ages 12 and older: One single dose of 2 g PO.
➤ **Trichomoniasis**
Adults and children ages 12 and older: One single dose of 2 g PO. Treat sexual partners at same dose at same time.

secukinumab

sek-ue-KIN-ue-mab

Cosentyx

Therapeutic class: Immunomodulators
Pharmacologic class: Human IgG1 monoclonal antibodies

AVAILABLE FORMS
Injection (IV): 125 mg/5 mL in single-dose vials
Injection: 75 mg/0.5 mL prefilled syringe, 150 mg/mL, 300 mg/2 mL autoinjector or prefilled syringe

INDICATIONS & DOSAGES
➤ **Moderate to severe plaque psoriasis in patients who are candidates for systemic therapy or phototherapy; psoriatic arthritis in patients with coexistent moderate to severe plaque psoriasis**
Adults: 300 mg as two subcut injections of 150 mg each on weeks 0, 1, 2, 3, and 4; then 300 mg every 4 weeks thereafter. If clinically indicated, a 150-mg dose may be acceptable for some patients with plaque psoriasis.

➤ **Moderate to severe plaque psoriasis in patients who are candidates for systemic therapy or phototherapy**
Children ages 6 and older weighing 50 kg or more: 150 mg subcut at weeks 0, 1, 2, 3, and 4; then 150 mg every 4 weeks thereafter.
Children ages 6 and older weighing less than 50 kg: 75 mg subcut at weeks 0, 1, 2, 3, and 4; then 75 mg every 4 weeks thereafter.
➤ **Active psoriatic arthritis**
Adults: To use with loading dose, give 150 mg subcut or 6 mg/kg IV infusion over 30 minutes once weekly at weeks 0, 1, 2, 3, and 4; then 150 mg subcut or 1.75 mg/kg IV every 4 weeks. To use without loading dose, give 150 mg subcut or 1.75 mg/kg IV infusion every 4 weeks. May consider increasing dosage to 300 mg subcut every 4 weeks. Maximum IV maintenance dose is 300 mg per infusion.
Children ages 2 and older weighing 50 kg or more: 150 mg subcut at weeks 0, 1, 2, 3, and 4; then 150 mg every 4 weeks thereafter.
Children ages 2 and older weighing 15 to less than 50 kg: 75 mg subcut at weeks 0, 1, 2, 3, and 4; then 75 mg every 4 weeks thereafter.
➤ **Active ankylosing spondylitis; active nonradiographic axial spondyloarthritis with objective signs of inflammation**
Adults: To use with loading dose, give 150 mg subcut or 6 mg/kg IV infusion over 30 minutes once weekly at weeks 0, 1, 2, 3, and 4; then 150 mg subcut or 1.75 mg/kg IV every 4 weeks. To use without loading dose, give 150 mg subcut or 1.75 mg/kg IV infusion every 4 weeks. For active psoriatic arthritis, consider increasing dosage to 300 mg subcut every 4 weeks. Maximum IV maintenance dose is 300 mg per infusion.
➤ **Enthesitis-related arthritis**
Adults and children ages 4 and older weighing 50 kg or more: 150 mg subcut at weeks 0, 1, 2, 3, and 4; then 150 mg every 4 weeks thereafter.
Adults and children ages 4 and older weighing 15 to less than 50 kg: 75 mg subcut at weeks 0, 1, 2, 3, and 4; then 75 mg every 4 weeks thereafter.

selexipag

se-LEX-i-pag

Uptravi

Therapeutic class: Vasodilators
Pharmacologic class: Prostacyclin receptor agonists

AVAILABLE FORMS
Injection (lyophilized powder): 1,800-mcg vial
Tablets (extended-release) ⓞⓡⓒ*:* 200 mcg, 400 mcg, 600 mcg, 800 mcg, 1,000 mcg, 1,200 mcg, 1,400 mcg, 1,600 mcg

INDICATIONS & DOSAGES
➤ **PAH (WHO Group I) to delay disease progression and reduce risk of hospitalization**
Adults: Initially, 200 mcg PO b.i.d. Increase dosage by increments of 200 mcg b.i.d. at weekly intervals to

highest tolerated dose. If dose isn't tolerated, decrease dosage to previous tolerated dose. Maximum dosage, 1,600 mcg b.i.d. If patient can't take oral form, may temporarily give by IV infusion at patient's current dose of tablets over 80 minutes b.i.d. Refer to manufacturer's instructions for IV dosing table.

Adjust-a-dose: For patients with Child-Pugh class B liver impairment, initiate therapy at 200 mcg once daily and increase by 200-mcg increments once daily at weekly intervals, as tolerated. Avoid use in patients with Child-Pugh class C liver impairment. If administered with moderate CYP2C8 inhibitor, reduce dosing to once daily.

SAFETY ALERT!

selinexor
sel-i-NEX-or

Xpovio

Therapeutic class: Antineoplastics
Pharmacologic class: Nuclear export inhibitors

AVAILABLE FORMS
Tablets ⓞⓝⓒ: 20 mg, 40 mg, 50 mg, 60 mg

INDICATIONS & DOSAGES
Adjust-a-dose (for all indications): Follow manufacturer's instructions for toxicity-related dosage adjustments.

➤ **Relapsed or refractory multiple myeloma in combination with dexamethasone in patients who have received at least four prior therapies and whose disease is refractory to at least two proteasome inhibitors, at least two immunomodulatory agents, and an anti-CD38 monoclonal antibody**
Adults: 80 mg PO with dexamethasone 20 mg PO on days 1 and 3 of each week until disease progresses or unacceptable toxicity occurs.

➤ **Relapsed or refractory diffuse large B-cell lymphoma after at least two lines of systemic therapy**
Adults: 60 mg PO on days 1 and 3 of each week until disease progresses or unacceptable toxicity occurs.

➤ **Multiple myeloma, in combination with bortezomib and dexamethasone, in patients who have received at least one prior therapy**
Adults: 100 mg once weekly in combination with bortezomib and dexamethasone until disease progresses or unacceptable toxicity occurs. Refer to manufacturer's instructions for bortezomib and dexamethasone for additional dosing information.

SAFETY ALERT!

selumetinib
sel-ue-ME-ti-nib

Koselugo

Therapeutic class: Antineoplastics
Pharmacologic class: Kinase inhibitors

AVAILABLE FORMS
Capsules ⓞⓝⓒ: 10 mg, 25 mg

INDICATIONS & DOSAGES
➤ **Neurofibromatosis type 1 with symptomatic, inoperable plexiform neurofibromas**
Children ages 2 and older: 25 mg/m^2 PO b.i.d. until disease progresses or unacceptable toxicity occurs.

Adjust-a-dose: For patients with Child-Pugh class B liver impairment, reduce dose to 20 mg/m^2 b.i.d. If patient is taking selumetinib with strong or moderate CYP3A4 inhibitor or fluconazole and current dose is 25 mg/m^2 b.i.d., reduce to 20 mg/m^2 b.i.d.; if current dose is 20 mg/m^2 b.i.d., reduce to 15 mg/m^2 b.i.d. After discontinuing strong or moderate CYP3A4 inhibitor or fluconazole, wait for three elimination half-lives; then resume selumetinib at dose taken before initiation of the inhibitor or fluconazole. Refer to manufacturer's instructions for toxicity-related dosage adjustments.

sertaconazole nitrate
sir-tah-KAHN-uh-zole

Ertaczo

Therapeutic class: Antifungals
Pharmacologic class: Imidazoles

AVAILABLE FORMS
Topical cream: 2%

INDICATIONS & DOSAGES
➤ **Interdigital tinea pedis caused by *Trichophyton rubrum*, *T. mentagrophytes*, or *Epidermophyton floccosum* in patients who are immunocompetent**
Adults and children ages 12 and older: Apply cream b.i.d. to affected areas between toes and healthy surrounding areas for 4 weeks.

silver sulfadiazine
sul-fa-DYE-a-zeen

Flamazine ✦, Silvadene, SSD, Thermazene

Therapeutic class: Antibacterials (topical)
Pharmacologic class: Broad-spectrum sulfonamides

AVAILABLE FORMS
Cream: 1%

INDICATIONS & DOSAGES
➤ **To prevent or treat wound infection in second- and third-degree burns**
Adults: Apply one-sixteenth-inch thickness of cream to clean, debrided wound daily or b.i.d. Burn areas should be always covered with cream. Reapply to areas from which it has been removed by patient activity.

siponimod ⚡
si-PON-i-mod

Mayzent

Therapeutic class: MS drugs
Pharmacologic class: Sphingosine 1-phosphate receptor modulators

AVAILABLE FORMS
Tablets ⓞⓝⓒ: 0.25 mg, 1 mg, 2 mg

INDICATIONS & DOSAGES
➤ **Relapsing forms of MS with CYP2C9 genotype *1/*1, *1/*2, or *2/*2** ⌘

Adults: Start drug with a 5-day titration to help reduce cardiac effects. Initially, on days 1 and 2, give 0.25 mg PO once daily; on day 3, give 0.5 mg PO once daily; on day 4, give 0.75 mg PO once daily; on day 5, give 1.25 mg PO once daily; on day 6, begin maintenance dosage of 2 mg PO once daily.

➤ **Relapsing forms of MS with CYP2C9 genotype *1/*3 or *2/*3** ⌘

Adults: Start drug with a 4-day titration to help reduce cardiac effects. Initially, on days 1 and 2, give 0.25 mg PO once daily; on day 3, give 0.5 mg PO once daily; on day 4, give 0.75 mg PO once daily; on day 5, begin maintenance dosage of 1 mg PO once daily.

---

sodium bicarbonate

Therapeutic class: Antacids
Pharmacologic class: Alkalinizers

AVAILABLE FORMS
Injection: 4.2% (0.5 mEq/1 mL), 7.5% (0.9 mEq/1 mL), 8.4% (1 mEq/1 mL)
Powder: 2,616 mg/½ tsp ◇
Tablets: 325 mg ◇, 650 mg ◇

INDICATIONS & DOSAGES
➤ **Metabolic acidosis**
Adults and children: Dosage depends on blood carbon dioxide content, pH, and patient's condition; usually, 2 to 5 mEq/kg IV infused over 4- to 8-hour period. Base subsequent doses on patient's acid-base status.

➤ **Antacid**
Adults younger than age 60: 650 to 2,600 mg PO up to every 4 hours with a glass of water. Maximum, 15,600 mg/day.
Adults ages 60 and older: 650 to 1,300 mg PO up to every 4 hours with a glass of water. Maximum, 7,800 mg/day.
Adults and children older than age 6: ½ tsp (2,616 mg) oral powder in 120 mL water PO every 2 hours, up to six doses daily for patients younger than age 60 or three doses daily for patients older than age 60.

➤ **Cardiac arrest**
Adults and children ages 2 and older: Administer according to arterial blood pH, partial pressure of arterial carbon dioxide, and calculated base deficit. Initially, 44.6 to 100 mEq of bicarbonate IV. Then redetermine serum pH and bicarbonate concentration. May give 44.6 to 50 mEq every 5 to 10 minutes if necessary.
Children younger than age 2: 1 to 2 mEq/kg IV slowly followed by 1 mEq/kg every 10 minutes of arrest. Don't give more than 8 mEq/kg IV total; a 4.2% solution may be preferred.

SAFETY ALERT!

SORAfenib tosylate
sohr-uh-FEN-ib

NexAVAR

Therapeutic class: Antineoplastics
Pharmacologic class: Multi-kinase inhibitors

AVAILABLE FORMS
Tablets: 200 mg

INDICATIONS & DOSAGES
➤ **Advanced renal cell carcinoma; unresectable hepatocellular carcinoma; locally advanced or metastatic, progressive, differentiated thyroid carcinoma refractory to radioactive iodine treatment**
Adults: 400 mg PO b.i.d. at least 1 hour before or 2 hours after eating. Continue until disease progresses or unacceptable toxicity occurs.
Adjust-a-dose: Refer to manufacturer's instructions for dosage adjustments for dermatologic and other toxicities.

---

spinosad
SPIN-oh-sad

Natroba

Therapeutic class: Scabicides-pediculicides
Pharmacologic class: Topical actinomycete bacterium derivatives

AVAILABLE FORMS
Topical solution: 0.9%*

INDICATIONS & DOSAGES
➤ **Head lice infestation**
Adults and children ages 6 months and older: Apply only amount needed to adequately cover dry scalp and hair, up to 120 mL. Leave on for 10 minutes (start timing after scalp and hair have been completely covered); then thoroughly rinse off with warm water. If live lice are seen 7 days after first treatment, apply second treatment.
➤ **Scabies infestation**
Adults and children ages 4 and older: Apply to skin to completely cover body from neck to soles of feet. For patients with balding scalp, also apply to scalp, hairline, temples, and forehead. Allow skin to dry for 10 minutes before patient dresses. Leave on skin for 6 hours before patient showers or bathes.

---

stiripentol
stir-i-PEN-tol

Diacomit

Therapeutic class: Anticonvulsants
Pharmacologic class: Anticonvulsants

AVAILABLE FORMS
Capsules ⓒ: 250 mg, 500 mg
Powder for oral suspension: 250 mg, 500 mg

INDICATIONS & DOSAGES

➤ **Seizures associated with Dravet syndrome in patients taking clobazam**

Adults: 50 mg/kg/day PO in two or three divided doses with a meal.

Children ages 1 year and older weighing 10 kg or more: 25 mg/kg PO b.i.d. or 16.67 mg/kg PO t.i.d. *Children ages 1 year and older weighing 7 to less than 10 kg:* 25 mg/kg PO b.i.d.

Children ages 6 months to younger than 1 year weighing 7 kg or more: 25 mg/kg PO b.i.d.

Adjust-a-dose: If exact dosage can't be achieved with the available strengths, round to nearest dosage, which is usually within 50 to 150 mg of the recommended 50 mg/kg/day. Maximum, 3,000 mg/day. If somnolence occurs, consider reducing clobazam dosage by 25%. If somnolence persists, consider decreasing clobazam dosage by an additional 25%. Consider adjusting the dosage of other concomitant anticonvulsants with sedating properties.

tacrolimus ☒
tack-ROW-lim-us

Advagraf♣, Astagraf XL, Envarsus XR, Prograf

Therapeutic class: Immunosuppressants
Pharmacologic class: Calcineurin inhibitors

AVAILABLE FORMS

Capsules ⓞ: 0.5 mg, 1 mg, 5 mg
Capsules (extended-release) ⓞ: 0.5 mg, 1 mg, 3 mg ♣, 5 mg
Granules for oral suspension: 0.2 mg, 1 mg unit-dose packets
Injection: 5 mg/mL*
Tablets (extended-release) ⓞ: 0.75 mg, 1 mg, 4 mg

INDICATIONS & DOSAGES

Boxed Warning Drug increases risk of serious infections and malignancies. Increased mortality reported in women with transplants using Astagraf XL. Astagraf XL isn't approved for use in liver transplantation. ∎

☒ *Adjust-a-dose (for all indications):* Give lowest recommended oral and IV dosages to older adults and patients with kidney or liver impairment. Patients who are Black with kidney transplants may need higher dosages than patients who are White to attain comparable trough concentrations.

↻ *Alert:* Extended-release capsules aren't interchangeable or substitutable with other tacrolimus extended-release or immediate-release products.

➤ **Prevention of organ rejection in allogenic liver, kidney, heart, or lung transplant (with other immunosuppressants)**

Adults: Individualize dosing regimen for optimal therapy. Frequently monitor trough concentrations in the early transplant period to ensure adequate drug exposure. Patients able to tolerate oral therapy should begin treatment no sooner than 6 hours after liver, heart, or lung transplant or within 24 hours of kidney transplant if kidney function has recovered. For patients who

can't take drug PO, give 0.03 to 0.05 mg/kg/day (liver or kidney), 0.01 mg/kg/day (heart), or 0.01 to 0.03 mg/kg/day (lung) IV continuous infusion. Switch to oral therapy as soon as possible, with first dose 8 to 12 hours after stopping IV infusion. See manufacturer's instructions for dosing based on transplanted organ; coadministration with azathioprine, basiliximab, MMF-IL-2 receptor antagonists, or corticosteroids; and desired whole blood trough concentration range. Adjust dosages based on patient response.

To convert from immediate-release form to Astagraf XL, initiate ER treatment in a 1:1 ratio (mg:mg) using previously established total daily dose of immediate-release form. Give once daily. To convert from immediate-release form to Envarsus XR, initiate ER treatment with a once-daily dose that's 80% of the total daily dose of the immediate-release product.

Children: For kidney transplant, 0.3 mg/kg/day immediate-release capsules or oral suspension, divided in two doses, administered every 12 hours; or, within 24 hours of reperfusion, 0.3 mg/kg Astagraf XL PO once daily in combination with basiliximab induction, MMF, and corticosteroids. For liver transplant, 0.15 to 0.2 mg/kg/day immediate-release capsules or 0.2 mg/kg/day oral suspension, divided in two doses, administered every 12 hours. For heart or lung transplant, 0.3 mg/kg/day immediate-release capsules or oral suspension or 0.1 mg/kg/day if cell-depleting induction treatment is administered, divided in two doses, administered every 12 hours. Children unable to receive oral formulation may start IV infusion. For liver transplant, give 0.03 to 0.05 mg/kg IV daily as continuous infusion. Children in general need higher tacrolimus doses compared to adults: Higher dose requirements may decrease as the child ages. Patients with cystic fibrosis may require higher doses.

➤ **Prevention of organ rejection in patients with de novo kidney transplant, in combination with other immunosuppressants (Envarsus XR)**

Adults: Initially, 0.14 mg/kg/day PO. Titrate dosage based on clinical assessments of rejection and tolerability and to achieve tacrolimus whole blood trough concentration range of 6 to 11 ng/mL during the first month, then 4 to 11 ng/mL during all subsequent months.

tafamidis ☒
ta-FAM-id-is

Vyndamax

tafamidis meglumine
Vyndaqel

Therapeutic class: Endocrine-metabolic agents
Pharmacologic class: Transthyretin stabilizers

AVAILABLE FORMS

tafamidis
Capsules ⓞ: 61 mg
tafamidis meglumine
Capsules ⓞ: 20 mg

INDICATIONS & DOSAGES

➤ **Cardiomyopathy of wild-type or hereditary transthyretin-mediated amyloidosis to reduce CV mortality and CV-related hospitalization** ⧗
Adults: 61 mg tafamidis PO once daily or 80 mg tafamidis meglumine (four 20-mg capsules) PO once daily.

tafenoquine succinate ⧗
ta-FEN-oh-kwin

Arakoda, Krintafel

Therapeutic class: Antimalarials
Pharmacologic class: Aminoquinolines

AVAILABLE FORMS
Tablets ⓓⓝⓒ: 100 mg, 150 mg

INDICATIONS & DOSAGES
➤ **Prevention of relapse of *Plasmodium vivax* malaria in patients who have tested negative for G6PD deficiency and who are receiving chloroquine therapy for acute *P. vivax* infection (Krintafel)** ⧗
Adults and children ages 16 and older: Single dose of 300 mg PO given as two 150-mg tablets taken together. Coadminister on first or second day of chloroquine therapy for acute *P. vivax* malaria.
➤ **Malaria prophylaxis in patients who have tested negative for G6PD deficiency (Arakoda)** ⧗
Adults: 200 mg PO once daily for 3 days before travel to a malarious area. Then, while patient is in malarious area, 200 mg once weekly beginning 7 days after last dose of loading regimen. After patient leaves malarious area, 200 mg PO as single dose 7 days after last dose of maintenance regimen.

SAFETY ALERT!

tapentadol hydrochloride
tah-PEN-tah-dol

Nucynta, Nucynta ER, Nucynta IR✦

Therapeutic class: Opioid analgesics
Pharmacologic class: Centrally acting synthetic opioid analgesics
Controlled substance schedule: II

AVAILABLE FORMS
Tablets: 50 mg, 75 mg, 100 mg
Tablets (extended-release) ⓓⓝⓒ: 50 mg, 100 mg, 150 mg, 200 mg, 250 mg

INDICATIONS & DOSAGES
Boxed Warning Opioid use increases risk of addiction, abuse, and misuse. Opioids can cause fatal respiratory depression. Opioids can cause respiratory depression and death in children with ingestion of even one dose. Opioids combined with benzodiazepines or CNS depressants, including alcohol, can cause death. Use during pregnancy can cause neonatal opioid withdrawal. ■
Adjust-a-dose (for all indications): Use lowest effective dosage for shortest duration consistent with individual patient treatment goals. Don't stop drug abruptly; withdraw slowly and individualize gradual taper plan to prevent signs and symptoms of withdrawal.
➤ **Acute pain severe enough to require an opioid analgesic and for which alternative treatments are inadequate (immediate-release only)**
Adults: 50 to 100 mg PO every 4 to 6 hours, as needed, for pain. On day 1, may give second dose in 1 hour if first dose is ineffective. Adjust subsequent dosing to maintain adequate pain control. Maximum daily dose, 700 mg on day 1; 600 mg on subsequent days.
Adjust-a-dose: For adults with Child-Pugh class B liver impairment, initially give 50 mg PO every 8 hours. Maximum, three doses (150 mg) in 24 hours; the interval between doses should be no less than 8 hours.
Children ages 6 and older weighing 80 kg or more: 50 mg PO every 4 hours. May increase dosage to 75 mg every 4 hours, then 100 mg every 4 hours to maintain adequate analgesia as tolerated. Maximum single dose, 100 mg.
Children ages 6 and older weighing 60 to 79 kg: 50 mg PO every 4 hours. May increase dosage to 75 mg every 4 hours to maintain adequate analgesia as tolerated. Maximum single dose, 75 mg.
Children ages 6 and older weighing 40 to 59 kg: 50 mg PO every 4 hours. Maximum single dose, 50 mg.
Adjust-a-dose: For children, maximum dosage is 7.5 mg/kg/day (six 1.25-mg/kg doses over 24 hours). In children with high BMI, maximum daily dose must not exceed the maximum dose for body weight at the 97th percentile for given age. Reduce dosage over time as acute pain decreases. Duration of treatment for children shouldn't exceed 3 days. Use in children with liver or kidney impairment isn't recommended.
➤ **Severe chronic pain when continuous, around-the-clock opioid analgesia is needed for an extended period (extended-release); neuropathic pain associated with diabetic peripheral neuropathy (extended-release)**
Adults: Initially, 50 mg PO b.i.d. (approximately every 12 hours). Titrate with dosage increases of 50 mg no more than b.i.d. every 3 days. Therapeutic range, 100 to 250 mg PO b.i.d. Maximum, 500 mg daily.
Adjust-a-dose: For patients with Child-Pugh class B liver impairment, initially 50 mg (extended-release) PO once every 24 hours. Maximum is 100 mg (extended-release) once daily. Monitor patient closely for respiratory and CNS depression, particularly during initiation and titration.

tedizolid phosphate
ted-eye-ZOE-lid

Sivextro

Therapeutic class: Antibiotics
Pharmacologic class: Oxazolidinones

AVAILABLE FORMS
Injection: 200 mg/vial
Tablets: 200 mg

INDICATIONS & DOSAGES

➤ **Acute bacterial skin and skin-structure infections caused by susceptible gram-positive isolates (*Staphylococcus aureus* [including MRSA and methicillin-susceptible strains], *Streptococcus pyogenes*, *Streptococcus agalactiae*, *Streptococcus anginosus* group [including *S. anginosus*, *Streptococcus intermedius*, and *Streptococcus constellatus*], and *Enterococcus faecalis*)**

Adults and children ages 12 and older: 200 mg PO or IV once daily for 6 days.

SAFETY ALERT!

temozolomide
teh-moh-ZOH-loh-mide

Temodal✚, Temodar

Therapeutic class: Antineoplastics
Pharmacologic class: Alkylating drugs

AVAILABLE FORMS
Capsules ⦿: 5 mg, 20 mg, 100 mg, 140 mg, 180 mg, 250 mg
Injection: 100 mg/vial

INDICATIONS & DOSAGES

Adjust-a-dose (for all indications): Refer to manufacturer's instructions for toxicity-related dosage adjustments.

➤ **Newly diagnosed glioblastoma in combination with radiation therapy**

Adults: Initially, 75 mg/m² IV infusion or PO once daily for 42 days (up to 49 days if no toxicity). Maintenance dosage, 150 mg/m² IV infusion or PO once daily on days 1 to 5 of a 28-day cycle for six cycles; may increase to 200 mg/m² for cycles two to six if CTCAE is grade 2 or less, ANC is 1.5×10^9/L or more, and platelet count is 100×10^9/L or more. If dosage was increased in cycle two, maintain at 200 mg/m² for days 1 to 5 of subsequent cycles, unless toxicity occurs. If dosage wasn't increased in cycle two, don't increase in subsequent cycles.

➤ **Refractory anaplastic astrocytoma**

Adults: Initially, 150 mg/m² IV infusion or PO once daily for 5 days of a 28-day treatment cycle. May increase to 200 mg/m² for 5 days of a 28-day treatment cycle, if nadir and day 1 of next cycle ANC is 1.5×10^9/L or more and platelet count is 100×10^9/L or more. Continue until disease progresses or unacceptable toxicity occurs.

✳ *NEW INDICATION:* **Adjuvant treatment for newly diagnosed anaplastic astrocytoma**

Adults: Initiate drug 4 weeks after end of radiotherapy. Cycle 1, give 150 mg/m² PO daily on days 1 to 5 of a 28-day cycle. Then, cycles 2 to 12, give 200 mg/m² daily on days 1 to 5 of each 28-day cycle. If dosage wasn't increased at start of cycle 2 due to toxicity, don't increase during cycles 3 to 6.

SAFETY ALERT!

temsirolimus
tem-sir-OH-li-mus

Torisel

Therapeutic class: Antineoplastics
Pharmacologic class: Kinase inhibitors

AVAILABLE FORMS
IV solution: 25 mg/mL

INDICATIONS & DOSAGES

➤ **Advanced renal cell carcinoma**

Adults: 25 mg IV over 30 to 60 minutes once weekly until disease progresses or unacceptable toxicity occurs. Give diphenhydramine 25 to 50 mg IV 30 minutes before each dose.

Adjust-a-dose: Reduce dosage to 15 mg once weekly in patients with bilirubin level more than 1 to $1.5 \times$ ULN or AST level more than ULN with normal bilirubin level. Refer to manufacturer's instructions for toxicity-related dosage adjustments.

If use with a strong CYP3A4 inhibitor is necessary, consider dosage reduction to 12.5 mg once weekly. If use with a strong CYP3A4 inducer is necessary, increase dosage to 50 mg once weekly.

tenapanor hydrochloride
ten-A-pa-nor

Ibsrela

Therapeutic class: Miscellaneous GI drugs
Pharmacologic class: Sodium/hydrogen exchanger 3 inhibitors

AVAILABLE FORMS
Tablets: 50 mg

INDICATIONS & DOSAGES

Boxed Warning Due to risk of dehydration, drug is contraindicated in children younger than age 6. Avoid use in children ages 6 to younger than 12. Safety and effectiveness in patients younger than age 18 haven't been established. ■

➤ **IBS with constipation**

Adults: 50 mg PO b.i.d., immediately before first meal of the day and dinner.

SAFETY ALERT!

tepotinib ▨
tep-OH-ti-nib

Tepmetko

Therapeutic class: Antineoplastics
Pharmacologic class: Kinase inhibitors

AVAILABLE FORMS
Tablets: 225 mg

INDICATIONS & DOSAGES

➤ **Metastatic NSCLC harboring mesenchymal-epithelial transition (*MET*) exon 14 skipping alterations** ▨

Adults: 450 mg PO daily until disease progresses or unacceptable toxicity occurs.

Adjust-a-dose: Refer to manufacturer's instructions for toxicity-related dosage adjustments. Permanently discontinue drug if patient can't tolerate 225 mg PO once daily.

terbutaline sulfate
ter-BYOO-ta-leen

Therapeutic class: Bronchodilators
Pharmacologic class: Beta₂ agonists

AVAILABLE FORMS
Injection: 1 mg/mL
Tablets: 2.5 mg, 5 mg

INDICATIONS & DOSAGES
Boxed Warning Drug hasn't been approved and shouldn't be used for tocolysis. Serious adverse reactions may occur. ■
➤ **Prevention and reversal of bronchospasm in patients with asthma and reversible bronchospasm associated with bronchitis and emphysema**
Adults and children ages 12 and older: 0.25 mg subcut. If needed, repeat in 15 to 30 minutes. Maximum, 0.5 mg in 4 hours. If patient fails to respond to second dose, consider other measures.
Adults and adolescents older than age 15: 2.5 to 5 mg PO t.i.d. every 6 hours while awake. Maximum, 15 mg daily.
Children ages 12 to 15: 2.5 mg PO t.i.d. every 6 hours while awake. Maximum, 7.5 mg daily.

SAFETY ALERT!

teriflunomide
ter-i-FLOO-noe-mide

Aubagio

Therapeutic class: Immunomodulators
Pharmacologic class: Pyrimidine synthesis inhibitors

AVAILABLE FORMS
Tablets: 7 mg, 14 mg

INDICATIONS & DOSAGES
Boxed Warning Severe and fatal liver injury can occur. May cause major birth defects. Contraindicated during pregnancy. ■
➤ **Relapsing forms of MS**
Adults: 7 or 14 mg PO once daily.

tezacaftor–ivacaftor and ivacaftor ⌧
tez-a-KAF-tor/eye-va-KAF-tor

Symdeko

Therapeutic class: Metabolic agents
Pharmacologic class: Cystic fibrosis transmembrane conductance regulator (CFTR) facilitators (tezacaftor); CFTR potentiators (ivacaftor)

AVAILABLE FORMS
Tablets: 50 mg tezacaftor/75 mg ivacaftor fixed-dose combination tablets copackaged with ivacaftor 75-mg tablets;100 mg tezacaftor/150 mg ivacaftor fixed-dose combination tablets copackaged with ivacaftor 150-mg tablets

INDICATIONS & DOSAGES
➤ **Cystic fibrosis in patients homozygous for the F508del mutation or who have at least one mutation in the *CFTR* gene that's responsive to tezacaftor–ivacaftor based on in vitro data or clinical evidence ⌧**
Adults, children ages 12 and older, and children ages 6 to younger than 12 weighing 30 kg or more: 100 mg tezacaftor and 150 mg ivacaftor (1 combination tablet) PO in the morning and 150 mg ivacaftor (1 tablet) PO in the evening, approximately 12 hours apart.
Children ages 6 to younger than 12 weighing less than 30 kg: 50 mg tezacaftor and 75 mg ivacaftor (1 combination tablet) PO in the morning and 75 mg ivacaftor (1 tablet) PO in the evening, approximately 12 hours apart.
Adjust-a-dose: For patients with Child-Pugh class B or C liver impairment, omit the ivacaftor evening dose. For patients with Child-Pugh class C liver impairment, consider giving the morning ivacaftor dose less frequently. For patients also taking CYP3A inhibitors, refer to manufacturer's instructions for dosage adjustments.

theophylline
thee-OFF-i-lin

Elixophyllin*, Theo ER✢, Theo-24

Therapeutic class: Bronchodilators
Pharmacologic class: Xanthine derivatives

AVAILABLE FORMS
Capsules (extended-release) ⓓⓝⓒ: 100 mg, 200 mg, 300 mg, 400 mg
Infusion: 400 mg/500 mL
Syrup: 80 mg/15 mL*
Tablets (extended-release) ⓓⓝⓒ: 100 mg, 200 mg, 300 mg, 400 mg, 450 mg, 600 mg

INDICATIONS & DOSAGES
🔵 *Alert:* Individualize dosage based on serum concentration to achieve a dosage that provides maximum benefit with minimal risk. Marked individual differences in the rate of theophylline clearance occur. Don't use extended-release preparations to treat acute bronchospasm.
➤ **Acute bronchospasm in patients not currently receiving theophylline**
Loading dose: 4.6 mg/kg ideal body weight IV over 30 minutes; then maintenance infusion.
Nonsmoking adults younger than age 60 and children older than age 16: 0.4 mg/kg/hour IV (maximum 900 mg daily).
Nonsmoking children ages 12 to 16: 0.5 mg/kg/hour IV (maximum 900 mg daily).

✢Canada   ◇ OTC   ◆ Off-label use   ⓓⓝⓒ Do not crush   *Liquid contains alcohol   ⌧ Genetic

Children ages 12 to 16 who smoke and children ages 9 to 12: 0.7 mg/kg/hour IV.

Children ages 1 to 9: 0.8 mg/kg/hour IV.

Infants ages 6 weeks to 1 year: Calculate mg/kg/hour IV dosage as follows: $0.008 \times$ (age in weeks) + 0.21.

Neonates older than 24 days: 1.5 mg/kg IV every 12 hours to achieve target theophylline concentration of 7.5 mcg/mL.

Neonates 24 days old and younger: 1 mg/kg IV every 12 hours to achieve a target theophylline concentration of 7.5 mcg/mL.

Adjust-a-dose: For adults older than age 60, give 0.3 mg/kg/hour IV, up to a maximum of 17 mg/hour. For adults with HF, cor pulmonale, liver disease, sepsis with multiorgan failure, or shock, give 0.2 mg/kg/hour IV, up to a maximum infusion rate of 17 mg/hour, unless serum theophylline concentrations are monitored at 24-hour intervals. Maximum daily dose is 400 mg.

➤ **Oral theophylline for acute bronchospasm in patients not currently receiving theophylline**

Adults ages 60 and younger, children ages 16 and older, and children ages 1 to 15 weighing 45 kg or more: 5 mg/kg PO, then 300 mg (immediate-release syrup) PO daily in divided doses every 6 to 8 hours for 3 days. If tolerated, increase to 400 mg PO daily in divided doses every 6 to 8 hours. If necessary, dosage may be increased after 3 days to 600 mg PO daily in divided doses every 6 to 8 hours.

Children ages 1 to 15 weighing less than 45 kg: 5 mg/kg PO, then 12 to 14 mg/kg immediate-release (maximum 300 mg) PO daily in divided doses every 4 to 6 hours for 3 days. If tolerated, increase to 16 mg/kg (maximum 400 mg) PO daily in divided doses every 4 to 6 hours. After 3 days, if necessary, increase to 20 mg/kg (maximum 600 mg) PO daily in divided doses every 4 to 6 hours.

Adjust-a-dose: For children ages 1 to 15 with risk factors for reduced theophylline clearance or for whom serum concentrations can't be monitored, give 5 mg/kg PO, then 12 to 14 mg/kg (maximum 300 mg) PO daily in divided doses every 4 to 6 hours for 3 days. If tolerated, increase to 16 mg/kg (maximum 400 mg) PO daily in divided doses every 4 to 6 hours. For children ages 16 and older and adults with risk factors for reduced theophylline clearance or for whom serum concentrations can't be monitored, give 5 mg/kg PO, then 300 mg PO daily in divided doses every 6 to 8 hours for 3 days. If tolerated, increase to 400 mg PO daily in divided doses every 6 to 8 hours.

➤ **Chronic bronchospasm using extended-release preparations**

Adults ages 60 and younger, children ages 16 and older, and children ages 6 to 15 weighing more than 45 kg: 300 mg PO daily in divided doses every 8 to 12 hours or 300 to 400 mg (24-hour extended-release capsule) PO daily for 3 days. If tolerated, increase to 400 mg PO in divided doses every 8 to 12 hours or 400 to 600 mg (24-hour extended-release capsule) PO daily. After 3 more days, if necessary, increase to 600 mg PO daily in divided doses every 8 to 12 hours. Titrate dosages greater than 600 mg according to serum blood levels.

Children ages 6 to 15 weighing less than 45 kg: 12 to 14 mg/kg (maximum 300 mg extended-release tablet) daily in divided doses every 8 to 12 hours for 3 days. If tolerated, increase to 16 mg/kg (maximum 400 mg extended-release tablet) daily in divided doses every 8 to 12 hours. After 3 more days, if necessary, increase to 20 mg/kg (maximum 600 mg extended-release tablet) daily in divided doses every 8 to 12 hours.

Adjust-a-dose: For children ages 6 to 15 with risk factors for reduced theophylline clearance or for whom serum concentrations can't be monitored, give 12 to 14 mg/kg (maximum 300 mg) daily in divided doses for 3 days. If tolerated, increase to a maximum of 16 mg/kg (maximum 400 mg) PO daily in divided doses every 8 to 12 hours. For children ages 16 and older and adults ages 60 and younger or for whom serum concentrations can't be monitored, give 300 mg PO daily in divided doses every 8 to 12 hours. After 3 days, if necessary, increase to maximum of 400 mg PO daily in divided doses every 8 to 12 hours. For adults older than age 60, the recommended maximum daily dose is 400 mg PO per day in divided doses every 8 to 12 hours, unless symptoms continue and peak serum concentration is less than 10 mcg/mL. Administer dosages greater than 400 mg PO daily cautiously. See manufacturer's instructions for dosage adjustment guided by theophylline concentration.

---

thioridazine hydrochloride
thye-oh-RYE-da-zeen

Therapeutic class: Antipsychotics
Pharmacologic class: Phenothiazines

AVAILABLE FORMS
Tablets: 10 mg, 25 mg, 50 mg, 100 mg

INDICATIONS & DOSAGES
Boxed Warning Drug may prolong QTc interval, increasing risk of life-threatening ventricular arrhythmias. Older adults with dementia-related psychosis treated with antipsychotics are at increased risk of death. Drug isn't approved to treat patients with dementia-related psychosis. ■

➤ **Schizophrenia in patients who don't respond to treatment with at least two other antipsychotics**

Adults: Initially, 50 to 100 mg PO t.i.d.; increase gradually to 800 mg daily in divided doses, as needed. Daily maintenance dosage ranges from 200 to 800 mg into two to four divided doses.

Children: Initially, 0.5 mg/kg PO daily in two to four divided doses. Increase gradually to optimal therapeutic effect. Maximum, 3 mg/kg daily.

---

tigecycline
tye-gah-SYE-klin

Tygacil

Therapeutic class: Antibiotics
Pharmacologic class: Glycylcycline antibacterials

AVAILABLE FORMS
Lyophilized powder: 50-mg vial

INDICATIONS & DOSAGES

Boxed Warning Compared to other drugs used to treat serious infections, tigecycline has an increased mortality risk. Use only in situations in which alternative treatments aren't suitable. ■

Adjust-a-dose (for all indications): For adults with Child-Pugh class C liver impairment, give initial dose of 100 mg IV; then give 25 mg IV every 12 hours.

➤ **Community-acquired bacterial pneumonia**
Adults: Initially, 100 mg IV; then 50 mg IV every 12 hours for 7 to 14 days. Infuse drug over 30 to 60 minutes.
Children ages 12 to 17: 50 mg IV every 12 hours for 7 to 14 days.
Children ages 8 to 11: 1.2 mg/kg IV every 12 hours for 7 to 14 days. Maximum, 50 mg every 12 hours.

➤ **Complicated skin or skin-structure infection; complicated intra-abdominal infection**
Adults: Initially 100 mg IV; then 50 mg every 12 hours for 5 to 14 days. Infuse drug over 30 to 60 minutes.

tildrakizumab-asmn
til-dra-KIZ-ue-mab

Ilumya

Therapeutic class: Antipsoriatics
Pharmacologic class: Interleukin-23 antagonists

AVAILABLE FORMS
Injection: 100 mg/mL single-dose prefilled syringes

INDICATIONS & DOSAGES
➤ **Moderate to severe plaque psoriasis in patients who are candidates for systemic therapy or phototherapy**
Adults: 100 mg subcut at weeks 0 and 4 and then every 12 weeks thereafter.

tinidazole
teh-NID-ah-zol

Therapeutic class: Antiprotozoals
Pharmacologic class: Antiprotozoals

AVAILABLE FORMS
Tablets: 250 mg, 500 mg

INDICATIONS & DOSAGES
Boxed Warning Use tinidazole only for the conditions for which it's indicated. Avoid long-term use. ■
Adjust-a-dose (for all indications): For patients receiving hemodialysis, give an additional dose equal to half the recommended dose after the hemodialysis session.

➤ **Bacterial vaginosis in patients who aren't pregnant**
Adults: 2 g PO once daily for 2 days or 1 g PO once daily for 5 days.

➤ **Trichomoniasis caused by *Trichomonas vaginalis***
Adults: 2 g PO as single dose. Sexual partners should be treated at the same time with the same dose.

➤ **Giardiasis caused by *Giardia lamblia (Giardia duodenalis)***
Adults: 2 g PO as single dose.
Children older than age 3 years: Give 50 mg/kg (up to 2 g) PO as single dose.

➤ **Intestinal amebiasis caused by *Entamoeba histolytica***
Adults: 2 g PO daily for 3 days.
Children older than age 3 years: Give 50 mg/kg (up to 2 g) PO daily for 3 days.

➤ **Amebic liver abscess (amebiasis)**
Adults: 2 g PO daily for 3 to 5 days.
Children older than age 3 years: Give 50 mg/kg (up to 2 g) PO daily for 3 to 5 days.

SAFETY ALERT!

tirofiban hydrochloride
tye-row-FYE-ban

Aggrastat

Therapeutic class: Antiplatelet drugs
Pharmacologic class: Glycoprotein IIb/IIIa receptor antagonists

AVAILABLE FORMS
Injection (premixed bag): 50 mcg/mL in 100 mL, 250 mL
Injection (vials): 50 mcg/mL in 100 mL, 250 mcg/mL in 15 mL (bolus)

INDICATIONS & DOSAGES
➤ **To reduce rate of thrombotic CV events (combined endpoint of death, MI, or refractory ischemia or repeat cardiac procedure) in patients with non-ST elevation ACS**
Adults: IV loading dose of 25 mcg/kg administered within 5 minutes, followed by 0.15 mcg/kg/minute for up to 18 hours.
Adjust-a-dose: If CrCl is 60 mL/minute or less, use an IV loading dose of 25 mcg/kg administered within 5 minutes, followed by 0.075 mcg/kg/minute for up to 18 hours.

SAFETY ALERT!

tivozanib
tye-VOE-za-nib

Fotivda

Therapeutic class: Antineoplastics
Pharmacologic class: Kinase inhibitors

AVAILABLE FORMS
Capsules ⓄⓃⒸ: 0.89 mg, 1.34 mg

INDICATIONS & DOSAGES
➤ **Relapsed or refractory advanced renal cell carcinoma after two or more prior systemic therapies**
Adults: 1.34 mg PO once daily for 21 days, followed by 7 days off for a 28-day cycle. Continue until disease progresses or unacceptable toxicity occurs.

Adjust-a-dose: In patients with total bilirubin level greater than 1.5 to 3 × ULN with any AST level, decrease dose to 0.89 mg. Refer to manufacturer's instructions for toxicity-related dosage adjustments.

tolcapone
TOLE-ka-pone

Tasmar

Therapeutic class: Antiparkinsonian drugs
Pharmacologic class: Catechol-O-methyltransferase inhibitors

AVAILABLE FORMS
Tablets: 100 mg

INDICATIONS & DOSAGES
Boxed Warning Drug poses risk of liver injury. Stop drug if patient shows no benefit within 3 weeks. ■
➤ **Adjunct to levodopa–carbidopa for signs and symptoms of idiopathic Parkinson disease in patients who have symptom fluctuation or haven't responded to other adjunctive treatment**
Adults: Initially, 100 mg PO t.i.d. with levodopa–carbidopa. May increase dosage to 200 mg PO t.i.d. if clinical benefit is justified, as this dosage is associated with increased frequency of ALT elevation. Levodopa dosage may need to be reduced by about 30% to minimize risk of dyskinesias, especially when levodopa dose is over 600 mg daily.

SAFETY ALERT!

toremifene citrate
tore-EM-ah-feen

Fareston

Therapeutic class: Antineoplastics
Pharmacologic class: Nonsteroidal antiestrogens

AVAILABLE FORMS
Tablets: 60 mg

INDICATIONS & DOSAGES
Boxed Warning May prolong QTc interval and risk of fatal ventricular arrhythmias. ■
➤ **Metastatic breast cancer in patients who are postmenopausal with estrogen receptor-positive or estrogen receptor-unknown tumors**
Adults: 60 mg PO once daily. Continue until disease progresses.

trandolapril ⊠
tran-DOE-la-pril

Therapeutic class: Antihypertensives
Pharmacologic class: ACE inhibitors

AVAILABLE FORMS
Tablets: 1 mg, 2 mg, 4 mg

INDICATIONS & DOSAGES
Boxed Warning Drugs that act directly on the RAAS can cause fetal harm; when pregnancy is detected, discontinue drug as soon as possible. ■

Adjust-a-dose (for all indications): If CrCl is below 30 mL/minute or patient has cirrhosis, first dose is 0.5 mg daily.
➤ **HTN** ⊠
Adults: For patients not taking a diuretic, initially 2 mg PO once daily for a patient who is Black and 1 mg PO once daily for all other patients. If control isn't adequate, increase dosage at intervals of at least 1 week. Maintenance dosages for most patients: 2 to 4 mg daily. Some patients taking once-daily doses of 4 mg may need b.i.d. doses. For patients also taking a diuretic, initially, 0.5 mg PO once daily. Base subsequent dosage adjustment on BP response.
➤ **HF or left ventricular dysfunction after MI**
Adults: Initially, 1 mg PO daily, adjusted to 4 mg PO daily. If patient can't tolerate 4 mg, continue at highest tolerated dose.

treprostinil
tra-PROS-tin-ill

Remodulin, Tyvaso

treprostinil diolamine
Orenitram

Therapeutic class: Antihypertensives
Pharmacologic class: Vasodilators

AVAILABLE FORMS
Injection: 1 mg/mL, 2.5 mg/mL, 5 mg/mL, 10 mg/mL in 20-mL vials
Powder for inhalation: 16 mcg, 32 mcg, 48 mcg, 64 mcg single-dose cartridges
Solution for inhalation: 1.74 mg/2.9 mL ampule (0.6 mg/mL)
Tablets (extended-release) ⊙: 0.125 mg, 0.25 mg, 1 mg, 2.5 mg, 5 mg

INDICATIONS & DOSAGES
➤ **To reduce symptoms caused by exercise in patients with NYHA Class II to IV PAH**
Adults: Initially, 1.25 nanograms/kg/minute by continuous subcut infusion. If patient doesn't tolerate initial dose, reduce infusion rate to 0.625 nanogram/kg/minute. Increase by 1.25 nanograms/kg/minute each week for first 4 weeks and then by no more than 2.5 nanograms/kg/minute each week for remaining duration of infusion. Experience with treprostinil dosages exceeding 40 nanograms/kg/minute is limited. May be given IV through a central venous catheter if subcut route isn't tolerated.
Adjust-a-dose: For patients with Child-Pugh class A or B liver impairment, initially, 0.625 nanogram/kg ideal body weight/minute and increased cautiously. Avoid abrupt discontinuation or sudden large dosage reductions, which may worsen PAH symptoms.
➤ **To decrease rate of clinical deterioration in patients with NYHA Class II to IV PAH requiring transition from Flolan (epoprostenol sodium)**
Adults: Start treprostinil subcut or IV infusion at 10% of the current IV epoprostenol dose; increase dose as epoprostenol dose is reduced. Decrease epoprostenol dose in 20% increments and increase treprostinil

in 20% increments, always maintaining a total dose of 110% of epoprostenol starting dose. Once epoprostenol is at 20% of starting dose and treprostinil is at 90%, decrease epoprostenol to 5% and increase treprostinil to 110%. Finally, stop epoprostenol and maintain treprostinil dose at 110% of epoprostenol starting dose plus an additional 5% to 10% as needed. Change rate based on individual patient response. Treat worsening of PAH symptoms with increases in treprostinil dose. Treat adverse effects associated with prostacyclin and prostacyclin analogues with decreases in epoprostenol dose.

➤ **PAH in patients with WHO Group I signs and symptoms to improve exercise capacity**
Adults: 0.25 mg PO every 12 hours or 0.125 mg PO every 8 hours. May increase in increments of 0.25 or 0.5 mg every 12 hours or 0.125 mg every 8 hours every 3 to 4 days as tolerated to achieve optimal clinical response. If incremental increases aren't tolerated, consider slower titration. Maximum dosage is determined by tolerability. If patient is taking strong CYP2C8 inhibitors, initiate at 0.125 mg PO every 12 hours; increase in increments of 0.125 mg every 12 hours every 3 to 4 days.

For solution inhalation: Initially, 18 mcg (3 inhalations) q.i.d. every 4 hours while patient is awake. If 3 inhalations aren't tolerated, reduce to 1 or 2 inhalations; then increase to 3 inhalations as tolerated. For maintenance, increase each dose by 3 inhalations at approximately 1- to 2-week intervals; target and maximum dose is 9 to 12 inhalation per session q.i.d.

For powder inhalation: Initially, 16 mcg (1 inhalation) q.i.d. May increase by 16 mcg per treatment every 1 to 2 weeks as tolerated. Target maintenance dose is 48 to 64 mcg per treatment session q.i.d.

To transition from subcut or IV to PO administration, refer to manufacturer's instructions.
Adjust-a-dose: If intolerable adverse effects occur, decrease PO dose in 0.25-mg increments. To discontinue therapy, reduce dose in steps of 0.5 to 1 mg/day; avoid discontinuing drug abruptly. If patient is unable to continue oral treatment, consider a temporary infusion of subcut or IV treprostinil. For patients with Child-Pugh class A liver impairment, initiate drug at 0.125 mg PO every 12 hours and increase in increments of 0.125 mg every 12 hours every 3 to 4 days.

If patient is taking strong CYP2C8 inhibitors, initiate at 0.125 mg PO every 12 hours; increase in increments of 0.125 mg every 12 hours every 3 to 4 days.
➤ **PAH associated with ILD in patients (WHO Group 3) to improve exercise ability**
Adults: For solution inhalation: Initially, 3 breaths (18 mcg) per treatment session q.i.d., approximately 4 hours apart. Increase by 3 breaths in 1- to 2-week intervals, as tolerated, to target maintenance dose of 9 to 12 breaths per treatment session q.i.d. If 3 breaths aren't tolerated initially, decrease to 1 or 2 breaths and increase as tolerated.

For powder inhalation: Initially, 16 mcg (1 inhalation) q.i.d. May increase by 16 mcg per treatment every 1 to 2 weeks as tolerated. Target maintenance dose is 48 to 64 mcg per treatment session q.i.d.

triclabendazole
tri-kla-BEN-da-zole

Egaten

Therapeutic class: Anthelmintics
Pharmacologic class: Anthelmintics

AVAILABLE FORMS
Tablets: 250 mg

INDICATIONS & DOSAGES
➤ **Fascioliasis**
Adults and children ages 6 and older: 10 mg/kg PO every 12 hours for two doses.

trifarotene
trye-FAR-oh-teen

Aklief

Therapeutic class: Antiacne drugs
Pharmacologic class: Retinoids

AVAILABLE FORMS
Cream: 0.005%

INDICATIONS & DOSAGES
➤ **Acne vulgaris**
Adults and children ages 9 and older: Apply thin layer to affected areas of face or trunk once daily in the evening on clean, dry skin.

SAFETY ALERT!

trifluridine–tipiracil hydrochloride ⬚
trye-FLURE-i-deen/tye-PIR-a-sil

Lonsurf

Therapeutic class: Antineoplastics
Pharmacologic class: Pyrimidine analogues

AVAILABLE FORMS
Tablets: 15 mg trifluridine/6.14 mg tipiracil, 20 mg trifluridine/8.19 mg tipiracil

INDICATIONS & DOSAGES
Adjust-a-dose (for all indications): Refer to manufacturer's instructions for dosage adjustments for hematologic and nonhematologic toxicities.
➤ **Metastatic colorectal cancer as monotherapy or in combination with bevacizumab in patients previously treated with fluoropyrimidine-, oxaliplatin-, and irinotecan-based chemotherapy, an anti-vascular endothelial growth factor biological therapy and, if RAS wild-type, an anti-epidermal growth factor receptor therapy** ⬚
Adults: 35 mg/m^2 (based on trifluridine component) PO b.i.d. with food up to maximum of 80 mg/dose (based on trifluridine component) on days 1 through 5 and days 8 through 12 of a 28-day cycle. Round doses to nearest 5-mg increment. Continue until disease progresses or unacceptable toxicity occurs. Refer to bevacizumab prescribing information for more information.

➤ **Metastatic gastric or gastroesophageal junction adenocarcinoma previously treated with at least two lines of chemotherapy that included a fluoropyrimidine, a platinum, either a taxane or irinotecan and, if appropriate, HER2/neu-targeted therapy**

Adults: 35 mg/m² (based on trifluridine component) PO b.i.d. with food up to a maximum of 80 mg/dose (based on trifluridine component) on days 1 through 5 and days 8 through 12 of a 28-day cycle. Round doses to nearest 5-mg increment. Continue until disease progresses or unacceptable toxicity occurs.

SAFETY ALERT!

trilaciclib
trye-la-SYE-klib

Cosela

Therapeutic class: Antineoplastics
Pharmacologic class: Kinase inhibitors

AVAILABLE FORMS
Injection: 300 mg single-dose vial

INDICATIONS & DOSAGES
➤ **To decrease incidence of chemotherapy-induced myelosuppression when administered before platinum/etoposide-containing regimen or topotecan-containing regimen for extensive-stage SCLC**

Adults: 240 mg/m² IV infusion over 30 minutes completed within 4 hours before start of chemotherapy on each day of chemotherapy. If given on sequential days, interval between trilaciclib doses shouldn't be greater than 28 hours.

Adjust-a-dose: Refer to manufacturer's instructions for toxicity-related dosage adjustments. If trilaciclib is discontinued, wait 96 hours from last dose before resuming chemotherapy only.

trimethobenzamide hydrochloride
trye-meth-oh-BEN-za-mide

Tigan

Therapeutic class: Antiemetics
Pharmacologic class: Anticholinergics

AVAILABLE FORMS
Capsules: 300 mg
Injection: 100 mg/mL

INDICATIONS & DOSAGES
➤ **Postoperative nausea and vomiting; nausea associated with gastroenteritis**

Adults: 300 mg PO or 200 mg IM t.i.d. or q.i.d.
Adjust-a-dose: Dosage reduction or increased dosing interval is recommended in older adults and patients with CrCl of 70 mL/minute/1.73 m² or less.

triptorelin pamoate
trip-toe-REL-in

Trelstar Mixject, Triptodur

Therapeutic class: Hormone analogues
Pharmacologic class: Gonadotropin releasing hormone agonists

AVAILABLE FORMS
Injectable suspension (Trelstar Mixject): 3.75 mg, 11.25 mg, 22.5 mg in Mixject single-dose delivery systems
Injectable suspension (extended-release) (Triptodur): 22.5 mg single-dose vials packaged with 2 mL of diluent sterile water for injection

INDICATIONS & DOSAGES
➤ **Palliative treatment of advanced prostate cancer (Trelstar Mixject only)**

Adults: 3.75 mg IM once every 4 weeks, or 11.25 mg IM once every 12 weeks, or 22.5 mg IM once every 24 weeks. Because of different release characteristics, dosing schedule depends on the product selected.

➤ **Central precocious puberty (Triptodur only)**

Children ages 2 and older: 22.5 mg IM once every 24 weeks. Treatment should be discontinued at appropriate age of onset of puberty at prescriber's discretion.

ubrogepant
ue-BROE-je-pant

Ubrelvy

Therapeutic class: Antimigraine drugs
Pharmacologic class: Calcitonin gene-related peptide antagonists

AVAILABLE FORMS
Tablets: 50 mg, 100 mg

INDICATIONS & DOSAGES
➤ **Acute treatment of migraine with or without aura**

Adults: 50 or 100 mg PO, as needed. May repeat once at least 2 hours after initial dose, if needed. Maximum, 200 mg a day.

Adjust-a-dose: For patients with Child-Pugh class C liver impairment or CrCl of 15 to 29 mL/minute, give 50 mg; if needed, may give a second 50-mg dose at least 2 hours after initial dose. For patients receiving moderate and weak CYP3A inhibitors, moderate and weak CYP3A4 inducers, BCRP or P-gp only inhibitors, refer to manufacturer's instructions for dosage adjustments.

upadacitinib
ue-pad-a-SYE-ti-nib

Rinvoq

Therapeutic class: Antirheumatics
Pharmacologic class: Janus kinase inhibitors

AVAILABLE FORMS

Tablets (extended release) 🔵 15 mg

INDICATIONS & DOSAGES

Boxed Warning Drug increases risk of TB and invasive fungal, bacterial, viral, and opportunistic infections. Prescreen patients for latent TB. Drug increases risk of CV events, all-cause mortality, malignancies, and thrombotic events, some resulting in death. ■

🔵 *Alert:* Drug isn't recommended for use in combination with other JAK inhibitors, biologic DMARDs, biologic therapies for Crohn disease or with potent immunosuppressants such as azathioprine and cyclosporine.

Adjust-a-dose (all indications): If serious infection develops, interrupt drug until the infection is controlled. Interrupt therapy if ANC is less than 1,000 cells/mm³, absolute lymphocyte count (ALC) is less than 500 cells/mm³, or Hb level is less than 8 g/dL. May restart drug once ANC, ALC, or Hb level returns above this value. If transaminase levels rise and drug-induced liver injury is suspected, interrupt treatment.

➤ **Moderate to severe active RA in patients who have had an inadequate response or intolerance to one or more TNF blockers**
Adults: 15 mg PO once daily.

➤ **Psoriatic arthritis in patients with inadequate response or intolerance to one or more TNF blockers**
Adults: 15 mg PO once daily.

➤ **Refractory, moderate to severe atopic dermatitis not adequately controlled with other systemic drugs, including biologicals, or when use of those therapies is inadvisable**
Adults and children ages 12 and older weighing at least 40 kg: Initially, 15 mg PO once daily. May increase to 30 mg once daily. If adequate response isn't achieved with 30-mg dose, stop therapy. Use lowest effective dose needed to maintain response.
Adjust-a-dose: In older adults or patients with CrCl less than 30 mL/minute, give 15 mg once daily. If used concomitantly with strong CYP3A4 inhibitors, give 15 mg once daily. Not recommended for patients with Child-Pugh class C liver impairment.

➤ **Moderate to severe ulcerative colitis after inadequate response or intolerance to one or more TNF blockers**
Adults: 45 mg PO once daily for 8 weeks, followed by maintenance dose of 15 mg once daily. May increase maintenance dose to 30 mg once daily for patients with refractory, severe, or extensive disease. If patient response to 30-mg dose is inadequate, discontinue drug. Use lowest effective dose needed to maintain response.
Adjust-a-dose: If patient has eGFR of 15 to 29 m/L/minute/1.73m² or Child-Pugh class A or B liver impairment or is taking a strong CYP3A4 inhibitor, give induction dose, 30 mg once daily for 8 weeks; then maintenance dose, 15 mg once daily.

➤ **Ankylosing spondylitis after inadequate response to or intolerance of one or more TNF blockers**
Adults: 15 mg PO once daily.

✱ *NEW INDICATION:* **Active nonradiographic axial spondyloarthritis in patients with inadequate response to or intolerance of TNF blocker therapy**
Adults: 15 mg PO once daily.

✱ *NEW INDICATION:* **Moderate to severely active Crohn disease in patients with inadequate response to or intolerance of one or more TNF blockers**
Adults: 45 mg PO once daily for 12 weeks, followed by maintenance dosage of 15 mg once daily. May increase maintenance dosage to 30 mg once daily for patients with refractory, severe, or extensive disease. If patient response to 30-mg dose is inadequate, discontinue drug. Use lowest effective dose needed to maintain response.
Adjust-a-dose: If patient has eGFR of 15 to 29 m/L/minute/1.73m² or Child-Pugh class A or B liver impairment or is taking a strong CYP3A4 inhibitor, give induction dose, 30 mg once daily for 12 weeks; then maintenance dose, 15 mg once daily.

valbenazine 🔀
val-BEN-a-zeen

Ingrezza

Therapeutic class: Neuromuscular transmission blockers
Pharmacologic class: Vesicular monoamine transporter 2 inhibitors

AVAILABLE FORMS
Capsules: 40 mg, 60 mg, 80 mg

INDICATIONS & DOSAGES
➤ **Tardive dyskinesia**
Adults: Initially, 40 mg PO once daily for 1 week, then 80 mg once daily; for some patients, 40 or 60 mg once daily may be appropriate.
Adjust-a-dose: For patients with Child-Pugh class B or C liver impairment or when drug is administered with a strong CYP3A4 inhibitor, give 40 mg once daily. If drug is administered with a strong CYP2D6 inhibitor and for patients who are known poor metabolizers of CYP2D6, consider a dosage reduction.

✱ *NEW INDICATION:* **Chorea associated with Huntington disease**
Boxed Warning Drug may increase risk of depression and suicidality in patients with Huntington disease. ■
Adults: Initially, 40 mg PO once daily. Increase dose in 20 mg increments every 2 weeks to recommended dosage of 80 mg once daily; for some patients, 40 or 60 mg once daily may be appropriate based on response and tolerability.
Adjust-a-dose: For patients with Child-Pugh class B or C liver impairment, for those who are known poor metabolizers of CYP2D6, or if drug is administered with a strong CYP2D6 or CYP3A4 inhibitor, give 40 mg once daily.

🍁Canada ◇ OTC ◆ Off-label use 🔵Do not crush *Liquid contains alcohol 🔀 Genetic

valGANciclovir hydrochloride
val-gan-SYE-kloe-veer

Valcyte

Therapeutic class: Antivirals
Pharmacologic class: Nucleosides-nucleotides

AVAILABLE FORMS
Oral solution: 50 mg/mL
Tablets ⓓ: 450 mg

INDICATIONS & DOSAGES
Boxed Warning Drug can cause severe bone marrow suppression and suppression of fertility in both males and females. Animal data suggest fetal harm and potential carcinogenic effects in humans. ■
Adjust-a-dose (for all indications): For adults with CrCl of 40 to 59 mL/minute, induction dosage is 450 mg b.i.d.; maintenance dosage is 450 mg daily. If CrCl is 25 to 39 mL/minute, induction dosage is 450 mg daily; maintenance dosage is 450 mg every 2 days. If CrCl is 10 to 24 mL/minute, induction dosage is 450 mg every 2 days; maintenance dosage is 450 mg twice weekly. Drug isn't recommended for patients with CrCl less than 10 mL/minute.
➤ **Prevention of CMV disease in heart, kidney, and kidney-pancreas transplantation patients at high risk (donor CMV-seropositive or recipient CMV-seronegative)**
Adults: For patients with a heart or kidney-pancreas transplant, 900 mg PO once daily starting within 10 days of transplantation until 100 days posttransplantation. For patients with a kidney transplant, 900 mg PO daily starting within 10 days of transplantation until 200 days posttransplantation.
➤ **Prevention of CMV disease in children with kidney transplant who are at high risk**
Children ages 4 months to 16 years: Once-daily dose starting within 10 days of transplantation until 200 days posttransplantation of kidney, based on BSA and CrCl (modified Schwartz formula):
$$Dose\ (mg) = 7 \times BSA \times CrCl$$
Adjust-a-dose: For children, maximum calculated CrCl (modified Schwartz formula) to be used is 150 mL/minute/1.73 m². even if calculated value is greater. The maximum pediatric dose is 900 mg, even if the calculated dose is greater.
➤ **Prevention of CMV disease in children with heart transplant who are at high risk**
Children ages 1 month to 16 years: Once-daily dose starting within 10 days of transplantation until 100 days posttransplantation of heart, based on BSA and CrCl (modified Schwartz formula):
$$Dose\ (mg) = 7 \times BSA \times CrCl$$
Maximum, 900 mg once daily.
➤ **CMV retinitis in patients with AIDS**
Adults: For active disease, 900 mg PO b.i.d. for 21 days; maintenance dosage, 900 mg PO daily. For inactive disease, 900 mg PO once daily.

vandetanib
van-DET-a-nib

Caprelsa

Therapeutic class: Antineoplastics
Pharmacologic class: Kinase inhibitors

AVAILABLE FORMS
Tablets ⓓ: 100 mg, 300 mg

INDICATIONS & DOSAGES
Boxed Warning May prolong QTc interval and increase risk of fatal ventricular arrhythmias. ■
➤ **Symptomatic or progressive medullary thyroid cancer in patients with unresectable locally advanced or metastatic disease**
Adults: 300 mg PO daily until disease progresses or unacceptable toxicity occurs.
Adjust-a-dose: In patients with CrCl of 30 to less than 50 mL/minute, initiate therapy at 200 mg PO daily. Refer to manufacturer's instructions for toxicity-related dosage adjustments.

vedolizumab
ve-doe-LIZ-ue-mab

Entyvio

Therapeutic class: Immune response modifiers
Pharmacologic class: Humanized IgG1 monoclonal antibodies

AVAILABLE FORMS
Injection (IV): 300 mg single-use vials
Injection (subcut): 108 mg/0.68 mL in single-dose prefilled pen or syringe

INDICATIONS & DOSAGES
➤ **Moderate to severe Crohn disease or ulcerative colitis**
Adults: 300 mg IV infusion over 30 minutes, administered at weeks 0, 2, and 6, then every 8 weeks thereafter. Patients with ulcerative colitis may be switched to 108 mg subcut injection at week 6, continued every 2 weeks thereafter. Discontinue use if no evidence of therapeutic benefit by week 14.

vemurafenib ▨
vem-ue-RAF-e-nib

Zelboraf

Therapeutic class: Antineoplastics
Pharmacologic class: Kinase inhibitors

AVAILABLE FORMS
Tablets ⓓ: 240 mg

INDICATIONS & DOSAGES
➤ **Unresectable or metastatic melanoma with *BRAF* V600E mutation; Erdheim-Chester disease with *BRAF* V600 mutation ▨**

Adults: 960 mg PO every 12 hours. Continue until disease progresses or unacceptable toxicity occurs.
Adjust-a-dose: Avoid concomitant use of strong CYP3A4 inducers. If use together is unavoidable, increase vemurafenib dosage by 240 mg (1 tablet) as tolerated. After discontinuation of a strong CYP3A4 inducer for 2 weeks, resume prior vemurafenib dosage. Refer to manufacturer's instructions for toxicity-related dosage adjustments.

SAFETY ALERT! ■

voclosporin
vok-loe-SPOR-in

Lupkynis

Therapeutic class: Immunomodulators
Pharmacologic class: Calcineurin inhibitors

AVAILABLE FORMS
Capsules ⓓⓝⓒ: 7.9 mg

INDICATIONS & DOSAGES
Boxed Warning Drug may increase risk of serious infections and malignancies. ■
➤ **Active lupus nephritis in combination with a background immunosuppressive therapy regimen**
Adults: 23.7 mg PO b.i.d. in combination with mycophenolate mofetil and corticosteroids.
Adjust-a-dose: If eGFR is less than 60 mL/minute/1.73 m² and reduced from baseline by more than 20% and less than 30%, reduce dosage by 7.9 mg b.i.d.; if eGFR is still reduced from baseline by more than 20% within 2 weeks, reduce dosage again by 7.9 mg b.i.d. If eGFR is less than 60 mL/minute/1.73 m² and reduced from baseline by 30% or more, discontinue drug. Consider restarting at 7.9 mg b.i.d. only if eGFR has returned to 80% or more of baseline within 2 weeks.

If a dosage decrease due to eGFR was made, consider increasing dosage by 7.9 mg b.i.d. for each eGFR measurement that is 80% or more of baseline; don't exceed starting dose. Avoid use in patients with baseline eGFR less than 45 mL/minute/1.73 m² unless benefit exceeds risk.

If used in patients with eGFR of 45 mL/minute/1.73 m² or less at baseline, give 15.8 mg b.i.d. For patients with Child-Pugh class B and B liver impairment, give 15.8 mg b.i.d. If concomitantly used with moderate CYP3A4 inhibitors, give 15.8 mg in the morning and 7.9 mg in the evening.

voxelotor
vox-EL-oh-tor

Oxbryta

Therapeutic class: Miscellaneous hematologic drugs
Pharmacologic class: Hemoglobin S polymerization inhibitors

AVAILABLE FORMS
Tablets ⓓⓝⓒ: 300 mg, 500 mg
Tablets for suspension: 300 mg

INDICATIONS & DOSAGES
➤ **Sickle cell disease with or without hydroxyurea**
Adults and children ages 12 and older: 1,500 mg PO once daily.
Children ages 4 to younger than 12 weighing 40 kg or more: 1,500 mg PO once daily.
Children ages 4 to younger than 12 weighing 20 to less than 40 kg: 900 mg PO once daily.
Children ages 4 to younger than 12 weighing 10 to less than 20 kg: 600 mg PO once daily.
Adjust-a-dose: For adults and children ages 12 and older with Child-Pugh class C liver impairment, reduce dosage to 1,000 mg PO once daily. For adults and children ages 12 and older currently receiving a strong CYP3A4 inducer, increase dosage to 2,500 mg once daily; moderate CYP3A4 inducer, increase dosage to 2,000 mg once daily.

For children ages 4 to younger than 12 with Child-Pugh class C liver impairment, reduce dosage based on body weight: If 40 kg or more, give 1,000 mg (two 500-mg tablets) or 900 mg (three 300-mg tablets for oral suspension) daily; if 20 to less than 40 kg, give 600 mg daily; if 10 to less than 20 kg, give 300 mg daily.

For children ages 4 to younger than 12 currently receiving a strong or moderate CYP3A4 inducer, see manufacturer's instructions for dosage adjustment based on weight.

zanamivir
zan-AM-ah-veer

Relenza Diskhaler

Therapeutic class: Antiretrovirals
Pharmacologic class: Selective neuraminidase inhibitors

AVAILABLE FORMS
Powder for inhalation: 5 mg/blister

INDICATIONS & DOSAGES
➤ **Uncomplicated acute illness caused by influenza virus A and B in patients who have had symptoms for no longer than 2 days**
Adults and children ages 7 and older: 2 oral inhalations (one 5-mg blister per inhalation for total dose of 10 mg) b.i.d. using the dry-powder inhalation device for 5 days. Give two doses on first day of treatment, allowing at least 2 hours to elapse between doses. Give subsequent doses about 12 hours apart (in the morning and evening) at about the same time each day. Some guidelines suggest that longer treatment duration may be considered in patients who remain severely ill after 5 days.
➤ **Prevention of influenza in a household setting**
Adults and children ages 5 and older: 2 oral inhalations (one 5-mg blister per inhalation for total dose of 10 mg) once daily for 10 days.
➤ **Prevention of influenza in a community setting**
Adults and adolescents ages 12 to 16: 2 oral inhalations (one 5-mg blister per inhalation for total dose of 10 mg) once daily for 28 days.

zanubrutinib
zan-ue-BROO-ti-nib

Brukinsa

Therapeutic class: Antineoplastic agents
Pharmacologic class: Tyrosine kinase inhibitors

AVAILABLE FORMS
Capsules (DNC): 80 mg

INDICATIONS & DOSAGES
➤ **Mantle cell lymphoma in patients who have received at least one prior therapy; Waldenström macroglobulinemia; marginal zone lymphoma; chronic lymphocytic leukemia or small lymphocytic lymphoma**
Adults: 160 mg PO b.i.d. or 320 mg PO once daily. Continue treatment until disease progresses or unacceptable toxicity occurs.
Adjust-a-dose: For patients with Child-Pugh class C liver impairment, reduce dosage to 80 mg PO b.i.d. If given with strong CYP3A inhibitor, decrease dosage to 80 mg PO once daily. If given with moderate CYP3A inhibitor, decrease dosage to 80 mg PO b.i.d. After discontinuation of a CYP3A inhibitor, resume previous zanubrutinib dosage. Avoid use with strong CYP3A inducers; if moderate CYP3A inducers cannot be avoided, increase dosage to 320 mg PO b.i.d. Refer to manufacturer's instructions for toxicity-related dosage adjustments.

ziv-aflibercept
ziv-a-FLIB-er-sept

Zaltrap

Therapeutic class: Antineoplastics
Pharmacologic class: Vascular endothelial growth factor inhibitors

AVAILABLE FORMS
Injection: 100 mg/4 mL, 200 mg/8 mL in single-use vials

INDICATIONS & DOSAGES
➤ **Metastatic colorectal cancer that is resistant or has progressed after an oxaliplatin-containing regimen in combination with FOLFIRI regimen**
Adults: 4 mg/kg IV infusion over 1 hour every 2 weeks until disease progresses or unacceptable toxicity occurs. Give before any component of FOLFIRI regimen on day of treatment.
Adjust-a-dose: Refer to manufacturer's instructions for toxicity-related dosage adjustments.

Index

A

abacavir sulfate, 23–24
abacavir sulfate–lamiVUDine, 1525
abacavir sulfate–lamiVUDine–zidovudine, 1526
abatacept, 24–27
Abelcet, 90–91
abemaciclib, 27–29
Abilify, 108–112
Abilify Maintena, 108–112
Abilify MyCite, 108–112
abiraterone acetate, 29–31
Abraxane, 1066–1068
Abrilada, 46–48
abrocitinib, 31–33
Absorica, 756–759
Absorica LD, 756–759
acalabrutinib, 1552
acamprosate calcium, 33–34
acarbose, 1552
Accolate, 1449–1450
Accupril, 1173–1175
Accuretic, 1524
ACET, 35–38
Acetadote, 40–42
acetaminophen, 35–38
acetaZOLAMIDE, 38–40
acetaZOLAMIDE sodium, 38–40
acetylcysteine, 40–42
acetylsalicylic acid, 117–120
Acid Gone, 1498
Aciphex, 1175–1177
aclidinium bromide, 1552
ACT, 1510–1511
Actemra, 1356–1359
Actidose-Aqua, 1531
Actidose with Sorbitol, 1531
Actimmune, 1590
Actiq, 554–560
Activase, 70–73
activated charcoal, 1531
Activella, 527–532
Actonel, 1213–1215
ActoPlus Met, 1520
Actos, 1121–1123
Acular, 1542
Acular LS, 1542
Acuvail, 1542
acyclovir, 43–45
acyclovir sodium, 43–45
adagrasib, 1467–1468

Adakveo, 1570
Adalat OROS, 970–972
Adalat XL, 970–972
adalimumab, 46–48
adalimumab-aacf, 46–48
adalimumab-adaz, 46–48
adalimumab-adbm, 46–48
adalimumab-afzb, 46–48
adalimumab-aqvh, 46–48
adalimumab-atto, 46–48
adalimumab-bwwd, 46–48
adalimumab-fkjp, 46–48
Adcetris, 175–177
Adcirca, 1315–1317
Adderall, 369–372
Adderall XR, 369–372
Addyi, 1583
Adempas, 1613–1614
adenosine, 49–50
Adipex-P, 1111–1113
Adlarity, 399–401
Admelog, 726–731
ado-trastuzumab emtansine, 50–53
Adrenaclick, 464–467
Adrenalin, 464–467
adrenaline, 464–467
Adriamycin, 406–409
Advagraf, 1619
Advair Diskus, 591–593
Advair HFA, 591–593
Advate, 1547
Adverse drug reactions, 3–4
Advil, 680–683
Adynovate, 1547
Aemcolo, 1613
Afinitor, 539–542
Afinitor Disperz, 539–542
Afirmelle, 527–532
aflibercept, 1538
Afrezza, 726–731
Afrin 12 Hour, 1515
Afstyla, 1547
Aggrastat, 1624
AHF, 1547
Aimovig, 475–476
AirDuo Digihaler, 591–593
AirDuo RespiClick, 591–593
Airomir, 53–55
Ajovy, 1585
Aklief, 1626

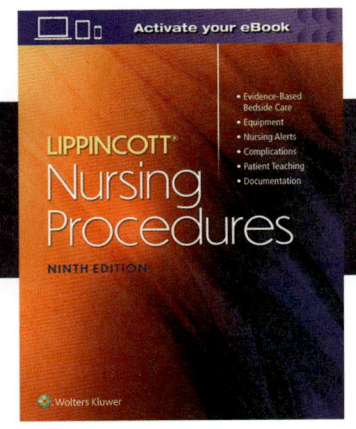

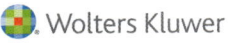